2007 LANGE

CURRENT
Medical
Diagnosis &
Treatment

FORTY-SIXTH EDITION

Edited by

Stephen J. McPhee, MD
Professor of Medicine
Division of General Internal Medicine
Department of Medicine
University of California, San Francisco

Maxine A. Papadakis, MD
Professor of Clinical Medicine
Associate Dean for Student Affairs
School of Medicine
University of California, San Francisco

Senior Editor

Lawrence M. Tierney, Jr., MD
Professor of Medicine
University of California, San Francisco
Associate Chief of Medical Service
Veterans Affairs Medical Center, San Francisco

With Associate Authors

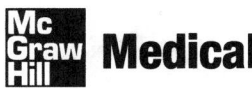 **Medical**

New York   Chicago   San Francisco   Lisbon   London   Madrid   Mexico City
Milan   New Delhi   San Juan   Seoul   Singapore   Sydney   Toronto

Current Medical Diagnosis & Treatment 2007, Forty-Sixth Edition

2 3 4 5 6 7 8 9 0   DOW/DOW   0 9 8 7

ISBN-13: 978-0-07-147247-0; ISBN-10: 0-07-147247-9

ISSN: 0092-8682

Notice

Medicine is an ever-changing science. As new research and clinical experience broaden our knowledge, changes in treatment and drug therapy are required. The authors and the publisher of this work have checked with sources believed to be reliable in their efforts to provide information that is complete and generally in accord with the standards accepted at the time of publication. However, in view of the possibility of human error or changes in medical sciences, neither the authors nor the publisher nor any other party who has been involved in the preparation or publication of this work warrants that the information contained herein is in every respect accurate or complete, and they disclaim all responsibility for any errors or omissions or for the results obtained from use of the information contained in this work. Readers are encouraged to confirm the information contained herein with other sources. For example and in particular, readers are advised to check the product information sheet included in the package of each drug they plan to administer to be certain that the information contained in this work is accurate and that changes have not been made in the recommended dose or in the contraindications for administration. This recommendation is of particular importance in connection with new or infrequently used drugs.

This book was set by Silverchair Science + Communications, Inc.
The editors were Jason O. Malley, Harriet Lebowitz, and Barbara Holton.
The production supervisor was Phil Galea.
The illustration manager was Charissa Baker.
The cover designer was Mary McKeon.
The index was prepared by Kathy Pitcoff.
RR Donnelley was printer and binder.

Cover photos clockwise from top left: Woman getting flu shot: LADA/Photo Researchers, Inc.; Streptococcus bacteria: Dr. Gary Gaugler/Photo Researchers, Inc.; Stethoscope: Photodisc

This book is printed on acid-free paper.

International Edition ISBN-13: 978-0-07-110449-4; ISBN-10: 0-07-110449-6

Contents

6. Skin, Hair, & Nails 87
Timothy G. Berger, MD

7. Eye 151
Paul Riordan-Eva, FRCS, FRCOphth

8. Ear, Nose, & Throat 182
Robert K. Jackler, MD, & Michael J. Kaplan, MD

24. Nervous System 998
Michael J. Aminoff, DSc, MD, FRCP

25. Psychiatric Disorders 1063
Stuart J. Eisendrath, MD, & Jonathan E. Lichtmacher, MD

26. Endocrinology 1123
Paul A. Fitzgerald, MD

Online-Only Chapters

Diagnostic Testing & Medical Decision Making
C. Diana Nicoll, MD, PhD, MPA, & Michael Pignone, MD, MPH

Benefits; Costs & Risks
Performance of Diagnostic Tests
Test Characteristics

Use of Tests in Diagnosis & Management
Odds-Likelihood Ratios

Basic Genetics
Reed E. Pyeritz, MD, PhD

Introduction to Medical Genetics
 Genes & Chromosomes
 Mutation
 Genes in Individuals
 Genes in Families
 Disorders of Multifactorial Causation
 Chromosomal Aberrations

The Techniques of Medical Genetics
 Family History & Pedigree Analysis
 Cytogenetics
 Biochemical Genetics
 DNA Analysis
 Prenatal Diagnosis
 Neoplasia: Chromosomal & DNA Analysis

Basic Immunology
Jeffrey L. Kishiyama, MD, & Daniel C. Adelman, MD

Allergic Diseases
Atopic Disease
Clinical Immunology
 Cells Involved in Immunity

Tests for Cellular Immunity
Immunoglobulin Structure and Function
Immunogenetics & Transplantation
 Genetic Control of the Immune Response

Authors

Daniel C. Adelman, MD
Adjunct Professor of Medicine, Division of Allergy and Immunology, University of California, San Francisco
dadelman@sunesis.com
Allergic & Immunologic Disorders; CMDT Online only—Basic Immunology

Joshua S. Adler, MD
Associate Professor of Clinical Medicine, Division of General Internal Medicine, University of California, San Francisco; Medical Director, Ambulatory Care, UC San Francisco Medical Center
josh.adler@ucsf.edu
Preoperative Evaluation & Perioperative Management

Michael J. Aminoff, MD, DSc, FRCP
Professor of Neurology, University of California, San Francisco; Attending Physician, University of California Medical Center, San Francisco
aminoffm@neurology.ucsf.edu
Nervous System

David M. Barbour, PharmD, BCPS
Adjunct Clinical Faculty, School of Pharmacy, University of Colorado Health Sciences Center, Denver; Lead Pharmacist, Acute Care, University of Colorado Hospital, Denver
david.barbour@uch.edu
Drug References

Robert B. Baron, MD, MS
Professor of Medicine; Associate Dean for Graduate and Continuing Medical Education; Vice Chief and Director, Educational Programs, Division of General Internal Medicine; University of California, San Francisco
baron@medicine.ucsf.edu
Lipid Abnormalities; Nutrition

Thomas Bashore, MD
Professor of Medicine; Director of Cardiology Fellowship Program, Duke University Medical Center, Durham, North Carolina
thomas.bashore@duke.edu
Heart

Timothy G. Berger, MD
Professor of Clinical Dermatology, Department of Dermatology, University of California, San Francisco
bergert@derm.ucsf.edu
Skin, Hair, & Nails

Brian M. Berman, MD
Professor of Family Medicine and Director, Center for Integrative Medicine, University of Maryland School of Medicine, Baltimore
bberman@compmed.umm.edu
Complementary & Alternative Medicine

Peter R. Carroll, MD, FACS
Professor and Chair, Department of Urology; Ken and Donna Derr-Chevron Distinguished Professor; University of California, San Francisco
pcarroll@urology.ucsf.edu
Urology

Henry F. Chambers, MD
Professor of Medicine, University of California, San Francisco; Chief, Division of Infectious Diseases, San Francisco General Hospital
hchambers@medsfgh.ucsf.edu
Infectious Diseases: Bacterial & Chlamydial

Mark S. Chesnutt, MD
Associate Professor of Medicine, Pulmonary & Critical Care Medicine, Oregon Health & Science University, Portland; Chief, Critical Care, Portland Veterans Affairs Medicine Center
chesnutm@ohsu.edu
Lung

Peter V. Chin-Hong, MD
Assistant Professor of Medicine; Co-leader, Doris Duke Clinical Research Fellowship for Medical Students, University of California, San Francisco; Attending Physician, Positive Health Practice, San Francisco General Hospital, San Francisco, California
phong@php.ucsf.edu
General Problems in Infectious Diseases

Richard Cohen, MD, MPH
Clinical Professor, Division of Occupational and Environmental Medicine, University of California, San Francisco
rcohenmd@pacbell.net
Disorders Due to Physical Agents

William R. Crombleholme, MD
Professor of Clinical Obstetrics & Gynecology, Columbia University College of Physicians and Surgeons, New York; Chairman, Department of Obstetrics and Gynecology, The Stamford Hospital, Stamford, Connecticut
wcrombleholme@stamhealth.org
Obstetrics

Stuart J. Eisendrath, MD
Professor of Clinical Psychiatry, University of California, San Francisco
stuart.eisendrath@ucsf.edu
Psychiatric Disorders

Paul A. Fitzgerald, MD
Clinical Professor of Medicine, Department of Medicine, Division of Endocrinology, University of California, San Francisco
paul.fitzgerald@ucsf.edu
Endocrinology

Lawrence S. Friedman, MD
Professor of Medicine, Harvard Medical School, Boston, Massachusetts; Chair, Department of Medicine, Newton-Wellesley Hospital, Newton, Massachusetts; Assistant Chief of Medicine, Massachusetts General Hospital, Boston, Massachusetts
lfriedman@partners.org
Liver, Biliary Tract, & Pancreas

Masafumi Fukagawa, MD, PhD, FJSIM, FASN
Associate Professor and Director, Division of Nephrology and Dialysis Center, Kobe University School of Medicine, Japan
fukagawa@med.kobe-u.ac.jp
Fluid & Electrolyte Disorders

Rebekah Gardner, MD
Fellow, Division of General Internal Medicine, Department of Medicine, University of California, San Francisco
rgardner@medicine.ucsf.edu
References

Armando E. Giuliano, MD
Chief of Science and Medicine, John Wayne Cancer Institute; Director, Joyce Eisenberg Keefer Breast Center, Saint John's Health Center, Santa Monica, California
giulianoa@jwci.org
Breast

Lee Goldman, MD, MPH
Executive Vice President for Health and Biomedical Sciences; Dean of the Faculty of Medicine; Dean of the Faculties of Health Sciences; Harold and Margaret Hatch Professor of the University; Professor of Medicine, College of Physicians and Surgeons; Professor of Epidemiology, Mailman School of Public Health; Columbia University Medical Center, New York, New York
lgoldman@columbia.edu
Preoperative Evaluation & Perioperative Management

Robert S. Goldsmith, MD, MPH, DTM&H
Professor Emeritus of Tropical Medicine and Epidemiology, Department of Epidemiology and Biostatistics, University of California, San Francisco
robert.goldsmith@ucsf.edu
Infectious Diseases: Protozoal & Helminthic

Antonio D. Gomez, MD
Fellow, Division of Pulmonary and Critical Care Medicine, Department of Medicine, University of California San Francisco
agomez@medsfgh.ucsf.edu
References

Ralph Gonzales, MD, MSPH
Associate Professor of Medicine, Epidemiology & Biostatistics, Division of General Internal Medicine, Department of Medicine, University of California, San Francisco
ralphg@medicine.ucsf.edu
Common Symptoms

Christopher B. Granger, MD
Associate Professor, Department Of Medicine, Division of Cardiology, Duke University Medical Center, Durham, North Carolina
grang001@mc.duke.edu
Heart

B. Joseph Guglielmo, PharmD
Professor and Chair, Department of Clinical Pharmacy, School of Pharmacy, University of California, San Francisco
guglielmoj@pharmacy.ucsf.edu
Anti-Infective Chemotherapeutic & Antibiotic Agents

Jennifer E. Guy, MD
Chief Medical Resident, San Francisco Veterans Administration Medical Center, Department of Medicine, University of California, San Francisco
jennifer.guy@ucsf.edu
References

Sadia Haider, MD
Clinical Fellow in Family Planning, Department of Obstetrics & Gynecology, University of California, San Francisco
haiders@obgyn.ucsf.edu
References

Richard J. Hamill, MD
Professor, Division of Infectious Diseases, Departments of Medicine and Molecular Virology & Microbiology, Baylor College of Medicine, Houston, Texas
richard.hamill@med.va.gov
Infectious Diseases: Mycotic

G. Michael Harper, MD
Associate Clinical Professor of Medicine, Geriatric Medicine, University of California, San Francisco; Director of Geriatrics Fellowship Training Program, San Francisco Veterans Affairs Medical Center, San Francisco, California
michael.harper3@med.va.gov
Geriatric Medicine

David B. Hellmann, MD, FACP
Aliki Perroti Professor of Medicine; Vice Dean for Johns Hopkins Bayview; Chairman, Department of Medicine, Johns Hopkins Bayview Medical Center, Johns Hopkins University School of Medicine, Baltimore, Maryland
hellmann@jhmi.edu
Arthritis & Musculoskeletal Disorders

Patrick M. Hranitzky, MD
Assistant Professor of Medicine, Duke University Medical Center; Director, Cardiac Electrophysiology, Durham VA Medical Center, Durham, North Carolina
patrick.hranitzky@duke.edu
Heart

Ellen F. Hughes, MD, PhD
Clinical Professor of Medicine, Division of General Internal Medicine, Department of Medicine, University of California, San Francisco
ehughes@medicine.ucsf.edu
Complementary & Alternative Medicine

Robert K. Jackler, MD
Sewall Professor and Chair, Department of Otolaryngology-Head and Neck Surgery, Stanford University School of Medicine, Stanford, California
jackler@stanford.edu
Ear, Nose, & Throat

Bradly P. Jacobs, MD, MPH
Chief of Integrative Medicine; Senior Medical Director, Care Division; Revolution Health Group, Washington, District of Columbia
bradly.jacobs@revolution.com
Complementary & Alternative Medicine

Richard A. Jacobs, MD, PhD
Clinical Professor of Medicine and Clinical Pharmacy, Division of Infectious Diseases, Department of Medicine, University of California, San Francisco
jacobsd@medicine.ucsf.edu
General Problems in Infectious Diseases; Infectious Diseases: Spirochetal; Anti-Infective Chemotherapeutic & Antibiotic Agents

C. Bree Johnston, MD
Associate Professor of Clinical Medicine, Division of Geriatrics, Department of Medicine, Veterans Affairs Medical Center, University of California, San Francisco
bree.johnston@ucsf.edu
Geriatric Medicine

Christopher J. Kane, MD, FACS
Associate Professor and Vice-Chair of Urology, University of California, San Francisco
ckane@urology.ucsf.edu
Urology

Michael J. Kaplan, MD
Professor, Department of Otolaryngology-Head and Neck Surgery; Professor, Neurosurgery and Surgery, Stanford University School of Medicine, Stanford, California
mjkaplan@stanford.edu
Ear, Nose, & Throat

Mitchell H. Katz, MD
Clinical Professor of Medicine, Epidemiology & Biostatistics, University of California, San Francisco; Director of Health, San Francisco Department of Public Health
mitch.katz@sfdph.org
HIV Infection

Jeffrey L. Kishiyama, MD
Associate Clinical Professor of Medicine, Division of Immunology, Department of Medicine, University of California, San Francisco
jeff.kishiyama@ucsf.edu
Allergic & Immunologic Disorders; CMDT Online only—Basic Immunology

Hoonmo L. Koo, MD
Infectious Diseases Fellow, Department of Internal Medicine, Baylor College of Medicine, Houston, Texas
koo@bcm.tmc.edu
Infectious Diseases: Viral & Rickettsial

Kiyoshi Kurokawa, MD, MACP
Adjunct Professor, Division of Health Policy, Research Center for Advanced Science, The University of Tokyo, Tokyo, Japan
kurokawa@is.icc.u-tokai.ac.jp
Fluid & Electrolyte Disorders

C. Seth Landefeld, MD
Professor; Chief, Division of Geriatrics; Director, UCSF-Mt. Zion Center on Aging, University of California, San Francisco; Director, Quality Scholars Fellowship Program, San Francisco Veterans Affairs Medical Center
sethl@medicine.ucsf.edu
Geriatric Medicine

Jonathan E. Lichtmacher, MD
Health Sciences Associate Clinical Professor of Psychiatry; Associate Director, Adult Psychiatry Clinic, Langley Porter Hospitals and Clinics, University of California, San Francisco
jonathanl@lppi.ucsf.edu
Psychiatric Disorders

Grace A. Lin, MD
Fellow, Division of General Internal Medicine, University of California, San Francisco
glin@medsfgh.ucsf.edu
References

Charles A. Linker, MD
Clinical Professor of Medicine; Director, Bone Mar-
row Transplant Program, Division of Hematology/
Oncology, University of California, San Francisco
linkerc@medicine.ucsf.edu
Blood

H. Trent MacKay, MD, MPH
Professor of Obstetrics and Gynecology, Uniformed
Services University of the Health Sciences, Be-
thesda, Maryland; Associate Director of Women's
Health Services, National Naval Medical Center,
Bethesda, Maryland
mackayt@mail.nih.gov
Gynecology

Umesh Masharani, MD, MB, MRCP(UK)
Clinical Professor of Medicine, Division of Endocri-
nology and Metabolism, Department of Medicine,
University of California, San Francisco
umesh.masharani@ucsf.edu
Diabetes Mellitus & Hypoglycemia

Stephen J. McPhee, MD
Professor of Medicine, Division of General Internal
Medicine, Department of Medicine, University of
California, San Francisco
smcphee@medicine.ucsf.edu
Approach to the Patient & Health Maintenance

Kenneth R. McQuaid, MD
Professor of Clinical Medicine, University of Califor-
nia, San Francisco; Director of Endoscopy, San
Francisco Veterans Affairs Medicine Center
kenneth.mcquaid@med.va.gov
Alimentary Tract

Louis M. Messina, MD
Professor of Surgery, Division of Vascular Surgery,
Department of Surgery, University of California,
San Francisco
messina@surgery.ucsf.edu
Blood Vessels & Lymphatics

Brent R.W. Moelleken, MD, FACS
Assistant Clinical Professor, Division of Plastic Surgery;
Attending Physician, University of California, Los
Angeles Medical Center; Private Practice in Plastic
and Reconstructive Surgery, Beverly Hills, California
drbrent@drbrent.com
Disorders Due to Physical Agents

Gail Morrison, MD
Vice Dean for Education; Director of Academic Programs; Professor of Medicine, School of Medicine,
Renal-Electrolyte and Hypertension Division, University of Pennsylvania Health System, Philadelphia, Pennsylvania
morrisog@mail.med.upenn.edu
Kidney

C. Diana Nicoll, MD, PhD, MPA
Clinical Professor and Interim Chair, Department
of Laboratory Medicine; Associate Dean,
University of California, San Francisco; Chief
of Staff and Chief, Laboratory Medicine Service,
San Francisco Veterans Affairs Medical
Center
diana.nicoll@med.va.gov
*Appendix: Therapeutic Drug Monitoring & Laboratory
Reference Ranges; CMDT Online only—Diagnostic
Testing & Medical Decision Making*

Kent R. Olson, MD
Clinical Professor of Medicine, Pediatrics, and Pharmacy, University of California, San Francisco;
Medical Director, San Francisco Division, California Poison Control System
kent.olson@ucsf.edu
Poisoning

Steven Z. Pantilat, MD
Associate Professor of Clinical Medicine, Department
of Medicine; Director, Palliative Care Service, University of California, San Francisco
stevep@medicine.ucsf.edu
Care at the End of Life

Maxine A. Papadakis, MD
Professor of Clinical Medicine and Associate Dean for
Student Affairs, School of Medicine, University of
California, San Francisco
papadakm@medsch.ucsf.edu
Fluid & Electrolyte Disorders

Michael Pignone, MD, MPH
Associate Professor of Medicine, University of North
Carolina, Chapel Hill
pignone@med.unc.edu
*Approach to the Patient & Health Maintenance; CMDT
Online only—Diagnostic Testing & Medical
Decision-Making*

Thomas J. Prendergast, MD
Associate Professor of Medicine and Anesthesiology,
Section of Pulmonary and Critical Care Medicine,
Dartmouth-Hitchcock Medical Center, Lebanon,
New Hampshire
thomas.j.prendergast@hitchcock.org
Lung

Reed E. Pyeritz, MD, PhD
Professor of Medicine and Genetics; Chief,
Division of Medical Genetics, University of
Pennsylvania Health System and School of Medi-
cine, Philadelphia
reed.pyeritz@uphs.upenn.edu
Genetic Disorders; CMDT Online only—Basic Genetics

Michael W. Rabow, MD
Associate Professor of Clinical Medicine, Division of General Internal Medicine, University of California, San Francisco
mrabow@medicine.ucsf.edu
Care at the End of Life

Paul Riordan-Eva, FRCS, FRCOphth
Consultant Ophthalmologist, King's College Hospital, London, United Kingdom
Paul.riordan-eva@kingsch.nhs.uk
Eye

Hope S. Rugo, MD
Clinical Professor of Medicine and Director, Breast Oncology Clinical Trials Program, University of California, San Francisco Comprehensive Cancer Center
hrugo@medicine.ucsf.edu
Cancer

Hilary K. Seligman, MD, MAS
Assistant Professor of Medicine, San Francisco General Hospital, University of California, San Francisco
hseligman@medsfgh.ucsf.edu
References

Wayne X. Shandera, MD
Assistant Professor, Department of Internal Medicine, Baylor College of Medicine, Houston, Texas
shandera@bcm.tmc.edu
Infectious Diseases: Viral & Rickettsial

Samuel A. Shelburne, MD
Assistant Professor, Department of Internal Medicine, Baylor College of Medicine, Houston, Texas
samuels@bcm.tmc.edu
Infectious Diseases: Mycotic

Marshall L. Stoller, MD
Professor and Vice Chairman, Department of Urology, University of California, San Francisco
mstoller@urology.ucsf.edu
Urology

John H. Stone, MD, MPH
Associate Professor of Medicine, Division of Rheumatology, Johns Hopkins University; Director, Johns Hopkins Vasculitis Center, Baltimore, Maryland
jstone@jhmi.edu
Arthritis & Musculoskeletal Disorders

Michael Sutters, MD, MRCP(UK)
Assistant Professor of Medicine, Division of Nephrology, Johns Hopkins Bayview Medical Center, Johns Hopkins University School of Medicine, Baltimore, Maryland
msutters@jhmi.edu
Systemic Hypertension

Suzanne Watnick, MD
Assistant Professor of Medicine, Division of Nephrology and Hypertension, Oregon Health & Science University, Portland; Director, Dialysis Unit, Portland VA Medical Center, Portland, Oregon
watnicks@ohsu.edu
Kidney

Andrew R. Zolopa, MD
Associate Professor of Medicine, Division of Infectious Diseases and Geographic Medicine, Stanford University, Stanford, California
azolopa@stanford.edu
HIV Infection

Preface

Current Medical Diagnosis & Treatment 2007 is the 46th annual volume of this single-source reference for practitioners in both hospital and ambulatory settings. It emphasizes the practical features of clinical diagnosis and patient management in all fields of internal medicine and in specialties of interest to primary care practitioners and to subspecialists who provide generalist care.

OUTSTANDING FEATURES

- Medical advances up to time of annual publication
- Detailed presentation of all primary care topics, including gynecology, obstetrics, dermatology, ophthalmology, otolaryngology, psychiatry, neurology, toxicology, urology, geriatrics, preventive medicine, and palliative care
- Concise format, facilitating efficient use in any practice setting
- More than 1000 diseases and disorders
- Only text with annual update on HIV infection
- Prevention and cost information
- Easy access to drug dosages, with trade names indexed and prices updated in each edition
- Annotated recent references, with unique identifiers (PubMed, PMID, numbers)

INTENDED AUDIENCE

House officers, medical students, and all other health professions students will find the descriptions of diagnostic and therapeutic modalities, with citations to the current literature, of everyday usefulness in patient care.

Internists, family physicians, hospitalists, nurse practitioners, physicians' assistants, and all primary care providers will appreciate *CMDT* as a ready reference and refresher text. Physicians in other specialties, surgeons, pharmacists, and dentists will find the book a basic internal medicine reference. Nurses, nurse-practitioners, and physicians' assistants will welcome the format and scope of the book as a means of learning medical diagnosis and treatment.

Patients and their family members who seek information about the nature of specific diseases and their diagnosis and treatment may also find this book to be a valuable resource.

SPECIAL TO THIS EDITION

- Major revisions of the heart chapter, including extensive updating of valvular heart disease
- Updated immunization tables presenting the latest guidelines for adults
- New drug regimens for lipid disorders
- Expanded discussion of antiphospholipid syndrome
- Enhanced description of squamous cell carcinoma of the larynx
- Updates on emerging infectious diseases such as West Nile virus, avian influenza, and severe acute respiratory syndrome (SARS)
- Palliative care information integrated throughout the text
- Developments in HIV infection, including new treatment regimens and the role of antiretroviral drug resistance assays
- New information on alternative medicine and complementary therapies
- Drug information, bibliographies, and Web sites updated through June 2006
- Update on antibiotics, including new antiviral and antifungal agents
- List of key Internet addresses for current peer-reviewed medical information, including:
  - Centers for Disease Control and Prevention traveler's and immunization information
  - National Institutes of Health Consensus Statements
  - Agency for Healthcare Research and Quality of the United States Public Health Service Clinical Guidelines

CMDT IS ONLINE

The online version of *CMDT* is now available through www.AccessMedicine.com. *CMDT Online* includes the following:

- Full electronic access to the content of *CMDT* 2007 anytime and anyplace you need it
- Quarterly updates by the *CMDT* editors
- Topic-based presentation of more than 1,000 diseases and disorders
- 1,200+ color and black-and-white images not available in the print version
- Instant access to all of the critical information through a sophisticated search engine, custom-designed for medical information
- *Practice Guidelines in Primary Care*, covering screening, prevention, and disease management
- Thorough coverage of all US prescription drugs provided by *Clinical Pharmacology* by Gold Standard Multimedia
- Patient Handouts
- A-Z topic index
- Links to related Web sites
- References hyperlinked to PubMed
- *Clip and Go* for instant downloading of dynamically indexed content to your handheld
- Ability to personalize your subscription to include bookmarking, managing PDA downloads, and e-mailing topics to colleagues

ACKNOWLEDGMENTS

We wish to thank our associate authors for participating once again in the annual updating of this important book. Many students and physicians also have contributed useful suggestions to this and previous editions, and we are grateful. We continue to welcome comments and recommendations for future editions in writing or via electronic mail. The editors' and authors' institutional and Internet e-mail addresses are given in the Authors section.

Stephen J. McPhee, MD
Maxine A. Papadakis, MD
Lawrence M. Tierney, Jr., MD

San Francisco, California
September 2006

From inability to let alone; from too much zeal for the new and contempt for what is old; from putting knowledge before wisdom, and science before art and cleverness before common sense; from treating patients as cases; and from making the cure of the disease more grievous than the endurance of the same, Good Lord, deliver us.

—Sir Robert Hutchison

Approach to the Patient & Health Maintenance

Michael Pignone, MD, MPH, & Stephen J. McPhee, MD

1

■ GENERAL APPROACH TO THE PATIENT

The approach to diagnosis begins with the history and pertinent physical examination—both susceptible to errors of omission and commission. The medical interview serves several functions. It is used to collect information of help in diagnosis (the "history" of the present illness), to assess and communicate prognosis, to establish a therapeutic relationship, and to reach agreement with the patient about further diagnostic procedures and therapeutic options. It also serves as an opportunity to influence patient behavior, such as in motivational discussions about smoking cessation or medication adherence. Interviewing techniques that avoid domination by the clinician increase patient involvement in care and patient satisfaction. Effective clinician-patient communication and increased patient involvement can improve health outcomes.

Patient Adherence

For many illnesses, treatment depends on difficult fundamental behavioral changes, including alterations in diet, taking up exercise, giving up smoking, cutting down drinking, and adhering to medication regimens that are often complex. Adherence is a problem in every practice; up to 50% of patients fail to achieve full adherence, and one-third never take their medicines. Many patients with medical problems, even those with access to care, do not seek appropriate care or may drop out of care prematurely. Adherence rates for short-term, self-administered therapies are higher than for long-term therapies and are inversely correlated with the number of interventions, their complexity and cost, and the patient's perception of overmedication.

As an example, in HIV-infected patients, adherence to antiretroviral therapy is a crucial determinant of treatment success. Studies have unequivocally demonstrated a close relationship between patient adherence and plasma HIV RNA levels, CD4 cell counts, and mortality. Adherence levels of > 95% are needed to maintain virologic suppression. However, studies show that over 60% of patients are < 90% adherent and that adherence tends to decrease over time. Patient reasons for nonadherence include simple forgetfulness, being away from home, being busy, and changes in daily routine. Other reasons include psychiatric disorders (depression or substance abuse), uncertainty about the effectiveness of treatment, lack of knowledge about the consequences of poor adherence, regimen complexity, and treatment side effects.

Patients seem better able to take prescribed medications than to comply with recommendations to change their diet, exercise habits, or alcohol intake or to perform various self-care activities (such as monitoring blood glucose levels at home). For short-term regimens, adherence to medications can be improved by giving clear instructions. Writing out advice to patients, including changes in medication, may be helpful. Because low functional health literacy is common (almost half of English-speaking patients are unable to read and understand standard health education materials), other forms of communication—such as illustrated simple text, videotapes, or oral instructions—may be more effective. For non–English-speaking patients, clinicians and health care delivery systems can work to provide culturally and linguistically appropriate health services.

To help improve adherence to long-term regimens, clinicians can work with patients to reach agreement on the goals for therapy, provide information about the regimen, ensure understanding by using the "teach-back" method, counsel about the importance of adherence and how to organize medication-taking, reinforce self-monitoring, provide more convenient care, prescribe a simple dosage regimen for all medications (preferably one or two doses daily), suggest ways to help in remembering to take doses (time of day, mealtime, alarms) and to keep appointments, and provide ways to simplify dosing (medication boxes). Single-unit doses supplied in foil-backed wrappers can increase adherence but should be avoided for patients who have difficulty opening them. Medication boxes with compartments (eg, Medisets) that are filled weekly are useful. Microelectronic devices can provide feedback to show patients whether they have taken doses as scheduled or to notify patients within a day if doses are skipped. The clinician can also enlist social support from family and friends, recruit an adherence monitor, and provide rewards and recognition for the patient's efforts to follow the regimen.

Adherence is also improved when a trusting doctor-patient relationship has been established and when patients actively participate in their care. Clinicians can improve patient adherence by inquiring specifically about the behaviors in question. When asked, many patients admit to incomplete adherence with medication regimens, with advice about giving up cigarettes, or with engaging only in "safe sex" practices. Although difficult, sufficient time must be made available for communication of health messages. Other ways of assessing medication adherence include pill counts and refill records; monitoring serum, urine, or saliva levels of drugs or metabolites; watching for appointment nonattendance and treatment nonresponse; and assessing predictable drug effects such as weight changes with diuretics or bradycardia from β-blockers. In some conditions, even partial adherence, as with drug treatment of hypertension and diabetes mellitus, improves outcomes compared with nonadherence; in other cases, such as HIV antiretroviral therapy or treatment of tuberculosis, partial adherence may be worse than complete nonadherence.

Guiding Principles of Care

Ethical decisions are often called for in medical practice, at both the "micro" level of the individual patient-clinician relationship and at the "macro" level of the allocation of resources. Ethical principles that guide the successful approach to diagnosis and treatment are honesty, beneficence, justice, avoidance of conflict of interest, and the pledge to do no harm. Increasingly, Western medicine involves patients in important decisions about medical care, including how far to proceed with treatment of patients who have terminal illnesses (see Chapter 5).

The clinician's role does not end with diagnosis and treatment. The importance of the empathic clinician in helping patients and their families bear the burden of serious illness and death cannot be overemphasized. "To cure sometimes, to relieve often, and to comfort always" is a French saying as apt today as it was five centuries ago—as is Francis Peabody's admonition: "The secret of the care of the patient is in caring for the patient."

Aliotta SL et al: Enhancing adherence to long-term medical therapy: a new approach to assessing and treating patients. Adv Ther 2004;21:214. [PMID: 15605616]

Connor J et al: Do fixed-dose combination pills or unit-of-use packaging improve adherence? A systematic review. Bull World Health Organ 2004;82:935. [PMID: 15654408]

DeWalt DA et al: Literacy and health outcomes: a systematic review of the literature. J Gen Intern Med 2004;19:1228. [PMID: 15610334]

Domino FJ: Improving adherence to treatment for hypertension. Am Fam Physician 2005;71:2089. [PMID: 15952435]

Haynes RB et al: Helping patients follow prescribed treatment: clinical applications. JAMA 2002;288:2880. [PMID: 12472330]

McDonald HP et al: Interventions to enhance patient adherence to medication prescriptions: scientific review. JAMA 2002; 288:2868. [PMID: 12472329]

Van Wijk BL et al: Effectiveness of interventions by community pharmacists to improve patient adherence to chronic medication: a systematic review. Ann Pharmacother 2005;39:319. [PMID: 15632223]

Vermeire E et al: Interventions for improving adherence to treatment recommendations in people with type 2 diabetes mellitus. Cochrane Database Syst Rev 2005;(2):CD003638. [PMID: 15846672]

■ HEALTH MAINTENANCE & DISEASE PREVENTION

Preventive medicine can be categorized as primary, secondary, or tertiary. Primary prevention aims to remove or reduce disease risk factors (eg, immunization, giving up or not starting smoking). Secondary prevention techniques promote early detection of disease or precursor states (eg, routine cervical Papanicolaou screening to detect carcinoma or dysplasia of the cervix). Tertiary prevention measures are aimed at limiting the impact of established disease (eg, partial mastectomy and radiation therapy to remove and control localized breast cancer). Table 1–1 gives data for deaths from preventable causes in the United States. Table 1–2 compares recommendations for periodic health examinations as developed by the United States Preventive Services Task Force, the

Table 1–1. Estimated annual deaths from preventable causes in the United States in 2000.

Preventable Cause	Estimated Number of Deaths (% total deaths)
Tobacco	435,000 (18%)
Poor diet and physical inactivity	365,000 (15%)
Alcohol	85,000 (3%)
Motor vehicle	43,000 (2%)
Firearms	29,000 (1%)
Illicit drug use	17,000 (0.7%)

From Mokdad AH et al: Actual causes of death in the United States, 2000. JAMA 2004;291:1238. Errata in: JAMA 2005;293:293,298.

Table 1–2. Expert recommendations for preventive care for asymptomatic, low-risk adults.

Preventive Service	USPSTF[1]	CTF[2]	Other Organizations
Screening tests			
Blood pressure	Recommended for all adults; interval not stated	Fair evidence for inclusion in routine care	Joint National Committee VII: Recommended for all adults at each clinical encounter
Serum lipids	Recommended for all middle-aged and older adults and for young adults with multiple risk factors	Insufficient evidence for or against inclusion	National Cholesterol Education Panel Adult Treatment Panel III: Recommended for all adults age 21 and older
Depression screening	Recommended (B recommendation)[3]	Fair evidence for *exclusion* from routine care	
Counseling			
Healthy diet	Recommended for patients with increased risk; insufficient evidence for or against in average-risk patients	Fair evidence for inclusion	
Physical activity	Recommended	Fair evidence for inclusion	
Immunizations and chemoprevention			
Aspirin chemoprevention	Recommended for adults at increased risk for coronary heart disease (CHD)	Insufficient evidence for or against use	American Heart Association: Recommended for adults at increased risk for CHD
Influenza vaccination	Recommended for all adults 65 and older and for selected high-risk groups	Not addressed	
Pneumococcal vaccination	Recommended for immunocompetent adults older than age 65 or for adults younger than age 65 at increased risk	Insufficient evidence for or against in immunocompetent free-living adults older than age 55	

[1]United States Preventive Services Task Force; recommendations available at http://www.ahrq.gov
[2]Canadian Task Force on Preventive Health Care; recommendations available at http://www.ctfphc.org/
[3]The USPSTF recommends that clinicians routinely provide the service to eligible patients. (The USPSTF found at least fair evidence that the service improves important health outcomes and concludes that benefits outweigh harms.)

American College of Physicians, and the Canadian Task Force on the Periodic Health Examination. Despite emerging consensus on many of the services, controversy persists for others. Many effective preventive services are underutilized. One analysis concluded that the following services had the most potential for improvement, based on their effectiveness and underuse: counseling about smoking cessation; screening older adults for vision impairment; screening and counseling adults and adolescents about alcohol abuse; screening older adults for colorectal cancer; screening young women for chlamydia infection; and vaccinating older adults against pneumococcal disease.

Jemal A et al: Trends in the leading cause of death in the United States, 1970–2002. JAMA 2005;294;1255. [PMID: 16160134]

Prochazka AV et al: Support of evidence-based guidelines for the annual physical examination: a survey of primary care providers. Arch Intern Med 2005;165:1347. [PMID: 15983282]

PREVENTION OF INFECTIOUS DISEASES

Much of the decline in the incidence and fatality rates of infectious diseases is attributable to public health measures—especially immunization, improved sanitation, and better nutrition.

Immunization remains the best means of preventing many infectious diseases. In the United States, childhood immunization has resulted in near elimination of measles, mumps, rubella, poliomyelitis, diphtheria, pertussis, and tetanus. *Haemophilus influenzae* type b invasive disease has been reduced by more than 95% since the introduction of the first conjugate vaccines. However, substantial vaccine-preventable morbidity and mortality continue to occur among adults from vaccine-preventable diseases, such as hepatitis A, hepatitis B, influenza, and pneumococcal infections. For example, in adults in the United States, there are an estimated 50,000–70,000 deaths annually from influenza, hepatitis B, and invasive pneumococcal disease. Yet in 2002, only about 65% of elderly persons reported receiving influenza and pneumococcal vaccines. The American College of Physicians recommends that clinicians should review each adult's immunization status at age 50; assess risk factors that would indicate a need for pneumococcal vaccination and annual influenza immunizations; reimmunize at age 65 those who received an immunization against pneumococcus more than 6 years before; ensure that all adults have completed a primary diphtheria-tetanus immunization series, and administer a single booster at age 50; and assess the postvaccination serologic response to hepatitis B vaccination in all recipients who have ongoing risks of exposure to blood or body fluids (eg, sharp injuries, blood splashes).

Recently, strategies have also been proposed to improve influenza, pneumococcal polysaccharide, and hepatitis B targeted vaccination; in other words, improve coverage among those adults aged 65 years or younger who are at high risk for exposure or disease. Strategies to enhance vaccinations in general include increasing community demand for vaccinations; enhancing access to vaccination services; and provider- or system-based interventions, such as reminder systems. Clinicians can substantially improve immunization rates by use of standing orders and algorithms, expanded nurse decision-making, patient education and incentives, and partnership with community pharmacies. Increasing reports of pertussis among US adolescents, adults, and their infant contacts have stimulated vaccine development for older age groups. A safe and effective tetanus-diphtheria 5-component acellular pertussis vaccine (Tdap) is now available for use in adolescents and adults. On October 26, 2005, the Advisory Committee on Immunization Practices (ACIP) recommended routine use of a single dose of Tdap for adults aged 19–64 years to replace the next booster dose of tetanus and diphtheria toxoids vaccine (Td). The ACIP also recommended Tdap for adults who have close contact with infants younger than 12 months, for pregnant women, and women who are planning a pregnancy.

In 2002, the ACIP approved a schedule for the routine vaccination of persons aged 19 years and older. Recommended immunization schedules for children and adolescents are set forth in Table 30–4. Persons traveling to countries where infections are endemic should take precautions described in Chapter 30. Immunization registries—confidential, population-based, computerized information systems that collect vaccination data about all residents of a geographic area—can be used to increase and sustain high vaccination coverage.

Skin testing for tuberculosis and treating selected patients reduce the risk of reactivation tuberculosis (see Table 9–12). Attention to technique helps separate negative from positive results. A more precise measurement of induration from the PPD can be obtained by drawing a line on the skin with a medium ballpoint pen, starting 1–2 cm away from the skin reaction and then stopping when resistance is felt. Patients with HIV infection are at an especially high risk

for tuberculosis. This is discussed in Chapter 31, as is multidrug-resistant tuberculosis.

HIV infection is now the major infectious disease problem in the world, and it affects 850,000–950,000 persons in the United States. Since sexual contact is a common mode of transmission, primary prevention relies on eliminating unsafe sexual behavior by promoting abstinence, later onset of first sexual activity, decreased number of partners, and use of latex condoms. Appropriately used, condoms can reduce the rate of HIV transmission by nearly 70%. In one study, couples with one infected partner who used condoms inconsistently had a considerable risk of infection: the rate of seroconversion was estimated to be 13% after 24 months. No seroconversions were noted with consistent condom use. Unfortunately, as many as one-third of HIV-positive individuals continue unprotected sexual practices after learning that they are HIV-infected. Tailored group educational intervention focused on practicing "safer sex" can reduce their transmission-risk behaviors with partners who are not HIV-positive. Other approaches to prevent HIV infection include treatment of sexually transmitted diseases, development of vaginal microbicides, and vaccine development. Increasingly, cases of HIV infection are transmitted by injection drug use. HIV prevention activities should include provision of sterile injection equipment for these individuals.

With regard to secondary prevention, many HIV-infected persons in the US currently receive the diagnosis at advanced stages of immunosuppression, and almost all will progress to AIDS if untreated. On the other hand, highly active antiretroviral therapy (HAART) substantially reduces the risk of clinical progression or death in patients with advanced immunosuppression. Screening tests for HIV are extremely (> 99%) accurate. While the benefits of HIV screening appear to outweigh its harms, current screening is generally based on individual patient risk factors. Such screening can identify persons at risk for AIDS but misses a substantial proportion of those infected. Nonetheless, the yield from screening higher prevalence populations is substantially greater than that from screening the general population, and more widespread screening of the population remains controversial.

In immunocompromised patients, live vaccines are contraindicated but many killed or component vaccines are safe and recommended. *Asymptomatic* HIV-infected patients have not shown adverse consequences when given live MMR and influenza vaccinations as well as tetanus, hepatitis B, *H influenzae* type b, and pneumococcal vaccinations—all should be given. However, if poliomyelitis immunization is required, the inactivated poliomyelitis vaccine is indicated. In *symptomatic* HIV-infected patients, live virus vaccines such as MMR should generally be avoided, but annual influenza vaccination is safe.

Whenever possible, immunizations should be completed before procedures that require or induce immunosuppression (organ transplantation or chemotherapy), or that reduce immunogenic responses (splenectomy). However, if this is not possible, the patient may mount only a partial immune response, yet even this partial response can be of benefit. Patients who undergo allogeneic bone marrow transplantation lose preexisting immunities and should be revaccinated. In many situations, family members should also be vaccinated to protect the immunocompromised patient, although oral live polio vaccine should be avoided because of the risk of infecting the patient.

New cases of poliomyelitis have been reported in the United States, Haiti, and the Dominican Republic recently, slowing its eradication in the Western Hemisphere.

The 2001 anthrax attacks in the United States have raised concern about the nation's vulnerability to a smallpox attack. Resumption of smallpox vaccination was undertaken for some health care workers, police and firemen, etc. However, smallpox vaccine has a higher complication rate than any other vaccine currently being used. Expected adverse events in a mass smallpox vaccination campaign include fever (less than one case per five vaccine recipients), rash (less than one case per one hundred recipients), encephalitis (less than three cases per million), and death (less than two cases per million). Careful prevaccination exclusion of high-risk individuals (those with eczema or immunosuppression or coronary artery disease) is essential to minimize such complications.

During the 2002–2004 smallpox vaccination campaign, only 214 neurologic events were reported among 665,000 persons vaccinated against smallpox, and these were generally mild and self-limited. Serious neurologic events, such as postvaccinal encephalitis, Bell's palsy, and Guillain-Barré syndrome, occurred with expected incidences. No neurologic sequelae were identified at a rate above baseline estimates. In terms of overall complications, among 37,901 volunteers receiving 38,885 doses of smallpox vaccine in 2003, there were 100 serious adverse events reported, resulting in 85 hospitalizations, 10 life-threatening illnesses, 2 permanent disabilities, and 3 deaths. Among the serious adverse events, there were 21 cases of myocarditis, pericarditis, and ischemic cardiac events. Serious adverse events were more common among older persons being revaccinated than among younger persons being vaccinated for the first time. Rigorous smallpox vaccine safety screening and educational programs contributed to low rates of preventable life-threatening adverse reactions.

The current epidemic of highly pathogenic H5N1 avian influenza within duck and poultry populations in Southeast Asia raises serious concerns that genetic reassortment will result in a human influenza pandemic. In 2003 through 2005, there were 138 confirmed cases of human infection with H5N1 avian influenza in Vietnam, Thailand, Indonesia, China, and Cambodia, with a mortality rate of > 50%. To prevent and prepare for an increase in human cases, public health officials are working to improve detection methods and to stockpile effective antivirals, such as oseltamivir. While vaccines are the mainstay of prophylaxis against influenza, there are technical and safety issues that must be overcome in the development of an avian influenza vaccine for use in humans.

Burns IT et al: Immunization barriers and solutions. J Fam Pract 2005;54(1 Suppl):S58. [PMID: 15623395]

Casey CG et al: Adverse events associated with smallpox vaccination in the United States, January-October 2003. JAMA 2005;294:2734. [PMID: 16333009]

Chou R et al: US Preventive Services Task Force: Screening for HIV: a review of the evidence for the U.S. Preventive Services Task Force. Ann Intern Med 2005;143:55. [PMID: 15998755]

Middleton DB et al: Vaccine schedules and procedures. J Fam Pract 2005;54(1 Suppl):S37. [PMID: 15623393]

Pichichero ME et al: Combined tetanus, diphtheria, and 5-component pertussis vaccine for use in adolescents and adults. JAMA 2005;293:3003. [PMID: 15933223]

Sejvar JJ et al: Neurologic adverse events associated with smallpox vaccination in the United States, 2002-2004. JAMA 2005; 294:2744. [PMID: 16333010]

Willis BC et al: Task Force on Community Preventive Services: Improving influenza, pneumococcal polysaccharide, and hepatitis B vaccination coverage among adults aged < 65 years at high risk: a report on recommendations of the Task Force on Community Preventive Services. MMWR Recomm Rep 2005;54(RR-5):1. [PMID: 15800472]

Zeitlin GA et al: Avian influenza. Curr Infect Dis Rep 2005; 7:193. [PMID: 15847721]

PREVENTION OF CARDIOVASCULAR DISEASE

Cardiovascular diseases, including coronary heart disease and stroke, represent two of the most important causes of morbidity and mortality in developed countries. Several risk factors increase the risk for coronary disease and stroke. They can be divided into those that are modifiable (eg, lipid disorders, hypertension, cigarette smoking) and those that are not (eg, gender, age, family history of early coronary disease). This section considers the role of screening for and treating modifiable risk factors.

Impressive declines in age-specific mortality rates from heart disease and stroke have been achieved in all age groups in North America during the past 2 decades. The chief reasons for this favorable trend appear to be modification of risk factors, especially cigarette smoking and hypercholesterolemia, plus more aggressive detection and treatment of hypertension and better care for patients with heart disease. In addition, it now appears that screening for abdominal aortic aneurysm in men aged 65–75 years is associated with a significant reduction in mortality (odds ratio, 0.57 [95% CI, 0.45 to 0.74]); this benefit has not been found for women.

Fleming C et al: Screening for abdominal aortic aneurysm: a best-evidence systematic review for the U.S. Preventive Services Task Force. Ann Intern Med 2005;142:203. [PMID: 15684209]

Cigarette Smoking

Cigarette smoking remains the most important cause of preventable morbidity and early mortality. In 2000, there were an estimated 4.8 million premature deaths in the world attributable to smoking, 2.4 million in developing countries and 2 million in industrialized countries. More than three-quarters (3.8 million) of these deaths were in men. The leading causes of death from smoking were cardiovascular diseases (1.7 million deaths), chronic obstructive pulmonary disease (COPD) (1 million deaths), and lung cancer (0.9 million deaths). Nicotine is highly addictive, raises brain levels of dopamine, and produces withdrawal symptoms on discontinuation. Cigarettes are responsible for one in every five deaths in the United States, yet smoking prevalence rates have been increasing among high school and college students. Cigar smoking has also increased; there is also continued use of smokeless tobacco (chewing tobacco and snuff), particularly among young people. Tobacco dependence may have a genetic component.

Smokers have twice the risk of fatal heart disease, 10 times the risk of lung cancer, and several times the risk of cancers of the mouth, throat, esophagus, pancreas, kidney, bladder, and cervix; a twofold to threefold higher incidence of stroke and peptic ulcers (which heal less well than in nonsmokers); a twofold to fourfold greater risk of fractures of the hip, wrist, and vertebrae; four times the risk of invasive pneumococcal disease; and a twofold increase in cataracts. In the United States, over 90% of cases of COPD occur among current or former smokers. Both active smoking and passive smoking are associated with deterioration of the elastic properties of the aorta (increasing the risk of aortic aneurysm) and with progression of carotid artery atherosclerosis. Smoking has also been associated with increased risks of leukemia, of colon and prostate cancers, of breast cancer among postmenopausal women who are slow acetylators of N-acetyltransferase-2 enzymes, osteoporosis, and Alzheimer's disease. In cancers of the head and neck, lung, esophagus, and bladder, smoking is linked to mutations of the *P53* gene, the most common genetic change in human cancer. Patients with head and neck cancer who continue to smoke during radiation therapy have lower rates of response than those who do not smoke. Olfaction and taste are impaired in smokers, and facial wrinkles are increased. Heavy smokers have a 2.5 greater risk of age-related macular degeneration. Smokers die 5–8 years earlier than never-smokers.

The children of smokers have lower birth weights, are more likely to be mentally retarded, have more frequent respiratory infections and less efficient pulmonary function, have a higher incidence of chronic ear infections than children of nonsmokers, and are more likely to become smokers themselves.

In addition, exposure to environmental tobacco smoke has been shown to increase the risk of cervical cancer, lung cancer, invasive pneumococcal disease, and heart disease; to promote endothelial damage and platelet aggregation; and to increase urinary excretion of tobacco-specific lung carcinogens. The incidence of breast cancer may be increased as well. Of approximately 450,000 smoking-related deaths in the United States annually, as many as 53,000 are attributable to environmental tobacco smoke.

Smoking cessation lessens the risks of death and of myocardial infarction in people with coronary artery disease; reduces the rate of death and acute myocardial infarction in patients who have undergone percutaneous coronary revascularization; lessens the risk of stroke; slows the rate of progression of carotid atherosclerosis; and is associated with improvement of COPD symptoms. On average, women smokers who quit smoking by age 35 add about 3 years to their life expectancy, and men add more than 2 years to theirs. Smoking cessation can increase life expectancy even for those who stop after the age of 65. Fortunately, adult rates in the United States are now at an all-time low—23%—but rates are climbing for young people.

Although tobacco use constitutes the most serious common medical problem, it is undertreated. Over 70% of smokers see a physician each year, but only 20% of them receive any medical quitting advice or assistance. (Persons whose physicians advise them to quit are 1.6 times as likely to attempt quitting.) About 4% of smokers are able to quit each year.

The five steps for helping smokers quit are summarized in Table 1–3. Common elements of supportive smoking cessation treatments are reviewed in Table 1–4. A system should be implemented to identify smokers, and advice to quit should be tailored to the patient's level of readiness to change. Pharmacotherapy to reduce cigarette consumption is ineffective in smokers who are unwilling or not ready to quit. Conversely, all patients trying to quit should be offered pharmacotherapy except those with medical contraindications, women who are pregnant or breast-feeding, and adolescents. Nicotine replacement therapy doubles the chance of successful quitting. Guidelines for its use are presented in Table 1–5. Suggestions for the nicotine patch are listed in Table 1–6 and for nicotine gum in Table 1–7. The nicotine patch, gum, and lozenges are available over-the-counter, and nicotine nasal spray and inhalers by prescription. When the spray is combined with the patch, cessation rates are substantially higher. The sustained-release antidepressant drug bupropion (150–300 mg/d orally) is an effective smoking cessation agent and is associated with minimal weight gain, although seizures are a contraindication. It acts by boosting brain levels of dopamine and norepinephrine, mimicking the effect of nicotine. Bupropion, either alone or in combination with a nicotine patch, has been shown to produce significantly higher abstinence rates (30–35% at 1 year) than either a patch alone or placebo. Weight gain was less in the combined program (Table 1–8).

Weight gain occurs in most patients (80%) following smoking cessation. For many it averages 2 kg, but for others (10–15%) major weight gain—over 13 kg—may occur.

Clinicians should not show disapproval of patients who have not stopped smoking or who are not ready to make a quit attempt. Thoughtful advice that emphasizes the benefits of cessation and recognizes common barriers to success can increase motivation to quit and quit rates. An intercurrent illness such as acute bronchitis or acute myocardial infarction may motivate even the most addicted smoker to quit. Individualized or group counseling is very cost-effective, even more so than treating hypertension. Smoking cessa-

Table 1–3. Actions and strategies for the primary care clinician to help patients quit smoking.

Action	Strategies for Implementation
Step 1. Ask—Systematically Identify All Tobacco Users at Every Visit	
Implement an officewide system that ensures that for *every* patient at *every* clinic visit, tobacco-use status is queried and documented[1]	Expand the vital signs to include tobacco use. Data should be collected by the health care team. The action should be implemented using preprinted progress note paper that includes the expanded vital signs, a vital signs stamp or, for computerized records, an item assessing tobacco-use status. Alternatives to the vital signs stamp are to place tobacco-use status stickers on all patients' charts or to indicate smoking status using computerized reminder systems.
Step 2. Advise—Strongly Urge All Smokers to Quit	
In a *clear, strong,* and *personalized* manner, urge every smoker to quit	Advice should be *Clear:* "I think it is important for you to quit smoking now, and I will help you. Cutting down while you are ill is not enough." *Strong:* "As your clinician, I need you to know that quitting smoking is the most important thing you can do to protect your current and future health." *Personalized:* Tie smoking to current health or illness and/or the social and economic costs of tobacco use, motivational level/readiness to quit, and the impact of smoking on children and others in the household. Encourage clinic staff to reinforce the cessation message and support the patient's quit attempt.
Step 3. Attempt—Identify Smokers Willing to Make a Quit Attempt	
Ask every smoker if he or she is willing to make a quit attempt at this time	If the patient is willing to make a quit attempt at this time, provide assistance (see step 4). If the patient prefers a more intensive treatment or the clinician believes more intensive treatment is appropriate, refer the patient to interventions administered by a smoking cessation specialist and follow up with him or her regarding quitting (see step 5). If the patient clearly states he or she is not willing to make a quit attempt at this time, provide a motivational intervention.
Step 4. Assist—Aid the Patient in Quitting	
A. Help the patient with a quit plan	*Set a quit date.* Ideally, the quit date should be within 2 weeks, taking patient preference into account. *Help the patient prepare for quitting.* The patient must: *Inform* family, friends, and coworkers of quitting and request understanding and support. *Prepare the environment* by removing cigarettes from it. Prior to quitting, the patient should avoid smoking in places where he or she spends a lot of time (eg, home, car). *Review* previous quit attempts. What helped? What led to relapse? *Anticipate* challenges to the planned quit attempt, particularly during the critical first few weeks.
B. Encourage nicotine replacement therapy except in special circumstances	Encourage the use of the nicotine patch or nicotine gum therapy for smoking cessation (see Table 1–5, Table 1–6, and Table 1–7 for specific instructions and precautions).
C. Give key advice on successful quitting	*Abstinence:* Total abstinence is essential. Not even a single puff after the quit date. *Alcohol:* Drinking alcohol is highly associated with relapse. Those who stop smoking should review their alcohol use and consider limiting or abstaining from alcohol use during the quit process. *Other smokers in the household:* The presence of other smokers in the household, particularly a spouse, is associated with lower success rates. Patients should consider quitting with their significant others and/or developing specific plans to maintain abstinence in a household where others still smoke.

(continued)

Table 1–3. Actions and strategies for the primary care clinician to help patients quit smoking. (continued)

Action	Strategies for Implementation
D. Provide supplementary materials	*Source:* Federal agencies, including the National Cancer Institute and the Agency for Health Care Policy and Research; nonprofit agencies (American Cancer Society, American Lung Association, American Heart Association); or local or state health departments. *Selection concerns:* The material must be culturally, racially, educationally, and age appropriate for the patient. *Location:* Readily available in every clinic office.
Step 5. Arrange—Schedule Follow-Up Contact	
Schedule follow-up contact, either in person or via telephone[1]	*Timing:* Follow-up contact should occur soon after the quit date, preferably during the first week. A second follow-up contact is recommended within the first month. Schedule further follow-up contacts as indicated. *Actions during follow-up:* Congratulate success. If smoking occurred, review the circumstances and elicit recommitment to total abstinence. Remind the patient that a lapse can be used as a learning experience and is not a sign of failure. Identify the problems already encountered and anticipate challenges in the immediate future. Assess nicotine replacement therapy use and problems. Consider referral to a more intense or specialized program.

[1]Repeated assessment is not necessary in the case of the adult who has never smoked or not smoked for many years and for whom the information is clearly documented in the medical record.

Modified and reproduced, with permission, from: The Agency for Health Care Policy and Research. Smoking Cessation Clinical Practice Guideline. JAMA 1996;275:1270.

tion counseling by telephone ("quitlines") has proved effective. An additional strategy is to recommend that any smoking take place out of doors to limit the effects of passive smoke on housemates and coworkers. This can lead to smoking reduction and quitting. The clinician's role in smoking cessation is summarized in Table 1–3.

Critchley JA et al: Mortality risk reduction associated with smoking cessation in patients with coronary heart disease: a systematic review. JAMA 2003;290:86. [PMID: 12837716]

Murphy-Hoefer R et al: A review of interventions to reduce tobacco use in colleges and universities. Am J Prev Med 2005; 28:188. [PMID: 15710275]

Parmet S et al: JAMA patient page. Smoking and the heart. JAMA 2003;290:146. [PMID: 12837726]

Schroeder SA: What to do with a patient who smokes. JAMA 2005;294:482. [PMID: 16046655]

Stead LF et al: Telephone counselling for smoking cessation. Cochrane Database Syst Rev 2003;(1):CD002850. [PMID: 12535442]

Stevens LW: JAMA patient page. Kicking the habit. JAMA 2002; 288:532. [PMID: 12141319]

Ziedalski TM et al: Smoking cessation: techniques and potential benefits. Thorac Surg Clin 2005;15:189. [PMID: 15999516]

Lipid Disorders

Lower low-density lipoprotein (LDL) cholesterol concentrations and higher high-density lipoprotein (HDL) levels are associated with a reduced risk of coronary heart disease. Elevated triglyceride levels and elevated plasma lipoprotein(a) are independent risk factors for coronary heart disease. The absolute benefits of screening for—and treating—abnormal lipid levels depend on the presence of other cardiovascular risk factors. If other risk factors are present, cardiovascular risk is higher and the benefits of therapy are greater. Patients with diabetes mellitus or known cardiovascular disease are at still higher risk and benefit from treatment even when lipid levels are normal.

Evidence for the effectiveness of statin-type drugs is better than for the other classes of lipid-lowering agents. Multiple large randomized, placebo-controlled trials have demonstrated important reductions in total mortality, major coronary events, and strokes with lowering levels of LDL cholesterol by statin therapy for patients with known cardiovascular disease. Statins also reduce cardiovascular events for patients with diabetes. For patients with no previous history of cardiovascular events, statins reduce coronary events for men, but less evidence is available for women.

Guidelines for therapy are discussed in Chapter 28.

Collins R et al: MRC/BHF Heart Protection Study of cholesterol-lowering with simvastatin in 5963 people with diabetes: a randomized placebo-controlled trial. Lancet 2003;361:2005. [PMID: 12814710]

Law MR et al: Quantifying effect of statins on low density lipoprotein cholesterol, ischaemic heart disease, and stroke: systematic review and meta-analysis. BMJ 2003;326:1423. [PMID: 12829554]

Walsh JM et al: Drug treatment of hyperlipidemia in women. JAMA 2004;291:2243. [PMID: 15138247]

Table 1–4. Common elements of supportive smoking treatments.

Component	Examples
Encouragement of the patient in the quit attempt	Note that effective cessation treatments are now available. Note that half the people who have *ever* smoked have now quit. Communicate belief in the patient's ability to quit.
Communication of caring and concern	Ask how the patient feels about quitting. Directly express concern and a willingness to help. Be open to the patient's expression of fears of quitting, difficulties experienced, and ambivalent feelings.

Encouragement of the patient to talk about the quitting process	Ask about
	  Reasons that the patient wants to quit.
	  Difficulties encountered while quitting.
	  Success the patient has achieved.
	  Concerns or worries about quitting.

Provision of basic information about smoking and successful quitting	Inform the patient about
	  The nature and time course of withdrawal.
	  The addictive nature of smoking.
	  The fact that any smoking (even a single puff) increases the likelihood of full relapse.

Modified, with permission, from: The Agency for Health Care Policy and Research. Smoking Cessation Clinical Practice Guideline. JAMA 1996;275:1270.

Hyperhomocysteinemia

Elevated plasma homocysteine may be an independent risk factor for coronary artery disease. Elevated levels can be reduced with folate and pyridoxine treatment and with smoking cessation (although not smoking reduction), but their clinical significance is unknown. Randomized trials of vitamin supplementation in patients with prior cardiovascular disease have generally yielded negative results. At this time, there is insufficient evidence to justify screening for elevated serum homocysteine, but patients should be encouraged to maintain an adequate dietary intake of folate, pyridoxine (vitamin B_6), and vitamin B_{12}.

Homocysteine Studies Collaboration: Homocysteine and risk of ischemic heart disease and stroke: a meta-analysis. JAMA 2002;288:2015. [PMID: 12387654]

Tice JA et al: Cost-effectiveness of vitamin therapy to lower plasma homocysteine levels for the prevention of coronary heart disease: effect of grain fortification and beyond. JAMA 2001;286:936. [PMID: 11509058]

Table 1–5. Clinical guidelines for prescribing nicotine replacement products.

1. Who should receive nicotine replacement therapy?

Available research shows that nicotine replacement therapy generally increases rates of smoking cessation. Therefore, except in special circumstances, the clinician should encourage the use of nicotine replacement with patients who smoke. Little research is available on the use of nicotine replacement with light smokers (ie, those smoking ≤ 10–15 cigarettes/d). If nicotine replacement is to be used with light smokers, a lower starting dose of the nicotine patch or nicotine gum should be considered.

2. Should nicotine replacement therapy be tailored to the individual smoker?

Research does not support the tailoring of nicotine patch therapy (except with light smokers as noted above). Patients should be prescribed the patch dosages outlined in Table 1–6.

Research supports tailoring nicotine gum treatment. Specifically, research suggests that 4-mg gum rather than 2-mg gum be used with patients who are highly dependent on nicotine (eg, those smoking > 20 cigarettes/d, those who smoke immediately upon awakening, and those who report histories of severe nicotine withdrawal symptoms). Clinicians may also recommend the higher gum dose if patients request it or have failed to quit using the 2-mg gum.

Modified with permission, from: The Agency for Health Care Policy and Research. Smoking Cessation Clinical Practice Guideline. JAMA 1996;275:1270.

Toole JF et al: Lowering homocysteine in patients with ischemic stroke to prevent recurrent stroke, myocardial infarction, and death: the Vitamin Intervention for Stroke Prevention (VISP) randomized controlled trial. JAMA 2004;291:565. [PMID: 14762035]

Hypertension

Over 43 million adults in the United States have hypertension, but 31% are unaware of their elevated blood pressure; 17% are aware but untreated; 29% are being treated but have not controlled their blood pressure (still greater than 140/90 mm Hg); and only 23% are well controlled. In every adult age group, higher values of systolic and diastolic blood pressure carry greater risks of stroke and congestive heart failure. Systolic blood pressure is a better predictor of morbid events than diastolic blood pressure. Clinicians can apply specific blood pressure criteria, such as those of the Joint National Committee, to decide at what levels treatment should be considered in individual cases. Table 11–1 presents a classification of hypertension based on blood pressures. Primary prevention of hypertension can be accomplished by strategies aimed at both the general population and special high-risk populations. The latter include per-

Table 1–6. Suggestions for the clinical use of the nicotine patch.

Parameter of Clinical Use	Suggestions
Patient selection	Appropriate as a primary pharmacotherapy for smoking cessation.
Precautions	*Pregnancy:* Pregnant smokers should first be encouraged to attempt cessation without pharmacologic treatment. The nicotine patch should be used during pregnancy only if the increased likelihood of smoking cessation, with its potential benefits, outweighs the risk of nicotine replacement and potential concomitant smoking. Similar factors should be considered in lactating women. *Cardiovascular diseases:* While not an independent risk factor for acute myocardial events, the nicotine patch should be used only after consideration of risks and benefits among particular cardiovascular patient groups: those in the immediate (within 2 weeks) post-myocardial infarction period, those with serious arrhythmias, and those with severe or worsening angina pectoris. *Skin reactions:* Up to 50% of patients using the nicotine patch will have a local skin reaction. Skin reactions are usually mild and self-limiting but may worsen over the course of therapy. Local treatment with hydrocortisone cream (2.5%) or triamcinolone cream (0.5%) and rotating patch sites may ameliorate such local reactions. In fewer than 5% of patients do such reactions require the discontinuation of nicotine patch treatment.
Dosage[1]	Treatment of 8 weeks or less has been shown to be as efficacious as longer treatment periods. Based on this finding, we suggest the following treatment schedules as reasonable for most smokers. Clinicians should consult the package insert for other treatment suggestions. Finally, clinicians should consider individualizing treatment based on specific patient characteristics such as previous experience with the patch, number of cigarettes smoked, and degree of addiction.

	Brand	Duration (weeks)	Dosage (mg/h)
	Nicoderm and Habitrol	4 then 2 then 2	21/24 14/24 7/24
	Prostep	4 then 4	22/24 11/24
	Nicotrol	4 then 2 then 2	15/16 10/16 5/16

Parameter of Clinical Use	Suggestions
Prescribing instructions	*Abstinence from smoking:* The patient should refrain from smoking while using the patch. *Location:* At the start of each day, the patient should place a new patch on a relatively hairless location between the neck and the waist. *Activities:* There are no restrictions while using the patch. *Time:* Patches should be applied as soon as patients awaken on their quit day.

[1]These dosage recommendations are based on a review of the published research literature and do not necessarily conform to package insert information.

Reproduced, with permission, from: The Agency for Health Care Policy and Research. Smoking Cessation Clinical Practice Guideline. JAMA 1996;275:1270. Updated and revised, with permission, from Treating Tobacco Use and Dependence. U.S. Public Health Service. www.surgeongeneral.gov/tobacco/default.htm

sons with high-normal blood pressure or a family history of hypertension, blacks, and individuals with various behavioral risk factors such as physical inactivity; excessive consumption of salt, alcohol, or calories; and deficient intake of potassium. Effective interventions for primary prevention of hypertension include reduced sodium and alcohol consumption, weight loss, and regular exercise. Potassium supple-

mentation lowers blood pressure modestly, and a diet high in fresh fruits and vegetables and low in fat, red meats, and sugar-containing beverages also reduces blood pressure. Interventions of unproved efficacy include pill supplementation of potassium, calcium, magnesium, fish oil, or fiber; macronutrient alteration; and stress management. A major cause of the recent impressive decline in stroke deaths has been

Table 1–7. Suggestions for the clinical use of nicotine gum.

Parameter of Clinical Use	Suggestions
Patient selection	Appropriate as a primary pharmacotherapy for smoking cessation.
Precautions	*Pregnancy:* Pregnant smokers should first be encouraged to attempt cessation without pharmacologic treatment. Nicotine gum should be used during pregnancy only if the increased likelihood of smoking cessation, with its potential benefits, outweighs the risk of nicotine replacement and potential concomitant smoking. *Cardiovascular diseases:* Although not an independent risk factor for acute myocardial events, nicotine gum should be used only after consideration of risks and benefits among particular cardiovascular patient groups: those in the immediate (within 2 weeks) post-myocardial infarction period, those with serious arrhythmias, and those with serious or worsening angina pectoris. *Adverse effects:* Common adverse effects of nicotine chewing gum include mouth soreness, hiccups, dyspepsia, and jaw ache. These effects are generally mild and transient and can often be alleviated by correcting the patient's chewing technique (see "Prescribing instructions" below).
Dosage	*Dosage:* Nicotine gum is available in doses of 2 mg and 4 mg per piece. Patients who smoke less than 25 cigarettes per day should be prescribed the 2-mg gum initially. The 4-mg gum should be prescribed to patients who express a preference for it, have failed with the 2-mg gum but remain motivated to quit, and/or smoke more than 25 cigarettes per day. The gum is most commonly prescribed for the first few months of a quit attempt. Clinicians should tailor the duration of therapy to fit the needs of each patient. Patients using the 2-mg strength should use not more than 30 pieces per day, whereas those using the 4-mg strength should not exceed 20 pieces per day.
Prescribing instructions	*Abstinence from smoking:* The patient should refrain from smoking while using the gum. *Chewing technique:* The gum should be chewed slowly until a "peppery" taste emerges, then "parked" between cheek and gum to facilitate nicotine absorption through the oral mucosa. Gum should be slowly and intermittently chewed and parked for about 30 minutes. *Absorption:* Acidic beverages (eg, coffee, juices, soft drinks) interfere with the buccal absorption of nicotine, so eating and drinking anything except water should be avoided for 15 minutes before and during chewing. *Scheduling of dose:* A common problem is that patients do not use enough gum to get the maximum benefit: they chew too few pieces per day and do not use the gum for a sufficient number of weeks. Instructions to chew the gum on a fixed schedule (at least 1 piece every 1 to 2 hours) for at least 1 to 3 months may be more beneficial than ad lib use.

Reproduced, with permission, from: The Agency for Health Care Policy and Research. Smoking Cessation Clinical Practice Guideline. JAMA 1996;275:1270. Updated and revised, with permission, from Treating Tobacco Use and Dependence. U.S. Public Health Service. www.surgeongeneral.gov/tobacco/default.htm

improved diagnosis and treatment of hypertension. Diets rich in fruits and vegetables may also protect against stroke. Pharmacologic management of hypertension is discussed in Chapter 11.

Chobanian AV et al: The Seventh Report of the Joint National Committee on Prevention, Detection, Evaluation, and Treatment of High Blood Pressure: the JNC 7 report. JAMA 2003;289:2560. [PMID: 12748199]

Law MR et al: Value of low dose combination treatment with blood pressure lowering drugs: analysis of 354 randomised trials. BMJ 2003;326:1427. [PMID: 12829555]

Sheridan S et al: Screening for high blood pressure: a review of the evidence for the U.S. Preventive Services Task Force. Am J Prev Med 2003;25:151. [PMID: 12880884]

Chemoprevention

As discussed in Chapters 10 and 24, regular use of low-dose aspirin (81–325 mg) can reduce the incidence of myocardial infarction in men. Low-dose aspirin reduces stroke but not myocardial infarction in middle-aged women. Antioxidant vitamin (vitamin E, vitamin C, and beta-carotene) supplementation produced no significant reductions in the 5-year incidence of—or mortality from—vascular disease, cancer, or other major outcomes in high-risk individuals with coronary artery disease, other occlusive arterial disease, or diabetes mellitus.

Hayden M et al: Aspirin for the primary prevention of cardiovascular events: a summary of the evidence for the U.S. Preventive Services Task Force. Ann Intern Med 2002; 136:161. [PMID: 11790072]

Heart Protection Study Collaborative Group: MRC/BHF Heart Protection Study of antioxidant vitamin supplementation in 20,536 high-risk individuals: a randomised placebo-controlled trial. Lancet 2002;360:23. [PMID: 12114037]

Ridker PM et al: A randomized trial of low-dose aspirin in the primary prevention of cardiovascular disease in women. N Engl J Med 2005;352:1293. [PMID: 15753114]

Table 1–8. Suggestions for the clinical use of bupropion SR.

Parameter of Clinical Use	Suggestions
Patient selection	Appropriate as a first-line pharmacotherapy for smoking cessation.
Precautions	*Pregnancy:* Pregnant smokers should be encouraged to quit first without pharmacologic treatment. Bupropion SR should be used during pregnancy only if the increased likelihood of smoking abstinence, with its potential benefits, outweighs the risk of bupropion SR treatment and potential concomitant smoking. Similar factors should be considered in lactating women (FDA Class B). *Cardiovascular diseases:* Generally well tolerated; infrequent reports of hypertension. *Side effects:* The most common side effects reported by bupropion SR users were insomnia (35–40%) and dry mouth (10%). *Contraindications:* Bupropion SR is contraindicated in individuals with a history of seizure disorder, a history of an eating disorder, who are using another form of bupropion (Wellbutrin or Wellbutrin SR), or who have used an MAO inhibitor in the past 14 days.
Dosage	Patients should begin with a dose of 150 mg every morning for 3 days, then increase to 150 mg bid. Dosing at 150 mg bid should continue for 7–12 weeks following the quit date. Unlike nicotine replacement products, patients should begin bupropion SR treatment 1–2 weeks before they quit smoking. For maintenance therapy, consider bupropion SR 150 mg bid for up to 6 months.
Prescribing instructions	*Cessation prior to quit date:* Recognize that some patients will lose their desire to smoke prior to their quit date, or will spontaneously reduce the amount they smoke. *Scheduling of dose:* If insomnia is marked, taking the evening dose earlier (in the afternoon, at least 8 hours after the first dose) may provide some relief. *Alcohol:* Use alcohol only in moderation.

MAO = monoamine oxidase inhibitor.
Modified, with permission, from Treating Tobacco Use and Dependence. U.S. Public Health Service. www.surgeongeneral.gov/tobacco/default.htm

Vivekananthan DP et al: Use of antioxidant vitamins for the prevention of cardiovascular disease: meta-analysis of randomised trials. Lancet 2003;361:2017. [PMID: 12814711]

PREVENTION OF PHYSICAL INACTIVITY

Lack of sufficient physical activity is the second most important contributor to preventable deaths, trailing only tobacco use. A sedentary lifestyle has been linked to 28% of deaths from leading chronic diseases. The Centers for Disease Control and Prevention (CDC) has recommended that every adult in the United States should engage in 30 minutes or more of moderate-intensity physical activity on most days of the week. This guideline complements previous advice urging at least 20–30 minutes of more vigorous aerobic exercise three to five times a week.

Patients who engage in regular moderate to vigorous exercise have a lower risk of myocardial infarction, stroke, hypertension, hyperlipidemia, type 2 diabetes mellitus, diverticular disease, and osteoporosis. The benefits of exercise appear to be dose-dependent, with a major difference in benefit between no and mild to moderate exercise and a smaller difference in benefit between moderate and vigorous exercise. Current evidence supports the recommended guidelines of 30 minutes of moderate physical activity on most days of the week in both the primary and secondary prevention of coronary heart disease (CHD). In fact, there appears to be a linear dose-response relationship between physical activity and CHD, at least up to a certain level of activity. Leisure time physical activity is associated with about a 30–50% reduction in risk of CHD in both men and women, in middle-aged and older persons, and in men with established CHD.

In older nonsmoking men, walking 2 miles or more per day is associated with an almost 50% lower age-related mortality. The relative risk of stroke was found to be less than one-sixth in men who exercised vigorously compared with those who were inactive; the risk of type 2 diabetes mellitus was about half among men who exercised five or more times weekly compared with those who exercised once a week. Glucose control is improved in diabetics who exercise regularly, even at a modest level. In sedentary individuals with dyslipidemia, high amounts of high-intensity exercise produce significant beneficial effects on serum lipoprotein profiles. Physical activity is associated with a lower risk of colon cancer (although not rectal cancer) in men and women and of breast and reproductive organ cancer in women. Finally, weight-bearing exercise (especially resistance and high-impact activities) increases bone mineral content and retards development of osteoporosis in women and contributes to a reduced risk of falls in older persons.

Exercise may also confer benefits on those with chronic illness. Men and women with chronic symptomatic osteoarthritis of one or both knees benefited from a supervised walking program, with improved self-reported functional status and decreased pain and use of pain medication. Exercise produces sustained lowering of both systolic and diastolic blood pressure in patients with mild hypertension. In addition, physical activity can help patients maintain ideal body weight. Individuals who maintain ideal body weight have a 35–55% lower risk for myocardial infarction than with those who are obese. Physical activity reduces depression and anxiety; improves adaptation to stress; improves sleep quality; and enhances mood, self-esteem, and overall performance.

In longitudinal cohort studies, individuals who report higher levels of leisure time physical activity are less likely to gain weight. Conversely, individuals who are overweight are less likely to stay active. However, the amount of physical activity necessary to control body weight may be > 30 minutes per day; at least 45–60 minutes of daily moderate-intensity physical activity may be necessary to maximize weight loss and prevent significant weight regain. Moreover, adequate levels of physical activity appear to be important for the prevention of weight gain and the development of obesity. Physical activity also appears to have an independent effect on health-related outcomes when compared with body weight, suggesting that adequate levels of activity may counteract the negative influence of body weight on health outcomes.

However, physical exertion can rarely trigger the onset of acute myocardial infarction, particularly in persons who are habitually sedentary. Increased activity increases the risk of musculoskeletal injuries, which can be minimized by proper warm-up and stretching, and by gradual rather than sudden increase in activity. Other potential complications of exercise include angina pectoris, arrhythmias, sudden death, and asthma. In insulin-requiring diabetics who undertake vigorous exercise, the need for insulin is reduced; hypoglycemia may be a consequence.

Only about 20% of adults in the United States are active at the moderate level—and only 8% currently exercise at the more vigorous level—recommended for health benefits. Instead, 60% report irregular or no leisure time physical activity.

The value of routine electrocardiography stress testing prior to initiation of an exercise program in middle-aged or older adults remains controversial. Patients with ischemic heart disease or other cardiovascular disease require medically supervised, graded exercise programs. Medically supervised exercise prolongs life in patients with congestive heart failure. Exercise should not be prescribed for patients with decompensated congestive heart failure, complex ventricular arrhythmias, unstable angina pectoris, hemodynamically significant aortic stenosis, or significant aortic aneurysm. Five- to 10-minute warm-up and cool-down periods, stretching exercises, and gradual increases in exercise intensity help prevent musculoskeletal and cardiovascular complications.

Physical activity can be incorporated into any person's daily routine. For example, the clinician can advise a patient to take the stairs instead of the elevator, to walk or bike instead of driving, to do housework or yard work, to get off the bus one or two stops earlier and walk the rest of the way, to park at the far end of the parking lot, or to walk during the lunch hour. The basic message should be the more the better and anything is better than nothing.

To be more effective in counseling about exercise, clinicians can also incorporate motivational interviewing techniques, adopt a whole practice approach (eg, use practice nurses to assist), and establish linkages with community agencies. Clinicians can incorporate the "5 As" approach:

1. Ask (identify those who can benefit).
2. Assess (current activity level).
3. Advise (individualize plan).
4. Assist (provide a written exercise prescription and support material).
5. Arrange (appropriate referral and follow up).

Such interventions have a moderate effect on self-reported physical activity and cardiorespiratory fitness, even if they do not always help patients to achieve a predetermined level of physical activity. In their counseling, clinicians should advise patients about both the benefits and risks of exercise, prescribe an exercise program appropriate for each patient, and provide advice to help prevent injuries or cardiovascular complications.

Hillsdon M et al: Interventions for promoting physical activity. Cochrane Database Syst Rev 2005;(1):CD003180. [PMID: 15674903]

Huang N: Motivating patients to move. Aust Fam Physician 2005;34:413. [PMID: 15931398]

Jakicic JM et al: Physical activity considerations for the treatment and prevention of obesity. Am J Clin Nutr 2005;82(1 Suppl):226S. [PMID: 16002826]

Wannamethee SG et al: Physical activity and cardiovascular disease. Semin Vasc Med 2002;2:257. [PMID: 16222619]

Wareham NJ et al: Physical activity and obesity prevention: a review of the current evidence. Proc Nutr Soc 2005; 64:229. [PMID: 15960868]

PREVENTION OF OVERWEIGHT & OBESITY

Obesity is now a true epidemic and public health crisis that both clinicians and patients must face. Normal body weight is defined as a body mass index (BMI), calculated as the weight in kilograms divided by the height in meters squared, of < 25 kg/m^2; overweight is defined as a BMI = 25.0–29.9 kg/m^2, and obesity as a BMI > 30 kg/m^2. The prevalence of obesity in US children, adolescents, and adults has grown dramatically since 1990. Currently, 59 million Americans (16%) are overweight or obese. Prevalence varies by race and age, with older

African American and Latina women having the greatest prevalence of obesity. This trend has been linked both to declines in physical activity and to increased caloric intake in diets rich in fats and carbohydrates. As noted above, only about 20% of Americans are physically active at a moderate level, and only 8% at a more vigorous level, and 60% report irregular or no leisure time physical activity. In addition, only 3% of Americans meet four of the five recommendations for the intake of grains, fruits, vegetables, dairy products, and meat of the Food Guide Pyramid. Only one of four Americans eats the recommended five or more fruits and vegetables per day.

Obesity is clearly associated with type 2 diabetes mellitus, hypertension, cancer, osteoarthritis, cardiovascular disease, obstructive sleep apnea, and asthma. One of the most important sequelae of the rapid surge in prevalence of overweight and obesity between 1990 and 2000 has been a dramatic 30–40% increase in the prevalence of type 2 diabetes mellitus. In addition, almost one-quarter of the US population currently has the metabolic syndrome, putting them at high risk for the development of coronary heart disease. The relationship between overweight and obesity and diabetes, hypertension, and coronary artery disease is thought to be due to insulin resistance and compensatory hyperinsulinemia. Persons with a BMI ≥ 40 have death rates from cancers that are 52% higher for men and 62% higher for women than the rates in men and women of normal weight. Significant trends of increasing risk of death with higher BMIs are observed for cancers of the stomach and prostate in men and for cancers of the breast, uterus, cervix, and ovary in women, and for cancers of the esophagus, colon and rectum, liver, gallbladder, pancreas, and kidney, non-Hodgkin's lymphoma, and multiple myeloma in both men and women.

In the Framingham Heart Study, overweight and obesity were associated with large decreases in life expectancy. For example, 40-year-old female nonsmokers lost 3.3 years and 40-year-old male nonsmokers lost 3.1 years of life expectancy because of overweight, and 7.1 years and 5.8 years of life expectancy, respectively, because of obesity. Obese female smokers lost 7.2 years and obese male smokers lost 6.7 years of life expectancy compared with normal-weight smokers, and 13.3 years and 13.7 years, respectively, compared with normal-weight nonsmokers. Clinicians must work to identify and provide the best prevention and treatment strategies for patients who are overweight and obese. Patients with abdominal obesity (high waist to hip size ratio) are at particularly increased risk.

Prevention of overweight and obesity involves both increasing physical activity and dietary modification to reduce caloric intake. Clinicians can help guide patients to develop personalized eating plans to reduce energy intake, particularly by recognizing the contributions of fat, concentrated carbohydrates, and large portion sizes (see Chapter 29). To prevent the long-term chronic disease sequelae of overweight or obesity, clinicians must work with patients to modify other risk factors, eg, by smoking cessation (see above) and strict glycemic and blood pressure control (see Chapters 27 and 11).

Treatment of obesity involves dietary counseling and therapy, pharmacotherapy (see Chapter 29), and surgery. Counseling interventions or pharmacotherapy can produce modest (3 to 5 kg) sustained weight loss over 6–12 months. Pharmacotherapy appears safe in the short term; long-term safety is still not established. Counseling appears to be most effective when intensive and combined with behavioral therapy. Maintenance strategies can help preserve weight loss.

In dietary therapy, one randomized trial comparing a low-carbohydrate, high-protein, high-fat (Atkins) diet to a low-calorie, high-carbohydrate, low-fat (conventional) diet, the low-carbohydrate diet produced a greater weight loss (absolute difference, approximately 4%) than did the conventional diet for the first 6 months, but the differences were not significant at 1 year. In a second randomized trial, severely obese persons with a high prevalence of diabetes or the metabolic syndrome lost more weight during 6 months on a carbohydrate-restricted diet than on a calorie- and fat-restricted diet. Adherence was poor and attrition was high in both studies. Longer and larger studies are required to determine the long-term safety and efficacy of low-carbohydrate, high-protein, high-fat diets. Finally, a recent randomized trial comparing four popular diets (Atkins, Ornish, Weight Watchers, and Zone diets) assessed both adherence rates to and effectiveness of the diets for weight loss and cardiac risk factor reduction. Individual participants were randomly assigned to Atkins (carbohydrate restriction), Zone (macronutrient balance), Weight Watchers (calorie restriction), or Ornish (fat restriction) diets. At 1 year, each of the diets modestly reduced body weight (by a mean of 2.1–3.3 kg), LDL/HDL cholesterol ratio (by approximately 10%), and serum levels of C-reactive protein and insulin, but overall self-reported dietary adherence rates were low (50–65%).

Weight loss strategies using dietary, physical activity, or behavioral interventions can produce significant improvements in weight among persons with prediabetes and a significant decrease in diabetes incidence. Multicomponent interventions including very-low-calorie or low-calorie diets hold promise for achieving weight loss in adults with type 2 diabetes mellitus.

Bariatric surgical procedures, eg, vertical banded gastroplasty and Roux-en-Y gastric bypass, are reserved for patients with morbid obesity whose BMI exceeds 40, or for less severely obese patients (with BMIs between 35 and 40) with high-risk comorbid conditions such as life-threatening cardiopulmonary problems (eg, severe sleep apnea, Pickwickian syndrome, and obesity-related cardiomyopathy) or severe diabetes mellitus. In selected patients, surgery can produce substantial weight loss (10 to 159 kg) over 1 to 5 years, with rare but sometimes severe complications.

Avenell A et al: What are the long-term benefits of weight reducing diets in adults? A systematic review of randomized controlled trials. J Hum Nutr Diet 2004;17:317. [PMID: 15250842]

Buchwald H et al: Bariatric surgery: a systematic review and meta-analysis. JAMA 2004;292:1724. [PMID: 15479938]

Dansinger ML et al: Comparison of the Atkins, Ornish, Weight Watchers, and Zone diets for weight loss and heart disease risk reduction: a randomized trial. JAMA 2005;293:43. [PMID: 15632335]

McTigue KM et al: Screening and interventions for obesity in adults: summary of the evidence for the U.S. Preventive Services Task Force. Ann Intern Med 2003;139:933. [PMID: 14644897]

Norris SL et al: Long-term non-pharmacological weight loss interventions for adults with prediabetes. Cochrane Database Syst Rev 2005;(2):CD005270. [PMID: 15846748]

Norris SL et al: Long-term non-pharmacologic weight loss interventions for adults with type 2 diabetes. Cochrane Database Syst Rev 2005;(2):CD004095. [PMID: 15846698]

Olsen J et al: Cost-effectiveness of nutritional counseling for obese patients and patients at risk of ischemic heart disease. Int J Technol Assess Health Care 2005;21:194. [PMID: 15921059]

Reaven GM: Importance of identifying the overweight patient who will benefit the most by losing weight. Ann Intern Med 2003;138:420. [PMID: 12614095]

Snow V et al: Clinical Efficacy Assessment Subcommittee of the American College of Physicians: Pharmacologic and surgical management of obesity in primary care: a clinical practice guideline from the American College of Physicians. Ann Intern Med 2005;142:525. [PMID: 15809464]

Torpy JM et al: JAMA patient page. Obesity. JAMA 2003;289:1880. [PMID: 12684367]

CANCER PREVENTION

Primary Prevention

Cigarette smoking is the most important preventable cause of cancer. Primary prevention of skin cancer consists of restricting exposure to ultraviolet light by wearing appropriate clothing and use of sunscreens. In the past 2 decades, there has been a threefold increase in the incidence of squamous cell carcinoma and a fourfold increase in melanoma in the United States. Individuals who engage in regular physical exercise and avoid obesity have lower rates of breast and colon cancer. Prevention of occupationally induced cancers involves minimizing exposure to carcinogenic substances such as asbestos, ionizing radiation, and benzene compounds. Chemoprevention may be an important part of primary cancer prevention (see Chapter 40). Use of tamoxifen, raloxifene, and aromatase inhibitors for breast cancer prevention is discussed in Chapters 16 and 40. Hepatitis B vaccination can prevent hepatocellular carcinoma, and the recent development of a human papillomavirus vaccine holds promise for prevention of cervical cancer.

Screening & Early Detection

Screening has been shown to prevent death from cancers of the breast, colon, and cervix. Current cancer screening recommendations from the American Cancer Society, the Canadian Task Force on Preventive Health Care, and the United States Preventive Services Task Force are shown in Table 1–9.

The appropriate form and frequency of screening for breast cancer is controversial. A large randomized trial of breast self-examination conducted among factory workers in Shanghai found no benefit. A systematic review performed for the United States Preventive Services Task Force found that mammography was moderately effective in reducing breast cancer mortality for women 40–74 years of age. The absolute benefit was greater for older women, and the risk of false-positive results was high for all women.

All current recommendations call for cervical and colorectal cancer screening. Prostate cancer screening, however, is controversial, as no completed studies have answered the question whether early detection and treatment after screen detection produce sufficient benefits to outweigh harms of treatment. Providers and patients are advised to discuss how to proceed in light of this uncertainty. Single serum prostate-specific antigen (PSA) measurements appear to offer relatively high sensitivity and specificity to detect prostate cancer. The sensitivity is about 65%, the specificity about 80%, and the positive predictive value for prostate cancer is about 45%. When both the digital rectal examination and serum PSA are abnormal, PSA specificity increases, but sensitivity falls (to 30%) and predictive value rises only slightly. Whether early detection through screening and subsequent treatment alter the natural course of the disease remains to be seen. There are still no data on the morbidity and mortality benefits of screening. Unlike the American College of Physicians, the American Cancer Society recommends that providers offer annual PSA testing for men over age 50. Screening is not recommended by any group for men who have estimated life expectancies of less than 10 years. Decision aids have been developed to help men weigh the arguments for and against PSA screening.

Annual or biennial fecal occult blood testing reduces mortality from colorectal cancer by 16–33%. The risk of death from colon cancer among patients undergoing at least one sigmoidoscopic examination is reduced by 60–80% compared with that among those not having sigmoidoscopy. Colonoscopy has also been advocated as a screening examination. While it is more accurate than flexible sigmoidoscopy for detecting cancer and polyps, its value in reducing colon cancer mortality has not been studied. Recent studies have shown that CT colography (virtual colonoscopy) is also able to detect cancers and polyps with reasonable accuracy.

Screening for cervical cancer with a Papanicolaou smear is indicated in sexually active adolescents and in adult women every 1–3 years. Screening for vaginal cancer with a Papanicolaou smear is not indicated in women who have undergone hysterectomies for benign disease with removal of the cervix—except in diethylstilbestrol (DES)-exposed women (see Chapter 17). Women over age 70 who have had normal results on three or more previous Papanicolaou smears may elect to stop screening.

Table 1–9. Cancer screening recommendations for average-risk adults, 2003.

	Test	ACS[1]	CTF[2]	USPSTF[3]
Breast	Self-examination (BSE)	Monthly for women over age 20.	Fair evidence that BSE *should not* be used.	Insufficient evidence to recommend for or against.
	Clinical breast examination	Every 3 years age 20–40 and annually thereafter.	Every 1–2 years in women aged 40–59.	Insufficient evidence to recommend for or against.
	Mammography	Annually age 40 and older.	Every 1–2 years in women aged 40–59. Current evidence does not support the recommendation that screening mammography be included in or excluded from the periodic health examination of women aged 40–49.	Recommended every 1–2 years for women aged 40 and over (B).
Cervix	Papanicolaou test	Annually beginning within 3 years after first vaginal intercourse or no later than age 21.	Annually at age of first intercourse or by age 18; can move to every-2-year screening after two normal results.	Every 3 years beginning at onset of sexual activity.
		After age 30, women with three normal tests may be screened every 2–3 years.		
		Women may choose to stop screening after age 70 if they have had three normal (and no abnormal) results within the last 10 years.		
Colon	Stool test for occult blood[4]	Screening recommended, with the combination of fecal occult blood test and sigmoidoscopy preferred over stool test or sigmoidoscopy alone. Barium enema and colonoscopy also considered reasonable alternatives.	Good evidence for screening every 1–2 years over age 50.	Screening strongly recommended (A), but insufficient evidence to determine best test.
	Sigmoidoscopy		Fair evidence for screening over age 50 (insufficient evidence about combining stool test and sigmoidoscopy).	
	Double-contrast barium enema		Not addressed.	
	Colonoscopy		Insufficient evidence for or against use in screening.	
	Digital rectal exam (DRE)	Not recommended.	No recommendation.	Not recommended.
Prostate	DRE	DRE and PSA should be offered annually to men age 50 and older who have at least a 10-year life expectancy. Information should be provided to men about the benefits and risks, and they should be allowed to participate in the decision. Men without a clear preference should be screened.	Insufficient evidence for or against including in routine care.	Insufficient evidence to recommend for or against.
	Prostate-specific antigen (PSA) blood test		Fair evidence *against* including in routine care.	
Other	Cancer-related checkup	Every 3 years for men 20–40 and annually thereafter; should include counseling and perhaps oral cavity, thyroid, lymph node, or testicular examinations.	Not assessed.	Not assessed.

[1]American Cancer Society recommendations, available at http://www.cancer.org
[2]Canadian Task Force on Preventive Health Care recommendations available at http://www.ctfphc.org
[3]United States Preventive Services Task Force recommendations available at http://www.ahrq.gov
[4]Home test with three samples.

Recommendation A: The USPSTF strongly recommends that clinicians routinely provide the service to eligible patients. (The USPSTF found good evidence that the service improves important health outcomes and concludes that benefits substantially outweigh harms.)

Recommendation B: The USPSTF recommends that clinicians routinely provide the service to eligible patients. (The USPSTF found at least fair evidence that the service improves important health outcomes and concludes that benefits substantially outweigh harms.)

Andriole GL et al: PLCO Project Team: Prostate Cancer Screening in the Prostate, Lung, Colorectal and Ovarian (PLCO) Cancer Screening Trial: findings from the initial screening round of a randomized trial. J Natl Cancer Inst 2005; 97:433. [PMID: 15770007]

Anthonisen NR et al: Lung Health Study Research Group: The effects of a smoking cessation intervention on 14.5-year mortality: a randomized clinical trial. Ann Intern Med 2005;142:233. [PMID: 15710956]

Aus G et al: Individualized screening interval for prostate cancer based on prostate-specific antigen level: results of a prospective, randomized, population-based study. Arch Intern Med 2005;165:1857. [PMID: 16157829]

Bill-Axelson A et al: Radical prostatectomy versus watchful waiting in early prostate cancer. N Engl J Med 2005;352:1977. [PMID: 15888698]

Denny L et al: Screen-and-treat approaches for cervical cancer prevention in low-resource settings: a randomized controlled trial. JAMA 2005;294:2173. [PMID: 16264158]

Harper DM et al: GlaxoSmithKline HPV Vaccine Study Group: Efficacy of a bivalent L1 virus-like particle vaccine in prevention of infection with human papillomavirus types 16 and 18 in young women: a randomized controlled trial. Lancet 2004;364:1757. [PMID: 15541448]

Harris R et al: Screening for prostate cancer: an update of the evidence for the U.S. Preventive Services Task Force. Ann Intern Med 2002;137:917. [PMID: 12458993]

Humphrey LL et al: Breast cancer screening: a summary of the evidence for the U.S. Preventive Services Task Force. Ann Intern Med 2002;137:347. [PMID: 12204020]

Pignone M et al: Screening for colorectal cancer in adults at average risk: a summary of the evidence for the U.S. Preventive Services Task Force. Ann Intern Med 2002; 137:132. [PMID: 12118972]

Prochaska JO et al: Stage-based expert systems to guide a population of primary care patients to quit smoking, eat healthier, prevent skin cancer, and receive regular mammograms. Prev Med 2005;41:406. [PMID: 15896835]

Saraiya M et al: Interventions to prevent skin cancer by reducing exposure to ultraviolet radiation: a systematic review. Am J Prev Med 2004;27:422. [PMID: 15556744]

Sawaya GF et al: Risk of cervical cancer associated with extending the interval between cervical-cancer screenings. N Engl J Med 2003;349:1501. [PMID: 14561792]

Torpy JM et al: JAMA patient page. Colon cancer screening. JAMA 2003;289:1334. [PMID: 12633198]

Villa LL et al: Prophylactic quadrivalent human papillomavirus (types 6, 11, 16, and 18) L1 virus-like particle vaccine in young women: a randomised double-blind placebo-controlled multicentre phase II efficacy trial. Lancet Oncol 2005;6:271. [PMID: 15863374]

Weissfeld JL et al: PLCO Project Team: Flexible sigmoidoscopy in the PLCO cancer screening trial: results from the baseline screening examination of a randomized trial. J Natl Cancer Inst 2005;97:989. [PMID: 15998952]

PREVENTION OF INJURIES & VIOLENCE

Injuries remain the most important cause of loss of potential years of life before age 65. Road traffic injuries, self-inflicted injuries, falls, and interpersonal violence are the major sources of injuries. Injuries affect mostly older women and young men, often causing long-term disability. Although there has been a steady decline in motor vehicle accident deaths per miles driven, road traffic injuries remain the tenth leading cause of death and the ninth leading cause of the burden of disease. Although seat belt use protects against serious injury and death in motor vehicle accidents, at least one-fourth of adults and one-third of teenagers do not use seat belts routinely. Air bags are protective for adults but not for small children.

Each year in the United States, more than 500,000 people are nonfatally injured while riding bicycles. The rate of helmet use by bicyclists and motorcyclists is significantly increased in states with helmet laws. By the end of 2000, bicycle helmet use in 15 communities monitored by the CDC's National Center for Injury Prevention and Control had risen from 40% to 55%, exceeding the Healthy People 2000 goal. Young men appear most likely to resist wearing helmets. Clinicians should try to educate their patients about seat belts, safety helmets, the risks of using cellular telephones while driving, drinking and driving—or using other intoxicants or long-acting benzodiazepines and then driving—and the risks of having guns in the home.

Long-term alcohol abuse adversely affects outcome from trauma and increases the risk of readmission for new trauma. Alcohol and illicit drug use are associated with an increased risk of violent death. There is a causal link between alcohol intoxication and injury due to assault. Harm reduction can be achieved through practical measures, such as using plastic glasses and bottles in licensed premises; controlling prices of drinks; and targeted policing based on police, accident, and emergency data.

Males aged 16–35 are at especially high risk for serious injury and death from accidents and violence, with blacks and Latinos at greatest risk. For 16- and 17-year-old drivers, the risk of fatal crashes increases with the number of passengers. Deaths from firearms have reached epidemic levels in the United States and will soon surpass the number of deaths from motor vehicle accidents. Having a gun in the home increases the likelihood of homicide nearly threefold and of suicide fivefold. In 2002, an estimated 877,000 individuals successfully committed suicide. Educating physicians to recognize and treat depression as well as restricting access to lethal methods have been found to reduce suicide rates.

In elderly patients, the risk of hip fracture when falling can be reduced by as much as 80% by wearing hip protectors, but only about half of patients use them regularly. Oral vitamin D supplementation with 700–800 IU/d appears to reduce the risk of hip and other nonvertebral fractures in both ambulatory and institutionalized elderly persons, but 400 IU/d is not sufficient for fracture prevention.

Finally, clinicians have a critical role in detection, prevention, and management of physical or sexual abuse—in particular, routine assessment of women for risk of domestic violence. Inclusion of a single question about domestic violence in the medical history— "At any time, has a partner ever hit you, kicked you, or otherwise physically hurt you?"—increased identification of this common problem from nil to 11.6%. Another screening device consists of three questions: (1) "Have you ever been hit, kicked, punched, or otherwise hurt by someone within the past year? If so, by whom?" (2) "Do you feel safe in your current relationship?" (3) "Is there a partner from a previous relationship who is making you feel unsafe now?" Asking these questions increased identification of domestic violence to 30% of women in an emergency department. The effect of screening and identifying intimate partner violence on health outcomes has not been well studied to date.

Physical and psychological abuse, exploitation, and neglect of older adults are serious underrecognized problems. Clues to elder mistreatment include the patient's appearance, recurrent urgent-care visits, missed appointments, suspicious physical findings, and implausible explanations for injuries.

Bischoff-Ferrari HA et al: Fracture prevention with vitamin D supplementation: a meta-analysis of randomized controlled trials. JAMA 2005;293:2257. [PMID: 15886381]

Cusens B et al: Prevention of alcohol-related assault and injury. Hosp Med 2005;66:346. [PMID: 15974163]

JAMA patient page. Partner violence. JAMA 2002;288:662. [PMID: 12171057]

Mann JJ et al: Suicide prevention strategies: a systematic review. JAMA 2005;294:2064. [PMID: 16249421]

McClure R et al: Population-based interventions for the prevention of fall-related injuries in older people. Cochrane Database Syst Rev 2005;(1):CD004441. [PMID: 15674948]

Nelson HD et al: Screening women and elderly adults for family and intimate partner violence: a review of the evidence for the U. S. Preventive Services Task Force. Ann Intern Med 2004;140:387. [PMID: 14996681]

Rivara FP et al: Injury prevention. (Two parts.) N Engl J Med 1997;337:543, 613. [PMID: 9262499, 9271485]

SUBSTANCE ABUSE: ALCOHOL & ILLICIT DRUGS

Substance abuse is a major public health problem in the United States and is estimated to be a factor in 41% of highway fatality accidents. The lifetime prevalence of alcoholism is estimated to be between 12% and 16%. Approximately two-thirds of high school seniors are regular users of alcohol. Underdiagnosis of alcohol abuse is substantial, both because of patient denial and lack of detection of clinical clues. A substantial decline in alcohol-related fatalities testifies to the success of educational and law-enforcement efforts to stop drinking and driving. Even so, alcohol-impaired driving remains prevalent, especially among men aged 18–34 years. Binge drinking among college students has recently increased.

As with cigarette use, clinician identification and counseling about alcoholism may improve the chances of recovery. About 10% of all adults seen in medical practices are problem drinkers. An estimated 15–30% of hospitalized patients have problems with alcohol abuse or dependence, but the connection between patients' presenting complaints and their alcohol abuse is often missed. The CAGE test (see Table 1–10) is both sensitive and specific for chronic alcoholism. However, it is less sensitive in detecting heavy or binge drinking in elderly patients and has been criticized for being less applicable to minority groups or to women. Others recommend asking three questions: (1) How many days per week do you drink (frequency)? (2) On a day when you drink alcohol, how many drinks do you have in one day (quantity)? (3) On how many occasions in the last month did you drink more than five drinks (binge drinking)? The Alcohol Use Disorder Identification Test (AUDIT) consists of questions on the quantity and frequency of alcohol consumption, on alcohol dependence symptoms, and on alcohol-related problems (Table 1–10). It has been found to accurately detect hazardous drinking, harmful drinking, and alcohol dependence and does not seem to be affected by ethnic or gender bias. Choice of therapy remains controversial. However, use of screening procedures and brief intervention methods (see Table 1–11 and Chapter 25) can produce a 10–30% reduction in long-term alcohol use and alcohol-related problems. However, brief advice and counseling without regular follow-up and reinforcement cannot sustain significant long-term reductions in unhealthy drinking behaviors. Several pharmacologic agents are effective in reducing alcohol consumption. In acute alcohol detoxification, standard treatment regimens use long-acting benzodiazepines, the preferred medications for alcohol detoxification, because they can be given on a fixed schedule or through "front-loading" or "symptom-triggered" regimens. Adjuvant sympatholytic medications can be used to treat hyperadrenergic symptoms that persist despite adequate sedation. For maintenance, persons who receive short-term treatment with naltrexone have a lower chance of alcoholism relapse. Compared with placebo, naltrexone can lower the risk of treatment withdrawal in alcohol-dependent patients. Nalmefene is not recommended for treatment of alcohol dependence.

Use of illegal drugs—including cocaine, methamphetamine, and so-called "designer drugs"—either sporadically or episodically remains an important problem. Disturbing trends include an increase in use of marijuana and inhalants among eighth graders and high school students and an increase in abuse of prescription pain medications. Many drug users are employed, and many use drugs during pregnancy. Cocaine or tobacco use during early pregnancy substantially increases the risk of miscarriage. Abuse of anabolic-androgenic steroids has been associated with use of other illicit drugs, alcohol, and cigarettes and with violence and criminal behavior. As with alcohol abuse, the recognition of drug abuse presents special problems and requires that the clinician actively consider the diagnosis. Clinical aspects of substance abuse are discussed in Chapter 25.

Currently, evidence does not support the use of carbamazepine, disulfiram, mazindol, phenytoin, ni-

Table 1–10. Screening for alcohol abuse.

---

1. **CAGE screening test**[1]

Have you ever felt the need to	**C**ut down on drinking?
Have you ever felt	**A**nnoyed by criticism of your drinking?
Have you ever felt	**G**uilty about your drinking?
Have you ever taken a morning	**E**ye opener?

   INTERPRETATION: Two "yes" answers are considered a positive screen. One "yes" answer should arouse a suspicion of alcohol abuse.

2. **The Alcohol Use Disorder Identification Test (AUDIT).**[2] (Scores for response categories are given in parentheses. Scores range from 0 to 40, with a cutoff score of ≥ 5 indicating hazardous drinking, harmful drinking, or alcohol dependence.)

1. How often do you have a drink containing alcohol?

(0) Never	(1) Monthly or less	(2) Two to four times a month	(3) Two or three times a week	(4) Four or more times a week

2. How many drinks containing alcohol do you have on a typical day when you are drinking?

(0) 1 or 2	(1) 3 or 4	(2) 5 or 6	(3) 7 to 9	(4) 10 or more

3. How often do you have six or more drinks on one occasion?

(0) Never	(1) Less than monthly	(2) Monthly	(3) Weekly	(4) Daily or almost daily

4. How often during the past year have you found that you were not able to stop drinking once you had started?

(0) Never	(1) Less than monthly	(2) Monthly	(3) Weekly	(4) Daily or almost daily

5. How often during the past year have you failed to do what was normally expected of you because of drinking?

(0) Never	(1) Less than monthly	(2) Monthly	(3) Weekly	(4) Daily or almost daily

6. How often during the past year have you needed a first drink in the morning to get yourself going after a heavy drinking session?

(0) Never	(1) Less than monthly	(2) Monthly	(3) Weekly	(4) Daily or almost daily

7. How often during the past year have you had a feeling of guilt or remorse after drinking?

(0) Never	(1) Less than monthly	(2) Monthly	(3) Weekly	(4) Daily or almost daily

8. How often during the past year have you been unable to remember what happened the night before because you had been drinking?

(0) Never	(1) Less than monthly	(2) Monthly	(3) Weekly	(4) Daily or almost daily

9. Have you or has someone else been injured as a result of your drinking?

(0) No	(2) Yes, but not in the past year	(4) Yes, during the past year

10. Has a relative or friend or a doctor or other health worker been concerned about your drinking or suggested you cut down?

(0) No	(2) Yes, but not in the past year	(4) Yes, during the past year

---

[1]Modified from Mayfield D et al: The CAGE questionnaire: validation of a new alcoholism screening instrument. Am J Psychiatry 1974; 131:1121.

[2]From Piccinelli M et al: Efficacy of the alcohol use disorders identification test as a screening tool for hazardous alcohol intake and related disorders in primary care: a validity study. BMJ 1997;314:420.

modipine, lithium, antidepressants, or dopamine agonists in the treatment of cocaine dependence. Buprenorphine has potential as a medication to ameliorate the signs and symptoms of withdrawal from opioids and has been shown to be effective in reducing concomitant cocaine and opiate abuse. Slow tapering with temporary substitution of methadone and buprenorphine—accompanied by medical supervision and ancillary medications—can reduce withdrawal severity, but most patients relapse to heroin use. Cessation of methadone maintenance is possible using buprenorphine by transfer from methadone to buprenorphine and subsequent buprenorphine reductions. Evidence does not support the use of naltrexone in maintenance treatment of opioid addiction. Rapid opioid detoxification with opioid antagonist induction using general anesthesia has emerged as an approach to treat opioid dependence. However, a randomized comparison of buprenorphine-assisted rapid opioid detoxification with naltrexone induction and clonidine-assisted opioid detoxification with delayed naltrexone induction found no significant differences in rates of completion of inpatient detoxification, treatment retention, or proportions of opioid-posi-

Table 1–11. Basic counseling steps for patients who abuse alcohol.

Establish a therapeutic relationship
Make the medical office or clinic off-limits for substance
  abuse
Present information about negative health consequences
Emphasize personal responsibility and self-efficacy
Convey a clear message and set goals
Involve family and other supports
Establish a working relationship with community treatment
  resources
Provide follow-up

From the United States Department of Health Human Services, U.S. Public Health Service, Office of Disease Prevention Health Promotion. Clinician's Handbook of Preventive Services: Put Prevention Into Practice. U.S. Government Printing Office, 1994.

tive urine specimens, and the anesthesia procedure was associated with more potentially life-threatening adverse events.

Blondell RD: Ambulatory detoxification of patients with alcohol dependence. Am Fam Physician 2005;71:495. [PMID: 15712624]

Breen CL et al: Cessation of methadone maintenance treatment using buprenorphine: transfer from methadone to buprenorphine and subsequent buprenorphine reductions. Drug Alcohol Depend 2003;71:49. [PMID: 12821205]

Collins ED et al: Anesthesia-assisted vs buprenorphine- or clonidine-assisted heroin detoxification and naltrexone induction: a randomized trial. JAMA 2005;294:903. [PMID: 16118380]

Fudala PJ et al: Office-based treatment of opiate addiction with a sublingual-tablet formulation of buprenorphine and naloxone. N Engl J Med 2003;349:949. [PMID: 12954743]

Isaacson JH et al: Prescription drug use and abuse. Risk factors, red flags, and prevention strategies. Postgrad Med 2005; 118:19. [PMID: 16106916]

JAMA patient page. Cocaine addiction. JAMA 2002;287:146. [PMID: 11797622]

Montoya ID et al: Randomized trial of buprenorphine for treatment of concurrent opiate and cocaine dependence. Clin Pharmacol Ther 2004;75:34. [PMID: 14749690]

Saitz R et al: Addressing alcohol problems in primary care: a cluster randomized, controlled trial of a systems intervention. The screening and intervention in primary care (SIP) study. Ann Intern Med 2003;138:372. [PMID: 12614089]

Sofuoglu M et al: Novel approaches to the treatment of cocaine addiction. CNS Drugs 2005;19:13. [PMID: 15651902]

Srisurapanont M et al: Opioid antagonists for alcohol dependence. Cochrane Database Syst Rev 200525;(1):CD001867. [PMID: 15674887]

Whitlock EP et al: Behavioral counseling interventions in primary care to reduce risky/harmful alcohol use by adults: a summary of the evidence for the U.S. Preventive Services Task Force. Ann Intern Med 2004;140:557. [PMID: 15068985]

Common Symptoms

Ralph Gonzales, MD, MSPH

New or unexplained symptoms account for about half of all office visits; the remainder of visits are for ongoing care of established medical conditions. Evidence-based symptom evaluation combines knowledge of a symptom's clinical epidemiology with disease candidates according to Bayesian principles (see Chapter 42), such that the likelihood of a specific disease is a function of patient demographics, comorbidities, and clinical features. This knowledge can help support decisions about further testing or treatment or whether to perform additional testing before treatment, or to treat without further testing.

In addition to epidemiologic factors, biological, psychological, social, and cultural factors affect how patients process, filter, and interpret symptoms. Patients vary in deciding when symptoms are sufficiently bothersome or worrisome to cause them to seek medical attention, and in what they expect from the office visit.

Many symptoms defy diagnosis. If symptom relief is not easily achieved, treatment of these patients becomes challenging. The shift toward evidence-based principles of medicine, which encourage narrow study questions in homogeneous study populations, inadvertently ignores syndromes that are not readily explained by current biomedical models of disease. Conversely, even when the cause of a disease is known, host and environmental factors can influence the symptoms that are manifested. For example, in 1967, Evans proposed five "realities" that reflect the conundrum clinicians face when associating an acute respiratory syndrome with an etiologic pathogen: (1) The same clinical syndrome may be produced by a variety of infectious pathogens; (2) the same pathogen may produce a variety of syndromes; (3) the most likely cause of a syndrome may vary by patient age, year, geography, and setting; (4) diagnosis of the pathogen is frequently impossible on the basis of clinical findings alone; and (5) the causes of a large proportion of infectious disease syndromes are still unknown.

COUGH

 ESSENTIAL INQUIRIES

- *Duration of cough.*
- *Dyspnea (at rest or with exertion).*
- *Constitutional symptoms.*

- *Tobacco use history.*
- *Vital signs (heart rate, respiratory rate, body temperature).*
- *Chest examination.*
- *Chest radiography when unexplained cough lasts more than 3–6 weeks.*

General Considerations

Cough adversely affects personal and work-related interactions, disrupts sleep, and often causes discomfort of the throat and chest wall. Most people seeking medical attention for acute cough desire symptom relief; few are worried about serious illness. Cough results from stimulation of mechanical or chemical afferent nerve receptors in the bronchial tree. Effective cough depends on an intact afferent–efferent reflex arc, adequate expiratory and chest wall muscle strength, and normal mucociliary production and clearance.

Clinical Findings

A. SYMPTOMS

Distinguishing acute (< 3 weeks) and persistent (> 3 weeks) cough illness syndromes is a useful first step in evaluation. In healthy adults, most acute cough syndromes are due to viral respiratory tract infections. Additional features of infection such as fever, nasal congestion, and sore throat help confirm the diagnosis. Dyspnea (at rest or with exertion) may reflect a more serious condition, and further evaluation should include assessment of oxygenation (pulse oximetry or arterial blood gas measurement), airflow (peak flow or spirometry), and pulmonary parenchymal disease (chest radiography). The timing and character of the cough have not been found to be useful in establishing the cause of acute or persistent cough syndromes, although cough-variant asthma should be considered in adults with prominent nocturnal cough. Uncommon causes of acute cough illness should be suspected in those with heart disease (congestive heart failure [CHF]) or hay fever (allergic rhinitis) and those with environmental risk factors.

Cough due to acute respiratory tract infection resolves within 3 weeks in the vast majority of patients (over

90%). Pertussis infection should be considered in previously immunized adults with persistent or severe cough lasting more than 2–3 weeks and approaches a prevalence of 20% when cough has persisted beyond 3 weeks.

When angiotensin-converting enzyme (ACE) inhibitor therapy, acute respiratory tract infection, and chest radiograph abnormalities are absent, up to 90% of cases of persistent cough are due to postnasal drip, asthma, or gastroesophageal reflux disease (GERD). A history of nasal or sinus congestion, wheezing, or heartburn should direct subsequent evaluation and treatment, though these conditions frequently cause persistent cough in the absence of typical symptoms. Bronchogenic carcinoma is suspected when cough is accompanied by unexplained weight loss and fevers with night sweats, particularly in persons with significant tobacco or occupational exposures. Persistent cough accompanied by excessive mucus secretions suggests chronic bronchitis in a smoker, or bronchiectasis in a patient with a history of recurrent or complicated pneumonia; chest radiographs are helpful in diagnosis. Dyspnea at rest or with exertion is not commonly reported among patients with persistent cough. The report of dyspnea requires assessment for other evidence of chronic lung disease or CHF.

B. Physical Examination

Examination can direct subsequent diagnostic testing for acute and persistent cough. Pneumonia is suspected when acute cough is accompanied by vital sign abnormalities (tachycardia, tachypnea, fever) or findings suggestive of airspace consolidation (rales, decreased breath sounds, fremitus, egophony). Purulent sputum is a poor predictor of pneumonia in the otherwise healthy adult. In the outpatient setting, pneumonia was present in 4% of adults with purulent sputum compared with 2% of adults without purulent sputum (relative risk = 2.0). In addition, antibiotic treatment of adults with purulent sputum production shows no benefit. Wheezing and rhonchi are frequent findings in adults with acute bronchitis and do not represent adult-onset asthma in most cases.

Physical examination of adults with persistent cough may also reveal evidence of chronic sinusitis, contributing to postnasal drip syndrome or asthma. Chest and cardiac signs may distinguish chronic obstructive pulmonary disease (COPD) from CHF. In patients with cough and dyspnea, a normal match test (ability to blow out a match from 25 cm away) and maximum laryngeal height > 4 cm (measured from the sternal notch to the cricoid cartilage at end expiration) substantially decrease the likelihood of COPD. Similarly, normal jugular venous pressure and negative hepatojugular reflux decrease the likelihood of biventricular CHF.

Differential Diagnosis

A. Acute Cough

Acute cough may be a symptom of acute respiratory tract infection, asthma, allergic rhinitis, and CHF, as well as a myriad of other less common causes.

B. Persistent Cough

Causes of persistent cough include postnasal drip syndrome, asthma (including cough-variant asthma), GERD, chronic bronchitis, bronchiectasis, tuberculosis or other chronic infection, interstitial lung disease, and bronchogenic carcinoma. Persistent cough may also be psychogenic.

Diagnostic Studies

A. Acute Cough

Chest radiography should be considered for any adult with acute cough who shows abnormal vital signs or in whom the chest examination is suggestive of pneumonia. The relationship between specific clinical findings and the probability of pneumonia is shown in Figure 2–1. In patients with dyspnea, pulse oximetry and peak flow help exclude hypoxemia or obstructive airway disease. However, a normal pulse oximetry value (eg, > 93%) does not rule out a significant alveolar–arterial (A–a) gradient when patients have effective respiratory compensation.

B. Persistent Cough

Chest radiography is indicated when ACE inhibitor therapy–related and postinfectious cough are excluded by history or further diagnostic testing. Pertussis infection should be evaluated with polymerase chain reaction tests as well as culture from a nasopharyngeal swab specimen. When the chest film is normal, evaluation for postnasal drip, asthma, and GERD should be initiated. The presence of typical symptoms of these conditions directs further evaluation or empiric therapy, though typical symptoms are often absent. Definitive procedures for determining the presence of each are available (Table 2–1). However, empiric treatment with a maximum-strength regimen for postnasal drip, asthma, or GERD for 2–4 weeks is the recommended approach since documenting the presence of postnasal drip, asthma, and GERD does not mean they are the cause of the cough illness. In about 25% of cases,

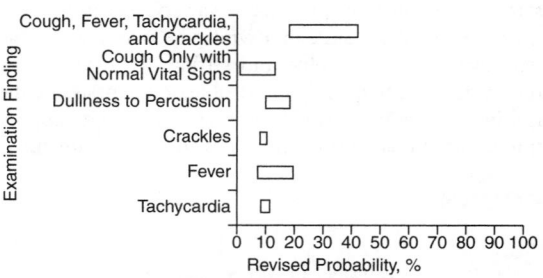

Figure 2–1. Revised pneumonia probabilities based on history and physical examination findings. (Reproduced, with permission, from Metlay JP et al: Testing strategies in the initial management of patients with community-acquired pneumonia. Ann Intern Med 2003;138:109.)

Table 2–1. Empiric treatments or tests for persistent cough.

Suspected Condition	Step 1 (Empiric Therapy)	Step 2 (Diagnostic Testing)
Postnasal drip	Therapy for allergy or chronic sinusitis	ENT referral; sinus CT scan
Asthma	β_2-Agonist	Spirometry; consider methacholine challenge if normal
GERD	Proton pump inhibitors	Esophageal pH monitoring

ENT = ear, nose, and throat; GERD = gastroesophageal reflux disease.

persistent cough has multiple contributors. Spirometry may help identify large airway obstruction in patients who have persistent cough and wheezing and who are not responding to asthma treatment.

Haque RA et al: Chronic idiopathic cough: a discrete clinical entity? Chest 2005;127:1710. [PMID: 15888850]

Hewlett EL et al: Clinical practice. Pertussis—not just for kids. N Engl J Med 2005;352:1215. [PMID: 15788498]

Irwin RS et al: The persistently troublesome cough. Am J Respir Crit Care Med 2002;165:1469. [PMID: 12045118]

Lin DA et al: Asthma or not? The value of flow volume loops in evaluating airflow obstruction. Allergy Asthma Proc 2003; 24:107. [PMID: 12776443]

Madison MD et al: Pharmacotherapy of chronic cough in adults. Expert Opin Pharmacother 2003;4:1039. [PMID: 12831332]

Metlay JP et al: Testing strategies in the initial management of patients with community-acquired pneumonia. Ann Intern Med 2003;138:109. [PMID: 12529093]

Schroeder K et al: Over-the-counter medications for acute cough in children and adults in ambulatory settings. Cochrane Database Syst Rev 2004;(4):CD001831. [PMID: 15495019]

DYSPNEA

 ESSENTIAL INQUIRIES

- *Fever.*
- *Cough.*
- *Chest pain.*
- *Vital sign measurements.*
- *Pulse oximetry.*
- *Chest examination.*
- *Cardiac examination.*
- *Chest radiography.*
- *Arterial blood gas measurement.*

General Considerations

Dyspnea is a subjective experience or *perception* of uncomfortable breathing. However, the relationship between level of dyspnea and the severity of underlying disease varies widely across individuals. Dyspnea can result from conditions that increase the mechanical effort of breathing (eg, COPD, restrictive lung disease, respiratory muscle weakness), from conditions that produce compensatory tachypnea (eg, hypoxemia or acidosis), or from psychogenic origins. Rate of onset, previous dyspnea, medications, comorbidities, psychological profile, and severity of underlying disorder play a role in how and when persons present with dyspnea. Nonetheless, in patients with established COPD, the severity of dyspnea is superior to forced expiratory volume in 1 second (FEV_1) in predicting quality of life and 5-year mortality.

Dyspnea commonly accompanies a multitude of acute and chronic medical conditions. Acute dyspnea, particularly as the chief complaint, demands urgent evaluation. Urgent/emergent conditions causing acute dyspnea include pneumonia, COPD, asthma, pneumothorax, pulmonary embolism, cardiac disease (eg, CHF, acute myocardial infarction, valvular dysfunction, arrhythmia, cardiac shunt), metabolic acidosis, cyanide toxicity, methemoglobinemia, and carbon monoxide poisoning.

With two notable exceptions (carbon monoxide poisoning and cyanide toxicity), routine arterial blood gas measurement distinguishes increased mechanical effort causes of dyspnea (respiratory acidosis with or without hypoxemia) from compensatory tachypnea (respiratory alkalosis with or without hypoxemia or metabolic acidosis) from psychogenic dyspnea (respiratory alkalosis). Carbon monoxide and cyanide impair oxygen delivery with minimal alterations in P_{O_2}; percent carboxyhemoglobin identifies carbon monoxide toxicity. Cyanide poisoning should be considered in a patient with profound lactic acidosis following a theater fire.

Clinical Findings

A. SYMPTOMS

The duration, severity, and periodicity of dyspnea influence the tempo of the clinical evaluation. Rapid onset, severe dyspnea in the absence of other clinical features should raise concern for pneumothorax, pulmonary embolism, or increased left ventricular end-diastolic pressure (LVEDP). Spontaneous pneumothorax is usually accompanied by chest pain and occurs most often in thin, young males, or in those with underlying lung disease. Pulmonary embolism should always be suspected when a patient reports a recent history (previous 4 weeks) of prolonged immobilization, estrogen therapy, or other risk factors for deep venous thrombosis (DVT) (eg, previous history of thromboembolism, cancer, obesity) and when the cause of dyspnea is not apparent. Silent myocardial infarction, which occurs more frequently in diabetic persons and women, can result in acute heart failure and dyspnea.

Accompanying symptoms provide important clues to various etiologies of dyspnea. When cough and fever are present, pulmonary disease (particularly infections) is the primary concern, although myocarditis, pericarditis, and septic emboli can also present in this manner. Chest pain should be further characterized as acute or chronic, pleuritic or exertional. Although acute pleuritic chest pain is the rule in acute pericarditis and pneumothorax, most patients with pleuritic chest pain in the outpatient clinic have pleurisy due to acute viral respiratory tract infection. Periodic chest pain that precedes the onset of dyspnea is suspicious for myocardial ischemia as well as pulmonary embolism. Most cases of dyspnea associated with wheezing are due to acute bronchitis; however, when acute bronchitis seems unlikely, the clinician should also consider new-onset asthma, foreign body, and vocal cord dysfunction.

When a patient reports prominent dyspnea with mild or no accompanying features, consider noncardiopulmonary causes of impaired oxygen delivery (anemia, methemoglobinemia, cyanide ingestion, carbon monoxide), pulmonary embolism, metabolic acidosis due to a variety of conditions, and panic attacks.

B. PHYSICAL EXAMINATION

A focused physical examination should include evaluation of the head and neck, chest, heart, and lower extremities. Visual inspection of the patient's respiratory pattern can suggest obstructive airway disease (pursed-lip breathing, use of extrarespiratory muscles, barrel-shaped chest), pneumothorax (asymmetric excursion), or metabolic acidosis (Kussmaul respirations). Patients with impending upper airway obstruction (eg, epiglottitis, foreign body), or severe asthma exacerbation, sometimes assume a tripod position. Focal wheezing raises the suspicion for a foreign body or other bronchial obstruction. Maximum laryngeal height (the distance between the top of the thyroid cartilage and the suprasternal notch at end expiration) is a measure of hyperinflation. Obstructive airway disease is virtually nonexistent when a nonsmoking patient younger than 45 years has a maximum laryngeal height < 4 cm (Table 2–2).

Because arterial blood gas testing is impractical in most outpatient settings, **pulse oximetry** has assumed a central role in the office evaluation of dyspnea. Oxygen saturation values above 96% almost always correspond with a $PO_2 > 70$ mm Hg, and values less than 94% almost always represent clinically significant hypoxemia. Important exceptions to this rule include carbon monoxide toxicity, which leads to a normal oxygen saturation (due to the similar wavelengths of oxyhemoglobin and carboxyhemoglobin), and methemoglobinemia, which results in an oxygen saturation of about 85%. Supplemental oxygen fails to improve desaturation due to methemoglobinemia. A normal or mildly abnormal oxygen saturation (< 90%) in a delirious or obtunded patient

Table 2–2. Clinical findings suggesting obstructive airway disease.

	Adjusted Likelihood Ratios	
	Factor Present	Factor Absent
> 40 pack-years smoking	11.6	0.9
Age ≥ 45 years	1.4	0.5
Maximum laryngeal height ≤ 4 cm	3.6	0.7
All three factors	58.5	0.3

Reprinted with permission from Straus SE et al: The accuracy of patient history, wheezing, and laryngeal measurements in diagnosing obstructive airway disease. CARE-COAD1 Group. Clinical Assessment of the Reliability of the Examination—Chronic Obstructive Airways Disease. JAMA 2000;283:1853.

with obstructive lung disease warrants immediate measurement of arterial blood gases to exclude hypercapnia and the need for intubation. When pulse oximetry yields equivocal results, assessment of desaturation with ambulation (eg, a brisk walk around the clinic) can be a useful finding (eg, when *Pneumocystis jiroveci* [formerly *P carinii*] pneumonia is suspected).

A systematic review has identified several clinical predictors of increased LVEDP useful in the evaluation of dyspneic patients with no prior history of CHF (Table 2–3). When none is present, there is a very low probability (< 10%) of increased LVEDP, and when two or more are present, there is a very high probability (> 90%) of increased LVEDP.

Table 2–3. Clinical findings suggesting increased left ventricular end-diastolic pressure.

Tachycardia
Systolic hypotension
Jugular venous distention (> 5–7 cm H_2O)[1]
Hepatojugular reflux (> 1 cm)[2]
Crackles, especially bibasilar
Third heart sound[3]
Lower extremity edema
Radiographic pulmonary vascular redistribution or cardiomegaly[1]

[1]These findings are particularly helpful.
[2]Proper abdominal compression for evaluating hepatojugular reflux requires > 30 seconds of sustained upper quadrant abdominal compression.
[3]Cardiac auscultation of the patient at 45-degree angle in left lateral decubitus position doubles the detection rate of third heart sounds.
Modified with permission from Badgett RG et al: Can the clinical examination diagnose left-sided heart failure in adults? JAMA 1997;277:1712.

Diagnostic Studies

Causes of dyspnea that can be managed without chest radiography are few: ingestions causing lactic acidosis, methemoglobinemia, and carbon monoxide poisoning. The diagnosis of pneumonia should be confirmed by chest radiography in most patients. When COPD exacerbation is severe enough to require hospitalization, results of chest radiography influence management decisions in up to 20% of patients. Chest radiography (detection of redistribution of pulmonary venous circulation) is fairly sensitive and specific for new-onset CHF and can help guide treatment decisions in patients with dyspnea secondary to cardiac disease. End-expiratory chest radiography enhances detection of a small pneumothorax.

A normal chest radiograph has substantial diagnostic value. In the absence of physical examination evidence of COPD or CHF, the major remaining causes of dyspnea include pulmonary embolism, upper airway obstruction, foreign body, and metabolic acidosis. If a patient has tachycardia and hypoxemia but a normal chest radiograph and ECG, then further tests to exclude pulmonary emboli are warranted (see Chapter 9), provided blood tests exclude significant anemia or metabolic acidosis. High-resolution chest CT is particularly useful in the evaluation of pulmonary embolism and interstitial lung disease. Suspected carbon monoxide poisoning or methemoglobinemia can be confirmed with either arterial or venous carboxyhemoglobin or methemoglobin levels.

Serum or whole blood brain natriuretic peptide (BNP) testing can be useful in the evaluation of dyspnea in the emergency department, since elevated BNP levels are both sensitive and specific for increased LVEDP in symptomatic persons.

Clinical examination and routine diagnostic testing will identify the cause of dyspnea in most cases. Persistent uncertainty warrants arterial blood gas measurement. Spirometry is very helpful in further classifying patients with obstructive airway disease, but is rarely needed in the initial or emergent evaluation of patients with acute dyspnea.

Episodic dyspnea can be challenging if an evaluation cannot be performed during symptoms. Life-threatening causes include recurrent pulmonary embolism, myocardial ischemia, and reactive airway disease. When associated with audible wheezing, vocal cord dysfunction should be considered, particularly in a young woman who does not respond to asthma therapy.

Treatment

The treatment of urgent or emergent causes of dyspnea should aim to relieve the underlying cause. Pending diagnosis, patients with hypoxemia should be immediately provided supplemental oxygen unless significant hypercapnia is present. Dyspnea frequently occurs in patients nearing the end of life, and opioid and oxygen therapy can be very effective in providing relief (see Chapter 5).

Collins SP et al: Diagnostic and prognostic usefulness of natriuretic peptides in emergency department patients with dyspnea. Ann Emerg Med 2003;41:532. [PMID: 12658254]

Jennings AL et al: A systematic review of the use of opioids in the management of dyspnea. Thorax 2002;57:929. [PMID: 12403875]

Karnani NG et al: Evaluation of chronic dyspnea. Am Fam Physician 2005;71:1529. [PMID: 15864893]

Luce JM et al: Management of dyspnea in patients with far-advanced lung disease: "once I lose it, it's kind of hard to catch it...." JAMA 2001;285:1331. [PMID: 11255389]

Mahler DA et al: Evaluation of dyspnea in the elderly. Clin Geriatr Med 2003;19:19. [PMID: 12735113]

Straus SE et al: The accuracy of patient history, wheezing, and laryngeal measurements in diagnosing obstructive airway disease. JAMA 2000;283:1853. [PMID: 10770147]

LOWER EXTREMITY EDEMA

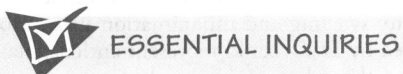

ESSENTIAL INQUIRIES

- *History of venous thromboembolism.*
- *Symmetry.*
- *Pain.*
- *Dependence.*

General Considerations

Acute and chronic lower extremity edema present important diagnostic and treatment challenges. Lower extremities can swell in response to increased venous or lymphatic pressures, decreased intravascular oncotic pressure, increased capillary leak, and local injury or infection. Chronic venous insufficiency is by far the most common cause, affecting up to 2% of the population, and the incidence of venous insufficiency has not changed during the past 25 years. Venous insufficiency is a common complication of DVT; however, only a small number of patients with chronic venous insufficiency report a history of this disorder. Venous ulcer formation commonly affects patients with chronic venous insufficiency, and management of venous ulceration is labor intensive and expensive.

Clinical Findings

A. SYMPTOMS AND SIGNS

Normal lower extremity venous pressure (in the erect position: 80 mm Hg in deep veins, 20–30 mm Hg in superficial veins) and cephalad venous blood flow require competent bicuspid venous valves, effective muscle contractions, and normal respirations. When one or more of these components fail, venous hypertension may result. Chronic exposure to elevated venous pressure by the postcapillary venules in the legs leads to leakage of fibrinogen and growth factors into the interstitial space, leukocyte aggregation and activation, and obliteration of the cutaneous lymphatic network. These changes account for the brawny, fibrotic skin changes observed in patients with chronic venous insufficiency, and the predisposition toward skin ulceration, particularly in the medial malleolar area.

Among common causes of lower extremity swelling, DVT is the most life-threatening. Clues suggesting DVT include a history of cancer, recent limb immobilization, or confinement to bed for at least 3 days following major surgery within the past month (Table 2–4). A search for alternative explanations is equally important in excluding DVT. Bilateral involvement and significant improvement upon awakening favor systemic causes (eg, venous insufficiency, CHF, and cirrhosis). "Heavy legs" are the most frequent symptom among patients with chronic venous insufficiency, followed by itching. Pain, particularly if severe, is uncommon in uncomplicated venous insufficiency. Lower extremity swelling and inflammation in a limb recently affected by DVT could represent anticoagulation failure and thrombus recurrence but more often are caused by postphlebitic syndrome with valvular incompetence. Other causes of a painful, swollen calf include ruptured popliteal cyst, calf strain or trauma, and cellulitis. Lower extremity swelling is a familiar

Table 2–4. Risk stratification of adults referred for ultrasound to rule out DVT.

Step 1: Calculate risk factor score
Score 1 point for each
Untreated malignancy
Paralysis, paresis, or recent plaster immobilization
Recently bedridden for > 3 days due to major surgery within 4 weeks
Localized tenderness along distribution of deep venous system
Entire leg swelling
Swelling of one calf > 3 cm more than the other (measured 10 cm below tibial tuberosity)
Pitting edema
Collateral superficial (nonvaricose) veins
Alternative diagnosis as likely as or more likely than DVT: subtract 2 points

	Step 2: Obtain ultrasound	
Score	**Ultrasound Positive**	**Ultrasound Negative**
≤ 0	Confirm with venogram	DVT ruled out
1–2	Treat for DVT	Repeat ultrasound in 3–7 days
≥ 3	Treat for DVT	Confirm with venogram

DVT = deep venous thrombosis.

complication of therapy with calcium channel blockers (particularly felodipine and amlodipine), thioglitazones, and minoxidil. Prolonged airline flights (>10 hours) are associated with increased risk of edema. In those with low to medium risk of thromboembolism (eg, women taking oral contraceptives), long flights are associated with a 2% incidence of asymptomatic popliteal DVT.

B. PHYSICAL EXAMINATION

Physical examination should include assessment of the heart, lungs, and abdomen for evidence of pulmonary hypertension (primary, or secondary to chronic lung disease), CHF, or cirrhosis. Some patients with the latter have pulmonary hypertension without lung disease. There is a spectrum of skin findings related to chronic venous insufficiency that depends on the severity and chronicity of the disease, ranging from hyperpigmentation and stasis dermatitis to abnormalities highly specific for chronic venous insufficiency: lipodermatosclerosis (thick brawny skin; in advanced cases, the lower leg resembles an inverted champagne bottle) and atrophie blanche (small depigmented macules within areas of heavy pigmentation). The size of both calves should be measured 10 cm below the tibial tuberosity and elicitation of pitting and tenderness performed. Swelling of the entire leg or swelling of one leg 3 cm more than the other suggests deep venous obstruction. In normal persons, the left calf is slightly larger than the right as a result of the left common iliac vein coursing under the aorta.

An ulcer located over the medial malleolus is a hallmark of chronic venous insufficiency but can be due to other causes. Shallow, large, modestly painful ulcers are characteristic of venous insufficiency, whereas small, deep, and more painful ulcers are more apt to be due to arterial insufficiency, vasculitis, or infection (including cutaneous diphtheria). Diabetic vascular ulcers, however, may be painless. When an ulcer is on the foot or above the mid calf, causes other than venous insufficiency should be considered.

C. DIAGNOSTIC STUDIES

Most causes of lower extremity swelling can be demonstrated with color duplex ultrasonography. Patients without an obvious cause of acute lower extremity swelling (eg, calf strain) should have an ultrasound performed, since DVT is difficult to exclude on clinical grounds. Assessment of the ankle-brachial pressure index (ABPI) is important in the management of chronic venous insufficiency, since peripheral arterial disease may be exacerbated by compression therapy. This can be performed at the same time as ultrasound. Caution is required in interpreting the results of ABPI in older patients and diabetics due to decreased compressibility of their arteries.

Differential Diagnosis

Possible causes include chronic venous insufficiency, DVT, cellulitis, musculoskeletal disorders (Baker's cyst rupture, gastrocnemius tear or rupture), lymphedema, CHF, cirrhosis, and nephrotic syndrome, as well as side effects from calcium channel blockers, minoxidil, or thioglitazones.

Treatment

In patients with chronic venous insufficiency without a comorbid volume overload state (eg, CHF), it is best to avoid diuretic therapy. These patients have relatively decreased intravascular volume, and administration of diuretics may result in acute renal insufficiency and oliguria. The most effective treatment involves (1) leg elevation, above the level of the heart, for 30 minutes three to four times daily, and during sleep; and (2) compression therapy. A wide variety of stockings and devices are effective in decreasing swelling and preventing ulcer formation. They should be put on with awakening, before hydration forces result in edema. Horse chestnut seed extract has been shown in several randomized trials to be equivalent to compression stockings, and can be quite useful in nonambulatory patients. Patients with decreased ABPI should be managed in concert with a vascular surgeon. Compression stockings (12–18 mm Hg at the ankle) are effective in preventing edema and asymptomatic thrombosis associated with long airline flights in low- to medium-risk persons.

Barwell JR et al: Comparison of surgery and compression with compression alone in chronic venous ulceration (ESCHAR study): randomised controlled trial. Lancet 2004;363:1854. [PMID: 15183623]

Belcaro G et al: Prevention of edema, flight microangiopathy and venous thrombosis in long flights with elastic stockings. A randomized trial: the LONFLIT 4 Concorde Edema-SSL Study. Angiology 2002;53:635. [PMID: 12463616]

Criqui MH et al: Chronic venous disease in an ethnically diverse population: the San Diego Population Study. Am J Epidemiol 2003;158:448. [PMID: 12936900]

Eberhardt RT et al: Chronic venous insufficiency. Circulation 2005;111:2398. [PMID: 15883226]

Felty CL et al: Compression therapy for chronic venous insufficiency. Semin Vasc Surg 2005;18:36. [PMID: 15791552]

Kahn SR et al: Relationship between deep venous thrombosis and the postthrombotic syndrome. Arch Intern Med 2004; 164:17. [PMID: 14718318]

FEVER & HYPERTHERMIA

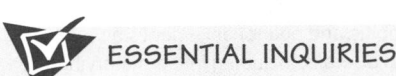 ESSENTIAL INQUIRIES

- Localizing symptoms.
- Weight loss.
- Joint pain.
- Injection substance use.
- Immunosuppression or neutropenia.
- History of cancer.
- Medications.
- Travel.

General Considerations

The average normal oral body temperature taken in mid-morning is 36.7 °C (range 36–37.4 °C). This spectrum includes a mean and 2 standard deviations, thus encompassing 95% of a normal population, measured in mid-morning (normal diurnal temperature variation is 0.5–1 °C). The normal rectal or vaginal temperature is 0.5 °C higher than the oral temperature, and the axillary temperature is correspondingly lower. Rectal temperature is more reliable than oral temperature, particularly in mouth breathers or in tachypneic states.

Fever is a regulated rise to a new "set point" of body temperature. When proper stimuli act on appropriate monocyte-macrophages, these cells elaborate pyrogenic cytokines, causing elevation of the set point through effects in the hypothalamus. These cytokines include interleukin-1 (IL-1), tumor necrosis factor (TNF), interferon-γ, and interleukin-6 (IL-6). The elevation in temperature results from either increased heat production (eg, shivering) or decreased loss (eg, peripheral vasoconstriction). Body temperature in cytokine-induced fever seldom exceeds 41.1 °C unless there is structural damage to hypothalamic regulatory centers.

Hyperthermia

Hyperthermia—not mediated by cytokines—occurs when body metabolic heat production or environmental heat load exceeds normal heat loss capacity or when there is impaired heat loss; heat stroke is an example. Body temperature may rise to levels (> 41.1 °C) capable of producing irreversible protein denaturation and resultant brain damage; no diurnal variation is observed.

Neuroleptic malignant syndrome is a rare and potentially lethal idiosyncratic reaction to major tranquilizers, particularly haloperidol and fluphenazine. It has clinical and pathophysiologic similarities to malignant hyperthermia of anesthesia (see Chapters 25 and 39).

Fever as a symptom provides important information about the presence of illness—particularly infections—and about changes in the clinical status of the patient. The fever pattern, however, is of marginal value for most specific diagnoses except for the relapsing fever of malaria, borreliosis, and occasional cases of lymphoma, especially Hodgkin's disease. Furthermore, the degree of temperature elevation does not necessarily correspond to the severity of the illness. In general, the febrile response tends to be greater in children than in adults. In older persons, neonates, and in persons receiving certain medications (eg, nonsteroidal anti-inflammatory drugs [NSAIDs] or corticosteroids), a normal temperature or even hypothermia may be observed.

Markedly elevated body temperature may result in profound metabolic disturbances. High temperature during the first trimester of pregnancy may cause birth defects, such as anencephaly. Fever increases insulin requirements and alters the metabolism and disposition of drugs used for the treatment of the diverse diseases associated with fever.

Prolonged Fever

Most febrile illnesses are due to common infections, are short-lived, and are relatively easy to diagnose. In certain instances, however, the origin of the fever may remain obscure ("fever of undetermined origin," FUO) even after protracted diagnostic examination. In upper respiratory tract infections, fever typically lasts no more than 3–5 days, beyond which additional evaluation is warranted. The term "FUO" has traditionally been reserved for unexplained cases of fever exceeding 38.3 °C on several occasions for at least 3 weeks in patients without neutropenia or immunosuppression (see Chapter 30).

After extensive evaluation, 25% of these patients are judged to have chronic or indolent infection, about 25% autoimmune diseases, and about 10% a malignancy; the remainder have miscellaneous other disorders or no diagnosis is reached. With improved imaging and microbiology testing, fewer cases are being attributed to infectious disease and more are being attributed to cancer and autoimmune disease (particularly among the elderly). Long-term follow-up of patients with initially undiagnosed FUO demonstrates that 50% become symptom free during evaluation. In the remainder, a definitive diagnosis is established in 20%, usually within 2 months after investigation, and 30% have persistent or recurring fever for months or even years.

Approach to the Patient with Fever of Undetermined Origin

Standardized algorithms for FUO are difficult to extrapolate to the individual patient. Nevertheless, the results of a history, physical examination, routine laboratory tests, and blood cultures provide important diagnostic clues that lead to a definitive diagnosis in most cases. Chest radiography, abdominal ultrasound, and CT scans, often repeated after previous nondiagnostic studies, are most helpful. Radionuclide agents include labeled leukocytes, gallium-67, and radiolabeled human immunoglobulin; however, these tests appear to be most useful in patients with localizing signs of inflammation. There is little or no value to be derived from undirected immunologic, microbiologic, serologic, or endocrinologic studies. In older patients, a temporal artery biopsy is occasionally of use. Newer imaging modalities that may be useful in challenging cases include fluorodeoxyglucose-positron emission tomography imaging.

FUO is commonly associated with AIDS and HIV-related infections, though uncomplicated HIV infection is not a cause of prolonged fever. When FUO is observed in HIV-infected individuals, it usually occurs in the late stages. The most common causes are disseminated *Mycobacterium avium* infection, *P jiroveci* pneumonia, cytomegalovirus infection, disseminated histoplasmosis, and lymphoma.

The differential diagnosis of a febrile illness in the returned traveler is extensive but most commonly includes tropical infections such as malaria, dysentery, hepatitis, and dengue fever. A substantial number of febrile illnesses in travelers are never diagnosed.

Differential Diagnosis

See Table 2–5.

Treatment

Most fever is well tolerated. When the temperature is greater than 40 °C, symptomatic treatment may be required. A reading over 41 °C is likely to be hyperthermia and thus not cytokine mediated, and emergent management is indicated. (See Heat Stroke, Chapter 38.)

A. MEASURES FOR REMOVAL OF HEAT

Alcohol sponges, cold sponges, ice bags, ice-water enemas, and ice baths will lower body temperature. They are more useful in hyperthermia, since patients with cytokine-related fever will attempt to override these therapies.

B. ANTIPYRETIC DRUGS

Antipyretic therapy is not needed except for patients with marginal hemodynamic status. Aspirin or aceta-

Table 2–5. Differential diagnosis of fever and hyperthermia.

Fever—common causes
  Infections: bacterial, viral, rickettsial, fungal, parasitic
  Autoimmune diseases
  Central nervous system disease, including head trauma and mass lesions
  Malignant disease, especially renal cell carcinoma, primary or metastatic liver cancer, leukemia, and lymphoma

Fever—less common causes
  Cardiovascular diseases, including myocardial infarction, thrombophlebitis, and pulmonary embolism
  Gastrointestinal diseases, including inflammatory bowel disease, alcoholic hepatitis, and granulomatous hepatitis
  Miscellaneous diseases, including drug fever, sarcoidosis, familial Mediterranean fever, tissue injury, hematoma, and factitious fever

Hyperthermia
  Peripheral thermoregulatory disorders, including heat stroke, malignant hyperthermia of anesthesia, and malignant neuroleptic syndrome

minophen, 325–650 mg every 4 hours, is effective in reducing fever. These drugs are best administered continuously rather than as needed, since "prn" dosing results in periodic chills and sweats due to fluctuations in temperature caused by varying levels of drug.

C. ANTIMICROBIAL THERAPY

In most febrile patients, empiric antibiotic therapy should be deferred pending further evaluation. However, empiric antibiotic therapy is sometimes warranted. Prompt broad-spectrum antimicrobials are indicated for febrile patients who are clinically unstable, even before infection can be documented. These include patients with hemodynamic instability, those with neutropenia (neutrophils < 500/mcL), others who are asplenic (surgically or secondary to sickle cell disease) or immunosuppressed (including individuals taking systemic corticosteroids, azathioprine, cyclosporine, or other immunosuppressive medications), and those who are HIV infected (see Chapter 31). For treatment of fever during neutropenia following chemotherapy, outpatient parenteral antimicrobial therapy with an agent such as ceftriaxone can be provided effectively and safely. If a fungal infection is suspected in patients with prolonged fever and neutropenia, fluconazole is an equally effective but less toxic alternative to amphotericin B.

Carapetis JR et al: Acute rheumatic fever. Lancet 2005;366:155. [PMID: 16005340]

Marik PE: Fever in the ICU. Chest 2000;117:855. [PMID: 10713016]

Roth AR et al: Approach to the adult patient with fever of unknown origin. Am Fam Physician 2003;68:2223. [PMID: 14677667]

Rusyniak DE et al: Toxin-induced hyperthermic syndromes. Med Clin North Am 2005;89:1277. [PMID: 16227063]

Sipsas NV et al: Perspectives for the management of febrile neutropenic patients with cancer in the 21st century. Cancer 2005;103:1103. [PMID: 15666328]

Vanderschueren S et al: From prolonged febrile illness to fever of unknown origin: the challenge continues. Arch Intern Med 2003;163:1033. [PMID: 12742800]

Watson JT et al: Clinical characteristics and functional outcomes of West Nile Fever. Ann Intern Med 2004;141:360. [PMID: 15353427]

Woolery WA et al: Fever of unknown origin: keys to determining the etiology in older patients. Geriatrics 2004;59:41. [PMID: 15508555]

INVOLUNTARY WEIGHT LOSS

 ESSENTIAL INQUIRIES

- *Age.*
- *Caloric intake.*
- *Fever.*
- *Change in bowel habits.*
- *Secondary confirmation (eg, changes in clothing size).*
- *Substance use.*
- *Age-appropriate cancer screening history.*

General Considerations

Body weight is determined by a person's caloric intake, absorptive capacity, metabolic rate, and energy losses. The metabolic rate can be affected by a multitude of medical conditions through the release of various cytokines such as cachectin and interleukins. Body weight normally peaks by the fifth or sixth decade and then gradually declines at a rate of 1–2 kg per decade. In NHANES II, a national survey of community-dwelling elders (age 50–80 years), recent involuntary weight loss (> 5% usual body weight) was reported by 7% of respondents, and this was associated with a 24% higher mortality.

Clinical Findings

Involuntary weight loss is regarded as clinically significant when it exceeds 5% or more of usual body weight over a 6- to 12-month period and often indicates serious physical or psychological illness. Physical causes are usually evident during the initial evaluation. Cancer (about 30%), gastrointestinal disorders (about 15%), and dementia or depression (about 15%) are the most common causes. When an adequately nourished-appearing patient complains of weight loss, inquiry should be made about exact weight changes (with approximate dates) and about changes in clothing size. Family members can provide confirmation of weight loss, as can old documents such as driver's licenses.

Once the weight loss is established, the history, medication profile, physical examination, and conventional laboratory and radiologic investigations such as complete blood count, serologic tests, thyroid-stimulating hormone (TSH) level, urinalysis, fecal occult blood test, chest radiography, and upper gastrointestinal series usually reveal the cause. When these tests are normal, the second phase of evaluation should focus on more definitive gastrointestinal investigation (eg, tests for malabsorption; endoscopy) and cancer screening (eg, Papanicolaou smear, mammography, prostate specific antigen [PSA]).

If the initial evaluation is unrevealing, follow-up is preferable to further diagnostic testing. Death at 2-year follow-up was not nearly as high in patients with unexplained involuntary weight loss (8%) as in those with weight loss due to malignant (79%) and established nonmalignant diseases (19%). Psychiatric consultation should be considered when there is evidence of depression, dementia, anorexia nervosa, or other emotional problems. Ultimately, in approximately 15–25% of cases, no cause for the weight loss can be found.

A mild, gradual weight loss occurs in some older individuals. It is due to changes in body composition, including loss of height and lean body mass and lower basal metabolic rate, leading to decreased energy requirements. However, rapid unintentional weight loss is predictive of morbidity and mortality in any population. In addition to various disease states, causes in older individuals include loss of teeth and consequent difficulty with chewing, alcoholism, and social isolation.

Differential Diagnosis

Malignancy, gastrointestinal disorders (eg, malabsorption, pancreatic insufficiency), dementia, depression, anorexia nervosa, hyperthyroidism, alcoholism, and social isolation are all established causes.

Treatment

Weight stabilization occurs in most surviving patients with both established and unknown causes of weight loss through treatment of the underlying disorder and caloric supplementation. Nutrient intake goals are established in relation to the severity of weight loss, in general ranging from 30 to 40 kcal/kg/d. In order of preference, route of administration options include oral, temporary nasojejunal tube, or percutaneous gastric or jejunal tube. Parenteral nutrition is reserved for patients with serious associated problems. A variety of pharmacologic agents have been proposed for the treatment of weight loss. These can be categorized into appetite stimulants (corticosteroids, progestational agents, dronabinol, and serotonin antagonists); anabolic agents (growth hormone and testosterone derivatives); and anticatabolic agents (omega-3 fatty acids, pentoxifylline, hydrazine sulfate, and thalidomide).

Alibhai SM et al: An approach to the management of unintentional weight loss in elderly people. CMAJ 2005;172:773. [PMID: 15767612]

Collins N: Protein-energy malnutrition and involuntary weight loss: nutritional and pharmacological strategies to enhance wound healing. Expert Opin Pharmacother 2003; 4:1121. [PMID: 12831338]

Hernandez JL et al: Clinical evaluation for cancer in patients with involuntary weight loss without specific symptoms. Am J Med 2003;114:631. [PMID: 12798450]

Lankisch P et al: Unintentional weight loss: diagnosis and prognosis. The first prospective follow-up study from a secondary referral centre. J Intern Med 2001;249:41. [PMID: 11168783]

Sahyoun NR et al: The epidemiology of recent involuntary weight loss in the United States population. J Nutr Health Aging 2004;8:510. [PMID: 15543425]

FATIGUE & CHRONIC FATIGUE SYNDROME

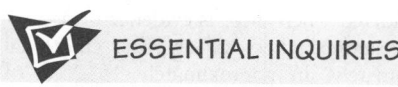

ESSENTIAL INQUIRIES

- *Weight loss.*
- *Fever.*
- *Sleep-disordered breathing.*
- *Medications.*
- *Substance use.*

General Considerations

As an isolated symptom, fatigue accounts for 1–3% of visits to generalists. The symptom of fatigue may be less well defined and explained by patients than symptoms associated with specific functions. Fatigue or lassitude and the closely related complaints of weakness, tiredness, and lethargy are often attributed to overexertion, poor physical conditioning, sleep disturbance, obesity, undernutrition, and emotional problems. A history of the patient's daily living and working habits may obviate the need for extensive and unproductive diagnostic studies.

Clinical Findings

Important diseases that can cause fatigue include hyperthyroidism and hypothyroidism, CHF, infections (endocarditis, hepatitis), COPD, sleep apnea, anemia, autoimmune disorders, and cancer. Alcoholism, drug side effects such as from sedatives and β-blockers, and psychological conditions (such as insomnia, depression, and somatization disorder) are other causes. The lifetime prevalence of significant fatigue (present for at least 2 weeks) is about 25%. Fatigue of unknown cause or related to psychiatric illness exceeds that due to physical illness, injury, medications, drugs, or alcohol. Psychiatric disorders associated with fatigue include depression, dysthymia, somatoform disorders, panic attack, and alcohol abuse. Prolonged fatigue is a central feature of several syndromes, such as irritable bowel syndrome and anxiety (Figure 2–2). Exercise and treatment of anemia are the two most established interventions for cancer-related fatigue. Psychostimulants appear promising based on early studies.

Chronic Fatigue Syndrome

A working case definition of chronic fatigue syndrome indicates that it is not a homogeneous abnormality, and there is no single pathogenic mechanism (Figure 2–3). No physical finding or laboratory test can be used to confirm the diagnosis of this disorder.

With regard to its pathophysiology, early theories postulated an infectious or immune dysregulation mechanism, and it appears that neurologic, affective, and cognitive symptoms also occur frequently. Neuropsychological, neuroendocrine, and brain imaging studies have confirmed the occurrence of neurobiologic abnormalities in most patients. Sleep disorders have been reported in 40–80% of patients with chronic fatigue syndrome, but their treatment has provided only modest benefit, suggesting that it is an effect rather than a cause of the fatigue. MRI scans may show brain abnormalities on T2-weighted images—chiefly small, punctate, subcortical white matter hyperintensities, predominantly in the frontal lobes. Veterans of the Gulf War

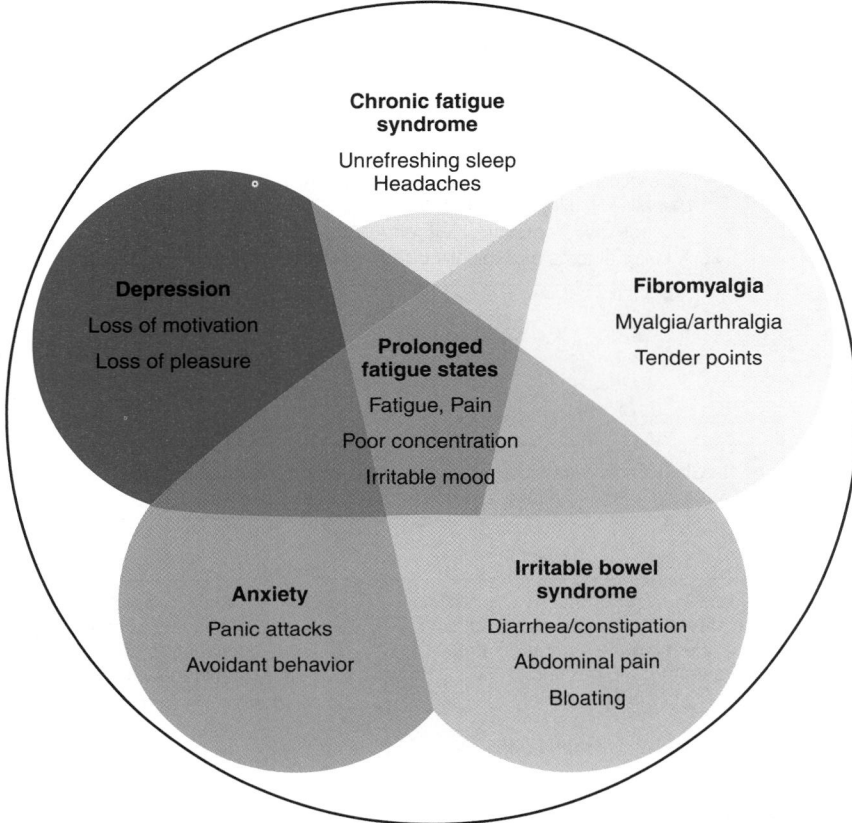

Figure 2–2. Overlapping diagnoses. Prolonged fatigue states are found in fibromyalgia, irritable bowel syndrome, anxiety, and depression as well as chronic fatigue syndrome. (Reproduced, with permission, from Chronic fatigue syndrome. Clinical practice guidelines–2002. Med J Aust 2002;176:S17.)

show a tenfold greater incidence of chronic fatigue syndrome compared with nondeployed military personnel.

In evaluating chronic fatigue, after the history and physical examination process is completed, standard investigation includes complete blood count, erythrocyte sedimentation rate, serum chemistries—blood urea nitrogen (BUN), electrolytes, glucose, creatinine, and calcium; liver and thyroid function tests—antinuclear antibody, urinalysis, and tuberculin skin test; and screening questionnaires for psychiatric disorders. Other tests to be performed as clinically indicated are serum cortisol, rheumatoid factor, immunoglobulin levels, Lyme serology in endemic areas, and tests for HIV antibody. More extensive testing is usually unhelpful, including antibody to Epstein-Barr virus. There may be an abnormally high rate of postural hypotension; some of these patients report response to increases in dietary sodium as well as antihypotensive agents such as fludrocortisone, 0.1 mg/d.

In treatment, a variety of agents and modalities have been tried. Acyclovir, intravenous immunoglobulin, nystatin, and low-dose hydrocortisone/fludro-

cortisone do not improve symptoms. There is a greater prevalence of past and current psychiatric diagnoses in patients with this syndrome. Affective disorders are especially common, but fluoxetine alone, 20 mg daily, is not beneficial. Patients with chronic fatigue syndrome have benefited from a comprehensive multidisciplinary intervention, including optimal medical management, treating any ongoing affective or anxiety disorder pharmacologically, and implementing a comprehensive cognitive-behavioral treatment program. **Cognitive-behavioral therapy,** a form of nonpharmacologic treatment emphasizing self-help and aiming to change perceptions and behaviors that may perpetuate symptoms and disability, is helpful. Although few patients are cured, the treatment effect is substantial. Response to cognitive-behavioral therapy is not predictable on the basis of severity or duration of chronic fatigue syndrome, although patients with low interest in psychotherapy rarely benefit. Graded exercise has also been shown to improve functional work capacity and physical function. At present, intensive individual cognitive-behavioral therapy ad-

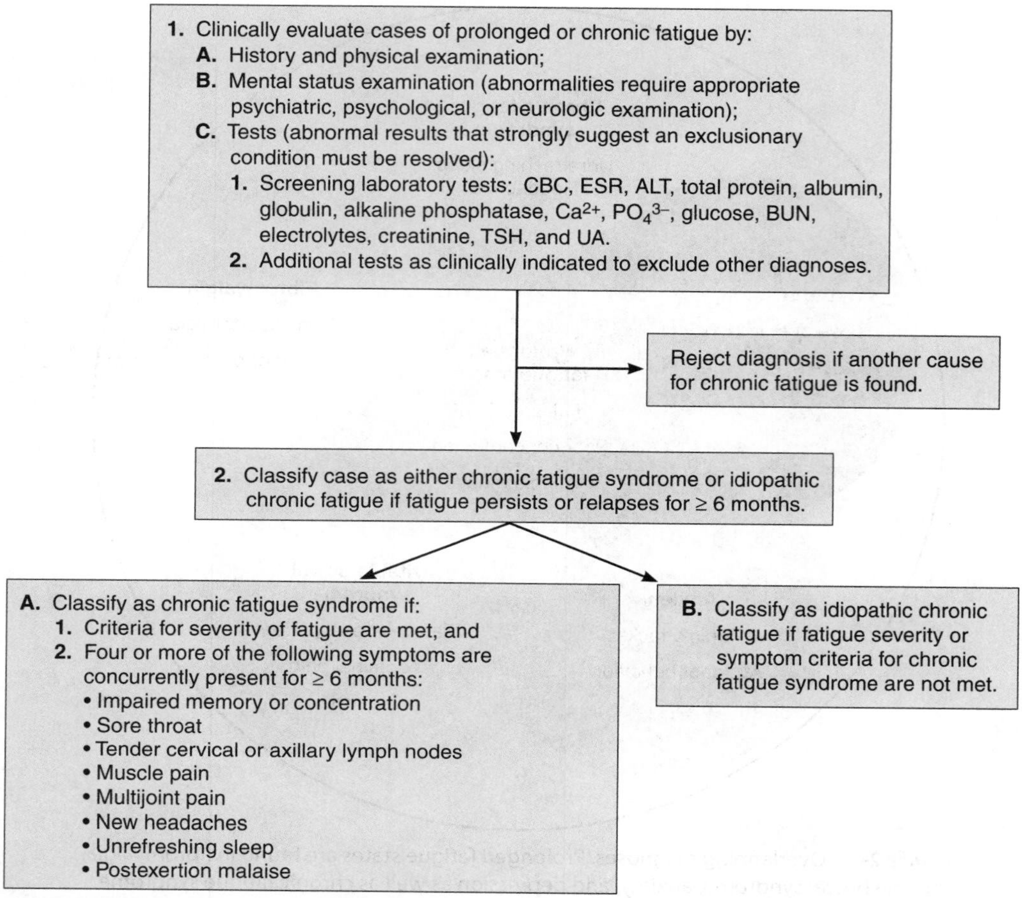

1. Clinically evaluate cases of prolonged or chronic fatigue by:
   A. History and physical examination;
   B. Mental status examination (abnormalities require appropriate psychiatric, psychological, or neurologic examination);
   C. Tests (abnormal results that strongly suggest an exclusionary condition must be resolved):
      1. Screening laboratory tests: CBC, ESR, ALT, total protein, albumin, globulin, alkaline phosphatase, Ca^{2+}, PO_4^{3-}, glucose, BUN, electrolytes, creatinine, TSH, and UA.
      2. Additional tests as clinically indicated to exclude other diagnoses.

Reject diagnosis if another cause for chronic fatigue is found.

2. Classify case as either chronic fatigue syndrome or idiopathic chronic fatigue if fatigue persists or relapses for ≥ 6 months.

A. Classify as chronic fatigue syndrome if:
   1. Criteria for severity of fatigue are met, and
   2. Four or more of the following symptoms are concurrently present for ≥ 6 months:
      • Impaired memory or concentration
      • Sore throat
      • Tender cervical or axillary lymph nodes
      • Muscle pain
      • Multijoint pain
      • New headaches
      • Unrefreshing sleep
      • Postexertion malaise

B. Classify as idiopathic chronic fatigue if fatigue severity or symptom criteria for chronic fatigue syndrome are not met.

Figure 2–3. Evaluation and classification of unexplained chronic fatigue. (CBC, complete blood count; ESR, erythrocyte sedimentation rate; ALT, alanine aminotransferase; Ca^{2+}, calcium; PO_4^{3-}, phosphate; BUN, blood urea nitrogen; TSH, thyroid-stimulating hormone; UA, urinalysis.) (Modified and reproduced, with permission, from Fukuda K et al: The chronic fatigue syndrome: a comprehensive approach to its definition and study. Ann Intern Med 1994;121:953.)

ministered by a skilled therapist and graded exercise are the treatments of choice for patients with chronic fatigue syndrome.

In addition, the clinician's sympathetic listening and explanatory responses can help overcome the patient's frustrations and debilitation by this still mysterious illness. All patients should be encouraged to engage in normal activities to the extent possible and should be reassured that full recovery is eventually possible in most cases.

Chalder T et al: Predictors of outcome in a fatigued population in primary care following a randomized controlled trial. Psychol Med 2003;33:283. [PMID: 12622306]

Chronic fatigue syndrome. Clinical practice guidelines—2002. Med J Aust 2002;176(Suppl):S23. [PMID: 12056987]

Reyes M et al: Prevalence and incidence of chronic fatigue syndrome in Wichita, Kansas. Arch Intern Med 2003;163:1530. [PMID: 12860574]

Sood A et al: Cancer-related fatigue: an update. Curr Oncol Rep 2005;7:277. [PMID: 15946587]

Viner R et al: Fatigue and somatic symptoms. BMJ 2005;330:1012. [PMID: 15860829]

Whiting P et al: Interventions for the treatment and management of chronic fatigue syndrome: a systematic review. JAMA 2001;286:1360. [PMID: 11560542]

ACUTE HEADACHE

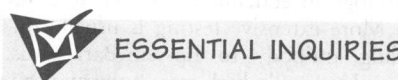 ESSENTIAL INQUIRIES

- *Age > 50 years.*
- *Rapid onset and severe intensity.*
- *Fever.*
- *Trauma.*
- *Vision changes.*

- *Past medical history of hypertension or HIV infection.*
- *Hypertension.*
- *Neurologic findings (mental status changes, motor or sensory deficits).*

General Considerations

Headache is a common reason that adults seek medical care, accounting for approximately 13 million visits each year in the United States to physicians' offices, urgent care clinics, and emergency departments. A broad range of disorders can lead to headache. This chapter will deal only with the approach to a new acute headache—not due to trauma—in adolescents and adults. The challenge in the initial evaluation of acute headache is to identify those conditions that are life-threatening. In the emergency department setting, approximately 1% of patients seeking medical attention for acute headache will have a life-threatening condition, whereas the prevalence of life-threatening conditions in the office practice setting is considerably lower.

Regardless of the underlying cause, headache is currently believed to occur as a result of the release of neuropeptides from trigeminal nerve endings that encapsulate the blood vessels of the pia mater and dura mater, resulting in neurogenic inflammation. Because this represents a final common pathway, diminution of headache in response to typical migraine therapies (such as serotonin receptor antagonists or ketorolac tromethamine) does not rule out critical conditions such as subarachnoid hemorrhage or meningitis as the underlying cause.

Clinical Findings

A careful history and physical examination should be aimed at identifying causes of acute headache that require immediate treatment. These causes can be broadly classified as imminent or completed **vascular events** (intracranial hemorrhage, thrombosis, vasculitis, malignant hypertension, arterial dissection, or aneurysm), **infections** (abscess, encephalitis, meningitis), **intracranial masses** causing intracranial hypertension, **preeclampsia,** and **carbon monoxide poisoning**. The natural history of the onset of headache can be helpful. Report of a sudden-onset headache that reaches maximal and severe intensity within seconds or a few minutes is the classic description of a "thunderclap headache" and should precipitate workup for subarachnoid hemorrhage. A new headache in a patient of advanced age or with a history of HIV disease under most circumstances (including a normal neurologic examination) warrants neuroimaging immediately (Table 2–6). When the patient has a medical history of hypertension—particularly uncontrolled hypertension—a complete search for criteria satisfying a diagnosis of "malig-

Table 2–6. Clinical features associated with acute headache that warrant urgent or emergent neuroimaging.

Prior to lumbar puncture
Abnormal neurologic examination
Abnormal mental status
Abnormal funduscopic examination (papilledema; loss of venous pulsations)
Meningeal signs
Emergent (conduct prior to leaving office or emergency department)
Abnormal neurologic examination
Abnormal mental status
Thunderclap headache
Urgent (scheduled prior to leaving office or emergency department)
HIV-positive patient[1]
Age > 50 years (normal neurologic examination)

[1]Use CT with or without contrast or MRI if HIV positive.
Adapted from American College of Emergency Physicians. Clinical Policy: critical issues in the evaluation and management of patients presenting to the emergency department with acute headache. Ann Emerg Med 2002;39:108.

nant hypertension" is appropriate to determine the correct urgency level of hypertension management (see Chapter 11). Headache and hypertension associated with pregnancy may be due to preeclampsia. Episodic headache associated with the triad of hypertension, heart palpitations, and sweats should suggest the possibility of pheochromocytoma. In the absence of thunderclap headache, advanced age, and HIV disease, findings on physical examination will usually determine the time course and need for further diagnostic testing.

Critical components of the physical examination of the patient with acute headache include vital sign measurements, neurologic examination, and vision testing with funduscopic examination. The finding of fever with acute headache should suggest additional maneuvers to elicit evidence of meningeal inflammation, such as Kernig and Brudzinski signs. Besides malignant hypertension, significant hypertension can also be a sign of intracranial hemorrhage, preeclampsia, and pheochromocytoma. Patients over 60 years of age should be examined for scalp or temporal artery tenderness.

Careful assessment of visual acuity, ocular gaze, visual fields, pupillary defects, the optic disk, and retinal vein pulsations is crucial. Diminished visual acuity is suggestive of glaucoma, temporal arteritis, or optic neuritis. Ophthalmoplegia or visual field defects may be signs of venous sinus thrombosis, tumor, or aneurysm. Afferent pupillary defects can be due to intracranial masses or optic neuritis. Ipsilateral ptosis and miosis suggest Horner's syndrome and in conjunction with acute headache may signify carotid artery dissection. Finally, papilledema or absent retinal venous pulsations are signs of elevated intracranial pressure—findings that should be followed by neuroimaging prior to performing lumbar puncture (Table 2–6).

Mental status and complete neurologic evaluations are also critical and should include assessment of motor and sensory systems, reflexes, gait, cerebellar function, and pronator drift. Any abnormality on mental status or neurologic evaluation warrants emergent neuroimaging (Table 2–6).

Diagnostic Studies

Under most circumstances, a noncontrast head CT is sufficient to exclude intracranial hypertension with impending herniation, intracranial hemorrhage, and many types of intracranial masses (notable exceptions include lymphoma and toxoplasmosis in HIV-positive patients, herpes simplex encephalitis, and brain abscess). When appropriate, a contrast study can often be ordered to follow a normal noncontrast study. A normal neuroimaging study does not sufficiently exclude subarachnoid hemorrhage and should be followed by lumbar puncture. In patients for whom there is a high level of suspicion for subarachnoid hemorrhage or aneurysm, a normal CT and lumbar puncture should be followed by angiography within the next few days (provided the patient is medically stable). Lumbar puncture is also indicated to exclude infectious causes of acute headache, particularly in patients with fever or meningeal signs. Cerebrospinal fluid tests should routinely include Gram stain, white blood cell count with differential, red blood cell count, glucose, total protein, and bacterial culture. In appropriate patients, also consider testing cerebrospinal fluid for VDRL (syphilis), cryptococcal antigen (HIV-positive patients), acid-fast bacillus stain and culture, and complement fixation and culture for coccidioidomycosis. Storage of an extra tube with 5 mL of cerebrospinal fluid is also prudent for conducting unanticipated tests in the immediate future. Consultation with infectious disease experts regarding local availability of newer polymerase chain reaction tests for specific infectious pathogens (eg, herpes simplex 2) should also be considered in patients with evidence of central nervous system infection but no identifiable pathogen.

In addition to neuroimaging and lumbar puncture, additional diagnostic tests for exclusion of life-threatening causes of acute headache include erythrocyte sedimentation rate (temporal arteritis; endocarditis), urinalysis (malignant hypertension; preeclampsia), and sinus CT or x-ray (bacterial sinusitis, independently or as a cause of venous sinus thrombosis).

Treatment

Treatment should be based on determination of the cause of acute headache.

Beck E et al: Management of cluster headache. Am Fam Physician 2005;71:717. [PMID: 15742909]

Colman I et al: Parenteral dihydroergotamine for acute migraine headache: a systematic review of the literature. Ann Emerg Med 2005;45:393. [PMID: 15795718]

Evans RW: New daily persistent headache. Curr Pain Headache Rep 2003;7:303. [PMID: 12828880]

Ryan RE: Common headache misdiagnoses. Prim Care 2004;31:395. [PMID: 15172514]

Silberstein SD: Migraine. Lancet 2004;363:381. [PMID: 15070571]

van de Beek D et al: Clinical features and prognostic factors in adults with bacterial meningitis. N Engl J Med 2004;351:1849. [PMID: 15509818]

DYSURIA

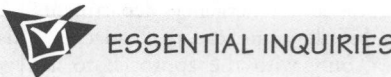

ESSENTIAL INQUIRIES

- *Fever.*
- *Nausea/Vomiting.*
- *New back or flank pain.*
- *Vaginal discharge.*
- *Pregnancy risk.*
- *Structural abnormalities.*
- *Instrumentation of urethra or bladder.*

General Considerations

Dysuria (painful urination) is a common reason for adolescents and adults to seek urgent medical attention. An inflammatory process (eg, infection; autoimmune disorder) underlies most causes of dysuria. In women, cystitis will be diagnosed in up to 50–60% of cases and has an incidence of 0.5–0.7% per year in sexually active young women. The key objective in evaluating women with dysuria is to exclude serious upper urinary tract disease, such as acute pyelonephritis, and sexually transmitted diseases. In contrast, in men, urethritis accounts for the vast majority of cases of dysuria.

Clinical Findings

A. Symptoms

Well-designed cohort studies have shown that some women can be reliably diagnosed with uncomplicated cystitis without a physical examination or urinalysis, and randomized controlled trials show that telephone management of uncomplicated cystitis is safe and effective. An increased likelihood of cystitis is present when women report multiple irritative voiding symptoms (dysuria, urgency, frequency), fever, or back pain (likelihood ratios = 1.6–2.0). Inquiring about symptoms of vulvovaginitis is important, since the presence of vaginal discharge or itching substantially decreases the likelihood of cystitis (likelihood ratios = 0.2–0.3). When women report dysuria and urinary frequency, and deny vaginal discharge and irritation, the likeli-

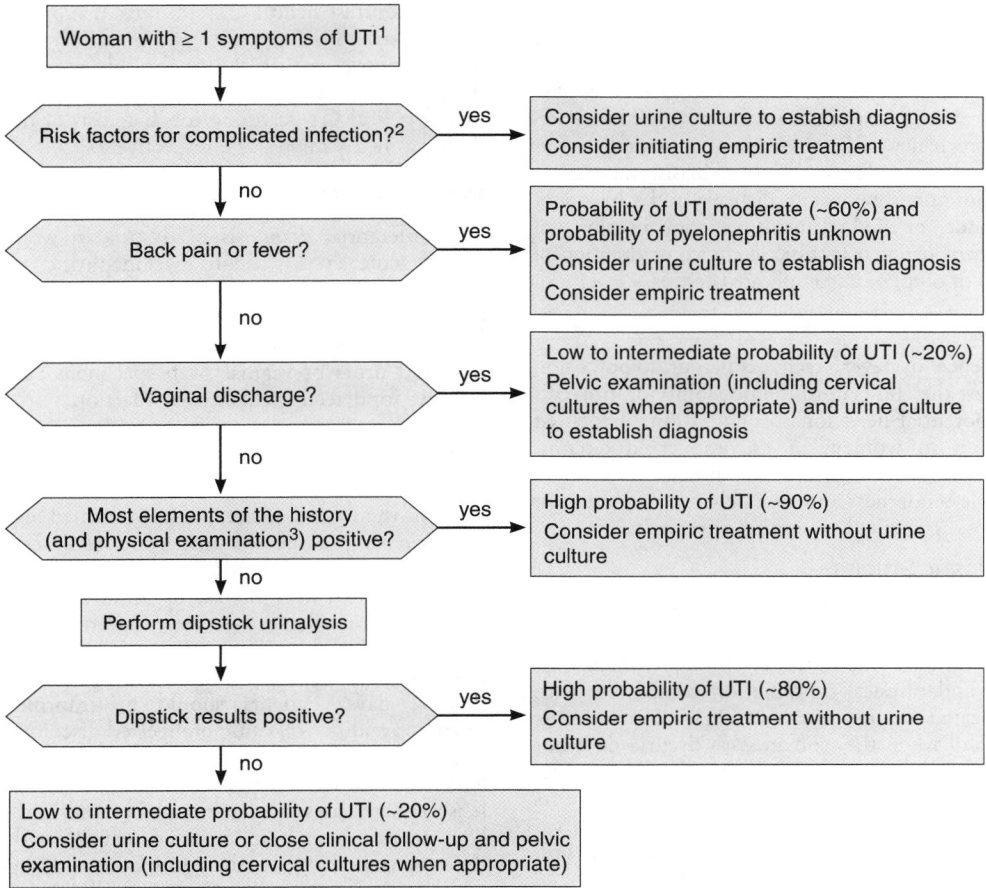

Figure 2–4. Proposed algorithm for evaluating women with symptoms of acute urinary tract infection (UTI). (Modified and reproduced, with permission, from Bent S et al: Does this woman have an acute uncomplicated urinary tract infection? JAMA 2002;297:2701.)

[1]In women who have risk factors for sexually transmitted diseases, consider testing for chlamydia. The US Preventive Services Task Force recommends screening for chlamydia for all women 25 years or younger and women of any age with more than one sexual partner, a history of sexually transmitted disease, or inconsistent use of condoms.

[2]A complicated UTI is one in an individual with a functional or anatomic abnormality of the urinary tract, including a history of polycystic renal disease, nephrolithiasis, neurogenic bladder, diabetes mellitus, immunosuppression, pregnancy, indwelling urinary catheter, or recent urinary tract instrumentation.

[3]The only physical examination finding that increases the likelihood of UTI is costovertebral angle tenderness, and clinicians may consider not performing this test in patients with typical symptoms of acute uncomplicated UTI (as in telephone management).

hood ratio for culture-confirmed cystitis is 24.5. In contrast, when vaginal discharge or irritation is present, as well as dysuria or urinary frequency, the likelihood ratio is 0.7. Gross hematuria in women with voiding symptoms usually represents hemorrhagic cystitis, but can also be a sign of bladder cancer (particularly in older patients) or upper tract disease. Failure of hematuria to resolve with antibiotic treatment should prompt further evaluation of the bladder and kidneys. Finally, chlamydial infection should be

strongly considered among women age 25 years or younger who are sexually active and who are seeking medical attention for a suspected urinary tract infection for the first time.

Because fever and back pain, as well as nausea and vomiting, are considered harbingers of (or clinical criteria for) acute pyelonephritis, women with these symptoms should usually be examined by a clinician prior to treatment in order to exclude coexistent urosepsis, hydronephrosis, or nephrolithiasis. Other major risk factors for acute pyelonephritis (among women 18–49 years of age) relate to sexual behaviors (frequency of sexual intercourse three or more times per week, new sexual partner in previous year, recent spermicide use), as well as diabetes mellitus and recent urinary tract infection or incontinence. Finally, pregnancy risk, underlying structural factors (polycystic kidney disease, nephrolithiasis, neurogenic bladder), immunosuppression, diabetes, and a history of recent bladder or urethral instrumentation usually alter the treatment regimen (antibiotic choice or duration of treatment, or both) of uncomplicated cystitis.

B. Physical Examination

The presence of fever, tachycardia, or hypotension should alert the clinician to the possibility of urosepsis and the potential need for hospitalization. A focused examination in women, in uncomplicated circumstances, could be limited to ascertainment of costovertebral angle tenderness and to a pelvic examination, if the history suggests vulvovaginitis or cervicitis.

C. Diagnostic Studies

1. Urinalysis—Urinalysis is probably overutilized in the evaluation of dysuria. The probability of culture-confirmed urinary tract infection among women with a history and physical examination compatible with uncomplicated cystitis is about 90%. Urinalysis is most helpful when the woman with dysuria does not have other typical features of cystitis. Dipstick detection (> trace) of leukocytes, nitrites, or blood supports a diagnosis of cystitis. When both leukocyte and nitrite tests are positive, the likelihood ratio is 4.2, and when both are negative, the likelihood ratio is 0.3.

2. Urine culture—Urine culture should be considered for all women with upper tract symptoms (prior to initiating antibiotic therapy), as well as those with dysuria and a negative urine dipstick test. In symptomatic women, a clean-catch urine culture is considered positive when 10^2–10^3 colony-forming units/mL of a uropathogenic organism is detected.

3. Renal imaging—When severe flank or back pain is present, the possibility of complicated kidney infection (perinephric abscess, nephrolithiasis) or of hydronephrosis should be considered. Depending on local availability, acceptable imaging options to assess for hydronephrosis include abdominal radiographs, renal ultrasound, or CT scanning. To exclude nephrolithiasis, noncontrast helical CT scanning is more accurate than intravenous urography and is rapidly becoming the diagnostic test of choice for this purpose. In a meta-analysis, the positive and negative likelihood ratios of helical CT scanning for diagnosis of nephrolithiasis were 23.2 and 0.05, respectively.

D. Differential Diagnosis

The differential diagnosis of dysuria in women includes acute cystitis, acute pyelonephritis, vaginitis (*Candida*, bacterial vaginosis, *Trichomonas*, herpes simplex), urethritis/cervicitis (*Chlamydia*, gonorrhea), and interstitial cystitis. Nucleic acid amplification tests from first-void urine or vaginal swab specimens are highly sensitive for detecting chlamydial infection.

E. Treatment

Definitive treatment is directed to the underlying cause of the dysuria. An evidence-informed algorithm for managing suspected urinary tract infection in women is shown in Figure 2–4. Symptomatic relief can be provided with phenazopyridine, a urinary analgesic that is available over-the-counter; it is used in combination with antibiotic therapy (when a urinary tract infection has been confirmed) but for no more than 2 days. Patients should be informed that phenazopyridine will cause orange/red discoloration of their urine and other bodily fluids (eg, some contact lens wearers have reported discoloration of their lenses). Rare cases of methemoglobinemia and hemolytic anemia have been reported, usually with overdoses or underlying renal dysfunction. Although current convention is to consider noninfectious causes of dysuria in women with negative urine dipstick tests, a recent randomized trial showed more rapid symptom resolution associated with antibiotic therapy.

Bent S et al: Does this woman have an acute uncomplicated urinary tract infection? JAMA 2002;287:2701. [PMID: 12020306]

Fihn S: Acute uncomplicated urinary tract infection in women. N Engl J Med 2003;349:259. [PMID: 12867610]

Richards D et al: Response to antibiotics of women with symptoms of urinary tract infection but negative dipstick urine test results: double blind randomised controlled trial. BMJ 2005;331:143. [PMID: 15972728]

Sholes D et al: Risk factors associated with acute pyelonephritis in healthy women. Ann Intern Med 2005;142:20. [PMID: 15630106]

Preoperative Evaluation & Perioperative Management

3

Joshua S. Adler, MD, & Lee Goldman, MD, MPH

Each year, tens of millions of patients in the United States undergo a surgical procedure requiring general or spinal-epidural anesthesia. A disproportionate and increasing number of these patients are over age 65. Recent estimates suggest that 15–23% of Americans over the age of 65 undergo surgery in any given year. Operative mortality has declined over the past 10–20 years, probably because of improvements in surgical, anesthetic, and monitoring techniques. Furthermore, most patients do not suffer significant morbidity as a result of the surgical procedure or the anesthetic. The rate of major complications varies from less than 1% to nearly 20% depending on the patient's age, the presence of underlying disease, and the type of surgery. Postoperative complications have significant impact. In patients over 70 years of age, the occurrence of a postoperative complication is associated with decreased long-term functional status and survival. Cardiac, pulmonary, infectious, and neurologic complications account for most of the perioperative morbidity and mortality.

The role of the medical consultant includes evaluating the severity and stability of the patient's medical conditions and providing a surgical risk assessment. The consultant's most important contribution, however, is recommending perioperative measures to reduce surgical risk.

Centers for Disease Control and Prevention National Center for Health Statistics: www.cdc.gov/nchs

Fleischmann KE et al: Association between cardiac and noncardiac complications in patients undergoing noncardiac surgery; outcomes and effects on length of stay. Am J Med 2003;115:515. [PMID: 14599629]

Lawrence VA et al: Functional independence after major abdominal surgery in the elderly. J Am Coll Surg 2004; 199:762. [PMID: 15501119]

Manku K et al: Prognostic significance of postoperative in-hospital complications in elderly patients. I. Long-term survival. Anesth Analg 2003;96:583. [PMID: 12538216]

PHYSIOLOGIC EFFECTS OF ANESTHESIA & SURGERY

Both general and spinal or epidural anesthetic agents usually cause peripheral vasodilation, and most of the commonly used general anesthetic regimens also decrease myocardial contractility. These effects often result in transient mild hypotension or, less frequently, prolonged or more severe hypotension. The decrease in tidal volume caused by general and spinal-epidural anesthesia can close small airways and lead to atelectasis. Epinephrine, norepinephrine, and cortisol levels increase during surgery and remain elevated for 1–3 days. Serum antidiuretic hormone levels may be elevated for up to 1 week postoperatively. There is mounting evidence that anesthesia and surgery may be associated with a relative hypercoagulable and inflammatory state mediated by increases in plasminogen activator-1, factor VIII, and platelet reactivity, and increased levels of tumor necrosis factor, interleukins 1 and 6, and C-reactive protein. These effects may be less evident with spinal or epidural anesthesia compared with general anesthesia. The degree to which these hypercoagulable or inflammatory states contribute to perioperative morbidity is not known.

There is no definitive evidence that spinal or epidural anesthesia is preferable to general anesthesia in terms of overall surgical outcomes in large clinical trials. However, subgroup analyses in patients undergoing thoracic, abdominal, and vascular surgery have consistently demonstrated superior analgesia in the spinal/epidural group and a reduction in specific adverse outcomes (cardiac, pulmonary, or neurologic). Similarly, routine use of invasive hemodynamic monitoring with pulmonary artery catheters does not improve surgical outcomes. There are now two randomized trials that have shown a reduction in postoperative cardiac outcomes through the maintenance of normothermia during the perioperative period. In general, the choice of anesthetic technique or agent, the decision to use invasive hemodynamic monitoring, and the regulation of body temperature should be left to the anesthesiologist.

Harvey S et al: Assessment of the clinical effectiveness of pulmonary artery catheters in management of patients in intensive care (PAC-Man): a randomised controlled trial. Lancet 2005;366:472. [PMID: 16084255]

Sandham JD et al: A randomized controlled trial of pulmonary artery catheters in high risk surgical patients. N Engl J Med 2003;348:5. [PMID: 12510037]

EVALUATION OF THE ASYMPTOMATIC PATIENT

Patients without significant medical problems—especially those under age 50—are at very low risk for perioperative complications. The preoperative evaluation of these patients should include a complete history and physical examination. Special emphasis is placed on the assessment of functional status, exercise tolerance, and cardiopulmonary symptoms and signs in an effort to reveal previously unrecognized disease (especially cardiopulmonary disease) that may require further evaluation prior to surgery. In addition, a directed bleeding history (Table 3–1) should be taken to uncover disorders of hemostasis that could contribute to excessive surgical blood loss. Routine preoperative testing of asymptomatic healthy patients under age 50 has not been found to predict risk or to aid in reducing adverse perioperative outcomes.

Patients who are older than 50 years and those with risk factors for coronary artery disease should have a 12-lead ECG because evidence of clinically silent coronary artery disease should prompt further cardiac evaluation. Minor ECG abnormalities such as bundle branch block, T wave changes, and premature ventricular contractions do not predict adverse postoperative outcomes.

Garcia-Miguel FJ et al: Preoperative assessment. Lancet 2003; 362:1749. [PMID: 14643127]

Liu LL et al: Preoperative electrocardiogram abnormalities do not predict postoperative cardiac complications in geriatric surgical patients. J Am Geriatr Soc 2002;50:1186. [PMID: 12133011]

CARDIAC RISK ASSESSMENT

The cardiac complications of noncardiac surgery are a major cause of perioperative morbidity and mortality. The most important perioperative cardiac complications are myocardial infarction (MI), congestive heart failure (CHF), and cardiac death. Older age, preexisting coronary artery disease, and CHF are the principal risk factors for development of these complications.

Major abdominal, thoracic, and vascular surgical procedures (especially abdominal aortic aneurysm repair) tend to carry a higher risk of postoperative cardiac complications than other procedures. Emergency

Table 3–1. Factors suggestive of a bleeding disorder.

Unprovoked bruising on the trunk of > 5 cm in diameter
Frequent unprovoked epistaxis or gingival bleeding
Menorrhagia with iron deficiency
Hemarthrosis with mild trauma
Prior excessive surgical blood loss or reoperation for bleeding
Family history of abnormal bleeding
Presence of severe kidney or liver disease

Table 3–2. Characteristics defining patients with known or suspected coronary artery disease.

1. History of myocardial infarction
2. Angiographic evidence of coronary artery disease
3. Evidence of ischemia on prior noninvasive testing
4. Typical angina pectoris
5. Peripheral vascular disease

Adapted, with permission, from Ashton CM et al: The incidence of perioperative myocardial infarction in men undergoing noncardiac surgery. Ann Intern Med 1993;118:504.

operations are generally associated with more cardiac complications than elective operations. These high-risk procedures are more often associated with major fluid shifts, hemorrhage, and hypoxemia, which may predispose to cardiac complications.

Coronary Artery Disease

Prior to the routine use of preoperative prophylactic β-blocking agents and the widespread use of less invasive surgical techniques, there were approximately 50,000 perioperative MIs annually. Current rates of perioperative MI are likely to be lower. Patients without coronary artery disease are at extremely low risk (< 0.5%) for perioperative ischemic cardiac complications. Patients with known or suspected coronary artery disease, as defined in Table 3–2, have a threefold to 25-fold increased risk of cardiac complications.

The estimated risk of cardiac complications in patients with coronary artery disease can be refined through an assessment of the severity of anginal symptoms, the use of multifactorial indices, and the judicious use of noninvasive tests for ischemia. The severity of anginal symptoms is most accurately assessed using a standardized scale such as that shown in Table 3–3. Multifactorial indices combine several clinical parameters to estimate an overall risk of cardiac complications. The Revised Cardiac Risk Index (RCRI), presented in Table 3–4, is the most recently developed and has been validated in several subsequent studies.

Preoperative Noninvasive Ischemia Testing

Noninvasive tests for myocardial ischemia such as exercise treadmill testing, dipyridamole-thallium scintigraphy, and dobutamine stress echocardiography have been shown to improve upon the clinical risk assessment and help optimize perioperative management in selected patients. Most patients can be accurately stratified through an assessment of anginal symptoms and use of a multifactorial index. Patients who have mild symptoms, defined as Canadian Cardiovascular Society (CCS) class I or II angina, and a low or intermediate multifactorial index score are at low risk for cardiac complications. Noninvasive testing in these patients is

Table 3–3. Canadian Cardiovascular Society angina class.

I. Ordinary physical activity, such as walking and climbing stairs, does not cause angina. Angina occurs with strenuous or rapid or prolonged exertion at work or recreation.

II. Slight limitation of ordinary activity. Angina occurs with walking or climbing stairs rapidly, walking uphill, walking or stair climbing after meals, or only during the few hours after awakening. Angina occurs when walking more than two blocks on the level or climbing more than one flight of stairs at a normal pace and in normal conditions.

III. Marked limitation of ordinary physical activity. Angina occurs with walking one to two blocks on the level and climbing one flight of stairs in normal conditions and at a normal pace.

IV. Inability to carry on any physical activity without discomfort; angina may be present at rest.

Reproduced, with permission, from Campeau L: Grading of angina pectoris (Letter). Circulation 1975;54:522.

generally unnecessary. Patients with severe symptoms, CCS class III or IV angina, or a high multifactorial index score are likely to be at high risk for cardiac complications. Stress echocardiography in this group of patients may be able to identify a low-risk subgroup. In the case of high-clinical-risk vascular surgery patients, the absence of a regional wall motion abnormality on stress echocardiography predicts a low risk of perioperative cardiac death or MI.

Noninvasive cardiac testing may also be useful in patients with known or suspected coronary artery disease and an unknown functional status. In patients who are able to walk, jog, or use a supine bicycle, the absence of ischemia at or above 85% of their maximal predicted heart rate on exercise ECG predicts a low risk for perioperative cardiac complications.

In patients who cannot exercise, a normal dipyridamole-thallium scan or stress echocardiogram predicts a low risk of complications (comparable to that of pa-

tients with a low-risk clinical assessment), whereas evidence of thallium redistribution—or stress-induced echocardiographic wall motion abnormalities—predicts a much higher risk (comparable to that of patients with a high-risk clinical assessment).

Of note—in patients with known coronary artery disease who cannot exercise but have other clinical indicators predicting a high risk of cardiac complications (such as a high multifactorial index score), dobutamine stress echocardiography is the preferred noninvasive test.

Any patient who is considered a candidate for noninvasive ischemia testing independent of the planned noncardiac surgery should generally have such testing prior to surgery if the test result may lead to coronary revascularization. This is particularly true for patients found to be at high risk on clinical assessment.

Left ventricular systolic dysfunction, moderate or severe left ventricular hypertrophy, and a peak aortic gradient greater than 40 mm Hg on resting echocardiography are associated with an increased risk of cardiac complications in selected patients. Resting echocardiography and radionuclide ventriculography, however, are not recommended for routine perioperative risk assessment.

Preoperative Management of Patients with Coronary Artery Disease

Patients with stable coronary disease have a 1–5% risk of MI and about a 1% mortality rate whereas patients with unstable symptoms or signs are at much higher risk. An approach to the assessment and management of patients with known or suspected coronary artery disease is shown in Figure 3–1.

A. MEDICATIONS

Preoperative antianginal medications, including β-blockers, calcium channel blockers, and nitrates, should be continued preoperatively and during the postoperative period. There have been several clinical trials demonstrating a reduction in perioperative cardiac morbidity with prophylactic β-blocking agents. Atenolol, metoprolol,

Table 3–4. Revised cardiac risk index (RCRI).

Independent Predictors of Postoperative Cardiac Complications	Scoring (Number of Predictors Present)	Risk of Major Cardiac Complications[1]
1. Intrathoracic, intraperitoneal, or infrainguinal vascular surgery		
2. History of ischemic heart disease	None	0.4%
3. History of congestive heart failure	One	0.9%
4. Insulin treatment for diabetes mellitus	Two	7.0%
5. Serum creatinine level > 2 mg/dL	More than two	11%
6. History of cerebrovascular disease		

[1]Myocardial infarction, pulmonary edema, ventricular fibrillation, cardiac arrest, and complete heart block.
Adapted from Lee TH et al: Derivation and prospective validation of a simple index for prediction of cardiac risk of major noncardiac surgery. Circulation 1999;100:1043.

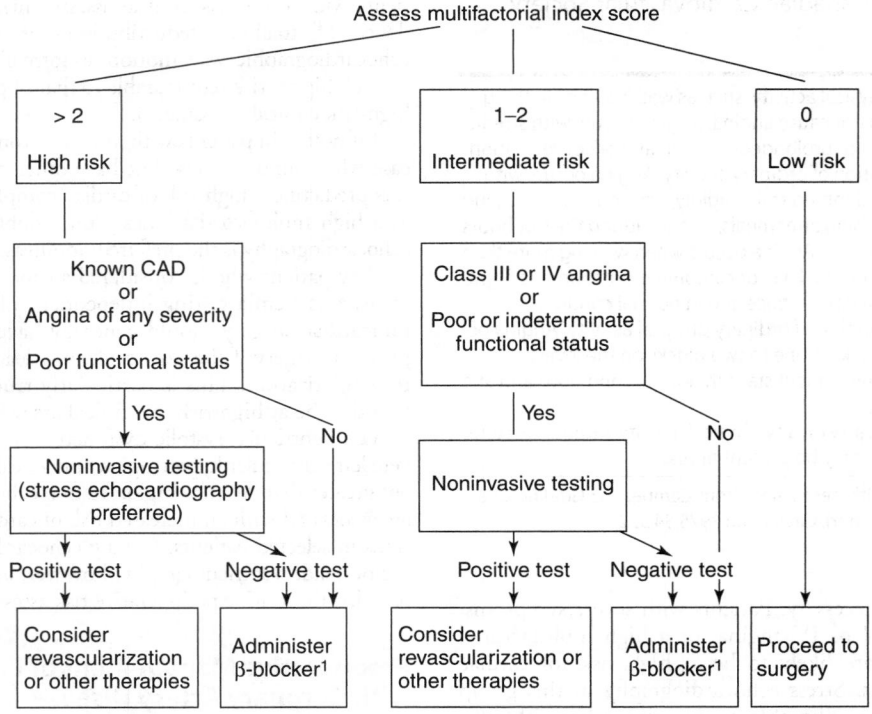

Assess multifactorial index score

| > 2
High risk | 1–2
Intermediate risk | 0
Low risk |

High risk: Known CAD or Angina of any severity or Poor functional status — Yes → Noninvasive testing (stress echocardiography preferred) → Positive test → Consider revascularization or other therapies; Negative test → Administer β-blocker[1]; No → Administer β-blocker[1]

Intermediate risk: Class III or IV angina or Poor or indeterminate functional status — Yes → Noninvasive testing → Positive test → Consider revascularization or other therapies; Negative test → Administer β-blocker[1]; No → Proceed to surgery

Low risk: Proceed to surgery

[1]Administer α-agonist if β-blockers are contraindicated. Consider using a statin medication for vascular surgery.

Figure 3–1. Assessment and management of patients with known or suspected coronary artery disease (CAD) undergoing major noncardiac surgery.

and bisoprolol have been the most frequently studied agents. Comparative trials are lacking, and these drugs are currently believed to be equally effective. The optimal dosing schedules have not been determined. Suggested regimens based on the available clinical trials are presented in Table 3–5. It is thought that heart rate control is one mechanism by which β-blockers reduce cardiac morbidity. The β-blocker dosage and route of administration should be adjusted to maintain a heart rate of 50–60 beats per minute. The patients most likely to benefit have two or more RCRI criteria.

A meta-analysis of six randomized trials that studied the use of prophylactic α_2-agonists (clonidine or mivazerol) showed that perioperative cardiac mortality was reduced. The effect was statistically significant only in vascular surgery patients. In the most recent trial, patients were randomized to receive clonidine (0.2 mg/d orally or via transdermal patch) or placebo for 4 days beginning the night before a variety of noncardiac procedures. There were no statistically significant differences in the groups during the original hospitalization. However, the 2-year mortality in the clonidine group was 15%, compared with 29% in the placebo group. Based on these data, an α_2-agonist should be considered in patients undergoing vascular surgery who are unable to take β-blocking agents. Suggested dosing for these agents is shown in Table 3–5.

Data from four retrospective studies showed an association between the use of statin medications during the perioperative period and lower rates of nonfatal MI and cardiac death. In the only published randomized trial, patients received either atorvastatin (20 mg/d) or placebo for 45 days, beginning at least 2 weeks before vascular surgery. At 6 months, the combined endpoint of nonfatal MI or cardiac death occurred in 8% of the atorvastatin group and 26% of the placebo group. Although there are insufficient data to make a general recommendation regarding the use of prophylactic statin medications, it seems reasonable to use them in vascular surgery patients.

Prophylactic intraoperative intravenous nitroglycerin may decrease the frequency of ischemia but has not been shown to reduce the rate of postoperative complications. This medication may be considered for high-risk patients. Too little is known about the effects of the prophylactic use of calcium channel blockers to make any recommendations.

B. Coronary Revascularization

The potential value of preoperative coronary revascularization in high-risk coronary artery disease patients has been a controversial issue. Studies of registries of patients who had previously undergone revasculariza-

Table 3–5. Preoperative prophylactic cardioprotective medications.

	Dosage	Timing
β-Blocking Agents		
Atenolol	50–100 mg orally daily or 5–10 mg intravenously every 12 hours	Start 3–30 days before surgery and continue for 3–7 days after surgery
Metoprolol	50–100 mg orally twice daily	Start 3–30 days before surgery and continue for 3–7 days after surgery
Bisoprolol	5–10 mg orally daily	Start 1–4 weeks before surgery and continue for 7 days after surgery
α₂-Agonists		
Clonidine	0.2–0.3 mg orally daily or transdermally, or 2–5 mcg/kg/d intravenously	Begin 90 min before surgery and continue for 3–4 days after surgery
Mivazerol	IV: 2–4 mcg/kg as a bolus, then 1.5 mcg/kg/h PO: 5–10 mg daily	IV: Begin 90 min before surgery and continue for 72 hours after surgery PO: Start 3–30 days before surgery and continue for 3–7 days after surgery
HMG CoA Reductase Inhibitors (Statins)		
Atorvastatin	PO: 20 mg daily	Start 2–4 weeks before surgery and continue for a total of 45 days

tion with coronary artery bypass grafting (CABG) surgery or percutaneous coronary interventions (PCI) have shown that such patients may undergo subsequent noncardiac surgery with a relatively low risk of cardiac morbidity and mortality. However, the use of intracoronary stents in the immediate preoperative period actually may increase the risk of perioperative cardiac complications. When the interval between intracoronary stenting and noncardiac surgery is less than 6 weeks, perioperative mortality is significantly higher than that observed when the interval is more than 6 weeks. The presumed mechanism of this increased mortality is acute stent thrombosis that results from discontinuation of anticoagulant therapy before the standard 4–6 week period. Therefore, it is prudent to delay elective surgery for at least 6 weeks after intracoronary stenting. However, these data do not support a strategy of prophylactic coronary revascularization, especially since the mortality rate for CABG surgery is roughly 1.5% and that for percutaneous transluminal coronary angioplasty (PTCA) ranges from 0.5% to 1.5%. For example, a recent trial randomized over 500 patients with definitive coronary artery disease on angiography to two groups: preoperative prophylactic revascularization with either CABG or PCI and no revascularization before vascular surgery. Postoperative nonfatal MI, 30-day mortality, and mortality at 2.7 years were similar in the two groups, suggesting that truly prophylactic revascularization before noncardiac surgery does not reduce the risk of cardiac complications. However, it seems prudent that patients who are candidates for coronary revascularization independent of the planned surgery undergo the revascularization before the elective noncardiac surgery.

C. PATIENTS WITH UNSTABLE CORONARY ARTERY DISEASE

Surgery should be postponed in this group of patients, except in emergency situations, to allow for stabilization of ischemic symptoms. For patients with a recent MI and evidence of ongoing ischemia, delaying surgery allows for appropriate stabilization, and therapy may significantly reduce perioperative mortality and morbidity rates. Patients with unstable angina should be evaluated and treated as indicated by their cardiac status prior to surgery and then reevaluated with respect to severity of symptoms and functional status. Patients with severe stable angina or worsening angina may be managed in a variety of ways. Like patients with less severe angina, those who are potential candidates for coronary revascularization independent of the planned noncardiac surgery should certainly undergo this procedure before the noncardiac surgery. For patients who are not obvious candidates for revascularization, one approach is to optimize their antianginal medications and reevaluate their symptoms. This approach assumes that an improvement in symptoms correlates with a reduction in perioperative cardiac complication rates—an assumption that is without clear validation at present. All high-risk patients should be treated with a prophylactic β-blocking medication, and perhaps a statin medication if they are not already taking one and if it is not otherwise contraindicated. If a β-blocker is contraindicated, an α₂-agonist, should be considered.

CHF & Left Ventricular Dysfunction

Decompensated CHF, manifested by an elevated jugular venous pressure, an audible third heart sound, or evidence of pulmonary edema on physical examination or chest radiography, significantly increases the risk of perioperative pulmonary edema (roughly 15%) and cardiac death (2–10%). It has been estimated that roughly one-third of perioperative cardiac deaths are a result of CHF. Similarly, patients who were hospitalized for CHF within 1 year prior to noncardiac surgery had a twofold increase in perioperative mortality compared with patients without a recent hospital stay for CHF. Preoperative control of CHF, including the use of diuretics and afterload reducing agents, is likely to reduce the perioperative risk. Clinicians must be cautious not to give too much diuretic, since the volume-depleted patient will be much more susceptible to intraoperative hypotension. Although spironolactone, β-adrenergic blocking agents, and angiotensin receptor-blocking agents have been shown to reduce long-term mortality in patients with heart failure, starting these medications in the immediate preoperative period has not been studied and is not recommended as routine practice.

Patients with compensated left ventricular dysfunction are at increased risk for perioperative pulmonary edema but are not at excess risk for other cardiac complications. One large study found that patients with a left ventricular ejection fraction of less than 50% had an absolute risk of 12% for postoperative CHF compared with 3% for patients with an ejection fraction greater than 50%. Such patients should continue taking all medications for chronic heart failure up to and including the day of surgery. Patients receiving digoxin and diuretics should routinely have serum electrolyte and digoxin levels measured prior to surgery because abnormalities in these levels may increase the risk of perioperative arrhythmias. Preoperative echocardiography or radionuclide angiography to assess left ventricular function should be considered for patients with evidence of left ventricular dysfunction who have not had an objective assessment of left ventricular function, and in patients for whom the cause of left ventricular dysfunction is in question. The surgeon and anesthesiologist should be made aware of the presence and severity of left ventricular dysfunction so that appropriate decisions can be made regarding perioperative fluid management and intraoperative monitoring.

Valvular Heart Disease

There are few data available regarding the perioperative risks of valvular heart disease independent of associated coronary artery disease or CHF. Patients with severe symptomatic aortic stenosis are clearly at increased risk for cardiac complications. Such patients who are candidates for valve replacement surgery or, if only short-term relief is needed, for balloon valvuloplasty independent of the planned noncardiac surgery should have the corrective procedure performed prior to noncardiac surgery. In the most recent series of patients with aortic stenosis who underwent noncardiac surgery, the combined endpoint of death or nonfatal MI was 31% in patients with severe aortic stenosis (aortic valve area < 0.7 cm²), 11% in those with moderate aortic stenosis (aortic valve area 0.7–1.0 cm²), and 2% in those without aortic stenosis. Other studies have found that patients with asymptomatic aortic stenosis appeared to be at lower risk than patients with symptomatic aortic stenosis. Noncardiac surgery in patients with severe aortic stenosis must be approached with great caution and requires close consultation with the anesthesiologist.

The severity of valvular lesions should be defined prior to surgery to allow for appropriate fluid management and consideration of invasive intraoperative monitoring. Echocardiography should also be considered in patients with a previously unexplained heart murmur for those procedures in which a valvular abnormality would require antibiotic prophylaxis. For specific recommendations regarding antibiotic prophylaxis, see Chapter 33.

Arrhythmias

Several early studies on cardiac risk factors reported that both atrial and ventricular arrhythmias were independent predictors of an increased risk of perioperative complications. Subsequent data have shown these rhythm disturbances to be frequently associated with underlying structural heart disease, especially coronary artery disease and left ventricular dysfunction. The finding of a rhythm disturbance on preoperative evaluation should prompt consideration of further cardiac evaluation, particularly when the finding of structural heart disease would alter perioperative management. Patients found to have a rhythm disturbance without evidence of underlying heart disease are at very low risk for perioperative cardiac complications.

Management of patients with arrhythmias in the preoperative period should be guided by factors independent of the planned surgery. In patients with atrial fibrillation, adequate rate control should be established. Symptomatic supraventricular and ventricular tachycardia must be controlled prior to surgery. There is no evidence that the use of antiarrhythmic medications to suppress an asymptomatic arrhythmia alters perioperative risk.

It seems prudent for patients who have indications for a permanent pacemaker to have it placed prior to noncardiac surgery. When surgery is urgent, these patients may be managed perioperatively with temporary transvenous pacing. Patients with bundle branch block who do not meet recognized criteria for a permanent pacemaker do not require pacing during surgery.

Hypertension

Severe hypertension, defined as a systolic pressure greater than 180 mm Hg or diastolic pressure greater than 110 mm Hg, appears to be an independent predictor of perioperative cardiac complications, including MI and CHF. Mild to moderate hypertension immediately preoperatively is associated with intraoperative blood pressure lability and asymptomatic myocardial ischemia but does not appear to be an independent risk factor for adverse cardiac outcomes. It seems wise to delay surgery in patients with severe hypertension until blood pressure can be controlled, although it is not known whether the risk of cardiac complications is reduced with this approach. It is unlikely that treatment of mild to moderate hypertension in the immediate preoperative period will significantly reduce the risk of cardiac complications. However, medications for chronic hypertension should be continued up to and including the day of surgery.

Auerbach A et al: Assessing and reducing the cardiac risk of noncardiac surgery. Circulation 2006;113:1361. [PMID: 16534031]

Boersma E et al: Perioperative cardiovascular mortality in noncardiac surgery: Validation of the Lee cardiac risk index. Am J Med 2005;118:1134. [PMID: 16194645]

Devereaux PJ et al: Perioperative cardiac events in patients undergoing noncardiac surgery: a review of the magnitude of the problem, the pathophysiology of the events and the methods to estimate and communicate risk. CMAJ 2005;173:627. [PMID: 16157727]

Devereaux PJ et al: Surveillance and prevention of major perioperative ischemic cardiac events in patients undergoing noncardiac surgery: a review. CMAJ 2005;173:779. [PMID: 16186585]

Durazzo AE et al: Reduction in cardiovascular events after vascular surgery with atorvastatin: a randomized trial. J Vasc Surg 2004;39:967. [PMID: 15111846]

Hernandez AF et al: Outcomes in heart failure patients after major noncardiac surgery. J Am Coll Cardiol 2004;44:1446. [PMID: 15464326]

Kertai MD et al: Aortic stenosis: an underestimated risk factor for perioperative complications in patients undergoing noncardiac surgery. Am J Med 2004;116:8. [PMID: 14706659]

McFalls EO et al: Coronary-artery revascularization before elective major vascular surgery. N Engl J Med 2004;351:2795. [PMID: 15625331]

Sandham JD et al: A randomized controlled trial of the use of pulmonary artery catheters in high risk surgical patients. N Engl J Med 2003;348:5. [PMID: 12510037]

Wallace AW et al: Effect of clonidine on cardiovascular morbidity and mortality after noncardiac surgery. Anesthesiol 2004; 101:284. [PMID: 15277909]

Wilson SH et al: Clinical outcomes of patients undergoing noncardiac surgery in the two months following coronary stenting. J Am Coll Cardiol 2003;42:234. [PMID: 12875757]

PULMONARY EVALUATION IN NON–LUNG RESECTION SURGERY

Pneumonia and respiratory failure requiring prolonged mechanical ventilation are the most important postoperative pulmonary complications and occur in 2–19% of surgical procedures. The occurrence of a postoperative pulmonary complication has been associated with a significant increase in hospital length of stay.

Risk Factors for the Development of Postoperative Pulmonary Complications

Numerous series have investigated the risk factors for the development of postoperative pulmonary complications. The risk of developing a pulmonary complication is highest in patients undergoing cardiac, thoracic, and upper abdominal surgery, with reported complication rates ranging from 9% to 19%. The risk in patients undergoing lower abdominal or pelvic procedures ranges from 2% to 5%, and for extremity procedures the range is less than 1–3%. The pulmonary complication rate for laparoscopic procedures appears to be much lower than that for open procedures. In one series of over 1500 patients who underwent laparoscopic cholecystectomy, the pulmonary complication rate was less than 1%.

Three patient-specific factors have been repeatedly found to increase the risk of postoperative pulmonary complications: chronic lung disease, morbid obesity, and tobacco use. Patients with chronic obstructive pulmonary disease (COPD) have a twofold to fourfold increased risk compared with patients without COPD. In a single large prospective cohort of US military veterans, additional risk factors for the development of postoperative pneumonia included age over 60 years, dependent functional status, impaired sensorium, and prior stroke. In addition, three studies found that placement of a nasogastric tube postoperatively increases the risk of pneumonia. In two studies, a positive cough test was associated with an increased risk of complications. The cough test is performed by asking the patient to take a deep inspiration and cough once. A positive test is defined as recurrent coughing after the first cough.

Patients with asthma are at increased risk for bronchospasm during tracheal intubation and extubation and during the postoperative period. However, if patients are at their optimal pulmonary function (as determined by symptoms, physical examination, or spirometry) at the time of surgery, they do not appear to be at increased risk for other pulmonary complications.

Postoperative pneumonia is approximately twice as likely to develop in morbidly obese patients—those weighing over 113 kg (250 lb)—than in patients weighing less. Mild obesity does not appear to increase the risk of clinically important pulmonary complications.

Several studies have shown that current cigarette smoking is associated with an increased risk of postoperative atelectasis. In a single study, cigarette smoking was also found to double the risk of postoperative pneumonia, even when controlling for underlying lung disease. A summary of the known risk factors for pulmonary complications is presented in Table 3–6.

Pulmonary Function Testing & Arterial Blood Gas Analysis

The majority of studies have shown that preoperative pulmonary function testing in unselected patients is not helpful in predicting postoperative pulmonary complications. The data are conflicting regarding the usefulness of preoperative pulmonary function testing in certain selected groups of patients: the morbidly

Table 3–6. Risk factors for postoperative pulmonary complications.

Upper abdominal or cardiothoracic surgery
Anesthetic time > 4 hours
Morbid obesity
Chronic obstructive pulmonary disease or asthma
Tobacco use > 20 pack-years
Cognitive impairment or impaired sensorium
Prior stroke
Postoperative nasogastric tube
Positive cough test

obese, those with COPD, and those undergoing upper abdominal or cardiothoracic surgery. Assessment of the severity of COPD using pulmonary function tests has not been shown to improve upon the clinical risk assessment with the exception that patients with a forced expiratory volume in 1 second (FEV_1) under 500 mL or an FEV_1 below 50% of the predicted value appear to be at particularly high risk. At present, definitive recommendations regarding the indications for preoperative pulmonary function testing cannot be made. In general terms, such testing may be helpful to confirm the diagnosis of COPD or asthma, to assess the severity of known pulmonary disease, and perhaps as part of the risk assessment for patients undergoing upper abdominal surgery, cardiac surgery, or thoracic surgery.

Arterial blood gas measurement is not routinely recommended except in patients with known lung disease and suspected hypoxemia or hypercapnia.

Perioperative Management

The goal of perioperative management is to reduce the likelihood of postoperative pulmonary complications. Smoking cessation for at least 4 weeks prior to thoracic surgery reduced the incidence of pulmonary complications by 25%. Incentive spirometry (IS), continuous positive airway pressure (CPAP), intermittent positive-pressure breathing (IPPB), and deep breathing exercises (DBE) have all been shown to reduce the incidence of postoperative atelectasis and, in a small number of studies, to reduce the incidence of postoperative pulmonary complications. In most comparative trials, these methods were equally effective. However, in a randomized trial of patients undergoing resection of the esophagus or stomach, those who received postoperative CPAP had a lower risk of prolonged mechanical ventilation or reintubation compared with those who did IS or DBE. Given the higher cost of CPAP and IPPB, IS and DBE are the preferred methods for most patients. CPAP may be preferable for patients undergoing esophageal or gastric resection. IS must be performed for 15 minutes every 2 hours. DBE must be performed hourly and consist of 3-second breath-holding, pursed lip breathing, and cough-

ing. These measures should be started preoperatively and be continued for 1–2 days postoperatively. Most studies suggest that postoperative epidural opioid and local anesthetic agents provide excellent pain control but do not appreciably reduce pulmonary complication rates.

There is some evidence that the incidence of postoperative pulmonary complications in patients with COPD or asthma may be reduced by preoperative optimization of pulmonary function. Patients who are wheezing will probably benefit from preoperative therapy with bronchodilators and, in certain cases, corticosteroids. Antibiotics may be of benefit for patients who cough with purulent sputum if the sputum can be cleared prior to surgery. On the other hand, the use of antibiotics in unselected patients undergoing head and neck cancer surgery did not reduce the occurrence of pulmonary complications. Patients receiving oral theophylline should continue taking the drug during the intraoperative and postoperative periods, using intravenous theophylline when necessary.

Block BM et al: Efficacy of postoperative epidural anesthesia: a meta-analysis. JAMA 2003;290:2455. [PMID: 14612482]

Fagevik Olsen M et al: Randomized clinical study of the prevention of pulmonary complications after thoracoabdominal resection by two different breathing techniques. Br J Surg 2002;89:1228. [PMID: 12296888]

Fisher BW et al: Predicting pulmonary complications after nonthoracic surgery: a systematic review of blinded studies. Am J Med 2002;112:219. [PMID: 11893349]

McAlister FA et al: Incidence of and risk factors for pulmonary complications after nonthoracic surgery. Am J Respir Crit Care Med 2005;171:514. [PMID: 15563632]

Ong SK et al: Pulmonary complications following major head and neck surgery with tracheostomy: a prospective, randomized, controlled trial of prophylactic antibiotics. Arch Otolaryngol Head Neck Surg 2004;130:1084. [PMID: 15381595]

EVALUATION OF THE PATIENT WITH LIVER DISEASE

Patients with serious liver disease are generally thought to be at increased risk for perioperative morbidity and demise. Appropriate preoperative evaluation requires consideration of the effects of anesthesia and surgery on postoperative liver function and of the complications associated with anesthesia and surgery in patients with preexisting liver disease.

The Effects of Anesthesia & Surgery on Liver Function

Postoperative elevation of serum aminotransferase levels is a relatively common finding after major surgery. Most of these elevations are transient and not associated with hepatic dysfunction. Studies in the 1960s and early 1970s showed that patients with liver disease are at increased relative risk for postoperative deterioration in hepatic function, although the absolute risk is not known. General anesthetic agents may cause deterioration of hepatic function via intraoperative reduction in hepatic blood flow leading to ischemic injury. It is important to remember that medications used for spinal and epidural anesthesia produce similar reductions in hepatic blood flow and thus may be equally likely to lead to ischemic liver injury. Intraoperative hypotension, hemorrhage, and hypoxemia may also contribute to liver injury.

Risk Factors for Surgical Complications

Surgery in the patient with serious liver disease has been associated in several series with a variety of significant complications, including hemorrhage, infection, renal failure, and encephalopathy, and with a substantial mortality rate. A key limitation in interpreting these data is our inability to determine the contribution of the liver disease to the observed complications independent of the surgical procedure.

In three small series of patients with acute viral hepatitis who underwent abdominal surgery, the mortality rate was roughly 10%. Cirrhotic patients undergoing portosystemic shunt surgery who have evidence of alcoholic hepatitis on the preoperative liver biopsy have a significantly increased surgical mortality rate compared with patients without alcoholic hepatitis. Although data are quite limited, it seems reasonable to delay elective surgery in patients with acute viral or alcoholic hepatitis, at least until the acute episode has resolved. These data are not sufficient to warrant substantial delays in urgent or emergent surgery.

There are few data regarding the risks of surgery in patients with chronic hepatitis. In a series of 272 patients with chronic hepatitis undergoing a variety of surgical procedures for variceal hemorrhage, the in-hospital mortality rate was less than 2%. It is of note that patients with Child-Turcotte-Pugh class C cirrhosis (see Chapter 15) or with serum aminotransferase levels over 150 units/L were excluded. In a study of patients undergoing hepatectomy for hepatocellular carcinoma, patients with both cirrhosis and active hepatitis on the preoperative liver biopsy had a fourfold increase in mortality (8.7%) compared with patients with cirrhosis alone or active hepatitis alone. In a study of patients with chronic viral hepatitis who underwent liver resection for cancer, a preoperative hyaluronic acid level greater than 200 ng/mL was associated with a substantially increased risk of postoperative hepatic failure.

Substantial data exist regarding surgery in patients with cirrhosis. In several series from the 1960s and 1970s, patients with cirrhosis undergoing abdominal surgery had substantial mortality rates. Biliary surgery was especially risky. Patients with Child-Turcotte-Pugh class C cirrhosis who underwent portosystemic shunt surgery, biliary surgery, or trauma surgery during the 1970s and 1980s had a 50–85% mortality rate. Patients with Child-Turcotte-Pugh class A or B cirrhosis who underwent abdominal surgery during the 1990s, however, had relatively low mortality rates (hepatectomy 0–8%, open cholecystectomy 0–1%, laparoscopic chole-

cystectomy 0–1%). In the most recent study of patients with cirrhosis who underwent major abdominal nonhepatic surgery, the Child-Turcotte-Pugh class was the most important predictor of perioperative complications and mortality. Patients with Child-Turcotte-Pugh class A cirrhosis were similar to noncirrhotic patients with respect to postoperative complications, mortality, and length of hospital stay. Patients with Child-Turcotte-Pugh class B and C cirrhosis had substantially higher complication and mortality rates. Cirrhosis-related complications (ascites, encephalopathy, gastrointestinal bleeding, renal and hepatic failure) were far more common in these patients. However, pulmonary, cardiac, and infectious complications were no more frequent than in the noncirrhotic patients. In recent years, the Model for End Stage Liver Disease (MELD) score has been used to predict survival in patients awaiting liver transplantation. The MELD score has now been compared to the Child-Turcotte-Pugh class in several series of cirrhotic patients undergoing abdominal surgery. In general, these scoring systems are comparable in predicting postoperative decompensation of liver function or mortality. A MELD score of > 7 seems to identify a very high risk group. A conservative approach would be to avoid elective surgery in patients with class C cirrhosis, those with class A or B cirrhosis and concomitant active hepatitis, and those with a MELD score > 7. In addition, when surgery is elective, it is prudent to attempt to reduce the severity of ascites, encephalopathy, and coagulopathy preoperatively.

Befeler AS et al: The safety of intra-abdominal surgery in patients with cirrhosis: model for end-stage liver disease score is superior to Child-Turcotte-Pugh classification in predicting outcome. Arch Surg 2005;140:650. [PMID: 16027329]

del Olmo JA et al: Risk factors for nonhepatic surgery in patients with cirrhosis. World J Surg 2003;27:647. [PMID: 12732995]

Nanashima A et al: Preoperative serum hyaluronic acid level as a good predictor of posthepatectomy complications. Surg Today 2004;34:913. [PMID: 15526125]

Perkins L et al: Utility of preoperative scores for predicting morbidity after cholecystectomy in patients with cirrhosis. Clin Gastroenterol Hepatol 2004;12:1123. [PMID 15625658]

PREOPERATIVE HEMATOLOGIC EVALUATION

Several hematologic disorders may have an impact on the outcomes of surgery. A detailed discussion of the preoperative management of patients with complicated hematologic disorders is beyond the scope of this section. Two of the more common clinical situations faced by the medical consultant are the patient with preexisting anemia and the assessment of bleeding risk.

The key issues in the anemic patient are to determine the need for preoperative diagnostic evaluation and the need for transfusion. When feasible, the diagnostic evaluation of the patient with previously unrecognized anemia should be done prior to surgery because certain types of anemia (particularly sickle cell disease and immune hemolytic anemias) may have implications for perioperative management. Anemia is common before surgery, with a prevalence of 5–75%. Most data suggest that morbidity and mortality increase as the preoperative hemoglobin level decreases, although none of these data were corrected for the presence of preexisting diseases. Hemoglobin levels below 7 or 8 g/dL appear to be associated with significantly more perioperative complications than higher levels. In patients with ischemic heart disease and with Child-Turcotte-Pugh class B or C cirrhosis, a preoperative hemoglobin level below 10 g/dL has been associated with an increased perioperative mortality rate. It is not known, however, whether preoperative transfusion reduces the risk for perioperative complications. Determination of the need for preoperative transfusion in an individual patient must consider factors other than the absolute hemoglobin level, including the presence of cardiopulmonary disease, the type of surgery, and the likelihood of surgical blood loss.

The most important component of the bleeding risk assessment is a directed bleeding history (see Table 3–1). Patients who are reliable historians and who reveal no suggestion of abnormal bleeding on directed bleeding history and physical examination are at very low risk for having an occult bleeding disorder. Laboratory tests of hemostatic parameters in these patients are generally not needed. When the directed bleeding history is unreliable or incomplete or when abnormal bleeding is suggested, a formal evaluation of hemostasis should be done prior to surgery and should include measurement of the prothrombin time, the activated partial thromboplastin time, the platelet count, and the bleeding time.

Armas-Loughran B et al: Evaluation and management of anemia and bleeding disorders in surgical patients. Med Clin North Am 2003;87:229. [PMID: 12575892]

Shander A et al: Prevalence and outcomes of anemia in surgery: a systematic review of the literature. Am J Med 2004;116 (Suppl 7A):58S. [PMID: 15050887]

NEUROLOGIC EVALUATION

Delirium occurs after major surgery in approximately 9% of patients over the age of 50 years. Postoperative delirium has been associated with higher rates of major postoperative cardiac and pulmonary complications, poor functional recovery, and increased length of hospital stay. In addition, postoperative delirium may be associated with an increased risk of subsequent dementia. Several prospective series of hip fracture patients have shown that postoperative delirium is associated with an increased likelihood of functional and cognitive decline in the 3–12 months following surgery and an increased mortality at 1 and 5 years. There were similar findings in a series of older patients undergoing abdominal surgery. Several preoperative and postoperative factors, particularly age and preoperative dementia, have been associated with the development of postoperative delir-

Table 3–7. Risk factors for the development of postoperative delirium.

Preoperative factors
Age > 70 years
Alcohol abuse
Poor cognitive status
Poor physical function status
Markedly abnormal serum sodium, potassium, or glucose level[1]
Aortic aneurysm surgery
Noncardiac thoracic surgery
Normal white blood cell count
Postoperative factors
Use of meperidine or benzodiazepines, anticholinergics, antihistamines
Increased pain at rest
Postoperative hematocrit < 30%
Use of urinary catheters

[1]Defined as follows: sodium < 130 or > 150 mmol/L, potassium < 3 or > 6 mmol/L, glucose < 60 or > 300 mg/dL.
Adapted, with permission, from Marcantonio ER et al: A clinical prediction rule for delirium after elective noncardiac surgery. JAMA 1994;271:134; and from Marcantonio ER et al: The relationship of postoperative delirium with psychoactive medications. JAMA 1994;272:1518.

ium (Table 3–7). Patients with multiple risk factors are at especially high risk.

Delirium is particularly common after hip fracture repair, occurring in 35–65% of patients. In a randomized controlled trial of hip fracture surgery patients, those who received daily visits and targeted recommendations from a geriatrician had a lower risk of postoperative delirium (32%) than the control patients (50%). The most frequent interventions to prevent delirium were maintenance of the hematocrit greater than 30%; minimizing the use of benzodiazepines and anticholinergic and antihistamine medications; maintenance of regular bowel function; and early discontinuation of urinary catheters.

Stroke may occur in 1–6% of patients undergoing cardiac or carotid artery surgery, but it occurs in less than 1% of all other surgical procedures. Most of the available data on postoperative stroke are in cardiac surgery patients. Stroke after cardiac surgery is associated with significantly increased mortality, up to 22% in some studies. The risk factors for stroke after cardiac surgery include age > 60 years, a calcified aorta, prior stroke, carotid stenosis > 50%, peripheral vascular disease, cigarette smoking, diabetes mellitus, and renal failure. Most studies suggest that asymptomatic carotid bruits are associated with little or no increased risk of stroke in noncardiac, noncarotid surgery. The importance of asymptomatic carotid artery stenoses > 50% is not known.

Prophylactic carotid endarterectomy in most patients with asymptomatic carotid artery disease is unlikely to be beneficial. On the other hand, patients with carotid disease who are candidates for carotid endarterectomy anyway (see Chapter 12) should probably have the carotid surgery prior to the elective surgery. Some patients require both cardiac and carotid surgery. The ideal timing of these two procedures is not certain and must be decided individually for each patient. In general, the more symptomatic and threatening condition should be addressed first. In a recent observational study of 1566 patients who underwent carotid endarterectomy, the use of a statin medication was associated with a significant reduction in the rate of perioperative stroke and overall mortality. Given the broad indications for statin therapy in patients with vascular disease, it is prudent to begin statin treatment in patients with appropriate indications prior to their undergoing carotid surgery. Nonstroke neurologic complications including coma, seizures, memory loss, and diminished intellectual function occur in up to 7% of patients after cardiac surgery. The risk factors for these complications include a calcified aorta, age > 70 years, pulmonary disease, diabetes, and neurologic disease.

Bitsch MS et al: Pathogenesis of and management strategies for postoperative delirium after hip fracture. Acta Orthop Scand 2004;75:378. [PMID: 15370579]

Lundstrom M et al: Dementia after delirium in patients with femoral neck fractures. J Am Geriatr Soc 2003;51:1002. [PMID: 12834522]

McGirt MJ et al: 3-Hydroxy-3-methylglutaryl coenzyme A reductase inhibitors reduce the risk of perioperative stroke and mortality after carotid endarterectomy. J Vasc Surg 2005; 42:829. [PMID: 16275430]

McKhann GM et al: Encephalopathy and stroke after coronary artery bypass grafting: incidence, consequences, and prediction. Arch Neurol 2002;59:1422. [PMID: 12223028]

MANAGEMENT OF ENDOCRINE DISEASES

Diabetes Mellitus

Patients with diabetes are at increased risk for postoperative infections, particularly those involving the surgical site. Furthermore, diabetic patients are more likely to have cardiovascular disease and thus are at increased risk for postoperative cardiac complications. The most challenging issue in diabetics, however, is the maintenance of glucose control during the perioperative period.

The increased secretion of cortisol, epinephrine, glucagon, and growth hormone during surgery is associated with insulin resistance and hyperglycemia in diabetic patients. The goal of management is the prevention of severe hyperglycemia or hypoglycemia in the perioperative period.

The ideal blood glucose level during surgery is not known. In vitro studies have shown that cellular immunity may be impaired when the blood glucose level exceeds 250 mg/dL. In several trials of patients under-going cardiac surgery, patients with mean postoperative glucose levels < 180 mg/dL had fewer serious surgical site infections, a lower risk of renal failure, and a shorter hospital stay than patients with higher mean levels. Based on these data, it is advisable to maintain perioperative glucose levels between 100 mg/dL and 180 mg/dL.

All diabetic patients should have serum electrolyte levels measured and abnormalities in any of these levels corrected prior to surgery. Serum creatinine and urea nitrogen levels should also be measured to assess renal function. The specific pharmacologic management of diabetes during the perioperative period depends on the type of diabetes (insulin-dependent or not), the level of glycemic control, and the type and length of surgery. In general, patients who require insulin to control the diabetes (whether type 1 or type 2) will need intraoperative insulin with any surgical procedure. Patients with type 2 diabetes who take oral agents generally require insulin during major or prolonged surgery.

Perioperative management of all diabetic patients requires frequent blood glucose monitoring to prevent hypoglycemia and to ensure prompt treatment of hyperglycemia (Tables 3–8 and 3–9). Specific recommendations for glycemic control in patients who do not need intraoperative insulin are shown in Table 3–8. For patients who require intraoperative insulin, no single regimen has been found to be superior in comparative trials. Three commonly used insulin administration methods are shown in Table 3–9. The subcutaneous route is used most often because it is easier to access and

Table 3–8. Management of patients who do not need insulin during surgery.

Patient	Recommended Management
Diabetes well controlled on diet alone	Avoid glucose-containing solutions during surgery Measure blood glucose level every 4–6 hours during surgery
Diabetes well controlled on an oral sulfonylurea, metformin, or a thiazolidinedione	The last dose of medication should be taken on the evening before surgery Measure glucose every 6 hours in the perioperative period and give subcutaneous regular insulin as needed to maintain blood sugar below 100–200 mg/dL While the patient is fasting, infuse 5% glucose-containing solution at approximately 100 mL/h and continue until the patient is eating Measure blood glucose level every 4–6 hours (or more frequently as indicated) during surgery Resume oral hypoglycemic therapy when the patient returns to baseline diet

Table 3–9. Intraoperative insulin administration methods.

Method	Intravenous Insulin Administration	Glucose Administration	Blood Glucose Monitoring
Subcutaneous insulin	One-half to two-thirds of the usual dose of insulin is administered on the morning of surgery	Infuse 5% glucose-containing solution at a rate of at least 100 mL/h beginning on the morning of surgery and continuing until the patient begins eating	Every 2–4 hours beginning the morning of surgery
Continuous intravenous insulin infusion in glucose-containing solution	On the morning of surgery, infuse 5–10% glucose solution containing 5–15 units regular insulin per liter of solution at a rate of 100 mL/h. This provides 0.5–1.5 units of insulin per hour. Additional insulin may be added as needed to keep blood sugar 100–200 mg/dL.		Every 2–4 hours during intravenous insulin infusion
Separate intravenous insulin and glucose infusions	Infuse intravenous regular insulin at a rate of 0.5–1.5 units/h, adjusting as needed to keep blood sugar 100–200 mg/dL	Infuse 5–10% glucose-containing solution at a rate of 100 mL/h	Every 2–4 hours during intravenous insulin infusion

is less expensive. Intravenous insulin, which offers more rapid onset, shorter duration of action, and ease of dose titration, may be preferable in patients with poorly controlled diabetes, patients in the intensive care unit, and in those undergoing cardiac surgery.

Corticosteroid Replacement

Perioperative complications (predominantly hypotension) resulting from primary or secondary adrenocortical insufficiency are rare. It is not known whether the administration of high-dose corticosteroids during the perioperative period in patients at risk for adrenocortical insufficiency decreases the risk of these complications. In a trial comparing high-dose corticosteroid therapy with simply administering long-term corticosteroid medications in patients with secondary adrenal suppression, there were no differences in perioperative complications. Therefore, definitive recommendations regarding perioperative corticosteroid therapy cannot be made. The most conservative approach would be to consider any patient to be at risk for having adrenocortical insufficiency who has received either the equivalent of 20 mg of prednisone daily for 3 weeks or the equivalent of 7.5 mg of prednisone daily for 1 month within the past year. A commonly used regimen is 50–100 mg of hydrocortisone given intravenously every 8 hours beginning on the morning of surgery and continuing for 48–72 hours. Tapering the dose is not necessary. Patients being maintained on long-term corticosteroids should then resume their usual dose.

Hypothyroidism

Severe symptomatic hypothyroidism has been associated with several perioperative complications, including intraoperative hypotension, CHF, cardiac arrest, and death. Elective surgery should be delayed in patients with severe hypothyroidism until adequate thy-

roid hormone replacement can be achieved. If emergency surgery is required in such patients, intravenous T3 or T4 and corticosteroids should be administered perioperatively. Conversely, patients with asymptomatic or mild hypothyroidism generally tolerate surgery well, with only a slight increase in the incidence of intraoperative hypotension; surgery need not be delayed for the month or more required to ensure adequate thyroid hormone replacement.

Coursin DB et al: Perioperative diabetic and hyperglycemic management issues. Crit Care Med 2004;32(4 Suppl):S116. [PMID: 15064670]

Lazar HL et al: Tight glycemic control in diabetic coronary artery bypass graft patients improves perioperative outcomes and decreases recurrent ischemic events. Circulation 2004; 109:1497. [PMID: 15006999]

Schiff RL et al: Perioperative evaluation and management of the patient with endocrine dysfunction. Med Clin North Am 2003;87:175. [PMID: 12575889]

RENAL DISEASE

The risk for development of a significant reduction in renal function, including dialysis-requiring acute renal failure, after major surgery has been estimated to be between 2% and 20%. The mortality associated with the development of postoperative acute renal failure that requires dialysis after general, vascular, or cardiac surgery exceeds 50%. Risk factors that have been associated with postoperative deterioration in renal function are shown in Table 3–10. Several medications, including "renal dose" dopamine, mannitol, N-acetylcysteine, and furosemide, have been evaluated in an attempt to preserve renal function during the perioperative period. None of these, however, have proved effective in clinical trials. Maintenance of adequate intravascular volume is likely to be the most effective method to reduce the risk of perioperative deterioration in renal function.

Table 3–10. Risk factors for the development of postoperative acute renal failure.

Preoperative chronic renal insufficiency
Aortic surgery
Cardiac surgery
Peripheral vascular disease
Severe heart failure
Preoperative jaundice
Age > 70 years
Diabetes

Although the mortality rate for elective major surgery is low (1–4%) in patients with dialysis-dependent chronic renal failure, the risk for perioperative complications, including postoperative hyperkalemia, pneumonia, fluid overload, and bleeding, is substantially increased. Postoperative hyperkalemia requiring emergent hemodialysis has been reported to occur in 20–30% of patients, and postoperative pneumonia may occur in up to 20% of patients. Patients should undergo dialysis preoperatively within 24 hours before surgery, and their serum electrolyte levels should be measured just prior to surgery and monitored closely during the postoperative period.

Bove T et al: The incidence and risk of acute renal failure after cardiac surgery. J Cardiovasc Anesth 2004;18:442. [PMID: 15365924]

Burns KE et al: Perioperative N-acetylcysteine to prevent renal dysfunction in high-risk patients undergoing CABG surgery: a randomized controlled trial. JAMA 2005;294:342. [PMID: 16030279]

ANTIBIOTIC PROPHYLAXIS OF SURGICAL SITE INFECTIONS

The development of a postoperative surgical site infection is a common and extremely important cause of morbidity and prolonged hospital stays. There are an estimated 0.5–1 million postoperative surgical site infections annually in the United States. For most major procedures, the use of prophylactic antibiotics has been demonstrated to reduce the incidence of postoperative wound infections significantly. For example, antibiotic prophylaxis in colorectal surgery reduces the

Table 3–11. Recommended antibiotic prophylaxis for selected surgical procedures.

Procedure	Recommended Antibiotic	Adult Dose
Superficial cutaneous	None	
Head and neck	Cefazolin	1–2 g intravenously
Neurologic	Cefazolin	1–2 g intravenously
Thoracic	Cefazolin	1–2 g intravenously
Noncardiac vascular	Cefazolin	1–2 g intravenously
Orthopedic, clean, without implantation of foreign material	None	
Orthopedic, all other	Cefazolin	1–2 g intravenously
Cesarean delivery	Cefazolin	2 g intravenously
Hysterectomy	Cefazolin or cefotetan	1–2 g intravenously
Gastroduodenal	Cefazolin (high risk only)[1]	1–2 g intravenously
Biliary	Cefazolin (high risk only)[1]	1–2 g intravenously
Urologic	Cefazolin (high risk only)[2]	1–2 g intravenously
Appendectomy for uncomplicated appendicitis	Cefotetan or cefoxitin	1–2 g intravenously
Colorectal[3]	Neomycin sulfate plus erythromycin base	1 g of each agent given orally at 19, 18, and 9 hours before surgery
	–or–	
	Cefotetan or cefoxitin	1–2 g intravenously
Breast and hernia	Cefazolin (high risk only)[1]	1–2 g intravenously

[1]High risk defined as patients with risk factors for wound infection such as older age, diabetes, or multiple medical comorbidities.
[2]High risk defined as prolonged postoperative catheterization or positive urine cultures.
[3]All patients should have mechanical bowel preparation with polyethylene glycol, mannitol, or magnesium citrate.

incidence of wound infection from 25–50% to below 9%. In addition, in a case control study of Medicare beneficiaries, the use of preoperative antibiotics within 2 hours of surgery was associated with a twofold reduction in 60-day mortality. Prophylactic antibiotics are considered standard care for all but "clean" surgical procedures. Clean procedures are those that are elective, nontraumatic, and not associated with acute inflammation and that do not enter the respiratory, gastrointestinal, biliary, or genitourinary tract. The postoperative wound infection rate for clean procedures is thought to be roughly 2%. However, in certain clean procedures, such as those that involve the insertion of a foreign body, antibiotic prophylaxis is still recommended because the consequences of infection are serious.

Multiple studies have evaluated the effectiveness of different antibiotic regimens for various surgical procedures. In most cases, no single antibiotic regimen has been shown to be superior. Several general conclusions can be drawn from these data. First, there is substantial evidence to suggest that a single dose of an appropriate intravenous antibiotic—or combination of antibiotics—is as effective as multiple-dose regimens that extend into the postoperative period. For longer procedures, the dose should be repeated every 3–4 hours to ensure maintenance of a therapeutic serum level. One important exception is cardiac surgery, in which at least 24 hours of postoperative therapy is recommended. Second, for most procedures, a first-generation cephalosporin is as effective as later-generation agents. Third, with the exception of colorectal surgery, all prophylactic antibiotics should be given intravenously at induction of anesthesia or roughly 30–60 minutes prior to the skin incision. Although the type of procedure is the main factor determining the risk of developing a postoperative wound infection, certain patient factors have been associated with increased risk, including diabetes, older age, obesity, heavy alcohol consumption, and multiple medical comorbidities. In addition, recent evidence suggests that nasal carriage with *Staphylococcus aureus* is associated with a twofold to ninefold increased risk of surgical site and catheter-related infections in surgical patients. Treatment of nasal carriers of *S aureus* with 2% mupirocin ointment (twice daily for 3 days) prior to cardiac surgery decreases the risk of surgical site infections. Current antibiotic prophylaxis recommendations for a variety of procedures are shown in Table 3–11.

Data on the use of supplemental oxygen to prevent surgical site infections are mixed. The most recent study found an increased risk of surgical site infections with the use of 80% oxygen compared with 35% in the immediate postoperative period. At present, however, high-flow supplemental oxygen specifically to prevent these infections is not recommended.

Perl TM: Prevention of *Staphylococcus aureus* infections among surgical patients: beyond traditional perioperative prophylaxis. Surgery 2003;134(5 Suppl):S10. [PMID: 14647028]

Pryor KO: Surgical site infection and the routine use of perioperative hyperoxia in a general surgical population: a randomized controlled trial. JAMA 2004;291:79. [PMID: 14709579]

Silber JH et al: Preoperative antibiotics and mortality in the elderly. Ann Surg 2005;242:107. [PMID: 15973108]

Smith RL et al: Wound infections after elective colorectal resection. Ann Surg 2004;239:599. [PMID: 15082963]

Geriatric Medicine

4

C. Bree Johnston, MD, G. Michael Harper, MD , & C. Seth Landefeld, MD

The impressive successes of medicine and public health over the past century have made it possible for elderly persons to live longer and healthier than ever before. Persons over the age of 65 account for about 13% of the population, which will swell to about 20% by 2030 as the "baby boomers" age. Thus, most physicians will spend a significant portion of their professional lives dealing with older adults' health care.

Older persons are remarkably heterogeneous. Many persons in their 60s are healthy and can expect to live another 30 years or longer. Yet, chronic diseases that will cause disability and ultimately death will develop in nearly all older persons. While age alone is a strong predictor of risk for disease, disability, and death, the health status, prognosis, and preferences of care of persons in their 70s, 80s, and 90s vary widely. Therefore, physicians caring for older adults must have skills in managing multiple comorbidities and wisely guiding the patient in both "curative" and "palliative care."

GENERAL PRINCIPLES OF GERIATRIC MEDICINE

The following principles are helpful to keep in mind while caring for older adults:

1. Many disorders are multifactorial in origin.
2. Diseases often present atypically.
3. Not all abnormalities require evaluation and treatment.
4. Complex medication regimens, adherence problems, and polypharmacy are common challenges.

Comorbidities are common in older people, and the diagnostic "law of parsimony" often does not apply. For example, fever, anemia, and a heart murmur are almost always diagnostic of endocarditis in a younger patient; however, in an older patient, three different explanations—a viral illness, colon cancer, and aortic sclerosis—might be equally likely than the unifying diagnosis of endocarditis.

Disease presentation is often atypical in elderly patients. A disorder in one organ system may lead to symptoms in another, especially one that is compromised by preexisting disease. Because these organ systems are often the brain, the lower urinary tract, and the cardiovascular or musculoskeletal systems, a limited number of presenting symptoms—ie, confusion, falling, incontinence, dizziness, and functional decline—predominate irrespective of the underlying disease. Thus, regardless of the presenting symptom in older people, the differential diagnosis is often similar. An 80-year-old person with new falls and confusion could have pneumonia, an acute myocardial infarction, a stroke, or a urinary tract infection. Furthermore, because many geriatric syndromes have multiple causes, multiple targeted interventions may be a more realistic approach than trying to find a "cure." For example, dizziness is often multifactorial in older adults. A practitioner who focuses on finding a diagnosis and treatment may become frustrated, while a practitioner who works on multiple problems, such as correcting vision, prescribing physical therapy focused on strength and balance, and reducing sedating medications, might meet with more success.

Many abnormal findings in younger patients are relatively common in older people and may not be responsible for a particular symptom. Such findings may include asymptomatic bacteriuria, premature ventricular contractions, and slowed reaction time. In addition, many older patients with multiple comorbidities may have laboratory abnormalities that, while pathologic, may not be clinically important. A complete workup for a mild anemia of chronic disease in a person with multiple other issues might be burdensome to the patient with little chance of impacting quality of life or longevity. While abnormalities should not be ignored, they can be addressed in order of priority, with the patient's goals (symptom management, desire for longevity) dictating the evaluation strategy.

Many older patients have to manage complex medication regimens, particularly those who have multiple comorbidities. Drug side effects can occur with low doses of drugs that usually produce no side effects in younger people. For instance, a mild anticholinergic agent (eg, diphenhydramine) may cause confusion, loop diuretics may precipitate urinary incontinence, digoxin may induce anorexia even with normal serum levels, and nonprescription sympathomimetics may result in urinary retention in older men with mild prostatic obstruction.

■ GENERAL APPROACH TO THE OLDER PATIENT

Therapy in elders should be guided by the estimated life expectancy and the patients' values and goals (Figure 4–1). Interventions that are likely to help elders who are well may differ from those that will benefit elders who are frail. Estimating life expectancy can help a health care provider focus on those issues most likely to be beneficial in a given patient. A mammogram would be appropriate for a healthy older woman with a life expectancy of 12 years, but not for a woman with congestive heart failure and chronic obstructive pulmonary disease with a life expectancy of less than 5 years.

Detecting and treating some conditions produce almost immediate benefit, and those may be useful at any age. These include visual impairment, hearing loss, falls, depression, incontinence, immobility, and pain. Smoking cessation and initiating an exercise program can also produce very rapid benefits, even in the oldest old.

An awareness of a patient's goals, values, and preferences can help the health care provider focus the patient's visits appropriately. For example, many evaluations and interventions can be avoided in an elderly patient who is interested in receiving symptomatic, but not life prolonging, care.

Certain strategies can make the care of older people in a busy outpatient practice a little more manageable. Such strategies include using brief assessment instruments for common geriatric conditions when appropriate, training nonprovider personnel in administering some of these assessments (hearing screen, vision screen), having portable amplifiers ("pocket talkers") available, and designing protocols for following up abnormal screening assessments. For example, a medical assistant might perform the simple geriatric screen (Figure 4–2) on all patients older than 75 years, and prompt the provider by having follow up instruments such as the Mini-Mental State Examination (MMSE) and the geriatric depression scale available when the screen was positive.

Many practitioners question which elders should be referred to geriatric care, home care, or team care. The answer depends on the resources of the community, but a good rule of thumb is that if it feels like the patient cannot be treated adequately in the setting where they are receiving care or if the coordination of care is taking so much time that it is detracting from the care of other patients, it may be time to explore a different level of care.

Fried TR et al: Understanding the treatment preferences of seriously ill patients. N Engl J Med 2002;346:1061. [PMID: 11932474]

ASSESSMENT OF OLDER ADULTS

Functional Assessment

Functional assessment gauges a patient's ability to manage tasks of self-care, household management, and mobility.

About one-fourth of patients over 65 have impairments in their IADLs (instrumental activities of daily living: transportation, shopping, cooking, using the telephone, managing money, taking medications, housecleaning, laundry) or ADLs (basic activities of daily living: bathing, dressing, eating, transferring from bed to chair, continence, toileting). Half of those persons older than 85 years have these latter impairments. Persons who are unable to perform IADLs independently are far more likely to have dementia than their independent counterparts.

Information about function can be used in a number of ways: (1) as baseline information, (2) as a measure of the patient's need for support services or placement, (3) as an indicator of possible caregiver burden,

Women

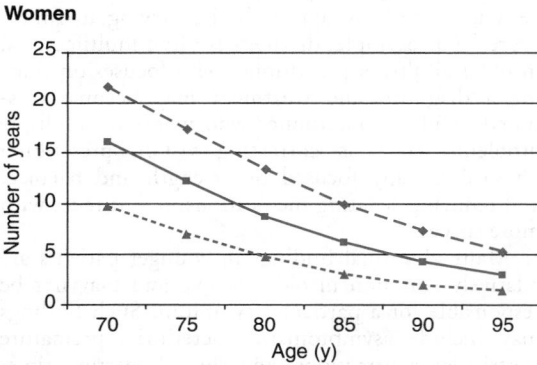

Men

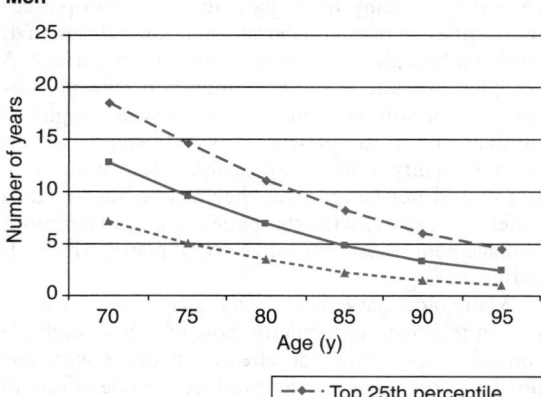

- –◆– Top 25th percentile
- –■– 50th percentile
- ––▲–– Lowest 25th percentile

Figure 4–1. Median life expectancy of older women and men. (Adapted from Walter LC et al: Screening for colorectal, breast, and cervical cancer in the elderly: a review of the evidence. Am J Med 2005;118:1078.)

Patient Name _____ Date _____

Source: Pt _____ Other _____

HISTORY ITEMS	ABNORMAL	ACTION	RESULT AND COMMENTS
Have you had any falls in the last year?	Yes	Gait assessment Further exam, home evaluation and PT Osteoporosis and injury risk assessment	_____
Do you have trouble with stairs, lighting, bathroom hazards, or other home hazards?	Yes to any	Home evaluation or PT	_____
Do you have a problem with urine leaks or accidents?	Yes	Rule out transient (DIAPPERS) History (stress, urge), exam, PVR	_____
Over the past month, have you often been bothered by feeling sad, depressed, or hopeless?	Yes to any	GDS or other depression assessment	_____
During the past month, have you often been bothered by little interest or pleasure in doing things?	Yes to either		
Do you ever feel unsafe where you live?	Yes	Explore further, social work, APS	_____
Does anyone threaten you or hurt you?	Yes		
Is pain a problem for you?	Yes	Evaluate _____	

Do you have any problems with any of the following areas? Who assists? Do you use any devices? (for "yes" answers, consider causes, social services, and home eval/PT/OT)

Doing strenuous activities like fast walking/bicycling? _____

Cooking? _____

Shopping? _____

Doing heavy housework like washing windows? _____

Doing laundry? _____

Getting to a place beyond walking distance by driving or taking a bus? _____

Managing finances? _____

Getting out of bed/transfer? _____

Dressing? _____

Toilet? _____

Eating? _____

Walking? _____

Bathing (sponge bath, tub, or shower)? _____

Review medications that the patient brought in	Confusion about medications	Consider simplification	_____
Also ask about herbs, vitamins, supplements, and nonprescription medications	> 5 medications Doesn't bring in	Medi-set or other aid Consider home visit	

PHYSICAL EXAM ITEMS (The next few items may be performed by nursing staff in some settings)

Weight/BMI	BMI < 21	Alert provider or nutrition evaluation	_____
And ask "have you lost weight?"	Loss of 5% since last visit		
If so, how much?	Or 10% over 1 year	Consider medical, dental, social causes	
Jaeger Card or Snellen eye chart Test each eye (with glasses)	Can't read 20/40	Alert provider or refer	_____
Whisper short sentences at 6–12 inches (out of visual view) OR audioscopy	Unable to hear Retest/refer	Cerumen check Hearing handicap inventory	_____
Name three objects/re-ask in 5 minutes Clock draw test	Misses any or unable	MMSE	_____
Rise from the chair (do not use arms to get up), walk 10 feet, turn, walk back to the chair and sit down	Observed problem or unable in < 10 seconds	Further gait and neurologic exam Home evaluation and PT	_____
Touch the back of your head with your hands Pick up the pencil	Unable to do either	Further exam Consider OT	_____

(Remember to ask about the 3 items!)

Other areas of concern: caregiver stress, alcohol use, social isolation, exercise, driving, advance directives and health care wishes.

Figure 4–2. Simple geriatric screen. PT = physical therapy; DIAPPERS = delirium, infection, atrophic urethritis or vaginitis, pharmaceuticals, psychological factors, excess urinary output, restricted mobility, stool impaction; PVR = postvoid residual; GDS = Geriatric Depression Screen; APS = Adult Protective Services; OT = occupational therapy; BMI = body mass index; MMSE = Mini-Mental State Exam. (Modified from Lachs M et al: A simple procedure for general screening for functional disability in elderly patients. Ann Intern Med 1990;112:699 and Moore AA et al: Screening for common problems in ambulatory elderly: clinical confirmation of a screening instrument. Am J Med 1996;100:438.)

(4) as a potential marker of specific disease activity, (5) to determine the need for therapeutic interventions, and (6) to indicate prognosis.

In general, persons who need help only with IADLs can usually live independently with minimal supports, such as financial services (eg, a representative payee) or a chore worker. If institutional care is needed, residential care, board-and-care, or assisted living is usually sufficient. While many persons who need help with ADLs may require a nursing home level of care, most live at home with caregivers and other community services (eg, day care).

Screening for Vision Impairment

An appreciable minority of elders have severe visual loss. Visual impairment is an independent risk factor for falls; it also has a significant impact on quality of life. Although administering direct visual testing with a Snellen chart or Jaeger card in most primary care settings is relatively easy, the prevalence of serious eye disease and visual impairment in elders is sufficient to warrant a complete eye examination by an ophthalmologist or optometrist annually or biannually for most elders. Many patients with visual loss benefit from a referral to a low vision program, and primary care practitioners should not assume that an ophthalmologist or optometrist will automatically make this referral.

Screening for Hearing Impairment

Over one-third of persons over age 65 and half of those over age 85 have some hearing loss. This deficit is correlated with social isolation and depression. Although the optimal screening method for hearing loss in older adults is undetermined, the whispered voice test is easy to perform and has sensitivities and specificities ranging from 70% to 100%. To determine the degree to which the impairment interferes with functioning, the provider may ask if the patient becomes frustrated when conversing with family members, is embarrassed when meeting new people, has difficulty listening to the radio or watching TV, or has problems understanding conversations in noisy restaurants. Caregivers or family members often have important information on the impact of hearing loss on the patient's social interactions.

Compliance with hearing amplification can be a challenge because of the stigma associated with hearing aid use as well as the cost of such devices, which are not paid for under most Medicare plans. High compliance rates can be achieved with a proactive approach such as the use of loaner aids for low-income persons. In addition to standard hearing aids, other devices are available. For example, portable amplifiers are small radio-sized units with earphones attached; they can be purchased inexpensively at many electronics stores and are well accepted by many patients. Special telephones, amplifiers for the television, and many other devices are available to aid the person with hearing loss.

Screening for Falls & Gait Impairment

Falls are the leading cause of nonfatal injuries in older persons, and their complications are the leading cause of death from injury in persons over age 65. Hip fractures are common precursors to functional impairment, nursing home placement, and death. Furthermore, fear of falling may lead some elders to restrict their activities. About one-third of people over 65 fall each year, and the frequency increases markedly with advancing age.

Every older person should be asked about falls; many will not volunteer such information. Clinicians should ask about home hazards that might be remediable. A thorough gait assessment should be performed in all older people. Gait and balance can be readily assessed by the "Up and Go Test," in which the patient is asked to stand up from a sitting position without use of hands, walk 10 feet, turn around, walk back, and sit down. Patients who take less than 10 seconds are usually normal, patients who take longer than 30 seconds tend to need assistance with many mobility tasks, and those in between tend to vary widely with respect to gait, balance, and function. The ability to recognize common patterns of gait disorders is an extremely useful clinical skill to develop. Examples of gait abnormalities and their causes are listed in Table 4–1.

Screening for Cognitive Impairment

The prevalence of dementia doubles every 5 years after age 60, so that by age 85 about 30–50% of individuals have some degree of impairment. Patients with mild or early dementia frequently remain undiagnosed because their social graces are retained.

Although there is no consensus at present on whether older patients should be screened for dementia, the benefits of early detection include identification of potentially reversible causes, planning for the future (including advance directives), providing support and counseling for the caregiver, modification of interventions for other diseases as appropriate (eg, simplifying drug regimens, minimizing anticholinergic drug use), and beginning acetylcholinesterase inhibitor drugs.

The combination of a clock drawing task with a three-item word recall is fairly quick to administer. Although a number of different methods for administering and scoring the clock draw test have been described, the authors of this chapter favor the approach of pre-drawing a four inch circle on a sheet of paper and instructing the patient to "draw a clock" with the time set at 10 minutes after 11. Scores are classified as normal, almost normal, or abnormal. When a patient is able to draw a clock normally and can remember all 3 objects, dementia is unlikely. When a patient fails this simple screen, further cognitive evaluation with

Table 4–1. Evaluation of gait abnormalities.

Gait Abnormality	Possible Cause
Inability to stand without use of hands	Deconditioning Myopathy (hyperthyroidism, alcohol, statin-induced) Hip or knee pain
Unsteadiness upon standing	Orthostatic hypotension Balance problem (peripheral neuropathy, vision problem, vestibular, other central nervous system causes) Generalized weakness
Stagger with eyes closed	Often indicates that vision is compensating for another deficit
Short steps	Weakness Parkinson's disease or related condition
Asymmetry	Cerebrovascular accident Focal pain or arthritis
Wide-based gait	Fear, balance problems
Flexed knees	Contractures, quadriceps weakness
Slow gait	Fear of falling, weakness, deconditioning, peripheral vascular disease, chronic obstructive pulmonary disease, congestive heart failure, angina

the MMSE (see Figure 25–1), neuropsychological testing, or other instruments is warranted.

Borson S et al: The Mini-Cog as a screen for dementia: Validation in a population based sample. J Am Geriatr Soc 2003; 51:1451. [PMID: 14511167]

Screening for Incontinence

Incontinence in older adults is common, and interventions can improve most patients. Many patients fail to tell their providers about it. A simple question about involuntary leakage of urine is a reasonable screen: "Do you have a problem with urine leaks or accidents?"

Screening for Depression

Although major depressive disorder has a slightly lower prevalence in older adults than in younger populations, depressive symptoms are actually more common. Its prevalence in ill and hospitalized elders is particularly high. A simple two-question screen (Figure 4–2) has shown 96% sensitivity for detecting major depression in a general population and may have even higher sensitivity in those over age 65. Positive responses can be followed up with more comprehensive, structured interviews, eg, Yesavage's Geriatric Depression Scale (Table 4–2).

Assessment of Decision-Making Capacity

It is common for a cognitively impaired elder to face a serious medical decision and for the clinicians involved in his care to ascertain whether the capacity exists to make the choice. There are five components of a thorough assessment: (1) ability to express a choice; (2) understanding relevant information about the risks and benefits of planned therapy and the alternatives, including no treatment; (3) comprehension of the problem and its consequences; and (4) ability to reason; and (5) consistency. A patient's choice should follow rationally from an understanding of the consequences.

Cultural sensitivity must be used in applying these five components to people of various cultural backgrounds. In performing such assessments, it is to be remembered that decision-making capacity varies over time: A delirious patient may regain his capacity after an infection is treated, and so reassessments are often appropriate. Furthermore, the capacity to make a decision is a function of the decision in question. A mildly demented woman may lack the capacity to consent to coronary artery bypass grafting yet retain the capacity

Table 4–2. Yesavage's Geriatric Depression Scale (short form).

1. Are you basically satisfied with your life? (no)
2. Have you dropped many of your activities and interests? (yes)
3. Do you feel that your life is empty? (yes)
4. Do you often get bored? (yes)
5. Are you in good spirits most of the time? (no)
6. Are you afraid that something bad is going to happen to you? (yes)
7. Do you feel happy most of the time? (no)
8. Do you often feel helpless? (yes)
9. Do you prefer to stay home at night, rather than go out and do new things? (yes)
10. Do you feel that you have more problems with memory than most? (yes)
11. Do you feel it is wonderful to be alive now? (no)
12. Do you feel pretty worthless the way you are now? (yes)
13. Do you feel full of energy? (no)
14. Do you feel that your situation is hopeless? (yes)
15. Do you think that most persons are better off than you are? (yes)

Score one point for each response that matches the yes or no answer after the question.
Key: Scores: 3 ± 2 = normal; 7 ± 3 = mildly depressed; 12 ± 2 = very depressed.

to designate a surrogate decision maker or allow removal of a suspicious nevus.

Caregiver Issues

Most elders with functional impairment live in the community with the help of an "informal" caregiver, most commonly a spouse or daughter. The health and well-being of the patient and caregiver are closely linked. High levels of functional dependency place an enormous burden on a caregiver, and may result in caregiver burnout, depression, morbidity, and even increased mortality.

An older patient's need for nursing home placement is often better predicted from assessment of the caregiver characteristics and stress than the severity of the patient's illness. Therefore, part of caring for a frail elder involves paying attention to the well-being of the caregiver. The older patient who is also a caregiver is at risk for depression and should be screened for it. For the stressed caregiver, a social worker may help identify programs such as caregiver support groups, respite programs, adult day care, or hired home health aides.

Elder Abuse

It is helpful to observe and talk with every older person alone for at least part of a visit in order to question directly about possible abuse and neglect (Table 4–3). Clues to the possibility of elder abuse include behavioral changes in the presence of the caregiver, delays between injuries and sought treatment, inconsistencies between an observed injury and associated explanation, lack of appropriate clothing or hygiene, and not filling prescriptions.

Functional Screening Instrument

Figure 4–2 gives a simple functional screening list. In addition to ADL and IADL assessment, it looks for evidence of health problems that affect function: sensory impairment, limited upper extremity range of motion, mobility, falls, weight loss, incontinence, depressed mood, and cognitive impairment.

Table 4–3. Questions that may elicit a history of elder abuse.

---

1. Has anyone ever hurt you?
2. Has anyone ever touched you without your consent?
3. Has anyone ever made you do things you didn't want to do?
4. Has anyone taken anything of yours without asking?
5. Has anyone ever scolded or threatened you?
6. Have you signed any papers that you didn't understand?
7. Is there anyone at home you are fearful of?
8. Are you alone much?
9. Has anyone ever refused to help you take care of yourself when you needed help?

Standard functional screening measures may not be useful in capturing subtle impairments in highly functional independent elders. One technique for these patients is to identify and regularly ask about a target activity, such as playing bridge, bowling, or working outside the home. If the patient begins to have trouble with or discontinues such an "advanced activity of daily living," it may indicate early impairment, such as dementia, incontinence, or worsening hearing loss, which additional gentle questioning or assessment may uncover.

SELECTED PREVENTIVE MEASURES IN GERIATRIC PRACTICE

Exercise

Inactive elders are at greater risk for becoming functionally dependent than their more physically active counterparts. Higher levels of physical activity are associated with reduced risks of future disability, disease-related morbidity, and mortality. Even sedentary elders should be urged to increase their level of physical activity. By writing out an exercise prescription, a provider demonstrates the importance of the activity and may improve compliance. Components that have been demonstrated to improve outcomes in elders include strength training (isolated muscle group contractions), endurance training (walking, cycling, swimming), and balance (tai chi, dance). Ideally, the patient should aim for a total of 30–60 minutes of activity daily. Recent data suggests that even short spurts of activity throughout the day are beneficial. The greatest increase in benefit is experienced by those going from a completely sedentary lifestyle to participating in some physical activity.

Gill TM et al: A program to prevent functional decline in physically frail, elderly persons who live at home. N Engl J Med 2002;347:1068. [PMID: 12362007]

Gill TM et al: Exercise stress testing for older persons starting an exercise program. JAMA 2000;284:2591. [PMID: 11086356]

Manson JE et al: Walking compared with vigorous exercise for the prevention of cardiovascular events in women. N Engl J Med 2002;347:716. [PMID: 12213942]

Hypertension

Treatment of hypertension is of substantial benefit in older adults, and the absolute benefit of treatment may be greater in older than in younger patients. The role of aggressive antihypertensive therapy in the persons over age 85 is still being debated. Treatment of hypertension and isolated systolic hypertension reduces the incidence of strokes, heart failure, and cardiovascular events but not overall mortality in this age group. Lifestyle modifications (weight loss for overweight patients, alcohol and sodium limitation, increased aerobic physical activity) are reasonable to recommend for all hypertensive patients for whom treatment is appropriate. For those who require pharmacologic treatment, thiazides are the drugs of choice unless a comorbid condition makes another choice preferable.

Cancer Screening

The authors of this chapter recommend against routinely screening elderly men for prostate cancer, since there is no evidence that the practice prolongs life, and the burdens of treatment can be considerable. An older woman is likely to benefit from breast cancer screening until her life expectancy falls below 5–10 years (Figure 4–1). Screening for colon cancer can be stopped when a patient's life expectancy is less than 5–10 years. Cervical cancer is uncommon in older women, and screening can usually be discontinued at age 65 if the woman has had a history of regular screening and normal Pap smears.

Walter LC et al: Screening for colorectal, breast, and cervical cancer in the elderly: a review of the evidence. Am J Med 2005;118:1078. [PMID: 16194635]

Immunizations

Individuals over age 65—and health care workers who are in contact with them—should receive annual influenza vaccinations. Although data from randomized controlled trials are scarce, observational studies suggest that flu vaccination decreases mortality and pneumonia in elders. Similarly, persons over 65 should receive at least one pneumococcal immunization; some experts recommend revaccination in those over 75 or with severe chronic disease and who were vaccinated more than 5 years previously, although data are lacking. The Centers for Disease Control and Prevention recommends primary vaccination for tetanus and diphtheria (Td) in elders who are previously unvaccinated. The historical recommendation has been to give booster doses of Td every 10 years. An alternative approach is to give a single booster dose of Td at midlife (age 50 years) to those who have received full pediatric immunizations (see Chapter 30).

PPD for Congregate Living

Older adults are a significant reservoir of tuberculosis, both primary and reactivation. The disease develops in over 20% of elderly patients who live in nursing homes. Long-term care facilities should routinely perform a tuberculin skin test (PPD) on all entering patients, using the two-step approach in which a second dose is administered to persons whose first was negative. If the second reaction is also negative, the patient is uninfected or anergic; if positive, a boosted response is likely, signifying a tuberculin reactor but not a recent converter. Whether these reactors need treatment is controversial, but their positive-PPD status should be noted. Prophylaxis and treatment regimens are described in Chapter 9. Skin testing is repeated annually in congregate settings or if an active case is identified in the group.

■ COMMON PROBLEMS OF THE FRAIL OLDER PERSON

DEMENTIA

 ESSENTIALS OF DIAGNOSIS

- *Progressive impairment of intellectual function, including loss of short-term memory.*
- *Deficits in at least one other area, including aphasia, apraxia, agnosia, or a disturbance in executive functioning.*
- *Deficit severe enough to cause impairment of function.*
- *Psychiatric manifestations common.*
- *Not delirious.*
- *Alzheimer's disease is most common cause, followed by vascular dementia and dementia with Lewy bodies.*

Older individuals experience occasional difficulty retrieving items from memory (usually manifested as word-finding complaints) and experience a slowing in their rate of information processing. By contrast, dementia is an acquired persistent and progressive impairment in intellectual function, with compromise of memory and at least one other cognitive domain. The diagnosis of dementia requires a significant decline in function that is severe enough to interfere with work or social life.

Intellectual impairments in older patients are frequently the result of two other syndromes, each of which frequently coexists with dementia: depression and delirium. Depression is a common concomitant of dementia, but it can also masquerade as dementia. Moreover, a patient with depression and cognitive impairment whose intellectual function improves with treatment of the mood disorder has an almost fivefold greater risk of suffering irreversible dementia later in life. Delirium, characterized by acute confusion, occurs much more commonly in patients with underlying dementia.

General Considerations

Alzheimer's disease is the eighth leading cause of death in the United States and sixth leading cause among the elderly. It has a prevalence that doubles every 5 years in the older population, reaching 30–50% at age 85. Women suffer disproportionately, both as patients (even after age adjustment) and as caregivers. Alzheimer's disease accounts for roughly two-thirds of cases in the

United States, with vascular dementia (either alone or combined with Alzheimer's disease) accounting for much of the rest. Risk factors for Alzheimer's disease are older age, family history, lower education level, and female gender. Some epidemiologic studies suggest that head injury, hypertension, higher homocysteine levels, and higher low-density lipoprotein (LDL) cholesterol levels are risk factors for dementia, while nonsteroidal anti-inflammatory drug (NSAID) use, HMG-CoA reductase inhibitor use, moderate alcohol intake, and strong social supports may decrease the risk. However, these studies of risk factors for dementia do not provide an adequate basis for treatment recommendations. Risk factors for vascular dementia are those for stroke, ie, older age, male sex, black race, hypertension, cigarette use, previous myocardial infarction, atrial fibrillation, diabetes, and hyperlipidemia.

Causes of potentially reversible cognitive impairment include drug effect, depression, thyroid disease, vitamin B_{12} deficiency, hypercalcemia, subdural hematoma, HIV infection, and normal-pressure hydrocephalus. The prevalence of fully reversible dementias is well under 5%, and the correction of these suspected causes leads only to partial improvement in most cases.

Clinical Features

Demented patients have memory impairment and at least one or more of the following: language impairment (initially just word finding; later, difficulty following a conversation; finally, mutism), apraxia (inability to perform previously learned tasks, such as cutting a loaf of bread, despite intact sensory and motor function), agnosia (inability to recognize objects), and impaired executive function (poor abstraction, mental flexibility, planning, and judgment). Alzheimer's disease typically presents with early problems in memory and visuospatial abilities (eg, becoming lost in familiar surroundings, inability to copy a geometric design on paper), yet social graces may be retained despite advanced cognitive decline. Personality changes and behavioral difficulties (wandering, inappropriate sexual behavior, agitation) may develop as the disease progresses. Hallucinations are not typically observed except in moderate-to-severe dementia. End-stage disease is characterized by near-mutism; inability to sit up, hold up the head, or track objects with the eyes; difficulty with eating and swallowing; weight loss; bowel or bladder incontinence; and recurrent respiratory or urinary infections.

"Subcortical" dementias (eg, the dementia of Parkinson's disease, and some cases of vascular dementia) are characterized by psychomotor slowing, reduced attention, early loss of executive function, and personality changes, and benefit from cuing-in tests of memory.

Dementia with Lewy bodies may be confused with delirium, as fluctuating cognitive impairment is frequently observed. Rigidity and bradykinesia are the primary signs, and tremor is rare. Response to dopaminergic agonist therapy is poor. Complex visual hallucinations—typically of people or animals—may be an early feature that can help distinguish dementia with Lewy bodies from Alzheimer's disease. These patients demonstrate a hypersensitivity to neuroleptic therapy, and attempts to treat the hallucinations may lead to marked worsening of extrapyramidal symptoms.

Frontotemporal dementias are a group of diseases that include Pick's disease, dementia associated with amyotrophic lateral sclerosis, and others. Patients manifest personality change (euphoria, disinhibition, apathy) and compulsive behaviors (often peculiar eating habits or hyperorality). In contrast to Alzheimer's disease, visuospatial function is relatively preserved.

Dementia in association with motor findings, such as extrapyramidal features or ataxia, may represent a less common disorder (eg, progressive supranuclear palsy, corticobasal ganglionic degeneration, olivopontocerebellar atrophy).

Differential Diagnosis

In addition to depression and delirium, apparent cognitive impairment in older adults may be the result of drug effects or uncorrected sensory deficits; these problems more often exacerbate dementia than mimic it.

Many medications have been associated with diminished mentation in older patients. Anticholinergic agents, hypnotics, neuroleptics, and opioids are well-established causes, but NSAIDs, antihistamines (including H_2-antagonists), and corticosteroids have been implicated as well.

An elderly patient with intact cognition but with severe impairments in vision or hearing commonly becomes confused in an unfamiliar medical setting and consequently may be falsely labeled as demented. Cognitive testing is best performed after optimal correction of the sensory deficits.

Diagnosis

Historical questions in an evaluation for dementia include those directed at the rate of progression of the deficits, their nature (including any personality or behavioral change), motor problems, risk factors for HIV, family history, medication list, functional disabilities, and degree of social support.

The neurologic examination emphasizes assessment of mental status (see Figure 25–1) but should also include evaluation for deficits related to previous strokes, parkinsonism, or peripheral neuropathy. The remainder of the physical examination should focus on identifying comorbid conditions that may aggravate the individual's disability.

Laboratory studies for most patients are intended to uncover treatable causes of cognitive impairment and include a complete blood count, electrolytes, calcium, creatinine, glucose, thyroid-stimulating hormone (TSH), and vitamin B_{12} levels. HIV testing, RPR (rapid plasma reagin) test, heavy metal screen, and liver function tests may be informative in selected patients but should not be considered part of routine testing.

Although consensus is lacking with respect to which patients benefit from head CT or MRI, those who are younger and those who have focal neurologic symptoms or signs, seizures, gait abnormalities, and an acute or subacute onset are most likely to yield positive findings.

Referral for neuropsychological testing may be helpful in the following circumstances: to distinguish dementia from depression, to diagnose dementia in persons of very poor education or very high premorbid intellect, and to aid diagnosis when impairment is mild.

Treatment

Soon after diagnosis, patients and families should be made aware of the Alzheimer's Association as well as the wealth of helpful publications available for advice in coping with behavioral problems, financial worries, and other matters. Caregiver support, education, and counseling can prevent or delay nursing home placement. Education includes the manifestations and natural history of dementia as well as the availability of local support services such as respite care. Even under the best of circumstances, caregiver stress can be substantial.

Because demented patients have greatly diminished cognitive reserve, they are at high risk for experiencing acute cognitive or functional decline in the setting of new medical illness. Consequently, fragile cognitive status may be best maintained by ensuring that comorbid diseases such as congestive heart failure and infections are detected and treated.

Most experts recommend considering a trial of acetylcholinesterase inhibitors (eg, donepezil, galantamine, rivastigmine) in most patients with mild to moderate Alzheimer's disease. These medications produce statistically significant but modest improvements in cognitive function. Acetylcholinesterase inhibitors may also benefit patients with vascular dementia or dementia with Lewy bodies. Starting doses, respectively, of donepezil, galantamine, and rivastigmine, are 5 mg orally once daily (maximum 10 mg once daily), 4 mg orally twice daily (maximum 12 mg twice daily), and 1.5 mg orally twice daily (maximum 6 mg twice daily). The doses are increased gradually as tolerated. The most bothersome side effects include diarrhea, nausea, anorexia, and weight loss.

Evidence from a recent long-term randomized controlled trial of donepezil versus placebo in community-dwelling patients with Alzheimer's disease confirmed the modest cognitive improvement seen in previous trials but found no difference in the rates of institutionalization or progression of disability at 3 years between the two groups. Some experts have been concerned that stopping these drugs may lead to irreversible worsening, but this trial did not substantiate this concern. Therefore, in those patients who have had no apparent benefit, experience side effects or for whom the financial outlay is a burden, the authors of this chapter recommend a trial of discontinuation.

In clinical trials, patients with more advanced disease have been shown to have statistical benefit from the use of memantine, a N-methyl-D-aspartate (NMDA) antagonist, with or without concomitant use of an acetylcholinesterase inhibitor. Long-term and meaningful functional outcomes have yet to be demonstrated.

Other agents have been studied. *Ginkgo biloba* has shown mixed results in clinical trials. Vitamin E demonstrated some efficacy in one randomized controlled trial, but the results are difficult to interpret. Estrogen and NSAIDs have shown no benefits in randomized trials.

Behavioral problems in demented patients are often best managed with a nonpharmacologic approach. Initially, it should be established that the problem is not unrecognized delirium, pain, urinary obstruction, or fecal impaction. It also helps to inquire whether the caregiver or institutional staff can tolerate the behavior, as it is often easier to find ways to accommodate to the behavior than to modify it. If not, the caregiver is asked to keep a brief, informal journal in which the behavior is described along with antecedent events and consequences. Recurring precipitants of the behavior are often found to be present or it may be that the behavior is rewarded—for example, by increased attention. Caregivers are taught to use simple language when communicating with the patient, to break down activities into simple component tasks, and to use a "distract, not confront" approach when the patient seems disturbed by a troublesome issue. Additional steps to address behavioral problems include the discontinuation of all medications except those considered absolutely necessary and correction, if possible, of sensory deficits.

There is no clear consensus about a pharmacologic approach to treatment of behavioral problems in patients who have not benefited from nonpharmacologic therapies. The target symptoms—depression, anxiety, psychosis—may suggest which class of medications might be most helpful in a given patient. Patients with depressive symptoms may show improvement with antidepressant therapy.

The efficacy of acetylcholinesterase inhibitors for behavioral disturbances in Alzheimer's dementia is still undetermined, but a meta-analysis suggested that they may exert a modest benefit on neuropsychiatric outcomes. Patients with dementia with Lewy bodies have shown clinically significant improvement in behavioral symptoms when treated with rivastigmine. Neuroleptics are commonly used for behavioral disturbances, but the literature on their efficacy is mixed. One review suggested that haloperidol may be modestly useful in reducing aggression—but not agitation—in dementia and that it is associated with significant adverse effects. The newer atypical agents (risperidone, olanzapine, quetiapine, aripiprazole, clozapine, ziprasidone) are reported to be better tolerated than older agents, but they are considerably more expensive. The US Food and Drug Administration recently issued a public health advisory warning that these agents, when used to treat elderly demented patients with behavioral disturbances, increased the mortality rates 1.6–1.7 times compared with placebo. A separate meta-analysis reached similar conclusions and also found a nonstatistically significant trend toward increased mortality with haloperidol. Because of limited efficacy data and safety concerns, caution should be used when prescribing neuroleptic agents for treating behavioral disturbances in dementia. When the choice is made to use these agents, starting and target dosages should be much lower than those used in schizophrenia (eg, haloperidol, 0.5–2 mg orally; risperidone, 0.25–2 mg orally). Federal regulations require that if antipsychotic agents are used in treatment of a nursing home patient, drug reduction efforts must be made at least every 6 months.

Anecdotal data suggest that some patients improve with agents such as mood stabilizers or trazodone, but randomized trials show mixed results. In one trial, haloperidol, trazodone, behavioral management techniques, and placebo produced comparable if modest reductions in agitation in patients with dementia.

Prognosis

Life expectancy after a diagnosis of Alzheimer's disease is typically 3–15 years; it may be shorter than previously reported. Other neurodegenerative dementias, such as dementia with Lewy bodies, show more rapid decline.

Courtney C et al: Long-term donepezil treatment in 565 patients with Alzheimer's disease (AD2000): randomised double-blind trial. Lancet 2004;363:2105. [PMID 15220031]

Lonergan E et al: Haloperidol for agitation in dementia. Cochrane Database Syst Rev 2002;(2):CD002852. [PMID: 12076456]

Schneider LS et al: Risk of death with atypical antipsychotic drug treatment for dementia; meta-analysis of randomized placebo controlled trials. JAMA 2005;294:1934. [PMID: 16234500]

Trinh NH et al: Efficacy of cholinesterase inhibitors in the treatment of neuropsychiatric symptoms and functional impairment in Alzheimer disease: a meta-analysis. JAMA 2003; 289:210. [PMID: 12517232]

Wilkinson D et al: Donepezil in vascular dementia: a randomized placebo controlled trial. Neurology 2003;61:479. [PMID: 12939421]

DEPRESSION

Geriatric patients with depression are more likely than younger ones to have somatic complaints, less likely to report depressed mood or feelings of guilt, and more likely to experience delusions.

Depressive syndromes that arise late in life are heterogeneous, and a significant number may represent persons with neurodegenerative disorders (eg, dementia). Consequently, close follow-up of a newly diagnosed patient, with frequent assessment of mental status and neurologic examination, may disclose an additional or alternative diagnosis.

Depression in older adults is associated with disability, increased rates of hospitalization and nursing home admission, and higher mortality. Medical illness

and disability—more common in older adults—are risk factors for depression. In particular, stroke and Parkinson's disease appear to predispose to depression. Suicide is most common in older men. Although the presence of comorbid medical illnesses and cognitive disorders may interfere with diagnosis, use of the Geriatric Depression Scale (see Table 4–2) with candidate cases may provide the data needed to make a treatment decision.

Elderly patients with depressive symptoms should be questioned about medication use, as many drugs (benzodiazepines, cimetidine, corticosteroids, and clonidine, to name a few) may contribute to the clinical picture. Similarly, several medical problems can cause fatigue, lethargy, or hypoactive delirium, all of which may be mistaken for depression. Laboratory requests should include a complete blood count; liver, thyroid, and renal function tests; and serum calcium. The workup to exclude an organic explanation calls for urinalysis and an electrocardiogram.

Choice of antidepressant agent in elders is usually based on side effect profile and cost. In general, fluoxetine is avoided because of its long duration of action and tricyclic antidepressants are avoided because of their high anticholinergic side effects. Regardless of the drug chosen, many experts recommend starting elders at a relatively low dose, titrating to full dose slowly, and continuing for a longer trial (at least 9 weeks) before trying a different medication. Cognitive behavioral therapy can improve outcomes alone or in combination with medication therapy. Depressed elders may do better with a collaborative care model than with usual care.

Unutzer J et al: Collaborative care management of late life depression in the primary care setting: a randomized controlled trial. JAMA 2002;288:2836. [PMID: 12472325]

DELIRIUM

 ESSENTIALS OF DIAGNOSIS

- *Rapid onset and fluctuating course.*
- *Primary deficit in attention rather than memory.*
- *May be hypoactive or hyperactive.*
- *Dementia frequently coexists.*

Delirium is an acute, fluctuating disturbance of consciousness, associated with a change in cognition or the development of perceptual disturbances (see also Chapter 25). It is the pathophysiologic consequence of an underlying general medical condition such as infection, coronary ischemia, hypoxemia, or metabolic derangement. Delirium persists in up to 25% of patients and is associated with worse clinical outcomes (higher in-hospital and postdischarge mortality, longer lengths of stay, greater probability of placement in a nursing facility).

Although the acutely agitated, "sundowning" elderly patient often comes to mind when considering delirium, many episodes are more subtle. Such quiet, or hypoactive, delirium may only be suspected if one notices new cognitive slowing or inattention.

Cognitive impairment is an important risk factor for delirium. Approximately 25% of delirious patients are demented, and 40% of demented hospitalized patients are delirious. Other risk factors are male sex, severe illness, hip fracture, fever or hypothermia, hypotension, malnutrition, polypharmacy and use of psychoactive medications, sensory impairment, use of restraints, use of intravenous lines or urinary catheters, metabolic disorders, depression, and alcoholism.

Assessment

A key component of a delirium workup is review of medications because a large number of drugs, the addition of a new drug, or the discontinuation of a medication known to cause withdrawal symptoms are all associated with the development of delirium. Laboratory evaluation of most patients should include a complete blood count, electrolytes, blood urea nitrogen (BUN) and serum creatinine, glucose, calcium, albumin, liver function studies, urinalysis, and electrocardiography. In selected cases, serum magnesium, serum drug levels, arterial blood gas measurements, blood cultures, chest radiography, and urinary toxin screens may be helpful.

Management

Prevention is the best approach. Measures include improving cognition (frequent reorientation, activities), sleep (massage, noise reduction), mobility, vision (visual aids and adaptive equipment), hearing (portable amplifiers, cerumen disimpaction), and hydration status (volume repletion). Management of established episodes of delirium is supportive, entailing treatment of the underlying cause, eliminating unnecessary medications, and avoidance of restraints. Antipsychotic agents (such as haloperidol, 0.5–1 mg, or quetiapine, 25 mg, at bedtime or twice daily) are considered the medication of choice when drug treatment of delirium is necessary. In emergency situations, starting haloperidol at 0.5 mg by mouth or intramuscularly and repeating every 30 minutes until the agitation is controlled may be necessary, but such treatment is often followed by prolonged sedation or other complications. Other medications (eg, trazadone, donepezil, mood stabilizers) have also been used, but clinical trials that support these approaches are lacking.

Most episodes of delirium clear in a matter of days after correction of the precipitant, but some patients suffer episodes of longer duration. These individuals merit closer follow-up for the development of dementia if not already diagnosed.

Cole MG et al: Systematic detection and multidisciplinary care of delirium in older medical inpatients: a randomized trial. CMAJ 2002;167:753. [PMID: 12389836]

Inouye SK et al: A multicomponent intervention to prevent delirium in hospitalized older patients. N Engl J Med 1999; 340:669. [PMID: 10053175]

Kalisvaart KJ et al: Haloperidol prophylaxis for elderly hip-surgery patients at risk for delirium: a randomized placebo-controlled study. J Am Geriatr Soc 2005;53:1658. [PMID: 16181163]

Marcantonio ER et al: Reducing delirium after hip fracture: a randomized trial. J Am Geriatr Soc 2001;49:516. [PMID: 11380742]

IMMOBILITY

Although common in older people, reduced mobility is never normal and is often treatable if its causes are identified. It is an important cause of hospital-induced functional decline. Among hospitalized medical patients over 70, about 10% experience a decline in their ability to perform ADLs, much of which results from preventable reductions in mobility.

The hazards of bed rest in older adults are multiple, serious, quick to develop, and slow to reverse. Deconditioning of the cardiovascular system occurs within days and involves fluid shifts, decreased cardiac output, decreased peak oxygen uptake, and increased resting heart rate. More striking changes occur in skeletal muscle, with loss of contractile velocity and strength. Pressure sores are a third serious complication; mechanical pressure, moisture, friction, and shearing forces all predispose to their development. Thrombophlebitis and pulmonary embolism are additional serious risks. Within days after being confined to bed, the risk of postural hypotension, falls, skin breakdown, and pulmonary embolism rises rapidly in the older patient. Moreover, recovery from these changes usually takes weeks to months.

Common causes of immobility are weakness, stiffness, pain, dizziness, and comorbid illness. Weakness may result from disuse of muscles, malnutrition, electrolyte disturbances, anemia, neurologic disorders, or myopathies. The most common cause of stiffness in older adults is osteoarthritis, but Parkinson's disease and inflammatory arthritides such as rheumatoid arthritis also are possible in this age group, and drugs such as haloperidol may also contribute. Polymyalgia rheumatica should be strongly considered in older patients with pain and stiffness, particularly of the pelvic and shoulder girdle, associated with systemic symptoms (see Chapter 20).

Pain, whether from bone (eg, osteoporosis, osteomalacia, Paget's disease, metastatic bone cancer, trauma), joints (eg, osteoarthritis, rheumatoid arthritis, hip fractures, gout), bursae, or muscle (polymyalgia rheumatica, intermittent claudication, or "pseudoclaudication"), may immobilize the patient. Painful foot problems are common as well and include plantar warts, ulcerations, bunions, corns, and ingrown and overgrown toenails. Poorly fitting shoes are a frequent cause of these disorders.

Imbalance and fear of falling are major causes of immobilization. Imbalance often results from several causes concurrently, including neurologic disorders (eg, stroke, cervical myelopathy, peripheral neuropathy due to diabetes or alcohol, and vestibulocerebellar abnormalities), orthostatic or postprandial hypotension, or drugs (eg, diuretics, antihypertensives, sedatives, neuroleptics, and antidepressants). It may also occur following prolonged bed rest.

Psychological conditions such as severe anxiety or depression may contribute to immobilization.

Prevention & Treatment

When immobilization cannot be avoided, several measures can be used to minimize its consequences. Adequate nutrition should be ensured, and the skin over pressure points should be inspected frequently; if the patient is unable to shift position, staff should do so every 2 hours. To minimize cardiovascular deconditioning, patients should be positioned as close to the upright position as possible, several times daily. To reduce the risks of contracture and weakness, range of motion exercises should be started immediately and isometric and isotonic exercises performed while the patient is in bed. Whenever possible, patients should assist with their own positioning, transferring, and self-care. As long as the patient remains immobilized, pharmacologic (eg, low-dose heparin) or nonpharmacologic means (eg, graduated compression stockings) should be used to reduce the risk of thrombosis if that is consistent with the patient's goals of care.

Avoiding restraints and discontinuing invasive devices (intravenous lines, urinary catheters) may increase an elderly patient's prospects for early mobility. Once this becomes feasible, graduated ambulation should begin. Advice from a physical therapist is often helpful. Installing handrails, lowering the bed, and providing chairs of proper height with arms and rubber skid guards may make the patient safely mobile in the home. A properly fitted cane or walker may also be useful.

If pain is contributing to immobility, it should be addressed (see section below on analgesics). If depression is preventing a patient from participating in physical therapy, it may prove necessary to start with a short course of stimulant medication (eg, methylphenidate; see Chapter 25), at least until a more traditional antidepressant has had time to take effect.

van Baar ME et al: Effectiveness of exercise therapy in patients with osteoarthritis of the hip or knee. Arthritis Rheum 1999;42:1361. [PMID: 104032263]

FALLS & GAIT DISORDERS

Thirty percent of community-dwelling elderly persons fall each year, including half of people over age 80. About 1% of falls result in hip fracture, and hip fracture is associated with significant increases in functional dependence, morbidity, and mortality. Fear of falling may contribute to loss of independence and other negative health effects. Falls are thought to be a contributing factor to almost half of nursing home admissions. Nonetheless, falls are not inevitable or untreatable.

Causes of Falls

Balance and ambulation require a complex interplay of cognitive, neuromuscular, and cardiovascular function. With age, balance becomes impaired and postural sway increases. This predisposes the older person to a fall when challenged by an additional insult to any of these systems.

A fall may be the clinical manifestation of an occult problem, such as pneumonia or myocardial infarction, but much more commonly falls are due to the interaction between an impaired patient and an environmental risk factor. While a warped floorboard may pose little problem for a vigorous, cognitively intact person, it may be sufficient to precipitate a fall and hip fracture in the patient with impaired vision, balance, muscle tone, or cognition. Thus, falls in older people are rarely due to a single cause, and effective intervention entails a comprehensive assessment of the patient's intrinsic deficits (usually diseases and medications), the activity engaged in at the time of the fall, and environmental obstacles.

Intrinsic deficits are those that impair sensory input, judgment, blood pressure regulation, reaction time, and balance and gait. Dizziness may be closely related to the deficits associated with falls and gait abnormalities. While it may be impossible to isolate a sole "cause" or a "cure" for falls, gait abnormalities, or dizziness, it is often possible to identify and ameliorate some of the underlying contributory conditions and improve the patient's overall function.

As for most geriatric conditions, medications and alcohol use are among the most common, significant, and reversible causes of falling. Benzodiazepines, sedative-hypnotics, antidepressants, neuroleptics, and the use of four or more medications simultaneously have been associated with an increased fall risk. Other often overlooked but treatable contributors include postprandial hypotension (which peaks 30–60 minutes after a meal), insomnia, urinary urgency, and peripheral edema (which can burden impaired leg strength and gait because of the additional weight).

Since most falls occur in or around the home, a visit by a visiting nurse, physical therapist, or health care provider reaps substantial benefits in identifying environmental obstacles and is generally reimbursed by third-party payers, including Medicare. Insufficient lighting is an underappreciated factor in many cases. In addition to the number and location of lamps, noting their wattage is also important; because of a loss of contrast sensitivity, older people often need twice the wattage to maximize visual acuity. Replacement of 60-watt bulbs with 100-watt bulbs may be cost-effective.

Complications of Falls

The most common fractures resulting from falls are of the wrist, hip, and vertebrae. There is a high mortality rate (approximately 20% in 1 year) in elderly women with hip fractures, particularly if they were debilitated prior to the time of the fracture.

Fear of falling again is a common, serious, but treatable factor in the elderly person's loss of confidence and independence. Referral to a physical therapist for gait training with special devices is often all that is required.

Chronic subdural hematoma is an easily overlooked complication of falls that must be considered in any elderly patient presenting with new neurologic symptoms or signs, particularly obtundation. Headache is uncommonly present. In many cases there is no history of trauma.

Patients who are unable to get up from a fall are at risk for dehydration, electrolyte imbalance, pressure sores, rhabdomyolysis, and hypothermia.

Prevention & Management

The risk of falling and consequent injury, disability, and potential institutionalization can be reduced by modifying those factors outlined in Table 4–4. Emphasis is placed on treating all contributory medical conditions, minimizing environmental hazards, and

Table 4–4. Fall risk factors and targeted interventions.

Risk Factor	Targeted Intervention
Postural hypotension (> 20 mm Hg drop in systolic blood pressure, or systolic blood pressure < 90 mm Hg)	Behavioral recommendations, such as hand clenching, elevation of head of bed; discontinuation or substitution of high-risk medications
Use of benzodiazepine or sedative-hypnotic agent	Education about sleep hygiene; discontinuation or substitution of medications
Use of three prescription medications	Review of medications
Environmental hazards	Appropriate changes; installation of safety equipment (eg, grab bars)
Gait impairment	Gait training, assistive devices, balance or strengthening exercises
Impairment in transfer or balance	Balance exercises, training in transfers, environmental alterations (eg, grab bars)
Impairment in leg or arm muscle strength or limb range of motion	Exercise with resistance bands or putty, with graduated increases in resistance

reducing the number of medications—particularly those that induce parkinsonism, orthostasis (eg, α-blockers, calcium channel blockers, nitrates, antiparkinsonism agents, antipsychotics, tricyclic antidepressants), peripheral edema, and confusion. Also important are strength, balance, and gait training as well as steps to improve bone density (with calcium and vitamin D supplementation in most older adults and other medications as indicated). There is some evidence that vitamin D may help prevent falls.

Assistive devices, such as canes and walkers, are useful for many older adults but are often used incorrectly. Canes should be used on the "good" side. The height of walkers and canes should generally be about the level of the wrist. Physical therapists are invaluable in assessing the need for an assistive device, selecting the best device, and training a patient in its correct use.

Patients with repeated falls are often reassured by the availability of phones at floor level, a portable phone, or a lightweight radio call system. Their therapy should also include training in techniques for arising after a fall. Use of an anatomically designed external hip protector reduces hip fracture risk in frail older people but is often poorly tolerated.

Bischoff-Ferrari HA et al: Effect of Vitamin D on falls: a meta-analysis. JAMA 2004;291:1999. [PMID: 15113819]

Guideline for the prevention of falls in older persons. American Geriatrics Society, British Geriatrics Society, and American Academy of Orthopaedic Surgeons Panel on Falls Prevention. J Am Geriatr Soc 2001;49:664. [PMID: 11380764]

Tinetti ME: Clinical practice. Preventing falls in elderly persons. N Engl J Med 2003;348:42. [PMID: 12510042]

URINARY INCONTINENCE

 ESSENTIALS OF DIAGNOSIS

- *Involuntary loss of urine.*
- *Stress incontinence presents with leakage of urine upon coughing, sneezing, or standing.*
- *Urge incontinence presents with symptoms of urgency and inability to delay urination.*
- *Overflow incontinence may have variable presentation.*

Classification

Because continence requires adequate mobility, mentation, motivation, and manual dexterity, problems outside the bladder often result in geriatric incontinence. In general, the authors of this chapter find it useful to differentiate between "transient" or "potentially reversible" causes of incontinence and more "established" causes.

A. Transient Causes

Use of the mnemonic "DIAPPERS" may be helpful in remembering the categories of transient incontinence.

1. Delirium—A clouded sensorium impedes recognition of both the need to void and the location of the nearest toilet. Delirium is the most common cause of incontinence in hospitalized patients; once it clears, incontinence usually resolves.

2. Infection—Symptomatic urinary tract infection commonly causes or contributes to urgency and incontinence. Asymptomatic bacteriuria does not.

3. Atrophic urethritis or vaginitis—Because it usually coexists with atrophic vaginitis, atrophic urethritis can be diagnosed presumptively by the presence of vaginal mucosal telangiectasia, petechiae, erosions, erythema, or friability. Urethral inflammation, if symptomatic, may contribute to incontinence in some women.

4. Pharmaceuticals—Drugs are one of the most common causes of transient incontinence. Typical offending agents include potent diuretics, anticholinergics, psychotropics, opioid analgesics, α-blockers (in women), α-agonists (in men), and calcium channel blockers.

5. Psychological factors—Severe depression with psychomotor retardation may impede the ability or motivation to reach a toilet.

6. Excess urinary output—Excess urinary output may also overwhelm the ability of an older person to reach a toilet in time. In addition to diuretics, common causes include excess fluid intake; metabolic abnormalities (eg, hyperglycemia, hypercalcemia, diabetes insipidus); and disorders associated with peripheral edema, with its associated heavy nocturia when previously dependent legs assume a horizontal position in bed. Edema may be due to heart failure, venous insufficiency, malnutrition, cirrhosis, and use of calcium channel blockers or NSAIDs.

7. Restricted mobility—(See Immobility section, above.) If mobility cannot be improved, access to a urinal or commode (eg, at the bedside) may improve continence.

8. Stool impaction—This is a common cause of urinary incontinence in hospitalized or immobile patients. Although the mechanism is still unknown, a clinical clue to its presence is the onset of both urinary and fecal incontinence. Disimpaction restores urinary continence.

B. Established Causes

Causes of established incontinence should be addressed after the transient causes have been uncovered and managed appropriately.

1. Detrusor overactivity (urge incontinence)—Detrusor overactivity refers to uninhibited bladder contractions that cause leakage. It is the most common cause of established geriatric incontinence, accounting for two-thirds of cases, and is usually idiopathic. Women will complain of urinary leakage after the onset of an intense urge to urinate that cannot be forestalled. In men the symptoms are similar, but detrusor overactivity commonly coexists with urethral obstruction from benign prostatic hyperplasia. Because detrusor overactivity also may be due to bladder stones or tumor, the abrupt onset of otherwise unexplained urge incontinence—especially if accompanied by perineal or suprapubic discomfort or sterile hematuria—should be investigated by cystoscopy and cytologic examination of a urine specimen.

2. Urethral incompetence (stress incontinence)—Urethral incompetence is the second most common cause of established urinary incontinence in older women. Urinary incontinence is most commonly seen in men after radical prostatectomy. Stress incontinence is characterized by instantaneous leakage of urine in response to a stress maneuver. It commonly coexists with detrusor overactivity. Typically, urinary loss occurs with laughing, coughing, or lifting heavy objects. Leakage is worse or occurs only during the day, unless another abnormality (eg, detrusor overactivity) is also present. To test for stress incontinence, have the patient relax her perineum and cough vigorously (a single cough) while standing with a full bladder. Instantaneous leakage indicates stress incontinence if urinary retention has been excluded by postvoiding residual determination using ultrasound. A delay of several seconds or persistent leakage suggests that the problem is instead caused by an uninhibited bladder contraction induced by coughing.

3. Urethral obstruction—Urethral obstruction (due to prostatic enlargement, urethral stricture, bladder neck contracture, or prostatic cancer) is a common cause of established incontinence in older men but is rare in older women. It can present as dribbling incontinence after voiding, urge incontinence due to detrusor overactivity (which coexists in two-thirds of cases), or overflow incontinence due to urinary retention. Renal ultrasound is required to exclude hydronephrosis in men whose postvoiding residual urine exceeds 150 mL.

4. Detrusor underactivity (overflow incontinence)—Detrusor underactivity is the least common cause of incontinence. It may be idiopathic or due to sacral lower motor nerve dysfunction ("neurogenic bladder"). When it causes incontinence, detrusor underactivity is associated with urinary frequency, nocturia, and frequent leakage of small amounts. The elevated postvoiding residual urine (generally over 450 mL) distinguishes it from detrusor overactivity and stress incontinence, but only urodynamic testing differentiates it from urethral obstruction in men. Such testing usually is not required in women, in whom obstruction is rarely present.

Treatment

A. Transient Causes

Each identified transient cause should be treated regardless of whether an established cause coexists. For patients with urinary retention induced by an anticholinergic agent, discontinuation of the drug should first be considered. If this is not feasible, substituting a less anticholinergic agent (eg, sertraline instead of desipramine for depression) may be useful.

B. ESTABLISHED CAUSES

1. Detrusor overactivity—The cornerstone of treatment is behavioral therapy. Patients are instructed to void every 1–2 hours while awake. Once daytime continence is restored, the interval is increased by 30 minutes until the interval is 4–5 hours. Most patients who become continent during the day on this regimen become continent at night as well. For patients who are unable to manage on their own, caregivers should ask whether they need to void at suitable intervals.

Pelvic floor exercises, behavioral approaches, and biofeedback can be extremely helpful in training cognitively intact, motivated patients. Results superior to those achieved with use of bladder relaxants are possible.

If behavioral approaches prove insufficient, drug therapy with oxybutynin (2.5–5 mg three or four times daily), long-acting oxybutynin (5–15 mg daily), tolterodine (1–2 mg twice daily), or long-acting tolterodine (2–4 mg daily) appear modestly effective at reducing episodes of incontinence in some patients. All of these agents can produce delirium, dry mouth, or urinary retention; long-acting preparations may be better tolerated. In men with both benign prostatic hyperplasia and detrusor overactivity, a postvoiding residual or urodynamic testing should be done if prescription of a bladder relaxant is planned in order to avoid precipitating urinary retention. In refractory cases, where intermittent catheterization is feasible, the provider may choose intentionally to induce urinary retention with a bladder relaxant and have the patient empty the bladder three or four times daily. Clean but not sterile technique is required.

2. Urethral incompetence (stress incontinence)—Although a last resort, surgery is the most effective treatment for stress incontinence, resulting in a cure rate of 75–85% even in older women. For women who wish to avoid surgery and who can employ them indefinitely, pelvic muscle exercises are effective for mild to moderate stress incontinence; they can be combined, if necessary, with biofeedback, electrical stimulation, or vaginal cones. Pelvic floor exercises can be taught during bimanual vaginal examination or by asking the patient to try to contract the muscle that they use to stop the flow of urine. It is often necessary to perform 30–60 exercises daily for 6 weeks before significant improvement will be noticed. Pessaries or vaginal cones may be helpful in some women but should be prescribed by practitioners who are experienced with using these modalities.

Drug therapy is limited. There is no evidence that topical or oral estrogens are helpful, although some experts prescribe a trial of topical estrogen in women with symptomatic atrophic urethritis. α-Agonists, such as pseudoephedrine, may have modest efficacy but are often poorly tolerated. Some new agents are under investigation.

3. Urethral obstruction—Surgical decompression is the most effective treatment for obstruction, especially in the setting of urinary retention. A variety of newer, less invasive techniques make decompression feasible even for frail men. For the nonoperative candidate with urinary retention, intermittent or indwelling catheterization is used. For a man with prostatic obstruction who does not require or desire immediate surgery, treatment with α-blocking agents (eg, terazosin, 1–10 mg daily; prazosin, 1–5 mg orally twice daily; tamsulosin, 0.4–0.8 mg daily) can improve symptoms and delay obstruction. Finasteride, 5 mg daily, can also improve outcomes and provides additional benefits to an α-blocking agent. However, finasteride may carry a risk of increasing high-grade prostate cancer.

4. Detrusor underactivity—For the patient with a poorly contractile bladder, augmented voiding techniques (eg, double voiding, suprapubic pressure) often prove effective. If further emptying is needed, intermittent or indwelling catheterization is the only option. Antibiotics should be used only for symptomatic upper urinary tract infection or as prophylaxis against recurrent symptomatic infections in a patient using intermittent catheterization; they should not be used as prophylaxis with an indwelling catheter.

Assessment and treatment of urinary incontinence. Scientific Committee of the First International Consultation on Incontinence. Lancet 2000;355:2153. [PMID: 10902644]

WEIGHT LOSS & MALNUTRITION

Undernutrition affects substantial numbers of elderly persons and often precedes hospitalization for "failure to thrive." The degree of unintended weight loss that deserves evaluation is not agreed upon, although a reasonable threshold is loss of 5% of body weight in 1 month or 10% of body weight in 6 months. Commonly overlooked causes of weight loss in elders include dental problems or poorly fitting dentures, new functional decline with loss of ability to shop or prepare meals, worsening dementia, occult depression, or lack of caregiver support.

Useful laboratory and radiologic studies include complete blood count, serum chemistries (including glucose, TSH, creatinine, calcium), urinalysis, and chest film. These studies are intended to uncover an occult metabolic or neoplastic cause but are not exhaustive.

Oral nutritional supplements of 200–1000 kcal/d can increase weight and improve outcomes in malnourished elders. Megestrol acetate as an appetite stimulant has not been shown to increase body mass or lengthen life in the elderly population. For those who have lost the ability to feed themselves, assiduous hand feeding may allow maintenance of weight. Although artificial nutrition and hydration ("tube feeding") may seem a more convenient alternative, it deprives the patient of the taste and texture of food as well as the social milieu typically associated with mealtime; before this option is chosen, the patient or his or her surrogate will wish to review the benefits and burdens of the treatment in light of overall goals of care. If the patient makes repeated attempts to pull out the tube during a trial of artificial nutrition, the treatment burden becomes substantial, and the utility of tube feeding should be reconsidered. Although commonly used, there is no evidence that tube feeding prolongs life in patients with end-stage dementia.

"Failure to thrive" is a syndrome lacking a consensus definition but generally representing a constellation of weight loss, weakness, and progressive functional decline. The label is typically applied when some triggering event—loss of social support, a bout of depression or pneumonia, the addition of a new medication—pulls a struggling elderly person below the threshold of successful independent living. Ideally, use of the preventive measures recommended earlier in this chapter will reduce the patient's chances of reaching this stage of frailty.

Finucane TE et al: Tube feeding in patients with advanced dementia: a review of the evidence. JAMA 1999;282:1365. [PMID: 10527184]

Milne AC et al: Meta-analysis: Protein and energy supplementation in older people. Ann Intern Med 2006;144:37. [PMID: 16389253]

PRESSURE ULCERS

ESSENTIALS OF DIAGNOSIS

- *Examine at-risk patients daily.*
- *Blanchable hyperemia (stage I).*
- *Extension through epidermis (stage II).*
- *Full thickness skin loss (stage III).*
- *Full thickness wounds with extension into muscle, bone, or supporting structures (stage IV).*
- *If eschar overlies the wound, staging cannot be done.*

General Considerations

The majority of pressure ulcers develop during a hospital stay for an acute illness. Incident rates range from 3% to 30% and vary according to patient characteristics. The primary risk factor for pressure ulcers is immobility. Other contributing risk factors include reduced sensory perception, moisture (urinary and fecal incontinence), poor nutritional status, and friction and shear forces.

A number of risk assessment instruments including the Braden Scale and the Norton score can be used to assess the risk of developing pressure ulcers; both have reasonable performance characteristics. These instruments can be used to identify the highest risk patients who might benefit most from scarce resources such as mattresses that reduce or relieve pressure.

Prevention

Pressure ulcers are often used as an indicator of quality of care; whether or not high quality preventive measures can eliminate pressure ulcers entirely is controversial. Mainstays of preventive therapy include promoting mobility and turning and repositioning immobile patients every 2 hours. For moderate- to high-risk patients, surfaces that reduce tissue pressure beyond a standard mattress but not to < 32 mm Hg (eg, air-fluid beds and low air loss beds) appear to be superior to standard mattresses. The literature comparing specific products is sparse and inconclusive.

Treatment

Treatment is aimed toward removing necrotic debris and maintaining a moist wound bed that will promote healing and formation of granulation tissue. The type of dressing that is recommended depends on the location and depth of the wound, whether necrotic tissue or dead space is present, and the amount of exudate (Table 4–5). Pressure-reducing devices (eg, air-fluid beds and

Table 4–5. Treatment of pressure ulcers.

Ulcer Type	Dressing Type and Considerations
Stage I	Polyurethane film Hydrocolloid wafer Semipermeable foam dressing
Stage II	Hydrocolloid wafers Semipermeable foam dressing Polyurethane film
Stage III/IV	For highly exudative wounds, use highly absorptive dressing or packing, such as calcium alginate Wounds with necrotic debris must be debrided Debridement can be autolytic, mechanical (wet to moist), or surgical Shallow, clean wounds can be dressed with hydrocolloid wafers, semipermeable foam, or polyurethane Deep wounds can be packed with gauze; if the wound is deep and highly exudative, an absorptive packing should be used
Heel ulcer	Do not remove eschar on heel ulcers because it can help promote healing (eschar in other locations should be debrided)

low air loss beds) are associated with improved healing rates. Although poor nutritional status is a risk factor for the development of pressure ulcers, the results of trials of nutritional supplementation in the treatment of pressure ulcers have been disappointing.

Practitioners can become easily overwhelmed by the array of products available for treatment of established pressure ulcers. Most institutions should designate a wound care expert or wound care team to select a streamlined wound care product line that has simple guidelines.

Complications

Pressure ulcers are associated with increased mortality rates, although a causal link has not been proven. Complications include pain, cellulitis, osteomyelitis, systemic sepsis, and prolongation of lengths of stay in the inpatient or nursing home setting.

PHARMACOTHERAPY & POLYPHARMACY

There are several reasons for the greater incidence of iatrogenic drug reactions in the elderly population, the most important of which is the high number of medications that are taken by elders, especially those with multiple comorbidities. Drug metabolism is often impaired in this group, due to a decrease in glomerular filtration rate as well as reduced hepatic clearance. The latter is due to decreased activity of microsomal enzymes and reduced hepatic perfusion with aging. The volume of distribution of drugs is also affected. Since older adults have a decrease in total body water and a relative increase in body fat, water-soluble drugs become more concentrated and fat-soluble drugs have longer half-lives. Serum albumin levels decrease, especially in acutely ill patients, with reduction in protein binding of some drugs (eg, warfarin, phenytoin), leaving more free (active) drug available.

Older individuals often have varying responses to a given serum drug level. Thus, they are more sensitive to some drugs (eg, opioids) and less sensitive to others (eg, β-blocking agents).

Precautions in Administering Drugs

The symptom requiring treatment may be due to another drug, leading to a "prescribing cascade," in which adverse drug effects are attributed to new medical conditions, in time resulting in prescription of still more medications.

Nonpharmacologic interventions can often be a first-line alternative to drugs (eg, mild hypertension or type 2 diabetes mellitus). Pharmacotherapy is not necessarily indicated in some common clinical situations. In asymptomatic bacteriuria, for example, antibiotics need not be given unless the disorder is associated with obstructive uropathy, other anatomic abnormalities, or stones. Ankle edema is often due to venous insuffi-

ciency, drugs (NSAIDs, calcium channel blockers), malnutrition, or inactivity in chair-bound patients and need not be treated with diuretics unless associated with heart failure. Leg elevation in the evening or fitted pressure-gradient stockings are often helpful.

Therapy is begun with less than the usual adult dosage and the dosage increased slowly, consistent with its pharmacokinetics in older patients. However, age-related changes in drug distribution and clearance are variable among individuals, and some require full doses. After determining acceptable measures of success and toxicity, the dose is increased until one or the other is reached.

Despite the importance of beginning new drugs in a slow, measured fashion, all too often an inadequate trial is permitted (in terms of duration of course, or ultimate dose) before they are discontinued. Angiotensin-converting enzyme inhibitors and antidepressants, in particular, are frequently stopped before therapeutic dosages are reached.

Steps are taken to improve adherence to the prescribed medical regimen. The following increase the odds of nonadherence: The patient lives alone; uses more than one pharmacy or provider; is prescribed medications with multiple daily doses; has a drug regimen that is changed frequently; is prescribed a large number of drugs; has difficulty reaching a pharmacy; and has poor cognition, vision, or dexterity. When possible, the provider should keep the dosing schedule simple, the number of pills low, and the medication changes infrequent.

The patient or caregiver is asked to bring in all medications at each visit for reinforcing instructions regarding reasons for drug use, dosage, frequency of administration, and possible adverse effects.

Although serum drug levels may be useful for monitoring certain drugs with narrow therapeutic windows (eg, digoxin), toxicity can still occur even with "normal" therapeutic levels of many drugs. The risk of toxicity goes up with the number of medications prescribed. Certain combinations of medications (eg, warfarin and many types of antibiotics, digoxin and clarithromycin, angiotensin-converting enzyme inhibitors and NSAIDs) are particularly likely to cause drug-drug interactions, and should be watched carefully.

Trials of individual drug discontinuation should be considered (including sedative-hypnotics, digoxin, proton pump inhibitors, NSAIDs) when the original indication is unclear, the goals of care have changed, or the patient might be experiencing side effects.

The Medicare prescription drug benefit in the United States certainly helps many elders with burdensome prescription drug costs. However, it is unclear how successful the program will be overall. Its benefits are complex and difficult to understand, particularly for those elders with limited cognition, literacy, and Internet access. Information is available at www.medicare.gov.

Care at the End of Life

5

Michael W. Rabow, MD, & Steven Z. Pantilat, MD

■ THE END OF LIFE

THE DEFINITION OF THE END OF LIFE

In the United States, approximately 2.4 million people die each year. While death itself remains a mystery and while caring for the dying traditionally has not been well researched or adequately taught as part of medical training, caring for patients at the end of life is an important responsibility and a rewarding opportunity for clinicians. Clinicians battling to prolong life must recognize when life is ending in order to continue caring properly for their patients. Unfortunately, end-of-life practices do not always meet the standards set by professional organizations and most clinical practice guidelines do not include significant attention to end-of-life care. End-of-life care refers to focusing care for those approaching death on the goals of relieving distressing symptoms and promoting quality of life rather than attempting to cure underlying disease. From the medical perspective, the end of life may be defined as that time when death—whether due to terminal illness, acute or chronic illness, or age itself—is expected within weeks to months and can no longer be reasonably forestalled by medical intervention. Yet, the palliative approach to caring for patients facing the end of life outlined in this chapter applies equally well to any patient with a serious, chronic illness at any point in their illness trajectory and should be provided simultaneously with all other appropriate medical treatments.

PROGNOSIS AT THE END OF LIFE

Clinicians play an important role in helping patients understand that their lives are ending. This information influences patients' treatment decisions and may change how they spend their remaining time. While certain diseases such as cancer are more amenable to prognostic estimates regarding the time course to death, the other common causes of mortality in the United States—including heart disease, stroke, chronic lung disease, and dementia—have more variable trajectories and difficult to predict prognoses (Figure 5–1). Even for patients with cancer, clinician estimates of prognosis are often inaccurate and generally overly optimistic. Nonetheless, clinical experience, epidemiologic data, guidelines from professional organizations,* and computer modeling and pre-

diction tools† may be used to help patients identify the end period of their lives. Clinicians can also ask themselves "Would I be surprised if this patient died in the next year?" to determine whether a discussion of prognosis and provision of end-of-life care would be appropriate. If the answer is "no," then the clinician should initiate a discussion. Recognizing that patients may have different levels of comfort with prognostic information, clinicians can introduce the topic by simply saying, "I have information about the likely time course of your illness. Would you like to talk about it?"

EXPECTATIONS ABOUT THE END OF LIFE

Patients' experiences of the end of life are influenced by their expectations about how they will die and the meaning of death. Many people fear how they will die more than death itself. Patients report fear of dying in pain or of suffocation, of loss of control, indignity, isolation, and being a burden to their families. All of these anxieties may be alleviated with good supportive care provided by an attentive group of caretakers.

Since medical advances can often forestall the end of life, death has become "medicalized." No longer seen clearly as a natural and profound personal and spiritual event basic to the human condition, death is often regarded by clinicians, patients, and families as a failure of medical science. This attitude can create or heighten a sense of guilt about the failure to prevent dying. Both the general public and clinicians are complicit in denying death, treating dying persons as patients and death as an enemy to be battled furiously in hospitals rather than as an inevitable outcome to be experienced as a part of life at home. As a result, approximately 75–80% of people in the United States die in hospitals or long-term care facilities.

The clinician may continue to pursue cure of potentially reversible disease for some patients. For all, however, offering comfort and helping the patient prepare for death are foremost considerations. Patients at the end of life and their families identify a number of ele-

---

*For example, the National Hospice Organization.
†For example, the Acute Physiology and Chronic Health Evaluation (APACHE) system, the Study to Understand Prognoses and Preferences for Outcomes and Risks of Treatment (SUPPORT) model, or the Palliative Performance Scale.

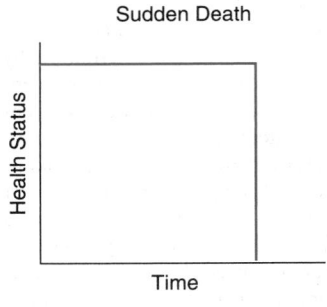
Sudden Death

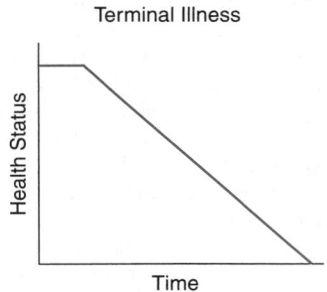
Terminal Illness

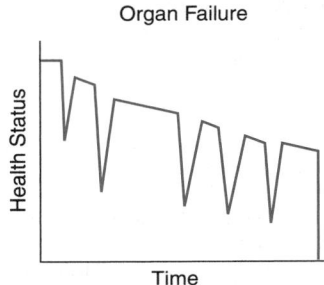
Organ Failure

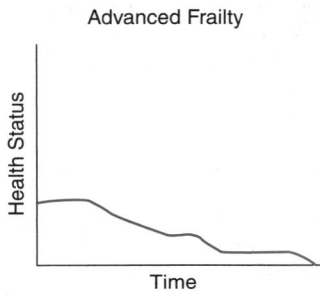
Advanced Frailty

Figure 5–1. Theoretical trajectories of dying. (Adapted, with permission, from Lunney JR et al: Profiles of older Medicare decedents. J Am Geriatr Soc 2002;50:1108.)

ments as important to quality end-of-life care: adequate pain and symptom management, avoiding inappropriate prolongation of dying, preserving dignity, preparing for death, achieving a sense of control, relieving the burden on others, and strengthening relationships with loved ones. Clinicians can help patients pursue their care goals in a process called advance care planning.

COMMUNICATION & CARE OF THE PATIENT

Caring for patients at the end of life requires the same skills clinicians use in other tasks of medical care: diagnosing treatable conditions, providing patient education, facilitating decision-making, and expressing understanding and caring. Communication skills are vitally important. In particular, clinicians must become experts at delivering bad news and then dealing with its consequences (Table 5–1). Higher-quality communication is associated with greater satisfaction and awareness of patient wishes. Three further obligations are central to the clinician's role at this time. First, he or she must work to identify, understand, and relieve suffering, which may include physical, psychological, social, or spiritual distress. Disease and disability at the end of life can threaten a person's sense of integrity or "intactness" and thereby cause suffering. In assisting with redirection and growth, providing support, assessing meaning, and fostering transcendence, clinicians can help ameliorate their patients' suffering and help the patient live fully during this stage of life. Second, clinicians can serve as facilitators or catalysts for hope. While a particular outcome may be extremely unlikely (such as cure of advanced cancer following exhaustive conventional and experimental treatments), hope may be defined as the patient's belief in what is *still* possible. Although expecting a "miraculous cure" may be simplistic and even harmful, hope for relief of pain, for reconciliation with loved ones, for discovery of meaning, and for spiritual transformation is realistic at the end of life. With questions such as "What is still possible now for you?"—"What do you wish for before you die?"—"What good might come of this?" clinicians can help patients uncover hope, explore meaningful and realistic goals, and develop strategies to realize them.

Third, dying patients' feelings of isolation and fear demand that clinicians assert that care will continue to be provided throughout the final stage of life. The promise of nonabandonment is perhaps the central principle of end-of-life care and is a clinician's pledge to an individual patient to serve as a caring partner, a resource for creative problem-solving and relief of suffer-

Table 5–1. Suggestions for the delivery of bad news.

Prepare an appropriate place and time.
Address basic information needs.
Be direct; avoid jargon and euphemisms.
Allow for silence and emotional ventilation.
Assess and validate patient reactions.
Respond to immediate discomforts and risks.
Listen actively and express empathy.
Achieve a common perception of the problem.
Reassure about pain relief.
Ensure basic follow-up and make specific plans for the future.

ing, a guide during uncertain times, and a witness to the patient's experiences—no matter what happens. Clinicians can say to a patient, "I will care for you whatever happens." Dying patients need their clinicians to offer their presence—not necessarily the ability to solve all problems but rather a commitment to recognize and receive the patients' difficulties and experiences with respect and empathy. At its best, the patient-clinician relationship can be a covenant of compassion and a recognition of common humanity.

CARING FOR THE FAMILY

In caring for patients at the end of life, clinicians must appreciate the central role played by family, friends, and romantic partners and often must deal with strong emotions of fear, anger, shame, sadness, and guilt experienced by those individuals. While significant others may support and comfort a patient at the end of life, the threatened loss of a loved one may also create or reveal dysfunctional or painful family dynamics. Furthermore, clinicians must be attuned to the potential impact of illness on the patient's family: substantial physical caregiving responsibilities and financial burdens as well as increased rates of anxiety, depression, chronic illness, and even mortality. Family caregivers, typically women, commonly provide the bulk of care for patients at the end of life, yet their work is often not acknowledged or compensated.

Clinicians can help families confront the imminent loss of a loved one (Table 5–2) and often must negotiate amid complex and changing family needs. Identifying a spokesperson for the family, conducting family meetings, allowing all to be heard, and providing time for consensus may help the clinician work effectively with the family.

CLINICIAN SELF-CARE

Many clinicians find caring for patients at the end of life to be one of the most rewarding aspects of practice. However, working with the dying requires tolerance of great uncertainty, ambiguity, and existential challenges.

Table 5–2. Clinician behaviors helpful to families of dying patients.

Timely, frequent, and consistent communication
Adapting communication to need
Focusing on patient's wishes
Attending to the comfort of the patient
Being aware of family conflict
Accommodating family's grief
Refocusing hope
Encouraging planning
Remaining available
Following up with family after death

Adapted, with permission, from Bascom PB, Tolle SW: Care of the family when the patient is dying. West J Med 1995;163:292.

Clinicians must recognize and respect their own limitations and attend to their own needs in order to avoid being overburdened, overly distressed, or emotionally depleted. Open recognition of their own feelings enables clinicians to process their emotions and take steps to care for themselves: conferring and consulting with colleagues, retreating, relaxing and recuperating, obtaining informal or professional support, or even—under extraordinary circumstances—transferring the care of a patient to another clinician when it is no longer possible for the original clinician to meet the patient's needs. Moreover, care of patients at the end of life is not solely the responsibility of physicians. Ideally, physicians, nurses, social workers, chaplains, pharmacists, and other clinicians should coordinate their efforts as part of an interdisciplinary team to care for patients and support one another.

Lamont EB et al: Complexities in prognostication in advanced cancer: "To help them live their lives the way they want to." JAMA 2003;290:98. [PMID: 12837717]

Lunney JR et al: Patterns of functional decline at the end of life. JAMA 2003;289:2387. [PMID: 12746362]

Mast KR et al: End-of-life content in treatment guidelines for life-limiting diseases. J Palliat Med 2004;7:754. [PMID: 15684843]

Mularski RA et al: Quality of dying in the ICU: ratings by family members. Chest 2005;128:28. [PMID: 16002947]

Rabow MW et al: Supporting family caregivers at the end of life: "they don't know what they don't know." JAMA 2004; 291:483. [PMID: 14747506]

Stevens LM et al: JAMA patient page. Palliative care. JAMA 2005; 293:1410. [PMID: 15769975]

■ THE SETTING & STRUCTURE OF CARE

ETHICAL & LEGAL BACKGROUND

Clinicians may be limited in caring for persons at the end of life not only by their emotional responses but by a sense of moral obligation as well. While the ethical, legal, and professional controversies over assisted suicide are beyond the scope of this chapter, clinicians should be aware of the "right to die" movement as an expression, at least in part, of patient dissatisfaction with how people are cared for at the end of life. In the United States, assisted suicide is illegal in every state but Oregon—and legal there only with careful restrictions. While individual clinicians must decide for themselves within the evolving legal context what their personal limits may be in caring for patients who request aid in dying (eg, assisted suicide), all clinicians can reclaim their long-privileged and universally accepted role of caring for the dying. They can do so by dedicating themselves not to abandon their patients and by providing appropriate attention to symptom management, sensitivity to psychological and social stresses, and unconditional presence and openness to spiritual challenges at the end of life. Research has demonstrated that palliative care interventions can cause some patients who have requested assisted suicide to withdraw their request.

Clinicians' care of patients at the end of life is guided by the same ethical and legal principles that inform other types of medical care. Foremost are truthtelling, nonmaleficence, beneficence, autonomy, confidentiality, proportionality, and distributive justice. These principles must guide clinicians in helping patients make difficult decisions about care, including decisions about palliative sedation and the withdrawal and withholding of life-prolonging interventions.

Important ethical principles may be in conflict. For example, while a patient may desire a particular medical intervention, the clinician may decline to undertake the intervention if it is of no therapeutic benefit (ie, futile) or violates the clinician's own moral code. Clinicians must use caution in invoking futility, since what constitutes futility is often a matter of controversy. Studies confirm that most disagreements can be resolved through repeated discussions between clinicians and families. Although clinicians and family members often feel differently about withholding versus withdrawing support, there is consensus among ethicists, supported by legal precedent, of their ethical equivalence. Patients and their surrogates have the same right to stop unwanted medical treatments once begun as they do to refuse those treatments in the first place, including nutrition and hydration. The ethical principle of "double effect" argues that the potential to hasten imminent death is acceptable if it comes as the unintended consequence of a primary intention to provide comfort and relieve suffering. For example, sufficient doses of morphine should be provided to control pain even if there is the potential unintended secondary effect of depressing respiration. The ethical argument for the practice of palliative sedation is based on this principle. In practice, one can almost always find an effective pain regimen without rendering a patient unconscious.

DECISION-MAKING, ADVANCE CARE PLANNING, & ADVANCE DIRECTIVES

Well-informed, competent adults have a right to refuse medical intervention even if this is likely to result in death. Many are willing to sacrifice some quantity of life in exchange for protecting a certain quality of life. In order to further patient autonomy, clinicians are obligated to inform patients about the risks, benefits, alternatives, and expected outcomes of end-of-life medical interventions such as cardiopulmonary resuscitation (CPR), intubation and mechanical ventilation, vasopressor medication, hospitalization and ICU care, and nutrition and hydration. Advance directives are oral or written statements made by patients when they are competent that are intended to guide care should they become incompetent. Advance directives allow patients to project their autonomy into the future and are an important part of advance care planning—a process whereby patients consider various paths their illness may take and contingencies for responding to these possible developments based on their care goals and values. While oral statements about these matters are ethically binding, they are not legally binding in all states. State-specific advance directive forms are available from a number of sources, including the Web site www.caringinfo.org.

In addition to documenting patient preferences for care, the Durable Power of Attorney for Health Care (DPOA-HC) allows the patient to designate a surrogate decision-maker. The DPOA-HC is important since it is often difficult to anticipate what decisions will need to be made. The responsibility of the surrogate is to provide "substituted judgment"—to decide as the *patient* would, not as the *surrogate* wants. In the absence of a designated surrogate, clinicians usually turn to family members or next of kin. Unfortunately, surveys demonstrate that clinicians and families often are no better than chance at predicting patient wishes, so it is imperative to have these discussions with all patients.

Clinicians should educate all patients—ideally, well before the end of life—about the opportunity to formulate an advance directive. Most patients have already thought about end-of-life issues, want to discuss them with their clinician, want the clinician to bring up the subject, and feel better for having had the discussion. Despite regulations requiring health care institutions to inform patients of their rights to formulate an advance directive, only about 10% of people in the United States (including clinicians themselves) actually have completed them, and studies have shown that clinicians are often unaware of or actually ignore their patients' advance directives.

DNAR ORDERS

As part of advance care planning, clinicians can encourage patients to express their preferences for the use of CPR. Most patients and many clinicians are uninformed or misinformed about the nature and success of CPR. Only about 15% of all patients who undergo CPR in the hospital survive to hospital discharge. Moreover, among certain populations—especially those with serious systemic noncardiac disease, metastatic cancer, and sepsis—the likelihood of survival to hospital discharge following CPR is virtually nil.

Patients may ask their clinician to write an order that CPR not be attempted on them. Although this order initially was referred to as a DNR ("do not resuscitate") order, many clinicians prefer the term DNAR ("do not attempt resuscitation") to emphasize the low likelihood of success.

Patients deciding about CPR preferences should also be informed about the sequelae of surviving CPR. It may result in fractured ribs, lacerated internal organs, and neurologic disability, and there is a high likelihood of a need for other aggressive interventions, such as ICU care, if CPR is successful.

For some patients at the end of life, decisions about CPR may be not about whether they will live but about how they will die. Clinicians should correct the misconception that withholding CPR in appropriate circumstances is tantamount to "not doing everything" or "just letting someone die." Typically, CPR does not improve the quality of a dying patient's life or alter the patient's underlying prognosis. While respecting the patient's right ultimately to make the decision—and keeping in mind their own biases and prejudices—clinicians should offer explicit recommendations about DNAR orders and protect dying patients and their families from feelings of guilt and from the sorrow associated with vain hopes. Finally, clinicians should encourage patients and their families to make proactive decisions about what is wanted in end-of-life care rather than focusing only on what is not to be done.

HOSPICE & OTHER PALLIATIVE CARE INSTITUTIONS

While most patients die in hospitals and while the number of hospital-based palliative care services is growing, good care of the dying may not be the central goal of most hospitals. Hospice is an approach to end-of-life care where the most urgent objective is to address the physical and emotional needs of the dying. Hospice care focuses on the patient and family rather than the disease and on providing comfort and pain relief rather than on treating illness or prolonging life. Hospices provide intensive caring with the goal of helping people live well until they die.

Hospice embodies the palliative care philosophy that emphasizes individualized attention, human contact, and an interdisciplinary team approach. Hospice care can include arranging for respite for family caregivers and providing legal, financial, and other services. While some hospice care is provided in hospitals and institutional residences, about 80% of patients receiving hospice care remain at home where they can be cared for by the family and visiting hospice staff. Primary care clinicians are strongly encouraged to continue caring for their patients during the time they are receiving hospice care.

Hospice care is highly rated by families and has been shown to increase patient satisfaction, to reduce costs (depending on when patients are referred to hospice care), and even to decrease family caregiver mortality. More than 25% of all patients who die in the United States receive hospice care, and about 50% of these people have end-stage cancer. Hospice care tends to be utilized late in the course of the end of life. The median length of stay in hospices in the United States is just 26 days, with 34% of patients dying within 7 days after beginning hospice care.

Most hospice organizations require clinicians to estimate the patient's probability of survival to be less than 6 months, since this is a criterion for eligibility to receive Medicare or other insurance coverage. Regrettably, the hospice benefit can be difficult to provide to people who are homeless or isolated or who have terminal prognoses that are difficult to quantify.

While the initiation of hospice care is often described as a transition from aggressive care to comfort care, hospice care also provides "aggressive" care, though not directed at achieving a cure or prolonging life. It is more appropriate to consider hospice care as one among many health care resources available to patients at the end of life. For the dying, it may be appropriate to "treat" pneumonia with morphine and antipyretics rather than with antibiotics. Helping patients decide when to avail themselves of the resources of hospice or inpatient palliative care is an important function even for clinicians providing the most aggressive and intensive curative medical interventions. While most people prefer to die at home, inpatient palliative care may be more appropriate for patients with complex, severe symptoms that are difficult to manage at home.

While the numbers of Americans dying in nursing homes is increasing, many long-term care facilities do not have staff trained in palliative care or provide formal palliative care services. Increasingly, however, long-term care facilities are recognizing their need to become experts in end-of-life care and a number of quality improvement programs show promise.

CULTURAL ISSUES

The individual's experience of dying occurs in the context of a complex interaction of personal, philosophic, and cultural influences. Various religious, ethnic, gender, class, and cultural traditions inform patients' styles of communication, comfort in discussing particular topics, expectations about dying and medical interventions, and attitudes about the appropriate disposition of dead bodies. There are differences in knowledge and beliefs regarding advance directives, autopsy, organ donation, hospice care, and withdrawal of support among patients of different ethnic groups. Clinicians must appreciate recent evidence suggesting that palliative care is susceptible to some of the same racial biases previously documented in other medical disciplines. While each patient must be considered an individual, understanding a person's cultural assumptions and beliefs and respecting ethnic traditions are important responsibilities of the clinician caring for a patient at the end of life, especially when the cultures of origin of the clinician and patient differ. A clinician may ask a patient, "What do I need to know about you and your beliefs that will help me take care of you?"

Christakis NA et al: The health impact of health care on families: a matched cohort study of hospice use by decedents and mortality outcomes in surviving, widowed spouses. Soc Sci Med 2003;57:465. [PMID: 12791489]

Hanson LC et al: Meeting palliative care needs in post-acute care settings: "to help them live until they die." JAMA 2006; 295:681. [PMID: 16467237]

Lo B et al: Palliative sedation in dying patients: "we turn to it when everything else hasn't worked." JAMA 2005;29:1810. [PMID: 16219885]

Morrison RS et al: The growth of palliative care programs in United States hospitals. J Palliat Med 2005;8:1127. [PMID: 16351525]

Teno JM et al: Family perspectives on end-of-life care at the last place of care. JAMA 2004;291:88. [PMID: 14709580]

Tulsky JA: Beyond advance directives: importance of communication skills at the end of life. JAMA 2005;294:359. [PMID: 16030281]

Weissman DE: Decision making at a time of crisis near the end of life. JAMA 2004;292:1738. [PMID: 15479939]

■ MANAGEMENT OF PAIN & OTHER COMMON SYMPTOMS

For patients at the end of life, maximizing the quality of life—rather than postponing death—is often the first priority of care. In this context, symptoms that cause disability and suffering must be considered medical emergencies and managed aggressively by frequent elicitation, continuous reassessment, and individualized treatment. While patients at the end of life may experience a host of distressing symptoms, pain, dyspnea, and delirium are reported to be among the most feared and burdensome. The palliative care of pain and a selected number of other common symptoms is described below. Throughout, the principles of good end-of-life care dictate that comfort is the main focus of palliative care and that properly informed patients or their surrogates may decide to pursue aggressive symptom relief even if, as a known but unintended consequence, the treatments hasten demise or preclude curative attempts. There is even a growing awareness that scrupulous symptom control for patients with end-stage illness may prolong life.

PAIN AT THE END OF LIFE

Definition & Prevalence

Pain is a common problem for patients at the end of life—up to 75% of patients dying of cancer experience pain—and it is what many people say they fear most about dying. Pain is a common complaint among patients with noncancer diagnoses as well. Pain is undertreated at the end of life. Up to 50% of severely ill hospitalized patients spent half of their time during the last 3 days of life in moderate to severe pain. The Joint Commission on Accreditation of Healthcare Organizations (JCAHO) includes pain management standards for all patient care organizations it accredits.

The experience of pain includes the patient's emotional reaction to it and is influenced by many factors, including the patient's prior experiences with pain, the meaning of the pain, emotional stresses, and the influence of family and culture. Pain is a subjective phenomenon, and clinicians cannot reliably detect its existence or quantify its severity without asking the patient directly. A useful means of assessing pain and evaluating the effectiveness of analgesia is to ask the patient to rate the degree of pain along a numerical or visual pain scale (Table 5–3).

Barriers to Good Care

Poor management of pain at the end of life has been documented in many settings. Some clinicians refer pain management to others when they believe that a patient's pain is not due to the disease for which they are treating the patient. Even oncologists often misperceive the origin of their patients' pain and inappropriately ignore complaints of pain.

Many clinicians have limited training and clinical experience with pain management and thus are understandably reluctant to attempt to manage severe pain. Lack of knowledge about the proper selection and dosing of analgesic medications carries with it attendant and typically exaggerated fears about the side effects of pain medications, including the possibility of respiratory depression with an overdose of opioids. Most clinicians, however, can develop good pain management skills, and nearly all pain, even at the end of life, can be managed without hastening death through respiratory depression.

Fears of the physiologic effects of opioids are often coupled with concerns on the part of clinician, patient, or family that patients will become addicted to opioid pain medications. While physiologic **tolerance** (requiring increasing dosage to achieve the same analgesic effect) and **dependence** (requiring continued dosing to prevent symptoms of medication withdrawal) are expected with opioid use, at the end of life the use of opioids for relief of pain and dyspnea is not associated with a risk of psychological **addiction** (misuse of a substance for purposes other than one for which it was prescribed and despite negative consequences in health, employment, or legal and social spheres). Even patients who demonstrate some of the behaviors sometimes associated with addiction (demand for specific medications and doses, anger and irritability, poor cooperation or disturbed interpersonal reactions) may in fact not be addicted. The term **pseudoaddiction** has been used when patients exhibit behaviors associated with addiction but only because their pain is inadequately treated. Once they achieve pain relief, these behaviors cease. In all cases, clinicians must be willing to use appropriate doses of opioids in order to relieve distressing symptoms for patients at the end of life.

Finally, some clinicians fear legal repercussions from prescribing the high doses of opioids sometimes necessary to control pain at the end of life. Some states have enacted special licensing and documentation requirements for opioid prescribing. However, governmental and professional medical groups, regulators, and the US Supreme Court are making it clear that appropriate treatment of pain is the right of the patient and a fundamental responsibility of the clinician. In fact, clinicians have been successfully sued for undertreatment of pain. Although clinicians may feel trapped between conse-

Table 5–3. Pain assessment scales.

A. Numeric Rating Scale

No pain   Worst pain

0   1   2   3   4   5   6   7   8   9   10

B. Numeric Rating Scale Translated into Word and Behavior Scales

Pain intensity	Word scale	Nonverbal behaviors
0	No pain	Relaxed, calm expression
1–2	Least pain	Stressed, tense expression
3–4	Mild pain	Guarded movement, grimacing
5–6	Moderate pain	Moaning, restless
7–8	Severe pain	Crying out
9–10	Excruciating pain	Increased intensity of above

C. Wong Baker FACES Pain Rating Scale[1]

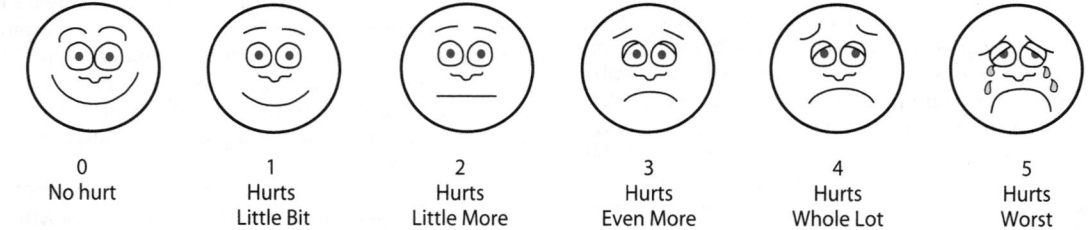

0	1	2	3	4	5
No hurt	Hurts Little Bit	Hurts Little More	Hurts Even More	Hurts Whole Lot	Hurts Worst

[1]Especially useful for patients who cannot read English and for pediatric patients. Wong DL, Hockenberry-Eaton M, Wilson D, Winkelstein ML, Ahmann E, DeVito-Thomas PA: *Whaley and Wong's Nursing Care of Infants and Children*, ed. 6. St. Louis, 1999, Mosby, p. 1153. Copyrighted by Mosby-Year Book, Inc. Reprinted by permission.

---

quences of overprescribing or underprescribing opioids, there remains a wide range of practice in which clinicians can appropriately treat pain. Referral to pain management experts is appropriate whenever pain cannot be controlled expeditiously by the primary clinician.

Principles of Pain Management

General guidelines for management of pain are recommended for the treatment of all patients with pain (Table 5–4). Because pain is so common at the end of life, all patients should be asked about its presence. Clinicians should ask about the nature, severity, timing, location, quality, and aggravating and relieving factors of the pain. Distinguishing between somatic, visceral, and neuropathic pain is essential to proper tailoring of pain treatments. The goal of pain management is properly decided by the patient. Some patients may wish to be completely free of pain even at the cost of significant sedation, while others will wish to control pain to a level that still allows maximal functioning.

Chronic severe pain should be treated continuously. For ongoing pain, one can give a long-acting analgesic around the clock plus a short-acting drug as needed for "breakthrough" pain. At the end of life, the oral route of administration is preferred because it is easier to adminis-

ter at home, is not painful, and imposes no risk from needle exposure. Rectal, transdermal, and subcutaneous administration are also frequently used, as is intravenous or intrathecal administration when necessary. Patient-controlled analgesia (PCA) of intravenous medications is appreciated by patients, may lead to less medication use, and has been adapted for use with oral administration.

When possible, the cause of pain should be diagnosed and treated, assuming that the burden of these efforts does not increase the patient's suffering. Removing the underlying cause of pain can preempt the need for ongoing treatment with analgesic medications along with their side effects. Regardless of decisions about seeking and treating the underlying cause of pain, however, prompt symptomatic relief of pain should be offered to every patient.

Pharmacologic Pain Management Strategies

Typically, pain can be well controlled with analgesic medications—both opioid and nonopioid. Evidence-based summaries and guidelines are available from the Agency for Healthcare Research and Quality (http://www.ncbi.nlm.nih.gov/books/bv.fcgi?rid=hstat1.chapter.86205) and other organizations (http://www.nccn.

Table 5–4. Recommended clinical approach to pain management.

Ask about pain regularly. Assess pain systematically (quality, description, location, intensity or severity, aggravating and ameliorating factors, cognitive responses). Ask about goals for pain control, management preferences.

Believe the patient and family in their reports of pain and what relieves it.

Choose pain control options appropriate for the patient, family, and setting. Consider drug type, dosage, route, contraindications, side effects. Consider nonpharmacologic adjunctive measures.

Deliver interventions in a timely, logical, coordinated manner.

Empower patients and their families. Enable patients to control their course to the greatest extent possible.

Follow up to reassess persistence of pain, changes in pain pattern, development of new pain.

Modified from Jacox AK et al: *Management of Cancer Pain: Quick Reference Guide No. 9.* AHCPR Publication No. 94–0593. Rockville, MD: Agency for Health Care Policy and Research, Public Health Service, U.S. Department of Health and Human Services. March 1994.

org/professionals/physician_gls/PDF/pain.pdf). For mild to moderate pain, acetaminophen, aspirin, and nonsteroidal anti-inflammatory drugs (NSAIDs) may be sufficient. For moderate to severe pain, analgesics that include those agents combined with opioids may be helpful. Severe pain typically requires full opioid agonists.

A. ACETAMINOPHEN AND NSAIDs

Appropriate doses of acetaminophen may be just as effective as an analgesic and antipyretic as NSAIDs but without anti-inflammatory effects and without the risk of gastrointestinal bleeding or ulceration. Acetaminophen can be given at a dosage of 500–1000 mg orally every 6 hours, although it can be taken every 4 hours as long as the risk of hepatotoxicity is kept in mind. Hepatotoxicity is a concern at doses greater than 4 g/d long-term, and doses for older patients and those with liver disease generally should not exceed 2 g/d.

Aspirin (325–650 mg orally every 4 hours) is an effective analgesic, antipyretic, and anti-inflammatory medication. Gastrointestinal irritation and bleeding, bleeding from other sources, allergy, and an association with Reye's syndrome in children and teenagers limit its use.

Commonly used NSAIDs and their dosages are listed in Table 5–5. Like aspirin, the other NSAIDs are antipyretic, analgesic, and anti-inflammatory. NSAIDs inhibit prostaglandin synthesis, inhibiting platelet aggregation and consequently increasing the risk of gastrointestinal bleeding by 1.5 times normal. The risks of bleeding and nephrotoxicity from NSAIDs are both increased in elders. Gastrointestinal bleeding and ulceration may be decreased with the concurrent use of proton pump inhibitors (eg, omeprazole, 20–40 mg orally daily)

or with the class of NSAIDs that inhibit only cyclooxygenase (COX)-2. Serious concerns about the safety of COX-2 inhibitors have led to the withdrawal of both rofecoxib and valdecoxib by their manufacturers; the Food and Drug Administration is conducting an ongoing review of this drug class. The only currently available COX-2 inhibitor is celecoxib (100 mg/d to 200 mg twice daily orally), which clinicians should use with caution in patients with cardiac disease because of its possible association with an increased risk of myocardial infarction. The NSAIDs, including COX-2 inhibitors, can lead to exacerbations of congestive heart failure and should be used with caution in patients with that disorder.

B. OPIOID MEDICATIONS

For many patients at the end of life, opioids are the mainstay of pain management. Opioids are appropriate for severe pain due to any cause. Opioid medications are listed in Table 5–6. Full opioid agonists such as morphine, hydromorphone, oxycodone, methadone, fentanyl, hydrocodone, and codeine are used most commonly. Hydrocodone and codeine are typically combined with acetaminophen or an NSAID. Short-acting formulations of oral morphine sulfate (starting dosage 4 mg orally every 3–4 hours), hydromorphone (1 mg orally every 3–4 hours), or oxycodone (5 mg orally every 3–4 hours) are useful for acute pain and as rescue treatment for patients experiencing pain that breaks through long-acting medications. For chronic stable pain, one should give sustained-release morphine (one to three times a day) or oxycodone (two or three times a day), methadone (three or four times a day), or transdermal fentanyl (starting dose 25 mcg every 3 days, with 24–40 hours required to achieve full analgesia).

Meperidine is not useful for chronic pain because it has a short half-life and a toxic metabolite that can cause irritability and seizures. Partial agonists such as buprenorphine are limited by a dose-related ceiling effect. Mixed agonist-antagonists such as pentazocine and butorphanol tartrate also have a ceiling effect and are contraindicated in patients already receiving full agonist opioids since they may reverse the pain control achieved by the full agonist and cause a withdrawal effect.

A useful technique for opioid management of chronic pain at the end of life is equianalgesic dosing (Table 5–6). The dosages of any full opioid agonists used to control pain can be translated into an equivalent dose of any other opioid. In this way, 24-hour opioid requirements and dosing regimens established initially using shorter-acting opioid medications can be translated into equivalent dosages of longer-acting medications or formulations. Cross-tolerance is often incomplete, however, so less than the full calculated equianalgesic dosage is generally administered initially when switching between opioid formulations. In addition, equianalgesic dosing for methadone is somewhat more complex and varies by dose.

While some clinicians and patients inexperienced with the management of severe chronic pain may feel more comfortable with combined nonopioid-opioid

Table 5–5. Acetaminophen, COX-2 inhibitors, and useful nonsteroidal anti-inflammatory drugs.

Drug	Usual Dose for Adults ≥ 50 kg	Usual Dose for Adults < 50 kg[1]	Cost per Unit	Cost for 30 Days[2]	Comments[3]
Acetaminophen[4] (Tylenol, Datril, etc)	650 mg q4h or 975 mg q6h	10–15 mg/kg q4h (oral); 15–20 mg/kg q4h (rectal)	$0.02/325 mg (oral) OTC; $0.39/650 mg (rectal) OTC	$7.20 (oral); $70.20 (rectal)	Not an NSAID because it lacks peripheral anti-inflammatory effects. Equivalent to aspirin as analgesic and antipyretic agent.
Aspirin[5]	650 mg q4h or 975 mg q6h	10–15 mg/kg q4h (oral); 15–20 mg/kg q4h (rectal)	$0.02/325 mg OTC; $0.26/600 mg (rectal) OTC	$7.20 (oral); $46.80 (rectal)	Available also in enteric-coated form that is more expensive and more slowly absorbed but better tolerated.
Celecoxib[4] (Celebrex)	200 mg qd (osteoarthritis); 100–200 mg bid (rheumatoid arthritis)	100 mg qd–bid	$1.91/100 mg; $3.14/200 mg	$94.20 OA; $188.40 RA	Cyclooxygenase-2 inhibitor. No antiplatelet effects. Lower doses for elderly who weigh < 50 kg. Lower incidence of endoscopic gastrointestinal ulceration. Not known if true lower incidence of gastrointestinal bleeding. Possible link to cardiovascular toxicity. Celecoxib is contraindicated in sulfonamide allergy.
Choline magnesium salicylate[6] (Trilasate, others)	1000–1500 mg tid	25 mg/kg tid	$0.57/500 mg	$153.90	Salicylates cause less gastrointestinal distress and renal impairment than NSAIDs but are probably less effective in pain management than NSAIDs.
Diclofenac (Voltaren, Cataflam, others)	50–75 mg bid–tid		$1.16/50 mg; $1.41/75 mg	$104.40; $126.90	May impose higher risk of hepatotoxicity. Low incidence of gastrointestinal side effects. Enteric-coated product; slow onset.
Diclofenac Sustained Release (Voltaren-XR, others)	100–200 mg qd		$2.81/100 mg	$168.60	
Diflunisal[7] (Dolobid, others)	500 mg q12h		$1.29/500 mg	$77.40	Fluorinated acetylsalicylic acid derivative.
Etodolac (Lodine, others)	200–400 mg q6–8h		$1.26/300 mg	$151.20	Perhaps less gastrointestinal toxicity.
Fenoprofen calcium (Nalfon, others)	300–600 mg q6h		$0.51/300 mg or 600 mg	$61.20	Perhaps more side effects than others, including tubulointerstitial nephritis.
Flurbiprofen (Ansaid)	50–100 mg tid–qid		$0.79/50 mg; $1.19/100 mg	$94.80; $142.80	Adverse gastrointestinal effects may be more common among elderly.
Ibuprofen (Motrin, Advil, Rufen, others)	400–800 mg q6h	10 mg/kg q6–8h	$0.28/600 mg Rx; $0.05/200 mg OTC	$33.60; $9.00	Relatively well tolerated. Less gastrointestinal toxicity.
Indomethacin (Indocin, Indometh, others)	25–50 mg bid–qid		$0.38/25 mg; $0.64/50 mg	$45.60; $76.80	Higher incidence of dose-related toxic effects, especially gastrointestinal and bone marrow effects.

(continued)

Table 5–5. Acetaminophen, COX-2 inhibitors, and useful nonsteroidal anti-inflammatory drugs. (continued)

Drug	Usual Dose for Adults ≥ 50 kg	Usual Dose for Adults < 50 kg[1]	Cost per Unit	Cost for 30 Days[2]	Comments[3]
Ketoprofen (Orudis, Oruvail, others)	25–75 mg q6–8h (max 300 mg/d)		$0.96/50 mg Rx; $1.07/75 mg Rx; $0.09/ 12.5 mg OTC	$172.80; $128.40; $16.20	Lower doses for elderly.
Ketorolac tromethamine (Toradol)	10 mg q4–6h to a maximum of 40 mg/d PO		$0.93/10 mg	Not recommended	Short-term use (< 5 days) only; otherwise, increased risk of gastrointestinal side effects.
Ketorolac tromethamine[8] (Toradol)	60 mg IM or 30 mg IV initially, then 30 mg q6h IM or IV		$3.89/30 mg	Not recommended	Intramuscular or intravenous NSAID as alternative to opioid. Lower doses for elderly. Short-term use (< 5 days) only.
Magnesium salicylate (various)	650 mg q4h		$0.17/325 mg OTC	$40.80	
Meclofenamate sodium[9] (Meclomen)	50–100 mg q6h		$3.40/100 mg	$408.00	Diarrhea more common.
Mefenamic acid (Ponstel)	250 mg q6h		$2.28/250 mg	$273.60	
Nabumetone (Relafen)	500–1000 mg once daily (max dose 2000 mg/d)		$1.30/500 mg; $1.53/ 750 mg	$91.80	May be less ulcerogenic than ibuprofen, but overall side effects may not be less.
Naproxen (Naprosyn, Anaprox, Aleve [OTC], others)	250–500 mg q6–8h	5 mg/kg q8h	$1.16/500 mg Rx; $0.09/220 mg OTC	$104.40; $8.10 OTC	Generally well tolerated. Lower doses for elderly.
Oxaprozin (Daypro, others)	600–1200 mg once daily		$1.51/600 mg	$90.60	Similar to ibuprofen. May cause rash, pruritus, photosensitivity.
Piroxicam (Feldene, others)	20 mg daily		$2.64/20 mg	$79.20	Single daily dose convenient. Long half-life. May cause higher rate of gastrointestinal bleeding and dermatologic side effects. High adverse drug reaction rate in the elderly.
Sodium salicylate	325–650 mg q3–4h		$0.08/650 mg OTC	$19.20	
Sulindac (Clinoril, others)	150–200 mg bid		$0.98/150 mg; $1.21/ 200 mg	$58.80; $72.60	May cause higher rate of gastrointestinal bleeding. May have less nephrotoxic potential.
Tolmetin (Tolectin)	200–600 mg qid		$0.65/200 mg; $1.62/ 600 mg	$78.00; $194.40	Perhaps more side effects than others, including anaphylactic reactions.

[1]Acetaminophen and NSAID dosages for adults weighing less than 50 kg should be adjusted for weight.
[2]Average wholesale price (AWP, for AB-rated generic when available) for quantity listed. Source: *Red Book* Update, Vol. 25, No. 1, January 2006. AWP may not accurately represent the actual pharmacy cost because wide contractual variations exist among institutions.
[3]The adverse effects of headache, tinnitus, dizziness, confusion, rashes, anorexia, nausea, vomiting, gastrointestinal bleeding, diarrhea, nephrotoxicity, visual disturbances, etc, can occur with any of these drugs. Tolerance and efficacy are subject to great individual variations among patients. Note: All NSAIDs can increase serum lithium levels.
[4]Acetaminophen and celecoxib lack the antiplatelet activities of other NSAIDs.
[5]May inhibit platelet aggregation for 1 week or more and may cause bleeding.
[6]May have minimal antiplatelet activity.
[7]Administration with antacids may decrease absorption.
[8]Has the same gastrointestinal toxicities as oral NSAIDs.
[9]Coombs-positive autoimmune hemolytic anemia has been associated with prolonged use.
OTC = over-the-counter; Rx = prescription; OA = osteoarthritis; RA = rheumatoid arthritis.
Modified from Jacox AK et al: *Management of Cancer Pain: Quick Reference Guide for Clinicians No. 9.* AHCPR Publication No. 94–0593. Rockville, MD: Agency for Health Care Policy and Research, Public Health Service, U.S. Department of Health and Human Services. March 1994.

Table 5–6. Useful opioid agonist analgesics.

Drug	Approximate Equianalgesic Dose[1]		Usual Starting Dose				Potential Advantages	Potential Disadvantages
	Oral	Parenteral	Adults ≥ 50 kg Body Weight		Adults < 50 kg Body Weight			
			Oral	Parenteral	Oral	Parenteral		
			OPIOID AGONISTS[2]					
Fentanyl	Not available	0.1 (100 mcg) q1h	Not available	50–100 mcg IV/IM q1h or 0.5–1.5 mcg/kg/h IV infusion $0.94/100 mcg	Not available	0.5–1 mcg/kg IV q1–4h or 1–2 mcg/kg IV x1, then 0.5–1 mcg/kg/h infusion	Possibly less neuroexcitatory effects, including in renal failure. Oral transmucosal formulation also available.	
Fentanyl Transdermal	Not available orally but can use "2:1 Rule[2]" for transdermal formulation	Not available	Not available orally but 12.5–25 mcg patch q72h $14.42/25 mcg	Not available	Not available orally but 12.5–25 mcg patch q72h	Not available	Stable medication blood levels	Not for use in opioid-naïve patients
Hydromorphone[3] (Dilaudid)	7.5 mg q3–4h	1.5 mg q3–4h	6 mg q3–4h; $0.37/2 mg	1.5 mg q3–4h; $1.02/2 mg	0.06 mg/kg q3–4h	0.015 mg/kg q3–4h	Similar to morphine. Available in injectable high-potency preparation, rectal suppository.	Short duration. (Sales of extended release formulation (Palladone) recently suspended due to potentially fatal interactions with alcohol.)
Levorphanol (Levo-Dromoran)	4 mg q6–8h	2 mg q6–8h	4 mg q6–8h; $1.07/2 mg	2 mg q6–8h; $3.96/2 mg	0.04 mg/kg q6–8h	0.02 mg q6–8h	Longer-acting than morphine sulfate.	
Meperidine[4] (Demerol)	300 mg q2–3h; normal dose 50–150 mg q3–4h	100 mg q3h; $0.69/50 mg	Not recommended; $0.69/50 mg	100 mg q3h; $0.83/100 mg	Not recommended	0.75 mg/kg q2–3h	May be useful for acute pain if the patient is intolerant to morphine.	Short duration. Metabolite in high concentrations may cause seizures.
Methadone (Dolophine, others)	20 mg q6–8h	10 mg q6–8h	20 mg q6–8h; $0.15/10 mg	10 mg q6–8h; $4.03/10 mg	0.2 mg/kg q6–8h	0.1 mg/kg q6–8h	Somewhat longer-acting than morphine. Useful in cases of intolerance to morphine.	Analgesic duration shorter than plasma duration. May accumulate, requiring close monitoring during first weeks of treatment. Equianalgesic ratios vary with dose.
Morphine[3] Immediate release (Roxanol)	30 mg q3–4h (repeat around-the-clock dosing); 60 mg q3–4h (single or intermittent dosing)	10 mg q3–4h	30 mg q3–4h; $0.18/15 mg	10 mg q3–4h; $0.76/10 mg	0.3 mg/kg q3–4h	0.1 mg/kg q3–4h	Standard of comparison; multiple dosage forms available.	No unique problems when compared with other opioids.

(continued)

Table 5–6. Useful opioid agonist analgesics. (continued)

Drug	Approximate Equianalgesic Dose[1] Oral	Parenteral	Usual Starting Dose Adults ≥ 50 kg Body Weight Oral	Parenteral	Adults < 50 kg Body Weight Oral	Parenteral	Potential Advantages	Potential Disadvantages
Morphine Controlled-release[3] (MS Contin, Oramorph)	90–120 mg q12h	Not available	90–120 mg q12h; $1.69/30 mg	Not available	Not available	Not available		
Morphine Extended release (Kadian, Avinza)	180–240 mg q24h	Not available	20–30 mg q24h; $3.08/30 mg	Not available	Not available	Not available	Once-daily dosing.	
Oxycodone (Roxicodone, OxyIR)	30 mg q3–4h	Not available	10 mg q3–4h; $0.36/5 mg	Not available	0.2 mg/kg q3–4h	Not available	Similar to morphine.	
Oxycodone Controlled release (Oxycontin)	40 mg q12h	Not available	20–40 mg q12h; $3.12/20 mg					
Oxymorphone[5] (Numorphan)	Not available	1 mg q3–4h	Not available	1 mg q3–4h; $3.26/1 mg			Active metabolite of oxycodone.	
COMBINATION OPIOID-NSAID PREPARATIONS								
Codeine[6,7] (with aspirin or acetaminophen)[8]	180–200 mg q3–4h; normal dose, 15–60 mg q4–6h	130 mg q3–4h	60 mg q4–6h; $0.64/60 mg	60 mg q2h (IM/SC); $1.06/60 mg	0.5–1 mg/kg q3–4h	Not recommended	Similar to morphine.	Closely monitor for efficacy as patients vary in their ability to convert the prodrug codeine to morphine.
Hydrocodone[5] (in Lorcet, Lortab, Vicodin, others)[8]	30 mg q3–4h	Not available	10 mg q3–4h; $0.45/5 mg	Not available	0.2 mg/kg q3–4h	Not available		Combination with acetaminophen limits dosage titration.
Oxycodone[6] (in Percocet, Percodan, Tylox, others)[8]	30 mg q3–4h	Not available	10 mg q3–4h; $0.51/5 mg	Not available	0.2 mg/kg q3–4h	Not available	Similar to morphine.	Combination with acetaminophen and aspirin limits dosage titration.

[1]Published tables vary in the suggested doses that are equianalgesic to morphine. Clinical response is the criterion that must be applied for each patient; titration to clinical efficacy is necessary. Because there is not complete cross-tolerance among these drugs, it is usually necessary to use a lower than equianalgesic dose initially when changing drugs and to retitrate to response.

[2]Dosing of transdermal fentanyl can be based on the "2:1 Rule"—the approximate equianalgesic dose of transdermal fentanyl in mcg/h is half the 24 hour mg dose of oral morphine.

[3]*Caution:* For morphine, hydromorphone, and oxymorphone, rectal administration is an alternative route for patients unable to take oral medications. Equianalgesic doses may differ from oral and parenteral doses. A short-acting opioid should normally be used for initial therapy.

[4]Not recommended for chronic pain. Doses listed are for brief therapy of acute pain only. Switch to another opioid for long-term therapy.

[5]*Caution:* Recommended doses do not apply for adult patients with renal or hepatic insufficiency or other conditions affecting drug metabolism.

[6]*Caution:* Doses of aspirin and acetaminophen in combination products must also be adjusted to the patient's body weight (Table 5–5).

[7]*Caution:* Doses of codeine above 60 mg often are not appropriate because of diminishing incremental analgesia with increasing doses but continually increasing nausea, constipation, and other side effects.

[8]*Caution:* Monitor total acetaminophen dose carefully, including any OTC use. Total acetaminophen dose maximum 4 g/d. If liver impairment or heavy alcohol use, maximum is 2 g/d.

Note: Average wholesale price (AWP, generic when available) for quantity listed. Source: *Red Book* Update, Vol. 25, No. 1, January 2006. AWP may not accurately represent the actual pharmacy cost because wide contractual variations exist among institutions.

Modified from Jacox AK et al: *Management of Cancer Pain: Quick Reference Guide for Clinicians No. 9.* AHCPR Publication No. 94–0593. Rockville, MD. Agency for Health Care Policy and Research, Public Health Service, U.S. Department of Health and Human Services. March 1994. Reproduced in part from Hosp Formul 1994;29(8 Part 2):586. (Erstad BL: A rational approach to the management of acute pain states.) Copyright by Advanstar Communications, Inc.

agents, full agonist opioids are typically a better choice in patients with severe pain because the dose of opioid is not limited by the toxicities of the acetaminophen or NSAID component of combination preparations. There is no maximal allowable or effective dose for full opioid agonists. The dose should be increased to whatever is necessary to relieve pain, remembering that certain types of pain may respond better to agents other than opioids.

While physiologic tolerance is possible with opioids, failure of a previously effective opioid dose to adequately relieve pain is usually due to an increase in the underlying pain. In this case, for moderate unrelieved pain, the dosage of opioid can be increased by 25–50%. For severe unrelieved pain, a dosage increase of 50–100% may be appropriate. The frequency of dosing should be adjusted so that pain control is continuous. In addition, long-term dosing may be adjusted by adding the amount of short-acting opioid necessary for breakthrough pain over the preceding 24 hours to the long-acting medication dose. In establishing or reestablishing adequate dosing, frequent reassessment of the patient's pain and medication side effects is necessary.

As opioids are titrated upwards, increasing difficulty with the side effects of can be expected. Constipation is common and should be anticipated and prevented in all patients. The prophylaxis and management of opioid-induced constipation are outlined below.

Sedation can be expected with opioids, although tolerance to this effect typically develops within 24–72 hours at a stable dose. Sedation typically appears well before significant respiratory depression. If treatment for sedation is desired, dextroamphetamine (2.5–7.5 mg orally at 8 AM and noon) or methylphenidate (2.5–10 mg orally at 8 AM and noon) may be helpful. Some patients even use caffeinated beverages to help manage minor opioid sedation.

Although sedation is more common, patients may experience euphoria when first taking opioids or when the dosage is increased. However, tolerance to this effect often develops after a few days at a stable dose. At very high doses of opioids, multifocal myoclonus may develop. This symptom may resolve after lowering the dose or switching opioids. While waiting for the level of the offending medication to fall, low doses of lorazepam or dantrolene may be helpful for treating myoclonus.

Nausea due to opioids may occur with initiation of therapy and resolve after a few days. If it is severe or persistent, it can be treated with prochlorperazine, 10 mg orally or intravenously every 8 hours or 25 mg rectally every 6 hours. The most common cause of nausea in patients taking opioids is constipation.

Although clinicians may worry about respiratory depression with opioids, that effect is uncommon when a low dose is given initially and titrated upward slowly. Even patients with pulmonary disease can tolerate low-dose opioids, although they should be monitored carefully. Clinicians should not allow concerns about respiratory depression to prevent them from treating pain adequately.

True allergy (with urticaria) to opioids is rare. More commonly, patients will describe an intolerance due to side effects such as nausea, pruritus, or urinary retention in response to a particular opioid. If such symptoms develop, they can usually be relieved by lowering the dose or switching to another opioid.

C. Neuropathic Pain

It is essential when taking a patient's history to listen for such descriptions as burning, shooting, pins and needles, or electricity, and for pain associated with numbness. Such a history suggests neuropathic pain, which is treated with some medications not typically used for other types of pain. Opioids are effective for neuropathic pain as are tricyclic antidepressants [TCAs], gabapentin, tramadol, and the lidocaine patch. These five medications have been found to be effective in multiple randomized trials and are considered first-line agents in the pharmacologic management of neuropathic pain (Table 5–7). The TCAs are a good first choice and usually have an effect within days and at lower doses than are needed for an antidepressant effect. Desipramine, 10–150 mg/d orally, and nortriptyline, 10–150 mg/d orally, are good first choices as they cause less orthostatic hypotension and have fewer anticholinergic effects than amitriptyline. One can start with a low dosage (10 mg orally daily) and titrate upward every 4 or 5 days.

The anticonvulsant gabapentin can be used in the same dosages that are used to prevent seizures. Gabapentin can cause sedation, dizziness, ataxia, and gastrointestinal side effects and therefore should be started at low dosages of 100–300 mg orally three times a day. The dose of gabapentin can be titrated upward by 300 mg/d every 4 or 5 days to a dosage of 3600 mg/d or higher. Gabapentin is relatively safe in accidental overdosage and may be preferred over TCAs for a patient with a history of congestive heart failure or arrhythmia or if there is a risk of suicide. Gabapentin and morphine in combination are more effective at lower doses of each than as single agents. Carbamazepine can also be effective for neuropathic pain, but because it can cause bone marrow suppression, a complete blood count is obtained periodically in patients taking this drug.

The 5% lidocaine patch is effective in postherpetic neuralgia and may be effective in other types of neuropathic pain also. A new patch is applied to the painful region daily for up to 12 hours. Tramadol should be started at 50 mg orally daily and can be titrated up to 100 mg orally four times daily. Successful management of neuropathic pain often requires the use of more than one effective medication. Duloxetine (60 mg/d), a norepinephrine and serotonin reuptake inhibitor, is approved for the treatment of diabetic neuropathy.

D. Adjuvant Pain Medications and Treatments

If pain cannot be controlled without uncomfortable medication side effects, clinicians should consider using lower doses of multiple medications rather than larger doses of one or two medications as is common for neuropathic pain. For bone pain, the anti-inflammatory ef-

Table 5–7. Pharmacologic management of neuropathic pain.

Drug[1]	Starting Dose	Typical Dose
Tricyclic antidepressants[2]		
Amitriptyline	25 mg orally at bedtime	10–150 mg orally at bedtime
Nortriptyline	25 mg orally at bedtime	10–150 mg orally at bedtime
Desipramine	25 mg orally at bedtime	10–200 mg orally at bedtime
Anticonvulsants		
Gabapentin	100–300 mg orally qd–tid	300–1200 mg orally tid
Carbamazepine[1,3]	100 mg orally bid	200 mg orally bid-qid
Opioids	(see Table 5–6)	(see Table 5–6)
Other medications		
Lidocaine transdermal	5% patch applied daily, for a maximum of 12 hours	1–3 patches applied daily for a maximum of 12 hours
Tramadol hydrochloride	50 mg orally qid	100 mg orally bid-qid

[1]Begin at the starting dose and titrate up every 4 or 5 days.
[2]Begin with a low dose. Pain relief can often be achieved at doses far below antidepressant doses, thereby minimizing adverse side effects.
[3]Periodically monitor blood counts, as drug can cause bone marrow suppression.

fect of NSAIDs can be particularly helpful. Radiation therapy and bisphosphonates may also relieve bone pain. For some patients, such as those with pain from pancreatic cancer, a nerve block—in this case, block of the celiac plexus—can provide relief. Intrathecal pumps may be useful for patients with severe pain responsive to opioids but who require such large doses that systemic side effects such as sedation and constipation become limiting. Neurolysis, rhizotomy, or ablative surgery and neurosurgery may be tried in selected patients. Cannabinoids have not been proven to work as analgesics. Chemotherapeutic agents are sometimes used for symptom management with palliative intent.

Corticosteroids such as dexamethasone or prednisone can be helpful for patients with headache due to increased intracranial pressure, pain from spinal cord compression, metastatic bone pain, and neuropathic pain due to invasion or infiltration of nerves by tumor. Because of the side effects of long-term corticosteroid administration, they are most appropriate in patients with end-stage disease.

Nonpharmacologic Treatments

Nonpharmacologic therapies are also valuable in treating pain. Hot or cold packs, massage, and physical therapy can be helpful for musculoskeletal pain. Similarly, biofeedback, acupuncture, chiropractic, meditation, music therapy, cognitive behavioral therapy, guided imagery, cognitive distraction, and framing may be of help in treating pain. Because mood and psychological issues play an important role in the patient's perception of and response to pain, psychotherapy, support groups, prayer, and pastoral counseling can also help in the management of pain. Major depression, which may be instigated by chronic pain or may alter the response to pain, should be treated aggressively.

DYSPNEA

Dyspnea is the subjective experience of difficulty in breathing and may be characterized by patients as tightness in the chest, shortness of breath, or a feeling of suffocation. Dyspnea is common among dying patients—up to 50% of severely ill patients may experience severe dyspnea.

Treatment of dyspnea is usually first directed at the cause, which may be related to pneumonia, pulmonary embolism, pleural effusion, bronchospasm, tracheal obstruction, neuromuscular disease, restriction of movement of the chest or abdominal walls, cardiac ischemia, congestive heart failure, superior vena cava syndrome, or severe anemia.

At the end of life, dyspnea is often treated nonspecifically with opioids. Immediate-release morphine orally or intravenously treats dyspnea effectively and typically at doses lower than would be necessary for the relief of moderate pain. Nebulized morphine provides no advantage over other routes of administration and the mask used for administration may exacerbate dyspnea. Supplemental oxygen may be useful for the dyspneic patient who is hypoxic and may provide subjective benefit to other dyspneic patients as well. However, a nasal cannula and face mask are sometimes not well tolerated, and fresh air from a window or fan may provide relief. Judicious use of nonpharmacologic relaxation techniques such as meditation and guided imagery may be beneficial for some patients. Benzodiazepines may be useful for the anxiety associated with dyspnea but do not appear to act directly to relieve dyspnea.

NAUSEA & VOMITING

Nausea and vomiting are common and distressing symptoms. As with pain, the management of nausea may be maximized by continuous dosing. An understanding of the four major inputs to the vomiting center may help direct treatment (see Chapter 14).

The chemoreceptor trigger zone may be stimulated by certain drugs (eg, opioids, NSAIDs), metabolic derangements, and chemotherapeutic agents. Vomiting associated with a particular opioid may be relieved by substitution with an equianalgesic dose of another opioid or a sustained-release formulation. In addition to the other dopamine receptor antagonist antiemetics listed in Table 14–2 that block the trigger zone, haloperidol (0.5–5 mg orally every 4–6 hours) is commonly used. Vomiting associated with chemotherapy may respond to agents such as ondansetron, granisetron, and dolasetron.

Vomiting may be due to stimulation of peripheral afferent nerves from the gut. Offering patients small amounts of food only when they are hungry may prevent nausea and vomiting. Nasogastric suction may provide rapid, short-term relief for vomiting associated with constipation, gastroparesis, or gastric outlet obstruction, with the addition of laxatives, prokinetic agents (only in the setting of partial not complete obstruction) metoclopramide (10–20 mg orally or intravenously four times a day), scopolamine (1.5-mg patch every 3 days), and high-dose corticosteroids as more definitive treatment. Treatment with high-dose corticosteroids (eg, dexamethasone, 20 mg orally or intravenously) or cyclizine (5 mg orally every 8 hours) may be useful for nausea and vomiting due to disease of intra-abdominal or pelvic organs.

Increased intracranial pressure may cause vomiting and may be relieved with high-dose corticosteroids or palliative cranial radiation. Vomiting due to disturbance of the vestibular apparatus may be treated with anticholinergic and antihistaminic agents (including diphenhydramine, 25 mg orally or intravenously every 8 hours, or scopolamine, 1.5-mg patch every 3 days).

Benzodiazepines can be effective in preventing the anticipatory nausea associated with chemotherapy but are otherwise not indicated for nausea and vomiting. Because they are sedating, these agents may increase the risk of aspiration in patients who vomit and therefore should rarely be used alone for the relief of nausea.

Finally, many patients find dronabinol (2.5–20 mg orally every 4–6 hours) helpful in the management of nausea and vomiting.

CONSTIPATION

Given the frequent use of opioids, poor dietary intake, and physical inactivity, constipation is a common

problem among the dying. Clinicians must inquire about any difficulty with hard or infrequent stools. Constipation is an easily preventable and treatable cause of discomfort, distress, and nausea and vomiting (see Chapter 14).

Constipation may be prevented or relieved if patients can increase their activity and their intake of dietary fiber and fluids. Simple considerations such as privacy, undisturbed toilet time, and a bedside commode rather than a bedpan may be important for some patients.

For patients taking opioids, anticipating and preventing constipation is important. A prophylactic bowel regimen of stool softeners (docusate) and stimulants (bisacodyl or senna) should be started when opioid treatment is begun. Lactulose, sorbitol, magnesium citrate, and enemas can be added as needed (see Table 14–4).

DELIRIUM & AGITATION

Many terminally ill patients die in a state of delirium—a disturbance of consciousness and a change in cognition that develops over a short time and is manifested by misinterpretations, illusions, hallucinations, disturbances in the sleep-wake cycle, psychomotor disturbances (eg, lethargy, restlessness), and mood disturbance (eg, fear, anxiety). Delirium complicated by myoclonus or convulsions at the end of life has been called **terminal restlessness.**

Careful attention to patient safety and nonpharmacologic strategies to help the patient remain oriented (clocks, calendars, a familiar environment, reassurance and redirection from caregivers) may be sufficient to prevent or manage minor delirium. Some delirious patients may be "pleasantly confused," and a decision by the patient's family and the clinician not to treat delirium may be justified.

More commonly, however, delirium at the end of life is distressing to patients and family and requires treatment. Delirium may interfere with the family's ability to feel comforting to the patient and may prevent a patient from being able to recognize and report important symptoms.

While there are many reversible causes of delirium (see Chapter 25), identifying and correcting the underlying cause at the end of life is often simply a question of attention to the choice and dosing of psychoactive medications.

When the cause of delirium cannot be identified, treated, or corrected rapidly enough, delirium may be treated symptomatically with neuroleptics. Haloperidol (1–10 mg orally, subcutaneously, intramuscularly, or intravenously twice or three times a day) is used commonly, but extrapyramidal adverse effects may occur. Newer agents such as risperidone (1–3 mg orally twice a day) also may be helpful in delirium.

As an adjuvant to the above neuroleptics, especially in the setting of significant, unrelieved anxiety, benzodiazepines such as lorazepam (0.5–2 mg orally, sublingually, subcutaneously, or intravenously every 4–6 hours) may be useful. When delirium is refractory to treatment and remains intolerable, sedation may be required to provide relief and may be achieved rapidly with midazolam (0.5–5 mg/h subcutaneously or intravenously) or barbiturates.

Bruera E et al: Nebulized versus subcutaneous morphine for patients with cancer dyspnea: a preliminary study. J Pain Symptom Manage 2005;29:613. [PMID: 15963870]

Dworkin et al: Advances in neuropathic pain: diagnosis, mechanisms, and treatment recommendations. Arch Neurol 2003; 60:1524. [PMID: 14623723]

Gilron I et al: Morphine, gabapentin, or their combination for neuropathic pain. N Engl J Med 2005;352:1324. [PMID: 15800228]

Hallenbeck J: Palliative care in the final days of life: "they were expecting it at any time." JAMA 2005;293:2265. [PMID: 15886382]

Pantilat SZ et al: Palliative care for patients with heart failure. JAMA 2004;291:2476. [PMID: 15161899]

■ OTHER SPECIFIC TASKS OF CARING

NUTRITION & HYDRATION

Tube feedings do not prevent aspiration pneumonia, and there is debate about whether artificial nutrition prolongs life in the terminally ill. In fact, there has been a growing awareness of the potential medical benefits of forgoing unwanted or artificial nutrition and hydration (including tube feedings, parenteral nutrition, and intravenous hydration) at the end of life.

Eating without hunger and artificial nutrition are associated with a number of potential complications. Force feeding may cause nausea and vomiting in ill patients, and eating will lead to diarrhea in the setting of malabsorption. Nutrition may increase oral and airway secretions and the risk of choking, aspiration, and dyspnea. Nasogastric and gastrostomy tube feeding and parenteral nutrition impose risks of infection, epistaxis, pneumothorax, electrolyte imbalance, and aspiration—as well as the need to physically restrain the delirious patient to prevent dislodgment of catheters and tubes.

Withholding nutrition at the end of life causes remarkably little hunger or distress. Ill people often have no hunger with total caloric deprivation, and the associated ketonemia produces a sense of well-being, analgesia, and mild euphoria. However, carbohydrate intake even in small amounts (such as that provided by 5% intravenous dextrose solution) blocks ketone production and may blunt the positive effects of total caloric deprivation.

Withholding hydration may lead to death in a few days to a month. The quality of life for those at the end of life may be adversely affected by supplemental hydration because of its contribution to oral and airway secretions (leading to aspiration or the "death rattle"), polyuria, and the development or worsening of ascites, pleural or other effusions, and peripheral and pulmonary edema.

Although it is unclear to what extent withholding hydration at the end of life creates an uncomfortable sensation of thirst, any such sensation is usually relieved by simply moistening the dry mouth. Ice chips, hard candy, swabs, or a solution of equal parts nystatin solution, viscous lidocaine, diphenhydramine, and minted mouthwash are effective.

Individuals at the end of life have a right to refuse nutrition and hydration. However, providing or withholding oral food and water is not simply a medical decision because feeding may have profound social and cultural significance for patients, families, and clinicians themselves. Withholding supplemental enteral or parenteral nutrition and hydration challenges the assumption that offering food is an expression of compassion and love and invokes distressing images of starvation. In fact, individuals at the end of life who choose to forgo nutrition and hydration are unlikely to suffer from hunger or thirst. Family and friends can be encouraged to express their love and caring in ways other than intrusive attempts at forced feeding or hydration.

WITHDRAWAL OF CURATIVE EFFORTS

Requests from appropriately informed and competent patients or their surrogates for withdrawal of life-sustaining interventions must be respected. The clinician receiving such requests should recognize and explore the significance of this change in health care goals. Alternatively, clinicians may determine unilaterally that further intervention is medically inappropriate—eg, continuing renal dialysis in a patient dying of multiorgan failure. In such cases, the clinician's intention to withdraw a specific intervention should be communicated to the patient and family. If differences of opinion exist about the appropriateness of what is being done, the assistance of an institutional palliative care service or ethics committee should be sought.

Limitation of life support prior to death is an increasingly common practice in intensive care units. The withdrawal of life-sustaining interventions such as mechanical ventilation must be approached carefully to avoid needless patient suffering and distress for those in attendance. Clinicians should educate the patient and family about the expected course of events and the difficulty of determining the precise timing of death after withdrawal of support. Sedative and analgesic agents should be administered to ensure patient comfort even at the risk of respiratory depression or hypotension. Scopolamine (10 mcg/h subcutaneously or intravenously, or a 15-mg patch every 3 days) or atropine (1% ophthalmic solution, 1 or 2 drops sublingually as often as every hour) can be used for controlling airway secretions and the resultant "death rattle."

Table 5–8. Guidelines for withdrawal of mechanical ventilation.

1. Stop neuromuscular blocking agents.
2. Administer opioids or sedatives to eliminate distress.
   If not already sedated, begin with fentanyl 100 mcg (or morphine sulfate 10 mg) by intravenous bolus and infusion of fentanyl 100 mcg/hour intravenously (or morphine sulfate 10 mg/hour intravenously).
   Distress is indicated by RR > 24, nasal flaring, use of accessory muscles of respiration, HR increase > 20%, MAP increase > 20%, grimacing, clutching.
3. Discontinue vasoactive agents and other agents unrelated to patient comfort, such as antibiotics, intravenous fluids, and diagnostic procedures.
4. Decrease FIO_2 to room air and PEEP to 0 cm H_2O.
5. Observe patient for distress.
   If patient is distressed, increase opioids by repeating bolus dose and increasing hourly infusion rate by 50 mcg fentanyl (or 5 mg morphine sulfate),[1] then return to observation.
   If patient is not distressed, place on T piece and observe.
   If patient continues without distress, extubate patient and continue to observe for distress.

[1]Ventilatory support may be increased until additional opioids have effect.
RR = respiratory rate; HR = heart rate; MAP = mean airway pressure; FIO_2 = fraction of inspired oxygen; PEEP = positive endexpiratory pressure.
Adapted, with permission, from San Francisco General Hospital Guidelines for Withdrawal of Mechanical Ventilation/Life Support.

A guideline for withdrawal of mechanical ventilation is provided in Table 5–8.

PSYCHOLOGICAL, SOCIAL, & SPIRITUAL ISSUES

Dying is not exclusively or even primarily a biomedical event. It is an intimate personal experience with profound psychological, interpersonal, and existential meanings. For many people at the end of life, the prospect of impending death stimulates a deep and urgent assessment of their identity, the quality of their relationships, and the meaning and purpose of their existence.

Psychological Challenges

In 1969, Elisabeth Kübler-Ross identified five psychological stages or patterns of emotions that patients at the end of life may experience: denial and isolation, anger, bargaining, depression, and acceptance. Not every patient will experience all these emotions, and not necessarily in an orderly progression. In addition to these five stages are the perpetual challenges of anxiety and fear of the unknown. Simple information, listening, assurance, and support may help patients with these psychological challenges. In fact, patients and families rank emotional support as one of the most important aspects of good end-of-life care. Psychotherapy and group support may be beneficial as well.

Despite the significant emotional stress of facing death, clinical depression is not normal at the end of life and should be treated. Cognitive and affective signs of depression (such as hopelessness) may help distinguish depression from the low energy and other vegetative signs common with end-stage illness. Although traditional antidepressant treatments such as selective serotonin reuptake inhibitors are effective, more rapidly acting medications such as dextroamphetamine or methylphenidate may be particularly useful when the end of life is near.

Social Challenges

At the end of life, patients should be encouraged to discharge personal, professional, and business obligations. This might include completing important work or personal projects, distributing possessions, writing a will, and making funeral and burial arrangements. The prospect of death often prompts patients to examine the quality of their interpersonal relationships, including the relationship with the clinician. Dying may intensify a patient's need to feel cared for by the doctor, highlighting the clinician's obligation of nonabandonment and the need for clinician empathy and compassion. Concern about estranged relationships or "unfinished business" with significant others and interest in reconciliation may become paramount at this time. At the end of life, even healthy interpersonal relationships must reach completion (Table 5–9).

Spiritual Challenges

Spirituality is the attempt to understand or accept the underlying meaning of life, one's relationships to oneself and other people, one's place in the universe, and the possibility of a "higher power" in the universe. Spirituality is distinguished from particular religious practices or beliefs and is generally considered a universal human concern.

Perhaps because of an inappropriately exclusive attention to the biologic challenge of forestalling death or perhaps from feelings of discomfort or incompetence, clinicians frequently ignore their patients' spiritual concerns or reflexively refer these

Table 5–9. Five statements often necessary for the completion of important interpersonal relationships.

(1) "Forgive me."	(An expression of regret)
(2) "I forgive you."	(An expression of acceptance)
(3) "Thank you."	(An expression of gratitude)
(4) "I love you."	(An expression of affection)
(5) "Good-bye."	(Leave-taking)

Courtesy of Ira R. Byock, MD.

important issues to psychiatrists or other caretakers (nurses, social workers, clergy). However, the existential challenges of dying are central to the well-being of people at the end of life and are the proper concern of clinicians. Within a biologic, psychosocial, and spiritual model of medical care, clinicians may work to provide more than simple physical comfort and control of bothersome symptoms. Clinicians can help dying patients by providing care to the whole person—by providing physical comfort and social support and by helping patients discover their own unique meaning in the world and an acceptance of death as a part of life.

Unlike physical ailments such as infections and fractures, which usually require a clinician's intervention to be treated, the patient's spiritual concerns often require only a clinician's attention, listening, and witness. Clinicians might choose to inquire about the patient's spiritual concerns and ask whether the patient wishes to discuss them. For example, asking, "How are you within yourself?" communicates that the clinician is interested in the patient's whole experience and provides an opportunity for the patient to share perceptions about his or her inner life. Questions that might constitute an existential "review of systems" are presented in Table 5–10.

Attending to the spiritual concerns of patients calls for listening to their stories. Story-telling gives patients the opportunity to verbalize what is meaningful to them and to leave something of themselves behind—the promise of being remembered. Story-telling may be facilitated by suggesting that the patient share his or her life story with family members, record it on audio or video tape, assemble a photo album, organize a scrapbook, or write an autobiography.

While dying may be a period of inevitable loss of physical functioning, the end of life also offers an opportunity for psychological, interpersonal, and spiritual development. Individuals may grow—even achieve a heightened sense of well-being or transcendence—in the process of dying. Through listening, support, and presence, clinicians may help foster this learning and be a catalyst for this transformation. Rather than thinking of dying simply as the termination of life, clinicians and patients may be guided by a developmental model of dying that recognizes a series of lifelong developmental tasks and landmarks and allows for growth at the end of life.

Chochinov HM: Dignity-conserving care—a new model for palliative care: helping people feel valued. JAMA 2002;287:2253. [PMID: 11980525]

Lo B et al: Discussing religious and spiritual issues at the end of life: a practical guide for physicians. JAMA 2002;287:749. [PMID: 11851542]

Monroe MH et al: Primary care physician preferences regarding spiritual behavior in medical practice. Arch Intern Med 2003;163:2751. [PMID: 14662629]

Murphy LM et al: Percutaneous endoscopic gastrostomy does not prolong survival in patients with dementia. Arch Intern Med 2003;163:1351. [PMID: 12796072]

Rubenfeld GD: Principles and practice of withdrawing life-sustaining treatments. Crit Care Clin 2004;20:435. [PMID: 15183212]

■ TASKS AFTER DEATH

After the death of a patient, the clinician is called upon to perform a number of tasks, both required and recommended. The clinician must plainly and directly inform the family of the death. Providing words of sympathy and reassurance, time for questions and initial grief, and a quiet private room for the family at this time is appropriate and much appreciated.

THE PRONOUNCEMENT & DEATH CERTIFICATE

In the United States, state policies direct clinicians to confirm the death of a patient in a formal process called "pronouncement." The clinician must verify the absence of spontaneous respirations and cardiac activity. A note describing these findings and the time of death is entered in the patient's chart. In many states, when a patient whose death is expected dies outside of the hospital (at home or in prisons, for example) nurses may be authorized to report the death over the telephone to a physician who must then sign the death certificate within 24 hours. For traumatic deaths, some states allow emergency medical technicians to

Table 5–10. An existential review of systems.

Intrapersonal
How are you within yourself?[1]
What does your illness/dying mean to you?
What do you think caused your illness?
How have you been healed in the past?
What do you think is needed for you to be healed now?
What is right with you now?
What do you hope for?
Interpersonal
Who is important to you?
To whom does your illness/dying matter?
Do you have any unfinished business with significant others?
Transpersonal
What is your source of strength, help, or hope?
Do you have spiritual concerns or a spiritual practice?
If so, how does your spirituality relate to your illness/dying, and how can I help integrate your spirituality into your health care?[1]
What do you think happens after we die?
What purpose might your illness/dying serve?
What do you think is trying to happen here?[1]

[1]Courtesy of IR Byock, MD, DB Larson, MD, and AL Suchman, MD.

pronounce a patient dead at the scene based on clearly defined criteria and with physician telephonic or radio supervision.

While the pronouncement may often seem like an awkward and unnecessary formality, clinicians may use this time to reassure the patient's loved ones at the bedside that the patient died peacefully and that all appropriate care had been given. Both clinicians and families may use the ritual of the pronouncement as an opportunity to begin to process emotionally the death of the patient.

Physicians are legally required to accurately report the underlying cause of death on the death certificate. This reporting is important both for patients' families (for insurance purposes and the need for an accurate family medical history) and for the epidemiologic study of disease and public health. Physicians are untrained in and unskilled at correctly completing death certificates. The physician should be specific about the major cause of death (eg, "decompensated cirrhosis") and its contributory cause (eg, "hepatitis B and hepatitis C infections and chronic alcoholic hepatitis") as well as any associated conditions (eg, "acute renal failure")—and not simply put down "cardiac arrest" as the cause of death.

AUTOPSY & ORGAN DONATION

Discussing the options and obtaining consent for autopsy and organ donation with patients themselves prior to death is usually the best practice. This advances the principle of patient autonomy and lessens the responsibilities of distressed family members during the period immediately following the death. After a patient dies, however, designated organ transplant personnel are more successful than the treating clinicians at obtaining consent for organ donation from surviving family members. Federal regulations now require that a designated representative of an organ procurement organization approach the family about organ donation. Most people in the United States support the donation of organs for transplants. Currently, however, organ transplantation is severely limited by the availability of donor organs. Many potential donors and the families of actual donors experience a sense of reward in contributing, even through death, to the lives of others.

Clinicians must be sensitive to ethnic and cultural differences in attitudes about autopsy and organ donation. Patients or their families should be reminded of their right to limit autopsy or organ donation in any way they choose. Pathologists can perform autopsies without interfering with funeral plans or the appearance of the deceased.

The results of an autopsy may help surviving family members (and clinicians) understand the exact cause of a patient's death and foster a sense of closure.

A clinician-family conference to review the results of the autopsy provides a good opportunity for clinicians to assess how well families are grieving and to answer questions. Despite the advantages of conducting postmortem examinations, autopsy rates have fallen drastically to less than 15% today. Families report refusing autopsies out of fear of disfigurement of the body or delay of the funeral—or say they were simply not asked. They allow autopsies in order to advance medical knowledge, to identify the exact cause of their loved one's death, and to be reassured that appropriate care was given. Routinely addressing these issues when discussing autopsy may help increase the autopsy rate; the most important mistake is the failure to ask for permission to perform it.

FOLLOW-UP & GRIEVING

Proper care of patients at the end of life includes following up with surviving family members after the patient has died. Following up enables the clinician to assess how families are grieving, to reassure them about the nature of normal grieving, and to identify complicated grief or depression. Clinicians can recommend support groups and counseling as needed. A card or telephone call from the clinician to the family days to weeks after the patient's death (and perhaps on the anniversary of the death) allows the clinician to express concern for the family and the deceased.

After a patient dies, the clinician too may need to grieve. Although clinicians may be relatively unaffected by the deaths of some patients, other deaths may cause distressing feelings of sadness, loss, and guilt. These emotions should be recognized as the first step toward processing them or preventing them in the future.

For clinicians, grieving the loss of a patient is normal. Each clinician may find personal or communal resources that help with the process of grieving. Shedding tears, the support of colleagues, time for reflection, and traditional or personal mourning rituals all may be effective. Attending the funeral of a patient who has died can be a satisfying personal experience that is almost universally appreciated by families and that may be the final element in caring well for people at the end of life.

Lakkireddy DR et al: Death certificate completion: how well are physicians trained and are cardiovascular causes overstated? Am J Med 2004;117:492. [PMID: 15464706]

Marchand L et al: Death pronouncements: using the teachable moment in end-of-life care residency training. J Palliat Med 2004;7:80. [PMID: 15000790]

Penson RT et al: When does the responsibility of our care end: bereavement. Oncologist 2002;7:251. [PMID: 12065799]

Shear K et al: Treatment of complicated grief: a randomized controlled trial. JAMA 2005;293:2601. [PMID: 15928281]

Skin, Hair, & Nails

6

Timothy G. Berger, MD

DIAGNOSIS OF SKIN DISORDERS

Morphology

Every skin disease produces a characteristic primary skin lesion. This chapter will group diseases according to the types of lesions they cause and guide the reader through the history, physical findings, and laboratory tests that discriminate among the differential diagnoses.

History

A detailed history is important, though in the case of skin cancer or moles (nevi) the physical examination takes precedence. Important components of a history include systemic disorders; prescription, over-the-counter, and alternative systemic and topical medications; and exposure to physical and chemical agents in the home and work environments.

Physical Examination

It is best to examine the entire skin surface, including the nails, scalp, palms, soles, and mucous membranes, in bright light. Total skin examination allows recognition of typical disease patterns and ensures that no potentially important lesions are overlooked. In examining the head for skin cancer, special attention should be paid to the lid margins, nose, ears, and lips—areas of sun exposure.

PRINCIPLES OF DERMATOLOGIC THERAPY

Frequently Used Treatment Measures

A. BATHING

Soap should be used only in the axillae and groin and on the feet by persons with dry or inflamed skin. Soaking in water for 10–15 minutes before applying topical corticosteroids enhances their efficacy.

B. TOPICAL THERAPY

In general, topical agents used by prescription are supplied in only one strength. Exceptions include hydrocortisone (1% and 2.5%); triamcinolone acetonide cream and ointment (0.025% and 0.1%) or solution (0.1%); and fluocinolone cream, ointment, or solution (0.01%), or cream and ointment (0.025%). There is little evidence that one concentration has clinical effects that are significantly different from another. Nondermatologists should become familiar with a few agents and use them properly rather than try to master the universe of topical agents.

1. **Corticosteroids**—Representative topical corticosteroid creams, lotions, ointments, gels, and sprays are presented in Table 6–1. Specific indications for topical corticosteroid therapy will be discussed in the context of specific dermatologic entities. Topical corticosteroids are divided into classes based on their potency. There is little (except price) to recommend one agent over another within the same class. For a given agent, an ointment is more potent than a cream; however, ointments are generally more greasy. The potency of a topical corticosteroid may be dramatically increased by applying an occlusive dressing over the corticosteroid. At least 4 hours of occlusion is required to enhance penetration. Such dressings may include gloves, plastic wrap, or plastic occlusive suits for patients with generalized erythroderma or atopy. Caution should be used in applying topical corticosteroids to areas of thin skin (face, scrotum, vulva, skin folds). Topical corticosteroid use on the eyelids may result in glaucoma or cataracts. One may estimate the amount of topical corticosteroid needed by using the "rule of nines" (as in burn evaluation; see Figure 38–2). In general, it takes an average of 20–30 g to cover the body surface of an adult once. Systemic absorption does occur, but adrenal suppression, diabetes, hypertension, osteoporosis, and other complications of systemic corticosteroids are very rare with topical corticosteroid therapy.

2. **Emollients for dry skin ("moisturizers")**— Dry skin is not related to water intake but to abnormal function of the epidermis. Many types of emollients are available. Petrolatum, mineral oil, Aquaphor, and Eucerin cream are the heaviest and best. Emollients are most effective when applied to wet skin immediately after a bath. They should be applied with the "grain" of the hairs rather than by rubbing up and down to avoid folliculitis. If the skin is too greasy after application, pat dry with a damp towel.

Table 6–1. Useful topical dermatologic therapeutic agents.

Agent	Formulations, Strengths, and Prices[1]	Apply	Potency Class	Common Indications	Comments
Corticosteroids					
Hydrocortisone acetate	Cream 1%: $3.60/30 g Ointment 1%: $3.72/30 g Lotion 1%: $20.20/120 mL	bid	Low	Seborrheic dermatitis Pruritus ani Intertrigo	Not the same as hydrocortisone butyrate or valerate! Not for poison oak! OTC lotion (Aquinil HC) OTC solution (Scalpicin, T Scalp)
	Cream 2.5%: $8.95/30 g	bid	Low	As for 1% hydrocortisone	Perhaps better for pruritus ani Not clearly better than 1% More expensive Not OTC
Alclometasone dipropionate (Aclovate)	Cream 0.05%: $22.67/15 g Ointment 0.05%: $46.29/45 g	bid	Low	As for hydrocortisone	More efficacious than hydrocortisone Perhaps causes less atrophy
Desonide	Cream 0.05%: $15.47/15 g Ointment 0.05%: $39.88/60 g Lotion 0.05%: $33.39/60 mL	bid	Low	As for hydrocortisone For lesions on face or body folds resistant to hydrocortisone	More efficacious than hydrocortisone Can cause rosacea or atrophy Not fluorinated
Prednicarbate (Dermatop)	Emollient cream 0.1%: $21.83/15 g Ointment 0.1%: $21.65/15 g	bid	Medium	As for triamcinolone	May cause less atrophy No generic formulations Preservative-free
Triamcinolone acetonide	Cream 0.1%: $3.60/15 g Ointment 0.1%: $3.60/15 g Lotion 0.1%: $42.44/60 mL	bid	Medium	Eczema on extensor areas Used for psoriasis with tar Seborrheic dermatitis and psoriasis on scalp	Caution in body folds, face Economical in 0.5-lb and 1-lb sizes for treatment of large body surfaces Economical as solution for scalp
	Cream 0.025%: $3.00/15 g Ointment 0.025%: $6.25/80 g	bid	Medium	As for 0.1% strength	Possibly less efficacy and few advantages over 0.1% formulation
Fluocinolone acetonide	Cream 0.025%: $3.05/15 g Ointment 0.025%: $4.20/15 g	bid	Medium	As for triamcinolone	
	Solution 0.01%: $11.00/60 mL	bid	Medium	As for triamcinolone solution	
Mometasone furoate (Elocon)	Cream 0.1%: $26.90/15 g Ointment 0.1%: $23.90/15 g Lotion 0.1%: $63.96/60 mL	qd	Medium	As for triamcinolone	Often used inappropriately on the face or in children Not fluorinated
Diflorasone diacetate	Cream 0.05%: $36.78/15 g Ointment 0.05%: $51.86/30 g	bid	High	Nummular dermatitis Allergic contact dermatitis Lichen simplex chronicus	
Amcinonide (Cyclocort)	Cream 0.1%: $18.42/15 g Ointment 0.1%: $27.46/30 g	bid	High	As for betamethasone	

(continued)

Table 6–1. Useful topical dermatologic therapeutic agents. (continued)

Agent	Formulations, Strengths, and Prices[1]	Apply	Potency Class	Common Indications	Comments
Fluocinonide (Lidex)	Cream 0.05%: $10.61/15 g Gel 0.05%: $21.01/15 g Ointment 0.05%: $21.25/15 g Solution 0.05%: $27.27/60 mL	bid	High	As for betamethasone Gel useful for poison oak	Economical generics Lidex cream can cause stinging on eczema Lidex emollient cream preferred
Betamethasone dipropionate (Diprolene)	Cream 0.05%: $7.80/15 g Ointment 0.05%: $9.40/15 g Lotion 0.05%: $30.49/60 mL	bid	Ultra-high	For lesions resistant to high-potency corticosteroids Lichen planus Insect bites	Economical generics available
Clobetasol propionate (Temovate)	Cream 0.05%: $24.71/15 g Ointment 0.05%: $24.71/15 g Lotion 0.05%: $53.10/50 mL	bid	Ultra-high	As for betamethasone dipropionate	Somewhat more potent than diflorasone Limited to 2 continuous weeks of use Limited to 50 g or less per week Cream may cause stinging; use "emollient cream" formulation Generic available
Halobetasol propionate (Ultravate)	Cream 0.05%: $31.49/15 g Ointment 0.05%: $31.49/15 g	bid	Ultra-high	As for clobetasol	Same restrictions as clobetasol Cream does not cause stinging Compatible with calcipotriene (Dovonex)
Flurandrenolide (Cordran)	Tape: $54.65/80" × 3" roll Lotion 0.05%: $45.42/60 mL	q12h	Ultra-high	Lichen simplex chronicus	Protects the skin and prevents scratching
Nonsteroidal anti-inflammatory agents					
Tacrolimus[2] (Protopic)	Ointment 0.1%: $74.06/30 g Ointment 0.03%: $69.29/30 g	bid	N/A	Atopic dermatitis	Steroid substitute not causing atrophy or striae Burns in ≥ 40% of patients with eczema
Pimecrolimus[2] (Elidel)	Cream 1%: $67.40/30 g	bid	N/A	Atopic dermatitis	Steroid substitute not causing atrophy or striae
Antibiotics (for acne)					
Clindamycin phosphate	Solution 1%: $12.09/30 mL Gel 1%: $38.13/30 mL Lotion 1%: $53.06/60 mL Pledget 1%: $46.40/60	bid	N/A	Mild papular acne	Lotion is less drying for patients with sensitive skin
Erythromycin	Solution 2%: $7.53/60 mL Gel 2%: $24.73/30 g Pledget 2%: $26.07/60	bid	N/A	As for clindamycin	Many different manufacturers Economical
Erythromycin/ Benzoyl peroxide (Benzamycin)	Gel: $68.60/23.3 g Gel: $128.00/46.6 g	bid	N/A	As for clindamycin Can help treat comedonal acne	No generics More expensive More effective than other topical antibiotic Main jar requires refrigeration
Clindamycin/ Benzoyl peroxide (Benzeclin)	Gel: $70.81/25 g Gel: $128.99/50 g	bid		As for benzamycin	No generic More effective than either agent alone

(continued)

Table 6–1. Useful topical dermatologic therapeutic agents. (continued)

Agent	Formulations, Strengths, and Prices[1]	Apply	Potency Class	Common Indications	Comments
Antibiotics (for impetigo)					
Mupirocin (Bactroban)	Ointment 2%: $44.85/22 g Cream 2%: $36.80/15 g	tid	N/A	Impetigo, folliculitis	Because of cost, use limited to tiny areas of impetigo Used in the nose twice daily for 5 days to reduce staphylococcal carriage
Antifungals					
Clotrimazole	Cream 1%: $4.25/15 g OTC Solution 1%: $7.40/10 mL	bid	N/A	Dermatophyte and *Candida* infections	Available OTC Inexpensive generic cream available
Miconazole	Cream 2%: $3.20/30 g OTC	bid	N/A	As for clotrimazole	As for clotrimazole
Other imidazoles					
Econazole (Spectazole)	Cream 1%: $22.06/15 g	qd	N/A	As for clotrimazole	No generic Somewhat more effective than clotrimazole and miconazole
Ketoconazole	Cream 2%: $16.46/15 g	qd	N/A	As for clotrimazole	No generic Somewhat more effective than clotrimazole and miconazole
Oxiconazole (Oxistat)	Cream 1%: $30.10/15 g Lotion 1%: $50.66/30 mL	bid	N/A		
Sulconazole (Exelderm)	Cream 1%: $12.56/15 g Solution 1%: $27.05/30 mL	bid	N/A	As for clotrimazole	No generic Somewhat more effective than clotrimazole and miconazole
Other antifungals					
Butenafine (Mentax)	Cream 1%: $40.27/15 g	qd	N/A	Dermatophytes	Fast response; high cure rate; expensive Available OTC
Ciclopirox (Loprox) (Penlac)	Cream 0.77%: $72.02/30 g Lotion 0.77%: $146.12/60 mL Solution 8%: $144.34/6.6 mL	bid	N/A	As for clotrimazole	No generic Somewhat more effective than clotrimazole and miconazole
Naftifine (Naftin)	Cream 1%: $48.66/30 g Gel 1%: $79.72/60 mL	qd	N/A	Dermatophytes	No generic Somewhat more effective than clotrimazole and miconazole
Terbinafine (Lamisil)	Cream 1%: $8.15/12 g OTC	qd	N/A	Dermatophytes	Fast clinical response OTC
Antipruritics					
Camphor/ menthol	Compounded lotion (0.5% of each)	bid–tid	N/A	Mild eczema, xerosis, mild contact dermatitis	
Pramoxine hydrochloride (Prax)	Lotion 1%: $14.78/120 mL	qid	N/A	Dry skin, varicella, mild eczema, pruritus ani	OTC formulations (Prax, Aveeno Anti-Itch Cream or Lotion; Itch-X Gel) By prescription mixed with 1% or 2% hydrocortisone
Doxepin (Zonalon)	Cream 5%: $64.19/30 g	qid	N/A	Topical antipruritic, best used in combination with appropriate topical corticosteroid to enhance efficacy	Can cause sedation

(continued)

Table 6–1. Useful topical dermatologic therapeutic agents. (continued)

Agent	Formulations, Strengths, and Prices[1]	Apply	Potency Class	Common Indications	Comments
Emollients					
Aveeno	Cream, lotion, others	qd–tid	N/A	Xerosis, eczema	Choice is most often based on personal preference by patient
Aqua glycolic	Cream, lotion, shampoo, others	qd–tid	N/A	Xerosis, ichthyosis, keratosis pilaris Mild facial wrinkles Mild acne or sebor- rheic dermatitis	Contains 8% glycolic acid Available from other makers, eg, Alpha Hydrox, or generic 8% glycolic acid lotion May cause stinging on eczematous skin
Aquaphor	Ointment: $7.50/50 g	qd–tid	N/A	Xerosis, eczema For protection of area in pruritus ani	Not as greasy as petrolatum
Carmol	Lotion 10%: $9.52/180 mL Cream 20%: $9.38/90 g	bid	N/A	Xerosis	Contains urea as humectant Nongreasy hydrating agent (10%); debrides keratin (20%)
Complex 15	Lotion: $6.48/240 mL Cream: $4.82/75 g	qd–tid	N/A	Xerosis Lotion or cream rec- ommended for split or dry nails	Active ingredient is a phos- pholipid
DML	Cream, lotion, facial mois- turizer: $5.32/240 mL	qd–tid	N/A	As for Complex 15	Face cream has sunscreen
Eucerin	Cream: $5.10/120 g Lotion: $5.10/240 mL	qd–tid	N/A	Xerosis, eczema	Many formulations made Eucerin Plus contains alphahy- droxy acid and may cause stinging on eczematous skin Facial moisturizer has SPF 25 sunscreen
Lac-Hydrin-Five	Lotion: $10.12/240 mL OTC	bid	N/A	Xerosis, ichthyosis, keratosis pilaris	Rx product is 12%
Lubriderm	Lotion: $5.03/300 mL	qd–tid	N/A	Xerosis, eczema	Unscented usually preferred
Neutrogena	Cream, lotion, facial mois- turizer: $7.39/240 mL	qd–tid	N/A	Xerosis, eczema	Face cream has titanium- based sunscreen
SBR Lipocream	Cream: $8.23/30 g	qd–tid	N/A	Xerosis, eczema	Less greasy but effective moisturizer
Ceratopic Cream	Cream: $39.50/4 oz	bid	N/A	Xerosis, eczema	Contains ceramide; anti- inflammatory and non- greasy moisturizer
U-Lactin	Lotion: $7.13/240 mL	qd	N/A	Hyperkeratotic heels	Moisturizes and removes keratin

[1]Average wholesale price (AWP, for AB-rated generic when available) for quantity listed. AWP may not accurately represent the actual pharmacy cost because wide contractual variations exist among institutions. Source: *Red Book Update*, Vol. 25, No. 5, May 2006.
[2]Topical tacrolimus and pimecrolimus should only be used when other topical treatments are ineffective. Treatment should be limited to an area and duration to be as brief as possible. Treatment with these agents should be avoided in persons with known immunosuppression, HIV infec- tion, bone marrow and organ transplantation, lymphoma, at high risk for lymphoma, and those with a prior history of lymphoma.
OTC = over-the-counter; N/A = not applicable.

In some cases, lotions may be useful and are not as greasy as creams and ointments. The appearance of dry skin and ichthyosis may be improved by lactic acid products or glycolic acid-containing lotions provided no inflammation (erythema or pruritus) is present. Moisturizers that mimic the skin's normal lipids and thus feel less greasy than ointments include SBR Lipocream and Ceratopic cream.

3. Drying agents for weepy dermatoses—If the skin is weepy from infection or inflammation, drying agents may afford relief. The best drying agent is water, and repeated compresses may be applied for 15–30 minutes alone or with aluminum salts (Burow's solution, Domeboro tablets) or colloidal oatmeal (Aveeno).

4. Topical antipruritics—Lotions that contain 0.5% each of camphor and menthol (Sarna) are effective for mild pruritic dermatoses. Pramoxine hydrochloride, 1% cream or lotion, with or without 0.5% menthol, is an effective antipruritic agent (eg, Prax, PrameGel, Aveeno Anti-Itch lotion). Hydrocortisone, 1% or 2.5%, may be incorporated for its anti-inflammatory effect (Pramosone cream, lotion, or ointment). Doxepin cream 5% may reduce pruritus due to eczematous dermatoses. Drowsiness may occur. Pramoxine and doxepin are most effective when applied with topical corticosteroids. Monoamine oxidase inhibitors should be discontinued at least 2 weeks before treatment with doxepin.

5. Systemic antipruritic drugs—

a. Antihistamines—H$_1$-blockers are the agents of choice for pruritus when due to histamine, such as in urticaria. Otherwise, they appear to relieve pruritus only by their sedating and not their antihistamine effects. Except in the case of urticaria, nonsedating antihistamines are of little or no value in inflammatory skin diseases such as atopic dermatitis and are rarely indicated.

Hydroxyzine 25–50 mg nightly is typically used for its sedative effect in pruritic diseases. Sedation can limit daytime use. The least sedating antihistamines are loratadine and famotidine. Cetirizine causes drowsiness in about 15% of patients. Some antidepressants, such as doxepin, mirtazapine, and paroxetine can be effective antipruritics.

b. Systemic corticosteroids—(See Chapter 26.)

Clarke P: Why am I so itchy? Aust Fam Physician 2004;33:489. [PMID: 15301164]

Lonsdale-Eccles A et al: Treatment of pruritus with systemic disorders in the elderly: a review of the role of new therapies. Drugs Aging 2003;20:197. [PMID: 12578400]

Yosipovitch G et al: Practical guidelines for relief of itch. Dermatol Nurs 2004;16:325. [PMID: 15471044]

Sunscreens

Protection from ultraviolet light should begin at birth but will reduce the incidence of actinic keratoses and some nonmelanoma skin cancers when initiated at any age. The best protection is shade, but protective clothing, avoidance of direct sun exposure during the peak hours of the day, and the assiduous use of chemical sunscreens are important.

A number of highly effective sunscreens are available in cream, lotion, and nongreasy gel and liquid formulations. Fair-complexioned persons should use a sunscreen with an SPF (sun protective factor) of at least 15 and preferably 30–40 every day. For those who are sensitive to PABA (*p*-aminobenzoic acid), PABA-free formulations are available. Sunscreens with high SPF values (> 30) afford some protection against UVA as well as UVB light exposure and may be helpful in managing photosensitivity disorders. Physical blockers (titanium dioxide and zinc oxide) are available in vanishing formulations. Aggressive sunscreen use should be accompanied by vitamin D supplementation in persons at risk for osteopenia (eg, organ transplant recipients).

Jorgensen CM: Scientific recommendations and human behaviour: sitting out in the sun. Lancet 2002;360:351. [PMID: 12241770]

Vatour LM et al: Long-term fracture risk following renal transplantation: a population-based study. Osteoporos Int 2004; 15:160. [PMID: 14666400]

Complications of Topical Dermatologic Therapy

Complications of topical therapy can be largely avoided. They fall into several categories:

A. ALLERGY

Of the topical antibiotics, neomycin and bacitracin have the greatest potential for sensitization. Diphenhydramine, benzocaine, vitamin E, aromatic essential oils, and bee pollen are potential sensitizers in topical medications. Preservatives and even the topical steroids themselves can cause allergic contact dermatitis.

B. IRRITATION

Preparations of tretinoin, benzoyl peroxide, and other acne medications should be applied sparingly to the skin. Sunscreens may cause irritation or an acne-like eruption.

C. ABSORPTION

Drugs may be absorbed through the skin, especially through broken or inflamed skin, or from under occlusive dressings. Notable examples of topical drugs to be avoided in pregnancy include podophyllum resin, and tretinoin (Retin-A). Consult a pharmacology reference source when prescribing medications for pregnant or nursing women.

D. OVERUSE

Topical corticosteroids may induce acne-like lesions on the face (steroid rosacea) and atrophic striae in body folds.

■ COMMON DERMATOSES

Dermatologic diseases will be discussed according to the types of lesions they cause. Therefore, in order to make a diagnosis, it is best to (1) focus on the type of individual lesion the patient exhibits; (2) choose the morphologic category the lesions seem to fit; and then (3) identify the specific features of the history, physical examination, and laboratory tests that will establish the diagnosis.

The major morphologic types of skin lesion are listed in Table 6–2 along with the disorders with which they are most prominently associated. Miscellaneous skin, hair, and nail disorders and drug eruptions are discussed at the end of the chapter.

PIGMENTED LESIONS

Deaths from **malignant melanoma** are prevented by early diagnosis followed by excision. The nonderma-tologist clinician must be able to evaluate pigmented lesions and appropriately refer for evaluation all potential malignant melanomas. In order to avoid missing some malignant melanomas, it is understood that many patients will be referred for what ultimately prove to be benign lesions.

In general, a **benign mole** is a small (< 6 mm), well-circumscribed lesion with a well-defined border and a single shade of pigment from beige or pink to dark brown. The physical examination must take precedence over the history, though a reliable history that a lesion has been present without change for decades is obviously a comfort.

Moles have a normal natural history. In the patient's first decade of life, moles often appear as flat, small, brown lesions. They are called **junctional nevi** because the nevus cells are at the junction of the epidermis and dermis. Over the next 2 decades, these moles grow in size and often become raised, reflecting the appearance of a dermal component, giving rise to **compound nevi.** Moles may darken and grow during pregnancy. As white patients enter their seventh and

Table 6–2. Morphologic categorization of skin lesions and diseases.

Pigmented	Freckle, lentigo, seborrheic keratosis, nevus, blue nevus, halo nevus, dysplastic nevus, melanoma
Scaly	Psoriasis, dermatitis (atopic, stasis, seborrheic, chronic allergic contact or irritant contact), xerosis (dry skin), lichen simplex chronicus, tinea, tinea versicolor, secondary syphilis, pityriasis rosea, discoid lupus erythematosus, exfoliative dermatitis, actinic keratoses, Bowen's disease, Paget's disease, intertrigo
Vesicular	Herpes simplex, varicella, herpes zoster, dyshidrosis (vesicular dermatitis of palms and soles), vesicular tinea, dermatophytid, dermatitis herpetiformis, miliaria, scabies, photosensitivity
Weepy or encrusted	Impetigo, acute contact allergic dermatitis, any vesicular dermatitis
Pustular	Acne vulgaris, acne rosacea, folliculitis, candidiasis, miliaria, any vesicular dermatitis
Figurate ("shaped") erythema	Urticaria, erythema multiforme, erythema migrans, cellulitis, erysipelas, erysipeloid, arthropod bites
Bullous	Impetigo, blistering dactylitis, pemphigus, pemphigoid, porphyria cutanea tarda, drug eruptions, erythema multiforme, toxic epidermal necrolysis
Papular	Hyperkeratotic: warts, corns, seborrheic keratoses Purple-violet: lichen planus, drug eruptions, Kaposi's sarcoma Flesh-colored, umbilicated: molluscum contagiosum Pearly: basal cell carcinoma, intradermal nevi Small, red, inflammatory: acne, miliaria, candidiasis, scabies, folliculitis
Pruritus[1]	Xerosis, scabies, pediculosis, bites, systemic causes, anogenital pruritus
Nodular, cystic	Erythema nodosum, furuncle, cystic acne, follicular (epidermal) inclusion cyst
Photodermatitis (photodistributed rashes)	Drug, polymorphic light eruption, lupus erythematosus
Morbilliform	Drug, viral infection, secondary syphilis
Erosive	Any vesicular dermatitis, impetigo, aphthae, lichen planus, erythema multiforme
Ulcerated	Decubiti, herpes simplex, skin cancers, parasitic infections, syphilis (chancre), chancroid, vasculitis, stasis, arterial disease

[1]Not a morphologic class but included because it is one of the most common dermatologic presentations.

eighth decades, most moles have lost their junctional component and dark pigmentation and undergo fibrosis or other degenerative changes. Still, at every stage of life, normal moles should be well-demarcated, symmetric, and uniform in contour and color.

Abbasi NR et al: Early diagnosis of cutaneous melanoma: Revisiting the ABCD criteria. JAMA 2004;292:2771. [PMID: 15585738]

ATYPICAL NEVI

The term "atypical nevus" or "atypical mole" has supplanted "dysplastic nevus." The diagnosis of atypical moles is made clinically and not histologically, and moles should be removed only if they are suspected to be melanomas. Clinically, these moles are large (> 5 mm in diameter), with an ill-defined, irregular border and irregularly distributed pigmentation. It is estimated that 5–10% of the United States population have one or more atypical nevi. Studies have defined an increased risk of melanoma in the following populations: patients with 50 or more nevi with one or more atypical moles and one mole at least 8 mm or larger, and patients with a few to many definitely atypical moles. These patients deserve education and regular (usually every 6–12 months) follow-up. Kindreds with familial melanoma (numerous atypical nevi and a strong family history) deserve even closer attention, as the risk of developing single or even multiple melanomas in these individuals approaches 50% by age 50.

Naeyaert JM et al: Clinical practice. Dysplastic nevi. N Engl J Med 2003;349:2233. [PMID: 14657431]

CONGENITAL NEVI

The management of small congenital nevi—less than a few centimeters in diameter—is controversial. The vast majority will never become malignant, but some experts believe that the risk of melanoma in these lesions may be somewhat increased. Since 1% of whites are born with these lesions, management should be conservative and excision advised only for lesions in cosmetically nonsensitive areas where the patient cannot easily see the lesion and note any suspicious changes. Excision should be considered for congenital nevi whose contour (bumpiness, nodularity) or color (different shades) makes it difficult for examiners to note early signs of malignant change. Giant congenital melanocytic nevi (> 5% body surface area [BSA]) are at greater risk for development of melanoma, and surgical removal is often recommended.

BLUE NEVI

Blue nevi are small, slightly elevated, and blue-black lesions. They are common in persons of Asian descent, and an individual patient may have several of them. If present without change for many years, they may be considered benign, since malignant blue nevi are rare. However, blue-black papules and nodules that are new or growing must be evaluated to rule out nodular melanoma.

FRECKLES & LENTIGINES

Freckles (ephelides) and lentigines are flat brown spots. Freckles first appear in young children, darken with ultraviolet exposure, and fade with cessation of sun exposure. In adults, depending on the fairness of the complexion, flat brown spots (lentigines), often with sharp borders, gradually appear in sun-exposed areas, particularly the dorsa of the hands. They do not fade with cessation of sun exposure. They should be evaluated like all pigmented lesions: If the pigmentation is homogeneous and they are symmetric and flat, they are most likely benign. Solar lentigines, also called liver spots, can be treated with topical 0.1% tretinoin, 2% 4-hydroxyanisole with tretinoin 0.01% (Solage), laser therapy, and cryotherapy.

Chan HH et al: The use of lasers and intense pulsed light sources of the treatment of primary lesions. Skin Therapy Lett 2004;9:5. [PMID: 15550991]

Ortonne JP et al: Safety and efficacy of combined use of 4-hydroxyanisole (mequinol) 2%/tretinoin 0.01% solution and sunscreen in solar lentigines. Cutis 2004,74:261. [PMID: 15551721]

SEBORRHEIC KERATOSES

Seborrheic keratoses are benign plaques, beige to brown or even black, 3–20 mm in diameter, with a velvety or warty surface. They appear to be stuck or pasted onto the skin. They are common—especially in the elderly—and may be mistaken for melanomas or other types of cutaneous neoplasms. Although they may be frozen with liquid nitrogen or curetted if they itch or are inflamed, no treatment is needed.

Herron MD et al: Seborrheic keratoses: a study comparing the standard cryosurgery with topical calcipotriene, topical tazarotene, and topical imiquimod. Int J Dermatol 2004; 43:300. [PMID: 15090020]

MALIGNANT MELANOMA

 ESSENTIALS OF DIAGNOSIS

- *May be flat or raised.*
- *Should be suspected in any pigmented skin lesion with recent change in appearance.*
- *Examination with good light may show varying colors, including red, white, black, and bluish.*
- *Borders typically irregular.*

General Considerations

Malignant melanoma is the leading cause of death due to skin disease. There were 55,000 cases of melanoma in the United States in 2004, with 7900 deaths. One in four cases of melanoma occur before the age of 40.

Overall survival for melanomas in whites rose from 60% in 1960–1963 to 85% in 1983–1990, due primarily to earlier detection of lesions.

Tumor thickness is the single most important prognostic factor. Ten-year survival rates—related to thickness in millimeters—are as follows: < 1 mm, 95%; 1–2 mm, 80%; 2–4 mm, 55%; and > 4 mm, 30%. With lymph node involvement, the 5-year survival rate is 30%; with distant metastases, it is less than 10%. More accurate prognoses can be made on the basis of site, histologic features, and gender of the patient.

Clinical Findings

Primary malignant melanomas may be classified into various clinicohistologic types, including lentigo maligna melanoma (arising on chemically sun-exposed skin of older individuals); superficial spreading malignant melanoma (two-thirds of all melanomas arising on intermittently sun-exposed skin); nodular malignant melanoma; acral-lentiginous melanomas (arising on palms, soles, and nail beds); malignant melanomas on mucous membranes; and miscellaneous forms such as amelanotic (nonpigmented) melanoma and melanomas arising from blue nevi (rare) and congenital nevi.

Clinical features of pigmented lesions suspicious for melanoma are an irregular notched border where the pigment appears to be leaking into the normal surrounding skin; a topography that may be irregular, ie, partly raised and partly flat. Color variegation is present, and colors such as pink, blue, gray, white, and black are indications for referral. The American Cancer Society has proposed the mnemonic "ABCD = Asymmetry, Border irregularity, Color variegation, and Diameter greater than 6 mm." "E" for Evolution can be added. The history of a changing mole (evolution) is the single most important historical reason for close evaluation and possible referral. Bleeding and ulceration are ominous signs. A mole that stands out from the patient's other moles deserves special scrutiny, "ugly duckling sign." A patient with a large number of moles is statistically at increased risk for melanoma and deserves careful and periodic examination, particularly if the lesions are atypical. Referral of suspicious pigmented lesions is always appropriate.

While superficial spreading melanoma is largely a disease of whites, persons of other races are at risk for other types of melanoma, particularly acral lentiginous melanoma. These occur as dark, sometimes irregularly shaped lesions on the palms and soles and as new, often broad and solitary, darkly pigmented longitudinal streaks in the nails. Acral lentiginous melanoma may be a difficult diagnosis because benign pigmented lesions of the hands, feet, and nails occur commonly in more darkly pigmented persons and clinicians may hesitate to biopsy the palms, soles, and nail beds. As a result, the diagnosis is often delayed until the tumor has become clinically obvious and histologically thick. Clinicians should give special attention to new or changing lesions in these areas.

Dermoscopy—use of a special magnifying device to evaluate pigmented lesions—helps select suspicious lesions that require biopsy. In experienced hands, the specificity is 85% and the sensitivity 95%.

Treatment

Treatment of melanoma consists of excision. After histologic diagnosis, the area is usually reexcised with margins dictated by the thickness of the tumor. Thin low-risk and intermediate-risk tumors require only conservative margins of 1–3 cm. More specifically, surgical margins of 0.5 cm for melanoma in situ and 1 cm for lesions less than 1 mm in thickness are recommended.

Sentinel lymph node biopsy (selective lymphadenectomy) using preoperative lymphoscintigraphy and intraoperative lymphatic mapping is effective for staging melanoma patients with intermediate risk without clinical adenopathy and is recommended for all patients with lesions over 1 mm in thickness or with high-risk histologic features. α-Interferon and vaccine therapy may reduce recurrences in patients with high-risk melanomas. Referral of intermediate-risk and high-risk patients to centers with expertise in melanoma is strongly recommended.

Bafounta M et al: Is dermoscopy (epiluminescence microscopy) useful for the diagnosis of melanoma? Arch Dermatol 2001; 137:1343. [PMID: 11594860]

Cochran AJ et al: Update on lymphatic mapping and sentinel node biopsy in the management of patients with melanocytic tumours. Pathology 2004;36:478. [PMID: 15370119]

Curtin JA et al: Distinct sets of genetic alterations in melanoma. N Engl J Med 2005;353:2135. [PMID: 16291983]

McCarthy WH: The Australian experience in sun protection and screening for melanoma. J Surg Oncol 2004;86:236. [PMID: 15221930]

Rager EL et al: Cutaneous melanoma: update on prevention, screening, diagnosis, and treatment. Am Fam Physician 2005;72:269. [PMID: 16050450]

Tsao H et al: Management of cutaneous melanoma. N Engl J Med 2004;351:998. [PMID: 15342808]

SCALING DISORDERS
ATOPIC DERMATITIS
(Eczema)

ESSENTIALS OF DIAGNOSIS

- *Pruritic, exudative, or lichenified eruption on face, neck, upper trunk, wrists, and hands and in the antecubital and popliteal folds.*
- *Personal or family history of allergic manifestations (eg, asthma, allergic rhinitis, atopic dermatitis).*
- *Tendency to recur.*

General Considerations

Atopic dermatitis looks different at different ages and in people of different races. Because most patients have scaly dry skin at some point, this disease is being discussed under scaly dermatoses. However, acute flares may present with red patches that are weepy, shiny, or licheni-fied (ie, thickened, with more prominent skin markings) and plaques and papules. Diagnostic criteria for atopic dermatitis must include pruritus, typical morphology and distribution (flexural lichenification in adults), and a tendency toward chronic or chronically relapsing dermatitis. Also helpful are (1) a personal or family history of atopic disease (asthma, allergic rhinitis, atopic dermatitis), (2) xerosis-ichthyosis, (3) facial pallor with infraorbital darkening, (4) elevated serum IgE, (5) fissures under the ear lobes, (6) a tendency toward nonspecific hand dermatitis, (7) a tendency toward repeated skin infections, and (8) nipple eczema.

Clinical Findings

A. SYMPTOMS AND SIGNS

Itching may be severe and prolonged. Rough, red patches usually without the thickening and discrete de-marcation of psoriasis affect the face, neck, and upper trunk ("monk's cowl"). The bends of the elbows and knees are involved. In chronic cases, the skin is dry, leathery, and lichenified. Pigmented persons may have a papular eruption, and poorly demarcated hypopig-mented patches (pityriasis alba) are commonly seen on the cheeks and extremities. In black patients with severe disease, pigmentation may be lost in lichenified areas.

B. LABORATORY FINDINGS

Food allergy is an uncommon cause of flares of atopic dermatitis in adults. Blinded food challenges are the most reliable method of diagnosing suspected food allergy. Radioallergosorbent tests (RASTs) or skin tests may suggest dust mite allergy. Eosinophilia and increased serum IgE levels may be present but are nonspecific.

Differential Diagnosis

Atopic dermatitis must be distinguished from sebor-rheic dermatitis (less pruritic, frequent scalp and face involvement, greasy and scaly lesions, and quick response to therapy). Contact dermatitis and impetigo may be in the differential, especially for hyperacute, weepy flares of atopic dermatitis (although typically these diseases do not have a chronic course and characteristic distribution). Patients with active lesions are almost always colonized with *Staphylococcus aureus*, and impetiginization of atopic skin should be considered and treated when an acute flare is present.

Treatment

Treatment is most effective if the patient is instructed about the general principles of skin care and exactly how to use medications.

A. GENERAL MEASURES

Atopic patients have hyperirritable skin. Anything that dries or irritates the skin will potentially trigger dermatitis. Atopic individuals are sensitive to low humidity and often get worse in the winter, when the air is dry. Adults with atopic disorders should not bathe more than once daily. Soap should be confined to the armpits, groin, scalp and feet. Washcloths and brushes should not be used. Soaps should not be drying, and Dove, Eucerin, Aveeno, Basis, Alpha Keri, Purpose, and other soaps or cleansers, such as Cetaphil or Aquanil, may be recommended. After rinsing, the skin should be patted dry (not rubbed) and then immediately—within three minutes—covered with a thin film of an emollient such as Aquaphor, Eucerin, Vaseline, or a corticosteroid as needed. Ceratopic cream, a therapeutic moisturizer, will reduce inflammation as well as moisturize without a greasy or occlusive feel. It is much more expensive than traditional moisturizers. Atopic patients may be irritated by scratchy fabrics, including wools and acrylics. Cottons are preferable, but synthetic blends also are tolerated. Other triggers of eczema in some patients include sweating, ointments, hot bathing, and animal danders.

To determine the potential effect of foods, the patient may eliminate one food at a time for several months and monitor the severity of the disease. Dairy products and wheat are the most common offenders. Foods that are a problem typically cause itching within minutes to a few hours after ingestion.

B. LOCAL TREATMENT

Corticosteroids should be applied sparingly to the dermatitis twice daily and rubbed in well. Their potency should be appropriate to the severity of the dermatitis. In general, one should begin with triamcinolone 0.1% or a stronger corticosteroid then taper to hydrocortisone or another slightly stronger mild corticosteroid (Aclovate, Desonide). It is vital that patients taper corticosteroids and substitute emollients when the dermatitis clears to avoid the side effects of corticosteroids. Tapering is also important to avoid rebound flares of the dermatitis that may follow their abrupt cessation. Doxepin cream 5% may be used up to four times daily and is best applied simultaneously with the topical corticosteroid. Stinging and drowsiness occur in 25%. Tacrolimus ointment (Protopic 0.03% or 0.1%) and pimecrolimus ointment (Elidel 1%) can be effective in managing atopic dermatitis when applied twice daily. Burning on application occurs in about 50% of patients using Protopic and in 10–25% of Elidel users, but it may resolve with continued treatment. These medications do not appear to cause skin atrophy, striae, or other topical corticosteroid-associated side effects and are safe for application on the face and even the eyelids.

The US Food and Drug Administration (FDA) has issued a black box warning for both topical tacrolimus and pimecrolimus due to concerns about the development of T-cell lymphoma. The agents should be used sparingly and only when less expensive corticosteroids cannot be used. Tacrolimus and pimecrolimus should be avoided in patients at high risk for lymphoma (ie, those with HIV, iatrogenic immunosuppression, prior lymphoma). The treatment of atopic dermatitis is dictated by the stage of the dermatitis.

1. Acute weeping lesions—Use water or aluminum subacetate solution (Domeboro tablets, one in a pint of cool water) or colloidal oatmeal (Aveeno; dispense one box, and use as directed on box) as soothing or astringent soaks, baths, or wet dressings for 10–30 minutes two to four times daily. Lesions on extremities particularly may be bandaged for protection at night. Corticosteroid lotions or creams are preferred to ointments for this stage. Use high-potency corticosteroids after bathing but spare the face and body folds. Tacrolimus may not be tolerated at this stage. Systemic corticosteroids may be required (see below).

2. Subacute or scaly lesions—At this stage, the lesions are dry but still red and pruritic. Mid- to high-potency corticosteroids in ointment form should be continued until scaling and elevated skin lesions are cleared and itching is decreased substantially. At that point, patients should begin a 2- to 4-week taper from twice-daily to daily to alternate-day dosing with topical corticosteroids to reliance on emollients, with occasional use of corticosteroids on specific itchy areas. Instead of tapering the frequency of usage of a more potent corticosteroid, it may be preferable to switch to a low-potency corticosteroid. Tacrolimus and pimecrolimus are more expensive alternatives and may be added if corticosteroids cannot be stopped to avoid the complications of long-term topical corticosteroid use.

3. Chronic, dry, lichenified lesions—Thickened and usually well-demarcated, they are best treated with high-potency to ultra-high-potency corticosteroid ointments. Nightly occlusion for 2–6 weeks may enhance the initial response. Occasionally, adding tar preparations such as LCD (liquor carbonis detergens) 10% in Aquaphor or 2% crude coal tar may be beneficial.

4. Maintenance treatment—Once symptoms have improved, constant application of effective moisturizers is recommended to prevent flares. In patients with moderate disease, weekend only use of topical corticosteroids can prevent flares.

C. SYSTEMIC AND ADJUVANT THERAPY

Systemic corticosteroids are indicated only for severe acute exacerbations. Oral prednisone dosages should be high enough to suppress the dermatitis quickly, usually starting with 40–60 mg daily for adults. The dosage is then tapered to nil over a period of 2–4 weeks. Owing to the chronic nature of atopic dermatitis and the side effects of chronic systemic corticosteroids, long-term use of these agents is not recommended for maintenance therapy. Classic antihistamines may relieve severe pruritus. Hydroxyzine, diphenhydramine, or doxepin may be use-

ful—the dosage increased gradually to avoid drowsiness. Fissures, crusts, erosions, or pustules indicate staphylococcal infection clinically. Therefore, antistaphylococcal antibiotics given systemically—such as dicloxacillin or first-generation cephalosporins—may be helpful in management. Cultures to exclude methicillin-resistant *S aureus* are recommended. Phototherapy can be an important adjunct for severely affected patients, and the properly selected patient with recalcitrant disease may benefit greatly from therapy with UVB with or without coal tar or PUVA (psoralen plus ultraviolet A). Oral cyclosporine, mycophenolate mofetil, or azathioprine may be used for the most severe and recalcitrant cases.

Complications of Treatment

The clinician should monitor for skin atrophy. **Eczema herpeticum,** a generalized herpes simplex infection manifested by monomorphic vesicles, crusts, or erosions superimposed on atopic dermatitis or other extensive eczematous processes, is treated successfully with oral acyclovir, 200 mg five times daily, or intravenous acyclovir in a dose of 10 mg/kg intravenously every 8 hours (500 mg/m^2 every 8 hours). Tacrolimus and pimecrolimus increase the risk of eczema herpeticum.

Smallpox vaccination is absolutely contraindicated in patients with atopic dermatitis or a history thereof because of the risk of eczema vaccinatum. Generalized vaccinia may develop in patients with atopic dermatitis who have contact with recent vaccine recipients who still have pustular or crusted vaccination sites. Eczema vaccinatum and generalized vaccinia are indications for vaccinia immune globulin.

Prognosis

Atopic dermatitis runs a chronic or intermittent course. Affected adults may have only hand dermatitis. Poor prognostic factors for persistence into adulthood in atopic dermatitis include onset early in childhood, early generalized disease, and asthma. Only 40–60% of these patients have lasting remissions.

Leung DY et al: Atopic dermatitis. Lancet 2003;361:151. [PMID: 12531593]

Roos TC et al: Recent advances in treatment strategies for atopic dermatitis. Drugs 2004;64:2639. [PMID: 15537368]

Williams HC: Twice-weekly topical corticosteroid therapy may reduce atopic dermatitis relapses. Arch Dermatol 2004;140: 1151. [PMID: 15381558]

Williams HC: Clinical practice. Atopic dermatitis. N Engl J Med 2005;352:2314. [PMID: 15930422]

LICHEN SIMPLEX CHRONICUS (Circumscribed Neurodermatitis)

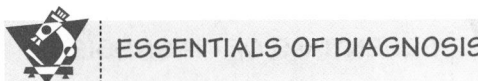

ESSENTIALS OF DIAGNOSIS

• *Chronic itching and scratching.*

- *Lichenified lesions with exaggerated skin lines overlying a thickened, well-circumscribed scaly plaque.*
- *Predilection for nape of neck, wrists, external surfaces of forearms, lower legs, scrotum, and vulva.*

General Considerations

Lichen simplex chronicus represents a self-perpetuating scratch-itch cycle.

Clinical Findings

Intermittent itching incites the patient to scratch the lesions. Itching may be so intense as to interfere with sleep. Dry, leathery, hypertrophic, lichenified plaques appear on the neck, ankles, perineum, or almost anywhere. The patches are rectangular, thickened, and hyperpigmented. The skin lines are exaggerated.

Differential Diagnosis

This disorder can be differentiated from plaque-like lesions such as psoriasis (redder lesions having whiter scales on the elbows, knees, and scalp and nail findings), lichen planus (violaceous, usually smaller polygonal papules), and nummular (coin-shaped) dermatitis. Lichen simplex chronicus may complicate chronic atopic dermatitis.

Treatment

For lesions in extra-genital regions, clobetasol, halobetasol, diflorasone, and betamethasone dipropionate are effective without occlusion and are used twice daily for several weeks. In some patients, flurandrenolide (Cordran) tape may be more effective, since it prevents scratching and rubbing of the lesion. These superpotent corticosteroids are probably the treatment of choice but must be used with careful follow-up to avoid local side effects. The injection of triamcinolone acetonide suspension (5–10 mg/mL) into the lesions may occasionally be curative. Use of tars, such as 10% LCD (liquor carbonis detergens) with topical corticosteroids, or continuous occlusion with a flexible hydrocolloid dressing for 7 days at a time for 1–2 months, may also be helpful. The area should be protected and the patient encouraged to become aware of when he or she is scratching. For genital lesions, see the section Pruritus Ani.

Prognosis

The disease tends to remit during treatment but may recur or develop at another site.

PSORIASIS

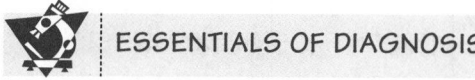

ESSENTIALS OF DIAGNOSIS

- *Silvery scales on bright red, well-demarcated plaques, usually on the knees, elbows, and scalp.*
- *Nail findings including pitting and onycholysis (separation of the nail plate from the bed).*
- *Mild itching (usually).*
- *May be associated with psoriatic arthritis.*
- *Histopathology is not often useful and can be confusing.*

General Considerations

Psoriasis is a common benign, chronic inflammatory skin disease with a genetic basis. Injury or irritation of normal skin tends to induce lesions of psoriasis at the site (Koebner's phenomenon). Psoriasis has several variants—the most common is the plaque type. Eruptive (guttate) psoriasis consisting of myriad lesions 3–10 mm in diameter occurs occasionally after streptococcal pharyngitis. Rarely, grave, occasionally life-threatening forms (generalized pustular and erythrodermic psoriasis) may occur. Plaque type or extensive erythrodermic psoriasis with abrupt onset may accompany HIV infection.

Clinical Findings

There are often no symptoms, but itching may occur. Although psoriasis may occur anywhere, the scalp, elbows, knees, palms and soles, and nails should be examined. The lesions are red, sharply defined plaques covered with silvery scales. The glans penis and vulva may be affected. Occasionally, only the flexures (axillae, inguinal areas) are involved. Fine stippling ("pitting") in the nails is highly suggestive of psoriasis. Psoriatics often have a pink or red intergluteal fold. Not all patients have findings in all locations, but the occurrence of a few may help make the diagnosis when other lesions are not typical. Some patients have mainly hand or foot dermatitis and only minimal findings elsewhere. There may be associated arthritis that is most commonly distal and oligoarticular, although the rheumatoid variety with a negative rheumatoid factor may occur.

Differential Diagnosis

The combination of red plaques with silvery scales on elbows and knees, with scaliness in the scalp or nail findings, is diagnostic. Psoriasis lesions are well demarcated and affect extensor surfaces—in contrast to atopic dermatitis, with poorly demarcated plaques in flexural distribution. In body folds, scraping and culture for candida and examination of scalp and nails will distinguish psoriasis from intertrigo and candidiasis. Dystrophic changes in nails may simulate onychomycosis, but again, the general examination combined with a potassium hydroxide (KOH) or fungal culture will be valuable in diagnosis. The cutaneous features of reactive arthritis (Reiter's syndrome) mimic psoriasis.

Treatment

There are many therapeutic options in psoriasis to be chosen according to the extent and severity of disease and with a clear understanding of the risks and benefits of therapy. Certain drugs, such as β-blockers, antimalarials, statins, and lithium, may flare or worsen psoriasis.

A. LIMITED DISEASE

For many patients, the easiest regimen is to use a high-potency to ultra-high-potency topical corticosteroid cream or ointment. It is best to restrict the ultra-high-potency corticosteroids to 2–3 weeks of twice-daily use and then use them in a pulse fashion three or four times on weekends or switch to a midpotency corticosteroid. Topical corticosteroids rarely induce a lasting remission. They may induce tachyphylaxis or cause psoriasis to become unstable. Additional measures are therefore commonly added to topical corticosteroid therapy. Calcipotriene ointment 0.005%, a vitamin D analog, is used twice daily for plaque psoriasis. Initially, patients are treated with twice-daily corticosteroids plus calcipotriene twice daily. This rapidly clears the lesions. Calcipotriene is then used alone once daily and with the corticosteroid once daily for several weeks. Eventually, the topical corticosteroids are stopped, and once- or twice-daily calcipotriene is continued long-term. Calcipotriene usually cannot be applied to the groin or on the face because of irritation. Treatment of extensive psoriasis with calcipotriene may result in hypercalcemia. Calcipotriene is incompatible with many topical corticosteroids (but not halobetasol), so if used concurrently it must be applied at a different time. Tar preparations such as Fototar cream, LCD (liquor carbonis detergens) 10% in Nutraderm lotion, alone or mixed directly with triamcinolone 0.1%, are useful adjuncts when applied twice daily. Occlusion alone has been shown to clear isolated plaques in 30–40% of patients. Occlusive hydrocolloid dressings such as thin DuoDerm are placed on the lesions and left undisturbed for as long as possible (a minimum of 5 days, up to 7 days) and then replaced. Responses may be seen within several weeks.

Tazarotene gel, a topical retinoid, is useful for the treatment of mild to moderate plaque psoriasis. About 50% of patients obtained at least 75% improvement of their skin lesions with twice-daily application, though fewer than 10% of plaques completely clear with 8 weeks of treatment. Tazarotene gel is available in 0.05% and 0.1% formulations. There is no difference between once-daily and twice-daily applications of the 0.1% formulation, but the 0.05% formulation is less effective when used once daily. Tazarotene gel appears to be similar to calcipotriene in that it may be used to augment the benefits of other forms of treatment. It is more expensive than calcipotriene and more irritating. Tazarotene gel is compatible with topical corticosteroids and may be applied simultaneously.

For the scalp, start with a tar shampoo, used daily if possible. For thick scales, use 6% salicylic acid gel (eg, Keralyt), P & S solution (phenol, mineral oil, and glycerin), or fluocinolone acetonide 0.01% in oil (Derma-Smoothe/FS) under a shower cap at night, and shampoo in the morning. In order of increasing potency, triamcinolone 0.1%, or fluocinolone, betamethasone dipropionate, fluocinonide or amcinonide, and clobetasol are available in solution form for use on the scalp twice daily. Clobetasol is also available as a shampoo. For psoriasis in the body folds, treatment is difficult, since potent corticosteroids cannot be used and other agents are poorly tolerated. Tacrolimus ointment 0.1% or 0.03% or pimecrolimus cream 1% may be effective in penile, groin, and facial psoriasis.

B. GENERALIZED DISEASE

If psoriasis involves more than 30% of the body surface, it is difficult to treat with topical agents. The treatment of choice is outpatient UVB light exposure three times weekly. Clearing occurs in an average of 7 weeks, but maintenance may be required. Severe psoriasis unresponsive to outpatient ultraviolet light may be treated in a psoriasis day care center with the Goeckerman regimen, which involves use of crude coal tar for many hours and exposure to UVB light. Such treatment may offer the best chance for prolonged remissions.

PUVA may be effective even in patients who have not responded to standard UVB treatment. Long-term use of PUVA is associated with an increased risk of skin cancer (especially squamous cell carcinoma and perhaps melanoma), particularly in persons with fair complexions. Thus, periodic examination of the skin is imperative. Atypical lentigines are a common complication. There can be rapid aging of the skin in fair individuals. Cataracts have not been reported with proper use of protective glasses. PUVA may be used in combination with other therapy, such as acitretin or methotrexate.

Parenteral corticosteroids should not be used because of the possibility of induction of pustular lesions. Methotrexate is very effective for severe psoriasis in doses up to 25 mg once weekly. It should be used according to published protocols. Liver biopsy is performed initially after methotrexate has been used long enough by the patient to demonstrate that it is effective and well tolerated, and then at intervals depending on the cumulative dose, usually 1.5–2 g. Administration of folic acid, 1–2 mg daily, will eliminate nausea caused by methotrexate without compromising efficacy.

Acitretin, a synthetic retinoid, is most effective for pustular psoriasis in dosages of 0.5–0.75 mg/kg/d, but it also improves erythrodermic and plaque types and psoriatic arthritis. Liver enzymes and serum lipids must be checked periodically. Because acitretin is a teratogen and persists for long periods in fat, women of childbearing age must wait at least 3 years after completing acitretin treatment before considering pregnancy. When used as single agents, retinoids will flatten psoriatic plaques, but will rarely result in complete clearing. Retinoids find their greatest use when combined with phototherapy—either UVB or PUVA, with which they are synergistic.

Cyclosporine dramatically improves psoriasis and may be used to control severe cases. Rapid relapse (rebound) is the rule after cessation of therapy, so another agent must be added if cyclosporine is stopped. Systemic immunomodulators can be effective in treating psoriasis. The tumor necrosis factor (TNF) inhibitors etanercept (Enbrel), 50 mg twice weekly, and infliximab (Remicade) have shown antipsoriatic activity. Infliximab provides the most rapid response and can be used for severe pustular or erythrodermic flares. Etanercept is used more frequently for long-term treatment at a dose of 50 mg twice weekly for 3 months, then 25 mg twice weekly. Alefacept (Amevive) also improves psoriasis. Efalizumab (Raptiva), an anti-CD11a monoclonal antibody has moderate efficacy. Treatment with these agents is usually effective, but in some patients the psoriasis may be worsened upon their withdrawal. High cost and potential toxicity are current limitations in the use of these new agents.

Prognosis

The course tends to be chronic and unpredictable, and the disease may be refractory to treatment.

Jacobi TC et al: A clinical dilemma while treating hypercholesterolaemia in psoriasis. Br J Dermatol 2003;149:1292. [PMID: 14674922]

Lebwohl M et al: Psoriasis treatment: traditional therapy. Ann Rheum Dis 2005;64:ii83. [PMID: 15708945]

Mallbris L et al: Psoriasis phenotype at disease onset: clinical characterization of 400 adult cases. J Invest Dermatol 2005; 124:499. [PMID: 15737189]

Mason J et al: Topical preparations for the treatment of psoriasis: a systematic review. Br J Dermatol 2002;146:351. [PMID: 11952534]

Yosipovitch G et al: Practical management of psoriasis in the elderly: epidemiology, clinical aspects, quality of life, patient education and treatment options. Drugs Aging 2002;19: 847. [PMID: 12428994]

PITYRIASIS ROSEA

ESSENTIALS OF DIAGNOSIS

- *Oval, fawn-colored, scaly eruption following cleavage lines of trunk.*
- *Herald patch precedes eruption by 1–2 weeks.*
- *Occasional pruritus.*

General Considerations

This is a common mild, acute inflammatory disease that is 50% more common in females. Young adults are principally affected, mostly in the spring or fall. Concurrent household cases have been reported.

Clinical Findings

Itching is common but is usually mild. The diagnosis is made by finding one or more classic lesions. The lesions consist of oval, fawn-colored plaques up to 2 cm in diameter. The centers of the lesions have a crinkled or "cigarette paper" appearance and a collarette scale, ie, a thin bit of scale that is bound at the periphery and free in the center. Only a few lesions in the eruption may have this characteristic appearance, however. Lesions follow cleavage lines on the trunk (so-called Christmas tree pattern), and the proximal portions of the extremities are often involved. A variant that affects the flexures (axillae and groin), so called inverse pityriasis rosea, and a papular variant, especially in black patients, also occur. An initial lesion ("herald patch") that is often larger than the later lesions often precedes the general eruption by 1–2 weeks. The eruption usually lasts 6–8 weeks and heals without scarring.

Differential Diagnosis

A serologic test for syphilis should be performed if at least a few perfectly typical lesions are not present and especially if there are palmar and plantar or mucous membrane lesions or adenopathy, features that are suggestive of secondary syphilis. For the nonexpert, an RPR (rapid plasma reagin) test in all cases is not unreasonable. Tinea corporis may present with red, slightly scaly plaques, but rarely are there more than a few lesions of tinea corporis compared to the many lesions of pityriasis rosea. A scraping of scale for a KOH test will rapidly make the diagnosis. Seborrheic dermatitis on occasion presents on the body with poorly demarcated patches over the sternum, in the pubic area, and in the axillae. The classic lesions of pityriasis rosea are not present. Tinea versicolor, viral exanthems, and drug eruptions may simulate pityriasis rosea.

Treatment

Pityriasis rosea often requires no treatment. In Asians, Hispanics, or blacks, in whom lesions may remain hyperpigmented for some time, more aggressive management may be indicated. The most effective management consists of daily UVB treatments, or prednisone as used for contact dermatitis. Topical corticosteroids of medium strength (triamcinolone 0.1%) may also be used if pruritus is bothersome. Oral erythromycin for 14 days was reported to clear 73% of patients within 2 weeks (compared with none of the patients on placebo).

Prognosis

Pityriasis rosea is usually an acute self-limiting illness that disappears in about 6 weeks.

Karnath B et al: Pityriasis rosea. Appearance and distribution of macules aid diagnosis. Postgrad Med 2003;113:93. [PMID: 12764899]

Stulberg DL et al: Pityriasis rosea. Am Fam Physician 2004; 69:87. [PMID: 14727822]

SEBORRHEIC DERMATITIS & DANDRUFF

 ESSENTIALS OF DIAGNOSIS

- *Dry scales and underlying erythema.*
- *Scalp, central face, presternal, interscapular areas, umbilicus, and body folds.*

General Considerations

Seborrheic dermatitis is an acute or chronic papulosquamous dermatitis. Seborrheic dermatitis may represent an inflammatory reaction to *Malassezia* yeasts.

Clinical Findings

Pruritus is an inconstant finding. The scalp, face, chest, back, umbilicus, eyelid margins, and body folds have dry scales or oily yellowish scurf. Fissuring and secondary infection are occasionally present. Patients with Parkinson's disease, patients who become acutely ill and are hospitalized, and patients with HIV infection often have seborrheic dermatitis.

Differential Diagnosis

There is a spectrum from seborrheic dermatitis to scalp psoriasis. Extensive seborrheic dermatitis may simulate intertrigo in flexural areas, but scalp, face, and sternal involvement suggests seborrheic dermatitis.

Treatment

A. Seborrhea of the Scalp

Shampoos that contain zinc pyrithione or selenium are used daily if possible. These may be alternated with ketoconazole shampoo (1% or 2%) used twice weekly. A combination of shampoos is used in refractory cases. Tar shampoos are also effective for milder cases and for scalp psoriasis. Topical corticosteroid solutions or lotions are then added if necessary and are used twice daily. (See treatment for scalp psoriasis, above.)

B. Facial Seborrheic Dermatitis

The mainstay of therapy is a mild corticosteroid (hydrocortisone 1%, alclometasone, desonide) used intermittently and not near the eyes. Potent fluorinated corticosteroids used on the face may produce steroid rosacea or atrophy and telangiectasia. These are rarely indicated for seborrheic dermatitis. If the disorder cannot be controlled with intermittent use of a topical corticosteroid alone, ketoconazole (Nizoral) 2% cream is added twice daily. Topical tacrolimus (Protopic) and pimecrolimus (Elidel) are steroid-sparing alternatives.

C. Seborrheic Dermatitis of Nonhairy Areas

Low-potency corticosteroid creams—ie, 1% or 2.5% hydrocortisone, desonide, or alclometasone dipropionate—are highly effective.

D. Seborrhea of Intertriginous Areas

Avoid greasy ointments. Apply low-potency corticosteroid lotions or creams twice daily for 5–7 days and then once or twice weekly for maintenance as necessary. Ketoconazole cream may be a useful adjunct. Tacrolimus or pimecrolimus topically may avoid corticosteroid atrophy in chronic cases.

E. Involvement of Eyelid Margins

"Marginal blepharitis" usually responds to gentle cleaning of the lid margins nightly as needed, with undiluted Johnson and Johnson Baby Shampoo using a cotton swab.

Prognosis

The tendency is for lifelong recurrences. Individual outbreaks may last weeks, months, or years.

Gupta AK et al: Seborrheic dermatitis. J Eur Acad Dermatol Venereol 2004;18:13. [PMID: 14678527]

FUNGAL INFECTIONS OF THE SKIN

Mycotic infections are traditionally divided into two principal groups—superficial and deep. In this chapter, we will discuss only the superficial infections: tinea corporis and tinea cruris; dermatophytosis of the feet and dermatophytid of the hands; tinea unguium (onychomycosis); and tinea versicolor. See Chapter 36 for discussion of deep mycoses.

The diagnosis of fungal infections of the skin is usually based on the location and characteristics of the lesions and on the following laboratory examinations: (1) Direct demonstration of fungi in 10% KOH of scrapings from suspected lesions. "If it's scaly, scrape it" is a time-honored maxim. (2) Cultures of organisms from skin scrapings. (3) Histologic sections of nails stained with periodic acid-Schiff (Hotchkiss-McManus) technique may be diagnostic if scrapings and cultures are negative.

Principles of Treatment

In general, treatment follows a diagnosis confirmed by KOH preparation or culture, especially if systemic antifungal therapy is to be used. Many other diseases cause scaling, and use of an antifungal agent without a firm diagnosis makes subsequent diagnosis more difficult. In general, fungal infections are treated topically except for those involving the nails or those deep in hair follicles on the face or body.

Griseofulvin is safe and effective for treating dermatophyte infections of the skin (except for the scalp and nails). Itraconazole, an azole antifungal, and terbinafine, an allylamine oral antifungal, have excellent activity against dermatophytes and can be used in shorter courses than griseofulvin.

Fluconazole has excellent activity against yeasts and may be the treatment of choice for many forms of mucocutaneous candidiasis. Fluconazole is less effective than itraconazole or terbinafine for the treatment of dermatophytosis.

Itraconazole, fluconazole, and terbinafine can all cause elevation of liver function tests and—though rarely in the dosing regimens used for the treatment of dermatophytosis—clinical hepatitis. Ketoconazole is no longer recommended for the treatment of dermatophytosis (except for tinea versicolor) because of the higher rate of hepatitis when it is used for more than a month.

General Measures & Prevention

Since moist skin favors the growth of fungi, dry the skin carefully after bathing or after perspiring heavily. Talc or other drying powders may be useful. The use of topical corticosteroids for other diseases may be complicated by intercurrent tinea or candidal infection, and topical antifungals are often used in intertriginous areas with corticosteroids to prevent this.

1. Tinea Corporis or Tinea Circinata (Body Ringworm)

  ESSENTIALS OF DIAGNOSIS

- Ring-shaped lesions with an advancing scaly border and central clearing or scaly patches with a distinct border.
- On exposed skin surfaces or the trunk.
- Microscopic examination of scrapings or culture confirms the diagnosis.

General Considerations

The lesions are often on exposed areas of the body such as the face and arms. A history of exposure to an infected cat may occasionally be obtained, usually indicating microsporum infection. All species of dermatophytes may cause this disease, but *Trichophyton rubrum* is the most common pathogen, usually representing extension onto the trunk or extremities of tinea cruris, pedis, or manuum.

Clinical Findings

A. SYMPTOMS AND SIGNS

Itching may be present. In classic lesions, rings of erythema have an advancing scaly border and central clearing, occasionally with hyperpigmentation.

B. LABORATORY FINDINGS

Hyphae can be demonstrated by removing scale and examining it microscopically using KOH. The diagnosis may be confirmed by culture.

Differential Diagnosis

Positive fungal studies distinguish tinea corporis from other skin lesions with annular configuration, such as the annular lesions of psoriasis, lupus erythematosus, syphilis, granuloma annulare, and pityriasis rosea. Psoriasis has typical lesions on elbows, knees, scalp, and nails. Secondary syphilis is often manifested by characteristic palmar, plantar, and mucous membrane lesions. Tinea corporis rarely has the large number of lesions seen in pityriasis rosea. Granuloma annulare lacks scales.

Complications

Complications include extension of the disease down the hair follicles (in which case it becomes much more difficult to cure) and pyoderma.

Prevention

Treat infected household pets (microsporum infections).

Treatment

A. LOCAL MEASURES

The following applied topically are effective against dermatophyte infections: miconazole, 2% cream; clotrimazole, 1% solution, cream, or lotion; econazole, 1% cream or lotion; sulconazole, 1% cream; oxiconazole, 1% cream; ciclopirox, 1% cream; naftifine, 1% cream or gel; butenafine cream; and terbinafine, 1% cream. Miconazole, clotrimazole, butenafine and terbinafine are available over the counter. Allylamines (especially terbinafine and butenafine) require shorter courses and lead to the most rapid response and prolonged remissions. Treatment should be continued for 1–2 weeks after clinical clearing. Betamethasone dipropionate with clotrimazole (Lotrisone) is not recommended. Long-term improper use may result in side effects from the high-potency corticosteroid component, especially in body folds. Cases of tinea that are clinically resistant to this combination have been reported.

B. SYSTEMIC MEASURES

Griseofulvin (ultramicrosize), 250–500 mg twice daily, is used. Typically, only 4–6 weeks of therapy are required. Itraconazole as a single week-long pulse of 200 mg daily is also effective in tinea corporis. Terbinafine, 250 mg daily for 1 month, is an alternative.

Prognosis

Body ringworm usually responds promptly to conservative topical therapy or to an oral agent within 4 weeks.

2. Tinea Cruris (Jock Itch)

 ESSENTIALS OF DIAGNOSIS

- Marked itching in intertriginous areas, usually sparing the scrotum.
- Peripherally spreading, sharply demarcated, centrally clearing erythematous lesions.
- May have associated tinea infection of feet or toenails.
- Laboratory examination with microscope or culture confirms diagnosis.

General Considerations

Tinea cruris lesions are confined to the groin and gluteal cleft. Intractable pruritus ani may occasionally be caused by a tinea infection.

Clinical Findings

A. SYMPTOMS AND SIGNS

Itching may be severe, or the rash may be asymptomatic. The lesions have sharp margins, cleared centers, and active, spreading scaly peripheries. Follicular pustules are sometimes encountered. The area may be hyperpigmented on resolution.

B. LABORATORY FINDINGS

Hyphae can be demonstrated microscopically in KOH preparations. The organism may be cultured.

Differential Diagnosis

Tinea cruris must be distinguished from other lesions involving the intertriginous areas, such as candidiasis, seborrheic dermatitis, intertrigo, psoriasis of body folds ("inverse psoriasis"), erythrasma, and rarely tinea versicolor. Candidiasis is generally bright red and marked by satellite papules and pustules outside of the main border of the lesion. Candida typically involves the scrotum. Tinea versicolor can be diagnosed by the KOH preparation. Seborrheic dermatitis also often involves the face, sternum, and axillae. Intertrigo tends to be more red, less scaly, and present in obese individuals in moist body folds with less extension onto the thigh. Inverse psoriasis is characterized by distinct plaques. Other areas of typical psoriatic involvement should be checked, and the KOH examination will be negative. Erythrasma is best diagnosed with Wood's light—a brilliant coral-red fluorescence is seen.

Treatment

A. GENERAL MEASURES

Drying powder (eg, miconazole nitrate [Zeasorb-AF]) should be dusted into the involved area in patients with excessive perspiration or occlusion of skin due to obesity. Underwear should be loose-fitting.

B. LOCAL MEASURES

Any of the preparations listed in the section on tinea corporis may be used. There is great variation in expense, with miconazole, clotrimazole, butenafine, and terbinafine available over the counter and usually at a lower price. Terbinafine cream is curative in over 80% of cases after once-daily use for 7 days.

C. SYSTEMIC MEASURES

Griseofulvin ultramicrosize is reserved for severe cases. Give 250–500 mg orally twice daily for 1–2 weeks. One week of either itraconazole, 200 mg daily, or terbinafine, 250 mg daily, is also effective.

Prognosis

Tinea cruris usually responds promptly to topical or systemic treatment. It may leave behind postinflammatory hyperpigmentation.

3. Tinea Manuum & Tinea Pedis (Dermatophytosis, Tinea of Palms & Soles, "Athlete's Foot")

 ESSENTIALS OF DIAGNOSIS

- Most often presenting with asymptomatic scaling.
- May progress to fissuring or maceration in toe web spaces.
- Common cofactor in lower leg cellulitis.
- Itching, burning, and stinging of interdigital web; scaling palms, and soles; vesicles of soles in inflammatory cases.
- The fungus is shown in skin scrapings examined microscopically or by culture of scrapings.

General Considerations

Tinea of the feet is an extremely common acute or chronic dermatosis. Certain individuals appear to be more susceptible than others. Most infections are caused by *Trichophyton* species.

Clinical Findings

A. SYMPTOMS AND SIGNS

The presenting symptom may be itching, burning, or stinging. Pain may indicate secondary infection with complicating cellulitis. Interdigital tinea pedis is the most common cause of leg cellulitis in healthy individuals. Tinea pedis has several presentations that vary with the location. On the sole and heel, tinea may appear as chronic noninflammatory scaling, occasionally with thickening and fissuring. This may extend over the sides of the feet in a "moccasin" distribution. The KOH preparation is usually positive. Tinea pedis often appears as a scaling or fissuring of the toe webs, perhaps with sodden maceration. As the web spaces become more macerated, the KOH preparation and fungal culture are less often positive because bacterial species begin to dominate. Finally, there may also be grouped vesicles distributed anywhere on the soles, generalized exfoliation of the skin of the soles, or nail involvement in the form of discoloration and thickening and crumbling of the nail plate.

B. LABORATORY FINDINGS

Hyphae can be demonstrated microscopically in skin scales treated with 10% KOH. KOH and culture does not always demonstrate pathogenic fungi from macerated areas.

Differential Diagnosis

Differentiate from other skin conditions involving the same areas, such as interdigital erythrasma (use Wood's light). Psoriasis may be a cause of chronic scaling on the palms or soles and may cause nail changes. Repeated fungal cultures should be negative, and the condition will not respond to antifungal therapy. Contact dermatitis (from shoes) will often involve the dorsal surfaces and will respond to topical or systemic corticosteroids. Vesicular lesions should be differentiated from pompholyx (dyshidrosis) and scabies by proper scraping of the roofs of individual vesicles. Rarely, gram-negative organisms may cause toe web infections in the setting of prior tinea or in its absence. Culture is not very specific, because gram-negative organisms can be cultured from normal toe webs. This entity is treated with aluminum salts (see below) and imidazole antifungal agents or ciclopirox.

Prevention

The essential factor in prevention is personal hygiene. Wear open-toed sandals if possible. Use of rubber or wooden sandals in community showers and bathing places is often recommended, though the effectiveness of this practice has not been studied. Careful drying between the toes after showering is essential. A hair dryer used on low setting may be used. Socks should be changed frequently, and absorbent nonsynthetic socks are preferred. Apply dusting and drying powders as necessary. The use of powders containing antifungal agents (eg, Zeasorb-AF) or chronic use of antifungal creams may prevent recurrences of tinea pedis.

Treatment

A. LOCAL MEASURES

1. Macerated stage—Treat with aluminum subacetate solution soaks for 20 minutes twice daily. Broadspectrum antifungal creams and solutions (containing

imidazoles or ciclopirox instead of tolnaftate and haloprogin) will help combat diphtheroids and other gram-positive organisms present at this stage and alone may be adequate therapy. If topical imidazoles fail, 1 week of once-daily topical allylamine treatment (terbinafine or butenafine) will often result in clearing.

2. Dry and scaly stage—Use any of the agents listed in the section on tinea corporis. The addition of urea 10% lotion or cream may increase the efficacy of topical treatments in thick ("moccasin") tinea of the soles.

B. SYSTEMIC MEASURES

Griseofulvin should be used only for severe cases or those recalcitrant to topical therapy. If the infection is cleared by systemic therapy, the patient should be encouraged to begin maintenance with topical therapy, since recurrence is common. Itraconazole, 200 mg daily for 2 weeks or 400 mg daily for 1 week, or terbinafine, 250 mg daily for 2–4 weeks, may be used in refractory cases.

Prognosis

For many individuals, tinea pedis is a chronic affliction, temporarily cleared by therapy only to recur.

Gupta AK et al: Optimal management of fungal infections of the skin, hair, and nails. Am J Clin Dermatol 2004;5:225. [PMID: 15301570]

Roujeau JC et al: Chronic dermatomycoses of the foot as risk factors for acute bacterial cellulitis of the leg: a case-control study. Dermatology 2004;209:301. [PMID: 15539893]

Zuber TJ et al: Superficial fungal infection of the skin. Where and how it appears help determine therapy. Postgrad Med 2001; 109:117, 123, 131. [PMID: 11198246]

4. Tinea Versicolor (Pityriasis Versicolor)

 ESSENTIALS OF DIAGNOSIS

- Velvety, tan, or pink macules or white macules that do not tan.
- Fine scales that are not visible but are seen by scraping the lesion.
- Central upper trunk the most frequent site.
- Yeast and short hyphae observed on microscopic examination of scales.

General Considerations

Tinea versicolor is a mild, superficial *Malassezia furfur* infection of the skin (usually of the trunk). This yeast is a colonizer of all humans, which accounts for the high recurrence rate after treatment. It is not understood why some patients manifest the spore and hyphal form of the organism and the clinical disease. The eruption is often called to patients' attention by the fact that the involved areas will not tan, and the resulting hypopigmentation may be mistaken for vitiligo. A hyperpigmented form is not uncommon.

Clinical Findings

A. SYMPTOMS AND SIGNS

Lesions are asymptomatic, but a few patients note itching. The lesions are velvety, tan, pink, or white macules that vary from 4–5 mm in diameter to large confluent areas. The lesions initially do not look scaly, but scales may be readily obtained by scraping the area. Lesions may appear on the trunk, upper arms, neck, face, and groin.

B. LABORATORY FINDINGS

Large, blunt hyphae and thick-walled budding spores ("spaghetti and meatballs") may be seen when skin scales have been cleared in 10% KOH. Fungal culture is not useful.

Differential Diagnosis

Vitiligo usually presents with larger periorificial lesions. Vitiligo (and not tinea versicolor) is characterized by total depigmentation, not just a lessening of pigmentation. Vitiligo does not scale. Pink and red-brown lesions on the chest are differentiated from seborrheic dermatitis of the same areas by the KOH preparation.

Treatment & Prognosis

Topical treatments include selenium sulfide lotion, which may be applied from neck to waist daily and left on for 5–15 minutes for 7 days; this treatment is repeated weekly for a month and then monthly for maintenance. Ketoconazole shampoo, 1% or 2%, lathered on the chest and back and left on for 5 minutes may also be used weekly for maintenance. Clinicians must stress to the patient that the raised and scaly aspects of the rash are being treated; the alterations in pigmentation may take months to fade or fill in. Tinver lotion (contains sodium thiosulfate) is effective. Irritation and odor are common complaints from patients. Relapses are common.

Sulfur-salicylic acid soap or shampoo or zinc pyrithrone-containing shampoos used on a continuing basis may be effective prophylaxis.

Ketoconazole, 200 mg daily orally for 1 week or 400 mg as a single oral dose, results in short-term cure of 90% of cases. Patients should be instructed not to shower for 8–12 hours after taking ketoconazole, because it is delivered in sweat to the skin. The single dose may not work in more hot and humid areas, and more protracted therapy carries a small but finite risk of drug-induced hepatitis for a completely benign disease. Without maintenance therapy, recurrences will occur in over 80% of "cured" cases over the subsequent 2 years. Treatment with a single dose of 400 mg of oral fluconazole is also effective but more expensive.

Newer imidazole creams, solutions, and lotions are quite effective for localized areas but are too expensive for use over large areas such as the chest and back.

Schwartz RA: Superficial fungal infections. Lancet 2004;364: 1173. [PMID: 15451228]

DISCOID LUPUS ERYTHEMATOSUS (Chronic Cutaneous Lupus Erythematosus)

 ESSENTIALS OF DIAGNOSIS

- *Localized red plaques, usually on the face.*
- *Scaling, follicular plugging, atrophy, dyspigmentation, and telangiectasia of involved areas.*
- *Histology distinctive.*
- *Photosensitive.*

General Considerations

Two forms of chronic cutaneous lupus erythematosus (LE) occur: chronic scarring (discoid) lesions (DLE) and erythematous non-scarring red plaques (subacute cutaneous LE) (SCLE). Both occur most frequently in areas exposed to solar irradiation. Permanent hair loss and loss of pigmentation are common sequelae of discoid lesions. Systemic lupus erythematosus (SLE) is discussed in Chapter 20. Patients with SLE may have DLE or SCLE lesions.

Clinical Findings

A. SYMPTOMS AND SIGNS

Symptoms are usually mild. The lesions consist of dusky red, well-localized, single or multiple plaques, 5–20 mm in diameter, usually on the face. The scalp, external ears, and oral mucous membranes may be involved. In discoid lesions there is atrophy, telangiectasia, depigmentation, and follicular plugging. Discoid lesions may be covered by dry, horny, adherent scales. On the scalp, significant hair loss may occur.

B. LABORATORY FINDINGS

If antinuclear antibody (ANA) is positive in high titer or when the clinical picture suggests systemic involvement, the findings of antibody to double-stranded DNA and hypocomplementemia suggest the diagnosis of SLE. Rare patients with marked photosensitivity and a picture otherwise suggestive of lupus have negative ANA tests but are positive for antibodies against Ro/SSA (SCLE). A direct immunofluorescence test reveals basement membrane antibody but may be falsely positive in sun-exposed skin.

Differential Diagnosis

The diagnosis is based on the clinical appearance confirmed by skin biopsy in all cases. In DLE, the scales are dry and "thumbtack-like" and can thus be distinguished from those of seborrheic dermatitis and psoriasis. Older lesions that have left depigmented scarring (classically in the concha of the ear) or areas of hair loss will also differentiate lupus from these diseases. Ten percent of patients with SLE have discoid skin lesions, and 5% of patients with discoid lesions have SLE. Medications (hydrochlorothiazide, calcium channel blockers, terbinafine) may induce chronic cutaneous LE with a positive Ro.

Treatment

A. GENERAL MEASURES

Protect from sunlight. Use high-SPF (> 30) sunblock with UVB and UVA coverage daily. **Caution:** Do not use any form of radiation therapy. Avoid using drugs that are potentially photosensitizing when possible.

B. LOCAL TREATMENT

The following should be tried before systemic therapy: high-potency corticosteroid creams applied each night and covered with airtight, thin, pliable plastic film (eg, Saran Wrap); or Cordran tape; or ultra-high-potency corticosteroid cream or ointment applied twice daily without occlusion.

C. LOCAL INFILTRATION

Triamcinolone acetonide suspension, 2.5–10 mg/mL, may be injected into the lesions once a month. This should be tried before systemic therapy.

D. SYSTEMIC TREATMENT

1. Antimalarials—**Caution:** These drugs should be used only when the diagnosis is secure because they have been associated with flares of psoriasis, which may be in the differential diagnosis. They may also cause ocular changes, and ophthalmologic evaluation is required every 6 months.

a. Hydroxychloroquine sulfate—0.2–0.4 g orally daily for several months may be effective and is often used prior to chloroquine. A 3-month trial is recommended.

b. Chloroquine sulfate—250 mg daily may be effective in some cases where hydroxychloroquine is not.

c. Quinacrine (Atabrine)—100 mg daily may be the safest of the antimalarials, since eye damage has not been reported. It colors the skin yellow and is therefore not acceptable to some patients. It may be added to the above antimalarials for incomplete responses.

2. Isotretinoin—Isotretinoin, 1 mg/kg/d, is effective in chronic or subacute cutaneous LE. Recurrences are prompt and predictable on discontinuation of therapy. Because of teratogenicity, the drug is used with caution in women of childbearing age using effective contraception with negative pregnancy tests before and during therapy.

3. Thalidomide—Thalidomide is a potent teratogen but very effective in refractory cases in doses of up to 300 mg daily. Monitor for neuropathy.

Prognosis

The disease is persistent but not life-endangering unless systemic lupus intervenes, which is uncommon. Treatment with antimalarials is effective in perhaps 60% of cases. Although the only morbidity may be cosmetic, this can be of overwhelming significance in more darkly pigmented patients with widespread disease. Scarring alopecia can be prevented or lessened with close attention and aggressive therapy.

Patel P et al: Cutaneous lupus erythematosus: a review. Dermatol Clin 2002;20:373. [PMID: 12170873]

CUTANEOUS T CELL LYMPHOMA (Mycosis Fungoides)

 ESSENTIALS OF DIAGNOSIS

- *Localized or generalized erythematous scaling patches and plaques.*
- *Pruritus.*
- *Lymphadenopathy.*
- *Distinctive histology.*

General Considerations

Mycosis fungoides is a cutaneous T cell lymphoma that begins on the skin and may involve only the skin for years or decades. Certain medications (including selective serotonin reuptake inhibitors) may produce eruptions clinically and histologically identical to those of mycosis fungoides, so this possibility must always be considered.

Clinical Findings

A. SYMPTOMS AND SIGNS

Localized or generalized erythematous patches or plaques are present usually on the trunk. Plaques are almost always over 5 cm in diameter. Pruritus is a frequent complaint. The lesions often begin as nondescript or nondiagnostic patches, and it is not unusual for the patient to have skin lesions for more than a decade before the diagnosis can be confirmed. In more advanced cases, tumors appear. Lymphadenopathy may occur locally or widely. Lymph node enlargement may be due to benign expansion of the node (dermatopathic lymphadenopathy) or by specific involvement with mycosis fungoides.

B. LABORATORY FINDINGS

The skin biopsy remains the basis of diagnosis, though at times numerous biopsies are required before the diagnosis can be confirmed. In addition, circulating atypical cells (Sézary cells) can be detected in the blood by sensitive methods. Eosinophilia may be present.

Differential Diagnosis

Mycosis fungoides may be confused with psoriasis, a drug eruption, an eczematous dermatitis, Hansen's disease (leprosy), or tinea corporis. Histologic examination can distinguish these conditions.

Treatment

The treatment of mycosis fungoides is complex. Early and aggressive treatment has not been proved to cure or prevent progression of the disease. Topical mechlorethamine ointment or solution, topical corticosteroids, UVB and PUVA are all used for early patches and plaques. Radiation therapy is effective for local lesions. Photopheresis is used at some centers. Systemic agents such as retinoids and immunomodulatory agents such as α-interferon are used alone or in various combinations for more advanced disease or in patients who fail topical therapy. Standard chemotherapeutic agents, except methotrexate, are used only when other approaches fail.

Prognosis

Mycosis fungoides is usually slowly progressive (over decades). Prognosis is better in patients with patch or plaque stage disease and worse in patients with erythroderma, tumors, and lymphadenopathy. Survival is not reduced in patients with limited patch disease. Elderly patients with patch and plaque stage disease commonly die of other causes. Overly aggressive treatment may lead to complications and premature demise.

Berger CL et al: Advances in understanding the immunobiology and immunotherapy of cutaneous T-cell lymphoma. Adv Dermatol 2004;20:217. [PMID: 15544202]

Foss F: Mycosis fungoides and the Sezary syndrome. Curr Opin Oncol 2004;16:421. [PMID: 15314509]

Singh F et al: Cutaneous T-cell lymphoma treatment using bexarotene and PUVA: a case series. J Am Acad Dermatol 2004; 51:570. [PMID: 15389192]

EXFOLIATIVE DERMATITIS (Exfoliative Erythroderma)

ESSENTIALS OF DIAGNOSIS

- Scaling and erythema over most of the body.
- Itching, malaise, fever, chills, weight loss.

General Considerations

A preexisting dermatosis is the cause of exfoliative dermatitis in up to 63% of cases, including psoriasis, atopic dermatitis, contact dermatitis, pityriasis rubra pilaris, and seborrheic dermatitis. Reactions to topical or systemic drugs (eg, sulfonamides) account for perhaps 20–40% of cases and cancer (cutaneous T cell lymphoma, Sézary syndrome) for 10–20%. Causation of the remainder is indeterminable. At the time of acute presentation, without a clear-cut prior history of skin disease or drug exposure, it may be impossible to make a specific diagnosis of the underlying condition, and diagnosis may require observation.

Clinical Findings

A. SYMPTOMS AND SIGNS

Symptoms may include itching, weakness, malaise, fever, and weight loss. Chills are prominent. Redness and scaling may be generalized and sometimes include loss of hair and nails. Generalized lymphadenopathy may be due to lymphoma or leukemia or may be part of the clinical picture of the skin disease (dermatopathic lymphadenitis). The mucosa is spared.

B. LABORATORY FINDINGS

A skin biopsy is required and may show changes of a specific inflammatory dermatitis or cutaneous T cell lymphoma or leukemia. Peripheral leukocytes may show clonal rearrangements of the T cell receptor in Sézary syndrome.

Differential Diagnosis

It may be impossible to identify the cause of exfoliative dermatitis early in the course of the disease, so careful follow-up is necessary. Psoriasis, severe seborrheic dermatitis, and drug eruptions may have an erythrodermic phase.

Complications

Debility (protein loss) and dehydration may develop in patients with generalized inflammatory exfoliative erythroderma; or sepsis may occur.

Treatment

A. TOPICAL THERAPY

Home treatment is with cool to tepid baths and application of mid-potency corticosteroids under wet dressings or with the use of an occlusive plastic suit. If the exfoliative erythroderma becomes chronic and is not manageable in an outpatient setting, hospitalize the patient. Keep the room at a constant warm temperature and provide the same topical treatment as for an outpatient.

B. SPECIFIC MEASURES

Stop all drugs, if possible. Systemic corticosteroids may provide spectacular improvement in severe or fulminant exfoliative dermatitis, but long-term therapy should be avoided (see Chapter 26). In addition, systemic corticosteroids must be used with caution because some patients with erythroderma have psoriasis and could develop pustular psoriasis. For cases of psoriatic erythroderma and pityriasis rubra pilaris, either acitretin or methotrexate may be indicated. Erythroderma secondary to lymphoma or leukemia requires specific topical or systemic chemotherapy. Suitable antibiotic drugs with coverage for staphylococcus should be given when there is evidence of bacterial infection.

Prognosis

Most patients recover completely or improve greatly over time but may require long-term therapy. Deaths are rare in the absence of cutaneous T cell lymphoma. A minority of patients will suffer from undiminished erythroderma for indefinite periods.

Balasubramaniam P et al: Erythroderma: 90% skin failure. Hosp Med 2004;65:100. [PMID: 14997777]

Gallelli L et al: Generalized exfoliative dermatitis induced by interferon alfa. Ann Pharmacother 2004;38:2173. [PMID: 15522975]

Jaffer AN et al: Exfoliative dermatitis. Erythroderma can be a sign of a significant underlying disorder. Postgrad Med 2005; 117:49. [PMID: 15672891]

Shegal VN et al: Erythroderma/exfoliative dermatitis: a synopsis. Int J Dermatol 2004;43:39. [PMID: 14693020]

MISCELLANEOUS SCALING DERMATOSES

Isolated scaly patches may represent actinic (solar) keratoses, nonpigmented seborrheic keratoses, or Bowen's or Paget's disease.

Actinic Keratoses

Actinic keratoses are small (0.2–0.6 cm) patches—flesh-colored, pink, or slightly hyperpigmented—that feel like sandpaper and are tender when the finger is drawn over them. They occur on sun-exposed parts of the body in persons of fair complexion. Actinic keratoses are considered premalignant, but only 1:1000 lesions per year progress to become squamous cell carcinomas.

Application of liquid nitrogen is a rapid and effective method of eradication. The lesions crust and disappear in 10–14 days. An alternative treatment is the use of fluorouracil cream. This agent may be rubbed into the lesions morning and night until they become first red and sore and then crusted and eroded (usually 2–3 weeks), and then stopped. Carac (0.5% fluorouracil) may be used once daily for a longer period (4 weeks to several months). Keratoses may clear with less irritation. Imiquimod 5% cream applied two to three times weekly for 3–6 weeks is the more costly alternative to topical fluorouracil (5FU). Any lesions that persist should be evaluated for possible biopsy.

Jorizzo JL: Current and novel treatment options for actinic keratoses. J Cutan Med Surg 2004;8 (Suppl 3):13. [PMID: 15647860]

Silapunt S et al: Topical and light-based treatments for actinic keratoses. Semin Cutan Med Surg 2003;22:162. [PMID: 14649583]

Weiss J et al: Effective treatment of actinic keratosis with 0.5% fluorouracil cream for 1, 2, or 4 weeks. Cutis 2002;70(2 Suppl):22. [PMID: 12353677]

Bowen's Disease & Paget's Disease

Bowen's disease (intraepidermal squamous cell carcinoma) occurs either on sun-exposed or sun-protected cutaneous surfaces. The lesion is usually a small (1–3 cm), well-demarcated, slightly raised, pink to red, scaly plaque and may resemble psoriasis or a large actinic keratosis. While it may take some time, these lesions may progress to invasive squamous cell carcinoma. Excision or other definitive treatment is indicated.

Extramammary Paget's disease, a manifestation of intraepidermal carcinoma or underlying genitourinary or gastrointestinal cancer, resembles chronic eczema and usually involves apocrine areas such as the genitalia. Mammary Paget's disease of the nipple, a unilateral or rarely bilateral red scaling plaque that may ooze, is associated with an underlying intraductal mammary carcinoma.

Nishimura Y et al: Bilateral Bowen's disease. Br J Dermatol 2004; 151:227. [PMID: 15270896]

Shepherd V et al: Extramammary Paget's disease. BJOG 2005; 112:273. [PMID: 15713139]

INTERTRIGO

Intertrigo is caused by the macerating effect of heat, moisture, and friction. It is especially likely to occur in obese persons and in humid climates. The symptoms are itching, stinging, and burning. The body folds develop fissures, erythema, and sodden epidermis, with superficial denudation. Candidiasis may complicate intertrigo. "Inverse psoriasis," tinea cruris, erythrasma, and candidiasis must be ruled out.

Maintain hygiene in the area, and keep it dry. Compresses may be useful acutely. Hydrocortisone 1% cream plus an imidazole or nystatin cream is effective. Recurrences are common.

VESICULAR DERMATOSES

HERPES SIMPLEX (Cold or Fever Sore; Genital Herpes)

 ESSENTIALS OF DIAGNOSIS

- *Recurrent small grouped vesicles on an erythematous base, especially in the orolabial and genital areas.*

- May follow minor infections, trauma, stress, or sun exposure; regional lymph nodes may be swollen and tender.
- Tzanck smear is positive for multinucleated epithelial giant cells; viral cultures and direct fluorescent antibody tests are positive.

General Considerations

Over 85% of adults have serologic evidence of herpes simplex type 1 (HSV-1) infections, most often acquired asymptomatically in childhood. Occasionally, primary infections may be manifested as severe gingivostomatitis. Thereafter, the patient may have recurrent self-limited attacks, provoked by sun exposure, orofacial surgery, fever, or a viral infection.

About 25% of the United States population has serologic evidence of infection with herpes simplex type 2 (HSV-2). HSV-2 causes lesions whose morphology and natural history are similar to those caused by HSV-1 on the genitalia of both sexes. The infection is acquired by sexual contact. In monogamous heterosexual couples where one partner has HSV-2 infection, seroconversion of the noninfected partner occurs in 10% over a 1-year period. Up to 70% of such infections appeared to be transmitted during periods of asymptomatic shedding. Owing to changes in sexual behavior, up to 40% of newly acquired cases of genital herpes are due to HSV-1.

Clinical Findings

A. SYMPTOMS AND SIGNS

The principal symptoms are burning and stinging. Neuralgia may precede or accompany attacks. The lesions consist of small, grouped vesicles that can occur anywhere but which most often occur on the vermilion border of the lips, the penile shaft, the labia, the perianal skin, and the buttocks. Regional lymph nodes may be swollen and tender. The lesions usually crust and heal in 1 week. Patients can be educated to recognize attacks that they previously did not identify as recurrent herpes simplex. Herpes simplex is the most common cause of painful genital ulcerations in patients with HIV infection.

B. LABORATORY FINDINGS

Lesions of herpes simplex must be distinguished from chancroid, syphilis, pyoderma, or trauma. Direct immunofluorescent antibody slide tests offer rapid, sensitive diagnosis. Viral culture may also be helpful. The Tzanck smear, which demonstrates multinucleated cells, is the least sensitive test. Herpes simplex and varicella-zoster viruses cannot be distinguished on the Tzanck smear. Herpes serology is not used in the diagnosis of an acute genital ulcer. However, specific HSV-2 serology by Western blot assay or enzyme-linked immunosorbent assay (ELISA) can determine who is HSV-infected and potentially infectious. Such testing is very useful in couples in which only one partner reports a history of genital herpes.

Complications

Complications include pyoderma, eczema herpeticum, herpetic whitlow, herpes gladiatorum (epidemic herpes in wrestlers transmitted by contact), esophagitis, neonatal infection, keratitis, and encephalitis.

Prevention

Sunscreens are useful adjuncts in preventing sun-induced recurrences. Prophylactic use of oral acyclovir may prevent recurrences. Acyclovir should be started at a dosage of 200 mg four times daily beginning 24 hours prior to ultraviolet light exposure, dental surgery, or orolabial cosmetic surgery. Comparable doses are 500 mg twice daily for valacyclovir and 250 mg twice daily for famciclovir.

Treatment

A. SYSTEMIC THERAPY

Three systemic agents are available for the treatment of herpes infections: acyclovir, its valine analog valacyclovir, and famciclovir. All three agents are very effective and, when used properly, virtually nontoxic. Only acyclovir is available for intravenous administration. In the immunocompetent, with the exception of severe orolabial herpes, only genital disease is treated. For first clinical episodes of herpes simplex, the dosage of acyclovir is 200 mg orally five times daily (or 800 mg three times daily); of valacyclovir, 1000 mg twice daily; and of famciclovir, 250 mg three times daily. The duration of treatment is from 7 to 10 days depending on the severity of the outbreak. Most cases of recurrent herpes are mild and do not require therapy. In addition, pharmacotherapy of recurrent HSV is of limited benefit, with studies finding a reduction in the average outbreak by only 12–24 hours. If treatment is desired, recurrent genital herpes outbreaks may be treated with 3 days of valacyclovir, 500 mg twice daily, or with 5 days of acyclovir, 200 mg five times a day; or famciclovir, 125 mg twice daily. Valacyclovir, 2 g twice daily for 1 day, or penciclovir, 1 g once or twice, can be effective for recurrences of orolabial or genital herpes. The addition of a potent topical corticosteroid three times daily reduces the duration, size, and pain of orolabial herpes treated with an oral antiviral agent.

In patients with frequent or severe recurrences, suppressive therapy is most effective in controlling disease. Suppressive treatment will reduce outbreaks by 85% and reduces viral shedding by more than 90%. This results in about a 50% reduced risk of transmissions. The recommended suppressive doses, taken continuously, are acyclovir, 400 mg twice daily; valacyclovir, 500 mg once daily; or famciclovir, 125–250 mg twice daily. Long-term suppression appears very safe, and after 5–7 years a substantial proportion of patients can discontinue treatment. The use of condoms, patient education, and long-term suppressive oral antiviral therapy are all effective in reducing transmission of genital herpes. However, there is nothing—alone or in combination—that absolutely prevents transmission.

B. LOCAL MEASURES

In general, topical therapy is not effective. It is strongly urged that 5% acyclovir ointment, if used at all, be limited to the restricted indications for which it has been approved, ie, initial herpes genitalis and mucocutaneous herpes simplex infections in immunocompromised patients. Penciclovir cream, to be applied at the first symptom every 2 hours while awake for 4 days for recurrent orolabial herpes, reduces the average attack duration from 5 days to 4.5 days.

Prognosis

Aside from the complications described above, recurrent attacks last several days, and patients recover without sequelae.

Corey L et al: Once-daily valacyclovir to reduce the risk of transmission of genital herpes. N Engl J Med 2004; 350:67. [PMID: 14702423]

Spruance SL et al: Combination treatment with famciclovir and a topical corticosteroid gel versus famciclovir alone for experimental ultraviolet radiation-induced herpes simplex labialis: a pilot study. J Infect Dis 2000;181:1906. [PMID: 10837169]

HERPES ZOSTER (Shingles)

 ESSENTIALS OF DIAGNOSIS

- *Pain along the course of a nerve followed by grouped vesicular lesions.*
- *Involvement is unilateral; some lesions (< 20) may occur outside the affected dermatome.*
- *Lesions are usually on face or trunk.*
- *Direct fluorescent antibody positive, especially in vesicular lesions.*

General Considerations

Herpes zoster is an acute vesicular eruption due to the varicella-zoster virus. It usually occurs in adults. With rare exceptions, patients suffer only one attack. Dermatomal herpes zoster does not imply the presence of a visceral malignancy. Generalized disease, however, raises the suspicion of an associated immunosuppressive disorder such as Hodgkin's disease or HIV infection. HIV-infected patients are 20 times more likely to develop zoster, often before other clinical findings of HIV disease are present. A history of HIV risk factors and HIV testing when appropriate should be considered, especially in patients with zoster who are younger than 55 years.

Clinical Findings

Pain usually precedes the eruption by 48 hours or more and may persist and actually increase in intensity after the lesions have disappeared. The lesions consist of grouped, tense, deep-seated vesicles distributed unilaterally along a dermatome. The most common distributions are on the trunk or face. Up to 20 lesions may be found outside the affected dermatomes. Regional lymph glands may be tender and swollen.

Differential Diagnosis

Since poison oak and poison ivy dermatitis can occur unilaterally, they must be differentiated at times from herpes zoster. Allergic contact dermatitis is pruritic; zoster is painful. One must differentiate herpes zoster from lesions of herpes simplex, which occasionally occurs in a dermatomal distribution. Doses of antivirals appropriate for zoster should be used in the absence of a clear diagnosis. Facial zoster may simulate erysipelas initially, but zoster is unilateral and shows vesicles after 24–48 hours. The pain of preeruptive herpes zoster may lead the clinician to diagnose migraine, myocardial infarction, acute abdomen, herniated nucleus pulposus, etc, depending on the dermatome involved.

Complications

Sacral zoster may be associated with bladder and bowel dysfunction. Persistent neuralgia, anesthesia or scarring of the affected area following healing, facial or other nerve paralysis, and encephalitis may occur. Postherpetic neuralgia is most common after involvement of the trigeminal region, and in patients over the age of 55. Early (within 72 hours after onset) and aggressive antiviral treatment of herpes zoster reduces the severity and duration of postherpetic neuralgia. Zoster ophthalmicus (V_1) can result in visual impairment.

Treatment

A. GENERAL MEASURES

1. **Immunocompetent host**—Since early treatment of zoster reduces postherpetic neuralgia, those with a risk of developing this complication should be treated, ie, those over age 55. In addition, younger patients with acute moderate to severe pain may benefit from effective antiviral therapy. Treatment can be given with oral acyclovir, 800 mg five times daily; famciclovir, 500 mg three times daily; or valacyclovir, 1 g three times daily—all for 7 days (see Chapter 37). For reasons of increased bioavailability and ease of dosing schedule, the preferred agents are those given three

times daily. Patients should maintain good hydration. The dose of antiviral should be adjusted for renal function as recommended. Nerve blocks may be important in the management of initial severe pain. Ophthalmologic consultation is vital for involvement of the first branch of the trigeminal nerve. Systemic corticosteroids are effective in reducing acute pain, improving quality of life, and returning patients to normal activities much more quickly. They do not increase the risk of dissemination in immunocompetent hosts. If not contraindicated, a tapering 3-week course of prednisone, starting at 60 mg/d, should be considered for its adjunctive benefit in immunocompetent patients. Oral corticosteroids do not reduce the prevalence, severity, or duration of postherpetic neuralgia beyond that achieved by effective antiviral therapy.

2. Immunocompromised host—Given the safety and efficacy of currently available antivirals, most immunocompromised patients with herpes zoster are candidates for antiviral therapy. The dosage schedule is as listed above, but treatment should be continued until the lesions have completely crusted and are healed or almost healed (up to 2 weeks). Because corticosteroids increase the risk of dissemination, they should not be given adjunctively in immunosuppressed patients. Progression of disease may necessitate intravenous therapy with acyclovir, 10 mg/kg intravenously, three times daily. After 3–4 days, oral therapy may be substituted if there has been a good response to intravenous therapy. Adverse effects include decreased renal function from crystallization, nausea and vomiting, and abdominal pain.

Foscarnet, administered in a dosage of 40 mg/kg two or three times daily intravenously, is indicated for treatment of acyclovir-resistant varicella-zoster virus infections.

B. Local Measures

Calamine or starch shake lotions may be of some help.

C. Postherpetic Neuralgia

The most effective treatment is prevention with early and aggressive antiviral therapy. Once established, postherpetic neuralgia may be treated with capsaicin ointment, 0.025–0.075%, or lidocaine (Lidoderm) topical patches. Chronic postherpetic neuralgia may be relieved by regional blocks (stellate ganglion, epidural, local infiltration, or peripheral nerve), with or without corticosteroids added to the injections. Amitriptyline, 25–75 mg as a single nightly dose, is the first-line oral therapy beyond simple analgesics. Gabapentin, up to 3600 mg daily (starting at 300 mg three times daily), may be added for additional pain relief.

Prognosis

The eruption persists 2–3 weeks and usually does not recur. Motor involvement in 2–3% of patients may lead to temporary palsy.

Vanhems P et al: The incidence of herpes zoster is less likely than other opportunistic infections to be reduced by highly active antiretroviral therapy. J Acquir Immune Defic Syndr 2005; 38:111. [PMID: 15608535]

Wareham D: Postherpetic neuralgia. Clin Evid 2003;10:942. [PMID: 15555130]

Wassilew S; Collaborative Brivudin PHN Study Group: Brivudin compared with famciclovir in the treatment of herpes zoster: effects in acute disease and chronic pain in immunocompetent patients. A randomized, double-blind, multinational study. J Eur Acad Dermatol Venereol 2005;19:47. [PMID: 15649191]

VARIOLA (Smallpox) & VACCINIA

ESSENTIALS OF DIAGNOSIS

- *Prodromal high fever.*
- *Eruption progressing from papules to vesicles to pustules, then crusts.*
- *All lesions in the same stage.*
- *Face and distal extremities (including palms and soles) favored.*

General Considerations

Concern for the use of smallpox virus as a bioterrorist weapon has led to the reintroduction of vaccination in some segments of the population (first responders and the military).

Clinical Findings

The incubation period for variola averages 12 days (7–17 days). The prodrome begins with abrupt onset of high fever, severe headaches, and backaches. At this stage, the infected person appears quite ill. The infectious phase begins with the appearance of an enanthem, followed in 1–2 days by a skin eruption. The lesions begin as macules, progressing to papules, then pustules, and finally crusts over 14–18 days. The face and distal extremities are favored. The face is affected first, followed by the upper extremities, then the lower extremities and trunk, completely evolving over 1 week. Lesions are relatively monomorphous, especially in each anatomic region.

Inoculation with vaccinia produces a papular lesion on day 2–3 that progresses to an umbilicated papule by day 4 and a pustular lesion by the end of the first week. The lesion then collapses centrally, and crusts. The crust eventually detaches up to a month after the inoculation. Persons with eczema should not be immunized as they may suffer widespread vaccinia (eczema vaccinatum) whose lesions might resemble those of smallpox. Vaccinia is moderately contagious, and patients with atopic dermatitis and Darier's disease may acquire severe generalized disease by exposure to a recently vaccinated person. Generalized vaccinia may be fatal. Prior vaccination does not prevent generalized vaccinia, but previously vaccinated individuals have milder disease. Progressive vaccinia (vaccinia gangrenosum)—progression of the primary inoculation site to a large ulceration—occurs in persons with systemic immune deficiency. It can have a fatal outcome.

Differential Diagnosis

Smallpox and vaccinia are to be distinguished from generalized varicella zoster virus infection or generalized herpes simplex. The latter two viral infections are not associated with a severe febrile prodrome. Lesions are at various stages at each anatomic site. Varicella usually appears in waves or crops. Multiple palm and sole lesions are common in variola and uncommon in generalized varicella-zoster and herpes simplex infection.

Direct fluorescent antibody testing for HSV and varicella zoster virus are the first-line diagnostic tests to differentiate varicella zoster virus, HSV, vaccinia, and variola. Until the diagnosis is confirmed, strict isolation of the patient is indicated. Similar fluorescent testing for variola can be performed in special laboratories.

Treatment

There is no specific and proven antiviral therapy for vaccinia or variola. Vaccinia immune globulin is used to treat eczema vaccinatum and progressive vaccinia. Cidofovir may have some activity against these poxviruses.

Breman J et al: Diagnosis and management of smallpox. N Engl J Med 2002;346:1300. [PMID: 11923491]

Sepkowitz K: How contagious is vaccinia? N Engl J Med 2003; 348:439. [PMID: 12496351]

POMPHOLYX; VESICULOBULLOUS HAND ECZEMA (Dyshidrosis, Dyshidrotic Eczema)

ESSENTIALS OF DIAGNOSIS

- "Tapioca" vesicles of 1–2 mm on the palms, soles, and sides of fingers, associated with pruritus.
- Vesicles may coalesce to form multiloculated blisters.
- Scaling and fissuring may follow drying of the blisters.
- Appearance in the third decade, with lifelong recurrences.

General Considerations

"Dyshidrotic eczema" is a misnomer, suggesting that the vesicles of this condition are related to eccrine sweat ducts and sweating, which they are not. This is an extremely common form of hand dermatitis, preferably called pompholyx (Gr "bubble") or vesiculobullous dermatitis of the palms and soles. Patients often have an atopic background and report flares with stress. Patients with widespread dermatitis due to any cause may develop pompholyx-like eruptions as a part of an autoeczematization response.

Clinical Findings

Small clear vesicles stud the skin at the sides of the fingers and on the palms or soles. They look like the grains in tapioca. They may be associated with intense itching. Later, the vesicles dry and the area becomes scaly and fissured.

Differential Diagnosis

Unroofing the vesicles and examining the blister roof with a KOH preparation will reveal hyphae in cases of bullous tinea. Blisters extending onto the dorsum of the hands may represent allergic contact dermatitis, and the culprit must be sought by history or by patch testing. Patients with inflammatory tinea pedis may have a vesicular dermatophytid of the palms. Always examine the feet of a patient with a hand eruption. Nonsteroidal anti-inflammatory drugs (NSAIDs) may produce an eruption very similar to that of dyshidrosis on the hands.

Prevention

There is no known way to prevent attacks.

Treatment

Topical and systemic corticosteroids help some patients dramatically. Since this is a chronic problem, systemic corticosteroids are generally not appropriate therapy. A high-potency topical corticosteroid used early in the attack may help abort the flare and ameliorate pruritus. Topical corticosteroids are also important in treating the scaling and fissuring that are seen after the vesicular phase. It is essential that patients avoid anything that irritates the skin; they should wear cotton gloves inside vinyl gloves when doing dishes or other wet chores, use long-handled brushes instead of sponges, and use a hand cream after washing the hands. Patients respond to PUVA therapy and injection of botulinum toxin into the palms as for hyperhidrosis.

Prognosis

For most patients, the disease is an inconvenience. For some, vesiculobullous hand eczema can be incapacitating.

Swartling C et al: Treatment of dyshidrotic hand dermatitis with intradermal botulinum toxin. J Am Acad Dermatol 2002; 47:667. [PMID: 12399757]

PORPHYRIA CUTANEA TARDA

 ESSENTIALS OF DIAGNOSIS

- *Noninflammatory blisters on sun-exposed sites, especially the dorsal surfaces of the hands.*
- *Hypertrichosis, skin fragility.*
- *Associated liver disease.*
- *Elevated urine porphyrins.*

General Considerations

Porphyria cutanea tarda is the most common type of porphyria. Cases are sporadic or hereditary. The disease is associated with ingestion of certain medications (eg, estrogens), and liver disease from alcoholism or hepatitis C. In patients with liver disease, hemosiderosis is often present.

Clinical Findings

A. SYMPTOMS AND SIGNS

Patients complain of painless blistering and fragility of the skin of the dorsal surfaces of the hands. Facial hypertrichosis and hyperpigmentation are common.

B. LABORATORY FINDINGS

Urinary uroporphyrins are elevated twofold to fivefold above coproporphyrins. Patients may also have abnormal liver function tests, evidence of hepatitis C infection, increased liver iron stores, and hemochromatosis gene mutations. Multiple triggering factors are often discovered.

Differential Diagnosis

Skin lesions identical to those of porphyria cutanea tarda may be seen in patients who receive maintenance dialysis and in those who take certain medications (tetracyclines and NSAIDs, especially naproxen). In this so-called pseudoporphyria, the biopsy results are identical to those associated with porphyria cutanea tarda, but urine porphyrins are normal.

Prevention

Although the lesions are triggered by sun exposure, the wavelength of light triggering the lesions is beyond that absorbed by sunscreens, which for that reason are ineffective. Barrier sun protection with clothing is required.

Treatment

Stopping all triggering medications and substantially reducing or stopping alcohol consumption may alone lead to improvement. Phlebotomy without oral iron supplementation at a rate of 1 unit every 2–4 weeks will gradually lead to improvement. Very low dose antimalarials (as low as 200 mg of hydroxychloroquine twice weekly), alone or in combination with phlebotomy, will increase the excretion of porphyrins, improving the skin disease. Treatment is continued until the patient is asymptomatic. Urine porphyrins may be monitored.

Prognosis

Most patients improve with treatment. Sclerodermoid skin lesions may develop on the trunk, scalp, and face.

Aziz Ibrahim A et al: Porphyria cutanea tarda in pregnancy: a case report. J Obstet Gynaecol 2004;24:574. [PMID: 15369945]

Dolan CK et al: Pseudoporphyria as a result of voriconazole use: a case report. Int J Dermatol 2004;43:768. [PMID: 15485539]

Hsu S: Skin fragility of the hands. Am Fam Physician 2004; 15:753. [PMID: 15338789]

Mehrany K et al: Association of porphyria cutanea tarda with hereditary hemochromatosis. J Am Acad Dermatol 2004;51: 205. [PMID: 15280838]

Phung TL et al: Beta-lactam antibiotic-induced pseudoporphyria. J Am Acad Dermatol 2004;51(2 Suppl):S80. [PMID: 15280819]

DERMATITIS HERPETIFORMIS

Dermatitis herpetiformis is an uncommon disease manifested by pruritic papules, vesicles, and papulovesicles mainly on the elbows, knees, buttocks, posterior neck, and scalp. It appears to have its highest prevalence in Scandinavia and is associated with HLA antigens -B8, -DR3, and -DQ2. The diagnosis is made by light microscopy, which demonstrates neutrophils at the dermal papillary tips. Direct immunofluorescence studies show granular deposits of IgA in the dermal papillae. Circulating antiendomysium antibodies and antibodies to tissue transglutaminase are present in 70% of cases. Patients have gluten-sensitive enteropathy, but for the great majority it is subclinical. However, ingestion of gluten is the cause of the disease, and strict long-term avoidance of dietary gluten has been shown to decrease the dose of dapsone (usually 100–200 mg/d) required to control the disease and may even eliminate the need for drug treatment. Although adherence to a gluten-free diet is difficult, the availability of many gluten-free foods makes this easier to accomplish. Patients with dermatitis herpetiformis are at increased risk for development of gastrointestinal lymphoma, and this risk is reduced by a gluten-free diet.

Borghi-Scoazec G et al: Onset of dermatitis herpetiformis after treatment by interferon and ribavirin for chronic hepatitis C. J Hepatol 2004;40:871. [PMID: 15094241]

Stroubou E et al: Ursodeoxycholic acid causing exacerbation of dermatitis herpetiformis. J Am Acad Dermatol 2001;45: 319. [PMID: 11464204]

Zone JJ et al: Warning: Bread may be harmful to your health. J Am Acad Dermatol 2004;51:27. [PMID: 15243499]

WEEPING OR CRUSTED LESIONS

IMPETIGO

ESSENTIALS OF DIAGNOSIS

- Superficial blisters filled with purulent material that rupture easily.
- Crusted superficial erosions.
- Positive Gram stain and bacterial culture.

General Considerations

Impetigo is a contagious and autoinoculable infection of the skin caused by staphylococci or streptococci (or both). Classically, two forms have been recognized: (1) a vesiculopustular type, with thick golden-crusted lesions caused by *S aureus* or group A β-hemolytic streptococci; and (2) a bullous type, associated with phage group II *S aureus*. However, most cases of impetigo of either presentation now appear to be due to staphylococci.

Clinical Findings

A. SYMPTOMS AND SIGNS

Itching is the only symptom. The lesions consist of macules, vesicles, bullae, pustules, and honey-colored gummy crusts that when removed leave denuded red areas. The face and other exposed parts are most often involved. **Ecthyma** is a deeper form of impetigo caused by staphylococci or streptococci, with ulceration and scarring. It occurs frequently on the extremities.

B. LABORATORY FINDINGS

Gram stain and culture confirm the diagnosis.

Differential Diagnosis

The main differential diagnoses are acute allergic contact dermatitis and herpes simplex. Contact dermatitis may be suggested by the history or by linear distribution of the lesions, and culture should be negative for staphylococci and streptococci. Herpes simplex infection usually presents with grouped vesicles or discrete erosions and may be associated with a history of recurrences. Viral cultures are positive.

Treatment

Topical antibiotics are not as effective as systemic antibiotics. In most cases, systemic antibiotics are indicated. Cephalexin, 250 mg four times daily, is usually effective. Doxycycline, 100 mg twice daily, is a reasonable alterna-

tive. Community-acquired methicillin-resistant *S aureus* (CA-MRSA) may cause impetigo, and initial coverage for MRSA could include doxycycline, clindamycin, or trimethoprim-sulfamethoxazole. Quinolones have poor activity against streptococci. About 50% of CA-MRSA are quinolone resistant. Recurrent impetigo is associated with nasal carriage of *S aureus*, treated with rifampin, 600 mg daily, or intranasal mupirocin ointment twice daily for 5 days.

Crusts and weepy areas may be treated with compresses, and washcloths and towels must be segregated and washed separately.

Hirschmann JV: Impetigo: etiology and therapy. Curr Clin Top Infect Dis 2002:22:42. [PMID: 12520646]

Levine N: Eruption on the face. Bulla formation and crusting on the forehead and nose can be easily treated. Geriatrics 2002; 57:17. [PMID: 12271824]

ALLERGIC CONTACT DERMATITIS

ESSENTIALS OF DIAGNOSIS

- Erythema and edema, with pruritus, often followed by vesicles and bullae in an area of contact with a suspected agent.
- Later, weeping, crusting, or secondary infection.
- A history of previous reaction to suspected contactant.
- Patch test with agent positive.

General Considerations

Contact dermatitis is an acute or chronic dermatitis that results from direct skin contact with chemicals or allergens. Eighty percent of cases are due to excessive exposure to or additive effects of primary or universal irritants (eg, soaps, detergents, organic solvents) and are called irritant contact dermatitis; only a small number of cases are due to actual contact allergy. The most common causes of allergic contact dermatitis are poison ivy or poison oak; topically applied antimicrobials (especially bacitracin and neomycin), antihistamines, and anesthetics (benzocaine); hair dyes; preservatives (eg, parabens); jewelry (nickel); latex; vitamin E; essential oils; and adhesive tape. Occupational exposure is an important cause of allergic contact dermatitis. Weeping and crusting are typically due to allergic and not irritant dermatitis, which often appears red and scaly. Contact dermatitis due to latex rubber in gloves is of special concern in health care workers.

Clinical Findings

A. SYMPTOMS AND SIGNS

In allergic contact dermatitis, the acute phase is characterized by tiny vesicles and weepy and crusted lesions, whereas resolving or chronic contact dermatitis presents with scaling, erythema, and possibly thickened skin. Itching, burning, and stinging may be severe. The lesions, distributed on exposed parts or in bizarre asymmetric patterns, consist of erythematous macules, papules, and vesicles. The affected area is often hot and swollen, with exudation and crusting, simulating—and at times complicated by—infection. The pattern of the eruption may be diagnostic (eg, typical linear streaked vesicles on the extremities in poison oak or ivy dermatitis). The location will often suggest the cause: Scalp involvement suggests hair tints, sprays, or tonics; face involvement, creams, cosmetics, soaps, shaving materials, nail polish; and neck involvement, jewelry, hair dyes, etc.

B. LABORATORY FINDINGS

Gram stain and culture will rule out impetigo or secondary infection (impetiginization). If itching is generalized and impetiginized scabies is considered, a scraping for mites should be done. After the episode has cleared, the patch test may be useful if the triggering allergen is not known. In suspected photocontact dermatitis—involvement of face, "V" (suprasternal notch) of the upper chest, and hands, sparing the skin under the nose, chin, and inner upper eyelid—photopatch tests may be done by exposing the traditional patch test site to ultraviolet light after 24 hours.

Differential Diagnosis

Asymmetric distribution, blotchy erythema around the face, linear lesions, and a history of exposure help distinguish acute contact dermatitis from other skin lesions. The most commonly mistaken diagnosis is impetigo. Chronic allergic contact dermatitis must be differentiated from scabies, atopic dermatitis, pompholyx, and other eczemas.

Prevention

Prompt and thorough removal of allergens by washing with water or solvents or other chemical agents may be effective if done very shortly after exposure to poison oak or ivy. Several over-the-counter barrier creams (eg, Stokogard, Ivy Shield) offer some protection to patients at high risk for poison oak and ivy dermatitis if applied before exposure. Iodoquinol cream may benefit nickel allergic patients in a similar manner. Ingestion of rhus antigen is of limited clinical value for the induction of tolerance.

The mainstay of prevention is identification of agents causing the dermatitis and avoidance of exposure or use of protective clothing and gloves. In industry-related cases, prevention may be accomplished by moving or retraining the worker.

Treatment

A. OVERVIEW

While local measures are important, severe or widespread involvement is difficult to manage without systemic corticosteroids because even the highest-potency topical corticosteroids seem not to work well on vesicular and weepy lesions. Localized involvement (except on the face) can often be managed solely with topical agents. Irritant contact dermatitis is treated by protection from the irritant and use of topical corticosteroids as for atopic dermatitis (described above). The treatment of allergic contact dermatitis is detailed below.

B. LOCAL MEASURES

1. Acute weeping dermatitis—Compresses are most often used. It is unwise to scrub lesions with soap and water. Calamine lotion may be used between wet dressings, especially for involvement of intertriginous areas or when oozing is not marked. Lesions on the extremities may be bandaged with wet dressings for 30–60 minutes several times a day. Potent topical corticosteroids in gel or cream form may help suppress acute contact dermatitis and relieve itching. In cases where weeping is marked or in intertriginous areas, ointments will make the skin even more macerated and should be avoided. Suggested preparations are fluocinonide gel, 0.05%, used two or three times daily with compresses, or clobetasol or halobetasol cream, used twice daily for a maximum of 2 weeks—not in body folds or on the face. This should be followed by tapering of the number of applications per day or use of a mid-potency corticosteroid such as triamcinolone 0.1% cream to prevent rebound of the dermatitis. A soothing formulation is 2 oz of 0.1% triamcinolone acetonide cream in 7.5 oz Sarna lotion (0.5% camphor, 0.5% menthol, 0.5% phenol) mixed by the patient.

2. Subacute dermatitis (subsiding)—Mid-potency (triamcinolone 0.1%) to high-potency corticosteroids (amcinonide, fluocinonide, desoximetasone) are the mainstays of therapy.

3. Chronic dermatitis (dry and lichenified)—High- to highest-potency corticosteroids are used in ointment form.

C. SYSTEMIC THERAPY

For acute severe cases, prednisone may be given orally for 12–21 days. Prednisone, 60 mg for 4–7 days, 40 mg for 4–7 days, and 20 mg for 4–7 days without a further taper is one useful regimen. Another is to dispense seventy-eight 5-mg pills to be taken 12 the first day, 11 the second day, and so on. The key is to use enough corticosteroid (and as early as possible) to achieve a clinical effect and to taper slowly enough to avoid rebound. A Medrol Dosepak (methylprednisolone) with 5 days of medication is inappropriate on both counts. (See Chapter 26.)

Prognosis

Allergic contact dermatitis is self-limited if reexposure is prevented but often takes 2–3 weeks for full resolution.

Arbogast JW et al: Effectiveness of a hand care regimen with moisturizer in manufacturing facilities where workers are prone to occupation irritant dermatitis. Dermatitis 2004; 15:10. [PMID: 15573643]

Goodall J: Oral corticosteroids for poison ivy dermatitis. CMAJ 2002;166:300. [PMID: 11868634]

Kist JM et al: The contact allergen replacement database and treatment of allergic contact dermatitis. Arch Dermatol 2004;140:1448. [PMID: 15611421]

PUSTULAR DISORDERS

ACNE VULGARIS

ESSENTIALS OF DIAGNOSIS

- *Occurs at puberty, though onset may be delayed into the third or fourth decade.*
- *Open and closed comedones are the hallmark of acne vulgaris.*
- *The most common of all skin conditions.*
- *Severity varies from purely comedonal to papular or pustular inflammatory acne to cysts or nodules.*
- *Face and trunk may be affected.*
- *Scarring may be a sequela of the disease or picking and manipulating by the patient.*

General Considerations

Acne vulgaris is polymorphic. Open and closed comedones, papules, pustules, and cysts are found. The disease is activated by androgens in those who are genetically predisposed.

Acne vulgaris is more common and more severe in males. It does not always clear spontaneously when maturity is reached. Twelve percent of women and 3% of men over age 25 have acne vulgaris. This rate does not decrease until after age 44. The skin lesions parallel sebaceous activity. Pathogenic events include plugging of the infundibulum of the follicles, retention of sebum, overgrowth of the acne bacillus (*Propionibacterium acnes*) with resultant release of and irritation by accumulated fatty acids, and foreign body reaction to extrafollicular sebum. The mechanism of antibiotics in controlling acne is not clearly understood, but they may work because of their antibacterial or anti-inflammatory properties.

When a resistant case of acne is encountered in a woman, hyperandrogenism may be suspected. This may or may not be accompanied by hirsutism, irregular menses, or other signs of virilism.

Clinical Findings

There may be mild soreness, pain, or itching. The lesions occur mainly over the face, neck, upper chest, back, and shoulders. Comedones are the hallmark of acne vulgaris. Closed comedones are tiny, flesh-colored, noninflamed bumps that give the skin a rough texture or appearance. Open comedones typically are a bit larger and have black material in them. Inflammatory papules, pustules, ectatic pores, acne cysts, and scarring are also seen.

Acne may have different presentations at different ages. Preteens often present with comedones as their first lesions. Inflammatory lesions in young teenagers are often found in the middle of the face, extending outward as the patient becomes older. Women in their third and fourth decades (often with no prior history of acne) commonly present with papular lesions on the chin and around the mouth—so-called perioral dermatitis.

Differential Diagnosis

In adults, acne rosacea presents with papules and pustules in the middle third of the face, but telangiectasia, flushing, and the absence of comedones distinguish this disease from acne vulgaris. A pustular eruption on the face in patients receiving antibiotics or with otitis externa should be investigated with culture to rule out an uncommon gram-negative folliculitis. Acne may develop in patients who use systemic corticosteroids or topical fluorinated corticosteroids on the face. Acne may be exacerbated or caused by irritating creams or oils. Pustules on the face can also be caused by tinea infections. Lesions on the back are more problematic. When they occur alone, staphylococcal folliculitis, miliaria ("heat rash") or, uncommonly, malassezia folliculitis should be suspected. Bacterial culture, trial of an antistaphylococcal antibiotic, and observing the response to therapy will help in the differential diagnosis. In patients with HIV infection, folliculitis is common and may be either staphylococcal folliculitis or eosinophilic folliculitis.

Complications

Cyst formation, pigmentary changes in pigmented patients, severe scarring, and psychological problems may result.

Treatment

A. GENERAL MEASURES

1. Education of the patient—When scarring seems out of proportion to the severity of the lesions, clinicians must suspect that the patient is manipulating the lesions. It is essential that the patient be educated in a supportive way about this complication. Although there are exceptions, it is wise to let the patient know that at least 4–6 weeks will be required to see improvement and that old lesions may take months to fade. Therefore, improvement will be judged according to the number of new lesions forming after 6–8 weeks of therapy. Additional time will be required to see improvement on the back and chest, as these areas are slowest to respond. If hair pomades are used, they should contain glycerin and not oil. Avoid topical exposure to oils, cocoa butter (theobroma oil), and greases.

2. Diet—Foods do not cause or exacerbate acne.

B. Comedonal Acne

Treatment of acne is based on the type and severity of lesions. Comedones require treatment different from that of pustules and cystic lesions. In assessing severity, take the sequelae of the lesions into account. Therefore, an individual who gets only two new lesions per month that scar or leave postinflammatory hyperpigmentation must be treated much more aggressively than a comparable patient whose lesions clear without sequelae. Soaps play little role in acne treatment, and unless the patient's skin is exceptionally oily, a mild soap should be used to avoid irritation that will limit the usefulness of other topicals, all of which are themselves somewhat irritating.

1. Topical retinoids—Tretinoin is very effective for comedonal acne or for treatment of the comedonal component of more severe acne, but its usefulness is limited by irritation. Start with 0.025% cream (not gel) and have the patient use it at first twice weekly at night, then build up to as often as nightly. A few patients cannot use even this low-strength preparation more than three times weekly but even that may cause improvement. A lentil-sized amount is sufficient to cover the entire face. To avoid irritation, have the patient wait 20 minutes after washing to apply. Adapalene gel 0.1% and reformulated tretinoin (Renova, Retin A Micro, Avita) are other options for patients irritated by standard tretinoin preparations. Some patients—especially teenagers—do best on 0.01% gel. Although the absorption of tretinoin is minimal, its use during pregnancy is contraindicated. Some patients report photosensitivity with tretinoin. Patients should be warned that they may flare in the first 4 weeks of treatment. Tazarotene gel (0.05% or 0.1%) (Tazorac) is a topical retinoid approved for treatment of psoriasis and acne.

2. Benzoyl peroxide—Benzoyl peroxide products are available in concentrations of 2.5%, 4%, 5%, 8%, and 10%, but it appears that 2.5% is as effective as 10% and less irritating. In general, water-based and not alcohol-based gels should be used to decrease irritation.

3. Antibiotics—Use of topical antibiotics (see below) has been demonstrated to decrease comedonal lesions.

4. Comedo extraction—Open and closed comedones may be removed with a comedo extractor but will recur if not prevented by treatment.

C. Papular Inflammatory Acne

Antibiotics are the mainstay for treatment of inflammatory acne. They may be used topically or orally. The oral antibiotics of choice are tetracycline and doxycycline. Minocycline is often effective in acne unresponsive or resistant to treatment with these antibiotics but it is expensive. Rarely, other antibiotics such as trimethoprim-sulfamethoxazole (one double-strength tablet twice daily), clindamycin (150 mg twice daily), or a cephalosporin (cefadroxil or cephalexin) may be used. Topical clindamycin phosphate and erythromycin are also used (see below). Topicals are probably the equivalent of about 500 mg/d of tetracycline given orally, which is half the usual starting dose. Topical antibiotics are used in three situations: for mild papular acne that can be controlled by topicals alone, for patients who refuse or cannot tolerate oral antibiotics, or to wean patients under good control from oral to topical preparations. It has been recommended that switching or rotating antibiotics be avoided to decrease resistance and that courses of benzoyl peroxide be used on occasion.

1. Mild acne—The first choice of topical antibiotics in terms of efficacy and relative lack of induction of resistant *P acnes* is the combination of erythromycin or clindamycin with benzoyl peroxide topical gel. Clindamycin (Cleocin T) lotion (least irritating), gel, or solution, or one of the many brands of topical erythromycin gel or solution, may be used twice daily and the benzoyl peroxide in the morning. (A combination of erythromycin or clindamycin with benzoyl peroxide is available as a prescription item.) The addition of tretinoin 0.025% cream or 0.01% gel at night may be effective, since it works via a different mechanism.

2. Moderate acne—Tetracycline, 500 mg twice daily, doxycycline, 100 mg twice daily, and minocycline, 50–100 mg twice daily, are all effective though minocycline is more expensive. When initiating minocycline therapy, start at 100 mg in the evening for 4–7 days, then 100 mg twice daily, to decrease the incidence of vertigo. Plan a return visit in 6 weeks and at 3–4 months after that. If the patient's skin is quite clear, instructions should be given for tapering the dose by 250 mg for tetracycline and erythromycin, by 100 mg for doxycycline, or by 50 mg for minocycline every 6–8 weeks—while treating with topicals—to arrive at the lowest systemic dose needed to maintain clearing. In general, lowering the dose to zero without other therapy results in prompt recurrence of acne. Tetracycline, minocycline, and doxycycline are contraindicated in pregnancy, but oral erythromycin may be used.

It is important to discuss the issue of contraceptive failure when prescribing antibiotics for women taking oral contraceptives. Women may need to consider using barrier methods as well, and should report breakthrough bleeding. Oral contraceptives or spironolactone (50–200 mg daily) may be added as an antiandrogen in women with antibiotic-resistant acne or in women in whom relapse occurs after isotretinoin therapy.

3. Severe acne—

a. Isotretinoin (Accutane)—A vitamin A analog, isotretinoin is used for the treatment of severe cystic acne that has not responded to conventional therapy. Informed consent must be obtained before its use and patients must be enrolled in a monitoring program (iPledge). A dosage of 0.5–1 mg/kg/d for 20 weeks for a cumulative dose of at least 120 mg/kg is usually adequate for severe cystic acne. Patients should be offered isotretinoin therapy before they experience significant scarring if they are not promptly and adequately controlled by antibiotics. The drug is *absolutely contraindicated during pregnancy* because of its teratogenicity; two serum pregnancy tests should be obtained before starting the drug in a female and every month thereafter. Sufficient medication for only 1 month should be dispensed. Two forms of effective contraception must be used. Side effects occur in most patients, usually related to dry skin and mucous membranes (dry lips, nosebleed, and dry eyes). If headache occurs, pseudotumor cerebri must be considered. Depression has been reported. Hypertriglyceridemia will develop in about 25% of patients, hypercholesterolemia in 15%, and a lowering of high-density lipoproteins in 5%. Minor elevations in liver function tests may develop in some patients. Fasting blood sugar may be elevated. Miscellaneous adverse reactions include decreased night vision, musculoskeletal or bowel symptoms, dry skin, thinning of hair, exuberant granulation tissue in lesions, and bony hyperostoses (seen only with very high doses or with long duration of therapy). Moderate to severe myalgias rarely necessitate decreasing the dosage or stopping the drug. Laboratory tests to be performed in all patients before treatment and after 4 weeks on therapy include cholesterol, triglycerides, and liver function studies.

Elevations of liver enzymes and triglycerides return to normal upon conclusion of therapy. The drug may induce long-term remissions in 40–60%, or acne may recur that is more easily controlled with conventional therapy. Occasionally, acne does not respond or promptly recurs after therapy, but it may clear after a second course.

b. Intralesional injection—In otherwise moderate acne, intralesional injection of dilute suspensions of triamcinolone acetonide (2.5 mg/mL, 0.05 mL per lesion) will often hasten the resolution of deeper papules and occasional cysts.

c. Laser, dermabrasion—Cosmetic improvement may be achieved by excision and punch-grafting of deep scars and by abrasion of inactive acne lesions, particularly flat, superficial scars. The technique is not without untoward effects, since hyperpigmentation, hypopigmentation, grooving, and scarring have been known to occur. Dark-skinned individuals do poorly. Corrective surgery within 12 months after isotretinoin therapy may not be advisable. Active acne of all types can be treated with certain laser and photodynamic therapies. This can be considered when standard treatments are contraindicated or fail.

Prognosis

Acne vulgaris eventually remits spontaneously, but when this will occur cannot be predicted. The condition may persist throughout adulthood and may lead to severe scarring if left untreated. Patients treated with antibiotics continue to improve for the first 3–6 months of therapy. Relapse during treatment may suggest the emergence of resistant *P acnes.* The disease is chronic and tends to flare intermittently in spite of treatment. Remissions following systemic treatment with isotretinoin may be lasting in up to 60% of cases. Relapses after isotretinoin usually occur within 3 years and require a second course in up to 20% of patients.

James WD: Clinical practice. Acne. N Engl J Med 2005;352: 1463. [PMID: 15814882]

Ozolins M et al: Comparison of five antimicrobial regimens for treatment of mild to moderate inflammatory facial acne vulgaris in the community randomised controlled trial. Lancet 2004;364:2188. [PMID: 15610805]

Shalita AR et al: Effects of tazarotene 0.1% cream in the treatment of facial acne vulgaris: pooled results from two multicenter, double-blind, randomized, vehicle-controlled, parallel-group trials. Clin Ther 2004;26:1865. [PMID: 15639698]

Thiboutot D: Acne: hormonal concepts and therapy. Clin Dermatol 2004;22:419. [PMID: 15556729]

van Vloten WA et al: Selecting an oral contraceptive agent for the treatment of acne in women. Am J Clin Dermatol 2004; 5:435. [PMID: 15663340]

ROSACEA

 ESSENTIALS OF DIAGNOSIS

- A chronic facial disorder.
- A vascular component (erythema and telangiectasis) and a tendency to flush easily.
- An acneiform component (papules and pustules) may also be present.
- A glandular component accompanied by hyperplasia of the soft tissue of the nose (rhinophyma).

General Considerations

The pathogenesis of this disorder is not known. Topical corticosteroids can change trivial dermatoses of the face into **perioral dermatitis** and **steroid rosacea.** These occur predominantly in young women.

Clinical Findings

The cheeks, nose, and chin—at times the entire face— may have a rosy hue. No comedones are seen. Inflammatory papules are prominent, and there may be pustules. Associated seborrhea may be found. The patient often complains of burning or stinging with episodes of flushing. Patients may have associated ophthalmic disease, including blepharitis and keratitis, that often requires systemic antibiotic therapy.

Differential Diagnosis

Rosacea is distinguished from acne by the presence of the vascular component and the absence of comedones. The rosy hue of rosacea and telangiectasis will pinpoint the diagnosis.

Treatment

Medical management is effective only for the inflammatory papules and pustules and the erythema that surrounds them. The only satisfactory treatment for the telangiectasis is surgery. Rhinophyma (soft tissue and sebaceous hyperplasia of the nose) responds to surgical debulking. Rosacea is usually a lifelong condition, so maintenance therapy is required.

A. LOCAL THERAPY

Metronidazole, 0.75% gel applied twice daily or 1% cream once daily, is the topical treatment of choice. If metronidazole is not tolerated, topical clindamycin (solution, gel, or lotion) used twice daily is effective. Response is noted in 4–8 weeks.

B. SYSTEMIC THERAPY

Tetracycline, 250 or 500 mg orally twice daily on an empty stomach, should be used when topical therapy is inadequate. Minocycline or doxycycline, 50–100 mg daily to twice daily, is also effective. Metronidazole or amoxicillin, 250–500 mg twice daily, may be used in refractory cases. Side effects are few, although metronidazole may produce a disulfiram-like effect when the patient ingests alcohol. Isotretinoin may succeed where other measures fail. A dosage of 0.5–1 mg/kg/d orally for 12–28 weeks is recommended. See precautions above.

Prognosis

Rosacea tends to be a persistent process. With the regimens described above, it can usually be controlled adequately.

Powell FC: Rosacea. N Engl J Med 2005;352:793. [PMID: 15728812]

FOLLICULITIS
(Including Sycosis)

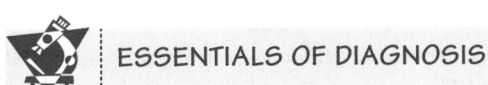

ESSENTIALS OF DIAGNOSIS

- *Itching and burning in hairy areas.*
- *Pustules in the hair follicles.*

General Considerations

Folliculitis has multiple causes. It is frequently caused by staphylococcal infection and may be more common in the diabetic patient. When the lesion is deep-seated, chronic, and recalcitrant on the head and neck, it is called sycosis. Sycosis is usually propagated by the autoinoculation and trauma of shaving. The upper lip is particularly susceptible to involvement in men.

Gram-negative folliculitis, which may develop during antibiotic treatment of acne, may present as a flare of acne pustules or nodules. *Klebsiella, Enterobacter, Escherichia coli,* and *Proteus* have been isolated from these lesions.

"Hot tub folliculitis," caused by *Pseudomonas aeruginosa,* is characterized by pruritic or tender follicular, pustular lesions occurring within 1–4 days after bathing in a hot tub, whirlpool, or public swimming pool. Rarely, systemic infections may result. Neutropenic patients should avoid these exposures.

Nonbacterial folliculitis may also be caused by oils that are irritating to the follicle, and these may be encountered in the workplace (machinists) or at home (various cosmetics and cocoa butter or coconut oils).

Folliculitis may also be caused by occlusion, perspiration, and rubbing, such as that resulting from tight jeans and other heavy fabrics on the upper legs.

Folliculitis on the back that looks like acne but does not respond to acne therapy may be caused by the yeast *M furfur.* Biopsy may be required for diagnosis.

Steroid acne may be seen during topical or systemic corticosteroid therapy.

A form of sterile folliculitis called eosinophilic folliculitis consisting of urticarial papules with prominent eosinophilic infiltration is common in patients with AIDS. It may appear first with institution of highly active antiretroviral therapy (HAART) and be mistaken for a drug eruption.

Pseudofolliculitis is caused by ingrowing hairs in the beard area. In this entity, the papules and pustules are located at the side of and not in follicles. It may be treated by growing a beard, by using chemical depilatories, or by shaving with a foil-guard razor. Laser hair removal is dramatically beneficial in patients with pseudofolliculitis, requires limited maintenance, and can be done on patients of any skin color. Pseudofolliculitis is a true medical indication for such a procedure and should not be considered cosmetic.

Clinical Findings

The symptoms range from slight burning and tenderness to intense itching. The lesions consist of pustules of hair follicles.

Differential Diagnosis

It is important to differentiate bacterial from nonbacterial folliculitis. The history is important for pinpointing the causes of nonbacterial folliculitis, and a

Gram stain and culture are indispensable. One must differentiate folliculitis from acne vulgaris or pustular miliaria (heat rash) and from infections of the skin such as impetigo or fungal infections. Pseudomonas folliculitis is often suggested by the history of hot tub use. Eosinophilic folliculitis in AIDS often requires biopsy for diagnosis.

Complications

Abscess formation is the major complication of bacterial folliculitis.

Prevention

Correct any predisposing local causes (eg, irritations of a mechanical or chemical nature). Control of blood glucose in diabetes may reduce the number of these infections. Be sure that the water in hot tubs and spas is treated properly with chlorine. If staphylococcal folliculitis is persistent, treatment of nasal or perineal carriage with rifampin, 600 mg daily for 5 days, or with topical mupirocin ointment 2% twice daily for 5 days, may help. Chronic oral clindamycin, 150–300 mg/d, is also effective in preventing recurrent staphylococcal folliculitis and furunculosis.

Treatment

A. LOCAL MEASURES

Anhydrous ethyl alcohol containing 6.25% aluminum chloride (Xerac AC), applied to lesions and environs, may be helpful, especially for chronic folliculitis of the buttocks.

B. SPECIFIC MEASURES

Systemic antibiotics may be tried if the skin infection is resistant to local treatment, if it is extensive or severe and accompanied by a febrile reaction, if it is complicated, or if it involves the nose or upper lip. Extended periods of treatment (4–8 weeks or more) with anti-staphylococcal antibiotics are required in some cases.

Hot tub pseudomonas folliculitis virtually always resolves without treatment but may be treated in adults with ciprofloxacin, 500 mg twice daily for 5 days.

Gram-negative folliculitis in acne patients may be treated with isotretinoin in compliance with all precautions discussed above (see Acne Vulgaris).

Folliculitis due to *M furfur* is treated with topical 2.5% selenium sulfide, 15 minutes daily for 3 weeks, or with oral ketoconazole, 200 mg daily for 7–14 days.

Eosinophilic folliculitis may be treated initially by the combination of potent topical corticosteroids and oral antihistamines. In more severe cases, treatment is with one of the following: topical permethrin (application for 12 hours every other night for 6 weeks); itraconazole, 200–400 mg daily; UVB or PUVA phototherapy; or isotretinoin, 0.5 mg/kg/d for up to 5 months. A remission may be induced by some of these therapies, but chronic treatment may be required.

Prognosis

Bacterial folliculitis is occasionally stubborn and persistent, requiring prolonged or intermittent courses of antibiotics. Corticosteroid folliculitis is treatable by acne therapy and resolves as corticosteroids are discontinued.

Cook-Bolden FE et al: Twice-daily applications of benzoyl peroxide 5%/clindamycin 1% gel versus vehicle in the treatment of pseudofolliculitis barbae. Cutis 2004;73:18. [PMID: 15228130]

Stulberg DL et al: Common bacterial skin infections. Am Fam Physician 2002;66:119. [PMID: 12126026]

MILIARIA
(Heat Rash)

 ESSENTIALS OF DIAGNOSIS

- *Burning, itching, superficial aggregated small vesicles, papules, or pustules on covered areas of the skin, usually the trunk.*
- *More common in hot, moist climates.*
- *Rare forms associated with fever and even heat prostration.*

General Considerations

Miliaria is an acute dermatitis that occurs most commonly on the trunk and intertriginous areas. A hot, moist environment is the most frequent cause. Bedridden febrile patients are susceptible. Plugging of the ostia of sweat ducts occurs, with ultimate rupture of the sweat duct, producing an irritating, stinging reaction. Increase in numbers of resident aerobes, notably cocci, apparently plays a role. Drugs that enhance sweat gland function (eg, clonidine, β-blockers, opiates), may contribute.

Clinical Findings

The usual symptoms are burning and itching. In severe cases, fever, heat prostration, and even death may result. The lesions consist of small, superficial, red, thin-walled, discrete but closely aggregated vesicles (miliaria crystallina), papules (miliaria rubra), or vesicopustules or pustules (miliaria pustulosa). The reaction occurs most commonly on covered areas of the skin and virtually always affects the back in a hospitalized patient.

Differential Diagnosis

Miliaria is to be distinguished from drug rash and folliculitis.

Prevention

Use of an antibacterial preparation such as chlorhexidine prior to exposure to heat and humidity may help prevent the condition. Susceptible persons should avoid exposure to hot, humid environments.

Treatment

The patient should keep cool and wear light clothing. Triamcinolone acetonide, 0.1% in Sarna lotion, or a mid-potency corticosteroid in a lotion or cream—but not ointment—base, should be applied two to four times daily. Secondary infections (superficial pyoderma) are treated with dicloxacillin, 250 mg four times daily by mouth. Anticholinergic drugs given by mouth may be helpful in severe cases, eg, glycopyrrolate, 1 mg twice daily.

Prognosis

Miliaria is usually a mild disorder, but severe forms (tropical anhidrosis and asthenia) result from interference with the heat-regulating mechanism.

Haas N et al: Miliaria crystallina in an intensive care setting. Clin Exp Dermatol 2004;29:32. [PMID: 14723716]

MUCOCUTANEOUS CANDIDIASIS

ESSENTIALS OF DIAGNOSIS

- *Severe pruritus of vulva, anus, or body folds.*
- *Superficial denuded, beefy-red areas with or without satellite vesicopustules.*
- *Whitish curd-like concretions on the oral and vaginal mucous membranes.*
- *Yeast on microscopic examination of scales or curd.*

General Considerations

Mucocutaneous candidiasis is a superficial fungal infection that may involve almost any cutaneous or mucous surface of the body. It is particularly likely to occur in diabetics, during pregnancy, and in obese persons who perspire freely. Antibiotics and oral contraceptive agents may be contributory. Oral candidiasis may be the first sign of HIV infection (see Chapter 31).

Clinical Findings

A. Symptoms and Signs

Itching may be intense. Burning is reported, particularly around the vulva and anus. The lesions consist of superficially denuded, beefy-red areas in the depths of the body folds such as in the groin and the intergluteal cleft, beneath the breasts, at the angles of the mouth, and in the umbilicus. The peripheries of these denuded lesions are superficially undermined, and there may be satellite vesicopustules. Whitish, curd-like concretions may be present on mucosal lesions. Paronychia may occur.

B. Laboratory Findings

Clusters of budding cells and pseudohyphae can be seen under high power when skin scales or curd-like lesions have been cleared in 10% KOH. Culture can confirm the diagnosis.

Differential Diagnosis

Intertrigo, seborrheic dermatitis, tinea cruris, "inverse psoriasis," and erythrasma involving the same areas may mimic mucocutaneous candidiasis.

Complications

Systemic invasive candidiasis with candidemia may be seen with immunosuppression and in patients receiving broad-spectrum antibiotic and hypertonic glucose solutions, as in hyperalimentation. There may or may not be clinically evident mucocutaneous candidiasis.

Treatment

A. General Measures

Affected parts should be kept dry and exposed to air as much as possible. If possible, discontinue systemic antibiotics. For treatment of systemic invasive candidiasis, see Chapter 36.

B. Local Measures

1. Nails and paronychia—Apply clotrimazole solution 1% three or four times daily. Thymol 4% in ethanol applied once daily is an alternative. Nipple pain during breastfeeding may be due to candidiasis.

2. Skin—Apply nystatin ointment or clotrimazole cream 1% with hydrocortisone cream 1% twice daily.

3. Vulvar and anal mucous membranes—For vaginal candidiasis, single-dose fluconazole (150 mg) is effective. Intravaginal clotrimazole, miconazole, terconazole, or nystatin may also be used. Long-term suppressive therapy may be required for recurrent or "intractable" cases. Non-*albicans* candidal species may be identified by culture in some refractory cases and may respond to oral itraconazole, 200 mg twice daily for 2–4 weeks.

4. Balanitis—This is most frequent in uncircumcised men, and candida usually plays a role. Topical nystatin ointment is the initial treatment if the lesions are mildly erythematous or superficially erosive. Soaking with dilute aluminum acetate for 15 minutes twice daily may quickly relieve burning or itching. Chronicity and relapses, especially after sexual contact, suggest reinfection from a sexual partner who should be treated. Severe purulent balanitis is usually due to bacteria. If it is so severe that phimosis occurs, oral antibiotics—some with activity against anaerobes—are required; if rapid improvement does not occur, urologic consultation is indicated.

Prognosis

Cases of cutaneous candidiasis range from the easily cured to the intractable and prolonged.

Amir L: Test your knowledge. Nipple pain in breastfeeding. Aust Fam Physician 2004;33:44. [PMID: 14988960]

Bielan B: What's your assessment? *Candida balanitis.* Dermatol Nurs 2003;15:134, 170. [PMID: 12751348]

Bielan B: What's your assessment? Candidiasis. Dermatol Nurs 2004;16:62. [PMID: 15022506]

ERYTHEMAS

REACTIVE ERYTHEMAS

1. URTICARIA & ANGIOEDEMA

 ESSENTIALS OF DIAGNOSIS

- *Eruptions of evanescent wheals or hives.*
- *Itching is usually intense but may on rare occasions be absent.*
- *Special forms of urticaria have special features (dermographism, cholinergic urticaria, solar urticaria, or cold urticaria).*
- *Most incidents are acute and self-limited over a period of 1–2 weeks.*
- *Chronic urticaria (episodes lasting > 6 weeks) may have an autoimmune basis.*

General Considerations

Urticaria can result from many different stimuli on an immunologic or nonimmunologic basis. The most common immunologic mechanism is hypersensitivity mediated by IgE, seen for most patients with acute urticaria; another involves activation of the complement cascade. Some patients with chronic urticaria demonstrate autoantibodies directed against mast cell IgE receptors. Angiotensin-converting enzyme inhibitor and angiotensin II receptor antagonist therapy may be complicated by urticaria or angioedema. In general, extensive costly workups are not indicated in patients who have urticaria. A careful history and physical examination are more helpful.

Clinical Findings

A. Symptoms and Signs

Lesions are itchy red swellings of a few millimeters to many centimeters. The morphology of the lesions may vary over a period of minutes to hours, resulting in geographic or bizarre patterns. Individual lesions in true urticaria last less than 24 hours, and often only 2–4 hours. Angioedema is involvement of deeper subcutaneous tissue with swelling of the lips, eyelids, palms, soles, and genitalia. Angioedema is no more likely than urticaria to be associated with systemic complications such as laryngeal edema or hypotension. In cholinergic urticaria, triggered by a rise in core body temperature (hot showers, exercise), wheals are 2–3 mm in diameter with a large surrounding red flare. Cold urticaria is acquired or inherited and triggered by exposure to cold and wind (see Chapter 38).

B. Laboratory Findings

Laboratory studies are not likely to be helpful in the evaluation of acute or chronic urticaria. The most common causes of acute urticaria are foods, infections, and medications. The cause of chronic urticaria is often not found. In patients with individual slightly purpuric lesions that persist past 24 hours, skin biopsy may confirm urticarial vasculitis. An autologous serum test may detect patients with an autoimmune basis for their chronic urticaria.

Differential Diagnosis

Papular urticaria resulting from insect bites persists for days. A central punctum can usually be seen. Streaked urticarial lesions may be seen in acute allergic plant dermatitis, eg, poison ivy, oak, or sumac. Contact urticaria may be caused by a host of substances, including chemicals, foods, and medications, and may be one type of reaction to latex. Urticarial response to heat, sun, water, and pressure are quite rare. Urticarial vasculitis may be seen as part of serum sickness, associated with fever and arthralgia.

In hereditary angioedema, there is generally a positive family history and gastrointestinal or respiratory symptoms. Urticaria is not part of the syndrome, and lesions are not pruritic.

Treatment

A. General Measures

A detailed search by history for a cause of acute urticaria should be undertaken, and treatment may then be tailored to include the provocative condition. The chief causes are drugs—eg, aspirin, NSAIDs, morphine, and codeine; arthropod bites—eg, insect bites and bee stings (though the latter may cause anaphylaxis as well as angioedema); physical factors such as heat, cold, sunlight, and pressure; and, presumably, neurogenic factors, as in cholinergic urticaria induced by exercise, excitement, hot showers, etc.

Other causes may include penicillins and other medications; inhalants such as feathers and animal danders; ingestion of shellfish, tomatoes, or strawberries; injections of sera biologic response modifiers and vaccines; external contactants, including various chemicals and cosmetics; and infections such as viral hepatitis.

B. Systemic Treatment

The mainstay of treatment initially includes H_1 antihistamines (see above). Hydroxyzine, 10 mg twice daily to 25 mg three times daily, may be very useful if tolerated. Giving hydroxyzine as one dose of 50–75 mg at night may reduce sedation and other side effects. Cyproheptadine, 4 mg four times daily, may be especially useful for cold urticaria. "Nonsedating" or less sedating antihistamines are added if the generic sedating antihistamines are not effective. Fexofenadine is given in a dosage of 60 mg twice a day, or loratadine is given in a dosage of 10 mg/d. Cetirizine, a metabolite of hydroxyzine, is less sedating (13% of patients) and is given in a dosage of 10 mg/d.

Doxepin (a tricyclic antidepressant), 25–75 mg at bedtime, can be very effective in chronic urticaria. It has anticholinergic side effects.

H_2-antihistamines in combination with H_1-blockers may be helpful in patients with symptomatic dermatographism and to a lesser degree in chronic urticaria.

A few patients with chronic urticaria may respond to elimination of salicylates and tartrazine (coloring agent). Asymptomatic foci of infection—sinusitis, vaginal candidiasis, cholecystitis, and intestinal parasites—may rarely cause chronic urticaria. Systemic corticosteroids in a dose of about 40 mg daily will usually suppress acute and chronic urticaria. However, the use of corticosteroids is rarely indicated, since properly selected combinations of antihistamines with less toxicity are usually effective. Once corticosteroids are withdrawn, the urticaria virtually always returns if it had been chronic. Rather than using systemic corticosteroids in difficult cases, consultation should be sought from a dermatologist or allergist with experience in managing severe urticaria. Cyclosporine (3–5 mg/kg/d) may be effective in severe cases of autoimmune chronic urticaria.

C. LOCAL TREATMENT

Local treatment is rarely rewarding.

Prognosis

Acute urticaria usually lasts only a few days to 6 weeks. Half of patients whose urticaria persists for more than 6 weeks will have it for years.

Caproni M et al: Chronic idiopathic and chronic autoimmune urticaria: clinical and immunopathological features of 68 subjects. Acta Derm Venereol 2004;84:288. [PMID: 15339073]

Gaig P et al: Epidemiology of urticaria in Spain. J Investig Allergol Clin Immunol 2004;14:214. [PMID: 15552715]

Grattan CE et al: Chronic urticaria. J Am Acad Dermatol 2002; 46:657. [PMID: 12004303]

Hennino A et al: Pathophysiology of urticaria. Clin Rev Allergy Immunol 2006;30:3. [PMID: 16461989]

Kaplan AP et al: Angioedema. J Am Acad Dermatol 2005;53:373. [PMID: 16112343]

Nikas SN et al: Urticaria and angioedema-like skin reactions in a patient treated with adalimumab. Clin Rheumatol 2006 [Epub ahead of print]. [PMID: 16421645]

Tilles SA: Approach to therapy in chronic urticaria: when Benadryl is not enough. Allergy Asthma Proc 2005;26:9. [PMID: 15813282]

2. ERYTHEMA MULTIFORME

 ESSENTIALS OF DIAGNOSIS

- *Sudden onset of symmetric erythematous skin lesions with history of recurrence.*
- *May be macular, papular, urticarial, bullous, or purpuric.*
- *"Target" lesions with clear centers and concentric erythematous rings or "iris" lesions may be noted in erythema multiforme minor. These are rare in drug-associated erythema multiforme major (Stevens-Johnson syndrome).*
- *Erythema multiforme minor on extensor surfaces, palms, soles, or mucous membranes. Erythema multiforme major favors the trunk.*
- *Herpes simplex is the most common cause of erythema multiforme minor.*
- *Drugs are the most common cause of erythema multiforme major.*

General Considerations

Erythema multiforme is an acute inflammatory skin disease. Erythema multiforme is divided clinically into minor and major types based on the clinical findings. Approximately 90% of cases of erythema multiforme minor follow outbreaks of herpes simplex. Erythema multiforme major (Stevens-Johnson syndrome) is marked by toxicity and involvement of two or more mucosal surfaces (often oral and conjunctival) and is most often caused by drugs, especially sulfonamides, NSAIDs, and anticonvulsants such as phenytoin. *Mycoplasma pneumoniae* may trigger erythema multiforme major. Immunization for smallpox and acute HIV infection may also cause erythema multiforme. Erythema multiforme may also present as recurring oral ulceration, with skin lesions present in only half of the cases, and is diagnosed by oral biopsy. Since erythema multiforme may have its own prodrome, many medications taken for such symptoms have been implicated in its pathogenesis without definitive proof. As in all drug eruptions, the exposure to drugs associated with erythema multiforme may be systemic or topical; any agent should be considered a potential offender.

Clinical Findings

A. SYMPTOMS AND SIGNS

A classic target lesion, found most commonly in herpes-associated erythema multiforme, consists of three concentric zones of color change, most often found acrally on the hands and feet. Not all lesions will have this appearance. Drug-associated erythema multiforme is manifested by raised target-like lesions, with only two zones of color change and a central blister, or nondescript reddish or purpuric macules. In erythema multiforme major, mucous membrane ulcerations are present at two or more sites, causing pain on eating, swallowing, and urination.

B. LABORATORY FINDINGS

Blood tests are not useful for diagnosis. Skin biopsy is diagnostic. Direct immunofluorescence studies are negative.

Differential Diagnosis

Urticaria and drug eruptions are the chief entities that must be differentiated from erythema multiforme minor. Individual lesions of true urticaria itch should come and go within 24 hours, are usually responsive to antihistamines, and do not affect the mucosa. In erythema multiforme major, the main differential diagnosis is paraneoplastic pemphigus. The presence of blisters is always worrisome and dictates the need for consultation. The differential diagnosis of blisters includes pemphigus, pemphigoid, and bullous drug eruptions. Skin biopsy is the mainstay of diagnosis.

Complications

The tracheobronchial mucosa and conjunctiva may be involved in severe cases with resultant scarring (Stevens-Johnson syndrome). Ophthalmologic consultation is required if ocular involvement is present.

Treatment

A. GENERAL MEASURES

Erythema multiforme major (Stevens-Johnson syndrome) with extensive denudation of skin is best treated in a burn unit. Otherwise, patients need not be admitted unless mucosal involvement interferes with hydration and nutrition. Patients who begin to blister should be seen daily. Immediate discontinuation of the inciting medication (before blistering occurs) improves prognosis and reduces the risk of death in erythema multiforme major.

B. SPECIFIC MEASURES

Although there are no good data to support the use of corticosteroids in erythema multiforme major, they are still often prescribed. If corticosteroids are to be tried in more severe cases, they should be used early, before blistering occurs, and in moderate to high doses (prednisone, 100–250 mg) and stopped within days if there is no dramatic response. Intravenous immunoglobulin (IGIV) (0.75 g/kg/d for 4 days) may be used in severe cases. Oral and topical corticosteroids are useful in the oral variant of erythema multiforme. Oral acyclovir prophylaxis of herpes simplex infections may be effective in preventing recurrent herpes-associated erythema multiforme minor.

C. LOCAL MEASURES

Topical therapy is not very effective in this disease. For oral lesions, 1% diphenhydramine elixir mixed with Kaopectate or with 1% dyclonine may be used as a mouth rinse several times daily.

Prognosis

Erythema multiforme minor usually lasts 2–6 weeks and may recur. Erythema multiforme major may be serious or even fatal in the most severe cases.

Bachot N et al: Intravenous immunoglobulin treatment for Stevens-Johnson syndrome and toxic epidermal necrolysis: a prospective noncomparative study showing no benefit on mortality or progression. Arch Dermatol 2003;139:33. [PMID: 12533161]

Faye O et al: Treatment of epidermal necrolysis with high-dose intravenous immunoglobulins (IV Ig): clinical experience to date. Drugs 2005;65:2085. [PMID: 16225365]

Fein JD et al: Images in clinical medicine. Stevens-Johnson syndrome. N Engl J Med 2005;352:1696. [PMID: 15843672]

Hynes AY et al: Controversy in the use of high-dose systemic steroids in the acute care of patients with Stevens-Johnson syndrome. Int Ophthalmol Clin 2005;45:25. [PMID: 16199965]

Letko E et al: Stevens-Johnson syndrome and toxic epidermal necrolysis: a review of the literature. Ann Allergy Asthma Immunol 2005;94:419. [PMID: 15875523]

3. ERYTHEMA MIGRANS (See also Chapter 34)

Erythema migrans is a unique cutaneous eruption that characterizes the localized or generalized early stage of Lyme disease. Three to 32 days (median: 7 days) after a tick bite, there is gradual expansion of redness around the papule representing the bite site. The advancing border is usually slightly raised, warm, red to bluish-red, and free of any scale. Centrally, the site of the bite may clear, leaving only a rim of peripheral erythema, or it may become indurated, vesicular, or necrotic. The annular erythema usually grows to a median diameter of 15 cm (range: 3–68 cm, but virtually always > 5 cm). It is accompanied by a burning sensation in half of patients; rarely, it is pruritic or painful. Multiple secondary annular lesions similar in appearance to the primary lesion but without indurated centers and generally of smaller size will develop in 20% of patients. In the southeastern United States, similar lesions are seen in patients without evidence of Lyme borreliosis. The etiology of these cases is unclear, but they are not due to *Borrelia*.

Without treatment, erythema migrans and the secondary lesions fade in a median of 28 days, though some may persist for months. Ten percent of untreated patients experience recurrences over the ensuing months. Treatment with systemic antibiotics (see Table 34–4) is necessary to prevent systemic involvement. However, only 60–70% of those with systemic involvement experience erythema migrans.

Stanek G et al: Lyme borreliosis. Lancet 2003;362:1639. [PMID: 14630446]

Weed B: Lyme disease presenting with multiple erythema migrans lesions, an illustrative case. Int J Dermatol 2003; 42:715. [PMID: 12956686]

Wormser GP et al: Microbiologic evaluation of patients from Missouri with erythema migrans. Clin Infect Dis 2005; 40:23. [PMID: 15668867]

INFECTIOUS ERYTHEMAS

1. ERYSIPELAS

 ESSENTIALS OF DIAGNOSIS

- *Edematous, spreading, circumscribed, hot, erythematous area, with or without vesicles or bullae.*
- *Central face frequently involved.*
- *Pain, chills, fever, and systemic toxicity may be striking.*

General Considerations

Erysipelas is a superficial form of cellulitis that occurs classically on the cheek, caused by β-hemolytic streptococci.

Clinical Findings

A. SYMPTOMS AND SIGNS

The symptoms are pain, malaise, chills, and moderate fever. A bright red spot appears first, very often near a fissure at the angle of the nose. This spreads to form a tense, sharply demarcated, glistening, smooth, hot area. The margin characteristically makes noticeable advances in days or even hours. The lesion is somewhat edematous and can be pitted slightly with the finger. Vesicles or bullae occasionally develop on the surface. The lesion does not usually become pustular or gangrenous and heals without scar formation. The disease may complicate any break in the skin that provides a portal of entry for the organism.

B. LABORATORY FINDINGS

Leukocytosis is almost invariably present; blood cultures may be positive.

Differential Diagnosis

Erysipeloid is a benign bacillary infection producing redness of the skin of the fingers or the backs of the hands in fishermen and meat handlers.

Complications

Unless erysipelas is promptly treated, death may result from extension of the process and systemic toxicity, particularly in the very young and in the aged.

Treatment

Place the patient at bed rest with the head of the bed elevated. Intravenous antibiotics effective against group A β-hemolytic streptococci and staphylococci are indicated for the first 48 hours in all but the mildest cases. A 7-day course is completed with penicillin VK, 250 mg, dicloxacillin, 250 mg, or a first-generation cephalosporin, 250 mg, orally four times a day. Alternatives in penicillin-allergic patients are clindamycin or erythromycin, the latter only if the infection is known to be due to streptococci.

Prognosis

Erysipelas was at one time a life-threatening infection. It can now usually be quickly controlled with systemic penicillin or erythromycin therapy.

See references in the next section.

2. CELLULITIS

 ESSENTIALS OF DIAGNOSIS

- *Edematous, expanding, erythematous, warm plaque with or without vesicles or bullae.*
- *Lower leg is frequently involved.*
- *Pain, chills, and fever are commonly present.*
- *Septicemia may develop.*

General Considerations

Cellulitis, a diffuse spreading infection of the dermis and subcutaneous tissue, is usually on the lower leg and most commonly due to gram-positive cocci, especially group A β-hemolytic streptococci and *S aureus*. Rarely, gram-negative rods or even fungi can produce a similar picture. In otherwise healthy persons, the most common portal of entry for lower leg cellulitis is tinea pedis of the toe web with fissuring. Injection drug use and open ulcerations may also be complicated by cellulitis. Cellulitis in the diabetic foot may be a major problem and is often associated with neuropathy and hyperkeratotic nodules from ill-fitting shoes and abnormal weight bearing.

Clinical Findings

A. SYMPTOMS AND SIGNS

Cellulitis begins as a small patch, which from its onset is tender. Swelling, erythema, and pain are often present. The lesion expands over hours, so that from onset to presentation is usually 6 to 36 hours. As the lesion grows, the patient becomes more ill with progressive chills, fever, and malaise. If septicemia develops, hypotension may develop followed by shock.

B. LABORATORY FINDINGS

Leukocytosis or at least a neutrophilia (left shift) is present from early in the course. Blood cultures may be positive. If a central ulceration, pustule, or abscess is present, culture may be of value. Aspiration of the advancing edge has a low yield (20%) and is usually not performed. Instead, if an unusual organism is suspected and there is no loculated site to culture, a full thickness skin biopsy taken before antibiotics are given can be useful. Part is cultured and part processed for histologic evaluation with Gram stain. This technique is particularly useful in the immunocompromised patient.

Differential Diagnosis

Two potentially life threatening entities that can mimic cellulitis (ie, present with a painful, red, swollen lower extremity) include deep venous thrombosis and necrotizing fasciitis. The diagnosis of necrotizing fasciitis should be suspected in a patient who has a very toxic appearance, bullae, crepitus or anesthesia of the involved skin, overlying skin necrosis, and laboratory evidence of rhabdomyolysis (elevated creatine phosphokinase [CPK]) or disseminated intravascular coagulation. While these findings may be present with severe cellulitis and bacteremia, it is essential to rule out necrotizing fasciitis because rapid surgical debridement is essential. Other skin lesions that may resemble cellulitis include sclerosing panniculitis, an acute, exquisitely tender red plaque on the medial lower legs above the malleolus in patients with venous stasis or varicosities, and acute severe contact dermatitis on a limb, which produces erythema, vesiculation, and edema as seen in cellulitis, but with itching instead of pain. The erythema and edema are also more superficial than in cellulitis.

Treatment

Intravenous or parenteral antibiotics may be required for the first 24–72 hours. In mild cases or following the initial parenteral therapy, dicloxacillin or cephalexin, 250–500 mg four times daily for 5–10 days, is usually adequate. In patients in whom intravenous treatment is not instituted, the first dose of oral antibiotic can be increased to 750–1000 mg to achieve rapid high blood levels.

Corwin P et al: Randomized controlled trial of intravenous antibiotic treatment for cellulitis at home compared with hospital. BMJ 2005;330:129. [PMID: 15604157]

Hepburn MJ et al: Comparison of short-course (5 days) and standard (10 days) treatment for uncomplicated cellulitis. Arch Intern Med 2004;164:1669. [PMID: 15302637]

Morris A: Cellulitis and erysipelas. Clin Evid 2004;(11):2133. [PMID: 15652104]

Roujeau JC et al: Chronic dermatomycoses of the foot as risk factors for acute bacterial cellulitis of the leg: a case-control study. Dermatology 2004;209:301. [PMID: 15539893]

Simonart T et al: The importance of serum creatine phosphokinase level in the early diagnosis and microbiological evalua-

tion of necrotizing fasciitis. J Eur Acad Dermatol Venereol 2004;18:687. [PMID: 15482296]

Swartz MN: Cellulitis. N Engl J Med 2004;350:904. [PMID: 14985488]

BLISTERING DISEASES

PEMPHIGUS

ESSENTIALS OF DIAGNOSIS

- *Relapsing crops of bullae.*
- *Often preceded by mucous membrane bullae, erosions, and ulcerations.*
- *Superficial detachment of the skin after pressure or trauma variably present (Nikolsky's sign).*
- *Acantholysis on biopsy.*
- *Immunofluorescence studies are confirmatory.*

General Considerations

Pemphigus is an uncommon intraepidermal blistering disease occurring on skin and mucous membranes. It is caused by autoantibodies to adhesion molecules expressed in the skin and mucous membranes (desmoglein 3, sometimes desmoglein 1 and plakoglobin in pemphigus vulgaris), and to a complex containing desmosomal proteins, including desmoglein 1 (in pemphigus foliaceus). These autoantibodies cause acantholysis, the separation of epidermal cells from each other. The cause is unknown, and in the preantibiotic, presteroid era the condition, if untreated, was usually fatal within 5 years. The bullae appear spontaneously and are tender and painful when they rupture. If the lesions become extensive, the complications of the disease lead to great toxicity and debility. Drug-induced pemphigus from drugs including penicillamine, captopril, and others has been reported. There are several forms of pemphigus: **pemphigus vulgaris** and its variant, **pemphigus vegetans;** and the more superficially blistering **pemphigus foliaceus** and its variant, **pemphigus erythematosus.** All forms may occur at any age but most commonly in middle age. The vulgaris form begins in the mouth in over 50% of cases. The foliaceus form is especially apt to be associated with other autoimmune diseases, or it may be drug-induced. Paraneoplastic pemphigus, a unique form of the disorder, is associated with numerous types of benign and malignant neoplasms but most frequently non-Hodgkin's lymphoma.

Clinical Findings

A. SYMPTOMS AND SIGNS

Pemphigus is characterized by an insidious onset of flaccid bullae in crops or waves. In pemphigus vulgaris, lesions often appear first on the oral mucous membranes, and these rapidly become erosive. In some cases, erosions and crusts predominate over blisters. The scalp is another site of early involvement. Rubbing a cotton swab or finger laterally on the surface of uninvolved skin may cause easy separation of the epidermis (**Nikolsky's sign**).

B. LABORATORY FINDINGS

The diagnosis is made by light microscopy and by direct and indirect immunofluorescence microscopy. Microscopically, acantholysis is the hallmark of pemphigus, but in some patients there may be eosinophilic spongiosis initially. Immunofluorescence microscopy shows intercellular deposits of IgG and C3 in the epidermis. Indirect immunofluorescence microscopy detects circulating pemphigus autoantibodies that correspond with disease activity and help in management.

Differential Diagnosis

Blistering diseases include erythema multiforme, drug eruptions, bullous impetigo, contact dermatitis, dermatitis herpetiformis, and bullous pemphigoid, but flaccid blisters are not typical of these diseases, and acantholysis is not seen. All of these diseases have clinical characteristics and different immunofluorescence test results that distinguish them from pemphigus.

Paraneoplastic pemphigus is clinically, histologically, and immunologically distinct from other forms of the disease. Oral erosions and erythematous plaques resembling erythema multiforme are seen. Survival rates are low because of the underlying malignancy.

Complications

Secondary infection commonly occurs; this is a major cause of morbidity and mortality. Disturbances of fluid, electrolyte, and nutritional intake can occur as a result of painful oral ulcers.

Treatment

A. GENERAL MEASURES

When the disease is severe, hospitalize the patient at bed rest and provide antibiotics and intravenous feedings as indicated. Anesthetic troches used before eating ease painful oral lesions.

B. SYSTEMIC MEASURES

Pemphigus very often requires systemic therapy as early in its course as possible. However, the main morbidity in this disease is due to the side effects of such therapy. Initial therapy is with systemic corticosteroids: prednisone, 60–80 mg daily. In all but the most mild cases, a steroid-sparing agent is added from the beginning, since the course of the disease is long and the steroid-sparing agents take several weeks to exert their activity. Azathioprine (100–200 mg daily) or mycophenolate mofetil (1–1.5 g twice daily) is used most frequently, the latter

seeming to be the most reliable and recommended for most cases. In refractory cases, monthly IGIV at 2 g/kg intravenously over 3 days is useful and has replaced high-dose corticosteroids plus cyclophosphamide and pulse intravenous corticosteroids as rescue therapy. Increased risk of thromboembolism is associated with IGIV therapy in these doses. In pemphigus foliaceus and mild cases of pemphigus vulgaris, tetracycline, 500 mg, and nicotinamide, 500 mg, three times daily, may be tried. Dapsone may also be tried as a steroid-sparing agent, especially in pemphigus foliaceus.

C. LOCAL MEASURES

In patients with limited disease, skin and mucous membrane lesions should be treated with topical corticosteroids. Complicating infection requires appropriate systemic and local antibiotic therapy.

Prognosis

The course tends to be chronic in most patients, though about one-third appear to experience remission. Infection is the most frequent cause of death, usually from *S aureus* septicemia.

Bystryn JC et al: Treatment of pemphigus with intravenous immunoglobulin. J Am Acad Dermatol 2002;47:358. [PMID: 12196744]

Sami N et al: Influence of IVIG therapy on autoantibody titers to desmoglein 1 in patients with pemphigus foliaceus. Clin Immunol 2002;105:192. [PMID: 12482393]

Sauret J et al: Rupturing bullae not responding to antibiotics. J Fam Pract 2004;53:981. Erratum in J Fam Pract 2005; 54:36. [PMID: 15581441]

OTHER BLISTERING DISEASES

Many other skin disorders are characterized by formation of bullae, or blisters. These include bullous pemphigoid, cicatricial pemphigoid, dermatitis herpetiformis, and pemphigoid gestationis.

Bullous Pemphigoid

Bullous pemphigoid is a relatively benign pruritic disease characterized by tense blisters in flexural areas, usually remitting in 5 or 6 years, with a course characterized by exacerbations and remissions. Most affected persons are over the age of 60 (often in their 70s or 80s), and men are affected twice as frequently as women. The appearance of blisters may be preceded by urticarial or edematous lesions for months. Oral lesions are present in about one-third of affected persons. The disease may occur in various forms, including localized, vesicular, vegetating, erythematous, erythrodermic, and nodular. There is no statistical association with internal malignant disease.

The diagnosis is made by biopsy and direct immunofluorescence examination. Light microscopy shows a subepidermal blister. With direct immunofluorescence, IgG and C3 are found at the dermal-epidermal junction. If the patient has mild disease, ultrapotent corticosteroids may be adequate. Prednisone at dosages of 0.75 mg/kg/d is often used to achieve rapid control of more widespread disease. Although slower in onset of action, tetracycline or erythromycin, 500 mg three times daily, alone or combined with nicotinamide—*not nicotinic acid or niacin!*—(up to 1.5 g/d), if tolerated, may control the disease in patients who cannot use corticosteroids or may allow decreasing or eliminating corticosteroids after control is achieved. Dapsone is particularly effective in mucous membrane pemphigoid. If these drugs are not effective, methotrexate, 5–25 mg weekly, or azathioprine, 50 mg one to three times daily, may be used as steroid-sparing agents. Mycophenolate mofetil (1 g twice daily) or IGIV as used for pemphigus vulgaris may be used in refractory cases.

Fernandez-Viadero C et al: Blisters in a nursing home: bullous pemphigoid more often than we think? J Am Geriatr Soc 2004;52:1405. [PMID: 15271141]

Khumalo N et al: Interventions for bullous pemphigoid. Cochrane Database Syst Rev 2005;(3):CD002292. [PMID: 16034874]

Mockenhaupt M et al: Daclizumab: a novel therapeutic option in severe bullous pemphigoid. Acta Derm Venereol 2005; 85:65. [PMID: 15848995]

Walsh SR et al: Bullous pemphigoid: from bench to bedside. Drugs 2005;65:905. [PMID: 15892587]

Herpes (Pemphigoid) Gestationis

Herpes gestationis occurs in about 1 in 50,000–60,000 pregnancies. The vesicles and bullae often appear first in periumbilical distribution, and there may be erythematous papules and plaques. It usually begins in the fifth or sixth month of pregnancy, or the onset may be delayed to the postpartum period. The disease is self-limited, but it may recur in subsequent pregnancies. Use of estrogens or progesterone or the onset of menses may trigger flare-ups. The risks to mother and fetus appear to be limited but include an increase in prematurity and small-for-gestational-age infants. Blisters are subepidermal, with eosinophils present. Direct immunofluorescence shows C3 at the basement membrane zone in most cases. IgG is found less often.

Corticosteroids are the treatment of choice and are sometimes effective when used topically only.

Wollina U et al: Itching stretch marks and bullous lesions in a pregnant woman. Int J Dermatol 2004;43:752. [PMID: 15485535]

PAPULES

WARTS

ESSENTIALS OF DIAGNOSIS

- *Verrucous papules anywhere on the skin or mucous membranes, usually no larger than 1 cm in diameter.*
- *Prolonged incubation period (average 2–18 months). Spontaneous "cures" are frequent (50% at 2 years for common warts).*
- *"Recurrences" (new lesions) are frequent.*

General Considerations

Warts are caused by human papillomaviruses (HPVs). The type of mucocutaneous surface infected and the morphology of the wart are closely related to the HPV type causing the infection. Especially in genital warts, simultaneous infection with numerous wart types is common. Genital HPVs are divided into low-risk and high-risk types depending on the likelihood of their association with cervical and anal cancer.

Clinical Findings

There are usually no symptoms. Tenderness on pressure occurs with plantar warts; itching occurs with anogenital warts. Occasionally a wart will produce mechanical obstruction (eg, nostril, ear canal, urethra).

Warts vary widely in shape, size, and appearance. Flat warts are most evident under oblique illumination. Subungual warts may be dry, fissured, and hyperkeratotic and may resemble hangnails or other nonspecific changes. Plantar warts resemble plantar corns or calluses.

Differential Diagnosis

Some warty-looking lesions are actually hypertrophic actinic keratoses or squamous cell carcinomas. Some genital warty lesions may be due to secondary syphilis (condylomata lata). The lesions of molluscum contagiosum may be mistaken for warts. Seborrheic keratosis may also be confused with warts. In AIDS, wart-like lesions may be caused by varicella zoster virus.

Prevention

The use of condoms may reduce transmission of genital warts. A person with flat warts should be educated about the infectivity of warts and advised not to scratch or traumatize the areas. Using an electric shaver may prevent autoinoculation.

Treatment

Treatment is aimed at inducing "wart-free" intervals for as long as possible without scarring, since no treatment can guarantee a remission or prevent recurrences. In immunocompromised patients, the goal is even more modest, ie, to control the size and number of lesions present.

A. REMOVAL

For common warts of the hands, patients are usually offered liquid nitrogen or keratolytic agents. The former may work in fewer treatments but requires office visits and is painful. Keratolytic agents are irritating but effective and usually painless if used correctly. They can be used at home but must be applied almost daily for 8–12 weeks for maximum effect.

1. Liquid nitrogen—Liquid nitrogen is applied to achieve a thaw time of 20–45 seconds. Two freeze-thaw cycles are given every 2–4 weeks for several visits. Scarring will occur if it is used incorrectly or too aggressively. For example, the face, dorsal hands, and legs are more sensitive than the palms. Improper use along the sides of the fingers has been reported to cause nerve damage and paresthesias. Liquid nitrogen may cause permanent depigmentation in pigmented individuals. It is useful on penile warts and on filiform warts involving the face and body. Liquid nitrogen may be used for condylomas, but snipping of lesions followed by light electrodesiccation is more effective.

2. Keratolytic agents and occlusion—Salicylic acid products may be used against common warts or plantar warts. They are applied then occluded. Plantar warts may be treated by applying a 40% salicylic acid plaster (Mediplast) after paring. The plaster may be left on for 5–6 days, then removed, the lesion pared down, and another plaster applied. Although it may take weeks or months to eradicate the wart, the method is safe and effective with almost no side effects. Chronic occlusion alone with water-impermeable tape (duct tape, adhesive tape) for months may be effective.

3. Podophyllum resin—Anogenital warts are often initially treated by painting each wart carefully (protecting normal skin) every 2–3 weeks with 25% podophyllum resin (podophyllin) in compound tincture of benzoin. Pregnant patients should not be so treated. The purified active component of the resin, podofilox, is available for use at home twice daily 3 consecutive days a week for cycles of 4–6 weeks. It is less irritating and more effective than podophyllum resin. After a single 4-week cycle, 45% of patients were wart-free; but of these, 60% relapsed at 6 weeks. Thus, multiple cycles of treatment are often necessary.

4. Imiquimod—A 5% cream of this local interferon inducer has moderate activity in clearing external genital warts. Seventy-seven percent of women and 40% of men with external genital warts had complete clearing of their lesions, and 90% and 74%, respectively, had greater than 50% reduction in their warts. The superior response in women may relate to enhanced penetration of the moist skin of the vulva as compared with the penile shaft. Treatment is once daily on 3 alternate days per week. Response may be slow, with patients who eventually cleared having responses at 8 weeks (44%) or 12 weeks (69%). Once cleared, about 13% had recurrences in the short term.

There is less pregnancy risk than with podophyllum resin (category B versus category X with podophyllin). It is more expensive than podophyllotoxin, but given the high rate of response in women and its safety and low relapse rate, it appears to be the "patient-administered" treatment of choice in women. In men, the more rapid response, lower cost, and similar efficacy make podophyllotoxin the initial treatment of choice, with imiquimod used for recurrences or refractory cases. Imiquimod has no demonstrated efficacy for—and should not be used to treat—plantar or common warts.

5. Operative removal—Plantar warts may be removed by blunt dissection. Local anesthetic is injected into the base, and the wart is then removed with a curette or scissors or by shaving off at the base of the wart with a scalpel. Trichloroacetic acid or Monsel's solution on a tightly wound cotton-tipped applicator may be painted on the wound, or light electrocautery may be used. Excision of warts, however, may result in a permanent painful scar on the foot and is not recommended. For genital warts, snip biopsy (scissors) removal followed by light electrocautery is more effective than cryotherapy but may scar. It is often preferred by patients with pedunculated or large lesions that require multiple cryotherapy or podophyllin treatments for removal.

6. Laser therapy—The CO_2 laser is effective for treating recurrent warts, periungual warts, plantar warts, and condylomata acuminata. It leaves open wounds that must fill in with granulation tissue over 4–6 weeks and is best reserved for warts resistant to all other modalities. Lasers with emissions of 585, 595, or 532 nm may also be used every 3–4 weeks to gradually ablate common or plantar warts. This is no more effective than cryotherapy in controlled trials. For genital warts, it has not been shown that laser therapy is more effective than electrosurgical removal.

7. Other agents—Bleomycin diluted to 1 unit/mL may be injected into warts. It has been shown to have a high cure rate for plantar and common warts. It should not be used on digital warts because of the potential complications of Raynaud's phenomenon, nail loss, and terminal digital necrosis.

B. IMMUNOTHERAPY

Squaric acid dibutylester may be effective. It is applied in a concentration of 0.2–2% directly to the warts from once weekly to five times weekly to induce a mild contact dermatitis. Between 60% and 80% of warts clear over 10–20 weeks. Injection of candida antigen may be used in the same way.

C. PHYSICAL MODALITIES

Soaking warts in hot (42.2 °C) water for 10–30 minutes daily for 6 weeks has resulted in dramatic involution in some cases.

Prognosis

There is a striking tendency to the development of new lesions. Warts may disappear spontaneously or may be unresponsive to treatment.

Focht DR 3rd et al: The efficacy of duct tape vs cryotherapy in the treatment of verruca vulgaris (the common wart). Arch Pediatr Adolesc Med 2002;156:971. [PMID: 12361440]

Gibbs S et al: Local treatments for cutaneous warts: systematic review. BMJ 2002;325:461. [PMID: 12202325]

Human papillomavirus infection. Am J Transplant 2004;4 Suppl 10:95. [PMID: 15504222]

Manhart LE et al: Do condoms prevent genital HPV infection, external genital warts or cervical neoplasia? A meta-analysis. Sex Transm Dis 2002;29:725. [PMID: 12438912]

Warren T et al: Counseling the patient who has genital herpes or genital human papillomavirus infection. Infect Dis Clin North Am 2005;19:459. [PMID: 15963883]

Wiley DJ et al: External genital warts: diagnosis, treatment and prevention. Clin Infect Dis 2002;35(Suppl 2):S210. [PMID: 12353208]

CALLOSITIES & CORNS OF FEET OR TOES

Callosities and corns are caused by pressure and friction due to faulty weight-bearing, orthopedic deformities, improperly fitting shoes, or neuropathies.

Tenderness on pressure and "after-pain" are the only symptoms. The hyperkeratotic well-localized overgrowths always occur at pressure points. Fingerprint lines are preserved over the surface (not so in warts). When the surface is shaved with a 15 blade, a glassy core is found (which differentiates these disorders from plantar warts, which have multiple capillary bleeding points or black dots when pared). A soft corn often occurs laterally on the proximal portion of the fourth toe as a result of pressure against the bony structure of the interphalangeal joint of the fifth toe.

Treatment consists of correcting mechanical abnormalities that cause friction and pressure. Shoes must be properly fitted and orthopedic deformities corrected. Callosities may be removed by careful paring of the callus after a warm water soak or with keratolytic agents as found in various brands of corn pads.

Plantar hyperkeratosis of the heels can be treated successfully by using 20% urea (Ureacin 20) or 12% lactic acid (Lac-Hydrin) or combinations nightly and a pumice stone after soaking in water.

Women who tend to form calluses and corns should not wear confining footgear and high-heeled shoes. Callosities on diabetic feet, especially in the setting of hyposensate neuropathy, can be a major problem and the value of early management to prevent complications is very important.

Filippo JS et al: The nonresponding "wart." Paring with a scalpel may reveal a different lesion. Postgrad Med 2003;114:57. [PMID: 12926177]

Pataky Z et al: The impact of callosities on the magnitude and duration of plantar pressure in patients with diabetes mellitus. A callus may cause 18,600 kilograms of excess plantar pressure per day. Diabetes Metab 2002;28:356. [PMID: 12461472]

MOLLUSCUM CONTAGIOSUM

Molluscum contagiosum, caused by a poxvirus, presents as single or multiple rounded, dome-shaped, waxy papules 2–5 mm in diameter that are umbilicated. Lesions at first are firm, solid, and flesh-colored but upon reaching maturity become softened, whitish, or pearly gray and may suppurate. The principal sites of involvement are the face, lower abdomen, and genitals.

The lesions are autoinoculable and spread by wet skin-to-skin contact. In sexually active individuals, they may be confined to the penis, pubis, and inner thighs and are considered a sexually transmitted disease.

Molluscum contagiosum is common in patients with AIDS, usually with a helper T cell count < 100/mcL. Extensive lesions tend to develop over the face and neck as well as in the genital area.

The diagnosis is easily established in most instances because of the distinctive central umbilication of the dome-shaped lesion. The best treatment is by curettage or applications of liquid nitrogen as for warts—but more briefly, since molluscum contagiosum is more responsive to therapy than warts. When lesions are frozen, the central umbilication often becomes more apparent. Light electrosurgery with a fine needle is also effective. It has been estimated that individual lesions persist for about 2 months. They are difficult to eradicate in patients with AIDS unless immunity improves, in which case spontaneous clearing may occur.

Baxter KF et al: Topical cidofovir and cryotherapy—combination treatment for recalcitrant molluscum contagiosum in a patient with HIV infection. J Eur Acad Dermatol Venereol 2004;18:330. [PMID: 15009318]

Lerbaek A et al: Facial eruption of molluscum contagiosum during topical treatment of atopic dermatitis with tacrolimus. Br J Dermatol 2004;150:1210. [PMID: 15214914]

Usatine RP: Pearly penile lesions. J Fam Prac 2004;53:885. [PMID: 15527725]

BASAL CELL CARCINOMA

 ESSENTIALS OF DIAGNOSIS

- *Pearly papule, erythematous patch > 6 mm, or nonhealing ulcer, in sun exposed areas (face, trunk, lower legs).*
- *History of bleeding.*
- *Fair-skinned person with a history of sun exposure (often intense, intermittent).*

General Considerations

Basal cell carcinomas are the most common form of cancer. They occur on sun-exposed skin in otherwise normal fair-skinned individuals; ultraviolet light is the cause. The most common presentation is a papule or nodule that may have a central scab or erosion. Occasionally the nodules have stippled pigment (pigmented basal cell carcinoma). Intradermal nevi without pigment on the face of older white individuals may resemble basal cell carcinomas. Basal cell carcinomas grow slowly, attaining a size of 1–2 cm or more in diameter, often after years of growth. There is a waxy, "pearly" appearance, with telangiectatic vessels easily visible. It is the pearly or translucent quality of these lesions that is most diagnostic, a feature best appreciated if the skin is stretched. Less common types include morpheaform or scar-like lesions. These are hypopigmented, somewhat thickened plaques. On the back and chest, basal cell carcinomas appear as reddish, somewhat shiny, scaly patches.

Clinicians should examine the skin routinely, looking for bumps, patches, and scabbed lesions. When examining the face, look at the eyelid margins and medial canthi, the nose and alar folds, the lips, and then around and behind the ears. While metastases almost never occur, therapy of basal cell carcinomas may cause significant cosmetic deformity in these areas, particularly for inadequately treated or recurrent lesions. Neglected lesions may ulcerate and produce great destruction. Basal cell carcinomas of the medial canthi are particularly dangerous. Recurrent lesions around the nose and ears may track along cartilage underneath the skin, requiring treatment of much more extensive areas than are apparent from inspection.

Treatment

Lesions suspected to be basal cell carcinomas should be biopsied, by shave or punch biopsy. Therapy is then aimed at eradication with minimal cosmetic deformity, often by excision and suturing with recurrence rates of 5% or less. The technique of three cycles of curettage and electrodesiccation depends on the skill of the operator and is not recommended for head and neck lesions. After 4–6 weeks of healing, it leaves a broad, hypopigmented, at times hypertrophic scar. Radiotherapy is effective and sometimes appropriate for older individuals (over 65), but recurrent tumors after radiation therapy are more difficult to treat and may be more aggressive. Radiation therapy is the most expensive method to treat basal cell carcinoma and should only be used if other treatment options are not appropriate. Mohs surgery—removal of the tumor followed by immediate frozen section histopathologic examination of margins with subsequent reexcision of tumor-positive areas and final closure of the defect—gives the highest cure rates (98%) and results in least tissue loss. It is appropriate therapy for tumors of the eyelids or for recurrent lesions, or where tissue sparing is needed for cosmesis. Patients with basal cell carcinomas must be followed to detect new or recurrent lesions.

Diepgen TL et al: The epidemiology of skin cancer. Br J Dermol 2002;146(Suppl 61):1. [PMID: 11966724]

Marks R et al: Efficacy and safety of 5% imiquimod cream in treating patients with multiple superficial basal cell carcinomas. Arch Dermatol 2004;140:1284. [PMID: 15492200]

SQUAMOUS CELL CARCINOMA

 ESSENTIALS OF DIAGNOSIS

- *Nonhealing ulcer or warty nodule.*
- *Skin damage due to long-term sun exposure.*
- *Common in fair-skinned organ transplant recipients.*

Squamous cell carcinoma usually occurs subsequent to prolonged sun exposure on exposed parts in fair-skinned individuals who sunburn easily and tan poorly. It may arise from an actinic keratosis. The lesions appear as small red, conical, hard nodules that occasionally ulcerate. The frequency of metastasis is not precisely known, though metastatic spread is said to be less likely with squamous cell carcinoma arising out of actinic keratoses than with those that arise de novo. In actinically induced squamous cell cancers, rates of metastasis are estimated from retrospective studies to be 3–7%. Squamous cell carcinomas of the lip, oral cavity, tongue, and genitalia have much higher rates of metastasis and require special management.

Keratoacanthomas most often act in benign fashion but resemble squamous cell carcinoma histologically and for all practical purposes should be treated as though they were skin cancers.

Examination of the skin and therapy are essentially the same as for basal cell carcinoma. The preferred treatment of squamous cell carcinoma is excision. Electrodesiccation and curettage and x-ray radiation may be used for some lesions, and fresh tissue microscopically controlled excision (Mohs) is recommended for high-risk lesions (lips, temples, ears, nose) and for recurrent tumors. Some keratoacanthomas respond to intralesional injection of fluorouracil or methotrexate, but they must be excised if they do not. Follow-up for squamous cell carcinoma must be more frequent and thorough than for basal cell carcinoma, starting at every 3 months, with careful examination of lymph nodes. In addition, palpation of the lips is essential to detect hard or indurated areas that represent early squamous cell carcinoma. All such cases must be biopsied. Multiple squamous cell carcinomas are very common on the sun-exposed skin of organ transplant patients. The intensity of immunosuppression, not the use of any particular immunosuppressive agent, is the primary risk factor in determining the development of skin cancer after transplant. The tumors begin to appear after 5 years of immunosuppression. Regular dermatologic evaluation in at-risk organ transplant recipients is recommended. Biologic behavior of skin cancer in organ transplant recipients may be aggressive, and careful management is required.

Fortina AB et al: Immunosuppressive level and other risk factors for basal cell carcinoma and squamous cell carcinoma in heart transplant recipients. Arch Dermatol 2004;140:1079. [PMID: 15381547]

Garner KL et al: Basal and squamous cell carcinoma. Prim Care 2000;27:447. [PMID: 10815054]

Ismail F et al: Unusual distribution of punctate dysplastic keratoses and skin cancers in sunbed users: a report of three cases. Br J Dermatol 2005;152:1374. [PMID: 15949021]

VIOLACEOUS TO PURPLE PAPULES & NODULES

LICHEN PLANUS

 ESSENTIALS OF DIAGNOSIS

- *Pruritic, violaceous, flat-topped papules with fine white streaks and symmetric distribution.*
- *Lacy lesions of the buccal mucosa.*
- *Commonly seen along linear scratch marks (Koebner phenomenon) on anterior wrists, penis, legs.*
- *Histopathologic examination is diagnostic.*

General Considerations

Lichen planus is an inflammatory pruritic disease of the skin and mucous membranes characterized by distinctive papules with a predilection for the flexor surfaces and trunk. The three cardinal findings are typical skin lesions, mucosal lesions, and histopathologic features of band-like infiltration of lymphocytes in the dermis. Drugs causing lichen planus-like reactions include gold, streptomycin, tetracycline, chloroquine, quinacrine, quinidine, NSAIDs, phenothiazines, and hydrochlorothiazide. Hepatitis C infection is found with greater frequency in lichen planus patients than in controls. Allergy to mercury amalgams can trigger oral lesions identical to lichen planus.

Clinical Findings

Itching is mild to severe. The lesions are violaceous, flat-topped, angulated papules, up to 1 cm in diameter, discrete or in clusters, with very fine white streaks (Wickham's striae) on the flexor surfaces of the wrists and on the penis, lips, tongue, and buccal and vaginal mucous membranes. The papules may become bullous or ulcerated. The disease may be generalized. Mucosal lichen planus has been reported in the genital and anorectal areas, the gastrointestinal tract, the bladder,

the larynx, and the conjunctiva. Mucous membrane lesions have a lacy white network overlying them that may be confused with leukoplakia. The Koebner phenomenon (appearance of lesions in areas of trauma) may be seen.

A special form of lichen planus is the erosive or ulcerative variety. On palms and soles, it can be disabling. It is a major problem in the mouth or genitalia, and squamous cell carcinoma develops in 5% of patients with erosive oral or genital lichen planus.

Differential Diagnosis

Lichen planus must be distinguished from similar lesions produced by medications (see above) and other papular lesions such as psoriasis, lichen simplex chronicus, and syphilis. Lichen planus on the mucous membranes must be differentiated from leukoplakia. Erosive oral lesions require biopsy and often direct immunofluorescence for diagnosis since lichen planus may simulate other erosive diseases. Histologic examination may make the distinction from graft-versus-host disease and in some cases from lichen planus-like drug eruptions.

Treatment

A. Topical Therapy

Superpotent topical corticosteroids applied twice daily are most helpful for localized disease in nonflexural areas. Alternatively, high-potency corticosteroid cream or ointment may be used nightly under thin pliable plastic film.

Topical tacrolimus appears effective in oral and vaginal erosive lichen planus, but long-term therapy is required to prevent relapse. If tacrolimus is used, lesions must be observed carefully for development of cancer. If the erosive lichen planus lesions are adjacent to a mercury containing amalgam, removal of the amalgam may result in clearing of the erosions.

B. Systemic Therapy

Corticosteroids (see Chapter 26) may be required in severe cases or in circumstances where the most rapid response to treatment is desired. Unfortunately, relapse almost always occurs as the corticosteroids are tapered, making systemic corticosteroid therapy an impractical option for the management of chronic lichen planus.

Isotretinoin and acitretin by mouth appear to be effective in some cases of oral and cutaneous lichen planus.

UV phototherapy may also be effective treatment.

Prognosis

Lichen planus is a benign disease, but it may persist for months or years and may be recurrent. Hypertrophic lichen planus and oral lesions tend to be especially persistent, and neoplastic degeneration has been described in chronically eroded lesions.

Byrd JA et al: Response of oral lichen planus to topical tacrolimus in 37 patients. Arch Dermatol 2004;140:1508. [PMID: 15611431]

Jensen JT et al: Patient satisfaction after the treatment of vulvovaginal erosive lichen planus with topical clobetasol and tacrolimus: a survey study. Am J Obstet Gynecol 2004; 190:1759. [PMID: 15284791]

Laeijendecker R et al: Oral lichen planus and allergy to dental amalgam restorations. Arch Dermatol 2004;140:1434. [PMID: 15611418]

Popkin DL et al: Widespread annular eruption in a black man—quiz case. Arch Dermatol 2005;141:93. [PMID: 15655155]

KAPOSI'S SARCOMA

General Considerations

Before 1980 in the United States, this rare malignant skin lesion was seen mostly in elderly white men, had a chronic clinical course, and was rarely fatal. Kaposi's sarcoma occurs endemically in an often aggressive form in young black men of equatorial Africa, but it is rare in American blacks. Kaposi's sarcoma continues to occur largely in homosexual men with HIV infection as an AIDS-defining illness. Kaposi's sarcoma may complicate immunosuppressive therapy, and stopping the immunosuppression may result in improvement. Human herpes virus 8 (HHV-8), or Kaposi's sarcoma-associated herpes virus (KSHV), is universally present in all forms of Kaposi's sarcoma. The virus is present in the skin lesions and circulating B lymphocytes of persons with Kaposi's sarcoma but uncommonly in their normal skin. A serologic test is available to detect infection with this virus, but its sensitivity is insufficient for commercial use.

Red or purple plaques or nodules on cutaneous or mucosal surfaces are characteristic. Kaposi's sarcoma commonly involves the gastrointestinal tract, but in asymptomatic patients these lesions are not sought or treated. Pulmonary Kaposi's sarcoma may be life-threatening and is managed aggressively. The incidence of AIDS-associated Kaposi's sarcoma is diminishing.

Treatment

For Kaposi's sarcoma in the elderly, palliative local therapy with intralesional chemotherapy or radiation is usually all that is required. In the setting of iatrogenic immunosuppression, the treatment of Kaposi's sarcoma is primarily reduction of doses of immunosuppressive medications. In AIDS-associated Kaposi's sarcoma, the patient should first be given effective anti-HIV antiretrovirals (including a protease inhibitor), because in most cases this treatment alone is associated with improvement. Other therapeutic options include cryotherapy or intralesional vinblastine (0.1–0.5 mg/mL) for cosmetically objectionable lesions; radiation therapy for accessible and space-occupying lesions; and laser surgery for certain intraoral and pharyngeal lesions. Systemic therapy is indicated in patients with rapidly progressive skin disease (more than ten new lesions per month), with edema or pain, and with symptomatic visceral disease or pulmonary disease. Liposomal doxorubicin is highly effective in controlling these cases and has considerably less toxicity—and greater efficacy—than anthracycline monotherapy or combination chemotherapeutic regimens. α-Interferon may also be used.

Antman K et al: Kaposi's sarcoma. N Engl J Med 2000;342:1027. [PMID: 10749966]

Bursics A et al: HHV-8 positive, HIV negative disseminated Kaposi's sarcoma complicating steroid dependent ulcerative colitis: a successfully treated case. Gut 2005;54:1049. [PMID: 15951561]

Cheung TW: AIDS-related cancer in the era of highly active antiretroviral therapy (HAART): a model of the interplay of the immune system, virus, and cancer. "On the offensive—the Trojan Horse is being destroyed"—Part A: Kaposi's sarcoma. Cancer Invest 2004;22:774. [PMID: 15581058]

Dal Maso L et al: Classic Kaposi's sarcoma in Italy, 1985–1998. Br J Cancer 2005;92:188. [PMID: 15570306]

Lim ST et al: Weekly docetaxel is safe and effective in the treatment of advanced-stage acquired immunodeficiency syndrome-related Kaposi sarcoma. Cancer 2005;103:417. [PMID: 15578686]

PRURITUS (Itching)

Pruritus is a disagreeable sensation that provokes a desire to scratch. It is modulated by central factors, including cortical ones. Not all cases of pruritus are mediated by histamine.

Although many cases of generalized pruritus can be attributed to dry skin—whether naturally occurring and precipitated or aggravated by climatic conditions or arising from disease states—there are many other causes: scabies, dermatitis herpetiformis, atopic dermatitis, genital pruritus, pruritus vulvae et ani, miliaria, insect bites, pediculosis, contact dermatitis, drug reactions, urticaria, psoriasis, lichen planus, lichen simplex chronicus, exfoliative dermatitis, folliculitis, bullous pemphigoid, and fiberglass dermatitis.

Persistent pruritus not explained by cutaneous disease should prompt a staged workup for systemic causes. Perhaps the most common cause of pruritus associated with systemic disease is uremia in conjunction with hemodialysis. Both this condition and the pruritus of liver disease may be helped by phototherapy with ultraviolet B or PUVA. Naltrexone and nalmefene have been shown to relieve the pruritus of liver disease. Naltrexone is not effective in pruritus associated with renal failure, but gabapentin may be effective. Endocrine disorders such as hypothyroidism or hyperthyroidism, psychiatric disturbances, lymphoma, leukemia, and other internal malignant disorders, iron deficiency anemia, and certain neurologic disorders may also cause pruritus. Antihistamines reduce pruritus only by their sedating effect (except in urticaria). Nonsedating, second generation antihistamines are of no value in nonurticarial pruritus.

Prognosis

Elimination of external factors and irritating agents may give complete relief from pruritus. Pruritus accompanying specific skin disease will subside when the disease is controlled. Pruritus accompanying serious internal disease may not respond to any type of therapy.

Bellmann R et al: Treatment of intractable pruritus in drug induced cholestasis with albumin dialysis: a report of two cases. ASAIO 2004;50:387. [PMID: 15307554]

Clarke P: Why am I so itchy? Aust Fam Physician 2004;33:489. [PMID: 15301164]

Crownover BK et al: Clinical inquiries. First- or second-generation antihistamines: which are more effective at controlling pruritus? J Fam Pract 2004;53:742. [PMID: 15353166]

Hiramanek N: Itch: a symptom of occult disease. Aust Fam Physician 2004;33:495. [PMID: 15301165]

Twycross R et al: Itch: scratching more than the surface. QJM 2003;96:7. [PMID: 12509645]

ANOGENITAL PRURITUS

ESSENTIALS OF DIAGNOSIS

- Itching, chiefly nocturnal, of the anogenital area.
- Examination is highly variable, ranging from no skin findings to excoriations and inflammation of any degree, including lichenification.

General Considerations

Many cases have no obvious cause, but multiple specific causes have been identified. Anogenital pruritus may be due to intertrigo, psoriasis, lichen simplex chronicus, or seborrheic or contact dermatitis (from soaps, colognes, douches, contraceptives, and perhaps scented toilet tissue), or it may be due to irritating secretions, as in diarrhea, leukorrhea, or trichomoniasis, or to local disease (candidiasis, dermatophytosis, erythrasma). Oxyuriasis (pinworm) is a rare cause in adults. Lichen sclerosus may at times be the cause. Erythrasma is easily diagnosed by demonstration of coral-red fluorescence with Wood's light; it is easily cured with erythromycin orally and topically.

Uncleanliness may be at fault. In pruritus ani, hemorrhoids are often found, and leakage of mucus and bacteria from the distal rectum onto the perianal skin may be important in cases in which no other skin abnormality is found.

Many women experience pruritus vulvae. In women, pruritus ani by itself is rare, and pruritus vulvae does not usually involve the anal area, though anal itching will usually spread to the vulva. In men, pruritus of the scrotum is most commonly seen in the absence of pruritus ani. Up to one-third of causes of ano-genital pruritus may be due to nerve impingements of the lumbosacral spine.

Clinical Findings

A. SYMPTOMS AND SIGNS

The only symptom is itching, which is chiefly nocturnal. Physical findings are usually not present, but there may be erythema, fissuring, maceration, lichenification, excoriations, or changes suggestive of candidiasis or tinea.

B. LABORATORY FINDINGS

Urinalysis and blood glucose testing may lead to a diagnosis of diabetes mellitus. Microscopic examination or culture of tissue scrapings may reveal yeasts or fungi. Stool examination may show pinworms. Radiologic studies may demonstrate spinal cord disease.

Differential Diagnosis

The etiologic differential diagnosis consists of *Candida* infection, parasitosis, local irritation from contact with drugs and irritants, nerve impingement and other primary skin disorders of the genital area such as psoriasis, seborrhea, intertrigo, or lichen sclerosus et atrophicus.

Prevention

Instruct the patient in proper anogenital hygiene after treating systemic or local conditions. If appropriate, physical therapy and exercises to support the lower spine are recommended.

Treatment

A. GENERAL MEASURES

Treating constipation, preferably with high-fiber management (psyllium), may help. Instruct the patient to use very soft or moistened tissue or cotton after bowel movements and to clean the perianal area thoroughly with cool water if possible. Women should use similar precautions after urinating. Instruct the patient regarding the harmful and pruritus-inducing effects of scratching.

B. LOCAL MEASURES

Pramoxine cream or lotion or hydrocortisone-pramoxine (Pramosone), 1% or 2.5% cream, lotion, or ointment, is helpful in managing pruritus in the anogenital area. The ointment or cream should be applied after a bowel movement. Topical doxepin cream 5% is similarly effective, but it may be sedating. Potent fluorinated topical corticosteroids may lead to atrophy and striae if used for more than a few days and should in general be avoided. This includes combinations with antifungals. The use of strong corticosteroids on the scrotum may lead to persistent severe burning upon withdrawal of the drug. Underclothing should be changed daily. Balneol Perianal Cleansing Lotion or Tucks premoistened pads, ointment, or cream (all Tucks preparations contain witch hazel) may be very useful for pruritus ani. About one-third of patients with scrotal or anal pruritus will respond to capsaicin 0.006%. Treatment for underlying spinal neurologic disease may be required. Squamous cell carcinoma of the anus and extramammary Paget's disease are rare causes of genital pruritus.

Prognosis

Although benign, anogenital pruritus may be persistent and recurrent.

Cohen AD et al: Neuropathic scrotal pruritus: anogenital pruritus is a symptom of lumbosacral radiculopathy. J Am Acad Dermatol 2005;52:61. [PMID: 15627082]

Handa Y et al: Squamous cell carcinoma of the anal margin with pruritus ani of long duration. Dermatol Surg 2003;29:108. [PMID: 12534524]

Heard S: Pruritus ani. Aust Fam Physician 2004;33:511. [PMID: 15301168]

Welsh B et al: Vulval itch. Aust Fam Physician 2004;33:505. [PMID: 15301167]

SCABIES

ESSENTIALS OF DIAGNOSIS

- *Generalized very severe itching.*
- *Pruritic vesicles and pustules in "runs" or "galleries," especially on finger webs and the heels of the palms and in wrist creases.*
- *Mites, ova, and brown dots of feces visible microscopically.*
- *Red papules or nodules on the scrotum and on the penile glans and shaft are pathognomonic.*

General Considerations

Scabies is caused by infestation with *Sarcoptes scabiei*. The infestation usually spares the head and neck (though even these areas may be involved in infants, in the elderly, and in patients with AIDS). Scabies is usually acquired by sleeping with or in the bedding of an infested individual or by other close contact. The entire household may be affected.

Clinical Findings

A. SYMPTOMS AND SIGNS

Itching is almost always present and can be quite severe. The lesions consist of more or less generalized excoriations with small pruritic vesicles, pustules, and "runs" or "burrows" in the web spaces and on the heels of the palms, wrists, elbows, and around the axillae. Often, burrows are found only on the feet, as they have been scratched off in other locations. The burrow appears as a short irregular mark, 2–3 mm long and the width of a hair. Characteristic lesions may occur on the nipples in females and as pruritic papules on the scrotum or penis in males. Pruritic papules may be seen over the buttocks.

B. LABORATORY FINDINGS

The diagnosis should be confirmed by microscopic demonstration of the organism, ova, or feces in a mounted specimen. The success of this procedure depends on choosing the best unexcoriated lesions from interdigital webs, wrists, elbows, or feet. A No. 15 blade is used to scrape the lesion until it is flat. Pinpoint bleeding may result from the scraping. The mite, ova, and feces can be seen under the light microscope.

Differential Diagnosis

Scabies must be distinguished from the various forms of pediculosis and from other causes of pruritus.

Treatment & Prognosis

Treatment is aimed at killing scabies mites and controlling the dermatitis, which can persist for months after effective eradication of the mites. Bedding and clothing should be laundered or cleaned or set aside for 14 days in plastic bags. If secondary pyoderma is present, it is treated with systemic antibiotics. Unless treatment is aimed at all infected persons in a family or institutionalized group, reinfestations will probably occur.

Permethrin 5% cream is highly effective and safe in the management of scabies. Treatment consists of a single application for 8–12 hours. It may be repeated in 1 week.

Pregnant patients should be treated only if they have documented scabies themselves. Permethrin 5% cream once for 12 hours—or 5% or 6% sulfur in petrolatum applied nightly for 3 nights from the collarbones down—may be used.

Patients will continue to itch for several weeks after treatment. Use of triamcinolone 0.1% cream will help resolve the dermatitis. Scabies in nursing home patients, institutionalized or mentally impaired (especially Down syndrome) patients, and AIDS patients may be much more difficult to treat.

Most failures in normal persons are related to incorrect use or incomplete treatment of the housing unit. In these cases, repeat treatment with permethrin once weekly for 2 weeks, with reeducation regarding the method and extent of application, is suggested. In immunocompetent individuals, ivermectin in a dose of 200 mcg/kg is effective in about 75% of cases with a single dose and 95% of cases with two doses 2 weeks apart. In immunosuppressed hosts and those with crusted (hyperkeratotic) scabies, multiple doses of ivermectin (every 2 weeks for two or three doses) plus topical therapy with permethrin once weekly may be effective when topical treatment and oral therapy alone fail.

Persistent pruritic postscabietic papules may be treated with mid- to high-potency corticosteroids or with intralesional triamcinolone acetonide (2.5–5 mg/mL).

Gimenez Garcia R et al: Scabies in the elderly. J Eur Acad Dermatol Venereol 2004;18:105. [PMID: 14678549]

Johnston G et al: Scabies: diagnosis and treatment. BMJ 2005; 331:619. [PMID: 16166133]

Krohn B: Scabies in long-term care settings. Expedient diagnosis and treatment are essential. Adv Nurse Pract 2004;12:35. [PMID: 15615219]

PEDICULOSIS

ESSENTIALS OF DIAGNOSIS

- *Pruritus with excoriation.*
- *Nits on hair shafts; lice on skin or clothes.*
- *Occasionally, sky-blue macules (maculae ceruleae) on the inner thighs or lower abdomen in pubic louse infestation.*

General Considerations

Pediculosis is a parasitic infestation of the skin of the scalp, trunk, or pubic areas. Body lice usually occur among people who live in overcrowded dwellings with inadequate hygiene facilities. Pubic lice may be acquired by sexual transmission. Head lice may be transmitted by shared use of hats or combs and are epidemic among children of all socioeconomic classes in elementary schools. Head lice are very uncommon among black children. Adults contacting children with head lice frequently acquire the infestation.

There are three different varieties: (1) pediculosis pubis, caused by *Phthirus pubis* (pubic louse, "crabs"); (2) pediculosis corporis, caused by *Pediculus humanus* var *corporis* (body louse); and (3) pediculosis capitis, caused by *Pediculus humanus* var *capitis* (head louse).

Head and body lice are similar in appearance and are 3–4 mm long. The body louse can seldom be found on the body, because the insect comes onto the skin only to feed and must be looked for in the seams of the clothing. Trench fever, relapsing fever, and typhus are transmitted by the body louse in countries where those diseases are endemic.

Clinical Findings

Itching may be very intense in body louse infestations, and scratching may result in deep excoriations, especially over the upper shoulders, posterior flanks, and neck. In some cases, only itching is present, with few excoriations seen. Pyoderma may be the presenting sign in any of these infestations. Head lice can be found on the scalp or may be manifested as small nits resembling pussy willow buds on the scalp hairs close to the skin. They are easiest to see above the ears and at the nape of the neck. Pubic louse infestations are occasionally generalized, particularly in hairy individuals; the lice may even be found on the eyelashes and in the scalp.

Differential Diagnosis

Head louse infestation must be distinguished from seborrheic dermatitis, body louse infestation from scabies, and pubic louse infestation from anogenital pruritus and eczema.

Treatment

Body lice are treated by disposing of the infested clothing. For pubic lice, permethrin rinse 1% for 10 minutes and permethrin cream 5% applied for 8 hours are effective. Sexual contacts should be treated. Clothes and bedclothes should be washed and dried at high temperature if possible.

Permethrin 1% cream rinse (Nix) is a topical over-the-counter pediculicide and ovicide and is the treatment of choice for head lice. It is applied to the scalp and hair and left on for 8 hours before being rinsed off. Permethrin resistance of head lice is common. Malathion lotion 1% (Ovide) is very effective, but it is highly volatile and flammable, so application must be done in a well-ventilated room or out of doors. For involvement of eyelashes, petrolatum is applied thickly twice daily for 8 days, and remaining nits are then plucked off. Adults with head lice virtually always acquire their infestation from elementary school-aged children, so a source of infection must always be sought. Head lice are extremely difficult to eradicate in the epidemic setting, probably because the currently available pediculicides are not uniformly ovicidal when applied as directed.

Dodd CS: Interventions for treating headlice. Cochrane Database Syst Rev 2001;(3):CD001165. [PMID: 11686980]

Huynh TH et al: Scabies and pediculosis. Dermatol Clin 2004; 22:7. [PMID: 15018005]

Thappa DM et al: Phthiriasis palpebrarum. Postgrad Med J 2003; 79:102. [PMID: 12612327]

SKIN LESIONS DUE TO OTHER ARTHROPODS

ESSENTIALS OF DIAGNOSIS

- *Localized rash with pruritus.*
- *Furuncle-like lesions containing live arthropods.*

• Tender erythematous patches that migrate ("larva migrans").

• Generalized urticaria or erythema multiforme in some patients.

General Considerations

Some arthropods (eg, mosquitoes and biting flies) are readily detected as they bite. Many others are not, eg, because they are too small, because there is no immediate reaction, or because they bite during sleep. Reactions are allergic and may be delayed for hours. Patients are most apt to consult a clinician when the lesions are multiple and pruritus is intense.

Many persons will react severely only to their earliest contacts with an arthropod, thus presenting pruritic lesions when traveling, moving into new quarters, etc. Body lice, fleas, bedbugs, and mosquitoes should be considered. Spiders are often incorrectly believed to be the source of bites; they rarely attack humans, though the brown spider (*Loxosceles laeta, Loxosceles reclusa*) may cause severe necrotic reactions and death due to intravascular hemolysis, and the black widow spider (*Latrodectus mactans*) may cause severe systemic symptoms and death. (See also Chapter 39.)

In addition to arthropod bites, the most common lesions are venomous stings (wasps, hornets, bees, ants, scorpions) or bites (centipedes), furuncle-like lesions due to fly maggots or sand fleas in the skin, and a linear creeping eruption due to a migrating larva.

Clinical Findings

The diagnosis may be difficult when the patient has not noticed the initial attack but suffers a delayed reaction. Individual bites are often in clusters and tend to occur either on exposed parts (eg, midges and gnats) or under clothing, especially around the waist or at flexures (eg, small mites or insects in bedding or clothing). The reaction is often delayed for 1–24 hours or more. Pruritus is almost always present and may be all but intolerable once the patient starts to scratch. Secondary infection may follow scratching. Urticarial wheals are common. Papules may become vesicular. The diagnosis is aided by searching for exposure to arthropods and by considering the patient's occupation and recent activities.

The principal arthropods are as follows:

1. **Fleas:** Fleas are bloodsucking ectoparasites that feed on dogs, cats, humans, and other species. Flea saliva produces papular urticaria in sensitized individuals. To break the life cycle of the flea, one must treat the home and pets, using quick-kill insecticides, residual insecticides, and a growth regulator.

2. **Bedbugs:** In crevices of beds or furniture; bites tend to occur in lines or clusters. Papular urticaria is a characteristic lesion of bedbug (*Cimex lectularius*) bites. The closely related kissing bug has a painful bite.

3. **Ticks:** Usually picked up by brushing against low vegetation. Ticks may transmit Rocky Mountain spotted fever, Lyme disease, relapsing fever, and ehrlichiosis.

4. **Chiggers or red bugs:** These are larvae of trombiculid mites. A few species confined to particular regions and locally recognized habitats (eg, berry patches, woodland edges, lawns, brush turkey mounds in Australia, poultry farms) attack humans, often around the waist, on the ankles, or in flexures, raising intensely itching erythematous papules after a delay of many hours. The red chiggers may sometimes be seen in the center of papules that have not yet been scratched.

5. **Bird and rodent mites:** Larger than chiggers, bird mites infest pigeon lofts or nests of birds in eaves. Bites are multiple anywhere on the body. Room air conditioning units may suck in bird mites and infest the inhabitants of the room. Rodent mites from mice or rats may cause similar effects. Pet gerbils may be infested with bird mites. The diagnosis of bird mites or rodent mites may easily be overlooked.

6. **Mites in stored products:** These are white and almost invisible and infest products such as copra, vanilla pods, sugar, straw, cottonseeds, and cereals. Persons who handle these products may be attacked, especially on the hands and forearms and sometimes on the feet. Infested bedding may occasionally lead to generalized dermatitis.

7. **Caterpillars of moths with urticating hairs:** The hairs are blown from cocoons or carried by emergent moths, causing severe and often seasonally recurrent outbreaks after mass emergence. The gypsy moth is a cause in the eastern United States.

8. **Tungiasis:** Tungiasis is due to the burrowing flea known as *Tunga penetrans* and is found in Africa, the West Indies, and South and Central America. The female burrows under the skin, sucks blood, swells to 0.5 cm, and then ejects her eggs onto the ground. Ulceration, lymphangitis, gangrene, and septicemia may result, in some cases with lethal effect. Ethyl chloride spray will kill the insect when applied to the lesion, and disinfestation may be accomplished with insecticide applied to the terrain. Simple surgical excision is usually performed.

Differential Diagnosis

Arthropods should be considered in the differential diagnosis of skin lesions showing any of the above symptoms.

Prevention

Arthropod infestations are best prevented by avoidance of contaminated areas, personal cleanliness, and disinfection of clothing, bedclothes, and furniture as indicated. Chiggers, bedbugs, and mites can be killed by permethrin applied to the head and clothing. (It is not necessary to remove clothing.)

Treatment

Living arthropods should be removed carefully with tweezers after application of alcohol and preserved in alcohol for identification. In endemic Rocky Mountain spotted fever areas, ticks should not be removed with the bare fingers.

Corticosteroid lotions or creams are helpful. Topical antibiotics may be applied if secondary infection is suspected. Localized persistent lesions may be treated with intralesional corticosteroids.

Stings produced by many arthropods may be alleviated by applying papain powder (Adolph's Meat Tenderizer) mixed with water, or aluminum chloride hexahydrate (Xerac AC).

Extracts from venom sacs of bees, wasps, yellow jackets, and hornets are available for immunotherapy of patients at risk for anaphylaxis.

Creel NB et al: Pet hamsters as a source of rat mite dermatitis. Cutis 2003;71:457. [PMID: 12839256]

Diba VC et al: Cutaneous larva migrans acquired in Britain. Clin Exp Dermatol 2004;29:555. [PMID: 15347353]

Whyte AS et al: Bats in the belfry, bugs in the bed? Lancet 2001; 357:604. [PMID: 11558488]

INFLAMMATORY NODULES

ERYTHEMA NODOSUM

ESSENTIALS OF DIAGNOSIS

- *Painful red nodules without ulceration on anterior aspects of legs.*
- *Slow regression over several weeks to resemble contusions.*
- *Women are predominantly affected by a ratio of 10:1 over men.*
- *Some cases associated with infection or drug sensitivity.*

General Considerations

Erythema nodosum is a symptom complex characterized by tender, erythematous nodules that appear most commonly on the extensor surfaces of the lower legs. It usually lasts about 6 weeks and may recur. The disease may be associated with various infections—streptococcosis, primary coccidioidomycosis, other deep fungal infections, tuberculosis, *Yersinia pseudotuberculosis* and *Yersinia enterocolitica* infection, or syphilis. It may accompany sarcoidosis, Behçet's disease, and in-

flammatory bowel disease. Erythema nodosum may be associated with pregnancy or with use of oral contraceptives or other medication.

Clinical Findings

A. Symptoms and Signs

The swellings are exquisitely tender and may be preceded by fever, malaise, and arthralgia. They are most often located on the anterior surfaces of the legs below the knees but may occur (rarely) on the arms, trunk, and face. The lesions, 1–10 cm in diameter, are at first pink to red; with regression, all the various hues seen in a contusion can be observed.

B. Laboratory Findings

The histologic finding of septal panniculitis is characteristic of erythema nodosum. Evaluation of patients presenting with acute erythema nodosum should include a careful history (including drug exposures) and physical examination for prior upper respiratory infection or diarrheal illness, symptoms of any deep fungal infection endemic to the area, a chest radiograph, a PPD, and two consecutive ASO/DNAseB titers at 2- to 4-week intervals. If no underlying cause is found, only a small percentage of patients will go on to develop a significant underlying illness (usually sarcoidosis) over the next year.

Differential Diagnosis

Erythema induratum from tuberculosis is seen on the posterior surfaces of the legs and may ulcerate. Lupus panniculitis presents as tender nodules on the buttocks and posterior arms that heal with depressed scars. Polyarteritis nodosa is less inflammatory, and the subcutaneous nodules are often associated with a fixed livedo. In the late stages, erythema nodosum must be distinguished from simple bruises and contusions.

Treatment

First, the underlying cause should be identified and treated. Primary therapy is with NSAIDs in usual doses. Saturated solution of potassium iodide, 5–15 drops three times daily, results in prompt involution in many cases. Side effects of potassium iodide include salivation, swelling of salivary glands, and headache. Complete bed rest may be advisable if the lesions are painful. Systemic therapy directed against the lesions themselves may include corticosteroid therapy (see Chapter 26) unless contraindicated by associated infection.

Prognosis

The lesions usually disappear after about 6 weeks, but they may recur.

Chew GY et al: Erythema induratum: a case of mistaken identity. Med J Aust 2005;183:534. [PMID: 16296968]

Kassutto S et al: Clinical problem-solving. Footprints. N Engl J Med 2004;351:1438. [PMID: 15459306]

Mert A et al: Erythema nodosum: an experience of 10 years. Scand J Infect Dis 2004;36:424. [PMID: 15307561]

FURUNCULOSIS (Boils) & CARBUNCLES

 ESSENTIALS OF DIAGNOSIS

- Extremely painful inflammatory swelling based on a hair follicle that forms an abscess.
- Predisposing condition (diabetes mellitus, HIV disease, injection drug use) sometimes present.
- Coagulase-positive Staphylococcus aureus is the causative organism.

General Considerations

A furuncle (boil) is a deep-seated infection (abscess) involving the entire hair follicle and adjacent subcutaneous tissue. The most common sites of occurrence are the hairy parts exposed to irritation and friction, pressure, or moisture. Because the lesions are autoinoculable, they are often multiple. Diabetes mellitus (especially if using insulin injections), injection drug use, allergy injections, and HIV disease all increase the risk of staphylococcal infections by increasing the rate of nasal carriage.

A carbuncle consists of several furuncles developing in adjoining hair follicles and coalescing to form a conglomerate, deeply situated mass with multiple drainage points.

Clinical Findings

A. SYMPTOMS AND SIGNS

Pain and tenderness may be prominent. The abscess is either rounded or conical. It gradually enlarges, becomes fluctuant, and then softens and opens spontaneously after a few days to 1–2 weeks to discharge a core of necrotic tissue and pus. The inflammation occasionally subsides before necrosis occurs. Infection of the soft tissue around the nails (paronychia) may be due to staphylococci when it is acute or candida when chronic.

B. LABORATORY FINDINGS

There may be slight leukocytosis, but a white blood cell count is rarely required. Pus should be cultured to rule out MRSA or other bacteria. Culture of the anterior nares may identify chronic staphylococcal carriage in cases of recurrent cutaneous infection.

Differential Diagnosis

The most common entity in the differential is an inflamed epidermal inclusion cyst that suddenly becomes red, tender, and expands greatly in size over one to a few days. The history of a prior cyst in the same location, the presence of a clearly visible cyst orifice, and the extrusion of malodorous cheesy rather than purulent material helps in the diagnosis. Tinea profunda (deep dermatophyte infection of the hair follicle) may simulate recurrent furunculosis. Furuncle is also to be distinguished from deep mycotic infections, such as sporotrichosis (often in gardeners); from other bacterial infections, such as anthrax and tularemia (rare); from atypical mycobacterial infections; and from acne cysts. Hidradenitis suppurativa presents with recurrent tender sterile abscesses in the axillae and groin, on the buttocks, or below the breasts. The presence of old scars or sinus tracts plus negative cultures suggests this diagnosis.

Complications

Serious and sometimes fatal complications of staphylococcal infection such as septicemia can occur.

Treatment

A. SPECIFIC MEASURES

Incision and drainage is recommended for all loculated suppurations and is the mainstay of therapy. Systemic antibiotics are usually given, although they offer little beyond adequate incision and drainage. Sodium dicloxacillin or cephalexin, 1 g daily in divided doses by mouth for 10 days, is usually effective. Doxycycline 100 mg twice daily, trimethoprim-sulfamethoxazole DS one tablet twice daily, and clindamycin 150–300 mg twice daily are effective in treating MRSA. Recurrent furunculosis may be effectively treated with a combination of cephalexin, 250–500 mg four times daily for 2–4 weeks, and rifampin, 300 mg twice daily for 5 days during this period. Chronic clindamycin, 150–300 mg daily for 1–2 months, may also cure recurrent furunculosis. Family members and intimate contacts may need evaluation for staphylococcal carrier state and perhaps concomitant treatment. Applications of topical 2% mupirocin to the nares, axillae, and anogenital areas twice daily for 5 days may eliminate the staphylococcal carrier state.

B. LOCAL MEASURES

Immobilize the part and avoid overmanipulation of inflamed areas. Use moist heat to help larger lesions "localize." Use surgical incision and debridement after the lesions are "mature." To incise and drain an acute staphylococcal paronychia, insert a flat metal spatula or sharpened hardwood stick into the nail fold where it adjoins the nail. This will release pus from a mature lesion. Inflamed epidermal cysts may be treated in the initial stages with intralesional injections of triamcinolone acetonide into the borders of the lesions. Drainage of fluctuant lesions results in rapid resolution and reduction of pain.

Prognosis

Recurrent crops may harass the patient for months or years.

Baggett HC et al: Community-onset methicillin-resistant *Staphylococcus aureus* associated with antibiotic use and the cytotoxin Panton-Valentin leukocidin during a furunculosis outbreak in rural Alaska. J Infect Dis 2004;189:1565. [PMID: 15116291]

Frazee BW et al: High prevalence of methicillin-resistant *Staphylococcus aureus* in emergency department skin and soft tissue infections. Ann Emerg Med 2005;45:311. [PMID: 15726056]

Leatherman M: What is causing a persistent skin boil? Adv Skin Wound Care 2005;18:30. [PMID: 15714034]

Stulberg DL et al: Common bacterial skin infections. Am Fam Physician 2002;66:119. [PMID: 12126026]

Winthrop KL et al: The clinical management and outcome of nail salon-acquired *Mycobacterium fortuitum* skin infection. Clin Infect Dis 2004;38:38. [PMID: 14679446]

Zetola N et al: Community-acquired methicillin-resistant *Staphylococcus aureus*: an emerging threat. Lancet 2005;5:275. [PMID: 15854883]

EPIDERMAL INCLUSION CYST

ESSENTIALS OF DIAGNOSIS

- *Firm dermal papule or nodule.*
- *Overlying black comedone or "punctum."*
- *Expressable foul-smelling cheesy material.*
- *May become red and drain, mimicking an abscess.*

General Considerations

Epidermal inclusion cysts (EICs) are common, benign growths of the upper portion of the hair follicle. They are common in Gardner's syndrome and may be the first stigmata of the condition.

Epidermal inclusion cysts favor the face and trunk and may complicate nodulocystic acne vulgaris. Individual lesions range in size from 0.3 cm to several centimeters. An overlying pore or punctum is characteristic. Lateral pressure may lead to extrusion of a foul-smelling, cheesy material.

Differential Diagnosis

EICs are distinguished from lipomas by being more superficial (in the dermis not the subcutaneous fat) and by their overlying punctum. Many other benign and malignant tumors may superficially resemble EICs, but all lack the punctum.

Complications

EICs may rupture, creating an acute inflammatory nodule very similar to an abscess. Cultures of the expressed material will be sterile.

Treatment

Treatment is not required if asymptomatic. Inflamed lesions may be treated with incision and drainage or intralesional triamcinolone acetomide 5–10 mg/mL. For large, symptomatic cysts, surgical excision is curative.

PHOTODERMATITIS

ESSENTIALS OF DIAGNOSIS

- *Painful or pruritic erythema, edema, or vesiculation on sun-exposed surfaces: the face, neck, hands, and "V" of the chest.*
- *Inner upper eyelids spared, as is the area under the chin.*

General Considerations

Photodermatitis is an acute or chronic skin reaction due to hypersensitivity to sunlight or other sources of radiation, photosensitization of the skin by certain drugs, or idiosyncrasy to actinic light as seen in some constitutional disorders including the porphyrias and many hereditary disorders (phenylketonuria, xeroderma pigmentosum, and others). Contact photosensitivity may occur with perfumes, antiseptics, and other chemicals.

Photodermatitis is manifested most commonly as phototoxicity—a tendency for the individual to sunburn more easily than expected—or, as photoallergy, a true immunologic reaction that often presents with dermatitis.

Clinical Findings

A. SYMPTOMS AND SIGNS

The acute inflammatory skin reaction, if severe enough, is accompanied by pain, fever, gastrointestinal symptoms, malaise, and even prostration, but this is very rare. Signs include erythema, edema, and possibly vesiculation and oozing on exposed surfaces. Peeling of the epidermis and pigmentary changes often result. The key to diagnosis is localization of the rash to photoexposed areas, though these eruptions may become generalized with time to involve even photoprotected areas. The lower lip is commonly involved in hereditary polymorphous light eruption (PMLE), a disorder seen in persons of Native American descent.

B. LABORATORY FINDINGS

Blood and urine tests are not helpful in diagnosis unless porphyria cutanea tarda is suggested by the presence of blistering, scarring, milia (white cysts 1–2 mm in diameter) and skin fragility of the dorsal hands, and facial hypertrichosis. Testing for photosensitivity may define the wavelengths of light triggering the reaction. This is critical in determining the form of photoprotection recommended.

Differential Diagnosis

The differential diagnosis is long. If a clear history of the use of a topical or systemic photosensitizer is not available and if the eruption is persistent, then a workup including biopsy and light testing may be required. Photodermatitis must be differentiated from contact dermatitis that may develop from one of the many substances in suntan lotions and oils, as these may often have a similar distribution. Sensitivity to actinic rays may also be part of a more serious condition such as porphyria cutanea tarda or lupus erythematosus. These disorders are diagnosed by appropriate blood or urine tests. Phenothiazines, quinine or quinidine, griseofulvin, sulfonylureas (especially hydrochlorothiazide), NSAIDs, and antibiotics (eg, some tetracyclines, quinolone, trimethoprim-sulfamethoxazole) may photosensitize the skin. PMLE is a very common idiopathic photodermatitis that affects both sexes equally and often has its onset in the third to fourth decades except in Native Americans and Latinos, in whom it may present in childhood. PMLE is chronic in nature. Transitory periods of spontaneous remission do occur. The action spectrum of PMLE usually lies in the short (below 320 nm) ultraviolet wavelengths but may also extend into the long ultraviolet wavelengths (320–400 nm). Drug-induced photosensitivity is most commonly in the longer UVA wavelengths.

Complications

Some individuals continue to be chronic light reactors even when they apparently are no longer exposed to photosensitizing drugs.

Prevention

While sunscreens are useful agents in general and should be used by persons with photosensitivity, patients may react to such low amounts of energy that sunscreens alone may not be sufficient. Sunscreens with an SPF of 30–50, usually containing avobenzone (Parasol 1789), titanium dioxide, and micronized zinc oxide, are especially useful in patients with photoallergic dermatitis.

Treatment

A. SPECIFIC MEASURES

Drugs should be suspected in cases of photoallergy even if the particular medication (such as hydrochlorothiazide) has been used for months.

B. LOCAL MEASURES

When the eruption is vesicular or weepy, treatment is similar to that of any acute dermatitis, using cooling and soothing wet dressing.

Sunscreens should be used as described above. Mid-potency to high-potency topical corticosteroids are of limited benefit in sunburn reactions but may help in PMLE and photoallergic reactions. Since the face is often involved, close monitoring is necessary to avoid side effects of potent corticosteroids.

C. SYSTEMIC MEASURES

Aspirin may have some value for fever and pain of acute sunburn. Systemic corticosteroids in doses as described for acute contact dermatitis may be required for severe photosensitivity reactions. Otherwise, different photodermatoses are treated in specific ways.

Patients with severe photodermatitis may require immunosuppressives, such as azathioprine, in the range of 50–150 mg/d, or cyclosporine, 3–5 mg/kg/d.

Prognosis

The most common phototoxic sunburn reactions are usually benign and self-limiting except when the burn is severe or when it occurs as an associated finding in a more serious disorder. PMLE and some cases of photoallergy can persist for years.

Bilu D et al: Clinical and epidemiologic characterization of photosensitivity in HIV-positive individuals. Photodermatol Photoimmunol Photomed 2004;20:175. [PMID: 15238095]

Brunner KL et al: Extreme photosensitivity. Mayo Clin Proc 2004;79:1316. [PMID: 15473416]

Dolan CK et al: Pseudoporphyria as a result of voriconazole use: a case report. Int J Dermatol 2004;43:768. [PMID: 15485539]

Morison WL: Clinical practice. Photosensitivity. N Engl J Med 2004;350:1111. [PMID: 15014184]

ULCERS

DECUBITUS ULCERS
(Bedsores, Pressure Sores)

Bedsores (pressure sores) are a special type of ulcer caused by impaired blood supply and tissue nutrition resulting from prolonged pressure over bony or cartilaginous prominences. The skin overlying the sacrum and hips is most commonly involved, but bedsores may also be seen over the occiput, ears, elbows, heels, and ankles. They occur most readily in aged, paralyzed, debilitated, and unconscious patients. Low-grade infection may occur as a complication.

Treatment costs for a pressure ulcer exceed $20,000 in most cases and hospital stay extensions due to severe pressure ulcers may cost in excess of $200,000. Standard staging systems are used to classify pressure ulcers (Table 6–3). In all nonhealing ulcerations, there is a

Table 6–3. Staging system for classifying pressure ulcers.

Grade	Description
1	Intact skin. Fixed erythema (pink, red, or mottled) after pressure is relieved.
2	Loss of epidermis or dermis. Resembles blister, abrasion, or shallow crater. Necrotic tissue may overlie ulcer.
3	Ulceration through the epidermis and dermis with damage to the underlying subcutaneous fat. Ulcer may extend to the fascia.
4	Full thickness skin loss with extension of the ulcer to bone, muscle, tendon, or joint.
5	Closed cavity communicating through a small sinus.

concern for underlying osteomyelitis. This is especially true for grade 3 to 5 ulcers.

Differential Diagnosis

Herpes simplex virus should be suspected in ulcers in immunocompromised patients, particularly if there is a scalloped border, representing the erosions of herpetic vesicles. Rarely, ulcerated lesions in the perianal area represent actual skin cancers. Rapidly expanding ulcers may also represent pyoderma gangrenosum associated with inflammatory bowel disease. Ecthyma gangrenosum is an ulcerating lesion, commonly due to *Pseudomonas,* and observed in neutropenic patients. All ulcerative lesions should be biopsied and cultured if suspicious or if they do not heal properly.

Prevention

The most important element of treatment of pressure ulcers is prevention. Good nursing care, good nutrition, and maintenance of skin hygiene are important preventive measures. The skin and the bed linens should be kept clean and dry. Bedfast, paralyzed, moribund, listless, or incontinent patients who are at risk for the development of decubiti must be turned *frequently* (at least every hour) and must be examined at pressure points for the appearance of small areas of redness and tenderness. Written schedules can be very helpful. Water-filled mattresses, rubber pillows, alternating-pressure mattresses, and thick papillated foam pads are useful in prevention and in the treatment of lesions. "Donut" devices should not be used. Avoidance of smoking and a "healthy lifestyle" are associated with avoiding pressure ulcers in spinal cord injury patients.

Treatment

A large number of treatments and protocols exist for management of decubiti. Early lesions should be treated with topical antibiotic powders and adhesive absorbent bandage (Gelfoam). Once clean, they may be treated with hydrocolloid dressings such as DuoDerm. Established lesions require surgery for debridement, cleansing, and dressing. A spongy foam pad placed under the patient may work best in some cases. It must be laundered often. In general, topical antiseptics are not recommended. Systemic antibiotics are required for deep infections.

Brem H et al: Protocol for the successful treatment of pressure ulcers. Am J Surg 2004;188:9. [PMID: 15223496]

Krause JS et al: Patterns of recurrent pressure ulcers after spinal cord injury: identification of risk and protective factors 5 or more years after onset. Arch Phys Med Rehabil 2004;85: 1257. [PMID: 15295750]

LEG ULCERS SECONDARY TO VENOUS INSUFFICIENCY

 ESSENTIALS OF DIAGNOSIS

- *Past history of varicosities, thrombophlebitis, or postphlebitic syndrome.*
- *Irregular ulceration, often on the medial aspect of the lower legs above the malleolus.*
- *Edema of the legs, varicosities, hyperpigmentation, and red and scaly areas (stasis dermatitis) and scars from old ulcers support the diagnosis.*

General Considerations

Patients at risk may have a history of venous insufficiency, either with obvious varicosities or with a past history of thrombophlebitis, or with immobility of the calf muscle group (paraplegics, etc). Red, pruritic patches of stasis dermatitis often precede ulceration. Because venous insufficiency is the most common cause of lower leg ulceration, testing of venous competence is a required part of the evaluation even when no changes of venous insufficiency are present.

Clinical Findings

A. SYMPTOMS AND SIGNS

Classically, chronic edema is followed by a dermatitis, which is often pruritic. These changes are followed by hyperpigmentation, skin breakdown, and eventually sclerosis of the skin of the lower leg. The ulcer base may be clean, but it often has a yellow fibrin eschar that may require surgical removal. Ulcers that appear on the feet, toes, or above the knees should be approached with other diagnoses in mind.

B. LABORATORY FINDINGS

Thorough evaluation of the patient's vascular system (including measurement of the ankle/brachial index) is essential. Doppler and light rheography examinations as office procedures are usually sufficient (except in the diabetic) to elucidate the cause of most vascular cases of lower leg ulceration.

Differential Diagnosis

The differential includes vasculitis, pyoderma gangrenosum, arterial ulcerations, infection, trauma, skin cancer, arachnid bites, and sickle cell anemia. When the diagnosis is in doubt, a punch biopsy from the border (not base) of the lesion may be helpful.

Prevention

Compression stockings to reduce edema are the most important means of prevention. Compression should achieve a pressure of 30 mm Hg below the knee and 40 mm Hg at the ankle. The stockings should not be used in patients with arterial insufficiency with an ankle-brachial pressure index less than 0.7. Pneumatic sequential compression devices may be of great benefit when edema is refractory to standard compression dressings.

Treatment

A. LOCAL MEASURES

Institution of compression therapy is begun after cleaning of the ulcer with saline or cleansers such as Saf-Clens. A curette or small scissors can be used to remove the yellow fibrin eschar; local anesthesia may be used if the areas are very tender.

The ulcer is treated with metronidazole gel to reduce bacterial growth and odor. Any red dermatitic skin is treated with a medium- to high-potency corticosteroid ointment. The ulcer is then covered with an occlusive hydroactive dressing (DuoDerm, Hydrasorb or Cutinova) or a polyurethane foam (Allevyn) followed by an Unna zinc paste boot. This is changed weekly. The ulcer should begin to heal within weeks, and healing should be complete within 4–6 months. If the patient is diabetic, becaplermin (Regranex) may be applied to those ulcers that are not becoming smaller or developing a granulating base. Some ulcerations require grafting. Full- or split-thickness grafts often do not take, and pinch grafts (small shaves of skin laid onto the bed) may be more effective. Cultured epidermal cell grafts may accelerate wound healing, but they are very expensive. They should be considered in refractory ulcers, especially those that have not healed after a year or more of conservative therapy.

B. SYSTEMIC THERAPY

Pentoxifylline, 400 mg three times daily administered with compression dressings, is beneficial in accelerating healing of leg ulcers. Zinc supplementation is occasionally beneficial in patients with low serum zinc levels. If cellulitis accompanies the ulcer, systemic antibiotics are recommended: dicloxacillin, 250 mg orally four times a day, or levofloxacin, 500 mg once daily for 1–2 weeks is usually adequate. If infection persists, an underlying osteomyelitis should be sought.

Prognosis

The combination of compression stockings and newer dressings enables venous stasis ulcers to heal within months. Topical growth factors, antibiotics, debriding agents, and xenografts and autografts have been shown to be effective in recalcitrant cases. Ongoing control of edema is essential to prevent recurrent ulceration.

Boulton AJ et al: Clinical practice. Neuropathic diabetic foot ulcers. N Engl J Med 2004;351:48. [PMID: 15229307]

Bonnetblanc JM: Leg ulcerations: a clinical appraisal. Eur J Dermatol 2005;15:127. [PMID: 15908292]

de Araujo T et al: Managing the patient with venous ulcers. Ann Intern Med 2003;138:326. [PMID: 12585831]

Jones JE et al: Skin grafting for venous leg ulcers. Cochrane Database Syst Rev 2005;(1):CD001737. [PMID: 15674883]

LayFlurrie K: Assessment and good technique are key to effective compression therapy. Prof Nurse 2005;20:31. [PMID: 15754720]

Sieggreen MY et al: Arterial insufficiency and ulceration: diagnosis and treatment options. Adv Skin Wound Care 2004;17 (5 Pt 1):242. [PMID: 15192492]

■ MISCELLANEOUS DERMATOLOGIC DISORDERS[1]

PIGMENTARY DISORDERS

Although the color of skin may be altered by many diseases and agents, the vast majority of patients have either an increase or decrease in pigment secondary to some inflammatory disease such as acne or atopic dermatitis.

Other pigmentary disorders include those resulting from exposure to exogenous pigments such as carotenemia, argyria, deposition of other metals (such as gold when given long-term for rheumatoid arthritis), and tattooing. Other endogenous pigmentary disorders are attributable to metabolic substances—including hemosiderin (iron)—in purpuric processes; or to homogentisic acid in ochronosis; bile pigments; and carotenes.

Classification

First, determine whether the disorder is hyperpigmentation or hypopigmentation, ie, an increase or decrease

---

[1]Hirsutism is discussed in Chapter 26.

in normal skin colors. Each may be considered to be primary or to be secondary to other disorders.

A. PRIMARY PIGMENTARY DISORDERS

1. Hyperpigmentation—The disorders in this category are nevoid, congenital or acquired, and include pigmented nevi, ephelides (juvenile freckles), and lentigines (senile freckles). Hyperpigmentation occurs also in arsenical melanosis or in association with Addison's disease (due to lack of the inhibitory influence of cortisol on the production of melanocyte-stimulating hormone by the pituitary gland). Axillary freckling and café au lait spots may be seen in neurofibromatosis. **Melasma (chloasma)** occurs as patterned hyperpigmentation of the face, usually as a direct effect of estrogens. It occurs not only during pregnancy but also in 30–50% of women taking oral contraceptives, and rarely in men. One report suggests that such men have low testosterone and elevated luteinizing hormone levels.

2. Hypopigmentation and depigmentation—The disorders in this category are vitiligo, albinism, and piebaldism. In vitiligo, pigment cells (melanocytes) are destroyed. Vitiligo, present in approximately 1% of the population, may be associated with hyperthyroidism and hypothyroidism, pernicious anemia, diabetes mellitus, and Addison's disease. Albinism represents a number of different genetically determined traits, with different phenotypes. These often affect the eye and vision. Piebaldism, a localized hypomelanosis manifested by a white forelock, is an autosomal dominant trait that in some cases may be associated with neurologic abnormalities. Hypopigmented halos are common around nevi and may occur around melanomas.

B. SECONDARY PIGMENTARY DISORDERS

Any damage to the skin (irritation, allergy, infection, excoriation, burns, or dermatologic therapy such as chemical peels and freezing with liquid nitrogen) may result in hyperpigmentation or hypopigmentation. Several disorders of clinical importance are described below.

1. Hyperpigmentation—The most common type of secondary hyperpigmentation occurs after another dermatologic condition, such as acne, and is most commonly seen in dark-skinned persons. It is called postinflammatory hyperpigmentation.

Pigmentation may be produced by certain drugs, eg, chloroquine, chlorpromazine, minocycline, and amiodarone. Irritation from benzoyl peroxide and tretinoin can result in hyperpigmentation, as may topical fluorouracil. Fixed drug eruptions to phenolphthalein in laxatives, to trimethoprim-sulfamethoxazole, to NSAIDs, and to tetracyclines, for example, are further causes. **Berloque hyperpigmentation** is the pigmentation due to phototoxicity from chemicals in the rinds of limes and other citrus fruits and to celery.

2. Hypopigmentation—**Leukoderma** is a disorder that may complicate atopic dermatitis, lichen planus, psoriasis, DLE, and lichen simplex chronicus. Practitioners must exercise special care in using liquid nitrogen on any patient with olive or darker complexions, since doing so may result in hypopigmentation or depigmentation, at times permanent. Intralesional or intra-articular injections of high concentrations of corticosteroids may also cause localized temporary hypopigmentation.

Differential Diagnosis

One must distinguish true lack of pigment from pseudoachromia, such as occurs in tinea versicolor, pityriasis simplex, and seborrheic dermatitis. The evaluation of pigmentary disorders in whites is helped by Wood's light, which accentuates epidermal pigmentation and highlights hypopigmentation.

Complications

Actinic keratoses and skin cancers are more likely to develop in persons with vitiligo and albinism. There may be severe emotional trauma in extensive vitiligo and other types of hypopigmentation and hyperpigmentation, particularly when they occur in naturally dark-skinned persons.

Treatment & Prognosis

A. HYPERPIGMENTATION

Therapeutic bleaching preparations generally contain hydroquinone. Hydroquinone has occasionally caused unexpected hypopigmentation, hyperpigmentation, or even secondary ochronosis and pigmented milia, particularly with prolonged use.

The role of exposure to ultraviolet light cannot be overstressed as a factor promoting or contributing to most disorders of hyperpigmentation, and such exposure should be minimized. Melasma, ephelides, and postinflammatory hyperpigmentation may be treated with varying success with 3–4% hydroquinone cream, gel, or solution and a sunscreen containing UVA photoprotectants (Avobenzone, zinc oxide, titanium dioxide). Tretinoin cream, 0.025–0.05%, may be added. Superficial melasma responds well, but if there is predominantly dermal deposition of pigment (does *not* enhance with Wood's light), the prognosis is poor. Response to therapy takes months and requires avoidance of sunlight. Hyperpigmentation often recurs after treatment if the skin is exposed to ultraviolet light. Solar lentigines respond to liquid nitrogen application. Tretinoin, 0.1% cream and tazarotene 0.1% used over 10 months, will fade solar lentigines (liver spots), hyperpigmented facial macules in Asians, and postinflammatory hyperpigmentation in blacks. New laser systems for the removal of epidermal and dermal pigments are available, and referral should be considered for patients whose responses to medical treatment are inadequate.

B. HYPOPIGMENTATION

In secondary hypopigmentation, repigmentation may occur spontaneously. Cosmetics such as Covermark and Dermablend are highly effective for concealing disfiguring patches. Therapy of vitiligo is long and tedious, and the patient must be strongly motivated. If less than 20% of the skin is involved (most cases), topical tacrolimus 0.1% twice daily is the first-line therapy. A superpotent corticosteroid may also be used, but local skin atrophy from prolonged use may ensue. With 20–25% involvement, narrowband UVB or oral PUVA is best. Severe phototoxic response (sunburn) may occur with oral PUVA. The face and upper chest respond best, and the fingertips and the genital areas do not respond as well to treatment. Years of treatment may be required. Newer techniques of using epidermal autografts and cultured epidermis combined with PUVA therapy give hope for surgical correction of vitiligo.

Czajkowski R: Comparison of melanocytes transplantation methods for the treatment of vitiligo. Dermatol Surg 2004;30: 1400. [PMID: 15522021]

Egli F et al: Images in clinical medicine. Vitiligo and pernicious anemia. N Engl J Med 2004;350:2698. [PMID: 15215486]

Stulberg DL et al: Common hyperpigmentation disorders in adults: Part II. Melanoma, seborrheic keratoses, acanthosis nigricans, melasma diabetic dermopathy, tinea versicolor and postinflammatory hyperpigmentation. Am Fam Physician 2003;68:1963. [PMID: 14655805]

Travis LB et al: Successful treatment of vitiligo with 0.1% tacrolimus ointment. Arch Dermatol 2003;139:571. [PMID: 12756092]

BALDNESS
(Alopecia)

Baldness Due to Scarring

Cicatricial baldness may occur following chemical or physical trauma, lichen planopilaris, bacterial or fungal infections, severe herpes zoster, chronic DLE, scleroderma, and excessive ionizing radiation. The specific cause is often suggested by the history, the distribution of hair loss, and the appearance of the skin, as in LE. Biopsy is useful in the diagnosis of scarring alopecia, but specimens must be taken from the active border and not from the scarred central zone.

Scarring alopecias are irreversible and permanent. It is important to diagnose and treat the scarring process as early in its course as possible.

Baldness Not Due to Scarring

Nonscarring alopecia may occur in association with various systemic diseases such as SLE, secondary syphilis, hyperthyroidism or hypothyroidism, iron deficiency anemia, and pituitary insufficiency. The only treatment necessary is prompt and adequate control of the underlying disorder, in which case hair loss may be reversible.

Androgenetic (pattern) baldness, the most common form of alopecia, is of genetic predetermination. The earliest changes occur at the anterior portions of the calvarium on either side of the "widow's peak" and on the crown (vertex) of the skull. The extent of hair loss is variable and unpredictable. Rogaine Extra Strength, a solution containing 50 mg/mL of minoxidil, is available over the counter. The best results are achieved in persons with recent onset (< 5 years) and smaller areas of alopecia. Approximately 40% of patients treated twice daily for a year will have moderate to dense growth. Finasteride (Propecia), 1 mg orally daily, has similar efficacy and may be additive to minoxidil. As opposed to minoxidil, finasteride is used only in males.

Hair loss or thinning of the hair in women results from the same cause as common baldness in men (androgenetic alopecia) and may be treated with minoxidil (Rogaine). A workup consisting of determination of serum testosterone, DHEAS, iron, total iron binding capacity, thyroid function tests, and a complete blood count will identify most other causes of hair thinning in premenopausal women. Women who complain of thin hair but show little evidence of alopecia need follow-up, because more than 50% of the scalp hair can be lost before the clinician can perceive it.

Telogen effluvium is transitory increase in the number of hairs in the telogen (resting) phase of the hair growth cycle. This may occur spontaneously, may appear at the termination of pregnancy, may be precipitated by "crash dieting," high fever, stress from surgery or shock, or malnutrition, or may be provoked by hormonal contraceptives. Whatever the cause, telogen effluvium usually has a latent period of 2–4 months. The prognosis is generally good. The condition is diagnosed by the presence of large numbers of hairs with white bulbs coming out upon gentle tugging of the hair. Counts of hairs lost by the patient on combing or shampooing often exceed 150 per day, compared to an average of 70–100. In one study, a major cause of telogen effluvium was found to be iron deficiency, and the hair counts bore a clear relationship to serum iron levels.

Alopecia areata is of unknown cause but is believed to be an immunologic process. Typically, there are patches that are perfectly smooth and without scarring. Tiny hairs 2–3 mm in length, called "exclamation hairs," may be seen. Telogen hairs are easily dislodged from the periphery of active lesions. The beard, brows, and lashes may be involved. Involvement may extend to all of the scalp hair (alopecia totalis) or to all scalp and body hair (alopecia universalis). Severe forms may be treated by systemic corticosteroid therapy, although recurrences follow discontinuation of therapy. Alopecia areata is occasionally associated with Hashimoto's thyroiditis, pernicious anemia, Addison's disease, and vitiligo.

Intralesional corticosteroids are frequently effective for alopecia areata. Triamcinolone acetonide in a concentration of 2.5–10 mg/mL is injected in aliquots of 0.1 mL at approximately 1- to 2-cm intervals, not exceeding a total dose of 30 mg per month for adults. Alternatively, anthralin 0.5% ointment, used daily, may help some patients. Alopecia areata is usually self-limiting, with complete regrowth of hair in 80% of patients with focal disease. Some mild cases are resistant to treatment, as are the extensive totalis and universalis types. Both topical diphencyprone and squaric acid dibutylester, have been used to treat persistent alopecia areata. The principle is to sensitize the skin, then intermittently apply weaker concentrations to produce and maintain a slight dermatitis. Hair regrowth in 3–6 months in some patients has been reported to be remarkable. Long-term safety and efficacy have not been established. Support groups for patients with extensive alopecia areata are very beneficial. In **trichotillomania** (the pulling out of one's own hair), the patches of hair loss are irregular and growing hairs are always present, since they cannot be pulled out until they are long enough. The patches are often unilateral, occurring on the same side as the patient's dominant hand. The patient may be unaware of the habit.

Drug-induced alopecia is becoming increasingly important. Incriminated drugs include excessive and prolonged use of vitamin A, retinoids, antimitotic agents, anticoagulants, antithyroid drugs, oral contraceptives, trimethadione, allopurinol, propranolol, indomethacin, amphetamines, salicylates, gentamicin, and levodopa. While chemotherapy-induced alopecia is very distressing, it must be emphasized to the patient before treatment that it is invariably reversible.

Chartier MB et al: Approach to the adult female patient with diffuse nonscarring alopecia. J Am Acad Dermatol 2002;47:809. [PMID: 12451364]

Dombrowski NC et al: Alopecia areata: what to expect from current treatments. Cleve Clin J Med 2005;72:758, 760, 765. [PMID: 16193824]

Ellis JA et al: Androgenetic alopecia: pathogenesis and potential for therapy. Expert Rev Mol Med 2002;2002:1. [PMID: 14585162]

Hunt N et al: The psychological impact of alopecia. BMJ 2005; 331:951. [PMID: 16239692]

Tosti A et al: Clobetasol propionate 0.05% under occlusion in the treatment of alopecia totalis/universalis. J Am Acad Dermatol 2003;49:96. [PMID: 12833016]

NAIL DISORDERS

1. Morphologic Abnormalities of the Nails

Classification

Acquired nail disorders may be classified as local or those associated with systemic or generalized skin diseases.

A. Local Nail Disorders

1. Onycholysis (distal separation of the nail plate from the nail bed, usually of the fingers) is caused by excessive exposure to water, soaps, detergents, alkalies, and industrial cleaning agents. Candidal infection of the nail folds and subungual area, nail hardeners, and drug-induced photosensitivity may cause onycholysis, as may hyperthyroidism and hypothyroidism and psoriasis.

2. Distortion of the nail occurs as a result of chronic inflammation of the nail matrix underlying the eponychial fold. Such changes may also be caused by warts, tumors, or cysts, impinging on the nail matrix.

3. Discoloration and crumbly thickened nails are noted in dermatophyte infection and psoriasis.

4. Allergic reactions (to resins in undercoats and polishes or to nail glues) are characterized by onycholysis or by grossly distorted, hypertrophic, and misshapen nails.

B. Nail Changes Associated with Systemic or Generalized Skin Diseases

1. Beau's lines (transverse furrows) may follow any serious systemic illness.

2. Atrophy of the nails may be related to trauma or to vascular or neurologic disease.

3. Clubbed fingers may be due to the prolonged hypoxemia associated with cardiopulmonary disorders. (See Chapter 9.)

4. Spoon nails may be seen in anemic patients.

5. Stippling or pitting of the nails is seen in psoriasis, alopecia areata, and hand eczema.

6. Nail hyperpigmentation may be caused by zidovudine, doxorubicin, cyclophosphamide, bleomycin, daunorubicin, fluorouracil, hydroxyurea, melphalan, mechlorethamine, and nitrosoureas.

Differential Diagnosis

Onychomycosis may cause nail changes identical to those seen in psoriasis. Careful examination for more characteristic lesions elsewhere on the body is essential to the diagnosis of the nail disorders. Cancer should be suspected (eg, Bowen's disease or squamous cell carcinoma) as the cause of any persistent solitary subungual or periungual lesion.

Complications

Toenail changes may lead to an ingrown nail—in turn often complicated by bacterial infection and occasionally by exuberant granulation tissue. Poor manicuring and poorly fitting shoes may contribute to this complication. Cellulitis may result.

Treatment & Prognosis

Treatment consists usually of careful debridement and manicuring and, above all, reduction of exposure to irritants (soaps, detergents, alkali, bleaches, solvents, etc). Longitudinal grooving due to temporary lesions of the matrix, such as warts, synovial cysts, and other impingements, may be cured by removal of the offending lesion.

If it is necessary to remove dystrophic nails for any reason (eg, fungal nails or severe psoriasis), a nonsurgical method is to apply urea 40%, anhydrous lanolin 20%, white wax 5%, white petrolatum 25%, and silica gel type H. The nail folds are painted with compound tincture of benzoin and covered with cloth adhesive tape. The urea ointment is applied generously to the nail surface and covered with plastic film, and then adhesive tape. The ointment is left on for 5–10 days; then the nail plate may be curetted off. Medication can then be applied that is appropriate for the condition being treated.

2. Tinea Unguium (Onychomycosis)

Tinea unguium is a trichophyton infection of one or more (but rarely all) fingernails or toenails. The species most commonly found is *T rubrum*. "Saprophytic" fungi may rarely (< 5%) cause onychomycosis.

The nails are lusterless, brittle, and hypertrophic, and the substance of the nail is friable. Laboratory diagnosis is mandatory since only 50% of dystrophic nails are due to dermatophytosis. Portions of the nail should be cleared with 10% KOH and examined under the microscope for hyphae. Fungi may also be cultured. Periodic acid-Schiff stain of a histologic section of the nail plate will also demonstrate the fungus readily. Each technique is positive in only 50% of cases so several different tests may need to be performed.

Onychomycosis is difficult to treat because of the long duration of therapy required and the frequency of recurrences. Fingernails respond more readily than toenails. For toenails, treatment is limited to patients with discomfort, inability to exercise, and immune compromise.

In general, systemic therapy is required to effectively treat nail onychomycosis. Topical therapy has limited value and the adjunctive value of surgical procedures is unproven. Fingernails can virtually always be cured and toenails are cured 35–50% of the time and are clinically improved about 75% of the time. In all cases, before treatment, the diagnosis should be confirmed. The costs of the various treatment options should be known and the most cost-effective treatment chosen. Drug interactions must be avoided. Ketoconazole, due to its higher risk for hepatotoxicity, is not recommended to treat any form of onychomycosis. For fingernails, ultramicronized griseofulvin 250 mg orally three times daily for 6 months can be effective. Alternative treatments are (in order of preference) oral terbinafine 250 mg/d for 6 weeks, oral itraconazole 400 mg/d for 7 days each month for 2 months, and oral itraconazole 200 mg/d for 2 months. Once clear, fingernails usually remain free of disease.

Onychomycosis of the toenails does not respond to griseofulvin therapy or topical treatments. The best treatment, which is also FDA approved, is oral terbinafine 250 mg daily for 12 weeks. Liver function tests and a complete blood count with platelets are performed monthly during treatment. A recently published alternative treatment schedule (but not confirmed by other workers) is oral terbinafine 250 mg/d for 1 week every 2 or 3 months for 1 year (four or six treatment pulses). Pulse oral itraconazole 200 mg twice daily for 1 week per month for 3 months is inferior to standard terbinafine treatments, but it is an acceptable alternative for those unable to take terbinafine.

For recurrent disease, terbinafine can be given as pulse therapy, 250 mg/d orally for 1 week every month for 12 months, or the standard 3 months of oral daily treatment of 250 mg/d can be given and repeated again 6 months following the first course (treat months 1 to 3 and 9 to 12).

Casciano J et al: Economic analysis of oral and topical therapies for onychomycosis of the toenails and fingernails. Manag Care 2003;12:47. [PMID: 12685377]

Hay R: Literature review. Onychomycosis. J Eur Acad Dermatol Venereol 2005;19 Suppl 1:1. [PMID: 16120198]

Heikkila H et al: Long-term results in patients with onychomycosis treated with terbinafine or itraconazole. Br J Dermatol 2002;146:250. [PMID: 11903235]

Wilcock M et al: Inappropriate use of oral terbinafine in family practice. Pharm World Sci 2003;25:25. [PMID: 12661473]

DERMATITIS MEDICAMENTOSA (Drug Eruption)

ESSENTIALS OF DIAGNOSIS

- Usually, abrupt onset of widespread, symmetric erythematous eruption.
- May mimic any inflammatory skin condition.
- Constitutional symptoms (malaise, arthralgia, headache, and fever) may be present.

General Considerations

As is well recognized, only a minority of cutaneous drug reactions result from allergy. True allergic drug reactions involve prior exposure, an "incubation" period, reactions to doses far below the therapeutic range, manifestations different from the usual pharmacologic effects of the drug, involvement of only a small portion of the population at risk, restriction to a limited number of syndromes (anaphylactic and anaphylactoid, urticarial, vasculitic, etc), and reproducibility.

Rashes are among the most common adverse reactions to drugs and occur in 2–3% of hospitalized patients. Amoxicillin, trimethoprim-sulfamethoxazole, and ampicillin or penicillin are the most common causes of urticarial and maculopapular reactions. Toxic epidermal necrolysis and Stevens-Johnson syndrome are most commonly produced by sulfonamides and anticonvulsants. Phenolphthalein, pyrazolone derivatives, tetracyclines, NSAIDs, trimethoprim-sulfa-

Table 6–4. Skin reactions due to systemic drugs.

Reaction	Appearance	Distribution and Comments	Common Offenders
Toxic erythema	Morbilliform, maculo-papular, exanthematous reactions.	The most common skin reaction to drugs. Often more pronounced on the trunk than on the extremities. In previously exposed patients, the rash may start in 2–3 days. In the first course of treatment, the eruption often appears about the seventh to ninth days. Fever may be present.	Antibiotics (especially ampicillin and trimethoprim-sulfamethoxazole), sulfonamides and related compounds (including thiazide diuretics, furosemide, and sulfonylurea hypoglycemic agents), and barbiturates.
Erythema multiforme major	Target-like lesions. Bullae may occur. Mucosal involvement.	Mainly on the extensor aspects of the limbs.	Sulfonamides, penicillamine, barbiturates, and NSAIDs.
Erythema nodosum	Inflammatory cutaneous nodules.	Usually limited to the extensor aspects of the legs. May be accompanied by fever, arthralgias, and pain.	Oral contraceptives.
Allergic vasculitis	Inflammatory changes may present as urticaria that lasts over 24 hours, hemorrhagic papules ("palpable purpura"), vesicles, bullae, or necrotic ulcers.	Most severe on the legs.	Sulfonamides, indomethacin, phenytoin, allopurinol, and ibuprofen.
Purpura	Itchy, petechial macular rash.	Dependent areas. Results most typically from thrombocytopenia.	Thiazides, sulfonamides, sulfonylureas, barbiturates, quinine, and sulindac.
Eczema	Similar to contact dermatitis.	A rare reaction in patients previously sensitized by external exposure who are given the same or a related substance systemically.	Penicillin, neomycin, phenothiazines, and local anesthetics.
Exfoliative dermatitis and erythroderma	Red and scaly.	Entire skin surface.	Allopurinol, sulfonamides, isoniazid, gold, or carbamazepine.
Photosensitivity: increased sensitivity to light, often of ultraviolet A wavelengths, but may be due to UVB or visible light as well	Sunburn, vesicles, papules in photodistributed pattern.	Exposed skin of the face, the neck, and the backs of the hands and, in women, the lower legs. Exaggerated response to ultraviolet light.	Sulfonamides and sulfonamide-related compounds (thiazide diuretics, furosemide, sulfonylureas), tetracyclines, phenothiazines, sulindac, amiodarone, and NSAIDs.
Drug-related lupus erythematosus	May present with a photosensitive rash accompanied by fever, polyarthritis, myalgia, and serositis.	Less severe than systemic lupus erythematosus, sparing the kidneys and central nervous system. Recovery often follows drug withdrawal.	Hydralazine, procainamide; less often, isoniazid, phenytoin, lisinopril, hydrochlorothiazide; diltiazem; may cause subacute lupus erythematosus.
Lichenoid and lichen planus–like eruptions	Pruritic, erythematous to violaceous polygonal papules that coalesce or expand to form plaques.	May be in photo- or nonphotodistributed pattern.	Bismuth, carbamazepine, chlordiazepoxide, chloroquine, chlorpropamide, dapsone, ethambutol, furosemide, gold salts, hydroxychloroquine, methyldopa, penicillamine, phenothiazines, propranolol, quinidine, quinine, quinacrine, streptomycin, sulfonylureas, tetracyclines, thiazides, and triprolidine.

(continued)

Table 6–4. Skin reactions due to systemic drugs. (continued)

Reaction	Appearance	Distribution and Comments	Common Offenders
Fixed drug eruptions	Single or multiple demarcated, round, erythematous plaques that often become hyperpigmented.	Recur at the same site when the drug is repeated. Hyperpigmentation, if present, remains after healing.	Numerous drugs, including antimicrobials, analgesics, barbiturates, cardiovascular drugs, heavy metals, antiparasitic agents, antihistamines, phenolphthalein, ibuprofen, and naproxen.
Toxic epidermal necrolysis	Large sheets of erythema, followed by separation, which looks like scalded skin.	Rare.	In adults, the eruption has occurred after administration of many classes of drugs, particularly anticonvulsants (lamotrigine and others), antibiotics, sulfonamides, and NSAIDs.
Urticaria	Red, itchy wheals that vary in size from < 1 cm to many centimeters. May be accompanied by angioedema.	Chronic urticaria is rarely caused by drugs.	Acute urticaria: penicillins, NSAIDs, sulfonamides, opiates, and salicylates. Angioedema is common in patients receiving ACE inhibitors.
Pruritus	Itchy skin without rash.		Pruritus ani may be due to overgrowth of *Candida* after systemic antibiotic treatment. NSAIDs may cause pruritus without a rash.
Hair loss		Hair loss most often involves the scalp, but other sites may be affected.	A predictable side effect of cytotoxic agents and oral contraceptives. Diffuse hair loss also occurs unpredictably with a wide variety of other drugs, including anticoagulants, antithyroid drugs, newer antimicrobials, cholesterol-lowering agents, heavy metals, corticosteroids, androgens, NSAIDs, retinoids (isotretinoin, etretinate), and β-blockers.
Pigmentary changes	Flat hyperpigmented areas.	Forehead and cheeks (chloasma, melasma). The most common pigmentary disorder associated with drug ingestion. Improvement is slow despite stopping the drug.	Oral contraceptives are the usual cause.
	Blue-gray discoloration.	Light-exposed areas.	Chlorpromazine and related phenothiazines.
	Brown or blue-gray pigmentation.	Generalized.	Heavy metals (silver, gold, bismuth, and arsenic). Arsenic, silver, and bismuth are not used therapeutically, but patients who receive gold for rheumatoid arthritis may show this reaction.
	Yellow color.	Generalized.	Usually quinacrine.
	Blue-black patches on the shins.		Minocycline, chloroquine.
	Blue-black pigmentation of the nails and palate and depigmentation of the hair.		Chloroquine.
	Slate-gray color.	Primarily in photoexposed areas.	Amiodarone.
	Brown discoloration of the nails.	Especially in more darkly pigmented patients.	Zidovudine (azidothymidine; AZT), hydroxyurea.

(continued)

Table 6–4. Skin reactions due to systemic drugs. (continued)

Reaction	Appearance	Distribution and Comments	Common Offenders
Psoriasiform eruptions	Scaly red plaques.	May be located on trunk and extremities. Palms and soles may be hyperkeratotic. May cause psoriasiform eruption or worsen psoriasis.	Chloroquine, lithium, β-blockers, and quinacrine.
Pityriasis rosea–like eruptions	Oval, red, slightly raised patches with central scale.	Mainly on the trunk.	Barbiturates, bismuth, captopril, clonidine, gold salts, methopromazine, metoprolol, metronidazole, and tripelennamine.

NSAIDs = nonsteroidal anti-inflammatory drugs; ACE = angiotensin-converting enzyme.

methoxazole, and barbiturates are the major causes of fixed drug eruptions.

Clinical Findings

A. SYMPTOMS AND SIGNS

The onset is usually abrupt, with bright erythema and often severe itching, but may be delayed. Fever and other constitutional symptoms may be present. The skin reaction usually occurs in symmetric distribution.

Table 6–4 summarizes the types of skin reactions, their appearance and distribution, and the common offenders in each case.

B. LABORATORY FINDINGS

Routinely ordered blood work is of no value in the diagnosis of drug eruptions. However, skin biopsies may be helpful in making the diagnosis.

Differential Diagnosis

Observation after discontinuation, which may be a slow process, helps establish the diagnosis. Rechallenge, though of theoretical value, may pose a danger to the patient and is best avoided.

Complications

Some cutaneous drug reactions may be associated with a clinical complex involving other organs (complex drug reactions). The organ systems involved depend on the individual medication or drug class. Most common is an infectious mononucleosis-like illness and hepatitis associated with administration of anticonvulsants.

Treatment

A. GENERAL MEASURES

Systemic manifestations are treated as they arise (eg, anemia, icterus, purpura). Antihistamines may be of value in urticarial and angioneurotic reactions. Epinephrine 1:1000, 0.5–1 mL intravenously or subcutaneously, should be used as an emergency measure. In severe cases, corticosteroids may be used at doses similar to those used for acute contact dermatitis.

B. LOCAL MEASURES

Extensive blistering eruptions resulting in erosions and superficial ulcerations demand hospitalization and nursing care as for burn patients.

Prognosis

Drug rash usually disappears upon withdrawal of the drug and proper treatment.

Baba M et al: The anticonvulsant hypersensitivity syndrome. J Eur Acad Dermatol Venereol 2003;17:399. [PMID: 12834448]

Devos SA et al: Adverse skin reactions to anti-TNF-alpha monoclonal antibody therapy. Dermatology 2003;206:388. [PMID: 12771494]

Dunn N: 10-minute consultation: adverse drug event. BMJ 2003; 326:1018. [PMID: 2742925]

Lerch M et al: The immunological and clinical spectrum of delayed drug-induced exanthems. Curr Opin Allergy Clin Immunol 2004;4:411. [PMID: 15349041]

Letko E et al: Stevens-Johnson syndrome and toxic epidermal necrolysis: a review of the literature. Ann Allergy Asthma Immunol 2005;94:419. [PMID: 15875523]

Wolf R et al: Treatment of toxic epidermal necrolysis syndrome with "disease modifying" drugs: the controversy goes on. Clin Dermatol 2004;22:267. [PMID: 15262313]

Eye

7

Paul Riordan-Eva, FRCS, FRCOphth

SYMPTOMS OF OCULAR DISEASE

Redness

Redness is the most frequently encountered symptom of ocular disorders. It is due to hyperemia of the conjunctival, episcleral, or ciliary vessels; erythema of the eyelids; or subconjunctival hemorrhage. The major differential diagnoses are conjunctivitis, corneal disorders, acute glaucoma, and acute uveitis (Table 7–1).

Hajj-Ali RA et al: Uveitis in the internist's office: are a patient's eye symptoms serious? Cleve Clin J Med 2005;72:329. [PMID: 15850244]

Ocular Discomfort

Ocular pain may be caused by trauma, infection, inflammation, or sudden increase in intraocular pressure.

Foreign body sensation may be due to corneal or conjunctival foreign bodies, disturbance of the corneal epithelium, or rubbing of eyelashes against the cornea (trichiasis).

Photophobia is usually due to corneal inflammation (keratitis) or anterior uveitis (iritis). Other causes are albinism, aniridia, cone dystrophy, or fever associated with various systemic infections.

Itching is characteristically associated with allergic eye disease.

Scratching and burning due to dryness of the eyes may be due to lacrimal gland hypofunction, including hypofunction caused by systemic disorders (eg, Sjögren's disease) or drugs (eg, atropine-like agents); ocular surface disease; or dry environment.

Watering is usually due to inadequate tear drainage through obstruction of the lacrimal drainage system or malposition of the lower lid. Reflex tearing occurs with any disturbance of the corneal epithelium.

"Eyestrain" & Headache

Refractive error including presbyopia, inadequate illumination, and latent ocular deviation are the usual causes of eyestrain. Headache is rarely due to ocular disorders but is a major symptom of giant cell arteritis, an important cause of visual loss in older individuals.

Conjunctival Discharge

Purulent discharge usually indicates bacterial infection of the conjunctiva, cornea, or lacrimal sac. Viral conjunctivitis or keratitis produces watery discharge; allergic conjunctivitis results in tearing, ropy discharge, and itching.

Visual Loss

Causes of blurred vision (reduced visual acuity) include refractive error, corneal opacities, cataract, intraocular inflammation (uveitis), vitreous hemorrhage, retinal detachment involving the macula, diabetic retinopathy, central retinal vein occlusion, central retinal artery occlusion, macular degeneration, and optic nerve disorders.

Monocular field loss usually indicates disease of the retina or optic nerve. Important causes are chronic glaucoma, retinal detachment, branch retinal artery or vein occlusion, optic neuritis, and anterior ischemic optic neuropathy, all of which, especially chronic glaucoma, may be bilateral. Lesions of the optic chiasm due to pituitary tumors usually result in bitemporal field loss. Retrochiasmal lesions cause contralateral homonymous field defects. The more posterior the lesion in the visual pathway, the more similar are the defects in the two eyes. Cerebrovascular disease and tumors are responsible for most lesions of the retrochiasmal visual pathways.

Visual Impairment & Blindness

The World Health Organization (WHO) defines low vision as best corrected distant visual acuity in the better eye less than 20/60 but 20/400 or better, or widest diameter of the visual field subtending an angle of less than 20 degrees but greater than 10 degrees, and blindness as best corrected distant visual acuity in the better eye of less than 20/400 or less or widest diameter of the visual field subtending an angle of less than 10 degrees. In 2002, an estimated 124 million people worldwide had low vision and about 37 million worldwide were blind. The most frequent causes of blindness worldwide are cataract, glaucoma, age-related macular degeneration, and diabetic retinopathy (all of which are increasing in prevalence, especially in older individuals) as well as trachoma. Overall, 75% of blindness worldwide is thought to be treatable or preventable.

Table 7–1. The inflamed eye: Differential diagnosis of common causes.

	Acute Conjunctivitis	Acute Uveitis	Acute Glaucoma[1]	Corneal Trauma or Infection
Incidence	Extremely common	Common	Uncommon	Common
Discharge	Moderate to copious	None	None	Watery or purulent
Vision	No effect on vision	Often blurred	Markedly blurred	Usually blurred
Pain	Mild	Moderate	Severe	Moderate to severe
Conjunctival injection	Diffuse; more toward fornices	Mainly circumcorneal	Mainly circumcorneal	Mainly circumcorneal
Cornea	Clear	Usually clear	Steamy	Clarity change related to cause
Pupil size	Normal	Small	Moderately dilated and fixed	Normal
Pupillary light response	Normal	Poor	None	Normal
Intraocular pressure	Normal	Commonly low but may be elevated	Elevated	Normal
Smear	Causative organisms	No organisms	No organisms	Organisms found only in corneal ulcers due to infection

[1]Angle-closure glaucoma.

In 2000, over 3 million US adults aged 40 years or older were blind or visually impaired, with large variation between racial and ethnic groups, and the numbers will increase by 70% by 2020. Most North American states require best corrected visual acuity with both eyes of 20/40 for an unrestricted driving license.

By definition, all the above prevalence figures do not take into account visual impairment due to uncorrected refractive error, which is an important treatable cause even in developed countries.

Centers for Disease Control and Prevention (CDC): Prevalence of visual impairment and selected eye diseases among persons aged ≥ 50 years with and without diabetes—United States, 2002. MMWR Morb Mortal Wkly Rep 2004;53: 1069. [PMID: 15549022]

Congdon N et al: Causes and prevalence of visual impairment among adults in the United States. Arch Ophthalmol 2004; 122:477. [PMID: 15078664]

Foster A et al: The impact of Vision 2020 on global blindness. Eye 2005;19:1133. [PMID: 16304595]

Taylor HR: Vision loss in Australia. Med J Aust 2005;182;565. [PMID: 15938683]

Wilson MR et al: Ophthalmologic disorders in minority populations. Med Clin North Am 2005;89:795. [PMID: 15925650]

Diplopia

Double vision typically results from acquired ocular misalignment. This may be caused by central disorders of eye movements or cranial nerve palsies due to head injury, vascular, neoplastic, or inflammatory intracranial disease, or Wernicke's syndrome; myasthenia gravis; or orbital disease including Graves' ophthalmopathy and muscle entrapment as a result of orbital blowout fracture. Monocular diplopia, which persists when the fellow eye is covered, is usually due to refractive error or lens opacities.

"Spots Before the Eyes" & "Flashing Lights"

Spots before the eyes (floaters) are often caused by benign vitreous opacities. However, they may also be caused by posterior vitreous detachment, vitreous hemorrhage, or posterior uveitis. Sudden onset of floaters, particularly when associated with flashing lights (photopsia), necessitates dilated fundal examination to exclude a retinal tear or detachment.

van Overdam KA et al: Symptoms and findings predictive for the development of new retinal breaks. Arch Ophthalmol 2005; 123:479. [PMID: 15824220]

OCULAR EXAMINATION

Abbreviations and symbols commonly used in ophthalmology are listed in the accompanying box.

Visual Acuity (VA)

Corrected distant visual acuity should be tested for each eye in turn, using a Snellen or logMAR (EDTRS) chart, annotated according to the distance at which each line can be read by a normal individual. It is traditionally measured at 20 feet (6 meters in Europe) or nearer if vision is poor, but other test distances may be used. Visual acuity is expressed as a fraction—the test distance over the figure assigned to the lowest line the patient can read. If the patient is unable to read the top line even when standing close to the chart, acuity is recorded as counting fingers (CF), hand movements (HM), perception of light (LP), or no light perception (NLP). A corrected acuity of less than 20/30 (6/9) is abnormal.

Near acuity is tested with a reduced Snellen chart or standardized reading test types. The patient must be wearing appropriate reading correction.

Visual Fields

Confrontation testing, preferably using a 5-mm red target, is valuable for rapid assessment of field defects. Amsler charts are the easiest method of detecting central field abnormalities due to macular disease.

Corbett JJ: The bedside and office neuro-ophthalmology examination. Semin Neurol 2003;23:63. [PMID: 12870107]

Pupils

The pupils are examined for absolute and relative size and reactions to both light and accommodation. A large, poorly reacting pupil may be due to third nerve palsy, iris damage caused by acute glaucoma, or pharmacologic mydriasis. A small, poorly reacting pupil is observed in Horner's syndrome, inflammatory adhesions between iris and lens (posterior synechiae), or neurosyphilis (Argyll Robertson pupils). Physiologic anisocoria is a common cause of unequal pupils that react normally.

A relative afferent pupillary defect, in which the pupillary light reaction is reduced when light is shined into the affected eye compared with the normal eye, generally indicates optic nerve disease. It is detected with the "swinging light test," in which the pupillary light reactions are compared as a bright light is moved from one eye to the other.

Extraocular Movements

Examination of extraocular movements begins with an assessment of whether the two eyes are correctly aligned. A misalignment of the visual axes under binocular viewing conditions is known as a manifest deviation, or **tropia**. A deviation when binocular function is disrupted is known as a latent deviation, or **phoria**. A manifest deviation may be apparent by comparing the relative positions of the corneal light reflexes. More reliable is the **cover test**, in which the deviated eye moves to take up fixation when the other eye is occluded. The correctional movement is in the direction opposite to that of the original manifest deviation. If no manifest deviation is present, occlusion of one eye will elicit any latent deviation because binocular function will have been disrupted. As the occluder is removed (**uncover test**), latent deviation is then detected by any correctional movement that occurs to reestablish the normal alignment of the eyes. Latent deviation is common among normal individuals.

Horizontal diplopia indicates dysfunction of the medial or lateral rectus muscles; vertical diplopia re-

ABBREVIATIONS & SYMBOLS USED IN OPHTHALMOLOGY

A or Acc	Accommodation
Ax or x	Axis of cylindric lens
BI or BO	Base-in or base-out (prism)
CF	Counting fingers
Cyl	Cylindric lens or cylinder
D	Diopter (lens strength)
E	Esophoria
EOG	Electro-oculography
EOM	Extraocular muscles or movements
ERG	Electroretinography
ET	Esotropia (with L or R)
H	Hyperphoria
HM	Hand movements
HT	Hypertrophia
IOP	Intraocular pressure
IPD	Interpupillary distance
J1–J20	Test types (Jaeger) for testing reading vision
KP	Keratic precipitate
LP	Light perception
L Proj	Light projection
NLP	No light perception
NPC	Near point of convergence
OD (R, or RE)	Oculus dexter (right eye)
OS (L, or LE)	Oculus sinister (left eye)
OU	Oculi unitas (both eyes)
PD	Prism diopter
PH	Pinhole
PRRE	Pupils round, regular, and equal
S or Sph	Spherical lens
VA	Visual acuity
VER	Visual evoked response
X	Exophoria
XT	Exotropia
+	Plus or convex lens
−	Minus or concave lens
⌒	Combined with
∞	Infinity (6 meters [20 feet] or more distance)
°	Degree (measurement of strabismus angle)
Δ	Prism diopter

sults from dysfunction of the superior or inferior recti or the obliques. The false outer image arises from the affected eye. If muscle contraction is impaired, the image separation will be greatest in its normal direction of action; if a muscle cannot relax, image separation will be greatest in the direction opposite to its normal action. For example, a paretic lateral rectus or a tethered medial rectus of the right eye will cause maximal image separation on looking to the right.

Nystagmus in the primary position is always abnormal. Minor degrees of nystagmus at the extremes of gaze are normal. Other forms of physiologic nystagmus include optokinetic nystagmus and nystagmus induced by rotation or caloric stimulation. Exaggerated gaze-evoked nystagmus may be due to drugs or posterior fossa disease.

Proptosis (Exophthalmos)

Proptosis is suspected when there is widening of the palpebral aperture, with exposure of sclera both superiorly and inferiorly. (Eyelid retraction causes more exposure superiorly than inferiorly.) By viewing from above while the patient is asked to look down and the upper lids are lifted by the examiner, a further estimate of the degree of proptosis can be made. Exophthalmometry provides objective assessment. In nonaxial proptosis, there is also horizontal or vertical displacement of the globe, indicating the presence of a mass lesion outside the extraocular muscle cone.

The most frequent cause of proptosis in adults is dysthyroid eye disease. Other causes include orbital cellulitis, tumors, and pseudotumor.

Ptosis

Ptosis is usually due to eyelid disease. Neurologic causes of ptosis include Horner's syndrome, in which the pupil is constricted, and third nerve palsy, in which there are abnormalities of eye movements and the pupil may be dilated and react poorly to light. In myasthenia gravis, the pupils are normal and characteristically the ptosis is fatiguable.

Anterior Segment Examination

Although slit-lamp examination is more sensitive, examination with a flashlight and loupe usually provides sufficient information for initial assessment. Patterns of redness indicate the site of the problem. In conjunctivitis, it extends diffusely across the globe and the inner surface of the lids. Keratitis, intraocular inflammation, and acute glaucoma lead to predominantly circumcorneal injection. Episcleritis and scleritis cause localized or diffuse deep injection, which in the case of scleritis is associated with blue discoloration.

Focal lesions of the cornea due to infection or trauma can be differentiated from the diffuse corneal haze of acute glaucoma and from the cloudiness of the anterior chamber and perhaps hypopyon (white cells within the anterior chamber) of iritis. Instillation of flu- orescein and examination with a blue light aid in detection of corneal epithelial defects.

Direct Ophthalmoscopy

Direct ophthalmoscopy, ideally following pupil dilation with tropicamide 0.5–1%, which rarely induces angle-closure glaucoma, is used for examining the retina. Assessment of the red reflex and clarity of fundal details indicate the degree of media opacity. Abnormalities may then be localized to the cornea, lens, or vitreous by variations of focus of the ophthalmoscope and use of parallax.

The optic disk is examined for swelling, pallor, and glaucomatous cupping. Macular lesions causing poor central vision are usually apparent. The retinal vessels are scrutinized for caliber and wall changes. Retinal hemorrhages, hard exudates, and cotton-wool spots are noted. In hospital patients, dilation should be noted in the record to avoid confusion on neurologic examination.

OPHTHALMOLOGIC REFERRALS

Sudden loss of vision requires emergency ophthalmologic consultation. Important causes in an uninflamed eye are vitreous hemorrhage, retinal detachment, exudative age-related macular degeneration, retinal artery or vein occlusion, anterior ischemic optic neuropathy, giant cell arteritis, and optic neuritis. In an inflamed eye, acute anterior uveitis, acute glaucoma, and corneal ulcer are possibilities. Other emergencies include orbital cellulitis, gonococcal keratoconjunctivitis, and ocular trauma.

Patients in whom gradual loss of vision develops should also be referred. The principal causes are cataract, atrophic age-related macular degeneration, chronic glaucoma, chronic uveitis, and intraorbital and intracranial tumors.

Patients with diabetes must undergo annual examination through dilated pupils. Any patient with myopia should be warned of the increased risk of retinal detachment and made aware of the importance of reporting relevant symptoms. First-degree adult relatives of patients with glaucoma should undergo screening annually.

REFRACTIVE ERRORS

Refractive errors are the most common cause of blurred vision and may be a treatable component of poor vision in patients with other diagnoses. In **emmetropia** (the normal state), objects at infinity are seen clearly with the unaccommodated eye. Objects nearer than infinity are seen with the aid of accommodation, which increases the refractive power of the lens. In **hyperopia**, objects at infinity are not seen clearly unless accommodation is used, and near objects may not be seen because accommodative capacity is finite. Hyperopia is corrected with plus (convex) lenses. In **myopia**, the unaccommodated eye focuses on objects closer than infinity; the distance of such objects from the patient becomes progressively shorter with increasing myopia. Thus, the high myope is able to focus on very near objects without glasses. Objects beyond this distance cannot be seen without the aid of corrective (minus, concave) lenses. In **astigmatism**, the refractive errors in the horizontal and vertical axes differ.

Various surgical techniques are available for the correction of refractive errors, particularly myopia, including photorefractive keratectomy (PRK), in which the excimer laser is used to reshape the anterior cornea; laser in situ keratomileusis (LASIK) and laser epithelial keratomileusis (LASEK), in which laser remodeling of the corneal stroma is performed after lifting away a flap of epithelium and stroma (LASIK) or just epithelium (LASEK), which is then replaced; intrastromal corneal ring segments (INTCS); extraction of the clear crystalline lens and insertion of an intraocular lens without removal of the crystalline lens. Overall visual outcomes from such procedures are impressive and many individuals seek treatment. However, outcomes for individual cases are not completely predictable, regression of effect from laser surgery may necessitate repeated treatment, and there is risk of complications with the possibility of severe permanent visual loss. Topical pirenzepine, a selective muscarinic antagonist, and rigid contact lens wear during sleep (orthokeratology) are also being investigated for myopia.

Presbyopia is the natural loss of accommodative capacity with age. Emmetropes usually notice inability to focus on objects at a normal reading distance at about age 45. Hyperopes experience symptoms at an earlier age. Presbyopia is corrected with plus lenses for near work. Various surgical techniques, particularly insertion of multifocal or accommodative intraocular lenses, are being evaluated.

Use of a pinhole will overcome most refractive errors and thus allows their exclusion as a cause of visual loss. Transient refractive errors occur in patients with diabetes—typically when diabetic control is erratic—and may be the presenting feature. Autoinoculation of scopolamine from seasickness patches or atropine from vials for parenteral use leads to inadvertent pupillary dilation and loss of accommodation.

Rad AS et al: Progressive keratectasia after laser in situ keratomileusis. J Refract Surg 2004;20(5 Suppl):S718. [PMID: 15521275]

Tahzib NG et al: Functional outcomes and patient satisfaction after laser in situ keratomileusis for correction of myopia. J Cataract Refract Surg 2005;31:1943. [PMID: 16338565]

Tan DT et al: One-year multicenter, double-masked, placebo-controlled, parallel safety and efficacy study of 2% pirenzepine ophthalmic gel in children with myopia. Ophthalmology 2005;112:84. [PMID: 15629825]

Walline JJ et al: A randomized trial of the effects of rigid contact lenses on myopia progression. Arch Ophthalmol 2004;122:1760. [PMID: 15596577]

Contact Lenses

Contact lenses are used mostly for correction of refractive errors, for which they often provide a better opti-cal correction than glasses, as well as for management of diseases of the cornea, conjunctiva, or lids. The various types are hard lenses, rigid gas-permeable lenses, and soft lenses. Hard lenses are much more durable and easier to care for than soft lenses but are more difficult to tolerate. Rigid gas-permeable lenses are an effective compromise.

Contact lens care includes cleaning and sterilization whenever the lenses are removed and removal of protein deposits as required. Sterilization is accomplished by thermal or chemical methods. For individuals developing reactions to preservatives in contact lens solutions, preservative-free systems are available. All contact lenses can be inserted in the morning and removed at night. Soft lenses are also available for extended wear. Disposable soft lenses to avoid the necessity for lens cleaning and sterilization are available for daily or extended wear.

The major risk from contact lens wear is corneal ulceration, potentially a blinding condition. Soft lenses present the major hazard, particularly with extended wear, for which there is an approximately eightfold increase in risk of corneal ulceration compared with daily wear. The increased risk from extended wear begins with the first night of overnight wear and increases progressively thereafter. Disposable lenses are also associated with corneal ulceration.

Contact lens wearers should be made aware of the risks they face and ways to minimize them, such as avoiding extended-wear soft lenses and maintaining meticulous lens hygiene, including not using tap water for lens cleaning. Whenever there is ocular discomfort or redness, contact lenses should be removed. Ophthalmologic care should be sought if symptoms persist.

Morgan PB et al: Incidence of keratitis of varying severity among contact lens wearers. Br J Ophthalmol 2005;89:430. [PMID: 15774919]

Verhelst D et al: Clinical, epidemiological and cost aspects of contact lens related infectious keratitis in Belgium: results of a seven-year retrospective study. Bull Soc Belge Ophtalmol 2005;297:7. [PMID: 16281729]

DISORDERS OF THE LIDS & LACRIMAL APPARATUS

Hordeolum

Hordeolum is a common staphylococcal abscess that is characterized by a localized red, swollen, acutely tender area on the upper or lower lid. Internal hordeolum is a meibomian gland abscess that points onto the conjunctival surface of the lid; external hordeolum or sty is smaller and on the margin.

Warm compresses are helpful. Incision may be indicated if resolution does not begin within 48 hours. An antibiotic ointment (bacitracin or erythromycin) applied to the eyelid every 3 hours may be beneficial during the acute stage. Internal hordeolum may lead to generalized cellulitis of the lid.

Chalazion

Chalazion is a common granulomatous inflammation of a meibomian gland that may follow an internal hordeolum. It is characterized by a hard, nontender swelling on the upper or lower lid with redness and swelling of the adjacent conjunctiva. If the chalazion is large enough to impress the cornea, vision will be distorted. Treatment is usually by incision and curettage but corticosteroid injection may also be effective.

Ben Simon GJ et al: Intralesional triamcinolone acetonide injection for primary and recurrent chalazia: is it really effective? Ophthalmology 2005;112:913. [PMID: 15878075]

Tumors

Verrucae and papillomas of the skin of the lids can often be excised by the general physician if they do not involve the lid margin; otherwise, surgery should be performed by an ophthalmologist so as to avoid permanent notching of the lid. Basal cell carcinoma, squamous cell carcinoma, meibomian gland carcinoma, and malignant melanoma should be excluded by microscopic examination of the excised material since 2% of lesions thought to be benign clinically are found to be malignant. Mohs' technique of intraoperative examination of excised tissue is particularly valuable in ensuring complete excision of eyelid tumors.

Malhotra R et al: The Australian Mohs database, part II: periocular basal cell carcinoma outcome at 5-year follow-up. Ophthalmology 2004;111:631. [PMID: 15051193]

Blepharitis

Blepharitis is a common chronic bilateral inflammatory condition of the lid margins. Anterior blepharitis involves the eyelid skin, eyelashes, and associated glands. It may be ulcerative, because of infection by staphylococci, or seborrheic dermatitis, and associated with seborrhea of the scalp, brows, and ears. Both types may be present. Posterior blepharitis results from inflammation of the meibomian glands. There may be bacterial infection, particularly with staphylococci, or primary glandular dysfunction, in which there is a strong association with acne rosacea.

Symptoms of blepharitis are irritation, burning, and itching. In anterior blepharitis, the eyes are "red-rimmed," and scales or granulations can be seen clinging to the lashes. In posterior blepharitis, the lid margins are hyperemic with telangiectasias; the meibomian glands and their orifices are inflamed, with dilation of the glands, plugging of the orifices, and abnormal secretions. The lid margin is frequently rolled inward to produce a mild entropion, and the tears may be frothy or abnormally greasy.

Blepharitis is a common cause of recurrent conjunctivitis. Both anterior and, more particularly, posterior blepharitis may be complicated by hordeola or chalazions; abnormal lid or lash positions, producing trichiasis; epithelial keratitis of the lower third of the cornea; marginal corneal infiltrates; and inferior corneal vascularization and thinning.

In anterior blepharitis, cleanliness of the scalp, eyebrows, and lid margins is effective local therapy. Scales must be removed from the lids daily with a damp cotton applicator and baby shampoo. An anti-staphylococcal antibiotic eye ointment such as bacitracin or erythromycin is applied daily to the lid margins with a cotton-tipped applicator. Antibiotic sensitivity studies may be required in severe staphylococcal blepharitis.

In mild posterior blepharitis, regular meibomian gland expression may be sufficient to control symptoms. Inflammation of the conjunctiva and cornea indicates a need for more active treatment, including long-term low-dose systemic antibiotic therapy, usually with tetracycline (250 mg twice daily), doxycycline (100 mg daily), minocycline (50–100 mg daily) or erythromycin (250 mg three times daily), and short-term topical corticosteroids, eg, prednisolone, 0.125% twice daily. Topical therapy with antibiotics such as ciprofloxacin 0.3% ophthalmic solution twice daily may be helpful but should be restricted to short courses.

Entropion & Ectropion

Entropion (inward turning of usually the lower lid) occurs occasionally in older people as a result of degeneration of the lid fascia, or may follow extensive scarring of the conjunctiva and tarsus. Surgery is indicated if the lashes rub on the cornea. Botulinum toxin injections may also be used for temporary correction of the involutional lower eyelid entropion of older people.

Ectropion (outward turning of the lower lid) is common with advanced age. Surgery is indicated if there is excessive tearing, exposure keratitis, or a cosmetic problem.

Dacryocystitis

Dacryocystitis is infection of the lacrimal sac due to obstruction of the nasolacrimal system. It may be acute or chronic and occurs most often in infants and in persons over 40 years. It is usually unilateral.

The usual infectious organisms are *Staphylococcus aureus* and β-hemolytic streptococci in acute dacryocystitis and *Staphylococcus epidermidis*, anaerobic streptococci, or *Candida albicans* in chronic dacryocystitis.

Acute dacryocystitis is characterized by pain, swelling, tenderness, and redness in the tear sac area; purulent material may be expressed. In chronic dacryocystitis, tearing and discharge are the principal signs, and mucus or pus may also be expressed.

Acute dacryocystitis responds well to systemic antibiotic therapy. Surgical relief of the underlying obstruction is usually done electively but may be performed urgently in acute cases. The chronic form may be kept latent with antibiotics, but relief of the obstruction is the only cure. In adults, the standard procedure for obstruction of the lacrimal drainage system is dacryocystorhinostomy, which involves surgical exploration of the lacrimal sac and formation of a fistula into the nasal cavity. Laser-assisted endoscopic dacryocystorhinostomy and balloon dilation or probing of the nasolacrimal system are alternatives. Congenital nasolacrimal duct obstruction often resolves spontaneously but, if necessary, can be treated by probing of the nasolacrimal system.

Ben Simon GJ et al: External versus endoscopic dacryocystorhinostomy for acquired nasolacrimal duct obstruction in a tertiary referral center. Ophthalmology 2005;112:1463. [PMID: 15953636]

CONJUNCTIVITIS

Conjunctivitis is the most common eye disease. It may be acute or chronic. Most cases are due to bacterial (including gonococcal and chlamydial) or viral infection. Other causes include keratoconjunctivitis sicca, allergy, chemical irritants, and deliberate self-harm. The mode of transmission of infectious conjunctivitis is usually direct contact via fingers, towels, handkerchiefs, etc, to the fellow eye or to other persons. It may be through contaminated eye drops.

Conjunctivitis must be differentiated from acute uveitis, acute glaucoma, and corneal disorders (Table 7–1).

Bacterial Conjunctivitis

The organisms isolated most commonly in bacterial conjunctivitis are staphylococci, streptococci (particularly *S pneumoniae*), *Haemophilus* species, *Pseudomonas*, and *Moraxella*. All may produce a copious purulent discharge. There is no blurring of vision and only mild discomfort. In severe cases, examination of stained conjunctival scrapings and cultures is recommended.

The disease is usually self-limited, lasting about 10–14 days if untreated. A sulfonamide (eg, sulfacetamide, 10% ophthalmic solution or ointment) instilled locally three times daily will usually clear the infection in 2–3 days. Povidone-iodine may also be effective. The use of topical fluoroquinolones is rarely justified for treatment of a generally self-limiting, benign infection.

Rose PW et al: Chloramphenicol treatment for acute infective conjunctivitis in children in primary care: a randomised double-blind placebo-controlled trial. Lancet 2005;366:37. [PMID: 15993231]

Sheik A et al: Topical antibiotics for acute bacterial conjunctivitis: Cochrane systematic review and meta-analysis update. Br J Gen Pract 2005;55:962. [PMID: 16378567]

A. GONOCOCCAL CONJUNCTIVITIS

Gonococcal conjunctivitis, usually acquired through contact with infected genital secretions, is manifested by a copious purulent discharge. It is an ophthalmologic emergency because corneal involvement may rapidly lead to perforation. The diagnosis should be confirmed by stained smear and culture of the discharge. A single 1-g dose of intramuscular ceftriaxone is usually adequate. Topical antibiotics such as erythromycin and bacitracin may be added. Other sexually transmitted diseases, including chlamydiosis, syphilis, and HIV infection, should be considered.

B. CHLAMYDIAL KERATOCONJUNCTIVITIS

1. Trachoma—(*Chlamydia trachomatis* serotypes A–C.) Trachoma is a major cause of blindness worldwide. Recurrent episodes of infection in childhood are manifest as bilateral follicular conjunctivitis, epithelial keratitis, and corneal vascularization (pannus). Cicatrization of the tarsal conjunctiva leads to entropion and trichiasis in adulthood, with secondary central corneal scarring.

Immunologic tests or polymerase chain reaction on conjunctival samples will confirm the diagnosis but treatment should be started on the basis of clinical findings. Single-dose therapy with oral azithromycin, 20 mg/kg, is effective. Alternatively, oral tetracycline or erythromycin, 250 mg four times a day, or doxycycline, 100 mg twice a day, is given for 3–4 weeks. Local treatment is not necessary. Surgical treatment includes correction of eyelid deformities and corneal transplantation.

Kumaresan J: Can blinding trachoma be eliminated by 20/20? Eye 2005;19:1067. [PMID: 16304586]

2. Inclusion conjunctivitis—(*C trachomatis* serotypes D–K.) The agent of inclusion conjunctivitis is a common cause of genital tract disease in adults. The eye is usually involved following accidental contact with genital secretions. Adult inclusion conjunctivitis thus occurs most frequently in sexually active young adults. The disease starts with acute redness, discharge, and irritation. The eye findings consist of follicular conjunctivitis with mild keratitis. A nontender preauricular lymph node can often be palpated. Healing usually leaves no sequelae. Diagnosis can be rapidly confirmed by immunologic tests or polymerase chain reaction on conjunctival samples. Treatment is with oral tetracycline or erythromycin, 500 mg four times a day, or doxycycline, 100 mg twice a day, for 1–2 weeks. Single-dose therapy with azithromycin, 1 g, may also be effective. Before treatment, all cases should be assessed for genital tract infection so that management can be adjusted accordingly, and other venereal diseases sought.

Melese M et al: Feasibility of eliminating ocular *Chlamydia trachomatis* with repeat mass antibiotic treatments. JAMA 2004;292:721. [PMID: 15304470]

Solomon AW et al: Mass treatment with single-dose azithromycin for trachoma. N Engl J Med 2004;351:1962. [PMID: 15525721]

Viral Conjunctivitis

One of the most common causes of viral conjunctivitis is adenovirus type 3. Conjunctivitis due to this agent is usually associated with pharyngitis, fever, malaise, and preauricular adenopathy (pharyngoconjunctival fever). Locally, the palpebral conjunctiva is red, and there is a copious watery discharge and scanty exudate. Children are more often affected than adults, and contaminated swimming pools are sometimes the source of infection. The disease usually lasts 10 days.

Epidemic keratoconjunctivitis is caused by adenovirus types 8, 19, 29, and 37. It is more likely to be complicated by visual loss due to corneal subepithelial infiltrates. The disease lasts at least 2 weeks. Local sulfonamide therapy prevents secondary bacterial infection and cold compresses reduce the discomfort of the associated lid edema.

Keratoconjunctivitis Sicca (Dry Eyes)

This is a common disorder, particularly in elderly women. A wide range of conditions predispose to or are characterized by dry eyes. Hypofunction of the lacrimal glands, causing loss of the aqueous component of tears, may be due to aging, hereditary disorders, systemic disease (eg, Sjögren's syndrome), or systemic and topical drugs. Excessive evaporation of tears may be due to environmental factors (eg, a hot, dry, or windy climate) or abnormalities of the lipid component of the tear film, as in blepharitis. Mucin deficiency may be due to malnutrition, infection, burns, or drugs. Hormone replacement therapy may increase the risk of dry eyes.

The patient complains of dryness, redness, or a scratchy feeling of the eyes. In severe cases, there is persistent marked discomfort, with photophobia, difficulty in moving the eyelids, and often excessive mucus secretion. In many cases, inspection reveals no abnormality, but on slit-lamp examination there are subtle abnormalities of tear film stability and reduced volume of the tear film meniscus along the lower lid. In more severe cases, damaged corneal and conjunctival cells stain with 1% rose bengal, which is to be avoided in severe cases because of the intense pain. In the most severe cases, there is marked conjunctival injection, loss of the normal conjunctival and corneal luster, epithelial keratitis that may progress to frank ulceration, and mucous strands. Schirmer's test, which measures the rate of production of the aqueous component of tears, may be helpful, but false-positive and false-negative results are frequent.

Treatment depends on cause. In most early cases, the corneal and conjunctival epithelial changes are reversible. Aqueous deficiency can be treated by replacement of the aqueous component of tears with various types of artificial tears. The simplest preparations are physiologic (0.9%) or hypo-osmotic (0.45%) solutions of sodium chloride. Balanced salt solution is more physiologic but also more expensive. All of these drop preparations can be used as frequently as every half-hour, but in most cases are needed only three or four times a day. More prolonged duration of action can be achieved with drop preparations containing methylcellulose (eg, Isopto Plain), polyvinyl alcohol (eg, Liquifilm Tears or HypoTears), or polyacrylic acid (carbomers) (eg, GelTears or Viscotears) or by using petrolatum ointment (Lacri-Lube). Such mucomimetics are particularly indicated when there is mucin deficiency. If there is tenacious mucus, mucolytic agents (eg, acetylcysteine, 20% six times daily) may be helpful. The presence of ocular surface and lacrimal gland inflammation in dry eyes has prompted trials of topical anti-inflammatory agents such as cyclosporine.

Lacrimal punctal occlusion by canalicular plugs or surgery is useful in severe cases. Blepharitis is treated as described above. Associated blepharospasm responds to botulinum toxin injections.

Artificial tear preparations are generally very safe and without side effects. However, the preservatives necessary to maintain their sterility are potentially toxic and allergenic and may cause keratitis and cicatrizing conjunctivitis in frequent users. Furthermore, the development of such reactions may be misinterpreted by both the patient and the doctor as a worsening of the dry eye state requiring more frequent use of the artificial tears and leading in turn to further deterioration, rather than being recognized as a need to change to a preservative-free preparation.

Sanchez-Guerrero J et al: Prevalence of Sjögren's syndrome in ambulatory patients according to the American-European Consensus Group criteria. Rheumatology (Oxford) 2005;44:235. [PMID: 15509625]

Stonecipher K et al: The impact of topical cyclosporine A emulsion 0.05% on the outcomes of patients with keratoconjunctivitis sicca. Curr Med Res Opin 2005;21:1057. [PMID: 16004673]

Allergic Eye Disease

Allergic eye disease takes a number of different forms but all are expressions of atopy, which may also manifest as atopic asthma, atopic dermatitis, or allergic rhinitis. Symptoms include itching, tearing, redness, stringy discharge and, occasionally, photophobia and visual loss.

Allergic conjunctivitis is a benign disease, occurring usually in late childhood and early adulthood. It may be seasonal, developing usually during the spring or summer, or perennial. Clinical signs are limited to conjunctival hyperemia and edema (chemosis), the latter at times being marked and sudden in onset. Vernal keratoconjunctivitis also tends to occur in late childhood and early adulthood. It is usually seasonal, with a predilection for the spring. Large "cobblestone" papillae are noted on the upper tarsal conjunctiva. There may be lymphoid follicles at the limbus. Atopic keratoconjunctivitis is a more chronic disorder of adulthood. Both the upper and the lower tarsal conjunctivas exhibit a fine papillary conjunctivitis with fibrosis, resulting in forniceal shortening and entropion with trichiasis. Staphylococcal blepharitis is a complicating factor. Corneal involvement, including refractory ulceration, is frequent during exacerbations of both vernal and atopic keratoconjunctivitis. They may also be complicated by herpes simplex keratitis.

For mild and moderately severe allergic eye disease, a topical histamine H_1-receptor antagonist, such as levocabastine hydrochloride 0.05% or emedastine difumarate 0.05%, or ketorolac tromethamine, a nonsteroidal anti-inflammatory agent, is applied topically four times daily. Ketotifen 0.025%, which has histamine H_1-receptor antagonist, mast cell stabilizer, and eosinophil inhibitor activity, is applied two to four times daily; olopatadine 0.1%, applied twice daily, reduces symptoms by a similar mechanism. Topical mast cell stabilizers, such as cromolyn sodium 4% or lodoxamide tromethamine 0.1%, applied four times daily, or nedocromil sodium 2%, applied twice daily, produce longer-term prophylaxis but the therapeutic response may be delayed. Topical vasoconstrictors and antihistamines are advocated in hay fever conjunctivitis but are of limited efficacy and may produce rebound hyperemia and follicular conjunctivitis. Systemic antihistamines may be useful in prolonged atopic keratoconjunctivitis. Topical corticosteroids are essential to the control of acute exacerbations of both vernal and atopic keratoconjunctivitis. Corticosteroid-induced side effects, including cataracts, glaucoma, and exacerbation of herpes simplex keratitis, are major problems. Topical cyclosporine may be effective. Systemic corticosteroid therapy and even plasmapheresis may be required in severe atopic keratoconjunctivitis. In allergic conjunctivitis, specific allergens may be identifiable and thus avoidable. In vernal keratoconjunctivitis, a cooler climate often provides significant benefit.

Bielory L et al: Efficacy and tolerability of newer antihistamines in the treatment of allergic conjunctivitis. Drugs 2005;65:215. [PMID: 15631542]

Butrus S et al: Ocular allergy: diagnosis and treatment. Ophthalmol Clin North Am 2005;18:485. [PMID: 16314214]

Ono SJ et al: Allergic conjunctivitis: update on pathophysiology and prospects for future treatment. J Allergy Clin Immunol 2005;115:118. [PMID: 15637556]

PINGUECULA & PTERYGIUM

Pinguecula is a yellow elevated nodule on either side of the cornea, more commonly the nasal side, in the area of the palpebral fissure. It is common in persons over age 35 years. Pterygium is a fleshy, triangular encroachment of the conjunctiva onto the nasal side of the cornea and is usually associated with constant exposure to wind, sun, sand, and dust. Pterygium may be either unilateral or bilateral.

Pingueculae rarely grow, but inflammation (pingueculitis) may occur. No treatment is usually required for pingueculitis or for inflammation of pterygium, but artificial tears are often beneficial, and short courses of topical nonsteroidal anti-inflammatory agents or weak corticosteroids (prednisolone, 0.125% three times a day) may be necessary.

The indications for excision of pterygium are growth threatening vision by approaching the visual axis, marked induced astigmatism, or severe ocular irritation. Recurrence is common and often more aggressive than the primary lesion.

Hirst LW: The treatment of pterygium. Surv Ophthalmol 2003; 48:145. [PMID: 12686302]

CORNEAL ULCER

Corneal ulcers are most commonly due to infection by bacteria, viruses, fungi, or amebas. Noninfectious causes—all of which may be complicated by infection—include neurotrophic keratitis (resulting from loss of corneal sensation), exposure keratitis (due to inadequate eyelid closure), severe dry eyes, severe allergic eye disease, and various inflammatory disorders that may be purely ocular or part of a systemic vasculitis. Delayed or ineffective treatment of corneal infection may lead to devastating consequences with intraocular infection or corneal scarring. Prompt referral is essential.

Patients present with pain, photophobia, tearing, and reduced vision. The eye is red, with predominantly circumcorneal injection, and there may be purulent or watery discharge. The corneal appearance varies according to the organisms involved.

Bacterial Keratitis

Bacterial keratitis pursues an aggressive course. Precipitating factors include contact lens wear—especially soft contact lenses worn overnight—and corneal trauma, including laser surgery. The pathogens most commonly isolated are *Pseudomonas aeruginosa*, *Pneumococcus*, *Moraxella* species, and staphylococci. The cornea is hazy, with a central ulcer and adjacent stromal abscess. Hypopyon is often present. The ulcer is scraped to recover material for Gram stain and culture prior to starting treatment with high-concentration topical antibiotics applied hourly day and night for at least the first 24 hours. Fluoroquinolones such as ciprofloxacin 0.3%, ofloxacin 0.3%, and norfloxacin 0.3% are commonly used as first-line agents. Experience with levofloxacin 0.5%, which is more effective against pneumococci than ciprofloxacin, and the fourth-generation fluoroquinolones (moxifloxacin 0.5% and gatifloxacin 0.3%), which are active against mycobacteria, is limited. Gram-positive cocci can also be treated with a cephalosporin such as cefazolin, 100 mg/mL; and gram-negative bacilli can be treated with an aminoglycoside such as tobramycin, 15 mg/mL. If no organisms are seen, these two agents can be used together.

Butler TK et al: Infective keratitis in older patients: a 4 year review, 1998-2002. Br J Ophthalmol 2005;89:591. [PMID: 15834091]

Keay L et al: Microbial keratitis predisposing factors and morbidity. Ophthalmology 2006;113:109. [PMID: 16360210]

Mah FS: Fourth-generation fluoroquinolones: new topical agents in the war on ocular bacterial infections. Curr Opin Ophthalmol 2004;15:316. [PMID: 15232471]

Parmar P et al: Microbial keratitis at extremes of age. Cornea 2006;25:153. [PMID: 16371773]

Herpes Simplex Keratitis

Herpes simplex keratitis is an important cause of ocular morbidity in adults. The ability of the virus to colonize the trigeminal ganglion leads to recurrences precipitated by fever, excessive exposure to sunlight, or immunodeficiency.

The dendritic (branching) ulcer is the most characteristic manifestation of this epithelial keratitis. More extensive ("geographic") ulcers also occur, particularly if topical corticosteroids have been used. These ulcers are most easily seen after instillation of fluorescein and examination with a blue light. Epithelial disease in itself does not lead to corneal scarring. It responds well to simple debridement and patching. More rapid healing can be achieved by the addition of topical antivirals such as trifluridine drops, vidarabine ointment, acyclovir ointment, or ganciclovir gel. Long-term oral acyclovir reduces the rate of recurrent epithelial disease, for which topical corticosteroids must not be used.

Stromal herpes simplex keratitis produces increasingly severe corneal opacity with each recurrence. Topical antivirals alone are insufficient to control stromal disease. Thus, topical corticosteroids are used in combination, but steroid dependence is a common consequence. Corticosteroids may also enhance viral replication, exacerbating epithelial disease. Oral acyclovir, 200–400 mg five times a day, may be helpful in the treatment of severe herpetic keratitis and for prophylaxis against recurrences, particularly in atopic or HIV-infected individuals. Corneal grafting is necessitated by severe stromal scarring, but the overall outcome is relatively poor. **Caution:** For patients with known or possible herpetic disease, topical corticosteroids should be prescribed only with ophthalmologic supervision.

Labetoulle M et al: Incidence of herpes simplex virus keratitis in France. Ophthalmology 2005;112:888. [PMID: 15878072]

Fungal Keratitis

Fungal keratitis tends to occur after corneal injury involving plant material or in an agricultural setting, in eyes with chronic ocular surface disease, and in contact lens wearers. It is an indolent process, with the cornea characteristically having multiple stromal abscesses and relatively little epithelial loss. Intraocular infection is common. Corneal scrapings are cultured on media suitable for fungi whenever the history or corneal appearance is suggestive of fungal disease.

Srinivasan M: Fungal keratitis. Curr Opin Ophthalmol 2004; 15:321. [PMID: 15232472]

Acanthamoeba Keratitis

Acanthamoeba is an important cause of suppurative keratitis in contact lens wearers. Although severe pain with perineural and ring infiltrates in the corneal stroma is characteristic, earlier forms with changes confined to the corneal epithelium are identifiable. Culture requires specialized media. Treatment is hampered by the organism's ability to encyst within the corneal stroma. Various agents have been used, including neomycin-polymyxin-gramicidin, chlorhexidine, the investigational agents propamidine isethionate and polyhexamethyl biguanide, and oral and topical imidazoles such as ketoconazole, miconazole, and itraconazole. Epithelial debridement may be useful in early infections. Corneal grafting may be required in the acute stage to arrest the progression of infection or after resolution to restore vision. Systemic immunosuppression may be needed if there is scleral involvement.

Awwad ST et al: Results of penetrating keratoplasty for visual rehabilitation after *Acanthamoeba* keratitis. Am J Ophthalmol 2005;140:1080. [PMID: 16376655]

Butler TK et al: Six-year review of *Acanthamoeba* keratitis in New South Wales, Australia: 1997-2002. Clin Experiment Ophthalmol 2005;33:41. [PMID: 15670077]

Herpes Zoster Ophthalmicus

Herpes zoster frequently involves the ophthalmic division of the trigeminal nerve. It presents with malaise, fever, headache, and periorbital burning and itching. These symptoms may precede the eruption by a day or more. The rash is initially vesicular, quickly becoming pustular and then crusting. Involvement of the tip of the nose or the lid margins predicts involvement of the eye. Ocular signs include conjunctivitis, keratitis, episcleritis, and anterior uveitis, often with elevated intraocular pressure. Recurrent anterior segment inflammation, neurotrophic keratitis, and posterior subcapsular cataract are long-term complications. Optic neuropathy, cranial nerve palsies, acute retinal necrosis, and cerebral angiitis are infrequent problems in the acute stage. HIV infection is an important risk factor for herpes zoster ophthalmicus and increases the likelihood of complications.

High-dose oral acyclovir (800 mg five times a day), valacyclovir (1 g three times a day), or famciclovir (250–500 mg three times a day) started within 72 hours after the appearance of the rash reduces the incidence of ocular complications but not of postherpetic neuralgia. Anterior uveitis requires treatment with topical corticosteroids and cycloplegics. Neurotrophic keratitis is an important cause of long-term morbidity.

Opstelten W et al: Managing ophthalmic herpes zoster in primary care. BMJ 2005;331:147. [PMID: 16020856]

ACUTE ANGLE-CLOSURE GLAUCOMA

 ESSENTIALS OF DIAGNOSIS

- *Rapid onset in older age groups, particularly hyperopes, Inuits, and Asians.*
- *Severe pain and profound visual loss with "halos around lights."*
- *Red eye, steamy cornea, dilated pupil.*
- *Hard eye to palpation.*

General Considerations

Primary acute angle-closure glaucoma occurs only with closure of a preexisting narrow anterior chamber angle, found in elderly persons (owing to enlargement of the lens), hyperopes, Inuits, and Asians. The value of prophylactic laser therapy in high-risk populations is being assessed. In the United States, about 1% of people over age 35 years have narrow anterior chamber angles but acute glaucoma rarely develops and prophylactic therapy is not generally indicated. Angle closure may be precipitated by pupillary dilation and thus can occur from sitting in a darkened theater, at times of stress or, rarely, from pharmacologic mydriasis. Anticholinergic or sympathomimetic agents (eg, nebulized bronchodilators, atropine for preoperative medication, antidepressants, nasal decongestants, or tocolytics) are also causes. Secondary acute angle-closure glaucoma may be observed with anterior uveitis, dislocation of the lens, or topiramate therapy. Symptoms are the same as in primary acute angle-closure glaucoma, but differentiation is important because of differences in management. Chronic angle-closure glaucoma is particularly common in eastern Asia. It presents in the same way as open-angle glaucoma (see below).

Clinical Findings

Patients with acute glaucoma usually seek treatment immediately because of extreme pain and blurred vision, though there are subacute cases. The blurred vision is associated with halos around lights. Nausea and abdominal pain may occur, and acute glaucoma must be remembered in the differential diagnosis of the acute abdomen. The eye is red, the cornea steamy, and the pupil moderately dilated and nonreactive to light. Intraocular pressure is usually over 40 mm Hg.

Differential Diagnosis

Acute glaucoma must be differentiated from conjunctivitis, acute uveitis, and corneal disorders (Table 7–1).

Treatment

A. PRIMARY

Initial treatment in primary angle-closure glaucoma is control of intraocular pressure. A single 500-mg intravenous dose of acetazolamide, followed by 250 mg orally four times a day, is usually sufficient. Osmotic diuretics such as oral glycerol and intravenous urea or mannitol—the dosage of all three being 1–2 g/kg—may be necessary if there is no response to acetazolamide. Laser therapy to the peripheral iris (iridoplasty) or anterior chamber paracentesis is also effective. Once the intraocular pressure has started to fall, topical 4% pilocarpine, 1 drop every 15 minutes for 1 hour and then four times a day, is used to reverse the underlying angle closure. The definitive treatment is laser peripheral iridotomy or surgical peripheral iridectomy, which should also be performed prophylactically on the fellow eye. Cataract extraction is a possible alternative. If it is not possible to control the intraocular pressure medically, glaucoma drainage surgery as for uncontrolled open-angle glaucoma (see below) may be required.

B. SECONDARY

In secondary acute angle-closure glaucoma, systemic acetazolamide is also used, with or without osmotic agents. Further treatment is determined by the cause.

Prognosis

Untreated acute angle-closure glaucoma results in severe and permanent visual loss within 2–5 days after onset of symptoms. Affected patients need to be observed for development of chronic glaucoma.

Guvendag Guven ES et al: Angle closure glaucoma induced by ritodrine. Acta Obstet Gynecol Scand 2005;84:489. [PMID: 15842216]

Johnson GJ et al: Can we prevent angle-closure glaucoma? Eye 2005;19:1119. [PMID: 16304593]

CHRONIC GLAUCOMA

 ESSENTIALS OF DIAGNOSIS

- *No symptoms in early stages.*
- *Gradual loss of peripheral vision over a period of years, resulting in tunnel vision.*
- *Insidious progression in older age groups.*
- *Pathologic cupping of the optic disks usually associated with persistent elevation of intraocular pressure.*

General Considerations

Chronic glaucoma is characterized by gradually progressive excavation ("cupping") and pallor of the optic disk with loss of vision varying from slight constriction of the peripheral fields to complete blindness. In chronic open-angle glaucoma, the intraocular pressure is elevated due to reduced drainage of aqueous through the trabecular meshwork. In chronic angle-closure glaucoma, flow of aqueous into the anterior chamber angle is obstructed. In normal-tension glaucoma, intraocular pressure is not elevated above the normal range but the same pattern of optic nerve damage occurs, probably due to vascular insufficiency.

The cause of the reduced drainage of aqueous in primary open-angle glaucoma has not been clearly established. The disease is bilateral, and there is an increased prevalence in first-degree relatives of affected individuals and in diabetics. In blacks, primary open-angle glaucoma is more frequent, occurs at an earlier age, and results in more severe optic nerve damage. Secondary open-angle glaucoma may result from uveitis or the effects of trauma. Elevation of intraocular pressure is also a complication of corticosteroid therapy, whether it be topical, systemic, inhaled, or administered by nasal spray.

In the United States, it is estimated that 2% of people over 40 years of age have glaucoma, affecting more than 2 million individuals and being three times more prevalent in blacks. At least 25% of cases are undetected. Over 90% of cases are of the open-angle type, either primary open-angle or normal-tension glaucoma. Worldwide, about 50% of all cases of glaucoma are due to acute (see above) or chronic angle closure due to the very high prevalence of angle closure in Asians.

Clinical Findings

Because patients with chronic glaucoma have no symptoms initially, diagnosis is often made incidentally at routine eye tests. On examination, there may be slight cupping of the optic disk observed as an absolute increase—or an asymmetry between the two eyes—of the ratio of the diameter of the optic cup to the diameter of the whole optic disk (cup-disk ratio). (Cup-disk ratio of greater than 0.5 or asymmetry of cup-disk ratio of 0.2 or more is suggestive.) The visual fields gradually constrict, but central vision remains good until late in the disease.

Diagnosis requires consistent and reproducible abnormalities in at least two out of three parameters—intraocular pressure, optic disk cupping, and central visual field. The normal range of intraocular pressure is 10–21 mm Hg. In many individuals, elevated intraocular pressure is not associated with optic disk or visual field abnormalities. These persons with ocular hypertension are at increased risk for glaucomatous damage. Treatment to reduce intraocular pressure is justified if there is a moderate to high risk of the development of glaucoma. Risk is determined by several factors, including age, optic disk appearance, level of intraocular pressure, and corneal thickness. Conversely, a significant proportion of patients with glaucoma have normal intraocular pressure when it is first measured, and only repeated measurements identify the abnormally high pressure. Furthermore, in patients with normal-tension glaucoma, the intraocular pressure is always within the normal range despite repeated measurement. There are many other causes of optic disk abnormalities or visual field changes that mimic glaucomatous damage, and visual field testing may prove unreliable in some patients, particularly the elderly. Taken together, these factors mean that the diagnosis of glaucoma is not always straightforward, hampering the effectiveness of screening programs.

Prevention

All persons over age 40 years should have intraocular pressure measurement and optic disk examination every 2–5 years. In persons with diabetes and in individuals with a family history of glaucoma, annual examination is indicated.

Treatment

The prostaglandin analogs (latanoprost 0.005%, bimatoprost 0.03%, and travoprost 0.004% once daily at night; or unoprostone isopropyl 0.15% twice daily) are commonly used as first-line therapy because of their efficacy, the convenience of once-daily administration, and their lack of systemic side effects. All may produce conjunctival hyperemia, permanent darkening of the iris and eyebrow color, and eyelash growth. Latanoprost has been associated with reactivation of uveitis and macular edema. Topical β-adrenergic blocking agents such as timolol 0.25% or 0.5%, carteolol 1%, levobunolol 0.5%, and metipranolol 0.3% solutions twice daily or timolol 0.5% gel once daily may be used alone or in combination with a prostaglandin analog. They are contraindicated in patients with reactive airway disease or heart failure. Betaxolol, 0.25% or 0.5%, a β-receptor selective blocking agent, is theoretically safer in reactive airway disease but less effective at reducing intraocular pressure. Brimonidine 0.2%, a selective α_2-agonist, and dorzolamide 2% or brinzolamide 1%, topical carbonic anhydrase inhibitors, also can be used in addition to a prostaglandin analog or a β-blocker (twice daily) or as initial therapy when prostaglandin analogs and β-blockers are contraindicated (brimonidine twice daily, dorzolamide and brinzolamide three times daily). Both are associated with allergic reactions. Combination drops Xalacom (latanoprost 0.005% and timolol 0.5%) used once daily in the morning, Cosopt (dorzolamide 2% and timolol 0.5%) used twice daily, and Combigan (brimonidine 0.2% and timolol 0.5%) used twice daily) improve compliance when multiple medications are required.

Apraclonidine, 0.5–1%, another α_2-agonist, can be used three times a day to postpone the need for surgery in patients receiving maximal medical therapy, but long-term use is limited by drug reactions. It is more commonly used to control acute rises in intraocular pressure such as after laser therapy. Epinephrine,

0.5–1%, and the prodrug dipivefrin, 0.1%, are being used much less frequently because of adverse effects on the outcome of subsequent glaucoma surgery. Pilocarpine 1–4% (and sometimes higher concentrations in patients with dark irides) four times a day is little used because of the induced myopia in younger patients and the pupillary constriction that compromises vision in patients with cataract. Oral carbonic anhydrase inhibitors (eg, acetazolamide) may still be used on a long-term basis if topical therapy is inadequate and surgical or laser therapy is inappropriate.

Laser trabeculoplasty is used as an adjunct to topical therapy to defer surgery and is also advocated as primary treatment. Surgery is generally undertaken when intraocular pressure is inadequately controlled by medical and laser therapy, but it may also be used as primary treatment. Trabeculectomy remains the standard procedure. Adjunctive treatment with subconjunctival mitomycin or fluorouracil is used perioperatively or postoperatively in difficult cases. Viscocanalostomy and deep sclerectomy with collagen implant—two alternative procedures that avoid a full-thickness incision into the eye—may be as effective as trabeculectomy but are more difficult to perform.

In chronic angle-closure glaucoma, laser peripheral iridotomy or surgical peripheral iridectomy may be helpful in the early stages.

Prognosis

Untreated chronic glaucoma that begins at age 40–45 years will probably cause complete blindness by age 60–65. Early diagnosis and treatment can preserve useful vision throughout life. In primary open-angle glaucoma—and if treatment is required in ocular hypertension—the aim is to reduce intraocular pressure to a level that will adequately reduce progression of visual field loss. In eyes with marked visual field or optic disk changes, intraocular pressure must be reduced to less than 16 mm Hg. In normal-tension glaucoma with progressive visual field loss, it is necessary to achieve even lower intraocular pressure such that surgery is often required.

Adatia FA et al: Chronic open-angle glaucoma. Review for primary care physicians. Can Fam Physician 2005;51:1229. [PMID: 16190176]

Burr J et al: Medical versus surgical interventions for open angle glaucoma. Cochrane Database Syst Rev 2005;2:CD004399. [PMID: 15846712]

Latina MA et al: Selective laser trabeculoplasty. Ophthalmol Clin North Am 2005;18:409. [PMID: 16054998]

Lee DA et al: Glaucoma and its treatment: a review. Am J Health Syst Pharm 2005;62:691. [PMID: 15790795]

Levin LA: Pathophysiology of the progressive optic neuropathy of glaucoma: Ophthalmol Clin North Am 2005;18:355. [PMID: 16054993]

Maier PC et al: Treatment of ocular hypertension and open angle glaucoma: meta-analysis of randomised controlled trials. BMJ 2005;331:134. [PMID: 1599465]

Singh A: Medical therapy of glaucoma: Ophthalmol Clin North Am 2005;18:397. [PMID: 16054997]

UVEITIS

Uveitis means inflammation of the uveal tract, which is formed by the iris (iritis), ciliary body (cyclitis), and choroid (choroiditis). Inflammatory eye disease may also originate primarily in the retina (retinitis) or retinal blood vessels (retinal vasculitis).

Intraocular inflammation is classified as anterior uveitis, posterior uveitis, or panuveitis. Uveitis may also be termed acute or chronic and granulomatous or nongranulomatous. In most cases, the pathogenesis of uveitis is primarily immunologic, but infection may be the cause, particularly in immunodeficiency states.

Clinical Findings

Anterior uveitis is characterized by inflammatory cells and flare within the aqueous. In severe cases, there may be hypopyon (layered collection of white cells) and fibrin within the anterior chamber. Cells may also be seen on the corneal endothelium as keratic precipitates (KPs). In granulomatous uveitis, these are large "mutton-fat" KPs, and iris nodules may be seen. In nongranulomatous uveitis, the KPs are smaller and iris nodules are not seen. The pupil is usually small, and with the development of posterior synechiae (adhesions between the iris and anterior lens capsule), it also becomes irregular.

Nongranulomatous anterior uveitis tends to present acutely with unilateral pain, redness, photophobia, and visual loss. Granulomatous anterior uveitis is more indolent, causing blurred vision in a mildly inflamed eye.

In posterior uveitis, there are cells in the vitreous. Inflammatory lesions may be present in the retina or choroid. Fresh lesions are yellow, with indistinct margins, whereas older lesions have more definite margins and are commonly pigmented. Retinal vessel sheathing may occur adjacent to such lesions or more diffusely. In severe cases, vitreous opacity precludes visualization of retinal details.

Posterior uveitis tends to present with gradual visual loss in a relatively quiet eye. Bilateral involvement is common. Visual loss may be due to vitreous haze and opacities, inflammatory lesions involving the macula, macular edema, retinal vein occlusion or, rarely, associated optic neuropathy.

Etiology

The systemic disorders associated with acute nongranulomatous anterior uveitis are the HLA-B27-related conditions ankylosing spondylitis, reactive arthritis, psoriasis, ulcerative colitis, and Crohn's disease. Behçet's syndrome produces both anterior uveitis, with recurrent hypopyon in 5% of patients, and posterior uveitis, with retinal vein occlusions on occasion. Both herpes simplex and herpes zoster infections may cause nongranulomatous anterior uveitis.

Diseases producing granulomatous anterior uveitis also tend to be causes of posterior uveitis. These include sarcoidosis, tuberculosis, syphilis, toxoplasmosis, Vogt-

Koyanagi-Harada syndrome (bilateral uveitis associated with alopecia, poliosis [depigmented eyelashes, eyebrows, or hair], vitiligo, and hearing loss), and sympathetic ophthalmia following penetrating ocular trauma. Syphilis produces a characteristic "salt and pepper" fundus, often with surprisingly little visual loss unless there is also primary syphilitic optic atrophy. In congenital toxoplasmosis, there is usually evidence of previous episodes of retinochoroiditis. The principal pathogens responsible for ocular inflammation in AIDS are cytomegalovirus (CMV), herpes simplex and herpes zoster viruses, mycobacteria, *Cryptococcus, Toxoplasma,* and *Candida.*

Autoimmune retinal vasculitis and pars planitis (intermediate uveitis) are idiopathic conditions that produce posterior uveitis.

Retinal detachment, intraocular tumors, and central nervous system lymphoma may all masquerade as uveitis.

Treatment

Anterior uveitis usually responds to topical corticosteroids. Occasionally, periocular corticosteroid injections or even systemic corticosteroids may be required. Dilation of the pupil is important to relieve discomfort and prevent posterior synechiae.

Posterior uveitis more commonly requires systemic corticosteroid therapy and occasionally systemic immunosuppression with agents such as azathioprine, tacrolimus, cyclosporine, or mycophenolate. Pupillary dilation is not usually necessary.

If an infectious cause is identified, specific antimicrobial therapy may be indicated. In general, the prognosis for anterior uveitis, particularly the nongranulomatous type, is better than that for posterior uveitis.

Becker MD et al: Management of sight-threatening uveitis: new therapeutic options. Drugs 2005;65:497. [PMID: 15733012]

Bonfioli AA et al: Sarcoidosis. Semin Ophthalmol 2005;20:177. [PMID: 16282152]

Chang JH et al: Acute anterior uveitis and HLA-B27. Surv Ophthalmol 2005;50:364. [PMID: 15967191]

Kiss S et al: Ocular manifestations and treatment of syphilis. Semin Ophthalmol 2005;20:161. [PMID: 16282150]

CATARACT

ESSENTIALS OF DIAGNOSIS

- *Blurred vision, progressive over months or years.*
- *No pain or redness.*
- *Lens opacities (may be grossly visible).*

General Considerations

Cataract is a lens opacity. Cataracts are usually bilateral. They may be congenital (owing to intrauterine infections such as rubella and CMV, or inborn errors of metabolism such as galactosemia); traumatic; or secondary to systemic disease (diabetes, myotonic dystrophy, atopic dermatitis), systemic or inhaled corticosteroid treatment, or uveitis. Senile cataract is by far the most common type; most persons over age 60 have some degree of lens opacity. Cigarette smoking increases the risk of cataract formation.

Clinical Findings

Even in its early stages, a cataract can be seen through a dilated pupil with an ophthalmoscope or slit lamp. As the cataract matures, the retina will become increasingly more difficult to visualize, until finally the fundus reflection is absent and the pupil is white.

Treatment

Functional visual impairment is the prime criterion for surgery. The cataract is usually removed by one of the techniques in which the posterior lens capsule remains (extracapsular). Laser treatment may be required subsequently if the posterior capsule opacifies. Ultrasonic fragmentation (phacoemulsification) of the lens nucleus allows cataract surgery to be performed through a small incision without the need for sutures, thus reducing the postoperative complication rate and accelerating visual rehabilitation.

It is routine practice to insert an intraocular lens at the time of surgery. This dispenses with the need for heavy cataract glasses or contact lenses. Multifocal and accommodative intraocular lenses have been used with some success to reduce the need for both distance and reading glasses.

Prognosis

If surgery is indicated, lens extraction improves visual acuity in 95% of cases and can have a profound impact on quality of life, although expectations must be realistic. The remainder either have preexisting retinal damage or develop perioperative or postoperative complications.

Asbell PA et al: Age-related cataract. Lancet 2005;365:599. [PMID: 15708105]

Dick HB: Accommodative intraocular lenses: current status. Curr Opin Ophthalmol 2005;16:8. [PMID: 15650575]

Harwood RH et al: Falls and health status in elderly women following first eye cataract surgery: a randomized controlled trial. Br J Ophthalmol 2005;89:53. [PMID: 15615747]

Lundstrom M et al: Duration of self assessed benefit of cataract extraction: a long term study. Br J Ophthalmol 2005;89:1017. [PMID: 16024857]

RETINAL DETACHMENT

ESSENTIALS OF DIAGNOSIS

- *Blurred vision in one eye becoming progressively worse.*

- *No pain or redness.*
- *Detachment seen by ophthalmoscopy.*

General Considerations

The primary event in rhegmatogenous retinal detachment is the development of a retinal tear. This is usually spontaneous, related to changes in the vitreous, but may be secondary to trauma. Spontaneous detachment occurs most frequently in persons over 50 years of age. Myopia and cataract extraction are the two most common predisposing causes. Once there is a tear in the retina, fluid vitreous is able to pass through the tear and lodge behind the sensory retina. This, combined with vitreous traction and the pull of gravity, results in progressive detachment. The superior temporal area is the most common site of detachment. The area involved rapidly increases, causing corresponding progressive visual loss. Central vision remains intact until the macula becomes detached.

The basis of traction retinal detachment is the development of preretinal fibrosis, such as in association with proliferative retinopathy secondary to diabetic retinopathy or retinal vein occlusion. Serous retinal detachment results from accumulation of subretinal fluid, such as in exudative age-related macular degeneration or secondary to choroidal tumors.

Clinical Findings

On ophthalmoscopic examination in rhegmatogenous retinal detachment, the retina is seen hanging in the vitreous like a gray cloud. One or more retinal tears will usually be found on further examination. In traction retinal detachment, there is irregular retinal elevation with fibrosis. With serous retinal detachment, the retina is dome-shaped and the subretinal fluid may shift position with changes in posture.

Treatment

All cases of retinal detachment must be referred immediately to an ophthalmologist. During transportation, the patient's head is positioned so that the detached portion of the retina will fall back with the aid of gravity. Treatment of rhegmatogenous retinal detachment is directed at closing the tears. A permanent adhesion between the neurosensory retina, the retinal pigment epithelium, and the choroid is produced in the region of the tears by applying cryotherapy to the sclera or laser photocoagulation to the retina. To achieve apposition of the neurosensory retina to the retinal pigment epithelium while this adhesion is developing, indentation of the sclera with a silicone sponge or buckle; subretinal fluid drainage via an incision in the sclera; and injection of an expansile gas into the vitreous cavity may be required. Certain types of uncomplicated retinal detachment may be treated by pneumatic retino-

pexy, in which an expansile gas is initially injected into the vitreous cavity followed by positioning of the patient's head to facilitate reattachment of the retina. Once the retina is repositioned, the tear is sealed by laser photocoagulation or cryotherapy. All the stages of pneumatic retinopexy can be performed under local anesthesia as an office procedure. The last stage is the same as is used to seal retinal tears without associated detachment as prophylaxis against recurrence.

In complicated retinal detachments—particularly those in which fibroproliferative tissue has developed on the surface of the retina or within the vitreous cavity, ie, traction retinal detachments—retinal reattachment can be accomplished only by removal of the vitreous, direct manipulation of the retina, and internal tamponade of the retina with air, expansile gases, or even silicone oil. (The presence of an expansile gas within the eye is a contraindication to air travel, mountaineering at high altitude, and nitrous oxide anesthesia. Such gases persist in the globe for weeks after surgery.) (See Chapter 38.) Treatment of serous retinal detachments is determined by the underlying cause.

Prognosis

About 80% of uncomplicated rhegmatogenous retinal detachments can be cured with one operation; an additional 15% will need repeated operations; and the remainder never reattach. The prognosis is worse if the macula is detached or if the detachment is of long duration. Without treatment, retinal detachment often becomes total within 6 months. Spontaneous detachments are ultimately bilateral in up to 25% of cases.

Gupta OP et al: The risk of fellow eyes in patients with rhegmatogenous retinal detachment. Curr Opin Ophthalmol 2005;16:175. [PMID: 15870575]

VITREOUS HEMORRHAGE

Patients with vitreous hemorrhage complain of sudden visual loss, abrupt onset of floaters that may progressively increase in severity or, occasionally, "bleeding within the eye." Visual acuity ranges from 20/20 to light perception only. The eye is not inflamed, and the clue to diagnosis is the inability to see fundal details clearly despite the presence of a clear lens. Causes of vitreous hemorrhage include diabetic retinopathy, retinal tears (with or without detachment), retinal vein occlusions, exudative age-related macular degeneration, blood dyscrasias, trauma, and subarachnoid hemorrhage. In all cases, examination by an ophthalmologist is essential. Retinal tears and detachments necessitate urgent treatment (see above).

AGE-RELATED MACULAR DEGENERATION

Age-related macular degeneration is the leading cause of permanent visual loss in the elderly. The exact cause is unknown, but the incidence increases with each decade over age 50 years (to almost 30% by age 75). Other associations in addition to age include race (usually white), sex (slight female predominance), family history, and a history of cigarette smoking.

Age-related macular degeneration includes a broad spectrum of clinical and pathologic findings that can be classified into two groups: atrophic ("dry") and exudative ("wet"). Although both are progressive and usually bilateral, they differ in manifestations, prognosis, and management. The precursor to age-related macular degeneration is age-related maculopathy, the hallmark of which is the development of retinal drusen. Hard drusen appear ophthalmoscopically as discrete yellow deposits, usually in the macular region. Soft drusen are larger, paler, and less distinct. Large, confluent soft drusen are particularly associated with exudative age-related macular degeneration.

Atrophic degeneration is characterized by gradually progressive bilateral visual loss of moderate severity due to atrophy and degeneration of the outer retina and retinal pigment epithelium. In exudative degeneration, visual loss is of more rapid onset and greater severity, and the two eyes are frequently affected sequentially over a period of a few years. The exudative form accounts for about 90% of all cases of legal blindness due to this disorder. Impairment of the barrier function of Bruch's membrane (between the retinal pigment epithelium and the choriocapillaris) allows serous fluid or blood to leak into the retina to produce elevation of the retinal pigment epithelium from Bruch's membrane (retinal pigment epithelial detachment) or separation of the neurosensory retina from the retinal pigment epithelium (serous retinal detachment). These changes may resolve spontaneously, with variable visual outcome, but are often associated with neovascularization arising from the choroidal vessels and extending between the retinal pigment epithelium and Bruch's membrane (subretinal neovascular membrane). This membrane produces permanent visual loss.

Sudden visual loss in patients with exudative age-related macular degeneration occurs at the time of pigment epithelial or sensory retinal detachment or hemorrhage from a subretinal neovascular membrane. All these changes may occur in previously undiagnosed patients, in patients known to have atrophic changes, and in the other eye of patients with exudative disease. Photodynamic laser therapy (PDT), involving intravenous injection of verteporfin activated by subsequent retinal laser irradiation to produce selective vascular damage, is particularly indicated when the neovascular membrane is well defined (whether it is subfoveal or extrafoveal) and may be helpful when it is not occult. Treatment often needs to be repeated. Intravitreal and periocular corticosteroid injections and intravitreal injections of inhibitors of vascular endothelial growth factor (VEGF) are being studied as alternative or adjuvant therapy to PDT. Conventional laser photocoagulation of subfoveal neovascular membranes is associated with an inevitable immediate reduction in vision because of associated retinal damage and is thus only suitable for extrafoveal membranes. Various surgical techniques to excise subfoveal neovascular membranes—or to reposition the macula away from them—continue to be investigated. Older patients developing sudden visual loss due to macular disease—particularly paracentral distortion or scotoma with preservation of central acuity—should be referred urgently to an ophthalmologist for assessment.

There is no specific treatment for atrophic age-related macular degeneration, but—as with the exudative form—patients often benefit from low vision aids. The disorder results in loss of central vision only. Peripheral fields and hence navigational vision are always maintained, though these may become impaired by cataract formation for which surgery may be helpful. The value of oral antioxidants and other dietary supplements in preventing visual loss in age-related macular degeneration continues to be assessed.

Augustin AJ et al: Verteporfin therapy combined with intravitreal triamcinolone in all types of choroidal neovascularization due to age-related macular degeneration. Ophthalmology 2006;113:14. [PMID: 16360209]

Azab M et al: Verteporfin therapy of subfoveal minimally classic choroidal neovascularization in age-related macular degeneration: 2-year results of a randomized clinical trial. Arch Ophthalmol 2005;123:448. [PMID: 15824216]

Childs AL et al: Surgery for hemorrhagic choroidal neovascular lesions of age-related macular degeneration: quality-of-life findings: SST report no. 14. Ophthalmology 2004;111: 2007. [PMID: 15522365]

Clemons TE et al: Risk factors for the incidence of Advanced Age-Related Macular Degeneration in the Age-Related Eye Disease Study (AREDS) AREDS report no. 19. Ophthalmology 2005;112:533. [PMID: 15808240]

Gragoudas ES et al: Pegaptanib for neovascular age-related macular degeneration. N Engl J Med 2004;351:2805. [PMID: 15625332]

Khan JC et al: Smoking and age related macular degeneration: the number of pack years of cigarette smoking is a major determinant of risk for both geographic atrophy and choroidal neovascularisation. Br J Ophthalmol 2006;90:75. [PMID: 16361672]

Pauleikhoff D: Neovascular age-related macular degeneration: Natural history and treatment outcomes. Retina 2005;5: 1065. [PMID: 16340538]

Slakter JS et al: Anecortave acetate (15 milligrams) versus photodynamic therapy for treatment of subfoveal neovascularization in age-related macular degeneration. Ophthalmology 2006;113:3. [PMID: 16368146]

Slakter JS et al: Quality of life in patients with age-related macular degeneration: impact of the condition and benefits of treatment. Surv Ophthalmol 2005;50:263. [PMID: 15850815]

Van de Moere A et al: Effect of posterior juxtascleral triamcinolone acetonide on choroidal neovascular growth after photodynamic therapy with verteporfin. Ophthalmology 2005; 112:1896. [PMID: 16214216]

CENTRAL & BRANCH RETINAL VEIN OCCLUSIONS

The visual impairment in central retinal vein occlusion is commonly first noticed upon waking. Ophthalmoscopic signs include disk swelling, venous dilation and tortuosity, retinal hemorrhages, and cotton-wool spots.

In those with initially good acuity (20/60 or better), the visual prognosis is good. With poor initial acuity (20/200 or worse), extensive hemorrhages and multiple cotton-wool spots indicate widespread retinal ischemia, which can be confirmed by demonstrating extensive areas of capillary closure on fluorescein angiography. These eyes are at high risk for developing neovascular (rubeotic) glaucoma, typically within 3 months after venous occlusion, and should be monitored by an ophthalmologist so that timely laser panretinal photocoagulation can be undertaken. Visual prognosis in such cases is poor. Improvement in vision has been reported in central retinal vein occlusion after direct injection of tissue plasminogen activator into the retinal venous system, incision of the sclera at the edge of the optic disk (radial optic neurotomy), and intravitreal corticosteroid injection when macular edema is present.

Branch retinal vein occlusions may present in a variety of ways. Sudden loss of vision may occur at the time of occlusion if the fovea is involved or some time afterward from vitreous hemorrhage due to retinal new vessels. More gradual visual loss may occur with development of macular edema.

In acute branch retinal vein occlusion there are signs similar to those of central retinal vein occlusion but affecting only the retina drained by the obstructed vein. If retinal neovascularization develops, the areas of ischemic retina should be laser photocoagulated. Macular edema may respond to laser treatment or possibly vitrectomy with surgical incision of the retinal vascular adventitia (arteriovenous sheathotomy) and injection of tissue plasminogen activator.

All patients with retinal vein occlusion should be referred urgently to an ophthalmologist. They should be screened for diabetes, systemic hypertension, hyperlipidemia, and glaucoma. In younger patients, antiphospholipid antibodies, inherited thrombophilia, and hyperhomocysteinemia should be considered. Hyperviscosity syndromes, including myeloproliferative disorders, are rarely associated with retinal vein occlusions but may worsen their prognosis.

Bashshur ZF et al: Intravitreal triamcinolone for the management of macular edema due to nonischemic central retinal vein occlusion. Arch Ophthalmol 2004;122:1137. [PMID: 15302653]

Charbonnel J et al: Management of branch retinal vein occlusion with vitrectomy and arteriovenous adventitial sheathotomy, the possible role of surgical posterior vitreous detachment. Graefes Arch Clin Exp Ophthalmol 2004;242:223. [PMID: 14685873]

Garcia-Arumi J: Management of macular edema in branch retinal vein occlusion with sheathotomy and recombinant tissue plasminogen activator. Retina 2004;24:530. [PMID: 15300073]

Wong TY et al: Cardiovascular risk factors for retinal vein occlusion and arteriolar emboli: the Atherosclerosis Risk in Communities & Cardiovascular Health studies. Ophthalmology 2005;112:540. [PMID: 15808241]

CENTRAL & BRANCH RETINAL ARTERY OCCLUSIONS

Central retinal artery occlusion presents as sudden profound monocular visual loss. Visual acuity is reduced to counting fingers or worse, and visual field is restricted to an island of vision in the temporal field. Ophthalmoscopy reveals pallid swelling of the retina, most obvious in the posterior segment, with a cherry-red spot at the fovea. The retinal arteries are attenuated, and "box-car" segmentation of blood in the veins may be seen. Occasionally, emboli are seen in the central retinal artery or its branches. The retinal swelling subsides over a period of 4–6 weeks, leaving a relatively normal retinal appearance but a pale optic disk and attenuated arterioles.

The patient is referred emergently to an ophthalmologist. If seen within a few hours after onset, emergency treatment—including laying the patient flat, ocular massage, high concentrations of inhaled oxygen, intravenous acetazolamide, and anterior chamber paracentesis—may influence the visual outcome. Studies of thrombolysis, particularly by local intra-arterial injection but also intravenously, have shown variable results.

Branch retinal artery occlusion may also present with sudden loss of vision if the fovea is involved, but more commonly sudden loss of visual field is the presenting complaint. Fundal signs of retinal swelling and adjacent cotton-wool spots are limited to the area of retina supplied by the occluded vessel. Patients with branch retinal artery occlusions should be referred urgently to an ophthalmologist.

Giant cell arteritis must be excluded in patients 55 years of age or older, especially because of the risk—highest in the first few days—of involvement of the other eye. If giant cell arteritis is suspected, either by clinical features, particularly jaw claudication, or markedly elevated serum inflammatory markers, usually erythrocyte sedimentation rate and C-reactive protein, immediately institute high-dose corticosteroids (oral prednisolone 1–1.5 mg/kg/d, if necessary preceded by intravenous hydrocortisone 250–500 mg stat) and proceed promptly to temporal artery biopsy. In patients with bilateral visual loss, initial treatment with methylprednisolone 1 g/d for 1–3 days should be considered.

In central and particularly in branch retinal artery occlusion, carotid and cardiac sources of emboli must be identified so that appropriate treatment is given to reduce the risk of stroke (see Chapter 12). Migraine, oral contraceptives, systemic vasculitis, congenital or acquired thrombophilia, and hyperhomocysteinemia should be considered in young patients, internal carotid artery dissection when there is neck pain or a recent history of neck trauma, and diabetes, hyperlipidemia, and systemic hypertension in all patients.

Azhar SS et al: Giant cell arteritis: diagnosing and treating inflammatory disease in older adults. Geriatrics 2005;60:26. [PMID: 16092890]

Danesh-Meyer H et al: Poor prognosis of visual outcome after visual loss from giant cell arteritis. Ophthalmology 2005; 112:1098. [PMID: 15885780]

Feltgen N et al: Multicenter study of the European Assessment Group for Lysis in the Eye (EAGLE) for the treatment of central retinal artery occlusion: design issues and implications. EAGLE Study report no. 1. Graefes Arch Clin Exp Ophthalmol 2005:1. [PMID: 16372192]

Rahman W et al: Giant cell (temporal) arteritis: an overview and update. Surv Ophthalmol 2005;50:415. [PMID: 16139037]

AMAUROSIS FUGAX

Amaurosis fugax ("fleeting blindness") is usually caused by retinal emboli from ipsilateral carotid disease. The visual loss is usually described as a curtain passing vertically across the visual field with complete monocular visual loss lasting a few minutes and a similar curtain effect as the episode passes. To reduce the risk of stroke, patients with high-grade stenosis (70–99%) of the ipsilateral internal carotid artery should be considered for carotid endarterectomy or angioplasty with stenting. Patients with medium-grade (30–69%) stenosis, unless there are other risk factors for stroke, or low-grade (up to 29%) stenosis are generally better treated medically with aspirin or other antiplatelet drugs. The most reliable method of evaluating carotid stenosis is intra-arterial angiography, but this is associated with a number of complications including stroke. The noninvasive techniques of duplex ultrasonography and magnetic resonance angiography are suitable screening methods. Emboli from cardiac sources may also be responsible for amaurosis fugax. Electrocardiography should be performed in all cases, particularly to identify atrial fibrillation. Echocardiography should be undertaken in young patients and in any patient with clinical evidence of a potential cardiac source of emboli. In younger patients without carotid or cardiac disease, amaurosis fugax may be due to choroidal or retinal vascular spasm, in which case calcium channel blockers such as slow-release nifedipine, 60 mg/d, appear to be effective. Antiphospholipid syndrome should be excluded.

Similar episodes of loss of vision, characteristically on exposure to bright light, may occur with poor ocular perfusion usually due to severe occlusive carotid disease. More transient episodes (lasting only a few seconds to 1 minute) affecting both eyes occur in patients with raised intracranial pressure. In all cases of episodic visual loss, early ophthalmologic consultation is advisable.

Alamowitch S et al: The risk and benefit of endarterectomy in women with symptomatic internal carotid artery disease. Stroke 2005;36:27.[PMID: 15569876]

RETINAL DISORDERS ASSOCIATED WITH SYSTEMIC DISEASES

Many systemic diseases are associated with retinal manifestations. These include diabetes mellitus, essential hypertension, preeclampsia-eclampsia of pregnancy, blood dyscrasias, and AIDS. The retinal changes caused by these disorders can be easily observed with an ophthalmoscope.

Diabetic Retinopathy

Diabetic retinopathy is the leading cause of new blindness among adults in the United States aged 20–65 years. It is broadly classified as nonproliferative or proliferative.

Nonproliferative retinopathy shows dilation of veins, microaneurysms, retinal hemorrhages, retinal edema, and hard exudates. A major subgroup includes those patients in whom visual loss develops owing to edema, exudates, or ischemia at the macula (diabetic maculopathy). This is the most common cause of legal blindness in maturity-onset diabetes.

Proliferative retinopathy is characterized by neovascularization, arising from either the optic disk or the major vascular arcades. Vitreous hemorrhage is a common sequela. Proliferation into the vitreous of blood vessels, with their associated fibrous component, leads to tractional retinal detachment. Without treatment, the visual prognosis with proliferative retinopathy is generally much worse than that with nonproliferative retinopathy. Severe proliferative retinopathy is often complicated by maculopathy.

Nonproliferative retinopathy is occasionally present at the time of diagnosis in type 2 diabetes. Treatment includes optimizing control of blood glucose, blood pressure, and serum lipids. Institution of intensive insulin therapy can be associated with temporary exacerbation of retinopathy, with multiple cotton-wool spots. Laser photocoagulation is helpful in the treatment of focal macular edema but may also be used when there is diffuse macular edema, which may also respond to intravitreal injection of corticosteroid or a VEGF inhibitor. The presence of macular edema can be detected only by stereoscopic examination of the retina or by fluorescein angiography. The level of visual acuity is a poor guide to the presence of treatable maculopathy—hence the need for regular ophthalmologic follow-up.

Proliferative retinopathy must be recognized early and treated by panretinal laser photocoagulation to prevent blindness. Neovascularization is all too often diagnosed only at the time of vitreous hemorrhage. In some patients, a "preproliferative" retinopathy may be identified. Whether panretinal laser photocoagulation should be undertaken at this time can be determined by the degree of retinal ischemia as assessed by fluorescein angiography. Regression of neovascularization has been demonstrated after intravitreal injection of a VEGF inhibitor.

Surgical treatment (vitrectomy) is used either to remove vitreous hemorrhage and thus allow perioperative panretinal laser photocoagulation for the underlying retinal neovascularization, to deal with retinal detachments involving the macula, to manage rapidly progressive proliferative disease, or to treat persistent macular edema.

Patients with diabetes should undergo yearly screening by fundal photography or ophthalmoscopic examination through dilated pupils. Examination by an ophthalmologist is advisable in type 1 diabetes of more than 5 years' duration; at the time of diagnosis in type 2 diabetes; prior to conception in women contemplating pregnancy, in early pregnancy and every 2–3 months throughout pregnancy; if ocular symptoms develop; or if there are suspicious findings of retinopathy, especially neovascularization or macular exudates. Failure to diagnose diabetic retinopathy by ophthalmoscopic examination is common, particularly if the pupils are not dilated. The severity of diabetic retinopathy can be decreased by control of blood glucose levels, but good diabetic control is more important in preventing the development of retinopathy than in influencing its subsequent course. Proliferative diabetic retinopathy, especially after successful laser treatment, is not a contraindication to treatment with thrombolytic agents, aspirin, or warfarin unless there has been recent vitreous or preretinal hemorrhage.

Bressler NM et al; Macugen Diabetic Retinopathy Study Group: Changes in retinal neovascularization after pegaptanib (Macugen) therapy in diabetic individuals. Ophthalmology 2006; 113:23. [PMID: 16343627]

Colucciello M: Diabetic retinopathy. Control of systemic factors preserves vision. Postgrad Med 2004;116:57. [PMID: 15274289]

Cunningham ET Jr et al: A phase II randomized double-masked trial of pegaptanib, an anti-vascular endothelial growth factor aptamer, for diabetic macular edema. Ophthalmology 2005;112:1747. [PMID: 16154196]

Matthews DR et al: Risks of progression of retinopathy and vision loss related to tight blood pressure control in type 2 diabetes mellitus: UKPDS 69. Arch Ophthalmol 2004; 122:1631. [PMID: 15534123]

Sjolie AK et al: Medical management of diabetic retinopathy. Diabet Med 2004;21:666. [PMID: 15209756]

Spandau UH et al: Dosage dependency of intravitreal triamcinolone acetonide as treatment for diabetic macular oedema. Br J Ophthalmol 2005;89:999. [PMID: 16024853]

Hypertensive Retinochoroidopathy

Systemic hypertension affects both the retinal and choroidal circulations. The clinical manifestations vary according to the degree and rapidity of rise in blood pressure and the underlying state of the ocular circulation. The most florid disease occurs in young patients with abrupt elevations of blood pressure, such as may occur in pheochromocytoma, malignant hypertension, or preeclampsia-eclampsia.

Chronic hypertension accelerates the development of atherosclerosis. The retinal arterioles become more tortuous and narrow and develop abnormal light reflexes ("silver-wiring" and "copper-wiring"). There is increased venous compression at the retinal arteriovenous crossings ("arteriovenous nicking"), an important factor predisposing to branch retinal vein occlusions. Flame-shaped hemorrhages occur in the nerve fiber layer of the retina.

Acute elevations of blood pressure result in loss of autoregulation in the retinal circulation, leading to the breakdown of endothelial integrity and occlusion of precapillary arterioles and capillaries. These pathologic changes are manifested as cotton-wool spots, retinal hemorrhages, retinal edema, and retinal exudates, often in a stellate appearance at the macula. In the choroid, vasoconstriction and ischemia result in serous retinal detachments and retinal pigment epithelial infarcts. These infarcts later develop into pigmented lesions that may be focal, linear, or wedge-shaped. The abnormalities in the choroidal circulation may also affect the optic nerve head, producing ischemic optic neuropathy with optic disk swelling. Malignant hypertensive retinopathy was the term previously used to describe the constellation of clinical signs resulting from the combination of abnormalities in the retinal, choroidal, and optic disk circulation. When there is such severe disease, there is likely to be permanent retinal, choroidal, or optic nerve damage. Precipitous reduction of blood pressure may exacerbate such damage.

Porta M et al: Hypertensive retinopathy: there's more than meets the eye. J Hypertens 2005;23:683. [PMID: 15775767]

Wong TY et al: Hypertensive retinopathy. N Engl J Med 2004; 351:2310. [PMID: 15564546]

Blood Dyscrasias

In conditions characterized by thrombocytopenia or severe anemia, various types of hemorrhages occur in both the retina and choroid and may lead to visual loss. If macular hemorrhages have not occurred, it is possible to regain normal vision with treatment.

Proliferative retinopathy (sickle cell retinopathy) is particularly common in hemoglobin SC disease but may also occur with other hemoglobin S variants. Severe visual loss is rare. Retinal photocoagulation reduces the frequency of vitreous hemorrhage. Surgery is occasionally needed for unresolving vitreous hemorrhage or tractional retinal detachment.

AIDS

Cotton-wool spots, retinal hemorrhages, and microaneurysms are the most common ophthalmic abnormalities in AIDS patients.

CMV retinitis occurs when CD4 counts are below 50/mcL. It is characterized by progressively enlarging yellowish-white patches of retinal opacification, which are accompanied by retinal hemorrhages; they usually begin adjacent to the major retinal vascular arcades. Patients are often asymptomatic until there is involvement of the fovea or optic nerve or until retinal detachment develops.

Alternatives for initial therapy follow: (1) intravenous—ganciclovir 5 mg/kg twice a day, foscarnet 60 mg/kg three times a day, or cidofovir 5 mg/kg once weekly, usually for 2 weeks; (2) oral—valganciclovir 900 mg twice daily; or (3) by local administration, using either intravitreal injection of ganciclovir, foscarnet, or fomivirsen or the sustained-release ganciclovir intravitreal implant. Intravitreal cidofovir is effective, but there is a high incidence of uveitis, low intraocular pressure, and ciliary body necrosis. Other major side effects are neutropenia and thrombocytopenia with systemic ganciclovir and nephrotoxicity with foscarnet and cidofovir. Doses of both ganciclovir and foscarnet are adjusted in patients with renal failure. Oral probenecid and intravenous hydration are used to minimize nephrotoxicity from cidofovir. All available agents are virostatic. Maintenance therapy can be conducted with lower-dose intravenous therapy (ganciclovir 3.75 mg/kg/d or foscarnet 60 mg/kg/d for 5 days each week, or cidofovir 5 mg/kg once every 2 weeks), with oral ganciclovir (3 g/d) or oral valganciclovir 900 mg once daily, or with intravitreal therapy. Local therapy tends to be more effective than systemic therapy and avoids systemic side effects, but there is a risk of intraocular complications, and the incidence of retinitis in the fellow eye and of extraocular CMV infection is higher. Unresponsive disease or reactivation during maintenance therapy can be managed by changing to a different agent or by use of combination therapy. Retinal detachment, either due to retinitis or as a complication of intravitreal therapy, requires vitrectomy and intravitreal silicone oil. Oral ganciclovir as prophylaxis against CMV retinitis in patients with low CD4 counts or high CMV burdens has not been found to be worthwhile.

Antiretroviral therapy may result in reduction of HIV virus load and increase in CD4 counts, and even regression of CMV retinitis without the use of anti-CMV therapy. If the CD4 count is maintained above 100/mcL, it may be possible to discontinue maintenance anti-CMV therapy. In patients with regressed CMV retinitis and restored CD4 counts, highly active antiretroviral therapy (HAART) commonly leads to "immune recovery" uveitis, which may lead to visual loss from cataract or retinal complications.

Other opportunistic ophthalmic infections occurring in AIDS patients include herpes simplex retinitis, toxoplasmic and candidal chorioretinitis, and herpes zoster ophthalmicus. Kaposi's sarcoma of the conjunctiva and orbital lymphoma may also be seen on rare occasions.

Chang M et al. Ganciclovir implant in the treatment of cytomegalovirus retinitis. Expert Rev Med Devices 2005;2: 421. [PMID: 16293081]

Cvetkovic RS et al: Valganciclovir: a review of its use in the management of CMV infection and disease in immunocompromised patients. Drugs 2005;65:859. [PMID: 15819597]

Goldberg DE et al: HIV-associated retinopathy in the HAART era. Retina 2005;25:633. [PMID: 16077362]

Jabs DA et al: Risk factors for mortality in patients with AIDS in the era of highly active antiretroviral therapy. Ophthalmology 2005;112:771. [PMID: 15878056]

Kempen JH et al: Incidence of cytomegalovirus (CMV) retinitis in second eyes of patients with the acquired immune deficiency syndrome and unilateral CMV retinitis. Am J Ophthalmol 2005;139:1028. [PMID: 15953432]

ANTERIOR ISCHEMIC OPTIC NEUROPATHY

Anterior ischemic optic neuropathy—due to inadequate perfusion of the posterior ciliary arteries that supply the anterior portion of the optic nerve—produces sudden visual loss, usually with an altitudinal field defect, and optic disk swelling. In older patients, it is often caused by giant cell arteritis, which necessitates high-dose systemic corticosteroid treatment to prevent visual loss in the fellow eye. (See Central and Branch Retinal Artery Occlusions, above.) The predominant factor predisposing to nonarteritic anterior ischemic optic neuropathy is congenitally small optic disks. Other causative factors include systemic hypertension, diabetes, hyperlipidemia, systemic vasculitis, inherited or acquired thrombophilia, and ingestion of sildenafil. Ischemic optic neuropathy, usually involving the retrobulbar optic nerve and thus not causing any optic disk swelling (posterior ischemic optic neuropathy), may complicate both ocular and nonocular surgery, particularly prolonged lumbar spine surgery.

Buono LM et al: Perioperative posterior ischemic optic neuropathy: review of the literature. Surv Ophthalmol 2005;50:15. [PMID: 15621075]

Chan CC et al: Predictors of recurrent ischemic optic neuropathy in giant cell arteritis. J Neuroophthalmol 2005;25:14. [PMID: 15756126]

Desai N et al: Nonarteritic anterior ischemic optic neuropathy. J Clin Hypertens 2005;7:130. [PMID: 15722660]

Pomeranz HD et al: Nonarteritic ischemic optic neuropathy developing soon after use of sildenafil (Viagra): a report of seven new cases. J Neuroophthalmol 2005;25:9. [PMID: 15756125]

OPTIC NEURITIS

Optic neuritis is characterized by unilateral loss of vision, which usually develops over a few days. Vision ranges from 20/30 to no perception of light. Commonly there is pain in the region of the eye, particularly on eye movements. Field loss is usually a central scotoma, but a wide range of monocular field defects is possible. There is marked loss of color vision and a relative afferent pupillary defect. In about two-thirds of cases, the optic nerve is normal during the acute stage (retrobulbar optic neuritis). In the remainder, the optic disk is swollen (papillitis) with occasional flame-shaped peripapillary hemorrhages. Visual acuity usually improves within 2–3 weeks and returns to 6/12 or better in 95% of previously unaffected eyes. Optic atrophy subsequently develops if there has been destruction of sufficient optic nerve fibers.

Optic neuritis is strongly associated with demyelinating disease, particularly multiple sclerosis. Among patients with clinically isolated optic neuritis, about 40% will develop multiple sclerosis within 10 years but the visual and neurologic prognosis is good. The major risk factors are female gender, multiple white matter lesions on brain MRI scan, and cerebrospinal fluid oligoclonal bands.

In acute demyelinating optic neuritis, intravenous methylprednisolone therapy followed by oral prednisolone accelerates visual recovery. Use in an individual patient is determined by the degree of visual loss, the state of the fellow eye, and the patient's visual requirements. In patients with a first episode of optic neuritis and multiple cerebral white matter lesions, long-term interferon therapy reduces the risk of subsequent development of multiple sclerosis by 25% at 2–3 years.

Optic neuritis also occurs with viral infections (including measles, mumps, influenza, and those caused by the varicella-zoster virus), with various autoimmune disorders, particularly systemic lupus erythematosus, and by spread of inflammation from meninges, orbital tissues, or paranasal sinuses. Optic neuritis due to herpes zoster or systemic lupus erythematosus generally has a poorer prognosis and requires high-dose intravenous corticosteroid therapy.

All patients with optic neuritis should be referred urgently for neuro-ophthalmologic assessment. Any patient with isolated optic neuritis in which visual recovery does not occur requires exclusion of a compressive lesion or an intrinsic optic nerve tumor.

Beck RW et al: Visual function more than 10 years after optic neuritis: experience of the optic neuritis treatment trial. Am J Ophthalmol 2004;137:77. [PMID: 14700647]

Frohman EM et al: The neuro-ophthalmology of multiple sclerosis. Lancet Neurol 2005;4:111. [PMID: 15664543]

Miller D et al: Clinically isolated syndromes suggestive of multiple sclerosis, part I: natural history, pathogenesis, diagnosis, and prognosis. Lancet Neurol 2005;4:281. [PMID: 15847841]

Tintore M et al: Is optic neuritis more benign than other first attacks in multiple sclerosis? Ann Neurol 2005;57:210. [PMID: 15668965]

OPTIC DISK SWELLING

Optic disk swelling may result from intraocular disease, orbital and optic nerve lesions, severe hypertensive retinochoroidopathy, or raised intracranial pressure. Intraocular causes include central retinal vein occlusion, posterior uveitis, and posterior scleritis. Optic nerve lesions causing disk swelling include optic neuritis; anterior ischemic optic neuropathy; optic disk drusen (pseudopapilledema); optic nerve sheath meningioma; and nerve infiltration by sarcoidosis, leukemia, or lymphoma. Any orbital lesion causing nerve compression may produce disk swelling.

Papilledema (optic disk swelling due to raised intracranial pressure) is usually bilateral and most commonly produces enlargement of the blind spot without loss of acuity. Chronic papilledema, as in idiopathic intracranial hypertension and dural venous sinus occlusion, may be associated with progressive visual field loss and occasionally with profound loss of acuity. All patients with chronic papilledema must be monitored carefully—especially their visual fields—and optic nerve sheath fenestration or lumboperitoneal shunt is considered in those with progressive visual failure not controlled by medical therapy (weight loss where appropriate and acetazolamide).

Optic disk drusen are a possibility when disk swelling is not associated with any visual disturbance or symptoms of raised intracranial pressure. Exposed optic disk drusen may be obvious clinically or can be demonstrated by their autofluorescence. Buried drusen are best detected by orbital ultrasound or CT scanning. Other family members may be similarly affected.

Friedman DI et al: Idiopathic intracranial hypertension. J Neuroophthalmol 2004;24:138. [PMID: 15179068]

Wilkins JM et al: Visual manifestations of visible and buried optic disc drusen. J Neuroophthalmol 2004;24:125. [PMID: 15179065]

OCULAR MOTOR PALSIES

In complete **third nerve paralysis**, there is ptosis with a divergent and slightly depressed eye. Extraocular movements are restricted in all directions except laterally (preserved lateral rectus function). Intact fourth nerve (superior oblique) function is detected by the presence of inward rotation on attempted depression of the eye.

Pupillary involvement (dilated pupil that does not react to accommodation or to light shone in either eye) is an important sign differentiating "surgical" from "medical" causes of isolated third nerve palsy. Compressive lesions of the third nerve—eg, aneurysm of the posterior communicating artery and uncal herniation due to a supratentorial mass lesion—characteristically have pupillary involvement. Patients with painful isolated third nerve palsy and pupillary involvement are assumed to have a posterior communicating artery aneurysm until this has been excluded. Medical causes of isolated third nerve palsy include diabetes, hypertension, and giant cell arteritis.

Fourth nerve paralysis causes upward deviation of the eye with failure of depression on adduction. There is vertical diplopia that becomes most apparent on attempted reading and descending stairs. Many cases of isolated fourth nerve palsy are due to a congenital lesion. Trauma is a major cause of acquired—particularly bilateral—fourth nerve palsy, but cerebral neoplasms and medical causes such as in third nerve palsies should also be considered.

Sixth nerve paralysis causes convergent squint in the primary position with failure of abduction of the affected eye, producing horizontal diplopia that increases on gaze to the affected side and on looking into the distance. It is an important sign of raised intracranial pressure. Sixth nerve palsy may also be due to trauma, neoplasms, brainstem lesions, or medical causes.

An intracranial or intraorbital mass lesion should be considered in any patient with an isolated ocular motor palsy. In patients with isolated ocular motor nerve palsies presumed to be due to medical causes, brain MRI is generally only necessary if recovery has not begun within 3 months, although a recent study suggests that it should be undertaken in all cases.

Ocular motor nerve palsies occurring in association with other neurologic signs may be due to lesions in the brainstem, the cavernous sinus, or in the orbit. Lesions around the cavernous sinus involve the upper divisions of the trigeminal nerve, the ocular motor nerves, and occasionally the optic chiasm. Orbital apex lesions involve the optic nerve and the ocular motor nerves.

Myasthenia and dysthyroid eye disease must always be considered in the differential diagnosis of disordered extraocular movements.

Chou KL et al: Acute ocular motor mononeuropathies: prospective study of the roles of neuroimaging and clinical assessment. J Neurol Sci 2004;219:35. [PMID: 15050435]

DYSTHYROID EYE DISEASE

Dysthyroid eye disease is a clinical syndrome caused by deposition of mucopolysaccharides and infiltration with chronic inflammatory cells of the orbital tissues, particularly the extraocular muscles. Patients may have clinical or laboratory evidence of thyroid dysfunction, elevated thyroid autoantibodies, or no detectable abnormality outside the orbit. Radioiodine therapy and cigarette smoking increase its severity.

The primary clinical features are proptosis, lid retraction and lid lag, conjunctival chemosis and episcleral inflammation, and extraocular muscle abnormalities due to restriction of their actions. Resulting symptoms are cosmetic abnormalities, surface irritation, which usually responds to artificial tears, and diplopia, which should be treated conservatively (eg, with prisms) in the active stages of the disease and only by surgery when the disease has been static for at least 6 months.

The important complications are corneal exposure and optic nerve compression, both of which may lead to marked visual loss. Treatment options are intravenous pulse methylprednisolone therapy (eg, 1 g daily for 3 days, repeated weekly for 3 weeks), oral prednisolone 80–100 mg/d, radiotherapy, or surgery (usually consisting of extensive removal of bone from the medial, inferior, and lateral walls of the orbit), either singly or in combination.

The optimal management of moderately severe dysthyroid eye disease without visual loss is controversial. Systemic corticosteroids and radiotherapy have not been shown to provide definite long-term benefit. Peribulbar corticosteroid injections have been advocated. Surgical decompression may be justified in patients with marked proptosis. Lateral tarsorrhaphy may be used for moderately severe corneal exposure. Other procedures are particularly useful for correcting lid retraction but should not be undertaken until the orbital disease is quiescent and orbital decompression

or extraocular muscle surgery has been undertaken. Establishing and maintaining euthyroidism are important in all cases.

Bartalena L et al: An update on medical management of Graves' ophthalmopathy. J Endocrinol Invest 2005;28:469. [PMID: 16075933]

Kahaly GJ et al: Randomized, single blind trial of intravenous versus oral steroid monotherapy in Graves' orbitopathy. Clin Endocrinol Metab 2005;90:5234. [PMID: 15998777]

Marcocci C et al: Comparison of the effectiveness and tolerability of intravenous or oral glucocorticoids associated with orbital radiotherapy in the management of severe Graves' ophthalmopathy: results of a prospective, single-blind, randomized study. J Clin Endocrinol Metab 2001;86:3562. [PMID: 11502779]

Wakelkamp IM et al: Surgical or medical decompression as a first-line treatment of optic neuropathy in Graves' ophthalmopathy? A randomized controlled trial. Clin Endocrinol 2005;63:323. [PMID: 16117821]

ORBITAL CELLULITIS

Orbital cellulitis is manifested by an abrupt onset of fever, proptosis, restriction of extraocular movements, and swelling with redness of the lids. Infection of the paranasal sinuses is the usual underlying cause. Immediate treatment with intravenous antibiotics is necessary to prevent optic nerve damage and spread of infection to the cavernous sinuses, meninges, and brain. The response to antibiotics is usually excellent, but abscess formation may necessitate surgical drainage. In immunocompromised patients, zygomycosis must be considered.

Greenberg RN et al: Zygomycosis (mucormycosis): emerging clinical importance and new treatments. Curr Opin Infect Dis 2004;17:517. [PMID: 15640705]

Howe L et al: Guidelines for the management of periorbital cellulitis/abscess. Clin Otolaryngol 2004;29:725. [PMID: 15533168]

OCULAR TRAUMA

Conjunctival & Corneal Foreign Bodies

If a patient complains of "something in my eye" and gives a consistent history, a foreign body is usually present on the cornea or under the upper lid even though it may not be visible. Visual acuity should be tested before treatment is instituted, as a basis for comparison in the event of complications.

After a local anesthetic (eg, proparacaine, 0.5%) is instilled, the eye is examined with a hand flashlight, using oblique illumination, and loupe. Corneal foreign bodies may be made more apparent by the instillation of sterile fluorescein. They are then removed with a sterile wet cotton-tipped applicator. Polymyxin-bacitracin ophthalmic ointment should be instilled. It is not necessary to patch the eye, but the patient must be examined 24 hours later for secondary infection of the crater. If a corneal foreign body cannot be removed in this manner, the patient should be referred to an ophthalmologist.

Steel foreign bodies usually leave a diffuse rust ring. This requires excision of the affected tissue and is best done under local anesthesia using a slit lamp. **Caution:** Anesthetic drops should not be given to the patient for self-administration.

If there is no infection, a layer of corneal epithelial cells will line the crater within 24 hours. The intact corneal epithelium forms an effective barrier to infection, but once it is disturbed the cornea becomes extremely susceptible to infection. Early infection is manifested by a white necrotic area around the crater and a small amount of gray exudate. These patients are referred immediately to an ophthalmologist; untreated corneal infection may lead to loss of the eye.

In the case of a foreign body under the upper lid, a local anesthetic is instilled and the lid is everted by grasping the lashes gently and exerting pressure on the mid portion of the outer surface of the upper lid with an applicator. If a foreign body is present, it can easily be removed by passing a wet sterile cotton-tipped applicator across the conjunctival surface.

Intraocular Foreign Body

Intraocular foreign body requires emergency treatment by an ophthalmologist. Patients giving a history of "something hitting the eye"—particularly while hammering on metal or using grinding equipment—must be assessed for this possibility, especially when no corneal foreign body is seen, a corneal or scleral wound is apparent, or there is marked visual loss or media opacity. Such patients must be treated as for corneal laceration (see below) and referred without delay. Intraocular foreign bodies significantly increase the risk of intraocular infection.

Corneal Abrasions

A patient with a corneal abrasion complains of severe pain and photophobia. There is often a history of trauma to the eye, commonly involving a fingernail, piece of paper, or contact lens. Visual acuity is recorded, and the cornea and conjunctiva are examined with a light and loupe to rule out a foreign body. If an abrasion is suspected but cannot be seen, sterile fluorescein is instilled into the conjunctival sac: the area of corneal abrasion will stain a deeper green than the surrounding cornea.

Treatment includes polymyxin-bacitracin ophthalmic ointment, mydriatic (cyclopentolate 1%), and analgesics either topical or oral nonsteroidal anti-inflammatory agents. Padding the eye is probably not helpful. The patient should be reviewed within 48 hours to be certain the cornea has healed. Recurrent corneal erosion may follow corneal abrasions.

Wilson SA et al: Management of corneal abrasions. Am Fam Physician 2004;70:123. [PMID: 15259527]

Contusions

Contusion injuries of the eye and surrounding structures may cause ecchymosis ("black eye"), subconjunctival hemorrhage, edema or rupture of the cornea, hemorrhage into the anterior chamber (hyphema), rupture of the root of the iris (iridodialysis), paralysis of the pupillary sphincter, paralysis of the muscles of accommodation, cataract, dislocation of the lens, vitreous hemorrhage, retinal hemorrhage and edema (most common in the macular area), detachment of the retina, rupture of the choroid, fracture of the orbital floor ("blowout fracture"), or optic nerve injury. Many of these injuries are immediately obvious; others may not become apparent for days or weeks. Patients with moderate to severe contusions should be seen by an ophthalmologist.

Any injury causing hyphema involves the danger of secondary hemorrhage, which may cause intractable glaucoma with permanent visual loss. The patient should be advised to rest until complete resolution has occurred. Daily ophthalmologic assessment is essential. Aspirin and any drugs inhibiting coagulation increase the risk of secondary hemorrhage and are to be avoided. Sickle cell anemia or trait adversely affects outcome.

Lacerations

A. Lids

If the lid margin is lacerated, the patient should be referred for specialized care, since permanent notching may result. Lacerations of the lower eyelid near the inner canthus often sever the lower canaliculus. Lid lacerations not involving the margin may be sutured like any skin laceration.

B. Conjunctiva

In lacerations of the conjunctiva, sutures are not necessary. To prevent infection, sulfonamides or other antibiotics are instilled into the eye until the laceration is healed.

C. Cornea or Sclera

Patients with suspected corneal or scleral lacerations must be seen promptly by an ophthalmologist. Manipulation is kept to a minimum, since pressure may result in extrusion of the intraocular contents. The eye is bandaged lightly and covered with a metal shield that rests on the orbital bones above and below. The patient should be instructed not to squeeze the eye shut and to remain still. The eye is routinely imaged by radiography, and CT scanning if necessary, to identify and localize any metallic intraocular foreign body. MRI is contraindicated because of the risk of movement of the foreign body in the magnetic field. Endophthalmitis occurs in over 5% of open globe injuries.

Essex RW et al: Post-traumatic endophthalmitis. Ophthalmology 2004;111:2015. [PMID: 15522366]

ULTRAVIOLET KERATITIS (Actinic Keratitis)

Ultraviolet burns of the cornea are usually caused by use of a sunlamp without eye protection, exposure to a welding arc, or exposure to the sun when skiing ("snow blindness"). There are no immediate symptoms, but about 6–12 hours later the patient complains of agonizing pain and severe photophobia. Slit-lamp examination after instillation of sterile fluorescein shows diffuse punctate staining of both corneas.

Treatment consists of binocular patching and instillation of 1–2 drops of 1% cyclopentolate (to relieve the discomfort of ciliary spasm). All patients recover within 24–48 hours without complications. Local anesthetics should not be prescribed.

Yen YL et al: Photokeratoconjunctivitis caused by different light sources. Am J Emerg Med 2004;22:511. [PMID: 15666251]

Chemical Conjunctivitis & Keratitis

Chemical burns are treated by irrigation of the eyes with saline solution or plain water as soon as possible after exposure. Neutralization of an acid with an alkali or vice versa generates heat and may cause further damage. Alkali injuries are more serious and require prolonged irrigation, since alkalies are not precipitated by the proteins of the eye as are acids. It is important to remove any retained particulate matter such as is typically present in injuries involving cement and building plaster. This may require double eversion of the upper lid. The pupil should be dilated with 1% cyclopentolate, 1 drop twice a day, to relieve discomfort and prophylactic topical antibiotics should be started. In moderate to severe injuries, intensive topical corticosteroids and topical and systemic vitamin C are also necessary. Complications include mucus deficiency, scarring of the cornea and conjunctiva, symblepharon (adhesions between the tarsal and bulbar conjunctiva), tear duct obstruction, and secondary infection. It can be difficult to assess severity of chemical burns without slit-lamp examination.

PRINCIPLES OF TREATMENT OF OCULAR INFECTIONS

Before determining the drug of choice for treatment of ocular infection, the causative organisms must be identified, but in most cases empiric treatment is used in the first instance. In the treatment of conjunctivitis and for prophylaxis against ocular infection, it is preferable to use a drug that is not given systemically. Although fluoroquinolones, including the fourth-generation fluoroquinolones, are advocated for the treatment of conjunctivitis, they should be reserved for treatment of bacterial keratitis and other serious infections. Of the available local antibacterial agents, the sulfonamides are effective and inexpensive; sulfisoxazole and sodium sulfacetamide are examples. The sulfonamides have the added advantages of low allergenicity and effectiveness against the chlamydial group of organisms. They are available in ointment or solution form. Combined bacitracin-polymyxin ointment is often used prophylactically after corneal foreign body removal for the protection it affords against both gram-positive and gram-negative organisms.

Among the most effective broad-spectrum antibiotics for ophthalmic use are fluoroquinolones (ciprofloxacin, ofloxacin, norfloxacin, levofloxacin, moxifloxacin, and gatifloxacin), gentamicin, tobramycin, and neomycin. For pneumococcus, one of the newer fluoroquinolones, penicillin G, or nafcillin (if β-lactamase resistance is present) is required. Allergic reactions to neomycin are common. Other antibiotics frequently used are erythromycin, the tetracyclines, and the cephalosporins.

Method of Administration

Most ocular anti-infective drugs are administered locally. Ointments have greater therapeutic effectiveness than solutions, since contact can be maintained longer. However, they do cause blurring of vision; if this must be avoided, solutions should be used.

Systemic administration is required for all intraocular infections, orbital cellulitis, dacryocystitis, gonococcal keratoconjunctivitis, inclusion conjunctivitis, and severe external infection that does not respond to local treatment.

TECHNIQUES USED IN THE TREATMENT OF OCULAR DISORDERS

Table 7–2 lists commonly used ophthalmic drugs and their indications and costs.

Instilling Medications

The patient is placed in a chair with head tilted back, both eyes open, and looking up. The lower lid is retracted slightly, and 2 drops of liquid are instilled into the lower cul-de-sac. The patient looks down while finger contact is maintained, so that the eyes are not squeezed shut. Ointments are instilled in the same general manner.

For self-medication, the same techniques are used except that medications are usually better instilled with the patient lying down.

Eye Bandage

Most eye bandages should be applied firmly enough to hold the lid securely against the cornea. An ordinary patch consisting of gauze-covered cotton is usually sufficient. Tape is applied from the cheek to the forehead.

Eyelid Taping

Eyelid taping, such as for corneal protection in facial palsy, is best achieved with 1-inch-width transparent plastic adhesive tape (eg, Transpore or even Sellotape) placed horizontally over the closed eyelids from the side of the nose to the temple.

Table 7–2. Topical ophthalmic agents.

Agent	Representative Cost/Size [1]	Recommended Regimen	Indications
AGENTS FOR GLAUCOMA AND OCULAR HYPERTENSION			
Sympathomimetics			
Apraclonidine HCl 0.5% solution (Iopidine)	$74.28/5 mL	1 drop three times daily	Reduction of intraocular pressure. Expensive. Reserve for treatment of resistant cases.
Apraclonidine HCl 1% solution (Iopidine)	$12.32/unit dose 0.1 mL	1 drop 1 hour before and immediately after anterior segment laser surgery	To control or prevent elevations of intraocular pressure after laser trabeculoplasty or iridotomy.
Brimonidine tartrate 0.2% solution (Alphagan)	$32.65/5 mL	1 drop two or three times daily	Reduction of intraocular pressure.
Dipivefrin HCl 0.1% solution (Propine)[2]	$14.07/5 mL	1 drop every 12 hours	Open-angle glaucoma.
β-Adrenergic blocking agents			
Betaxolol HCl 0.5% solution and 0.25% suspension (Betoptic S)[3]	0.5%: $44.56/10 mL 0.25%: $85.98/10 mL	1 drop twice daily	Reduction of intraocular pressure.
Levobunolol HCl 0.25% and 0.5% solution (Betagan)[4]	0.5%: $32.25/10 mL	1 drop once or twice daily	
Metipranolol HCl 0.3% solution (OptiPranolol)[4]	$26.85/10 mL	1 drop twice daily	
Timolol 0.25% and 0.5% solution (Betimol)[4]	0.5%: $42.84/10 mL	1 drop once or twice daily	
Timolol maleate 0.25% and 0.5% solution (Timoptic) and 0.25% and 0.5% gel (Timoptic-XE)[4]	0.5% solution: $32.35/10 mL 0.5% gel: $35.00/5 mL	1 drop once or twice daily	
Miotics			
Pilocarpine HCl (various)[5] 1–4%, 6%, 8%, and 10%	2%: $11.80/15 mL	1 drop three or four times daily	Reduction of intraocular pressure, treatment of acute or chronic angle-closure glaucoma, and pupillary constriction.
Pilocarpine HCl 4% gel (Pilopine HS)	$43.80/4 g	Apply 0.5-inch ribbon in lower conjunctival sac at bedtime	
Carbonic anhydrase inhibitors			
Dorzolamide HCl 2% solution (Trusopt)	$56.53/10 mL	1 drop three times daily	Reduction of intraocular pressure.
Brinzolamide 1% suspension (Azopt)	$71.76/10 mL	1 drop three times daily	
Prostaglandin analogs			
Bimatoprost 0.03% solution (Lumigan)	$66.45/2.5 mL	1 drop once daily at night	
Latanoprost 0.005% solution (Xalatan)	$58.84/2.5 mL	1 drop once or twice daily at night	
Travoprost 0.004% solution (Travatan)	$62.70/2.5 mL	1 drop once daily at night	Reduction of intraocular pressure.
Unoprostone 0.15% solution (Rescula)	Not available in United States	1 drop twice daily	

(continued)

Table 7–2. Topical ophthalmic agents. (continued)

Agent	Representative Cost/Size[1]	Recommended Regimen	Indications
Combined preparations			
Xalacom (latanoprost 0.005% and timolol 0.5%)	Not available in United States	1 drop daily in the morning	Reduction of intraocular pressure.
Cosopt (dorzolamide 2% and timolol 0.5%)	$53.51/5 mL	1 drop twice daily	Reduction of intraocular pressure.
Combigan (brimonidine 0.2% and timolol 0.5%)	Not available in United States	1 drop twice daily	Reduction of intraocular pressure.
ANTI-INFLAMMATORY AGENTS			
Nonsteroidal anti-inflammatory agents[6]			
Diclofenac sodium 0.1% solution (Voltaren)	$67.61/5 mL	1 drop to operated eye four times daily beginning 24 hours after cataract surgery and continuing through first 2 postoperative weeks	Treatment of postoperative inflammation following cataract extraction and laser corneal surgery.
Flurbiprofen sodium 0.03% solution (various)	$8.73/2.5 mL	1 drop every half hour beginning 2 hours before surgery; 1 drop to operated eye four times daily beginning 24 hours after cataract surgery	Inhibition of intraoperative miosis. Treatment of cystoid macular edema and inflammation after cataract surgery.
Ketorolac tromethamine 0.5% solution (Acular)	$71.53/5 mL	1 drop four times daily	Relief of ocular itching due to seasonal allergic conjunctivitis.
Corticosteroids[7]			
Dexamethasone sodium phosphate 0.1% solution (various)	$17.31/5 mL	1 or 2 drops as often as indicated by severity; use every hour during the day and every 2 hours during the night in severe inflammation; taper off as inflammation decreases	Treatment of steroid-responsive inflammatory conditions of anterior segment.
Dexamethasone sodium phosphate 0.05% ointment (various)	$6.34/3.5 g	Apply thin coating on lower conjunctival sac three or four times daily	
Fluorometholone 0.1% suspension (various)[8]	$26.16/10 mL	1 or 2 drops as often as indicated by severity; use every hour during the day and every 2 hours during the night in severe inflammation; taper off as inflammation decreases	
Fluorometholone 0.25% suspension (FML Forte)[8]	$37.60/10 mL		
Fluorometholone 0.1% ointment (FML S.O.P.)	$34.00/3.5 g	Apply thin coating on lower conjunctival sac three or four times daily	
Medrysone 1% suspension (HMS)	$33.24/10 mL	1 or 2 drops as often as indicated by severity of inflammation; use every hour during the day and every 2 hours during the night in severe inflammation; taper off as inflammation decreases	
Prednisolone acetate 0.12% suspension (Pred Mild)	$36.14/10 mL		
Prednisolone sodium phosphate 0.125% solution (various)	$30.90/10 mL		

(continued)

Table 7–2. Topical ophthalmic agents. (continued)

Agent	Representative Cost/Size [1]	Recommended Regimen	Indications
Corticosteroids[8] (continued)			
Prednisolone acetate 1% suspension (various)	$23.10/10 mL	1 or 2 drops as often as indicated by severity of inflammation; use every hour during the day and every 2 hours during the night in severe inflammation; taper off as inflammation decreases	Treatment of steroid-responsive inflammatory conditions of anterior segment.
Prednisolone sodium phosphate 1% solution (various)	$36.14/10 mL		
Rimexolone 1% suspension (Vexol)	$52.56/10 mL		
Mast cell stabilizers			
Cromolyn sodium 4% solution (Crolom)	$37.25/10 mL	1 drop four to six times daily	Allergic conjunctivitis.
Ketotifen fumarate 0.025% solution (Zaditor)	$66.80/5 mL	1 drop two to four times daily	Allergic conjunctivitis.
Lodoxamide tromethamine 0.1% solution (Alomide)	$77.28/10 mL	1 or 2 drops four times daily (up to 3 months)	Allergic conjunctivitis and vernal keratoconjunctivitis.
Nedocromil sodium 2% solution (Alocril)	$79.85/5 mL	1 drop twice daily	Allergic conjunctivitis.
Olopatadine hydrochloride 0.1% solution (Patanol)	$77.94/5 mL	1 drop twice daily	Allergic conjunctivitis.
ANTIBIOTIC OINTMENTS AND SOLUTIONS			
Bacitracin 500 units/g ointment (various)[9]	$4.75/3.5 g	Refer to package insert (instructions vary)	Infections involving lid, conjunctiva, or cornea.
Chloramphenicol 1% (10 mg/g) ointment (Ocu-chlor)[10]	$1.65/3.5 g		As above, with both gram-positive and gram-negative coverage.
Ciprofloxacin HCl (Ciloxan)	0.3% solution: $53.16/5 mL 0.3% ointment: $61.56/3.5 g		
Erythromycin 0.5% ointment (various)[11]	$5.73/3.5 g		
Gatifloxacin 0.3% solution (Zymar)	$56.42/5 mL		
Gentamicin sulfate 0.3% solution (various)	$8.17/5 mL		
Gentamicin sulfate 0.3% ointment (various)	$17.70/3.5 g		
Moxifloxacin sulfate 0.5% solution (Vigamox)	$54.18/3 mL		
Norfloxacin 0.3% solution (Chibroxin)	Not available in United States		
Ofloxacin 0.3% solution (Ocuflox)	$51.08/5 mL		
Polymyxin B sulfate 500,000 units, powder for solution (Polymyxin B Sulfate Sterile)[12]	$13.80/500,000 units		
Tobramycin 0.3% solution (various)	$15.00/5 mL	Refer to package insert (instructions vary)	As above, with both gram-positive and gram-negative coverage.
Tobramycin 0.3% ointment (Tobrex)	$53.88/3.5 g		

(continued)

Table 7–2. Topical ophthalmic agents. (continued)

Agent	Representative Cost/Size [1]	Recommended Regimen	Indications
SULFONAMIDES			
Sulfacetamide sodium 10% solution (various)	$3.53/15 mL	1 or 2 drops every 1–3 hours	Conjunctivitis, corneal ulcer, and other superficial ocular infections due to susceptible microorganisms.
Sulfacetamide sodium 10% ointment (various)	$8.10/3.5 g	Apply small amount (0.5 inch) into lower conjunctival sac once to four times daily and at bedtime	Conjunctivitis, corneal ulcer, and other superficial ocular infections due to susceptible microorganisms.
Note: Many combination products containing antibiotics, antibiotics and corticosteroids, or sulfonamides and corticosteroids are available as solutions, suspensions, or ointments.			
TOPICAL ANTIFUNGAL AGENTS			
Natamycin 5% suspension (Natacyn)	$164.58/15 mL	1 drop every 1–2 hours	Fungal blepharitis, conjunctivitis, and keratitis caused by susceptible organisms. Drug of choice for *Fusarium solani* keratitis.
TOPICAL ANTIVIRAL AGENTS			
Ganciclovir 4.5 mg surgical insert (Vitrasert)	$5000.00 each	1 implant every 5–8 months	Treatment of cytomegalovirus retinitis in patients with AIDS.
Trifluridine 1% solution (Viroptic)	$96.55/7.5 mL	1 drop onto cornea every 2 hours while awake for a maximum daily dose of 9 drops until resolution occurs; then an additional 7 days of 1 drop every 4 hours while awake (minimum five times daily)	Primary keratoconjunctivitis and recurrent epithelial keratitis due to herpes simplex virus types 1 or 2.[13]
TOPICAL ANTIHISTAMINES[14]			
Levocabastine HCl 0.05% ophthalmic solution (Livostin)	$94.59/10 mL	1 drop four times daily (up to 2 weeks)	Allergic conjunctivitis; temporary relief of seasonal allergic conjunctivitis.
Emedastine difumarate 0.05% solution (Emadine)	$61.08/5 mL	1 drop four times daily	Allergic conjunctivitis.

[1] Average wholesale price (AWP, for AB-rated generic when available) for quantity listed. Source: *Red Book Update*, Vol. 25, No. 1, January 2006. AWP may not accurately represent the actual pharmacy cost because wide contractual variations exist among institutions.
[2] Macular edema occurs in 30% of patients.
[3] Cardioselective (β_1) β-blocker.
[4] Nonselective (β_1 and β_2) β-blocker. Monitor all patients for systemic side effects, particularly exacerbation of asthma.
[5] Decreased night vision, headaches possible.
[6] Cross-sensitivity to aspirin and other nonsteroidal anti-inflammatory drugs.
[7] Long-term use may increase intraocular pressure or cause cataracts.

[8] May be less likely to elevate intraocular pressure.
[9] Little efficacy against gram-negative organisms (except *Neisseria*).
[10] Aplastic anemia has been reported with prolonged ophthalmic use. Use only in serious infections for which less toxic drugs are ineffective or contraindicated.
[11] Also indicated for prophylaxis of ophthalmia neonatorum due to *N gonorrhoeae* or *C trachomatis*. Increasing resistance of *S pneumoniae* and *P aeruginosa* has been noted.
[12] No gram-positive coverage.
[13] Recurrences are common and call for additional 7-day treatment.
[14] Antihistamines (topical) are potential sensitizers and may produce local reactions.

PRECAUTIONS IN MANAGEMENT OF OCULAR DISORDERS

Use of Local Anesthetics

Unsupervised self-administration of local anesthetics is dangerous because the patient may further injure an anesthetized eye without knowing it. The drug may also interfere with the normal healing process.

Pupillary Dilation

Dilating the pupil can very occasionally precipitate acute glaucoma if the patient has a narrow anterior chamber angle and should be undertaken with caution if the anterior chamber is obviously shallow (readily determined by oblique illumination of the anterior segment of the eye). A short-acting mydriatic such as tropicamide should be used and the patient warned to

Table 7–3. Adverse ocular effects of systemic drugs.

Drug	Possible Side Effects
Respiratory drugs	
Oxygen	Retinopathy of prematurity.
Anticholinergic bronchodilators	Angle-closure glaucoma due to mydriasis, blurring of vision due to cycloplegia.
Sympathomimetic bronchodilators and decongestants	Angle-closure glaucoma due to mydriasis
Cetirizine	Oculogyric crisis.
Cardiovascular system drugs	
Digitalis	Disturbance of color vision, photopsia.
Thiazides	Xanthopsia (yellow vision), myopia.
Carbonic anhydrase inhibitors (acetazolamide)	Stevens-Johnson syndrome, myopia.
Amiodarone	Corneal deposits, optic neuropathy, thyroid ophthalmopathy.
Sildenafil	Ischemic optic neuropathy.
Statins	Myasthenic syndrome.
Gastrointestinal drugs	
Anticholinergic agents	Angle-closure glaucoma due to mydriasis, blurring of vision due to cycloplegia.
Central nervous system drugs	
Anticholinergic agents including preoperative medications	Angle-closure glaucoma due to mydriasis, blurring of vision due to cycloplegia.
Phenothiazines	Deposits of pigment in conjunctiva, cornea, lens, and retina, oculogyric crises.
Haloperidol	Capsular cataract.
Lithium carbonate	Proptosis, oculogyric crisis, nystagmus.
Amphetamines	Widening of palpebral fissure, blurring of vision due to mydriasis.
Monoamine oxidase inhibitors	Nystagmus.
Tricyclic agents	Angle-closure glaucoma due to mydriasis, blurring of vision due to cycloplegia.
Phenytoin	Nystagmus.
Neostigmine	Nystagmus, miosis.
Morphine	Miosis.
Diazepam	Nystagmus.
Topiramate	Angle-closure glaucoma, myopia.
Paroxetine	Angle-closure glaucoma.
Vigabatrin	Visual field constriction.
Obstetric drugs	
Sympathomimetic tocolytics	Angle-closure glaucoma due to mydriasis

(continued)

Table 7–3. Adverse ocular effects of systemic drugs. (continued)

Drug	Possible Side Effects
Hormonal agents	
Corticosteroids	Cataract (posterior subcapsular); susceptibility to viral (herpes simplex), bacterial, and fungal infections; steroid-induced glaucoma.
Female sex hormones	Retinal artery occlusion, retinal vein occlusion, papilledema, extraocular muscle palsies, ischemic optic neuropathy.
Tamoxifen	Crystalline retinal deposits, optic neuropathy.
Immunosuppressants	
Cyclosporine	Optic neuropathy.
Tacrolimus	Optic neuropathy.
Antibacterials	
Chloramphenicol	Optic neuropathy.
Streptomycin	Optic neuropathy.
Tetracycline	Papilledema, myopia.
Doxycycline	Papilledema.
Minocycline	Papilledema.
Sulfonamides	Stevens-Johnson syndrome, myopia.
Ethambutol	Optic neuropathy.
Isoniazid	Optic neuropathy.
Antimalarial agents	
Chloroquine, hydroxychloroquine	Retinal degeneration principally involving the macula, keratopathy.
Amebicides	
Iodochlorhydroxyquin	Optic neuropathy.
Chemotherapeutic agents	
Chlorambucil	Optic neuropathy.
Vincristine	Optic neuropathy.
Heavy metals	
Gold salts	Deposits in the cornea and conjunctiva.
Lead compounds	Optic neuropathy, papilledema, ocular palsies.
Chelating agents	
Penicillamine	Ocular pemphigoid, optic neuropathy, myasthenic syndrome.
Desferrioxamine	Retinopathy, optic neuropathy, lens opacity.
Oral hypoglycemic agents	
Chlorpropamide	Refractive error, Stevens-Johnson syndrome, optic neuropathy.
Vitamins	
Vitamin A	Papilledema.
Vitamin D	Band-shaped keratopathy.
Antirheumatic agents	
Salicylates	Subconjunctival or retinal hemorrhages, nystagmus.
Indomethacin	Corneal deposits.
Phenylbutazone	Retinal hemorrhages.
Dermatologic agents	
Retinoids (isotretinoin, tretinoin, acitretin, and etretinate)	Papilledema, blepharoconjunctivitis, corneal opacities, decreased contact lens tolerance, decreased dark adaptation, teratogenic ocular abnormalities.
Bisphosphonates	
Pamidronate	Scleritis, uveitis, conjunctival hyperemia.
Alendronate	Scleritis.

report immediately if ocular discomfort or redness develops. Angle closure is more likely to occur if pilocarpine is used to overcome pupillary dilation than if the pupil is allowed to constrict naturally.

Corticosteroid Therapy

Repeated use of local corticosteroids presents several hazards: herpes simplex (dendritic) keratitis, fungal infection, open-angle glaucoma, and cataract formation. Furthermore, perforation of the cornea may occur when the corticosteroids are used for herpes simplex keratitis. Topical nonsteroidal anti-inflammatory agents are being used increasingly. The potential for causing or exacerbating systemic hypertension, diabetes mellitus, gastritis, or osteoporosis must always be borne in mind when systemic corticosteroids are prescribed, such as for uveitis or giant cell arteritis.

Garrott HM et al: Glaucoma from topical corticosteroids to the eyelids. Clin Exp Ophthalmol 2004;32:224. [PMID: 15068445]

Ross JJ et al: Facial eczema and sight-threatening glaucoma. J R Soc Med 2004;97:485. [PMID: 15459262]

Contaminated Eye Medications

Ophthalmic solutions are prepared with the same degree of care as fluids intended for intravenous administration, but once bottles are opened there is always a risk of contamination, particularly with solutions of tetracaine, proparacaine, fluorescein, and any preservative-free preparations. The most dangerous is fluorescein, as this solution is frequently contaminated with *P aeruginosa*, which can rapidly destroy the eye. Sterile fluorescein filter paper strips are recommended for use in place of fluorescein solutions.

Whether in plastic or glass containers, eye solutions should not remain in use for long periods after the bottle is opened. Four weeks after opening is an absolute maximal time to use a solution containing preservatives before discarding. Preservative-free preparations should be kept refrigerated and discarded within 1 week after opening.

If the eye has been injured accidentally or by surgical trauma, it is of the greatest importance to use freshly opened bottles of sterile medications or single-use eye-dropper units.

Toxic & Hypersensitivity Reactions to Topical Therapy

In patients receiving long-term topical therapy, local toxic or hypersensitivity reactions to the active agent or preservatives may develop, especially if there is inadequate tear secretion. Preservatives in contact lens cleaning solutions may produce similar problems. Burning and soreness are exacerbated by drop instillation or contact lens insertion; occasionally, fibrosis and scarring of the conjunctiva and cornea may occur.

An antibiotic instilled into the eye can sensitize the patient to that drug and cause an allergic reaction upon subsequent systemic administration.

Systemic Effects of Ocular Drugs

The systemic absorption of certain topical drugs (through the conjunctival vessels and lacrimal drainage system) must be considered when there is a systemic medical contraindication to the use of the drug. Ophthalmic solutions of the nonselective β-blockers, eg, timolol, may worsen patients with congestive heart failure or asthma. Atropine ointment should be prescribed for children rather than the drops, since absorption of the 1% topical solution may be toxic. Phenylephrine eye drops may precipitate hypertensive crises and angina. Also to be considered are adverse interactions between systemically administered and ocular drugs. Using only 1 or 2 drops at a time and a few minutes of nasolacrimal occlusion or eyelid closure ensure maximum efficacy and decrease systemic side effects of topical agents.

Fraunfelder FW et al: Adverse systemic effects from pledgets of topical ocular phenylephrine 10%. Am J Ophthalmol 2002; 134:624. [PMID: 12383833]

ADVERSE OCULAR EFFECTS OF SYSTEMIC DRUGS

Systemically administered drugs produce a wide variety of adverse effects on the visual system. Table 7–3 lists the major examples.

Flach AJ, Fraunfelder FW: Ocular and systemic side effects of drugs. In: *Vaughan & Asbury's General Ophthalmology,* 16th ed. Riordan-Eva P, Whitcher JP (editors). McGraw-Hill, 2004.

Fraunfelder FW et al: Adverse ocular drug reactions recently identified by the National Registry of Drug-Induced Ocular Side Effects. Ophthalmology 2004;111:1275. [PMID: 15234126]

Ear, Nose, & Throat

8

Robert K. Jackler, MD, & Michael J. Kaplan, MD

■ DISEASES OF THE EAR

HEARING LOSS

ESSENTIALS OF DIAGNOSIS

- Three main types of hearing loss: conductive, sensory, and neural.
- Most commonly due to cerumen impaction or transient auditory tube dysfunction associated with upper respiratory tract infection.

Classification & Epidemiology

A. CONDUCTIVE HEARING LOSS

Conductive hearing loss results from dysfunction of the external or middle ear. There are four mechanisms, each resulting in impairment of the passage of sound vibrations to the inner ear: (1) obstruction (eg, cerumen impaction), (2) mass loading (eg, middle ear effusion), (3) stiffness effect (eg, otosclerosis), and (4) discontinuity (eg, ossicular disruption). Conductive losses in adults are most commonly due to cerumen impaction or transient auditory tube dysfunction associated with upper respiratory tract infection. Persistent conductive losses usually result from chronic ear infection, trauma, or otosclerosis. Conductive hearing loss is generally correctable with medical or surgical therapy—or in some cases both.

B. SENSORY HEARING LOSS

Sensory hearing loss results from deterioration of the cochlea, usually due to loss of hair cells from the organ of Corti. Sensorineural losses in adults are common. A gradually progressive, predominantly high-frequency loss with advancing age (presbyacusis) is typical. Other than aging effects, common causes of sensorineural loss include excessive noise exposure, head trauma, and systemic diseases such as diabetes mellitus. Sensory hearing loss is not correctable with medical or surgical therapy but often may be prevented or stabilized.

Angeli SI et al: Etiologic diagnosis of sensorineural hearing loss in adults. Otolaryngol Head Neck Surg 2005;132:890. [PMID: 15944560]

C. NEURAL HEARING LOSS

Neural hearing loss occurs with lesions involving the eighth nerve, auditory nuclei, ascending tracts, or auditory cortex. It is the least common clinically recognized cause of hearing loss. Causes include acoustic neuroma, multiple sclerosis, and cerebrovascular disease.

Jackler RK: A 73-year-old man with hearing loss. JAMA 2003; 289:1557. [PMID: 12672773]

Evaluation of Hearing (Audiology)

In a quiet room, the hearing level may be estimated by having the patient repeat aloud words presented in a soft whisper, a normal spoken voice, or a shout. Tuning forks are useful in differentiating conductive from sensorineural losses. A 512-Hz tuning fork is used, since frequencies below this level elicit a tactile response. In the **Weber test**, the tuning fork is placed on the forehead or front teeth. In conductive losses, the sound appears louder in the poorer-hearing ear, whereas in sensorineural losses it radiates to the better side. In the **Rinne test**, the tuning fork is placed alternately on the mastoid bone and in front of the ear canal. In conductive losses, bone conduction exceeds air conduction; in sensorineural losses, the opposite is true.

Formal audiometric studies are performed in a soundproofed room. Pure-tone thresholds in decibels (dB) are obtained over the range of 250–8000 Hz (the main speech frequencies are between 500 and 3000 Hz) for both air and bone conduction. Conductive losses create a gap between the air and bone thresholds, whereas in sensorineural losses both air and bone thresholds are equally diminished. The threshold of normal hearing is from 0 to 20 dB, which corresponds to the loudness of a soft whisper. Mild hearing loss is indicated by a threshold of 20–40 dB (soft spoken voice), moderate loss by a threshold of 40–60 dB (normal spoken voice), severe loss by a threshold of 60–80 dB (loud spoken voice), and profound loss by a threshold of 80 dB (shout). The clarity of hearing is often impaired in sensorineural hearing loss. This is evaluated by speech discrimination testing, which is reported as percentage correct (90–100% is normal).

The site of the lesion responsible for sensorineural loss—whether it lies in the cochlea or in the central auditory system—may be determined with auditory brainstem-evoked responses.

Every patient who complains of a hearing loss should be referred for audiologic evaluation unless the cause is easily remediable (eg, cerumen impaction, otitis media). Audiologic screening is not recommended for adults with apparently normal hearing unless they are exposed to potentially injurious levels of noise or have reached the age of 65, after which screening evaluations should be done every few years.

Bagai A et al: Does this patient have hearing impairment? JAMA 2006;295:416. [PMID: 16434632]

Hearing Rehabilitation

Patients with hearing loss not correctable by medical therapy may benefit from hearing amplification. Contemporary hearing aids are comparatively free of distortion and have been miniaturized to the point where they often may be contained entirely within the ear canal. To optimize the benefit, a hearing aid must be carefully selected to conform to the nature of the hearing loss. Digitally programmable hearing aids are now becoming available that allow optimization of speech intelligibility and may be tuned to deal with difficult listening circumstances.

Currently, there is much interest focused on the development of semi-implantable and even fully implantable hearing aids. A variety of devices are under development that deliver vibrations—usually via either a rare earth magnet or a piezoceramic crystal—directly to the ossicular chain. Some of these devices are in clinical trials. An alternative strategy, the bone-anchored hearing aid, uses an oscillating post drilled into the mastoid. This technology shows promise in surgically uncorrectable conductive hearing loss as well as in unilateral sensorineural deafness.

Aside from hearing aids, many assistive devices are available to improve comprehension in individual and group settings, to help with hearing television and radio programs, and for telephone communication. In persons with profound sensory hearing loss, the cochlear implant—an electronic device that is surgically implanted to stimulate the auditory nerve—offers socially beneficial auditory rehabilitation to most adults with acquired deafness.

Copeland BJ et al: Cochlear implantation for the treatment of deafness. Annu Rev Med 2004;55:157. [PMID: 14746514]

Hol MK et al: Bone-anchored hearing aids in unilateral inner ear deafness: an evaluation of audiometric and patient outcome measurements. Otol Neurotol 2005;26:999. [PMID: 16151349]

Lesner SA: Candidacy and management of assistive listening devices: special needs of the elderly. Int J Audiol 2003;42 (Suppl 2):2S68. [PMID: 12918632]

Middlebrooks JC et al: Cochlear implants: the view from the brain. Curr Opin Neurobiol 2005;15:488. [PMID: 16009544]

Mo B et al: Cochlear implants and quality of life: a prospective study. Ear Hear 2005;26:186. [PMID: 15809544]

Palmer CV et al: Hearing loss and hearing aids. Neurol Clin 2005;23:901. [PMID: 16026682]

DISEASES OF THE AURICLE

Disorders of the external ear are for the most part dermatologic. Skin cancers due to sun exposure are common and may be treated with standard techniques. Traumatic auricular hematoma must be recognized and drained to prevent significant cosmetic deformity (cauliflower ear) resulting from dissolution of supporting cartilage. Similarly, cellulitis of the auricle must be treated promptly to prevent development of perichondritis and its resultant deformity. Relapsing polychondritis is a systemic disorder often associated with recurrent, frequently bilateral, painful episodes of auricular erythema and edema. Treatment with corticosteroids may help forestall cartilage dissolution. Respiratory compromise may occur as a result of progressive involvement of the tracheobronchial tree. Chondritis and perichondritis may be differentiated from auricular cellulitis by sparing of involvement of the lobule, which does not contain cartilage.

Silapunt S et al: Squamous cell carcinoma of the auricle and Mohs micrographic surgery. Dermatol Surg 2005;31(11 Pt 1): 1423. [PMID: 16416611]

DISEASES OF THE EAR CANAL

1. Cerumen Impaction

Cerumen is a protective secretion produced by the outer portion of the ear canal. In most persons, the ear canal is self-cleansing. Recommended hygiene consists of cleaning the external opening with a washcloth over the index finger without entering the canal itself. In most cases, cerumen impaction is self-induced through ill-advised attempts at cleaning the ear. It may be relieved with detergent ear drops (eg, 3% hydrogen peroxide; 6.5% carbamide peroxide), mechanical removal, suction, or irrigation. Irrigation is performed with water at body temperature to avoid a vestibular caloric response. The stream should be directed at the ear canal wall adjacent to the cerumen plug. Irrigation should be performed only when the tympanic membrane is known to be intact.

Use of jet irrigators designed for cleaning teeth (eg, WaterPik) for wax removal should be avoided since they may result in tympanic membrane perforations. Following professional irrigation, the ear canal should be thoroughly dried (eg, by instilling isopropyl alcohol or using a hair blow-dryer on low-power setting) to reduce the likelihood of inducing external otitis. Specialty referral for cleaning under microscopic guidance is indicated when the impaction has not responded to routine measures or if the patient has a history of chronic otitis media or tympanic membrane perforation.

Hobson JC et al: Use and abuse of cotton buds. J R Soc Med 2005;98:360. [PMID: 16055901]

Roland PS et al: Randomized, placebo-controlled evaluation of Cerumenex and Murine earwax removal products. Arch Otolaryngol Head Neck Surg 2004;130:1175. [PMID: 15492164]

2. Foreign Bodies

Foreign bodies in the ear canal are more frequent in children than in adults. Firm materials may be removed with a loop or a hook, taking care not to displace the object medially toward the tympanic membrane; microscopic guidance is helpful. Aqueous irrigation should not be performed for organic foreign bodies (eg, beans, insects), because water may cause them to swell. Living insects are best immobilized before removal by filling the ear canal with lidocaine.

Thompson SK et al: External auditory canal foreign body removal: management practices and outcomes. Laryngoscope 2003;113:1912. [PMID: 14603046]

3. External Otitis

ESSENTIALS OF DIAGNOSIS

- *Erythema and edema of the ear canal skin.*
- *Often with purulent exudates.*
- *Persistent external otitis in the diabetic or immunocompromised patient may evolve into osteomyelitis of the skull base, often called malignant external otitis.*

External otitis presents with otalgia, frequently accompanied by pruritus and purulent discharge. There is often a history of recent water exposure or mechanical trauma (eg, scratching, cotton applicators). External otitis is usually caused by gram-negative rods (eg, *Pseudomonas, Proteus*) or fungi (eg, *Aspergillus*), which grow in the presence of excessive moisture.

Examination reveals erythema and edema of the ear canal skin, often with a purulent exudate. Manipulation of the auricle often elicits pain. Because the lateral surface of the tympanic membrane is ear canal skin, it is often erythematous. However, in contrast to acute otitis media, it moves normally with pneumatic otoscopy. When the canal skin is very edematous, it may be impossible to visualize the tympanic membrane.

Fundamental to the treatment of external otitis is protection of the ear from additional moisture and avoidance of further mechanical injury by scratching. Otic drops containing a mixture of aminoglycoside antibiotic and anti-inflammatory corticosteroid in an acid vehicle are generally very effective (eg, neomycin sulfate, polymyxin B sulfate, and hydrocortisone). Purulent debris filling the ear canal should be gently removed to permit entry of the topical medication.

Drops should be used abundantly (five or more drops three or four times a day) to penetrate the depths of the canal. When substantial edema of the canal wall prevents entry of drops into the ear canal, a wick is placed to facilitate entry of the medication. In recalcitrant cases—particularly when cellulitis of the periauricular tissue has developed—oral fluoroquinolones (eg, ciprofloxacin, 500 mg twice daily for 1 week) are the drugs of choice because of their effectiveness against *Pseudomonas* species.

Block SL: Otitis externa: providing relief while avoiding complications. J Fam Pract 2005;54:669. [PMID: 16061052]

Roland PS et al: Ciprodex Otic AOE Study Group. Efficacy and safety of topical ciprofloxacin/dexamethasone versus neomycin/polymyxin B/hydrocortisone for otitis externa. Curr Med Res Opin 2004;20:1175. [PMID: 15324520]

4. Pruritus

Pruritus of the external auditory canal, particularly at the meatus, is a common problem. While it may be associated with external otitis or with dermatologic conditions such as seborrheic dermatitis and psoriasis, most cases are self-induced either from excoriation or by overly zealous ear cleaning. To permit regeneration of the protective cerumen blanket, patients should be instructed to avoid use of soap and water or cotton swabs in the ear canal. Patients with excessively dry canal skin may benefit from application of mineral oil, which helps counteract dryness and repel moisture. When an inflammatory component is present, topical application of a corticosteroid (eg, 0.1% triamcinolone) may be beneficial. It is axiomatic in persistent pruritus that the patient must cease scratching the ear. In stubborn cases, the fingernails must be kept short and the patient may need to wear cotton gloves at night to avoid manipulation during sleep. Symptomatic reduction of pruritus may be obtained by use of oral antihistamines (eg, diphenhydramine, 25 mg orally at bedtime). Topical application of isopropyl alcohol promptly relieves ear canal pruritus in many patients.

5. Malignant External Otitis

Persistent external otitis in the diabetic or immunocompromised patient may evolve into osteomyelitis of the skull base, often called malignant external otitis. Usually caused by *Pseudomonas aeruginosa*, osteomyelitis begins in the floor of the ear canal and may extend into the middle fossa floor, the clivus, and even the contralateral skull base. The patient usually presents with persistent foul aural discharge, granulations in the ear canal, deep otalgia, and progressive cranial nerve palsies involving nerves VI, VII, IX, X, XI, or XII. Diagnosis is confirmed by the demonstration of osseous erosion on CT and radionuclide scanning.

Treatment is chiefly medical, requiring prolonged antipseudomonal antibiotic administration, often for several months. Although intravenous therapy is often required, selected patients may be managed with ciprofloxacin

(500–1000 mg orally twice daily), which has proved effective against many of the causative *Pseudomonas* strains. To avoid relapse, antibiotic therapy should be continued, even in the asymptomatic patient, until gallium scanning indicates a marked reduction in the inflammatory process. Surgical debridement of infected bone is reserved for cases of deterioration despite medical therapy.

Rubin Grandis J et al: The changing face of malignant (necrotising) external otitis: clinical, radiological, and anatomic correlations. Lancet Infect Dis 2004;4:34. [PMID: 14720566]

Singh A et al: Skull base osteomyelitis: diagnostic and therapeutic challenges in atypical presentation. Otolaryngol Head Neck Surg 2005;133:121. [PMID: 16025065]

6. Exostoses & Osteomas

Bony overgrowths of the ear canal are a frequent incidental finding and occasionally have clinical significance. Clinically, they present as skin-covered mounds in the medial ear canal obscuring the tympanic membrane to a variable degree. Solitary osteomas are of no significance as long as they do not cause obstruction or infection. Multiple exostoses, which are generally acquired from repeated exposure to cold water, often progress and require surgical removal.

Vasama JP: Surgery for external auditory canal exostoses: a report of 182 operations. ORL J Otorhinolaryngol Relat Spec 2003;65:189. [PMID: 14564090]

7. Neoplasia

The most common neoplasm of the ear canal is squamous cell carcinoma (SCC). When an apparent otitis externa does not resolve on therapy, SCC should be suspected and biopsy performed. This disease carries a very high 5-year mortality rate because the tumor tends to invade the lymphatics of the cranial base and must be treated with wide surgical resection and radiation therapy. Adenomatous tumors, originating from the ceruminous glands, generally follow a more indolent course.

Devaney KO et al: Tumours of the external ear and temporal bone. Lancet Oncol 2005;6:411. [PMID: 15925819]

Yin M et al: Analysis of 95 cases of squamous cell carcinoma of the external and middle ear. Auris Nasus Larynx 2006 [Epub ahead of print]. [PMID: 16431060]

DISEASES OF THE AUDITORY TUBE

1. Auditory Tube Dysfunction

ESSENTIALS OF DIAGNOSIS

- Aural fullness.
- Fluctuating hearing.
- Discomfort with barometric pressure change.

The tube that connects the middle ear to the nasopharynx—the auditory tube, or eustachian tube—provides ventilation and drainage for the middle ear cleft. It is normally closed, opening only during the act of swallowing or yawning. When auditory tube function is compromised, air trapped within the middle ear becomes absorbed and negative pressure results. The most common causes of auditory tube dysfunction are diseases associated with edema of the tubal lining, such as viral upper respiratory tract infections and allergy. The patient usually reports a sense of fullness in the ear and mild to moderate impairment of hearing. When the tube is only partially blocked, swallowing or yawning may elicit a popping or crackling sound. Examination reveals retraction of the tympanic membrane and decreased mobility on pneumatic otoscopy. Following a viral illness, this disorder is usually transient, lasting days to weeks. Treatment with systemic and intranasal decongestants (eg, pseudoephedrine, 60 mg orally every 4 hours; oxymetazoline, 0.05% spray every 8–12 hours) combined with autoinflation by forced exhalation against closed nostrils may hasten relief. Autoinflation should not be recommended to patients with active intranasal infection, since this maneuver may precipitate middle ear infection. Allergic patients may also benefit from desensitization or intranasal corticosteroids (eg, beclomethasone dipropionate, two sprays in each nostril twice daily for 2–6 weeks). Air travel, rapid altitudinal change, and underwater diving should be avoided.

An overly patent auditory tube is a relatively uncommon problem that may be quite distressing. Typical complaints include fullness in the ear and autophony, an exaggerated ability to hear oneself breathe and speak. A patulous auditory tube may develop during rapid weight loss, or may be idiopathic. In contrast to a hypofunctioning auditory tube, the aural pressure is often made worse by exertion and may diminish during an upper respiratory tract infection. Although physical examination is usually normal, respiratory excursions of the tympanic membrane may occasionally be detected during vigorous breathing. Treatment includes avoidance of decongestant products, insertion of a ventilating tube to reduce the outward stretch of the eardrum during phonation, and, rarely, surgical narrowing of the auditory tube.

Grimmer JF et al: Update on eustachian tube dysfunction and the patulous eustachian tube. Curr Opin Otolaryngol Head Neck Surg 2005;13:277. [PMID: 16160520]

2. Serous Otitis Media

ESSENTIALS OF DIAGNOSIS

- Blocked auditory tube remains for a prolonged period.
- Resultant negative pressure will result in transudation of fluid.

When the auditory tube remains blocked for a prolonged period, the resultant negative pressure will result in transudation of fluid. This condition, known as serous otitis media, is especially common in children because their auditory tubes are narrower and more horizontal in orientation than those in adults. Serous otitis media is less common in adults, in whom it usually follows an upper respiratory tract infection or barotrauma. In an adult with persistent unilateral serous otitis media, nasopharyngeal carcinoma must be excluded. The tympanic membrane in serous otitis media is dull and hypomobile, occasionally accompanied by air bubbles in the middle ear and conductive hearing loss. The treatment of serous otitis media is similar to that for auditory tube dysfunction. A short course of oral corticosteroids (eg, prednisone, 40 mg/d for 7 days) has been advocated by some in the management of serous otitis media, as have oral antibiotics (eg, amoxicillin, 250 mg orally three times daily for 7 days)—or even a combination of the two. The role of these regimens remains controversial, but they are probably of little lasting benefit.

When medication fails to bring relief after several months, a ventilating tube placed through the tympanic membrane may restore hearing and alleviate the sense of aural fullness. Endoscopically guided laser expansion of the nasopharyngeal orifice of the auditory tube may improve function in recalcitrant cases.

Dogru H et al: Squamous cell metaplasia of the nasopharyngeal epithelium and its association with adult-onset otitis media with effusion. Acta Otolaryngol 2005;125:580. [PMID: 16076705]

Kujawski OB et al: Laser eustachian tuboplasty. Otol Neurotol 2004;25:1. [PMID: 14724483]

Satre TJ et al: Treatments for persistent otitis media with effusion. Am Fam Physician 2005;71:529. [PMID: 15712626]

3. Barotrauma

Persons with auditory tube dysfunction caused by either congenital narrowness or acquired mucosal edema may be unable to equalize the barometric stress exerted on the middle ear by air travel, rapid altitudinal change, or underwater diving. The problem is generally most acute during airplane descent, since the negative middle ear pressure tends to collapse and lock the auditory tube. Several measures are useful to enhance auditory tube function and avoid otic barotrauma. The patient should be advised to swallow, yawn, and autoinflate frequently during descent, which may be painful if the auditory tube collapses. Systemic decongestants (eg, pseudoephedrine, 60–120 mg) should be taken several hours before anticipated arrival time so that they will be maximally effective during descent. Topical decongestants such as 1% phenylephrine nasal spray should be administered 1 hour before arrival.

The treatment of acute negative middle ear pressure that persists on the ground is with decongestants and attempts at autoinflation. Myringotomy (creation of a small eardrum perforation) provides immediate relief and is appropriate in the setting of severe otalgia and hearing loss. Repeated episodes of barotrauma in persons who must fly frequently may be alleviated by insertion of ventilating tubes.

Underwater diving represents even a greater barometric stress to the ear than flying. The problem occurs most commonly during the descent phase, when pain develops within the first 15 feet if inflation of the middle ear via the auditory tube has not occurred. Divers must descend slowly and equilibrate in stages to avoid the development of severely negative pressures in the tympanum that may result in hemorrhage (hemotympanum) or perilymphatic fistulization. In the latter, the oval or round window ruptures, resulting in sensory hearing loss and acute vertigo. Emesis due to acute labyrinthine dysfunction can be very dangerous during an underwater dive. Sensory hearing loss or vertigo, which develops during the ascent phase of a saturation dive, may be the first (or only) symptom of decompression sickness. Immediate recompression will return intravascular gas bubbles to solution and restore the inner ear microcirculation. Patients should be warned to avoid diving when they have upper respiratory infections or episodes of nasal allergy. Tympanic membrane perforation is an absolute contraindication to diving, as the patient will experience an unbalanced thermal stimulus to the semicircular canals and may experience vertigo, disorientation, and even emesis. Finally, persons with only one hearing ear should be discouraged from diving because of the significant risk of otologic injury.

Mirza S et al: Otic barotrauma from air travel. J Laryngol Otol 2005;119:366. [PMID: 15949100]

DISEASES OF THE MIDDLE EAR

1. Acute Otitis Media

 ESSENTIALS OF DIAGNOSIS

- Otalgia, often with an upper respiratory tract infection.
- Erythema and hypomobility of tympanic membrane.

General Considerations

Acute otitis media is a bacterial infection of the mucosally lined air-containing spaces of the temporal bone. Purulent material forms not only within the middle ear cleft but also within the mastoid air cells and petrous apex when they are pneumatized. Acute otitis media is usually precipitated by a viral upper respiratory tract infection that causes auditory tube edema. This results in accumulation of fluid and mucus, which becomes secondarily infected by bacteria. The most common pathogens both in adults and in children are *Streptococcus pneumoniae, Haemophilus influenzae,* and *Streptococcus pyogenes.*

Clinical Findings

Acute otitis media is most common in infants and children, although it may occur at any age. Presenting symptoms and signs include otalgia, aural pressure, decreased hearing, and often fever. The typical physical findings are erythema and decreased mobility of the tympanic membrane. Occasionally, bullae will be seen on the tympanic membrane. Although it is taught that this represents infection with *Mycoplasma pneumoniae,* most cases involve more common pathogens.

Rarely, when middle ear empyema is severe, the tympanic membrane can be seen to bulge outward. In such cases, tympanic membrane rupture is imminent. Rupture is accompanied by a sudden decrease in pain, followed by the onset of otorrhea. With appropriate therapy, spontaneous healing of the tympanic membrane occurs in most cases. When perforation persists, chronic otitis media frequently evolves. Mastoid tenderness often accompanies acute otitis media and is due to the presence of pus within the mastoid air cells. This alone does not indicate suppurative (surgical) mastoiditis.

Treatment

The treatment of acute otitis media is specific antibiotic therapy, often combined with nasal decongestants. The first-choice oral antibiotic treatment is amoxicillin (20–40 mg/kg/d) or erythromycin (50 mg/kg/d) plus sulfonamide (150 mg/kg/d) for 10 days. Alternatives useful in resistant cases are cefaclor (20–40 mg/kg/d) or amoxicillin-clavulanate (20–40 mg/kg/d) combinations.

Tympanocentesis for bacterial (aerobic and anaerobic) and fungal culture may be performed by any experienced physician. A 20-gauge spinal needle bent 90 degrees to the hub attached to a 3-mL syringe is inserted through the inferior portion of the tympanic membrane. Interposition of a pliable connecting tube between the needle and syringe permits an assistant to aspirate without inducing movement of the needle. Tympanocentesis is useful for otitis media in immunocompromised patients and when infection persists or recurs despite multiple courses of antibiotics.

Surgical drainage of the middle ear (myringotomy) is reserved for patients with severe otalgia or when complications of otitis (eg, mastoiditis, meningitis) have occurred.

Recurrent acute otitis media may be managed with long-term antibiotic prophylaxis. Single daily oral doses of sulfamethoxazole (500 mg) or amoxicillin (250 or 500 mg) are given over a period of 1–3 months. Failure of this regimen to control infection is an indication for insertion of ventilating tubes.

Rovers MM et al: Otitis media. Lancet 2004;363:465. [PMID: 14962529]

2. Chronic Otitis Media & Cholesteatoma

Chronic infection of the middle ear and mastoid generally develops as a consequence of recurrent acute otitis media, although it may follow other diseases and trauma. Perforation of the tympanic membrane is usually present. This may be accompanied by mucosal changes such as polypoid degeneration and granulation tissue and osseous changes such as osteitis and sclerosis. The bacteriology of chronic otitis media differs from that of acute otitis media. Common organisms include *P aeruginosa, Proteus* species, *Staphylococcus aureus,* and mixed anaerobic infections. The clinical hallmark of chronic otitis media is purulent aural discharge. Drainage may be continuous or intermittent, with increased severity during upper respiratory tract infection or following water exposure. Pain is uncommon except during acute exacerbations. Conductive hearing loss results from destruction of the tympanic membrane and ossicular chain. The medical treatment of chronic otitis media includes regular removal of infected debris, use of earplugs to protect against water exposure, and topical antibiotic drops for exacerbations. The activity of ciprofloxacin against *Pseudomonas* may help dry a chronically discharging ear when given in a dosage of 500 mg orally twice a day for 1–6 weeks.

Definitive management is surgical in most cases. Tympanic membrane repair may be accomplished with temporalis muscle fascia or with homograft middle ear structures. Successful reconstruction of the tympanic membrane may be achieved in about 90% of cases, often with elimination of infection and significant improvement in hearing. When the mastoid air cells are involved by irreversible infection, they should be exenterated through mastoidectomy.

Cholesteatoma is a special variety of chronic otitis media. The most common cause is prolonged auditory tube dysfunction, with resultant chronic negative middle ear pressure that draws inward the upper flaccid portion of the tympanic membrane. This creates a squamous epithelium-lined sac, which—when its neck becomes obstructed—may fill with desquamated keratin and become chronically infected. Cholesteatomas typically erode bone, with early penetration of the mastoid and destruction of the ossicular chain. Over time they may erode the inner ear, involve the facial nerve, and on rare occasions spread intracranially. Physical examination reveals an epitympanic retraction pocket or marginal tympanic membrane perforation that exudes keratin debris. The treatment of cholesteatoma is surgical marsupialization of the sac or its complete removal. This often requires creation of a "mastoid bowl" in which the ear canal and mastoid are joined into a large common cavity that must be periodically cleaned.

Bance M et al: Topical treatment for otorrhea: issues and controversies. J Otolaryngol 2005;34 (Suppl 2):S52. [PMID: 16076416]

Gardner EK et al: Results with titanium ossicular reconstruction prostheses. Laryngoscope 2004;114:65. [PMID: 14709997]

Olszewska E et al: Etiopathogenesis of cholesteatoma. Eur Arch Otorhinolaryngol 2004;261:6. [PMID: 12835944]

3. Complications of Otitis Media

Mastoiditis

Acute suppurative mastoiditis usually evolves following several weeks of inadequately treated acute otitis media. It is characterized by postauricular pain and erythema accompanied by a spiking fever. Radiography reveals coalescence of the mastoid air cells due to destruction of their bony septa. Initial treatment consists of intravenous antibiotics and myringotomy for culture and drainage. Failure of medical therapy indicates the need for surgical drainage (mastoidectomy).

Agrawal S et al: Complications of otitis media: an evolving state. J Otolaryngol 2005;34(Suppl 1):S33. [PMID: 16089238]

Leskinen K et al: Acute complications of otitis media in adults. Clin Otolaryngol 2005;30:511. [PMID: 16402975]

Petrous Apicitis

The medial portion of the petrous bone between the inner ear and clivus may become a site of persistent infection when the drainage of its pneumatic cell tracts becomes blocked. This may cause foul discharge, deep ear and retro-orbital pain, and sixth nerve palsy (Gradenigo's syndrome); meningitis may be a complication. Treatment is with prolonged antibiotic therapy (based on culture results) and surgical drainage via petrous apicectomy.

Lee YH et al: CT, MRI and gallium SPECT in the diagnosis and treatment of petrous apicitis presenting as multiple cranial neuropathies. Br J Radiol 2005;78:948. [PMID: 16177020]

Otogenic Skull Base Osteomyelitis

Infections originating in the external or middle ear may result in osteomyelitis of the skull base, usually due to *P aeruginosa*. The diagnosis and management of this disease are discussed in the section on malignant external otitis.

Facial Paralysis

Facial palsy may be associated with either acute or chronic otitis media. In the acute setting, it results from inflammation of the seventh nerve in its middle ear segment, perhaps mediated through bacterially secreted neurotoxins. Treatment consists of myringotomy for drainage and culture, followed by intravenous antibiotics (based on culture results). The use of corticosteroids is controversial. The prognosis is excellent, with complete recovery in most cases.

Facial palsy associated with chronic otitis media usually evolves slowly due to chronic pressure on the seventh nerve in the middle ear or mastoid by cho-lesteatoma. Treatment requires surgical correction of the underlying disease. The prognosis is less favorable than for facial palsy associated with acute otitis media.

Popovtzer A et al: Facial palsy associated with acute otitis media. Otolaryngol Head Neck Surg 2005;132:327. [PMID: 1569254]

Sigmoid Sinus Thrombosis

Trapped infection within the mastoid air cells adjacent to the sigmoid sinus may cause septic thrombophlebitis. This is heralded by signs of systemic sepsis (spiking fevers, chills), at times accompanied by signs of increased intracranial pressure (headache, lethargy, nausea and vomiting, papilledema). Diagnosis can be made noninvasively by magnetic resonance venography. Treatment is with intravenous antibiotics (based on culture results), surgical drainage, and—when embolization is suspected—ligation of the internal jugular vein in the neck.

Manolidis S et al: Diagnosis and management of lateral sinus thrombosis. Otol Neurotol 2005;26:1045. [PMID: 16151357]

Central Nervous System Infection

Otogenic meningitis is by far the most common intracranial complication of ear infection. In the setting of acute suppurative otitis media, it arises from hematogenous spread of bacteria, most commonly *H influenzae* and *S pneumoniae*. In chronic otitis media, it results either from passage of infections along preformed pathways such as the petrosquamous suture line or from direct extension of disease through the dural plates of the petrous pyramid.

Epidural abscesses arise from direct extension of disease in the setting of chronic infection. They are usually asymptomatic but may present with deep local pain, headache, and low-grade fever. They are often discovered as an incidental finding at surgery. Brain abscess may arise in the temporal lobe or cerebellum as a result of septic thrombophlebitis adjacent to an epidural abscess. The predominant causative organisms are *S aureus, S pyogenes,* and *S pneumoniae.* Rupture into the subarachnoid space results in meningitis and often death. (See Chapter 30.)

Migirov L et al: Otogenic intracranial complications: a review of 28 cases. Acta Otolaryngol 2005;125:819. [PMID: 16158527]

Penido Nde O et al: Intracranial complications of otitis media: 15 years of experience in 33 patients. Otolaryngol Head Neck Surg 2005;132:37. [PMID: 15632907]

4. Otosclerosis

Otosclerosis is a progressive disease with a marked familial tendency that affects bone surrounding the inner ear. Lesions involving the footplate of the stapes result in increased impedance to the passage of sound through the ossicular chain, producing conductive hearing loss. This may be corrected through surgical replacement of the stapes with a prosthesis (stapedectomy). When otosclerotic lesions impinge on the cochlea, permanent sensory hearing loss occurs. Some evidence suggests that this level of hearing loss may be stabilized by treatment with oral sodium fluoride over prolonged periods of time (Florical—8.3 mg sodium fluoride and 364 mg calcium carbonate—two tablets orally each morning). Fluorides have minimal adverse effects other than occasional mild gastric irritation, which may be eliminated by ingesting the drug with meals.

Chandarana S et al: Quality of life following small fenestra stapedotomy. Ann Otol Rhinol Laryngol 2005;114:472. [PMID: 16042105]

Massey BL et al: Stapedectomy outcomes: titanium versus teflon wire prosthesis. Laryngoscope 2005;115:249. [PMID: 15689744]

5. Trauma to the Middle Ear

Tympanic membrane perforation may result from impact injury or explosive acoustic trauma. Spontaneous healing occurs in the great majority of cases. Persistent perforation may result from secondary infection brought on by exposure to water. Patients should be advised to wear earplugs while swimming or bathing during the healing period. Hemorrhage behind an intact tympanic membrane (hemotympanum) may follow blunt trauma or extreme barotrauma. Spontaneous resolution over several weeks is the usual course. When a conductive hearing loss greater than 30 dB persists for more than 3 months following trauma, disruption of the ossicular chain should be suspected. Middle ear exploration with reconstruction of the ossicular chain, combined with repair of the tympanic membrane when required, will usually restore hearing.

Ohlrogge M et al: Temporal bone fracture. Otol Neurotol 2004;25:195. [PMID: 15021784]

6. Middle Ear Neoplasia

Primary middle ear tumors are rare. Glomus tumors arise either in the middle ear (glomus tympanicum) or in the jugular bulb with upward erosion into the hypotympanum (glomus jugulare). They present clinically with pulsatile tinnitus and hearing loss. A vascular mass may be visible behind an intact tympanic membrane. Large glomus jugulare tumors are often associated with multiple cranial neuropathies, especially involving nerves VII, IX, X, XI, and XII. Treatment may require surgery, radiotherapy, or both.

Durvasula VS et al: Laser excision of glomus tympanicum tumours: long-term results. Eur Arch Otorhinolaryngol 2005; 262:325. [PMID: 15316822]

EARACHE

External otitis and acute otitis media are the two most common causes of earache. In external otitis, there is often a recent history of swimming, Q-tip use, or physical trauma, while in acute otitis media there is usually an antecedent or concurrent upper respiratory infection. The physical findings also differ. In external otitis, the ear canal skin is erythematous, while in acute otitis media this generally occurs only if the tympanic membrane has ruptured, spilling purulent material into the ear canal. Also, in external otitis the tympanic membrane may be erythematous, but it retains its mobility owing to the normal aeration of the middle ear cavity. Pain out of proportion to the physical findings may be due to herpes zoster oticus, especially when vesicles appear in the ear canal or concha. Chronic otitis media is usually not painful except during acute exacerbations. Persistent pain and discharge from the ear suggest osteomyelitis of the skull base or cancer.

The sensory innervation of the ear is derived from the trigeminal, facial, glossopharyngeal, vagal, and upper cervical nerves. Because of this rich innervation, referred otalgia is quite frequent. Temporomandibular joint dysfunction is a common cause of ear pain. It is often made worse by chewing or psychogenic grinding of the teeth (bruxism) and may be associated with dental malocclusion. Management includes soft diet, local heat to the masticatory muscles, massage, analgesics, and dental referral. Repeated episodes of severe lancinating otalgia may occur in glossopharyngeal neuralgia. Treatment with carbamazepine (100–300 mg orally every 8 hours) often confers substantial symptomatic relief. Severe glossopharyngeal neuralgia, which is refractory to medical management, may respond to microvascular decompression of the ninth nerve. Infections and neoplasia that involve the oropharynx, hypopharynx, and larynx frequently cause otalgia. Persistent earache demands specialty referral to exclude cancer of the upper aerodigestive tract.

Scarbrough TJ et al: Referred otalgia in head and neck cancer: a unifying schema. Am J Clin Oncol 2003;26:e157. [PMID: 14528091]

Tuz HH et al: Prevalence of otologic complaints in patients with temporomandibular disorder. Am J Orthod Dentofacial Orthop 2003;123:620. [PMID: 12806339]

DISEASES OF THE INNER EAR

1. Sensory Hearing Loss

Diseases of the cochlea result in sensory hearing loss, a condition that is usually irreversible. Most cochlear diseases result in bilateral symmetric hearing loss. The presence of unilateral or asymmetric sensorineural hearing loss suggests a lesion proximal to the cochlea. Lesions affecting the eighth nerve and central auditory system are discussed in the section on neural hearing loss. The primary goals in the management of sensory hearing loss are prevention of further losses and functional improvement with amplification and auditory rehabilitation.

Presbyacusis

Presbyacusis, the most frequent cause of sensory hearing loss, is the progressive, predominantly high-frequency symmetric hearing loss of advancing age. It is difficult to separate the various etiologic factors (eg, noise trauma) that may contribute to presbyacusis, but genetic predisposition appears to play a role. Most patients notice a loss of speech discrimination that is especially pronounced in noisy environments. About 25% of people between the ages of 65 and 75 years and almost 50% of those over 75 experience hearing difficulties.

Gates GA et al: Presbycusis. Lancet 2005;366:1111. [PMID: 16182900]

Noise Trauma

Noise trauma is the second most common cause of sensory hearing loss. Sounds exceeding 85 dB are potentially injurious to the cochlea, especially with prolonged exposures. The loss typically begins in the high frequencies (especially 4000 Hz) and progresses to involve the speech frequencies with continuing exposure. Among the more common sources of injurious noise are industrial machinery, weapons, and excessively loud music. Personal music devices (eg, MP3 and CD players) used at excessive loudness levels may also be potentially injurious. In recent years, monitoring of noise levels in the workplace by regulatory agencies has led to preventive programs that have reduced the frequency of occupational losses. Individuals of all ages, especially those with existing hearing losses, should wear earplugs when exposed to moderately loud noises and specially designed earmuffs when exposed to explosive noises.

Nelson DI et al: The global burden of occupational noise-induced hearing loss. Am J Ind Med 2005;48:446. [PMID: 16299704]

Williams W: Noise exposure levels from personal stereo use. Int J Audiol 2005;44:231. [PMID: 16011051]

Physical Trauma

Head trauma has effects on the inner ear similar to those of severe acoustic trauma. Some degree of sensory hearing loss may occur following simple concussion and is frequent after skull fracture. Deployment of air bags during an automobile accident has been associated with hearing loss.

Ishman SL et al: Temporal bone fractures: traditional classification and clinical relevance. Laryngoscope 2004;114:1734. [PMID: 15454763]

Ototoxicity

Ototoxic substances may affect both the auditory and vestibular systems. The most common ototoxic medications are salicylates; aminoglycosides; loop diuretics;

and several antineoplastic agents, notably cisplatin. The latter three categories may cause irreversible hearing loss even when administered in therapeutic doses. When using these medications, it is important to identify high-risk patients such as those with preexisting hearing losses or renal insufficiency. Patients simultaneously receiving multiple ototoxic agents are at particular risk owing to ototoxic synergy. Useful measures to reduce the risk of ototoxic injury include serial audiometry and monitoring of serum peak and trough levels and substitution of equivalent nonototoxic drugs whenever possible. Efforts are underway to develop strategies, known as ototoxic chemoprotection, using drugs that shield the inner ear from damage during ototoxic exposure.

It is possible for topical agents that enter the middle ear to be absorbed into the inner ear via the round window. When the tympanic membrane is perforated, use of potentially ototoxic ear drops (eg, neomycin, gentamicin) is best avoided.

Black FO et al: Permanent gentamicin vestibulotoxicity. Otol Neurotol 2004;25:559. [PMID: 15241236]

Roland PS: New developments in our understanding of ototoxicity. Ear Nose Throat J 2004;83(9 Suppl 4):15. [PMID: 15543837]

Unal OF et al: Prevention of gentamicin induced ototoxicity by trimetazidine in animal model. Int J Pediatr Otorhinolaryngol 2005;69:193. [PMID: 15656952]

Sudden Sensory Hearing Loss

Sudden loss of hearing in one ear may occur at any age but is more common in the elderly. It most probably is the result of sudden vascular occlusion of the internal auditory artery or of a viral inner ear infection. Prognosis is mixed, with many patients suffering permanent deafness in the involved ear while others have complete recovery. Although treatment with oral corticosteroids is controversial, many clinicians believe that such treatment improves the odds of recovery. A common regimen is prednisone, 80 mg/d, followed by a tapering dose over a 10-day period. For patients who have not responded to oral corticosteroid therapy, some clinicians advocate using supplemental intratympanic administration of corticosteroids.

Cadoni G et al: Sudden sensorineural hearing loss: our experience in diagnosis, treatment, and outcome. J Otolaryngol 2005; 34:395. [PMID: 16343399]

Mamak A et al: A study of prognostic factors in sudden hearing loss. Ear Nose Throat J 2005;84:641. [PMID: 16382746]

Wei B et al: Steroids for idiopathic sudden sensorineural hearing loss. Cochrane Database Syst Rev 2006;(1):CD003998. [PMID: 16437471]

Hereditary Hearing Loss

Sensory hearing loss with onset during adult life often runs in families. The mode of inheritance may be either autosomal dominant or recessive. The age at onset, the rate of progression of hearing loss, and the audiometric pattern (high-frequency, low-frequency, or flat) can often be predicted by studying family members. In recent years, great strides have been made in identifying the molecular genetic errors associated with hereditary hearing loss. Over 100 genes have now been identified, many of which have been cloned. The connexin-26 mutation, a particularly prevalent form of autosomal recessive nonsyndromic hearing loss may be tested clinically. Hearing loss is also frequently found in hereditary mitochondrial disorders. Progress is being made toward the development of methods to restore lost hair cells in genetic and other forms of deafness. Both insertion of the hair cell regulatory gene Math-1 via gene therapy as well as stem cell–mediated techniques show considerable promise.

Aggarwal R et al: The genetics of hearing loss. Hosp Med 2005;66:32. [PMID: 15686164]

Bayazit YA et al: An overview of hereditary hearing loss. ORL J Otorhinolaryngol Relat Spec 2006;68:57. [PMID: 16428895]

Finsterer J et al: Nuclear and mitochondrial genes mutated in nonsyndromic impaired hearing. Int J Pediatr Otorhinolaryngol 2005;69:621. [PMID: 15850684]

Izumikawa M et al: Auditory hair cell replacement and hearing improvement by Atoh1 gene therapy in deaf mammals. Nat Med 2005;11:271. [PMID: 15711559]

Li H et al: Stem cells as therapy for hearing loss. Trends Mol Med 2004;10:309. [PMID: 15242678]

Maiorana CR et al: Advances in inner ear gene therapy: exploring cochlear protection and regeneration. Curr Opin Otolaryngol Head Neck Surg 2005;13:308. [PMID: 16160526]

Autoimmune Hearing Loss

Sensory hearing loss may be associated with a wide array of systemic autoimmune disorders such as systemic lupus erythematosus, Wegener's granulomatosis, and Cogan's syndrome (hearing loss, keratitis, aortitis). The loss is most often bilateral and progressive. The hearing level often fluctuates, with periods of deterioration alternating with partial or even complete remission. The tendency is for the gradual evolution of permanent hearing loss, which usually stabilizes with some remaining auditory function but occasionally proceeds to complete deafness. Vestibular dysfunction, particularly dysequilibrium and postural instability, may accompany the auditory symptoms. A syndrome resembling Meniere's disease may also occur with intermittent attacks of severe vertigo.

In the majority of cases, the autoimmune pattern of audiovestibular dysfunction presents in the absence of recognized systemic autoimmune disease. Use of laboratory tests to screen for autoimmune disease (eg, antinuclear antibody, rheumatoid factor, erythrocyte sedimentation rate) may be informative. Specific tests of immune reactivity against inner ear antigens (anticochlear antibodies, lymphocyte transformation tests) are available but are currently of interest for research purposes only. Responsiveness to oral corticosteroid treatment is helpful in making the diagnosis and constitutes first-line ther-

apy. If stabilization of hearing becomes dependent on long-term corticosteroid use, steroid-sparing immunosuppressive regimens may become necessary.

Broughton SS et al: Immune-mediated inner ear disease: 10-year experience. Semin Arthritis Rheum 2004;34:544. [PMID: 15505770]

Niparko JK et al: Serial audiometry in a clinical trial of AIED treatment. Otol Neurotol 2005;26:908. [PMID: 16151337]

Other Causes of Sensory Hearing Loss

There are numerous less common causes of sensory hearing loss. Metabolic derangements (eg, diabetes, hypothyroidism, hyperlipidemia, and renal failure), infections (eg, measles, mumps, syphilis), and physical factors (eg, radiation therapy) are some of the chief examples. Identification of metabolic or infectious sensory hearing losses is especially important, as these may occasionally be reversible with medical therapy. Meniere's syndrome and labyrinthitis are discussed in the section on vestibular disorders.

Kakarlapudi V et al: The effect of diabetes on sensorineural hearing loss. Otol Neurotol 2003;24:382. [PMID: 12806288]

2. Tinnitus

Tinnitus is the perception of abnormal ear or head noises. Persistent tinnitus usually indicates the presence of sensory hearing loss. Intermittent periods of mild, high-pitched tinnitus lasting for several minutes are common in normal-hearing persons. When severe and persistent, tinnitus may interfere with sleep and the ability to concentrate, resulting in considerable psychological distress.

The most important treatment of tinnitus is avoidance of exposure to excessive noise, ototoxic agents, and other factors that may cause cochlear damage. Masking the tinnitus with music or through amplification of normal sounds with a hearing aid may also bring some relief. Although intravenous treatment with antiarrhythmic drugs (eg, lidocaine) suppresses tinnitus in some individuals, evidence suggests no benefit with oral agents that are potentially suitable for long-term symptom relief. Among the numerous drugs that have been tried, oral antidepressants (eg, nortriptyline at an initial dosage of 50 mg orally at bedtime) have proved to be the most effective. Habituation techniques, such as tinnitus retraining therapy, may prove beneficial in those with refractory symptoms.

Pulsatile tinnitus—often described by the patient as listening to one's own heartbeat—should be distinguished from tonal tinnitus. Although often ascribed to conductive hearing loss, this symptom may be far more serious and indicates a vascular abnormality such as glomus tumor, venous sinus stenosis, carotid vasoocclusive disease, arteriovenous malformation, or aneurysm. MR angiography and venography should be considered to establish the diagnosis.

A staccato "clicking" tinnitus may result from middle ear muscle spasm, sometimes associated with palatal myoclonus. The patient typically perceives a rapid series of popping noises, lasting seconds to a few minutes, accompanied by a fluttering feeling in the ear.

Folmer RL et al: Long-term effectiveness of ear-level devices for tinnitus. Otolaryngol Head Neck Surg 2006;134:132. [PMID: 16399193]

Henry JA et al: General review of tinnitus: prevalence, mechanisms, effects, and management. J Speech Lang Hear Res 2005;48:1204. [PMID: 16411806]

Herraiz C et al: Long-term clinical trial of tinnitus retraining therapy. Otolaryngol Head Neck Surg 2005;133:774. [PMID: 16274808]

Liyanage SH et al: Pulsatile tinnitus. J Laryngol Otol 2006; 120:93. [PMID: 16359136]

3. Hyperacusis

Excessive sensitivity to sound may occur in normal-hearing individuals either for psychological reasons or in association with ear disease. Patients with cochlear dysfunction commonly experience recruitment, an abnormal sensitivity to loud sounds despite a reduced sensitivity to softer ones. Fitting hearing aids and other amplification devices to patients with recruitment requires use of compression circuitry to avoid uncomfortable overamplification. For normal-hearing individuals with hyperacusis, use of an earplug in noisy environments is often beneficial.

Baguley DM: Hyperacusis. J R Soc Med 2003;96:582. [PMID: 14645606]

4. Vertigo

ESSENTIALS OF DIAGNOSIS

- Either a sensation of motion when there is no motion or an exaggerated sense of motion in response to a given bodily movement.
- Cardinal symptom of vestibular disease.
- Must differentiate peripheral from central etiologies of vestibular dysfunction.
- Peripheral: Onset of vertigo is sudden; tinnitus, hearing loss, and horizontal nystagmus may be present.
- Central: Onset of vertigo is gradual; when nystagmus is present, it is usually vertical. Brain MRI helpful in evaluation.

Clinical Findings

A. SYMPTOMS AND SIGNS

Vertigo is the cardinal symptom of vestibular disease. It is either a sensation of motion when there is no mo-

tion or an exaggerated sense of motion in response to a given bodily movement. Thus, vertigo is not just "spinning" but may present, for example, as a sense of tumbling, of falling forward or backward, or of the ground rolling beneath one's feet ("earthquake-like"). It should be distinguished from imbalance, light-headedness, and syncope, all of which are usually nonvestibular in origin. The vertigo that results from peripheral vestibulopathy is usually of sudden onset, may be so severe that the patient is unable to walk or stand, and is frequently accompanied by nausea and vomiting. Tinnitus and hearing loss may be associated and provide strong support for a peripheral origin.

A minimal physical examination of the patient with vertigo includes the Romberg test, an evaluation of gait, and observation for the presence of nystagmus. In peripheral lesions, nystagmus is usually horizontal with a rotatory component; the fast phase usually beats away from the diseased side. Visual fixation tends to inhibit nystagmus except in very acute peripheral lesions or with central nervous system disease. The Nylen-Bárány maneuvers are performed as follows: Put the patient in a sitting position on the examination table with the head turned to the right. Quickly lower the patient to the supine position with the head extending over the edge and placed 30 degrees lower than the body. Watch for nystagmus for 30 seconds. Repeat with the head turned to the left. Lastly, perform the maneuver without turning the head.

These maneuvers are intended to induce positioning nystagmus but are of limited use when the patient is able to visually fixate. This objection may be overcome either by placing +2-diopter lenses (Fresnel glasses) over the eyes or by making observations in the dark by means of electronystagmographic recording. The Fukuda test, in which the patient walks in place with eyes closed, is useful for detecting subtle defects. A positive response is observed when the patient rotates, usually toward the side of the diseased labyrinth. Vertigo arising from central lesions tends to develop gradually and then become progressively more severe and debilitating. Nystagmus is not always present but can occur in any direction and may be dissociated in the two eyes. The associated nystagmus is often nonfatigable, vertical rather than horizontal in orientation, without latency, and unsuppressed by visual fixation. Electronystagmography is useful in documenting these characteristics. The evaluation of central audiovestibular dysfunction usually requires imaging of the brain with MRI.

Episodic vertigo can occur in patients with diplopia from external ophthalmoplegia and is maximal when the patient looks in the direction where the separation of images is greatest. Cerebral lesions involving the temporal cortex may also produce vertigo, which is sometimes the initial symptom of a seizure. Finally, vertigo may be a feature of a number of systemic disorders and can occur as a side effect of certain anticonvulsant, antibiotic, hypnotic, analgesic, and tranquilizing drugs or of alcohol.

B. Laboratory Findings

Laboratory investigations such as audiologic evaluation, caloric stimulation, electronystagmography, CT scan or MRI, and brain stem auditory evoked potential studies are indicated in patients with persistent vertigo or when central nervous system disease is suspected. These studies will help distinguish between central and peripheral lesions and to identify causes requiring specific therapy. Electronystagmography consists of objective recording of the nystagmus induced by head and body movements, gaze, and caloric stimulation. It is helpful in quantifying the degree of vestibular hypofunction and may help with the differentiation between peripheral and central lesions. Computer-driven rotatory chairs and posturography platforms offer improved diagnostic abilities but are not widely available.

Brandt T et al: General vestibular testing. Clin Neurophysiol 2005;116:406. [PMID: 15661119]

Guilemany JM et al: Clinical and epidemiological study of vertigo at an outpatient clinic. Acta Otolaryngol 2004;124:49. [PMID: 14977078]

Lempert T et al: Episodic vertigo. Curr Opin Neurol 2005;18:5. [PMID: 15655395]

Vertigo Syndromes Due to Peripheral Lesions

A. Endolymphatic Hydrops (Meniere's Syndrome)

Meniere's syndrome results from distention of the endolymphatic compartment of the inner ear. The primary lesion appears to be in the endolymphatic sac, which is thought to be responsible for endolymph filtration and excretion. Although a precise cause of hydrops cannot be established in most cases, two known causes are syphilis and head trauma. The classic syndrome consists of episodic vertigo, usually lasting 1–8 hours; low-frequency sensorineural hearing loss, often fluctuating; tinnitus, usually low-tone and "blowing" in quality; and a sensation of aural pressure. Symptoms wax and wane as the endolymphatic pressure rises and falls. Caloric testing commonly reveals loss or impairment of thermally induced nystagmus on the involved side.

Episodic vertigo resembling that of Meniere's syndrome but without accompanying auditory symptoms is known as recurrent vestibulopathy. The pathogenic mechanism of this symptom complex is unknown in most cases, although a few patients suffer from a variant of migraine. Others will go on to develop the classic syndrome of endolymphatic hydrops.

Kim HH et al: Trends in the diagnosis and the management of Meniere's disease: results of a survey. Otolaryngol Head Neck Surg 2005;132:722. [PMID: 15886625]

Onuki J et al: Comparative study of the daily lifestyle of patients with Meniere's disease and controls. Ann Otol Rhinol Laryngol 2005;114:927. [PMID: 16425558]

B. Labyrinthitis

Patients with labyrinthitis suffer from acute onset of continuous, usually severe vertigo lasting several days to a week, accompanied by hearing loss and tinnitus. During a recovery period that lasts for several weeks, rapid head movements may bring on transient vertigo. Hearing may return to normal or remain permanently impaired in the involved ear. The cause of labyrinthitis is unknown, although it frequently follows an upper respiratory tract infection.

C. Positioning Vertigo

This form of vertigo is usually peripheral in origin. Transient vertigo following changes in head position is a frequent complaint. The term "positioning vertigo" is more accurate than "positional vertigo" because it is provoked by changes in head position rather than by the maintenance of a particular posture. Use of the term "*benign* position*al* vertigo" is discouraged except for cases known to be unassociated with central nervous system disorders. True positional vertigo suggests either vertebrobasilar insufficiency or dysfunction of the cervical spine.

The typical symptoms of positioning vertigo occur in clusters that persist for several days. Typically with peripheral lesions, there is a latency period of several seconds following a head movement before symptoms develop, and they subside within 10–60 seconds. Constant repetition of the positional change leads to habituation. In central lesions, there is no latent period, fatigability, or habituation of the sign and symptoms. Single-session physical therapy protocols, based on the theory that peripheral positioning vertigo results from free-floating otoconia within a semicircular canal, have recently been developed. These strive to reposition the offending crystals through a series of head manipulations. New surgical procedures are also being explored which, by interrupting the posterior semicircular canal, attempt to prevent the exaggerated response to angular head motion.

Salvinelli F et al: Benign paroxysmal positional vertigo: diagnosis and treatment. Clin Ter 2004;155:395. [PMID: 15700633]

von Brevern M et al: Benign paroxysmal positional vertigo: current status of medical management. Otolaryngol Head Neck Surg 2004;130:381. [PMID: 15054387]

D. Vestibular Neuronitis

In vestibular neuronitis, a paroxysmal, usually single attack of vertigo occurs without accompanying impairment of auditory function and may persist for several days to weeks before clearing. Examination reveals nystagmus and absent responses to caloric stimulation on one or both sides. The cause of the disorder is unclear. Treatment is symptomatic.

E. Traumatic Vertigo

The most common cause of vertigo following head injury is labyrinthine concussion. Symptoms generally diminish within several days but may linger for a month or more. Basilar skull fractures that traverse the inner ear usually result in severe vertigo lasting several days to a week and deafness in the involved ear. Chronic posttraumatic vertigo may result from cupulolithiasis. This occurs when traumatically detached statoconia (otoconia) settle on the ampulla of the posterior semicircular canal and cause an excessive degree of cupular deflection in response to head motion. Clinically, this presents as episodic positioning vertigo.

Ernst A et al: Management of posttraumatic vertigo. Otolaryngol Head Neck Surg 2005;132:554. [PMID: 15806044]

F. PERILYMPHATIC FISTULA

Leakage of perilymphatic fluid from the inner ear into the tympanic cavity via the round or oval window is often discussed as a cause of vertigo and sensory hearing loss but is actually very rare. Most cases result from either physical injury (eg, blunt head trauma, hand slap to ear); extreme barotrauma during airflight, scuba diving, etc; or vigorous Valsalva maneuver (eg, during weight lifting). Treatment may require middle ear exploration and window sealing with a tissue graft; however, this is seldom indicated without a clear-cut history of a precipitating traumatic event.

G. CERVICAL VERTIGO

Position receptors located in the facets of the cervical spine are important physiologically in the coordination of head and eye movements. Cervical proprioceptive dysfunction is a common cause of vertigo triggered by neck movements. This disturbance often commences after neck injury, particularly hyperextension. An association also exists with degenerative cervical spine disease. Although symptoms vary, vertigo may be triggered by assuming a particular head position as opposed to moving to a new head position (the latter typical of labyrinthine dysfunction). Management consists of neck movement exercises to the extent permitted by orthopedic considerations.

Endo K et al: Cervical vertigo and dizziness after whiplash injury. Eur Spine J 2006;15:886. [PMID: 16432749]

H. MIGRAINOUS VERTIGO

Episodic vertigo is frequently associated with a migraine type of headache. Most commonly, the vertigo is temporally related to the headache and lasts up to several hours. Some patients experience a positioning vertigo pattern. Occasionally, vertigo occurs independently of the head pain. The importance of recognizing this association is that antimigraine pharmacotherapy often relieves the vestibular symptoms.

Crevits L et al: Migraine-related vertigo: towards a distinctive entity. Clin Neurol Neurosurg 2005;107:82. [PMID: 1570822]

Neuhauser HK et al: Diagnostic criteria for migrainous vertigo. Acta Otolaryngol 2005;125:1247. [PMID: 16353420]

I. SUPERIOR SEMICIRCULAR CANAL DEHISCENCE

Deficiency in the bony covering of the superior semicircular canal may be associated with vertigo triggered by loud noise exposure and an apparent conductive hearing loss. Diagnosis is with coronal high-resolution CT scan. Symptoms can be improved in selected cases by operatively sealing the dehiscent canal.

Banerjee A et al: Superior canal dehiscence: review of a new condition. Clin Otolaryngol 2005;30:9. [PMID: 15748182]

Vertigo Syndromes Due to Central Lesions

Central nervous system causes of vertigo include brainstem vascular disease, arteriovenous malformations, tumor of the brainstem and cerebellum, multiple sclerosis, and vertebrobasilar migraine. Vertigo of central origin often becomes unremitting and disabling. The associated nystagmus is often nonfatigable, vertical rather than horizontal in orientation, without latency, and unsuppressed by visual fixation. Electronystagmography is useful in documenting these characteristics. There are commonly other signs of brainstem dysfunction (eg, cranial nerve palsies; motor, sensory, or cerebellar deficits in the limbs) or of increased intracranial pressure. Auditory function is generally spared. The underlying cause should be treated.

Baloh RW: Episodic vertigo: central nervous system causes. Curr Opin Neurol 2002;15:17. [PMID: 11796946]

Bruzzone MG et al: Neuroradiological features of vertigo. Neurol Sci 2004;25(Suppl 1):S20. [PMID: 15045615]

Treatment of the Patient with Vertigo

Few specific treatments for labyrinthine disorders have been designed to reverse a known pathogenic mechanism. In Meniere's disease, treatment is intended to lower endolymphatic pressure. A low-salt diet (< 2 g sodium daily), at times supplemented by diuretics, adequately controls symptoms in the great majority of patients. A typical diuretic regimen is hydrochlorothiazide, 50–100 mg orally daily. Other specific treatments are antibiotics as required and surgical repair of perilymphatic fistulas.

Symptomatic treatment is useful in the vertiginous patient to lessen the abnormal sensation and to alleviate vegetative symptoms such as nausea and vomiting. The most common drug classes used are the antihistamines, anticholinergics, and sedative-hypnotics. Ample evidence exists that vestibular suppressant medications adversely affect the process of central compensation following acute vestibular disease. For this reason, these drugs should be used only for brief periods. Generally, they are best administered to patients with prominent vegetative symptoms and are best tapered and halted when symptoms are resolved, usually within 1–2 weeks.

In acute severe vertigo, vestibular suppressants such as diazepam, 2.5–5 mg sublingually, orally, or intravenously, may abate an attack. Relief from nausea and vomiting usually requires an antiemetic delivered intramuscularly or by rectal suppository (eg, prochlorperazine, 10 mg intramuscularly, or 25 mg rectally every 6 hours). Less severe vertigo may often be successfully alleviated with antihistamines such as meclizine, 25 mg, or cyclizine or dimenhydrinate, 25–50 mg, orally every 6 hours. Scopolamine, administered in low dosage transdermally (0.5 mg/d), has proved beneficial to many patients with recurrent vertigo, although side effects (dry mouth, blurred vision, urinary obstruction) often limit its usefulness. Sometimes using half or even one-fourth of a patch may allow therapeutic effect without the usual adverse consequences. A combination of drugs sometimes helps when the response to one drug is disappointing.

Bed rest may reduce the severity of acute vertigo. Conversely, in chronic or recurrent vertigo, one of the most important therapies is exercise. Physical activity substantially enhances the central nervous system's ability to compensate for labyrinthine dysfunction and should be encouraged once nausea and vomiting have resolved. In general, the patient should be instructed to repeatedly perform maneuvers that provoke vertigo—up to the point of nausea or fatigue—in an effort to habituate them. Patients with vertigo and imbalance refractory to conventional therapy may benefit from a formal rehabilitation program under the guidance of a physical therapist. Substantial success has been reported in such patients through use of customized habituation protocols and specialized equipment, including tilt tables. A series of head maneuvers (theoretically intended to reposition free-floating otolithic particles) may help in the management of positioning vertigo. Such protocols have been shown to be at least as effective as vestibular habituation exercises, and they are less time-consuming.

For patients with recalcitrant vertigo or clusters of attacks, specialty referral may be useful. Prednisone has been used for clusters refractory to diuretics, low-salt diet, and vestibular suppressants.

Permanent therapy in medically refractory unilateral peripheral vestibular dysfunction is selective chemical destruction of the vestibular hair cell population by infusion of ototoxins transtympanically into the middle ear. Absorption into perilymph occurs via the round window. The most frequently used drug is gentamicin (80 mg/mL diluted 50:50 with bicarbonate), which is injected into the middle ear via a spinal needle. Results in patients with Meniere's syndrome have been impressive, with about 80–90% of patients relieved of severe episodic vertigo. An additional management option of endolymphatic hydrops (Meniere's disease) is a device that applies intermittent pressure pulses to the inner ear via a tympanostomy tube. Preliminary results for this minimally invasive technique have been promising. Surgical remedies are reserved for those who remain substantially disabled despite a prolonged and varied trial of medical therapy and exercises. Selective section of the vestibular portion of the eighth nerve brings relief of vertigo in over 90% of such patients. Surgical removal of the semicircular canals (labyrinthectomy) is also highly effective but is appropriate only for patients with little or no hearing in the involved ear.

Cohen HS: Disability and rehabilitation in the dizzy patient. Curr Opin Neurol 2006;1:49. [PMID: 16415677]

Longridge NS: Meta-analysis of intratympanic gentamicin. Otol Neurotol 2005;26:554. [PMID: 15891674]

Morales-Luckie E et al: Oral administration of prednisone to control refractory vertigo in Meniere's disease: a pilot study. Otol Neurotol 2005;26:1022. [PMID: 16151353]

Steenerson RL et al: Effectiveness of treatment techniques in 923 cases of benign paroxysmal positional vertigo. Laryngoscope 2005;115:226. [PMID: 15689740]

Straube A: Pharmacology of vertigo/nystagmus/oscillopsia. Curr Opin Neurol 2005;18:11. [PMID: 15655396]

Thomsen J et al: Local overpressure treatment reduces vestibular symptoms in patients with Meniere's disease: a clinical, randomized, multicenter, double-blind, placebo-controlled study. Otol Neurotol 2005;26:68. [PMID: 15699722]

DISEASES OF THE CENTRAL AUDITORY & VESTIBULAR SYSTEMS (Table 8–1)

Lesions of the eighth cranial nerve and central audiovestibular pathways produce neural hearing loss and vertigo. One characteristic of neural hearing loss is deterioration of speech discrimination out of proportion to the decrease in pure tone thresholds. Another is auditory adaptation, wherein a steady tone appears to the

Table 8–1. Common vestibular disorders: Differential diagnosis based on classic presentations.

Duration of Typical Vertiginous Episodes	Auditory Symptoms Present	Auditory Symptoms Absent
Seconds	Perilymphatic fistula	Positioning vertigo (cupulolithiasis), vertebrobasilar insufficiency, cervical vertigo
Hours	Endolymphatic hydrops (Meniere's syndrome, syphilis)	Recurrent vestibulopathy, vestibular migraine
Days	Labyrinthitis, labyrinthine concussion	Vestibular neuronitis
Months	Acoustic neuroma, ototoxicity	Multiple sclerosis, cerebellar degeneration

listener to decay and eventually disappear. Auditory evoked responses are useful in distinguishing cochlear from neural losses and may give insight into the site of lesion within the central pathways.

The evaluation of central audiovestibular disorders usually requires imaging of the internal auditory canal, cerebellopontine angle, and brain with enhanced MRI.

Jackler RK et al: *Neurotology,* 2nd ed. Mosby, 2004.

1. Vestibular Schwannoma (Acoustic Neuroma)

Eighth nerve schwannomas are among the most common of intracranial tumors. Most are unilateral, but about 5% are associated with the hereditary syndrome, neurofibromatosis type 2, in which bilateral eighth nerve tumors may be accompanied by meningiomas and other intracranial and spinal tumors. Although recent concern over the role of cell phones in the origin of these tumors has appeared in the popular press, the evidence of an association is in doubt. These benign lesions arise within the internal auditory canal and gradually grow to involve the cerebellopontine angle, eventually compressing the pons and resulting in hydrocephalus. Their typical auditory symptoms are unilateral hearing loss with a deterioration of speech discrimination exceeding that predicted by the degree of pure tone loss. Nonclassic presentations, such as sudden unilateral hearing loss, are fairly common. Any individual with a unilateral or asymmetric sensorineural hearing loss should be evaluated for an intracranial mass lesion. Vestibular dysfunction more often takes the form of continuous dysequilibrium than episodic vertigo. Other lesions of the cerebellopontine angle such as meningioma and epidermoids may have similar audiovestibular manifestations. Diagnosis is made by enhanced MRI, although auditory evoked responses may have a role in screening. Microsurgical excision is often indicated, although small tumors in older persons may be managed with stereotactic radiotherapy or simply monitored with serial imaging studies.

Betchen SA et al: Long-term hearing preservation after surgery for vestibular schwannoma. J Neurosurg 2005;102:6. [PMID: 15658089]

Lunsford LD et al: Radiosurgery of vestibular schwannomas: summary of experience in 829 cases. J Neurosurg 2005;102 Suppl:195. [PMID: 15662809]

Neff BA et al: Current concepts in the evaluation and treatment of neurofibromatosis type II. Otolaryngol Clin North Am 2005;38:671. [PMID: 16005725]

Schoemaker MJ et al: Mobile phone use and risk of acoustic neuroma: results of the Interphone case-control study in five North European countries. Br J Cancer 2005;93:842. [PMID: 16136046]

Yoshimoto Y: Systematic review of the natural history of vestibular schwannoma. J Neurosurg 2005;103:59. [PMID: 16121974]

2. Vascular Compromise

Vertebrobasilar insufficiency is a common cause of vertigo in the elderly. It is often triggered by changes in posture or extension of the neck. Reduced flow in the vertebrobasilar system may be demonstrated noninvasively through magnetic resonance angiography. Empiric treatment is with vasodilators and aspirin.

Vascular loops that impinge upon the brainstem root entry zone of cranial nerves have been shown to cause dysfunction. Widely recognized examples are hemifacial spasm and tic douloureux. It has been suggested that hearing loss, tinnitus, and disabling positioning vertigo may result from a vascular loop abutting the eighth nerve.

Sauvaget E et al: Vertebrobasilar occlusive disorders presenting as sudden sensorineural hearing loss. Laryngoscope 2004;114: 327. [PMID: 14755213]

3. Multiple Sclerosis

Patients with multiple sclerosis may suffer from episodic vertigo and chronic imbalance. Hearing loss in this disease is most commonly unilateral and of rapid onset. Spontaneous recovery may occur.

Frohman EM et al: Benign paroxysmal positioning vertigo in multiple sclerosis: diagnosis, pathophysiology and therapeutic techniques. Mult Scler 2003;9:250. [PMID: 12814171]

OTOLOGIC MANIFESTATIONS OF AIDS

The otologic manifestations of AIDS are protean. The pinna and external auditory canal may be affected by Kaposi's sarcoma as well as persistent and potentially invasive fungal infections, particularly due to *Aspergillus fumigatus.* The most common middle ear manifestation of AIDS is serous otitis media due to auditory tube dysfunction arising from adenoidal hypertrophy (HIV lymphadenopathy), recurrent mucosal viral infections, or an obstructing nasopharyngeal tumor (eg, lymphoma). For middle ear effusions, ventilating tubes are seldom helpful and may trigger profuse watery otorrhea. Acute otitis media is usually caused by the typical bacterial organisms that occur in nonimmunocompromised patients, although *Pneumocystis jiroveci* (formerly *Pneumocystis carinii*) otitis has been reported. Sensorineural hearing loss is common and in some cases appears to result from viral central nervous system infection. In cases of progressive hearing loss, it is important to evaluate for cryptococcal meningitis and syphilis. Acute facial paralysis due to herpes zoster infection (Ramsay Hunt's syndrome) is quite common and follows a clinical course similar to that in nonimmunocompromised patients. Treatment is primarily with high-dose acyclovir (see Chapters 6 and 32). Corticosteroids may also be effective.

Gurney TA: Otolaryngologic manifestations of human immunodeficiency virus infection. Otolaryngol Clin North Am 2003; 36:607. [PMID: 14567056]

■ DISEASES OF THE NOSE & PARANASAL SINUSES

INFECTIONS OF THE NOSE & PARANASAL SINUSES

1. Viral Rhinitis (Common Cold)

The nonspecific symptoms of the ubiquitous common cold are present in the early phases of many diseases that affect the upper aerodigestive tract. Because there are numerous serologic types of rhinoviruses, adenoviruses, and other viruses, patients remain susceptible throughout life. Headache, nasal congestion, watery rhinorrhea, sneezing, and a scratchy throat accompanied by general malaise are typical in viral infections. Nasal examination usually shows reddened, edematous mucosa and a watery discharge. The presence of purulent nasal discharge suggests bacterial infection.

There is no curative treatment for a cold. There is a common misperception among patients that antibiotics are helpful. Supportive measures such as decongestants (pseudoephedrine, 30–60 mg every 4–6 hours or 120 mg twice daily) may provide some relief of rhinorrhea and nasal obstruction.

Nasal sprays such as oxymetazoline or phenylephrine are rapidly effective. They should not be used for more than a few days at a time, since chronic use leads to a rebound congestion that is often worse than the original symptoms. This chronic nasal stuffiness is known as rhinitis medicamentosa. Treatment requires complete cessation of the sprays. This triggers a period of severe nasal congestion that usually lasts 1–2 weeks. Topical intranasal corticosteroids (flunisolide, two sprays in each nostril twice daily) or a short tapering course of oral prednisone may help during the process of withdrawal.

Other than transient middle ear effusion, complications of viral rhinitis are unusual. Secondary bacterial infection may occur and is suggested by persistence of symptoms beyond a week accompanied both by purulent green or yellow nasal secretions and unilateral facial or tooth pain. The most common pathogens are the same as those responsible for acute otitis media, ie, *S pneumoniae*, other streptococci, *H influenzae*, *S aureus*, and *Moraxella catarrhalis*. (See Acute Sinusitis, below.)

Eccles R: Understanding the symptoms of the common cold and influenza. Lancet Infect Dis 2005;5:718. [PMID: 16253889]

Hirschmann JV: Antibiotics for common respiratory tract infections in adults. Arch Intern Med 2002;162:256. [PMID: 11822917]

Steinman MA et al: Predictors of broad-spectrum antibiotic prescribing for acute respiratory tract infections in adult primary care. JAMA 2003;289:719. [PMID: 12585950]

Wright ED et al: Infectious adult rhinosinusitis: etiology, diagnosis, and management principles. J Otolaryngol 2005;34 (Suppl 1): S7. [PMID: 16089234]

2. Acute Sinusitis

 ESSENTIALS OF DIAGNOSIS

- *Pain is usually unilateral over the maxillary sinus or is toothache-like.*
- *Symptoms usually last for more than 1 week but less than 4 weeks.*
- *Change of secretions from mucoid to purulent green or yellow.*
- *Occasional visible swelling or erythema over a sinus.*
- *Postnasal drainage, headache, and cough may also be present.*
- *Diseases that swell the nasal mucous membrane, such as viral or allergic rhinitis, are usually the underlying cause.*

General Considerations

Acute sinus infections are uncommon compared with viral rhinitis, but they still affect over 14% of the population, accounting for over 2 billion dollars in health care expenditures for sinusitis annually. Because sinusitis usually has followed an acute respiratory infection and because media advertisements often use the term "sinusitis" when "rhinitis" would be more accurate, it is understandable that patients and clinicians alike sometimes confuse these entities. Sinusitis is suggested when symptoms have persevered for more than a week and pain is reported unilaterally, either as toothache or as pain over the maxillary sinus. Objective signs include a change of secretions from watery or mucoid to purulent green or yellow, or (occasionally) visible swelling or erythema over a sinus.

Sinusitis usually is a result of impaired mucociliary clearance and obstruction of the osteomeatal complex. Diseases that swell the nasal mucous membrane, such as viral or allergic rhinitis, are usually the underlying cause. Edematous mucosa causes obstruction of the sinus drainage tract, resulting in the accumulation of mucous secretion in the sinus cavity that becomes secondarily infected by bacteria. The typical pathogens of bacterial sinusitis are the same as those that cause acute otitis media: *S pneumoniae*, other streptococci, *H influenzae*, and, less commonly, *S aureus* and *M catarrhalis*. It should be kept in mind that about 25% of healthy asymptomatic individuals may, if sinus aspirates are cultured, harbor such bacteria as well.

Clinical Findings

A. SYMPTOMS AND SIGNS

Because the maxillary sinus is the largest of the paranasal sinuses and its ostia into the nose is superiorly placed, thereby failing to take advantage of gravity, it is the most commonly affected sinus. Pain and pressure over the cheek are the usual symptoms. Pain may refer to the upper incisor and canine teeth via branches of the trigeminal nerve, which traverse the floor of the sinus. It is not uncommon for maxillary sinusitis to result from dental infection, and teeth that are tender should be carefully examined for signs of abscess. Discolored nasal discharge and poor response to decongestants may also suggest sinusitis. Other possible causes for facial pain, such as trigeminal neuralgia and optic neuritis, should be kept in mind as well.

Acute ethmoiditis in adults is usually accompanied by maxillary sinusitis. In such cases, the symptoms of maxillary sinusitis generally predominate. Ethmoidal infection presents with pain and pressure over the high lateral wall of the nose that may radiate to the orbit. Periorbital cellulitis may be present.

Sphenoid sinusitis is usually seen in the setting of pansinusitis. The patient may complain of a headache "in the middle of the head" and often points to the vertex. Sixth nerve palsy may occur as the abducens nerve courses just lateral to the sinus.

Acute frontal sinusitis usually causes pain and tenderness of the forehead. This is most easily elicited by palpation of the orbital roof just below the medial end of the eyebrow. Palpation here is more accurate than percussion of the supraorbital area or forehead.

B. IMAGING

It is usually possible to make the diagnosis of sinusitis on clinical grounds alone. Although more sensitive than clinical examination, routine radiographs are not cost-effective and are not recommended by the Agency for Health Care Policy and Research. However, they may be helpful when clinically based criteria are difficult to evaluate. The hallmarks of acute sinusitis radiologically are soft tissue density without bone destruction. An air-fluid level may also be seen.

Limited coronal CT scans have replaced conventional sinus films. CT is no more expensive, is more sensitive to both inflammatory changes and bone destruction (which would raise the possibility of an underlying tumor), and identifying anatomic blockage of the ostiomeatal complex may also help guide endoscopic sinus surgery in recurrent or chronic sinusitis. In critically ill intubated patients, where the prevalence of nosocomial sinusitis is as high as 40%, CT identification and subsequent antibiotic treatment appear to reduce the incidence of bronchopneumonia. Occasionally, a CT scan may be indicated to demonstrate that a patient with midface pain does *not* have sinusitis.

While reasonably sensitive, CT scans are not specific. Sinus abnormalities can be seen in the majority of patients with an upper respiratory infection, while only 2% develop bacterial sinusitis. Thus, sinusitis is a clinical diagnosis for which CT may be helpful in confirming, denying, or monitoring.

If malignancy is suspected, MRI with gadolinium should be ordered instead of CT. MRI will distinguish tumor from inflammation and inspissated mucus far better than CT, as well as better delineating tumor extent with respect to adjacent structures such as the orbit, skull base, and palate. Bone destruction can be demonstrated as well by MRI as by CT.

Treatment

As two-thirds of untreated patients will improve symptomatically within 2 weeks, appropriate criteria for the use of antibiotics are symptoms lasting more than 10–14 days or severe symptoms, including fever, facial pain, and periorbital swelling. Administration of antibiotics does, however, reduce by 50% the incidence of clinical failure and, coupled with clinical criteria-based diagnosis, represents the most cost-effective treatment strategy. Symptoms may be improved with oral or nasal decongestants (or both)—eg, oral pseudoephedrine, 30–120 mg per dose, up to 240 mg/d; nasal oxymetazoline, 0.05%, or xylometazoline, 0.05–0.1%, one or two sprays in each nostril every 6–8 hours for up to 3 days.

Double-blinded studies exist to support any of the following antibiotic choices, with the choice generally based on predicted efficacy, cost, and side effects:

Amoxicillin (500 mg orally three times a day), possibly with clavulanate (125 mg three times a day)

Trimethoprim-sulfamethoxazole (4 mg/kg TMP and 20 mg/kg SMZ twice daily; available as tablets with 80 or 160 mg TMP and 160 or 800 mg SMZ)

Cephalexin (250–500 mg orally four times a day)

Cefuroxime (250 mg orally twice daily)

Cefaclor (250 mg orally three times a day)

Cefixime (400 mg orally daily)

Quinolones, such as ciprofloxacin (500 mg twice daily), levofloxacin (500 mg once daily), moxifloxacin (400 mg once daily), and sparfloxacin (200 mg once daily after an initial dose of 400 mg)

Macrolides, such as azithromycin (500 mg once daily, possibly for only 3 days) or clarithromycin (500 mg orally twice daily, for 14 days)

Usually, amoxicillin or TMP-SMZ is adequate and most cost-effective and covers the common pathogens discussed earlier. Treatment is usually for 10 days (or as stated above), although longer courses are sometimes required to prevent relapses. Recurrent sinusitis or sinusitis that does not appear to respond clinically warrants evaluation by a specialist. Selection of antibiotics is usually empiric, but if symptoms persist, obtaining a culture endoscopically or via maxillary sinus puncture may help narrow the choice based on culture and sensitivity tests. Resistance by *H influenzae* and *S pneumoniae* is a public health concern. Culture may also be helpful in nosocomial sinusitis, where the bacterial spectrum may be less typical and the potential complications greater.

Failure of sinusitis to resolve after an adequate course of oral antibiotics may necessitate hospital admission for intravenous antibiotics and possible surgical drainage. Frontal sinusitis that does not promptly respond to outpatient care should be managed aggressively because the posterior sinus wall is adjacent to the dura and because undertreated infection may lead to intracranial extension. If intravenous antibiotics fail to ameliorate symptoms, it may be necessary to surgically drill a small opening into the floor of the frontal sinus to drain and irrigate the sinus. Persistent maxillary empyema may be cultured and relieved with a needle inserted through the lateral wall of the nose or anterior wall of the antrum through the gingivobuccal sulcus.

Complications

Local complications of sinusitis include osteomyelitis and mucocele. Mucoceles, a consequence of long-standing ductal obstruction, are more common in the supraorbital ethmoids and frontal sinuses and may become secondarily infected. They appear radiologically as a smoothly expanded sinus filled with homogeneous soft tissue density. Treatment is surgical, requiring either drainage of the mucocele intranasally or its complete excision with fat ablation of the sinus cavity.

Osteomyelitis requires prolonged antibiotics as well as removal of necrotic bone. The frontal sinus is most commonly affected, with bone involvement suggested by a tender puffy swelling of the forehead. Following treatment, secondary cosmetic reconstructive procedures may be necessary.

Intracranial complications of sinusitis occur either through hematogenous spread, as in cavernous sinus thrombosis and meningitis, or by direct extension, as in epidural and intraparenchymal brain abscesses. Fortunately, they are rare today. Cavernous sinus thrombosis is heralded by ophthalmoplegia, chemosis, and visual loss. Frontal epidural abscess is usually quiescent. It may be detected on CT scan, a study recommended in all cases of atypical or complicated sinusitis.

It should always be kept in mind that paranasal sinus cancer is in the differential diagnosis of sinusitis. The presence of bone destruction radiologically, cranial neuropathies (especially V_2), persistent pain, epistaxis, or a prolonged clinical course should raise the suspicion of possible cancer.

Merenstein D et al: Are antibiotics beneficial for patients with sinusitis complaints? A randomized double-blind clinical trial. J Fam Pract 2005;54:144. [PMID: 15689289]

Piccirillo JF: Clinical practice. Acute bacterial sinusitis. N Engl J Med 2004;351:902. [PMID: 15329428]

Scheid EC et al: Acute bacterial rhinosinusitis in adults: part I. Evaluation. Am Fam Physician 2004;70:1685. [PMID: 15554486]

Scheid EC et al: Acute bacterial rhinosinusitis in adults: part II. Treatment. Am Fam Physician 2004;70:1697. [PMID: 15554487]

Slavin RG et al; American Academy of Allergy, Asthma and Immunology; American College of Allergy, Asthma and Immunology; Joint Council of Allergy, Asthma and Immunology: The diagnosis and management of sinusitis: a practice parameter update. J Allergy Clin Immunol 2005; 116(6 Suppl):S13. [PMID: 16416688]

Werning JW et al: Physician specialty is associated with differences in the evaluation and management of acute bacterial rhinosinusitis. Arch Otolaryngol Head Neck Surg 2002; 128:123. [PMID: 11843718]

Williams JW Jr et al: Antibiotics for acute maxillary sinusitis. Cochrane Database Syst Rev 2003;(2):CD00024. [PMID: 12804392]

3. Nasal Vestibulitis

Inflammation of the nasal vestibule commonly results from folliculitis of the hairs that line this orifice. Systemic antibiotics effective against S aureus (such as dicloxacillin, 250 mg orally four times daily for 7–10 days) are indicated. Topical mupirocin (applied two or three times daily) may be a helpful addition. If recurrent, the addition of rifampin (10 mg/kg orally twice daily for the last 4 days of treatment) may eliminate the S aureus carrier state. If a furuncle exists, it should be incised and drained, preferably intranasally. Adequate treatment of these infections is important to prevent retrograde spread of infection through valveless veins into the cavernous sinus and intracranial structures.

4. Rhinocerebral Mucormycosis

Although mucormycosis is rare, any clinician seeing patients in a primary care setting must be aware of its presenting signs and symptoms. The fungus (*Mucor, Absidia, Rhizopus*) spreads rapidly through vascular channels and may be lethal if not detected early. Patients with mucormycosis almost invariably have an underlying disease, often diabetes mellitus or end-stage renal disease. It also occurs following bone marrow transplantation, in patients with lymphoma, in patients who are immunosuppressed for other reasons, and in patients receiving deferoxamine (a metal chelator). Occasional cases have been reported in patients with AIDS, although *Aspergillus* is more common in this setting. The initial symptoms may be similar to those of bacterial sinusitis, although facial pain is often more severe. Examination of the nasal mucosa is likely to show black, necrotic eschar adherent to the inferior turbinate, although this may not be present in early stages. Cranial neuropathies and black necrotic skin overlying the ethmoid sinuses are advanced signs. Early diagnosis requires suspicion of the disease and nasal or sinus biopsy, which reveals broad nonseptate hyphae within tissues. Because CT or MRI may initially show only soft tissue changes, intervention should be based on the clinical setting and not on radiologic demonstration of bony destruction or intracranial changes.

Mucormycosis represents a medical and surgical emergency. Once recognized, prompt wide surgical debridement and amphotericin B by intravenous infusion are indicated. Lipid-based amphotericin B may be used in patients who have renal insufficiency or in those in whom it develops secondary to nephrotoxic doses of nonlipid amphotericin. When there appears to be sufficiently little orbital involvement that orbital preservation is a realistic therapeutic objective, conservative debridement of the orbit may be supplemented with adjunctive amphotericin B irrigation. There is evidence that suggests that iron chelator therapy may also be a useful adjunct. Close management of the underlying disease is also of great importance. Even with early diagnosis and immediate appropriate intervention, the prognosis is guarded. In diabetics, the mortality rate is about 20%; in patients with renal failure, it is over 50%; in AIDS, it is close to 100%.

Case records of the Massachusetts General Hospital. Weekly clinicopathological exercises. Case 22-1999. A 68-year-old woman with multiple myeloma, diabetes mellitus, and an inflamed eye. N Engl J Med 1999;41:265. [PMID: 10413740]

Mondy KE et al: Rhinocerebral mucormycosis in the era of lipid-based amphotericin B: case report and literature review. Pharmacotherapy 2002;22:519. [PMID: 11939688]

O'Neill BM et al: Disseminated rhinocerebral mucormycosis: a case report and review of the literature. J Oral Maxillofac Surg 2006;64:326. [PMID: 16413907]

Spellberg B et al: Novel perspectives on mucormycosis: pathophysiology, presentation, and management. Clin Microbiol Rev 2005;18:556. [PMID: 1602069]

ALLERGIC RHINITIS

The symptoms of "hay fever" are similar to those of viral rhinitis but are usually persistent and show seasonal variation. Nasal symptoms are often accompanied by eye irritation, which causes pruritus, erythema, and excessive tearing. Numerous allergens may cause these symptoms: pollens are most common in the spring, grasses in the summer, and ragweed in the fall. Dust and household mites may produce year-round symptoms.

On physical examination, the mucosa of the turbinates is usually pale or violaceous because of venous engorgement. This is in contrast to the erythema of viral rhinitis. Nasal polyps, which are yellowish boggy masses of hypertrophic mucosa, may be seen.

Treatment of allergic and perennial rhinitis has improved in recent years. Numerous over-the-counter antihistamines, such as brompheniramine or chlorpheniramine (4 mg orally every 6–8 hours, or 8–12 mg orally every 8–12 hours as a sustained-release tablet) and clemastine (1.34–2.68 mg orally twice daily) offer the benefit of reduced cost though usually associated with higher rates of drowsiness compared with the newer prescription antihistamines. These oral H_1-receptor antagonists include cetirizine (10 mg orally once daily), fexofenadine (60 mg orally twice daily or

120 mg once daily), and loratadine (10 mg orally once daily). Fexofenadine appears to be nonsedating; the other two minimally sedating. Also shown to be effective in randomized trials are ebastine (10–20 mg orally once daily) and misolastine (10 mg once daily). Two H_1-receptor antagonist antihistamine nasal sprays have also been shown to be effective in randomized trials: levocabastine (0.2 mg twice daily) and azelastine (two sprays per nostril, 1.1 mg/d).

Intranasal corticosteroid sprays are a mainstay of treatment of allergic rhinitis. Evidence-based literature reviews show that these are more effective—and frequently less expensive—than nonsedating antihistamines. Patients should be reminded that there may be a delay in onset of relief of 1–2 weeks. Corticosteroid sprays may also shrink nasal polyps, thereby providing an improved nasal airway and delaying or eliminating the indications for endoscopic sinus surgery. Available preparations include beclomethasone (42 mcg/spray twice daily each nostril), flunisolide (25 mcg/spray twice daily each nostril), mometasone furoate (200 mcg once daily per nostril), and fluticasone propionate (200 mcg once daily per nostril). The latter two synthetic corticosteroids appear to have higher topical potencies and lipid solubility and reduced systemic bioavailability, suggesting possible practical advantages.

In addition to intranasal corticosteroid sprays and antihistamines, including H_1-receptor antagonists, literature supports the use of antileukotriene medications such as montelukast (10 mg/d orally) alone or with cetirizine (10 mg/d orally) or with loratadine (10 mg/d orally). There are proinflammatory effects of cysteinyl leukotrienes in upper and lower airway disease, including asthma, allergic rhinitis, and hyperplastic sinusitis and polyposis. Improved nasal rhinorrhea, sneezing, and congestion are seen with the use of leukotriene receptor antagonists, often in conjunction with antihistamines.

Maintaining an allergen-free environment by covering pillows and mattresses with plastic covers, substituting synthetic materials (foam mattress, acrylics) for animal products (wool, horsehair), and removing dust-collecting household fixtures (carpets, drapes, bedspreads, wicker) is worth the attempt to help more troubled patients. Air purifiers and dust filters (such as Bionaire models) may also aid in maintaining an allergen-free environment. When symptoms are extremely bothersome, a search for offending allergens may prove helpful. This can either be done by skin testing or by serum RAST testing. Desensitization by gradually increasing subdermal exposure to identified allergens may be tried in selected patients, with variable results.

Adjunctive options include intranasal anticholinergic agents such as ipratropium bromide 0.03% sprays (42 mcg per nostril three times daily) when rhinorrhea is a major symptom and intranasal cromolyn spray prior to the onset of seasonal symptoms.

For more information on allergic rhinitis, see Chapter 19.

Gendo K et al: Evidence-based diagnostic strategies for evaluating suspected allergic rhinitis. Ann Intern Med 2004;140:278. [PMID: 14970151]

Haberal I et al: The role of leukotrienes in nasal allergy. Otolaryngol Head Neck Surg 2003;129:274. [PMID: 12958580]

Nielsen LP et al: Comparison of intranasal corticosteroids and antihistamines in allergic rhinitis: a review of randomized, controlled trials. Am J Respir Med 2003;2:55. [PMID: 14720022]

Portnoy JM et al: Evidence-based strategies for treatment of allergic rhinitis. Curr Allergy Asthma Rep 2004;4:439. [PMID: 15462709]

Prenner ME et al: Allergic rhinitis: treatment based on patient profiles. Am J Med 2006;119:230. [PMID: 16490466]

Simons FE: Advances in H₁-antihistamines. N Engl J Med 2004; 351:2203. [PMID: 15548781]

Wilson DR et al: Sublingual immunotherapy for allergic rhinitis. Cochrane Database Syst Rev 2003;(2):CD002893. [PMID: 12804442]

OLFACTORY DYSFUNCTION

The physiology of olfaction is less well understood than that of the other special senses. The taste of foods is strongly affected by our sense of smell, and studies have shown a moderate correlation between taste discrimination ability and odor discrimination ability. In the past few years, discovery of the family of odor-receptor genes as well as inositol phosphate and cyclic nucleotide signaling pathways has led to a molecular basis of olfactory reception. Clinically, odorant molecules traverse the nasal vault to reach the cribriform area and become soluble in the mucus overlying the exposed dendrites of receptor cells. Anatomic blockage of the nares is the most common cause of olfactory dysfunction (hyposmia or anosmia). Polyps, septal deformities, and nasal tumors may prevent air from reaching the area of the cribriform plate high in the nose where these receptors are located. Transient olfactory dysfunction often accompanies the common cold, nasal allergies, and perennial rhinitis. About 20% of olfactory dysfunction is idiopathic, although it often follows a viral illness. Some have suggested administering large doses of vitamin A and zinc to such patients, although little evidence supports their use. Central nervous system neoplasms, especially those that involve the olfactory groove or temporal lobe, may affect olfaction. Head trauma accounts for less than 5% of cases of hyposmia. Absent, diminished, or distorted smell or taste has been reported in a wide variety of endocrine, nutritional, and nervous disorders. In particular, olfactory dysfunction in Parkinson's disease and Alzheimer's disease has been the subject of recent research. A great many medications have also been implicated.

Evaluation of olfactory dysfunction should include a thorough history of systemic illnesses and medication use as well as a physical examination focusing on the nose and nervous system. Most clinical offices are not set up to test olfaction, but such tests may at times be worthwhile if only to assess whether a patient possesses any sense of smell at all. Odor identification and discrimination can be tested using standardized choices (see references). Odor threshold can be tested using increasing concentrations of various materials. In permanent hyposmia, counseling should be offered about seasoning foods with spices (eg, pepper) that stimulate the trigeminal as well as olfactory chemoreceptors and about safety issues such as the use of smoke alarms and electric rather than gas home appliances.

Hawkes C: Olfaction in neurodegenerative disorder. Mov Disord 2003;18:364. [PMID: 12671941]

Kovacs T: Mechanisms of olfactory dysfunction in aging and neurodegenerative disorders. Ageing Res Rev 2004;3:215. [PMID: 15177056]

Moberg PJ et al: Scent of a disorder: olfactory functioning in schizophrenia. Curr Psychiatry Rep 2003;5:311. [PMID: 12857535]

Murphy C et al: Prevalence of olfactory impairment in older adults. JAMA 2002;288:2307. [PMID: 12425708]

Wrobel BB et al: Smell and taste disorders. Facial Plast Surg Clin North Am 2004;12:459i. [PMID: 15337114]

EPISTAXIS

 ESSENTIALS OF DIAGNOSIS

- *Bleeding from the anterior nasal cavity is by far the most common type of epistaxis encountered.*
- *Most cases may be successfully treated by direct pressure on the bleeding site. When this is inadequate, various nasal tamponade methods are usually effective.*

Predisposing factors include nasal trauma (nose picking, foreign bodies, forceful nose blowing), rhinitis, drying of the nasal mucosa from low humidity, deviation of the nasal septum, alcohol use, and antiplatelet medications. Most cases of anterior epistaxis may be successfully treated by direct pressure on the bleeding site. The nasal alae should be firmly compressed for at least 10 minutes. Venous pressure is reduced in the sitting position, and leaning forward lessens the swallowing of blood. Short-acting topical nasal decongestants (eg, phenylephrine, 0.125–1% solution, one or two sprays), which act as vasoconstrictors, may also be helpful. When the bleeding does not readily subside, the nose should be examined, using good illumination and suction, in an attempt to locate the bleeding site. Topical 4% cocaine applied either as a spray or on a cotton strip serves both as an anesthetic and as a vasoconstricting agent. If cocaine is unavailable, a topical decongestant (eg, oxymetazoline) and a topical anesthetic (eg, tetracaine) provide equivalent results. When visible, the bleeding site may be cauterized with silver nitrate, diathermy, or electrocautery. A supplemental patch of Surgicel or Gelfoam may be helpful.

Occasionally, a site of bleeding may be inaccessible to direct control, or attempts at direct control may be unsuccessful. In such cases there are a number of alternatives. When the site of bleeding is anterior, a hemostatic sealant, pneumatic nasal tamponade, or anterior packing may suffice. There are a number of ways to do this, such as with several feet of lubricated iodoform packing systematically placed in the floor of the nose and then the vault of the nose, or with various manufactured products designed for nasal tamponade.

About 5% of nasal bleeding originates in the **posterior nasal cavity.** If an anteriorly placed pneumatic nasal tamponade is unsuccessful, it may be necessary to place a pack to occlude the choana before placing a pack anteriorly. Because this is uncomfortable and because it may require oxygen supplementation to prevent hypoxia, hospitalization for several days is indicated. Opioid analgesics are needed to reduce the considerable discomfort and elevated blood pressure caused by a posterior pack. Ligation of the nasal arterial supply (internal maxillary artery and ethmoid arteries) is an alternative to posterior nasal packing, as is endovascular embolization of the internal maxillary artery. This is certainly necessary when packing fails to control life-threatening hemorrhage. On rare occasions, ligation of the external carotid artery may be necessary.

After control of epistaxis, the patient is advised to avoid vigorous exercise for several days. Avoidance of hot or spicy foods and tobacco is also advisable, as they may cause vasodilation. Avoiding nasal trauma, including nose picking, is an obvious necessity. Lubrication with petroleum jelly or bacitracin ointment and increased home humidity may also be useful ancillary measures.

It is important in all patients with epistaxis to consider underlying causes of the bleeding. Laboratory assessment of bleeding parameters may be indicated, especially in recurrent cases. Other causes of recurrent epistaxis, such as hereditary hemorrhagic telangiectasia (Osler-Weber-Rendu syndrome), should also be considered. Similarly, once the acute episode has passed, careful examination of the nose and paranasal sinuses to rule out neoplasia is wise.

Patients presenting with epistaxis often have higher blood pressures than control patients. Continued management of patients with epistaxis should therefore include follow-up investigation of possible hypertension.

Herkner H et al: Active epistaxis at ED presentation is associated with arterial hypertension. Am J Emerg Med 2002;20:92. [PMID: 11880870]

Jones GL et al: The value of coagulation profiles in epistaxis management. Int J Clin Pract 2003;57:577. [PMID: 14529056]

Klotz DA et al: Surgical management of posterior epistaxis: a changing paradigm. Laryngoscope 2002;112:1577. [PMID: 12352666]

Mathiasen RA et al: Prospective, randomized, controlled clinical trial of a novel matrix hemostatic sealant in patients with acute anterior epistaxis. Laryngoscope 2005;115:899. [PMID: 15867662]

Singer AJ et al: Comparison of nasal tampons for the treatment of epistaxis in the emergency department: a randomized controlled trial. Ann Emerg Med 2005;45:134. [PMID: 15671968]

NASAL TRAUMA

The nasal pyramid is the most frequently fractured bone in the body. Fracture is suggested by crepitance or palpably mobile bony segments. Epistaxis and pain are common, as are soft tissue hematomas ("black eye"). It is important to make certain that there is no palpable step-off of the infraorbital rim, which would indicate the presence of a zygomatic complex fracture. Radiologic confirmation may at times be helpful but is not necessary in uncomplicated nasal fractures. It is also important to assess for possible concomitant additional facial, pulmonary, or intracranial injuries when the circumstances of injury are suggestive, as in the case of automobile and motorcycle accidents.

Treatment is aimed at maintaining long-term nasal airway patency and nasal aesthetics. Closed reduction, using topical 4% cocaine and locally injected 1% lidocaine, should be attempted within 1 week of injury. In the presence of marked nasal swelling, it is best to wait several days for the edema to subside before undertaking reduction. Persistent functional or cosmetic defects may be repaired by delayed reconstructive nasal surgery.

Intranasal examination should be performed in all cases to rule out septal hematoma, which appears as a widening of the anterior septum, visible just posterior to the columella. The septal cartilage receives its only nutrition from its closely adherent mucoperichondrium. An untreated subperichondrial hematoma will result in loss of the nasal cartilage with resultant saddlenose deformity. Septal hematomas may become infected, with *S aureus* the predominant organism. Treatment consists of incision and drainage via an intranasal septal mucosal incision. It is important to be sure that both sides of the septal cartilage are adequately drained. A small Penrose drain sutured in place is helpful. Antibiotics should be given and the drained fluid sent for culture.

Alvi A et al: Facial fractures and concomitant injuries in trauma patients. Laryngoscope 2003;113:102. [PMID: 12514391]

Green KM: Reduction of nasal fractures under local anaesthetic. Rhinology 2001;39:43. [PMID: 11340695]

Gur E et al: Walk-through injuries: glass door facial injuries. Ann Plast Surg 2001;46:613. [PMID: 11405360]

Kraus JF et al: Facial trauma and the risk of intracranial injury in motorcycle riders. Ann Emerg Med 2003;41:18. [PMID: 12514678]

Ridder GJ et al: Technique and timing for closed reduction of isolated nasal fractures: a retrospective study. Ear Nose Throat J 2002;81:49. [PMID: 11816391]

TUMORS & GRANULOMATOUS DISEASE

1. Benign Nasal Tumors

Nasal Polyps

Nasal polyps are pale, edematous, mucosally covered masses commonly seen in patients with allergic rhinitis, but compelling evidence argues against a purely allergic pathogenesis. They may result in chronic nasal obstruction and a diminished sense of smell. In patients with nasal polyps and a history of asthma, aspirin should be avoided as it may precipitate a severe episode of bronchospasm. The presence of polyps in children should suggest the possibility of cystic fibrosis.

Initial treatment with topical nasal corticosteroids (see Allergic Rhinitis section for specific drugs) for 1–3 months is usually successful for small polyps and may reduce the need for operation. A short course of oral corticosteroids (eg, prednisone, 6-day course using 21 5-mg tablets: 30 mg on day 1 and tapering by 5 mg each day) may also be of benefit. When medical management is unsuccessful, polyps should be removed surgically. In healthy persons, this is a minor outpatient procedure. In recurrent cases or when surgery itself is associated with increased risk (such as in patients with asthma), a more complete procedure, such as ethmoidectomy, may be advisable. In recurrent polyposis, it may be necessary to remove polyps from the ethmoid, sphenoid, and maxillary sinuses to provide longer-lasting relief.

Alobid I et al: Nasal polyposis and its impact on quality of life: comparison between the effects of medical and surgical treatments. Allergy 2005;60:452. [PMID: 15727575]

Badia L et al: Topical corticosteroids in nasal polyposis. Drugs 2001;61:573. [PMID: 11368283]

Grigoreas C et al: Nasal polyps in patients with rhinitis and asthma. Allergy Asthma Proc 2002;23:169. [PMID: 12125503]

Slavin RG: Nasal polyps and sinusitis. Clin Allergy Immunol 2002;16:295. [PMID: 11577544]

Stjarne P et al: A randomized controlled trial of mometasone furoate nasal spray for the treatment of nasal polyposis. Arch Otolaryngol Head Neck Surg 2006;132:179. [PMID: 16490876]

Inverted Papilloma

Inverted papillomas are benign tumors that usually arise in the common wall between the nose and maxillary sinus. They present with unilateral nasal obstruction and occasionally hemorrhage. Because SCC is seen in about 10% of inverted or schneiderian papillomas, complete excision is strongly recommended. This usually requires a medial maxillectomy, but in selected cases an endoscopic approach may be possible. Because recurrence rates for inverted papilloma are reported to be as high as 20%, subsequent clinical and radiologic follow-up is imperative. All excised tissue (not just a portion) should be carefully reviewed by the pathologist to be sure no carcinoma is present.

Kasa S et al: Endoscopic resection of inverted papilloma: University of Miami experience. Am J Rhinol 2003;17:185. [PMID: 1296218]

Lawson W et al: Treatment outcomes in the management of inverted papilloma: an analysis of 160 cases. Laryngoscope 2003;113:1548. [PMID: 12972932]

Tomenzoli D et al: Different endoscopic surgical strategies in the management of inverted papilloma of the sinonasal tract: experience with 47 patients. Laryngoscope 2004;114:193. [PMID: 14755188]

Juvenile Angiofibroma

These highly vascular tumors arise in the nasopharynx, typically in adolescent males. Initially, they cause nasal obstruction and hemorrhage. Any adolescent male with recurrent epistaxis should be evaluated for an angiofibroma. Although benign, these tumors expand locally from the sphenopalatine foramen to the pterygopalatine fossa at the pterygoid canal and extend to the pterygoid base, the greater wing of the sphenoid, the nasal cavity, and the paranasal sinuses. They may involve the skull base, usually extradurally, and extend into the superior clivus. Treatment consists of preoperative embolization followed by surgical excision via an approach appropriate for the tumor extent. Small angiofibromas that do not involve the infratemporal fossa may be resected endoscopically. Extensive ones may require skull base approaches. Recurrences are not uncommon and should be resected if possible. Unresectable recurrences that do not appear to grow significantly may be followed radiologically with serial MR scans in expectation of possible eventual involution stabilization or involution of tumor. Low-dose (30 Gy) irradiation may be helpful in nonresectable, continually growing tumors.

Hofmann T et al: Endoscopic resection of juvenile angiofibromas—long term results. Rhinology 2005;43:282. [PMID: 16405273]

Lee JT: The role of radiation in the treatment of advanced juvenile angiofibroma. Laryngoscope 2002;112(7 Part 1):1213. [PMID: 12169902]

Mann WJ et al: Juvenile angiofibromas: changing surgical concept over the last 20 years. Laryngoscope 2004;114:291. [PMID: 14755205]

Nicolai P et al: Endoscopic surgery for juvenile angiofibroma: when and how. Laryngoscope 2003;113:775. [PMID: 12792310]

Wormald PJ et al: Endoscopic removal of juvenile angiofibromas. Otolaryngol Head Neck Surg 2003;129:684. [PMID: 14663436]

2. Malignant Nasopharyngeal & Paranasal Sinus Tumors

Unfortunately, malignant tumors of the nose, nasopharynx, and paranasal sinuses tend to remain asymptomatic until late in their course. Although the prognosis is poor for advanced tumors, the results of treating resectable tumors of paranasal sinus origin have improved with the wider use of skull base resections and intensity-modulated radiation therapy. Cure rates are often 45–60%. Early symptoms are nonspecific, mimicking those of rhinitis or sinusitis. Unilateral nasal obstruction and discharge are common, with pain and recurrent hemorrhage often clues to the diagnosis of cancer. Any patient with unilateral or persistent nasal symptoms should be thoroughly evaluated. A high index of suspicion remains a key to the earlier diagnosis of these tumors. Patients often present with advanced symptoms such as proptosis, expansion of a cheek, or ill-fitting maxillary dentures. Malar hypesthesia, due to involvement of the infraorbital nerve, is common in maxillary sinus tumors. Biopsy is necessary for definitive diagnosis, and MRI is the best imaging study to delineate the extent of disease and plan appropriate surgery and radiation.

SCC is the most common cancer found. It is especially common in the nasopharynx, where it obstructs the auditory tube and results in serous otitis media. Nasopharyngeal carcinoma (poorly differentiated SCC, nonkeratinizing SCC, or lymphoepithelioma) is usually associated with elevated IgA antibody to the viral capsid antigen of the Epstein-Barr virus (EBV). It is particularly common in patients of southern Chinese descent. Any adult with persistent serous otitis media, especially when unilateral, requires careful evaluation of the nasopharynx. Adenocarcinomas, mucosal melanomas, sarcomas, and non-Hodgkin's lymphomas are less commonly encountered neoplasms of this area.

Treatment depends on the tumor type and the extent of disease. Nasopharyngeal carcinoma at this time is best treated by concomitant radiation and cisplatin followed by adjuvant chemotherapy with cisplatin and fluorouracil—this protocol significantly decreased local, nodal, and distant failures and increased progression-free and overall survival. Locally recurrent nasopharyngeal carcinoma may in selected cases be treated with repeat irradiation protocols or surgery with moderate success and a high degree of concern about local wound healing. Other SCCs are best treated—when resectable—with a combination of surgery and irradiation. Numerous protocols investigating the role of chemotherapy are under evaluation. Cranial base surgery appears to be an effective modality in improving the overall prognosis in paranasal sinus malignancies eroding the ethmoid roof.

Duthoy W et al: Postoperative intensity-modulated radiotherapy in sinonasal carcinoma: clinical results in 39 patients. Cancer 2005;104:71. [PMID: 15915466]

Fee WE Jr et al: Nasopharyngectomy for recurrent nasopharyngeal cancer: a 2- to 17-year follow-up. Arch Otolaryngol Head Neck Surg 2002;128:280. [PMID: 11886344]

Ganly I et al: Craniofacial resection for malignant paranasal sinus tumors: Report of an International Collaborative Study. Head Neck 2005;27:575. [PMID: 15825201]

Maghami E et al: Cancer of the nasal cavity and paranasal sinuses. Expert Rev Anticancer Ther 2004;4:411. [PMID: 15161440]

Myers LL et al: Differential diagnosis and treatment options in paranasal sinus cancers. Surg Oncol Clin N Am 2004; 13:167. [PMID: 15062368]

Resto VA et al: Sinonasal malignancies. Otolaryngol Clin North Am 2004;37:473. [PMID: 15064075]

3. Wegener's Granulomatosis, NK Cell & T Cell EBV-Positive Lymphoma, & Sarcoidosis

The nose and paranasal sinuses are involved in over 90% of cases of Wegener's granulomatosis. It is often not realized that involvement at these sites is more common than involvement of lungs or kidneys. Examination shows bloodstained crusts and friable mucosa. Biopsy classically shows necrotizing granulomas and vasculitis, but the diagnosis may be difficult. Sarcoidosis also commonly involves the paranasal sinuses and is clinically similar to other chronic sinonasal inflammatory processes. Biopsy shows noncaseating granulomas.

Polymorphic reticulosis (midline malignant reticulosis, idiopathic midline destructive disease, lethal midline granuloma), as the multitude of apt descriptive terms suggest, is not well understood but appears to be a nasal lymphoma. In contrast to Wegener's granulomatosis, involvement is limited to the mid face, and there may be extensive bone destruction. Its progression in time to a lymphoma is being described with increasing frequency.

Many destructive lesions of the mucosa and nasal structures labeled as polymorphic reticulosis are in fact non-Hodgkin's lymphoma of either NK cell or T cell origin. Immunophenotyping, especially for CD56 expression, is essential in the histologic evaluation. Even when apparently localized, these lymphomas have a poor prognosis, with progression and death within a year the rule.

For treatment of Wegener's granulomatosis, see Chapter 20.

Abdou NI et al: Wegener's granulomatosis: survey of 701 patients in North America. Changes in outcome in the 1990s. J Rheumatol 2002;29:309. [PMID: 11838848]

Cheung MM et al: Early stage nasal NK/T-cell lymphoma: clinical outcome, prognostic factors, and the effect of treatment modality. Int J Radiat Oncol Biol Phys 2002;54:182. [PMID: 12182990]

Cox CE et al: Sarcoidosis. Med Clin North Am 2005;89:817. [PMID: 15925652]

Lee J et al: Extranodal natural killer T-cell lymphoma, nasal-type: a prognostic model from a retrospective multicenter study. J Clin Oncol 2006;24:612. [PMID: 16380410]

Lloyd G et al: Rhinologic changes in Wegener's granulomatosis. J Laryngol Otol 2002;116:565. [PMID: 12238684]

Merkel PA: Current status of outcome measures in vasculitis: focus on Wegener's granulomatosis and microscopic polyangiitis. Report from OMERACT 7. J Rheumatol 2005;32: 2488. [PMID: 1633179]

Nagai H et al: Clinical review of Wegener's granulomatosis. Acta Otolaryngol Suppl 2002;(547):50. [PMID: 12212594]

■ DISEASES OF THE ORAL CAVITY & PHARYNX

LEUKOPLAKIA, ERYTHROPLAKIA, ORAL LICHEN PLANUS, & ORAL CANCER

 ESSENTIALS OF DIAGNOSIS

- **Leukoplakia**—A white lesion that, unlike oral candidiasis, cannot be removed by rubbing the mucosal surface.

- *Erythroplakia*—Similar to leukoplakia except that it has a definite erythematous component.
- *Oral Lichen Planus*—Most commonly presents as lacy leukoplakia but may be erosive; definitive diagnosis requires biopsy.
- *Oral Cancer*—Early lesions appear as leukoplakia or erythroplakia; more advanced lesions will be larger, with invasion into tongue such that a mass lesion is palpable.
- Ulceration may be present.

The areas of leukoplakia are usually small but may be several centimeters in diameter. Histologically, they are often hyperkeratoses occurring in response to chronic irritation (eg, from dentures, tobacco, lichen planus); about 2–6%, however, represent either dysplasia or early invasive SCC.

Distinguishing between erythroplakia and leukoplakia is important because about 90% of cases of erythroplakia are either dysplasia or carcinoma. SCC accounts for 90% of oral cancer. Alcohol and tobacco use are the major epidemiologic risk factors. The differential diagnosis may include oral candidiasis, necrotizing sialometaplasia, pseudoepitheliomatous hyperplasia, median rhomboid glossitis, and vesiculoerosive inflammatory disease such as erosive lichen planus. This should not be confused with the brown-black gingival melanin pigmentation—diffuse or speckled—common in nonwhites, blue-black embedded fragments of dental amalgam, or other systemic disorders associated with general pigmentation (neurofibromatosis, familial polyposis, Addison's disease). Intraoral melanoma is extremely rare.

Oral lichen planus is a relatively common (0.5–2% of the population) chronic inflammatory autoimmune disease that may be difficult to diagnose clinically because of its numerous distinct phenotypic subtypes. For example, the reticular pattern may mimic candidiasis or hyperkeratosis, while the erosive pattern may mimic SCC. Management begins with distinguishing it from other oral lesions. Exfoliative cytology or a small incisional or excisional biopsy is indicated, especially if SCC is suspected. Therapy is aimed at managing pain and discomfort. Corticosteroids have been used widely both locally and systemically. Cyclosporines and retinoids have also been used. Many think there is a low rate (1%) of SCC arising within lichen planus (in addition to the possibility of clinical misdiagnosis).

Any area of erythroplakia, enlarging area of leukoplakia, or a lesion that has submucosal depth on palpation should have an incisional biopsy or an exfoliative cytologic examination. Specialty referral should be sought early both for diagnosis and treatment. Intraoral staining with 1% toluidine blue may aid in selection of the most suspicious biopsy site. A systematic intraoral examination—including the lateral tongue, floor of the mouth, gingiva, buccal area, palate, and tonsillar fossae—and palpation of the neck for enlarged lymph nodes should be part of any general physical examination, especially in patients over the age of 45 who smoke tobacco or drink immoderately. Indirect or fiberoptic examination of the nasopharynx, oropharynx, hypopharynx, and larynx by an otolaryngologist, head and neck surgeon, or radiation oncologist should also be considered for such patients when there is unexplained or persistent throat or ear pain, oral or nasal bleeding, or oral erythroplakia. Fine-needle aspiration (FNA) biopsy may be indicated if an enlarged lymph node is found.

Early detection of SCC is the key to successful management. Lesions less than 4 mm in depth have a low propensity to metastasize. Most patients in whom the tumor is detected before it is 2 cm in diameter are cured. Small lesions are best treated with surgical excision, sometimes with a laser. Radiation is an alternative but is associated with xerostomia, osteonecrosis of the mandible, and inability to use a curative dose again in the treatment field. Large tumors are usually treated with a combination of resection and irradiation. Reconstruction, if required, is done at the time of resection and can involve the use of myocutaneous flaps or vascularized free flaps with or without bone.

Molecular and genetic analysis of premalignant and malignant tissue has produced increasing evidence of genetic instability (including microsatellite instability, cell cycle-regulatory gene *P16* and *P14* deletions and hypermethylation, and mutations in *P53*); and clonal alterations, such as loss of retinoic acid β-receptor expression, occur during the early stage of aerodigestive tract carcinogenesis. These molecular and epidemiologic studies provide the foundation on which clinical trials have been designed to evaluate the role of retinoids and other compounds in the reversal of premalignancy and the possible reduction in the 4–5% annual rate of second primary tumors.

A number of clinical trials have suggested a role for beta-carotene, vitamin E, and retinoids in producing regression of leukoplakia and reducing the incidence of recurrent SCCs. Retinoids suppress head and neck and lung carcinogenesis in animal models and inhibit carcinogenesis in individuals with premalignant lesions. They also seem to reduce the incidence of second primary cancers in head and neck and lung cancer patients previously treated for a primary. Sudbo has demonstrated clearly that aneuploidy in leukoplakic lesions is associated with an increased propensity to develop malignancy. If validated, increased screening for genomic instability may become plausible in the future.

Bromwich M: Retrospective study of the progression of oral premalignant lesions to squamous cell carcinoma: a South Wales experience. J Otolaryngol 2002;31:150. [PMID: 12121018]

Eisen D et al: Number V Oral lichen planus: clinical features and management. Oral Dis 2005;11:338. [PMID: 16269024]

Hegarty AM et al: Fluticasone propionate spray and betamethasone sodium phosphate mouthrinse: a randomized crossover study for the treatment of symptomatic oral lichen planus. J Am Acad Dermatol 2002;47:271. [PMID: 12140475]

Neville BW et al: Oral cancer and precancerous lesions. CA Cancer J Clin 2002;52:195. [PMID: 12139232]

Sudbo J et al: Which putatively pre-malignant oral lesions become oral cancers? J Oral Pathol Med 2003;32:63. [PMID: 12542827]

CANDIDIASIS

Oral candidiasis (thrush) is usually painful and looks like creamy-white curd-like patches overlying erythematous mucosa. Because these white areas are easily rubbed off (eg, by a tongue depressor)—unlike leukoplakia or lichen planus—only the underlying irregular erythema may be seen. Oral candidiasis is commonly encountered among denture wearers; in debilitated patients, diabetes patients, anemia patients, patients undergoing chemotherapy or local irradiation; and in patients receiving corticosteroids or broad-spectrum antibiotics. Candidiasis is often seen as the first manifestation of HIV infection. Angular cheilitis is another manifestation of candidiasis, although it is also seen in nutritional deficiencies.

The diagnosis is made clinically. A wet preparation using potassium hydroxide will reveal spores and may show nonseptate mycelia. Biopsy will show intraepithelial pseudomycelia of *Candida albicans.*

Effective antifungal therapy may be achieved with any of the following: fluconazole (100 mg/d for 7–14 days), ketoconazole (200–400 mg with breakfast [requires acidic gastric environment for absorption] for 7–14 days), clotrimazole troches (10 mg dissolved orally five times daily), or nystatin vaginal troches (100,000 units dissolved orally five times daily) or mouth rinses (500,000 units [5 mL of 100,000 units/mL] held in the mouth before swallowing three times daily). Shorter-duration therapy has proved effective, using fluconazole. In patients with HIV infection, however, longer courses may be needed, and oral itraconazole (200 mg/d) may be indicated in fluconazole-refractory cases. In addition, 0.12% chlorhexidine or half-strength hydrogen peroxide mouth rinses may provide local relief. Nystatin powder (100,000 units/g) applied to dentures three or four times daily for several weeks may help denture wearers.

Lefebvre JL et al: A comparative study of the efficacy and safety of fluconazole oral suspension and amphotericin B oral suspension in cancer patients with mucositis. Oral Oncol 2002;38:337. [PMID: 12076696]

Pankhurst C: Candidiasis (oropharyngeal). Clin Evid 2005;(13): 1701. [PMID: 16135307]

Patton LL et al: A systematic review of the effectiveness of antifungal drugs for the prevention and treatment of oropharyngeal candidiasis in HIV-positive patients. Oral Surg Oral Med Oral Pathol Oral Radiol Endod 2001;92:170. [PMID: 11505264]

Vazquez JA et al: Mucosal candidiasis. Infect Dis Clin North Am 2002;16:793. [PMID: 12512182]

GLOSSITIS, GLOSSODYNIA, DYSGEUSIA, & BURNING MOUTH SYNDROME

Inflammation of the tongue with loss of filiform papillae leads to a red, smooth-surfaced tongue (glossitis). Rarely painful, it may be secondary to nutritional deficiencies (eg, niacin, riboflavin, iron, or vitamin E), drug reactions, dehydration, irritants, and possibly autoimmune reactions or psoriasis. If the primary cause cannot be identified and corrected, empiric nutritional replacement therapy may be of value.

Glossodynia is burning and pain of the tongue; it may occur with or without glossitis. It has been associated with diabetes, drugs (eg, diuretics), tobacco, xerostomia, and candidiasis as well as the listed causes of glossitis. Periodontal disease is not apt to be a factor. Treating possible underlying causes, changing chronic medications to alternative ones, and smoking cessation may resolve symptoms. Glossodynia is benign, and reassurance that there is no infection or tumor is likely to be appreciated. Anxiolytic medications and evaluation of possible psychological status may be considered as well. Symptoms that cannot be related to a specific medication or other cause may be neuropathic in origin. An empiric trial of gabapentin for symptom control may be used.

Clark GT et al: Orofacial pain and sensory disorders in the elderly. Dent Clin North Am 2005;49:343. [PMID: 15755409]

Grushka M et al: Burning mouth syndrome. Am Fam Physician 2002;65:615. [PMID: 11871678]

Lamey PJ et al: Vulnerability and presenting symptoms in burning mouth syndrome. Oral Surg Oral Med Oral Pathol Oral Radiol Endod 2005;99:48. [PMID: 15599348]

Tanaka M et al: Incidence and treatment of dysgeusia in patients with glossodynia. Acta Otolaryngol Suppl 2002;(546):142. [PMID: 12132612]

INTRAORAL ULCERATIVE LESIONS

1. Necrotizing Ulcerative Gingivitis (Trench Mouth, Vincent's Infection)

Necrotizing ulcerative gingivitis, often caused by an infection of both spirochetes and fusiform bacilli, is common in young adults under stress (classically at examination time). Underlying systemic diseases may also predispose to this disorder. Clinically, there is painful acute gingival inflammation and necrosis, often with bleeding, halitosis, fever, and cervical lymphadenopathy. Warm half-strength peroxide rinses and oral penicillin (250 mg three times daily for 10 days) may help. Dental gingival curettage may prove necessary.

Necrotizing ulcerative periodontitis is discussed later in this chapter in the section on AIDS.

2. Aphthous Ulcer (Canker Sore, Ulcerative Stomatitis)

Aphthous ulcers are very common and easy to recognize. Their cause remains uncertain, although an association with human herpesvirus 6 has been suggested. Found on nonkeratinized mucosa (eg, buccal and labial mucosa and not gingiva or palate), they may be single or multiple, are usually recurrent, and appear as painful small (usually 1–2 mm, but sometimes 1–2 cm) round ulcerations with yellow-gray fibrinoid centers surrounded by red halos. The painful stage lasts 7–10 days; healing is completed in 1–3 weeks.

Treatment is nonspecific. Topical corticosteroids (triamcinolone acetonide, 0.1%, or fluocinonide ointment, 0.05%) in an adhesive base (Orabase Plain) do appear to provide symptomatic relief. Other topical therapies shown to be effective in controlled studies include diclofenac 3% in hyaluronan 2.5%, doxymycine-cyanoacrylate, mouthwashes containing the enzymes amyloglucosidase and glucose oxidase, and amlexanox 5% oral paste. A 1-week tapering course of prednisone (40–60 mg/d) has also been used successfully. Thalidomide has been used selectively in recurrent aphthous ulcerations in HIV-positive patients.

Large or persistent areas of ulcerative stomatitis may be secondary to erythema multiforme or drug allergies, acute herpes simplex, pemphigus, pemphigoid, bullous lichen planus, Behçet's disease, or inflammatory bowel disease. SCC may occasionally present in this fashion. When the diagnosis is not clear, incisional biopsy is indicated.

Akintoye SO et al: Recurrent aphthous stomatitis. Dent Clin North Am 2005;49:31, vii. [PMID: 15567359]

Letsinger JA et al: Complex aphthosis: a large case series with evaluation algorithm and therapeutic ladder from topicals to thalidomide. J Am Acad Dermatol 2005;52(3 Pt 1):500. [PMID: 15761429]

Muzio LL et al: The treatment of oral aphthous ulceration or erosive lichen planus with topical clobetasol propionate in three preparations: a clinical and pilot study on 54 patients. J Oral Pathol Med 2001;30:611. [PMID: 11722711]

Tilliss TS et al: Differential diagnosis: is it herpes or aphthous? J Contemp Dent Pract 2002;3:1. [PMID: 12167909]

3. Herpetic Stomatitis

Herpetic gingivostomatitis is common, mild, and short-lived and requires no intervention in most adults. In immunocompromised persons, however, reactivation of herpes simplex virus infection is frequent and may be severe. Clinically, there is initial burning, followed by typical small vesicles that rupture and form scabs. Acyclovir (200–800 mg five times daily for 7–14 days) may shorten the course and reduce postherpetic pain. Differential diagnosis includes ulcerative stomatitis (see above), erythema multiforme, syphilitic chancre, and carcinoma. Coxsackievirus-caused lesions (grayish white tonsillar and palatal ulcers of herpangina or buccal and lip ulcers in hand-foot-and-mouth disease) are seen more commonly in children under age 6.

Holbrook WP et al: Herpetic gingivostomatitis in otherwise healthy adolescents and young adults. Acta Otol Scand 2001;59:113. [PMID: 11501877]

Whitley RJ: Herpes simplex virus infection. Semin Pediatr Infect Dis 2002;13:6. [PMID: 12118847]

PHARYNGITIS & TONSILLITIS

ESSENTIALS OF DIAGNOSIS

- Sore throat.
- Fever.
- Anterior cervical adenopathy.
- Tonsillar exudate.
- Focus is to treat group A β-hemolytic streptococcus infection to prevent rheumatic sequelae.

General Considerations

Pharyngitis and tonsillitis account for over 10% of all office visits to primary care clinicians and 50% of outpatient antibiotic use. The most appropriate management continues to be debated because some of the issues are deceptively complex, but consensus has increased in recent years. The main concern is determining who is likely to have a group A β-hemolytic streptococcal infection (GABHS), as this can lead to subsequent complications such as rheumatic fever and glomerular nephritis. A second public health policy concern is reducing the extraordinary cost (both in dollars and in the development of antibiotic-resistant S pneumoniae) in the United States associated with unnecessary and unrecommended antibiotic use. Questions now being asked: Is there still a role for culturing a sore throat, or have the rapid antigen tests supplanted this procedure under most circumstances? Are clinical criteria alone a sufficient basis for decisions about which patients should be given antibiotics? Should any patient receive any antibiotic other than penicillin (or erythromycin if penicillin-allergic)? For how long should treatment be continued? Numerous well-done studies in the past few years as well as increasing experience with rapid laboratory tests for detection of streptococci (eliminating the delay caused by culturing) appear to make a consensus approach more possible.

Clinical Findings

The clinical features most suggestive of group A β-hemolytic streptococcal pharyngitis include fever over 38°C, tender anterior cervical adenopathy, lack of a cough, and a pharyngotonsillar exudate. These four features (the Centor criteria), when present, strongly suggest GABHS, and some would treat regardless of laboratory results. When three of the four are present, laboratory sensitivity of rapid antigen testing exceeds 90%. When only one criterion is present, GABHS is unlikely. Sore throat may be severe, with odynophagia, tender adenopathy, and a scarlatiniform rash. An elevated white count and left shift are also possible.

Hoarseness, cough, and coryza are not suggestive of this disease.

Marked lymphadenopathy and a shaggy white-purple tonsillar exudate, often extending into the nasopharynx, suggest mononucleosis, especially if present in a young adult. Hepatosplenomegaly and a positive heterophil agglutination test or elevated anti-EBV titer are corroborative. However, about one-third of patients with infectious mononucleosis have secondary streptococcal tonsillitis, requiring treatment. Ampicillin should routinely be avoided if mononucleosis is suspected because it induces a rash. Diphtheria (extremely rare but described in the alcoholic population) presents with low-grade fever and an ill patient with a gray tonsillar pseudomembrane.

The most common pathogens other than group A β-hemolytic streptococci in the differential diagnosis of "sore throat" are viruses, *Neisseria gonorrhoeae, Mycoplasma,* and *Chlamydia trachomatis.* Rhinorrhea and lack of exudate would suggest a virus, but in practice it is not possible to confidently distinguish viral upper respiratory infection from GABHS on clinical grounds alone. Infections with *Corynebacterium diphtheriae,* anaerobic streptococci, and *Corynebacterium haemolyticum* (which responds better to erythromycin than penicillin) may also mimic pharyngitis due to group A β-hemolytic streptococci.

Treatment

Treatment strategies for pharyngitis and tonsillitis range from "treat all comers" to "test all comers, reserving treatment for those with positive results." Issues that affect this decision include the reliability of cultures and rapid tests for streptococci (latex agglutination antigen tests and solid-phase enzyme immunoassays [ELISA]), the incidence of pharyngitis not due to group A β-hemolytic streptococci in the community, patient follow-up and medical compliance, and cost. The advantage of the "treat all" approach is the initial short-term cost, savings from elimination of diagnostic tests, and prevention of rheumatic fever, but such an approach necessarily causes the highest rate of antibiotic use and side effects and therefore overall the highest cost. At the other extreme is the "culture all" approach, which is associated with the fewest side effects but is dependent on excellent and rapid follow-up to prevent postinfectious complications. The sensitivity of current GABHS rapid antigen tests is now excellent, exceeding 90% in appropriately selected patients. It thus appears appropriate to screen for the four Centor criteria and use them in one of the following ways: (1) test patients who satisfy two or more criteria, and treat only those with positive results; (2) test those who satisfy two or three criteria, and treat both those with positive results and all patients who satisfy all four criteria without testing them; or (3) test nobody and treat all who satisfy three or four criteria. Routine cultures arc not needed. Webb and colleagues, using this approach, found no

increase in rates of complications among 7500 patients annually, about 75% of whom had high-specificity antigen tests without culture confirmation of negative results.

Given the availability of many well-documented studies in recent years, one would think that a consensus might develop as to the most appropriate way to treat a sore throat. The Infectious Diseases Society of America recommends laboratory confirmation of the clinical diagnosis by means of either throat culture or a rapid antigen detection test. The American College of Physicians–American Society of Internal Medicine (ACP-ASIM), in collaboration with the Centers for Disease Control and Prevention, advocates use of a clinical algorithm alone—in lieu of microbiologic testing—for confirmation of the diagnosis in adults for whom the suspicion of streptococcal infection is high. Others examine the assumptions of the ACP-ASIM guideline for using a clinical algorithm alone and question whether those recommendations will achieve the stated objective of dramatically decreasing excess antibiotic use. Convincing clinical trials as well as clinician reminders and patient-based interventions may be needed before clinicians are likely to abandon long-held teachings (even as different clinicians appear to have been taught different strategies) regarding diagnosis and management of group A streptococcal pharyngitis. The Cochrane review concluded that multifaceted interventions where educational interventions occur on many levels were the only interventions whose effects were of sufficient magnitude to potentially reduce the incidence of antibiotic-resistant bacteria.

Thirty years ago, a single injection of benzathine penicillin or procaine penicillin was standard antibiotic treatment. This remains effective, but the injections are painful. If compliance is an issue, it may be the best choice. Oral treatment is also effective. Antibiotic choice aims to reduce the already low (10–20%) incidence of treatment failures (positive culture after treatment despite symptomatic resolution) and recurrences. A review of recent controlled studies suggests that penicillin V potassium (250 mg orally three times daily or 500 mg twice daily for 10 days) or cefuroxime axetil (250 mg orally twice daily for 5–10 days) are both effective. The efficacy of a 5-day regimen of penicillin V appears to be similar to a that of a 10-day course, with a 94% clinical response rate and an 84% streptococcal eradication rate. Erythromycin (active against *Mycoplasma* and *Chlamydia*) is a reasonable alternative to penicillin in allergic patients. Cephalosporins are somewhat more effective than penicillin in producing bacteriologic cures; 5-day administration has been successful for cefpodoxime and cefuroxime. The macrolide antibiotics have also been reported to be successful in shorter-duration regimens. Azithromycin (500 mg once daily), because of its long half-life, need be taken for only 3 days.

Adequate antibiotic treatment usually avoids the streptococcal complications of scarlet fever, glomerulonephritis, rheumatic myocarditis, and local abscess formation.

Antibiotics for treatment failures are also somewhat controversial. Surprisingly, penicillin-tolerant strains are not isolated more frequently in those who fail treatment than in those treated successfully with penicillin. The reasons for failure appear to be complex, and a second course of treatment with the same drug is not unreasonable. Alternatives to penicillin include cefuroxime and other cephalosporins, dicloxacillin (which is β-lactamase-resistant), and amoxicillin with clavulanate. When there is a history of penicillin allergy, alternatives should be used, such as erythromycin. Erythromycin resistance—with failure rates of about 25%—is an increasing problem in many areas. In cases of severe penicillin allergy, cephalosporins should be avoided as the cross-reaction is common (8% or more).

Ancillary treatment of pharyngitis includes analgesics and anti-inflammatory agents, such as aspirin or acetaminophen. Some patients find that salt water gargling is soothing. In severe cases, anesthetic gargles and lozenges (eg, benzocaine) may provide additional symptomatic relief. Occasionally, odynophagia is so intense that hospitalization for intravenous hydration and antibiotics is necessary. (See Chapter 33.)

Arnold SR et al: Interventions to improve antibiotic prescribing practices in ambulatory care. Cochrane Database Syst Rev 2005;(4):CD003539. [PMID: 16235325]

Bisno AL et al: Practice guidelines for the diagnosis and management of group A streptococcal pharyngitis. Infectious Diseases Society of America. Clin Infect Dis 2002;35:113. [PMID: 12087516]

Carapetis JR et al: The global burden of group A streptococcal diseases. Lancet Infect Dis 2005;5:685. [PMID: 16253886]

Colletti T et al: Strep throat: guidelines for diagnosis and treatment. JAAPA 2005;18:38; quiz 45. [PMID: 16184870]

Hirschmann JV: Antibiotics for common respiratory tract infections in adults. Arch Intern Med 2002;162:256. [PMID: 11822917]

Johnson BC et al: Cost-effective workup for tonsillitis. Testing, treatment, and potential complications. Postgrad Med 2003;113:115. [PMID: 12647478]

Tewfik TL et al: Tonsillopharyngitis: clinical highlights. J Otolaryngol 2005;34 Suppl 1:S45. [PMID: 16089240]

PERITONSILLAR ABSCESS & CELLULITIS

When infection penetrates the tonsillar capsule and involves the surrounding tissues, peritonsillar cellulitis results. Peritonsillar abscess and cellulitis present with severe sore throat, odynophagia, trismus, medial deviation of the soft palate and peritonsillar fold, and an abnormal muffled ("hot potato") voice. Following therapy, peritonsillar cellulitis usually either resolves over several days or evolves into peritonsillar abscess. The existence of an abscess may be confirmed by aspirating pus from the peritonsillar fold just superior and medial to the upper pole of the tonsil. A No. 19 or No. 21 needle should be passed no deeper than 1 cm, because the internal carotid artery may lie more medially than its usual location and pass posterior and deep

to the tonsillar fossa. There is controversy regarding the three ways to treat a peritonsillar abscess: needle aspiraton, incision and drainage, or tonsillectomy. Some clinicians incise and drain the area and continue with parenteral antibiotics, whereas others aspirate only and monitor as an outpatient. To drain the abscess and avoid recurrence, it may be appropriate to consider immediate tonsillectomy (quinsy tonsillectomy). About 10% of patients with peritonsillar abscess exhibit relative indications for tonsillectomy. All three approaches are effective and have support in the literature. Regardless of the method used, one must be sure the abscess is adequately treated, since complications such as extension to the retropharyngeal, deep neck, and posterior mediastinal spaces are possible. Bacteria may also be aspirated into the lungs, resulting in pneumonia. While there is controversy about whether a single abscess is sufficient indication for tonsillectomy, most would agree that patients with recurrent abscesses should have a tonsillectomy.

Dunne AA et al: Peritonsillar abscess—critical analysis of abscess tonsillectomy. Clin Otolaryngol 2003;28:420. [PMID: 12969344]

Franzese CB et al: Peritonsillar and parapharyngeal space abscess in the older adult. Am J Otolaryngol 2003;24:169. [PMID: 12761704]

Johnson RF et al: The contemporary approach to diagnosis and management of peritonsillar abscess. Curr Opin Otolaryngol Head Neck Surg 2005;13:157. [PMID: 1590881]

Khayr W et al: Management of peritonsillar abscess: needle aspiration versus incision and drainage versus tonsillectomy. Am J Ther 2005;12:344. [PMID: 1604119]

Matsuda A et al: Peritonsillar abscess: a study of 724 cases in Japan. Ear Nose Throat J 2002;81:384. [PMID: 12092281]

TONSILLECTOMY

Despite the frequency with which tonsillectomy is performed, the indications for the procedure remain controversial. Most clinicians would agree that airway obstruction causing sleep apnea or cor pulmonale is an absolute indication for tonsillectomy. Similarly, persistent marked tonsillar asymmetry should prompt an excisional biopsy to rule out lymphoma. Relative indications include recurrent streptococcal tonsillitis, causing considerable loss of time from school or work, recurrent peritonsillar abscess, and chronic tonsillitis.

Tonsillectomy is not an entirely benign procedure. The pros and cons of tonsillectomy need to be discussed with each prospective patient. Postoperative bleeding occurs in 2–4% of cases and on rare occasions can lead to laryngospasm and airway obstruction. Pain may be considerable, especially in the adult. Protracted emesis or fever may also occasionally occur. Secondary bleeding 5–8 days postoperatively is far more common than bleeding in the first 24 hours. There is increasing economic pressure for these procedures to be done as outpatient surgery. At present it seems clear that outpatient tonsillectomy is usually safe when followed by a 6-hour period of uneventful observation, but individual circumstances may mandate hospitalization.

Although reports in the 1970s suggested an association of tonsillectomy with Hodgkin's disease, careful review of this literature reveals no conclusively causative association.

Bhattacharyya N et al: Economic benefit of tonsillectomy in adults with chronic tonsillitis. Ann Otol Rhinol Laryngol 2002;111:983. [PMID: 12450171]

Darrow DH et al: Indications for tonsillectomy and adenoidectomy. Laryngoscope 2002;112:6. [PMID: 12172229]

Dhiwakar M et al: Antibiotics to improve recovery following tonsillectomy: a systematic review. Otolaryngol Head Neck Surg 2006;134:357. [PMID: 16500427]

Windfuhr JP et al: Incidence of post-tonsillectomy hemorrhage in children and adults: a study of 4,848 patients. Ear Nose Throat J 2002;81:626. [PMID: 12353439]

DEEP NECK INFECTIONS

Deep neck abscesses usually present with marked neck pain and swelling in a toxic febrile patient. They are emergencies because they may rapidly compromise the airway. They may also spread to the mediastinum or cause septicemia. Most commonly, they originate from odontogenic infections. Other causes include suppurative lymphadenitis, direct spread of pharyngeal infection, penetrating trauma, pharyngoesophageal foreign bodies, cervical osteomyelitis, and intravenous injection of the internal jugular vein, especially in drug abusers. Recurrent deep neck infection may suggest an underlying congenital lesion such as a branchial cleft cyst.

Fundamentals of treatment include securing the airway, intravenous antibiotics, and incision and drainage. In highly selected patients without airway compromise, needle aspiration and catheter drainage or even conservative management without antibiotics alone has been reported to be successful in uniloculated abscesses. The airway may be secured, when indicated, either by intubation or tracheotomy. Tracheotomy is preferable in the patients with substantial pharyngeal edema, since attempts at intubation may precipitate acute airway obstruction. Bleeding in association with a deep neck abscess suggests the possibility of carotid artery or internal jugular vein involvement and requires prompt neck exploration both for drainage of pus and for vascular control.

Contrast-enhanced CT usually augments the clinical examination in defining the extent of the infection. It often will distinguish inflammation (requiring antibiotics) from abscess (requiring drainage) and define for the surgeon the extent of an abscess. CT with MRI may also identify thrombophlebitis of the internal jugular vein secondary to oropharyngeal inflammation. This condition, known as Lemierre's syndrome, may be associated with septic emboli and requires prompt institution of antibiotics appropriate for *Fusobacterium necrophorum* as well as the more usual upper airway pathogens. The presence of pulmonary infiltrates (or septic arthritis) in the setting of a neck abscess should lead one to suspect Lemierre's syndrome.

Ludwig's angina is the most commonly encountered neck space infection. It is a cellulitis of the sublingual and submaxillary spaces, often arising from infection of the mandible. Clinically, there is edema and erythema of the upper neck under the chin and often of the floor of the mouth. The tongue may be displaced upward and backward by the posterior spread of cellulitis. This may lead to occlusion of the airway and necessitate tracheotomy. Microbiologic isolates include streptococci, staphylococci, *Bacteroides,* and *Fusobacterium.* Usual doses of penicillin plus metronidazole, ampicillin-sulbactam, clindamycin, or selective cephalosporins are good initial choices. Culture and sensitivity data will then refine the choice. Dental consultation is advisable. External drainage via bilateral submental incisions is required if the airway is threatened or when medical therapy has not reversed the process.

Brook I: Microbiology and management of deep facial infections and Lemierre syndrome. ORL J Otorhinolaryngol Relat Spec 2003;65:117. [PMID: 12824734]

Chirinos JA et al: The evolution of Lemierre syndrome: report of 2 cases and review of the literature. Medicine (Baltimore) 2002;81:458. [PMID: 12441902]

Dool H et al: Lemierre's syndrome: three cases and a review. Eur Arch Otorhinolaryngol 2005;262:651. [PMID: 15599753]

Lin D et al: Internal jugular vein thrombosis and deep neck infection from intravenous drug use: management strategy. Laryngoscope 2004;114:56. [PMID: 14709995]

Parhiscar A et al: Deep neck abscess: a retrospective review of 210 cases. Ann Otol Rhinol Laryngol 2001;110:1051. [PMID: 11713917]

Ridder GJ et al: Spectrum and management of deep neck space infections: an 8-year experience of 234 cases. Otolaryngol Head Neck Surg 2005;133:709. [PMID: 16274797]

Wang LF et al: Space infection of the head and neck. Kaohsiung J Med Sci 2002;18:386. [PMID: 12476681]

■ DISEASES OF THE SALIVARY GLANDS

The salivary glands are divided into the two large parotid glands, two submandibular glands, several sublingual glands, and 600–1000 minor salivary glands located throughout the upper aerodigestive tract.

ACUTE INFLAMMATORY SALIVARY GLAND DISORDERS

1. Sialadenitis

Acute bacterial sialadenitis in the adult most commonly affects either the parotid or submandibular gland. It typically presents with acute swelling of the gland, increased pain and swelling with meals, and tenderness and erythema of the duct opening. Pus often can be massaged from the duct. Sialadenitis often occurs in the setting of dehydration or in association with chronic illness. Underlying Sjögren's syndrome may contribute. Ductal obstruction, often by an inspissated mucous plug, is followed by salivary stasis and secondary infection. The most common organism recovered from purulent draining saliva is *S aureus*. Treatment consists of intravenous antibiotics such as nafcillin (1 g intravenously every 4–6 hours) and measures to increase salivary flow, including hydration, warm compresses, sialagogues (eg, lemon drops), and massage of the gland. Usually one can switch to an oral agent based on clinical and microbiologic improvement to complete a 10-day course. Failure of the process to resolve on this regimen suggests abscess formation, ductal stricture, stone, or tumor causing obstruction. Ultrasound or CT scan may be helpful in establishing the diagnosis. Sialography is best avoided in acute cases.

2. Sialolithiasis

Calculus formation is more common in Wharton's duct (draining the submandibular glands) than in Stensen's duct (draining the parotid glands). Clinically, a patient may note postprandial pain and local swelling, often with a history of recurrent acute sialadenitis. Stones in Wharton's duct are usually large and radiopaque, whereas those in Stensen's duct are usually radiolucent and smaller. Those very close to the orifice of Wharton's duct may be palpated manually in the anterior floor of the mouth and removed intraorally by dilating or incising the distal duct. The duct proximal to the stone must be temporarily clamped (using, for instance, a single throw of a suture) to keep manipulation of the stone from pushing it back toward the submandibular gland. Those more than 1.5–2 cm from the duct are too close to the lingual nerve to be removed safely in this manner. Similarly, dilation of Stensen's duct, located on the buccal surface opposite the second maxillary molar, may relieve distal stricture or allow a small stone to pass. In addition to intraoral stone removal, both extracorporeal shock-wave lithotripsy and fluoroscopically guided basket retrieval have been used successfully in recent years, with success rates between 40% and 80%.

Repeated episodes of sialadenitis are usually associated with stricture and chronic infection. If the obstruction cannot be safely removed or dilated, excision of the gland may be necessary to relieve recurrent symptoms.

Baurmash HD: Submandibular salivary stones: current management modalities. J Oral Maxillofac Surg 2004;62:369. [PMID: 15015173]

Brook I: Aerobic and anaerobic microbiology of suppurative sialadenitis. J Med Microbiol 2002;51:526. [PMID: 12018662]

McGurk M et al: Modern management of salivary calculi. Br J Surg 2005;92:107. [PMID: 15573365]

Ziegler CM et al: Endoscopy as minimal invasive routine treatment for sialolithiasis. Acta Odontol Scand 2003;61:137. [PMID: 12868686]

CHRONIC INFLAMMATORY & INFILTRATIVE DISORDERS OF THE SALIVARY GLANDS

Numerous infiltrative disorders may cause unilateral or bilateral parotid gland enlargement. Sjögren's disease and sarcoidosis are examples of lymphoepithelial and granulomatous diseases that may affect the salivary glands. Metabolic disorders, including alcoholism, diabetes mellitus, and vitamin deficiencies, may also cause diffuse enlargement. Several drugs have been associated with parotid enlargement, including thioureas, iodine, and drugs with cholinergic effects (eg, phenothiazines), which stimulate salivary flow and cause more viscous saliva.

SALIVARY GLAND TUMORS

Approximately 80% of salivary gland tumors occur in the parotid gland. In adults, about 80% of these are benign. In the submandibular triangle, it is sometimes difficult to distinguish a primary submandibular gland tumor from a metastatic submandibular space node. Only 50–60% of primary submandibular tumors are benign. Tumors of the minor salivary glands are most likely to be malignant, with adenoid cystic carcinoma predominating.

Most parotid tumors present as an asymptomatic mass in the superficial part of the gland. Their presence may have been noted by the patient for months or years. Facial nerve involvement correlates strongly with malignancy. Tumors may extend deep to the plane of the facial nerve or may originate in the parapharyngeal space. In such cases, medial deviation of the soft palate is visible on intraoral examination. MRI and CT scans have largely replaced sialography in defining the extent of tumor.

When the clinician encounters a patient with an otherwise asymptomatic salivary gland mass where tumor is the most likely diagnosis, the choice is whether to simply excise the mass via a parotidectomy with facial nerve dissection or submandibular gland excision or to obtain an FNA biopsy first. Although the accuracy of FNA biopsy for malignancy has been reported to be quite high, results vary among institutions. If a negative FNA biopsy would lead to a decision not to proceed to surgery, then it should be considered. Poor overall health of the patient and the possibility of inflammatory disease as the cause of the mass are situations where FNA biopsy might be helpful. In otherwise straightforward nonrecurrent cases, excision is indicated. In benign and small low-grade malignant tumors, no additional treatment is needed. Postoperative irradiation is indicated for larger and high-grade cancers.

Bajaj Y et al: Critical clinical appraisal of the role of ultrasound guided fine needle aspiration cytology in the management of parotid tumours. J Laryngol Otol 2005;119:289. [PMID: 15949083]

Bhattacharyya N et al: Nodal metastasis in major salivary gland cancer: predictive factors and effects on survival. Arch Otolaryngol Head Neck Surg 2002;128:904. [PMID: 12162768]

Bhattacharyya N et al: Determinants of survival in parotid gland carcinoma: a population-based study. Am J Otolaryngol 2005;26:39. [PMID: 15635580]

Guzzo M et al: Mucoepidermoid carcinoma of the salivary glands: clinicopathologic review of 108 patients treated at the National Cancer Institute of Milan. Ann Surg Oncol 2002; 9:688. [PMID: 12167584]

Luukkaa H et al: Salivary gland cancer in Finland 1991–96: an evaluation of 237 cases. Acta Otolaryngol 2005;125:207. [PMID: 15880955]

Seethala RR et al: Relative accuracy of fine-needle aspiration and frozen section in the diagnosis of lesions of the parotid gland. Head Neck 2005;27:217. [PMID: 15672359]

Wahlberg P et al: Carcinoma of the parotid and submandibular glands—a study of survival in 2465 patients. Oral Oncol 2002;38:706. [PMID: 12167424]

Witt RL: Minimally invasive surgery for parotid pleomorphic adenoma. Ear Nose Throat J 2005;84:308, 310. [PMID: 15971755]

■ DISEASES OF THE LARYNX

DYSPHONIA, HOARSENESS, & STRIDOR

The primary symptoms of laryngeal disease are hoarseness and stridor. Hoarseness is caused by an abnormal flow of air past the vocal cords. The voice is "breathy" when too much air passes incompletely apposed vocal cords, as in unilateral vocal cord paralysis. The voice is harsh when turbulence is created by irregularity of the vocal cords, as in laryngitis or a mass lesion. Stridor, a high-pitched sound, is produced by lesions that narrow the airway. Airway narrowing above the vocal cords produces predominantly inspiratory stridor. Airway narrowing below the vocal cord level produces either expiratory or mixed stridor.

Evaluation of an abnormal voice begins with obtaining a history of the circumstances preceding its onset and an examination of the airway. Any patient with hoarseness that has persisted beyond a few weeks should be evaluated by indirect fiberoptic laryngoscopy. Especially when the patient has a history of tobacco use, laryngeal cancer or lung cancer (leading to paralysis of a recurrent laryngeal nerve) must be strongly considered. Laryngitis, voice abuse, and vocal cord nodules are among the most common causes of hoarseness.

Altman KW et al: Current and emerging concepts in muscle tension dysphonia: a 30-month review. J Voice 2005;19:261. [PMID: 15907440]

Garrett CG et al: Hoarseness. Med Clin North Am 1999;83:115. [PMID: 9927964]

MacKenzie K et al: Is voice therapy an effective treatment for dysphonia? A randomized controlled trial. BMJ 2001;323:658. [PMID: 11566828]

Merati AL et al: Common movement disorders affecting the larynx: a report from the neurolaryngology committee of the AAO-HNS. Otolaryngol Head Neck Surg 2005;133:654. [PMID: 16274788]

Sataloff RT: Professional voice users: the evaluation of voice disorders. Occup Med 2001;16:633. [PMID: 11567923]

COMMON LARYNGEAL DISORDERS

1. Epiglottitis

Epiglottitis (or, more correctly, supraglottitis) in adults should be suspected when a patient presents with a rapidly developing sore throat or when odynophagia (pain on swallowing) is out of proportion to apparently minimal oropharyngeal findings on examination. It is more common in diabetics and may be viral or bacterial in origin. Rarely in the era of *H influenzae* type b vaccine is this bacterium isolated in adults. Unlike in children, indirect laryngoscopy is generally safe and may demonstrate a swollen, erythematous epiglottis. Initial treatment is hospitalization for intravenous antibiotics—eg, ceftizoxime, 1–2 g intravenously every 8–12 hours; or cefuroxime, 750–1500 mg intravenously every 8 hours; and dexamethasone, usually 4–10 mg as initial bolus, then 4 mg intravenously every 6 hours—and observation of the airway. Corticosteroids may be tapered as signs and symptoms resolve. Similarly, substitution of oral antibiotics may be appropriate to complete a 10-day course. Less than 10% of adults require intubation. Indications for intubation are dyspnea or rapid pace of sore throat (where progression to airway compromise may occur before the effects of corticosteroids and antibiotics). If the patient is not intubated, prudence suggests monitoring oxygen saturation with continuous pulse oximetry and initial admission to a monitored unit.

Berger G et al: The rising incidence of adult acute epiglottitis and epiglottic abscess. Am J Otolaryngol 2003;24:374. [PMID: 14608569]

Chang YL et al: Adult acute epiglottitis: experiences in a Taiwanese setting. Otolaryngol Head Neck Surg 2005;132: 689. [PMID: 15886619]

Cohen B: The death of George Washington (1732–99) and the history of cynanche. J Med Biogr 2005;13:225. [PMID: 16244717]

Katori H et al: Acute epiglottitis: analysis of factors associated with airway intervention. J Laryngol Otol 2005;119:967. [PMID: 16354360]

Sack JL et al: Identifying acute epiglottitis in adults. High degree of awareness, close monitoring are key. Postgrad Med 2002; 112:81. [PMID: 12146095]

2. Recurrent Respiratory Papillomatosis

Papillomas are common lesions of the larynx and other sites where ciliated and squamous epithelia meet. Unlike oral papillomas, recurrent respiratory papillomatosis (RRP) is likely to be symptomatic, with hoarseness that progresses to stridor over weeks to months. The disease is more common in children. Repeated laser vaporizations via microdirect laryngoscopy are usually the mainstay of treatment. Tracheotomy should be avoided, if possible, since it introduces an additional squamociliary junction where papillomas appear to preferentially grow. Interferon treatment has been under investigation for over two decades; rare cases of malignant transformation (often in smokers) have been reported. Cidofovir (a cytosine nucleotide analog in use to treat cytomegalovirus retinitis) is also being investigated as intralesional therapy for RRP; its potential for carcinogenesis is being monitored. Antiviral vaccines to HPV 11 and 6 are being investigated as well.

Chadha NK et al: Adjuvant antiviral therapy for recurrent respiratory papillomatosis. Cochrane Database Syst Rev 2005;(4): CD005053. [PMID: 16235390]

Derkay CS et al: Recurrent respiratory papillomatosis. Ann Otol Rhinol Laryngol 2006;115:1. [PMID: 1646609]

Gerein V et al: Use of interferon-alpha in recurrent respiratory papillomatosis: 20-year follow-up. Ann Otol Rhinol Laryngol 2005;114:463. [PMID: 16042104]

Lee JH et al: Recurrent respiratory papillomatosis: pathogenesis to treatment. Curr Opin Otolaryngol Head Neck Surg 2005; 13:354. [PMID: 16282764]

Naiman AN et al: Natural history of adult-onset laryngeal papillomatosis following multiple cidofovir injections. Ann Otol Rhinol Laryngol 2006;115:175. [PMID: 16572605]

Shehab N et al: Cidofovir for the treatment of recurrent respiratory papillomatosis: a review of the literature. Pharmacotherapy 2005;25:977. [PMID: 1600627]

3. Acute Laryngitis

Acute laryngitis is probably the most common cause of hoarseness, which may persist for a week or so after other symptoms of an upper respiratory infection have cleared. The patient should be warned to avoid vigorous use of the voice (singing, shouting) while laryngitis is present, since this may foster the formation of vocal nodules. Although thought to be usually viral in origin, both *M catarrhalis* and *H influenzae* may be isolated from the nasopharynx at higher than expected frequencies. Erythromycin may reduce the severity of hoarseness and cough.

4. Gastroesophageal Reflux & Hoarseness

Gastroesophageal reflux into the larynx (laryngopharyngeal reflux) is considered a possible cause of chronic hoarseness when other causes of abnormal laryngeal airflow (such as tumor) have been excluded by indirect or direct laryngoscopy. Gastroesophageal reflux disease (GERD) has also been suggested as a contributing factor to other symptoms such as throat clearing, throat discomfort, chronic cough, a sensation of postnasal drip, and esophageal spasm; as well as in many cases of posterior laryngitis and some cases of asthma. Since less than half of patients with documented laryngopharyngeal reflux have typical symptoms of heartburn and regurgitation, the lack of such symptoms should not be construed as eliminating this cause.

Management should initially exclude other causes of hoarseness, laryngitis, or chronic cough; consultation with an otolaryngologist is advisable. Many clinicians opt next for an empiric trial of a proton pump inhibitor at twice-daily dosing (eg, omeprazole 20 mg twice daily) for 2–3 months as a practical alternative to an initial pH study. If symptoms improve and cessation of therapy leads to symptoms again, then a proton pump inhibitor is resumed at the lowest dose effective for remission, usually daily but at times on a demand basis. Although H_2-receptor antagonists are an alternative to proton pump inhibitors, they are generally both less clinically effective and less cost-effective. Nonresponders should undergo pH testing and manometry. Twenty-four-hour pH monitoring of the pharynx should best document laryngopharyngeal reflux and is advocated by some as the initial management step but it is costly, more difficult, and less available than lower esophageal monitoring alone. Lower esophageal pH monitoring does not correlate well with laryngopharyngeal reflux symptoms.

Ahmed TF et al: Chronic laryngitis associated with gastroesophageal reflux: prospective assessment of differences in practice patterns between gastroenterologists and ENT physicians. Am J Gastroenterol 2006;101:470. [PMID: 16542282]

Hopkins C et al: Acid reflux treatment for hoarseness. Cochrane Database Syst Rev 2006;(1):CD005054. [PMID: 16437513]

Noordzij JP et al: Correlation of pH probe-measured laryngopharyngeal reflux with symptoms and signs of reflux laryngitis. Laryngoscope 2002;112:2192. [PMID: 12461340]

Oelschlager BK et al: Typical GERD symptoms and esophageal pH monitoring are not enough to diagnose pharyngeal reflux. J Surg Res 2005;128:55. [PMID: 16115493]

Williams RB et al: Predictors of outcome in an open label, therapeutic trial of high-dose omeprazole in laryngitis. Am J Gastroenterol 2004;99:777. [PMID: 15128336]

TUMORS OF THE LARYNX

1. Benign Tumors of the Larynx

Vocal cord nodules are smooth, paired lesions that form at the junction of the anterior one-third and posterior two-thirds of the vocal cords. They are a common cause of hoarseness resulting from vocal abuse. In adults, they are referred to as "singer's nodules"; in children, "screamer's nodules." Treatment requires modification of voice habits, and referral to a speech therapist is indicated. Recalcitrant nodules may require surgical excision.

Polypoid changes in the vocal cords may result from vocal abuse, smoking, chemical industrial irritants, or hypothyroidism. Attention to the underlying problem may resolve the polypoid changes. Inhaled corticosteroid spray (eg, beclomethasone, 42 mcg/spray, or dexamethasone, 84 mcg/spray, two or three times a day) may hasten resolution. At times, removal of the hyperplastic vocal cord mucosa may be indicated.

A common but often unrecognized cause of hoarseness is contact ulcers on the vocal processes of the arytenoid cartilages secondary to esophageal reflux. Treatment may be with H_2-receptor blockers or proton pump inhibitors (see Gastroesophageal Reflux and Hoarseness, above). Intubation granulomas may also be seen posteriorly between the vocal processes.

2. Laryngeal Leukoplakia

Leukoplakia is a frequent cause of chronic hoarseness, most commonly arising in smokers. Direct laryngoscopy with biopsy is advised. Histologic examination usually demonstrates mild, moderate, or severe dysplasia. Cessation of smoking may reverse dysplastic changes. A certain percentage of patients—estimated to be less than 5% of those with mild dysplasia and about 35–60% of those with severe dysplasia—will subsequently develop SCC. In some cases, invasive SCC is present in the initial biopsy specimen.

3. Squamous Cell Carcinoma of the Larynx

 ESSENTIALS OF DIAGNOSIS

- Persistent (more than 2 weeks duration) hoarseness.
- Persistent throat pain.
- Unexplained ear pain (referred otalgia).
- Neck mass.
- Hemoptysis.
- Stridor or other symptoms of a compromised airway.
- More common in smokers.
- If a neck mass is present, an FNA biopsy is usually adequate for initial diagnosis.

Clinical Findings

A. SYMPTOMS AND SIGNS

SCC of the larynx, the most common malignancy of the larynx, occurs almost exclusively in patients with a history of significant tobacco use, and often with alcohol. SCC is usually seen in persons age 50–70 years; about 13,000 new cases are seen in United States each year. A change in voice quality is almost always noted, although throat or ear pain, hemoptysis, dysphagia, weight loss, and airway compromise may occur. Neck metastases are not common in early glottic (true vocal cord [TVC]) cancer in which the vocal cords are mobile, but a third of patients in whom there is impaired

cord mobility will also have involved nodes. Supraglottic carcinoma (false vocal cords, aryepiglottic folds, epiglottis), on the other hand, often metastasizes to both sides of the neck early. Complete head and neck examination, including indirect or fiberoptic laryngoscopy, by an experienced clinician is mandated for any person with the concerning symptoms listed under Essentials of Diagnosis.

B. IMAGING AND LABORATORY STUDIES

Radiologic evaluation is helpful in assessing tumor extent. In contrast to other head and neck sites, CT scanning is preferable to MRI for the larynx. CT scan evaluates neck nodes, tumor volume, and cartilage sclerosis or destruction. A chest CT scan is indicated if there are level VI enlarged nodes (around the trachea and the thyroid gland) or IV enlarged nodes (inferior to the cricoid cartilage along the internal jugular vein) or if a chest film is concerning for a second primary lesion or metastases. Laboratory evaluation includes complete blood count and liver function tests. Formal cardiopulmonary evaluation may be indicated, especially if partial laryngeal surgery is being considered. A positron emission tomography (PET) scan or CT-PET scan may be indicated to assess for distant metastases when there appears to be advanced local or regional disease.

C. BIOPSY

Diagnosis is made by biopsy at the time of laryngoscopy. At that time, true cord mobility and arytenoid fixation, as well as surface tumor extent, can be evaluated. Most otolaryngologists recommend flexible esophagoscopy and flexible bronchoscopy at that time. Although an FNA biopsy of an enlarged neck node may have already been done, it is generally acceptable to assume radiologically enlarged neck nodes are neck metastases; rarely is an open biopsy necessary.

D. TUMOR STAGING

Staging is helpful in discussing laryngeal cancer, but a number of factors that are not included in the TNM staging are also important in deciding treatment recommendations. Table 8–2 outlines (slightly abbreviated) the current American Joint Committee on Cancer (AJCC) tumor staging for the glottis and supraglottis.

Treatment

Treatment of laryngeal carcinoma has four goals: cure, preservation of safe effective swallowing, preservation of useful voice, and avoidance of a permanent tracheostoma. Early tumors (T1 and many T2 lesions, without involved nodes) may be treated with either radiation therapy or partial laryngeal surgery assuming at least one cricoarytenoid unit is normal (transoral endoscopic laser resection, classic open vertical hemilaryngectomy for glottic tumors, or classic horizontal supraglottic laryngectomy). Five-year loco-regional cure rates exceed 80–90%, and patient-reported satisfac-

Table 8–2. Staging of glottis and supraglottis tumors.

Stage	Glottis	Supraglottis
T1	Limited to true vocal cords	One site, with normal true vocal cord mobility
T2	Extends to supraglottis or subglottis; or impaired true vocal cord mobility	Two sites, with normal true vocal cord mobility
T3	True vocal cord fixation	True vocal cord fixation, or extension to preepiglottic space, medial pyriform sinus, or postcricoid area
T4	Extralaryngeal (eg, invasion of thyroid cartilage or strap muscles)	
N[1]		
N0	No nodes (includes information from physical examination, CT and MRI scans, and positron emission tomography)	
N1	Ipsilateral node < 3 cm	
N2a	Ipsilateral node ≥ 3 cm but < 6 cm	
N2b	Ipsilateral multiple nodes, all < 6 cm	
N2c	Bilateral (or contralateral nodes only) < 6 cm	
N3	Node(s) ≥ 6 cm	

[1]N staging is the same for all head and neck squamous cell carcinoma except nasopharyngeal carcinoma.

tion is excellent. In supraglottic tumors, even when clinically N0, selective neck dissection or irradiation is indicated because of the high risk of neck node involvement.

For more advanced tumors, cisplatin-based chemoradiation protocols are used. Twenty-five years ago, total laryngectomy was often recommended for such patients. However, the 1994 VA study (with induction cisplatin and 5-fluorouracil followed by irradiation alone in responders) demonstrated that two-thirds of patients could preserve their larynx. Since that study, cisplatin-based chemotherapy concomitant with radiation therapy has been shown to be superior to either irradiation alone or induction chemotherapy followed by radiation. However, chemoradiation is associated with prolonged gastrostomy-dependent dysphagia. This high rate of chemoradiation-associated dysphagia has prompted a reevaluation of the role of extended, but less-than-total, laryngeal surgery for selected advanced laryngeal carcinoma in which at least one cricoarytenoid unit is intact. Supracricoid laryngectomy (with cricoepiglottohyoidpexy for glottic tumors or cricohyoidpexy for supraglottic tumors) as well as endoscopic resection of selected more advanced tumors, should be discussed as an alternative to chemoradiation. Supracricoid laryngectomy and chemoradiation have similar cure rates; the risk of permanent tracheostoma may be less with supracricoid laryngectomy, but the voice quality may be superior without surgery. Patient comorbidities and patient choice, after thorough discussion, play an important role in the choice between surgery and chemoradiation. A patient and his or her physicians must carefully consider *different* side effects and complications associated with different treatment modalities. These include the risks of chemotherapy, the likelihood of avoiding irradiation side effects, the likelihood of surgical complications, the likelihood of avoiding a permanent tracheostoma, the quality of posttreatment voice, and the likelihood of cure.

The presence of malignant adenopathy in the neck affects the prognosis greatly. Supraglottic tumors metastasize early and bilaterally to the neck, and this must be included in the treatment plans even when the neck is apparently uninvolved. Glottic tumors in which the TVCs are mobile have less than a 5% rate of nodal involvement; when a cord is immobile, the rate of ipsilateral nodal involvement climbs to about 30%. An involved neck is treated by surgery or chemoradiation, or both. This decision will depend on the treatment chosen for the larynx and the extent of neck involvement.

Total laryngectomy is largely reserved for far-advanced resectable tumors with extralaryngeal spread, those with persistent tumor following chemoradiation, and for recurrent disease. Voice rehabilitation via a primary (or at times secondary) tracheoesophageal puncture produces good speech in about 75–85% of patients. Indwelling prostheses that are changed every 3–6 months are a common alternative to patient-inserted prostheses, which need changing more frequently.

Long-term follow-up is critical in head and neck cancer patients. In addition to the 3–4% annual rate of second tumors and monitoring for recurrence, psychosocial aspects of treatment are common. Dysphagia, impaired communication, and altered appearance, may result in patient difficulties adapting to the workplace and to social interactions. In addition, smoking cessation and alcohol abatement are common challenges. Nevertheless, about 65% of patients with larynx cancer are cured, most have useful speech, and many resume their prior livelihoods, albeit with adaptations.

Bernier J et al: Postoperative irradiation with or without concomitant chemotherapy for locally advanced head and neck cancer. N Eng J Med 2004;350:1945. [PMID: 15128894]

Forastiere AA et al: Concurrent chemotherapy and radiotherapy for organ preservation in advanced laryngeal cancer. N Engl J Med 2003;349:2091. [PMID: 14645636]

Gallo A et al: Supracricoid partial laryngectomy in the treatment of laryngeal cancer: univariate and multivariate analysis of prognostic factors. Arch Otolaryngol Head Neck Surg 2005;131:620. [PMID: 16027286]

Ganly I et al: Results of surgical salvage after failure of definitive radiation therapy for early-stage squamous cell carcinoma of the glottic larynx. Arch Otolaryngol Head Neck Surg 2006;132:59. [PMID: 16415431]

Gilbert J et al: Organ preservation for cancer of the larynx: current indications and future directions. Semin Radiat Oncol 2004;14:167. [PMID: 15095262]

Hanna E et al: Quality of life for patients following total laryngectomy vs chemoradiation for laryngeal preservation. Arch Otolaryngol Head Neck Surg 2004;130:875. [PMID: 15262766]

Jones AS et al: The treatment of early laryngeal cancers (T1-T2 N0): surgery or irradiation? Head Neck 2004;26:127. [PMID: 14762881]

Loughran S et al: Quality of life and voice following endoscopic resection or radiotherapy for early glottic cancer. Clin Otolaryngol 2005;30:42. [PMID: 15748189]

Mendenhall WM et al: Management of T1-T2 glottic carcinomas. Cancer 2004;100:1786. [PMID: 15112257]

Sessions DG et al: Supraglottic laryngeal cancer: analysis of treatment results. Laryngoscope 2005;115:1402. [PMID: 16094113]

Smith JC et al: Quality of life, functional outcome, and costs of early glottic cancer. Laryngoscope 2003;113:68. [PMID: 12514385]

van Gogh CD et al: The efficacy of voice therapy in patients after treatment for early glottic carcinoma. Cancer 2006;106:95. [PMID: 16323175]

Yamazaki H et al: Radiotherapy for early glottic carcinoma (T1N0M0): results of prospective randomized study of radiation fraction size and overall treatment time. Int J Radiat Oncol Biol Phys 2006;64:77. [PMID: 16169681]

VOCAL CORD PARALYSIS

Most cases of vocal cord paralysis result from involvement of a recurrent laryngeal nerve; others arise more proximally along the vagus nerve itself. Common causes of recurrent laryngeal nerve involvement include thyroid surgery (and occasionally thyroid cancer), other neck surgery (anterior discectomy and carotid endarterectomy), and mediastinal or apical involvement by lung cancer. Skull base tumors often involve cranial nerves IX, X, and XI. Occasionally, no cause can be identified. When either no cause is found or the paresis follows surgical trauma in which the nerve was not divided, spontaneous recovery commonly occurs, usually within a year.

Unlike unilateral cord paralysis, which produces a breathy hoarseness, bilateral cord paralysis usually causes inspiratory and expiratory stridor if acute, in which case intervention to create an emergency airway may be needed. If insidious in onset, it may be asymptomatic at rest, including a normal voice, although there is usually dyspnea on exertion. Causes of bilateral cord paralysis include thyroid surgery, esophageal cancer, and ventricular shunt malfunction. Unilateral or bilateral cord immobility may also be seen in cricoarytenoid arthritis secondary to advanced rheumatoid arthritis, intubation injuries, glottic and subglottic stenosis and, of course, laryngeal cancer. The goal of intervention is the creation of a safe airway with minimal reduction in voice quality and airway protection from aspiration. A number of cord lateralization procedures have been advocated as a means of removing the tracheotomy tube.

Surgical management of persistent or irrecoverable symptomatic unilateral vocal cord paralysis has evolved over the last several decades. The primary goal is medialization of the paralyzed cord in order to rehabilitate the voice. Additional goals include eliminating aspiration, improving diet, and aiding in the subsequent decannulation of individuals with glottic insufficiency. Success has been reported for years with injection medialization using predominantly Teflon, but other materials as well have been used, such as fat or Gelfoam. An alternative to injection medialization of the vocal fold is to medialize the soft tissue and arytenoid via an endoscopically monitored transcutaneous injection or a small incision overlying the thyroid cartilage under local anesthesia. A section of the cartilage is removed, providing access to the soft tissue of the larynx and the arytenoid cartilage. An implant is inserted that displaces this soft tissue and arytenoid medially.

Abraham MT et al: Type I thyroplasty for acute unilateral vocal fold paralysis following intrathoracic surgery. Ann Otol Rhinol Laryngol 2002;111:667. [PMID: 12184585]

Baron EM et al: Dysphagia, hoarseness, and unilateral true vocal fold motion impairment following anterior cervical diskectomy and fusion. Ann Otol Rhinol Laryngol 2003;112:9. [PMID: 14653359]

Bhattacharyya N et al: Dysphagia and aspiration with unilateral vocal cord immobility: incidence, characterization, and response to surgical treatment. Ann Otol Rhinol Laryngol 2002;111:672. [PMID: 12184586]

Jung A et al: Recurrent laryngeal nerve palsy during anterior cervical spine surgery: a prospective study. J Neurosurg Spine 2005;2:123. [PMID: 15739522]

Nayak VK et al: Patterns of swallowing failure following medialization in unilateral vocal fold immobility. Laryngoscope 2002;112:1840. [PMID: 12368626]

Ollivere B et al: Swallowing dysfunction in patients with unilateral vocal fold paralysis: aetiology and outcomes. J Laryngol Otol 2006;120:38. [PMID: 16359143]

Urquhart AC et al: Idiopathic vocal cord palsies and associated neurological conditions. Arch Otolaryngol Head Neck Surg 2005;131:1086. [PMID: 16365222]

■ TRACHEOSTOMY & CRICOTHYROTOMY

There are two primary indications for tracheostomy: airway obstruction at or above the level of the larynx and respiratory failure requiring prolonged mechanical ventilation. In an acute emergency, cricothyrotomy secures an airway more rapidly than tracheostomy, with fewer potential immediate complications such as pneumothorax and hemorrhage. Although classically it has been recommended that one should change a cricothyrotomy to a tracheostomy as soon as it is convenient and safe, recent studies have questioned this if decannulation can be expected soon. Percutaneous dilation tracheostomy as an elective bedside (or intensive care unit) procedure has undergone scrutiny in recent years as an alternative to tracheostomy. In experienced hands, the various methods of percutaneous dilation tracheostomy have been documented to be safe, although complications do occur. When a patient is not intubated, simultaneous bronchoscopy may reduce complications. The major cost reduction comes from not using the main operating room. Bedside tracheostomy (in the intensive care unit) achieves similar cost reduction and is advocated by some as slightly less costly than the percutaneous dilation procedure.

The most common indication for elective tracheostomy is the need for prolonged mechanical ventilation. There is no firm rule about how many days a patient must be intubated before conversion to tracheostomy should be advised. The incidence of serious complications such as subglottic stenosis increases with extended endotracheal intubation. As soon as it is apparent that the patient will require protracted ventilatory support, tracheostomy should replace the endotracheal tube. Less frequent indications for tracheostomy are life-threatening aspiration pneumonia, the need to improve pulmonary toilet to correct problems related to insufficient clearing of tracheobronchial secretions, and sleep apnea.

Posttracheostomy care requires humidified air to prevent secretions from crusting and occluding the inner cannula of the tracheostomy tube. The tracheostomy tube should be cleaned several times daily. The most frequent early complication of tracheostomy is dislodgment of the tracheostomy tube. Surgical creation of an inferiorly based tracheal flap sutured to the inferior neck skin may make reinsertion of a dislodged tube easier. It should be recalled that the act of swallowing requires elevation of the larynx, which is prevented by tracheostomy. Therefore, frequent tracheal and bronchial suctioning is often required to clear the aspirated saliva as well as the increased tracheobronchial secretions. Care of the skin around the stoma is important to prevent maceration and secondary infection.

Durbin CG Jr: Early complications of tracheostomy. Respir Care 2005;50:511. [PMID: 15807913]

Epstein SK: Late complications of tracheostomy. Respir Care 2005;50:542. [PMID: 15807919]

Homewood J et al: Tracheostomy care. Br J Hosp Med (Lond) 2005;66:M72. [PMID: 16308953]

Melker JS et al: Melker cricothyrotomy kit: an alternative to the surgical technique. Ann Otol Rhinol Laryngol 2005;114:525. [PMID: 16134347]

Thatcher GW et al: The long-term evaluation of tracheostomy in the management of severe obstructive sleep apnea. Laryngoscope 2003;113:201. [PMID: 12567068]

■ FOREIGN BODIES IN THE UPPER AERODIGESTIVE TRACT

FOREIGN BODIES OF THE TRACHEA & BRONCHI

Aspiration of foreign bodies occurs less frequently in adults than in children. The elderly and denture wearers appear to be at greatest risk. Wider familiarity with the Heimlich maneuver has reduced deaths. If the maneuver is unsuccessful, cricothyrotomy may be necessary. Plain chest radiographs may reveal a radiopaque foreign body. Detection of radiolucent foreign bodies may be aided by inspiration-expiration films that demonstrate air trapping distal to the obstructed segment. Atelectasis and pneumonia may occur later.

Tracheal and bronchial foreign bodies should be removed under general anesthesia by a skilled endoscopist working with an experienced anesthesiologist.

Eroglu A et al: Tracheobronchial foreign bodies: a 10 year experience. Ulus Travma Derg 2003;9:262. [PMID: 14569482]

Swanson KL et al: Tracheobronchial foreign bodies. Chest Surg Clin N Am 2001;11:861. [PMID: 11780300]

Tariq SM et al: Inhaled foreign bodies in adolescents and adults. Monaldi Arch Chest Dis 2005;63:193. [PMID: 16454218]

ESOPHAGEAL FOREIGN BODIES

Foreign bodies in the esophagus create urgent but not life-threatening situations as long as the airway is not compromised. There is probably time to consult an experienced clinician for management. Patients are likely to have difficulty handling secretions and may be spitting out their saliva. It is a useful diagnostic sign of complete obstruction if the patient is drooling or cannot handle secretions. They may often point to the exact level of the obstruction. Indirect laryngoscopy often shows pooling of saliva at the esophageal inlet. Plain films may detect radiopaque foreign bodies such as chicken bones. Coins tend to align in the coronal plane in the esophagus and sagittally in the trachea. If a foreign body is suspected, a barium swallow may help make the diagnosis.

The treatment of an esophageal foreign body depends very much on identification of its nature. In children, swallowed nonfood objects are common. In adults, however, food foreign bodies are more common, and there is the greater possibility of underlying esophageal pathology. Endoscopic removal and examination is usually best, via flexible esophagoscopy or rigid laryngoscopy-esophagoscopy. If there is nothing sharp such as a bone, some clinicians advocate a hospitalized 24-hr observation period prior to esophagoscopy, noting that spontaneous passage of the foreign body will occur in 50% of adult patients. Obstruction may sometimes occur from a metal stent placed in the treatment of esophageal cancer.

Athanassiadi K et al: Management of esophageal foreign bodies: a retrospective review of 400 cases. Eur J Cardiothorac Surg 2002;21:653. [PMID: 11932163]

Lam HC et al: Management of ingested foreign bodies: a retrospective review of 5240 patients. J Laryngol Otol 2001; 115:954. [PMID: 11779322]

Mosca S et al: Endoscopic management of foreign bodies in the upper gastrointestinal tract: report on a series of 414 adult patients. Endoscopy 2001;33:692. [PMID: 11490386]

Tsikoudas A et al: The management of acute oesophageal obstruction from a food bolus. Can we be more conservative? Eur Arch Otorhinolaryngol 2005;262:528. [PMID: 15592861]

■ DISEASES PRESENTING AS NECK MASSES

The differential diagnosis of neck masses is heavily dependent on the location in the neck, the age of the patient, and the presence of associated disease processes. Rapid growth and tenderness suggest an inflammatory process, while firm, painless, and slowly enlarging masses are often neoplastic. In young adults, most neck masses are benign (branchial cleft cyst, thyroglossal duct cyst, reactive lymphadenitis), although malignancy should always be considered (lymphoma, metastatic thyroid carcinoma). Lymphadenopathy is common in HIV-positive persons, but a growing or dominant mass may well be malignant. In adults over age 40, cancer is the most common cause of persistent neck mass. A metastasis from SCC arising within the mouth, pharynx, larynx, or upper esophagus should be suspected, especially if there is a history of tobacco or significant alcohol use. Especially among patients younger than 30 or older than 70, lymphoma should be considered. In any case, a comprehensive otolaryngologic examination is needed. Cytologic evaluation of the neck mass via FNA biopsy is likely to be the next step if an obvious primary tumor is not visible or palpable on physical examination.

CONGENITAL LESIONS PRESENTING AS NECK MASSES IN ADULTS

1. Branchial Cleft Cysts

Branchial cleft cysts usually present as a soft cystic mass along the anterior border of the sternocleidomastoid muscle. These lesions are usually recognized in the second or third decades of life, often when they suddenly swell or become infected. To prevent recurrent infection and possible carcinoma, they should be completely excised, along with their fistulous tracts.

First branchial cleft cysts present high in the neck, sometimes just below the ear. A fistulous connection with the floor of the external auditory canal may be present. Second branchial cleft cysts, which are far more common, may communicate with the tonsillar fossa. Third branchial cleft cysts, which may communicate with the piriform sinus, are rare.

Bloch R: Images in emergency medicine. Branchial cleft cyst. Ann Emerg Med 2006;47:291, 308. [PMID: 16492498]

Enepekides DJ: Management of congenital anomalies of the neck. Facial Plast Surg Clin North Am 2001;9:131. [PMID: 11465000]

Eskey CJ et al: Imaging of benign and malignant soft tissue tumors of the neck. Radiol Clin North Am 2000;38: 1091. [PMID: 11054971]

Palacios E et al: Branchial cleft cyst. Ear Nose Throat J 2001; 80:302. [PMID: 11393908]

Prakash PK et al: Differential diagnosis of neck lumps. Practitioner 2002;246:252. [PMID: 11961991]

Schwetschenau E et al: The adult neck mass. Am Fam Physician 2002;66:831. [PMID: 12322776]

2. Thyroglossal Duct Cysts

Thyroglossal duct cysts occur along the embryologic course of the thyroid's descent from the tuberculum impar of the tongue base to its usual position in the low neck. Although they may occur at any age, they are most common before age 20. They present as a midline neck mass, often just below the hyoid bone, which moves with swallowing. Surgical excision is recommended to prevent recurrent infection. This requires removal of the entire fistulous tract along with the middle portion of the hyoid bone.

Ahuja AT et al: Imaging for thyroglossal duct cyst: the bare essentials. Clin Radiol 2005;60:141. [PMID: 15664568]

Dedivitis RA et al: Thyroglossal duct: a review of 55 cases. J Am Coll Surg 2002;194:274. [PMID: 11893130]

Ewing CA et al: Presentations of thyroglossal duct cysts in adults. Eur Arch Otorhinolaryngol 1999;256:136. [PMID: 10234482]

Mohan PS et al: Thyroglossal duct cysts: a consideration in adults. Am Surg 2005;71:508. [PMID: 16044932]

INFECTIOUS & INFLAMMATORY NECK MASSES

1. Reactive Cervical Lymphadenopathy

Normal lymph nodes in the neck are usually less than 1 cm in length. Infections involving the pharynx, salivary glands, and scalp often cause tender enlargement of neck nodes. Enlarged nodes are common in HIV-infected persons. Except for the occasional node that suppurates and requires incision and drainage, treatment is directed against the underlying infection. An enlarged node unassociated with an obvious infection should be further evaluated, especially if the patient has a history of smoking or alcohol use (common etiologic factors in head and neck SCC) or a history of cancer. Other common indications for FNA biopsy of a node include its persistence or continued enlargement. Common causes of cervical adenopathy include tumor (SCC, lymphoma, occasional metastases from non-head and neck sites) and infection (eg, reactive nodes, mycobacteria [discussed below], and cat scratch disease). Rare causes of adenopathy include Kikuchi's disease (histiocytic necrotizing lymphadenitis) and autoimmune adenopathy.

Murakami K et al: Cat scratch disease: analysis of 130 seropositive cases. J Infect Chemother 2002;8:349. [PMID: 12525897]

Ridder GJ et al: Role of cat-scratch disease in lymphadenopathy in the head and neck. Clin Infect Dis 2002;35:643. [PMID: 12203159]

2. Tuberculous & Nontuberculous Mycobacterial Lymphadenitis

Granulomatous neck masses are not uncommon. The differential diagnosis includes mycobacterial adenitis, sarcoidosis, and cat-scratch disease due to *Bartonella henselae*. Although mycobacterial adenitis can extend to the skin and drain externally (as described for atypical mycobacteria and referred to as scrofula), this late presentation is no longer common. The usual presentation of granulomatous disease in the neck is simply single or matted nodes. FNA biopsy is usually the best initial diagnostic approach: cytology, smear for acid-fast bacilli, culture, and sensitivity test; and polymerase chain reaction (PCR) can all be done.

Mycobacterial lymphadenitis is on the rise both in immunocompromised and immunocompetent individuals. Identification of *Mycobacterium tuberculosis* can usually be confirmed by a combination of FNA smear and culture, but excisional biopsy of a node may be needed. PCR from FNA (or from excised tissue) is the single most sensitive test and is particularly useful when conventional methods have not been diagnostic but clinical impression remains consistent for tuberculous infection.

Short-course therapy (6 months) consisting of an initial 4 months of streptomycin, isoniazid, rifampin, and pyrazinamide followed by 2 months of rifampin is the current recommended treatment for tuberculous lymphadenopathy. For atypical (nontuberculous) lymphadenopathy, treatment depends on sensitivity results of culture, but antibiotics likely to be useful include 6 months of isoniazid and rifampin and, for at least the first 2 months, ethambutol—all in standard dosages (see Table 9–14). Some would totally excise the involved nodes prior to chemotherapy, depending on location and other factors.

Golden MP et al: Extrapulmonary tuberculosis: an overview. Am Fam Physician 2005;72:1761. [PMID: 16300038]

Jawahar MS et al: Treatment of lymph node tuberculosis—a randomized clinical trial of two 6-month regimens. Trop Med Int Health 2005;10:1090. [PMID: 16262733]

Koo V et al: Fine needle aspiration cytology (FNAC) in the diagnosis of granulomatous lymphadenitis. Ulster Med J 2006; 75:59. [PMID: 16457406]

Pahwa R et al: Assessment of possible tuberculous lymphadenopathy by PCR compared to non-molecular methods. J Med Microbiol 2005;54:873. [PMID: 16091440]

Polesky A et al: Peripheral tuberculous lymphadenitis: epidemiology, diagnosis, treatment, and outcome. Medicine (Baltimore) 2005;84:350. [PMID: 16267410]

3. Lyme Disease

Lyme disease, caused by the spirochete *Borrelia burgdorferi* and transmitted by ticks of the *Ixodes* genus, may have protean manifestation, but over 75% of patients have symptoms involving the head and neck. Facial paralysis, dysesthesias, dysgeusia, or other cranial neuropathies are most common. Headache, pain, and cervical lymphadenopathy may occur. See Chapter 34 for a more thorough discussion.

Bunikis J et al: Laboratory testing for suspected Lyme disease. Med Clin North Am 2002;86:311. [PMID: 11982304]

DePietropaolo DL et al: Diagnosis of lyme disease. Am Fam Physician 2005;72:297. [PMID: 16050454]

Ljostad U et al: Acute peripheral facial palsy in adults. J Neurol 2005;252:672. [PMID: 15778908]

Lorenzi MC et al: Sudden deafness and Lyme disease. Laryngoscope 2003;113:312. [PMID: 12567088]

Steere AC: Lyme disease. N Engl J Med 2001;345:115. [PMID: 11450660]

TUMOR METASTASES

In older adults, 80% of firm, persistent, and enlarging neck masses are metastatic in origin. The great majority of these arise from SCC of the upper aerodigestive tract. A complete head and neck examination may reveal the tumor of origin, but examination under anesthesia with direct laryngoscopy, esophagoscopy, and bronchoscopy is usually required to fully evaluate the tumor and exclude second primaries.

It is often helpful to obtain a cytologic diagnosis if initial head and neck examination fails to reveal the primary tumor. An open biopsy should be done only when neither physical examination by an experienced clinician specializing in head and neck cancer nor FNA biopsy performed by an experienced cytopathologist yields a diagnosis. In such a setting, one should strongly consider obtaining an MRI or PET scan prior to open biopsy, as these methods may yield valuable information about a possible presumed primary site or another site for FNA.

Other than thyroid carcinoma, non-squamous cell metastases to the neck are infrequent. While tumors not involving the head and neck seldom metastasize to the middle or upper neck, the supraclavicular region is quite often involved by lung and breast tumors. Infradiaphragmatic tumors, with the exception of renal cell carcinoma, rarely metastasize to the neck.

Barzilai G et al: Pattern of regional metastases from cutaneous squamous cell carcinoma of the head and neck. Otolaryngol Head Neck Surg 2005;132:852. [PMID: 15944554]

Brockstein B et al: Patterns of failure, prognostic factors and survival in locoregionally advanced head and neck cancer treated with concomitant chemoradiotherapy: a 9-year, 337-patient, multi-institutional experience. Ann Oncol 2004;15:1179. [PMID: 15277256]

Cooper JS et al: Postoperative concurrent radiotherapy and chemotherapy for high-risk squamous-cell carcinoma of the head and neck. N Engl J Med 2004;305:1937. [PMID: 15128893]

Moore BA et al: Lymph node metastases from cutaneous squamous cell carcinoma of the head and neck. Laryngoscope 2005;115:1561. [PMID: 16148695]

Piccirillo JF et al: Development of a new head and neck cancer-specific comorbidity index. Arch Otolaryngol Head Neck Surg 2002;128:1172. [PMID: 12365889]

LYMPHOMA

About 10% of lymphomas present in the head and neck. Lymphoma arising in AIDS patients is an increasing concern. Multiple rubbery nodes, especially in the young adult, are suggestive of this disease. A thorough physical examination may demonstrate other sites of nodal or organ involvement. FNA biopsy may be diagnostic, but open biopsy is often required.

■ OTOLARYNGOLOGIC MANIFESTATIONS OF HIV INFECTION (See also Chapter 31)

ORAL CAVITY & PHARYNX

The evaluation of oral lesions is critically important in HIV-infected individuals and in patients at risk for HIV infection. Oral candidiasis and hairy leukoplakia, each occurring in 10–20% of HIV-infected patients, are frequently the presenting signs of HIV disease. Kaposi's sarcoma (prevalence about 1%) may similarly be the first indication of HIV infection—as may necrotizing ulcerative periodontitis (occurring in 2–5%), but less predictively. The course of candidiasis and hairy leukoplakia in known HIV-infected patients may correlate with the degree of immune suppression and overall disease progression, heralding the subsequent development of AIDS. For these reasons, oral lesions are useful in

staging HIV disease and in designing entry criteria and end points for antiretroviral clinical trials. The United States Department of Health Services Clinical Practice Guideline for Evaluation and Management of Early HIV Infection recommends examination of the oral mucosa with each physician visit as well as dental examination at least every 6 months.

When CD4 cell counts drop below 200/mcL, the incidence of intraoral lesions rises dramatically. In the past few years, the severity of these lesions has lessened, but their incidence has increased. Candidiasis is common and may require treatment for longer than the usual 1-week course with fluconazole (100 mg daily) or ketoconazole (200–400 mg daily). Clotrimazole and topical nystatin are less effective. Itraconazole (200 mg daily) is often helpful in fluconazole-resistant cases, or some cases due to non-albicans species, which are frequently azole-unresponsive. Giant intraoral ulcers have been seen in some patients.

Hairy leukoplakia occurring on the lateral border of the tongue is another common early finding. It may develop quickly and appears as slightly raised leukoplakic areas with a corrugated or "hairy" surface. Histologically, parakeratosis and koilocytes are seen with little or no underlying inflammation. Among HIV-positive patients with oral lesions, hairy leukoplakia was seen in 19% in one study. Clinical response following administration of zidovudine or acyclovir has been reported, and treatment is under active investigation. The appearance of hairy leukoplakia may herald subsequent more ominous manifestations of AIDS.

Kaposi's sarcoma is most common on the hard palate but may be seen anywhere in the oral cavity and pharynx. It usually appears as a raised violaceous lesion beneath an intact mucosa, although it may be ulcerated, erythematous, and bleeding. Radiation therapy may control the tumor. A brisk mucositis can be expected following radiation therapy.

In addition to Kaposi's sarcoma, an increased incidence of non-Hodgkin's lymphoma is seen in AIDS. An increase in SCC is also seen in the homosexual population, perhaps related to HIV infection.

Birnbaum W et al: Prognostic significance of HIV-associated oral lesions and their relation to therapy. Oral Dis 2002;8(Suppl 2):110. [PMID: 12164643]

Campo J et al: Oral candidiasis as a clinical marker related to viral load, CD4 lymphocyte count and CD4 lymphocyte percentage in HIV-infected patients. J Oral Pathol Med 2002; 31:5. [PMID: 11896816]

Cattaneo C et al: Oral cavity lymphomas in immunocompetent and human immunodeficiency virus infected patients. Leuk Lymphoma 2005;46:77. [PMID: 15621784]

Challacombe SJ et al: Overview of the Fourth International Workshop on the Oral Manifestations of HIV Infection. Oral Dis 2002;8(Suppl 2):9. [PMID: 12164668]

Coogan MM et al: Oral lesions in infection with human immunodeficiency virus. Bull World Health Organ 2005;83:700. [PMID: 1621116]

de Faria PR et al: Tongue disease in advanced AIDS. Oral Dis 2005;11:72. [PMID: 15752079]

Eyeson JD et al: Oral manifestations of an HIV positive cohort in the era of highly active anti-retroviral therapy (HAART) in South London. J Oral Pathol Med 2002;31:169. [PMID: 11903824]

Kroidl A et al: Prevalence of oral lesions and periodontal diseases in HIV-infected patients on antiretroviral therapy. Eur J Med Res 2005;10:448. [PMID: 16287607]

Patton LL et al: Prevalence and classification of HIV-associated oral lesions. Oral Dis 2002;8(Suppl 2):98. [PMID: 12164670]

Ramirez-Amador V et al: Synchronous kinetics of CD4+ lymphocytes and viral load before the onset of oral candidosis and hairy leukoplakia in a cohort of Mexican HIV-infected patients. AIDS Res Hum Retroviruses 2005;21:981. [PMID: 16379600]

Singh B et al: The epidemiology of the oral lesions of HIV infection in the developed world. Oral Dis 2002;8(Suppl 2):34. [PMID: 12164657]

THE NECK

Persistent generalized lymphadenopathy is extremely common in HIV infection. A tender or growing node may represent secondary infection, lymphoma, or other tumor. FNA for culture and cytology is the best initial diagnostic step. Open biopsy will often be needed if granulomatous disease or lymphoma is suspected, although FNA biopsy may be diagnostic of *M tuberculosis* infection in seropositive patients.

Parotid cysts and benign lymphoepithelial lesions in HIV-positive patients may be seen, often in association with cervical adenopathy.

Diamond C et al: Changes in acquired immunodeficiency syndrome-related non-Hodgkin lymphoma in the era of highly active antiretroviral therapy: incidence, presentation, treatment, and survival. Cancer 2006;106:128. [PMID: 16329140]

Owotade FJ et al: Clinical experience with parotid gland enlargement in HIV infection: a report of five cases in Nigeria. J Contemp Dent Pract 2005;6:136. [PMID: 15719085]

PARANASAL SINUSES

Sinusitis is common in HIV infection and the causative organisms are diverse. The same pathogens encountered in nonimmunocompromised patients remain the most common. Early sinus irrigation, with aspirates sent for cytologic examination as well as fungal, viral, *Legionella,* and aerobic and anaerobic culture may be helpful in severe cases. Guaifenesin (600 mg orally four times daily), a mucolytic agent, may offer some adjunctive symptomatic relief. Functional endoscopic surgery to provide sinus drainage is often helpful.

Invasive *Aspergillus* sinusitis is an increasingly reported complication in AIDS. Although this infection is more indolent than mucormycosis, most patients with AIDS and *Aspergillus* sinusitis die as a result of intracranial extension.

Rosen EJ et al: Alterations of nasal mucociliary clearance in association with HIV infection and the effect of guaifenesin therapy. Laryngoscope 2005;115:27. [PMID: 15630360]

Scheid DC et al: Head and neck manifestations of HIV infection: a preliminary study. J Indian Med Assoc 2003;101:93. [PMID: 12841491]

Lung

9

Mark S. Chesnutt, MD, & Thomas J. Prendergast, MD

■ COMMON MANIFESTATIONS OF LUNG DISEASE

DYSPNEA

Dyspnea is a common symptom. It is analogous to hunger or nausea in that sensory input from multiple sites is integrated in the cerebral cortex. In general, dyspnea increases with the level of functional impairment as measured by spirometry. However, there is only a weak correlation between the severity of dyspnea and quantitative measures of airflow limitation or exercise tolerance.

Several pathophysiologic processes contribute to dyspnea. The most important is the increased respiratory effort that accompanies many different diseases: airflow obstruction (asthma; chronic obstructive pulmonary disease [COPD]), changes in pulmonary compliance (interstitial fibrosis, congestive heart failure) or chest wall compliance (obesity, pleural disease), intrinsic respiratory muscle weakness (inanition, neuromuscular disease, chronic respiratory failure), or the weakness conveyed by the mechanical disadvantage of hyperinflation (asthma or emphysema). Dyspnea is magnified by increased respiratory drive. Acute hypercapnia is therefore a potent stimulus to dyspnea, while hypoxemia is usually a weak one. Stimulation of irritant receptors in the airways intensifies dyspnea, while stimulation of pulmonary stretch receptors decreases it. In mechanically ventilated patients, failure to provide adequate inspiratory flow rates to patients with heightened respiratory drive commonly results in dyspnea that may present as agitation.

Clinical Findings

The history should focus on onset and timing of symptoms, the patient's position at onset of symptoms, the relationship of symptoms to activity, and any factors that may improve or exacerbate symptoms. The clinician can assess dyspnea and response to treatment with a numeric rating scale by asking the patient, "On a scale of zero to ten, with zero being no shortness of breath and ten being the worst shortness of breath you can imagine, how short of breath are you?" Exertional dyspnea should be quantified, but the absolute level of exertion that precipitates dyspnea is less important than acute changes in the threshold level of activity. Complete allergic, occupational, and smoking histories are essential.

Acute dyspnea has a short list of causes, most of which are readily identified: asthma, pulmonary infection, pulmonary edema, pneumothorax, pulmonary embolus, metabolic acidosis, or acute respiratory distress syndrome (ARDS). Panic attacks may present as a respiratory complaint. **Orthopnea** (dyspnea on recumbency) and nocturnal dyspnea suggest asthma, gastroesophageal reflux disease (GERD), left ventricular dysfunction, or obstructive sleep apnea. Rapid onset of severe dyspnea when supine suggests phrenic nerve impairment leading to diaphragmatic weakness or paralysis. **Platypnea** (dyspnea that worsens in the upright position) is a rare complaint associated with arteriovenous malformations at the lung bases or with hepatopulmonary syndrome, resulting in increased shunting and hypoxemia in the upright position (orthodeoxia).

Chronic dyspnea is invariably progressive. Symptoms often first appear during exertion; patients learn to limit their activity to accommodate their diminished pulmonary reserve until dyspnea occurs with minimal activity or at rest. Episodic dyspnea suggests congestive heart failure, asthma, acute or chronic bronchitis, or recurrent pulmonary emboli. Constant dyspnea is most commonly due to COPD but may indicate interstitial lung disease (eg, pulmonary fibrosis), pulmonary vascular disease, or fixed airflow obstruction from severe asthma.

Evaluation should include a complete blood count, renal function tests, chest radiograph, spirometry, and noninvasive oximetry. Patients over 40 years of age or with a family history of early coronary disease should have an electrocardiogram. Arterial blood gases, measurement of lung volumes, ventilation-perfusion (V/Q) scanning, echocardiography, and cardiopulmonary exercise testing are reserved for cases that elude diagnosis on initial evaluation.

Treatment

In patients with advanced lung disease, the responsible condition may be easily identified but treatment only partially effective. Oxygen improves survival in those who are hypoxemic and can improve the exercise tolerance of all patients. Its effect on dyspnea is variable.

Opioids reduce respiratory drive and blunt dyspnea. They can be titrated safely even in patients with advanced lung disease. Anxiety can play an important role in the distress caused by dyspnea and may be relieved by judicious use of benzodiazepines such as lorazepam, 0.5–1 mg orally every 6–8 hours. Pulmonary rehabilitation can improve respiratory function and train patients in energy conservation and breathing techniques that help moderate their sense of respiratory effort. Finally, fresh air or a fan may offer additional relief. Smokers with progressive exertional dyspnea should know that they can limit future loss of function through smoking cessation.

Dyspnea is increasingly being recognized as a major issue in the care of dying patients, and clinicians typically undertreat this symptom. See Chapter 5.

Dyspnea. Mechanisms, assessment, and management: a consensus statement. American Thoracic Society. Am J Respir Crit Care Med 1999;159:321. [PMID: 9872857]

Karnani NG et al: Evaluation of chronic dyspnea. Am Fam Physician 2005;71:1529. [PMID: 15864893]

Luce JM et al: Management of dyspnea in patients with far-advanced lung disease: "once I lose it, it's kind of hard to catch it…" JAMA 2001;285:1331. [PMID: 11255389]

COUGH

Cough is an important physiologic mechanism that defends against respiratory pathogens and helps clear the tracheobronchial tree of mucus, foreign particles, and noxious aerosols. Excessive cough is one of the most common symptoms for which patients seek medical care and may represent up to one-third of a pulmonologist's outpatient practice referrals. Persistent severe cough, seen in interstitial lung disease or bronchiectasis, may impair respiration as well as disrupt sleep and social functioning. Bronchospasm (brought on by repetitive forced exhalation), syncope, rib fractures, and urinary incontinence are all potential complications. A reduced or absent cough, seen in some postoperative patients or those with neuromuscular disease, will reduce clearance of secretions and may impair oxygenation.

Cough may be voluntary or involuntary. Involuntary cough is stimulated by vagal afferent receptors in the trachea, especially at the carina, and the larynx but also from others throughout the head and neck. Stimulation of cough receptors may be mechanical, as in cases of aspiration, or irritative.

Clinical Findings

It is important to distinguish acute (< 3 weeks) from subacute (3–8 weeks) and chronic (> 8 weeks) cough. **Acute cough** most commonly follows viral or bacterial upper respiratory tract infection. Within 2 days after onset of the common cold, 85% of untreated patients cough; 25% are still coughing 14 days later; in a few, cough will persist for 6–8 weeks. Many patients with persistent cough following upper respiratory tract infection have underlying asthma. Other causes of acute cough include aspiration, pneumonia, pulmonary embolism, and pulmonary edema.

The most common cause of **chronic cough** is a low-grade chronic bronchitis secondary to exposure to tobacco smoke, though smokers do not commonly seek medical attention for this problem. Over 90% of non-smokers presenting for evaluation of chronic cough suffer from postnasal drip, GERD, or asthma (even without other symptoms). Angiotensin-converting enzyme (ACE) inhibitors have become another common cause. In primary care settings, single causes predominate.

The character and timing of chronic cough and the presence or absence of sputum production do not permit an etiologic diagnosis and should not be used as the sole basis for empiric therapy. The history and physical examination should attempt to identify anatomic locations of the afferent limb of the cough reflex in light of the common causes listed above. A nasal discharge, frequent need to clear the throat, and mucoid or mucopurulent secretions in the posterior pharynx suggest postnasal drip. Sinus radiographs may be diagnostic of acute or chronic sinusitis. Wheezing on chest auscultation or airflow obstruction on pulmonary function tests suggests asthma. In cough-variant asthma, methacholine bronchoprovocation testing may be positive in the absence of clinical findings of asthma. GERD is an important cause of chronic cough but is associated with the fewest clinical clues; cough, in the absence of heartburn, may be the only symptom. Barium swallow is specific but insensitive, and esophageal pH monitoring may be necessary for diagnosis. **Chest radiographs** are best reserved for evaluation of cough in smokers and patients with hemoptysis or constitutional symptoms such as fever and weight loss.

Treatment

The first step is to eliminate irritant exposures such as tobacco smoke (primary or secondary) and occupational agents and to discontinue medications such as ACE inhibitors or β-blockers, including eyedrops. Cough due to ACE inhibitors should subside within 1–4 days after discontinuing the medication, though it may take several weeks. Postnasal drip syndrome due to allergic rhinitis that does not respond to antihistamines should be treated with intranasal corticosteroids. Chronic sinusitis may require prolonged antibiotics directed against *Haemophilus influenzae*. Cough caused by asthma that does not respond after 2 weeks of bronchodilators and corticosteroids suggests another contributing condition. Cough due to GERD is difficult to treat and may require proton pump inhibitors since H_2 blockers may be inadequate. Patients whose cough began after an upper respiratory tract infection usually respond to treatment with an antihistamine-decongestant combination or treatment for asthma.

Chang AB et al: Gastro-oesophageal reflux treatment for prolonged non-specific cough in children and adults. Cochrane Database Syst Rev 2005;(2):CD004823. [PMID: 15846735]

Hewlett EL et al: Clinical practice. Pertussis—not just for kids. N Engl J Med 2005;352:1215. [PMID: 15788498]

Morice AH et al; ERS Task Force: The diagnosis and management of chronic cough. Eur Respir J 2004;24:481. [PMID: 15358710]

Pratter MR et al: An empiric integrative approach to the management of cough: ACCP evidence-based clinical practice guidelines. Chest 2006;129(1 Suppl):222S. [PMID: 16428715]

HEMOPTYSIS

Hemoptysis is the expectoration of blood that originates below the vocal cords. It is commonly classified as trivial, mild, or massive—the latter defined as more than 200–600 mL in 24 hours. The dividing lines are arbitrary, since the amount of blood is rarely quantified with precision. Massive hemoptysis can be usefully defined as any amount that is hemodynamically significant or threatens ventilation, in which case the initial management goal is not diagnostic but therapeutic.

The lungs are supplied with a dual circulation. The pulmonary arteries arise from the right ventricle to supply the pulmonary parenchyma in a low-pressure circuit. The bronchial arteries arise from the aorta or intercostal arteries and carry blood under systemic pressure to the airways, blood vessels, hila, and visceral pleura. The bronchial arterial circulation is a high-pressure circuit that provides the blood supply to the airways and lesions within those airways. Although the bronchial circulation represents only 1–2% of total pulmonary blood flow, it can increase dramatically under conditions of chronic inflammation—eg, chronic bronchiectasis—and is frequently the source of hemoptysis.

The causes of hemoptysis can be classified anatomically. Blood may arise from the airways in chronic bronchitis, bronchiectasis, and bronchogenic carcinoma; from the pulmonary vasculature in left ventricular failure, mitral stenosis, pulmonary emboli, and arteriovenous malformations; or from the pulmonary parenchyma in pneumonia, inhalation of crack cocaine, or autoimmune diseases such as Goodpasture's disease or Wegener's granulomatosis. Iatrogenic hemorrhage may follow transbronchial lung biopsies, anticoagulation, or pulmonary artery rupture due to distal placement of a balloon-tipped catheter.

Clinical Findings

Blood-tinged sputum in the setting of acute bronchitis in an otherwise healthy nonsmoker does not warrant an extensive diagnostic evaluation if the hemoptysis subsides with resolution of the infection. However, hemoptysis is frequently a sign of serious disease, especially in patients with a high prior probability of underlying pulmonary pathology. The goal of the history is to identify patients at risk for one of the disorders listed above. Pertinent features include past or current tobacco use, duration of symptoms, or the presence of respiratory infection. Nonpulmonary sources of hemorrhage—from the nose or the gastrointestinal tract—should be excluded.

Laboratory evaluation should include a chest radiograph and complete blood count, including platelet count. Renal function tests, urinalysis, and coagulation studies are appropriate in specific circumstances. Flexible bronchoscopy reveals endobronchial cancer in 3–6% of patients with hemoptysis who have a normal (non-lateralizing) chest radiograph. Nearly all of these patients are smokers over the age of 40, and most will have had symptoms for more than a week. Bronchoscopy is indicated in such patients. High-resolution CT of the chest is complementary to bronchoscopy. It can diagnose unsuspected bronchiectasis and arteriovenous malformations and will show central endobronchial lesions in many cases. It is the test of choice for suspected small peripheral malignancies.

Treatment

The management of mild hemoptysis consists of identifying and treating the specific cause. Massive hemoptysis is life-threatening. The airway must be protected, ventilation ensured, and effective circulation maintained. If the location of the bleeding site is known, the patient should be placed in the decubitus position with the involved lung dependent. Uncontrollable hemorrhage warrants rigid bronchoscopy and surgical consultation. In stable patients, flexible bronchoscopy may localize the site of bleeding, and angiography can embolize the involved bronchial arteries. Embolization is effective initially in 85% of cases, though rebleeding may occur in up to 20% of patients over the following year. The anterior spinal artery arises from the bronchial artery in up to 5% of people, and paraplegia may result if it is inadvertently cannulated.

Bidwell JL et al: Hemoptysis: diagnosis and management. Am Fam Physician 2005;72:1253. [PMID: 16225028]

Flume PA et al: Massive hemoptysis in cystic fibrosis. Chest 2005; 128:729. [PMID: 16100161]

Yoon YC et al: Hemoptysis: bronchial and nonbronchial systemic arteries at 16-detector row CT. Radiology 2005; 234:292. [PMID: 15550375]

■ APPROACH TO THE PATIENT

PHYSICAL EXAMINATION

Examination of the patient with suspected pulmonary disease includes inspection, palpation, percussion, and auscultation of the chest. An efficient approach begins with observing the pattern of breathing, auscultation of the chest, and inspection for extrapulmonary signs of pulmonary disease. More detailed examination follows from initial findings.

The pattern of breathing refers to the respiratory rate and rhythm, the depth of breathing or tidal volume, and the relative amount of time spent in inspiration and expiration. Normal values are a rate of 12–14 breaths per minute, tidal volumes of 5 mL/kg, and a ratio of inspiratory to expiratory time of 2:3. **Tachypnea** is an increased rate of breathing and is commonly associated with a decrease in tidal volume. Respiratory rhythm is normally regular, with a sigh (1.5–2 times normal tidal volume) every 90 breaths or so to prevent collapse of alveoli and atelectasis. Alterations in the rhythm of breathing include rapid, shallow breathing, seen in restrictive lung disease and as a precursor to respiratory failure; **Kussmaul** breathing, rapid large-volume breathing indicating intense stimulation of the respiratory center, seen in metabolic acidosis; and **Cheyne-Stokes** respiration, a rhythmic waxing and waning of both rate and tidal volumes that includes regular periods of apnea. This last pattern is seen in patients with end-stage left ventricular failure or neurologic disease and in many normal persons at high altitude, especially during sleep.

During normal quiet breathing, the primary muscle of respiration is the diaphragm. Movement of the chest wall is minimal. The use of accessory muscles of respiration, the intercostal and sternocleidomastoid muscles, indicates high work of breathing. At rest, the use of accessory muscles is a sign of significant pulmonary impairment. As the diaphragm contracts, it pushes the abdominal contents down. Hence, the chest and abdominal wall normally expand simultaneously. Expansion of the chest but collapse of the abdomen on inspiration indicates weakness of the diaphragm. The chest normally expands symmetrically. Asymmetric expansion suggests unilateral volume loss, as in atelectasis or pleural effusion, unilateral airway obstruction, asymmetric pulmonary or pleural fibrosis, or splinting from chest pain.

The examiner may palpate as follows: the trachea at the suprasternal notch, to detect shifts in the mediastinum; on the posterior chest wall, to gauge fremitus and the transmission through the lungs of vibrations of spoken words; and on the anterior chest wall to assess the cardiac impulse. All these maneuvers are characterized by low interobserver agreement.

Chest percussion identifies dull areas that correspond to lung consolidation or pleural effusion or hyperresonant areas suggesting emphysema or pneumothorax. Percussion has a low sensitivity (10–20% in several studies) compared with chest radiographs to detect abnormalities. Specificity is high (85–99%). Since an insensitive test is a poor screening examination, percussion and palpation are not necessary in every patient. These techniques do serve as important confirmatory tests in specific patients when the prior probability of a finding is increased. For example, in a patient with a suspected tension pneumothorax, the finding of tracheal shift and hyperresonance can be lifesaving, permitting immediate decompression of the affected side.

Auscultation of the chest depends on a reliable and consistent classification of auditory findings. Normal lung sounds heard over the periphery of the lung are called **vesicular**. They have a gentle, rustling quality heard throughout inspiration that fades during expiration. Normal sounds heard over the suprasternal notch are called tracheal or **bronchial** lung sounds. They are louder, higher-pitched, and have a hollow quality that tends to be louder on expiration. Bronchial lung sounds heard over the periphery of the lung are abnormal and imply consolidation. Globally diminished lung sounds are an important finding predictive of significant airflow obstruction.

Abnormal lung sounds ("adventitious" breath sounds) may be continuous (> 80 ms in duration) or discontinuous (< 20 ms). Continuous lung sounds are divided into **wheezes**, which are high-pitched, musical, and have a distinct whistling quality; and **rhonchi**, which are lower-pitched, sonorous, and may have a gurgling quality. Wheezes occur in the setting of bronchospasm, mucosal edema, or excessive secretions. In each case, the airway is narrowed to the point where adjacent airway walls flutter as airflow is limited. Rhonchi originate in the larger airways when excessive secretions and abnormal airway collapsibility cause repetitive rupture of fluid films. Rhonchi frequently clear after cough.

Discontinuous lung sounds are called **crackles**— brief, discrete, nonmusical sounds with a popping quality. Fine crackles are soft, high-pitched, and crisp (< 10 ms in duration). They are formed by the explosive opening of small airways previously held closed by surface forces and are heard in interstitial diseases or early pulmonary edema. Coarse crackles are louder, lower-pitched, and slightly longer in duration (< 20 ms) and probably result from gas bubbling through fluid. Coarse crackles are heard in pneumonia, obstructive lung disease, and late pulmonary edema.

Interobserver agreement regarding auscultatory findings is good. The clinical usefulness of these findings is also well established. The presence of wheezes on physical examination is a powerful predictor of obstructive lung disease. The absence of wheezes is not helpful since patients may have significant airflow limitation without wheezing. Such patients will have globally diminished lung sounds as the clinical clue to their obstructive lung disease. Normal lung sounds exclude significant airway obstruction. The timing and character of crackles can reliably distinguish different pulmonary disorders. Fine, late inspiratory crackles suggest pulmonary fibrosis, while early coarse crackles suggest pneumonia or heart failure.

Extrapulmonary signs of intrinsic pulmonary disease include digital clubbing, cyanosis, elevation of central venous pressures, and lower extremity edema.

Digital clubbing refers to structural changes at the base of the nails that include softening of the nail bed and loss of the normal 150-degree angle between the nail and the cuticle. The distal phalanx is convex and enlarged: its thickness is equal to or greater than the thickness of the distal interphalangeal joint. Symmetric clubbing may be a normal variant but more commonly is a sign of underlying disease. Clubbing is seen in patients with chronic infections of the lungs and pleura (lung abscess, empyema, bronchiectasis, cystic fibrosis), malignancies of the lungs and pleura, chronic interstitial lung disease (idiopathic pulmonary fibrosis), and arteriovenous malformations. It does not normally accompany asthma or COPD; when seen in the latter, concomitant lung cancer should be suspected. It is observed less often in small-cell cancer than in other histologic types. Clubbing is not specific to pulmonary disorders; it is also seen in cyanotic congenital heart disease, infective endocarditis, cirrhosis, and inflammatory bowel disease. **Hypertrophic pulmonary osteoarthropathy** is a syndrome of digital clubbing, chronic proliferative periostitis of the long bones, and synovitis. It is seen in the same conditions as digital clubbing but is particularly common in bronchogenic carcinoma. The cause of clubbing and hypertrophic osteoarthropathy is not known with certainty, but the disorder may reflect platelet clumping and local release of platelet-derived growth factor at the nail bed. Both clubbing and osteoarthropathy may resolve with appropriate treatment of the underlying disease. **Cyanosis** is a blue or bluish-gray discoloration of the skin and mucous membranes caused by increased amounts (> 5 g/dL) of unsaturated hemoglobin in capillary blood. Since the oxygen saturation at which cyanosis becomes clinically apparent is a function of hemoglobin concentration, anemia may prevent cyanosis from appearing while polycythemia may lead to cyanosis in the setting of mild hypoxemia. Cyanosis is therefore not a reliable indicator of hypoxemia but should prompt direct measurement of arterial PO_2 or of hemoglobin saturation.

Estimation of **central venous pressure** (CVP) and assessment of lower extremity edema are indirect measures of pulmonary hypertension, the major cardiovascular complication of chronic lung disease. Estimation of CVP can be done with precision in many patients. Elevated CVP is a pathologic finding associated with impaired ventricular function, pericardial effusion or restriction, valvular heart disease, and chronic obstructive or restrictive lung disease. Peripheral edema is a nonspecific finding that, in the setting of chronic lung disease, suggests right ventricular failure.

Bettencourt PE et al: Clinical utility of chest auscultation in common pulmonary diseases. Am J Respir Crit Care Med 1994; 150(5 Pt 1):1291. [PMID: 7952555]

Lichtenstein D et al: Comparative diagnostic performances of auscultation, chest radiography, and lung ultrasonography in acute respiratory distress syndrome. Anesthesiology 2004; 100:9. [PMID: 14695718]

Myers KA et al: Does this patient have clubbing? JAMA 2001; 286:341. [PMID: 11466101]

PULMONARY FUNCTION TESTS

Standard pulmonary function tests measure airflow rates, lung volumes, and the ability of the lung to transfer gas across the alveolar-capillary membrane. Indications for pulmonary function testing include assessment of the type and extent of lung dysfunction; diagnosis of causes of dyspnea and cough; detection of early evidence of lung dysfunction; longitudinal surveillance in occupational settings; follow-up of response to therapy; preoperative assessment; and disability evaluation.

Contraindications to pulmonary function testing include acute severe asthma, respiratory distress, angina aggravated by testing, pneumothorax, ongoing hemoptysis, and active tuberculosis. Many test results are effort-dependent, and some patients may be too impaired to make a maximal effort. Suboptimal effort limits validity and is a common cause of misinterpretation of results. All pulmonary function tests are measured against predicted values derived from large studies of healthy subjects. In general, these predictions vary with age, gender, height and, to a lesser extent, weight and ethnicity.

Spirometry (see box, p. 227) and measurement of lung volumes allow measurement of the presence and severity of obstructive and restrictive pulmonary dysfunction. Obstructive dysfunction is marked by a reduction in airflow rates judged by a fall in the ratio of FEV_1 (forced expiratory volume in the first second) to FVC (forced vital capacity). Causes include asthma, COPD (chronic bronchitis and emphysema), bronchiectasis, bronchiolitis, and upper airway obstruction. Restrictive dysfunction is marked by a reduction in lung volumes with a normal to increased FEV_1/FVC ratio. Severity is graded by the reduction in total lung capacity. A reduced FVC suggests pulmonary restriction but is not diagnostic. Causes include decreased lung compliance from infiltrative disorders such as pulmonary fibrosis; reduced muscle strength from phrenic nerve injury, diaphragm dysfunction, or neuromuscular disease; pleural disease, including large pleural effusion or marked pleural thickening; and prior lung resection. The flow-volume loop combines the maximal expiratory and inspiratory flow-volume curves and is especially helpful in determining the site of airway obstruction. (See Figure 9–1.)

Spirometry is adequate for evaluation of most patients with suspected respiratory disease. If airflow obstruction is evident, spirometry may be repeated 10–20 minutes after an inhaled bronchodilator is administered. This doubles the cost of the study. The absence of improvement in spirometry after inhaled bronchodilator in the pulmonary function laboratory does *not* preclude a successful clinical response to bronchodilator therapy. Measurements of lung volumes and diffusing capacity are useful in selected patients, but these tests are expensive and should not be ordered routinely with spirometry.

Measurement of the single-breath **diffusing capacity** for carbon monoxide (DL_{CO}), which reflects the ability of the lung to transfer gas across the alveolar/capillary interface, is particularly helpful in evaluation of patients with diffuse infiltrative lung disease or emphysema. The total pulmonary diffusing capacity depends on the diffusion properties of the alveolar-capillary membrane and the amount of hemoglobin occupying the pulmonary capillaries. The diffusing capacity should therefore be corrected for the blood hemoglobin concentration.[1]

---

[1]Corrected DL_{CO} = Measured $DL_{CO} \times \dfrac{[Hb] + 10.22}{1.7\,[Hb]}$

where [Hb] is the measured hemoglobin concentration (g/dL).

LUNG VOLUMES, CAPACITIES, AND THE NORMAL SPIROGRAM

The volume of gas in the lungs is divided into volumes and capacities as shown in the bars to the left of the figure below. Lung volumes are primary: they do not overlap each other. Tidal volume (Vt) is the amount of gas inhaled and exhaled with each resting breath. Residual volume (RV) is the amount of gas remaining in the lungs at the end of a maximal exhalation. The vital capacity (VC) is the total amount of gas that can be exhaled following a maximal inhalation. The vital capacity and the residual volume together constitute the total lung capacity (TLC), or the total amount of gas in the lungs at the end of a maximal inhalation. The functional residual capacity (FRC) is the amount of gas in the lungs at the end of a resting tidal breath. (IC = inspiratory capacity; IRV = inspiratory reserve volume; ERV = expiratory reserve volume; RV = residual volume.)

The forced vital capacity (FVC) maneuver begins with an inhalation from FRC to TLC (lasting about 1 second) followed by a forceful exhalation from TLC to RV (lasting about 5 seconds). The amount of gas exhaled during the first second of this maneuver is the forced expiratory volume in the first second (FEV_1). Normal subjects expel approximately 80% of the FVC in the first second. The ratio of the FEV_1 to the FVC (often referred to as the FEV_1%) is diminished in patients with obstructive lung disease. It may be increased in patients with restrictive physiology.

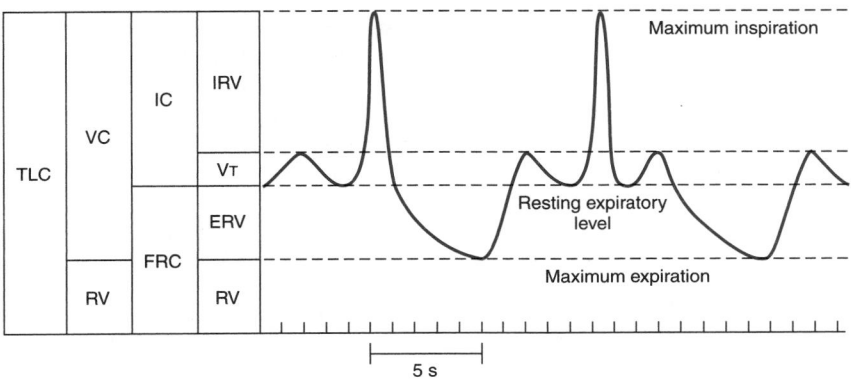

Modified, with permission, from Comroe JH et al: *The Lung: Clinical Physiology and Pulmonary Function Tests,* 2nd ed. Year Book Medical Publishers, 1962.

Elevated DL_{CO} is observed in pulmonary hemorrhage and may be seen in acute congestive heart failure and asthma due to an increase in pulmonary capillary blood volume. A diffusing capacity of 6 mL CO/mm Hg or more below the predicted value in women or 8.1 mL CO/mm Hg in men is considered abnormally low (Intermountain Thoracic Society guidelines). Reporting the ratio of measured diffusing capacity to alveolar volume (DL_{CO}/VA) is helpful, because a diminished diffusing capacity may only reflect a reduction in lung volume. In patients with emphysema, the diffusing capacity is characteristically low, the alveolar volume normal or increased, and the DL_{CO}/VA ratio is low. In patients with diffuse infiltrative lung disease, both the diffusing capacity and the alveolar volume are characteristically reduced, and the DL_{CO}/VA ratio is normal or low.

In patients with AIDS, DL_{CO} is a highly sensitive screening test for the presence of pulmonary disease, especially *Pneumocystis jiroveci* (formerly *P carinii*) pneumonia, but it lacks specificity. A normal DL_{CO} in an AIDS patient is strong evidence against *Pneumocystis* pneumonia. An abnormal result indicates the need for further diagnostic evaluation. Routine measurement of DL_{CO} and other pulmonary function tests in AIDS patients with pulmonary disease is not advised, because of expense and lack of specificity.

Arterial blood gas analysis is indicated whenever a clinically important acid-base disturbance, hypoxemia, or hypercapnia is suspected. Oximetry provides an inexpensive, noninvasive alternative means of monitoring hemoglobin saturation with oxygen. Oximeters monitor hemoglobin saturation and not oxygen tension. Figure 9–2 displays the normal relationship between hemoglobin saturation and partial pressure of oxygen in blood. This relationship is not linear. The clinical accuracy of pulse oximeters is reduced in such conditions as severe anemia (< 5 g/dL hemoglobin), the presence of abnormal hemoglobin moieties (carboxyhemoglobin, methemoglobin, fetal hemoglobin), the presence of intravascular dyes, motion artifact, and lack of pulsatile arterial blood flow (hypotension, hypothermia, cardiac arrest, simultaneous use of a blood pressure cuff, and cardiopulmonary bypass). The normal arterial PO_2 falls with increasing altitude (Table 9–1).

Nonspecific **bronchial provocation testing** may aid the evaluation of suspected asthma, when baseline spirometry is normal, and in unexplained cough. The subject inhales a nebulized solution containing metha-

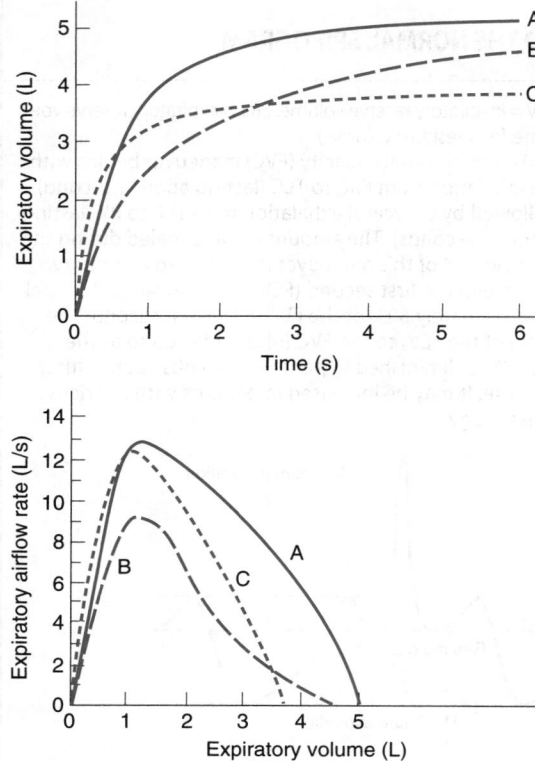

Figure 9–1. Representative spirograms (upper panel) and expiratory flow-volume curves (lower panel) for normal (A), obstructive (B), and restrictive (C) patterns.

choline or histamine. These agents cause bronchial smooth muscle constriction in asthmatic patients at much lower doses than in nonasthmatics. If the FEV_1 falls by more than 20% at a dose of 16 mg/mL or less, the test is positive. Bronchial provocation testing is 95% sensitive for the diagnosis of asthma. A negative result therefore makes asthma unlikely. Specificity is lower—about 70%—since false positives may occur in several common conditions, including COPD, congestive heart failure, recent viral respiratory infection, cystic fibrosis, and sarcoidosis.

Evans SE et al: Current practice in pulmonary function testing. Mayo Clin Proc 2003;78:758. [PMID: 12934788]

Miller MR et al; ATS/ERS Task Force: General considerations for lung function testing. Eur Respir J 2005;26:153. [PMID: 15994402]

Cardiopulmonary Exercise Stress Testing

Cardiopulmonary exercise testing is usually performed to evaluate patients with unexplained exertional dyspnea. A bicycle ergometer or treadmill is used. Minute ventilation, expired oxygen and carbon dioxide tension, heart rate, blood pressure, and respiratory rate are monitored. The exercise protocol is determined by

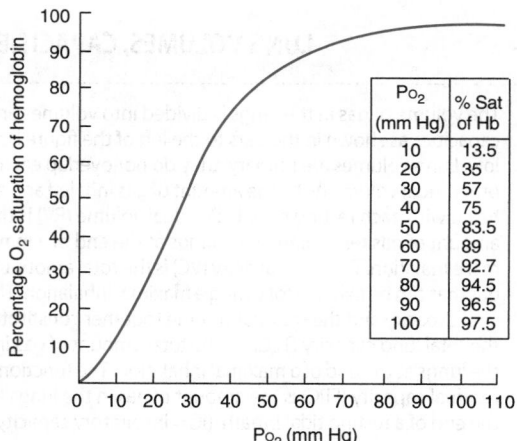

Figure 9–2. Oxygen-hemoglobin dissociation curve, pH 7.40, temperature 38 °C. (Reproduced, with permission, from Comroe JH Jr et al: *The Lung: Clinical Physiology and Pulmonary Function Tests*, 2nd ed. Year Book Medical Publishers, 1962.)

the indications for the test and the ability of the patient to exercise. Complications are rare.

American Thoracic Society; American College of Chest Physicians: ATS/ACCP statement on cardiopulmonary exercise testing. Am J Respir Crit Care Med 2003;167:211. [PMID: 12524257]

Bronchoscopy

Flexible bronchoscopy is an essential tool in the diagnosis and management of many pulmonary diseases. Bron-

Table 9–1. The effect of altitude on Po_2 in normal adults.

Altitude (feet)	Barometric Pressure (mm Hg)	Atmospheric[1] Po_2 (mm Hg)	Tracheal[2] Po_2 (mm Hg)	Arterial[3] Po_2 (mm Hg)
Sea level	760	159	149	99
2000	707	148	138	88
4000	656	137	127	77
6000	609	127	118	68
8000	564	118	108	58
10,000	523	109	100	50
15,000	426	90	80	30

[1]Dry gas.
[2]Saturated with water vapor.
[3]Actual values at altitude will be higher, depending on the degree of adaptation (ventilatory response to hypoxia).

choscopy is indicated for evaluation of the airway, diagnosis and staging of bronchogenic carcinoma, evaluation of hemoptysis, and diagnosis of pulmonary infections. It allows transbronchial lung biopsy, bronchoalveolar lavage, and removal of retained secretions and foreign bodies from the airway. The procedure is contraindicated in severe bronchospasm or a bleeding diathesis. Complications include hemorrhage, fever, and transient hypoxemia. The rate of major complications is less than 1% but increases to about 7% when transbronchial lung biopsy is performed. Deaths are rare. Hospitalization for flexible bronchoscopy is not necessary.

Rigid bronchoscopy is performed for massive bleeding, extraction of large obstructing objects (foreign bodies, blood clots, tumor masses, broncholiths), biopsy of tracheal or main stem bronchus tumors and bronchial carcinoids, and facilitation of laser therapy. Unlike flexible bronchoscopy, which can usually be performed with only topical anesthesia and low-dose conscious sedation (an opioid or a benzodiazepine or both), rigid bronchoscopy usually requires general anesthesia.

Advances in techniques including endobronchial laser therapy, electrocautery, tracheobronchial stenting, and endobronchial ultrasound guidance to locate lymph nodes prior to transbronchial needle aspiration biopsy ("Wang" biopsy) promise to expand diagnostic and therapeutic avenues available to the bronchoscopist significantly. This is an area of rapid technological advancement and emerging clinical research study.

Peikert T et al: Safety, diagnostic yield, and therapeutic implications of flexible bronchoscopy in patients with febrile neutropenia and pulmonary infiltrates. Mayo Clin Proc 2005; 80:1414. [PMID: 16295020]

Seijo LM et al: Interventional pulmonology. N Engl J Med 2001; 344:740. [PMID: 11236779]

■ DISORDERS OF THE AIRWAYS

Airway disorders have diverse causes but share certain common pathophysiologic and clinical features. Airflow limitation is characteristic and frequently causes dyspnea and cough. Other symptoms are common and typically disease-specific. Disorders of the airways can be classified as those that involve the upper airways—loosely defined as those above and including the vocal cords—and those that involve the lower airways.

DISORDERS OF THE UPPER AIRWAYS

Upper airway obstruction may occur acutely or present as a chronic condition. **Acute upper airway obstruction** can be immediately life-threatening and must be relieved promptly to avoid asphyxia. Causes of acute upper airway obstruction include foreign body aspiration, laryngospasm, laryngeal edema from airway burns, angioedema, trauma to the larynx or pharynx, infec-

tions (Ludwig's angina, pharyngeal or retropharyngeal abscess, acute epiglottis), and acute allergic laryngitis.

Chronic obstruction of the upper airway may be caused by carcinoma of the pharynx or larynx, laryngeal or subglottic stenosis, laryngeal granulomas or webs, or bilateral vocal cord paralysis. Laryngeal or subglottic stenosis may become evident weeks or months following a period of translaryngeal endotracheal intubation. Inspiratory stridor, intercostal retractions on inspiration, a palpable inspiratory thrill over the larynx, and wheezing localized to the neck or trachea on auscultation are characteristic findings. Flow-volume loops may show flow limitations characteristic of obstruction. Soft tissue radiographs of the neck may show supraglottic or infraglottic narrowing. CT and MRI scans can reveal exact sites of obstruction. Flexible endoscopy may be diagnostic, but caution is necessary to avoid exacerbating upper airway edema and precipitating critical airway narrowing.

Vocal cord dysfunction syndrome is a condition characterized by paradoxical vocal cord adduction, resulting in both acute and chronic upper airway obstruction. It can cause dyspnea and wheezing that may present as asthma; it may be distinguished from asthma by the lack of response to bronchodilator therapy, normal spirometry immediately after an attack, spirometric evidence of upper airway obstruction, a negative bronchial provocation test, or direct visualization of adduction of the vocal cords on both inspiration and expiration. Bronchodilators are of no therapeutic benefit. Treatment consists of speech therapy.

Ernst A et al: Central airway obstruction. Am J Respir Crit Care Med 2004;169:1278. [PMID: 15187010]

Gose JE: Acute workup of vocal cord dysfunction. Ann Allergy Asthma Immunol 2003;91:318. [PMID: 14533667]

Soli CG et al: Vocal cord dysfunction: An uncommon cause of stridor. J Emerg Med 2005;28:31. [PMID: 15657001]

DISORDERS OF THE LOWER AIRWAYS

Tracheal obstruction may be intrathoracic (below the suprasternal notch) or extrathoracic. Fixed tracheal obstruction may be caused by acquired or congenital tracheal stenosis, primary or secondary tracheal neoplasms, extrinsic compression (tumors of the lung, thymus, or thyroid; lymphadenopathy; congenital vascular rings; aneurysms, etc), foreign body aspiration, tracheal granulomas and papillomas, and tracheal trauma.

Acquired **tracheal stenosis** is usually secondary to previous tracheotomy or endotracheal intubation. Dyspnea, cough, and inability to clear pulmonary secretions occur weeks to months after tracheal decannulation or extubation. Physical findings may be absent until tracheal diameter is reduced 50% or more, when wheezing, a palpable tracheal thrill, and harsh breath sounds may be detected. The diagnosis is usually confirmed by plain films or CT of the trachea. Complications include recurring pulmonary infection and life-threatening respiratory failure. Management is directed toward ensuring adequate ventilation and oxygenation and avoiding manipulative procedures that may increase edema of the tracheal mucosa. Surgical reconstruction, endotracheal stent placement, or laser photoresection may be required.

Bronchial obstruction may be caused by retained pulmonary secretions, aspiration, foreign bodies, bronchogenic carcinoma, compression by extrinsic masses, and tumors metastatic to the airway. Clinical and radiographic findings vary depending on the location of the obstruction and the degree of airway narrowing. Symptoms include dyspnea, cough, wheezing, and, if infection is present, fever and chills. A history of recurrent pneumonia in the same lobe or segment or slow resolution (> 3 months) of pneumonia on successive radiographs suggests the possibility of bronchial obstruction and the need for bronchoscopy. Complete obstruction of a main stem bronchus may be obvious on physical examination (asymmetric chest expansion, mediastinal shift, absence of breath sounds on the affected side, and dullness to percussion), but partial obstruction is often difficult or impossible to detect. Prolonged expiration and localized wheezing may be the only clues. Segmental or subsegmental bronchial obstruction may produce no abnormalities on physical examination.

Roentgenographic findings include **atelectasis** (local parenchymal collapse), postobstructive infiltrates, and air trapping caused by unidirectional expiratory obstruction. CT scanning may demonstrate the nature and the exact location of obstruction of the central bronchi. MRI may be superior to CT for delineating the extent of the underlying disease in the hilum, but it is usually reserved for cases in which CT findings are equivocal. Bronchoscopy is the definitive diagnostic study, particularly if tumor or foreign body aspiration is suspected. The finding of tubular breath sounds on physical examination or an air bronchogram on chest radiograph in an area of atelectasis rules out complete airway obstruction. Bronchoscopy is unlikely to be of therapeutic benefit in this situation.

Right middle lobe syndrome is recurrent or persistent atelectasis of the right middle lobe. This collapse is related to the relatively long length and narrow diameter of the right middle lobe bronchus and the oval ("fish mouth") opening to the lobe, in the setting of impaired collateral ventilation. Fiberoptic bronchoscopy or CT scan is often necessary to rule out obstructing tumor. Foreign body or other benign causes are common.

Duggan M et al: Pulmonary atelectasis: a pathogenic perioperative entity. Anesthesiology 2005;102:838. [PMID: 15791115]

Kwon KY et al: Middle lobe syndrome: a clinicopathological study of 21 patients. Hum Pathol 1995;26:302. [PMID: 7890282]

ASTHMA

 ESSENTIALS OF DIAGNOSIS

- *Episodic or chronic symptoms of airflow obstruction: breathlessness, cough, wheezing, and chest tightness.*

- *Symptoms frequently worse at night or in the early morning.*

- *Prolonged expiration and diffuse wheezes on physical examination.*

- *Limitation of airflow on pulmonary function testing or positive bronchoprovocation challenge.*

- *Complete or partial reversibility of airflow obstruction, either spontaneously or following bronchodilator therapy.*

General Considerations

Asthma is a common disease, affecting approximately 5% of the population. Men and women appear to be equally affected. Each year, approximately 470,000 hospital admissions and 5000 deaths in the United States are attributed to asthma. Hospitalization rates have been highest among blacks and children, and death rates for asthma are consistently highest among blacks aged 15–24 years. Prevalence, hospitalizations, and fatal asthma have all increased in the United States over the past 20 years.

Definition & Pathogenesis

Asthma is a chronic inflammatory disorder of the airways. The histopathologic features include denudation of airway epithelium, collagen deposition beneath the basement membrane, airway edema, mast cell activation, and inflammatory cell infiltration with neutrophils, eosinophils, and lymphocytes (especially T lymphocytes). Hypertrophy of bronchial smooth muscle and hypertrophy of mucous glands with plugging of small airways with thick mucus can occur. This airway inflammation underlies disease chronicity and contributes to airway hyperresponsiveness, airflow limitation, and respiratory symptoms (including recurrent episodes of wheezing, breathlessness, chest tightness, and cough, particularly during the nighttime and early morning hours).

A genetic predisposition to asthma is recognized. The strongest identifiable predisposing factor for the development of asthma is atopy. Exposure of sensitive patients to inhaled allergens increases airway inflammation, airway hyperresponsiveness, and symptoms. Symptoms may develop immediately (immediate asthmatic response) or 4–6 hours after allergen exposure (late asthmatic response). Common aeroallergens include house dust mites (often found in pillows, mattresses, upholstered furniture, carpets, and drapes), cockroaches, cats, and seasonal pollens. Substantially reducing exposure reduces pathologic findings and clinical symptoms.

Nonspecific precipitants of asthma include exercise, upper respiratory tract infections, rhinitis, sinusitis, postnasal drip, aspiration, gastroesophageal reflux, changes in the weather, and stress. Exposure to environmental tobacco smoke increases asthma symptoms and the need for medications and reduces lung function. In-

Table 9–2. Classification of severity of chronic stable asthma.

	Symptoms	Nighttime Symptoms	Lung Function
Mild intermittent	Symptoms ≤ 2 times a week Asymptomatic and normal PEF between exacerbations Exacerbations brief (few hours to few days); intensity may vary	≤ 2 times a month	FEV_1 or PEF ≥ 80% predicted PEF variability ≤ 20%
Mild persistent	Symptoms > 2 times a week but < 1 time a day Exacerbations may affect activity	> 2 times a month	FEV_1 or PEF > 80% predicted PEF variability 20–30%
Moderate persistent	Daily symptoms Daily use of inhaled short-acting β_2-agonist Exacerbations affect activity Exacerbations ≥ 2 times a week; may last days	> 1 time a week	FEV_1 or PEF > 60% to < 80% predicted PEF variability > 30%
Severe persistent	Continual symptoms Limited physical activity Frequent exacerbations	Frequent	FEV_1 or PEF ≤ 60% predicted PEF variability > 30%

PEF = peak expiratory flow; FEV_1 = forced expiratory volume in the first second.
Adapted from National Asthma Education and Prevention Program. Expert Panel Report 2: Guidelines for the Diagnosis and Management of Asthma. National Institutes of Health Pub. No. 97-4051. Bethesda, MD, 1997.

creased air levels of respirable particles, ozone, SO_2, and NO_2 precipitate asthma symptoms and increase emergency department visits and hospitalizations. Selected individuals may experience asthma symptoms after exposure to aspirin, nonsteroidal anti-inflammatory drugs, or tartrazine dyes. Certain other medications may also precipitate asthma symptoms (Table 9–28). Occupational asthma is triggered by various agents in the workplace and may occur weeks to years after initial exposure and sensitization. Women may experience catamenial asthma at predictable times during the menstrual cycle. Exercise-induced bronchoconstriction usually begins within 3 minutes after the end of exercise, peaks within 10–15 minutes, and then resolves by 60 minutes. This phenomenon is thought to be a consequence of the airways' attempt to warm and humidify an increased volume of expired air during exercise. "Cardiac asthma" is wheezing precipitated by uncompensated congestive heart failure.

Clinical Findings

Symptoms and signs vary widely from patient to patient as well as individually over time. General clinical findings in stable asthma patients are listed below (Table 9–2); findings seen during asthma exacerbations are listed in Table 9–3.

A. SYMPTOMS AND SIGNS

Asthma is characterized by episodic wheezing, difficulty in breathing, chest tightness, and cough. The frequency of asthma symptoms is highly variable. Some patients may have only a chronic dry cough and others a productive cough. Some patients have infrequent, brief attacks of asthma and others may suffer nearly continuous symptoms. Asthma symptoms may occur spontaneously or may be precipitated or exacerbated by many different triggers as discussed above. Asthma symptoms are frequently worse at night; circadian variations in bronchomotor tone and bronchial reactivity reach their nadir between 3 AM and 4 AM, increasing symptoms of bronchoconstriction.

Some physical findings increase the probability of asthma. Nasal mucosal swelling, increased nasal secretions, and nasal polyps are often seen in patients with allergic asthma. Eczema, atopic dermatitis, or other manifestations of allergic skin disorders may also be present. Hunched shoulders and use of accessory muscles of respiration suggest an increased work of breathing. Chest examination may be normal between exacerbations in patients with mild asthma. Wheezing during normal breathing or a prolonged forced expiratory phase correlates well with the presence of airflow obstruction. Wheezing during forced expiration does not. During severe asthma exacerbations, airflow may be too limited to produce wheezing, and the only diagnostic clue on auscultation may be globally reduced breath sounds with prolonged expiration.

B. PULMONARY FUNCTION TESTING

Clinicians are able to identify airflow obstruction on examination, but they have limited ability to assess it

Table 9–3. Classification of severity of asthma exacerbations.

	Mild	Moderate	Severe	Impending Respiratory Failure
Symptoms				
Breathlessness	With activity	With talking	At rest	At rest
Speech	Sentences	Phrases	Words	Mute
Signs				
Body position	Able to recline	Prefers sitting	Unable to recline	Unable to recline
Respiratory rate	Increased	Increased	Often > 30/min	> 30/min
Use of accessory respiratory muscles	Usually not	Commonly	Usually	Paradoxical thoracoabdominal movement
Breath sounds	Moderate wheezing at mid- to end-expiration	Loud wheezes throughout expiration	Loud inspiratory and expiratory wheezes	Little air movement without wheezes
Heart rate (beats/min)	< 100	100–120	> 120	Relative bradycardia
Pulsus paradoxus (mm Hg)	< 10	10–25	Often > 25	Often absent
Mental status	May be agitated	Usually agitated	Usually agitated	Confused or drowsy
Functional assessment				
PEF (% predicted or personal best)	> 80	50–80	< 50 or response to therapy lasts < 2 hours	< 50
Sao_2 (%, room air)	> 95	91–95	< 91	< 91
Pao_2 (mm Hg, room air)	Normal	> 60	< 60	< 60
$Paco_2$ (mm Hg)	< 42	< 42	≥ 42	≥ 42

PEF = peak expiratory flow.
Adapted from National Asthma Education and Prevention Program. Expert Panel Report 2: Guidelines for the Diagnosis and Management of Asthma. National Institutes of Health Pub. No. 97-4051. Bethesda, MD, 1997.

or to predict whether it is reversible. The evaluation for asthma should therefore include spirometry (FEV_1, FVC, FEV_1/FVC) before and after the administration of a short-acting bronchodilator. These measurements help determine the presence and extent of airflow obstruction and whether it is immediately reversible. Airflow obstruction is indicated by a reduced FEV_1/FVC ratio (< 75%). In severe airflow obstruction with significant air trapping, the FVC may also be reduced, resulting in a pattern that suggests a restrictive ventilatory defect. Significant reversibility of airflow obstruction is defined by an increase of ≥ 12% and 200 mL in FEV_1 or ≥ 15% and 200 mL in FVC after inhaling a short-acting bronchodilator. However, the absence of improvement in airflow after administration of a bronchodilator is not proof of irreversible airflow obstruction.

Peak expiratory flow (PEF) meters are handheld devices designed as home monitoring tools. PEF monitoring can establish peak flow variability, quantify asthma severity, and provide both the patient and the clinician with objective measurements on which to base treatment decisions. There are conflicting data about whether measuring PEF improves asthma outcomes, but doing so is recommended as part of a comprehensive approach to asthma management in Expert Panel Report 2 of the National Asthma Education and Prevention Program (NAEPP) of the National Heart, Lung and Blood Institute.

Predicted values for PEF vary with age, height, and gender but are poorly standardized. Comparison with reference values is less helpful than comparison with the patient's best baseline. PEF shows diurnal variation. It is generally lowest on first awakening and highest several hours before the midpoint of the waking day. PEF should be measured in the morning before the administration of a bronchodilator and in the afternoon after taking a bronchodilator. A 20% change in PEF values from morning to afternoon or from day to day suggests inadequately controlled asthma. PEF values less than 200 L/min indicate severe airflow obstruction.

Bronchial provocation testing with histamine or methacholine—or exercise challenge testing—may be useful when asthma is suspected and spirometry is nondiagnostic. Bronchial provocation is not generally recommended if the FEV_1 is less than 65% of predicted. A positive test is defined as a decrease in FEV_1 of at least 20% at exposure to a dose of 16 mg/mL or less. A negative test has a negative predictive value for asthma of 95%.

Arterial blood gas measurements may be normal during a mild asthma exacerbation, but respiratory alkalosis and an increase in the alveolar-arterial oxygen difference (A–a–DO_2) are common. During severe exacerbations, hypoxemia develops and the $PaCO_2$ returns to normal. The combination of an increased $PaCO_2$ and respiratory acidosis is a harbinger of respiratory failure and may indicate the need for mechanical ventilation.

C. ADDITIONAL TESTING

Routine chest radiographs in patients with asthma usually show only hyperinflation. Other findings may include bronchial wall thickening and diminished peripheral lung vascular shadows. Chest radiographs are indicated when pneumonia, another disorder mimicking asthma, or a complication of asthma such as pneumothorax is suspected. The diagnostic usefulness of measurements of biologic markers of inflammation such as cell counts and mediator titers in blood and sputum is being investigated. Skin testing or in vitro testing to assess sensitivity to relevant environmental allergens may be useful in patients with persistent asthma. Evaluations for paranasal sinus disease or gastroesophageal reflux should be considered in patients with pertinent symptoms and in those who have severe or refractory asthma.

Complications

Complications of asthma include exhaustion, dehydration, airway infection, cor pulmonale, and tussive syncope. Pneumothorax occurs but is rare. Acute hypercapnic and hypoxic respiratory failure occurs in severe disease.

Differential Diagnosis

Disorders that mimic asthma typically fall into one of three categories: upper and lower airway disorders, systemic vasculitides, and psychiatric disorders. It is prudent to consider these conditions in patients who have atypical asthma symptoms or response to therapy. Upper airway disorders that mimic asthma include vocal cord paralysis, vocal cord dysfunction syndrome, foreign body aspiration, laryngotracheal masses, tracheal narrowing, tracheomalacia, and airway edema as in the setting of angioedema or inhalation injury. Lower airway disorders include nonasthmatic COPD (chronic bronchitis or emphysema), bronchiectasis, allergic bronchopulmonary mycosis, cystic fibrosis, eosinophilic pneumonia, and bronchiolitis obliterans. Systemic vasculitides that often have an asthmatic component include Churg-Strauss syndrome and other systemic vasculitides with pulmonary involvement. Psychiatric causes include conversion disorders, which have been variably referred to as functional asthma, emotional laryngeal wheezing, vocal cord dysfunction, or episodic laryngeal dyskinesis. Munchausen syndrome or malingering may rarely explain the patient's complaints.

Classification of Asthma Severity

The Expert Panel of the NAEPP has developed asthma classification schemes that are useful in directing asthma therapy and identifying patients at high risk for developing life-threatening asthma attacks. Table 9–2 is used to classify the severity of chronic, stable asthma; Table 9–3 is used to classify the severity of asthma exacerbations. A patient's clinical features before treatment are used to classify the patient. The presence of only one of the severity features is sufficient to place a patient in that category; patients should be assigned to the most severe grade in which any feature occurs.

Approach to Long-Term Treatment

The goals of asthma therapy are to minimize chronic symptoms that impair normal activity (including exercise), to prevent recurrent exacerbations, to minimize the need for emergency department visits or hospitalizations, and to maintain near-normal pulmonary function. These goals should be met while providing optimal pharmacotherapy with the fewest adverse effects and while meeting patients' and families' expectations of satisfaction with asthma care.

Current approaches to persistent asthma focus on daily anti-inflammatory therapy with inhaled corticosteroids. Treatment algorithms are based on both the severity of a patient's baseline asthma and the severity of asthma exacerbations. Expert Panel Report 2 from the NAEPP recommends a stepwise approach to therapy (Table 9–4). The amount of medication and frequency of dosing are dictated by asthma severity and directed toward suppression of increasing airway inflammation. To establish prompt control, therapy should be initiated early at a higher intensity level than anticipated for long-term therapy. Pharmacotherapy can then be cautiously stepped down once asthma control is achieved and sustained; this allows for identification of the minimum medication necessary to maintain long-term control.

Pharmacologic Agents for Asthma

Asthma medications can be divided into two categories: agents that offer quick relief of symptoms and agents taken to promote long-term asthma control. Quick-relief medications are taken to promote prompt reversal of acute airflow obstruction and relieve accompanying symptoms by direct relaxation of bronchial smooth muscle. Long-term control medications are taken daily independent of symptoms to achieve and maintain control of persistent asthma. These agents—also known as maintenance, controller, or preventive medications—act primarily to attenuate airway inflammation.

Table 9–4. Stepwise approach for managing asthma.[1]

	Long-Term Control	Quick Relief	Education
Step 1: Mild intermittent	No daily medication needed.	Short-acting bronchodilator: **inhaled β_2-agonists** as needed for symptoms. Intensity of treatment will depend on severity of exacerbation. Use of short-acting **inhaled β_2-agonists** > 2 times a week may indicate the need for long-term control therapy.	Teach basic facts about asthma Teach inhaler/inhalation chamber technique Discuss roles of medications Develop self-management and action plans Discuss appropriate environmental control measures
Step 2: Mild persistent	One daily medication: **Anti-inflammatory: either inhaled corticosteroid** (low doses) or **cromolyn** or **nedocromil** Less desirable alternatives: sustained-release **theophylline** or **leukotriene modifier**	Step 1 actions plus: Use of short-acting **inhaled β_2-agonists** on a daily basis, or increasing use, indicates the need for additional long-term control therapy.	Step 1 actions plus: Teach self-monitoring Refer to group education if available Review and update self-management plan
Step 3: Moderate persistent	Daily medication: Either **Anti-inflammatory: inhaled corticosteroid** (medium dose) or **Inhaled corticosteroid** (low-medium dose) and a **long-acting bronchodilator** (long-acting **inhaled β_2-agonist,** sustained-release **theophylline** or long-acting **β_2-agonist tablets**) If needed: **Anti-inflammatory: inhaled corticosteroid** (medium-high dose) and **Long-acting bronchodilator** (long-acting **inhaled β_2-agonist,** sustained-release **theophylline** or long-acting **β_2-agonist tablets**)	As for step 2.	Step 1 actions plus: Teach self-monitoring Refer to group education if available Review and update self-management plan
Step 4: Severe persistent	Daily medication: **Anti-inflammatory: inhaled corticosteroid** (high dose) and **Long-acting bronchodilator** (long-acting **inhaled β_2-agonist,** sustained release **theophylline** or long-acting **inhaled β_2-agonist tablets**) and **Corticosteroid tablets or syrup** (1–2 mg/kg/d, generally not to exceed 60 mg/d)	As for step 2.	Step 2 and 3 actions plus: Refer to individual education, counseling

Step down: Review treatment every 1–6 months; a gradual stepwise reduction in treatment may be possible.

Step up: If asthma control is not maintained, consider step up to next treatment level after reviewing medication technique, adherence, and environmental control.

[1]Preferred treatments are in bold text; however, specific medication plans should be tailored to individual patients.
Modified from National Asthma Education and Prevention Program. Expert Panel Report 2: Guidelines for the Diagnosis and Management of Asthma. National Institutes of Health Pub. No. 97-4051. Bethesda, MD, 1997.

Many asthma medications are administered orally or by inhalation. Inhalation of an appropriate agent results in a more rapid onset of pulmonary effects as well as fewer systemic effects compared with oral administration of the same dose. Metered-dose inhalers (MDIs) propelled by chlorofluorocarbons (CFCs) have been the most widely used delivery system, but non-CFC propellant systems and dry powder inhalers are available. These alternatives are effective and well tolerated. Proper MDI technique and the use of an inhalation chamber improve drug delivery to the lung and decrease oropharyngeal deposition. Nebulizer therapy is reserved for acutely ill patients and those who cannot use MDIs because of difficulties with coordination or cooperation.

A. LONG-TERM CONTROL MEDICATIONS

Anti-inflammatory agents, long-acting bronchodilators, and leukotriene modifiers comprise the important medications in this group of agents (see Table 9–5). Other classes of agents are mentioned briefly below.

1. Anti-inflammatory agents—Corticosteroids are the most potent and consistently effective anti-inflammatory agents currently available. They reduce both acute and chronic inflammation, resulting in fewer asthma symptoms, improvement in airflow, decreased airway hyperresponsiveness, fewer asthma exacerbations, and less airway remodeling. These agents may also potentiate the action of β-adrenergic agonists.

Inhaled corticosteroids are preferred for the long-term control of asthma and are first-line agents for patients with persistent asthma. Patients with persistent symptoms or asthma exacerbations who are not taking inhaled corticosteroids should be started on an inhaled corticosteroid; symptomatic patients already taking an inhaled corticosteroid should have the dose increased. Dosages for inhaled corticosteroids vary depending on the specific agent and delivery device. The most important determinants of agent selection and appropriate dosing are the patient's status and response to treatment. For most patients, twice-daily dosing provides adequate control of asthma. Once-daily dosing may be sufficient in selected patients with mild persistent asthma. Maximum responses from inhaled corticosteroids may not be observed for months. The use of an inhalation chamber coupled with mouth washing after inhalation decreases local side effects (cough, dysphonia, oropharyngeal candidiasis) and systemic absorption. Systemic effects (adrenal suppression, osteoporosis, skin thinning, easy bruising, and cataracts) may occur with high-dose inhalation therapy.

Systemic corticosteroids (oral or parenteral) are most effective in achieving prompt control of asthma during exacerbations or when initiating long-term asthma therapy. In patients with severe persistent asthma, systemic corticosteroids are often required for the long-term suppression of symptoms. Repeated efforts should be made to reduce the dose to the minimum needed to control symptoms. Alternate-day treatment is preferred to daily treatment. Rapid discontinuation of systemic corticosteroids after chronic use may precipitate adrenal insufficiency. Concurrent treatment with calcium supplements and vitamin D should be initiated to prevent corticosteroid-induced bone mineral loss in long-term administration. Bisphosphonates may offer additional protection to these patients (see Table 26–18).

2. Long-acting bronchodilators—

a. Mediator inhibitors—Cromolyn sodium and nedocromil are long-term control medications that prevent asthma symptoms and improve airway function in patients with mild persistent asthma or exercise-induced asthma. Both of these agents modulate mast cell mediator release and eosinophil recruitment and inhibit both early and late asthmatic responses to allergen challenge and exercise-induced bronchospasm. The clinical response to these agents is less predictable than the response to inhaled corticosteroids. Nedocromil may help reduce the dose requirements for inhaled corticosteroids. Both agents have excellent safety profiles.

b. β-Adrenergic agents—Long-acting β₂-agonists provide bronchodilation for up to 12 hours after a single dose. However, because their onset of action is delayed, they are not effective—and should not be used—in the treatment of acute bronchoconstriction. Salmeterol and formoterol are the two agents in this class available in the United States. They are administered via dry powder delivery devices. They are indicated for long-term prevention of asthma symptoms, nocturnal symptoms, and for prevention of exercise-induced bronchospasm. They should not be used in place of anti-inflammatory therapy. When added to standard doses of inhaled corticosteroids, salmeterol provides control equivalent to what is achieved by doubling the inhaled corticosteroid dose. Side effects are minimal at standard doses.

c. Phosphodiesterase inhibitors—Theophylline provides mild bronchodilation in asthmatic patients. This drug may also have anti-inflammatory properties, enhance mucociliary clearance, and strengthen diaphragmatic contractility. Sustained-release theophylline preparations are effective in controlling nocturnal asthma and are usually reserved for use as adjuvant therapy in patients with moderate or severe persistent asthma. They can also be used as alternative long-term preventive therapy in patients with mild persistent asthma. Theophylline serum concentrations need to be monitored closely owing to the drug's narrow toxic-therapeutic range, individual differences in metabolism, and the effects of many factors on drug absorption and metabolism. Decreases in theophylline clearance accompany the use of cimetidine, macrolide and quinolone antibiotics, and oral contraceptives. Increases in theophylline clearance are caused by rifampin, phenytoin, barbiturates, and tobacco.

Adverse effects at therapeutic doses include insomnia, upset stomach, aggravation of dyspepsia and gastroesophageal reflux symptoms, and urination difficulties in elderly men with prostatism. Dose-related toxicities are common and include nausea, vomiting,

Table 9–5. Long-term control medications for asthma.[1]

Drug	Important Formulations	Usual Adult Dosage	Cost[2]	Comments
Inhaled corticosteroids[3]				
Beclomethasone dipropionate (QVAR)	40 mcg/puff 80 mcg/puff	Two or three puffs BID One to two puffs BID	$61.54/7.30 g $77.44/7.30 g	Chlorofluorocarbon-free; hydrofluoralkane propellant
Budesonide (Pulmicort Turbuhaler)	Dry powder delivery system: 200 mcg/puff; 200 puffs/inhaler	One inhalation twice a day	$158.15/inhaler	Dry powder
Flunisolide (AeroBid)	MDI: 250 mcg/puff; 100 puffs/inhaler	Two to four puffs twice a day	$77.57/7 g	Chlorofluorocarbon propellant
Fluticasone (Flovent HFA)	MDI: 44, 110, or 220 mcg/puff; 120 puffs/inhaler	Two or three puffs (of 110 mcg) twice a day	$103.98/13 g (110 µg)	Chlorofluorocarbon propellant
Fluticasone (Flovent Rotadisk)	Dry powder delivery system: 44, 88, 220 mcg/blister; 4 blisters/Rotadisk, 15 Rotadisks per tube	One or two puffs (of 88 mcg) twice a day	Not available in the U.S.	Dry powder
Triamcinolone acetonide (Azmacort)	MDI: 100 mcg/puff; 240 puffs/inhaler	Two or three puffs four times a day, or four to six puffs twice daily	$92.58/20 g	Chlorofluorocarbon propellant
Systemic corticosteroids				
Methylprednisolone (many)	Tablets: 4 mg	5–60 mg daily to every other day as needed	$0.54/4 mg	
Prednisolone (many)	Tablets: 5 mg	5–60 mg daily to every other day as needed	$0.04/5 mg	
Prednisone (many)	Tablets: 1, 2.5, 5, 10, 20, 50 mg	5–60 mg daily to every other day as needed	$0.04/5 mg	
Combination inhaled corticosteroid and long-acting β₂-agonist				
Fluticasone and salmeterol (Advair Diskus)	Dry powder delivery system: 100, 250, or 500 mcg fluticasone per dose and 50 mcg salmeterol per dose	One puff twice a day of 250/50; cannot use more than one puff twice a day due to salmeterol component	$177.71/60 250/ 60 disks	Dry powder
Cromolyn (Intal)	MDI: 800 mcg per puff; 200 puffs/inhaler Nebulizer solution: 20 mg/2 mL ampule	2–4 puffs 4 times a day 20 mg (2 mL) four times a day	$102.12/14.2 g $1.26/2 mL	Chlorofluorocarbon propellant Administer with powered nebulizer
Nedocromil (Tilade)	MDI: 1.75 mg/puff; 112 puffs/inhaler	Two puffs four times a day	$79.68/16.2 g	Chlorofluorocarbon propellant

Long-acting β_2 agonists[4] Salmeterol (Serevent Diskus)	Dry powder: 50 mcg/blister; 60 blisters per pack	One blister every 12 hours	$100.16/60	Dry powder
Formoterol (Foradil Aerolizer)	Dry powder: 12 mcg/capsule; 60 capsules/Aerolizer	One capsule every 12 hours	$79.83/60	Dry powder
Sustained-release albuterol (Proventil Repetab)	Sustained-release tablet, 4 mg	One tablet every 12 hours	$1.24/4 mg	Usually reserved for nocturnal symptoms not improved with other therapies
Theophylline (many)	Sustained-release tablets and capsules	Initially 10 mg/kg/d up to 300 mg maximum; then 200–600 mg every 8–24 hours	$0.33/200 mg	Maintenance dose guided by serum drug level. Absorption and dosing vary with brand
Leukotriene modifiers Montelukast (Singulair)	Tablet, 10 mg	One tablet each evening	$3.47/10 mg $104.10/mo	
Zafirlukast (Accolate)	Tablet, 20 mg	One tablet twice a day	$1.46/20 mg $88.10/mo	Administration with meals decreases bioavailability; take at least 1 hour before or 2 hours after meals
Zileuton (Zyflo)	Tablet, 600 mg	One tablet four times a day	$2.28/600 mg $273.75/mo	Monitor hepatic enzymes

[1]Only drugs available in the United States are listed.

[2]Average wholesale price (AWP, for AB-rated generic when available) for quantity listed. Source: *Red Book Update*, Vol. 25, No. 5. May 2006. AWP may not accurately represent actual pharmacy cost because wide contractual variations exist among institutions.

[3]Dosing should be individualized. See text.

[4]Not for acute relief of symptoms.

MDI = metered-dose inhaler.

tachyarrhythmias, headache, seizures, hyperglycemia, and hypokalemia.

3. Leukotriene modifiers—This is the newest class of medications for long-term control of asthma. Leukotrienes are potent biochemical mediators that contribute to airway obstruction and asthma symptoms by contracting airway smooth muscle, increasing vascular permeability and mucus secretion, and attracting and activating airway inflammatory cells. Zileuton is a 5-lipoxygenase inhibitor that decreases leukotriene production, and zafirlukast and montelukast are cysteinyl leukotriene receptor antagonists. They cause modest improvements in lung function and reductions in asthma symptoms and lessen the need for β-agonist rescue therapy. These agents may be considered as alternatives to low-dose inhaled corticosteroids in patients with mild persistent asthma. Zileuton can cause reversible elevations in plasma aminotransferase levels, and Churg-Strauss syndrome has been diagnosed in a small number of patients who have taken montelukast or zafirlukast.

4. Desensitization—Immunotherapy for specific allergens may be considered in selected asthma patients who have exacerbations of asthma symptoms when exposed to allergens to which they are sensitive and who do not respond to environmental control measures or other forms of conventional therapy. Studies show a reduction in asthma symptoms in patients treated with single-allergen immunotherapy. Because of the risk of immunotherapy-induced bronchoconstriction, it should be administered only in a setting where such complications can be treated.

5. Miscellaneous agents—Oral sustained-release β₂-agonists are reserved for patients with bothersome nocturnal asthma symptoms or moderate to severe persistent asthma who do not respond to other therapies. Omalizumab is a recombinant antibody that binds IgE without activating mast cells. In clinical trials, it reduces the need for corticosteroids in moderate to severe asthmatic patients with elevated IgE levels. Corticosteroid-sparing anti-inflammatory agents such as troleandomycin, methotrexate, cyclosporine, intravenous immunoglobulin, and gold should be used only in selected severe asthmatic patients. These and other agents have variable benefit and worrisome toxicities.

B. QUICK-RELIEF MEDICATIONS

Short-acting bronchodilators and systemic corticosteroids comprise the important medications in this group of agents (Table 9–6).

1. β-Adrenergic agents—Short-acting inhaled β-adrenergic agonists are clearly the most effective bronchodilators during exacerbations. β-Adrenergic agonists should be used in all patients to treat acute symptoms. These agents relax airway smooth muscle and cause a prompt increase in airflow and reduction of symptoms. Administration before exercise effectively prevents exercise-induced bronchoconstriction. There is no convincing evidence to support the use of one agent over another. However, β₂-selective agents produce less cardiac stimulation than those with mixed β₁ and β₂ activities. Currently available short-acting β₂-selective adrenergic agonists include albuterol, bitolterol, pirbuterol, and terbutaline.

Inhaled β-adrenergic agonist therapy is as effective as oral or parenteral therapy in relaxing airway smooth muscle and improving acute asthma and offers the advantages of rapid onset of action (< 5 minutes) with fewer systemic side effects. Repetitive administration produces incremental bronchodilation. Intravenous and subcutaneous routes of administration should be reserved for patients who because of age or mechanical factors are unable to inhale medications.

One or two inhalations of a short-acting inhaled β₂-agonist from an MDI are usually sufficient for mild to moderate symptoms. Severe exacerbations frequently require higher doses: equivalent bronchodilation can be achieved by high doses (6–12 puffs every 30–60 minutes) of a β₂-agonist by MDI with an inhalation chamber or by nebulizer therapy. Administration by wet nebulization does not offer more effective delivery than MDIs but it is given in higher doses. With most β₂-agonists, the recommended dose by nebulizer for acute asthma (albuterol, 2.5 mg) is 25–30 times that delivered by a single activation of the MDI (albuterol, 0.09 mg). This difference suggests that the standard use of inhalations from an MDI will often be insufficient in the setting of an acute exacerbation. Independent of dose, nebulizer therapy may be more effective in patients who are unable to coordinate inhalation of medication from an MDI because of age, agitation, or severity of the exacerbation.

Scheduled daily use of short-acting β₂-agonists is not generally recommended. Increased use (more than one canister a month) or lack of expected effect indicates diminished asthma control and dictates the need for additional long-term control therapy.

2. Anticholinergics—Anticholinergic agents reverse vagally mediated bronchospasm but not allergen- or exercise-induced bronchospasm. They may decrease mucus gland hypersecretion seen in asthma. Ipratropium bromide, a quaternary derivative of atropine free of atropine's side effects, reverses acute bronchospasm and is the inhaled alternative for patients with intolerance to β₂-agonists. Ipratropium bromide may be a useful adjunct to inhaled short-acting β₂-agonists and considered in patients with moderate to severe asthma exacerbations. High doses of inhaled ipratropium bromide (0.5 mg) cause additional bronchodilation in some patients with severe airway obstruction, but the role in long-term management of asthma has not been clarified. It is the drug of choice for bronchospasm due to β-blocker medications.

3. Phosphodiesterase inhibitors—Methylxanthines are not recommended for therapy of asthma exacerbations. Aminophylline has clearly been shown to be less

Table 9–6. Quick-relief medications for asthma.[1]

Drug	Important Formulations	Usual Adult Dosage	Cost[2]	Comments
Short-acting Inhaled β_2-agonists				
Albuterol (Proventil, Ventolin)	MDI: 90 mcg/puff, 200 puffs/canister	Two puffs 5 minutes before exercise Two puffs every 4–6 hours as needed	$29.79/17 g	Preferred formulation in most cases. Chlorofluorocarbon propellant.
	Nebulizer solutions: 5 mg/mL (0.5%)	1.25–5 mg (0.25–1 mL) in 2–3 mL of normal saline every 4–8 hours as needed	$16.50/20 mL	Administer with powered nebulizer. More frequent dosing is acceptable for acute or severe exacerbations.
	Unit dose: 0.083%, 3 mL	One dose every 4–8 hours as needed	$1.24/unit	May mix with cromolyn or ipratropium nebulizer solutions.
	Tablets: 2 mg, 4 mg	2–4 mg orally every 6–8 hours	$31.14/100 2-mg tablets	Extended-release 4-mg tablet (Proventil Repetab) available for use every 12 hours.
Albuterol HFA (Proventil HFA)	MDI: 90 mcg/puff, 200 puffs/canister	Two puffs 5 minutes before exercise Two puffs every 4–6 hours as needed	$42.20/6.7 g	Nonchlorofluorocarbon propellant.
Pirbuterol (Maxair Autoinhaler)	MDI 200 mcg/puff, 400 puffs/canister	Two puffs every 4–6 hours as needed	$96.78/14 g	Breath-activated MDI system. Chlorofluorocarbon propellant.
Terbutaline (Brethine)	Tablets: 2.5 mg, 5 mg	2.5–5 mg orally three times a day	$62.21/100 5-mg tablets	Tremor, nervousness, palpitations common; therefore not recommended.
	Injection solution, 1 mg/mL	0.25 mg (0.25 mL) subcutaneously; may be repeated once in 30 minutes	$22.49/1 mg	Onset of action 30 minutes. Not limited to β_2-agonist effects.
Anticholinergics				
Ipratropium bromide (Atrovent HFA)	MDI: 18 mcg/puff, 200 puffs/canister	Two to four puffs every 6 hours	$84.60/14 g	Non-chlorofluorocarbon propellant.
	Unit dose nebulizer solution, 0.2 mg/mL (0.02%), 2.5 mL (0.5 mg)	0.25–0.5 mg (1–2 mL) every 6 hours	$1.76/unit	
Systemic corticosteroids				
Methylprednisolone (many)	Tablets: 4 mg	40–60 mg/d as single dose or in two divided doses for 3–10 days	$11.00/4-mg dose-pack	
Methylprednisolone sodium succinate (many)	Intravenous injection solution vials: 40, 125, 500 mg	0.5–1 mg/kg every 6 hours	$3.75/125-mg vial	
Prednisolone (many)	Tablets: 5 mg Syrup: 15 mg/5 mL	40–60 mg/d as single dose or in two divided doses for 3–10 days	$0.04/5-mg tablet $6.21/240 mL syrup	
Prednisone (many)	Tablets: 1, 2.5, 5, 10, 20, 50 mg	40–60 mg/d as single dose or in two divided doses for 3–10 days	$0.04/5 mg	

[1]Only drugs available in the United States are listed.
[2]Average wholesale price (AWP, for AB-rated generic when available) for quantity listed. Source: *Red Book Update,* Vol. 25., No. 5, May 2006. AWP may not accurately represent the actual pharmacy cost because wide contractual variations exist among institutions.
MDI = metered-dose inhaler.

effective than β_2-agonists when used as single-drug therapy for acute asthma and adds little except toxicity to the acute bronchodilator effects achieved by nebulized metaproterenol alone. Patients with exacerbations who are currently taking a theophylline-containing preparation should have their serum theophylline concentration measured to exclude theophylline toxicity.

4. Corticosteroids—Systemic corticosteroids are effective primary treatment for patients with moderate to severe exacerbations or for patients who do not respond promptly and completely to inhaled β_2-agonist therapy. Systemic corticosteroids are one of the mainstays of the treatment of patients with severe asthma. These medications speed the resolution of airflow obstruction and reduce the rate of relapse. Delays in administering corticosteroids may result in delayed benefits from these important agents. Therefore, oral corticosteroids should be available for early administration at home in many patients with moderate to severe asthma.

It may be prudent to administer corticosteroids to critically ill patients via the intravenous route in order to avoid concerns about altered gastrointestinal absorption. The minimal effective dose of systemic corticosteroids for asthma patients has not been identified. Outpatient prednisone "burst" therapy is 0.5–1 mg/kg/d (typically 40–60 mg) as a single or in two divided doses for 3–10 days. Severe exacerbations requiring hospitalization typically require 1 mg/kg of prednisone equivalent every 6–12 hours for 48 hours or until the FEV_1 (or PEF rate) returns to 50% of predicted (or 50% of baseline). The dose is then decreased to 60–80 mg/d until the PEF reaches 70% of predicted or personal best. No clear advantage has been found for higher doses of corticosteroids in severe exacerbations.

5. Antimicrobials—Antibiotics have no role in routine asthma exacerbations. They may be useful if bacterial respiratory tract infections are thought to contribute. Thus, patients with fever and purulent sputum and evidence of pneumonia or bacterial sinusitis are reasonable candidates.

Approach to Treatment of Asthma Exacerbations

The principal goals in the treatment of asthma exacerbations are correction of hypoxemia, reversal of airflow obstruction, and reduction of the likelihood of recurrence of obstruction. Early intervention may lessen the severity and duration of an exacerbation. Of paramount importance is correction of hypoxemia through the use of supplemental oxygen. At the same time, rapid reversal of airflow obstruction should be attempted by repetitive or continuous administration of an inhaled short-acting β_2-agonist and the early administration of systemic corticosteroids to patients with moderate to severe asthma exacerbations or to patients who do not respond promptly and completely to an inhaled short-acting β_2-agonist.

Serial measurements of lung function to quantify the severity of airflow obstruction and its response to treatment are especially useful. The improvement in FEV_1 after 30 minutes of treatment correlates significantly with a broad range of indices of the severity of asthma exacerbations. Serial measurement of airflow in the emergency department is an important factor in disposition and may reduce the rate of hospital admissions for asthma exacerbations.

The postexacerbation care plan is an important aspect of management. Regardless of the severity, all patients should be provided with necessary medications and education in how to use them, instruction in self-assessment, a follow-up appointment, and instruction in an action plan for managing recurrence.

Approach to Treatment of Mild Asthma Exacerbations

Mild asthma exacerbations are characterized by only minor changes in airway function (PEF > 80%) and minimal symptoms and signs of airway dysfunction (Table 9–3). The majority of exacerbations can be managed with home-based therapies. Most patients respond quickly and fully to an inhaled short-acting β_2-agonist alone. However, an inhaled short-acting β_2-agonist may need to be continued every 3–4 hours for 24–48 hours. For mild exacerbations in patients already taking an inhaled corticosteroid, the dose is doubled until peak flow returns to predicted or personal best. In patients not already taking an inhaled corticosteroid, initiation of this agent should be considered. A 3- to 10-day course of oral corticosteroids may be necessary for mild exacerbations that persist despite an increase in the dose of inhaled corticosteroids. See Table 9–6.

Approach to Treatment of Moderate & Severe Asthma Exacerbations

Some patients with moderate asthma exacerbations can be managed at home with the telephone assistance of a clinician. However, most such patients require a more comprehensive evaluation and treatment program such as that outlined below for severe asthma exacerbations. A course of oral corticosteroids is usually necessary.

Owing to the life-threatening nature of severe exacerbations of asthma, treatment should be started immediately once the exacerbation is recognized. All patients with a severe exacerbation should immediately receive oxygen, high doses of an inhaled short-acting β_2-agonist, and systemic corticosteroids. A brief history pertinent to the exacerbation can be completed while treatment is given. More detailed assessments, including laboratory studies, usually add little in the early phase of evaluation and management and should be delayed until after initial therapy has been completed.

Asphyxia is a common cause of death, and oxygen therapy is therefore very important. Supplemental oxygen should be given to maintain an $SaO_2 > 90\%$ or a $PaO_2 > 60$ mm Hg. Oxygen-induced hypoventilation is extremely rare, and concern for hypercapnia should never delay correction of hypoxemia.

Frequent high-dose delivery of an inhaled short-acting β_2-agonist is indicated and is usually well tolerated in the setting of severe airway obstruction. Some studies suggest that continuous therapy is more efficacious than intermittent administration of these agents, but there is no clear consensus as long as similar doses are administered. At least three MDI or nebulizer treatments should be given in the first hour of therapy. Thereafter, the frequency of administration varies according to the improvement in airflow and associated symptoms and the occurrence of side effects.

Systemic corticosteroids are administered as detailed above. Mucolytic agents (eg, acetylcysteine, potassium iodide) may worsen cough or airflow obstruction. Anxiolytic and hypnotic drugs are contraindicated in critically ill asthma patients because of their respiratory depressant effects.

Repeat assessment of patients with severe exacerbations should be made after the initial dose of inhaled bronchodilator and after three doses of inhaled bronchodilators (60–90 minutes after initiating treatment). The response to initial treatment is a better predictor of the need for hospitalization than is the severity of an exacerbation on presentation. The decision to hospitalize a patient should be based on the duration and severity of symptoms, severity of airflow obstruction, course and severity of prior exacerbations, medication use at the time of the exacerbation, access to medical care and medications, adequacy of social support and home conditions, and presence of psychiatric illness. In general, discharge to home is appropriate if the PEF or FEV_1 has returned to $\geq 70\%$ of predicted or personal best and symptoms are minimal or absent. Patients with a rapid response to treatment should be observed for 30 minutes after the most recent dose of bronchodilator to ensure stability of response before discharge to home.

A small minority of patients will not respond well to treatment and will show signs of impending respiratory failure due to a combination of worsening airflow obstruction and respiratory muscle fatigue (Table 9–3). Such patients can deteriorate rapidly and thus should be monitored in a critical care setting. Intubation of an acutely ill asthma patient is technically difficult and is best done semielectively, before the crisis of a respiratory arrest. At the time of intubation, close attention should be given to maintaining intravascular volume because hypotension commonly accompanies the administration of sedation and the initiation of positive-pressure ventilation in patients dehydrated due to poor recent oral intake and high insensible losses.

The main goals of mechanical ventilation are to ensure adequate oxygen and to avoid barotrauma. Controlled hypoventilation with permissive hypercapnia is often required to limit airway pressures. Frequent high-dose delivery of inhaled short-acting β_2-agonists should be continued along with anti-inflammatory agents as discussed above. Many questions remain regarding the optimal delivery of inhaled β_2-agonists to intubated, mechanically ventilated patients. Further studies are needed to determine the comparative efficacy of MDIs and nebulizers, optimal ventilator settings to use during drug delivery, ideal site along the ventilator circuit for introduction of the delivery system, and maximal acceptable drug doses. In acute severe asthma ($FEV_1 < 25\%$ of predicted), intravenous magnesium sulfate produces a detectable but clinically insignificant improvement in airflow. Unconventional therapies such as helium-oxygen mixtures and inhalational anesthetic agents are of unclear benefit but may be appropriate in selected patients.

Assessment, Monitoring, & Prevention

Periodic assessments and ongoing monitoring of asthma are essential to determine if the goals of therapy are being met. Clinical assessment and patient self-assessment are the primary methods for monitoring asthma. Patients should be given a written action plan based on signs and symptoms or expiratory flow rates. An action plan is especially important for patients with moderate to severe asthma or those with a history of severe exacerbations. Patients should be taught to recognize symptoms—especially patterns indicating inadequate asthma control or predicting the need for additional therapy. The written asthma action plan should direct the asthma patient to adjust medications in response to particular signs, symptoms, and peak flow measurements and should state when to seek medical help.

Spirometry is recommended at the time of initial assessment, once treatment is initiated and symptoms and peak flows have stabilized, and at least every 1–2 years thereafter. Regular follow-up visits (at least every 6 months, or more frequently based on patient status) are essential to help maintain asthma control and to reevaluate medication requirements. Patients with asthma should receive the pneumococcal vaccine (Pneumovax) and annual influenza vaccinations.

Barnes PJ et al: How do corticosteroids work in asthma? Ann Intern Med 2003;139:359. [PMID: 12965945]

Busse WW et al: Asthma. N Engl J Med 2001;344:350. [PMID: 11172168]

Kallstrom TJ: Evidence-based asthma management. Respir Care 2004;49:783. [PMID: 15222910]

National Asthma Education and Prevention Program: Expert Panel Report: Guidelines for the Diagnosis and Management of Asthma Update on Selected Topics—2002. J Allergy Clin Immunol 2002;110(5 Suppl):S141. [PMID: 12542074]

Sin DD et al: Pharmacological management to reduce exacerbations in adults with asthma: a systematic review and meta-analysis. JAMA 2004;292:367. [PMID: 15265853]

Walker S et al: Anti-IgE for chronic asthma in adults and children. Cochrane Database Syst Rev 2004;3:CD003559. [PMID: 15266491]

Wenzel S: Severe asthma in adults. Am J Respir Crit Care Med 2005;172:149. [PMID: 15849323]

CHRONIC OBSTRUCTIVE PULMONARY DISEASE

ESSENTIALS OF DIAGNOSIS

- *History of cigarette smoking.*
- *Chronic cough and sputum production (in chronic bronchitis) and dyspnea (in emphysema).*
- *Rhonchi, decreased intensity of breath sounds, and prolonged expiration on physical examination.*
- *Airflow limitation on pulmonary function testing that is not fully reversible and most often progressive.*

General Considerations

COPD is a disease state characterized by the presence of airflow obstruction due to chronic bronchitis or emphysema; the airflow obstruction is generally progressive, may be accompanied by airway hyperreactivity, and may be partially reversible (American Thoracic Society). The National Heart, Lung, and Blood Institute estimates that 14 million Americans have been diagnosed with COPD; an equal number are thought to be afflicted but remain undiagnosed. Grouped together, COPD and asthma now represent the fourth leading cause of death in the United States, with over 120,000 deaths reported annually. The death rate from COPD is increasing rapidly, especially among elderly men.

Most patients with COPD have features of both emphysema and chronic bronchitis. **Chronic bronchitis** is a clinical diagnosis defined by excessive secretion of bronchial mucus and is manifested by daily productive cough for 3 months or more in at least 2 consecutive years. **Emphysema** is a pathologic diagnosis that denotes abnormal permanent enlargement of air spaces distal to the terminal bronchiole, with destruction of their walls and without obvious fibrosis.

Cigarette smoking is clearly the most important cause of COPD. Nearly all smokers suffer an accelerated decline in lung function that is dose- and duration-dependent. Fifteen percent develop progressively disabling symptoms in their 40s and 50s. It is estimated that 80% of patients seen for COPD have significant exposure to tobacco smoke. The remaining 20% frequently have a combination of exposures to environmental tobacco smoke, occupational dusts and chemicals, and indoor air pollution from biomass fuel used for cooking and heating in poorly ventilated buildings. Outdoor air pollution, airway infection, familial factors, and allergy have also been implicated in chronic bronchitis, and hereditary factors (deficiency of α_1-antiprotease) have been implicated in COPD. The pathogenesis of emphysema may involve excessive lysis of elastin and other structural proteins in the lung matrix by elastase and other proteases derived from lung neutrophils, macrophages, and mononuclear cells. Atopy and the tendency for bronchoconstriction to develop in response to nonspecific airway stimuli may be important risks for COPD.

Clinical Findings

A. Symptoms and Signs

Patients with COPD characteristically present in the fifth or sixth decade of life complaining of excessive cough, sputum production, and shortness of breath. Symptoms have often been present for 10 years or more. Dyspnea is noted initially only on heavy exertion, but as the condition progresses it occurs with mild activity. In severe disease, dyspnea occurs at rest. A hallmark of COPD is frequent exacerbations of illness that result in absence from work and eventual disability. Pneumonia, pulmonary hypertension, cor pulmonale, and chronic respiratory failure characterize the late stage of COPD. Death usually occurs during an exacerbation of illness in association with acute respiratory failure.

Clinical findings may be completely absent early in the course of COPD. As the disease progresses, two symptom patterns tend to emerge, historically referred to as "pink puffers" and "blue bloaters" (Table 9–7). These patterns have been thought to represent pure forms of emphysema and bronchitis, respectively, but this is a simplification of the anatomy and pathophysiology. Most COPD patients have pathologic evidence of both disorders, and their clinical course may reflect other factors such as central control of ventilation and concomitant sleep-disordered breathing.

B. Laboratory Findings

Spirometry provides objective information about pulmonary function and assesses the results of therapy. Pulmonary function tests early in the course of COPD reveal only evidence of abnormal closing volume and reduced midexpiratory flow rate. Reductions in FEV_1 and in the ratio of forced expiratory volume to vital capacity ($FEV_1\%$ or FEV_1/FVC ratio) occur later. In severe disease, the FVC is markedly reduced. Lung volume measurements reveal a marked increase in residual volume (RV), an increase in total lung capacity (TLC), and an elevation of the RV/TLC ratio, indicative of air trapping, particularly in emphysema.

Arterial blood gas measurements characteristically show no abnormalities early in COPD other than an increased $A–a–DO_2$. Indeed, they are unnecessary unless (1) hypoxemia or hypercapnia is suspected, (2) the FEV_1 is < 40% of predicted, or (3) there are clinical signs of right heart failure. Hypoxemia occurs in advanced disease, particularly when chronic bronchitis predominates. Compensated respiratory acidosis occurs in patients with chronic respiratory failure, particularly in chronic bronchitis, with worsening of acidemia during acute exacerbations.

Table 9-7. Patterns of disease in advanced COPD.

	Type A: Pink Puffer (Emphysema Predominant)	Type B: Blue Bloater (Bronchitis Predominant)
History and physical examination	Major complaint is dyspnea, often severe, usually presenting after age 50. Cough is rare, with scant clear, mucoid sputum. Patients are thin, with recent weight loss common. They appear uncomfortable, with evident use of accessory muscles of respiration. Chest is very quiet without adventitious sounds. No peripheral edema.	Major complaint is chronic cough, productive of mucopurulent sputum, with frequent exacerbations due to chest infections. Often presents in late 30s and 40s. Dyspnea usually mild, though patients may note limitations to exercise. Patients frequently overweight and cyanotic but seem comfortable at rest. Peripheral edema is common. Chest is noisy, with rhonchi invariably present; wheezes are common.
Laboratory studies	Hemoglobin usually normal (12–15 g/dL). Pao_2 normal to slightly reduced (65–75 mm Hg) but Sao_2 normal at rest. $Paco_2$ normal to slightly reduced (35–40 mm Hg). Chest radiograph shows hyperinflation with flattened diaphragms. Vascular markings are diminished, particularly at the apices.	Hemoglobin usually elevated (15–18 g/dL). Pao_2 reduced (45–60 mm Hg) and $Paco_2$ slightly to markedly elevated (50–60 mm Hg). Chest radiograph shows increased interstitial markings ("dirty lungs"), especially at bases. Diaphragms are not flattened.
Pulmonary function tests	Airflow obstruction ubiquitous. Total lung capacity increased, sometimes markedly so. DL_{CO} reduced. Static lung compliance increased.	Airflow obstruction ubiquitous. Total lung capacity generally normal but may be slightly increased. DL_{CO} normal. Static lung compliance normal.
Special evaluations V/Q matching	Increased ventilation to high V/Q areas, ie, high dead space ventilation	Increased perfusion to low V/Q areas.
Hemodynamics	Cardiac output normal to slightly low. Pulmonary artery pressures mildly elevated and increase with exercise.	Cardiac output normal. Pulmonary artery pressures elevated, sometimes markedly so, and worsen with exercise.
Nocturnal ventilation	Mild to moderate degree of oxygen desaturation not usually associated with obstructive sleep apnea.	Severe oxygen desaturation, frequently associated with obstructive sleep apnea.
Exercise ventilation	Increased minute ventilation for level of oxygen consumption. Pao_2 tends to fall, $Paco_2$ rises slightly.	Decreased minute ventilation for level of oxygen consumption. Pao_2 may rise; $Paco_2$ may rise significantly.

DL_{CO} = single-breath diffusing capacity for carbon monoxide; V/Q = ventilation-perfusion.

Examination of the sputum may reveal *Streptococcus pneumoniae*, *H influenzae*, or *Moraxella catarrhalis*. Positive sputum cultures are poorly correlated with acute exacerbations, and research techniques demonstrate evidence of preceding viral infection in a majority of patients with exacerbations. The ECG may show sinus tachycardia, and in advanced disease, chronic pulmonary hypertension may produce electrocardiographic abnormalities typical of cor pulmonale. Supraventricular arrhythmias (multifocal atrial tachycardia, atrial flutter, and atrial fibrillation) and ventricular irritability also occur.

C. IMAGING

Radiographs of patients with chronic bronchitis typically show only nonspecific peribronchial and perivascular markings. Plain radiographs are insensitive for the diagnosis of emphysema; they show hyperinflation with flattening of the diaphragm or peripheral arterial deficiency in about half of cases. Parenchymal bullae in the setting of either of these findings are diagnostic of emphysema. Pulmonary hypertension becomes evident as enlargement of central pulmonary arteries in advanced disease. Doppler echocardiography is an effective way to estimate pulmonary artery pressure if pulmonary hypertension is suspected.

Differential Diagnosis

Clinical, roentgenographic, and laboratory findings should enable the clinician to distinguish COPD from other obstructive pulmonary disorders such as bronchial asthma, bronchiectasis, cystic fibrosis, bronchopulmonary mycosis, and central airflow obstruction. Simple asthma is characterized by complete or near-complete reversibility of airflow obstruction. Bronchiectasis is distinguished from COPD by features such as recurrent pneumonia and hemoptysis, digital clubbing, and radiographic abnormalities. Patients with severe α_1-antiprotease deficiency are recognized by the appearance of panacinar, bibasilar emphysema early in life, usually in the third or fourth decade, and hepatic cirrhosis and hepatocellular carcinoma may occur. Cystic fibrosis occurs in children and younger adults. Rarely, mechanical obstruction of the central airways simulates COPD. Flow-volume loops may help separate patients with central airway obstruction from those with diffuse intrathoracic airway obstruction characteristic of COPD.

Complications

Acute bronchitis, pneumonia, pulmonary thromboembolism, and concomitant left ventricular failure may worsen otherwise stable COPD. Pulmonary hypertension, cor pulmonale, and chronic respiratory failure are common in advanced COPD. Spontaneous pneumothorax occurs in a small fraction of patients with emphysema. Hemoptysis may result from chronic bronchitis or may signal bronchogenic carcinoma.

Prevention

COPD is largely preventable through elimination of long-term exposure to tobacco smoke. Smokers with early evidence of airflow limitation can alter their disease by smoking cessation. Smoking cessation slows the decline in FEV_1 in middle-aged smokers with mild airways obstruction. Vaccination against influenza and pneumococcal infection may also be of benefit.

Treatment

Standards for the management of patients with COPD have been published by the American Thoracic Society and the Global Initiative for Obstructive Lung Disease (GOLD), a joint expert committee of the National Heart, Lung, and Blood Institute and the World Health Organization. See Chapter 38 for a discussion of air travel in patients with lung disease.

A. AMBULATORY PATIENTS

1. Smoking cessation—The single most important intervention in smokers with COPD is to encourage smoking cessation. Simply telling a patient to quit succeeds 5% of the time. The Lung Health Study reported 22% sustained abstinence at 5 years in their intervention group (behavior modification plus nicotine gum). Nicotine transdermal patch, nicotine gum, and bupropion increase cessation rates in motivated smokers (see Chapter 1).

2. Oxygen therapy—The only drug therapy that is documented to improve the natural history of COPD is supplemental oxygen in those patients with resting hypoxemia. Proved benefits of home oxygen therapy in advanced COPD include longer survival, reduced hospitalization needs, and better quality of life. Survival in hypoxemic patients with COPD treated with supplemental oxygen therapy is directly proportionate to the number of hours per day oxygen is administered: in patients treated with continuous oxygen, the survival after 36 months is about 65%—significantly better than the survival rate of about 45% in those who are treated with only nocturnal oxygen. Oxygen by nasal prongs must be given at least 15 hours a day unless therapy is intended only for exercise or sleep.

Requirements for Medicare coverage for a patient's home use of oxygen and oxygen equipment are listed in Table 9–8. Arterial blood gas analysis is preferred over oximetry to guide initial oxygen therapy. Hypoxemic patients with pulmonary hypertension, chronic cor pulmonale, erythrocytosis, impaired cognitive function, exercise intolerance, nocturnal restlessness, or morning headache are particularly likely to benefit from home oxygen therapy.

Home oxygen may be supplied by liquid oxygen systems (LOX), compressed gas cylinders, or oxygen concentrators. Most patients benefit from having both stationary and portable systems. For most patients, a flow rate of 1–3 L/min achieves a PaO_2 greater than 55 mm Hg. The monthly cost of home oxygen therapy ranges from $300.00 to $500.00 or more, being higher for liquid oxygen systems. Medicare covers approximately 80% of home oxygen expenses. **Transtracheal oxygen** is an alternative method of delivery and may be useful for patients who require higher flows of oxygen than can be delivered via the nose or who are experiencing troublesome side effects from nasal delivery such as nasal drying or epistaxis. Reservoir nasal cannulas or "pendants" and demand (pulse) oxygen delivery systems are also available to conserve oxygen.

3. Bronchodilators—Bronchodilators are the most important agents in the pharmacologic management of patients with COPD. Bronchodilators do not alter the inexorable decline in lung function that is a hallmark of the disease, but they offer some patients improvement in symptoms, exercise tolerance, and overall health status. Aggressiveness of bronchodilator therapy should be matched to the severity of the patient's disease. In patients who experience no symptomatic improvement, bronchodilators should be discontinued.

The two most commonly prescribed bronchodilators are the anticholinergic ipratropium bromide and short-acting β_2-agonists (eg, albuterol, metaproterenol), delivered by MDI or as an inhalation solution by nebulizer. Ipratropium bromide is generally preferred to the short-acting β_2-agonists as a first-line agent because of its longer duration of action and absence of sympathomimetic side effects. Some studies have suggested that ipratropium achieves superior bronchodilation in COPD patients. Typical doses are two to four puffs (36–72 mcg) every 6 hours. There is a dose response above this level without additional side effects. Short-acting β_2-agonists are less expensive and have a more rapid onset of action, commonly leading to

Table 9–8. Home oxygen therapy: requirements for Medicare coverage.[1]

Group I (any of the following):

1. $PaO_2 \leq 55$ mm Hg or $SaO_2 \leq 88\%$ taken at rest breathing room air, while awake.

2. During sleep (prescription for nocturnal oxygen use only):
   a. $PaO_2 \leq 55$ mm Hg or $SaO_2 \leq 88\%$ for a patient whose awake, resting, room air PaO_2 is ≥ 56 mm Hg or $SaO_2 \geq 89\%$,

      or

   b. Decrease in $PaO_2 > 10$ mm Hg or decrease in $SaO_2 > 5\%$ associated with symptoms or signs reasonably attributed to hypoxemia (eg, impaired cognitive processes, nocturnal restlessness, insomnia).

3. During exercise (prescription for oxygen use only during exercise):
   a. $PaO_2 \leq 55$ mg Hg or $SaO_2 \leq 88\%$ taken during exercise for a patient whose awake, resting, room air PaO_2 is ≥ 56 mm Hg or $SaO_2 \geq 89\%$,

      and

   b. There is evidence that the use of supplemental oxygen during exercise improves the hypoxemia that was demonstrated during exercise while breathing room air.

Group II[2]:

$PaO_2 = 56$–59 mm Hg or $SaO_2 = 89\%$ if there is evidence of any of the following:

1. Dependent edema suggesting congestive heart failure.
2. P pulmonale on ECG (P wave > 3 mm in standard leads II, III, or aVF).
3. Hematocrit > 56%.

---

[1]Health Care Financing Administration, 1989.
[2]Patients in this group must have a second oxygen test 3 months after the initial oxygen set-up.

---

greater patient satisfaction. At maximal doses, β_2-agonists have bronchodilator action equivalent to that of ipratropium but may cause tachycardia, tremor, or hypokalemia. There does not appear to be any advantage of scheduled use of short-acting β_2-agonists compared with as-needed administration. Use of both short-acting β_2-agonists and anticholinergics at submaximal doses leads to improved bronchodilation compared with either agent alone but does not improve dyspnea.

Long-acting β_2-agonists (eg, formoterol, salmeterol) and anticholinergics (tiotropium) appear to achieve bronchodilation that is equivalent or superior to what is experienced with ipratropium in addition to similar improvements on health status. They are currently more expensive than short-acting agents. Their role in management of stable COPD is an area of active research.

Oral **theophylline** is a third-line agent in COPD patients who fail to achieve adequate symptom control with anticholinergics and β_2-agonists. Sustained-release theophylline improves arterial oxygen hemoglobin satu-ration during sleep in COPD patients and is a first-line agent for those with sleep-related breathing disorders. Theophylline has fallen out of favor because of its narrow toxic therapeutic window and the availability of potent inhaled bronchodilators. Nonetheless, theophylline does improve dyspnea, exercise performance, and pulmonary function in many stable COPD patients. Its benefits may result from anti-inflammatory properties and extrapulmonary effects on diaphragm strength, myocardial contractility, and renal function.

4. Corticosteroids—Apart from acute exacerbations, COPD is not generally a corticosteroid-responsive disease. Only 10% of stable outpatients with COPD given oral corticosteroids will have a greater than 20% increase in FEV_1 compared with patients receiving placebo. Since there are no clear predictors of which patients will respond, empiric trials of oral (equivalent to 0.5 mg/kg/d of prednisone for 14–21 days) and inhaled (6–12 weeks of therapy) corticosteroids are common. Such trials should be guided by the following principles: The baseline FEV_1 should be stable, ie, not measured during an exacerbation, and documented on maximal bronchodilator therapy. The postbronchodilator FEV_1 value is considered the appropriate baseline. The drug should be discontinued unless there is a 20% or greater increase in FEV_1 after the trial of therapy. Patients who feel better without spirometric evidence of improvement are nonresponders. Responders to oral agents are usually switched to inhaled corticosteroids, but there are few data to guide this practice.

Several large clinical trials have reported no effect of inhaled corticosteroids on the characteristic decline in lung function experienced by COPD patients. Some clinical trials have reported a small reduction in the frequency of COPD exacerbations and an increase in self-reported functional status in patients treated with inhaled agents. Typically, these effects are small and occur with long-term, high-dose inhaled therapy.

5. Antibiotics—Antibiotics are commonly prescribed to outpatients with COPD for the following indications: (1) to treat an acute exacerbation, (2) to treat acute bronchitis, and (3) to prevent acute exacerbations of chronic bronchitis (prophylactic antibiotics). There is evidence from clinical studies that antibiotics improve outcomes slightly in the first two situations. There is no convincing evidence to support the use of prophylactic antibiotics in patients with COPD. Patients with a flare of COPD associated with dyspnea and a change in the quantity or character of sputum benefit the most from antibiotic therapy. Common agents include trimethoprim-sulfamethoxazole (160/800 mg every 12 hours), amoxicillin or amoxicillin-clavulanate (500 mg every 8 hours), or doxycycline (100 mg every 12 hours) given for 7–10 days. Broader-spectrum therapy may be indicated in patients with more severe baseline airflow obstruction. There are few controlled trials of antibiotics in severe COPD exacerbations; prompt administration of parenteral antibiotics seems reasonable as long as the decision is reevaluated frequently.

6. Other measures—In patients with chronic bronchitis, increased mobilization of secretions may be accomplished through the use of adequate systemic hydration, effective cough training methods, or use of a hand-held flutter device and postural drainage, sometimes with chest percussion or vibration. Postural drainage and chest percussion should be used only in selected patients with excessive amounts of retained secretions that cannot be cleared by coughing and other methods; these measures are of no benefit in pure emphysema. Expectorant-mucolytic therapy has generally been regarded as unhelpful in patients with chronic bronchitis. Cough suppressants and sedatives should be avoided as routine measures.

Human α_1-antitrypsin is available for replacement therapy in emphysema due to congenital deficiency of α_1-antitrypsin. Patients over 18 years of age with airflow obstruction by spirometry and levels less than 11 mcmol/L are potential candidates for replacement therapy. α_1-Antitrypsin is administered intravenously in a dose of 60 mg/kg body weight once weekly.

Graded aerobic physical exercise programs (eg, walking 20 minutes three times weekly, or bicycling) are helpful to prevent deterioration of physical condition and to improve the patient's ability to carry out daily activities. Training of inspiratory muscles by inspiring against progressively larger resistive loads improves exercise tolerance in some but not all patients. Pursed-lip breathing to slow the rate of breathing and abdominal breathing exercises to relieve fatigue of accessory muscles of respiration may reduce dyspnea in some patients.

Severe dyspnea in spite of optimal medical management may warrant a clinical trial of an opioid. Sedative-hypnotic drugs (eg, diazepam, 5 mg three times daily) are controversial in intractable dyspnea but may benefit very anxious patients. Intermittent negative-pressure (cuirass) ventilation and transnasal positive-pressure ventilation at home to rest the respiratory muscles are promising approaches to improve respiratory muscle function and reduce dyspnea in patients with severe COPD. A bilevel transnasal ventilation system has been reported to reduce dyspnea in ambulatory patients with severe COPD, but the long-term benefits of this approach and compliance with it have not been defined.

B. HOSPITALIZED PATIENTS

Hospitalization is indicated for acute worsening of COPD that fails to respond to measures for ambulatory patients. Patients with acute respiratory failure or complications such as cor pulmonale and pneumothorax should also be hospitalized.

Management of the hospitalized patient with an acute exacerbation of COPD includes supplemental oxygen, inhaled ipratropium bromide and inhaled β_2-agonists, and broad-spectrum antibiotics, corticosteroids and, in selected cases, chest physiotherapy. Theophylline should not be initiated in the acute setting, but patients taking theophylline prior to acute hospitalization should have their theophylline serum levels measured and maintained in the therapeutic range. Oxygen therapy should not be withheld for fear of worsening respiratory acidemia; hypoxemia is more detrimental than hypercapnia. Cor pulmonale usually responds to measures that reduce pulmonary artery pressure, such as supplemental oxygen and correction of acidemia; bed rest, salt restriction, and diuretics may add some benefit. Cardiac arrhythmias, particularly multifocal atrial tachycardia, usually respond to aggressive treatment of COPD itself. Atrial flutter may require DC cardioversion after initiation of the above therapy. If progressive respiratory failure ensues, tracheal intubation and mechanical ventilation are necessary. In clinical trials of COPD patients with hypercapnic acute respiratory failure, noninvasive positive- pressure ventilation (NPPV) delivered via face mask reduced the need for intubation and shortened lengths of stay in the intensive care unit (ICU). Other studies have suggested a lower risk of nosocomial infections and less use of antibiotics in COPD patients treated with NPPV. These benefits do not appear to extend to hypoxemic respiratory failure or to patients with acute lung injury or ARDS.

C. SURGERY FOR COPD

1. Lung transplantation—Experience with both single and bilateral sequential lung transplantation for severe COPD is extensive. Requirements for lung transplantation are severe lung disease, limited activities of daily living, exhaustion of medical therapy, ambulatory status, potential for pulmonary rehabilitation, limited life expectancy without transplantation, adequate function of other organ systems, and a good social support system. Average total charges for lung transplantation through the end of the first postoperative year exceed $250,000. The two-year survival rate after lung transplantation for COPD is 75%. Complications include acute rejection, opportunistic infection, and obliterative bronchiolitis. Substantial improvements in pulmonary function and exercise performance have been noted after transplantation.

2. Lung volume reduction surgery—Lung volume reduction surgery (LVRS), or reduction pneumoplasty, is a surgical approach to relieve dyspnea and improve exercise tolerance in patients with advanced diffuse emphysema and lung hyperinflation. Bilateral resection of 20–30% of lung volume in selected patients results in modest improvements in pulmonary function, exercise performance, and dyspnea. The duration of any improvement as well as any mortality benefit remains uncertain. Prolonged air leaks occur in up to 50% of patients postoperatively. Mortality rates in centers with the largest experience with LVRS range from 4% to 10%.

The National Emphysema Treatment Trial compared LVRS with medical treatment in a randomized, multicenter clinical trial of 1218 patients with severe emphysema. Overall, surgery improved exercise capacity but not mortality when compared with medical therapy. The persistence of this benefit remains to be defined. Subgroup analysis suggested that certain patient groups might have improved survival while other groups suffered excess mortality when randomized to surgery.

3. Bullectomy—Bullectomy is an older surgical procedure for palliation of severe dyspnea in patients with severe bullous emphysema. In this procedure, the surgeon removes a very large emphysematous bulla that demonstrates no ventilation or perfusion on lung scanning and compresses adjacent lung that has preserved function. Bullectomy can now be performed with a CO_2 laser via thoracoscopy.

Prognosis

The outlook for patients with clinically significant COPD is poor. The median survival of patients with severe COPD ($FEV_1 \leq 1$ L) is about 4 years. The degree of pulmonary dysfunction (as measured by FEV_1) at the time the patient is first seen is probably the most important predictor of survival. Comprehensive care programs, cessation of smoking, and supplemental oxygen may reduce the rate of decline of pulmonary function, but therapy with bronchodilators and other approaches probably has little, if any, impact on the natural course of COPD.

Dyspnea at the end of life can be extremely uncomfortable and distressing to the patient and family. Dyspnea can be effectively managed with a combination of medications and mechanical interventions (see Dyspnea, Treatment, above). As patients near the end of life, meticulous attention to palliative care is essential. (See Chapter 5.)

Bach PB et al: Management of acute exacerbations of chronic obstructive pulmonary disease: a summary and appraisal of published evidence. Ann Intern Med 2001;134:600. [PMID: 11296189]

Cote CG et al: New treatment strategies for COPD. Pairing the new with the tried and true. Postgrad Med 2005;117:27. [PMID: 15782671]

Gluck O et al: Recognizing and treating glucocorticoid-induced osteoporosis in patients with pulmonary diseases. Chest 2004; 125:1859. [PMID: 15136401]

Hersh CP et al: Predictors of survival in severe, early onset COPD. Chest 2004;126:1443. [PMID: 15539711]

Hogg JC et al: The nature of small-airway obstruction in chronic obstructive pulmonary disease. N Engl J Med 2004;350:2645. [PMID: 15215480]

Pauwels RA et al: Global strategy for the diagnosis, management, and prevention of chronic obstructive pulmonary disease. NHLBI/WHO Global Initiative for Chronic Obstructive Lung Disease (GOLD) Workshop summary. Am J Respir Crit Care Med 2001;163:1256. [PMID: 11316667]

Shapiro SD: COPD unwound. N Engl J Med 2005;352:2016. [PMID: 15888704]

Sin DD et al: Contemporary management of chronic obstructive pulmonary disease: scientific review. JAMA 2003;290:2301. [PMID: 14600189]

Wouters EF: Management of severe COPD. Lancet 2004;364:883. [PMID: 15351196]

BRONCHIECTASIS

 ESSENTIALS OF DIAGNOSIS

- Chronic productive cough with dyspnea and wheezing.
- Recurrent pulmonary infections requiring antibiotics.
- A preceding history of recurrent pulmonary infections or inflammation, or a predisposing condition.
- Radiographic findings of dilated, thickened airways and scattered, irregular opacities.

General Considerations

Bronchiectasis is a congenital or acquired disorder of the large bronchi characterized by permanent, abnormal dilation and destruction of bronchial walls. It may be caused by recurrent inflammation or infection of the airways and may be localized or diffuse. Cystic fibrosis causes about half of all cases of bronchiectasis. Other causes include lung infection (tuberculosis, fungal infections, lung abscess, pneumonia), abnormal lung defense mechanisms (humoral immunodeficiency, α_1-antiprotease deficiency with cigarette smoking, mucociliary clearance disorders, rheumatic diseases), and localized airway obstruction (foreign body, tumor, mucoid impaction). Immunodeficiency states that may lead to bronchiectasis include congenital or acquired panhypogammaglobulinemia; common variable immunodeficiency; selective IgA, IgM, and IgG subclass deficiencies; and acquired immunodeficiency from cytotoxic therapy, AIDS, lymphoma, multiple myeloma, leukemia, and chronic renal and hepatic diseases. However, most patients with bronchiectasis have panhypergammaglobulinemia, presumably reflecting an immune system response to chronic airway infection. Acquired primary bronchiectasis is now uncommon in the United States because of improved control of bronchopulmonary infections.

Clinical Findings

A. SYMPTOMS AND SIGNS

Symptoms of bronchiectasis include chronic cough with production of copious amounts of purulent sputum, hemoptysis, and pleuritic chest pain. Dyspnea and wheezing occur in 75% of patients. Weight loss, anemia, and other systemic manifestations are common. Physical findings are nonspecific, but persistent crackles at the lung bases are common. Clubbing is infrequent in mild cases but is common in severe disease. Copious, foul-smelling, purulent sputum is characteristic. Obstructive pulmonary dysfunction with hypoxemia is seen in moderate or severe disease.

B. Imaging

Radiographic abnormalities include dilated and thickened bronchi that may appear as "tram-tracks" or as ring-like markings. Scattered irregular opacities, atelectasis, and focal consolidation may be present. High-resolution CT is the diagnostic study of choice.

Treatment

Treatment of acute exacerbations consists of antibiotics (selected on the basis of sputum smears and cultures), daily chest physiotherapy with postural drainage and chest percussion, and inhaled bronchodilators. Hand-held flutter valve devices may be as effective as chest physiotherapy in clearing secretions. Empiric oral antibiotic therapy for 10–14 days with amoxicillin or amoxicillin-clavulanate (500 mg every 8 hours), ampicillin or tetracycline (250–500 mg four times daily), or trimethoprim-sulfamethoxazole (160/800 mg every 12 hours) is reasonable therapy in an acute exacerbation if a specific bacterial pathogen cannot be isolated. Preventive or suppressive treatment is sometimes given to stable outpatients with bronchiectasis who have copious purulent sputum. Clinical trial data to guide this practice are scant. Common regimens include macrolides (azithromycin, 500 mg three times a week; erythromycin, 500 mg twice daily), high-dose (3 g/d) amoxicillin or alternating cycles of the antibiotics listed above given orally for 2–4 weeks. Inhaled aerosolized aminoglycosides reduce colonization by *Pseudomonas* species. In patients with underlying cystic fibrosis, inhaled antibiotics improve FEV$_1$ and reduce hospitalizations, but these benefits are not consistently seen in the non–cystic fibrosis population. Complications of bronchiectasis include hemoptysis, cor pulmonale, amyloidosis, and secondary visceral abscesses at distant sites (eg, brain). Bronchoscopy is sometimes necessary to evaluate hemoptysis, remove retained secretions, and rule out obstructing airway lesions. Massive hemoptysis may require embolization of bronchial arteries or surgical resection. Surgical resection is otherwise reserved for the few patients with localized bronchiectasis and adequate pulmonary function in whom conservative management fails.

Barker AF: Bronchiectasis. N Engl J Med 2002;346:1383. [PMID: 11986413]

Evans DJ et al: Prolonged antibiotics for purulent bronchiectasis. Cochrane Database Syst Rev 2003;(4):CD001392. [PMID: 14583934]

Noone PG et al: Primary ciliary dyskinesia: diagnostic and phenotypic features. Am J Respir Crit Care Med 2004;169: 459. [PMID: 14656747]

ALLERGIC BRONCHOPULMONARY MYCOSIS

Allergic bronchopulmonary mycosis is a pulmonary hypersensitivity disorder caused by allergy to fungal antigens that colonize the tracheobronchial tree. It usually occurs in atopic asthmatic individuals who are 20–40 years of age, in response to antigens of *Aspergillus* species. For this reason, the disorder is commonly referred to as allergic bronchopulmonary aspergillosis (ABPA). Primary criteria for the diagnosis of ABPA include (1) a clinical history of asthma, (2) peripheral eosinophilia, (3) immediate skin reactivity to *Aspergillus* antigen, (4) precipitating antibodies to *Aspergillus* antigen, (5) elevated serum IgE levels, (6) pulmonary infiltrates (transient or fixed), and (7) central bronchiectasis. If the first six of these seven primary criteria are present, the diagnosis is almost certain. Secondary diagnostic criteria include identification of *Aspergillus* in sputum, a history of brown-flecked sputum, and late skin reactivity to *Aspergillus* antigen. High-dose prednisone (0.5–1 mg/kg orally per day) for at least 2 months is the treatment of choice, and the response in early disease is usually excellent. Depending on the overall clinical situation, prednisone can then be cautiously tapered. Relapses are frequent, and protracted or repeated treatment with corticosteroids is not uncommon. Patients with corticosteroid-dependent disease may benefit from itraconazole (200 mg orally once or twice daily) without added toxicity. Bronchodilators (Table 9–6) are also helpful. Complications include hemoptysis, severe bronchiectasis, and pulmonary fibrosis.

Greenberger PA: Allergic bronchopulmonary aspergillosis. J Allergy Clin Immunol 2002;110:685. [PMID: 12417875]

Wark P: Pathogenesis of allergic bronchopulmonary aspergillosis and an evidence-based review of azoles in treatment. Respir Med 2004;98:915. [PMID: 15481266]

CYSTIC FIBROSIS

 ESSENTIALS OF DIAGNOSIS

- Chronic or recurrent cough, sputum production, dyspnea, and wheezing.
- Recurrent infections or chronic colonization of the airways with nontypeable H influenzae, mucoid and nonmucoid Pseudomonas aeruginosa, Staphylococcus aureus, or Burkholderia cepacia.
- Pancreatic insufficiency, recurrent pancreatitis, distal intestinal obstruction syndrome, chronic hepatic disease, nutritional deficiencies, or male urogenital abnormalities.
- Bronchiectasis and scarring on chest radiographs.
- Airflow obstruction on spirometry.
- Sweat chloride concentration above 60 mEq/L on two occasions or gene mutation known to cause cystic fibrosis.

General Considerations

Cystic fibrosis is the most common cause of severe chronic lung disease in young adults and the most common fatal hereditary disorder of whites in the United States. It is an autosomal recessive disorder affecting about 1 in 3200 whites; 1 in 25 is a carrier. Cystic fibrosis is caused by abnormalities in a membrane chloride channel (the cystic fibrosis transmembrane conductance regulator [CFTR] protein) that results in altered chloride transport and water flux across the apical surface of epithelial cells. Almost all exocrine glands produce an abnormal mucus that obstructs glands and ducts. Obstruction results in glandular dilation and damage to tissue. In the respiratory tract, inadequate hydration of the tracheobronchial epithelium impairs mucociliary function. High concentration of DNA in airway secretions (due to chronic airway inflammation and autolysis of neutrophils) increases sputum viscosity. Over 1000 mutations in the gene that encodes CFTR have been described, and at least 230 mutations are known to be associated with clinical abnormalities. The mutation referred to as ΔF508 accounts for about 60% of cases of cystic fibrosis.

Over one-third of the nearly 30,000 cystic fibrosis patients in the United States are adults. Because of the wide range of alterations seen in the CFTR protein structure and function, cystic fibrosis in adults may present with a variety of pulmonary and nonpulmonary manifestations. Pulmonary manifestations in adults include acute and chronic bronchitis, bronchiectasis, pneumonia, atelectasis, and peribronchial and parenchymal scarring. Pneumothorax and hemoptysis are common. Hypoxemia, hypercapnia, and cor pulmonale occur in advanced cases. Biliary cirrhosis and gallstones may occur. Nearly all men with cystic fibrosis have congenital bilateral absence of the vas deferens with azoospermia. Patients with cystic fibrosis have an increased risk of malignancies of the gastrointestinal tract, osteopenia, and arthropathies.

Clinical Findings

A. SYMPTOMS AND SIGNS

Cystic fibrosis should be suspected in a young adult with a history of chronic lung disease (especially bronchiectasis), pancreatitis, or infertility. Cough, sputum production, decreased exercise tolerance, and recurrent hemoptysis are typical complaints. Patients also often complain of facial (sinus) pain or pressure and purulent nasal discharge. Steatorrhea, diarrhea, and abdominal pain are also common. Digital clubbing, increased anteroposterior chest diameter, hyperresonance to percussion, and apical crackles are noted on physical examination. Sinus tenderness, purulent nasal secretions, and nasal polyps may also be seen.

B. LABORATORY FINDINGS

Arterial blood gas studies often reveal hypoxemia and, in advanced disease, a chronic, compensated respiratory acidosis. Pulmonary function studies show a mixed obstructive and restrictive pattern. There is a reduction in FVC, airflow rates, and TLC. Air trapping (high ratio of RV to TLC) and reduction in pulmonary diffusing capacity are common.

C. IMAGING

Hyperinflation is seen early in the disease process. Peribronchial cuffing, mucus plugging, bronchiectasis (ring shadows and cysts), increased interstitial markings, small rounded peripheral opacities, and focal atelectasis may be seen separately or in various combinations. Pneumothorax can also be seen. Thin-section CT scanning may confirm the presence of bronchiectasis.

D. DIAGNOSIS

The quantitative pilocarpine iontophoresis sweat test reveals elevated sodium and chloride levels (> 60 mEq/L) in the sweat of patients with cystic fibrosis. Two tests on different days are required for accurate diagnosis. Facilities must perform enough tests to maintain laboratory proficiency and quality. A normal sweat chloride test does not exclude the diagnosis. Genotyping or other alternative diagnostic studies (such as measurement of nasal membrane potential difference, semen analysis, or assessment of pancreatic function) should be pursued if the test is repeatedly negative but there is a high clinical suspicion of cystic fibrosis. Standard genotyping is a limited diagnostic tool because it screens for only a fraction of the known cystic fibrosis mutations.

Treatment

Early recognition and comprehensive multidisciplinary therapy improve symptom control and the chances of survival. Referral to a regional cystic fibrosis center is strongly recommended. Conventional treatment programs focus on the following areas: clearance and reduction of lower airway secretions, reversal of bronchoconstriction, treatment of respiratory tract infections and airway bacterial burden, pancreatic enzyme replacement, and nutritional and psychosocial support (including genetic and occupational counseling).

Clearance of lower airway secretions can be promoted by postural drainage, chest percussion or vibration techniques, positive expiratory pressure (PEP) or flutter valve breathing devices, directed cough, and other breathing techniques; these approaches require detailed patient instruction by experienced personnel. Sputum viscosity in cystic fibrosis is increased by the large quantities of extracellular DNA that result from chronic airway inflammation and autolysis of neutrophils. Inhaled recombinant human deoxyribonuclease (rhDNase) cleaves extracellular DNA in sputum; when administered long-term at a daily nebulized dose of 2.5 mg, this therapy leads to improved FEV_1 and reduces the risk of cystic fibrosis–related respiratory exacerbations and the need for intravenous antibiotics. Pharyngitis, laryngitis, and voice alterations are common adverse effects. Antibiotics are used to treat active airway infections based on results of culture and susceptibility testing of sputum. S aureus (including methicillin-resistant strains) and a mucoid variant of *Pseudomonas aeruginosa* are commonly present. *H influenzae, Stenotrophomonas maltophilia,* and *B cepacia* (which is a highly drug-resistant organism) are occasionally isolated. Azithromycin (500 mg orally three times a week) may slow progression of disease in patients with *P aeruginosa.* The use of aerosolized antibiotics (inhalation tobramycin solution and others) for prophylaxis or treatment of lower respiratory tract infections is sometimes helpful. Although some studies of inhaled antibiotics demonstrate reduced exacerbations and increased FEV_1 in patients chronically infected with *P aeruginosa,* there is concern about the emergence of drug-resistant organisms, equipment contamination with *B cepacia,* and side effects such as bronchospasm.

Inhaled bronchodilators (eg, albuterol, two puffs every 4 hours as needed) should be considered in patients who demonstrate an increase of at least 12% in FEV_1 after an inhaled bronchodilator. Vaccination against pneumococcal infection and annual influenza vaccination are advised. Screening of family members and genetic counseling are suggested.

Lung transplantation is currently the only definitive treatment for advanced cystic fibrosis. Double-lung or heart-lung transplantation is required. A few transplant centers offer living lobar lung transplantation to selected patients. The 3-year survival rate following transplantation for cystic fibrosis is about 55%.

Investigational therapies for cystic fibrosis include anti-inflammatory agents (eg, ibuprofen, pentoxifylline, antiproteases), protein modification agents (eg, milrinone, phenylbutyrate), ion transport agents (eg, amiloride), and gene therapy.

Prognosis

The longevity of patients with cystic fibrosis is increasing, and the median survival age is over 30 years. Death occurs from pulmonary complications (eg, pneumonia, pneumothorax, or hemoptysis) or as a result of terminal chronic respiratory failure and cor pulmonale.

Elkins MR et al; National Hypertonic Saline in Cystic Fibrosis (NHSCF) Study Group: A controlled trial of long-term inhaled hypertonic saline in patients with cystic fibrosis. N Engl J Med 2006;354:229. [PMID: 16421364]

Ellaffi M et al: One-year outcome after severe pulmonary exacerbation in adults with cystic fibrosis. Am J Respir Crit Care Med 2005;171:158. [PMID: 15502116]

Gibson RL et al: Pathophysiology and management of pulmonary infections in cystic fibrosis. Am J Respir Crit Care Med 2003;168:918. [PMID: 14555458]

Rowe SM et al: Cystic fibrosis. N Engl J Med 2005;352:1992. [PMID: 15888700]

Yankaskas JR et al: Cystic fibrosis adult care: consensus conference report. Chest 2004;125(1 Suppl):1S. [PMID: 14734689]

BRONCHIOLITIS

Bronchiolitis is nonspecific inflammation of terminal and respiratory bronchioles. In infants and children, bronchiolitis is a common and often severe acute respiratory illness, usually caused by respiratory syncytial virus or adenovirus. Acute infectious bronchiolitis is rare in adults. In adults, bronchiolitis is a chronic, frequently progressive nonspecific response of the distal small airways to injury.

Bronchiolitis has two pathologic variants, either of which may be associated with obliteration of bronchioles. **Constrictive bronchiolitis** (formerly referred to as bronchiolitis obliterans) is characterized by chronic inflammation, concentric scarring, and smooth muscle hypertrophy causing luminal obstruction. These patients have airflow obstruction on spirometry, minimal radiographic abnormalities, and a progressive clinical course unresponsive to corticosteroids. **Proliferative bronchiolitis** occurs when intraluminal polyps consisting of fibroblasts, foamy macrophages, and lymphocytes partially or completely obstruct the bronchioles. When this exudate extends to the alveolar space, the pattern is referred to as bronchiolitis obliterans with organizing pneumonia (see below). The most common clinical patterns are described below.

Toxic fume bronchiolitis obliterans follows 1–3 weeks after exposure to oxides of nitrogen, phosgene, and other noxious gases. The chest radiograph shows diffuse nonspecific alveolar or "ground-glass" densities.

Postinfectious bronchiolitis obliterans is a late response to mycoplasmal or viral lung infection in adults and has a highly variable radiographic appearance.

Constrictive bronchiolitis may occur in association with rheumatoid arthritis, polymyositis, and dermatomyositis. Penicillamine therapy has been implicated as a possible cause in patients with rheumatoid arthritis. Constrictive bronchiolitis also occurs in up to 70% of patients following lung transplantation and 10% of patients undergoing allogeneic bone marrow transplantation, the latter occurring in the setting of chronic graft-versus-host disease.

Bronchiolitis obliterans with organizing pneumonia (BOOP), now more commonly referred to as **cryptogenic organizing pneumonitis (COP),** affects men and women equally. Most patients are between the ages of 50 and 70. Dry cough, dyspnea, and a flu-like illness, ranging in duration from a few days to several months, are typical. Fever and weight loss are common. Physical examination demonstrates crackles in most patients, and wheezing is present in about a third. Clubbing is uncommon. Pulmonary function studies demonstrate restrictive dysfunction and hypoxemia. The chest radiograph typically shows patchy, bilateral, ground glass or alveolar infiltrates. Solitary pneumonia-like infiltrates and a diffuse interstitial pattern have also been described (see Table 9–19).

COP is usually a difficult diagnosis to make on clinical grounds alone. The presence of fever and weight loss, abrupt onset of symptoms (often following an upper respiratory tract infection), a relatively short duration of symptoms, the absence of clubbing, and the presence of alveolar infiltrates help the clinician distinguish this entity from idiopathic interstitial pneumonia. Surgical lung biopsy may be necessary.

Buds of loose connective tissue and inflammatory cells fill alveoli and distal bronchioles. Corticosteroid therapy is effective in two-thirds of cases, often abruptly. Relapses are common if corticosteroids are stopped prematurely, and most patients require at least 6 months of therapy. Prednisone is usually given initially in doses of 1 mg/kg/d for 2–3 months. The dose is then tapered slowly to 20–40 mg/d, depending on response, and eventually to an alternate-day regimen.

Two other well-described disorders are not usually associated with obliteration of bronchioles. **Respiratory bronchiolitis** is a disorder of small airways in cigarette smokers. Clinically and radiographically, this disorder resembles desquamative interstitial pneumonia (DIP). (See Table 9–19.) Cough, dyspnea, and crackles on chest auscultation are typical. However, the reduction in lung compliance seen in pulmonary fibrosis is not found in this disorder. The condition may be recognized only on surgical lung biopsy, which demonstrates characteristic metaplasia of terminal and respiratory bronchioles and filling of respiratory and terminal bronchioles, alveolar ducts, and alveoli by pigmented alveolar macrophages. The prognosis is good if the patient stops smoking.

Diffuse panbronchiolitis is an idiopathic disorder of respiratory bronchioles frequently diagnosed in Japan. The condition appears to be less common in the United States or Europe. Men are affected about twice as often as women and are usually between ages 20 and 80. About two-thirds of patients are nonsmokers. The large majority have a history of chronic pansinusitis. Marked dyspnea, cough, and sputum production are cardinal features. Crackles and rhonchi are noted on physical examination. Pulmonary function tests reveal obstructive abnormalities. The chest radiograph shows a distinct pattern of diffuse small nodular shadows and hyperinflation. Surgical lung biopsy is necessary for diagnosis.

Boehler A et al: Post-transplant bronchiolitis obliterans. Eur Respir J 2003;22:1007. [PMID: 14680094]

Cordier JF: Cryptogenic organizing pneumonia. Clin Chest Med 2004;25:727. [PMID: 15564018]

Oymak FS et al: Bronchiolitis obliterans organizing pneumonia. Clinical and roentgenological features in 26 cases. Respiration 2005;72:254. [PMID: 15942294]

Ryu JH et al: Bronchiolar disorders. Am J Respir Crit Care Med 2003;168:1277. [PMID: 14644923]

■ PULMONARY INFECTIONS

PNEUMONIA

Lower respiratory tract infections continue to be a major health problem despite advances in the identification of etiologic organisms and the availability of potent antimicrobial drugs. In addition, there is still much controversy regarding diagnostic approaches and treatment choices for pneumonia.

Characteristics of pneumonia caused by specific agents and appropriate antimicrobial therapy are presented in Table 9–9. Pneumonias are typically classified as being either community-acquired or hospital-acquired (nosocomial). Anaerobic pneumonias and lung abscess can occur in both settings and warrant separate consideration.

This section sets forth the evaluation and management of immunocompetent hosts separately from the approach to the evaluation and management of pulmonary infiltrates in immunocompromised hosts—defined as patients with HIV disease, absolute neutrophil counts < 1000/mcL, current or recent exposure to myelosuppressive or immunosuppressive drugs, or those currently taking prednisone in a dosage of over 5 mg/d.

1. Community-Acquired Pneumonia

 ESSENTIALS OF DIAGNOSIS

- *Symptoms and signs of an acute lung infection: fever or hypothermia, cough with or without sputum, dyspnea, chest discomfort, sweats, or rigors.*
- *Bronchial breath sounds or rales are frequent auscultatory findings.*
- *Parenchymal infiltrate on chest radiograph.*
- *Occurs outside of the hospital or less than 48 hours after admission in a patient who is not hospitalized or residing in a long-term care facility for more than 14 days before the onset of symptoms.*

General Considerations

Community-acquired pneumonia is a common disorder, with approximately 2–3 million cases diagnosed each year in the United States. It is the most deadly infectious disease in the United States and the sixth leading cause of death. Mortality is estimated to be approximately 14% among hospitalized patients and less than 1% for patients who do not require hospitalization. Important risk factors for increased morbidity and mortality from community-acquired pneumonia include advanced age, alcoholism, comorbid medical conditions, altered mental status, respiratory rate ≥ 30 breaths/min, hypotension (defined by systolic blood pressure < 90 mm Hg or diastolic blood pressure < 60 mm Hg), and blood urea nitrogen (BUN) > 30 mg/dL.

A predictor of patient risk and mortality from community-acquired pneumonia has been developed and validated by the Pneumonia Patient Outcomes Research Team (PORT). The PORT prediction scheme uses 19 clinical variables to stratify patients into five

Table 9–9. Characteristics and treatment of selected pneumonias.

Organism; Appearance on Smear of Sputum	Clinical Setting	Complications	Laboratory Studies	Antimicrobial Therapy[1,2]
Streptococcus pneumoniae (pneumococcus). Gram-positive diplococci.	Chronic cardiopulmonary disease; follows upper respiratory tract infection	Bacteremia, meningitis, endocarditis, pericarditis, empyema	Gram stain and culture of sputum, blood, pleural fluid	Preferred[3]: Penicillin G, amoxicillin. Alternative: Macrolides, cephalosporins, doxycycline, fluoroquinolones, clindamycin, vancomycin, TMP-SMZ, linezolid.
Haemophilus influenzae. Pleomorphic gram-negative coccobacilli.	Chronic cardiopulmonary disease; follows upper respiratory tract infection	Empyema, endocarditis	Gram stain and culture of sputum, blood, pleural fluid	Preferred[3]: Cefotaxime, ceftriaxone, cefuroxime, doxycycline, azithromycin, TMP-SMZ. Alternative: Fluoroquinolones, clarithromycin.
Staphylococcus aureus. Plump gram-positive cocci in clumps.	Residence in chronic care facility, nosocomial, influenza epidemics; cystic fibrosis, bronchiectasis, injection drug use	Empyema, cavitation	Gram stain and culture of sputum, blood, pleural fluid	For methicillin-susceptible strains: Preferred: A penicillinase-resistant penicillin with or without rifampin, or gentamicin. Alternative: A cephalosporin; clindamycin, TMP-SMZ, vancomycin, a fluoroquinolone. For methicillin-resistant strains: Vancomycin with or without gentamicin or rifampin, linezolid.
Klebsiella pneumoniae. Plump gram-negative encapsulated rods.	Alcohol abuse, diabetes mellitus; nosocomial.	Cavitation, empyema	Gram stain and culture of sputum, blood, pleural fluid	Preferred: Third-generation cephalosporin. For severe infections, add an aminoglycoside. Alternative: Aztreonam, imipenem, meropenem, β-lactam/β-lactamase inhibitor, an aminoglycoside, or a fluoroquinolone.
Escherichia coli. Gram-negative rods.	Nosocomial; rarely, community-acquired	Empyema	Gram stain and culture of sputum, blood, pleural fluid	Same as for *Klebsiella pneumoniae*.
Pseudomonas aeruginosa. Gram-negative rods.	Nosocomial; cystic fibrosis, bronchiectasis	Cavitation	Gram stain and culture of sputum, blood	Preferred: An antipseudomonal β-lactam plus an aminoglycoside. Alternative: Ciprofloxacin plus an aminoglycoside or an antipseudomonal β-lactam.
Anaerobes. Mixed flora.	Aspiration, poor dental hygiene	Necrotizing pneumonia, abscess, empyema	Culture of pleural fluid or of material obtained by transtracheal or transthoracic aspiration	Preferred: Clindamycin, β-lactam/β-lactamase inhibitor, imipenem.

Organism and Gram stain	Epidemiology	Complications	Diagnostic evaluation	Antimicrobial therapy[1,2]
Mycoplasma pneumoniae. PMNs and monocytes; no bacteria.	Young adults; summer and fall	Skin rashes, bullous myringitis; hemolytic anemia	PCR. Culture.[4] Complement fixation titer.[5] Cold agglutinin serum titers are not helpful as they lack sensitivity and specificity.	Preferred: Doxycycline or erythromycin. Alternative: Clarithromycin; azithromycin, or a fluoroquinolone.
Legionella species. Few PMNs; no bacteria.	Summer and fall; exposure to contaminated construction site, water source, air conditioner; community-acquired or nosocomial	Empyema, cavitation, endocarditis, pericarditis	Direct immunofluorescent examination or PCR of sputum or tissue; culture of sputum or tissue.[4] Urinary antigen assay for *L pneumophila* serogroup 1.	Preferred: A macrolide with or without rifampin; a fluoroquinolone. Alternative: Doxycycline with or without rifampin, TMP-SMZ.
Chlamydia pneumoniae. Nonspecific.	Clinically similar to *M pneumoniae,* but prodromal symptoms last longer (up to 2 weeks). Sore throat with hoarseness common. Mild pneumonia in teenagers and young adults.	Reinfection in older adults with underlying COPD or heart failure may be severe or even fatal	Isolation of the organism is very difficult. Serologic studies include microimmunofluorescence with TWAR antigen. PCR at selected laboratories.	Preferred: Doxycycline. Alternative: Erythromycin, clarithromycin, azithromycin, or a fluoroquinolone.
Moraxella catarrhalis. Gram-negative diplococci.	Preexisting lung disease; elderly; corticosteroid or immunosuppressive therapy	Rarely, pleural effusions and bacteremia	Gram stain and culture of sputum, blood, pleural fluid	Preferred: A second- or third-generation cephalosporin; a fluoroquinolone. Alternative: TMP-SMZ, amoxicillin-clavulanic acid, or a macrolide.
Pneumocystis jiroveci. Nonspecific.	AIDS, immunosuppressive or cytotoxic drug therapy, cancer	Pneumothorax, respiratory failure, ARDS, death	Methenamine silver, Giemsa, or DFA stains of sputum or bronchoalveolar lavage fluid	Preferred: TMP-SMZ or pentamidine isethionate plus prednisone. Alternative: Dapsone plus trimethoprim; clindamycin plus primaquine; trimetrexate plus folinic acid.

[1] Antimicrobial sensitivities should guide therapy when available. (Modified from: The choice of antibacterial drugs. Med Lett Drugs Ther 2004;43:69, and from Bartlett JG et al: Practice guidelines for the management of community-acquired pneumonia in adults. Clin Infect Dis 2000;31:347.)

[2] For additional antimicrobial therapy information, see Infectious Disease: Antimicrobial Therapy: Tables 37–1 (drugs of choice), 37–5 and 37–7 (doses per day), and 37–4, 37–8, and 37–9 (pharmacology and dosage adjustment for renal dysfunction).

[3] Consider penicillin resistance when choosing therapy. See text.

[4] Selective media are required.

[5] Fourfold rise in titer is diagnostic.

TMP-SMZ = trimethoprim-sulfamethoxazole; PCR = polymerase chain reaction; COPD = chronic obstructive pulmonary disease; ARDS = acute respiratory distress syndrome.

Table 9–10. Scoring system for risk class assignment for PORT prediction rule.

Patient Characteristic	Points Assigned[1]
Demographic factor	
Age: men	Number of years
Age: women	Number of years minus 10
Nursing home resident	10
Comorbid illnesses	
Neoplastic disease[2]	30
Liver disease[3]	20
Congestive heart failure[4]	10
Cerebrovascular disease[5]	10
Renal disease[6]	10
Physical examination finding	
Altered mental status[7]	20
Respiratory rate ≥ 30 breaths/min	20
Systolic blood pressure < 90 mm Hg	20
Temperature ≤ 35°C or ≥ 40°C	15
Pulse ≥ 125 beats/min	10
Laboratory or radiographic finding	
Arterial pH < 7.35	30
Blood urea nitrogen ≥ 30 mg/dL	20
Sodium < 130 mEq/L	20
Glucose > 250 mg/dL	10
Hematocrit < 30%	10
Arterial P_{O_2} < 60 mm Hg	10
Pleural effusion	10

[1]A total point score for a given patient is obtained by summing the patient's age in years (age minus 10 for women) and the points for each applicable characteristic.
[2]Any cancer except basal or squamous cell of the skin that was active at the time of presentation or diagnosed within 1 year before presentation.
[3]Clinical or histologic diagnosis of cirrhosis or another form of chronic liver disease.
[4]Systolic or diastolic dysfunction documented by history, physical examination and chest radiograph, echocardiogram, MUGA scan, or left ventriculogram.
[5]Clinical diagnosis of stroke or transient ischemic attack or stroke documented by MRI or CT scan.
[6]History of chronic renal disease or abnormal blood urea nitrogen and creatinine concentration documented in the medical record.
[7]Disorientation (to person, place, or time, not known to be chronic), stupor, or coma.
Modified and reproduced, with permission, from Fine MJ et al: A prediction rule to identify low-risk patients with community-acquired pneumonia. N Engl J Med 1997;336:243. Copyright © 1997 Massachusetts Medical Society. All rights reserved.

mortality risk classes. (See Table 9–10.) Patients under 50 years of age without those comorbid conditions and specific physical examination abnormalities listed in Table 9–10 are assigned to risk class I. All other patients are assigned to risk categories based on the scoring system in Table 9–11. Thirty-day mortality by category is listed in Table 9–11. The PORT model can be used along with clinical judgment in the initial decision about whether to hospitalize a patient with community-acquired pneumonia.

In immunocompetent patients, the history, physical examination, radiographs, and sputum examination are neither sensitive nor specific for identifying the microbiologic cause of community-acquired pneumonia. While helpful in selected patients, these modalities do not consistently differentiate bacterial from viral causes or distinguish "typical" from "atypical" causes. As a result, the American Thoracic Society recommends empiric treatment based on epidemiologic data. In contrast, practice guidelines proposed by the Infectious Disease Society of America advocate systematic use of the microbiology laboratory in an attempt to administer pathogen-directed antimicrobial therapy whenever possible, especially in hospitalized patients.

Definition & Pathogenesis

Community-acquired pneumonia begins outside of the hospital or is diagnosed within 48 hours after admission to the hospital in a patient who has not resided in a long-term care facility for 14 days or more before the onset of symptoms.

Pulmonary defense mechanisms (cough reflex, mucociliary clearance system, immune responses) normally prevent the development of lower respiratory tract infections following aspiration of oropharyngeal

Table 9–11. PORT risk class 30-day mortality rates and recommendations for site of care.

Number of Points	Risk Class	Mortality at 30 days (%)	Recommended Site of Care
Absence of predictors	I	0.1–0.4	Outpatient
≤ 70	II	0.6–0.7	Outpatient
71–90	III	0.9–2.8	Outpatient or brief inpatient
91–130	IV	8.2–9.3	Inpatient
≥ 130	V	27.0–31.1	Inpatient

Data from Fine MJ et al: A prediction rule to identify low-risk patients with community-acquired pneumonia. N Engl J Med 1997; 336:243. Copyright © 1997 Massachusetts Medical Society. All rights reserved.

secretions containing bacteria or inhalation of infected aerosols. Community-acquired pneumonia occurs when there is a defect in one or more of the normal host defense mechanisms or when a very large infectious inoculum or a highly virulent pathogen overwhelms the host.

Prospective studies have failed to identify the cause of community-acquired pneumonia in 40–60% of cases; two or more causes are identified in up to 5% of cases. Bacteria are more commonly identified than viruses. The most common bacterial pathogen identified in most studies of community-acquired pneumonia is *S pneumoniae*, accounting for approximately two-thirds of bacterial isolates. Other common bacterial pathogens include *H influenzae, Mycoplasma pneumoniae, Chlamydia pneumoniae, S aureus, Neisseria meningitidis, M catarrhalis, Klebsiella pneumoniae*, other gram-negative rods, and *Legionella* species. Common viral causes of community-acquired pneumonia include influenza virus, respiratory syncytial virus, adenovirus, and parainfluenza virus. A detailed assessment of epidemiologic risk factors may aid in diagnosing pneumonias due to the following causes: *Chlamydia psittaci* (psittacosis), *Coxiella burnetii* (Q fever), *Francisella tularensis* (tularemia), endemic fungi (*Blastomyces, Coccidioides, Histoplasma*), and sin nombre virus (hantavirus pulmonary syndrome).

Clinical Findings

A. Symptoms and Signs

Most patients with community-acquired pneumonia experience an acute or subacute onset of fever, cough with or without sputum production, and dyspnea. Other common symptoms include rigors, sweats, chills, chest discomfort, pleurisy, hemoptysis, fatigue, myalgias, anorexia, headache, and abdominal pain.

Common physical findings include fever or hypothermia, tachypnea, tachycardia, and mild arterial oxygen desaturation. Many patients will appear acutely ill. Chest examination is often remarkable for altered breath sounds and rales. Dullness to percussion may be present if a parapneumonic pleural effusion is present.

The differential diagnosis of lower respiratory tract symptoms and signs is extensive and includes upper respiratory tract infections, reactive airway diseases, congestive heart failure, BOOP, lung cancer, pulmonary vasculitis, pulmonary thromboembolic disease, and atelectasis.

B. Laboratory Findings

Controversy surrounds the role of Gram stain and culture analysis of expectorated sputum in patients with community-acquired pneumonia. Most reports suggest that these tests have poor positive and negative predictive value in most patients. Some argue, however, that the tests should still be performed to try to identify etiologic organisms in the hope of reducing microbial resistance to drugs, unnecessary drug costs, and avoidable

side effects of empiric antibiotic therapy. Expert panel guidelines suggest that sputum Gram stain should be attempted in all patients with community-acquired pneumonia and that sputum culture should be obtained for all patients who require hospitalization. Sputum should be obtained before antibiotics are initiated except in a case of suspected antibiotic failure. The specimen is obtained by deep cough and should be grossly purulent. Culture should be performed only if the specimen meets strict cytologic criteria, eg, more than 25 neutrophils and fewer than 10 squamous epithelial cells per low power field. These criteria do not apply to cultures of legionella or mycobacteria.

Additional testing is generally recommended for patients who require hospitalization: preantibiotic blood cultures (at least two sets with needle sticks at separate sites), arterial blood gases, complete blood count with differential, and a chemistry panel (including serum glucose, electrolytes, urea nitrogen, creatinine, bilirubin, and liver enzymes). The results of these tests help assess the severity of the disease and guide evaluation and therapy. HIV serology should be obtained from all hospitalized patients.

C. Imaging

Chest radiography may confirm the diagnosis and detect associated lung diseases. It can also be used to help assess severity and response to therapy over time. Radiographic findings can range from patchy airspace infiltrates to lobar consolidation with air bronchograms to diffuse alveolar or interstitial infiltrates. Additional findings can include pleural effusions and cavitation. No pattern of radiographic abnormalities is pathognomonic of a specific cause of pneumonia.

Progression of pulmonary infiltrates during antibiotic therapy or lack of radiographic improvement over time are poor prognostic signs and also raise concerns about secondary or alternative pulmonary processes. Clearing of pulmonary infiltrates in patients with community-acquired pneumonia can take 6 weeks or longer and is usually fastest in young patients, nonsmokers, and those with only single lobe involvement.

D. Special Examinations

Sputum induction is reserved for patients who cannot provide expectorated sputum samples or who may have *P jiroveci* or *Mycobacterium tuberculosis* pneumonia. Transtracheal aspiration, fiberoptic bronchoscopy, and transthoracic needle aspiration techniques to obtain samples of lower respiratory secretions or tissues are reserved for selected patients.

Thoracentesis with pleural fluid analysis (Gram stain and cultures; glucose, lactate dehydrogenase (LDH), and total protein levels; leukocyte count with differential; pH determination) should be performed on most patients with pleural effusions to assist in diagnosis of the etiologic agent and assess for empyema or complicated parapneumonic process. Serologic assays, polymerase chain reaction tests, specialized culture tests, and other new diagnostic tests for organisms such as *Legionella, M pneumoniae,* and *C pneumoniae* are performed when these diagnoses are suspected. Limitations of many of these tests include delay in obtaining test results and poor sensitivity and specificity.

Treatment

Antimicrobial therapy should be initiated promptly after the diagnosis of pneumonia is established and appropriate specimens are obtained, especially in patients who require hospitalization. Delays in obtaining diagnostic specimens or the results of testing should not preclude the early administration of antibiotics to acutely ill patients. Decisions regarding hospitalization should be based on prognostic criteria as outlined above in the section on general considerations. Treatment recommendations can be divided into those for patients who can be treated as outpatients and those for patients who require hospitalization.

Special consideration must be given to penicillin-resistant strains of *S pneumoniae.* Intermediate resistance to penicillin is defined as a minimum inhibitory concentration (MIC) of 0.1–1 mcg/mL. Strains with high-level resistance usually require an MIC ≥ 2 mcg/mL for penicillin. Resistance to other antibiotics (β-lactams, trimethoprim-sulfamethoxazole, macrolides, others) often accompanies resistance to penicillin. The prevalence of resistance varies by patient group, geographic region, and over time. Local resistance pattern data should therefore guide empiric therapy of suspected or documented *S pneumoniae* infections until specific susceptibility test results are available.

A. Treatment of Outpatients

Empiric antibiotic options for patients with community-acquired pneumonia who do not require hospitalization include the following: (1) Macrolides (clarithromycin, 500 mg orally twice a day, or azithromycin, 500 mg orally as a first dose and then 250 mg once a day for 4 days). (2) Doxycycline (100 mg orally twice a day). (3) Fluoroquinolones (with enhanced activity against *S pneumoniae,* such as gatifloxacin 400 mg orally once a day, levofloxacin 500 mg orally once a day, or moxifloxacin 400 mg orally once a day). Some experts prefer doxycycline or macrolides for patients under 50 years of age without comorbidities and a fluoroquinolone for patients with comorbidities or who are older than 50 years of age. Alternatives include erythromycin (250–500 mg orally four times daily), amoxicillin-potassium clavulanate—especially for suspected aspiration pneumonia—500 mg orally three times a day or 875 mg orally twice a day, and some second- and third-generation cephalosporins such as cefuroxime axetil (250–500 mg orally twice a day), cefpodoxime proxetil (100–200 mg orally twice a day), or cefprozil (250–500 mg orally twice a day).

There are limited data to guide recommendations for duration of treatment. The decision is influenced by the severity of illness, the etiologic agent, response to therapy, other medical problems, and complications. Therapy until the patient is afebrile for at least 72 hours is usually sufficient for pneumonia due to *S pneumoniae.* A minimum of 2 weeks of therapy is appropriate for pneumonia due to *S aureus, P aeruginosa, Klebsiella,* anaerobes, *M pneumoniae, C pneumoniae,* or *Legionella* species.

B. Treatment of Hospitalized Patients

Empiric antibiotic options for patients with community-acquired pneumonia who require hospitalization can be divided into those for patients who can be cared for on a general medical ward and those for patients who require care in an ICU. Patients who only require general medical ward care usually respond to an extended-spectrum β-lactam (such as ceftriaxone or cefotaxime) with a macrolide (clarithromycin or azithromycin is preferred if *H influenzae* infection is suspected) or a fluoroquinolone (with enhanced activity against *S pneumoniae*) such as gatifloxacin, levofloxacin, or moxifloxacin. Alternatives include a β-lactam/β-lactamase inhibitor (ampicillin-sulbactam or piperacillin-tazobactam) with a macrolide.

Patients requiring admission to the ICU require a macrolide or a fluoroquinolone (with enhanced activity against *S pneumoniae*) plus an extended-spectrum cephalosporin (ceftriaxone, cefotaxime) or a β-lactam/β-lactamase inhibitor (ampicillin-sulbactam or piperacillin-tazobactam). Patients with penicillin allergies can be treated with a fluoroquinolone (with enhanced activity against *S pneumoniae*) with or without clindamycin. Patients with suspected aspiration pneumonia should receive a fluoroquinolone (with enhanced activity against *S pneumoniae*) with or without clindamycin, metronidazole, or a β-lactam/β-lactamase inhibitor. Patients with structural lung diseases such as bronchiectasis or cystic fibrosis benefit from empiric therapy with an antipseudomonal penicillin, carbapenem, or cefepime plus a fluoroquinolone (including high-dose ciprofloxacin) until sputum culture and sensitivity results are available. Expanded discussions of specific antibiotics are provided in Chapter 37.

Almost all patients who are admitted to a hospital for therapy of community-acquired pneumonia receive intravenous antibiotics. Despite this preference, no studies demonstrate superior outcomes when hospitalized patients are treated intravenously instead of orally if patients can tolerate oral therapy and the drug is well absorbed. Duration of antibiotic treatment is the same as for outpatients with community-acquired pneumonia.

Prevention

Polyvalent pneumococcal vaccine (containing capsular polysaccharide antigens of 23 common strains of *S pneumoniae*) has the potential to prevent or lessen the severity of the majority of pneumococcal infections in immunocompetent patients. Indications for pneumococcal vaccination include the following: age ≥ 65 years or any chronic illness that increases the risk of community-acquired pneumonia (see Chapter 30). Immunocompromised patients and those at highest risk of fatal pneumococcal infections should receive a single revaccination 6 years after the first vaccination. Immunocompetent persons 65 years of age or older should receive a second dose of vaccine if the patient first received the vaccine 6 or more years previously and was under 65 years old at the time of vaccination.

The influenza vaccine is effective in preventing severe disease due to influenza virus with a resulting positive impact on both primary influenza pneumonia and secondary bacterial pneumonias. The influenza vaccine is administered annually to persons at risk for complications of influenza infection (age ≥ 65 years, residents of long-term care facilities, patients with pulmonary or cardiovascular disorders, patients recently hospitalized with chronic metabolic disorders) as well as health care workers and others who are able to transmit influenza to high-risk patients.

Hospitalized patients who would benefit from pneumococcal and influenza vaccines should be vaccinated during hospitalization. The vaccines can be given simultaneously, and there are no contraindications to use immediately after an episode of pneumonia.

Bodi M et al; Community-Acquired Pneumonia Intensive Care Units (CAPUCI) Study Investigators: Antibiotic prescription for community-acquired pneumonia in the intensive care unit: impact of adherence to IDSA guidelines on survival. Clin Infect Dis 2005;41:1709. [PMID: 16288392]

File TM Jr et al: Guidelines for empiric antimicrobial prescribing in community-acquired pneumonia. Chest 2004;125:1888. [PMID: 15136404]

Metlay JP et al: Testing strategies in the initial management of patients with community-acquired pneumonia. Ann Intern Med 2003;138:109. [PMID: 12529093]

Niederman MS et al: Guidelines for the management of adults with community-acquired pneumonia. Diagnosis, assessment of severity, antimicrobial therapy, and prevention. Am J Respir Crit Care Med 2001;163:1730. [PMID: 11401897]

Wunderink RG et al: Community-acquired pneumonia: pathophysiology and host factors with focus on possible new approaches to management of lower respiratory tract infections. Infect Dis Clin North Am 2004;18:743. [PMID: 15555822]

2. Hospital-Acquired Pneumonia

 ESSENTIALS OF DIAGNOSIS

- *Occurs more than 48 hours after admission to the hospital and excludes any infection present at the time of admission.*
- *At least two of the following: fever, cough, leukocytosis, purulent sputum.*
- *New or progressive parenchymal infiltrate on chest radiograph.*
- *Especially common in patients requiring intensive care or mechanical ventilation.*

General Considerations

Hospital-acquired (nosocomial) pneumonia is an important cause of morbidity and mortality despite widespread use of preventive measures, advances in diagnostic testing, and potent new antimicrobial agents. Nosocomial pneumonia is the second most common cause of hospital-acquired infection and is the leading cause of death due to nosocomial infection with mortality rates ranging from 20% to 50%. While the majority of cases occur in patients who are not in the ICU, the highest-risk patients are those in such units or who are being mechanically ventilated; these patients also experience higher morbidity and mortality from nosocomial pneumonias.

Definition & Pathogenesis

Hospital-acquired pneumonia is defined as pneumonia developing more than 48 hours after admission to the hospital. Ventilator-associated pneumonia develops in a mechanically ventilated patient more than 48 hours after intubation.

Colonization of the pharynx and possibly the stomach with bacteria is the most important step in the pathogenesis of nosocomial pneumonia. Pharyngeal colonization is promoted by exogenous factors (instrumentation of the upper airway with nasogastric and endotracheal tubes, contamination by dirty hands and equipment, and treatment with broad-spectrum antibiotics that promote the emergence of drug-resistant organisms) and patient factors (malnutrition, advanced age, altered consciousness, swallowing disorders, and underlying pulmonary and systemic diseases). Aspiration of infected pharyngeal or gastric secretions delivers bacteria directly to the lower airway. Impaired cellular and mechanical defense mechanisms in the lungs of hospitalized patients raise the risk of infection after aspiration has occurred. Tracheal intubation increases the risk of lower respiratory infection by mechanical obstruction of the trachea, impairment of mucociliary clearance, trauma to the mucociliary escalator system, and interference with coughing. Tight adherence of bacteria such as *Pseudomonas* to the tracheal epithelium and the biofilm that lines the endotracheal tube makes clearance of these organisms from the lower airway difficult. Less important pathogenetic mechanisms of nosocomial pneumonia include inhalation of contaminated aerosols and hematogenous dissemination of microorganisms.

The role of the stomach in the pathogenesis of nosocomial pneumonia remains controversial. Observational studies have suggested that elevations of gastric pH due to antacids, H_2-receptor antagonists, or enteral feeding is associated with gastric microbial overgrowth, tracheobronchial colonization, and nosocomial pneumonia. Sucralfate, a cytoprotective agent that does not alter gastric pH, is associated with a trend toward a lower incidence of ventilator-associated pneumonia.

The most common organisms responsible for nosocomial pneumonia are *P aeruginosa, S aureus, Enterobacter, K pneumoniae,* and *Escherichia coli. Proteus, Serratia marcescens, H influenzae,* and streptococci account for most of the remaining cases. Infection by *P aeruginosa* and *Acinetobacter* tend to cause pneumonia in the most debilitated patients, those with previous antibiotic therapy, and those requiring mechanical ventilation. Anaerobic organisms (bacteroides, anaerobic streptococci, fusobacterium) may also cause pneumonia in the hospitalized patient; when isolated, they are commonly part of a polymicrobial flora. Mycobacteria, fungi, chlamydiae, viruses, rickettsiae, and protozoal organisms are uncommon causes of nosocomial pneumonia.

Clinical Findings

A. Symptoms and Signs

The signs and symptoms associated with nosocomial pneumonia are nonspecific; however, one or more clinical findings (fever, leukocytosis, purulent sputum, and a new or progressive pulmonary infiltrate on chest radiograph) are present in most patients. Other findings associated with nosocomial pneumonia include those listed above for community-acquired pneumonia.

The differential diagnosis of new lower respiratory tract symptoms and signs in hospitalized patients includes congestive heart failure, atelectasis, aspiration, ARDS, pulmonary thromboembolism, pulmonary hemorrhage, and drug reactions.

B. Laboratory Findings

The minimum evaluation for suspected nosocomial pneumonia includes blood cultures from two different sites and an arterial blood gas or pulse oximetry determination. Blood cultures can identify the pathogen in up to 20% of all patients with nosocomial pneumonia; positivity is associated with increased risk for complications and other sites of infection. The assessment of oxygenation helps define the severity of illness and determines the need for supplemental oxygen. Blood counts and clinical chemistry tests are not helpful in establishing a specific diagnosis of nosocomial pneumonia; however, they can help define the severity of illness and identify complications. Thoracentesis for pleural fluid analysis (stains, cultures; glucose, LDH, and total protein levels; leukocyte count with differential; pH determination) should be performed in patients with pleural effusions.

Examination of sputum is attended by the same disadvantages as in community-acquired pneumonia. Gram stains and cultures of sputum are neither sensitive nor specific in the diagnosis of nosocomial pneumonia. The identification of a bacterial organism by culture of sputum does not prove that the organism is a lower respiratory tract pathogen. However, it can be used to help identify antibiotic sensitivity patterns of bacteria and as a guide to therapy. If nosocomial pneumonia from *Legionella pneumophila* is suspected, direct

fluorescent antibody staining can be performed. Sputum stains and cultures for mycobacteria and certain fungi may be diagnostic.

C. Imaging

Radiographic findings are nonspecific and can range from patchy airspace infiltrates to lobar consolidation with air bronchograms to diffuse alveolar or interstitial infiltrates. Additional findings can include pleural effusions and cavitation. Progression of pulmonary infiltrates during antibiotic therapy and lack of radiographic improvement over time are poor prognostic signs and also raise concerns about secondary or alternative pulmonary processes. Clearing of pulmonary infiltrates can take 6 weeks or longer.

D. Special Examinations

Endotracheal aspiration using a sterile suction catheter and fiberoptic bronchoscopy with bronchoalveolar lavage or a protected specimen brush can be used to obtain lower respiratory tract secretions for analysis, most commonly in patients with ventilator-associated pneumonias. Endotracheal aspiration cultures have significant negative predictive value but limited positive predictive value in the diagnosis of specific etiologic agents in patients with nosocomial pneumonia. An invasive diagnostic approach using quantitative culture of bronchoalveolar lavage samples or protected specimen brush samples in patients suspected of having ventilator-associated pneumonia leads to significantly less antibiotic use, earlier attenuation of organ dysfunction, and fewer deaths at 14 days.

Treatment

Treatment of nosocomial pneumonia, like treatment of community-acquired pneumonia, is usually empiric. Because of the high mortality rate, therapy should be started as soon as pneumonia is suspected. Initial regimens must be broad in spectrum and tailored to the specific clinical setting. There is no uniform consensus on the best regimens.

Recommendations for the treatment of hospital-acquired pneumonia have been proposed by many organizations, including the American Thoracic Society. Initial empiric therapy with antibiotics is determined by the severity of illness, risk factors, and the length of hospitalization. Empiric therapy for mild to moderate nosocomial pneumonia in a patient without unusual risk factors or a patient with severe early-onset (within 5 days after hospitalization) hospital-acquired pneumonia may consist of a second-generation cephalosporin, a nonantipseudomonal third-generation cephalosporin, or a combination of a β-lactam and β-lactamase inhibitor.

Empiric therapy for patients with severe, late-onset (≥ 5 days after hospitalization) hospital-acquired pneumonia or with ICU- or ventilator-associated pneumonia should include a combination of antibiotics directed against the most virulent organisms, particularly *P aerugi-*

nosa, *Acinetobacter* species, and *Enterobacter* species. The antibiotic regimen should include an aminoglycoside or fluoroquinolone plus one of the following: an antipseudomonal penicillin, an antipseudomonal cephalosporin, a carbapenem, or aztreonam—aztreonam alone with an aminoglycoside will be inadequate if coverage for gram-positive organisms or *H influenzae* is required. Vancomycin is added if infection with methicillin-resistant *S aureus* is of concern (especially in patients with coma, head trauma, diabetes mellitus, or renal failure, or who are in the ICU). Anaerobic coverage with clindamycin or a β-lactam/β-lactamase inhibitor combination may be added for patients who have risk factors for anaerobic pneumonia, including aspiration, recent thoracoabdominal surgery, or an obstructing airway lesion. A macrolide is added when patients are at risk for *Legionella* infection, such as those receiving high-dose corticosteroids. After results of sputum, blood, and pleural fluid cultures have been obtained, it may be possible to switch to a regimen with a narrower spectrum. Duration of antibiotic therapy should be individualized based on the pathogen, severity of illness, response to therapy, and comorbid conditions. Therapy for gram-negative bacterial pneumonia should continue for at least 14–21 days.

Expanded discussions of specific antibiotics are provided in Chapter 37. Antibiotic dosage suggestions are provided in Chapter 37.

Fagon JY et al: Antimicrobial treatment of hospital-acquired pneumonia. Clin Chest Med 2005;26:97. [PMID: 15802171]

Mehta RM et al: Nosocomial pneumonia in the intensive care unit: controversies and dilemmas. J Inten Care Med 2003; 18:175. [PMID: 15035764]

Sopena N et al: Multicenter study of hospital-acquired pneumonia in non-ICU patients. Chest 2005;127:213. [PMID: 15653986]

3. Anaerobic Pneumonia & Lung Abscess

ESSENTIALS OF DIAGNOSIS

- *History of or predisposition to aspiration.*
- *Indolent symptoms, including fever, weight loss, malaise.*
- *Poor dentition.*
- *Foul-smelling purulent sputum (in many patients).*
- *Infiltrate in dependent lung zone, with single or multiple areas of cavitation or pleural effusion.*

General Considerations

Aspiration of small amounts of oropharyngeal secretions occurs during sleep in normal individuals but rarely causes disease. Sequelae of aspiration of larger amounts of material include nocturnal asthma, chemical pneumonitis, mechanical obstruction of airways by particulate matter, bronchiectasis, and pleuropulmo-

nary infection. Individuals predisposed to disease induced by aspiration include those with depressed levels of consciousness due to drug or alcohol use, seizures, general anesthesia, or central nervous system disease; those with impaired deglutition due to esophageal disease or neurologic disorders; and those with tracheal or nasogastric tubes, which disrupt the mechanical defenses of the airways.

Periodontal disease and poor dental hygiene, which increase the number of anaerobic bacteria in aspirated material, are associated with a greater likelihood of anaerobic pleuropulmonary infection. Aspiration of infected oropharyngeal contents initially leads to pneumonia in dependent lung zones, such as the posterior segments of the upper lobes and superior and basilar segments of the lower lobes. Body position at the time of aspiration determines which lung zones are dependent. The onset of symptoms is insidious. By the time the patient seeks medical attention, necrotizing pneumonia, lung abscess, or empyema may be apparent.

Most aspiration patients with necrotizing pneumonia, lung abscess, and empyema are found to be infected with multiple species of anaerobic bacteria. Most of the remainder are infected with both anaerobic and aerobic bacteria. *Prevotella melaninogenica, Peptostreptococcus, Fusobacterium nucleatum,* and *Bacteroides* species are commonly isolated anaerobic bacteria.

Clinical Findings

A. SYMPTOMS AND SIGNS

Patients with anaerobic pleuropulmonary infection usually present with constitutional symptoms such as fever, weight loss, and malaise. Cough with expectoration of foul-smelling purulent sputum suggests anaerobic infection, though the absence of productive cough does not rule out such an infection. Dentition is often poor. Patients are rarely edentulous; if so, an obstructing bronchial lesion is usually present.

B. LABORATORY FINDINGS

Expectorated sputum is inappropriate for culture of anaerobic organisms because of contaminating mouth flora. Representative material for culture can be obtained only by transthoracic aspiration, thoracentesis, or bronchoscopy with a protected brush. Transthoracic aspiration is rarely indicated, because drainage occurs via the bronchus and anaerobic pleuropulmonary infections usually respond well to empiric therapy.

C. IMAGING

The different types of anaerobic pleuropulmonary infection are distinguished on the basis of their radiographic appearance. **Lung abscess** appears as a thick-walled solitary cavity surrounded by consolidation. An air-fluid level is usually present. Other causes of cavitary lung disease (tuberculosis, mycosis, cancer, infarction, Wegener's granulomatosis) should be excluded. **Necrotizing pneumonia** is distinguished by multiple areas of cavitation within an area of consolidation. **Empyema** is characterized by the presence of purulent pleural fluid and may accompany either of the other two radiographic findings. Ultrasonography is of value in locating fluid and may also reveal pleural loculations.

Treatment

Penicillins have been the standard treatment for anaerobic pleuropulmonary infections. However, an increasing number of anaerobic organisms produce β-lactamases, and up to 20% of patients do not respond to penicillins. Improved responses have been documented with clindamycin (600 mg intravenously every 8 hours until improvement, then 300 mg orally every 6 hours) or amoxicillin-clavulanate (875 mg orally every 12 hours). Penicillin (amoxicillin, 500 mg every 8 hours, or penicillin G, 1–2 million units intravenously every 4–6 hours) plus metronidazole (500 mg orally or intravenously every 8–12 hours) is another option. Antibiotic therapy should be continued until the chest radiograph improves, a process that may take a month or more; patients with lung abscesses should be treated until radiographic resolution of the abscess cavity is demonstrated. Anaerobic pleuropulmonary disease requires adequate drainage with tube thoracostomy for the treatment of empyema. Open pleural drainage is sometimes necessary because of the propensity of these infections to produce loculations in the pleural space.

Marik PE: Aspiration pneumonitis and aspiration pneumonia. N Engl J Med 2001;344:665. [PMID: 11228282]

PULMONARY INFILTRATES IN THE IMMUNOCOMPROMISED HOST

Pulmonary infiltrates in immunocompromised patients may arise from infectious or noninfectious causes. Infection may be due to bacterial, mycobacterial, fungal, protozoal, helminthic, or viral pathogens. Noninfectious processes such as pulmonary edema, alveolar hemorrhage, drug reactions, pulmonary thromboembolic disease, malignancy, and radiation pneumonitis may mimic infection.

Although almost any pathogen can cause pneumonia in a compromised host, two clinical tools help the clinician narrow the differential diagnosis. The first is knowledge of the underlying immunologic defect. Specific immunologic defects are associated with particular infections. Defects in humoral immunity predispose to bacterial infections; defects in cellular immunity lead to infections with viruses, fungi, mycobacteria, and protozoa. Neutropenia and impaired granulocyte function predispose to infections from *S aureus, Aspergillus,* gram-negative bacilli, and *Candida.* Second, the time course of infection also provides clues to the etiology of pneumonia in immunocompromised patients. A fulminant pneumonia is often caused by bacterial infection, whereas an insidious pneumonia is more apt to be

caused by viral, fungal, protozoal, or mycobacterial infection. Pneumonia occurring within 2–4 weeks after organ transplantation is usually bacterial, whereas several months or more after transplantation *P jiroveci*, viruses (eg, cytomegalovirus), and fungi (eg, *Aspergillus*) are encountered more often.

Chest radiography is rarely helpful in narrowing the differential diagnosis. Examination of expectorated sputum for bacteria, fungi, mycobacteria, *Legionella,* and *P jiroveci* is important and may preclude the need for expensive, invasive diagnostic procedures. Sputum induction is often necessary for diagnosis. The sensitivity of induced sputum for detection of *P jiroveci* depends on institutional expertise, number of specimens analyzed, and detection methods.

Routine evaluation frequently fails to identify a causative organism. The clinician may begin empiric antimicrobial therapy and proceed to invasive procedures such as bronchoscopy, transthoracic needle aspiration, or open lung biopsy. The approach to management must be based on the severity of the pulmonary infection, the underlying disease, the risks of empiric therapy, and local expertise and experience with diagnostic procedures. Bronchoalveolar lavage using the flexible bronchoscope is a safe and effective method for obtaining representative pulmonary secretions for microbiologic studies. It involves less risk of bleeding and other complications than bronchial brushing and transbronchial biopsy. Bronchoalveolar lavage is especially suitable for the diagnosis of *P jiroveci* pneumonia in patients with AIDS when induced sputum analysis is negative. Open lung biopsy, now often performed by video-assisted thoracoscopy, provides the best opportunity for diagnosis of pulmonary infiltrates in the immunocompromised host. However, a specific diagnosis is obtained in only about two-thirds of cases, and the information obtained rarely affects the outcome. Therefore, empiric treatment is often preferred.

Hohenthal U et al: Bronchoalveolar lavage in immunocompromised patients with haematological malignancy—value of new microbiological methods. Eur J Hematol 2005;74:203. [PMID: 15693789]

Jain P et al: Role of flexible bronchoscopy in immunocompromised patients with lung infiltrates. Chest 2004;125:712. [PMID: 14769756]

Shorr AF et al: Pulmonary infiltrates in the non-HIV-infected immunocompromised patient: etiologies, diagnostic strategies, and outcomes. Chest 2004;125:260. [PMID: 14718449]

Yen KT et al: Pulmonary complications in bone marrow transplantation: a practical approach to diagnosis and treatment. Clin Chest Med 2004;25:189. [PMID: 15062610]

PULMONARY TUBERCULOSIS

 ESSENTIALS OF DIAGNOSIS

• *Fatigue, weight loss, fever, night sweats, and cough.*

- *Pulmonary infiltrates on chest radiograph, most often apical.*
- *Positive tuberculin skin test reaction (most cases).*
- *Acid-fast bacilli on smear of sputum or sputum culture positive for M tuberculosis.*

General Considerations

Tuberculosis is one of the world's most widespread and deadly illnesses. *M tuberculosis*, the organism that causes tuberculosis infection and disease, infects an estimated 20–43% of the world's population. Each year, 3 million people worldwide die of the disease. In the United States, it is estimated that 15 million people are infected with *M tuberculosis*. Tuberculosis occurs disproportionately among disadvantaged populations such as the malnourished, homeless, and those living in overcrowded and substandard housing. There is an increased occurrence of tuberculosis among HIV-positive individuals.

Infection with *M tuberculosis* begins when a susceptible person inhales airborne droplet nuclei containing viable organisms. Tubercle bacilli that reach the alveoli are ingested by alveolar macrophages. Infection follows if the inoculum escapes alveolar macrophage microbicidal activity. Once infection is established, lymphatic and hematogenous dissemination of tuberculosis typically occurs before the development of an effective immune response. This stage of infection, **primary tuberculosis**, is usually clinically and radiographically silent. In most persons with intact cell-mediated immunity, T cells and macrophages surround the organisms in granulomas that limit their multiplication and spread. The infection is contained but not eradicated, since viable organisms may lie dormant within granulomas for years to decades.

Individuals with this **latent tuberculosis infection** do not have active disease and cannot transmit the organism to others. However, reactivation of disease may occur if the host's immune defenses are impaired. Active tuberculosis will develop in approximately 10% of individuals with latent tuberculosis infection who are not given preventive therapy; half of these cases occur in the 2 years following primary infection. Up to 50% of HIV-infected patients will develop active tuberculosis within 2 years after infection with tuberculosis. Diverse conditions such as gastrectomy, silicosis, and diabetes mellitus and disorders associated with immunosuppression (eg, HIV infection or therapy with corticosteroids or other immunosuppressive drugs) are associated with an increased risk of reactivation.

In approximately 5% of cases, the immune response is inadequate and the host develops **progressive primary tuberculosis**, accompanied by both pulmonary and constitutional symptoms that are described below.

Standard teaching has held that 90% of tuberculosis in adults represents activation of latent disease. New diagnostic technologies such as DNA fingerprinting suggest that as many as one-third of new cases of tuberculosis in urban populations are primary infections resulting from person-to-person transmission.

The percentage of patients with atypical presentations—particularly elderly patients, patients with HIV infection, and those in nursing homes—has increased. Extrapulmonary tuberculosis is especially common in patients with HIV infection, who often display lymphadenitis or miliary disease.

Strains of *M tuberculosis* resistant to one or more first-line antituberculous drugs are being encountered with increasing frequency. Risk factors for drug resistance include immigration from parts of the world with a high prevalence of drug-resistant tuberculosis, close and prolonged contact with individuals with drug-resistant tuberculosis, unsuccessful previous therapy, and patient noncompliance. Resistance to one or more antituberculous drugs has been found in 15% of tuberculosis patients in the United States. Outbreaks of multidrug-resistant tuberculosis in hospitals and correctional facilities in Florida and New York have been associated with mortality rates of 70–90% and median survival rates of 4–16 weeks.

Clinical Findings

A. SYMPTOMS AND SIGNS

The patient with pulmonary tuberculosis typically presents with slowly progressive constitutional symptoms of malaise, anorexia, weight loss, fever, and night sweats. Chronic cough is the most common pulmonary symptom. It may be dry at first but typically becomes productive of purulent sputum as the disease progresses. Blood-streaked sputum is common, but significant hemoptysis is rarely a presenting symptom; life-threatening hemoptysis may occur in advanced disease. Dyspnea is unusual unless there is extensive disease. Rarely, the patient is asymptomatic. On physical examination, the patient appears chronically ill and malnourished. On chest examination, there are no physical findings specific for tuberculosis infection. The examination may be normal or may reveal classic findings such as posttussive apical rales.

B. LABORATORY FINDINGS

Definitive diagnosis depends on recovery of *M tuberculosis* from cultures or identification of the organism by DNA or RNA amplification techniques. Three consecutive morning sputum specimens are advised. Sputum induction may be helpful in patients who cannot voluntarily produce satisfactory specimens. Fluorochrome staining with rhodamine-auramine of concentrated, digested sputum specimens is performed initially as a screening method, with confirmation by the Kinyoun or Ziehl-Neelsen stains. Demonstration of acid-fast bacilli on sputum smear does not confirm a diagnosis of tuberculosis, since saprophytic nontuberculous mycobacteria may colonize the airways and rarely may cause pulmonary disease.

In patients thought to have tuberculosis despite negative sputum smears, fiberoptic bronchoscopy can be considered. Bronchial washings are helpful; however, transbronchial lung biopsies increase the diagnostic yield. Postbronchoscopy expectorated sputum specimens may also be useful. Early morning aspiration of gastric contents after an overnight fast is an alternative to bronchoscopy but is suitable only for culture and not for stained smear, because nontuberculous mycobacteria may be present in the stomach in the absence of tuberculous infection. M tuberculosis may be cultured from blood in up to 15% of patients with tuberculosis.

Cultures on solid media to identify M tuberculosis may require 12 weeks. Liquid medium culture systems allow detection of mycobacterial growth in several days. Once mycobacteria have been grown in culture, nucleic acid probes or high-performance liquid chromatography can be used to identify the species within hours. The results of nucleic acid (DNA and RNA) amplification tests for tuberculosis should be interpreted in the clinical context and on the basis of local laboratory performance. Drug susceptibility testing of culture isolates is considered routine for the first isolate of M tuberculosis, when a treatment regimen is failing, and when sputum cultures remain positive after 2 months of therapy.

DNA fingerprinting using the restriction fragment length polymorphism analysis is available to identify individual strains of M tuberculosis, thereby revealing if infection has been transmitted from person to person. In addition, this method can be used to detect laboratory cross-contamination.

Needle biopsy of the pleura reveals granulomatous inflammation in approximately 60% of patients with pleural effusions caused by M tuberculosis. Pleural fluid cultures for M tuberculosis are positive in less than 25% of cases of pleural tuberculosis. Culture of three pleural biopsy specimens combined with microscopic examination of a pleural biopsy yields a diagnosis in up to 90% of patients with pleural tuberculosis.

C. Imaging

Radiographic abnormalities in primary tuberculosis include small homogeneous infiltrates, hilar and paratracheal lymph node enlargement, and segmental atelectasis. Pleural effusion may be present, especially in adults, sometimes as the sole radiographic abnormality. Cavitation may be seen with progressive primary tuberculosis. Ghon (calcified primary focus) and Ranke (calcified primary focus and calcified hilar lymph node) complexes are seen in a minority of patients and represent residual evidence of healed primary tuberculosis.

Reactivation tuberculosis is associated with various radiographic manifestations, including fibrocavitary apical disease, nodules, and pneumonic infiltrates. The usual location is in the apical or posterior segments of the upper lobes or in the superior segments of the lower lobes; up to 30% of patients may present with radiographic evidence of disease in other locations. This is especially true in elderly patients, in whom lower lobe infiltrates with or without pleural effusion are encountered with increasing frequency. Lower lung tuberculosis may masquerade as pneumonia or lung cancer. A "miliary" pattern (diffuse small nodular densities) can be seen with hematologic or lymphatic dissemination of the organism. Resolution of reactivation tuberculosis leaves characteristic radiographic findings. Dense nodules in the pulmonary hila, with or without obvious calcification, upper lobe fibronodular scarring, and bronchiectasis with volume loss are common findings.

In patients with early HIV infection, the radiographic features of tuberculosis resemble those in patients without HIV infection. In contrast, atypical radiographic features predominate in patients with late stage HIV infection. These patients often display lower lung zone, diffuse, or miliary infiltrates, pleural effusions, and involvement of hilar and, in particular, mediastinal lymph nodes.

D. Special Examinations

The tuberculin **skin test** identifies individuals who have been infected with M tuberculosis but does not distinguish between active and latent infection. The test is used to evaluate a person who has symptoms of tuberculosis, an asymptomatic person who may be infected with M tuberculosis (eg, after contact exposure), or to establish the prevalence of tuberculous infection in a population. Routine testing of individuals at low risk for tuberculosis is not recommended. The Mantoux test is the preferred method: 0.1 mL of purified protein derivative (PPD) containing 5 tuberculin units is injected intradermally on the volar surface of the forearm using a 27-gauge needle on a tuberculin syringe. The transverse width in millimeters of induration at the skin test site should be measured after 48–72 hours. Table 9–12 summarizes the criteria established by the Centers for Disease Control and Prevention (CDC) for interpretation of the Mantoux tuberculin skin test. In patients who have serial testing, a **tuberculin skin test conversion** is defined as an increase of ≥ 10 mm of induration within a 2-year period regardless of patient age.

In general, it takes 2–10 weeks after tuberculosis infection for an immune response to PPD to develop. Both false-positive and false-negative results occur. False-positive tuberculin skin test reactions occur in persons previously vaccinated against M tuberculosis with bacillus Calmette-Guérin (BCG) (extract of Mycobacterium bovis) and in those infected with nontuberculous mycobacteria. False-negative tuberculin skin test reactions may result from improper testing technique, concurrent infections, malnutrition, advanced age, immunologic disorders, lymphoreticular malig-

Table 9–12. Classification of positive tuberculin skin test reactions.[1]

Reaction Size	Group
≥ 5 mm	1. HIV-positive persons. 2. Recent contacts of individuals with active tuberculosis. 3. Persons with fibrotic changes on chest x-rays suggestive of prior tuberculosis. 4. Patients with organ transplants and other immunosuppressed patients (receiving the equivalent of > 15 mg/d of prednisone for 1 month or more).
≥ 10 mm	1. Recent immigrants (< 5 years) from countries with a high prevalence of tuberculosis (eg, Asia, Africa, Latin America). 2. HIV-negative injection drug users. 3. Mycobacteriology laboratory personnel. 4. Residents of and employees[2] in the following high-risk congregate settings: correctional institutions; nursing homes and other long-term facilities for the elderly; hospitals and other health care facilities; residential facilities for AIDS patients; and homeless shelters. 5. Persons with the following medical conditions that increase the risk of tuberculosis: gastrectomy, ≥ 10% below ideal body weight, jejunoileal bypass, diabetes mellitus, silicosis, chronic renal failure, some hematologic disorders, (eg, leukemias, lymphomas), and other specific malignancies (eg, carcinoma of the head or neck and lung). 6. Children < 4 years of age or infants, children, and adolescents exposed to adults at high risk.
≥ 15 mm	1. Persons with no risk factors for tuberculosis.

[1]A tuberculin skin test reaction is considered positive if the transverse diameter of the *indurated* area reaches the size required for the specific group. All other reactions are considered negative.

[2]For persons who are otherwise at low risk and are tested at entry into employment, a reaction of > 15 mm induration is considered positive.

Adapted from: Screening for tuberculosis and tuberculosis infection in high-risk populations: recommendations of the Advisory Council for the Elimination of Tuberculosis. MMWR Morb Mortal Wkly Rep 1995;44(RR-11):19.

nancies, corticosteroid therapy, chronic renal failure, HIV infection, and fulminant tuberculosis. Some individuals with latent tuberculosis infection may have a negative skin test reaction when tested many years after exposure.

Serial testing may create a false impression of skin test conversion. Dormant mycobacterial sensitivity is sometimes restored by the antigenic challenge of the initial skin test. This phenomenon is called "boosting." A two-step testing procedure is used to reduce the likelihood that a boosted tuberculin reaction will be misinterpreted as a recent infection. Following a negative tuberculin skin test, the person is retested in 1–3 weeks. If the second test is negative, the person is uninfected or anergic; if positive, a boosted reaction is likely. Two-step testing should be used for the initial tuberculin skin testing of individuals who will be tested repeatedly, such as health care workers. Anergy testing is not recommended for routine use to distinguish a true-negative result from anergy. Poor anergy test standardization and lack of outcome data limit the evaluation of its effectiveness. Interpretation of the tuberculin skin test in persons who have previously received BCG vaccination is the same as in those who have not had BCG.

Novel in vitro methods promise significant changes in the identification of persons with latent *M tuberculosis* infection. Potential advantages of in vitro testing include reduced variability and subjectivity associated with placing and reading the PPD, fewer false-positive results from prior BCG vaccination, and better discrimination of positive responses due to nontuberculous mycobacteria.

Persons with concomitant HIV and tuberculosis infection usually respond best when the HIV infection is treated concurrently. In some cases, prolonged antituberculous therapy may be warranted. Therefore, all patients with tuberculosis infection should be tested for HIV within 2 months after diagnosis.

Treatment

A. General Measures

The goals of therapy are to eliminate all tubercle bacilli from an infected individual while avoiding the emergence of clinically significant drug resistance. The basic principles of antituberculous treatment are (1) to administer multiple drugs to which the organisms are susceptible; (2) to add at least two new antituberculous agents to a regimen when treatment failure is suspected; (3) to provide the safest, most effective therapy in the shortest period of time; and (4) to ensure adherence to therapy.

All suspected and confirmed cases of tuberculosis should be reported promptly to local and state public health authorities. Public health departments will perform case investigations on sources and patient contacts to determine if other individuals with untreated, infectious tuberculosis are present in the community. They can identify infected contacts eligible for treatment of latent tuberculous infection, and ensure that a plan for monitoring adherence to therapy is established for each patient with tuberculosis. Patients with tuberculosis should be treated by physicians who are

Table 9–13. Characteristics of antituberculous drugs.[1]

Drug	Most Common Side Effects	Tests for Side Effects	Drug Interactions	Remarks
Isoniazid	Peripheral neuropathy, hepatitis, rash, mild CNS effects.	AST and ALT; neurologic examination.	Phenytoin (synergistic); disulfiram.	Bactericidal to both extracellular and intracellular organisms. Pyridoxine, 10 mg orally daily as prophylaxis for neuritis; 50–100 mg orally daily as treatment.
Rifampin	Hepatitis, fever, rash, flu-like illness, gastrointestinal upset, bleeding problems, renal failure.	CBC, platelets, AST and ALT.	Rifampin inhibits the effect of oral contraceptives, quinidine, corticosteroids, warfarin, methadone, digoxin, oral hypoglycemics; aminosalicyclic acid may interfere with absorption of rifampin. Significant interactions with protease inhibitors and nonnucleoside reverse transcriptase inhibitors.	Bactericidal to all populations of organisms. Colors urine and other body secretions orange. Discoloring of contact lenses.
Pyrazinamide	Hyperuricemia, hepatotoxicity, rash, gastrointestinal upset, joint aches.	Uric acid, AST, ALT.	Rare.	Bactericidal to intracellular organisms.
Ethambutol	Optic neuritis (reversible with discontinuance of drug; rare at 15 mg/kg); rash.	Red-green color discrimination and visual acuity (difficult to test in children under 3 years of age).	Rare.	Bacteriostatic to both intracellular and extracellular organisms. Mainly used to inhibit development of resistant mutants. Use with caution in renal disease or when ophthalmologic testing is not feasible.
Streptomycin	Eighth nerve damage, nephrotoxicity.	Vestibular function (audiograms); BUN and creatinine.	Neuromuscular blocking agents may be potentiated and cause prolonged paralysis.	Bactericidal to extracellular organisms. Use with caution in older patients or those with renal disease.

[1]See also Chapter 37.
Key: AST = aspartate aminotransferase; ALT = alanine aminotransferase; CBC = complete blood count; BUN = blood urea nitrogen.

skilled in the management of this infection. Clinical expertise is especially important in cases of drug-resistant tuberculosis.

Nonadherence to antituberculous treatment is a major cause of treatment failure, continued transmission of tuberculosis, and the development of drug resistance. Adherence to treatment can be improved by providing detailed patient education about tuberculosis and its treatment in addition to a case manager who oversees all aspects of an individual patient's care. **Directly observed therapy (DOT)**, which requires that a health care worker physically observe the patient ingest antituberculous medications in the home, clinic, hospital, or elsewhere, also improves adherence to treatment. The importance of direct observation of therapy cannot be overemphasized. The CDC recommends DOT for all patients with drug-resistant tuberculosis and for those receiving intermittent (twice- or thrice-weekly) therapy.

Hospitalization for initial therapy of tuberculosis is not necessary for most patients. It should be considered if a patient is incapable of self-care or is likely to expose new, susceptible individuals to tuberculosis. Hospitalized patients with active disease require a private room with appropriate ventilation until tubercle bacilli are no longer found in their sputum ("smear-negative") on three consecutive smears taken on separate days.

Additional treatment considerations can be found in Chapter 33. Characteristics of antituberculous drugs are provided in Table 9–13 and in Chapter 37. More complete information can be obtained from the CDC's Division of Tuberculosis Elimination Web site at http://www.cdc.gov/nchstp/tb/.

B. TREATMENT OF TUBERCULOSIS IN HIV-NEGATIVE PERSONS

Most patients with previously untreated pulmonary tuberculosis can be effectively treated with either a 6-month or a 9-month regimen, though the 6-month regimen is preferred. The initial phase of a 6-month regimen consists of 2 months of daily isoniazid, rifampin, pyrazinamide, and ethambutol. Once the isolate is determined to be isoniazid-sensitive, ethambutol may be discontinued. If the *M tuberculosis* isolate is susceptible to isoniazid and rifampin, the second phase of therapy consists of isoniazid and rifampin for a minimum of 4 additional months, with treatment to extend at least 3 months beyond documentation of conversion of sputum cultures to negative for *M tuberculosis*. If DOT is used, medications may be given intermittently using one of three regimens: (1) Daily isoniazid, rifampin, pyrazinamide, and ethambutol for 2 months, followed by isoniazid and rifampin two or three times each week for 4 months if susceptibility to isoniazid and rifampin is demonstrated. (2) Daily isoniazid, rifampin, pyrazinamide, and ethambutol for 2 weeks, then administration of the same agents twice weekly for 6 weeks followed by administration of isoniazid and rifampin twice each week for 4 months if susceptibility to isoniazid and rifampin is demonstrated. (3) Thrice-weekly administration of isoniazid, rifampin, pyrazinamide, and ethambutol for 6 months.

Patients who cannot or should not (eg, pregnant women) take pyrazinamide should receive daily isoniazid and rifampin along with ethambutol for 4–8 weeks. If susceptibility to isoniazid and rifampin is demonstrated or drug resistance is unlikely, ethambutol can be discontinued and isoniazid and rifampin may be given twice a week for a total of 9 months of therapy. If drug resistance is a concern, patients should receive isoniazid, rifampin, and ethambutol for 9 months. Patients with smear- and culture-negative disease (eg, pulmonary tuberculosis diagnosed on clinical grounds) and patients for whom drug susceptibility testing is not available can be treated with 6 months of isoniazid and rifampin combined with pyrazinamide for the first 2 months. This regimen assumes low prevalence of drug resistance. Previous guidelines have used streptomycin interchangeably with ethambutol. Increasing worldwide streptomycin resistance has made this drug less useful as empiric therapy.

When a twice-weekly or thrice-weekly regimen is used instead of a daily regimen, the dosages of isoniazid, pyrazinamide, and ethambutol or streptomycin must be increased. Recommended dosages for the initial treatment of tuberculosis are listed in Table 9–14. Fixed-dose combinations of isoniazid and rifampin (Rifamate) and of isoniazid, rifampin, and pyrazinamide (Rifater) are available to simplify treatment. Single tablets improve compliance but are more expensive than the individual drugs purchased separately.

C. TREATMENT OF TUBERCULOSIS IN HIV-POSITIVE PERSONS

Management of tuberculosis is rendered even more complex in patients with concomitant HIV disease. Experts in the management of both tuberculosis and HIV disease should be involved in the care of such patients. The CDC has published detailed recommendations for the treatment of tuberculosis in HIV-positive patients. These documents can be obtained by accessing the CDC Division of Tuberculosis Elimination Web site at http://www.cdc.gov/nchstp/tb/pubs/mmwrhtm/Maj_guide/HIV_AIDS.htm

The basic approach to HIV-positive patients with tuberculosis is similar to that detailed above for patients without HIV disease. Additional considerations in HIV-positive patients include (1) longer duration of therapy and (2) drug interactions between rifamycin derivatives

Table 9–14. Recommended dosages for the initial treatment of tuberculosis.

Drugs	Daily	Cost[1]	Twice a Week[2]	Cost[1]/wk	Three Times a Week[2]	Cost[1]/wk
Isoniazid	5 mg/kg Max: 300 mg/dose	$0.13/300 mg	15 mg/kg Max: 900 mg/dose	$0.78	15 mg/kg Max: 900 mg/dose	$1.17
Rifampin	10 mg/kg Max: 600 mg/dose	$3.80/600 mg	10 mg/kg Max: 600 mg/dose	$7.60	10 mg/kg Max: 600 mg/dose	$11.40
Pyrazinamide	15–30 mg/kg Max: 2 g/dose	$4.40/2 g	50–70 mg/kg Max: 4 g/dose	$17.60	50–70 mg/kg Max: 3 g/dose	$19.80
Ethambutol	5–25 mg/kg Max: 2.5 g/dose	$11.27/2.5 g	50 mg/kg Max: 2.5 g/dose	$22.54	25–30 mg/kg Max: 2.5 g/dose	$33.81
Streptomycin	15 mg/kg Max: 1 g/dose	$9.75/1 g	25–30 mg/kg Max: 1.5 g/dose	$39.00	25–30 mg/kg Max: 1.5 g/dose	$58.50

[1]Average wholesale price (AWP, for AB-rated generic when available) for quantity listed. Source: *Red Book Update,* Vol. 25, No. 5, May 2006. AWP may not accurately represent the actual pharmacy cost because wide contractual variations exist among institutions.
[2]All intermittent dosing regimens should be used with directly observed therapy.

such as rifampin and rifabutin, used to treat tuberculosis, and some of the protease inhibitors and nonnucleoside reverse transcriptase inhibitors (NNRTIs), used to treat HIV (see above Web site). DOT should be used for all HIV-positive tuberculosis patients. Pyridoxine (vitamin B_6), 25–50 mg orally each day, should be administered to all HIV-positive patients being treated with isoniazid to reduce central and peripheral nervous system side effects.

D. Treatment of Drug-Resistant Tuberculosis

Patients with drug-resistant *M tuberculosis* infection require careful supervision and management. Clinicians who are unfamiliar with the treatment of drug-resistant tuberculosis should seek expert advice. Tuberculosis resistant only to isoniazid can be successfully treated with a 6-month regimen of rifampin, pyrazinamide, and ethambutol or streptomycin or a 12-month regimen of rifampin and ethambutol. When isoniazid resistance is documented during a 9-month regimen without pyrazinamide, isoniazid should be discontinued. If ethambutol was part of the initial regimen, rifampin and ethambutol should be continued for a minimum of 12 months. If ethambutol was not part of the initial regimen, susceptibility tests should be repeated and two other drugs to which the organism is susceptible should be added. Treatment of *M tuberculosis* isolates resistant to agents other than isoniazid and treatment of drug resistance in HIV-infected patients require expert consultation.

Multidrug-resistant tuberculosis (MDRTB) calls for an individualized daily directly observed treatment plan under the supervision of a clinician experienced in the management of this entity. Treatment regimens are based on the patient's overall status and the results of susceptibility studies. Most MDRTB isolates are resistant to at least isoniazid and rifampin and require a minimum of three drugs to which the organism is susceptible. These regimens are continued until culture conversion is documented, and then a two-drug regimen is then continued for at least another 12 months. Some experts recommend at least 18–24 months of a three-drug regimen.

E. Treatment of Extrapulmonary Tuberculosis

In most cases, regimens that are effective for treating pulmonary tuberculosis are also effective for treating extrapulmonary disease. However, many experts recommend 9 months of therapy when miliary, meningeal, or bone and joint disease is present. Treatment of skeletal tuberculosis is enhanced by early surgical drainage and debridement of necrotic bone. Corticosteroid therapy has been shown to help prevent cardiac constriction from tuberculous pericarditis and to reduce neurologic complications from tuberculous meningitis.

F. Treatment of Pregnant or Lactating Women

Tuberculosis in pregnancy is usually treated with isoniazid, rifampin, and ethambutol. Ethambutol can be excluded if isoniazid resistance is unlikely. Therapy is continued for 9 months. Since the risk of teratogenic-ity with pyrazinamide has not been clearly defined, pyrazinamide should be used only if resistance to other drugs is documented and susceptibility to pyrazinamide is likely. Streptomycin is contraindicated in pregnancy because it may cause congenital deafness. Pregnant women taking isoniazid should receive pyridoxine (vitamin B_6), 10–25 mg orally once a day, to prevent peripheral neuropathy.

Small concentrations of antituberculous drugs are present in breast milk and are not known to be harmful to nursing newborns. Therefore, breastfeeding is not contraindicated while receiving antituberculous therapy.

G. Treatment Monitoring

Adults should have measurements of serum bilirubin, hepatic enzymes, urea nitrogen, creatinine, and a complete blood count (including platelets) before starting chemotherapy for tuberculosis. Visual acuity and red-green color vision tests are recommended before initiation of ethambutol and serum uric acid before starting pyrazinamide. Audiometry should be performed if streptomycin therapy is initiated.

Routine monitoring of laboratory tests for evidence of drug toxicity during therapy is not recommended. Monthly questioning for symptoms of drug toxicity is advised. Patients should be educated about common side effects of antituberculous medications and instructed to seek medical attention should these symptoms occur. Monthly follow-up of outpatients is recommended, including sputum smear and culture for *M tuberculosis* until cultures convert to negative. Patients with negative sputum cultures after 2 months of treatment should have at least one additional sputum smear and culture performed at the end of therapy. Patients with MDRTB should have sputum cultures performed monthly during the entire course of treatment. A chest radiograph at the end of therapy provides a useful baseline for any future films.

Patients whose cultures do not become negative or whose symptoms do not resolve despite 3 months of therapy should be evaluated for drug-resistant organisms and for nonadherence to the treatment regimen. DOT is required for the remainder of the treatment regimen, and the addition of at least two drugs not previously given should be considered pending repeat drug susceptibility testing. The clinician should seek expert assistance if drug resistance is newly found, if the patient remains symptomatic, or if smears or cultures remain positive.

Patients with only a clinical diagnosis of pulmonary tuberculosis (smears and cultures negative for *M tuberculosis*) whose symptoms and radiographic abnormalities are unchanged after 3 months of treatment usually either have another process or have had tuberculosis in the past.

H. Treatment of Latent Tuberculosis

Treatment of latent tuberculous infection is essential to controlling and eliminating tuberculosis in the

United States. Treatment of latent tuberculous infection substantially reduces the risk that infection will progress to active disease. Targeted testing is used to identify persons who are at high risk for tuberculosis and who stand to benefit from treatment of latent infection. Table 9–12 defines high-risk groups and gives the tuberculin skin test criteria for treatment of latent tuberculous infection. It is essential that each person who meets the criteria for treatment of latent tuberculous infection undergo a careful assessment to exclude active disease. A history of past treatment for tuberculosis and contraindications to treatment should be sought. All patients at risk for HIV infection should be tested for HIV. Patients suspected of having tuberculosis should receive one of the recommended multidrug regimens for active disease until the diagnosis is confirmed or excluded.

Some close contacts of persons with active tuberculosis should be evaluated for treatment of latent tuberculous infection despite a negative tuberculin skin test reaction (< 5 mm induration). These include immunosuppressed persons and those who may develop disease quickly after tuberculous infection. Close contacts who have a negative tuberculin skin test reaction on initial testing should be retested 10–12 weeks later.

Several treatment regimens for both HIV-negative and HIV-positive persons are available for the treatment of latent tuberculous infection: (1) **Isoniazid:** A 9-month regimen (minimum of 270 doses administered within 12 months) is considered optimal. Dosing options include a daily dose of 300 mg or twice-weekly doses of 15 mg/kg. Persons at risk for developing isoniazid-associated peripheral neuropathy (diabetes mellitus, uremia, malnutrition, alcoholism, HIV infection, pregnancy, seizure disorder) may be given supplemental pyridoxine (vitamin B_6), 10–50 mg/d. (2) **Rifampin and pyrazinamide:** A 2-month regimen (60 doses administered within 3 months) of daily rifampin (10 mg/kg up to a maximum dose of 600 mg) and pyrazinamide (15–20 mg/kg up to a maximum dose of 2 g) is recommended. (3) **Rifampin:** Patients who cannot tolerate isoniazid or pyrazinamide can be considered for a 4-month regimen (minimum of 120 doses administered within 6 months) of rifampin. HIV-positive patients given rifampin who are receiving protease inhibitors or NNRTIs require management by experts in both tuberculosis and HIV disease (see Treatment of Tuberculosis in HIV-Positive Persons, above).

Contacts of persons with isoniazid-resistant, rifampin-sensitive tuberculosis should receive a 2-month regimen of rifampin and pyrazinamide or a 4-month regimen of daily rifampin alone. Contacts of persons with MDRTB should receive two drugs to which the infecting organism has demonstrated susceptibility. Tuberculin skin test-negative and HIV-negative contacts may be observed without treatment or treated for 6 months. HIV-positive contacts should be treated for 12 months. All contacts of persons with MDRTB should have 2 years of follow-up regardless of treatment.

Persons with a positive tuberculin skin test (≥ 5 mm of induration) and fibrotic lesions suggestive of old tuberculosis on chest radiographs who have no evidence of active disease and no history of treatment for tuberculosis should receive 9 months of isoniazid, or 2 months of rifampin and pyrazinamide, or 4 months of rifampin (with or without isoniazid). Pregnant or breastfeeding women with latent tuberculosis should receive either daily or twice-weekly isoniazid with pyridoxine (vitamin B_6).

Baseline laboratory testing is indicated for patients at risk for liver disease, patients with HIV infection, women who are pregnant or within 3 months of delivery, and persons who use alcohol regularly. Patients receiving treatment for latent tuberculous infection should be evaluated once a month to assess for signs and symptoms of active tuberculosis and hepatitis and for adherence to their treatment regimen. Routine laboratory testing during treatment is indicated for those with abnormal baseline laboratory tests and for those at risk for developing liver disease.

Vaccine BCG is an antimycobacterial vaccine developed from an attenuated strain of *M bovis*. Millions of individuals worldwide have been vaccinated with BCG. However, it is not generally recommended in the United States because of the low prevalence of tuberculous infection, the vaccine's interference with the ability to determine latent tuberculous infection using tuberculin skin test reactivity, and its variable effectiveness against pulmonary tuberculosis. BCG vaccination in the United States should only be undertaken after consultation with local health officials and experts in the management of tuberculosis. Vaccination of health care workers should be considered on an individual basis in settings in which a high percentage of tuberculosis patients are infected with strains resistant to both isoniazid and rifampin, in which transmission of such drug-resistant *M tuberculosis* and subsequent infection are likely, and in which comprehensive tuberculous infection-control precautions have been implemented but have not been successful. The BCG vaccine is contraindicated in persons with impaired immune responses due to disease or medications.

Prognosis

Almost all properly treated patients with tuberculosis can be cured. Relapse rates are less than 5% with current regimens. The main cause of treatment failure is nonadherence to therapy.

American Thoracic Society; Centers for Disease Control and Prevention; Infectious Diseases Society of America: controlling tuberculosis in the United States. Am J Respir Crit Care Med 2005;172:1169. [PMID: 16249321]

Blumberg HM et al: American Thoracic Society/Centers for Disease Control and Prevention/Infectious Diseases Society of America: treatment of tuberculosis. Am J Respir Crit Care Med 2003;167:603. [PMID: 12588714]

Blumberg HM et al: Update on the treatment of tuberculosis and latent tuberculosis infection. JAMA 2005;293:2776. [PMID: 15941808]

Brodie D et al: The diagnosis of tuberculosis. Clin Chest Med 2005;26:247. [PMID: 15837109]

Burman WJ: Issues in the management of HIV-related tuberculosis. Clin Chest Med 2005;26:283. [PMID: 15837111]

Diagnostic Standards and Classification of Tuberculosis in Adults and Children. American Thoracic Society and Centers for Disease Control and Prevention. Am J Respir Crit Care Med 2000;161(4 Part 1):1376. [PMID: 10764337]

Frieden TR et al: Tuberculosis. Lancet 2003;362:887. [PMID: 13678977]

PULMONARY DISEASE CAUSED BY NONTUBERCULOUS MYCOBACTERIA

 ESSENTIALS OF DIAGNOSIS

- *Chronic cough, sputum production, and fatigue; less commonly: malaise, dyspnea, fever, hemoptysis, and weight loss.*
- *Parenchymal infiltrates on chest radiograph, often with thin-walled cavities, that spread contiguously and often involve overlying pleura.*
- *Isolation of nontuberculous mycobacteria in a sputum culture.*

General Considerations

Mycobacteria other than *M tuberculosis*—nontuberculous mycobacteria (NTM), sometimes referred to as "atypical" mycobacteria—are ubiquitous in water and soil and have been isolated from tap water. There appears to be a continuing increase in the number and prevalence of NTM species. Marked geographic variability exists, both in the NTM species responsible for disease and in the prevalence of disease. These organisms are not considered communicable from person to person, have distinct laboratory characteristics, and are often resistant to most antituberculous drugs. See Chapter 33 for further information.

Definition & Pathogenesis

The diagnosis of lung disease caused by NTM is based on a combination of clinical, radiographic, and bacteriologic criteria and the exclusion of other diseases that can resemble the condition. Specific diagnostic criteria are discussed below. Complementary data are important for diagnosis because NTM organisms can reside in or colonize the airways without causing clinical disease, especially in patients with AIDS, and many patients have preexisting lung disease that may make their chest radiographs abnormal.

Mycobacterium avium complex (MAC) is the most frequent cause of NTM pulmonary disease in humans in the United States. *Mycobacterium kansasii* is the next most frequent pulmonary pathogen. Other NTM causes of pulmonary disease include *Mycobacterium abscessus*, *Mycobacterium xenopi*, and *Mycobacterium malmoense;* the list of more unusual etiologic NTM species is long. Most NTM cause a chronic, slowly progressive pulmonary infection that resembles tuberculosis but tends to progress

more slowly. Disseminated disease is rare in immunocompetent hosts; however, disseminated MAC disease is common in patients with AIDS.

Clinical Findings

A. SYMPTOMS AND SIGNS

Most patients with NTM infection experience a chronic cough, sputum production, and fatigue. Less common symptoms include malaise, dyspnea, fever, hemoptysis, and weight loss. Symptoms from coexisting lung disease (commonly COPD, bronchiectasis, previous mycobacterial disease, cystic fibrosis, and pneumoconiosis) may confound the evaluation.

Common physical findings include fever and altered breath sounds, including rales or rhonchi.

B. LABORATORY FINDINGS

The diagnosis of NTM infection rests on recovery of the pathogen from cultures. Sputum cultures positive for atypical mycobacteria do not in themselves prove infection because NTM may exist as saprophytes colonizing the airways or may be environmental contaminants. Bronchial washings are considered to be more sensitive than expectorated sputum samples; however, their specificity for clinical disease is not known.

Bacteriologic criteria have been proposed based on studies of patients with cavitary disease with MAC or *M kansasii*. Diagnostic criteria in HIV-seronegative or immunocompetent hosts include the following: (1) at least three sputum or bronchial wash samples within a 1-year period with the following findings: three positive cultures with negative acid-fast bacilli (AFB) smears or two positive cultures and one positive AFB smear; (2) if expectorated sputum samples are not available, a single bronchial wash culture with 2+ to 4+ growth or any positive culture plus a 2+ to 4+ AFB smear. The diagnosis can also be established by demonstrating NTM in a lung biopsy or bronchial wash plus histopathologic changes such as granulomatous inflammation in a lung biopsy. Rapid species identification of some NTM is possible using DNA probes or high-pressure liquid chromatography.

Diagnostic criteria are less stringent for patients with severe immune suppression. HIV-infected patients may show significant MAC growth on culture of bronchial washings without clinical infection, and, therefore, HIV patients being evaluated for MAC infection must be considered individually.

In general, drug susceptibility testing on cultures of NTM is not recommended except for the following NTM: (1) *M kansasii* and rifampin; (2) rapid growers (such as *Mycobacterium fortuitum*, *Mycobacterium chelonei*, *M abscessus*) and amikacin, doxycycline, imipenem, fluoroquinolones, clarithromycin, cefoxitin, and a sulfonamide.

C. IMAGING

Chest radiographic findings include infiltrates that are progressive or persist for at least 2 months, cavitary lesions, and multiple nodular densities. The cavities are often thin-walled and have less surrounding parenchymal infiltrate than is commonly seen with MTB infections. Evidence of contiguous spread and pleural involvement is often present. High-resolution CT of the chest may show multiple small nodules with or without multifocal bronchiectasis. Progression of pulmonary infiltrates during therapy or lack of radiographic improvement over time are poor prognostic signs and also raise concerns about secondary or alternative pulmonary processes. Clearing of pulmonary infiltrates due to NTM is slow.

Treatment

Treatment regimens and responses vary with the species of NTM. Disease caused by *M kansasii* responds well to drug therapy. A daily regimen of rifampin, isoniazid, and ethambutol for at least 18 months with a minimum of 12 months of negative cultures is usually successful.

The treatment of the immunocompetent patient with MAC infection is controversial and largely empiric. Traditional chemotherapeutic regimens have taken an aggressive approach using a combination of agents, but these have been associated with a high incidence of drug-induced side effects. Adherence to such regimens is also difficult. Non-HIV-infected patients with MAC pulmonary disease usually receive a combination of daily clarithromycin or azithromycin, rifampin or rifabutin, and ethambutol. Streptomycin is considered for the first 2 months as tolerated. The optimal duration of treatment is unknown, but therapy should be continued for 12 months after sputum conversion. Medical treatment is initially successful in about two-thirds of cases, but relapses after treatment are common; long-term benefit is demonstrated in about half of all patients. Those who do not respond favorably generally have active but stable disease. Surgical resection is an alternative for the patient with progressive disease that responds poorly to chemotherapy; the success rate with surgical therapy is good.

Field SK et al: *Mycobacterium avium* complex pulmonary disease in patients without HIV infection. Chest 2004;126:566. [PMID: 15302746]

Kim JS et al: Nontuberculous mycobacterial infection: CT scan findings, genotype, and treatment responsiveness. Chest 2005;128:3863. [PMID: 16354855]

Wagner D et al: Nontuberculous mycobacterial infections: a clinical review. Infection 2004;32:257. [PMID: 15624889]

■ PULMONARY NEOPLASMS

SCREENING FOR LUNG CANCER

Periodic evaluation of asymptomatic people at high risk for lung cancer is an attractive strategy without demonstrated benefit. Available evidence from the Mayo Lung Project suggests that serial chest radiographs can identify a significant number of early stage malignancies but that neither disease-specific mortality from lung cancer nor all-cause mortality is affected by screening. The illusory benefits of screening have been attributed to lead time, length time, and overdiagnosis biases. Since three large randomized clinical trials published between 1984 and 1986 came to similar conclusions, screening for lung cancer has not been recommended by any major advisory group.

The availability of rapid-acquisition, low-dose helical computed tomography (LDCT) has rekindled enthusiasm for lung cancer screening. LDCT is a very sensitive test. Compared with chest radiography, LDCT identifies between four and ten times the number of asymptomatic lung malignancies. LDCT may also increase the number of false-positive tests, unnecessary diagnostic procedures, and overdiagnosis. A mortality benefit remains to be proved. The National Lung Cancer Screening Trial is an ongoing NCI-funded multicenter trial to determine whether using LDCT to screen current or former heavy smokers for lung cancer will improve mortality in this population. Information is available at http://www.cancer.gov/NLST/.

Humphrey LL et al: Lung cancer screening with sputum cytologic examination, chest radiography, and computed tomography: an update for the U.S. Preventive Services Task Force. Ann Intern Med 2004;140:740. [PMID: 15126259]

Mulshine JL et al: Clinical practice. Lung cancer screening. N Engl J Med 2005;352:2714. [PMID: 15987920]

SOLITARY PULMONARY NODULE

A solitary pulmonary nodule, sometimes referred to as a "coin lesion," is a < 3 cm isolated, rounded opacity on the chest radiograph outlined by normal lung and not associated with infiltrate, atelectasis, or adenopathy. Most are asymptomatic and represent an unexpected finding on chest radiography. The finding is important because it carries a significant risk of malignancy. The frequency of malignancy in surgical series ranges from 10% to 68% depending on patient population. Most benign nodules are infectious granulomas. **Benign neoplasms** such as hamartomas account for less than 5% of solitary nodules.

The goals of evaluation are to identify and resect malignant tumors in patients who stand to benefit from resection while avoiding invasive procedures in benign disease. The task is to identify nodules with a sufficiently high probability of malignancy to warrant biopsy or resection or a sufficiently low probability of malignancy to justify observation.

Symptoms alone rarely establish the cause, but clinical and radiographic data can be used to assess the probability of malignancy. The patient's age is important. Malignant nodules are rare in persons under age 30. Above age 30, the likelihood of malignancy increases with age. Smokers are at increased risk, and the likelihood of malignancy increases with the number of cigarettes smoked daily. Patients with a prior malignancy have a higher likelihood of having a malignant solitary nodule.

The first and most important step in the radiographic evaluation is to review old radiographs. Comparison with prior studies allows estimation of doubling time, which is an important marker for malignancy. Rapid progression (doubling time less than 30 days) suggests infection; long-term stability (doubling time over 465 days) suggests benignity. Certain radiographic features help in estimating the probability of malignancy. Increasing size is correlated with malignancy. A recent study of solitary nodules identified by CT scan showed a 1% malignancy rate in those measuring 2–5 mm, 24% in 6–10 mm, 33% in 11–20 mm, and 80% in 21–45 mm. The appearance of a smooth, well-defined edge is characteristic of a benign process. Ill-defined margins or a lobular appearance suggest malignancy. A high-resolution CT finding of spiculated margins and a peripheral halo are both highly associated with malignancy. Calcification and its pattern are also helpful clues. Benign lesions tend to have dense calcification in a central or laminated pattern. Malignant lesions are associated with sparser calcification that is typically stippled or eccentric. Cavitary lesions with thick (> 16 mm) walls are much more likely to be malignant. High-resolution CT offers better resolution of these characteristics than chest radiography and is more likely to detect lymphadenopathy or the presence of multiple lesions. High-resolution CT is indicated in any suspicious solitary pulmonary nodule.

Treatment

Based on clinical and radiologic data, the clinician should assign a specific probability of malignancy to the lesion. The decision whether and how to obtain a diagnostic biopsy depends on the interpretation of this probability in light of the patient's unique clinical situation. The probabilities in parentheses below represent guidelines only and should not be interpreted as prescriptive.

In the case of solitary pulmonary nodules, a continuous probability function may be grouped into three categories. In patients with a low probability (< 8%) of malignancy (eg, age under 30, lesions stable for more than 2 years, characteristic pattern of benign calcification), watchful waiting is appropriate. Management consists of serial radiographs every 3 months for 1 year and then every 6 months for a second year. Three-dimensional reconstruction of high-resolution CT images may provide a more sensitive test for growth. These techniques are in research trials.

Patients with a high probability (> 70%) of malignancy should proceed directly to resection following staging, provided there are no contraindications to surgery. Biopsies rarely yield a specific benign diagnosis and are not indicated.

Optimal management of patients with an intermediate probability of malignancy (8–70%) remains contro-versial. The traditional approach is to obtain a diagnostic biopsy either through transthoracic needle aspiration (TTNA) or bronchoscopy. Bronchoscopy yields a diagnosis in 10–80% of procedures depending on the size of the nodule and its location. Complications are generally rare. TTNA has a higher diagnostic yield, reported to be between 50% and 97%. The yield is strongly operator-dependent, however, and is affected by the location and size of the lesion. Complications are higher than bronchoscopy, with pneumothorax occurring in up to 30% of patients.

Disappointing diagnostic yields and a high false-negative rate (up to 25–30% in TTNA) have prompted alternative approaches. Several new imaging techniques may help improve the specificity of high-resolution CT in excluding malignancy. Malignant nodules tend to be more highly vascularized and therefore show increased enhancement on high-resolution CT following the intravenous infusion of iodine-containing contrast media. Sensitivity and specificity appear promising but await validation. Positron emission tomography (PET) detects increased glucose metabolism within malignant lesions with high sensitivity (85–97%) and specificity (70–85%). Many diagnostic algorithms have incorporated PET into the assessment of patients with inconclusive high-resolution CT findings. PET has several drawbacks, however: resolution below 1 cm is poor, the test is expensive, and availability remains limited. Sputum cytology is highly specific but lacks sensitivity. It is used in central lesions and in patients who are poor candidates for invasive diagnostic procedures. Researchers have attempted to improve the sensitivity of sputum cytology through the use of monoclonal antibodies to proteins that are up-regulated in pulmonary malignancies. Such tests offer promise but remain research tools at this time.

Video-assisted thoracoscopic surgery (VATS) offers a more aggressive approach to diagnosis. VATS is more invasive than bronchoscopy or TTNA but is associated with less postoperative pain, shorter hospital stays, and more rapid return to function than traditional thoracotomy. These advantages have led some centers to recommend VATS resection of all solitary pulmonary nodules with intermediate probability of malignancy. In some cases, surgeons will remove the nodule and evaluate it in the operating room with frozen section. If the nodule is malignant, they will proceed to lobectomy and lymph node sampling, either thoracoscopically or through conversion to standard thoracotomy.

Gurney JW: Determining the likelihood of malignancy in solitary pulmonary nodules with Bayesian analysis. Part I. Theory. Radiology 1993;186:405. [PMID: 8421743]

MacMahon H et al: Guidelines for management of small pulmonary nodules detected on CT scans: a statement from the Fleischner Society. Radiology 2005;237:395. [PMID: 16244247]

Ost D et al: Clinical practice. The solitary pulmonary nodule. N Engl J Med 2003;348:2535. [PMID: 12815140]

BRONCHOGENIC CARCINOMA

ESSENTIALS OF DIAGNOSIS

- *New cough, or change in chronic cough.*
- *Dyspnea, hemoptysis, anorexia, weight loss.*
- *Enlarging nodule or mass; persistent infiltrate, atelectasis, or pleural effusion on chest radiograph or CT scan.*
- *Cytologic or histologic findings of lung cancer in sputum, pleural fluid, or biopsy specimen.*

General Considerations

Lung cancer is the leading cause of cancer deaths in both men and women. The American Cancer Society estimates 172,570 new diagnoses and 163,510 deaths from lung cancer in the United States in 2005, accounting for approximately 13% of new cancer diagnoses and 28% of all cancer deaths. More Americans now die of lung cancer than of colorectal, breast, and prostate cancers combined. This dramatic increase in a previously reportable disease is causally related to exposure to carcinogens through inhalation of tobacco smoke. The causal connection between cigarettes and lung cancer is now established not only epidemiologically but also through identification of carcinogens in tobacco smoke and analysis of the effect of these carcinogens on specific oncogenes expressed in lung cancer. Even cigarette manufacturers no longer dispute the role of tobacco in this epidemic.

Cigarette smoking causes more than 80% of cases of lung cancer. Through the 1990s, mortality from lung cancer fell among men while it increased among women, reflecting changing patterns of tobacco use over the past 30 years (see Chapter 1). Other environmental risk factors for the development of lung cancer include exposure to environmental tobacco smoke, radon gas (among uranium miners and in areas where radium in the soil causes significant indoor air contamination), asbestos (60- to 100-fold increased risk in smokers with asbestos exposure), metals (arsenic, chromium, nickel, iron oxide), and industrial carcinogens (bis-chloromethyl ether). A familial predisposition to lung cancer is recognized. Certain diseases are associated with an increased risk of lung cancer, including pulmonary fibrosis, COPD, and sarcoidosis. Second primary lung cancers are more frequent in patients who survive their initial lung cancer.

The mean age at diagnosis of lung cancer is 60; it is unusual under the age of 40. After the diagnosis of lung cancer is made, approximately 40% of patients survive 1 year. The combined 5-year survival rate for all stages of lung cancer is now approximately 15%, improved from 12% in 1974–1976.

Four histologic types of bronchogenic carcinoma account for more than 90% of cases of primary lung cancer. **Squamous cell carcinoma** (25–35% of cases) arises from the bronchial epithelium, typically as a centrally located, intraluminal sessile or polypoid mass. Squamous cell tumors are more likely to present with hemoptysis and more frequently are diagnosed by sputum cytology. They spread locally and may be associated with hilar adenopathy and mediastinal widening on chest radiography. **Adenocarcinoma** (35–40% of cases) arises from mucus glands or, in the case of the **bronchioloalveolar cell carcinoma** (2% of cases), from any epithelial cell within or distal to the terminal bronchioles. Adenocarcinomas usually present as peripheral nodules or masses. Bronchioloalveolar cell carcinoma spreads intra-alveolarly and may present as an infiltrate or as single or multiple pulmonary nodules. **Large cell carcinoma** (5–10% of cases) is a heterogeneous group of relatively undifferentiated tumors that share large cells and do not fit into other categories. Large cell carcinomas typically have rapid doubling times and an aggressive clinical course. They present as central or peripheral masses. **Small cell carcinoma** (15–20% of cases) is a tumor of bronchial origin that typically begins centrally, infiltrating submucosally to cause narrowing or obstruction of the bronchus without a discrete luminal mass. Hilar and mediastinal abnormalities are common on chest radiography.

For purposes of staging and treatment, bronchogenic carcinoma is divided into small cell lung cancer (SCLC) and the other three types, conveniently labeled non–small cell lung cancer (NSCLC). This practical classification reflects different natural histories and different treatment. SCLC is prone to early hematogenous spread. It is rarely amenable to surgical resection and has a very aggressive course with a median survival (untreated) of 6–18 weeks. The three histologic categories comprising NSCLC spread more slowly. They may be cured in the early stages following resection, and they respond similarly to chemotherapy.

Clinical Findings

Lung cancer is symptomatic at diagnosis in 75–90% of patients. The clinical presentation depends on the type and location of the primary tumor, the extent of local spread, and the presence of distant metastases and any paraneoplastic syndromes.

A. SYMPTOMS AND SIGNS

Anorexia, weight loss, or asthenia occurs in 55–90% of patients presenting with a new diagnosis of lung cancer. Up to 60% of patients have a new cough or a change in a chronic cough; 6–31% have hemoptysis; and 25–40% complain of pain, sometimes nonspecific chest pain but often referable to bony metastases to the vertebrae, ribs, or pelvis. Local spread may cause endobronchial obstruction with atelectasis and postobstructive pneumonia, pleural effusion (12–33%), change in voice (compromise of the recurrent laryngeal nerve), superior vena cava syndrome (obstruction of the superior vena cava with supraclavicular venous engorgement), and Horner's syndrome (ipsilateral ptosis, miosis, and anhidrosis from involvement of the inferior cervical ganglion and the paravertebral sympathetic chain). Distant metastases to the liver are associated with asthenia and weight loss. Brain metastases (10%; more common in adenocarcinoma) may present with headache, nausea, vomiting, seizures, or altered mental status.

Paraneoplastic syndromes are incompletely understood patterns of organ dysfunction related to immune-mediated or secretory effects of neoplasms (see Chapter 40). These syndromes occur in 10–20% of lung cancer patients. They may precede, accompany, or follow the diagnosis of lung cancer. They do not necessarily indicate metastatic disease. Fifteen percent of patients with small cell carcinoma will develop syndrome of inappropriate antidiuretic hormone (SIADH); 10% of patients with squamous cell carcinoma will develop hypercalcemia. Digital clubbing is seen in up to 20% of patients at diagnosis. Other common paraneoplastic syndromes include increased ACTH production, anemia, hypercoagulability, peripheral neuropathy, and the Eaton-Lambert myasthenia syndrome. Their recognition is important because treatment of the primary tumor may improve or resolve symptoms even when the cancer is not curable.

B. LABORATORY FINDINGS

The diagnosis of lung cancer rests on examination of a tissue or cytology specimen. Sputum cytology is highly specific but insensitive; the yield is highest when there are lesions in the central airways. Thoracentesis (sensitivity 50–65%) can be used to establish a diagnosis of lung cancer in patients with malignant pleural effusions. If cytologic examination of an adequate sample (50–100 mL) of pleural fluid is nondiagnostic, the procedure should be repeated once. If results remain negative, thoracoscopy is preferred to blind pleural biopsy. Fine-needle aspiration of palpable supraclavicular or cervical lymph nodes is frequently diagnostic. Serum tumor markers are neither sensitive nor specific enough to aid in diagnosis.

Fiberoptic bronchoscopy allows visualization of the major airways, cytology brushing of visible lesions or lavage of lung segments with cytologic evaluation of specimens, direct biopsy of endobronchial abnormalities, blind transbronchial biopsy of the pulmonary parenchyma or peripheral nodules, and fine-needle aspiration biopsy of mediastinal lymph nodes. Diagnostic yield varies widely (10–90%) depending on the size of the lesion and its location. Recent advances include fluorescence bronchoscopy, which improves the ability to identify early endobronchial lesions; and endoscopic ultrasound, which permits more accurate direction of fine-needle aspiration. TTNA has a sensitivity between 50% and 97%. Mediastinoscopy, VATS, and thoracotomy are necessary in cases where less invasive techniques fail to yield a diagnosis.

C. IMAGING

Nearly all patients with lung cancer have abnormal findings on chest radiography or CT scan. These findings are rarely specific for a particular diagnosis. Interpretation of characteristic findings in isolated nodules is described above (see Solitary Pulmonary Nodule).

D. SPECIAL EXAMINATIONS

1. Staging—Accurate staging (Table 9–15) is crucial (1) to provide the clinician with information to guide treatment, (2) to provide the patient with accurate information regarding prognosis, and (3) to standardize entry criteria for clinical trials to allow interpretation of results.

There are two essential principles of staging NSCLC. First, the more extensive the disease, the worse the prognosis; second, surgical resection offers the best and perhaps the only realistic hope for cure. Staging of NSCLC uses two integrated systems. The **TNM international staging system** attempts a physical description of the neoplasm: T describes the size and location of the primary tumor; N describes the presence and location of nodal metastases; and M refers to the presence or absence of distant metastases. These TNM stages are grouped into prognostic categories (stages I–IV) using the results of clinical trials. This classification is used to guide therapy. Many patients with stage I and stage II disease are cured through surgery. Patients with stage IIIB and stage IV disease do not benefit from surgery. Patients with stage IIIA disease have locally invasive disease that may benefit from surgery in certain circumstances.

SCLC is not staged using the TNM system because micrometastases are assumed to be present on diagnosis. SCLC is divided into two categories: **limited disease** (30%), when the tumor is limited to the unilateral hemithorax (including contralateral mediastinal nodes); or **extensive disease** (70%), when the tumor extends beyond the hemithorax (including pleural effusion). This scheme also guides therapy. Patients with limited SCLC benefit from thoracic radiation therapy in addition to chemotherapy and may benefit from prophylactic cranial radiation therapy.

For both SCLC and NSCLC, staging begins with a thorough history and physical examination. A complete examination is essential to exclude obvious metastatic disease to lymph nodes, skin, and bone. A detailed history is essential because the patient's performance status is a powerful predictor of disease course. All patients should have measurement of a complete blood count, electrolytes including calcium, creatinine, liver tests including LDH and alkaline phosphatase, and a chest radiograph. Further evaluation will follow the results of these tests. In general, screening asymptomatic lung cancer patients with CT and MRI imaging of the brain, radionuclide bone imaging, and abdominal CT imaging does not change patient outcomes. These tests should be targeted to specific symptoms and signs (see Table 9–16).

NSCLC patients being considered for surgery require meticulous evaluation to identify those with resectable disease. CT imaging is the most important modality for staging candidates for resection. A chest CT scan precisely defines the size of parenchymal lesions

Table 9–15. TNM staging for lung cancer.

Stage	T	N	M	Description
0	Tis			Carcinoma in situ
IA	T1	N0	M0	Limited local disease without nodal or distant metastases
IB	T2	N0	M0	
IIA	T1	N1	M0	Limited local disease with ipsilateral hilar or peribronchial nodal involvement but not distant metastases *or*
IIB	T2	N1	M0	
	T3	N0	M0	Locally invasive disease without nodal or distant metastases
IIIA	T3	N1	M0	Locally invasive disease with ipsilateral or peribronchial nodal involvement but not distant metastases *or*
	T1–3	N2	M0	Limited or locally invasive disease with ipsilateral mediastinal or subcarinal nodal involvement but not distant metastases
IIIB	Any T	N3	M0	Any primary with contralateral mediastinal or hilar nodes, or ipsilateral scalene or supraclavicular nodes *or*
	T4	Any N	M0	Unresectable local invasion with any degree of adenopathy but no distant metastases; malignant pleural effusion
IV	Any T	Any N	M1	Distant metastases
Primary Tumor (T)				
TX	Primary tumor cannot be assessed; or tumor proved by the presence of malignant cells in sputum or bronchial washings but not visualized by imaging or bronchoscopy.			
T0	No evidence of primary tumor.			
Tis	Carcinoma in situ.			
T1	A tumor ≤ 3 cm in greatest dimension, surrounded by lung or visceral pleura, and without evidence of invasion proximal to a lobar bronchus at bronchoscopy.			
T2	A tumor > 3.0 cm in greatest dimension, or a tumor of any size that either involves a main bronchus (but is ≥ 2 cm distal to the carina), invades the visceral pleura, or has associated atelectasis or obstructive pneumonitis extending to the hilar region. Any associated atelectasis or obstructive pneumonitis must involve less than an entire lung.			
T3	A tumor of any size with direct extension into the chest wall (including superior sulcus tumors), the diaphragm, the mediastinal pleura, or the parietal pericardium; or a tumor in the main bronchus < 2 cm distal to the carina without involving the carina; or associated atelectasis or obstructive pneumonitis of the entire lung.			
T4	A tumor of any size with invasion of the mediastinum, heart, great vessels, trachea, esophagus, vertebral body, or carina; or with a malignant pleural or pericardial effusion; or with satellite tumor nodules within the ipsilateral lobe of the lung containing the primary tumor.			
Regional Lymph Nodes (N)				
NX	Regional lymph nodes cannot be assessed.			
N0	No demonstrable metastasis to regional lymph nodes.			
N1	Metastasis to lymph nodes in the peribronchial or the ipsilateral hilar region, or both, including direct extension.			
N2	Metastasis to ipsilateral mediastinal lymph nodes and/or subcarinal lymph nodes.			
N3	Metastasis to contralateral mediastinal lymph nodes, contralateral hilar lymph nodes, ipsilateral or contralateral scalene or supraclavicular lymph nodes.			
Distant Metastases (M)				
MX	Presence of distant metastasis cannot be assessed.			
M0	No (known) distant metastasis.			
M1	Distant metastasis present.			

Adapted from Mountain CF: Revisions in the international system for staging lung cancer. Chest 1997;111:1710.

Table 9–16. Approach to staging of patients with lung cancer.

Part A: Recommended tests for all patients
  Complete blood count
  Electrolytes, calcium, alkaline phosphatase, albumin, AST, ALT, total bilirubin, creatinine
  Chest radiograph
  CT of chest through the adrenal glands[1,2]
  Pathologic confirmation of malignancy[3]

Part B: Recommended tests for selected but not all patients

Test	Indication
CT with contrast of liver or liver ultrasound	Elevated liver function tests; abnormal non-contrast-enhanced CT of liver or abnormal clinical evaluation
CT with contrast of brain or MRI of brain	CNS symptoms or abnormal clinical evaluation
Whole body ^{18}F-fluoro-deoyx-D-glucose positron emission tomography scan (FDG-PET)	To evaluate the mediastinum in patients who are candidates for surgery
Radionuclide bone scan	Elevated alkaline phosphatase (bony fraction), elevated calcium, bone pain, or abnormal clinical evaluation
Pulmonary function tests	If lung resection or thoracic radiotherapy planned
Quantitative radionuclide perfusion lung scan or exercise testing to evaluate maximum oxygen consumption	Patients with borderline resectability due to limited cardiovascular status

[1]May not be necessary if patient has obvious M1 disease on chest x-ray or physical examination.
[2]Intravenous iodine contrast enhancement is not essential but is recommended in probable mediastinal invasion.
[3]While optimal in most cases, tissue diagnosis may not be necessary prior to surgery in some cases where the lesion is enlarging or the patient will undergo surgical resection regardless of the outcome of a biopsy.
Modified and reproduced, with permission, from: Pretreatment evaluation of non-small cell lung cancer. Consensus Statement of the American Thoracic Society and the European Respiratory Society. Am J Respir Crit Care Med 1997;156:320.

and identifies atelectatic lung or pleural effusions. However, CT imaging is less accurate at determining invasion of the chest wall (sensitivity 62%) or mediastinum (sensitivity 60–75%). The sensitivity and specificity of CT imaging for identifying lung cancer metastatic to the mediastinal lymph nodes are 57% (49–66%) and 82% (77–86%), respectively. Therefore, chest CT imaging does not provide definitive information on staging. CT imaging does help in making the decision about whether to proceed to resection of the primary tumor and sample the mediastinum at thoracotomy (common if there are no lymph nodes > 1 cm) or to use TTNA, mediastinoscopy, esophageal ultrasound with transesophageal needle aspiration, or limited thoracotomy to biopsy suspected metastatic disease (common where there are lymph nodes > 1–2 cm).

PET using 2-[18F]fluoro-2-deoxyglucose (FDG) is a noninvasive alternative for identifying metastatic foci in the mediastinum or distant sites. The sensitivity and specificity of PET for detecting mediastinal spread of primary lung cancer depend on the size of mediastinal nodes or masses. When only normal-sized (< 1 cm) mediastinal lymph nodes are present, the sensitivity and specificity of PET for tumor involvement of nodes are 74% and 96%, respectively. When CT shows enlarged (> 1 cm) lymph nodes, the sensitivity and specificity are 95% and 76%, respectively.

PET imaging is being incorporated into diagnostic algorithms that take advantage of both its positive and negative predictive values. Many lung cancer specialists find PET most useful to confirm lack of metastatic disease in NSCLC patients who are candidates for surgical resection. There is also evidence that PET imaging reduces futile thoracotomies by identifying mediastinal and distant metastases in patients with NSCLC. Disadvantages of PET imaging include limited resolution below 1 cm; the expense of FDG; limited availability; and false-positive scans due to sarcoidosis, tuberculosis, or fungal infections.

2. Preoperative assessment—See Chapter 3.

3. Pulmonary function testing—Many patients with NSCLC have moderate to severe chronic lung disease that increases the risk of perioperative complications as well as long-term pulmonary insufficiency following lung resection. All patients considered for surgery require spirometry. In the absence of other comorbidities, patients with good lung function (preoperative $FEV_1 > 2$ L) are at low risk for complications from lobectomy or pneumonectomy. If the FEV_1 is less than 2 L, then an estimated postoperative FEV_1 should be calculated. The postresection FEV_1 may be estimated from considering preoperative spirometry and the amount of lung to be resected; in severe obstructive disease, a quantitative lung perfusion scan may improve the estimate. A predicted post-lung resection $FEV_1 > 800$ mL (or > 40% of predicted FEV_1) is associated with a low incidence of perioperative complications. High-risk patients include those with a predicted postoperative $FEV_1 < 700$ mL (or < 40% of predicted FEV_1). In these patients—and in those with borderline spirometry—cardiopulmonary exercise testing may be helpful. A maximal oxygen uptake ($\dot{V}O_2$) of > 15 mL/kg/min identifies patients with an acceptable incidence of complications and mortality. Patients with an $\dot{V}O_2$ of < 10 mL/kg/min have a very high mortality rate at thoracotomy. Hypoxemia and hypercapnia are not independent predictors of outcome.

Treatment

A. NON–SMALL CELL CARCINOMA

Cure of NSCLC is unlikely without resection. Therefore, the initial approach to the patient is determined by the answers to two questions: (1) Is complete surgical resection technically feasible? (2) If yes, is the patient able to tolerate the surgery with acceptable morbidity and mortality? Clinical features that preclude complete resection include extrathoracic metastases or a malignant pleural effusion; or tumor involving the heart, pericardium, great vessels, esophagus, recurrent laryngeal or phrenic nerves, trachea, main carina, or contralateral mediastinal lymph nodes. Accordingly, stage I and stage II patients are treated with surgical resection where possible. Stage IIIA patients have poor outcomes when treated with resection alone. They should be referred to multimodality protocols, including chemotherapy and radiotherapy. Stage IIIB patients treated with combined chemotherapy and radiation therapy have improved survival. Selected stage IIIB patients taken to resection following multimodality therapy have shown long-term survival and may be cured. Stage IV patients are treated with symptom-based palliative therapy, which may include outpatient chemotherapy (see below).

Surgical approach affects outcome. In a prospective trial of stage I patients randomized to lobectomy versus limited resection, there was a threefold increased rate of local recurrence in the limited resection group and a trend toward mortality benefit at 5 years in the lobectomy patients (56% versus 73% mortality, P = .09). There are inadequate outcome data on which to base a comparison of VATS with standard thoracotomy. Radiation therapy following surgery improves local control but does not improve survival.

Neoadjuvant chemotherapy consists of giving antineoplastic drugs in advance of surgery or radiation therapy. There is no consensus on the impact of neoadjuvant therapy on survival in stage I and stage II NSCLC. Such therapy is not recommended outside of ongoing clinical trials. Neoadjuvant therapy is more widely used in selected patients with stage IIIA or stage IIIB disease. Some studies suggest a survival advantage. This remains an area of active research.

Adjuvant chemotherapy consists of administering antineoplastic drugs following surgery or radiation therapy. Adjuvant chemotherapy with alkylating agents such as cyclophosphamide increases mortality. In stage I and N0 stage II disease, patients treated with multidrug platinum-based chemotherapy show a trend toward improved survival—on the order of 3 months at 5 years. Toxicity may be significant, however, and such therapy is not recommended. Newer antineoplastic agents with less toxicity are in clinical trials in these patients. In patients with stage IIIA disease and node positive stage II disease, the data are conflicting whether chemotherapy following surgery improves survival. Patients with locally advanced disease (stages IIIA and IIIB) who are not surgical candidates have improved survival when treated with combination chemotherapy and radiation therapy compared with no therapy or radiation alone.

Multidrug platinum-based chemotherapy is associated with an increase in survival equivalent to a mean gain of 6 weeks at 1 year in patients with advanced disease (stage IIIB and stage IV) but good performance status (Karnofsky performance status ≥ 60, < 5% weight loss in the past 6 months; see Chapter 40). There is no evidence of a survival benefit in patients with poor performance status.

Multiple clinical trials evaluating quality of life suggest that there is better overall performance status and symptom control in patients with stage IIIB and stage IV NSCLC receiving chemotherapy plus good supportive care versus supportive care alone. Several trials suggest an increase in median survival of from 5 months to 7 months. These trials compare small numbers of patients; they are unblinded; they are supported by the pharmaceutical companies that make the drugs used—all of which suggests caution in interpreting the results. Nonetheless, the reported findings are consistent. Furthermore, newer antineoplastic agents show increased effectiveness in advanced NSCLC along with favorable side effect profiles. It remains to be seen which patients stand to benefit most from what combination of agents. At this time, outpatient chemotherapy for advanced NSCLC should be offered on protocol to patients with good performance status.

B. SMALL CELL CARCINOMA

Response rates of SCLC to cisplatin and etoposide are excellent: 80–100% response in limited-stage disease (50–70% complete response), and 60–80% response in extensive stage disease (15–40% complete response). However, remissions tend to be short-lived with a median duration of 6–8 months. Once the disease has recurred, median survival is 3–4 months. Overall 2-year survival is 20% in limited-stage disease and 5% in extensive-stage disease. Thoracic radiation therapy improves survival in patients with limited SCLC but not those with extensive disease. Whole brain radiation therapy decreases the incidence of central nervous system disease but does not affect survival. Its effect on symptoms is controversial.

Occasionally, a patient may have a peripheral nodule resected that turns out to be SCLC. Five-year survival following resection of the equivalent of stage I and stage II SCLC is higher than in patients treated with chemotherapy.

C. PALLIATIVE THERAPY

Photoresection with the Nd:YAG laser is sometimes performed on central tumors to relieve endobronchial obstruction, improve dyspnea, and control hemoptysis. External beam radiation therapy is also used to control dyspnea and hemoptysis, pain from bony metastases, obstruction from superior vena cava syndrome, and symptomatic brain metastases. Resection of *solitary* brain metastases does not affect survival but may improve quality of life when combined with radiation therapy. Intraluminal radiation (brachytherapy) is an alternative approach to endobronchial disease. Pain syndromes are very common in advanced disease. As patients approach the end of life, meticulous efforts at pain control are essential (see Chapter 5). Consultation with or referral to a palliative care specialist is recommended in advanced disease to aid in symptom management and to facilitate referrals to hospice programs.

Prognosis

The overall 5-year survival rate for lung cancer is 15%. Predictors of survival are the type of tumor (SCLC versus NSCLC), the stage of the tumor, and the patient's performance status, including weight loss in the past 6 months. These are independent predictors in both early and late stage disease. Most data suggest that there is no difference among non–small cell carcinomas when adjusted for stage and performance status. However, squamous cell carcinoma may have a better prognosis than adenocarcinoma or large cell carcinoma at the same TNM stage. (See Table 9–17.)

American College of Chest Physicians; Health and Science Policy Committee: Diagnosis and management of lung cancer: ACCP evidence-based guidelines. Chest 2003;123(1 Suppl): 1S. [PMID: 12527560]

Barnes DJ: The changing face of lung cancer. Chest 2004;126:1718. [PMID: 15596660]

Hamilton W et al: Diagnosis of lung cancer in primary care: a structured review. Fam Pract 2004;21:605. [PMID: 15520035]

Jackman DM et al: Small-cell lung cancer. Lancet 2005;366:1385. [PMID: 16226617]

Macbeth F et al: Palliative treatment for advanced non-small cell lung cancer. Hematol Oncol Clin North Am 2004;18: 115. [PMID: 15005285]

Mazzone PJ et al: Lung cancer: Preoperative pulmonary evaluation of the lung resection candidate. Am J Med 2005; 118:578. [PMID: 15922686]

Patel JD et al: Lung cancer in US women: a contemporary epidemic. JAMA 2004;291:1763. [PMID: 15082704]

Spira A et al: Multidisciplinary management of lung cancer. N Engl J Med 2004;350:379. [PMID: 14736930]

Yang P et al: Clinical features of 5,628 primary lung cancer patients: experience at Mayo Clinic from 1997 to 2003. Chest 2005;128:452. [PMID: 16002972]

Table 9–17. Approximate survival rates following treatment for lung cancer.

Non-Small Cell Lung Cancer: Mean 5-Year Survival Following Resection		
Stage	Clinical Staging	Surgical Staging
IA (T1N0M0)	60%	74%
IB (T2N0M0)	38%	61%
IIA (T1N1M0)	34%	55%
IIB (T2N1M0, T3N0M0)	23%	39%
IIIA	9–13%	22%
IIIB[1]	3–12%	
IV[1]	4%	

Small Cell Lung Cancer: Survival Following Chemotherapy		
	Mean 2-Year	
Stage	Survival	Median Survival
Limited	15–20%	14–20 months
Extensive	< 3%	8–13 months

[1]Independent of therapy, generally not surgical patients.
Data from multiple sources. Modified and reproduced, with permission, from Reif MS et al: Evidence-based medicine in the treatment of non-small cell cancer. Clin Chest Med 2000;21:107.

BRONCHIAL CARCINOID TUMORS

Carcinoid and bronchial gland tumors are sometimes termed "bronchial adenomas." This term should be avoided because it implies that the lesions are benign, when in fact carcinoid tumors and bronchial gland carcinomas are low-grade malignant neoplasms.

Carcinoid tumors are about six times more common than bronchial gland carcinomas, and most of them occur as pedunculated or sessile growths in central bronchi. Men and women are equally affected. Most patients are under 60 years of age. Common symptoms of bronchial carcinoid tumors are hemoptysis, cough, focal wheezing, and recurrent pneumonia. Peripherally located bronchial carcinoid tumors are rare and present as asymptomatic solitary pulmonary nodules. Carcinoid syndrome (flushing, diarrhea, wheezing, hypotension) is rare. Fiberoptic bronchoscopy may reveal a pink or purple tumor in a central airway. These lesions have a well-vascularized stroma, and biopsy may be complicated by significant bleeding. CT scanning is helpful to localize the lesion and to follow its growth over time. Octreotide scintigraphy is also available for localization of these tumors.

Bronchial carcinoid tumors grow slowly and rarely metastasize. Complications involve bleeding and airway obstruction rather than invasion by tumor and metastases. Surgical excision is necessary in some cases, and the prognosis is generally favorable. Most bronchial carcinoid tumors are resistant to radiation and chemotherapy.

Fink G et al: Pulmonary carcinoid: presentation, diagnosis, and outcome in 142 cases in Israel and review of 640 cases from the literature. Chest 2001;119:1647. [PMID: 11399686]

Hage R et al: Update in pulmonary carcinoid tumors: a review article. Ann Surg Onc 2003;10:697. [PMID: 12839856]

Schnirer II et al: Carcinoid—a comprehensive review. Acta Oncolog 2003;42:672. [PMID: 14690153]

SECONDARY LUNG CANCER

Secondary lung cancers represent metastases from extrapulmonary malignant neoplasms that spread to the lungs through vascular or lymphatic channels or by direct extension. Almost any cancer can metastasize to the lung. Metastases usually occur via the pulmonary artery and typically present as multiple nodules or masses on chest radiography. The radiographic differential diagnosis of multiple pulmonary nodules also includes pulmonary arteriovenous malformation, pulmonary abscesses, granulomatous infection, sarcoidosis, rheumatoid nodules, and Wegener's granulomatosis. Metastases to the lungs are found in 20–55% of patients dying of various malignancies. Most are intraparenchymal. Endobronchial metastases occur in fewer than 5% of patients dying of nonpulmonary cancer; carcinoma of the kidney, breast, colon, and cervix and malignant melanoma are the most likely primary tumors.

Lymphangitic carcinomatosis denotes diffuse involvement of the pulmonary lymphatic network by primary or secondary lung cancer, probably a result of extension of tumor from lung capillaries to the lymphatics. **Tumor embolization** from extrapulmonary cancer (renal cell carcinoma, hepatocellular carcinoma, choriocarcinoma) is an uncommon route for tumor spread to the lungs. Secondary lung cancer may also present as malignant pleural effusion (see below).

Clinical Findings

A. SYMPTOMS AND SIGNS

Symptoms are uncommon but include cough, hemoptysis and, in advanced cases, dyspnea and hypoxemia. Symptoms are more often referable to the site of the primary tumor.

B. LABORATORY FINDINGS

The diagnosis of secondary lung cancer is usually established by identifying a primary tumor. Appropriate studies should be ordered if there is a suspicion of any primary cancer, such as breast, thyroid, testis, or prostate, for which specific treatment is available. Mammography should be considered unless one has been performed recently. If the history and physical examination fail to reveal the site of the primary tumor, attention is better focused on the lung, where tissue samples obtained by bronchoscopy, percutaneous needle biopsy, or thoracotomy may establish the histologic diagnosis and suggest the most likely primary. Occasionally, cytologic studies of pleural fluid or pleural biopsy reveal the diagnosis. Sputum cytology is rarely helpful.

C. IMAGING

Chest radiographs usually show multiple spherical densities with sharp margins. The size of metastatic lesions varies from a few millimeters (miliary densities) to large masses. Nearly all are less than 5 cm in diameter. The lesions are usually bilateral, pleural or subpleural in location, and more common in lower lung zones. Cavitation suggests primary squamous cell tumor; calcification suggests osteosarcoma. Lymphangitic spread and solitary pulmonary nodule are less common radiographic presentations of secondary lung cancer. Conventional chest radiography is less sensitive than CT scan in detecting pulmonary metastases.

Treatment

Once the diagnosis has been established, management consists of treatment of the primary neoplasm and any pulmonary complications. Surgical resection of a *solitary* pulmonary nodule is often prudent in the patient with known current or previous extrapulmonary cancer. Local resection of one or more pulmonary metastases is feasible in a few carefully selected patients with various sarcomas and carcinomas (breast, testis, colon, kidney, and head and neck). Surgical resection should be considered only if the primary tumor is under control, if the patient is a good surgical risk, if all of the metastatic tumor can be resected, if nonsurgical approaches are not available, and if there are no metastases elsewhere in the body. Relative contraindications to resection of pulmonary metastases include (1) malignant melanoma primary, (2) requirement for pneumonectomy, (3) pleural involvement, and (4) simultaneous appearance of two or more metastases. The overall 5-year survival rate in secondary lung cancer treated surgically is 20–35%. For patients with progressive disease, diligent attention to palliative care is essential (see Chapter 5).

Avdalovic M et al: Thoracic manifestations of common nonpulmonary malignancies of women. Clin Chest Med 2004;25:379. [PMID: 15099897]

Greelish JP et al: Secondary pulmonary malignancy. Surg Clin North Am 2000;80:633. [PMID: 10836010]

MESOTHELIOMA

 ESSENTIALS OF DIAGNOSIS

- *Unilateral, nonpleuritic chest pain and dyspnea.*
- *Distant (> 20 years earlier) history of exposure to asbestos.*

• *Pleural effusion or pleural thickening or both on chest radiographs.*
• *Malignant cells in pleural fluid or tissue biopsy.*

General Considerations

Mesotheliomas are primary tumors arising from the surface lining of the pleura (80% of cases) or peritoneum (20% of cases). About three-fourths of pleural mesotheliomas are diffuse (usually malignant) tumors, and the remaining one-fourth are localized (usually benign). Men outnumber women by a 3:1 ratio. Numerous studies have confirmed the association of **malignant pleural mesothelioma** with exposure to asbestos (particularly the crocidolite form). The lifetime risk to asbestos workers of developing malignant pleural mesothelioma is about 8%. Sixty to 80 percent of patients with malignant mesothelioma report a history of asbestos exposure. The latent period between exposure and onset of symptoms ranges from 20 to 40 years. The clinician should inquire about asbestos exposure through mining, milling, manufacturing, shipyard work, insulation, brake linings, building construction and demolition, roofing materials, and a variety of asbestos products (pipe, textiles, paint, tile, gaskets, panels). Although cigarette smoking significantly increases the risk of bronchogenic carcinoma in asbestos workers and aggravates asbestosis, there is no association between smoking and mesothelioma.

Clinical Findings

A. SYMPTOMS AND SIGNS

The mean age at onset of symptoms of malignant pleural mesothelioma is about 60 years. Symptoms include the insidious onset of shortness of breath, nonpleuritic chest pain, and weight loss. Physical findings include dullness to percussion, diminished breath sounds and, in some cases, digital clubbing.

B. LABORATORY FINDINGS

Pleural fluid is exudative and often hemorrhagic. VATS biopsy is usually necessary to obtain an adequate specimen for histologic diagnosis; even then, distinction from benign inflammatory conditions and from metastatic adenocarcinoma may be difficult. The histologic variants of malignant pleural mesothelioma are epithelial and fibrous (sarcomatous). Special stains and electron microscopy may be needed to confirm the diagnosis.

C. IMAGING

Radiographic abnormalities consist of nodular, irregular, unilateral pleural thickening and varying degrees of unilateral pleural effusion. There may be scoliosis toward the side of the lesion. CT scan helps demonstrate the extent of pleural involvement.

Complications

Malignant pleural mesothelioma progresses rapidly as the tumor spreads along the pleural surface to involve the pericardium, mediastinum, and contralateral pleura. The tumor may eventually extend beyond the thorax to involve abdominal lymph nodes and organs. Progressive pain and dyspnea are characteristic. Local invasion of thoracic structures may cause superior vena cava syndrome, hoarseness, Horner's syndrome, and dysphagia. Paraneoplastic syndromes associated with mesothelioma include thrombocytosis, hemolytic anemia, disseminated intravascular coagulopathy, and migratory thrombophlebitis.

Treatment

Treatment with surgery, radiotherapy, chemotherapy, and a combination of methods has been attempted but is generally unsuccessful. Some surgeons believe that extrapleural pneumonectomy is the preferred surgical approach for patients with early stage disease. Drainage of pleural effusions, pleurodesis, radiation therapy, and even surgical resection may offer palliative benefit in some patients.

Prognosis

Most patients die of respiratory failure and complications of local extension. Median survival time from onset of symptoms ranges from 4 months in extensive disease to 16 months in localized disease. Five-year survival is less than 5%.

Robinson BW et al: Advances in malignant mesothelioma. N Engl J Med 2005;353:1591. [PMID: 16221782]

van Ruth S et al: Surgical treatment of malignant pleural mesothelioma: a review. Chest 2003;123:551. [PMID: 12576380]

MEDIASTINAL MASSES

Various developmental, neoplastic, infectious, traumatic, and cardiovascular disorders may cause masses that appear in the mediastinum on chest radiograph. A useful convention arbitrarily divides the mediastinum into three compartments—anterior, middle, and posterior—in order to classify mediastinal masses and assist in differential diagnosis. Specific mediastinal masses have a predilection for one or more of these compartments; most are located in the anterior or middle compartment. The differential diagnosis of an anterior mediastinal mass includes thymoma, teratoma, thyroid lesions, lymphoma, and mesenchymal tumors (lipoma, fibroma). The differential diagnosis of a middle mediastinal mass includes lymphadenopathy, pulmonary artery enlargement, aneurysm of the aorta or innominate artery, developmental cyst (bronchogenic, enteric, pleuropericardial), dilated azygous or hemiazygous vein, and foramen of Morgagni hernia. The differential diagnosis of a posterior mediastinal mass includes hiatus hernia, neurogenic tumor, meningocele, esophageal tumor, foramen of Bochdalek hernia, thoracic spine disease, and extramedullary hematopoiesis. The neurogenic tumor group includes neurilemmoma, neurofibroma, neurosarcoma, ganglioneuroma, and pheochromocytoma.

Symptoms and signs of mediastinal masses are nonspecific and are usually caused by the effects of the mass on surrounding structures. Insidious onset of retrosternal chest pain, dysphagia, or dyspnea is often an important clue to the presence of a mediastinal mass. In about half of cases, symptoms are absent, and the mass is detected on routine chest radiograph. Physical findings vary depending on the nature and location of the mass.

CT scanning is helpful in management; additional radiographic studies of benefit include barium swallow if esophageal disease is suspected, Doppler sonography or venography of brachiocephalic veins and the superior vena cava, and arteriography. MRI is useful; its advantages include better delineation of hilar structures and distinction between vessels and masses. MRI also allows imaging in multiple planes, whereas CT permits only axial imaging. Tissue diagnosis is necessary if a neoplastic disorder is suspected. Treatment and prognosis depend on the underlying cause of the mediastinal mass.

Aquino SL et al: Reconciliation of the anatomic, surgical, and radiographic classifications of the mediastinum. J Comp Assist Tomogr 2001;25:489. [PMID: 11351204]

Duwe BV et al: Tumors of the mediastinum. Chest 2005; 128:2893. [PMID: 16236967]

■ INTERSTITIAL LUNG DISEASE (Diffuse Parenchymal Lung Disease)

Interstitial lung disease, or diffuse parenchymal lung disease, comprises a heterogeneous group of disorders that share a common response of the lung to injury: alveolitis, or inflammation, and fibrosis of the interalveolar septum. The term "interstitial" is misleading since the pathologic process usually begins with injury to the alveolar epithelial or capillary endothelial cells. Persistent alveolitis may lead to obliteration of alveolar capillaries and reorganization of the lung parenchyma, accompanied by irreversible fibrosis. The process does not affect the airways proximal to the respiratory bronchioles. At least 180 disease entities may present as interstitial lung disease (Table 9–18). In most patients, no specific cause can be identified. In the remainder, drugs and a variety of organic and inorganic dusts are the principal causes.

The clinical consequence of widespread lung fibrosis is diminished lung compliance, which presents as restrictive lung disease. Patients usually describe an in-

Table 9–18. Differential diagnosis of interstitial lung disease.

Drug-related
  Antiarrhythmic agents (amiodarone)
  Antibacterial agents (nitrofurantoin, sulfonamides)
  Antineoplastic agents (bleomycin, cyclophosphamide, methotrexate, nitrosoureas)
  Antirheumatic agents (gold salts, penicillamine)
  Phenytoin
Environmental and occupational (inhalation exposures)
  Dust, inorganic (asbestos, silica, hard metals, beryllium)
  Dust, organic (thermophilic actinomycetes, avian antigens, *Aspergillus* species)
  Gases, fumes, and vapors (chlorine, isocyanates, paraquat, sulfur dioxide)
  Ionizing radiation
  Talc (injection drug users)
Infections
  Fungus, disseminated (*Coccidioides immitis, Blastomyces dermatitidis, Histoplasma capsulatum*)
  Mycobacteria, disseminated
  Pneumocystis jiroveci
  Viruses
Primary pulmonary disorders
  Cryptogenic organizing pneumonitis (COP)
  Idiopathic fibrosing interstitial pneumonia: Acute interstitial pneumonitis, desquamative interstitial pneumonitis, nonspecific interstitial pneumonitis, usual interstitial pneumonitis, respiratory bronchiolitis-associated interstitial lung disease
  Pulmonary alveolar proteinosis
Systemic disorders
  Acute respiratory distress syndrome
  Amyloidosis
  Ankylosing spondylitis
  Autoimmune disease: Dermatomyositis, polymyositis, rheumatoid arthritis, systemic sclerosis (scleroderma), systemic lupus erythematosus
  Chronic eosinophilic pneumonia
  Goodpasture's syndrome
  Idiopathic pulmonary hemosiderosis
  Inflammatory bowel disease
  Langerhans cell histiocytosis (eosinophilic granuloma)
  Lymphangitic spread of cancer (lymphangitic carcinomatosis)
  Lymphangioleiomyomatosis
  Pulmonary edema
  Pulmonary venous hypertension, chronic
  Sarcoidosis
  Wegener's granulomatosis

sidious onset of exertional dyspnea and cough. Sputum production is minimal. Chest examination reveals fine, late inspiratory crackles at the lung bases. Digital clubbing is seen in 25–50% of patients at diagnosis.

Pulmonary function testing shows a loss of lung volume with normal to increased airflow rates. The diffusing capacity for carbon monoxide is decreased, and hypoxemia with exercise is common. In advanced cases, resting hypoxemia may be present. The chest radiograph is normal on presentation in up to 10% of patients. More typically, it shows patchy distribution of ground-glass, reticular, or reticulonodular infiltrates. In advanced disease, there are multiple small, thick-walled cystic spaces in the lung periphery ("honeycomb" lung). Honeycombing indicates the presence of locally advanced fibrosis with destruction of normal lung architecture. Conventional CT and high-resolution CT imaging reveal in greater detail the findings described on chest radiograph. In some cases, high-resolution CT may be strongly suggestive of a specific pathologic process.

The history—particularly the occupational and medication history—may provide evidence of a specific cause. Serologic tests for antinuclear antibodies and rheumatoid factor are positive in 20–40% of patients but are rarely diagnostic. Antineutrophil cytoplasmic antibodies (ANCAs) may be diagnostic in some clinical settings. Invasive diagnostic testing is frequently necessary to make a specific diagnosis. Three diagnostic techniques are in common use: bronchoalveolar lavage, transbronchial biopsy, and surgical lung biopsy, either through an open procedure or using VATS.

Bronchoalveolar lavage may provide a specific diagnosis in cases of infection, particularly with *P jiroveci* or mycobacteria, or when cytologic examination reveals the presence of malignant cells. The findings may be suggestive if not diagnostic of eosinophilic pneumonia, Langerhans cell histiocytosis, and alveolar proteinosis. Analysis of the cellular constituents of lavage fluid may suggest a specific disease, but these findings are not diagnostic.

Transbronchial biopsy through the flexible bronchoscope is easily performed in most patients. The risks of pneumothorax (5%) and hemorrhage (1–10%) are low. However, the tissue specimens recovered are small, sampling error is common, and crush artifact may complicate diagnosis. Transbronchial biopsy can make a definitive diagnosis of sarcoidosis, lymphangitic spread of carcinoma, pulmonary alveolar proteinosis, miliary tuberculosis, and Langerhans cell histiocytosis. Transbronchial biopsy cannot establish a specific diagnosis of idiopathic interstitial pneumonia. These patients generally require surgical lung biopsy.

Surgical lung biopsy is the standard for diagnosis of interstitial lung disease. Two or three biopsies taken from multiple sites in the same lung, including apparently normal tissue, may yield a specific diagnosis as well as prognostic information regarding the extent of fibrosis versus active inflammation. Patients under age 60 without a specific diagnosis generally should undergo surgical lung biopsy. In older and sicker patients, the risks and benefits must be weighed carefully for three reasons: (1) the morbidity of the procedure can be significant;

(2) a definitive diagnosis may not be possible even with surgical lung biopsy; and (3) when a specific diagnosis is made, there may be no effective treatment. Empiric therapy or no treatment may be preferable to surgical lung biopsy in some patients.

Known causes of interstitial lung disease are dealt with in their specific sections. The important idiopathic forms are discussed below.

IDIOPATHIC FIBROSING INTERSTITIAL PNEUMONIA (Formerly: Idiopathic Pulmonary Fibrosis)

The most common diagnosis among patients presenting with interstitial lung disease is idiopathic pulmonary fibrosis, known in Britain as cryptogenic fibrosing alveolitis. Historically, this diagnosis was based on clinical and radiographic criteria with only a minority of patients undergoing surgical lung biopsy. When biopsies were obtained, the common element of fibrosis led to the grouping together of several histologic patterns under the category of idiopathic pulmonary fibrosis. We now recognize that these distinct histopathologic features are associated with different natural histories and responses to therapy (see Table 9–19). Therefore, in the evaluation of patients with idiopathic interstitial lung disease, clinicians should attempt to identify specific disorders and reserve the terms "idiopathic pulmonary fibrosis" or "cryptogenic fibrosing alveolitis" to denote only the histologic pattern of usual interstitial pneumonitis (UIP).

Patients with idiopathic fibrosing interstitial pneumonia may present with any of the histologic patterns described in Table 9–19. The first step in evaluation is to identify patients whose disease is truly idiopathic. As indicated in Table 9–18, most identifiable causes of interstitial lung disease are infectious, drug-related, or environmental or occupational agents. Interstitial lung diseases associated with other medical conditions (pulmonary-renal syndromes, collagen-vascular disease) may be identified through a careful medical history. Apart from acute interstitial pneumonia, the clinical presentations of the idiopathic interstitial pneumonias are sufficiently similar to preclude a specific diagnosis. Chest radiographs and high-resolution CT scans are occasionally diagnostic. Ultimately, many patients with apparently idiopathic disease require surgical lung biopsy to make a definitive diagnosis. The importance of accurate diagnosis is twofold. First, it allows the clinician to provide accurate information about the cause and natural history of the illness. Second, accurate diagnosis helps distinguish patients most likely to benefit from therapy. Surgical lung biopsy may spare patients with UIP treatment with potentially morbid therapies.

The diagnosis of UIP can be made on clinical grounds alone in selected patients. A diagnosis of UIP can be made with 90% confidence in patients over 65 years of age who have idiopathic disease by history and who demonstrate inspiratory crackles on physical ex-

Table 9–19. Idiopathic fibrosing interstitial pneumonias.

Name and Clinical Presentation	Histopathology	Radiographic Pattern	Response to Therapy and Prognosis
Usual interstitial pneumonia (UIP) Age 55–60, slight male predominance. Insidious dry cough and dyspnea lasting months to years. Clubbing present at diagnosis in 25–50%. Diffuse fine late inspiratory crackles on lung auscultation. Restrictive ventilatory defect and reduced diffusing capacity on pulmonary function tests. ANA and RF positive in 25% in the absence of documented collagen-vascular disease.	Patchy, temporally and geographically nonuniform distribution of fibrosis, honeycomb change, and normal lung. Type I pneumocytes are lost, and there is proliferation of alveolar type II cells. "Fibroblast foci" of actively proliferating fibroblasts and myofibroblasts. Inflammation is generally mild and consists of small lymphocytes. Intra-alveolar macrophage accumulation is present but is not a prominent feature.	Diminished lung volume. Increased linear or reticular bibasilar and subpleural opacities. Unilateral disease is rare. High-resolution CT scanning shows minimal ground-glass and variable honeycomb change. Areas of normal lung may be adjacent to areas of advanced fibrosis. Between 2% and 10% have normal chest radiographs and high-resolution CT scans on diagnosis.	No randomized study has demonstrated improved survival compared with untreated patients. Inexorably progressive. Response to corticosteroids and cytotoxic agents at best 15%, and these probably represent misclassification of histopathology. Median survival approximately 3 years, depending on stage at presentation. Current interest in antifibrotic agents.
Respiratory bronchiolitis-associated interstitial lung disease (RB-ILD)[1] Age 40–45. Presentation similar to that of UIP though in younger patients. Similar results on pulmonary function tests, but less severe abnormalities. Patients with respiratory bronchiolitis are invariably heavy smokers.	Increased numbers of macrophages evenly dispersed within the alveolar spaces. Rare fibroblast foci, little fibrosis, minimal honeycomb change. In RB-ILD the accumulation of macrophages is localized within the peribronchiolar air spaces; in DIP,[1] it is diffuse. Alveolar architecture is preserved.	May be indistinguishable from UIP. More often presents with a nodular or reticulonodular pattern. Honeycombing rare. High-resolution CT more likely to reveal diffuse ground-glass opacities and upper lobe emphysema.	Spontaneous remission occurs in up to 20% of patients, so natural history unclear. Smoking cessation is essential. Prognosis clearly better than that of UIP: median survival greater than 10 years. Corticosteroids thought to be effective, but there are no randomized clinical trials to support this view.
Acute interstitial pneumonitis (AIP) Clinically known as Hamman-Rich syndrome. Wide age range, many young patients. Acute onset of dyspnea followed by rapid development of respiratory failure. Half of patients report a viral syndrome preceding lung disease. Clinical course indistinguishable from that of idiopathic ARDS.	Pathologic changes reflect acute response to injury within days to weeks. Resembles organizing phase of diffuse alveolar damage. Fibrosis and minimal collagen deposition. May appear similar to UIP but more homogeneous and there is no honeycomb change—though this may appear if the process persists for more than a month in a patient on mechanical ventilation.	Diffuse bilateral airspace consolidation with areas of ground-glass attenuation on high-resolution CT scan.	Supportive care (mechanical ventilation) critical but effect of specific therapies unclear. High initial mortality: Fifty to 90 percent die within 2 months after diagnosis. Not progressive if patient survives. Lung function may return to normal or may be permanently impaired.
Nonspecific interstitial pneumonitis (NSIP) Age 45–55. Slight female predominance. Similar to UIP but onset of cough and dyspnea over months, not years.	Nonspecific in that histopathology does not fit into better-established categories. Varying degrees of inflammation and fibrosis, patchy in distribution but uniform in time, suggesting response to single injury. Most have lymphocytic and plasma cell inflammation without fibrosis. Honeycombing present but scant. Some have advocated division into cellular and fibrotic subtypes.	May be indistinguishable from UIP. Most typical picture is bilateral areas of ground-glass attenuation and fibrosis on high-resolution CT. Honeycombing is rare.	Treatment thought to be effective, but no prospective clinical studies have been published. Prognosis overall good but depends on the extent of fibrosis at diagnosis. Median survival greater than 10 years.

(contin᾽

Table 9–19. Idiopathic fibrosing interstitial pneumonias. (continued)

Name and Clinical Presentation	Histopathology	Radiographic Pattern	Response to Therapy and Prognosis
Cryptogenic organizing pneumonitis (formerly bronchiolitis obliterans organizing pneumonia [BOOP]) Typically age 50–60 but wide variation. Abrupt onset, frequently weeks to a few months following a flu-like illness. Dyspnea and dry cough prominent, but constitutional symptoms are common: fatigue, fever, and weight loss. Pulmonary function tests usually show restriction, but up to 25% show concomitant obstruction.	Included in the idiopathic interstitial pneumonias on clinical grounds. Buds of loose connective tissue (Masson bodies) and inflammatory cells fill alveoli and distal bronchioles.	Lung volumes normal. Chest radiograph typically shows interstitial and parenchymal disease with discrete, peripheral alveolar and ground-glass infiltrates. Nodular opacities common. High-resolution CT shows subpleural consolidation and bronchial wall thickening and dilation.	Rapid response to corticosteroids in two-thirds of patients. Long-term prognosis generally good for those who respond. Relapses are common.

[1]Includes desquamative interstitial pneumonia (DIP).
ANA = antinuclear antibody; RF = rheumatoid factor; UIP = usual interstitial pneumonia; ARDS = acute respiratory distress syndrome.

amination; restrictive physiology on pulmonary function testing; characteristic radiographic evidence of progressive fibrosis over several years; and diffuse, patchy fibrosis with pleural-based honeycombing on high-resolution CT scan. Such patients do not need surgical lung biopsy. Note that the diagnosis of UIP cannot be confirmed on transbronchial lung biopsy since the histologic diagnosis requires a pattern of changes rather than a single pathognomonic finding. Transbronchial biopsy may exclude UIP by confirming a specific alternative diagnosis.

Treatment of idiopathic fibrosing interstitial pneumonia is controversial. No randomized study has demonstrated that any treatment improves survival or quality of life compared with no treatment. Clinical experience suggests that patients with desquamative interstitial pneumonia (DIP; or respiratory bronchiolitis-associated interstitial lung disease, RB-ILD), nonspecific interstitial pneumonia (NSIP), or COP (see Table 9–19) frequently respond to corticosteroids and should be given a trial of therapy—typically prednisone, 1–2 mg/kg/d for a minimum of 2 months. The same therapy is almost uniformly ineffective in patients with UIP. Since this therapy carries significant morbidity, the pulmonary community does not recommend routine use of corticosteroids in patients with UIP. Antifibrotic therapy is an area of intense research. A clinical trial of interferon gamma-1b in UIP did not demonstrate statistically significant improvement in the primary end point of progression-free survival. No significant treatment effect was observed on measures of lung function, gas exchange, or quality of life. Subgroup analysis suggested improved survival in patients with mild to moderate disease.

American Thoracic Society; European Respiratory Society: American Thoracic Society/European Respiratory Society International Multidisciplinary Consensus Classification of the Idiopathic Interstitial Pneumonias. Am J Respir Crit Care Med 2002;165:277. [PMID: 11790668]

Collard HR et al: Demystifying idiopathic interstitial pneumonia. Arch Intern Med 2003;163:17. [PMID: 12523913]

King TE Jr: Clinical advances in the diagnosis and therapy of the interstitial lung diseases. Am J Respir Crit Care Med 2005; 172:268. [PMID: 15879420]

Leslie KO: Pathology of interstitial lung disease. Clin Chest Med 2004;25:657. [PMID: 15564015]

Lynch DA et al: Idiopathic interstitial pneumonias: CT features. Radiology 2005;236:10. [PMID: 15987960]

Swigris JJ et al: Idiopathic pulmonary fibrosis: challenges and opportunities for the clinician and investigator. Chest 2005; 127:275. [PMID: 15653995]

SARCOIDOSIS

 ESSENTIALS OF DIAGNOSIS

- *Symptoms related to the lung, skin, eyes, peripheral nerves, liver, kidney, heart, and other tissues.*
- *Demonstration of noncaseating granulomas in a biopsy specimen.*
- *Exclusion of other granulomatous disorders.*

General Considerations

Sarcoidosis is a systemic disease of unknown etiology characterized in about 90% of patients by granulomatous inflammation of the lung. The incidence is highest in North American blacks and northern European whites; among blacks, women are more frequently affected than men. Onset of disease is usually in the third or fourth decade.

Clinical Findings

A. SYMPTOMS AND SIGNS

Patients may present with malaise, fever, and dyspnea of insidious onset. Symptoms referable to the skin, eyes, peripheral nerves, liver, kidney, or heart may also cause the patient to seek care. Some individuals are asymptomatic and come to medical attention after abnormal findings (typically bilateral hilar and right paratracheal lymphadenopathy) on chest radiographs. Physical findings are atypical of interstitial lung disease: crackles are uncommon on chest examination. Other findings may include erythema nodosum, parotid gland enlargement, hepatosplenomegaly, and lymphadenopathy.

B. LABORATORY FINDINGS

Laboratory tests may show leukopenia, an elevated erythrocyte sedimentation rate, and hypercalcemia (about 5% of patients) or hypercalciuria (20%). Angiotensin-converting enzyme (ACE) levels are elevated in 40–80% of patients with active disease. This finding is neither sensitive nor specific enough to have diagnostic significance. Physiologic testing may reveal evidence of airflow obstruction, but restrictive changes with decreased lung volumes and diffusing capacity are more common. Skin test anergy is present in 70%. ECG may show conduction disturbances and dysrhythmias.

C. IMAGING

Radiographic findings are variable and include bilateral hilar adenopathy alone (radiographic stage I), hilar adenopathy and parenchymal involvement (radiographic stage II), or parenchymal involvement alone (radiographic stage III). Parenchymal involvement is usually manifested radiographically by diffuse reticular infiltrates, but focal infiltrates, acinar shadows, nodules and, rarely, cavitation may be seen. Pleural effusion is noted in fewer than 10% of patients.

D. SPECIAL EXAMINATIONS

The diagnosis of sarcoidosis generally requires histologic demonstration of noncaseating granulomas in biopsies from a patient with other typical associated manifestations. Other granulomatous diseases (eg, berylliosis, tuberculosis, fungal infections) and lymphoma must be excluded. Biopsy of easily accessible sites (eg, palpable lymph nodes, skin lesions, or salivary glands) is likely to be positive. Transbronchial lung biopsy has a high yield (75–90%) as well, especially in patients with radiographic evidence of parenchymal involvement. Some clinicians believe that tissue biopsy is not necessary when stage I radiographic findings are detected in a

clinical situation that strongly favors the diagnosis of sarcoidosis (eg, a young black woman with erythema nodosum). Biopsy is essential whenever clinical and radiographic findings suggest the possibility of an alternative diagnosis such as lymphoma. Bronchoalveolar lavage fluid in sarcoidosis is usually characterized by an increase in lymphocytes and a high CD4/CD8 cell ratio. Bronchoalveolar lavage does not establish a diagnosis but may be useful in following the activity of sarcoidosis in selected patients. All patients require a complete ophthalmologic evaluation.

Treatment

Indications for treatment with oral corticosteroids (prednisone, 0.5–1.0 mg/kg/d) include disabling constitutional symptoms, hypercalcemia, iritis, uveitis, arthritis, central nervous system involvement, cardiac involvement, granulomatous hepatitis, cutaneous lesions other than erythema nodosum, and progressive pulmonary lesions. Long-term therapy is usually required over months to years. Serum ACE levels usually fall with clinical improvement. Immunosuppressive drugs and cyclosporine have been tried, primarily when corticosteroid therapy has been exhausted, but experience with these drugs is limited.

Prognosis

The outlook is best for patients with hilar adenopathy alone; radiographic involvement of the lung parenchyma is associated with a worse prognosis. Erythema nodosum portends a good outcome. About 20% of patients with lung involvement suffer irreversible lung impairment, characterized by progressive fibrosis, bronchiectasis, and cavitation. Pneumothorax, hemoptysis, mycetoma formation in lung cavities, and respiratory failure often complicate this advanced stage. Myocardial sarcoidosis occurs in about 5% of patients, sometimes leading to restrictive cardiomyopathy, cardiac dysrhythmias, and conduction disturbances. Death from pulmonary insufficiency occurs in about 5% of patients.

Patients require long-term follow-up; at a minimum, yearly physical examination, pulmonary function tests, chemistry panel, ophthalmologic evaluation, chest radiograph, and ECG.

Baughman RP: Pulmonary sarcoidosis. Clin Chest Med 2004; 25:521. [PMID: 15331189]

Paramothayan NS et al: Corticosteroids for pulmonary sarcoidosis. Cochrane Database Syst Rev 2005;(2):CD001114. [PMID: 15846612]

Statement on sarcoidosis. Joint Statement of the American Thoracic Society (ATS), the European Respiratory Society (ERS) and the World Association of Sarcoidosis and Other Granulomatous Disorders (WASOG) adopted by the ATS Board of Directors and by the ERS Executive Committee, February 1999. Am J Respir Crit Care Med 1999;160: 736. [PMID: 10430755]

Thomas KW et al: Sarcoidosis. JAMA 2003;289:3300. [PMID: 12824213]

PULMONARY ALVEOLAR PROTEINOSIS

Pulmonary alveolar proteinosis is a disease in which phospholipids accumulate within alveolar spaces. The condition may be primary (idiopathic) or secondary (occurring in immune deficiency; hematologic malignancies; inhalation of mineral dusts; or following lung infections, including tuberculosis and viral infections). Progressive dyspnea is the usual presenting symptom, and chest radiograph shows bilateral alveolar infiltrates suggestive of pulmonary edema. The diagnosis is based on demonstration of characteristic findings on bronchoalveolar lavage (milky appearance and PAS-positive lipoproteinaceous material) in association with typical clinical and radiographic features. In some cases, transbronchial or surgical lung biopsy (revealing amorphous intra-alveolar phospholipid) is necessary.

The course of the disease varies. Some patients experience spontaneous remission; others develop progressive respiratory insufficiency. Pulmonary infection with nocardia or fungi may occur. Therapy for alveolar proteinosis consists of periodic whole lung lavage.

Trapnell BC et al: Pulmonary alveolar proteinosis. N Engl J Med 2003;349:2527. [PMID: 14695413]

EOSINOPHILIC PULMONARY SYNDROMES

Eosinophilic pulmonary syndromes are a diverse group of disorders typically characterized by eosinophilic pulmonary infiltrates, peripheral blood eosinophilia, and pulmonary symptoms such as dyspnea and cough. Many patients have constitutional symptoms, including fever. **Chronic eosinophilic pneumonia** is predominantly a disorder of women characterized by fever, night sweats, weight loss, and dyspnea. Pulmonary infiltrates on chest radiography are invariably peripheral. Therapy with oral prednisone (1 mg/kg daily for 1–2 weeks followed by a gradual taper over many months) usually results in dramatic improvement; however, most patients require at least 10–15 mg of prednisone every other day for a year or more (sometimes indefinitely) to prevent relapses.

Other eosinophilic pulmonary syndromes demonstrate a variety of patterns of pulmonary infiltrates associated with exposure to various drugs (common drugs include nitrofurantoin, phenytoin, ampicillin, acetaminophen, and ranitidine) or infection with helminths (eg, ascaris, hookworms, strongyloides) or filariae (eg, *Wuchereria bancrofti, Brugia malayi*, tropical pulmonary eosinophilia). Löffler's syndrome is **acute eosinophilic pneumonia** with transient pulmonary infiltrates. Pulmonary eosinophilia can also be a feature of many other processes, including ABPA, Churg-Strauss syndrome, systemic hypereosinophilic syndromes, eosinophilic granuloma of the lung (properly referred to as pulmonary Langerhans cell histiocytosis), neoplasms, and numerous interstitial lung diseases. No precipitating cause may be apparent in as many as one-

third of cases. If an extrinsic cause is identified, therapy consists of removal of the offending drug or treatment of the underlying parasitic infection. Corticosteroid treatment (prednisone, 1 mg/kg body weight orally per day) should be instituted if no treatable extrinsic cause is discovered. The response to corticosteroids is usually dramatic. Recurrences are common.

Milbrandt EB et al: Progressive infiltrates and eosinophilia with multiple possible causes. Chest 2000;118:230. [PMID: 10893384]

Mochimaru H et al: Clinicopathological differences between acute and chronic eosinophilic pneumonia. Respirology 2005;10:76. [PMID: 15691242]

■ DISORDERS OF THE PULMONARY CIRCULATION

PULMONARY VENOUS THROMBOEMBOLISM

ESSENTIALS OF DIAGNOSIS

- *Predisposition to venous thrombosis, usually of the lower extremities.*
- *One or more of the following: dyspnea, chest pain, hemoptysis, syncope.*
- *Tachypnea and a widened alveolar-arterial Po_2 difference.*
- *Characteristic defects on ventilation-perfusion lung scan, helical CT scan of the chest, or pulmonary arteriogram.*

General Considerations

Pulmonary venous thromboembolism, often referred to as pulmonary embolism, is a common, serious, and potentially fatal complication of thrombus formation within the deep venous circulation. Pulmonary venous thromboembolism is estimated to cause 200,000 deaths each year in the United States and is the third leading cause of death among hospitalized patients. Despite this prevalence, the majority of cases are not recognized antemortem, and fewer than 10% of patients with fatal emboli have received specific treatment for the condition. Management demands a vigilant systematic approach to diagnosis and an understanding of risk factors so that appropriate preventive therapy can be given.

Many substances can embolize to the pulmonary circulation, including air (during neurosurgery, from central venous catheters), amniotic fluid (during active labor), fat (long bone fractures), foreign bodies (talc in injection drug users), parasite eggs (schistosomiasis), septic emboli (acute infectious endocarditis), and tumor cells (renal cell carcinoma). The most common embolus is thrombus, which may arise anywhere in the venous circulation or heart but most often originates in the deep veins of the major calf muscles. Thrombi confined to the calf rarely embolize to the pulmonary circulation. However, about 20% of calf vein thrombi propagate proximally to the popliteal and ileofemoral veins, at which point they may break off and embolize to the pulmonary circulation. Pulmonary emboli will develop in 50–60% of patients with proximal deep venous thrombosis (DVT); half of these embolic events will be asymptomatic. Nearly 70% of patients who have symptomatic pulmonary emboli will have lower extremity DVT when evaluated.

Pulmonary embolism and DVT are two manifestations of the same disease. The risk factors for pulmonary emboli are the risk factors for thrombus formation within the venous circulation: venous stasis, injury to the vessel wall, and hypercoagulability (Virchow's triad). Venous stasis increases with immobility (bed rest—especially postoperative—obesity, stroke), hyperviscosity (polycythemia), and increased central venous pressures (low cardiac output states, pregnancy). Vessels may be damaged by prior episodes of thrombosis, orthopedic surgery, or trauma. Hypercoagulability can be caused by medications (oral contraceptives, hormonal replacement therapy) or disease (malignancy, surgery) or may be the result of inherited gene defects. The most common inherited cause in white populations is resistance to activated protein C, also known as factor V Leiden. The trait is present in approximately 3% of healthy American men and in 20–40% of patients with idiopathic venous thrombosis. Other major risks for hypercoagulability include the following: deficiencies or dysfunction of protein C, protein S, and antithrombin III; prothrombin gene mutation; and the presence of antiphospholipid antibodies (lupus anticoagulant and anticardiolipin antibody).

Pulmonary thromboembolism has multiple physiologic effects. Physical obstruction of the vascular bed and vasoconstriction from neurohumoral reflexes both increase pulmonary vascular resistance. Massive thrombus may cause right ventricular failure. Vascular obstruction increases physiologic dead space (wasted ventilation) and leads to hypoxemia through right-to-left shunting, decreased cardiac output, and surfactant depletion causing atelectasis. Reflex bronchoconstriction promotes wheezing and increased work of breathing.

Clinical Findings

A. Symptoms and Signs

The clinical diagnosis of pulmonary thromboembolism is notoriously difficult for two reasons. First, the clinical findings depend on both the size of the embolus and the patient's preexisting cardiopulmonary status. Second, common symptoms and signs of pulmonary emboli are not specific to this disorder (Table 9–20).

Indeed, no single symptom or sign or combination of clinical findings is specific to pulmonary thromboembolism. Some findings are fairly sensitive: dyspnea and pain on inspiration occur in 75–85% and 65–75% of patients, respectively. Tachypnea is the only sign reliably found in more than half of patients. A common clinical strategy is to use combinations of clinical findings to identify patients at low risk for pulmonary thromboembolism. For example, 97% of patients in the Prospective Investigation of Pulmonary Embolism Diagnosis (PIOPED) study with angiographically proved pulmonary emboli had one or more of three findings: dyspnea, chest pain with breathing, or tachypnea. Such a sensitive screen allows exclusion of the diagnosis on clinical grounds in a small number of patients. To establish the diagnosis or to exclude it definitively, further testing is required in the majority of patients.

B. Laboratory Findings

The **ECG** is abnormal in 70% of patients with pulmonary thromboembolism. However, the most common abnormalities are sinus tachycardia and nonspecific ST and T wave changes, each seen in approximately 40% of patients. Five percent or less of patients in the PIOPED study had P pulmonale, right ventricular hypertrophy, right axis deviation, and right bundle branch block.

Arterial blood gases usually reveal acute respiratory alkalosis due to hyperventilation. The arterial PO_2 and the alveolar-arterial oxygen difference (A–a–DO_2) are most often abnormal in patients with pulmonary thromboembolism compared with healthy, age-matched controls. However, arterial blood gases are not diagnostic: among patients who presented for evaluation in the PIOPED study, neither the PO_2 nor the A–a–DO_2 differentiated between those with and those without pulmonary emboli. Profound hypoxia with a normal chest radiograph in the absence of preexisting lung disease is highly suspicious for pulmonary thromboembolism.

Plasma levels of **D-dimer**, a degradation product of cross-linked fibrin, are elevated in the presence of thrombus. Using a D-dimer threshold between 300 and 500 ng/mL, the quantitative enzyme-linked immunosorbent assay (ELISA) has shown a sensitivity for venous thromboembolism of 95–97% and a specificity of 45%. Therefore, a D-dimer < 500 ng/mL using ELISA provides strong evidence against venous thromboembolism, with a likelihood ratio of 0.11–0.13. Two considerations have delayed widespread inclusion of plasma D-dimer assays into diagnostic algorithms. First, the accurate quantitative ELISA used in clinical research takes several hours to perform and is not widely available. Commonly used latex agglutination assays are much less sensitive and are difficult to standardize. Second, the D-dimer is elevated in most hospitalized patients, particularly those with malignancies or following surgery. Appropriate diagnostic thresholds are not yet established for inpatients.

Table 9–20. Frequency of specific symptoms and signs in patients at risk for pulmonary thromboembolism.

	UPET[1] PE+ (n = 327)	PIOPED[2] PE+ (n = 117)	PIOPED[2] PE– (n = 248)
Symptoms			
Dyspnea	84%	73%	72%
Respirophasic chest pain	74%	66%	59%
Cough	53%	37%	36%
Leg pain	nr	26%	24%
Hemoptysis	30%	13%	8%
Palpitations	nr	10%	18%
Wheezing	nr	9%	11%
Anginal pain	14%	4%	6%
Signs			
Respiratory rate ≥ 16 UPET, ≥ 20 PIOPED	92%	70%	68%
Crackles (rales)	58%	51%	40%[3]
Heart rate ≥ 100/min	44%	30%	24%
Fourth heart sound (S_4)	nr	24%	13%[3]
Accentuated pulmonary component of second heart sound (S_2P)	53%	23%	13%[3]
T ≥ 37.5 °C UPET, ≥ 38.5 °C PIOPED	43%	7%	12%
Homans' sign	nr	4%	2%
Pleural friction rub	nr	3%	2%
Third heart sound (S_3)	nr	3%	4%
Cyanosis	19%	1%	2%

[1]Data from the Urokinase-Streptokinase Pulmonary Embolism Trial, as reported in Bell WR, Simon TL, DeMets DL: The clinical features of submassive and massive pulmonary emboli. Am J Med 1977;62:355.
[2]Data from patients enrolled in the PIOPED study, as reported in Stein PD et al: Clinical, laboratory, roentgenographic, and electrocardiographic findings in patients with acute pulmonary embolism and no preexisting cardiac or pulmonary disease. Chest 1991;100:598.
[3]$P < .05$ comparing patients in the PIOPED study.
PE+ = confirmed diagnosis of pulmonary embolism; PE– = diagnosis of pulmonary embolism ruled out; nr = not reported.

C. IMAGING AND SPECIAL EXAMINATIONS

1. Chest radiography—The chest radiograph is necessary to exclude other common lung diseases and to permit interpretation of the ventilation-perfusion (V/Q) scan, but it does not establish the diagnosis by itself. The chest radiograph was normal in only 12% of patients with confirmed pulmonary thromboembolism in the PIOPED study. The most frequent findings were atelectasis, parenchymal infiltrates, and pleural effusions. However, the prevalence of these findings was the same in hospitalized patients without pulmonary thromboembolism. A prominent central pulmonary artery with local oligemia (Westermark's sign) or pleural-based areas of increased opacity that represent intraparenchymal hemorrhage (Hampton's hump) are uncommon. Paradoxically, the chest radiograph may be most helpful when normal in the setting of hypoxemia.

2. Lung scanning—A perfusion scan is performed by injecting radiolabeled microaggregated albumin into the venous system, allowing the particles to embolize to the pulmonary capillary bed. To perform a ventilation scan, the patient breathes a radioactive gas or aerosol while the distribution of radioactivity in the lungs is recorded.

A defect on perfusion scanning represents diminished blood flow to that region of the lung. This finding is not specific for pulmonary embolism. Defects in the perfusion scan are interpreted in conjunction with the ventilation scan to give a high, low, or intermediate (indeterminate) probability that pulmonary thromboembolism is the cause of the abnormalities. Criteria for the combined interpretation of ventilation and perfusion scans (commonly referred to as a single test, the V̇/Q̇ scan) are complex, confusing, and not completely standardized. A normal perfusion scan excludes the diagnosis of clinically significant pulmonary thromboembolism (negative predictive value of 91% in the PIOPED study). A high-probability V̇/Q̇ scan is most often defined as having two or more segmental perfusion defects in the presence of normal ventilation and is sufficient to make the diagnosis of pulmonary thromboembolism in most instances (positive predictive value of 88% among PIOPED patients). In the presence of abnormal pulmonary vasculature, as commonly happens in prior pulmonary thromboembolism, or if the clinical pretest probability for embolism is low, angiography may be indicated even in the presence of a high-probability V̇/Q̇ scan.

V̇/Q̇ scans are most helpful when they are either normal or indicate a high probability of pulmonary thromboembolism. Such readings are reliable—interobserver agreement is best for normal and high-probability scans, and they carry predictive power. The likelihood ratios associated with normal and high-probability scans are 0.10 and 18, respectively, indicating significant and frequently conclusive changes from pretest to posttest probability.

However, 75% of PIOPED V̇/Q̇ scans were nondiagnostic, ie, of low or intermediate probability. At angiography, these patients had an overall incidence of pulmonary thromboembolism of 14% and 30%, respectively. The likelihood ratios associated with low-probability and intermediate scans are 0.36 and 1.2, respectively, confirming the clinical impression that these studies add little diagnostic information. One of the most important findings of PIOPED was that the clinical assessment of pretest probability could be used to aid the interpretation of the V̇/Q̇ scan. For those patients with low-probability V̇/Q̇ scans and a low (20% or less) clinical pretest probability of pulmonary thromboembolism, the diagnosis was confirmed in only 4%. Such patients may reasonably be observed without angiography. All other patients with nondiagnostic V̇/Q̇ scans require further testing to determine the presence of venous thromboembolism.

3. CT—Helical CT arteriography is rapidly supplanting V̇/Q̇ scanning as the initial diagnostic study for suspected pulmonary thromboembolism. Helical CT arteriography requires administration of intravenous radiocontrast dye but is otherwise noninvasive. It is very sensitive for the detection of thrombus in the proximal pulmonary arteries but less so in the segmental and subsegmental arteries. Test results vary widely by study and facility. Factors influencing results include patient size and cooperation, the type and quality of the scanner, the imaging protocol, and the experience of the radiologist. One report comparing helical CT with standard arteriography reported sensitivity of 53–60% and specificity of 81–97%. Comparing helical CT to the V̇/Q̇ scan as the initial test for pulmonary thromboembolism, detection of thrombi is com-

parable, but more nonthromboembolism pulmonary diagnoses are made with CT scanning. Independent of cost and availability, helical CT may offer advantages as a screening examination, especially in hospitalized patients and in patients with significant comorbidities. A contentious issue is whether a negative helical CT requires any further evaluation. False-negative results may occur in up to 20% of helical CTs. Advocates contend that these false-negatives represent small peripheral thromboemboli and that such patients can be monitored off anticoagulation without undue risk. One study reported a venous thromboembolism rate of 0.8% in 3-month follow-up of 376 patients with negative helical CT scans, but the mortality rate at 3 months was 10.1%. Further study is required to clarify the role of this diagnostic modality, especially in view of ongoing advances in CT technology and the increasing availability of multi-detector-row scanners.

4. Venous thrombosis studies—Seventy percent of patients with pulmonary thromboembolism will have DVT on evaluation, and approximately half of patients with DVT will have pulmonary thromboembolism on angiography. Since the history and physical examination are neither sensitive nor specific for pulmonary thromboembolism and since the results of V̇/Q̇ scanning are frequently equivocal, documentation of DVT in a patient with suspected pulmonary thromboembolism establishes the need for treatment and may preclude pulmonary arteriography.

Commonly available diagnostic techniques include venous ultrasonography, impedance plethysmography, and contrast venography. In most centers, venous ultrasonography is the test of choice to detect proximal DVT. Inability to compress the common femoral or popliteal veins in symptomatic patients is diagnostic of first-episode DVT (positive predictive value of 97%); full compressibility of both sites excludes proximal DVT (negative predictive value of 98%). The test is less accurate in distal thrombi, recurrent thrombi, or in asymptomatic patients. Impedance plethysmography relies on changes in electrical impedance between patent and obstructed veins to determine the presence of thrombus. Accuracy is comparable though not quite as high as ultrasonography. Both ultrasonography and impedance plethysmography are useful in the serial examination of patients with high clinical suspicion of venous thromboembolism but negative leg studies. In patients with suspected first-episode DVT and a negative ultrasound or impedance plethysmography examination, multiple studies have confirmed the safety of withholding anticoagulation while conducting two sequential studies on days 1–3 and 7–10. Similarly, patients with nondiagnostic V̇/Q̇ scans and an initial negative venous ultrasound or impedance plethysmography examination may be monitored off therapy with serial leg studies over 2 weeks. When serial examinations are negative for proximal DVT, the risk of subsequent venous thromboembolism over the following 6 months is less than 2%.

Contrast venography remains the reference standard for the diagnosis of DVT. An intraluminal filling defect is diagnostic of venous thrombosis. However, venography has significant shortcomings and has been replaced by venous ultrasound as the diagnostic procedure of choice. Difficulties include patient discomfort, expense, allergic reactions to radiocontrast media, contrast-induced phlebitis, and technical difficulties in cannulation of dorsal foot veins and in the interpretation of studies. There is a significant (2–4%) risk of developing venous thrombosis from the procedure—a risk that may be higher than the false-negative rate of noninvasive studies. Venography is used principally in complex situations where there is discrepancy between clinical suspicion and noninvasive testing.

5. Pulmonary arteriography—Pulmonary arteriography remains the reference standard for the diagnosis of pulmonary thromboembolism. An intraluminal filling defect in more than one projection establishes a definitive diagnosis. Secondary findings highly suggestive of pulmonary thromboembolism include abrupt arterial cutoff, asymmetry of blood flow—especially segmental oligemia—or a prolonged arterial phase with slow filling. Pulmonary arteriography was performed in 755 patients in the PIOPED study. A definitive diagnosis was established in 97%; in 3% the studies were nondiagnostic. Four patients (0.8%) with negative arteriograms subsequently had pulmonary thromboemboli at autopsy. Serial arteriography has demonstrated minimal resolution of thrombus prior to day 7 following presentation. Thus, negative arteriography within 7 days of presentation excludes the diagnosis.

Pulmonary arteriography is a safe but invasive procedure with well-defined morbidity and mortality data. Minor complications occur in approximately 5% of patients. Most are allergic contrast reactions, transient renal dysfunction, or related to percutaneous catheter insertion; cardiac perforation and arrhythmias are reported but rare. Among the PIOPED patients who underwent arteriography, there were five deaths (0.7%) directly related to the procedure. Pulmonary hypertension is thought to increase the risk of serious complications, though a study of patients with average pulmonary arterial pressures of 74/34 mm Hg developed no major complications or deaths associated with pulmonary arteriography.

The appropriate role of pulmonary arteriography in the diagnosis of pulmonary thromboembolism remains a subject of active debate. There is wide agreement that arteriography is indicated in several specific situations: in patients with nondiagnostic V/Q scans, intermediate or high clinical pretest probability of pulmonary thromboembolism, and negative noninvasive leg studies; in any patient in whom the diagnosis is in doubt when there is a high clinical pretest probability of pulmonary thromboembolism; and when the diagnosis of pulmonary thromboembolism must be established with certainty, as when anticoagulation is con-

traindicated or placement of an inferior vena cava filter is contemplated.

6. MRI—MRI has sensitivity and specificity equivalent to contrast venography in the diagnosis of DVT. It has improved sensitivity when compared with venous ultrasound in the diagnosis of DVT, without loss of specificity. The test is noninvasive and avoids the use of potentially nephrotoxic radiocontrast dye. However, it remains expensive and not widely available. Artifacts introduced by respiratory and cardiac motion have limited the use of MRI in the diagnosis of pulmonary thromboembolism. New techniques have improved sensitivity and specificity to levels comparable with helical CT, but MRI remains primarily a research tool for pulmonary thromboembolism.

7. Integrated approach—The integrated approach uses the clinical likelihood of venous thromboembolism along with the overlapping results of noninvasive testing to come to one of three decision points: to establish venous thromboembolism (pulmonary thromboembolism or DVT) as the diagnosis, to exclude venous thromboembolism with sufficient confidence to follow the patient without therapy, or to refer the patient for pulmonary arteriography. An ideal diagnostic algorithm would proceed in a stepwise fashion to come to these decision points in a cost-effective way at minimal risk to the patient. We present two such algorithms in Figure 9–3.

Prevention

Venous thromboembolism is often clinically silent until it presents with significant morbidity or mortality. It is a prevalent disease, clearly associated with identifiable risk factors. For example, the incidence of proximal DVT, pulmonary thromboembolism, and fatal pulmonary thromboembolism in untreated patients undergoing hip fracture surgery is reported to be 10–20%, 4–10%, and 0.2–5%, respectively. There is unambiguous evidence of the efficacy of prophylactic therapy in this and other clinical situations, yet it remains underused. Only about 50% of surgical deaths from pulmonary thromboembolism had received any form of preventive therapy. Tables 9–21 and 9–22 provide overviews of strategies for the prevention of venous thromboembolism.

Options for therapy begin with mechanical devices such as graduated-compression stockings and intermittent pneumatic compression. The latter improves venous return and may increase endogenous fibrinolysis by stimulating the vascular endothelium. Standard pharmacologic therapy in medical patients is low-dose unfractionated heparin, 5000 units subcutaneously every 8–12 hours. Low-molecular-weight (LMW) heparins are more expensive but have several advantages compared with unfractionated heparin: better bioavailability, once- or twice-daily dosing, and a lower incidence of heparin-associated thrombocytopenia. In high-risk surgical patients, LMW heparins can be administered without the need for

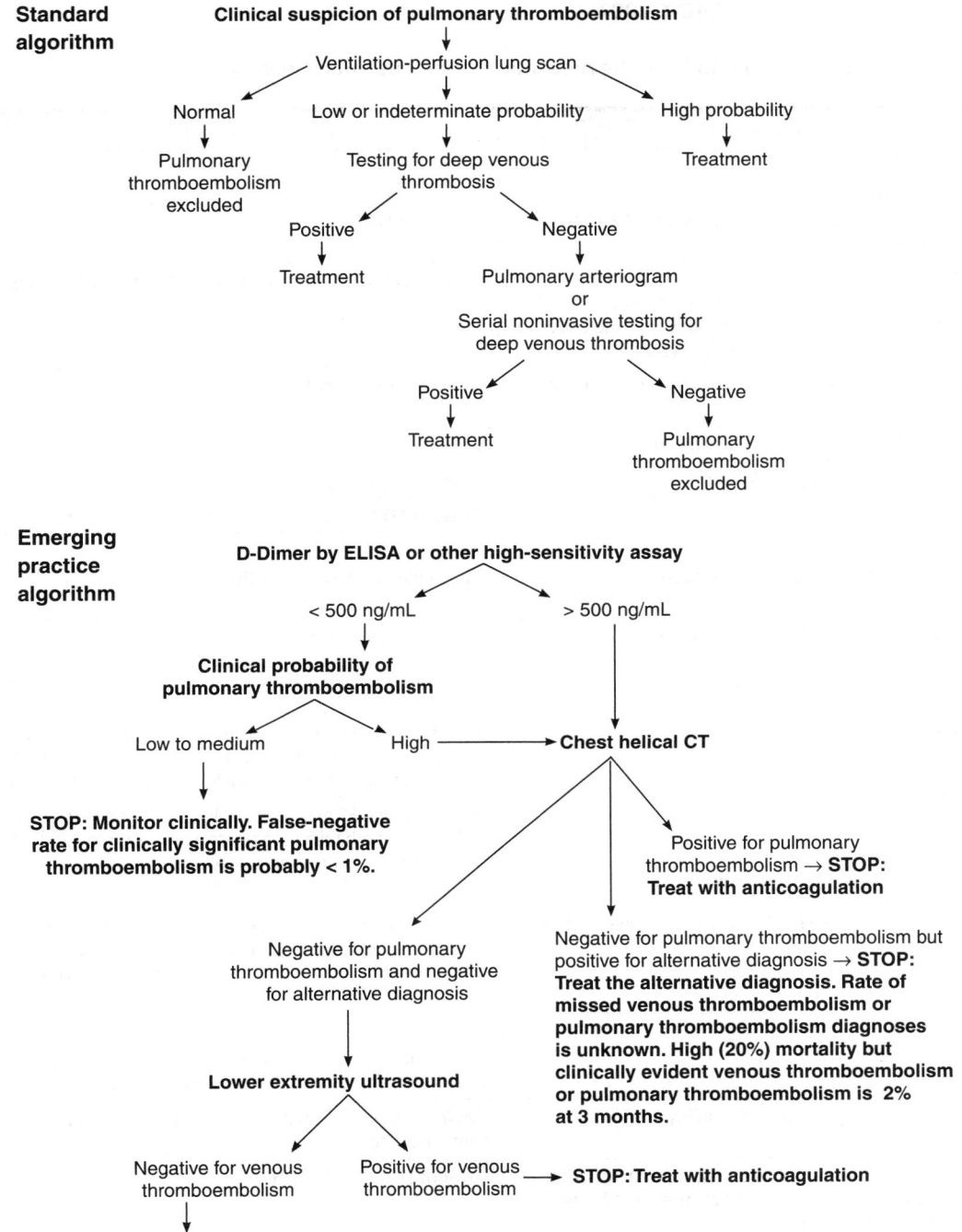

Figure 9–3. Two simple algorithms to guide evaluation of suspected venous thromboembolism. The standard algorithm is based on the results of ventilation-perfusion lung scanning using PIOPED data. Management of patients with ventilation-perfusion lung scans of low and indeterminate probability must always be guided by clinical judgment based upon cumulative clinical information and the degree of suspicion of pulmonary thromboembolism. The second algorithm uses D-dimer, helical CT, and venous ultrasonography to describe an evidence-based, efficient evaluation that reflects emerging practice. This second algorithm is not based on the experience of the standard ventilation-perfusion approach but anticipates a shift toward use of helical CT as the primary diagnostic test in pulmonary thromboembolism.

Table 9–21. Selected methods for the prevention of venous thromboembolism.

Risk Group	Recommendations for Prophylaxis
Surgical patients	
General surgery	
Low-risk: Minor procedures, age under 40, and no clinical risk factors	Early ambulation
Moderate risk: Minor procedures with additional thrombosis risk factors; age 40–60, and no other clinical risk factors; or major operations with age under 40 without additional clinical risk factors	ES, or LDUH, or LMWH, or IPC; plus early ambulation if possible
Higher risk: Major operation, over age 40 or with additional risk factors	LDUH, or LMWH, or IPC
Higher risk plus increased risk of bleeding	ES or IPC
Very high risk: Multiple risk factors	LDUH, or higher-dose LMWH, plus ES or IPC
Selected very high risk	Consider ADPW, INR 2.0–3.0, or postdischarge LMWH
Orthopedic surgery	
Elective total hip replacement surgery	Subcutaneous LMWH, or ADPW, or adjusted-dose heparin started preoperatively; plus IPC or ES
Elective total knee replacement surgery	LMWH, or ADPW, or IPC
Hip fracture surgery	LMWH or ADPW
Neurosurgery	
Intracranial neurosurgery	IPC with or without ES; LDUH and postoperative LMWH are acceptable alternatives; IPC or ES plus LDUH or LMWH may be more effective than either modality alone in high-risk patients.
Acute spinal cord injury	LMWH; IPC and ES may have additional benefit when used with LMWH. In the rehabilitation phase, conversion to full-dose warfarin may provide ongoing protection.
Trauma	
With an identifiable risk factor for thromboembolism	LMWH; IPC or ES if there is a contraindication to LMWH; consider duplex ultrasound screening in very high risk patients; IVC filter insertion if proximal DVT is identified and anticoagulation is contraindicated.
Medical patients	
Acute myocardial infarction	Subcutaneous LDUH, or full-dose heparin; if heparin is contraindicated, IPC and ES may provide some protection.
Ischemic stroke with impaired mobility	LMWH or LDUH or danaparoid; IPC or ES if anticoagulants are contraindicated
General medical patients with clinical risk factors; especially patients with cancer, congestive heart failure, or severe pulmonary disease	Low-dose LMWH, or LDUH
Cancer patients with indwelling central venous catheters	Warfarin, 1 mg/d, or LMWH

ADPW = adjusted-dose perioperative warfarin: begin 5–10 mg the day of or the day following surgery; adjust dose to INR 2.0–3.0; DVT = deep venous thrombosis; ES = elastic stockings; IPC = intermittent pneumatic compression; IVC = inferior vena cava; LDUH = low-dose unfractionated heparin: 5000 units subcutaneously every 8–12 hours starting 1–2 hours before surgery; LMWH = low-molecular-weight heparin. See Table 9–24 for dosing regimens.
Recommendations assembled from Geerts WH et al: Prevention of venous thromboembolism. Chest 2001;119(Suppl):132.

Table 9–22. Selected low-molecular-weight heparin and heparinoid regimens to prevent venous thromboembolism.

Risk Group	Drug	Subcutaneous Dose[1]	Administration Regimen	Cost[2]
General surgery, moderate risk	Dalteparin (Fragmin)	2500 units	1–2 h preop and qd postop	$18.08/dose
	Enoxaparin (Lovenox)	20 mg	1–2 h preop and qd postop	$22.26/dose
	Nadroparin (Fraxiparin)	2850 units	2–4 h preop and qd postop	No price available: Not available in USA
	Tinzaparin (Innohep)	3500 units	2 h preop and qd postop	$28.22/dose
General surgery, high risk	Dalteparin (Fragmin)	5000 units	8–12 preop and qd postop	$29.34/dose
	Danaparoid (Orgaran)	750 units	1–4 h preop and q12 h postop	No price available: Not available in USA
	Enoxaparin (Lovenox)	40 mg	1–2 h preop and qd postop	$29.68/dose
	Enoxaparin (Lovenox)	30 mg	q12 h starting 8–12 h postop	$22.26/dose
Orthopedic surgery	Dalteparin (Fragmin)	5000 units	8–12 h preop and qd starting 12–24 h postop	$29.34/dose
	Dalteparin (Fragmin)	2500 units	6–8 h postop then 5000 units qd	$18.08/dose
	Danaparoid (Orgaran)	750 units	1–4 preop and q12 h postop	No price available: Not available in USA
	Enoxaparin (Lovenox)	30 mg	q12 h starting 12–24 h postop	$22.26/dose
	Enoxaparin (Lovenox)	40 mg	qd starting 10–12 h preop	$29.68/dose
	Nadroparin (Fraxiparin)	38 units/kg	12 h preop, 12 h postop, and qd on postop days 1, 2, 3; then increase to 57 units/kg qd	No price available: Not available in USA
	Tinzaparin (Innohep)	75 units/kg	qd starting 12–24 h postop	$36.29/dose (60 kg pt)
	Tinzaparin (Innohep)	4500 units	12 h preop and qd postop	$36.29/dose
Major trauma	Enoxaparin (Lovenox)	30 mg	q12h starting 12–36 h postinjury if hemostatically stable	$21.41/dose
Acute spinal cord injury	Enoxaparin (Lovenox)	30 mg	q12h	$21.41/dose
Medical conditions	Dalteparin (Fragmin)	2500 units	qd	$17.22/dose
	Danaparoid (Orgaran)	750 units	q12h	No price available: Not available in USA
	Enoxaparin (Lovenox)	40 mg	qd	$28.54/dose
	Nadroparin (Fraxiparin)	2850 units	qd	No price available: Not available in USA

[1]Dose expressed in anti-Xa units; for enoxaparin, 1 mg = 100 anti-Xa units.
[2]Average wholesale price (AWP, for AB-rated generic when available) for quantity listed. Source: *Red Book* Update, Vol. 24, No. 4, April 2005. AWP may not accurately represent the actual pharmacy cost because wide contractual variations exist among institutions.
Preop = preoperatively; Postop = postoperatively; qd = once daily.
Modified and reproduced with permission, from Geerts WH et al: Prevention of venous thromboembolism. Chest 2001;119:132S.

coagulation monitoring and dose adjustments, as would be the case with unfractionated heparin.

Treatment

A. ANTICOAGULATION

Anticoagulation is not definitive therapy but a form of secondary prevention. Heparin binds to and accelerates the ability of antithrombin III to inactivate thrombin, factor Xa, and factor IXa. It thus retards additional thrombus formation, allowing endogenous fibrinolytic mechanisms to lyse existing clot. The standard regimen of heparin followed by 6 months of oral warfarin results in an 80–90% reduction in the risk of both recurrent venous thrombosis and death from pulmonary thromboembolism.

Heparin has troublesome pharmacokinetics. Its clearance is dose-dependent; it is highly protein-bound; and a minimum or threshold level is necessary to achieve an antithrombotic effect. It is necessary to monitor the activated partial thromboplastin time (aPTT) and adjust dosing to maintain the aPTT 1.5–2.5 times control. In patients with a moderate to high clinical likelihood of pulmonary thromboembolism and no contraindications, full anticoagulation with heparin should begin with the diagnostic evaluation. Once the diagnosis of proximal DVT or pulmonary thromboembolism is established, it

Table 9–23. Intravenous heparin dosing based on body weight.

Initial dosing

1. Load with 80 units/kg IV, then
2. Initiate a maintenance infusion at 18 units/kg/h
3. Check activated partial thromboplastin time (aPTT) in 6 hours

Dose adjustment schedule based on aPTT results

< 35 s (< 1.2 × control)	Rebolus with 80 units/kg; increase infusion by 4 units/kg/h
35–45 s (1.2–1.5 × control)	Rebolus with 40 units/kg; increase infusion by 2 units/kg/h
46–70 s (1.5–2.3 × control)	No change
71–90 s (2.3–3 × control)	Decrease infusion rate by 2 units/kg/h
> 90 s (> 3 × control)	Stop infusion for 1 hour, then decrease infusion by 3 units/kg/h

Repeat aPTT every 6 hours for the first 24 hours. If the aPTT is 46–70 s after 24 hours, then recheck once daily every morning. If the aPTT is outside this therapeutic range at 24 hours, continue checking every 6 hours until it is 46–70 s. Once it has been in the therapeutic range on two consecutive measurements after 24 hours, check once daily every morning.

Adapted from Raschke RA et al: The weight-based heparin dosing nomogram compared with a "standard care" nomogram. Ann Intern Med 1993;119:874.

Table 9–24. Selected low-molecular-weight heparin anticoagulation regimens.

Drug	Suggested Treatment Dose [1] (Subcutaneous)
Dalteparin	200 units/kg once daily (not to exceed 18,000 units/dose)
Enoxaparin	1.5 mg/kg once daily (single dose not to exceed 180 mg)
Nadroparin	86 units/kg twice daily for 10 days, or 171 units/kg once daily (single dose not to exceed 17,000 units)
Tinzaparin	175 units/kg once daily

[1]Dose expressed in anti-Xa units; for enoxaparin, 1 mg = 100 anti-Xa units.
Modified and reproduced with permission, from Hyers TM et al: Antithrombotic therapy for venous thromboembolic disease. Chest 2001;119(Suppl):176S.

is critical to ensure adequate therapy. Failure to achieve therapeutic heparin levels within 24 hours is associated with a fivefold-increased risk of clot propagation. The weight-based regimen in Table 9–23 is superior to standard dosing. Heparin causes immune-mediated thrombocytopenia in 3% of patients; therefore, the platelet count should be determined frequently for the first 14 days of therapy.

LMW heparins are depolymerized preparations of heparin with multiple advantages over unfractionated heparin. They exhibit less binding to cells and proteins and have superior bioavailability, a longer plasma half-life, and more predictable dose-response characteristics. They appear to carry an equivalent or lower risk of hemorrhage, and immune-mediated thrombocytopenia is less common. LMW heparins are as effective as unfractionated heparin in the treatment of venous thromboembolism. They are administered in dosages determined by body weight once or twice daily without the need for coagulation monitoring, and subcutaneous administration appears to be as effective as the intravenous route. This profile makes LMW heparins ideal for home-based therapy of venous thromboembolism. Home-based therapy appears safe and efficacious in a small number of selected patients. Table 9–24 sets forth selected LMW heparin anticoagulation regimens.

Anticoagulation therapy for venous thromboembolism is continued for a minimum of 3 months, so oral anticoagulant therapy with warfarin is usually initiated concurrently with heparin. Warfarin affects hepatic synthesis of vitamin K-dependent coagulant proteins. It usually requires 5–7 days to become therapeutic; therefore, heparin is generally continued for 5 days. Warfarin is safe if begun concurrently with heparin, initially at a dose of 2.5–10 mg/d. The lower dose is preferred in elderly patients. Maintenance therapy usually requires 2–15 mg/d. Adequacy of therapy must be monitored by following the prothrombin time, most often adjusted for differences in reagents and reported as the international normalized ratio (INR). The target INR is 2.5, with the acceptable range from 2.0 to 3.0; below 2.0, there is an increased risk of thrombosis; above 4.0, there is an increased risk of hemorrhage. Warfarin has interactions with many drugs. Meticulous attention to medications is part of the routine management of every patient receiving warfarin. Warfarin is a pregnancy category X medication, indicating known fetopathic and teratogenic effects. When oral anticoagulation with warfarin is contraindicated, LMW heparin is a convenient alternative.

The optimal duration of anticoagulation therapy for venous thromboembolism is unknown. There appears to be a protective benefit to continued anticoagulation in first-episode venous thromboembolism (twice the rate of recurrence in 6 weeks compared with 6 months of therapy) and recurrent disease (eightfold risk of recurrence in 6 months compared with 4 years of therapy). These studies do not distinguish patients with reversible risk factors, such as surgery or transient immobility, from patients who have a nonreversible hypercoagulable state such as factor V Leiden, inhibitor deficiency, antiphospholipid syndrome, or malignancy. A randomized controlled trial of low-dose warfarin (INR 1.5–2.0) versus no therapy following 6 months of standard therapy in patients with idiopathic DVT was stopped early. The protective benefits of continued anticoagulation include fewer DVTs in addition to a trend toward lower mortality despite more hemorrhage in the warfarin group. Risk reductions were consistent across groups with and without inherited thrombophilia.

For many patients, venous thrombosis is a recurrent disease, and continued therapy will result in a lower rate of recurrence at the cost of an increased risk of hemorrhage. Therefore, the appropriate duration of therapy will need to take into consideration potentially reversible risk factors, the individual's age, the likelihood and potential consequences of hemorrhage, and patient preferences for continued therapy. It is reasonable to continue therapy for 6 months after a first episode when there is a reversible risk factor, 12 months after a first-episode idiopathic thrombus, and 6–12 months to indefinitely in patients with nonreversible risk factors or recurrent disease. If confirmed, these data may lead to lifelong low-dose anticoagulation.

The major complication of anticoagulation is hemorrhage. Risk factors for hemorrhage include the intensity of the anticoagulant effect; the duration of therapy; concomitant administration of drugs such as aspirin that interfere with platelet function; and patient characteristics, particularly increased age, previous gastrointestinal hemorrhage, and coexistent renal insufficiency.

The reported incidence of major hemorrhage following intravenous administration of unfractionated heparin is nil to 7%; that of fatal hemorrhage is nil to 2%. The incidence with LMW heparins is not statistically different. There is no information comparing hemorrhage rates at different doses of heparin. The risk of subtherapeutic heparin administration in the first 24–48 hours after diagnosis is significant; it appears to outweigh the risk of short-term supratherapeutic heparin levels. The incidence of hemorrhage during therapy with warfarin is reported to be between 3% and 4% per patient year. The frequency varies with the target INR and is consistently higher when the INR exceeds 4.0. There is no apparent additional antithrombotic benefit in venous thromboembolism with a target INR above 2.0–3.0.

B. THROMBOLYTIC THERAPY

Streptokinase, urokinase, and recombinant tissue plasminogen activator (rt-PA; alteplase) increase plasmin levels and thereby directly lyse intravascular thrombi. In patients with established pulmonary thromboembolism, thrombolytic therapy accelerates resolution of emboli within the first 24 hours compared with standard heparin therapy. This is a consistent finding using angiography, V̇/Q̇ scanning, echocardiography, and direct measurement of pulmonary artery pressures. However, at 1 week and 1 month after diagnosis, these agents show no difference in outcome compared with heparin and warfarin. There is no evidence that thrombolytic therapy improves mortality. Subtle improvements in pulmonary function, including improved single-breath diffusing capacity and a lower incidence of exercise-induced pulmonary hypertension, have been observed. The reliability and clinical importance of these findings is unclear. The major disadvantages of thrombolytic therapy compared with heparin are its greater cost and a significant increase in major hemorrhagic complications. The incidence of intracranial hemorrhage in patients with pulmonary thromboemboli treated with alteplase is 2.1% compared with 0.2% in patients treated with heparin.

Current evidence supports thrombolytic therapy for pulmonary thromboembolism in patients at high risk for death in whom the more rapid resolution of thrombus may be lifesaving. Such patients are usually hemodynamically unstable despite heparin therapy. Absolute contraindications to thrombolytic therapy include active internal bleeding and stroke within the past 2 months. Major contraindications include uncontrolled hypertension and surgery or trauma within the past 6 weeks.

C. ADDITIONAL MEASURES

Interruption of the inferior vena cava may be indicated in patients with a major contraindication to anticoagulation who have or are at high risk for development of proximal DVT or pulmonary embolus. Placement of an inferior vena cava filter is also recommended for recurrent thromboembolism despite adequate anticoagulation, for chronic recurrent embolism with pulmonary hypertension, and with the concurrent performance of surgical pulmonary embolectomy or pulmonary thromboendarterectomy. Percutaneous transjugular placement of a mechanical filter is the preferred mode of inferior vena cava interruption. These devices reduce the short-term incidence of pulmonary thromboemboli in patients presenting with proximal lower extremity DVT. However, they are associated with a two-fold increased risk of recurrent DVT in the first 2 years following placement.

In rare critically ill patients for whom thrombolytic therapy is contraindicated or unsuccessful, mechanical or surgical extraction of thrombus may be indicated. Pulmonary embolectomy is an emergency procedure of last resort with a very high mortality rate. It is now performed only in a few specialized centers. Several catheter devices to fragment and extract thrombus through a transvenous approach have been reported in small numbers of patients. Comparative outcomes with surgery, thrombolytic therapy, or heparin have not been studied.

Prognosis

Pulmonary thromboembolism is estimated to cause more than 50,000 deaths annually. In the majority of deaths, pulmonary thromboembolism is not recognized antemortem or death occurs before specific treatment can be initiated. These statistics highlight the importance of preventive therapy in high-risk patients. The outlook for patients with diagnosed and appropriately treated pulmonary thromboembolism is generally good. Overall prognosis depends on the underlying disease rather than the pulmonary thromboembolism itself. Death from recurrent thromboemboli is uncommon, occurring in less than 3% of cases. Perfusion defects resolve in most survivors. Approximately 1% of patients develop chronic thromboembolic pulmonary hypertension. Selected patients may benefit from pulmonary endarterectomy.

Blom JW et al: Malignancies, prothrombotic mutations, and the risk of venous thrombosis. JAMA 2005;293:715. [PMID: 15701913]

Buller HR et al: Antithrombotic therapy for venous thromboembolic disease: the Seventh ACCP Conference on Antithrombotic and Thrombolytic Therapy. Chest 2004;126(3 Suppl): 401S. [PMID: 15383479]

Geerts WH et al: Prevention of venous thromboembolism: the Seventh ACCP Conference on Antithrombotic and Thrombolytic Therapy. Chest 2004;126(3 Suppl):338S. [PMID: 15383478]

Hirsh J et al: New anticoagulants. Blood 2005;105:453. [PMID: 15191946]

Hull RD: Revisiting the past strengthens the present: an evidence-based medicine approach for the diagnosis of deep venous thrombosis. Ann Intern Med 2005;142:583. [PMID: 15809468]

Nijkeuter M et al: Resolution of thromboemboli in patients with acute pulmonary embolism: a systematic review. Chest 2006;129:192. [PMID: 16424432]

Perrier A et al: Multidetector-row computed tomography in suspected pulmonary embolism. N Engl J Med 2005;352:1760. [PMID: 15858185]

Quiroz R et al: Clinical validity of a negative computed tomography scan in patients with suspected pulmonary embolism: a systematic review. JAMA 2005;293:2012. [PMID: 15855435]

Roy PM et al: Systematic review and meta-analysis of strategies for the diagnosis of suspected pulmonary embolism. BMJ 2005;331:259. [PMID: 16052017]

van Belle A et al; Christopher Study Investigators: Effectiveness of managing suspected pulmonary embolism using an algorithm combining clinical probability, D-dimer testing, and computed tomography. JAMA 2006;295:172. [PMID: 16403929]

Wells PS et al: Does this patient have deep vein thrombosis? JAMA 2006;295:199. [PMID: 16403932]

PULMONARY HYPERTENSION

 ESSENTIALS OF DIAGNOSIS

- Dyspnea, fatigue, chest pain, and syncope on exertion.
- Narrow splitting of second heart sound with loud pulmonary component; findings of right ventricular hypertrophy and cardiac failure in advanced disease.
- Hypoxemia and increased wasted ventilation on pulmonary function tests.
- Electrocardiographic evidence of right ventricular strain or hypertrophy and right atrial enlargement.
- Enlarged central pulmonary arteries on chest radiograph.

General Considerations

The pulmonary circulation is unique because of its high blood flow, low pressure (normally 25/8 mm Hg, mean 12), and low resistance (normally 200–250 dynes/sec/cm^{-5}). It can accommodate large increases in blood flow during exercise with only modest increases in pressure because of its ability to recruit and distend lung blood vessels. Contraction of smooth muscle in the walls of pulmonary arteriolar resistance vessels becomes an important factor in numerous pathologic states. Pulmonary hypertension is present when pulmonary artery pressure rises to a level inappropriate for a given cardiac output. Once present, pulmonary hypertension is self-perpetuating. It introduces secondary structural abnormalities in pulmonary vessels, including smooth muscle hypertrophy and intimal proliferation, and these may eventually stimulate atheromatous changes and in situ thrombosis, leading to further narrowing of the arterial bed.

Primary (idiopathic) pulmonary hypertension (see Chapter 10) is a rare disorder of the pulmonary circulation occurring mostly in young and middle-aged women. Untreated, it is characterized by progressive dyspnea, a rapid downhill course, and an invariably fatal outcome. This condition is also called plexogenic pulmonary arteriopathy, in reference to the character-

Table 9–25. Mechanisms of pulmonary hypertension and examples of corresponding clinical conditions.

Reduction in cross-sectional area of pulmonary arterial bed
  Vasoconstriction
    Hypoxemia from any cause (chronic lung disease, sleep-disordered breathing, etc)
    Acidosis
  Loss of vessels
    Lung resection
    Emphysema
    Vasculitis
    Interstitial lung disease
    Collagen-vascular disease
  Obstruction of vessels
    Pulmonary embolism (thromboemboli, tumor emboli, etc)
    In situ thrombosis
    Schistosomiasis
    Sickle cell disease
  Narrowing of vessels
    Secondary structural changes due to pulmonary hypertension
Increased pulmonary venous pressure
  Constrictive pericarditis
  Left ventricular failure or reduced compliance
  Mitral stenosis
  Left atrial myxoma
  Pulmonary veno-occlusive disease
  Mediastinal diseases compressing pulmonary veins
Increased pulmonary blood flow
  Congenital left-to-right intracardiac shunts
Increased blood viscosity
  Polycythemia
Miscellaneous
  Pulmonary hypertension occurring in association with hepatic cirrhosis and portal hypertension
  HIV infection

---

istic histopathologic plexiform lesion found in muscular pulmonary arteries. It has been observed in occasional patients with HIV infection.

Selected mechanisms responsible for **secondary pulmonary hypertension** and examples of corresponding clinical conditions are set forth in Table 9–25. Pulmonary arteriolar vasoconstriction due to chronic hypoxemia may complicate any chronic lung disease and compound the effects of loss of pulmonary blood vessels (as seen with disorders such as emphysema and pulmonary fibrosis) and obstruction of the pulmonary vascular bed (as seen with disorders such as chronic pulmonary thromboembolic disease). Sustained increases in pulmonary venous pressure from disorders such as left ventricular failure (systolic, diastolic, or both), mitral stenosis, and pulmonary veno-occlusive disease may cause "postcapillary" pulmonary hypertension. Increased pulmonary blood flow due to intracardiac shunts and increased blood viscosity due to polycythemia can also cause pulmonary hypertension. Pulmonary hypertension has also been associated with hepatic cirrhosis and portal hypertension.

Pulmonary veno-occlusive disease is a rare cause of postcapillary pulmonary hypertension occurring in children and young adults. The cause is unknown, but associations with various conditions such as viral infection, bone marrow transplantation, chemotherapy, and malignancy have been described. The disease is characterized by progressive fibrotic occlusion of pulmonary veins and venules, along with secondary hypertensive changes in the pulmonary arterioles and muscular pulmonary arteries. Nodular areas of pulmonary congestion, edema, hemorrhage, and hemosiderosis are found. Chest radiography reveals prominent, symmetric interstitial markings, Kerley B lines, pulmonary artery dilation, and normally sized left atrium and left ventricle. Antemortem diagnosis is often difficult but is occasionally established by open lung biopsy. There is no effective therapy, and most patients die within 2 years as a result of progressive pulmonary hypertension.

Clinical Findings

A. SYMPTOMS AND SIGNS

Secondary pulmonary hypertension is difficult to recognize clinically in the early stages, when symptoms and signs are primarily those of the underlying disease. Pulmonary hypertension may cause or contribute to dyspnea, present initially on exertion and later at rest. Dull, retrosternal chest pain resembling angina pectoris may be present. Fatigue and syncope on exertion also occur, presumably a result of reduced cardiac output related to elevated pulmonary artery pressures or bradycardia.

The signs of pulmonary hypertension include narrow splitting of the second heart sound, accentuation of the pulmonary component of the second heart sound, and a systolic ejection click. In advanced cases, tricuspid and pulmonary valve insufficiency and signs of right ventricular failure and cor pulmonale are found.

B. LABORATORY FINDINGS

Polycythemia is found in many cases of pulmonary hypertension that are associated with chronic hypoxemia. Electrocardiographic changes are those of right axis deviation, right ventricular hypertrophy, right ventricular strain, or right atrial enlargement.

C. IMAGING AND SPECIAL EXAMINATIONS

Radiographs and high-resolution CT scans of the chest can assist in the diagnosis of pulmonary hypertension and determination of the cause. In chronic disease, dilation of the right and left main and lobar pulmonary arteries and enlargement of the pulmonary outflow tract are seen; in advanced disease, right ventricular and right atrial enlargement are seen. Peripheral "pruning" of large pulmonary arteries is characteristic of pulmonary hypertension in severe emphysema.

Echocardiography is helpful in evaluating patients thought to have mitral stenosis, left atrial myxoma, and pulmonary valvular disease and may also reveal right ventricular enlargement and paradoxical motion of the interventricular septum. Doppler ultrasonography is a reliable noninvasive means of estimating pulmonary artery systolic pressure. However, precise hemodynamic measurements can only be obtained with right heart catheterization, which is helpful when postcapillary pulmonary hypertension, intracardiac shunting, or thromboembolic disease is considered as part of the differential diagnosis.

The diagnosis of pulmonary hypertension cannot be made on routine pulmonary function tests. Some results may help identify the cause; eg, diminution of the pulmonary capillary bed may cause reduction in the single breath diffusing capacity.

The following studies may be useful to exclude causes of secondary pulmonary hypertension: liver function tests, HIV test, collagen-vascular serologic studies, polysomnography, V/Q lung scanning, pulmonary angiography, and surgical lung biopsy. V/Q lung scanning is very helpful in identifying patients with pulmonary hypertension caused by recurrent pulmonary thromboemboli, a condition that is often difficult to recognize clinically.

Treatment

Treatment of primary pulmonary hypertension is discussed in Chapter 10. Treatment of secondary pulmonary hypertension consists mainly of treating the underlying disorder. Early recognition of pulmonary hypertension is crucial to interrupt the self-perpetuating cycle responsible for rapid clinical progression. By the time most patients present with signs and symptoms of pulmonary hypertension, however, the condition is far advanced. If hypoxemia or acidosis is detected, corrective measures should be started immediately. Supplemental oxygen administered for at least 15 hours per day has been demonstrated to slow the progression of pulmonary hypertension in patients with hypoxemic COPD.

Permanent anticoagulation is indicated in primary pulmonary hypertension but should be given only to those patients with secondary pulmonary hypertension at high risk for thromboembolism. Vasodilator therapy using various pharmacologic agents (eg, calcium antagonists, hydralazine, isoproterenol, diazoxide, nitroglycerin) has shown disappointing results in secondary pulmonary hypertension. Patients most likely to benefit from long-term pulmonary vasodilator therapy are those who respond favorably to a vasodilator challenge at right heart catheterization. It is clear that long-term oral vasodilator therapy should be used only if hemodynamic benefit is documented. Complications of pulmonary vasodilator therapy include systemic hypotension, hypoxemia, and even death.

Continuous long-term intravenous infusion (using a portable pump) of prostacyclin (PGI_2; epoprostenol), a potent pulmonary vasodilator, has been shown to confer hemodynamic and symptomatic benefits in selected patients with primary or secondary pulmonary hypertension. This is the first therapy to demonstrate improved survival of patients with primary pulmonary hypertension. Limitations of continuous infusion prostacyclin are difficulties in titration, technical problems with portable delivery systems, and the high cost of the drug. Newer agents in research trials include subcutaneous (treprostinil), inhaled (iloprost), and oral (beraprost) prostacyclin analogues, endothelin receptor antagonists (bosentan), and phosphodiesterase inhibitors (sildenafil).

Patients with marked polycythemia (hematocrit > 60%) should undergo repeated phlebotomy in an attempt to reduce blood viscosity. Cor pulmonale complicating pulmonary hypertension is treated by managing the underlying pulmonary disease and by using diuretics, salt restriction and, in appropriate patients, supplemental oxygen. The use of digitalis in cor pulmonale remains controversial. Pulmonary thromboendarterectomy may benefit selected patients with pulmonary hypertension secondary to chronic thrombotic obstruction of major pulmonary arteries.

Single or double lung transplantation may be performed on patients with end-stage primary pulmonary hypertension. The 2-year survival rate is 50%.

Prognosis

The prognosis in secondary pulmonary hypertension depends on the course of the underlying disease. Patients with pulmonary hypertension due to fixed obliteration of the pulmonary vascular bed generally respond poorly to therapy; development of cor pulmonale in these cases implies a poor prognosis. The prognosis is favorable when pulmonary hypertension is detected early and the conditions leading to it are readily reversed.

Doyle RL et al: American College of Chest Physicians. Surgical treatments/interventions for pulmonary arterial hypertension: ACCP evidence-based clinical practice guidelines. Chest 2004;126(1 Suppl):63S. [PMID: 15249495]

Farber HW et al: Pulmonary arterial hypertension. N Engl J Med 2004;351:1655. [PMID: 15483284]

Pengo V et al: Thromboembolic Pulmonary Hypertension Study Group. Incidence of chronic thromboembolic pulmonary hypertension after pulmonary embolism. N Engl J Med 2004;350:2257. [PMID: 15163775]

Rubin LJ et al: Evaluation and management of the patient with pulmonary arterial hypertension. Ann Intern Med 2005; 143:282. [PMID: 16103472]

Wright JL et al: Pulmonary hypertension in chronic obstructive pulmonary disease: current theories of pathogenesis and their implications for treatment. Thorax 2005;60: 605. [PMID: 15994270]

PULMONARY VASCULITIS

Wegener's granulomatosis is an idiopathic disease manifested by a combination of glomerulonephritis, necrotizing granulomatous vasculitis of the upper and lower respiratory tracts, and varying degrees of small vessel vasculitis. Chronic sinusitis, arthralgias, fever, skin rash, and weight loss are frequent presenting symptoms. Specific pulmonary complaints occur less often. The most common sign of lung disease is nodular pulmonary infiltrates, often with cavitation, seen on chest radiography. Tracheal stenosis and endobronchial disease are sometimes seen. The diagnosis is most often based on serologic testing and biopsy of lung, sinus tissue, or kidney with demonstration of necrotizing granulomatous vasculitis. See Chapter 20.

Allergic angiitis and granulomatosis (Churg-Strauss syndrome) is an idiopathic multisystem vasculitis of small and medium-sized arteries that occurs in patients with asthma. Histologic features include fibrinoid necrotizing epithelioid and eosinophilic granulomas. The skin and lungs are most often involved, but other organs, including the heart, gastrointestinal tract, liver, and peripheral nerves, may also be affected. Marked peripheral eosinophilia is the rule. Abnormalities on chest radiographs range from transient infiltrates to multiple nodules. This illness may be part of a spectrum that includes polyarteritis nodosa.

Treatment of pulmonary vasculitis consists of combination therapy with corticosteroids and cyclophosphamide. Oral prednisone (1 mg/kg ideal body weight per day initially, tapering slowly to alternate-day therapy over 3–6 months) is the corticosteroid of choice; in Wegener's granulomatosis, some clinicians may omit the use of corticosteroids. For fulminant vasculitis, therapy may be initiated with intravenous methylprednisolone (up to 1 g intravenously per day) for several days. Cyclophosphamide (1–2 mg/kg ideal body weight per day initially, with dosage adjustments to avoid neutropenia) is given daily by mouth for at least 1 year after complete remission is obtained and then is slowly tapered.

Five-year survival rates in patients with these vasculitis syndromes have been improved by the combination therapy. Complete remissions can be achieved in over 90% of patients with Wegener's granulomatosis. The addition of trimethoprim-sulfamethoxazole (one double-strength tablet by mouth twice daily) to standard therapy may help prevent relapses, but its role as sole therapy or as part of combination therapy in patients with active disease remains uncertain.

Langford CA: Update on Wegener granulomatosis. Cleve Clin J Med 2005;72:689. [PMID: 16122054]

Noth I et al: Churg-Strauss syndrome. Lancet 2003;361:587. [PMID: 12598156]

Seo P et al: The antineutrophil cytoplasmic antibody-associated vasculitides. Am J Med 2004;117:39. [PMID: 15210387]

ALVEOLAR HEMORRHAGE SYNDROMES

Diffuse alveolar hemorrhage may occur in a variety of immune and nonimmune disorders. Hemoptysis, alveolar infiltrates on chest radiograph, anemia, dyspnea, and occasionally fever are characteristic. Rapid clearing of diffuse lung infiltrates within 2 days is a clue to the diagnosis of diffuse alveolar hemorrhage. Pulmonary hemorrhage can be associated with an increased DL_{CO}.

Causes of **immune alveolar hemorrhage** have been classified as anti-basement membrane antibody disease (Goodpasture's syndrome), vasculitis and collagen vascular disease (systemic lupus erythematosus, Wegener's granulomatosis, systemic necrotizing vasculitis, and others), and pulmonary capillaritis associated with idiopathic rapidly progressive glomerulonephritis. **Nonimmune causes** of diffuse hemorrhage include coagulopathy, mitral stenosis, necrotizing pulmonary infection, drugs (penicillamine), toxins (trimellitic anhydride), and idiopathic pulmonary hemosiderosis.

Goodpasture's syndrome is idiopathic recurrent alveolar hemorrhage and rapidly progressive glomerulonephritis. The disease is mediated by anti-glomerular basement membrane antibodies. Goodpasture's syndrome occurs mainly in men who are in their 30s and 40s. Hemoptysis is the usual presenting symptom, but pulmonary hemorrhage may be occult. Dyspnea, cough, hypoxemia, and diffuse bilateral alveolar infiltrates are typical features. Iron deficiency anemia and microscopic hematuria are usually present. The diagnosis is based on characteristic linear IgG deposits in glomeruli or alveoli by immunofluorescence and on the presence of anti-glomerular basement membrane antibody in serum. Combinations of immunosuppressive drugs (initially methylprednisolone, 30 mg/kg intravenously over 20 minutes every other day for three doses, followed by daily oral prednisone, 1 mg/kg/d; with cyclophosphamide, 2 mg/kg by mouth per day) and plasmapheresis have yielded excellent results.

Idiopathic pulmonary hemosiderosis is a disease of children or young adults characterized by recurrent pulmonary hemorrhage; in contrast to Goodpasture's syndrome, renal involvement and anti-glomerular basement membrane antibodies are absent, but iron deficiency is typical. Treatment of acute episodes of hemorrhage with corticosteroids may be useful. Recurrent episodes of pulmonary hemorrhage may result in interstitial fibrosis and pulmonary failure.

Collard HR et al: Diffuse alveolar hemorrhage. Clin Chest Med 2004;25:583. [PMID: 15331194]

■ ENVIRONMENTAL & OCCUPATIONAL LUNG DISORDERS

SMOKE INHALATION

The inhalation of products of combustion may cause serious respiratory complications. As many as one-third of patients admitted to burn treatment units have pulmonary injury from smoke inhalation. Morbidity and mortality due to smoke inhalation exceed those attributed to the burns themselves. The death rate of patients with both severe burns and smoke inhalation exceeds 50%.

All patients suspected of having significant smoke inhalation must be assessed for three consequences of smoke inhalation: impaired tissue oxygenation, thermal injury to the upper airway, and chemical injury to the lung. Impaired tissue oxygenation results from inhalation of carbon monoxide or cyanide and is an immediate threat to life. The management of patients with carbon monoxide and cyanide poisoning is discussed in Chapter 39. The clinician must recognize that patients with carbon monoxide poisoning display a normal partial pressure of oxygen in arterial blood (PaO_2) but have a low *measured* (ie, not oximetric) hemoglobin saturation (SaO_2). Immediate treatment with 100% oxygen is essential and should be continued until the measured carboxyhemoglobin level falls to less than 10% and concomitant metabolic acidosis has resolved.

Thermal injury to the mucosal surfaces of the upper airway occurs from inhalation of hot gases. Complications become evident by 18–24 hours. These include edema, impaired ability to clear oral secretions, and upper airway obstruction, producing inspiratory stridor. Respiratory failure occurs in severe cases. Early management (see also Chapter 38) includes the use of a high-humidity face mask with supplemental oxygen, gentle suctioning to evacuate oral secretions, elevation of the head 30 degrees to promote clearing of secretions, and topical epinephrine to reduce edema of the oropharyngeal mucous membrane. Helium-oxygen gas mixtures (Heliox) may reduce labored breathing due to upper airway narrowing. Close monitoring with arterial blood gases and later with oximetry is important. Examination of the upper airway with a fiberoptic laryngoscope or bronchoscope is superior to routine physical examination. Endotracheal intubation is often necessary to establish airway patency and is likely to be necessary in patients with deep facial burns or oropharyngeal or laryngeal edema. Tracheotomy should be avoided if possible because of an increased risk of pneumonia and death from sepsis.

Chemical injury to the lung results from inhalation of toxic gases and products of combustion, including aldehydes and organic acids. The site of lung injury depends on the solubility of the gases inhaled, the duration of exposure, and the size of inhaled particles that transport noxious gases to distal lung units. Bronchorrhea and bronchospasm are seen early after exposure along with dyspnea, tachypnea, and tachycardia. Labored breathing and cyanosis may follow. Physical examination at this stage reveals diffuse wheezing and rhonchi. Bronchiolar and alveolar edema (eg, ARDS) may develop within 1–2 days after exposure. Sloughing of the bronchiolar mucosa may occur within 2–3 days, leading to airway obstruction, atelectasis, and worsening

hypoxemia. Bacterial colonization and pneumonia are common by 5–7 days after the exposure.

Treatment of smoke inhalation consists of supplemental oxygen, bronchodilators, suctioning of mucosal debris and mucopurulent secretions via an indwelling endotracheal tube, chest physical therapy to aid clearance of secretions, and adequate humidification of inspired gases. Positive end-expiratory pressure (PEEP) has been advocated to treat bronchiolar edema. Judicious fluid management and close monitoring for secondary bacterial infection with daily sputum Gram stains round out the management protocol.

The routine use of corticosteroids for chemical lung injury from smoke inhalation has been shown to be ineffective and may even be harmful. Routine or prophylactic use of antibiotics is not recommended.

Patients who survive should be watched for the late development of bronchiolitis obliterans.

Miller K et al: Acute inhalation injury. Emerg Med Clin North Am 2003;21:533. [PMID: 12793627]

Sheridan R: Specific therapies for inhalation injury. Crit Care Med 2002;30:718. [PMID: 11990950]

PULMONARY ASPIRATION SYNDROMES

Aspiration of foreign material into the tracheobronchial tree results from various disorders that impair normal deglutition, especially disturbances of consciousness and esophageal dysfunction.

Aspiration of Inert Material

Aspiration of inert material may cause asphyxia if the amount aspirated is massive and if cough is impaired, in which case immediate tracheobronchial suctioning is necessary. Most patients suffer no serious sequelae from aspiration of inert material.

Aspiration of Toxic Material

Aspiration of toxic material into the lung usually results in clinically evident pneumonia. **Hydrocarbon pneumonitis** is caused by aspiration of ingested petroleum distillates, eg, gasoline, kerosene, furniture polish, and other household petroleum products. Lung injury results mainly from vomiting and secondary aspiration. Therapy is supportive. The lung should be protected from repeated aspiration with a cuffed endotracheal tube if necessary. **Lipoid pneumonia** is a chronic syndrome related to the repeated aspiration of oily materials, eg, mineral oil, cod liver oil, and oily nose drops; it often occurs in elderly patients with impaired swallowing. Patchy infiltrates in dependent lung zones and lipid-laden macrophages in expectorated sputum are characteristic findings.

"Café Coronary"

Acute obstruction of the upper airway by food is associated with difficulty in swallowing, old age, dental problems that impair chewing, and use of alcohol and sedative drugs. The Heimlich procedure is lifesaving in many cases.

Retention of an Aspirated Foreign Body

Retention of an aspirated foreign body in the tracheobronchial tree may produce both acute and chronic conditions, including recurrent pneumonia, bronchiectasis, lung abscess, atelectasis, and postobstructive hyperinflation. Occasionally, a misdiagnosis of asthma, COPD, or lung cancer is made in adult patients who have aspirated a foreign body. The plain chest radiograph usually suggests the site of the foreign body. In some cases, an expiratory film, demonstrating regional hyperinflation due to a check-valve effect, is helpful. Bronchoscopy is usually necessary to establish the diagnosis and attempt removal of the foreign body.

Baharloo F et al: Tracheobronchial foreign bodies: presentation and management in children and adults. Chest 1999;115: 1357. [PMID: 10334153]

Chronic Aspiration of Gastric Contents

Chronic aspiration of gastric contents may result from primary disorders of the larynx or the esophagus, such as achalasia, esophageal stricture, systemic sclerosis (scleroderma), esophageal carcinoma, esophagitis, and gastroesophageal reflux. In the last condition, relaxation of the tone of the lower esophageal sphincter allows reflux of gastric contents into the esophagus and predisposes to chronic pulmonary aspiration, especially at night. Cigarette smoking, consumption of alcohol, and use of theophylline are known to relax the lower esophageal sphincter. Pulmonary disorders linked to gastroesophageal reflux and chronic aspiration include bronchial asthma, pulmonary fibrosis, and bronchiectasis. Even in the absence of aspiration, acid in the esophagus may trigger bronchospasm through reflex mechanisms.

The diagnosis of chronic aspiration is difficult. Ambulatory monitoring of esophageal pH for 24 hours detects esophageal reflux. Esophagogastroscopy and barium swallow are sometimes necessary to rule out esophageal disease. Management consists of elevation of the head of the bed, cessation of smoking, weight reduction, and antacids, H_2-receptor antagonists (eg, cimetidine, 300–400 mg), or proton pump inhibitors (eg, omeprazole, 20 mg) at night. Metoclopramide (10–15 mg orally four times daily or 20 mg at bedtime) or bethanechol (10–25 mg at bedtime) may also be helpful in some patients with gastroesophageal reflux.

Acute Aspiration of Gastric Contents (Mendelson's Syndrome)

Acute aspiration of gastric contents is often catastrophic. The pulmonary response depends on the characteristics and amount of the gastric contents aspirated. The more acidic the material, the greater the degree of chemical pneumonitis. Aspiration of pure gastric acid (pH < 2.5) causes extensive desquamation of the bronchial epithelium, bronchiolitis, hemorrhage, and pulmonary edema. Acute gastric aspiration is one of the most common causes of ARDS. The clinical picture is one of abrupt onset of respiratory distress, with cough, wheezing, fever, and tachypnea. Crackles are audible at the bases of the lungs. Hypoxemia may be noted immediately after aspiration occurs. Radiographic abnormalities, consisting of patchy alveolar infiltrates in dependent lung zones, appear within a few hours. If particulate food matter has been aspirated along with gastric acid, radiographic features of bronchial obstruction may be observed. Fever and leukocytosis are common even in the absence of superinfection.

Treatment of acute aspiration of gastric contents consists of supplemental oxygen, measures to maintain the airway, and the usual measures for treatment of acute respiratory failure. There is no evidence to support the routine use of corticosteroids or prophylactic antibiotics after gastric aspiration has occurred. Secondary pulmonary infection, which occurs in about one-fourth of patients, typically appears 2–3 days after aspiration. Management of this complication depends on the observed flora of the tracheobronchial tree. Hypotension secondary to alveolocapillary membrane injury and intravascular volume depletion is common and is managed with the judicious administration of intravenous fluids.

Marik PE: Aspiration pneumonitis and aspiration pneumonia. N Engl J Med 2001;344:665. [PMID: 11228282]

OCCUPATIONAL PULMONARY DISEASES

Many acute and chronic pulmonary diseases are directly related to inhalation of noxious substances encountered in the workplace. Disorders that are due to chemical agents may be classified as follows: (1) pneumoconioses, (2) hypersensitivity pneumonitis, (3) obstructive airway disorders, (4) toxic lung injury, (5) lung cancer, (6) pleural diseases, and (7) miscellaneous disorders.

Pneumoconioses

Pneumoconioses are chronic fibrotic lung diseases caused by the inhalation of coal dust and various other inert, inorganic, or silicate dusts (Table 9–26). Pneumoconioses due to inhalation of inert dusts may be asymptomatic disorders with diffuse nodular infiltrates on chest radiograph. Clinically important pneumoconioses include coal workers' pneumoconiosis, silicosis, and asbestosis. Treatment for each is supportive.

A. COAL WORKER'S PNEUMOCONIOSIS

In coal worker's pneumoconiosis, ingestion of inhaled coal dust by alveolar macrophages leads to the formation

Table 9–26. Selected pneumoconioses.

Disease	Agent	Occupations
Metal dusts		
Siderosis	Metallic iron or iron oxide	Mining, welding, foundry work
Stannosis	Tin, tin oxide	Mining, tin-working, smelting
Baritosis	Barium salts	Glass and insecticide manufacturing
Coal dust		
Coal worker's pneumoconiosis	Coal dust	Coal mining
Inorganic dusts		
Silicosis	Free silica (silicon dioxide)	Rock mining, quarrying, stone cutting, tunneling, sandblasting, pottery, diatomaceous earth
Silicate dusts		
Asbestosis	Asbestos	Mining, insulation, construction, shipbuilding
Talcosis	Magnesium silicate	Mining, insulation, construction, shipbuilding
Kaolin pneumoconiosis	Sand, mica, aluminum silicate	Mining of china clay; pottery and cement work
Shaver's disease	Aluminum powder	Manufacture of corundum

of coal macules, usually 2–5 mm in diameter, which appear on chest radiograph as diffuse small opacities that are especially prominent in the upper lung. Simple coal worker's pneumoconiosis is usually asymptomatic; pulmonary function abnormalities are unimpressive. Cigarette smoking does not increase the prevalence of coal worker's pneumoconiosis but may have an additive detrimental effect on ventilatory function. In complicated coal worker's pneumoconiosis (**"progressive massive fibrosis"**), conglomeration and contraction in the upper lung zones occur, with radiographic features resembling complicated silicosis. **Caplan's syndrome** is a rare condition characterized by the presence of necrobiotic rheumatoid nodules (1–5 cm in diameter) in the periphery of the lung in coal workers with rheumatoid arthritis.

B. SILICOSIS

In silicosis, extensive or prolonged inhalation of free silica (silicon dioxide) particles in the respirable range (0.3–5 mcm) causes the formation of small rounded opacities (silicotic nodules) throughout the lung. Calcification of the periphery of hilar lymph nodes ("egg-

shell" calcification) is an unusual radiographic finding that strongly suggests silicosis. Simple silicosis is usually asymptomatic and has no effect on routine pulmonary function tests; in complicated silicosis, large conglomerate densities appear in the upper lung and are accompanied by dyspnea and obstructive and restrictive pulmonary dysfunction. The incidence of pulmonary tuberculosis is increased in patients with silicosis. All patients with silicosis should have a tuberculin skin test and a current chest radiograph. If old, healed pulmonary tuberculosis is suspected, multidrug treatment for tuberculosis (not single-agent preventive therapy) should be instituted.

C. ASBESTOSIS

Asbestosis is a nodular interstitial fibrosis occurring in workers exposed to asbestos fibers (shipyard and construction workers, pipefitters, insulators) over many years (typically 10–20 years). Patients with asbestosis usually seek medical attention at least 15 years after exposure with the following symptoms and signs: progressive dyspnea, inspiratory crackles, and in some cases, clubbing and cyanosis. The radiographic features of asbestosis include linear streaking at the lung bases, opacities of various shapes and sizes, and honeycomb changes in advanced cases. The presence of pleural calcifications may be a clue to diagnosis. High-resolution CT scanning is the best imaging method for asbestosis because of its ability to detect parenchymal fibrosis and define the presence of coexisting pleural plaques. Cigarette smoking in asbestos workers increases the prevalence of radiographic pleural and parenchymal changes and markedly increases the incidence of lung carcinoma. It may also interfere with the clearance of short asbestos fibers from the lung. Pulmonary function studies show restrictive dysfunction and reduced diffusing capacity. The presence of a ferruginous body in tissue suggests significant asbestos exposure; however, other histologic features must be present for diagnosis. There is no specific treatment.

Cugell DW et al: Asbestos and the pleura: a review. Chest 2004; 125:1103. [PMID: 15006974]

Kuschner WG et al: Occupational lung disease. Part 2. Discovering the cause of diffuse parenchymal lung disease. Postgrad Med 2003;113:81. [PMID: 12718237]

Scarisbrick D: Silicosis and coal workers' pneumoconiosis. Practitioner 2002;246:114. [PMID: 11852619]

Hypersensitivity Pneumonitis

Hypersensitivity pneumonitis (extrinsic allergic alveolitis) is a nonatopic, nonasthmatic allergic pulmonary disease. It is manifested mainly as an occupational disease (Table 9–27), in which exposure to inhaled organic agents leads to acute and eventually chronic pulmonary disease. Acute illness is characterized by sudden onset of malaise, chills, fever, cough, dyspnea, and nausea 4–8 hours after exposure to the offending agent. This may occur after the patient has left work or even at night and

Table 9–27. Selected causes of hypersensitivity pneumonitis.

Disease	Antigen	Source
Farmer's lung	*Micropolyspora faeni, Thermo-actinomyces vulgaris*	Moldy hay
"Humidifier" lung	Thermophilic actinomycetes	Contaminated humidifiers, heating systems, or air conditioners
Bird fancier's lung ("pigeon-breeder's disease")	Avian proteins	Bird serum and excreta
Bagassosis	*Thermoactino-myces sacchari* and *T vulgaris*	Moldy sugar cane fiber (bagasse)
Sequoiosis	Graphium, aureobasidium, and other fungi	Moldy redwood sawdust
Maple bark stripper's disease	*Cryptostroma (Coniosporium) corticale*	Rotting maple tree logs or bark
Mushroom picker's disease	Same as farmer's lung	Moldy compost
Suberosis	*Penicillium frequentans*	Moldy cork dust
Detergent worker's lung	*Bacillus subtilis* enzyme	Enzyme additives

thus may mimic paroxysmal nocturnal dyspnea. Bibasilar crackles, tachypnea, tachycardia, and (occasionally) cyanosis are noted. Small nodular densities sparing the apices and bases of the lungs are noted on chest radiograph. Pulmonary function studies reveal restrictive dysfunction and reduced diffusing capacity. Laboratory studies reveal an increase in the white blood cell count with a shift to the left, hypoxemia, and the presence of precipitating antibodies to the offending agent in serum. Hypersensitivity pneumonitis antibody panels against common offending antigens are available.

Acute hypersensitivity pneumonitis is characterized by interstitial infiltrates of lymphocytes and plasma cells, with noncaseating granulomas in the interstitium and air spaces. A subacute hypersensitivity pneumonitis syndrome (15% of cases) has been described that is characterized by the insidious onset of chronic cough and slowly progressive dyspnea, anorexia, and weight loss. Chronic respiratory insufficiency and the appearance of pulmonary fibrosis on radiographs may occur after repeated exposure to the offending agent. Surgical lung biopsy is occasionally necessary for diagnosis.

Diffuse fibrosis is the hallmark of the subacute and chronic phases.

Treatment of hypersensitivity pneumonitis consists of identification of the offending agent, avoidance of further exposure, and, in severe acute or protracted cases, oral corticosteroids (prednisone, 0.5 mg/kg daily as a single morning dose, tapered to nil over 4–6 weeks). Change in occupation is often unavoidable.

Jacobs RL et al: Hypersensitivity pneumonitis: beyond classic occupational disease-changing concepts of diagnosis and management. Ann Allergy Asthma Immunol 2005;95:115. [PMID: 16136760]

Lacasse Y et al: Clinical diagnosis of hypersensitivity pneumonitis. Am J Respir Crit Care Med 2003;168:952. [PMID: 12842854]

Obstructive Airway Disorders

Occupational pulmonary diseases manifested as obstructive airway disorders include occupational asthma, industrial bronchitis, and byssinosis.

A. OCCUPATIONAL ASTHMA

It has been estimated that from 2% to 5% of all cases of asthma are related to occupation. Offending agents in the workplace are numerous; they include grain dust, wood dust, tobacco, pollens, enzymes, gum arabic, synthetic dyes, isocyanates (particularly toluene diisocyanate), rosin (soldering flux), inorganic chemicals (salts of nickel, platinum, and chromium), trimellitic anhydride, phthalic anhydride, formaldehyde, and various pharmaceutical agents. Diagnosis of occupational asthma depends on a high index of suspicion, an appropriate history, spirometric studies before and after exposure to the offending substance, and peak flow rate measurements in the workplace. Bronchial provocation testing may be helpful in some cases. Treatment consists of avoidance of further exposure to the offending agent and bronchodilators, but symptoms may persist for years after workplace exposure has been terminated.

B. INDUSTRIAL BRONCHITIS

Industrial bronchitis is chronic bronchitis found in coal miners and others exposed to cotton, flax, or hemp dust. Chronic disability from industrial bronchitis is infrequent.

C. BYSSINOSIS

Byssinosis is an asthma-like disorder in textile workers caused by inhalation of cotton dust. The pathogenesis is obscure. Chest tightness, cough, and dyspnea are characteristically worse on Mondays or the first day back at work, with symptoms subsiding later in the week. Repeated exposure leads to chronic bronchitis.

Toxic Lung Injury

Toxic lung injury from inhalation of irritant gases is discussed in the section on smoke inhalation. **Silo-filler's disease** is acute toxic high-permeability pulmonary edema caused by inhalation of nitrogen dioxide encountered in recently filled silos. Bronchiolitis obliterans is a common late complication, which may be prevented by early treatment of the acute reaction with corticosteroids. Extensive exposure to silage gas may be fatal.

Lung Cancer

Many industrial pulmonary carcinogens have been identified, including asbestos, radon gas, arsenic, iron, chromium, nickel, coal tar fumes, petroleum oil mists, isopropyl oil, mustard gas, and printing ink. Cigarette smoking acts as a cocarcinogen with asbestos and radon gas to cause bronchogenic carcinoma. Asbestos alone causes malignant mesothelioma. Almost all histologic types of lung cancer have been associated with these carcinogens. Chloromethyl methyl ether specifically causes small cell carcinoma of the lung.

Pleural Diseases

Occupational diseases of the pleura may result from exposure to asbestos (see above) or talc. Inhalation of talc causes pleural plaques that are similar to those caused by asbestos. Benign asbestos pleural effusion occurs in some asbestos workers and may cause chronic blunting of the costophrenic angle on chest radiograph.

Other Occupational Pulmonary Diseases

Occupational agents are also responsible for other pulmonary disorders. These include **berylliosis**, an acute or chronic pulmonary disorder related to exposure to beryllium, which is absorbed through the lungs or skin and widely disseminated throughout the body. Acute berylliosis is a toxic, ulcerative tracheobronchitis and chemical pneumonitis following intense and severe exposure to beryllium. Chronic berylliosis, a systemic disease closely resembling sarcoidosis, is more common. Chronic pulmonary beryllium disease is thought to be an alveolitis mediated by the proliferation of beryllium-specific helper-inducer T cells in the lung. Exposure to beryllium now occurs in machining and handling of beryllium products and alloys. Beryllium miners are not at risk for berylliosis. Beryllium is no longer used in fluorescent lamp production, which was a source of exposure before 1950.

American Thoracic Society Statement: Occupational contribution to the burden of airway disease. Am J Respir Crit Care Med 2003;167:787. [PMID: 12598220]

Glazer CS et al: Occupational interstitial lung disease. Clin Chest Med 2004;25:467. [PMID: 15331187]

Kim JS et al: Imaging of nonmalignant occupational lung disease. J Thorac Imaging 2002;17:238. [PMID: 12362064]

Mapp CE et al: Occupational asthma. Am J Respir Crit Care Med 2005;172:280. [PMID: 15860754]

Singh N et al: Review: occupational and environmental lung disease. Curr Opin Pulm Med 2002;8:117. [PMID: 11845007]

DRUG-INDUCED LUNG DISEASE

Typical patterns of pulmonary response to drugs implicated in drug-induced respiratory disease are summarized in Table 9–28. Pulmonary injury due to drugs occurs as a result of allergic reactions, idiosyncratic reactions, overdose, or undesirable side effects. In most patients, the mechanism of pulmonary injury is unknown.

Precise diagnosis of drug-induced pulmonary disease is often difficult, because results of routine laboratory studies are not helpful and radiographic findings

Table 9–28. Pulmonary manifestations of selected drug toxicities.

Asthma	Pulmonary edema
β-Blockers	Noncardiogenic
Aspirin	Aspirin
Nonsteroidal anti-inflammatory drugs	Chlordiazepoxide
	Cocaine
Histamine	Ethchlorvynol
Methacholine	Heroin
Acetylcysteine	Cardiogenic
Aerosolized pentamidine	β-Blockers
Any nebulized medication	**Pleural effusion**
Chronic cough	Bromocriptine
Angiotensin-converting enzyme inhibitors	Nitrofurantoin
	Any drug inducing systemic lupus erythematosus
Pulmonary infiltration	
Without eosinophilia	
Amitriptyline	Methysergide
Azathioprine	Chemotherapeutic agents
Amiodarone	**Mediastinal widening**
With eosinophilia	Phenytoin
Sulfonamides	Corticosteroids
L-Tryptophan	Methotrexate
Nitrofurantoin	**Respiratory failure**
Penicillin	Neuromuscular blockade
Methotrexate	Aminoglycosides
Crack cocaine	Succinylcholine
Drug-induced systemic lupus erythematosus	Gallamine
Hydralazine	Dimethyltubocurarine (metocurine)
Procainamide	Central nervous system depression
Isoniazid	
Chlorpromazine	Sedatives
Phenytoin	Hypnotics
Interstitial pneumonitis/ fibrosis	Opioids
	Alcohol
Nitrofurantoin	Tricyclic antidepressants
Bleomycin	Oxygen
Busulfan	
Cyclophosphamide	
Methysergide	
Phenytoin	

are not specific. A high index of suspicion and a thorough medical history of drug usage are critical to establishing the diagnosis of drug-induced lung disease. The clinical response to cessation of the suspected offending agent is also helpful. Acute episodes of drug-induced pulmonary disease usually disappear 24–48 hours after the drug has been discontinued, but chronic syndromes may take longer to resolve. Challenge tests to confirm the diagnosis are risky and rarely performed.

Treatment of drug-induced lung disease consists of discontinuing the offending agent immediately and managing the pulmonary symptoms appropriately.

Inhalation of crack cocaine may cause a spectrum of acute pulmonary syndromes, including pulmonary infiltration with eosinophilia, pneumothorax and pneumomediastinum, bronchiolitis obliterans, and acute respiratory failure associated with diffuse alveolar damage and alveolar hemorrhage. Corticosteroids have been used with variable success to treat alveolar hemorrhage.

Babu KS et al: Drug-induced airway diseases. Clin Chest Med 2004;25:113. [PMID: 15062603]

Huggins JT et al: Drug-induced pleural disease. Clin Chest Med 2004;25:141. [PMID: 15062606]

RADIATION LUNG INJURY

The lung is an exquisitely radiosensitive organ that can be damaged by external beam radiation therapy. The degree of pulmonary injury is determined by the volume of lung irradiated, the dose and rate of exposure, and potentiating factors (eg, concurrent chemotherapy, previous radiation therapy in the same area, and simultaneous withdrawal of corticosteroid therapy). Symptomatic radiation lung injury occurs in about 10% of patients treated for carcinoma of the breast, 5–15% of patients treated for carcinoma of the lung, and 5–35% of patients treated for lymphoma. Two phases of the pulmonary response to radiation are apparent: an acute phase (radiation pneumonitis) and a chronic phase (radiation fibrosis).

Radiation Pneumonitis

Radiation pneumonitis usually occurs 2–3 months (range 1–6 months) after completion of radiotherapy and is characterized by insidious onset of dyspnea, intractable dry cough, chest fullness or pain, weakness, and fever. The pathogenesis of acute radiation pneumonitis is unknown, but there is speculation that hypersensitivity mechanisms are involved. The dominant histopathologic findings are a lymphocytic interstitial pneumonitis progressing to an exudative alveolitis. Inspiratory crackles may be heard in the involved area. In severe disease, respiratory distress and cyanosis occur that are characteristic of ARDS. An increased white blood cell count and elevated sedimentation rate are common. Pulmonary function studies reveal reduced lung volumes, reduced lung compliance, hypoxemia, reduced diffusing capacity, and reduced maximum voluntary ventilation. Chest radiography, which correlates poorly with the presence of symptoms, usually demonstrates an alveolar or nodular infiltrate limited to the irradiated area. Air bronchograms are often observed. Sharp borders of the infiltrate may help distinguish radiation pneumonitis from other conditions such as infectious pneumonia, lymphangitic spread of carcinoma, and recurrent tumor. No specific therapy is proved to be effective in radiation pneumonitis, but prednisone (1 mg/kg/d orally) is commonly given immediately for about 1 week. The dose is then reduced and maintained at 20–40 mg/d for several weeks, then slowly tapered. Radiation pneumonitis may improve in 2–3 weeks following onset of symptoms as the exudative phase resolves. Acute respiratory failure, if present, is treated supportively. Death from ARDS is unusual.

Pulmonary Radiation Fibrosis

Pulmonary radiation fibrosis occurs in nearly all patients who receive a full course of radiation therapy for cancer of the lung or breast. Patients who experience radiation pneumonitis develop pulmonary fibrosis after an intervening period (6–12 months) of well-being. Most patients are asymptomatic, though slowly progressive dyspnea may occur. Radiation fibrosis may occur with or without antecedent radiation pneumonitis. Cor pulmonale and chronic respiratory failure are rare. Radiographic findings include obliteration of normal lung markings, dense interstitial and pleural fibrosis, reduced lung volumes, tenting of the diaphragm, and sharp delineation of the irradiated area. No specific therapy is proved effective, and corticosteroids have no value.

Other Complications of Radiation Therapy

Other complications of radiation therapy directed to the thorax include pericardial effusion, constrictive pericarditis, tracheoesophageal fistula, esophageal candidiasis, radiation dermatitis, and rib fractures. Small pleural effusions, radiation pneumonitis outside the irradiated area, spontaneous pneumothorax, and complete obstruction of central airways are unusual occurrences.

Abratt RP et al: Pulmonary complications of radiation therapy. Clin Chest Med 2004;25:167. [PMID: 15062608]

Camus P et al: Interstitial lung disease induced by drugs and radiation. Respiration 2004;71:301. [PMID: 15316202]

■ PLEURAL DISEASES

PLEURITIS

Pain due to acute pleural inflammation is caused by irritation of the parietal pleura. Such pain is localized, sharp, and fleeting; it is made worse by coughing, sneezing, deep breathing, or movement. When the central portion of the diaphragmatic parietal pleura is irritated, pain may be referred to the ipsilateral shoulder. There are numerous causes of pleuritis. The setting in which pleuritic pain develops helps narrow the differential diagnosis. In young, otherwise healthy individuals, pleuritis is usually caused by viral respiratory infections or pneumonia. The presence of pleural effusion, pleural thickening, or air in the pleural space requires further diagnostic and therapeutic measures. Simple rib fracture may cause severe pleurisy.

Treatment of pleuritis consists of treating the underlying disease. Analgesics and anti-inflammatory drugs (eg, indomethacin, 25 mg orally two or three times daily) are often helpful for pain relief. Codeine (30–60 mg orally every 8 hours) may be used to control cough associated with pleuritic chest pain if retention of airway secretions is not a likely complication. Intercostal nerve blocks are sometimes helpful but the benefit is usually transient.

PLEURAL EFFUSION

ESSENTIALS OF DIAGNOSIS

- *May be asymptomatic; chest pain frequently seen in the setting of pleuritis, trauma, or infection; dyspnea is common with large effusions.*
- *Dullness to percussion and decreased breath sounds over the effusion.*
- *Radiographic evidence of pleural effusion.*
- *Diagnostic findings on thoracentesis.*

General Considerations

There is constant movement of fluid from parietal pleural capillaries into the pleural space at a rate of 0.01 mL/kg body weight/h. Absorption of pleural fluid occurs through parietal pleural lymphatics. The resultant homeostasis leaves 5–15 mL of fluid in the normal pleural space. A pleural effusion is an abnormal accumulation of fluid in the pleural space. Pleural effusions may be classified by differential diagnosis (Table 9–29) or by underlying pathophysiology. Five pathophysiologic processes account for most pleural effusions: increased production of fluid in the setting of normal capillaries due to increased hydrostatic or decreased oncotic pressures (transudates); increased production of fluid due to abnormal capillary permeability (exudates); decreased lymphatic clearance of fluid from the pleural space (exudates); infection in the pleural space (empyema); and bleeding into the pleural space (hemothorax).

Diagnostic thoracentesis should be performed whenever there is a new pleural effusion and no clini-

Table 9–29. Causes of pleural fluid transudates and exudates.

Transudates	Exudates
Congestive heart failure (≈90% of cases)	Pneumonia (parapneumonic effusion)
Cirrhosis with ascites	Cancer
Nephrotic syndrome	Pulmonary embolism
Peritoneal dialysis	Bacterial infection
Myxedema	Tuberculosis
Acute atelectasis	Connective tissue disease
Constrictive pericarditis	Viral infection
Superior vena cava obstruction	Fungal infection
Pulmonary embolism	Rickettsial infection
	Parasitic infection
	Asbestos
	Meigs' syndrome
	Pancreatic disease
	Uremia
	Chronic atelectasis
	Trapped lung
	Chylothorax
	Sarcoidosis
	Drug reaction
	Post-myocardial infarction syndrome

cally apparent cause. Observation is appropriate in some situations (eg, symmetric bilateral pleural effusions in the setting of congestive heart failure), but an atypical presentation or failure of an effusion to resolve as expected warrants thoracentesis. Sampling allows visualization of the fluid in addition to chemical and microbiologic analyses to identify the pathophysiologic processes listed above. A definitive diagnosis is made through positive cytology or identification of a specific causative organism in approximately 25% of cases. In another 50–60% of patients, identification of relevant pathophysiology in the appropriate clinical setting greatly narrows the differential diagnosis and leads to a presumptive diagnosis.

Clinical Findings

A. SYMPTOMS AND SIGNS

Patients with pleural effusions most often report dyspnea, cough, or respirophasic chest pain. Symptoms are more common in patients with existing cardiopulmonary disease. Small pleural effusions are less likely to be symptomatic than larger effusions. Physical findings are usually absent in small effusions. Larger effusions may present with dullness to percussion and diminished or absent breath sounds over the effusion. Compressive atelectasis may cause bronchial breath sounds and egophony just above the effusion. A massive effusion with increased intrapleural pressure may cause contralateral shift of the trachea and bulging of the intercostal spaces. A pleural friction rub indicates infarction or pleuritis.

B. LABORATORY FINDINGS

The gross appearance of pleural fluid helps identify several types of pleural effusion. Grossly purulent fluid signifies empyema, an infection of the pleural space. Milky white pleural fluid should be centrifuged. A clear supernatant above a pellet of white cells indicates empyema, whereas a persistently turbid supernatant suggests a chylous effusion. Analysis of this supernatant reveals chylomicrons and a high triglyceride level (> 100 mg/dL), often from traumatic disruption of the thoracic duct. Hemorrhagic pleural effusion is a mixture of blood and pleural fluid. Ten thousand red cells per milliliter create blood-tinged pleural fluid; 100,000/mL create grossly bloody pleural fluid. Hemothorax is the presence of gross blood in the pleural space, usually following chest trauma or instrumentation. It is defined as a ratio of pleural fluid hematocrit to peripheral blood hematocrit > 0.5.

Pleural fluid samples should be sent for measurement of protein, glucose, and LDH in addition to total and differential white blood cell counts. Chemistry determinations are used to classify effusions as transudates or exudates. This classification is important because the differential diagnosis for each entity is vastly different (Table 9–29). A pleural exudate is an effusion that has *one or more* of the following laboratory features: (1) ratio of pleural fluid protein to serum protein > 0.5; (2) ratio of pleural fluid LDH to serum LDH > 0.6; (3) pleural fluid LDH greater than two-thirds the upper limit of normal serum LDH.

Transudates have none of these features. Transudates occur in the setting of normal capillary integrity and suggest the *absence* of local pleural disease. Distinguishing laboratory findings include a glucose equal to serum glucose, pH between 7.40 and 7.55, and fewer than 1000 white blood cells/mcL with a predominance of mononuclear cells. Causes include increased hydrostatic pressure (congestive heart failure accounts for 90% of transudates), decreased oncotic pressure (hypoalbuminemia, cirrhosis), and greater negative pleural pressure (acute atelectasis). Exudates form as a result of pleural disease associated with increased capillary permeability or reduced lymphatic drainage. Bacterial pneumonia and cancer are the most common causes of exudative effusion, but there are many other causes with characteristic laboratory findings. These findings are summarized in Table 9–30.

Pleural fluid pH is useful in the assessment of parapneumonic effusions. A pH below 7.30 suggests the need for drainage of the pleural space. An elevated amylase level in pleural fluid suggests pancreatitis, pancreatic pseudocyst, adenocarcinoma of the lung or pancreas, or esophageal rupture.

Thoracentesis with culture and pleural biopsy is indicated in suspected tuberculous pleural effusion. Pleural fluid culture is 44% sensitive, and the combination of closed pleural biopsy with culture and histologic examination for granulomas is 70–90% sensitive for the diagnosis of pleural tuberculosis.

Pleural fluid specimens should be sent for cytologic examination in all cases of exudative effusions in patients suspected of harboring an underlying malignancy. The diagnostic yield depends on the nature and extent of the underlying malignancy. Sensitivity is between 50% and 65%. A negative cytologic examination in a patient with a high prior probability of malignancy should be followed by one repeat thoracentesis. If that examination is negative, thoracoscopy (by a pulmonologist or by VATS) is preferred to closed pleural biopsy. The sensitivity of thoracoscopy is 92–96%.

C. IMAGING

The lung is less dense than water and floats on pleural fluid that accumulates in dependent regions. Subpulmonary fluid may appear as lateral displacement of the apex of the diaphragm with an abrupt slope to the costophrenic sulcus or a greater than 2-cm separation between the gastric air bubble and the lung. On a standard upright chest radiograph, approximately 75–100 mL of pleural fluid must accumulate in the posterior costophrenic sulcus to be visible on the lateral view, and 175–200 mL must be present in the lateral costophrenic sulcus to be visible on the frontal view. Chest CT scans may identify as little as 10 mL of fluid. At least 1 cm of fluid on the decubitus view is necessary to permit blind thoracentesis. Ultrasonography is useful to guide thoracentesis in the setting of smaller effusions.

Pleural fluid may become trapped (loculated) by pleural adhesions, thereby forming unusual collections along the lateral chest wall or within lung fissures. Round or oval fluid collections in fissures that resemble intraparenchymal masses are called pseudotumors. Massive pleural effusion causing opacification of an entire hemithorax is most commonly caused by cancer but may be seen in tuberculosis and other diseases.

Treatment

A. TRANSUDATIVE PLEURAL EFFUSION

Transudative pleural effusions characteristically occur in the absence of pleural disease. Treatment is directed at the underlying condition. Therapeutic thoracentesis for severe dyspnea typically offers only transient benefit. Pleurodesis and tube thoracostomy are rarely indicated.

B. MALIGNANT PLEURAL EFFUSION

Approximately 15% of patients dying of cancer are reported to have malignant pleural effusions. Almost any form of cancer may cause effusions, but the most common causes are lung cancer (one-third of cases) and breast cancer. In 5–10% of malignant pleural effusions, no primary tumor is identified.

Between 40% and 80% of exudative pleural effusions are malignant, while over 90% of malignant pleural effusions are exudative. The most common mecha-

Table 9–30. Characteristics of important exudative pleural effusions.

Etiology or Type of Effusion	Gross Appearance	White Blood Cell Count (cells/mcL)	Red Blood Cell Count (cells/mcL)	Glucose	Comments
Malignant effusion	Turbid to bloody; occasionally serous	1000 to < 100,000 M	100 to several hundred thousand	Equal to serum levels; < 60 mg/dL in 15% of cases	Eosinophilia uncommon; positive results on cytologic examination
Uncomplicated parapneumonic effusion	Clear to turbid	5000–25,000 P	< 5000	Equal to serum levels	Tube thoracostomy unnecessary
Empyema	Turbid to purulent	25,000–100,000 P	< 5000	Less than serum levels; often very low	Drainage necessary; putrid odor suggests anaerobic infection
Tuberculosis	Serous to serosanguineous	5000–10,000 M	< 10,000	Equal to serum levels; occasionally < 60 mg/dL	Protein > 4.0 g/dL and may exceed 5 g/dL; eosinophils (> 10%) or mesothelial cells (> 5%) make diagnosis unlikely
Rheumatoid effusion	Turbid; greenish yellow	1000–20,000 M or P	< 1000	< 40 mg/dL	Secondary empyema common; high LDH, low complement, high rheumatoid factor, cholesterol crystals are characteristic
Pulmonary infarction	Serous to grossly bloody	1000–50,000 M or P	100 to > 100,000	Equal to serum levels	Variable findings; no pathognomonic features
Esophageal rupture	Turbid to purulent; red-brown	< 5000 to > 50,000 P	1000–10,000	Usually low	High amylase level (salivary origin); pneumothorax in 25% of cases; effusion usually on left side; pH < 6.0 strongly suggests diagnosis
Pancreatitis	Turbid to serosanguineous	1000–50,000 P	1000–10,000	Equal to serum levels	Usually left-sided; high amylase level

Key: M = mononuclear cell predominance; P = polymorphonuclear leukocyte predominance; LDH = lactate dehydrogenase.

nisms contributing to the formation of malignant effusions include direct tumor involvement of the pleura, local inflammation in response to tumor spread, and impairment or disruption of lymphatics. The term "paramalignant pleural effusion" refers to an effusion in a patient with cancer when repeated attempts to identify tumor cells in the pleura or pleural fluid are nondiagnostic but when there is a presumptive relation to the underlying malignancy. For example, superior vena cava syndrome with elevated systemic venous pressures causing a transudative effusion would be "paramalignant."

Most patients with malignant effusions have advanced disease and multiple symptoms. Dyspnea occurs in over half of patients with malignant pleural effusions. The cause of dyspnea is probably related to mechanical distortion of the lung and chest wall. Hypoxemia from intrapulmonary shunting and V/Q mismatching is common and may be severe. Treatment may be systemic, with therapy for the underlying ma-

lignancy; or local, to address specific symptoms related to the effusion itself. Local treatment usually involves drainage through repeated thoracentesis or placement of a chest tube. Pleurodesis is a procedure by which an irritant is placed into the pleural space following chest tube drainage and lung reexpansion. The goal is to form fibrous adhesions between the visceral and parietal pleura, resulting in obliteration of the pleural space to prevent or significantly reduce reaccumulation of pleural fluid. Multiple agents have been used for pleurodesis, but the two in most common use are doxycycline (500 mg in 50–100 mL saline) and sterile, asbestos-free talc (by poudrage at thoracoscopy using 5 g or instillation of talc slurry through a chest tube using 4–5 g in 50 mL saline). Doxycycline and talc are associated with a 70–75% and a 90% success rate, respectively. Major side effects are pain and fever, which appear to be less common with talc. Pain associated with pleurodesis can be extreme. Patients should be premedicated with an anxiolytic-amnestic agent in addition to opioid analgesics.

C. PARAPNEUMONIC PLEURAL EFFUSION

Parapneumonic pleural effusions are exudates that accompany approximately 40% of bacterial pneumonias. They are divided into three categories: simple or uncomplicated, complicated, and empyema. Uncomplicated parapneumonic effusions are free-flowing sterile exudates of modest size that resolve quickly with antibiotic treatment of pneumonia. They do not need drainage. Empyema is gross infection of the pleural space indicated by positive Gram stain or culture. Empyema should always be drained by tube thoracostomy to facilitate clearance of infection and to reduce the probability of fibrous encasement of the lung, causing permanent pulmonary impairment.

Complicated parapneumonic effusions present the most difficult management decisions. They tend to be larger than simple parapneumonic effusions and to show more evidence of inflammatory stimuli such as low glucose level, low pH, or evidence of loculation. Inflammation probably reflects ongoing bacterial invasion of the pleural space despite rare positive bacterial cultures. The morbidity associated with complicated effusions is due to their tendency to form a fibropurulent pleural "peel," trapping otherwise functional lung and leading to permanent impairment. Tube thoracostomy is indicated when pleural fluid glucose is < 60 mg/dL or the pH is < 7.2. These thresholds have not been prospectively validated and should not be interpreted strictly. The clinician should consider drainage of a complicated effusion if the pleural fluid pH is between 7.2 and 7.3 or the LDH is > 1000 units/mL. Pleural fluid cell count and protein have little diagnostic value in this setting.

Tube thoracostomy drainage of empyema or parapneumonic effusions is frequently complicated by loculation that prevents adequate drainage. Intrapleural injection of fibrinolytic agents (streptokinase, 250,000 units, or urokinase, 100,000 units, in 50–100 mL of normal saline once or twice daily) has been reported to improve drainage, shorten hospitalization, and reduce the need for surgery. Reported success rates in small studies are between 70% and 90%.

D. HEMOTHORAX

A small-volume hemothorax that is stable or improving on chest radiographs may be managed by close observation. In all other cases, hemothorax is treated by immediate insertion of a large-bore thoracostomy tube to (1) drain existing blood and clot, (2) quantify the amount of bleeding, (3) reduce the risk of fibrothorax, and (4) permit apposition of the pleural surfaces in an attempt to reduce hemorrhage. Thoracotomy may be indicated to control hemorrhage, remove clot, and treat complications such as bronchopleural fistula formation.

Colice GL et al: Medical and surgical treatment of parapneumonic effusions: an evidence-based guideline. Chest 2000; 118:1158. [PMID: 11035692]

Shaw P et al: Pleurodesis for malignant pleural effusions. Cochrane Database Syst Rev 2004;(1):CD002916. [PMID: 14973997]

Yataco JC et al: Pleural effusions: evaluation and management. Cleve Clin J Med 2005;72:854. [PMID: 16231684]

SPONTANEOUS PNEUMOTHORAX

 ESSENTIALS OF DIAGNOSIS

- *Acute onset of unilateral chest pain and dyspnea.*
- *Minimal physical findings in mild cases; unilateral chest expansion, decreased tactile fremitus, hyperresonance, diminished breath sounds, mediastinal shift, cyanosis and hypotension in tension pneumothorax.*
- *Presence of pleural air on chest radiograph.*

General Considerations

Pneumothorax, or accumulation of air in the pleural space, is classified as spontaneous (primary or secondary) or traumatic. Primary spontaneous pneumothorax occurs in the absence of an underlying lung disease, whereas secondary spontaneous pneumothorax is a complication of preexisting pulmonary disease. Traumatic pneumothorax results from penetrating or blunt trauma. Iatrogenic pneumothorax may follow procedures such as thoracentesis, pleural biopsy, subclavian or internal jugular vein catheter placement, percutaneous lung biopsy, bronchoscopy with transbronchial biopsy, and positive-pressure mechanical ventilation. Tension pneumothorax usually occurs in the setting of penetrating trauma, lung infection, cardiopulmonary resuscitation, or positive-pressure mechanical ventilation. In tension pneumothorax, the pressure of air in the pleural space exceeds ambient pressure throughout the respiratory cycle. A check-valve mechanism allows air to enter the pleural space on inspiration and prevents egress of air on expiration.

Primary pneumothorax affects mainly tall, thin boys and men between the ages of 10 and 30 years. It is thought to occur from rupture of subpleural apical blebs in response to high negative intrapleural pressures. Family history and cigarette smoking may also be important factors.

Secondary pneumothorax occurs as a complication of COPD, asthma, cystic fibrosis, tuberculosis, *Pneumocystis* pneumonia, menstruation (catamenial pneumothorax), and a wide variety of interstitial lung diseases including sarcoidosis, lymphangioleiomyomatosis, Langerhans cell histiocytosis, and tuberous sclerosis. Aerosolized pentamidine and a prior history of *Pneumocystis* pneumonia are considered risk factors for the development of pneumothorax. One-half of patients with pneumothorax in the setting of recurrent *Pneumocystis* pneumonia will develop pneumothorax on the contralateral side. The mortality rate of pneumothorax in *Pneumocystis* pneumonia is high.

Clinical Findings

A. SYMPTOMS AND SIGNS

Chest pain ranging from minimal to severe on the affected side and dyspnea occur in nearly all patients. Symptoms usually begin during rest and usually resolve within 24 hours even if the pneumothorax persists. Alternatively, pneumothorax may present with life-threatening respiratory failure if underlying COPD or asthma is present.

If pneumothorax is small (less than 15% of a hemithorax), physical findings, other than mild tachycardia, are unimpressive. If pneumothorax is large, diminished breath sounds, decreased tactile fremitus, and decreased movement of the chest are often noted. Tension pneumothorax should be suspected in the presence of marked tachycardia, hypotension, and mediastinal or tracheal shift.

B. LABORATORY FINDINGS

Arterial blood gas analysis is often unnecessary but reveals hypoxemia and acute respiratory alkalosis in most patients. Left-sided primary pneumothorax may produce QRS axis and precordial T wave changes on the ECG that may be misinterpreted as acute myocardial infarction.

C. IMAGING

Demonstration of a visceral pleural line on chest radiograph is diagnostic and may only be seen on an expiratory film. A few patients have secondary pleural effusion that demonstrates a characteristic air-fluid level on chest radiography. In supine patients, pneumothorax on a conventional chest radiograph may appear as an abnormally radiolucent costophrenic sulcus (the "deep sulcus" sign). In patients with tension pneumothorax, chest radiographs show a large amount of air in the affected hemithorax and contralateral shift of the mediastinum.

Differential Diagnosis

If the patient is a young, tall, thin, cigarette-smoking man, the diagnosis of primary spontaneous pneumothorax is usually obvious and can be confirmed by chest radiograph. In secondary pneumothorax, it is sometimes difficult to distinguish loculated pneumothorax from an emphysematous bleb. Occasionally, pneumothorax may mimic myocardial infarction, pulmonary embolization, or pneumonia.

Complications

Tension pneumothorax may be life-threatening. Pneumomediastinum and subcutaneous emphysema may occur as complications of spontaneous pneumothorax. If pneumomediastinum is detected, rupture of the esophagus or a bronchus should be considered.

Treatment

Treatment depends on the severity of pneumothorax and the nature of the underlying disease. In a reliable patient with a small (< 15% of a hemithorax), stable spontaneous primary pneumothorax, observation alone may be appropriate. Many small pneumothoraces resolve spontaneously as air is absorbed from the pleural space; supplemental oxygen therapy may increase the rate of reabsorption. Simple aspiration drainage of pleural air with a small-bore catheter (eg, 16 gauge angiocatheter or larger drainage catheter) can be performed for spontaneous primary pneumothoraces that are large or progressive. Placement of a small-bore chest tube (7F to 14F) attached to a one-way Heimlich valve provides protection against development of tension pneumothorax and may permit observation from home. The patient should be treated symptomatically for cough and chest pain, and followed with serial chest radiographs every 24 hours.

Patients with secondary pneumothorax, large pneumothorax, tension pneumothorax, or severe symptoms or those who have a pneumothorax on mechanical ventilation should undergo chest tube placement (tube thoracostomy). The chest tube is placed under water-seal drainage, and suction is applied until the lung expands. The chest tube can be removed after the air leak subsides.

All patients who smoke should be advised to discontinue smoking and warned that the risk of recurrence is 50%. Future exposure to high altitudes, flying in unpressurized aircraft, and scuba diving should be avoided.

Indications for thoracoscopy or open thoracotomy include recurrences of spontaneous pneumothorax, any occurrence of bilateral pneumothorax, and failure of tube thoracostomy for the first episode (failure of lung to reexpand or persistent air leak). Surgery permits resection of blebs responsible for the pneumothorax and pleurodesis by mechanical abrasion and insufflation of talc.

Management of pneumothorax in patients with *Pneumocystis* pneumonia is challenging because of a tendency toward recurrence, and there is no consensus on the best approach. Use of a small chest tube attached to a Heimlich valve has been proposed to allow the patient to leave the hospital. Some clinicians favor its insertion early in the course.

Prognosis

An average of 30% of patients with spontaneous pneumothorax experience recurrence of the disorder after either observation or tube thoracostomy for the first episode. Recurrence after surgical therapy is less frequent. Following successful therapy, there are no long-term complications.

Baumann MH et al: Management of spontaneous pneumothorax: an American College of Chest Physicians Delphi consensus statement. Chest 2001;119:590. [PMID: 11171742]

Sahn SA et al: Spontaneous pneumothorax. N Engl J Med 2000; 342:868. [PMID: 10727592]

■ DISORDERS OF CONTROL OF VENTILATION

The principal influences on ventilatory control are arterial P_{CO_2}, pH, P_{O_2}, and brainstem tissue pH. These variables are monitored by peripheral and central chemoreceptors. Under normal conditions, the ventilatory control system maintains arterial pH and P_{CO_2} within narrow limits; arterial P_{O_2} is more loosely controlled.

Abnormal control of ventilation can be seen with a variety of conditions ranging from rare disorders such as Ondine's curse, neuromuscular disorders, myxedema, starvation, and carotid body resection to more common disorders such as asthma, COPD, obesity, congestive heart failure, and sleep-related breathing disorders. A few of these disorders will be discussed in this section.

Caruana-Montaldo B et al: The control of breathing in clinical practice. Chest 2000;117:205. [PMID: 10631221]

Perrin C et al: Pulmonary complications of chronic neuromuscular diseases and their management. Muscle Nerve 2004; 29:5. [PMID: 14694494]

Prabhakar NR et al: Peripheral chemoreceptors in health and disease. J Appl Physiol 2004;96:359. [PMID: 14660497]

PRIMARY ALVEOLAR HYPOVENTILATION

Primary alveolar hypoventilation ("Ondine's curse") is a rare syndrome of unknown cause characterized by inadequate alveolar ventilation despite normal neurologic function and normal airways, lungs, chest wall, and ventilatory muscles. Hypoventilation is even more marked during sleep. Individuals with this disorder are usually nonobese males in their third or fourth decades who have lethargy, headache, and somnolence. Dyspnea is absent. Physical examination may reveal cyanosis and evidence of pulmonary hypertension and cor pulmonale. Hypoxemia and hypercapnia are present and improve with voluntary hyperventilation. Erythrocytosis is common. Treatment with ventilatory stimulants is usually unrewarding. Augmentation of ventilation by mechanical methods (phrenic nerve stimulation, rocking bed, mechanical ventilators) has been helpful to some patients. Adequate oxygenation should be maintained with supplemental oxygen, but nocturnal oxygen therapy should be prescribed only if diagnostic nocturnal polysomnography has demonstrated its efficacy and safety. Primary alveolar hy-

poventilation resembles—but should be distinguished from—**central alveolar hypoventilation**, in which impaired ventilatory drive with chronic respiratory acidemia and hypoxemia follows an insult to the brainstem (eg, bulbar poliomyelitis, infarction, meningitis, encephalitis, trauma).

OBESITY-HYPOVENTILATION SYNDROME (Pickwickian Syndrome)

In obesity-hypoventilation syndrome, alveolar hypoventilation appears to result from a combination of blunted ventilatory drive and increased mechanical load imposed upon the chest by obesity. Voluntary hyperventilation returns the P_{CO_2} and the P_{O_2} toward normal values, a correction not seen in lung diseases causing chronic respiratory failure such as COPD. Most patients with obesity-hypoventilation syndrome also suffer from obstructive sleep apnea (see below), which must be treated aggressively if identified as a comorbid disorder. Therapy of obesity-hypoventilation syndrome consists mainly of weight loss, which improves hypercapnia and hypoxemia as well as the ventilatory responses to hypoxia and hypercapnia. NPPV is helpful in some patients. Respiratory stimulants may be helpful and include theophylline, acetazolamide, and medroxyprogesterone acetate, 10–20 mg every 8 hours orally. Improvement in hypoxemia, hypercapnia, erythrocytosis, and cor pulmonale are goals of therapy.

Buchwald H et al: Bariatric surgery: a systematic review and meta-analysis. JAMA 2004;292:1724. [PMID: 15479938]

Olson AL et al: The obesity hypoventilation syndrome. Am J Med 2005;118:948. [PMID: 16164877]

HYPERVENTILATION SYNDROMES

Hyperventilation is an increase in alveolar ventilation that leads to hypocapnia. It may be caused by a variety of conditions, such as pregnancy, hypoxemia, obstructive and infiltrative lung diseases, sepsis, hepatic dysfunction, fever, and pain. The term "central neurogenic hyperventilation" denotes a monotonous, sustained pattern of rapid and deep breathing seen in comatose patients with brainstem injury of multiple causes. Functional hyperventilation may be acute or chronic. **Acute** hyperventilation presents with hyperpnea, paresthesias, carpopedal spasm, tetany, and anxiety. **Chronic** hyperventilation may present with various nonspecific symptoms, including fatigue, dyspnea, anxiety, palpitations, and dizziness. The diagnosis of chronic hyperventilation syndrome is established if symptoms are reproduced during voluntary hyperventilation. Once organic causes of hyperventilation have been excluded, treatment of acute hyperventilation consists of rebreathing expired gas from a paper bag held over the face in order to decrease respiratory alkalemia and its associated symptoms. Anxiolytic drugs may also be useful.

Foster GT et al: Respiratory alkalosis. Respir Care 2001;46:384. [PMID: 11262557]

Laffey JG et al: Hypocapnia. N Engl J Med 2002;347:43. [PMID: 12097540]

SLEEP-RELATED BREATHING DISORDERS

Abnormal ventilation during sleep is manifested by apnea (breath cessation for at least 10 seconds) or hypopnea (decrement in airflow with drop in hemoglobin saturation of at least 4%). Episodes of apnea are **central** if ventilatory effort is absent for the duration of the apneic episode, **obstructive** if ventilatory effort persists throughout the apneic episode but no airflow occurs because of transient obstruction of the upper airway, and **mixed** if absent ventilatory effort precedes upper airway obstruction during the apneic episode. Pure central sleep apnea is uncommon; it may be an isolated finding or may occur in patients with primary alveolar hypoventilation or with lesions of the brainstem. Obstructive and mixed sleep apneas are more common and may be associated with life-threatening cardiac arrhythmias, severe hypoxemia during sleep, daytime somnolence, pulmonary hypertension, cor pulmonale, systemic hypertension, and secondary erythrocytosis.

Definitive diagnostic evaluation for suspected sleep apnea should include otolaryngologic examination and overnight polysomnography (the monitoring of multiple physiologic factors during sleep). Electroencephalography, electro-oculography, electromyography, electrocardiography, pulse oximetry, and measurement of respiratory effort and airflow are performed in a complete evaluation. Screening may be performed using home nocturnal pulse oximetry, which when normal has a high negative predictive value in ruling out significant sleep apnea.

OBSTRUCTIVE SLEEP APNEA

ESSENTIALS OF DIAGNOSIS

- *Daytime somnolence or fatigue.*
- *A history of loud snoring with witnessed apneic events.*
- *Overnight polysomnography demonstrating apneic episodes with hypoxemia.*

General Considerations

Upper airway obstruction during sleep occurs when loss of normal pharyngeal muscle tone allows the pharynx to collapse passively during inspiration. Patients with anatomically narrowed upper airways (eg, micrognathia, macroglossia, obesity, tonsillar hypertrophy) are predisposed to the development of obstructive sleep apnea.

Ingestion of alcohol or sedatives before sleeping or nasal obstruction of any type, including the common cold, may precipitate or worsen the condition. Hypothyroidism and cigarette smoking are additional risk factors for obstructive sleep apnea. Before making the diagnosis of obstructive sleep apnea, a drug history should be obtained and a seizure disorder, narcolepsy, and depression should be excluded.

Clinical Findings

A. SYMPTOMS AND SIGNS

Most patients with obstructive or mixed sleep apnea are obese, middle-aged men. Systemic hypertension is common. Patients may complain of excessive daytime somnolence, morning sluggishness and headaches, daytime fatigue, cognitive impairment, recent weight gain, and impotence. Bed partners usually report loud cyclical snoring, breath cessation, witnessed apneas, restlessness, and thrashing movements of the extremities during sleep. Personality changes, poor judgment, work-related problems, depression, and intellectual deterioration (memory impairment, inability to concentrate) may also be observed.

Physical examination may be normal or may reveal systemic and pulmonary hypertension with cor pulmonale. The patient may appear sleepy or even fall asleep during the evaluation. The oropharynx is frequently found to be narrowed by excessive soft tissue folds, large tonsils, pendulous uvula, or prominent tongue. Nasal obstruction by a deviated nasal septum, poor nasal airflow, and a nasal twang to the speech may be observed. A "bull neck" appearance is common.

B. LABORATORY FINDINGS

Erythrocytosis is common. A hemoglobin level and thyroid function tests should be obtained. Observation of the sleeping patient reveals loud snoring interrupted by episodes of increasingly strong ventilatory effort that fail to produce airflow. A loud snort often accompanies the first breath following an apneic episode. **Polysomnography** reveals apneic episodes lasting as long as 60 seconds. Oxygen saturation falls, often to very low levels. Bradydysrhythmias such as sinus bradycardia, sinus arrest, or atrioventricular block may occur. Tachydysrhythmias, including paroxysmal supraventricular tachycardia, atrial fibrillation, and ventricular tachycardia, may be seen once airflow is reestablished.

Treatment

Weight loss and strict avoidance of alcohol and hypnotic medications are the first steps in management. Weight loss may be curative, but most patients are unable to lose the 10–20% of body weight required. **Nasal continuous positive airway pressure (nasal CPAP)** at night is curative in many patients. Polysomnography is frequently necessary to determine the level of CPAP (usually 5–15 cm H_2O) necessary to abolish obstructive apneas. Unfortunately, only about 75% of patients continue to use nasal CPAP after 1 year. Pharmacologic therapy for obstructive sleep apnea is disappointing. Supplemental oxygen may lessen the severity of nocturnal desaturation but may also lengthen apneas. Polysomnography is necessary to assess the effects of oxygen therapy; it should not be routinely prescribed. Mechanical devices inserted into the mouth at bedtime to hold the jaw forward and prevent pharyngeal occlusion have modest effectiveness in relieving apnea; however, patient compliance is not optimal.

Uvulopalatopharyngoplasty (UPPP), a procedure consisting of resection of pharyngeal soft tissue and amputation of approximately 15 mm of the free edge of the soft palate and uvula, is helpful in approximately 50% of selected patients. It is more effective in eliminating snoring than apneic episodes. UPPP may now be performed on an outpatient basis with a laser. **Nasal septoplasty** is performed if gross anatomic nasal septal deformity is present. **Tracheotomy** relieves upper airway obstruction and its physiologic consequences and represents the definitive treatment for obstructive sleep apnea. However, it has numerous adverse effects, including granuloma formation, difficulty with speech, and stoma and airway infection. Furthermore, the long-term care of the tracheotomy, especially in obese patients, can be difficult. Tracheotomy and other maxillo-facial surgery approaches are reserved for patients with life-threatening arrhythmias or severe disability who have not responded to conservative therapy.

Some patients with sleep apnea have nocturnal bradycardia. A pilot study in 15 patients with either central or obstructive sleep apnea showed some improvement in oxygen saturation with atrial pacing. This single study must be considered preliminary.

Bao G et al: Upper airway resistance syndrome—one decade later. Curr Opin Pulm Med 2004;10:461. [PMID: 15510051]

Caples SM et al: Obstructive sleep apnea. Ann Intern Med 2005; 142:187. [PMID: 15684207]

Shamsuzzaman AS et al: Obstructive sleep apnea: implications for cardiac and vascular disease. JAMA 2003;290:1906. [PMID: 14532320]

White DP: Pathogenesis of obstructive and central sleep apnea. Am J Respir Crit Care Med 2005;172:1363. [PMID: 16100008]

■ ACUTE RESPIRATORY FAILURE

Respiratory failure is defined as respiratory dysfunction resulting in abnormalities of oxygenation or ventilation (CO_2 elimination) severe enough to threaten the function of vital organs. Arterial blood gas criteria for respiratory failure are not absolute but may be arbitrarily established as a PO_2 under 60 mm Hg or a PCO_2 over 50 mm Hg. Acute respiratory failure may occur in a variety of pulmonary and nonpulmonary disorders (Table 9–31). A complete discussion of treatment of acute respiratory failure is

beyond the scope of this chapter. Only a few selected general principles of management will be reviewed here.

Clinical Findings

Symptoms and signs of acute respiratory failure are those of the underlying disease combined with those of hypoxemia or hypercapnia. The chief symptom of hypoxemia is dyspnea, though profound hypoxemia may exist in the absence of complaints. Signs of hypoxemia include cyanosis, restlessness, confusion, anxiety, delirium, tachypnea, bradycardia or tachycardia, hypertension, cardiac dysrhythmias, and tremor. Dyspnea and headache are the cardinal symptoms of hypercapnia. Signs of hypercapnia include peripheral and conjunctival hyperemia, hypertension, tachycardia, tachypnea, impaired consciousness, papilledema, and asterixis. The symptoms and signs of acute respiratory failure are both insensitive and nonspecific; therefore, the physician must maintain a high index of suspicion and obtain arterial blood gas analysis if respiratory failure is suspected.

Treatment

Treatment of the patient with acute respiratory failure consists of (1) specific therapy directed toward the underlying disease; (2) respiratory supportive care directed toward the maintenance of adequate gas exchange; and (3) general supportive care. Only the last two aspects are discussed below.

A. RESPIRATORY SUPPORT

Respiratory support has both nonventilatory and ventilatory aspects.

1. Nonventilatory aspects—The main therapeutic goal in acute hypoxemic respiratory failure is to ensure adequate oxygenation of vital organs. Inspired oxygen concentration should be the lowest value that results in an arterial hemoglobin saturation of $\geq$ 90% ($PO_2 \geq$ 60 mm Hg). Higher arterial oxygen tensions are of no proven benefit. Restoration of normoxia may rarely cause hypoventilation in patients with chronic hypercapnia; however, *oxygen therapy should not be withheld for fear of causing progressive respiratory acidemia*. Hypoxemia in patients with obstructive airway disease is usually easily corrected by administering low-flow oxygen by nasal cannula (1–3 L/min) or Venturi mask (24–40%). Higher concentrations of oxygen are necessary to correct hypoxemia in patients with ARDS, pneumonia, and other parenchymal lung diseases.

2. Ventilatory aspects—Ventilatory support consists of maintaining patency of the airway and ensuring adequate alveolar ventilation. Mechanical ventilation may be provided via face mask (noninvasive) or through tracheal intubation.

a. Noninvasive positive-pressure ventilation—NPPV delivered via a full face mask or nasal mask has become first-line therapy in COPD patients with hypercapnic respiratory failure who can protect and main-

Table 9–31. Selected causes of acute respiratory failure in adults.

Airway disorders	**Neuromuscular and related disorders**
Asthma	Primary neuromuscular diseases
Acute exacerbation of chronic bronchitis or emphysema	Guillain-Barré syndrome
Obstruction of pharynx, larynx, trachea, main stem bronchus, or lobar bronchus by edema, mucus, mass, or foreign body	Myasthenia gravis
	Poliomyelitis
	Polymyositis
Pulmonary edema	Drug- or toxin-induced
Increased hydrostatic pressure	Botulism
Left ventricular dysfunction (eg, myocardial ischemia, heart failure)	Organophosphates
Mitral regurgitation	Neuromuscular blocking agents
Left atrial outflow obstruction (eg, mitral stenosis)	Aminoglycosides
Volume overload states	Spinal cord injury
Increased pulmonary capillary permeability	Phrenic nerve injury or dysfunction
Acute respiratory distress syndrome	Electrolyte disturbances: hypokalemia, hypophosphatemia
Acute lung injury	Myxedema
Unclear etiology	**Central nervous system disorders**
Neurogenic	Drugs: sedative, hypnotic, opioid, anesthetics
Negative pressure (inspiratory airway obstruction)	Brain stem respiratory center disorders: trauma, tumor, vascular disorders, hypothyroidism
Reexpansion	Intracranial hypertension
Tocolytic-associated	Central nervous system infections
Parenchymal lung disorders	**Increased CO_2 production**
Pneumonia	Fever
Interstitial lung diseases	Infection
Diffuse alveolar hemorrhage syndromes	Hyperalimentation with excess caloric and carbohydrate intake
Aspiration	Hyperthyroidism
Lung contusion	Seizures
Pulmonary vascular disorders	Rigors
Thromboembolism	Drugs
Air embolism	
Amniotic fluid embolism	
Chest wall, diaphragm, and pleural disorders	
Rib fracture	
Flail chest	
Pneumothorax	
Pleural effusion	
Massive ascites	
Abdominal distention and abdominal compartment syndrome	

tain the patency of their airway, handle their own secretions, and tolerate the mask apparatus. Several studies have demonstrated the effectiveness of this therapy in reducing intubation rates and ICU stays in patients with ventilatory failure. Patients with acute lung injury or ARDS or those who suffer from severely impaired oxygenation do not benefit and should be intubated if they require mechanical ventilation. A bilevel positive pressure ventilation mode is preferred for most patients.

b. Tracheal intubation—Indications for tracheal intubation include (1) hypoxemia despite supplemental oxygen, (2) upper airway obstruction, (3) impaired airway protection, (4) inability to clear secretions, (5) respiratory acidosis, (6) progressive general fatigue, tachypnea, use of accessory respiratory muscles, or mental status deterioration, and (7) apnea. In general, orotracheal intubation is preferred to nasotracheal intubation in urgent or emergency situations because it is easier, faster, and less traumatic. The position of the tip of the endotracheal tube at the level of the aortic arch should be verified by chest radiograph immediately following intubation, and auscultation should be performed to verify that both lungs are being inflated. Only tracheal tubes with high-volume, low-pressure air-filled cuffs should be used. Cuff inflation pressure should be kept below 20 mm Hg if possible to minimize tracheal mucosal injury.

c. Mechanical ventilation—Indications for mechanical ventilation include (1) apnea, (2) acute hypercapnia that is not quickly reversed by appropriate specific therapy, (3) severe hypoxemia, and (4) progressive patient fatigue despite appropriate treatment.

Several modes of positive-pressure ventilation are available. Controlled mechanical ventilation (CMV; also known as assist-control or A-C) and synchronized intermittent mandatory ventilation (SIMV) are ventilatory modes in which the ventilator delivers a minimum number of breaths of a specified tidal volume each minute. In both CMV and SIMV, the patient may trigger the ventilator to deliver additional breaths. In CMV, the ventilator responds to breaths initiated by the patient above the set rate by delivering additional full tidal volume breaths. In SIMV, additional breaths are not supported by the ventilator unless the pressure support mode is added. Numerous alternative modes of mechanical ventilation now exist, the most popular being pressure support ventilation (PSV), pressure control ventilation (PCV), and CPAP.

PEEP is useful in improving oxygenation in patients with diffuse parenchymal lung disease such as ARDS. It should be used cautiously in patients with localized parenchymal disease, hyperinflation, or very high airway pressure requirements during mechanical ventilation.

d. Complications of mechanical ventilation— Potential complications of mechanical ventilation are numerous. Migration of the tip of the endotracheal tube into a main bronchus can cause atelectasis of the contralateral lung and overdistention of the intubated lung. **Barotrauma** (alternatively referred to as "volutrauma"), manifested by subcutaneous emphysema, pneumomediastinum, subpleural air cysts, pneumothorax, or systemic gas embolism, may occur in patients whose lungs are overdistended by excessive tidal volumes, especially those with hyperinflation caused by airflow obstruction. Subtle parenchymal lung injury due to overdistention of alveoli is another potential hazard. Strategies to avoid barotrauma include deliberate hypoventilation through the use of low mechanical tidal volumes and respiratory rates, resulting in "permissive hypercapnia."

Acute respiratory alkalosis caused by overventilation is common. Hypotension induced by elevated intrathoracic pressure that results in decreased return of systemic venous blood to the heart may occur in patients treated with PEEP, those with severe airflow obstruction, and those with intravascular volume depletion. Ventilator-associated pneumonia is another serious complication of mechanical ventilation.

B. General Supportive Care

Maintenance of adequate nutrition is vital; parenteral nutrition should be used only when conventional enteral feeding methods are not possible. Overfeeding, especially with carbohydrate-rich formulas, should be avoided, because it can increase CO_2 production and may potentially worsen or induce hypercapnia in patients with limited ventilatory reserve. However, failure to provide adequate nutrition is more common. Hypokalemia and hypophosphatemia may worsen hypoventilation due to respiratory muscle weakness. Sedative-hypnotics and opioid analgesics are frequently used. They should be titrated carefully to avoid oversedation, leading to prolongation of intubation. Temporary paralysis with a nondepolarizing neuromuscular blocking agent is occasionally used to facilitate mechanical ventilation and to lower oxygen consumption. Prolonged muscle weakness due to an acute myopathy is a potential complication of these agents. Myopathy is more common in patients with renal dysfunction and in those given concomitant corticosteroids.

Psychological and emotional support of the patient and family, skin care to avoid decubitus ulcers, and meticulous avoidance of nosocomial infection and complications of tracheal tubes are vital aspects of comprehensive care for patients with acute respiratory failure.

Attention must also be paid to preventing complications associated with serious illness. Stress gastritis and ulcers may be avoided by administering sucralfate, histamine H_2-receptor antagonists, or proton pump inhibitors. There is some concern that the latter two agents, which raise the gastric pH, may permit increased growth of gram-negative bacteria in the stomach, predisposing to pharyngeal colonization and ultimately nosocomial pneumonia; many clinicians therefore prefer sucralfate. The risk of DVT and pulmonary embolism may be reduced by subcutaneous administration of heparin (5000 units every 12 hours), the use of LMW heparin, or placement of a sequential compression device on an extremity.

Course & Prognosis

The course and prognosis of acute respiratory failure vary and depend on the underlying disease. The prognosis of acute respiratory failure caused by uncomplicated sedative or narcotic drug overdose is excellent. Acute respiratory failure in patients with COPD who do not require intubation and mechanical ventilation has a good immediate prognosis. On the other hand, ARDS associated with sepsis has an extremely poor prognosis, with mortality rates of about 90%. Overall, adults requiring mechanical ventilation for all causes of acute respiratory failure have survival rates of 62% to weaning, 43% to hospital discharge, and 30% to 1 year after hospital discharge.

Calfee CS et al: Recent advances in mechanical ventilation. Am J Med 2005;118:584. [PMID: 15922687]

Esteban A et al: Noninvasive positive-pressure ventilation for respiratory failure after extubation. N Engl J Med 2004;350:2452. [PMID: 15190137]

Garland A et al: Outcomes up to 5 years after severe, acute respiratory failure. Chest 2004;126:1897. [PMID: 15596690]

Honrubia T et al: Noninvasive vs conventional mechanical ventilation in acute respiratory failure: a multicenter, randomized controlled trial. Chest 2005;128:3916. [PMID: 16354864]

MacIntyre NR et al; National Association for Medical Direction of Respiratory Care: Management of patients requiring prolonged mechanical ventilation: report of a NAMDRC consensus conference. Chest 2005;128:3937. [PMID:16354866]

Perrin C et al: Pulmonary complications of chronic neuromuscular diseases and their management. Muscle Nerve 2004; 29:5. [PMID: 14694494]

Raju P et al: The pathogenesis of respiratory failure: an overview. Respir Clin N Am 2000;6:195. [PMID: 10757961]

■ ACUTE RESPIRATORY DISTRESS SYNDROME

 ESSENTIALS OF DIAGNOSIS

- *Acute onset of respiratory failure.*
- *Bilateral radiographic pulmonary infiltrates.*
- *Absence of elevated left atrial pressure (if measured, pulmonary capillary wedge pressure ≤ 18 mm Hg).*
- *Ratio of partial pressure of oxygen in arterial blood (Pao$_2$) to fractional concentration of inspired oxygen (Fio$_2$) < 200, regardless of the level of PEEP.*

General Considerations

ARDS denotes acute hypoxemic respiratory failure following a systemic or pulmonary insult without evidence of heart failure. ARDS is the most severe form of acute lung injury and is characterized by bilateral, widespread radiographic pulmonary infiltrates, normal pulmonary capillary wedge pressure (≤ 18 mm Hg) and a Pao$_2$/Fio$_2$ ratio < 200. ARDS may follow a wide variety of clinical events (Table 9–32). Common risk factors for ARDS include sepsis, aspiration of gastric contents, shock, infection, lung contusion, nonthoracic trauma, toxic inhalation, near-drowning, and multiple blood transfusions. About one-third of ARDS patients initially have sepsis syndrome. Pro-inflammatory cytokines released from stimulated inflammatory cells appear to be pivotal in lung injury. Although the mechanism of lung injury varies with the cause, damage to capillary endothelial cells and alveolar epithelial cells is common to ARDS regardless of cause. Damage to these cells causes increased vascular permeability and decreased production and activity of surfactant; these abnormalities lead to interstitial and alveolar pulmonary edema, alveolar collapse, and hypoxemia.

Table 9–32. Selected disorders associated with ARDS.

Systemic Insults	Pulmonary Insults
Trauma	Aspiration of gastric contents
Sepsis	Embolism of thrombus, fat, air, or amniotic fluid
Pancreatitis	
Shock	Miliary tuberculosis
Multiple transfusions	Diffuse pneumonia (eg, SARS)
Disseminated intravascular coagulation	Acute eosinophilic pneumonia
Burns	Cryptogenic organizing pneumonitis
Drugs and drug overdose	
Opioids	Upper airway obstruction
Aspirin	Free-base cocaine smoking
Phenothiazines	Near-drowning
Tricyclic antidepressants	Toxic gas inhalation
Amiodarone	Nitrogen dioxide
Chemotherapeutic agents	Chlorine
Nitrofurantoin	Sulfur dioxide
Protamine	Ammonia
Thrombotic thrombocytopenic purpura	Smoke
	Oxygen toxicity
Cardiopulmonary bypass	Lung contusion
Head injury	Radiation exposure
Paraquat	High-altitude exposure
	Lung reexpansion or reperfusion

ARDS = acute respiratory distress syndrome; SARS = severe acute respiratory syndrome.

Clinical Findings

ARDS is marked by the rapid onset of profound dyspnea that usually occurs 12–48 hours after the initiating event. Labored breathing, tachypnea, intercostal retractions, and crackles are noted on physical examination. Chest radiography shows diffuse or patchy bilateral infiltrates that rapidly become confluent; these characteristically spare the costophrenic angles. Air bronchograms occur in about 80% of cases. Upper lung zone venous engorgement is distinctly uncommon. Heart size is normal, and pleural effusions are small or nonexistent. Marked hypoxemia occurs that is refractory to treatment with supplemental oxygen. Many patients with ARDS demonstrate multiple organ failure, particularly involving the kidneys, liver, gut, central nervous system, and cardiovascular system.

Differential Diagnosis

Since ARDS is a physiologic and radiographic syndrome rather than a specific disease, the concept of differential diagnosis does not strictly apply. Normal-permeability ("cardiogenic" or hydrostatic) pulmonary edema must be excluded, however, because specific therapy is available for that disorder. Measurement of pulmonary capillary wedge pressure by means of a flow-directed pulmonary artery catheter may be required in selected patients with suspected cardiac dysfunction. Routine use of the Swan-Ganz catheter in ARDS is discouraged.

Prevention

No measures that effectively prevent ARDS have been identified; specifically, prophylactic use of PEEP in patients at risk for ARDS has not been shown to be effective. Intravenous methylprednisolone does not prevent ARDS when given early to patients with sepsis syndrome or septic shock.

Treatment

Treatment of ARDS must include identification and specific treatment of the underlying precipitating and secondary conditions (eg, sepsis). Meticulous supportive care must then be provided to compensate for the severe dysfunction of the respiratory system associated with ARDS and to prevent complications (see above).

Treatment of the hypoxemia seen in ARDS usually requires tracheal intubation and positive-pressure mechanical ventilation. The lowest levels of PEEP (used to recruit atelectatic alveoli) and supplemental oxygen required to maintain the PaO_2 above 60 mm Hg or the SaO_2 above 90% should be used. Efforts should be made to decrease FIO_2 to less than 60% as soon as possible in order to avoid oxygen toxicity. PEEP can be increased as needed as long as cardiac output and oxygen delivery do not decrease and airway pressures do not increase excessively. Prone positioning may transiently improve oxygenation in selected patients by helping recruit atelectatic alveoli; however, great care must be taken during the maneuver to avoid dislodging catheters and tubes.

A variety of mechanical ventilation strategies are available. A multicenter study of 800 patients demonstrated that a protocol using volume-cycled ventilation with small tidal volumes (6 mL/kg of ideal body weight) resulted in a 10% absolute mortality reduction over standard therapy; this trial reported the lowest mortality (31%) of any intervention to date for ARDS.

Cardiac output that falls when PEEP is used may be improved by reducing the level of PEEP or by the judicious use of inotropic drugs (eg, norepinephrine); administering fluids to increase intravascular volume should be done only with great caution because increases in pulmonary capillary pressure worsen pulmonary edema in the presence of increased capillary permeability. Therefore, the goal of fluid management is to maintain pulmonary capillary wedge pressure at the lowest level compatible with adequate cardiac output. Crystalloid solutions should be used when intravascular volume expansion is necessary. Diuretics should be used to reduce intravascular volume if pulmonary capillary wedge pressure is elevated.

Oxygen delivery can be increased in anemic patients by ensuring that hemoglobin concentrations are at least 7 g/dL; patients are not likely to benefit from higher levels. Increasing oxygen delivery to supranormal levels through the use of inotropes and high hemoglobin concentrations is not clinically useful and may be harmful. Strategies to decrease oxygen consumption include the appropriate use of sedatives, analgesics, and antipyretics.

A large number of innovative therapeutic interventions to improve outcomes in ARDS patients have been or are being investigated. Unfortunately, to date, none have consistently shown benefit in clinical trials. Systemic corticosteroids have been studied extensively with variable and inconsistent results. While recent studies suggest a benefit in late-phase ARDS, confirmatory studies are required before they can be recommended for use on a routine basis.

Course & Prognosis

The mortality rate associated with ARDS is 30–40%. If ARDS is accompanied by sepsis, the mortality rate may reach 90%. The major causes of death are the primary illness and secondary complications such as multiple organ system failure or sepsis. Median survival is about 2 weeks. Many patients who succumb to ARDS and its complications die after withdrawal of support (see Withdrawal of Support in Chapter 5). Most survivors of ARDS are left with some pulmonary symptoms (cough, dyspnea, sputum production), which tend to improve over time. Mild abnormalities of oxygenation, diffusing capacity, and lung mechanics persist in some individuals.

Adhikari N et al: Pharmacologic therapies for adults with acute lung injury and acute respiratory distress syndrome. Cochrane Database Syst Rev 2004;(4):CD004477. [PMID: 15495113]

Bernard GR: Acute respiratory distress syndrome: a historical perspective. Am J Respir Crit Care Med 2005;172:798. [PMID: 16020801]

Hager DN et al: Tidal volume reduction in patients with acute lung injury when plateau pressures are not high. Am J Respir Crit Care Med 2005;172:1241. [PMID: 16081547]

Matthay MA et al: Acute lung injury and the acute respiratory distress syndrome: four decades of inquiry into pathogenesis and rational management. Am J Respir Cell Mol Biol 2005; 33:319. [PMID: 16172252]

Richard C et al: Early use of the pulmonary artery catheter and outcomes in patients with shock and acute respiratory distress syndrome: a randomized controlled trial. JAMA 2003; 290:2713. [PMID: 14645314]

Rubenfeld GD et al: Incidence and outcomes of acute lung injury. N Engl J Med 2005;353:1685. [PMID: 16236739]

Schwarz MI et al: "Imitators" of the ARDS: implications for diagnosis and treatment. Chest 2004;125:1530. [PMID: 15078770]

Ventilation with lower tidal volumes as compared with traditional tidal volumes for acute lung injury and the acute respiratory distress syndrome. The Acute Respiratory Distress Syndrome Network. N Engl J Med 2000;342:1301. [PMID: 10793162]

Heart

10

Thomas M. Bashore, MD, Christopher B. Granger, MD, & Patrick Hranitzky, MD

■ SYMPTOMS & SIGNS

COMMON SYMPTOMS

The most common symptoms of heart disease are chest pain, dyspnea, palpitations, syncope or presyncope, and fatigue. None is specific, and interpretation depends on the entire clinical picture and, in many cases, diagnostic testing.

Chest Pain or Discomfort

Chest pain and other forms of discomfort are common symptoms that can occur as a result of pulmonary, pleural, or musculoskeletal disease, esophageal or other gastrointestinal disorders, or anxiety states, as well as many cardiovascular diseases. Myocardial ischemia is a frequent cause of cardiac chest pain and the most important to identify to prevent complications, but it is often experienced more as a sensation of discomfort than actual pain, thereby increasing the potential for being ignored by the patient or misdiagnosed by the physician. This is usually described as dull, aching, or as a sensation of "pressure," "tightness," "squeezing," or "gas," rather than as sharp or spasmodic. **Ischemic symptoms** usually subside within 5–20 minutes but may last longer. Progressive symptoms or symptoms at rest may represent unstable angina due to coronary plaque rupture and thrombosis. Protracted episodes often represent **myocardial infarction**, although one-third of patients with acute myocardial infarction do not have chest pain. When present, the pain is commonly accompanied by a sense of anxiety or uneasiness. The location is usually retrosternal or left precordial. Because there are not the appropriate sensory nerves on the heart, the central nervous system (CNS) interpretation of pain location often results in pressure or "heaviness" being referred to the throat, lower jaw, shoulders, inner arms, upper abdomen, or back. Ischemic pain may be precipitated by exertion, cold temperature, meals, stress, or combinations of these factors and is usually relieved by rest, but many episodes do not conform to these patterns. It is not related to position or respiration and is usually not elicited by chest palpation. In myocardial infarction, a precipitating factor is frequently not apparent. One clue that the pain may be ischemic is other symptoms associated with the pain, such as shortness of breath, dizziness,

a feeling of impending doom, and vagal symptoms, such as nausea and diaphoresis.

Hypertrophy of either ventricle or stenotic aortic valvular disease may also give rise to ischemic pain or pain with less typical features. Myocarditis, pulmonary hypertension, and mitral valve prolapse are also associated with chest pain atypical for angina pectoris. Pericarditis may produce pain that is greater supine than upright, and may increase with respiration, or swallowing. Pleuritic chest pain is not ischemic, and pain on palpation should signal a musculoskeletal etiology. Aortic dissection classically produces an abrupt onset of tearing pain of great intensity that often radiates to the back.

Boie ET: Initial evaluation of chest pain. Emerg Med Clin North Am 2005;23:937. [PMID: 16199332]

Canto JG et al: Prevalence, clinical characteristics, and mortality among patients with myocardial infarction presenting without chest pain. JAMA 2000;283:3223. [PMID: 10866870]

Kohn MA et al: Prevalence of acute myocardial infarction and other serious diagnoses in patients presenting to an urban emergency department with chest pain. J Emerg Med 2005;29:383. [PMID: 16243193]

Lee TH et al: Evaluation of the patient with acute chest pain. N Engl J Med 2000;342:1187. [PMID: 10770985]

Dyspnea

Dyspnea due to heart disease is generally precipitated or exacerbated by exertion and usually results from elevated left atrial (LA) and pulmonary venous pressures or from hypoxia, though some patients with purely right heart disease complain of dyspnea as well. The former are most commonly caused by left ventricular (LV) systolic dysfunction, LV diastolic dysfunction (due to hypertrophy, fibrosis, or pericardial disease), or valvular stenosis or regurgitation. Exertional dyspnea may be an anginal equivalent. The acute onset or worsening of LA hypertension may result in **pulmonary edema. Hypoxia** may be a consequence of pulmonary edema, inherent lung disease, or shunting. Dyspnea should be quantified by the amount of activity that precipitates it. It is important to ask if commonly performed tasks can precipitate it, such as climbing stairs, housework, grocery shopping, mowing the lawn, vacuuming, etc. It is also a common symptom of primary and secondary pulmonary disease, and the etiologic distinction may be difficult. The diagnosis of congestive heart failure (CHF) may be aided by measurement of B-type natriuretic peptide (BNP), though high levels of BNP may also result from right ventricular (RV) dysfunction and pulmonary embolism. Shortness of breath may also occur in sedentary or obese individuals and is associated with anxiety states, anemia, and many other illnesses.

Orthopnea is dyspnea that occurs in recumbency and results from an increase in central blood volume. It may also result from pulmonary disease and obesity. **Paroxysmal nocturnal dyspnea** is shortness of breath that occurs abruptly 30 minutes to 4 hours after going to bed and is relieved (after 10 or 20 minutes) by sitting up or standing up; this symptom is more specific for cardiac disease.

Palpitations, Dizziness, Syncope

Palpitations, or awareness of the heartbeat, may be a normal phenomenon or may reflect increased cardiac or stroke output in patients with many noncardiac conditions (eg, exercise, thyrotoxicosis, anemia, anxiety). It may also be due to cardiac abnormalities that increase stroke volume (regurgitant valvular disease, bradycardia) or may be a manifestation of cardiac dysrhythmias. Ventricular premature beats may be sensed as extra or "skipped" beats. Supraventricular or ventricular tachycardia may be felt as rapid, regular or irregular palpitations or "fluttering"; many patients are asymptomatic, however.

If the abnormal rhythm is associated with a sufficient decline in arterial pressure or cardiac output, it may—especially in the upright position—impair cerebral blood flow, causing lightheadedness, blurring of vision, loss of consciousness (syncope), or other symptoms. However, **dizziness** in particular is nonspecific and is an uncommon symptom of cardiac disease or dysrhythmia.

Cardiogenic syncope most commonly results from bradyarrhythmias (sinus node arrest or exit block, atrioventricular [AV] conduction block), very rapid supraventricular rhythms or ventricular tachycardia or fibrillation. The absence of premonitory symptoms helps distinguish cardiogenic syncope from vasovagal faints, postural hypotension, or seizure, but is not a reliable screening tool. Although recovery is often immediate, some patients may exhibit seizure-like movements. Aortic stenosis and hypertrophic obstructive cardiomyopathy may also cause syncope, which is usually exertional or postexertional. Another form of syncope is termed **neurocardiogenic syncope**, commonly known as vasovagal syncope. In this syndrome, there is an inappropriate increase in vagal efferent activity, often resulting from a precedent increase in sympathetic cardiac stimulation. Syncope may follow presyncopal symptoms and may accompany a brief period of nausea and/or diaphoresis, or it may be abrupt in onset, mimicking arrhythmia-induced syncope. Autonomic dysfunction due to venous insufficiency or peripheral neuropathy can result in a positional fall in blood pressure (BP), and supine and upright BPs should be checked in all patients with syncope. Carotid sinus hypersensitivity may also result in syncope that is related to stimulation of the baroreceptors in the carotid sinus. Gentle carotid massage while monitoring the BP and cardiac rhythm usually can elicit the response.

Grubb BP: Clinical practice. Neurocardiogenic syncope. N Engl J Med 2005;352:1004. [PMID: 15758011]

Kapoor WN: Syncope. N Engl J Med 2000;343:1856. [PMID: 11117979]

Masotti G et al; Task Force on Syncope, European Society of Cardiology: Guidelines on management (diagnosis and treatment) of syncope—update 2004. Europace 2004;6: 467. [PMID: 15519256]

Schnipper JL et al: Diagnostic evaluation and management of patients with syncope. Med Clin North Am 2001;85:423, xi. [PMID: 11233954]

Sloane PD et al: Dizziness: state of the science. Ann Intern Med 2001;134:823. [PMID: 11346317]

See also references in the section on syncope.

FUNCTIONAL CLASSIFICATION OF HEART DISEASE

In the management of patients with heart disease, it is important to quantify and monitor the severity of symptoms. A commonly used classification system is that of the New York Heart Association, shown below. However, in following individual patients, it is better to document specific activities that produce symptoms, such as walking distance, stairs climbed, or activities of daily living.

Class I: No limitation of physical activity. Ordinary physical activity does not cause undue fatigue, dyspnea, or anginal pain.

Class II: Slight limitation of physical activity. Ordinary physical activity results in symptoms.

Class III: Marked limitation of physical activity. Comfortable at rest, but less than ordinary activity causes symptoms.

Class IV: Unable to engage in any physical activity without discomfort. Symptoms may be present even at rest.

Other classifications have been proposed, but these are universally accepted, and clinically can be applied to both heart failure and anginal symptoms.

SIGNS OF HEART DISEASE

Although the cardiovascular examination centers on the heart, peripheral signs often provide important information.

Appearance

Although cardiac patients may appear healthy and comfortable at rest, many with acute myocardial infarction appear anxious and restless. **Diaphoresis** suggests hypotension or a hyperadrenergic state, such as during pericardial tamponade, tachyarrhythmias, or myocardial infarction. Cold and clammy skin or pallor suggests low cardiac output and may be a sign of cardiogenic shock or anemia. Patients with severe chronic CHF or other long-standing low cardiac output states may appear **cachectic**.

Cyanosis may be central, due to arterial desaturation, or peripheral, reflecting impaired tissue delivery of adequately saturated blood in low-output states, polycythemia, or peripheral vasoconstriction. Clubbing may be present in chronic cyanotic states. Central cyanosis may be caused by pulmonary disease, left heart failure, or right-to-left intracardiac or intrapulmonary shunting; the latter will not be improved by increasing the inspired oxygen concentration. Edema may be present and its pitting nature and extent quantified. Note if presacral edema is present. Severe right heart failure may also present with ascites and scrotal edema.

Vital Signs

Although the normal resting **heart rate** usually ranges from 50 to 90 beats/min, both slower and more rapid rates may occur in normal individuals or may reflect noncardiac conditions such as anxiety or pain, medication effect, fever, thyroid disease, pulmonary disease, anemia, or hypovolemia. If symptoms or clinical suspicion warrants, an electrocardiogram (ECG) should be performed to diagnose arrhythmia, conduction disturbance, or other abnormalities. The range of normal BP is wide, but even in asymptomatic individuals systolic pressures below 90 mm Hg or above 140 mm Hg and diastolic pressures above 90 mm Hg warrant further clinical evaluation and follow-up. BP may vary between the upper extremities (often the left brachial is slightly lower than the right) and the BP measurement in the leg is usually higher than in the arm. Anxiety may increase the BP, and the patient should be asked if it has been checked in other settings. The ready availability of home BP monitoring or drugstore monitoring units should be considered before beginning antihypertensive therapy if the BP is borderline elevated. **Tachypnea** is also nonspecific, but pulmonary disease and heart failure should be considered when respiratory rates exceed 16/min under resting conditions. Cheyne–Stokes respiration, a form of **periodic breathing**, is not uncommon in severe heart failure.

Peripheral Pulses & Venous Pulsations

The quality of the pulses palpated is a reflection of the pulse pressure. **Diminished peripheral pulses** most commonly result from arteriosclerotic peripheral vascular disease and may be accompanied by localized **bruits**. Asymmetry of pulses should also arouse suspicion of coarctation of the aorta or aortic dissection, especially if a delay is noted between the brachial or radial pulse and the femoral pulse. **Exaggerated upper extremity pulses** may indicate aortic regurgitation, coarctation, patent ductus arteriosus (PDA), or other conditions that increase stroke volume. The carotid pulse is a valuable aid to assessment

of LV ejection. It has a **delayed upstroke** in aortic stenosis and a **bisferiens** quality (two palpable peaks) in mixed aortic stenosis and regurgitation or hypertrophic obstructive cardiomyopathy. It may be difficult to feel in significant aortic stenosis or in low output states. **Pulsus paradoxus** (a decrease in systolic BP during inspiration) is a normal sign unless exaggerated to > 10 mm Hg. The most common cause of pulsus paradoxus is asthma and chronic obstructive pulmonary disease, though its presence may be a critical component to the diagnosis of pericardial tamponade. **Pulsus alternans**, in which the amplitude of the pulse alternates every other beat during sinus rhythm, occurs when cardiac contractility is very depressed. It is volume dependent and at times can be elicited by feeling the pulse on standing.

Jugular venous pulsations (JVP) provide insight into right atrial (RA) pressure and function. To identify the waveforms, it is important to palpate the opposite carotid pulse while simultaneously observing the JVP. During ventricular systole (a positive carotid pulse wave), the normal RA pressure falls due to both atrial diastole and the pulling of the tricuspid valve into the RV cavity (the x descent). In the JVP, a prominent waveform just prior to systole is the a wave. A prominent waveform just after systole is the v wave. A waveform during systole is the c-v wave. **Prominent a waves** imply poor RV compliance or atrial contraction against a closed tricuspid valve (due to AV dissociation associated with ventricular arrhythmias, pacing, or tricuspid stenosis). **A prominent v wave** implies rapid filling of the RA, such as in an atrial septal defect (ASD) or mild tricuspid regurgitation, and a **c-v wave** implies significant tricuspid regurgitation. The height of the JVP provides a measure of RA pressure with an **elevated central venous pressure** if it is visible above the angle of Louis with the patient upright. An increased central blood volume and reduced RV compliance can also be assumed if the JVP rise more than 1 cm and are sustained (> 200 seconds) by right upper quadrant abdominal pressure (**hepatojugular reflux**). **Kussmaul's sign** (failure of jugular venous pressure to decrease with inspiration) is commonly seen with RV infarction, postoperatively after cardiac surgery, with tricuspid regurgitation, and with constrictive pericarditis.

Abidov A et al: Prognostic significance of dyspnea in patients referred for cardiac stress testing. N Engl J Med 2005;353: 1889. [PMID: 16267320]

Constant J: Using internal jugular pulsations as a manometer for right atrial pressure measurements. Cardiology 2000;93:26. [PMID: 10894903]

Drazner MH et al: Prognostic importance of elevated jugular venous pressure and a third heart sound in patients with heart failure. N Engl J Med 2001;345:574. [PMID: 11529211]

Maisel A et al; Rapid Emergency Department Heart Failure Outpatient Trial investigators: Primary results of the Rapid Emergency Department Heart Failure Outpatient Trial (RED-HOT). A multicenter study of B-type natriuretic peptide levels, emergency department decision making, and outcomes in patients presenting with shortness of breath. J Am Coll Cardiol 2004;44:1328. [PMID: 15364340]

Pulmonary Examination

Rales heard at the lung bases are a sign of CHF but may be caused by similarly localized pulmonary disease. Cardiac rales tend to occur late in inspiration and be fine in nature, while pulmonary rales tend to be more coarse and appear in early or mid inspiration. Rales are loudest at the bases in heart failure, and the examiner should note how far up from the diaphragm they are audible. **Wheezing** suggests obstructive pulmonary disease and only rarely occurs in left heart failure. **Pleural effusions** with bibasilar percussion dullness and reduced breath sounds are common in CHF and are more frequent or larger on the right. Egophony may be present due to pulmonary compression over a pleural effusion or to a pulmonary infiltration.

Precordial Pulsations

A **parasternal lift** usually indicates right ventricular hypertrophy (RVH), pulmonary hypertension (pulmonary artery [PA] systolic pressure > 50 mm Hg), or LA enlargement; PA pulsations may also be visible. The examiner should feel the LV apical impulse in the left lateral position and note if it is sustained or enlarged and whether an early impulse (*A* wave) precedes the main apical thrust. The *A* wave implies poor LV compliance and corresponds to a fourth heart sound. If the second heart sound is palpable along the left sternal border, it may imply an increased P_2 and pulmonary hypertension.

Heart Sounds & Murmurs

Auscultation is helpful in the diagnosis of many heart diseases, and provides evidence for cardiac failure. Specific findings are discussed under individual diseases below.

The **first heart sound** (S_1), the closing of the mitral valve and tricuspid valve, may be diminished with severe LV dysfunction or accentuated with mitral stenosis or short PR intervals. Separation of the components of S_2 is due to the normally compliant lung, allowing for continuing forward cardiac output with systole compared to the stiffer arterial system. The pulmonary valve closes later than the aortic valve for that reason (splitting). Inspiration increases flow to the lung and reduces flow to the left heart, and splitting is increased. **Splitting** may be *fixed* in atrial septal defect, *wide* with right bundle branch block, and *absent* or *reversed* (**paradoxic splitting**) with aortic stenosis, LV failure, or left bundle branch block. With normal splitting, an accentuated P_2 is an important sign of pulmonary hypertension. **Third and fourth heart sounds** (ventricular and atrial gallops, respectively) indicate ventricular volume overload or impaired compliance and may be heard over either ventricle. A right-sided gallop may increase with inspiration or may be confirmed if heard in the right subclavicular area (where a left-sided gallop does not usually radiate). A palpable *A* wave helps confirm an S_4. An apical S_3 is a normal finding in younger individuals and in high output states, such as pregnancy. Additional auscultatory findings include sharp, high-pitched sounds classified as **"clicks."** These may be early systolic and represent **ejection sounds** (as with a bicuspid aortic valve or pulmonary stenosis) or may occur in mid or late systole, indicating myxomatous changes in the mitral valve.

Although many **murmurs** indicate valvular disease, a soft, short systolic murmur, usually localized along the left sternal border or toward the apex, may be innocent, reflecting pulmonary or aortic flow. **Innocent murmurs** often vary with inspiration, diminish in the upright position, and are most frequently heard in thin individuals. **Systolic murmurs** should be classified as **"holosystolic"** when they merge with S_1 and persist through S_2 or **"ejection"** when they begin after S_1 and end before S_2. Holosystolic murmurs tend to have a uniform intensity during systole, while ejection murmurs have a peak at some part of the systolic cycle. Holosystolic murmurs usually represent mitral regurgitation if maximal at the apex or in the axilla and tricuspid regurgitation or ventricular septal defect (VSD) if best heard at the sternal border. Short aortic ejection murmurs with a preserved A_2 are common in older individuals, especially when hypertension has been present, and even if they are moderately loud they usually reflect thickening (sclerosis) of the valve rather than stenosis. Association of murmurs with palpable vibrations (**"thrills"**) is always clinically significant, as are **diastolic murmurs**. High-pitched diastolic murmurs imply flow from a high-pressure to low-pressure chamber (ie, pulmonic regurgitation in pulmonary hypertension, aortic regurgitation, or VSD) while low-pitched diastolic "rumbles" imply filling across an AV valve (ie, mitral stenosis). Further evaluation is warranted when the patient has symptoms of possible cardiac origin. An echocardiogram should be ordered when a murmur is heard that is of unclear etiology or significance.

Attenhofer Jost CG et al: Echocardiography in the evaluation of systolic murmurs of unknown cause. Am J Med 2000;108: 614. [PMID: 10856408]

Chun AA et al: Bedside diagnosis of coronary artery disease: a systematic review. Am J Med 2004;117:334. [PMID: 15336583]

Kobal SL et al: Comparison of effectiveness of hand-carried ultrasound to bedside cardiovascular physical examination. Am J Cardiol 2005;96:1002. [PMID: 16188532]

Richardson TR et al: Bedside cardiac examination: constancy in a sea of change. Curr Probl Cardiol 2000;25:783. [PMID: 11082789]

Edema

Subcutaneous fluid collections appear first in the lower extremities in ambulatory patients or in the sacral region of bedridden individuals. In heart disease, edema primarily results from elevated RA pressures or associated peripheral venous disease. Right heart failure most commonly results from left heart failure, pulmonary disease, or RV dysfunction and tricuspid regurgitation, or constrictive pericarditis. Edema may also be due to nephrotic syndrome, low serum albumin, cirrhosis, premenstrual fluid retention, or drugs (especially vasodilators such as calcium channel blockers or salt-retaining medications such as nonsteroidal anti-inflammatory agents or thiazolidinedione diabetic agents), or it may be idiopathic. Ascites may predominate, especially in constrictive pericarditis or following aggressive diuretic usage (where peripheral edema is mobilized more readily than intra-abdominal fluid).

Cho S et al: Peripheral edema. Am J Med 2002;113:580. [PMID: 12459405]

O'Brien JG et al: Treatment of edema. Am Fam Physician 2005; 71:2111. [PMID: 15952439]

Rasool A et al: Treatment of edematous disorders with diuretics. Am J Med Sci 2000;319:25. [PMID: 10653442]

■ DIAGNOSTIC TESTING

The **chest radiograph** provides information about heart size (with cardiomegaly being a poor prognostic sign in chronic heart failure), the pulmonary circulation (with characteristic signs suggesting both pulmonary arterial or pulmonary venous hypertension), primary pulmonary disease, and aortic abnormalities. Individual chamber sizes can be estimated, and the presence of pleural effusions noted. The **echocardiogram**, though, provides much more reliable information about chamber size and hypertrophy, and the presence of pericardial effusions, valvular abnormalities, and congenital abnormalities and has replaced the radiograph for evaluation of structural cardiac disease. The **ECG** indicates cardiac rhythm, reveals conduction abnormalities, and provides evidence of ventricular hypertrophy, myocardial infarction, or ischemia. Nonspecific ST segment and T wave changes may reflect these processes but are also noted with electrolyte imbalance, drug effects, and many other conditions. Routine radiographs and ECGs are not recommended to screen for heart disease. **Stress testing** is useful in eliciting ischemia due to fixed coronary lesions, but its use in the typical asymptomatic patient is limited. For instance, it is useful to recall Bayes' theorem when contemplating stress testing patients as part of an "executive physical." Bayes' theorem states that the results of a test depend on the risk of disease. If the patient is at low risk for coronary artery disease (CAD), for instance, one can expect a high number of false-positive stress results. If the patient is at high risk for CAD, one can expect a high number of false-negative results. Stress studies are most effective in those with an intermediate risk for CAD. The clinician's goal is to help define the CAD risk using the history, physical examination, and other available laboratory tests (see below). Stress testing may also be useful in non-CAD whenever symptoms seem disproportionate to anatomic defects. For instance, in valvular disease, if the patient is complaining of major symptoms but has only minor anatomic disease, a stress study may help define exercise capacity. Similarly, if there is significant disease by echocardiography, but few or no symptoms, the stress study may define an unrecognized disability. **Blood chemistry tests** play a major role in defining cardiac risk factors (ie, serum lipid levels, serum human C-reactive protein [hCRP] level, creatinine) and can help with determining etiology of symptoms (ie, BNP level).

NONINVASIVE DIAGNOSTIC IMAGING FOR NONCORONARY HEART DISEASE

The diagnostic procedures for CAD will be discussed in the following section on Coronary Heart Disease. Reviewed here is the use of noninvasive testing for noncoronary heart disease.

Echocardiography & Doppler Ultrasound Imaging

Echocardiography provides information regarding all four chamber sizes, regional and global systolic function, and chamber wall thickness. Excellent images of valve motion, intracardiac masses, abnormal or absent cardiac structures, and pericardial fluid can all be distinguished. **Pulsed Doppler ultrasound** provides a semiquantitative or qualitative estimation of the severity of transvalvular gradients, RV systolic pressure, PA pressure, valvular regurgitation, and intracardiac shunts. The Doppler mitral inflow pattern can help confirm diastolic dysfunction and can help verify a restrictive cardiomyopathic picture or constrictive pericarditis. **Color flow Doppler ultrasound** provides a visual pattern of blood flow velocities superimposed over the anatomic two-dimensional (2-D) echocardiographic image. This allows for the demonstration of turbulence from stenotic or regurgitant valves, and for the visualization of intracardiac defects. Since some regurgitant flow occurs normally, especially when the AV valves close, the presence of minor amounts of regurgitant color flow should not be construed as pathology. **Tissue Doppler** methods are now being explored as a means of defining the extent of either mitral annular or ventricular wall motion independent of intracardiac flow velocity, and the relationship between the two may prove useful for defining diastolic pressure elevation, identifying abnormalities in ventricular contraction or relaxation, or evaluating pacemaker therapy.

Transesophageal echocardiography (TEE) with Doppler ultrasound is used to obtain echocardiographic data when surface sound transmission is poor, to derive information about posterior structures (especially the atria and AV valves), prosthetic heart valves, and intracardiac masses not seen on chest wall echocardiography (eg, vegetations in endocarditis or thrombi on pacemaker leads), and to monitor patients during surgery. It can confirm the location of the pulmonary veins and define septal defects or the presence of a patent foramen ovale (PFO). It is superior to surface echocardiography in diagnosing LA appendage thrombi and regurgitant lesions associated with prosthetic valves. The absence of atrial thrombi identifies patients in atrial fibrillation at low risk for embolization, thus facilitating early cardioversion. It is also quite sensitive in detecting aortic dissection and severe atherosclerosis of the ascending aorta, which may be the source for transient ischemic attacks or embolic strokes.

Stress echocardiography can be used in valvular as well as ischemic heart disease. Echocardiograms may be performed during or immediately following exercise. Valvular gradient changes after exercise or during dobutamine or nitroprusside infusion can be evaluated. Transient segmental wall motion abnormalities during or immediately following exercise or pharmacologic stress suggest ischemia. Improvement in wall motion during low-dose dobutamine infusions is an indicator of myocardial viability.

Cheitlin MD et al: ACC/AHA/ASE 2003 guideline update for the clinical application of echocardiography—summary article: a report of the American College of Cardiology/American Heart Association Task Force on Practice Guidelines (ACC/AHA/ASE Committee to Update the 1997 Guidelines for the Clinical Application of Echocardiography). J Am Coll Cardiol 2003;42:954. [PMID: 12957449]

Biagini E et al: The use of stress echocardiography for prognostication in coronary artery disease: an overview. Curr Opin Cardiol 2005;20:386. [PMID: 16093757]

Goldman ME et al: Echocardiography in search of a cardioembolic source. Curr Probl Cardiol 2002;27:342. [PMID: 12237620]

Gottdiener JS: Overview of stress echocardiography: uses, advantages, and limitations. Prog Cardiovasc Dis 2001;43:315. [PMID: 11235847]

Lerakis S et al: Part I: use of echocardiography in the evaluation of patients with suspected cardioembolic stroke. Am J Med Sci 2005;329:310. [PMID: 15958873]

Cardiac MRI & Multislice CT

Cardiac **MRI** continues to evolve rapidly. Currently available systems provide high-quality and high-resolution images of cardiac and adjacent vascular structures. MRI also provides excellent images that can be used to quantify cardiac function and structure. It is particularly useful for defining myocardial diseases such as sarcoidosis or amyloidosis. Flow measurements, valve orifice sizes, and shunt sizes can all be determined. With the use of gadolinium contrast agents, MRI can be used to assess myocardial perfusion during adenosine pharmacologic stress and viability. Contrast-enhanced images can provide accurate measurement of myocardial infarction size and location. MRI can also provide accurate 3-D reconstruction of the great vessels and abdominal aorta. The study can also be used to screen for renal artery stenosis in patients with hypertension. However, patients with metal pacemakers or defibrillators are not candidates for MRI.

Cardiac multislice CT (fast CT) is a new modality. At lower resolution, it has primarily been used to screen patients for CAD. The extent of calcium within the coronary vessels was found to correlate with the extent of atherosclerotic CAD. More recently, higher resolution imaging modes and faster acquisition have enabled noninvasive coronary angiography. At this stage, cardiac multislice CT is still undergoing investigation, but the predictive value of a negative study is high (around 95%), suggesting that it is an excellent test to confirm normal coronaries. Calcium in the arterial wall may limit its ability to define the severity of coronary disease, but the inherent resolution of fast CT allows it to better visualize coronaries than cardiac MRI. Multislice CT, with its impressive three-dimensional (3-D) reconstruction algorithms, also provides outstanding images in valvular, myocardial, and congenital heart disease. However, there is some concern regarding the radiation dose with multislice CT, which is not an issue with MRI. For most individuals, however, the effective dose equivalent is around 20 milliSieverts, about the same as a rest and exercise thallium study.

Becker CR et al: Past, present, and future perspective of cardiac computed tomography. J Magn Reson Imaging 2004;19:676. [PMID: 15170776]

Berman DS et al: Roles of nuclear cardiology, cardiac computed tomography, and cardiac magnetic resonance: assessment of patients with suspected coronary artery disease. J Nucl Med 2006;47:74. [PMID: 16391190]

Constantine G et al: Role of MRI in clinical cardiology. Lancet 2004;363:2162. [PMID: 15220041]

Heatlie GJ et al: Cardiac magnetic resonance imaging. Postgrad Med J 2004;80:19. [PMID: 14760173]

Lima JA et al: Cardiovascular magnetic resonance imaging: current and emerging applications. J Am Coll Cardiol 2004;44:1164. [PMID: 15364314]

Mahnken AH et al: Multislice spiral computed tomography of the heart: technique, current applications, and perspective. Cardiovasc Intervent Radiol 2005;28:388. [PMID: 15959701]

Raggi P et al: Computed tomography coronary calcium screening and myocardial perfusion imaging. J Nucl Cardiol 2005;12:96. [PMID: 15682370]

CARDIAC CATHETERIZATION & ANGIOGRAPHY

Cardiac catheterization is evolving from a diagnostic procedure to a therapeutic one, as more and more types of cardiac lesions are approached with percutaneous techniques.

Right heart catheterization is convenient to perform in the laboratory, at the bedside, or in the operating room. It allows measurement of RA, RV, PA, and pulmonary capillary wedge pressures (PCWP; the latter an indicator of LA pressure), oxygen saturation, and cardiac output. These data may diagnose intracardiac shunts, physiologically significant pericardial disease, and right-sided valve lesions and can distinguish between cardiac and pulmonary disease. It is useful in pulmonary hypertension to document whether the elevated pressures are related to pulmonary disease or to left heart disease. In those with pulmonary vascular disease, vasodilators can be administered to test for vasoactivity. Hemodynamic monitoring with a PA catheter may be very helpful in the assessment and treatment of shock, heart failure, complicated myocardial infarction, respiratory failure, and postoperative hemodynamic instability. However, this procedure is not without risk—complications include pneumothorax, bleeding, arrhythmias, PA rupture, pulmonary emboli, infection, and patient immobility. Therefore, the role of this procedure remains unsettled, although it is still commonly used to monitor cardiac patients in surgery and in critical care settings. Bedside echocardiography can often fulfill this role for most situations.

Left heart catheterization is performed to assess the cardiac valves and LV function plus the presence and severity of CAD. Mitral stenosis and aortic stenosis are quantified by measuring the pressure gradients across the valves and, taking flow into account, the estimated valve areas. Mitral and aortic regurgitation are assessed semiquantitatively from contrast injections in the LV and aorta, respectively. The ejection fraction (EF) and regional wall motion are assessed by contrast left ventriculography. Stenotic valvular disease is well defined by echocardiography with Doppler ultrasound, but assessing the consequences of regurgitant valvular disease is more difficult and cardiac catheterization with hemodynamics is often more helpful.

Both coronary and noncoronary interventions are now common in the cardiac catheterization laboratory. Acute interventions include plain old balloon angioplasty (POBA) and stenting (now often with stents coated with agents to reduce restenosis). Coronary interventions are now done routinely in the acute as well as chronic setting. Other novel interventional procedures include balloon valvuloplasty (primarily for pulmonic or mitral valve stenosis); stenting of coarctation or branch PA stenosis; percutaneous occlusion of intracardiac defects, such as ASD, PFO or PDA; or alcohol ablation of the subaortic septum in hypertrophic cardiomyopathy.

Bernard GR et al: Pulmonary artery catheterization and clinical outcomes: National Heart, Lung, and Blood Institute and Food and Drug Administration Workshop Report. Consensus Statement. JAMA 2000;283:2568. [PMID: 10815121]

Harvey S et al; PAC-Man study collaboration: Assessment of the clinical effectiveness of pulmonary artery catheters in management of patients in intensive care (PAC-Man): a randomised controlled trial. Lancet 2005;366:472. [PMID: 16084255]

Ivanov R et al: The incidence of major morbidity in critically ill patients managed with pulmonary artery catheters: a meta-analysis. Crit Care Med 2000;28:615. [PMID: 10752803]

Shah MR et al: Impact of the pulmonary artery catheter in critically ill patients: meta-analysis of randomized clinical trials. JAMA 2005;294:1664. [PMID: 16204666]

Scanlon PJ et al: ACC/AHA guidelines for coronary angiography. A report of the American College of Cardiology/American Heart Association Task Force on practice guidelines (Committee on Coronary Angiography). Developed in collaboration with the Society for Cardiac Angiography and Interventions. J Am Coll Cardiol 1999;33:1756. [PMID: 10334456]

■ CONGENITAL HEART DISEASE

Congenital lesions account for only about 2% of heart disease that presents in adulthood. As surgical and medical techniques have improved, more and more children are now reaching adulthood, and it is estimated that up to a million adults may now be surviving with congenital heart disease.

Bolger AP et al: Congenital heart disease: the original heart failure syndrome. Eur Heart J 2003;24:970. [PMID: 12714029]

Brickner ME et al: Congenital heart disease in adults. N Engl J Med 2000;342:256, 334. [PMID: 10648769, 10655533]

Corno AF: Surgery for congenital heart disease. Curr Opin Cardiol 2000;15:238. [PMID: 11139086]

Ellis CR et al: Clinical presentations of unoperated and operated adults with congenital heart disease. Curr Cardiol Rep 2005;7:291. [PMID: 15987627]

Krasuski RA et al: The emerging role of percutaneous intervention in adults with congenital heart disease. Rev Cardiovasc Med 2005;6:11. [PMID: 15741921]

Moodie DS: Diagnosis and management of congenital heart disease in the adult. Cardiol Rev 2001;9:276. [PMID: 11520451]

Perloff JK et al: Challenges posed by adults with repaired congenital heart disease. Circulation 2001;103:2637. [PMID: 11382736]

PULMONARY STENOSIS

 ESSENTIALS OF DIAGNOSIS

- *No symptoms in patients with mild or moderately severe lesions.*
- *Severe cases may present with right-sided heart failure.*
- *High-pitched systolic ejection murmur maximal in the second left interspace with radiation to the left shoulder.*
- *P_2 delayed and soft or absent. Ejection click often present and decreases with inspiration—the only right heart auscultatory event that decreases with inspiration, all others increase.*
- *Increased RV impulse.*
- *Palpable thrill at second left intercostal space.*
- *RVH on ECG; PA dilation on radiograph.*
- *Echocardiography/Doppler is diagnostic.*
- *Patients with peak pulmonic valve gradients > 50 mm Hg should undergo intervention regardless of symptoms.*

General Considerations

Stenosis of the pulmonary valve or RV infundibulum increases the resistance to RV outflow, raises the RV pressure, and limits pulmonary blood flow. Pulmonic stenosis is often associated with other cardiac lesions. Pulmonary blood flow preferentially goes to the left lung in valvular pulmonic stenosis. Most patients with valvular pulmonic stenosis have a domed valve, though some patients have a dysplastic valve. Patients with Noonan's syndrome have a high likelihood of a dysplastic pulmonary valve. The phenotype of Noonan's syndrome includes short stature, web neck, dental malocclusion, antimongoloid slanting of the eyes, mental retardation, and hypogonadism. Unlike those with a domed valve, patients with a dysplastic valve do not have a dilated main PA or commissural fusion. In the absence of associated shunts, arterial saturation is normal. Infundibular stenosis may be so severe that the RV is divided into a low-pressure and high-pressure chamber (double-chambered RV). Peripheral pulmonic stenosis can accompany valvular pulmonic stenosis and may be part of a variety of clinical syndromes, including the congenital rubella syndrome. Patients who have had the Ross procedure (transfer of the pulmonary valve to the aortic position with a homograft pulmonary valve placed in the pulmonary position) may experience postoperative pulmonic stenosis due to an immune response in the homograft.

Clinical Findings

A. Symptoms and Signs

Mild cases (RV-PA gradient < 30 mm Hg) are asymptomatic. Moderate pulmonic stenosis (gradients between 30 mm Hg and 50 mm Hg) to severe stenosis (gradients > 50 mm Hg) may cause symptoms of dyspnea on exertion, syncope, chest pain, and eventually RV failure.

There is often a palpable parasternal lift due to RVH and the pulmonary outflow tract may be palpable if it is enlarged. A loud, harsh systolic murmur and occasionally a prominent thrill are present in the left second and third interspaces parasternally. The murmur radiates toward the left shoulder and increases with inspiration. In mild to moderate pulmonic stenosis, a loud ejection click can be heard to precede the murmur; this sound decreases with inspiration as the increased RV filling from inspiration prematurely opens the valve during atrial systole. The valve excursion in systole, therefore, is less with inspiration, and the click diminishes in intensity. The second sound is obscured by the murmur in severe cases; the pulmonary component may be diminished, delayed, or absent. A right-sided S_4 and a prominent a wave in the venous pulse are present when there is RV diastolic dysfunction or a c-v wave if there is tricuspid regurgitation present. Right-sided S_4 gallops may be best heard in the right subclavicular area (where left-sided gallops would be distinctly uncommon). Pulmonic valve regurgitation is relatively uncommon in pulmonic stenosis and may be very difficult to hear, as the gradient between the reduced PA diastolic pressure and the elevated RV diastolic pressure may be quite small (low-pressure pulmonic regurgitation).

B. ECG and Chest Radiography

Right axis deviation or RVH is noted; peaked P waves provide evidence of RA overload. Heart size may be normal on radiographs, or there may be a prominent RV and RA or gross cardiac enlargement, depending on the severity. There is often poststenotic dilation of the main and left pulmonary arteries. Pulmonary vascularity is usually normal. A careful look at the chest radiograph may reveal greater vascular perfusion of the left than the right base (Chen's sign). In the adult, calcium may also be present in the main PA or pulmonic valve.

C. Diagnostic Studies

Echocardiography/Doppler is key to the diagnosis, can provide evidence for a doming valve versus a dysplastic valve, can determine the gradient across the valve, and can provide information regarding subvalvular obstruction. Echocardiography also helps define RV function and the presence or absence of tricuspid or pulmonic valvular regurgitation. Catheterization is usually unnecessary for the diagnosis, but is performed when percutaneous valvuloplasty is necessary. MRI and CT do not add additional information unless there is concern regarding associated cardiac lesions or peripheral pulmonary arterial stenosis.

Prognosis & Treatment

Patients with mild pulmonic stenosis (peak gradient < 30 mm Hg) may have a normal life span. Moderate stenosis may be asymptomatic in childhood and adolescence, but symptoms may appear as patients grow older. The degree of stenosis does worsen with time in many patients, so serial follow-up is important. Severe stenosis is associated with sudden death and can cause right heart failure in patients as early as in their 20s and 30s.

Class I indications for intervention include all symptomatic patients and all those with a resting gradient over 50 mm Hg, regardless of symptoms. The 2006 Class II guidelines from the American College of Cardiology/American Heart Association (ACC/AHA) suggest that intervention is reasonable in symptomatic patients when the peak gradient is > 30 mm Hg or in asymptomatic patients when the peak gradient is > 40 mm Hg. Percutaneous balloon valvuloplasty is highly successful in domed valve patients and is the treatment of choice. Surgical commissurotomy can also be done, or pulmonary valve replacement (with either a bioprosthetic valve or homograft) when pulmonic regurgitation is more severe or the valve is dysplastic.

Earing MG et al: Long-term follow-up of patients after surgical treatment for isolated pulmonary valve stenosis. Mayo Clin Proc 2005;80:871. [PMID: 16007892]

Khambadkone S et al: Percutaneous pulmonary valve implantation in humans: results in 59 consecutive patients. Circulation 2005;112:1189. [PMID: 16103239]

Latson LA: Critical pulmonary stenosis. J Interv Cardiol 2001; 14:345. [PMID: 12053395]

COARCTATION OF THE AORTA

ESSENTIALS OF DIAGNOSIS

- *Infants may have severe heart failure; children and adults are usually asymptomatic, presenting with hypertension.*
- *At least 50% of patients with coarctation have an associated bicuspid aortic valve.*
- *Some patients have a webbed neck (XO karyotype, Turner's syndrome).*
- *Absent or weak femoral pulses. Delay of the palpable pulse between the femoral and brachial artery.*
- *In some patients, the coarctation murmur can be heard in the back. In severe coarctation, the continuous murmurs of collaterals around the coarctation can be heard in the back.*
- *Systolic pressure is higher in upper extremities than in lower extremities; diastolic pressures are similar.*
- *ECG shows LV hypertrophy; chest radiograph shows rib notching; echocardiography/Doppler is diagnostic.*

General Considerations

Coarctation of the aorta consists of localized narrowing of the aortic arch just distal to the origin of the left subclavian artery. Its development is thought to be related to accessory ductal material that contracts soon after birth. Therefore, it is not usually present in the fetus. Collateral circulation develops around the coarctation through the intercostal arteries and the branches of the subclavian arteries. Coarctation is one of the causes of secondary hypertension and should be considered in young patients with elevated BP. A bicuspid valve is seen in over 50% of the cases and there is an increased incidence of cerebral berry aneurysms. The renin–angiotensin system is reset and this contributes to the hypertension noted. Elevated BP may not return to normal after coarctation repair.

Clinical Findings

A. SYMPTOMS AND SIGNS

If cardiac failure does not occur in infancy, there are usually no symptoms until the hypertension produces LV failure or cerebral hemorrhage; the latter may also occur from the associated cerebral aneurysms. Strong arterial pulsations are seen in the neck and suprasternal notch. Hypertension is present in the arms, but the pressure is normal or low in the legs. This difference is exaggerated by exercise. Femoral pulsations are weak and are delayed in comparison with the brachial pulse. Patients may have severe coarctation, but with large collaterals may have relatively small gradients because of high flow through the collaterals to the aorta distal to the coarctation. Late systolic ejection murmurs at the base are often heard better posteriorly, especially over the spinous processes. There may be an associated aortic insufficiency or stenosis murmur due to the bicuspid aortic valve.

B. ECG AND CHEST RADIOGRAPHY

The ECG usually shows LV hypertrophy (LVH). Radiography shows scalloping of the ribs due to enlarged collateral intercostal arteries, dilation of the left subclavian artery and poststenotic aortic dilation, and LV enlargement. The coarctation region and the poststenotic dilation of the descending aorta may result in a "3" sign along aortic shadow on the PA chest radiograph (the notch in the "3" representing the area of coarctation).

C. DIAGNOSTIC STUDIES

Echocardiography/Doppler is usually confirmatory and may provide additional evidence for a bicuspid aortic valve. Both MRI and CT can also provide excellent images of the coarctation region to assess involvement of contiguous branch vessels. MRI and echocardiography/Doppler can provide estimates of the gradient across the lesion. Cardiac catheterization provides definitive gradient information and is necessary if percutaneous stenting is to be considered.

Prognosis & Treatment

Cardiac failure is common in infancy and in older untreated patients; it is uncommon in late childhood and young adulthood. Patients with a demonstrated gradient of > 20 mm Hg should be considered for intervention. Most untreated patients with the adult form of coarctation die before age 50 years from the complications of hypertension, rupture of the aorta, infective endarteritis, or cerebral hemorrhage. Aortic dissection also occurs with increased frequency in coarctation. Coarctation may be poorly tolerated in pregnancy because of the inability to support the placental flow.

Resection of the coarctation site has a surgical mortality rate of 1–4% and includes risk of spinal cord injury. Balloon angioplasty of the stenosis has been accomplished successfully, especially in coarctation restenosis after surgery, but the interventional procedure of choice is percutaneous stenting when feasible. Otherwise, surgical resection (usually with end-to-end anastomosis) should be performed. About 25% of surgically corrected patients continue to be hypertensive years after surgery because of the changes in the renin–angiotensin system described above, and they have all the complications associated with hypertension.

Hornung TS et al: Interventions for aortic coarctation. Cardiol Rev 2002;10:139. [PMID: 12047792]

Mahadevan V et al: Endovascular management of aortic coarctation. Int J Cardiol 2004;97(Suppl 1):75. [PMID: 15590082]

Oliver JM et al: Risk factors for aortic complications in adults with coarctation of the aorta. J Am Coll Cardiol 2004;44: 1641. [PMID: 15489097]

Ramnarine I: Role of surgery in the management of the adult patient with coarctation of the aorta. Postgrad Med J 2005; 81:243. [PMID: 15811888]

Toro-Salazar OH et al: Long-term follow-up of patients after coarctation of the aorta repair. Am J Cardiol 2002;89:541. [PMID: 11867038]

Vriend JW et al: Late complications in patients after repair of aortic coarctation: implications for management. Int J Cardiol 2005;101:399. [PMID: 15907407]

ATRIAL SEPTAL DEFECT & PATENT FORAMEN OVALE

 ESSENTIALS OF DIAGNOSIS

- *Often asymptomatic and discovered on routine physical examination.*
- *RV lift; S_2 widely split and fixed.*
- *Grade I–III/VI systolic ejection murmur at pulmonary area.*
- *ECG shows RV conduction delay; radiograph shows dilated pulmonary arteries and increased vascularity; echocardiography/Doppler diagnostic.*
- *A PFO is present in 25% of the population but can lead to paradoxic emboli and cerebrovascular events. Suspicion should be highest in patients who had cryptogenic stroke before age 55 years.*

General Considerations

Knowing how the atrial septum forms helps in understanding the different anatomic lesions that create a communication between the atria. Embryologically, the septum primum separates the two atria first, moving inferiorly toward the endocardial cushions. The ventricular septum forms by moving upward from the ventricles to the endocardial cushions at the same time. If the atrial septum does not make it all the way, the residual defect in the septum primum (ostium primum) results in the primum ASD. If the septum primum makes it all the way, a hole or holes (fenestrations) form in the middle of the septum (forming the ostium secundum). A second septum then moves down the right side of the first and normally covers the ostium secundum hole. If it does not cover the hole, a secundum ASD is present. The septum secundum normally completely covers the right side of the atrial septum except for an ovale hole in it (the foramen ovale). If the septae do not fuse, a patent path from the RA to the LA persists (the patent foramen ovale). The most common form of ASD (80% of cases) is persistence of the ostium secundum in the mid septum; less commonly, the ostium primum (which is low in the septum) persists. In many patients with an ostium primum defect, there are mitral or tricuspid valve clefts as part of the AV canal defect. A third form of ASD is the sinus venosus defect, a hole usually at of the upper part of the atrial septum due to failure of the embryonic superior vena cava (SVC) to merge with the atria properly. This latter lesion is often associated with anomalous drainage of the right upper pulmonary vein into the SVC. Rarer forms of ASD include a sinus venosus defect associated with failure of the inferior vena cava (IVC) to merge with the atria and a coronary sinus ASD that is basically an unroofed coronary sinus. In all cases, normally oxygenated blood from the higher-pressure LA passes into the RA, increasing RV output and pulmonary blood flow. In children, the degree of shunting across these defects may be quite large (3:1 or so). As the RV diastolic pressure rises from the chronic volume overload, the RA pressure may rise and the degree of left-to-right shunting may decrease. Eventually, the shunt may even be right-to-left and cyanosis appears.

The pulmonary pressures are modestly elevated in most patients with an ASD due to the high pulmonary blood flow, but severe pulmonary hypertension (Eisenmenger's physiology) is actually rare, occurring in only about 15% of the patients. Eventual RV failure may occur, and most shunts should be corrected unless they are quite small (< 1.5:1 right-to-left shunt). In adults, a large right-to-left shunt may have begun to reverse, so the absolute size at the time the patient is studied may underestimate what it was some years ago. In addition, in most patients the LV compliance normally declines more over time than the RV, and the natural history of small atrial septal shunts is to increase as the patient ages (unless RV failure ensues).

ASDs also predispose to atrial fibrillation due to RA enlargement, and paradoxic right-to-left emboli do occur. Interestingly, paradoxic emboli may be more common in patients with a PFO than a true ASD, as the eustachian valve in the RA directs flow from the inferior vena cava (IVC) toward the septum, and the usual significant left-to-right flow from an ASD is often not present with a simple PFO. An aneurysm of the atrial septum is when there is redundancy of the septum primum through the foramen ovale; it may include the septum secundum. When present with a PFO, there is more shunting right to left as the atrial septum swings back and forth. This latter anatomic issue may explain why more right to left shunting occurs in patients with an atrial septal aneurysm and PFO than in those with a PFO alone.

Clinical Findings

A. SYMPTOMS AND SIGNS

Patients with small or moderate ASDs and with a PFO are asymptomatic unless a complication occurs. With large shunts, exertional dyspnea or cardiac failure may develop, most commonly in the fourth decade of life or later. Prominent RV and PA pulsations are readily visible and palpable. A moderately loud systolic ejection murmur can be heard in the second and third interspaces parasternally as a result of increased PA flow. S_2 is widely split and does not vary with breathing due to the fact that the left-to-right shunt decreases as the RA pressure increases with inspiration.

B. ECG AND CHEST RADIOGRAPHY

Right axis deviation or RVH may be present depending on the size of the RV volume overload. Incomplete or complete right bundle branch block is present in nearly all cases of ASD, and superior axis deviation is noted in the AV canal defect, where complete heart block is often seen as well. With sinus venosus defects, the P axis is leftward of +15° due to abnormal atrial activation with loss of the upper RA tissue from around the sinus node. The chest radiograph shows large pulmonary arteries, increased pulmonary vascularity, an enlarged RA and RV, and a small aortic knob with all pre-tricuspid cardiac left-to-right shunts.

C. DIAGNOSTIC STUDIES

Echocardiography demonstrates evidence of RA and RV volume overload. The atrial defect is usually observed, though sinus venosus defects may be elusive. Many patients with a PFO also have a redundant atrial septum (atrial septal aneurysm) that promotes right-to-left shunting. Echocardiography with agitated saline bubble contrast can demonstrate a right-to-left shunt and both pulsed and colorflow Doppler flow studies can demonstrate shunting in either direction. A TEE is helpful when transthoracic echocardiography quality is not optimal, and it improves the sensitivity for small shunts and provides a better assessment of PFO anatomy. Radionuclide flow studies quantify left-to-right shunting by observing the bolus of contrast within the lung fields and demonstrating early recirculation. Both CT and MRI can also elucidate the atrial septal anatomy as well, and allow for observation of associated lesions. Cardiac catheterization is often helpful, especially if there are associated anomalous pulmonary veins. The size and location of the shunt can be determined and the pulmonary pressure and pulmonary vascular resistance (PVR) measured. Cardiac catheterization is required if percutaneous closure is to be contemplated.

Prognosis & Treatment

Patients with small atrial shunts may live a normal life span. Large shunts usually cause disability by age 40 years. Because left-to-right shunts tend to increase with age-related changes in LV compliance, most clinicians believe that closure of all shunts over 1.5:1 should be accomplished. Increased PVR and hypertension secondary to pulmonary vascular disease rarely occur in childhood or young adult life in secundum defects but are more common in primum defects. Significant pulmonary hypertension rarely develops in older patients. After age 40 years, cardiac arrhythmias

(especially atrial fibrillation) and heart failure may occur due to the chronic right heart volume overload. Paradoxical systemic arterial embolization becomes more of a concern as RV compliance is lost and the left-to-right shunt begins to reverse.

PFOs are not associated with significant shunting, and therefore the patients are asymptomatic and the heart size is normal. However, PFOs are responsible for most paradoxical emboli and are one of the most frequent causes of cryptogenic strokes in patients under age 55 years. That is likely because there is often right-to-left or bidirectional shunting, and the IVC blood is directed toward the foramen ovale by the eustachian valve.

Small ASDs do not require intervention. The easiest way to decide if a shunt is small is by echocardiography. If the shunt is not creating an RV volume overload, then one can assume the shunt needs no further evaluation. For larger deficits (those with an RV volume overload), surgery can be done at very low risk. Surgery involves anything from simple stitching of the foramen closed to patching of the hole with Dacron or a pericardial patch. Anomalous pulmonary venous connections are baffled to the LA through the sinus venosus defect when such anomalous veins are present. For ostium secundum ASDs, percutaneous closure by use of a variety of devices is now preferred over surgery. The percutaneous closure devices often resemble double umbrellas that lock the septum between the Dacron umbrellas when opened.

Patients with a PFO may have symptoms related to stroke or transient ischemic attack (especially if the age is under 55) or have hypoxemia (especially upon standing—so called platypnea orthodeoxia). There are data that suggest that migraine headaches may be more common in patients with a PFO, suggesting some unknown substance normally metabolized in the lung is entering the systemic circulation through the PFO. For patients with cryptogenic stroke or transient ischemic attack, it is uncertain whether closure of the PFO, either by open surgical or percutaneous techniques, has any advantage over anticoagulation with either warfarin or aspirin. Although there are no data yet suggesting that PFO closure is better than medical therapy, ongoing randomized trials should help settle this issue.

Azarbal B et al: Association of interatrial shunts and migraine headaches: impact of transcatheter closure. J Am Coll Cardiol 2005;45:489. [PMID: 15708691]

Diener HC et al: Patent foramen ovale: paradoxical connection to migraine and stroke. Curr Opin Neurol 2005;18:299. [PMID: 15891416]

Hara H et al: Patent foramen ovale: current pathology, pathophysiology, and clinical status. J Am Coll Cardiol 2005;46:1768. [PMID: 16256883]

Martin F et al: Percutaneous transcatheter closure of patent foramen ovale in patients with paradoxical embolism. Circulation 2002;106:1121. [PMID: 12196339]

Mas JL et al: Recurrent cerebrovascular events associated with patent foramen ovale, atrial septal aneurysm, or both. N Engl J Med 2001;345:1740. [PMID: 11742048]

Messe SR et al: Practice parameter: recurrent stroke with patent foramen ovale and atrial septal aneurysm: report of the Quality Standards Subcommittee of the American Academy of Neurology. Neurology 2004;62:1042. [PMID: 15078999]

Wahl A et al: Transcatheter treatment of atrial septal aneurysm associated with patent foramen ovale for prevention of recurrent paradoxical embolism in high-risk patients. J Am Coll Cardiol 2005;45:377. [PMID:15680715]

VENTRICULAR SEPTAL DEFECT

 ESSENTIALS OF DIAGNOSIS

- A restrictive VSD is small and makes a louder murmur than an unrestricted one.
- Adults may remain asymptomatic if the defect is small.
- Larger defects may result in pulmonary hypertension (Eisenmenger physiology) if not repaired.
- A grade II–VI/VI pansystolic murmur maximal at the left sternal border is heard; an associated thrill is common.
- ECG may show LVH, RVH, or both; radiograph shows increased pulmonary vascularity, and increased PA and LA size.
- Echocardiography/Doppler is diagnostic. The higher the gradient across the septum, the smaller the left-to-right shunt.

General Considerations

De novo VSDs are uncommon in adults. Congenital VSDs occur in various parts of the ventricular septum, but in adults most are in the membranous septum. Others occur high where both ventricles may be committed to the defect or in the muscular septum. Membranous and muscular septal defects may spontaneously close in childhood as the septum grows and hypertrophies. A left-to-right shunt is present unless there is associated RV hypertension. The smaller the defect, the greater the gradient from the LV to the RV and the louder the murmur. The presentation in adults is dependent on the size of the shunt and whether there is associated pulmonic or subpulmonic stenosis that has protected the lung from the systemic pressure and volume. Unprotected lungs with large shunts invariably lead to pulmonary vascular disease and severe pulmonary hypertension (Eisenmenger physiology).

Clinical Findings

A. SYMPTOMS AND SIGNS

The clinical features depend on the size of the defect and the presence or absence of increased pulmonary vascular resistance. Small shunts are associated with loud, harsh holosystolic murmurs in the left third and fourth inter-spaces along the sternum. Larger shunts may create RV volume and pressure overload. If pulmonary hypertension occurs, high-pressure pulmonic regurgitation may result. A systolic thrill is common. Right heart failure may gradually become evident late in the course, and the shunt will begin to reverse as RV and LV systolic pressures equalize with the advent of pulmonary hypertension. Cyanosis from right-to-left shunting may then occur.

B. ECG AND CHEST RADIOGRAPHY

The ECG may be normal or may show right, left, or biventricular hypertrophy, depending on the size of the defect and the pulmonary vascular resistance. With large shunts, the RV, the LV the LA, and the pulmonary arteries are enlarged, and pulmonary vascularity is increased on chest radiographs. If pulmonary vascular disease (pulmonary hypertension) evolves, an enlarged PA with pruning of the distal pulmonary vascular bed is seen. In rare cases of a very high VSD, an aortic cusp may prolapse into the VSD and reduce the VSD shunt but result in acute aortic regurgitation.

C. DIAGNOSTIC STUDIES

Echocardiography can demonstrate the size of the overloaded chambers (RV, PA, LA, and LV) and can readily define the defect anatomy. Doppler ultrasound can qualitatively assess the magnitude of shunting by noting the gradient from LV to RV and, if some tricuspid regurgitation is present, the RV systolic pressure can be estimated. Colorflow Doppler helps delineate the shunt defect and the presence of valvular regurgitation. MRI and cardiac CT can often visualize the defect and describe any other anatomic abnormalities. MRI can provide quantitative shunt data as well. Radionuclide flow studies are sometimes used to quantify the relative size of the left-to-right shunt. Cardiac catheterization is usually reserved for those with at least moderate shunting to determine the PVR and the degree of pulmonary hypertension. A PVR of > 7.0 absolute units or a PVR/SVR ratio of > 0.7 usually implies inoperability.

Prognosis & Treatment

Patients with the typical murmur as the only abnormality have a normal life expectancy except for the threat of infective endocarditis. Endocarditis is more typical of smaller shunts due to the high velocity of the jet lesion. Antibiotic prophylaxis is recommended. With large shunts, CHF may develop early in life, and survival beyond age 40 years is unusual.

Small shunts (pulmonary-to-systemic flow ratio < 1.5) in asymptomatic patients do not require surgery or other intervention. Defects causing large shunts should be repaired to prevent pulmonary hypertension or late heart failure. The presence of RV infundibular stenosis distal or pulmonary valve stenosis may protect the pulmonary circuit such that some patients even with a large VSD may still be operable as adults.

Surgical repair of a VSD is generally a low risk procedure unless there is significant Eisenmenger physiology as noted above. Currently, several new percutaneous closure devices are under review for nonsurgical closure of VSDs; devices for muscular VSDs are now approved and those for membranous VSDs are being implanted with promising results.

Ammash NM et al: Ventricular septal defects in adults. Ann Intern Med 2001;135:812. [PMID: 11694106]

Fu YC et al: Transcatheter closure of perimembranous ventricular septal defects using the new Amplatzer membranous VSD occluder: results of the U.S. phase I trial. J Am Coll Cardiol 2006;47:319. [PMID:16412854]

Gabriel HM et al: Long-term outcome of patients with ventricular septal defect considered not to require surgical closure during childhood. J Am Coll Cardiol 2002;39:1066. [PMID: 11897452]

Knauth AL et al: Transcatheter device closure of congenital and postoperative residual ventricular septal defects. Circulation 2004;110:501. [PMID: 15262841]

TETRALOGY OF FALLOT

 ESSENTIALS OF DIAGNOSIS

- *Four features are characteristic: VSD, RVH, RV outflow obstruction from infundibular stenosis, and an overriding aorta (< 50%). A right-sided aortic arch is common (seen in 25%).*

- *Most adult patients with tetralogy of Fallot have been operated upon, usually with an RV ouflow patch and VSD closure.*

- *Physical examination may be deceptive after classic tetralogy repair, with wide-open pulmonic regurgitation often present if a transannular patch was used.*

- *Echocardiography/Doppler may underestimate significant pulmonic regurgitation. Be wary if the RV is enlarged.*

- *Arrhythmias are common and periodic Holter monitoring is recommended.*

- *If the QRS width is > 180 msec, then the patient is subject to serious arrhythmias and sudden death.*

General Considerations

Patients with tetralogy of Fallot have a VSD, RV infundibular stenosis, RVH, and a dilated aorta (in about 50% of patients it overrides the septum). There may or may not be pulmonary valve stenosis as well, usually due to a bicuspid pulmonary valve. The aorta can be quite enlarged and aortic regurgitation may occur. If more than 50% of the aorta overrides into the RV outflow tract, the situation is not unlike a double outlet RV. Two vascular abnormalities are common: a right-sided aortic arch and anomalous left anterior descending coronary artery from the right cusp. The lat-

ter is important in that surgical correction must avoid cutting this vessel and producing an anterior myocardial infarction. A right-sided aortic arch occurs in 25% of patients and has no functional significance.

Most adult patients have undergone prior surgery. If significant RV outflow obstruction is present in infancy, a Blalock-Taussig (or similar) shunt is often the initial surgical procedure to improve pulmonary blood flow. This procedure enables blood to reach the underperfused lung either by directly attaching one of the subclavian arteries to the PA (classic Blalock shunt) or by creating a conduit between the two (modified Blalock shunt). Other types of systemic to pulmonary shunts no longer in use include a window between the right PA and the aorta (Waterston-Cooley shunt) or a window between the left PA and the descending aorta (Potts shunt). In the adult, there may be a reduced upper extremity pulse on the side used for the Blalock procedure. Total repair of the tetralogy of Fallot generally includes a VSD patch and usually a larger RV outflow tract patch, as well as a take-down of the Blalock shunt. Often the RV outflow tract patch extends through the pulmonary valve into the PA (transannular patch), and the patient is left with wide-open pulmonic regurgitation. Over the years, the volume overload from the severe pulmonary regurgitation becomes the major hemodynamic problem. Patients with tetralogy of Fallot should be monitored to ensure the RV volume does not increase. If it does, then pulmonary valve replacement should be done to correct the pulmonary insufficiency. Ventricular arrhythmias can also originate from the edge of the patch, and tend to correlate with the size of the RV.

Clinical Findings

Most patients are relatively asymptomatic unless right heart failure occurs or arrhythmias become an issue. Patients can be active and generally require no specific therapy except endocarditis prophylaxis. However, low-pressure pulmonic regurgitation is difficult to diagnose except at cardiac catheterization due to the fact that the RV diastolic pressures tend to be high and the pulmonary arterial diastolic pressure is low. This means there is little gradient between the PA and the RV in diastole, so that there may be little murmur or evidence for turbulence on colorflow Doppler. If the RV begins to enlarge, it must be assumed that this is due to pulmonic regurgitation until proven otherwise. Patients often do well into their 40s and 50s.

A. SYMPTOMS AND SIGNS

Physical examination should include checking both arms for any loss of pulse from a prior shunt procedure in infancy. The JVP may reveal an increased *a* wave from poor RV compliance or a *c-v* wave due to tricuspid regurgitation. The right-sided arch has no consequence. The precordium may be active, often with a persistent pulmonary outflow murmur. P$_2$ may or may not be present. A right-sided gallop may be heard. A residual VSD or aortic regurgitation may also be present. At times, the insertion site of a prior Blalock or other shunt may create a stenotic area in the PA and a continuous murmur occurs as a result.

B. ECG AND CHEST RADIOGRAPHY

The ECG reveals RVH and right axis deviation; in repaired tetralogy, there is often a right bundle branch block pattern. The chest radiograph shows a classic boot-shaped heart with prominence of the RV and a concavity in the RV outflow tract. This may be less impressive following repair. The aorta may be enlarged and right-sided. Importantly, the width of the QRS should be examined yearly. There are data that persons at greatest risk for sudden death are those with a QRS width of greater than 180 msec. The width of the QRS corresponds to the RV size, and in many patients, the QRS width actually decreases following repair of the pulmonary insufficiency.

C. DIAGNOSTIC STUDIES

Echocardiography/Doppler usually establishes the diagnosis by noting the unrestricted (large) VSD, the RV infundibular stenosis, and the enlarged aorta. In patients who have had tetralogy of Fallot repaired, echocardiography/Doppler also provides data regarding the amount of pulmonic regurgitation, RV and LV function, and the presence of aortic regurgitation.

Cardiac MRI and CT are evolving to have more major diagnostic roles, since they can quantitate both the pulmonary insufficiency and the RV volumes. In addition, cardiac MRI and CT can identify whether there is either a native pulmonary arterial branch stenosis or a stenosis at the distal site of a prior Blalock or other shunt. Cardiac catheterization is sometimes required to document the degree of pulmonic regurgitation because noninvasive studies depend on velocity gradients. Pulmonary angiography demonstrates the degree of pulmonic regurgitation, and RV angiography helps assess any postoperative outflow tract aneurysm.

Prognosis & Treatment

A few patients with "just the right amount" of pulmonic stenosis enter adulthood without having had surgery. However, most patients have had surgical repair of tetralogy of Fallot, including VSD closure, resection of infundibular muscle, and insertion of an outflow tract patch. Many have a transannular patch resulting in pulmonic regurgitation. If an anomalous coronary is present, then an extracardiac conduit around it from the RV to the PA may be necessary. By 20-year follow-up, reoperation is needed in about 10–15%, not only for severe pulmonic regurgitation but also for residual infundibular stenosis. Usually the pulmonary valve is replaced with a pulmonary homograft, though a porcine bioprosthetic valve is also suitable. Cryoablation of tissue giving rise to arrhythmias is sometimes performed at the time of reoperation. Branch pulmonary stenosis may be percutaneously opened by stenting. All patients require endocarditis prophylaxis.

Atik FA et al: Long-term results of correction of tetralogy of Fallot in adulthood. Eur J Cardiothorac Surg 2004;25:250. [PMID: 14747122]

Therrien J et al: Pulmonary valve replacement in adults late after repair of tetralogy of Fallot: are we operating too late? J Am Coll Cardiol 2000;36:1670. [PMID: 11079675]

Warnes CA: The adult with congenital heart disease: born to be bad? J Am Coll Cardiol 2005;46:1. [PMID: 15992627]

PATENT DUCTUS ARTERIOSUS

 ESSENTIALS OF DIAGNOSIS

- *Rare in adults.*
- *Adults with small or moderate size PDA are usually asymptomatic, at least until middle age.*
- *Widened pulse pressure; loud S_2.*
- *Continuous murmur over left pulmonary area; thrill common.*
- *Echocardiography/Doppler is helpful, but the lesion is best visualized by MRI, CT, or contrast angiography.*

General Considerations

The embryonic ductus arteriosus allows shunting of blood from the PA to the aorta in utero. The ductus arteriosus normally closes immediately after birth so that pulmonary blood flows to the pulmonary arteries. Failure to close normally results in a persistent shunt connecting the left PA and aorta, usually near the origin of the left subclavian artery. Prior to birth, the ductus is kept patent by the effect of circulating prostaglandins; in the neonate, a patent ductus can often be closed by administration of a prostaglandin inhibitor such as indomethacin. The effect of the persistent left-to-right shunt on the pulmonary circuit is dependent on the size of the ductus. If large enough, pulmonary hypertension (Eisenmenger physiology) may occur. A small ductus may be well tolerated until adulthood.

Clinical Findings

A. SYMPTOMS AND SIGNS

There are no symptoms unless LV failure or pulmonary hypertension develops. The heart is of normal size or slightly enlarged, with a hyperdynamic apical impulse. The pulse pressure is wide, and diastolic pressure is low. A continuous rough "machinery" murmur, accentuated in late systole at the time of S_2, is heard best in the left first and second interspaces at the left sternal border. Thrills are common. If pulmonary hypertension is present, the shunt may reverse and the lower body receives desaturated blood, while the upper body receives saturated blood. Thus, the hands appear normal while the toes are cyanotic and clubbed.

B. ECG AND CHEST RADIOGRAPHY

A normal tracing or LVH is found, depending on the magnitude of shunting. On chest radiographs, the heart is normal in size and contour, or there may be LV and LA enlargement. The PA, aorta, and LA are prominent because they all are in the shunt pathway.

C. DIAGNOSTIC STUDIES

Echocardiography/Doppler can determine LV, RV, and atrial dimensions. Colorflow Doppler allows visualization of the high velocity shunt jet into the proximal left PA. Cardiac MRI and CT can demonstrate the abnormality and assess the size of the pulmonary arteries. Cardiac catheterization can establish the shunt size and direction, and define the size of the ductus. It can also help determine whether pulmonary hypertension has occurred. If percutaneous closure is feasible, catheterization can be therapeutic.

Prognosis & Treatment

Large shunts cause a high mortality rate from cardiac failure early in life. Smaller shunts are compatible with long survival, CHF being the most common complication. Infective endocarditis or endarteritis may also occur, and antibiotic prophylaxis is recommended.

Surgical ligation of the patent ductus can be accomplished with excellent results in patients with few complications, even in very young children. If the lumen size of the ductus is small enough (< 4 mm), percutaneous approaches using either coils or occluder devices can be used with excellent results. Duct closure is usually feasible unless pulmonary hypertension and right-to-left shunting is present.

Arora R: Transcatheter closure of patent ductus arteriosus. Expert Rev Cardiovasc Ther 2005;3:865. [PMID: 16181031]

Bilkis AA et al: The Amplatzer duct occluder: experience in 209 patients. J Am Coll Cardiol 2001;37:258. [PMID: 11153748]

Pass RH et al: Multicenter USA Amplatzer patent ductus arteriosus occlusion device trial: initial and one-year results. J Am Coll Cardiol 2004;44:513. [PMID: 15358013]

■ VALVULAR HEART DISEASE

Although most cases of valvular disease in the United States were at one time due to rheumatic heart disease (still true in developing countries), other causes are now much more common. In the elderly, "degenerative" aortic valvular disease appears to be due to the same process that produces atherosclerosis, and studies have suggested that about 25% of adults over age 65 have some thickening of their aortic valve (aortic sclerosis) while 2–3% have frank aortic stenosis. Aortic sclerosis alone is a marker for future cardiovascular events and death. Calcium deposition may also occur in the mitral annulus creating enough

dysfunction of the valve that either stenosis or regurgitation (or both) results. Endocarditis remains a serious problem and its incidence has risen over the last 10 years. Mitral valve prolapse is still frequently seen and may be associated with the hyperadrenergic syndrome in younger patients. Valvular regurgitation may be due to LV dysfunction (mitral regurgitation) or RV dysfunction (tricuspid regurgitation).

The typical findings of each native lesion are described in Table 10–1. Table 10–2 shows how to use bedside maneuvers to distinguish the various murmurs.

Echocardiography yields key information about valve morphology, LV mass and function, and atrial and ventricular chamber size. Doppler ultrasound provides quantitative measurements of transvalvular gradients and RV systolic pressure (a surrogate for peak PA pressure when there is no pulmonic stenosis) and gives more qualitative estimates of the presence and severity of valvular regurgitation. TEE often provides improved image quality and valve morphology (particularly prosthetic valves), vegetations, thrombi, and eccentric regurgitant jets are more easily identified with TEE. Cardiac MRI and CT generally add only confirmatory information, though abnormalities of the great vessels are best seen by these modalities; the procedures are useful in tracking the size of ascending aortic aneurysms in patients with bicuspid aortic valve and in quantitating RV function.

Bach DS et al: Perioperative assessment and management of patients with valvular heart disease undergoing noncardiac surgery. Minerva Cardioangiol 2004;52:255. [PMID: 15284676]

Bonow RO et al: Guidelines for the management of patients with valvular heart disease. Circulation 1998;98:1949. [PMID: 9799219]

Boon NA: The medical management of valvar heart disease. Heart 2002;87:395. [PMID: 11907022]

Botkin NF et al: Asymptomatic valvular disease: who benefits from surgery? Curr Cardiol Rep 2005;7:87. [PMID: 15717953]

Elkayam U et al: Valvular heart disease and pregnancy part I: native valves. Am Coll Cardiol 2005;46:223. [PMID: 16022946]

Elkayam U et al: Valvular heart disease and pregnancy: part II: prosthetic valves. J Am Coll Cardiol 2005;46:403. [PMID: 16053950]

Rahimtoola SH: The year in valvular heart disease. J Am Coll Cardiol 2006;47:427. [PMID: 16412873]

Rahimtoola SH: Valvular heart disease/cardiac surgery. J Am Coll Cardiol 2005;45(11 Suppl B):20B. [PMID: 15936638]

Sachdev M et al: Effect of fenfluramine-derivative diet pills on cardiac valves: a meta-analysis of observational studies. Am Heart J 2002;44:1065. [PMID: 12486432]

Seiler C: Management and follow up of prosthetic heart valves. Heart 2004;90:818. [PMID: 15201262]

MITRAL STENOSIS

 ESSENTIALS OF DIAGNOSIS

• *Exertional dyspnea, orthopnea, and paroxysmal nocturnal dyspnea when the stenosis becomes severe.*

Table 10-1. Differential diagnosis of valvular heart disease.

	Mitral Stenosis	Mitral Regurgitation	Aortic Stenosis	Aortic Regurgitation	Tricuspid Stenosis	Tricuspid Regurgitation
Inspection	Malar flush, precordial bulge, and diffuse pulsation in young patients.	Usually prominent and hyperdynamic apical impulse to left of MCL.	Sustained PMI, prominent atrial filling wave.	Hyperdynamic PMI to left of MCL and down. Visible carotid pulsations.	Giant a wave in jugular pulse with sinus rhythm. Often olive-colored skin (mixed jaundice and local cyanosis).	Large v wave in jugular pulse.
Palpation	"Tapping" sensation over area of expected PMI. Middiastolic or presystolic thrill at apex. Small pulse. Right ventricular pulsation left third to fifth ICS parasternally when pulmonary hypertension is present.	Forceful, brisk PMI; systolic thrill over PMI. Pulse normal, small, or slightly collapsing.	Powerful, heaving PMI to left and slightly below MCL. Systolic thrill over aortic area, sternal notch, or carotids. Small and slowly rising carotid pulse.	Apical impulse forceful and displaced significantly to left and down. Prominent carotid pulses. Rapidly rising and collapsing pulses.	Middiastolic thrill between lower left sternal border and PMI. Presystolic pulsation of liver (sinus rhythm only).	Right ventricular pulsation. Occasionally systolic thrill at lower left sternal edge. Systolic pulsation of liver.
Heart sounds, rhythm, and blood pressure	Loud snapping M_1. Opening snap following S_2 along left sternal border or at apex. Atrial fibrillation common. Blood pressure normal.	M_1 normal or buried in murmur. Prominent third heart sound. Atrial fibrillation common. Blood pressure normal. Midsystolic clicks may be present.	A_2 normal, soft, or absent. Paradox splitting of S_2 if A_2 is audible. Prominent S_4. Blood pressure normal or systolic pressure normal with high diastolic pressure.	S_1 normal or reduced, A_2 loud. Wide pulse pressure with diastolic pressure < 60 mm Hg.	S_1 often loud.	Atrial fibrillation is usually present.
Murmurs						
Location and transmission	Localized at or near apex. Rarely, short diastolic (Graham Steell) murmur along lower left sternal border in severe pulmonary hypertension.	Loudest over PMI; transmitted to left axilla, left infrascapular area. With posterior papillary muscle dysfunction, may transmit to base.	Right second ICS parasternally or at apex, heard in carotids and occasionally in upper interscapular area.	Diastolic: louder along left sternal border in third to fourth interspace. Heard over aortic area and apex. May be associated with low-pitched middiastolic murmur at apex (Austin Flint) in nonrheumatic disease.	Third to fifth ICS along left sternal border out to apex.	As for tricuspid stenosis.
Timing	Onset at opening snap ("middiastolic") with presystolic accentuation if in sinus rhythm. Graham Steell begins with P_2 (early diastole).	Pansystolic: begins with M_1 and ends at or after A_2. May be late systolic in papillary muscle dysfunction.	Midsystolic: begins after M_1, ends before A_2, reaches maximum intensity in mid systole.	Begins immediately after aortic second sound and ends before first sound.	As for mitral stenosis.	As for mitral regurgitation.

(continued)

Table 10–1. Differential diagnosis of valvular heart disease. (continued)

	Mitral Stenosis	Mitral Regurgitation	Aortic Stenosis	Aortic Regurgitation	Tricuspid Stenosis	Tricuspid Regurgitation
Character	Low-pitched, rumbling; presystolic murmur merges with loud M₁, and ends at or after A₂. May be late systolic in papillary muscle dysfunction.	Blowing, high-pitched; occasionally harsh or musical.	Harsh, rough.	Blowing, often faint.	As for mitral regurgitation.	Blowing, coarse, or musical.
Optimum auscultatory conditions	After exercise, left lateral recumbency. Bell chest piece lightly applied.	After exercise, diaphragm chest piece. In prolapse, findings most prominent while standing.	Patient resting, leaning forward, breath held in full expiration.	Patient leaning forward, breath held in expiration.	Murmur usually louder and at peak during inspiration. Patient recumbent.	Murmur usually becomes louder during inspiration.
Radiography	Straight left heart border. Large left atrium sharply indenting esophagus. Elevation of left mainstem bronchus. Large right ventricle and pulmonary artery if pulmonary hypertension is present. Calcification occasionally seen in mitral valve.	Enlarged left ventricle and left atrium.	Concentric left ventricular hypertrophy. Prominent ascending aorta, small knob. Calcified valve common.	Moderate to severe left ventricular enlargement. Prominent aortic knob.	Enlarged right atrium only.	Enlarged right atrium and ventricle.
Electrocardiography	Broad P waves in standard leads; broad negative phase of diphasic P in V₁. If pulmonary hypertension is present, tall peaked P waves, right axis deviation, or right ventricular hypertrophy appears.	Left axis deviation or frank left ventricular hypertrophy. P waves broad, tall, or notched in standard leads. Broad negative phase of diphasic P in V₁.	Left ventricular hypertrophy.	Left ventricular hypertrophy.	Tall, peaked P waves. Normal axis.	Right axis usual.
Echocardiography M mode	Thickened, immobile mitral valve with anterior and posterior leaflets moving together. Slow early diastolic filling slope, left atrial enlargement, normal to small left ventricle.	Thickened mitral valve in rheumatic disease; mitral valve prolapse; flail leaflet or vegetations may be seen. Enlarged left ventricle with above-normal, normal, or decreased function.	Dense persistent echoes from the aortic valve with poor leaflet excursion, left ventricular hypertrophy with preserved contractile function.	Diastolic vibrations of the anterior leaflet of the mitral valve and septum, early closure of the mitral valve when severe, dilated left ventricle with normal or decreased contractility.	Tricuspid valve thickening, decreased early diastolic filling slope of the tricuspid valve. Mitral valve also usually abnormal.	Enlarged right ventricle, prolapsing valve, mitral valve often abnormal.

Two-dimensional	Maximum diastolic orifice size reduced, subvalvular apparatus foreshortened, variable thickening of other valves.	Same as M mode but more reliable.	Above plus poststenotic dilation of the aorta, restricted opening of the aortic leaflets, bicuspid aortic valve in about 30%.	Above plus may show vegetations in endocarditis, bicuspid valve, root dilation.	Above plus enlargement of the right atrium.	Same as above.
Doppler	Prolonged pressure half-time across mitral valve; indirect evidence of pulmonary hypertension.	Regurgitant flow mapped into left atrium; indirect evidence of pulmonary hypertension.	Increased transvalvular flow velocity, yielding calculated gradient. Valve area estimate using continuity equation.	Demonstrates regurgitation and qualitatively estimates severity.	Prolonged pressure half-time across tricuspid valve.	Regurgitant flow mapped into right atrium and venae cavae; right ventricular systolic pressure estimated.

A_2 = aortic second sound; ICS = intercostal space; M_1= mitral first sound; MCL = midclavicular line; P_2 = pulmonary second sound; PMI = point of maximal impulse; S_2 = second heart sound; S_4 = fourth heart sound; V_1 = chest ECG lead 1.

Table 10–2. Effect of various interventions on systolic murmurs.

Intervention	Hypertrophic Obstructive Cardiomyopathy	Aortic Stenosis	Mitral Regurgitation	Mitral Prolapse
Valsalva	↑	↓	↓ or ↔	↑ or ↓
Standing	↑	↑ or ↔	↓ or ↔	↑
Handgrip or squatting	↓	↓ or ↔	↑	↓
Supine position with legs elevated	↓	↑ or ↔	↔	↓
Exercise	↑	↑ or ↔	↓	↑
Amyl nitrite	↑↑	↑	↓	↑
Isoproterenol	↑↑	↑	↓	↑

↑ = increased; ↑↑ = markedly increased; ↓ = decreased; ↔ = unchanged.
Modified from Paraskos JA: Combined valvular disease. In: *Valvular Heart Disease.* Dalen JE, Alpert JS (editors). Little, Brown, 1987.

- *Symptoms often precipitated by onset of atrial fibrillation or pregnancy.*
- *Two syndromes occur; one with moderate mitral stenosis and pulmonary edema, and one with severe mitral stenosis, pulmonary hypertension, and low cardiac output.*
- *Prominent mitral first sound, opening snap (usually), and apical diastolic rumble.*
- *ECG shows LA abnormality and, commonly, atrial fibrillation. Echocardiography/Doppler confirms diagnosis and quantitates severity.*
- *Surgery indicated for symptoms or evidence of pulmonary hypertension. Most symptomatic patients have a valve area less than 1.5 cm².*

General Considerations

Patients with mitral stenosis are usually presumed to have underlying rheumatic heart disease, though a history of rheumatic fever is usually noted in only about one-third. Rheumatic mitral stenosis results in thickening of the leaflets, fusion of the mitral commissures, retraction, thickening and fusion of the chordae, and calcium deposition in the valve. Mitral stenosis can also occur due to congenital disease due to chordal fusion or papillary muscle malposition. The papillary muscles may be abnormally close together, sometimes so close they merge into a single papillary muscle (the parachute mitral valve). In these patients, the chordae and/or valvular tissue may also be fused. In other patients, mitral annular calcification may build up enough to produce a mitral gradient, most often in the elderly or patients with end-stage renal disease. Calcium in the mitral annulus virtually invades the mitral leaflet from the annulus inward. Mitral valve obstruction may also develop in patients who have had mitral valve repair with a ring that is too small, or in patients who have had a surgical valve replacement.

Clinical Findings

A. SYMPTOMS AND SIGNS

A characteristic finding of mitral stenosis is a localized mid-diastolic murmur low in pitch whose duration increases with the severity of the stenosis and the heart rate (Table 10–1). Because the valve is stiff and the LA pressure is high relative to the LV diastolic pressure, the valve opens in early diastole with a snap. The sound is sharp and widely distributed over the chest. The interval between the opening snap and aortic closure sound is long when the LA pressure is low but shortens as the LA pressure rises and approaches the aortic diastolic pressure. The gradient across the mitral valve produces a low-pitched rumble, best heard at the apex with the patient in the left lateral position. Brief exercise, such as sit ups, increase the heart rate and cardiac output resulting in increased flow across the mitral valve and increased audibility of the mitral rumble. Mitral regurgitation may accompany mitral stenosis. Generally, if a regurgitant murmur is audible, there is too much mitral regurgitation to allow either percutaneous valvuloplasty or surgical commissurotomy and valve replacement is the only alternative.

Two clinical syndromes occur with mitral stenosis. In mild to moderate stenosis, LA pressure and cardiac output may be essentially normal and the patient is either asymptomatic or symptomatic only with extreme exertion. The measured valve area is usually between 1.8 cm² and 1.3 cm² in those cases. In severe mitral stenosis (valve area < 1.0 cm²), severe pulmonary hypertension develops due to a "secondary stenosis" of the pulmonary vasculature. In this condition, pulmonary edema is uncommon, but symptoms of low cardiac output and right heart failure predominate.

Paroxysmal or chronic atrial fibrillation develops in 50–80% of patients. Any increase in the heart rate reduces diastolic time and increases the mitral gradient. A sudden increase in heart rate may precipitate pulmonary edema. Therefore, heart rate control is important to maintain, with slow heart rates preferred.

B. Diagnostic Studies

Echocardiography is the most valuable technique for assessing mitral stenosis. A scoring system is used to help define which patients are eligible for valvuloplasty. One to four points are assigned to each of four observed parameters, with one being the least involvement and four the greatest: mitral leaflet thickening, mitral leaflet mobility, submitral scarring, and commissural calcium. Patients with a total valve score of 8 or less respond better to balloon valvuloplasty techniques than patients with scores less than 8. LA size can also be determined by echocardiography: increased size denotes an increased likelihood of atrial fibrillation and thrombus formation. The effective mitral valve area can be determined by planimetering the smallest mitral orifice or by using the continuous-wave Doppler gradient. Some determination of the pulmonary pressure can also be quantitated by measuring the peak RV pressure from the tricuspid velocity jet signal.

Because echocardiography and careful symptom evaluation provide most of the needed information, cardiac catheterization is used primarily to detect associated valve, coronary, or myocardial disease—usually after the decision to intervene has been made.

Treatment & Prognosis

Mitral stenosis may be present for a lifetime with few or no symptoms, or it may become severe in a few years. In most cases, there is a long asymptomatic phase, followed by subtle limitation of activity. Pregnancy and its associated increase in cardiac output and the increased transmitral pressure gradient that results often precipitate symptoms. Toward the end of pregnancy, the cardiac output is also maintained by an increase in heart rate, further increasing the mitral gradient. The onset of atrial fibrillation often precipitates more severe symptoms, which usually improve with control of the ventricular rate or restoration of sinus rhythm. Conversion to and subsequent maintenance of sinus rhythm are most commonly successful when the duration of atrial fibrillation is brief (< 6–12 months) and the LA is not severely dilated (diameter < 4.5 cm). Once atrial fibrillation occurs, the patient should receive warfarin anticoagulation therapy even if sinus rhythm is restored, since atrial fibrillation often recurs even with antiarrhythmic therapy and 20–30% of these patients will have systemic embolization if untreated. Systemic embolization in the presence of only mild to moderate disease is not an indication for surgery but should be treated with warfarin anticoagulation.

Indications for intervention focus on symptoms such as an episode of pulmonary edema, a decline in exercise capacity, or evidence for pulmonary hypertension.

Open mitral commissurotomy is now rarely performed and has given way to percutaneous balloon valvuloplasty. Ten-year follow-up data comparing surgery to balloon valvuloplasty suggest no real difference in outcome between the two modalities. Replacement of the valve is indicated when combined stenosis and regurgitation are present or when the mitral valve echo score is > 8. Percutaneous mitral valvuloplasty has a very low mortality rate (< 0.5%) and low morbidity rate (3–5%). Operative mortality rates are also low: 1–3% in most institutions. Repeat valvuloplasty can be done if the morphology of the valve is suitable.

Mechanical mitral prosthetic valves are more prone to thrombosis than aortic valves. Bioprosthetic valves degenerate after about 10–12 years and percutaneous balloon valvuloplasty procedures cannot be done on bioprosthetic valves should stenosis occur. Younger patients and those with end-stage renal disease do least well with bioprosthetic heart valves. Endocarditis prophylaxis is always indicated. Percutaneous balloon valvuloplasty can safely be done during pregnancy if symptoms warrant.

Arora R et al: Percutaneous transvenous mitral commissurotomy: immediate and long-term follow-up results. Catheter Cardiovasc Interv 2002;55:450. [PMID: 11948890]

Fawzy ME et al: Immediate and long-term results of mitral balloon valvotomy for restenosis following previous surgical or balloon mitral commissurotomy. Am J Cardiol 2005;96:971. [PMID: 16188526]

Guerios EE et al: Mitral stenosis and percutaneous mitral valvuloplasty (part 1). J Invasive Cardiol 2005;17:382. [PMID: 16003027]

Guerios EE et al: Mitral stenosis and percutaneous mitral valvuloplasty (part 2). J Invasive Cardiol 2005;17:440. [PMID: 16079452]

Krasuski RA et al. Comparison of results of percutaneous balloon mitral commissurotomy in patients aged ≥ 65 years with those in patients aged < 65 years. Am J Cardiol 2001;88:994. [PMID: 11703995]

Iung B et al: The long-term outcome of balloon valvuloplasty for mitral stenosis. Curr Cardiol Rep 2002;4:118. [PMID: 11827634]

Rahimtoola SH: Current evaluation and management of patients with mitral stenosis. Circulation 2002;106;1183. [PMID: 12208789]

MITRAL REGURGITATION (Mitral Insufficiency)

 ESSENTIALS OF DIAGNOSIS

- Variable causes determine clinical presentation.
- May be asymptomatic for many years (or for life) or may cause left-sided heart failure.
- Pansystolic murmur at the apex, radiating into the axilla; associated with S_3 when regurgitant volume is great.
- ECG shows LA abnormality or atrial fibrillation and LVH; radiograph shows LA and LV enlargement.
- Echocardiographic findings can help decide when to operate.

- *For primary mitral regurgitation, surgery is indicated for symptoms or when LV EF is < 60% or the echocardiographic LV end-systolic diameter is > 4.5 cm.*

General Considerations

The components of the mitral valve apparatus include the myocardium below the papillary muscles, the papillary muscles themselves, the chordae, the leaflets, and the mitral annulus. Chordae from both the anterior and posterior leaflets attach to both papillary muscles. When ventricular contraction occurs, the papillary muscles contract first and pull the leaflets toward each other. As the LV pressure rises, the leaflets touch and the rising pressure in the LV pushes the leaflets together (so-called "keystone" effect). The chordae continue to rein in the mitral valve as systole commences and the annulus contracts. All of these components keep the mitral valve from leaking. Failure of any of these components results in mitral regurgitation. Thus, if the papillary muscles are displaced (as in dilated cardiomyopathy), the chordae are too long, the leaflets are too baggy (as in mitral prolapse), or the annulus does not contract (as in annular calcification or cardiomyopathy), then mitral regurgitation will result. Mitral regurgitation places a volume load on the heart (increases preload), but reduces afterload. The result is an enlarged LV with an increased EF. Over time, the stress of the volume overload weakens the LV; when this occurs, there is a drop in EF and a rise in end-systolic volume.

Clinical Findings

A. SYMPTOMS AND SIGNS

During LV systole, the mitral leaflets do not close normally, and blood is ejected into the LA as well as through the aortic valve. In acute mitral regurgitation, LA pressure rises abruptly, leading to pulmonary edema if severe. When chronic, the LA enlarges progressively and the increased volume can be handled without a major rise in the LA pressure; the pressure in pulmonary veins and capillaries may rise only transiently during exertion. Exertional dyspnea and fatigue progress gradually over many years.

Mitral regurgitation leads to LA enlargement and may cause subsequent atrial fibrillation. Systemic embolization is relatively unusual compared with other conditions causing atrial fibrillation. Mitral regurgitation may predispose to infective endocarditis.

Clinically, mitral regurgitation is characterized by a pansystolic murmur maximal at the apex, radiating to the axilla and occasionally to the base; a hyperdynamic LV impulse and a brisk carotid upstroke; and a prominent third heart sound due to the increased volume returning to the LV in early diastole. LA enlargement is at times considerable in chronic mitral regurgitation;

the degree of LV enlargement usually reflects the severity of regurgitation. Calcification of the mitral valve is less common than in pure mitral stenosis. Hemodynamically, LV volume overload may ultimately lead to LV failure and reduced cardiac output, but for many years the LV end-diastolic pressure and the cardiac output may be normal at rest.

Nonrheumatic mitral regurgitation may develop abruptly, such as with papillary muscle dysfunction following myocardial infarction, valve perforation in infective endocarditis, or ruptured chordae tendineae in mitral valve prolapse.

Mitral valve prolapse ("floppy" or myxomatous mitral valve) is usually asymptomatic but may be associated with nonspecific chest pain, dyspnea, fatigue, or palpitations. Most patients are female, many are thin, and some have skeletal deformities such as pectus excavatum or scoliosis. A hyperadrenergic syndrome has been described, especially in young females, that may be responsible for some of the noncardiac symptoms observed. This syndrome attenuates with age. Some patients have findings of a systemic collagen abnormality (Marfan or Ehler-Danlos syndrome). In these conditions, a dilated aortic root and aortic regurgitation may coexist with the mitral valve prolapse.

On auscultation, there are characteristic mid-systolic clicks that emanate from the chordae or redundant valve tissue and that may be multiple. If leaflets fail to come together properly, the clicks will be followed by a late systolic murmur. As the mitral regurgitation worsens, the murmur is heard more and more throughout systole. The smaller the LV chamber, the greater the degree of prolapse, and thus auscultatory findings are often accentuated in the standing position. The diagnosis is primarily clinical but can be confirmed echocardiographically.

The significance of mitral valve prolapse is in dispute because of the frequency with which it is diagnosed in healthy young women (up to 10%), but in occasional patients this lesion is not benign. Patients who have only a mid-systolic click usually have no sequelae, but significant mitral regurgitation may develop, occasionally due to rupture of chordae tendineae (flail leaflet), in patients with a late or pansystolic murmur. The need for valve repair or replacement is most common in men and increases with aging, so that approximately 2% of patients with clinically significant regurgitation over age 60 years will require surgery. Mitral valve repair is favored over valve replacement, and its efficacy has led many to recommend intervention earlier and earlier in the course of the disease process. Mitral repair may include shortening of chordae, chordae transfers, wedge resection of redundant valve tissue, and mitral annular ring to reduce the annular size. Stitching of the leaflets together to create a double orifice mitral valve is also used at times (Alfieri procedure). Mitral repair or replacement can be done through a right minithoracotomy. Robotic devices are also being used to repair these valves. A variety of new percutaneous methods for repair of the regurgitant mitral valve are being investigated. These methods include devices to create a double orifice mitral valve by clipping the anterior and posterior leaflets together, devices that are inserted in the coronary sinus to cinch the annulus and make it smaller, and devices that can be inserted onto the annulus from the ventricular side that can pull the annulus inward and reduce annular circumference. Most of these percutaneous methods are in phase 1 or phase 2 trials.

Infective endocarditis may occur, primarily in patients with murmurs; such patients should have antibiotic prophylaxis prior to dental work and surgical procedures, though the data supporting the use of antibiotic prophylaxis are actually quite poor. New guidelines regarding prophylaxis for endocarditis are due out by the end of 2006. β-Adrenergic blocking agents are often effective for supraventricular arrhythmias and may be useful if there are symptoms of the hyperadrenergic syndrome. Sudden death is rare in mitral prolapse, but when symptomatic ventricular tachycardia is present, aggressive management with an implantable cardioverter-defibrillator is usually indicated. An association between mitral prolapse and embolic cerebrovascular events has also been reported but has not been confirmed in subsequent studies. Echocardiographic evidence of marked thickening or redundancy of the valve is associated with a higher incidence of most complications.

Papillary muscle dysfunction or infarction following acute myocardial infarction is less common. When mitral regurgitation is due to papillary dysfunction, it may subside as the infarction heals or LV dilation diminishes. The cause of the regurgitation in most situations is displacement of the papillary muscles and an enlarged mitral annulus rather than true papillary muscle ischemia. In acute infarction, rupture of the papillary muscle may occur with catastrophic results. Transient—but sometimes severe—mitral regurgitation may occur during episodes of myocardial ischemia and contribute to flash pulmonary edema. Patients with dilated cardiomyopathies of any origin may have **secondary mitral regurgitation** due to papillary muscle displacement or dilation of the mitral annulus. In patients with ischemic cardiomyopathy, ventricular reconstructive surgery to restore the mitral apparatus anatomy is under investigation (eg, the Dor procedure). If mitral valve replacement is performed, preservation of the chordae to the native valve helps prevent further ventricular dilation following surgery. Several groups have reported good results with mitral valve repair in patients with LV EFs greater than 30% and secondary mitral insufficiency.

B. DIAGNOSTIC STUDIES

Echocardiography is useful in demonstrating the underlying pathologic process (rheumatic, prolapse, flail leaflet, cardiomyopathy), and Doppler techniques provide qualitative and semiquantitative estimates of the severity of mitral regurgitation. It should be noted that a minor degree of retrograde flow from the closing of the mitral valve occurs almost uniformly and echocardiography/Doppler detects this clinically insignificant regurgita-

tion in many normal individuals. Echocardiographic information concerning LV size and function, LA size, PA pressure, and RV function can be invaluable in planning treatment as well as in recognizing associated lesions. TEE may help reveal the cause of regurgitation and is especially useful in patients who have had mitral valve replacement, in endocarditis, and in identifying candidates for valvular repair. Echocardiographic dimensions and measures of systolic function are critical in deciding the timing of surgery. In the past, exercise radionuclide angiography for measurements of exercise EF or determination of myocardial stress–EF relationships was recommended, but this is now not often done. Cardiac MRI is occasionally useful, for example, if specific myocardial causes are being sought (such as amyloid or myocarditis) or if myocardial viability is needed prior to deciding whether to add coronary artery bypass grafting to mitral repair in patients with chronic ischemic mitral regurgitation.

Cardiac catheterization provides a further assessment of regurgitation and its hemodynamic impact along with LV function, resting cardiac output, and PA pressure. Coronary angiography is often indicated to determine the presence of CAD prior to valve surgery in patients with risk factors or those older than age 45 years. In the near future, it may be that multidetector CT methods will be adequate to screen patients with valvular heart disease for asymptomatic CAD.

Treatment & Prognosis

Acute mitral regurgitation due to endocarditis, myocardial infarction, and ruptured chordae tendineae often requires emergency surgery. Some patients can be stabilized with vasodilators or intra-aortic balloon counterpulsation, which reduce the amount of regurgitant flow by lowering systemic vascular resistance. Patients with chronic lesions may remain asymptomatic for many years. Surgery is necessary when symptoms develop. However, because progressive and irreversible deterioration of LV function may occur prior to the onset of symptoms, early operation is indicated even in asymptomatic patients with a reduced EF (< 60%) or marked LV dilation (end-systolic dimension > 4.5 cm on echocardiography). There is controversy regarding the role of afterload reduction in mitral regurgitation, since the lesion inherently results in a reduction in afterload. A heightened sympathetic state has led some to suggest β-blockade as well. Most clinicians who monitor patients with chronic mitral regurgitation do prescribe medications, eg, angiotensin-converting enzyme (ACE) inhibitors, to reduce afterload, extrapolating data from studies of patients with cardiomyopathy or aortic regurgitation. In mitral regurgitation, studies suggest that such afterload reduction reduces chamber sizes and the amount of regurgitation, but there has yet to be prospective studies that show a definite long-term benefit.

Badhwar V et al: Mitral valve surgery: when is it appropriate? Congest Heart Fail 2002;8:210. [PMID: 12147944]

Block PC: Percutaneous mitral valve repair for mitral regurgitation. J Interv Cardiol 2003;16:93. [PMID: 12664822]

Feldman T et al: Percutaneous mitral valve repair using the edge-to-edge technique: six-month results of the EVEREST Phase I Clinical Trial. J Am Coll Cardiol 2005;46:2134. [PMID: 16325053]

Freed LA et al: Mitral valve prolapse in the general population: the benign nature of echocardiographic features in the Framingham Heart Study. J Am Coll Cardiol 2002;40:1298. [PMID: 12383578]

Hayek E et al: Mitral valve prolapse. Lancet 2005;365:507. [PMID: 15705461]

Mohty D et al: The long-term outcome of mitral valve repair for mitral valve prolapse. Curr Cardiol Rep 2002;4:104. [PMID: 11827632]

Otto CM: Timing of surgery in mitral regurgitation. Heart 2003; 89:100. [PMID: 12482807]

Webb JG et al: Percutaneous transvenous mitral annuloplasty: initial human experience with device implantation in the coronary sinus. Circulation 2006;113:851. [PMID: 16461812]

AORTIC STENOSIS

ESSENTIALS OF DIAGNOSIS

- *In adults with a bicuspid aortic valve, usually asymptomatic until middle or old age.*
- *Growing evidence that "degenerative" or calcific aortic stenosis is related to the same process as atherosclerosis.*
- *Delayed and diminished carotid pulses.*
- *Soft, absent, or paradoxically split S_2.*
- *Harsh systolic murmur, sometimes with thrill along left sternal border, often radiating to the neck; may be louder at apex in older patients.*
- *ECG usually shows LVH; calcified valve on radiography or fluoroscopy; echocardiography/Doppler is diagnostic.*
- *Surgery indicated for symptoms. Surgical risk is typically low even in the very elderly.*
- *Symptoms likely once the peak echo gradient is > 64 mm Hg.*
- *Surgery often considered for asymptomatic patients when severe aortic stenosis is documented by echocardiography/Doppler.*

General Considerations

There are two common clinical scenarios in which aortic stenosis is prevalent. The first is due to a congenitally abnormal valve, usually bicuspid rather than tricuspid. Symptoms at times occur in young or adolescent individuals if severe, but more often symptoms emerge at age 50–65 years when calcification and degeneration of the valve becomes manifest. A dilated ascending aorta, primarily due to an intrinsic defect in the aortic media, may accompany the bicuspid valve. Coarctation of the aorta is also seen in a small number of patients with aortic stenosis. A second group develops what has traditionally been called degenerative or calcific aortic stenosis, which is thought to be related to calcium deposition due to processes similar to what occurs in atherosclerotic vascular disease. Approximately 25% of patients over age 65 years and 35% of those over age 70 years have echocardiographic evidence of aortic sclerosis. About 10–20% of these will progress to hemodynamically significant aortic stenosis over a period of 10–15 years. Thus, aortic stenosis has become the most common surgical valve lesion in developed countries, and many patients are elderly. The risk factors for aortic stenosis in the elderly are similar to those for atherosclerosis, including hypertension, hypercholesterolemia, and smoking. LV outflow tract obstruction may also be caused by other rare congenital lesions, such as supravalvular aortic stenosis (seen in Williams' syndrome) or by subvalvular obstruction such as a subvalvular membrane. Hypertrophic obstructive cardiomyopathy may also coexist with valvular aortic stenosis.

Clinical Findings

A. SYMPTOMS AND SIGNS

Aortic stenosis produces a progressive afterload increase on the LV. To reduce wall stress, the ventricle hypertrophies by laying sarcomeres on top of each other, and increasing the wall thickness. At times, severe LVH ensues. Eventually, the hypertrophy may lead to myocardial dysfunction. Since the EF measurement is afterload dependent, at times it is difficult to sort out whether the low EF is due to increased afterload or to myocardial dysfunction.

Slightly narrowed, thickened, or roughened valves (aortic sclerosis) or aortic dilation may produce the typical ejection murmur of aortic stenosis. In mild or moderate cases where the valve is still pliable, an ejection click may precede the murmur. The characteristic systolic ejection murmur is heard at the aortic area and is usually transmitted to the neck and apex. In some cases, only the high-pitched components of the murmur are heard at the apex, and the murmur may sound like mitral regurgitation (so-called Gallaverdin phenomenon). In severe cases, a palpable LV heave or thrill, a weak to absent aortic second sound, or reversed splitting of the second sound is present (see Table 10–1). When the valve area is less than 0.8–1 cm² (normal, 3–4 cm²), ventricular systole becomes prolonged and the typical carotid pulse pattern of delayed upstroke and low amplitude is present. This may be an unreliable finding, however, in older patients with extensive arteriosclerotic vascular disease. LVH increases progressively, with resulting elevation in ventricular end-diastolic pressure, and consequently LA and PCWPs. Cardiac output is maintained until the stenosis is severe (with a valve area < 0.8 cm²). LV failure, angina pectoris, or syncope may be presenting symptoms and signs of aortic stenosis; importantly, all occur with exertion.

Symptoms of failure may be sudden in onset or may progress gradually. Angina pectoris frequently occurs in aortic stenosis due to underperfusion of the endocardium. Of patients with calcific aortic stenosis and angina, 50% have significant associated CAD, whereas CAD is noted at only half this rate in the absence of angina. Syncope is typically exertional and a late finding. Very rarely, it is a presenting symptom in otherwise asymptomatic patients. Syncope occurs with exertion due to stimulation of reflex baroreceptors. With exertion, the LV pressures rise, stimulating these LV baroreceptors to peripherally vasodilate. This results in an increase in stroke volume in an attempt to further increase cardiac output, which increases the LV systolic pressure again due to the obstructed aortic valve; a cycle of vasodilation and stimulation of the baroreceptors thus occurs and eventually the stenotic valve will not allow an adequate increase in cardiac output and systemic BP falls. Less commonly, syncope may be due to arrhythmias (usually ventricular tachycardia but sometimes sinus bradycardia as calcific invasion of the conduction system from the aortic valve may occur).

B. DIAGNOSTIC STUDIES

The clinical assessment of the severity of aortic stenosis may be difficult, especially when there is reduced cardiac output or significant associated aortic regurgitation. The ECG reveals LVH or suggestive repolarization changes in most patients, but can be normal in up to 10%. The chest radiograph may show a normal or enlarged cardiac silhouette, calcification of the aortic valve, and dilation and calcification of the ascending aorta. The echocardiogram provides useful data about aortic valve calcification and opening and LV thickness and function, while Doppler can provide a good estimate of the aortic valve gradient. These data can usually reliably exclude or diagnose severe stenosis. The maximal Doppler gradient reflects the peak instantaneous gradient across the aortic valve and this differs from the catheterization peak-to-peak gradient. The mean gradients from Doppler and catheterization are more often in agreement. The peak Doppler gradient is derived by multiplying the maximal flow velocity through the valve orifice squared (m/s) times 4; thus, a 4 m/s maximum velocity gradient translates into a 64 mm Hg peak Doppler gradient. Valve area estimation by echocardiography is less reliable. With improvement in the reliability of echocardiography/Doppler, cardiac catheterization mostly provides confirmatory data, an assessment of the hemodynamic consequence of the aortic stenosis, and a look at the coronary arteries. In younger patients, and in patients with high aortic gradients the aortic valve need not be crossed at catheterization. If it is crossed, the valve gradient can be measured at catheterization and an estimated valve area calculated; a valve area below 1.0 cm^2 indicates significant stenosis

in the newest ACC/AHA guidelines. Aortic regurgitation can be semiquantified by aortic root angiography. In patients with a low EF and both low output and a low valve gradient, the valve area calculations may erroneously indicate significant aortic stenosis, and it may be unclear if an increased afterload is responsible for the low EF or if there is an associated cardiomyopathy. To sort this out, the patient should be studied at baseline and then during an intervention that increases cardiac output (eg, dobutamine or nitroprusside infusion). If the valve area calculation increases, the flow-limiting problem is not the valve, but rather the cardiomyopathy, and surgery is not warranted. If the valve area remains unchanged at the higher outputs, then the valve is considered flow limiting and surgery is indicated.

Prognosis & Treatment

Following the onset of heart failure, angina, or syncope, the prognosis without surgery is poor (50% 3-year mortality rate). Medical treatment may stabilize patients in heart failure, but surgery is indicated for all symptomatic patients with evidence of significant aortic stenosis, as described above. Valve replacement is usually not indicated in asymptomatic individuals, though a Class II indication is to operate once the peak valve gradient by Doppler exceeds 64 mm Hg or the mean exceeds 40 mm Hg because of the high likelihood of symptoms developing over the next 2 years.

The surgical mortality rate for valve replacement is remarkably low even in the elderly, and ranges from 2% to 5%. This low risk is due to the dramatic hemodynamic improvement that occurs with relief of the increased afterload. Mortality rates are substantially higher when there is an associated ischemic cardiomyopathy. Severe coronary lesions are usually bypassed at the same time and bypass adds only a small amount to the overall mortality and morbidity.

The interventional options in patients with aortic stenosis are variable and dependent on the patient's lifestyle and age. In the young and adolescent patient, percutaneous valvuloplasty still has a role. Balloon valvuloplasty is less effective and is associated with early restenosis in the elderly, and thus is rarely used. Data suggest aortic balloon valvuloplasty has an advantage only in those with preserved LV function, and such patients are usually excellent candidates for surgical aortic valve replacement (AVR). There is continuing interest in using the Ross procedure in younger patients. The Ross procedure is performed by moving the patient's own pulmonary valve to the aortic position and replacing the pulmonary valve with a homograft (or rarely a bioprosthetic valve). However, dilation of the pulmonary valve autograft and consequent aortic regurgitation, plus early stenosis of the pulmonary homograft in the pulmonary position, has reduced the enthusiasm for this approach in some institutions. Middle-aged adults generally can take the anticoagulation necessary for the use of mechanical AVR, so most undergo AVR with a bileaflet mechanical valve. If the aortic root is severely dilated as well (> 5.5 cm), then the valve may be housed in a Dacron sheath (Bentall procedure) and the root replaced as well. Alternatively, a human homograft root and valve replacement may be used. In the elderly, bioprosthetic (either porcine or bovine pericardial) valves with a life expectancy of about 10–15 years are routinely used to avoid need for anticoagulation. Recent data favor the bovine over the porcine pericardial valve. If the aortic anulus is small, a bioprosthetic valve with a short sheath can be sewn to the aortic wall (the stentless AVR) rather than sewing the prosthetic annulus to the aortic annulus.

Anticoagulation is required with the use of mechanical valves, and the international normalized ratio (INR) should be maintained between 2.0 and 2.5. Mechanical aortic valves are less subject to thrombosis than mechanical mitral valves.

Recently, there has been interest in developing a percutaneous approach to AVR. Both a retrograde approach (from the aorta) and an antegrade approach (from the ventricles by way of a transseptal catheter across the atrial septum) are being investigated. The devices being tested use either a stent with a trileaflet bovine pericardial valve constructed in it, or a stent with a large valve from a cow's jugular vein mounted inside. Preliminary data are encouraging.

Alborino D et al: Value of exercise testing to evaluate the indication for surgery in asymptomatic patients with valvular aortic stenosis. J Heart Valve Dis 2002;11:204. [PMID: 12000161]

Carabello B: Clinical practice. Aortic stenosis. N Engl J Med 2002; 346:677. [PMID: 11870246]

Cosmi JE et al: The risk of the development of aortic stenosis in patients with "benign" aortic valve thickening. Arch Intern Med 2002;162:2345. [PMID: 12418948]

Cowell SJ et al; Scottish Aortic Stenosis and Lipid Lowering Trial, Impact on Regression (SALTIRE) Investigators: A randomized trial of intensive lipid-lowering therapy in calcific aortic stenosis. N Engl J Med 2005;352:2389. [PMID: 15944423]

Palta S et al: New insights into the progression of aortic stenosis: implications for secondary prevention. Circulation 2000; 101:2497. [PMID: 10831524]

Park MH: Timely intervention in asymptomatic aortic stenosis. Emerging clinical parameters may help predict outcomes. Postgrad Med 2001;110:28. [PMID: 11787414]

Pereira JJ et al: Survival after aortic valve replacement for severe aortic stenosis with low transvalvular gradients and severe left ventricular dysfunction. J Am Coll Cardiol 2002;39: 1356. [PMID: 11955855]

Touati GD et al: Management of patients with asymptomatic moderate aortic stenosis undergoing coronary artery bypass grafting. J Heart Valve Dis 2002;11:210. [PMID: 12000162]

AORTIC REGURGITATION (Chronic Regurgitation)

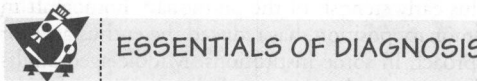 ESSENTIALS OF DIAGNOSIS

- Usually asymptomatic until middle age; presents with left-sided failure or chest pain.

- Wide pulse pressure with associated peripheral signs.
- Hyperactive, enlarged LV.
- Diastolic murmur along left sternal border.
- ECG shows LVH; radiograph shows LV dilation. Echocardiography/Doppler confirms diagnosis and estimates severity.
- Afterload reduction proven to be of benefit if the LV is dilated (LV end-diastolic dimension > 5.0 cm).
- Surgery indicated for symptoms or EF < 55% or LV end-systolic dimension by echocardiography > 5.0 cm.

General Considerations

Rheumatic aortic regurgitation has become much less common than in the preantibiotic era, and nonrheumatic causes now predominate. These include congenitally bicuspid valves, infective endocarditis, and hypertension. Many patients have aortic regurgitation secondary to aortic root diseases such as cystic medial necrosis, Marfan syndrome, or aortic dissection. Rarely, inflammatory diseases, such as ankylosing spondylitis or Reiter's syndrome, may be causative.

Chronic aortic regurgitation presents both an increased preload and an increased afterload to the LV. The response to these effects is to hypertrophy by laying sarcomeres end to end, increasing the LV chamber size greater than the wall thickness (eccentric hypertrophy). The amount of hypertrophy is substantial and greater than that seen in aortic stenosis or mitral regurgitation.

Clinical Findings

A. SYMPTOMS AND SIGNS

The clinical presentation is determined by the rapidity with which regurgitation develops. In chronic regurgitation, the only sign for many years may be a soft aortic diastolic murmur. As the valve deformity increases, the severity of the aortic regurgitation increases, diastolic BP falls, and the LV progressively enlarges. Most patients remain asymptomatic even at this point, and an often prolonged plateau phase, characterized by stable LV dilation, occurs. LV failure is a late event and may be sudden in onset. Exertional dyspnea and fatigue are the most frequent symptoms, but paroxysmal nocturnal dyspnea and pulmonary edema may also occur. Angina pectoris or atypical chest pain may occasionally be present. Associated CAD and presyncope or syncope are less common than in aortic stenosis.

Hemodynamically, because of compensatory LV dilation, patients eject a large stroke volume, which is adequate to maintain forward cardiac output until late in the course of the disease. LV diastolic pressure remains normal also but may rise when heart failure occurs. Abnormal LV systolic function, as manifested by reduced EF and increasing end-systolic LV volume, is a sign that surgical intervention is warranted.

The major physical findings in chronic aortic regurgitation relate to the high stroke volume being ejected into the systemic vascular system with rapid runoff as the regurgitation takes place. This results in a wide arterial pulse pressure. The pulse has a rapid rise and fall (water-hammer pulse or Corrigan's pulse), with an elevated systolic and low diastolic pressure. The large stroke volume is also responsible for characteristic findings such as Quincke's pulses (subungual capillary pulsations), Duroziez's sign (to and fro murmur over a partially compressed peripheral artery, commonly the femoral), and Musset's sign (head bob with each pulse). In younger patients, the increased stroke volume may summate with the reflected wave from the periphery and create an even higher systolic pressure in the extremity compared with the central aorta. Since the peripheral bed is much larger in the leg than the arm, the BP in the leg may be over 40 mm Hg higher than in the arm (Hill's sign). The apical impulse is prominent, laterally displaced, usually hyperdynamic, and may be sustained. A systolic murmur is usually present and may be quite soft and localized; the aortic diastolic murmur is usually high-pitched and decrescendo. A mid or late diastolic low-pitched mitral murmur (Austin Flint murmur) may be heard in advanced aortic regurgitation, owing to obstruction of mitral flow produced by partial closure of the mitral valve by the regurgitant jet and the rapidly rising LV diastolic pressure.

When aortic regurgitation develops acutely (as in aortic dissection or infective endocarditis), LV failure, manifested primarily as pulmonary edema, may develop rapidly, and surgery is urgently required. Patients with acute aortic regurgitation do not have the dilated LV of chronic aortic regurgitation and the extra volume is handled poorly. For the same reason, the diastolic murmur is shorter and may be minimal in intensity, and the pulse pressure may not be widened, making clinical diagnosis difficult. The mitral valve may close prematurely before systole has been initiated (pre-closure) due to the rapid rise in the LV diastolic pressure and the first heart sound is thus diminished or inaudible.

B. DIAGNOSTIC STUDIES

The ECG usually shows moderate to severe LVH. Radiographs show cardiomegaly with LV prominence and sometimes dilated aorta.

Echocardiography demonstrates the major diagnostic features, including whether the lesion involves the proximal aortic root and what valvular disease is present. Serial assessments of LV size and function are critical in determining the timing for valve replacement. Color Doppler techniques can qualitatively estimate the severity of regurgitation, though some "mild" regurgitation due to aortic valve closure is not uncommon and should not be overinterpreted. Cardiac MRI and CT have a role in estimating aortic root size, particularly when there is concern for an ascending aneurysm. MRI can provide a regurgitant fraction to help confirm severity. Scintigraphic studies are infrequently used but can quantify LV function and functional reserve during exercise. Exercise increases the heart rate and reduces the diastolic time, resulting in less aortic regurgitation per beat; this complicates interpretation of the exercise EF. Cardiac catheterization may be unnecessary in younger patients, particularly those with acute aortic regurgitation, but can help define hemodynamics, aortic root abnormalities, and associated CAD preoperatively in older patients.

Treatment & Prognosis

Aortic regurgitation that appears or worsens during or after an episode of infective endocarditis or aortic dissection may lead to acute severe LV failure or subacute progression over weeks or months. The former usually presents as pulmonary edema; surgical replacement of the valve is indicated even during active infection. These patients may be transiently improved or stabilized by vasodilators.

Chronic regurgitation has a long natural history, but the prognosis without surgery becomes poor when symptoms occur. Since aortic regurgitation places both a volume and afterload increase on the LV, vasodilators, such as hydralazine, nifedipine, and ACE inhibitors, can reduce the severity of regurgitation, and prophylactic treatment, which may postpone or avoid surgery in asymptomatic patients with severe regurgitation and dilated LVs, is indicated. Most clinicians prescribe ACE inhibitors whenever the LV diastolic size is increased > 5.0 cm as shown on echocardiogram. β-Blocker therapy may slow the rate of aortic dilation in Marfan syndrome by reducing the dP/dt, though the slower heart rates that result may theoretically increase the diastolic time and the amount of regurgitation per beat. Patients with aortic regurgitation need to be monitored serially by echocardiography. Surgery is indicated once symptoms emerge or for any evidence of LV dysfunction. LV dysfunction in this situation can be defined by echocardiography if the EF is < 55% or if the LV end-systolic dimension is > 5.0 cm, even in the asymptomatic patient. In addition, aortic root diameters of > 5.0 cm in Marfan or > 5.5 cm in non-Marfan patients are indications for surgery to avoid rapid expansion. Although the operative mortality rate is higher when LV function is severely impaired, valve replacement or repair is still indicated, since LV function often improves and the long-term prognosis is thereby enhanced even in this situation. The issues with AVR covered in the above section concerning aortic stenosis pertain here. Currently, however, there are no percutaneous approaches to aortic regurgitation. The choice of prosthetic valve for AVR depends on the patient's age and compatibility with warfarin anticoagulation.

The operative mortality rate is usually in the 3–5% range. Aortic regurgitation due to aortic root disease requires repair or replacement of the root. Though valve-sparing operations have improved recently, most patients with root replacement undergo valve replacement at the same time. Root replacement procedures include the Ross procedure (moving the pulmonary valve to the aortic position and replacing the pulmonary valve with a homograft or, less commonly, bioprosthetic valve), the direct homograft for the aortic root and valve, and the Bentall procedure (the use of a Dacron sheath with a mechanical or bioprosthetic valve sewn in place). Root replacement in association with valve replacement requires reanastomosis of the coronary arteries, and thus the procedure is more complex than valve replacement alone. Following surgery, LV size usually decreases and LV function generally improves even when the baseline EF is depressed. For that reason, a surgical approach is often recommended. However, the improvement in EF is generally much less, and the surgical risk is higher than in aortic stenosis patients with a similar EF.

Chaliki HP et al: Outcomes after aortic valve replacement in patients with severe aortic regurgitation and markedly reduced left ventricular function. Circulation 2002;106:2687. [PMID: 12438294]

Enriquez-Sarano M et al: Clinical practice. Aortic regurgitation. N Engl J Med 2004;351:1539. [PMID: 15470217]

Evangelista A et al: Long-term vasodilator therapy in patients with severe aortic regurgitation. N Engl J Med 2005;353: 1342. [PMID: 16192479]

Ha JW et al: Is prophylactic aortic valve replacement indicated during mitral valve surgery for mild to moderate aortic valve disease? Ann Thorac Surg 2002;74:1115. [PMID: 12400754]

Hicks GL Jr et al: Update on indications for surgery in aortic insufficiency. Curr Opin Cardiol 2002;17:172. [PMID: 11981251]

Scognamiglio R et al: Long-term survival and functional results after aortic valve replacement in asymptomatic patients with chronic severe aortic regurgitation and left ventricular dysfunction. J Am Coll Cardiol 2005;45:1025. [PMID: 15808758]

TRICUSPID STENOSIS

 ESSENTIALS OF DIAGNOSIS

- *Female predominance.*
- *History of rheumatic heart disease. Carcinoid disease more common in the United States.*
- *Elevated JVP with prominent a wave.*
- *Right heart failure after tricuspid surgery or in rheumatic disease or carcinoid syndrome.*
- *Echocardiography/Doppler key to diagnosis.*
- *Mean valve gradient > 5 mm Hg by echocardiography indicates severe tricuspid stenosis.*

General Considerations

Tricuspid stenosis is usually rheumatic in origin, though in the United States, tricuspid stenosis is more com-monly due to tricuspid valve repair or replacement or to carcinoid syndrome than to rheumatic fever. Tricuspid regurgitation frequently accompanies the lesion. It should be suspected when "right heart failure" appears in the course of mitral valve disease without significant pulmonary hypertension, or in the postoperative period after tricuspid valve repair or replacement.

Clinical Findings

Tricuspid stenosis is characterized by right heart failure and hepatomegaly, ascites, and dependent edema. A giant *a* wave is seen in the JVP, which is elevated. The typical diastolic rumble along the lower left sternal border mimics mitral stenosis, with the rumble increasing upon inspiration. In sinus rhythm, a presystolic liver pulsation may be found.

Diagnostic Studies

In the absence of atrial fibrillation, the ECG reveals RA enlargement. The chest radiograph may show marked cardiomegaly with a normal PA size. A dilated SVC and azygous vein may be evident.

The normal valve area of the tricuspid valve is 10 cm², so significant stenosis must be present to produce a gradient. Hemodynamically, a mean diastolic pressure gradient of > 5 mm Hg is considered significant, though even a 2 mm Hg gradient can be considered abnormal. This can be demonstrated by echocardiography or at cardiac catheterization. The echocardiogram reveals constricted motion and often thickening of the leaflets. At catheterization, the RA pressures demonstrate prominent *a* waves and with a slow *y* descent because of the slow RV filling. If there is associated tricuspid regurgitation a *c-v* wave will be observed.

Treatment & Prognosis

Tricuspid stenosis may be progressive, eventually causing severe right heart failure. Initial therapy is directed at reducing the fluid congestion, with diuretics the mainstay. When there is considerable bowel edema, torsemide may have an advantage over other loop diuretics, such as furosemide. Aldactone may also help if there is ascites. Neither surgical nor percutaneous valvuloplasty is effective for residual tricuspid regurgitation after tricuspid valve procedures, and tricuspid valve replacement is clearly the preferred surgical approach. Opening the commissure between the anterior and posterior leaflets is particularly prone to producing tricuspid regurgitation. Mechanical tricuspid valve replacement is rarely done because the low flow predisposes to thrombosis and because the mechanical valve cannot be crossed should the need arise for right heart catheterization or pacemaker implantation. Therefore, bioprosthetic valves are almost always used. Often tricuspid valve replacement is done in conjunction with mitral valve replacement for mitral stenosis.

Garcia-Pinilla JM et al: Reversible tricuspid stenosis secondary to massive ascites in hepatic cirrhosis. Ann Intern Med 2004; 140:233. [PMID: 14757628]

Staicu I et al: Tricuspid stenosis: a rare cause of heart failure in the United States. Congest Heart Fail 2002;8:281. [PMID: 12368592]

Thatipelli MR et al: Isolated tricuspid stenosis and heart failure: a focus on carcinoid heart disease. Congest Heart Fail 2003; 9:294. [PMID: 14564150]

TRICUSPID REGURGITATION

 ESSENTIALS OF DIAGNOSIS

- *Frequently occurs in patients with pulmonary or cardiac disease, especially if pulmonary hypertension is present (functional tricuspid regurgitation).*
- *Systolic c-v wave in jugular venous pulsations.*
- *Holosystolic murmur along left sternal border, which increases with inspiration.*
- *Echocardiography useful in determining cause (low- or high-pressure tricuspid regurgitation).*

General Considerations

The tricuspid valve apparatus differs in many ways from the mitral valve apparatus. Besides having three leaflets rather than two, the tricuspid valve has many chordae that attach to the RV endocardium rather than to discrete papillary muscles, and chordal attachments to the RV septum. The result of this anatomic feature is that tricuspid valvular incompetence often occurs whenever there is RV dilation from any cause. As tricuspid regurgitation increases, the RV size increases further, and this in turn worsens the tricuspid regurgitation. The causes of tricuspid regurgitation thus relate to anatomic issues with either the valve itself or to the RV geometry. An enlarged, dilated RV may be present if there is pulmonary hypertension for any reason, in severe pulmonic regurgitation, or in cardiomyopathy. The RV may be injured from myocardial infarction or may be inherently dilated due to infiltrative diseases (RV dysplasia or sarcoidosis). Usually the RV dilation is secondary to left heart failure. Inherent abnormalities of the tricuspid valve include Ebstein's anomaly (displacement of the septal and posterior leaflets into the RV), tricuspid valve prolapse, carcinoid plaque formation, collagen disease inflammation, tricuspid endocarditis, or RV pacemaker catheter injury.

Clinical Findings

The symptoms and signs of tricuspid regurgitation are identical to those resulting from RV failure due to any cause. As a generality, the diagnosis can be made by careful inspection of the JVP. The JVP waveform should decline during ventricular systole (the x descent). The tim-

ing of this decline can be observed by palpating the opposite carotid artery. As tricuspid regurgitation worsens, more and more of this valley in the JVP is filled with the regurgitant wave until all of the x descent is obliterated and a positive systolic waveform will be noted in the JVP. An associated tricuspid regurgitation murmur may or may not be present and can be distinguished from mitral regurgitation by the left parasternal location and increase with inspiration. An S_3 may accompany the murmur. Cyanosis may be present if the increased RA pressure stretches the atrial septum and opens a PFO or there is a true ASD (eg, in about 50% of patients with Ebstein's anomaly).

The ECG is usually nonspecific, though atrial fibrillation is not uncommon. The chest radiograph may reveal evidence for an enlarged RA or dilated azygous vein and pleural effusion. The echocardiogram helps assess severity of tricuspid regurgitation, PA pressure, and RV size and function. A paradoxically moving interventricular septum may be present. Catheterization confirms the presence of the regurgitant wave in the RA and elevated RA pressures. If the PA or RV systolic pressure is < 40 mm Hg, primary tricuspid regurgitation should be suspected.

Treatment & Prognosis

Minor tricuspid regurgitation is well tolerated. Severe tricuspid regurgitation results in hepatomegaly, edema, and ascites. In patients in the intensive care unit, tricuspid regurgitation may result in erroneous thermodilution cardiac output measurements because the recirculation of the saline bolus back to the RA reduces the temperature signal to noise required to perform the measurement. When present, bowel edema may reduce the effectiveness of oral furosemide, and intravenous diuretics should initially be used. Torsemide is better absorbed in this situation. Aldosterone antagonists have a role as well, particularly if ascites is present. At times, the efficacy of loop diuretics can be enhanced by adding a thiazide diuretic.

Definitive treatment usually requires elimination of the cause of the tricuspid regurgitation. If the problem is left heart disease (cardiomyopathy, aortic or mitral valve disease), then its treatment may lower pulmonary pressures, reduce RV size, and resolve the tricuspid regurgitation. Other causes for pulmonary hypertension, such as hypoxemia or pneumonia, may also need to be addressed and treated appropriately. Treatment for primary and secondary causes of pulmonary hypertension will generally reduce the tricuspid regurgitation. If surgery is contemplated for other reasons, especially mitral valve disease, then tricuspid annuloplasty is generally performed at the same time. Annuloplasty without insertion of a prosthetic ring (DeVega annuloplasty) may be effective to reduce the annular dilation. The valve can occasionally be repaired in tricuspid valve endocarditis. In heroin addicts with tricuspid regurgitation due to endocarditis, the tricuspid valve may be temporarily removed to aid in cure of the endocarditis, though it must eventually be replaced (usually by 6 months). If there is an inherent defect in the tricuspid apparatus that cannot be repaired, then replacement of the tricuspid valve is warranted. Generally, a bioprosthetic valve, and not a mechanical valve, is used. Anticoagulation is not required unless there is associated atrial fibrillation.

Behm CZ et al: Clinical correlates and mortality of hemodynamically significant tricuspid regurgitation. J Heart Valve Dis 2004;13:784. [PMID: 15473480]

Filsoufi F et al: Long-term outcomes of tricuspid valve replacement in the current era. Ann Thorac Surg 2005;80:845. [PMID: 16122441]

Hung MJ et al: Reversible left ventricular function after tricuspid valve replacement for a patient with congenital isolated severe tricuspid regurgitation. Echocardiography 2002;19:517. [PMID: 12356349]

Koelling TM et al: Prognostic significance of mitral regurgitation and tricuspid regurgitation in patients with left ventricular systolic dysfunction. Am Heart J 2002;144:524. [PMID: 12228791]

Nath J et al: Impact of tricuspid regurgitation on long-term survival. J Am Coll Cardiol 2004;43:405. [PMID: 15013122]

PULMONIC REGURGITATION

 ESSENTIALS OF DIAGNOSIS

- *Most cases are due to pulmonary hypertension.*
- *Loud diastolic (Graham–Steell) murmur in high-pressure pulmonic regurgitation.*
- *Soft or no murmur in low-pressure pulmonic regurgitation.*
- *Echocardiogram is definitive in high-pressure but may be less helpful in low-pressure pulmonic regurgitation.*
- *Low-pressure pulmonic regurgitation is well tolerated.*

General Considerations

Pulmonary valve regurgitation can be divided into high-pressure causes (due to pulmonary hypertension) and low-pressure causes (usually due to a dilated pulmonary annulus [idiopathic or traumatic] or to plaque from carcinoid disease or following surgical repair). It may be iatrogenic, eg, frequently occurring after repair of tetralogy of Fallot. Because the RV tolerates a volume load more than a pressure load, it tends to tolerate pulmonic regurgitation well.

Clinical Findings

On examination, a hyperdynamic RV can usually be palpated. If the PA is enlarged, it may be palpated along the left sternal border. P₂ will be palpable in pulmonary hypertension and both systolic and diastolic thrills are occasionally noted. On auscultation, the second heart sound may sound widely split due to prolonged RV systole. Systolic clicks may be noted as well as a right-sided gallop. In high-pressure pulmonic regurgitation, the pulmonary diastolic (Graham–Steell) murmur is readily audible. It is often due to a dilated pulmonary annulus. The murmur increases with inspiration and diminishes with the Valsalva maneuver. It is often confused with the murmur of aortic regurgitation. In low-pressure pulmonic regurgitation, the PA diastolic pressure may be only a few mm Hg higher than the RV diastolic pressure and there is little diastolic gradient to produce a murmur or characteristic echocardiography/Doppler findings. At times, only contrast angiography of the main PA will show the free flowing pulmonic regurgitation in this situation.

The ECG is generally of little value. The chest radiograph may show only the enlarged RV and PA. Echocardiography may demonstrate evidence of RV volume overload (paradoxic septal motion), and Doppler can determine peak systolic RV pressure and reveal any associated tricuspid regurgitation. The size of the main PA can be determined and colorflow Doppler can demonstrate the pulmonic regurgitation, particularly in the high-pressure situation. Cardiac MRI and CT can be useful for assessing the size of the PA, for imaging the jet lesion, for excluding other causes of pulmonary hypertension (eg, thromboembolic disease, peripheral PA stenosis), and for evaluating RV function.

Treatment & Prognosis

Pulmonic regurgitation rarely needs specific therapy other than treatment of the primary cause. In low-pressure pulmonic regurgitation due to surgical patch repair of tetralogy of Fallot, pulmonary valve replacement may be indicated if RV enlargement or dysfunction is present. In carcinoid heart disease, pulmonary valve replacement with a porcine bioprosthesis may be undertaken, though the plaque from this disorder eventually covers the prosthetic valve and this tends to limit the lifespan of these valves. In high-pressure pulmonic regurgitation, treatment to control the cause of the pulmonary hypertension is key.

Backer CL: Severe pulmonary valvar insufficiency should be aggressively treated. Cardiol Young 2005;15(Suppl 1):64. [PMID: 15934694]

Bouzas B et al: Pulmonary regurgitation: not a benign lesion. Eur Heart J 2005;26:433. [PMID: 15640261]

Gaynor JW: Severe pulmonary insufficiency should be conservatively treated. Cardiol Young 2005;15(Suppl 1):68. [PMID: 15934695]

CHOICE & MANAGEMENT OF PROSTHETIC VALVES & PERCUTANEOUS APPROACHES

In general, surgical results for valve replacement have improved over the past few decades. There is clearly interest, particularly among patients, for less invasive surgical procedures. This interest has led to mini-incisional approaches to aortic, mitral, and tricuspid valve replacement and repair. Percutaneous valvuloplasty has replaced surgical commissurotomy for mitral stenosis in most cases. However, percutaneous valvuloplasty is effective in aortic stenosis only in children and adolescents; it has a very limited role in adults. Neither surgical nor percutaneous tricuspid valvuloplasty is very effective.

Repair of the mitral valve is successful in appropriate patients and has lowered the threshold for intervention in mitral regurgitation. Some experts recommend that all mitral prolapse patients with mitral regurgitation undergo mitral valve repair even when other indications are not present. However, to recommend this option, the surgeon performing the procedure must have extensive experience with excellent results. When tricuspid regurgitation is present and mitral valve repair or replacement is planned, tricuspid repair is now commonplace. Aortic valve sparing procedures are also improving and may obviate the need for AVR, especially in patients undergoing root replacement. Early experience, though, with aortic valve repair is mixed. Direct valvular repair and removal of vegetations are also viable options in some patients with endocarditis.

The choice of prosthetic valve depends on a variety of considerations, including the expected survival of the patient versus the durability of the valve and the safety of warfarin for the patient. Bioprosthetic valves usually have a life expectancy of 10–15 years, but less in young patients and those on dialysis. The lifespan of bovine pericardial valves is somewhat longer than porcine valves in some series. Bioprosthetic valves, homografts, and the Ross procedure do not require anticoagulation with warfarin. Mechanical valves have a much longer lifespan, but all require use of warfarin (and frequently aspirin as an adjunct). The long-term risk of warfarin depends on patient compliance and whether there is coexisting disease that may predispose to bleeding.

Mechanical mitral valve prostheses pose a greater risk for thrombosis than mechanical aortic valves. For that reason, the INR should be kept between 2.5 and 3.5 for mechanical mitral prosthetic valves but can be kept between 2.0 and 2.5 for mechanical aortic prosthetic valves. Enteric-coated aspirin 81 mg once daily is given to patients with both types of mechanical valves, but appears to be more important for mitral valve prostheses.

Warfarin causes fetal skeletal abnormalities in about 2% of women who become pregnant while taking warfarin, so every effort is made to defer valve replacement in women until after childbearing age. However, if a woman with a mechanical valve becomes pregnant while taking warfarin, the risk of stopping warfarin is higher for the mother than the risk of continuing warfarin for the fetus. The risk of warfarin to the fetal skeleton is greatest during the first trimester, so if pregnancy is planned in a woman with a mechanical valve, unfractionated heparin is often used

temporarily during the first trimester. After the first trimester, warfarin use is safe again until 2 weeks before planned delivery, when the patient should be switched back to unfractionated heparin. Low-molecular-weight heparin has not been shown to be effective and should not be substituted for unfractionated heparin in the pregnant patient.

When patients with mechanical valves must undergo noncardiac surgery, the risk of thrombosis from stopping warfarin versus the risk of excessive bleeding from continuing it must be weighed. In general, for bileaflet aortic mechanical valves, warfarin can be stopped 3–4 days ahead of the surgical procedure and resumed the night of the procedure without "bridging" by use of unfractionated or low-molecular-weight heparin. In patients with a bileaflet mitral valve, warfarin may be stopped 3–4 days ahead of time and bridging low-molecular-weight heparin used until the warfarin is restarted and the INR is > 1.9. The highest risk for thromboembolic events occurs in patients with a ball-in-cage mechanical valve in any position, and in patients with a bileaflet mitral valve prosthesis and concurrent atrial fibrillation. In this latter group, bridging with either unfractionated or low-molecular-weight heparin is warranted once the INR has dropped below 2.0 before surgery; heparin is continued until warfarin is restarted and the INR is once again > 1.9.

Block PC et al: Percutaneous approaches to valvular heart disease. Curr Cardiol Rep 2005;7:108. [PMID: 15717957]

Bloomfield P: Choice of heart valve prosthesis. Heart 2002;87: 583. [PMID: 12010950]

Puvimanasinghe JP et al: Comparison of outcomes after aortic valve replacement with a mechanical valve or a bioprosthesis using microsimulation. Heart 2004;90:1172. [PMID: 15367517]

Salem DN et al: Antithrombotic therapy in valvular heart disease— native and prosthetic: the Seventh ACCP Conference on Antithrombotic and Thrombolytic Therapy. Chest 2004; 126(3 Suppl):457S. [PMID: 15383481]

Thamilarasan M: Choosing the most appropriate valve operation and prosthesis. Cleve Clin J Med 2002;69:688. [PMID: 12222973]

Thistlethwaite PA et al: Tricuspid valvular disease in the patient with chronic pulmonary thromboembolic disease. Curr Opin Cardiol 2003;18:111. [PMID: 12652215]

■ CORONARY HEART DISEASE (Atherosclerotic CAD; Ischemic Heart Disease)

Coronary heart disease, or atherosclerotic CAD, is the number one killer in the United States and worldwide. Every minute, an American dies of coronary heart disease. About 40% of people who experience a coronary attack will die of it in the same year. Coronary heart disease is responsible for more than one in five deaths and nearly 700,000 deaths per year in the United States. More than 10 times the number of women die each year from cardiovascular disease than from breast cancer. Coronary heart disease afflicts over 13 million Americans and the prevalence rises steadily with age; thus, the aging of the U.S. population promises to increase the overall burden of coronary heart disease.

Risk Factors for CAD

Epidemiologic studies have identified a number of important risk factors for CAD. Most patients with coronary heart disease have some identifiable risk factor. These include a positive family history (the younger the onset in a first-degree relative, the greater the risk), male gender, blood lipid abnormalities, diabetes mellitus, hypertension, physical inactivity and obesity, and cigarette smoking. A recent large international epidemiologic study of myocardial infarction shows that most of the population-attributable risk is explained by eight factors: abnormal lipids, smoking, hypertension, diabetes mellitus, abdominal obesity, psychosocial factors, consumption of too few fruits and vegetables and too much alcohol, and lack of regular physical activity. Smoking remains the number one preventable cause of cardiovascular disease worldwide. Although smoking rates have declined in the United States in recent decades, 21% of women and 25% of men smoke. According to the World Health Organization, 1 year after quitting, the risk of coronary heart disease decreases by 50%. Various interventions, including physician counseling, formal smoking cessation programs, nicotine replacement therapy, and bupropion, have been shown to increase the likelihood of successful cessation (see Chapter 1).

Overwhelming evidence indicates that hypercholesterolemia and other lipid abnormalities provide an important modifiable risk factor for coronary heart disease. Risk increases progressively with higher levels of low-density lipoprotein (LDL) cholesterol and declines with higher levels of high-density lipoprotein (HDL) cholesterol. Composite risk scores, such as the Framingham score (see Table 28–2), provide estimates of 10-year probability of development of coronary heart disease that can guide primary prevention strategies.

The metabolic syndrome is defined as a constellation of three or more of the following: abdominal obesity, triglycerides ≥ 150 mg/dL, HDL cholesterol < 40 mg/dL for men and < 50 mg/dL for women, fasting glucose ≥ 110 mg/dL, and hypertension. This syndrome, recognized as a major contributor to coronary heart disease risk, is increasing in prevalence at an alarming rate. Related to the metabolic syndrome, the epidemic of obesity in the United States is likewise a major factor contributing to coronary heart disease risk. In 2001, over 20% of the population was obese (body mass index [BMI] > 30 kg/m^2), a 74% increase compared to 1991. Particularly alarming is the rapidly increasing incidence of obesity in adolescents in the United States. Increasing physical activity is an impor-

tant goal to help combat obesity and its consequences. Although the American Heart Association continues to promote a diet based largely on low saturated fat, more information is needed on the health consequences of all diets, especially given the lack of protection from a low-fat diet in the largest randomized study ever done, the Women's Health Initiative trial. Surprisingly, low carbohydrate diets, even when high in saturated fat, may improve the cholesterol profile in overweight men, at least temporarily. Fish, rich in omega-3 fatty acids, may help protect against vascular disease and it is recommended that it be eaten three times a week by patients at risk.

It is now clear that markers of inflammation are strong risk factors for CAD. High sensitivity CRP is the best-characterized inflammatory marker and is available for clinical use, but others include interleukin-6, CD-40 ligand, myelopyroxidase, and placental growth factor. Although CRP levels > 10 mcg/mL are often found in systemic inflammation, levels < 1, 1–3, and > 3 mcg/mL, respectively, identify patients at low, intermediate, and high risk for future cardiovascular events. The prognostic value of CRP levels is independent and additive to lipid levels. Use of CRP may be helpful in determining which patients at intermediate risk according to the Framingham 10-year risk of coronary heart disease calculation (score of 10–20%) are at high enough risk to warrant more intensive primary prevention, including use of statins to lower LDL cholesterol. CRP levels are often elevated in patients who have other conditions associated with accelerated atherosclerosis, such as diabetes, the metabolic syndrome, and obesity. In patients presenting with acute coronary syndromes, these elevations identify a group that is at high risk for early recurrent events.

Pathophysiology

Knowledge concerning the pathophysiology of atherosclerosis has accumulated rapidly. Abnormal lipid metabolism or excessive intake of cholesterol and saturated fats—especially when superimposed on a genetic predisposition—is important in early stages of the atherosclerotic process. The initial step is the "fatty streak," or subendothelial accumulation of lipids and lipid-laden monocytes (macrophages). LDLs are the major atherogenic lipid. HDLs, in contrast, are protective by virtue of their role in reverse cholesterol transport, removing cholesterol from the vascular wall. The pathogenetic role of other lipids, including triglycerides, is less clear. LDLs undergo in situ oxidation, which makes them more difficult to mobilize as well as locally cytotoxic.

Macrophages migrate into the subendothelial space and take up lipids, giving them the appearance of "foam" cells. As the plaque progresses, smooth muscle cells also migrate into the lesion. At this stage, the lesion may be hemodynamically insignificant, but endothelial function is abnormal and its ability to limit the entry of lipoproteins into the vessel wall is impaired. If the plaque remains stable, a fibrous cap forms, the lesion becomes calcified, remodeling of the vessel wall occurs, and ultimately the vessel lumen may become narrowed, although extensive atherosclerosis may be present even before this occurs.

Although many atherosclerotic plaques remain stable or progress only gradually, others may rupture, often related to the inflammatory process and metalloproteinase activity. The rupture causes turbulent flow, extrusion of lipids and fatty gruel, and exposure of tissue factor that result in a cascade of events culminating in intravascular thrombosis. The outcome of these events is determined in large part by whether the vessel becomes occluded, which depends on the lesion anatomy as well as the balance of pro- and antithrombotic and pro- and antifibrinolytic forces. The result may be partial or complete vessel occlusion (causing the symptoms of unstable angina or myocardial infarction), or the plaque may become restabilized, often with more severe stenosis. Transient occlusion and/or embolization of platelet and thrombin debris, which may result in elevation in serum troponin, predispose to clinical events and portend a worse prognosis.

Several features are associated with enhanced plaque vulnerability, including a higher lipid content, a higher concentration of macrophages, especially in the plaque shoulder, and a very thin fibrous cap. Lesions with these characteristics are often relatively early lesions that can be responsible for acute myocardial infarction or sudden death as the first manifestation of coronary disease. Such lesions may occur in up to 50% of cases. This abrupt progression explains why most infarctions do not occur at the site of preexisting critical stenosis. Conversely, the relatively greater reduction in clinical events than in lesion severity in lipid-lowering treatment trials is probably explained by the stabilization of these early nonfibrotic lesions.

American Heart Association: Heart Disease and Stroke Statistics—2006 Update. Dallas, TX: American Heart Association, 2006. (www.aha.org)

Centers for Disease Control and Prevention. Overweight and Obesity: Home (www.cdc.gov/nccdphp/dnpa/obesity; accessed March 2006)

Haffner SM: Insulin resistance, inflammation, and the prediabetic state. Am J Cardiol 2003;92:18J. [PMID: 12957323]

Howard BV et al: Low-fat dietary pattern and risk of cardiovascular disease: the Women's Health Initiative Randomized Dietary Modification Trial. JAMA 2006;295:655. [PMID: 16467234]

Libby P: Current concepts of the pathogenesis of the acute coronary syndromes. Circulation 2001;104:365. [PMID: 11457759]

Libby P et al: Inflammation and atherosclerosis. Circulation 2002;105:1135. [PMID: 11877368]

Nissen SE et al: Intravascular ultrasound: novel pathophysiological insights and current clinical applications. Circulation 2001;103:604. [PMID: 11157729]

Pearson TA et al; Centers for Disease Control and Prevention; American Heart Association: Markers of inflammation and cardiovascular disease: application to clinical and public health practice: A statement for healthcare professionals from the Centers for Disease Control and Prevention and the American Heart Association. Circulation 2003;107:499. [PMID: 12551878]

Resnick HE et al: Diabetes and cardiovascular disease. Annu Rev Med 2002;53:245. [PMID: 11818473]

Ridker PM: Clinical application of C-reactive protein for cardiovascular disease detection and prevention. Circulation 2003; 107:363. [PMID: 12551853]

Yusuf S et al; INTERHEART Study Investigators: Effect of potentially modifiable risk factors associated with myocardial infarction in 52 countries (the INTERHEART study): case-control study. Lancet 2004;364:937. [PMID: 15364185]

Primary & Secondary Prevention of Coronary Heart Disease

Although many risk factors for CAD are not modifiable, it is now clear that interventions such as smoking cessation, treatment of dyslipidemia, and lowering of BP can both prevent coronary disease and delay its progression and complications after it is manifest. Treatment of lipid abnormalities delays the progression of atherosclerosis and in some cases may produce regression. Even in the absence of regression, fewer new lesions develop, endothelial function may be restored, and coronary event rates are markedly reduced in patients with clinical evidence of vascular disease.

A series of clinical trials has demonstrated the efficacy of hydroxymethylglutaryl coenzyme A (HMG-CoA) reductase inhibitors (statins) in preventing death, coronary events, and strokes. Beneficial results have been found in patients who have already experienced coronary events (secondary prevention), in those at particularly high risk for events (diabetics and patients with peripheral artery disease), and those with elevated LDL cholesterol without multiple risk factors. Benefits occurred regardless of age, race, or the presence of hypertension. There is now clear evidence that treatment with statins can prevent coronary events and stroke in patients without clinically manifest atherosclerosis (primary prevention) and LDL levels as low as 130 mg/dL. It is also clear that for patients with vascular disease, statins provide benefit for those with normal cholesterol levels, and that more aggressive LDL lowering is associated with greater benefits. The Heart Protection Study demonstrated that simvastatin 40 mg a day reduces vascular events by more than 20% in patients with prior myocardial infarction, stroke, peripheral vascular disease, or diabetes with total cholesterol levels as low as 135 mg/dL. The treatment benefit was similar regardless of baseline LDL cholesterol, with equal benefit above or below 100 mg/dL. This result suggests that all patients at significant risk for vascular events should receive a statin regardless of their cholesterol levels. The PROVE-IT trial showed that vascular events were reduced with more aggressive lipid lowering (atorvastatin 80 mg/d compared to pravastatin 40 mg/d following an acute coronary syndrome), providing more evidence of "lower is better" for patients with vascular disease. The TNT (Treating to New Targets) trial likewise found greater benefit with more aggressive LDL lowering (atorvastatin 80 mg versus 10 mg) in a population of patients with coronary heart disease and LDL cholesterol < 130 mg/dL.

The IDEAL (Incremental Decrease in End Points Through Aggressive Lipid Lowering) trial provided only modest support for very aggressive lipid lowering, showing a nonstatistically significant reduction in major coronary events with 80 mg/d of atorvastatin compared with 20 mg/d of simvastatin in patients with prior myocardial infarction. Although true regression of plaque is uncommon even with intensive lipid therapy (as in the REVERSAL and ASTEROID trials), progression can be prevented at least in the short run in most patients.

Treatment of abnormally low HDL levels or elevations of lipoprotein(a) and small, dense LDL particles is more difficult, but oral niacin in high dosages (2–3 g/d or more) may be effective. A trial in postinfarction patients has demonstrated that an increase in HDL levels with gemfibrozil (600 mg twice daily) in patients with relatively low LDL levels prolongs reinfarction-free survival, although the larger FIELD trial failed to show prevention of nonfatal myocardial infarction or coronary heart disease death with fenofibrate for patients with type 2 diabetes mellitus. The value of reducing elevated triglyceride levels is less clear, but since elevated triglycerides are often associated with other lipid abnormalities, treatment of high-risk patients with niacin, gemfibrozil, or fenofibrate for levels above 400 mg/dL is appropriate.

Because LDL oxidation appears to play a role in the atherogenicity of lipid molecules that have passed into the vessel wall, antioxidant therapy has been advocated as a preventive measure. Thus far, however, there are few data to support this popular concept, and many large, well-controlled studies have failed to demonstrate a benefit with vitamin E therapy. In fact, the Heart Protection Study and the Heart Outcomes Prevention Evaluation (HOPE) trial found that vitamin E may even be harmful by increasing the likelihood of heart failure and other trials have suggested that vitamin E may hinder the effectiveness of statin therapy.

Elevated plasma homocysteine levels are associated with an increased risk of vascular events. Although homocysteine levels can be reduced with dietary supplements of folic acid (1 mg/d) in combination with vitamin B_6 and vitamin B_{12}, two randomized clinical trials have shown that they are of little or no value in preventing vascular events.

Antiplatelet therapy is another very effective preventive measure. Aspirin (325 mg every other day) in males over the age of 50 years reduces the incidence of myocardial infarction. A similar approach (100 mg every other day), however, did not prevent myocardial infarction in women age 45 years or older, although stroke did appear to be reduced. Thus, the role of aspirin in primary prevention, including the dose, remains controversial. A prudent approach would be to administer 81–325 mg daily to men with multiple coronary risk factors or concomitant diabetes starting at age 45–50 years if no contraindication is present. While clopidogrel was found to be effective at preventing vascular events for 9–12 months after acute coronary syndromes, it was not found to be effective at preventing vascular events in the CHARISMA trial. This large trial included patients with clinically evident stable atherothrombosis or with multiple risk factors; all were treated with aspirin and observed for a median of 28 months.

The previously mentioned GISSI Prevention Trial found a significant reduction in mortality with administration of omega-3 fatty acid (1 g daily)—which has an antiplatelet effect in addition to other purported mechanisms—in postinfarction patients.

The effect of hormone replacement therapy in postmenopausal women has now been clarified, and it is clear that neither combined estrogen–progesterone nor estrogen alone therapy is protective (in fact both cause harm). Control of BP has been shown to prevent infarctions. Individuals who exercise for at least 30 minutes a week are at lower risk for subsequent coronary events, and 30 minutes of exercise five times a week reduces the risk of developing diabetes in half among patients at risk.

The HOPE and the EUROPA trials demonstrated that ACE inhibitors (ramipril 10 mg/d and perindopril 8 mg/d, respectively) reduce fatal and nonfatal vascular events (cardiovascular deaths, nonfatal myocardial infarctions, and nonfatal strokes) by 20–25% in patients at high risk, including diabetics with additional risk factors or patients with clinical coronary, cerebral, or peripheral arterial atherosclerotic disease. The PEACE trial did not show benefit of the ACE inhibitor trandolapril in a lower-risk population of patients with coronary heart disease, most of whom had been treated aggressively with medical and revascularization therapies. Therefore, while low-risk patients may not derive substantial benefits from ACE inhibitors, higher-risk patients with vascular disease, even in the absence of heart failure or LV dysfunction, should be treated with an ACE inhibitor.

Bhatt DL et al: Clopidogrel and aspirin versus aspirin alone for the prevention of atherothrombotic events. N Engl J Med 2006;354:1706. [PMID: 16531616]

Bonaa KH et al; NORVIT Trial Investigators: Homocysteine lowering and cardiovascular events after acute myocardial infarction. N Engl J Med 2006;354:1578. [PMID: 16531614]

Braunwald E et al; PEACE Trial Investigators: Angiotensin-converting-enzyme inhibition in stable coronary artery disease. N Engl J Med 2004;351:2058. [PMID: 15531767]

Cannon CP et al: Intensive versus moderate lipid lowering with statins after acute coronary syndromes. N Engl J Med 2004; 350:1495. [PMID: 15007110]

Collaborative meta-analysis of randomised trials of antiplatelet therapy for prevention of death, myocardial infarction, and stroke in high-risk patients. BMJ 2002;324:71. [PMID: 11786451]

Fox KM et al: Efficacy of perindopril in reduction of cardiovascular events among patients with stable coronary artery disease: randomised, double-blind, placebo-controlled, multicentre trial (the EUROPA study). Lancet 2003;362:782. [PMID: 13678872]

Grundy SM et al; National Heart, Lung, and Blood Institute; American College of Cardiology Foundation; American Heart Association: Implications of recent clinical trials for the National

Cholesterol Education Program Adult Treatment Panel III guidelines. Circulation 2004;110:227. [PMID: 15249516]

Hu FB et al: Optimal diets for prevention of coronary heart disease. JAMA 2002;288:2569. [PMID: 12444864]

Keech A et al; FIELD study investigators: Effects of long-term fenofibrate therapy on cardiovascular events in 9795 people with type 2 diabetes mellitus (the FIELD study): randomised controlled trial. Lancet 2005;366:1849. [PMID: 16310551]

Khot UN et al: Prevalence of conventional risk factors in patients with coronary heart disease. JAMA 2003;290:898. [PMID: 12928466]

Larosa JC et al: Intensive lipid lowering with atorvastatin in patients with stable coronary disease. N Engl J Med 2005;352:1423. [PMID: 15755765]

Lauer MS: Clinical practice. Aspirin for primary prevention of coronary events. N Engl J Med 2002;346:1468. [PMID: 12000818]

Lonn E et al; Heart Outcomes Prevention Evaluation (HOPE) 2 Investigators: Homocysteine lowering with folic acid and B vitamins in vascular disease. N Engl J Med 2006;354:1567. [PMID: 16531613]

MRC/BHF Heart Protection Study of cholesterol lowering with simvastatin in 20,536 high-risk individuals: a randomised placebo-controlled trial. Lancet 2002;360:7. [PMID: 12114036]

Nelson HD et al: Postmenopausal hormone replacement therapy: scientific review. JAMA 2002;288:872. [PMID: 12186605]

Nissen SE et al: Effect of intensive compared with moderate lipid-lowering therapy on progression of coronary atherosclerosis: a randomized controlled trial. JAMA 2004;291:1071. [PMID: 14996776]

Pearson TA et al: AHA Guidelines for Primary Prevention of Cardiovascular Disease and Stroke: 2002 Update: Consensus Panel Guide to Comprehensive Risk Reduction for Adult Patients Without Coronary or Other Atherosclerotic Vascular Diseases. American Heart Association Science Advisory and Coordinating Committee. Circulation 2002; 106:388. [PMID: 12119259]

Pedersen TR et al; Incremental Decrease in End Points Through Aggressive Lipid Lowering (IDEAL) Study Group: High-dose atorvastatin vs usual-dose simvastatin for secondary prevention after myocardial infarction: the IDEAL study: a randomized controlled trial. JAMA 2005;294:2437. [PMID: 16287954]

Ridker PM et al: A randomized trial of low-dose aspirin in the primary prevention of cardiovascular disease in women. N Engl J Med 2005;352:1293. [PMID: 15753114]

Third Report of the National Cholesterol Education Program (NCEP) Expert Panel on Detection, Evaluation, and Treatment of High Blood Cholesterol in Adults (Adult Treatment Panel III) final report. Circulation 2002;106:3143. [PMID: 12485966]

van den Hoogen PC et al: The relation between blood pressure and mortality due to coronary heart disease among men in different parts of the world. Seven Countries Study Research Group. N Engl J Med 2000;342:1. [PMID: 10620642]

Women's Health Initiative Investigators: Risks and benefits of estrogen plus progestin in healthy post-menopausal women: principal results from the Women's Health Initiative randomized controlled trial. JAMA 2002;288:321. [PMID: 12117397]

Pathophysiology of Chronic Ischemia & Acute Coronary Syndromes

Chronic ischemia, including stable angina, is classically caused by supply and demand mismatch, where significant fixed coronary stenosis and/or excess myocardial demand result in ischemia. Precipitants include exercise, eating, cold weather, and emotional stress.

The acute coronary syndromes of unstable angina and myocardial infarction are generally caused by a combination of plaque disruption, platelet and thrombin-mediated coronary thrombosis, coronary spasm, and microvascular dysfunction. Of interest is the predilection for these episodes to occur in the early morning or shortly after arising. Antithrombotic therapy is directed toward inhibition of platelet activity (aspirin, clopidogrel, IIb/IIIa receptor antagonists), inhibition of coagulation (unfractionated or low-molecular-weight heparin), and fibrinolysis for ST-segment elevation myocardial infarction.

Some episodes of myocardial ischemia are symptomatic, causing angina pectoris; others are completely silent. Many silent episodes are brought on by emotional and mental stress. In patients with diagnosed coronary disease, as evidenced by prior myocardial infarction or angina, silent ischemic episodes have the same prognostic import as symptomatic ones. The prognosis for patients with only silent ischemia is not well established, nor is the potential benefit of preventing silent ischemia.

Faxon DP; American Heart Association: Atherosclerotic Vascular Disease Conference: Writing Group III: pathophysiology. Circulation 2004;109:2617. [PMID: 15173044]

Servoss SJ et al: Triggers of acute coronary syndromes. Prog Cardiovasc Dis 2002;44:369. [PMID: 12024335]

Myocardial Hibernation & Stunning

Areas of myocardium that are persistently underperfused but still viable may develop sustained contractile dysfunction. This phenomenon, which is termed "myocardial hibernation," appears to represent an adaptive response but may lead to LV failure. It is important to recognize this phenomenon, since this form of dysfunction is reversible following coronary revascularization. Hibernating myocardium can be identified by radionuclide testing, positron emission tomography (PET), contrast-enhanced MRI, or its retained response to inotropic stimulation with dobutamine. A related phenomenon, termed "myocardial stunning," is the occurrence of persistent contractile dysfunction following prolonged or repetitive episodes of myocardial ischemia.

ANGINA PECTORIS

 ESSENTIALS OF DIAGNOSIS

- *Precordial chest pain, usually precipitated by stress or exertion, relieved rapidly by rest or nitrates.*
- *ECG or scintigraphic evidence of ischemia during pain or stress testing.*

• *Angiographic demonstration of significant obstruction of major coronary vessels.*

General Considerations

Angina pectoris is usually due to atherosclerotic heart disease. Coronary vasospasm may occur at the site of a lesion or, less frequently, in apparently normal vessels. Other unusual causes of coronary artery obstruction such as congenital anomalies, emboli, arteritis, or dissection may cause ischemia or infarction. Angina may also occur in the absence of coronary artery obstruction as a result of severe myocardial hypertrophy, severe aortic stenosis or regurgitation, or in response to increased metabolic demands, as in hyperthyroidism, marked anemia, or paroxysmal tachycardias with rapid ventricular rates. Rarely, angina occurs with angiographically normal coronary arteries and without other identifiable causes. This presentation has been labeled syndrome X and is most likely due to inadequate flow reserve in the resistance vessels (microvasculature). Although treatment is often not very successful in relieving symptoms, the prognosis of syndrome X is good.

Clinical Findings

A. History

The diagnosis of angina pectoris depends principally upon the history, which should specifically include the following information: circumstances that precipitate and relieve angina, characteristics of the discomfort, location and radiation, duration of attacks, and effect of nitroglycerin.

1. Circumstances that precipitate and relieve angina—Angina occurs most commonly during activity and is relieved by resting. Patients may prefer to remain upright rather than lie down, as increased preload in recumbency increases myocardial work. The amount of activity required to produce angina may be relatively consistent under comparable physical and emotional circumstances or may vary from day to day. The threshold for angina is usually less after meals, during excitement, or on exposure to cold. It is often lower in the morning or after strong emotion; the latter can provoke attacks in the absence of exertion. In addition, discomfort may occur during sexual activity, at rest, or at night as a result of coronary spasm.

2. Characteristics of the discomfort—Patients often do not refer to angina as "pain" but as a sensation of tightness, squeezing, burning, pressing, choking, aching, bursting, "gas," indigestion, or an ill-characterized discomfort. It is often characterized by clenching a fist over the mid chest. The distress of angina is rarely sharply localized and is not spasmodic.

3. Location and radiation—The distribution of the distress may vary widely in different patients but is usually the same for each patient unless unstable angina or myocardial infarction supervenes. In most cases, the discomfort is felt behind or slightly to the left of the mid sternum. When it begins farther to the left or, uncommonly, on the right, it characteristically moves centrally substernally. Although angina may radiate to any dermatome from C8 to T4, it radiates most often to the left shoulder and upper arm, frequently moving down the inner volar aspect of the arm to the elbow, forearm, wrist, or fourth and fifth fingers. Radiation to the right shoulder and distally is less common, but the characteristics are the same. Occasionally, angina may be felt initially in the lower jaw, the back of the neck, the interscapular area, high in the left back, or in the volar aspect of the wrist.

4. Duration of attacks—Angina is of short duration and subsides completely without residual discomfort. If the attack is precipitated by exertion and the patient promptly stops to rest, it usually lasts less than 3 minutes. Attacks following a heavy meal or brought on by anger often last 15–20 minutes. Attacks lasting more than 30 minutes are unusual and suggest the development of unstable angina, myocardial infarction, or an alternative diagnosis.

5. Effect of nitroglycerin—The diagnosis of angina pectoris is strongly supported if sublingual nitroglycerin promptly and invariably shortens an attack and if prophylactic nitrates permit greater exertion or prevent angina entirely.

B. Signs

Examination during a spontaneous or induced attack frequently reveals a significant elevation in systolic and diastolic BP, although hypotension may also occur, and may reflect more severe ischemia or inferior ischemia (especially with bradycardia) due to a Bezold–Jarisch reflex. Occasionally, a gallop rhythm and an apical systolic murmur due to transient mitral regurgitation from papillary muscle dysfunction are present during pain only. Supraventricular or ventricular arrhythmias may be present, either as the precipitating factor or as a result of ischemia.

It is important to detect signs of diseases that may contribute to or accompany atherosclerotic heart disease, eg, diabetes mellitus (retinopathy or neuropathy), xanthelasma, tendinous xanthomas, hypertension, thyrotoxicosis, myxedema, or peripheral vascular disease. Aortic stenosis or regurgitation, hypertrophic cardiomyopathy, and mitral valve prolapse should be sought, since they may produce angina or other forms of chest pain.

Differential Diagnosis

Angina can usually be diagnosed from a proper history. When atypical features are present—such as prolonged duration (hours or days) or darting, knifelike pains at the apex or over the precordium—ischemia is less likely.

Anterior chest wall syndrome is characterized by sharply localized tenderness of intercostal muscles. Inflammation of the chondrocostal junctions, which may be warm, swollen, and red, may result in diffuse chest pain that is also reproduced by local pressure (Tietze's syndrome). Intercostal neuritis (due to herpes zoster, diabetes mellitus, etc) also mimics angina.

Cervical or thoracic spine disease involving the dorsal roots produces sudden sharp, severe chest pain suggesting angina in location and "radiation" but related to specific movements of the neck or spine, recumbency, and straining or lifting. Pain due to cervical or thoracic disk disease involves the outer or dorsal aspect of the arm and the thumb and index fingers rather than the ring and little fingers.

Peptic ulcer, chronic cholecystitis, esophageal spasm, and functional gastrointestinal disease may produce pain suggestive of angina pectoris. Reflux esophagitis is characterized by lower chest and upper abdominal pain after heavy meals, occurring in recumbency or upon bending over, and awakening patients several hours after eating. The pain is relieved by antacids, sucralfate, H_2-receptor antagonists, or proton pump inhibitors. The picture may be especially confusing because ischemic pain may also be associated with upper gastrointestinal symptoms, and esophageal motility disorders may be improved by nitrates and calcium channel blockers. Assessment of esophageal motility may be helpful.

Degenerative and inflammatory lesions of the left shoulder and thoracic outlet syndromes may cause chest pain due to nerve irritation or muscular compression; the symptoms are usually precipitated by movement of the arm and shoulder and are associated with paresthesias.

Spontaneous pneumothorax may cause chest pain as well as dyspnea and may create confusion with angina as well as myocardial infarction. The same is true of pneumonia and pulmonary embolism. Dissection of the thoracic aorta can cause severe chest pain that is commonly felt in the back; it is sudden in onset, reaches maximum intensity immediately, and may be associated with changes in pulses. Other cardiac disorders such as mitral valve prolapse, hypertrophic cardiomyopathy, myocarditis, pericarditis, aortic valve disease, or RVH may cause atypical chest pain or even myocardial ischemia. Noninvasive testing and, in many cases, cardiac catheterization may be required to establish the diagnosis.

Evaluation of Patients with Angina Pectoris

A. LABORATORY FINDINGS

Serum lipid levels should be determined in all patients with suspected angina. Anemia and diabetes may also be investigated if clinically appropriate.

B. ECG

The resting ECG is normal in about 25% of patients with angina. In the remainder, abnormalities include old myocardial infarction, nonspecific ST–T changes, AV or intraventricular conduction defects, and changes of LVH. During anginal episodes, the characteristic ECG change is horizontal or downsloping ST-segment depression that reverses after the ischemia disappears. T wave flattening or inversion may also occur. Less frequently, ST-segment elevation is observed; this finding suggests severe (transmural) ischemia and often occurs with coronary spasm.

C. EXERCISE ECG

Exercise testing is the most useful noninvasive procedure for evaluating the patient with angina. Ischemia that is not present at rest is detected by precipitation of typical chest pain or ST-segment depression (or, rarely, elevation). Exercise testing is often combined with imaging studies (nuclear, echocardiography, or MRI [see below]), but in patients without baseline ST segment abnormalities or in whom anatomic localization is not necessary, the exercise ECG remains the recommended initial procedure because of considerations of cost and convenience.

Exercise testing can be done on a motorized treadmill or with a bicycle ergometer. A variety of exercise protocols are utilized, the most common being the Bruce protocol, which increases the treadmill speed and elevation every 3 minutes until limited by symptoms. At least two ECG leads should be monitored continuously.

1. Precautions and risks—The usually quoted risk of exercise testing is one infarction or death per 1000 tests, but individuals who continue to have pain at rest or minimal activity are at higher risk and should not be tested. Many of the traditional exclusions, such as recent myocardial infarction or CHF, are no longer used *if the patient is stable and ambulatory*, but aortic stenosis remains a contraindication. Although most tests are carried to a symptom-limited end point (except submaximal testing early postinfarction), the test should be terminated when hypotension, significant ventricular or supraventricular arrhythmias, more than mild to moderate angina, or more than 3- to 4-mm ST-segment depression occurs.

2. Indications—Exercise testing is used (1) to confirm the diagnosis of angina; (2) to determine the severity of limitation of activity due to angina; (3) to assess prognosis in patients with known coronary disease, including those recovering from myocardial infarction, by detecting groups at high or low risk; (4) to evaluate responses to therapy; and (5) less successfully, to screen asymptomatic populations for silent coronary disease. The latter application is controversial. Because false-positive tests often exceed true positives, leading to much patient anxiety and self-imposed or mandated disability, exercise testing of asymptomatic individuals should be done only for those at high risk (usually a strong family history of premature coronary disease or hyperlipidemia), those whose occupations place them or others at special risk (eg, airline pilots), and older individuals commencing strenuous activity.

3. Interpretation—The usual ECG criterion for a positive test is 1 mm (0.1 mV) horizontal or downsloping ST-segment depression (beyond baseline) measured 80 milliseconds after the J point. By this criterion, 60–80% of patients with anatomically significant coronary disease will have a positive test, but 10–30% of those without significant disease will also be positive. False positives are uncommon when a 2-mm depression is present. Additional information is inferred from the time of onset and duration of the ECG changes, their magnitude and configuration, BP and heart rate changes, the duration of exercise, and the presence of associated symptoms. In general, patients exhibiting more severe ST-segment depression (> 2 mm) at low workloads (< 6 minutes on the Bruce protocol) or heart rates (< 70% of age-predicted maximum)—especially when the duration of exercise and rise in BP are limited or when hypotension occurs during the test—have more severe disease and a poorer prognosis. Depending on symptom status, age, and other factors, such patients should be referred for coronary arteriography and possible revascularization. On the other hand, less impressive positive tests in asymptomatic patients are often "false positives." Therefore, exercise testing results that do not conform to the clinical picture should be confirmed by stress scintigraphy or echocardiography.

D. Scintigraphic Assessment of Ischemia

Two nuclear medicine studies provide additional information about the presence, location, and extent of CAD.

1. Myocardial perfusion scintigraphy—This test provides images in which radionuclide uptake is proportionate to blood flow at the time of injection. Thallium-201, technetium-99m sestamibi, and tetrafosmin are most frequently used. Areas of diminished uptake reflect relative hypoperfusion (compared with other myocardial regions). If the radiotracer is injected during exercise or dipyridamole- or adenosine-induced coronary vasodilation, scintigraphic defects indicate a zone of hypoperfusion that may represent either ischemia or scar. If the myocardium is viable, as relative blood flow equalizes over time or during a scintigram performed under resting conditions, these defects tend to "fill in" or reverse, indicating reversible ischemia. Defects observed when the radiotracer is injected at rest or still present 3–4 hours after an injection during exercise or pharmacologic vasodilation (intravenous adenosine or dipyridamole) usually indicate myocardial infarction (old or recent) but may be present with severe ischemia. Occasionally, other conditions, including infiltrative diseases (sarcoidosis, amyloidosis), left bundle branch block, and dilated cardiomyopathy, may produce resting or persistent perfusion defects.

In experienced laboratories, stress perfusion scintigraphy is positive in 75–90% of patients with anatomically significant coronary disease and in 20–30% of those without it. False-positive tests may occur as a result of diaphragmatic attenuation or, in women, attenuation through breast tissue. Tomographic imaging (single-photon emission computed tomography, SPECT) can reduce the severity of artifacts. Gated imaging allows for analysis of ventricular size, EF, and regional wall motion.

Myocardial scintigraphy is indicated (1) when the resting ECG makes an exercise ECG difficult to interpret (left bundle branch block, baseline ST–T changes, low voltage, etc); (2) for confirmation of the results of the exercise ECG when they are contrary to the clinical impression (eg, a positive test in an asymptomatic patient); (3) to localize the region of ischemia; (4) to distinguish ischemic from infarcted myocardium; (5) to assess the completeness of vascularization following bypass surgery or coronary angioplasty; or (6) as a prognostic indicator in patients with known coronary disease.

2. Radionuclide angiography—This procedure images the LV and measures its EF and wall motion. In coronary disease, resting abnormalities usually represent infarction, and those that occur only with exercise usually indicate stress-induced ischemia. Normal subjects usually exhibit an increase in EF with exercise or no change; patients with coronary disease may exhibit a decrease. Exercise radionuclide angiography has approximately the same sensitivity as thallium-201 scintigraphy, but it is less specific in older individuals and those with other forms of heart disease. The indications are similar to those for thallium-201 scintigraphy.

3. Positron emission tomography—PET scanning uses positron-emitting agents to demonstrate either perfusion or metabolism of myocardium. PET can accurately distinguish transiently dysfunctional ("stunned") myocardium from scar by showing persistent glycolytic metabolism with the tracer fluorodeoxyglucose (FDG) in regions with reduced blood flow. A nearby cyclotron is required to produce this tracer. The newer SPECT camera can provide acceptable images without the more expensive PET technology.

E. Echocardiography

Echocardiography can image the LV and reveal segmental wall motion abnormalities, which may indicate ischemia or prior infarction. It is a convenient technique for assessing LV function, which is an important indicator of prognosis and determinant of therapy. Echocardiograms performed during supine exercise or immediately following upright exercise may demonstrate exercise-induced segmental wall motion abnormalities as an indicator of ischemia. This technique requires considerable expertise; however, in experienced laboratories, the test accuracy is comparable to that obtained with scintigraphy—though a higher proportion of tests is technically inadequate. Pharmacologic stress with high-dose (20–40 mcg/kg/min) dobutamine can be used as an alternative to exercise. Echocardiography contrast agents allow for perfusion imaging and may improve the diagnostic accuracy of this form of testing.

F. CT AND MRI SCANNING

Many new imaging techniques have been developed, but their application in cardiovascular disease remains to be determined. **CT scan** can image the heart and, with contrast medium and thin slice technology, the coronary arteries with increasing resolution, but with a need for relatively large radiation exposure and contrast load. An important application of CT is the evaluation of pericardial disease. **Ultrafast** or **electron beam CT (EBCT)** involves a specially designed instrument with high temporal resolution. Its availability is limited, but it provides excellent assessments of cardiac structure and function. EBCT is increasingly being used to detect and quantify coronary artery calcification, but proper application of this highly sensitive test is uncertain. False-negative studies may occur in patients under 50 years of age, and positive studies in older patients do not necessarily provide a quantitative assessment of the severity of coronary arteriosclerosis. Thus, although this test can stratify patients into lower and higher risk groups, the appropriate management of individual patients with asymptomatic coronary artery calcification—beyond aggressive risk factors modification—is unclear.

Cardiac MRI provides high-resolution images of the heart and great vessels without radiation exposure or use of iodinated contrast media. It provides excellent anatomic definition, permitting assessment of pericardial disease, neoplastic disease of the heart, myocardial thickness, chamber size, and many congenital heart defects. It is an excellent noninvasive test for nonemergently evaluating dissection of the aorta. Rapid acquisition sequences can produce excellent cine-mode images demonstrating LV function and wall motion, and it is thus a useful alternative when the echocardiogram is suboptimal. Perfusion imaging can be done with gadolinium first pass perfusion using dobutamine or adenosine to produce pharmacologic stress. Recent advances have been made in imaging the proximal coronary arteries, but this application remains investigational.

G. AMBULATORY ECG MONITORING

With current ambulatory ECG recorders and with trained technicians, episodes of ischemic ST-segment depression can be monitored. In patients with CAD, these episodes usually signify ischemia, even when asymptomatic ("silent"). In many, silent episodes are more frequent than symptomatic ones. In most cases, they occur in patients with other evidence of ischemia, and they respond to the same treatments, so that the role of ambulatory monitoring is unclear, as is the benefit of abolishing all such episodes in patients who are otherwise being managed properly.

H. CORONARY ANGIOGRAPHY

Selective coronary arteriography is the definitive diagnostic procedure for CAD. It can be performed with low mortality (about 0.1%) and morbidity (1–5%), but the cost is high, and with currently available noninvasive techniques it is usually not indicated solely for diagnosis.

Coronary arteriography should be performed in the following groups:

1. Patients being considered for coronary artery revascularization because of limiting stable angina who have not improved on an adequate medical regimen.

2. Patients in whom coronary revascularization is being considered because the clinical presentation (unstable angina, postinfarction angina, etc) or noninvasive testing suggests high-risk disease (see Indications for Revascularization).

3. Patients with aortic valve disease who also have angina pectoris, to determine whether the angina is due to accompanying coronary disease. Coronary angiography is also performed in asymptomatic older patients undergoing valve surgery so that concomitant bypass may be done if the anatomy is propitious.

4. Patients who have had coronary revascularization with subsequent recurrence of symptoms, to determine whether bypass grafts or native vessels are occluded.

5. Patients with cardiac failure in whom a surgically correctable lesion, such as LV aneurysm, mitral regurgitation, or reversible ischemic dysfunction, is suspected.

6. Patients surviving sudden death or with symptomatic or life-threatening arrhythmias in whom CAD may be a correctable cause.

7. Patients with chest pain of uncertain cause or cardiomyopathy of unknown cause.

Coronary arteriography visualizes the location and severity of stenoses. Narrowing greater than 50% of the luminal diameter is considered clinically significant, although most lesions producing ischemia are associated with narrowing in excess of 70%. This information has important prognostic value, since mortality rates are progressively higher in patients with one-, two-, and three-vessel disease and those with left main coronary artery obstruction (ranging from 1% per year to 25% per year). In those with strongly positive exercise ECGs or scintigraphic studies, three-vessel or left main disease may be present in 75–95% depending on the criteria used. Coronary arteriography also shows whether the obstructions are amenable to bypass surgery or percutaneous transluminal coronary angioplasty.

Coronary angiography may underestimate the degree of atherosclerosis because it images only the lumen of the vessel. If there is concentric plaque with arterial enlargement (remodeling), then the lumen may appear relatively normal. Intravascular ultrasound (IVUS) uses a small ultrasound transducer that can be positioned within the artery and image beneath the endothelial surface. This technique is useful when the angiogram is equivocal as well as for assessing the results of angioplasty or stenting.

I. LV Angiography

LV angiography is usually performed at the same time as coronary arteriography. Global and regional LV function are visualized, as well as mitral regurgitation if present. LV function is a major determinant of prognosis in coronary heart disease.

Acampa W et al: Nuclear medicine procedures in cardiovascular diseases. An evidence based approach. Q J Nucl Med 2002; 46:323. [PMID: 12411873]

ACC/AHA 2002 guideline update for exercise testing: summary article. Circulation 2002;106:1833. [PMID: 12356646]

ACC/AHA 2002 guideline update for the management of patients with chronic stable angina—summary article. Circulation 2003;107:149. [PMID: 12515758]

Botoman VA: Noncardiac chest pain. J Clin Gastroenterol 2002; 34:6. [PMID: 11743240]

Gottdiener JS: Overview of stress echocardiography: uses, advantages, and limitations. Prog Cardiovasc Dis 2001;43:315. [PMID: 11235847]

Kim WY et al: Coronary magnetic resonance angiography for the detection of coronary stenoses. N Engl J Med 2001;345: 1863. [PMID: 11756576]

Lee TH et al: Clinical practice. Noninvasive tests in patients with stable coronary artery disease. N Engl J Med 2001;344:1840. [PMID: 11407346]

O'Rourke RA et al: American College of Cardiology/American Heart Association Expert Consensus Document on electron-beam computed tomography for the diagnosis and prognosis of coronary artery disease. J Am Coll Cardiol 2000;36:326. [PMID: 10898458]

Paetsch I et al: Comparison of dobutamine stress magnetic resonance, adenosine stress magnetic resonance, and adenosine stress magnetic resonance perfusion. Circulation 2004;110: 835. [PMID: 15289384]

Scanlon PJ et al: ACC/AHA guidelines for coronary angiography: executive summary and recommendations. A report of the American College of Cardiology/American Heart Association Task Force on Practice Guidelines (Committee on Coronary Angiography) developed in collaboration with the Society for Cardiac Angiography and Interventions. Circulation 1999;99:2345. [PMID: 10226103]

Williams SV et al: Guidelines for the management of patients with chronic stable angina: diagnosis and risk stratification. Ann Intern Med 2001;135:530. [PMID: 11578158]

Coronary Vasospasm & Angina with Normal Coronary Arteriograms

Although most symptoms of myocardial ischemia result from fixed stenosis of the coronary arteries or intraplaque hemorrhage or thrombosis at the site of lesions, some ischemic events may be precipitated or exacerbated by coronary vasoconstriction.

Spasm of the large coronary arteries with resulting decreased coronary blood flow may occur spontaneously or may be induced by exposure to cold, emotional stress, or vasoconstricting medications, such as ergot derivative drugs. Spasm may occur both in normal and in stenosed coronary arteries and may be silent or result in angina pectoris. Even myocardial infarction may occur as a result of spasm in the absence of visible obstructive coronary heart disease, although

most instances of such coronary spasm occur in the presence of coronary stenosis.

Cocaine can induce myocardial ischemia and infarction by causing coronary artery vasoconstriction or by increasing myocardial energy requirements.

Prinzmetal's (variant) angina is a clinical syndrome in which chest pain occurs without the usual precipitating factors and is associated with ST-segment elevation rather than depression. It often affects women under 50 years of age. It characteristically occurs in the early morning, awakening patients from sleep, tends to involve the right coronary artery, and is apt to be associated with arrhythmias or conduction defects. There may be no fixed stenoses. Ischemia usually results from coronary vasoconstriction and may be diagnosed by challenge with ergonovine (a vasoconstrictor), although such provocation entails risk.

Patients with this pattern of pain or any chest pain syndrome associated with ST-segment elevation should undergo coronary arteriography to determine whether fixed stenotic lesions are present. If they are, aggressive medical therapy or revascularization is indicated, since this may represent an unstable phase of the disease. If significant lesions are not seen and spasm is suspected, avoidance of precipitants such as cigarette smoking and cocaine is the top priority. Episodes of coronary spasm generally respond well to nitrates, and both nitrates and calcium channel blockers (including long-acting nifedipine, diltiazem, or amlodipine) are effective prophylactically. By allowing unopposed α_1-mediated vasoconstriction, β-blockers have exacerbated coronary vasospasm, but they may have a role in management of patients in whom spasm is associated with fixed stenoses.

There is a growing consensus that myocardial ischemia may also occur in patients with normal coronary arteries as a result of disease of the coronary microcirculation or abnormal vascular reactivity. This has been termed "syndrome X."

Al Suwaidi J et al: Pathophysiology, diagnosis, and current management strategies for chest pain in patients with normal findings on angiography. Mayo Clin Proc 2001;76:813. [PMID: 11499821]

Frishman WH et al: Cardiovascular manifestations of substance abuse part 1: cocaine. Heart Dis 2003;5:187. [PMID: 12783633]

Lange RA et al: Cardiovascular complications of cocaine use. N Engl J Med 2001;345:351. [PMID: 11484693]

Treatment

A. Treatment of Anginal Episodes

Sublingual nitroglycerin is the drug of choice; it acts in about 1–2 minutes. Nitrates decrease arteriolar and venous tone, reduce preload and afterload, and lower the oxygen demand of the heart. Nitrates may also improve myocardial blood flow by dilating collateral channels and, in the presence of increased vasomotor tone, coronary stenoses. As soon as the attack begins, one fresh tablet is placed under the tongue. This may be repeated at 3- to 5-minute intervals. The dosage (0.3, 0.4, or 0.6 mg) and the number of tablets to be used before seeking further medical attention must be individualized. Nitroglycerin buccal spray is also available as a metered (0.4 mg) delivery system. It has the advantage of being more convenient for patients who have difficulty handling the pills and of being more stable. Nitroglycerin can also be used prophylactically before activities likely to precipitate angina. Pain not responding to three tablets or lasting more than 20 minutes may represent evolving infarction, and the patient should be instructed to seek immediate medical attention.

B. PREVENTION OF FURTHER ATTACKS

1. Aggravating factors—Angina may be aggravated by hypertension, LV failure, arrhythmia (usually tachycardias), strenuous activity, cold temperatures, and emotional states. These factors should be identified and treated when possible.

2. Nitroglycerin—Nitroglycerin, 0.3–0.6 mg sublingually or 0.4–0.8 mg translingually by spray, should be taken 5 minutes before any activity likely to precipitate angina. Sublingual isosorbide dinitrate (2.5–10 mg) is only slightly longer-acting than sublingual nitroglycerin.

3. Long-acting nitrates—A number of longer-acting nitrate preparations are available. These include isosorbide dinitrate, 10–40 mg orally three times daily; isosorbide mononitrate, 10–40 mg orally twice daily or 60–120 mg once daily in a sustained-release preparation; oral sustained-release nitroglycerin preparations, 6.25–12.5 mg two to four times daily; nitroglycerin ointment, 6.25–25 mg applied two to four times daily; and transdermal nitroglycerin patches that deliver nitroglycerin at a predetermined rate (usually 5–20 mg/24 h). The main limitation to long-term nitrate therapy is tolerance, which occurs to some degree in most patients. The degree of tolerance can be limited by using a regimen that includes a minimum 8- to 10-hour period per day without nitrates. Isosorbide dinitrate can be given three times daily, with the last dose after dinner, or longer-acting isosorbide mononitrate once daily. Transdermal nitrate preparations should be removed overnight in most patients.

Nitrate therapy is often limited by headache. Other side effects include nausea, light-headedness, and hypotension.

4. β-Blockers—β-Blockers prevent angina by reducing myocardial oxygen requirements during exertion and stress. This is accomplished by reducing the heart rate, myocardial contractility, and, to a lesser extent, BP. The β-blockers are the only antianginal agents that have been demonstrated to prolong life in patients with coronary disease (post-myocardial infarction). They are at least as effective at relieving angina as alternative agents in studies employing exercise testing, ambulatory monitoring, and symptom assessment. As a result, they should be considered for first-line therapy in most patients with chronic angina.

β-Blockers with intrinsic sympathomimetic activity, such as pindolol, are less desirable because they may exacerbate angina in some individuals and have not been effective in secondary prevention trials. The pharmacology and side effects of the β-blockers are discussed in Chapter 11 (see Table 11–7). The dosages of all these drugs when given for angina are similar. The major contraindications are severe bronchospastic disease, bradyarrhythmias, and decompensated heart failure.

5. Calcium channel blocking agents—Verapamil, diltiazem, and the dihydropyridine group of calcium blockers are chemically and pharmacologically heterogeneous agents that prevent angina by reducing myocardial oxygen requirements and by inducing coronary artery vasodilation. Myocardial oxygen demand is decreased by reducing BP, LV wall stress and, in the case of verapamil and diltiazem, resting or exercise heart rate. Though these agents are all potent coronary vasodilators, it is unclear whether they improve myocardial blood flow in most patients with stable exertional angina. In those with coronary vasospasm, the calcium channel blockers may be the agents of choice.

Most calcium channel blockers have negative inotropic, chronotropic, and dromotropic properties in vitro, but the reflex sympathetic response may obscure these effects in vivo (except in the presence of β-blockade or severely depressed LV function). Unlike the β-blockers, calcium channel blockers have not been shown to reduce mortality postinfarction and in some cases have increased ischemia and mortality rates. This appears to be the case with some dihydropyridines and with diltiazem and verapamil in patients with clinical heart failure or moderate to severe LV dysfunction. Meta-analyses have suggested that short-acting nifedipine in moderate to high doses causes an increase in mortality. It is uncertain whether these findings are relevant to longer-acting dihydropyridines. Nevertheless, considering the uncertainties and the lack of demonstrated favorable effect on outcomes, calcium channel blockers should be considered third-line anti-ischemic drugs in the postinfarction patient. Similarly, with the exception of amlodipine, which in the PRAISE trial proved safe in patients with heart failure, these agents should be avoided in patients with CHF or low EFs.

The pharmacologic effects and side effects of the calcium channel blockers are discussed in Chapter 11 and summarized in Table 11–9. Although all have been shown to be efficacious for angina, not all preparations and agents are approved for this indication. By and large, diltiazem and verapamil are preferable as first-line agents because they produce less reflex tachycardia and because the former, at least, may cause fewer side effects. Nifedipine, nicardipine, and amlodipine are also approved agents for angina. Isradipine, felodipine, and nisoldipine are not approved for angina but probably are as effective as the other dihydropyridines.

6. Alternative and combination therapies—Patients who do not respond to one class of antianginal medication often respond to another. It may, therefore, be worthwhile to use an alternative agent before progressing to combinations. If the patient remains symptomatic, a β-blocker and a long-acting nitrate or a β-blocker and a calcium channel blocker (other than verapamil, where the risk of AV block or heart failure is higher) are the most appropriate combinations. A few patients will have a further response to a regimen including all three agents.

7. Ranolazine—Ranolazine, an agent that involves selective inhibition of the late sodium current, has been approved by the US Food and Drug Administration to prevent angina, the first such new drug in more than 10 years. The approval was based on two trials showing that ranolazine reduced angina compared with β-blockers or calcium channel blockers.

The usual dose is 500 mg orally twice a day. Because it can cause QT prolongation, it is contraindicated in patients with existing QT prolongation, concurrent use of QT prolonging drugs such as class I or III antiarrhythmics (eg, quinidine, dofetilide, sotalol), and potent and moderate CYP450 3A inhibitors. An ECG is recommended both at baseline and during treatment. It is also contraindicated in patients with significant liver and renal disease. Ranolazine is not to be used for treatment of acute anginal episodes.

8. Platelet-inhibiting agents—Coronary thrombosis is responsible for most episodes of myocardial infarction and many unstable ischemic syndromes. Several studies have demonstrated the benefit of antiplatelet drugs following unstable angina and infarction. Therefore, unless contraindicated, small doses of aspirin (81–325 mg daily) should be prescribed for patients with angina. Clopidogrel is an antiplatelet agent that acts by blocking the ADP receptor and resulting platelet aggregation. Unlike its older congener ticlopidine, clopidogrel does not cause agranulocytosis but may rarely induce thrombotic thrombocytopenic purpura. It can reduce cardiac events in patients with acute coronary syndromes and is an appropriate alternative in aspirin-intolerant patients.

9. Risk reduction—As discussed above, patients with coronary disease should undergo aggressive risk factor modification. This approach, with a particular focus on lowering LDL cholesterol, treating hypertension, stopping smoking, and exercise and weight loss (especially for patients with metabolic syndrome or at risk for diabetes), may markedly improve outcome.

10. Revascularization—The indications for coronary artery revascularization and the choice of procedure are discussed below.

11. Mechanical extracorporeal counterpulsation—Extracorporeal counterpulsation (ECP) entails repetitive inflation of a high-pressure chamber surrounding the lower half of the body during the diastolic phase of the cardiac cycle for daily 1-hour sessions over a period of 7 weeks. Randomized trials have shown that ECP reduces angina, improves exercise tolerance, and can reduce symptoms of heart failure. However, the response has been variable, often time limited, and not shown to be associated with improved myocardial perfusion—so a placebo effect may be responsible.

Table 10–3. Duke treadmill score: calculation and interpretation.

Time in minutes on Bruce protocol	=	_____
–5 % amount of depression (in mm)	=	_____
–4 % angina index (0 = no angina on test; 1 = angina, not limiting; 2 = limiting angina)	=	Total score

Total Score	Risk Group	Annual Mortality
≥5	Low	0.25%
–10 to +4	Intermediate	1.25%
≤–11	High	5.25%

Prognosis

The prognosis of angina pectoris has improved with development of therapies aimed at secondary prevention. Mortality rates vary depending on the number of vessels diseased, the severity of obstruction, the status of LV function, and the presence of complex arrhythmias. The outlook in individual patients is unpredictable, and nearly half of the deaths are sudden. Therefore, risk stratification is often attempted. Patients with accelerating symptoms have a poorer outlook. Among stable patients, those whose exercise tolerance is severely limited by ischemia (less than 6 minutes on the Bruce treadmill protocol) and those with extensive ischemia by exercise ECG or scintigraphy have more severe anatomic disease and a poorer prognosis. The Duke Treadmill Score, based on a standard Bruce protocol exercise treadmill test, provides an estimate of risk of death at 1 year. The score uses time on the treadmill, amount of ST-segment depression, and presence of angina (Table 10–3).

Chaitman BR et al; Combination Assessment of Ranolazine In Stable Angina (CARISA) Investigators: Effects of ranolazine with atenolol, amlodipine, or diltiazem on exercise tolerance and angina frequency in patients with severe chronic angina: a randomized controlled trial. JAMA 2004;291:309. [PMID: 14734593]

Gibbons RJ et al: ACC/AHA 2002 guideline update for the management of patients with chronic stable angina—summary article: a report of the American College of Cardiology/American Heart Association Task Force on practice guidelines (Committee on the Management of Patients With Chronic Stable Angina). J Am Coll Cardiol 2003;41:159. [PMID: 12570960]

U.S. Food and Drug Administration: FDA Approves New Treatment for Chest Pain. http://www.fda.gov/bbs/topics/news/2006/NEW01306.html

REVASCULARIZATION PROCEDURES FOR PATIENTS WITH ANGINA PECTORIS

Indications

There is general agreement that otherwise healthy patients in the following groups should undergo revascularization: (1) Patients with unacceptable symptoms despite medical therapy to its tolerable limits. (2) Patients with left main coronary artery stenosis greater than 50% with or without symptoms. (3) Patients with three-vessel disease with LV dysfunction (EF < 50% or previous transmural infarction). (4) Patients with unstable angina who after symptom control by medical therapy continue to exhibit ischemia on exercise testing or monitoring. (5) Post-myocardial infarction patients with continuing angina or severe ischemia on noninvasive testing. (See sections on Acute Coronary Syndromes and Myocardial Infarction.)

In addition, many cardiologists believe that patients with less severe symptoms should be revascularized if they have two-vessel disease associated with underlying LV dysfunction, anatomically critical lesions (> 90% proximal stenoses, especially of the proximal left anterior descending artery), or physiologic evidence of severe ischemia (early positive exercise tests, large exercise-induced thallium scintigraphic defects, or frequent episodes of ischemia on ambulatory monitoring). This trend toward aggressive intervention has accelerated as a result of the growing use of coronary angioplasty and stenting. Although such patients are at increased risk, it has not been proved that their prognosis is better after coronary revascularization by either surgery or angioplasty.

Type of Procedure

A. CORONARY ARTERY BYPASS GRAFTING

Coronary artery bypass grafting (CABG) can be accomplished with a very low mortality rate (1–3%) in otherwise healthy patients with preserved cardiac function. However, the mortality rate of this procedure rises to 4–8% in older individuals and in patients who have had a prior CABG. Increasingly, younger individuals with focal lesions of one or several vessels are undergoing coronary angioplasty as the initial revascularization procedure.

Grafts using one or both internal mammary arteries (usually to the left anterior descending artery or its branches) provide the best long-term results in terms of patency and flow. Segments of the saphenous vein (or, less optimally, other veins) or the radial artery interposed between the aorta and the coronary arteries distal to the obstructions are also used. One to five distal anastomoses are commonly performed. After successful surgery, symptoms generally abate. The need for antianginal medications diminishes, and LV function may improve.

Minimally invasive surgical techniques utilize different approaches to the heart than standard sternotomy and cardiopulmonary bypass. The surgical approach may involve a limited sternotomy, lateral thoracotomy (MIDCAB), or thoracoscopy (port-access). These approaches may be used in conjunction with standard cardiopulmonary bypass, with peripheral cardiopulmonary bypass, or with operating on the beating heart utilizing a mechanical coronary stabilizer. Avoiding bypass may decrease the risk of cerebral complications. These techniques allow earlier postoperative mobilization and discharge. They are more technically demanding, usually not suitable for more than two grafts, and do not have established durability.

The operative mortality rate is increased in patients with poor LV function (LV EF < 35%) or those requiring additional procedures (valve replacement or ventricular aneurysmectomy). Patients over 70 years of age, patients undergoing repeat procedures, or those with important noncardiac disease (especially renal insufficiency and diabetes) or poor general health also have higher operative mortality and morbidity rates, and full recovery is slow. Thus, CABG should be reserved for more severely symptomatic patients in this group. Early (1–6 months) graft patency rates average 85–90% (higher for internal mammary grafts), and subsequent graft closure rates are about 4% annually. Early graft failure is common in vessels with poor distal flow, while late closure is more frequent in patients who continue smoking and those with untreated hyperlipidemia. Antiplatelet therapy with aspirin improves graft patency rates. Smoking cessation and vigorous treatment of blood lipid abnormalities are necessary, with a goal for LDL cholesterol of 100 mg/dL and of HDL cholesterol 45 mg/dL. Repeat revascularization (see below) is often necessitated by progressive native vessel disease and graft occlusions. Reoperation is technically demanding and less often fully successful than the initial operation.

B. PERCUTANEOUS CORONARY INTERVENTION INCLUDING STENTING

Coronary artery stenoses can be effectively dilated by inflation of a balloon under high pressure. This procedure is performed in the cardiac catheterization laboratory under local anesthesia either at the same time as diagnostic coronary arteriography or at a later time. The mechanism of dilation involves both rupture of the atheromatous plaque and remodeling of the vessel.

This procedure was at one time reserved for proximal single-vessel disease, but now it is widely used in multivessel disease with multiple lesions, though only rarely in left main disease. Percutaneous transluminal coronary angioplasty (PTCA) is possible but often less successful in bypass graft stenoses. Bypass graft patients with multivessel disease have lower mortality rates and fewer nonfatal myocardial infarctions with surgery than with percutaneous interventions. Optimal lesions for PTCA are relatively proximal, noneccentric, free of significant calcification or plaque dissection, and removed from the origin of large branches. With improved catheter systems, experienced operators are able to successfully dilate 90% of lesions attempted. The major early complication is intimal dissection with vessel occlusion. This can usually be treated by repeat PTCA or by deployment of an intracoronary stent. The use of platelet glycoprotein IIb/IIIa inhibitors (abciximab, eptifibatide, tirofiban) has substantially reduced the rate of acute vessel closure, and placement of intracoronary stents has markedly improved initial and long-term angiographic results, especially with complex and long lesions. Although the early experience with stents was complicated by an unacceptable rate of acute thrombosis, this problem has largely been prevented by aggressive antithrombotic therapy (long-term aspirin plus clopidogrel for between 30 days and 1 year, with acute use of platelet glycoprotein IIb/IIIa inhibitors in high-risk patients). Restenosis rates have fallen with the use of stents. Stents are now used in the majority of patients undergoing percutaneous revascularization.

The major limitation with PTCA has been restenosis, which occurs in the first 6 months in 30–40% of vessels dilated, though it can often be treated successfully by repeat PTCA. Factors associated with higher restenosis rates include diabetes, small luminal diameter, longer and more complex lesions, and lesions at coronary ostia or in the left anterior descending coronary artery. The use of stents has reduced the restenosis rate by 50%. Drug-eluting stents that elute antiproliferative agents such as sirolimus or paclitaxel have substantially reduced restenosis to rates of < 10%. These devices have had a significant impact on clinical practice, leading to increased use of percutaneous interventions in patients with multiple and less favorable lesions. However, because prevention of tissue proliferation around the stent may leave exposed stent and predispose to thrombosis, drug-eluting stents are associated with a small but poorly defined incidence of late stent thrombosis. Full stent deployment as well as use of clopidogrel for at least 3 (for sirolimus) to 6 (for paclitaxel) months are important to prevent stent thrombosis.

Currently, in-stent restenosis is often treated with either brachytherapy or restenting with drug-eluting stents.

The number of PTCA and stenting procedures now exceeds the number of CABG operations, but the justification for many of the procedures performed in patients with stable angina is unclear. Several studies have shown PTCA to be superior to medical therapy for symptom relief but not in preventing infarction or death. In patients with no or only mild symptoms, aggressive lipid-lowering and antianginal therapy may be preferable to PTCA.

Several studies of PTCA versus CABG in patients with multivessel disease have been reported. The consistent finding has been comparable mortality and infarction rates over follow-up periods of 1–3 years but a high rate (approximately 40%) of repeat procedures following PTCA. As a result, the choice of revascularization procedure is often a matter of patient preference. However, it should be noted that less than 20% of patients with multivessel disease met the entry criteria, so these results cannot be generalized to all multivessel disease patients. Outcomes with percutaneous revascularization in diabetics have been inferior to those with CABG. However, these trials preceded the widespread use of stenting.

C. EXPERIMENTAL APPROACHES

Several experimental approaches have been studied in patients with refractory angina who are not candidates for percutaneous or surgical revascularization procedures. Laser transmyocardial revascularization has been used ei-

ther from the epicardial surface of the LV during surgery or from the ventricular cavity by catheter-based techniques. Several studies reporting an improvement in symptoms have not shown objective evidence of improvement in perfusion, raising the possibility of a placebo effect, and clinical outcomes are either not improved or worsened. Other studies have evaluated intracoronary injections of growth factors, such as vascular endothelial growth factor (VEGF) or fibroblast growth factors, or cell therapy using endothelial progenitor cells, but thus far there is inconclusive evidence of benefit.

Summary of Results of Treatment

Several randomized trials have shown that over follow-up periods of several years, the mortality and infarction rates with percutaneous revascularization and CABG are generally comparable. An exception may be diabetic patients, who have had better outcomes with CABG. Recovery after PTCA is obviously faster, but the intermediate-term success rate of CABG is higher both because of the high restenosis rate with PTCA and, less importantly, with stenting. The increasing popularity of PTCA and stenting primarily reflects the lower cost and shorter hospitalization, the perception that CABG is best done only once and can be reserved for later, and the preference of patients for less invasive treatment. These arguments make PTCA the procedure of choice for revascularization of single-vessel disease. The situation is less clear with multivessel disease. It should also be noted that the excellent outcome of patients treated medically has made it difficult to show an advantage with either revascularization approach except in patients who remain symptom limited or have left main lesions or three-vessel disease and LV dysfunction. The availability of drug-eluting stents is shifting the balance toward percutaneous revascularization.

Arora RR et al: The multicenter study of enhanced external counterpulsation (MUST-EECP): effect of EECP on exercise-induced myocardial ischemia and anginal episodes. J Am Coll Cardiol 1999;33:1833. [PMID: 10362181]

Eagle KA et al: ACC/AHA Guidelines for Coronary Artery Bypass Graft Surgery: a Report of the American College of Cardiology/American Heart Association Task Force on Practice Guidelines (Committee to Revise the 1991 Guidelines for Coronary Artery Bypass Graft Surgery). American College of Cardiology/American Heart Association. J Am Coll Cardiol 1999;34:1262. [PMID: 10520819]

Kim MC: Refractory angina pectoris. J Am Coll Cardiol 2002; 39:923. [PMID: 11897431]

Lowe HC: Coronary in-stent restenosis: current status and future strategies. J Am Coll Cardiol 2002;39:183. [PMID: 11788206]

Moses JW et al; SIRIUS Investigators: Sirolimus-eluting stents versus standard stents in patients with stenosis in a native coronary artery. N Engl J Med 2003;349:1315. [PMID: 14523139]

O'Shea JC et al: Platelet glycoprotein IIb/IIIa integrin blockade with eptifibatide in coronary stent intervention. JAMA 2001;285:2468. [PMID: 11368699]

Schofield PM: Indications for percutaneous and surgical revascularisation: how far does the evidence base guide us? Heart 2003;89:565. [PMID: 12695476]

Steinhubl SR et al: Early and sustained dual oral antiplatelet therapy following percutaneous coronary intervention. A randomized controlled trial. JAMA 2002;288:2411. [PMID: 11297702]

Stone GW et al; TAXUS-IV Investigators: One-year clinical results with the slow-release, polymer-based, paclitaxel-eluting TAXUS stent: the TAXUS-IV trial. Circulation 2004; 109:1942. [PMID: 15078803]

Trial of invasive versus medical therapy in elderly patients with chronic symptomatic coronary-artery disease (TIME): a randomised trial. Lancet 2001;358:951. [PMID: 11583747]

ACUTE CORONARY SYNDROMES

Acute coronary syndromes comprise the spectrum of unstable cardiac ischemia from unstable angina to acute myocardial infarction. Rather than the traditional nomenclature of unstable angina, non-Q wave and Q wave myocardial infarction, acute coronary syndromes are now classified based on the presenting ECG as either "ST elevation" or "non-ST elevation." This allows for immediate classification and guides determination of whether patients should be considered for acute reperfusion therapy. The evolution of cardiac markers then allows determination of whether myocardial infarction has occurred. Acute coronary syndromes represent a dynamic state in which patients frequently shift from one category to another, as new ST elevation can develop after presentation and cardiac markers can become abnormal with recurrent ischemic episodes.

Diagnosis

Many patients with acute coronary syndromes will exhibit ECG changes during pain—either ST-segment elevation, ST-segment depression, or T wave flattening or inversion. They may exhibit signs of LV dysfunction during pain and for a time thereafter.

Chest pain is one of the most frequent reasons for emergency department visits. Algorithms have been developed to aid in determining the likelihood that a patient has an acute coronary syndrome, and for those patients that do have an acute coronary syndrome, the risk of death or death and ischemic events.

Many hospitals have developed **chest pain observation units** to provide a systematic approach toward serial risk stratification to improve the triage process. In many cases those who have not experienced new chest pain and have no ECG changes or cardiac enzyme elevations undergo treadmill exercise tests or imaging procedures to exclude ischemia at the end of an 8- to 24-hour period and are discharged directly from the emergency department if these tests are negative.

Treatment

Table 10–4 provides a summary of the ACC/AHA Guideline recommendations for selected medical treatments.

A. GENERAL MEASURES

Treatment of acute coronary syndromes without ST elevation should be multifaceted and vigorous. Patients who are at high risk should be hospitalized, maintained at bed rest or at very limited activity, monitored, and given supplemental oxygen. Sedation with a benzodiazepine agent may help if anxiety is present.

B. ANTICOAGULATION, ANTIPLATELET, AND THROMBOLYTIC THERAPY

Coronary thrombosis plays a prominent role in the pathophysiology of unstable angina and its progression to myocardial infarction, and antithrombotic therapy plays an important role in treatment. Patients should receive a combination of antiplatelet and anticoagulant agents. Aspirin, 81–325 mg daily, and heparin (low-molecular-weight or unfractionated) should be commenced on presentation. Several trials have shown that low-molecular-weight heparin (and specifically enoxaparin 1 mg/kg subcutaneously every 12 hours) is somewhat more effective than unfractionated heparin in preventing recurrent ischemic events in the setting of acute coronary syndromes. However, the SYNERGY trial showed that unfractionated heparin and enoxaparin had similar rates of death or (re)infarction in the setting of frequent early coronary intervention. Fondaparinux, a specific factor Xa inhibitor given in a dose of 2.5 mg subcutaneously once a day, was found in the OASIS-6 trial to be equally effective as enoxaparin among 20,000 patients at preventing early death, myocardial infarction, and refractory ischemia, and resulted in a 50% reduction in major bleeding. This reduction in major bleeding appeared to translate into a reduction in mortality (and in death and/or myocardial infarction) at 30 days. While catheter-related thrombosis was more common during coronary intervention procedures with fondaparinux, it appears that this can be controlled by adding unfractionated heparin during the procedure. This trial not only established fondaparinux as an excellent treatment for acute coronary syndromes but also highlighted the importance of bleeding and its prevention.

The ACUITY trial showed that the direct thrombin inhibitor bivalirudin appears to be a reasonable alternative to heparin or enoxaparin plus a glycoprotein IIb/IIIa antagonist for many patients with acute coronary syndromes who are undergoing early coronary intervention.

The Clopidogrel in Unstable Angina to Prevent Recurrent Events (CURE) trial demonstrated a 20% reduction in the composite end point of cardiovascular death, myocardial infarction, and stroke with the addition of clopidogrel (300 mg loading dose, 75 mg/d for 9–12 months) in patients with non–ST-segment elevation acute coronary syndromes. When treated with clopidogrel, the optimal aspirin dose appears to be 81 mg/d (versus 160 mg/d or 325 mg/d) based on similar thrombotic event rates and lower rates of bleeding.

Small molecule inhibitors of the platelet glycoprotein IIb/IIIa receptor are useful adjuncts in high-risk patients (usually defined by fluctuating ST-segment depression or positive biomarkers) with acute coronary syndromes, particularly when they are undergoing PTCA or stenting.

Table 10–4. Summary of the current ACC/AHA guideline recommendations for medical management of acute coronary syndromes (ACS) and acute myocardial infarction (AMI).[1]

Medication	Acute Therapies ACS	Acute Therapies AMI	Discharge Therapies
Aspirin (ASA)	IA	IA	IA
Clopidogrel in ASA-allergic patients	IA	IC	IA
Clopidogrel, intended medical management	IA	—	IA
Clopidogrel, early catheterization/percutaneous coronary intervention (catheterization/percutaneous coronary intervention [cath/PCI])	IA (prior to or at time of PCI)	IB	IA
Heparin (unfractionated or low-molecular-weight)	IA	IA[2]	—
β-Blockers	IB	IA	IB
Angiotensin-converting enzyme (ACE) inhibitors	IB[3]	IA/IIaB[4]	IA
Glycoprotein (GP) IIb/IIIa inhibitors for intended early cath/PCI			
Eptifibatide/tirofiban	IA	—	—
Abciximab	IA	IIaB[5]	—
GP IIb/IIIa inhibitors for high-risk patients without intended early cath/PCI			
Eptifibatide/tirofiban	IIaA	—	—
Abciximab	IIIA	—	—
Lipid-lowering agent[6]	—	—	IA
Smoking cessation counseling	—	—	IB

[1]Class I indicates treatment is useful and effective, IIa indicates weight of evidence is in favor of usefulness/efficacy, class IIb indicates weight of evidence is less well established, and class III indicates intervention is not useful/effective and may be harmful. Type A recommendations are derived from large-scale randomized trials, and B recommendations are derived from smaller randomized trials or carefully conducted observational analyses. ACC/AHA = American College of Cardiology/American Heart Association.
[2]As a class IIb, low-molecular-weight heparin (best studied is enoxaparin with tenecteplase) can be considered an acceptable alternative to unfractionated heparin for patients less than 75 years old who are receiving fibrinolytic therapy provided significant renal dysfunction is not present.
[3]For patients with persistent hypertension despite treatment, diabetes mellitus, congestive heart failure, or any left ventricular dysfunction.
[4]IA for patients with congestive heart failure or ejection fraction < 0.40, IIa for others, in absence of hypotension (systolic blood pressure < 100 mm Hg); angiotensin receptor blocker (valsartan or candesartan) for patients with ACE inhibitor intolerance.
[5]As early as possible before primary PCI.
[6]For patients with a low-density lipoprotein cholesterol level > 100 mg/dL.

Tirofiban, 0.4 mcg/kg/min for 30 minutes, followed by 0.1 mcg/kg/min, and eptifibatide, 180 mcg/kg bolus followed by a continuous infusion of 0.1 mcg/kg/min, have both been shown to be effective when added to heparin. Downward dose adjustments are required in patients with reduced renal function. For example, if the estimated creatinine clearance is below 50 mL/min, the eptifibatide infusion should be cut in half to 1 mcg/kg/min.

Fibrinolytic therapy should be avoided in patients without ST-segment elevation since they generally have a patent culprit artery, and since the risk of such therapy appears to outweigh the benefit.

C. NITROGLYCERIN

The nitrates are first-line anti-ischemic therapy for acute coronary syndromes. Nonparenteral therapy with sub-lingual or oral agents or nitroglycerin ointment is usually sufficient. If pain persists or recurs, intravenous nitroglycerin should be started. The usual initial dosage is 10 mcg/min. The dosage should be titrated upward by 10–20 mcg/min (to a maximum of 200 mcg/min) until angina disappears or mean arterial pressure drops by 10%. Careful—usually continuous—BP monitoring is required when intravenous nitroglycerin is used. Avoid hypotension (systolic BP < 100 mm Hg). Tolerance to continuous nitrate infusion is common.

D. β-BLOCKERS

These agents are also a part of the initial treatment of unstable angina unless otherwise contraindicated. If the patient has no physical findings of heart failure, these agents can usually be started without measurements of

LV function. Patients with evidence of large or multiple old infarctions are an exception. The pharmacology of these agents is discussed in Chapter 11 and summarized in Table 11–7. Use of agents with intrinsic sympathomimetic activity should be avoided in this setting. The goal of acute treatment is to reduce the heart rate below 60–70 beats/min. Oral medication is adequate in most patients, but intravenous treatment with metoprolol, given as three 5 mg doses 5 minutes apart, achieves a more rapid effect. Oral therapy should be aggressively titrated upward as BP permits.

E. CALCIUM CHANNEL BLOCKERS

Calcium channel blockers have not been shown to favorably affect outcome in unstable angina, and they should be used primarily as third-line therapy in patients with continuing symptoms on nitrates and β-blockers or those who are not candidates for these drugs. In the presence of nitrates and without accompanying β-blockers, diltiazem or verapamil is preferred, since nifedipine and the other dihydropyridines are more likely to cause reflex tachycardia or hypotension. The initial dosage should be low, but upward titration should proceed rapidly (see Table 11–9).

F. STATINS

The PROVE-IT trial provides evidence for starting a statin in the days immediately following an acute coronary syndrome. In this trial, more intensive therapy with atorvastatin 80 mg a day, regardless of total or LDL cholesterol level, improved outcome compared to pravastatin 40 mg a day, with the curves of death or major cardiovascular event separating as early as 3 months after starting therapy.

G. INTRA-AORTIC BALLOON COUNTERPULSATION

Intra-aortic balloon counterpulsation (IABC) can both reduce myocardial energy requirements (systolic unloading) and improve diastolic coronary blood flow. This approach is sometimes used to stabilize patients prior to angiography or revascularization, but with modern techniques it is rarely necessary.

Prognosis & Indications for Revascularization

Risk stratification is important for determining intensity of care. Several therapies, including glycoprotein IIb/IIIa receptor antagonists, low-molecular-weight heparin, and early invasive catheterization, have been shown to have the greatest benefit in higher-risk patients. As outlined in the ACC/AHA guidelines, patients with any high-risk feature (Table 10–5) warrant an early invasive strategy with catheterization and revascularization. For patients without these high-risk features, either an invasive or noninvasive approach, using exercise (or pharmacologic stress for patients unable to exercise) stress testing to identify patients who have residual ischemia and/or high risk, can be used.

Table 10–5. Indications for catheterization and percutaneous coronary intervention.

Acute coronary syndromes (unstable angina and non-ST elevation MI)

Class I	Early invasive strategy for any of the following high-risk indicators: Recurrent angina/ischemia at rest or with low-level activity; Elevated troponin; ST-segment depression; Recurrent ischemia with evidence of CHF; High-risk stress test result; EF < 0.40; Hemodynamic instability; Sustained ventricular tachycardia; PCI within 6 months; Prior CABG. In the absence of these findings, either an early conservative or early invasive strategy
Class IIa	Early invasive strategy for patients with repeated presentations for ACS despite therapy
Class III	Extensive comorbidities in patients in whom benefits of revascularization are not likely to outweigh the risks; Acute chest pain with low likelihood of ACS

Acute MI after fibrinolytic therapy (2004 ACC/AHA AMI Guideline)

Class I	Recurrent ischemia (spontaneous or provoked); Recurrent MI; Cardiogenic shock or hemodynamic instability
Class IIa	LV EF ≤ 0.40, CHF (even transient), serious ventricular arrhythmias
Class IIb	Routine PCI as part of invasive strategy after fibrinolytic therapy

MI = myocardial infarction; CHF = congestive heart failure; EF = ejection fraction; PCI = percutaneous coronary intervention; CABG = coronary artery bypass grafting; ACS = acute coronary syndrome; ACC/AHA = American College of Cardiology/American Heart Association; AMI = acute myocardial infarction; LV EF = left ventricular ejection fraction.

Two risk-stratification tools are available that can be used at the bedside, the TIMI Risk Score and the GRACE Risk Score. The TIMI Risk Score includes nine variables: age ≥ 65, three or more cardiac risk factors, prior coronary stenosis ≥ 50%, ST-segment deviation, two anginal events in prior 24 hours, acetylsalicylic acid in prior 7 days, and elevated cardiac markers. The GRACE risk score, which applies to patients with or without ST elevation, includes Killip class, BP, ST-segment deviation, cardiac arrest at presentation, serum creatinine, elevated creatine kinase (CK)-MB or troponin, and heart rate. The TIMI

Risk Score is available for PDA download at http://www.timi.org.

ACC/AHA 2002 guideline update for the management of patients with unstable angina and non-ST-segment elevation myocardial infarction—summary article. J Am Coll Cardiol 2002;40:1366. [PMID: 12383588]

Boden WE et al: Optimizing management of non-ST segment elevation acute coronary syndromes. J Am Coll Cardiol 2003; 41(Suppl):1S. [PMID: 12644334]

Boersma E et al: Platelet glycoprotein IIb/IIIa inhibitors in acute coronary syndromes: a meta-analysis of all major randomised clinical trials. Lancet 2002;359:189. [PMID: 11812552]

Cannon CP et al: Comparison of early invasive and conservative strategies in patients with unstable coronary syndromes treated with the glycoprotein IIb/IIIa inhibitor tirofiban. N Engl J Med 2001;344:1879. [PMID: 11419424]

de Feyter PJ et al: Bypass surgery versus stenting for the treatment of multivessel disease in patients with unstable angina compared with stable angina. Circulation 2002;105:2367. [PMID: 12021222]

Eagle KA et al; GRACE Investigators: A validated prediction model for all forms of acute coronary syndrome: estimating the risk of 6-month postdischarge death in an international registry. JAMA 2004;291:2727. [PMID: 15187054]

Fox KA et al: Interventional versus conservative treatment for patients with unstable angina or non-ST-elevation myocardial infarction: the British Heart Foundation RITA 3 randomised trial. Lancet 2002;360:743. [PMID: 12241831]

Granger CB et al; Global Registry of Acute Coronary Events Investigators: Predictors of hospital mortality in the global registry of acute coronary events. Arch Intern Med 2003; 163:2345. [PMID: 14581255]

Hamm CW et al: Acute coronary syndrome without ST elevation: implementation of new guidelines. Lancet 2001;358: 1533. [PMID: 11705583]

Levine GN et al: Antithrombotic therapy in patients with acute coronary syndromes. Arch Intern Med 2001;161:937. [PMID: 11295956]

Mahoney EM et al: Cost and cost-effectiveness of an early invasive vs conservative strategy for the treatment of unstable angina and non-ST-segment elevation myocardial infarction. JAMA 2002;288:1851. [PMID: 12377083]

Schofield PM: Indications for percutaneous and surgical revascularisation: how far does the evidence base guide us? Heart 2003;89:565. [PMID: 12695476]

Stone GW: ACUITY Trial. Presented at Scientific Sessions of American College of Cardiology Late Breaking Clinical Trial. March 2006, Atlanta, GA. http://www.medscape.com/viewarticle/529634

Udelson JE et al: Myocardial perfusion imaging for evaluation and triage of patients with suspected acute cardiac ischemia: a randomized controlled trial. JAMA 2002;288:2693. [PMID: 12460092]

Wong GC et al: Use of low-molecular-weight heparins in the management of acute coronary artery syndromes and percutaneous coronary intervention. JAMA 2003;289:331. [PMID: 12525234]

Yusuf S et al: Effects of clopidogrel in addition to aspirin in patients with acute coronary syndromes without ST-segment elevation. N Engl J Med 2001;345:494. [PMID: 11519503]

Yusuf S et al; Fifth Organization to Assess Strategies in Acute Ischemic Syndromes Investigators: Comparison of fondaparinux and enoxaparin in acute coronary syndromes. N Engl J Med 2006;354:1464. [PMID: 16537663]

ACUTE MYOCARDIAL INFARCTION

 ESSENTIALS OF DIAGNOSIS

- *Sudden but not instantaneous development of prolonged (> 30 minutes) anterior chest discomfort (sometimes felt as "gas" or pressure) that may produce arrhythmias, hypotension, shock, or cardiac failure.*
- *Sometimes painless, masquerading as acute CHF, syncope, stroke, or shock.*
- *ECG: ST-segment elevation or depression, evolving Q waves, symmetric inversion of T waves.*
- *Elevation of cardiac markers (CK-MB, troponin T, or troponin I).*
- *Appearance of segmental wall motion abnormality by imaging techniques.*

General Considerations

Myocardial infarction results from prolonged myocardial ischemia, precipitated in most cases by an occlusive coronary thrombus at the site of a preexisting (though not necessarily severe) atherosclerotic plaque. More rarely, infarction may result from prolonged vasospasm, inadequate myocardial blood flow (eg, hypotension), or excessive metabolic demand. Very rarely, myocardial infarction may be caused by embolic occlusion, vasculitis, aortic root or coronary artery dissection, or aortitis. Cocaine is a cause of infarction, which should be considered in young individuals without risk factors.

A condition that may mimic ST elevation acute myocardial infarction is stress cardiomyopathy (also referred to as Tako-Tsubo cardiomyopathy or apical ballooning syndrome). This is a reversible acute cardiomyopathy involving the cardiac apex, without angiographic evidence of coronary obstruction. It is often associated with emotional stress in older women and is generally associated with small increases in cardiac biomarkers.

The location and extent of infarction depend on the anatomic distribution of the occluded vessel, the presence of additional stenotic lesions, and the adequacy of collateral circulation. Thrombosis in the anterior descending branch of the left coronary artery results in infarction of the anterior LV and interventricular septum. Occlusion of the left circumflex artery produces anterolateral or posterolateral infarction. Right coronary thrombosis leads to infarction of the posteroinferior portion of the LV and generally involves the RV myocardium if the obstruction is proximal. The arteries supplying the AV node and the sinus node more commonly arise from the right coronary artery; thus, AV block at the nodal level and sinus node dysfunction occur more frequently during inferior or right-sided infarctions. Individual variation in coronary anatomy and the presence of collateral vessels can make the prediction of coronary anatomy from infarct location imperfect.

Infarctions are often classified as Q wave versus non-Q wave infarction. This classification is generally related to whether there was ST-segment elevation on the presenting ECG, and whether there is transmural or subendocardial involvement. However, Q waves may be transient, and the relationships among Q waves, ST elevation, and extent of infarction are often misleading. Patients presenting without ST elevation are more likely to be older, have multivessel disease, and more vascular disease in general, and thus this population is at higher risk for adverse outcomes following hospital discharge.

The size and anatomic location of an infarction influence the acute course, the early complications, and the long-term prognosis. Hemodynamic stability is related to both noninfarct zone LV function and extent of acute necrosis. Patients with LV dysfunction or clinical heart failure are an important population because of their poor prognosis and the availability of several medical treatments able to improve their survival. The complications of acute infarction are discussed below.

Boersma E et al: Acute myocardial infarction. Lancet 2003;361: 847. [PMID: 12642064]

Myocardial infarction redefined—a consensus document of The Joint European Society of Cardiology/American College of Cardiology Committee for the redefinition of myocardial infarction. J Am Coll Cardiol 2000;36:959. [PMID: 10987628]

Sharkey SW et al: Acute and reversible cardiomyopathy provoked by stress in women from the United States. Circulation 2005;111:472. [PMID: 15687136]

Clinical Findings

A. Symptoms

1. Premonitory pain—Many patients give a history of alteration in the pattern of angina preceding the time of onset of symptoms of myocardial infarction, classically the onset of angina with minimal exertion or at rest.

2. Pain of infarction—Unlike anginal episodes, most infarctions occur at rest, and more commonly in the early morning. The pain is similar to angina in location and radiation but it may be more severe, and it builds up rapidly or in waves to maximum intensity over a few minutes or longer. Nitroglycerin has little effect; even opioids may not relieve the pain.

3. Associated symptoms—Patients may break out in a cold sweat, feel weak and apprehensive, and move about, seeking a position of comfort. They prefer not to lie quietly. Light-headedness, syncope, dyspnea, orthopnea, cough, wheezing, nausea and vomiting, or abdominal bloating may be present singly or in any combination.

4. Painless infarction—One-third of patients with acute myocardial infarction present without chest pain, and these patients tend to be undertreated and have poor outcomes. Older patients, women, and patients with diabetes mellitus are more likely to present without classic chest pain. As many as 25% of infarctions are detected on routine ECG without any recallable acute episode.

5. Sudden death and early arrhythmias—Of all deaths from myocardial infarction, about 50% occur before the patients arrive at the hospital, with death presumably caused by ventricular fibrillation.

B. Signs

1. General—Patients may appear anxious and sometimes are sweating profusely. The heart rate may range from marked bradycardia (most commonly in inferior infarction) to tachycardia resulting from increased sympathetic nervous system activity, low cardiac output, or arrhythmia. The BP may be high, especially in former hypertensives, or low in patients with shock. Respiratory distress usually indicates heart failure. Fever, usually low grade, may appear after 12 hours and persist for several days.

2. Chest—Listening for rales on lung examination as evidence for pulmonary edema is a very important part of the physical examination. The Killip classification is a common way to classify heart failure in patients with acute myocardial infarction and has powerful prognostic value. Killip Class I is absence of rales and S_3, Class II is rales that do not clear with coughing over one-third or less of the lung fields or presence of an S_3, Class III is rales that do not clear with coughing over more than one-third of the lung fields, and Class IV is cardiogenic shock (rales, hypotension, and signs of hypoperfusion).

3. Heart—The cardiac examination may be unimpressive or very abnormal. An abnormally located ventricular impulse often represents the dyskinetic infarcted region. Jugular venous distention reflects RA hypertension, which may indicate RV infarction or elevated LV filling pressures. The absence of elevated central venous pressure, however, does not indicate normal LA or LV diastolic pressures. Soft heart sounds may indicate LV dysfunction. Atrial gallops (S_4) are the rule, whereas ventricular gallops (S_3) are less common and indicate significant LV dysfunction. Mitral regurgitation murmurs are not uncommon and usually indicate papillary muscle dysfunction or, rarely, rupture. Pericardial friction rubs are uncommon in the first 24 hours but may appear later.

4. Extremities—Edema is usually not present. Cyanosis and cold temperature indicate low output. The peripheral pulses should be noted, since later shock or emboli may alter the examination.

C. Laboratory Findings

The most valuable laboratory tests are cardiac-specific markers of myocardial damage, including quantitative determinations of CK-MB, troponin I, and troponin T. Troponins are more sensitive and specific but stay elevated for days and, therefore, are generally not useful for evaluating suspected early reinfarction. Each of these tests may become positive as early as 4–6 hours after the onset of a myocardial infarction and should be abnormal by 8–12 hours. Circulating levels of troponins may remain elevated for 5–7 days or longer.

D. ECG

Most patients with acute infarction have ECG changes, and a normal tracing is uncommon. The extent of the ECG abnormalities, especially the sum of the total amount of ST-segment deviation, is a good indicator of extent of acute infarction and risk of subsequent adverse events. The classic evolution of changes is from peaked ("hyperacute") T waves, to ST-segment elevation, to Q wave development, to T wave inversion. This may occur over a few hours to several days. The evolution of new Q waves (> 30 milliseconds in duration and 25% of the R wave amplitude) is diagnostic, but Q waves do not occur in 30–50% of acute infarctions (non-Q wave infarctions).

E. Chest Radiography

The chest radiograph may demonstrate signs of CHF, but these changes often lag behind the clinical findings. Signs of aortic dissection, including mediastinal widening, should be sought as a possible alternative diagnosis.

F. Echocardiography

Echocardiography provides convenient bedside assessment of LV global and regional function. This can help with the diagnosis and management of infarction; echocardiography has been used successfully to make judgments about admission and management of patients with suspected infarction, since normal wall motion makes an infarction unlikely. Doppler echocardiography is probably the most convenient procedure for diagnosing postinfarction mitral regurgitation or VSD.

G. Scintigraphic Studies

Technetium-99m pyrophosphate scintigraphy can be used to diagnose acute myocardial infarction. When injected at least 18 hours postinfarction, the radiotracer complexes with calcium in necrotic myocardium to provide a "hot spot" image of the infarction. This test is insensitive to small infarctions, and false-positive studies occur, so its use is limited to patients in whom the diagnosis by ECG and enzymes is not possible—principally those who present several days after the event or have intraoperative infarctions. **Radiolabeled antimyosin antibody fragments** are more sensitive and specific imaging agents, but scintigraphy must be performed 24 and 48 hours postinjection, so this test has limited clinical usefulness in the diagnosis of acute myocardial infarction.

Scintigraphy with thallium-201 or the newer technetium-based perfusion tracers will demonstrate "cold spots" in regions of diminished perfusion, which usually represent infarction when the radiotracer is administered at rest, but abnormalities do not distinguish recent from old damage.

Radionuclide angiography demonstrates akinesis or dyskinesis in areas of infarction and also measures EF, which can be valuable. RV dysfunction may indicate infarction of this chamber.

MRI with gadolinium contrast enhancement has emerged as one of the most sensitive tests to detect and quantitate extent of infarction.

H. Hemodynamic Measurements

These can be helpful in managing the patient with suspected cardiogenic shock. Their use is described below and in Table 10–6. Use of PA catheters, however, has generally not been associated with better outcomes and should be limited to patients with severe hemodynamic compromise.

Ammann P et al: Characteristics and prognosis of myocardial infarction in patients with normal coronary arteries. Chest 2000;117:333. [PMID: 10669671]

Cohen MG et al: Pulmonary artery catheterization in acute coronary syndromes: insights from the GUSTO IIb and GUSTO III trials. Am J Med 2005;18:482. [PMID: 15866250]

Mahrholdt H et al: Relationship of contractile function to transmural extent of infarction in patients with chronic coronary artery disease. J Am Coll Cardiol 2003;42:505. [PMID: 12906981]

Myocardial infarction redefined—a consensus document of The Joint European Society of Cardiology/American College of Cardiology Committee for the redefinition of myocardial infarction. J Am Coll Cardiol 2000;36:959. [PMID: 10987628]

Zimetbaum PJ et al: Current concepts. Use of the electrocardiogram in acute myocardial infarction. N Engl J Med 2003; 348:933. [PMID: 12621138]

Treatment

Table 10–4 provides a summary of the ACC/AHA Guideline recommendations for selected medical treatments.

A. Aspirin and Clopidogrel

All patients with definite or suspected myocardial infarction should receive aspirin at a dose of 162 mg or 325 mg at once regardless of whether thrombolytic therapy is being considered or the patient has been taking aspirin. Chewable aspirin provides more rapid blood levels. Patients with a definite aspirin allergy should be treated with clopidogrel; a 300 mg (or 600 mg) loading dose will result in faster onset of action than the standard 75 mg dose.

Clopidogrel, in addition to aspirin, has also been shown to provide important benefits in patients with acute ST elevation myocardial infarction. In the CLARITY trial, a loading dose of 300 mg of clopidogrel given with thrombolytic therapy, followed by 75 mg a day, led to substantial improvement in coro-

Table 10–6. Hemodynamic subsets in acute myocardial infarction.

Category	CI or SWI	PCWP	Treatment	Comment
Normal	> 2.2, < 30	< 15	None	Mortality rate < 5%.
Hyperdynamic	> 3.0, > 40	< 15	β-Blockers	Characterized by tachycardia; mortality rate < 5%.
Hypovolemic	< 2.5, < 30	< 10	Volume expansion	Hypotension, tachycardia, but preserved left ventricular function by echocardiography; mortality rate 4–8%.
Left ventricular failure	< 2.2, < 30	> 15	Diuretics	Mild dyspnea, rales, normal blood pressure; mortality rate 10–20%.
Severe failure	< 2.0, < 20	> 18	Diuretics, vasodilators	Pulmonary edema, mild hypotension; inotropic agents, IABC may be required; mortality rate 20–40%.
Shock	< 1.8, < 30	> 20	Inotropic agents, IABC	IABC early unless rapid reversal occurs; mortality rate > 60%.

CI = cardiac index (L/min/m²); SWI = stroke work index (g-m/m², calculated as [mean arterial pressure – PCWP] × stroke volume index × 0.0136); PCWP = pulmonary capillary wedge pressure (in mm Hg; pulmonary artery diastolic pressure may be used instead); IABC = intra-aortic balloon counterpulsation.

nary patency on catheterization 3.5 days following thrombolysis. Moreover, there was no increase in serious bleeding in this population of patients up to 75 years of age. The COMMIT/CCS-2 trial randomized over 45,000 patients in China with acute myocardial infarction to clopidogrel 75 mg a day or placebo, and found a small but statistically significant reduction in early death, myocardial reinfarction, and stroke, with no excess in major bleeding. For patients who have received thrombolytic therapy but will undergo angiography in the first day or two, the early benefits of clopidogrel need to be weighed against the need to delay bypass surgery for approximately 5 days for those patients found to require surgical revascularization.

B. THROMBOLYTIC THERAPY

Thrombolytic therapy reduces mortality and limits infarct size in patients with acute myocardial infarction associated with ST-segment elevation (defined as ≥ 0.1 mV in two inferior or lateral leads or two contiguous precordial leads), or with left bundle branch block. The greatest benefit occurs if treatment is initiated within the first 3 hours, when up to a 50% reduction in mortality rate can be achieved. The magnitude of benefit declines rapidly thereafter, but a 10% relative mortality reduction can be achieved up to 12 hours after the onset of chest pain. The survival benefit is greatest in patients with large—usually anterior—infarctions. Patients without ST-segment elevation (previously labeled "non-Q wave" infarctions) do not benefit, and may derive harm, from thrombolysis.

Major bleeding complications occur in 0.5–5% of patients, the most serious of which is intracranial hemorrhage. The major risk factors for intracranial bleeding are age over 65 years, hypertension at presentation, low body weight (< 70 kg), and the use of clot-specific thrombolytic agents (alteplase, reteplase, tenecteplase). Although patients over age 75 years have a much higher mortality rate with acute myocardial infarction and therefore may derive greater benefit, the risk of severe bleeding is also higher, particularly among patients with risk factors from bleeding or intracranial hemorrhage, such as severe hypertension or recent stroke. Patients presenting more than 12 hours after the onset of chest pain may also derive a small benefit, particularly if pain and ST-segment elevation persist, but rarely does this benefit outweigh the attendant risk.

Therefore, the current recommendation is to treat patients with ST-segment elevation infarction who seek medical attention within 6–12 hours of the onset of symptoms with reperfusion therapy, either primary percutaneous coronary intervention (PCI) or thrombolytic therapy. Contraindications include previous hemorrhagic stroke, other strokes or cerebrovascular events within 1 year, known intracranial neoplasm, active internal bleeding (excluding menstruation), or suspected aortic dissection. Relative contraindications are BP > 180/110 mm Hg at presentation, other intracerebral pathology not listed above as a contraindication, known bleeding diathesis, trauma within 2–4 weeks, major surgery within 3 weeks, prolonged (> 10 minutes) or traumatic cardiopulmonary resuscitation, recent (within 2–4 weeks) internal bleeding, noncompressible vascular punctures, active diabetic retinopathy, pregnancy, active peptic ulcer disease, a history of severe hypertension, current use of anticoagulants (INR > 2.0–3.0), and prior allergic reaction or exposure to streptokinase or anistreplase within 2 years.

The following thrombolytic agents are available for acute myocardial infarction and are characterized in Table 10–7.

Streptokinase is not commonly used for treatment of acute myocardial infarction since it is less effective at opening occluded arteries and less effective at reducing mortality. It is non-fibrin-specific, causes depletion of circulating fibrinogen, and has a tendency to induce hypotension, particularly if infused rapidly.

Table 10–7. Thrombolytic therapy for acute myocardial infarction.

	Streptokinase	Alteplase; Tissue Plasminogen Activator (t-PA)	Reteplase	Tenecteplase (TNK-t-PA)
Source	Group C streptococcus	Recombinant DNA	Recombinant DNA	Recombinant DNA
Half-life	20 minutes	5 minutes	15 minutes	20 minutes
Usual dose	1.5 million units	100 mg	20 units	40 mg
Administration	750,000 units over 20 minutes followed by 750,000 units over 40 minutes	Initial bolus of 15 mg, followed by 50 mg infused over the next 30 minutes and 35 mg over the following 60 minutes	10 units as a bolus over 2 minutes, repeated after 30 minutes	Single weight-adjusted bolus, 0.5 mg/kg
Anticoagulation after infusion	Aspirin, 325 mg daily; there is no evidence that adjunctive heparin improves outcome following streptokinase	Aspirin, 325 mg daily; heparin, 5000 units as bolus, followed by 1000 units per hour infusion, subsequently adjusted to maintain PTT 1.5–2 times control	Aspirin, 325 mg; heparin as with t-PA	Aspirin, 325 mg daily
Clot selectivity	Low	High	High	High
Fibrinogenolysis	+++	+	+	+
Bleeding	+	+	+	+
Hypotension	+++	+	+	+
Allergic reactions	++	0	0	+
Reocclusion	5–20%	10–30%	—	5–20%
Approximate cost[1]	$562.50	$3609.06	$2895.48	$2917.48

[1]Average wholesale price (AWP, for AB-rated generic when available) for quantity listed. Source: *Red Book Update*, Vol. 25, No. 5, May 2006. AWP may not accurately represent the actual pharmacy cost because wide contractual variations exist among institutions. PTT = partial thromboplastin time.

This can be managed by slowing or interrupting the infusion and administering fluids. There is controversy as to whether adjunctive heparin is beneficial in patients given streptokinase, unlike its administration with the more clot-specific agents. Allergic reactions, including anaphylaxis, occur in 1–2% of patients, and this agent should generally not be administered to patients with prior exposure.

Alteplase (recombinant tissue plasminogen activator; t-PA) is a naturally occurring plasminogen activator that is modestly fibrin specific, resulting in about a 50% reduction in circulating fibrinogen. In the first GUSTO trial, which compared t-PA (with unfractionated heparin) with streptokinase, the 30-day mortality rate with t-PA was one absolute percentage point lower (one additional life saved per 100 patients treated), though there was also a small *increase* in the rate of intracranial hemorrhage. An angiographic substudy confirmed a higher 90-minute patency rate and a higher rate of normal (TIMI grade 3) flow in patients.

Reteplase is a recombinant deletion mutant of t-PA that is slightly less fibrin specific. In comparative trials, it appears to have efficacy similar to that of alteplase, but it has a longer duration of action and can be administered as two boluses 30 minutes apart.

Tenecteplase (TNK-t-PA) is a genetically engineered substitution mutant of native t-PA that has reduced plasma clearance, increased fibrin sensitivity, and increased resistance to plasminogen activator inhibitor-1. It can be given as a single weight-adjusted bolus. In a large comparative trial, this agent was equivalent to t-PA with regard to efficacy and resulted in significantly less noncerebral bleeding.

1. Selection of a thrombolytic agent—In the United States, most patients are treated with alteplase, reteplase, or tenecteplase. The differences in efficacy between them are small compared with the potential benefit of treating a greater proportion of appropriate candidates in a more prompt manner. The principal objective should be to administer a thrombolytic agent within 30 minutes of presentation—or even during transport. The ability to administer tenecteplase as a single bolus is an attractive feature that may facilitate earlier treatment. The combination of a reduced-dose thrombolytic given with a platelet glycoprotein IIb/IIIa antagonist has been investigated in several trials, with no evidence of reduction in mortality but a modest increase in bleeding complications.

2. Postthrombolytic management—After completion of the thrombolytic infusion, aspirin should be continued. Anticoagulation with intravenous heparin (initial dose of 60 units/kg bolus to a maximum of 4000 units, followed by an infusion of 12 units/kg/min to a maximum of 1000 units, then adjusted to maintain an activated partial thromboplastin time [aPTT] of 50–75 seconds beginning with an aPTT drawn 3 hours after thrombolytic) is continued for at least 24 hours after alteplase, reteplase, or tenecteplase.

With tenecteplase, enoxaparin, a 30 mg intravenous bolus, followed by 1 mg/kg every 12 hours, resulted in a lower incidence of the composite of death, myocardial infarction, refractory ischemia, and disabling stroke in the ASSENT-3 trial, but bleeding rates were increased in the elderly. In the larger EXTRACT trial, enoxaparin reduced death and myocardial infarction at day 30 (compared with unfractionated heparin), at the expense of a modest increase in bleeding. In patients younger than age 75, enoxaparin was given as a 30 mg intravenous bolus and 1 mg/kg every 12 hours; in patients age 75 years and older, it was given with no bolus and 0.75 mg/kg intravenously every 12 hours. Another antithrombotic option is fondaparinux, given at a dose of 2.5 mg subcutaneously once a day. In the OASIS-6 trial, it resulted in significant reductions in death and reinfarction when compared with control (unfractionated heparin when indicated, otherwise placebo). Similar to the findings of the OASIS-5 trial, fondaparinux tended to result in less bleeding, despite its longer duration compared with heparin and despite its comparison to placebo in about half of the enrolled patients. There was no benefit of fondaparinux among patients undergoing primary PCI.

For all patients with acute myocardial infarction treated with intensive antithrombotic therapy, prophylactic treatment with antacids and an H$_2$-blocker is advisable.

Myocardial reperfusion can be recognized clinically by the early cessation of pain and the resolution of ST-segment elevation. Although at least 50–70% resolution of ST-segment elevation by 90 minutes may occur without coronary reperfusion, ST resolution is a strong predictor of better outcome. Even with anticoagulation, 10–20% of reperfused vessels will reocclude during hospitalization, although reocclusion and reinfarction appear to be reduced following intervention. Reinfarction, indicated by recurrence of pain and ST-segment elevation, can be treated by readministration of a thrombolytic agent or immediate angiography and PCI. The role of catheterization and intervention after thrombolysis is controversial. For patients who do not reperfuse based on lack of at least 50% resolution of ST elevation, rescue angioplasty has been shown to reduce the composite of death, reinfarction, stroke, or severe heart failure. Many cardiologists advocate routine catheterization and revascularization following acute myocardial infarction, in otherwise suitable candidates, although the data to support this are inconclusive. Patients with recurrent ischemic pain prior to discharge should undergo catheterization and, if indicated, revascularization. Asymptomatic, clinically stable patients should undergo predischarge evaluation to determine whether residual jeopardized myocardium is present. This can be accomplished by submaximal exercise or pharmacologic stress scintigraphy. Those with significantly positive tests or a low threshold for symptomatic ischemia should undergo angiography and revascularization where feasible.

C. Primary Percutaneous Coronary Intervention for ST Segment Elevation Myocardial Infarction

Immediate coronary angiography and primary PCI (including stenting) of the infarct-related artery have been shown to be superior to thrombolysis when done by experienced operators in high-volume centers with rapid time from first medical contact to intervention ("door-to-balloon"). U.S. and European guidelines call for first medical contact or "door-to-balloon" times of < 90 minutes. Several trials have shown that if efficient transfer systems are in place, transfer of patients with acute myocardial infarction from hospitals without to hospitals with primary PCI capability can improve outcome compared with thrombolytic therapy at the presenting hospital, although this requires sophisticated systems to ensure rapid identification, transfer, and PCI. Primary PCI is the approach of choice in patients with absolute and many relative contraindications to thrombolytic therapy. The results of this approach in specialized centers are excellent, exceeding those obtainable by thrombolytic therapy even in good candidates, but this experience may not be generalizable to centers and operators with less experience or expertise. Stenting—in conjunction with the platelet glycoprotein IIb/IIIa antagonist abciximab—is now widely used in patients with acute myocardial infarction. In the subgroup of patients with cardiogenic shock, early catheterization and percutaneous or surgical revascularization are the preferred management. Because an acute interventional approach carries a lower risk of hemorrhagic complications, it may also be the preferred strategy in many older patients (see Tables 10–4 and 10–5 for factors to consider in choosing thrombolytic therapy or primary PCI).

In part because patients in the United States who are transferred for primary PCI tend to have long delays from first hospital arrival to balloon inflation, there has been interest in developing "facilitated" PCI whereby a combination of medications (full or reduced dose fibrinolytic agents with or without glycoprotein IIb/IIIa inhibitors) is given to establish patency followed by immediate PCI. While this approach has been shown to establish patency at the time of catheterization laboratory arrival in a substantial portion of patients, it has not yet been shown to improve outcome. In fact, in the ASSENT-4 PCI trial, patients with a delay in median time to PCI balloon inflation did better if they did not receive full-dose tenecteplase on the way to the catheterization laboratory. Thus, for the time being, patients should be treated either with fibrinolytic agents (and immediate rescue PCI for reperfusion failure) or with primary PCI, if it can be done in the rapid timecourse outlined in the ACC/AHA guidelines.

D. GENERAL MEASURES

Cardiac care unit monitoring should be instituted as soon as possible. Patients without complications can be transferred to a telemetry unit after 24–48 hours. Activity should initially be limited to bed rest but can be advanced within 24 hours. Progressive ambulation should be started after 24–72 hours if tolerated. For patients without complications, discharge by day 4 appears to be appropriate. Low-flow oxygen therapy (2–4 L/min) should be given if oxygen saturation is reduced.

E. ANALGESIA

An initial attempt should be made to relieve pain with sublingual nitroglycerin. However, if no response occurs after two or three tablets, intravenous opioids provide the most rapid and effective analgesia and may also reduce pulmonary congestion. Morphine sulfate, 4–8 mg, or meperidine, 50–75 mg, should be given. Subsequent small doses can be given every 15 minutes until pain abates.

F. β-ADRENERGIC BLOCKING AGENTS

Although trials have shown modest short-term benefit from intravenous β-blockers given immediately after acute myocardial infarction, it has not been clear that this provides a major advantage over simply beginning an oral β-blocker. The Chinese COMMIT/CCS-2 trial involving 45,000 patients found no overall benefit to intravenous followed by oral metoprolol; the aggressive dosing (three 5 mg intravenous boluses followed by 200 mg/d orally) appeared to prevent reinfarction at the cost of increasing shock in patients presenting with heart failure. Thus, β-blockade should be avoided in patients with decompensated heart failure, decompensated asthma, or high degrees of AV block. The CAPRICORN trial showed the benefits of carvedilol following the acute phase of large myocardial infarction with contemporary care.

G. NITRATES

Nitroglycerin is the agent of choice for continued or recurrent ischemic pain and is useful in lowering BP or relieving pulmonary congestion. However, routine nitrate administration is not recommended, since no improvement in outcome has been observed in the ISIS-4 or GISSI-3 trials, in which a total of over 70,000 patients were randomized to nitrate treatment or placebo. Nitrates should be avoided in patients who received phosphodiesterase inhibitors (sildenafil, vardenafil, and tadalafil) in the prior 24 hours.

H. ACE INHIBITORS

A series of trials (SAVE, AIRE, SMILE, TRACE, GISSI-III, and ISIS-4) have shown both short- and long-term improvement in survival with ACE inhibitor therapy. The benefits are greatest in patients with low EFs, large infarctions, or clinical evidence of heart failure. Because substantial amounts of the survival benefit occur on the first day, ACE inhibitor treatment should be commenced early in patients without hypotension, especially patients with large or anterior myocardial infarction.

I. ANGIOTENSIN RECEPTOR BLOCKERS

Although there has been inconsistency in the effects of different angiotensin receptor blockers (ARBs) on mortality for patients post-myocardial infarction with heart failure and/or LV dysfunction, the VALIANT trial showed that valsartan 160 mg twice a day is equivalent to captopril in reducing mortality. Thus, valsartan should be used for all patients with ACE inhibitor intolerance, and is a reasonable, albeit more expensive, alternative to captopril. The combination of captopril and valsartan (at reduced dose) was no better than either agent alone and resulted in more side effects.

J. ALDOSTERONE ANTAGONISTS

The RALES trial showed that spironolactone can reduce the mortality rate of patients with advanced heart failure, and the EPHESUS trial showed a 15% relative risk reduction in mortality with eplerenone for patients post-myocardial infarction with LV dysfunction and heart failure. Patients must be monitored carefully for development of hyperkalemia.

K. ANTIARRHYTHMIC PROPHYLAXIS

The incidence of ventricular fibrillation in hospitalized patients is approximately 5%, with 80% of episodes occurring in the first 12–24 hours. Prophylactic lidocaine infusions (1–2 mg/min) prevent most episodes, but this therapy has not reduced the mortality rate and it increases the risk of asystole, so this approach is no longer recommended except in patients with sustained ventricular tachycardia.

L. CALCIUM CHANNEL BLOCKERS

There are no studies to support the routine use of calcium channel blockers in most patients with acute myocardial infarction—and indeed, they have the potential to exacerbate ischemia and cause death from reflex tachycardia or myocardial depression. Long-acting calcium channel blockers should generally be reserved for management of hypertension or ischemia as second- or third-line drugs after β-blockers and nitrates.

M. LONG-TERM ANTITHROMBOTIC THERAPY

Discharge on aspirin, since it is highly effective, inexpensive, and well tolerated, is a key quality indicator of myocardial infarction care. In the WARIS-II trial, long-term anticoagulation with warfarin post-myocardial infarction was associated with a reduction in the composite of death, reinfarction, and stroke. However, whether the results of this trial are transferable to the United States where anticoagulation services may be less organized and effective than in Norwegian hospitals is unknown. In the CURE trial, clopidogrel for 3–12 months for non-ST elevation acute coronary syndromes resulted in a similar 20% relative risk reduction in cardiovascular death, myocardial infarction, and stroke.

Antman EM et al; ExTRACT-TIMI 25 Investigators: Enoxaparin versus unfractionated heparin with fibrinolysis for ST-elevation myocardial infarction. N Engl J Med 2006;354:1477. [PMID: 16537665]

Assessment of the Safety and Efficacy of a New Thrombolytic Regimen (ASSENT-3) Investigators: Efficacy and safety of tenecteplase in combination with enoxaparin, abciximab, or unfractionated heparin: the ASSENT-3 randomised trial in acute myocardial infarction. Lancet 2001;358:605. [PMID: 11530146]

Assessment of the Safety and Efficacy of a New Treatment Strategy with Percutaneous Coronary Intervention (ASSENT-4 PCI) investigators. Primary versus tenecteplase-facilitated percutaneous coronary intervention in patients with ST-segment elevation acute myocardial infarction (ASSENT-4 PCI): randomised trial. Lancet 2006;367:569. [PMID: 16488800]

Chen Z: Results of the COMMIT/CCS-2 Trial. American College of Cardiology, Orlando, FL, March 2005. Results online at http://www.ctsu.ox.ac.uk/~ccs2/live/content/presentations/slideshow/ (accessed March 28, 2005).

Collins R: Results of the COMMIT/CCS-2 Trial. American College of Cardiology, Orlando, FL, March 2005. Results online at http://www.ctsu.ox.ac.uk/~ccs2/live/content/presentations/slideshow/ (accessed March 28, 2005).

Hurlen M et al: Warfarin, aspirin, or both after myocardial infarction. N Engl J Med 2002;347:969. [PMID: 12324552]

Keeley EC et al: Primary coronary intervention for acute myocardial infarction. JAMA 2004;291:736. [PMID: 14871919]

Lincoff AM et al: Mortality at 1 year with combination platelet glycoprotein IIb/IIIa inhibition and reduced-dose fibrinolytic therapy vs conventional fibrinolytic therapy for acute myocardial infarction: GUSTO V randomized trial. JAMA 2002;288:2130. [PMID: 12413372]

Pfeffer MA et al: Valsartan, captopril, or both in myocardial infarction complicated by heart failure, left ventricular dysfunction, or both. N Engl J Med 2003;349:1893. [PMID: 14610160]

Rapaport E: ACC/AHA American College of Cardiology/American Heart Association. Guidelines for the acute coronary syndromes. Curr Cardiol Rep 2001;3:289. [PMID: 11406086]

Ryan TJ et al: 1999 update: ACC/AHA guidelines for the management of acute myocardial infarction: a report of the American College of Cardiology/American Heart Association Task Force on Practice Guidelines (Committee on Management of Acute Myocardial Infarction). J Am Coll Cardiol 1999;34:890. [PMID: 10483976]

Sabatine MS et al; CLARITY-TIMI 28 Investigators: Addition of clopidogrel to aspirin and fibrinolytic therapy for myocardial infarction with ST-segment elevation. N Engl J Med 2005;352:1179. [PMID: 15758000]

Stone GW et al: Comparison of angioplasty with stenting, with or without abciximab, in acute myocardial infarction. N Engl J Med 2002;346:957. [PMID: 11919304]

Yusuf S et al; OASIS-6 Trial Group: Effects of fondaparinux on mortality and reinfarction in patients with acute ST-segment elevation myocardial infarction: the OASIS-6 randomized trial. JAMA 2006;295:1519. [PMID: 16537725]

Complications

A variety of complications can occur after myocardial infarction even when treatment is initiated promptly.

A. POSTINFARCTION ISCHEMIA

In recent clinical trials of thrombolysis, recurrent ischemia occurred in about one-third of patients, was more common following non-ST elevation than ST elevation myocardial infarction, and had important short- and long-term prognostic implications. Vigorous medical therapy should be instituted, including nitrates and β-blockers as well as aspirin, heparin, and consideration of platelet glycoprotein IIb/IIIa antagonists. Most patients with postinfarction angina—and all who are refractory to medical therapy—should undergo early catheterization and revascularization by PTCA or CABG.

B. ARRHYTHMIAS

Abnormalities of rhythm and conduction are common.

1. Sinus bradycardia—This is most common in inferior infarctions or may be precipitated by medications. Observation or withdrawal of the offending agent is usually sufficient. If accompanied by signs of low cardiac output, atropine, 0.5–1 mg intravenously, is usually effective. Temporary pacing is rarely required.

2. Supraventricular tachyarrhythmias—Sinus tachycardia is common and may reflect either increased adrenergic stimulation or hemodynamic compromise due to hypovolemia or pump failure. In the latter, β-blockade is contraindicated. Supraventricular premature beats are common and may be premonitory for atrial fibrillation. Electrolyte abnormalities and hypoxia should be corrected and causative agents (especially aminophylline) stopped. Atrial fibrillation should be rapidly controlled or converted to sinus rhythm. Intravenous β-blockers such as metoprolol (2.5–5 mg/h) or short-acting esmolol (50–200 mcg/kg/min) are the agents of choice if cardiac function is adequate. Intravenous diltiazem (5–15 mg/h) may be used if β-blockers are contraindicated or ineffective. Digoxin (0.5 mg as initial dose, then 0.25 mg every 90–120 minutes [up to 1–1.25 mg] for a loading dose, followed by 0.25 mg daily if renal function is normal) is preferable if heart failure is present with atrial fibrillation, but the onset of action is delayed. Electrical cardioversion (commencing with 100 J) may be necessary if atrial fibrillation is complicated by hypotension, heart failure, or ischemia, but the arrhythmia often recurs. Amiodarone (150 mg intravenous bolus and then 15–30 mg/h intravenously, or rapid oral loading with 400 mg three times daily) may be helpful to restore or maintain sinus rhythm.

3. Ventricular arrhythmias—Ventricular arrhythmias are most common in the first few hours after infarction. Ventricular premature beats may be premonitory for ventricular tachycardia or fibrillation but generally should not be treated in the absence of frequent nonsustained ventricular tachycardia (usually more than six consecutive beats). Lidocaine is recommended as a prophylactic measure. Toxicity (tremor, anxiety, confusion, seizures) is common, especially in older patients and those with hypotension, heart failure, or liver disease.

Sustained ventricular tachycardia should be treated with a 1 mg/kg bolus of lidocaine if the patient is stable or by electrical cardioversion (100–200 J) if not. If the arrhythmia cannot be suppressed with lidocaine, procainamide (100 mg boluses over 1–2 minutes every 5 minutes to a cumulative dose of 750–1000 mg) or intravenous amiodarone (150 mg over 10 minutes, which may be repeated as needed, followed by 360 mg over 6 hours and then 540 mg over 18 hours) should be initiated, followed by an infusion of 20–80 mg/kg/min. Ventricular fibrillation is treated electrically (300–400 J). Unresponsive ventricular fibrillation should be treated with additional amiodarone and repeat cardioversion while cardiopulmonary resuscitation (CPR) is administered.

Accelerated idioventricular rhythm is a regular, wide-complex rhythm at a rate of 70–100/min. It may occur with or without reperfusion and does not require specific therapy.

4. Conduction disturbances—All degrees of AV block may occur in the course of acute myocardial infarction. Block at the level of the AV node is more common than infranodal block and occurs in approximately 20% of inferior myocardial infarctions. First-degree block is the most common and requires no treatment. Second-degree block is usually of the Mobitz type I form (Wenckebach), is often transient, and requires treatment only if associated with a heart rate slow enough to cause symptoms. Complete AV block occurs in up to 5% of acute inferior infarctions, usually is preceded by Mobitz I second-degree block, and generally resolves spontaneously, though it may persist for hours to several weeks. The escape rhythm originates in the distal AV node or AV junction and hence has a narrow QRS complex and is reliable, albeit often slow (30–50 beats/min). Treatment is often necessary because of resulting hypotension and low cardiac output. Intravenous atropine (1 mg) usually restores AV conduction temporarily, but if the escape complex is wide or if repeated atropine treatments are needed, temporary ventricular pacing is indicated. The prognosis for these patients is only slightly worse than for patients in whom AV block did not develop.

In anterior infarctions, the site of block is distal, below the AV node, and usually a result of extensive damage of the His-Purkinje system and bundle branches. New first-degree block (prolongation of the PR interval) is unusual in anterior infarction; Mobitz type II AV block or complete heart block may be preceded by intraventricular conduction defects or may occur abruptly. The escape rhythm, if present, is an unreliable wide-complex idioventricular rhythm. Urgent ventricular pacing is mandatory, but even with successful pacing, morbidity and mortality are high because of the extensive myocardial damage. New conduction abnormalities such as right or left bundle branch block or fascicular blocks may presage progression, often sudden, to second- or third-degree AV block. Temporary ventricular pacing is recommended for new-onset alternating bilateral bundle branch block, bifascicular block, or bundle branch block with worsening first-degree AV block. Patients with anterior infarction who progress to second- or third-degree block even transiently should be considered for insertion of a prophylactic permanent ventricular pacemaker before discharge.

C. MYOCARDIAL DYSFUNCTION

The severity of cardiac dysfunction is proportionate to the extent of myocardial necrosis but is exacerbated by preexisting dysfunction and ongoing ischemia. Patients who have normal BP, no signs of heart failure, and normal urinary output have a good prognosis. Those with hypotension or evidence of more than mild heart failure should have bedside right heart catheterization and continuous measurements of arterial pressure. These measurements permit the accurate assessment of cardiac function, facilitate the correct choice of therapy, and provide important prognostic information. Table 10–6 categorizes patients based on these hemodynamic findings.

1. Acute LV failure—Basilar rales are common in acute myocardial infarction, but dyspnea, more diffuse rales, and arterial hypoxemia usually indicate LV failure. Because both the physical examination and chest radiograph correlate poorly with hemodynamic measurements and because the central venous pressure does not correlate with the PCWP, right heart catheterization may be useful in cases of suspected cardiogenic shock. General measures include supplemental oxygen to increase arterial saturation to above 95% and elevation of the trunk. Diuretics are usually the initial therapy unless RV infarction is present. Intravenous furosemide (10–40 mg) or bumetanide (0.5–1 mg) is preferred because of the reliably rapid onset and short duration of action of these drugs. Higher dosages can be given if an inadequate response occurs. Morphine sulfate (4 mg intravenously followed by increments of 2 mg) is valuable in acute pulmonary edema.

Diuretics are usually effective; however, because most patients with acute infarction are not volume overloaded, the hemodynamic response may be limited and may be associated with hypotension. Vasodilators will reduce PCWP and improve cardiac output by a combination of venodilation (increasing venous capacitance) and arteriolar dilation (reducing afterload and LV wall stress). In mild heart failure, sublingual isosorbide dinitrate (2.5–10 mg every 2 hours) or nitroglycerin ointment (6.25–25 mg every 4 hours) may be adequate to lower PCWP. In more severe failure, especially if cardiac output is reduced, sodium nitroprusside is the preferred agent. It should be initiated only with arterial pressure monitoring; the initial dosage should be low (0.25 mcg/kg/min) to avoid excessive hypotension, but the dosage can be increased by increments of 0.5 mcg/kg/min every 5–10 minutes up to 5–10 mcg/kg/min until the desired hemodynamic response is obtained. Excessive hypotension (mean BP < 65–75 mm Hg) or tachycardia (> 10/min increase) should be avoided.

Intravenous nitroglycerin (starting at 10 mcg/min) also may be effective but may lower PCWP with less hypotension. Oral or transdermal vasodilator therapy with nitrates or ACE inhibitors is often necessary after the initial 24–48 hours (see below).

Inotropic agents should be avoided if possible, because they often increase heart rate and myocardial oxygen requirements and worsen clinical outcomes. Dobutamine has the best hemodynamic profile, increasing cardiac output and modestly lowering PCWP, usually without excessive tachycardia, hypotension, or arrhythmias. The initial dosage is 2.5 mcg/kg/min, and it may be increased by similar increments up to 15–20 mcg/kg/min at intervals of 5–10 minutes. Dopamine is more useful in the presence of hypotension (see below), since it produces peripheral vasoconstriction, but it has a less beneficial effect on PCWP. Amrinone is a positive inotrope and vasodilator that produces hemodynamic effects similar to those of dobutamine but with a greater decrease in PCWP. However, its longer duration of action makes it less useful in unstable situations. Milrinone is a more potent and newer congener of amrinone with fewer side effects. It should be commenced in a loading dose of 50 mcg/kg over 10 minutes, followed by an infusion of 0.375–0.75 mcg/kg/min. Digoxin has not been helpful in acute infarction except to control the ventricular response in atrial fibrillation, but it may be beneficial if chronic heart failure persists.

2. Hypotension and shock—Patients with hypotension (systolic BP < 100 mm Hg, individualized depending on prior BP) and signs of diminished perfusion (low urinary output, confusion, cold extremities) that does not respond to fluid resuscitation should be considered for hemodynamic monitoring with a PA catheter. Up to 20% will have findings indicative of intravascular hypovolemia (due to diaphoresis, vomiting, decreased venous tone, medications—such as diuretics, nitrates, morphine, β-blockers, calcium channel blockers, and thrombolytic agents—and lack of oral intake). These should be treated with successive boluses of 100 mL of normal saline until PCWP reaches 15–18 mm Hg to determine whether cardiac output and BP respond. Pericardial tamponade due to hemorrhagic pericarditis (especially after thrombolytic therapy or cardiopulmonary resuscitation) or ventricular rupture should be considered and excluded by echocardiography if clinically indicated. RV infarction, characterized by a normal PCWP but elevated RA pressure, can produce hypotension. This is discussed below.

Most patients with cardiogenic shock will have moderate to severe LV systolic dysfunction, with a mean EF of 30% in the SHOCK trial. If hypotension is only modest (systolic pressure > 90 mm Hg) and the PCWP is elevated, diuretics and an initial trial of nitroprusside (see above for dosing) are indicated. If the BP falls, inotropic support will need to be added or substituted. Such patients may also be treated with IABC. This device unloads the LV during systole and increases diastolic coronary artery filling pressure. It often facilitates the use of vasodilators in patients who previously did not tolerate them.

Dopamine is the most appropriate pressor for cardiogenic hypotension. It should be initiated at a rate of 2–4 mcg/kg/min and increased at 5-minute intervals to the appropriate hemodynamic end point. At low dosages (< 5 mcg/kg/min), it improves renal blood flow; at intermediate dosages (2.5–10 mcg/kg/min), it stimulates myocardial contractility; at higher dosages (> 8 mcg/kg/min), it is a potent α_1-adrenergic agonist. In general, BP and cardiac index rise, but PCWP does not fall. Dopamine may be combined with nitroprusside or dobutamine (see above for dosing), or the latter may be used in its place if hypotension is not severe. Milrinone has hemodynamic effects similar to those of dobutamine, but the longer duration of action precludes rapid dosage adjustment. Norepinephrine (0.1–0.5 mcg/kg/min) is the usual pressor of last resort, since isoproterenol and epinephrine produce less vasoconstriction and do not increase coronary perfusion pressure (aortic diastolic pressure), but both tend to worsen the balance between myocardial oxygen delivery and utilization.

Patients with cardiogenic shock not due to hypovolemia have a poor prognosis, with 30-day mortality rates of 50–80%. If they do not respond rapidly, IABC should be instituted. Surgically implanted ventricular assist devices may be used in extreme cases. Emergent cardiac catheterization and coronary angiography followed by percutaneous or surgical revascularization offer the best chance of survival, particularly in patients under 75 years of age.

D. RV INFARCTION

RV infarction is present in one-third of patients with inferior wall infarction but is clinically significant in less than 50% of these. It presents as hypotension with relatively preserved LV function and should be considered whenever patients with inferior infarction exhibit low BP, raised venous pressure, and clear lungs. Hypotension is often exacerbated by medications that decrease intravascular volume or produce venodilation, such as diuretics, nitrates, and narcotics. RA pressure and jugular venous pulsations are high, while PCWP is normal or low and the lungs are clear. The diagnosis is suggested by ST-segment elevation in right-sided anterior chest leads, particularly RV_4. The diagnosis can be confirmed by echocardiography or hemodynamic measurements. Treatment consists of fluid loading to improve LV filling, and inotropic agents if necessary.

E. MECHANICAL DEFECTS

Partial or complete rupture of a papillary muscle or of the interventricular septum occurs in less than 1% of acute myocardial infarctions and carries a poor prognosis. These complications occur in both anterior and inferior infarctions, usually 3–7 days after the acute event. They are detected by the appearance of a new systolic murmur and clinical deterioration, often with pulmonary edema. The two lesions are distinguished by the location of the murmur (apical versus parasternal) and by Doppler echocardiography. Hemodynamic monitoring is essential for appropriate management and demonstrates an increase in oxygen saturation between the RA and PA in VSD and, often, a large *v* wave with mitral regurgitation. Treatment by nitroprusside and, preferably, IABC reduces the regurgitation or shunt, but surgical correction is mandatory. In patients remaining hemodynamically unstable or requiring continuous parenteral pharmacologic treatment or counterpulsation, early surgery is recommended, though mortality rates are high (15% to nearly 100%), depending on residual ventricular function and clinical status). Patients who are stabilized medically can have delayed surgery with lower risks (10–25%), although this may be due to the death of sicker patients, some of whom may have been saved by earlier surgery.

F. MYOCARDIAL RUPTURE

Complete rupture of the LV free wall occurs in less than 1% of patients and usually results in immediate death. It occurs 2–7 days postinfarction, usually involves the anterior wall, and is more frequent in older women. Incomplete or gradual rupture may be sealed off by the pericardium, creating a **pseudoaneurysm**. This may be recognized by echocardiography, radionuclide angiography, or LV angiography, often as an incidental finding. It demonstrates a narrow-neck connection to the LV. Early surgical repair is indicated, since delayed rupture is common.

G. LV ANEURYSM

An LV aneurysm, a sharply delineated area of scar that bulges paradoxically during systole, develops in 10–20% of patients surviving an acute infarction. This usually follows anterior Q wave infarctions. Aneurysms are recognized by persistent ST-segment elevation (beyond 4–8 weeks), and a wide neck from the LV can be demonstrated by echocardiography, scintigraphy, or contrast angiography. They rarely rupture but may be associated with arterial emboli, ventricular arrhythmias, and CHF. Surgical resection may be performed for these indications if other measures fail. The best results (mortality rates of 10–20%) are obtained when the residual myocardium contracts well

and when significant coronary lesions supplying adjacent regions are bypassed.

H. PERICARDITIS

The pericardium is involved in approximately 50% of infarctions, but pericarditis is often not clinically significant. Twenty percent of patients with Q wave infarctions will have an audible friction rub if examined repetitively. Pericardial pain occurs in approximately the same proportion after 2–7 days and is recognized by its variation with respiration and position (improved by sitting). Often, no treatment is required, but aspirin (650 mg every 4–6 hours) will usually relieve the pain. Indomethacin and corticosteroids can cause impaired infarct healing and predispose to myocardial rupture, and therefore should generally be avoided in the early post-myocardial infarction period. Likewise, anticoagulation should be used cautiously, since hemorrhagic pericarditis may result.

One week to 12 weeks after infarction, Dressler's syndrome (post-myocardial infarction syndrome) occurs in less than 5% of patients. This is an autoimmune phenomenon and presents as pericarditis with associated fever, leukocytosis and, occasionally, pericardial or pleural effusion. It may recur over months. Treatment is the same as for other forms of pericarditis. A short course of nonsteroidal agents or corticosteroids may help relieve symptoms.

I. MURAL THROMBUS

Mural thrombi are common in large anterior infarctions but not in infarctions at other locations. Arterial emboli occur in approximately 2% of patients with known infarction, usually within 6 weeks. Anticoagulation with heparin followed by short-term (3-month) warfarin therapy prevents most emboli and should be considered in all patients with large anterior infarctions. Mural thrombi can be detected by echocardiography or CT scan (MRI has yielded frequent false-positive results) but with only moderate reliability, and only a small percentage (up to 25%) embolize, so these procedures should not be relied upon for determining the need for anticoagulation.

Brady WJ et al: Diagnosis and management of bradycardia and atrioventricular block associated with acute coronary ischemia. Emerg Med Clin North Am 2001;19:371. [PMID: 11373984]

Crenshaw BS et al: Risk factors, angiographic patterns, and outcomes in patients with ventricular septal defect complicating acute myocardial infarction. Circulation 2000;101:27. [PMID: 10618300]

Goldstein JA: Pathophysiology and management of right heart ischemia. J Am Coll Cardiol 2002;40:841. [PMID: 12225706]

Hochman JS et al: Early revascularization in acute myocardial infarction complicated by cardiogenic shock. SHOCK Investigators. Should We Emergently Revascularize Occluded Coronaries for Cardiogenic Shock. N Engl J Med 1999;341:625. [PMID: 10460813]

Mangrum JM: Tachyarrhythmias associated with acute myocardial infarction. Emerg Med Clin North Am 2001;19:385. [PMID: 11373985]

Menon V et al: Management of cardiogenic shock complicating acute myocardial infarction. Heart 2002;88:531. [PMID: 12381652]

Pfisterer M: Right ventricular involvement in myocardial infarction and cardiogenic shock. Lancet 2003;362:392. [PMID: 12907014]

Prieto A et al: Nonarrhythmic complications of acute myocardial infarction. Emerg Med Clin North Am 2001;19:397. [PMID: 11373986]

Rathore SS et al: Acute myocardial infarction complicated by heart block in the elderly: prevalence and outcomes. Am Heart J 2001;141:47. [PMID: 11136486]

Sayer JW et al: Prognostic implications of ventricular fibrillation in acute myocardial infarction: new strategies required for mortality reduction. Heart 2000;84:258. [PMID: 10956285]

Postinfarction Management

After the first 24 hours, the focus of patient management is to prevent recurrent ischemia, improve infarct healing and prevent remodeling, and prevent recurrent vascular events. Patients with hemodynamic compromise, who are at high risk for death, need careful monitoring and management of volume status.

A. RISK STRATIFICATION

Just as for non–ST-segment elevation acute coronary syndrome, risk stratification is important for management of ST-segment elevation acute myocardial infarction. GRACE and TIMI risk scores can be helpful tools. Patients with recurrent ischemia (spontaneous or provoked), hemodynamic instability, impaired LV function, heart failure, or serious ventricular arrhythmias should undergo cardiac catheterization (Table 10–5). ACE inhibitor (or ARB) therapy is indicated in patients with clinical heart failure or LV EF < 40%.

For patients not undergoing cardiac catheterization, submaximal exercise (or pharmacologic stress testing for patients unable to exercise) before discharge or a maximal test after 3–6 weeks (the latter being more sensitive for ischemia) helps patients and physicians plan the return to normal activity. Imaging in conjunction with stress testing adds additional sensitivity for ischemia and provides localizing information. Both exercise and pharmacologic stress imaging have successfully predicted subsequent outcome. One of these tests should be used prior to discharge in patients who have received thrombolytic therapy as a means of selecting appropriate candidates for coronary angiography.

B. SECONDARY PREVENTION

Postinfarction management should begin with identification and modification of risk factors. Treatment of hyperlipidemia and smoking cessation both prevent recurrent infarction and death. LDL cholesterol levels should be lowered below 100 mg/dL, and probably to a goal of 70 mg/dL, with a statin commencing prior to discharge. BP control and cardiac rehabilitation or exercise are also recommended.

β-Blockers improve survival rates, primarily by reducing the incidence of sudden death in high-risk subsets of patients, though their value may be less in patients without complications with small infarctions and normal exercise tests. While a variety of β-blockers have been shown to be beneficial, for patients with LV dysfunction managed with contemporary treatment, carvedilol has been shown to reduce mortality. β-Blockers with intrinsic sympathomimetic activity have not proved beneficial in postinfarction patients.

Antiplatelet agents are beneficial; aspirin (81–325 mg daily) is recommended, and adding clopidogrel (75 mg daily) has been shown to provide additional benefit short term after ST-segment elevation myocardial infarction and for up to 1 year after non-ST elevation acute coronary syndromes. Warfarin anticoagulation for 3 months reduces the incidence of arterial emboli after large anterior infarctions, and according to the results of at least one study it improves long-term prognosis. An advantage to combining low-dose aspirin and warfarin has not been demonstrated, except perhaps in patients with atrial fibrillation.

Calcium channel blockers have not been shown to improve prognoses overall and should not be prescribed purely for secondary prevention. Antiarrhythmic therapy other than with β-blockers has not been shown to be effective except in patients with symptomatic arrhythmias. Amiodarone has been studied in several trials of postinfarct patients with either LV dysfunction or frequent ventricular ectopy. Although survival was not improved, amiodarone was not harmful—unlike other agents in this setting. Therefore, it is the agent of choice for individuals with symptomatic postinfarction supraventricular arrhythmias. While implantable defibrillators improve survival for patients with postinfarction LV dysfunction and heart failure, the DINAMIT trial found no benefit to implantable defibrillators implanted in the 40 days following acute myocardial infarction.

Cardiac rehabilitation programs and exercise training can be of considerable psychological benefit and appear to improve prognosis.

C. ACE INHIBITORS AND ANGIOTENSIN RECEPTOR BLOCKERS IN PATIENTS WITH LV DYSFUNCTION

Patients who sustain substantial myocardial damage often experience subsequent progressive LV dilation and dysfunction, leading to clinical heart failure and reduced long-term survival. In patients with EFs less than 40%, long-term ACE inhibitor (or ARB) therapy prevents LV dilation and the onset of heart failure and prolongs survival. The HOPE trial also demonstrated a reduction of approximately 20% in mortality rates and the occurrence of nonfatal myocardial infarction and stroke with ramipril treatment of postinfarction patients without confirmed LV systolic dysfunction. Therefore, ACE inhibitor therapy should be strongly considered in this broader group of patients—and especially in diabetics and patients with even mild systolic hypertension, in whom the greatest benefit was observed.

D. REVASCULARIZATION

Because of the increasing use of thrombolytic therapy and accumulating experience with PTCA, the indications for revascularization are rapidly evolving. Postinfarction patients who appear likely to benefit from early revascularization if the anatomy is appropriate are (1) those who have undergone thrombolytic therapy and have residual symptoms or laboratory evidence of ischemia; (2) patients with LV dysfunction (EF < 30–40%) and evidence of ischemia; (3) patients with non-Q wave infarction and evidence of more than mild ischemia; and (4) patients with markedly positive exercise tests and multivessel disease. The value of revascularization in the following groups is less clear: (1) patients treated with thrombolytic agents, with little evidence of reperfusion or residual ischemia; (2) patients with LV dysfunction but no detectable ischemia; and (3) patients with preserved LV function who have mild ischemia and are not symptom limited. Patients who survive infarctions without complications, have preserved LV function (EF > 50%), and have no exercise-induced ischemia have an excellent prognosis and do not require invasive evaluation.

Ades PA: Cardiac rehabilitation and secondary prevention of coronary heart disease. N Engl J Med 2001;345:892. [PMID: 11565523]

Dargie HJ et al: Effect of carvedilol on outcome after myocardial infarction in patients with left ventricular dysfunction: the CAPRICORN randomized trial. Lancet 2001;357:1385. [PMID: 11356434]

Hohnloser SH et al; DINAMIT Investigators: Prophylactic use of an implantable cardioverter-defibrillator after acute myocardial infarction. N Engl J Med 2004;351:2481. [PMID: 15590950]

Hurlen M et al: Warfarin, aspirin, or both after myocardial infarction. N Engl J Med 2002;347:969. [PMID: 12324552]

JAMA patient page: Heart attack. JAMA 1998;280:1462. [PMID: 9801010]

Michaels AD et al: Risk stratification after acute myocardial infarction in the reperfusion era. Prog Cardiovasc Dis 2000; 42:273. [PMID: 10661780]

Sutton MGS et al: Left ventricular remodeling after myocardial infarction: pathophysiology and therapy. Circulation 2000; 101:2981. [PMID: 10869273]

See also references for section on Primary and Secondary Prevention of Ischemic Heart Disease.

■ DISTURBANCES OF RATE & RHYTHM

Abnormalities of cardiac rhythm and conduction can be lethal (sudden cardiac death), symptomatic (syncope, near syncope, dizziness, fatigue, or palpitations), or asymptomatic. They are dangerous to the extent that they reduce cardiac output, so that perfusion of the brain or myocardium is impaired, or tend to deteriorate into more serious arrhythmias with the same consequences. Stable supraventricular tachycardia is generally well tolerated in patients without underlying heart disease but may lead to myocardial ischemia or CHF in patients with coronary disease, valvular abnormalities, and systolic or diastolic myocardial dysfunction. Ventricular tachycardia, if prolonged (lasting more than 10–30 seconds), often results in hemodynamic compromise and is more likely to deteriorate into ventricular fibrillation.

Whether slow heart rates produce symptoms at rest or on exertion depends on whether cerebral perfusion can be maintained, which is generally a function of whether the patient is upright or supine and whether LV function is adequate to maintain stroke volume. If the heart rate abruptly slows, as with the onset of complete heart block or sinus arrest, syncope or convulsions may result.

Arrhythmias are detected either because they present with symptoms or because they are detected during the course of monitoring. Arrhythmias causing sudden death, syncope, or near syncope require further evaluation and treatment unless they are related to conditions that are unlikely to recur (eg, electrolyte abnormalities or acute myocardial infarction). In contrast, there is controversy over when and how to evaluate and treat rhythm disturbances that are not symptomatic but are possible markers for more serious abnormalities (eg, nonsustained ventricular tachycardia). This uncertainty reflects two issues: (1) the difficulty of reliably stratifying patients into high-risk and low-risk groups; and (2) the lack of treatments that are both effective and safe. Thus, screening patients for these so-called "premonitory" abnormalities is often not productive.

A number of procedures are used to evaluate patients with symptoms who are believed to be at risk for life-threatening arrhythmias, including in-hospital and ambulatory ECG monitoring, event recorders (instruments that can be used for prolonged periods to record or transmit rhythm tracings when infrequent episodes occur), exercise testing, intracardiac electrophysiologic studies (to assess sinus node function, AV conduction, and inducibility of arrhythmias), signal-averaged ECGs, and tests of autonomic nervous system function (especially tilt-table testing). These are discussed below and in the subsequent sections on individual rhythm disturbance and symptomatic presentation. In general, these techniques are more successful in diagnosing symptomatic arrhythmias than in predicting the outcome of asymptomatic ones.

MECHANISMS OF ARRHYTHMIAS

Susceptibility to arrhythmias results from genetic abnormalities (most often affecting ion channels) and acquired structural heart disease. Susceptibility may be increased by electrolyte abnormalities, hormonal imbalances (thyrotoxicosis, hypercatecholaminergic states), hypoxia, drug effects (such as QT interval prolongation or changes in automaticity, conduction, and refractoriness), and myocardial ischemia. Ongoing research has given us important information on the genetic basis of arrhythmias and knowledge in this arena is expanding rapidly. Most arrhythmias can be classified as (1) disorders of impulse formation or automaticity, (2) abnormalities of impulse conduction, (3) reentry, and (4) triggered activity.

Altered automaticity is the mechanism for sinus node arrest, many premature beats, and automatic rhythms as well as an initiating factor in reentry arrhythmias.

Abnormalities of impulse conduction can occur at the sinus or AV node, in the intraventricular conduction system, and within the atria or ventricles. These are responsible for sinoatrial exit block, for AV block at the node or below, and for establishing reentry circuits.

Reentry is the underlying mechanism for many arrhythmias, including premature beats, most paroxysmal supraventricular tachycardias, atrial flutter, and infarct-related ventricular tachycardia. For reentry to occur, there must be an area of unidirectional block with an appropriate delay to allow repeat depolarization at the site of origin. Reentry is confirmed if the arrhythmia can be terminated by interruption of the circuit by a spontaneous or induced premature beat.

Triggered activity occurs when afterdepolarizations (abnormal electrical activity persisting after repolarization) reach the threshold level required to trigger a new depolarization. Triggered activity can be divided into two different categories: pause-dependent and catecholamine-dependent. Pause-dependent triggered activity is caused by early afterdepolarizations in phase 3 of the action potential. These ventricular tachycardias are usually polymorphic.

Catecholamine-dependent triggered activity is caused by late afterdepolarizations in phase 4 of the action potential. They may be seen in patients with digitalis toxicity, cardiac ischemia, or congenitally prolonged QT intervals. Increased sympathetic tone also plays a part in these arrhythmias. RV outflow tract ventricular tachycardia is attributed to this mechanism.

Eckardt L et al: Arrhythmias in heart failure: current concepts of mechanisms and therapy. J Cardiovasc Electrophysiol 2000; 11:106. [PMID: 10695472]

Napolitano C et al: Genetics of ventricular tachycardia. Curr Opin Cardiol 2002;17:222. [PMID: 12015470]

Wall TS et al: Ventricular tachycardia in structurally normal hearts. Curr Cardiol Rep 2002;4:388. [PMID: 12169235]

Wilde AA et al: Genetics of cardiac arrhythmias. Heart 2005; 91:1352. [PMID: 16162633]

TECHNIQUES FOR EVALUATING RHYTHM DISTURBANCES

ECG Monitoring

The ideal way of establishing a causal relationship between a symptom and a rhythm disturbance is to demonstrate the presence of the rhythm during the symptom. Unfortunately, this is not always easy because symptoms are usually sporadic.

Patients with aborted sudden death and recent or recurrent syncope are often monitored in the hospital. Those with less ominous symptoms may be monitored as outpatients. When episodes are infrequent, use of an event recorder (either implantable or external) is preferable to 24-hour continuous monitoring. Exercise testing may be helpful when the symptoms are associated with exertion or stress. If symptomatic bradyarrhythmias or supraventricular tachyarrhythmias are detected, therapy can usually be initiated without additional diagnostic studies. Further electrophysiologic studies may be useful in evaluating ventricular tachyarrhythmias.

Caution is required before attributing a patient's symptom to rhythm or conduction abnormalities observed during monitoring without concomitant symptoms. In many cases, the symptoms are due to a different arrhythmia or to noncardiac causes. For instance, dizziness or syncope in older patients may be unrelated to concomitantly observed bradycardia, sinus node abnormalities, and ventricular ectopy. Ambulatory monitoring is frequently used to quantify ventricular ectopy and detect asymptomatic ventricular tachycardia in post-myocardial infarction or heart failure patients.

Abbott AV: Diagnostic approach to palpitations. Am Fam Physician 2005;71:743. [PMID: 15742913]

Kadish AH et al: ACC/AHA clinical competence statement on electrocardiography and ambulatory electrocardiography: a report of the ACC/AHA/ACP-ASIM task force on clinical competence (ACC/AHA Committee to develop a clinical competence statement on electrocardiography and ambulatory electrocardiography) endorsed by the International Society for Holter and Noninvasive Electrocardiology. Circulation 2001;104:3169. [PMID: 11748119]

Sarasin FP et al: Usefulness of 24-h Holter monitoring in patients with unexplained syncope and a high likelihood of arrhythmias. Int J Cardiol 2005;101:203. [PMID: 15882664]

Heart Rate Variability

Although it has long been appreciated that there are periodical fluctuations in heart rate even under basal conditions, considerable recent interest has been focused on measurements of **heart rate variability**. These measurements can be made under controlled conditions in the ECG laboratory or from recordings obtained during ambulatory monitoring. Greater fluctuations in heart rate correspond to greater parasympathetic activity, and several studies have indicated that greater heart rate variability is associated with a better prognosis and fewer life-threatening arrhythmias in a variety of cardiac conditions More recently, analyses have used frequency transformation of RR cycle length variability to provide indices of the relative balance between parasympathetic and sympathetic activity, with the greater contribution of the parasympathetic system being considered to confer a better prognosis. In studies of postinfarction patients and patients with symptomatic arrhythmias, these indices have had some prognostic value. More recent studies of heart rate variability in patients with CHF have shown that decreases in heart rate variability are associated with worse outcomes.

De Jong MJ: Heart rate variability analysis in the assessment of autonomic function in heart failure. J Cardiovasc Nurs 2005;20:186. [PMID: 15870589]

Jouven X et al: Heart-rate profile during exercise as a predictor of sudden death. N Engl J Med 2005;352:1951. [PMID: 15888695]

Pumprla J et al: Functional assessment of heart rate variability: physiological basis and practical applications. Int J Cardiol 2002;84:1. [PMID: 12104056]

Sugiura H et al: Heart rate variability is a useful parameter for evaluation of anticholinergic effect associated with inducibility of atrial fibrillation. Pacing Clin Electrophysiol 2005; 28:1208. [PMID: 16359288]

Signal-Averaged ECG

Another technique is the **signal-averaged ECG**. Most commonly, an orthogonal three-lead system is used to record 300 consecutive beats during basal conditions. Using appropriate electrical filtering and computer averaging of the signal, very low frequency signals called "late potentials" can be identified in the period following the QRS complex. Abnormal late potentials are considered markers for potential ventricular arrhythmias. Adequate data are not yet available to define the role of this technique with confidence, but it may be useful in detecting groups of patients at increased risk for arrhythmic events after myocardial infarction. Approximately one-third of post-myocardial infarction patients will have abnormal late potentials, and these individuals are at higher risk for arrhythmic events, though the positive predictive value of this finding is relatively low (10–15%). More importantly, the absence of late potentials identifies a group of patients at low risk for arrhythmic events, so post-myocardial infarction patients found to have frequent ventricular ectopy or nonsustained ventricular tachycardia in the absence of late potentials may not require further investigation or treatment. The prognostic value of late potentials in patients with chronic ischemic heart disease who are more than 6–12 months removed from myocardial infarction and in patients with other forms of heart disease is not yet known.

Gomes JA et al: Prediction of long-term outcomes by signal-averaged electrocardiography in patients with unsustained ventricular tachycardia, coronary artery disease and left ventricular dysfunction. Circulation 2001;104:436. [PMID: 11468206]

Iravanian S et al: Role of electrophysiologic studies, signal-averaged electrocardiography, heart rate variability, T-wave alternans, and loop recorders for risk stratification of ventricular arrhythmias. Am J Geriatr Cardiol 2005;14:16. [PMID: 15654148]

Electrophysiologic Testing

Electrophysiologic testing using intracardiac ECG recordings and programmed atrial or ventricular (or both) stimulation is useful in the diagnosis and management of complex arrhythmias. The primary indications for electrophysiologic testing are (1) evaluation of recurrent syncope of possible cardiac origin, when the ambulatory ECG has not provided the diagnosis; (2) differentiation of supraventricular from ventricular arrhythmias; (3) evaluation of therapy in patients with accessory atrioventricular pathways; and (4) evaluation of patients for catheter ablation procedures or antitachycardia devices.

Autonomic Testing (Tilt-Table Testing)

In many patients with recurrent syncope or near syncope, arrhythmias are not the cause. This is particularly true when the patient has no evidence of associated heart disease by history, examination, standard ECG, or noninvasive testing. Syncope may be neurocardiogenic in origin, mediated by excessive vagal stimulation or an imbalance between sympathetic and parasympathetic autonomic activity. With assumption of upright posture, there is venous pooling in the lower limbs. However, instead of the normal response, which consists of an increase in heart rate and vasoconstriction, a sympathetically mediated increase in myocardial contractility activates mechanoreceptors that trigger reflex bradycardia and vasodilation. Autonomic testing can be an important component of the evaluation in these individuals and, if performed, should usually precede invasive electrophysiologic procedures. Carotid sinus massage in patients who do not have carotid bruits or a history of cerebral vascular disease can precipitate sinus node arrest or AV block in patients with carotid sinus hypersensitivity. Head-up tilt-table testing can identify patients whose syncope may be on a vasovagal basis. Although different testing protocols are used, passive tilting to at least 70 degrees for 10–40 minutes—in conjunction with isoproterenol infusion, if necessary—is typical. Syncope due to bradycardia, hypotension, or both will occur in approximately one-third of patients with recurrent syncope. Some recent studies have suggested that, at least with some of the more extreme protocols, false-positive responses may occur.

Fitzpatrick AP et al: Tilt methodology in reflex syncope: emerging evidence. J Am Coll Cardiol 2000;36:179. [PMID: 10898431]

Sheldon R: Tilt testing for syncope: a reappraisal. Curr Opin Cardiol 2005;20:38 [PMID: 15596958]

Antiarrhythmic Drugs (Table 10–8)

Antiarrhythmic drugs have variable efficacy and produce frequent side effects. They are often divided into classes based upon their electropharmacologic actions. Some have multiple actions. The most frequently used classification scheme is the Vaughn-Williams classification, which consists of four classes.

Class I agents block membrane sodium channels. Three subclasses are further defined by the effect of agents on the Purkinje fiber action potential. Class Ia drugs (ie, quinidine, procainamide, disopyramide,

Table 10–8. Antiarrhythmic drugs.

Agent	Intravenous Dosage	Oral Dosage	Therapeutic Plasma Level	Route of Elimination	Side Effects
Class Ia: Action: Sodium channel blockers: Depress phase 0 depolarization; slow conduction; prolong repolarization. **Indications:** Supraventricular tachycardia, ventricular tachycardia, prevention of ventricular fibrillation, symptomatic ventricular premature beats.					
Quinidine	6–10 mg/kg (intramuscularly or intravenously) over 20 min (rarely used parenterally)	200–400 mg every 4–6 h or every 8 h (long-acting)	2–5 mg/mL	Hepatic	GI, ↓LVF, ↑Dig
Procainamide	100 mg/1–3 min to 500–1000 mg; maintain at 2–6 mg/min	50 mg/kg/d in divided doses every 3–4 h or every 6 h (long-acting)	4–10 mg/mL; NAPA (active metabolite), 10–20 mcg/mL	Renal	SLE, hypersensitivity, ↓LVF
Disopyramide		100–200 mg every 6–8 h	2–8 mg/mL	Renal	Urinary retention, dry mouth, markedly ↓LVF
Moricizine		200–300 mg every 8 h	***Note:*** Active metabolites	Hepatic	Dizziness, nausea, headache, ↓theophylline level, ↓LVF
Class Ib: Action: Shorten repolarization. **Indications:** Ventricular tachycardia, prevention of ventricular fibrillation, symptomatic ventricular beats.					
Lidocaine	1–2 mg/kg at 50 mg/min; maintain at 1–4 mg/min		1–5 mg/mL	Hepatic	CNS, GI
Mexiletine		100–300 mg every 6–12 h; maximum: 1200 mg/d	0.5–2 mg/mL	Hepatic	CNS, GI, leukopenia
Phenytoin	50 mg/5 min to 1000 mg (12 mg/kg); maintain at 200–400 mg/d	200–400 mg every 12–24 h	5–20 mg/mL	Hepatic	CNS, GI
Class Ic: Action: Depress phase 0 repolarization; slow conduction. *Propafenone* is a weak calcium channel blocker and β-blocker and prolongs action potential and refractoriness. **Indications:** Life-threatening ventricular tachycardia or fibrillation, refractory supraventricular tachycardia.					
Flecainide		100–200 mg twice daily	0.2–1 mg/mL	Hepatic	CNS, GI, ↓↓LVF, incessant VT, sudden death
Propafenone		150–300 mg every 8–12 h	***Note:*** Active metabolites	Hepatic	CNS, GI, ↓↓LVF, ↑Dig
Class II: Action: β-blocker, slows AV conduction. ***Note:*** Other β-blockers may also have antiarrhythmic effects but are not yet approved for this indication in the United States. **Indications:** Supraventricular tachycardia; may prevent ventricular fibrillation.					
Esmolol	500 mcg/kg over 1–2 min; maintain at 25–200 mcg/kg/min	Other β-blockers may be used concomitantly	Not established	Hepatic	↓LVF, bronchospasm
Propranolol	1–5 mg at 1 mg/min	40–320 mg in 1–4 doses daily (depending on preparation)	Not established	Hepatic	↓LVF, bradycardia, AV block, bronchospasm
Metoprolol	2.5–5 mg	50–200 mg daily	Not established	Hepatic	↓LVF, bradycardia, AV block

(continued)

Table 10–8. Antiarrhythmic drugs. (continued)

Agent	Intravenous Dosage	Oral Dosage	Therapeutic Plasma Level	Route of Elimination	Side Effects
Class III: Action: Prolong action potential. **Indications:** *Amiodarone:* refractory ventricular tachycardia, supraventricular tachycardia, prevention of ventricular tachycardia, atrial fibrillation, ventricular fibrillation; *dofetilide:* atrial fibrillation and flutter; *sotalol:* ventricular tachycardia, atrial fibrillation; *bretylium:* ventricular fibrillation, ventricular tachycardia; *ibutilide:* conversion of atrial fibrillation and flutter.					
Amiodarone	150 mg infused rapidly, followed by 1-mg/min infusion for 6 h (360 mg) and then 0.5 mg/min; additional 150 mg as needed	800–1600 mg/d for 7–21 days; maintain at 100–400 mg/d (higher doses may be needed)	1–5 mg/mL	Hepatic	Pulmonary fibrosis, hypothyroidism, hyperthyroidism, corneal and skin deposits, hepatitis, ↑Dig, neurotoxicity, GI
Sotalol		80–160 mg every 12 h (higher doses may be used for life-threatening arrhythmias)		Renal (dosing interval should be extended if creatinine clearance is < 60 mL/min)	Early incidence of torsades de pointes, ↓LVF, bradycardia, fatigue (and other side effects associated with β-blockers)
Dofetilide		500 mg twice daily		Renal (dose must be reduced with renal dysfunction)	Torsades de pointes in 3%; interaction with cytochrome P-450 inhibitors
Ibutilide	1 mg over 10 min, followed by a second infusion of 0.5–1 mg over 10 min			Hepatic and renal	Torsades de pointes in up to 5% of patients within 3 h after administration; patients must be monitored with defibrillator nearby
Bretylium	5–10 mg/kg over 5–10 min; maintain at 0.5–2 mg/min; maximum: 30 mg/kg		0.5–1.5 mg/mL	Renal	Hypotension, nausea
Class IV: Action: Slow calcium channel blockers. **Indications:** Supraventricular tachycardia.					
Verapamil	10–20 mg over 2–20 min; maintain at 5 mg/kg/min	80–120 mg every 6–8 h; 240–360 mg once daily with sustained-release preparation	0.1–0.15 mg/mL	Hepatic	↓LVF, constipation, ↑Dig, hypotension
Diltiazem	0.25 mg/kg over 2 min; second 0.35-mg/kg bolus after 15 min if response is inadequate; infusion rate, 5–15 mg/h	180–360 mg daily in 1–3 doses depending on preparation (oral forms not approved for arrhythmias)		Hepatic metabolism, renal excretion	Hypotension, ↓LVF

(continued)

Table 10–8. Antiarrhythmic drugs. (continued)

Agent	Intravenous Dosage	Oral Dosage	Therapeutic Plasma Level	Route of Elimination	Side Effects
Miscellaneous: Indications: Supraventricular tachycardia.					
Adenosine	6 mg rapidly followed by 12 mg after 1–2 min if needed; use half these doses if administered via central line.			Adenosine receptor stimulation, metabolized in blood	Transient flushing, dyspnea, chest pain, AV block, sinus bradycardia; effect ↓ by theophylline, ↑ by dipyridamole
Digoxin	0.5 mg over 20 min followed by increment of 0.25 or 0.125 mg to 1–1.5 mg over 24 h	1–1.5 mg over 24–36 h in 3 or 4 doses; maintenance, 0.125–0.5 mg/d	0.7–2 mg/mL	Renal	AV block, arrhythmias, GI, visual changes

AV = atrioventricular; CNS = central nervous system; ↑Dig = elevation of serum digoxin level; GI = gastrointestinal (nausea, vomiting, diarrhea); ↓LVF = reduced left ventricular function; NAPA = *N*-acetylprocainamide; SLE = systemic lupus erythematosus; VT = ventricular tachycardia.

moricizine) slow the rate of rise of the action potential (V_{max}) and prolong its duration, thus slowing conduction and increasing refractoriness (moderate depression of phase 0 upstroke of the action potential). Class Ib agents (ie, lidocaine, mexiletine, tocainide, phenytoin) shorten action potential duration; they do not affect conduction or refractoriness (minimal depression of phase 0 upstroke of the action potential). Class Ic agents (ie, flecainide, propafenone) prolong V_{max} and slow repolarization, thus slowing conduction and prolonging refractoriness, but more so than class Ia drugs (maximal depression of phase 0 upstroke of the action potential).

Class II agents are the β-blockers, which decrease automaticity, prolong AV conduction, and prolong refractoriness.

Class III agents (ie, amiodarone, sotalol, dofetilide, azimilide, ibutilide) block potassium channels and prolong repolarization, widening the QRS and prolonging the QT interval. They decrease automaticity and conduction and prolong refractoriness.

Class IV agents are the calcium channel blockers, which decrease automaticity and AV conduction.

Although the in vitro electrophysiologic effects of most of these agents have been defined, their use remains largely empirical. All can exacerbate arrhythmias (proarrhythmic effect), and most depress LV function.

The risk of antiarrhythmic agents has been highlighted by the Coronary Arrhythmia Suppression Trial (CAST), in which two class Ic agents (flecainide, encainide) and a class Ia agent (moricizine) increased mortality rates in patients with asymptomatic ventricular ectopy after myocardial infarction. A similar result has been reported in the Mortality in the Survival With Oral D-sotalol (SWORD) study with D-sotalol

class III agent without the β-blocking activity of D,L-sotalol, the currently marketed formulation. Therefore, these agents (and perhaps any antiarrhythmic drug) should not be used except for life-threatening ventricular arrhythmias and symptomatic supraventricular tachyarrhythmias and patients receiving these agents should be monitored regularly.

The use of antiarrhythmic agents for specific arrhythmias is discussed below.

Cordina J et al: Pharmacological cardioversion for atrial fibrillation and flutter. Cochrane Database Syst Rev 2005;(2): CD003713. [PMID: 15846675]

Khan MH: Oral class III antiarrhythmics: what is new? Curr Opin Cardiol 2004;19:47. [PMID: 14688634]

Kowey PR et al: Classification and pharmacology of antiarrhythmic drugs. Am Heart J 2000;140:12. [PMID: 10874257]

Roden DM: Antiarrhythmic drugs: from mechanisms to clinical practice. Heart 2000;84:339. [PMID: 10956304]

Radiofrequency Ablation for Cardiac Arrhythmias

Catheter ablation techniques have become first-line therapy for treatment of many arrhythmias. This growing trend reflects the increasing ability to localize the origin or conduction pathways of many arrhythmias and safely deliver lesions to destroy the arrhythmia focus, the improved technology for delivering radiofrequency energy, and the growing dissatisfaction with the efficacy and safety of pharmacologic therapy. Ablation has become the primary modality of therapy for many symptomatic supraventricular arrhythmias, including AV nodal reentry tachycardia, reentry tachycardias involving accessory pathways, paroxysmal atrial tachycardia, inappropriate sinus tachycardia, atrial flutter and automatic junctional tachycardia. Ablation of atrial fibrillation is more complex and involves electrical isolation of the pulmonary veins, which are often the site of initiation of atrial fibrillation, or placing linear lesions within the atria to prevent spread of the rhythm. This technique has become mainstream and is considered a reasonable second-line therapy for certain patients with symptomatic atrial fibrillation. Catheter ablation of ventricular arrhythmias has proved more difficult, but experienced centers have had reasonable success with all types of ventricular tachycardias including: bundle-branch reentry, tachycardia originating in the ventricular outflow tract, tachycardias originating in the left side of the interventricular septum (also called fascicular ventricular tachycardia), and even ventricular tachycardias occurring in patients with CAD and dilated cardiomyopathy.

These procedures are generally safe, though there is a low incidence of perforation of the atria or RV that results in pericardial tamponade and sufficient damage to the AV node to require permanent cardiac pacing in less than 5% of patients. In addition, some procedures involve transseptal or retrograde LV catheterization, with the attendant potential complications of aortic perforation, damage to the heart valves, or left-sided emboli. A potentially lethal complication during the ablation of atrial fibrillation is the development of an atrio-esophageal fistula resulting from ablation lesions placed on the posterior wall of the LA just overlying the esophagus.

Oral H et al: Catheter ablation for paroxysmal atrial fibrillation: segmental pulmonary vein ostial ablation versus left atrial ablation. Circulation 2003;108:2355. [PMID: 14557355]

Pappone C et al: Atrio-esophageal fistula as a complication of percutaneous transcatheter ablation of atrial fibrillation. Circulation 2004;109:2724. [PMID: 15159294]

Saad EB et al: Ablation of atrial fibrillation. Curr Cardiol Rep 2002;4:379. [PMID: 12169234]

Wu RC et al: Catheter ablation of atrial flutter and macroreentrant atrial tachycardia. Curr Opin Cardiol 2002;17:58. [PMID: 11790935]

See also references in sections devoted to specific rhythm disturbances.

SUPRAVENTRICULAR ARRHYTHMIAS

1. Sinus Arrhythmia, Bradycardia, & Tachycardia

Sinus arrhythmia is a cyclic increase in normal heart rate with inspiration and decrease with expiration. It results from reflex changes in vagal influence on the normal pacemaker and disappears with breath holding or increase of heart rate due to any cause. It has no clinical significance. It is common in both the young and the elderly.

Sinus bradycardia is a heart rate slower than 50 beats/min due to increased vagal influence on the normal pacemaker or organic disease of the sinus node. The rate usually increases during exercise or administration of atropine. In healthy individuals, and especially in patients who are in excellent physical condition, sinus bradycardia to a rate of 50 beats/min or even lower is a normal finding. However, severe sinus bradycardia may be an indication of sinus node pathology (see below), especially in elderly patients and individuals with heart disease. It may cause weakness, confusion, or syncope if cerebral perfusion is impaired. Atrial, junctional and ventricular ectopic rhythms are more apt to occur with slow sinus rates. Pacing may be required if symptoms correlate with the bradycardia.

Sinus tachycardia is defined as a heart rate faster than 100 beats/min that is caused by rapid impulse formation from the normal pacemaker; it occurs with fever, exercise, emotion, pain, anemia, heart failure, shock, thyrotoxicosis, or in response to many drugs. Alcohol and alcohol withdrawal are common causes of sinus tachycardia and other supraventricular arrhythmias. The onset and termination are usually gradual, in contrast to paroxysmal supraventricular tachycardia due to reentry. The rate infrequently exceeds 160 beats/min but may reach 180 beats/min in young persons. The rhythm is basically regular, but serial 1-minute counts of the heart rate indicate that it varies five or more beats per minute with changes in position, with breath holding, or with sedation. Rare individuals have persistent or episodic "inappropriate" sinus tachycardia that may be very symptomatic or may lead to LV contractile dysfunction. Radiofrequency modification of the sinus node has mitigated this problem.

Still AM et al: Prevalence, characteristics and natural course of inappropriate sinus tachycardia. Europace 2005;7:104. [PMID: 15763524]

Yusuf S et al: Deciphering the sinus tachycardias. Clin Cardiol 2005;28:267. [PMID: 16028460]

2. Atrial Premature Beats (Atrial Extrasystoles)

Atrial premature beats occur when an ectopic focus in the atria fires before the next sinus node impulse or a reentry circuit is established. The contour of the P wave usually differs from the patient's normal complex, unless the ectopic focus is near the sinus node. The subsequent RR cycle length is usually unchanged or only slightly prolonged. Such premature beats occur frequently in normal hearts and are never a sufficient basis for a diagnosis of heart disease. Speeding of the heart rate by any means usually abolishes most premature beats. Early atrial premature beats may cause aberrant QRS complexes (wide and bizarre) or may be nonconducted to the ventricles because the latter are still refractory.

3. Differentiation of Aberrantly Conducted Supraventricular Beats from Ventricular Beats

This distinction can be very difficult in patients with a wide QRS complex; it is important because of the differing prognostic and therapeutic implications of each type. Findings favoring a ventricular origin include (1) AV dissociation; (2) a QRS duration exceeding 0.14 second; (3) capture or fusion beats (infrequent); (4) left axis deviation with right bundle branch block morphology; (5) monophasic (R) or biphasic (qR, QR, or RS) complexes in V_1; and (6) a qR or QS complex in V_6. Supraventricular origin is favored by (1) a triphasic QRS complex, especially if there was initial negativity in leads I and V_6; (2) ventricular rates exceeding 170 beats/min; (3) QRS duration longer than 0.12 second but not longer than 0.14 second; and (4) the presence of preexcitation syndrome.

The relationship of the P waves to the tachycardia complex is helpful. A 1:1 relationship usually means a supraventricular origin, except in the case of ventricular tachycardia with retrograde P waves.

4. Paroxysmal Supraventricular Tachycardia

This is the most common paroxysmal tachycardia and often occurs in patients without structural heart disease. Episodes begin and end abruptly and may last a few seconds to several hours or longer. The heart rate may be 140–240 beats/min (usually 160–220 beats/min) and is perfectly regular (despite exercise or change in position). The P wave usually differs in contour from sinus beats. Patients may be asymptomatic except for awareness of rapid heart action, but some experience mild chest pain or shortness of breath, especially when episodes are prolonged, even in the absence of associated cardiac abnormalities. Paroxysmal supraventricular tachycardia may result from digitalis toxicity and then is commonly associated with AV block.

The most common mechanism for paroxysmal supraventricular tachycardia is reentry, which may be initiated or terminated by a fortuitously timed atrial or ventricular premature beat. The reentry circuit most commonly involves dual pathways (a slow and a fast pathway) within the AV node. This is referred to as AV nodal reentry tachycardia (AVNRT). Less commonly, reentry is due to an accessory pathway between the atria and ventricles (AVRT). Approximately one-third of patients with supraventricular tachycardia have aberrant pathways to the ventricles. The pathophysiology and management of arrhythmias due to accessory pathways differ in important ways and are discussed separately below.

Treatment of the Acute Attack

In the absence of heart disease, serious effects are rare, and most attacks break spontaneously. Particular effort should be made to terminate the attack quickly if cardiac failure, syncope, or anginal pain develops or if there is underlying cardiac or (particularly) coronary disease. Because reentry is the most common mechanism for paroxysmal atrial tachycardia, effective therapy requires that conduction be interrupted at some

point in the reentry circuit and the majority of these circuits involve the AV node.

A. MECHANICAL MEASURES

A variety of methods have been used to interrupt attacks, and patients may learn to perform these themselves. These include Valsalva's maneuver, stretching the arms and body, lowering the head between the knees, coughing, splashing cold water on the face, and breath holding. Carotid sinus massage is often performed by physicians but should be avoided if the patient has carotid bruits or a history of transient cerebral ischemic attacks. Firm but gentle pressure and massage are applied first over the right carotid sinus for 10–20 seconds and, if unsuccessful, then over the left carotid sinus. *Pressure should not be exerted on both sides at the same time!* Continuous ECG or auscultatory monitoring of the heart rate is essential so that pressure can be relieved as soon as the rhythm is broken or if excessive bradycardia occurs. Carotid sinus pressure will interrupt up to half of the attacks, especially if the patient has received a digitalis glycoside or other agent (such as adenosine or a calcium channel blocker) that delays AV conduction. These maneuvers stimulate the vagus nerve, delay AV conduction, and block the reentry mechanism, terminating the arrhythmia.

B. DRUG THERAPY

If mechanical measures fail, two rapidly acting intravenous agents will terminate more than 90% of episodes. Intravenous adenosine has a very brief duration of action and minimal negative inotropic activity. Initially, a 6 mg bolus is administered. If no response is observed after 1–2 minutes, a second 12 mg bolus should be given, followed by a third if necessary. Because the half-life of adenosine is less than 10 seconds, the drug must be given rapidly (in 1–2 seconds from a peripheral intravenous line); use half the dose if given through a central line. Adenosine causes block of electrical conduction through the AV node. Adenosine is very well tolerated, but nearly 20% of patients will experience transient flushing, and some patients experience severe chest discomfort. Caution must be taken when adenosine is given to elderly patients because the resulting pause can be prolonged. Adenosine must also be used with caution in patients with reactive airways disease because it can promote bronchospasm.

Calcium channel blockers also rapidly induce AV block and break most episodes of reentry supraventricular tachycardia. Intravenous verapamil may be given as a 2.5 mg bolus, followed by additional doses of 2.5–5 mg every 1–3 minutes up to a total of 20 mg if blood pressure and rhythm are stable. If the rhythm recurs, further doses can be given. Oral verapamil, 80–120 mg every 4–6 hours, can be used as well in stable patients who are tolerating the rhythm without difficulty, but avoid it if there is any concern that the arrhythmia may be ventricular in origin. Intravenous diltiazem (0.25 mg/kg over 2 minutes, followed by a second bolus of 0.35 mg/kg if necessary and then an infusion of 5–15 mg/h) may cause less hypotension and myocardial depression.

Esmolol, a short-acting β-blocker, may also be effective; the initial dose is 500 mcg/kg intravenously over 1 minute followed by an infusion of 25–200 mcg/min. Metoprolol is also effective and can be given in 5 mg boluses every 5 minutes and repeated up to two times. Digoxin is effective, but it often requires several hours to safely administer an adequate dose. An initial dose of 0.5–0.75 mg intravenously over 20 minutes, followed by 0.25-mg or 0.125-mg increments every 2–4 hours up to a total of 1–1.25 mg, is used. If the tachycardia is believed to be mediated by an accessory pathway, intravenous procainamide may terminate supraventricular tachycardia by prolonging refractoriness in the accessory pathway; however, because it facilitates AVconduction and an initial increase in rate may occur, it is usually not given until after digoxin, verapamil, or a β-blocker has been administered. Although intravenous amiodarone is safe, it is usually not required and often ineffective for treatment of these arrhythmias.

C. CARDIOVERSION

If the patient is hemodynamically unstable or if adenosine and verapamil are contraindicated or ineffective, synchronized electrical cardioversion (beginning at 100 J) is almost universally successful. If digitalis toxicity is present or strongly suspected, as in the case of paroxysmal tachycardia with block, electrical cardioversion should be avoided.

Prevention of Attacks

A. RADIOFREQUENCY ABLATION

Because of concerns about the safety and the intolerability of antiarrhythmic medications, radiofrequency ablation is the preferred approach to patients with recurrent symptomatic reentry supraventricular tachycardia, whether it is due to dual pathways within the AV node or to accessory pathways.

B. DRUGS

AV nodal blocking agents are the drugs of choice as first-line medical therapy. Non-dihydropyridine calcium channel blockers, such as diltiazem and verapamil, or β-blockers are typically used first. For patients with heart failure, digoxin can be effective as initial treatment. Patients who do not respond to agents that increase refractoriness of the AV node may be treated with antiarrhythmics. The class Ic agents (flecainide, propafenone) can be used in patients without underlying structural heart disease. In patients with evidence of structural heart disease, class III agents, such as sotalol or amiodarone, are probably a better choice because of the lower incidence of ventricular proarrhythmia during long-term therapy.

Blomstrom-Lundqvist C et al; European Society of Cardiology Committee, NASPE-Heart Rhythm Society: ACC/AHA/ESC guidelines for the management of patients with supraventricular arrhythmias—executive summary. A report of the American college of cardiology/American heart association task force on practice guidelines and the European society of cardiology committee for practice guidelines (writing committee to develop guidelines for the management of patients with supraventricular arrhythmias) developed in collaboration with NASPE-Heart Rhythm Society. J Am Coll Cardiol 2003;42:1493. [PMID: 14563598]

Chauhan VS et al: Supraventricular tachycardia. Med Clin North Am 2001;85:193. [PMID: 11233946]

Hebbar AK et al: Management of common arrhythmias: Part I. Supraventricular arrhythmias. Am Fam Physician 2002;65:2479. [PMID: 12086237]

5. Supraventricular Tachycardias Due to Accessory AV Pathways (Preexcitation Syndromes)

Pathophysiology & Clinical Findings

Accessory pathways between the atria and the ventricle that avoid the conduction delay of the AV node predispose to reentry tachycardias, such as AVRT, atrial flutter, and atrial fibrillation. These may be wholly or partly within the node (Mahaim fibers), yielding a short PR interval and normal QRS morphology (**Lown-Ganong-Levine syndrome**). More commonly, they make direct connections between the atria and ventricle through Kent bundles (**Wolff-Parkinson-White syndrome**). This produces a short PR interval but an early delta wave at the onset of the wide, slurred QRS complex owing to early ventricular depolarization of the region adjacent to the pathway. Although the morphology and polarity of the delta wave can suggest the location of the bypass tract, mapping by intracardiac recordings is required for precise anatomic localization.

Accessory pathways occur in 0.1–0.3% of the population and facilitate reentry arrhythmias owing to the disparity in refractory periods of the AV node and accessory pathway. Whether the tachycardia is associated with a narrow or wide QRS complex is determined by whether antegrade conduction is through the node (narrow) or the bypass tract (wide). Many patients with Wolff-Parkinson-White syndrome never conduct in an antegrade direction through the bypass tract, which is therefore "concealed." Orthodromic tachycardia is a reentrant rhythm that conducts antegrade down the AV node and retrograde up the accessory pathway, resulting in a narrow QRS complex unless an underlying bundle branch block or interventricular conduction delay is present. Antidromic tachycardia conducts down the accessory pathway and retrograde through the AV node, resulting in a wide QRS complex. Because accessory pathways are less refractory than specialized conduction tissue, tachycardias proceeding in this direction have the potential to be more rapid. Up to 30% of patients with Wolff-Parkinson-White syndrome will develop atrial fibrillation or flutter with antegrade conduction down the accessory pathway and a rapid ventricular response.

If this conduction is very rapid, it can potentially degenerate to ventricular fibrillation

Treatment

Some patients have a delta wave found incidentally on ECG. In the absence of palpitations, light-headedness, or syncope, these patients do not require specific therapy. They should be advised to report the onset of any of these symptoms. Patients found incidentally to have delta waves who have jobs that could potentially put others at risk (ie, pilot, bus driver, etc) may need to undergo electrophysiologic testing and prophylactic catheter ablation to ensure that they are not at risk for sudden death.

A. RADIOFREQUENCY ABLATION

As with AVNRT, radiofrequency ablation has become the procedure of choice in patients with accessory pathways and recurrent symptoms. Patients with pre-excitation syndromes who have episodes of atrial fibrillation or flutter should be tested by induction of atrial fibrillation in the electrophysiologic laboratory, noting duration of the RR cycle; if it is less than 220 ms, a short refractory period is present. These individuals are at highest risk for sudden death, and prophylactic ablation is indicated. Success rates for ablation of accessory pathways with radiofrequency catheters exceed 90% in appropriate patients.

B. PHARMACOLOGIC THERAPY

Narrow-complex reentry rhythms involving a bypass tract can be managed as discussed for AVNRT. Atrial fibrillation and flutter must be managed differently, since agents such as digoxin, calcium channel blockers, and even β-blockers may decrease the refractoriness of the accessory pathway or increase that of the AV node, leading to sometimes faster ventricular rates. Therefore, these agents should be avoided. The class Ia, class Ic, and class III antiarrhythmic agents will increase the refractoriness of the bypass tract and are the drugs of choice for wide-complex tachycardias. If hemodynamic compromise is present, electrical cardioversion is warranted.

Long-term therapy often involves a combination of agents that increases refractoriness in the bypass tract (class Ia or Ic agents) and in the AV node (verapamil, digoxin, and β-blockers), provided that atrial fibrillation or flutter with short RR cycle lengths is not present (see above). The class III agents sotalol and amiodarone are effective in refractory cases. Patients who are difficult to manage should undergo electrophysiologic evaluation.

Antz M et al: Risk of sudden death after successful accessory atrioventricular pathway ablation in resuscitated patients with Wolff-Parkinson-White syndrome. J Cardiovasc Electrophysiol 2002;13:231. [PMID: 11942588]

Hamada T et al: Mechanisms for atrial fibrillation in patients with Wolff-Parkinson-White syndrome. J Cardiovasc Electrophysiol 2002;13:223. [PMID: 11942586]

Jezior MR et al: Exercise testing in Wolff-Parkinson-White syndrome: case report with ECG and literature review. Chest 2005;127:1454. [PMID: 15821231]

Keating L et al: Electrocardiographic features of Wolff-Parkinson-White syndrome. Emerg Med J 2003;20:491. [PMID: 12954704]

Pappone C et al: A randomized study of prophylactic catheter ablation in asymptomatic patients with the Wolff-Parkinson-White syndrome. N Engl J Med 2003;349:1803. [PMID: 14602878]

6. Atrial Fibrillation

Atrial fibrillation is the most common chronic arrhythmia, with an incidence and prevalence that rise with age, so that it affects nearly 10% of individuals over age 80 years. It occurs in rheumatic and other forms of valvular heart disease, dilated cardiomyopathy, ASD, hypertension, and coronary heart disease as well as in patients with no apparent cardiac disease; it may be the initial presenting sign in thyrotoxicosis, and this condition should be excluded with the initial episode. Atrial fibrillation often appears paroxysmally before becoming the established rhythm. Pericarditis, chest trauma, thoracic or cardiac surgery, or pulmonary disease (as well as medications such as theophylline and β-adrenergic agonists) may cause attacks in patients with normal hearts. Acute alcohol excess and alcohol withdrawal—and, in predisposed individuals, even consumption of small amounts of alcohol—may precipitate atrial fibrillation. This latter presentation, which is often termed "holiday heart," is usually transient and self-limited. Short-term rate control usually suffices as treatment.

Atrial fibrillation is the only common arrhythmia in which the ventricular rate is rapid and the rhythm very irregular. Because of the varying stroke volumes resulting from varying periods of diastolic filling, not all ventricular beats produce a palpable peripheral pulse. The difference between the apical rate and the pulse rate is the "pulse deficit"; this deficit is greater when the ventricular rate is high.

Atrial fibrillation itself is rarely life-threatening; however, it can have serious consequences if the ventricular rate is sufficiently rapid to precipitate hypotension, myocardial ischemia, or tachycardia-induced myocardial dysfunction. Although many patients—particularly older or inactive individuals—have relatively few symptoms if the rate is controlled, some patients are aware of the irregular rhythm and may experience it as very uncomfortable. Most patients will complain of fatigue whether they experience other symptoms or not. Perhaps the most serious consequence of atrial fibrillation is the propensity for thrombus formation due to stasis in the atria (particularly the atrial appendages) and consequent embolization, most devastatingly to the cerebral circulation. Overall, the rate of stroke is approximately five events per 100 patient-years of follow-up. However, patients with significant obstructive valvular disease, chronic heart failure or LV dysfunction, diabetes, hypertension, or age over 75 years and those with a history of prior embolic events are at substantially higher risk (up to nearly 20 events per 100 patient-years in patients with multiple risk factors) (Table 10–9). A simple score derived from the Framingham study to estimate risk of stroke is avail-

Table 10–9. Risk factors for ischemic stroke and systemic embolism in patients with nonvalvular atrial fibrillation.

Risk Factors[1]	Relative Risk
Previous stroke or TIA	2.5
Diabetes mellitus	1.7
History of hypertension	1.6
Congestive heart failure	1.4
Advanced age (continuous, per decade)	1.4

[1]Data derived from collaborative analysis of five untreated control groups in primary prevention trials. As a group, patients with nonvalvular atrial fibrillation have about a sixfold increased risk of thromboembolism compared with patients in normal sinus rhythm.

TIA = transient ischemic attack.

Reprouced, with permission from ACC/AHA/ESC 2006 guidelines for the management of patients with atrial fibrillation. ©2006, American Heart Association, Inc.

able for PDA download at http://www.statcoder.com/a-fib_stroke.htm. Patients with one or more risk factors for stroke should be treated with warfarin. Patients with none of these factors may be treated with aspirin if conditions are present that increase the risk of warfarin. While there was hope that clopidogrel and aspirin might be reasonable alternatives for warfarin for some patients, the ACTIVE trial was stopped early because of substantially lower rates of stroke with warfarin compared with clopidogrel. Anticoagulation clinics with systematic management of warfarin dosing and adjustment have been shown to result in better maintanance of target anticoagulation. Patients below the age of 60–65 years without any of these stroke risk factors ("lone atrial fibrillation") may be treated with aspirin or no antithrombotic therapy.

Newly Diagnosed Atrial Fibrillation

A. INITIAL MANAGEMENT

The approach to the initial management of atrial fibrillation depends on the clinical presentation. If, as is often the case—particularly in older individuals—the patient has no symptoms, hemodynamic instability, or evidence of important precipitating conditions (such as silent myocardial infarction or ischemia, decompensated heart failure, pulmonary embolism, or hemodynamically significant valvular disease), hospitalization is usually not necessary. In most of these cases, atrial fibrillation is an unrecognized chronic or paroxysmal condition and should be managed accordingly (see below). For new onset atrial fibrillation, thyroid function tests and assessment for occult valvular or myocardial disease should be performed.

In contrast, if the patient is hemodynamically unstable—usually as a result of a rapid ventricular rate or associated cardiac or noncardiac conditions—hospitalization and immediate treatment of atrial fibrillation are required. Urgent cardioversion is usually indicated in patients with shock or severe hypotension, pulmonary edema, or ongoing myocardial infarction or ischemia. Although if atrial fibrillation has been present for more than 48 hours, there is a potential risk of thromboembolism; however, the need for immediate rate control in these very unstable patients outweighs that risk. Electrical cardioversion is usually preferred in unstable patients. An initial shock with 100–200 J is administered in synchrony with the R wave. If sinus rhythm is not restored, an additional attempt with 360 J is indicated. If this fails, cardioversion may be successful after loading with intravenous ibutilide (1 mg over 10 minutes, repeated in 10 minutes if necessary) or intravenous procainamide (500–1000 mg administered at a rate of 20 mg/min with careful monitoring of blood pressure).

In less unstable patients or those at particularly high risk for embolism (underlying mitral stenosis, a history of prior emboli, or severe heart failure), a strategy of rate control is appropriate. A rate control strategy is appropriate both when the conditions that precipitated atrial fibrillation are likely to persist (such as following cardiac or noncardiac surgery, respiratory failure, or pericarditis) and when these conditions might resolve spontaneously over a period of hours to days (such as alcohol-induced atrial fibrillation, electrolyte or fluid imbalances, excessive exposure to theophylline or sympathomimetic agents, or some of the same previously cited conditions). The choice of agent is guided by the hemodynamic status of the patient, associated conditions, and the urgency of achieving rate control. Although both hypotension and heart failure may improve when the ventricular rate is slowed, calcium channel blockers and β-blockers may themselves precipitate hemodynamic deterioration. Digoxin is less risky, but even when used aggressively (0.5 mg intravenously over 30 minutes, followed by increments of 0.25 mg every 1–2 hours to a total dose of 1–1.5 mg over 24 hours in patients not previously receiving this agent), rate control is rather slow and may be inadequate, particularly in patients with sympathetic activation. In the setting of myocardial infarction or ischemia, β-blockers are the preferred agent. The most frequently used agents are either metoprolol (administered as a 5 mg intravenous bolus, repeated twice at intervals of 5 minutes and then given as needed by repeat boluses or orally at total daily doses of 50–400 mg) or, in very unstable patients, esmolol (0.5 mg/kg intravenously, repeated if necessary, followed by a titrated infusion of 0.05–0.2 mg/kg/min). If hypertension is present or β-blockers are contraindicated, calcium channel blockers are immediately effective. Diltiazem (20 mg bolus, repeated after 15 minutes if necessary, followed by a maintenance infusion of 5–15 mg/h) is the preferred calcium blocker if hypotension or LV dysfunction is present. Otherwise, verapamil (5–10 mg intravenously over 2–3 minutes, repeated after 30 minutes if necessary) may be used. Amiodarone, even when administered intravenously, has a relatively slow onset but is often a useful adjunct when rate control with the previously cited agents is incomplete or contraindicated or when cardioversion is planned in the near future. However, amiodarone should not be used in this setting if long-term therapy is planned with other antiarrhythmic agents.

If rate control proves unsuccessful or early cardioversion is considered necessary and the duration of atrial fibrillation exceeds 2–3 days or is unknown, a strategy of transesophageal echocardiography-guided cardioversion should be considered. By this approach, the presence of atrial thrombus is excluded and electrical cardioversion can be attempted while the patient remains under sedation. If thrombus is present, the cardioversion is delayed until after a 3- to 4-week period of therapeutic anticoagulation. In any case, because atrial contractile activity may not recover for several weeks after restoration of sinus rhythm in patients who have been in atrial fibrillation for more than several days, cardioversion is usually followed by anticoagulation for at least 1 month unless it is contraindicated.

B. Subsequent Management

Up to two-thirds of patients experiencing a first episode of atrial fibrillation will spontaneously revert to sinus rhythm within 24 hours. If atrial fibrillation persists or has been present for more than a week, spontaneous conversion is unlikely. In most cases early cardioversion is not required, so management consists of rate control and anticoagulation whether or not the patient has been admitted to hospital. Rate control is usually relatively easy to achieve with β-blockers, rate-slowing calcium blockers, and digoxin, used as single agents or more often in combination. Good rate control should consist of a ventricular rate between 50 and 100 beats/min with usual daily activities and a ventricular rate not exceeding 120 beats/min except with moderate to strenuous activity. In older patients, who often have diminished AV nodal function and relatively limited activity, this can often be achieved with a single agent. Most younger or more active individuals require a combination of two agents. Choice of the initial medication is best based on the presence of accompanying conditions: Hypertensive patients should be given β-blockers or calcium blockers; coronary patients should usually receive a β-blocker; and patients with heart failure should be given a β-blocker with consideration of adding digoxin. Adequacy of rate control should be evaluated by recording the apical pulse rate both at rest and with an appropriate level of activity (such as after brisk walking around the corridor or climbing stairs).

For patients with atrial fibrillation, even when it is paroxysmal or occurs rarely, anticoagulation with warfarin to an INR target of 2.0–3.0 should be established and maintained indefinitely, at least for patients with at least one risk factor for stroke (Table 10–9). An exception is the patient with "lone atrial fibrillation" (eg, no evidence of associated heart disease, hypertension, atherosclerotic vascular disease, or diabetes) who is under age 60 years. Cardioversion, if planned, should be performed after at least 3 weeks of anticoagulation at a therapeutic level.

C. Rate Control or Elective Cardioversion

Two recent large randomized controlled trials (the 4060-patient Atrial Fibrillation Follow-up Investigation of Rhythm Management, or AFFIRM trial; and the Rate Control Versus Electrical Cardioversion for Persistent Atrial Fibrillation, or RACE trial) compared strategies of rate control and rhythm control. In both, a strategy of rate control and long-term anticoagulation was associated with no higher rates of death or stroke—both, if anything, favored rate control—and only a modestly increased risk of hemorrhagic events than a strategy of restoring sinus rhythm and maintaining it with antiarrhythmic drug therapy. Of note is that exercise tolerance and quality of life were not significantly better in the rhythm control group. Nonetheless, the decision as to whether to attempt to restore sinus rhythm following the initial episode remains controversial. Elective cardioversion following an appropriate period of anticoagulation is generally recommended for the initial episode in patients in whom atrial fibrillation is thought to be of recent onset and when there is an identifiable precipitating factor. Similarly, cardioversion is appropriate in patients who remain symptomatic from the rhythm despite aggressive efforts to achieve rate control. However, it should be noted that even in patients for whom this is the initial episode of atrial fibrillation, the recurrence rate is sufficiently high that longer-term anticoagulation is generally appropriate until persistence of sinus rhythm can be confirmed for at least 6 months.

In cases in which elective cardioversion is required, it may be accomplished electrically (as described above) or pharmacologically. Intravenous ibutilide may also be used as described above in a setting in which the patient can undergo continuous ECG monitoring for at least 3 hours following administration. In patients in whom a decision has been made to continue antiarrhythmic therapy to maintain sinus rhythm (see next paragraph), cardioversion can be attempted with an agent that is being considered for long-term use. For instance, after therapeutic anticoagulation has been established, amiodarone can be initiated on an outpatient basis (300–400 mg twice daily for 2 weeks, followed by 200 mg twice daily for at least a 2–4 weeks and then a maintenance dose of 200 mg daily). Because amiodarone increases the prothrombin time in patients taking warfarin and digoxin levels, careful monitoring of anticoagulation and drug levels is required. Other agents that may be used for both cardioversion and maintenance therapy include propafenone (150–300 mg twice daily; should be avoided in patients with structural heart disease), flecainide (50–150 mg twice daily; should be avoided in patients with structural heart disease and should be used in conjunction with an AV nodal blocking drug if there is a history of atrial flutter), and dofetilide (0.5 mg twice daily; downward dose adjustment is required with renal dysfunction and dosing must be initiated in hospital because of risk of torsades de pointes). Sotalol (80–160 mg twice daily; should be initiated in hospital in patients with structural heart disease because of risk of torsades de pointes) is not very effective for converting atrial fibrillation but can be used to maintain sinus rhythm following cardioversion.

Unfortunately, sinus rhythm will persist in only 25% of patients who have had a sustained (lasting more than several days) or recurrent episode of atrial fibrillation. However, if the patient is treated long-term with an antiarrhythmic agent, sinus rhythm will persist in approximately 50%. The most commonly used medications are amiodarone, sotalol, propafenone, flecainide, and dofetilide, but the latter four agents are associated with a clear risk of proarrhythmia, and amiodarone frequently causes other adverse effects. Therefore, it may be prudent to determine whether atrial fibrillation recurs during a period of 6 months without antiarrhythmic drugs during which anticoagulation is maintained. If it does recur, the decision as to whether to restore sinus rhythm and initiate long-term antiarrhythmic therapy can be based on how well the patient tolerates atrial fibrillation. In such a patient, long-term anticoagulation is probably indicated in any case, because of the high rate of recurrence and the likely occurrence of asymptomatic paroxysmal episodes.

Paroxysmal & Refractory Atrial Fibrillation

A. RECURRENT PAROXYSMAL ATRIAL FIBRILLATION

It is now well established that patients with recurrent paroxysmal atrial fibrillation are at similar stroke risk as those who are in atrial fibrillation chronically. Although these episodes may be apparent to the patient, many are not recognized and may be totally asymptomatic. Thus, ambulatory ECG monitoring or event recorders are indicated in those in whom paroxysmal atrial fibrillation is suspected. Antiarrhythmic agents are usually not successful in preventing all paroxysmal atrial fibrillation episodes. However, dofetilide has been shown to be as effective as amiodarone in maintaining sinus rhythm in certain patients and does not have as many untoward effects. Long-term anticoagulation is indicated except in those who are under 60–65 years of age and have no additional stroke risk factors (see above).

B. REFRACTORY ATRIAL FIBRILLATION

Because of trial results indicating that important adverse clinical outcomes (death, stroke, hemorrhage, heart failure) are no more common with rate control than rhythm control, atrial fibrillation should generally be considered refractory if it causes persistent symptoms or limits activity. This is much more likely in younger individuals and those who are very active or engage in strenuous exercise. Even in such individuals, two-drug or three-drug combinations of a β-blocker, rate-slowing calcium blocker, and digoxin usually can prevent excessive ventricular rates, though in some cases they are associated with excessive bradycardia during sedentary periods.

If no drug works, radiofrequency AV node ablation and permanent pacing ensure rate control and may facilitate a more physiologic rate response to activity, but this is used only as a last resort. There is growing experience with focal ablation of foci in and around the pulmonary veins that initiate atrial fibrillation, following which sinus rhythm may be restored or maintained. This therapy has become more widely accepted and is a reasonable second-line therapy for individuals with symptomatic atrial fibrillation that is refractory to pharmacologic therapy. This procedure is routinely performed in the electrophysiology laboratory using a catheter-based approach and can also be performed thorascopically in the operating room by experienced surgeons.

Aasbo JD et al: Amiodarone prophylaxis reduces major cardiovascular morbidity and length of stay after cardiac surgery: a meta-analysis. Ann Intern Med 2005;143:327. [PMID: 16144891]

Corley SD et al; AFFIRM Investigators: Relationships between sinus rhythm, treatment, and survival in the Atrial Fibrillation Follow-Up Investigation of Rhythm Management (AFFIRM) Study. Circulation 2004;109:1509. [PMID: 15007003]

Daoud EG: Management of atrial fibrillation in the post-cardiac surgery setting. Cardiol Clin 2004;22:159. [PMID: 14994855]

de Denus S et al: Rate vs rhythm control in patients with atrial fibrillation: a meta-analysis. Arch Intern Med 2005;165:258. [PMID: 15710787]

Fang MC et al: Anticoagulation for atrial fibrillation. Cardiol Clin 2004;22:47. [PMID: 14994847]

Finta B et al: Catheter ablation therapy for atrial fibrillation. Cardiol Clin 2004;22:127. [PMID: 14994853]

Gage BF et al: Selecting patients with atrial fibrillation for anticoagulation: stroke risk stratification in patients taking aspirin. Circulation 2004;110:2287. [PMID: 15477396]

Gillinov AM et al: Advances in the surgical treatment of atrial fibrillation. Cardiol Clin 2004;22:147. [PMID: 14994854]

Joglar JA et al: Electrical cardioversion of atrial fibrillation. Cardiol Clin 2004;22:101. [PMID: 14994851]

McKeown PP et al; American College of Chest Physicians: Executive summary: American College of Chest Physicians guidelines for the prevention and management of postoperative atrial fibrillation after cardiac surgery. Chest 2005;128(2 Suppl):1S. [PMID: 16167657]

McNamara RL et al: Management of atrial fibrillation: review of the evidence for the role of pharmacologic therapy, electrical cardioversion, and echocardiography. Ann Intern Med 2003;139:1018. [PMID: 14678922]

Rockson SG et al: Comparing the guidelines: anticoagulation therapy to optimize stroke prevention in patients with atrial fibrillation. J Am Coll Cardiol 2004;43:929. [PMID: 15028346]

Singh BN et al; Sotalol Amiodarone Atrial Fibrillation Efficacy Trial (SAFE-T) Investigators: Amiodarone versus sotalol for atrial fibrillation. N Engl J Med 2005;352:1861. [PMID: 15872201]

Tamariz LJ et al: Pharmacological rate control of atrial fibrillation. Cardiol Clin 2004;22:35. [PMID: 14994846]

VerNooy RA et al: Antiarrhythmic drug therapy of atrial fibrillation. Cardiol Clin 2004;22:21. [PMID: 14994845]

Wang TJ et al: A risk score for predicting stroke or death for individuals with new-onset atrial fibrillation in the community: the Framingham Heart Study. JAMA 2003;290:1049. [PMID: 12941677]

Wazni OM et al: Radiofrequency ablation vs antiarrhythmic drugs as first-line treatment of symptomatic atrial fibrillation: a randomized trial. JAMA 2005;293:2634. [PMID: 15928285]

Wijffels MC et al: Rate versus rhythm control in atrial fibrillation. Cardiol Clin 2004;22:63. [PMID: 14994848]

7. Atrial Flutter

Atrial flutter is less common than fibrillation. It occurs most often in patients with chronic obstructive pulmonary disease (COPD) but may be seen also in those with rheumatic or coronary heart disease, CHF, ASD, or surgically repaired congenital heart disease. Ectopic impulse formation occurs at atrial rates of 250–350 beats/min, with transmission of every second, third, or fourth impulse through the AV node to the ventricles. Ventricular rate control is accomplished using the same agents used in atrial fibrillation, but it is much more difficult with atrial flutter than with atrial fibrillation. Conversion of atrial flutter to sinus rhythm with class I antiarrhythmic agents is also difficult to achieve, and administration of these drugs has been associated with slowing of the atrial flutter rate to the point at which 1:1 AV conduction can occur at rates in excess of 200 beats/min, with subsequent hemodynamic collapse. The intravenous class III antiarrhythmic agent ibutilide has been significantly more successful in converting atrial flutter. About 50–70% of patients return to sinus rhythm within 60–90 minutes following the infusion of 1–2 mg of this agent. Electrical cardioversion is also very effective for atrial flutter, with approximately 90% of patients converting following shocks of as little as 25–50 J.

The persistence of atrial contractile function in this arrhythmia provides some protection against thrombus formation, though the risk of systemic embolization remains increased. Precardioversion anticoagulation is not necessary for atrial flutter of less than 48 hours duration except in the setting of mitral valve disease. However, anticoagulation is prudent in chronic atrial flutter, particularly since transient periods of atrial fibrillation are common in these patients.

Chronic atrial flutter is often a difficult management problem, as rate control is difficult. If pharmacologic therapy is chosen, amiodarone and dofetilide are the antiarrhythmics of choice. Dofetilide is often given in conjunction with an AV nodal blocker.

Atrial flutter can follow a typical or atypical reentry circuit around the atrium. The anatomy of the typical circuit has been well defined and allows for catheter ablation within the atrium to interrupt the circuit and eliminate atrial flutter. Catheter ablation has become the preferred treatment for recurrent typical atrial flutter.

Ghali WA et al: Atrial flutter and the risk of thromboembolism: a systematic review and meta-analysis. Am J Med 2005;118: 101. [PMID: 15694889]

Lee KW et al: Atrial flutter: a review of its history, mechanisms, clinical features, and current therapy. Curr Probl Cardiol 2005;30:121. [PMID: 15711509]

Knight BP et al; American Heart Association Council on Clinical Cardiology (Subcommittee on Electrocardiography and Arrhythmias); Quality of Care and Outcomes Research Interdisciplinary Working Group; Heart Rhythm Society; AHA Writing Group: Role of permanent pacing to prevent atrial fibrillation: science advisory from the American Heart Association Council on Clinical Cardiology (Subcommittee on Electrocardiography and Arrhythmias) and the Quality of Care and Outcomes Research Interdisciplinary Working Group, in collaboration with the Heart Rhythm Society. Circulation 2005;111: 240. [PMID: 15657388]

Sun JL et al: Clinical comparison of ibutilide and propafenone for converting atrial flutter. Cardiovasc Drugs Ther 2005;19:57. [PMID: 15883757]

Wu RC et al: Catheter ablation of atrial flutter and macroreentrant atrial tachycardia. Curr Opin Cardiol 2002;17:58. [PMID: 11790935]

8. Multifocal (Chaotic) Atrial Tachycardia

This is a rhythm characterized by varying P wave morphology (by definition, three or more foci) and markedly irregular PP intervals. The rate is usually between 100 and 140 beats/min, and AV block is unusual. Most patients have severe associated COPD. Treatment of the underlying condition is the most effective approach; verapamil, 240–480 mg daily in divided doses, is also of value in some patients, but this particular arrhythmia is very difficult to manage.

Spodick DH: Multifocal atrial arrhythmia. Am J Geriatr Cardiol 2005;14:162. [PMID: 15886545]

9. AV Junctional Rhythm

The atrial-nodal junction or the nodal-His bundle junctions may assume pacemaker activity for the heart, usually at a rate of 40–60 beats/min. This may occur in patients with myocarditis, CAD, and digitalis toxicity as well as in individuals with normal hearts. The rate responds normally to exercise, and the diagnosis is often an incidental finding on ECG monitoring, but it can be suspected if the jugular venous pulse shows cannon *a* waves. Junctional rhythm is often an escape rhythm because of depressed sinus node function with sinoatrial block or delayed conduction in the AV node. **Nonparoxysmal junctional tachycardia** results from increased automaticity of the junctional tissues in digitalis toxicity or ischemia and is associated with a narrow QRS complex and a rate usually less than 120–130 beats/min. It is usually considered benign when it occurs in acute myocardial infarction, but the ischemia that induces it may also cause ventricular tachycardia and ventricular fibrillation.

VENTRICULAR ARRHYTHMIAS

1. Ventricular Premature Beats (Ventricular Extrasystoles)

Ventricular premature beats are characterized by wide QRS complexes that differ in morphology from the patient's normal beats. They are usually not preceded by a P wave, although retrograde ventriculoatrial conduction may occur. Unless the latter is present, there is a fully compensatory pause (ie, without change in the PP interval). Bigeminy and trigeminy are arrhythmias in which every second or third beat is premature; these patterns confirm a reentry mechanism for the ectopic beat. Exercise generally abolishes premature beats in normal hearts, and the rhythm becomes regular. The patient may or may not sense the irregular beat, usually as a skipped beat. Ambulatory ECG monitoring or monitoring during graded exercise may reveal more frequent and complex ventricular premature beats than occur in a single routine ECG. An increased frequency of ventricular premature beats during exercise is associated with a higher risk of cardiovascular mortality, though there is no evidence that specific therapy has a role.

Sudden death occurs more frequently (presumably as a result of ventricular fibrillation) when ventricular premature beats occur in the presence of organic heart disease but not in individuals with no known cardiac disease. If no associated cardiac disease is present and if the ectopic beats are asymptomatic, no therapy is indicated. If they are frequent, electrolyte abnormalities (especially hypokalemia or hyperkalemia and hypomagnesemia), hyperthyroidism, and occult heart disease should be excluded. Pharmacologic treatment is indicated only for patients who are symptomatic. Because of concerns about worsening arrhythmia and sudden death with most antiarrhythmic agents, β-blockers are the agents of first choice. If the underlying condition is mitral prolapse, hypertrophic cardiomyopathy, LVH, or coronary disease—or if the QT interval is prolonged—β-blocker therapy is appropriate. The class I and III agents (see Table 10–8) are all effective in reducing ventricular premature beats but often cause side effects and may exacerbate serious arrhythmias in 5–20% of patients. Therefore, every attempt should be made to avoid using class I or III antiarrhythmic agents in patients without symptoms.

Conti CR: Ventricular arrhythmias: a general cardiologist's assessment of therapies in 2005. Clin Cardiol 2005;28:314. [PMID: 16075822]

Morshedi-Meibodi A et al: Clinical correlates and prognostic significance of exercise-induced ventricular premature beats in the community: the Framingham Heart Study. Circulation 2004;109:2417. [PMID: 15148273]

O'Neill JO et al: Severe frequent ventricular ectopy after exercise as a predictor of death in patients with heart failure. J Am Coll Cardiol 2004;44:820. [PMID: 15312865]

2. Ventricular Tachycardia

Ventricular tachycardia is defined as three or more consecutive ventricular premature beats. The usual rate is 160–240 beats/min and is moderately regular but less so than atrial tachycardia. The distinction from aberrant conduction of supraventricular tachycardia may be difficult. The usual mechanism is reentry, but abnormally triggered rhythms occur. Ventricular tachycardia is either nonsustained (lasting less than 30 seconds) or sustained. It may be asymptomatic or associated with syncope or milder symptoms of impaired cerebral perfusion.

Ventricular tachycardia is a frequent complication of acute myocardial infarction and dilated cardiomyopathy but may occur in chronic coronary disease, hypertrophic cardiomyopathy, mitral valve prolapse, myocarditis, and in most other forms of myocardial disease. **Torsades de pointes**, a form of ventricular tachycardia in which QRS morphology twists around the baseline, may occur spontaneously in the setting of hypokalemia or hypomagnesemia or after any drug that prolongs the QT interval; it has a particularly poor prognosis. In nonacute settings, most patients with ventricular tachycardia have known or easily detectable cardiac disease, and the finding of ventricular tachycardia is an unfavorable prognostic sign.

Treatment

A. ACUTE VENTRICULAR TACHYCARDIA

The treatment of acute ventricular tachycardia is determined by the degree of hemodynamic compromise and the duration of the arrhythmia. The management of ventricular tachycardia in acute infarction has been discussed. In other patients, if ventricular tachycardia causes hypotension, heart failure, or myocardial ischemia, synchronized DC cardioversion with 100–360 J should be performed immediately. If the patient is tolerating the rhythm, lidocaine, 1 mg/kg as an intravenous bolus injection, or amiodarone 150 mg as a slow intravenous bolus over 10 minutes, followed by a slow infusion of 1 mg/min for 6 hours and then a maintenance infusion of 0.5 mg/min for an additional 18–42 hours can be used. If the ventricular tachycardia recurs, supplemental amiodarone infusions of 150 mg over 10 minutes can be given. If the patient is stable, intravenous procainamide, 20 mg/min intravenously (up to 1000 mg), followed by an infusion of 20–80 mcg/kg/min could also be tried. Empiric magnesium replacement (1 g intravenously) may help. Ventricular tachycardia can also be terminated by ventricular overdrive pacing, and this approach is useful when the rhythm is recurrent.

B. CHRONIC RECURRENT VENTRICULAR TACHYCARDIA

1. Sustained ventricular tachycardia—Patients with symptomatic or sustained ventricular tachycardia in the absence of a reversible precipitating cause (acute myocardial infarction or ischemia, electrolyte imbalance, drug toxicity, etc) are at high risk for recurrence. In those with significant LV dysfunction, subsequent sudden death is common. Several trials, including the Antiarrhythmic Drug Versus Implantable Defibrillator (AVID) and the Canadian Implantable Defibrillator trials, strongly suggest that these patients should be managed with implantable cardioverter-defibrillator devices (ICDs). In those with preserved LV function, the mortality rate is lower and the etiology is often different than in those with depressed ventricular function. Treatment with amiodarone, optimally in combination with a β-blocker, may be adequate. Sotalol may be an alternative, though there is less supporting evidence. However, many times if ventricular tachycardia occurs in a patient with preserved ventricular function, it is either an outflow tract tachycardia or a fascicular ventricular tachycardia, and these arrhythmias will often respond to AV nodal blockers and can be effectively treated with catheter ablation. The role of electrophysiologic studies in this group is less clear than was previously thought, but they may help identify patients who are candidates for radiofrequency ablation of a ventricular tachycardia focus. This is particularly the case for arrhythmias that originate in the RV outflow tract (appearing as left bundle branch block with inferior axis on the surface ECG), the posterior fascicle (right bundle branch block, superior axis morphology), or sustained bundle branch reentry. Catheter ablation can be used as a palliative therapy for those patients with recurrent tachycardia who receive ICD shocks despite antiarrhythmic therapy.

2. Nonsustained ventricular tachycardia (NSVT)— NSVT is defined as runs of three or more ventricular beats lasting less than 30 seconds. These may be symptomatic (usually experienced as light-headedness) or asymptomatic. In individuals without heart disease, NSVT is not clearly associated with a poor prognosis. However, in patients with structural heart disease, particularly when they have reduced EFs, there is an increased risk of subsequent symptomatic ventricular tachycardia or sudden death. β-Blockers reduce these risks in patients who have coronary disease with significant LV systolic dysfunction (EFs < 35–40%), but if sustained ventricular tachycardia has been induced during electrophysiologic testing, an implantable defibrillator may be indicated. In patients with chronic heart failure and reduced EFs—whether due to coronary disease or primary cardiomyopathy and regardless of the presence of asymptomatic ventricular arrhythmias—β-blockers reduce the incidence of sudden death by 40–50% and should be routine therapy (see section on Heart Failure).

Although there are no definitive data with amiodarone in this group, trends from a number of studies suggest that it may be beneficial. Other antiarrhythmic agents should generally be avoided because their proarrhythmic risk appears to outweigh any benefit, even in patients with inducible arrhythmias

that are successfully suppressed in the electrophysiology laboratory.

Brodsky MA et al: Prognostic value of baseline electrophysiology studies in patients with sustained ventricular tachyarrhythmia: the Antiarrhythmics Versus Implantable Defibrillators (AVID) trial. Am Heart J 2002;144:478. [PMID: 12228785]

Ermis C et al: Comparison of ventricular arrhythmia frequency in patients with ischemic cardiomyopathy versus nonischemic cardiomyopathy treated with implantable cardioverter defibrillators. Am J Cardiol 2005;96:233. [PMID: 16018849]

Kadish A et al; Defibrillators in Non-Ischemic Cardiomyopathy Treatment Evaluation (DEFINITE) Investigators: Prophylactic defibrillator implantation in patients with nonischemic dilated cardiomyopathy. N Engl J Med 2004;350: 2151. [PMID: 15152060]

Katritsis DG et al: Nonsustained ventricular tachycardia: where do we stand? Eur Heart J 2004;25:1093. [PMID: 15231366]

Klein RC et al: Analysis of implantable cardioverter defibrillator therapy in the Antiarrhythmics Versus Implantable Defibrillators (AVID) Trial. J Cardiovasc Electrophysiol 2003;14: 940. [PMID: 12950538]

Sarkozy A et al: Advances in the acute pharmacologic management of cardiac arrhythmias. Curr Cardiol Rep 2003;5:387. [PMID: 12917054]

Wall TS et al: Ventricular tachycardia in structurally normal hearts. Curr Cardiol Rep 2002;4:388. [PMID: 12169235]

Wietholt D et al: Prevention of sustained ventricular tachyarrhythmias in patients with implantable cardioverter-defibrillators—the PREVENT study. J Interv Card Electrophysiol 2003;9:383. [PMID: 14618061]

Zimetbaum PJ et al: Electrocardiographic predictors of arrhythmic death and total mortality in the multicenter unsustained tachycardia trial. Circulation 2004;110:766. [PMID: 15289365]

3. Ventricular Fibrillation & Sudden Death

Sudden cardiac death is defined as unexpected nontraumatic death in clinically well or stable patients who die within 1 hour after onset of symptoms. The causative rhythm in most cases is ventricular fibrillation, which is usually preceded by ventricular tachycardia except in the setting of acute ischemia or infarction. Complete heart block and sinus node arrest may also cause sudden death. A disproportionate number of sudden deaths occur in the early morning hours. Over 75% of victims of sudden cardiac death have severe CAD. Many have old infarctions. Sudden death may be the initial manifestation of coronary disease in up to 20% of patients and accounts for approximately 50% of deaths from coronary disease. When ventricular fibrillation occurs in the initial 24 hours after infarction, long-term management is no different from that of other patients with acute infarction. Other conditions that predispose to sudden death include severe LVH, hypertrophic cardiomyopathy, congestive cardiomyopathy, aortic stenosis, pulmonary stenosis, primary pulmonary hypertension, cyanotic congenital heart disease, atrial myxoma, mitral valve prolapse, hypoxia, electrolyte abnormalities, prolonged QT interval syndrome, the Brugada syndrome and conduction system disease. Late potentials (after the QRS complex) on a signal-averaged surface ECG in patients with prior myocardial infarction may identify a group of patients at risk for ventricular arrhythmias and sudden death.

Unless ventricular fibrillation occurred shortly after myocardial infarction, is associated with ischemia, or is seen with an unusual correctable process (such as an electrolyte abnormality, drug toxicity, or aortic stenosis), surviving patients require evaluation and intervention since recurrences are frequent. Exercise testing or coronary arteriography should be performed to exclude coronary disease as the underlying cause, since revascularization may prevent recurrence. Conduction disturbances should be managed as described in the next section. If prodromal supraventricular arrhythmias or ventricular arrhythmias, such as sustained or nonsustained ventricular tachycardia, are found by ambulatory ECG monitoring, their elimination by pharmacologic therapy or ablation may prevent further episodes. There is growing consensus that if myocardial infarction or ischemia, other precipitating causes of ventricular fibrillation, or bradyarrhythmias and conduction disturbances are not found to be the cause of the sudden death episode, an implantable defibrillator is the treatment of choice for appropriate patients. In addition, evidence from the MADIT II study and Sudden Cardiac Death in Heart Failure Trial (SCD-HeFT) suggest that patients with severe LV dysfunction—whether due to an ischemic cause such as a remote myocardial infarction or a nonischemic cause of advanced heart failure—have a reduced risk of death with the prophylactic implantation of a implantable cardioverter-defibrillator. However, there is also evidence that implanting prophylactic ICDs in patients early after myocardial infarction is associated with a trend toward worse outcomes.

ACC/AHA/NASPE 2002 guideline update for implantation of cardiac pacemakers and antiarrhythmia devices: summary article. J Am Coll Cardiol 2002;40:1703. [PMID: 12427427]

Bardy GH et al; Sudden Cardiac Death in Heart Failure Trial (SCD-HeFT) Investigators. Amiodarone or an implantable cardioverter-defibrillator for congestive heart failure. N Engl J Med 2005;352:225. Erratum in: N Engl J Med 2005;352:2146. [PMID: 15659722]

Bokhari F et al: Long-term comparison of the implantable cardioverter defibrillator versus amiodarone: eleven-year follow-up of a subset of patients in the Canadian Implantable Defibrillator Study (CIDS). Circulation 2004;110:112. [PMID: 15238454]

Brodine WN et al; MADIT-II Research Group: Effects of beta-blockers on implantable cardioverter defibrillator therapy and survival in the patients with ischemic cardiomyopathy (from the Multicenter Automatic Defibrillator Implantation Trial-II). Am J Cardiol 2005;96:691. [PMID: 16125497]

Dorian P et al: Amiodarone as compared with lidocaine for shock-resistant ventricular fibrillation. N Engl J Med 2002; 346:884. [PMID: 11907287]

Eckardt L et al: Long-term prognosis of individuals with right precordial ST-segment-elevation Brugada syndrome. Circulation 2005;111:257. [PMID: 15642768]

Hohnloser SH et al; DINAMIT Investigators: Prophylactic use of an implantable cardioverter-defibrillator after acute myocardial infarction. N Engl J Med 2004;351:2481. [PMID: 15590950]

Kadish A et al; Defibrillators in Non-Ischemic Cardiomyopathy Treatment Evaluation (DEFINITE) Investigators: Prophylactic defibrillator implantation in patients with nonischemic dilated cardiomyopathy. N Engl J Med 2004;350: 2151. [PMID: 15152060]

Klein RC et al: Analysis of implantable cardioverter defibrillator therapy in the Antiarrhythmics Versus Implantable Defibrillators (AVID) Trial. J Cardiovasc Electrophysiol 2003;14: 940. [PMID: 12950538]

Moss AJ: Prophylactic implantation of a defibrillator in patients with myocardial infarction and reduced ejection fraction. N Engl J Med 2002;346:877. [PMID: 11907286]

Sanders GD et al: Cost-effectiveness of implantable cardioverter-defibrillators. N Engl J Med 2005;353:1471. [PMID: 16207849]

Wilde AA et al: Proposed diagnostic criteria for the Brugada syndrome: consensus report. Circulation 2002;106:2514. [PMID: 12417552]

4. Accelerated Idioventricular Rhythm

Accelerated idioventricular rhythm is a regular wide complex rhythm with a rate of 60–120 beats/min, usually with a gradual onset. Because the rate is often similar to the sinus rate, fusion beats and alternating rhythms are common. Two mechanisms have been invoked: (1) an escape rhythm due to suppression of higher pacemakers resulting from sinoatrial and AV block or from depressed sinus node function; and (2) slow ventricular tachycardia due to increased automaticity or, less frequently, reentry. It occurs commonly in acute infarction and following reperfusion after thrombolytic drugs. The incidence of associated ventricular fibrillation is much less than that of ventricular tachycardia with a rapid rate, and treatment is not indicated unless there is hemodynamic compromise or more serious arrhythmias. This rhythm also is common in digitalis toxicity.

Accelerated idioventricular rhythm must be distinguished from the idioventricular or junctional rhythm with rates less than 40–45 beats/min that occurs in the presence of complete AV block. AV dissociation—where ventricular rate exceeds sinus—but not AV block occurs in most cases of accelerated idioventricular rhythm.

5. Long QT Syndrome

Congenital long QT syndrome is an uncommon disease that is characterized by recurrent syncope, a long QT interval (usually 0.5–0.7 second), documented ventricular arrhythmias, and sudden death. It may occur in the presence (Jervell syndrome, Lange-Nielsen syndrome) or absence (Romano-Ward syndrome) of congenital deafness. Inheritance may be autosomal recessive or autosomal dominant (Romano-Ward). Specific genetic mutations affecting membrane potassium and sodium channels have been identified and help delineate the mechanisms of susceptibility to arrhythmia.

Because this is a primary electrical disorder, usually with no evidence of structural heart disease or LV dysfunction, the long-term prognosis is excellent if arrhythmia is controlled. Long-term treatment with β-blockers, permanent pacing, or left cervicothoracic sympathectomy is frequently effective. ICD implantation is recommended for patients in whom recurrent syncope, sustained ventricular arrhythmias, or sudden cardiac death occurs despite drug therapy. The ICD should be considered as primary therapy in certain patients, such as those in whom aborted sudden cardiac death is the initial presentation of the long-QT syndrome, when there is a strong family history of sudden cardiac death, or when compliance or intolerance to drugs is a concern.

Acquired long QT interval secondary to use of antiarrhythmic agents or antidepressant drugs, electrolyte abnormalities, myocardial ischemia, or significant bradycardia may result in ventricular tachycardia (particularly torsades de pointes, ie, twisting about the baseline into varying QRS morphology). Notably, many drugs that are in some settings effective for the treatment of ventricular arrhythmias prolong the QT interval. Prudence dictates that drug therapy that prolongs the QT interval beyond 500 ms be discontinued.

The management of **torsades de pointes** differs from that of other forms of ventricular tachycardia. Class I, Ic, or III antiarrhythmics, which prolong the QT interval, should be avoided—or withdrawn immediately if being used. Intravenous β-blockers may be effective, especially in the congenital form; intravenous magnesium should be given acutely. An effective approach is temporary ventricular or atrial pacing, which can both break and prevent the rhythm.

Chiang CE: Congenital and acquired long QT syndrome. Current concepts and management. Cardiol Rev 2004;12:222. [PMID: 15191637]

Goldenberg I et al: Sudden cardiac death without structural heart disease: update on the long QT and Brugada syndromes. Curr Cardiol Rep 2005;7:349. [PMID: 16105490]

Monnig G et al: Implantable cardioverter-defibrillator therapy in patients with congenital long-QT syndrome: a long-term follow-up. Heart Rhythm 2005;2:497.[PMID: 15840474]

Passman R et al: Polymorphic ventricular tachycardia, long Q-T syndrome, and torsades de pointes. Med Clin North Am 2001;85:321. [PMID: 11233951]

Priori SG et al: Association of long QT syndrome loci and cardiac events among patients treated with beta-blockers. JAMA 2004;292:1341. [PMID: 15367556]

Wehrens XH et al: Novel insights in the congenital long QT syndrome. Ann Intern Med 2002;137:981. [PMID: 12484714]

Welde AA: Is there a role for implantable cardioverter defibrillators in long QT syndrome? J Cardiovasc Electrophysiol 2002;13(1 Suppl):S110. [PMID: 11852886]

■ BRADYCARDIAS & CONDUCTION DISTURBANCES

Abnormalities of conduction can occur between the sinus node and atrium, within the AV node, and in the intraventricular conduction pathways.

SICK SINUS SYNDROME

This imprecise diagnosis is applied to patients with sinus arrest, sinoatrial exit block (recognized by a pause equal to a multiple of the underlying PP interval or progressive shortening of the PP interval prior to a pause), or persistent sinus bradycardia. These rhythms are often caused or exacerbated by drug therapy (digitalis, calcium channel blockers, β-blockers, sympatholytic agents, antiarrhythmics), and agents that may be responsible should be withdrawn prior to making the diagnosis. Another presentation is of recurrent supraventricular tachycardias (paroxysmal re-entry tachycardias, atrial flutter, and atrial fibrillation), associated with bradyarrhythmias ("tachy-brady syndrome"). The long pauses that often follow the termination of tachycardia cause the associated symptoms.

Sick sinus syndrome occurs most commonly in elderly patients. The pathologic changes are usually nonspecific, characterized by patchy fibrosis of the sinus node and cardiac conduction system. Sick sinus syndrome may be caused by other conditions, including sarcoidosis, amyloidosis, Chagas' disease, and various cardiomyopathies. Coronary disease is an uncommon cause.

Most patients with ECG evidence of sick sinus syndrome are asymptomatic, but rare individuals may experience syncope, dizziness, confusion, palpitations, heart failure, or angina. Because these symptoms are either nonspecific or are due to other causes, it is essential that they be demonstrated to coincide temporally with arrhythmias. This may require prolonged ambulatory monitoring or the use of an event recorder. Pharmacologic therapy for sick sinus syndrome has been difficult, but recent studies have indicated that oral theophylline may be effective, especially when sinus bradycardia is the major manifestation. Most symptomatic patients will require permanent pacing. Dual-chamber pacing is preferred because ventricular pacing is associated with a higher incidence of subsequent atrial fibrillation, and subsequent atrioventricular block occurs at a rate of 2% per year. Treatment of associated tachyarrhythmias is often difficult without first instituting pacing, since digoxin and other antiarrhythmic agents may exacerbate the bradycardia. Unfortunately, symptomatic relief following pacing has not been consistent, largely because of inadequate documentation of the etiologic role of bradyarrhythmias in producing the symptom. Furthermore, many of these patients may have associated ventricular arrhythmias that may require treatment; however, carefully selected patients may become asymptomatic with permanent pacing alone.

Adan V et al: Diagnosis and treatment of sick sinus syndrome. Am Fam Physician 2003;67:1725. [PMID: 12725451]

Brignole M: Sick sinus syndrome. Clin Geriatr Med 2002;18: 211. [PMID: 12180244]

Dretzke J et al: Dual chamber versus single chamber ventricular pacemakers for sick sinus syndrome and atrioventricular block. Cochrane Database Syst Rev 2004;(2):CD003710. [PMID: 15106214]

Lamas GA et al: Quality of life and clinical outcomes in elderly patients treated with ventricular pacing as compared with dual-chamber pacing. Pacemaker Selection in the Elderly Investigators. N Engl J Med 1998;338:1097. [PMID: 9545357]

AV BLOCK

AV block is categorized as first-degree (PR interval > 0.21 second with all atrial impulses conducted), second-degree (intermittent blocked beats), or third-degree (complete heart block, in which no supraventricular impulses are conducted to the ventricles).

Second-degree block is subclassified. In **Mobitz type I (Wenckebach)** AV block, the AV conduction time (PR interval) progressively lengthens, with the RR interval shortening, before the blocked beat; this phenomenon is almost always due to abnormal conduction within the AV node. In **Mobitz type II** AV block, there are intermittently nonconducted atrial beats not preceded by lengthening AV conduction. It is usually due to block within the His bundle system. The classification as Mobitz type I or Mobitz type II is only partially reliable because patients may appear to have both types on the surface ECG, and the site of origin of the 2:1 AV block cannot be predicted from the ECG. The width of the QRS complexes assists in determining whether the block is nodal or infranodal. When they are narrow, the block is usually nodal; when they are wide, the block is usually infranodal. Electrophysiologic studies may be necessary for accurate localization. Management of AV block in acute myocardial infarction has already been discussed. This section deals with patients in the nonischemic setting.

First-degree and **Mobitz type I block** may occur in normal individuals with heightened vagal tone. They may also occur as a drug effect (especially digitalis, calcium channel blockers, β-blockers, or other sympatholytic agents), often superimposed on organic disease. These disturbances also occur transiently or chronically due to ischemia, infarction, inflammatory processes, fibrosis, calcification, or infiltration. The prognosis is usually good, since reliable alternative pacemakers arise from the AV junction below the level of block if higher degrees of block occur.

Mobitz type II block is almost always due to organic disease involving the infranodal conduction system. In the event of progression to complete heart block, alternative pacemakers are not reliable. Thus, prophylactic ventricular pacing is required.

Complete (third-degree) heart block is a more advanced form of block often due to a lesion distal to the His bundle and associated with bilateral bundle branch block. The QRS is wide and the ventricular rate is slower, usually less than 50 beats/min. Transmission of atrial impulses through the AV node is completely blocked, and a ventricular pacemaker maintains a slow, regular ventricular rate, usually less than 45 beats/min. Exercise does not increase the rate. The first heart sound varies in intensity; wide pulse pressure, a changing systolic blood pressure level, and cannon venous pulsations in the neck are also present. Patients may be asymptomatic or may complain of weakness or dyspnea if the rate is less than 35 beats/min; symptoms may occur at higher rates if the left ventricle cannot increase its stroke output. During periods of transition from partial to complete heart block, some patients have ventricular asystole that lasts several seconds to minutes. Syncope occurs abruptly.

Patients with episodic or chronic infranodal complete heart block require permanent pacing, and temporary pacing is indicated if implantation of a permanent pacemaker is delayed.

Barold SS: Atrioventricular block revisited. Compr Ther 2002; 28:74. [PMID: 11894446]

Bourke JP: Atrioventricular block and problems with atrioventricular conduction. Clin Geriatr Med 2002;18:229. [PMID: 12180245]

Toff WD et al; United Kingdom Pacing and Cardiovascular Events Trial Investigators: Single-chamber versus dual-chamber pacing for high-grade atrioventricular block. N Engl J Med 2005;353:145. [PMID: 16014884]

AV DISSOCIATION

When a ventricular pacemaker is firing at a rate faster than or close to the sinus rate (accelerated idioventricular rhythm, ventricular premature beats, or ventricular tachycardia), atrial impulses arriving at the AV node when it is refractory may not be conducted. This phenomenon is AV dissociation but does not necessarily indicate AV block. No treatment is required aside from management of the causative arrhythmia.

INTRAVENTRICULAR CONDUCTION DEFECTS

Intraventricular conduction defects, including bundle branch block, are common in individuals with otherwise normal hearts and in many disease processes, including ischemic heart disease, inflammatory disease, infiltrative disease, cardiomyopathy, and postcardiotomy. Below the AV node and bundle of His, the conduction system trifurcates into a right bundle and anterior and posterior fascicles of the left bundle. Conduction block in each of these fascicles can be recognized on the surface ECG. Although such conduction abnormalities are often seen in normal hearts, they are more commonly due to organic heart disease—either an isolated process of fibrosis and calcification or more generalized myocardial disease. Bifascicular block is present when two of these—right bundle, left anterior and posterior hemibundle—are involved. Trifascicular block is defined as right bundle branch block with alternating left hemiblock, alternating right and left bundle branch block, or bifascicular block with documented prolonged infranodal conduction (long His-ventricular interval).

The prognosis of intraventricular block is generally that of the underlying myocardial process. Patients with no apparent heart disease have an overall survival rate similar to that of matched controls. However, left bundle branch block—but not right—is associated with a higher risk of development of overt cardiac disease and cardiac mortality. Even in bifascicular block, the incidence of occult complete heart block or progression to it is low, and pacing is not usually warranted. In patients with symptoms (eg, syncope) consistent with heart block and intraventricular block, pacing should be reserved for those with documented concomitant complete heart block on monitoring or those with a very prolonged HV interval (> 90 ms) with no other cause for symptoms. Even in the latter group, prophylactic pacing has not improved the prognosis significantly, probably because of the high incidence of ventricular arrhythmias in the same population.

PERMANENT PACING

The indications for permanent pacing have been discussed: symptomatic bradyarrhythmias, asymptomatic Mobitz II AV block, or complete heart block. The versatility of pacemaker generator units has increased markedly, and dual-chamber multiple programmable units are being implanted with increasing frequency. A standardized nomenclature for pacemaker generators is used, usually consisting of four letters. The first letter refers to the chamber that is stimulated (A = atrium, V = ventricle, D = dual, for both). The second letter refers to the chamber in which sensing occurs (also A, V, or D). The third letter refers to the sensory mode (I = inhibition by a sensed impulse, T = triggering by a sensed impulse, D = dual modes of response). The fourth letter refers to the programmability or rate modulation capacity (usually P for programming for two functions, M for programming more than two, and R for rate modulation).

A pacemaker that senses and paces in both chambers is the most physiologic approach to pacing patients who remain in sinus rhythm. AV synchrony is particularly important in patients in whom atrial contraction produces a substantial increment in stroke volume and in those in whom sensing the atrial rate to provide rate-responsive ventricular pacing is useful. Dual-chamber pacing is most useful for individuals with LV systolic or—perhaps more importantly—diastolic dysfunction and for physically active individuals. In patients with single-chamber pacemakers, the lack of an atrial kick may lead to the so-called pacemaker syndrome, in which the patient experiences signs of low cardiac output while upright.

Pulse generators are also available that can increase their rate in response to motion or respiratory rate when the atrial rate is not an indication of the optimal heart rate. These are most useful in active individuals. Follow-up after pacemaker implantation, usually by telephonic monitoring, is essential. All pulse generators and lead systems have an early failure rate that is now below 5% and an expected battery life varying from 4 years to 10 years.

ACC/AHA/NASPE 2002 guideline update for implantation of cardiac pacemakers and antiarrhythmia devices: summary article. J Am Coll Cardiol 2002;40:1703. [PMID: 12427427]

Bryce M et al: Evolving indications for permanent pacemakers. Ann Intern Med 2001;134:1130. [PMID: 11412054]

Faddis MN et al: Pacing interventions for falls and syncope in the elderly. Clin Geriatr Med 2002;18:279. [PMID: 12180248]

Gregoratos G: Indications and recommendations for pacemaker therapy. Am Fam Physician 2005;71:1563. [PMID: 15864898]

JAMA patient page: Heart pacemakers. JAMA 2001;286:878. [PMID: 11519499]

Trohman RG et al: Cardiac pacing: the state of the art. Lancet 2004;364:1701. [PMID: 15530632]

Vlietstra RE et al: Choice of pacemakers in patients aged 75 years and older: ventricular pacing mode vs. dual-chamber pacing mode. Am J Geriatr Cardiol 2005;14:35. [PMID: 15654152]

Wong GC et al: Single chamber ventricular compared with dual chamber pacing: a review. Can J Cardiol 2002;18:301. [PMID: 11907619]

EVALUATION OF SYNCOPE

Syncope, defined as a transient loss of consciousness and postural tone due to inadequate cerebral blood flow with prompt recovery without resuscitative measures, is a common clinical problem, especially in the elderly. Thirty percent of the adult population will experience at least one episode, and syncope accounts for approximately 3% of emergency department visits. Causes include cardiac abnormalities (either disturbances of rhythm or hemodynamics), vascular disorders, or neurologic processes. A specific cause is identified in about 50% of cases during the initial evaluation. The prognosis is relatively benign except when accompanying cardiac disease is present. Syncope is more likely to occur in patients with known heart disease, older men, and young women (who are prone to vasovagal episodes). Syncope is characteristically abrupt in onset, often resulting in injury, transient (lasting for seconds to a few minutes), and followed by prompt recovery of full consciousness.

Vasomotor syncope may be due to excessive vagal tone or impaired reflex control of the peripheral circulation. The most frequent type of vasodepressor syncope is vasovagal hypotension or the "common faint," which is often initiated by a stressful, painful, or claustrophobic experience, especially in young women. Premonitory symptoms, such as nausea, diaphoresis, tachycardia, and pallor, are usual. Episodes can be aborted by lying down or removing the inciting stimulus. Enhanced vagal tone with resulting hypotension is the cause of syncope in carotid sinus hypersensitivity and postmicturition syncope; vagal-induced sinus bradycardia, sinus arrest, and AV block are common accompaniments and may themselves be the cause of syncope. Carotid sinus massage under carefully monitored conditions or tilt-table testing may be diagnostic (see above under Autonomic Testing). Treatment consists largely of counseling patients to avoid predisposing situations. Paradoxically, β-blockers have been used in patients with altered autonomic function uncovered by head-up tilt testing but they have provided only minimal benefit. Permanent pacing has little benefit except in patients with documented severe pauses and bradycardiac responses.

Volume expanders, such as fludrocortisone, or vasoconstrictors, such as midodrine, have also been tried but with minimal benefit. Selective serotonin reuptake inhibitors have shown some benefit in select patients.

Orthostatic (postural) hypotension is another common cause of vasomotor syncope, especially in the elderly, in diabetics or other patients with autonomic neuropathy, in patients with blood loss or hypovolemia, and in patients taking vasodilators, diuretics, and adrenergic-blocking drugs. In addition, a syndrome of chronic idiopathic orthostatic hypotension exists primarily in older men. In most of these conditions, the normal vasoconstrictive response to assuming upright posture, which compensates for the abrupt decrease in venous return, is impaired. A greater than normal decline (20 mm Hg) in blood pressure immediately upon arising from the supine to the standing position is observed, with or without tachycardia depending on the status of autonomic (baroreceptor) function. Studying patients with a tilt table can establish the diagnosis with more certainty. Autonomic function can be assessed by observing blood pressure and heart rate responses to Valsalva's maneuver and by tilt testing. In older patients, vasoconstrictor abnormalities and autonomic insufficiency are perhaps the most common causes of syncope. Thus, tilt testing should be done before proceeding to invasive studies unless clinical and ambulatory ECG evaluation suggests a cardiac abnormality.

Cardiogenic syncope can occur on a mechanical or arrhythmic basis. Mechanical problems that can cause syncope include aortic stenosis (where syncope may occur from autonomic reflex abnormalities or ventricular tachycardia), pulmonary stenosis, hypertrophic obstructive cardiomyopathy, congenital lesions associated with pulmonary hypertension or right-to-left shunting, and LA myxoma obstructing the mitral valve. Episodes are commonly exertional or postexertional. More commonly, cardiac syncope is due to disorders of automaticity (sick sinus syndrome), conduction disorders (AV block), or tachyarrhythmias (especially ventricular tachycardia and supraventricular tachycardia with rapid ventricular rate).

The evaluation for syncope depends on findings from the history and physical examination (especially orthostatic blood pressure evaluation, examination of carotid and other arteries, cardiac examination, and, if appropriate, carotid sinus massage). The resting ECG may reveal arrhythmias, evidence of accessory pathways, prolonged QT interval, and other signs of heart disease (such as infarction or hypertrophy). If the history is consistent with syncope, ambulatory ECG monitoring is essential. This may need to be repeated several times, since yields increase with longer periods of monitoring, at least up to 3 days. Event recorder and transtelephone ECG monitoring may be helpful in patients with intermittent presyncopal episodes. Electrophysiologic studies to assess sinus node function and AV conduction and to induce supraventricular or ventricular tachycardia are indicated in patients with recurrent episodes and nondiagnostic ambulatory ECGs. They reveal an arrhythmic cause in 20–

50% of patients, depending on the study criteria, and are most often diagnostic when the patient has had multiple episodes and has identifiable cardiac abnormalities.

Faddis MN et al: Pacing interventions for falls and syncope in the elderly. Clin Geriatr Med 2002;18:279. [PMID: 12180248]

Goldschlager N: Etiologic considerations in the patient with syncope and an apparently normal heart. Arch Intern Med 2003;163:151. [PMID: 12546605]

Grubb BP: Neurocardiogenic syncope. N Engl J Med 2005;352: 1004. [PMID: 15758011]

Kapoor WN: Current evaluation and management of syncope. Circulation 2002;106:1606. [PMID: 12270849]

Kenny RA: Syncope in the elderly: diagnosis, evaluation, and treatment. J Cardiovasc Electrophysiol 2003;14(9 Suppl): S74. [PMID: 12950524]

Weimer LH et al: Syncope and orthostatic intolerance. Med Clin North Am 2003;87:835. [PMID: 12834151]

RECOMMENDATIONS FOR RESUMPTION OF DRIVING

An important management problem in patients who have experienced syncope, symptomatic ventricular tachycardia, or aborted sudden death is to provide recommendations concerning automobile driving. According to a survey published in 1991, only eight states had specific laws dealing with this issue, whereas 42 had laws restricting driving in patients with seizure disorders. Patients with syncope or aborted sudden death thought to have been due to temporary factors (acute myocardial infarction, bradyarrhythmias subsequently treated with permanent pacing, drug effect, electrolyte imbalance) should be strongly advised after recovery not to drive for at least 1 month. Other patients with symptomatic ventricular tachycardia or aborted sudden death, whether treated pharmacologically, with antitachycardia devices, or with ablation therapy, should not drive for at least 6 months. Longer restrictions are warranted in these patients if spontaneous arrhythmias persist. The physician should comply with local regulations and consult local authorities concerning individual cases.

Akiyama T et al: Resumption of driving after life-threatening ventricular tachyarrhythmia. N Engl J Med 2001;345:391. [PMID: 11496849]

Baessler C et al; DAVID Investigators: Time to resumption of driving after implantation of an automatic defibrillator (from the Dual chamber and VVI Implantable Defibrillator [DAVID] trial). Am J Cardiol 2005;95:665. [PMID: 15721116]

■ CONGESTIVE HEART FAILURE

  ESSENTIALS OF DIAGNOSIS

- *LV failure: Exertional dyspnea, cough, fatigue, orthopnea, paroxysmal nocturnal dyspnea,*

cardiac enlargement, rales, gallop rhythm, and pulmonary venous congestion.

- *RV failure: Elevated venous pressure, hepatomegaly, dependent edema; usually due to LV failure.*
- *Assessment of LV function is a crucial part of diagnosis and management.*

Epidemiology

Heart failure is a common syndrome that is increasing in incidence and prevalence. Approximately 5 million patients in the United States have heart failure, and there are nearly 500,000 new cases each year. It is primarily a disease of aging, with over 75% of existing and new cases occurring in individuals over 65 years of age. The prevalence of heart failure rises from < 1% in individuals below 60 years to nearly 10% in those over 80 years of age.

Pathophysiology

Systolic function of the heart is governed by four major determinants: the contractile state of the myocardium, the preload of the ventricle (the end-diastolic volume and the resultant fiber length of the ventricles prior to onset of the contraction), the afterload applied to the ventricles (the impedance to LV ejection), and the heart rate.

Cardiac function may be inadequate as a result of alterations in any of these determinants. In most instances, the primary derangement is depression of myocardial contractility caused either by loss of functional muscle (due to myocardial infarction, etc) or by processes diffusely affecting the myocardium. However, the heart may fail as a pump because preload is excessively elevated, such as in valvular regurgitation, or when afterload is excessive, such as in aortic stenosis or in severe hypertension. Pump function may also be inadequate when the heart rate is too slow or too rapid. Whereas the normal heart can tolerate wide variations in preload, afterload, and heart rate, the diseased heart often has limited reserve for such alterations. Finally, cardiac pump function may be supranormal but nonetheless inadequate when metabolic demands or requirements for blood flow are excessive. This situation is termed **high-output heart failure** and, though uncommon, tends to be specifically treatable. Causes of high output include thyrotoxicosis, severe anemia, arteriovenous shunting (including dialysis fistulas), Paget's disease of bone, and thiamine deficiency (beriberi).

Manifestations of cardiac failure can also occur as a result of isolated or predominant **diastolic dysfunction** of the heart. In these cases, filling of the LV or RV is abnormal, either because myocardial relaxation is impaired or because the chamber is noncompliant ("stiff") due to excessive hypertrophy or changes in composition of the myocardium. Even though contractility may be preserved, diastolic pressures are elevated and cardiac output may be reduced, potentially causing fluid retention, dyspnea, and exercise intolerance.

When the heart fails, a number of adaptations occur both in the heart and systemically. If the stroke volume of either ventricle is reduced by depressed contractility or excessive afterload, end-diastolic volume and pressure in that chamber will rise. This increases end-diastolic myocardial fiber length, resulting in a greater systolic shortening (Starling's law of the heart). If the condition is chronic, ventricular dilation will occur. Although this may restore resting cardiac output, the resulting chronic elevation of diastolic pressures will be transmitted to the atria and to the pulmonary and systemic venous circulation. Ultimately, increased capillary pressure may lead to transudation of fluid with resulting pulmonary or systemic edema. Reduced cardiac output, particularly if associated with reduced arterial pressure or perfusion of the kidneys, will also activate several neural and humoral systems. Increased activity of the sympathetic nervous system will stimulate myocardial contractility, heart rate, and venous tone; the latter change results in a rise in the effective central blood volume, which serves to further elevate preload. Though these adaptations are designed to increase cardiac output, they may themselves be deleterious. Thus, tachycardia and increased contractility may precipitate ischemia in patients with underlying CAD, and the rise in preload may worsen pulmonary congestion. Sympathetic nervous system activation also increases peripheral vascular resistance; this adaptation is designed to maintain perfusion to vital organs, but when it is excessive it may itself reduce renal and other tissue blood flow. Peripheral vascular resistance is also a major determinant of LV afterload, so that excessive sympathetic activity may further depress cardiac function.

One of the more important effects of lower cardiac output is reduction of renal blood flow and glomerular filtration rate, which leads to sodium and fluid retention. The renin–angiotensin–aldosterone system is also activated, leading to further increases in peripheral vascular resistance and LV afterload as well as sodium and fluid retention. Heart failure is associated with increased circulating levels of arginine vasopressin, which also serves as a vasoconstrictor and inhibitor of water excretion. Whereas release of atrial natriuretic peptide is increased in heart failure owing to the elevated atrial pressures, there is evidence of resistance to its natriuretic and vasodilating effects.

Myocardial failure is characterized by two hemodynamic derangements, and the clinical presentation is determined by their severity. The first is reduction in cardiac reserve, ie, the ability to increase cardiac output in response to increased demands imposed by exercise or even ordinary activity. The second abnormality, elevation of ventricular diastolic pressures, is primarily a result of the compensatory processes in systolic heart failure but is the primary derangement in diastolic heart failure.

Heart failure may be right sided or left sided. Patients with **left heart failure** have symptoms of low cardiac output and elevated pulmonary venous pressure; dyspnea is the predominant feature. Signs of fluid retention predominate in **right heart failure**, with the patient exhibiting edema, hepatic congestion, and, on occasion, ascites. Most patients exhibit symptoms or signs of both right- and left-sided failure, and LV dysfunction is the primary cause of RV failure. Surprisingly, some individuals with severe LV dysfunction will display few signs of left heart failure and appear to have isolated right heart failure. Indeed, they may be clinically indistinguishable from patients with cor pulmonale, who have right heart failure secondary to pulmonary disease.

Although this section primarily concerns cardiac failure due to systolic LV dysfunction, patients with **diastolic heart failure** experience many of the same symptoms and may be difficult to distinguish clinically. Diastolic pressures are elevated even though diastolic volumes are normal or small. These pressures are transmitted to the pulmonary and systemic venous systems, resulting in dyspnea and edema. The most frequent cause of diastolic cardiac dysfunction is LVH, commonly resulting from hypertension, but conditions such as hypertrophic or restrictive cardiomyopathy, diabetes, and pericardial disease can produce the same clinical picture. Although diuretics are often useful in these patients, the other therapies discussed in this section (digitalis, vasodilators, inotropic agents) may be inappropriate.

Causes & Prevention of Cardiac Failure

The syndrome of cardiac failure can be produced by many diseases. In developed countries, CAD with resulting myocardial infarction and loss of functioning myocardium (ischemic cardiomyopathy) is the most common cause. Systemic hypertension remains an important cause of CHF and, even more commonly in the United States, an exacerbating factor in patients with cardiac dysfunction due to other causes such as CAD. A number of other processes may present with dilated or congestive cardiomyopathy, which is characterized by LV or biventricular dilation and generalized systolic dysfunction. These are discussed elsewhere in this chapter, but the most common are alcoholic cardiomyopathy, viral myocarditis (including infections by HIV), and dilated cardiomyopathies with no obvious underlying cause (idiopathic cardiomyopathy). Rare causes of dilated cardiomyopathy include infiltrative diseases (hemochromatosis, sarcoidosis, amyloidosis, etc), other infectious agents, metabolic disorders, cardiotoxins, and drug toxicity. Valvular heart diseases—particularly degenerative aortic stenosis and chronic aortic or mitral regurgitation—are not infrequent causes of heart failure.

Because many of the processes leading to heart failure are of long standing and progress gradually, heart failure is often preventable by early detection of patients at risk and early intervention. The importance of these approaches is emphasized by guidelines that have incorporated a classification of heart failure that includes four stages (Table 10–10). Stage A includes patients at risk for developing heart failure (such as patients with hypertension or CAD without current or previous symptoms or identifiable structural abnormalities of the myocardium). In the majority of these patients, development of heart failure can be prevented with interventions such as the aggressive treatment of hypertension, modification of coronary risk factors, and reduction of excessive alcohol intake (Figure 10–1). Stage B includes patients who have structural heart disease but no current or previously recognized symptoms of heart failure. Examples include patients with previous myocardial infarction, other causes of reduced systolic function, LVH, or asymptomatic valvular disease. Both ACE inhibitors and β-blockers prevent heart failure in the first two of these conditions, and more aggressive treatment of hypertension and early surgical intervention are effective in the latter two. Stages C and D include patients with clinical heart failure and the relatively small group of patients that has become refractory to the usual therapies, respectively. These are discussed below.

Prognosis

Once manifest, heart failure carries a poor prognosis. The 5-year survival rate is less than 50% overall. Mortality rates vary from < 5% per year in those with no or few symptoms to > 30% per year in those with severe and refractory symptoms. In general, men have a poorer prognosis than women because they are more likely to have CAD, which is associated with a higher mortality rate, and are less likely to have diastolic heart failure, which has a lower mortality rate. These figures emphasize the critical importance of early detection and intervention. The prognosis of heart failure has improved in the past two decades, probably at least in part because of the more widespread use of ACE inhibitors and β-blockers, which markedly improve survival.

Brozena SC et al: The new staging system for heart failure. What every primary care physician should know. Geriatrics 2003; 58:31. [PMID: 12813870]

Gottdiener JS et al: Outcome of congestive heart failure in elderly patients: influence of left ventricular systolic function. Ann Intern Med 2002;137:631. [PMID: 12379062]

Hunt SA et al: ACC/AHA Guidelines for the evaluation and management of chronic heart failure in the adult: executive summary. A report of the American College of Cardiology/ American Heart Association Task Force on Practice Guidelines (Committee to revise the 1995 Guidelines for the Evaluation and Management of Heart Failure). J Am Coll Cardiol 2001;38:2101. [PMID: 11738322]

Massie BM: Pathophysiology of heart failure. In: *Cecil Textbook of Medicine,* 21st ed. Saunders, 2001.

McMurray JJ et al: Epidemiology, aetiology, and prognosis of heart failure. Heart 2000;83:596. [PMID: 10768918]

Zile MR et al: New concepts in diastolic dysfunction and diastolic heart failure. Circulation 2002;105:1387, 1503. [PMID: 11901053, 11914262]

Table 10–10. Stages of heart failure.

Stage	Description	Examples
A	Patients at high risk for developing heart failure because of the presence of conditions that are strongly associated with the development of heart failure. Such patients have no identified structural or functional abnormalities of the pericardium, myocardium, or cardiac valves and have never shown symptoms or signs of heart failure.	Systemic hypertension; coronary artery disease; diabetes mellitus; history of cardiotoxic drug therapy or alcohol abuse; personal history of rheumatic fever; family history of cardiomyopathy.
B	Patients who have developed structural heart disease that is strongly associated with the development of heart failure but who have never shown symptoms or signs of heart failure.	Left ventricular hypertrophy or fibrosis; left ventricular dilation or hypocontractility; asymptomatic valvular heart disease; previous myocardial infarction.
C	Patients who have current or prior symptoms of heart failure associated with underlying structural heart disease.	Dyspnea or fatigue due to left ventricular systolic dysfunction; asymptomatic patients who are undergoing treatment for prior symptoms of heart failure.
D	Patients with advanced structural heart disease and marked symptoms of heart failure at rest despite maximal medical therapy and who require specialized interventions.	Patients who are frequently hospitalized for heart failure and cannot be safely discharged from the hospital; patients in the hospital awaiting heart transplantation; patients at home receiving continuous intravenous support for symptom release or being supported with a mechanical circulatory assist device; patients in a hospice setting for the management of heart failure.

Derived from Hunt SA et al: ACC/AHA 2005 guideline update for the diagnosis and treatment of chronic heart failure in the adult. Circ 2005;112:154.

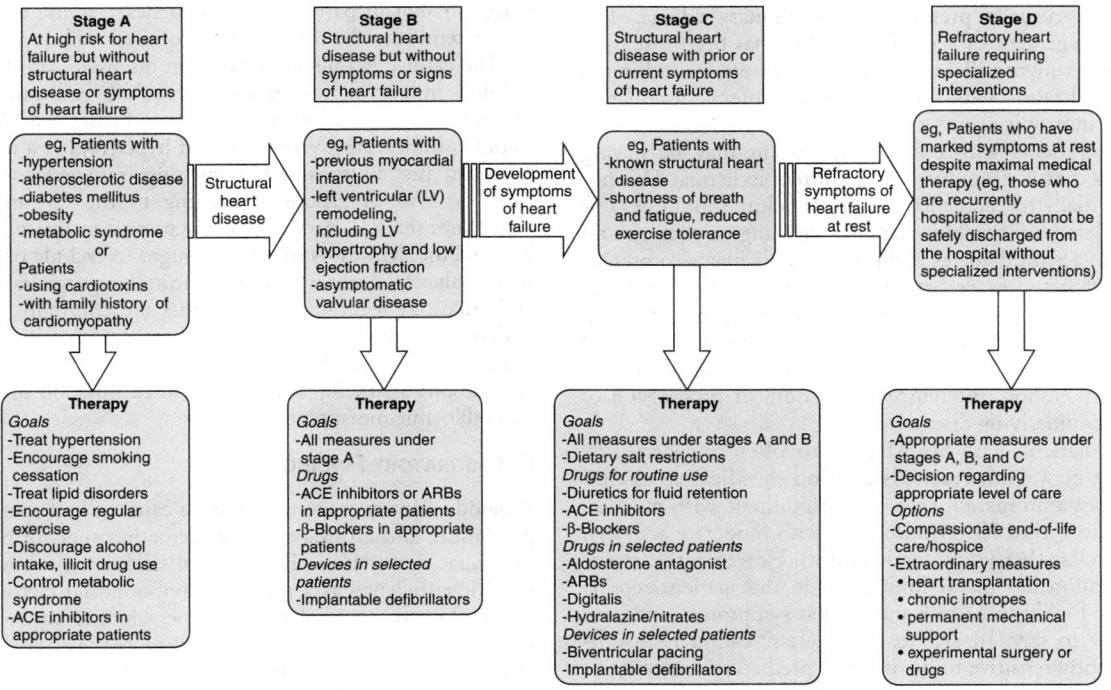

Figure 10–1. Stages in the evolution of heart failure and recommended therapy by stage. ACE = angiotensin-converting enzyme. (Reproduced, with permission, from Hunt SA et al: ACC/AHA 2005 Guidelines Update for the evaluation and management of chronic heart failure in the adult: A report of the American College of Cardiology/American Heart Association Task Force on Practice Guidelines [Writing Committee to Update the 2001 Guidelines for the Evaluation and Management of Heart Failure]. ACC/AHA 2005 Guidelines Update for the diagnosis and management of chronic heart failure in the adult. ©2005, American Heart, Inc.)

Clinical Findings

A. SYMPTOMS

The symptoms of CHF have been discussed in part in earlier sections. The most common complaint is short-ness of breath, chiefly exertional dyspnea at first and then progressing to orthopnea, paroxysmal nocturnal dyspnea, and rest dyspnea. A more subtle and often overlooked symptom of heart failure is a chronic non-productive cough, which is often worse in the recum-bent position. Nocturia due to excretion of fluid re-tained during the day and increased renal perfusion in the recumbent position is a common nonspecific symptom of heart failure. Patients with heart failure also complain of fatigue and exercise intolerance. These symptoms correlate poorly with the degree of cardiac dysfunction and result in part from changes in peripheral blood flow and blood flow to skeletal mus-cle, which are part of the syndrome of heart failure. Patients with right heart failure may experience right upper quadrant pain due to passive congestion of the liver, loss of appetite and nausea due to edema of the gut or impaired gastrointestinal perfusion, and periph-eral edema.

Cardiac failure may present acutely in a previously asymptomatic patient. Causes include myocardial in-farction, myocarditis, and acute valvular regurgitation due to endocarditis or other conditions. These pa-tients usually present with pulmonary edema. The management of acute heart failure has been discussed under myocardial infarction and centers around initial stabilization with diuretics and parenteral vasodilators or inotropic agents.

Patients with episodic symptoms may be having LV dysfunction due to intermittent ischemia. This po-tentially reversible form of heart failure should be con-sidered, especially in patients with angina pectoris and those with diabetes mellitus. Patients may also present with acute exacerbations of chronic, stable heart fail-ure. Exacerbations are usually caused by alterations in therapy (or patient noncompliance), excessive salt and fluid intake, arrhythmias, excessive activity, pulmo-nary emboli, intercurrent infection, or progression of the underlying disease.

Patients with heart failure are often categorized by the New York Heart Association classification as class I (asymptomatic), class II (symptomatic with mild ac-tivity), class III (symptomatic with moderate activity), or class IV (symptomatic at rest). However, this classi-fication has major limitations in that patient reports are highly subjective and in that symptoms vary from day to day. In any case, the classification is insuffi-ciently sensitive to be useful in predicting outcomes or assessing the results of treatment.

B. SIGNS

Many patients with heart failure, including some with severe symptoms, appear comfortable at rest. Others will be dyspneic during conversation or minor activity, and those with long-standing severe heart failure may appear cachectic or cyanotic. The vital signs may be normal, but tachycardia, hypotension, and reduced pulse pressure may be present. Patients often show signs of increased sympathetic nervous system activity, including cold extremities and diaphoresis. Important peripheral signs of heart failure can be detected by ex-amination of the neck, the lungs, the abdomen, and the extremities. RA pressure may be estimated through the height of the pulsations in the jugular venous sys-tem. In addition to the height of the venous pressure, abnormal pulsations such as regurgitant v waves should be sought. Examination of the carotid pulse may allow estimation of pulse pressure as well as de-tection of aortic stenosis. The thyroid examination is important, since occult hyperthyroidism and hypothy-roidism are readily treatable causes of heart failure. In the lungs, crackles at the lung bases reflect transuda-tion of fluid into the alveoli. Pleural effusions may cause bibasilar dullness to percussion. Expiratory wheezing and rhonchi may be signs of heart failure. Patients with severe right heart failure may have he-patic enlargement—tender or nontender—due to pas-sive congestion. Systolic pulsations may be felt in tri-cuspid regurgitation. Sustained moderate pressure on the liver may increase jugular venous pressure (a posi-tive hepatojugular reflux is an increase of > 1 cm). As-cites may also be present. Peripheral pitting edema is a common sign in patients with right heart failure and may extend into the thighs and abdominal wall.

The cardiac examination has been discussed. Cardi-nal signs in heart failure are a parasternal lift, indicating pulmonary hypertension; an enlarged and sustained LV impulse, indicating LV dilation and hypertrophy; a di-minished first heart sound, suggesting impaired con-tractility; and S_3 gallops originating in the LV and sometimes the RV. An S_4 is usually present in diastolic heart failure. Murmurs should be sought to exclude pri-mary valvular disease; secondary mitral regurgitation and tricuspid regurgitation murmurs are common in patients with dilated ventricles. In chronic heart failure, many of the expected signs of heart failure may be ab-sent despite markedly abnormal cardiac function and hemodynamic measurements.

C. LABORATORY FINDINGS

A blood count may reveal anemia, a cause of high-out-put failure and an exacerbating factor in other forms of cardiac dysfunction. Biochemical studies may show renal insufficiency as a possible compounding factor. Renal function tests also determine whether cardiac failure is associated with prerenal azotemia. Serum electrolytes may disclose hypokalemia, which increases the risk of arrhythmias; hyperkalemia, which may limit the use of inhibitors of the renin–angiotensin system; or hyponatremia, an indicator of marked acti-vation of the renin–angiotensin system and a poor prognostic sign. Thyroid function should be assessed in older patients to detect occult thyrotoxicosis or myxedema. In unexplained cases, appropriate biopsies may lead to a diagnosis of amyloidosis, and additional assessment should include iron studies to exclude hemochromatosis. Myocardial biopsy may exclude specific causes of dilated cardiomyopathy but rarely reveals specific reversible diagnoses.

Assays of serum BNP or amino terminal pro-BNP can be a useful adjunct to the clinical history and physical examination in the diagnosis of heart failure. Measurement of serum BNP has been shown to add to clinical assessment in differentiating dyspnea due to heart failure from noncardiac causes. BNP is expressed primarily in the ventricles and is elevated when ventricular filling pressures are high. It is quite sensitive in patients with symptomatic heart failure—whether due to systolic or to diastolic dysfunction—but less specific in older patients, women, and patients with COPD. The roles of these assays in screening asymptomatic individuals or as a guide to management have not been established.

D. ECG and Chest Radiography

ECG may indicate an underlying or secondary arrhythmia, myocardial infarction, or nonspecific changes that often include low voltage, intraventricular conduction defects, LVH, and nonspecific repolarization changes. Chest radiographs provide information about the size and shape of the cardiac silhouette. Cardiomegaly is an important finding. Evidence of pulmonary venous hypertension includes relative dilation of the upper lobe veins, perivascular edema (haziness of vessel outlines), interstitial edema, and alveolar fluid. In acute heart failure, these findings correlate moderately well with pulmonary venous pressure. However, patients with chronic heart failure may show relatively normal pulmonary vasculature despite markedly elevated pressures. Pleural effusions are common and tend to be bilateral or right sided.

E. Additional Studies

Many studies have indicated that the clinical diagnosis of systolic myocardial dysfunction is often inaccurate. The primary confounding conditions are diastolic dysfunction of the heart with decreased relaxation and filling of the LV (particularly in hypertension and in hypertrophic states) and pulmonary disease. Because patients with heart failure usually have significant resting ECG abnormalities, stress imaging procedures such as perfusion scintigraphy or dobutamine echocardiography are often indicated.

The most useful test is the echocardiogram. This will reveal the size and function of both ventricles and of the atria. It will also allow detection of pericardial effusion, valvular abnormalities, intracardiac shunts, and segmental wall motion abnormalities suggestive of old myocardial infarction as opposed to more generalized forms of dilated cardiomyopathy.

Radionuclide angiography measures LV EF and permits analysis of regional wall motion. This test is especially useful when echocardiography is technically suboptimal, such as in patients with severe pulmonary disease. When myocardial ischemia is suspected as a cause of LV dysfunction, stress testing should be performed.

F. Cardiac Catheterization

In most patients with heart failure, clinical examination and noninvasive tests can determine LV size and function well enough to confirm the diagnosis. Left heart catheterization is necessary when significant valvular disease must be excluded and when the presence and extent of CAD must be determined. The latter is particularly important when LV dysfunction may be partially reversible by revascularization. The combination of angina or noninvasive evidence of significant myocardial ischemia with symptomatic heart failure is often an indication for coronary angiography if the patient is a potential candidate for revascularization. Right heart catheterization may be useful to select and monitor therapy in patients refractory to standard therapy.

Angeja BG et al: Evaluation and management of diastolic heart failure. Circulation 2003;107:659. [PMID: 12578862]

Cowie MR et al: BNP and congestive heart failure. Prog Cardiovasc Dis 2002;44:293. [PMID: 12007084]

Davies MK et al: ABC of heart failure. BMJ 2000;320:297. [PMID: 10650030]

Drazner MH et al: Prognostic importance of elevated jugular venous pressure and a third heart sound in patients with heart failure. N Engl J Med 2001;345:574. [PMID: 11529211]

Maisel AS et al: Rapid measurement of B-type natriuretic peptide in the emergency diagnosis of heart failure. N Engl J Med 2002;347:161. [PMID: 12124404]

Pharmacologic Treatment

The treatment of chronic heart failure is discussed here. Acute heart failure and pulmonary edema are discussed in the next section.

A. Correction of Reversible Causes

The major reversible causes of chronic heart failure include valvular lesions, myocardial ischemia, uncontrolled hypertension, arrhythmias (especially persistent tachycardias), alcohol- or drug-induced myocardial depression, intracardiac shunts, and high-output states. Calcium channel blockers, antiarrhythmic drugs, and nonsteroidal anti-inflammatory agents are important causes of worsening heart failure. Some metabolic and infiltrative cardiomyopathies may be partially reversible, or their progression may be slowed; these include hemochromatosis, sarcoidosis, and amyloidosis. Reversible causes of diastolic dysfunction include pericardial disease and LVH due to hypertension. Once it is established that there is no reversible component, the measures outlined below are appropriate.

B. Diuretic Therapy

Diuretics are the most effective means of providing symptomatic relief to patients with moderate to severe CHF.

Few patients with symptoms or signs of fluid retention can be optimally managed without a diuretic. However, excessive diuresis can lead to electrolyte imbalance and neurohormonal activation. A combination of a diuretic and an ACE inhibitor should be the initial treatment in most symptomatic patients. When fluid retention is mild, thiazide diuretics or a similar type of agent (hydrochlorothiazide, 25–100 mg; metolazone, 2.5–5 mg; chlorthalidone, 25–50 mg; etc) may be sufficient. These agents block sodium reabsorption in the cortical diluting segment at the terminal portion of the loop of Henle and in the proximal portion of the distal convoluted tubule. The result is natriuresis and kaliuresis. These agents also have weak carbonic anhydrase inhibitor activity, which results in proximal tubule inhibition of sodium reabsorption. Thiazide or related diuretics often provide better control of hypertension than short-acting loop agents.

The thiazides are generally ineffective when the glomerular filtration rate falls below 30–40 mL/min, a not infrequent occurrence in patients with severe heart failure. Metolazone maintains its efficacy down to a glomerular filtration rate of approximately 20–30 mL/min. Adverse reactions include hypokalemia and intravascular volume depletion with resulting prerenal azotemia, skin rashes, neutropenia and thrombocytopenia, hyperglycemia, hyperuricemia, and hepatic dysfunction.

Patients with more severe heart failure should be treated with one of the loop diuretics. These include furosemide (20–320 mg daily), bumetanide (1–8 mg daily), and torsemide (20–200 mg daily). These agents have a rapid onset and a relatively short duration of action. In patients with preserved renal function, two or more doses are preferable to a single larger dose. In acute situations or when gastrointestinal absorption is in doubt, they should be given intravenously. The loop diuretics inhibit chloride reabsorption in the ascending limb of the loop of Henle, which results in natriuresis, kaliuresis, and metabolic alkalosis. They are active even in severe renal insufficiency, but larger doses (up to 500 mg of furosemide or equivalent) may be required. The major adverse reactions include intravascular volume depletion, prerenal azotemia, and hypotension. Hypokalemia, particularly with accompanying digitalis therapy, is a major problem. Less common side effects include skin rashes, gastrointestinal distress, and ototoxicity (the latter more common with ethacrynic acid and possibly less common with bumetanide).

The potassium-sparing agents spironolactone, triamterene, and amiloride are often useful in combination with the loop diuretics and thiazides. Triamterene and amiloride act on the distal tubule to reduce potassium secretion. Their diuretic potency is only mild and not adequate for most patients with heart failure, but they may minimize the hypokalemia induced by more potent agents. Side effects include hyperkalemia, gastrointestinal symptoms, and renal dysfunction. Spironolactone is a specific inhibitor of aldosterone, which is often increased in CHF and has important effects beyond potassium retention (see below). Its onset

of action is slower than the other potassium-sparing agents, and its side effects include gynecomastia. Combinations of potassium supplements or ACE inhibitors and potassium-sparing drugs can produce hyperkalemia but have been used with success in patients with persistent hypokalemia.

Patients with refractory edema may respond to combinations of a loop diuretic and thiazide-like agents. Metolazone, because of its maintained activity with renal insufficiency, is the most useful agent for such a combination. Extreme caution must be observed with this approach, since massive diuresis and electrolyte imbalances often occur; 2.5 mg of metolazone should be added to the previous dosage of loop diuretic. In many cases this is necessary only once or twice a week, but dosages up to 10 mg daily have been used in some patients.

C. Inhibitors of the Renin–Angiotensin–Aldosterone System

The renin–angiotensin–aldosterone system is activated early in the course of heart failure and plays an important role in the progression of this syndrome. Inhibition of this system with ACE inhibitors should be considered part of the initial therapy of this syndrome based on their favorable effects on prognosis.

1. ACE inhibitors—ACE inhibitors block the renin–angiotensin–aldosterone system by inhibiting the conversion of angiotensin I to angiotensin II, producing vasodilation by limiting angiotensin II-induced vasoconstriction, and decreasing sodium retention by reducing aldosterone secretion. Because ACE is also involved in the degradation of bradykinin, ACE inhibitors result in higher bradykinin levels, which in turn stimulate the synthesis of prostaglandins and nitric oxide. Experimental data and hemodynamic studies in patients indicate that these latter actions may be important. Although the other vasodilators tend to stimulate the renin–angiotensin system and often lose part of their effect due to the resulting fluid retention, tolerance to the ACE inhibitors is uncommon.

Many ACE inhibitors are available, and at least seven have been shown to be effective for the treatment of heart failure or the related indication of postinfarction LV dysfunction (see Table 11–8). ACE inhibitors reduce mortality by approximately 20% in patients with symptomatic heart failure and have been shown also to prevent hospitalizations, increase exercise tolerance, and reduce symptoms in these patients. As a result, ACE inhibitors should be part of first-line treatment of patients with symptomatic LV systolic dysfunction (EF < 40%), usually in combination with a diuretic. They are also indicated for the management of patients with reduced EFs without symptoms because they prevent the progression to clinical heart failure.

Because ACE inhibitors may induce significant hypotension, particularly following the initial doses, they must be started with caution. Hypotension is most prominent in patients with already low BPs (systolic pressure < 100 mm Hg), hypovolemia, prerenal azotemia (especially if it is diuretic induced), and hyponatremia (an indicator of activation of the renin–angiotensin system). These patients should generally be started at low dosages (captopril 6.25 mg three times daily, enalapril 2.5 mg daily, or the equivalent), but other patients may be started at twice these dosages. Within several days (for those with the markers of higher risk) or at most 2 weeks, patients should be questioned about symptoms of hypotension, and both renal function and K^+ levels should be monitored.

ACE inhibitors should be titrated to the dosages proved effective in clinical trials (captopril 50 mg three times daily, enalapril 10 mg twice daily, lisinopril 10 mg daily, or the equivalent) over a period of 1–3 months. Most patients will tolerate these doses. Asymptomatic hypotension is not a contraindication to up-titrating or continuing ACE inhibitors. Some patients exhibit increases in serum creatinine or K^+, but they do not require discontinuation if the levels stabilize—even at values as high as 3 mg/dL and 5.5 mEq/L, respectively. Renal dysfunction is more frequent in diabetics, older patients, and those with low systolic pressures, and these groups should be monitored more closely. The most common side effects of ACE inhibitors in heart failure patients are dizziness (often not related to the level of BP) and cough, though the latter is often due as much to heart failure or intercurrent pulmonary conditions as to the ACE inhibitor.

2. Angiotensin II receptor blockers—Another approach to inhibiting the renin–angiotensin–aldosterone system is the use of specific ARBs (see Table 11–8), which will block or decrease most of the effects of the system. In addition, because there are alternative pathways of angiotensin II production in many tissues, the receptor blockers may provide more complete system blockade.

However, these agents do not share the effects of ACE inhibitors on other potentially important pathways that produce increases in bradykinin, prostaglandins, and nitric oxide in the heart, blood vessels, and other tissues. The Valsartan in Heart Failure Trial (Val-HeFT) examined the efficacy of adding valsartan (titrated to a dose of 160 mg twice a day) to ACE inhibitor therapy. While valsartan did not reduce mortality, the composite of death or hospitalization for heart failure was significantly reduced. The CHARM trial randomized 7601 patients with chronic heart failure with or without LV systolic dysfunction and with or without background ACE inhibitor therapy to candesartan (titrated to 32 mg a day) or placebo. Among patients with an LV EF of < 40%, there was an 18% reduction in cardiovascular death or heart failure hospitalization and a statistically significant 12% reduction in all-cause mortality. The benefits were similar among patients on ACE inhibitors, including among patients on full-dose ACE inhibitors. Thus, ARBs, specifically candesartan or valsartan, provide impor-

tant benefits as an alternative, and in addition, to ACE inhibitors in chronic heart failure.

3. Spironolactone—There is growing evidence that aldosterone may mediate some of the major effects of renin–angiotensin–aldosterone system activation, such as myocardial remodeling and fibrosis, as well as sodium retention and potassium loss at the distal tubules. Thus, spironolactone should be considered as a neurohormonal antagonist rather than narrowly as a potassium-sparing diuretic. The RALES trial compared spironolactone 25 mg daily with placebo in patients with advanced heart failure already receiving ACE inhibitors and diuretics and showed a 29% reduction in mortality as well as similar decreases in other clinical end points. Hyperkalemia was uncommon in this severe heart failure clinical trial population, which was maintained on high doses of diuretic, but hyperkalemia with spironolactone appears to be common in general practice. Potassium levels should be monitored closely during initiation of spironolcatone (after 1 and 4 weeks of therapy), particularly for patients with even mild degrees of renal insufficiency, and in patients receiving ACE inhibitors. Neither the efficacy nor the safety of spironolcatone has been established in the large majority of patients with mild or moderate heart failure who are taking low doses of diuretics, though this agent may be considered in patients who require potassium supplementation. It is not known whether the more selective aldosterone inhibitor, eplerenone, is effective in improving outcome in chronic heart failure.

D. β-BLOCKERS

Although β-blockers have traditionally been considered to be contraindicated in patients with heart failure because they may block the compensatory actions of the sympathetic nervous system, there is now strong evidence that these agents have important beneficial effects in this patient population. The mechanism of this benefit remains unclear, but it is likely that chronic elevations of catecholamines and sympathetic nervous system activity cause progressive myocardial damage, leading to worsening LV function and dilation. The primary evidence for this hypothesis is that over a period of 3–6 months, β-blockers produce consistent substantial rises in EF (averaging 10% absolute increase) and reductions in LV size and mass.

Clinical trial results have been reported in nearly 14,000 patients (ranging from asymptomatic post-myocardial infarction LV dysfunction to severe heart failure with LV EFs < 35–40%) receiving ACE inhibitors and diuretics randomized to β-blockers or placebo. Carvedilol, a nonselective β_1- and β_2-receptor blocker with additional weak α-blocking activity, was the first β-blocker approved for heart failure in the United States after showing a reduction in death and hospitalizations in four smaller studies with a total of nearly 1100 patients. Subsequently, trials with two β_1-selective agents, bisoprolol (CIBIS II, with 2647 patients) and sustained-release metoprolol succinate (MERIT, with nearly 4000 patients), showed 35% reductions in mortality as well as fewer hospitalizations. Recently, a trial using carvedilol in 2200 patients with severe (New York Heart Association [NYHA] class III/IV) heart failure was terminated ahead of schedule because of a 35% reduction in mortality. In these trials, there were reductions in sudden deaths and deaths from worsening heart failure, and benefits were seen in patients with underlying coronary disease and those with primary cardiomyopathies. In all these studies, the β-blockers were generally well tolerated, with similar numbers of withdrawals in the active and placebo groups. This has led to a strong recommendation that *stable* patients (defined as having no recent deterioration or evidence of volume overload) with mild, moderate, and even severe heart failure should be treated with a β-blocker unless there is a noncardiac contraindication. In the COPERNICUS trial, carvedilol was both well tolerated and highly effective in reducing both mortality and heart failure hospitalizations in a group of patients with severe (NYHA class III or IV) symptoms, but care was taken to ensure that they were free of fluid retention at the time of initiation. In this study, one death was prevented for every 13 patients treated for 1 year—as dramatic an effect as has been seen with a pharmacologic therapy in the history of cardiovascular medicine. One trial comparing carvedilol and (short-acting) metoprolol tartrate (COMET) found significant reductions in all-cause mortality and cardiovascular mortality with carvedilol, and thus patients should be treated with extended-release metoprolol, bisoprolol, or carvedilol, but not short-acting metoprolol.

Because even apparently stable patients may deteriorate when β-blockers are initiated, initiation must be done gradually and with great care. Carvedilol is initiated at a dosage of 3.125 mg twice daily and may be increased to 6.25, 12.5, and 25 mg twice daily at intervals of approximately 2 weeks. The protocols for sustained-release metoprolol use were started at 12.5 or 25 mg daily and doubled at intervals of 2 weeks to a target dose of 200 mg daily (using the Toprol XL sustained-release preparation). Bisoprolol was administered at a dosage of 1.25, 2.5, 3.75, 5, 7.5, and 10 mg daily, with increments at 1- to 4-week intervals. More gradual up-titration is often more convenient and may be better tolerated.

Patients should be instructed to monitor their weights at home as an indicator of fluid retention and to report any increase or change in symptoms immediately. Before each dose increase, the patient should be seen and examined to ensure that there has not been fluid retention or worsening of symptoms. If heart failure worsens, this can usually be managed by increasing diuretic doses and delaying further increases in β-blocker doses, though downward adjustments or discontinuation is sometimes required. Carvedilol, because of its α-blocking activity, may cause dizziness or hypotension. This can usually be managed by reducing the doses of other vasodilators and by slowing the pace of dose increases.

E. DIGITALIS GLYCOSIDES

The digitalis glycosides (primarily digoxin) are the only orally active positive inotropic agents currently available. They bind to the sodium–potassium ATPase on the sarcolemmal membrane, inhibiting the sodium pump and thereby increasing intracellular sodium. This facilitates sodium–calcium exchange, with a resultant increase in cytosolic calcium, which enhances contractile protein cross-bridge formation and force generation. The digitalis glycosides also have electrophysiologic effects that may be beneficial or deleterious in individual patients. The primary therapeutic effect is an enhancement of cardiac parasympathetic tone, which delays AV conduction and reduces sinus node automaticity, thereby decreasing the ventricular response in patients with atrial fibrillation and slightly slowing the rate of patients in sinus rhythm. However, the increase in intracellular calcium and sodium may enhance automaticity of latent pacemakers, increasing the excitability of ventricular myocytes and inducing ventricular arrhythmias, especially when hypokalemia or myocardial ischemia is present.

Although the digitalis glycosides were once the mainstay of treatment of CHF, their use in patients who are in sinus rhythm has declined because they lack the benefits of the neurohormonal antagonists on prognosis and because safety concerns persist. However, their efficacy in reducing the symptoms of heart failure has been established in at least four multicenter trials that have demonstrated that digoxin withdrawal is associated with worsening symptoms and signs of heart failure, more frequent hospitalizations for decompensation, and reduced exercise tolerance. This was also seen in the 6800-patient Digitalis Investigators Group (DIG) trial, though that study found no benefit (or harm) with regard to survival. A reduction in deaths due to progressive heart failure was balanced by an increase in deaths due to ischemic and arrhythmic events. Based on these results, digoxin should be used for patients who remain symptomatic when taking diuretics and ACE inhibitors as well as for patients with heart failure who are in atrial fibrillation and require rate control.

Digoxin, the only widely used digitalis preparation, has a half-life of 24–36 hours and is eliminated almost entirely by the kidneys. The oral maintenance dose may range from 0.125 mg three times weekly to 0.5 mg daily. It is lower in patients with renal dysfunction, in older patients, and in those with smaller lean body mass. Although a loading dose of 0.75–1.25 mg (depending primarily on lean body size) over 24–48 hours may be given if an early effect is desired, in most patients with chronic heart failure it is sufficient to begin with the expected maintenance dose (usually 0.125–0.25 mg daily). Amiodarone, quinidine, propafenone, and verapamil are among the drugs that may increase digoxin levels up to 100%. It is prudent to measure a blood level after 7–14 days (and at least 6 hours after the last dose was administered). Most of the positive inotropic effect is apparent with serum digoxin levels between 0.7 ng/mL and 1.2 ng/mL, and levels above this range may be associated with a higher risk of arrhythmias and lower survival rates, though clinically evident toxicity is rare with levels below 1.8 ng/mL. Once an appropriate maintenance dose is established, subsequent levels are usually not indicated unless there is a change in renal function or medications that affects digoxin levels or a significant deterioration in cardiac status that may be associated with reduced clearance.

Digoxin toxicity has become less frequent as there has been a better appreciation of its pharmacology, but the therapeutic-to-toxic ratio is quite narrow. Symptoms of digitalis toxicity include anorexia, nausea, headache, blurring or yellowing of vision, and disorientation. Cardiac toxicity may take the form of AV conduction or sinus node depression; junctional, atrial, or ventricular premature beats or tachycardias; or ventricular fibrillation. Potassium administration (following serum potassium measurement, since severe toxicity may be associated with hyperkalemia) is usually indicated for the tachyarrhythmias even when levels are in the normal range, but may worsen conduction disturbances. Lidocaine or phenytoin may be useful for ventricular arrhythmias, as is overdrive pacing, but quinidine, amiodarone, and propafenone should be avoided because they will increase digoxin levels. Electrical cardioversion should be avoided if possible, as it may cause intractable ventricular fibrillation or cardiac standstill. Pacing is indicated for third-degree AV block (complete heart block) and symptomatic or severe block (heart rate < 40 beats/min) if they persist after treatment with atropine. Digoxin immune fab (ovine) is available for life-threatening toxicity or large overdoses, but it should be remembered that its half-life is shorter than that of digoxin and so repeat administration may be required.

F. Vasodilators

Agents that dilate arteriolar smooth muscle and lower peripheral vascular resistance reduce LV afterload. Medications that diminish venous tone and increase venous capacitance reduce the preload of both ventricles as their principal effect. Because most patients with moderate to severe heart failure have both elevated preload and reduced cardiac output, the maximum benefit of vasodilator therapy can be achieved by an agent or combination of agents with both actions. Many patients with heart failure have mitral or tricuspid regurgitation; agents that reduce resistance to ventricular outflow tend to redirect regurgitant flow in a forward direction.

Although vasodilators that are also neurohumoral antagonists—specifically, the ACE inhibitors—improve prognosis, such a benefit is less clear with the direct-acting vasodilators. The combination of hydralazine and isosorbide dinitrate has also improved survival, but to a lesser extent than ACE inhibitors. The A-HeFT trial studied hydralazine (75 mg) and isosorbide dinitrate (40 mg) three times a day in 1050 African Americans with NYHA class III or IV chronic heart failure, most of whom were treated with ACE inhibitors and β-blockers. The primary endpoint was a clinical compos-

ite. The trial was stopped early because of a significant 43% reduction in all-cause mortality with hydralazine and nitrates. Whether the benefits of this approach are limited to African Americans, who may have a less active renin–angiotensin system and less available nitric oxide, is not known, but it is now prudent to use this combination in addition to other effective therapies in African Americans with severe heart failure.

The intravenous vasodilating drugs and their dosages have been discussed elsewhere in this chapter (in the section on complications in acute myocardial infarction).

1. Nitrates—Intravenous vasodilators (sodium nitroprusside or nitroglycerin) are used primarily for acute or severely decompensated chronic heart failure, especially when accompanied by hypertension or myocardial ischemia. If neither of the latter is present, therapy is best initiated and adjusted based on hemodynamic measurements. The starting dosage for nitroglycerin is generally about 10 mcg/min, which is titrated upward by 10–20 mcg/min (to a maximum of 200 mcg/min) until mean arterial pressure drops by 10%. Hypotension (BP < 100 mm Hg systolic) should be avoided. For sodium nitroprusside, the starting dosage is 0.3–0.5 mcg/kg/min with upward titration to a maximum dose of 10 mcg/kg/min.

Isosorbide dinitrate, 20–80 mg orally three times daily, has proved effective in several small studies. Nitroglycerin ointment, 12.5–50 mg (1–4 inches) every 6–8 hours, appears to be equally effective although somewhat inconvenient for long-term therapy. The nitrates are moderately effective in relieving shortness of breath, especially in patients with mild to moderate symptoms, but less successful—probably because they have little effect on cardiac output—in advanced heart failure. Nitrate therapy is generally well tolerated, but headaches and hypotension may limit the dose of all agents. The development of tolerance to long-term nitrate therapy is now generally acknowledged. This is minimized by intermittent therapy, especially if a daily 8- to 12-hour nitrate-free interval is used, but probably develops to some extent in most patients receiving these agents. Transdermal nitroglycerin patches have no sustained effect in patients with heart failure and should not be used for this indication.

2. Nesiritide—This agent, a recombinant form of human brain natriuretic peptide, is a potent vasodilator that reduces ventricular filling pressures and improves cardiac output. Its hemodynamic effects resemble those of intravenous nitroglycerin with a more predictable dose–response curve and a longer duration of action. In clinical studies, nesiritide (administered as 2 mcg/kg by intravenous bolus injection followed by an infusion of 0.01 mcg/kg/min, which may be uptitrated if needed) produced a rapid improvement in both dyspnea and hemodynamics. The primary adverse effect is hypotension, which may be symptomatic and sustained. Because most patients with acute heart failure respond well to conventional therapy, the role of nesiritide may be primarily in patients who continue to be symptomatic after initial treatment with diuretics and nonparenteral nitrates.

3. Hydralazine—Oral hydralazine is a potent arteriolar dilator and markedly increases cardiac output in patients with CHF. However, as a single agent, it has not been shown to improve symptoms or exercise tolerance during long-term treatment. The combination of nitrates and oral hydralazine produces greater hemodynamic effects.

Hydralazine therapy is frequently limited by side effects. Approximately 30% of patients are unable to tolerate the relatively high doses required to produce hemodynamic improvement in heart failure (200–400 mg daily in divided doses). The major side effect is gastrointestinal distress, but headaches, tachycardia, and hypotension are relatively common. ARBs have largely supplanted the use of the hydralazine–isosorbide dinitrate combination in ACE-intolerant patients.

G. Positive Inotropic Agents

The digitalis derivatives are the only available oral inotropic agents in the United States. A number of other oral positive inotropic agents have been investigated for the long-term treatment of heart failure, but all have increased mortality without convincing evidence of improvement in symptoms. Intravenous agents, such as the β_1-agonist dobutamine and the phosphodiesterase inhibitor milrinone, are sometimes used on a long-term or intermittent basis. The limited available data suggest that continuous therapy is also likely to increase mortality; intermittent inotropic therapy has never been evaluated in controlled trials, and its use is largely based on anecdotal experience. A recent randomized placebo-controlled trial of 950 patients evaluating intravenous milrinone in patients admitted for decompensated heart failure who had no definite indications for inotropic therapy showed no benefit in terms of survival, decreasing length of admission, or preventing readmission—and significantly increased rates of sustained hypotension and atrial fibrillation. Thus, the role of positive inotropic agents appears to be limited to patients with symptoms and signs of low cardiac output (primarily hypoperfusion and deteriorating renal function) and those who do not respond to intravenous diuretics. In some cases, dobutamine or milrinone may help maintain patients who are awaiting cardiac transplantation.

H. Calcium Channel Blockers

First-generation calcium channel blockers may accelerate the progression of CHF. However, two trials with amlodipine in patients with severe heart failure showed that this agent was safe, though not superior to placebo. These agents should be avoided unless they are being utilized to treat associated angina or hypertension, and for these indications amlodipine is the drug of choice.

I. Anticoagulation

Patients with LV failure and reduced EFs are at somewhat increased risk for developing intracardiac thrombi and systemic arterial emboli. However, this risk appears to be primarily in patients who are in atrial fibrillation or who have large recent (within 3–6 months) myocardial infarctions. These groups should be anticoagulated. Other patients with heart failure have embolic rates of approximately two per 100 patient-years of follow-up, which approximates the rate of major bleeding, and routine anticoagulation does not appear warranted except in patients with prior embolic events or mobile LV thrombi.

J. Antiarrhythmic Therapy

Patients with moderate to severe heart failure have a high incidence of both symptomatic and asymptomatic arrhythmias. Although fewer than 10% of patients have syncope or presyncope resulting from ventricular tachycardia, ambulatory monitoring reveals that up to 70% of patients have asymptomatic episodes of nonsustained ventricular tachycardia. These arrhythmias indicate a poor prognosis independent of the severity of LV dysfunction, but many of the deaths are probably not arrhythmia related. β-Blockers, because of their marked favorable effect on prognosis in general and on the incidence of sudden death specifically, should be initiated in these as well as all other patients with heart failure. Empiric antiarrhythmic therapy with amiodarone did not improve outcome in the SCD-HeFT trial, and most other agents are contraindicated because of their proarrhythmic effects in this population and their adverse effect on cardiac function.

K. Implantable Cardioverter Defibrillators

Randomized clinical trials have extended the indications for ICDs beyond patients with symptomatic or asymptomatic arrhythmias to the broad population of patients with chronic heart failure and LV systolic dysfunction. In the second Multicenter Automatic Defibrillator Implantation Trial (MADIT II), 1232 patients with prior myocardial infarction and an EF < 30% were randomized to an ICD or a control group. Mortality was 31% lower in the ICD group, which translated into nine lives saved for each 100 patients who received a device and were monitored for 3 years. The Sudden Cardiac Death in Heart Failure Trial (SCD-HeFT) reinforced and extended these results, showing a 23% relative (7.2% absolute) reduction in mortality over 5 years with a simple single-lead ICD in a population of patients with symptomatic chronic heart failure and an EF of ≤ 35%. These patients were well-managed with contemporary heart failure treatments, including β-blockers. Based on these results, the United States Centers for Medicare and Medicaid Services have expanded reimbursement coverage to include patients with chronic heart failure and ischemic or nonischemic cardiomyopathy with an EF ≤ 35%.

Nonpharmacologic Treatment

A. Case Management, Diet, and Exercise Training

Thirty to 50 percent of CHF patients who are hospitalized will be readmitted within 3–6 months. Strategies to prevent clinical deterioration, such as case management, home monitoring of weight and clinical status, and patient adjustment of diuretics, can prevent rehospitalizations and should be part of the treatment regimen of advanced heart failure.

Patients should routinely practice moderate salt restriction (2–2.5 g sodium or 5–6 g salt per day). More severe sodium restriction is usually difficult to achieve and unnecessary because of the availability of potent diuretic agents.

Exercise training improves activity tolerance in significant part by reversing the peripheral abnormalities associated with heart failure and deconditioning. In severe heart failure, restriction of activity may facilitate temporary recompensation. However, in stable patients, a prudent increase in activity or a regular exercise regimen can be encouraged. Indeed, a gradual exercise program is associated with diminished symptoms and substantial increases in exercise capacity.

B. Coronary Revascularization

Since underlying CAD is the cause of heart failure in the majority of patients, coronary revascularization may both improve symptoms and prevent progression. However, trials have not been performed in patients with symptomatic heart failure. Nonetheless, patients with angina who are candidates for surgery should be evaluated for revascularization, usually by coronary angiography. Noninvasive testing for ischemic but viable myocardium may be a more appropriate first step in patients with known coronary disease but no current clinical evidence of ischemia. The benefit of evaluating patients with heart failure of new onset without angina or prior myocardial infarction is limited. In general, bypass surgery is preferable to PTCA in the setting of heart failure because it provides more complete revascularization.

C. Biventricular Pacing (Resynchronization)

Many patients with heart failure due to systolic dysfunction have abnormal intraventricular conduction that results in dyssynchronous and hence inefficient contractions. Several studies have evaluated the efficacy of "multisite" pacing, using leads that stimulate the RV from the apex and the LV from the lateral wall via the coronary sinus. Patients with wide QRS complexes (generally ≥ 120 milliseconds), reduced EFs, and moderate to severe symptoms have been evaluated. Results from trials with up to 2 years of follow-up have shown an increase in EF, improvement in symptoms and exercise tolerance, and reduction in death and hospitalization. The COMPANION trial included 1520 patients with NYHA class III or IV heart failure, EF of ≤ 35%, and QRS duration ≥ 120 milliseconds. In addition to optimal medical therapy, resynchronization therapy with biventricular pacing with or without implantable defibrillator capability reduced death and hospitalization from any cause by about 20%. The CARE-HF trial randomized 813 similar patients, who also required mechanical evidence of dyssynchrony if QRS duration was 120–149 milliseconds, to resynchronization therapy. Over a mean follow-up of 29 months, death or hospitalization for cardiac cause was reduced by 37% and mortality was reduced by 36%. Thus, resynchronization therapy is indicated for patients with moderate to severe heart failure and LV dyssynchrony.

D. Cardiac Transplantation

Because of the poor prognosis of patients with advanced heart failure, cardiac transplantation has become widely used. Since the advent of cyclosporine immunosuppressive therapy and more careful screening of donor hearts, the survival of patients after cardiac transplantation has increased considerably. Many centers now have 1-year survival rates exceeding 80–90%, and 5-year survival rates above 70%. Infections, hypertension and renal dysfunction caused by cyclosporine, rapidly progressive coronary atherosclerosis, and immunosuppressant-related cancers have been the major complications. The high cost and limited number of donor organs require careful patient selection early in the course.

E. Other Surgical Treatment Options

Several surgical procedures for severe heart failure have received considerable publicity. Cardiomyoplasty is a procedure in which the latissimus dorsi muscle is wrapped around the heart and stimulated to contract synchronously with it. In ventricular reduction surgery, a large part of the anterolateral wall is resected to make the heart function more efficiently. Both approaches are too risky in end-stage patients and have not been shown to improve prognosis or symptoms in controlled studies, and for these reasons they have largely been dropped. Externally powered and implantable ventricular assist devices can be used in patients who require ventricular support either to allow the heart to recover or as a bridge to transplantation. The latest generation devices are small enough to allow patients unrestricted mobility and even discharge from the hospital. However, complications are frequent, including bleeding, thromboembolism, and infection, and the cost is very high, exceeding $200,000 in the initial 1–3 months.

Although 1-year survival was improved in a recent randomized trial, all patients died by 26 months.

F. Palliative Care

Despite the technologic advances of recent years, including cardiac resynchronization, implantable defibrillators, LV assist devices, and totally implantable artificial hearts, it should be remembered that many patients with chronic heart failure are elderly and have multiple comorbidities. Many of them will not experience meaningful improvements in survival with aggressive therapy, and the goal of management should be symptomatic improvement and palliation (see Chapter 5).

Adams KF Jr et al: B-type natriuretic peptide: from bench to bedside. Am Heart J 2003;145(2 Suppl):S34. [PMID: 12594450]

Albert NM et al: Improving the care of patients dying of heart failure. Cleve Clin J Med 2002;69:321. [PMID: 11996202]

Bardy GH; Sudden Cardiac Death in Heart Failure Trial (SCD-HeFT) Investigators: Amiodarone or an implantable cardioverter-defibrillator for congestive heart failure. N Engl J Med 2005;352:225. [PMID: 15659722]

Bettencourt P: Brain natriuretic peptide (nesiritide) in the treatment of heart failure. Cardiovasc Drug Rev 2002;20:27. [PMID: 12070532]

Bradley DJ et al: Cardiac resynchronization and death from progressive heart failure: a meta-analysis of randomized controlled trials. JAMA 2003;289:730. [PMID: 12585952]

Bristow MR et al: Comparison of Medical Therapy, Pacing, and Defibrillation in Heart Failure (COMPANION) Investigators: Cardiac-resynchronization therapy with or without an implantable defibrillator in advanced chronic heart failure. N Engl J Med 2004;350:2140. [PMID: 15152059]

Cleland JG et al: The effect of cardiac resynchronization on morbidity and mortality in heart failure. N Engl J Med 2005;352:1539. [PMID: 15753115]

Cuffe MS et al: Short-term intravenous milrinone for acute exacerbation of chronic heart failure: a randomized controlled trial. JAMA 2002;287:1541. [PMID: 11911756]

Eichhorn EJ et al: Digoxin. Prog Cardiovasc Dis 2002;44:251. [PMID: 12007081]

Fonarow GC: Pharmacologic therapies for acutely decompensated heart failure. Rev Cardiovasc Med 2002;3(Suppl 4):S18. [PMID: 12439427]

Hunt SA et al: ACC/AHA Guidelines for the evaluation and management of chronic heart failure in the adult: executive summary. A report of the American College of Cardiology/American Heart Association Task Force on Practice Guidelines (Committee to Revise the 1995 Guidelines for the Evaluation and Management of Heart Failure). J Am Coll Cardiol 2001;38:2101. [PMID: 11738322]

Kukin ML: Beta-blockers in chronic heart failure: considerations for selecting an agent. Mayo Clin Proc 2002;77:1199. [PMID: 12440556]

Moller JE et al: Effects of losartan and captopril on left ventricular systolic and diastolic function after acute myocardial infarction: results of the Optimal Trial in Myocardial Infarction with Angiotensin II Antagonist Losartan (OPTIMAAL) echocardiographic substudy. Am Heart J 2004;147:494. [PMID: 14999200]

Moss AJ et al: Prophylactic implantation of a defibrillator in patients with myocardial infarction and reduced ejection fraction. N Engl J Med 2002;346:877. [PMID: 11907286]

Mueller C et al: Use of B-type natriuretic peptide in the evaluation and management of acute dyspnea. N Engl J Med 2004;350:647. [PMID: 14960741]

Nohria A et al: Medical management of advanced heart failure. JAMA 2002;287:628. [PMID: 11829703]

Pepine CJ et al: A calcium antagonist vs a non-calcium antagonist hypertension treatment strategy for patients with coronary artery disease. The International Verapamil-Trandolapril Study (INVEST): a randomized controlled trial. JAMA 2003;290:2805. [PMID: 14657064]

Pfeffer MA et al: Valsartan, captopril, or both in myocardial infarction complicated by heart failure, left ventricular dysfunction, or both. N Engl J Med 2003;349:1893. [PMID: 14610160]

Taylor AL et al; African-American Heart Failure Trial Investigators: Combination of isosorbide dinitrate and hydralazine in blacks with heart failure. N Engl J Med 2004;351:2049. [PMID: 15533851]

Williams M et al: Cardiac assist devices for end-stage heart failure. Heart Dis 2001;3:109. [PMID: 11975779]

Young JB et al; Candesartan in Heart failure Assessment of Reduction in Mortality and morbidity (CHARM) Investigators and Committees: Mortality and morbidity reduction with candesartan in patients with chronic heart failure and left ventricular systolic dysfunction: results of the CHARM low-left ventricular ejection fraction trials. Circulation 2004;110:2618. [PMID: 15492298]

ACUTE HEART FAILURE & PULMONARY EDEMA

 ESSENTIALS OF DIAGNOSIS

- *Acute onset or worsening of dyspnea at rest.*
- *Tachycardia, diaphoresis, cyanosis.*
- *Pulmonary rales, rhonchi; expiratory wheezing.*
- *Radiograph shows interstitial and alveolar edema with or without cardiomegaly.*
- *Arterial hypoxemia.*

General Considerations

Typical causes of acute cardiogenic pulmonary edema include acute myocardial infarction or severe ischemia, exacerbation of chronic heart failure, acute volume overload of the LV (valvular regurgitation), and mitral stenosis. By far the most common presentation in developed countries is one of acute or subacute deterioration of chronic heart failure, precipitated by discontinuation of medications, excessive salt intake, myocardial ischemia, tachyarrhythmias (especially rapid atrial fibrillation), or intercurrent infection. Often in the latter group, there is preceding volume overload with worsening edema and progressive shortness of breath for which earlier intervention can usually avoid the need for hospital admission.

Clinical Findings

Acute pulmonary edema presents with a characteristic clinical picture of severe dyspnea, the production of pink, frothy sputum, and diaphoresis and cyanosis. Rales are present in all lung fields, as are generalized wheezing and rhonchi. Pulmonary edema may appear acutely or subacutely in the setting of chronic heart failure or may be the first manifestation of cardiac disease, usually acute myocardial infarction, which may be painful or silent. Less severe decompensations usually present with dyspnea at rest and rales and other evidence of fluid retention but without severe hypoxia.

A number of noncardiac conditions can also produce pulmonary edema. This occurs either because of imbalance in the Starling forces (either a decrease in plasma proteins or an increase in pulmonary venous pressure) or a functional or anatomic abnormality of the alveolar–capillary membrane. Causes include intravenous opioids, increased intracerebral pressure, high altitude, sepsis, several medications, inhaled toxins, transfusion reactions, shock, and disseminated intravascular coagulation. These are distinguished from cardiogenic pulmonary edema by the clinical setting, the history, and the physical examination. Conversely, in most patients with cardiogenic pulmonary edema, an underlying cardiac abnormality can usually be detected clinically or by the ECG, chest radiograph, or echocardiogram.

The chest radiograph reveals signs of pulmonary vascular redistribution, blurriness of vascular outlines, increased interstitial markings, and, characteristically, the butterfly pattern of distribution of alveolar edema. The heart may be enlarged or normal in size depending on whether heart failure was previously present. Assessment of cardiac function by echocardiography is important, since a substantial proportion of patients has normal EFs with elevated atrial pressures due to diastolic dysfunction. In cardiogenic pulmonary edema, the PCWP is invariably elevated, usually over 25 mm Hg. In noncardiogenic pulmonary edema, the wedge pressure may be normal or even low.

Treatment

In full-blown pulmonary edema, the patient should be placed in a sitting position with legs dangling over the side of the bed; this facilitates respiration and reduces venous return. Oxygen is delivered by mask to obtain an arterial PO_2 greater than 60 mm Hg. Noninvasive pressure support ventilation may improve oxygenation and prevent severe CO_2 retention while pharmacologic interventions take effect. However, if respiratory distress remains severe, endotracheal intubation and mechanical ventilation may be necessary.

Morphine is highly effective in pulmonary edema and may be helpful in less severe decompensations when the patient is uncomfortable. The initial dosage is 2–8 mg intravenously (subcutaneous administration is effective in milder cases) and may be repeated after 2–4 hours. Morphine increases venous capacitance, lowering LA pressure, and relieves anxiety, which can reduce the efficiency of ventilation. However, morphine may lead to CO_2 retention by reducing the ventilatory drive. It should be avoided in patients with opioid-induced pulmonary edema, who may improve with opioid-antagonists, and in those with neurogenic pulmonary edema.

Intravenous diuretic therapy (furosemide, 40 mg, or bumetanide, 1 mg—or higher doses if the patient has been receiving long-term diuretic therapy) is usually indicated even if the patient has not exhibited prior fluid retention. These agents produce venodilation prior to the onset of diuresis.

Nitrate therapy accelerates clinical improvement by reducing both BP and LV filling pressures. Sublingual nitroglycerin or isosorbide dinitrate, topical nitroglycerin, or intravenous nitrates will ameliorate dyspnea rapidly prior to the onset of diuresis, and these agents are particularly valuable in patients with accompanying hypertension. Intravenous nesiritide (recombinant BNP), when given as a bolus followed by an infusion, improves dyspnea more rapidly than intravenous nitroglycerin, though this may reflect the cautious way in which nitroglycerin is up-titrated by many practitioners. This agent, as well as nitrates, may precipitate hypotension, especially since these agents are used in combination with multiple drugs that lower BP. In patients with low-output states—particularly when hypotension is present—positive inotropic agents are indicated. These approaches to treatment have been discussed previously.

Bronchospasm may occur in response to pulmonary edema and may itself exacerbate hypoxemia and dyspnea. Treatment with inhaled β-adrenergic agonists or intravenous aminophylline may be helpful, but both may also provoke tachycardia and supraventricular arrhythmias.

In most cases, pulmonary edema responds rapidly to therapy. When the patient has improved, the cause or precipitating factor should be ascertained. In patients without prior heart failure, evaluation should include echocardiography and in many cases cardiac catheterization and coronary angiography. Patients with acute decompensation of chronic heart failure should be treated to achieve a euvolemic state and have their medical regimen optimized. Generally, an oral diuretic and an ACE inhibitor should be initiated, with efficacy and tolerability confirmed prior to discharge. In selected patients, early but careful initiation of β-blockers in low doses should be considered.

Cotter G et al: Pulmonary edema: new insight on pathogenesis and treatment. Curr Opin Cardiol 2001;16:159. [PMID: 11357010]

Fonarow GC: Pharmacologic therapies for acutely decompensated heart failure. Rev Cardiovasc Med 2002;3(Suppl 4):S18. [PMID: 12439427]

Gandhi SK et al: The pathogenesis of acute pulmonary edema associated with hypertension. N Engl J Med 2001;344:17. [PMID: 11136955]

Jain P et al: Current medical treatment for the exacerbation of chronic heart failure resulting in hospitalization. Am Heart J 2003;145(2 Suppl):S3. [PMID: 12594447]

Young JB et al: Intravenous nesiritide vs nitroglycerin for treatment of decompensated congestive heart failure: a randomized controlled trial. JAMA 2002;287:1531. [PMID: 11911755]

■ MYOCARDITIS & THE CARDIOMYOPATHIES

ACUTE MYOCARDITIS

Acute myocarditis causes focal or diffuse inflammation of the myocardium. Most cases are infectious, caused by viral, bacterial, rickettsial, spirochetal, fungal, or parasitic agents; but toxins, drugs, and immunologic disorders can also cause myocarditis.

1. Infectious Myocarditis

 ESSENTIALS OF DIAGNOSIS

- *Often follows an upper respiratory infection.*
- *May present with chest pain (pleuritic or nonspecific) or signs of heart failure.*
- *ECG may show sinus tachycardia, other arrhythmias, nonspecific repolarization changes, and intraventricular conduction abnormalities.*
- *Echocardiogram documents cardiomegaly and contractile dysfunction.*
- *Myocardial biopsy, though not sensitive, may reveal a characteristic inflammatory pattern.*

General Considerations

Cardiac dysfunction due to primary myocarditis is presumed to be caused by either an acute viral infection or a postviral immune response. Secondary myocarditis is the result of inflammation caused by nonviral pathogens, drugs, chemicals, physical agents, or inflammatory diseases such as systemic lupus erythematosus. The list of infectious causes of myocarditis is extensive and includes viruses with DNA and RNA cores. The coxsackie virus is the predominant agent, but many others have been implicated. Rickettsial myocarditis occurs with scrub typhus, Rocky Mountain spotted fever, and Q fever. Diphtheritic myocarditis is caused by the exotoxin and is often manifested by conduction abnormalities as well as heart failure.

Chagas' disease, caused by the insect-borne protozoan *Trypanosoma cruzi,* is a common form of myocarditis in Central and South America; the major clinical manifestations appear after a latent period of more than a decade. At this stage, patients present with cardiomyopathy, conduction disturbances, and sudden death. Associated gastrointestinal involvement (megaesophagus and megacolon) is the rule. Toxoplasmosis causes myocarditis that is usually asymptomatic but can lead to heart failure. Among parasitic infections, trichinosis is the most common cause of cardiac involvement. The potential for the HIV virus to cause myocarditis is now well recognized, though the prevalence of this complication is not known and it appears related to the level of viral load and CD4 count. In addition, other infectious causes of myocarditis are more common in patients with AIDS. A complete list of infectious causes of myocarditis is shown in Table 10–11.

Giant cell myocarditis is a rare idiopathic disorder characterized by giant cell and lymphocyte infiltration of the heart muscle. Patients usually die of ventricular arrhythmias or heart failure but occasionally respond to immunosuppressive therapy or early transplantation.

Table 10–11. Major causes of infectious myocarditis.

Viral

Adenovirus, arbovirus (dengue fever, yellow fever), arenavirus (Lassa fever), coxsackie virus, cytomegalovirus, echovirus, encephalomyocarditis virus, Epstein–Barr virus, hepatitis B, herpesvirus, HIV-1, influenza virus, mumps virus, poliomyelitis virus, rabies, respiratory syncytial virus, rubella and rubeola virus, vaccinia virus, varicella virus, variola virus

Bacterial

Brucellosis, clostridia, diphtheria, *Francisella* (tularemia), gonococcus, *Haemophilus, Legionella,* meningococcus, *Mycobacterium, Mycoplasma, Pneumococcus,* psittacosis, *Salmonella, Staphylococcus, Streptococcus,* Whipple's disease

Fungal

Actinomyces, Aspergillus, Blastomyces, Candida, Cryptococcus, Histoplasma, Nocardia, Sporothrix

Rickettsial

Rocky Mountain spotted fever, Q fever, scrub typhus, typhus

Spirochetal

Borrelia (Lyme disease and relapsing fever), *Leptospira,* syphilis

Helminthic

Cysticercus, Echinococcus, Schistosoma, Toxocara (visceral larva migrans), *Trichinella*

Protozoal

Entamoeba, Leishmania, Tryponosoma (Chagas' disease), toxoplasmosis

Modified from Pisani B et al: Inflammatory myocardial disease and cardiomyopathies. Am J Med 1997;102:459.

Clinical Findings

A. SYMPTOMS AND SIGNS

Patients may present several days to a few weeks after the onset of an acute febrile illness or a respiratory infection or with heart failure without antecedent symptoms. The onset of heart failure may be gradual or may be abrupt and fulminant. Emboli may occur due to the procoagulant effect of cytokines combined with decreased myocardial contractility and blood pooling. Pleural-pericardial chest pain is common. Examination reveals tachycardia, gallop rhythm, and other evidence of heart failure or conduction defect. Many acute infections are subclinical, though they may present later as idiopathic cardiomyopathy or with ventricular arrhythmias. At times, the presentation may mimic an acute myocardial infarction with ST changes, positive cardiac markers, and regional wall motion abnormalities despite normal coronaries. Microaneurysms may also occur and may be associated with serious ventricular arrhythmias. Patients may present in a variety of ways with fulminant, subacute, or chronic myocarditis.

B. ECG AND CHEST RADIOGRAPHY

Nonspecific ST–T changes and conduction disturbances are common. Ventricular ectopy may be the initial and only clinical finding. Chest radiograph is nonspecific, but cardiomegaly is frequent, though not universal. Evidence for pulmonary venous hypertension is common and frank pulmonary edema may be present.

C. DIAGNOSTIC STUDIES

There is no specific laboratory study that is consistently present, though the white blood cell count is usually elevated and the sedimentation rate may increase. Troponin I levels are elevated in about one-third of patients, but CK-MB is elevated in only 10%. Echocardiography provides the most convenient way of evaluating cardiac function and can exclude many other processes. Gallium-67 scintigraphy may reveal increased cardiac uptake in acute or subacute myocarditis, but it is not very sensitive. MRI with gadolinium enhancement reveals spotty areas of injury throughout the myocardium. Paired serum viral titers and serologic tests for other agents may indicate the cause.

D. ENDOMYOCARDIAL BIOPSY

Pathologic examinations may reveal a lymphocytic inflammatory response with necrosis, but the patchy distribution of abnormalities makes this relatively insensitive. By biopsy, the diagnosis of myocarditis has been established by the 1986 "Dallas" criteria. The diagnosis is dependent on describing the severity of an inflammatory infiltrate with necrosis and degeneration of adjacent myocytes. The type of infiltrate is dependent on the causal agent; usually this is lymphocytic in viral disease, but it may be neutrophilic, eosinophilic, giant cell, granulomatous, or mixed.

Treatment & Prognosis

Patients with fulminant myocarditis may present with acute cardiogenic shock. Their ventricles are usually not dilated, but thickened (possibly due to myoedema). There is a high death rate, but if the patients recover, they are usually left with no residual cardiomyopathy. Patients who present with subacute disease have a dilated cardiomyopathy and generally make an incomplete recovery. Those who present with chronic disease tend to have only mild dilation of the LV and eventually present with a more restrictive cardiomyopathy.

Specific antimicrobial therapy is indicated when an infecting agent is identified. All patients should receive standard heart failure therapy and have arrhythmias suppressed. Exercise should be limited during the recovery phase. Some believe digoxin should be avoided. Immunosuppressive therapy with corticosteroids and intravenous immunoglobulins may improve the outcome when the process is acute (< 6 months) and if the biopsy suggests ongoing inflammation. However, controlled trials have not been positive, so the value of routine myocardial biopsies in patients presenting with an acute myocarditic picture is uncertain; immunosuppressive therapy without histologic confirmation is clearly unwise, and there are few data to support its use. Patients with fulminant myocarditis require aggressive short-term support including an intra-aortic balloon pump or an LV assist device. Ongoing studies are addressing whether patients with giant cell myocarditis may be responsive to immunosuppressive agents, as a special case. Overall, if improvement does not occur, many patients may be eventual candidates for cardiac transplantation.

Barbaro G: Cardiovascular manifestations of HIV infection. Circulation 2002;106:1420. [PMID: 12221062]

Brady WJ et al: Myocarditis: emergency department recognition and management. Emerg Med Clin North Am 2004;22:865. [PMID: 15474774]

Feldman AM et al: Myocarditis. N Engl J Med 2000;343:1388. [PMID: 11070105]

Liu PP et al: Advances in the understanding of myocarditis. Circulation 2001;104:1076. [PMID: 11524405]

Magnani JW et al: Myocarditis: current trends in diagnosis and treatment. Circulation 2006;113:876. [PMID: 16476862]

Veinot JP: Diagnostic endomyocardial biopsy pathology—general biopsy considerations, and its use for myocarditis and cardiomyopathy: a review. Can J Cardiol 2002;18:55. [PMID: 11826329]

Wijetunga M et al: Myocarditis in systemic lupus erythematosus. Am J Med 2002;113:419. [PMID: 12401537]

2. Drug-Induced & Toxic Myocarditis

A variety of medications, illicit drugs, and toxic substances can produce acute or chronic myocardial injury; the clinical presentation varies widely. Doxorubicin and other cytotoxic agents, emetine, and catecholamines (especially with pheochromocytoma) can produce a pathologic picture of inflammation and necrosis together with clinical heart failure and arrhythmias; toxicity of the first two is dose related. The phenothiazines, lithium, chloroquine, disopyramide, antimony-containing compounds, and arsenicals can also cause ECG changes, arrhythmias, or heart failure. Hypersensitivity reactions to sulfonamides, penicillins, and aminosalicylic acid as well as other drugs can result in cardiac dysfunction. Radiation can cause an acute inflammatory reaction as well as a chronic fibrosis of heart muscle, usually in conjunction with pericarditis.

The incidence of cocaine cardiotoxicity has increased markedly. Cocaine can cause coronary artery spasm, myocardial infarction, arrhythmias, and myocarditis. Because many of these processes are believed to be mediated by cocaine's inhibitory effect on norepinephrine reuptake by sympathetic nerves, β-blockers have been used therapeutically. In documented coronary spasm, calcium channel blockers and nitrates may be effective.

Floyd JD et al: Cardiotoxicity of cancer therapy. J Clin Oncol 2005;23:7685. [PMID: 16234530]

Gharib MI et al: Chemotherapy-induced cardiotoxicity: current practice and prospects of prophylaxis. Eur J Heart Fail 2002;4:235. [PMID: 12034146]

Yeh ET et al: Cardiovascular complications of cancer therapy: diagnosis, pathogenesis, and management. Circulation 2004; 109:3122. [PMID: 15226229]

THE CARDIOMYOPATHIES

The cardiomyopathies are a heterogeneous group of entities affecting the myocardium primarily and not associated with the major causes of cardiac disease, ie, ischemic heart disease, hypertension, pericardial disease, valvular disease, or congenital defects. Although some have specific causes, many cases are idiopathic. There is now general agreement on a classification based upon features of presentation and pathophysiology (Table 10–12).

Ardehali H et al: Endomyocardial biopsy plays a role in diagnosing patients with unexplained cardiomyopathy. Am Heart J 2004;147:919. [PMID: 15131552]

Bowles KR et al: Genetics of inherited cardiomyopathies. Expert Rev Cardiovasc Ther 2004;2:683. [PMID: 15350170]

Davies MJ: The cardiomyopathies: an overview. Heart 2000; 83:469. [PMID: 10722553]

Franz WM et al: Cardiomyopathies: from genetics to the prospect of treatment. Lancet 2001;358:1627. [PMID: 11716909]

Torpy JM et al: JAMA patient page. Cardiomyopathy JAMA 2004;292:2936. [PMID: 15598925]

1. Primary Dilated Cardiomyopathy

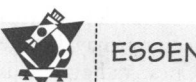 ESSENTIALS OF DIAGNOSIS

- Symptoms and signs of heart failure.
- Examination often reveals cardiomegaly, elevated JVP, S_3, S_4, mitral and tricuspid regurgitation, low systemic BP and pulse width, occasionally pulsus alternans.
- ECG may show low QRS voltage, nonspecific repolarization abnormalities, intraventricular conduction abnormalities.
- Radiograph shows cardiomegaly.
- Echocardiogram confirms LV dilation, thinning, and global dysfunction.

General Considerations

Dilated cardiomyopathies cause about 25% of all cases of CHF. It usually presents with symptoms and signs of CHF (most commonly dyspnea). Occasionally, symptomatic ventricular arrhythmias are the presenting event. LV dilation and systolic dysfunction (EF < 50%) are essential for diagnosis. Dilated cardiomyopathy occurs more often in blacks than whites and in

Table 10–12. Classification of the cardiomyopathies.

	Dilated	Hypertrophic	Restrictive
Frequent causes	Idiopathic, alcoholic, myocarditis, postpartum, doxorubicin, endocrinopathies, genetic diseases	Hereditary syndrome, possibly chronic hypertension	Amyloidosis, post-radiation, post-open heart surgery, diabetes, endomyocardial fibrosis
Symptoms	Left or biventricular congestive heart failure	Dyspnea, chest pain, syncope	Dyspnea, fatigue, right-sided congestive heart failure
Physical examination	Cardiomegaly, S_3, elevated jugular venous pressure, rales	Sustained point of maximal impulse, S_4, variable systolic murmur, bisferiens carotid pulse	Elevated jugular venous pressure, Kussmaul's sign
Electrocardiogram	ST–T changes, conduction abnormalities, ventricular ectopy	Left ventricular hypertrophy, exaggerated septal Q waves	ST–T changes, conduction abnormalities, low voltage
Chest radiograph	Enlarged heart, pulmonary congestion	Mild cardiomegaly	Mild to moderate cardiomegaly
Echocardiogram, nuclear studies, MRI	Left ventricular dilation and dysfunction	Left ventricular hypertrophy, asymmetric septal hypertrophy, small left ventricular size, normal or supranormal function, systolic anterior mitral motion, diastolic dysfunction	Small or normal left ventricular size, normal or mildly reduced left ventricular function
Cardiac catheterization	Left ventricular dilation and dysfunction, high diastolic pressures, low cardiac output	Small, hypercontractile left ventricle, dynamic outflow gradient, diastolic dysfunction	High diastolic pressure, "square root" sign, normal or mildly reduced left ventricular function

men more than women. A growing number of cardiomyopathies due to genetic abnormalities are being recognized, and these may represent up to 25–30% of cases. Often no cause can be identified, but chronic alcohol abuse and unrecognized myocarditis are probably frequent causes. Chronic tachycardia may also precipitate a dilated cardiomyopathy. Amyloidosis, sarcoidosis, hemochromatosis, and diabetes may rarely present as dilated cardiomyopathies, as well as the more classic restrictive picture. The RV may be primarily involved in arrhythmogenic RV dysplasia, an unusual cardiomyopathy with displacement of myocardial cells by adipose tissue, or in Uhl's disease, in which there is extreme thinning of the RV walls. Intraventricular thrombus is not uncommon. Histologically, the picture is one of extensive fibrosis unless a specific diagnosis is established. Myocardial biopsy is rarely useful in establishing the diagnosis, though occasionally the underlying cause (eg, sarcoidosis, hemochromatosis) can be discerned.

Clinical Findings

A. Symptoms and Signs

In most patients, symptoms of heart failure develop gradually. Cardiomyopathy may be recognized because of asymptomatic cardiomegaly or ECG abnormalities, including arrhythmias. The initial presentation may be severe biventricular failure. The physical examination reveals rales, an elevated JVP, cardiomegaly, S_3 gallop rhythm, often the murmurs of functional mitral or tricuspid regurgitation, peripheral edema, or ascites. In severe CHF, Cheyne-Stokes breathing, pulsus alternans, pallor, and cyanosis may be present.

B. ECG and Chest Radiography

The major findings are listed in Table 10–12. Sinus tachycardia is common. Other common abnormalities include left bundle branch block and ventricular or atrial arrhythmias. The chest radiograph reveals cardiomegaly, evidence for left and/or right heart failure, and pleural effusions (right > left).

C. Diagnostic Studies

An echocardiogram is indicated to exclude unsuspected valvular or other lesions and confirm the presence of dilated cardiomyopathy and reduced systolic function. Mitral Doppler inflow patterns also help in the diagnosis of diastolic dysfunction. Colorflow Doppler can reveal tricuspid or mitral regurgitation, and continuous Doppler can help define PA pressures. Exercise or pharmacologic stress myocardial perfusion imaging may suggest the possibility of underlying coronary disease. Radionuclide ventriculography provides a noninvasive measure of the EF and both RV and LV wall motion. Cardiac MRI is particularly helpful in infiltrative processes, such as sarcoidosis or hemochromatosis, and is probably the diagnostic study of choice for RV dysplasia. MRI can also help exclude an ischemic etiology by noting gadolinium enhancement consistent with myocardial scar. Cardiac catheterization is seldom of specific value unless myocardial ischemia or LV aneurysm is suspected. The serum ferritin is an adequate screening study for hemochromatosis. The erythrocyte sedimentation rate may be low due to liver congestion. The serum level of BNP or pro-BNP can be used to help quantitate the severity of CHF.

Treatment

Standard therapy for heart failure should include ACE inhibitor, β-blockers, diuretics, and an aldosterone antagonist. Digoxin is a second-line drug but remains favored as an adjunct by some clinicians. Calcium channel blockers should generally be avoided. Sodium restriction is helpful, especially in acute cardiomyopathy. When atrial fibrillation is present, heart rate control is important if sinus rhythm cannot be established or maintained. Many patients may now be candidates for cardiac synchronization therapy with biventricular pacing and an implantable defibrillator. Few cases of cardiomyopathy are amenable to specific therapy for the underlying cause. Alcohol use should be discontinued. There is often marked recovery of cardiac function following a period of abstinence in alcoholic cardiomyopathy. Endocrine causes (thyroid dysfunction, acromegaly, and pheochromocytoma) should be treated. Immunosuppressive therapy is not indicated in chronic dilated cardiomyopathy. The management of CHF is outlined in the section on heart failure.

Prognosis

The prognosis of dilated cardiomyopathy without clinical heart failure is variable, with some patients remaining stable, some deteriorating gradually, and others declining rapidly. Once heart failure is manifest, the natural history is similar to that of other causes of heart failure, with an annual mortality around 11–13%. Arterial and pulmonary emboli are more common in dilated cardiomyopathy than in ischemic cardiomyopathy. Suitable candidates may benefit from long-term anticoagulation, and all patients with atrial fibrillation should be so treated. Some patients may be candidates for cardiac transplantation.

Burkett EL et al: Clinical and genetic issues in familial dilated cardiomyopathy. J Am Coll Cardiol 2005;45:969. [PMID: 15808750]

Corrado D et al: Arrhythmogenic right ventricular cardiomyopathy: diagnosis, prognosis, and treatment. Heart 2000;83:588. [PMID: 10768917]

Felker GM et al: Underlying causes and long-term survival in patients with initially unexplained cardiomyopathy. N Engl J Med 2000;342:1077. [PMID: 10760308]

Maisch B et al: Dilated cardiomyopathies as a cause of congestive heart failure. Herz 2002;27:113. [PMID: 12025458]

Mohan SB et al: Idiopathic dilated cardiomyopathy: a common but mystifying cause of heart failure. Cleve Clin J Med 2002;69:481. [PMID: 12061463]

Piano MR: Alcoholic cardiomyopathy: incidence, clinical characteristics, and pathophysiology. Chest 2002;121:1638. [PMID: 12006456]

Sen-Chowdhry S et al: Arrhythmogenic right ventricular cardiomyopathy: clinical presentation, diagnosis, and management. Am J Med 2004;117:685. [PMID: 15501207]

Wu LA et al: Current role of endomyocardial biopsy in the management of dilated cardiomyopathy and myocarditis. Mayo Clin Proc 2001;76:1030. [PMID: 11605687]

2. Hypertrophic Cardiomyopathy

 ESSENTIALS OF DIAGNOSIS

- *May present with dyspnea, chest pain, syncope.*
- *Though outflow gradient is classic, symptoms are primarily related to diastolic dysfunction.*
- *Examination shows sustained apical impulse, S₄ systolic ejection murmur that increases with Valsalva.*
- *ECG shows LVH, occasionally septal Q waves in the absence of infarction.*
- *Echocardiogram shows hypertrophy, which is usually asymmetric, and enhanced contractility. Systolic anterior motion of the anterior mitral valve is present if there is outflow tract obstruction.*
- *Echocardiography/Doppler confirms outflow tract gradient.*

General Considerations

Myocardial hypertrophy unrelated to any pressure or volume overload reduces LV systolic stress, increases the EF, and can result in an "empty ventricle" at end-systole. The interventricular septum may be disproportionately involved (asymmetric septal hypertrophy), but in some cases the hypertrophy is localized to the apex (the apical form of hypertrophic cardiomyopathy). The LV outflow tract is often narrowed during systole between the bulging septum and an anteriorly displaced anterior mitral valve leaflet, causing a dynamic obstruction (hence the name idiopathic hypertrophic subaortic stenosis; IHSS). The obstruction is worsened by factors that increase myocardial contractility (sympathetic stimulation, digoxin, postextrasystolic beat) or that decrease LV filling (Valsalva's maneuver, peripheral vasodilators). The amount of obstruction is variable even from day to day. The consequence of the hypertrophy is elevated diastolic pressures rather than systolic dysfunction. The LV is usually more involved than the RV and the atria are frequently significantly enlarged. When the septum is primarily involved, the term "asymmetric septal hypertrophy" has been applied. Hypertrophic cardiomyopathy in some cases is inherited as an autosomal dominant trait with variable penetrance; the inherited form is caused by mutations of a number of genes, most of which code for myosin heavy chains or proteins regulating calcium handling. The prognosis is related to the specific gene mutation. These patients usually present in early adulthood. Elite athletes may demonstrate considerable hypertrophy that can be confused with hypertrophic cardiomyopathy, but generally diastolic dysfunction is not present. The apical variety is particularly common in those of Asian descent. A hypertrophic cardiomyopathy in the elderly (usually in association with hypertension) has also been defined as a distinct entity. Mitral annular calcification is often present.

Clinical Findings

A. SYMPTOMS AND SIGNS

The most frequent symptoms are dyspnea and chest pain. Syncope is also common and is typically postexertional, when diastolic filling diminishes and outflow obstruction increases. Arrhythmias are an important problem. Atrial fibrillation is a long-term consequence of chronically elevated LA pressures and is a poor prognostic sign. Ventricular arrhythmias are also common, and sudden death may occur, often in athletes after extraordinary exertion.

Features on physical examination are a bisferiens carotid pulse, triple apical impulse (due to the prominent atrial filling wave and early and late systolic impulses), and a loud S₄. The JVP may reveal a prominent a wave due to reduced RV compliance. In cases with outflow obstruction, a loud systolic murmur is present along the left sternal border that increases with upright posture or Valsalva's maneuver and decreases with squatting. These maneuvers help differentiate the murmur of hypertrophic cardiomyopathy from that of aortic stenosis. Mitral regurgitation is frequently present as well.

B. ECG AND CHEST RADIOGRAPHY

LVH is nearly universal in symptomatic patients, though entirely normal ECGs are present in up to 25%, usually in those with localized hypertrophy. Exaggerated septal Q waves inferolaterally may suggest myocardial infarction. The chest radiograph is often unimpressive. Unlike aortic stenosis, the ascending aorta is not dilated.

C. DIAGNOSTIC STUDIES

The echocardiogram is diagnostic, revealing asymmetric LVH, systolic anterior motion of the mitral valve, early closing followed by reopening of the aortic valve, a small and hypercontractile LV, and delayed relaxation and filling of the LV during diastole. The septum is usually 1.3–1.5 times the thickness of the posterior wall. Septal motion tends to be reduced. Doppler ultrasound reveals turbulent flow and a dynamic gradient in the LV outflow tract and, commonly, mitral regurgitation. Abnormalities in the diastolic filling pattern are present in 80% of patients. Myocardial perfusion imaging may suggest septal ischemia in the presence of normal coronary arteries. Cardiac MRI confirms the hypertrophy and contrast enhancement frequently reveals evidence for scar at the junction of the RV attachment to the septum. Cardiac catheterization confirms the diagnosis and assesses the presence of CAD. Frequently, coronary arterial bridging (squeezing in systole) occurs, especially of the septal arteries. Alcohol in small doses can be injected into these septal perforators to create a septal infarction that reduces the outflow tract gradient.

Treatment

β-Blockers should be the initial drug in symptomatic individuals, especially when dynamic outflow obstruction is noted on the echocardiogram. The resulting slower heart rates assist with diastolic filling of the stiff LV. Dyspnea, angina, and arrhythmias respond in about 50% of patients. Calcium channel blockers, especially verapamil, have also been effective in symptomatic patients. Their effect is due primarily to improved diastolic function, but their vasodilating actions can also increase outflow obstruction. Disopyramide (Norpace) is also used because of its negative inotropic effects; it is usually used in addition to the other therapies. Diuretics are frequently necessary due to the high diastolic pressure and PCWP. Patients do best in sinus rhythm, and atrial fibrillation should be aggressively treated with antiarrhythmics. Dual-chamber pacing may prevent the progression of hypertrophy and obstruction. Nonsurgical septal ablation has been performed by injection of alcohol into septal branches of the left coronary artery with good results in small series of patients. Patients with malignant ventricular arrhythmias and unexplained syncope in the presence of a positive family history for sudden death are probably best managed with an implantable defibrillator. Excision of part of the outflow myocardial septum (myotomy–myomectomy) by surgeons experienced with the procedure has been successful in patients with severe symptoms. Some experts advocate mitral valve replacement, as this results in resolution of the gradient as well, and prevents associated mitral regurgitation.

Prognosis

The natural history of hypertrophic cardiomyopathy is highly variable. Several specific mutations are associated with a higher incidence of early malignant arrhythmias and sudden death, and definition of the genetic abnormality provides the best estimate of prognosis. Some patients remain asymptomatic for many years or for life. Sudden death, especially during exercise, may be the initial event. Indeed, hypertrophic cardiomyopathy is the pathologic feature most frequently associated with sudden death in athletes. Those athletes with marked hypertrophy are at greatest risk. Other patients have a history of gradually progressive symptoms. Preg-

nancy is generally well tolerated. Endocarditis prophylaxis is indicated. A final stage may be a transition into dilated cardiomyopathy in 5–10% of patients.

Abbas AE et al: Alcohol septal ablation for hypertrophic obstructive cardiomyopathy. J Interv Cardiol 2005;18:155. [PMID: 15966918]

Elliott P et al: Hypertrophic cardiomyopathy. Lancet 2004;363: 1881. [PMID: 15183628]

Ly HQ et al: Sudden death and hypertrophic cardiomyopathy: a review. Can J Cardiol 2005;21:441. [PMID: 15861263]

Maron BJ: Hypertrophic cardiomyopathy: a systematic review. JAMA 2002;287:1308. [PMID: 11886323]

Maron BJ: Risk stratification and prevention of sudden death in hypertrophic cardiomyopathy. Cardiol Rev 2002;10:173. [PMID: 12047795]

Maron MS et al: Effect of left ventricular outflow tract obstruction on clinical outcome in hypertrophic cardiomyopathy. N Engl J Med 2003;348:295. [PMID: 12540642]

Qin JX et al: Outcome of patients with hypertrophic obstructive cardiomyopathy after percutaneous transluminal septal myocardial ablation and septal myectomy surgery. J Am Coll Cardiol 2001;38:1994. [PMID: 11738306]

3. Restrictive Cardiomyopathy

ESSENTIALS OF DIAGNOSIS

- Right heart failure tends to dominate over left heart failure.
- Pulmonary hypertension present.
- Amyloidosis is the most common cause.
- Echocardiography is key to diagnosis. Rapid early filling is present with diastolic dysfunction. Normal or near normal EF.
- MRI and cardiac catheterization are helpful. Myocardial biopsy can confirm.

Restrictive cardiomyopathy is characterized by impaired diastolic filling with preserved contractile function. The diastolic filling pattern in restrictive cardiomyopathy differs from other diseases with diastolic dysfunction in that the early diastolic filling is accentuated rather than inhibited. Once the rapid early filling occurs, then filling is restricted and the pressure waveform reflects this by rising rapidly, demonstrating a "square root" sign. The LV systolic function may be mildly depressed and the atria are enlarged; if present, hypertrophy of the interatrial septum is a helpful additional finding diagnostically. The condition is relatively uncommon, with the most frequent causes being amyloidosis. In Africa, endomyocardial fibrosis, a specific entity in which there is severe fibrosis of the endocardium, often with eosinophilia (Löffler's syndrome), is common. Other causes of restrictive cardiomyopathy are infiltrative cardiomyopathies (eg, hemochromatosis, carcinoid syndrome) and connective tissue diseases (eg, scleroderma).

Amyloidosis results from deposition of various proteins within the myocardium. Primary amyloidosis is caused by deposition of immunoglobulin light chains (AL) by monoclonal plasma cells, often as a consequence of multiple myeloma. The heart may be the only organ involved at times. Systemic amyloidosis is due to production of AA light chains. Familial amyloidosis results from production of a carrier protein called transthyretin. Systemic amyloidosis may affect any organ but is particularly associated with significant pulmonary and renal involvement and with a peripheral neuropathy (that often results in orthostatic hypotension).

Conduction disturbances are frequently present. Low voltages on the ECG combined with ventricular hypertrophy revealed by echocardiography are suggestive. Cardiac MRI presents a distinctive pattern in amyloidosis and is a useful screening test. The echocardiogram reveals a small thickened LV with bright myocardium, rapid early diastolic filling revealed by Doppler, and biatrial enlargement. Atrial septal thickening may also be evident. Rectal, abdominal fat, or gingival biopsies can confirm systemic involvement, but myocardial involvement may still be present if these are negative. Myocardial amyloidosis can be confirmed by myocardial biopsy.

Restrictive cardiomyopathy must be distinguished from constrictive pericarditis. The clinical differentiation is described below, but the key feature is that ventricular interaction is accentuated with respiration in constrictive pericarditis, and that interaction is absent in restrictive cardiomyopathy. Pulmonary pressure is invariably elevated in restrictive cardiomyopathy and is normal in uncomplicated constrictive pericarditis.

Unfortunately, little useful therapy is available for either the causative conditions or the restrictive cardiomyopathy itself. Diuretics can help, but excessive diuresis can produce worsening symptoms. As with most patients with severe right heart failure, loop diuretics, thiazides, and aldosterone antagonists are all useful. Digoxin may precipitate arrhythmias and generally should not be used. β-Blockers help slow heart rates and improve filling. Corticosteroids may be helpful in sarcoidosis but relieve conduction abnormalities more often than heart failure. Chemotherapy for amyloidosis with alkylating agents or with interferon is sometimes used, but unless the underlying diagnosis is multiple myeloma, there is little cardiac improvement. Bone marrow stem cell replacement for amyloidosis is under investigation and some of the best results to date have been attributed to this process. Cardiac transplantation is an option in patients with primary cardiac amyloidosis. Liver transplantation has been used as well in the familial form in an attempt to prevent the production of transthyretin.

Ammash NM et al: Clinical profile and outcome of idiopathic restrictive cardiomyopathy. Circulation 2000;101:2490. [PMID: 10831523]

Asher CR et al: Diastolic heart failure: restrictive cardiomyopathy, constrictive pericarditis, and cardiac tamponade: clinical and echocardiographic evaluation. Cardiol Rev 2002;10:218. [PMID: 12144733]

Gertz MA et al: Primary systemic amyloidosis. Curr Treat Options Oncol 2002;3:261. [PMID: 12057072]

Goldstein JA: Cardiac tamponade, constrictive pericarditis, and restrictive cardiomyopathy. Curr Probl Cardiol 2004;29:503. [PMID: 15365561]

Hancock EW: Differential diagnosis of restrictive cardiomyopathy and constrictive pericarditis. Heart 2001;86:343. [PMID: 11514495]

Yazdani K et al: Differentiating constrictive pericarditis from restrictive cardiomyopathy. Rev Cardiovasc Med 2005;6:61. [PMID: 15976729]

■ ACUTE RHEUMATIC FEVER & RHEUMATIC HEART DISEASE

 ESSENTIALS OF DIAGNOSIS

- *Uncommon in the United States (approximately 2 cases/100,000 population); more common (100 cases/100,000 population) in developing countries.*
- *Peak incidence ages 5–15 years.*
- *Diagnosis based on Jones criteria and confirmation of streptococcal infection.*
- *May involve mitral and other valves acutely, rarely leading to heart failure.*

General Considerations

Rheumatic fever is a systemic immune process that is a sequela to β-hemolytic streptococcal infection of the pharynx. Pyodermic infections are not associated with rheumatic fever. Signs of rheumatic fever usually commence 2–3 weeks after infection but may appear as early as 1 week or as late as 5 weeks. In recent years, the disease has become quite uncommon in the United States, except in immigrants. However, there have been reports of new outbreaks in several regions of the United States. The peak incidence is between ages 5 and 15 years; rheumatic fever is rare before age 4 years or after age 40 years. Rheumatic carditis and valvulitis may be self-limited or may lead to slowly progressive valvular deformity. The characteristic lesion is a perivascular granulomatous reaction with vasculitis. The mitral valve is attacked in 75–80% of cases, the aortic valve in 30% (but rarely as the sole valve), and the tricuspid and pulmonary valves in under 5% of cases.

Clinical Findings

The diagnostic criteria first described by Jones were updated in 1992. The presence of two major criteria—or one major and two minor criteria—establishes the diagnosis.

A. MAJOR CRITERIA

1. Carditis—Carditis is most likely to be evident in children and adolescents. Any of the following suggests the presence of carditis: (1) pericarditis; (2) cardiomegaly, detected by physical signs, radiography, or echocardiography; (3) CHF, right- or left-sided—the former perhaps more prominent in children, with painful liver engorgement due to tricuspid regurgitation; and (4) mitral or aortic regurgitation murmurs, indicative of dilation of a valve ring with or without associated valvulitis. The Carey–Coombs short mid-diastolic mitral murmur may be present.

In the absence of any of the above definitive signs, the diagnosis of carditis depends on the following less specific abnormalities: (1) ECG changes, including changing contour of P waves or inversion of T waves; (2) changing quality of heart sounds; and (3) sinus tachycardia, arrhythmia, or ectopic beats.

2. Erythema marginatum and subcutaneous nodules—Erythema marginatum begins as rapidly enlarging macules that assume the shape of rings or crescents with clear centers. They may be raised, confluent, and either transient or persistent.

Subcutaneous nodules are uncommon except in children. They are small (≤ 2 cm in diameter), firm, and nontender and are attached to fascia or tendon sheaths over bony prominences. They persist for days or weeks, are recurrent, and are indistinguishable from rheumatoid nodules.

3. Sydenham's chorea—Sydenham's chorea—involuntary choreoathetoid movements primarily of the face, tongue, and upper extremities—may be the sole manifestation; only 50% of cases have other overt signs of rheumatic fever. Girls are more frequently affected, and occurrence in adults is rare. This is the least common (3% of cases) but most diagnostic of the manifestations of rheumatic fever.

4. Polyarthritis—This is a migratory polyarthritis that involves the large joints sequentially. In adults, only a single joint may be affected. The arthritis lasts 1–5 weeks and subsides without residual deformity. Prompt response of arthritis to therapeutic doses of salicylates or nonsteroidal agents is characteristic.

B. MINOR CRITERIA

These include fever, polyarthralgias, reversible prolongation of the PR interval, and an elevated erythrocyte sedimentation rate or CRP. Supporting evidence includes positive throat culture or rapid streptococcal antigen test and elevated or rising streptococcal antibody titer.

C. LABORATORY FINDINGS

There is nonspecific evidence of inflammatory disease, as shown by a rapid sedimentation rate. High or in-creasing titers of antistreptococcal antibodies (antistreptolysin O and anti-DNase B) are used to confirm recent infection; 10% of cases lack this serologic evidence.

Differential Diagnosis

Rheumatic fever may be confused with the following: rheumatoid arthritis, osteomyelitis, endocarditis, chronic meningococcemia, systemic lupus erythematosus, Lyme disease, sickle cell anemia, "surgical abdomen," and many other diseases.

Complications

CHF occurs in severe cases. In the longer term, the development of rheumatic heart disease is the major problem. Other complications include arrhythmias, pericarditis with effusion, and rheumatic pneumonitis.

Treatment

A. GENERAL MEASURES

The patient should be kept at strict bed rest until the temperature returns to normal (without the use of antipyretic medications) and the sedimentation rate, plus the resting pulse rate, and the ECG have all returned to baseline.

B. MEDICAL MEASURES

1. Salicylates—The salicylates markedly reduce fever and relieve joint pain and swelling. They have no effect on the natural course of the disease. Adults may require large doses of aspirin, 0.6–0.9 g every 4 hours; children are treated with lower doses. Toxicity includes tinnitus, vomiting, and gastrointestinal bleeding.

2. Penicillin—Penicillin (benzathine penicillin, 1.2 million units intramuscularly once, or procaine penicillin, 600,000 units intramuscularly daily for 10 days) is used to eradicate streptococcal infection if present. Erythromycin may be substituted (40 mg/kg/d).

3. Corticosteroids—There is no proof that cardiac damage is prevented or minimized by corticosteroids. A short course of corticosteroids (prednisone, 40–60 mg orally daily, with tapering over 2 weeks) usually causes rapid improvement of the joint symptoms and is indicated when response to salicylates has been inadequate.

Prevention of Recurrent Rheumatic Fever

The initial episode of rheumatic fever can usually be prevented by early treatment of streptococcal pharyngitis. (See Chapter 33.) Prevention of recurrent episodes is critical. Recurrences of rheumatic fever are most common in patients who have had carditis during their initial episode and in children, 20% of whom will have a second episode within 5 years. Recurrences are uncommon after 5 years following the first episode, and in patients over 25 years of age. Prophylaxis is usually discontinued after these times except in groups with a high risk of streptococcal infection—parents or teachers of young children, nurses, military recruits, etc. Secondary prevention of rheumatic fever depends on whether carditis has occurred. If there is no evidence for carditis, preventive therapy can be stopped at age 21 years. If carditis has occurred but there is no residual valvular disease, it can be stopped at 10 years after the episode. If carditis has occurred with residual valvular involvement, it should be continued for 10 years after the last episode or until age 40 years if the patient is in a situation in which reexposure would be expected.

A. PENICILLIN

The preferred method of prophylaxis is with benzathine penicillin G, 1.2 million units intramuscularly every 4 weeks. Oral penicillin (200,000–250,000 units twice daily) is less reliable.

B. ALTERNATIVES FOR PENICILLIN-ALLERGIC PATIENTS

If the patient is allergic to penicillin, sulfadiazine (or sulfisoxazole), 1 g daily, or erythromycin, 250 mg orally twice daily, may be substituted. The macrolide azithromycin is similarly effective against group A streptococcal infection. If the patient has not had an immediate hypersensitivity (anaphylactic-type) reaction to penicillin, then cephalosporin may also be used.

Prognosis

Initial episodes of rheumatic fever may last months in children and weeks in adults. The immediate mortality rate is 1–2%. Persistent rheumatic carditis with cardiomegaly, heart failure, and pericarditis implies a poor prognosis; 30% of children thus affected die within 10 years after the initial attack. After 10 years, two-thirds of patients will have detectable valvular abnormalities (usually thickened valves with limited mobility), but significant symptomatic valvular heart disease or persistent cardiomyopathy occurs in less than 10% of patients with a single episode. In developing countries, acute rheumatic fever occurs earlier in life, recurs more frequently, and the evolution to chronic valvular disease is both accelerated and more severe.

Rheumatic Heart Disease

Chronic rheumatic heart disease results from single or repeated attacks of rheumatic fever that produce rigidity and deformity of valve cusps, fusion of the commissures, or shortening and fusion of the chordae tendineae. Stenosis or insufficiency results, and the two often coexist. The mitral valve alone is affected in 50–60% of cases; combined lesions of the aortic and mitral valves occur in 20%; pure aortic lesions are less common. Tricuspid involvement occurs in about 10% of cases but only in association with mitral or aortic disease and is thought to be more common when recurrent infections have occurred. The pulmonary valve is rarely affected. A history of rheumatic fever is

obtainable in only 60% of patients with rheumatic heart disease.

Recurrences of acute rheumatic fever can be prevented (see above). The patient should also receive prophylactic antibiotics preceding dental extraction, urologic and surgical procedures, etc, to prevent endocarditis (Table 33–4). With mitral valve disease, it is important to identify the onset of atrial fibrillation to institute anticoagulation. The important findings in each of the major valve lesions are summarized in Table 10–1.

Carapetis JR et al: Acute rheumatic fever. Lancet 2005;366:155. [PMID: 16005340]

Cilliers AM et al: Anti-inflammatory treatment for carditis in acute rheumatic fever. Cochrane Database Syst Rev 2003; (2):CD003176. [PMID: 12804454]

Guilherme L et al: Rheumatic fever: from sore throat to autoimmune heart lesions. Int Arch Allergy Immunol 2004;134: 56. [PMID: 15103230]

McDonald M et al: Acute rheumatic fever: a chink in the chain that links the heart to the throat? Lancet Infect Dis 2004; 4:240. [PMID: 15050943]

Narula J et al: Diagnosis of active rheumatic carditis. Circulation 1999;100:1576. [PMID: 10510063]

Rullan E et al: Rheumatic fever. Curr Rheumatol Rep 2001; 3:445. [PMID: 11564377]

Stollerman GH: Rheumatic fever in the 21st century. Clin Infect Dis 2001;33:806. [PMID: 11512086]

■ DISEASES OF THE PERICARDIUM

ACUTE PERICARDITIS

Anatomic & Physiologic Considerations

The pericardium consists of two layers: the inner visceral layer, which is attached to the epicardium, and an outer parietal layer. About 50 mL of serous fluid is normally present and provides lubrication between the two layers. The pericardial reflection encompasses the heart and great vessels. The pericardium stabilizes the heart in anatomic position and reduces contact between the heart and the surrounding structures. It is composed of fibrous tissue, and although it will permit moderate changes in cardiac size, it cannot stretch rapidly enough to accommodate rapid dilation of the heart or accumulation of fluid without increasing intrapericardial (and, therefore, intracardiac) pressure.

The pericardium is often involved by processes that affect the heart, but it may also be affected by diseases of adjacent tissues and may itself be a primary site of disease.

INFLAMMATORY PERICARDITIS

Acute (< 2 weeks) inflammation of the pericardium may be infectious in origin or may be due to systemic diseases (autoimmune syndromes, uremia), neoplasm, radiation, drug toxicity, hemopericardium, postcardiac surgery, or contiguous inflammatory processes in the myocardium or lung. In many of these conditions, the pathologic process involves both the pericardium and the myocardium.

The presentation and course of inflammatory pericarditis depend on its cause, but all syndromes are often (not always) associated with chest pain, which is usually pleuritic and postural (relieved by sitting). The pain is substernal but may radiate to the neck, shoulders, back, or epigastrium. Dyspnea may also be present. A pericardial friction rub is characteristic, with or without evidence of fluid accumulation or constriction (see below). Fever and leukocytosis are often present. The ECG usually shows generalized ST and T wave changes and may manifest a characteristic progression beginning with diffuse ST elevation, followed by a return to baseline and then to T wave inversion. Atrial injury is often present and manifested by PR depression especially in the limb leads. The chest radiograph is frequently normal, but may show cardiac enlargement if fluid has collected, as well as signs of related pulmonary disease. Mass lesions and enlarged lymph nodes may suggest a neoplastic process. The echocardiogram is often normal or reveals only a trivial amount of fluid during the acute inflammatory process.

Viral Pericarditis

Viral infections (especially infections with coxsackieviruses and echoviruses but also influenza, Epstein–Barr, varicella, hepatitis, mumps, and HIV viruses) are the most common cause of acute pericarditis and probably are responsible for many cases classified as idiopathic. Males—usually under age 50 years—are most commonly affected. Pericardial involvement often follows upper respiratory infection. The diagnosis is usually clinical, but rising viral titers in paired sera may be obtained for confirmation. Cardiac enzymes may be slightly elevated, reflecting a myocarditic component. The differential diagnosis is primarily with myocardial infarction.

Treatment is generally symptomatic. Aspirin (650 mg every 3–4 hours) or other nonsteroidal agents (eg, indomethacin, 100–150 mg daily in divided doses) are usually effective. Corticosteroids may be beneficial in unresponsive cases. In general, symptoms subside in several days to weeks. The major early complication is tamponade, which occurs in less than 5% of patients. There may be recurrences in the first few weeks or months. Rare patients will continue to experience recurrences chronically. These patients may require long-term anti-inflammatory medications, either corticosteroids or colchicine. Rarely, acute pericarditis may lead to constrictive pericarditis, when pericardial resection may be necessary (see below).

Tuberculous Pericarditis

Tuberculous pericarditis has become rare in developed countries but remains common in other areas. It re-sults from direct lymphatic or hematogenous spread; clinical pulmonary involvement may be absent or minor, although associated pleural effusions are common. The presentation tends to be subacute, but nonspecific symptoms (fever, night sweats, fatigue) may be present for days to months. One to 8 percent of patients with pulmonary tuberculosis develop pericardial involvement. Pericardial effusions are usually small or moderate but may be large. The diagnosis can be inferred if acid-fast bacilli are found elsewhere. The yield of organisms by pericardiocentesis is low; pericardial biopsy has a higher yield but may also be negative, and pericardiectomy may be required. Standard antituberculous drug therapy is usually successful (see Chapter 9), but constrictive pericarditis can occur.

Other Infectious Pericarditides

Bacterial pericarditis has become rare and usually results from direct extension from pulmonary infections. Pneumococci can cause a primary pericardial infection. Symptoms and signs of bacterial pericarditis are similar to those of other types of inflammatory pericarditides, but patients appear toxic and are often critically ill. *Borrelia burgdorferi*, the organism responsible for Lyme disease, can also cause myopericarditis. If bacterial pericarditis is suspected on clinical grounds, diagnostic pericardiocentesis may be of value.

Uremic Pericarditis

Uremic pericarditis is a common complication of renal failure. The pathogenesis is uncertain; it occurs both with untreated uremia and in otherwise stable dialysis patients. In uremic patients not on dialysis, the incidence correlates roughly with the level of blood urea nitrogen (BUN) and creatinine. The pericardium is characteristically "shaggy," and the effusion is hemorrhagic and exudative. Uremic pericarditis can present with or without symptoms; fever is absent. The pericarditis usually resolves with the institution of—or with more aggressive—dialysis. Tamponade is fairly common, and partial pericardiectomy (pericardial window) may be necessary. Whereas anti-inflammatory agents may relieve the pain and fever associated with uremic pericarditis, indomethacin and systemic corticosteroids do not affect its natural history. Most uremic patients with pericarditis respond to intensive dialysis, although patients who have progressed to tamponade do so less well and usually require drainage.

Neoplastic Pericarditis

Spread of adjacent lung cancer as well as invasion by breast cancer, renal cell carcinoma, Hodgkin's disease, and lymphomas are the most common neoplastic processes involving the pericardium and have become the most frequent causes of pericardial tamponade in many countries. Often the process is painless, and the presenting symptoms relate to hemodynamic compromise or the primary disease. Pericardial effusions develop over a long period of time and may become quite huge (> 2 L). The diagnosis can occasionally be made by cytologic examination of the effusion or by pericardial biopsy, but it may be difficult to establish clinically if the patient has received mediastinal radiation within the previous year. MRI and CT scan can visualize neighboring tumor when present. The prognosis with neoplastic effusion is dismal, with only a small minority surviving 1 year. If it is compromising the clinical comfort of the patient, the effusion is initially drained percutaneously. Early attempts at ballooning the pericardium from a subxiphoid approach have been mostly abandoned in favor of surgical approaches. A pericardial window, either by a subxiphoid approach or via video-assisted thoracic surgery, allows for partial pericardiectomy. Instillation of chemotherapeutic agents or tetracycline may occasionally be used to reduce the recurrence rate.

Postmyocardial Infarction or Postcardiotomy Pericarditis (Dressler's Syndrome)

Pericarditis may occur 2–5 days after infarction due to an inflammatory reaction to transmural myocardial necrosis. It usually presents as a recurrence of pain with pleural-pericardial features. A rub is often audible, and repolarization changes may be confused with ischemia. Large effusions are uncommon, and spontaneous resolution usually occurs in a few days. Aspirin or nonsteroidal agents in the dosages given in the section on viral pericarditis provide symptomatic relief.

Dressler's syndrome occurs weeks to several months after myocardial infarction or open heart surgery, may be recurrent, and probably represents an autoimmune syndrome. Patients present with typical pain, fever, malaise, and leukocytosis. Occasionally, the syndrome will occur within days of surgery. The sedimentation rate is high. Large pericardial effusions and accompanying pleural effusions are frequent. Rarely, other symptoms of an autoimmune disorder, such as joint pain and fever, may occur. Tamponade is rare with Dressler's syndrome after myocardial infarction but not when it occurs postoperatively. Nonsteroidal anti-inflammatory agents given for 2–4 weeks are usually effective. In more severe cases, corticosteroids should be given in rapidly tapering doses. Relapses do occur and may require slow withdrawal of anti-inflammatory therapy over several months. Colchicine may be required for months to help prevent recurrences.

Radiation Pericarditis

Radiation can initiate a fibrinous and fibrotic process in the pericardium, presenting as subacute pericarditis or constriction. The clinical onset is usually within the first year but may be delayed for many years. Radiation pericarditis usually follows treatments of more than 4000 cGy delivered to ports including more than 30% of the heart. Symptomatic therapy is the initial approach, but recurrent effusions and constriction often require surgery.

Other Causes of Pericarditis

These include connective tissue diseases, such as lupus erythematosus and rheumatoid arthritis, drug-induced pericarditis (minoxidil, penicillins), and myxedema. Myxedema pericardial effusions usually are characterized by the presence of cholesterol crystals.

Imazio M et al: Management, risk factors, and outcomes in recurrent pericarditis. Am J Cardiol 2005;96:736. [PMID: 16125506]

Lee PJ et al: Cardiovascular effects of radiation therapy: practical approach to radiation therapy-induced heart disease. Cardiol Rev 2005;13:80. [PMID: 15705258]

Ross AM et al: Acute pericarditis. Evaluation and treatment of infectious and other causes. Postgrad Med 2004;115: 67. [PMID: 15038256]

Talreja DR et al: Constrictive pericarditis in 26 patients with histologically normal pericardial thickness. Circulation 2003; 108:1852. [PMID: 14517161]

Troughton RW et al: Pericarditis. Lancet 2004;363:717. [PMID: 15001332]

PERICARDIAL EFFUSION

Pericardial effusion can develop during any of the processes previously discussed. The speed of accumulation determines the physiologic importance of the effusion. Because the pericardium stretches, large effusions (> 1000 mL) that develop slowly may produce no hemodynamic effects. Smaller effusions that appear rapidly can cause tamponade. Tamponade is characterized by elevated intrapericardial pressure (> 15 mm Hg), which restricts venous return and ventricular filling. As a result, the stroke volume and pulse pressure fall, and the heart rate and venous pressure rise. Shock and death may result.

Clinical Findings

A. Symptoms and Signs

Pericardial effusions may be associated with pain if they occur as part of an acute inflammatory process or may be painless, as is often the case with neoplastic or uremic effusion. Dyspnea and cough are common, especially with tamponade. Other symptoms may result from the primary disease.

A pericardial friction rub may be present even with large effusions. In cardiac tamponade, tachycardia, tachypnea, a narrow pulse pressure, and a relatively preserved systolic pressure are characteristic. Pulsus paradoxus—a greater than 10 mm Hg decline in systolic pressure during inspiration due to further impairment of LV filling—is the classic finding, but it may also occur with obstructive lung disease. Central venous pressure is elevated and there is no evident y descent in the RA, RV, or LV hemodynamic tracings. Edema or ascites are rarely present; these signs favor a more chronic process.

B. LABORATORY FINDINGS

Laboratory tests tend to reflect the underlying processes (see causes of pericarditis above).

C. DIAGNOSTIC STUDIES

Chest radiograph can suggest effusion by an enlarged cardiac silhouette with a globular configuration but may appear normal. The ECG often reveals nonspecific T wave changes and low QRS voltage. Electrical alternans is present uncommonly but is pathognomonic. It is due to the heart swinging within the large effusion. Echocardiography is the primary method for demonstrating pericardial effusion and is quite sensitive. If tamponade is present, the high intrapericardial pressure may collapse lower pressure cardiac structures, such as the RA and RV. In tamponade, the normal inspiratory reduction in LV filling is accentuated due to RV/LV interaction and there is a > 25% reduction in mitral inflow velocities. Cardiac CT and MRI also demonstrate pericardial fluid and lesions. Diagnostic pericardiocentesis or biopsy is often indicated for microbiologic and cytologic studies; a pericardial biopsy may be performed relatively simply through a small subxiphoid incision.

Treatment

Small effusions can be followed clinically by careful observations of the JVP and by testing for a paradoxical pulse. Serial echocardiograms are indicated if no intervention is immediately contemplated. When tamponade is present, urgent pericardiocentesis is required. Because the pressure–volume relationship in the pericardial fluid is curvilinear and upsloping, removal of a small amount of fluid often produces a dramatic fall in the intrapericardial pressure and immediate hemodynamic benefit; but complete drainage with a catheter is preferable. Continued or repeat drainage may be indicated, especially in malignant effusions. Pericardial windows via video-assisted thorascopy have been particularly effective in preventing recurrences.

Additional therapy is determined by the nature of the primary process. Recurrent effusion in neoplastic disease and uremia, in particular, may require partial pericardiectomy as noted earlier.

Burgess LJ et al: Role of biochemical tests in the diagnosis of large pericardial effusions. Chest 2002;121:495. [PMID: 11834663]

Rienmuller R et al: CT and MR imaging of pericardial disease. Radiol Clin North Am 2004;42:587. [PMID: 15193931]

Shabetai R: Pericardial effusion: haemodynamic spectrum. Heart 2004;90:255. [PMID: 14966038]

Soler-Soler J et al: Management of pericardial effusion. Heart 2001;86:235. [PMID: 11454853]

Tsang TS: Outcomes of primary and secondary treatment of pericardial effusion in patients with malignancy. Mayo Clin Proc 2000;75:248. [PMID: 10725950]

Wang ZJ et al: CT and MR imaging of pericardial disease. Radiographics 2003;23 Spec No:S167. [PMID: 14557510]

CONSTRICTIVE PERICARDITIS

Inflammation can lead to a thickened, fibrotic, adherent pericardium that restricts diastolic filling and produces chronically elevated venous pressures. In the past, tuberculosis was the most common cause of constrictive pericarditis, but the process now more often occurs after radiation therapy, cardiac surgery, or viral pericarditis; histoplasmosis is another uncommon cause.

The principal symptoms are slowly progressive dyspnea, fatigue, and weakness. Chronic edema, hepatic congestion, and ascites are usually present. Ascites often seems out of proportion to the degree of peripheral edema. The examination reveals these signs and a characteristically elevated jugular venous pressure with a rapid y descent. This can be detected at bedside by careful observation of the jugular pulse and noting an apparent increased pulse wave at the end of systole (due to accentuation of the v wave by the rapid y descent). Kussmaul's sign—a failure of the JVP to fall with inspiration—is also a frequent finding. The apex may actually retract with systole and a pericardial "knock" may be heard in early diastole. Pulsus paradoxus is unusual. Atrial fibrillation is common.

The chest radiograph may show normal heart size or cardiomegaly. Pericardial calcification is best seen on the lateral view and is uncommon. It rarely involves the LV apex, and finding of calcification at the LV apex is more consistent with myocardial aneurysm. Echocardiography rarely demonstrates a thickened pericardium. A septal "bounce" reflecting the rapid early filling is common, though. RV/LV interaction may be demonstrated by a reduction in the mitral inflow pattern of > 25%, much as in tamponade. Cardiac CT and MRI are only occasionally helpful. Pericardial thickening of > 4 mm must be present to establish the diagnosis, yet no pericardial thickening is demonstrated in 20–25% of patients with constrictive pericarditis. At times constrictive pericarditis is extremely difficult to differentiate from restrictive cardiomyopathy. When unclear, the use of noninvasive testing and cardiac catheterization is required to sort out the difference. As a generality, the pulmonary pressure is lower in constriction and there must be signs of RV/LV interaction (reduced LV filling pattern with inspiration) on echocardiography/Doppler. In constrictive pericarditis, because of the need to demonstrate RV/LV interaction, cardiac catheterization should include simultaneous measurement of both the LV and RV. Hemodynamically, patients with constriction have equalization of end-diastolic pressures throughout their cardiac chambers, there is rapid early filling then an abrupt increase in diastolic pressure ("square-root" sign), the RV end-diastolic pressure is more than one-third the systolic pressure, simultaneous measurements of RV and LV systolic pressure reveal a discordance with inspiration (the RV rises as the LV falls), and there is usually a Kussmaul's sign (failure of the RA pressure to fall with inspiration). The width of the RV pressure tracing may also be narrow in expiration and greater during inspiration, reflecting the wide variation in filling of the RV with respiration. In restrictive cardiomyopathy, the LV diastolic pressure is usually greater than the RV diastolic pressure by 5 mm Hg, there is pulmonary hypertension, and simultaneous measurements of the RV and LV systolic pressure reveal a concordant drop in both with inspiration. Initial treatment consists of diuresis. As in other disorders of right heart failure, the diuresis should be aggressive, using loop diuretics (torsemide if bowel edema is suspected), thiazides, and aldosterone antagonists (especially if ascites is present). Surgical pericardiectomy should be done when diuretics are unable to control symptoms. Pericardiectomy removes the pericardium between the phrenic nerves only, however, and most patients still require diuretics after the procedure, though symptoms are usually dramatically improved. Morbidity and mortality after pericardiectomy are high (up to 15%) and are greatest in those with the most disability prior to the procedure. For that reason, most experts recommend earlier rather than later pericardiectomy if symptoms are present.

Asher CR et al: Diastolic heart failure: restrictive cardiomyopathy, constrictive pericarditis, and cardiac tamponade: clinical and echocardiographic evaluation. Cardiol Rev 2002;10: 218. [PMID: 12144733]

Bertog SC et al: Constrictive pericarditis: etiology and cause-specific survival after pericardiectomy. J Am Coll Cardiol 2004; 43:1445. [PMID: 15093882]

Hoit BD: Management of effusive and constrictive pericardial heart disease. Circulation 2002;105:2939. [PMID: 12081983]

Nishimura RA: Constrictive pericarditis in the modern era: a diagnostic dilemma. Heart 2001;86:619. [PMID: 11711451]

Sagrista-Sauleda J et al: Effusive-constrictive pericarditis. N Engl J Med 2004;350:469. [PMID: 14749455]

Wang A et al: Clinical problem-solving. Undercover and overlooked. N Engl J Med 2004;351:1014. [PMID: 15342810]

■ PULMONARY HYPERTENSION & PULMONARY HEART DISEASE

PRIMARY PULMONARY HYPERTENSION

The normal pulmonary bed offers about one-tenth as much resistance to blood flow as the systemic arterial system. Pulmonary hypertension is defined as mild if the mean PA pressure is > 20 mm Hg, moderate if > 30 mm Hg, and severe if > 45 mm Hg. As opposed to the systemic circulation, the pulmonary resistance is influenced by local vascular mediators much more than the adrenergic nervous system, even though both α- and β-receptors are present on pulmonary vascular smooth muscle. The normal pulmonary endothelial cell maintains the vascular smooth muscle in a state of relaxation. Pulmonary vasoconstriction is mediated by hypoxia and by endothelin

and angiotensin II. Vasodilation can be affected by certain prostaglandins, endothelin receptor blockers, smooth muscle relaxants and by nitric oxide.

Primary pulmonary hypertension is defined as pulmonary hypertension and elevated PVR in the absence of other disease of the lungs or heart. Its cause is unknown, though there are clear genetic patterns that have been identified, and it likely represents a derangement in one or more of the biologic pathways described above. Pathologically, it is characterized by diffuse narrowing of the pulmonary arterioles. Circumstantial evidence suggests that unrecognized recurrent pulmonary emboli or in situ thrombosis may play a role in some cases. However, the latter may well be an exacerbating factor (precipitated by local endothelial injury) rather than a cause of the syndrome. Primary pulmonary hypertension must be distinguished from other causes of severe secondary pulmonary hypertension, such as systemic sclerosis, HIV-related pulmonary hypertension, cirrhosis, and congenital heart defects (primarily those with a shunt distal to the level of the tricuspid valve). Rarely, pulmonary venous disease (pulmonary veno-occlusive disease) or peripheral PA stenosis may be present. Left heart disease, in particular mitral stenosis, or any reason for an elevated LA pressure must be excluded as well. Table 10–13 includes clinical disorders causing pulmonary hypertension.

The laboratory evaluation of primary pulmonary hypertension must exclude a secondary cause. A hypercoagulable state should be sought and chronic pulmonary emboli excluded (usually by lung scan or contrast CT). The chest radiograph helps exclude a primary pulmonary etiology—evidence for patchy edema may raise the suspicion of pulmonary veno-occlusive disease. The ECG is generally consistent with RVH and RA enlargement. Echocardiography/Doppler demonstrates an enlarged RV and RA—at times they may be huge and hypocontractile. Severe pulmonic or tricuspid regurgitation may be present. Septal flattening is consistent with pulmonary hypertension. Doppler interrogation of the tricuspid regurgitation jet helps provide an estimate of RV systolic pressure. Pulmonary function tests help exclude other disorders, though primary pulmonary hypertension may present with a reduced carbon monoxide diffusing capacity of the lung ($D_{L_{CO}}$) and severe desaturation (particularly if a PFO has been stretched open and a right-to-left shunt is present). Chest CT demonstrates enlarged pulmonary arteries and excludes other causes (such as emphysema or interstitial lung disease). Pulmonary angiography (or MR angiography or CT angiography) reveals loss of the smaller acinar pulmonary vessels and tapering of the larger ones. Catheterization allows measurement of pulmonary pressures and testing for vasoreactivity using a variety of agents, including 100% oxygen, adenosine, epoprostenol, and nitric oxide. A positive response is one that decreases the pulmonary mean pressure by > 25% (ideally below 30 mm Hg).

The clinical picture is similar to that of pulmonary hypertension from other causes. Patients—characteristically young women—present with evidence of right heart failure that is usually progressive, leading to

Table 10–13. Causes of pulmonary hypertension.

Pulmonary arterial hypertension
    Primary pulmonary hypertension
    Persistent pulmonary hypertension of the newborn
    Secondary causes
        Connective tissue disease
        Eisenmenger physiology (congenital heart disease)
        Portal hypertension
        HIV
        Drugs/toxins (especially anorexigens)
Pulmonary venous hypertension
    Left-sided heart disease
    Pulmonary venous obstruction
        Veno-occlusive disease
        Fibrosing mediastinitis (usually related to histoplasmosis or radiation)
Disorders of the lung or hypoxemia
    Chronic obstructive pulmonary disease
    Interstitial lung disease
    Sleep apnea
    High altitude (chronic exposure)
    Alveolar-capillary dysplasia
Chronic thromboembolic disease
    Thrombotic obstruction (clot)
    Pulmonary emboli (tumor, foreign material)
Disorders of pulmonary vasculature
    Schistosomiasis
    Sarcoidosis
    Histiocytosis X
    Other

Modified from Rich S (editor): Primary pulmonary hypertension: Executive summary from the World Symposium–Primary Pulmonary Hypertension, 1998. Available from the World Health Organization (www.who.int/ncd/cvd/pph.html).

death in 2–8 years. This is a decidedly different prognosis than patients with Eisenmenger physiology due to a left-to-right shunt; 40% of Eisenmenger patients are alive 25 years after the diagnosis has been made. Patients have manifestations of low cardiac output, with weakness and fatigue, as well as edema and ascites as right heart failure advances. Peripheral cyanosis is present, and syncope on effort may occur.

Until recently, there was no therapy for primary pulmonary hypertension, except lung transplantation. Currently, a variety of therapeutic options are being investigated. Some authorities advocate long-term oral anticoagulation and this is given in most patients with primary pulmonary hypertension. Supplemental oxygen, particularly at night, appears to improve symptoms and helps reduce pulmonary pressures. Diuretics help with right heart edema. Calcium channel blockers, at times in large doses, have been used with mixed results. Some patients respond well, especially if they are proven responders to vasodilators. However, calcium channel blockers can worsen RV function by their negative inotropic effects.

Other agents are now available for direct treatment of pulmonary hypertension. Epoprostenol (Flolan) is administered by continuous infusion and has been shown to improve functional capacity and survival. Analogs of epoprostenol are also available, including trepostinol (Remodulin), beraprost, and iloprost. Treprostinil is given by subcutaneous injection, beraprost by mouth, and iloprost by inhalation. Endothelin antagonists are also available orally, such as bosentan (Tracleer) and sitaxentan (Thelin). Finally, phosphodiesterase inhibitors, such as sildenafil, are also being carefully investigated. The cost of all of these agents, except for sildenafil and calcium channel blockers, is quite high.

Pulmonary transplantation is a viable option in selected centers, though the operative mortality is high (around 20–25%) and 2-year survival only about 55%.

Chatterjee K et al: Pulmonary hypertension: hemodynamic diagnosis and management. Arch Intern Med 2002;162:1925. [PMID: 12230414]

McLauglin VV: Survival in primary pulmonary hypertension: the impact of epoprostenol therapy. Circulation 2002;15:1477. [PMID: 12234951]

Olschewski H et al: Inhaled iloprost for severe pulmonary hypertension. N Engl J Med 2002;347:322. [PMID: 12151469]

Rubin LJ et al: Bosentan therapy for pulmonary arterial hypertension. N Engl J Med 2002;346:806. [PMID: 11907289]

Rubin LJ et al: Evaluation and management of the patient with pulmonary arterial hypertension. Ann Intern Med 2005;143:282. [PMID: 16103472]

Sitbon O et al: Primary pulmonary hypertension: current therapy. Prog Cardiovasc Dis 2002;45:115.[PMID: 12411973]

PULMONARY HEART DISEASE (Cor Pulmonale)

 ESSENTIALS OF DIAGNOSIS

- *Symptoms and signs of chronic bronchitis and pulmonary emphysema.*
- *Elevated jugular venous pressure, parasternal lift, edema, hepatomegaly, ascites.*
- *ECG shows tall, peaked P waves (P pulmonale), right axis deviation, and RVH.*
- *Chest radiograph: Enlarged RV and PA.*
- *Echocardiogram or radionuclide angiography excludes primary LV dysfunction.*

General Considerations

The term "cor pulmonale" denotes RV hypertrophy and eventual failure resulting from pulmonary disease and attendant hypoxia or from pulmonary vascular disease. Its clinical features depend upon both the primary underlying disease and its effects on the heart.

Cor pulmonale is most commonly caused by COPD. Less frequent causes include pneumoconiosis, pulmonary fibrosis, kyphoscoliosis, primary pulmonary hypertension, repeated episodes of subclinical or clinical pulmonary embolization, Pickwickian syndrome, schistosomiasis, and obliterative pulmonary capillary or lymphangitic infiltration from metastatic carcinoma.

Clinical Findings

A. Symptoms and Signs

The predominant symptoms of compensated cor pulmonale are related to the pulmonary disorder and include chronic productive cough, exertional dyspnea, wheezing respirations, easy fatigability, and weakness. When the pulmonary disease causes RV failure, these symptoms may be intensified. Dependent edema and right upper quadrant pain may also appear. The signs of cor pulmonale include cyanosis, clubbing, distended neck veins, RV heave or gallop (or both), prominent lower sternal or epigastric pulsations, an enlarged and tender liver, and dependent edema.

B. Laboratory Findings

Polycythemia is often present in cor pulmonale secondary to COPD. The arterial oxygen saturation is often below 85%; PCO_2 may or may not be elevated.

C. ECG and Chest Radiography

The ECG may show right axis deviation and peaked P waves. Deep S waves are present in lead V_6. Right axis deviation and low voltage may be noted in patients with pulmonary emphysema. Frank RVH is uncommon except in primary pulmonary hypertension. The ECG often mimics myocardial infarction; Q waves may be present in leads II, III, and aVF because of the vertically placed heart, but they are rarely deep or wide, as in inferior myocardial infarction. Supraventricular arrhythmias are frequent and nonspecific.

The chest radiograph discloses the presence or absence of parenchymal disease and a prominent or enlarged RV and PA.

D. Diagnostic Studies

Pulmonary function tests usually confirm the underlying lung disease. The echocardiogram should show normal LV size and function but RV and RA dilation. Perfusion lung scans are rarely of value, but, if negative, they help to exclude chronic pulmonary emboli, an occasional cause of cor pulmonale. Multislice CT has replaced pulmonary angiography as the most specific method of diagnosis for the pulmonary emboli.

Differential Diagnosis

In its early stages, cor pulmonale can be diagnosed on the basis of radiologic, echocardiographic, or ECG evidence. Catheterization of the right heart will establish a definitive diagnosis but is more often performed to exclude left-sided heart failure, which may in some patients be an inapparent cause of right-sided failure. Differential diagnostic considerations relate primarily to the specific pulmonary disease that has produced RV failure (see above).

Treatment

The details of the treatment of chronic pulmonary disease (chronic respiratory failure) are discussed in Chapter 9. Otherwise, therapy is directed at the pulmonary process responsible for right heart failure. Oxygen, salt and fluid restriction, and diuretics are mainstays, with combination diuretic therapy (loop diuretics, thiazides and spironolactone) often useful, as described above for other causes of right heart failure.

Prognosis

Compensated cor pulmonale has the same prognosis as the underlying pulmonary disease. Once congestive signs appear, the average life expectancy is 2–5 years, but survival is significantly longer when uncomplicated emphysema is the cause.

Lehrman S et al: Primary pulmonary hypertension and cor pulmonale. Cardiol Rev 2002;10:265. [PMID: 12215190]

Morrison LK et al: Utility of a rapid B-natriuretic peptide assay in differentiating congestive heart failure from lung disease in patients presenting with dyspnea. J Am Coll Cardiol 2002; 39:202. [PMID: 11788208]

Vizza CD et al: Right and left ventricular dysfunction in patients with severe pulmonary disease. Chest 1998;113:576. [PMID: 9515827]

■ NEOPLASTIC DISEASES OF THE HEART

Primary cardiac tumors are rare and constitute only a small fraction of all tumors that involve the heart or pericardium. The most common primary tumor is atrial myxoma; it comprises about 50% of all tumors in adult case series. It is generally attached to the atrial septum and is more likely to affect the LA than the RA. Familial myxomas occur as part of the Carney complex—that consists of myxomas, pigmented skin lesions, and endocrine neoplasia. Patients with myxoma can present with the characteristics of a systemic illness, with obstruction of blood flow through the heart, or with signs of peripheral embolization. The characteristics include fever, malaise, weight loss, leukocytosis, elevated sedimentation rate, and emboli (peripheral or pulmonary, depending on the location of the tumor). This is often confused with infective endocarditis, lymphoma, other cancers, or autoimmune diseases. In other cases, the tumor may grow to considerable size and produce symptoms by obstructing mitral flow. Episodic pulmonary edema (classically occurring when an upright posture is assumed) and signs of low output may result.

Physical examination may reveal a diastolic sound related to motion of the tumor ("tumor plop") or a diastolic murmur similar to that of mitral stenosis. Right-sided myxomas may cause symptoms of right-sided failure. The diagnosis is established by echocardiography or by pathologic study of embolic material. Cardiac MRI is useful as an adjunct only. Contrast angiography is frequently not necessary. Surgical excision is usually curative, though recurrences do occur and serial echocardiographic follow-up, on at least a yearly basis, is recommended.

The second most common cardiac tumors are valvular papillary fibroelastomas and atrial septal lipomas. These tend to be benign and usually require no therapy. Other primary cardiac tumors include rhabdomyomas (that often appear multiple in both the RV and LV), fibrous histiocytomas, hemangiomas, and a variety of unusual sarcomas. The diagnosis may be supported by an abnormal cardiac contour on radiograph. Echocardiography is usually helpful but may miss tumors infiltrating the ventricular wall. It is likely that MRI will prove useful as well.

Metastases from malignant tumors can also affect the heart. Most often this occurs in malignant melanoma, but other tumors involving the heart include bronchogenic carcinoma, carcinoma of the breast, the lymphomas, renal cell carcinoma, and, in patients with AIDS, Kaposi's sarcoma. These are often clinically silent but may lead to pericardial tamponade, arrhythmias and conduction disturbances, heart failure, and peripheral emboli. The diagnosis is often made by echocardiography, but cardiac MRI and CT scanning are also helpful. ECG may reveal regional Q waves. The prognosis is dismal; effective treatment is not available. On rare occasions, surgical resection or chemotherapy is warranted.

Bennett KR et al: The Carney complex: unusual skin findings and recurrent cardiac myxoma. Arch Dermatol 2005;141:916. [PMID: 16027322]

Butany J et al: Cardiac tumours: diagnosis and management. Lancet Oncol 2005;6:219. [PMID: 15811617]

Restrepo CS et al: CT and MR imaging findings of benign cardiac tumors. Curr Probl Diagn Radiol 2005;34:12. [PMID: 15644859]

Reynen K et al: Metastases to the heart. Ann Oncol 2004;15:375. [PMID: 14998838]

Roberts WC: Primary and secondary neoplasms of the heart. Am J Cardiol 1997;80:671. [PMID: 9295010]

Sun JP et al: Clinical and echocardiographic characteristics of papillary fibroelastomas: a retrospective and prospective study in 162 patients. Circulation 2001;103:2687. [PMID: 11390338]

■ CARDIAC INVOLVEMENT IN MISCELLANEOUS SYSTEMIC DISEASES

The heart may be involved in a number of systemic syndromes. Many of these have been mentioned briefly in this chapter. The pericardium, myocardium, heart valves, and coronary arteries may be involved either singly or in various combinations. In most cases the cardiac manifestations are not the dominant feature, but in some it is the primary cause of symptoms and may be fatal.

The most common type of myocardial involvement is an infiltrative cardiomyopathy, such as systemic amyloidosis, sarcoidosis, hemochromatosis, Fabry's or glycogen storage disease. These result in a restrictive cardiomyopathy (see above). Cardiac calcinosis can occur in hyperparathyroidism (usually the secondary form) and in primary oxalosis. A number of muscular dystrophies can cause a cardiomyopathic picture (particularly Duchenne's, less frequently myotonic dystrophy, and several rarer forms). Involvement of the heart in Duchenne's dystrophy results in a focal cardiomyopathy of the posterior wall; the classic ECG has prominent anterior precordial forces. In addition to LV dysfunction and heart failure, all of these conditions frequently cause conduction abnormalities, which may be the presenting or only feature. The myocardium may also be involved in inflammatory and autoimmune diseases. It is commonly affected in polymyositis and dermatomyositis, but usually this is subclinical. Systemic lupus erythematosus, scleroderma, and mixed connective tissue disease may cause myocarditis, but these more commonly involve the pericardium, coronary arteries, or valves. Several endocrinopathies, including acromegaly, thyrotoxicosis, myxedema, and pheochromocytoma, can produce dilated cardiomyopathies that resolve when the underlying disease is appropriately treated.

Pericardial involvement is quite common in many of the connective tissue diseases. Systemic lupus erythematosus may present with pericarditis, and pericardial involvement is not uncommon (but is less frequently symptomatic) in active rheumatoid arthritis, systemic sclerosis, and mixed connective tissue disease. Endocardial involvement takes the form of patchy fibrous—predominantly on the right side—or inflammatory or sclerotic changes of the heart valves. Carcinoid heart disease results from the layering of plaque-like material over the tricuspid valve, RV endocardium, and pulmonic valve and presents with right heart failure due to tricuspid and pulmonic regurgitation. The hypereosinophilic syndromes involve the endocardium, leading to restrictive cardiomyopathy. A variety of arthritic syndromes are associated with aortic valvulitis or aortitis with resulting aortic regurgitation. These include ankylosing spondylitis, rheumatoid arthritis, and Reiter's syndrome. Disorders of collagen (Marfan syndrome is the most frequent, followed by Ehlers–Danlos syndrome) often affect the ascending aorta, with resulting aneurysmal dilation and aortic regurgitation. Mitral valve prolapse is also a common finding in these disorders.

Almost any vasculitic syndrome can involve the coronary arteries, leading to myocardial infarction. This is most common with polyarteritis nodosa and systemic lupus erythematosus. Two vasculitic syndromes have a particular predilection for the coronary arteries—Kawasaki's disease and Takayasu's disease. Kawasaki's disease can result in coronary aneurysms, occasionally of huge size. Takayasu's disease affects the great vessels more than the coronaries and smooth, tapering lesions are usually seen, particularly at the vessel ostia. In these, myocardial infarction may be the presenting symptom.

Biondi M: Effects of subclinical thyroid dysfunction on the heart. Ann Intern Med 2002;137:904. [PMID: 12458990]

Kulke MH et al: Carcinoid tumors. N Engl J Med 1999;340:858. [PMID: 10080850]

Magnani JW et al: Myocarditis: current trends in diagnosis and treatment. Circulation 2006;113:876. [PMID: 16476862]

Moder KG et al: Cardiac involvement in systemic lupus erythematosus. Mayo Clin Proc 1999;74:275. [PMID: 10089998]

Riboldi P et al: Cardiac involvement in systemic autoimmune diseases. Clin Rev Allergy Immunol 2002;23:247. [PMID: 12402411]

Steen V: The heart in systemic sclerosis. Curr Rheumatol Rep 2004;6:137. [PMID: 15016344]

Wijetunga M et al: Myocarditis in systemic lupus erythematosus. Am J Med 2002;113:419. [PMID: 12401537]

■ TRAUMATIC HEART DISEASE

Penetrating wounds to the heart are, of course, usually lethal unless surgically repaired. Stab wounds to the RV occasionally lead to hemopericardium without progressing to tamponade.

Blunt trauma is a more frequent cause of cardiac injuries, particularly outside of the emergency department setting. This type of injury is quite frequent in motor vehicle accidents and may occur with any form of chest trauma, including CPR efforts. The most common injuries are myocardial contusions or hematomas. Other forms of nonischemic cardiac injury include metabolic injury due to burns, electrical current, or sepsis. These may be asymptomatic (particularly in the setting of more severe injuries) or may present with chest pain of a nonspecific nature or, not uncommonly, with a pericardial component. Elevations of cardiac enzymes are frequent but the levels do not correlate with prognosis. Echocardiography may reveal an akinetic segment or pericardial effusion. Pericardiocentesis is warranted if tamponade is evident. Heart failure is uncommon if there are no associated cardiac or pericardial injuries, and conservative management is usually sufficient.

Severe trauma may also cause cardiac or valvular rupture. Cardiac rupture may involve any chamber, but survival is most likely if injury is to one of the atria or the RV. Hemopericardium or pericardial tamponade is the usual clinical presentation, and surgery is almost always necessary. Mitral and aortic valve rupture may occur during severe blunt trauma—the former presumably if the impact occurs during systole and the latter if during diastole. Patients reach the hospital in shock or severe heart failure. Immediate surgical repair is essential. The same types of injuries may result in transection

of the aorta, either at the level of the arch or distal to the takeoff of the left subclavian artery. Transthoracic echocardiography and TEE are the most helpful and immediately available diagnostic techniques.

Blunt trauma may also result in damage to the coronary arteries. Acute or subacute coronary thrombosis is the most common presentation. The clinical syndrome is one of acute myocardial infarction with attendant ECG, enzymatic, and contractile abnormalities. Emergent revascularization is sometimes feasible, either by the percutaneous route or by coronary artery bypass surgery. LV aneurysms are common outcomes of traumatic coronary occlusions. Coronary artery dissection or rupture may also occur in the setting of blunt cardiac trauma.

Bansal MK et al: Myocardial contusion injury: redefining the diagnostic algorithm. Emerg Med J 2005;22:465. [PMID: 15983078]

Geddes LA et al: Evolution of our knowledge of sudden death due to commotio cordis. Am J Emerg Med 2005;23:67. [PMID: 15672341]

Harada H et al: Traumatic coronary artery dissection. Ann Thorac Surg 2002;74:236. [PMID: 12118767]

Lindstaedt M et al: Acute and long-term clinical significance of myocardial contusion following blunt thoracic trauma: results of a prospective study. J Trauma 2002;52:479. [PMID: 11901323]

Schultz JM et al: Blunt cardiac injury. Crit Care Clin 2004;20:57. [PMID: 14979329]

Wall MJ Jr et al: Trauma to cardiac valves. Curr Opin Cardiol 2002;17:188. [PMID: 11981254]

■ THE CARDIAC PATIENT & SURGERY

Patients with known or suspected cardiac disease undergoing general surgery present a common management problem. Anesthesia and surgery are often associated with marked fluctuations of heart rate and BP, changes in intravascular volume, myocardial ischemia or depression, arrhythmias, decreased oxygenation, increased sympathetic nervous system activity, and alterations in medical regimens and pharmacokinetics. Even with careful monitoring and management, the perioperative period can be very stressful to cardiac patients.

The risk of surgery in patients with heart disease depends primarily on three factors: the type of operation, the nature of the heart disease, and the degree of preoperative stability. The type of anesthesia is less important, though halothane, enflurane, and barbiturates are more severe myocardial depressants, whereas opioids have little depressive effect. Spinal and epidural anesthesia were previously thought to be preferable in patients with heart disease, but this has not proved to be the case.

The highest-risk procedures are surgery of the aorta and vascular procedures, in part because these patients often have associated severe coronary disease but also because marked BP and volume changes are common. Major abdominal and thoracic surgery are also associated with substantial cardiovascular risk, particularly in older patients with associated cardiovascular disease.

Numerous studies have evaluated the excess risk of surgery in patients with various cardiac diseases. Recent (within 3 months) myocardial infarction, unstable angina, CHF, and significant aortic stenosis are associated with substantial increases in operative morbidity and mortality rates. Any degree of instability in these conditions magnifies the potential risk. Stable angina, particularly in an inactive individual, is also associated with a higher operative risk. Although less common, cyanotic congenital heart disease and severe primary or secondary pulmonary hypertension pose great risks during major surgery. In patients with any of these problems, the risk-to-benefit ratio of the planned surgery should be carefully examined. If the procedure is necessary but elective, consideration should be given to delaying it until full recovery postinfarction and correction or optimal stabilization of the other conditions are achieved. Hypertension should be at least moderately controlled. Patients with severe angina should have increased medical therapy initiated or be considered for revascularization before noncardiac surgery. Symptomatic arrhythmias, nonsustained ventricular tachycardia, or high-grade AV block and cardiac failure should be treated optimally.

Clinical assessment provides the most useful guidance in determining the risk of noncardiac surgery. Important indicators of high risk have been discussed above. A multifactorial cardiac risk index is included in Chapter 3 (Table 3–4). Patients with known but clinically stable heart disease, such as angina pectoris or prior myocardial infarction, are at intermediate risk, particularly for major operations such as vascular surgery. If a history or symptoms of heart failure are present, assessment of LV function can be very helpful in perioperative management. Although frequently advocated, further noninvasive testing for myocardial ischemia for the purpose of risk stratification is probably overutilized. Tests such as stress myocardial perfusion scintigraphy or dobutamine echocardiography should be reserved for situations in which the results may alter patient management. There is no evidence that prophylactic revascularization by either PCI or coronary artery bypass surgery alters long-term outcome in patients undergoing noncardiac surgical procedures without the usual indications for PCI or CABG. Only in the case of major vascular operations is perioperative mortality and morbidity high enough that prophylactic PCI or CABG should be considered.

However, it should be noted that many patients undergoing surgery have not had recent medical follow-up, and this may be an appropriate opportunity to perform a more complete evaluation. Thus, stress testing may be indicated for selected patients with symptomatic angina or prior myocardial infarction with a view to instituting more comprehensive medical management or performing coronary revascularization to reduce long-term (rather than perioperative) mortality and morbidity. At the least, such patients should not be discharged without a plan for an appropriate follow-up and institution of antihyperlipidemic, aspirin, and β-blocker therapy as indicated.

Once the decision to operate is made, careful management is essential. Most cardiac medications should be continued preoperatively and postoperatively. In patients judged to be at high risk or medium risk, β-blockers should be initiated preoperatively unless contraindicated. If practical, oral therapy with atenolol or metoprolol should be started several days prior to surgery with the dosage gradually increased to 100 mg in single or divided doses. Otherwise, 15 mg of metoprolol or 10 mg of atenolol may be administered intravenously in 5 mg increments separated by 5–10 minutes prior to induction. These doses should be repeated every 12 hours—or more frequently if excessive tachycardia occurs—until oral therapy can be commenced. Monitoring is an important prophylactic measure in high-risk individuals; hemodynamic monitoring can facilitate early intervention in patients with heart failure, severe valve disease, or easily induced myocardial ischemia. Excessive hypertension, hypotension, and myocardial ischemia should be identified and appropriately treated using rapidly acting agents. TEE can also be used for intraoperative monitoring of ischemia, but its value has never been established in well-designed studies. Ischemic events, whether symptomatic or silent, should be vigorously treated.

Auerbach AD et al: Beta-blockers and reduction of cardiac events in noncardiac surgery: scientific review. JAMA 2002;287:1435. [PMID: 11903031]

Boersma E et al: Predictors of cardiac events after major vascular surgery: role of clinical characteristics, dobutamine echocardiography, and beta-blocker therapy. JAMA 2001;285:1865. [PMID: 11308400]

Devereaux PJ et al: How strong is the evidence for the use of perioperative beta blockers in non-cardiac surgery? Systematic review and meta-analysis of randomised controlled trials. BMJ 2005;331:313. [PMID: 15996966]

Eagle KA et al: ACC/AHA guideline update for perioperative cardiovascular evaluation for noncardiac surgery—executive summary: a report of the American College of Cardiology/American Heart Association Task Force on Practice Guidelines (Committee to Update the 1996 Guidelines on Perioperative Cardiovascular Evaluation for Noncardiac Surgery). J Am Coll Cardiol 2002;39:542. [PMID: 11823097]

Fleisher LA et al: Clinical practice. Lowering cardiac risk in non-cardiac surgery. N Engl J Med 2001;345:1677. [PMID: 11759647]

Hernandez AF et al: Preoperative evaluation for major noncardiac surgery: focusing on heart failure. Arch Intern Med 2004; 164:1729. [PMID: 15364665]

■ THE CARDIAC PATIENT & PREGNANCY

The management of cardiac disease in pregnancy is discussed in detail in the references listed below. Only a few major points can be covered in this brief section.

CARDIOVASCULAR CHANGES DURING PREGNANCY

Normal physiologic changes during pregnancy can exacerbate symptoms of underlying cardiac disease even in previously asymptomatic individuals. Maternal blood volume rises progressively until the end of the sixth or seventh month. Stroke volume increases over the same time course as a result of the volume change and an increase in EF. The latter reflects predominantly a decline in peripheral resistance due to vasodilation and the low-resistance shunting through the placenta. The heart rate tends to rise in the third trimester to further increase the cardiac output as the stroke volume levels out. Overall, cardiac output increases by 30–50%; systolic BP tends to rise slightly or remain unchanged, but diastolic pressure falls significantly. Venocaval compression of the IVC from the gravid uterus can lead to reduced venous return and a lower cardiac output in the supine position.

High cardiac output causes alterations in the cardiac examination. A third heart sound is prominent and normal, and a pulmonary flow murmur is common. ECG changes include rate-related decreases in PR and QT intervals, a leftward axis shift, inferior Q waves due to the more horizontal position of the heart, and nonspecific ST–T wave changes. Normal echocardiographic findings include slightly increased chamber sizes, functional valvular regurgitation, and occasionally small pericardial effusions.

MANAGEMENT OF PREEXISTING CONDITIONS

The physiologic changes imposed by pregnancy can cause cardiac decompensation in patients with any significant cardiac abnormality, but the most severe problems are encountered in patients with valvular stenosis (especially mitral and aortic stenosis), congenital or acquired abnormalities associated with pulmonary hypertension or right-to-left shunting, CHF due to any cause, coronary heart disease, and hypertension. Valvular insufficiency or left-to-right shunting often diminishes because of the fall in peripheral resistance and is better tolerated than other lesions.

Mitral stenosis becomes more hemodynamically severe because of the increase in diastolic flow and the rate-related shortening of diastole. LA pressures rise, and dyspnea or pulmonary edema can occur in previously asymptomatic individuals. The onset of atrial fibrillation often leads to acute decompensation. Patients with moderate to severe mitral or aortic stenosis should have the condition corrected prior to becoming pregnant if possible. Patients who become symptomatic can undergo successful surgery, preferably in the third trimester, although balloon valvuloplasty is the treatment of choice if the mitral valve is amenable. Coarctation of the aorta is usually well tolerated unless severe, when perfusion of the gravid uterus and upper extremity hypertension become an issue. Patients with

symptoms or significant upper extremity hypertension before pregnancy should have corrective surgery before embarking on a pregnancy. Patients with severe pulmonary hypertension and cyanotic congenital heart disease and those with severe aortic stenosis are at extremely high risk and should avoid pregnancy. Balloon valvuloplasty of severe aortic stenosis is feasible and preferable to surgical intervention during pregnancy if possible. Patients with most right-sided lesions do well with pregnancy, including those with ASD, pulmonic stenosis, pulmonic regurgitation, operated tetralogy of Fallot, and Ebstein's anomaly. Those with an RV that supports the systemic circulation can usually tolerate pregnancy unless symptomatic heart failure has already occurred. Most adult patients with a systemic RV have transposition of the great vessels that has been surgically corrected or is congenitally corrected (L-transposition of the great vessels). Patients with hypertrophic cardiomyopathy generally do well, though the risk of pregnancy is higher than normal.

In Marfan syndrome, there are two issues, the risk of transmission of the disease to the child and the risk of cardiovascular complications with pregnancy. Marfan patients tolerate pregnancy well if the aorta is 4.0 cm or less. If the aorta is significantly dilated and/or there has been prior dissection, the pregnancy may not be tolerated. If the Marfan patient becomes pregnant, then physical activity should be limited and β-blockers used throughout the pregnancy. Cesarean section is favored over vaginal delivery.

Asymptomatic arrhythmias should be closely observed unless underlying heart disease is present, in which case they should be treated with drugs. Paroxysmal supraventricular arrhythmias are quite common. Patients with Wolff–Parkinson–White syndrome may have more problems during pregnancy. Therapy is similar to that required for nonpregnant women. Issues related to pregnancy and the use of anticoagulation are discussed above under Prosthetic Valve Management.

Preexisting systemic hypertension is usually well tolerated and controllable, though the fetal morbidity rate is slightly increased. The incidence of preeclampsia and eclampsia (see Chapter 18) is increased.

Hydralazine and methyldopa are the antihypertensive agents for which there has been the greatest experience during pregnancy. Diuretics have also been used frequently, but concern has been raised that intravascular hypovolemia might impair uterine blood flow. Nonetheless, these agents are relatively safe. More recently, there has been considerable use of the combined α-β-blocker labetalol and of calcium channel blockers, which have proved to be effective and safe to both the mother and fetus. On the other hand, atenolol has been associated with lower fetal weights. ACE inhibitors and angiotensin II blockers are contraindicated in pregnancy because of the risk of fetal injury. β-Blockers may retard fetal growth, but experience with them has been generally favorable. Little is known about the safety of most other antihypertensive agents.

A comprehensive review of the safety of drugs in pregnancy and during breast-feeding can be found at www.perinatology.com/exposures/druglist.htm.

CARDIOVASCULAR COMPLICATIONS OF PREGNANCY

Pregnancy-related hypertension (eclampsia and pre-eclampsia) is discussed in Chapter 18.

Cardiomyopathy of Pregnancy (Peripartum Cardiomyopathy)

In approximately one of 4000–15,000 patients, dilated cardiomyopathy develops in the final month of pregnancy or within 6 months after delivery. The cause is unclear, but immune and viral causes have been postulated. The disease occurs more frequently in women over age 30 years, is generally related to the first or second pregnancy, and is associated with gestational hypertension and drugs used to stop uterine contractions. The course of the disease is variable; many cases improve or resolve completely over several months, but others progress to refractory heart failure. About 60% of patients make a complete recovery. Immunosuppressive therapy has been advocated, but few supportive data are available. Recently, β-blockers have been administered judiciously to these patients, with at least anecdotal success. Some advocate anticoagulation because of an increased risk for thrombotic events. Recurrence in subsequent pregnancies is common, particularly if cardiac function has not recovered.

Coronary Artery & Other Vascular Abnormalities

There have been a number of reports of myocardial infarction during pregnancy. It is known that pregnancy predisposes to dissection of the aorta and other arteries, perhaps because of the accompanying connective tissue changes. The risk may be particularly high in patients with Marfan or Ehlers-Danlos syndromes. However, coronary artery dissection is responsible for only a minority of the infarctions; most are caused by atherosclerotic CAD or coronary emboli. Most of the events occur near term or shortly following delivery, and paradoxical emboli through a PFO has been implicated in some cases. Clinical management is essentially similar to that of other patients with acute infarction, unless there is a connective tissue disorder. If nonatherosclerotic dissection is present, coronary intervention is risky as further dissection can be aggravated. In most instances, conservative management is warranted.

SPECIAL PROBLEMS

Prophylaxis for Infective Endocarditis

Although there is no universal agreement, many authorities recommend antibiotic prophylaxis during labor for patients at risk for endocarditis, especially if forceps delivery is anticipated or episiotomy is performed. Ampicillin (2 g intravenously or intramuscularly) plus gentamicin (1.5 mg/kg intravenously or intramuscularly [up to 80 mg]) followed by amoxicillin, 1.5 g orally every 6 hours, is the recommended regimen.

Management of Labor

Although vaginal delivery is usually well tolerated, unstable patients (including patients with severe hypertension and worsening heart failure) should have planned cesarean section. An increased risk of aortic rupture has been noted during delivery in patients with coarctation of the aorta and severe aortic root dilation with Marfan syndrome, and vaginal delivery should be avoided in these conditions. For most patients, even those with congenital heart disease, vaginal delivery is preferred.

Elkayam U et al: Maternal and fetal outcomes of subsequent pregnancies in women with peripartum cardiomyopathy. N Engl J Med 2001;344:1567. [PMID: 11372007]

Elkayam U et al: Valvular heart disease and pregnancy part I: native valves. J Am Coll Cardiol 2005;46:223. [PMID: 16022946]

Elkayam U et al: Valvular heart disease and pregnancy: part II: prosthetic valves. J Am Coll Cardiol 2005;46:403. [PMID: 16053950]

Ginsberg JS et al: Use of antithrombotic agents during pregnancy. Chest 2001;119:122S. [PMID: 11157646]

Head CE et al: Congenital heart disease in pregnancy. Postgrad Med J 2005;81:292. [PMID: 15879040]

Lupton M et al: Cardiac disease in pregnancy. Curr Opin Obstet Gynecol 2002;14:137. [PMID: 11914690]

Pearson GD et al: Peripartum cardiomyopathy: NHLBI workshop recommendations and review. JAMA 2000;283:1183. [PMID: 10703781]

Report of the National High Blood Pressure Education Program Working Group on High Blood Pressure in Pregnancy. Am J Obstet Gynecol 2000;183:S1. [PMID: 10920346]

Sliwa K et al: Outcome of subsequent pregnancy in patients with documented peripartum cardiomyopathy. Am J Cardiol 2004;93:1441. [PMID: 15165937]

Tidswell M: Peripartum cardiomyopathy. Crit Care Clin 2004; 20:777. [PMID: 15388202]

CARDIOVASCULAR SCREENING OF ATHLETES

The sudden death of a competitive athlete inevitably becomes an occasion for local if not national publicity. On each occasion, the public and the medical community ask whether such events could be prevented by more careful or complete screening. Although each event is tragic, it must be appreciated that there are approximately 5 million competitive athletes at the high school level or above in any given year. The number of cardiac deaths occurring during athletic participation is unknown, but estimates at the high school level range from one in 300,000 to one in 100,000 participants. Death rates among more mature athletes increase as the prevalence of CAD rises. These numbers highlight the problem of how to screen individual participants. Even an inexpensive test such as an ECG would generate an enormous cost if required of all athletes, and it is likely that few at-risk individuals would be detected. Echocardiography, either as a routine test or as a follow-up examination for abnormal ECGs, would be prohibitively expensive except for the elite professional athlete. Thus, the most feasible approach is that of a careful medical history and cardiac examination performed by personnel aware of the conditions responsible for most sudden deaths in competitive athletes. In a series of 158 athletic deaths in the United States between 1985 and 1995, hypertrophic cardiomyopathy (36%) and coronary anomalies (19%) were by far the most frequent underlying conditions. LV hypertrophy was present in another 10%, ruptured aorta (presumably due to Marfan syndrome or cystic medial necrosis) in 6%, myocarditis or dilated cardiomyopathy in 6%, aortic stenosis in 4%, and arrhythmogenic RV dysplasia in 3%. In addition, commotio cordis, or sudden death due to direct myocardial injury, may occur. More common in children, it may occur even after a minor direct blow to the heart; it is thought to be due to the precipitation of a premature ventricular contraction just prior to the peak of the T wave on ECG.

It is likely that a careful family and medical history and cardiovascular examination will identify some individuals at risk. A family history of premature sudden death or cardiovascular disease or of any of these predisposing conditions should mandate further workup, including an ECG and echocardiogram. Symptoms of chest pain, syncope, or near-syncope also warrant further evaluation. A Marfan-like appearance, significant elevation of BP or abnormalities of heart rate or rhythm, and pathologic heart murmurs or heart sounds should also be investigated before clearance for athletic participation is given. Such an evaluation is recommended before participation at the high school and college levels and every 2 years during athletic competition.

Stress-induced syncope or chest pressure may be the first clue to an anomalous origin of a coronary artery. Anatomically, this lesion occurs most often when the left anterior descending artery arises from the right coronary cusp and traverses between the aorta and pulmonary trunks. The "slit-like" orifice that results from the angulation at the vessel origin is thought to cause ischemia when the aorta and pulmonary arteries enlarge during rigorous exercise.

The toughest distinction may be in sorting out the healthy athlete with LVH from the athlete with hypertrophic cardiomyopathy. In general, the healthy athlete's heart is *less* likely to have an unusual pattern of LVH, LA enlargement, an abnormal ECG, an LV cavity < 45 mm in diameter at end-diastole, an abnormal diastolic filling pattern, a family history of hypertrophic cardiomyopathy, and the athlete is more likely to be male than the individual with hypertrophic cardiomyopathy.

Selective use of routine ECG and stress testing is recommended in men above age 40 years and women above age 50 years who continue to participate in vigorous exercise and at earlier ages when there is a positive family history for premature CAD, hypertrophic cardiomyopathy, or multiple risk factors.

Corrado D et al: Screening for hypertrophic cardiomyopathy in young athletes. N Engl J Med 1998;339:364. [PMID: 9691102]

Hosey RG: Sudden cardiac death. Clin Sports Med 2003;22:51. [PMID: 12613086]

Maron BJ et al: Working Groups of the American Heart Association Committee on Exercise, Cardiac Rehabilitation, and Prevention; Councils on Clinical Cardiology and Cardiovascular Disease in the Young: Recommendations for physical activity and recreational sports participation for young patients with genetic cardiovascular diseases. Circulation 2004;109:2807. [PMID: 15184297]

Pelliccia A et al: Clinical significance of abnormal electrocardiographic patterns in trained athletes. Circulation 2000;102:278. [PMID: 10899089]

Pfister GC et al: Preparticipation cardiovascular screening for US collegiate student-athletes. JAMA 2000;283:1597. [PMID: 10735397]

Pluim BM et al: The athlete's heart. A meta-analysis of cardiac structure and function. Circulation 2000;101:336. [PMID: 10645932]

Seto CK: Preparticipation cardiovascular screening. Clin Sports Med 2003;22:23. [PMID: 12613084]

Systemic Hypertension

11

Michael Sutters, MD

Fifty million Americans have elevated blood pressure (systolic blood pressure ≥ 140 mm Hg or diastolic blood pressure ≥ 90 mm Hg); of these, 70% are aware of their diagnosis, but only 50% are receiving treatment and only 25% are under control using a threshold criterion of 140/90 mm Hg. The prevalence of hypertension increases with age and is more common in blacks than in whites. The mortality rates for stroke and coronary heart disease, two of the major complications of hypertension, have declined by up to 60% over the past three decades but have recently leveled off. The numbers of patients with end-stage renal disease and heart failure—two other conditions in which hypertension plays a major causative role—continue to rise.

Cardiovascular morbidity and mortality increase as both systolic and diastolic blood pressures rise, but in individuals over age 50 years, the systolic pressure and pulse pressure are better predictors of complications than diastolic pressure. Table 11–1 provides a summary of the classification and management of blood pressure in adults from the 7th Report of the U.S. Joint National Commission on Prevention, Detection, Evaluation, and Treatment of High Blood Pressure (JNC 7).

How Is Blood Pressure Measured and Hypertension Diagnosed?

Blood pressure should be measured with a well-calibrated sphygmomanometer. The bladder width within the cuff should encircle at least 80% of the arm circumference. Readings should be taken after the patient has been resting comfortably, back supported in the sitting or supine position, for at least 5 minutes and at least 30 minutes after smoking or coffee ingestion. Hypertension is diagnosed when blood pressure is consistently elevated above 140/90 mm Hg; a single elevated blood pressure reading is not sufficient to establish the diagnosis of hypertension. The major exceptions to this rule are hypertensive presentations with unequivocal evidence of life-threatening end-organ damage, as seen in hypertensive emergency, or in hypertensive urgency where blood pressure is > 220/125 mm Hg but life-threatening end-organ damage is absent. In less severe cases, the diagnosis of hypertension depends on a series of measurements of blood pressure, since readings can vary and tend to regress toward the mean with time. Patients whose blood pressure is in a hypertensive range initially typically exhibit the greatest fall toward the

normal range between the first and second encounters. Although blood pressure readings may still show variability after the third visit, these later changes are mostly random. However, the concern for diagnostic precision needs to be balanced by an appreciation of the importance of establishing the diagnosis of hypertension as quickly as possible, since a 3-month delay in treatment of hypertension in high-risk patients is associated with a twofold increase in cardiovascular morbidity and mortality. The guidelines of the 2005 Canadian Hypertension Education Program provide an algorithm designed to expedite the diagnosis of hypertension (Figure 11–1). To this end, they recommend short intervals between the initial office visits and the early identification of target organ damage which, if present, obviates the need for protracted confirmation of blood pressure elevation prior to pharmacologic intervention. In addition, the Canadian guidelines exploit the less volatile ambulatory and home blood pressure measurements as complements to office-based evaluations; hypertension is diagnosed at lower levels when based on measurements taken outside the office environment.

Prehypertension

Data from the Framingham cohort indicate that blood pressure bears a linear relationship with cardiovascular risk down to a systolic blood pressure of 115 mm Hg; based on these data, it is recommended that individuals with blood pressures in the gray area of 120–139/80–89 mm Hg be categorized as having prehypertension (Table 11–1). This demonstrates a trend away from defining hypertension as a simple numerical threshold and toward a more subtle appreciation of blood pressure as a component of overall cardiovascular risk. Although data concerning the treatment of prehypertension are lacking, the JNC guidelines suggest that antihypertensive medications be offered to persons with prehypertension with compelling indications (Table 11–1).

The British Hypertension Society (BHS) guidelines make similar recommendations but go further by suggesting that antihypertensive medication also be offered to patients with prehypertension who have an elevated projected cardiovascular risk based on Framingham criteria (discussed below). Consequently, a low-risk patient with blood pressure between 120–139/80–89 mm Hg may be advised to make lifestyle modifications (Table

Table 11–1. Classification and management of blood pressure for adults aged 18 years or older.

BP Classification	Systolic BP, mm Hg[1]		Diastolic BP, mm Hg[1]	Lifestyle Modification	Management	
					Initial Drug Therapy	
					Without Compelling Indication	With Compelling Indications[2]
Normal	< 120	and	< 80	Encourage		
Prehypertension	120–139	or	80–89	Yes	No antihypertensive drug indicated	Drugs for the compelling indications[3]
Stage 1 hypertension	140–159	or	90–99	Yes	Thiazide-type diuretics for most; may consider ACE inhibitor, ARB, β-blocker, CCB, or combination	Drug(s) for the compelling indications Other antihypertensive drugs (diuretics, ACE inhibitor, ARB, β-blocker, CCB) as needed
Stage 2 hypertension	≥ 160	or	≥ 100	Yes	Two-drug combination for most (usually thiazide-type diuretic and ACE inhibitor or ARB or β-blocker or CCB)[4]	Drug(s) for the compelling indications Other antihypertensive drugs (diuretics, ACE inhibitor, ARB, β-blocker, CCB) as needed

[1]Treatment determined by highest BP category.
[2]See Table 11–4.
[3]Treat patients with chronic kidney disease or diabetes to BP goal of < 130/80 mm Hg.
[4]Initial combined therapy should be used cautiously in those at risk for orthostatic hypotension.
ACE = angiotensin-converting enzyme; ARB = angiotensin receptor blocker; BP = blood pressure; CCB = calcium channel blocker.
From Chobanian AV et al: The Seventh Report of the Joint National Committee on Prevention, Detection, Evaluation, and Treatment of High Blood Pressure: the JNC 7 report. JAMA 2003;289:2560.

11–2) and be monitored without receiving an absolute diagnosis of prehypertension. Circumspection about labeling patients is warranted since there is evidence that simply telling someone that he or she is hypertensive has unintended consequences, transforming a perception of general health into one of general ill-health. Nonetheless, because prehypertension often develops into hypertension (50% of people within 4 years), even low-risk prehypertensive patients should be monitored annually. To summarize, the diagnosis of hypertension is less important than deciding which patients will benefit from blood pressure reduction as part of a comprehensive risk reduction strategy.

Bolli P et al; Canadian Hypertension Education Program: Applying the 2005 Canadian Hypertension Education Program recommendations: 1. Diagnosis of hypertension. CMAJ 2005;173:480. [PMID: 16129865]

Chaudhry SI et al: Systolic hypertension in older persons. JAMA 2004;292:1074. [PMID: 15339901]

Chobanian AV et al: The Seventh Report of the Joint National Committee on Prevention, Detection, Evaluation, and Treatment of High Blood Pressure: the JNC 7 Report. JAMA 2003;289:2560. [PMID: 12748199]

European Society of Hypertension-European Society of Cardiology Guidelines Committee: 2003 European Society of Hypertension-European Society of Cardiology guidelines for the management of arterial hypertension J Hypertens 2003;21:1011. [PMID: 12777938]

Hart PD et al: Hypertension control rates: time for translation of guidelines into clinical practice. Am J Med 2004;117:62. [PMID: 15210392]

Kaplan NM et al: *Clinical Hypertension,* 8th ed. Lippincott Williams & Wilkins, 2002.

Pepine C: What is the optimal blood pressure and drug therapy for patients with coronary artery disease? JAMA 2004;292:2271. [PMID: 15536116]

Pickering TG: Now we are sick: labeling and hypertension. J Clin Hypertens (Greenwich) 2006;8:57. [PMID: 16407691]

Sheridan S et al: Screening for high blood pressure: a review of the evidence for the U.S. Preventive Services Task Force. Am J Prev Med 2003;25:151. [PMID: 12880884]

Williams B et al; British Hypertension Society: Guidelines for management of hypertension: report of the fourth working party of the British Hypertension Society, 2004-BHS IV. J Hum Hypertens 2004;18:139. [PMID: 14973512]

APPROACH TO HYPERTENSION

Etiology & Classification

A. PRIMARY (ESSENTIAL) HYPERTENSION

Primary (essential) hypertension is the term applied to the 95% of cases in which no cause for hypertension can be identified. This occurs in 10–15% of white

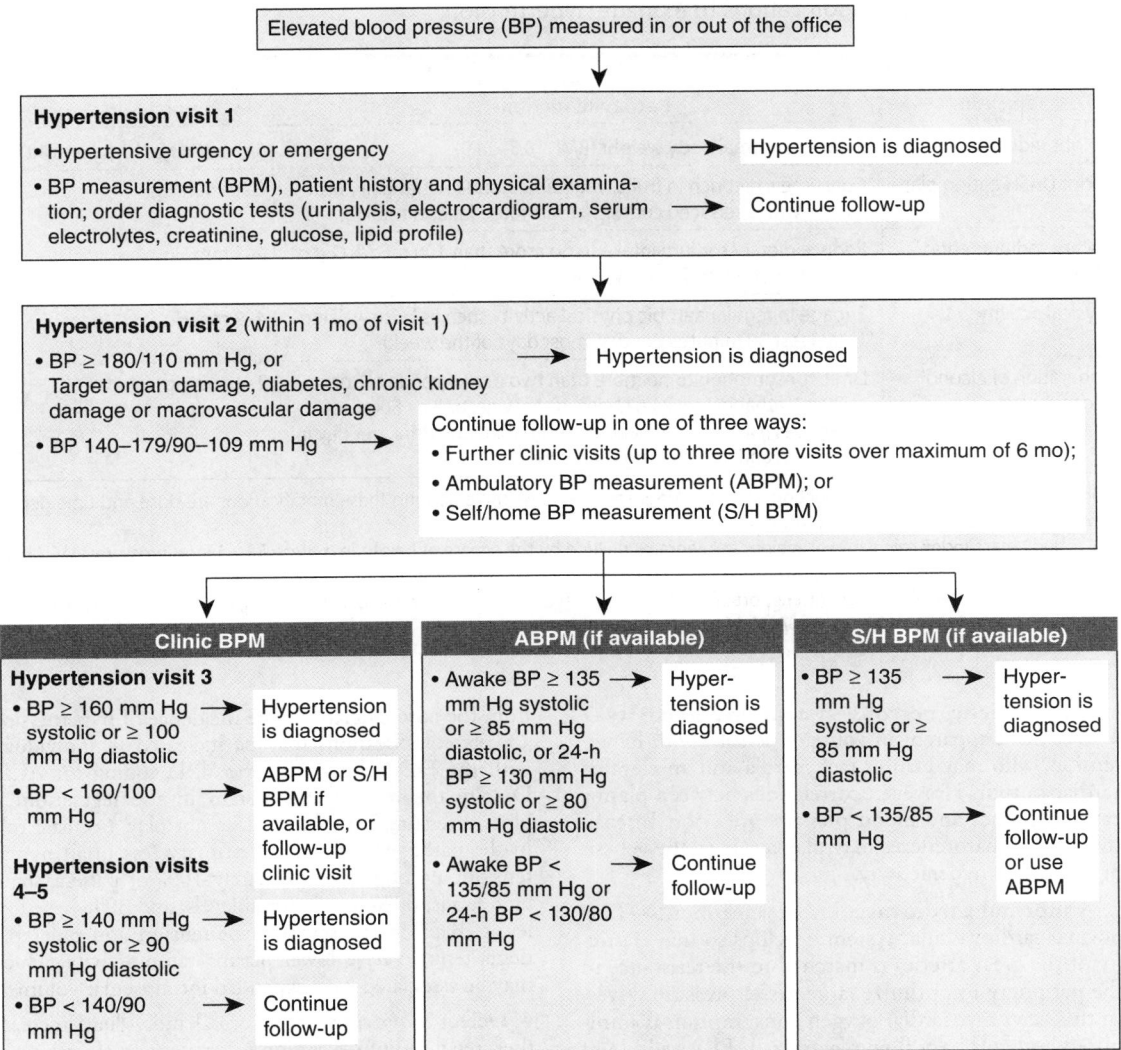

Figure 11–1. The 2005 Canadian Hypertension Education Program recommendations for the assessment and diagnosis of hypertension. Patients with an elevated blood pressure measured during visits 4–5 may still have white-coat (office-induced) hypertension. (Applying the 2005 Canadian Hypertension Education Program recommendations: 1. Diagnosis of hypertension — Reprinted from, CMAJ 30-Aug-05; 173(5), Page(s) 480-483 by permission of the publisher. © 2005 CMA Media Inc.)

adults and 20–30% of black adults in the United States. The onset is usually between ages 25 and 55 years; it is uncommon before age 20 years. Much less commonly, hypertension arises from an identifiable cause, in which case it is called secondary hypertension (see below). The secondary form should be suspected in children or young adults and in older persons in whom onset of hypertension is new or in whom hypertension suddenly worsens.

The pathogenesis of primary (essential) hypertension is multifactorial. Genetic factors play an important role. Children have higher blood pressure when one parent is hypertensive (and more so when both parents are hypertensive). Environmental factors also are significant. Increased salt intake and obesity have long been incriminated. These factors alone are probably not sufficient to raise blood pressure to abnormal levels but are synergistic with a genetic predisposition. Other factors that may be involved in the pathogenesis of primary (essential) hypertension are sympathetic nervous system hyperactivity, abnormal cardiovascular development, renin-angiotensin system activity, defect in natriuresis, intracellular sodium and calcium, as well as exacerbating factors (including obesity, alcohol, cigarette smoking, and polycythemia).

Table 11–2. Lifestyle modifications to manage hypertension.[1]

Modification	Recommendation	Approximate Systolic BP Reduction, Range
Weight reduction	Maintain normal body weight (BMI, 18.5–24.9)	5–20 mm Hg/10-kg weight loss
Adopt DASH eating plan	Consume a diet rich in fruits, vegetables, and low-fat dairy products with a reduced content of saturated fat and total fat	8–14 mm Hg
Dietary sodium reduction	Reduce dietary sodium intake to no more than 100 mEq/L (2.4 g sodium or 6 g sodium chloride)	2–8 mm Hg
Physical activity	Engage in regular aerobic physical activity such as brisk walking (at least 30 minutes per day, most days of the week)	4–9 mm Hg
Moderation of alcohol consumption	Limit consumption to no more than two drinks per day (1 oz or 30 mL ethanol [eg, 24 oz beer, 10 oz wine, or 3 oz 80-proof whiskey]) in most men and no more than one drink per day in women and lighter-weight persons	2–4 mm Hg

[1]For overall cardiovascular risk reduction, stop smoking. The effects of implementing these modifications are dose and time dependent and could be higher for some individuals.
BMI = body mass index calculated as weight in kilograms divided by the square of height in meters; BP = blood pressure; DASH = Dietary Approaches to Stop Hypertension.
From Chobanian AV et al: The Seventh Report of the Joint National Committee on Prevention, Detection, Evaluation, and Treatment of High Blood Pressure: the JNC 7 report. JAMA 2003;289:2560.

1. Sympathetic nervous system hyperactivity— This is most apparent in younger persons with hypertension, who may exhibit tachycardia and an elevated cardiac output. However, correlations between plasma catecholamines and blood pressure are poor. Insensitivity of the baroreflexes may play a role in the genesis of adrenergic hyperactivity.

2. Abnormal cardiovascular development—The normal cardiovascular system develops so that elasticity of the great arteries is matched to the resistance in the periphery to optimize large vessel pressure waves. In this way, myocardial oxygen consumption is minimized and coronary flow maximized. Elevated blood pressure later in life could arise from abnormal development of aortic elasticity or reduced development of the microvascular network. This has been postulated as the sequence of events in low birth weight infants who have an increased risk of hypertension developing in adulthood.

3. Renin–angiotensin system activity—Renin, a proteolytic enzyme, is secreted by the juxtaglomerular cells surrounding afferent arterioles in response to a number of stimuli, including reduced renal perfusion pressure, diminished intravascular volume, circulating catecholamines, increased sympathetic nervous system activity, increased arteriolar stretch, and hypokalemia. Plasma renin levels are classified in relation to dietary sodium intake or urinary sodium excretion. Renin acts on angiotensinogen to cleave off the ten-amino-acid peptide angiotensin I. This peptide is then acted upon by angiotensin-converting enzyme (ACE) to create the eight-amino-acid peptide angiotensin II, a potent vasoconstrictor and a major stimulant of aldosterone release

from the adrenal glands. The incidence of hypertension and its complications may be increased in individuals with the DD genotype of the allele coding for ACE. Despite the role of this system in the regulation of blood pressure, it probably does not play a central role in the pathogenesis of most primary (essential) hypertension; although approximately 10% of patients have high levels, 60% have normal levels, and 30% have low levels. Black persons with hypertension and older patients tend to have lower plasma renin activity, which may be associated with expanded intravascular volume.

4. Defect in natriuresis—Normal individuals increase their renal sodium excretion in response to elevations in arterial pressure and to a sodium or volume load. Hypertensive patients, particularly when their blood pressure is controlled, exhibit a diminished ability to excrete a sodium load. This defect may result in increased plasma volume and hypertension. During chronic hypertension, a sodium load is usually handled normally.

5. Intracellular sodium and calcium—Intracellular Na^+ is elevated in blood cells and other tissues in primary (essential) hypertension. This may result from abnormalities in Na^+–K^+ exchange and other Na^+ transport mechanisms. An increase in intracellular Na^+ may lead to increased intracellular Ca^{2+} concentrations as a result of facilitated exchange and might explain the increase in vascular smooth muscle tone that is characteristic of established hypertension.

6. Exacerbating factors—A number of conditions elevate blood pressure, especially in predisposed individuals. **Obesity** is associated with an increase in intravascular volume and an elevated cardiac output. Weight reduction lowers blood pressure modestly. The relationship between **sodium intake** and hypertension remains controversial, and some—not all—persons with hypertension respond to high salt intake with substantial increases in blood pressure. Patients with high normal or elevated blood pressures should consume no more than 100 mmol/d of salt (2.4 g of sodium, 6 g of sodium chloride daily).

Excessive use of **alcohol** also raises blood pressure, perhaps by increasing plasma catecholamines. Hypertension can be difficult to control in patients who consume more than 40 g of ethanol (two drinks) daily or drink in "binges." **Cigarette smoking** raises blood pressure, again by increasing plasma norepinephrine. Although the long-term effect of smoking on blood pressure is less clear, the synergistic effects of smoking and high blood pressure on cardiovascular risk are well documented. The relationship of **exercise** to hypertension is variable. Aerobic exercise lowers blood pressure in previously sedentary individuals, but increasingly strenuous exercise in already active subjects has less effect. The relationship between stress and hypertension is not established. **Polycythemia**, whether primary or due to diminished plasma volume, increases blood viscosity and may raise blood pressure. **Nonsteroidal anti-inflammatory drugs (NSAIDs)** produce increases in blood pressure averaging 5 mm Hg and are best avoided in patients with borderline or elevated blood pressures. Low **potassium intake** is associated with higher blood pressure in some patients; an intake of 90 mmol/d is recommended.

There is a growing recognition that the complex of abnormalities termed the "metabolic syndrome" is associated with both the development of hypertension and an increased risk of adverse cardiovascular outcomes. The metabolic syndrome (sometimes also called syndrome X or the "deadly quartet") consists of upper body obesity, hyperinsulinemia and insulin resistance, hypertriglyceridemia, and hypertension. Affected patients usually also have low high-density lipoprotein (HDL) cholesterol levels and have been found to have elevated catecholamines and inflammatory markers such as C-reactive protein. Patients with hypertension should be encouraged to follow the lifestyle changes listed in Table 11–2.

B. SECONDARY HYPERTENSION

Approximately 5% of patients with hypertension have specific causes (Table 11–3). The history, examination, and routine laboratory tests may identify such patients. In particular, patients in whom hypertension develops at an early age, those who first exhibit hypertension when over age 50 years, or those previously well controlled who become refractory to treatment are more likely to have secondary hypertension. Causes include renal disease, genetic causes, renal vascular hypertension, primary hyperaldosteronism, Cushing's syndrome, pheochromocytoma, coarctation of the aorta (uncommon), hypertension associated with pregnancy, estrogen use, as well as other causes (eg, hypercalcemia and medications).

1. Renal disease—Renal parenchymal disease is the most common cause of secondary hypertension. Hyper-

Table 11–3. Identifiable causes of hypertension.

Sleep apnea
Drug-induced or drug-related
Chronic kidney disease
Primary aldosteronism
Renovascular disease
Long-term corticosteroid therapy and Cushing's syndrome
Pheochromocytoma
Coarctation of the aorta
Thyroid or parathyroid disease

From Chobanian AV et al: The Seventh Report of the Joint National Committee on Prevention, Detection, Evaluation, and Treatment of High Blood Pressure: the JNC 7 report. JAMA 2003;289:2560.

tension may result from diabetic and inflammatory glomerular diseases, tubular interstitial disease, and polycystic kidneys. Most cases are related to increased intravascular volume or increased activity of the renin–angiotensin–aldosterone system.

2. Genetic causes—Hypertension can be caused by mutations in single genes, inherited on a mendelian basis. Although rare, these conditions provide important insight into blood pressure regulation and possibly, the genetic basis of essential hypertension. **Glucocorticoid remediable aldosteronism** is an autosomal dominant cause of early-onset hypertension with normal or high aldosterone and low renin levels. It is caused by the formation of a chimeric gene encoding both the enzyme responsible for the synthesis of aldosterone (transcriptionally regulated by AII) and an enzyme responsible for synthesis of cortisol (transcriptionally regulated by ACTH). As a consequence, aldosterone synthesis becomes driven by ACTH, which can be suppressed by exogenous cortisol. In the **syndrome of apparent mineralocorticoid excess**, early-onset hypertension with hypokalemic metabolic alkalosis is inherited on an autosomal recessive basis. Although plasma renin is low and plasma aldosterone level is very low in these patients, aldosterone antagonists are effective in controlling hypertension. This disease is caused by loss of the enzyme 11β-hydroxysteroid dehydrogenase, which normally protects the otherwise promiscuous mineralocorticoid receptor in the distal nephron from inappropriate glucocorticoid activation, by metabolism of cortisol. Similarly, glycyrrhetinic acid, found in licorice, causes increased blood pressure through inhibition of 11β-hydroxysteroid dehydrogenase. The syndrome of **hypertension exacerbated in pregnancy** is inherited as an autosomal dominant trait. In these patients, a mutation in the mineralocorticoid receptor makes it abnormally responsive to progesterone and, paradoxically, to spironolactone. **Liddle's syndrome** is an autosomal dominant condition characterized by early-onset hypertension, hypokalemic alkalosis, low renin and low aldosterone levels. This is caused by a mutation that results in constitutive activation of the epithelial sodium channel of the distal nephron, with resultant unregulated sodium reabsorption and volume expansion.

3. Renal vascular hypertension—Renal artery stenosis is present in 1–2% of hypertensive patients. Its cause in most younger individuals is fibromuscular hyperplasia, particularly in women under 50 years of age. The remainder of renal vascular disease is due to atherosclerotic stenoses of the proximal renal arteries. The mechanism of hypertension is excessive renin release due to reduction in renal blood flow and perfusion pressure. Renal vascular hypertension may occur when a single branch of the renal artery is stenotic, but in as many as 25% of patients both arteries are obstructed.

Renal vascular hypertension should be suspected in the following circumstances: (1) if the documented onset is before age 20 or after age 50 years, (2) hypertension is resistant to three or more drugs, (3) if there are epigastric or renal artery bruits, (4) if there is atherosclerotic disease of the aorta or peripheral arteries (15–25% of patients with symptomatic lower limb atherosclerotic vascular disease have renal artery stenosis), (5) if there is abrupt deterioration in renal function after administration of ACE inhibitors, or (6) if episodes of pulmonary edema are associated with abrupt surges in blood pressure. There is no ideal screening test for renal vascular hypertension. If suspicion is sufficiently high, renal arteriography, the definitive diagnostic test, is the best approach. Renal arteriography is not recommended as a routine adjunct to coronary studies. Where suspicion is moderate to low, radioisotope renography, duplex ultrasound, magnetic resonance angiography (MRA) or CT angiography have all been used successfully, but the results vary greatly among institutions. The extent of preexisting parenchymal damage to the affected and contralateral kidney has the greatest influence on blood pressure and renal function outcomes following revascularization. Correction of the lesion should be considered in young individuals and in low-risk patients of any age with blood pressure that is resistant to medical therapy. Percutaneous intervention with stent placement is the preferred approach for fibromuscular hyperplasia and for discrete stenotic arteriosclerotic lesions that do not involve the renal artery ostium. In older individuals with arteriosclerosis, only a minority experience complete normalization without continued drug therapy. Thus, it is reasonable to manage these patients medically if renal function does not deteriorate. Although ACE inhibitors have improved the success rate of medical therapy of hypertension due to renal artery stenosis, they have been associated with marked hypotension and (usually reversible) renal dysfunction in individuals with bilateral renal artery stenosis. Thus, renal function and blood pressure should be closely monitored during the first weeks of therapy in patients in whom this is a consideration.

4. Primary hyperaldosteronism—Primary hyperaldosteronism occurs because of excessive secretion of aldosterone by the adrenal cortex. It may, in fact, be the most common potentially curable and specifically treatable cause of hypertension. In the past, the diagnosis was often suspected when hypokalemia prior to diuretic therapy associated with excessive urinary potassium excretion (usually > 40 mEq/L on a spot specimen) and

suppressed levels of plasma renin activity presented in hypertensive patients. However, the development and application of new screening tests to the population of hypertensive persons have resulted in a marked increase in the detection rate for primary hyperaldosteronism. It now appears that up to 5–15% of patients in whom primary (essential) hypertension is diagnosed actually have primary hyperaldosteronism, with most having normal serum potassium levels. Currently, the best screening test for primary hyperaldosteronism involves determinations of plasma aldosterone concentration (normal: 1–16 ng/dL) and plasma renin activity (normal: 1–2.5 ng/mL/h) and calculation of the plasma aldosterone/renin ratio (normal: < 25). Medications that alter renin and aldosterone levels, including ACE inhibitors, angiotensin receptor blockers (ARBs), and diuretics (especially spironolactone), should be discontinued at least a week before sampling. Patients with aldosterone/renin ratios of ≥ 25 require further evaluation for primary hyperaldosteronism. The lesion responsible is an adrenal adenoma, though some patients have bilateral adrenal hyperplasia. The lesion can be demonstrated by CT or MRI scanning.

5. Cushing's syndrome—Less commonly, hypertension presents in patients with Cushing's syndrome (glucocorticoid excess). However, among those with spontaneous Cushing's syndrome, hypertension occurs in about 75–85% of patients. The exact pathogenesis of the hypertension is unclear. It may be related to salt and water retention from the mineralocorticoid effects of the excess glucocorticoid. Alternatively, it may be due to increased secretion of angiotensinogen. While plasma renin activity and concentrations are generally normal or suppressed in Cushing's syndrome, angiotensinogen levels are elevated to approximately twice normal because of a direct effect of glucocorticoids on its hepatic synthesis, and angiotensin II levels are increased by about 40%. Administration of the angiotensin II antagonist saralasin to patients with Cushing's syndrome causes a prompt 8- to 10-mm Hg drop in systolic and diastolic blood pressure. In addition, glucocorticoids exert permissive effects on vascular tone by a variety of mechanisms.

Diagnosis and treatment of Cushing's syndrome are discussed in Chapter 26.

6. Pheochromocytoma—Pheochromocytomas are uncommon; they are probably found in less than 0.1% of all patients with hypertension and in approximately two individuals per million population. In about 50% of patients with pheochromocytoma, hypertension is sustained but the blood pressure shows marked fluctuations, with peak pressures during symptomatic paroxysms. During a hypertensive episode, the systolic blood pressure can rise to as high as 300 mm Hg. In about one-third of cases, hypertension is truly intermittent. In some cases, hypertension is absent. The blood pressure elevation caused by the catecholamine excess results from two mechanisms: α-receptor-mediated vasoconstriction of arterioles, leading to an increase in peripheral resistance, and β_1-receptor-mediated increases in cardiac output and in renin release, leading to increased circulating levels of angiotensin II. The increased total peripheral vascular resistance is probably primarily responsible for the maintenance of high arterial pressures. Chronic vasoconstriction of the arterial and venous beds leads to a reduction in plasma volume and predisposes to postural hypotension.

Indeed, the majority of patients have orthostatic decreases in blood pressure, the converse of primary (essential) hypertension. Glucose intolerance develops in some patients. Hypertensive crisis in pheochromocytoma may be precipitated by a variety of drugs, including tricyclic antidepressants, antidopaminergic agents, metoclopramide, and naloxone. The diagnosis and treatment of pheochromocytoma are discussed in Chapter 26.

7. Coarctation of the aorta—This uncommon cause of hypertension is discussed in Chapter 10.

8. Hypertension associated with pregnancy—Hypertension occurring de novo or worsening during pregnancy, including preeclampsia and eclampsia, is one of the most common causes of maternal and fetal morbidity and mortality (see Chapter 18).

9. Estrogen use—A small increase in blood pressure occurs in most women taking oral contraceptives, but considerable increases are noted occasionally. This is caused by volume expansion due to increased activity of the renin–angiotensin–aldosterone system. The primary abnormality is an increase in the hepatic synthesis of renin substrate. Five percent of women taking oral contraceptives chronically exhibit a rise in blood pressure above 140/90 mm Hg, twice the expected prevalence. Contraceptive-related hypertension is more common in women over 35 years of age, in those who have taken contraceptives for more than 5 years, and in obese individuals. It is less common in those taking low-dose estrogen tablets. In most, hypertension is reversible by discontinuing the contraceptive, but it may take several weeks. Postmenopausal estrogen does not generally cause hypertension, but rather maintains endothelium-mediated vasodilation.

10. Other causes of secondary hypertension—Hypertension has also been associated with hypercalcemia due to any cause: acromegaly, hyperthyroidism, hypothyroidism, and a variety of neurologic disorders causing increased intracranial pressure. A number of other medications may cause or exacerbate hypertension—most importantly cyclosporine and NSAIDs.

August P: Overview: mechanisms of hypertension: cells, hormones, and the kidney. J Am Soc Nephrol 2004;15:1971. [PMID: 15284282]

Bravo EL: Pheochromocytoma. Cardiol Rev 2002;10:44. [PMID: 11790269]

Failor RA et al: Hyperaldosteronism and pheochromocytoma: new tricks and tests. Prim Care 2003;30:801. [PMID: 15024897]

Freel EM et al: Mechanisms of hypertension: the expanding role of aldosterone. J Am Soc Nephrol 2004;15:1993. [PMID: 15284285]

Hartman RP et al: Evaluation of renal causes of hypertension. Radiol Clin North Am 2003;41:909. [PMID: 14521201]

Lifton RP et al: Molecular mechanisms of human hypertension. Cell 2001;104:545. [PMID: 11239411]

Loney EL et al: Renovascular hypertension. Q J Nucl Med 2002; 46:283. [PMID: 12411868]

Nordmann AJ et al: Balloon angioplasty versus medical therapy for hypertensive patients with renal artery obstruction. Cochrane Database Syst Rev 2003;(3):CD002944. [PMID: 12917937]

Nussberger J: Investigating mineralocorticoid hypertension. J Hypertens Suppl 2003;21(Suppl 2):S25. [PMID: 12929904]

Onusko E: Diagnosing secondary hypertension. Am Fam Physician 2003;67:67. [PMID: 12537168]

Oparil S et al: Pathogenesis of hypertension. Ann Intern Med 2003;139:761. [PMID: 14597461]

Radermacher J et al: Techniques for predicting a favourable response to renal angioplasty in patients with renovascular disease. Curr Opin Nephrol Hypertens 2001;10:799. [PMID: 11706308]

Reaven G: Insulin resistance, hypertension, and coronary heart disease. J Clin Hypertens 2003;5:269. [PMID: 12939567]

Safar ME et al: Vascular development, pulse pressure, and the mechanisms of hypertension. Hypertension 2005;46:205. [PMID: 15911744]

Stas SN et al: Pathogenesis of hypertension in diabetes. Rev Endocr Metab Disord 2004;5:221. [PMID: 15211093]

Strazzullo P et al: Altered renal handling of sodium in human hypertension: short review of the evidence. Hypertension 2003;41:1000. [PMID: 12668589]

Textor SC: Managing renal arterial disease and hypertension. Curr Opin Cardiol 2003;18:260. [PMID: 12858123]

Young WF Jr: Minireview: primary aldosteronism—changing concepts in diagnosis and treatment. Endocrinology 2003;144: 2208. [PMID: 12746276]

Complications of Untreated Hypertension

Complications of hypertension are related either to sustained elevations of blood pressure, with consequent changes in the vasculature and heart, or to atherosclerosis that accompanies and is accelerated by long-standing hypertension. Most of the adverse outcomes in hypertension are associated with thrombosis rather than bleeding, and there is evidence that increased vascular shear stress converts the normally anticoagulant endothelium to a prothrombotic state. The excess morbidity and mortality related to hypertension are progressive over the whole range of systolic and diastolic blood pressures; the risk approximately doubles for each 6 mm Hg increase in diastolic blood pressure. However, target-organ damage varies markedly between individuals with similar levels of office hypertension. Ambulatory pressures are superior to office readings in the prediction of end-organ damage.

A. HYPERTENSIVE CARDIOVASCULAR DISEASE

Cardiac complications are the major causes of morbidity and mortality in primary (essential) hypertension, and preventing them is a major goal of therapy. Electrocardiographic evidence of left ventricular hypertrophy is found in up to 15% of persons with chronic hypertension. For any level of blood pressure, its presence is associated with incremental cardiovascular risk. Echocardiographic left ventricular hypertrophy is a powerful predictor of prognosis. Left ventricular hypertrophy may cause or facilitate many cardiac complications of hypertension, including congestive heart failure, ventricular arrhythmias, myocardial ischemia, and sudden death.

Left ventricular diastolic dysfunction, which may present with all of the symptoms and signs of congestive heart failure, is common in patients with long-standing hypertension. The occurrence of heart failure is reduced by 50% with antihypertensive therapy. Hypertensive left ventricular hypertrophy regresses with therapy and is most closely related to the degree of systolic blood pressure reduction. Diuretics have produced equal or greater reductions of left ventricular mass when compared with other drug classes. β-Blockers are less effective in reducing left ventricular hypertrophy but play a specific role in patients with established coronary artery disease or impaired left ventricular function.

B. Hypertensive Cerebrovascular Disease and Dementia

Hypertension is the major predisposing cause of hemorrhagic and ischemic stroke. Cerebrovascular complications are more closely correlated with systolic than diastolic blood pressure. The incidence of these complications is markedly reduced by antihypertensive therapy. Preceding hypertension is associated with a higher incidence of subsequent dementia of both vascular and Alzheimer types. Effective blood pressure control may modify the risk or rate of progression of cognitive dysfunction.

C. Hypertensive Renal Disease

Chronic hypertension leads to nephrosclerosis, a common cause of renal insufficiency; aggressive blood pressure control attenuates the process. In patients with hypertensive nephropathy, the blood pressure should be 130/80 mm Hg or lower, especially when proteinuria is present. Secondary renal disease is more common in blacks, particularly when accompanied by diabetes mellitus. Hypertension also plays an important role in accelerating the progression of other forms of renal disease, most commonly diabetic nephropathy. ACE inhibitors are particularly effective in preventing the latter complication, but these agents also appear to prevent the progression of other forms of nephropathy.

D. Aortic Dissection

Hypertension is a contributing factor in many patients with dissection of the aorta. Its diagnosis and treatment are discussed in Chapter 12.

E. Atherosclerotic Complications

Most Americans with hypertension die of complications of atherosclerosis, but the linkage between hypertension and atherosclerotic cardiovascular disease is not as clear as that with the previously discussed complications. Effective antihypertensive therapy is thus less successful in preventing complications of coronary heart disease.

Dielis AW et al: The prothrombotic paradox of hypertension: role of the renin-angiotensin and kallikrein-kinin systems. Hypertension 2005;46:1236. [PMID: 16286563]

Forette F et al: The prevention of dementia with antihypertensive treatment. Arch Intern Med 2002;162:2046. [PMID: 12374512]

Izzo JL et al: Mechanisms and management of hypertensive heart disease: from left ventricular hypertrophy to heart failure. Med Clin North Am 2004;88:1257. [PMID: 15331316]

Lapu-Bula R et al: Diastolic heart failure: the forgotten manifestation of hypertensive heart disease. Curr Hypertens Rep 2004; 6:164. [PMID: 15128466]

Luft FC: Hypertensive nephrosclerosis: update. Curr Opin Nephrol Hypertens 2004;13:147. [PMID: 15202608]

Manolio TA et al: Hypertension and cognitive function: pathophysiologic effects of hypertension on the brain. Curr Hypertens Rep 2003;5:255. [PMID: 12724059]

Persu A et al: Recent insights in the development of organ damage caused by hypertension. Acta Cardiol 2004;59:369. [PMID: 15368798]

Clinical Findings

The clinical and laboratory findings are mainly referable to involvement of the target organs: heart, brain, kidneys, eyes, and peripheral arteries.

A. Symptoms

Mild to moderate primary (essential) hypertension is largely asymptomatic for many years. The most frequent symptom, headache, is also very nonspecific. Suboccipital pulsating headaches, occurring early in the morning and subsiding during the day, are said to be characteristic, but any type of headache may occur. Accelerated hypertension is associated with somnolence, confusion, visual disturbances, and nausea and vomiting (hypertensive encephalopathy).

Hypertension in patients with pheochromocytomas that secrete predominantly norepinephrine is usually sustained but may be episodic. The typical attack lasts from minutes to hours and is associated with headache, anxiety, palpitation, profuse perspiration, pallor, tremor, and nausea and vomiting. Blood pressure is markedly elevated, and angina or acute pulmonary edema may occur. In primary aldosteronism, patients may have muscular weakness, polyuria, and nocturia due to hypokalemia; malignant hypertension is rare. Chronic hypertension often leads to left ventricular hypertrophy, which may be associated with diastolic or, in late stages, systolic dysfunction. Exertional and paroxysmal nocturnal dyspnea may result, and ischemic heart disease is more common (especially when concomitant coronary artery disease is present). Cerebral involvement causes (1) stroke due to thrombosis or (2) small or large hemorrhage from microaneurysms of small penetrating intracranial arteries. Hypertensive encephalopathy is probably caused by acute capillary congestion and exudation with cerebral edema. The findings are usually reversible if adequate treatment is given promptly. There is no strict correlation of diastolic blood pressure with hypertensive encephalopathy; but it usually exceeds 130 mm Hg.

B. Signs

Like symptoms, physical findings depend on the cause of hypertension, its duration and severity, and the degree of effect on target organs.

1. Blood pressure—On initial examination, pressure is taken in both arms and, if lower extremity pulses are diminished or delayed, in the legs to exclude coarctation of the aorta. An orthostatic drop is present in pheochromocytoma. Older patients may have falsely elevated readings by sphygmomanometry because of noncompressible vessels. This may be suspected in the presence of Osler's sign—a palpable brachial or radial artery when the cuff is inflated above systolic pressure. Occasionally, it may be necessary to make direct measurements of intra-arterial pressure, especially in patients with apparent severe hypertension who do not tolerate therapy.

2. Retinas—Narrowing of arterial diameter to less than 50% of venous diameter, copper or silver wire appearance, exudates, hemorrhages, or papilledema are associated with a worse prognosis.

3. Heart and arteries—Left ventricular enlargement with a left ventricular heave indicates severe or longstanding hypertrophy. Older patients frequently have systolic ejection murmurs resulting from calcific aortic sclerosis, and these may evolve to significant aortic stenosis in some individuals. Aortic insufficiency may be auscultated in up to 5% of patients, and hemodynamically insignificant aortic insufficiency can be detected by Doppler echocardiography in 10–20%. A presystolic (S_4) gallop due to decreased compliance of the left ventricle is quite common in patients with sinus rhythm.

4. Pulses—The timing of upper and lower extremity pulses should be compared to exclude coarctation of the aorta. All major peripheral pulses should be evaluated to exclude aortic dissection and peripheral atherosclerosis, which may be associated with renal artery involvement.

C. Laboratory Findings

Recommended testing includes the following: hemoglobin; urinalysis and renal function studies, to detect hematuria, proteinuria, and casts, signifying primary renal disease or nephrosclerosis; fasting blood sugar level, since hyperglycemia is noted in diabetes and pheochromocytoma; plasma lipids, as an indicator of atherosclerosis risk and an additional target for therapy; serum uric acid which, if elevated, is a relative contraindication to diuretic therapy; and basal electrolytes. Measurement of the plasma aldosterone/renin ratio is indicated to screen for mineralocorticoid excess in hypertensive patients with hypokalemic alkalosis

(even if they are taking diuretics), resistant hypertension, or an adrenal "incidentaloma."

D. Electrocardiography and Chest Radiographs

Electrocardiographic criteria are highly specific but not very sensitive for left ventricular hypertrophy. The "strain" pattern of ST–T wave changes is a sign of more advanced disease and is associated with a poor prognosis. A chest radiograph is not necessary in the workup for uncomplicated hypertension since it usually does not yield additional information.

E. Echocardiography

Although echocardiography has been advocated to determine the need for drug therapy in patients with borderline or mildly elevated pressures, it is unusual to find left ventricular mass readings above the upper 75% confidence limits in the absence of systolic hypertension. The primary role of echocardiography should be to evaluate patients with clinical symptoms or signs of cardiac disease.

F. Diagnostic Studies

Additional diagnostic studies are indicated only if the clinical presentation or routine tests suggest secondary or complicated hypertension. These may include tests such as 24-hour urine free cortisol, plasma metanephrine and the plasma aldosterone/renin ratio for endocrine causes of hypertension, renal ultrasound to diagnose primary renal disease (polycystic kidneys, obstructive uropathy), and testing for renal artery stenosis. Further evaluation may include abdominal imaging studies (ultrasound, CT scan, or MRI) or renal arteriography.

G. Summary

Since most hypertension is "primary," few studies are necessary beyond those listed above. If conventional therapy is unsuccessful or if symptoms suggest a secondary cause, further studies are indicated.

Nonpharmacologic Therapy

Lifestyle modification may have an impact on morbidity and mortality. A diet rich in fruits, vegetables, and low-fat dairy foods and low in saturated and total fats (DASH diet) has been shown to lower blood pressure. Additional measures can prevent or mitigate hypertension or its cardiovascular consequences as shown in Table 11–2.

All patients with high-normal or elevated blood pressures, those who have a family history of cardiovascular complications of hypertension, and those who have multiple coronary risk factors should be counseled about nonpharmacologic approaches to lowering blood pressure. Approaches of proved but modest value include weight reduction, reduced alcohol consumption and, in some patients, reduced salt intake. Gradually increasing activity levels should be encouraged in previously sedentary patients, but strenuous exercise training programs in already active individuals may have less benefit. Calcium and potassium supplements have been advocated, but their ability to lower blood pressure is limited.

Smoking cessation will reduce overall cardiovascular risk.

Bray GA et al: A further subgroup analysis of the effects of the DASH diet and three dietary sodium levels on blood pressure: results of the DASH-Sodium Trial. Am J Cardiol 2004;94:222. [PMID: 15246908]

Hooper L et al: Advice to reduce dietary salt for prevention of cardiovascular disease. Cochrane Database Syst Rev 2004;(1): CD003656. [PMID: 14974027]

Krousel-Wood MA et al: Primary prevention of essential hypertension. Med Clin North Am 2004;88:223. [PMID: 14871061]

Stewart KJ: Exercise training and the cardiovascular consequences of type 2 diabetes and hypertension: plausible mechanisms for improving cardiovascular health. JAMA 2002;288:1622. [PMID: 12350193]

Whelton SP et al: Effect of aerobic exercise on blood pressure: a meta-analysis of randomized controlled trials. Ann Intern Med 2002;136:493. [PMID: 11926784]

Wilburn AJ et al: The natural treatment of hypertension. J Clin Hypertens (Greenwich) 2004;6:242. [PMID: 15133406]

Who Should Be Treated with Medications?

Many excellent trials have shown that drug therapy of patients with stage 2 hypertension reduces the incidence of stroke by 30–50%, congestive heart failure by 40–50%, and progression to accelerated hypertension syndromes. The decreases in fatal and nonfatal coronary heart disease and cardiovascular and total mortality have been less dramatic, ranging from 10% to 15%. This lesser decrease in coronary heart disease has generated controversy. Some experts have attributed the decreased benefit to characteristics of the drugs (primarily diuretics and β-blockers), such as their adverse effect on lipid profiles and electrolyte balance. Others believe it is due to the more chronic and multifactorial nature of coronary artery disease, the generally low-risk populations included in trials, and the large number of crossovers from placebo to active therapy. Several studies in older persons with predominantly systolic hypertension have confirmed that antihypertensive therapy prevents fatal and nonfatal myocardial infarction and overall cardiovascular mortality. These trials have also placed the focus on control of systolic blood pressure—in contrast to the historical emphasis on diastolic blood pressures.

The decision to initiate drug therapy is relatively straightforward once hypertension has been unequivocally diagnosed (Table 11–1 and Figure 11–1), but less clear in persons with prehypertension (blood pressure of 120–139/80–89 mm Hg). In the latter group, treatment decisions should be based on an assessment of overall cardiovascular risk rather than the level of blood pressure alone. The JNC criteria for institution of therapy (Table 11–1) suggest that patients with prehypertension should be treated if they exhibit at least one additional high-risk condition with compelling indications (listed in Table 11–4), such as chronic kidney disease or diabetes mellitus. In the presence of compelling indications, the target blood pressure should be < 130/80 mm Hg in persons with prehypertension just as in those with hypertension. Table 11–5 lists the major risk factors for cardiovascular morbidity and mortality and the cardiovascular manifestations that predispose to further complications. The BHS promotes a similar approach but goes further by introducing a consideration of overall predicted cardiovascular risk (Figure 11–2). According to the BHS recommendations, risk analysis should be used to target treatment to patients with borderline hypertension who are most likely to benefit, particularly individuals at high combined risk of coronary heart or stroke event (> 20–30% within 10 years). A risk calculation tool can be downloaded from the BHS web site at http://www.bhsoc.org/Cardiovascular_Risk_Charts_and_Calculators.htm (in using this tool, convert cholesterol from mmol/L to mg/dL by multiplying by 38.7). A free PDA-based coronary heart disease risk calculator is available at http://www.statcoder.com/cholesterol.htm. In general, 20% total cardiovascular risk (which includes stroke) is equivalent to 15% coronary heart disease risk.

Goals of Treatment

Treatment should ideally be offered to all persons in whom blood pressure reduction, irrespective of initial blood pressure levels, will reduce overall cardiovascular risk (see above). Blood pressure targets for hypertensive patients at the greatest risk for cardiovascular events, particularly diabetic patients, should be lower (< 130/80 mm Hg) than for individuals at lower total cardiovascular risk (< 140/90 mm Hg). As discussed below, hypertensive patients with chronic kidney disease should also be treated until blood pressure is < 130/80 mm Hg. However, since there does not seem to be a blood pressure level below which risk plateaus, these recommendations should be taken as reasonable goals pending further information on optimal targets, which may be even lower. There is no clear consensus on blood pressure goals in the treatment of prehypertension.

Large-scale trials in hypertension have focused on discrete end points occurring over relatively short intervals, thereby placing the emphasis on the prevention of catastrophic events in advanced disease. More recently, in parallel with a new emphasis on hypertension in the context of overall cardiovascular risk, attention is turning to the importance of the long view. Accordingly, treatment of persons with hypertension should focus on comprehensive risk reduction. More careful consideration should be given to the possible long-term adverse consequences of the metabolic derangements linked to some antihypertensives (particularly conventional β-blockers and thiazide diuretics).

Statins should be more widely used. In this respect, there is now evidence from the Anglo-Scandinavian

Table 11–4. Clinical trial and guideline basis for compelling indications for individual drug classes.

High-Risk Conditions with Compelling Indication[1]	Recommended Drugs						Clinical Trial Basis[2]
	Diuretic	β-Blocker	ACE Inhibitor	ARB	CCB	Aldosterone Antagonist	
Heart failure	•	•	•			•	ACC/AHA Heart Failure Guideline, MERIT-HF, COPERNICUS, CIBIS, SOLVD, AIRE, TRACE, ValHEFT, RALES
Post-myocardial infarction		•	•			•	ACC/AHA Post-MI Guideline, BHAT, SAVE, Capricorn, EPHESUS
High coronary disease risk	•	•	•		•		ALLHAT, HOPE, ANBP2, LIFE, CONVINCE
Diabetes mellitus	•	•	•	•	•		NKF-ADA Guideline, UKPDS, ALLHAT
Chronic kidney disease			•	•			NKF Guideline, Captopril Trial, RENAAL, IDNT, REIN, AASK
Recurrent stroke prevention	•		•				PROGRESS

AASK = African American Study of Kidney Disease and Hypertension; ACC/AHA = American College of Cardiology/American Heart Association; ACE = angiotensin converting enzyme; AIRE = Acute Infarction Ramipril Efficacy; ALLHAT = Antihypertensive and Lipid-Lowering Treatment to Prevent Heart Attack Trial; ANBP2 = Second Australian National Blood Pressure Study; ARB = angiotensin receptor blocker; BHAT = β-Blocker Heart Attack Trial; CCB = calcium channel blocker; CIBIS = Cardiac Insufficiency Bisoprolol Study; CONVINCE = Controlled Onset Verapamil Investigation of Cardiovascular End Points; COPERNICUS = Carvedilol Prospective Randomized Cumulative Survival Study; EPHESUS = Eplerenone Post-Acute Myocardial Infarction Heart Failure Efficacy and Survival Study; HOPE = Heart Outcomes Prevention Evaluation Study; IDNT = Irbesartan Diabetic Nephropathy Trial; LIFE = Losartan Intervention For Endpoint Reduction in Hypertension Study; MERIT-HF = Metoprolol CR/XL Randomized Intervention Trial in Congestive Heart Failure; NKF-ADA = National Kidney Foundation–American Diabetes Association; PROGRESS = Perindopril Protection Against Recurrent Stroke Study; RALES = Randomized Aldactone Evaluation Study; REIN = Ramipril Efficacy in Nephropathy Study; RENAAL = Reduction of Endpoints in Non-Insulin-Dependent Diabetes Mellitus with the Angiotensin II Antagonist Losartan Study; SAVE = Survival and Ventricular Enlargement Study; SOLVD = Studies of Left Ventricular Dysfunction; TRACE = Trandolapril Cardiac Evaluation Study; UKPDS = United Kingdom Prospective Diabetes Study; ValHEFT = Valsartan Heart Failure Trial.

[1]Compelling indications for antihypertensive drugs are based on benefits from outcome studies or existing clinical guidelines; the compelling indication is managed in parallel with the blood pressure.

[2]Conditions for which clinical trials demonstrate benefit of specific classes of antihypertensive drugs.

From Chobanian AV et al: The Seventh Report of the Joint National Committee on Prevention, Detection, Evaluation, and Treatment of High Blood Pressure: the JNC 7 report. JAMA 2003;289:2560.

Cardiac Outcomes Trial (ASCOT) that statins can significantly improve outcomes in persons with hypertension (with modest background cardiovascular risk) whose total cholesterol is < 250 mg/dL. The BHS guidelines recommend that statins be offered as secondary prevention to patients whose total cholesterol exceeds 135 mg/dL if they have documented coronary artery disease or a history of ischemic stroke. In addition, statins should be considered as primary prevention in patients with long-standing type 2 diabetes mellitus or in those with type 2 diabetes mellitus who are older than age 50 years, and perhaps in all persons with type 2 diabetes mellitus. Ideally, total and low-density lipoprotein (LDL) cholesterol should be reduced by 30% and 40% respectively, or to approximately < 155 mg/dL and < 77 mg/dL, whichever is the greatest reduction. However, total and LDL cholesterol levels of < 194 mg/dL and < 116 mg/dL respectively, or reductions of 25% and 30% are regarded as clinically acceptable objectives. Primary prevention with statins might also be reasonably extended to all patients with total cholesterol > 135 mg/dL and a total cardiovascular risk > 20% (to similar target cholesterol levels), but trial evidence for this is not currently available.

Low-dose aspirin (81 mg/day) is likely to be beneficial in patients older than age 50 with either target organ damage or elevated total cardiovascular risk (> 20–30%). Care should be taken to ensure that blood pressure is controlled to the recommended levels in patients receiving aspirin to minimize the risk of bleeding.

Table 11–5. Cardiovascular risk factors.

Major risk factors
  Hypertension[1]
  Cigarette smoking
  Obesity (BMI ≥ 30)[1]
  Physical inactivity
  Dyslipidemia[1]
  Diabetes mellitus[1]
  Microalbuminuria or estimated GFR < 60 mL/min
  Age (> 55 years for men, > 65 years for women)
  Family history of premature cardiovascular disease (men
    < 55 years or women 65 years)
Target-organ damage
  Heart
    Left ventricular hypertrophy
    Angina or prior myocardial infarction
    Prior coronary revascularization
    Heart failure
  Brain
    Stroke or transient ischemic attack
  Chronic kidney disease
  Peripheral arterial disease
  Retinopathy

[1]Components of the metabolic syndrome.
BMI indicates body mass index calculated as weight in kilo-grams divided by the square of height in meters; GFR = glomer-ular filtration rate.
From Chobanian AV et al: The Seventh Report of the Joint National Committee on Prevention, Detection, Evaluation, and Treatment of High Blood Pressure: the JNC 7 report. JAMA 2003;289:2560.

Friday G et al: Control of hypertension and risk of stroke recurrence. Stroke 2002;33:2652. [PMID: 12411656]

Lawes CM et al: Blood pressure and stroke: an overview of published reviews. Stroke 2004;35:776. [PMID: 14976329]

Sever PS et al; ASCOT investigators: Prevention of coronary and stroke events with atorvastatin in hypertensive patients who have average or lower-than-average cholesterol concentrations, in the Anglo-Scandinavian Cardiac Outcomes Trial—Lipid Lowering Arm (ASCOT-LLA): a multicentre randomised controlled trial. Lancet 2003;361:1149. [PMID: 12686036]

Snow V et al: The evidence base for tight blood pressure control in the management of type 2 diabetes mellitus. Ann Intern Med 2003;138:587. [PMID: 12667031]

Whelton PK et al: Strategies for improvement of awareness, treatment and control of hypertension: results of a panel discussion. J Hum Hypertens 2004;18:563. [PMID: 15116145]

Whitworth JA: 2003 World Health Organization (WHO)/International Society of Hypertension (ISH) statement on management of hypertension. J Hypertens 2003;21:1983. [PMID: 14597836]

DRUG THERAPY

General Principles

There are now many classes of potentially antihypertensive drugs of which five (diuretics, β-blockers, ACE inhibitors, calcium channel blockers, and ARBs) are suitable for initial or single-drug therapy based on efficacy and tolerability. A number of considerations enter into the selection of the initial drug for a given patient. These include the weight of evidence for beneficial effects on clinical outcomes, the safety and tolerability of the drug, its cost, demographic differences in response, concomitant medical conditions, and lifestyle issues. The specific classes of antihypertensive medications are discussed below, and guidelines for the choice of initial medications are offered.

Current Antihypertensive Agents

A. DIURETICS

Diuretics are the antihypertensives that have been most extensively studied and most consistently effective in clinical trials. They lower blood pressure initially by decreasing plasma volume (by suppressing tubular reabsorption of sodium, thus increasing the excretion of sodium and water) and cardiac output, but during long-term therapy their major hemodynamic effect is reduction of peripheral vascular resistance. Most of the antihypertensive effect of these agents is achieved at lower dosages than used previously (typically, 12.5 or 25 mg of hydrochlorothiazide or equivalent), but their biochemical and metabolic effects are dose related. The thiazide diuretics are the most widely used (Table 11–6). During long-term therapy, hydrochlorothiazide may be administered every other day with undiminished efficacy. The loop diuretics (such as furosemide) may lead to electrolyte and volume depletion more readily than the thiazides and have short durations of action; therefore, loop diuretics should not be used in hypertension except in the presence of renal dysfunction (serum creatinine above 2.5 mg/dL). Relative to the β-blockers and the ACE inhibitors, diuretics are more potent in blacks, older individuals, the obese, and other subgroups with increased plasma volume or low plasma renin activity. Interestingly, they are relatively more effective in smokers than in nonsmokers. Long-term diuretic administration also mitigates the loss of bone mineral content in older women at risk for osteoporosis.

Overall, diuretics administered alone control blood pressure in 50% of patients with mild to moderate hypertension and can be used effectively in combination with all other agents. They are also useful for lowering isolated or predominantly systolic hypertension. Some observations suggest that the use of thiazide diuretics as initial therapy has been associated with greater reductions in myocardial infarction than β-blockers.

The adverse effects of diuretics relate primarily to the metabolic changes listed in Table 11–6. Impotence, skin rashes, and photosensitivity are less frequent. Hypokalemia has been a concern but is uncommon at the recommended dosages (12.5–25 mg hydrochlorothiazide). The risk can be minimized by limiting dietary salt or increasing dietary potassium; potassium replacement is not usually required to maintain serum K+ at > 3.5 mmol/L. Higher serum levels are prudent in patients at special risk from intracellular potassium depletion, such as those taking digoxin or with a history of ventricular arrhyth-

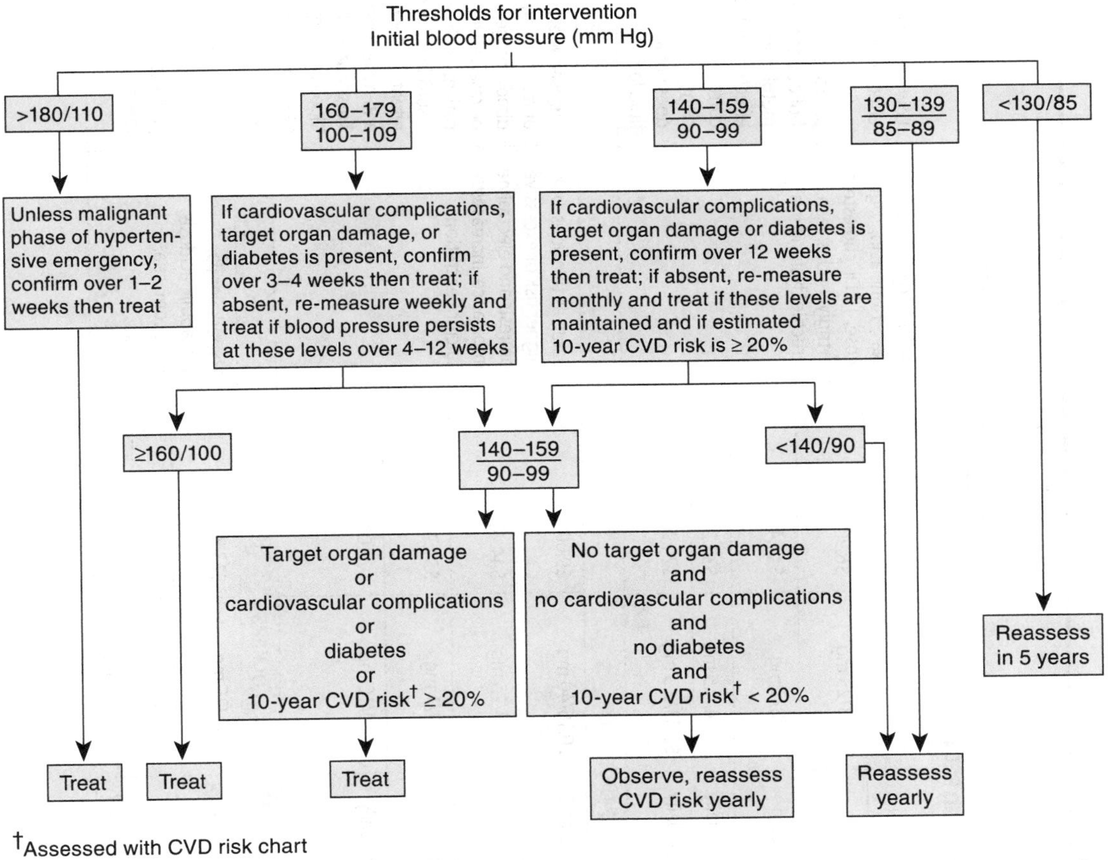

Thresholds for intervention
Initial blood pressure (mm Hg)

†Assessed with CVD risk chart

Figure 11–2. British Hypertension Society algorithm for diagnosis and treatment of hypertension, incorporating total cardiovascular risk in deciding which "prehypertensive" patients to treat. (CVD = cardiovascular disease.) (Reproduced with permission from: Guidelines for management of hypertension: report of the Fourth Working Party of the British Hypertension Society, 2004-BHS IV. J Hum Hypertens 2004;18:139–185.)

mias. If higher doses of diuretic are required, the drug should be used in combination with a potassium-sparing agent or with an ACE inhibitor or ARB. Diuretics reduce insulin sensitivity and cause modest increases in blood glucose. Compared with ACE inhibitors and ARBs, diuretic therapy is associated with a slightly higher incidence of new-onset diabetes. Diuretics also increase serum uric acid and may precipitate gout. Increases in blood glucose, triglycerides, LDL cholesterol, and plasma insulin may occur but are relatively minor during long-term low-dose therapy.

B. β-ADRENERGIC BLOCKING AGENTS

These drugs are effective in hypertension because they decrease the heart rate and cardiac output. Even after continued use of β-blockers, cardiac output remains lower and systemic vascular resistance higher with agents that do not have intrinsic sympathomimetic or α-blocking activity. The β-blockers also decrease renin release and are more efficacious in populations with elevated plasma renin activity, such as younger white patients. They neutralize the reflex tachycardia caused by vasodilators and are especially useful in patients with associated conditions that benefit from the cardioprotective effects of these agents. These include individuals with angina pectoris, previous myocardial infarction, and stable congestive heart failure as well as those with migraine headaches and somatic manifestations of anxiety. In some clinical trials, β-blockers have not been as effective as diuretics in preventing first myocardial infarctions.

Although all β-blockers appear to be similar in antihypertensive potency, controlling approximately 50% of patients, they differ in a number of pharmacologic properties (these differences are summarized in Table 11–7), including those relatively specific to the cardiac β_1-receptors (cardioselectivity) and whether they also block the β_2-receptors in the bronchi and vasculature; at higher dosages, however, all agents are nonselective. The β-blockers also differ in their pharmacokinetics and lipid solubility—which determines whether they cross the blood–brain barrier and affect the incidence of cen-

Table 11–6. Antihypertensive drugs: diuretics.

Drug	Proprietary Name	Initial Dosage	Dosage Range	Cost per Unit	Cost of 30 Days Treatment[1] (Average Dosage)	Adverse Effects	Comments
THIAZIDES AND RELATED DIURETICS							
Hydrochlorothiazide	Esidrix, Hydro-Diuril	12.5 or 25 mg once daily	12.5–50 mg once daily	$0.08/25 mg	$2.40	$\downarrow K^+$, $\downarrow Mg^{2+}$, $\uparrow Ca^{2+}$, $\downarrow Na^+$, $\uparrow$ uric acid, $\uparrow$ glucose, $\uparrow$ LDL cholesterol, $\uparrow$ triglycerides; rash, erectile dysfunction.	Low dosages effective in many patients without associated metabolic abnormalities; metolazone more effective with concurrent renal insufficiency; indapamide does not alter serum lipid levels.
Chlorthalidone	Hygroton, Thaliton	12.5 or 25 mg once daily	12.5–50 mg once daily	$0.23/25 mg	$6.90		
Metolazone	Zaroxolyn	1.25 or 2.5 mg once daily	1.25–5 mg once daily	$1.48/5 mg	$44.40		
	Mykrox	0.5 mg once daily	0.5–1 mg once daily	$1.24/0.5 mg	$37.20		
Indapamide	Lozol	2.5 mg once daily	2.5–5 mg once daily	$0.83/2.5 mg	$24.90		
LOOP DIURETICS							
Furosemide	Lasix	20 mg twice daily	40–320 mg in 2 or 3 doses	$0.16/40 mg	$9.60	Same as thiazides, but higher risk of excessive diuresis and electrolyte imbalance. Increases calcium excretion.	**Furosemide:** Short duration of action a disadvantage; should be reserved for patients with renal insufficiency or fluid retention. Poor anti-hypertensive. **Torsemide:** Effective blood pressure medication at low dosage.
Ethacrynic acid	Edecrin	50 mg once daily	50–100 mg once or twice daily	$0.37/25 mg	$44.40		
Bumetanide	Bumex	0.25 mg twice daily	0.5–10 mg in 2 or 3 doses	$0.52/1 mg	$31.20		
Torsemide	Demadex	2.5 mg once daily	5–10 mg once daily	$0.70/10 mg	$21.00		
ALDOSTERONE RECEPTOR BLOCKERS							
Spironolactone	Aldactone	12.5 or 25 mg once daily	12.5–100 mg once daily	$0.46/25 mg	$13.80	Hyperkalemia, metabolic acidosis, gynecomastia.	Can be useful add-on therapy in patients with refractory hypertension.
Amiloride	Midamor	5 mg once daily	5–10 mg once daily	$0.48/5 mg	$14.40		
Eplerenone	Inspra	25 mg once daily	25–100 mg once daily	$3.78/25 mg	$113.40		

COMBINATION PRODUCTS

Hydrochlorothiazide and triamterene	Dyazide (25/50 mg); Maxzide (25/37.5 mg)	1 tab once daily	1 or 2 tabs once daily	$0.36	$10.80	Same as thiazides plus GI disturbances, hyperkalemia rather than hypokalemia, headache; triamterene can cause kidney stones and renal dysfunction; spironolactone causes gynecomastia. Hyperkalemia can occur if this combination is used in patients with renal failure or those taking ACE inhibitors.	Use should be limited to patients with demonstrable need for a potassium-sparing agent.
Hydrochlorothiazide and amiloride	Moduretic (50/5 mg)	1/2 tab once daily	1 or 2 tabs once daily	$0.33	$9.90		
Hydrochlorothiazide and spironolactone	Aldactazide (25/25 mg)	1 tab once daily	1 or 2 tabs once daily	$0.50	$15.00		

[1]Average wholesale price (AWP, for AB-rated generic when available) for quantity listed. Source: *Red Book Update*, Vol. 25, No. 1, January 2006. AWP may not accurately represent the actual pharmacy cost because wide contractual variations exist among institutions.

LDL = low-density lipoprotein; GI = gastrointestinal; ACE = angiotensin-converting enzyme.

Table 11–7. Antihypertensive drugs: β-adrenergic blocking agents.

Drug	Proprietary Name	Initial Dosage	Dosage Range	Cost per Unit	Cost of 30 Days Treatment (Based on Average Dosage)[1]	β₁ Selectivity[2]	ISA[3]	MSA[4]	Lipid Solubility	Renal vs Hepatic Elimination	Comments[5]
						Special Properties					
Acebutolol	Sectral	200 mg once daily	200–1200 mg in 1 or 2 doses	$1.34/400 mg	$40.20	+	+	+	+	H > R	Positive ANA; rare LE syndrome; also indicated for arrhythmias. Doses > 800 mg have β₁ and β₂ effects.
Atenolol	Tenormin	25 mg once daily	25–200 mg once daily	$0.83/50 mg	$24.90	+	0	0	0	R	Also indicated for angina pectoris and post-MI. Doses > 100 mg have β₁ and β₂ effects.
Betaxolol	Kerlone	10 mg once daily	10–40 mg once daily	$1.10/10 mg	$33.00	+	0	0	+	H > R	
Bisoprolol and hydrochlorothiazide	Ziac	5 mg/6.25 mg	2.5–10 mg plus 6.25 mg	$1.14/2.5/6.25 mg	$34.20	+	0	0	+	R = H	Low-dose combination approved for initial therapy. Bisoprolol also effective for heart failure.
Carteolol	Cartrol	2.5 mg once daily	2.5–10 mg once daily	$1.37/5 mg	$41.10	0	+	0	+	R > H	
Carvedilol	Coreg	6.25 mg	12.5–100 mg in 2 doses	$1.83/25 mg	$109.80 (25 mg twice a day)	0	0	0	+++	H > R	α:β-Blocking activity 1:9; may cause orthostatic symptoms; effective for congestive heart failure.
Labetalol	Normodyne, Trandate	100 mg twice daily	200–1200 mg in 2 doses	$0.71/200 mg	$42.60	0	0/+	0	++	H	α:β-Blocking activity 1:3; more orthostatic hypotension, fever, hepatotoxicity.

Metoprolol	Lopressor	50 mg in 1 or 2 doses	50–200 mg in 1 or 2 doses	$0.55/50 mg	$33.00	+	0	+	+++	H	Also indicated for angina pectoris and post-MI. Approved for heart failure. Doses > 100 mg have β₁ and β₂ effects.
	Toprol XL (SR preparation)	50 mg once daily	50–200 mg once daily	$1.36/100 mg	$40.80						
Nadolol	Corgard	20 mg once daily	20–160 mg once daily	$1.05/40 mg	$31.50	0	0	0	0	R	
Penbutolol	Levatol	20 mg once daily	20–80 mg once daily	$1.87/20 mg	$56.10	0	+	0	++	R > H	
Pindolol	Visken	5 mg twice daily	10–60 mg in 2 doses	$0.70/5 mg	$42.00	0	++	+	+	H > R	In adults, 35% renal clearance.
Propranolol	Inderal	20 mg twice daily	40–320 mg in 2 doses	$0.51/40 mg	$30.60	0	0	++	+++	H	Once-daily SR preparation also available. Also indicated for angina pectoris and post-MI.
Timolol	Blocadren	5 mg twice daily	10–40 mg in 2 doses	$0.38/10 mg	$22.80	0	0	0	++	H > R	Also indicated for post-MI. 80% hepatic clearance.

[1] Average wholesale price (AWP, for AB-rated generic when available) for quantity listed. Source: *Red Book Update*, Vol. 25, No. 1, January 2006. AWP may not accurately represent the actual pharmacy cost because wide contractual variations exist among institutions.

[2] Agents with β₁ selectivity are less likely to precipitate bronchospasm and decreased peripheral blood flow *in low doses*, but selectivity is only relative.

[3] Agents with ISA cause less resting bradycardia and lipid changes.

[4] MSA generally occurs at concentrations greater than those necessary for β-adrenergic blockade. The clinical importance of MSA by β-blockers has not been defined.

[5] Adverse effects of all β-blockers: bronchospasm, fatigue, sleep disturbance and nightmares, bradycardia and atrioventricular block, worsening of congestive heart failure, cold extremities, gastrointestinal disturbances, impotence, ↑triglycerides, ↓HDL cholesterol, rare blood dyscrasias.

ISA = intrinsic sympathomimetic activity; MSA = membrane-stabilizing activity; ANA = antinuclear antibody; LE = lupus erythematosus; MI = myocardial infarction; SR = sustained release; 0 = no effect; +, ++, +++ = some, moderate, most effect.

tral nervous system side effects—and route of metabolism. Labetalol and carvedilol are combined α- and β-blockers and, unlike most β-blockers, decrease peripheral vascular resistance.

The side effects of all β-blockers include inducing or exacerbating bronchospasm in predisposed patients (eg, those with asthma and some patients with chronic obstructive pulmonary disease [COPD]); sinus node dysfunction and atrioventricular (AV) conduction depression (resulting in bradycardia or AV block); precipitating or worsening clinically important left ventricular failure; nasal congestion; Raynaud's phenomenon; and central nervous system symptoms with nightmares, excitement, depression, and confusion. Fatigue, lethargy, and impotence may occur. All β-blockers tend to increase plasma triglycerides. The nonselective and, to a lesser extent, the cardioselective (β_1-selective) β-blockers tend to depress the protective HDL fraction of plasma cholesterol. As with diuretics, the changes are blunted with time and dietary changes.

β-Blockers have traditionally been considered contraindicated in patients with congestive heart failure. Evolving experience suggests that they have a propitious effect on the natural history of patients with chronic stable heart failure and reduced ejection fraction (see Chapter 10). β-Blockers are used cautiously in patients with type 1 diabetes, since they can mask the symptoms of hypoglycemia and prolong these episodes by inhibiting gluconeogenesis. Although they may increase blood glucose levels in type 2 diabetics, the prognosis of these patients on balance is improved. These drugs should also be used with caution in patients with advanced peripheral vascular disease associated with rest pain or nonhealing ulcers, but they are generally well tolerated in patients with mild claudication. In treatment of pheochromocytoma, β-blockers should not be administered until α-blockade has been established. Otherwise, blockade of vasodilatory β_2-adrenergic receptors will allow unopposed vasoconstrictor α-adrenergic receptor activation with worsening of hypertension.

Because of the lack of efficacy in prevention of myocardial infarction and inferiority compared with other drugs in prevention of stroke and left ventricular hypertrophy, there is now increasing doubt whether β-blockers should still be regarded as ideal first-line agents in the treatment of hypertension without specific compelling indications (such as active coronary artery disease). In addition to the adverse metabolic changes associated with their use, some experts have suggested that the therapeutic shortcomings of β-blockers are the consequence of the particular hemodynamic profile associated with these drugs. Pressure peaks in the aorta are augmented by reflection of pressure waves from the peripheral circulation. These reflected waves are delayed in patients taking ACE inhibitors and thiazide diuretics, resulting in decreased systolic and pulse pressures. By contrast, β-blockers have no effect on reflection of pressure waves, possibly because peripheral resistance vessels are a reflection

point and peripheral resistance is not decreased by β-blockers. This might explain why β-blockers are less effective at control of systolic and pulse pressure.

The ASCOT trial showed that the atenolol/bendroflumethiazide combination was inferior to the amlodipine/perindopril combination in predominantly white patients with modestly elevated cardiovascular risk. Subsequent analyses indicated that differences in blood pressure and HDL cholesterol accounted for the excess risk of stroke and coronary events respectively in the β-blocker group. Despite these concerns, the compelling indications for β-blockers remain, such as active coronary artery disease and impaired left ventricular function. Great care should be exercised if the decision is made, in the absence of compelling indications, to remove β-blockers from the treatment regimen since abrupt withdrawal can precipitate acute coronary events and severe increases in blood pressure.

C. ANGIOTENSIN-CONVERTING ENZYME INHIBITORS

ACE inhibitors are being increasingly used as the initial medication in mild to moderate hypertension (Table 11–8). Their primary mode of action is inhibition of the renin–angiotensin–aldosterone system, but they also inhibit bradykinin degradation, stimulate the synthesis of vasodilating prostaglandins and, sometimes, reduce sympathetic nervous system activity. These latter actions may explain why they exhibit some effect even in patients with low plasma renin activity. ACE inhibitors appear to be more effective in younger white patients. They are relatively less effective in blacks and older persons and in predominantly systolic hypertension. Although as single therapy they achieve adequate antihypertensive control in only about 40–50% of patients, the combination of an ACE inhibitor and a diuretic or calcium channel blocker is potent.

ACE inhibitors are the agents of choice in persons with type 1 diabetes with frank proteinuria or evidence of renal dysfunction because they delay the progression to end-stage renal disease. Many authorities have expanded this indication to include persons with type 2 diabetes and those who have type 1 diabetes with microalbuminuria, even when they do not meet the usual criteria for antihypertensive therapy. The Heart Outcomes Prevention Evaluation (HOPE) trial demonstrated that the ACE inhibitor ramipril reduces the number of cardiovascular deaths, nonfatal myocardial infarctions, and nonfatal strokes and also reduces the incidence of new-onset heart failure, renal dysfunction, and new-onset diabetes in a population of patients at high risk for vascular events. Although this was not specifically a hypertensive population, the benefits were associated with a modest reduction in blood pressure, and the results inferentially support the use of ACE inhibitors in similar hypertensive patients. ACE inhibitors may also delay the progression of other forms of renal disease. They are a drug of choice (usually in conjunction with a diuretic and a β-blocker) in patients with congestive heart failure and are indicated also in asymptomatic patients with reduced ejection fractions whether due to myocardial infarction or to other causes.

Table 11–8. Antihypertensive drugs: ACE inhibitors and angiotensin II receptor blockers.

Drug	Proprietary Name	Initial Dosage	Dosage Range	Cost per Unit	Cost of 30 Days Treatment (Average Dosage)[1]	Adverse Effects	Comments
ACE INHIBITORS							
Benazepril	Lotensin	10 mg once daily	5–40 mg in 1 or 2 doses	$1.05/20 mg	$31.50	Cough, hypotension, dizziness, renal dysfunction, hyperkalemia, angioedema; taste alteration and rash (may be more frequent with captopril); rarely, proteinuria, blood dyscrasia. Contraindicated in pregnancy.	More fosinopril is excreted by the liver in patients with renal dysfunction (dose reduction may or may not be necessary). Captopril and lisinopril are active without metabolism. Captopril, enalapril, lisinopril, and quinapril are approved for congestive heart failure.
Captopril	Capoten	25 mg twice daily	50–300 mg in 2 or 3 doses	$0.65/25 mg	$39.00		
Enalapril	Vasotec	5 mg once daily	5–40 mg in 1 or 2 doses	$1.52/20 mg	$45.60		
Fosinopril	Monopril	10 mg once daily	10–80 mg in 1 or 2 doses	$1.19/20 mg	$35.70		
Lisinopril	Prinivil, Zestril	5–10 mg once daily	5–40 mg once daily	$1.06/20 mg	$31.80		
Moexipril	Univasc	7.5 mg once daily	7.5–30 mg in 1 or 2 doses	$1.33/7.5 mg	$39.90		
Perindopril	Aceon	4 mg once daily	4–16 mg in 1 or 2 doses	$2.07/8 mg	$62.10		
Quinapril	Accupril	10 mg once daily	10–80 mg in 1 or 2 doses	$1.22/20 mg	$36.60		
Ramipril	Altace	2.5 mg once daily	2.5–20 mg in 1 or 2 doses	$1.67/5 mg	$50.10		
Trandolapril	Mavik	1 mg once daily	1–8 mg once daily	$1.20/4 mg	$36.00		
ANGIOTENSIN II RECEPTOR BLOCKERS							
Candesartan cilexitil	Atacand	16 mg once daily	8–32 mg once daily	$1.68/16 mg	$50.40	Hyperkalemia, renal dysfunction, rare angioedema. Combinations have additional side effects. Contraindicated in pregnancy.	Losartan has a very flat dose-response curve. Valsartan and irbesartan have wider dose-response ranges and longer durations of action. Addition of low-dose diuretic (separately or as combination pills) increases the response.
Candesartan cilexitil/ HCTZ	Atacand HCT	16 mg/ 12.5 mg once daily	8–32 mg of candesartan once daily	$2.27/16 mg/12.5 mg	$68.10		
Eprosartan	Teveten	600 mg once daily	400–800 mg in 1–2 doses	$1.51/ 600 mg	$45.30		
Eprosartan/ HCTZ	Teveten HCT	600 mg/ 12.5 mg once daily	600 mg/12.5 mg or 600 mg/25 mg once daily	$1.51/ 600 mg/ 12.5 mg	$45.30		
Irbesartan	Avapro	150 mg once daily	150–300 mg once daily	$1.69/ 150 mg	$50.70		
Irbesartan and hydrochlorothiazide	Avalide	150 mg/ 12.5 mg once daily	150–300 mg irbesartan daily	$2.09/ 150 mg	$62.70		
Losartan	Cozaar	50 mg once daily	25–100 mg in 1 or 2 doses	$1.77/50 mg	$53.10		

(continued)

Table 11–8. Antihypertensive drugs: ACE inhibitors and angiotensin II receptor blockers. (continued)

Drug	Proprietary Name	Initial Dosage	Dosage Range	Cost per Unit	Cost of 30 Days Treatment (Average Dosage)[1]	Adverse Effects	Comments
ANGIOTENSIN II RECEPTOR BLOCKERS (continued)							
Losartan and hydrochlorothiazide	Hyzaar	50 mg/ 12.5 mg once daily	One or 2 tablets once daily	$1.77/50 mg/12.5 mg/tablet	$53.10	Hyperkalemia, renal dysfunction, rare angioedema. Combinations have additional side effects. Contraindicated in pregnancy.	Losartan has a very flat dose-response curve. Valsartan and irbesartan have wider dose-response ranges and longer durations of action. Addition of low-dose diuretic (separately or as combination pills) increases the response.
Olmesartan	Benicar	20 mg once daily	20–40 mg daily	$1.68/20 mg	$50.40		
Olmesartan and HCTZ	Benicar HCT	20 mg/ 12.5 mg daily	20–40 mg olmesartan daily	$1.81/20 mg/12.5 mg	$54.30		
Telmisartan	Micardis	40 mg once daily	20–80 mg once daily	$1.84/40 mg	$55.20		
Telmisartan and HCTZ	Micardis HCT	40 mg/ 12.5 mg once daily	20–80 mg telmisartan daily	$1.97/40 mg/12.5 mg	$59.10		
Valsartan	Diovan	80 mg once daily	80–320 mg once daily	$2.04/ 160 mg	$61.20		
Valsartan and HCTZ	Diovan HCT	80 mg/ 12.5 mg once daily	80–320 mg valsartan daily	$2.22/ 160 mg/ 12.5 mg	$66.60		

[1]Average wholesale price (AWP, for AB-rated generic when available) for quantity listed. Source: *Red Book Update,* Vol. 25, No. 1, January 2006. AWP may not accurately represent the actual pharmacy cost because wide contractual variations exist among institutions. ACE = angiotensin-converting enzyme; HCTZ = hydrochlorothiazide.

ACE inhibitors have effects on mortality and most cardiovascular outcomes similar to those achieved with diuretics and β-blockers. However, compared with calcium channel blockers, ACE inhibitors are associated with lower incidences of coronary events and heart failure.

An advantage of the ACE inhibitors is their relative freedom from troublesome side effects. Severe hypotension can occur in patients with bilateral renal artery stenosis; acute renal failure may ensue but is usually reversible with discontinuation of ACE inhibition. Hyperkalemia may develop in patients with intrinsic renal disease and type IV renal tubular acidosis (commonly seen in diabetics) and in the elderly. A chronic dry cough is common, seen in 10% of patients or more, and may require stopping the drug. Dizziness occurs but may not be related to the degree of blood pressure lowering. Skin rashes are observed with any ACE inhibitor. Taste alterations are seen more often with captopril than with the non-sulfhydryl-containing agents (enalapril and lisinopril) but often disappear with continued therapy. Angioedema is an uncommon but potentially dangerous side effect of all agents of this class because of their inhibition of kininase.

D. ANGIOTENSIN II RECEPTOR BLOCKERS

Although losartan, the first member of this group, was less potent than high doses of ACE inhibitors in reducing blood pressure, the newer ARBs (valsartan, irbesartan, candesartan, telmisartan, and eprosartan) appear to be equipotent to ACE inhibitors (Table 11–8). A growing body of data indicates that ARBs can improve cardiovascular outcomes in patients with hypertension as well as in patients with related conditions such as heart failure and type 2 diabetes with nephropathy. ARBs have not been compared with ACE inhibitors in randomized controlled trials in patients with hypertension, but two trials comparing losartan with captopril in heart failure and post-myocardial infarction left ventricular dysfunction showed trends toward worse outcomes in the losartan group. Whether this suggestion of reduced efficacy is specific to losartan or may also be true for other ARBs is as yet unknown. However, the Losartan Intervention for Endpoints (LIFE) trial in nearly 9000 hypertensive patients with electrocardiographic evidence of left ventricular hypertrophy—comparing losartan with the β-blocker atenolol as initial therapy—demonstrated a significant reduction in stroke with losartan. Of note is that in diabetic patients, death and myocardial infarction were also reduced, and there was a lower occurrence of new-onset diabetes. In this trial, as in the Antihypertensive and Lipid-Lowering Treatment to Prevent Heart Attack Trial (ALLHAT) with an ACE inhibitor, blacks exhibited less blood pressure reduction and less benefit with regard to clinical end points.

Unlike ACE inhibitors, the ARBs do not cause cough and are only infrequently associated with skin rashes, the most common side effects of the ACE inhibitors. However, they still present a risk of hypotension and renal failure in patients with bilateral renal artery stenosis and hyperkalemia, and, rarely—but much less frequently than with ACE inhibitors—angioedema.

E. Calcium Channel Blocking Agents

These agents act by causing peripheral vasodilation but with less reflex tachycardia and fluid retention than other vasodilators. They are effective as single-drug therapy in approximately 60% of patients in all demographic groups and all grades of hypertension (Table 11–9). As a result, they may be preferable to β-blockers and ACE inhibitors in blacks and older subjects. Calcium channel blockers and diuretics are less additive when given together than when either is combined with β-blockers or ACE inhibitors. However, verapamil and diltiazem should be combined cautiously with β-blockers because of their potential for depressing AV conduction and sinus node automaticity as well as contractility.

Initial concerns about possible adverse cardiac effects of calcium channel blockers have been convincingly allayed by several subsequent large studies which have demonstrated that calcium channel blockers are equivalent to ACE inhibitors, thiazide diuretics, and β-blockers in prevention of coronary heart disease, major cardiovascular events, cardiovascular death, and total mortality. Diabetic patients receiving calcium channel blockers may have higher rates of heart failure and myocardial infarction than those receiving ACE inhibitors, and in other studies, heart failure has been more common than in patients treated with diuretics or ACE inhibitors. Whether these outcomes reflect beneficial effects of the comparators or specific risks of calcium channel blockers is uncertain. A protective effect against stroke with calcium blockers is well established, and in two trials (ALLHAT and the Systolic Hypertension in Europe trial), these agents appeared to be more effective than diuretic-based therapy.

The most common side effects of calcium channel blockers are headache, peripheral edema, bradycardia, and constipation (especially with verapamil in the elderly). The dihydropyridine agents—nifedipine, nicardipine, isradipine, felodipine, nisoldipine, and amlodipine—are more likely to produce symptoms of vasodilation, such as headache, flushing, palpitations,

and peripheral edema. Calcium channel blockers have negative inotropic effects and may cause or exacerbate heart failure in patients with cardiac dysfunction. Amlodipine is the only calcium channel blocker with established safety in patients with severe heart failure. Most calcium channel blockers are now available in preparations that can be administered once daily.

F. α-Adrenoceptor Antagonists

Prazosin, terazosin, and doxazosin (Table 11–10) block postsynaptic α-receptors, relax smooth muscle, and reduce blood pressure by lowering peripheral vascular resistance. These agents are effective as single-drug therapy in some individuals, but tachyphylaxis may appear during long-term therapy and side effects are relatively common. These include marked hypotension and syncope after the first dose which, therefore, should be small and be given at bedtime. Postdosing palpitations, headache, and nervousness may continue to occur during long-term therapy; they may be less frequent or severe with doxazosin because of its more gradual onset of action.

Unlike the β-blockers and diuretics, the α-blockers have no adverse effect on serum lipid levels—in fact, they increase HDL cholesterol while reducing total cholesterol. Whether this is beneficial in the long term has not been established. In ALLHAT, persons receiving doxazosin as initial therapy had a significant increase in heart failure hospitalizations and a higher incidence of stroke relative to the persons receiving diuretics and were removed from the study. To summarize, α-blockers should generally not be used as initial agents to treat hypertension—except perhaps in men with symptomatic prostatism.

G. Drugs with Central Sympatholytic Action

Methyldopa, clonidine, guanabenz, and guanfacine (Table 11–10) lower blood pressure by stimulating α-adrenergic receptors in the central nervous system, thus reducing efferent peripheral sympathetic outflow. These agents are effective as single therapy in some patients, but they are usually used as second- or third-line agents because of the high frequency of drug intolerance, including sedation, fatigue, dry mouth, postural hypotension, and impotence. An important concern is rebound hypertension following withdrawal. Methyldopa also causes hepatitis and hemolytic anemia and is avoided except in individuals who have already tolerated long-term therapy. There is considerable experience with methyldopa in pregnant women, and it is still used for this population. Clonidine is available in patches and may have particular value in patients in whom compliance is a troublesome issue.

H. Arteriolar Dilators

Hydralazine and minoxidil (Table 11–10) relax vascular smooth muscle and produce peripheral vasodilation. When given alone, they stimulate reflex tachycardia, increase myocardial contractility, and cause headache, pal-

Table 11–9. Antihypertensive drugs: calcium channel blocking agents.

Drug	Proprietary Name	Initial Dosage	Dosage Range	Cost of 30 Days Treatment (Average Dosage)[1]	Special Properties Peripheral Vasodilation	Special Properties Cardiac Automaticity and Conduction	Special Properties Contractility	Adverse Effects	Comments
NONDIHYDROPYRIDINE AGENTS									
Diltiazem	Cardizem SR	90 mg twice daily	180–360 mg in 2 doses	$69.60 (120 mg twice daily)	++	↓↓	↓↓	Edema, headache, bradycardia, GI disturbances, dizziness, AV block, congestive heart failure, urinary frequency.	Also approved for angina.
	Cardizem CD; Cartia XT	180 mg daily	180–360 mg daily	$61.50 (240 mg daily)					
	Dilacor XR	180 or 240 mg daily	180–480 mg daily	$34.50 (240 mg daily)					
	Tiazac SA	240 mg daily	180–540 mg daily	$53.27 (240 mg daily)					
Verapamil	Calan SR, Isoptin SR, Verelan	180 mg daily	180–480 mg in 1 or 2 doses	$46.80 (240 mg daily)	++	↓↓↓	↓↓↓	Same as diltiazem but more likely to cause constipation and congestive heart failure.	Also approved for angina and arrhythmias.
	Covera HS			$66.00 (240 mg daily)					
DIHYDROPYRIDINES									
Amlodipine	Norvasc	5 mg daily	5–20 mg daily	$68.55 (10 mg daily)	+++	↓/0	↓/0	Edema, dizziness, palpitations, flushing, headache, hypotension, tachycardia, GI disturbances, urinary frequency, worsening of congestive heart failure (may be less common with felodipine, amlodipine).	Amlodipine, nicardipine, and nifedipine also approved for angina.
Felodipine	Plendil	5 mg daily	5–20 mg daily	$75.00 (10 mg daily)	+++	↓/0	↓/0		
Isradipine	DynaCirc	2.5 mg twice daily	2.5–5 mg twice daily	$133.50 (5 mg twice daily)	+++	↓/0	→		
	DynaCirc CR	5 mg daily	5–10 mg daily	$95.40 (10 mg daily)					
Nicardipine	Cardene	20 mg three times daily	20–40 mg three times daily	$41.20 (20 mg three times daily)	+++	↓/0	→		
	Cardene SR	30 mg twice daily	30–60 mg twice daily	$62.66 (30 mg twice daily)					
Nifedipine	Adalat CC	30 mg daily	30–120 mg daily	$65.10 (60 mg daily)	+++	→	↓↓		
	Procardia XL	30 mg daily	30–120 mg daily	$68.70 (60 mg daily)					
Nisoldipine	Sular	20 mg/d	20–60 mg/d	$62.10 (40 mg daily)	+++	↓/0	→		

[1]Average wholesale price (AWP, for AB-rated generic when available) for quantity listed. Source: *Red Book Update*, Vol. 25, No. 1, January 2006. AWP may not accurately represent the actual pharmacy cost because wide contractual variations exist among institutions.

GI = gastrointestinal; AV = atrioventricular.

Table 11–10. α-Adrenoceptor blocking agents, sympatholytics, and vasodilators.

Drug	Proprietary Name	Initial Dosage	Dosage Range	Cost per Unit	Cost of 30 Days Treatment (Average Dosage)[1]	Adverse Effects	Comments
α-ADRENOCEPTOR BLOCKERS							
Prazosin	Minipress	1 mg hs	2–20 mg in 2 or 3 doses	$0.78/5 mg	$46.80 (5 mg twice daily)	Syncope with first dose; postural hypotension, dizziness, palpitations, headache, weakness, drowsiness, sexual dysfunction, anticholinergic effects, urinary incontinence; first-dose effects may be less with doxazosin.	May ↑ HDL and ↓ LDL cholesterol. May provide short-term relief of obstructive prostatic symptoms. Less effective in preventing cardiovascular events than diuretics.
Terazosin	Hytrin	1 mg hs	1–20 mg in 1 or 2 doses	$1.60/1, 2, 5, 10 mg	$48.00 (5 mg daily)		
Doxazosin	Cardura	1 mg hs	1–16 mg daily	$0.97/4 mg	$29.10 (4 mg daily)		
CENTRAL SYMPATHOLYTICS							
Clonidine	Catapres	0.1 mg twice daily	0.2–0.6 mg in 2 doses	$0.22/0.1 mg	$13.20 (0.1 mg twice daily)	Sedation, dry mouth, sexual dysfunction, headache, bradyarrhythmias; side effects may be less with guanfacine. Contact dermatitis with clonidine patch. Methyldopa also causes hepatitis, hemolytic anemia, fever.	"Rebound" hypertension may occur even after gradual withdrawal. Methyldopa should be avoided in favor of safer agents.
	Catapres TTS	0.1 mg/d patch weekly	0.1–0.3 mg/d patch weekly	$28.07/0.2 mg	$112.26 (0.2 mg weekly)		
Guanabenz	Wytensin	4 mg twice daily	8–64 mg in 2 doses	$0.98/4 mg	$58.80 (4 mg twice daily)		
Guanfacine	Tenex	1 mg once daily	1–3 mg daily	$0.87/1 mg	$26.10 (1 mg daily)		
Methyldopa	Aldomet	250 mg twice daily	500–2000 mg in 2 doses	$0.63/500 mg	$37.80 (500 mg twice daily)		
PERIPHERAL NEURONAL ANTAGONISTS							
Reserpine	Serpasil	0.05 mg once daily	0.05–0.25 mg daily	$0.32/0.1 mg	$9.60 (0.1 mg daily)	Depression (less likely at low dosages, ie, < 0.25 mg), night terrors, nasal stuffiness, drowsiness, peptic disease, gastrointestinal disturbances, bradycardia.	
DIRECT VASODILATORS							
Hydralazine	Apresoline	25 mg twice daily	50–300 mg in 2–4 doses	$0.51/25 mg	$30.60 (25 mg twice daily)	GI disturbances, tachycardia, headache, nasal congestion, rash, LE-like syndrome.	May worsen or precipitate angina.
Minoxidil	Loniten	5 mg once daily	5–40 mg qd	$1.29/10 mg	$38.70 (10 mg qd)	Tachycardia, fluid retention, headache, hirsutism, pericardial effusion, thrombocytopenia.	Should be used in combination with β-blocker and diuretic.

[1]Average wholesale price (AWP, for AB-rated generic when available) for quantity listed. Source: *Red Book Update*, Vol. 25, No. 1, January 20065. AWP may not accurately represent the actual pharmacy cost because wide contractual variations exist among institutions.

GI = gastrointestinal; LE = lupus erythematosus.

pitations, and fluid retention. They are usually given in combination with diuretics and β-blockers in resistant patients. Hydralazine produces frequent gastrointestinal disturbances and may induce a lupus-like syndrome. Minoxidil causes hirsutism and marked fluid retention; this agent is reserved for the most refractory of cases.

I. PERIPHERAL SYMPATHETIC INHIBITORS

These agents are now used infrequently and usually in refractory hypertension. Reserpine remains a cost-effective antihypertensive agent (Table 11–10). Its reputation for inducing mental depression and its other side effects—sedation, nasal stuffiness, sleep disturbances, and peptic ulcers—has made it unpopular, though these problems are uncommon at low dosages. Guanethidine and guanadrel inhibit catecholamine release from peripheral neurons but frequently cause orthostatic hypotension (especially in the morning or after exercise), diarrhea, and fluid retention.

Developing an Antihypertensive Regimen

Historically, data from a number of large trials support the overall conclusion that antihypertensive therapy with diuretics and β-blockers has a major beneficial effect on a broad spectrum of cardiovascular outcomes. Similar placebo-controlled data pertaining to the newer agents are generally lacking, except for stroke reduction with the calcium channel blocker nitrendipine in the Systolic Hypertension in Europe trial. However, there is substantial evidence that ACE inhibitors, and to a lesser extent ARBs, reduce adverse cardiovascular outcomes in other related populations (eg, patients with diabetic nephropathy, heart failure, or postmyocardial infarction and individuals at high risk for cardiovascular events). Most large clinical trials that have compared outcomes in relatively unselected patients have failed to show a difference between newer agents—such as ACE inhibitors, calcium channel blockers, and ARBs—and the older diuretics and β-blockers with regard to survival, myocardial infarction, and stroke. Therefore, experts recommend diuretics as the first-line treatment of most older patients with hypertension because these agents are less expensive than the newer agents. Exceptions are appropriate for individuals who have specific indications for another class of agent, such as postmyocardial infarction patients (β-blockers, ACE inhibitors), patients with diabetic nephropathy (ACE inhibitors, ARBs), or other comorbid conditions. Table 11–4 provides suggestions for individualizing first-line treatment based on compelling indications.

More recently, the perception that all antihypertensive drugs are equally effective at controlling cardiovascular risk has been challenged by the results of the ASCOT trial, which suggest that more modern agents (amlodipine/perindopril) are superior to the older combination (atenolol/bendroflumethiazide). For the reasons discussed above, many experts

would suggest that β-blockers no longer be considered ideal first-line drugs in the treatment of hypertension without compelling indications for their use and would tend to restrict the use of thiazide diuretics to older patients in whom they are particularly effective, The predominant use of thiazides in older patients would also limit exposure to the cumulative metabolic consequences of these drugs, a particular concern in young persons with hypertension who are subject to lifelong therapy.

For the purpose of devising an optimal treatment regimen, drugs can be divided into two complementary groups easily remembered as AB and CD. A and B refer to drugs that interrupt the renin-angiotensin system (**A**CE /ARB and β-**b**lockers) and C and D refer to those that do not (**c**alcium channel blockers and thiazide **di**uretics). Combinations of drugs between these groups are likely to be more potent in lowering blood pressure than combinations within a group. Drugs A/B are more effective in young, white persons, in whom renins tend to be higher, and drugs C/D are more effective in old or black persons, in whom renin levels are generally lower. It is also important to note that antihypertensive treatment is effective at reducing cardiovascular risk at all ages, including the very elderly.

Figure 11–3 illustrates guidelines established by the BHS for developing a rational antihypertensive regimen. In these guidelines, "B" is placed in parentheses. This reflects the increasingly prevalent view that β-blockers should no longer be considered an ideal first-line agent. In trials that include patients with systolic

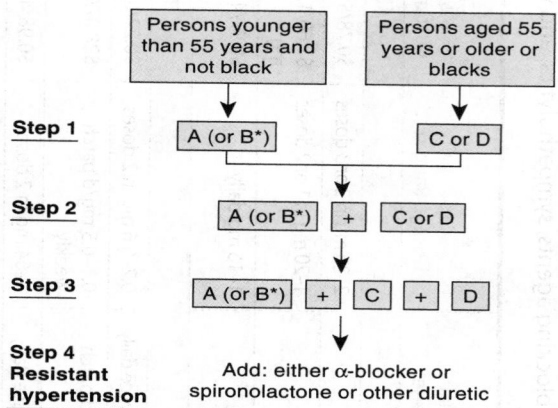

Figure 11–3. The British Hypertension Society's recommendations for combining blood pressure lowering drugs. The "ABCD" rule. A = Angiotensin-converting enzyme inhibitor or angiotensin receptor blocker; B = β-blocker (the parentheses indicate that β-blockers should no longer be considered ideal first-line agents); C = calcium channel blockers; D = diuretic (thiazide). (Reproduced with permission from: Guidelines for management of hypertension: report of the Fourth Working Party of the British Hypertension Society, 2004-BHS IV. J Hum Hypertens 2004;18:139–185.)

hypertension, most patients require two or more medications and even then a substantial proportion of patients does not achieve the goal systolic blood pressure of < 140 mm Hg (< 130 mm Hg in high-risk individuals). In diabetic patients, three or four drugs are usually required to reduce systolic blood pressure to < 140 mm Hg. In many patients, blood pressure cannot be maintained at the recommended goal of < 130 mm Hg with any combination. As a result, debating the appropriate first-line agent is less relevant than determining the most appropriate combinations of agents. This has led many experts and practitioners to reconsider the use of fixed-dose combination antihypertensive agents as first-line therapy in patients with substantially elevated systolic pressures (> 160 mm Hg) or difficult-to-control hypertension (associated diabetes or renal dysfunction). Based both on antihypertensive efficacy and complementarity, combinations of a diuretic and an ACE inhibitor (or an ARB if patient is intolerant of ACE inhibitor) or a diuretic and a β-blocker are recommended. In younger white patients, the best choice is probably a combination of an ACE inhibitor and a calcium channel blocker. The initial use of low-dose combinations allows faster blood pressure reduction without substantially higher intolerance rates and is likely to be better accepted by patients.

When an initial agent is selected, the patient should be informed of common side effects and the need for diligent compliance. Treatment should start at a low dose, and unless the initial blood pressure is very high (> 160/100 mm Hg), follow-up visits should usually be at 4- to 6-week intervals to allow for full medication effects to be established (especially with diuretics) before further titration or adjustment. If, after titration to usual doses, the patient has shown a discernible but incomplete response and a good tolerance of the initial drug, a second medication should be added.

Hypertension can be controlled in most patients with one-drug or two-drug regimens that combine complementary agents. A small number of patients require three, four, or even more medications in combination. Patients who are compliant with their medications and who do not respond to these combinations should usually be evaluated for secondary hypertension before proceeding to more complex regimens.

Special Considerations in the Treatment of Diabetic Hypertensive Patients

Hypertensive patients with diabetes are at particularly high risk for cardiovascular events. More aggressive treatment of hypertension in these patients prevents progressive nephropathy, myocardial infarction, and stroke. Treatment recommendations suggest a target of < 130/80 mm Hg. Because of their beneficial effects in diabetic nephropathy, ACE inhibitors (and ARBs in intolerant patients) should be part of the initial treatment regimen. However, most diabetics require combinations of three to five agents to achieve these goals, usually including a diuretic and a calcium channel blocker or β-blocker. In addition to rigorous blood pressure control, treatment of persons with diabetes should include aggressive treatment of other risk factors and early intervention for coronary disease and left ventricular dysfunction.

Treatment of Hypertension in Chronic Kidney Disease

Hypertension is present in 40% of patients with a glomerular filtration rate (GFR) of 60–90 mL/min, and 75% of patients with a GFR < 30 mL/min. Many factors play a role in the hypertension of renal failure, including volume; the renin-angiotensin system; renal artery disease; activation of the sympathetic nervous system; and increased arterial stiffness and changes in vasoactive mediators, such as prostaglandins, endothelin, and parathyroid hormone. ACE inhibitors and ARBs have been shown to delay progression of renal impairment in persons with type 1 and type 2 diabetes, respectively. It is also likely that inhibition of the renin-angiotensin system protects renal function in nondiabetic renal disease associated with significant proteinuria.

As discussed above, hypertension should be treated until blood pressure reaches < 130/80 mm Hg in patients with chronic kidney disease. There is a lack of definitive data to show that tighter blood pressure control slows the decline of GFR in persons with hypertensive chronic kidney disease without high-grade proteinuria. However, since all patients with chronic kidney disease are at high risk for cardiovascular damage, treatment of blood pressure to the < 130/80 mm Hg target is appropriate, and interruption of the renin-angiotensin system would seem a reasonable approach. Furthermore, it has recently been demonstrated that ACE inhibitors remain protective and safe in renal disease associated with significant proteinuria and creatinine as high as 5 mg/dL. It should be noted that such treatment would likely result in acute worsening of renal function in patients with significant renal artery stenosis, so renal function and electrolytes should be monitored carefully after introduction of ACE inhibitors.

Hypertension Management in Blacks

Substantial evidence indicates that blacks are not only more likely to become hypertensive and more susceptible to the cardiovascular complications of hypertension—they also respond differently to many antihypertensive medications. This may reflect genetic differences in the cause of hypertension or the subsequent responses to it, differences in occurrence of comorbid conditions such as diabetes or obesity, or environmental factors such as diet, activity, stress, or access to health care services. In any case, as in all persons with hypertension, a multifaceted program of education and lifestyle modification is warranted. Because it appears that ACE inhibitors and ARBs—in the absence of concomitant diuretics—are less effective in blacks than in whites, initial therapy should generally be a diuretic or a diuretic combination, with the use of additional agents as discussed above. Some experts have recommended a goal blood pressure of 130/80 mm Hg for blacks at high risk for cardiovascular events as well as those with diabetes.

Treatment of Additional Cardiovascular Risk Factors

Because the goal is to reduce cardiovascular morbidity and mortality, attention must be paid to the management of other risk factors. Elevated LDL cholesterol should be aggressively treated (see above), and patients should be urged to stop smoking, exercise regularly, and lose weight.

Follow-Up of the Treated Hypertensive Patient

Once blood pressure is controlled on a well-tolerated regimen, follow-up visits can be infrequent and laboratory testing limited to tests appropriate for the patient and the medications used. Yearly monitoring of blood lipids is recommended, and an electrocardiogram should be repeated at 2- to 4-year intervals depending on whether initial abnormalities are present, the presence of coronary risk factors, and age.

Patients who have had excellent blood pressure control for several years, especially if they have lost weight and initiated favorable lifestyle modifications, should be considered for "step-down" of therapy to determine whether lower doses or discontinuation of medications are feasible.

August P: Initial treatment of hypertension. N Engl J Med 2003;348:620. [PMID: 12584370]

Barzilay JI et al; ALLHAT Collaborative Research Group: Cardiovascular outcomes using doxazosin vs. chlorthalidone for the treatment of hypertension in older adults with and without glucose disorders: a report from the ALLHAT study. J Clin Hypertens (Greenwich) 2004;6:116. [PMID: 15010644]

Brewster LM et al: Systematic review: antihypertensive drug therapy in black patients. Ann Intern Med 2004;14:614. [PMID: 15492341]

Chobanian AV et al: The Seventh Report of the Joint National Committee on Prevention, Detection, Evaluation, and Treatment of High Blood Pressure: The JNC 7 Report. JAMA 2003;289:2560. [PMID: 12748199]

Dahlof B et al: Cardiovascular morbidity and mortality in the Losartan Intervention For Endpoint reduction in hypertension study (LIFE): a randomised trial against atenolol. Lancet 2002;359:995. [PMID: 11937178]

Dahlof B et al; ASCOT Investigators: Prevention of cardiovascular events with an antihypertensive regimen of amlodipine adding perindopril as required versus atenolol adding bendroflumethiazide as required, in the Anglo-Scandinavian Cardiac Outcomes Trial-Blood Pressure Lowering Arm (ASCOT-BPLA): a multicentre randomised controlled trial. Lancet 2005;366:895. [PMID: 16154016]

Iino Y et al; Japanese Losartan Therapy Intended for the Global Renal Protection in Hypertensive Patients (JLIGHT) Study Investigators: Renoprotective effect of losartan in comparison to amlodipine in patients with chronic kidney disease and hypertension. Hypertens Res 2004;27:21. [PMID: 15055252]

Julius S et al; VALUE trial group: Outcomes in hypertensive patients at high cardiovascular risk treated with regimens based on valsartan or amlodipine: the VALUE randomised trial. Lancet 2004;363:2022. [PMID: 15207952]

Khan NA et al; Canadian Hypertension Education Program: The 2004 Canadian recommendations for the management of hypertension: Part II—Therapy. Can J Cardiol 2004;20:41. [PMID: 14968142]

Kuschnir E et al: Effects of the combination of low-dose nifedipine GITS 20 mg and losartan 50 mg in patients with mild to moderate hypertension. J Cardiovasc Pharmacol 2004;43:300. [PMID: 14716221]

Lindholm LH et al: Should beta blockers remain first choice in the treatment of primary hypertension? A meta-analysis. Lancet 2005;366:1545. [PMID: 16257341]

London GM et al; REASON Project Investigators: Mechanism(s) of selective systolic blood pressure reduction after a low-dose combination of perindopril/indapamide in hypertensive subjects: comparison with atenolol. J Am Coll Cardiol 2004;43:92. [PMID: 14715189]

Major outcomes in high-risk hypertensive patients randomized to angiotensin-converting enzyme inhibitor or calcium channel blocker vs diuretic. The Antihypertensive and Lipid-Lowering Treatment to Prevent Heart Attack Trial (ALLHAT). JAMA 2002;288:2981. [PMID: 12479763]

Papademetriou V et al: Stroke prevention with the angiotensin II type 1-receptor blocker candesartan in elderly patients with isolated systolic hypertension: the Study on Cognition and Prognosis in the Elderly (SCOPE). J Am Coll Cardiol 2004;44:1175. [PMID: 15364316]

Psaty BM et al: Health outcomes associated with various antihypertensive therapies used as first-line agents: a network meta-analysis. JAMA 2003;289:2534. [PMID: 12759325]

Sehgal AR: Overlap between whites and blacks in response to antihypertensive drugs. Hypertension 2004;43:566. [PMID: 14757779]

Staessen JA et al; Treatment of Hypertension Based on Home or Office Blood Pressure (THOP) Trial Investigators: Antihypertensive treatment based on blood pressure measurement at home or in the physician's office: a randomized controlled trial. JAMA 2004;291:955. [PMID: 14982911]

Stergiou GS et al; World Health Organization-International Society of Hypertension (WHO-ISH); USA Joint National Committee on Prevention, Detection, Evaluation, and Treatment of High Blood Pressure (JNC-7); European Society of Hypertension-European Society of Cardiology (ESH-ESC): New European, American and International guidelines for hypertension management: agreement and disagreement. Expert Rev Cardiovasc Ther 2004;2:359. [PMID: 15151482]

Verberk WJ et al: Home versus Office blood pressure Measurements: Reduction of Unnecessary treatment Study: rationale and study design of the HOMERUS trial. Blood Press 2003;12:326. [PMID: 14763665]

Vijan S et al: Treatment of hypertension in type 2 diabetes mellitus: blood pressure goals, choice of agents, and setting priorities in diabetes care. Ann Intern Med 2003;138:593. [PMID: 12667032]

Wing LM et al: A comparison of outcomes with angiotensin-converting-enzyme inhibitors and diuretics for hypertension in the elderly. N Engl J Med 2003;348:583. [PMID: 12584366]

RESISTANT HYPERTENSION

Resistant hypertension is defined in JNC 7 as the failure to reach blood pressure control in patients who are adherent to full doses of an appropriate three-drug

Table 11–11. Causes of resistant hypertension.

Improper blood pressure measurement
Volume overload and pseudotolerance
    Excess sodium intake
    Volume retention from kidney disease
    Inadequate diuretic therapy
Drug-induced or other causes
    Nonadherence
    Inadequate doses
    Inappropriate combinations
    Nonsteroidal anti-inflammatory drugs; cyclooxygenase-
      2 inhibitors
    Cocaine, amphetamines, other illicit drugs
    Sympathomimetics (decongestants, anorectics)
    Oral contraceptives
    Adrenal steroids
    Cyclosporine and tacrolimus
    Erythropoietin
    Licorice (including some chewing tobacco)
    Selected over-the-counter dietary supplements and
      medicines (eg, ephedra, ma haung, bitter orange)
Associated conditions
    Obesity
    Excess alcohol intake
Identifiable causes of hypertension (see Table 11–3)

From Chobanian AV et al: The Seventh Report of the Joint National Committee on Prevention, Detection, Evaluation, and Treatment of High Blood Pressure: the JNC 7 report. JAMA 2003;289:2560.

regimen (including a diuretic). In this situation, the clinician should first exclude potential identifiable causes of hypertension (Table 11–3), and then carefully explore reasons why the patient might not be at goal blood pressure (Table 11–11). The clinician should pay particular attention to the type of diuretic being used in relation to the patient's renal function. If goal blood pressure cannot be achieved by these measures, consultation with a hypertension specialist should be considered.

HYPERTENSIVE URGENCIES & EMERGENCIES

Hypertensive emergencies have become less frequent in recent years but still require prompt recognition and aggressive but careful management. A spectrum of urgent presentations exists, and the appropriate therapeutic approach varies accordingly.

Hypertensive urgencies are situations in which blood pressure must be reduced within a few hours. These include patients with asymptomatic severe hypertension (systolic blood pressure > 220 mm Hg or diastolic pressure > 125 mm Hg that persists after a period of observation) and those with optic disk edema, progressive target organ complications, and severe perioperative hypertension. Elevated blood pressure levels alone—in the absence of symptoms or new or progressive target organ damage—rarely require

emergency therapy. Parenteral drug therapy is not usually required, and partial reduction of blood pressure with relief of symptoms is the goal.

Hypertensive emergencies require substantial reduction of blood pressure within 1 hour to avoid the risk of serious morbidity or death. Although blood pressure is usually strikingly elevated (diastolic pressure > 130 mm Hg), the correlation between pressure and end-organ damage is often poor. It is the latter that determines the seriousness of the emergency and the approach to treatment. Emergencies include hypertensive encephalopathy (headache, irritability, confusion, and altered mental status due to cerebrovascular spasm), hypertensive nephropathy (hematuria, proteinuria, and progressive renal dysfunction due to arteriolar necrosis and intimal hyperplasia of the interlobular arteries), intracranial hemorrhage, aortic dissection, preeclampsia-eclampsia, pulmonary edema, unstable angina, or myocardial infarction. **Malignant hypertension** is by historical definition characterized by encephalopathy or nephropathy with accompanying papilledema. Progressive renal failure usually ensues if treatment is not provided. The therapeutic approach is identical to that used with other antihypertensive emergencies.

Parenteral therapy is indicated in most hypertensive emergencies, especially if encephalopathy is present. The initial goal in hypertensive emergencies is to reduce the pressure by no more than 25% (within minutes to 1 or 2 hours) and then toward a level of 160/100 mm Hg within 2–6 hours. Excessive reductions in pressure may precipitate coronary, cerebral, or renal ischemia. To avoid such declines, the use of agents that have a predictable, dose-dependent, transient, and not precipitous antihypertensive effect is preferable. In that regard, the use of sublingual or oral fast-acting nifedipine preparations is best avoided.

Acute ischemic stroke is often associated with marked elevation of blood pressure, which will usually fall spontaneously. In such cases, antihypertensives should only be used if the blood pressure exceeds 220/120 mm Hg, and blood pressure should be reduced cautiously by 10–15%. If thrombolytics are to be given, blood pressure should be maintained at < 185/110 mm Hg during treatment and for 24 hours following treatment.

In hemorrhagic stroke, the aim is to minimize bleeding with a target mean arterial pressure of < 130 mm Hg. In acute subarachnoid hemorrhage, as long as the bleeding source remains uncorrected, a compromise must be struck between preventing further bleeding and maintaining cerebral perfusion in the face of cerebral vasospasm. In this situation, blood pressure goals depend on the patient's usual blood pressure. In normotensive patients, the target should be a systolic blood pressure of 110–120 mm Hg; in hypertensive patients, blood pressure should be treated to 20% below baseline pressure. In the treatment of hypertensive emergencies complicated by (or precipitated by) central nervous system injury, labetalol or nicardipine are good choices, since they are nonsedating and do not cause significant cerebral vasodilation, which can increase intracranial pressure (a potential problem with sodium nitroprusside). In hypertensive emergencies arising from catecholaminergic mechanisms, such as pheochromocytoma or cocaine use, β-blockers can worsen the hypertension because of unopposed peripheral vasoconstriction; phentolamine is a better choice. Labetalol is useful in these patients if the heart rate must be controlled.

Pharmacologic Management

A. Parenteral Agents

A growing number of agents are available for management of acute hypertensive problems. (Table 11–12 lists drugs, dosages, and adverse effects.) Sodium nitroprusside is the agent of choice for the most serious emergencies because of its rapid and easily controllable action, but continuous monitoring is essential when this agent is used. In the presence of myocardial ischemia, intravenous nitroglycerin or an intravenous β-blocker, such as labetalol or esmolol, is preferable.

1. Nitroprusside sodium—This agent is given by controlled intravenous infusion gradually titrated to the desired effect. It lowers the blood pressure within seconds by direct arteriolar and venous dilation. Monitoring with an intra-arterial line avoids hypotension. Nitroprusside—in combination with a β-blocker—is especially useful in patients with aortic dissection.

2. Nitroglycerin, intravenous—This agent is a less potent antihypertensive than nitroprusside and should be reserved for patients with accompanying acute ischemic syndromes.

3. Labetalol—This combined β- and α-blocking agent is the most potent adrenergic blocker for rapid blood pressure reduction. Other β-blockers are far less potent. Excessive blood pressure drops are unusual. Experience with this agent in hypertensive syndromes associated with pregnancy has been favorable.

4. Esmolol—This rapidly acting β-blocker is approved only for treatment of supraventricular tachycardia but is often used for lowering blood pressure. It is less potent than labetalol and should be reserved for patients in whom there is particular concern about serious adverse events related to β-blockers.

5. Nicardipine—Intravenous nicardipine is the most potent antihypertensive agent and the longest acting of the parenteral calcium channel blockers. As a primarily arterial vasodilator, it has the potential to precipitate reflex tachycardia, and for that reason it should not be used without a β-blocker in patients with coronary artery disease.

6. Fenoldopam—Fenoldopam is a peripheral dopamine-1 (DA$_1$) receptor agonist that causes a dose-dependent reduction in arterial pressure without evidence of tolerance, rebound, or withdrawal or deterioration of renal function. In higher dosage ranges, tachycardia may occur.

7. Enalaprilat—This is the active form of the oral ACE inhibitor enalapril. The onset of action is usually within 15 minutes, but the peak effect may be delayed for up to 6 hours. Thus, enalaprilat is used primarily as an adjunctive agent.

8. Diazoxide—Diazoxide acts promptly as a vasodilator without decreasing renal blood flow. To avoid hypotension, it should be given in small boluses or as an infusion rather than as the previously recommended large bolus. One use of diazoxide has been in pre-eclampsia-eclampsia. Hyperglycemia and sodium and water retention may occur. The drug should be used only for short periods and is best combined with a loop diuretic.

9. Hydralazine—Hydralazine can be given intravenously or intramuscularly, but its effect is less predictable than that of other drugs in this group. It produces reflex tachycardia and should not be given without β-blockers in patients with possible coronary disease or aortic dissection. Hydralazine is now used primarily in pregnancy and in children, but even in these situations, newer agents are supplanting it.

10. Trimethaphan—The ganglionic blocking agent trimethaphan is titrated with the patient sitting; its activity depends on this. The patient can be placed supine if the hypotensive effect is excessive. The effect occurs within a few minutes and persists for the duration of the infusion. This agent has largely been replaced by nitroprusside and newer medications.

11. Diuretics—Intravenous loop diuretics can be very helpful when the patient has signs of heart failure or fluid retention, but the onset of their hypotensive response is slow, making them an adjunct rather than a primary agent for hypertensive emergencies. Low dosages should be used initially (furosemide, 20 mg or bumetanide, 0.5 mg). They facilitate the response to vasodilators, which often stimulate fluid retention.

B. Oral Agents

Patients with less severe acute hypertensive syndromes can often be treated with oral therapy. Abrupt blood pressure lowering is not usually necessary in asymptomatic individuals, and the use of agents such as rapid-acting nifedipine probably causes more adverse effects than benefits.

1. Clonidine—Clonidine, 0.2 mg orally initially, followed by 0.1 mg every hour to a total of 0.8 mg, will usually lower blood pressure over a period of several hours. Sedation is frequent, and rebound hypertension may occur if the drug is stopped.

2. Captopril—Captopril, 12.5–25 mg orally, will also lower blood pressure in 15–30 minutes. The response is variable and may be excessive.

3. Nifedipine—Fast-acting nifedipine capsules are commonly used in the emergency department or urgent care setting because they usually provide a rapid reduction in blood pressure. However, the nifedipine

Table 11–12. Drugs for hypertensive emergencies and urgencies.

Agent	Action	Dosage	Onset	Duration	Adverse Effects	Comments
PARENTERAL AGENTS (INTRAVENOUSLY UNLESS NOTED)						
Nitroprusside (Nipride)	Vasodilator	0.25–10 mcg/kg/min	Seconds	3–5 minutes	GI, CNS; thiocyanate and cyanide toxicity, especially with renal and hepatic insufficiency; hypotension.	Most effective and easily titratable treatment. Use with β-blocker in aortic dissection.
Nitroglycerin	Vasodilator	0.25–5 mcg/kg/min	2–5 minutes	3–5 minutes	Headache, nausea, hypotension, bradycardia.	Tolerance may develop. Useful primarily with myocardial ischemia.
Labetalol (Normodyne, Trandate)	β- and α-Blocker	20–40 mg every 10 minutes to 300 mg; 2 mg/min infusion	5–10 minutes	3–6 hours	GI, hypotension, bronchospasm, bradycardia, heart block.	Avoid in congestive heart failure, asthma. May be continued orally.
Esmolol (Brevibloc)	β-Blocker	Loading dose 500 mcg/kg over 1 minute; maintenance, 25–200 mcg/kg/min	1–2 minutes	10–30 minutes	Bradycardia, nausea.	Avoid in congestive heart failure, asthma. Weak antihypertensive.
Fenoldopam (Corlopam)	Dopamine receptor agonist	0.1–1.6 mcg/kg/min	4–5 minutes	< 10 minutes	Reflex tachycardia, hypotension, ↑ intraocular pressure.	May protect renal function.
Nicardipine (Cardene)	Calcium channel blocker	5 mg/h; may increase by 1–2.5 mg/h every 15 minutes to 15 mg/h	1–5 minutes	3–6 hours	Hypotension, tachycardia, headache.	May precipitate myocardial ischemia.
Enalaprilat (Vasotec)	ACE inhibitor	1.25 mg every 6 hours	15 minutes	6 hours or more	Excessive hypotension.	Additive with diuretics; may be continued orally.
Furosemide (Lasix)	Diuretic	10–80 mg	15 minutes	4 hours	Hypokalemia, hypotension.	Adjunct to vasodilator.
Hydralazine (Apresoline)	Vasodilator	5–20 mg intravenously or intramuscularly (less desirable); may repeat after 20 minutes	10–30 minutes	2–6 hours	Tachycardia, headache, GI.	Avoid in coronary artery disease, dissection. Rarely used except in pregnancy.
Diazoxide (Hyperstat)	Vasodilator	50–150 mg repeated at intervals of 5–15 minutes, or 15–30 mg/min by intravenous infusion to a maximum of 600 mg	1–2 minutes	4–24 hours	Excessive hypotension, tachycardia, myocardial ischemia, headache, nausea, vomiting, hyperglycemia. Necrosis with extravasation.	Avoid in coronary artery disease and dissection. Use with β-blocker and diuretic. Mostly obsolete.
Trimethaphan (Arfonad)	Ganglionic blocker	0.5–5 mg/min	1–3 minutes	10 minutes	Hypotension, ileus, urinary retention, respiratory arrest. Liberates histamine; use caution in allergic individuals.	Useful in aortic dissection. Otherwise rarely used.

(continued)

Table 11–12. Drugs for hypertensive emergencies and urgencies. (continued)

Agent	Action	Dosage	Onset	Duration	Adverse Effects	Comments
			ORAL AGENTS			
Nifedipine (Adalat, Procardia)	Calcium channel blocker	10 mg initially; may be repeated after 30 minutes	15 minutes	2–6 hours	Excessive hypotension, tachycardia, headache, angina, myocardial infarction, stroke.	Response unpredictable.
Clonidine (Catapres)	Central sympatholytic	0.1–0.2 mg initially; then 0.1 mg every hour to 0.8 mg	30–60 minutes	6–8 hours	Sedation.	Rebound may occur.
Captopril (Capoten)	ACE inhibitor	12.5–25 mg	15–30 minutes	4–6 hours	Excessive hypotension.	

GI = gastrointestinal; CNS = central nervous system; ACE = angiotensin-converting enzyme.

458

effect is unpredictable and may be excessive, resulting in hypotension and reflex tachycardia. Because myocardial infarction and stroke have been reported in this setting, the use of nifedipine without concomitant β-blocker therapy is not advised.

C. SUBSEQUENT THERAPY

When the blood pressure has been brought under control, combinations of oral antihypertensive agents can be added as parenteral drugs are tapered off over a period of 2–3 days. Most subsequent regimens should include a diuretic.

Cherney D et al: Management of patients with hypertensive urgencies and emergencies. J Gen Intern Med 2002;17:947. [PMID: 12372930]

Devlin JW et al: Fenoldopam versus nitroprusside for the treatment of hypertensive emergency. Ann Pharmacother 2004; 38:755. [PMID: 15039472]

Khanna A et al: Malignant hypertension presenting as hemolysis, thrombocytopenia, and renal failure. Rev Cardiovasc Med 2003;4:255. [PMID: 14674379]

Migneco A et al: Hypertensive crises: diagnosis and management in the emergency room. Eur Rev Med Pharmacol Sci 2004; 8:143. [PMID: 15636400]

Phillips RA et al: Hypertensive emergencies: diagnosis and management. Prog Cardiovasc Dis 2002;45:33. [PMID: 12138413]

Blood Vessels & Lymphatics

12

Louis M. Messina, MD

Most arterial occlusive disease is produced by atherosclerosis. Atherosclerosis is a generalized response of the artery wall to injury. Atherosclerotic plaques are characterized by smooth muscle migration into the intima and subsequent proliferation and extracellular lipid deposition. Complex lesions are composed of a fibrous cap containing smooth muscle and inflammatory cells overlying a central core of lipid-rich necrotic debris. Clinical symptoms are produced by progressive stenosis, calcification, intraplaque hemorrhage, distal embolization, and luminal thrombosis after cap rupture. Atherosclerosis is a systemic disease, associated with some degree of involvement of all major arteries, but its most common clinical manifestations involve a limited number of arteries at areas of turbulent flow and low sheer stress: the carotid bifurcation, the infrarenal aorta and the iliac, superficial femoral, and tibial arteries, and the ostia of the renal and visceral arteries.

Most arterial aneurysms are classified as atherosclerotic or degenerative, because atheromas are found in the aneurysm wall and many patients have typical atherosclerotic risk factors. Both occlusive disease and aneurysms may be present in the same individual. However, the exact role of atherosclerosis in the causation of aneurysms is poorly defined. An imbalance of tissue metalloproteinases and metalloproteinase inhibitors is responsible for elastin and collagen degradation. Genetic predisposition, inflammation, and hemodynamic factors may also play a permissive role in aneurysm formation.

Atherosclerosis has been associated with increasing age, hypercholesterolemia, diabetes mellitus, smoking, a positive family history, hypertension, elevated levels of lipoprotein(a) and C-reactive protein, sedentary lifestyle, obesity, and homocystinuria. Control of risk factors by use of antihypertensive and lipid-lowering medications, regulation of blood sugar, tobacco cessation, and regular exercise remain the mainstays of treatment. Aspirin and clopidogrel (and potentially glycoprotein IIb/IIIa inhibitors) may prevent microemboli by impairing platelet aggregation; clopidogrel reduces the relative risk of stroke, myocardial infarction, and vascular death by 24% over aspirin alone in at-risk patients. Preliminary studies suggest that antioxidants, particularly dietary vitamin E, may also be beneficial in slowing the progression of disease.

Bhatt DL et al; REACH Registry Investigators: International prevalence, recognition, and treatment of cardiovascular risk factors in outpatients with atherothrombosis. JAMA 2006; 295:180. [PMID: 16403930]

Chapman MJ: Beyond the statins: new therapeutic perspectives in cardiovascular disease prevention. Cardiovasc Drugs Ther 2005;19:135. [PMID: 16025232]

■ ARTERIAL ANEURYSMS

ANEURYSMS OF THE ABDOMINAL AORTA

 ESSENTIALS OF DIAGNOSIS

- *Most aortic aneurysms are asymptomatic, detected during a routine physical examination or a diagnostic study.*
- *Severe back or abdominal pain, a pulsatile mass, and hypotension indicate rupture.*
- *Concomitant atherosclerotic occlusive disease of the lower extremities is present in 25% of patients.*

General Considerations

Over 90% of abdominal aneurysms originate below the renal arteries, and many extend into the common iliac arteries. The infrarenal aorta is normally 2 cm in diameter; an aneurysm is defined by an aortic diameter that exceeds 3 cm. An aortic aneurysm is present in 5–8% of men over the age of 65 years. The reported incidence has tripled over the past 30 years. Routine ultrasound screening of high-risk groups is associated with a 53% reduction in aneurysm-related deaths. Half of all newly detected aneurysms are under 5 cm in diameter, and nearly two-thirds of these will increase sufficiently in size to require repair. β-Blockers and, more recently, oral roxithromycin (300 mg daily for 30 days) have been shown to decrease the expansion rate of small aneurysms. Patients with chronic obstructive pulmonary disease appear more likely to rupture smaller aneurysms.

Clinical Findings

A. SYMPTOMS AND SIGNS

1. Asymptomatic aneurysms—An aneurysm may be suspected on routine physical examination by detection of a prominent aortic pulsation. More often, asymptomatic aneurysms are discovered as incidental findings on abdominal ultrasound or CT scan. Peripheral pulses are often normal, but coexisting renal or lower extremity arterial occlusive disease is present in 25% of patients. Popliteal artery aneurysms are present in 15% of patients with aneurysms of the abdominal aorta, and, conversely, more than one-third of patients with popliteal aneurysms have abdominal aortic aneurysms.

2. Symptomatic aneurysms—Midabdominal or lower back pain (or both) in the presence of a prominent aortic pulsation may indicate rapid aneurysmal growth, rupture, or an inflammatory aortic aneurysm. Inflammatory aneurysms account for fewer than 5% of aortic aneurysms and are characterized by extensive periaortic and retroperitoneal inflammation of unknown cause. These patients may have low-grade fever, elevated sedimentation rate, and a history of recent upper respiratory tract infection; they are often active smokers. Infected aortic aneurysms (either caused by septic emboli to a normal aorta or bacterial colonization of an existing aneurysm) are rare but should be suspected in patients with saccular aneurysms or aneurysms in conjunction with fever of unknown origin, particularly if blood cultures are positive for *Salmonella*. Peripheral emboli can also be a symptom of aneurysmal disease.

3. Ruptured aneurysms—Patients with ruptured aortic aneurysms present with severe back, abdominal, or flank pain and hypotension. Posterior rupture confined to the retroperitoneum carries a better prognosis than anterior rupture into the peritoneal cavity. As many as 90% of patients die either before they reach the hospital or in the immediate perioperative period. The only chance for survival is emergent surgical repair.

B. LABORATORY FINDINGS

ECG, serum creatinine, hematocrit and hemoglobin, and type and cross-match should be obtained routinely in all patients.

C. IMAGING

Abdominal ultrasonography is the screening study of choice and is valuable also for following aneurysm growth in patients with small (< 5 cm) aneurysms. Aneurysms typically grow by about 10% of their diameter per year; annual ultrasound examinations are recommended for aneurysms greater than 3.5 cm. In about 75% of patients, size can be estimated by measurement of curvilinear calcifications in the aneurysm wall on an abdominal radiograph, but this is much less accurate than ultrasonography.

Contrast-enhanced CT scanning not only precisely sizes the aneurysm but also defines its relationship to the renal arteries. MRI is as sensitive and specific as CT and is useful if renal insufficiency precludes contrast-enhanced CT. Aortography is indicated prior to elective aneurysm repair when arterial occlusive disease of the visceral or lower extremity arteries is suspected or when endograft repair is being considered.

Treatment

A. STANDARD THERAPY

Unless contraindicated, all patients should receive perioperative β-blockade to reduce cardiac complications. Surgical excision and synthetic graft replacement are the treatment of choice for most aneurysms of the infrarenal abdominal aorta that are greater than 5 cm. The maximum diameter of the aneurysm correlates best with the risk of rupture. Yearly rupture risk is 2% for 4- to 5.5-cm aneurysms, 7% for 6- to 6.9-cm aneurysms, and 25% for 7-cm aneurysms. Recommendation of an elective repair must be balanced with the risk of rupture. In asymptomatic good-risk patients, surgery is advised when the aneurysm exceeds 5 cm, whereas poor-risk patients may not be considered for repair until the aneurysm exceeds 6 cm. Urgent repair is indicated for symptomatic patients irrespective of aneurysm size.

Preoperative evaluation must include a detailed assessment of cardiac risk and examination of the carotid arteries since acute myocardial infarction, arrhythmia, and stroke remain the most frequent perioperative complications. In patients with asymptomatic aneurysms and a history of angina or of carotid stenosis greater than 80%, coronary angioplasty, coronary bypass grafting, or carotid endarterectomy may be indicated before repair of the aneurysm.

B. ENDOVASCULAR REPAIR

Endovascular stent grafts, or "covered stents," have evolved over the past decade for treatment of aortic aneurysms. Aortic stent grafts are configured to be uni-iliac or bifurcated depending on the particular anatomy of the aneurysm. Uni-iliac grafts are combined with endovascular occlusion of the contralateral common iliac artery and femoral–femoral bypass grafting. Both types of grafts are deployed via the common femoral arteries; in most cases, this involves bilateral inguinal incisions. The operation can be performed under epidural anesthesia, often in less than 2 hours and with minimal blood loss, which has made repair of aortic aneurysms feasible in high-risk patients previously deemed inoperable. Additional advantages include reduced incisional pain, fewer cardiopulmonary complications, and avoidance of postoperative ileus; most patients are discharged from the hospital on the second postoperative day. Endografts have been used successfully for repair of ruptured aneurysms, using balloon catheter control of the supraceliac aorta to facilitate intraoperative angiography and stent deployment.

Not all patients are candidates for standard endovascular repair. The proximal neck of the aneurysm must be adequate (at least 1.5 cm in length and less than 3 cm in width) to allow fixation and sufficient tissue apposition below the renal arteries. Iliac artery aneurysms, iliac stenoses, and iliac tortuosity or calcification all increase the complexity of stent deployment. The newest technology includes use of smaller introducer sheaths for percutaneous deployment. Long-term durability of endovascular grafts needs to be established before comparison can be made with open repair for use in the good-risk patient with asymptomatic aortic aneurysm. Objective comparison with open surgical repair has been complicated by the multiplicity of continually evolving stent graft designs.

Complications

Complications after aneurysm resection include myocardial infarction, bleeding, respiratory insufficiency, ischemic colitis, limb ischemia, renal insufficiency, and stroke. Bowel infarction, liver dysfunction, acalculous cholecystitis, and renal failure are more common with emergent aneurysm repair or when repair of the aneurysm requires supraceliac or suprarenal cross-clamping. However, renal insufficiency can occur even when the clamp is infrarenal and there is no reported intraoperative hypotension, presumably because of renal artery vasoconstriction, atheroemboli, preoperative contrast administration for CT scan, and dehydration from fasting or bowel preparation. For this reason, mannitol (25-g intravenous bolus) is given as a diuretic and free-radical scavenger prior to cross-clamping, and dopamine (3 mcg/kg/min) or fenoldopam (0.05–0.1 mcg/kg/min) is continued in the immediate postoperative period to increase renal perfusion and glomerular filtration rate. Rarely (0.1% of cases), lower extremity paralysis complicates repair of abdominal aortic aneurysm because of occlusion of the spinal artery from atheroemboli, shock, or aortic cross-clamping. Graft infection and graft-enteric fistulas are late complications, occurring more often after emergent aneurysm repair. One complication specific to endovascular repair is persistent filling of the aneurysm (endoleak). Endoleaks are classified as type 1 (leak around the top or bottom of the stent graft), type 2 (leak from a back-bleeding patent lumbar artery or inferior mesenteric artery), and type 3 (leak through the graft material). They are detected by contrast CT obtained routinely on postoperative day 30, and at 6-month or yearly intervals thereafter. Type 1 endoleaks are restented to allow adequate proximal or distal fixation. Type 2 endoleaks are not uncommon (20–30% of patients) in the immediate postoperative period but usually disappear by the 1-month CT scan.

Persistent type 2 endoleaks occur in 5% of patients and are correlated with the use of warfarin and the presence of a patent inferior mesenteric artery preoperatively. They can be eliminated by endovascular coil embolization of the feeding arteries.

Renal failure from contrast nephropathy, intraoperative atheroemboli, or graft impingement on the main or accessory renal arteries is another possible complication of endovascular repair. Conversion to open repair because of aortic or iliac rupture, inability to gain access, error in positioning, inadequate fixation, or stent malfunction is rare (1–3%) if patients are properly screened preoperatively.

Prognosis

Mortality following elective open or endovascular repair is 1–5%. In general, a patient with an aortic aneurysm greater than 5 cm has a threefold greater chance of dying as a consequence of rupture of the aneurysm than of dying from surgical resection. Five-year survival after surgical repair is 60–80%. Another aortic aneurysm will develop adjacent to the graft or in the thoracic aorta in 5–10% of patients.

Brewster DC et al: Guidelines for the treatment of abdominal aortic aneurysms. Report of a subcommittee of the Joint Council of the American Association for Vascular Surgery and Society for Vascular Surgery. J Vasc Surg 2003;37:1106. [PMID: 12756363]

Fleming C et al: Screening for abdominal aortic aneurysm: a best-evidence systematic review for the U.S. Preventive Services Task Force. Ann Intern Med 2005;142:203. [PMID: 15684209]

Gorham TJ et al: Endovascular treatment of abdominal aortic aneurysm. Br J Surg 2004;91:815. [PMID: 15227687]

Greenhalgh RM et al; EVAR trial participants: Comparison of endovascular aneurysm repair with open repair in patients with abdominal aortic aneurysm (EVAR trial 1), 30-day operative mortality results: randomised controlled trial. Lancet 2004;364:843. [PMID: 15351191]

Lederle FA et al: Rupture rate of large abdominal aortic aneurysms in patients refusing or unfit for elective repair. JAMA 2002;287:2968. [PMID: 12052126]

Prinssen M et al: Dutch Randomized Endovascular Aneurysm Management (DREAM) Trial Group: a randomized trial comparing conventional and endovascular repair of abdominal aortic aneurysms. N Engl J Med 2004;351:1607. [PMID: 15483279]

ANEURYSMS OF THE THORACIC AORTA

Aneurysms of the thoracic aorta account for fewer than 10% of aortic aneurysms. Medial degeneration, chronic dissection, vasculitis, and collagen-vascular disease (Marfan's syndrome or Ehlers–Danlos syndrome) are common causes; syphilis is now a rare cause of thoracic aneurysm. Traumatic aneurysms occur at the ligamentum arteriosus just beyond the left subclavian artery and result from shearing injury during rapid-deceleration automobile accidents.

Thoracoabdominal aneurysms are categorized by the Crawford classification: type I extends from the left subclavian artery to the renal arteries, type II from the left subclavian artery to the iliac bifurcation, type III from the midthoracic to the infrarenal region, and type IV from the distal thoracic aorta to the infrarenal region. The prevalence of each type of thoracoabdominal aneurysm is roughly equal, but type IV aneurysms have the lowest operative mortality (2–5%) and the lowest risk of postoperative neurologic deficits (2–10%).

Clinical Findings

A. SYMPTOMS AND SIGNS

Clinical manifestations depend largely on the size and position of the aneurysm and its rate of growth. Most are asymptomatic and are discovered during a diagnostic procedure undertaken for other reasons. Some patients complain of substernal, back, or abdominal pain. Others experience dyspnea, stridor, or a brassy cough from pressure on the trachea, dysphagia from pressure on the esophagus, hoarseness from pressure on the left recurrent laryngeal nerve, or neck and arm edema from external compression of the superior vena cava. Aortic regurgitation due to distortion of the aortic valve annulus may occur with aneurysms of the ascending aorta.

B. IMAGING

An aneurysm suspected on chest radiography must be differentiated from other anterior mediastinal masses, including lung neoplasm, thymoma, cyst, and substernal goiter. CT scan and MRI are the most sensitive and accurate means of imaging thoracic aneurysms. Aortography may be necessary to assess involvement of the arch vessels. The coronary vessels and the aortic valve should also be studied if aortic root replacement is anticipated.

Treatment

Control of hypertension and use of β-blockers may slow aneurysmal growth. Indications for surgical treatment include the presence of symptoms, rapid expansion, or size greater than 5 cm. Operative risk from comorbid medical conditions must be considered when recommending repair of asymptomatic aneurysms. Morbidity and mortality are higher than with abdominal aortic aneurysms; the 30-day operative mortality is 8–20% with repair of type I and type II thoracoabdominal aneurysms. The thoracotomy incision is associated with a higher risk of pulmonary complications and more challenging postoperative pain management. Proximity to the recurrent laryngeal nerve, the phrenic nerve, and the carotid and subclavian arteries makes injury to these structures possible. The great radicular artery (artery of Adamkiewicz) arises from an intercostal artery between T8 and L1 and is the dominant artery to the spinal cord in 80% of patients, imposing a 5–30% risk of paraplegia during thoracic aneurysm repair. Use of left heart bypass to femoral bypass to preserve retrograde perfusion below the level of the cross-clamp or antegrade perfusion by direct cannulation of selected arteries reduces end-organ ischemia. Lumbar drains have been proven to reduce the rate of paraplegia.

Endovascular repair of thoracic aortic aneurysms reduces cardiopulmonary risk, but the location of the aneurysm may preclude endovascular repair by current methods. Recent investigations involve development of branched stent grafts for repair of arch and thoracoabdominal aneurysms.

Prognosis

Five-year survival for patients with unrepaired thoracic aneurysms greater than 6 cm is 20–25%. Most deaths are due to rupture or to the complications of generalized atherosclerosis.

Hansen CJ et al: Complications of endovascular repair of high-risk and emergent descending thoracic aortic aneurysms and dissections. J Vasc Surg 2004;40:228. [PMID: 15297815]

Leurs LJ et al: EUROSTAR; UK Thoracic Endograft Registry collaborators: endovascular treatment of thoracic aortic diseases: combined experience from the EUROSTAR and United Kingdom Thoracic Endograft registries. J Vasc Surg 2004;40:670. [PMID: 15472593]

PERIPHERAL ARTERY ANEURYSMS (Popliteal & Femoral)

Most lower extremity aneurysms occur in men over age 50 years. Half are bilateral. One-third of patients with popliteal aneurysms and one-half of those with femoral aneurysms have an associated aortoiliac aneurysm.

Popliteal Aneurysms

Popliteal aneurysms account for approximately 85% of all peripheral artery aneurysms. Symptoms are rarely due to rupture but result rather from arterial thrombosis, peripheral embolization, or compression of adjacent structures with resultant venous thrombosis or neuropathy. Arterial thrombosis can be limb-threatening if all outflow vessels are occluded, leading to amputation in up to 30% of patients.

Ultrasound is the diagnostic study of choice to measure the diameter of the aneurysm as well as to search for other arterial aneurysms. Magnetic resonance angiography (MRA) or conventional arteriography is required to define the anatomy of the outflow arteries in preparation for operative repair.

Surgery is recommended for all asymptomatic aneurysms larger than 2 cm and for all symptomatic aneurysms regardless of size. If preoperative angiography reveals no patent distal vessels for bypass, catheter-directed thrombolysis can be attempted. If a patent outflow vessel is identified or is recanalized with thrombolytic therapy, a saphenous vein bypass graft with proximal and distal ligation of the aneurysm is performed. In large aneurysms producing popliteal vein or nerve compression, resection of the aneurysm in addition to grafting is required.

Femoral Aneurysms

Femoral aneurysms present as pulsatile groin masses. They have the potential for the same complications as popliteal aneurysms. Because the incidence of complications is lower than with popliteal aneurysms, patients with combined disease undergo repair of aortoiliac and popliteal aneurysms before repair of the femoral aneurysm.

Femoral pseudoaneurysms may result from injury produced by injection drug abuse, femoral artery puncture for angiography, or femoral line insertion. Mycotic aneurysms must be widely debrided with proximal and distal ligation or interposition grafting using an autologous vein. Uninfected, small (< 5 cm) traumatic pseudoaneurysms can often be treated by ultrasound-guided compression of the neck of the aneurysm or by thrombin injection, which has a reported success rate of 90%. If these techniques are not successful, open repair is required. Pseudoaneurysms may also develop at the distal anastomosis of an aortofemoral bypass graft. They should be repaired if graft infection is suspected or if their diameter exceeds 2 cm.

Antonello M et al: Open repair versus endovascular treatment for asymptomatic popliteal artery aneurysm: results of a prospective randomized study. J Vasc Surg 2005;42:185. [PMID: 16102611]

Aulivola B et al: Popliteal artery aneurysms: a comparison of outcomes in elective versus emergent repair. J Vasc Surg 2004; 39:1171. [PMID: 15192554]

Kruger K et al: Femoral pseudoaneurysms: management with percutaneous thrombin injections—success rates and effects on systemic coagulation. Radiology 2003;226:452. [PMID: 12563139]

Marty B et al: Success of thrombolysis as a predictor of outcome in acute thrombosis of popliteal aneurysms. J Vasc Surg 2002;35:487. [PMID: 11877696]

Pittathankal AA et al: Expansion rates of asymptomatic popliteal artery aneurysms. Eur J Vasc Endovasc Surg 2004;27:382. [PMID: 15015187]

VISCERAL ANEURYSMS

Mesenteric, Hepatic, & Splenic Artery Aneurysms

Historically, mesenteric aneurysms had a high mortality rate because of delay in diagnosis. High-resolution CT scanning has increased the ability to detect incidental mesenteric aneurysms and has broadened our understanding of the disease. In the last decade, hepatic artery aneurysms have become the most common of the visceral artery aneurysms, superseding splenic artery aneurysms, which now comprise less than 40% of the total. Superior mesenteric, celiac, gastric, and gastroepiploic artery aneurysms each represents about 5% of visceral aneurysms. Aneurysms of mesenteric branch vessels are rare and are often associated with connective tissue disease or vasculitis.

Medial degeneration is the most commonly cited cause of hepatic aneurysms. Increasingly, however, injury during cholangiography, hepatic biopsy, or blunt abdominal trauma is implicated—particularly in intrahepatic aneurysms, which account for about half of all hepatic aneurysms. Splenic artery aneurysms are most commonly related to medial fibroplasia, though portal hypertension, splenomegaly, pregnancy, and local inflammation (eg, pancreatitis) have all been implicated as possible risk factors. These aneurysms occur four times more frequently in women than in men, underscoring possible hormonal influences. Most superior mesenteric artery aneurysms are associated with infective endocarditis and suspected septic emboli. Atherosclerosis may play a role in the pathogenesis of celiac artery aneurysms—and a secondary role in development of other mesenteric aneurysms.

Surgical (aneurysmectomy or aneurysmorrhaphy with ligation of branches) or endovascular (embolization or stent graft repair) management is warranted for symptomatic aneurysms and aneurysms over 2 cm in diameter. Asymptomatic splenic aneurysms less than 2 cm in diameter rarely rupture, and treatment is not generally advised unless the patient is pregnant or anticipates becoming pregnant since the highest risk of rupture is in young women during pregnancy.

Abbas MA et al: Hepatic artery aneurysm: factors that predict complications. J Vasc Surg 2003;38:41. [PMID: 12844087]

Grego FG et al: Visceral artery aneurysms: a single center experience. Cardiovasc Surg 2003;11:19. [PMID: 12543567]

Morimoto N et al: Inferior mesenteric artery aneurysm in Behcet syndrome. J Vasc Surg 2003;38:1434. [PMID: 14681655]

Stambo GW et al: Coil embolization of multiple hepatic artery aneurysms in a patient with undiagnosed polyarteritis nodosa. J Vasc Surg 2004;39:1122. [PMID: 15111872]

Renal Artery Aneurysms

Renal artery aneurysms have a reported incidence of about 1% in the adult population. Many renal artery aneurysms are asymptomatic and diagnosed as an incidental finding on CT scan or angiography performed for another purpose. Others are found during evaluation for hematuria, renal infarct, flank pain, or suspected renovascular hypertension. Five percent of renal artery aneurysms present with rupture. Fibromuscular dysplasia is present in about 40% of patients; another 25% have atherosclerosis. Medial degeneration, trauma, and injury after renal biopsy or percutaneous nephrolithostomy are other potential causes. Indications for treatment include size greater than 2 cm, local symptoms, renovascular hypertension, distal embolization, growth on serial imaging, or aneurysms in women of childbearing age.

The standard surgical approach for renal artery aneurysms is excision with interposition grafting; infrequently, the aneurysm extends into the branch vessels, and ex vivo reconstruction may be required. Autologous and prosthetic materials have been equally effective for interposition grafting of main renal arteries greater than 5 mm in diameter, with a 5-year primary patency rate approaching 90%. Recently, polytetrafluoroethylene-covered stent grafts have been used for treatment of saccular aneurysms of the main renal artery. Interlobar aneurysms can be treated by endovascular embolization with microcoils.

English WP et al: Surgical management of renal artery aneurysms. J Vasc Surg 2004;40:53. [PMID: 15218462]

Pershad A et al: Renal artery aneurysm: successful exclusion with a stent graft. Catheter Cardiovasc Interv 2004;61:314. [PMID: 14988886]

AORTIC DISSECTION

ESSENTIALS OF DIAGNOSIS

- *A history of hypertension or Marfan's syndrome is often present.*
- *Sudden severe chest pain with radiation to the back, occasionally migrating to the abdomen and hips.*
- *Patient appears to be in shock, but blood pressure is normal or elevated; pulse discrepancy in many patients.*
- *Acute aortic regurgitation may develop.*

General Considerations

Aortic dissection is the most common aortic catastrophe requiring admission to a hospital. It is caused by an intimal tear, which allows creation of a false lumen between the media and adventitia. Over 95% of intimal tears occur either in the ascending aorta just distal to the aortic valve (Stanford type A) or just distal to the left subclavian artery (Stanford type B). These are points where the aorta is fixed and allow for intimal injury during shear stress. The false lumen can rupture into the pericardial sac, left pleural space, or retroperitoneum. More commonly, the dissection propagates distally to involve aortic branch vessels, producing acute spinal cord (3%), visceral (9%), renal (12%), or lower extremity (9%) ischemia. Proximal extension of a type A dissection can stretch the aortic annulus or occlude a coronary artery orifice, producing acute aortic regurgitation, myocardial infarction, and intrapericardial rupture with tamponade. Both blood pressure and the rate of acceleration of pulsatile flow (dP/dt) are important in propagation of dissection; 80% of patients with acute dissection are hypertensive. Other risk factors for dissection are Marfan's syndrome, pregnancy, bicuspid aortic valve, and coarctation of the aorta.

When not appropriately diagnosed and treated, type A aortic dissection is a lethal disease. Untreated type A dissections are associated with 50% mortality at 48 hours and 90% mortality at 1 month—due to free rupture, tamponade, or acute left ventricular failure. Mortality with untreated type B dissection is 10–20%, usually secondary to free rupture into the pleural space, acute mesenteric ischemia, or renal failure.

Clinical Findings

A. SYMPTOMS AND SIGNS

Eighty-five percent of patients report sudden excruciating ("ripping") pain in the chest or upper back. The pain may radiate into the abdomen, neck, or groin. Many patients are hypertensive at presentation. Some present with syncope, hemiplegia, or lower extremity paralysis. On physical examination, peripheral pulses and blood pressures may be diminished or unequal. A diastolic murmur of aortic insufficiency may be heard.

B. LABORATORY FINDINGS

The ECG may be normal but often reveals left ventricular hypertrophy from long-standing hypertension. Acute ischemic changes suggest coronary artery involvement. Because dissections preferentially extend into the right coronary ostium, inferior wall abnormalities predominate.

C. IMAGING

Chest radiographs often reveal—in comparison with previous films—an abnormal aortic contour or a widened superior mediastinum. Pleural or pericardial effusion may be present. Dynamic CT scanning, angiography, MRI, and transesophageal echocardiography (TEE) have all been used to diagnose acute dissection. TEE is favored because of its high sensitivity (98%) and specificity (99%) and because it can be performed rapidly and at the bedside. The best initial study is the one most readily available that can be interpreted accurately in a given hospital setting. MRI has not played a major role in the initial diagnosis but is useful for serial follow-up.

Differential Diagnosis

Acute myocardial infarction, pulmonary embolism, esophageal disruption, strangulated paraesophageal hernia, mesenteric ischemia, and symptomatic aortic aneurysm may all be considered in the differential diagnosis of acute aortic dissection.

Treatment

A. MEDICAL TREATMENT

Aggressive blood pressure control should be initiated immediately. Treatment is targeted to reduce aortic pressure and pulsatile flow (dP/dt). This is accomplished by lowering systemic vascular resistance and cardiac output (primarily heart rate).

Systemic vascular resistance is reduced by means of a rapid-acting antihypertensive agent titrated by intravenous infusion to maintain a systolic blood pressure of 100–120 mm Hg. Possible medications include ni-troprusside (0.3–10 mcg/kg/min), which causes direct vasodilation by its action on smooth muscle nitric oxide pathways, or fenoldopam (0.1–1.6 mcg/kg/min), which acts as an agonist of D_1-dopamine receptors. When nitroprusside is continued for 48 hours or more, thiocyanate levels should be checked and the infusion stopped if the level is over 10 mg/dL (to avoid toxicity).

The heart rate is decreased by administering the selective β_1-adrenergic antagonist esmolol (50–300 mcg/kg/min intravenously) and by intermittent administration of metoprolol (5–10 mg intravenously every 15 minutes) or the α_1- and nonselective β-antagonist labetalol (20–80 mg intravenously every 10 minutes or 1–2 mg/min).

Long-term drug therapy for aortic dissections involves use of a β-antagonist (eg, metoprolol, 25–100 mg orally twice daily; atenolol, 50–100 mg orally daily), often in combination with another antihypertensive agent such as the centrally acting α_2-agonist clonidine (0.1–0.3 mg orally twice daily or 0.1–0.3 mg transdermal patch topically every 24 hours) or the direct vasodilator hydralazine (10–50 mg orally four times daily); the calcium channel blocker amlodipine (2.5–10 mg orally daily); or the angiotensin-converting enzyme inhibitor enalapril (2.5–20 mg orally daily).

B. SURGICAL TREATMENT

All patients with type A dissection should undergo emergent surgical repair. Most patients with type B dissection can be managed initially with aggressive drug therapy. Indications for surgical treatment of type B dissections are aortic rupture; severe intractable pain; mesenteric, renal, or limb ischemia; and progression of the dissection. For type A dissection, the ascending aorta and, if necessary, the aortic valve and arch are replaced with reimplantation of the coronary and brachiocephalic vessels. The mortality rate for such operations approaches 20%. Type B dissection with ischemic complications is treated by obliteration of the false lumen and/or secondary arterial bypass if this fails to restore blood flow to the ischemic organs. Several different techniques have been described for obliteration of the false lumen: resection of the entry point of the dissection and prosthetic tube graft interposition, open or endovascular fenestration of the dissection flap, or stent graft deployment to cover the entry point. Use of felt strips or instillation of tissue glue into the false lumen during open repair can strengthen the dissected aortic wall.

Surgical indications and risks for chronic type B dissections are the same as for degenerative thoracoabdominal aneurysms. Repair is considered in symptomatic patients or patients with aneurysms larger than 5 cm. Reported surgical mortality is 5–30%. For this reason, long-term drug therapy may be the preferred treatment for patients with significant comorbidities.

Prognosis

Because of comorbid illnesses, operative mortality of patients with type B dissection is twice that of patients with type A dissection. After hospital discharge, 5-year survival is 70–80% for repaired type A and 50–70% for repaired type B dissections. In some medically treated type B dissections, the false lumen thromboses and eventually heals with minimal dilation. In others, a chronic dissection results in a progressively enlarging aneurysm requiring eventual repair in up to 30% of patients. For this reason, all unoperated patients should be monitored with annual CT scan or MRI.

Aziz S et al: Acute dissection of the thoracic aorta. Hosp Med 2004;65:136. [PMID: 15052903]

Clouse WD et al: Acute aortic dissection: population-based incidence compared with degenerative aortic aneurysm rupture. Mayo Clin Proc 2004;79:176. [PMID: 14959911]

Hansen CJ et al: Complications of endovascular repair of high-risk and emergent descending thoracic aortic aneurysms and dissections. J Vasc Surg 2004;40:228. [PMID: 15297815]

Knaut AL et al: Aortic emergencies. Emerg Med Clin North Am 2003;21:817. [PMID: 14708810]

Mehta RH et al: International Registry of Acute Aortic Dissection Investigators: acute type B aortic dissection in elderly patients: clinical features, outcomes, and simple risk stratification rule. Ann Thorac Surg 2004;77:1622. [PMID: 15111153]

Roseborough G et al: Twenty-year experience with acute distal thoracic aortic dissections. J Vasc Surg 2004;40:235. [PMID: 15297816]

Suzuki T et al: Clinical profiles and outcomes of acute type B aortic dissection in the current era: lessons from the International Registry of Aortic Dissection (IRAD). Circulation 2003;108(Suppl 1):II312. [PMID: 12970252]

Tan ME et al: Operative risk factors of type A aortic dissection: analysis of 252 consecutive patients. Cardiovasc Surg 2003; 11:277. [PMID: 12802263]

Yu HY et al: Late outcome of patients with aortic dissection: study of a national database. Eur J Cardiothorac Surg 2004; 25:683. [PMID: 15082267]

■ LOWER EXTREMITY OCCLUSIVE DISEASE

Occlusive disease of the lower extremities is present in 8–12 million persons in the United States and is an important cause of disability. It is also a predictor of all-cause mortality and an independent risk factor for cardiovascular morbidity and mortality; patients with intermittent claudication have a 2.5 times higher risk of cardiac events than that of an age-matched population. Severe triple-vessel coronary artery disease is found in almost 30% of patients undergoing routine coronary catheterization prior to peripheral bypass. Vascular endothelial dysfunction is a systemic phenomenon and a marker for atherosclerosis; impairment of flow-mediated dilation in the peripheral arteries has been shown to correlate with the presence of coronary artery disease. It is essential for the primary care clinician to emphasize prevention of disease, particularly in light of what is known about etiologic factors.

DeBakey first characterized the distribution of atherosclerotic disease in the lower extremity. Plaque formation predominates at the aortic bifurcation, at the tibial trifurcation, and in the superficial femoral artery at the adductor hiatus. Interestingly, occlusive disease often spares the internal iliac, profunda, and peroneal arteries. Three distinct patterns of disease have since been described. Type 1 disease affects about 10–15% of patients and is limited to the aorta and common iliac arteries. It is most commonly found in younger men and women (ages 40–55 years) who are heavy smokers or who have hyperlipidemia. Type 2 disease (25% of patients) involves the aorta, the common iliac artery, and the external iliac artery. Type 3 disease is the most common (60–70% of patients) and is multilevel disease, affecting the aorta and the iliac, femoral, popliteal, and tibial arteries. Patients with type 2 and type 3 patterns of disease have typical risk factors for atherosclerosis: older age, male gender, diabetes, and hypertension. They also have a high incidence of coexisting cerebrovascular and coronary artery disease.

Clinical Findings

A. SYMPTOMS AND SIGNS

Lower extremity occlusive disease is manifested by several different clinical presentations: erectile dysfunction, claudication, rest pain, and gangrene. The symptoms and physical examination predict the location and severity of disease. Occlusive disease of the iliac arteries can produce male erectile dysfunction. The triad of bilateral hip and buttock claudication, erectile dysfunction, and absent femoral pulses is known as Leriche's syndrome.

Claudication is characterized by fatigue, pain, or weakness in the calves, thighs, or buttocks brought on by walking and completely relieved after a few minutes of rest. The reproducibility of these symptoms helps differentiate claudication from other causes of leg pain such as radiculopathy and musculoskeletal disorders. Ischemic rest pain, defined as pain in the absence of exertion, is usually described as a nocturnal pain located across the dorsum of the foot at the metatarsal heads. It can be reduced by placing the legs in the dependent position, usually by hanging them over the side of the bed. Rest pain, ischemic ulceration, or gangrene implies impending limb loss.

Examination of the pulses indicates the level of disease. Absent or weak femoral pulses or the presence of an iliac or femoral bruit suggests inflow disease. Similarly, normal femoral pulses but a diminished or absent popliteal pulse is indicative of superficial femoral artery stenosis and normal femoral and popliteal pulses and nonpalpable dorsalis pedis or posterior tib-

ial pulse indicate tibial disease. An ankle–brachial index (ABI) is useful in gauging the degree of arterial insufficiency. A normal ratio of ankle to brachial systolic blood pressures is 1.0; less than 0.8 is consistent with claudication. Exercise, which lowers the ABI by exaggerating the difference in brachial and ankle blood pressures, can sometimes aid in detection of occlusive disease. Rest pain and nonhealing ulcers are common with an ABI less than 0.4. A toe–brachial index (TBI) can be used in diabetic or renal failure patients when an ABI cannot be obtained because the tibial arteries are calcified and noncompressible. A penile–brachial index (PBI) is obtained when vasogenic impotence is suspected. A PBI less than 0.6 suggests significant arterial disease. These measurements can also be used to monitor progression of disease and to assess the effect of therapeutic intervention.

Other findings on physical examination include atrophy of the skin, subcutaneous tissues, and muscles of the calf. Dependent rubor, hair loss, and coolness of the skin are signs of advanced ischemia. Ulcers from arterial occlusive disease are painful, well-circumscribed lesions generally located over pressure points, such as the first metatarsal head or heel. Ulcers that have failed to heal with 3 months of appropriate local wound care and ulcers associated with an ABI less than 0.3 are unlikely to heal without treatment to improve arterial blood flow and tissue perfusion.

B. IMAGING

Catheter or MRA demonstrates the extent of the disease and the condition of the distal target vessels for potential bypass operation. The standard study images the infrarenal aorta and iliacs (including oblique views of the pelvis and groin to visualize the origins of the hypogastric and profunda arteries), the runoff vessels, and the foot in a lateral position. Angiography is undertaken only for percutaneous treatment or in preparation for surgical intervention. Gadolinium-enhanced MRA is used in the evaluation of lower extremity occlusive disease, particularly in patients with renal insufficiency. Ultrasound is also used in routine followup of infrainguinal bypass grafts to screen for graft stenoses amenable to prophylactic angioplasty or segmental replacement. Radiographs of the lower leg and foot are often obtained to rule out osteomyelitis underlying an infected ulcer or to identify severe calcification of potential runoff vessels.

Treatment

A. CONSERVATIVE MEASURES

Treatment of claudication begins with identification and control of risk factors and initiation of an exercise program. Tobacco cessation slows the rate of progression of arterial occlusive disease and reduces cardiovascular mortality. Lipid-lowering medications have been shown to produce a 40% risk reduction for new-onset claudication or worsening of claudication. A supervised, dedicated walking program sustained over 3–6 months has been shown to increase pain-free walking distance by as much as 150%. Exercise improves symptoms by increasing muscle anaerobic metabolism and shifting the energy of walking to muscles with higher oxygen delivery. A standard program is structured as four 30-minute sessions per week: walking along flat ground until discomfort occurs, resting until it subsides, and then resuming walking.

The main drug used in therapy is the phosphodiesterase inhibitor, cilostazol (100 mg orally twice daily), which impairs platelet aggregation, increases calcium-mediated vasodilation, and has been shown to increase walking distance by 34% more than placebo. It is contraindicated in patients with heart failure and is not well tolerated in about 20% of patients due to side effects of headache, dizziness, and diarrhea. Propionyl-L-carnitine (1000 mg orally twice daily) has also been correlated with increased walking distance in patients with claudication. Its mechanism of action is unknown; it may improve skeletal muscle metabolism. *Ginkgo biloba* extract (120 mg/d) is an herbal medication with some reported benefit in claudication (see Chapter 42). It has been correlated with an increased risk of bleeding and so should be used with caution in patients on warfarin or clopidogrel. Aspirin (325 mg orally daily) is routinely prescribed for all patients who do not have drug allergy or intolerance. It is continued indefinitely after angioplasty or surgery to decrease thrombotic complications and impede progression of intimal hyperplasia. Clopidogrel (75 mg orally daily) or warfarin (dosed to maintain an INR of 2.0–3.0) may be selected for postoperative patients perceived to have a higher risk of graft thrombosis due to a hypercoagulable state, suboptimal conduit, or poor distal runoff.

Treatment of male erectile dysfunction requires evaluation of its possible causes (medications, diabetes mellitus, psychogenic factors, and arterial occlusive disease). Iliac or dorsal penile artery revascularization can be beneficial in some cases of vasculogenic impotence. Other patients may respond to sildenafil, 25–50 mg 30 minutes to 4 hours prior to sexual activity. It is contraindicated in patients taking nitroglycerin because of the risk of myocardial ischemia due to hypotension (see Chapter 23).

B. SURGERY

Percutaneous or open operation is considered for good-risk patients with short-distance (less than two blocks) claudication that impairs their ability to work or perform activities of daily living. Development of rest pain or tissue loss indicates progression of disease and also warrants evaluation for limb revascularization.

Because many of these patients have coexisting ischemic heart disease, medical management should be optimized preoperatively. The roles of exercise testing and coronary angiography are discussed in Chapters 3 and 10. The carotid arteries should be imaged by ul-

trasound; endarterectomy may be indicated to minimize perioperative risk of stroke.

1. Endovascular techniques—Common iliac artery stenoses are often amenable to percutaneous treatment. Stent angioplasty has been shown to decrease recurrence rates seen with angioplasty alone; most recent studies report a 70–80% 3-year patency rate with self-expanding (Wall) stents or balloon-expandable (Palmaz) stents. Stenting of distal lesions (external iliac or infrainguinal arteries) is not as successful, with reported 3-year primary patency rates of 55–60%. Stents do not appear to confer added benefits over angioplasty alone for femoral–popliteal lesions except in cases of postangioplasty arterial dissection or successfully recanalized short-segment arterial occlusion. Ideal lesions for angioplasty are discrete, short-segment (< 5 cm in length), concentric lesions in noncalcified large-diameter vessels. Often, endovascular techniques are used in conjunction with surgery for treatment of multifocal lower extremity occlusive disease such as an iliac stent being placed at the time of an ipsilateral femoral popliteal bypass. Some surgeons are evaluating long-segment closed superficial femoral artery endarterectomy combined with distal stenting as an alternative to femoral popliteal bypass in high-risk surgical patients with suboptimal vein available for bypass conduit. Few groups have achieved favorable results with percutaneous atherectomy devices or laser probes.

2. Open surgery—Aortobifemoral bypass grafting using a synthetic prosthesis is the standard treatment for complex aortoiliac occlusive disease. In general, a bifurcated polytetrafluoroethylene or Dacron graft is anastomosed end to end with the infrarenal abdominal aorta and end to side to each common femoral artery. If both external iliac arteries are occluded, an end-to-side aortic anastomosis preserves inflow into the internal iliac arteries. For high-risk patients, an axillary–femoral or femoral–femoral bypass graft can be considered, though such extra-anatomic grafts have lower long-term patency than bypass grafting (50% versus 80% at 10 years).

For infrainguinal occlusive disease, the bypass conduit of choice is the autogenous greater saphenous vein. Five-year patency rates of 75–80% can be achieved with vein bypasses to the dorsalis pedis artery or the posterior tibial artery at the ankle. By contrast, the 5-year patency of femoral–tibial bypasses performed with synthetic conduit is less than 40%. Some surgeons prefer prosthetic graft for femoral-to-above-knee-popliteal artery bypasses, as the reported long-term patency in this position is almost equivalent to that of vein graft. Others maintain an "all autogenous" policy for all infrainguinal bypass grafts. In as many as 30% of patients, the greater saphenous vein is inadequate because it is sclerotic, thrombosed, or less than 3 mm in diameter or because the patient has undergone varicose vein stripping or saphenous vein harvesting for coronary artery bypass or previous leg bypass. Alternative conduits in these patients include the lesser saphenous vein, arm vein, cryopreserved homologous vein, or prosthetic graft with a distal vein cuff.

Other determinants of long-term graft patency include quality of arterial inflow, patency of runoff arteries, and length of the bypass conduit. It is imperative to address any flow-limiting aortoiliac disease before performing any infrainguinal bypass.

Thromboendarterectomy involves resecting the thickened intima and media from the diseased artery and is an alternative to bypass for short-segment lesions in larger arteries. It can be used in type 1 disease to obviate the need for prosthetic graft. Common femoral or profunda femoral thromboendarterectomy is combined with distal bypass to improve inflow.

Operative mortality is 2–5% for open aortic surgery and 1–3% for infrainguinal bypass, largely attributable to cardiac complications. Risks specific to aortic surgery include renal insufficiency, bowel ischemia, impotence or retrograde ejaculation, and blue toe syndrome secondary to distal emboli. Late complications include graft thrombosis, graft infection, and aortoduodenal fistula. Complications of percutaneous techniques include problems at the puncture site (hematoma, pseudoaneurysm, arteriovenous fistula, retroperitoneal hemorrhage, occlusion), dissection or rupture of the artery during angioplasty, distal emboli from catheter manipulation, and contrast nephropathy. Patients with chronic renal insufficiency (serum creatinine > 1.5 mg/dL) undergoing angiography may be pretreated with intravenous hydration and acetylcysteine, 400 mg orally twice daily for 48 hours before and after contrast administration.

Prognosis

Ischemic rest pain or ulceration will eventually develop in 25% of patients with claudication; approximately 10% will require amputation. In part, the high rate of limb salvage reflects a high mortality rate from comorbid disease. Because of coronary artery disease, patients with claudication have a 5-year survival of 50%. For this reason, surgery is generally deferred until failure of drug therapy and exercise programs and impairment of activities of daily living.

The overall 5-year patency rate for infrainguinal saphenous vein grafts is 60–80%. Higher graft patency and limb salvage rates are achieved with suprageniculate bypasses and with patients presenting with claudication rather than rest pain or gangrene. Graft occlusion may convert a patient with claudication to one with limb-threatening ischemia because of loss of collateral flow. Conversely, a patient who undergoes bypass for distal gangrene may have a clinically silent graft occlusion after the ulcer heals. Surveillance duplex ultrasound is advised at 6-month intervals to detect stenotic, or "threatened," grafts before they progress.

Bachoo P et al: Endovascular stents for intermittent claudication. Cochrane Database Syst Rev 2003;(1):CD003228. [PMID: 12535463]

Gey DC et al: Management of peripheral arterial disease. Am Fam Physician 2004;69:525. Erratum in Am Fam Physician 2004;69:1863. [PMID: 14971833]

McDermott MM et al: Functional decline in peripheral arterial disease: associations with the ankle brachial index and leg symptoms. JAMA 2004;292:453. [PMID: 15280343]

Peripheral Arterial Diseases Antiplatelet Consensus Group: Antiplatelet therapy in peripheral arterial disease. Consensus statement. Eur J Vasc Endovasc Surg 2003;26:1. [PMID: 12819642]

Raines JK et al: Ankle/brachial index in the primary care setting. Vasc Endovasc Surg 2004;38:131. [PMID: 15064843]

Tran H et al: Oral antiplatelet therapy in cerebrovascular disease, coronary artery disease, and peripheral arterial disease. JAMA 2004;292:1867. [PMID: 15494585]

UNUSUAL CAUSES OF POPLITEAL ARTERY OCCLUSION

The most common cause of popliteal artery occlusion is athero-occlusive disease. Thrombosis of a popliteal aneurysm can also cause popliteal occlusion and acute leg ischemia. Claudication in a young, athletic individual with no risk factors for atherosclerosis and normal pedal pulses may suggest popliteal entrapment syndrome, popliteal adventitial cystic disease, trauma, or extrinsic compression by a Baker cyst.

Popliteal entrapment syndrome is a group of anatomic anomalies that leads to popliteal arterial compression. Type 1 (20% of patients) is produced by an abnormal course of the popliteal artery, passing medial to the medial head of the gastrocnemius muscle. Type 2 (25%) is caused by medial insertion of the medial head of the gastrocnemius muscle. The popliteal artery is compressed by an abnormal accessory slip of gastrocnemius muscle in type 3 (30%) or popliteus muscle in type 4 (8%). Almost 30% of patients have bilateral disease. Claudication symptoms may be atypical, such as pain with walking but not with running. Diagnosis is made by MRA or by positional angiography; the patent artery becomes impinged with passive dorsiflexion or active plantar flexion of the ankle. Treatment is surgical and involves transection of the abnormal muscle; if the artery is injured or occluded, short-segment bypass with the greater saphenous vein is required.

Popliteal adventitial disease is a rare disorder of unknown cause characterized by formation of cysts within the wall of the popliteal artery. The cysts compress the arterial lumen, causing stenosis or occlusion. Their contents resemble synovial fluid, and some may be in continuity with the joint space. The disease most often affects healthy men 40–50 years of age. Larger cysts are amenable to ultrasound-guided aspiration, but most are small and appear only as a thickening of the popliteal artery wall on MRA. In these cases, bypass or interposition grafting is curative.

Elias DA et al: Clinical evaluation and MR imaging features of popliteal artery entrapment and cystic adventitial disease. AJR Am J Roentgenol 2003;180:627. [PMID: 12591664]

OCCLUSIVE CEREBROVASCULAR DISEASE

Every year, half a million people in the United States suffer a stroke. Fifteen to 30 percent of these episodes are fatal, making stroke the third leading cause of death in this country. Carotid artery stenosis is responsible for as many as 25% of these strokes in the elderly. Most neurologic events are caused by emboli occluding small cerebral arteries. Emboli from the carotid bifurcation may consist of platelet aggregates that form on irregular or ulcerated surfaces or plaque debris liberated by turbulent flow and intraplaque hemorrhage. Less commonly (less than 10% of cases), emboli arise from the heart (eg, mural thrombus or atrial myxoma) or from the aortic arch. Stroke can also be caused by intracerebral hemorrhage (from trauma or a ruptured cerebral aneurysm) or by small vessel occlusive disease in the pons, basal ganglia, and internal capsule of the brain (lacunar infarcts).

A transient ischemic attack (TIA) is defined as the sudden onset of a neurologic deficit that resolves completely within 24 hours. A stroke is a neurologic deficit that persists beyond 24 hours. A single TIA or stroke is associated with a 30% risk of subsequent stroke.

Risk factors for carotid disease include hypertension, diabetes mellitus, hypercholesterolemia, advanced age, smoking, and coronary artery disease.

Clinical Findings

A. Symptoms and Signs

Clinical manifestations of carotid artery occlusive disease include contralateral weakness or sensory loss, expressive aphasia, and amaurosis fugax (transient partial or complete loss of vision in the ipsilateral eye). Vertebrobasilar TIAs are characterized by brainstem and cerebellar symptoms, including dysarthria, diplopia, vertigo, ataxia, and hemiparesis or quadriparesis.

Dizziness and unsteadiness, particularly when associated with a quick change in position, are nonspecific symptoms and more often the result of postural hypotension than of vertebrobasilar insufficiency. Syncope is rarely a manifestation of carotid artery occlusive disease. Rather, it is usually a result of a cardiac arrhythmia.

Occlusive disease of the brachiocephalic arteries may be accompanied by cervical bruits, diminished or absent pulses in the neck or arms, Hollenhorst plaques (bright, refractile cholesterol emboli) in the retinal arteries, or a blood pressure difference between the two arms of more than 10 mm Hg. The common carotid pulsation can be examined qualitatively by palpation at the base of the neck. The presence of superficial temporal artery pulsation confirms patency of the ipsilateral external carotid artery. A carotid bruit is a high-pitched, blowing noise localized in the mid neck close to the angle of the mandible. Heart sounds must be auscultated to make certain that the bruit is not caused by a referred murmur of aortic stenosis. Only 30% of patients with cervical bruits have carotid stenosis greater than 60%. The absence of a bruit also does not preclude the possibility of a hemodynamically significant lesion—thus, bruits are neither sensitive nor specific for carotid occlusive disease. In fact, asymptomatic carotid bruits are stronger predictors of death from coronary artery disease than of death from stroke.

B. Imaging Studies

Duplex ultrasonography has become the study of choice for evaluation of carotid occlusive disease. It provides both physiologic and anatomic information. Percent stenosis is derived from measurement of blood flow velocities, with sensitivity and specificity greater than 90%. Ultrasound also provides some characterization of the plaque itself, including its location and the presence of calcification, ulceration, and intraplaque hemorrhage. Patients with adequate ultrasound studies may be offered surgery without further imaging. Patients with suboptimal ultrasound studies or in whom intracranial tandem lesions may be suspected are referred for gadolinium-enhanced MRA, which provides more detailed information about plaque composition and characterizes the intracranial circulation and the brain parenchyma. When compared with en bloc resected specimens, correlation of percent stenosis is better with ultrasound and MRA than with conventional angiography. This can be explained by the fact that MRA and ultrasound both produce cross-sectional imaging of vessels whose stenotic regions may be eccentric. Symptomatic patients with ipsilateral carotid occlusion by ultrasound should be referred for conventional or CT angiography before electing nonoperative management because a small percentage of these patients will have an internal carotid artery "string sign" and should be revascularized. Catheter angiography carries a 1% risk of procedure-related stroke and is reserved for patients with greatly disparate ultrasound and MRA findings, those suspected of vertebrobasilar insufficiency or intracranial lesions unable to undergo MRA, and those potentially requiring endovascular intervention. As ultrasound is highly operator dependent, whereas MRA is highly equipment dependent, selection of the most accurate imaging modality may vary by institution.

Treatment

A. Medical Measures

Acute or evolving strokes and strokes associated with major neurologic deficits are initially managed medically, delaying surgery for 5–8 weeks until the deficit is stable, as discussed in the section on cerebrovascular accidents in Chapter 24. Patients with TIAs may be treated initially with an oral antiplatelet medication (aspirin, 81 mg daily, or clopidogrel, 75 mg daily) to reduce the likelihood of thrombosis and microemboli and then scheduled for elective surgery. However, if the attacks are of increasing frequency, the patient is admitted, and intravenous heparin is started while the patient is evaluated for surgery. Postoperatively, most patients are maintained on aspirin indefinitely to reduce the incidence of thrombosis or recurrent disease in the newly endarterectomized vessel.

For patients in whom neurologic symptoms are thought to be secondary to intracerebral disease not amenable to surgical reconstruction, warfarin or clopidogrel may be indicated.

B. SURGERY

1. TIAs and stroke—Carotid endarterectomy plus optimal drug therapy and risk factor modification are highly effective in preventing stroke and death in symptomatic patients with carotid stenosis greater than 70%—as demonstrated by the North American Symptomatic Carotid Endarterectomy Trial (NASCET). A more modest risk-benefit ratio has been demonstrated for carotid endarterectomy in symptomatic 50–69% stenoses. Surgical success is maximized when preoperative symptoms are related to ischemia of the ipsilateral hemisphere and when the surgery is done by a vascular surgeon who performs carotid endarterectomies regularly with a mortality-complication rate less than 5%. Placement of a temporary carotid shunt during surgery may be necessary to allow cerebral perfusion during cross-clamping. Indications for intraoperative shunting vary by surgeon. Most surgeons shunt patients with previous stroke; some selectively shunt for a measured stump pressure (internal carotid back pressure) under 50 mm Hg or for patients with electroencephalogram (EEG) changes, and others shunt all patients.

2. Asymptomatic carotid stenosis—Patients with asymptomatic carotid stenosis greater than 80% have a 12% risk of stroke. This statistic helps form the basis for the American Heart Association's recommendation of upper limits of acceptable combined morbidity and mortality for carotid endarterectomy: 3% for asymptomatic patients, 5–7% for those with TIAs or stroke, and 10% for those with recurrent carotid stenosis. The Asymptomatic Carotid Artery Stenosis (ACAS) trial demonstrated that in good-risk asymptomatic patients with greater than 60% stenosis, surgery afforded an overall relative risk reduction of 53% over aspirin alone. These findings are supported by a smaller Veterans Administration Hospital study of patients with asymptomatic carotid artery stenosis. Most vascular surgeons offer surgery to good-risk asymptomatic patients with greater than 80% stenosis in the ipsilateral carotid artery.

3. Percutaneous techniques—Patients who are not good candidates for surgery because of medical comorbidities can be considered for carotid angioplasty and stenting. This is also an option in patients with a history of previous neck surgery or irradiation, in whom there is a higher risk of cranial nerve injury because of fibrosis and scarring. Carotid stenting is associated with a 2–18% risk of periprocedural stroke or TIA and an 8–14% per year incidence of recurrent stenosis (compared with less than 4% per year with surgery). Recent trials suggest that complications after carotid stenting may be similar to those after open endarterectomy.

Prognosis

Carotid endarterectomy carries a reported average 1–2% mortality rate and a 1–5% risk of neurologic complication, though institutional variation exists. In symptomatic patients, endarterectomy reduces stroke risk fivefold to tenfold at 5 years. The 5–15% incidence of late stroke after uncomplicated endarterectomy is often related to contralateral carotid or intracranial disease.

Restenosis occurring less than 2 years after carotid endarterectomy is usually not symptomatic because it is due to intimal hyperplasia, which produces a smooth, nonfriable luminal surface. These lesions respond well to angioplasty and stenting, and the risk of procedural neurologic events is lower than for atherosclerotic lesions. Such lesions may regress and intervention is reserved for stenoses of 80% or greater. After 2 years, restenosis is more often related to progression of atherosclerotic disease. These lesions can be friable and prone to intraplaque hemorrhage, just like the original plaque. In general, repeat surgery or stenting is advised for symptomatic restenoses or stenoses greater than 80%.

Albers GW et al: Antithrombotic and thrombolytic therapy for ischemic stroke: the Seventh ACCP Conference on Antithrombotic and Thrombolytic Therapy. Chest 2004;126(3 Suppl):483S. [PMID: 15383482]

Collins R et al: Heart Protection Study Collaborative Group: effects of cholesterol-lowering with simvastatin on stroke and other major vascular events in 20536 people with cerebrovascular disease or other high-risk conditions. Lancet 2004;363:757. [PMID: 15016485]

Coward LJ et al: Percutaneous transluminal angioplasty and stenting for carotid artery stenosis. Cochrane Database Syst Rev 2004;(2):CD000515. [PMID: 15106153]

Halliday A et al: MRC Asymptomatic Carotid Surgery Trial (ACST) Collaborative Group: prevention of disabling and fatal strokes by successful carotid endarterectomy in patients without recent neurological symptoms: randomised controlled trial. Lancet 2004;363:1491. Erratum in Lancet 2004;364:416. [PMID: 15135594]

Mas JL et al: EVA-3S Investigators: carotid angioplasty and stenting with and without cerebral protection: clinical alert from the Endarterectomy Versus Angioplasty in Patients With Symptomatic Severe Carotid Stenosis (EVA-3S) trial. Stroke 2004;35:e18. [PMID: 14657456]

Meyers PM et al: Use of stents to treat extracranial cerebrovascular disease. Ann Rev Med 2006;57:437. [PMID: 16409159]

Rothwell PM et al: Carotid Endarterectomy Trialists Collaboration: endarterectomy for symptomatic carotid stenosis in relation to clinical subgroups and timing of surgery. Lancet 2004;363:915. [PMID: 15043958]

Yadav JS et al: Stenting and Angioplasty with Protection in Patients at High Risk for Endarterectomy Investigators: protected carotid-artery stenting versus endarterectomy in high-risk patients. N Engl J Med 2004;351:1493. [PMID: 15470212]

OTHER DISEASES OF THE CAROTID ARTERY

Carotid Dissection

Carotid dissection is a false channel in the wall of the carotid artery produced by a tear in the intima. The classic triad of symptoms is unilateral neck pain or headache, stroke or TIA, and an incomplete Horner syndrome (miosis and ptosis without anhidrosis). Dissections can be spontaneous or traumatic, caused by shearing of the internal carotid artery between the C2 and C3 transverse processes during deceleration injuries such as car accidents, wrestling, or chiropractic maneuvers. The primary treatment of dissection is drug therapy. With warfarin anticoagulation (to an INR of 2.0–3.0), 60–85% of carotid dissections will heal in 3–6 months with complete or near-complete neurologic recovery. Recurrent dissection is estimated at 3% at 3 years and 12% at 10 years and most often involves a different cervical vessel, which justifies the use of long-term aspirin. Surgery (usually carotid interposition) or carotid stenting is indicated for persistent symptoms despite optimal drug therapy.

Carotid Body Tumors

The carotid body is a chemoreceptor derived from embryonic neural crest cells located at the carotid bifurcation. Carotid body tumors (also called paragangliomas or chemodectomas) are rare and usually present as painless neck masses. Most of these tumors are slow growing and benign, but lymph node metastases have been reported. If untreated, they are locally invasive; a large tumor may cause vagus or hypoglossal nerve deficit from mass effect or may encircle the internal carotid artery to the skull base. The tumor is hypervascular and splays the internal and external carotid arteries, giving it a classic angiographic appearance of a tumor blush in the center of a widened carotid bifurcation. Biopsy is contraindicated; diagnosis is made by CT angiography or MRA. Preoperative angiography for tumor embolization and test occlusion of the internal carotid artery may be considered for tumors over 4 cm in diameter. Using the same approach as for carotid endarterectomy, the tumor is resected from the carotid artery, with care to preserve the artery wall adventitia. Many small arteries arising from the external and internal carotid arteries supply the tumor and must be ligated individually. The incidence of cranial nerve injury with resection of large tumors approaches 40%. Prognosis after complete resection is excellent, with survival equal to that of age-matched controls and long-term recurrence of 6%.

Carotid Artery Aneurysms

Carotid aneurysms are much more common in the intracerebral than in the cervical portion of the carotid arteries. Most often, cervical aneurysms arise in the common carotid artery and are fusiform; these are associated with atherosclerosis. Traumatic aneurysms can be related to healing of an internal carotid dissection or to penetrating trauma. Mycotic aneurysms can be caused by staphylococcal, *Escherichia coli*, or tuberculous infections. Many other vasculitides are associated with carotid aneurysms, such as Behçet's disease, Takayasu's disease, fibromuscular dysplasia, and segmental arterial mediolysis. Anytime a mass in the neck is pulsatile, an aneurysm should be considered and diagnosis confirmed by angiography. Other symptoms include neck pain, cranial nerve dysfunction, and TIA or stroke. Surgery should be considered for aneurysms resulting from penetrating trauma, aneurysms associated with neurologic deficit, mycotic aneurysms, and aneurysms over 2 cm in diameter. Primary repair of the artery may be accomplished for most penetrating injuries. Carotid resection and interposition grafting are performed for most other aneurysms.

Assadian A et al: Long-term results of covered stent repair of internal carotid artery dissections. J Vasc Surg 2004;40:484. [PMID: 15337877]

Bergeron P et al: Long-term results of endovascular exclusion of extracranial internal carotid artery aneurysms and dissecting aneurysm. J Interv Cardiol 2004;17:245. [PMID: 15318896]

Luna-Ortiz K et al: Carotid body tumors: review of a 20-year experience. Oral Oncol 2005;41:56. [PMID: 15598586]

Thanvi B et al: Carotid and vertebral artery dissection syndromes. Postgrad Med J 2005;81:383. [PMID: 15937204]

VISCERAL ARTERY INSUFFICIENCY

Chronic intestinal ischemia results from atherosclerotic occlusive lesions at the origins of the superior mesenteric artery (SMA), celiac artery, and inferior mesenteric artery (IMA). Because of collateral flow via the middle colic artery branch of the SMA and the ascending colic artery of the IMA, the superior and inferior pancreaticoduodenal arteries, and the superior and inferior hemorrhoidal arteries, bowel ischemia does not occur until two of the three main visceral arteries are diseased severely. In fact, almost 30% of patients with peripheral vascular disease have asymptomatic occlusive disease of the mesenteric arteries. Symptoms consist of postprandial epigastric pain, and at later stages, food avoidance (sitophobia), resulting in weight loss. Chronic intestinal ischemia is a diagnosis of exclusion, derived after a negative workup for peptic ulcer disease, gastroesophageal reflux, pancreatitis, irritable bowel syndrome, and malignancy. A suggestive history in a person over 45 years of age who appears chronically ill, has risk factors for arterial occlusive disease, and has no other identifiable cause for abdominal symptoms is an indication for arteriography. Intravenous hydration must be provided to avoid acute bowel ischemia from catheter-induced or contrast-associated arterial spasm. Surgical or endovascular management is directed toward restoration of antegrade visceral arterial flow. Transaortic endarterectomy and mesenteric artery bypass are associated with a 5–9% mortality rate and a 10–25% recurrence rate at long-term follow-up. A higher recurrence rate is observed with stenting of short-segment lesions; these patients require routine angiographic follow-up. Survivors have an unexpectedly good long-term life expectancy.

Celiac axis compression syndrome (stenosis of the celiac artery caused by external compression of the arcuate ligament) has been described as a variant of chronic mesenteric ischemia. As an isolated entity, it is occasionally associated with cramping abdominal pain, nausea, vomiting, and diarrhea. Division of the arcuate ligament may be combined with celiac artery dilation. The pathophysiological basis for this disease remains elusive.

Acute intestinal ischemia may result from (1) embolic occlusion of a visceral branch of the abdominal aorta, generally in patients with mitral valvular disease, atrial fibrillation, or left ventricular mural thrombus; (2) thrombosis of an atherosclerotic mesenteric vessel; (3) low-flow or shock state due to cardiac failure or arterial spasm induced by ergot or cocaine intoxication; or (4) postcoarctectomy syndrome, producing nonocclusive mesenteric vascular insufficiency. Emboli are responsible for almost half of all cases. Symptoms include sudden onset of severe epigastric and periumbilical abdominal pain with minimal appreciable findings on abdominal examination ("pain out of proportion to physical findings") and a high leukocyte count. Lactic acidosis, hypotension, and abdominal distention indicate bowel infarction. Mortality approaches 80% despite aggressive surgical management.

Visceral angiography can be performed in the stable patient; duplex ultrasound is of less diagnostic value in this setting. Mesenteric thrombosis causes occlusion at the origin of the vessel, while emboli most often lodge within the superior mesenteric artery usually at the first jejunal branch. In hypoperfusion-related mesenteric ischemia, the vessels are pruned but patent. Angiography also allows delivery of catheter-directed therapy: thrombolytics (alteplase, 0.5–1 mg/h) for thrombotic disease or vasodilators (papaverine, 30–60 mg/h) for nonocclusive disease. Broad-spectrum antibiotics are administered to all patients. Embolic disease, acidosis, hemodynamic instability, or severe or progressive abdominal pain mandate emergent laparotomy. Mesenteric flow is first reestablished with thromboembolectomy or bypass, and the bowel resection margins are then determined by gross inspection or examination with fluorescein. A second-look operation is planned if any bowel is of questionable viability at the close of the case.

Mesenteric vein occlusion is responsible for 5–15% of cases of acute mesenteric ischemia. Risk factors include hypercoagulable state (malignancy; protein C, protein S, or antithrombin III deficiency; presence of anticardiolipin or antiphospholipid antibody; polycythemia vera), intra-abdominal sepsis, previous splenectomy or portal angiography or sclerotherapy, portal hypertension, and cirrhosis. Diagnosis is made by contrast-enhanced abdominal CT scan or arterial portography. Patients should be treated with long-term anticoagulation. Surgery is reserved for those suspected of having bowel infarction and consists of

bowel resection and occasionally venous thrombectomy. In some cases, percutaneous transhepatic administration of thrombolytics has been successful.

Ischemic colitis can develop as a result of acute or chronic colonic ischemia and is characterized by bouts of crampy lower abdominal pain and mild—often bloody—diarrhea. This picture may be indistinguishable from inflammatory bowel disease. Colonoscopy reveals segmental inflammatory changes, most prominent in the watershed areas of the rectosigmoid junction and splenic flexure. Conservative management is usually adequate. Surgery may be indicated for progressive symptoms or stricture formation.

Angelelli G et al: Acute bowel ischemia: CT findings. Eur J Radiol 2004;50:37. [PMID: 15093234]

Baixauli J et al: Investigation and management of ischemic colitis. Cleve Clin J Med 2003;70:920. [PMID: 14650467]

Brown DJ et al: Mesenteric stenting for chronic mesenteric ischemia. J Vasc Surg 2005;42:268. [PMID: 16102625]

Burns BJ et al: Intestinal ischemia. Gastroenterol Clin North Am 2003;32:1127. [PMID: 14696300]

Edwards MS et al: Acute occlusive mesenteric ischemia: surgical management and outcomes. Ann Vasc Surg 2003;17:72. [PMID: 12522695]

Oldenburg WA et al: Acute mesenteric ischemia: a clinical review. Arch Intern Med 2004;164:1054. [PMID: 15159262]

RENAL ARTERY STENOSIS

Renal artery stenosis is produced predominantly by atherosclerotic occlusive disease (80–90% of patients) or fibromuscular dysplasia (10–15% of patients). Characteristically, patients with occlusive disease have common risk factors for atherosclerosis, and their lesions are focal proximal or ostial calcific plaques, often described as "spillover" aortic disease. Patients with fibromuscular dysplasia tend to be women 30–50 years of age with distal renal artery disease that often extends into the branch vessels in a classic "string of beads" pattern of alternating stenoses and dilations.

Renal artery stenosis has two important clinical manifestations: renovascular hypertension and ischemic nephropathy. Renovascular hypertension accounts for about 5% of all cases of hypertension. In certain subsets of patients, the incidence is much higher. Seventy percent of patients over 60 years of age with diastolic blood pressure greater than 105 mm Hg and serum creatinine greater than 2 mg/dL have renovascular hypertension. In hypertensive children, the incidence of this disease approaches 80%. Evaluation should be considered in patients with poorly controlled or acutely worsening hypertension that was previously well controlled by drug therapy (three or more antihypertensive medications), particularly when renal insufficiency, lateral abdominal bruit, or noncardiogenic "flash" pulmonary edema present in conjunction. A history of acute renal failure when starting an angiotensin-converting enzyme inhibitor is highly suggestive.

An incidental finding of renal artery stenosis greater than 50% is noted in as many as 45% of patients undergoing angiography for aortoiliac occlusive disease. Infrequently, it is associated with progressive renal insufficiency. High-grade (over 70%) bilateral stenoses or stenosis in a solitary kidney warrant close follow-up. Renal artery occlusive disease is suspected in patients with rapidly progressive renal insufficiency and no evidence of obstructive uropathy or intrinsic renal disease (no proteinuria on urinalysis, no polycystic disease on ultrasound).

Initial screening tests include duplex ultrasound, captopril renal scintigraphy, and MRA. Sensitivity and specificity of detecting renal artery stenosis greater than 60% are over 90% for each of these modalities, but the tests are highly operator dependent and equipment dependent—the most reliable examination varies by institution. An assessment should also be made of the kidney parenchyma: renal length, cortical thickness, and presence of infarcts. One pitfall of these modalities is failure to identify small accessory renal arteries, which when diseased can contribute to renovascular hypertension.

Indications for treatment include renovascular hypertension refractory to aggressive drug therapy or renal artery stenosis with progressive renal failure or sudden-onset noncardiogenic pulmonary edema. Severe stenosis unaccompanied by renal insufficiency or poorly controlled hypertension may be considered for therapy to prevent loss of renal mass.

Angiography is generally required for planning an operative strategy and in many cases discloses a lesion amenable to angioplasty and stenting. Ideal lesions for endovascular treatment are focal, proximal, nonostial plaques that do not extend into the branch vessels. Primary stenting is advised for stenoses in renal arteries greater than 5 mm in diameter because of improved patency over angioplasty alone. One exception to this rule is fibromuscular dysplasia, in which a durable clinical effect is often produced by angioplasty alone. In patients with renal insufficiency, use of nonionized contrast, preprocedure intravenous hydration, and administration of the antioxidant acetylcysteine, 600 mg orally twice daily for 2 days before and 2 days after examination, are advised. The long-term patency of renal artery stents is yet undefined, but a 20% restenosis rate from intimal hyperplasia is noted at 6–36 months. Overall, 3–13% of initially stented patients ultimately require surgery.

Surgery is indicated for threatened loss of total renal mass (bilateral renal artery stenosis greater than 75%), for treatment of progressive renal failure or uncontrolled renovascular hypertension in patients with lesions refractory to angioplasty, for complex lesions extending into the branch vessels, or for concomitant aortic disease requiring surgical reconstruction. Because of superior long-term patency, surgery may be preferred over angioplasty for primary treatment of renal artery occlusive disease in good-risk younger surgical candidates. Surgical options include transaortic renal endarterectomy, renal artery bypass, or extra-anatomic (hepatorenal, splenorenal, or ilorenal) bypass. Mannitol (25 g intravenously) and fenoldopam (0.5–1

mcg/kg/min) have been beneficial in the perioperative management of these patients. Nephrectomy is considered for patients with renovascular hypertension and irreversible renal atrophy (kidney length less than 7 cm, severe cortical thinning, less than 10% of total renal function by split function testing). Endarterectomy and aortorenal bypass have 5-year patency greater than 80%, with beneficial blood pressure response in 70–90% of patients and improvement or stabilization in renal function in 70–80%.

Bax L et al: STAR Study Group: the benefit of Stent placement and blood pressure and lipid-lowering for the prevention of progression of renal dysfunction caused by Atherosclerotic ostial stenosis of the Renal artery. The STAR-study: rationale and study design. J Nephrol 2003;16:807. [PMID: 14736007]

Gill KS et al: Atherosclerotic renal arterial stenosis: clinical outcomes of stent placement for hypertension and renal failure. Radiology 2003;226:821. [PMID: 12601202]

Marekovic Z et al: Long-term outcome after surgical kidney revascularization for fibromuscular dysplasia and atherosclerotic renal artery stenosis. J Urol 2004;171:1043. [PMID: 14767266]

Olin JW: Renal artery disease: diagnosis and management. Mt Sinai J Med 2004;71:73. [PMID: 15029399]

Rao RK et al: Current endovascular management of atherosclerotic renal artery stenosis. Surg Clin North Am 2004;84:1353. [PMID: 15364559]

Zhang H et al: Renal MR angiography. Magn Reson Imaging Clin North Am 2004;12:487. [PMID: 15271367]

ACUTE LIMB ISCHEMIA

Acute limb ischemia can be embolic, thrombotic, or traumatic. Symptoms and signs are related to the location of the occlusion, the duration of ischemia, and the degree of development of collateral circulation. Baseline pulse examination and assessment of motor and sensory function are imperative. Characteristically, acute ischemia is described by the six Ps: pain, pallor, pulselessness, paresthesias, poikilothermia, and paralysis. Pain and paresthesias are the most common symptoms.

The following differential points should be considered: (1) Are there manifestations of advanced occlusive arterial disease in other areas, especially the opposite extremity (bruit, absent pulses, secondary skin changes), and is there a history of intermittent claudication? These findings suggest primary arterial thrombosis. (2) Is there a history of rheumatic heart disease, atrial fibrillation, or myocardial infarction? These findings suggest embolism.

1. Arterial Embolism

Eighty to 90 percent of arterial emboli arise from the heart. Atrial fibrillation is present in 60–70% of patients with arterial emboli and is associated with formation of thrombus in the left atrial appendage. Thrombus within a postinfarct ventricular aneurysm may also be a potential embolic source. Emboli arising from rheumatic heart disease are decreasing in incidence and now comprise less than 20% of arterial emboli. Cardiac valvular prostheses and cardiac tumors (myxomas) can also produce emboli. Noncardiac emboli arise from atherosclerotic lesions in proximal vessels, tumors, and foreign bodies. Paradoxic emboli deriving from deep venous thrombosis (DVT) in the leg can also occur.

Emboli tend to lodge at the bifurcation of major arteries, with 40% going to the aortic, femoral, or popliteal bifurcations. Thirty percent lodge in the cerebrovascular vessels, 10% in the visceral vessels, and 15% in the upper extremity vessels. Noncardiac emboli from arterial ulcerations are usually small (> 400 mcm), giving rise to peripheral ulceration and digital ischemia or occasionally to a systemic illness resembling vasculitis.

Treatment

Heparin sodium should be given as soon as the diagnosis of acute arterial occlusion is made and continued intraoperatively to prevent distal thrombosis. Emergent embolectomy is performed by introducing a balloon catheter through a small arteriotomy. An embolus at the aortic bifurcation or in the iliac artery can often be removed under local anesthesia through unilateral or bilateral common femoral arteriotomies. Smaller balloon catheters passed distally from the femoral artery can be used to extract popliteal or tibial emboli, though these often require popliteal arteriotomy. Percutaneous catheter techniques (aspiration, mechanical thrombolysis, or thrombolytic therapy) have some reported success in treatment of peripheral embolic disease. Lifelong anticoagulation is recommended because of the high frequency of recurrent emboli. Surface or TEE should be performed to exclude the possibility of atrial thrombus, valvular disease, or cardiac tumor.

Embolectomy performed more than 6 hours following onset of symptoms is often accompanied by development of a compartment syndrome. In mild cases, fasciotomy performed at the time of embolectomy can result in full functional recovery of the limb. The most common persistent major neurologic deficit is foot drop secondary to peroneal nerve ischemia. Myoglobinuria and renal failure can result from rhabdomyolysis and can be minimized with aggressive hydration, induced diuresis, and alkalinization of the urine. These measures decrease the risk of myoglobin precipitation in the renal tubules. One regimen involves initial infusion of 250 mL/h of crystalloid, half as 0.45 normal saline and the rest as D_5W, with two ampules of sodium bicarbonate and 12.5 g of mannitol per liter of fluid taken if the diagnosis is delayed. Severe cases of compartment syndrome may result in anuric renal failure and systemic inflammatory response syndrome. In these patients, primary amputation may be lifesaving.

Prognosis

Arterial embolism is associated with a 5–25% risk of limb loss and a 25–30% in-hospital mortality. Heart disease is responsible for the majority of these deaths.

In patients with atrial fibrillation, mechanical or pharmacologic cardioversion or long-term anticoagulant therapy may decrease the risk of further emboli.

If no heart disease exists, prognosis is dependent on identification and exclusion of the embolic source. Cholesterol emboli from proximal arterial aneurysm or ulceration may occlude small distal vessels, producing digital ischemia. One common scenario is "blue toes" after aortography or aortic cross-clamping for coronary artery bypass or aneurysm repair. However, atheroemboli can also produce TIAs, acute renal insufficiency, or bowel ischemia depending on their location. Microhematuria, eosinophilia, and an elevated sedimentation rate are detectable transiently on laboratory testing. Biopsy of the infarcted tissue reveals cholesterol clefts in the small vessels under polarized light. These lesions are not treatable by embolectomy because the vessels involved are so small, and heparinization may worsen the problem by liberating more fragments from an ulcerated atherosclerotic plaque. Aortic or iliac lesions can be treated by endarterectomy, by resection and interposition graft, or by placement of a covered stent.

2. Acute Arterial Thrombosis

Acute arterial thrombosis is most commonly a complication of chronic atherosclerotic occlusive disease but can also occur as a consequence of trauma, low-flow states such as hypovolemic or cardiogenic shock, or an inflammatory arteritis. Polycythemia, dehydration, and hypercoagulable states also increase the risk of thrombosis. Generally, thrombus starts at the point of greatest stenosis and propagates distally to the next open branch point, such as a patent collateral vessel.

Treatment

Nonoperative treatment is the initial approach for many patients with acute arterial thrombosis. Because thrombosis develops in the setting of chronic occlusive disease, there are usually well-developed collaterals and little arterial spasm. The extremity is able to tolerate the longer periods of ischemia required for catheter-directed thrombolysis. Instillation of alteplase (0.5–1 mg/h) directly into the thrombus through a multiside-holed catheter may allow recanalization of distal vessels that are less amenable to surgical thrombectomy. It also helps disclose the underlying stenotic lesion, which can then be treated with angioplasty, endarterectomy, or bypass grafting. Thrombolysis is successful in 50–80% of cases, with a limb salvage rate approaching 90%.

Less commonly, arterial thrombosis follows penetrating trauma, such as arterial transection and foreign body embolization, or blunt trauma, such as posterior knee dislocation and crush injury. These patients require surgical treatment. The vessel involved may be previously undiseased, with only a few small collaterals. Thrombolysis is generally not indicated because of the more advanced state of limb ischemia on presentation and the high incidence of bleeding complications.

Prognosis

Limb salvage is usually possible with acute thrombosis of the iliac or superficial femoral arteries but is less likely with popliteal thrombosis because of the paucity of available collaterals. Acute thrombosis of a popliteal aneurysm is associated with a 10–25% risk of amputation.

Clagett GP et al: Antithrombotic therapy in peripheral arterial occlusive disease: the Seventh ACCP Conference on Antithrombotic and Thrombolytic Therapy. Chest 2004;126(3 Suppl):609S. [PMID: 15383487]

Earnshaw JJ et al: National Audit of Thrombolysis for Acute Leg Ischemia (NATALI): clinical factors associated with early outcome. J Vasc Surg 2004;39:1018. [PMID: 15111854]

Kessel DO et al: Infusion techniques for peripheral arterial thrombolysis. Cochrane Database Syst Rev 2004;(1): CD000985. [PMID: 14973961]

■ OTHER ARTERIOPATHIES

THROMBOANGIITIS OBLITERANS (Buerger's Disease)

Buerger's disease is an episodic and segmental inflammatory and thrombotic process of the peripheral arteries and veins. The cause is not known. It is seen most commonly in men under 40 years of age who smoke, and particularly in those of Eastern European or Asian background. It is characterized by occlusion of distal arteries, producing claudication, rest pain, and tissue necrosis. The inflammatory process is intermittent, with quiescent periods lasting weeks, months, or years. Different arterial segments may become occluded in successive episodes; recanalization can occur during periods of disease remission.

There are no pathognomonic signs, but several findings are characteristic of Buerger's disease. (1) The typical patient is a man under 40 years of age who smokes. Fewer than 20% of patients are women. (2) There is a history of migratory superficial segmental thrombophlebitis, eg, red, tender nodules in the branches of the saphenous vein. Biopsy of the affected vein may show inflammatory infiltrate in the vessel wall, microabscesses, and thrombus or recanalization with perivascular fibrosis, depending on the stage of disease. (3) Intermittent claudication typically begins in the arch of the foot and progresses to the calf; instep claudication is not typical of atherosclerotic occlusive disease. Rest pain and diminished sensation from ischemic neuropathy are present in over 70% of patients at presentation. (4) Proximal pulses are normal, whereas distal pulses are absent. Digital disease is often asymmetric: Not all of the toes are affected to the same degree. The affected digits may be pale, cyanotic, erythematous, or gangrenous. (5) Ul-

cers are present in 75% of patients and are typically located at the nail margins. (6) The disease is never confined to one limb. Although not all limbs may be symptomatic, an abnormal Allen test or distal pulse examination can usually be demonstrated. (7) There is often a history of cold sensitivity or Raynaud's phenomenon. (8) The clinical course is usually episodic, with acute exacerbations followed by rather definite remissions. By contrast, steadily progressive symptoms are typical in atherosclerotic occlusive disease.

Atherosclerotic occlusive disease, emboli, and autoimmune disorders are included in the differential diagnosis. Several angiographic findings can be helpful in making these distinctions. Buerger's disease involves the distal arteries and spares the proximal arteries; it is segmental in appearance, with skip areas of disease; there is no vascular calcification; and extensive collateralization via tortuous "corkscrew" vessels is typical. Peripheral ultrasound or angiography and echocardiography are helpful in excluding an embolic source. Blood tests (complete blood count, coagulation studies, sedimentation rate, antinuclear antibody, lupus anticoagulant, rheumatoid factor, anticentromere antibody, and antiphospholipid antibody) are obtained to rule out vasculitis, lupus erythematosus, scleroderma, rheumatoid vascular disease, or a hypercoagulable state due to antiphospholipid antibody syndrome. A careful history is generally sufficient to exclude other rare disorders that may mimic Buerger's disease, such as ergotamine intoxication, cannabis arteritis, or small vessel occlusive disease secondary to the use of vibratory tools (hypothenar hammer syndrome).

Smoking cessation is imperative. The disease can remain active with as little as a single cigarette a day; chewing tobacco, marijuana, nicotine patches, nicotine gum, and exposure to second-hand smoke must all be eliminated to arrest the disease process. Local wound care of ulcers consists of limited debridement, appropriate dressings, and intravenous antibiotics for cellulitis. Nonulcerated skin should be kept moisturized. Lamb's wool between the toes and heel protectors or sheepskin-lined boots (Rooke boots) help reduce further trauma to the skin. Warming pads must be used judiciously, as burns are possible in patients with diminished sensation from peripheral neuropathy. Supplementary oxygen by nasal cannula is often used to increase oxygen supply to the wound. Some ulcers may respond to hyperbaric oxygen.

Nonsteroidal anti-inflammatory medications and opioids are used for pain control. Aspirin (81 mg daily) or another antiplatelet agent is generally prescribed to reduce thrombotic complications. Calcium channel blockers are often used to promote vasodilation. Preliminary trials have shown intravenous infusion of the prostaglandin analog iloprost to be efficacious in healing of ischemic ulcers, but the drug is not yet available in the United States. Vascular endothelial growth factor (VEGF) is also being investigated for use in Buerger's disease.

Rarely do distal target vessels exist for arterial bypass. Sympathectomy may at least transiently reduce the vasospastic manifestations of the disease and aid in the establishment of collateral circulation to the skin. It is indicated for relief of intractable rest pain and healing of ulcers refractory to other treatment. Sympathectomy is often performed in conjunction with digital amputation. Amputation is reserved for patients with wet gangrene or severe rest pain.

Prognosis depends on the success of smoking cessation. Over 90% of patients who quit smoking avoid further amputation.

Calguneri M et al: Buerger's disease with multisystem involvement. A case report and a review of the literature. Angiology 2004;55:325. [PMID: 15156267]

Ohta T et al: Clinical and social consequences of Buerger disease. J Vasc Surg 2004;39:176. [PMID: 14718836]

Olin JW: Current concepts: thromboangiitis obliterans (Buerger's disease). N Engl J Med 2000;343:864. [PMID: 10995867]

IDIOPATHIC ARTERITIS OF TAKAYASU ("Pulseless Disease")

Takayasu's disease is a rare polyarteritis of unknown cause with a special predilection for the branches of the aortic arch. It results in segmental stenoses, occlusions, and aneurysms. It is seen frequently in Asian women under the age of 40 years. There are a myriad of clinical presentations depending on the stage of disease (early "inflammatory" or late "occlusive") and the arteries involved. Early stages of disease are often accompanied by fever, myalgias, arthralgias, and pain over the involved artery as well as leukocytosis and elevated sedimentation rate. Other symptoms are related to arterial insufficiency: syncope, dizziness, amaurosis fugax, stroke, angina, pulmonary hypertension, and claudication. Hypertension related to proximal renal artery stenosis or aortic coarctation is present in over 25% of patients. Vascular bruits, diminished peripheral pulses, or asymmetric blood pressure measurements are common findings on physical examination.

Angiography is essential for diagnosis and most often will reveal combined occlusive and aneurysmal disease. The most commonly involved vessels are the subclavian artery, descending thoracic aorta, renal artery, carotid artery, and mesenteric arteries, although the ascending and abdominal aorta and the vertebral, coronary, pulmonary, iliac, and brachial arteries can also be affected. In cases of upper extremity stenoses, aortic root pressure should be measured by manometry at the time of angiography to assess for essential hypertension. MRA can also be used for routine surveillance of patients with suspected Takayasu's disease.

Pulseless disease must be differentiated from vascular lesions of the aortic arch due to atherosclerosis, though in the latter instance concomitant lower extremity disease is invariably present. Histologically, the arterial lesions are indistinguishable from those of giant cell arteritis. In the early, active stage, corticosteroids (prednisone, 1 mg/kg/d) are used to control symptoms and limit the progression of disease; cyto-

toxic agents may be added if corticosteroids are ineffectual. Surgical or percutaneous intervention is not advised until the disease becomes indolent. Bypass of the occluded or aneurysmal segments is the usual surgical approach. Histologic examination of the resected artery may show nonspecific transmural inflammation or chronic fibrosis. Percutaneous angioplasty or stenting is possible for short-segment stenoses, but there is a high recurrence rate in these usually noncompliant vessels.

Kissin EY et al: Diagnostic imaging in Takayasu arteritis. Curr Opin Rheumatol 2004;16:31. [PMID: 14673386]

Liang P et al: Takayasu's arteritis: vascular interventions and outcomes. J Rheumatol 2004;31:102. [PMID: 14705227]

Vanoli M et al; Itaka Study Group: Takayasu's arteritis: A study of 104 Italian patients. Arthritis Rheum 2005; 53:100. [PMID: 15696576]

FIBROMUSCULAR DYSPLASIA

Fibromuscular dysplasia is a nonatherosclerotic, noninflammatory disease of unknown cause characterized by segmental irregularity of small and medium-sized muscular arteries. Typically, it affects white women 30–50 years of age; a family history of disease is not unusual. The most frequently involved vessels (in descending order) are the renal, carotid, and common iliac arteries. Fibromuscular dysplasia presents with renovascular hypertension and, less often, with renal insufficiency, TIAs, or claudication. Angiography reveals a "string of beads" pattern of disease. There are four recognized histologic types of fibromuscular dysplasia: medial fibrodysplasia, intimal fibroplasia, medial hyperplasia, and perimedial dysplasia, though the first type is responsible for over 80% of all cases. Aspirin is advised for most patients. Percutaneous or surgical intervention is reserved for symptomatic patients. Most lesions respond well to percutaneous angioplasty; stents do not appear to offer any advantage over angioplasty alone. More complex lesions extending into branch vessels may require interposition grafting. It is important to recognize that intracranial aneurysms are present in up to 50% of patients with internal carotid fibromuscular dysplasia.

Birrer M: Treatment of renal artery fibromuscular dysplasia with balloon angioplasty: a prospective follow-up study. Eur J Vasc Endovasc Surg 2002;23:146. [PMID: 11863332]

Guill CK et al: Fatal mesenteric fibromuscular dysplasia: a case report and review of the literature. Arch Intern Med 2004; 164:1148. [PMID: 15159274]

Olin JW: Renal artery disease: diagnosis and management. Mt Sinai J Med 2004;71:73. [PMID: 15029399]

VASCULITIS

The term vasculitis describes a diverse group of inflammatory disorders characterized by multiorgan system vascular involvement, systemic markers of disease (fever, malaise, weight loss, elevated white blood cell count and sedimentation rate), and suspected immunologic origin. Often there are accompanying rheumatologic or cutaneous manifestations such as arthralgias, conjunctivitis, or erythema nodosum. Drugs (amphetamines, cocaine, hydralazine, procainamide), infections (hepatitis B, gonococcus, streptococcus), chronic inflammatory diseases, and cancer are cited as inciting causes for vasculitis. These diseases can be grouped into disorders that affect medium and large blood vessels (polyarteritis nodosa, scleroderma, systemic lupus erythematosus, temporal arteritis, Behçet's disease, Kawasaki syndrome, rheumatoid arteritis, relapsing polychondritis) and those that affect smaller vessels (Churg–Strauss syndrome, Wegener's granulomatosis, Henoch–Schönlein purpura, essential mixed cryoglobulinemia). These are discussed in detail in Chapter 20. In general, the vascular lesions are treated with anti-inflammatory medications. Surgery is indicated for acute complications (bowel infarction, gangrene, or aneurysm rupture) and for chronic ischemic symptoms or large aneurysms in patients with quiescent disease.

■ VASOMOTOR DISORDERS

RAYNAUD'S DISEASE & RAYNAUD'S PHENOMENON

ESSENTIALS OF DIAGNOSIS

- Episodic bilateral digital pallor, cyanosis, and rubor.
- Precipitated by cold or emotional stress; relieved by warmth.
- Seventy to 80 percent of patients are women.

General Considerations

Raynaud's syndrome is an episodic vasospastic disorder characterized by digital color change (white-blue-red) with exposure to cold environment or emotional stress. If idiopathic, it is called Raynaud's disease. If associated with a possible precipitating systemic or regional disorder (autoimmune diseases, myeloproliferative disorders, multiple myeloma, cryoglobulinemia, myxedema, macroglobulinemia, or arterial occlusive disease), it is called Raynaud's phenomenon. The incidence of disease is estimated to be as high as 10% in the general population. Other vasospastic disorders, such as variant angina and migraine headache, are common in patients with Raynaud's syndrome. An abnormality of the sympathetic nervous system has long been implicated in the etiology of Raynaud's disease; recently, research has focused on the theory of up-regulation of vascular smooth muscle α_2-adrenergic receptors.

Clinical Findings

Classically, Raynaud's disease and Raynaud's phenomenon are characterized by intermittent attacks of pallor of the hands or fingers brought on by cold or emotional stress, progressing to cyanosis and then rubor on rewarming. Mild discomfort, paresthesias, numbness, and trace edema often accompany the color changes. In Raynaud's disease, the disease is symmetric, by rule; in Raynaud's phenomenon, the changes may be most noticeable in one hand or even in one or two fingers only. Infrequently, the feet and toes are involved. Between attacks, the affected extremities may be entirely normal.

The distinction between Raynaud's disease and Raynaud's phenomenon is meant to reflect a difference in prognosis. Whereas Raynaud's disease is benign and often controllable, Raynaud's phenomenon may progress to atrophy of the terminal fat pads and development of fingertip gangrene. However, because many inciting diseases may not be clinically suspected at the time the diagnosis of Raynaud's disease is made, there is a large degree of crossover between groups. The diagnosis is based on clinical criteria. Raynaud's disease appears first between ages 15 and 45, almost always in women. A patient with suggestive symptoms that persist for over 3 years without evidence of an associated disease is given the diagnosis of Raynaud's disease.

Differential Diagnosis

A patient with Raynaud's syndrome must be evaluated for possible inciting systemic disorders. Directed history and physical examination and serologic testing may be helpful in excluding the collagen-vascular disorders, which include scleroderma, systemic lupus erythematosus, dermatomyositis, and rheumatoid arthritis. It is estimated that Raynaud's phenomenon ultimately develops in 80% of patients with scleroderma. Likewise, cryoglobulinemia can be excluded by appropriate testing. Raynaud's phenomenon is also occasionally seen in patients with neurogenic thoracic outlet syndrome or carpal tunnel syndrome. Frostbite, ergotamine toxicity, and use of chemotherapeutic agents, which can also be associated with Raynaud's phenomenon, can usually be excluded by a careful history; symptomatic vasospastic disease develops in up to one-third of patients receiving combined bleomycin and vincristine (such as for testicular cancer). An abnormal or asymmetric pulse examination, differential blood pressure cuff measurements, gangrene, or a positive Allen test are suggestive of arterial occlusive disease and should prompt upper extremity angiography to exclude stenosis or occlusion from atherosclerosis, Buerger's disease, arterial thoracic outlet syndrome, embolic disease, or repetitive motion injury of the small vessels of the hand. Even undiseased upper extremity vessels often show intense vasospasm with contrast injection, so the arm is wrapped for warmth and prophylactic use of a vasodilator (papaverine or nitroglycerin, 30 mg, injected through the angiography catheter) is advised; both arms are imaged for side-by-side comparison.

Other vasospastic disorders that should be included in the differential but are usually easily distinguishable by physical examination are acrocyanosis and livedo reticularis.

Treatment

A. GENERAL MEASURES

Warmth and protection of the hands are the basic tenets of therapy. In Raynaud's phenomenon, wounds heal slowly, and infections are consequently hard to control. Gloves should be worn in cold environments and during activities that may cause trauma to the skin, such as dishwashing, gardening, woodworking, or office filing. Moisturizing lotion should be applied frequently to avoid fissured dry skin. Smoking cessation is imperative, as nicotine is a known vasoconstrictor. Stress management should be addressed when appropriate. Oral contraceptives, β-blockers, and ergotamines are associated with exacerbation of symptoms and ideally should be discontinued. Aspirin is prescribed to decrease the risk of thrombotic complications.

B. VASODILATORS

Vasodilator drugs may be of some benefit in patients whose symptoms are not adequately controlled with simpler measures. Low-dose nifedipine (sustained release, 30 mg/d) or diltiazem (sustained release, 30 mg/d) has superseded topical or oral nitroglycerin for treatment of vasospasm. Use of prostaglandins has been disappointing, but the serotonin reuptake inhibitor and antidepressant fluoxetine (20 mg daily) shows some promise in reduction of the frequency and severity of attacks.

C. SURGERY

Sympathectomy is indicated for pure vasospastic disease refractory to medical management. In the lower extremity, sympathectomy may produce complete and permanent relief of symptoms; however, for unclear reasons, the beneficial effects are often transient in the upper extremity. Limited improvement is seen in advanced ischemia, particularly if significant digital artery obstructive disease is present.

Prognosis

Raynaud's disease is usually benign, causing mild discomfort on exposure to cold and progressing very slightly over the years. The prognosis of Raynaud's phenomenon is that of the associated disease.

Grader-Beck T et al: Raynaud's phenomenon in mixed connective tissue disease. Rheum Dis Clin North Am 2005;31: 465. [PMID: 16084319]

Thompson AE et al: Calcium channel blockers for primary Raynaud's phenomenon: a meta-analysis. Rheumatology (Oxford) 2005;44:145. [PMID: 15546967]

LIVEDO RETICULARIS

Livedo reticularis is a vasospastic disorder of unknown cause that results in a painless, mottled discoloration on large areas of the extremities, generally in a fishnet pattern with reticulated cyanotic areas surrounding a paler central core. It occurs in men and women of all ages. In most instances, livedo reticularis is entirely benign; infrequently, it is associated with an occult malignancy, polyarteritis nodosa, atherosclerotic microemboli, or antiphospholipid antibody syndrome. The disorder is characterized by arteriolar vasoconstriction with capillary and venous dilation; the particular pattern is believed to represent arborization of capillaries surrounding the feeding arteriole.

Livedo reticularis is most apparent on the thighs but can occur on the forearms or lower abdomen and is most pronounced in cold weather. In warm environments, the reticular pattern may fade but does not entirely disappear. A few patients report paresthesias, coldness, or numbness in the involved areas. Peripheral pulses are normal. The affected regions may be cool. Skin ulceration is rare. Treatment consists of protection from exposure to cold; use of vasodilators is seldom indicated. In the rare patient in whom ulcerations or gangrene develops, an underlying systemic disease should be excluded.

ACROCYANOSIS

Acrocyanosis is an uncommon vasospastic disorder characterized by persistent cyanosis of the hands and feet and, to a lesser degree, the forearms and legs. It is associated with arteriolar vasoconstriction combined with dilation of the subcapillary venous plexus of the skin, through which deoxygenated blood slowly circulates. It is worse in cold weather but does not completely disappear during the warm season. It occurs primarily in women, is most common in the teens and twenties, and may improve with advancing age or during pregnancy. It is characterized by symmetric coldness, sweating, slight edema, and cyanotic discoloration of the hands or feet. Peripheral pulses are normal, and pain, trophic lesions, and disability do not occur.

ERYTHROMELALGIA

Erythromelalgia is a paroxysmal bilateral vasodilatory disorder of unknown cause. Idiopathic (primary) erythromelalgia occurs in otherwise healthy persons and affects men and women equally. A secondary type is occasionally seen in patients with polycythemia vera, hypertension, gout, and neurologic diseases.

The primary symptoms are erythema, warmth, and bilateral burning pain that lasts minutes to hours, at first involving circumscribed areas on the balls of the feet or palms and often progressing to involve the entire extremity. Symptoms occur in response to vasodilation produced by exercise or heat and can be prominent at night when the extremities are warmed under bedclothes. Relief may be obtained by cooling and elevating the affected extremity.

No findings are generally present between attacks. With onset of an attack, skin temperature and arterial pulsations are increased and the involved areas are warm, erythematous, and sweaty.

In primary erythromelalgia, aspirin (650 mg every 4–6 hours) often provides excellent relief and may in fact be diagnostic. Warm environments are to be avoided. β-Blockers, epidural corticosteroid injections, and lidocaine patches have reported anecdotal success. Secondary erythromelalgia may improve with treatment of the primary disease process.

Orstavik K et al: Pain in primary erythromelalgia—a neuropathic component? Pain 2004;110:531. [PMID: 15288393]

Waxman SG et al: Erythromelalgia: a hereditary pain syndrome enters the molecular era. Ann Neurol 2005;57:785. [PMID: 15929046]

COMPLEX REGIONAL PAIN SYNDROME TYPE 1 (Reflex Sympathetic Dystrophy)

 ESSENTIALS OF DIAGNOSIS

- *Burning or aching pain of greater severity and longer duration than expected following trauma to an extremity.*
- *Manifestations of localized vasomotor instability are generally present.*

General Considerations

The syndrome is characterized by burning or aching pain in an injured extremity that is more severe than would be expected given the inciting trauma. It occurs in all age groups and equally in both sexes and can involve either the arms or the legs. The degree of trauma is in some cases surprisingly minor (phlebotomy), but most cases follow crushing injuries with lacerations and soft tissue destruction. Closed fractures, simple lacerations, burns (especially electric burns), elective operative procedures, and myocardial infarction with referred left arm pain are other reported causes.

Clinical Findings

In the early stages, the pain, tenderness, and hyperesthesia are localized to the injured area, and the extremity is warm, dry, swollen, and red or slightly cyanotic. With time, muscle spasm and joint stiffness limit mobility, and the nails may become ridged. In advanced stages, the pain is more diffuse, and nocturnal pain may become extreme; the extremity becomes cool and clammy and intolerant of temperature changes (particularly cold); and the skin becomes glossy and atrophic.

The patient's dominant concern is to avoid external stimuli, particularly in trigger point areas. Pain and disuse lead to loss of function. Radiographs reveal asymmetric osteopenia more severe than anticipated from immobility alone.

Prevention

Trauma to peripheral nerves during surgery is avoided by knowledge of their anatomy and careful mobilization by handling of the perineural tissue only. Splinting and adequate analgesia followed by early mobilization of an injured extremity minimize the occurrence of reflex sympathetic dystrophy.

Treatment & Prognosis

A. CONSERVATIVE MEASURES

Early recognition and treatment are essential to preserve function of the limb. In the early stages, when major secondary changes have not yet developed, physical therapy involving active and passive exercises combined with a mild anxiolytic (diazepam, 2 mg twice daily, or alprazolam, 0.125–0.25 mg twice daily) may relieve symptoms. Opioids have been a mainstay of treatment; recently, however, gabapentin (beginning at 200–900 mg twice daily) has been used with success. Sympathetic blocks (stellate ganglion or lumbar) can be combined with intensive physical therapy for cases refractory to more conservative treatment. Protection from further injury and avoidance of irritating stimuli are imperative.

B. SURGERY

Patients who achieve significant temporary relief of symptoms after sympathetic blocks may be cured by sympathectomy. With advanced disease and in cases with significant psychological overlay, however, the prognosis for improvement with sympathectomy is poor. Implantable spinal cord biostimulator devices have had limited success.

Quisel A et al: Complex regional pain syndrome: which treatments show promise? J Fam Pract 2005;54:599. [PMID: 16009087]

Teasdall RD et al: Complex regional pain syndrome (reflex sympathetic dystrophy). Clin Sports Med 2004;23:145. [PMID: 15062588]

THORACIC OUTLET SYNDROME

Thoracic outlet syndrome can be subdivided into neurogenic, venous, and arterial types depending on which structures are compressed in the interscalene triangle or costoclavicular space.

Neurogenic thoracic outlet syndrome is the most common (over 90% of patients) and often the most difficult to diagnose and treat effectively. Patients most often present with supraclavicular and anterior chest pain often burning in nature and with segmental pain and paresthesias of the arm and hand in an ulnar nerve distribution. Weakness and atrophy of the forearm and of the intrinsic muscles of the hand secondary to disease are not uncommon. Thenar or hypothenar muscle wasting is rare. There is usually a history of whiplash trauma (motor vehicle accident, fall, assault) or repetitive activity of the upper extremity (word processing, filing), particularly overhead activities (lifting). Physical examination will often disclose supraclavicular tenderness and positive brachial plexus tension testing. A positive Adson test (obliteration of the radial pulse on inspiration while turning the head away from the affected side), or a positive Roos test (reproduction of symptoms with rapid opening and closing of the hand with the arm 90 degrees abducted at the shoulder and 90 degrees flexed at the elbow), or a positive Tinel sign (tingling in the distribution of the nerve produced by tapping in the supraclavicular interscalene region) may also be elicited. Presence of a cervical rib or other bony anomalies should be excluded by chest radiograph. Electrophysiologic testing is usually negative. The cornerstone of treatment is specific physical therapy such as the Edgelow Neurovascular Entrapment Self-Treatment (ENVEST) program, beginning with breathing exercises and attention to posture. Transcutaneous electrical nerve stimulation (TENS) can be helpful. Surgery is indicated in severe refractory cases and involves resection of the hypertrophied anterior and middle scalene muscles, brachial plexus neurolysis, and resection of muscular or fibrous bands and any bony abnormalities. Although in carefully selected patients the initial surgical outcome is excellent, symptoms return within a year in as many as 25% of patients, presumably due to late postoperative scarring around the nerve roots.

Venous thoracic outlet syndrome involves external compression of the subclavian vein by the first rib, anterior scalene muscle, clavicle, and costocoracoid ligament. A history of repetitive upper arm exercises or clavicular fracture is common. Positional venography is essential in the diagnosis of venous thoracic outlet syndrome; external compression of the vein and filling of venous collaterals are demonstrated by abduction of the arm. Thrombosis of the involved vein segment is known as Paget–Schroetter syndrome, or effort thrombosis, and often presents as acute unilateral arm edema, axillary fullness, hand cyanosis, and enlarged shoulder and chest wall collateral veins in an otherwise healthy patient. Evaluation for hypercoagulable state, including plasma levels of antithrombin III, factor V Leiden, cardiolipin antibody, and proteins C and S, is recommended, as an abnormality can be detected in some patients presenting with acute axillary-subclavian vein thrombosis. Treatment for symptomatic venous thoracic outlet syndrome involves anterior and middle scalenectomy and first rib resection with venolysis, which can be performed through a supraclavicular, a combined supraclavicular and infraclavicular, or a transaxillary approach. Intraoperative venography confirms relief of extrinsic compression. Residual stenosis can be dilated. If the vein is thrombosed, multimodal-

ity therapy is used: preoperative thrombolysis followed immediately by surgery with intraoperative angioplasty of any residual venous stenosis. If the vein cannot be recannulated preoperatively, surgical thrombectomy may be required. The prognosis is excellent with appropriate treatment.

Arterial thoracic outlet syndrome is the least common of these disorders and involves compression of the subclavian artery between the anterior and middle scalene muscles. It most often produces subclavian artery stenosis and poststenotic dilation, which result in digital ischemia due to atheroemboli. These lesions can be subtle, often requiring magnified multiplanar views to be shown angiographically. Arm claudication is a less common presentation. The Wylie–Allen test (performed by exsanguinating the arm with elevation, occluding the radial and ulnar arteries at the wrist, and observing capillary refill of the hand when these arteries are released) may reveal occult digital artery occlusions that can be confirmed by angiography. Treatment involves removal of the anterior and middle scalene muscles, first rib resection, and resection of the affected subclavian artery with replacement by a polytetrafluoroethylene interposition graft.

Crosby CA et al: Conservative treatment for thoracic outlet syndrome. Hand Clin 2004;20:43. [PMID: 15005383]

Sanders RJ et al: Venous thoracic outlet syndrome. Hand Clin 2004;20:113. [PMID: 15005393]

Schneider DB et al: Combination treatment of venous thoracic outlet syndrome: open surgical decompression and intraoperative angioplasty. J Vasc Surg 2004;40:599. [PMID: 15472583]

■ VENOUS DISEASES

VARICOSE VEINS

ESSENTIALS OF DIAGNOSIS

- *Dilated, tortuous superficial veins in the lower extremities.*
- *May be asymptomatic or associated with fatigue, aching discomfort, bleeding, or localized pain.*
- *Edema, pigmentation, and ulceration suggest concomitant venous stasis disease.*
- *Increased frequency after pregnancy.*

General Considerations

Abnormally dilated veins develop in several locations, giving rise to varicoceles, esophageal varices, and hemorrhoids. However, varicose veins are most commonly found in the legs as abnormally dilated, elongated, and tortuous alterations in the saphenous veins and their tributaries. Saphenous vein varicosities develop in 15% of adults. Risk factors include female gender, pregnancy, family history, prolonged standing, and history of phlebitis.

The long saphenous vein and its tributaries are most commonly involved, but the short saphenous vein may also be affected. These vessels lie immediately beneath the skin and superficial to the deep fascia.

An inherited vein wall or valvular defect appears to play a role in the development of most primary varicosities. Secondary varicosities may result from valve damage following thrombophlebitis, trauma, DVT, arteriovenous fistula, or nontraumatic proximal venous obstruction (pregnancy, pelvic tumor). Venous reflux caused by valvular incompetence is characteristic of both primary and secondary varicose veins. At the saphenofemoral junction and the perforating veins of the medial calf and thigh, the superficial and deep veins of the leg communicate; valve incompetence in these segments permits blood flow to be bidirectional. Thus, high venous pressures (> 300 mm Hg) from within the deep system that occur during calf compression associated with walking are transmitted to these superficial veins, which dilate. With long-standing disease, the surrounding tissue and skin may develop secondary changes such as fibrosis, chronic edema, and skin pigmentation and atrophy.

Clinical Findings

A. SYMPTOMS

The severity of the symptoms is not necessarily correlated with the number and size of the varicosities. Dull, aching heaviness or a feeling of fatigue brought on by periods of standing is the most common complaint. Itching from an associated eczematoid dermatitis may occur above the ankle.

B. SIGNS

Dilated, tortuous, elongated veins on the medial aspect of the thigh and leg are usually readily visible with the patient standing. Smaller, flat, blue-green reticular veins, telangiectasias, and spider veins may accompany varicose veins and are further evidence of venous dysfunction. Secondary tissue changes may be absent even in the presence of extensive large varicosities; however, with superficial or deep venous insufficiency and long-standing varicose veins, the signs of chronic venous insufficiency appear. These may include brownish pigmentation and thinning of the skin above the ankle, edema, fibrosis, scaling dermatitis, and venous ulceration. Duplex ultrasonography is used to detect the precise location of incompetent valves. The Brodie–Trendelenburg test can help differentiate saphenofemoral valve incompetence from perforator vein incompetence. With the patient lying supine, the leg is elevated until all varicosities collapse. A tourniquet is placed at the mid thigh to exclude reflux secondary to incompetence at the saphenofemoral

junction. With the tourniquet in place, the patient is asked to stand. Varicosities that remain collapsed indicate valvular insufficiency at the saphenofemoral junction. However, if the varicosities rapidly refill, perforator vein incompetence is implicated. The tourniquet can then be moved more distally to identify the location of the incompetent perforator.

Differential Diagnosis

Primary varicose veins should be differentiated from secondary varicose veins to exclude the possibility of chronic venous insufficiency of the superficial or deep system of veins, obstruction of the pelvic veins, arteriovenous fistula (congenital or acquired), or congenital venous malformation. If extensive varicose veins are encountered in a young patient—especially if unilateral and in an atypical distribution (lateral leg)—Klippel–Trénaunay syndrome must be considered. The classic triad of Klippel–Trénaunay syndrome is varicose veins, limb hypertrophy, and a cutaneous birthmark (port wine stain or venous malformation). Because the deep veins are often anomalous or absent, saphenous vein stripping is contraindicated. Standard treatment for patients with Klippel–Trénaunay syndrome is graduated support stockings and surgery for correction of leg length discrepancy.

Pain or discomfort secondary to arthritis, radiculopathy, or arterial insufficiency should be distinguished from symptoms associated with coexistent varicose veins.

Complications

Complications of varicose veins include secondary ulceration, bleeding, chronic stasis dermatitis, superficial venous thrombosis, and thrombophlebitis.

Treatment

A. NONSURGICAL MEASURES

Knee-high or thigh-high elastic graduated compression stockings give external support to the superficial veins. For most patients, a gradient of compression of 20–30 mm Hg is appropriate. The stockings are worn all day to reduce venous hypertension due to pooling of blood and are removed at night. Periodic leg elevation and regular exercise are encouraged. In many patients, this program may provide relief of symptoms and discourage progression of disease sufficient to avoid surgery.

Small venous ulcers generally heal with leg elevation and compression bandages (Ace wrap or Unna boot). Varicose vein excision should be postponed until infection and edema are controlled.

B. SURGICAL MEASURES

Indications for surgical treatment include persistent or disabling pain, recurrent superficial thrombophlebitis, erosion of the overlying skin with bleeding, and manifestations of chronic venous insufficiency (particularly ulceration).

The operative plan is dependent on determination of the competency of the superficial, deep, or perforating veins and the location of sites of venous reflux. Preoperative duplex ultrasound is essential in the identification of incompetent perforating veins and in the assessment of the saphenofemoral junction. Surgery can then be tailored to the pattern of disease. Stab avulsion surgery is combined with prevention of reflux by high ligation of the saphenofemoral junction or ligation of perforator branches. Endovenous radiofrequency ablation of the proximal saphenous vein alone or combined with stab avulsion of calf varicosities is more frequently being used. Stripping of the entire saphenous system is rarely required and may be complicated by hematoma formation, infection, and saphenous nerve irritation.

C. Compression Sclerotherapy

Compression sclerotherapy can be used for telangiectasias, spider veins, and small (< 4 mm) varicosities that persist after vein stripping. With patients in a supine position, small volumes of a sclerosing solution (23.4% hypertonic saline or 2.5% sodium morrhuate) are injected, and direct pressure is then maintained with compression stockings. The goal is to obliterate the abnormal vein by inducing localized endothelial destruction and fibrosis. More than one treatment is often required. Complications—including allergic reactions, thrombophlebitis, neoangiogenesis, skin necrosis, or hyperpigmentation—are rare.

Prognosis

With careful patient selection and properly selected operative techniques, most patients experience relief of symptoms, and the recurrence rate is about 10%. Patients should be informed that this is a chronic disease and that prevention of new varicosities is dependent on continued use of the compression stockings, leg elevation, and exercise. If extensive varicosities reappear after surgery, the completeness of the high ligation should be questioned, and reexploration of the saphenofemoral area may be necessary. Even after adequate treatment, secondary tissue changes may not regress.

Kahle B et al: Efficacy of sclerotherapy in varicose veins—prospective, blinded, placebo-controlled study. Dermatol Surg 2004;30:723. [PMID: 15099314]

Lurie F et al: Prospective randomized study of endovenous radiofrequency obliteration (closure procedure) versus ligation and stripping in a selected patient population (EVOLVeS Study). J Vasc Surg 2003;38:207. [PMID: 12891099]

Mundy L et al: Systematic review of endovenous laser treatment for varicose veins. Br J Surg 2005;92:1189. [PMID: 16175538]

THROMBOPHLEBITIS OF THE DEEP VEINS

ESSENTIALS OF DIAGNOSIS

- *Pain in the calf or thigh, often associated with edema. Fifty percent of patients are asymptomatic.*
- *History of congestive heart failure, recent surgery, trauma, neoplasia, oral contraceptive use, or prolonged inactivity.*
- *Physical signs unreliable.*
- *Duplex ultrasound is diagnostic.*

General Considerations

Acute DVT affects as many as 800,000 new patients per year. Treatment of this disease is estimated to cost $1–2.5 billion per year, not including costs associated with long-term sequelae.

Although the cause is often multifactorial, Virchow's triad (stasis, vascular injury, and hypercoagulability) defines the events that predispose a vein to the development of thrombophlebitis. Trauma to the endothelium of the vein wall results in exposure of subendothelial tissues to platelets. With venous stasis, platelet aggregates form on the vein wall and deposition of fibrin, leukocytes, and erythrocytes results in a free-floating thrombus. Within 7–10 days, this thrombus becomes adherent to the vein wall and secondary inflammatory changes develop, though a free-floating tail may persist. The thrombus is ultimately invaded by fibroblasts, resulting in neovascularization and scarring of the vein wall and destruction of the valves. Central recanalization usually follows, with restoration of flow through the vein; however, because the valves are damaged irreparably, chronic venous insufficiency with postphlebitis syndrome occurs in approximately 35% of patients. In 80% of cases, the thrombosis begins in the deep veins of the calf. Propagation into the popliteal and femoral veins takes place in approximately 25% of these cases.

Clinical manifestations of thrombophlebitis develop in about 3% of patients undergoing major general surgical procedures, and asymptomatic DVT develops in up to 30%. Certain operations, such as total hip replacement, are associated with appreciably higher incidences of thromboembolic complications. Prolonged bed rest or immobility caused by cardiac failure, stroke, ventilatory support, pelvic bone or limb fracture, paralysis, extended air travel, or a lengthy operative procedure is one contributing factor. A hypercoagulable state resulting from malignancy, nephrotic syndrome, inherited deficiency in protein C or S or antithrombin III, homocystinuria, factor V Leiden mutation, or paroxysmal nocturnal hemoglobinuria may also play a role. Other risk factors for DVT include advanced age, type A blood group, obesity, previous thrombosis, multiparity, use of oral contraceptives, inflammatory bowel disease, and lupus erythematosus. Oral contraceptives should be avoided in women who smoke or who have a history of phlebitis because of the high associated risk of thrombotic disease.

Clinical Findings

A. Symptoms and Signs

Fifty percent of patients with thrombophlebitis and 60–70% with acute pulmonary embolism have no symptoms or signs in the involved extremity. Symptomatic patients with DVT may complain of a dull ache, tightness, or pain in the calf or leg, especially when walking. Physical examination may disclose slight edema of the involved calf, a palpable cord, distention of the superficial venous collaterals, or low-grade fever and tachycardia. Homans' sign (pain on passive dorsiflexion of the ankle) is positive in only 50% of cases. Iliofemoral venous thrombosis can result in cyanosis of the skin (phlegmasia cerulea dolens) or a pale, cool extremity if reflex arterial spasm is superimposed (phlegmasia alba dolens).

B. Diagnostic Techniques

Because of the difficulty in making a precise diagnosis by history and physical examination and because of the morbidity associated with treatment, diagnostic studies should be used liberally.

1. Duplex ultrasonography—Duplex ultrasonography, because of its high sensitivity, specificity, and reproducibility, has supplanted venography as the most widely used diagnostic test in the initial evaluation of patients in whom this disorder is suspected. The examination includes both a B mode image and Doppler flow analysis. Each venous segment is assessed for the presence of thrombosis, indicated by venous dilation and incompressibility during light probe pressure. Doppler findings suggestive of acute thrombosis are absence of spontaneous flow, loss of flow variation with respiration, and failure to increase flow velocity with distal augmentation. The criteria for the presence of chronic venous thrombosis are less well established. The chronically occluded vein is often narrowed, and there are prominent nearby collaterals. Chronic thrombi are highly echogenic, whereas acute thrombi are anechoic (and therefore not visible) on the B mode image.

2. Ascending contrast venography—This study is used rarely because it is invasive and exposes the patient to ionizing radiation and the risks of contrast allergy, contrast-induced nephropathy, and phlebitis. Patients in whom DVT is strongly suspected but ultrasound is equivocal are now being referred for gadolinium-enhanced magnetic resonance venography. In experienced hands, this examination has a sensitivity of 100% and a specificity of 96% and may provide some information about the age of the thrombus.

3. D-dimer test—Recent evidence suggests that a negative D-dimer test in a patient in whom DVT is suspected is sufficient to omit ultrasound testing.

Differential Diagnosis

Localized muscle strain or contusion or Achilles tendon rupture can often mimic thrombophlebitis. Cellulitis can have a similar clinical presentation: edema, localized pain, and erythema. Other causes of unilateral leg edema (lymphedema, rupture of a Baker cyst, obstruction of the popliteal vein by a Baker cyst, obstruction of the iliac vein by tumor or fibrosis, or external compression of the left iliac vein by the right common

iliac artery, known as May–Thurner syndrome) and bilateral leg edema (heart, liver, or kidney failure, or vena caval obstruction by tumor, retroperitoneal fibrosis, or pregnancy) must be excluded.

Complications

Complications of DVT include pulmonary embolism (see Chapter 9), varicose veins, and chronic venous insufficiency.

Prevention

Prophylactic measures may diminish the incidence of venous thrombosis in hospitalized patients. Choice of therapy is dependent on stratification of individual patient risk factors.

A. Nonpharmacologic Measures

Venous stasis can be minimized by several simple maneuvers. Elevation of the foot of the bed 15–20 degrees encourages venous outflow. Slight flexion of the knees is desirable. A footboard enables the patient to perform leg exercises (ankle flexion and extension) while in bed. Sitting in a chair for long periods in the early postoperative period should be avoided. Early ambulation is ideal. Graduated compression stockings and sequential compression devices have proven efficacy in reducing risk of calf vein thrombosis and are particularly useful in moderate-risk and high-risk patients in whom anticoagulation is contraindicated. They function by increasing venous flow, decreasing venous stasis, and increasing the release of endothelial fibrinolytic factors and are safe for use on almost all patients. They have not been shown to decrease the incidence of pulmonary emboli.

B. Anticoagulation

Low-dose unfractionated heparin, 5000 units subcutaneously twice daily, and low-molecular-weight heparin (LMWH), eg, with enoxaparin, 30 mg subcutaneously twice daily, have both been shown to reduce significantly the incidence of postoperative DVT and pulmonary embolism. LMWH appears to be more effective in the orthopedic surgery patient and is associated also with a lower risk of bleeding complications (1–5% with enoxaparin versus 2–12% with unfractionated heparin). Use of heparin products is contraindicated in patients with recent craniotomy, intracranial bleeding, or severe gastrointestinal bleeding. Either medication must be withheld 12 hours prior to placement or removal of an epidural catheter to avoid epidural hematoma. Coagulation studies are unaffected with prophylactic dosing, but the platelet count must be monitored for early detection of heparin-induced thrombocytopenia, which occurs with peak incidence at 5–10 days of treatment. Warfarin is seldom used for perioperative DVT prophylaxis except for orthopedic surgery, but may be indicated for long-term management of minimally ambulatory patients. Lifetime anticoagulation with low-dose warfarin or prophylactic vena caval filter placement is considered in patients with hypercoagulable state or paralysis.

Treatment

The standard treatment of DVT is systemic anticoagulation with heparin (initial bolus 100 units/kg followed by 10 units/kg/h, dosed to a goal partial thromboplastin time of 1.5–2 times normal). This reduces the risk of pulmonary embolism and decreases the rate of thrombophlebitis recurrence by 80%. Systemic anticoagulation does not directly lyse thrombi but stops propagation and allows natural fibrinolysis to occur.

Warfarin is started after therapeutic heparinization. The two therapies should overlap to diminish the possibility of a hypercoagulable state, which can occur during the first few days of warfarin administration because warfarin also inhibits synthesis of the natural anticoagulant proteins C and S. The recommended treatment for the first episode of uncomplicated DVT is 3–6 months of warfarin to maintain a goal INR of 2.0–3.0. After a second episode, warfarin is continued indefinitely. The risk for recurrent venous thrombosis is increased markedly in the presence of factor V Leiden mutations, homozygous activated protein C resistance, antiphospholipid antibody, and deficiencies of antithrombin III and of protein C or protein S, so lifelong anticoagulation is also recommended for these conditions.

Recently, enoxaparin at therapeutic dosing (1 mg/kg subcutaneously twice daily) has been shown to be equally safe and effective for treatment of DVT. Enoxaparin does not require monitoring of its anticoagulant effect because of its predictable dose–response relationship, so it has been promoted for use in outpatient treatment. Unfractionated heparin inhibits thrombin by complexing thrombin and antithrombin III. The enoxaparin molecule is too small to inhibit thrombin in this manner; its main therapeutic effect comes from inhibition of factor Xa activity, which accounts for its lower risk of bleeding complications and thrombocytopenia. It has also demonstrated less protein C and S inhibition, less complement activation, and a lower risk of osteoporosis.

Current research efforts are directed toward creation of an oral thrombin inhibitor. This is expected to have a more favorable dose–response curve and side effect profile than warfarin.

Many studies have evaluated the efficacy of fibrinolytic agents in the treatment of acute DVT. Although faster clot lysis and increased venous patency are observed with alteplase versus heparin, this has not translated to a decreased incidence of postphlebitis syndrome. Risk of bleeding complications is higher with alteplase and does not appear to be reduced by selective catheterization for local administration. To be effective, it is felt that alteplase should be instituted within 1 week after clot formation, before extensive fibrin cross-linking can occur. One indication for alteplase is acute iliofemoral venous thrombosis complicated by massive extremity edema and cyanosis. In this setting, iliofemoral thrombectomy is unsuccessful in as many as 50% of patients, often because of an inability to effectively treat distal thrombosis.

Treatment of isolated calf vein thrombosis is controversial, as it is associated with a low risk of pulmonary emboli. However, if untreated, 25% progress to the proximal deep veins, where the incidence of chronic venous insufficiency is 25% and that of fatal pulmonary embolism is 10%. Patients with symptomatic calf vein thrombosis should be anticoagulated; asymptomatic patients may be monitored expectantly with serial ultrasound examination.

Prognosis

With early and effective treatment, prognosis in most cases is good. Mortality is related to pulmonary embolism, which occurs in 60% of patients with inadequately treated proximal lower extremity thrombosis.

Goodacre S et al: Meta-analysis: The value of clinical assessment in the diagnosis of deep venous thrombosis. Ann Intern Med 2005;143:129. [PMID: 16027455]

Merli G: Anticoagulants in the treatment of deep vein thrombosis. Am J Med 2005;118(Suppl 8A):13S. [PMID: 16125510]

Wells PS et al: Evaluation of D-dimer in the diagnosis of suspected deep-vein thrombosis. N Engl J Med 2003;349:1203. [PMID: 14507948]

Winter M et al; Haemostoasis and Thrombosis Task Force of the British Committee for Standards in Haematology: Procedures for the outpatient management of patients with deep venous thrombosis. Clin Lab Haematol 2005;27:61. [PMID: 15686510]

THROMBOPHLEBITIS OF THE SUPERFICIAL VEINS

 ESSENTIALS OF DIAGNOSIS

- Induration, redness, and tenderness along a superficial vein.
- Often a history of recent intravenous line or trauma. No significant swelling of the extremity.

General Considerations

Superficial thrombophlebitis may occur spontaneously in patients with varicose veins, in pregnant or postpartum women, or in patients with thromboangiitis obliterans or Behçet's disease. It can also occur after trauma, such as a blow to the leg, or after intravenous infusion. A migratory thrombophlebitis may be a manifestation of abdominal cancer such as carcinoma of the pancreas (Trousseau's syndrome). The long saphenous vein and its tributaries are most often involved. Superficial thrombophlebitis is associated with occult DVT in about 20% of cases. Pulmonary emboli are rare unless extension into the deep venous system occurs.

Clinical Findings

The patient usually experiences a dull pain in the region of the involved vein. Induration, redness, and tenderness correspond to dilated, thrombosed superficial veins. Edema of the extremity and deep calf tenderness are absent unless the deep veins are involved. Chills and high fever suggest septic or suppurative phlebitis, which is most often encountered as a complication of an indwelling intravenous catheter. Plastic intravenous catheters should be observed daily for signs of local inflammation and removed if a local reaction develops to avoid serious thrombotic or septic complications.

Differential Diagnosis

The linear rather than circular nature of the lesion and the distribution along the course of a superficial vein help differentiate superficial phlebitis from cellulitis, erythema nodosum, erythema induratum, panniculitis, and fibrositis. Lymphangitis and deep thrombophlebitis must also be considered.

Treatment

The primary treatment of superficial venous thrombophlebitis is the administration of nonsteroidal antiinflammatory drugs, local heat, and elevation. Ambulation is encouraged. In the majority of circumstances, symptoms will resolve within 7–10 days. Excision of the involved vein is recommended for symptoms that persist over 2 weeks on treatment, or for recurrent phlebitis in the same vein segment. If there is progressive proximal extension to the saphenofemoral junction or cephalic–subclavian junction, ligation and resection of the vein at the junction should be performed. Anticoagulation is reserved for rapidly progressing disease or extension into the deep vein system.

Septic thrombophlebitis requires treatment with intravenous antibiotics. As the causative organism is often *Staphylococcus* or a gram-negative rod, broad-spectrum antibiotic coverage should be instituted until blood culture results become available. If rapid resolution of the phlebitis occurs, no treatment beyond a 7- to 10-day course of antibiotics is required. However, if the patient becomes septic, immediate excision of the infected vein is required.

Prognosis

The course is generally benign and brief, and the prognosis depends on the underlying pathologic process. Phlebitis of a saphenous vein occasionally extends to the deep veins, in which case pulmonary emboli may occur.

Leon L et al: Clinical significance of superficial vein thrombosis. Eur J Vasc Endovasc Surg 2005;29:10. [PMID: 15570265]

CHRONIC VENOUS INSUFFICIENCY

 ESSENTIALS OF DIAGNOSIS

- History of phlebitis or leg injury.
- Ankle edema is the earliest sign.
- Late signs are stasis pigmentation, dermatitis, subcutaneous induration, varicosities, and ulceration.

General Considerations

Chronic venous insufficiency is most often secondary to DVT, although a history of phlebitis is not obtainable in about 25% of patients. Other possible causes are leg trauma, varicose veins, neoplastic obstruction of the pelvic veins, or congenital or acquired arteriovenous fistula.

The basic physiologic abnormality in patients with chronic venous insufficiency is chronic elevation in venous pressure. The normal venous capacitance can accommodate large-volume changes that occur during exercise with only minimal changes in venous pressure. However, when valves in the deep or perforating veins are destroyed by thrombophlebitis, valvular reflux and bidirectional blood flow result in abnormally high ambulatory venous pressures. Proximal venous obstruction also results in venous hypertension. High ambulatory venous pressure transmitted through perforating veins of the calf and ankle results in superficial varicosities, edema and fibrosis of the subcutaneous tissue and skin, hyperpigmentation and, later, dermatitis and ulceration.

Clinical Findings

Chronic venous insufficiency is characterized by progressive edema of the leg that begins at the ankle and calf and is accompanied by a dull aching discomfort. Typically, the edema is worst at the end of the day and improves with leg elevation. Varicosities are often present. Stasis dermatitis, brownish pigmentation, brawny induration, and ulceration develop with long-standing disease. The skin is usually thin, shiny, atrophic, and cyanotic. Cellulitis may appear in scaly, dry, itchy regions with skin breakdown; in other areas, a weeping dermatitis may develop. Venous stasis ulcers are large, painless, and irregular in outline. They have a shallow, moist granulation bed and occur in the gaiter area on the medial or lateral aspects of the ankle. Healing of these ulcers results in a thin scar on a fibrotic base that often breaks down with minor trauma.

Differential Diagnosis

Congestive heart failure and chronic renal disease may result in bilateral edema of the lower extremities. Lymphedema is associated with a brawny thickening in the subcutaneous tissue that does not respond readily to elevation; edema is particularly prominent on the dorsum of the feet and in the toes; varicosities are absent, and there is often a history of recurrent cellulitis.

Primary varicose veins or acute DVT may be difficult to differentiate from chronic venous insufficiency without diagnostic tests.

Other conditions associated with chronic ulcers of the leg include autoimmune diseases (eg, Felty's syndrome), arterial insufficiency (often painful, well circumscribed, and located over pressure points), sickle cell anemia, erythema induratum (bilateral and usually on the posterior aspect of the lower part of the leg), and fungal infections (cultures specific; no chronic swelling or varicosities).

Prevention

The irreversible tissue changes that accompany chronic venous stasis disease can be minimized by early and aggressive management of conditions associated with deep venous reflux such as acute DVT and varicose veins.

Treatment

A. General Measures

The key to successful management of chronic venous stasis disease is the realization that it is an incurable but manageable problem. Most patients respond to a conservative treatment program. The causes of complications of chronic venous insufficiency are largely mechanical, and so the solutions are mechanical. Bed rest with leg elevation is fundamental in the treatment of the acute complications. Similarly, long-term care of the leg includes (1) intermittent elevation of the legs during the day and elevation of the legs at night (kept above the level of the heart with pillows under the mattress), (2) avoidance of long periods of sitting or standing, (3) the daily use of fitted knee-high or thigh-high graduated compression stockings (20–30 mm Hg), and (4) regular exercise.

B. Management of Stasis Dermatitis

Eczematous eruption may be acute or chronic; treatment varies accordingly. The simplest treatment for acute weeping dermatitis is strict bed rest, leg elevation, and wet saline compresses. Antiseptic solutions containing peroxide, boric acid, or buffered aluminum acetate (Burow's solution) are not recommended because they impede wound healing. Cadexomer iodine is an iodine-containing starch powder dressing that has been shown to speed healing of weepy ulcers. Alginate dressings are also effective in this setting. In general, however, no definitive advantage has emerged of occlusive over semiocclusive dressings or of topical antibiotics, growth factors, or free radical scavengers over simple inert dressings.

Systemic antibiotics and topical antifungal agents (1% clotrimazole or 2% miconazole cream) are indicated only if active infection is suspected. With reduction of the acute edema, 0.5% hydrocortisone cream is applied to the area for 1–2 weeks or until no further improvement is noted. Cordran tape, a plastic tape impregnated with flurandrenolide, is a convenient way to apply both medication and dressing. Zinc oxide ointment with ichthammol, 3%, applied once or twice daily, is an alternative treatment for chronic dermatitis.

C. Ulceration

Venous ulcerations can be treated by wet-to-dry normal saline dressings and Ace wrap compression, or with an Unna boot. The Unna boot is a layered dressing composed of a medicated bandage (such as the original Dome paste composed of calamine, zinc oxide, glycerin, sorbitol, gelatin, and magnesium aluminum silicate), followed by a gauze dressing, followed by an elastic wrap. It must be kept dry and is usually changed weekly. Occasionally, the ulcer is so large and chronic that wide debridement and skin grafting are the best approach. This can be combined with open or endoscopic ligation of incompetent perforating veins contributing to elevated venous pressure in the ulcer bed. Venous reconstructive surgery is performed in some centers for intractable chronic venous stasis disease. The goal of the surgery is to increase venous outflow and decrease venous hypertension in the limb by repairing or replacing incompetent valves in the deep system. Valvuloplasty, venous segment transposition, and valvular transplantation have been performed with variable reported success rates.

Prognosis

Recurrent venous stasis ulcers and progressive venous stasis changes of the skin are not uncommon, particularly if patients do not adhere to a lifelong routine of intermittent leg elevation, regular exercise, and use of graduated compression stockings.

Barwell JR et al: Comparison of surgery and compression with compression alone in chronic venous ulceration (ESCHAR study): randomised controlled trial. Lancet 2004;363:1854. [PMID: 15183623]

Beebe-Dimmer JL et al: The epidemiology of chronic venous insufficiency and varicose veins. Ann Epidemiol 2005;15:175. [PMID: 15723761]

Kahn SR et al: Relationship between deep venous thrombosis and the postthrombotic syndrome. Arch Intern Med 2004;164:17. [PMID: 14718318]

SUPERIOR VENA CAVA OBSTRUCTION

Superior vena cava syndrome is a rare disorder caused by partial or complete obstruction of the superior vena cava. The most frequent causes are (1) superior mediastinal tumors (responsible for over 80% of cases), such as adenocarcinoma of the lung, lymphoma, thyroid carcinoma, thymoma, teratoma, synovial cell carcinoma, or angiosarcoma; (2) chronic fibrotic mediastinitis, either idiopathic or secondary to tuberculosis, histoplasmosis, pyogenic infections, or drugs (such as methysergide); (3) thrombophlebitis secondary to indwelling central venous catheters or pacemaker wires; (4) aneurysm of the aortic arch; and (5) constrictive pericarditis.

Clinical Findings

A. Symptoms and Signs

Symptoms include swelling of the neck and face, headache, dizziness, visual disturbances, stupor, and syncope related to progressive obstruction of the venous drainage of the head, neck, and upper extremities. Bending over or lying down accentuates the symptoms; sitting quietly is generally preferred. The severity of symptoms is dependent on the degree and duration of stenosis and the development of venous collateral circulation. Dilated anterior chest wall veins and facial flushing ultimately can progress to brawny edema and cyanosis of the face and arms. Cerebral and laryngeal edema result in impaired mental status and respiratory insufficiency.

B. DIAGNOSIS

Diagnosis is usually suggested by the history and physical examination. Duplex ultrasound can be suggestive, but more specific anatomic information is obtained with CT scan or MRA, which can also disclose etiologic causes. Contrast venography is reserved for cases in which surgical or endoscopic treatment is anticipated.

Treatment

Therapy is dictated by the cause of the disease and the severity of symptoms. Benign thrombosis is treated with central venous catheter removal, head elevation, and short-course warfarin anticoagulation or thrombolysis and venous angioplasty. Venous bypass (left atrial appendage to internal jugular or innominate vein) has good patency rates in selected patients refractory to more conservative measures. Surgical excision of the fibrous tissue encasing the great vessels may reestablish flow in patients with mediastinal fibrosis or pericardial constriction. Unless concomitant tumor resection is planned, superior vena cava syndrome secondary to malignant disease is preferentially treated by endovascular stenting. Chemotherapy or external beam radiation may also achieve symptomatic improvement in patients with malignancy.

Bays S et al: Fibrosing mediastinitis as a cause of superior vena cava syndrome. Eur J Cardiothorac Surg 2004;26:453. [PMID: 15296918]

Urruticoechea A et al: Treatment of malignant superior vena cava syndrome by endovascular stent insertion. Experience on 52 patients with lung cancer. Lung Cancer 2004;43:209. [PMID: 14739042]

■ DISEASES OF THE LYMPHATIC CHANNELS

LYMPHANGITIS & LYMPHADENITIS

ESSENTIALS OF DIAGNOSIS

- *Red streak extending from an infected area toward enlarged, tender regional lymph nodes.*
- *Chills, fever, and malaise may be present.*

General Considerations

Lymphangitis and lymphadenitis frequently accompany a streptococcal or staphylococcal infection in the distal arm or leg. The inciting wound may be a superficial scratch with cellulitis, an insect bite, or an established abscess. A prominent red streak extending toward tender, enlarged regional lymph nodes is diagnostic. Systemic manifestations include fever, chills, tachycardia, and malaise. If untreated, the infection can progress rapidly, often in a matter of hours.

Clinical Findings

A. SYMPTOMS AND SIGNS

Throbbing pain at the site of the inciting wound is usually present. Malaise, anorexia, sweating, chills, and fever of 37.8–40 °C develop rapidly. The red streak may be faint initially and easily missed, especially in dark-skinned patients. The involved regional lymph nodes may be significantly enlarged and tender.

B. LABORATORY FINDINGS

Leukocytosis with a left shift is usually present. Blood cultures are often positive for staphylococcal or streptococcal species. Wound cultures may be helpful in the treatment of more severe or refractory infections but are often difficult to interpret because of skin contaminants.

Differential Diagnosis

Superficial thrombophlebitis is distinguished from lymphangitis by the pattern of erythema (localized to an indurated thrombosed vein) and the lack of lymphadenitis. Cat-scratch disease caused by *Bartonella henselae* typically presents with enlarged but nontender lymph nodes. Lymphangitis must also be differentiated from cellulitis and from severe soft tissue infections such as acute streptococcal hemolytic gangrene and necrotizing fasciitis requiring emergent debridement. These infections are nonlinear and are characterized by induration and subcutaneous crepitus.

Treatment

The extremity is elevated, and warm compresses are applied to the involved area. Analgesics and intravenous antibiotics (penicillin G, 4 million units every 6 hours, or cefazolin, 1 g every 8 hours) should be instituted immediately. Examination of the wound will determine the need for debridement or incision and drainage of an abscess.

Prognosis

Early institution of appropriate antibiotic therapy and wound care will usually control the infection in 48–72 hours. Delayed or inadequate therapy can result in rapidly progressive infection, septicemia, and death.

Badger C et al: Antibiotics/anti-inflammatories for reducing acute inflammatory episodes in lymphoedema of the limbs. Cochrane Database Syst Rev 2004;(2):CD003143. [PMID: 15106193]

LYMPHEDEMA

ESSENTIALS OF DIAGNOSIS

- *Painless edema of upper or lower extremities.*
- *Involves the dorsal surfaces of the hands and fingers or the feet and toes.*
- *Developmental or acquired, unilateral or bilateral.*
- *Edema is pitting initially and becomes brawny and nonpitting with time.*
- *Ulceration, varicosities, and stasis pigmentation do not occur. There may be episodes of lymphangitis and cellulitis.*

General Considerations

The underlying mechanism in lymphedema is impairment of the flow of lymph from an extremity. When due to congenital developmental abnormalities consisting of hypoplastic or hyperplastic changes of the proximal or distal lymphatics, it is referred to as primary lymphedema. Familial lymphedema developing before 1 year of age is called Milroy's disease; it is usually bilateral and affects boys more often than girls. More commonly, lymphedema develops during adolescence (lymphedema praecox) and is unilateral; there is a 3.5:1 female predominance. Lymphedema occurring after age 35 years is referred to as lymphedema tarda. The secondary form of lymphedema results from an inflammatory or mechanical obstruction of the lymphatics following trauma, regional lymph node resection, irradiation, bacterial or fungal infections, lymphoproliferative diseases, or filariasis.

Lymphatic obstruction results in stasis of a protein-rich fluid, with slowly progressive, painless edema and secondary fibrosis that may be exacerbated by superimposed episodes of acute infection. The edema is usually centered around the ankle and involves the toes and the dorsum of the foot. Hypertrophy of the limb results, with markedly thickened skin and subcutaneous tissue. Rarely, lymphangiosarcoma or angiosarcoma may develop as a complication of chronic lymphedema. This neoplastic transformation of blood vessels and lymphatics is called the Stewart–Treves syndrome.

Diagnosis is usually made on the basis of clinical findings. Venous duplex ultrasonography is performed to exclude venous insufficiency or vascular malformations. Lymphangiography and radioactive isotope studies are indicated only if surgical reconstruction is anticipated.

Treatment

Lymphedema is a chronic disease for which there is no complete cure. However, a variety of conservative measures can substantially reduce the risk of further complications and disability. No drug therapy is effective. Use of benzopyrones (eg, dicumarol) and corticosteroid injections to increase lymphatic transport has not shown consistent benefit. Diuretics can be useful for acute exacerbation of edema secondary to infection or for coexisting venous stasis disease but are not recommended for long-term use.

The mainstay of treatment is external compression and meticulous skin care. Mechanical reduction of lymphedema can best be achieved with a program of frequent leg elevation, manual lymphatic drainage massage, and external compression. Sequential pneumatic compression devices are traditionally the first line of treatment for limb reduction. Many different devices are available for use on the leg, and Reid sleeves can be custom fit for patients with postmastectomy arm lymphedema. Graduated compression stockings (20–30 mm Hg) maintain the limb after reduction by pneumatic compression.

Good skin care is imperative to prevent infection. Moisturizing lotions should be applied regularly, especially after showering or bathing. Drying and cracking of the skin can create portals of entry for bacteria. Infection is difficult to eradicate because of disordered lymphatic drainage and can be a threat to limb survival.

In carefully selected cases, surgery may improve limb function. The goal is to reduce limb bulk, either by ablative techniques (excision of excess tissue) or by physiologic techniques (lymphatic reconstruction). Microsurgical lymphaticovenous anastomosis has yielded some satisfactory cosmetic and functional results, though long-term efficacy is as yet unknown.

Hinrichs CS et al: Lymphedema secondary to postmastectomy radiation: incidence and risk factors. Ann Surg Oncol 2004; 11:573. [PMID: 15172932]

Kligman L et al: The treatment of lymphedema related to breast cancer: a systematic review and evidence summary. Support Care Cancer 2004;12:421. [PMID: 15095073]

Northup KA et al: Syndromic classification of hereditary lymphedema. Lymphology 2003;36:162. [PMID: 14992570]

Ozaslan C et al: Lymphedema after treatment of breast cancer. Am J Surg 2004;187:69. [PMID: 14706589]

Sieggreen MY et al: Current concepts in lymphedema management. Adv Skin Wound Care 2004;17(4 Pt 1):174. [PMID: 15360026]

Taylor MJ et al: Macrofilaricidal activity after doxycycline treatment of *Wuchereria bancrofti*: a double-blind, randomised placebo-controlled trial. Lancet. 2005;365:2116. [PMID: 15964448]

■ HYPOTENSION & SHOCK

 ESSENTIALS OF DIAGNOSIS

- *Hypotension, tachycardia, oliguria, altered mental status.*
- *Peripheral hypoperfusion and hypoxia.*

General Considerations

Shock occurs when the rate of arterial blood flow is inadequate to meet tissue metabolic needs. Tissue oxygen delivery is dependent on cardiac output, hemoglobin saturation, and peripheral microcirculation—some or all of these factors are altered in the shock state. The physiologic response to shock is mediated by the neuroendocrine system through release of catecholamines, renin, antidiuretic hormone, glucagon, cortisol, and growth hormone. These hormones are responsible for many of the clinical manifestations of shock: tachycardia, oliguria, delayed capillary refill, increasing agitation, and insulin resistance. Treatment must be directed both at the manifestations of shock and at its cause.

Classification

A. HYPOVOLEMIC SHOCK

Decreased intravascular volume resulting from loss of blood, plasma, or fluids and electrolytes may be obvious (eg, external hemorrhage) or subtle (eg, sequestration in a "third space") (Table 12–1). Compensatory vasoconstriction temporarily reduces the size of the vascular bed and may transiently maintain the blood pressure, but unreplaced ongoing losses of over 15% of the blood volume result in hypotension, increased peripheral resistance, collapse of capillary and venous beds, and progressive tissue hypoxia. Even a moderate sudden loss of circulating fluids can result in severe damage to vital organs.

B. CARDIOGENIC SHOCK

Pump failure can be related to myocardial infarction, cardiomyopathy, myocardial contusion, valvular incompetence or stenosis, or arrhythmias (Table 12–1). See discussion in Chapter 10.

C. OBSTRUCTIVE SHOCK

Cardiac tamponade, tension pneumothorax, and massive pulmonary embolism can cause an acute decrease in cardiac output resulting in shock (Table 12–1). These are medical emergencies requiring prompt diagnosis and treatment. Pericardiocentesis or pericardial window, chest tube placement, or catheter-directed thrombolytic therapy can be lifesaving.

Table 12–1. Classification of shock by mechanism and common causes.

Hypovolemic shock
  Loss of blood (hemorrhagic shock)
    External hemorrhage
      Trauma
      Gastrointestinal tract bleeding
    Internal hemorrhage
      Hematoma
      Hemothorax or hemoperitoneum
  Loss of plasma
    Burns
    Exfoliative dermatitis
  Loss of fluid and electrolytes
    External
      Vomiting
      Diarrhea
      Excessive sweating
      Hyperosmolar states (diabetic ketoacidosis, hyperosmolar nonketotic coma)
    Internal ("third spacing")
      Pancreatitis
      Ascites
      Bowel obstruction
Cardiogenic shock
  Dysrhythmia
    Tachyarrhythmia
    Bradyarrhythmia
  "Pump failure" (secondary to myocardial infarction or other cardiomyopathy)
  Acute valvular dysfunction (especially regurgitant lesions)
  Rupture of ventricular septum or free ventricular wall
Obstructive shock
  Tension pneumothorax
  Pericardial disease (tamponade, constriction)
  Disease of pulmonary vasculature (massive pulmonary emboli, pulmonary hypertension)
  Cardiac tumor (atrial myxoma)
  Left atrial mural thrombus
  Obstructive valvular disease (aortic or mitral stenosis)
Distributive shock
  Septic shock
  Anaphylactic shock
  Neurogenic shock
  Vasodilator drugs
  Acute adrenal insufficiency

Reproduced, with permission, from Saunders CE, Ho MT (editors): *Current Emergency Diagnosis & Treatment*, 4th ed. McGraw-Hill, 1992.

D. DISTRIBUTIVE SHOCK

Reduction in systemic vascular resistance from sepsis, anaphylaxis, systemic inflammatory response syndrome (SIRS) produced by severe pancreatitis or burns, or acute adrenal insufficiency may result in inadequate cardiac output despite normal circulatory volume (Table 12–1). Elevated nitric oxide levels may explain many of the physiologic aspects of the disease.

1. Septic shock—Sepsis is the most common cause of distributive shock and carries a mortality of 40–80%. Typically, patients present with fever, chills, hypotension, hyperglycemia, and altered mental status due to gram-negative bacteremia (*E coli, Klebsiella, Proteus,* and *Pseudomonas*). Gram-positive cocci and gram-negative anaerobes (*Bacteroides*) are less often implicated. Risk factors include extremes of age, diabetes, immunosuppression, and recent urinary, biliary, or gynecologic manipulation, such as placement of a percutaneous nephrostomy or biliary drain in an obstructed system.

2. Neurogenic shock—Neurogenic shock is caused by traumatic spinal cord injury or effects of an epidural or spinal anesthetic. Reflex vagal parasympathetic stimulation evoked by pain, gastric dilation, or fright may simulate neurogenic shock, producing hypotension, bradycardia, and syncope.

Diagnosis of Shock & Impending Shock

The different types of shock are characterized by the same clinical signs.

A. HYPOTENSION

Hypotension in adults is traditionally defined as a systolic blood pressure of 90 mm Hg or less but must be evaluated relative to the patient's normal blood pressure. Whereas a systolic blood pressure of 90 mm Hg may be normal in a healthy, athletic adult, a pressure of 100 mm Hg may indicate shock in a patient who is normally hypertensive. A drop in systolic pressure of more than 10–20 mm Hg and an increase in pulse of more than 15 with positional change suggest depleted intravascular volume. Orthostatic hypotension resulting from peripheral neuropathy or use of β-blockers is usually not associated with an increase in pulse rate.

B. END-ORGAN HYPOPERFUSION

Patients in shock often have cool or mottled extremities and weak or absent peripheral pulses. Splanchnic vasoconstriction leads to oliguria, bowel ischemia, and hepatic dysfunction, which can ultimately result in multiorgan failure.

C. ALTERED MENTAL STATUS

Patients may demonstrate normal mental status or may be restless, agitated, confused, lethargic, or comatose as a result of inadequate perfusion of the brain.

Treatment

A. GENERAL MEASURES

Treatment depends on prompt diagnosis and an accurate appraisal of inciting conditions. Initial therapy consists of basic life support: airway maintenance, oxygen, cardiopulmonary resuscitation, intravenous access, and fluid resuscitation. Cardiac monitoring can detect myocardial ischemia requiring cardiac catheterization and thrombolytic therapy or malignant arrhythmias treated by standard advanced cardiac life support (ACLS) protocols. A thorough history and physical examination, including stool guaiac testing, is helpful in locating potential sources of sepsis or hemorrhage and excluding immediately reversible causes such as tamponade or tension pneumothorax. Unresponsive or minimally responsive patients are immediately given 50% dextrose (one ampule intravenously) and naloxone (2 mg intravenously or intramuscularly) followed by neurologic assessment (Glasgow Coma Scale) and are then intubated for airway protection. Specimens should be sent for complete blood count, electrolytes, glucose, arterial blood gas determinations, coagulation parameters, and typing and cross-matching. An arterial line is placed for continuous blood pressure measurement and a Foley catheter for assessment of urine volume. Urinary output should be maintained at > 0.5 mL/kg/h.

Early consideration is given to placement of a pulmonary artery catheter for hemodynamic pressure measurements or transthoracic echocardiography. This is helpful in distinguishing cardiogenic and septic shock and in monitoring the effects of volume resuscitation or pressor medications. Because of the attendant risks associated with pulmonary artery catheters (infection, arrhythmias, vein thrombosis, pulmonary artery rupture), the value of the information they might provide must be carefully weighed in each patient. They are useful in the management of patients with cardiogenic shock; in other types of shock, a central venous line may be adequate. Central lines may also be useful in the administration of medications and in the measurement of central venous oxygen saturation. In general, a central venous pressure (CVP) or pulmonary capillary wedge pressure (PCWP) under 5 mm Hg suggests hypovolemia and over 18 mm Hg suggests volume overload, cardiac failure, tamponade, or pulmonary hypertension. A cardiac index < 2 L/min/m^2 indicates a need for pharmacologic or mechanical pressor support. A high cardiac index (> 4 L/min/m^2) in a hypotensive patient is consistent with early septic shock. The systemic vascular resistance (SVR) is a derived value and is low (< 800 dyn · s/cm^5) in early sepsis and neurogenic shock and high (> 1500 dyn · s/cm^5) in hypovolemic and cardiogenic shock. Treatment is directed at maintaining a CVP of 8–12 mm Hg, a mean arterial pressure of 65–90 mm Hg, a cardiac index of 2–4 L/min/m^2, and central venous oxygen saturation of greater than 70%.

B. VOLUME REPLACEMENT

Hypovolemic shock is treated with fluid resuscitation. Initial response is gauged after bolus administration of 2 L of crystalloid, and additional fluid requirements are then estimated from measurement of ongoing losses, CVP or PCWP, and urinary output.

Selection of the proper fluid for restoration and maintenance of hemodynamic stability is controversial. Blood products are indicated in hemorrhagic shock; type-specific or type O negative packed red blood cells (PRBC) are given to maintain the hematocrit above 30%. Whole blood provides extra volume and clotting factors. Each unit of PRBC or whole blood is expected to raise the hematocrit by 3%. With abnormal coagulation studies, platelet count less than 10,000/mcL, or transfusion of over six units of PRBC, fresh frozen plasma and platelets should be administered. When hematocrit is greater than 30% and CVP is less than 8 mm Hg, crystalloid solutions are generally the preferred resuscitation fluid. Isotonic (0.9%) sodium chloride or lactated Ringer's solution (which contains potassium, calcium, and bicarbonate as well as sodium chloride) is given in boluses of 500 mL or 1000 mL. Dextrose-containing solutions are generally not needed initially except in the treatment of hypoglycemic shock. Hypertonic (7.5%) saline is being investigated for use in the prehospital setting and in the hypotensive patient with closed head injury.

Plasma expanders—or colloids such as albumin, dextran, and hetastarch—are high-molecular-weight substances that increase plasma oncotic pressure. Increased capillary permeability in the lung accompanying septic shock or SIRS may result in increased pulmonary edema in patients administered colloids, so use of these agents warrants careful consideration. Side effects include coagulopathy and anaphylaxis. Oxygen-carrying synthetic plasma expanders ("artificial blood") have been used with success in some trauma centers for treatment of hypovolemic shock.

Large-volume resuscitation with unwarmed fluids produces hypothermia, which must be treated to avoid hypothermia-induced coagulopathy.

C. Medications

Calcium should be administered to maintain an ionized calcium level greater than 1.15 mmol/L. Sodium bicarbonate may be considered in patients with arterial pH less than 7.20.

Pressors are administered only after adequate fluid resuscitation. Dopamine hydrochloride has variable effects according to dosage. At low doses (2–3 mcg/kg/min), stimulation of dopaminergic and β-agonist receptors produces increased glomerular filtration rate, heart rate, and contractility. At higher doses (> 5 mcg/kg/min), α-adrenergic effects predominate, resulting in peripheral vasoconstriction.

Dobutamine (2–20 mcg/kg/min), a synthetic catecholamine with greater inotropic effect and afterload reduction than dopamine, is the first-line drug for cardiogenic shock. Because tachyphylaxis can occur after 48 hours, the phosphodiesterase inhibitor amrinone (5–15 mcg/kg/min) is often substituted. Diuretics, thrombolytics, morphine, nitroglycerin, antiarrhythmics, and antiplatelet agents may be part of a multimodality approach to treatment of cardiogenic shock secondary to acute myocardial infarction.

Distributive shock or neurogenic shock may require peripheral vasoconstrictors such as epinephrine (2–10 mcg/min) or norepinephrine (0.5–30 mcg/min). Phenylephrine is avoided in neurogenic shock because of the potential for reflex bradycardia.

Vasopressin (antidiuretic hormone [ADH]) is gaining widespread acceptance in the treatment of distributive shock and has been added to the ACLS algorithm for ventricular fibrillation cardiac arrest. Shock due to sepsis or SIRS is associated with low levels of endogenous vasopressin; in hemorrhagic shock, vasopressin is initially elevated and then drops to subnormal levels. Vasopressin has multiple therapeutic effects: peripheral vasoconstriction, decreased heart rate, hemostasis, increased serum cortisol, and coronary, cerebral, and pulmonary vasodilation. It has also been shown to potentiate the effects of other peripheral vasoconstrictors. Paradoxically, at low doses (0.01–0.04 units/min), it acts as a diuretic. The dose is regulated to maintain normal physiologic serum levels of 20–30 pg/mL. The effect on mortality rate in septic shock is as yet unknown. Vasopressin-induced vasoconstriction may be mediated by effects on nitric oxide synthesis.

Methylene blue is another inhibitor of the nitric oxide pathway being investigated for use in distributive shock.

Broad-spectrum antibiotics are administered in septic shock until blood cultures and sensitivities become available. Sedation, anxiolytics, and pain medications are tailored for each individual case. Corticosteroids are lifesaving in the treatment of shock associated with acute adrenal insufficiency (see Chapter 26) and decrease inflammation associated with acute spinal shock, but they are of no benefit in other types of shock. Research has focused on regulation of specific inhibitors of the inflammatory response. Protein C levels are diminished in septic shock, and recombinant protein C (drotrecogin alfa) is now in phase 3 trials. It has been shown to significantly decrease 28-day mortality in septic shock when given as a continuous infusion of 24 mcg/kg/h for 96 hours. Its mechanism of action is reduction of systemic inflammation by inhibition of thrombosis. Administration of recombinant protein C has been correlated with lower D-dimer and interleukin-6 levels in this setting.

Other Treatment Modalities

Cardiac failure may require use of transcutaneous or transvenous pacing or placement of an intra-arterial balloon pump. Emergent revascularization by stent angioplasty or coronary artery bypass appears to improve long-term outcome. Urgent hemodialysis or continuous venovenous hemofiltration may be indicated for maintenance of fluid and electrolyte balance during acute renal insufficiency resulting from shock.

Annane D et al: Septic shock. Lancet 2005;365:63. [PMID: 15639681]

Duvernoy CS et al: Management of cardiogenic shock attributable to acute myocardial infarction in the reperfusion era. J Intensive Care Med 2005;20:188. [PMID: 16061902]

Gluck T et al: Advances in sepsis therapy. Drugs 2004;64:837. [PMID: 15059039]

Graham CA et al: Critical care in the emergency department: shock and circulatory support. Emerg Med J 2005;22:17. [PMID: 15611535]

Minneci PC et al: Meta-analysis: the effect of steroids on survival and shock during sepsis depends on the dose. Ann Intern Med 2004;141:47. [PMID: 15238370]

Weigand MA et al: The systemic inflammatory response syndrome. Best Pract Res Clin Anaesthesiol 2004;18:455. [PMID: 15212339]

Blood

13

Charles A. Linker, MD

■ ANEMIAS

General Approach to Anemias

Anemia is present in adults if the hematocrit is less than 41% (hemoglobin < 13.5 g/dL) in males or less than 37% (hemoglobin < 12 g/dL) in females. Congenital anemia is suggested by the patient's personal and family history. Poor diet results in folic acid deficiency and contributes to iron deficiency, but bleeding is much more commonly the cause of iron deficiency in adults. Physical examination includes attention to signs of primary hematologic diseases (lymphadenopathy, hepatosplenomegaly, or bone tenderness). Mucosal changes such as a smooth tongue suggest megaloblastic anemia.

Anemias are classified according to their pathophysiologic basis, ie, whether related to diminished production or accelerated loss of red blood cells (Table 13–1), or according to cell size (Table 13–2). The diagnostic possibilities in microcytic anemia are iron deficiency, thalassemia, and anemia of chronic disease. A severely microcytic anemia (mean cell volume [MCV] < 70 fL) is due either to iron deficiency or thalassemia. Macrocytic anemia may be due to megaloblastic (folate or vitamin B$_{12}$ deficiency) or nonmegaloblastic causes, in particular myelodysplasia and the use of antiretroviral drugs. A severely macrocytic anemia (MCV > 125 fL) is almost always megaloblastic; exceptions are the myelodysplastic syndromes.

IRON DEFICIENCY ANEMIA

 ESSENTIALS OF DIAGNOSIS

- Serum ferritin < 12 mcg/L.
- Caused by bleeding in adults unless proved otherwise.
- Responds to iron therapy.

General Considerations

Iron deficiency is the most common cause of anemia worldwide. The causes are listed in Table 13–3. Iron is necessary for the formation of heme and other enzymes. Total body iron ranges between 2 and 4 g: approximately 50 mg/kg in men and 35 mg/kg in women. Most (70–95%) of the iron is present in hemoglobin in circulating red blood cells. One milliliter of packed red blood cells (not whole blood) contains approximately 1 mg of iron. In men, red blood cell volume is approximately 30 mL/kg. A 70-kg man will therefore have approximately 2100 mL of packed red blood cells and consequently 2100 mg of iron in his circulating blood. In women, the red cell volume is about 27 mL/kg; a 50-kg woman will thus have 1350 mg of iron circulating in her red blood cells. Only 200–400 mg of iron is present in myoglobin and nonheme enzymes. Aside from circulating red blood cells, the major location of iron in the body is the storage pool, as ferritin or as hemosiderin and in macrophages. The range for storage iron is wide (0.5–2 g); approximately 25% of women in the United States have none.

The average American diet contains 10–15 mg of iron per day. About 10% of this amount is absorbed. Absorption occurs in the stomach, duodenum, and upper jejunum. Dietary iron present as heme is efficiently absorbed (10–20%) but nonheme iron less so (1–5%), largely because of interference by phosphates, tannins, and other food constituents. Small amounts of iron—approximately 1 mg/d—are normally lost though exfoliation of skin and mucosal cells. There is no physiologic mechanism for increasing normal body iron losses.

Menstrual blood loss in women plays a major role in iron metabolism. The average monthly menstrual blood loss is approximately 50 mL, or about 0.7 mg/d. However, menstrual blood loss may be five times the average. To maintain adequate iron stores, women with heavy menstrual losses must absorb 3–4 mg of iron from the diet each day. This strains the upper limit of what may reasonably be absorbed, and women with menorrhagia of this degree will almost always become iron deficient without iron supplementation.

In general, iron metabolism is balanced between absorption of 1 mg/d and loss of 1 mg/d. Pregnancy may also upset the iron balance, since requirements increase to 2–5 mg of iron per day during pregnancy and lactation. Normal dietary iron cannot supply these requirements, and medicinal iron is needed during pregnancy and lacta-

Table 13–1. Classification of anemias by pathophysiology.

Decreased production
  Hemoglobin synthesis: iron deficiency, thalassemia, anemia of chronic disease
  DNA synthesis: megaloblastic anemia
  Stem cell: aplastic anemia, myeloproliferative leukemia
  Bone marrow infiltration: carcinoma, lymphoma
  Pure red cell aplasia
Increased destruction
  Blood loss
  Hemolysis (intrinsic)
    Membrane: hereditary spherocytosis, elliptocytosis
    Hemoglobin: sickle cell, unstable hemoglobin
    Glycolysis: pyruvate kinase deficiency, etc
    Oxidation: glucose-6-phosphate dehydrogenase deficiency
  Hemolysis (extrinsic)
    Immune: warm antibody, cold antibody
    Microangiopathic: thrombotic thrombocytopenic purpura, hemolytic-uremic syndrome, mechanical cardiac valve, paravalvular leak
    Infection: clostridial
    Hypersplenism

tion. Repeated pregnancy (especially with breast-feeding) may cause iron deficiency if increased requirements are not met with supplemental medicinal iron. Decreased iron absorption can on very rare occasions cause iron deficiency and usually occurs after gastric surgery, though concomitant bleeding is frequent.

By far the most important cause of iron deficiency anemia is blood loss, especially gastrointestinal blood loss. Chronic aspirin use may cause it even without a documented structural lesion. Iron deficiency demands a search for a source of gastrointestinal bleeding if other sites of blood loss (menorrhagia, other uterine bleeding, and repeated blood donations) are excluded.

Table 13–2. Classification of anemias by mean cell volume.

Microcytic
  Iron deficiency
  Thalassemia
  Anemia of chronic disease
Macrocytic
  Megaloblastic
    Vitamin B_{12} deficiency
    Folate deficiency
  Nonmegaloblastic
    Myelodysplasia, chemotherapy
    Liver disease
    Increased reticulocytosis
    Myxedema
Normocytic
  Many causes

Table 13–3. Causes of iron deficiency.

Deficient diet
Decreased absorption
Increased requirements
  Pregnancy
  Lactation
Blood loss
  Gastrointestinal
  Menstrual
  Blood donation
Hemoglobinuria
Iron sequestration
  Pulmonary hemosiderosis

Chronic hemoglobinuria may lead to iron deficiency since iron is lost in the urine; traumatic hemolysis due to a prosthetic cardiac valve and other causes of intravascular hemolysis (eg, paroxysmal nocturnal hemoglobinuria) should also be considered.

Clinical Findings

A. SYMPTOMS AND SIGNS

As a rule, the only symptoms of iron deficiency anemia are those of the anemia itself (easy fatigability, tachycardia, palpitations and tachypnea on exertion). Severe deficiency causes skin and mucosal changes, including a smooth tongue, brittle nails, and cheilosis. Dysphagia because of the formation of esophageal webs (Plummer–Vinson syndrome) also occurs. Many iron-deficient patients develop pica, craving for specific foods (ice chips, etc) often not rich in iron.

B. LABORATORY FINDINGS

Iron deficiency develops in stages. The first is depletion of iron stores. At this point, there is anemia and no change in red blood cell size. The serum ferritin will become abnormally low. A ferritin value less than 30 mcg/L is a highly reliable indicator of iron deficiency. The serum total iron-binding capacity (TIBC) rises. Bone marrow biopsy for evaluation of iron stores is now rarely performed because of intraobserver variation in its interpretation.

After iron stores have been depleted, red blood cell formation will continue with deficient supplies of iron. Serum iron values decline to less than 30 mcg/dL and transferrin saturation to less than 15%.

In the early stages, the MCV remains normal. Subsequently, the MCV falls and the blood smear shows hypochromic microcytic cells. With further progression, anisocytosis (variations in red blood cell size) and poikilocytosis (variation in shape of red cells) develop. Severe iron deficiency will produce a bizarre peripheral blood smear, with severely hypochromic cells, target cells, hypochromic pencil-shaped cells, and occasionally small numbers of nucleated red blood cells. The platelet count is commonly increased.

Differential Diagnosis

Other causes of microcytic anemia include anemia of chronic disease, thalassemia, and sideroblastic anemia. Anemia of chronic disease is characterized by normal or increased iron stores in the bone marrow and a normal or elevated ferritin level; the serum iron is low, often drastically so, and the TIBC is either normal or low. Thalassemia produces a greater degree of microcytosis for any given level of anemia than does iron deficiency. Red blood cell morphology on the peripheral smear is abnormal earlier in the course of thalassemia.

Treatment

The diagnosis of iron deficiency anemia can be made either by demonstrating an iron-deficient state or by evaluating the response to a therapeutic trial of iron replacement.

Since the anemia itself is rarely life-threatening, the most important part of treatment is identification of the cause—especially a source of occult blood loss.

A. ORAL IRON

Ferrous sulfate, 325 mg three times daily, which provides 180 mg of iron daily of which up to 10 mg is absorbed (though absorption may exceed this amount in cases of severe deficiency), is the preferred therapy. Compliance is improved by introducing the medicine more slowly in a gradually escalating dose with food. Alternatively, in cases of poor tolerance, one pill of ferrous sulfate can be taken at bedtime on an empty stomach. It is preferable to prescribe a lower dose of iron or to allow ingestion concurrent with food than to insist on a more rigorous schedule that will not be followed. An appropriate response is a return of the hematocrit level halfway toward normal within 3 weeks with full return to baseline after 2 months. Iron therapy should continue for 3–6 months after restoration of normal hematologic values to replenish iron stores. Failure of response to iron therapy is usually due to noncompliance, although occasional patients may absorb iron poorly. Other reasons for failure to respond include incorrect diagnosis (anemia of chronic disease, thalassemia) and ongoing gastrointestinal blood loss that exceeds the rate of new erythropoiesis.

B. PARENTERAL IRON

The indications are intolerance to oral iron, refractoriness to oral iron, gastrointestinal disease (usually inflammatory bowel disease) precluding the use of oral iron, and continued blood loss that cannot be corrected. Because of the possibility of anaphylactic reactions, parenteral iron therapy should be used only in cases of persistent anemia after a reasonable course of oral therapy. Until recently, iron dextran had been the only form of parenteral iron available in the United States. Now, sodium ferric gluconate is available and has been shown to result in a lower incidence of severe anaphylaxis. To date, no deaths have been reported with the use of this preparation.

The dose (total 1.5–2 g) may be calculated by estimating the decrease in volume of red blood cell mass and then supplying 1 mg of iron for each milliliter of volume of red blood cells below normal. Approximately 1 g should then be added for storage iron. The entire dose may be given as an intravenous infusion over 4–6 hours. A test dose of a dilute solution is given first, and the patient should be observed during the entire infusion for anaphylaxis.

Capurso G et al: Can patient characteristics predict the outcome of endoscopic evaluation of iron deficiency anemia: a multiple logistic regression analysis. Gastrointest Endosc 2004; 59:766. [PMID: 15173787]

Cook JD et al: The quantitative assessment of body iron. Blood 2003;101:3359. [PMID: 12521995]

Eichbaum Q et al: Is iron gluconate really safer than iron dextran? Blood 2003;101:3756. [PMID: 12707229]

Makrides M et al: Efficacy and tolerability of low-dose iron supplements during pregnancy: a randomized controlled trial. Am J Clin Nutr 2003;78:145. [PMID: 12816784]

Yates JM et al: Iron deficiency anaemia in general practice: clinical outcomes over three years and factors influencing diagnostic investigations. Postgrad Med J 2004;80:405. [PMID: 15254305]

ANEMIA OF CHRONIC DISEASE

Many chronic systemic diseases are associated with mild or moderate anemia. Common causes include chronic infection or inflammation, cancer, and liver disease. The anemia of chronic renal failure is somewhat different in pathophysiology and is usually more severe.

Red blood cell survival is modestly reduced, and the bone marrow fails to compensate adequately by increasing red blood cell production. Failure to increase red cell production is largely due to sequestration of iron within the reticuloendothelial system. Decrease in erythropoietin is rarely an important cause of underproduction of red cells except in renal failure.

Clinical Findings

A. SYMPTOMS AND SIGNS

The clinical features are those of the causative condition. The diagnosis should be suspected in patients with known chronic diseases; it is confirmed by the findings of low serum iron, low TIBC, and normal or increased serum ferritin (or normal or increased bone marrow iron stores). In cases of significant anemia, coexistent iron deficiency or folic acid deficiency should be suspected. Decreased dietary intake of folate or iron is common in these ill patients, and many will also have ongoing gastrointestinal blood losses. Patients undergoing hemodialysis regularly lose both iron and folate during dialysis.

B. LABORATORY FINDINGS

The hematocrit rarely falls below 60% of baseline (except in renal failure). The MCV is usually normal or slightly reduced. Red blood cell morphology is nondiagnostic, and the reticulocyte count is neither strikingly reduced nor increased. Serum iron values may be unmeasurable, and transferrin saturation may be extremely low, leading to an erroneous diagnosis of iron deficiency. In contrast to iron deficiency, serum ferritin values should be normal or increased. A serum ferritin value of less than 30 mcg/L should suggest coexistent iron deficiency.

Treatment

In most cases, no treatment is necessary. Purified recombinant erythropoietin (epoetin alfa) is effective for treatment of the anemia of renal failure and other secondary anemias, such as anemia related to cancer or inflammatory disorders (eg, rheumatoid arthritis). In renal failure, optimal response to epoetin alfa requires adequate intensity of dialysis. Epoetin alfa must be injected subcutaneously and is very expensive. One effective schedule is 30,000 units once weekly. This agent is used only when the patient is transfusion dependent or when the quality of life is clearly improved by the hematologic response.

Ganz T: Hepcidin, a key regulator of iron metabolism and mediator of anemia of inflammation. Blood 2003;102:783. [PMID: 12663437]

Smith RE Jr et al: A dose- and schedule-finding study of darbepoetin alpha for the treatment of chronic anaemia of cancer. Br J Cancer 2003;88:1851. [PMID: 12799626]

Weiss G et al: Anemia of chronic disease. N Engl J Med 2005; 352:1011. [PMID: 15758012]

Weiss G et al: Possible role of cytokine-induced tryptophan degradation in anaemia of inflammation. Eur J Haematol 2004; 72:130. [PMID: 14962250]

THE THALASSEMIAS

ESSENTIALS OF DIAGNOSIS

- Microcytosis out of proportion to the degree of anemia.
- Positive family history or lifelong personal history of microcytic anemia.
- Abnormal red blood cell morphology with microcytes, acanthocytes, and target cells.
- In β-thalassemia, elevated levels of hemoglobin A_2 or F.

General Considerations

The thalassemias are hereditary disorders characterized by reduction in the synthesis of globin chains (α or β). Reduced globin chain synthesis causes reduced hemoglobin synthesis and eventually produces a hypochromic microcytic anemia because of defective hemoglobinization of red blood cells. Thalassemias can be considered among the hypoproliferative anemias, the hemolytic anemias, and the anemias related to abnormal hemoglobin, since all of these factors play a role in pathogenesis.

Normal adult hemoglobin is primarily hemoglobin A, which represents approximately 98% of circulating hemoglobin. Hemoglobin A is formed from a tetramer—two α chains and two β chains—and can be designated $\alpha_2\beta_2$. Two copies of the α-globin gene are located on chromosome 16, and there is no substitute for α-globin in the formation of hemoglobin. The β-globin gene resides on chromosome 11 adjacent to genes encoding the β-like globin chains, δ and γ. The tetramer of $\alpha_2\delta_2$ forms hemoglobin A_2, which normally comprises 1–2% of adult hemoglobin. The tetramer $\alpha_2\gamma_2$ forms hemoglobin F, which is the major hemoglobin of fetal life but which comprises less than 1% of normal adult hemoglobin.

α-Thalassemia is due primarily to gene deletion causing reduced α-globin chain synthesis (Table 13–4). Since all adult hemoglobins are α containing, α-thalassemia produces no change in the percentage distribution of hemoglobins A, A_2, and F. In severe forms of α-thalassemia, excess β chains may form a β_4 tetramer called hemoglobin H.

β-Thalassemias are usually caused by point mutations rather than deletions (Table 13–5). These mutations result in premature chain termination or in problems with transcription of RNA and ultimately result in reduced or absent β-globin chain synthesis. The molecular defects leading to β-thalassemia are numerous and heterogeneous. Defects that result in absent globin chain expression are termed β^0, whereas those causing reduced synthesis are termed β^+. The reduced β-globin chain synthesis in β-thalassemia results in a relative increase in the percentages of hemoglobins A_2 and F compared to hemoglobin A, as the β-like globins (γ and δ) substitute for the missing β chains. In the presence of reduced β chains, the excess α chains are unstable and precipitate, leading to damage of red blood cell membranes. This leads to intramedullary and peripheral hemolysis. The bone marrow becomes hyperplastic under the drive of anemia and ineffective erythropoiesis resulting from the intramedullary destruction of the developing erythroid

Table 13–4. α-Thalassemia syndromes.

α-Globin Genes	Syndrome	Hematocrit	MCV
4	Normal	Normal	
3	Silent carrier	Normal	
2	Thalassemia minor	28–40%	60–75 fL
1	Hemoglobin H disease	22–32%	60–70 fL
0	Hydrops fetalis		

MCV = mean cell volume.

Table 13–5. β-Thalassemia syndromes.

	β-Globin Genes	Hb A	Hb A$_2$	Hb F
Normal	Homozygous β	97–99%	1–3%	< 1%
Thalassemia major	Homozygous β^0	0%	4–10%	90–96%
Thalassemia major	Homozygous β$^+$	0–10%	4–10%	90–96%
Thalassemia intermedia	Homozygous β$^+$ (mild)	0–30%	0–10%	6–100%
Thalassemia minor	Heterozygous β^0	80–95%	4–8%	1–5%
	Heterozygous β$^+$	80–95%	4–8%	1–5%

Hb = hemoglobin.

cells. In cases of severe thalassemia, the marked expansion of the erythroid element in the bone marrow may cause severe bony deformities, osteopenia, and pathologic fractures.

Clinical Findings

A. SYMPTOMS AND SIGNS

The α-thalassemia syndromes are seen primarily in persons from southeast Asia and China and, less commonly, in blacks. Normally, adults have four copies of the α-globin chain. When three α-globin genes are present, the patient is hematologically normal (silent carrier). When two α-globin genes are present, the patient is said to have α-thalassemia trait, one form of thalassemia minor. These patients are clinically normal and have a normal life expectancy and performance status, with a mild microcytic anemia. When only one α-globin chain is present, the patient has hemoglobin H disease. This is a chronic hemolytic anemia of variable severity (thalassemia minor or intermedia). Physical examination will reveal pallor and splenomegaly. Although affected individuals do not usually require transfusions, they may do so during periods of hemolytic exacerbation caused by infection or other stresses. When all four α-globin genes are deleted, the affected fetus is stillborn as a result of hydrops fetalis.

β-Thalassemia primarily affects persons of Mediterranean origin (Italian, Greek) and to a lesser extent Chinese, other Asians, and blacks. Patients homozygous for β-thalassemia have thalassemia major. Affected children are normal at birth, but after 6 months, when hemoglobin synthesis switches from hemoglobin F to hemoglobin A, severe anemia requiring transfusion develops. Numerous clinical problems ensue, including growth failure, bony deformities (abnormal facial structure, pathologic fractures), hepatosplenomegaly, and jaundice. The clinical course is modified significantly by transfusion therapy, but the transfusional iron overload (hemosiderosis) results in a clinical picture similar to hemochromatosis, with heart failure, cirrhosis, and endocrinopathies, usually after more than 100 units of red blood cells. These problems develop because of the body's inability to excrete the iron (see above) from transfused red cells. Before the application of allogeneic stem cell transplantation and the development of more effective forms of iron chelation, death from cardiac failure usually occurred between the ages of 20 and 30 years.

Patients homozygous for a milder form of β-thalassemia (allowing a higher rate of globin gene synthesis) have thalassemia intermedia. These patients have chronic hemolytic anemia but do not require transfusions except under periods of stress. Iron overload because of periodic transfusion may also develop. They survive into adult life but with hepatosplenomegaly and bony deformities. Patients heterozygous for β-thalassemia have thalassemia minor and a clinically insignificant microcytic anemia.

Prenatal diagnosis is available, and genetic counseling should be offered and the opportunity for prenatal diagnosis discussed.

B. LABORATORY FINDINGS

1. α-Thalassemia trait—Patients with two α-globin genes have mild anemia, with hematocrits between 28% and 40%. The MCV is strikingly low (60–75 fL) despite the modest anemia, and the red blood count is normal or increased. The peripheral blood smear shows microcytes, hypochromia, occasional target cells, and acanthocytes (cells with irregularly spaced bulbous projections). The reticulocyte count and iron parameters are normal. Hemoglobin electrophoresis will show no increase in the percentage of hemoglobins A$_2$ or F and no hemoglobin H. α-Thalassemia trait is thus usually diagnosed by exclusion. Genetic testing to demonstrate α-globin gene deletion is available in research laboratories.

2. Hemoglobin H disease—These patients have a more marked hemolytic anemia, with hematocrits between 22% and 32%. The MCV is remarkably low (60–70 fL) and the peripheral blood smear is markedly abnormal, with hypochromia, microcytosis, target cells, and poikilocytosis. The reticulocyte count is elevated. Hemoglobin electrophoresis will show the presence of a fast migrating hemoglobin (hemoglobin H), which comprises 10–40% of the hemoglobin. A peripheral blood smear can be stained with supravital dyes to demonstrate the presence of hemoglobin H.

3. β-Thalassemia minor—As in α-thalassemia trait, these patients have a modest anemia with hematocrit between 28% and 40%. The MCV ranges from 55 to 75 fL, and the red blood cell count is normal or increased. The peripheral blood smear is mildly abnormal, with hypochromia, microcytosis, and target cells. In contrast to α-thalassemia, basophilic stippling may be present. The reticulocyte count is normal or slightly elevated. Hemoglobin electrophoresis (using quantitative techniques) may show an elevation of hemoglobin A_2 to 4–8% and occasional elevations of hemoglobin F to 1–5%.

4. β-Thalassemia major—β-Thalassemia major produces severe anemia, and without transfusion the hematocrit may fall to less than 10%. The peripheral blood smear is bizarre, showing severe poikilocytosis, hypochromia, microcytosis, target cells, basophilic stippling, and nucleated red blood cells. Little or no hemoglobin A is present. Variable amounts of hemoglobin A_2 are seen, and the major hemoglobin present is hemoglobin F.

Differential Diagnosis

Mild forms of thalassemia must be differentiated from iron deficiency. Compared to iron deficiency anemia, patients with thalassemia have a lower MCV, a more normal red blood count, and a more abnormal peripheral blood smear at modest levels of anemia. Iron studies are normal. Severe forms of thalassemia may be confused with other hemoglobinopathies. The diagnosis is made by hemoglobin electrophoresis.

Treatment

Patients with mild thalassemia (α-thalassemia trait or β-thalassemia minor) require no treatment and should be identified so that they will not be subjected to repeated evaluations and treatment for iron deficiency. Patients with hemoglobin H disease should take folate supplementation and avoid medicinal iron and oxidative drugs such as sulfonamides. Patients with severe thalassemia are maintained on a regular transfusion schedule and receive folate supplementation. Splenectomy is performed if hypersplenism causes a marked increase in the transfusion requirement. Deferoxamine is routinely given as an iron-chelating agent to avoid or postpone hemosiderosis. Deferipone is a new oral iron chelator that has been approved for clinical use in Europe, but is not currently available in the United States. A diet low in iron may help in all of these patients.

Allogeneic bone marrow transplantation has become the treatment of choice for β-thalassemia major. Children who have not yet experienced iron overload and chronic organ toxicity do well, with long-term survival in more than 80% of cases.

Chaidos A et al: Treatment of beta-thalassemia patients with recombinant human erythropoietin: effect on transfusion requirements and soluble adhesion molecules. Acta Haematol 2004;111:189. [PMID: 15153710]

Chui D et al: Hemoglobin H disease: not necessarily a benign disorder. Blood 2003;101:791. [PMID: 12393486]

Cunningham MJ et al: Thalassemia Clinical Research Network. Complications of beta-thalassemia major in North America. Blood 2004;104:34. [PMID: 14988152]

Hoffbrand AV et al: Role of deferiprone in chelation therapy for transfusional iron overload. Blood 2003;102:17. [PMID: 12637334]

Rund D et al: β-Thalassemia. N Engl J Med 2005;353:1135. [PMID: 16162884]

SIDEROBLASTIC ANEMIA

The sideroblastic anemias are a heterogeneous group of disorders in which hemoglobin synthesis is reduced because of failure to incorporate heme into protoporphyrin to form hemoglobin. Iron accumulates, particularly in the mitochondria. A Prussian blue stain of the bone marrow will reveal ringed sideroblasts, cells with iron deposits encircling the red cell nucleus. The disorder is usually acquired. Sometimes it represents a stage in evolution of a generalized bone marrow disorder (myelodysplasia) that may ultimately terminate in acute leukemia. Other causes include chronic alcoholism and lead poisoning.

Patients have no specific clinical features other than those related to anemia. The anemia is usually moderate, with hematocrits of 20–30%, but transfusions may occasionally be required. Although the MCV is usually normal or slightly increased, it may occasionally be low, leading to confusion with iron deficiency. The peripheral blood smear characteristically shows a dimorphic population of red blood cells, one normal and one hypochromic. In cases of lead poisoning, coarse basophilic stippling of the red cells is seen.

The diagnosis is made by examination of the bone marrow. Characteristically, there is marked erythroid hyperplasia, a sign of ineffective erythropoiesis (expansion of the erythroid compartment of the bone marrow that does not result in the production of reticulocytes in the peripheral blood). The iron stain of the bone marrow shows a generalized increase in iron stores and the presence of ringed sideroblasts. Other characteristic laboratory features include a high serum iron and a high transferrin saturation. In lead poisoning, serum lead levels will be elevated.

Occasionally, the anemia is so severe that support with transfusion is required. These patients usually do not respond to erythropoietin therapy.

Germing U et al: Two types of acquired idiopathic sideroblastic anaemia (AISA): a time-tested distinction. Br J Haematol 2000;108:724. [PMID: 10792275]

VITAMIN B_{12} DEFICIENCY

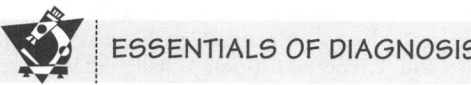 ESSENTIALS OF DIAGNOSIS

- *Macrocytic anemia.*

- Macro-ovalocytes and hypersegmented neutrophils on peripheral blood smear.
- Serum vitamin B_{12} level less than 100 pg/mL.

General Considerations

Vitamin B_{12} belongs to the family of cobalamins and serves as a cofactor for two important reactions in humans. As methylcobalamin, it is a cofactor for methionine synthetase in the conversion of homocysteine to methionine, and as adenosylcobalamin for the conversion of methylmalonyl-coenzyme A (CoA) to succinyl-CoA. All vitamin B_{12} comes from the diet and is present in all foods of animal origin. The daily absorption of vitamin B_{12} is 5 mcg.

After being ingested, vitamin B_{12} is bound to intrinsic factor, a protein secreted by gastric parietal cells. Other cobalamin-binding proteins (called R factors) compete with intrinsic factor for vitamin B_{12}. Vitamin B_{12} bound to R factors cannot be absorbed. The vitamin B_{12}–intrinsic factor complex travels through the intestine and is absorbed in the terminal ileum by cells with specific receptors for the complex. It is then transported through plasma and stored in the liver. Three plasma transport proteins have been identified. Transcobalamins I and III (differing only in carbohydrate structure) are secreted by white blood cells. Although approximately 90% of plasma vitamin B_{12} circulates bind to these proteins, only transcobalamin II is capable of transporting vitamin B_{12} into cells. The liver contains 2000–5000 mcg of stored vitamin B_{12}. Since daily losses are 3–5 mcg/d, the body usually has sufficient stores of vitamin B_{12} so that vitamin B_{12} deficiency develops more than 3 years after vitamin B_{12} absorption ceases.

Since vitamin B_{12} is present in all foods of animal origin, dietary vitamin B_{12} deficiency is extremely rare and is seen only in vegans—strict vegetarians who avoid all dairy products as well as meat and fish (Table 13–6). Abdominal surgery may lead to vitamin B_{12} de-

Table 13–6. Causes of vitamin B_{12} deficiency.

Dietary deficiency (rare)
Decreased production of intrinsic factor
    Pernicious anemia
    Gastrectomy
Helicobacter pylori infection
Competition for vitamin B_{12} in gut
    Blind loop syndrome
    Fish tapeworm (rare)
Pancreatic insufficiency
Decreased ileal absorption of vitamin B_{12}
    Surgical resection
    Crohn's disease
Transcobalamin II deficiency (rare)

---

ficiency in several ways. Gastrectomy will eliminate that site of intrinsic factor production; blind loop syndrome will cause competition for vitamin B_{12} by bacterial overgrowth in the lumen of the intestine; and surgical resection of the ileum will eliminate the site of vitamin B_{12} absorption. Rare causes of vitamin B_{12} deficiency include fish tapeworm (*Diphyllobothrium latum*) infection, in which the parasite uses luminal vitamin B_{12}, pancreatic insufficiency (with failure to inactivate competing cobalamin-binding proteins), and severe Crohn's disease, causing sufficient destruction of the ileum to impair vitamin B_{12} absorption.

The most common cause of vitamin B_{12} deficiency is associated with pernicious anemia. Although the disease is hereditary, it is rare clinically before age 35 years. Pernicious anemia produces a number of clinical findings in addition to vitamin B_{12} deficiency. Atrophic gastritis is invariably present and results in histamine-fast achlorhydria. These patients may also have a number of other autoimmune diseases, including immunoglobulin (Ig) A deficiency, as well as polyglandular endocrine insufficiency. The atrophic gastritis is associated with an increased risk of gastric carcinoma.

Clinical Findings

A. SYMPTOMS AND SIGNS

The hallmark of symptomatic vitamin B_{12} deficiency is megaloblastic anemia. However, subclinical cobalamin deficiency is an increasingly recognized condition, especially in those with predisposing conditions such as ileal disease or gastric surgery. In advanced cases, the anemia may be severe, with hematocrits as low as 10–15%, and may be accompanied by leukopenia and thrombocytopenia. The megaloblastic state also produces changes in mucosal cells, leading to glossitis, as well as other vague gastrointestinal disturbances such as anorexia and diarrhea. Vitamin B_{12} deficiency also leads to a complex neurologic syndrome. Peripheral nerves are usually affected first, and patients complain initially of paresthesias. The posterior columns next become impaired, and patients complain of difficulty with balance. In more advanced cases, cerebral function may be altered as well, and on occasion dementia and other neuropsychiatric changes may precede hematologic changes.

Patients are usually pale and may be mildly icteric. Neurologic examination may reveal decreased vibration and position sense but is more commonly normal in early stages of the disease.

B. LABORATORY FINDINGS

The megaloblastic state produces an anemia of variable severity that on occasion may be very severe. The MCV is usually strikingly elevated, between 110 and 140 fL. However, it is possible to have vitamin B_{12} deficiency with a normal MCV. Occasionally, the normal MCV may be explained by coexistent thalassemia or iron deficiency, but in other cases the reason is obscure. Patients with neurologic symptoms and signs that suggest possible vitamin B_{12} deficiency should be evaluated for that deficiency despite a normal MCV and the absence of anemia. The peripheral blood smear is usually strikingly abnormal, with anisocytosis and poikilocytosis. A characteristic finding is the macro-ovalocyte, but numerous other abnormal shapes are usually seen. The neutrophils are hypersegmented. Typical features include a mean lobe count greater than four or the finding of six-lobed neutrophils. The reticulocyte count is reduced. Because vitamin B_{12} deficiency affects all hematopoietic cell lines, in severe cases the white blood cell count and the platelet count are reduced, and pancytopenia is present.

Bone marrow morphology is characteristically abnormal. Marked erythroid hyperplasia is present as a response to defective red blood cell production (ineffective erythropoiesis). Megaloblastic changes in the erythroid series include abnormally large cell size and asynchronous maturation of the nucleus and cytoplasm—ie, cytoplasmic maturation continues while impaired DNA synthesis causes retarded nuclear development. In the myeloid series, giant metamyelocytes are characteristically seen.

Other laboratory abnormalities include elevated serum lactate dehydrogenase (LDH) and a modest increase in indirect bilirubin. These two findings are a reflection of intramedullary destruction of developing abnormal erythroid cells and are similar to those observed in peripheral hemolytic anemias.

The diagnosis of vitamin B_{12} deficiency is made by finding an abnormally low vitamin B_{12} (cobalamin) serum level. Whereas the normal vitamin B_{12} level is > 240 pg/mL, most patients with overt vitamin B_{12} deficiency will have serum levels < 170 pg/mL, with symptomatic patients usually having levels < 100 pg/mL. A level of 170–240 pg/mL is borderline. When the serum level of vitamin B_{12} is borderline, the diagnosis is best confirmed by finding an elevated level of serum methylmalonic acid (> 1000 nmol/L). However, elevated levels of serum methylmalonic acid can be due to renal insufficiency. The Schilling test is now rarely used.

Differential Diagnosis

Vitamin B_{12} deficiency should be differentiated from folic acid deficiency, the other common cause of megaloblastic anemia, in which red blood cell folate is low while vitamin B_{12} levels are normal. The distinction between vitamin B_{12} deficiency and myelodysplasia (the other common cause of macrocytic anemia with abnormal morphology) is based on the characteristic morphology and the low vitamin B_{12} level.

Treatment

Patients with pernicious anemia have historically been treated with parenteral therapy. Intramuscular injections of 100 mcg of vitamin B_{12} are adequate for each dose. Replacement is usually given daily for the first week, weekly for the first month, and then monthly for life. It is a lifelong disorder, and if patients discontinue their monthly therapy the vitamin deficiency will recur. Oral cobalamin may be used instead of parenteral therapy and can provide equivalent results. The dose is 1000 mcg/d and must be continued indefinitely.

Patients respond to therapy with an immediate improvement in their sense of well-being. Hypokalemia may complicate the first several days of therapy, particularly if the anemia is severe. A brisk reticulocytosis occurs in 5–7 days, and the hematologic picture normalizes in 2 months. Central nervous system symptoms and signs are reversible if they are of relatively short duration (less than 6 months) but become permanent if treatment is not initiated promptly.

Andres E et al: Vitamin B_{12} (cobalamin) deficiency in elderly patients. CMAJ 2004;171:251. [PMID: 15289425]

Bolaman Z et al: Oral versus intramuscular cobalamin treatment in megaloblastic anemia: a single-center, prospective, randomized, open-label study. Clin Ther 2003;25:3124. [PMID: 14749150]

Carmel R: Current concepts in cobalamin deficiency. Annu Rev Med 2000;51:357. [PMID: 10774470]

FOLIC ACID DEFICIENCY

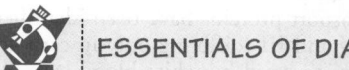 ESSENTIALS OF DIAGNOSIS

- *Macrocytic anemia.*
- *Macro-ovalocytes and hypersegmented neutrophils on peripheral blood smear.*
- *Normal serum vitamin B_{12} levels.*
- *Reduced folate levels in red blood cells or serum.*

General Considerations

Folic acid is the term commonly used for pteroylmonoglutamic acid. In its reduced form of tetrahydrofolate, it serves as an important mediator of many reactions involving one-carbon transfers. Important reactions include the conversion of homocysteine to methionine and of deoxyuridylate to thymidylate, an important step in DNA synthesis.

Folic acid is present in most fruits and vegetables (especially citrus fruits and green leafy vegetables) and daily requirements of 50–100 mcg/d are usually met in the diet. Total body stores of folate are approximately 5000 mcg, enough to supply requirements for 2–3 months.

By far the most common cause of folate deficiency is inadequate dietary intake (Table 13–7). Alcoholics, anorectic patients, persons who do not eat fresh fruits and vegetables, and those who overcook their food are candidates for folate deficiency. Reduced folate absorption is rarely seen, since absorption occurs from the entire gastrointestinal tract. However, drugs such as pheny-

Table 13–7. Causes of folate deficiency.

Dietary deficiency
Decreased absorption
   Tropical sprue
   Drugs: phenytoin, sulfasalazine, trimethoprim-sulfameth-
     oxazole
Increased requirement
   Chronic hemolytic anemia
   Pregnancy
   Exfoliative skin disease
Loss: dialysis
Inhibition of reduction to active form
   Methotrexate

toin, trimethoprim-sulfamethoxazole, or sulfasalazine may interfere with folate absorption. Folic acid requirements are increased in pregnancy, hemolytic anemia, and exfoliative skin disease, and in these cases the increased requirements (five to ten times normal) may not be met by a normal diet. Patients with increased folate requirements should receive supplementation with 1 mg/d of folic acid.

Clinical Findings

A. SYMPTOMS AND SIGNS

The features are similar to those of vitamin B_{12} deficiency, with megaloblastic anemia and megaloblastic changes in mucosa. However, there are none of the neurologic abnormalities associated with vitamin B_{12} deficiency.

B. LABORATORY FINDINGS

Megaloblastic anemia is identical to anemia resulting from vitamin B_{12} deficiency (see above). However, the serum vitamin B_{12} level is normal. A red blood cell folate level of less than 150 ng/mL is diagnostic of folate deficiency.

Differential Diagnosis

The megaloblastic anemia of folate deficiency should be differentiated from vitamin B_{12} deficiency by the finding of a normal vitamin B_{12} level and a reduced red blood cell folate or serum folate level. Alcoholics, who often have folate deficiency, may also have anemia of liver disease. This latter macrocytic anemia does not cause megaloblastic morphologic changes but rather produces target cells in the peripheral blood. Hypothyroidism is associated with mild macrocytosis but also with pernicious anemia.

Treatment

Folic acid deficiency is treated with folic acid, 1 mg/d orally. The response is similar to that seen in the treatment of vitamin B_{12} deficiency, with rapid improvement and a sense of well-being, reticulocytosis in 5–7 days, and total correction of hematologic abnormalities within 2 months. Large doses of folic acid may produce hematologic responses in cases of vitamin B_{12} deficiency but will allow neurologic damage to progress.

Clarke R et al: Vitamin B_{12} and folate deficiency in later life. Age Ageing 2004;33:34. [PMID: 14695861]

PURE RED CELL APLASIA

Adult acquired pure red cell aplasia is rare. It appears to be an autoimmune disease mediated either by T lymphocytes or (rarely) by an IgG antibody against erythroid precursors. In adults, the disease is usually idiopathic. However, cases have been seen in association with systemic lupus erythematosus, chronic lymphocytic leukemia (CLL), lymphomas, or thymoma. Some drugs (phenytoin, chloramphenicol) may cause red cell aplasia. Transient episodes of red cell aplasia are probably common in response to viral infections, especially parvovirus infections. However, these acute episodes will go unrecognized unless the patient has a chronic hemolytic disorder, in which case the hematocrit may fall precipitously.

The only signs are those of anemia unless the patient has an associated autoimmune or lymphoproliferative disorder. The anemia is often severe and normochromic, with low or absent reticulocytes. Red blood cell morphology is normal, and the myeloid and platelet lines are unaffected. The bone marrow is normocellular. All elements present are normal, but erythroid precursors are markedly reduced or absent. In some cases, chest imaging studies will reveal a thymoma.

The disorder is distinguished from aplastic anemia (in which the marrow is hypocellular and all cell lines are affected) and from myelodysplasia. This latter disorder is recognized by the presence of morphologic abnormalities that should not be present in pure red cell aplasia.

Possible offending drugs should be stopped. With thymoma, resection results in amelioration of anemia in some instances. High-dose intravenous immune globulin has produced excellent responses in a small number of cases, especially in parvovirus-related cases. For most cases, the treatment of choice is immunosuppressive therapy with a combination of antithymocyte globulin and cyclosporine (or tacrolimus)—similar to therapy of aplastic anemia. Anti-CD20 monoclonal antibody (rituximab) has also had some success.

Casadevall N et al: Pure red-cell aplasia and antierythropoietin antibodies in patients treated with recombinant erythropoietin. N Engl J Med 2002;346:469. [PMID: 11844847]

Zecca M et al: Anti-CD20 monoclonal antibody for the treatment of severe immune-mediated pure red cell aplasia and hemolytic anemia. Blood 2001;97:3995. [PMID: 11389047]

HEMOLYTIC ANEMIAS

The hemolytic anemias are a group of disorders in which red blood cell survival is reduced, either episodically or continuously. The bone marrow has the ability to increase erythroid production up to eightfold in response to reduced red cell survival, so anemia will be present only when the ability of the bone marrow to compensate is outstripped. This will occur when red cell survival is extremely short or when the ability of the bone marrow to compensate is impaired for some second reason.

Since red blood cell survival is normally 120 days, in the absence of red cell production the hematocrit will fall at the rate of approximately 1/100 of the hematocrit per day, which translates to a decrease in the hematocrit reading of approximately 3% per week. For example, a fall of hematocrit from 45% to 36% over 3 weeks need not indicate hemolysis, since this rate of fall would result simply from cessation of red blood cell production. If the hematocrit is falling at a rate faster than that due to decreased production, blood loss or hemolysis is the cause.

Reticulocytosis is an important clue to the presence of hemolysis, since in most hemolytic disorders the bone marrow will respond with increased red blood cell production. However, hemolysis can be present without reticulocytosis when a second disorder (infection, folate deficiency) is superimposed on hemolysis; in these circumstances, the hematocrit will fall rapidly. However, reticulocytosis also occurs during recovery from hypoproliferative anemia or bleeding. Hemolysis is correctly diagnosed (when bleeding is excluded) if the hematocrit is either falling or stable despite reticulocytosis.

Hemolytic disorders are generally classified according to whether the defect is intrinsic to the red cell or due to some external factor (Table 13–8). Intrinsic defects have been described in all components of the red blood cell, including the membrane, enzyme systems, and hemoglobin; most of these disorders are heredi-

Table 13–8. Classification of hemolytic anemias.

Intrinsic
  Membrane defects: hereditary spherocytosis, hereditary elliptocytosis, paroxysmal nocturnal hemoglobinuria
  Glycolytic defects: pyruvate kinase deficiency, severe hypophosphatemia
  Oxidation vulnerability: glucose-6-phosphate dehydrogenase deficiency, methemoglobinemia
  Hemoglobinopathies: sickle cell syndromes, unstable hemoglobins, methemoglobinemia
Extrinsic
  Immune: autoimmune, lymphoproliferative disease, drug toxicity
  Microangiopathic: thrombotic thrombocytopenic purpura, hemolytic-uremic syndrome, disseminated intravascular coagulation, valve hemolysis, metastatic adenocarcinoma, vasculitis
  Infection: *Plasmodium*, *Clostridium*, *Borrelia*
  Hypersplenism
  Burns

---

tary. Hemolytic anemias due to external factors are the immune and microangiopathic hemolytic anemias.

Certain laboratory features are common to all the hemolytic anemias. Haptoglobin, a normal plasma protein that binds and clears hemoglobin released into plasma, may be depressed in hemolytic disorders. However, haptoglobin levels are influenced by many factors and, by themselves, are not a reliable indicator of hemolysis. When intravascular hemolysis occurs, transient hemoglobinemia occurs. Hemoglobin is filtered through the glomerulus and is usually reabsorbed by tubular cells. Hemoglobinuria will be present only when the capacity for reabsorption of hemoglobin by these cells is exceeded. In its absence, evidence for prior intravascular hemolysis is the presence of hemosiderin in shed renal tubular cells (positive urine hemosiderin). With severe intravascular hemolysis, hemoglobinemia and methemalbuminemia may be present. Hemolysis increases the indirect bilirubin, and the total bilirubin may rise to 4 mg/dL. Bilirubin levels higher than this may indicate some degree of hepatic dysfunction. Serum LDH levels are strikingly elevated in cases of microangiopathic hemolysis (thrombotic thrombocytopenic purpura [TTP], hemolytic-uremic syndrome [HUS]) and may be elevated in other hemolytic anemias.

HEREDITARY SPHEROCYTOSIS

 ESSENTIALS OF DIAGNOSIS

- *Positive family history.*
- *Splenomegaly.*
- *Spherocytes and increased reticulocytes on peripheral blood smear.*
- *Microcytic, hyperchromic indices.*

General Considerations

Hereditary spherocytosis is a disorder of the red blood cell membrane, leading to chronic hemolytic anemia. Normally, the red blood cell is a biconcave disk with a diameter of 7–8 mcm. The red blood cells must be both strong and deformable—strong to withstand the stress of circulating for 120 days and deformable so as to pass through capillaries 3 mcm in diameter and splenic fenestrations in the cords of the red pulp of approximately 2 mcm. The red blood cell skeleton, made up primarily of the proteins spectrin and actin, gives the red cells these characteristics of strength and deformability.

The membrane defect in hereditary spherocytosis is an abnormality in spectrin, the protein providing most of the scaffolding for the red blood cell membranes. The result is a decrease in surface-to-volume ratio that results in a spherical shape of the cell. These spherical cells are less deformable and unable to pass through 2-mcm fenestrations in the splenic red pulp. Hemolysis takes place because of trapping of red blood cells within the spleen.

Clinical Findings

A. SYMPTOMS AND SIGNS

Hereditary spherocytosis is an autosomal dominant disease of variable severity. It is often diagnosed during childhood, but milder cases may be discovered incidentally late in adult life. Anemia may or may not be present, since the bone marrow may be able to compensate for shortened red cell survival. Severe anemia (aplastic crisis) may occur in folic acid deficiency or when bone marrow compensation is temporarily impaired by infection. Chronic hemolysis causes jaundice and pigment (calcium bilirubinate) gallstones, leading to attacks of cholecystitis. Examination may reveal icterus and a palpable spleen.

B. LABORATORY FINDINGS

The anemia is of variable severity, and the hematocrit may be normal. Reticulocytosis is always present. The peripheral blood smear shows the presence of spherocytes, small cells that have lost their central pallor. Spherocytes usually make up only a small percentage of red blood cells on the peripheral smear. Hereditary spherocytosis is the only important disorder associated with microcytosis and an increased mean corpuscular hemoglobin concentration (MCHC), often greater than 36 g/dL. As with other hemolytic disorders, there may be an increase in indirect bilirubin. The Coombs test is negative.

Because spherocytes are red cells that have lost some membrane surface, they are abnormally vulnerable to swelling induced by hypotonic media. Increased osmotic fragility merely reflects the presence of spherocytes and does not distinguish hereditary spherocytosis from other spherocytic hemolytic disorders such as autoimmune hemolytic anemia. In some laboratories, the osmotic fragility test has been supplanted by ektacytometry, which has the advantages of better reliability and the ability to distinguish spherocytes from other red blood cell abnormalities such as elliptocytosis.

Treatment

These patients should receive uninterrupted supplementation with folic acid, 1 mg/d. The treatment of choice is splenectomy, which will correct neither the membrane defect nor the spherocytosis but will eliminate the site of hemolysis. In very mild cases discovered late in adult life, splenectomy may not be necessary.

Kimura F et al: Partial splenic embolization for the treatment of hereditary spherocytosis. AJR Am J Roentgenol 2003;181: 1021. [PMID: 14500222]

PAROXYSMAL NOCTURNAL HEMOGLOBINURIA

Paroxysmal nocturnal hemoglobinuria is an acquired clonal stem cell disorder that results in abnormal sensitivity of the red blood cell membrane to lysis by complement. The underlying cause is a defect in the gene for phosphatidylinositol class A (PICA), which results in a deficiency of the glycosylphosphatidylinositol (GPI) anchor for cellular membrane proteins. In particular, the complement-regulating proteins CD55 and CD59 are deficient. Paroxysmal nocturnal hemoglobinuria should be suspected in confusing cases of hemolytic anemia or pancytopenia. The best screening test is flow cytometry to demonstrate deficiency of CD59 on red blood cells. This test has largely replaced the classic sucrose hemolysis test.

Clinical Findings

A. SYMPTOMS AND SIGNS

Classically, patients report episodic hemoglobinuria resulting in reddish brown urine. Hemoglobinuria is most often noticed in the first morning urine, probably because of its increased concentration. In addition to being prone to anemia, these patients are prone to thrombosis, especially mesenteric and hepatic vein thromboses. Other common sites of thrombosis include the central nervous system (saggital vein) and the skin, with formation of painful nodules. This hypercoagulopathy may be related to platelet activation by complement. As this is a stem cell disorder, paroxysmal nocturnal hemoglobinuria may progress either to aplastic anemia, to myelodysplasia, or to acute myelogenous leukemia (AML).

B. LABORATORY FINDINGS

Anemia is of variable severity, and reticulocytosis may or may not be present. Abnormalities on the blood smear are nondiagnostic and may include macro-ovalocytes. Since the episodic hemolysis in paroxysmal nocturnal hemoglobinuria is intravascular, the finding of urine hemosiderin is a useful test. Serum LDH is characteristically elevated. Iron deficiency is commonly present and is related to chronic iron loss from hemoglobinuria, since hemolysis is primarily intravascular.

The white blood cell count and platelet count may be decreased. A decreased leukocyte alkaline phosphatase—evidence for a qualitative abnormality in the myeloid series—may be seen. Bone marrow morphology is variable and may show either generalized hypoplasia or erythroid hyperplasia. Flow cytometric assays may confirm the diagnosis by demonstrating the absence of CD59.

Treatment

Iron replacement is often indicated for treatment of iron deficiency. This may improve the anemia but may also cause a transient increase in hemolysis. For unclear reasons, prednisone is effective in decreasing hemolysis, and some patients can be managed effectively with alternate-day corticosteroids. In severe cases and cases of transformation to myelodysplasia, allogeneic bone marrow transplantation has been used to treat the disorder.

Hillmen P et al: Effect of eculizumab on hemolysis and transfusion requirements in patients with paroxysmal nocturnal hemoglobinuria. N Engl J Med 2004;350:552. [PMID: 14762182]

Moyo VM et al: Natural history of paroxysmal nocturnal haemoglobinuria using modern diagnostic assays. Br J Haematol 2004;126:133. [PMID: 15198744]

Parker C et al; International PNH Interest Group: Diagnosis and management of paroxysmal nocturnal hemoglobinuria. Blood 2005;106:3699. [PMID: 16051736]

Rosse WF et al: Clinical manifestations of paroxysmal nocturnal hemoglobinuria: present state and future problems. Int J Hematol 2003;77:113. [PMID: 12627845]

GLUCOSE-6-PHOSPHATE DEHYDROGENASE DEFICIENCY

ESSENTIALS OF DIAGNOSIS

- *X-linked recessive disorder seen commonly in American black men.*
- *Episodic hemolysis in response to oxidant drugs or infection.*
- *Minimally abnormal peripheral blood smear.*
- *Reduced levels of glucose-6-phosphate dehydrogenase between hemolytic episodes.*

General Considerations

Glucose-6-phosphate dehydrogenase (G6PD) deficiency is a hereditary enzyme defect that causes episodic hemolytic anemia because of the decreased ability of red blood cells to deal with oxidative stresses. The hexose monophosphate shunt is not an important source of energy in red cells but is important in generating reduced glutathione, which protects hemoglobin from oxidative denaturation. The first step in this pathway is the production of nicotinamide adenine dinucleotide phosphate (reduced) (NADPH) by the action of G6PD on glucose 6-phosphate. NADPH serves as a cofactor for glutathione reductase in generating reduced glutathione, which detoxifies hydrogen peroxide. In the absence of reduced glutathione, hemoglobin may become oxidized. Oxidized hemoglobin denatures and forms precipitants called Heinz bodies. These Heinz bodies cause membrane damage, which leads to removal of these cells by the spleen.

Numerous types of G6PD enzymes have been described. The normal type found in whites is designated G6PD-B. Most American blacks have G6PD-A, which is normal in function. Ten to 15 percent of American blacks have the variant G6PD designated A–, in which there is only 15% of normal enzyme activity, and enzyme activity declines rapidly as the red blood cell ages past 40 days, a fact that explains many of the clinical findings in this disorder. Many other G6PD variants have been described, including some Mediterranean variants with extremely low enzyme activity.

Clinical Findings

G6PD deficiency is an X-linked recessive disorder affecting 10–15% of American black males. Female carriers are rarely affected—only when an unusually high percentage of cells producing the normal enzyme is inactivated.

A. SYMPTOMS AND SIGNS

Patients are usually healthy, without chronic hemolytic anemia or splenomegaly. Hemolysis occurs as a result of oxidative stress on the red blood cells, generated either by infection or exposure to certain drugs. Common drugs initiating hemolysis include dapsone, primaquine, quinidine, quinine, sulfonamides, and nitrofurantoin. Even with continuous use of the offending drug, the hemolytic episode is self-limited because older red blood cells (with low enzyme activity) are removed and replaced with a population of young red blood cells with adequate functional levels of G6PD. Severe G6PD deficiency (as in Mediterranean variants) may produce a chronic hemolytic anemia.

B. LABORATORY FINDINGS

Between hemolytic episodes, the blood is normal. During episodes of hemolysis, there is reticulocytosis and increased serum indirect bilirubin. The red blood cell smear is not diagnostic but may reveal a small number of "bite" cells—cells that appear to have had a bite taken out of their periphery. This indicates pitting of hemoglobin aggregates by the spleen. Heinz bodies may be demonstrated by staining a peripheral blood smear with cresyl violet; they are not visible on the usual Wright-stained blood smear. Specific enzyme assays for G6PD may reveal a low level but may be misleading if they are performed shortly after a hemolytic episode when the enzyme-deficient cohort of cells has been removed. In these cases, the enzyme assays should be repeated weeks after hemolysis has resolved. In severe cases of G6PD deficiency, enzyme levels are always low.

Treatment

No treatment is necessary except to avoid known oxidant drugs.

Mehta A et al: Glucose-6-phosphate dehydrogenase deficiency. Baillieres Best Pract Res Clin Haematol 2000;13:21. [PMID: 10916676]

SICKLE CELL ANEMIA & RELATED SYNDROMES

ESSENTIALS OF DIAGNOSIS

- *Irreversibly sickled cells on peripheral blood smear.*
- *Positive family history and lifelong history of hemolytic anemia.*

- *Recurrent painful episodes.*
- *Hemoglobin S is the major hemoglobin seen on electrophoresis.*

General Considerations

Sickle cell anemia is an autosomal recessive disorder in which an abnormal hemoglobin leads to chronic hemolytic anemia with numerous clinical consequences. A single DNA base change leads to an amino acid substitution of valine for glutamine in the sixth position on the β-globin chain. The abnormal β chain is designated $β^s$ and the tetramer of $α_2β^s_2$ is designated hemoglobin S.

When in the deoxy form, hemoglobin S forms polymers that damage the red blood cell membrane. Both polymer formation and early membrane damage are reversible. However, red blood cells that have undergone repeated sickling are damaged beyond repair and become irreversibly sickled.

The rate of sickling is influenced by a number of factors, most importantly by the concentration of hemoglobin S in the individual red blood cell. Red cell dehydration makes the cell quite vulnerable to sickling. Sickling is also strongly influenced by the presence of other hemoglobins within the cell. Hemoglobin F cannot participate in polymer formation, and its presence markedly retards sickling. Other factors that increase sickling are those that lead to formation of deoxyhemoglobin S, eg, acidosis and hypoxemia, either systemic or locally in tissues.

Prenatal diagnosis is now available for couples at risk of producing a child with sickle cell anemia. DNA from fetal cells can be directly examined, and the presence of the sickle cell mutation can be accurately and definitively diagnosed. Genetic counseling should be made available to such couples.

Clinical Findings

A. Symptoms and Signs

The hemoglobin S gene is carried in 8% of American blacks, and one birth out of 400 in American blacks will produce a child with sickle cell anemia. The disorder has its onset during the first year of life, when hemoglobin F levels fall as a signal is sent to switch from production of γ-globin to β-globin.

Chronic hemolytic anemia produces jaundice, pigment (calcium bilirubinate) gallstones, splenomegaly, and poorly healing ulcers over the lower tibia. The chronic anemia may become life-threatening when severe anemia is produced by hemolytic or aplastic crises. The latter occur when the ability of the bone marrow to compensate is reduced by viral or other infection or by folate deficiency. Hemolytic crises may be related to splenic sequestration of sickled cells (primarily in childhood, before the spleen has been infarcted as a result of repeated sickling) or with coexistent disorders such as G6PD deficiency.

Acute painful episodes due to acute vaso-occlusion may occur spontaneously or be provoked by infection, dehydration, or hypoxia. Clusters of sickled red cells occlude the microvasculature of the organs involved. These episodes last hours to days and produce acute pain and low-grade fever. Common sites of acute painful episodes include the bones (especially the back and long bones) and the chest. Acute vaso-occlusion may also cause strokes due to sinus thrombosis and priapism. Vaso-occlusive episodes are not associated with increased hemolysis.

Repeated episodes of vascular occlusion affect a large number of organs, especially the heart and liver. Ischemic necrosis of bone occurs, rendering the bone susceptible to osteomyelitis due to staphylococci or (less commonly) salmonellae. Infarction of the papillae of the renal medulla causes renal tubular concentrating defects and gross hematuria, more often encountered in sickle cell trait than in sickle cell anemia. Retinopathy similar to that noted in diabetes is often present and may lead to blindness.

These patients are prone to delayed puberty. An increased incidence of infection is related to hyposplenism as well as to defects in the alternative pathway of complement.

On examination, patients are often chronically ill and jaundiced. There is hepatomegaly, but the spleen is not palpable in adult life. The heart is enlarged, with a hyperdynamic precordium and systolic murmurs. Nonhealing ulcers of the lower leg and retinopathy may be present.

Sickle cell anemia becomes a chronic multisystem disease, with death from organ failure. With improved supportive care, average life expectancy is now between 40 and 50 years of age.

B. Laboratory Findings

Chronic hemolytic anemia is present. The hematocrit is usually 20–30%. The peripheral blood smear is characteristically abnormal, with irreversibly sickled cells comprising 5–50% of red cells. Other findings include reticulocytosis (10–25%), nucleated red blood cells, and hallmarks of hyposplenism such as Howell–Jolly bodies and target cells. The white blood cell count is characteristically elevated to 12,000–15,000/mcL, and thrombocytosis may occur. Indirect bilirubin levels are high.

Most clinical laboratories offer a screening test for sickle cell hemoglobin, and the diagnosis of sickle cell anemia is then confirmed by hemoglobin electrophoresis (Table 13–9). Hemoglobin S has an abnormal migration pattern on electrophoresis and will usually comprise 85–98% of hemoglobin. In homozygous S disease, no hemoglobin A will be present. Hemoglobin F levels are variably increased, and high hemoglobin F levels are associated with a more benign clinical course.

Treatment

No specific treatment is available for the primary disease. Patients are maintained on folic acid supplementation and given transfusions for aplastic or hemolytic

Table 13–9. Hemoglobin distribution in sickle cell syndromes.

Genotype	Clinical Diagnosis	Hb A	Hb S	Hb A$_2$	Hb F
AA	Normal	97–99%	0	1–2%	< 1%
AS	Sickle trait	60%	40%	1–2%	< 1%
SS	Sickle cell anemia	0	86–98%	1–3%	5–15%
S β^0-thalassemia	Sickle β-thalassemia	0	70–80%	3–5%	10–20%
S β$^+$-thalassemia	Sickle β-thalassemia	10–20%	60–75%	3–5%	10–20%
AS, α-thalassemia	Sickle trait	70–75%	25–30%	1–2%	< 1%

Hb = hemoglobin.

crises. Pneumococcal vaccination reduces the incidence of infections with this pathogen.

When acute painful episodes occur, precipitating factors should be identified and infections treated if present. The patient should be kept well hydrated, and oxygen should be given if the patient is hypoxic.

Acute vaso-occlusive crises can be treated with exchange transfusion. These are primarily indicated for the treatment of intractable pain crises, priapism, and stroke.

Cytotoxic agents increase hemoglobin F levels by stimulating erythropoiesis in more primitive erythroid precursors. Hydroxyurea (500–750 mg/d) reduces the frequency of painful crises in patients whose quality of life is disrupted by frequent pain crises. Long-term safety is uncertain, and concern remains about the potential of secondary malignancies. Allogeneic bone marrow transplantation is being studied as a possible curative option for severely affected young patients.

Adams RJ et al; The Optimizing Primary Stroke Prevention in Sickle Cell Anemia (STOP 2) Trial Investigators: Discontinuing prophylactic transfusions used to prevent stroke in sickle cell disease. N Engl J Med 2005;353:2769. [PMID: 16382063]

Alexander N et al: Are there clinical phenotypes of homozygous sickle cell disease? Br J Haematol 2004;126:606. [PMID: 15287956]

Hankins JS et al: Long-term hydroxyurea therapy for infants with sickle cell anemia: the HUSOFT extension study. Blood 2005; 106:2269. [PMID: 16172253]

Steinberg MH et al: Effect of hydroxyurea on mortality and morbidity in adult sickle cell anemia: risks and benefits up to 9 years of treatment. JAMA 2003;289:1645. [PMID: 12672732]

Stuart MJ et al: Sickle-cell disease. Lancet 2004;364:1343. [PMID: 15474138]

SICKLE CELL TRAIT

Patients with the heterozygous genotype (AS) have sickle cell trait. These persons are clinically normal and have acute painful episodes only under extreme conditions such as vigorous exertion at high altitudes (or in unpressurized aircraft). The patients are hematologically normal, with no anemia and normal red blood cells on peripheral blood smear. They may, however, have a defect in renal tubular function, causing an inability to concentrate the urine, and experience episodes of gross hematuria. This appears to be caused by many years of sickling in the sluggish circulation of the renal medulla. A screening test for sickle hemoglobin will be positive, and hemoglobin electrophoresis will reveal that approximately 40% of hemoglobin is hemoglobin S (Table 13–9).

No treatment is necessary. Genetic counseling is a reasonable strategy.

SICKLE THALASSEMIA

Patients with homozygous sickle cell anemia and α-thalassemia have a somewhat milder form of hemolysis because of a slower rate of sickling related to reduced MCHC within the red blood cell.

Patients who are double heterozygotes for sickle cell anemia and β-thalassemia are clinically affected with sickle cell syndromes. Sickle β^0-thalassemia is clinically very similar to homozygous SS disease. Vaso-occlusive crises may be somewhat less severe, and the spleen is usually not infarcted. Hematologically, the MCV is usually low, in contrast to the normal MCV of sickle cell anemia. Hemoglobin electrophoresis (Table 13–9) reveals no hemoglobin A but will show an increase in hemoglobin A$_2$, which is not present in sickle cell anemia.

Sickle β$^+$-thalassemia is a milder disorder than homozygous SS disease, with fewer crises. The spleen is usually palpable. The hemolytic anemia is less severe, and the hematocrit is usually 30–38%, with reticulocytes of 5–10%. Hemoglobin electrophoresis shows the presence of some hemoglobin A.

HEMOGLOBIN C DISORDERS

Hemoglobin C is formed by a single amino acid substitution at the same site of substitution as in sickle hemoglobin but with lysine instead of valine substituted for glutamine at the β$_6$ position. Hemoglobin C is nonsickling but may participate in polymer formation in association with hemoglobin S. Homozygous hemoglobin C disease produces a mild hemolytic anemia with splenomegaly, mild jaundice, and pigment (calcium bilirubinate) gallstones. The peripheral blood smear shows generalized red cell targeting and occasional cells with rectangular crystals of hemoglobin C. Persons heterozygous for hemoglobin C are clinically normal.

Patients with hemoglobin SC disease are double heterozygotes for β S and β C. These patients, like those with sickle β⁺-thalassemia, have a milder hemolytic anemia and milder clinical course than those with homozygous SS disease. There are fewer vaso-occlusive events, and the spleen remains palpable in adult life. However, persons with hemoglobin SC disease have more retinopathy and more ischemic necrosis of bone than those with SS disease. The hematocrit is usually 30–38%, with 5–10% reticulocytes and few irreversibly sickled cells on the blood smear. Target cells are more numerous than in SS disease. Hemoglobin electrophoresis will show approximately 50% hemoglobin C, 50% hemoglobin S, and no increase in hemoglobin F levels.

Nagel RL et al: The paradox of hemoglobin SC disease. Blood Rev 2003;17:167. [PMID: 12818227]

UNSTABLE HEMOGLOBINS

Unstable hemoglobins are prone to oxidative denaturation even in the presence of a normal G6PD system. The disorder is autosomal dominant and of variable severity. Most patients have a mild chronic hemolytic anemia with splenomegaly, mild jaundice, and pigment (calcium bilirubinate) gallstones. Less severely affected patients are not anemic except under conditions of oxidative stress.

The diagnosis is made by the finding of Heinz bodies and a normal G6PD level. Hemoglobin electrophoresis is usually normal, since these hemoglobins characteristically do not have a change in their migration pattern. These hemoglobins precipitate in isopropanol. Usually no treatment is necessary. Patients with chronic hemolytic anemia should receive folate supplementation and avoid known oxidative drugs. In rare cases, splenectomy may be required.

AUTOIMMUNE HEMOLYTIC ANEMIA

 ESSENTIALS OF DIAGNOSIS

- *Acquired anemia caused by IgG autoantibody.*
- *Spherocytes and reticulocytosis on peripheral blood smear.*
- *Positive Coombs' test.*

General Considerations

Autoimmune hemolytic anemia is an acquired disorder in which an IgG autoantibody is formed that binds to the red blood cell membrane. The antibody is most commonly directed against a basic component of the Rh system present on most human red blood cells. When IgG antibodies coat the red blood cell, the Fc portion of the antibody is recognized by macrophages present in the spleen and other portions of the reticuloendothelial system. The interaction between splenic macrophage and the antibody-coated red blood cell results in removal of red blood cell membrane and the formation of a spherocyte because of the decrease in surface-to-volume ratio of the red blood cell. These spherocytic cells have decreased deformability and become trapped in the red pulp of the spleen because of their inability to squeeze through the 2-mcm fenestrations. When large amounts of IgG are present on red blood cells, complement may be fixed. Direct lysis of cells is rare, but the presence of C3b on the surface of red blood cells allows Kupffer cells in the liver to participate in the hemolytic process because of the presence of C3b receptors on Kupffer cells.

Approximately 50% of all cases of autoimmune hemolytic anemia are idiopathic. The disorder may also be seen in association with systemic lupus erythematosus, CLL, or lymphomas. It must be distinguished from drug-induced hemolytic anemia. Penicillin (and other drugs) coats the red blood cell membrane, and the antibody is directed against the membrane–drug complex.

The Coombs antiglobulin test forms the basis for diagnosis of these immune hemolytic disorders. The Coombs reagent is a rabbit IgM antibody raised against human IgG or human complement. The direct Coombs test is performed by mixing the patient's red blood cells with the Coombs reagent and looking for agglutination, which indicates the presence of antibody on the red blood cell surface. The indirect Coombs test is performed by mixing the patient's serum with a panel of type O red blood cells. After incubation of the test serum and panel red blood cells, the Coombs reagent is added. Agglutination in this system indicates the presence of free antibody in the patient's serum.

Clinical Findings

A. SYMPTOMS AND SIGNS

Autoimmune hemolytic anemia typically produces an anemia of rapid onset that may be life-threatening in severity. Patients complain of fatigue and may present with angina or congestive heart failure. On examination, jaundice and splenomegaly are usually present.

B. LABORATORY FINDINGS

The anemia is of variable severity but may be severe, with hematocrit of less than 10%. Reticulocytosis is usually present, and spherocytes are seen on the peripheral blood smear. In cases of severe hemolysis, the stressed bone marrow may also release nucleated red blood cells. As with other hemolytic disorders, indirect bilirubin is increased. Approximately 10% of patients with autoimmune hemolytic anemia have coincident immune thrombocytopenia (Evans's syndrome).

The direct Coombs test is positive, and the indirect Coombs test may or may not be positive. A positive indirect Coombs test indicates the presence of a large amount of autoantibody that has saturated binding sites in the red blood cell and consequently appears in the serum. Because the patient's serum usually contains the autoantibody, it may be difficult to obtain a compatible cross-match with donor's cells.

Treatment

Initial treatment consists of prednisone, 1–2 mg/kg/d in divided doses. Most transfused blood will survive similarly to the patient's own red blood cells. Because of difficulty in performing the cross-match, incompatible blood may be given. Decisions regarding transfusions should be made in consultation with a hematologist. If prednisone is ineffective or if the disease recurs on tapering the dose, splenectomy should be performed. Patients with autoimmune hemolytic anemia refractory to prednisone and splenectomy may be treated with a variety of agents. Treatment with rituximab, a monoclonal antibody against the B cell antigen CD20, is effective in some cases. The suggested dose is 375 mg/m^2 intravenously weekly for 4 weeks. Danazol, 600–800 mg/d, is less often effective than in immune thrombocytopenia but is well suited for long-term use because of its low toxicity. Immunosuppressive agents, including cyclophosphamide, azathioprine, or cyclosporine, may also be used. High-dose intravenous immune globulin (1 g daily for 1 or 2 days) may be highly effective in controlling hemolysis. The benefit is short-lived (1–3 weeks), and the drug is very expensive. The long-term prognosis for patients with this disorder is good, especially if there is no underlying autoimmune disorder or lymphoma. Splenectomy is often successful in controlling the disorder.

Petz LD: A physician's guide to transfusion in autoimmune haemolytic anaemia. Br J Haematol 2004;124:712. [PMID: 15009058]

Robak T: Monoclonal antibodies in the treatment of autoimmune cytopenias. Eur J Haematol 2004;72:79. [PMID: 14962245]

COLD AGGLUTININ DISEASE

ESSENTIALS OF DIAGNOSIS

- *Increased reticulocytes and spherocytes on peripheral blood smear.*
- *Coombs' test positive only for complement.*
- *Positive cold agglutinin test.*

General Considerations

Cold agglutinin disease is an acquired hemolytic anemia due to an IgM autoantibody usually directed against the I antigen on red blood cells. These IgM autoantibodies characteristically will not react with cells at 37°C but only at lower temperatures. Since the blood temperature (even in the most peripheral parts of the body)

rarely goes lower than 20°C, only antibodies active at higher temperatures will produce clinical effects. Hemolysis results indirectly from attachment of IgM, which in the cooler parts of the circulation (fingers, nose, ears) binds and fixes complement. When the red blood cell returns to a warmer temperature, the IgM antibody dissociates, leaving complement on the cell. Lysis of cells rarely occurs. Rather, C3b present on the red cells is recognized by Kupffer cells (which have receptors for C3b), and red blood cell sequestration ensues.

Most cases of chronic cold agglutinin disease are idiopathic. Others occur in association with Waldenström's macroglobulinemia, in which a monoclonal IgM paraprotein is produced. Acute postinfectious cold agglutinin disease occurs following mycoplasmal pneumonia or infectious mononucleosis (with antibody directed against antigen i rather than I).

Clinical Findings

A. SYMPTOMS AND SIGNS

In chronic cold agglutinin disease, symptoms related to red blood cell agglutination occur on exposure to cold, and patients may complain of mottled or numb fingers or toes. Hemolytic anemia is rarely severe, but episodic hemoglobinuria may occur on exposure to cold. The hemolytic anemia in acute postinfectious syndromes is rarely severe.

B. LABORATORY FINDINGS

Mild anemia is present with reticulocytosis and spherocytes. The direct Coombs test will be positive for complement only. Occasionally, a micro-Coombs test is necessary to reveal bound complement (low-titer cold agglutinin disease). A bedside cold agglutinin test may be performed by placing a glass slide in ice and then putting a few drops of heparinized blood on it. Inspection may reveal small clumps of agglutinated blood.

Treatment

Treatment is largely symptomatic, based on avoiding exposure to cold. Patients with severe involvement may be treated with alkylating agents such as cyclophosphamide or with immunosuppressive agents such as cyclosporine. Splenectomy and prednisone are usually ineffective since hemolysis takes place in the liver. High-dose intravenous immunoglobulin (2 g/kg) may be effective temporarily, but is rarely used because of the extreme cost and short duration of benefit. Rituximab, a monoclonal antibody directed against the CD20 antigen on B lymphocytes, is emerging as the treatment of choice. The dose is 375 mg/m^2 intravenously weekly for 4 weeks.

Berentsen S et al: Rituximab for primary chronic cold agglutinin disease: a prospective study of 37 courses of therapy in 27 patients. Blood 2004;103:2925. [PMID: 15070665]

MICROANGIOPATHIC HEMOLYTIC ANEMIAS

The microangiopathic hemolytic anemias are a group of disorders in which red blood cell fragmentation takes place. The anemia is intravascular, producing hemoglobinemia, hemoglobinuria, and, in severe cases, methemalbuminemia. The hallmark of the disorder is the finding of fragmented red blood cells (schistocytes, helmet cells) on the peripheral blood smear.

These fragmentation syndromes can be caused by a variety of disorders (Table 13–8). TTP is the most important of these and is discussed below. Clinical features are variable and depend on the underlying disorder. Coagulopathy and thrombocytopenia are variably present.

Chronic microangiopathic hemolytic anemia (such as is present with a malfunctioning cardiac valve prosthesis) may cause iron deficiency anemia because of continuous low-grade hemoglobinuria.

APLASTIC ANEMIA

 ESSENTIALS OF DIAGNOSIS

- *Pancytopenia.*
- *No abnormal cells seen.*
- *Hypocellular bone marrow.*

General Considerations

All hematopoietic cells are derived from a pluripotent stem cell that gives rise to precursors of erythroid, myeloid, and platelet forms. Injury to or suppression of this hematopoietic stem cell will result in pancytopenia. Aplastic anemia is a condition of bone marrow failure that arises from injury to or abnormal expression of the stem cell. The bone marrow becomes hypoplastic, and pancytopenia develops.

There are a number of causes of aplastic anemia (Table 13–10). Direct stem cell injury may be caused by radiation, chemotherapy, toxins, or pharmacologic agents. Systemic lupus erythematosus may rarely cause suppression of the hematopoietic stem cell by an IgG autoantibody directed against the stem cell. However, the most common pathogenesis of aplastic anemia appears to be autoimmune suppression of hematopoiesis by a T cell–mediated cellular mechanism.

Clinical Findings

A. SYMPTOMS AND SIGNS

Patients come to medical attention because of the consequences of bone marrow failure. Anemia leads to symptoms of weakness and fatigue, neutropenia causes vulnerability to bacterial infections, and thrombocytopenia results in mucosal and skin bleeding. Physical examination may reveal signs of pallor, purpura, and petechiae. Other abnormalities such as hepatosplenomegaly, lymphadenopathy, or bone tenderness should *not* be present, and their presence should lead to questioning the diagnosis.

B. LABORATORY FINDINGS

The hallmark of aplastic anemia is pancytopenia. However, early in the evolution of aplastic anemia, only one or two cell lines may be reduced.

Anemia may be severe and is always associated with decreased reticulocytes. Red blood cell morphology is unremarkable. The MCV is usually normal but occasionally may be increased. Neutrophils and platelets are reduced in number, and no immature or abnormal forms are seen. The bone marrow aspirate and the bone marrow biopsy appear hypocellular, with only scant amounts of normal hematopoietic progenitors. No abnormal cells are seen.

Differential Diagnosis

The diagnosis of aplastic anemia is made in cases of pancytopenia with a hypocellular marrow biopsy containing no abnormal cells. Aplastic anemia must be differentiated from other causes of pancytopenia (Table 13–11). Myelodysplastic disorders, especially hy-

Table 13–10. Causes of aplastic anemia.

Congenital (rare)
"Idiopathic" (probably autoimmune)
Systemic lupus erythematosus
Chemotherapy, radiotherapy
Toxins: benzene, toluene, insecticides
Drugs: chloramphenicol, phenylbutazone, gold salts, sulfonamides, phenytoin, carbamazepine, quinacrine, tolbutamide
Posthepatitis
Pregnancy
Paroxysmal nocturnal hemoglobinuria

Table 13–11. Causes of pancytopenia.

Bone marrow disorders
  Aplastic anemia
  Myelodysplasia
  Acute leukemia
  Myelofibrosis
  Infiltrative disease: lymphoma, myeloma, carcinoma, hairy cell leukemia
  Megaloblastic anemia
Nonmarrow disorders
  Hypersplenism
  Systemic lupus erythematosus
  Infection: tuberculosis, AIDS, leishmaniasis, brucellosis

pocellular forms of myelodysplasia, or acute leukemia may occasionally be confused with aplastic anemia. These are differentiated by the presence of morphologic abnormalities or increased blasts, or by the presence of abnormal cytogenetics in bone marrow cells. Hairy cell leukemia has been misdiagnosed as aplastic anemia and should be recognized by the presence of splenomegaly and by abnormal lymphoid cells on the bone marrow biopsy. Pancytopenia with a normocellular bone marrow is usually due to systemic lupus erythematosus, disseminated infection, or hypersplenism. Isolated thrombocytopenia may occur early as aplastic anemia develops and be confused with immune thrombocytopenia.

Treatment

Mild cases of aplastic anemia may be treated with supportive care. Red blood cell transfusions and platelet transfusions are given as necessary, and antibiotics are used to treat infections.

Severe aplastic anemia is defined by a neutrophil count of less than 500/mcL, platelets less than 20,000/mcL, reticulocytes less than 1%, and bone marrow cellularity less than 20%. When this constellation of features is present (or three of the four), the median survival without treatment is approximately 3 months, and only 20% of patients survive for 1 year. The treatment of choice for young adults (under age 50) who have HLA-matched siblings is allogeneic bone marrow transplantation. Children or young adults may also benefit from allogeneic transplantation using an unrelated donor. The use of reduced-intensity preparative regimens for allogeneic transplantation has reduced the toxicity of transplantation. Because of the increased risks associated with unrelated-donor transplantation, this treatment is usually reserved for patients who have not benefited from immunosuppressive therapy.

For adults over age 50 years or those without HLA-matched siblings, the treatment of choice for severe aplastic anemia is immunosuppression with antithymocyte globulin (ATG) plus cyclosporine. ATG is given in the hospital in conjunction with transfusion and antibiotic support. A useful regimen is 40 mg/kg/d for 4 days in combination with cyclosporine, 6 mg/kg orally twice daily. ATG must be used in combination with corticosteroids (prednisone 1–2 mg/kg/d initially, followed by a rapid taper) to avoid complications of serum sickness. Responses usually occur in 4–12 weeks and are usually only partial, but the blood counts rise high enough to give patients a safe and transfusion-free life.

High-dose immunosuppression with cyclophosphamide, 200 mg/kg, has produced remissions in refractory cases and should be considered for patients without suitable bone marrow donors. Androgens have been widely used in the past, with a low response rate. However, a few patients can be maintained successfully with this form of treatment. One regimen is oxymetholone, 2–3 mg/kg orally daily.

Course & Prognosis

Patients with severe aplastic anemia have a rapidly fatal illness if left untreated. Allogeneic bone marrow transplantation is highly successful in children and young adults, especially with HLA-matched siblings. For this group of patients, the durable complete response rate exceeds 80%. Advances in the field of unrelated donor transplantation have made this a more attractive option than in the past. ATG treatment leads to partial response in approximately 60% of adults, and the long-term prognosis of responders appears to be good. After many years of follow-up, there is increasing evidence that clonal hematologic disorders, such as paroxysmal nocturnal hemoglobinuria or myelodysplasia, may develop in some fraction (as many as 25%) of these nontransplanted patients.

Ades L et al: Long-term outcome after bone marrow transplantation for severe aplastic anemia. Blood 2004;103:2490. [PMID: 14656884]

Frickhofen N et al: Antithymocyte globulin with or without cyclosporin A: 11-year follow-up of a randomized trial comparing treatments of aplastic anemia. Blood 2003;101:1236. [PMID: 12393680]

Yamaguchi H et al: Mutations in TERT, the gene for telomerase reverse transcriptase, in aplastic anemia. N Engl J Med 2005; 352:1413. [PMID: 15814878]

Young NS: Acquired aplastic anemia. Ann Intern Med 2002; 136:534.[PMID: 11926789]

■ NEUTROPENIA

Neutropenia is present when the neutrophil count is below 1500/mcL, though blacks and other specific population groups may normally have neutrophil counts as low as 1200/mcL. The neutropenic patient is increasingly vulnerable to infection by gram-positive and gram-negative bacteria and by fungi. The risk of infection is related to the severity of neutropenia. Patients with "chronic benign neutropenia" are free of infection for years despite very low neutrophil levels.

A variety of bone marrow disorders and nonmarrow conditions may cause neutropenia (Table 13–12). All the causes of aplastic anemia (Table 13–10) and pancytopenia (Table 13–11) may cause neutropenia. Isolated neutropenia is often due to an idiosyncratic reaction to a drug, and agranulocytosis (complete absence of neutrophils in the peripheral blood) is almost always due to a drug reaction. In these cases, examination of the bone marrow shows an almost complete absence of myeloid precursors, with other cell lines undisturbed. **Felty's syndrome**—immune neutropenia associated with seropositive nodular rheumatoid arthritis and splenomegaly—is another cause. Neutropenia in the presence of a normal bone marrow may be due to immunologic peripheral destruction, sepsis,

Table 13–12. Causes of neutropenia.

Bone marrow disorders
  Aplastic anemia
  Pure white cell aplasia
  Congenital (rare)
  Cyclic neutropenia
  Drugs: sulfonamides, chlorpromazine, procainamide, pen-
    icillin, cephalosporins, cimetidine, methimazole,
    phenytoin, chlorpropamide, antiretroviral medications
  Benign chronic
Peripheral disorders
  Hypersplenism
  Sepsis
  Immune
  Felty's syndrome
  HIV infection
  Large granular lymphocytosis

or hypersplenism. Severe neutropenia may be associated with clonal disorders of T lymphocytes, often with the morphology of large granular lymphocytes.

Clinical Findings

Neutropenia results in stomatitis and in infections due to gram-positive or gram-negative aerobic bacteria or to fungi such as *Candida* or *Aspergillus*. The most common infections are septicemia, cellulitis, and pneumonia. In the presence of severe neutropenia, the usual signs of inflammatory response to infection may be absent. Nevertheless, fever in the neutropenic patient should always be assumed to be of infectious origin.

Treatment

Potential causative drugs are discontinued. Infections are treated with broad-spectrum antibiotics, but particular attention should be paid to enteric gram-negative bacteria. Effective antibiotics include the quinolones such as levofloxacin, 500 mg orally or intravenously daily, or new cephalosporins such as cefepime, 2 g intravenously every 8 hours. New antifungal agents such as voriconazole and caspofungin can provide both better efficacy and reduced toxicity compared to amphotericin.

Many cases of idiopathic or autoimmune neutropenia respond to myeloid growth factors such as granulocyte colony-stimulating factor (G-CSF). Once-weekly or twice-weekly dosage will often be sufficient to produce a protective neutrophil count.

When Felty's syndrome leads to repeated bacterial infections, splenectomy has been the treatment of choice, but it now appears that sustained use of G-CSF is effective and provides a nonsurgical alternative. The prognosis of patients with neutropenia depends on the underlying cause. Most patients with drug-induced agranulocytosis can be supported with broad-spectrum antibiotics and will recover completely. The myeloid growth factors G-CSF (filgrastim) and GM-CSF (sargramostim) may be useful in shortening the duration of neutropenia associated with chemotherapy. The neutropenia associated with large granular lymphocytes may respond to therapy with either cyclosporin or low-dose methotrexate.

Cullen M et al; Simple Investigation in Neutropenic Individuals of the Frequency of Infection after Chemotherapy +/– Antibiotic in a Number of Tumours (SIGNIFICANT) Trial Group: Antibacterial prophylaxis after chemotherapy for solid tumors and lymphomas. N Engl J Med 2005;353:988. [PMID: 16148284]

Walsh TJ et al: Caspofungin versus liposomal amphotericin B for empirical antifungal therapy in patients with persistent fever and neutropenia. N Engl J Med 2004;351:1391. [PMID: 15459300]

■ LEUKEMIAS & OTHER MYELOPROLIFERATIVE DISORDERS

Myeloproliferative disorders are due to acquired clonal abnormalities of the hematopoietic stem cell. Since the stem cell gives rise to myeloid, erythroid, and platelet cells, qualitative and quantitative changes are seen in all these cell lines. In some disorders (chronic myelogenous leukemia [CML]), specific characteristic chromosomal changes are seen. In others, no characteristic cytogenetic abnormalities are seen.

Classically, the myeloproliferative disorders produce characteristic syndromes with well-defined clinical and laboratory features (Tables 13–13 and 13–14). However, these disorders are grouped together because the disease may evolve from one form into another and because hybrid disorders are commonly seen. All of the myeloproliferative disorders may progress to AML.

POLYCYTHEMIA VERA

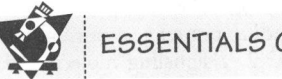

ESSENTIALS OF DIAGNOSIS

· *Increased red blood cell mass.*

Table 13–13. Classification of myeloproliferative disorders.

Myeloproliferative syndromes
  Polycythemia vera
  Myelofibrosis
  Essential thrombocytosis
  Chronic myeloid leukemia
Myelodysplastic syndromes
Acute myeloid leukemia

Table 13–14. Laboratory features of myeloproliferative disorders.

	White Count	Hematocrit	Platelet Count	Red Cell Morphology
Chronic myeloid leukemia	↑↑	N	N or ↑	N
Myelofibrosis	N or ↓ or ↑	N or ↓	↓ or N or ↑	Abn
Polycythemia vera	N or ↑	↑	N or ↑	N
Essential thrombocytosis	N or ↑	N	↑↑	N

* Splenomegaly.
* Normal arterial oxygen saturation.
* Usually elevated white blood count and platelet count.

General Considerations

Polycythemia vera is an acquired myeloproliferative disorder that causes overproduction of all three hematopoietic cell lines, most prominently the red blood cells. The hematocrit is elevated (at sea level) when values exceed 54% in males or 51% in females (Table 13–15).

When the hematocrit is elevated, the red blood cell mass should be measured to determine whether true polycythemia or relative polycythemia exists. Normal values for red blood cell mass are 26–34 mL/kg in men and 21–29 mL/kg in women. Relative ("spurious") polycythemia presents in middle-aged men who are overweight and hypertensive (often on diuretic therapy); the hematocrit is almost always less than 60%, and they have a high-normal red cell mass and a low-normal plasma volume.

If the red blood cell mass is increased, it is necessary to determine whether the increase is primary or secondary. Primary polycythemia (polycythemia vera) is a bone marrow disorder characterized by autonomous overproduction of erythroid cells. Erythroid production is independent of erythropoietin, and the serum erythropoietin level is low. In vitro, erythroid progenitor cells grow without added erythropoietin, a finding not seen in normal individuals. A mutation in JAK2, a signaling molecule, has been demonstrated in most cases and is likely involved in the pathogenesis.

Clinical Findings

A. Symptoms and Signs

Most presenting symptoms are related to expanded blood volume and increased blood viscosity. Common complaints include headache, dizziness, tinnitus, blurred vision, and fatigue. Generalized pruritus, especially following a warm shower or bath, may be a striking symptom and is related to histamine release from the increased number of basophils present. Patients may also initially complain of epistaxis. This is probably related to engorge-

ment of mucosal blood vessels in combination with abnormal hemostasis due to qualitative abnormalities in platelet function. Sixty percent of patients are men, and the median age at presentation is 60 years. Polycythemia rarely occurs in persons under age 40 years.

Physical examination reveals plethora and engorged retinal veins. The spleen is palpable in 75% of cases but is nearly always enlarged when imaged.

Thrombosis is the most common complication of polycythemia vera and the major cause of morbidity and death in this disorder. Thrombosis appears to be related to increased blood viscosity and abnormal platelet function. Uncontrolled polycythemia leads to a very high incidence of thrombotic complications of surgery, and elective surgery should be deferred until the condition has been treated. Paradoxically, in addition to thrombosis, increased bleeding also occurs. There is a high incidence of peptic ulcer disease.

B. Laboratory Findings

The hallmark of polycythemia vera is a hematocrit above normal, at times greater than 60%. Red blood cell morphology is normal. By definition, the red blood cell mass is elevated, but this is rarely measured. The white blood count is elevated to 10,000–20,000/mcL and the platelet count is variably increased, sometimes to counts exceeding 1,000,000/mcL. Platelet morphology is usually normal. White blood cells are usually normal, but basophilia and eosinophilia are frequently present.

The bone marrow is hypercellular, with panhyperplasia of all hematopoietic elements. Iron stores are usually absent from the bone marrow, having been transferred to the increased circulating red blood cell mass. Iron deficiency may also result from chronic gastrointestinal blood

Table 13–15. Causes of polycythemia.

Spurious polycythemia
Secondary polycythemia
    Hypoxia: cardiac disease, pulmonary disease, high altitude
    Carboxyhemoglobin: smoking
    Renal lesions
    Erythropoietin-secreting tumors (rare)
    Abnormal hemoglobins (rare)
Polycythemia vera

loss. Bleeding may lower the hematocrit to the normal range (or lower), creating diagnostic confusion.

Vitamin B_{12} levels are strikingly elevated because of increased levels of transcobalamin III (secreted by white blood cells). Overproduction of uric acid may lead to hyperuricemia.

Although red blood cell morphology is usually normal at presentation, microcytosis, hypochromia, and poikilocytosis may result from iron deficiency following treatment by phlebotomy (see below). Progressive hypersplenism may also lead to elliptocytosis.

Differential Diagnosis

Spurious polycythemia, in which an elevated hematocrit is due to contracted plasma volume rather than increased red cell mass, may be related to diuretic use or may occur without obvious cause.

A secondary cause of polycythemia should be suspected if splenomegaly is absent and the high hematocrit is not accompanied by increases in other cell lines. Arterial oxygen saturation should be measured to determine if hypoxia is the cause. A smoking history should be taken; carboxyhemoglobin levels may be elevated in smokers. A renal CT scan or sonogram may be considered to look for an erythropoietin-secreting cyst or tumor (see Figure 13–1). A positive family history should lead to investigation for congenital high-oxygen-affinity hemoglobin.

Polycythemia vera should be differentiated from other myeloproliferative disorders (Table 13–14). Marked elevation of the white blood count (above 30,000/mcL) suggests CML. This disorder is confirmed by the presence of the Philadelphia chromosome or the *bcr/abl* fusion gene. Abnormal red blood cell morphology and nucleated red blood cells in the peripheral blood are seen in myelofibrosis. This condition is diagnosed by bone marrow biopsy showing fibrosis of the marrow. Essential thrombocytosis is diagnosed when the platelet count is strikingly elevated and the red blood cell mass is normal.

Treatment

The treatment of choice is phlebotomy. One unit of blood (approximately 500 mL) is removed weekly until the hematocrit is less than 45%; the hematocrit is maintained at less than 45% by repeated phlebotomy as necessary. Because repeated phlebotomy intentionally produces iron deficiency, the requirement for phlebotomy should gradually decrease. It is important to avoid medicinal iron supplementation, as this can thwart the goals of a phlebotomy program. Maintaining the hematocrit at normal levels has been shown to decrease the incidence of thrombotic complications. A diet low in iron may also increase the intervals between phlebotomies.

Occasionally, myelosuppressive therapy is indicated. Indications include a high phlebotomy requirement, thrombocytosis, and intractable pruritus. There is evidence that reduction of the platelet count to less than 600,000/mcL will reduce the risk of thrombotic compli-

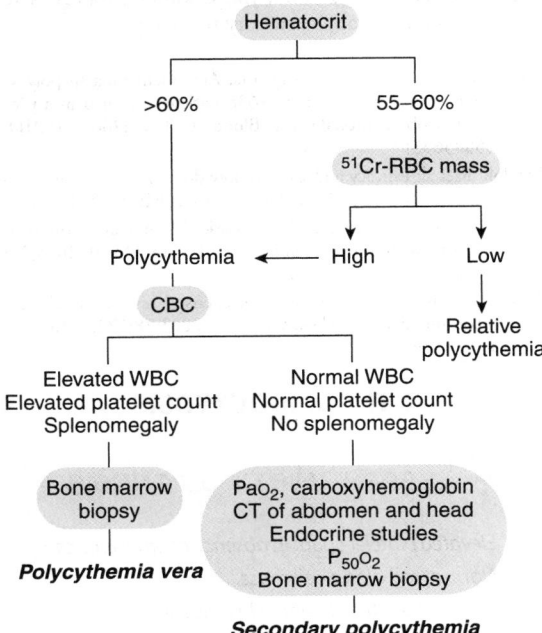

POLYCYTHEMIA SUSPECTED

Figure 13–1. Diagnostic evaluation of patients with suspected polycythemia. (RBC, red blood count; CBC, complete blood count; WBC, white blood count; Pao_2, partial pressure of oxygen in arterial blood; $P_{50}O_2$, partial pressure of oxygen at which hemoglobin is 50% saturated.) (From Nicoll D, McPhee SJ, Pignone M [editors]: *Pocket Guide to Diagnostic Tests*, 4th ed. McGraw-Hill, 2004. Modified from: Stein JH [editor]: *Internal Medicine*, 5th ed. 1998 with permission from Elsevier.)

cations. Alkylating agents have been shown to increase the risk of conversion of this disease to acute leukemia and should be avoided. Hydroxyurea is now being widely used when myelosuppressive therapy is indicated. The usual dose is 500–1500 mg/d orally, adjusted to keep platelets < 500,000/mcL without reducing the neutrophil count to < 2000/mcL. Anagrelide may be substituted or added when hydroxyurea is not well tolerated but is not the preferred initial agent. Low-dose aspirin (75–81 mg daily) has been shown to reduce the risk of thrombosis without excessive bleeding, and should be part of therapy for all patients without contraindications to aspirin.

Allopurinol may be indicated for hyperuricemia. Antihistamine therapy with diphenhydramine or other H_1-blockers may be helpful for control of pruritus, and some reports suggest the efficacy of selective serotonin reuptake inhibitors in refractory cases.

Prognosis

Polycythemia is an indolent disease with median survival of 11–15 years. The major cause of morbidity and mortality is arterial thrombosis. Over time, polycythemia vera may convert to myelofibrosis or to CML. In approximately 5% of cases, the disorder progresses to AML, which is usually refractory to therapy.

Finazzi G et al; ECLAP Investigators: Acute leukemia in polycythemia vera: an analysis of 1638 patients enrolled in a prospective observational study. Blood 2005;105:2664. [PMID: 15585653]

Landolfi R et al: Efficacy and safety of low-dose aspirin in polycythemia vera. N Engl J Med 2004;350:114. [PMID: 14711910]

Marchioli R et al: Vascular and neoplastic risk in a large cohort of patients with polycythemia vera. J Clin Oncol 2005;23: 2224. [PMID: 15710945]

Tefferi A: Polycythemia vera: a comprehensive review and clinical recommendations. Mayo Clin Proc 2003;78:174. [PMID: 12583529]

ESSENTIAL THROMBOCYTOSIS

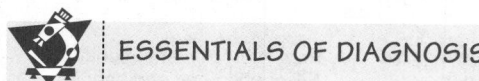

ESSENTIALS OF DIAGNOSIS

- *Elevated platelet count in absence of other causes.*
- *Normal red blood cell mass.*
- *Absence of Philadelphia chromosome.*

General Considerations

Essential thrombocytosis is an uncommon myeloproliferative disorder of unknown cause in which marked proliferation of the megakaryocytes in the bone marrow leads to elevation of the platelet count. As with polycythemia vera, the recent finding of a high frequency of mutations of JAK2 in these patients promises to advance the understanding of this disorder.

Clinical Findings

A. SYMPTOMS AND SIGNS

The median age at presentation is 50–60 years, and there is a slightly increased incidence in women. The disorder is often suspected when an elevated platelet count is found. Less frequently, the first sign is thrombosis, which is the most common clinical problem. The risk of thrombosis rises with age. Venous thromboses may occur in unusual sites such as the mesenteric, hepatic, or portal vein. Some patients experience erythromelalgia, painful burning of the hands accompanied by erythema; this symptom is reliably relieved by aspirin. Bleeding, typically mucosal, is less common and is related to a concomitant qualitative platelet defect. Splenomegaly is present in at least 25% of patients.

B. LABORATORY FINDINGS

An elevated platelet count is the hallmark of this disorder, and may be over 2,000,000/mcL. The white blood cell count is often mildly elevated, usually not above 30,000/mcL, but with some immature myeloid forms.

The hematocrit is normal. The peripheral blood smear reveals large platelets, but giant degranulated forms seen in myelofibrosis are not observed. Red blood cell morphology is normal. The bleeding time is prolonged in 20% of patients.

The bone marrow shows increased numbers of megakaryocytes but no other morphologic abnormalities. The Philadelphia chromosome is absent but should be assayed by molecular testing of peripheral blood for the *bcr/abl* fusion gene in all suspected cases to differentiate the disorder from chronic myeloid leukemia.

Differential Diagnosis

Essential thrombocytosis must be distinguished from secondary causes of an elevated platelet count. In reactive thrombocytosis, the platelet count seldom exceeds 1,000,000/mcL. Inflammatory disorders such as rheumatoid arthritis and ulcerative colitis cause significant elevations of the platelet count, as may chronic infection. The thrombocytosis of iron deficiency is observed only when anemia is significant. The platelet count is temporarily elevated after splenectomy.

Regarding other myeloproliferative disorders, the lack of elevated hematocrit and red blood cell mass distinguishes it from polycythemia vera. Unlike myelofibrosis, red blood cell morphology is normal, nucleated red blood cells are absent, and giant degranulated platelets are not seen. In chronic myeloid leukemia, the Philadelphia chromosome (or *bcr/abl* by molecular testing) establishes the diagnosis.

Treatment

The risk of thrombosis can be reduced by control of the platelet count, which should be kept at less than 500,000/mcL. The treatment of choice is hydroxyurea in a dose of 0.5–2 g/d. Hydroxyurea has been shown to be more effective than anagrelide in preventing thrombotic events, with no increase in toxicity. In cases in which hydroxyurea is not well tolerated because of anemia, low doses of anagrelide, 1–2 mg/d, may be added. Higher doses of anagrelide are often complicated by headache, peripheral edema, and congestive heart failure.

Vasomotor symptoms such as erythromelalgia and paresthesias respond rapidly to aspirin and eventually to control of the platelet count. The role of chronic low-dose aspirin therapy to reduce the risk of thrombosis remains unsettled. In the unusual event of severe bleeding, the platelet count can be lowered rapidly with plateletpheresis.

Course & Prognosis

Essential thrombocytosis is an indolent disorder and allows long-term survival. Average survival is longer than 15 years from diagnosis, and the survival of patients younger than 50 years does not appear different from matched controls. The major source of morbidity—thrombosis—can be reduced by appropriate platelet control. Late in the course of the disease, the bone marrow may become fibrotic, and massive splenomegaly may occur, sometimes with splenic infarction. There is a 10–15% risk of progression to myelofibrosis after 15 years, and a 1–5% risk of transformation to acute leukemia over 20 years.

Barbui T et al: Practice guidelines for the therapy of essential thrombocythemia. A statement from the Italian Society of Hematology, the Italian Society of Experimental Hematology, and the Italian Group for Bone Marrow Transplantation. Haematologica 2004;89:215. [PMID: 15003898]

Harrison CN et al; United Kingdom Medical Research Council Primary Thrombocythemia 1 Study: Hydroxyurea Compared with anagrelide in high-risk essential thrombocythemia. N Engl J Med 2005;353:33. [PMID: 16000354]

Harrison CN et al: Essential thrombocythemia. Hematol Oncol Clin North Am 2003;17:1175. [PMID: 14560781]

MYELOFIBROSIS

ESSENTIALS OF DIAGNOSIS

- *Striking splenomegaly.*
- *Teardrop poikilocytosis on peripheral smear.*
- *Leukoerythroblastic blood picture; giant abnormal platelets.*
- *Hypercellular bone marrow with reticulin or collagen fibrosis.*

General Considerations

Myelofibrosis (myelofibrosis with myeloid metaplasia, agnogenic myeloid metaplasia) is a myeloproliferative disorder characterized by fibrosis of the bone marrow, splenomegaly, and a leukoerythroblastic peripheral blood picture with teardrop poikilocytosis. It is widely believed that fibrosis occurs in response to increased secretion of platelet-derived growth factor (PDGF) and possibly other cytokines. In response to bone marrow fibrosis, extramedullary hematopoiesis takes place in the liver, spleen, and lymph nodes. In these sites, mesenchymal cells responsible for fetal hematopoiesis can be reactivated. As with other myeloproliferative diseases, abnormalities of JAK2 signalling pathways may be involved in the pathogenesis.

Clinical Findings

A. SYMPTOMS AND SIGNS

Myelofibrosis develops in adults over age 50 years and is usually insidious in onset. Patients most commonly present with fatigue due to anemia or abdominal fullness related to splenomegaly. Uncommon presentations include bleeding and bone pain. On examination, splenomegaly is almost invariably present and is commonly massive. The liver is enlarged in more than 50% of cases.

Later in the course of the disease, progressive bone marrow failure takes place as it becomes increasingly more fibrotic. Anemia becomes severe, requiring transfusion. Progressive thrombocytopenia leads to bleeding. The spleen continues to enlarge, which leads to early satiety. Painful episodes of splenic infarction may occur. Late in the course, the patient becomes cachectic and may experience severe bone pain, especially in the upper legs. Hematopoiesis in the liver leads to portal hypertension with ascites, esophageal varices, and occasionally transverse myelitis caused by myelopoiesis in the epidural space.

B. LABORATORY FINDINGS

Patients are almost invariably anemic at presentation. The white blood count is variable—either low, normal, or elevated—and may be increased to 50,000/mcL. The platelet count is variable. The peripheral blood smear is dramatic, with significant poikilocytosis and numerous teardrop forms in the red cell line. Nucleated red blood cells are present and the myeloid series is shifted, with immature forms including a small percentage of promyelocytes or myeloblasts. Platelet morphology may be bizarre, and giant degranulated platelet forms (megakaryocyte fragments) may be seen. The triad of teardrop poikilocytosis, leukoerythroblastic blood, and giant abnormal platelets is highly suggestive of myelofibrosis.

The bone marrow usually cannot be aspirated (dry tap), though early in the course of the disease it is hypercellular, with a marked increase in megakaryocytes. Fibrosis at this stage is detected by a silver stain demonstrating increased reticulin fibers. Later, biopsy reveals more severe fibrosis, with eventual replacement of hematopoietic precursors by collagen. There is no characteristic chromosomal abnormality.

Differential Diagnosis

A leukoerythroblastic blood picture from other causes may be seen in response to severe infection, inflammation, or infiltrative bone marrow processes. However, teardrop poikilocytosis and giant abnormal platelet forms will not be present. Bone marrow fibrosis may be seen in metastatic carcinoma, Hodgkin's disease, and hairy cell leukemia. These disorders are diagnosed by characteristic morphology of involved tissues.

Concerning other myeloproliferative disorders, CML is diagnosed when there is marked leukocytosis, normal red blood cell morphology, and the presence of the Philadelphia chromosome or *bcr/abl* fusion gene. Polycythemia vera is characterized by an elevated red blood cell mass. Essential thrombocytosis shows predominant and consistent platelet count elevations.

Treatment

Patients with mild forms of the disease may require no therapy or occasional transfusion support. Recently, biologic agents have shown some benefit. Thalidomide has produced definite responses with acceptable toxicity, and the investigational agent lenalidomide (Revlimid) may have equivalent efficacy with less toxicity. Allogeneic bone marrow transplantation has been performed successfully with 50% long-term survival and should be considered in younger patients. The use of less toxic, nonmyeloablative regimens for allogeneic transplantation has produced encouraging results. Anemic patients are supported with transfusion. Erythropoietin may increase red blood cell production and decrease transfusion requirements. Splenectomy is not routinely performed but is indicated for splenic enlargement causing recurrent painful episodes, severe thrombocytopenia, or an unacceptable transfusion requirement.

Course & Prognosis

It is difficult to date the onset of myelofibrosis, but the median survival from time of diagnosis is approximately 5 years. New therapies with biologic agents, such as thalidomide and lenalidomide, and the application of reduced-intensity allogeneic stem cell transplantation now appear to offer the possibility of improving the outcome for many patients. End-stage myelofibrosis is characterized by generalized debility, liver failure, and bleeding from thrombocytopenia, with some cases terminating in AML.

Deeg HJ et al: Allogeneic hematopoietic stem cell transplantation for myelofibrosis. Blood 2003;102:3912. [PMID: 12920019]

Dingli D et al: Myelofibrosis with myeloid metaplasia: new developments in pathogenesis and treatment. Intern Med 2004; 43:540. [PMID: 15335177]

Kralovics R et al: A gain-of-function mutation of JAK2 in myeloproliferative disorders. N Engl J Med 2005;352:1779. [PMID: 15858187]

Mesa RA et al: Durable responses to thalidomide-based drug therapy for myelofibrosis with myeloid metaplasia. Mayo Clin Proc 2004;79:883. [PMID: 15244384]

CHRONIC MYELOGENOUS LEUKEMIA

ESSENTIALS OF DIAGNOSIS

- *Strikingly elevated white blood count.*
- *Markedly left-shifted myeloid series but with a low percentage of promyelocytes and blasts.*
- *Presence of Philadelphia chromosome or bcr/abl gene.*

General Considerations

CML is a myeloproliferative disorder characterized by overproduction of myeloid cells. These myeloid cells retain the capacity for differentiation, and normal bone marrow function is retained during the early phases. The disease usually remains stable for years and then transforms to a more overtly malignant disease.

CML is characterized by a specific chromosomal abnormality, the Philadelphia chromosome, a reciprocal translocation between the long arms of chromosomes 9 and 22. A large portion of 22q is translocated to 9q, and a smaller piece of 9q is moved to 22q. The portion of 9q that is translocated contains *abl*, a protooncogene that is the cellular homolog of the Ableson murine leukemia virus. The *abl* gene is received at a specific site on 22q, the break point cluster (bcr). The fusion gene *bcr/abl* produces a novel protein that differs from the normal transcript of the *abl* gene in that it possesses tyrosine kinase activity (a characteristic activity of transforming genes). Evidence that the *bcr/abl* fusion gene is pathogenic is provided by transgenic mouse models in which introduction of the gene almost invariably leads to leukemia. Furthermore, targeted therapy with imatinib, which inhibits the tyrosine kinase activity of the *bcr/abl* protein, is remarkably effective as treatment.

Approximately 5% of cases of CML are Philadelphia chromosome negative at the level of light microscope cytogenetics, though molecular studies demonstrate the *bcr/abl* fusion gene, and these patients appear to have the same clinical outcome as those with the overt cytogenetic finding. The entity formerly known as Philadelphia chromosome-negative CML is now recognized as chronic myelomonocytic leukemia, a subtype of myelodysplasia.

Early CML ("chronic phase") does not behave like a malignant disease. Normal bone marrow function is retained, white blood cells differentiate, and, despite some qualitative abnormalities (low leukocyte alkaline phosphatase), the neutrophils combat infection normally. However, CML is inherently unstable, and the disease progresses to an accelerated phase and finally after several years, to blast crisis. This progression of the disease is often associated with added chromosomal defects superimposed on the Philadelphia chromosome. Blast crisis CML is morphologically indistinguishable from acute leukemia.

Clinical Findings

A. SYMPTOMS AND SIGNS

CML is a disorder of middle age (median age at presentation is 55 years). Patients usually present with fatigue, night sweats, and low-grade fever related to the hypermetabolic state caused by overproduction of white blood cells. At other times, the patient complains of abdominal fullness related to splenomegaly. In many cases, an elevated white blood count is discovered incidentally. Rarely, the patient will present with a clinical syndrome related to leukostasis with blurred vision, respiratory distress, or priapism. The white blood count in these cases is usually greater than 500,000/mcL.

On examination, the spleen is enlarged (often markedly so), and sternal tenderness may be present as a sign of marrow overexpansion. In cases discovered during routine laboratory monitoring, these findings are often absent.

Acceleration of the disease is often associated with fever in the absence of infection, bone pain, and splenomegaly. In blast crisis, patients may experience bleeding and infection related to bone marrow failure.

B. LABORATORY FINDINGS

The hallmark of CML is an elevated white blood count; the median white blood count at diagnosis is 150,000/mcL, although in some cases the white blood cell count is only modestly increased. The peripheral blood is characteristic. The myeloid series is left shifted, with mature forms dominating and with cells usually present in proportion to their degree of maturation. Blasts are usually less than 5%. Basophilia and eosinophilia of granulocytes may be present. At presentation, the patient is usually not anemic. Red blood cell morphology is normal, and nucleated red blood cells are rarely seen. The platelet count may be normal or elevated (sometimes to strikingly high levels). Platelet morphology is usually normal, but abnormally large forms may be seen.

The bone marrow is hypercellular, with left-shifted myelopoiesis. Myeloblasts comprise less than 5% of marrow cells.

The hallmark of the disease is that the *bcr/abl* gene is detected in the peripheral blood. This is best done by the polymerase chain reaction (PCR) test, which has now supplanted cytogenetics in looking for the Philadelphia chromosome. A bone marrow examination is not necessary for diagnosis, although it is useful for prognosis and for detecting additional chromosomal abnormalities in addition to the Philadelphia chromosome.

With progression to the accelerated and blast phases, progressive anemia and thrombocytopenia occur, and the percentage of blasts in the blood and bone marrow increases. Blast phase CML is diagnosed when blasts comprise more than 30% of bone marrow cells.

Differential Diagnosis

Early CML must be differentiated from the reactive leukocytosis associated with infection. In such cases, the white blood count is usually less than 50,000/mcL, splenomegaly is absent, and the *bcr/abl* gene is not present.

CML must be distinguished from other myeloproliferative disease (Table 13–14). The hematocrit should not be elevated, the red blood cell morphology is normal, and nucleated red blood cells are rare or absent. Definitive diagnosis is made by finding the *bcr/abl* gene.

Treatment

Treatment is usually not emergent even with white blood counts over 200,000/mcL, since the majority of circulating cells are mature myeloid cells that are smaller and more deformable than primitive leukemic blasts. In the rare instances in which symptoms result from extreme hyperleukocytosis (priapism, respiratory distress, visual blurring, altered mental status), emergent leukapheresis is performed in conjunction with myelosuppressive therapy.

The treatment of CML has been transformed by the introduction of imatinib mesylate. This drug is a specifically designed inhibitor of the tyrosine kinase activity of the *bcr/abl* oncogene. It is well tolerated and results in nearly universal (98%) hematologic control of chronic phase disease. It has now replaced both interferon and hydroxyurea as standard therapy. For patients with the chronic phase of CML, the standard dose is 400 mg orally daily. Higher doses, such as 600–800 mg daily, may overcome some degree of resistance and may produce more rapid initial responses, but side effects are more prominent with these doses. The most common toxicities are nausea, periorbital swelling, edema, rash, and myalgia, but most of these are modest. Fewer than 5% of patients discontinue the drug due to unacceptable side effects.

Response is assessed in several ways. First, the patient should enter hematologic complete remission, with normalization of blood counts and splenomegaly. This usually occurs within several weeks, but should occur within 3 months. Second, cytogenetic remission should be achieved, ideally within 6 months but certainly within 12 months. A "major cytogenetic response" is identified when < 35% of metaphases contain the Philadelphia chromosome, and a "complete cytogenetic response" indicates the absence of the abnormal chromosome. More recently, quantitative assessment of the *bcr/abl* gene using PCR assays has become the standard method of assessment. At this time, with lead patients out 5 years from start of imatinib, 100% of patients with the best response (complete cytogenetic response and > 3 log reduction in *bcr/abl*) remain free of progression. Others with lesser degrees of response have increased risk of early progression, and these patients are best treated with allogeneic stem cell transplantation. Although imatinib has been a remarkable new treatment, since almost all clinical experience with imatinib began in early 2000, the long-term outcome is uncertain.

Current clinical trials focus on new molecular targeted agents that can overcome resistance to imatinib. Dasatinib has been shown to produce responses in a high proportion of patients whose disease has become resistant to imatinib and is being evaluated as initial therapy. Other investigational agents are similarly being evaluated. It is possible that combinations of molecular targeted agents will be used in the future.

Hydroxyurea was formerly the standard treatment for this disease and can be used for patients who do not tolerate imatinib. Hydroxyurea is oral and very well tolerated. The usual dose is 0.5–2.5 g/d, adjusted to keep the white blood cell count ideally near 5000/mcL but in any case above 2000/mcL. It is given without interruption because of rapid white blood cell rebound.

The only available curative therapy for CML is allogeneic bone marrow transplantation. The best results (80% cure rate) are obtained in patients who are under 40 years of age and transplanted within 1 year after diagnosis from HLA-matched siblings. The introduction of imatinib has changed the approach to allogeneic transplant for CML. Patients with the best transplant outcomes (under 40 years of age with matched sibling donors) may be offered allogeneic transplant as initial therapy. An alternative approach is to initiate imatinib and to recommend transplant if there is a suboptimal response, either lack of a complete cytogenetic response, a suboptimal molecular response, or an increasing level of *bcr/abl* transcripts. These recommendations are in flux and may change as long-term experience with imatinib and other agents accumulates. For patients without sibling donors whose disease is not well controlled by imatinib, HLA-matched unrelated donors may be located through registries such as the National Marrow Donors Program. Results are somewhat inferior to those achieved with matched sibling transplants but offer a cure rate of 40–60% in an otherwise invariably fatal disease.

Allogeneic transplantation cures CML by initial cytoreduction followed by long-term immunologic control mediated by the donor's immune system. This alloimmune phenomenon has been called the "graft-versus-leukemia" effect. The most compelling evidence for its importance is that chronic phase disease that has recurred after allogeneic transplantation can usually be reversed without additional chemotherapy by the infusion of T lymphocytes from the initial bone marrow donor. This donor lymphocyte infusion can lead to long-term remission in 50–70% of cases. In response to appreciation of the importance of the graft-versus-leukemia effect, less toxic forms of allogeneic transplantation (nonmyeloablative) have been developed that require much less initial cytoreductive therapy and rely exclusively on the immune effect for long-term disease control. This approach has been encouraging and is likely to further expand the role of allogeneic transplant for CML, allowing transplant in selected patients up to age 70 years.

Course & Prognosis

In the past, median survival was 3–4 years. In the era of imatinib therapy, and with the recent development of new molecular targeted agents, more than 80% of patients remain alive and in remission at 4 years. It is impossible to predict at this time to what extent long-term survival will be impacted. At the current time, allogeneic stem cell transplantation remains the only proven curative treatment.

Crossman LC et al: Imatinib therapy in chronic myeloid leukemia. Hematol Oncol Clin North Am 2004;18:605. [PMID: 15271395]

Deininger M et al: The development of imatinib as a therapeutic agent for chronic myeloid leukemia. Blood 2005;105:2640. [PMID: 15618470]

Kantarjian HM et al: Long-term survival benefit and improved complete cytogenetic and molecular response rates with imatinib mesylate in Philadelphia chromosome-positive chronic-phase chronic myeloid leukemia after failure of interferon-alpha. Blood 2004;104:1979. [PMID: 15198956]

Or R et al: Nonmyeloablative allogeneic stem cell transplantation for the treatment of chronic myeloid leukemia in first chronic phase. Blood 2003;101:441. [PMID: 12393604]

Radich JP et al: HLA-matched related hematopoietic cell transplantation for chronic-phase CML using a targeted busulfan and cyclophosphamide preparative regimen. Blood 2003; 102:31. [PMID: 12595317]

Shah NP et al: Overriding imatinib resistance with a novel ABL kinase inhibitor. Science 2004;305:399. [PMID: 15256671]

MYELODYSPLASTIC SYNDROMES

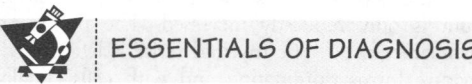 ESSENTIALS OF DIAGNOSIS

- *Cytopenias with a hypercellular bone marrow.*
- *Morphologic abnormalities in two or more hematopoietic cell lines.*

General Considerations

The myelodysplastic syndromes are a group of acquired clonal disorders of the hematopoietic stem cell. They are characterized by the constellation of cytopenias, a hypercellular marrow, and a number of morphologic and cytogenetic abnormalities. The disorders are usually idiopathic but may be seen after cytotoxic chemotherapy.

Despite the presence of adequate numbers of hematopoietic progenitor cells, "ineffective hematopoiesis" occurs, resulting in various cytopenias. Ultimately, the disorder may evolve into AML, and the term "preleukemia" has been used in the past to describe these disorders. Although no specific chromosomal abnormality is seen in myelodysplasia, there are frequently abnormalities involving the long arm of chromosome 5 (which contains a number of genes encoding both growth factors and receptors involved in myelopoiesis) as well as deletions of chromosomes 5 and 7.

Myelodysplasia encompasses several heterogeneous syndromes. Those without excess bone marrow blasts are termed "refractory anemia," with or without ringed sideroblasts. Syndromes with excess blasts are diagnosed as "refractory anemia with excess blasts" (RAEB 5–19% blasts). Those with a proliferative syndrome including peripheral blood monocytosis greater than 1000/mcL are termed "chronic myelomonocytic leukemia (CMML)." An International Prognostic Scoring System (IPSS) has been developed that classifies patients by risk status based on the percentage of bone marrow blasts, cytogenetics, and the severity of cytopenias.

Clinical Findings

A. Symptoms and Signs

Patients are usually over age 60 years. Many are diagnosed while asymptomatic because of the finding of abnormal blood counts. Patients usually present with fatigue, infection, or bleeding related to bone marrow failure. The course may be indolent, and the disease may present as a wasting illness with fever, weight loss, and general debility. On examination, splenomegaly may be present in combination with pallor, bleeding, and various signs of infection.

B. LABORATORY FINDINGS

Anemia may be marked and may require transfusion support. The MCV is normal or increased, and macroovalocytes may be seen on the peripheral blood smear. The reticulocyte count is usually reduced. The white blood cell count is usually normal or reduced, and neutropenia is common. The neutrophils may exhibit morphologic abnormalities, including deficient numbers of granules or a bilobed nucleus (Pelger–Huet). The myeloid series may be left shifted, and small numbers of promyelocytes or blasts may be seen. The platelet count is normal or reduced, and hypogranular platelets may be present.

The bone marrow is characteristically hypercellular, but may be hypocellular. Erythroid hyperplasia is common, and signs of abnormal erythropoiesis include megaloblastic features, nuclear budding, or multinucleated erythroid precursors. The Prussian blue stain may demonstrate ringed sideroblasts. The myeloid series is often left shifted, with variable increases in blasts. Deficient or abnormal granules may be seen. A characteristic abnormality is the presence of dwarf megakaryocytes with a unilobed nucleus. A variety of cytogenetic abnormalities in the bone marrow are characteristic of myelodysplasia. Some patients with an indolent form of the disease have an isolated partial deletion of chromosome 5 (5q– syndrome). The presence of other abnormalities such as monosomy 7 is associated with more aggressive disease.

Differential Diagnosis

In subtle cases, cytogenetic evaluation of the bone marrow may help distinguish this clonal disorder from other causes of cytopenias. As the number of blasts increases in the bone marrow, myelodysplasia is arbitrarily separated from AML by the presence of less than 20% blasts.

Treatment

Historically, there has been no effective therapy for this disorder, and patients have been managed with supportive care. However, this is now changing. Patients affected primarily by anemia may be supported with red blood cell transfusions. Erythropoietin (epoetin alfa), 30,000 units subcutaneously weekly, reduces the red cell transfusion requirement in some patients. The response rate is 20%, but a 4-week trial of epoetin alfa is reasonable since it will be of benefit and cost-effective for the subgroup of responders. The combination of myeloid growth factors and high doses of epoetin alfa produces a higher response rate, but the cost is very high. Lenalidomide has recently been approved for the treatment of transfusion-dependent anemia due to my-elodysplasia. It is remarkably effective in patients with the 5q- cytogenetic abnormality, with significant responses in 70% of patients. The recommended initial dose is 10 mg daily. The most common side effects are neutropenia and thrombocytopenia, but venous thrombosis is also seen. The cost of this new agent is extremely high. Patients affected primarily with severe neutropenia may benefit from the use of myeloid growth factors such as G-CSF or GM-CSF.

Azacitidine (5-azacytidine) has been approved as an effective treatment based on its ability to improve both symptoms and blood counts and to prolong the time to conversion to acute leukemia. It is now the treatment of choice for many patients, especially those with higher risk disease based on increased blasts in the bone marrow. Occasional patients can benefit from immunosuppressive therapy including ATG. Patients with hypocellular bone marrows and those with HLA A15 have an increased chance of response. Allogeneic stem cell transplantation is the only curative therapy for myelodysplasia, but its role is limited by the advanced age of many patients and the indolent course of disease in some subsets of patients. The optimal use and timing of allogeneic transplantation are controversial, but the use of reduced-intensity preparative regimens for transplantation has expanded the role of this therapy, using both family and matched unrelated donors.

Course & Prognosis

Myelodysplasia is an ultimately fatal disease, and allogeneic transplantation is the only curative therapy, with cure rates of 30–60% depending primarily on the risk status of the disease. Patients most commonly die of infections or bleeding. The risk of transformation to AML depends on the percentage of blasts in the bone marrow. Patients with refractory anemia may survive many years, and the risk of leukemia is low (< 10%). Those with excess blasts or CMML have short survivals (usually < 2 years) and have a higher (20–50%) risk of developing acute leukemia. The finding of full deletions of chromosomes 5 and 7 is associated with a poor prognosis.

Cortes J et al: Phase I Study of BMS-214662, a farnesyl transferase inhibitor in patients with acute leukemias and high-risk myelodysplastic syndromes. J Clin Oncol 2005;23:2805. [PMID: 15728224]

Ho AY et al: Reduced-intensity allogeneic hematopoietic stem cell transplantation for myelodysplastic syndrome and acute myeloid leukemia with multilineage dysplasia using fludarabine, busulphan, and alemtuzumab (FBC) conditioning. Blood 2004;104:1616. [PMID: 15059843]

Jädersten M et al: Long-term outcome of treatment of anemia in MDS with erythropoietin and G-CSF. Blood 2005;106:803. [PMID: 15840690]

List A et al: Efficacy of lenalidomide in myelodysplastic syndromes. N Engl J Med 2005;352:549. [PMID: 15703420]

Silverman LR et al: Randomized controlled trial of azacitidine in patients with the myelodysplastic syndrome: a study of the cancer and leukemia group B. J Clin Oncol 2002;20:2429. [PMID: 12011120]

ACUTE LEUKEMIA

ESSENTIALS OF DIAGNOSIS

- *Short duration of symptoms, including fatigue, fever, and bleeding.*
- *Cytopenias or pancytopenia.*
- *More than 20% blasts in the bone marrow.*
- *Blasts in peripheral blood in 90% of patients.*

General Considerations

Acute leukemia is a malignancy of the hematopoietic progenitor cell. The malignant cell loses its ability to mature and differentiate. These cells proliferate in an uncontrolled fashion and replace normal bone marrow elements. Most cases arise with no clear cause. However, radiation and some toxins (benzene) are leukemogenic. In addition, a number of chemotherapeutic agents (especially procarbazine, melphalan, other alkylating agents, and etoposide) may cause leukemia. The leukemias seen after toxin or chemotherapy exposure often develop from a myelodysplastic prodrome and are associated with abnormalities in chromosomes 5 and 7.

Much has been learned about the molecular biology of the leukemias. One subtype, acute promyelocytic leukemia, is characterized by chromosomal translocation t(15;17), which produces the fusion gene *PML-RARα*. This change in the retinoic acid receptor produces a block in differentiation that can be overcome with pharmacologic doses of retinoic acid (see below).

Most of the clinical findings in acute leukemia are due to replacement of normal bone marrow elements by the malignant cell. Less common manifestations result from organ infiltration (skin, gastrointestinal tract, meninges). Acute leukemia is potentially curable with combination chemotherapy.

Acute lymphoblastic leukemia (ALL) comprises 80% of the acute leukemias of childhood. The peak incidence is between 3 and 7 years of age. It is also seen in adults, causing approximately 20% of adult acute leukemias. AML is primarily an adult disease with a median age at presentation of 60 years and an increasing incidence with advanced age.

Clinical Findings

A. SYMPTOMS AND SIGNS

Most patients have been ill only for days or weeks. Bleeding (usually due to thrombocytopenia) occurs in the skin and mucosal surfaces, with gingival bleeding, epistaxis, or menorrhagia. Less commonly, widespread bleeding is seen in patients with disseminated intravascular coagulation (DIC) (in acute promyelocytic leukemia and monocytic leukemia). Infection is due to neutropenia, with the risk of infection rising as the neutrophil count falls below 500/mcL; with neutrophil counts less than 100/mcL, infection within days is the rule. The most common pathogens are gram-negative bacteria (*Escherichia coli*, *Klebsiella*, *Pseudomonas*) or fungi (*Candida*, *Aspergillus*). Common presentations include cellulitis, pneumonia, and perirectal infections; death within a few hours may occur if treatment with appropriate antibiotics is delayed.

Patients may also seek medical attention because of gum hypertrophy and bone and joint pain. The most dramatic presentation is hyperleukocytosis, in which a markedly elevated circulating blast count (usually > 200,000/mcL) leads to impaired circulation, presenting as headache, confusion, and dyspnea. Such patients require emergent leukapheresis and chemotherapy.

On examination, patients appear pale and have purpura and petechiae; signs of infection may not be present. Stomatitis and gum hypertrophy may be seen in patients with monocytic leukemia, as may rectal fissures. There is variable enlargement of the liver, spleen, and lymph nodes. Bone tenderness may be present, particularly in the sternum, tibia, and femur.

B. LABORATORY FINDINGS

The hallmark of acute leukemia is the combination of pancytopenia with circulating blasts. However, blasts may be absent from the peripheral smear in as many as 10% of cases ("aleukemic leukemia"). The bone marrow is usually hypercellular and dominated by blasts. More than 20% blasts are required to make a diagnosis of acute leukemia.

A number of other laboratory abnormalities are noted. Hyperuricemia may be seen. If DIC is present, the fibrinogen level will be reduced, the prothrombin time prolonged, and fibrin degradation products or fibrin D-dimers present. Patients with ALL (especially T cell) may have a mediastinal mass visible on chest radiograph. Meningeal leukemia will have blasts present in the spinal fluid, seen in approximately 5% of cases at diagnosis; it is more common in monocytic types of AML.

Acute leukemia should be classified as either ALL or AML. The Auer rod, an eosinophilic needle-like inclusion in the cytoplasm, is pathognomonic of AML. To confirm the myeloid nature of the cells, histochemical stains demonstrating myeloid enzymes such as peroxidase may be useful. Monocytic lineage can be established by the finding of butyrate esterase. ALL is considered when there is no morphologic or histochemical evidence of myeloid or monocytic lineage. The diagnosis is confirmed by demonstrating surface markers characteristic of primitive lymphoid cells, typically by flow cytometry; terminal deoxynucleotidyl transferase (TdT) is present in 95% of cases of ALL. A variety of monoclonal antibodies have been used to define other phenotypes of ALL. Primitive B lymphocyte antigens include CD19 and sometimes CD10. T cell ALL is diagnosed by the finding of CD2, CD5, and CD7.

AML is usually categorized on the basis of morphology and histochemistry as follows: acute undifferentiated leukemia (M0), acute myeloblastic leukemia (M1), acute myeloblastic leukemia with differentiation (M2), acute promyelocytic leukemia (M3), acute myelomonocytic leukemia (M4), acute monoblastic leukemia (M5), erythroleukemia (M6), and megakaryoblastic leukemia (M7). The World Health Organization (WHO) has sponsored a new classification of the leukemias and other hematologic malignancies that incorporates cytogenetic, molecular, and immunophenotype information.

ALL is most usefully classified by immunologic phenotype as follows: common, early B lineage, and T cell.

Cytogenetic studies are the most powerful prognostic factors in the acute leukemias. Favorable cytogenetics in AML include t(8;21), t(15;17), and inv(16)(p13;q22). These patients have a higher chance of achieving both short- and long-term disease control. In ALL, the hyperdiploid states are associated with a better prognosis. Unfavorable cytogenetics in AML are monosomy 5 and 7 and complex abnormalities; unfavorable cytogenetics in ALL are the Philadelphia chromosomes t(9;22) and t(4;11).

Differential Diagnosis

AML must be distinguished from other myeloproliferative disorders, CML, and myelodysplastic syndromes. Acute leukemia also resembles a left-shifted bone marrow recovering from a previous toxic insult. If the question is in doubt, a bone marrow study should be repeated in several days to see if maturation has taken place. ALL must be separated from other lymphoproliferative disease such as CLL, lymphomas, and hairy cell leukemia. It may also be confused with the atypical lymphocytosis of mononucleosis and pertussis.

Treatment

Most young patients with acute leukemia are treated with the objective of effecting a cure. The first step in treatment is to obtain complete remission, defined as normal peripheral blood with resolution of cytopenias, normal bone marrow with no excess blasts, and normal clinical status. The type of initial chemotherapy depends on the subtype of leukemia. Most patients with AML are treated with a combination of an anthracycline (daunorubicin or idarubicin) plus cytarabine, either alone or in combination with other agents. This therapy will produce complete remissions in 70–80% of patients under age 60 years and in 40–60% of older patients. Acute promyelocytic leukemia is treated differently from other forms of AML. Induction therapy includes an anthracycline plus all-*trans*-retinoic acid. This agent is an analog of vitamin A that leads to terminal differentiation of acute promyelocytic leukemia cells through an interaction with the abnormal retinoic acid receptor created by a specific chromosomal translocation, which is the hallmark of the subtype of leukemia. With this approach 90–95% of patients will achieve complete remission. Adults with ALL are treated with

combination chemotherapy, including daunorubicin, vincristine, prednisone, and asparaginase. This treatment produces complete remissions in 80–90% of patients. Those patients with Philadelphia chromsome-positive ALL (or *bcr-abl* plus ALL) should have imatinib added to their initial chemotherapy.

Once a patient has entered remission, postremission therapy is given with curative intent. Options include standard chemotherapy and autologous and allogeneic transplantation. The optimal treatment strategy depends on the patient's age and clinical status and the risk factor profile of the leukemia. Acute promyelocytic leukemia is generally treated with chemotherapy plus retinoic acid, and 70–80% of patients remain in long-term remission. Arsenic trioxide has been approved for treatment of relapsed disease, and is under investigation during primary therapy in the hope of increasing cure rates. For average-risk patients with AML, cure rates for postremission therapy are 35–40% for chemotherapy, 50% for autologous transplantation, and 50–60% for allogeneic transplantation. Some types of AML whose cytogenetics involved core-binding factors have a more favorable prognosis, with cure rates of 40–60% with chemotherapy and 70% with autologous transplantation. Patients who do not enter remission or who have high-risk cytogenetics (such as monosomy 7 and complex cytogenetics) do far more poorly and are rarely cured with chemotherapy. Allogeneic transplantation is the treatment of choice, but cure rates are only 20–30%.

Once leukemia has recurred after initial chemotherapy, the prognosis is much more guarded. For patients in second remission, transplantation (autologous or allogeneic) offers a 20–40% chance of cure. For those patients with acute promyelocytic leukemia who relapse, arsenic trioxide is a novel therapy that can produce second remissions, and autologous transplant in second remission produces cure rates of 60–70%.

ALL is treated initially with combination chemotherapy, including daunorubicin, vincristine, prednisone, and asparaginase. Remission induction therapy for ALL is less myelosuppressive than treatment for AML and does not necessarily produce marrow aplasia. After achieving complete remission, patients receive central nervous system prophylaxis so that meningeal sequestration of leukemic cells does not develop. As with AML, patients may be treated with either chemotherapy or high-dose chemotherapy plus bone marrow transplantation. Treatment decisions are made based on patient age and risk factors of the disease. High-risk patients with adverse cytogenetics or poor responses to chemotherapy are best treated with allogeneic transplantation. Autologous transplantation is a possibility in high-risk patients who lack a suitable donor.

Prognosis

Approximately 70–80% of adults with AML under age 60 years achieve complete remission. High-dose postremission chemotherapy leads to cure in 35–40%

of these patients, and high-dose cytarabine has been shown to be superior to therapy with lower doses. Allogeneic bone marrow transplantation (for younger adults with HLA-matched siblings) is curative in 50–60% of cases. Autologous bone marrow transplantation may be superior to nonablative chemotherapy. Older adults with AML achieve complete remission in up to 50% of instances. The cure rates for older patients with AML have been very low (approximately 10–15%), even if they achieve remission and are able to receive postremission chemotherapy. The use of reduced-intensity allogeneic transplantation is being explored in order to improve on these outcomes.

Berg SL et al; Children's Oncology Group: Phase II Study of nelarabine (compound 506U78) in children and young adults with refractory T-cell malignancies: a report from the Children's Oncology Group. J Clin Oncol 2005;23:3376. [PMID: 15908649]

Breems DA et al: Prognostic index for adult patients with acute myeloid leukemia in first relapse. J Clin Oncol 2005;23: 1969. [PMID: 15632409]

Farag S et al: Outcome if induction and postremission therapy in younger adults with acute myeloid leukemia with normal karyotype: A cancer and leukemia group b study. J Clin Oncol 2005;23:482. [PMID: 15534356]

Lee S et al: The effect of first-line imatinib interim therapy on the outcome of allogeneic stem cell transplantation in adults with newly diagnosed Philadelphia chromosome-positive acute lymphoblastic leukemia. Blood 2005;105:3449. [PMID: 15657178]

Mancini M et al: A comprehensive genetic classification of adult acute lymphoblastic leukemia (ALL): analysis of the GIMEMA 0496 protocol. Blood 2005;105:3434. [PMID: 15650057]

Pui CH et al: Treatment of acute lymphoblastic leukemia. N Engl J Med 2006;354:166. [PMID: 16407512]

Sanz MA et al: Tricks of the trade for the appropriate management of newly diagnosed acute promyelocytic leukemia. Blood 2005;105:3019. [PMID: 15604216]

CHRONIC LYMPHOCYTIC LEUKEMIA

 ESSENTIALS OF DIAGNOSIS

- *Most patients asymptomatic at presentation.*
- *Splenomegaly typical.*
- *Lymphocytosis > 5000/mcL.*
- *Mature appearance of lymphocytes.*
- *Coexpression of CD19, CD5.*

General Considerations

Chronic lymphocytic leukemia (CLL) is a clonal malignancy of B lymphocytes. The disease is usually indolent, with slowly progressive accumulation of long-lived small lymphocytes. These cells are immunoincompetent and respond poorly to antigenic stimulation.

CLL is manifested clinically by immunosuppression, bone marrow failure, and organ infiltration with lymphocytes. Immunodeficiency is also related to inadequate antibody production by the abnormal B cells. With advanced disease, CLL may cause damage by direct tissue infiltration.

Information about CLL is now evolving rapidly, with new findings in biology and new treatment options.

Clinical Findings

A. SYMPTOMS AND SIGNS

CLL is a disease of older patients, with 90% of cases occurring after age 50 years and a median age at presentation of 65 years. Many patients will be incidentally discovered to have lymphocytosis. Others present with fatigue or lymphadenopathy. On examination, 80% of patients will have lymphadenopathy and 50% will have enlargement of the liver or spleen.

A prognostically useful staging system (Rai system) has been developed as follows: stage 0, lymphocytosis only; stage I, lymphocytosis plus lymphadenopathy; stage II, organomegaly; stage III, anemia; stage IV, thrombocytopenia.

CLL usually pursues an indolent course; a variant, prolymphocytic leukemia, is more aggressive. The morphology of the latter is different, characterized by larger and more immature cells. In 5–10% of cases, CLL may be complicated by autoimmune hemolytic anemia or autoimmune thrombocytopenia. In approximately 5% of cases, while the systemic disease remains stable, an isolated lymph node transforms into an aggressive large cell lymphoma (**Richter's syndrome**).

B. LABORATORY FINDINGS

The hallmark of CLL is isolated lymphocytosis. The white blood count is usually greater than 20,000/mcL and may be markedly elevated to several hundred thousand. Usually 75–98% of the circulating cells are lymphocytes. Lymphocytes appear small and mature, with condensed nuclear chromatin, and are morphologically indistinguishable from normal small lymphocytes, but smaller numbers of larger and activated lymphocytes may be seen. The hematocrit and platelet count are usually normal at presentation. The bone marrow is variably infiltrated with small lymphocytes. The immunophenotype of CLL demonstrates coexpression of the B lymphocyte lineage marker CD19 with the T lymphocyte marker CD5; this finding is commonly observed only in CLL and mantle cell lymphoma. CLL is distinguished from mantle cell lymphoma by the expression of CD23 and the typical low expression of surface immunoglobulin and CD20. Patients whose CLL cells have mutated forms of the immunoglobulin gene (which can currently be tested only in research laboratories) appear to have a more indolent form of disease; these cells typically express low levels of the surface antigen CD38 and do not express the zeta-associated protein (ZAP-70). Conversely, patients whose cells have unmutated IgV genes and high levels of ZAP-70 expression do less well. The assessment of genomic changes by fluorescence in-situ hybridization (FISH) provides important prognostic information. The findings of deletions of chromosome 17p or 11q have a poor prognosis, whereas those whose only genomic change is deletion of 13q have a very favorable outcome.

Hypogammaglobulinemia is present in 50% of patients and becomes more common with advanced disease. In some, a small amount of IgM paraprotein is present in the serum. Pathologic changes in lymph nodes are the same as in diffuse small cell lymphocytic lymphoma.

Differential Diagnosis

Few syndromes can be confused with CLL. Viral infections producing lymphocytosis should be obvious from the presence of fever and other clinical findings; however, fever may occur in CLL from concomitant bacterial infection. Pertussis may cause a particularly high total lymphocyte count. Other lymphoproliferative diseases such as Waldenström's macroglobulinemia, hairy cell leukemia, or lymphoma (especially mantle cell) in the leukemic phase are distinguished on the basis of the morphology and immunophenotype of circulating lymphocytes and bone marrow.

Treatment

Most cases of early indolent CLL require no specific therapy, and the standard of care for early stage disease has been observation. However, with advances in therapy and with no information on biologic prognostic factors, new clinical trials will investigate whether there is a role for early intervention in subsets of patients with early stage disease. At the present time, indications for treatment include progressive fatigue, symptomatic lymphadenopathy, or anemia or thrombocytopenia. These patients have either symptomatic and progressive stage II disease or stage III/IV disease. The current treatment of choice is the combination of the chemotherapeutic drug fludarabine plus the antibody rituximab. Treatment is usually given monthly for 6 months and then stopped. Other combinations including fludarabine plus cyclophosphamide (and the three-drug combination adding rituximab) also produce high response rates and are being studied but produce somewhat more toxicity. Chlorambucil, 0.6–1 mg/kg orally every 3 weeks for approximately 6 months, was the standard treatment prior to the development of fludarabine. This treatment is convenient, well tolerated, and remains a reasonable first choice for elderly patients for whom frequent trips to the physician's office is a hardship. The monoclonal antibody alemtuzumab has been approved for treatment of refractory CLL and has been shown to reduce minimal residual disease during primary therapy. However, it produces significant immunosuppression, and its role in primary therapy remains to be determined.

Associated autoimmune hemolytic anemia or immune thrombocytopenia may require treatment with rituximab, prednisone, or splenectomy. Fludarabine should be avoided in patients with autoimmune hemolytic anemia since it may exacerbate this condition. Patients with recurrent bacterial infections and hypogammaglobulinemia benefit from prophylactic infusions of gamma globulin (0.4 g/kg/month), but this treatment is very expensive and can be justified only when these infections are severe.

Allogeneic transplantation offers potentially curative treatment for patients with CLL, but it should be used only in patients whose disease cannot be controlled by standard therapies. Nonmyeloablative allogeneic transplant has produced encouraging results and may expand the role of transplant in CLL.

Prognosis

New therapies appear to be changing the prognosis of CLL. In the past, median survival was approximately 6 years, and only 25% of patients lived more than 10 years. Patients with stage 0 or stage I disease have a median survival of 10–15 years, and these patients may be reassured that they can live a normal life for many years. Patients with stage III or stage IV disease had a median survival of less than 2 years in the past, but with new fludarabine-based combination therapies, 2-year survival is now greater than 90% and the long-term outlook appears to be substantially changed. Biologic markers, such as IgV gene mutation status, ZAP-70 expression, and genomic abnormalities, will better predict outcomes of subsets of patients with CLL and will help direct appropriate patients to reduced-intensity allogeneic transplant.

Byrd JC et al: Addition of rituximab to fludarabine may prolong progression-free survival and overall survival in patients with previously untreated chronic lymphocytic leukemia: an updated retrospective comparative analysis of CALGB 9712 and CALGB 9011. Blood 2005;105:49. [PMID: 15138165]

Chiorazzi N et al: Chronic lymphocytic leukemia. N Engl J Med 2005;352:804. [PMID: 15728813]

Keating MJ et al: Early results of a chemoimmunotherapy regimen of fludarabine, cyclophosphamide, and rituximab as initial therapy for chronic lymphocytic leukemia. J Clin Oncol 2005;23:4079. [PMID: 15767648]

Montserrat E et al: How I treat refractory CLL. Blood 2006;107:1276. [PMID: 16204307]

Moreno C et al: Allogeneic stem-cell transplantation may overcome the adverse prognosis of unmutated VH gene in patients with chronic lymphocytic leukemia. J Clin Oncol 2005;23:3433. [PMID: 15809449]

Moreton P et al: Eradication of minimal residual disease in b-cell chronic lymphocytic leukemia after alemtuzumab therapy is associated with prolonged survival. J Clin Oncol 2005;23:2971. [PMID: 15738539]

HAIRY CELL LEUKEMIA

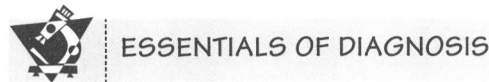

ESSENTIALS OF DIAGNOSIS

- *Pancytopenia.*
- *Splenomegaly, often massive.*

- *Hairy cells present on blood smear and especially in bone marrow biopsy.*

General Considerations

Hairy cell leukemia, an uncommon form of leukemia, is an indolent cancer of B lymphocytes.

Clinical Findings

A. SYMPTOMS AND SIGNS

The disease characteristically presents in middle-aged men. The median age at presentation is 55 years, and there is a striking 5:1 male predominance. Most patients present with gradual onset of fatigue, others complain of symptoms related to markedly enlarged spleen, and some come to attention because of infection.

Splenomegaly is almost invariably present and may be massive. The liver is enlarged in 50% of cases; lymphadenopathy is uncommon.

Hairy cell leukemia is usually an indolent disorder whose course is dominated by pancytopenia and recurrent infections, including mycobacterial infections.

B. LABORATORY FINDINGS

The hallmark of hairy cell leukemia is pancytopenia. Anemia is nearly universal, and 75% of patients have thrombocytopenia and neutropenia. Nearly all patients have striking monocytopenia, which is encountered in almost no other condition. The "hairy cells" are usually present in small numbers on the peripheral blood smear and have a characteristic appearance with numerous cytoplasmic projections. The bone marrow is usually inaspirable (dry tap), and the diagnosis is made by characteristic morphology on bone marrow biopsy. The hairy cells have a characteristic histochemical staining pattern, with tartrate-resistant acid phosphatase (TRAP). On immunophenotyping, the cells coexpress the antigens CD11c and CD22. Pathologic examination of the spleen shows marked infiltration of the red pulp with hairy cells. This is in contrast to the usual predilection of lymphomas to involve the white pulp of the spleen.

Differential Diagnosis

Hairy cell leukemia should be distinguished from other lymphoproliferative diseases such as Waldenström's macroglobulinemia and non-Hodgkin's lymphomas. It also may be confused with other causes of pancytopenia, including hypersplenism due to any cause, aplastic anemia, and paroxysmal nocturnal hemoglobinuria.

Treatment

The treatment of choice is cladribine (2-chlorodeoxyadenosine; CdA), 0.14 mg/kg daily for 7 days. This is a relatively nontoxic drug that produces benefit in 95% of cases

and complete remission in more than 80%. Responses are long-lasting, with few patients relapsing in the first few years. Treatment with pentostatin produces similar results, but that drug is more cumbersome to administer.

Course & Prognosis

The development of new therapies has changed the prognosis of this disease. Formerly, median survival was 6 years, and only one-third of patients survived longer than 10 years. It now appears that more than 90% of patients with hairy cell leukemia will live longer than 10 years.

Chadha P et al: Treatment of hairy cell leukemia with 2-chlorodeoxyadenosine (2-CdA): long-term follow-up of the Northwestern University experience. Blood 2005;106:241. [PMID: 15761021]

Jehn U et al: An update: 12-year follow-up of patients with hairy cell leukemia following treatment with 2-chlorodeoxyadenosine. Leukemia 2004;18:1476. [PMID: 15229616]

Robak T: Monoclonal antibodies in the treatment of chronic lymphoid leukemias. Leuk Lymphoma 2004;45:205. [PMID: 15101704]

■ LYMPHOMAS

NON-HODGKIN'S LYMPHOMAS

The non-Hodgkin's lymphomas are a heterogeneous group of cancers of lymphocytes. The disorders vary in clinical presentation and course from indolent to rapidly progressive.

Molecular biology has provided clues to the pathogenesis of these disorders. The best-studied example is Burkitt's lymphoma, in which a characteristic cytogenetic abnormality of translocation between the long arms of chromosomes 8 and 14 has been identified. The protooncogene c-*myc* is translocated from its normal position on chromosome 8 to the heavy chain locus on chromosome 14. Cells committed to B cell differentiation are likely to have enhanced expression of this heavy chain locus, and it is likely that overexpression of c-*myc* (in its new anomalous position) is related to malignant transformation. In the follicular lymphomas, the t(14,18) translocation is characteristic and results in overexpression of *bcl-2,* resulting in protection against apoptosis, the usual mechanism of cell death.

Classification of the lymphomas is a controversial area still undergoing evolution. The most recent grouping (see Table 13–16) separates diseases based on both clinical and pathologic features.

Clinical Findings

A. SYMPTOMS AND SIGNS

Patients with indolent lymphomas usually present with painless lymphadenopathy, which may be iso-

Table 13–16. World Health Organization proposed classification of non-Hodgkin's lymphomas.

Precursor B
    B cell lymphoblastic lymphoma
Mature B
    Diffuse large B cell lymphoma
    Mediastinal large B cell lymphoma
    Follicular lymphoma
    Small lymphocytic lymphoma
    Lymphoplasmacytic lymphoma
    Mantle cell lymphoma
    Burkitt's lymphoma
    Marginal zone lymphoma
        MALT type
        Nodal
        Splenic
    Mucosal tissue associated
Precursor T
    T cell lymphoblastic lymphoma
Mature T (and NK cell)
    Anaplastic T cell lymphoma
    Peripheral T cell lymphoma

lated or widespread. Involved lymph nodes may be present in the retroperitoneum, mesentery, and pelvis. The indolent lymphomas are usually disseminated at the time of diagnosis, and bone marrow involvement is frequent. Patients with intermediate and high-grade lymphomas also have constitutional symptoms such as fever, drenching night sweats, or weight loss.

On examination, lymphadenopathy may be isolated, or extranodal sites of disease (skin, gastrointestinal tract) may be found. Patients with Burkitt's lymphoma are noted to have abdominal pain or abdominal fullness because of the predilection of the disease for the abdomen.

Once a pathologic diagnosis is established, the patient is staged. Chest radiograph and CT scan of the abdomen and pelvis, bone marrow biopsy, and lumbar puncture (in selected cases with high-risk morphology) are performed.

B. LABORATORY FINDINGS

The peripheral blood is usually normal, but a number of lymphomas may present in a leukemic phase.

Bone marrow involvement is manifested as paratrabecular lymphoid aggregates. In some high-grade lymphomas, the meninges are involved and malignant cells are found with cerebrospinal fluid cytology. The chest radiograph may show a mediastinal mass in lymphoblastic lymphoma. The serum LDH has been shown to be a useful prognostic marker and is now incorporated in risk stratification of treatment.

The diagnosis of lymphoma is made by tissue biopsy. Needle aspiration may yield suspicious results, but a lymph node biopsy (or biopsy of involved extranodal tissue) is required for diagnosis and staging.

Molecular profiling based on the examination of gene expression may lead to a new classification of the lymphomas.

Treatment

The treatment of indolent lymphoma depends on the stage of disease and the clinical status of the patient. A small number of patients have limited disease with only one abnormal lymph node and may be treated with localized irradiation with curative intent. Most patients with indolent lymphoma have disseminated disease at the time of diagnosis. If the disease is not bulky and the patient not symptomatic, no initial therapy may be required. Some patients will have spontaneous remissions and may defer treatment for 1–3 years. There are an increasing number of reasonable treatment options for low-grade lymphomas, but no clear consensus has emerged on the best strategy. Treatment with the anti-CD20 antibody rituximab is a commonly used treatment because of its very low toxicity and avoidance of chemotherapy. Combinations of rituximab with chemotherapy may also be used. Radioimmunoconjugates that fuse anti-B cell antibodies with radiation may produce improved results with modest increases in toxicity compared with antibody alone, and one such agent (yttrium-90 ibritumomab tiuxetan) is in use. Some patients with clinically aggressive low-grade lymphomas may be appropriate candidates for allogeneic transplantation. As in other hematologic malignancies, the use of less toxic nonmyeloablative regimens for allogeneic transplant may expand the role of transplant in this disease. The role of autologous transplantation for follicular lymphoma remains uncertain, but some patients with recurrent disease appear to have prolonged remissions.

Patients with intermediate-grade lymphomas such as diffuse large cell lymphoma are treated with curative intent. Those with localized disease receive either short-course chemo-immunotherapy (such as three courses of rituximab, cyclophosphamide, doxorubicin [hydroxydaunomycin; Adriamycin], vincristine [Oncovin], and prednisone [R-CHOP]) plus localized radiation or six courses of chemotherapy without radiation. Most patients who have more advanced disease are treated with six to eight cycles of chemotherapy such as R-CHOP. Individuals with very high-risk lymphoma are best treated with autologous stem cell transplantation early in the course. Patients with intermediate-grade lymphoma who relapse after initial chemotherapy may still be cured by autologous stem cell transplantation if their disease remains responsive to chemotherapy.

Persons with special forms of lymphoma require individualized therapy. Burkitt's lymphoma is treated with intensive regimens specifically tailored for this histologic type. Those with lymphoblastic lymphoma receive regimens similar to those used for T cell ALL. Mantle cell lymphoma is not effectively treated with standard chemotherapy regimens. Intensive initial therapy including autologous stem cell transplantation has been shown to improve outcomes and is now the standard of care. Patients with mucosal associated lymphoid tumors (MALT lymphomas) of the stomach may be appropriately treated with combination antibiotics directed against *Helicobacter pylori* but require frequent endoscopic monitoring.

Prognosis

The median survival of patients with indolent lymphomas has been 6–8 years, but this appears to be changing for the better. These diseases ultimately become refractory to chemotherapy. This often occurs at the time of histologic progression of the disease to a more aggressive form of lymphoma.

The International Prognostic Index is now widely used to categorize patients with intermediate-grade lymphoma into risk groups. Factors that confer adverse prognosis are age over 60 years, elevated serum LDH, stage III or stage IV disease, and poor performance status. Patients with no risk factors or one risk factor have high complete response rates (80%) to standard chemotherapy, and most responses (80%) are durable. Patients with two risk factors have a 70% complete response rate, 70% being long-lasting. Patients with higher-risk disease have lower response rates and poor survival with standard regimens, and alternative treatments are needed. Early treatment with high-dose therapy and autologous stem cell transplantation improves the outcome.

For patients who relapse after initial chemotherapy, the prognosis depends on whether the lymphoma is still partially sensitive to chemotherapy. If it is, autologous transplantation offers a 50% chance of long-term salvage.

The treatment of older patients with lymphoma has been difficult because of poorer tolerance of aggressive chemotherapy. The use of myeloid growth factors and prophylactic antibiotics to reduce neutropenic complications may improve outcomes.

New techniques of molecular profiling using gene array technology are being studied to better define subsets of lymphomas with different biologic features and prognoses.

Abramson JS et al: Advances in the biology and therapy of diffuse large B-cell lymphoma: moving toward a molecularly targeted approach. Blood 2005;106:1164. [PMID: 15855278]

Dreyling M et al: Early consolidation by myeloablative radiochemotherapy followed by autologous stem cell transplantation in first remission significantly prolongs progression-free survival in mantle-cell lymphoma: results of a prospective randomized trial of the European MCL Network. Blood 2005;105:2677. [PMID: 15591112]

Escalon MP et al: Nonmyeloablative allogeneic hematopoietic transplantation: a promising salvage therapy for patients with non-Hodgkin's lymphoma whose disease has failed a prior autologous transplantation. J Clin Oncol 2004;22:2419. [PMID: 15197204]

Feugier P et al: Long-term results of the R-CHOP study in the treatment of elderly patients with diffuse large B-cell lymphoma: a study for the Groupe d'Etude des Lymphomes de l'Adulte. J Clin Oncol 2005;23:4117. [PMID: 15867204]

Fisher RI et al: New treatment options have changed the survival of patients with follicular lymphoma. J Clin Oncol 2005;23:8447. [PMID: 16230674]

Marcus R et al: CVP chemotherapy plus rituximab compared with CVP as first-line treatment for advanced follicular lymphoma. Blood 2005;105:1417. [PMID: 15494430]

Milpied N et al; Groupe Ouest-Est des Leucemies et des Autres Maladies du Sang: Initial treatment of aggressive lymphoma with high-dose chemotherapy and autologous stem-cell support. N Engl J Med 2004;350:1287. [PMID: 15044639]

Sehn LH et al: Introduction of combined CHOP plus rituximab therapy dramatically improved outcome of diffuse large B-cell lymphoma in British Columbia. J Clin Oncol 2005;23:5027. [PMID: 15955905]

HODGKIN'S DISEASE

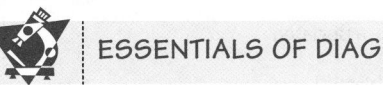

ESSENTIALS OF DIAGNOSIS

- *Painless lymphadenopathy.*
- *Constitutional symptoms may or may not be present.*
- *Pathologic diagnosis by lymph node biopsy.*

General Considerations

Hodgkin's disease is a group of cancers characterized by Reed–Sternberg cells in an appropriate reactive cellular background. The nature of the malignant cell is a subject of controversy.

Clinical Findings

There is a bimodal age distribution, with one peak in the 20s and a second over age 50 years. Most patients present because of a painless mass, commonly in the neck. Others may seek medical attention because of constitutional symptoms such as fever, weight loss, or drenching night sweats, or because of generalized pruritus. An unusual symptom of Hodgkin's disease is pain in an involved lymph node following alcohol ingestion.

An important feature of Hodgkin's disease is its tendency to arise within single lymph node areas and spread in an orderly fashion to contiguous areas of lymph nodes. Only late in the course of the disease will vascular invasion lead to widespread hematogenous dissemination.

Hodgkin's disease is divided into several subtypes: lymphocyte predominance, nodular sclerosis, mixed cellularity, and lymphocyte depletion. Hodgkin's disease should be distinguished pathologically from other malignant lymphomas and may occasionally be confused with reactive lymph nodes seen in infectious mononucleosis, cat-scratch disease, or drug reactions (eg, phenytoin).

Patients undergo a staging evaluation to determine the extent of disease. The staging nomenclature (Ann Arbor) is as follows: stage I, one lymph node region involved; stage II, involvement of two lymph node areas on one side of the diaphragm; stage III, lymph node regions involved on both sides of the diaphragm; and stage IV, disseminated disease with bone marrow or liver involvement. In addition, patients are designated stage A if they lack constitutional symptoms and stage B if 10% weight loss over 6 months, fever, or night sweats are present. If symptoms indicate careful evaluation for higher numerical stage, clinical stage IB (for example) is highly likely to emerge as stage II or stage IIIB.

Treatment

The treatment of Hodgkin's disease has evolved, with radiation therapy used as initial treatment only for patients with low-risk stage IA and IIA disease. Staging is usually clinical, and laparotomy is no longer routinely performed. The addition of limited chemotherapy for some patients treated with radiation appears promising.

Most patients with Hodgkin's disease (including all with stage IIIB and IV disease) are best treated with combination chemotherapy using doxorubicin (Adriamycin), bleomycin, vincristine, and dacarbazine (ABVD). New shorter and more intensive regimens have produced promising results and may supplant ABVD in the treatment of advanced disease.

Prognosis

All patients with both localized and disseminated disease should be treated with curative intent. The prognosis of patients with stage IA or IIA disease treated by radiotherapy is excellent, with 10-year survival rates in excess of 80%. Patients with disseminated disease (IIIB, IV) have 5-year survival rates of 50–60%. Poorer results are seen in patients who are older, those who have bulky disease, and those with lymphocyte depletion or mixed cellularity on histologic examination. Others whose disease recurs after initial radiotherapy treatment may still be curable with chemotherapy. The treatment of choice for patients who relapse after initial chemotherapy is high-dose chemotherapy with autologous stem cell transplantation. This offers a 35–50% chance of cure when disease is still chemotherapy sensitive.

Bonadonna G et al: ABVD plus subtotal nodal versus involved-field radiotherapy in early-stage Hodgkin's disease: long-term results. J Clin Oncol 2004;22:2835. [PMID: 15199092]

Engert A et al; German Hodgkin's Study Group: Hodgkin's lymphoma in elderly patients: a comprehensive retrospective analysis from the German Hodgkin's Study Group. J Clin Oncol 2005;23:5052. [PMID: 15955904]

Friedberg JW et al: FDG-PET is superior to gallium scintigraphy in staging and more sensitive in the follow-up of patients with de novo Hodgkin lymphoma: a blinded comparison. Leuk Lymphoma 2004;45:85. [PMID: 15061202]

le Maignan C et al: Three cycles of adriamycin, bleomycin, vinblastine, and dacarbazine (ABVD) or epirubicin, bleomycin, vin-

blastine, and methotrexate (EBVM) plus extended field radiation therapy in early and intermediate Hodgkin disease: 10-year results of a randomized trial. Blood 2004;103:58. [PMID: 12907440]

Re D et al: From Hodgkin disease to Hodgkin lymphoma: biologic insights and therapeutic potential. Blood 2005;105:4553. [PMID: 15728122]

MULTIPLE MYELOMA

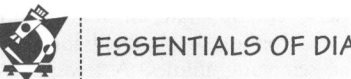 ESSENTIALS OF DIAGNOSIS

- Bone pain, often in the lower back.
- Monoclonal paraprotein by serum and urine protein electrophoresis or immunoelectrophoresis.
- Replacement of bone marrow by malignant plasma cells.

General Considerations

Multiple myeloma is a malignancy of plasma cells characterized by replacement of the bone marrow, bone destruction, and paraprotein formation. Myeloma causes clinical symptoms and signs through a variety of mechanisms.

Replacement of the bone marrow (and perhaps humoral suppression of myelopoiesis) leads initially to anemia and later to general bone marrow failure. Malignant plasma cells can form tumors (plasmacytomas) that may cause spinal cord compression. Bone involvement causes bone pain, osteoporosis, lytic lesions, pathologic fractures, and hypercalcemia. The pathogenesis of osteoclast activation in myeloma appears to involve osteoprotegerin ligand, and the decoy receptor osteoprotegerin may be able to interfere with this pathway.

The paraproteins secreted by the malignant plasma cells may cause problems in their own right. Very high paraprotein levels (either IgG or IgA) may cause hyperviscosity, though this is more often caused by IgM in Waldenström's macroglobulinemia. The light chain component of the immunoglobulin often leads to renal failure (often aggravated by hypercalcemia). Light chain components may be deposited in tissues as amyloid, worsening renal failure with albuminuria and causing a vast array of systemic symptoms.

Myeloma patients are prone to recurrent infections for a number of reasons, including neutropenia and the immunosuppressive effects of chemotherapy. More often, there is a failure of antibody production in response to antigen challenge, and myeloma patients are especially prone to infections with encapsulated organisms such as Streptococcus pneumoniae and Haemophilus influenzae.

Clinical Findings

A. SYMPTOMS AND SIGNS

Myeloma is a disease of older adults (median age at presentation, 65 years). The most common presenting complaints are those related to anemia, bone pain, and infection. Bone pain is most common in the back or ribs or may present as a pathologic fracture, especially of the femoral neck. Patients may also come to medical attention because of renal failure, spinal cord compression, or the hyperviscosity syndrome (mucosal bleeding, vertigo, nausea, visual disturbances, alterations in mental status). Equally as often, patients are diagnosed because of laboratory findings of hypercalcemia, proteinuria, elevated sedimentation rate, or abnormalities on serum protein electrophoresis obtained for symptoms or in routine screening studies. A few patients come to medical attention because of amyloidosis.

Examination may reveal pallor, bone tenderness, and soft tissue masses. Patients may have neurologic signs related to neuropathy and spinal cord compression. Patients with amyloidosis may have an enlarged tongue, neuropathy, congestive heart failure, or hepatomegaly. Splenomegaly is absent unless amyloidosis is present. Fever occurs only with infection.

B. LABORATORY FINDINGS

Anemia is nearly universal. Red blood cell morphology is normal, but rouleau formation is common and may be marked. The neutrophil and platelet counts are usually normal at presentation. Only rarely will plasma cells be visible on peripheral smear (plasma cell leukemia).

The hallmark of myeloma is the finding of a paraprotein on serum protein electrophoresis (SPEP). The majority of patients will have a monoclonal spike visible in the β- or γ-globulin region. Immunofixation (IF) will reveal this to be a monoclonal protein. Approximately 15% of patients will have no demonstrable paraprotein in the serum. In these, IF of the urine will reveal either complete immunoglobulin or light chains. Overall, approximately 60% of myeloma patients will have an IgG paraprotein, 25% an IgA, and 15% light chains only. In sporadic cases, no paraprotein is present ("nonsecretory myeloma"); these patients have particularly aggressive disease.

The bone marrow will be infiltrated by variable numbers of plasma cells ranging from 5% to 100%. The plasma cells will occasionally appear normal but more commonly are morphologically abnormal. Many benign processes can result in plasmacytosis, but the presence of highly atypical plasma cells or effacement of normal bone marrow elements helps to distinguish myeloma. Bone radiographs are important in establishing the diagnosis of myeloma. Lytic lesions are most commonly seen in the axial skeleton: skull, spine, proximal long bones, and ribs. At other times, only generalized osteoporosis is seen. The radionuclide bone scan is not useful in detecting bone lesions in myeloma, as there is usually no osteoblastic component. Positron emission tomography (PET) scans are being evaluated in the staging of myeloma, and may become routine.

The level of β$_2$-microglobulin has strong prognostic significance in myeloma, with levels > 3 mg/L associated with poor survival. Bone marrow cytogenetic characteristics have greater prognostic significance, with deletions of chromosome 13q associated with a dismal outcome. Other laboratory features include hypercalcemia, renal failure, and an elevated erythrocyte sedimentation rate; alkaline phosphatase is not elevated despite extensive bony involvement. Some patients have proximal renal tubular acidosis, with phosphaturia, glycosuria, uricosuria, and aminoaciduria. The urinalysis may reveal proteinuria, but the dipstick test (which detects primarily albumin) is unreliable for light chains. Often there is a narrow anion gap when the paraprotein is cationic (70% of cases).

The standard staging system for multiple myeloma, the Salmon-Durie system, has been based on the level of paraprotein, blood counts, bone radiographs, and serum calcium. A new International Staging System has been proposed based on serum albumin and β$_2$-microglobulin.

Differential Diagnosis

When a patient is discovered to have a monoclonal paraprotein, the distinction between myeloma and monoclonal gammopathy of unknown significance (MGUS) must be made. MGUS is present in 1% of all adults and 3% of adults over age 70 years. Thus, among all patients with paraproteins, MGUS is far more common than myeloma. Most commonly, patients with MGUS will have a monoclonal IgG spike less than 2.5 g/dL, and the height of the spike remains stable. In approximately 25% of cases, MGUS progresses to overt malignant disease, but this may take many years.

Myeloma is distinguished from MGUS by findings of replacement of the bone marrow, bone destruction, and progression. Although the height of the paraprotein spike should not be used by itself to distinguish benign from malignant disease, nearly all patients with IgG spikes greater than 3.5 g/dL prove to have myeloma; an IgA spike of > 2 g/dL is similarly suggestive. If there is doubt about whether paraproteinemia is benign or malignant, the patient should be observed without therapy, since there is no advantage to early treatment of asymptomatic multiple myeloma.

Myeloma must be distinguished from reactive polyclonal hypergammaglobulinemia. Myeloma may also be similar to other malignant lymphoproliferative diseases such as Waldenström's macroglobulinemia, lymphomas, and primary amyloidosis (with which it is commonly associated).

Treatment

Patients with minimal disease or in whom the diagnosis of malignancy is in doubt should be observed without treatment. Most commonly, patients require treatment at diagnosis because of bone pain or other symptoms related to the disease. The treatment of myeloma is rapidly changing, and the optimal initial treatment regimen is in flux. The most commonly used initial regimen is the combination of thalidomide plus dexamethasone. This combination has been shown to be more effective than vincristine-doxorubicin-dexamethasone (VAD) chemotherapy for initial disease control and is more convenient since the agents are given orally, although prophylaxis against deep venous thrombosis is warranted and not all patients tolerate thalidomide. Other combinations including the nonchemotherapeutic agents bortezomib and lenalidomide are being explored. Bortezomib, available only intravenously, is a proteosome inhibitor and has significant activity in myeloma, either as a single agent or in combination. Lenalidomide, an oral agent, is a derivative of thalidomide with both improved efficacy and greatly reduced toxicity. However, both of these new agents are extremely expensive.

After initial disease control ("induction therapy"), the optimal consolidation therapy for patients under age 70 years with myeloma is autologous stem cell transplantation. Early aggressive treatment prolongs both duration of remission and overall survival. Clinical trials are now evaluating the role of posttransplant maintenance therapy with agents such as lenalidomide. For young patients with aggressive disease, autologous transplant followed by a reduced-intensity allogeneic transplant is under active investigation.

Allogeneic transplantation is potentially curative in myeloma, but its role has been limited because of the unusually high mortality rate (40–50%) in myeloma patients. Newer and less toxic forms of allogeneic transplantation using nonmyeloablative regimens have produced encouraging results, especially when performed early in the course of disease, such as the minimal disease state following autologous stem cell transplantation.

Localized radiotherapy may be useful for palliation of bone pain or for eradicating tumor at the site of pathologic fracture. Hypercalcemia should be treated aggressively and immobilization and dehydration avoided. The bisphosphonates (pamidronate 90 mg or zoledronic acid 4 mg intravenously monthly) reduce pathologic fractures in patients with significant bony disease and are an important adjunct in this subset of patients.

Prognosis

The median survival of patients with myeloma has been 3 years, but the outlook appears to be changing with new treatment approaches. The prognosis is markedly affected by a number of prognostic features, with shorter survivals in those with high paraprotein spikes, renal failure, hypercalcemia, or extensive bony disease. Patients are said to have a low tumor burden (stage I) if the IgG spike is less than 5 g/dL, there is no more than one lytic bone lesion, and there is no evidence of hypercalcemia or renal failure. Such patients have a median survival of 5–6 years. Conversely, patients with a high tumor burden (stage III) have an IgG spike greater than 7 g/dL, hematocrit less than 25%, calcium greater than 12 mg/dL, or more than three lytic bone lesions. Me-

dian survival for this group was formerly 1–2 years, but early intervention with autologous stem cell transplantation prolongs median survival to 5–6 years in this group. A new staging system that incorporates β_2-microglobulin, serum albumin, and bone marrow cytogenetics has been proposed, and appears to predict outcome better than the traditional staging system. Broader use of immunotherapy with allogeneic transplantation may improve the outlook further, and it is likely that the new biologic agents will lead to additional therapeutic gains.

Barlogie B et al: Treatment of multiple myeloma. Blood 2004;103:20.[PMID: 12969978]

Cavo M et al: Superiority of thalidomide and dexamethasone over vincristine-doxorubicin-dexamethasone (VAD) as primary therapy in preparation for autologous transplantation for multiple myeloma. Blood 2005;106:35. [PMID: 15761019]

Crawley C et al: Outcome for reduced-intensity allogeneic transplantation for multiple myeloma: an analysis of prognostic factors from the Chronic Leukaemia Working Party of the EBMT. Blood 2005;105:4532. [PMID: 15731182]

Greipp PR et al: International staging system for multiple myeloma. J Clin Oncol 2005;23:3412. [PMID: 15809451]

Rajkumar SV et al: Combination therapy with lenalidomide plus dexamethasone (Rev/Dex) for newly diagnosed myeloma. Blood 2005;106:4050. [PMID: 16118317]

Richardson PG et al: Bortezomib or high-dose dexamethasone for relapsed multiple myeloma. N Engl J Med 2005;352:2487. [PMID: 15958804]

WALDENSTRÖM'S MACROGLOBULINEMIA

 ESSENTIALS OF DIAGNOSIS

- *Symptoms nonspecific; splenomegaly common on examination.*
- *Monoclonal IgM paraprotein.*
- *Infiltration of bone marrow by plasmacytic lymphocytes.*
- *Absence of lytic bone disease.*

General Considerations

Waldenström's macroglobulinemia is a malignant disease of B cells that appear to be a hybrid of lymphocytes and plasma cells. These cells characteristically secrete an IgM paraprotein, and many clinical manifestations of the disease are related to this macroglobulin.

Clinical Findings

A. SYMPTOMS AND SIGNS

This disease characteristically develops insidiously in patients in their 60s or 70s. Patients usually present with fatigue related to anemia. Hyperviscosity of serum may be manifested in a number of ways. Mucosal and gastrointestinal bleeding are related to engorged blood vessels and platelet dysfunction. Other complaints include nausea, vertigo, and visual disturbances. Alterations in consciousness vary from mild lethargy to stupor and coma. The IgM paraprotein may also cause symptoms of cold agglutinin disease or peripheral neuropathy.

On examination, there may be hepatosplenomegaly or lymphadenopathy. The retinal veins are engorged. Purpura may be present. There should be no bone tenderness.

B. LABORATORY FINDINGS

Anemia is nearly universal, and rouleau formation is common. The anemia is related in part to expansion of the plasma volume by 50–100% due to the presence of the paraprotein. Other blood counts are usually normal. The abnormal plasmacytic lymphocytes usually appear in small numbers on the peripheral blood smear. The bone marrow is characteristically infiltrated by the plasmacytic lymphocytes.

The hallmark of macroglobulinemia is the presence of a monoclonal IgM spike seen on SPEP in the β- or γ-globulin region. The serum viscosity is usually increased above the normal of 1.4–1.8 times that of water. Symptoms of hyperviscosity usually develop when the serum viscosity is over four times that of water, and marked symptoms usually arise when the viscosity is over six times that of water. Because paraproteins vary in their physicochemical properties, there is no strict correlation between the concentration of paraprotein and serum viscosity.

The IgM paraprotein may cause a positive Coombs test or have cold agglutinin or cryoglobulin properties. If macroglobulinemia is suspected but the SPEP shows only hypogammaglobulinemia, the test should be repeated while taking special measures to maintain the blood at 37°C, since the paraprotein may precipitate out at room temperature if it is cryoprecipitable.

Bone radiographs are normal, and there is no evidence of renal failure.

Differential Diagnosis

Waldenström's macroglobulinemia is differentiated from monoclonal gammopathy of unknown significance by the finding of bone marrow infiltration. It is distinguished from chronic lymphocytic leukemia and multiple myeloma by bone marrow morphology and the finding of the characteristic IgM spike, and also on clinical grounds.

Treatment

Patients with marked hyperviscosity syndrome (stupor or coma) should be treated on an emergency basis with plasmapheresis. On a chronic basis, some patients can be managed with periodic plasmapheresis alone. As with other indolent lymphoid diseases, fludarabine and rituximab have replaced alkylator-based chemotherapy for initial therapy.

As with multiple myeloma, autologous stem cell transplantation is playing a more important role in management and is considered in younger patients with more aggressive disease.

Prognosis

Waldenström's macroglobulinemia is an indolent disease with a median survival rate of 3–5 years. However, patients may survive 10 years or longer.

Dimopoulos MA et al: Diagnosis and management of Waldenström's macroglobulinemia. J Clin Oncol 2005;23:1564. [PMID: 15735132]

Kyle RA et al: Long-term follow-up of IgM monoclonal gammopathy of undetermined significance. Blood 2003;102: 3759. [PMID: 12881316]

Mitsiades CS et al: Novel biologically based therapies for Waldenström's macroglobulinemia. Semin Oncol 2003;30: 309. [PMID: 12720159]

Munshi NC et al: Role for high-dose therapy with autologous hematopoietic stem cell support in Waldenstrom's macroglobulinemia. Semin Oncol 2003;30:282. [PMID: 12720153]

■ DISORDERS OF HEMOSTASIS

Disorders of hemostasis may be due to defects in either platelet number or function or to problems in formation of a fibrin clot (coagulation). Bleeding due to platelet disorders is typically mucosal or dermatologic. Common problems include epistaxis, gum bleeding, menorrhagia, gastrointestinal bleeding, purpura, and petechiae. Petechiae are seen almost exclusively in conditions of thrombocytopenia and not platelet dysfunction. Bleeding due to coagulopathy may occur as deep muscle hematomas as well as skin bleeding. Spontaneous hemarthroses are seen only in severe hemophilia.

IDIOPATHIC (Autoimmune) THROMBOCYTOPENIC PURPURA

 ESSENTIALS OF DIAGNOSIS

- *Isolated thrombocytopenia.*
- *Other hematopoietic cell lines normal.*
- *No systemic illness.*
- *Spleen not palpable.*
- *Normal bone marrow with normal or increased megakaryocytes.*

General Considerations

Idiopathic thrombocytopenic purpura is an autoimmune disorder in which an IgG autoantibody is formed that binds to platelets. It is not clear which antigen on the platelet surface is involved. Although the antiplatelet antibody may bind complement, platelets are not destroyed by direct lysis. Rather, destruction takes place in the spleen, where splenic macrophages with Fc receptors bind to antibody-coated platelets. Since the spleen is the major site both of antibody production and platelet sequestration, splenectomy is highly effective therapy.

Clinical Findings

A. SYMPTOMS AND SIGNS

Idiopathic thrombocytopenic purpura occurs commonly in childhood, frequently precipitated by viral infection and usually self-limited. In contrast, the adult form is usually a chronic disease and only infrequently follows a viral infection. It is a disease of young persons, with peak incidence between ages 20 and 50 years, and there is a 2:1 female predominance.

Patients are systemically well and usually not febrile. The presenting complaint is mucosal or skin bleeding. Common types of bleeding are epistaxis, oral bleeding, menorrhagia, purpura, and petechiae.

On examination, the patient appears well, and there are no abnormal findings other than those related to bleeding. An enlarged spleen should lead one to doubt the diagnosis. Common signs of bleeding are purpura, petechiae, and hemorrhagic bullae in the mouth.

B. LABORATORY FINDINGS

The hallmark of the disease is thrombocytopenia, with platelet counts that may be less than 10,000/mcL. Other counts are usually normal except for occasional mild anemia, which can be explained by bleeding or associated hemolysis. Peripheral blood cell morphology is normal except that platelets are slightly enlarged (megathrombocytes). These larger platelets are young platelets produced in response to enhanced platelet destruction. Approximately 10% of patients will have coexistent autoimmune hemolytic anemia (**Evans's syndrome**), and in these cases anemia, reticulocytosis, and spherocytes are seen on peripheral smear. Red blood cell fragmentation should not be seen.

The bone marrow will appear normal, with a normal or increased number of megakaryocytes. Coagulation studies will be entirely normal.

Differential Diagnosis

Thrombocytopenia may be produced either by abnormal bone marrow function or by peripheral destruction (Table 13–17). Although most bone marrow disorders produce abnormalities in addition to isolated thrombocytopenia, diagnoses such as myelodysplasia can be excluded only by examining the bone marrow. Most causes of thrombocytopenia resulting from peripheral destruction can be ruled out by initial evaluation. Disorders such as DIC, TTP, HUS, hypersplenism, and

Table 13–17. Causes of thrombocytopenia.

Bone marrow disorders
Aplastic anemia
Hematologic malignancies
Myelodysplasia
Megaloblastic anemia
Chronic alcoholism
Nonmarrow disorders
Immune disorders
Idiopathic thrombocytopenic purpura
Drug-induced
Secondary (CLL, SLE)
Posttransfusion purpura
Hypersplenism
Disseminated intravascular coagulation
Thrombotic thrombocytopenic purpura
Hemolytic-uremic syndrome
Sepsis
Hemangiomas
Viral infections, AIDS
Liver failure

CLL = chronic lymphocytic leukemia; SLE = systemic lupus erythematosus.

sepsis are easily excluded by the absence of systemic illness. Thus, patients with isolated thrombocytopenia with no other abnormal findings almost certainly have immune thrombocytopenia. Patients should be questioned regarding drug use, especially sulfonamides, quinine, thiazides, cimetidine, gold, and heparin. Heparin is now the most common cause of drug-induced thrombocytopenia in hospitalized patients. Systemic lupus erythematosus and CLL are common causes of secondary thrombocytopenic purpura, hematologically identical to idiopathic thrombocytopenic purpura.

Treatment

Few adults with idiopathic thrombocytopenic purpura will have spontaneous remissions, and most will require treatment. Initial treatment is with prednisone, 1–2 mg/kg/d. Prednisone works primarily by decreasing the affinity of splenic macrophages for antibody-coated platelets. High-dose prednisone therapy also reduces the binding of antibody to the platelet surface, and long-term therapy may decrease antibody production. Bleeding will often diminish within 1 day after beginning prednisone—even before the platelet count begins to rise. This effect has been attributed to enhanced vascular stability. The platelet count will usually begin to rise within a week, and responses are almost always seen within 3 weeks. About 80% of patients will respond, and the platelet count will usually return to normal. High-dose therapy should be continued until the platelet count is normal, and the dose should then be gradually tapered. In most, thrombocytopenia will recur if prednisone is completely withdrawn, and the aim is to find a dose that will maintain an adequate platelet count. It is not necessary for the platelet count to be entirely normal; the risk of bleeding is small with platelet counts above 50,000/mcL. An alternative steroid regimen is the use of high-dose dexamethasone, 40 mg/d for 4 days.

Splenectomy is the most definitive treatment for idiopathic thrombocytopenic purpura, and most adult patients will ultimately undergo splenectomy. High-dose prednisone therapy should not be continued indefinitely in an attempt to avoid surgery. Splenectomy is indicated if patients do not respond to prednisone initially or require unacceptably high doses to maintain an adequate platelet count. Other patients may be intolerant of prednisone or may simply prefer the surgical alternative. Splenectomy can be performed safely even with platelet counts less than 10,000/mcL. Eighty percent of patients benefit from splenectomy with either complete or partial remission.

High-dose intravenous immunoglobulin, 1 g/kg for 1 or 2 days, is highly effective in rapidly raising the platelet count. The response rate is 90%, and the platelet count rises within 1–5 days. However, this treatment is expensive, and the beneficial effect lasts only 1–2 weeks. Immunoglobulin treatment should be reserved for bleeding emergencies or situations such as preparing a severely thrombocytopenic patient for surgery.

For patients who fail to respond to prednisone and splenectomy, danazol, 600 mg/d, has been used, with responses obtained in about 50% of cases. Immunosuppressive agents employed in refractory cases include vincristine, azathioprine, cyclosporine, and cyclophosphamide. Rituximab can produce good responses in some patients with refractory disease. Rare patients with severe and refractory disease are now being treated with high-dose immunosuppression and autologous stem cell transplantation.

Platelet transfusions are rarely used in the treatment of idiopathic thrombocytopenic purpura, since exogenous platelets will survive no better than the patient's own and will usually survive less than a few hours. Platelet transfusion should be reserved for cases of life-threatening bleeding in which even fleeting hemostasis may be of benefit.

Prognosis

The prognosis for remission is good. In most cases, the disease is initially controlled with prednisone, and splenectomy offers definitive therapy. The major concern during the initial phases is cerebral hemorrhage, which becomes a risk when the platelet count is less than 5000/mcL. These patients usually exhibit warning signs of mucosal bleeding. However, even at these very low platelet counts, fatal bleeding is rare.

Cines DB et al: How I treat idiopathic thrombocytopenic purpura (ITP). Blood 2005;106:2244. [PMID: 15941913]

Kojouri K et al: Splenectomy for adult patients with idiopathic thrombocytopenia purpura: a systematic review to assess long-term platelet count responses, prediction of response, and surgical complications. Blood 2004;104:2623. [PMID: 15217831]

Vesely SK et al: Management of adult patients with persistent idiopathic thrombocytopenic purpura following splenectomy: a systematic review. Ann Intern Med 2004;140:112. [PMID: 14734334]

HEPARIN-INDUCED THROMBOCYTOPENIA

 **ESSENTIALS OF DIAGNOSIS**

- *Thrombocytopenia occurring during heparin use.*
- *Positive test for antibodies to platelet factor 4, usually in a complex with heparin.*
- *Arterial and venous thrombosis.*

General Considerations

Heparin-induced thrombocytopenia (HIT) is the most common type of drug-induced thrombocytopenia, and one of the most common causes of thrombocytopenia in hospitalized patients. It is caused by an IgG autoantibody that reacts with platelet factor 4 (PF4) on the platelet surface, usually in a complex with heparin. The risk of HIT is significantly higher with the use of unfractionated heparin than with low-molecular-weight heparin and, for unclear reasons, is higher in surgical patients. The interaction of the antibody with PF4 is profoundly prothrombotic, possibly because of the release of platelet microparticles into the circulation.

Clinical Findings

HIT typically develops during heparin use, the risk rising after the first 4 days. Most often, the first finding is asymptomatic thrombocytopenia. However, both arterial and venous thromboses may occur. Laboratory testing can confirm the diagnosis, with the finding of HIT antibodies based on assays using either washed platelets or PF4 antigen.

Differential Diagnosis

HIT must be distinguished from other types of immune thrombocytopenia, including other drug-induced types. The HIT antibody assay is helpful in making this distinction.

Treatment

Once the HIT syndrome has been recognized, the heparin must be stopped. Because of the high risk of associated thrombosis and the high mortality rate of these events, alternative forms of anticoagulation are indicated. The direct thrombin inhibitors such as argatroban and lepirudin are effective.

Prognosis

The HIT syndrome is self-limited, and there is no anamnestic response to distant challenge with heparin. The key is the recognition of the syndrome and the discontinuation of heparin. However, the syndrome is serious, with a mortality rate of approximately 5% due to thrombosis.

Alving BM: How I treat heparin-induced thrombocytopenia and thrombosis. Blood 2003;101:31. [PMID: 12393689]

Di Nisio M et al: Direct thrombin inhibitors. N Engl J Med 2005;353:1028. [PMID: 16148288]

Hirsh J et al: Treatment of heparin-induced thrombocytopenia: a critical review. Arch Intern Med 2004;164:361. [PMID: 14980986]

Warkentin TE et al: Heparin-induced thrombocytopenia: recognition, treatment, and prevention: the Seventh ACCP Conference on Antithrombotic and Thrombolytic Therapy. Chest 2004;126(3 Suppl):311S. [PMID: 15383477]

THROMBOTIC THROMBOCYTOPENIC PURPURA

 ESSENTIALS OF DIAGNOSIS

- *Thrombocytopenia.*
- *Microangiopathic hemolytic anemia.*
- *Neurologic and renal abnormalities, fever.*
- *Reduced level of ADAMTS13.*
- *Normal coagulation tests.*
- *Elevated serum LDH.*

General Considerations

TTP is an uncommon syndrome with microangiopathic hemolytic anemia, thrombocytopenia, and a markedly elevated serum LDH. Noninfectious fever, neurologic disorders, and renal abnormalities are less commonly seen. The pathogenesis of sporadic adult TTP appears to involve a deficiency of a von Willebrand factor-cleaving protease, ADAMTS13, in some cases due to an antibody directed against the protease. In the absence of appropriate cleavage, ultralarge multimers of von Willebrand factor accumulate and lead to platelet agglutination and adhesion to endothelium. It is likely that the full expression of the syndrome involves an additional inciting factor.

TTP is seen primarily in young adults between ages 20 and 50 years, and there is a slight female predominance. The syndrome is occasionally precipitated by estrogen use, pregnancy, drugs, or infections. The most common drugs implicated are quinine and ticlopidine. The syndrome may also occur as a complication of bone marrow transplantation or the use of cyclosporine or tacrolimus. Familial cases occur, but are rare.

Clinical Findings

A. SYMPTOMS AND SIGNS

Patients come to medical attention because of anemia, bleeding, or neurologic abnormalities. The neurologic symptoms and signs are unusual in that they may wax and wane over minutes. Neurologic symptoms include headache, confusion, aphasia, and alterations in consciousness from lethargy to coma. With more advanced disease, hemiparesis and seizures may occur.

On examination, the patient appears acutely ill and is usually febrile. Pallor, purpura, petechiae, and signs of neurologic dysfunction may be detected. Patients may have abdominal pain and tenderness due to pancreatitis.

B. LABORATORY FINDINGS

Anemia is universal and may be marked. There is usually marked reticulocytosis and occasional circulating nucleated red blood cells. The hallmark is a microangiopathic blood picture with fragmented red blood cells (schistocytes, helmet cells, triangle forms) on the smear. The diagnosis cannot be made without significant red blood cell fragmentation. Thrombocytopenia is invariably present and may be severe.

Hemolysis may be manifested by increasing indirect bilirubin and occasionally hemoglobinemia and hemoglobinuria; methemalbuminemia may impart a brown color to the plasma. The LDH is markedly elevated in proportion to the severity of hemolysis; the Coombs test is negative.

Coagulation tests (prothrombin time, partial thromboplastin time, fibrinogen) are normal unless ischemic tissue damage causes secondary DIC. Elevated fibrin degradation products may be seen, as in other acutely ill patients. Renal insufficiency may be present, with an abnormal urinalysis. ADAMTS13 is usually absent during active disease. However, its absence should not deter diagnosis (and treatment) in a clinically compelling case, and its presence does not, by itself, define the syndrome.

Pathologically, there may be thrombi in capillaries and small arteries, with no evidence of inflammation.

Differential Diagnosis

The normal values of coagulation tests differentiate TTP from DIC. Other conditions causing microangiopathic hemolysis (Table 13–18) should be excluded. Evans's

Table 13–18. Causes of microangiopathic hemolytic anemia.

Thrombotic thrombocytopenic purpura
Hemolytic-uremic syndrome
Disseminated intravascular coagulation
Prosthetic valve hemolysis
Metastatic adenocarcinoma
Malignant hypertension
Vasculitis

syndrome is the combination of autoimmune thrombo-cytopenia and autoimmune hemolytic anemia, but the peripheral smear will show spherocytes and not red blood cell fragments. Skin biopsy is usually not necessary for diagnosis but may be helpful when vasculitis is a consideration. TTP and HUS are not distinct disease entities—rather, there is a spectrum of disease, with TTP characterized by more neurologic findings and more severe thrombocytopenia and HUS with more renal failure.

Treatment

TTP should be treated emergently with large-volume plasmapheresis. Sixty to 80 mL/kg of plasma should be removed and replaced with fresh-frozen plasma. Treatment should be continued daily until the patient is in complete remission. The optimal duration of plasmapheresis after remission is unknown. Prednisone and antiplatelet agents (aspirin [325 mg three times daily] and dipyridamole [75 mg three times daily]) have been used in addition to plasmapheresis, but their role is unclear.

The management of patients who do not respond to plasmapheresis or who have rapid recurrences is controversial. Increasing the volume or frequency of plasma exchange is often beneficial. The combination of splenectomy, corticosteroids, and dextran has been used with success. Splenectomy performed in remission may prevent subsequent relapses. Immunosuppression with drugs such as cyclophosphamide has also been effective.

Prognosis

With the advent of plasmapheresis, the formerly dismal prognosis of TTP has been dramatically changed; 80–90% of patients now recover completely. Neurologic abnormalities are almost always completely reversed. Most complete responses are durable, but in 20% of cases the disease will be chronic and relapsing.

Ahmad A et al: Rituximab for treatment of refractory/relapsing thrombotic thrombocytopenic purpura (TTP). Am J Hematol 2004;77:171. [PMID: 15389904]

Fakhouri F et al: Efficiency of curative and prophylactic treatment with rituximab in ADAMTS 13-deficient thrombotic thrombocytopenic purpura: a study of 11 cases. Blood 2005;106:1932. [PMID: 15933059]

Knovich MA et al: Simplified assay for VWF cleaving protease (ADAMTS13) activity and inhibitor in plasma. Am J Hematol 2004;76:286. [PMID: 15224369]

Zheng XL et al: Effect of plasma exchange on plasma ADAMTS13 metalloprotease activity, inhibitor level, and clinical outcome in patients with idiopathic and nonidiopathic thrombotic thrombocytopenic purpura. Blood 2004;103:4043. [PMID: 14982878]

HEMOLYTIC-UREMIC SYNDROME

 ESSENTIALS OF DIAGNOSIS

- *Microangiopathic hemolytic anemia.*

- *Thrombocytopenia and renal failure.*
- *Elevated serum LDH.*
- *Normal coagulation tests.*
- *Absence of neurologic abnormalities.*

General Considerations

HUS is an uncommon disorder consisting of microangiopathic hemolytic anemia, thrombocytopenia, and renal failure due to microangiopathy (with decreased glomerular filtration, proteinuria, and hematuria). The cause is unclear. The disease is similar to TTP except that different vascular beds are involved. In fact, the two diseases are probably best considered as part of a spectrum of HUS–TTP disorders. The pathogenesis of the two disorders is probably similar, and a platelet-agglutinating factor found in plasma may be involved. In children, HUS frequently occurs after a diarrheal illness secondary to infections with *Shigella, Salmonella, E coli* strain O157:H7, or viral agents. The mortality rate of this form is low (< 5%). In adults, this syndrome is often precipitated by estrogen use or by the postpartum state. HUS may be seen as a delayed complication of high-dose corticosteroid therapy and autologous bone marrow or stem cell transplantation, or of the use of cyclosporine or tacrolimus as immunosuppression in allogeneic transplantation. A familial (hereditary) type has been identified in which members of a family have recurrent episodes over several years.

Clinical Findings

A. SYMPTOMS AND SIGNS

Presenting symptoms include anemia, bleeding, or renal failure. The renal failure may or may not be oliguric. In contrast to TTP, there are no neurologic manifestations other than those due to the uremic state.

B. LABORATORY FINDINGS

As in TTP, there is microangiopathic hemolytic anemia and thrombocytopenia, but the thrombocytopenia is often less severe. The peripheral blood smear should show striking red blood cell fragmentation, and the diagnosis is untenable without this finding. The LDH is usually elevated out of proportion to the degree of hemolysis, and the Coombs test is negative. Coagulation tests are normal with the exception of elevated fibrin degradation products. As in TTP, levels of ADAMTS13 are usually low.

Kidney biopsy will show endothelial hyaline thrombi in the afferent arterioles and glomeruli. Ischemic necrosis in the renal cortex may occur with obstruction from intravascular coagulation.

Differential Diagnosis

DIC is excluded by normal coagulation results. Other causes of microangiopathic hemolytic anemia (Table

13–18) should be entertained. Occasionally, vasculitis or acute glomerulonephritis is considered, and in these cases renal biopsy may be necessary to establish the diagnosis if the platelet count will allow it.

HUS is arbitrarily distinguished from TTP by the consistent presence of renal failure and the lack of neurologic findings.

Treatment

In children, HUS is almost always self-limited and requires only conservative management of acute renal failure. In adults, however, without treatment, there is a high rate of permanent renal insufficiency and death. The treatment of choice (as in TTP) is large-volume plasmapheresis with fresh-frozen replacement (exchange of up to 80 mL/kg), repeated daily until remission is achieved.

Prognosis

The prognosis of HUS in adults remains unclear. Without effective therapy, up to 40% of patients have died, and 80% have had chronic renal insufficiency. Early institution of aggressive therapy with plasmapheresis promises to be beneficial. Survival and correction of hematologic abnormalities are the rule, but restoration of renal function requires that treatment be initiated early.

Garg AX et al: Long-term renal prognosis of diarrhea-associated hemolytic uremic syndrome: a systematic review, meta-analysis, and meta-regression. JAMA 2003;290:1360. [PMID: 12966129]

Vesely SK et al: ADAMTS13 activity in thrombotic thrombocytopenic purpura-hemolytic uremic syndrome: relation to presenting features and clinical outcomes in a prospective cohort of 142 patients. Blood 2003;102:60. [PMID: 12637323]

CONGENITAL QUALITATIVE PLATELET DISORDERS

Bleeding disorders characterized by prolonged bleeding times despite a normal platelet count are called qualitative platelet disorders. Patients have a family history or lifelong personal history of the defect. The disorders may be classified as (1) von Willebrand's disease, a congenital disorder of a plasma protein necessary for platelet adhesion, and (2) congenital disorders intrinsic to the platelet (Table 13–19). When an intrinsic qualitative platelet disorder is suspected, platelet aggregation studies should be evaluated to make a specific diagnosis.

1. von Willebrand's Disease

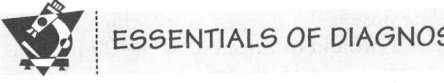 ESSENTIALS OF DIAGNOSIS

- *Family history with autosomal dominant pattern of inheritance.*

Table 13–19. Qualitative platelet disorders.

Congenital
Glanzmann's thrombasthenia
Bernard–Soulier syndrome
Storage pool disease
Acquired
Myeloproliferative disorders
Uremia
Drugs: aspirin, anti-inflammatory agents
Autoantibody
Paraproteins
Acquired storage pool disease
Fibrin degradation products
von Willebrand's disease

- *Prolonged bleeding time, either at baseline or after challenge with aspirin.*
- *Reduced levels of factor VIII antigen or ristocetin cofactor.*
- *Reduced levels of factor VIII coagulant activity in some patients.*

General Considerations

von Willebrand's disease is the most common congenital disorder of hemostasis. It is transmitted in an autosomal dominant pattern. It is a group of disorders characterized by deficient or defective von Willebrand factor (vWF), a protein that mediates platelet adhesion. Adhesion is a process separate from platelet aggregation. Platelets adhere to the subendothelium via vWF, which is bound to a specific receptor on the platelet composed of glycoprotein Ib (and missing in Bernard–Soulier syndrome). Platelets aggregate via fibrinogen, which binds to a different receptor composed of glycoproteins IIb and IIIa (deficient in Glanzmann's thrombasthenia). The platelet aggregation system is entirely normal in von Willebrand's disease.

vWF is synthesized in megakaryocytes and endothelial cells and circulates in plasma as multimers of varying size. Only the large multimeric forms are functional in mediating platelet adhesion. vWF has a separate function of binding the factor VIII coagulant protein and protecting it from degradation. The factor VIII coagulant protein (factor VIII:C), a protein encoded by a gene on the X chromosome, is the protein deficient in classic hemophilia. Any of the multimeric forms of vWF can bind and protect factor VIII:C. von Willebrand's disease, although primarily a disorder of platelet function, may secondarily cause a coagulation disturbance because of deficient levels of factor VIII:C. However, this coagulopathy is rarely severe.

There are several subtypes of von Willebrand's disease. The most common type (type I, 80% of all cases) is caused by a quantitative decrease in vWF. Type IIa is caused by a qualitative abnormality in protein that prevents multimer formation. Only small multimers are present, and both intermediate and large forms that mediate platelet adhesion are missing. Type IIb von Willebrand's disease is caused by a qualitative abnormality in the protein that causes rapid clearance of the large multimeric forms. Type III von Willebrand's disease is a rare autosomal recessive disorder in which vWF is nearly absent. Pseudo-von Willebrand disease is a rare disorder manifested as an abnormal platelet membrane with excessive avidity for the large multimeric forms of vWF, causing their clearance from plasma.

Clinical Findings

A. SYMPTOMS AND SIGNS

von Willebrand's disease is a common disorder affecting both men and women. Most cases are mild. Most bleeding is mucosal (epistaxis, gingival bleeding, menorrhagia), but gastrointestinal bleeding may occur. In most cases, incisional bleeding occurs after surgery or dental extractions. von Willebrand's disease is rarely as severe as hemophilia, and spontaneous hemarthroses do not occur (except in the rare type III). The bleeding tendency is exacerbated by aspirin. Characteristically, bleeding decreases during pregnancy or estrogen use.

B. LABORATORY FINDINGS

Platelet number and morphology are normal, and the bleeding time is usually (not always) prolonged. The bleeding time should be ascertained whenever this diagnosis is considered; it correlates most closely with clinical bleeding. When the bleeding time is normal, it is prolonged markedly by aspirin. Normal persons will prolong their bleeding time to a minor extent with aspirin but rarely out of the normal range. In the most common form of von Willebrand's disease (type I), vWF levels in plasma are reduced. This may be measured by factor VIII antigen, which measures the immunologic presence of vWF, or by ristocetin cofactor activity, which measures functional properties of vWF in mediating platelet adhesion.

When factor VIII antigen is reduced, factor VIII coagulant (factor VIII:C) levels may also decrease. When factor VIII:C levels are less than 25%, the partial thromboplastin time (PTT) will be prolonged. Platelet aggregation studies with standard agonists (adenosine diphosphate [ADP], collagen, thrombin) are normal, but platelet aggregation in response to ristocetin may be subnormal.

In difficult cases, it may be helpful to assay directly the multimeric composition of vWF.

Differential Diagnosis

When patients present with a prolonged bleeding time, von Willebrand's disease must be distinguished from other qualitative platelet disorders (Table 13–19). Acquired qualitative disorders are suggested by recent

Table 13–20. Causes of prolonged partial thromboplastin time.

Congenital factor deficiencies
Contact factors
Factor XII
Factor XI
Factor IX (hemophilia B)
Factor VIII
Hemophilia A
von Willebrand's disease
Anticoagulants
Anti-VIII
Lupus
Heparin

onset of the bleeding tendency. Congenital intrinsic platelet disorders may present with a positive family history and lifelong history of bleeding episodes. von Willebrand's disease is diagnosed by the finding of abnormal measurements of vWF and by normal results of platelet aggregation.

When patients present with a prolonged PTT, measurements of factor VIII:C will distinguish von Willebrand's disease from all disorders except hemophilia (Table 13–20). Hemophilia is diagnosed when factor VIII:C is reduced but all measurements of vWF (factor VIII antigen, ristocetin cofactor activity) are normal.

Patients with a suspicious bleeding history but with normal bleeding time and PTT pose a diagnostic problem. On occasion, the postaspirin bleeding time can be used to unmask a bleeding disorder. At other times, further plasma assays of vWF must be performed to make the diagnosis. von Willebrand's disease waxes and wanes in severity and may be difficult to diagnose, especially in a woman taking estrogens, which raise vWF levels.

It is often useful to distinguish between subtypes of von Willebrand's disease (Table 13–21), because type I usually responds to desmopressin and type IIb may be aggravated by its use.

Treatment

The bleeding disorder is characteristically mild, and no treatment is routinely given other than avoidance of aspirin. However, patients often need to be prepared for surgical or dental procedures. The bleeding time is probably the best indicator of the likelihood of bleeding, and prophylactic therapy may be reasonably withheld if the procedure is minor and the bleeding time is normal.

Desmopressin acetate (DDAVP) is useful for mild type I von Willebrand's disease and should be considered first. The dose is 0.3 mcg/kg, after which vWF levels usually rise twofold to threefold in 30–90 minutes. It can also be given as a nasal spray; levels peak 2 hours after use. DDAVP appears to cause release of stored vWF from endothelial cells. The treatment can be given

Table 13–21. Types of von Willebrand's disease.

	Bleeding Time	Factor VIII Antigen	Ristocetin Cofactor Activity	Factor VIII Coagulant Activity	Multimer
Type I	↑ or N[1]	↓ or N	↓ or N	↓ or N	N
Type IIa	↑	↓ or N	0	↓ or N	Abn
Type IIb	↑	↓ or N	↓ or N	↓ or N	Abn
Type III	↑	0	0	0	...
Pseudo-von Willebrand's disease	↑	↓ or N	↓ or N	↓	Abn
Hemophilia A	N	N	N	N	N

[1]Increases with aspirin.

only every 24 hours as stores of vWF become depleted. It is best to give a therapeutic trial of DDAVP before relying on it for effective hemostasis during surgery or procedures. The drug is not effective in type IIa von Willebrand's disease, in which no endothelial stores are present, and may be harmful in type IIb, leading to thrombocytopenia and increased bleeding.

Factor VIII concentrates are available that have replaced cryoprecipitate as the treatment of choice for von Willebrand's disease if factor replacement is required. Some (not all) of these products now contain functional vWF and do not transmit HIV or hepatitis. One appropriate product is Humate-P (Armour). The dose is 20–50 units/kg depending on disease severity.

The antifibrinolytic agent ε-aminocaproic acid (EACA) is useful as adjunctive therapy during dental procedures. After DDAVP, the patient is given 4 g every 4 hours to reduce the likelihood of bleeding.

Prognosis

The prognosis is excellent. In most cases, the bleeding disorder is mild, and in the more serious cases replacement therapy is effective.

Federici AB et al: Biologic response to desmopressin in patients with severe type 1 and type 2 von Willebrand disease: results of a multicenter European study. Blood 2004;103:2032. [PMID: 14630825]

Laffan M et al: The diagnosis of von Willebrand disease: a guideline from the UK Haemophilia Centre Doctors' Organization. Haemophilia 2004;10:199. [PMID: 15086318]

Sadler JE et al: Von Willebrand disease type 1: a diagnosis in search of a disease. Blood 2003;101:2089. [PMID: 12411289]

Vincentelli A et al: Acquired von Willebrand syndrome in aortic stenosis. N Engl J Med 2003;349:343. [PMID: 12878741]

2. Disorders Intrinsic to the Platelets

Glanzmann's Thrombasthenia

This is a rare autosomal recessive intrinsic platelet disorder causing bleeding. Platelets are unable to aggregate because of lack of receptors (containing glycoproteins IIb and IIIa) for fibrinogen, which form the bridges between platelets during aggregation. Clinically, it is manifested chiefly as mucosal (epistaxis, gingival bleeding, menorrhagia) and postoperative bleeding. The defect is of variable severity but may be severe.

Platelet numbers and morphology are normal, but the bleeding time is markedly prolonged. Platelets fail to aggregate in response to typical agonists (ADP, collagen, thrombin) but aggregate normally in response to ristocetin, which causes platelet clumping by a separate mechanism.

Patients are treated with platelet transfusions when necessary. Platelet transfusion therapy is limited by the tendency of these patients to develop multiple alloantibodies.

Bernard–Soulier Syndrome

This is a rare autosomal recessive intrinsic platelet disorder causing bleeding. Platelets cannot adhere to subendothelium because they lack receptors (composed of glycoprotein Ib) for von Willebrand factor, which mediates platelet adhesion. This is often a severe bleeding disorder with mucosal and postoperative bleeding.

Thrombocytopenia may be present, and platelets on smear are abnormally large. The bleeding time is markedly prolonged. Platelet aggregation is normal in response to standard agonists (collagen, ADP, thrombin), but platelets fail to aggregate in response to ristocetin. Measurements of von Willebrand factor in the plasma are normal. Patients are treated with platelet transfusion when necessary.

Storage Pool Disease

This is a group of mild bleeding disorders characterized by defective secretion of platelet granule contents (especially ADP) that stimulates platelet aggregation. Most patients are mildly affected and have increased bruising and postoperative bleeding.

Platelets are normal in number and morphology, but the bleeding time is slightly prolonged. In some cases, the baseline bleeding time is normal, but it becomes markedly prolonged after aspirin. There are variable abnormalities in platelet aggregation studies.

Most patients do not require treatment but should avoid aspirin. Platelet transfusions transiently correct the bleeding tendency. Some patients respond to DDAVP, 0.3 mcg/kg every 24 hours.

Beguin S et al: Fibrin polymerization is crucial for thrombin generation in platelet-rich plasma in a VWF-GPIb-dependent process, defective in Bernard-Soulier syndrome. J Thromb Haemost 2004;2:170. [PMID: 14717981]

Toogeh G et al: Presentation and pattern of symptoms in 382 patients with Glanzmann thrombasthenia in Iran. Am J Hematol 2004;77:198. [PMID: 15389911]

ACQUIRED QUALITATIVE PLATELET DISORDERS

A number of acquired disorders lead to abnormal platelet function (Table 13–19).

Uremia

Uremia causes abnormal platelet function by unknown mechanisms. The severity of the bleeding tendency is roughly proportional to the degree of renal insufficiency. Bleeding is most commonly mucosal and gastrointestinal and may occasionally be severe. Dialysis is effective in reducing the bleeding tendency but may not completely eliminate it. Patients respond to DDAVP, 0.3 mcg/kg every 24 hours.

Myeloproliferative Disorders

All the myeloproliferative disorders can produce abnormalities in platelet function. A number of biochemical abnormalities are present in these platelets, but the cause of the bleeding tendency is unclear. The severity of the bleeding tendency correlates roughly with the height of the platelet count, although conditions causing reactive thrombocytosis of normal platelets are not associated with abnormal function. Bleeding decreases when the platelet count is controlled with myelosuppressive therapy. In cases of life-threatening bleeding with high platelet counts, plateletpheresis may be necessary.

Other Disorders

Aspirin causes a mild bleeding tendency by irreversibly acetylating cyclooxygenase, an enzyme that participates in platelet aggregation. The effect lasts for the life of the platelet and may be manifest for 7–10 days, although the major effect lasts 3–5 days. The effect is not dose dependent, and 65 mg of aspirin is sufficient.

Aspirin by itself does not cause significant bleeding, but it may unmask bleeding disorders such as mild von Willebrand's disease or mild thrombocytopenia. Certain antibiotics (ticarcillin, some cephalosporins) cause a

mild bleeding tendency, presumably by coating the surface of platelets. Nonsteroidal anti-inflammatory drugs cause an aspirin-like effect that disappears when the drug leaves the system.

Patients with autoantibodies against platelets may have prolonged bleeding times even in the absence of thrombocytopenia. Platelet-associated IgG levels should be high, and the bleeding tendency responds quickly to modest doses of prednisone, eg, 20 mg/d. Acquired storage pool disease refers to the circulation of "exhausted platelets" that have been stimulated to release their granule contents and hence are no longer functional. Such granule release occurs in response to cardiopulmonary bypass and severe vasculitis.

Noris M et al: Uremic bleeding: closing the circle after 30 years of controversies? Blood 1999;94:2569. [PMID: 10515859]

HEMOPHILIA A

 ESSENTIALS OF DIAGNOSIS

- *X-linked recessive pattern of inheritance with only males affected.*
- *Low factor VIII coagulant (VIII:C) activity.*
- *Normal factor VIII antigen.*
- *Spontaneous hemarthroses.*

General Considerations

Hemophilia A (classic hemophilia, factor VIII deficiency hemophilia) is a hereditary disorder in which bleeding is due to deficiency of the coagulation factor VIII (VIII:C). In most cases, the factor VIII coagulant protein is quantitatively reduced, but in a small number of cases the coagulant protein is present by immunoassay but defective.

Hemophilia is an X-linked recessive disease, and as a rule only males are affected. In rare instances, female carriers are clinically affected if their normal X chromosomes are disproportionately inactivated. Females may also become affected if they are the offspring of a hemophiliac father and carrier mother.

Hemophilia is classified as severe if factor VIII:C levels are less than 1%, moderate if levels are 1–5%, and mild if levels are greater than 5%. Families tend to breed true in the severity of hemophilia produced.

Clinical Findings

A. SYMPTOMS AND SIGNS

Hemophilia A is the most common severe bleeding disorder and after von Willebrand's disease is the most common congenital bleeding disorder overall. Approximately one in 10,000 males is affected. The bleeding tendency is related to factor VIII:C levels. Bleeding may occur anywhere. The most common sites of bleeding are into joints (knees, ankles, elbows), into muscles, and from the gastrointestinal tract. Spontaneous hemarthroses are so characteristic of hemophilia that they are almost diagnostic of the disorder. Patients with mild hemophilia bleed only after major trauma or surgery, those with moderately severe hemophilia bleed with mild trauma or surgery, and those with severe disease bleed spontaneously.

Many hemophiliacs are now seropositive for HIV infection transmitted via factor VIII concentrate, and many already have AIDS. HIV-associated immune thrombocytopenia may aggravate the bleeding tendency.

B. LABORATORY FINDINGS

The PTT is prolonged, and other measures of coagulation, including prothrombin time, bleeding time, and fibrinogen level, are normal. Levels of factor VIII:C are reduced, but measurements of vWF are normal (Table 13–21).

If plasma from a hemophiliac patient is mixed with normal plasma, the PTT will become normal. Failure of the PTT to normalize in such a mixing test is diagnostic of the presence of a factor VIII inhibitor.

A low platelet count should raise a suspicion of HIV-associated immune thrombocytopenia.

Differential Diagnosis

The finding of a reduced factor VIII:C level will distinguish this disorder from other causes of prolonged PTT (Table 13–20). Clinically, factor VIII hemophilia is indistinguishable from factor IX hemophilia, and only specific factor assays can distinguish these disorders. In cases of mild hemophilia, the disorder needs to be distinguished from von Willebrand's disease by VIII:A assay, which shows normal levels of factor VIII antigen in the former.

An important issue for the families of hemophiliac patients is identifying which females are carriers. They can usually be identified by the presence of low or normal levels of factor VIII:C with normal levels of factor VIII antigen.

Treatment

Standard treatment is based on infusion of factor VIII concentrates, either recombinant or heat treated. The level of factor VIII achieved in plasma depends on the severity of the bleeding problem. In response to minor bleeding, it may be necessary to raise factor VIII:C levels to only 25% with one infusion. For moderate bleeding (such as deep muscle hematomas), it is adequate to raise the level initially to 50% and maintain the level at greater than 25% with repeated infusion for 2–3 days. When major surgery is to be performed, the factor VIII:C level is raised to 100% and then the factor level is maintained at greater than 50% continuously for 10–14 days. Head injuries (with or without neurologic signs) should be emergently treated as though major bleeding were present.

The dose of factor VIII concentrate is calculated assuming that one unit of factor VIII is the amount present in 1 mL of plasma. Plasma volume is 40 mL/kg, and the volume of distribution of factor VIII:C is 1.5 times the plasma volume. Thus, to raise the level 100%, the dose should be $40 \times 1.5 = 60$ units/kg, or approximately 4000 units for a 70-kg individual. To raise the levels to 25% would require 1000 units. The half-life of factor VIII:C is approximately 12 hours. Thus, during major surgery, to achieve an initial level of 100% and maintain it continuously at greater than 50%, a dose of 60 units/kg (approximately 4000 units) initially followed by 30 units/kg (approximately 2000 units) every 12 hours should be adequate. During surgery, initially verify that these doses give the anticipated factor VIII levels. If factor VIII levels fail to rise as expected, an inhibitor should be suspected.

For mild hemophiliacs, DDAVP, 0.3 mcg/kg every 24 hours, may be useful in preparing for minor surgical procedures. It causes release of factor VIII:C and will raise the factor VIII:C levels two- to threefold for several hours. In the management of persistent bleeding following use of either desmopressin acetate or factor VIII concentrate, patients may be treated with EACA (Amicar), 4 g orally every 4 hours for several days.

Aspirin should be avoided in these patients.

Prognosis

The prognosis of patients with hemophilia has been transformed by the availability of factor VIII replacement. Gene therapy is currently in the developmental phase, but could further transform the outlook for these patients. The major limiting factor is disability from recurrent joint bleeding. Hepatitis B and C and HIV infection from recurrent transfusion are diminishing in incidence. Approximately 15% of patients develop inhibitors to factor VIII, and these patents cannot be adequately supported with factor VIII.

Goudemand J et al: Influence of the type of factor VIII concentrate on the incidence of factor VIII inhibitors in previously untreated patients with severe hemophilia A. Blood 2006; 107:46. [PMID: 16166584]

Plug I et al: Thirty years of hemophilia treatment in the Netherlands, 1972-2001. Blood 2004;104:3494. [PMID: 15308570]

ACQUIRED FACTOR VIII ANTIBODIES

Antibodies to factor VIII may develop either postpartum or with no underlying illness. Factor VIII antibodies also occur in 15–20% of patients with factor VIII hemophilia who have received infusions of plasma concentrates. Inhibitors typically develop in patients with severe disease, and are thought to represent an immune response to a "foreign antigen" in the form of infused factor VIII. However, some cases of moderate hemophilia caused by mutations are also associated with inhibitor development. In cases of hemophilia A with inhibitors, one treatment approach is immune tolerance induction, based on the use of repeated exposure to low levels of antigen. The success rate is approximately 70%. Cases of life-threatening bleeding can be treated by removal of the antibody with plasma exchange combined with infusion of high doses of factor VIII. Another approach is the use of factor VIII bypassing agents or activated factor VIIa.

Factor VIII antibodies can also occur spontaneously, and then usually produce a severe bleeding disorder. The PTT is prolonged, and the fibrinogen level, prothrombin time, and platelet count are not affected. A plasma mixing test will usually reveal the presence of an inhibitor by the failure of normal plasma to correct the prolonged PTT. However, the mixing test may require incubation for 2–4 hours to reveal the inhibitor. Factor VIII coagulant levels are low.

Factor VIII antibodies should be suspected in any acquired severe bleeding disorder associated with a prolonged PTT. Factor VIII antibodies are distinguished from lupus anticoagulants both by the presence of clinical bleeding and more importantly by the reduced factor VIII:C level. The diagnosis is confirmed by mixing tests and in vivo by the failure of factor VIII concentrates to raise the factor VIII:C levels by the expected amount.

The treatment of choice is cyclophosphamide, usually combined with prednisone. In the interim, aggressive factor VIII replacement may be necessary. Products that bypass factor VIII, such as activated factor VII, may be effective but are expensive.

Hind D et al: Recombinant factor VIIa concentrate versus plasma derived concentrates for the treatment of acute bleeding episodes in people with haemophilia A and inhibitors. Cochrane Database Syst Rev 2004;(2):CD004449. [PMID: 15106253]

Stasi R et al: Selective B-cell depletion with rituximab for the treatment of patients with acquired hemophilia. Blood 2004;103:4424. [PMID: 14996701]

United Kingdom Haemophelia Centre Doctors' Organisation: Guidelines on the selection and use of therapeutic products to treat haemophilia and other hereditary bleeding disorders. Haemophilia 2003;9:1. [PMID: 12558775]

HEMOPHILIA B

 ESSENTIALS OF DIAGNOSIS

- X-linked recessive inheritance, with only males affected.
- Low levels of factor IX coagulant activity.
- Spontaneous hemarthroses.

General Considerations

Hemophilia B (Christmas disease, factor IX hemophilia) is a hereditary bleeding disorder due to defi-

ciency of coagulation factor IX. Most commonly, factor IX is quantitatively reduced, but in one-third of cases an abnormally functioning molecule is immunologically present. Factor IX deficiency is one-seventh as common as factor VIII deficiency hemophilia but is otherwise clinically and genetically identical.

The PTT is prolonged, and factor IX levels are reduced when measured by specific factor assays. Other laboratory features are the same as for factor VIII hemophilia.

Treatment

Factor IX hemophilia is managed with factor IX concentrates. Factor VIII concentrates are ineffective in this type of hemophilia. The same dosing considerations apply as in factor VIII hemophilia, with the exception that the volume of distribution of factor IX is twice the plasma volume, so that 80 units/kg is necessary to achieve a 100% level. In addition, the half-life of factor IX is 18 hours. Thus, to maintain a patient through major surgery, the dosage should be 80 units/kg (approximately 6000 units) initially followed by 40 units/kg (3000 units) every 18 hours. Factor IX levels should be measured to ensure that expected levels are achieved and that an inhibitor is not present.

Unlike factor VIII concentrates, factor IX concentrates contain a number of other proteins, including activated coagulating factors that appear to contribute to a risk of thrombosis with recurrent usage of factor IX concentrates. Because of the risk of thrombosis, more care is needed in deciding to use these concentrates. DDAVP is not useful in this disorder, and patients should be cautioned to avoid aspirin.

Prognosis

The prognosis for these patients is the same as for those with factor VIII hemophilia.

Shapiro AD et al: The safety and efficacy of recombinant human blood coagulation factor IX in previously untreated patients with severe or moderately severe hemophilia B. Blood 2005; 105:518. [PMID: 15383463]

OTHER CONGENITAL COAGULATION DISORDERS

Factor XI Deficiency

This disorder is seen primarily among Ashkenazi Jews and is autosomal recessive. The PTT may be markedly prolonged, and specific assays of factor XI will show reduced levels. This is usually a mild bleeding disorder manifested primarily by postoperative bleeding. Factor replacement is given with fresh-frozen plasma when necessary.

Afibrinogenemia

In this rare disorder, fibrinogen is absent and both prothrombin time and partial thromboplastin time are markedly prolonged. These patients may have a severe bleeding disorder similar to hemophilia. Fibrinogen is replaced with cryoprecipitate.

Other Coagulation Disorders

Bleeding disorders due to isolated deficiency of factors II, V, X, or VII are extremely rare. Deficiencies of factor XII and the contact pathway factors cause a markedly prolonged PTT but are not associated with any increased bleeding.

Factor XIII deficiency results in delayed bleeding after trauma or surgery. All coagulation tests are normal. The disorder is diagnosed by showing instability of the fibrin clot in 8 M urea. Factor XIII is replaced with cryoprecipitate or plasma. A rare cause of bleeding is deficiency of the normal inhibitors of fibrinolytic activity: α_2-antiplasmin and plasminogen activator inhibitor.

Roberts HR et al: The use of recombinant factor VIIa in the treatment of bleeding disorders. Blood 2004;104:3858. [PMID: 15328151]

COAGULOPATHY OF LIVER DISEASE

The liver is the site of synthesis of all the coagulation factors except factor VIII. As hepatic insufficiency develops, the vitamin K-dependent factors (factors II, VII, IX, X) and factor V are the first to be affected. Because of its rapid turnover (half-life 6 hours), factor VII levels are the first to decline. Conversely, fibrinogen levels are remarkably well conserved, and decreased fibrinogen synthesis does not occur unless liver disease is very severe.

Liver disease has a number of other effects on the hemostatic system. Increased fibrinolysis occurs because the liver synthesizes α_2-antiplasmin (the main inhibitor of fibrinolysis), which is responsible for the clearance of plasminogen activator. Biliary tract disease may lead to malabsorption of vitamin K, and congestive splenomegaly may produce mild thrombocytopenia. A variety of chronic liver diseases cause abnormal posttranslation modification of fibrinogen with resultant dysfibrinogenemia. The majority of patients with cirrhosis have very low levels of thrombopoietin, and this may contribute to the thrombocytopenia.

Long-term treatment of hepatic coagulopathy with factor replacement is usually ineffective. Fresh-frozen plasma is the treatment of choice, and volume overload will limit the ability to maintain hemostatic factor levels. For example, to maintain factor levels greater than 25%, the level must initially be raised to 50% with 50% of the plasma volume (20 mL/kg) and then 10 mL/kg must be replaced every 6 hours to maintain adequate factor VII levels. In average-sized persons, this will require transfusion of 1400 mL of plasma initially followed by 700 mL every 6 hours. Factor IX concentrates are contraindicated in liver disease because of their tendency to cause DIC. If thrombocytopenia is present, platelet transfusion may be of some help, but platelet recovery is usually disappointing because of hypersplenism.

The prognosis is that of the underlying liver disease.

Youssef WI et al: Role of fresh frozen plasma infusion in correction of coagulopathy of chronic liver disease: a dual phase study. Am J Gastroenterol 2003;98:1391. [PMID: 12818286]

VITAMIN K DEFICIENCY

 ESSENTIALS OF DIAGNOSIS

- *Underlying dietary deficiency or antibiotic use.*
- *Prothrombin time more prolonged than PTT.*
- *Rapid correction with vitamin K replacement.*

General Considerations

Vitamin K plays a role in coagulation by acting as a cofactor for the posttranslational γ-carboxylation of zymogens II, VII, IX, and X. The modified zymogens (with γ-carboxyglutamic acid residues) are able to bind to platelets in a calcium-dependent reaction and consequently better participate in the complex reactions that activate factors X and II. Without γ-carboxylation, these reactions on the platelet surface occur slowly and hemostasis is impaired.

Vitamin K is supplied in the diet primarily in leafy vegetables and endogenously from synthesis by intestinal bacteria. Factors that contribute to vitamin K deficiency include poor diet, malabsorption, and broad-spectrum antibiotics suppressing colonic flora. A characteristic setting for vitamin K deficiency is a postoperative patient who is not eating and who is receiving antibiotics. Body stores of vitamin K are small, and deficiency may develop in as little as 1 week.

Clinical Findings

A. SYMPTOMS AND SIGNS

There are no specific clinical features, and bleeding may occur at any site.

B. LABORATORY FINDINGS

The prothrombin time (PT) is prolonged to a greater extent than the PTT, and with mild vitamin K deficiency only the PT is defective (Tables 13–22 and 13–23). Fi-

Table 13–22. Causes of isolated prolonged prothrombin time.

Liver disease
Vitamin K deficiency
Warfarin therapy
Factor VII deficiency

Table 13–23. Causes of prolonged prothrombin time and partial thromboplastin time.

Liver disease
Vitamin K deficiency
Disseminated intravascular coagulation
Heparin
Warfarin
Isolated factor deficiencies (rare): II, V, X, I

brinogen level, thrombin time, and platelet count are not affected.

Differential Diagnosis

Vitamin K deficiency can be distinguished from hepatic coagulopathy only by assessing the response to vitamin K therapy. Surreptitious warfarin use will produce laboratory features indistinguishable from those of vitamin K deficiency.

Vitamin K deficiency differs from DIC by normal platelet count and fibrinogen levels in the former.

Treatment

Vitamin K deficiency responds rapidly to subcutaneous vitamin K, and a single dose of 15 mg will completely correct laboratory abnormalities in 12–24 hours.

Prognosis

The prognosis is excellent, as vitamin K deficiency can be completely corrected with replacement.

Crowther MA et al: Oral vitamin K lowers the international normalized ratio more rapidly than subcutaneous vitamin K in the treatment of warfarin-associated coagulopathy. A randomized, controlled trial. Ann Intern Med 2002;137:251. [PMID: 12186515]

DISSEMINATED INTRAVASCULAR COAGULATION

ESSENTIALS OF DIAGNOSIS

- *Underlying serious illness.*
- *Microangiopathic hemolytic anemia may be present.*
- *Hypofibrinogenemia, thrombocytopenia, fibrin degradation products, and prolonged PT.*

General Considerations

Coagulation is usually confined to a localized area by the combination of blood flow and circulating inhibitors of coagulation, especially antithrombin III. If the stimulus to coagulation is too great, these control mechanisms can be overwhelmed, leading to the syndrome of DIC. Antithrombin III levels may be low in DIC due to the combination of increased consumption and decreased synthesis. In pathophysiologic terms, DIC can be thought of as the consequence of the presence of circulating thrombin (normally confined to a localized area). The effects of thrombin are to cleave fibrinogen to fibrin monomer, stimulate platelet aggregation, activate factors V and VIII, and release plasminogen activator, which generates plasmin. Plasmin in turn cleaves fibrin, generating fibrin degradation products, and further inactivates factors V and VIII. Thus, the excess thrombin activity produces hypofibrinogenemia, thrombocytopenia, depletion of coagulation factors, and fibrinolysis.

Other physiologic mechanisms that contribute to the control of thrombin generation may also be disrupted in DIC. Activated protein C inhibits the activated forms of factors V and VIII, and activated protein C levels may be reduced both by consumption and by the downmodulation of thrombomodulin on endothelial cells (necessary for the activation of protein C) induced by high levels of tumor necrosis factor (TNF). Recent evidence demonstrates that much of the stimulus to thrombin activation in DIC comes from the tissue factor/factor VIIa pathway. It is possible that deficiencies in the tissue factor pathway inhibitor also contribute to the pathogenesis of DIC.

DIC can be caused by a number of serious illnesses, including sepsis (especially with gram-negative bacteria but possible with any widespread bacterial or fungal infection), severe tissue injury (especially burns and head injury), obstetric complications (amniotic fluid embolus, septic abortion, retained fetus), cancer (acute promyelocytic leukemia, mucinous adenocarcinomas), and major hemolytic transfusion reactions.

Clinical Findings

A. SYMPTOMS AND SIGNS

DIC leads to both bleeding and thrombosis. Bleeding is far more common than thrombosis, but the latter may dominate if coagulation is activated to a far greater extent than fibrinolysis. Bleeding may occur at any site, but spontaneous bleeding and oozing at venipuncture sites or wounds are important clues to the diagnosis. Thrombosis is most commonly manifested by digital ischemia and gangrene, but catastrophic events such as renal cortical necrosis and hemorrhagic adrenal infarction may occur. DIC may also secondarily produce microangiopathic hemolytic anemia.

Subacute DIC is seen primarily in cancer patients and is manifested primarily as recurrent superficial and deep venous thromboses (**Trousseau's syndrome**).

B. LABORATORY FINDINGS

DIC produces a complex coagulopathy with the characteristic constellation of hypofibrinogenemia, elevated fibrin degradation products, thrombocytopenia, and a prolonged PT. Of the fibrin degradation products, the D-dimer is the most sensitive, since its cross-linking implies origin from fibrin in a clot. All fibrin degradation products are cleared by the liver and thus may be elevated in hepatic dysfunction. Hypofibrinogenemia is another important diagnostic laboratory feature, because only a few other disorders (congenital hypofibrinogenemia, severe liver disease) will lower the fibrinogen level. In some cases of DIC, when the patient's baseline fibrinogen level is markedly elevated, the initial fibrinogen level may be normal. However, since the half-life of fibrinogen is approximately 4 days, a declining fibrinogen level will confirm the diagnosis of DIC.

Other laboratory abnormalities are variably present. The PTT may or may not be prolonged. In approximately 25% of cases, a microangiopathic hemolytic anemia is present, and fragmented red blood cells are seen on the peripheral smear. Antithrombin III levels may be markedly depleted. When fibrinolysis is activated, levels of plasminogen and α_2-antiplasmin may be low.

Subacute DIC produces a very different laboratory picture. Thrombocytopenia and elevated D-dimer are usually the only abnormalities. Fibrinogen levels are normal, and the PTT may be normal.

Differential Diagnosis

Liver disease may prolong both the PT and PTT, but fibrinogen levels are usually normal, and the platelet count is usually normal or only slightly reduced. However, severe liver disease may be difficult to distinguish from DIC. Vitamin K deficiency will not affect the fibrinogen level or platelet count and will be completely corrected by vitamin K replacement.

Sepsis may produce thrombocytopenia and digital ischemia, and coagulopathy may be present because of vitamin K deficiency. However, in these cases, the fibrinogen level should be normal.

TTP may produce fever and microangiopathic hemolytic anemia. However, fibrinogen levels and other coagulation studies should be normal.

Treatment

The primary focus should be the diagnosis and treatment of the underlying disorder that has given rise to DIC. In many cases, DIC will produce laboratory abnormalities with only mild clinical manifestations, and in these cases no specific therapy is required.

When the underlying cause of DIC is rapidly reversible (such as in obstetric cases), replacement therapy alone may be indicated. The role of heparin in the treatment of DIC is controversial. In some cases, when any increase in bleeding is unacceptable (neurosurgical procedures), heparin therapy is contraindicated. However, when DIC is producing serious clinical consequences and the underlying cause is not rapidly reversible, heparin may be helpful. One clear indication for heparin therapy is the presence of thrombosis or fibrin deposition leading to acral cyanosis. In using heparin, a dose of 500–750 units per hour is usually sufficient. Heparin cannot be effective if antithrombin III levels are markedly depleted. Antithrombin III levels should be measured, and fresh-frozen plasma or concentrates of antithrombin III used to raise levels to greater than 50%. In using heparin, it is not necessary to prolong the PTT. Successful therapy is indicated by a rising fibrinogen level. Fibrin degradation products will decline over 1–2 days. Improvement in the platelet count may lag as much as 1 week behind control of the coagulopathy.

In replacement therapy, platelet transfusion should be used to maintain a platelet count greater than 30,000/mcL, and 50,000/mcL if possible. Fibrinogen is replaced with cryoprecipitate, and the aim is for a plasma fibrinogen level of 150 mg/dL. One unit of cryoprecipitate usually raises the fibrinogen level by 6–8 mg/dL, so that 15 units of cryoprecipitate will raise the level from 50 to 150 mg/dL. Coagulation factor deficiency may require replacement with fresh-frozen plasma.

In some cases, when DIC is complicated by excessive fibrinolysis, even the combination of heparin and replacement therapy may not be adequate to control bleeding. In these cases, EACA, 1 g intravenously per hour, may be added to decrease the rate of fibrinolysis, raise the fibrinogen level, and control bleeding. EACA should not be used without heparin in DIC because of the risk of thrombosis.

Although infusions of large doses of antithrombin III have not reduced the mortality rate of severe sepsis complicated by DIC, one large trial has shown benefit for the use of activated protein C.

Prognosis

The prognosis is that of the underlying disease.

Franchini M et al: Update on the treatment of disseminated intravascular coagulation. Hematology 2004;9:81. [PMID: 15203862]

Hoffmann JN et al: Effect of long-term and high-dose antithrombin supplementation on coagulation and fibrinolysis in patients with severe sepsis. Crit Care Med 2004;32:1851. [PMID: 15343012]

■ HYPERCOAGULABLE STATES

Most cases of thromboembolism likely result from a convergence of an underlying genetic predisposition and acquired precipitating events such as immobilization, pregnancy, or surgery (Table 13–24).

Cancer is associated with an increased risk of both venous and arterial thrombosis. In some cases, low-grade DIC appears to be responsible. In unusual cases,

Table 13–24. Causes of hypercoagulability.

Acquired
Cancer
Inflammatory disorders: ulcerative colitis
Myeloproliferative disorders
Postoperative
Estrogens, pregnancy
Lupus anticoagulant
Heparin-induced thrombocytopenia
Anticardiolipin antibodies
Paroxysmal nocturnal hemoglobinuria
Congenital
Antithrombin III deficiency
Factor V Leiden
Protein C deficiency
Protein S deficiency
Dysfibrinogenemia
Abnormal plasminogen
Activated protein C resistance

a unique cancer procoagulant stimulates the clotting system. Myeloproliferative disorders such as polycythemia vera, essential thrombocytosis, and paroxysmal nocturnal hemoglobinuria are associated with a high incidence of thrombosis, caused by qualitative platelet abnormalities. Venous thrombosis may occur in unusual locations such as the mesenteric, hepatic, or splenic venous beds. Arterial thrombosis occurs as well and may be manifested as large vessel occlusion (stroke, myocardial infarction) or as microvascular events with burning in the hands and feet.

A number of congenital biochemical defects have also been associated with hypercoagulability (Table 13–24). A family history is usually present. The thromboses are almost always venous and may occur in the large veins of the abdomen. Thromboses often occur during early adulthood rather than in childhood and are often precipitated by factors such as trauma or pregnancy. The most common of these disorders is an abnormal factor V (factor V Leiden), which is resistant to degradation by activated protein C. Dysfibrinogenemia is diagnosed by a prolonged reptilase time.

The syndrome of **warfarin-induced skin necrosis** may occur in patients with undiagnosed protein C deficiency. Protein C is vitamin K dependent and has a shorter half-life than the coagulation proteins. Warfarin, by creating a vitamin K-dependent state, will transiently deplete protein C before it leads to anticoagulation. During the period of hypercoagulability due to unopposed protein C depletion, thrombosis of skin vessels may lead to infarction and necrosis. The syndrome can be prevented by the use of heparin for 5–7 days until warfarin induces anticoagulation.

Treatment

If a patient is recognized to be at increased risk of thrombosis, effective prophylactic therapy is usually available. Low-molecular-weight heparin has largely replaced unfractionated heparin because of improved efficacy and ease of monitoring. Warfarin has long been the standard outpatient therapy for prevention of thrombosis, except in cancer-associated thrombosis when low-grade DIC is a pathogenic mechanism. The investigational agent ximelagatran, a direct thrombin inhibitor, may come to replace current anticoagulants based on its ease of use (oral administration, fixed dose, no monitoring) as well as its efficacy and safety (see Chapter 9).

In patients with myeloproliferative disease who have had symptoms of thrombosis, antiplatelet therapy may be helpful. However, such therapy should not be used indiscriminately, because these patients are also at increased risk of bleeding. For patients with **erythromelalgia** (painful redness and burning of the hands), aspirin, 325 mg daily, is effective.

In congenital biochemical defects such as deficiency of antithrombin III or the vitamin K–dependent proteins C and S, warfarin is effective and is given indefinitely. Family members are screened for the presence of the defect.

Kovalevsky G et al: Evaluation of the association between hereditary thrombophilias and recurrent pregnancy loss: a meta-analysis. Arch Intern Med 2004;164:558. [PMID: 15006834]

Mann KG et al: Factor V: a combination of Dr Jekyll and Mr Hyde. Blood 2003;101:20. [PMID: 12393635]

Prandoni P: How I treat venous thromboembolism in patients with cancer. Blood 2005;106:4027. [PMID: 16076870]

Rieder MJ et al: Effect of VKORC1 haplotypes on transcriptional regulation and warfarin dose. N Engl J Med 2005;352:2285. [PMID: 15930419]

LUPUS ANTICOAGULANT

The lupus anticoagulant is an IgM or IgG immunoglobulin that produces a prolonged PTT by binding to the phospholipid used in the in vitro PTT assay. As such, it is a laboratory artifact and does not cause a clinical bleeding disorder. The "lupus anticoagulant" is seen in 5–10% of patients with systemic lupus erythematosus. More commonly, it is seen without an underlying disorder or in patients taking phenothiazines.

There is no bleeding defect unless a second disorder such as thrombocytopenia, hypoprothrombinemia, or a prolonged bleeding time is present. In fact, the lupus anticoagulant has been associated with an increased risk of thrombosis and of recurrent spontaneous abortions.

The PTT is prolonged and fails to correct when the patient's plasma is mixed in a 1:1 dilution with normal plasma. The PT is either normal or slightly prolonged. The fibrinogen level and thrombin time are normal. The Russell viper venom (RVV) time is a more sensitive assay and is specifically designed to demonstrate the presence of a lupus anticoagulant. An antiphospholipid, the lupus anticoagulant will cause a false-positive VDRL test for syphilis. A related autoantibody, anticardiolipin, can be detected by separate assays.

Lupus anticoagulant should be suspected in cases of a markedly prolonged PTT without clinical bleeding (other causes are factor XII or contact factor deficiency). The plasma mixing test will demonstrate the presence of an inhibitor by the failure of normal plasma to correct the PTT. When acquired factor VIII inhibitors are being considered, a factor VIII:C level may be measured; this will be normal in patients with lupus anticoagulant.

No specific treatment is necessary. Prednisone will usually rapidly eliminate the lupus anticoagulant, and it has been suggested that prednisone therapy reduces spontaneous abortions in this syndrome. It is not clear whether prednisone has any effect on the thrombotic tendency associated with lupus anticoagulant. Patients with thromboses should be treated with anticoagulation in standard doses. Because of the artificially prolonged PTT, heparin therapy is difficult to monitor properly, and low-molecular-weight heparin may be preferred. The dose of warfarin administered may also be inadequate if the baseline PT is prolonged.

Brouwer JL et al: The contribution of inherited and acquired thrombophilic defects, alone or combined with antiphospholipid antibodies, to venous and arterial thromboembolism in patients with systemic lupus erythematosus. Blood 2004;104:143. [PMID: 15026314]

Proven A et al: Clinical importance of positive test results for lupus anticoagulant and anticardiolipin antibodies. Mayo Clin Proc 2004;79:467. [PMID: 15065611]

■ BLOOD TRANSFUSIONS

RED BLOOD CELL TRANSFUSIONS

Red blood cell transfusions are given to raise the hematocrit levels in patients with anemia or to replace losses after acute bleeding episodes.

Sources of Red Cells for Transfusion

Several types of components containing red blood cells are available.

A. Fresh Whole Blood

The advantage of whole blood for transfusion is the simultaneous presence of red blood cells, plasma, and fresh platelets. Fresh whole blood is never absolutely necessary, since all the above components are available separately. The major indications for use of whole blood are cardiac surgery or massive hemorrhage when more than 10 units of blood are required in a 24-hour period.

B. Packed Red Blood Cells

Packed red cells are the component most commonly used to raise the hematocrit. Each unit has a volume of about 300 mL, of which approximately 200 mL consists of red blood cells. One unit of packed red cells will usually raise the hematocrit by approximately 4%. The expected rise in hematocrit can be calculated using an estimated red blood cell volume of 200 mL/unit and a total blood volume of about 70 mL/kg. For example, a 70-kg man will have a total blood volume of 4900 mL, and each unit of packed red blood cells will raise the hematocrit by $200 \div 4900$, or 4%.

C. Leukopoor Blood

Patients with severe leukoagglutinin reactions to packed red blood cells may require depletion of white blood cells and platelets from transfused units. White blood cells can be removed either by centrifugation or by washing. Preparation of leukopoor blood is expensive and leads to some loss of red cells.

D. Frozen Blood

Red blood cells can be frozen and stored for up to 3 years, but the technique is cumbersome and expensive, and frozen blood should be used sparingly. The major application is for the purpose of maintaining a supply of rare blood types. Patients with such types may donate units for autologous transfusion should the need arise. Frozen red cells are also occasionally needed for patients with severe leukoagglutinin reactions or anaphylactic reactions to plasma proteins, since frozen blood has essentially all white blood cells and plasma components removed.

E. Autologous Packed Red Blood Cells

Patients scheduled for elective surgery may donate blood for autologous transfusion. These units may be stored for up to 35 days.

Compatibility Testing

Before transfusion, the recipient's and the donor's blood are cross-matched to avoid hemolytic transfusion reactions. Although many antigen systems are present on red blood cells, only the ABO and Rh systems are specifically tested prior to all transfusions. The A and B antigens are the most important, because everyone who lacks one or both red cell antigens has isoantibodies against the missing antigen or antigens in his or her plasma. These antibodies activate complement and can cause rapid intravascular lysis of the incompatible red cells. In emergencies, type O blood can be given to any recipient, but only packed cells should be given to avoid transfusion of donor plasma containing anti-A or anti-B antibodies.

The other important antigen routinely tested for is the D antigen of the Rh system. Approximately 15% of the population lack this antigen. In patients lacking the antigen, anti-D antibodies are not naturally present, but the antigen is highly immunogenic. A recipient whose red cells lack D and who receives D-positive blood may develop anti-D antibodies that can cause severe lysis of subsequent transfusions of D-positive red cells.

Blood typing includes assay of recipient serum for unusual antibodies by mixing the serum with panels of red cells representing commonly occurring weak antigens. The screening is particularly important if the recipient has had previous transfusions.

Hemolytic Transfusion Reactions

The most severe reactions are those involving mismatches in the ABO system. Most of these cases are due to clerical errors and mislabeled specimens. Hemolysis is rapid and intravascular, releasing free hemoglobin into the plasma. The severity of these reactions depends on the dose of red blood cells given. The most severe reactions are those seen in surgical patients under anesthesia.

Hemolytic transfusion reactions caused by minor antigen systems are typically less severe. The hemolysis usually takes place at a slower rate and is extravascular. Sometimes these transfusion reactions may be delayed for 5–10 days after transfusion. In such cases, the recipient has received blood containing an immunogenic action, and in the time since transfusion, a new alloantibody has been formed. The most common antigens involved in such reactions are Duffy, Kidd, Kell, and C and E loci of the Rh system.

A. Symptoms and Signs

Major hemolytic transfusion reactions cause fever and chills, with backache and headache. In severe cases, there may be apprehension, dyspnea, hypotension, and vascular collapse. *The transfusion must be stopped immediately.* In severe cases, DIC, acute renal failure from tubular necrosis, or both can occur.

Patients under general anesthesia will not manifest such signs, and the first indication may be generalized bleeding and oliguria.

B. Laboratory Findings

Identification of the recipient and of the blood should be checked. The donor transfusion bag with its pilot tube must be returned to the blood bank, and a fresh sample of the recipient's blood must accompany the donor bag for retyping of donor and recipient blood samples and for repeat of the cross-match.

The hematocrit will fail to rise by the expected amount. Coagulation studies may reveal evidence of renal failure and DIC. Hemoglobinemia will turn the plasma pink and eventually result in hemoglobinuria. In cases of delayed hemolytic reactions, the hematocrit will fall and the indirect bilirubin will rise. In these cases, the new offending alloantibody is easily detected in the patient's serum.

C. Treatment

If a hemolytic transfusion reaction is suspected, the transfusion should be stopped at once. A sample of anticoagulated blood from the recipient should be centrifuged to detect free hemoglobin in the plasma. If hemoglobinemia is present, the patient should be vig-

orously hydrated to prevent acute tubular necrosis. Forced diuresis with mannitol may help prevent renal damage.

Leukoagglutinin Reactions

Most transfusion reactions are not hemolytic but represent reactions to antigens present on white blood cells in patients who have been sensitized to the antigens through previous transfusions or pregnancy. Most commonly, patients will develop fever and chills within 12 hours after transfusion. In severe cases, cough and dyspnea may occur and the chest x-ray may show transient pulmonary infiltrates. Because no hemolysis is involved, the hematocrit rises by the expected amount despite the reaction.

Leukoagglutinin reactions may respond to acetaminophen and diphenhydramine; corticosteroids are also of value. Removal of leukocytes by filtration before blood storage will reduce the incidence of these reactions.

Anaphylactic Reactions

Rarely, patients will develop urticaria or bronchospasm during a transfusion. These reactions are almost always due to plasma proteins rather than white blood cells. Patients who are IgA deficient may develop these reactions because of antibodies to IgA. Patients with such reactions may require transfusion of washed or even frozen red blood cells to avoid future severe reactions.

Contaminated Blood

Rarely, blood is contaminated with gram-negative bacteria. Transfusion can lead to septicemia and shock from endotoxin. If this is suspected, the offending unit should be cultured and the patient treated with antibiotics as indicated.

Diseases Transmitted Through Transfusion

Despite the use of only volunteer blood donors and the routine screening of blood, transfusion-associated viral diseases remain a problem. All blood products (red blood cells, platelets, plasma, cryoprecipitate) can transmit viral diseases. All blood donors are screened with questionnaires designed to detect donors at high risk of transmitting diseases. All blood is now screened for hepatitis B surface antigen, antibody to hepatitis B core antigen, syphilis, p24 antigen and antibody to HIV, antibody to hepatitis C virus (HCV), antibody to human T cell lymphotropic/leukemia virus (HTLV), and antibody to West Nile virus.

With improved screening, the risk of posttransfusion hepatitis has steadily decreased. The risk of hepatitis B is 1:200,000 per unit and of HIV 1:250,000 per unit. The risk of seroconversion to HTLV is 1:70,000, but clinical sequelae when this occurs are rare. The major infectious risk of blood products is hepatitis C, with a seroconversion rate of 1:3300 per unit transfused. Most of these cases are clinically silent, but there is a high incidence of chronic hepatitis.

Platelet Transfusion

Platelet transfusions are indicated in cases of thrombocytopenia due to decreased platelet production. They are not useful in immune thrombocytopenia, since transfused platelets will last no longer than the patient's endogenous platelets. The risk of spontaneous bleeding rises when the platelet count falls to less than 10,000/mcL, and the risk of life-threatening bleeding increases when the platelet count is less than 5000/mcL. Because of this, prophylactic platelet transfusions are often given at these very low levels. Platelet transfusions are also given prior to invasive procedures or surgery, and the goal should be to raise the platelet count to over 50,000/mcL.

Platelets are most commonly derived from donated blood units. One unit of platelets (derived from 1 unit of blood) usually contains $5–7 \times 10^{10}$ platelets suspended in 35 mL of plasma. Ideally, 1 platelet unit will raise the recipient's platelet count by 10,000/mcL, and transfused platelets will last for 2 or 3 days. However, responses are often suboptimal, with poor platelet increments and short survival times. This may be due to sepsis, splenomegaly, or alloimmunization. Most alloantibodies causing platelet destruction are directed at HLA antigens. Patients requiring long periods of platelet transfusion support should be monitored to document adequate responses to transfusions so that the most appropriate product can be used. Patients may benefit from HLA-matched platelets derived from either volunteer donors or family members, with platelets obtained by plateletpheresis. Techniques of cross-matching platelets have been developed and appear to identify suitable platelet donors (nonreactive with the patient's serum) without the need for HLA typing. Such single-donor platelets usually contain the equivalent of six units of random platelets, or $30–50 \times 10^{10}$ platelets suspended in 200 mL of plasma. Ideally, these platelet concentrates will raise the recipient's platelet count by 60,000/mcL. Leukocyte depletion of platelets has been shown to delay the onset of alloimmunization.

Granulocyte Transfusions

Granulocyte transfusions are seldom indicated and have largely been replaced by the use of myeloid growth factors (G-CSF and GM-CSF) that speed neutrophil recovery. However, they may be beneficial in patients with profound neutropenia (< 100/mcL) who have gram-negative sepsis or progressive soft tissue infection despite optimal antibiotic therapy. In these cases, it is clear that progressive infection is due to failure of host defenses. In such situations, daily granulocyte transfusions should be given and continued until the neutrophil count rises to above 500/mcL. Such granulocytes must be derived from ABO-matched donors. Although HLA matching is not necessary, it is preferred, since patients with alloantibodies to donor white blood cells will have severe reactions and no benefit.

The donor cells usually contain some immunocompetent lymphocytes capable of producing graft-versus-host disease in HLA-incompatible hosts whose immunocompetence may be impaired. Irradiation of the units of cells with 1500 cGy will destroy the lymphocytes without harm to the granulocytes or platelets.

Silliman CC et al: Transfusion-related acute lung injury. Blood 2005;105:2266. [PMID: 15572582]

Slichter SJ et al: Factors affecting posttransfusion platelet increments, platelet refractoriness, and platelet transfusion intervals in thrombocytopenic patients. Blood 2005;105:4106. [PMID: 15692069]

Stramer SL et al: West Nile virus among blood donors in the United States, 2003 and 2004. N Engl J Med 2005;353: 451. [PMID: 16079368]

TRANSFUSION OF PLASMA COMPONENTS

Fresh-frozen plasma is available in units of approximately 200 mL. Fresh plasma contains normal levels of all coagulation factors (about 1 unit/mL). Fresh frozen plasma is used to correct coagulation factor deficiencies and to treat TTP. The risk of transmitting viral disease is comparable to that associated with transfusion of red blood cells.

Cryoprecipitate is made from fresh plasma. One unit has a volume of approximately 20 mL and contains approximately 250 mg of fibrinogen and between 80 and 100 units of factor VIII and vWF. Cryoprecipitate is used to supplement fibrinogen in cases of congenital deficiency of fibrinogen or DIC. One unit of cryoprecipitate will raise the fibrinogen level by about 8 mg/dL.

Alimentary Tract

14

Kenneth R. McQuaid, MD

■ SYMPTOMS & SIGNS OF GASTROINTESTINAL DISEASE

DYSPEPSIA

Dyspepsia refers to acute, chronic, or recurrent pain or discomfort centered in the upper abdomen. The discomfort may be characterized by or associated with upper abdominal fullness, early satiety, burning, bloating, belching, nausea, retching, or vomiting. Heartburn (retrosternal burning) should be distinguished from dyspepsia. Patients with dyspepsia often have heartburn as an additional symptom. When heartburn is the dominant complaint, gastroesophageal reflux is nearly always present. Dyspepsia occurs in 25% of the adult population and accounts for 3% of general medical office visits.

Etiology

A. Food or Drug Intolerance

Acute, self-limited "indigestion" may be caused by overeating, eating too quickly, eating high-fat foods, eating during stressful situations, or drinking too much alcohol or coffee. Many medications cause dyspepsia, including aspirin, nonsteroidal anti-inflammatory drugs (NSAIDs), antibiotics (metronidazole, macrolides), various diabetes drugs (metformin, alpha-glucosidase inhibitors, amylin analogs, GLP-1 receptor antagonists), cholinesterase inhibitors (donepezil, rivastigmine), corticosteroids, digoxin, iron, and opioids.

B. Luminal Gastrointestinal Tract Dysfunction

Peptic ulcer disease is present in 5–15% of patients with dyspepsia. Gastroesophageal reflux disease is present in up to 20% of patients with dyspepsia, even without significant heartburn. Gastric cancer is identified in 1% but is rare in persons under age 45 years. Other causes include gastroparesis (especially in diabetes mellitus), lactose intolerance or malabsorptive conditions, and parasitic infection (*Giardia, Strongyloides*).

C. *Helicobacter pylori* Infection

Chronic gastric infection with *H pylori* as a cause of dyspepsia remains controversial. The prevalence of *H pylori*-associated chronic gastritis in patients with dyspepsia without peptic ulcer disease is 20–50%, the same as in the general population.

D. Pancreatic Disease

Pancreatic carcinoma, chronic pancreatitis.

E. Biliary Tract Disease

The abrupt onset of epigastric or right upper quadrant pain due to cholelithiasis or choledocholithiasis should be readily distinguished from dyspepsia.

F. Other Conditions

Diabetes, thyroid disease, renal insufficiency, myocardial ischemia, intra-abdominal malignancy, gastric volvulus or paraesophageal hernia, and pregnancy are sometimes accompanied by dyspepsia.

G. Functional Dyspepsia

This is the most common cause of chronic dyspepsia. Up to two-thirds of patients have no obvious organic cause for their symptoms after evaluation. Symptoms may arise from a complex interaction of increased visceral afferent sensitivity, gastric delayed emptying or impaired accommodation to food, or psychosocial stressors. Although benign, these symptoms may be chronic and difficult to treat.

Clinical Findings

A. Symptoms and Signs

Given the nonspecific nature of dyspeptic symptoms, the history has limited diagnostic utility. It should clarify the chronicity, location, and quality of the discomfort, its relationship to meals, and whether it is relieved by antacids. Concomitant weight loss, persistent vomiting, constant or severe pain, dysphagia, hematemesis, or melena warrants endoscopy or abdominal imaging. Potentially offending medications and excessive alcohol use should be identified and discontinued if possible. The patient's reason for seeking care should be determined. Recent changes in employment, marital discord, physical and sexual abuse, anxiety, depression, and fear of serious disease may all contribute to the development and reporting of symptoms. Patients with functional dyspepsia often are younger, report a variety of abdominal and extragastrointestinal complaints, show signs of anxiety or depression, or have a history of use of psychotropic medications.

The symptom profile alone does not differentiate between functional dyspepsia and organic gastrointestinal disorders. Based on the clinical history alone, primary care physicians misdiagnose nearly half of patients with peptic ulcers or gastroesophageal reflux and have < 25% accuracy in diagnosing functional dyspepsia.

The physical examination is rarely helpful. Signs of serious organic disease such as weight loss, organomegaly, abdominal mass, or fecal occult blood are further evaluated. In patients over age 50 years, initial laboratory work should include a blood count, electrolytes, liver enzymes, calcium, and thyroid function tests.

B. Special Examinations

1. Upper endoscopy—Upper endoscopy is the study of choice to diagnose gastroduodenal ulcers, erosive esophagitis, and upper gastrointestinal malignancy. Upper gastrointestinal barium radiography is inferior to endoscopy for the evaluation of dyspepsia. Upper endoscopy is indicated to look for gastric cancer or other serious organic disease in all patients over age 55 years with new-onset dyspepsia and in all patients with "alarm" features such as weight loss, dysphagia, recurrent vomiting, evidence of bleeding, or anemia. It is also helpful for patients who are concerned about serious underlying disease. For patients born in regions in which there is a higher incidence of gastric cancer, an age threshold of 45 years may be appropriate.

2. Empiric management—In patients younger than 55 years with uncomplicated dyspepsia (in whom gastric cancer is rare), initial noninvasive management strategies should be pursued. In most clinical settings, a noninvasive test for *H pylori* (IgG serology, fecal antigen test, or urea breath test) should be performed first. Although serologic tests are inexpensive, performance characteristics are poor in low-prevalence populations. If test results are negative in a patient not taking NSAIDs, peptic ulcer disease is virtually excluded. Most of these *H pylori*–negative patients have functional dyspepsia or atypical gastroesophageal reflux disease and can be treated with an antisecretory agent (proton pump inhibitor) for 4 weeks. For patients who have symptom relapse after discontinuation of the proton pump inhibitor, intermittent or long-term proton pump inhibitor therapy may be considered.

For patients in whom test results are positive for *H pylori*, antibiotic therapy proves definitive for over 90% of peptic ulcers and may improve symptoms in a small subset (< 10%) of infected patients with functional dyspepsia. Patients with persistent dyspepsia after *H pylori* eradication can be given a trial of proton pump inhibitor therapy. In clinical settings in which the prevalence of *H pylori* infection in the population is low (< 10%), it may be more cost-effective to initially treat all young patients with uncomplicated dyspepsia with a 4-week trial of a proton pump inhibitor. Patients who have symptom relapse after discontinua-

tion of the proton pump inhibitor should be tested for *H pylori* and treated if positive.

Endoscopic evaluation is warranted when symptoms fail to respond to initial empiric management strategies or frequent symptom relapse occurs after discontinuation of antisecretory therapy. Abdominal imaging (ultrasonography or CT scanning) is performed only when pancreatic or biliary tract disease is suspected. Gastric emptying studies are valuable only in patients with recurrent vomiting. Ambulatory esophageal pH testing may be of value when atypical gastroesophageal reflux is suspected.

Treatment of Functional Dyspepsia

Regardless of the initial strategy undertaken for patients with dyspepsia, a significant proportion will have persistent or recurrent symptoms requiring evaluation with endoscopy. Most patients will have no significant findings and will be given a diagnosis of functional dyspepsia.

A. General Measures

Most patients have mild, intermittent symptoms that respond to reassurance and lifestyle changes. Alcohol, caffeine, and fatty foods should be reduced or discontinued. A food diary, in which patients record their food intake, symptoms, and daily events, may reveal dietary or psychosocial precipitants of pain.

B. Pharmacologic Agents

Drugs have demonstrated limited efficacy in the treatment of functional dyspepsia. One-third of patients derive relief from placebo. Antisecretory therapy for 2–4 weeks with either H_2-receptor antagonists (ranitidine or nizatidine, 150 mg twice daily; famotidine, 20 mg twice daily; or cimetidine, 400–800 mg twice daily) or proton pump inhibitors (omeprazole, esomeprazole, or rabeprazole 20 mg, lansoprazole 30 mg, or pantoprazole 40 mg) may benefit 10–15% of patients, particularly those with dyspepsia and heartburn ("reflux-like dyspepsia"). Superiority of proton pump inhibitors to H_2-antagonists has not been established. Low doses of antidepressants (eg, desipramine or nortriptyline, 10–50 mg at bedtime) are believed to benefit some patients, possibly by moderating visceral afferent sensitivity. However, side effects are common and response is patient specific. Doses should be increased slowly. The prokinetic agent metoclopramide (5–10 mg three times daily) may improve symptoms, but improvement does not correlate with the presence or absence of gastric emptying delay. Long-term metoclopramide use is associated with a high incidence of neuropsychiatric side effects and cannot be recommended. Limited studies to date have not demonstrated efficacy for the prokinetic agent tegaserod.

C. Anti-*H pylori* Treatment

A meta-analysis has suggested that a small number of patients (< 10%) derive benefit from *H pylori* eradication therapy.

D. ALTERNATIVE THERAPIES

Psychotherapy and hypnotherapy may be of benefit in selected motivated patients. Herbal therapies (peppermint, caraway) may offer benefit with little risk of adverse effects.

Ford AC et al: *Helicobacter pylori* "test and treat" or endoscopy for managing dyspepsia: an individual patient data meta-analysis. Gastroenterology 2005;128:1838. [PMID: 15940619]

Gupta S et al: Management of nonsteroidal, anti-inflammatory, drug-associated dyspepsia. Gastroenterology 2005;129:1711. [PMID: 16285968]

Talley NJ et al; American Gastroenterological Association: American Gastroenterological Association Medical Position Statement: Evaluation of dyspepsia. Gastroenterology 2005;129: 1753. [PMID: 16285970]

Talley NJ et al; Practice Parameters Committee of the American College of Gastroenterology: Guidelines for the management of dyspepsia. Am J Gastroenterol 2005;100:2324. [PMID: 16181387]

Timmons S et al: Functional dyspepsia: motor abnormalities, sensory dysfunction, and therapeutic options. Am J Gastroenterol 2004;99:739. [PMID: 15089910]

NAUSEA & VOMITING

Nausea is a vague, intensely disagreeable sensation of sickness or "queasiness" that may or may not be followed by vomiting and is distinguished from anorexia. Vomiting often follows, as does retching (spasmodic respiratory and abdominal movements). Vomiting should be distinguished from regurgitation, the effortless reflux of liquid or food stomach contents; and from rumination, the chewing and swallowing of food that is regurgitated volitionally after meals.

The medullary vomiting center (which contains histamine H_1-receptors and muscarinic cholinergic receptors) may be stimulated by four different sources of afferent input: (1) Afferent vagal and splanchnic fibers from the gastrointestinal viscera are rich in serotonin 5-HT_3 receptors; these may be stimulated by biliary or gastrointestinal distention, mucosal or peritoneal irritation, or infections. (2) Fibers of the vestibular system, which have high concentrations of histamine H_1 and muscarinic cholinergic receptors. (3) Higher central nervous system centers; here, certain sights, smells, or emotional experiences may induce vomiting. For example, patients receiving chemotherapy may develop vomiting in anticipation of its administration. (4) The chemoreceptor trigger zone, located outside the blood-brain barrier in the area postrema of the medulla, which is rich in opioid, serotonin 5-HT_3, neurokinin 1 (NK_1) and dopamine D_2 receptors. This region may be stimulated by drugs and chemotherapeutic agents, toxins, hypoxia, uremia, acidosis, and radiation therapy. Although the causes of vomiting are many, a simplified list is provided in Table 14–1.

Complications of vomiting include dehydration, hypokalemia, metabolic alkalosis, aspiration, rupture of the esophagus (Boerhaave's syndrome), and bleeding secondary to a mucosal tear at the gastroesophageal junction (Mallory-Weiss syndrome).

Clinical Findings

A. SYMPTOMS AND SIGNS

Acute symptoms without abdominal pain are typically caused by food poisoning, infectious gastroenteritis, drugs, or systemic illness. Inquiry should be made into recent changes in medications, diet, other intestinal symptoms, or similar illnesses in family members. The acute onset of severe pain and vomiting suggests peritoneal irritation, acute gastric or intestinal obstruction, or pancreaticobiliary disease. Examination may reveal fever, focal tenderness or rigidity, guarding, or rebound tenderness. Persistent vomiting suggests pregnancy, gastric outlet obstruction, gastroparesis, intestinal dysmotility, psychogenic disorders, and central nervous system or systemic disorders. Vomiting that occurs in the morning before breakfast is common with pregnancy, uremia, alcohol intake, and increased intracranial pressure. Vomiting immediately after meals strongly suggests bulimia or psychogenic causes. Vomiting of undigested food one to several hours after meals is characteristic of gastroparesis or a gastric outlet obstruction; physical examination may reveal a succussion splash. Patients with acute or chronic symptoms should be asked about neurologic symptoms that suggest a central nervous system cause such as headache, stiff neck, vertigo, and focal paresthesias or weakness.

B. SPECIAL EXAMINATIONS

With vomiting that is severe or protracted, serum electrolytes should be obtained to look for hypokalemia, azotemia, or metabolic alkalosis resulting from loss of gastric contents. Flat and upright abdominal radiographs are obtained in patients with severe pain or suspicion of mechanical obstruction to look for free intraperitoneal air or dilated loops of small bowel. If mechanical small intestinal or gastric obstruction is thought likely, a nasogastric tube is placed for relief of symptoms. The cause of gastric outlet obstruction is best demonstrated by upper endoscopy, and the cause of small intestinal obstruction is best demonstrated with barium radiography or abdominal CT imaging. Gastroparesis is confirmed by nuclear scintigraphic studies or ^{13}C-octanoic acid breath tests, which show delayed gastric emptying and either upper endoscopy or barium upper gastrointestinal series showing no evidence of mechanical gastric outlet obstruction. Abnormal liver function tests or elevated amylase or lipase suggest pancreaticobiliary disease, which may be investigated with an abdominal sonogram or CT scan. Central nervous system causes are best evaluated with either head CT or MRI.

Treatment

A. GENERAL MEASURES

Most causes of acute vomiting are mild, self-limited, and require no specific treatment. Patients should in-

Table 14–1. Causes of nausea and vomiting.

Visceral afferent stimulation	**Infections**
	Mechanical obstruction
	Gastric outlet obstruction: peptic ulcer disease, malignancy, gastric volvulus
	Small intestinal obstruction: adhesions, hernias, volvulus, Crohn's disease, carcinomatosis
	Dysmotility
	Gastroparesis: diabetic, medications (metformin, acarbose, pramlintide, exenatide), postviral, postvagotomy
	Small intestine: scleroderma, amyloidosis, chronic intestinal pseudo-obstruction, familial myoneuropathies
	Peritoneal irritation
	Peritonitis: perforated viscus, appendicitis, spontaneous bacterial peritonitis
	Viral gastroenteritis: Norwalk agent, rotavirus
	"Food poisoning": toxins from *Bacillus cereus, Staphylococcus aureus, Clostridium perfringens*
	Hepatitis A or B
	Acute systemic infections
	Hepatobiliary or pancreatic disorders
	Acute pancreatitis
	Cholecystitis or choledocholithiasis
	Topical gastrointestinal irritants
	Alcohol, NSAIDs, oral antibiotics
	Postoperative
	Other
	Cardiac disease: acute myocardial infarction, congestive heart failure
	Urologic disease: stones, pyelonephritis
CNS disorders	**Vestibular disorders**
	Labyrinthitis, Meniere's syndrome, motion sickness, migraine
	Increased intracranial pressure
	CNS tumors, subdural or subarachnoid hemorrhage
	Migraine
	Infections
	Meningitis, encephalitis
	Psychogenic
	Anticipatory vomiting, bulimia, psychiatric disorders
Irritation of chemoreceptor trigger zone	**Antitumor chemotherapy**
	Drugs and medications
	Calcium channel blockers
	Opioids
	Anticonvulsants
	Antiparkinsonism drugs
	β-Blockers, antiarrhythmics, digoxin
	Nicotine
	Oral contraceptives
	Cholinesterase inhibitors
	Radiation therapy
	Systemic disorders
	Diabetic ketoacidosis
	Uremia
	Adrenocortical crisis
	Parathyroid disease
	Hypothyroidism
	Pregnancy
	Paraneoplastic syndrome

NSAIDs = nonsteroidal anti-inflammatory drugs; CNS = central nervous system.

gest clear liquids (broths, tea, soups, carbonated beverages) and small quantities of dry foods (soda crackers). For more severe acute vomiting, hospitalization may be required. Patients unable to eat and losing gastric fluids may become dehydrated, resulting in hypokalemia with metabolic alkalosis. Intravenous 0.45% saline solution with 20 mEq/L of potassium chloride is given in most cases to maintain hydration. A nasogastric suction tube for gastric decompression improves patient comfort and permits monitoring of fluid loss.

B. ANTIEMETIC MEDICATIONS

Medications may be given either to prevent or to control vomiting (see above). Combinations of drugs from different classes may provide better control of symptoms with less toxicity in some patients. All of these medications should be avoided in pregnancy. (For dosages, see Table 14–2.)

1. Serotonin 5-HT$_3$-receptor antagonists—Ondansetron, granisetron, dolasetron, and palonosetron are effective in preventing chemotherapy- and radiation-induced emesis when initiated prior to treatment. Single-dose administration schedules are as effective as multiple-dose regimens. Although serotonin antagonists are effective for the prevention of postoperative nausea and vomiting, less expensive alternatives (eg, dexamethasone or droperidol) are equally effective.

2. Corticosteroids—Corticosteroids (eg, dexamethasone) have antiemetic properties, but the basis for these effects is unknown. These agents enhance the efficacy of serotonin receptor antagonsists for preventing acute and delayed nausea and vomiting in patients receiving moderately to highly emetogenic chemotherapy regimens. For the prevention of postoperative nausea and vomiting, corticosteroids, serotonin antagonists, and droperidol have efficacy; however, combinations of these agents have additive benefit.

3. Neurokinin receptor antagonists—Aprepitant is a highly selective antagonist for NK$_1$-receptors in the area postrema. It is used in combination with corticosteroids and serotonin antagonists for the prevention of acute and delayed nausea and vomiting with highly emetogenic chemotherapy regimens. Combined therapy with aprepitant prevents acute emesis in 80–90% and delayed emesis in > 70% of patients treated with highly emetogenic regimens.

4. Dopamine antagonists—The phenothiazines, butyrophenones, and substituted benzamides have antiemetic properties that are due to dopaminergic blockade as well as to their sedative effects. High doses of these agents are associated with antidopaminergic side effects, including extrapyramidal reactions and depression. These agents are used in a variety of situations. Cases of QT prolongation leading to ventricular tachycardia (torsade de pointes) have been reported in several patients receiving droperidol, hence electrocardiographic monitoring is recommended before and after administration.

Table 14–2. Common antiemetic dosing regimens.

	Dosage	Route
Serotonin 5-HT$_3$ antagonists		
Ondansetron	8–32 mg or 0.15 mg/kg once daily	IV
	8 mg twice daily	PO
Granisetron	1 mg or 0.01 mg/kg once daily	IV
	2 mg once daily	PO
Dolasetron	100 mg or 1.8 mg/kg once daily	IV
	100 mg once daily	PO
Palonosetron	0.25 mg once as a single dose 30 min before start of chemotherapy	IV
Corticosteroids		
Dexamethasone	8–20 mg once daily	IV
	4–20 mg once or twice daily	PO
Methylprednisolone	40–100 mg once daily	IV
Dopamine receptor antagonists		
Metoclopramide	10–20 mg or 0.5 mg/kg every 6–8 hours	IV
	10–20 mg every 6–8 hours	PO
Prochlorperazine	5–10 mg every 4–6 hours	PO, IM, IV
	25 mg suppository every 6 hours	PR
Promethazine	25 mg every 4–6 hours	PO, PR, IM, IV
Trimethobenzamide	250 mg every 6–8 hours	PO
	200 mg every 6–8 hours	IM, PR
Sedatives		
Diazepam	2–5 mg every 4–6 hours	PO, IV
Lorazepam	1–2 mg every 4–6 hours	PO, IV

IV = intravenously; PO = orally; IM = intramuscularly; PR = per rectum.

5. Antihistamines and anticholinergics—These drugs (eg, meclizine, dimenhydrinate, transdermal scopolamine) may be valuable in the prevention of vomiting arising from stimulation of the labyrinth, ie, motion sickness, vertigo, and migraines. They may induce drowsiness.

6. Sedatives—Benzodiazepines are used in psychogenic and anticipatory vomiting.

7. Cannabinoids—Marijuana has been used widely as an appetite stimulant and antiemetic. Pure Δ^9-tetrahydrocannabinol (THC) is the major active ingredient in marijuana and is available by prescription as dronabinol. In doses of 5–15 mg/m^2, oral dronabinol is effective in treating nausea associated with chemotherapy, but it is associated with central nervous system side effects in most patients.

Apfel CC et al: A factorial trial of six interventions in the prevention of postoperative nausea and vomiting. N Engl J Med 2004;350:2441. [PMID: 15190136]

Hasler WL et al: Nausea and vomiting. Gastroenterology 2003; 125:1860. [PMID: 14724837]

Sharma R et al: Management of chemotherapy-induced nausea, vomiting, oral mucositis, and diarrhoea. Lancet Oncol 2005;6:93. [PMID: 15683818]

Tramer MR: Treatment of postoperative nausea and vomiting. BMJ 2003;327:762. [PMID: 14525850]

HICCUPS (Singultus)

Though usually a benign and self-limited annoyance, hiccups may be persistent and a sign of serious underlying illness. In patients on mechanical ventilation, hiccups can trigger a full respiratory cycle and result in respiratory alkalosis.

Causes of benign, self-limited hiccups include gastric distention (carbonated beverages, air swallowing, overeating), sudden temperature changes (hot then cold liquids, hot then cold shower), alcohol ingestion, and states of heightened emotion (excitement, stress, laughing). There are over 100 causes of recurrent or persistent hiccups, grouped into the following categories:

Central nervous system: Neoplasms, infections, cerebrovascular accident, trauma.

Metabolic: Uremia, hypocapnia (hyperventilation).

Irritation of the vagus or phrenic nerve: (1) Head, neck: Foreign body in ear, goiter, neoplasms. (2) Thorax: Pneumonia, empyema, neoplasms, myocardial infarction, pericarditis, aneurysm, esophageal obstruction, reflux esophagitis. (3) Abdomen: Subphrenic abscess, hepatomegaly, hepatitis, cholecystitis, gastric distention, gastric neoplasm, pancreatitis, or pancreatic malignancy.

Surgical: General anesthesia, postoperative.

Psychogenic and idiopathic.

Clinical Findings

Evaluation of the patient with persistent hiccups should include a detailed neurologic examination, serum creatinine, liver chemistry tests, and a chest radiograph. When the cause remains unclear, CT of the head, chest, and abdomen, echocardiography, bronchoscopy, and upper endoscopy may help. On occasion, hiccups may be unilateral; chest fluoroscopy will make the diagnosis.

Treatment

A number of simple remedies may be helpful in patients with acute benign hiccups. (1) Irritation of the nasopharynx by tongue traction, lifting the uvula with a spoon, catheter stimulation of the nasopharynx, or

eating 1 tsp of dry granulated sugar. (2) Interruption of the respiratory cycle by breath holding, Valsalva's maneuver, sneezing, gasping (fright stimulus), or rebreathing into a bag. (3) Stimulation of the vagus, carotid massage. (4) Irritation of the diaphragm by holding knees to chest or by continuous positive airway pressure during mechanical ventilation. (5) Relief of gastric distention by belching or insertion of a nasogastric tube.

A number of drugs have been promoted as being useful in the treatment of hiccups. Chlorpromazine, 25–50 mg orally or intramuscularly, is most commonly used. Other agents reported to be effective include anticonvulsants (phenytoin, carbamazepine), benzodiazepines (lorazepam, diazepam), metoclopramide, baclofen, gabapentin, and occasionally general anesthesia.

Krakauer EL et al: Case records of the Massachusetts General Hospital. Weekly clinicopathological exercises. Case 6-2005. A 58-year-old man with esophageal cancer and nausea, vomiting, and intractable hiccups. N Engl J Med 2005; 352:817. [PMID: 15728815]

Moretti R et al: Gabapentin as a drug therapy of intractable hiccup because of vascular lesion: a three-year follow up. Neurologist 2004;10:102. [PMID: 14998440]

CONSTIPATION

The first step in evaluating the patient is to determine what is meant by "constipation." Patients may define constipation as infrequent stools (fewer than 3 in a week), hard stools, excessive straining, or a sense of incomplete evacuation. Table 14–3 summarizes the many causes of constipation, which are discussed below.

Common Identifiable Causes of Constipation

A. POOR DIETARY AND BEHAVIORAL HABITS

The majority of constipated patients have mild symptoms that cannot be attributed to any structural abnormalities, intestinal motility disorders, or systemic disease. Dietary review will reveal that most of these patients do not consume adequate fiber and fluids. Ingestion of additional 10–12 g of fiber per day either by dietary changes or the addition of commercial fiber supplementation is often all that is needed. At least one or two glasses of fluid should be taken with meals. The elderly are predisposed because of poor eating habits, a variety of medications, decreased colonic motility and, in some cases, inability to sit on a toilet (bed-bound patients).

B. STRUCTURAL ABNORMALITIES

Constipation may be caused by colonic lesions, such as neoplasms and strictures, that obstruct fecal passage. Diagnostic studies to exclude such lesions are indicated in patients with a family history of colon cancer or inflammatory bowel disease; with alarm symptoms

Table 14–3. Causes of constipation in adults.

Most common
 Inadequate fiber or fluid intake
 Poor bowel habits
Systemic disease
 Endocrine: hypothyroidism, hyperparathyroidism, diabe-
  tes mellitus
 Metabolic: hypokalemia, hypercalcemia, uremia, porphyria
 Neurologic: Parkinson's, multiple sclerosis, sacral nerve
  damage (prior pelvic surgery, tumor), paraplegia, auto-
  nomic neuropathy
Medications
 Opioids
 Diuretics
 Calcium channel blockers
 Anticholinergics
 Psychotropics
 Calcium and iron supplements
 NSAIDs
 Clonidine
 Sucralfate
 Cholestyramine
Structural abnormalities
 Anorectal: rectal prolapse, rectocoele, rectal intussuscep-
  tion, anorectal stricture, anal fissure, solitary rectal ulcer
  syndrome
 Perineal descent
 Colonic mass with obstruction: adenocarcinoma
 Colonic stricture: radiation, ischemia, diverticulosis
 Hirschsprung's disease
 Idiopathic megarectum
Slow colonic transit
 Idiopathic: isolated to colon
 Psychogenic
 Eating disorders
 Chronic intestinal pseudo-obstruction
Pelvic floor dysfunction
Irritable bowel syndrome

NSAIDs = nonsteroidal anti-inflammatory drugs.

or signs, such as hematochezia, weight loss, anemia, or positive fecal occult blood tests (FOBT); and in patients older than 45–50 years with new-onset constipation. Defecatory difficulties also can be due to a variety of anorectal outlet problems that impede or obstruct flow (perineal descent, rectal prolapse, rectocele), some of which may require surgery, and Hirschsprung's disease (usually suggested by lifelong constipation).

C. SYSTEMIC DISEASES

Medical diseases can cause constipation due to neurologic gut dysfunction, myopathies, endocrine disorders, and electrolyte abnormalities such as hypercalcemia or hypokalemia.

D. MEDICATIONS

Anticholinergic and opioid agents are common causes of constipation.

Causes of Severe or Refractory Constipation

Patients whose constipation cannot be attributed to the above causes and who do not respond to conservative dietary management present difficult management problems. Conceptually, these patients can be divided into three classes.

A. SLOW COLONIC TRANSIT

Normal colonic transit time is approximately 35 hours; more than 72 hours is significantly abnormal. Slow colonic transit may be part of a more generalized gastrointestinal dysmotility syndrome but most commonly is idiopathic. Colonic inertia is more common in women, some of whom have a history of psychosocial problems or sexual abuse.

B. PELVIC FLOOR DYSFUNCTION

With normal defecation, the anal sphincter and puborectalis muscle relaxes. Patients with pelvic floor dysfunction—women more often than men—have a paradoxical contraction of the anal sphincter and pelvic floor during attempted defecation that impedes the bowel movement. They may complain of excessive straining with a sense of incomplete evacuation, the need for digital pressure on the vagina or perineum, or the need for digital disimpaction.

C. IRRITABLE BOWEL SYNDROME

Patients with primary complaints of abdominal pain, bloating, or a sense of incomplete evacuation may have irritable bowel syndrome. (See below.)

Evaluation

A. INITIAL MANAGEMENT

All patients should undergo a history and physical examination, including digital rectal examination and stool testing for occult blood. Digital examination should assess for anatomic abnormalities, such as anal stricture, rectocele, rectal prolapse, or perineal descent during straining. In otherwise healthy patients under age 50 without alarm symptoms or signs, it is reasonable to initiate a trial of empiric treatment. Further diagnostic tests should be performed in patients with any of the following: age 50 years or older, severe constipation, signs of an organic disorders, alarm symptoms (hematochezia, weight loss, positive FOBT), a family history of colon cancer or inflammatory bowel disease, and in patients whose symptoms have not responded to empiric management. Laboratory studies should include a complete blood count, serum electrolytes, serum calcium, serum glucose, and serum thyroid-stimulating hormone (TSH). A colonoscopy or flexible sigmoidoscopy and barium enema should be obtained to exclude a neoplasm, stricture, or inflammatory bowel disease.

B. SECOND LEVEL OF INVESTIGATION

Patients with refractory constipation not responding to conservative measures may require further investigation by means of colonic transit and pelvic floor function studies in order to distinguish slow colonic transit from outlet disorders. Colon transit time is measured by performing an abdominal radiograph 120 hours after ingestion of 24 radio-opaque markers. Retention of > 20% of the markers indicates prolonged transit. Pelvic floor dysfunction and anorectal disorders are assessed with balloon expulsion testing, anal manometry, and defecography.

Standard Treatment of Chronic Constipation

A. DIETARY MEASURES

Proper dietary fluid and fiber intake should be emphasized. Fiber may be given by means of dietary alterations or fiber supplements (Table 14–4). Increased dietary fiber may cause temporary distention or flatulence, which often diminishes over several days. Response to fiber therapy is not immediate, and increases in dosage should be made gradually over 7–10 days. Whereas fiber may benefit most patients, it normally does not benefit patients with severe colonic inertia or outlet disorders.

B. STOOL SURFACTANT AGENTS

Docusate sodium, 50–200 mg/d, or mineral oil, 14–45 mL/d, may be given orally or rectally to promote softening of stools. Aspiration of mineral oil can cause lipoid pneumonia.

C. OSMOTIC LAXATIVES

These agents, used to soften stools, may be given alone or in combination with fiber supplements (Table 14–4). They are commonly used in older nonambulatory patients to prevent constipation and fecal impaction. They are safe and are titrated to a dose that results in soft to semiliquid stools. The less expensive saline laxatives should be tried first before using more expensive osmotic agents, such as nonabsorbable carbohydrates or polyethylene glycol solution.

1. Saline laxatives—Magnesium-containing saline laxatives (milk of magnesia, magnesium sulfate) are the most commonly used agents for the prevention and treatment of chronic constipation. These agents should not be given to patients with renal insufficiency. Sodium phosphate or magnesium citrate may be used for aggressive treatment of acute constipation or as a purgative prior to surgical, endoscopic, or radiographic procedures.

2. Nonabsorbable carbohydrates—Either sorbitol (70%) or lactulose, 15–30 mL once or twice daily, is efficacious for the prevention or treatment of chronic constipation. These malabsorbed sugars are often limited by their propensity to induce bloating, cramps, and flatulence.

3. Polyethylene glycol solution—Polyethylene glycol is a component of solutions traditionally used for colonic lavage prior to colonoscopy (CoLyte, GoLYTELY, NuLytely). Polyethylene glycol 3350 powder (Miralax) is available for the treatment of acute or chronic constipation. Seventeen grams of powder may be mixed in water or juice and taken once or twice daily.

D. STIMULANT AGENTS

These agents stimulate fluid secretion and colonic contraction, resulting in a bowel movement within 6–12 hours after oral ingestion or 15–60 minutes after rectal administration. Common preparations include bisacodyl, senna, cascara, and castor oil (Table 14–4). Colchicine (0.6 mg) or misoprostol (200–400 mcg) two or three times daily may be helpful in some patients with refractory constipation. The prokinetic agent tegaserod (6 mg twice daily) is a $5-HT_4$-receptor agonist that is approved for the treatment of chronic constipation. In randomized trials of patients with chronic constipation (fewer than three spontaneous bowel movements per week), 40% of patients who received tegaserod experienced an increase in the number of spontaneous bowel movements compared with 25% of those who received placebo. At present, this drug should be reserved for patients who have suboptimal response or side effects with less expensive agents.

Treatment of Fecal Impaction

Severe impaction of stool in the rectal vault may result in obstruction to further fecal flow, leading to partial or complete large bowel obstruction. Predisposing factors include severe psychiatric disease, prolonged bed rest and debility, neurogenic disorders of the colon, and spinal cord disorders. Clinical presentation includes decreased appetite, nausea, and vomiting, and abdominal pain and distention. There may be paradoxical "diarrhea" as liquid stool leaks around the impacted feces. Firm feces are palpable on digital examination of the rectal vault. Initial treatment is directed at relieving the impaction with enemas (saline, mineral oil, or diatrizoate) or digital disruption of the impacted fecal material. Long-term care is directed at maintaining soft stools and regular bowel movements (as above).

American College of Gastroenterology Task Force: An evidence-based approach to the management of chronic constipation in North America. Am J Gastroenterol 2005;100 (Suppl 1):S1. [PMID: 16008640]

Cash BD et al: The role of serotonergic agents in the treatment of patients with primary constipation. Aliment Pharmacol Ther 2005;22:1047. [PMID: 16305718]

Table 14–4. Pharmacologic management of constipation.

Agent	Dosage	Onset of Action	Comments
Fiber laxatives			
Bran powder	1–4 tbsp orally twice daily	Days	Inexpensive; may cause gas, flatulence
Psyllium	1 tsp once or twice daily	Days	(Metamucil; Perdiem)
Methylcellulose	1 tsp once or twice daily	Days	(Citrucel) Less gas, flatulence
Calcium polycarbophil	1 or 2 tablets once or twice daily	12–24 hours	(FiberCon) Does not cause gas; pill form
Guargum	1 tbsp once or twice daily	Days	(Benefiber) non-gritty, tasteless, less gas
Stool surfactants			
Docusate sodium	100 mg once or twice daily	12–72 hours	(Colace) Marginal benefit
Mineral oil	15–45 mL once or twice daily	6–8 hours	May cause lipoid pneumonia if aspirated
Osmotic laxatives			
Magnesium hydroxide; magnesium sulfate	15–30 mL orally once or twice daily	3–12 hours	(Milk of magnesia; Epsom salts)
Lactulose or 70% sorbitol	15–60 mL orally once daily to three times daily	24–48 hours	Cramps, bloating, flatulence
Polyethylene glycol (PEG 3350)	17 g in 8 oz liquid once or twice daily	3–24 hours	(Miralax) Less bloating than lactulose, sorbitol
Stimulant laxatives			
Bisacodyl	5–15 mg orally as needed	6–8 hours	May cause cramps; avoid daily use if possible
Bisacodyl	10 mg per rectum as needed	1 hour	
Cascara	4–8 mL or 2 tablets as needed	8–12 hours	(Nature's Remedy) May cause cramps; avoid daily use if possible
Senna	8.6–17.2 mg orally one to three times daily	8–12 hours	(ExLax; Senekot) May cause cramps; avoid daily use if possible
Enemas			
Tap water	500 mL per rectum	5–15 minutes	
Phosphate enema	120 mL per rectum	5–15 minutes	Commonly used for acute constipation or to induce movement prior to medical procedures
Soapsuds enema	Up to 1500 mL per rectum	5–15 minutes	Impaction
Mineral oil enema	100–250 mL per rectum		To soften and lubricate fecal impaction
Agents used for acute purgative or to clean bowel prior to medical procedures			
Polyethylene glycol (PEG)	4 L orally administered over 2–4 hours	< 4 hours	(GoLYTELY; CoLYTE; NuLYTE) Used to cleanse bowel before colonoscopy
Sodium phosphate	45 mL in 12 oz water; may repeat in 10–12 hours	1–6 hours	Used before colonoscopy
Magnesium citrate	10 oz	3–6 hours	Lemon-flavored
Combination kits: sodium phosphate and bisacodyl			(Fleet) Commonly used prior to barium enema

Muller-Lissner SA et al: Myths and misconceptions about chronic constipation. Am J Gastroenterol 2005;100:232. [PMID: 15654804]

Rao SS et al: Clinical utility of diagnostic tests for constipation in adults: a systematic review. Am J Gastroenterol 2005;100: 1605. [PMID: 15984989]

Ramkumar D et al: Efficacy and safety of traditional medical therapies for chronic constipation: systematic review. Am J Gastroenterol 2005;100:936. [PMID: 15784043]

Wald A: Severe constipation. Clin Gastroenterol Hepatol 2005; 3:432. [PMID: 15880311]

GASTROINTESTINAL GAS

Belching

Belching (eructation) is the involuntary or voluntary release of gas from the stomach or esophagus. It occurs most frequently after meals, when gastric distention results in transient lower esophageal sphincter relaxation. Belching is a normal reflex and does not itself denote gastrointestinal dysfunction. Virtually all stomach gas comes from swallowed air. With each swallow, 2–5 mL of air is ingested, and excessive amounts may result in distention, flatulence, and abdominal pain. This may occur with rapid eating, gum chewing, smoking, and the ingestion of carbonated beverages. Chronic excessive belching is almost always caused by aerophagia, common in anxious individuals and institutionalized patients. Evaluation should be restricted to patients with other complaints such as dysphagia, heartburn, early satiety, or vomiting.

Once patients understand the relationship between aerophagia and belching, most can deal with the problem by behavioral modification. Physical defects that hamper normal swallowing (ill-fitting dentures, nasal obstruction) should be corrected. Antacids and simethicone are of no value.

Flatus

The rate and volume of expulsion of flatus is highly variable. Flatus is derived from two sources: swallowed air and bacterial fermentation of undigested carbohydrate. The majority of swallowed air not belched passes through the gut and leaves as flatus. Swallowed air may contribute up to 500 mL of flatus per day (primarily nitrogen). Bacterial fermentation of undigested carbohydrates leads to the additional production of gas, particularly H_2, CO_2, and methane. The majority of this fermentation takes place in the colon. Under normal circumstances, a small substrate of fermentable substances reaches the colon. These substances include fructose, lactose, sorbitol, trehalose (mushrooms), raffinose, and stachyose (legumes, cruciferous vegetables). Complex starches and fiber may also cause gas. Gas production may be increased with ingestion of these carbohydrates or with malabsorption.

Determining abnormal from normal amounts of flatus is difficult. An initial trial of a lactose-free diet is recommended. Common gas-producing foods should be reviewed and the patient given an elimination trial.

These include beans of all kinds, peas, lentils, brussels sprouts, cabbage, parsnips, leeks, onions, beer, and coffee. Fructose intolerance may be more common than previously appreciated. Fructose is present not only in many fruits but is also used commonly as a sweetener or as fructose corn syrup in candy, fruit juices, and soda. Foul odor may be caused by garlic, onion, eggplant, mushrooms, and certain herbs and spices. For patients with persistent complaints, complex starches, and fiber may be eliminated, but such restrictive diets are unacceptable to most patients. Of refined flours, only rice flour is gas-free.

The nonprescription agent Beano (α-d-galactosidase enzyme) reduces gas caused by foods containing raffinose and stachyose, ie, cruciferous vegetables, legumes, nuts, and some cereals. Activated charcoal may afford relief. Simethicone is of no proved benefit.

Complaints of chronic abdominal distention or bloating are common. Some of these patients may produce excess gas. However, many patients have impaired small bowel gas propulsion or enhance visceral sensitivity to gas distention. Many of these patients have an underlying functional gastrointestinal disorder such as irritable bowel syndrome or functional dyspepsia. Reduction of dietary fat, which delays intestinal gas clearance, may be helpful.

Azpiroz F et al: Abdominal bloating. Gastroenterology 2005; 129:1060. [PMID: 16143143]

Chitkara DK et al: Aerophagia in adults: a comparison with functional dyspepsia. Aliment Pharmacol Ther 2005;22:855. [PMID: 16225495]

DIARRHEA

Diarrhea can range in severity from an acute self-limited episode to a severe, life-threatening illness. To properly evaluate the complaint, the physician must determine the patient's normal bowel pattern and the nature of the current symptoms.

Approximately 10 L of fluid enter the duodenum daily, of which all but 1.5 L are absorbed by the small intestine. The colon absorbs most of the remaining fluid, with < 200 mL lost in the stool. Although diarrhea sometimes is defined as a stool weight of more than 200–300 g/24 h, quantification of stool weight is necessary only in some patients with chronic diarrhea. In most cases, the physician's working definition of diarrhea is increased stool frequency (more than three bowel movements per day) or liquidity of feces.

The causes of diarrhea are myriad. In clinical practice, it is helpful to distinguish acute from chronic diarrhea, as the evaluation and treatment are entirely different (Tables 14–5 and 14–7).

1. Acute Diarrhea

Etiology & Clinical Findings

Diarrhea acute in onset and persisting for less than 2 weeks is most commonly caused by infectious agents,

Table 14–5. Causes of acute infectious diarrhea.

Noninflammatory Diarrhea	Inflammatory Diarrhea
Viral Noroviruses Rotavirus	**Viral** Cytomegalovirus
Protozoal *Giardia lamblia* *Cryptosporidium* *Cyclospora*	**Protozoal** *Entamoeba histolytica*
Bacterial 1. Preformed enterotoxin production *Staphylococcus aureus* *Bacillus cereus* *Clostridium perfringens* 2. Enterotoxin production Enterotoxigenic *Escherichia coli* (ETEC) *Vibrio cholerae*	**Bacterial** 1. Cytotoxin production Enterohemorrhagic *E coli* O157:H5 (EHEC) *Vibrio parahaemolyticus* *Clostridium difficile* 2. Mucosal invasion *Shigella* *Campylobacter jejuni* *Salmonella* Enteroinvasive *E coli* (EIEC) *Aeromonas* *Plesiomonas* *Yersinia enterocolitica* *Chlamydia* *Neisseria gonorrhoeae* *Listeria monocytogenes*

bacterial toxins (either preformed or produced in the gut), or drugs. Community outbreaks (including nursing homes, schools, cruise ships) suggest a viral etiology or a common food source. Similar recent illnesses in family members suggest an infectious origin. Ingestion of improperly stored or prepared food implicates food poisoning. Day care attendance or exposure to unpurified water (camping, swimming) may result in infection with *Giardia* or *Cryptosporidium*. Large *Cyclospora* outbreaks have been traced to contaminated produce. Recent travel abroad suggests "traveler's diarrhea" (see Chapter 30). Antibiotic administration within the preceding several weeks increases the likelihood of *Clostridium difficile* colitis. Finally, risk factors for HIV infection or sexually transmitted diseases should be determined. (AIDS-associated diarrhea is discussed in Chapter 31; infectious proctitis is discussed in this chapter under Anorectal Disorders.) Persons engaging in anal intercourse or oral-anal sexual activities are at risk for a variety of infections that cause proctitis, including gonorrhea, syphilis, lymphogranuloma venereum, and herpes simplex.

The nature of the diarrhea helps distinguish among different infectious causes (Table 14–5).

A. NONINFLAMMATORY DIARRHEA

Watery, nonbloody diarrhea associated with periumbilical cramps, bloating, nausea, or vomiting suggests a small bowel source caused by either a toxin-producing bacterium (enterotoxigenic *Escherichia coli* [ETEC], *Staphylococcus aureus*, *Bacillus cereus*, *Clostridium perfringens*) or other agents (viruses, *Giardia*) that disrupt normal absorption and secretory process in the small intestine. Prominent vomiting suggests viral enteritis or *S aureus* food poisoning. Although typically mild, the diarrhea (which originates in the small intestine) can be voluminous and result in dehydration with hypokalemia and metabolic acidosis (eg, cholera). Because tissue invasion does not occur, fecal leukocytes are not present.

B. INFLAMMATORY DIARRHEA

The presence of fever and bloody diarrhea (dysentery) indicates colonic tissue damage caused by invasion (shigellosis, salmonellosis, *Campylobacter* or *Yersinia* infection, amebiasis) or a toxin (*C difficile*, *E coli* O157:H7). Because these organisms involve predominantly the colon, the diarrhea is small in volume (< 1 L/d) and associated with left lower quadrant cramps, urgency, and tenesmus. Fecal leukocytes or lactoferrin usually are present in infections with invasive organisms. *E coli* O157:H7 is a Shiga toxin-producing noninvasive organism most commonly acquired from contaminated meat that has resulted in several outbreaks of an acute, often severe hemorrhagic colitis. In immunocompromised and HIV-infected patients, cytomegalovirus (CMV) can cause intestinal ulceration with watery or bloody diarrhea.

Infectious dysentery must be distinguished from acute ulcerative colitis, which may also present acutely with fever, abdominal pain, and bloody diarrhea. Diarrhea that persists for more than 14 days is not attributable to bacterial pathogens (except for *C difficile*) and should be evaluated as chronic diarrhea.

Evaluation

In over 90% of patients with acute noninflammatory diarrhea, the illness is mild and self-limited, responding within 5 days to simple rehydration therapy or antidiarrheal agents; diagnostic investigation is unnecessary. The isolation rate of bacterial pathogens from stool cultures in patients with acute noninflammatory diarrhea is under 3%. Thus, the goal of initial evaluation is to distinguish patients with mild disease from those with more serious illness. If diarrhea worsens or persists for more than 7 days, stool should be sent for fecal leukocyte or lactoferrin determination, ovum and parasite evaluation, and bacterial culture.

Prompt medical evaluation is indicated in the following situations (Figure 14–1): (1) Signs of inflammatory diarrhea manifested by any of the following: fever (> 38.5 °C), bloody diarrhea, or abdominal pain. (2) The passage of six or more unformed stools in 24

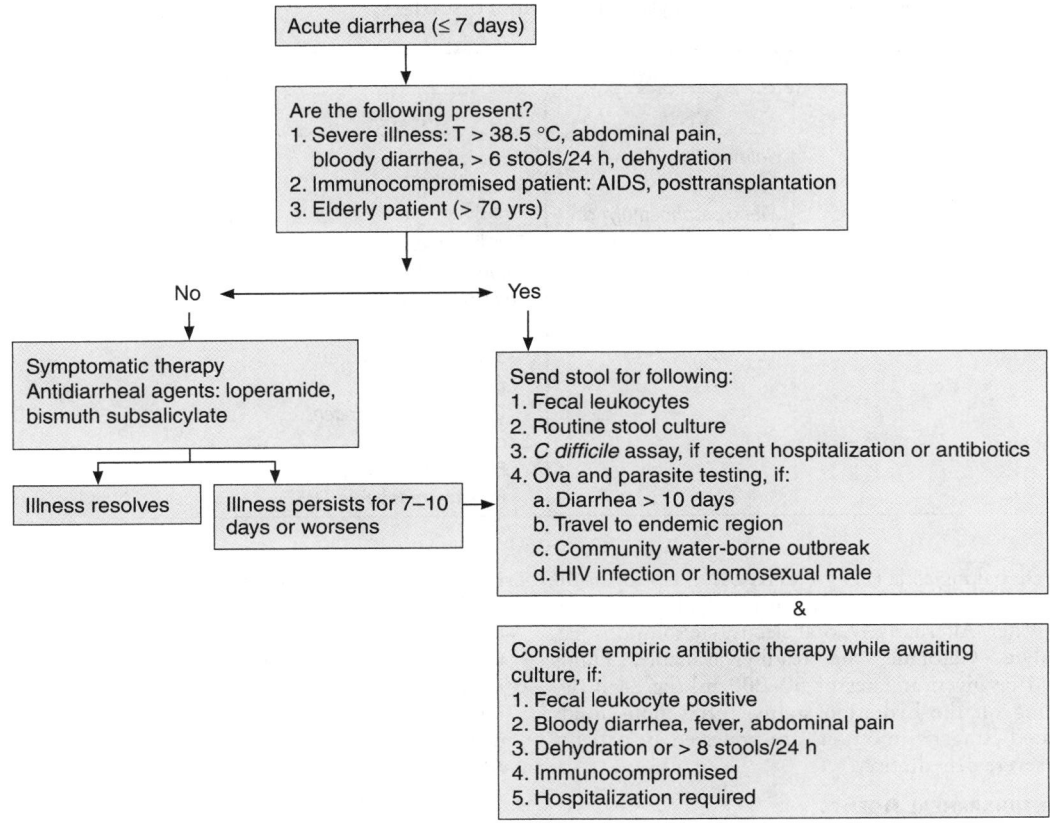

Figure 14–1. Evaluation of acute diarrhea.

hours. (3) Profuse watery diarrhea and dehydration. (4) Frail older patients. (5) Immunocompromised patients (AIDS, posttransplantation). (6) Nosocomial diarrhea (onset more than 3 days after hospitalization).

Physical examination pays note to the patient's level of hydration, mental status, and the presence of abdominal tenderness or peritonitis. Peritoneal findings may be present in infection with *C difficile* or enterohemorrhagic *E coli*. Hospitalization is required in patients with severe dehydration, toxicity, or marked abdominal pain. Stool specimens should be sent for examination for bacterial cultures (Table 14–6).

The rate of positive bacterial cultures in such patients is 60–75%. For bloody stools, the laboratory should be directed to perform serotyping for Shiga-producing *E coli* O157:H7. Special culture media are required for *Yersinia*, *Vibrio*, and *Aeromonas*. In patients who are hospitalized or who have a history of antibiotic exposure, a stool sample should be tested for *C difficile* toxin. In patients with diarrhea that persists for more than 10 days, who have a history of travel to areas where amebiasis is endemic, or who engage in oral-anal sexual practices, three stool examinations for ova and parasites should also be performed. The stool antigen detection tests for both *Giardia* and *Entam-*

oeba histolytica are more sensitive than stool microscopy for detection of these organisms. A serum antigen detection test for *E histolytica* is also available. *Cyclospora* and *Cryptosporidium* are detected by fecal acid-fast staining.

Treatment

A. DIET

Most mild diarrhea will not lead to dehydration provided the patient takes adequate oral fluids containing carbohydrates and electrolytes. Patients find it more comfortable to rest the bowel by avoiding high-fiber foods, fats, milk products, caffeine, and alcohol. Frequent feedings of tea, "flat" carbonated beverages, and soft, easily digested foods (eg, soups, crackers, bananas, applesauce, rice, toast) are encouraged.

B. REHYDRATION

In more severe diarrhea, dehydration can occur quickly, especially in children, the frail, and the elderly. Oral rehydration with fluids containing glucose, Na^+, K^+, Cl^-, and bicarbonate or citrate is preferred when feasible. A convenient mixture is $^1/_2$ tsp salt (3.5

Table 14–6. Fecal leukocytes in intestinal disorders.

Infectious			Noninfectious
Present	**Variable**	**Absent**	**Present**

Shigella
Campylobacter
Enteroinvasive
  Escherichia coli
  (EIEC)
	Salmonella
	Yersinia
	Vibrio parahaemolytica
	Clostridium difficile
	Aeromonas
		Noroviruses
		Rotavirus
		
		Giardia lamblia
		Entamoeba histolytica
		Cryptosporidium
		"Food poisoning"
		  Staphylococcus aureus
		  Bacillus cereus
		  Clostridium perfringens
		E coli
		  Enterotoxigenic (ETEC)
		  Enterohemorrhagic (EHEC)
			Ulcerative colitis
			Crohn's disease
			Radiation colitis
			Ischemic colitis

g), 1 tsp baking soda (2.5 g NaHCO$_3$), 8 tsp sugar (40 g), and 8 oz orange juice (1.5 g KCl), diluted to 1 L with water. Alternatively, oral electrolyte solutions (eg, Pedialyte, Gatorade) are readily available. Fluids should be given at rates of 50–200 mL/kg/24 h depending on the hydration status. Intravenous fluids (lactated Ringer's injection) are preferred in patients with severe dehydration.

C. Antidiarrheal Agents

Antidiarrheal agents may be used safely in patients with mild to moderate diarrheal illnesses to improve patient comfort. Opioid agents help decrease the stool number and liquidity and control fecal urgency. However, they should not be used in patients with bloody diarrhea, high fever, or systemic toxicity and should be discontinued in patients whose diarrhea is worsening despite therapy. With these provisos, such drugs provide excellent symptomatic relief. Loperamide is preferred, in a dosage of 4 mg initially, followed by 2 mg after each loose stool (maximum: 16 mg/24 h).

Bismuth subsalicylate (Pepto-Bismol), two tablets or 30 mL four times daily, reduces symptoms in patients with traveler's diarrhea by virtue of its antiinflammatory and antibacterial properties. It also reduces vomiting associated with viral enteritis. Anticholinergic agents (eg, diphenoxylate with atropine) are contraindicated in acute diarrhea because of the rare precipitation of toxic megacolon.

D. Antibiotic Therapy

1. Empiric treatment—Empiric antibiotic treatment of all patients with acute diarrhea is not indicated. Even patients with inflammatory diarrhea caused by invasive pathogens usually have symptoms that will resolve within several days without antimicrobials. Empiric treatment may be considered in patients with non-hospital-acquired diarrhea with moderate to severe fever, tenesmus, or bloody stools or the presence of fecal lactoferrin while the stool bacterial culture is incubating, provided that infection with *E coli* O157:H7 is not suspected. The drugs of choice for empiric treatment are the fluoroquinolones (eg, ciprofloxacin 500 mg, ofloxacin 400 mg, or norfloxacin 400 mg, twice daily, or levofloxacin 500 mg once daily) for 5–7 days. Alternatives include trimethoprim-sulfamethoxazole, 160/800 mg twice daily; or doxycycline, 100 mg twice daily. Macrolides and penicillins are no longer recommended because of widespread microbial resistance to these agents. Rifaximin, a nonabsorbed oral antibiotic, 200 mg three times daily for 3 days, is approved for empiric treatment of noninflammatory traveler's diarrhea (see Chapter 30).

2. Specific antimicrobial treatment—Antibiotics are not recommended in patients with nontyphoid *Salmonella*, *Campylobacter*, *E coli* O157:H7, *Aeromonas*, or *Yersinia*, except in severe disease, because they do not hasten recovery or reduce the period of fecal bacterial excretion. The infectious diarrheas for which treatment is recommended are shigellosis, cholera, extraintestinal salmonellosis, traveler's diarrhea, *C difficile* infection, giardiasis, and amebiasis. Therapy for traveler's diarrhea, infectious (sexually transmitted) proctitis, and AIDS-related diarrhea is presented in other chapters of this book.

Musher DM et al: Contagious acute gastrointestinal infections. N Engl J Med 2004;350:2417. [PMID: 15575058]

Thielman NM et al: Clinical practice. Acute infectious diarrhea. N Engl J Med 2004;350:38. [PMID: 14702426]

2. Chronic Diarrhea

Etiology

The causes of chronic diarrhea may be grouped into seven major pathophysiologic categories (Table 14–7).

Table 14–7. Causes of chronic diarrhea.

Osmotic diarrhea
CLUES: Stool volume decreases with fasting; increased stool osmotic gap
1. Medications: antacids, lactulose, sorbitol
2. Disaccharidase deficiency: lactose intolerance
3. Factitious diarrhea: magnesium (antacids, laxatives)

Secretory diarrhea
CLUES: Large volume (> 1 L/d); little change with fasting; normal stool osmotic gap
1. Hormonally mediated: VIPoma, carcinoid, medullary carcinoma of thyroid (calcitonin), Zollinger-Ellison syndrome (gastrin)
2. Factitious diarrhea (laxative abuse); phenolphthalein, cascara, senna
3. Villous adenoma
4. Bile salt malabsorption (ileal resection; Crohn's ileitis; postcholecystectomy)
5. Medications

Inflammatory conditions
CLUES: Fever, hematochezia, abdominal pain
1. Ulcerative colitis
2. Crohn's disease
3. Microscopic colitis
4. Malignancy: lymphoma, adenocarcinoma (with obstruction and pseudodiarrhea)
5. Radiation enteritis

Malabsorption syndromes
CLUES: Weight loss, abnormal laboratory values; fecal fat > 10 g/24h
1. Small bowel mucosal disorders: celiac sprue, tropical sprue, Whipple's disease, eosinophilic gastroenteritis, small bowel resection (short bowel syndrome), Crohn's disease
2. Lymphatic obstruction: lymphoma, carcinoid, infectious (tuberculosis, MAI), Kaposi's sarcoma, sarcoidosis, retroperitoneal fibrosis
3. Pancreatic disease: chronic pancreatitis, pancreatic carcinoma
4. Bacterial overgrowth: motility disorders (diabetes, vagotomy), scleroderma, fistulas, small intestinal diverticula

Motility disorders
CLUES: Systemic disease or prior abdominal surgery
1. Postsurgical: vagotomy, partial gastrectomy, blind loop with bacterial overgrowth
2. Systemic disorders: scleroderma, diabetes mellitus, hyperthyroidism
3. Irritable bowel syndrome

Chronic infections
1. Parasites: *Giardia lamblia, Entamoeba histolytica*
2. AIDS-related:
   Viral: Cytomegalovirus, HIV infection (?)
   Bacterial: *Clostridium difficile, Mycobacterium avium* complex
   Protozoal: Microsporida (*Enterocytozoon bieneusi*), *Cryptosporidium, Isospora belli*

Factitious
See Osmotic and Secretory diarrhea above.

MAI = *Mycobacterium avium-intracellulare.*

A. OSMOTIC DIARRHEAS

As stool leaves the colon, fecal osmolality is equal to the serum osmolality, ie, approximately 290 mosm/kg. Under normal circumstances, the major osmoles are Na^+, K^+, Cl^-, and HCO_3^-. The stool osmolality may be estimated by multiplying the stool ($Na^+ + K^+$) × 2. The **osmotic gap** is the difference between the *measured* osmolality of the stool (or serum) and the *estimated* stool osmolality and is normally less than 50 mosm/kg. An increased osmotic gap (> 125 mosm/kg) implies that the diarrhea is caused by ingestion or malabsorption of an osmotically active substance. The most common causes are disaccharidase deficiency (lactase deficiency), laxative abuse, and malabsorption syndromes (see below). Osmotic diarrheas resolve during fasting. Those caused by malabsorbed carbohydrates are characterized by abdominal distention, bloating, and flatulence due to increased colonic gas production.

Disaccharidase deficiencies are common and should be considered in all patients with chronic diarrhea. Lactase deficiency occurs in 75% of nonwhite adults and up to 25% of whites. It may also be acquired after an episode of viral gastroenteritis, medical illness, or gastrointestinal surgery. Sorbitol is commonly used as a sweetener in gums, candies, and some medications that may cause diarrhea in some patients. The diagnosis of sorbitol or lactose malabsorption may be established by an elimination trial for 2–3 weeks.

Ingestion of magnesium- or phosphate-containing compounds (laxatives, antacids) should be considered in enigmatic chronic diarrhea. Surreptitious use should be considered, especially in patients with a long history of undiagnosed medical ailments or employment in the medical field. The fat substitute olestra also causes diarrhea and cramps in occasional patients.

B. SECRETORY CONDITIONS

Increased intestinal secretion or decreased absorption results in a high-volume watery diarrhea with a normal osmotic gap. There is little change in stool output during the fasting state, and dehydration and electrolyte imbalance may develop. Causes include endocrine tumors (stimulating intestinal or pancreatic secretion), bile salt malabsorption (stimulating colonic secretion), and laxative abuse.

C. INFLAMMATORY CONDITIONS

Diarrhea is present in most patients with inflammatory bowel disease (ulcerative colitis, Crohn's disease, microscopic colitis). A variety of other symptoms may be present, including abdominal pain, fever, weight loss, and hematochezia. (See Inflammatory Bowel Disease, below.)

D. MALABSORPTIVE CONDITIONS

The major causes of malabsorption are small mucosal intestinal diseases, intestinal resections, lymphatic obstruction, small intestinal bacterial overgrowth, and pancreatic insufficiency. Its characteristics are weight loss, osmotic diarrhea, steatorrhea, and nutritional deficiencies. Significant diarrhea in the absence of weight loss is not likely to be due to malabsorption. The physical and laboratory abnormalities related to deficiencies of vitamins or minerals are discussed in Chapter 29.

E. MOTILITY DISORDERS

Abnormal intestinal motility secondary to systemic disorders or surgery may result in diarrhea due to rapid transit or to stasis of intestinal contents with bacterial overgrowth, resulting in malabsorption. Probably the most common cause of chronic diarrhea is irritable bowel syndrome (see Irritable Bowel Syndrome, below).

F. CHRONIC INFECTIONS

Chronic parasitic infections may cause diarrhea through a number of mechanisms. Pathogens most commonly associated with diarrhea include the protozoans *Giardia*, *E histolytica*, and *Cyclospora* as well as the intestinal nematodes. Bacterial infections with *Aeromonas* and *Plesiomonas* may uncommonly be a cause of chronic diarrhea.

Immunocompromised patients are susceptible to infectious organisms that can cause acute or chronic diarrhea (see Chapter 31), including Microsporida, *Cryptosporidium*, CMV, *Isospora belli*, *Cyclospora*, and *Mycobacterium avium* complex.

G. FACTITIOUS DIARRHEA

Fifteen percent of patients have factitious diarrhea caused by surreptitious laxative abuse or dilution of stool.

Evaluation

The history and physical examination commonly suggest the underlying pathophysiology that guides the subsequent diagnostic workup (Figure 14–2). Important tests are described here. AIDS-associated diarrhea is discussed in Chapter 31.

A. STOOL ANALYSIS

1. Twenty-four-hour stool collection for weight and quantitative fecal fat—A stool weight of more than 300 g/24 h confirms diarrhea. A weight > 500 g excludes irritable bowel syndrome, whereas a weight > 1000–1500 g suggests a secretory process. A fecal fat determination in excess of 10 g/24 h indicates a malabsorptive disorder. (See Celiac Sprue and specific tests for malabsorption, below.)

2. Stool osmolality—Stool osmolality less than serum osmolality implies that water or urine has been added to the specimen (factitious diarrhea). A stool pH < 5.6 is consistent with carbohydrate malabsorption.

3. Stool laxative screen—In cases of suspected laxative abuse, stool magnesium, phosphate, and sulfate levels may be measured. Phenolphthalein and bisacodyl can be analyzed in stool water, using chromatographic techniques. Anthraquinones and bisacodyl are sought for in the urine.

4. Fecal leukocytes—The presence of fecal leukocytes or lactoferrin implies inflammatory diarrhea.

5. Stool for ova and parasites—The presence of *Giardia* and *E histolytica* may be detected in wet mounts. However, fecal antigen detection tests for *Giardia* and *E histolytica* may be a more sensitive and specific method of detection. *Cryptosporidium* and *Cyclospora* are found with modified acid-fast staining.

B. BLOOD TESTS

1. Routine laboratory tests—Complete blood count, serum electrolytes, liver function tests, calcium, phosphorus, albumin, TSH, β-carotene, and prothrombin time may be of value. Anemia occurs in malabsorption syndromes (folate, iron deficiency [rare], or vitamin B_{12}) as well as inflammatory conditions. Hypoalbuminemia is present in malabsorption, protein-losing enteropathies, and inflammatory diseases. Hyponatremia and nonanion gap metabolic acidosis occur in secretory diarrheas.

2. Other laboratory tests—In patients with suspected malabsorption, serologic testing for celiac sprue includes IgG and IgA antigliadin or tissue transglutaminase antibodies. Secretory diarrheas due to neuroendocrine tumors are rare. When this is suspected, serum vasoactive intestinal peptide (VIP) (VIPoma), calcitonin (medullary thyroid carcinoma), gastrin (Zollinger-Ellison syndrome), and glucagon determinations may be diagnostic. Urine should be sent for 5-hydroxyindoleacetic acid (5-HIAA) (carcinoid), vanillylmandelic acid (VMA), metanephrine, and histamine determinations.

3. Endoscopic examination and mucosal biopsy—Either sigmoidoscopy or colonoscopy with mucosal biopsy is helpful in the detection of inflammatory bowel disease (including microscopic colitis) and melanosis coli (indicative of chronic anthraquinone laxative use). Upper endoscopy with small bowel biopsy is performed when a small intestinal malabsorptive disorder is suspected (celiac sprue, Whipple's disease) and in patients with AIDS to document *Cryptosporidium*, Microsporida, and *M avium-intracellulare* infection. If bacterial overgrowth is suspected, the diagnosis is confirmed with noninvasive breath tests (D-[^{14}C]xylose, glucose, or lactulose) or by obtaining an aspirate of small intestinal contents for quantitative aerobic and anaerobic bacterial culture.

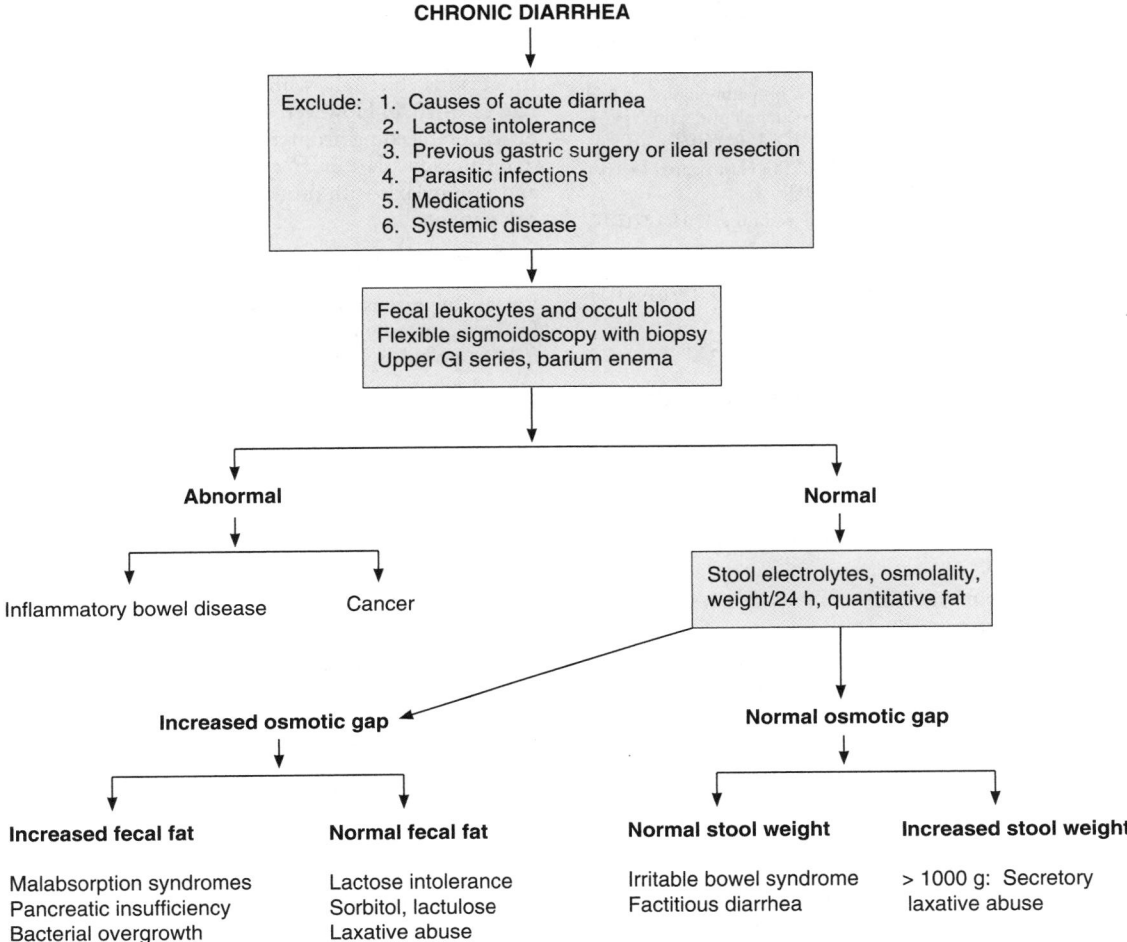

Figure 14–2. Decision diagram for diagnosis of causes of chronic diarrhea.

4. Other imaging studies—Calcification on a plain abdominal radiograph confirms a diagnosis of chronic pancreatitis, although abdominal CT and endoscopic ultrasonography are more sensitive for the diagnosis of chronic pancreatitis as well as pancreatic cancer. Small intestinal barium radiography is helpful in the diagnosis of Crohn's disease, small bowel lymphoma, carcinoid, and jejunal diverticula. Neuroendocrine tumors may be localized using somatostatin receptor scintigraphy.

Treatment

A number of antidiarrheal agents may be used in certain patients with chronic diarrheal conditions and are listed below. Opioids are safe in most patients with chronic, stable symptoms.

Loperamide: 4 mg initially, then 2 mg after each loose stool (maximum: 16 mg/d).

Diphenoxylate with atropine: One tablet three or four times daily as needed.

Codeine and deodorized tincture of opium: Because of potential habituation, these drugs are avoided except in cases of chronic, intractable diarrhea. Codeine may be given in a dosage of 15–60 mg every 4 hours; tincture of opium, 10–25 drops every 6 hours as needed.

Clonidine: α_2-Adrenergic agonists inhibit intestinal electrolyte secretion. Clonidine, 0.1–0.6 mg twice daily, or a clonidine patch, 0.1–0.2 mg/d, may help in some patients with secretory diarrheas, diabetic diarrhea, or cryptosporidiosis.

Octreotide: This somatostatin analog stimulates intestinal fluid and electrolyte absorption and inhibits intestinal fluid secretion and the release of gastrointestinal peptides. It is given for secretory diarrheas due to neuroendocrine tumors (VIPomas, carcinoid) and in some cases of AIDS-related diarrhea. Effective doses range from 50 to 250 mcg subcutaneously three times daily.

Cholestyramine: This bile salt-binding resin may be useful in patients with bile salt-induced diarrhea secondary to intestinal resection or ileal disease. A dosage of 4 g once to three times daily is recommended.

Camilleri M: Chronic diarrhea: a review on pathophysiology and management for the clinical gastroenterologist. Clin Gastroenterol Hepatol 2004;2:198. [PMID: 15017602]

Headstrom PD et al: Chronic diarrhea. Clin Gastroenterol Hepatol 2005;3:734. [PMID: 16234000]

Schiller L: Chronic diarrhea. Gastroenterology 2004;127:287. [PMID: 15236193]

Thomas PD et al: Guidelines for the investigation of chronic diarrhea, 2nd edition. Gut 2003;52(Suppl 5):v1. [PMID: 12801941]

GASTROINTESTINAL BLEEDING

1. Acute Upper Gastrointestinal Bleeding

 ESSENTIALS OF DIAGNOSIS

- *Hematemesis (bright red blood or "coffee grounds").*
- *Melena in most cases; hematochezia in massive upper gastrointestinal bleeds.*
- *Volume status to determine severity of blood loss; hematocrit is a poor early indicator of blood loss.*
- *Endoscopy diagnostic and may be therapeutic.*

General Considerations

There are over 250,000 hospitalizations a year in the United States for acute upper gastrointestinal bleeding, with a mortality rate of 7–10%. Approximately half of patients are over 60 years of age, and in this age group the mortality rate is even higher. Patients seldom die of exsanguination but rather from complications of an underlying disease.

The most common presentation of upper gastrointestinal bleeding is hematemesis or melena. Hematemesis may be either bright red blood or brown "coffee grounds" material. Melena develops after as little as 50–100 mL of blood loss in the upper gastrointestinal tract, whereas hematochezia requires a loss of more than 1000 mL. Although hematochezia generally suggests a lower bleeding source (eg, colonic), upper gastrointestinal bleeding may present with hematochezia in 10% of cases.

Upper gastrointestinal bleeding is self-limited in 80% of patients; urgent medical therapy and endoscopic evaluation are obligatory in the rest. Patients with bleeding more than 48 hours prior to presentation have a low risk of recurrent bleeding.

Etiology

Acute upper gastrointestinal bleeding may originate from a number of sources. These are listed in order of the frequency and discussed in detail below.

A. PEPTIC ULCER DISEASE

Peptic ulcers account for half of major upper gastrointestinal bleeding with an overall acute mortality rate of 6–10%. However, in North America the incidence of bleeding from ulcers is declining, perhaps due to eradication of *H pylori*, use of safer NSAIDs, and prophylaxis with proton pump inhibitors in high-risk patients.

B. PORTAL HYPERTENSION

Portal hypertension causes bleeding from varices (most commonly esophageal; rarely, gastric or duodenal) or portal hypertensive gastropathy. Acute bleeding develops in less than one-third of patients with portal hypertension and varices; however, these lesions account for 10–20% of significant gastrointestinal hemorrhages. If untreated, 50% of varices will rebleed during hospitalization. Due to improved care, the hospital mortality rate of has declined over the past 20 years from 40% to 15%. Nevertheless, a mortality rate of 60–80% is expected at 1–4 years due to recurrent bleeding or other complications of chronic liver disease.

C. MALLORY-WEISS TEARS

Lacerations of the gastroesophageal junction cause 5–10% of cases of upper gastrointestinal bleeding. Many patients report a history of heavy alcohol use or retching. Less than 10% have continued or recurrent bleeding.

D. VASCULAR ANOMALIES

Vascular anomalies are found throughout the gastrointestinal tract and may be the source of chronic or acute gastrointestinal bleeding. They account for 7% of cases of acute upper tract bleeding. **Vascular ectasias** (angiodysplasias) have a bright red stellate appearance. They may be part of systemic conditions (hereditary hemorrhagic telangiectasia, CREST syndrome) or may occur sporadically. There is an increased incidence in patients with chronic renal failure. Dieulafoy's lesion is an aberrant, large-caliber submucosal artery, most commonly in the proximal stomach that causes recurrent, intermittent bleeding.

E. GASTRIC NEOPLASMS

Gastric neoplasms result in 1% of upper gastrointestinal hemorrhages.

F. EROSIVE GASTRITIS

Because this process is superficial, it is a relatively unusual cause of severe gastrointestinal bleeding (< 5% of cases) and more commonly results in chronic blood loss. Gastric mucosal erosions are due to NSAIDs, alcohol, or severe medical or surgical illness (stress gastritis).

G. EROSIVE ESOPHAGITIS

Severe erosive esophagitis due to chronic gastroesophageal reflux may rarely cause significant upper gastrointestinal bleeding, especially in patients who are bed bound long-term.

H. OTHERS

An aortoenteric fistula complicates 2% of abdominal aortic grafts or can occur as the initial presentation of a previously untreated aneurysm. Usually located between the graft or aneurysm and the third portion of the duodenum, these fistulas characteristically present with a herald nonexsanguinating initial hemorrhage, with melena and hematemesis, or with chronic intermittent bleeding. The diagnosis may be suspected by upper endoscopy or abdominal CT. Surgery is mandatory to prevent exsanguinating hemorrhage. Unusual causes of upper gastrointestinal bleeding include hemobilia (from hepatic tumor, angioma, penetrating trauma), pancreatic malignancy, and pseudoaneurysm (hemosuccus pancreaticus).

Initial Evaluation & Management

A. STABILIZATION

The initial step is assessment of the hemodynamic status. A systolic blood pressure less than 100 mm Hg identifies a high-risk patient with severe acute bleeding. A heart rate over 100 beats/min with a systolic blood pressure over 100 mm Hg signifies moderate acute blood loss. A normal systolic blood pressure and heart rate suggest relatively minor hemorrhage. Postural hypotension and tachycardia are useful when present but may be due to causes other than blood loss. Because the hematocrit may take 24–72 hours to equilibrate with the extravascular fluid, it is not a reliable indicator of the severity of acute bleeding.

In patients with significant bleeding, two 18-gauge or larger intravenous lines should be started prior to further diagnostic tests. Blood is sent for complete blood count, prothrombin time with international normalized ratio (INR), serum creatinine, liver enzymes, and cross-matching for 2–4 units or more of packed red blood cells. In patients without hemodynamic compromise or overt active bleeding, aggressive fluid repletion can be delayed until the extent of the bleeding is further clarified. Patients with evidence of hemodynamic compromise are given 0.9% saline or lactated Ringer's injection and cross-matched blood. It is rarely necessary to administer type-specific or O-negative blood. Central venous pressure monitoring is desirable in some cases, but line placement should not interfere with rapid volume resuscitation.

A nasogastric tube should be placed in all patients with suspected active upper tract bleeding. The aspiration of red blood or "coffee grounds" confirms an upper gastrointestinal source of bleeding, though 10% of patients with confirmed upper tract sources of bleeding have nonbloody aspirates—especially when bleeding originates in the duodenum. An aspirate of bright red blood indicates active bleeding and is associated with the highest risk of further bleeding,

and complications, while a clear aspirate identifies patients at lower initial risk. Efforts to stop or slow bleeding by gastric lavage with large volumes of fluid are of no benefit and expose the patient to an increased risk of aspiration. Periodic reaspiration of the nasogastric tube serves as an indicator of ongoing bleeding or rebleeding.

B. BLOOD REPLACEMENT

The amount of fluid and blood products required is based on assessment of vital signs, evidence of active bleeding from nasogastric aspirate, and laboratory tests. Sufficient packed red blood cells should be given to maintain a hematocrit of 25–30%. In the absence of continued bleeding, the hematocrit should rise 4% for each unit of transfused packed red cells. Transfusion of blood should not be withheld from patients with brisk active bleeding regardless of the hematocrit. It is desirable to transfuse blood in anticipation of the nadir hematocrit. In actively bleeding patients, platelets are transfused if the platelet count is under 50,000/mcL and considered if there is impaired platelet function due to aspirin use (regardless of the platelet count). Uremic patients (who also have dysfunctional platelets) with active bleeding are given three doses of desmopressin (DDAVP), 0.3 mcg/kg intravenously, at 12-hour intervals. Fresh frozen plasma is administered for actively bleeding patients with a coagulopathy and an INR > 1.5. In the face of massive bleeding, 1 unit of fresh frozen plasma should be given for each 5 units of packed red blood cells transfused.

C. INITIAL TRIAGE

A preliminary assessment of risk based on several clinical factors aids in the resuscitation as well as the rational triage of the patient. Clinical predictors of increased risk of rebleeding and death include age over 65 years, comorbid illnesses, shock, and bright red blood in the nasogastric aspirate or on rectal examination.

1. Very low risk—Reliable patients without serious comorbid medical illnesses or advanced liver disease who have normal hemodynamics, no evidence of overt bleeding (hematemesis or melena) within 48 hours, a negative nasogastric lavage, and normal laboratory tests do not require hospital admission and can undergo further evaluation as outpatients as indicated.

2. High risk—Patients with active bleeding manifested by hematemesis or bright red blood on nasogastric aspirate, shock, persistent hemodynamic derangement despite fluid resuscitation, serious comorbid medical illness, or evidence of advanced liver disease require admission to an intensive care unit (ICU). Emergent endoscopy should be performed after adequate resuscitation, usually within 12 hours.

3. Low to moderate risk—All other patients are admitted to a step-down unit or medical ward after appropriate stabilization for further evaluation and treatment. Patients without evidence of active bleeding undergo nonemergent endoscopy usually within 12–24 hours. In some centers, these patients undergo urgent upper endoscopy to help decide appropriate triage. Based on the findings at endoscopy, patients deemed to be at low risk of rebleeding may be discharged and monitored as outpatients.

Subsequent Evaluation & Treatment

Specific treatment of the various causes of upper gastrointestinal bleeding is discussed elsewhere in this chapter. The following general comments apply to most patients with bleeding.

A. History and Physical Examination

The physician's impression of the bleeding source is correct in only 40% of cases. Signs of chronic liver disease implicate bleeding due to portal hypertension, but a different lesion is identified in 25% of patients with cirrhosis. A history of dyspepsia, NSAID use, or peptic ulcer disease suggests peptic ulcer. Acute bleeding preceded by heavy alcohol ingestion or retching suggests a Mallory-Weiss tear, though most of these patients have neither.

B. Upper Endoscopy

Virtually all patients with upper tract bleeding should undergo upper endoscopy. The benefits of endoscopy in this setting are threefold.

1. To identify the source of bleeding—The appropriate acute and long-term medical therapy is determined by the cause of bleeding. Patients with portal hypertension will be treated differently from those with ulcer disease. If surgery is required for uncontrolled bleeding, the source of bleeding as determined at endoscopy will determine the approach.

2. To determine the risk of rebleeding—Patients with a nonbleeding Mallory-Weiss tear, esophagitis, gastritis, and ulcers that have a clean, white base have a very low risk of rebleeding. It may be safe and cost-effective to discharge such patients from the emergency department or from the medical ward with subsequent outpatient follow-up. Patients with ulcers that are actively bleeding or have a visible vessel or who have variceal bleeding require closer observation in an ICU or step down unit.

3. To render endoscopic therapy—Hemostasis can be achieved in actively bleeding lesions with endoscopic modalities such as cautery, injection, or endoclips. About 90% of bleeding or nonbleeding varices can be effectively treated immediately with injection of a sclerosant or application of rubber bands to the varices. Similarly, 90% of bleeding ulcers, angiomas, or Mallory-Weiss tears can be controlled with either injection of epinephrine, direct cauterization of the vessel by a heater probe or multipolar electrocautery probe, or application of an endoclip. Certain nonbleeding lesions such ulcers with visible blood vessels, and angiomas are also treated with these therapies. Specific endoscopic

therapy of varices, peptic ulcers, and Mallory-Weiss tears is dealt with elsewhere in this chapter.

C. Acute Pharmacologic Therapies

1. Acid inhibitory therapy—H_2-receptor antagonists do not stop acute bleeding or reduce the incidence of rebleeding. Intravenous proton pump inhibitors (omeprazole, lansoprazole, or pantoprazole, 80 mg bolus, followed by 8 mg/h continuous infusion for 72 hours) reduce the risk of rebleeding in patients with peptic ulcers with high-risk features (active bleeding, visible vessel, or adherent clot) after endoscopic treatment. High doses of oral proton pump inhibitors (omeprazole 40 mg or lansoprazole 60 mg, twice daily for 5 days) may also be effective. Pending the results of endoscopic examination, it may be reasonable to initiate therapy with a high-dose proton pump inhibitor (intravenously or orally) in patients with suspected peptic ulcer bleeding.

2. Octreotide—Continuous intravenous infusion of octreotide (100 mcg bolus, followed by 50–100 mcg/h) reduces splanchnic blood flow and portal blood pressures and is effective in the initial control of bleeding related to portal hypertension. It is administered promptly to all patients with active upper gastrointestinal bleeding and evidence of liver disease or portal hypertension until the source of bleeding can be determined by endoscopy.

3. Vasoactive agents—Intravenous vasopressin is no longer used in the treatment of upper gastrointestinal bleeding. In countries where it is available, terlipressin may be preferred to octreotide for the treatment of bleeding related to portal hypertension because of its sustained reduction of portal and variceal pressures and its proven reduction in mortality.

D. Other Treatment

1. Intra-arterial embolization or vasopressin—Angiographic treatment is used rarely in patients with persistent bleeding from ulcers, angiomas, or Mallory-Weiss tears who have failed endoscopic therapy and are poor operative risks.

2. Transvenous intrahepatic portosystemic shunts (TIPS)—Placement of a wire stent from the hepatic vein through the liver to the portal vein provides effective decompression of the portal venous system and control of acute variceal bleeding. It is indicated in patients in whom endoscopic modalities have failed to control acute variceal bleeding.

Adler DG: ASGE Guideline: the role of endoscopy in acute nonvariceal upper-GI hemorrhage. Gastrointest Endosc 2004; 60;497. [PMID: 15472669]

Bardou M et al: Meta-analysis: proton-pump inhibition in high-risk patients with acute peptic ulcer bleeding. Aliment Pharmacol Ther 2005;21:677. [PMID: 15771753]

Barkun A et al: Consensus recommendations for managing patients with nonvariceal upper gastrointestinal bleeding. Ann Intern Med 2003;139:843. [PMID: 14623622]

Das A et al: Prediction of outcome of acute GI hemorrhage: a review of risk scores and predictive models. Gastrointest Endosc 2004;60:85. [PMID: 15229431]

Pavey DA: Endoscopic therapy for upper-GI vascular ectasias. Gastrointest Endosc 2004;59:233. [PMID: 14745397]

2. Acute Lower Gastrointestinal Bleeding

ESSENTIALS OF DIAGNOSIS

- *Hematochezia usually present.*
- *Ten percent of cases of hematochezia due to upper gastrointestinal source.*
- *Evaluation with colonoscopy in stable patients.*
- *Massive active bleeding calls for evaluation with sigmoidoscopy, upper endoscopy, angiography, or nuclear bleeding scan.*

General Considerations

Lower gastrointestinal bleeding is defined as that arising below the ligament of Treitz, ie, the small intestine or colon; however, over 95% of cases arise from the colon. The severity of lower gastrointestinal bleeding ranges from mild anorectal bleeding to massive, large-volume hematochezia. Bright red blood that drips into the bowl after a bowel movement or is mixed with solid brown stool signifies mild bleeding, usually from an anorectosigmoid source, and can be evaluated in the outpatient setting. Serious lower gastrointestinal bleeding is more common in older men. In patients hospitalized with gastrointestinal bleeding, lower tract bleeding is one-fourth as common as upper gastrointestinal hemorrhage and tends to have a more benign course. Patients hospitalized with lower gastrointestinal tract bleeding are less likely to present with shock or orthostasis (< 20%) or to require transfusions (< 40%). Spontaneous cessation of bleeding occurs in over 85% of cases, and hospital mortality is less than 3%.

Etiology

The cause of these lesions depends on both the age of the patient and the severity of the bleeding. In patients under 50 years of age, the most common causes are infectious colitis, anorectal disease, and inflammatory bowel disease. In older patients, significant hematochezia is most often seen with diverticulosis, vascular ectasias, malignancy, or ischemia. In 20% of acute bleeding episodes, no source of bleeding can be identified.

A. DIVERTICULOSIS

Hemorrhage occurs in 3–5% of all patients with diverticulosis and is the most common cause of major lower tract bleeding, accounting for 50% of cases. A significant percentage of cases are associated with the use of nonsteroidal anti-inflammatory agents. Although diverticula are more prevalent on the left side of the colon, bleeding more commonly originates on the right side. Diverticular bleeding usually presents as acute, painless, large-volume maroon or bright red hematochezia in patients over age 50 years. More than 95% of cases require less than 4 units of blood transfusion. Bleeding subsides spontaneously in 80% but may recur in up to 25% of patients.

B. VASCULAR ECTASIAS

Vascular ectasias (or angiodysplasias) occur throughout the upper and lower intestinal tracts and cause painless bleeding ranging from melena or hematochezia to occult blood loss. They are responsible for 5–10% of cases of lower gastrointestinal bleeding, where they are most often seen in the cecum and ascending colon. They are flat, red lesions (2–10 mm) with ectatic peripheral vessels radiating from a central vessel, and are most common in patients over 70 years and in those with chronic renal failure. Bleeding in younger patients more commonly arises from the small intestine.

Most colonic ectasias are degenerative lesions that are felt to arise from chronic colonic mucosal contraction obstructing venous mucosal drainage. Over time, the mucosal capillaries dilate and become incompetent. The cause of gastric and small intestinal ectasias is unknown. Some are congenital, part of an inherited syndrome such as hereditary hemorrhagic telangiectasia, or related to autoimmune disorders, typically scleroderma. Ectasias can be identified in up to 6% of subjects over age 60 years, so their mere presence does not prove that the lesion is the source of bleeding, as active bleeding is seldom seen.

C. NEOPLASMS

Benign polyps and carcinoma are associated with chronic occult blood loss or intermittent anorectal hematochezia. However, colonic neoplasms may cause up to 10% of acute lower gastrointestinal hemorrhage. After endoscopic removal of colonic polyps, important bleeding may occur up to 2 weeks later in 0.3% of patients. Although many patients can be treated conservatively (ie, without colonoscopy), prompt colonoscopy generally is recommended to treat postpolypectomy hemorrhage and minimize the need for transfusions.

D. INFLAMMATORY BOWEL DISEASE

Patients with inflammatory bowel disease (especially ulcerative colitis) often have diarrhea with variable amounts of hematochezia. Bleeding varies from occult blood loss to recurrent hematochezia usually mixed with stool. Symptoms of abdominal pain, tenesmus, and urgency are often present.

E. ANORECTAL DISEASE

Anorectal disease commonly results in small amounts of bright red blood noted on the toilet paper, streaking of the stool, or dripping into the toilet bowl. The bleeding is slight and seldom results in significant blood loss. Painless bleeding is commonly caused by internal hemorrhoids. Bleeding associated with pain during bowel movements suggests an anal fissure.

F. ISCHEMIC COLITIS

This condition is seen commonly in older patients, most of whom have atherosclerotic disease. Most cases occur spontaneously due to transient episodes of non-occlusive ischemia. Ischemic colitis may also occur in 5% of patients after surgery for ileoaortic or abdominal aortic aneurysm. In young patients, colonic ischemia may develop due to vasculitis, coagulation disorders, estrogen therapy, and long distance running. Ischemic colitis results in hematochezia or bloody diarrhea associated with mild cramps. In most patients, the bleeding is mild and self-limited.

G. OTHERS

Radiation-induced proctitis causes anorectal bleeding that may develop months to years after pelvic radiation. Endoscopy reveals multiple rectal telangiectasias. Acute infectious colitis (see Acute Diarrhea, above) commonly causes bloody diarrhea. Rare causes of lower tract bleeding include vasculitic ischemia, solitary rectal ulcer, NSAID-induced ulcers in the small bowel or right colon, small bowel diverticula, and colonic varices.

Evaluation & Management

The color of the stool helps distinguish upper from lower gastrointestinal bleeding, especially when observed by the physician. Brown stools mixed or streaked with blood predict a source in the rectosigmoid or anus. Large volumes of bright red blood suggest a colonic source; maroon stools imply a lesion in the right colon or small intestine; and black stools (melena) predict a source proximal to the ligament of Treitz. Although 10% of patients admitted with self-reported hematochezia have an upper gastrointestinal source of bleeding (eg, peptic ulcer), this almost always occurs in the setting of massive hemorrhage with hemodynamic instability. Painless large-volume bleeding usually suggests diverticular bleeding or vascular ectasias. Bloody diarrhea associated with cramping abdominal pain, urgency, or tenesmus is characteristic of inflammatory bowel disease, infectious colitis, or ischemic colitis.

Important considerations in management include exclusion of an upper tract source, anoscopy and sigmoidoscopy, colonoscopy, nuclear bleeding scans and angiography, and small intestine push enteroscopy or capsule imaging.

A. EXCLUSION OF AN UPPER TRACT SOURCE

A nasogastric tube with aspiration should be considered, especially in patients with hemodynamic compro-

mise. Aspiration of red blood or dark brown ("coffee grounds") guaiac-positive material strongly implicates an upper gastrointestinal source of bleeding. If blood is not seen and bile is aspirated, an upper source is found in only 1% of patients.

B. ANOSCOPY AND SIGMOIDOSCOPY

In otherwise healthy patients without anemia under age 45 years with small-volume bleeding, anoscopy and sigmoidoscopy are performed to look for evidence of anorectal disease, inflammatory bowel disease, or infectious colitis. If a lesion is found, no further evaluation is needed immediately unless the bleeding persists or is recurrent. In patients over age 45 years with small-volume hematochezia, the entire colon must be evaluated with colonoscopy to exclude tumor.

C. COLONOSCOPY

In those patients with stable vital signs whose lower gastrointestinal bleeding appears to have stopped (ie, no rectal bleeding within 4 hours of evaluation), elective colonoscopy should be performed to determine the probable site of bleeding within 24 hours of admission after adequate resuscitation and routine colonic lavage. For patients with signs of severe or active lower gastrointestinal bleeding (defined as pulse 100 beats/min or higher, systolic blood pressure < 100 mm Hg), urgent colonoscopy is performed within 6–12 hours of admission after administration of a rapid, high-volume colonic lavage solution, given until the effluent is clear of blood and clots (GoLYTELY, Co-LYTE, NuLYTE, 4–8 L given orally or by nasogastric tube over 3–5 hours). At urgent colonoscopy, the probable site of bleeding can be identified in 70–85% of patients, and a high-risk lesion can be identified and treated in up to 20%. Alternatively, many physicians choose first to obtain a nuclear bleeding scan to determine whether there is active bleeding. If no bleeding is detected on the scan, a colonoscopy should be done. If bleeding is detected, angiography should be performed.

D. NUCLEAR BLEEDING SCANS AND ANGIOGRAPHY

Significant continued bleeding occurs in only 15% of patients but may limit the diagnostic effectiveness of colonoscopy. In such patients, either angiographic embolization or surgery may become necessary to control the bleeding. Technetium-labeled red blood cell scanning can detect significant active bleeding and localize it to the small intestine, right colon, or left colon. Because bleeding may be slow or intermittent, less than half of studies are diagnostic, and the accuracy of a positive study is only 78%. Nuclear bleeding studies are more apt to be positive in patients who are passing bright red or maroon stools at the time of the scan. Selective mesenteric angiography requires more brisk bleeding (0.5–1 mL/min) for a positive result than technetium scans and leads to major complications in up to 3% of patients. Accordingly, angiograms are performed only in patients with positive technetium scans or with hemodynamically significant, ongoing bleeding. Localization of an actively bleeding vessel is possible in up to 80%.

E. SMALL INTESTINE PUSH ENTEROSCOPY OR CAPSULE IMAGING

Less than 5% of acute episodes of lower gastrointestinal bleeding arise from the small intestine, eluding diagnostic evaluation with upper endoscopy and colonoscopy. Because of the difficulty of examining the small intestine and its relative rarity as a source of acute bleeding, evaluation of the small bowel is not usually pursued in patients during the initial episode of acute lower gastrointestinal bleeding. However, the small intestine is investigated in patients with unexplained recurrent hemorrhage of obscure origin. (See Occult & Obscure Gastrointestinal Bleeding below.)

Treatment

A. DISCONTINUE ASPIRIN AND NSAIDS

Up to 80% of patients with lower gastrointestinal tract bleeding have recently ingested aspirin or NSAIDs, which may potentiate bleeding through inhibition of platelet function. These agents should be discontinued. Platelet transfusion (3–6 units) should be administered for persistent bleeding.

B. THERAPEUTIC COLONOSCOPY

Until recently, colonoscopy served a largely diagnostic role in the patient with lower gastrointestinal bleeding. High-risk lesions (eg, diverticulum with active bleeding or a visible vessel, or a vascular ectasia) may now be treated endoscopically with epinephrine injection, cautery (bipolar or heater probe), or application of metallic endoclips. In severe diverticular hemorrhage with high-risk lesions identified at colonoscopy, rebleeding occurs in half of untreated patients compared with virtually no rebleeding in patients treated endoscopically. Radiation proctitis is effectively treated with applications of cautery therapy to the rectal telangiectasias, preferably with an argon plasma coagulator.

C. INTRA-ARTERIAL VASOPRESSIN OR EMBOLIZATION

Selective mesenteric arterial infusion of vasoconstrictors (eg, vasopressin) may arrest bleeding in up to 80% of patients with active bleeding from a diverticulum or vascular ectasia, but bleeding recurs in up to 50%. Selective arterial embolization with microcoils is now preferred by most angiographers because it provides definitive control of bleeding in up to 90% with reduced risk of bowel ischemia (< 10%) compared with other embolic agents. Embolization may be preferred to surgery in patients with continued bleeding who are poor surgical candidates.

D. SURGICAL TREATMENT

Surgery is indicated in patients with ongoing bleeding that requires more than 4–6 units of blood within 24 hours or more than 10 total units. Most such hemorrhages are caused by a bleeding diverticulum or vascular ectasia. With increasing experience with urgent colonoscopy and angiographic embolization, the need for surgical treatment appears to be decreasing. Preoperative localization of the bleeding site by nuclear scan or angiography allows limited resection of the bleeding segment of small intestine or colon. When accurate localization is not possible or when emergency surgery is required for massive hemorrhage, total abdominal colectomy with ileorectal anastomosis is required—with significantly higher morbidity and mortality than limited resections.

Surgery may also be indicated in patients with two or more hospitalizations for diverticular hemorrhage depending on the severity of bleeding and the patient's other comorbid conditions.

Davila RE et al; Standards of Practice Committee: ASGE Guideline: the role of endoscopy in the patient with lower-GI bleeding. Gastrointest Endosc 2005;62:656. [PMID: 16246674]

Elta GH: Urgent colonoscopy for acute lower-GI bleeding. Gastrointest Endosc 2004;59:402. [PMID: 14997144]

Jensen D: Management of patients with severe hematochezia—with all current evidence available. Am J Gastroenterol 2005;100:2403. [PMID: 16279892]

Khanna A et al: Embolization as first-line therapy for diverticulosis-related massive lower gastrointestinal bleeding: evidence from a meta-analysis. J Gastrointest Surg 2005;9:343. [PMID: 15749594]

Simpson PW et al: Use of endoclips in the treatment of massive colonic diverticular bleeding. Gastrointest Endosc 2004;59: 433. [PMID: 14997150]

Strate LL et al: Validation of a clinical prediction rule for severe acute lower intestinal bleeding. Am J Gastroenterol 2005; 100:1821. [PMID: 16086720]

Villavicencio R et al: Efficacy and complications of argon plasma coagulation for hematochezia related to radiation therapy. Gastrointest Endosc 2002;55:70. [PMID: 11756918]

3. Occult & Obscure Gastrointestinal Bleeding

Occult gastrointestinal bleeding refers to bleeding that is not apparent to the patient. Chronic gastrointestinal blood loss of less than 100 mL/d may cause no appreciable change in stool appearance. Thus, occult bleeding in an adult is identified by a positive FOBT or iron deficiency anemia in the absence of visible blood loss. FOBT may be performed in patients with gastrointestinal symptoms or as a screening test for colorectal neoplasia (see Colorectal Cancer Screening, below). From 1% to 2.5% of patients in screening programs have a positive FOBT.

In the United States, 2% of men and 5% of women have iron deficiency anemia (serum ferritin < 30–45 mcg/L). In premenopausal women, iron deficiency anemia is most commonly attributable to menstrual and pregnancy-associated iron loss; however, a gastrointestinal source of chronic blood loss is present in 10%. Among men and postmenopausal women, a potential gastrointestinal cause of blood loss can be identified in the colon in 15–30% and in the upper gastrointestinal tract in 35–55%; a malignancy is present in 10%. Iron deficiency on rare occasions is caused by malabsorption (especially celiac disease) or malnutrition.

Obscure gastrointestinal bleeding refers to occult or overt bleeding of unknown origin that persists or recurs after initial endoscopic evaluation with upper endoscopy and colonoscopy. Obscure-occult bleeding is manifested by recurrent positive FOBTs or recurrent iron deficiency anemia, or both. Obscure-overt bleeding is manifested by persistent or recurrent visible evidence of gastrointestinal bleeding (hematemesis, hematochezia, or melena). Up to 5% of patients admitted to hospitals with clinically overt gastrointestinal bleeding do not have a cause identified on upper endoscopy or colonoscopy.

Causes of Occult or Obscure Gastrointestinal Blood Loss

Occult blood loss may arise from anywhere in the gastrointestinal tract. The most common causes are (1) neoplasms; (2) vascular abnormalities (vascular ectasias, portal hypertensive gastropathy); (3) acid-peptic lesions (esophagitis, peptic ulcer disease, erosions in hiatal hernia); (4) infections (nematodes, especially hookworm; tuberculosis); (5) medications (especially NSAIDs or aspirin); and (6) other causes such as inflammatory bowel disease.

Obscure bleeding (either occult or overt) most commonly arises from lesions in the small intestine. In up to one-third of cases, however, a source of bleeding has been overlooked in the upper or lower tract on prior endoscopic studies. Hematemesis or melena suggests a source proximal to the ligament of Treitz: vascular ectasias, Dieulafoy's vascular malformation, portal hypertensive gastropathy, gastroduodenal varices, or hepatic and pancreatic lesions. In the small intestine, the most common causes of occult or overt obscure bleeding are vascular ectasias and NSAID-induced erosions and ulcerations. Other causes include small bowel neoplasms (stromal tumors, carcinoid, lymphoma, adenocarcinoma) and Meckel's diverticula-associated ulceration.

Evaluation

All adults over age 40–45 years with positive FOBTs or iron deficiency anemia should undergo colonoscopy or upper endoscopy. Endoscopic evaluation is also recommended in premenopausal women and younger men with gastrointestinal symptoms (abdominal pain, dyspepsia or heartburn, change in bowel habits, weight loss), a positive family history of gastrointestinal cancer, or anemia that is disproportionate to the estimated menstrual blood loss. The presence and nature of gastrointestinal symptoms help guide the choice of initial study. After evaluation of the upper and lower gastrointestinal tract with upper endoscopy and colonos-

copy, the origin of positive FOBT or iron deficiency anemia remains unexplained in 30–50% of patients. Patients with occult bleeding who have a negative initial endoscopic evaluation may be given a trial of iron supplementation and closely observed. Most require no further evaluation. For recurrent or persistent chronic gastrointestinal blood loss or anemia that responds poorly to iron supplementation, further evaluation is pursued for a source of obscure bleeding (as described below). Where possible, NSAIDs and aspirin should be discontinued.

A. Colonoscopy

Unless patients have symptoms referable to the upper gastrointestinal tract, the colon should be evaluated first. Colonoscopy detects over 95% of colorectal polyps and cancer and permits polypectomy, tumor biopsy, or endoscopic cautery of vascular ectasias. The finding on colonoscopy of a significant lesion clearly consistent with chronic bleeding (mass lesion, large ulceration, bleeding ectasias) obviates the need for upper endoscopy. Barium enema examinations are less accurate than colonoscopy, missing up to 50% of significant adenomas. Furthermore, up to 30–40% of patients with a positive FOBT will have a polyp or mass lesion detected on barium enema, which then necessitates colonoscopic evaluation. For these reasons, barium enema can no longer be recommended except in patients in whom colonoscopy is contraindicated or where expertise in colonoscopy is not available.

B. Upper Endoscopy

Upper endoscopy should be performed first in patients with symptoms referable to the upper gastrointestinal tract (heartburn, dyspepsia, dysphagia, vomiting, weight loss). Upper endoscopy should also be performed in patients with iron deficiency anemia after colonoscopy. In asymptomatic patients with a positive FOBT without iron deficiency anemia whose colonoscopic examination is negative, significant abnormalities are found in almost 50% of patients on upper endoscopy. Although the cost-effectiveness of evaluation of the upper gastrointestinal tract in this setting is uncertain, upper endoscopy is recommended by many experts. Owing to its lower diagnostic accuracy, upper gastrointestinal radiography should be performed only in patients in whom upper endoscopy is contraindicated or where a gastroenterologist is unavailable.

C. Evaluation of Occult or Overt Obscure Bleeding

Upper endoscopy and colonoscopy should be repeated to ascertain that a lesion in these regions has not been overlooked. Abdominal CT may be considered to exclude an hepatic or pancreatic source of bleeding. Small bowel push enteroscopy permits visualization of the upper one-third of the small intestine and permits thermocoagulative treatment of vascular ectasias or bleeding ulcers, when identified. If enteroscopy is unrevealing, video capsule endoscopy of the small intestine should be performed. This device captures up to 8 hours of video images of the small intestine, which are transmitted to a portable recorder for subsequent viewing. Capsule endoscopy is superior to radiographic studies (standard small bowel follow through, enteroclysis, or CT enterography) for the detection of small bowel abnormalities, demonstrating possible sources of occult bleeding, most commonly vascular abnormalities and ulcers, in over 50% of patients in whom these studies were unrevealing. Capsule imaging is unable to provide precise localization and is obscured in the setting of significant active bleeding. Laparotomy with intraoperative enteroscopy of the entire small bowel is reserved for patients with obscure gastrointestinal bleeding that is believed to arise from a source in the small intestine, especially for those patients in whom a possible source has been identified on capsule imaging, and who have required multiple transfusions or repeated hospitalizations. A new double-balloon enteroscope is available that allows visualization of most or all of the small intestine via the oral or anal routes with the ability to obtain biopsies or apply thermocoagulation. As this technique becomes more widely available, it may obviate the need for intraoperative endoscopy in many patients.

For patients with hemodynamically significant acute bleeding, angiography may be helpful for localization and embolization of a bleeding vascular abnormality.

Gralnek I: Obscure-overt gastrointestinal bleeding. Gastroenterology 2005;128:1424. [PMID: 15887123]

Hartmann D et al: A prospective two-center study comparing wireless capsule endoscopy with intraoperative enteroscopy in patients with obscure GI bleeding. Gastrointest Endosc 2005;61:826. [PMID: 15933683]

May A et al: Double-balloon enteroscopy (push-and-pull enteroscopy) of the small bowel: feasibility and diagnostic and therapeutic yield in patients with suspected small bowel disease. Gastrointest Endosc 2005;62:62. [PMID: 15990821]

Pannazio M et al: Outcome of patients with obscure gastrointestinal bleeding after capsule endoscopy: report of 100 consecutive patients. Gastroenterology 2004;126:643. [PMID: 14988816]

Triester SL et al: A meta-analysis of the yield of capsule endoscopy compared to other diagnostic modalities in patients with obscure gastrointestinal bleeding. Am J Gastroenterol 2005;100:2407. [PMID: 16279893]

■ DISEASES OF THE PERITONEUM

APPROACH TO THE PATIENT WITH ASCITES

Etiology of Ascites

The term "ascites" denotes the pathologic accumulation of fluid in the peritoneal cavity. Healthy men have little or no intraperitoneal fluid, but women normally may have up to 20 mL depending on the phase of the menstrual cycle. The causes of ascites may be classified into two broad pathophysiologic categories: that which is associated with a normal peritoneum and that which occurs due to a diseased peritoneum (Table 14–8). The most common cause of ascites is portal hy-

Table 14–8. Causes of ascites.

NORMAL PERITONEUM
Portal hypertension (SAAG ≥ 1.1 g/dL)
1. Hepatic congestion[1]
Congestive heart failure
Constrictive pericarditis
Tricuspid insufficiency
Budd-Chiari syndrome
Veno-occlusive disease
2. Liver disease[2]
Cirrhosis
Alcoholic hepatitis
Fulminant hepatic failure
Massive hepatic metastases
Hepatic fibrosis
Acute fatty liver of pregnancy
3. Portal vein occlusion
Hypoalbuminemia (SAAG < 1.1 g/dL)
Nephrotic syndrome
Protein-losing enteropathy
Severe malnutrition with anasarca
Miscellaneous conditions (SAAG < 1.1 g/dL)
Chylous ascites
Pancreatic ascites
Bile ascites
Nephrogenic ascites
Urine ascites
Myxedema (SAAG ≥ 1.1 g/dL)
Ovarian disease
DISEASED PERITONEUM (SAAG < 1.1 G/DL)[2]
Infections
Bacterial peritonitis
Tuberculous peritonitis
Fungal peritonitis
HIV-associated peritonitis
Malignant conditions
Peritoneal carcinomatosis
Primary mesothelioma
Pseudomyxoma peritonei
Massive hepatic metastases
Hepatocellular carcinoma
Other conditions
Familial Mediterranean fever
Vasculitis
Granulomatous peritonitis
Eosinophilic peritonitis

[1]Hepatic congestion usually associated with SAAG ≥ 1.1 g/dL and ascitic fluid total protein > 2.5 g/dL.
[2]There may be cases of "mixed ascites" in which portal hypertensive ascites is complicated by a secondary process such as infection. In these cases, the SAAG is ≥ 1.1 g/dL.
SAAG = serum-ascites albumin gradient.

pertension secondary to chronic liver disease, which accounts for over 80% of patients with ascites. The management of portal hypertensive ascites is discussed in Chapter 15. The most common causes of nonportal hypertensive ascites include infections (tuberculous peritonitis), intra-abdominal malignancy, inflammatory disorders of the peritoneum, and ductal disruptions (chylous, pancreatic, biliary).

Clinical Features

A. SYMPTOMS AND SIGNS

The history usually is one of increasing abdominal girth, with the presence of abdominal pain depending on the cause. Because most ascites is secondary to chronic liver disease with portal hypertension, patients should be asked about risk factors for liver disease, especially alcohol consumption, transfusions, tattoos, injection drug use, a history of viral hepatitis or jaundice, and birth in an area endemic for hepatitis. A history of cancer or marked weight loss arouses suspicion of malignant ascites. Fevers may suggest infected peritoneal fluid, including bacterial peritonitis (spontaneous or secondary). Patients with chronic liver disease and ascites are at greatest risk for developing spontaneous bacterial peritonitis. In immigrants, immunocompromised hosts, or severely malnourished alcoholics, tuberculous peritonitis should be considered.

Physical examination should emphasize signs of portal hypertension and chronic liver disease. Elevated jugular venous pressure may suggest right-sided congestive heart failure or constrictive pericarditis. A large tender liver is characteristic of acute alcoholic hepatitis or Budd-Chiari syndrome. The presence of large abdominal wall veins with cephalad flow also suggests portal hypertension; inferiorly directed flow implies hepatic vein obstruction. Signs of chronic liver disease include palmar erythema, cutaneous spider angiomas, gynecomastia, and Dupuytren's contracture. Asterixis secondary to hepatic encephalopathy may be present. Anasarca results from cardiac failure or nephrotic syndrome with hypoalbuminemia. Finally, firm lymph nodes in the left supraclavicular region or umbilicus may suggest intra-abdominal malignancy.

The physical examination is relatively insensitive for detecting ascitic fluid. In general, patients must have at least 1500 mL of fluid to be detected reliably by this method. Even the experienced clinician may find it difficult to distinguish between obesity and small-volume ascites. Abdominal ultrasound establishes the presence of fluid.

B. LABORATORY TESTING

1. Abdominal paracentesis—Abdominal paracentesis is performed as part of the diagnostic evaluation in all patients with new onset of ascites to help determine the cause. It should also be performed to diagnose bacterial peritonitis in all patients admitted to the hospital with cirrhosis and ascites (in whom the prevalence of

bacterial peritonitis is 10–30%) and when patients with known ascites develop clinical deterioration (fever, abdominal pain, rapid worsening of renal function, or worsened hepatic encephalopathy).

a. Inspection—Cloudy fluid suggests infection. Milky fluid is seen with chylous ascites due to high triglyceride levels. Bloody fluid is most commonly attributable to a traumatic paracentesis, but up to 20% of cases of malignant ascites are bloody.

b. Routine studies—

(1) Cell count—A white blood cell count is the most important test. Normal ascitic fluid contains < 500 leukocytes/mcL and < 250 polymorphonuclear neutrophils (PMNs)/mcL. Any inflammatory condition can cause an elevated ascitic white count. A PMN count of > 250/mcL (neutrocytic ascites) with a percentage of > 75% of all white cells is highly suggestive of bacterial peritonitis, either spontaneous primary peritonitis or secondary peritonitis (ie, caused by an intra-abdominal source of infection, such as a perforated viscus or appendicitis). An elevated white count with a predominance of lymphocytes arouses suspicion of tuberculosis or peritoneal carcinomatosis.

(2) Albumin and total protein—The serum-ascites albumin gradient (SAAG) is the best single test for the classification of ascites into portal hypertensive and nonportal hypertensive causes (Table 14–8). Calculated by subtracting the ascitic fluid albumin from the serum albumin, the gradient correlates directly with the portal pressure. An SAAG ≥ 1.1 g/dL suggests underlying portal hypertension, while gradients < 1.1 g/dL implicate nonportal hypertensive causes.

The accuracy of the SAAG exceeds 95% in classifying ascites. It should be recognized, however, that approximately 4% of patients have "mixed ascites," ie, underlying cirrhosis with portal hypertension complicated by a second cause for ascites formation (such as malignancy or tuberculosis). Thus, a high SAAG is indicative of portal hypertension but does not exclude concomitant malignancy.

The ascitic fluid total protein provides some additional clues to the cause. An elevated SAAG and a high protein level (> 2.5 g/dL) are seen in most cases of hepatic congestion secondary to cardiac disease or Budd-Chiari syndrome. However, an increased ascitic fluid protein is also found in up to 20% of cases of uncomplicated cirrhosis. Two-thirds of patients with malignant ascites have a total protein level > 2.5 g/dL.

(3) Culture and Gram stain—The best technique consists of the inoculation of aerobic and anaerobic blood culture bottles with 5–10 mL of ascitic fluid at the patient's bedside, which increases the sensitivity for detecting bacterial peritonitis to over 85% in patients with neutrocytic ascites (> 250 PMNs/mcL), compared with approximately 50% sensitivity by conventional agar plate or broth cultures.

c. Optional studies—Other laboratory tests are of utility in some specific clinical situations. Glucose and lactate dehydrogenase (LDH) may be helpful in distinguishing spontaneous from secondary bacterial peritonitis (see below). Glucose levels are reduced in patients with tuberculous peritonitis. An elevated amylase may suggest pancreatic ascites or a perforation of the gastrointestinal tract with leakage of pancreatic secretions into the ascitic fluid. Perforation of the biliary tree is suspected with an ascitic bilirubin concentration that is greater than the serum bilirubin. An elevated ascitic creatinine suggests leakage of urine from the bladder or ureters. Ascitic fluid cytologic examination is ordered if peritoneal carcinomatosis is suspected.

C. IMAGING

Abdominal ultrasound is useful in confirming the presence of ascites and in the guidance of paracentesis. Both ultrasound and CT imaging are useful in distinguishing between causes of portal and nonportal hypertensive ascites. Doppler ultrasound and CT can detect thrombosis of the hepatic veins (Budd-Chiari syndrome) or portal veins. In patients with nonportal hypertensive ascites, these studies are useful in detecting lymphadenopathy and masses of the mesentery and of solid organs such as the liver, ovaries, and pancreas. Furthermore, they permit directed percutaneous needle biopsies of these lesions. Ultrasound and CT are poor procedures for the detection of peritoneal carcinomatosis.

D. LAPAROSCOPY

Laparoscopy is an important test in the evaluation of some patients with nonportal hypertensive ascites (low SAAG) or mixed ascites. It permits direct visualization and biopsy of the peritoneum, liver, and some intra-abdominal lymph nodes. Cases of suspected peritoneal tuberculosis or suspected malignancy with nondiagnostic CT imaging and ascitic fluid cytology are best evaluated by this method.

Krige JE et al: ABC of diseases of the liver, pancreas, and biliary system: portal hypertension 2. Ascites, encephalopathy, and other conditions. BMJ 2001;322:416. [PMID: 11179165]

Runyon BA: AASLD Practice Guideline. Management of adult patients with ascites due to cirrhosis. Hepatology 2004; 39:841. [PMID: 14999706]

SPONTANEOUS BACTERIAL PERITONITIS

 ESSENTIALS OF DIAGNOSIS

- *A history of chronic liver disease and ascites.*
- *Fever and abdominal pain.*
- *Peritoneal finding on examination uncommonly encountered.*
- *Neutrocytic ascites (> 250 white blood cells/mcL) with neutrophilic predominance.*

General Considerations

"Spontaneous" bacterial infection of ascitic fluid occurs in the absence of an apparent intra-abdominal source of infection. It is seen with few exceptions in patients with ascites caused by chronic liver disease. Translocation of enteric bacteria across the gut wall or mesenteric lymphatics leads to seeding of the ascitic fluid, as may bacteremia from other sites. Approximately 20–30% of cirrhotic patients with ascites develop spontaneous peritonitis; however, the incidence is greater than 40% in patients with ascitic fluid total protein < 1 g/dL, probably due to decreased ascitic fluid opsonic activity.

Virtually all cases of spontaneous bacterial peritonitis are caused by a monomicrobial infection. The most common pathogens are enteric gram-negative bacteria (*E coli, Klebsiella pneumoniae, Enterococcus* species) or gram-positive bacteria (*Streptococcus pneumoniae*, viridans streptococci). Anaerobic bacteria are not associated with spontaneous bacterial peritonitis.

Clinical Findings

A. SYMPTOMS AND SIGNS

Eighty to 90 percent of patients with spontaneous bacterial peritonitis are symptomatic; in many cases the presentation is subtle. Spontaneous bacterial peritonitis may be present in 20% of patients hospitalized with chronic liver disease in the absence of any suggestive symptoms or signs.

The most common symptoms are fever and abdominal pain, present in two-thirds of patients. Spontaneous bacterial peritonitis may also present with a change in mental status due to exacerbation or precipitation of hepatic encephalopathy, or sudden worsening of renal function. Physical examination typically demonstrates signs of chronic liver disease with ascites. Abdominal tenderness is present in less than 50% of patients, and its presence suggests other processes.

B. LABORATORY FINDINGS

The most important diagnostic test is abdominal paracentesis. Ascitic fluid should be sent for cell count, and blood culture bottles should be inoculated at the bedside; Gram stain is insensitive. An ascitic fluid total protein of more than 1 g/dL is evidence against spontaneous bacterial peritonitis.

In the proper clinical setting, an ascitic fluid PMN count of > 250 cells/mcL (neutrocytic ascites) is presumptive evidence of bacterial peritonitis. The percentage of PMNs is greater than 50–70% of the ascitic fluid white blood cells and commonly approximates 100%. Patients with neutrocytic ascites are presumed to be infected and should be started—regardless of symptoms—on antibiotics. Although 10–30% of patients with neutrocytic ascites have negative ascitic bacterial cultures ("culture-negative neutrocytic ascites"), it is presumed that these patients have bacterial peritonitis and should be treated empirically. Occasionally, a positive blood culture identifies the organism when ascitic fluid is sterile.

Differential Diagnosis

Spontaneous bacterial peritonitis must be distinguished from secondary bacterial peritonitis, in which ascitic fluid has become secondarily infected by an intra-abdominal infection. Even in the presence of perforation, clinical symptoms and signs of peritonitis may be lacking in up to 30% of patients owing to the separation of the visceral and parietal peritoneum by the ascitic fluid. Causes of secondary bacterial peritonitis include appendicitis, diverticulitis, perforated peptic ulcer, and perforated gallbladder. Secondary bacterial infection accounts for 3% of cases of infected ascitic fluid.

Ascitic fluid total protein, LDH, and glucose are useful in distinguishing spontaneous bacterial peritonitis from secondary infection. Up to two-thirds of patients with secondary bacterial peritonitis have at least two of the following: decreased glucose level (< 50 mg/dL), an elevated LDH level (greater than serum), and total protein > 1 g/dL. Ascitic neutrophil counts > 10,000/mcL also are suspicious; however, most patients with secondary peritonitis have neutrophil counts within the range of spontaneous peritonitis. The presence of multiple organisms on ascitic fluid Gram stain or culture is diagnostic of secondary peritonitis.

If secondary bacterial peritonitis is suspected, plain films, abdominal CT imaging, and water-soluble contrast studies of the upper and lower gastrointestinal tracts should be obtained to look for evidence of an intra-abdominal source of infection. If these studies are negative and secondary peritonitis still is suspected, repeat paracentesis should be performed after 48 hours of antibiotic therapy to confirm that the PMN count is decreasing. Secondary bacterial peritonitis should be suspected in patients in whom the PMN count is not below the pretreatment value at 48 hours.

Neutrocytic ascites may also be seen in some patients with peritoneal carcinomatosis, pancreatic ascites, or tuberculous ascites. In these circumstances, however, PMNs account for less than 50% of the ascitic white blood cells.

Prevention

Up to 70% of patients who survive an episode of spontaneous bacterial peritonitis will have another episode within 1 year. Prophylactic therapy—with norfloxacin, 400 mg/d; ciprofloxacin, 750 mg weekly; or trimethoprim-sulfamethoxazole, one double-strength tablet daily—has been shown to reduce the rate of recurrent infections to less than 20% and is recommended. Prophylaxis should be considered also in patients who have not had prior bacterial peritonitis but are at increased risk of infection due to low-protein ascites (total ascitic protein < 1 g/dL). Although im-

provement in survival in cirrhotic patients with ascites treated with prophylactic antibiotics has not been shown, decision analytic modeling suggests that in patients with prior bacterial peritonitis or low ascitic fluid protein, the use of prophylactic antibiotics is a cost-effective strategy.

Treatment

Empiric therapy for spontaneous bacterial peritonitis should be initiated with a third-generation cephalosporin such as cefotaxime (dosage: 2 g intravenously every 8–12 hours depending on renal function), which covers 98% of causative agents of this disorder. If enterococcus infection is suspected, ampicillin may be added. Because of a high risk of nephrotoxicity in patients with chronic liver disease, aminoglycosides should not be used. Although the optimal duration of therapy is unknown, a course of 5–10 days is sufficient in most patients, or until the ascites fluid PMN count decreases to < 250 cells/mcL. Renal failure develops in up to 40% of patients and is a major cause of death. In patients given intravenous albumin, 1.5 g/kg on day 1 and 1 g/kg on day 3, the incidence of renal failure and mortality are reduced both during hospitalization and at follow-up. Patients with suspected secondary bacterial peritonitis should be given broad-spectrum coverage for enteric aerobic and anaerobic flora with a third-generation cephalosporin and metronidazole pending identification and definitive (usually surgical) treatment of the cause. In fact, the most effective treatment for spontaneous bacterial peritonitis is liver transplant.

Prognosis

The mortality rate of spontaneous bacterial peritonitis exceeds 30%. However, if the disease is recognized and treated early, the rate is less than 10%. As the majority of patients have underlying severe liver disease, many may die of liver failure, hepatorenal syndrome, or bleeding complications from portal hypertension.

Gines P et al: Management of cirrhosis and ascites. N Engl J Med 2004;350:1646. [PMID: 15084697]

Runyon BA: AASLD Practice Guideline. Management of adult patients with ascites due to cirrhosis. Hepatology 2004; 39:841. [PMID: 14999706]

Runyon BA: The evolution of ascitic fluid analysis in the diagnosis of spontaneous bacterial peritonitis. Am J Gastroenterol 2003;98:1675. [PMID: 12907318]

Sheer TA et al: Spontaneous bacterial peritonitis. Dig Dis 2005; 23:39. [PMID: 15920324]

Soares-Weiser K et al: Evidence based case report. Antibiotic treatment for spontaneous bacterial peritonitis. BMJ 2002; 324:100. [PMID: 11786457]

TUBERCULOUS PERITONITIS

Tuberculosis occurs in extrapulmonary sites in 20% of non–HIV-infected people and up to 70% of those infected with HIV. Although tuberculous involvement of the peritoneum accounts for less than 2% of all causes of ascites in the United States, it remains a significant problem in the developing world. In Western countries, its incidence is higher among those with HIV disease, immigrants from underdeveloped countries, the urban poor, patients with cirrhosis, and nursing home residents.

The presenting symptoms include low-grade fever, abdominal pain, anorexia, and weight loss. Most patients have symptoms for months before the diagnosis is established. On physical examination, patients may have generalized abdominal tenderness and distention. There may be clinically evident ascites or suggestion of an abdominal mass. Ultrasonography or CT imaging of the abdomen reveals free or loculated ascites in > 80% of patients and also may demonstrate lymphadenopathy or peritoneal, mesenteric, or omental thickening.

The diagnosis thus can be difficult to establish, particularly in patients with underlying cirrhosis with ascites and in patients without ascites (in whom the diagnosis may not be suspected). Chest radiographs are abnormal in over 70%, but active tuberculous pulmonary disease is evident in less than 20% of patients. Skin tests are positive in 50%. Smears of ascitic fluid for acid-fast bacilli are usually negative, and cultures are positive in only 35%. Other findings are an ascitic fluid total protein > 3.0 g/dL, LDH > 90 units/L, or mononuclear cell-predominant leukocytosis > 500/mcL—each has a sensitivity of 70–80% but limited specificity. Several studies report that ascites adenosine deaminase activity $\geq$ 30 IU/L has sensitivity and specificity levels of > 90% for the diagnosis of tuberculous peritonitis.

In patients with suspected tuberculous peritonitis, laparoscopy establishes the diagnosis. In over 90% of patients, characteristic peritoneal nodules are visible, and granulomas are seen on peritoneal biopsy. Peritoneal cultures require at least 4–6 weeks and are positive in less than two-thirds of patients.

Treatment of tuberculosis is discussed in Chapter 9.

Sanai FM et al: Systematic review: tuberculous peritonitis—presenting features, diagnostic strategies and treatment. Aliment Pharmacol Ther 2005;22:685. [PMID: 16197489]

MALIGNANT ASCITES

Two-thirds of cases of malignant ascites are caused by peritoneal carcinomatosis. The most common tumors causing carcinomatosis are primary adenocarcinomas of the ovary, uterus, pancreas, stomach, colon, lung, or breast. The remaining one-third are due to lymphatic obstruction or portal hypertension due to hepatocellular carcinoma or diffuse hepatic metastases. Patients present with nonspecific abdominal discomfort and weight loss associated with increased abdominal girth. Nausea or vomiting may be caused by partial or complete intestinal obstruction. Abdominal CT may be useful to demonstrate the primary malignancy or hepatic metastases but seldom confirms the diagnosis of peritoneal carcinomatosis. In patients with carcinomatosis, paracentesis demonstrates a low serum ascites-albumin gradient (< 1.1 mg/dL), an increased total protein (> 2.5 g/dL), and an elevated white cell count (often both neutrophils and mononuclear cells) but with a lymphocyte predominance. Cytology is positive in over 95%, but laparoscopy may be required in patients with negative cytology to confirm the diagnosis and to exclude tuberculous peritonitis, with which it may be confused. Malignant ascites attributable to portal hypertension usually is associated with an increased serum ascites-albumin gradient (> 1.1 g/dL), a variable total protein, and negative ascitic cytology. Ascites caused by peritoneal carcinomatosis does not respond to diuretics.

Patients may be treated with periodic large-volume paracentesis for symptomatic relief. Intraperitoneal chemotherapy is sometimes used to shrink the tumor, but the overall prognosis is extremely poor, with only 10% survival at 6 months. Ovarian cancers represent an exception to this rule. With newer treatments consisting of surgical debulking and intraperitoneal chemotherapy, long-term survival from ovarian cancer is possible.

Adam RA et al: Malignant ascites: past, present, and future. J Am Coll Surg 2004;198:999. [PMID: 15194082]

FAMILIAL MEDITERRANEAN FEVER

This is a rare autosomal recessive disorder of unknown pathogenesis that almost exclusively affects people of Mediterranean ancestry, especially Sephardic Jews, Armenians, Turks, and Arabs. Patients lack a protease in serosal fluids that normally inactivates interleukin-8 and the chemotactic complement factor 5A. Symptoms present in most patients before the age of 20 years. It is characterized by episodic bouts of acute peritonitis that may be associated with serositis involving the joints and pleura. Peritoneal attacks are marked by the sudden onset of fever, severe abdominal pain, and abdominal tenderness with guarding or rebound tenderness. If left untreated, attacks resolve within 24–48 hours. Because symptoms resemble those of surgical peritonitis, patients may undergo unnecessary exploratory laparotomy. Colchicine, 0.6 mg two or three times daily, has been shown to decrease the frequency and severity of attacks. Secondary amyloidosis (AA protein) with renal or hepatic involvement may occur in 25% of cases and is the main cause of death. Colchicine prevents or arrests further progression of amyloidosis development. In the absence of amyloidosis, the prognosis is excellent. The diagnosis of familial Mediterranean fever still is based on clinical criteria. Although the gene responsible for familial Mediterranean fever (MEFV) has been identified, commercial genetic tests fail to identify one of the known gene mutations in up to one-third of patients. Genetic testing is most useful to confirm the diagnosis in patients with atypical symptoms.

Mor A et al: Abdominal and digestive system associations of familial Mediterranean fever. Am J Gastroenterol 2003;98: 2594. [PMID: 14687803]

Simon A et al: Mediterranean fever—a not so unusual cause of abdominal pain. Best Pract Res Clin Gastroenterol 2005; 19:199. [PMID: 15833688]

MESOTHELIOMA

Primary malignant mesothelioma is a rare tumor. Over 70% of cases have a history of asbestos exposure. Presenting symptoms and signs include abdominal pain or bowel obstruction, increased abdominal girth, and small to moderate ascites. The chest radiograph reveals pulmonary asbestosis in over 50%. The ascitic fluid is hemorrhagic, with a low serum-ascites albumin gradient. Cytology is often negative. Abdominal CT may reveal sheet-like masses involving the mesentery and omentum. Diagnosis is made at laparotomy or laparoscopy. The prognosis is extremely poor, but long-term survivors have been described with a combination of surgical debulking of tumor followed by heated intraoperative intraperitoneal chemotherapy and early postoperative intraperitoneal chemotherapy. Multicystic and well-differentiated papillary mesotheliomas are associated with a long survival with surgical treatment alone.

Hassan R et al: Nonpleural mesotheliomas: mesothelioma of the peritoneum, tunica vaginalis, and pericardium. Hematol Oncol Clin North Am 2005;19:1067. [PMID: 16325124]

MISCELLANEOUS PERITONEAL DISEASES

Chylous ascites is the accumulation of lipid-rich lymph in the peritoneal cavity. The ascitic fluid is characterized by a milky appearance with a triglyceride level > 1000 mg/dL. The usual cause in adults is lymphatic obstruction or leakage caused by malignancy, especially lymphoma. Nonmalignant causes include postoperative trauma, cirrhosis, tuberculosis, pancreatitis, and filariasis.

Pancreatic ascites is the intraperitoneal accumulation of massive amounts of pancreatic secretions due either to disruption of the pancreatic duct or to a pancreatic pseudocyst. It is most commonly seen in patients with chronic pancreatitis and complicates up to 3% of cases of acute pancreatitis. Because the pancreatic enzymes are not activated, pain often is absent. The ascitic fluid is characterized by a high protein level (> 2.5 g/dL) but a low SAAG. Ascitic fluid amylase levels are in excess of 1000 units/L. In nonsurgical cases, initial treatment consists of bowel rest, total parenteral nutrition (TPN), and octreotide to decrease pancreatic secretion. Persistent leakage requires treatment with either endoscopic placement of stents into the pancreatic duct or surgical drainage.

Bile ascites is caused most commonly by complications of biliary tract surgery, percutaneous liver biopsy, or abdominal trauma. Unless the bile is infected, bile ascites usually does not cause abdominal pain, fever, or leukocytosis. Paracentesis reveals yellow fluid with a ratio of ascites bilirubin to serum bilirubin greater than 1.0. Treatment depends on the location and rate of bile leakage. Postcholecystectomy cystic duct leaks may be treated with endoscopic sphincterotomy or biliary stent placement to facilitate bile flow across the sphincter of Oddi. Other leaks may be treated with percutaneous drainage by interventional radiologists or with surgical closure.

Le Moine O et al: Endoscopic management of pancreatic fistula after pancreatic and other abdominal surgeries. Best Pract Res Clin Gastroenterol 2004;18:957. [PMID: 15494289]

Leong RW et al: Chylous ascites caused by portal vein thrombosis treated with octreotide. J Gastroenterol Hepatol 2003;18: 1211. [PMID: 12974913]

■ DISEASES OF THE ESOPHAGUS

EVALUATION OF ESOPHAGEAL DISORDERS

Symptoms

Heartburn, dysphagia, and odynophagia almost always indicate a primary esophageal disorder.

A. HEARTBURN

Heartburn (pyrosis) is the feeling of substernal burning, often radiating to the neck. Caused by the reflux of acidic (or, rarely, alkaline) material into the esophagus, it is highly specific for gastroesophageal reflux disease.

B. DYSPHAGIA

Difficulties in swallowing may arise from problems in transferring the food bolus from the oropharynx to the upper esophagus (oropharyngeal dysphagia) or from impaired transport of the bolus through the body of the esophagus (esophageal dysphagia). The history usually leads to the correct diagnosis.

1. Oropharyngeal dysphagia—The oropharyngeal phase of swallowing is a complex process requiring elevation of the tongue, closure of the nasopharynx, relaxation of the upper esophageal sphincter, closure of the airway, and pharyngeal peristalsis. A variety of mechanical and neuromuscular conditions can disrupt this process (Table 14–9). Problems with the oral phase of swallowing cause drooling or spillage of food from the mouth, inability to chew or initiate swallowing, or dry mouth. Pharyngeal dysphagia is characterized by an immediate sense of the bolus catching in the neck, the need to swallow repeatedly to clear food from the pharynx, or coughing or choking during

Table 14–9. Causes of oropharyngeal dysphagia.

Neurologic disorders
  Brainstem cerebrovascular accident, mass lesion
  Amyotrophic lateral sclerosis, multiple sclerosis, pseudobul-
    bar palsy, post-polio syndrome, Guillain-Barré syndrome
  Parkinson's disease, Huntington's disease, dementia
  Tardive dyskinesia
Muscular and rheumatologic disorders
  Myopathies, polymyositis
  Oculopharyngeal dystrophy
  Sjögren's syndrome
Metabolic disorders
  Thyrotoxicosis, amyloidosis, Cushing's disease, Wilson's
    disease
  Medication side effects: anticholinergics, phenothiazines
Infectious disease
  Polio, diphtheria, botulism, Lyme disease, syphilis, mucosi-
    tis (*Candida*, herpes)
Structural disorders
  Zenker's diverticulum
  Cervical osteophytes, cricopharyngeal bar, proximal
    esophageal webs
  Oropharyngeal tumors
  Postsurgical or radiation changes
  Pill-induced injury
Motility disorders
  Upper esophageal sphincter dysfunction

meals. There may be associated dysphonia, dysarthria, or other neurologic symptoms.

2. Esophageal dysphagia—Esophageal dysphagia may be caused by **mechanical lesions** obstructing the esophagus or by **motility disorders** (Table 14–10). Patients with mechanical obstruction experience dysphagia, primarily for solids. This is recurrent, predictable, and, if the lesion progresses, will worsen as the lumen narrows. Patients with **motility disorders** have dysphagia for both solids and liquids. It is episodic, unpredictable, and nonprogressive.

C. ODYNOPHAGIA

Odynophagia is sharp substernal pain on swallowing that may limit oral intake. It usually reflects severe erosive disease. It is most commonly associated with infectious esophagitis due to *Candida*, herpesviruses, or CMV, especially in immunocompromised patients. It may also be caused by corrosive injury due to caustic ingestions and by pill-induced ulcers.

Diagnostic Studies

A. UPPER ENDOSCOPY

Endoscopy is the study of choice for evaluating persistent heartburn, odynophagia, and structural abnormalities detected on barium esophagography. In addition to direct visualization, it allows biopsy of mucosal abnormalities and dilation of strictures.

B. VIDEOESOPHAGOGRAPHY

Oropharyngeal dysphagia is best evaluated with rapid-sequence videoesophagography.

C. BARIUM ESOPHAGOGRAPHY

Patients with esophageal dysphagia often are evaluated first with a radiographic barium study to differentiate between mechanical lesions and motility disorders, providing important information about the latter in particular. In patients with esophageal dysphagia and a suspected motility disorder, barium esophagoscopy should be obtained first. In patients in whom there is a high suspicion of a mechanical lesion, many clinicians will proceed first to endoscopic evaluation because it better identifies mucosa lesions (eg, erosions) and permits mucosal biopsy and dilation. However, barium study is more sensitive for detecting subtle esophageal narrowing due to rings, achalasia, and proximal esophageal lesions.

D. ESOPHAGEAL MANOMETRY

Esophageal motility may be assessed using manometric techniques. They are indicated (1) to determine the location of the lower esophageal sphincter to allow precise placement of a conventional electrode pH probe; (2) to establish the etiology of dysphagia in patients in whom a mechanical obstruction cannot be found, especially if a diagnosis of achalasia is suspected by endoscopy or barium study; (3) for the preoperative assessment of patients being considered for antireflux surgery to exclude an alternative diagnosis (eg, achalasia) or possibly to assess peristaltic function in the esophageal body.

E. ESOPHAGEAL pH RECORDING

Esophageal pH may be monitored continuously by means of a small pH electrode that is passed transna-

Table 14–10. Causes of esophageal dysphagia.

Cause	Clues
Mechanical obstruction	**Solid foods worse than liquids**
Schatzki's ring	Intermittent dysphagia; not progressive
Peptic stricture	Chronic heartburn; progressive dysphagia
Esophageal cancer	Progressive dysphagia; age over 50 years
Eosinophilic esophagitis	Young adults; small-caliber lumen, proximal stricture, corrugated rings, or white papules
Motility disorder	**Solid and liquid foods**
Achalasia	Progressive dysphagia
Diffuse esophageal spasm	Intermittent; not progressive; may have chest pain
Scleroderma	Chronic heartburn; Raynaud's phenomenon

sally and placed 5 cm above the lower esophageal sphincter. The probe is attached to a portable pH device capable of recording pH for up to 24 hours. The recording provides information about the amount of esophageal acid reflux and on the temporal correlations between symptoms and reflux. A wireless system now is available in which a radiotelemetry pH capsule that is attached to the mucosa of the esophagus transmits data to a pager-sized receiver worn by the patient.

Traditional pH monitoring devices provide information about the amount of esophageal acid reflux but not nonacid reflux. New techniques using multichannel intraluminal impedance allow assessment of gas and nonacid liquid reflux. Although not yet widely available, they may be useful in evaluation of patients with atypical reflux symptoms or persistent symptoms despite therapy.

Achem SR et al: Dysphagia in aging. J Clin Gastroenterol 2005; 39:357. [PMID: 15815202]

Arora AS: Management strategies for dysphagia with a normal-appearing esophagus. Clin Gastroenterol Hepatol 2005;3:299. [PMID: 15765451]

Pandolfino JE et al; American Gastroenterological Association: American Gastroenterological Association medical position statement: Clinical use of esophageal manometry. Gastroenterology 2005;128:207. [PMID: 15633137]

Pandolfino JE et al; American Gastroenterological Association: AGA Technical review on the clinical use of esophageal manometry. Gastroenterology 2005;128:209. [PMID: 15633138]

Prakash C et al: Value of extended recording time with wireless pH monitoring in evaluating gastroesophageal reflux disease. Clin Gastroenterol Hepatol 2005;3:329. [PMID: 15822037]

Streets CG et al: Ambulatory 24-hour pH esophageal monitoring. Why, when, and what to do. J Clin Gastroenterol 2003;37: 14. [PMID: 12811203]

Tutuian R et al: Multichannel intraluminal impedance in esophageal function testing and gastroesophageal reflux monitoring. J Clin Gastroenterol 2003;37:206. [PMID: 12960718]

GASTROESOPHAGEAL REFLUX DISEASE

ESSENTIALS OF DIAGNOSIS

- *Heartburn; may be exacerbated by meals, bending, or recumbency.*
- *Typical uncomplicated cases do not require diagnostic studies.*
- *Endoscopy demonstrates abnormalities in < 50% of patients.*
- *Barium esophagography seldom helpful.*

General Considerations

Gastroesophageal reflux disease affects 20% of adults, who report at least weekly episodes of heartburn, and up to 10% complain of daily symptoms. Although most patients have mild disease, esophageal mucosal damage (re-

flux esophagitis) develops in up to 50% and more serious complications develop in a few others. Several factors may contribute to gastroesophageal reflux disease.

A. INCOMPETENT LOWER ESOPHAGEAL SPHINCTER

The antireflux barrier at the gastroesophageal junction depends on intrinsic lower esophageal sphincter pressure, the intra-abdominal location of the sphincter, and the extrinsic compression of the sphincter by the crural diaphragm. In most patients, baseline lower esophageal sphincter pressures are normal (10–30 mm Hg). In patients without hiatal hernias, about 70% of reflux episodes occur during relaxations of the lower esophageal sphincter that occur spontaneously ("transient relaxations") or as prolonged relaxation after swallowing. The remaining events occur during periods of low sphincter pressure ("hypotensive" sphincter). A small number of patients with more severe involvement (especially those with strictures) have chronically incompetent sphincters (< 10 mm Hg), resulting in free reflux or stress reflux during lifting, bending, or abdominal straining.

B. HIATAL HERNIA

Hiatal hernias are common and usually cause no symptoms. In patients with gastroesophageal reflux, however, they are associated with higher amounts of acid reflux and delayed esophageal acid clearance leading to more severe esophagitis, especially Barrett's esophagus. Increased reflux episodes occur during normal swallowing-induced relaxation, periods of sphincter hypotension, and straining due to reflux of acid from the hiatal hernia sac into the esophagus.

C. IRRITANT EFFECTS OF REFLUXATE

Esophageal mucosal damage is related to the potency of the refluxate and the amount of time it is in contact with the mucosa. Acidic gastric fluid (pH < 4.0) is extremely caustic to the esophageal mucosa and is the major injurious agent in the majority of cases. In some patients, reflux of bile or alkaline pancreatic secretions may be contributory.

D. ABNORMAL ESOPHAGEAL CLEARANCE

Acid refluxate normally is cleared and neutralized by esophageal peristalsis and salivary bicarbonate. During sleep, swallowing-induced peristalsis is infrequent, prolonging acid exposure to the esophagus. One-third of patients with severe gastroesophageal reflux disease also have diminished peristaltic clearance. Certain medical conditions such as scleroderma are associated with diminished peristalsis. Sjögren's syndrome, anticholinergic medications, and oral radiation therapy may exacerbate gastroesophageal reflux disease due to impaired salivation.

E. DELAYED GASTRIC EMPTYING

Impaired gastric emptying due to gastroparesis or partial gastric outlet obstruction potentiates gastroesophageal reflux disease.

Clinical Findings

A. SYMPTOMS AND SIGNS

The typical symptom is heartburn. This most often occurs 30–60 minutes after meals and upon reclining. Patients often report relief from taking antacids or baking soda. When this symptom is dominant, the diagnosis is established with a high degree of reliability. Many patients, however, have less specific dyspeptic symptoms with or without heartburn. Overall, a clinical diagnosis of gastroesophageal reflux has a sensitivity of 80% but a specificity of only 70%. Severity is not correlated with the degree of tissue damage. In fact, some patients with severe esophagitis are only mildly symptomatic. Patients may complain of regurgitation—the spontaneous reflux of sour or bitter gastric contents into the mouth. Dysphagia occurs in one-third of patients and may be due to erosive esophagitis, abnormal esophageal peristalsis, or the development of an esophageal stricture.

"Atypical" manifestations of gastroesophageal disease are being recognized with increasing frequency. These include asthma, chronic cough, chronic laryngitis, sore throat, and noncardiac chest pain. Gastroesophageal reflux may be either a causative or an exacerbating factor in up to 50% of these patients, especially those with refractory symptoms. Because many of these patients do not have heartburn or regurgitation, the diagnosis often is overlooked.

Physical examination and laboratory data are normal in uncomplicated disease.

B. SPECIAL EXAMINATIONS

Patients with typical symptoms of heartburn and regurgitation and with uncomplicated disease may be treated empirically for 4 weeks for gastroesophageal reflux disease without the need for diagnostic studies. Further investigation is required in patients with complicated disease and those unresponsive to empiric therapy.

1. Upper endoscopy—Upper endoscopy with biopsy is the standard procedure for documenting the type and extent of tissue damage in gastroesophageal reflux. Fifty percent of patients with proved acid reflux will have visible mucosal damage (known as reflux esophagitis), characterized by single or multiple erosions or ulcers in the distal esophagus at the squamocolumnar junction. However, endoscopy is normal in up to 50% of symptomatic patients with gastroesophageal reflux, a condition sometimes referred to as nonerosive reflux disease (NERD). The Los Angeles classification grades esophageal abnormalities on a scale of A (one or more isolated mucosal breaks ≤ 5 mm that do not extend between the tops of two mucosal folds) to D (one or more mucosal breaks that involve at least 75% of the esophageal circumference). Initial medical therapy for gastroesophageal reflux disease is guided by the presence of symptoms, not the endoscopic findings. Hence, endoscopy is not warranted for most patients with typical symptoms suggesting uncomplicated reflux disease. Endoscopy should be performed in patients whose symptoms have not responded after initial empiric therapy and patients with symptoms suggesting complicated disease (dysphagia, odynophagia, occult or overt bleeding, or iron deficiency anemia).

2. Barium esophagography—This study plays a limited role. In patients with severe dysphagia, it is sometimes obtained prior to endoscopy to identify a stricture.

3. Ambulatory esophageal pH monitoring—Ambulatory pH monitoring is the best study for documenting acid reflux, but it is unnecessary in most patients. Dual-channel transnasal probes are sometimes used to measure reflux in the proximal esophagus or hypopharynx in patients with atypical reflux symptoms, especially laryngitis, cough, and asthma. Esophageal pH monitoring is indicated in the following situations: (1) to document abnormal esophageal acid exposure in a patient being considered for antireflux surgery who has a normal endoscopy (ie, no evidence of reflux esophagitis); (2) to evaluate patients with a normal endoscopy who have reflux symptoms unresponsive to therapy with a proton pump inhibitor; (3) to detect either abnormal amounts of reflux or an association between reflux episodes and atypical symptoms such as noncardiac chest pain, asthma, chronic cough, laryngitis, and sore throat. It is recommended that most patients with atypical symptoms first be given an empiric trial of antireflux therapy with a double-dose proton pump inhibitor for 2–3 months. If symptoms fail to improve, a pH study is then performed.

Differential Diagnosis

Symptoms of gastroesophageal reflux disease may be similar to those of other diseases such as esophageal motility disorders, peptic ulcer, functional dyspepsia, and angina pectoris. Reflux erosive esophagitis may be confused with pill-induced damage, radiation esophagitis, or infections (CMV, herpes, *Candida*).

Complications

A. BARRETT'S ESOPHAGUS

This is a condition in which the squamous epithelium of the esophagus is replaced by metaplastic columnar epithelium containing goblet and columnar cells (specialized intestinal metaplasia). Present in up to 10% of patients with chronic reflux, it arises from chronic reflux-induced injury to the esophageal squamous epithelium. Barrett's esophagus is suspected at endoscopy from the presence of orange, gastric type epithelium that extends upward from the stomach into the distal tubular esophagus in a tongue-like or circumferential fashion. Biopsies obtained at endoscopy confirm the diagnosis. Three types of columnar epithelium may be identified: gastric cardiac, gastric fundic, and specialized intestinal metaplasia. Only the latter is believed to carry an increased risk of neoplasia.

Barrett's esophagus does not provoke specific symptoms but gastroesophageal reflux does. Most patients have a long history of reflux symptoms, such as heartburn and regurgitation. Dysphagia due to impaired motility is common. Paradoxically, one-third of patients report minimal or no symptoms of gastroesophageal reflux disease, suggesting decreased acid sensitivity of Barrett's epithelium. Indeed, over 90% of individuals with Barrett's esophagus in the general population do not seek medical attention. Barrett's esophagus may be complicated by stricture formation or acid-peptic ulceration, which can bleed.

Barrett's esophagus should be treated with long-term proton pump inhibitors. Surgical fundoplication may be desirable in some situations. Medical or surgical therapy may prevent progression, but there is no convincing evidence that regression occurs in most patients. Endoscopic ablation of Barrett's epithelium with cautery probes or photodynamic therapy (using photosensitizers and laser energy) results in partial or complete regression of columnar epithelium but is not recommended outside of clinical trials for uncomplicated disease.

The most serious complication of Barrett's esophagus is esophageal adenocarcinoma. It is believed that most adenocarcinomas of the esophagus and many such tumors of the gastric cardia arise from dysplastic epithelium in Barrett's esophagus. Current clinical guidelines recommend screening endoscopy in patients with longstanding reflux symptoms (over 5 years) to look for Barrett's esophagus and surveillance endoscopy every 3–5 years in patients with Barrett's esophagus to look for dysplasia or adenocarcinoma. Although there is a 40-fold increased risk compared with patients without Barrett's esophagus, adenocarcinoma of the esophagus remains a relatively uncommon malignancy in the United States (7000 cases/year). Given the large number of adults with chronic GERD relative to the small number in whom adenocarcinoma develops, it is unclear whether screening or surveillance for Barrett's esophagus is cost-effective. Among patients with Barrett's esophagus who do not have dysplasia at initial diagnosis, the estimated annual incidence of adenocarcinoma is < 0.5% per year. It is controversial whether these low-risk patients merit chronic surveillance.

In contrast, patients with low-grade dysplasia require repeat endoscopic surveillance in 3–6 months to screen for coexisting high-grade dysplasia or cancer. If low-grade dysplasia persists (which occurs in < 25% of patients), endoscopic surveillance should be repeated yearly. The treatment of patients with high-grade dysplasia or superficial mucosal cancers is controversial and evolving rapidly. Because 10–40% of patients may progress to (or already have) invasive adenocarcinoma, esophagectomy generally has been recommended for patients deemed to have a low operative risk. For patients with high-grade dysplasia who are deemed to be at high risk for esophagectomy, photodynamic therapy has been demonstrated to reduce the incidence of adenocarcinoma by 50% (28% vs 13%). Alternatively, patients with high-grade dysplasia may undergo close endoscopic surveillance with biopsy every 3–6 months, reserving surgery or photodynamic therapies for treatment of invasive adenocarcinoma.

The high morbidity and mortality rates (40% and 2–9%, respectively) associated with esophagectomy has led many centers to offer endoscopic mucosal resections rather than esophagectomy for selected patients with focal areas of high-grade dysplasia or even small (< 2 cm) mucosal adenocarcinomas that have undergone staging with endoscopic ultrasonography. Provided there is no evidence of invasion of the muscularis mucosa or submucosa, endoscopic mucosal snare resection of focal lesions can be safely performed. If pathologic assessment of the tissue specimen demonstrates submucosal invasion, esophagectomy should be recommended. Residual Barrett's epithelium may be treated with photodynamic therapy to reduce the risk of tumor recurrence.

B. Peptic Stricture

Stricture formation occurs in about 10% of patients with esophagitis. It is manifested by the gradual development of solid food dysphagia progressive over months to years. Often there is a reduction in heartburn because the stricture acts as a barrier to reflux. Most strictures are located at the gastroesophageal junction. Strictures located above this level usually occur with Barrett's metaplasia. Endoscopy with biopsy is mandatory in all cases to differentiate peptic stricture from malignant causes of esophageal stricture (esophageal carcinoma). Active erosive esophagitis is often present. Up to 90% of symptomatic patients are effectively treated with dilation with flexible weighted bougies (passed under fluoroscopic guidance), graduated polyvinyl catheters passed over a wire placed at the time of endoscopy or fluoroscopically, or balloons passed fluoroscopically or through an endoscope. Dilation is continued over one to several sessions. A luminal diameter of 13–17 mm is usually sufficient to relieve dysphagia. Long-term therapy with a proton pump inhibitor is required to decrease the likelihood of stricture recurrence. Some patients require intermittent dilation to maintain luminal patency, but operative management for strictures that do not respond to dilation is seldom required. Refractory strictures may benefit from endoscopic injection of triamcinolone into the stricture.

Treatment

A. Medical Treatment

The goal of treatment is to provide symptomatic relief, to heal esophagitis (if present), and to prevent complications. In the majority of patients with uncomplicated disease, empiric treatment is initiated based on a compatible history without the need for further confirmatory studies. Patients not responding and those with suspected complications undergo further evaluation with upper endoscopy or esophageal pH recording.

Patients with known erosive esophagitis, complications (such as a peptic stricture or Barrett's esophagus), or suspected atypical manifestations (such as asthma or laryngitis) are treated initially with a proton pump inhibitor (see below). In most other patients, treatment may proceed in the following stepwise fashion.

1. Mild, intermittent symptoms—Gastroesophageal reflux is a lifelong disease that requires lifestyle modifications as well as medical intervention. The best advice is to avoid lying down within 3 hours after meals, the period of greatest reflux. Elevating the head of the bed on 6-inch blocks or a foam wedge to reduce reflux and enhance esophageal clearance is recommended, especially for patients with nocturnal and atypical symptoms. Patients should be advised to avoid acidic foods (tomato products, citrus fruits, spicy foods, coffee) and agents that relax the lower esophageal sphincter or delay gastric emptying (fatty foods, peppermint, chocolate, alcohol, and smoking). Weight loss, avoidance of bending after meals, and reduction of meal size may also be helpful.

Antacids are the mainstay for rapid relief of occasional heartburn; however, their duration of action is less than 2 hours. Many are available over the counter. Those containing magnesium should not be used in renal failure, and patients with this condition should be cautioned appropriately. Gaviscon is an alginate-antacid combination that decreases reflux in the upright position.

All H_2-receptor antagonists are available in over-the-counter formulations: cimetidine 200 mg, ranitidine and nizatidine 75 mg, famotidine 10 mg—all of which are half of the typical prescription strength. When taken for active heartburn, these agents have a delay in onset of at least 30 minutes; antacids provide more immediate relief. However, once these agents take effect, they provide heartburn relief for up to 8 hours. When taken before meals known to provoke heartburn, these agents reduce the symptom. A combination agent containing famotidine 10 mg and antacid (calcium carbonate and magnesium hydroxide) is available.

2. Moderate symptoms—Patients with typical reflux symptoms that occur several times per week or daily and with uncomplicated disease should be treated empirically with an H_2-receptor antagonist or a proton pump inhibitor. Standard twice-daily prescription doses of H_2-receptor antagonists are ranitidine or nizatidine 150 mg, famotidine 20 mg, or cimetidine 400–800 mg. These agents reduce 24-hour acidity by over 60%. Ranitidine and cimetidine are available in less expensive generic formulations. Treatment twice daily affords improvement in up to two-thirds of patients. Given their superior efficacy and once-daily dosing, proton pump inhibitors increasingly are prescribed as first-line therapy for mild to moderate symptoms in preference to beginning with an H_2-receptor antagonist (see below for dosing). However, generic H_2-receptor antagonists are significantly less expensive than proton pump inhibitors and provide effective symptomatic relief in most patients with mild to moderate reflux symptoms.

Patients whose symptoms persist despite 6 weeks of standard doses of H_2-receptor antagonist therapy should be treated with a proton pump inhibitor (once daily omeprazole or rabeprazole 20 mg, lansoprazole 30 mg, esomeprazole or pantoprazole 40 mg). The decision to prescribe proton pump inhibitors is based on the presence of persistent symptoms, not endoscopic findings. Omeprazole 20 mg is now available both as an over-the-counter formulation and as a generic formulation available by prescription.

In those who achieve good symptomatic relief with either an H_2-receptor antagonist or a proton pump inhibitor, therapy should be discontinued after 8–12 weeks. Patients whose symptoms relapse may be treated with either continuous therapy, intermittent 2–4 week courses, or "on demand" therapy (ie, drug taken until symptoms abate) depending on symptom frequency and patient preference. Many patients have their symptoms controlled adequately with intermittent or on demand courses of therapy rather than continuous maintenance treatment.

3. Severe symptoms and erosive disease—For patients with severe symptoms and for patients who undergo endoscopy and have documented erosive esophagitis, Barrett's esophagus, or peptic stricture, the optimal initial therapy is a proton pump inhibitor (omeprazole or rabeprazole 20 mg, lansoprazole 30 mg, pantoprazole or esomeprazole 40 mg) once daily. Proton pump inhibitors given once daily provide symptom relief and healing of esophagitis in over 80% and given twice daily provide relief in over 95% of patients—compared with under 50% with standard doses of H_2-receptor antagonists—and are therefore the drugs of choice for severe or erosive disease. Because there appears to be little difference between these agents in efficacy or side effect profiles, the choice of agent is determined by cost. Esomeprazole, the S-isomer of omeprazole, provides slightly greater inhibition of 24-hour gastric acidity than the other agents, resulting in a small (5%) improvement in esophagitis healing rates compared with other proton pump inhibitors. Approximately 10–20% of patients fail to achieve symptom relief with a once-daily dose within 2–4 weeks and require a higher dosage (twice-daily) proton pump inhibitor. Therefore, some recommend initiating therapy with a twice-daily dose of proton pump inhibitor, reducing therapy after 2–4 weeks to a once-daily dose. The initial course of therapy is usually 8–12 weeks. As tissue healing correlates well with symptom resolution, repeat endoscopy is warranted in patients only if they fail to respond to once-daily or twice-daily proton pump inhibitor therapy.

After discontinuation of proton pump inhibitor therapy, relapse of symptoms occurs in 80% of patients within 1 year—the majority of relapses occurring within the first 3 months. Therefore, chronic therapy to maintain symptom remission is required in most but not all patients. Patients with severe erosive esophagitis, Barrett's esophagus, or peptic stricture should be maintained on chronic therapy with a proton pump inhibitor at a dose sufficient to provide complete symptom relief. In other patients, a trial off proton pump inhibitors should be considered. Patients with prolonged symptomatic remissions (over 3 months) may be treated effectively with intermittent 4- to 8-week courses of acute proton pump inhibitor therapy. Patients with prompt recurrence of symptoms (within 3 months) require chronic maintenance therapy with either a proton pump inhibitor or an H₂-receptor antagonist. The therapy should be stepped down to the lowest dose that is effective in controlling reflux symptoms.

The maintenance doses of proton pump inhibitors may escalate over time, with over 20% of patients eventually requiring double or triple doses of proton pump inhibitors to control symptoms.

4. Extraesophageal reflux manifestations—Establishing a causal relationship between gastroesophageal reflux and extraesophageal symptoms (eg, asthma, hoarseness, cough) can be difficult. Although ambulatory esophageal pH testing can document the presence of increased acid esophageal reflux, it does not prove a causative connection. A trial of a twice-daily proton pump inhibitor for 2–3 months helps determine whether these symptoms improve after acid suppression.

5. Unresponsive disease—Approximately 10–20% of patients with gastroesophageal reflux symptoms do not respond to once-daily doses of proton pump inhibitors, and 5% do not respond to twice-daily doses. These patients undergo endoscopy prior to escalation of therapy. The presence of active erosive esophagitis usually is indicative of inadequate acid suppression and can almost always be treated successfully with higher proton pump inhibitor doses (eg, omeprazole 40 mg twice daily). Truly refractory esophagitis may be caused by gastrinoma with gastric acid hypersecretion (Zollinger-Ellison syndrome), pill-induced esophagitis, resistance to proton pump inhibitors, and medical noncompliance. Patients without endoscopically visible esophagitis should undergo esophageal pH monitoring to determine the amount of esophageal acid reflux and to assess whether the symptoms are acid related. If the pH study shows a normal amount of acid reflux, treatment with a low-dose tricyclic antidepressant (eg, imipramine or nortriptyline 25 mg at bedtime) may be beneficial. Where clinically available, impedance monitoring may be useful to document nonacid reflux.

B. SURGICAL TREATMENT

Surgical fundoplication affords good to excellent relief of symptoms and healing of esophagitis in over 85% of properly selected patients and may now be performed laparoscopically with low complication rates in most instances. Cost-effectiveness studies suggest that aggregate medical costs exceed surgical costs after 10 years. Although patient satisfaction is high, over 50% of patients require intermittent or continuous acid-suppression medication after fundoplication. Furthermore, over 30% of patients develop new symptoms of dysphagia, bloating, increased flatulence, or dyspepsia. Within 5–10 years after surgery, typical reflux symptoms occur in 10–30% of patients. Surgical treatment is not recommended for patients who are well controlled with medical therapies but should be considered (1) for otherwise healthy patients with extraesophageal manifestations of reflux, as these symptoms often require high doses of proton pump inhibitors and may be more effectively controlled with antireflux surgery; (2) for those with severe reflux disease who are unwilling to accept lifelong medical therapy due to its expense, inconvenience, or theoretical risks; and (3) for patients with erosive disease who are intolerant of or resistant to proton pump inhibitors.

C. ENDOSCOPIC THERAPY

There are three types of endoscopic modalities that are approved for the treatment of mild to moderate gastroesophageal reflux disease, one of which was recently removed from the market by the manufacturer. It is believed that these techniques may decrease the frequency of reflux events or the volume of refluxate by changing the anatomic or mechanical properties of the gastroesophageal junction. The first uses an endoscopic "sewing machine" to place sutures below the gastroesophageal junction in the region of the gastric cardia, creating a mucosal plication that may mimic a surgical fundoplication. The second uses an intraesophageal balloon catheter from which needle electrodes are inserted through the mucosa and into the muscularis at multiple levels of the distal esophagus and cardia, permitting application of radiofrequency wave current. It is believed that this current may disrupt neural reflex pathways from the stomach to the esophagus, resulting in a decrease in transient relaxations of the lower esophageal sphincter. The third involves endoscopic injection of a biocompatible, sponge-like nonresorbable polymer to bolster the lower esophageal sphincter. This compound was recently removed from the marketplace by the manufacturer because of complications. To date, two prospective controlled studies have been performed, which compared radiofrequency wave energy and polymer injection to sham therapy. After 3–6 months, more patients in the active treatment groups had improvement in heartburn and quality of life, but there were no differences in esophageal acid exposure times. The polymer injection also resulted in a reduced usage of proton pump inhibitors. Uncontrolled studies demonstrate modest improvement in symptoms and reduction in use of antisecretory medications, but less impact on esophageal acid reflux as assessed by pH testing. With all techniques, minor, temporary post-procedure adverse events (chest pain) are common, and rare but serious complications have occurred, including esophageal perforation and death. Pending further controlled clinical studies, endoluminal therapies are not recommended for routine clinical practice.

Armstrong D et al: Heartburn dominant, uninvestigated dyspepsia: a comparison of 'PPI-start' and 'H2-RA-start' management strategies in primary care—the CADET-HR study. Aliment Pharmacol Ther 2005;21:1189. [PMID: 15882239]

Barlow WJ et al: The pathogenesis of heartburn in nonerosive reflux disease: a unifying hypothesis. Gastroenterology 2005; 128:771. [PMID: 15765412]

Behm BW et al: Endoluminal therapies for gastroesophageal reflux disease. J Clin Gastroenterol 2004;38:209. [PMID: 15128065]

Boyce HW: Dilation of difficult benign esophageal strictures. Am J Gastroenterol 2005;100:744. [PMID: 15784012]

Charbel S et al: The role of esophageal pH monitoring in symptomatic patients on PPI therapy. Am J Gastroenterol 2005; 100:283. [PMID: 15667483]

Dean BB et al: Effectiveness of proton pump inhibitors in nonerosive reflux disease. Clin Gastroenterol Hepatol 2004; 2:656. [PMID: 15290657]

Fass R et al: Systematic review: proton-pump inhibitor failure in the gastro-oesophageal reflux disease—where next? Aliment Pharmacol Ther 2005;22:79. [PMID: 16011666]

Inadomi JM et al: PPI use in the OTC era: who to treat, with what, and for how long? Clin Gastroenterol Hepatol 2005; 3:208. [PMID: 15765438]

Johnson D et al: Heartburn severity underestimates erosive esophagitis severity in elderly patients with gastroesophageal reflux disease. Gastroenterology 2004;126:660. [PMID: 14988819]

Larghi A et al: EUS followed by EMR for staging of high-grade dysplasia and early cancer in Barrett's esophagus. Gastrointest Endosc 2005;62:16. [PMID: 15990814]

Lee TJ et al: Systematic review: is there excessive use of proton pump inhibitors in gastro-oesophageal reflux disease? Aliment Pharmacol Ther 2004;20:1241. [PMID: 15606386]

Peters FP et al: Endoscopic treatment of high-grade dysplasia and early stage cancer in Barrett's esophagus. Gastrointest Endosc 2005;61:506. [PMID: 15812401]

Sampliner R: Endoscopic ablative therapy for Barrett's esophagus: current status. Gastrointest Endosc 2004;59:66. [PMID: 14722550]

Shaheen N: Advances in Barrett's esophagus and esophageal adenocarcinoma. Gastroenterology 2005;128:1554. [PMID: 15887151]

Shaheen N: Raising the bar in studies of endoscopic anti-reflux procedures. Gastroenterology 2005;128:779. [PMID: 15765413]

Spechler S: The management of patients who have "failed" antireflux surgery. Am J Gastroenterol 2004;99:552. [PMID: 15056101]

Spechler S: Dysplasia in Barrett's esophagus: limitations of current management strategies. Am J Gastroenterol 2005;100: 927. [PMID: 15784042]

Tack J et al: Gastroesophageal reflux disease poorly responsive to single-dose proton pump inhibitors in patients without Barrett's esophagus: acid reflux, bile reflux, or both? Am J Gastroenterol 2004;99:981. [PMID: 15180713]

Tytgat GN: Management of mild and severe gastro-oesophageal reflux disease. Aliment Pharmacol Ther 2003;17(Suppl 2): 52. [PMID: 12786613]

Wolfsen HC: Present status of photodynamic therapy for high-grade dysplasia in Barrett's esophagus. J Clin Gastroenterol 2005;39:189. [PMID: 15718860]

INFECTIOUS ESOPHAGITIS

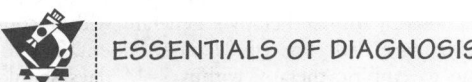

ESSENTIALS OF DIAGNOSIS

- Immunosuppressed patient.
- Odynophagia, dysphagia, and chest pain.
- Endoscopy with biopsy establishes diagnosis.

General Considerations

Infectious esophagitis occurs most commonly in immunosuppressed patients. Patients with AIDS, solid organ transplants, leukemia, lymphoma, and those receiving immunosuppressive drugs are at particular risk for opportunistic infections. *Candida albicans*, herpes simplex, and CMV are the most common pathogens. *Candida* infection may occur also in patients who have uncontrolled diabetes and those being treated with systemic corticosteroids, radiation therapy, or systemic antibiotic therapy. Herpes simplex can affect normal hosts, in which case the infection is generally self-limited.

Clinical Findings

A. Symptoms and Signs

The most common symptoms are odynophagia and dysphagia. Substernal chest pain occurs in some patients. Patients with candidal esophagitis are sometimes asymptomatic. Oral thrush is present in only 75% of patients with candidal esophagitis and 25–50% of patients with viral esophagitis and is therefore an unreliable indicator of the cause of esophageal infection. Patients with esophageal CMV infection may have infection at other sites such as the colon and retina. Oral ulcers (herpes labialis) are often associated with herpes simplex esophagitis.

B. Special Examinations

Treatment may be empiric. For diagnostic certainty, endoscopy with biopsy and brushings (for microbiologic and histopathologic analysis) is preferred because of its high diagnostic accuracy. The endoscopic signs of candidal esophagitis are diffuse, linear, yellow-white plaques adherent to the mucosa. CMV esophagitis is characterized by one to several large, shallow, superficial ulcerations. Herpes esophagitis results in multiple small, deep ulcerations.

Treatment

A. Candidal Esophagitis

Initial episodes of oropharyngeal candidiasis may be treated with clotrimazole troches (10 mg dissolved in mouth five times daily) or nystatin suspension (500,000 units five times daily), but systemic therapy is required for esophageal candidiasis. An empiric trial of antifungal therapy is often administered without performing diagnostic endoscopy. Initial therapy is generally with fluconazole, 100 mg/d orally for 14–21 days. Patients not responding to empiric therapy within 7–14 days should undergo endoscopy with brushings, biopsy, and culture to distinguish resistant fungal infection from other infections (eg, CMV, herpes). Esophageal candidiasis not responding to fluconazole therapy may be treated with itraconazole suspension (not capsules), 200 mg/d orally, or voriconazole, 200 mg twice daily. Refractory infection may be treated intravenously with caspofungin, 50 mg daily or amphotericin B, 0.3–0.7 mg/kg/d.

B. CYTOMEGALOVIRUS ESOPHAGITIS

In patients with HIV infection, immune restoration with highly active antiretroviral therapy (HAART) is the most effective means of controlling CMV disease. Initial therapy is with ganciclovir, 5 mg/kg intravenously every 12 hours for 3–6 weeks. Neutropenia is a frequent dose-limiting side effect. Once resolution of symptoms occurs, it may be possible to complete the course of therapy with oral valganciclovir, 900 mg once daily. Patients who either do not respond to or cannot tolerate ganciclovir are treated acutely with foscarnet, 90 mg/kg intravenously every 12 hours for 3–6 weeks. The principal toxicity is renal failure, hypocalcemia, and hypomagnesemia.

C. HERPETIC ESOPHAGITIS

Immunocompetent patients may be treated symptomatically and generally do not require specific antiviral therapy. Immunosuppressed patients may be treated with oral acyclovir, 400 mg orally five times daily, or 250 mg/m^2 intravenously every 8–12 hours, usually for 7–10 days. Famciclovir, 250 mg three times daily, and valacyclovir, 1 g twice daily, are effective but significantly more expensive than generic acyclovir. Nonresponders require therapy with foscarnet, 40 mg/kg intravenously every 8 hours for 21 days.

Prognosis

Most patients with infectious esophagitis can be effectively treated with complete symptom resolution. Depending on the patient's underlying immunodeficiency, relapse of symptoms off therapy can raise difficulties. Chronic suppressive therapy is sometimes required.

Bobak DA: Gastrointestinal infections caused by cytomegalovirus. Curr Infect Dis Rep 2003;5:101. [PMID: 12641994]

Pappas PG et al: Guidelines for the treatment of candidasis. Clin Infect Dis 2004;38:161. [PMID: 14699449]

Ramanathan J et al: Herpes simplex esophagitis in the immunocompetent host: an overview. Am J Gastroenterol 2000; 95: 2171. [PMID: 11007213]

Wilcox CM et al: Prospective comparison of brush cytology, viral culture, and histology for the diagnosis of ulcerative esophagitis in AIDS. Clin Gastroenterol Hepatol 2004;2:564. [PMID: 15224280]

PILL-INDUCED ESOPHAGITIS

A number of different medications may injure the esophagus, presumably through direct, prolonged mucosal contact. The most commonly implicated are the NSAIDs, potassium chloride pills, quinidine, zalcitabine, zidovudine, alendronate and risedronate, emepronium bromide, iron, vitamin C, and antibiotics (doxycycline, tetracycline, clindamycin, trimethoprim-sulfamethoxazole). Because injury is most likely to occur if pills are swallowed without water or while supine, hospitalized or bed-bound patients are at greater risk. Symptoms include severe retrosternal chest pain, odynophagia, and dysphagia, often beginning several hours after taking a pill. These may occur suddenly and persist for days. Some patients (especially the elderly) have relatively little pain, presenting with dysphagia. Endoscopy may reveal one to several discrete ulcers that may be shallow or deep. Chronic injury may result in severe esophagitis with stricture, hemorrhage, or perforation. Healing occurs rapidly when the offending agent is eliminated. To prevent pill-induced damage, patients should take pills with 4 oz of water and remain upright for 30 minutes after ingestion. Known offending agents should not be given to patients with esophageal dysmotility, dysphagia, or strictures.

Abid S et al: Pill-induced esophageal injury: endoscopic features and clinical outcomes. Endoscopy 2005;37:740. [PMID: 16032493]

Winstead NS et al: Pill esophagitis. Curr Treat Options Gastroenterol 2004;7:71. [PMID: 14723840]

CAUSTIC ESOPHAGEAL INJURY

Caustic esophageal injury occurs from accidental (usually children) or deliberate (suicidal) ingestion of liquid or crystalline alkali (drain cleaners, etc) or acid. Ingestion is followed almost immediately by severe burning and varying degrees of chest pain, gagging, dysphagia, and drooling. Aspiration results in stridor and wheezing. Initial examination should be directed to circulatory status and to prompt assessment of airway patency, including laryngoscopy. Subsequently, chest and abdominal radiographs are obtained looking for pneumonitis or free perforation. Initial treatment is supportive, with intravenous fluids and analgesics. Nasogastric lavage and oral antidotes may be dangerous and should generally not be administered. Most patients may be managed medically. Endoscopy is usually performed within the first 24 hours to assess the extent of injury. Many patients are discovered to have no mucosal injury to the esophagus or stomach, allowing prompt discharge and psychiatric referral. Patients with evidence of mild damage (edema, erythema, exudates or superficial ulcers) recover quickly, have low risk of developing stricture, and may be advanced from liquids to a regular diet over 24–48 hours. Nasoenteric feedings should be initiated after 24–48 hours and subsequent oral feedings when the patient is tolerating oral secretions. Patients with signs of severe injury—deep or circumferential ulcers or necrosis (black discoloration) have a high risk (up to 65%) of acute complications, including perforation with mediastinitis or peritonitis, bleeding, stricture, or esophageal-tracheal fistulas. These patients must be kept fasting and monitored closely for signs of deterioration that warrant emergency surgery with possible esophagectomy and colonic or jejunal interposition. A nasoenteric feeding tube is placed after 24 hours. Oral feedings of liquids may be initiated after 2–3 days if the patient is able to tolerate secretions. Neither corticosteroids nor antibiotics are recommended. Esophageal strictures develop in up to 70% of patients with serious esophageal injury weeks to months after the initial injury, requiring recurrent dilations. Endoscopic injection of intralesional corticosteroids (triamcinolone 40 mg) increases the interval between dilations. The risk of esophageal squamous carcinoma is 2–3%, warranting endoscopic surveillance 15–20 years after the caustic ingestion.

Ramasamy K et al: Corrosive ingestion in adults. J Clin Gastroenterol 2003;37:119. [PMID: 12869880]

Poley JW et al: Ingestion of acid and alkaline agents: outcome and prognostic value of early upper endoscopy. Gastrointest Endosc 2004;60:372. [PMID: 15332026]

BENIGN ESOPHAGEAL LESIONS

1. Mallory-Weiss Syndrome (Mucosal Laceration of Gastroesophageal Junction)

ESSENTIALS OF DIAGNOSIS

- *Hematemesis; usually self-limited.*
- *Prior history of vomiting, retching in 50%.*
- *Endoscopy establishes diagnosis.*

General Considerations

Mallory-Weiss syndrome is characterized by a nonpenetrating mucosal tear at the gastroesophageal junction that is hypothesized to arise from events that suddenly raise transabdominal pressure, such as lifting, retching, or vomiting. Alcoholism is a strong predisposing factor. Mallory-Weiss tears are responsible for approximately 5% of cases of upper gastrointestinal bleeding.

Clinical Findings

A. SYMPTOMS AND SIGNS

Patients usually present with hematemesis with or without melena. A history of retching, vomiting, or straining is obtained in about 50% of cases.

B. SPECIAL EXAMINATIONS

As with other causes of upper gastrointestinal hemorrhage, upper endoscopy should be performed after the patient has been appropriately resuscitated. The diagnosis is established by identification of a 0.5- to 4-cm linear mucosal tear usually located either at the gastroesophageal junction or, more commonly, just below the junction in the gastric mucosa.

Differential Diagnosis

At endoscopy, other potential causes of upper gastrointestinal hemorrhage are found in over 35% of patients with Mallory-Weiss tears, including peptic ulcer disease, erosive gastritis, arteriovenous malformations, and esophageal varices. Patients with underlying portal hypertension are at higher risk of continued or recurrent bleeding.

Treatment

Patients are initially treated as needed with fluid resuscitation and blood transfusions. Most patients stop bleeding spontaneously and require no therapy. Endoscopic hemostatic therapy is employed in patients who have continuing active bleeding. Injection with epinephrine (1:10,000), cautery with a bipolar or heater probe coagulation device, or mechanical compression of the artery by application of an endoclip or band is effective in 90–95% of cases. Angiographic arterial embolization or operative intervention is required in patients who fail endoscopic therapy.

Park CH et al: A prospective, randomized trial of endoscopic band ligation vs. epinephrine injection for actively bleeding Mallory-Weiss syndrome. Gastrointest Endosc 2004;60:22. [PMID: 15229420]

2. Esophageal Webs & Rings

Esophageal webs are thin, diaphragm-like membranes of squamous mucosa that typically occur in the mid or upper esophagus and may be multiple. They may be congenital but also occur with graft-versus-host disease, pemphigoid, epidermolysis bullosa, pemphigus vulgaris, and, rarely, in association with iron deficiency anemia (Plummer-Vinson syndrome). Esophageal "Schatzki" rings are smooth, circumferential, thin (< 4 mm in thickness) mucosal structures located in the distal esophagus at the squamocolumnar junction. Their pathogenesis is controversial. They are associated in nearly all cases with a hiatal hernia, and reflux symptoms are common, suggesting that acid gastroesophageal reflux may be contributory in many cases. Most webs and rings are over 20 mm in diameter and are asymptomatic. Solid food dysphagia most often occurs with rings less than 13 mm in diameter. Characteristically, dysphagia is intermittent and not progressive. Large poorly chewed food boluses such as beefsteak are most likely to cause symptoms. Obstructing boluses may pass by drinking extra liquids or after regurgitation. In some cases, an impacted bolus must be extracted endoscopically. Esophageal webs and rings are best visualized using a barium esophagogram with full esophageal distention. Endoscopy is less sensitive than barium esophagography.

The majority of symptomatic patients with a single ring or web can be effectively treated with the passage of a large (> 16-mm-diameter) bougie dilator to disrupt the lesion. A single dilation may suffice, but repeat dilations are required in many patients. Patients who have heartburn or who require repeated dilation should receive acid suppressive therapy with a chronic proton pump inhibitor.

Eosinophilic esophagitis is an entity that previously was recognized in children but is increasingly identified in young or middle-aged adults with dysphagia and food impactions. Barium swallowing studies may demonstrate a small-caliber esophagus, long and tapered strictures, or multiple concentric rings. Endoscopic appearances include multiple fine concentric rings, vertical furrowing, and whitish papules. Mucosal biopsy demonstrates multiple mucosal eosinophils. Optimal treatment is uncertain, but dietary restrictions and topical corticosteroids (fluticasone 220 mcg/puff swallow four puffs taken after inspiration, without a spacer twice daily after meals) are reported to be beneficial in uncontrolled trials. Graduated dilation of strictures should be conducted cautiously because there is an increased risk of perforation and postprocedural chest pain.

Arora AS et al: Eosinophilic esophagitis: asthma of the esophagus? Clin Gastroenterol Hepatol 2004;2:523. [PMID: 15224275]

Desai TK et al: Association of eosinophilic inflammation with esophageal food impaction in adults. Gastrointest Endosc 2005;61:795. [PMID: 15933677]

Ibrahim A et al: Schatzki's ring: to cut or break an unresolved problem. Dig Dis Sci 2004;49:379. [PMID: 15139484]

Sgouros SN et al: Long-term acid suppressive therapy may prevent the relapse of esophageal (Schatzki's) rings: a prospective, randomized, placebo-controlled study. Am J Gastroenterol 2005;100:1929. [PMID: 16128935]

3. Esophageal Diverticula

Zenker's Diverticulum

Zenker's diverticulum is a protrusion of pharyngeal mucosa that develops at the pharyngoesophageal junction between the inferior pharyngeal constrictor and the cricopharyngeus. The cause is believed to be loss of elasticity of the upper esophageal sphincter, resulting in restricted opening during swallowing. Symptoms of dysphagia and regurgitation tend to develop insidiously over years in older patients. Initial symptoms include vague oropharyngeal dysphagia with coughing or throat discomfort. As the diverticulum enlarges and retains food, patients may note halitosis, spontaneous regurgitation of undigested food, nocturnal choking, gurgling in the throat, or a protrusion in the neck. Complications include aspiration pneumonia, bronchiectasis, and lung abscess. The diagnosis is best established by a barium esophagogram.

Symptomatic patients require upper esophageal myotomy and, in most cases, surgical diverticulectomy. An intraluminal approach has been developed recently in which the septum between the esophagus and diverticulum is incised. Significant improvement occurs in over 90% of patients treated surgically. Small asymptomatic diverticula may be observed.

Altman JI et al: Fiberoptic endoscopic-assisted diverticulotomy: a novel technique for the management of Zenker's divertidulum. Ann Otol Rhinol Laryngol 2005;114:347. [PMID: 15966520]

Evrard S et al: Zenker's diverticulum: a new endoscopic treatment with a soft diverticulosope. Gastrointest Endosc 2003;58:116. [PMID: 12838237]

Van Overbeek JJ: Pathogenesis and methods of treatment of Zenker's diverticulum. Ann Otol Rhinol Laryngol 2003;112:583. [PMID: 12903677]

Esophageal Diverticula

Diverticula may occur in the mid or distal esophagus. These may arise secondary to motility disorders (diffuse esophageal spasm, achalasia) or may develop above esophageal strictures. Diverticula are seldom symptomatic. For patients with severe symptoms or pulmonary complications, surgical myotomy with or without diverticulectomy is the optimal treatment.

Cassivi SD et al: Diverticula of the esophagus. Surg Clin North Am 2005;85:494. [PMID: 15927646]

Michael H et al: Treatment of epiphrenic and mid-esophageal diverticula. Curr Treat Options Gastroenterol 2004;7:41. [PMID: 14723837]

4. Benign Esophageal Neoplasms

Benign tumors of the esophagus are quite rare. They are submucosal, the most common being leiomyoma. Most are asymptomatic and picked up incidentally on endoscopy or barium esophagography. Larger lesions can cause dysphagia, pain, and rarely ulceration with bleeding. The risk of malignant transformation is low. Therefore, the major clinical importance of these lesions is to distinguish them from malignant neoplasms. At endoscopy, a smooth, sessile nodule is observed with normal overlying mucosa. Because the lesion is submucosal, endoscopic biopsies are generally nonrevealing. Endoscopic ultrasonography is extremely helpful to confirm the submucosal origin of the tumor and to help distinguish benign leiomyomas from malignant leiomyosarcomas. Surgical (or in selected cases endoscopic) resection is indicated for lesions that are symptomatic, ulcerated, or increasing in size.

Lee LS et al: Current management of esophageal leiomyoma. J Am Coll Surg 2004;198:136. [PMID: 14698321]

5. Esophageal Varices

- *Develop secondary to portal hypertension.*
- *Found in 50% of patients with cirrhosis.*
- *One-third of patients with varices develop upper gastrointestinal bleeding.*
- *Diagnosis established by upper endoscopy.*

General Considerations

Esophageal varices are dilated submucosal veins that develop in patients with underlying portal hypertension and may result in serious upper gastrointestinal bleeding. The causes of portal hypertension are discussed in Chapter 15. Under normal circumstances, there is a 2–6 mm Hg pressure gradient between the portal vein and the inferior vena cava. When the gradient exceeds 12 mm Hg, significant portal hypertension exists. Esophageal varices are the most common cause of important gastrointestinal bleeding due to portal hypertension, though gastric varices and, rarely, intestinal varices may also bleed. Bleeding from esophageal varices most commonly occurs in the distal 5 cm of the esophagus.

The most common cause of portal hypertension is cirrhosis. Although approximately 50% of patients with cirrhosis have esophageal varices, only one-third of patients with varices develop serious bleeding from the varices. Bleeding esophageal varices have a higher morbidity and mortality rate than any other source of upper gastrointestinal bleeding. In the absence of treatment, the acute mortality from variceal hemorrhage is 30–50%; however, with current therapies, the mortality has been reduced to 20%.

A number of factors have been identified that may portend an increased risk of bleeding from esophageal varices. The most important are (1) the size of the varices; (2) the presence at endoscopy of red color signs on the varix (wale markings, hematocystic spots, or red spots); (3) the severity of liver disease (as assessed by Child scoring); and (4) active alcohol abuse—alcoholic cirrhotics who continue to drink have an extremely high risk of bleeding. The risk of bleeding correlates poorly with the absolute portosystemic pressure gradient, though bleeding almost never occurs with a gradient under 12 mm Hg.

Clinical Findings

A. Symptoms and Signs

Patients with bleeding esophageal varices present with symptoms and signs of acute gastrointestinal hemorrhage. (See Acute Upper Gastrointestinal Bleeding, above.) In some cases, there may be preceding retching or dyspepsia attributable to alcoholic gastritis or withdrawal. Varices per se do not cause symptoms of dyspepsia, dysphagia, or retching. Variceal bleeding usually is severe, resulting in hypovolemia manifested by postural vital signs or shock. Twenty percent of patients with chronic liver disease who develop bleeding—despite findings such as spider angiomas, asterixis, and ascites—do so from some other source.

B. Laboratory Findings

These are identical to those listed above in the section on acute upper gastrointestinal tract bleeding.

Initial Management

A. Acute Resuscitation

The initial management of patients with acute upper gastrointestinal bleeding is also discussed in the section on acute upper gastrointestinal bleeding (see above). Variceal hemorrhage is life-threatening; rapid assessment and resuscitation with fluids or blood products are essential. Overtransfusion should be avoided as it leads to increased central and portal venous pressures, increasing the risk of rebleeding. Many patients with bleeding esophageal varices have coagulopathy due to underlying cirrhosis; fresh frozen plasma (20 mL/kg loading dose, then 10 mg/kg every 6 hours) or platelets should be administered to patients with INRs > 1.8–2.0 or with platelet counts < 50,000/mcL in the presence of active bleeding. Patients with advanced liver disease are at high risk for poor outcome regardless of the bleeding source and should be transferred to an ICU. In 50% of cases, variceal hemorrhage stops spontaneously; without therapy, over half of these will rebleed within 1 week. The in-hospital mortality rate associated with bleeding esophageal varices is 15%.

B. Emergent Endoscopy

Emergent endoscopy is performed after the patient's hemodynamic status has been appropriately stabilized (usually within 2–12 hours). In patients with active bleeding, endotracheal intubation is commonly performed to protect against aspiration during endoscopy. An endoscopic examination is performed to exclude other or associated causes of upper gastrointestinal bleeding such as Mallory-Weiss tears, peptic ulcer disease, and portal hypertensive gastropathy. In many patients, variceal bleeding has stopped spontaneously by the time of endoscopy, and the diagnosis of variceal bleeding is made presumptively. Acute endoscopic treatment of the varices is performed with either banding or sclerotherapy. These techniques arrest active bleeding in 80–90% of patients and reduce by 50% (from 70%) the chance of early recurrent bleeding, but their impact on in-hospital mortality is less clear.

If banding is chosen, repeat sessions are scheduled at intervals of 1–3 weeks until the varices are obliterated or reduced to a small size. Banding achieves lower rates of rebleeding, complications, and death than sclerotherapy and should be considered the endoscopic treatment of choice.

Sclerotherapy is still preferred by some endoscopists in the actively bleeding patient (in whom visualization for banding may be difficult). Sclerotherapy is performed by injecting the variceal trunks with a sclerosing agent (eg, ethanolamine, tetradecyl sulfate). Complications occur in 20–30% of patients and include chest pain, fever, bacteremia, esophageal ulceration, stricture, and perforation. After initial treatment, band ligation therapy should be performed.

C. PHARMACOLOGIC THERAPY

1. Antibiotic prophylaxis—Cirrhotic patients admitted with upper gastrointestinal bleeding have a greater than 50% chance of developing a severe bacterial infection during hospitalization—such as bacterial peritonitis, pneumonia, or urinary tract infection—with or without sepsis. Most organisms causing infections are of gut origin. Prophylactic administration of antibiotics may reduce the risk of serious infection to 10–20% as well as hospital mortality. Although the optimal choice of antibiotic is uncertain, initial treatment with an intravenous quinolone antibiotic (ciprofloxacin 400 mg every 12 hours, levofloxacin 500 mg every 24 hours, or gatifloxacin 400 mg every 24 hours) followed after stabilization by an oral or nasogastric quinolone for 7–10 days may be recommended.

2.Vasoactive drugs—Somatostatin and octreotide infusions reduce portal pressures in ways that are poorly understood. Somatostatin (250 mcg/h)—not available in the United States—or octreotide (50 mcg intravenous bolus followed by 50 mcg/h) reduces splanchnic and hepatic blood flow and portal pressures in cirrhotic patients. Both agents appear to provide acute control of variceal bleeding in up to 80% of patients although neither has been shown to reduce mortality. Data about the absolute efficacy of both are conflicting, but they may be comparable in efficacy to endoscopic therapy. Combined treatment with octreotide or somatostatin infusion and endoscopic therapy (band ligation or sclerotherapy) is superior to either modality alone in controlling acute bleeding and early rebleeding, and it may improve survival. In patients with advanced liver disease and upper gastrointestinal hemorrhage, it is reasonable to initiate therapy with octreotide or somatostatin on admission and continue for 5 days. If bleeding is determined by endoscopy not to be secondary to portal hypertension, the infusion can be discontinued.

Terlipressin (not available in the United States) is a synthetic vasopressin analog that causes a significant and sustained reduction in portal and variceal pressures while preserving renal perfusion. It is superior to placebo in the control of acute variceal hemorrhage and reduces mortality by 34%. Where available, terlipressin may be preferred to somatostatin or octreotide.

Terlipressin is contraindicated in patients with significant coronary, cerebral, or peripheral vascular disease.

3. Vitamin K—In cirrhotic patients with an abnormal prothrombin time, vitamin K (10 mg) should be administered subcutaneously.

4. Lactulose—Encephalopathy may complicate an episode of gastrointestinal bleeding in patients with severe liver disease. In patients with encephalopathy, lactulose should be administered in a dosage of 30–45 mL/h orally until evacuation occurs, then reduced to 15–45 mL/h every 8–12 hours as needed to promote two or three bowel movements daily. (See Chapter 15.)

D. BALLOON TUBE TAMPONADE

Mechanical tamponade with specially designed nasogastric tubes containing large gastric and esophageal balloons (Minnesota or Sengstaken-Blakemore tubes) provides initial control of active variceal hemorrhage in 60–90% of patients; rebleeding occurs in 50%. The gastric balloon is inflated first, followed by the esophageal balloon if bleeding continues. After balloon inflation, tension is applied to the tube to directly tamponade the varices. Complications of prolonged balloon inflation include esophageal and oral ulcerations, perforation, aspiration, and airway obstruction (due to a misplaced balloon). Endotracheal intubation is recommended before placement. Given its high rate of complications, mechanical tamponade is used as a temporizing measure only in patients with bleeding that cannot be controlled with pharmacologic or endoscopic techniques until more definitive decompressive therapy (eg, TIPS; see below) can be provided.

E. PORTAL DECOMPRESSIVE PROCEDURES

In patients with variceal bleeding that cannot be controlled with pharmacologic or endoscopic therapy, emergency portal decompression may be considered.

1. Transvenous intrahepatic portosystemic shunts—Over a wire that is passed through the catheter inserted in the jugular vein, an expandable wire mesh stent (8–12 mm in diameter) is passed through the liver parenchyma, creating a portosystemic shunt from the portal vein to the hepatic vein. TIPS can control acute hemorrhage in over 90% of patients actively bleeding from gastric or esophageal varices. However, when TIPS is performed in the actively bleeding patient, the mortality approaches 40%, especially in patients requiring ventilatory support or blood pressure support and patients with renal insufficiency, bilirubin > 3.0 mg/dL, or encephalopathy. Therefore, TIPS should be considered in the 5–10% of patients with acute variceal bleeding that cannot be controlled with pharmacologic and endoscopic therapy, but it may not be warranted in patients with a poor prognosis.

2. Emergency portosystemic shunt surgery—Emergency portosystemic shunt surgery is associated with a 40–60% mortality rate. At centers where TIPS is available, that procedure has become the preferred means of providing emergency portal decompression.

Prevention of Rebleeding

Once the initial bleeding episode has been controlled, the risk of rebleeding is 50–70% without further therapy. The highest incidence of rebleeding is in the first 6 weeks. Several options are available to decrease the likelihood of rebleeding, though their relative merits are controversial. Use of these approaches varies in different medical centers.

A. Endoscopic Techniques

Long-term treatment with band ligation reduces the incidence of rebleeding to 20–50%; the mortality rate may also be reduced. Band ligation of the varix appears to be equal or superior to sclerotherapy in preventing rebleeding and is associated with a significantly lower complication rate. In most patients, four to six treatment sessions are needed to eradicate the varices.

B. β-Blockers and Nitrates

Nonselective β-adrenergic blockers (propranolol, nadolol) are effective in reducing the incidence of rebleeding from esophageal varices and portal hypertensive gastropathy compared with placebo. Some—but not all—studies demonstrate a lower incidence of rebleeding with band ligation than with β-adrenergic blockers. Thus, the choice between β-blockers and endoscopic therapy to prevent recurrent variceal bleeding is not established and depends on local experience. Compliant patients with well-compensated liver disease may be optimal candidates for therapy with β-blockers alone. Most others may be offered endoscopic variceal banding where available. A combination of band ligation plus β-blockers further reduces the rate of recurrent bleeding compared with ligation alone (14% vs 38%). Therefore, patients without contraindications to β-blockers may be given propranolol, 20–40 mg twice daily, long-acting propranolol, 60–80 mg once daily, or nadolol, 40 mg once daily, increasing the dosage every 1–2 weeks until the heart rate falls by 25% or reaches 55 beats/min, provided the systolic blood pressure remains above 90 mm Hg and the patient has no side effects. The average dosage of propranolol is 120 mg daily and for nadolol, 80 mg daily. One-third of patients with cirrhosis are intolerant of β-blockers, experiencing fatigue or hypotension. Drug administration at bedtime may reduce the frequency and severity of side effects.

C. Transvenous Intrahepatic Portosystemic Shunt

TIPS has resulted in a significant reduction in recurrent bleeding compared with endoscopic sclerotherapy or band ligation—either alone or in combination with β-blocker therapy. At 1 year, rebleeding rates in patients treated with TIPS versus various endoscopic therapies average 20% and 40%, respectively. However, TIPS was also associated with a higher incidence of encephalopathy (35% versus 15%) and did not result in a decrease in mortality. Another limitation of TIPS is that stenosis and thrombosis of the stents occur in the majority of patients over time with a consequent risk of rebleeding. Therefore, periodic monitoring with Doppler ultrasonography or hepatic venography is required. Stent patency usually can be maintained by balloon angioplasty or additional stent placement. Given these problems, TIPS should be reserved for patients who have recurrent (two or more) episodes of variceal bleeding that have failed endoscopic or pharmacologic therapies. TIPS is also useful in patients with recurrent bleeding from gastric varices or portal hypertensive gastropathy (for which endoscopic therapies cannot be used). TIPS is likewise considered in patients who are noncompliant with other therapies or who live in remote locations (without access to emergency care).

D. Surgical Portosystemic Shunts

Shunt surgery has a significantly lower rate of rebleeding compared with endoscopic therapy but also a higher incidence of encephalopathy. With the advent and widespread adoption of TIPS, surgical shunts are seldom performed.

E. Liver Transplantation

Candidacy for orthotopic liver transplantation should be assessed in all patients with chronic liver disease and bleeding due to portal hypertension. Transplant candidates should be treated with band ligation or TIPS to control bleeding pretransplant.

Prevention of First Episodes of Variceal Bleeding

Because of the high mortality rate associated with variceal hemorrhage, prevention of the initial bleeding episode is desirable. Therefore, patients with cirrhosis should undergo diagnostic endoscopy to determine whether varices are present. The risk of bleeding in patients with small varices (< 5 mm) is 5% per year and with large varices is 15–20% per year. Either nonselective β-adrenergic blockers (nadolol, propranolol) or prophylactic band ligation decrease the absolute risk of variceal bleeding by approximately 10% per year and reduce mortality by almost 5%. In meta-analysis of comparative studies of banding versus β-blockers, banding appears to reduce the risk of variceal bleeding slightly but not the risk of mortality. However, because endoscopy is invasive and more expensive, a trial of β-blockers is recommended as initial therapy for compliant patients with large varices or medium varices with red color markings. For patients with small or absent varices, no prophylaxis is necessary but endoscopy should be repeated in 1–2 years. For patients with contraindications to or intolerance of β-blockers, prophylactic treatment with band ligation should be considered.

Boyer T et al; American Association for the Study of Liver Diseases: The role of transjugular intrahepatic portosystemic shunt in the management of portal hypertension. Hepatology 2005;41:386. [PMID: 15660434]

De Franchis R: Incidental esophageal varices. Gastroenterology 2004;126:1860. [PMID: 15188180]

De la Pena J et al: Variceal ligation plus nadolol compared with ligation for prophylaxis of variceal rebleeding: a multicenter trial. Hepatology 2005;41:572. [PMID: 15726659]

Gotzsche PC et al: Somatostatin analogues for acute bleeding oesophageal varices. Cochrane Database Syst Rev 2005;(1): CD000193. [PMID: 15674868]

Ioannou G et al: Terlipressin for acute esophageal variceal hemorrhage. Cochrane Database Syst Rev 2003;(1):CD002147. [PMID: 12535432]

Jutabha R et al: Randomized study comparing banding and propranolol to prevent initial variceal hemorrhage in cirrhotics with high-risk esophageal varices. Gastroenterology 2005; 128:870. [PMID: 15825071]

Kamath PS: Esophageal variceal bleeding: primary prophylaxis. Clin Gastroenterol Hepatol 2005;3:90. [PMID: 15645410]

Khuroo MS et al: Meta-analysis: endoscopic variceal ligation for primary prophylaxis of oesophageal variceal bleeding. Aliment Pharmacol Ther 2005;21:347. [PMID: 15709985]

Mihas AA et al: Recurrent variceal bleeding despite endoscopic and medical therapy. Gastroenterology 2004;127:621. [PMID: 15300593]

Nevens F: Review article: a critical comparison of drug therapies in currently used therapeutic strategies for variceal hemorrhage. Aliment Pharmacol Ther 2004;20(Suppl 3):18. [PMID: 15335394]

Qureshi W et al; Standards of Practice Committee: ASGE Guideline: the role of endoscopy in the management of variceal hemorrhage, updated July 2005. Gastrointest Endosc 2005; 62:651. [PMID: 16246673]

Sarin SK et al: Endoscopic variceal ligation plus propranolol versus endoscopic variceal ligation alone in primary prophylaxis of variceal bleeding. Am J Gastroenterol 2005;100: 797. [PMID: 15784021]

ESOPHAGEAL CANCER

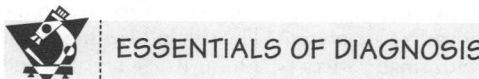

ESSENTIALS OF DIAGNOSIS

- *Progressive solid food dysphagia.*
- *Weight loss common.*
- *Endoscopy with biopsy establishes diagnosis.*

General Considerations

Esophageal cancer usually develops in persons between 50 and 70 years of age. The overall ratio of men to women is 3:1. There are two histologic types: squamous cell carcinoma and adenocarcinoma. In the United States, squamous cell cancer is much more common in blacks than in whites. Chronic alcohol and tobacco use are strongly associated with an increased risk of squamous cell carcinoma. The risk of squamous cell cancer is also increased in patients with tylosis (a rare disease transmitted by autosomal dominant inheritance and manifested by hyperkeratosis of the palms and soles), achalasia, caustic-induced esophageal stricture, and other head and neck cancers. Squamous cell cancer has a high incidence in certain regions of China and Southeast Asia. Half of all cases occur in the distal third of the esophagus. Adenocarcinoma is more common in whites. It is increasing dramatically in incidence and now is as common as squamous carcinoma. The majority of adenocarcinomas develop as a complication of Barrett's metaplasia due to chronic gastroesophageal reflux. Thus, most adenocarcinomas arise in the distal third of the esophagus. Obesity also is strongly associated with adenocarcinoma, even after controlling for gastroesophageal reflux; however, no causal relationship has been convincingly shown.

Clinical Findings

A. SYMPTOMS AND SIGNS

Most patients with esophageal cancer present with advanced, incurable disease. Over 90% have solid food dysphagia, which progresses over weeks to months. Odynophagia is sometimes present. Significant weight loss is common. Local tumor extension into the tracheobronchial tree may result in a tracheoesophageal fistula, characterized by coughing on swallowing or pneumonia. Chest or back pain suggests mediastinal extension. Recurrent laryngeal involvement may produce hoarseness. Physical examination is often unrevealing. The presence of supraclavicular or cervical lymphadenopathy or of hepatomegaly implies metastatic disease.

B. LABORATORY FINDINGS

Laboratory findings are nonspecific. Anemia related to chronic disease or occult blood loss is common. Elevated aminotransferase or alkaline phosphatase concentrations suggest hepatic or bony metastases. Hypoalbuminemia may result from malnutrition.

C. IMAGING

Chest x-rays may show adenopathy, a widened mediastinum, pulmonary or bony metastases, or signs of tracheoesophageal fistula such as pneumonia. A barium esophagogram is obtained as the first study to evaluate dysphagia. The appearance of a polypoid, infiltrative, or ulcerative lesion is suggestive of carcinoma and requires endoscopic evaluation. However, even lesions felt to be benign by radiography warrant endoscopic evaluation.

D. UPPER ENDOSCOPY

Endoscopy with biopsy establishes the diagnosis of esophageal carcinoma with a high degree of reliability. In some cases, significant submucosal spread of the tumor may yield nondiagnostic mucosal biopsies. Repeated biopsy may be necessary.

Differential Diagnosis

Esophageal carcinoma must be distinguished from other causes of progressive dysphagia, including peptic stricture, achalasia, and adenocarcinoma of the gastric cardia with esophageal involvement. Benign-appearing peptic strictures should be biopsied at presentation to exclude occult malignancy.

Staging of Disease

After confirmation of the diagnosis of esophageal carcinoma, the stage of the disease should be determined since doing so influences the choice of therapy. Patients should undergo evaluation with CT of the chest and liver to look for evidence of pulmonary or hepatic metastases, lymphadenopathy, and local tumor extension. If there is no evidence of distant metastases or extensive local spread on CT, endoscopic ultrasonography with guided fine-needle aspiration (FNA) biopsy of lymph nodes should be performed, which is superior to CT in demonstrating the level of local mediastinal extension and local lymph node involvement. Positron emission tomography imaging with fluorodeoxyglucose is used increasingly to look for regional or distant spread in patients thought to have localized disease after other diagnostic studies. Bronchoscopy is sometimes required in proximal esophageal cancer to exclude tracheobronchial extension. Apart from distant metastasis, the two most important predictors of poor survival are lymph node involvement and adjacent mediastinal spread.

Stages are determined by the TNM classification as set forth in the accompanying box.

Treatment

The approach to esophageal cancer depends on the tumor stage, patient preference and functional status, and the expertise of the attending surgeons, oncologists, gastroenterologists, and radiotherapists. There is no consensus about the optimal treatment approach. It is helpful, however, to classify patients into two general categories.

A. PALLIATIVE THERAPY

Patients with extensive local tumor spread (T4) or distant metastases (M1) are incurable, ie, patients with stage IIIB and stage IV tumors. Surgery is not warranted in these patients. The goal is to provide relief from dysphagia and pain, and the optimal palliative approach depends on the patient's expected survival, patient preference, and local institutional experience. None of the modalities prolongs survival, and many patients may prefer concerted efforts at pain relief and care directed at symptom management (see Chapter 5).

1. Radiation or chemoradiation therapy—Combined radiation therapy and chemotherapy may achieve palliation in two-thirds of patients but is associated with significant side effects. It should be consid-

---

STAGING CRITERIA FOR ESOPHAGEAL CANCER

Primary Tumor (T)

T1: Invasion of lamina propria or submucosa
T2: Invasion of muscularis propria
T3: Invasion of adventitia
T4: Invasion of adjacent structures

Regional Lymph Nodes

N0: No regional lymph node involvement
N1: Regional lymph node involvement

Distant Metastasis (M)

M0: No metastasis
M1: Distant metastasis
M1a: Cervical or celiac lymph nodes
M1b: Other distant metastasis

Based upon these parameters, the tumor is classified as:

Stage I: T1, N0, M0
Stage IIA: T2 or T3, and N0, M0
Stage IIB: T1 or T2, and N1, M0
Stage IIIA: T3, N1, M0
Stage IIIB: T4, Any N, M0
Stage IVA: Any T, Any N, M1a
Stage IVB: Any T, Any N, M1b

---

ered for patients with a good functional status without other significant medical problems. Radiation therapy alone may afford significant short-term relief of pain and dysphagia and may be suitable for patients with poor functional status or underlying medical problems. During therapy, esophagitis may lead to worsening of dysphagia and odynophagia.

2. Local antitumor therapy—Patients with advanced esophageal cancer may have a poor functional and nutritional status and an average survival of less than 12 weeks from diagnosis. Radiation or chemoradiation is poorly tolerated. Rapid palliation of dysphagia may be achieved by peroral placement of permanent expandable wire stents, application of endoscopic laser therapy, or photodynamic therapy. Although dysphagia and quality of life are improved significantly, patients can seldom eat normally. Complications of stents occur in 20–40% and include perforation, migration, and tumor ingrowth. These are most suitable for patients with a short life expectancy, patients with tracheoesophageal fistula, patients who have failed radiation therapy, or patients in locations where optimal surgical or radiation modalities are not available. Laser therapy (Nd:YAG laser) maintains luminal patency in up to 90% of patients but involves multiple treatment sessions and can be difficult to administer. Photodynamic therapy has been shown to be superior to laser therapy. A photosensitizing agent (porfimer sodium) in combination with a low-power 630-nm laser results in significant tumor necrosis. Side effects include sun sensitivity of the skin for 4–6 weeks and the development of esophageal stricture. Both laser therapy and photodynamic therapy require expensive equipment that is not available at many institutions.

B. "Curable" Disease

For a discussion of the treatment options for early-stage adenocarcinoma arising in Barrett's esophagus that appears on EUS to be limited to the mucosa, see the section on Barrett's Esophagus. For all other potentially "curable" esophageal cancers (stage I, II, or IIIA), the approach to therapy depends on institutional experience.

1. Surgery with or without neoadjuvant chemoradiation therapy—There is controversy over the optimal surgical approach. The procedure with the lowest morbidity is transhiatal esophagectomy with anastomosis of the stomach to the cervical esophagus; however, this approach does not involve sampling or removal of mediastinal lymph nodes. Alternatively, many surgeons recommend extended en bloc transthoracic excision of the esophagus extended dissection of lymph nodes in the mediastinum and upper abdomen. In a randomized controlled trial comparing these two approaches, en bloc resection was associated with higher perioperative morbidity but a nonsignificant trend toward improved 5-year survival (39% vs 27%). Transhiatal resection may be more appropriate for patients who are elderly or have comorbid illness and en bloc resection may be more appropriate in younger or healthier patients with a better prognosis.

Patients with stage I and stage IIA cancer have high cure rates with surgery alone and require no other radiation or chemotherapy. Lymph node spread is the most important preditor of survival. If lymph node metastases have occurred (stage IIB and stage IIIA), the rate of cure with surgery alone is reduced to less than 10%. Trials of adjuvant (postoperative) or neoadjuvant (preoperative) radiation therapy or chemotherapy have not demonstrated benefits over surgery alone. However, a combination radiation therapy and chemotherapy (cisplatin and fluorouracil) given before surgery results in complete pathologic remission (no evidence of tumor at the time of surgery) in up to 25% of patients. A meta-analysis of trials comparing neoadjuvant chemoradiation plus surgery to surgery alone concluded that neoadjuvant therapy decreased local and regional tumor recurrence and increased 3-year survival. However, there is significant morbidity associated with chemoradiation therapy. Therefore, multimodal treatment (neoadjuvant chemoradiation plus surgery) remains controversial but may be considered in young patients without other comorbid illnesses, preferably in the context of a clinical trial.

2. Chemotherapy plus radiation therapy—Combined therapy with chemotherapy and radiation therapy is superior to radiation therapy alone and has achieved overall survival rates that equal or exceed those of historical surgical cohorts, though there have been no trials specifically comparing these approaches. However, severe side effects occur commonly with combined therapy. The most promising chemotherapeutic agents have been cisplatin and fluorouracil. Chemoradiation therapy alone should be considered in patients with localized disease (stage II or IIIA) who are poor surgical candidates due to serious medical illness or poor functional status (ECOG score > 2).

Prognosis

The overall 5-year survival rate of esophageal carcinoma is less than 15%. Despite improvements in surgical mortality and increased surgical resectability rates, the prognosis of this disease has not changed for years, in part because most patients present with advanced disease. This suggests that surgical approaches alone are inadequate for most patients. For those patients whose disease progresses despite chemotherapy, meticulous efforts at palliative care are essential (see Chapter 5).

Enzinger PC et al: Esophageal cancer. N Engl J Med 2003; 349:2241. [PMID: 14657432]

Fiorica F et al: Preoperative chemoradiotherapy for oesophageal cancer: a systematic review and meta-analysis. Gut 2004; 53:925. [PMID: 15194636]

Hulscher JB et al: Extended transthoracic resection compared with limited transhiatal resection for adenocarcinoma of the esophagus. N Engl J Med 2002;347:1662. [PMID: 12444180]

Malthaner RA et al: Neoadjuvant or adjuvant therapy for resectable esophageal cancer: a clinical practice guideline. BMC Cancer 2004;4:67. [PMID: 15447791]

National Cancer Institute Esophageal Cancer home page: http://www.cancer.gov/cancerinfo/types/esophageal.

Vazquez-Sequeiros E et al: Impact of lymph node staging on therapy of esophageal carcinoma. Gastroenterology 2003; 125:1626. [PMID: 14724814]

Wang KK et al; American Gastroenterological Association: American Gastroenterological Association medical position statement: Role of the gastroenterologist in the management of esophageal carcinoma. Gastroenterology 2005;128:1468. [PMID: 15887128]

Wang KK et al: American Gastroenterological Association Technical Review on the role of the gastroenterologist in the management of esophageal carcinoma. Gastroenterology 2005;128:1471. [PMID: 15887129]

Weber WA et al: Imaging of esophageal and gastric cancer. Semin Oncol 2004;31:530. [PMID: 15297944]

ESOPHAGEAL MOTILITY DISORDERS

1. Achalasia

ESSENTIALS OF DIAGNOSIS

- *Gradual, progressive dysphagia for solids and liquids.*

- *Regurgitation of undigested food.*
- *Barium esophagogram with "bird's beak" distal esophagus.*
- *Esophageal manometry confirms diagnosis.*

General Considerations

Achalasia is an idiopathic motility disorder characterized by loss of peristalsis in the distal two-thirds (smooth muscle) of the esophagus and impaired relaxation of the lower esophageal sphincter. There appears to be denervation of the esophagus resulting primarily from loss of nitric oxide-producing inhibitory neurons in the myenteric plexus. The cause of the neuronal degeneration is unknown.

Clinical Findings

A. SYMPTOMS AND SIGNS

There is a steady increase in the incidence of achalasia with age; however, it can be seen in individuals as young as 25 years. Patients complain of the gradual onset of dysphagia for solid foods and, in the majority, of liquids also. Symptoms at presentation may have persisted for months to years. Substernal discomfort or fullness may be noted after eating. Many patients eat more slowly and adopt specific maneuvers such as lifting the neck or throwing the shoulders back to enhance esophageal emptying. Regurgitation of undigested food is common and may occur during meals or up to several hours later. Nocturnal regurgitation can provoke coughing or aspiration. Up to 50% of patients report substernal chest pain that is unrelated to meals or exercise and may last up to hours. Weight loss is common. Physical examination is unhelpful.

B. IMAGING

Chest x-rays may show an air-fluid level in the enlarged, fluid-filled esophagus. Barium esophagography discloses characteristic findings, including esophageal dilation, loss of esophageal peristalsis, poor esophageal emptying, and a smooth, symmetric "bird's beak" tapering of the distal esophagus. Without treatment, the esophagus may become markedly dilated ("sigmoid esophagus").

C. SPECIAL EXAMINATIONS

After esophagography, endoscopy is always performed to evaluate the distal esophagus and gastroesophageal junction to exclude a distal stricture or a submucosal infiltrating carcinoma. The diagnosis is confirmed by esophageal manometry. The typical manometric features are as follows: (1) Complete absence of peristalsis; swallowing results in simultaneous waves that are usually of low amplitude. (2) Incomplete lower esophageal sphincteric relaxation with swallowing. Whereas the normal sphincter relaxes by over 90%, relaxation with most swallows in patients with achalasia is less than 50%. In many patients, the baseline lower esophageal sphincteric pressure is quite elevated. (3) Intraesophageal pressures are greater than gastric pressures due to a fluid- and food-filled esophagus.

Differential Diagnosis

Chagas' disease is associated with esophageal dysfunction that is indistinguishable from idiopathic achalasia and should be considered in patients from endemic regions (Central and South America); it is becoming more common in the southern United States. Primary or metastatic tumors can invade the gastroesophageal junction, resulting in a picture resembling that of achalasia, called "pseudoachalasia." Endoscopic ultrasonography and chest CT may be required to examine the distal esophagus in suspicious cases. Tumors such as small cell lung cancer can cause a paraneoplastic syndrome resembling achalasia due to secretion of antineuronal nuclear antibodies (ANNA-1 or Anti-Hu) that affect the myenteric plexus. Achalasia must be distinguished from other motility disorders such as diffuse esophageal spasm and scleroderma esophagus with a peptic stricture.

Treatment

A. BOTULINUM TOXIN INJECTION

Endoscopically guided injection of botulinum toxin directly into the lower esophageal sphincter results in a marked reduction in lower esophageal sphincter pressure with initial improvement in symptoms in 65–85% of patients. However, symptom relapse occurs in over 50% of patients within 6–9 months and in all patients within 2 years. Three-fourths of initial responders who relapse have improvement with repeated injections. Because it is inferior to pneumatic dilation therapy and surgery in producing sustained symptomatic relief, this therapy is most appropriate for patients with comorbidities who are poor candidates for more invasive procedures.

B. PNEUMATIC DILATION

Between 75% and 85% of patients derive good to excellent relief of dysphagia after one to three sessions of pneumatic dilation of the lower esophageal sphincter and between 50% and 70% of patients achieve long-term relief. Perforations occur in less than 3% of dilations and may require operative repair.

C. SURGICAL MYOTOMY

A modified Heller cardiomyotomy of the lower esophageal sphincter and cardia results in good to excellent symptomatic improvement in over 85% of patients. Because gastroesophageal reflux may develop in up to 20% of patients after myotomy, most surgeons also perform an antireflux procedure (fundoplication). Myotomy is now performed with a laparoscopic approach and is preferred to the open surgical approach. Indeed, the low morbidity of laparoscopic surgery has led some experts to recommend it for initial treatment. In experienced hands, the initial efficacies of pneumatic dilation and laparoscopic myotomy are nearly equivalent. Analysis indicates that pneumatic dilation may be a more cost-effective strategy than either botulinum toxin injection or laparoscopic myotomy. The success of laparoscopic surgery is not compromised by prior therapy with either botulinum injection or pneumatic dilation.

Farhoomand K et al: Predictors of outcome of pneumatic dilation in achalsia. Clin Gastroenterol Hepatol 2004;2:389. [PMID: 15118976]

Karamanolis G et al: Long-term outcome of pneumatic dilation in the treatment of achalasia. Am J Gastroenterol 2005;100:270. [PMID: 15667481]

Mikaeli J et al: Pneumatic balloon dilation in achalasia: a prospective comparison of safety and efficacy with different balloon diameters. Aliment Pharmacol Ther 2004;20:431. [PMID: 15298637]

Park W et al: Etiology and pathogenesis of achalasia: the current understanding. Am J Gastroenterol 2005;100:1404. [PMID: 15929777]

Vela MF et al: Complexities of managing achalasia at a tertiary referral center: use of pneumatic dilation, Heller myotomy, and botulinum toxin injection. Am J Gastroenterol 2004; 99:1029. [PMID: 15180721]

2. Other Primary Esophageal Motility Disorders

Abnormalities in esophageal motility may cause dysphagia or chest pain. Dysphagia for liquids as well as solids tends to be intermittent and nonprogressive. Periods of normal swallowing may alternate with periods of dysphagia, which usually is mild though bothersome—rarely severe enough to result in significant alterations in lifestyle or weight loss. Dysphagia may be provoked by stress, large boluses of food, or hot or cold liquids. Some patients may experience anterior chest pain that may be confused with angina pectoris but usually is nonexertional. The pain generally is unrelated to eating. (See Chest Pain of Undetermined Origin, below.)

The evaluation of suspected esophageal motility disorders includes barium esophagography, upper endoscopy, and, in some cases, esophageal manometry. Barium esophagography is useful to exclude mechanical obstruction and to evaluate esophageal motility. The presence of simultaneous contractions (spasm), disordered peristalsis, or failed peristalsis supports a diagnosis of esophageal dysmotility. Upper endoscopy also is performed to exclude a mechanical obstruction (as a cause of dysphagia) and to look for evidence of erosive reflux esophagitis (a common cause of chest pain) or eosinophilic esophagitis (confirmed by esophageal biopsy).

The further evaluation of noncardiac chest pain is discussed in a subsequent section. Manometry should not be routinely used for mild to moderate symptoms because the findings seldom influence further medical management. For patients with disabling symptoms of dysphagia, stationary esophageal manometry should be performed. Based on the findings of esophageal manometry, the following conditions may be diagnosed: (1) Diffuse esophageal spasm: normal primary peristalsis with ≥ 20% simultaneous contractions of > 30 mm Hg contraction amplitude. (2) Nutcracker esophagus: normal peristalsis but increased duration and high amplitude of distal contractions (> 180 mm Hg). (3) Hypertensive lower esophageal sphincter: elevated lower esophageal sphincter pressure (> 45 mm Hg) with normal peristalsis. (4) Ineffective esophageal motility: > 30% of swallows resulting in failed or interrupted peristalsis or distal esophageal hypocontraction (< 30 mm Hg contraction amplitude).

For patients with mild symptoms, therapy is directed at symptom reduction and reassurance. Patients with dysphagia should be instructed to eat more slowly and take smaller bites of food. In some cases, a warm liquid at the start of a meal may facilitate swallowing. Gastroesophageal reflux should be identified and treated. Treatment of more severe cases with nitrates (isosorbide, 10–20 mg four times daily) or nitroglycerin (0.4 mg sublingually as needed) and calcium channel blockers (nifedipine 10 mg or diltiazem 60–90 mg, 30–45 minutes before meals) may be tried; their efficacy is unproved. Injection of botulinum toxin into the lower esophagus may improve chest pain and dysphagia in over 70% for a limited time. For unclear reasons, dilation with esophageal Maloney bougies provides symptomatic relief in some cases. In debilitated patients, a long surgical myotomy (which may be performed via a thoracoscopic approach) may lead to improvement in 70–80% of cases.

Bajaj JS et al: Esophageal veggie spasms: a food-specific cause of chest distress. Am J Gastroenterol 2004;99:1396. [PMID: 15233683]

Miller LS et al: Treatment of chest pain in patients with noncardiac, nonreflux, nonachalasia spastic esophageal motor disorders using botulinum toxin injection into the gastroesophageal junction. Am J Gastroenterol 2002;97:1640. [PMID: 12135012]

Richter JE: Oesophageal motility disorders. Lancet 2001;358: 823. [PMID: 11564508]

Spechler S et al: Classification of oesophageal motility abnormalities. Gut 2001;49:145. [PMID: 11413123]

Tutuian R et al: Combined multichannel intraluminal impedance and manometry clarifies esophageal function abnormalities: study in 350 patients. Am J Gastroenterol 2004; 99:1020. [PMID: 15180718]

CHEST PAIN OF UNDETERMINED ORIGIN

One-third of patients with chest pain undergo negative cardiac evaluation. Patients with recurrent noncardiac chest pain thus pose a difficult clinical problem. Because coronary artery disease is common and can present atypically, it must be excluded prior to evaluation for other causes.

Causes of noncardiac chest pain may include the following.

A. CHEST WALL AND THORACIC SPINE DISEASE

These are easily diagnosed by history and physical examination.

B. GASTROESOPHAGEAL REFLUX

Up to 50% of patients have increased amounts of gastroesophageal acid reflux or a correlation between acid reflux episodes and chest pain demonstrated on esophageal pH testing. An empiric 8-week trial of acid-suppressive therapy with a high-dose proton pump inhibitor is recommended (eg, omeprazole or rabeprazole, 40 mg twice daily; lansoprazole, 30–60 mg twice daily; or esomeprazole or pantoprazole, 40 mg twice-daily), especially in patients with reflux symptoms. Symptomatic improvement strongly suggests that the pain is due to acid esophageal reflux. The sensitivity and specificity of this treatment are 78% and 80%, respectively, compared with therapy based on results of esophageal pH testing. In patients with persistent symptoms, an ambulatory esophageal pH study while continuing antisecretory therapy is useful to definitively exclude a relationship between acid reflux episodes and chest pain events.

C. HEIGHTENED VISCERAL SENSITIVITY

Studies suggest that many patients with noncardiac chest pain report pain in response to a variety of minor noxious stimuli such as intraesophageal acid infusion, inflation of balloons within the esophageal lumen, injection of intravenous edrophonium (a cholinergic stimulus), or intracardiac catheter manipulation. Low doses of antidepressants such as trazodone 50 mg or imipramine 50 mg reduce chest pain symptoms and are thought to reduce visceral afferent awareness.

D. PSYCHOLOGICAL DISORDERS

A significant number of patients have underlying depression, anxiety, and panic disorder. Patients reporting dyspnea, sweating, tachycardia, suffocation, or fear of dying should be evaluated for panic disorder.

E. ESOPHAGEAL DYSMOTILITY

Esophageal motility abnormalities such as diffuse esophageal spasm or nutcracker esophagus are rare causes of noncardiac chest pain. In patients with chest pain and dysphagia, barium swallow x-ray should be obtained to look for evidence of achalasia or diffuse esophageal spasm. Stationary or ambulatory manometry is not routinely performed because of low specificity and the unlikelihood of finding a clinically significant disorder, but these procedures may be recommended in patients with frequent symptoms.

Bautista J et al: The effect of an empirical trial of high-dose lansoprazole on symptom response of patients with non-cardiac chest pain—a randomized, double-blind, placebo-controlled, crossover trial. Aliment Pharmacol Ther 2004;15:1123. [PMID: 15142202]

Cremonini F et al: Diagnostic and therapeutic use of proton pump inhibitors in non-cardiac chest pain: a meta-analysis. Am J Gastroenterol 2005;100:1226. [PMID: 15929749]

Dekel R et al: Assessment of oesophageal motor function in patients with dysphagia or chest pain—the Clinical Outcomes Research Initiative experience. Aliment Pharmacol Ther 2003;18:1083. [PMID: 14653827]

Eslick GD: Noncardiac chest pain: epidemiology, natural history, health care seeking, and quality of life. Gastroenterol Clin North Am 2004;33:1. [PMID: 15062433]

■ DISEASES OF THE STOMACH & DUODENUM

GASTRITIS & GASTROPATHY

The term "gastropathy" should be used to denote conditions in which there is epithelial or endothelial damage without inflammation, and "gastritis" should be used to denote conditions in which there is histologic evidence of inflammation. In clinical practice, the term "gastritis" is commonly applied to three categories: (1) erosive and hemorrhagic "gastritis" (gastropathy); (2) nonerosive, nonspecific (histologic) gastritis; and (3) specific types of gastritis, characterized by distinctive histologic and endoscopic features diagnostic of specific disorders.

1. Erosive & Hemorrhagic "Gastritis" (Gastropathy)

 ESSENTIALS OF DIAGNOSIS

- *Most commonly seen in alcoholics, critically ill patients, or patients taking NSAIDs.*
- *Often asymptomatic; may cause epigastric pain, nausea, and vomiting.*
- *May cause hematemesis; usually not significant bleeding.*

General Considerations

The most common causes of erosive gastropathy are drugs (especially NSAIDs), alcohol, stress due to severe medical or surgical illness, and portal hypertension ("portal gastropathy"). Uncommon causes include caustic ingestion and radiation. Erosive and hemorrhagic gastropathy typically are diagnosed at endoscopy, often being performed because of dyspepsia or upper gastrointestinal bleeding. Endoscopic findings include subepithelial hemorrhages, petechiae, and erosions. These lesions are superficial, vary in size and number, and may be focal or diffuse. There usually is no significant inflammation on histologic examination.

Clinical Findings

A. SYMPTOMS AND SIGNS

Erosive gastropathy is usually asymptomatic. Symptoms, when they occur, include anorexia, epigastric pain, nausea, and vomiting. There is poor correlation between symptoms and the number or severity of endoscopic abnormalities. The most common clinical manifestation of erosive gastritis is upper gastrointestinal bleeding, which presents as hematemesis, "coffee grounds" emesis, or bloody aspirate in a patient receiving nasogastric suction, or as melena. Because erosive gastritis is superficial, hemodynamically significant bleeding is rare.

B. LABORATORY FINDINGS

The laboratory findings are nonspecific. The hematocrit is low if significant bleeding has occurred; iron deficiency may be found.

C. SPECIAL EXAMINATIONS

Upper endoscopy is the most sensitive method of diagnosis. Although bleeding from gastritis is usually insignificant, it cannot be distinguished on clinical grounds from more serious lesions such as peptic ulcers or esophageal varices. Hence, endoscopy is generally performed within 24 hours in patients with upper gastrointestinal bleeding to identify the source. An upper gastrointestinal series is sometimes obtained in lieu of endoscopy in patients with hemodynamically insignificant upper gastrointestinal bleeds to exclude serious lesions but is insensitive for the detection of gastritis.

Differential Diagnosis

Epigastric pain may be due to peptic ulcer, gastroesophageal reflux, gastric cancer, biliary tract disease, food poisoning, viral gastroenteritis, and functional dyspepsia. With severe pain, one should consider a perforated or penetrating ulcer, pancreatic disease, esophageal rupture, ruptured aortic aneurysm, gastric volvulus, and myocardial colic. Causes of upper gastrointestinal bleeding include peptic ulcer disease, esophageal varices, Mallory-Weiss tear, and arteriovenous malformations.

Specific Causes & Treatment

A. STRESS GASTRITIS

1. Prophylaxis—Stress-related mucosal erosions and subepithelial hemorrhages develop within 72 hours in the majority of critically ill patients. Clinically overt bleeding occurs in 6%, but clinically important bleed-

ing in less than 3%. Bleeding is associated with a higher mortality rate but is seldom the cause of death. Major risk factors include mechanical ventilation, coagulopathy, trauma, burns, shock, sepsis, central nervous system injury, hepatic or renal failure, and multiorgan failure. The use of enteral nutrition reduces the risk of stress-related bleeding.

Pharmacologic prophylaxis with intravenous H_2-receptor antagonists, oral proton pump inhibitors such as omeprazole suspension, or sucralfate in critically ill patients has been shown to reduce the incidence of clinically overt and significant bleeding by 50%. The optimal, cost-effective regimen is unclear. Prophylaxis should be routinely administered upon admission to critically ill patients with risk factors for significant bleeding. Two of the most important risk factors are coagulopathy and respiratory failure with the need for mechanical ventilation for over 48 hours. When these two risk factors are absent, the risk of significant bleeding is only 0.1%.

Although most critically ill patients have normal or decreased acid secretion, numerous studies have shown that maintaining intragastric pH > 4 reduces the incidence of clinically significant stress-related bleeding. Continuous infusions of H_2-receptor antagonists provide adequate control of intragastric pH in most patients in the following doses over 24 hours: cimetidine (900–1200 mg), ranitidine (150 mg), or famotidine (20 mg). After 4 hours of infusion, the pH should be checked by nasogastric aspirate and the dose doubled if the pH is under 4.0.

Sucralfate suspension (1 g orally every 4–6 hours) is effective also for the prevention of stress-related bleeding, and a reduction of nosocomial pneumonia had been observed compared with H_2-receptor antagonists. However, there is a higher incidence of clinically important upper gastrointestinal bleeding with sucralfate (4%) versus H_2-receptor antagonists (2%) with no difference in nosocomial pneumonia in more recent studies. In most ICUs, intravenous H_2-receptor antagonists or proton pump inhibitors are preferred because of their ease of administration.

At this time, the optimal agent for the reduction of stress-related mucosal bleeding is uncertain. For patients with nasoenteric tubes, immediate-release omeprazole may be preferred to intravenous H_2-receptor antagonists because of lower cost, ease of administration, and comparable efficacy. For patients without a nasogastric tube or with significant ileus, intravenous H_2-receptor antagonists may be preferred to intravenous proton pump inhibitors because of lower cost, established dosing regimens, and proven efficacy.

2. Treatment—Once bleeding occurs, patients should receive continuous infusions of a proton pump inhibitor (esomeprazole, lansoprazole, or pantoprazole 80 mg intravenous bolus, followed by 8 mg/h continuous infusion) as well as sucralfate suspension. Endoscopy should be performed in patients with clinically significant bleeding to look for treatable causes, especially stress-related peptic ulcers with active bleeding or visible vessels. When bleeding arises from diffuse gastritis, endoscopic hemostasis techniques are not helpful.

B. NSAID GASTRITIS

Of patients receiving NSAIDs in clinical trials, 25–50% have gastritis and 10–20% have ulcers at endoscopy; however, symptoms of significant dyspepsia develop in about 5%. In population surveys, the rate of dyspepsia is increased 1.5- to 2-fold with NSAID use. However, dyspeptic symptoms correlate poorly with significant mucosal abnormalities or the development of adverse clinical events (ulcer bleeding or perforation). Given the frequency of dyspeptic symptoms in patients taking NSAIDs, it is neither feasible nor desirable to investigate all such cases. Patients with alarm symptoms or signs, such as severe pain, weight loss, vomiting, gastrointestinal bleeding, or anemia, should undergo diagnostic upper endoscopy. For other patients, symptoms may improve with discontinuation of the agent, reduction to the lowest effective dose, or administration with meals. Proton pump inhibitors have demonstrated efficacy in controlled trials for the treatment NSAID-related dyspepsia. Although superiority to H_2-receptor antagonists for relief of NSAID-related dyspepsia has not been established, proton pump inhibitors have demonstrated superiority for healing of NSAID-related ulcers in the setting of continued NSAID use. Therefore, an empiric 2–4 week trial of a proton pump inhibitor (omeprazole, rabeprazole, or esomeprazole 20–40 mg/d; lansoprazole, 30 mg/d; pantoprazole, 40 mg/d) is recommended for patients with NSAID-related dyspepsia, especially those in whom continued NSAID treatment is required. If symptoms do not improve, diagnostic upper endoscopy should be conducted.

C. ALCOHOLIC GASTRITIS

Excessive alcohol consumption may lead to dyspepsia, nausea, emesis, and minor hematemesis—a condition sometimes labeled "alcoholic gastritis." However, it is not proven that alcohol alone actually causes significant erosive gastritis. Therapy with H_2-receptor antagonists, proton pump inhibitors, or sucralfate for 2–4 weeks often is empirically prescribed.

D. PORTAL HYPERTENSIVE GASTROPATHY

Portal hypertension commonly results in gastric mucosal and submucosal congestion of capillaries and venules, which is correlated with the severity of the portal hypertension and underlying liver disease. Usually asymptomatic, it may cause chronic gastrointestinal bleeding in 10% of patients and, less commonly, clinically significant bleeding with hematemesis. Treatment with propranolol or nadolol reduces the incidence of recurrent acute bleeding by lowering portal pressures. Patients who fail propranolol therapy may be successfully treated with portal decompressive procedures (see section on treatment of esophageal varices).

Conrad SA et al: Randomized, double-blind comparison of immediate-release omeprazole suspension versus intravenous cimetidine for the prevention of upper gastrointestinal bleeding in critically ill patients. Crit Care Med 2005;33: 760. [PMID: 15818102]

Gupta S et al: Management of nonsteroidal, anti-inflammatory, drug-associated dyspepsia. Gastroenterology 2005;129:1711. [PMID: 16285968]

Hawkey C et al; NASA1 SPACE1 Study Group: Improvement with esomeprazole in patients with upper gastrointestinal symptoms taking non-steroidal antiinflammatory drugs, including selective COX-2 inhibitors. Am J Gastroenterol 2005;100:1028. [PMID: 15842575]

Merli M et al: The natural history of portal hypertensive gastropathy in patients with liver cirrhosis and mild portal hypertension. Am J Gastroenterol 2004;99:1959. [PMID: 15447756]

Stollman N et al: Pathophysiology and prophylaxis of stress ulcer in intensive care unit patients. J Crit Care 2005;20:35. [PMID: 16015515]

2. Nonerosive, Nonspecific Gastritis

The diagnosis of nonerosive gastritis is based on histologic assessment of mucosal biopsies. Endoscopic findings are normal in many cases and do not reliably predict the presence of histologic inflammation. The main types of nonerosive gastritis are those due to *H pylori* infection, those associated with pernicious anemia, and lymphocytic gastritis. (See Specific Types of Gastritis below.)

Helicobacter pylori Gastritis

H pylori is a spiral gram-negative rod that resides beneath the gastric mucous layer adjacent to gastric epithelial cells. Although not invasive, it causes gastric mucosal inflammation with PMNs and lymphocytes. The mechanisms of injury and inflammation may in part be related to the products of two genes, *vacA* and *cagA*.

In developed countries the prevalence of *H pylori* is rapidly declining. In the United States, the prevalence rises from less than 10% in non-immigrants under age 30 years to over 50% in those over age 60 years. The prevalence is higher in non-whites and immigrants from developing countries and is correlated inversely with socioeconomic status. Transmission is from person to person, mainly during infancy and childhood; however, the mode of transmission is unknown.

Acute infection with *H pylori* may cause a transient clinical illness characterized by nausea and abdominal pain that may last for several days and is associated with acute histologic gastritis with PMNs. After these symptoms resolve, the majority progress to chronic infection with chronic, diffuse mucosal inflammation characterized by PMNs and lymphocytes. Inflammation may be confined to the superficial gastric epithelium or may extend deeper into the gastric glands, resulting in varying degrees of gland atrophy (atrophic gastritis) and metaplasia of the gastric epithelium to intestinal type epithelium. Eradication of *H pylori* may be achieved with antibiotics in over 85% of patients and leads to resolution of the chronic gastritis (see section on peptic ulcer disease).

Although chronic *H pylori* infection with gastritis is present in 30–50% of the population, the majority are asymptomatic and suffer no sequelae. *H pylori* infection is strongly associated with peptic ulcer disease; however, only 15% of people with chronic infection develop a peptic ulcer (see section on peptic ulcer disease). Chronic *H pylori* gastritis is associated with a 3.5- to 20-fold increased risk of gastric adenocarcinoma and low-grade B cell gastric lymphoma (mucosa-associated lymphoid tissue lymphoma; MALToma). There is little evidence that chronic *H pylori*-associated gastritis is a cause of dyspeptic symptoms. (See Dyspepsia at the beginning of this chapter.)

Testing is indicated for patients with either active or a past history of documented peptic ulcer disease or gastric MALToma and probably for patients with a family history of gastric carcinoma, especially if they are of Asian descent. Testing and empiric treatment may also be cost-effective in young patients (< 55 years of age) with uncomplicated dyspepsia prior to further medical evaluation. The role of testing and treating *H pylori* in patients with functional dyspepsia remains controversial (see Dyspepsia, above). Because *H pylori* is a common organism but infrequently causes disease, screening of the general population is not indicated.

A. Noninvasive Testing for *H pylori*

Although serologic tests are easily obtained and widely available, most clinical guidelines no longer endorse their use for testing for *H pylori* infection because they are less accurate than other noninvasive tests that measure active infection. Laboratory-based quantitative serologic ELISA tests have an overall accuracy of only 80%. Qualitative office-based kits using whole blood from a finger-stick have a lower sensitivity (< 75%) but can be performed within 10 minutes at a cost of $10. In comparison, the fecal antigen immunoassay and [^{13}C] urea test have excellent sensitivity and specificity (> 95%) at a cost of less than $60. Although more expensive and cumbersome to perform, these tests of active infection are more cost-effective in most clinical settings because they reduce unnecessary treatment for patients without active infection.

Proton pump inhibitors significantly reduce the sensitivity of urea breath tests and fecal antigen assays (but not serologic tests) and should be discontinued 7–14 days prior to testing.

B. Endoscopic Testing for *H pylori*

Endoscopy is not indicated to diagnose *H pylori* infection in most circumstances. However, when it is performed for another reason, gastric biopsy specimens can be obtained for detection of *H pylori* and tested for active infection by urease production. This simple, inexpensive ($10) test has excellent sensitivity and specificity (90%). In patients with active upper gastrointestinal bleeding or patients taking proton pump

inhibitors, histologic assessment for *H pylori* is preferred. Histologic assessment of biopsies from the gastric antrum and body is more definitive but more expensive ($150–$250) than a rapid urease test. Histologic assessment is also indicated in patients with suspected MALTomas and, possibly, in patients with suspected infection whose rapid urease test is negative. However, serologic testing is the most cost-effective means of confirming *H pylori* infection in patients with a negative rapid urease test.

Axon A: *Helicobacter pylori*. What do we still need to know? J Clin Gastroenterol 2006;40:15. [PMID: 16340627]

Byzer P et al: Treatment of *Helicobacter pylori*. Helicobacter 2005; 10 (Suppl 1):40. [PMID: 16178970]

Gillen D et al: Gastroduodenal disease, *Helicobacter pylori*, and genetic polymorphisms. Clin Gastroenterol Hepatol 2005; 3:1180. [PMID: 16361041]

Moayyedi P et al: Eradication of *Helicobacter pylori* for non-ulcer dyspepsia. Cochrane Database Syst Rev 2005;(1):CD002096. [PMID: 15674892]

Vakil N et al: Non-invasive tests for the diagnosis of *H pylori* infection. Rev Gastroenterol Disord 2004;4:1. [PMID: 15029105]

Vakil N: Primary and secondary treatment for *Helicobacter pylori* in the United States. Rev Gastroenterol Disord 2005;5:67. [PMID: 15976737]

Pernicious Anemia Gastritis

Pernicious anemia gastritis is an autoimmune disorder involving the fundic glands with resultant achlorhydria and vitamin B_{12} malabsorption. Of patients with B_{12} deficiency, less than half have pernicious anemia. The majority have malabsorption secondary to aging or chronic *H pylori* infection that results in atrophic gastritis, hypochlorhydria, and impaired release of B_{12} from food. Fundic histology in pernicious anemia is characterized by severe gland atrophy and intestinal metaplasia caused by autoimmune destruction of the gastric fundic mucosa. Parietal cell antibodies directed against the H^+-K^+-ATPase pump are present in 90% of patients. Inflammation and autoimmune destruction of the acid-secreting parietal cells leads to secondary loss of fundic zymogen cells, which secrete intrinsic factor. Achlorhydria leads to pronounced hypergastrinemia (> 1000 pg/mL) due to loss of acid inhibition of gastrin G cells. Hypergastrinemia may induce hyperplasia of gastric enterochromaffin-like cells that may lead to the development of small, multicentric carcinoid tumors in 5% of patients. Metastatic spread is uncommon in lesions smaller than 2 cm. The risk of adenocarcinoma is increased threefold, with a prevalence of 1–3%. Endoscopy with biopsy is indicated in patients with pernicious anemia at the time of diagnosis. Patients with dysplasia or small carcinoids require periodic endoscopic surveillance. Pernicious anemia is discussed in detail in Chapter 13.

Andres E et al: Vitamin B_{12} (cobalamin) deficiency in elderly patients. CMAJ 2004;171:251. [PMID: 15289425]

3. Specific Types of Gastritis

A number of disorders are associated with specific mucosal histologic features.

Infections

Acute bacterial infection of the gastric submucosa and muscularis with a variety of aerobic or anaerobic organisms produces a rare, rapidly progressive, life-threatening condition known as phlegmonous or necrotizing gastritis, which requires broad-spectrum antibiotic therapy and, in many cases, emergency gastric resection. Viral infection with CMV is commonly seen in patients with AIDS and after bone marrow or solid organ transplantation. Endoscopic findings include thickened gastric folds and ulcerations. Fungal infection with *Candida* may occur in immunocompromised patients. Larvae of *Anisakis marina* ingested in raw fish or sushi may become embedded in the gastric mucosa, producing severe abdominal pain. Pain persists for several days until the larvae die. Endoscopic removal of the larvae provides rapid symptomatic relief.

Kim GY et al: Phlegmonous gastritis: case report and review. Gastrointest Endosc 2005;61:168. [PMID: 15672083]

Granulomatous Gastritis

Chronic granulomatous inflammation may be caused by a variety of systemic diseases, including Crohn's disease, *H pylori* infection, tuberculosis, syphilis, fungal infections, or sarcoidosis. These may be asymptomatic or associated with a variety of gastrointestinal complaints.

Maeng L et al: Granulomatous gastritis: a clinicopathological analysis of 18 biopsy cases. Am J Surg Pathol 2004;28:941. [PMID: 15223966]

Eosinophilic Gastritis

This is a rare disorder in which eosinophils infiltrate the antrum and sometimes the proximal intestine. Infiltration may involve the mucosa, muscularis, or serosa. Peripheral eosinophilia is prominent. Symptoms include anemia from mucosal blood loss, abdominal pain, early satiety, and postprandial vomiting. Treatment with corticosteroids is beneficial in the majority of patients.

Lymphocytic Gastritis

This is an idiopathic condition characterized by fluctuating abdominal pain, nausea, and vomiting. Endoscopic features include mucosal erosions and a varioliform ("pox-like") appearance. Biopsies reveal a diffuse lymphocytic gastritis. There is no established effective therapy.

Ménétrier's Disease (Hypertrophic Gastropathy)

This is an idiopathic entity characterized by giant thickened gastric folds involving predominantly the body of the stomach. Patients complain of nausea, epigastric pain, weight loss, and diarrhea. Because of chronic protein loss, patients may develop severe hypoproteinemia and anasarca. The cause is unknown. Treatment is directed at symptoms. There are case reports of resolution of symptoms and improvement in histologic appearance after *H pylori* eradication. Dramatic improvement recently has been reported in a small number of patients with cetuximab, an antibody that binds epidermal growth factor receptor (EGFR). Gastric resection is required in severe cases.

Settle SH et al: Chronic treatment of Menetrier's disease with Erbitux: clinical efficacy and insight into pathophysiology. Clin Gastroenterol Hepatol 2005;3:654. [PMID: 16206497]

PEPTIC ULCER DISEASE

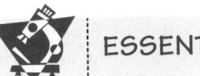 ESSENTIALS OF DIAGNOSIS

- *History of nonspecific epigastric pain present in 80–90% of patients with variable relationship to meals.*
- *Ulcer symptoms characterized by rhythmicity and periodicity.*
- *Ten to 20 percent of patients present with ulcer complications without antecedent symptoms.*
- *Of NSAID-induced ulcers, 30–50% are asymptomatic.*
- *Upper endoscopy with antral biopsy for* H pylori *is the diagnostic procedure of choice in most patients.*
- *Gastric ulcer biopsy or documentation of complete healing necessary to exclude gastric malignancy.*

General Considerations

Peptic ulcer is a break in the gastric or duodenal mucosa that arises when the normal mucosal defensive factors are impaired or are overwhelmed by aggressive luminal factors such as acid and pepsin. By definition, ulcers extend through the muscularis mucosae and are usually over 5 mm in diameter. In the United States, there are about 500,000 new cases per year of peptic ulcer and 4 million ulcer recurrences; the lifetime prevalence of ulcers in the adult population is approximately 10%. Ulcers occur five times more commonly in the duodenum, where over 95% are in the bulb or pyloric channel. In the stomach, benign ulcers are located most commonly in the antrum (60%) and at the junction of the antrum and body on the lesser curvature (25%).

Ulcers occur slightly more commonly in men than in women (1.3:1). Although ulcers can occur in any age group, duodenal ulcers most commonly occur in patients between the ages of 30 and 55 years, whereas gastric ulcers are more common in patients between the ages of 55 and 70 years. Ulcers are more common in smokers and in patients taking NSAIDs on a chronic basis (see below). Alcohol, dietary factors, and stress do not appear to cause ulcer disease. The incidence of duodenal ulcer disease has been declining dramatically for the past 30 years, but the incidence of gastric ulcers appears to be increasing as a result of the widespread use of NSAIDs and low-dose aspirin.

Etiology

Three major causes of peptic ulcer disease are now recognized: NSAIDs, chronic *H pylori* infection, and acid hypersecretory states such as Zollinger-Ellison syndrome. Evidence of *H pylori* infection or NSAID ingestion should be sought in all patients with peptic ulcer. NSAID- and *H pylori*–associated ulcers will be considered in the present section; Zollinger-Ellison syndrome will be discussed subsequently. Uncommon causes of ulcer disease include CMV (especially in transplant recipients), systemic mastocytosis, Crohn's disease, lymphoma, and medications (eg, alendronate). Up to 10% of ulcers are idiopathic.

A. *H PYLORI*–ASSOCIATED ULCERS

H pylori appears to be a necessary cofactor for the majority of duodenal and gastric ulcers not associated with NSAIDs. Overall, it is estimated that one in six infected patients will develop ulcer disease. The prevalence of *H pylori* infection in duodenal ulcer patients is 75–90%. Most *H pylori*–infected duodenal ulcer patients have infection predominantly in the gastric antrum, which is associated with increased gastric acid secretion and decreased duodenal mucosal bicarbonate secretion. It is hypothesized that increased acid exposure can give rise to small islands of gastric metaplasia in the duodenal bulb. Colonization of these islands by *H pylori* may lead to duodenitis or duodenal ulcer. The association with gastric ulcers is lower, but *H pylori* is found in the majority of patients in whom NSAIDs cannot be implicated. *H pylori*–associated gastric ulcers tend to form at the junction of the gastric body and antrum—the site of transition from oxyntic to pyloric epithelium. Most *H pylori*–infected gastric ulcer patients have infection that predominates in the gastric body and is associated with decreased acid secretion. It is hypothesized that chronic inflammation overwhelms the gastric mucosal defense mechanisms.

The natural history of *H pylori*–associated peptic ulcer disease is well defined. In the absence of specific antibiotic treatment to eradicate the organism, 85% of patients will have an endoscopically visible recurrence within 1 year. Half of these will be symptomatic. After successful eradication of *H pylori* with antibiotics, ulcer recurrence rates are reduced dramatically to 5–20% at 1 year. Some of these ulcer recurrences may be due to NSAID use or reinfection with *H pylori*.

B. NSAID-INDUCED ULCERS

There is a 10–20% prevalence of gastric ulcers and a 2–5% prevalence of duodenal ulcers in long-term NSAID users. The relative risk of gastric ulcers is increased 40-fold, but the risk of duodenal ulcers is only slightly increased. Users of NSAIDs are at least three times more likely than nonusers to suffer serious gastrointestinal complications from these ulcers such as bleeding, perforation, or death. It is noteworthy that gastric ulcers and duodenal ulcers cause about the same number of complications. Approximately 1–2% of long-term NSAID users will have a major complication within 1 year. The risk of NSAID complications is greater within the first 3 months of therapy and in patients who are older, patients who take higher doses of NSAIDs, as well as patients with a prior history of ulcer disease, concomitant corticosteroid or anticoagulation administration, or serious medical illness. Aspirin is the most ulcerogenic NSAID. Use of even low-dose aspirin (81–162 mg/d) leads to complications in 0.6–1.2% of patients each year. *H pylori* infection increases the risk of ulcer disease and complications over threefold in patients taking NSAIDs or low-dose aspirin. It is hypothesized that NSAID initiation may potentiate or aggravate ulcer disease in susceptible infected individuals.

Celecoxib (and the other "coxibs") are NSAIDs that preferentially inhibit cyclooxygenase-2 (COX-2)—the principal enzyme involved in prostaglandin production at sites of inflammation—while providing relative sparing of cyclooxygenase-1 (COX-1), the principal enzyme involved with prostaglandin production in the gastroduodenal mucosa and gastric cytoprotection. Two other NSAIDs—etodolac and meloxicam—have COX-2/COX-1 selectivity that is similar to celecoxib but have undergone limited study to confirm their safety. The generic etodolac is significantly less expensive than other coxib agents. The incidence of endoscopically visible ulcers after 6–12 weeks of coxib therapy is reduced by approximately 75% compared with nonselective NSAIDs. Of greater clinical importance, the risk of significant clinical events (obstruction, perforation, or severe bleeding) is approximately 0.7% in patients taking coxibs and 1.4% in patients taking nonselective NSAIDs—a relative risk reduction of 50%. Concurrent use of low-dose aspirin appears to partially negate the mucosal-sparing effects of coxibs. Among patients taking low-dose aspirin, the risk of a serious clinical event was not significantly different between patients taking coxibs and standard NSAIDs.

A twofold increase in the incidence in cardiovascular complications (myocardial infarction, cerebrovascular infarction, and death) was detected in patients taking rofecoxib and valdecoxib compared with placebo, prompting its voluntary withdrawal from the market by the manufacturers. It is hypothesized that selective inhibition of COX-2 leads to decreased vascular prostacyclin, reduced arterial vasodilation, enhanced atherogenesis, and enhanced platelet adhesion. A review by a Food and Drug Administration (FDA) panel concluded that celecoxib, which has less COX-2 selectivity than rofecoxib and valdecoxb, does not have a higher incidence of cardiovascular complications compared with other nonselective NSAIDs. Nonetheless, pending further clinical information, celecoxib should be restricted to short-term use (< 3 months) in patients at increased risk for NSAID-induced complications and deemed to have a low risk of cardiovascular disease.

Clinical Findings

A. SYMPTOMS AND SIGNS

Epigastric pain (dyspepsia), the hallmark of peptic ulcer disease, is present in 80–90% of patients. However, this complaint is not sensitive or specific enough to serve as a reliable diagnostic criterion for peptic ulcer disease. The clinical history cannot accurately distinguish duodenal from gastric ulcers. Less than 25% of patients with dyspepsia have ulcer disease at endoscopy. Twenty percent of patients with ulcer complications such as bleeding have no antecedent symptoms ("silent ulcers"). Nearly 60% of patients with NSAID-related ulcer complications do not have prior symptoms.

Pain is typically well localized to the epigastrium and not severe. It is described as gnawing, dull, aching, or "hunger-like." Approximately 50% of patients report relief of pain with food or antacids (especially duodenal ulcers) and a recurrence of pain 2–4 hours later. However, many patients deny any relationship to meals or report worsening of pain. Two-thirds of duodenal ulcers and one-third of gastric ulcers cause nocturnal pain that awakens the patient. A change from a patient's typical rhythmic discomfort to constant or radiating pain may reflect ulcer penetration or perforation. Most patients have symptomatic periods lasting up to several weeks with intervals of months to years in which they are pain free (periodicity).

Nausea and anorexia may occur with gastric ulcers. Significant vomiting and weight loss are unusual with uncomplicated ulcer disease and suggest gastric outlet obstruction or gastric malignancy.

The physical examination is often normal in uncomplicated peptic ulcer disease. Mild, localized epigastric tenderness to deep palpation may be present. FOBT is positive in one-third of patients.

B. LABORATORY FINDINGS

Laboratory tests are normal in uncomplicated peptic ulcer disease but are ordered to exclude ulcer complications or confounding disease entities. Anemia may occur with acute blood loss from a bleeding ulcer or less commonly from chronic blood loss. Leukocytosis suggests ulcer penetration or perforation. An elevated serum amylase in a patient with severe epigastric pain suggests ulcer penetration into the pancreas. A fasting serum gastrin level to screen for Zollinger-Ellison syndrome is obtained in some patients (see below). Because acid inhibition may raise serum gastrin levels, H_2-receptor antagonists should be withheld for 24 hours and proton pump inhibitors for 1 week before a gastrin level is measured.

C. ENDOSCOPY

Upper endoscopy is the procedure of choice for the diagnosis of duodenal and gastric ulcers. Endoscopy provides better diagnostic accuracy than barium radiography and the ability to biopsy for the presence of malignancy and H pylori infection. Duodenal ulcers are virtually never malignant and do not require biopsy. Three to 5 percent of benign-appearing gastric ulcers prove to be malignant. Hence, biopsies of the ulcer margin are almost always performed. Provided that the gastric ulcer appears benign to the endoscopist and adequate biopsy specimens reveal no evidence of cancer, dysplasia, or atypia, the patient may be followed without further endoscopy. If these conditions are not fulfilled, follow-up endoscopy should be performed 12 weeks after the start of therapy to document complete healing; nonhealing ulcers are suspicious for malignancy.

D. IMAGING

Barium upper gastrointestinal series is an acceptable alternative to screening of patients with uncomplicated dyspepsia. However, because it has limited accuracy in distinguishing benign from malignant gastric ulcers, all gastric ulcers in patients younger than 45 years diagnosed by x-ray should be reevaluated with endoscopy after 8–12 weeks of therapy.

E. TESTING FOR H PYLORI

In patients in whom an ulcer is diagnosed by endoscopy, gastric mucosal biopsies should be obtained both for a rapid urease test and for histologic examination. The specimens for histology are discarded if the urease test is positive.

In patients with a history of peptic ulcer or when an ulcer is diagnosed by upper gastrointestinal series, noninvasive assessment for H pylori with fecal antigen assay or urea breath testing should be done. Proton pump inhibitors may cause false-negative urea breath tests and fecal antigen tests and should be withheld for at least 7 days before testing. Because of its lower sensitivity and specificity, serologic testing should not be performed unless fecal antigen testing or urea breath testing is unavailable.

Differential Diagnosis

Peptic ulcer disease must be distinguished from other causes of epigastric distress (dyspepsia). Over 50% of patients with dyspepsia have no obvious organic explanation for their symptoms and are classified as having functional dyspepsia (see sections above on dyspepsia and functional dyspepsia). Atypical gastroesophageal reflux may be manifested by epigastric symptoms. Biliary tract disease is characterized by discrete, intermittent episodes of pain that should not be confused with other causes of dyspepsia. Severe epigastric pain is atypical for peptic ulcer disease unless complicated by a perforation or penetration. Other causes include acute pancreatitis, acute cholecystitis or choledocholithiasis, esophageal rupture, gastric volvulus, and ruptured aortic aneurysm.

Pharmacologic Agents

The pharmacology of several agents that enhance the healing of peptic ulcers is briefly discussed here. They may be divided into three categories: (1) acid-antisecretory agents, (2) mucosal protective agents, and (3) agents that promote healing through eradication of *H pylori*. Recommendations for their use are provided in subsequent sections.

A. Acid-Antisecretory Agents

1. Proton pump inhibitors—Proton pump inhibitors covalently bind the acid-secreting enzyme H^+-K^+-ATPase, or "proton pump," permanently inactivating it. Restoration of acid secretion requires synthesis of new pumps, which have a half-life of 18 hours. Thus, although these agents have a serum half-life of less than 60 minutes, their duration of action exceeds 24 hours. The available agents—omeprazole or rabeprazole 20 mg, lansoprazole 30 mg, esomeprazole or pantoprazole 40 mg—inhibit over 90% of 24-hour acid secretion, compared with under 65% for H_2-receptor antagonists in standard dosages. Proton pump inhibitors should be administered 30 minutes before meals (usually breakfast).

Each of the four proton pump inhibitors results in over 90% healing of duodenal ulcers after 4 weeks and 90% of gastric ulcers after 8 weeks when given once daily. Compared with H_2-receptor antagonists, proton pump inhibitors provide faster pain relief and more rapid ulcer healing. However, nearly equivalent overall healing rates may be achieved with longer courses of H_2-receptor antagonists.

The proton pump inhibitors are remarkably safe in short-term therapy. Serum gastrin levels rise significantly (> 500 pg/mL) in 3% of patients receiving long-term therapy, which is associated with the development of gastric enterochromaffin-like cell hyperplasia in humans and gastric carcinoid tumors in rats. Clinical experience with these agents for over 10 years has not detected any significant toxicity in humans. Long-term use may lead to a mild decrease in vitamin B_{12} and iron absorption of unclear significance. Long-term use is unnecessary in peptic ulcer disease but is frequently required in gastroesophageal reflux disease.

2. H_2-receptor antagonists—Although H_2-receptor antagonists are effective in the treatment of peptic ulcer disease, proton pump inhibitors are now the pre-ferred agents because of their ease of use and superior efficacy. Four H_2-receptor antagonists are available: cimetidine, ranitidine, famotidine, and nizatidine. All four agents effectively inhibit nocturnal acid output, but they are less effective at inhibiting meal-stimulated acid secretion. For uncomplicated peptic ulcers, H_2-receptor antagonists may be administered once daily at bedtime as follows: ranitidine and nizatidine 300 mg, famotidine 40 mg, and cimetidine 800 mg. Ulcer symptom relief usually occurs within 2 weeks. Duodenal and gastric ulcer healing rates of 85–90% are obtained within 6 weeks and 8 weeks, respectively. All four agents are well tolerated, and serious adverse effects are rare. Cimetidine is rarely used because it inhibits hepatic cytochrome P-450 metabolism (raising the serum concentration of theophylline, warfarin, lidocaine, and phenytoin) and may cause gynecomastia or impotence. Ranitidine binds P-450 with 10% of the avidity of cimetidine; famotidine and nizatidine have negligible effects.

B. Agents Enhancing Mucosal Defenses

Bismuth, misoprostol, and low doses of aluminum-containing antacids all have been shown to promote ulcer healing through the enhancement of mucosal defensive mechanisms. Given the greater efficacy and safety of antisecretory agents and better compliance of patients, these other agents are no longer used as first-line therapy for active ulcers in most clinical settings. Because of the rapid relief of ulcer symptoms they provide, antacids are commonly used as needed to supplement antisecretory agents during the first few days of treatment. Bismuth has direct antibacterial action against *H pylori* and may be used in combination with antibiotics for eradication (see below). Misoprostol is a prostaglandin analog that stimulates gastroduodenal mucus and bicarbonate secretion. It is effective as a prophylactic agent in reducing the incidence of gastroduodenal ulcers in patients taking nonselective NSAIDs but must be given three or four times daily and causes diarrhea in 10–20% of patients; however, it is not commonly used for this indication because of the advent of proton pump inhibitors and COX-2 selective NSAIDs.

C. *H Pylori* Eradication Therapy

Eradication of *H pylori* has proved difficult. Combination regimens that use two antibiotics with a proton pump inhibitor or bismuth are required to achieve adequate rates of eradication and to reduce the number of failures due to antibiotic resistance. Resistance develops rapidly to metronidazole and clarithromycin but not to amoxicillin or tetracycline. In the United States, up to 50% of strains are resistant to metronidazole and 7% are resistant to clarithromycin. It is advisable to include amoxicillin in first-line therapy in most patients, reserving metronidazole for penicillin-allergic patients. Recommended regimens are listed in Table 14–11. All currently recommended regimens achieve

Table 14–11. Treatment options for peptic ulcer disease.

Active *Helicobacter pylori*–associated ulcer

1. Treat with anti-*H pylori* regimen for 7–14 days. Treatment options:

   Proton pump inhibitor twice daily[1]
   Clarithromycin 500 mg twice daily
   Amoxicillin 1 g twice daily (or metronidazole 500 mg twice daily, if penicillin allergic)

   Proton pump inhibitor twice daily[1]
   Bismuth subsalicylate two tablets four times daily
   Tetracycline 500 mg four times daily
   Metronidazole 250 mg four times daily

   Ranitidine bismuth citrate 400 mg twice daily (not available in the United States)
   Clarithromycin 500 mg twice daily
   Amoxicillin 1 g or tetracycline 500 mg or metronidazole 500 mg twice daily

   (Proton pump inhibitors administered before meals. Avoid metronidazole regimens in areas of known high resistance or in patients who have failed a course of treatment that included metronidazole.)

2. After completion of 7–14-day course of *H pylori* eradication therapy, continue treatment with proton pump inhibitor[1] once daily or H$_2$-receptor antagonist (as below) for 4–8 weeks to promote healing.

Active ulcer not attributable to *H pylori*

1. Consider other causes: NSAIDs, Zollinger-Ellison syndrome, gastric malignancy. Treatment options:

   Proton pump inhibitors[1]:
     Uncomplicated duodenal ulcer: treat for 4 weeks
     Uncomplicated gastric ulcer: treat for 8 weeks
   H$_2$-receptor antagonists:
     Uncomplicated duodenal ulcer: cimetidine 800 mg, ranitidine or nizatidine 300 mg, famotidine 40 mg, once daily at bed-
       time for 6 weeks
     Uncomplicated gastric ulcer: cimetidine 400 mg, ranitidine or nizatidine 150 mg, famotidine 20 mg, twice daily for 8 weeks
     Complicated ulcers: proton pump inhibitors are the preferred drugs

Prevention of ulcer relapse

1. NSAID-induced ulcer: prophylactic therapy for high-risk patients (prior ulcer disease or ulcer complications, use of corticosteroids or anticoagulants, age > 70 years, serious comorbid illnesses).
   Treatment options:

   Proton pump inhibitor once daily
   COX-2 selective NSAID (celecoxib)
   (In special circumstances: misoprostol 200 mcg 3–4 times daily)

2. Long-term "maintenance" therapy indicated in patients with recurrent ulcers who either are *H pylori*-negative or who have
   failed attempts at eradication therapy: once-daily proton pump inhibitor[1] or H$_2$-receptor antagonist at bedtime (cimetidine 400–800 mg, nizatidine or ranitidine 150–300 mg, famotidine 20–40 mg)

---

[1]Proton pump inhibitors: omeprazole 20 mg, rabeprazole 20 mg, lansoprazole 30 mg, pantoprazole 40 mg, esomeprazole 40 mg.
All proton pump inhibitors are given twice daily except esomeprazole (once daily).
NSAIDs = nonsteroidal anti-inflammatory drugs; COX-2 = cyclooxygenase-2.

rates of eradication greater than 85% after 7–14 days of treatment. In most centers in the United States, the preferred regimen is with a 10-day course of treatment with a proton pump inhibitor—omeprazole or ra-beprazole 20 mg twice daily, lansoprazole 30 mg twice daily, pantoprazole 40 mg twice daily, or esomeprazole 40 mg once daily—plus amoxicillin 1 g twice daily and clarithromycin 500 mg twice daily. In patients whose infection persists after an initial course of anti-biotic therapy, the optimal regimen may be quadruple therapy with a proton pump inhibitor, bismuth sub-salicylate, tetracycline, and metronidazole for 14 days (Table 14–11).

Medical Treatment

Patients should be encouraged to eat balanced meals at regular intervals. There is no justification for bland or restrictive diets. Moderate alcohol intake is not harm-ful. Smoking retards the rate of ulcer healing and increases the frequency of recurrences and should be discouraged.

A. TREATMENT OF *H PYLORI*–ASSOCIATED ULCERS

1. Treatment of active ulcer—The goals of treat-ment of active *H pylori*–associated ulcers are to relieve dyspeptic symptoms, to promote ulcer healing, and to eradicate *H pylori* infection. Uncomplicated *H pylori*–associated ulcers should be treated for the first 10 days with one of the proton pump inhibitor-based *H pylori* eradication regimens listed in Table 14–11. An antisecretory agent must be administered for an additional 2–4 weeks (duodenal ulcer) or 4–6 weeks (gastric ulcer) after completion of the antibiotic regimen to ensure complete ulcer healing. A once-daily proton pump inhibitor (omeprazole or rabeprazole 20 mg, lansoprazole 30 mg, pantoprazole or esomeprazole 40 mg) is most convenient, but H$_2$-receptor antagonists may be chosen as less expensive therapy. Confirmation of *H pylori* eradication in patients with uncomplicated ulcers is not necessary. Confirmation is required in all patients with ulcers complicated by bleeding, perforation, or obstruction.

2. Therapy to prevent recurrence—Successful eradication reduces ulcer recurrences to less than 20% after 1–2 years. Therefore, antisecretory therapy can be discontinued after 4–8 weeks in patients with uncomplicated ulcers and the patient observed for recurrence of symptoms. The most common cause of recurrence after antibiotic therapy is failure to achieve successful eradication, which must be evaluated. Once cure has been achieved, reinfection rates are less than 0.5% per year. Although *H pylori* eradication has reduced the need for chronic maintenance antisecretory therapy to prevent ulcer recurrences, there remains a subset of patients who require chronic therapy with either a proton pump inhibitor once daily or an H$_2$-receptor antagonist at bedtime. This subset includes patients with *H pylori*–positive ulcers who have failed recurrent attempts at eradication therapy, patients with a history of *H pylori*–positive ulcers who have recurrent ulcers despite successful eradication, and patients with idiopathic ulcers (ie, *H pylori*–negative and not taking NSAIDs). In all patients with recurrent ulcers, NSAID usage (unintentional or surreptitious) and hypersecretory states (including gastrinoma) should be excluded.

B. TREATMENT OF NSAID-ASSOCIATED ULCERS

1. Treatment of active ulcers—In patients with NSAID-induced ulcers, the offending agent should be discontinued whenever possible. Both gastric and duodenal ulcers respond rapidly to therapy with H$_2$-receptor antagonists or proton pump inhibitors (Table 14–11) once NSAIDs are eliminated. In some patients with severe inflammatory diseases, it may not be feasible to discontinue NSAIDs. These patients should be treated with proton pump inhibitors once daily, which results in ulcer healing rates of approximately 80% at 8 weeks in patients continuing to take NSAIDs. All patients with NSAID-associated ulcers should undergo testing for *H pylori* infection. Antibiotic eradication therapy should be given if *H pylori* tests are positive.

2. Prevention of NSAID-induced ulcers—The goal of prophylactic therapy is to prevent ulcer complications, which occur in only 1–2% of NSAID-treated patients per year. Therefore, prophylactic therapy should be reserved for patients at high risk for developing complications. High-risk factors include a history of ulcer disease or complications, concurrent therapy with corticosteroids or anticoagulants, concurrent use of NSAID plus low-dose aspirin, serious underlying medical illness, and age over 60 years. Such patients have a 2–10% chance per year of developing a complicated ulcer from taking a nonselective NSAID. Whenever possible, NSAIDs should be avoided in this high-risk population. If NSAIDs must be given, the following options can be considered. (At this time, the optimal cost-effective approach has not been determined.)

a. Test for and treat *H pylori* infection—All patients who are started on nonselective NSAIDs should have noninvasive testing for *H pylori* infection followed by treatment, if positive. Eradication of *H pylori* reduces the incidence of endoscopic ulcers in acute NSAID users from 26–34% to 7–12% within 12 weeks.

b. Proton pump inhibitor—Treatment with a proton pump inhibitor given once daily (omeprazole or rabeprazole 20 mg, lansoprazole 30 mg, or pantoprazole or esomeprazole 40 mg) appears to be effective in the prevention of NSAID-induced gastric and duodenal ulcers and is approved by the FDA for this indication. For patients taking a daily proton pump inhibitor for another indication (such as gastroesophageal reflux disease), use of a generic nonselective NSAID is an attractive, cost-effective option.

c. Misoprostol—The prostaglandin analog misoprostol is effective in the prevention of NSAID-induced gastric and duodenal ulcers when given at a dosage of 100–200 mcg four times daily. However, misoprostol is less commonly used as a prophylactic agent against NSAID-induced complications than either concurrent therapy with a proton pump inhibitor or COX-2 selective agent because of its high side effect profile and the need for dosing four times daily. With increased restriction on long-term use of COX-2 selective drugs, usage of misoprostol in conjunction with nonselective NSAIDs may increase.

d. COX-2 selective agents—As discussed above, there is an increased risk of major cardiovascular events in patients taking rofecoxib or valdecoxib compared with nonselective NSAIDs or placebo—an absolute increase of approximately 1.6% in patients taking rofecoxib, which led to the voluntary withdrawal of these agents from the market. Although celecoxib does not appear to have an increased risk of cardiovascular events compared with nonselective NSAIDs, one long-term polyp prevention study has shown an increased risk of such adverse events with celecoxib compared with placebo. Pending further outcomes data, celecoxib should be restricted to < 90 days of therapy in patients deemed at increased risk for NSAID-induced complications and at low risk for cardiovascular complications. In patients who require concurrent therapy with low-dose aspirin for cardiovascular prophylaxis, the gastrointestinal safety of a COX-2 selective agent is partially or completely negated.

e. Multiple NSAID risk factors—Patients with prior ulcer complications or with multiple risk factors are at particularly high risk for NSAID-induced complications (10–20% per year). The optimal cost-effective approach to management of these patients is unknown. All patients should undergo noninvasive testing for *H pylori*, and if results are positive, treatment should be given. If NSAID therapy is deemed to be clinically required despite the increased risks, treatment options include a COX-2 selective agent (celecoxib, etodolac, or meloxicam) plus a prophylactic agent (proton pump inhibitor or misoprostol) or—in patients with increased risk of cardiovascular disease—a standard NSAID and a prophylactic agent (double-dose proton pump inhibitor or misoprostol).

D. REFRACTORY ULCERS

Ulcers that are truly refractory to medical therapy are now uncommon. Less than 5% of ulcers are unhealed after 8 weeks of therapy with proton pump inhibitors. Noncompliance is the most common cause of ulcer nonhealing. Cigarettes retard ulcer healing and should be proscribed. NSAID and aspirin use, sometimes surreptitious, are commonly implicated in refractory ulcers and must be stopped. *H pylori* eradication enhances healing and decreases the high recurrence rates of refractory ulcers. Therefore, evidence of *H pylori* infection should be sought and the infection treated, if present, in all refractory ulcer patients. Fasting serum gastrin levels should be obtained to exclude gastrinoma with acid hypersecretion (Zollinger-Ellison syndrome). Nonhealing gastric ulcers raise concerns that an undiagnosed gastric malignancy may be masquerading as a benign gastric ulcer. Repeat ulcer biopsies are mandatory after 2–3 months of therapy in all nonhealed gastric ulcers, and they should be followed with serial endoscopies to verify complete healing. Almost all benign refractory ulcers heal within 8 weeks with a proton pump inhibitor twice daily (omeprazole or rabeprazole 20 mg twice daily, lansoprazole 30 mg twice daily). Patients with persistent nonhealing ulcers are referred for surgical therapy after exclusion of NSAID use and persistent *H pylori* infection.

Chan FK et al: Peptic-ulcer disease. Lancet 2002;360:933. [PMID: 12354485]

Fitzgerald GA: Coxibs and cardiovascular disease. N Engl J Med 2004;351:1709. [PMID: 15470192]

Ford AD et al: Eradication therapy in *Helicobacter pylori* positive peptic ulcer disease: systematic review and economic analysis. Am J Gastroenterol 2004;99:1833. [PMID: 15330927]

Gisbert JP et al: Systematic review and meta-analysis: is 1-week proton pump inhibitor-based triple therapy sufficient to heal peptic ulcer? Aliment Pharmacol Ther 2005;21:795. [PMID: 15801914]

Gatta L et al: A 10-day levofloxacin-based triple therapy in patients who have failed two eradication courses. Aliment Pharmacol Ther 2005;22:45. [PMID: 15963079]

Laine L et al: Ulcer formation with low-dose enteric-coasted aspirin and the effect of COX-2 selective inhibition: a double-blind trial. Gastroenterology 2004;127:395. [PMID: 15300570]

Lanas A: Gastrointestinal complications from NSAID therapy. How to reduce the risk of complications. Postgrad Med 2005;117:23. [PMID: 16001765]

Vakil N: Primary and secondary treatment for *Helicobacter pylori* in the United States. Rev Gastroenterol Disord 2005;5:67. [PMID: 15976737]

Vergara M et al: Meta-analysis: role of *Helicobacter pylori* eradication in the prevention of peptic ulcer in NSAID users. Aliment Pharmacol Ther 2005;21:1411. [PMID: 15948807]

Zullo A et al: High rate of *Helicobacter pylori* eradication with sequential therapy in elderly patients with peptic ulcer: a prospective controlled study. Aliment Pharmacol Ther 2005; 21:1419. [PMID: 15948808]

COMPLICATIONS OF PEPTIC ULCER DISEASE

1. Gastrointestinal Hemorrhage

 ESSENTIALS OF DIAGNOSIS

- *"Coffee grounds" emesis, hematemesis, melena, or hematochezia.*
- *Emergent upper endoscopy is diagnostic and therapeutic.*

General Considerations

Approximately 50% of all episodes of upper gastrointestinal bleeding are due to peptic ulcer. Clinically significant bleeding occurs in 10% of ulcer patients. About 80% of patients stop bleeding spontaneously and generally have an uneventful recovery; the remaining 20% have more severe bleeding. The overall mortality rate for ulcer bleeding is 6–10%, but it is higher in the elderly, in patients with comorbid medical problems, and in patients with nosocomial bleeding. Mortality is also higher in patients who present with persistent hypotension or shock, bright red blood in the vomitus or nasogastric lavage fluid, or severe coagulopathy.

Clinical Findings

A. SYMPTOMS AND SIGNS

Up to 20% of patients have no antecedent symptoms of pain; this is particularly true of patients receiving NSAIDs. Common presenting signs include melena and hematemesis. Massive upper gastrointestinal bleeding or rapid gastrointestinal transit may result in hematochezia rather than melena; this may be misinterpreted as signifying a lower tract bleeding source. Nasogastric lavage that demonstrates "coffee grounds" or bright red blood confirms an upper tract source. Recovered nasogastric lavage fluid that is negative for blood does not exclude active bleeding from a duodenal ulcer.

B. Laboratory Findings

The hematocrit may fall as a result of bleeding or expansion of the intravascular volume with intravenous fluids. The blood urea nitrogen (BUN) may rise as a result of absorption of blood nitrogen from the small intestine and prerenal azotemia.

Treatment

The assessment and initial management of upper gastrointestinal tract bleeding are discussed elsewhere in this chapter. Specific issues pertaining to peptic ulcer bleeding are described below.

A. Medical Therapy

1. Antisecretory agents—Intravenous proton pump inhibitors or high-dose oral proton pump inhibitors should be administered for 3 days in patients with ulcers whose endoscopic appearance suggests a high risk of rebleeding after endoscopic therapy. Intravenous or high-dose oral proton pump inhibitors have been associated with a reduction in rebleeding, transfusions, the need for further endoscopic therapy, and surgery in the subset of patients with high-risk ulcers, ie, an ulcer with active bleeding, visible vessel, or adherent clot (see below). Intravenous omeprazole (80 mg bolus injection, followed by 8 mg/h continuous infusion for 72 hours) has undergone the most clinical testing but is not available in the United States. After initial successful endoscopic treatment of ulcer hemorrhage, intravenous omeprazole reduces the rebleeding rate from approximately 20% to < 10%. In the United States, intravenous esomeprazole, lansoprazole, and pantoprazole are available and commonly used at comparable dosing (80 mg bolus injection, followed by 8 mg/h) for this indication, although published data confirming their efficacy are unavailable. High-dose oral proton pump inhibitors (omeprazole 40 mg twice daily) also appear to be effective in reducing rebleeding but have not been compared to the intravenous regimen. Many physicians choose to administer a high-dose proton pump inhibitor prior to endoscopy in all patients admitted to the hospital with gastrointestinal bleeding suspected to be due to peptic ulcer, discontinuing therapy after endoscopy in patients with ulcers deemed to be at low risk of rebleeding. Intravenous H_2-receptor antagonists have not been demonstrated to be of any benefit in the treatment of acute ulcer bleeding.

2. Long-term prevention of rebleeding—Recurrent ulcer bleeding develops within 3 years in one-third of patients if no specific therapy is given. In patients with bleeding ulcers who are *H pylori* positive, successful eradication effectively prevents recurrent ulcer bleeding in almost all cases. It is therefore recommended that all patients with bleeding ulcers be tested for *H*

pylori infection and treated if positive. Four to 8 weeks after completion of antibiotic therapy, a urea breath or fecal antigen test for *H pylori* should be administered or endoscopy performed with biopsy for histologic confirmation of successful eradication. In patients in whom *H pylori* persists or the small subset of patients whose ulcers are not associated with NSAIDs or *H pylori*, chronic acid suppression with a bedtime dose of an H_2-antagonist (ranitidine 150 mg) or a once-daily proton pump inhibitor should be prescribed to reduce the likelihood of recurrence of bleeding.

B. Endoscopy

Endoscopy is the preferred diagnostic procedure in almost all cases of upper gastrointestinal bleeding because of its high diagnostic accuracy, its ability to predict the likelihood of recurrent bleeding, and its availability for therapeutic intervention in high-risk lesions. Endoscopy should be performed within 12–24 hours in most cases. In cases of severe active bleeding, endoscopy is performed as soon as patients have been appropriately resuscitated and are hemodynamically stable.

On the basis of clinical and endoscopic criteria, it is possible to predict which patients are at a higher risk of rebleeding and therefore to make more rational use of hospital resources. Nonbleeding ulcers under 2 cm in size with a base that is clean have a less than 5% chance of rebleeding. Most young (under age 60), otherwise healthy patients with clean-based ulcers may be safely discharged from the emergency or hospital after endoscopy. Ulcers that have a flat red or black spot have a less than 10% chance of significant rebleeding. Patients who are hemodynamically stable with these findings should be admitted to a hospital ward for 24–72 hours and may begin immediate oral feedings and antiulcer (or anti-*H pylori*) medication.

By contrast, the risk of rebleeding or continued bleeding in ulcers with a firmly adherent clot is 12–33%, with a nonbleeding visible vessel is 50%, and with active bleeding it is 80–90%. Endoscopic therapy with dilute epinephrine (1:10,000) injection, thermocoagulation (bipolar or heater probes), or application of endoscopic clips (akin to a staple) is the standard of care for such lesions because it reduces the risk of rebleeding, the number of transfusions, and the need for subsequent surgery. Using any of these techniques, successful hemostasis of actively bleeding lesions is achieved in 90%. For actively bleeding ulcers, a combination of epinephrine injection followed by thermocoagulation yields better control of bleeding than either modality alone. Significant rebleeding occurs in 10–20% of cases, of which over 70% can be managed successfully with repeat endoscopic treatment. In limited comparative studies, hemoclipping appears to be as effective as injection and thermocoagulation techniques. Patients with these high-risk lesions should receive a high-dose intravenous or oral proton pump inhibitor regimen for 72 hours. After endoscopic treatment, high-risk patients should be monitored in an ICU setting for at least 24 hours and should remain hospitalized for at least 72 hours, when the risk of rebleeding is < 3%.

C. SURGICAL TREATMENT

Patients with recurrent bleeding or bleeding that cannot be controlled by endoscopic techniques should be evaluated by a surgeon. However, less than 5% of patients treated with hemostatic therapy require surgery for continued or recurrent bleeding. Overall surgical mortality for emergency ulcer bleeding is less than 6%. The prognosis is poorer for patients over age 60 years, those with serious underlying medical illnesses or chronic renal failure, and those who require more than 10 units of blood transfusion.

2. Ulcer Perforation

Perforations develop in < 5% of ulcer patients, usually from ulcers on the anterior wall of the stomach or duodenum. The incidence of perforations may be increasing, perhaps as a consequence of using NSAIDs or crack cocaine. Perforation results in a chemical peritonitis that causes sudden, severe generalized abdominal pain that prompts most patients to seek immediate attention. Elderly or debilitated patients and those receiving long-term corticosteroid therapy may experience minimal initial symptoms, presenting late with bacterial peritonitis, sepsis, and shock. On physical examination, patients appear ill, with a rigid, quiet abdomen and rebound tenderness. Hypotension develops later after bacterial peritonitis has developed. If hypotension is present early with the onset of pain, other abdominal emergencies should be considered such as a ruptured aortic aneurysm, mesenteric infarction, or acute pancreatitis. Leukocytosis is almost always present. A mildly elevated serum amylase (less than twice normal) is sometimes seen. Upright or decubitus films of the abdomen reveal free intraperitoneal air in 75% of cases, and in most cases this establishes the diagnosis without need for further studies. The absence of free air may lead to a misdiagnosis of pancreatitis, cholecystitis, or appendicitis. Upper gastrointestinal or CT radiography with water-soluble contrast may be useful in this setting. Barium studies are contraindicated in patients with possible perforation.

Traditional surgical dogma held that the majority of patients with perforated ulcers should undergo emergency laparotomy. Closure of the perforation was performed with an omental ("Graham") patch and, in stable patients, a proximal gastric vagotomy was performed to decrease the chance of ulcer recurrence. This approach is changing as a result of two factors. The first is minimally invasive surgical technique. Laparoscopic perforation closure can be performed in many centers, significantly reducing operative morbidity. Second is the recognition that *H pylori* infection is associated with most ulcers and ulcer perforations. Postoperative treatment of *H pylori* reduces the risk of ulcer recurrence, obviating the need for intraoperative

vagotomy. The overall mortality rate in patients treated surgically is 5%.

Up to 40% of ulcer perforations seal spontaneously by the adherence of omentum or adjacent organs to the lesion and do not have significant intraperitoneal spillage. Thus, initial nonoperative management may be suitable for patients whose onset of symptoms is less than 12 hours and whose upper gastrointestinal series with water-soluble contrast medium does not demonstrate leakage. Such conservative therapy is most appropriate for patients who are poor operative candidates. Patients should be monitored closely while receiving fluids, nasogastric suction, intravenous proton pump inhibitors, and broad-spectrum antibiotics. If their condition deteriorates over the first 12 hours (as evidenced by increasing pain, rising pulse or temperature, or worsening peritonitis), they should be taken to the operating room.

3. Ulcer Penetration

An ulcer located along the posterior wall of the duodenum or stomach may perforate into contiguous structures such as the pancreas, liver, or biliary tree. Patients complain of a change in the intensity and rhythmicity of their ulcer symptoms. The pain becomes more severe and constant, may radiate to the back, and is unresponsive to antacids or food. Physical examination and laboratory tests are nonspecific. Mild amylase elevations may sometimes occur. Endoscopy and barium x-ray studies confirm the ulceration but are not diagnostic of an actual penetration. Patients should be given intravenous proton pump inhibitors and monitored closely. Those who do not improve should be considered for surgery.

4. Gastric Outlet Obstruction

Gastric outlet obstruction occurs in 2% of patients with ulcer disease and is due to edema or cicatricial narrowing of the pylorus or duodenal bulb. Most patients have a prior known history of ulcer disease. Obstruction is less commonly caused by gastric neoplasms or extrinsic duodenal obstruction by intra-abdominal neoplasms. The most common symptoms are early satiety, vomiting, and weight loss. Early symptoms are epigastric fullness or heaviness after meals. Later, vomiting may develop that typically occurs one to several hours after eating and consists of partially digested food contents. Chronic obstruction may result in a grossly dilated, atonic stomach, severe weight loss, and malnutrition. Patients may develop dehydration, metabolic alkalosis, and hypokalemia. On physical examination, a succussion splash may be heard in the epigastrium. In most cases, nasogastric aspiration will result in evacuation of a large amount (> 200 mL) of foul-smelling fluid, which establishes the diagnosis. More subtle obstruction is diagnosed by a saline load test or by a nuclear gastric emptying study. Patients are treated initially with intravenous isotonic saline and KCl to correct fluid and electrolyte disorders, an intravenous proton pump inhibitor, and nasogastric decompression of the stomach. Severely malnourished patients should receive TPN. Upper endoscopy is performed after 24–72 hours to define the nature of the obstruction and to exclude gastric neoplasm. Patients whose symptoms fail to improve within 5–7 days on nasogastric suction require endoscopic or surgical treatment. Upper endoscopy with dilation of the gastric obstruction by hydrostatic balloons passed through the instrument improves symptoms in up to two-thirds of patients and may be attempted in patients with milder symptoms. Surgical treatment with vagotomy and either pyloroplasty or antrectomy is required in patients with inadequate response or symptom relapse after endoscopic dilation.

ASGE guideline: the role of endoscopy in acute non-variceal upper-GI hemorrhage. Gastrointest Endosc 2004;60:497. [PMID: 15472669]

Barkun A et al: Consensus guidelines for managing patients with nonvariceal upper gastrointestinal bleeding. Ann Intern Med 2003;139:843. [PMID: 14623622]

Bardou M et al: Meta-analysis: proton-pump inhibition in high-risk patients with acute peptic ulcer bleeding. Aliment Pharmacol Ther 2005;21:677. [PMID: 15771753]

Calvet X et al: Addition of a second endoscopic treatment following epinephrine injection improves outcome in high-risk bleeding ulcers. Gastroenterology 2004;126:441. [PMID: 14762781]

Hung LC et al: Long-term outcome of Helicobacter pylori–negative idiopathic bleeding ulcers: a prospective cohort study. Gastroenterology 2005;128:1845. [PMID: 15940620]

Julapalli VR et al: Appropriate use of intravenous proton pump inhibitors in the management of bleeding peptic ulcer. Dig Dis Sci 2005;50:1185. [PMID: 16047458]

Lanas A et al: A nationwide study of mortality associated with hospital admission due to severe gastrointestinal events and those associated with nonsteroidal antiinflammatory drug use. Am J Gastroenterol 2005;100:1685. [PMID: 16086703]

Park CH et al: A prospective, randomized trial comparing mechanical methods of hemostasis plus epinephrine injection to epinephrine injection alone for bleeding peptic ulcer. Gastrointest Endosc 2004;60:173. [PMID: 15278040]

Ramsoekh D et al: Outcome of peptic ulcer bleeding, nonsteroidal anti-inflammatory drug use, and Helicobacter pylori infection. Clin Gastroenterol Hepatol 2005;3:859. [PMID: 16234022]

Saltzman JR et al: Prospective trial of endoscopic clips versus combination therapy in upper GI bleeding (PROTECCT—UGI Bleeding). Am J Gastroenterol 2005;100:1503. [PMID: 15984972]

ZOLLINGER-ELLISON SYNDROME (Gastrinoma)

ESSENTIALS OF DIAGNOSIS

- Peptic ulcer disease; may be severe and atypical.
- Gastric acid hypersecretion.
- Diarrhea common, relieved by nasogastric suction.
- Most cases are sporadic; 25% with multiple endocrine neoplasia type 1 (MEN 1).

General Considerations

Zollinger-Ellison syndrome is caused by gastrin-secreting gut neuroendocrine tumors (gastrinomas), which result in hypergastrinemia and acid hypersecretion. Less than 1% of peptic ulcer disease is caused by gastrinomas. Primary gastrinomas may arise in the pancreas (25%), duodenal wall (45%), or lymph nodes (5–15%), and in other locations or of unknown primary in 20%. Approximately 80% arise within the "gastrinoma triangle" bounded by the porta hepatis, the neck of the pancreas, and the third portion of the duodenum. Most gastrinomas are solitary or multifocal nodules that are potentially resectable. Over two-thirds of gastrinomas are malignant, and one-third have already metastasized to the liver at initial presentation. Approximately 25% of patients have small multicentric gastrinomas associated with MEN 1 that are more difficult to resect.

Clinical Findings

A. Symptoms and Signs

Over 90% of patients with Zollinger-Ellison syndrome develop peptic ulcers. In most cases, the symptoms are indistinguishable from other causes of peptic ulcer disease and therefore may go undetected for years. Ulcers usually are solitary and located in the duodenal bulb, but they may be multiple or occur more distally in the duodenum. Isolated gastric ulcers do not occur. Gastroesophageal reflux symptoms occur often. Diarrhea occurs in one-third of patients, in some cases in the absence of peptic symptoms. Gastric acid hypersecretion can cause direct intestinal mucosal injury and pancreatic enzyme inactivation, resulting in diarrhea, steatorrhea, and weight loss; nasogastric aspiration of stomach acid stops the diarrhea. Screening for Zollinger-Ellison syndrome with fasting gastrin levels should be obtained in patients with ulcers that are refractory to standard therapies, giant ulcers (> 2 cm), ulcers located distal to the duodenal bulb, multiple duodenal ulcers, frequent ulcer recurrences, ulcers associated with diarrhea, ulcers occurring after ulcer surgery, and patients with ulcer complications. Ulcer patients with hypercalcemia or family histories of ulcers (suggesting MEN 1) should also be screened. Finally, patients with peptic ulcers who are H pylori negative and who are not taking NSAIDs should be screened.

B. Laboratory Findings

The most sensitive and specific method for identifying Zollinger-Ellison syndrome is demonstration of an increased fasting serum gastrin concentration (> 150 pg/mL). Levels should be obtained with patients not taking H_2-receptor antagonists for 24 hours or proton pump inhibitors for 6 days. The median gastrin level is 500–700 pg/mL, and 60% of patients have levels less than 1000 pg/mL. Hypochlorhydria with increased gastric pH is a much more common cause of hypergastrinemia than is gastrinoma. Therefore, a measurement of gastric pH (and, where available, gastric secretory studies) is performed in patients with fasting hypergastrinemia. Most patients have a basal acid output of over 15 mEq/h. A gastric pH of > 3.0 implies hypochlorhydria and excludes gastrinoma. In a patient with a serum gastrin level of > 1000 pg/mL and acid hypersecretion, the diagnosis of Zollinger-Ellison syndrome is established. With lower gastrin levels (150–1000 pg/mL) and acid secretion, a secretin stimulation test is performed to distinguish Zollinger-Ellison syndrome from other causes of hypergastrinemia. Intravenous secretin (2 units/kg) produces a rise in serum gastrin of over 200 pg/mL within 2–30 minutes in 85% of patients with gastrinoma. An elevated serum calcium suggests hyperparathyroidism and MEN 1 syndrome. In all patients with Zollinger-Ellison syndrome, a serum parathyroid hormone (PTH), prolactin, luteinizing hormone-follicle-stimulating hormone (LH-FSH), and growth hormone (GH) level should be obtained to exclude MEN 1.

C. IMAGING

Imaging studies are obtained in an attempt to determine whether there is metastatic disease and, if not, to identify the site of the primary tumor. Gastrinomas express somatostatin receptors that bind radiolabeled octreotide. Somatostatin receptor scintigraphy (SRS) with single photon emission computed tomography (SPECT) allows total body imaging for detection of primary gastrinomas in the pancreas and lymph nodes, primary gastrinomas in unusual locations, and metastatic gastrinomas (liver and bone). SRS has a sensitivity (> 80%) for tumor detection that exceeds all other imaging studies combined. If SRS is positive for tumor localization, further imaging studies are not necessary. In patients with negative SRS, endoscopic ultrasonography (EUS) may be useful to detect small gastrinomas in the duodenal wall, pancreas, or peripancreatic lymph nodes. CT and MRI scans are commonly obtained to look for large hepatic metastases and primary lesions, but they have low sensitivity for small lesions. With a combination of SRS and EUS, more than 90% of primary gastrinomas can be localized preoperatively.

Differential Diagnosis

Gastrinomas are one of several gut neuroendocrine tumors that have similar histopathologic features and arise either from the gut or pancreas. These include carcinoid, insulinoma, VIPoma, glucagonoma, and somatostatinoma. These tumors usually are differentiated by the gut peptides that they secrete; however, poorly differentiated neuroendocrine tumors may not secrete any hormones. Patients may present with symptoms caused by tumor metastases (jaundice, hepatomegaly) rather than functional symptoms. Once a diagnosis of a neuroendocrine tumor is established

from the liver biopsy, the specific type of tumor can subsequently be determined. Both carcinoids and gastrinomas may be detected incidentally during endoscopy after biopsy of a submucosal nodule and must be distinguished by subsequent studies.

Hypergastrinemia due to gastrinoma must be distinguished from other causes of hypergastrinemia. Atrophic gastritis with decreased acid secretion is detected by gastric secretory analysis. Other conditions associated with hypergastrinemia (eg, gastric outlet obstruction, vagotomy, chronic renal failure) are associated with a negative secretin stimulation test.

Treatment

A. METASTATIC DISEASE

The most important predictor of survival is the presence of hepatic metastases. In patients with multiple hepatic metastases, initial therapy should be directed at controlling hypersecretion. Proton pump inhibitors (omeprazole, esomeprazole, rabeprazole, pantoprazole, or lansoprazole) are given at a dose of 40–120 mg/d, titrated to achieve a basal acid output of < 10 mEq/h. At this level, there is complete symptomatic relief and ulcer healing. In patients with isolated hepatic metastases, surgical resection or cryoablation may decrease the need for antisecretory medications and may prolong survival. Owing to the slow growth of these tumors, 30% of patients with hepatic metastases have a survival of 10 years.

B. LOCALIZED DISEASE

Cure can be achieved only if the gastrinoma can be resected before hepatic metastatic spread has occurred. Lymph node metastases do not adversely affect prognosis. Laparotomy should be considered in all patients in whom preoperative studies fail to demonstrate hepatic or other distant metastases. A combination of preoperative studies, duodenotomy with careful duodenal inspection, and intraoperative palpation and sonography allows successful localization and resection in the majority of cases. The 15-year survival of patients who do not have liver metastases at initial presentation is over 95%. The role of surgery in patients with MEN 1 is controversial. Surgical cure in patients with MEN 1 rarely occurs, and long-term survival is common in the absence of surgery. Some experts recommend surgery only in patients with MEN 1 whose tumors are larger than 2 cm, in whom the risk of hepatic metastases is increased.

Norton J et al: Resolved and unresolved controversies in the surgical management of patients with Zollinger-Ellison syndrome. Ann Surg 2004;240:757. [PMID: 15492556]

BENIGN TUMORS OF THE STOMACH

Gastric epithelial polyps are usually detected incidentally at endoscopy. The majority are fundic gland polyps or hyperplastic polyps, which are small, single or multiple, have no malignant potential, and do not require removal or endoscopic surveillance. Adenomatous polyps account for 10–20% of gastric polyps. They are usually solitary lesions. In rare instances they ulcerate, causing chronic blood loss. Because of their premalignant potential, endoscopic removal is indicated. Annual endoscopic surveillance is recommended to screen for further polyp development. Submucosal gastric polypoid lesions include benign gastric stromal tumors (commonly misclassified as leiomyomas) and pancreatic rests.

Burt R: Gastric fundic gland polyps. Gastroenterology 2003; 125:1462. [PMID: 14598262]

MALIGNANT TUMORS OF THE STOMACH

1. Gastric Adenocarcinoma

ESSENTIALS OF DIAGNOSIS

- Dyspeptic symptoms with weight loss in patients over age 40 years.
- Iron deficiency anemia; occult blood in stools.
- Abnormality detected on upper gastrointestinal series or endoscopy.

General Considerations

Although gastric adenocarcinoma is the most common cancer (other than skin cancer) worldwide, its incidence in the United States has declined by two-thirds over the last 30 years to 20,000 cases annually. Gastric cancer is uncommon in persons younger than 40 years; the mean age at diagnosis is 63 years. Men are affected twice as often as women. The incidence is higher in Latinos, African-Americans, and Asian-Americans. Certain regions such as Chile, Colombia, Central America, and Japan have rates as high as 80 per 100,000 population. Although most gastric cancers arise in the antrum, the incidence of proximal tumors of the cardia and fundus is increasing dramatically.

Chronic *H pylori* gastritis is a strong risk factor for gastric carcinoma of the distal (but not proximal) stomach, increasing the relative risk 3.5- to 20-fold. It is estimated that 60–90% of cases of distal gastric carcinoma may be attributable to *H pylori*. Patients infected with a virulent strain of *H pylori* (CagA-positive) and patients with gastritis associated with atrophy or intestinal metaplasia are at increased risk. During a mean of 7.5 years of follow-up, gastric cancer developed in approximately 1.4–2.9% of patients with chronic *H pylori* gastritis. Prospective controlled studies have not demonstrated a reduction in gastric cancer incidence after *H pylori* eradication, although a

decreased incidence has been observed in the subset of infected patients without precancerous lesions (atrophy or intestinal metaplasia) prior to therapy. Because of its unproven efficacy and cost-effectiveness, screening for *H pylori* infection and treating it to prevent gastric cancer is not recommended for asymptomatic adults in the general population but may be considered in patients who have immigrated from regions with a high incidence of gastric cancer or who have a family history of gastric cancer. Other risk factors for gastric cancer include pernicious anemia and a history of partial gastric resection more than 15 years previously.

Gastric cancer may occur in a variety of morphologic types: (1) polypoid or fungating intraluminal masses; (2) ulcerating masses; (3) diffusely spreading (linitis plastica), in which the tumor spreads through the submucosa, resulting in a rigid, atonic stomach with thickened folds (prognosis dismal); and (4) superficially spreading or "early" gastric cancer—confined to the mucosa or submucosa (with or without lymph node metastases) and associated with an excellent prognosis.

Clinical Findings

A. SYMPTOMS AND SIGNS

Gastric carcinoma is generally asymptomatic until the disease is quite advanced. Symptoms are nonspecific and are determined in part by the location of the tumor. Dyspepsia, vague epigastric pain, anorexia, early satiety, and weight loss are the presenting symptoms in most patients. Patients may derive initial symptomatic relief from over-the-counter remedies, further delaying diagnosis. Ulcerating lesions can lead to acute gastrointestinal bleeding with hematemesis or melena. Pyloric obstruction results in postprandial vomiting. Lower esophageal obstruction causes progressive dysphagia. Physical examination is rarely helpful. A gastric mass is palpated in less than 20% of patients. Signs of metastatic spread include a left supraclavicular lymph node (Virchow's node), an umbilical nodule (Sister Mary Joseph nodule), a rigid rectal shelf (Blumer's shelf), and ovarian metastases (Krukenberg tumor). Guaiac-positive stools may be detectable.

B. LABORATORY FINDINGS

Iron deficiency anemia due to chronic blood loss or anemia of chronic disease is common. Liver function test abnormalities may be present if there is metastatic liver spread. Other tumor markers are of no value.

C. ENDOSCOPY

Upper endoscopy should be obtained in all patients over age 55 years with new onset of epigastric symptoms (dyspepsia) and in anyone with dyspepsia that is persistent or fails to respond to a short trial of antisecretory therapy. Endoscopy with cytologic brushings and biopsies of suspicious lesions is highly sensitive for detecting gastric carcinoma. It can be difficult to obtain adequate biopsy specimens in linitis plastica lesions. Because of the high incidence of gastric carcinoma in Japan, screening upper endoscopy is performed to detect early gastric carcinoma. Approximately 40% of tumors detected by screening are early, with a 5-year survival rate of almost 90%. Screening programs are not recommended in the United States.

D. IMAGING

A barium upper gastrointestinal series is an acceptable alternative when endoscopy is not readily available but may not detect small or superficial lesions and cannot reliably distinguish benign from malignant ulcerations. Any abnormalities detected with this procedure require endoscopic confirmation.

Once a gastric cancer is diagnosed, preoperative evaluation with abdominal CT and EUS is indicated to delineate the local extent of the primary tumor as well as nodal or distant metastases. Abdominal CT is valuable in identifying distant metastases and direct invasion of adjacent structures. Endoscopic ultrasound imaging is superior to CT in determining the depth of tumor penetration and nodal metastases.

E. STAGING

Staging is defined according to the TNM system, in which T1 tumors invade the lamina propria (T1a) or submucosa (T1b), T2 invade the muscularis propria, T3 penetrate the serosa, and T4 invade adjacent structures. Nodes are graded as N0 if there is no involvement, N1 if there are metastases to perigastric nodes, and N2 if regional lymph nodes are involved. M1 signifies the presence of metastatic disease. The stages are defined in the accompanying box.

STAGING CRITERIA FOR GASTRIC ADENOCARCINOMA

Stage I: T1N0, T1N1, T2N0, all M0
Stage II: T1N2, T2N1, T3N0, all M0
Stage III: T2N2, T2N1, T4N0, all M0
Stage IV: T4N2M0, any M1

Differential Diagnosis

Ulcerating gastric adenocarcinomas are distinguished from benign gastric ulcers by biopsies. Approximately 3% of gastric ulcers initially believed to be benign later prove to be malignant. To exclude malignancy, all gastric ulcers identified at endoscopy should be biopsied. Ulcers that are suspicious for malignancy to the endoscopist or that have atypia or dysplasia on histologic examination warrant repeat endoscopy in 2–3 months to verify healing and exclude malignancy. Nonhealing

ulcers should be considered for resection. Infiltrative carcinoma with thickened gastric folds must be distinguished from lymphoma and other hypertrophic gastropathies such as Ménétrier's disease.

Treatment

A. CURATIVE SURGICAL RESECTION

After preoperative staging, about two-thirds of patients will be found to have localized disease (ie, stages I–III). In Japan and some centers in other countries, endoscopic mucosal resection is performed in selected patients with small (< 3 cm), early (intramucosal or T1aN0) gastric cancers after careful staging. For all other patients, surgical resection is the only therapy with curative potential. At surgery, approximately 25% of these patients will be found to have locally unresectable tumors or peritoneal, hepatic, or distant lymph node metastases for which "curative" surgical resection is not warranted (see below). The remaining patients with confirmed localized disease should undergo radical surgical resection with curative intent. For adenocarcinoma localized to the distal two-thirds of the stomach, a subtotal distal gastrectomy should be performed. For proximal gastric cancer or diffusely infiltrating disease, total gastrectomy is necessary. Although lymph node dissection should be performed for curative resections, there has been ongoing debate about whether an extended (perigastric and regional) lymph node dissection or a limited (perigastric) dissection is needed. However, there appears to be greater short-term morbidity and no long-term survival advantage for extended lymph node dissection. Neither preoperative nor postoperative (adjuvant) chemotherapy or radiochemotherapy appear to confer a survival benefit in most studies in patients who have undergone curative resection with careful nodal dissection. Nevertheless, adjuvant treatment may be considered in patients with stage III cancer, preferably as part of a clinical trial.

B. PALLIATIVE MODALITIES

Many patients will be found either preoperatively or at the time of surgical exploration to have advanced disease that is not amenable to "curative" surgery due to peritoneal or distant metastases or local invasion of other organs. In many of these cases, palliative resection of the tumor nonetheless may be indicated. Such resection removes the risk of bleeding and obstruction, leads to improved quality of life, and improves survival. For patients with unresectable disease, gastrojejunostomy may be indicated to prevent obstruction. Bleeding or obstruction from unresected tumors may be treated with endoscopic laser or stent therapy, radiation therapy, or angiographic embolization. Although chemotherapy has not been shown to prolong life, single-agent or combination therapies with fluorouracil, doxorubicin, and cisplatin or mitomycin may provide palliation in up to 30%.

Prognosis

The long-term survival of gastric carcinoma is less than 15%. However, 5-year survival in patients who undergo successful curative resection is over 45%. Survival is related to tumor stage, location, and histologic features. Stage I and stage II tumors resected for cure have a greater than 50% long-term survival. Patients with stage III tumors have a poor prognosis (< 20% long-term survival) and should be considered for enrollment in clinical trials. Tumors of the diffuse and signet ring type have a worse prognosis than the intestinal type. Tumors of the proximal stomach (fundus and cardia) carry a far worse prognosis than distal lesions. Even with apparently localized disease, proximal tumors have a 5-year survival of less than 15%. For those whose disease progresses despite therapy, meticulous efforts at palliative care are essential (see Chapter 5).

Dicken BJ et al: Gastric adenocarcinoma: review and considerations for future directions. Ann Surg 2005;241:27. [PMID: 15621988]

Genta RM: Screening for gastric cancer: does it make sense? Aliment Pharmacol Ther 2004;20(Suppl 2):42. [PMID: 15335412]

Hohenberger P et al: Gastric cancer. Lancet 2003;362:305. [PMID: 12892963]

Macdonald JS: Adjuvant therapy for gastric cancer. Semin Oncol 2003;30(suppl 11):19. [PMID: 14506600]

McCulloch P et al: Extended versus limited lymph node dissection technique for adenocarcinoma of the stomach. Cochrane Database Syst Rev 2004;(4):CD001964. [PMID: 15495024]

Melfertheiner P et al: *Helicobacter pylori* eradication has the potential to prevent gastric cancer: a state-of-the-art critique. Am J Gastroenterol 2005;100:2100. [PMID: 16128957]

2. Lymphoma

Lymphoma is the second most common gastric malignancy, accounting for 3–6% of gastric cancers. More than 95% of these are non-Hodgkin's B cell lymphomas. Gastric lymphomas may be primary (arising from the gastric mucosa) or may represent a site of secondary involvement in patients with nodal lymphomas. About 60% of primary gastric lymphomas are believed to arise from mucosa-associated lymphoid tissue (MALT). Distinguishing advanced primary gastric lymphoma with adjacent nodal spread from advanced nodal lymphoma with secondary gastric spread can be problematic. Because the prognosis and treatment of primary and secondary gastric lymphomas are entirely different, the distinction is important. B cells of nodal origin may be distinguished from those derived from MALT (CD19 and CD20 positive).

Infection with *H pylori* may be an important risk factor for the development of primary gastric lymphoma. Chronic infection with *H pylori* causes an intense lymphocytic inflammatory response that may lead to the development of lymphoid follicles. Over 85% of low-grade primary gastric lymphomas and 40% of high-grade lymphomas are associated with *H*

pylori infection. The risk of developing lymphoma is increased sevenfold in patients with chronic *H pylori* infection. It is hypothesized that chronic antigenic stimulation may result in a monoclonal lymphoproliferation that may culminate in a low-grade MALT lymphoma. At present, the relationship between high-grade primary lymphomas, MALT, and *H pylori* infection is unclear.

The clinical presentation and endoscopic appearance of gastric lymphoma are similar to those of adenocarcinoma. Most patients have abdominal pain, weight loss, or bleeding. Night sweats are absent in primary lymphoma. At endoscopy, lymphoma may appear as an ulcer, mass, or diffusely infiltrating lesion. The diagnosis is established with endoscopic biopsy. All patients should undergo staging with abdominal and chest CT. EUS is the most sensitive test for determining the presence of perigastric lymphadenopathy.

Nodal lymphomas with secondary gastrointestinal involvement usually present at an advanced stage with widely disseminated disease and are seldom curable. Their treatment is addressed in Chapter 13. By contrast, primary low-grade gastric lymphomas usually are localized to the stomach wall (stage IE) or adjacent lymph nodes (stage IIE) and have an excellent prognosis. Patients with primary low-grade gastric MALT-lymphoma should be tested for *H pylori* infection and treated if positive. Where available, EUS should be performed to accurately determine tumor stage. Complete lymphoma regression after successful *H pylori* eradication occurs in 75% of cases of stage IE low-grade lymphoma. Remission may take as long as a year. Patients with stage IE or IIE low-grade lymphomas who either are not infected with *H pylori* or fail to respond to eradication therapy can be treated successfully with surgical resection, local radiation therapy, or combination therapy. Stage IE or IIE high-grade lymphomas may be treated with resection and CHOP chemotherapy. Stage III and stage IV primary lymphomas are treated with combination chemotherapy. Because of a low risk of perforation with either radiation therapy or chemotherapy, surgical resection is no longer recommended. The long-term survival of primary gastric lymphoma for stage I is over 85% and for stage II is 35–65%.

Al-Akwaa AM et al: Primary gastric lymphoma. World J Gastroenterol 2004;10:5. [PMID: 14695759]

Bierman PJ: Gastrointestinal lymphoma. Curr Treat Options Oncol 2003;4:421. [PMID: 12941202]

Farinha P et al: *Helicobacter pylori* and MALT lymphoma. Gastroenterology 2005;128:1579. [PMID: 15887153]

Levy M et al: Conservative treatment of primary gastric low-grade B-cell lymphoma of mucosa-associated lymphoid tissue: predictive factors of response and outcome. Am J Gastroenterol 2002;97:292. [PMID: 11866264]

3. Carcinoid Tumors

Gastric carcinoids are rare neuroendocrine tumors that make up less than 1% of gastric neoplasms. They may occur sporadically or secondary to chronic hypergastrinemia that results in hyperplasia and transformation of enterochromaffin cells in the gastric fundus. Sporadic carcinoids account for 20% of gastric carcinoids. Most are solitary, over 2 cm in size, and have a strong propensity for metastatic spread. Most sporadic carcinoids already have carcinoid syndrome and hepatic or pulmonary metastatic involvement at initial presentation. Localized sporadic carcinoids should be treated with radical gastrectomy.

The majority of carcinoids caused by hypergastrinemia occur in association with either pernicious anemia (75%) or Zollinger-Ellison syndrome (5%). Carcinoids associated with Zollinger-Ellison syndrome occur almost exclusively in patients with MEN 1, in which loss of 11q13 has been reported. Carcinoids caused by hypergastrinemia tend to be multicentric, less than 1 cm in size, and have a low potential for metastatic spread or development of carcinoid syndrome. Small lesions may be successfully treated with endoscopic resection followed by periodic endoscopic surveillance. Antrectomy reduces serum gastrin levels and may lead to regression of small tumors. Patients with large or multiple carcinoids should undergo surgical tumor resection.

Modlin IM et al: Current status of gastrointestinal carcinoids. Gastroenterology 2005;128:1717. [PMID: 15887161]

4. Mesenchymal Tumors

Gastrointestinal mesenchymal tumors occur throughout the gastrointestinal tract, but approximately two-thirds occur in the stomach. These tumors (which include stromal tumors, leiomyomas, and schwannomas) derive from mesenchymal stem cells and have an epithelioid or spindle cell histologic pattern, resembling smooth muscle. The most common stromal tumors are gastrointestinal stromal tumors ("GIST"), which appear to originate from interstitial cells of Cajal, and which have a mutation in the protooncogene c-*kit* tyrosine kinase that leads to constitutive activation. Thus, stromal tumors stain positively for CD117 (part of the c-*kit* protein); most also stain positively for CD34. Other mesenchymal tumors such as leiomyomas, which derive from smooth muscle cells, stain negative for CD117. Mesenchymal tumors may grow quite large before causing symptoms, mainly acute or chronic bleeding due to central ulceration within the tumor. At endoscopy, they appear as a submucosal mass that may have central umbilication or ulceration. EUS (possibly with guided FNA biopsy) is the optimal study for diagnosing mesenchymal tumors and distinguishing them from other submucosal lesions. However, it is difficult to distinguish with certainty benign from malignant (sarcoma) tumors by EUS appearance, FNA, or even by histologic specimens obtained at surgery. Lesions that are smaller than 3 cm, have a smooth border, and have a homogeneous echo pattern on EUS are more likely benign.

Surgery is recommended for all patients with tumors that are symptomatic, ≥ 3 cm, are increasing in size, or have an EUS appearance suspicious for malignancy. The management of asymptomatic benign-appearing lesions 1–3 cm in size is problematic. Because of a low risk of malignancy, surgical resection should be considered in younger, otherwise healthy patients; however, other patients may be followed up with serial EUS examinations or, in selected cases, endoscopic resections. There is a high risk of metastasis or recurrence when tumors are larger than 5 cm, have an irregular border or cystic spaces, and have increased mitotic activity (more than five mitoses per high-power field). These high-risk tumors have a 50% 5-year survival rate after complete surgical resection. Metastatic tumors are aggressive and carry a poor prognosis. The tyrosine kinase inhibitor imatinib induces partial response and clinical improvement in up to half of patients with metastatic disease.

Davila R et al: GI stromal tumors. Gastrointest Endosc 2003; 58:80. [PMID: 12838226]

Hwang JH et al: The incidental upper gastrointestinal subepithelial mass. Gastroenterology 2004;126:301. [PMID: 14699508]

Lograno R et al: Recent advances in cell biology, diagnosis, and therapy of gastrointestinal stromal tumor (GIST). Cancer Cell Biol 2004;3:251. [PMID: 14726714]

Van Glabbeke M et al: Initial and late resistance to imatinib in advanced gastrointestinal stromal tumors are predicted by different prognostic factors: a European Organisation for Research and Treatment of Cancer-Italian Sarcoma Group-Australasian Gastrointestinal Trials Group study. J Clin Oncol 2005;20:5795. [PMID: 16110036]

■ DISEASES OF THE SMALL INTESTINE

MALABSORPTION

The term "malabsorption" denotes disorders in which there is a disruption of digestion and nutrient absorption. The clinical and laboratory manifestations of malabsorption are summarized in Table 14–12.

Normal Digestion

Normal digestion and absorption may be divided into three phases.

A. INTRALUMINAL PHASE

Dietary fats, proteins, and carbohydrates are hydrolyzed and solubilized by pancreatic and biliary secretions. Fats are broken down by pancreatic lipase to monoglycerides and fatty acids that form micelles with bile salts. Micelles are important for the solubilization and absorption of fat-soluble vitamins (A, D, E, K). Proteins are hydrolyzed by pancreatic proteases to di- and tripeptides and amino ac-

Table 14–12. Clinical and laboratory manifestations of malabsorption.

Manifestation	Laboratory Findings	Malabsorbed Nutrients
Steatorrhea (bulky, light-colored stools)	Increased fecal fat; decreased serum cholesterol	Fat
Diarrhea (increased fecal water)	Increased fecal fat or positive bile salt breath test	Fatty acids or bile salts
Weight loss; malnutrition (muscle wasting); weakness, fatigue, abdominal distention	Increased fecal fat and nitrogen; decreased glucose and xylose absorption	Calories (fat, protein, carbohydrates)
Iron deficiency anemia	Hypochromic anemia; low serum iron	Iron
Megaloblastic anemia	Macrocytosis; decreased vitamin B_{12} absorption (^{57}Co-labeled B_{12}); decreased serum vitamin B_{12} and red cell folate	Vitamin B_{12} or folic acid
Paresthesia; tetany; positive Trousseau and Chvostek signs	Decreased serum calcium, magnesium, and potassium	Calcium, vitamin D, magnesium, potassium
Bone pain; pathologic fractures; skeletal deformities	Osteoporosis on x-ray; osteomalacia on biopsy	Calcium, protein
Bleeding tendency (ecchymoses, melena, hematuria)	Prolonged prothrombin time	Vitamin K
Edema	Decreased serum albumin; increased fecal loss of α_1-antitrypsin (antiprotease)	Protein (or protein-losing enteropathy)
Nocturia; abdominal distention	Increased small bowel fluid on x-ray	Water
Milk intolerance (cramps, bloating, diarrhea)	Flat lactose tolerance test; decreased mucosal lactase levels	Lactose

Modified from Bayless TM: Malabsorption in the elderly. Hosp Pract (Aug) 1979;14:67.

ids. Impaired intraluminal digestion may be caused by insufficient intraluminal concentrations of pancreatic enzymes or bile salts. These conditions will not be covered in detail here (see Chapter 15).

Pancreatic insufficiency may be caused by chronic pancreatitis, cystic fibrosis, or pancreatic cancer. Pancreatic enzymes may also be inactivated within the intestinal lumen by acid hypersecretion (Zollinger-Ellison syndrome). Significant pancreatic enzyme insufficiency generally results in significant steatorrhea (due to malabsorption of triglycerides)—often more than 20–40 g/24 h—resulting in weight loss, gaseous distention and flatulence, and large, greasy, foul-smelling stools. The digestion of proteins and carbohydrates is affected to a far lesser degree and is generally not clinically significant. Because micellar function and intestinal absorption are normal, signs of other nutrient or vitamin deficiencies are rare.

Decreased bile salt concentrations may be due to biliary obstruction or cholestatic liver diseases. Because bile salts are resorbed in the terminal ileum, resection or disease of this area (eg, Crohn's disease) can lead to insufficient intraluminal bile salts. Finally, destruction or loss of bile salts may be caused by bacterial overgrowth, massive acid hypersecretion, or medications that bind bile salts (eg, cholestyramine). (Bacterial overgrowth is discussed below.)

Insufficient concentrations of intraluminal bile salts lead to mild steatorrhea (due to malabsorption of fatty acids and monoglycerides), though generally less than 20 g/d. Weight loss is minimal. Impaired absorption of fat-soluble vitamins (A, D, E, K) is common, resulting in bleeding tendencies, osteoporosis, and hypocalcemia (Table 14–12). Other nutrient absorption is intact. Intestinal loss of bile salts into the colon may cause a watery secretory diarrhea.

B. MUCOSAL PHASE

The mucosal phase requires a sufficient surface area of intact small intestinal epithelium. Brush border enzymes are important in the hydrolysis of disaccharides and di- and tripeptides. Malabsorption of specific nutrients may occur as a result of deficiency in an isolated brush border enzyme. With the exception of lactase deficiency, these are rare congenital disorders that are evident in childhood. Malabsorption due to primary mucosal diseases, extensive intestinal resections (short bowel syndrome), or lymphoma is discussed below. These disorders result in malabsorption of all nutrients: fats, proteins, and amino acids. Depending on the severity of malabsorption, patients may manifest a number of symptoms and signs, as outlined in Table 14–12.

C. ABSORPTIVE PHASE

Obstruction of the lymphatic system results in impaired absorption of chylomicrons and lipoproteins.

This may lead to steatorrhea and significant enteric protein losses or "protein-losing enteropathy," discussed below.

1. Celiac Disease

 ESSENTIALS OF DIAGNOSIS

- *Typical symptoms: weight loss, chronic diarrhea, abdominal distention, growth retardation.*
- *Atypical symptoms: dermatitis herpetiformis, iron deficiency anemia, osteoporosis.*
- *Abnormal serologic test results.*
- *Abnormal small bowel biopsy.*
- *Clinical improvement on gluten-free diet.*

General Considerations

Also known as gluten enteropathy or celiac sprue, celiac disease is characterized by diffuse damage to the proximal small intestinal mucosa that results in malabsorption of most nutrients. Although "typical" symptoms may manifest between 6 months and 24 months of age after the introduction of weaning foods, the majority of cases present with "atypical" symptoms in childhood or adulthood. Population screening with serologic tests suggests that the disease is present in 1:100 whites of Northern European ancestry, in whom a clinical diagnosis of celiac disease is made in only 10%, suggesting that most cases are undiagnosed or asymptomatic. Celiac disease only develops in people with the HLA-DQ2 (80%) or -DQ8 (20%) class II molecules, which are present in up to 50% of the population. Although the precise mechanism of damage is unknown, it is clear that removal of gluten from the diet results in resolution of symptoms and intestinal healing in most patients. Glutens are storage proteins that are present in certain grains such as wheat, rye, and barley but not oats, rice, or corn. It is hypothesized that in a small number of genetically susceptible dietary gluten stimulates an inappropriate T cell–mediated autoimmune response in the intestinal submucosa that results in destruction of mucosal enterocytes. One target of this autoimmune response is tissue transglutaminase (tTG), an enzyme that modifies a component of gluten (gliadin) to a form that more strongly stimulates T cells.

Clinical Findings

The most important step in diagnosing celiac disease is to consider the diagnosis. Symptoms are present for more than 10 years in most adults before the correct diagnosis is established. Because of its protean manifestations, celiac disease is grossly underdiagnosed in the adult population.

A. SYMPTOMS AND SIGNS

The gastrointestinal symptoms and signs of celiac disease depend on the length of small intestine involved and the patient's age when the disease presents. "Typical" symptoms of malabsorption, including diarrhea, steatorrhea, weight loss, abdominal distention, weakness, muscle wasting, or growth retardation, more commonly present in infants (< 2 years). Older children and adults are less likely to manifest signs of serious malabsorption. They may report chronic diarrhea, dyspepsia, or flatulence due to colonic bacterial digestion of malabsorbed nutrients, but the severity of weight loss is variable. Many adults have minimal or no gastrointestinal symptoms but present with extraintestinal manifestations, including fatigue, depression, anemia, osteoporosis, short stature, delayed puberty, amenorrhea or reduced fertility, dental enamel hypoplasia, or neurologic symptoms (epilepsy, peripheral neuropathy, ataxia). Approximately 40% of patients with positive serologic tests consistent with sprue have no symptoms of disease; the natural history of these patients with "silent" sprue is unclear.

Physical examination may be normal in mild cases or may reveal signs of malabsorption such as loss of muscle mass or subcutaneous fat, pallor due to anemia, easy bruising due to vitamin K deficiency, hyperkeratosis due to vitamin A deficiency, bone pain due to osteomalacia, or neurologic signs (peripheral neuropathy, ataxia) due to vitamin B_{12} or vitamin E deficiency. Abdominal examination may reveal distention with hyperactive bowel sounds.

Dermatitis herpetiformis is regarded as a cutaneous variant of celiac disease. It is a characteristic skin rash consisting of pruritic papulovesicles over the extensor surfaces of the extremities and over the trunk, scalp, and neck. Dermatitis herpetiformis occurs in less than 10% of patients with celiac disease; however, almost all patients who present with dermatitis herpetiformis have evidence of celiac disease on intestinal mucosal biopsy, though it may not be clinically evident.

B. LABORATORY FINDINGS

1. Routine laboratory tests—Depending on the severity of illness and the extent of intestinal involvement, nonspecific laboratory abnormalities may be present that may raise the suspicion of malabsorption and celiac disease. Limited proximal involvement may result only in microcytic anemia due to iron deficiency. More than 10% of adults with iron deficiency not due to gastrointestinal blood loss may have undiagnosed celiac disease. More extensive involvement results in a megaloblastic anemia due to folate or vitamin B_{12} deficiency. Low serum calcium or elevated alkaline phosphatase may reflect impaired calcium or vitamin D absorption with osteomalacia or osteoporosis. Dual-energy x-ray densitometry scanning is recommended for all patients with sprue to screen for osteoporosis. Elevations of prothrombin time, or decreased vitamin A or D levels reflect impaired fat-soluble vitamin absorption. A low serum albumin may reflect small intestine protein loss or poor nutrition. Severe diarrhea may result in a nonanion gap acidosis and hypokalemia. Mild elevations of aminotransferases are found in up to 40%.

2. Serologic tests—Serologic tests should be performed in all patients in whom there is a suspicion of celiac disease. The two tests with the highest diagnostic accuracy are the IgA endomysial antibody and IgA tTG antibody tests, both of which have a ≥ 90% sensitivity and ≥ 95% specificity for the diagnosis of celiac disease. A negative test reliably excludes the diagnosis of celiac disease. Antigliadin antibodies are no longer recommended because of their lower sensitivity and specificity. Because up to 3% of patients with celiac disease have IgA deficiency, an IgA level should be obtained. For the subset of patients with IgA deficiency, IgG tTG or endomysial antibodies can be obtained. Levels of all antibodies become undetectable after 6–12 months of dietary gluten withdrawal and may be used to monitor dietary compliance, especially in patients whose symptoms fail to resolve after institution of a gluten-free diet.

C. MUCOSAL BIOPSY

Endoscopic mucosal biopsy of the distal duodenum or proximal jejunum is the standard method for confirmation of the diagnosis in patients with a positive serologic test for celiac disease. Rarely, mucosal biopsy may be pursued in patients with negative serologies when symptoms and laboratory studies are suggestive of celiac disease. At endoscopy, atrophy or scalloping of the duodenal folds may be observed. Histology reveals loss or blunting of intestinal villi, hypertrophy of the intestinal crypts, and extensive infiltration of the lamina propria with lymphocytes and plasma cells. An adequate normal biopsy excludes the diagnosis. Reversion of these abnormalities on repeat biopsy after a patient is placed on a gluten-free diet establishes the diagnosis. However, if a patient with a compatible biopsy demonstrates prompt clinical improvement on a gluten-free diet and a decrease in antigliadin antibodies, a repeat biopsy is unnecessary.

Differential Diagnosis

Many patients with chronic diarrhea or flatulence are erroneously diagnosed as having irritable bowel syndrome. Celiac sprue must be distinguished from other causes of malabsorption, as outlined above. Severe panmalabsorption of multiple nutrients is almost always caused by mucosal disease. Other causes of steatorrhea include pancreatic insufficiency, reduced bile salts, bacterial overgrowth, or lymphatic obstruction. The histologic appearance of celiac sprue may resemble other mucosal diseases such as tropical sprue, bacterial overgrowth, cow's milk intolerance, viral gastroenteritis, eosinophilic gastroenteritis, and mucosal damage caused by acid hypersecretion associated with gastrinoma. Documentation of clinical response to gluten withdrawal therefore is essential to the diagnosis.

Treatment

Removal of all gluten from the diet is essential to therapy—all wheat, rye, and barley must be eliminated. Although oats appear to be safe, commercial products may be contaminated with wheat or barley during processing. Because of the pervasive use of gluten products in manufactured foods and additives, in medications, and by restaurants, it is imperative that patients and their families confer with a knowledgeable dietitian to comply satisfactorily with this lifelong diet. Several excellent dietary guides and patient support groups are available. Most patients with celiac disease also have lactose intolerance either temporarily or permanently and should avoid dairy products until the intestinal symptoms have improved on the gluten-free diet. Dietary supplements (folate, iron, calcium, and vitamins A, B_{12}, D, and E) should be provided in the initial stages of therapy but usually are not required long-term with a gluten-free diet. Patients with confirmed osteoporosis may require long-term calcium, vitamin D, and bisphosphonate therapy.

Improvement in symptoms should be evident within a few weeks on the gluten-free diet. The most common reason for treatment failure is incomplete removal of gluten.

Prognosis & Complications

If appropriately diagnosed and treated, patients with celiac disease have an excellent prognosis. Celiac disease may be associated with other autoimmune disorders, including Addison's disease, Graves' disease, type 1 diabetes mellitus, myasthenia gravis, scleroderma, Sjögren's syndrome, atrophic gastritis, and pancreatic insufficiency. In some patients, celiac disease may evolve and become refractory to the gluten-free diet. The most common cause is intentional or unintentional dietary noncompliance, which may be suggested by positive serologic tests. Celiac disease that is truly refractory to gluten withdrawal generally carries a poor prognosis. It may be caused by the development of ulcerative jejunitis or rarely of enteropathy associated T cell lymphoma. These conditions should be considered in patients previously responsive to the gluten-free diet in whom new weight loss, abdominal pain, and malabsorption develop. Many other patients with refractory symptoms have a "cryptic" intestinal lymphoma, ie, a monoclonal expansion of the intraepithelial T lymphocyte that may or may not progress. Patients with refractory sprue who do not have intestinal T cell lymphoma or ulcerative jejunitis may respond to corticosteroids or immunosuppression with azathioprine or cyclosporine.

Celiac Disease Foundation, 13251 Ventura Blvd, Suite #1, Studio City, CA 91604-1838; http://www.celiac.org

Celiac Disease and Gluten-Free Support Page: http://www.celiac.com

Chand N et al: Celiac disease. Current concepts in diagnosis and treatment. J Clin Gastroenterol 2006;40:3. [PMID: 16340626]

National Institutes of Health Consensus Development Conference Statement on Celiac Disease, June 28–30, 2004: Gastroenterology 2005;128:(4 Suppl 1):S1. [PMID: 15825115]

2. Whipple's Disease

ESSENTIALS OF DIAGNOSIS

- Multisystemic disease.
- Fever, lymphadenopathy, arthralgias.
- Weight loss, malabsorption, chronic diarrhea.
- Duodenal biopsy with periodic acid-Schiff (PAS)-positive macrophages with characteristic bacillus.

General Considerations

Whipple's disease is a rare multisystemic illness caused by infection with the bacillus *Tropheryma whippelii*. It may occur at any age but most commonly affects white men in the fourth to sixth decades. The source of infection is unknown, but no cases of human-to-human spread have been documented.

Clinical Findings

A. SYMPTOMS AND SIGNS

The clinical manifestations are protean. Arthralgias or a migratory, nondeforming arthritis occurs in 80% and is typically the first symptom experienced. Gastrointestinal symptoms occur in approximately 75% of cases. They include abdominal pain, diarrhea, and some degree of malabsorption with distention, flatulence, and steatorrhea. Weight loss is the most common presenting symptom—seen in almost all patients. Loss of protein due to intestinal or lymphatic involvement may result in protein-losing enteropathy with hypoalbuminemia and edema. In the absence of gastrointestinal symptoms, the diagnosis often is delayed for several years. Intermittent low-grade fever occurs in over 50% of cases. Chronic cough is common. There may be generalized lymphadenopathy that resembles sarcoidosis. Myocardial or valvular involvement may lead to congestive failure or valvular regurgitation. Ocular findings include uveitis, vitreitis, keratitis, retinitis, and retinal hemorrhages. Central nervous system involvement in approximately 10% of cases is manifested by a variety of findings such as dementia, lethargy, coma, seizures, myoclonus, or hypothalamic signs. Cranial nerve findings include ophthalmoplegia or nystagmus.

Physical examination may reveal hypotension (a late finding), low-grade fever, and evidence of malabsorption (see Table 14–12). Lymphadenopathy is present in 50%. Heart murmurs due to valvular involvement may be evident. Peripheral joints may be enlarged or warm, and peripheral edema may be present. Neurologic findings are cited above. Hyperpigmentation on sun-exposed areas is evident in up to 40%.

B. LABORATORY FINDINGS

If significant malabsorption is present, patients may have laboratory abnormalities as outlined in Table 14–12. There may be steatorrhea.

C. HISTOLOGIC EVALUATION

In most cases, the diagnosis of Whipple's disease is established by endoscopic biopsy of the duodenum with histologic evaluation, which demonstrates infiltration of the lamina propria with PAS-positive macrophages that contain gram-positive bacilli (which are not acid-fast) and dilation of the lacteals. The Whipple bacillus has a characteristic trimellar wall appearance on electron microscopy. In some patients who present with nongastrointestinal symptoms, the duodenal biopsy may be normal, and biopsy of other involved organs or lymph nodes may be necessary. Because the PAS stain is less sensitive and specific for extraintestinal Whipple's disease, polymerase chain reaction (PCR) is used to confirm the diagnosis by demonstrating the presence of 16S ribosomal RNA of *T whippelii* in blood, cerebrospinal fluid, vitreous fluid, synovial fluid, or cardiac valves. The sensitivity of PCR is 97% and the specificity 100%.

Differential Diagnosis

Whipple's disease should be considered in patients who present with signs of malabsorption, fever of unknown origin, lymphadenopathy, seronegative arthritis, culture-negative endocarditis, or multisystemic disease. Small bowel biopsy readily distinguishes Whipple's disease from other mucosal malabsorptive disorders, such as celiac sprue. Patients with AIDS and infection of the small intestine with *Mycobacterium avium* complex (MAC) may have a similar clinical and histologic picture; although both conditions are characterized by PAS-positive macrophages, they may be distinguished by the acid-fast stain, which is positive for MAC and negative for the Whipple bacillus. Other conditions that may be confused with Whipple's disease include sarcoidosis, Reiter's syndrome, familial Mediterranean fever, systemic vasculitides, Behçet's disease, intestinal lymphoma, and subacute infective endocarditis.

Treatment

Antibiotic therapy results in a dramatic clinical improvement within several weeks, even in some patients with neurologic involvement. The optimal regimen is unknown. Complete clinical response usually is evident within 1–3 months; however, relapse may occur in up to one-third of patients after discontinuation of treatment. Therefore, prolonged treatment for at least 1 year is required. Drugs that cross the blood-brain barrier are preferred. In severely ill patients, treatment should be initiated with intravenous ceftriaxone (2 g daily) for 2 weeks. Thereafter, trimethoprim-sulfamethoxazole (one double-strength tablet twice daily for 1 year) is recommended as first-line therapy. In patients allergic to sulfonamides or resistant to therapy, long-term treatment with cephalosporins or fluoroquinolones and interferon-γ has been proposed. After treatment, repeat duodenal biopsies may be obtained at 6 and 12 months for histologic evaluation. The absence of PAS-positive material predicts a low likelihood of clinical relapse.

Prognosis

If untreated, the disease is fatal. Because some neurologic signs may be permanent, the goal of treatment is to prevent this progression. Patients must be followed closely after treatment for signs of symptom recurrence.

Bai JC: Whipple's disease. Clin Gastroenterol Hepatol 2004; 2:849. [PMID: 15476147]

Marth T et al: Whipple's disease. Lancet 2003;361:239. [PMID: 12547551]

3. Bacterial Overgrowth

The small intestine normally contains a small number of bacteria. Bacterial overgrowth in the small intestine of whatever cause may result in malabsorption via a number of mechanisms. Bacterial deconjugation of bile salts may lead to inadequate micelle formation, resulting in decreased fat absorption with steatorrhea. Microbial uptake of specific nutrients reduces absorption of vitamin B_{12} and carbohydrates. Bacterial proliferation also causes direct damage to intestinal epithelial cells and the brush border, further impairing absorption of proteins and carbohydrates. Passage of the malabsorbed bile acids and carbohydrates into the colon leads to an osmotic and secretory diarrhea.

Causes of bacterial overgrowth include (1) gastric achlorhydria (especially if other predisposing conditions are present); (2) anatomic abnormalities of the small intestine with stagnation (afferent limb of Billroth II gastrojejunostomy, small intestine diverticula, obstruction, blind loop, radiation enteritis); (3) small intestine motility disorders (scleroderma, diabetic enteropathy, chronic intestinal pseudo-obstruction); (4) gastrocolic or coloenteric fistula (Crohn's disease, malignancy, surgical resection); and (5) miscellaneous disorders (AIDS, chronic pancreatitis). Bacterial overgrowth is an important cause of malabsorption in the elderly, perhaps because of decreased gastric acidity or impaired intestinal motility.

Clinical Findings

Many patients with bacterial overgrowth are asymptomatic. Patients with severe overgrowth have symptoms and signs of malabsorption, including distention, weight loss, and steatorrhea (Table 14–12). Watery diarrhea is common. Megaloblastic anemia or neurologic signs due to vitamin B_{12} deficiency are common findings and may be manifest at presentation. In patients with vitamin B_{12} deficiency, the Schilling test is diagnostic of bacterial overgrowth if it is abnormal in phase I and II (without and with intrinsic factor) but normalizes after a course of antibiotics. Qualitative or quantitative fecal fat assessment typically is abnormal. D-Xylose absorption is also abnormal due to bacterial uptake of the carbohydrate.

Bacterial overgrowth should be considered in any patient with diarrhea, steatorrhea, weight loss, or macrocytic anemia, especially if the patient has a predisposing cause (such as prior gastrointestinal surgery). A stool collection should be obtained to corroborate the presence of steatorrhea. A small bowel barium radiography study should be obtained to look for mechanical factors predisposing to intestinal stasis. A small intestinal biopsy may be necessary to exclude other mucosal malabsorptive conditions and to detect intestinal inflammation, commonly present with symptomatic bacterial overgrowth. A specific diagnosis can be established firmly only by an aspirate and culture of proximal jejunal secretion that demonstrates over 10^5 organisms/mL. However, this is an invasive and laborious test that requires careful collection and culturing techniques and therefore is not available in many clinical settings. Noninvasive breath tests have been developed that are easier to perform and have a sensitivity of 60–90% compared with jejunal cultures. The [^{14}C]xylose breath test is the most reliable. In this test, bacterial uptake and degradation of the isotope leads to the release of $^{14}CO_2$, which can be measured in exhaled breath. Breath hydrogen tests with glucose or lactulose as substrate are commonly done because of their ease of use, but they have lower sensitivity (< 65%) and specificity (< 85%).

Owing to the lack of an optimal test for bacterial overgrowth, many clinicians use an empiric antibiotic trial as a diagnostic and therapeutic maneuver in patients with predisposing conditions for bacterial overgrowth who develop unexplained diarrhea or steatorrhea.

Treatment

Where possible, the anatomic defect that has potentiated bacterial overgrowth should be corrected. Otherwise, treatment as follows for 1–2 weeks with broad-spectrum antibiotics effective against enteric aerobes and anaerobes usually leads to dramatic improvement: twice daily ciprofloxacin 500 mg, norfloxacin 400 mg, or amoxicillin clavulanate 875 mg, or a combination of metronidazole 250 mg three times daily plus either trimethoprim-sulfamethoxazole (one double-strength tablet) twice daily or cephalexin 250 mg four times daily. Rifaximin 400 mg three times daily is a nonabsorbable antibiotic that also appears to be effective but has fewer side effects than the other systemically absorbed antibiotics.

In patients in whom symptoms recur off antibiotics, cyclic therapy (eg, 1 week out of 4) may be sufficient. Continuous antibiotics should be avoided, if possible, to avoid development of bacterial antibiotic resistance.

In patients with severe intestinal dysmotility, treatment with small doses of octreotide may prove to be of benefit.

Lauritano EC et al: Rifaximin dose-finding study for the treatment of small intestinal bacterial overgrowth. Aliment Pharmacol Ther 2005;22:31. [PMID: 15963077]

Romagnuolo J et al: Using breath tests wisely in a gastroenterology practice: an evidence-based review of indications and pitfalls in interpretation. Am J Gastroenterol 2002;97:1113. [PMID: 12014715]

Singh VV et al: Small bowel bacterial overgrowth: presentation, diagnosis, and treatment. Curr Gastroenterol Rep 2003; 5:365. [PMID: 12959716]

4. Short Bowel Syndrome

Short bowel syndrome is the malabsorptive condition that arises secondary to removal of significant segments of the small intestine. The most common causes in adults are Crohn's disease, mesenteric infarction, radiation enteritis, volvulus, tumor resection, and trauma. The type and degree of malabsorption depend on the length and site of the resection and the degree of adaptation of the remaining bowel.

Terminal Ileal Resection

Resection of the terminal ileum results in malabsorption of bile salts and vitamin B_{12}, which are normally absorbed in this region. Patients with low serum vitamin B_{12} levels, an abnormal Schilling test, or resection of over 50 cm of ileum require monthly intramuscular vitamin B_{12} injections. In patients with less than 100 cm of ileal resection, bile salt malabsorption stimulates fluid secretion from the colon, resulting in watery diarrhea. This may be treated with bile salt binding resins (cholestyramine, 2–4 g three times daily with meals). Resection of over 100 cm of ileum leads to a reduction in the bile salt pool that results in steatorrhea and malabsorption of fat-soluble vitamins. Treatment is with a low-fat diet and vitamins supplemented with medium-chain triglycerides, which do not require micellar solubilization. Unabsorbed fatty acids bind with calcium, reducing its absorption and enhancing the absorption of oxalate. Oxalate kidney stones may develop. Calcium supplements should be administered to bind oxalate and increase serum calcium. Cholesterol gallstones due to decreased bile salts are common also. In patients with resection of the ileocolonic valve, bacterial overgrowth may occur in the small intestine, further complicating malabsorption (as outlined above).

Extensive Small Bowel Resection

Resection of 40–50% of the total length of small intestine usually is well tolerated. A more massive resection may result in "short-bowel syndrome," characterized by weight loss and diarrhea due to nutrient, water, and electrolyte malabsorption. After resection, the remaining small intestine has a remarkable ability to adapt, gradually increasing its absorptive capacity up to fourfold over 1 year. The colon also plays an important role in absorption of fluids, electrolytes, and digestion of complex carbohydrates (through bacterial fermentation to short-chain fatty acids) after small bowel resection. If the colon is preserved, 100 cm of proximal jejunum may be sufficient to maintain adequate oral nutrition with a low-fat, high complex-carbohydrate diet, though fluid and electrolyte losses may still be significant. In patients in whom the colon has been removed, at least 200 cm of proximal jejunum is typically required to maintain oral nutrition. Duodenal resection may result in folate, iron, or calcium malabsorption. Levels of other minerals such as zinc, selenium, and magnesium should be monitored. Parenteral vitamin supplementation may be necessary. Antidiarrheal agents (loperamide, 2–4 mg three times daily) slow transit and reduce diarrheal volume. Octreotide reduces intestinal transit time and fluid and electrolyte secretion. Gastric hypersecretion usually complicates intestinal resection and should be treated with proton pump inhibitors.

Patients with less than 100–200 cm of proximal jejunum remaining almost always require parenteral nutrition. Of patients who do, the estimated annual mortality rate is 2–5% per year. Death is most commonly due to TPN-induced liver disease, sepsis, or loss of venous access. Small intestine transplantation is now being performed with reported 5-year graft survival rates of 40%. Currently, it is performed chiefly in patients who develop serious problems due to parenteral nutrition.

Buchman AL: Short-bowel syndrome. Clin Gastroenterol Hepatol 2005;3:1066. [PMID: 16271335]

Buchman AL et al: AGA technical review on short bowel syndrome and intestinal transplantation. Gastroenterology 2003;124:1111. [PMID: 12671904]

DiBaise JK et al: Intestinal rehabilitation and short bowel syndrome: Part 2. Am J Gastroenterol 2004;99:1823. [PMID: 15330926]

5. Lactase Deficiency

Lactase is a brush border enzyme that hydrolyzes the disaccharide lactose into glucose and galactose. The concentration of lactase enzyme levels is high at birth but declines steadily in most people of non-European ancestry during childhood and adolescence and into adulthood. Thus, approximately 50 million people in the United States have partial to complete lactose intolerance. As many as 90% of Asian-Americans, 70% of African-Americans, 95% of Native Americans, 50% of Mexican-Americans, and 60% of Jewish Americans are lactose intolerant compared with less than 25% of white adults. Lactase deficiency may also arise secondary to other gastrointestinal disorders that affect the proximal small intestinal mucosa. These include Crohn's disease, sprue, viral gastroenteritis, giardiasis, short bowel syndrome, and malnutrition. Malabsorbed lactose is fermented by intestinal bacteria, producing gas and organic acids. The nonmetabolized lactose and organic acids result in an increased stool osmotic load with an obligatory fluid loss.

Clinical Findings

A. SYMPTOMS AND SIGNS

Patients have great variability in clinical symptoms, depending both on the severity of lactase deficiency and the amount of lactose ingested. Because of the nonspecific nature of these symptoms, there is a tendency for both lactose-intolerant and lactose-tolerant individuals to mistakenly attribute a variety of abdominal symptoms to lactose intolerance. Most patients with lactose intolerance can drink one or two 8 oz glasses of milk daily without symptoms if taken with food at wide intervals, though rare patients have almost complete intolerance. With mild to moderate amounts of lactose malabsorption, patients may experience bloating, abdominal cramps, and flatulence. With higher lactose ingestions, an osmotic diarrhea will result. Isolated lactase deficiency does not result in other signs of malabsorption or weight loss. If these findings are present, other gastrointestinal disorders should be pursued. Diarrheal specimens reveal an increased osmotic gap and a pH of less than 6.0.

B. LABORATORY FINDINGS

The most widely available test for the diagnosis of lactase deficiency is the hydrogen breath test. After ingestion of 50 g of lactose, a rise in breath hydrogen of greater than 20 ppm within 90 minutes is a positive test, indicative of bacterial carbohydrate metabolism. In clinical practice, many physicians prescribe an empiric trial of a lactose-free diet for 2 weeks. Resolution of symptoms (bloating, flatulence, diarrhea) is highly suggestive of lactase deficiency (though a placebo response cannot be excluded) and may be confirmed, if necessary, with a breath hydrogen study.

Differential Diagnosis

The symptoms of late-onset lactose intolerance are nonspecific and may mimic a number of gastrointestinal disorders, such as inflammatory bowel disease, mucosal malabsorptive disorders, irritable bowel syndrome, and pancreatic insufficiency. Furthermore, lactase deficiency frequently develops secondary to other gastrointestinal disorders (as listed above). Concomitant lactase deficiency should always be considered in these gastrointestinal disorders.

Treatment

The goal of treatment in patients with isolated lactase deficiency is achieving patient comfort. Patients usually find their "threshold" of intake at which symptoms will occur. Foods that are high in lactose include milk (12 g/cup), ice cream (9 g/cup), and cottage cheese (8 g/cup). Aged cheeses have a lower lactose content (0.5 g/oz). Unpasteurized yogurt contains bacteria that produce lactase and is generally well tolerated.

Many patients will choose simply to restrict or eliminate milk products. By spreading dairy product intake throughout the day in quantities of less than 12 g of lactose (one cup of milk), most patients can take dairy products without symptoms and do not require lactase supplements. Calcium supplementation should be considered in susceptible patients to prevent osteoporosis. Most food markets provide milk that has been pretreated with lactase, rendering it 70–100% lactose free. Lactase enzyme replacement is commercially available as a nonprescription formulation (Lactaid). Caplets of lactase may be taken with milk products, improving lactose absorption and eliminating symptoms. The number of caplets ingested depends on the degree of lactose intolerance.

Mathews SB et al: Systemic lactose intolerance: a new perspective on an old problem. Postgrad Med J 2005;81:167. [PMID: 15749792]

Swagerty DL Jr et al: Lactose intolerance. Am Fam Physician 2002;65:1845. [PMID: 12018807]

INTESTINAL MOTILITY DISORDERS

1. Acute Paralytic Ileus

 ESSENTIALS OF DIAGNOSIS

- *Precipitating factors: surgery, peritonitis, electrolyte abnormalities, medications, severe medical illness.*
- *Nausea, vomiting, obstipation, distention.*
- *Minimal abdominal tenderness; decreased bowel sounds.*
- *Plain abdominal radiography with gas and fluid distention in small and large bowel.*

General Considerations

Ileus is a condition in which there is neurogenic failure or loss of peristalsis in the intestine in the absence of any mechanical obstruction. It is commonly seen in hospitalized patients as a result of (1) intra-abdominal processes such as recent gastrointestinal or abdominal surgery or peritoneal irritation (peritonitis, pancreatitis, ruptured viscus, hemorrhage); (2) severe medical illness such as pneumonia, respiratory failure requiring intubation, sepsis or severe infections, uremia, diabetic ketoacidosis, and electrolyte abnormalities (hypokalemia, hypercalcemia, hypomagnesemia, hypophosphatemia); and (3) medications that affect intestinal motility (opioids, anticholinergics, phenothiazines). Following surgery, small intestinal motility usually normalizes first (often within hours), followed by the stomach (24–48 hours), and the colon (48–72 hours).

Clinical Findings

A. SYMPTOMS AND SIGNS

Patients who are conscious report mild diffuse, continuous abdominal discomfort with nausea and vomiting.

Generalized abdominal distention is present with minimal abdominal tenderness but no signs of peritoneal irritation (unless due to the primary disease). Bowel sounds are diminished to absent.

B. LABORATORY FINDINGS

The laboratory abnormalities are attributable to the underlying condition. Serum electrolytes, including potassium, magnesium, phosphorus, and calcium, should be obtained to exclude abnormalities as contributing factors.

C. IMAGING

Plain film radiography of the abdomen demonstrates distended gas-filled loops of small and large intestine. Air-fluid levels may be seen. Under some circumstances, it may be difficult to distinguish ileus from partial small bowel obstruction. A limited barium small bowel series or a CT scan may be useful in such instances to exclude mechanical obstruction, especially in postoperative patients.

Differential Diagnosis

Ileus must be distinguished from mechanical obstruction of the small bowel or proximal colon. Pain from small bowel mechanical obstruction is usually intermittent, cramping, and associated initially with profuse vomiting. Acute gastroenteritis, acute appendicitis, and acute pancreatitis may all present with ileus.

Treatment

The primary medical or surgical illness that has precipitated adynamic ileus should be treated. Most cases of ileus respond to restriction of oral intake with gradual liberalization of diet as bowel function returns. Severe or prolonged ileus requires nasogastric suction and parenteral administration of fluids and electrolytes.

Behm B et al: Postoperative ileus: etiologies and interventions. Clin Gastroenterol Hepatol 2003;1:71. [PMID: 15017498]

Luckey A et al: Mechanisms and treatment of postoperative ileus. Arch Surg 2003;138:206. [PMID: 12578422]

Taguchi A et al: Selective postoperative inhibition of gastrointestinal opioid receptors. N Engl J Med 2001;345:935. [PMID: 11575284]

2. Acute Colonic Pseudo-obstruction (Ogilvie's Syndrome)

ESSENTIALS OF DIAGNOSIS

- *Severe abdominal distention.*
- *Arises in postoperative state or with severe medical illness.*
- *May be precipitated by electrolyte imbalances, medications.*
- *Absent to mild abdominal pain; minimal tenderness.*
- *Massive dilation of cecum or right colon.*

General Considerations

Spontaneous massive dilation of the cecum and proximal colon may occur in a number of different settings in hospitalized patients. Progressive cecal dilation may lead to spontaneous perforation with dire consequences. The risk of perforation correlates poorly with absolute cecal size and duration of colonic distention. Early detection and management are important to reduce morbidity and mortality. Colonic pseudo-obstruction is most commonly detected in postsurgical patients (mean 3–5 days), after trauma, and in medical patients with respiratory failure, metabolic imbalance, malignancy, myocardial infarction, congestive heart failure, pancreatitis, or a recent neurologic event (stroke, subarachnoid hemorrhage, trauma). Liberal use of opioids or anticholinergic agents may precipitate colonic pseudo-obstruction in susceptible patients. It may also occur as a manifestation of colonic ischemia. The etiology of colonic pseudo-obstruction is unknown, but either an increase in gut sympathetic activity or a decrease in sacral parasympathetic activity of the distal colon, or both, is hypothesized to impair colonic motility.

Clinical Findings

A. SYMPTOMS AND SIGNS

Many patients are on ventilatory support or are unable to report symptoms due to altered mental status. Abdominal distention is frequently noted by the clinician as the first sign, often leading to a plain film radiograph that demonstrates colonic dilation. Some patients are asymptomatic, although most report constant but mild abdominal pain. Nausea and vomiting may be present. Bowel movements may be absent, but up to 40% of patients continue to pass flatus or stool. Abdominal tenderness with some degree of guarding or rebound tenderness may be detected; however, signs of peritonitis are absent unless perforation has occurred. Bowel sounds may be normal or decreased.

B. LABORATORY FINDINGS

Laboratory findings reflect the underlying medical or surgical problems. Serum sodium, potassium, magnesium, phosphorus, and calcium should be obtained. Significant fever or leukocytosis raises concern for colonic ischemia or perforation.

C. IMAGING

Radiographs demonstrate colonic dilation, usually confined to the cecum and proximal colon. The upper limits of normal for cecal size is 9 cm. A cecal diameter greater than 10–12 cm is associated with an increased risk of colonic perforation. Varying amounts of small intestinal dilation and air-fluid levels due to adynamic ileus may be seen. Because the dilated appearance of the colon may raise concern that there is a distal colonic mechanical obstruction due to malignancy, volvulus, or fecal impaction, a CT scan or water-soluble (diatrizoate meglumine) enema may sometimes be performed.

Differential Diagnosis

Colonic pseudo-obstruction should be distinguished from distal colonic mechanical obstruction (as above) and toxic megacolon, which is acute dilation of the colon due to inflammation (inflammatory bowel disease) or infection (*C difficile*–associated colitis, CMV). Patients with toxic megacolon manifest fever; dehydration; significant abdominal pain; leukocytosis; and diarrhea, which is often bloody.

Treatment

Conservative treatment is the appropriate first step for patients with no or minimal abdominal tenderness, no fever, no leukocytosis, and a cecal diameter less than 12 cm. The underlying illness is treated appropriately. A nasogastric tube and a rectal tube should be placed. Patients should be ambulated or periodically rolled from side to side and to the knee-chest position in an effort to promote expulsion of colonic gas. All drugs that reduce intestinal motility, such as opioids, anticholinergics, and calcium channel blockers, are discontinued if possible. Enemas may be administered judiciously if large amounts of stool are evident on radiography. Oral laxatives are not helpful and may cause perforation, pain, or electrolyte abnormalities.

Conservative treatment is successful in over 80% of cases within 1–2 days. Patients must be watched for signs of worsening distention or abdominal tenderness. Cecal size should be assessed by abdominal radiographs every 12 hours. Intervention should be considered in patients with any of the following: (1) no improvement or clinical deterioration after 24–48 hours of conservative therapy; (2) cecal dilation > 10 cm for a prolonged period (> 3–4 days); (3) patients with cecal dilation > 12 cm. Neostigmine injection should be given unless contraindicated. A single dose (2 mg intravenously) results in rapid (within 30 minutes) colonic decompression in 75–90% of patients. Cardiac monitoring during neostigmine infusion is indicated for possible bradycardia that may require atropine administration. Colonoscopic decompression is indicated in patients who fail to respond to neostigmine. Colonic decompression with aspiration of air or placement of a decompression tube is successful in 70% of patients. However, the procedure is technically difficult in an unprepared bowel and has been associated with perforations in the distended colon. Dilation recurs in up to 50% of patients. In patients in whom colonoscopy is unsuccessful, a tube cecostomy can be created through a small laparotomy or with percutaneous radiologically guided placement.

Prognosis

In most cases, the prognosis is related to the underlying illness. The risk of perforation or ischemia is increased with cecal diameter > 12 cm and when distention has been present for more than 6 days. With aggressive therapy, the development of perforation is unusual.

Kahi CJ et al: Bowel obstruction and pseudo-obstruction. Gastroenterol Clin North Am 2003;32:1229. [PMID: 14696305]

Saunders MD et al: Systematic review: acute colonic pseudo-obstruction. Aliment Pharmcol Ther 2005;22:917. [PMID: 16268965]

3. Chronic Intestinal Pseudo-obstruction & Gastroparesis

Gastroparesis and chronic intestinal pseudo-obstruction are chronic conditions characterized by intermittent, waxing and waning symptoms and signs of gastric or intestinal obstruction in the absence of any mechanical lesions to account for the findings. They are caused by a heterogeneous group of endocrine disorders (diabetes mellitus, hypothyroidism, cortisol deficiency), postsurgical conditions (vagotomy, partial gastric resection, fundoplication, gastric bypass, Whipple procedure), neurologic conditions (Parkinson's disease, muscular and myotonic dystrophy, autonomic dysfunction, multiple sclerosis, postpolio syndrome, porphyria), rheumatologic syndromes (progressive systemic sclerosis), infections (postviral, Chagas' disease), amyloidosis, paraneoplastic syndromes, medications, and eating disorders (anorexia); a cause may not always be identified. Gastric involvement leads to chronic or intermittent symptoms of gastroparesis with early satiety, nausea, and postprandial vomiting (1–3 hours after meals).

Patients with predominantly small bowel involvement may have abdominal distention, vomiting, diarrhea, and varying degrees of malnutrition. Abdominal pain is not common and should prompt investigation for structural causes of obstruction. Bacterial overgrowth in the stagnant intestine may result in malabsorption. Colonic involvement may result in constipation or alternating diarrhea and constipation.

Plain film radiography may demonstrate dilation of the esophagus, stomach, small intestine, or colon resembling ileus or mechanical obstruction. Mechanical obstruction of the stomach, small intestine, or colon is much more common than gastroparesis or intestinal pseudo-obstruction and must be excluded with endoscopy or barium radiography (upper gastrointestinal series with small bowel follow-through), especially in patients with prior surgery, recent onset of symptoms, or abdominal pain. In cases of unclear origin, studies based on the clinical picture are obtained to exclude underlying systemic disease. Gastric scintigraphy with a low-fat solid meal is the optimal means for assessing gastric emptying. Gastric retention of 60% after 2 hours or more than 10% after 4 hours is abnormal. Small bowel manometry is useful for distinguishing visceral from myopathic disorders and for excluding cases of mechanical obstruction that are otherwise difficult to diagnose by endoscopy or radiographic studies.

There is no specific therapy for gastroparesis or pseudo-obstruction. Acute exacerbations are treated with nasogastric suction and intravenous fluids. Long-term treatment is directed at maintaining nutrition. Patients should eat small, frequent meals that are low in fiber, milk, gas-forming foods, and fat. Some patients may require liquid enteral supplements. Agents that reduce gastrointestinal motility (opioids, anticholinergics) should be avoided. In diabetics, glucose levels should be maintained below 200 mg/dL, as hyperglycemia may slow gastric emptying even in the absence of diabetic neuropathy. Metoclopramide (5–20 mg orally or 5–10 mg intravenously or subcutaneously four times daily) and erythromycin (50–125 mg orally three times daily) before meals are of benefit in treatment of gastroparesis but not small bowel dysmotility. The 5-HT$_4$-receptor agonist, tegaserod 6–12 mg twice daily, enhances gastric emptying and colonic motility but has undergone limited testing for gastroparesis or chronic intestinal pseudo-obstruction. Unblinded studies in small numbers of patients with diabetic or idiopathic gastroparesis report improvement in symptoms and gastric emptying after injection of botulinum toxin into the pylorus, which is hypothesized to reduce pyloric spasm. Gastric pacing with internally implanted neurostimulators has shown benefit in small studies of patients with severe gastroparesis. Bacterial overgrowth should be treated with intermittent antibiotics (see above). Patients with predominant small bowel distention may require a venting gastrostomy to relieve distress. Some patients may require placement of a jejunostomy for long-term enteral nutrition. Patients unable to maintain adequate enteral nutrition require TPN or small bowel transplantation. Difficult cases should be referred to centers with expertise in this area.

Abell T et al: Gastric electrical stimulation for medically refractory gastroparesis. Gastroenterology 2003;125:421. [PMID: 12903891]

Friedenberg FK et al: Management of delayed gastric emptying. Clin Gastroenterol Hepatol 2005;3:642. [PMID: 16206495]

Jones M et al: A systematic review of surgical therapy for gastroparesis. Am J Gastroenterol 2003;98:2122. [PMID: 14572555]

Maganti K et al: Oral erythromycin and symptomatic relief of gastroparesis: a systematic review. Gastroenterology 2003;98:259. [PMID: 12591038]

Panganamamula KV et al: Chronic intestinal pseudo-obstruction. Curr Treat Options Gastroenterol 2005;8:3. [PMID: 15625029]

Parkman H et al: American Gastroenterological Association medical position statement: diagnosis and treatment of gastroparesis. Gastroenterology 2004;127:1589. [PMID: 15521125]

Talley NJ: Diabetic gastropathy and prokinetics. Am J Gastroenterol 2003;98:264. [PMID: 12591039]

TUMORS OF THE SMALL INTESTINE

Benign and malignant tumors of the small intestine are rare. They often cause no symptoms or signs. However, they may cause acute gastrointestinal bleeding with hematochezia or melena or chronic gastrointestinal blood loss resulting in fatigue and iron deficiency anemia. Small bowel tumors may cause obstruction due to luminal narrowing or intussusception of a polypoid mass. Small bowel tumors usually are identified by barium radiographic studies, either enteroclysis or a small bowel series. Visualization and biopsy of duodenal and proximal jejunal mass lesions are performed with a long upper endoscope known as an enteroscope.

1. Benign Tumors of Small Intestine

Benign polyps may be symptomatic or may be incidental findings detected on endoscopy or radiographic study. Most occur singly, and the presence of multiple polyps is suggestive of hereditary polyposis syndrome (discussed under Diseases of the Colon and Rectum). With the exception of lipomas, surgical or endoscopic excision usually is recommended. Adenomatous polyps are the most common benign mucosal tumor. The majority are asymptomatic, though acute or chronic bleeding may occur. Because malignant transformation does occur, endoscopic or surgical resection is warranted. Villous adenomas occur most commonly in the periampullary region of the duodenum (especially in patients with familial adenomatous polyposis) and carry a high risk for development of invasive cancer. Periodic endoscopic surveillance to detect early ampullary neoplasms is recommended in patients with familial adenomatous polyposis. Evaluation with endoscopic retrograde cholangiopancreatography (ERCP) and endoscopic ultrasound is required to exclude invasive carcinoma. Ampullary adenomas may be removed by endoscopic or surgical techniques. Lipomas occur commonly in the ileum. Most are asymptomatic and identified incidentally at endoscopy or radiography; however, they rarely may cause obstruction with intussusception. Benign stromal tumors (formerly called leiomyomas) are found at all levels of the intestine. These submucosal mesenchymal lesions may be intraluminal, intramural, or extraluminal. Although most are asymptomatic, they may ulcerate and cause acute or chronic bleeding or obstruction. It is difficult to distinguish benign from malignant stromal tumors (leiomyosarcomas) except by excision.

Catalano M et al: Endoscopic management of adenoma of the major duodenal papilla. Gastrointest Endosc 2004;59:225. [PMID: 15472678]

2. Malignant Tumors of Small Intestine

Malignant tumors of the small intestine are extremely rare, accounting for less than 2% of all gastrointestinal malignancies. They may present with anemia, bleeding, obstruction, or evidence of metastatic disease.

Adenocarcinoma

These are aggressive tumors that occur most commonly in the duodenum or proximal jejunum. The ampulla of Vater is the most common site of small bowel carcinoma, and the incidence of ampullary carcinoma is increased more than 200-fold in patients with familial adenomatous polyposis. Ampullary carcinoma may present with jaundice due to bile duct obstruction or bleeding. Surgical resection of early lesions is curative in up to 40% of patients. Periodic endoscopic surveillance to detect early ampullary neoplasms therefore is recommended in patients with this disorder. Nonampullary adenocarcinoma of the small intestine accounts for 30–40% of small bowel cancers. Most cases present with symptoms of obstruction, acute or chronic bleeding, or weight loss. Eighty percent of small bowel cancers have already metastasized at the time of diagnosis. Resection is recommended for control of symptoms. Patients with Crohn's disease have an increased risk of small intestine adenocarcinoma, most commonly in the ileum, which may be difficult to distinguish from disease-related fibrous strictures.

Lymphoma

Gastrointestinal lymphomas may arise in the gastrointestinal tract or involve it secondarily with disseminated disease. In Western countries, primary gastrointestinal lymphomas account for 5% of lymphomas and 20% of small bowel malignancies. They occur most commonly in the distal small intestine. The majority are non-Hodgkin's intermediate or high-grade B cell lymphomas. However, T cell lymphomas may arise in patients with celiac sprue. In the Middle East, lymphomas may arise also in the setting of immunoproliferative small intestinal disease. In this condition, there is diffuse lymphoplasmacytic infiltration with IgA-secreting B lymphocytes of the mucosa and submucosa that results in weight loss, diarrhea, and malabsorption, which may lead to lymphomatous transformation. A characteristic feature of the disease is the presence of α heavy chains in the serum in 70% produced by clones of IgA plasma cells. The early, premalignant phase may respond to antibiotic therapy for $H\ pylori$ alone (Table 14–11).

Presenting symptoms or signs of primary lymphoma include abdominal pain, weight loss, nausea and vomiting, distention, anemia, and occult blood in the stool. Fevers are unusual. Protein-losing enteropathy may result in hypoalbuminemia, but other signs of malabsorption are unusual. Barium radiography helps to localize the site of the lesion. The diagnosis requires endoscopic, percutaneous, or laparoscopic biopsy. To determine tumor stage, patients must undergo chest and abdominal CT, bone marrow biopsy, and, in some cases, lymphangiography.

Treatment depends on the stage of disease. Resection of primary intestinal lymphoma, if feasible, is usually recommended. Even in cases of stage III or stage IV disease, surgical debulking may improve survival. In patients with limited disease (stage IE) in whom resection is performed, the role of adjuvant chemotherapy is unclear. Most patients with more extensive disease are treated with systemic chemotherapy with or without radiation therapy (see Chapter 40).

Carcinoid Tumors

Gastrointestinal carcinoids are slow growing neuroendocrine tumors that may arise anywhere in the gastrointestinal tract but most commonly occur in the small intestine (30%), rectum (12%), colon (8%), appendix (8%), and stomach (10–30%; see above). Carcinoids have intracytoplasmic electron-dense secretory granules that may contain a variety of hormones, including serotonin, somatostatin, gastrin, and substance P (which may or may not be secreted), and usually display immunoreactivity to chromogranin A. Although many carcinoids behave in an indolent fashion, the overall 5-year survival rate for patients with carcinoids is 50%, suggesting that most are malignant. The risk of metastatic spread is closely related to tumor size and tumor location. Many small carcinoids are detected incidentally at endoscopy or autopsy. It is not possible by histologic examination to distinguish benign from malignant disease. The best indicator of prognosis is evidence of invasive growth and the presence of regional or distant metastasis.

Rectal carcinoids are usually detected incidentally as submucosal nodules during proctoscopic examination. Similarly, appendiceal carcinoids are identified in 0.3% of appendectomies. Almost 80% of these tumors are less than 1 cm in size, and 90% are less than 2 cm. Rectal carcinoids less than 1 cm and appendiceal carcinoids less than 2 cm virtually never metastasize and are treated effectively with local excision or simple appendectomy. Tumors larger than 2 cm are associated with the development of metastasis in over 20% of appendiceal carcinoids and 10% of rectal carcinoids. Hence, in younger patients who are good operative risks, a more extensive cancer resection operation is warranted.

Carcinoids account for up to one-third of small intestinal tumors. Approximately two-thirds of carcinoids of the duodenum secrete gastrin (gastrinomas) (see Zollinger-Ellison Syndrome). Small intestinal carcinoids most commonly arise in the ileum. Up to one-third are multicentric. Although 60% are less than 2 cm in size, even these small carcinoids may metastasize. Almost all tumors over 2 cm are associated with metastasis. Most smaller lesions are asymptomatic and difficult to detect by endoscopy or imaging studies. Therefore, most carcinoids present at an advanced and incurable stage. Through local extension or metastasis to mesenteric lymph nodes, carcinoids engender a fibroblastic reaction with contraction and kinking of the bowel. This may lead to symptoms of partial small bowel obstruction with intermittent abdominal pain or obstruction. Small bowel barium studies may reveal kinking, but because the lesion is extraluminal the diagnosis may be overlooked for several years. Encasement of the mesenteric vessels can lead to bowel infarction. Carcinoid involvement of the heart (resulting in right-sided valvular lesions) is a late manifestation of metastatic disease. Carcinoid syndrome occurs in less than 10% of patients (see Chapter 40) and only in patients with hepatic metastasis. It is caused by tumor secretion of hormonal mediators that cause cramps, flushing, diarrhea, cyanosis, or bronchospasm. Almost all patients with carcinoid syndrome have obvious signs of cancer with liver metastasis on abdominal imaging.

Plasma chromogranin A (CgA) is the most sensitive screening test for small intestine carcinoids, although its sensitivity for small, localized tumors is unknown. CgA is elevated in almost 90% of patients with advanced small bowel carcinoid. Urinary 5-HIAA or platelet serotonin levels are also elevated in patients with metastatic carcinoid; however, these tests are less sensitive than CgA. Abdominal CT may demonstrate a mesenteric mass with tethering of the bowel, lymphadenopathy, and hepatic metastasis. Somatostatin receptor scintigraphy, which is positive in over 90% of patients with metastatic carcinoid, is superior to all other imaging modalities for the diagnosis of primary and metastatic lesions.

Small intestinal carcinoids are extremely indolent tumors with slow spread. Patients with disease confined to the small intestine should have local excision, for which the cure rate exceeds 85%. In patients with resectable disease who have lymph node involvement, the 5-year disease-free survival is 80%; however, by 25 years, less than 25% remain disease free. Even patients with hepatic metastases may have an indolent course with a median survival of 3 years. In patients with advanced disease, therapy should be deferred until the patient is symptomatic. Surgery should be directed toward palliation of obstructive symptoms. In patients with carcinoid syndrome or diarrhea, resection of hepatic metastases may provide dramatic improvement. The somatostatin analog octreotide (150–500 mcg subcutaneously three times daily) inhibits hormone secretion from the carcinoid tumor, resulting in dramatic relief of diarrhea and symptoms of carcinoid syndrome in 90% of patients for a median period of 1 year. Thereafter, many patients escape from octreotide control. Hepatic artery occlusion and chemotherapy may provide symptomatic improvement in some patients with hepatic metastases.

Sarcoma

Most small intestine sarcomas arise from stromal tumors that stain positive for CD117; a minority arise from smooth muscle tumors (leiomyosarcomas) (see Malig-

nant Tumors of the Stomach: Mesenchymal Tumors). Tumors may grow quite large before causing symptoms due to obstruction, intussusception, or bleeding due to central ulceration within the tumor. Because many of these tumors cannot be reached by endoscopy for biopsy, surgery should be performed in patients with symptomatic tumors and asymptomatic tumors larger than 3 cm (in which the risk of malignancy is increased).

Kaposi's sarcoma was at one time a common complication in AIDS, but the incidence is declining with highly active antiretroviral therapy (HAART). It is strongly associated with infection with human herpesvirus 8. Lesions may be present anywhere in the intestinal tract. Visceral involvement usually is associated with cutaneous disease. Most lesions are clinically silent; however, large lesions may be symptomatic. Lesions of the gingiva, palate, and hypopharynx can lead to painful mastication and dysphagia. Lesions of the stomach or small intestine may lead to bleeding, obstruction, or even perforation. The diagnosis may be confirmed at endoscopy by the characteristic visual appearance and by biopsy. Oral complications can be treated with the CO_2 laser or radiation. Limited bleeding or obstructing lesions in the stomach or anus can be treated with the YAG laser or radiation therapy. Interferon-α induces regression in up to one-third of patients who have a CD4 cell count of > 200/mcL. Widespread involvement may be best treated by systemic chemotherapy using combinations of vincristine, bleomycin, or doxorubicin, to which the tumor is very responsive.

Bierman PJ: Gastrointestinal lymphoma. Curr Treat Options Oncol 2003;4:421. [PMID: 12941202]

Debaja BS et al: Adenocarcinoma of the small bowel: presentation, prognostic factors, and outcome of 217 patients. Cancer 2004;101:518. [PMID: 15274064]

Modlin IM et al: Current status of gastrointestinal carcinoids. Gastroenterology 2005;128:1717. [PMID: 15887161]

Torres M et al: Malignant tumors of the small intestine. J Clin Gastroenterol 2003;37:372. [PMID: 14564183]

APPENDICITIS

 ESSENTIALS OF DIAGNOSIS

- *Early: periumbilical pain; later: right lower quadrant pain and tenderness.*
- *Anorexia, nausea and vomiting, obstipation.*
- *Tenderness or localized rigidity at McBurney's point.*
- *Low-grade fever and leukocytosis.*

General Considerations

Appendicitis is the most common abdominal surgical emergency, affecting approximately 10% of the population. It occurs most commonly between the ages of 10 and 30 years. It is initiated by obstruction of the appendix by a fecalith, inflammation, foreign body, or neoplasm. Obstruction leads to increased intraluminal pressure, venous congestion, infection, and thrombosis of intramural vessels. If untreated, gangrene and perforation develop within 36 hours.

Clinical Findings

A. SYMPTOMS AND SIGNS

Appendicitis usually begins with vague, often colicky periumbilical or epigastric pain. Within 12 hours the pain shifts to the right lower quadrant, manifested as a steady ache that is worsened by walking or coughing. Almost all patients have nausea with one or two episodes of vomiting. Protracted vomiting or vomiting that begins before the onset of pain suggests another diagnosis. A sense of constipation is typical, and some patients administer cathartics in an effort to relieve their symptoms—though some report diarrhea. Low-grade fever (< 38 °C) is typical; high fever or rigors suggest another diagnosis or appendiceal perforation.

On physical examination, localized tenderness with guarding in the right lower quadrant can be elicited with gentle palpation with one finger. When asked to cough, patients may be able to precisely localize the painful area, a sign of peritoneal irritation. Light percussion may also elicit pain. Although rebound tenderness is also present, it is unnecessary to elicit this finding if the above signs are present. The psoas sign (pain on passive extension of the right hip) and the obturator sign (pain with passive flexion and internal rotation of the right hip) are indicative of adjacent inflammation and strongly suggestive of appendicitis.

B. LABORATORY FINDINGS

Moderate leukocytosis (10,000–20,000/mcL) with neutrophilia is common. Microscopic hematuria and pyuria are present in 25% of patients.

C. IMAGING

Both abdominal ultrasound and CT scanning are useful in diagnosing appendicitis as well as excluding other diseases presenting with similar symptoms, including adnexal disease in younger women. However, CT scanning appears to be more accurate (sensitivity 94%, specificity 95%, positive likelihood ratio 13.3, negative likelihood ratio 0.09). Abdominal CT scanning is also useful in cases of suspected appendiceal perforation to diagnose a periappendiceal abscess. In patients in whom there is a clinically high suspicion of appendicitis, some surgeons feel that preoperative diagnostic imaging is unnecessary. However, studies suggest that even in this group, imaging studies suggest an alternative diagnosis in up to 15%.

Atypical Presentations of Appendicitis

Owing to the variable location of the appendix, there are a number of "atypical" presentations. Because the retrocecal appendix does not touch the anterior abdominal wall, the pain remains less intense and poorly localized; abdominal tenderness is minimal and may be elicited in the right flank. The psoas sign may be positive. With pelvic appendicitis there is pain in the lower abdomen, often on the left, with an urge to urinate or defecate. Abdominal tenderness is absent, but tenderness is evident on pelvic or rectal examination; the obturator sign may be present. In the elderly, the diagnosis of appendicitis is often delayed because patients present with minimal, vague symptoms and mild abdominal tenderness. Appendicitis in pregnancy may present with pain in the right lower quadrant, periumbilical area, or right subcostal area owing to displacement of the appendix by the uterus.

Differential Diagnosis

Given its frequency and myriad presentations, appendicitis should be considered in the differential diagnosis of all patients with abdominal pain. It is difficult to reliably diagnose the disease in some cases. A several-hour period of close observation with reassessment usually clarifies the diagnosis. Absence of the classic migration of pain (from the epigastrium to the right lower abdomen), right lower quadrant pain, fever, or guarding makes appendicitis less likely. Ten to 20 percent of patients with suspected appendicitis have either a negative examination at laparotomy or an alternative surgical diagnosis. The widespread use of ultrasonography and CT has reduced the number of incorrect diagnoses. Still, in some cases diagnostic laparotomy or laparoscopy is required. The most common causes of diagnostic confusion are gastroenteritis and gynecologic disorders. Viral gastroenteritis presents with nausea, vomiting, low-grade fever, and diarrhea and can be difficult to distinguish from appendicitis. The onset of vomiting before pain makes appendicitis less likely. As a rule, the pain of gastroenteritis is more generalized and the tenderness less well localized. Acute salpingitis or tubo-ovarian abscess should be considered in young, sexually active women with fever and bilateral abdominal or pelvic tenderness. A twisted ovarian cyst may also cause sudden severe pain. The sudden onset of lower abdominal pain in the middle of the menstrual cycle suggests mittelschmerz. Sudden severe abdominal pain with diffuse pelvic tenderness and shock suggests a ruptured ectopic pregnancy. A positive pregnancy test and pelvic ultrasonography are diagnostic. Retrocecal or retroileal appendicitis (often associated with pyuria or hematuria) may be confused with ureteral colic or pyelonephritis. Other conditions that may resemble appendicitis are diverticulitis, Meckel's diverticulitis, carcinoid of the appendix, perforated colonic cancer, Crohn's ileitis, perforated peptic ulcer, cholecystitis, and mesenteric adenitis. It is virtually impossible to distinguish appendicitis from Meckel's diverticulitis, but both require surgical treatment.

Complications

Perforation occurs in 20% of patients and should be suspected in patients with pain persisting for over 36 hours, high fever, diffuse abdominal tenderness or peritoneal findings, a palpable abdominal mass, or marked leukocytosis. Localized perforation results in a contained abscess, usually in the pelvis. A free perforation leads to suppurative peritonitis with toxicity. Septic thrombophlebitis (pylephlebitis) of the portal venous system is rare and suggested by high fever, chills, bacteremia, and jaundice.

Treatment

The treatment of uncomplicated appendicitis is surgical appendectomy. This may be performed through a laparotomy or by laparoscopy. Prior to surgery, patients should be given systemic antibiotics, which reduce the incidence of postoperative wound infections. Emergency appendectomy is also required in patients with perforated appendicitis with generalized peritonitis.

The optimal treatment of stable patients with perforated appendicitis and a contained abscess is controversial. Surgery in this setting can be difficult. Many recommend percutaneous CT-guided drainage of the abscess with intravenous fluids and antibiotics to allow the inflammation to subside. An interval appendectomy may be performed after 6 weeks to prevent recurrent appendicitis.

Prognosis

The mortality rate from uncomplicated appendicitis is extremely low. Even with perforated appendicitis, the mortality rate in most groups is only 0.2%, though it approaches 15% in the elderly.

Rettenbacher T et al: Appendicitis: should diagnostic imaging be performed if the clinical presentation is highly suggestive of the disease? Gastroenterology 2002;123:992. [PMID: 12360459]

Sauerland S et al: Laparoscopic versus open surgery for suspected appendicitis. Cochrane Database Syst Rev 2004;(4):CD0001546. [PMID: 15495014]

Terasawa T et al: Systematic review: computed tomography and ultrasonography to detect acute appendicitis in adults and adolescents. Ann Intern Med 2004;141:537. [PMID: 15466771]

INTESTINAL TUBERCULOSIS

Intestinal tuberculosis is common in underdeveloped countries. Previously rare in the United States, its incidence has been rising in immigrant groups and patients with AIDS. It is caused by both *Mycobacterium tuberculosis* and *M bovis*. Active pulmonary disease is present in less than 50% of patients. The most frequent site of involvement is the ileocecal region; however, any region of the gastrointestinal tract may be involved. Intestinal tuberculosis may cause mucosal ulcerations or scarring and fibrosis with narrowing of the lumen. Patients may be without symptoms or complain of chronic abdominal pain, obstructive symptoms, weight loss, and diarrhea. An abdominal mass may be palpable. Complications include intesti-

nal obstruction, hemorrhage, and fistula formation. The purified protein derivative (PPD) skin test may be negative, especially in patients with weight loss or AIDS. Barium radiography may demonstrate mucosal ulcerations, thickening, or stricture formation. Colonoscopy may demonstrate an ulcerated mass, multiple ulcers with steep edges and adjacent small sessile polyps, small ulcers or erosions, or small diverticula, most commonly in the ileocecal region. The differential diagnosis includes Crohn's disease, carcinoma, and intestinal amebiasis. The diagnosis is established by either endoscopic or surgical biopsy revealing acid-fast bacilli, caseating granuloma, or positive cultures from the organism. Detection of tubercle bacilli in biopsy specimens by PCR is now the most sensitive means of diagnosis.

Treatment with standard antituberculous regimens is effective.

Sato S et al: Colonoscopy in the diagnosis of intestinal tuberculosis. Gastrointest Endosc 2004;59:362. [PMID: 14997132]

Villanueva Saenz E et al: Colonic tuberculosis. Dig Dis Sci 2002; 47:2045. [PMID: 12353853]

PROTEIN-LOSING ENTEROPATHY

Protein-losing enteropathy comprises a number of conditions that result in excessive loss of serum proteins into the gastrointestinal tract. The essential diagnostic features are hypoalbuminemia and an elevated fecal α_1-antitrypsin level.

The normal intact gut epithelium prevents the loss of serum proteins. Proteins may be lost through one of three mechanisms: (1) mucosal disease with ulceration, resulting in the loss of proteins across the disrupted mucosal surface; (2) lymphatic obstruction, resulting in the loss of protein-rich chylous fluid from mucosal lacteals; and (3) idiopathic change in permeability of mucosal capillaries and conductance of interstitium, resulting in "weeping" of protein-rich fluid from the mucosal surface (Table 14–13).

Hypoalbuminemia is the sine qua non of protein-losing enteropathy. However, a number of other serum proteins such as α_1-antitrypsin also are lost from the gut epithelium. In protein-losing enteropathy caused by lymphatic obstruction, loss of lymphatic fluid commonly results in lymphocytopenia (< 1000/ mcL), hypoglobulinemia, and hypocholesterolemia.

In most cases, protein-losing enteropathy is recognized as a sequela of a known gastrointestinal disorder. In patients in whom the cause is unclear, evaluation is indicated and is guided by the clinical suspicion. Protein-losing enteropathy must be distinguished from other causes of hypoalbuminemia, which include liver disease and nephrotic syndrome; and from congestive heart failure. Protein-losing enteropathy is confirmed by determining the gut α_1-antitrypsin clearance (24-hour volume of feces × stool concentration of α_1-antitrypsin ÷ serum α_1-

Table 14–13. Causes of protein-losing
enteropathy.

Mucosal disease with ulceration
   Chronic gastric ulcer
   Gastric carcinoma
   Lymphoma
   Inflammatory bowel disease
   Idiopathic ulcerative jejunoileitis
Lymphatic obstruction
   Primary intestinal lymphangiectasia
   Secondary obstruction
      Cardiac disease: constrictive pericarditis, congestive
         heart failure
      Infections: tuberculosis, Whipple's disease
      Neoplasms: lymphoma, Kaposi's sarcoma
      Retroperitoneal fibrosis
      Sarcoidosis
Idiopathic mucosal transudation
   Ménétrier's disease
   Zollinger-Ellison syndrome
   Acute viral gastroenteritis
   Celiac sprue
   Eosinophilic gastroenteritis
   Allergic protein-losing enteropathy
   Parasite infection: giardiasis, hookworm
   Amyloidosis
   Common variable immunodeficiency
   Systemic lupus erythematosus

antitrypsin concentration). A clearance of more than 13 mL/24 h is abnormal.

Laboratory evaluation of protein-losing enteropathy includes serum protein electrophoresis, lymphocyte count, and serum cholesterol to look for evidence of lymphatic obstruction. Serum ANA and C3 levels are useful to screen for autoimmune disorders. Stool samples should be examined for ova and parasites. Evidence of malabsorption is evaluated by means of a stool qualitative fecal fat determination. Intestinal imaging is performed with an upper endoscopy with small bowel biopsy and a small bowel barium series. Colonic diseases are excluded with barium enema or colonoscopy. A CT scan of the abdomen is performed to look for evidence of neoplasms or lymphatic obstruction. Rarely, lymphangiography is helpful. In some situations, laparotomy with full-thickness intestinal biopsy is required to establish a diagnosis.

Treatment is directed at the underlying cause. Patients with lymphatic obstruction benefit from low-fat diets supplemented with medium-chain triglycerides. Case reports suggest that octreotide may lead to symptomatic and nutritional improvement in some patients.

Landzberg BR et al: Protein-losing enteropathy and gastropathy. Curr Treat Options Gastroenterol 2001;4:39. [PMID: 11177680]

■ DISEASES OF THE COLON & RECTUM

IRRITABLE BOWEL SYNDROME

 ESSENTIALS OF DIAGNOSIS

- *Chronic functional disorder characterized by abdominal pain or discomfort with alterations in bowel habits.*
- *Symptoms usually begin in late teens to early twenties.*
- *Limited evaluation to exclude organic causes of symptoms.*

General Considerations

The functional gastrointestinal disorders are characterized by a variable combination of chronic or recurrent gastrointestinal symptoms *not explicable by the presence of structural or biochemical abnormalities.* Several clinical entities are included under this broad rubric, including chest pain of unclear origin (noncardiac chest pain), functional dyspepsia, and biliary dyskinesia (sphincter of Oddi dysfunction). There is a large overlap among these entities. For example, over 50% of patients with noncardiac chest pain and over one-third with functional dyspepsia also have symptoms compatible with irritable bowel syndrome. In none of these disorders is there a definitive diagnostic study. Rather, the diagnosis is a subjective one based on the presence of a compatible profile and the exclusion of similar disorders.

Irritable bowel syndrome can be defined, therefore, as an idiopathic clinical entity characterized by some combination of chronic (more than 3 months) lower abdominal symptoms and bowel complaints that may be continuous or intermittent. Consensus definition of irritable bowel syndrome is abdominal discomfort or pain that has two of the following three features: (1) relieved with defecation, (2) onset associated with a change in frequency of stool, or (3) onset associated with a change in form (appearance) of stool. Other symptoms supporting the diagnosis include abnormal stool frequency (more than three bowel movements per day or fewer than three per week); abnormal stool form (lumpy or hard; loose or watery); abnormal stool passage (straining, urgency, or feeling of incomplete evacuation); passage of mucus; and bloating or a feeling of abdominal distention.

Patients may have other somatic or psychological complaints such as dyspepsia, heartburn, chest pain, headaches, fatigue, myalgias, urologic dysfunction, gynecologic symptoms, anxiety, or depression.

The disorder is a common problem presenting to both gastroenterologists and primary care physicians. Up to 20% of the adult population have symptoms compatible with the diagnosis, but most never seek medical attention. Approximately two-thirds of patients with irritable bowel syndrome are women.

Pathogenesis

A number of pathophysiologic mechanisms have been identified and may have varying importance in different individuals.

A. ABNORMAL MOTILITY

A variety of abnormal myoelectrical and motor abnormalities have been identified in the colon and small intestine. In some cases, these are temporally correlated with episodes of abdominal pain or emotional stress. Whether they represent a primary motility disorder or are secondary to psychosocial stress is debated. Differences between patients with constipation-predominant and diarrhea-predominant syndromes are reported.

B. VISCERAL HYPERSENSITIVITY

Patients often have a lower visceral pain threshold, reporting abdominal pain at lower volumes of colonic gas insufflation or colonic balloon inflation than controls. Although many patients complain of bloating and distention, their absolute intestinal gas volume is normal. Many patients report rectal urgency despite small rectal volumes of stool.

C. ENTERIC INFECTION

Symptoms compatible with irritable bowel syndrome develop in up to 30% of patients after an episode of bacterial gastroenteritis. Women and patients with increased life stressors at the onset of gastroenteritis appear to be at increased risk for developing "postinfectious" irritable bowel syndrome. Increased inflammatory cells have been found in the mucosa, submucosa, and muscularis of some patients with irritable bowel syndrome, but their importance is unclear. Chronic inflammation is postulated by some investigators to contribute to alterations in motility or visceral hypersensitivity. Some recent investigations report an increase in breath hydrogen excretion after lactulose ingestion in up to 80% of patients with irritable bowel syndrome, believed to be suggestive of small intestinal bacterial overgrowth, although other investigators have not confirmed these findings. It is hypothesized that bacterial overgrowth may lead to alterations in immune alterations that affect motility or visceral sensitivity. In addition, bacterial degradation of carbohydrates in the small intestine could cause increased postprandial gas, bloating and distention, which may improve after antibiotic treatment. However, other studies dispute these findings.

D. PSYCHOSOCIAL ABNORMALITIES

More than 50% of patients with irritable bowel who seek medical attention have underlying depression, anxiety, or somatization. By contrast, those who do not seek medical attention are similar psychologically to normal individuals. Psychological abnormalities may influence how the patient perceives or reacts to illness and minor visceral sensations. Chronic stress may alter intestinal motility or modulate pathways that affect central and spinal processing of visceral afferent sensation.

Clinical Findings

A. SYMPTOMS AND SIGNS

Irritable bowel is a chronic condition. Symptoms usually begin in the late teens to twenties. Symptoms should be present for at least 3 months before the diagnosis can be considered. The diagnosis is established in the presence of compatible symptoms and the judicious use of tests to exclude organic disease.

Abdominal pain usually is intermittent, crampy, and in the lower abdominal region. As previously stated, the onset of pain typically is associated with a change in stool frequency or form and commonly is relieved by defecation. It does not usually occur at night or interfere with sleep. Patients with irritable bowel syndrome may be classified into one of three categories: those who have predominant problems with constipation, diarrhea, or alternating constipation and diarrhea. It is important to clarify what the patient means by these complaints. Patients with irritable bowel and constipation report infrequent bowel movements (less than three per week), hard or lumpy stools, or straining. Patients with irritable bowel syndrome with diarrhea refer to loose or watery stools, frequent stools (more than three per day), urgency, or fecal incontinence. Many patients report that they have a firm stool in the morning followed by progressively looser movements. Mucus is commonly seen. Complaints of visible distention and bloating are common, though these are not always clinically evident.

The patient should be asked about "alarm symptoms" that suggest a diagnosis other than irritable bowel syndrome and warrant further investigation. The acute onset of symptoms raises the likelihood of organic disease, especially in patients aged > 40–50 years. Nocturnal diarrhea, severe constipation or diarrhea, hematochezia, weight loss, and fever are incompatible with a diagnosis of irritable bowel syndrome and warrant investigation for underlying disease. Patients who have a family history of cancer, inflammatory bowel disease, or celiac disease should undergo additional evaluation.

A physical examination should be performed to look for evidence of organic disease and to allay the patient's anxieties. The physical examination usually is normal. Abdominal tenderness, especially in the lower abdomen, is common but not pronounced. A new onset of symptoms in a patient over age 40 years warrants further examination.

B. LABORATORY FINDINGS AND SPECIAL EXAMINATIONS

In patients whose symptoms fulfill the diagnostic criteria for irritable bowel syndrome and who have no other alarm symptoms, evidence-based consensus guidelines do not support further diagnostic testing, as the likelihood of serious organic diseases does not appear to be increased. Although the vague nature of symptoms and patient anxiety may prompt clinicians to consider a variety of diagnostic studies, overtesting should be avoided. A complete blood count, chemistry panel, and serum albumin should be obtained in most patients. However, erythrocyte sedimentation rate, thyroid function tests, stool occult blood test, stool for ova and parasites, sigmoidoscopy or colonoscopy, or barium enema in patients with symptoms of irritable bowel syndrome are not recommended for patients without alarm symptoms or abnormal hematology or chemistry studies. In patients with diarrhea, serologic tests for celiac disease may be performed. In all patients age 50 years or older who have not had a previous evaluation, barium enema or colonoscopy should be considered to exclude malignancy. Pending further clinical studies, routine testing for bacterial overgrowth cannot be recommended.

Differential Diagnosis

A number of disorders may present with similar symptoms. Examples include colonic neoplasia, inflammatory bowel disease (ulcerative colitis, Crohn's disease, microscopic colitis), hyperthyroidism or hypothyroidism, parasites, malabsorption (especially celiac disease, bacterial overgrowth, lactase deficiency), causes of chronic secretory diarrhea (carcinoid), and endometriosis. Psychiatric disorders such as depression, panic disorder, and anxiety must be considered as well. Women with refractory symptoms have an increased incidence of prior sexual and physical abuse. These diagnoses should be excluded in patients with presumed irritable bowel syndrome who do not improve within 2–4 weeks of empiric treatment or in whom subsequent alarm symptoms develop.

Treatment

A. GENERAL MEASURES

As with other functional disorders, the most important interventions the physician can offer are reassurance, education, and support. An ongoing therapeutic relationship may be the most important factor in successful management of this disorder. This includes identifying and responding to the patient's concerns, careful explanation of the pathophysiology and natural history of the disorder, setting realistic treatment goals, and involving the patient in the treatment process. Because irritable bowel symptoms are chronic, the patient's reasons for seeking consultation at this time should be determined. These may include major life events or recent psychosocial stressors, dietary or medication changes, concerns about serious underlying disease, or reduced quality of life and impairment of daily activities. In discussing with the patient the importance of the mind-gut interaction, it may be helpful to explain that alterations in visceral motility and sensitivity may be exacerbated by environmental, social, or psychological factors such as foods, medications, hormones, and stress. Symptoms such as pain, bloating, and altered bowel habits may lead to anxiety and distress, which in turn may further exacerbate bowel disturbances due to disordered communication between the gut and the central nervous system. A symptom diary in which patients record the time and severity of symptoms, food intake, and life events may help uncover aggravating dietary or psychosocial factors. Physicians will earn the confidence of their patients by being nonjudgmental and attentive. Fears that the symptoms will progress, require surgery, or degenerate into serious illness should be allayed. The patient should understand that irritable bowel syndrome is a chronic disorder characterized by periods of exacerbation and quiescence. The physician can help but cannot "cure" such a disorder. The emphasis should be shifted from finding the cause of the symptoms to finding a way to cope with them. Physicians must resist the temptation to chase chronic complaints with new or repeated diagnostic studies.

B. DIETARY THERAPY

Patients commonly report dietary intolerances, although a role for dietary triggers in irritable bowel syndrome has never been convincingly demonstrated. Fatty foods and caffeine are poorly tolerated by many patients with irritable bowel syndrome. In patients with diarrhea, bloating, and flatulence, lactose intolerance should be excluded with a breath hydrogen test or a trial of a lactose-free diet. Malabsorption of dietary fructose or sorbitol (contained in fruits and artificially sweetened foods) may exacerbate bloating, flatulence, and diarrhea. A variety of foods are flatulogenic, producing pain and distention in some patients. These include brown beans, Brussels sprouts, cabbage, cauliflower, raw onions, grapes, plums, raisins, coffee, garlic, red wine, and beer.

A high-fiber diet appears to be of little value in patients with irritable bowel syndrome. Many patients report little change in bowel frequency but increased gas and distention with high-fiber diets or fiber supplementation.

C. PHARMACOLOGIC MEASURES

More than two-thirds of patients with irritable bowel syndrome have mild symptoms that respond readily to education, reassurance, and dietary interventions. Drug therapy should be reserved for patients with moderate to severe symptoms that do not respond to conservative measures. These agents should be viewed as being adjunctive rather than curative. Given the wide spectrum of symptoms, no single agent is expected to provide relief in all or even most patients. Nevertheless, therapy targeted at the specific dominant symptom (pain, constipation, or diarrhea) may be beneficial.

1. Antispasmodic agents—Anticholinergic agents are used by some practitioners for treatment of acute episodes of pain or bloating despite a lack of well-designed trials demonstrating efficacy. Available agents include hyoscyamine, 0.125 mg orally (or sublingually as needed) or sustained-release, 0.037 mg or 0.75 mg orally twice daily; dicyclomine, 10–20 mg orally; or methscopolamine 2.5–5 mg orally before meals and at bedtime. Anticholinergic side effects are common, including urinary retention, constipation, tachycardia, and dry mouth. Hence, these agents should be used with caution in the elderly and in patients with constipation.

2. Antidiarrheal agents—Loperamide (2 mg orally three or four times daily) is effective for the treatment of patients with diarrhea, reducing stool frequency, liquidity, and urgency. It may best be used "prophylactically" in situations in which diarrhea is anticipated (such as stressful situations) or would be inconvenient (social engagements).

3. Anticonstipation agents—Treatment with osmotic laxatives (milk of magnesia or polyethylene glycol) may increase stool frequency, improve stool consistency, and reduce straining. Lactulose or sorbitol produces increased flatus and distention, which are poorly tolerated in patients with irritable bowel syndrome. Patients with intractable constipation should undergo further assessment for slow colonic transit and pelvic floor dysfunction (see Constipation, above).

4. Psychotropic agents—Patients with predominant symptoms of pain or bloating may benefit from low doses of tricyclic antidepressants, which are believed to have effects on motility, visceral sensitivity, and central pain perception that are independent of their psychotropic effects. Because of their anticholinergic effects, these agents may be more useful in patients with diarrhea-predominant than constipation-predominant symptoms. Nortriptyline, desipramine, or imipramine, may be started at a low dosage of 10 mg at bedtime and increased gradually to 50–150 mg as tolerated. Response rates do not correlate with dosage, and many patients respond to doses of ≤ 50 mg daily. Side effects are common, and lack of efficacy with one agent does not preclude benefit from another. Improvement should be evident within 4 weeks. The serotonin reuptake inhibitors (sertraline, 50–150 mg daily; paroxetine 10–20 mg daily; or fluoxetine, 20–40 mg daily) may lead to improvement in overall sense of well-being but have little impact on abdominal pain or bowel symptoms. Anxiolytics should not be used chronically in irritable bowel syndrome because of their habituation potential. Patients with major depression or anxiety disorders should be identified and treated with therapeutic doses of appropriate agents.

5. Serotonin receptor agonists and antagonists—Serotonin is an important mediator of gastrointestinal motility and sensation. Two agents approved for treatment of irritable bowel syndrome that modulate serotonin pathways are tegaserod and alosetron. Although both of these agents have some effect on visceral sensation, they have very different effects on intestinal motility.

Tegaserod is a selective partial 5-HT$_4$-receptor agonist that has been approved recently for treatment of women who have irritable bowel syndrome with predominant constipation. Through stimulation of neurons in the intestinal mucosa, tegaserod stimulates intestinal peristalsis, inhibits visceral afferents involved in pain sensation, and stimulates colonic chloride and water secretion. In humans it acts as a prokinetic agent, accelerating gastric emptying and small and large bowel transit. Tegaserod (6 mg twice daily) results in modest but significant improvement compared with placebo in global irritable bowel symptoms in women. Efficacy in men has not been established. Tegaserod leads to an increase in stool frequency, improvement of stool consistency, and a reduction in abdominal pain and bloating. Symptom improvement is evident within 1 week in responsive patients. Diarrhea occurs in about 10% but usually resolves with continued therapy. The drug is otherwise extremely well tolerated and without significant drug interactions. For patients who demonstrate symptomatic improvement, it may be continued for 4–12 weeks and used intermittently for symptomatic flares.

Alosetron is a 5-HT$_3$ antagonist that has been approved for the treatment of women with severe irritable bowel syndrome with predominant diarrhea. It appears to alter visceral sensation through blockade of peripheral 5-HT$_3$-receptors on enteric afferent neurons as well as central receptors. It also inhibits enteric cholinergic motor neurons, resulting in inhibition of colonic motility. In humans, it increases the pain threshold in response to intestinal distention and slows colonic transit time. Alosetron (1 mg twice daily) results in improvement in 50–60% of women compared with 30–40% treated with placebo. Alosetron reduces symptoms of pain, discomfort, cramps, urgency, and diarrhea. Efficacy in men has not been demonstrated. In contrast to the excellent safety profile of other 5-HT$_3$ antagonists (eg, ondansetron), alosetron may cause constipation in 30% of patients, frequently requiring discontinuation. Severe constipation (requiring hospitalization) and ischemic colitis may occur in 4:1000 patients. Given the seriousness of these side effects, alosetron is restricted to women with severe irritable bowel syndrome with diarrhea who have failed conventional therapies and who have been educated about the relative risks and benefits of the agent. It should not be used in patients with constipation.

6. Antibiotics—Controlled clinical trials from some centers report symptoms in up to half of patients with irritable bowel syndrome who were given antibiotics for presumed small intestinal bacterial overgrowth. Pending further clinical investigation, routine testing and treatment for small intestinal bacterial overgrowth cannot be recommended.

7. Probiotics—Small controlled clinical trials report improved symptoms in some patients treated with one probiotic, *Bifidobacterium infantis*, but not with another probiotic, *Lactobacillus salivarius*, or placebo. Results of further clinical trials are awaited before probiotic therapy can be recommended for irritable bowel syndrome.

D. PSYCHOLOGICAL THERAPIES

Cognitive-behavioral therapies, relaxation techniques, and hypnotherapy appear to be beneficial in some patients. Patients with underlying psychological abnormalities may benefit from evaluation by a psychiatrist or psychologist. Patients with severe disability should be referred to a pain treatment center.

Prognosis

The majority of patients with irritable bowel syndrome learn to cope with their symptoms and lead productive lives.

Chey WD et al: Long-term safety and efficacy of alosetron in women with severe diarrhea-predominant irritable bowel syndrome. Am J Gastroenterol 2004;99:2195. [PMID: 1555502]

Evidence-based position statement on the management of irritable bowel syndrome in North America. Am J Gastroenterol 2002;97(11 Suppl):S1. [PMID: 12425585]

Halpert A et al: Clinical response to tricyclic antidepressants in functional bowel disorders is not related to dosage. Am J Gastroenterol 2005;100:664. [PMID: 15743366]

Lesbros-Pantoflickova D et al: Meta-analysis: the treatment of irritable bowel syndrome. Aliment Pharmacol Ther 2004; 20:1253. [PMID: 15606387]

Lin HC: Small intestinal bacterial overgrowth: a framework for understanding irritable bowel syndrome. JAMA 2004;292: 852. [PMID: 15316000]

Muller-Lissner S et al: Tegaserod is effective in the initial and retreatment of irritable bowel syndrome with constipation. Aliment Pharmacol Ther 2005;21:11. [PMID: 15644040]

O'Mahony L et al: *Lactobacillus* and *Bifidobacterium* in irritable bowel syndrome: symptom responses and relationship to cytokine profiles. Gastroenterology 2005;128:541. [PMID: 15765388]

Spiller RC: Infection, immune function, and functional gut disorders. Clin Gastroenterol Hepatol 2004;2:445. [PMID: 15181610]

Walters B et al: Detection of bacterial overgrowth in IBS using the lactulose H₂ breath test: comparison with 14C-D-xylose and healthy controls. Am J Gastroenterol 2005;100:1566. [PMID: 15984983]

Whorwell PJ: Review article: the history of hypnotherapy and its role in the irritable bowel syndrome. Aliment Pharmacol Ther 2005;22:1061. [PMID: 16305719]

ANTIBIOTIC-ASSOCIATED COLITIS

 ESSENTIALS OF DIAGNOSIS

- *Most cases of antibiotic-associated diarrhea are not attributable to C difficile and are usually mild and self-limited.*
- *Symptoms of antibiotic-associated colitis vary from mild to fulminant; almost all colitis is attributable to C difficile.*
- *Diagnosis in mild to moderate cases established by stool toxin assay.*
- *Flexible sigmoidoscopy provides most rapid diagnosis in severe cases.*

General Considerations

Antibiotic-associated diarrhea is a common clinical occurrence. Characteristically, the diarrhea occurs during the period of antibiotic exposure, is dose related, and resolves spontaneously after discontinuation of the antibiotic. In most cases, this diarrhea is mild, self-limited, and does not require any specific laboratory evaluation or treatment. Stool examination usually reveals no fecal leukocytes, and stool cultures reveal no pathogens. Although *C difficile* is identified in the stool of 15–25% of cases of antibiotic-associated diarrhea, it is also identified in 5–10% of patients treated with antibiotics who do not have diarrhea. Most cases of antibiotic-associated diarrhea are due to changes in colonic bacterial fermentation of carbohydrates and are not due to *C difficile*.

Antibiotic-associated colitis is a significant clinical problem almost always caused by *C difficile* infection. Hospitalized patients are most susceptible, especially those who are severely ill or malnourished or who are receiving chemotherapy. *C difficile*–colitis is the major cause of diarrhea in patients hospitalized for more than 3 days, affecting 22 patients of every 1000. This anaerobic bacterium colonizes the colon of 3% of healthy adults. However, it is acquired in approximately 20% of hospitalized patients, most of whom have received antibiotics that disrupt the normal bowel flora and thus allow the bacterium to flourish. Although almost all antibiotics have been implicated, colitis most commonly develops after use of ampicillin, clindamycin, third-generation cephalosporins, and flouroquinolones. *C difficile*–colitis will develop in approximately one-third of infected patients. Symptoms usually begin during or shortly after antibiotic therapy but may be delayed for up to 8 weeks. All patients with acute diarrhea should be asked about recent antibiotic exposure. Patients who are elderly, debilitated, immunocompromised, receiving multiple antibiotics or prolonged (> 10 days) antibiotic therapy, or receiving enteral tube feedings have a higher risk of acquiring *C difficile* and developing *C difficile*–associated diarrhea. The organism is spread by fecal-oral transmission. It is found throughout hospitals in patient rooms and bathrooms and is readily transmitted from patient to patient by hospital personnel. Fastidious hand washing and use of disposable gloves are helpful in minimizing transmission.

The incidence and severity of *C difficile*–colitis in hospitalized patients appear to be increasing, which is attributable to the emergence of a more virulent strain of *C difficile* (BI/NAP1) that contains an 18-base pair deletion of the tcdC gene, resulting in higher toxin production. This toxin-gene variant strain has been associated with several hospital outbreaks. The 30-day mortality attributed to infection with this strain is 7% but is 14% in the elderly.

Clinical Findings

A. SYMPTOMS AND SIGNS

Most patients report mild to moderate greenish, foul-smelling watery diarrhea with lower abdominal cramps. Physical examination is normal or reveals mild left lower quadrant tenderness. With more serious illness, there is abdominal pain and profuse watery diarrhea with up to 30 stools per day. The stools may have mucus but seldom gross blood. There may be fever up to 40 °C, abdominal tenderness, and leukocytosis as high as 50,000/mcL. *C difficile*–colitis should be considered in all hospitalized patients with unexplained leukocytosis. In most patients, colitis is most severe in the distal colon and rectum. When colitis is more severe in the right side of the colon, there may be little or no diarrhea. In such cases, fever, abdominal distention, pain and tenderness, and leukocytosis suggest the presence of infection.

B. SPECIAL EXAMINATIONS

1. Stool studies—Pathogenic strains of *C difficile* produce two toxins: toxin A is an enterotoxin and toxin B is a cytotoxin. In most patients, the diagnosis of antibiotic-associated colitis is established by the demonstration of *C difficile* toxins in the stool. A cytotoxicity assay (toxin B) performed in cell cultures has a specificity of 90% and a sensitivity of 95%. This is the definitive test, but it is expensive and results are not available for 24–48 hours. Rapid enzyme immunoassays (EIA) (2–4 hours) for toxins A and B are now widely used and have an 80–90% sensitivity with a single stool specimen but > 90% with two specimens. Some toxic strains of *C difficile* do not produce a functional toxin A (and therefore have a negative EIA); therefore, testing for toxin A and B is preferred. When *C difficile* is suspected but the EIA is negative, a cytotoxicity assay should be performed. Culture for *C difficile* is the most sensitive test, but 25% of isolates are not pathogenic. Because it is slower (2–3 days), more costly, and less specific than toxin assays, it is not used in most clinical settings. Fecal leukocytes are present in only 50% of patients with colitis.

2. Flexible sigmoidoscopy—Flexible sigmoidoscopy is performed in patients with more severe symptomatology when a rapid diagnosis is desired so that therapy can be initiated. In patients with mild to moderate symptoms, there may be no abnormalities or only patchy or diffuse, nonspecific colitis indistinguishable from other causes. In patients with severe illness, true **pseudomembranous colitis** is seen. This has a characteristic appearance, with yellow adherent plaques 2–10 mm in diameter scattered over the colonic mucosa interspersed with hyperemic mucosa. Biopsies reveal epithelial ulceration with a classic "volcano" exudate of fibrin and neutrophils. In 10% of cases, pseudomembranous colitis is confined to the proximal colon and may be missed at sigmoidoscopy.

3. Imaging studies—Abdominal radiographs are obtained in patients with fulminant symptoms to look for evidence of toxic dilation or megacolon but are of no value in mild disease. Mucosal edema or "thumbprinting" may be evident. Abdominal CT scan may be very useful in detecting colonic edema, especially in patients with predominantly right-sided colitis or abdominal pain without significant diarrhea (in whom the diagnosis may be unsuspected). CT scanning is also useful in the evaluation of possible complications.

Differential Diagnosis

In the hospitalized patient in whom acute diarrhea develops after admission, the differential diagnosis includes simple antibiotic-associated diarrhea (not related to *C difficile*), enteral feedings, medications, and ischemic colitis. Other infectious causes are unusual in hospitalized patients in whom diarrhea develops more than 72 hours after admission, and it is not cost-effective to obtain stool cultures unless tests for *C difficile* are negative. Rarely, other organisms (staphylococci, *Clostridium perfringens*) have been associated with pseudomembranous colitis.

Complications

Fulminant disease may result in dehydration, electrolyte imbalance, toxic megacolon, perforation, and death. Chronic untreated colitis may result in weight loss and protein-losing enteropathy.

Treatment

A. IMMEDIATE TREATMENT

If possible, antibiotic therapy should be discontinued. In patients with mild symptoms, doing so may result in prompt resolution of symptoms without specific treatment. If diarrhea is severe or persistent, specific therapy is warranted. The drug of choice is metronidazole, 500 mg orally three times daily. The duration of therapy is usually 10–14 days. However, in patients requiring long-term systemic antibiotics, it may be appropriate to continue metronidazole therapy until the antibiotics can be discontinued. Vancomycin, 125 mg orally four times daily, is as effective as metronidazole but significantly more expensive, and it promotes the emergence of vancomycin-resistant nosocomial infections. Therefore, metronidazole is the preferred first-line therapy in most patients. Vancomycin should be reserved for patients who are intolerant of metronidazole, pregnant women, and children. Symptomatic improvement occurs in most patients within 72 hours. For patients with severe disease who do not respond rapidly to initial metronidazole therapy, therapy should be switched to vancomycin, 125 mg orally four times daily, escalating the dose to 500 mg four times daily if diarrhea and leukocytosis fail to improve. In patients who are unable to take oral medications and those with toxic megacolon, intravenous metronidazole, 500–750 mg every 6 hours, should be given—sometimes supplemented by oral vancomycin administered per nasoenteric tube or enema. Intravenous vancomycin does not penetrate the bowel and should not be used. Total abdominal colectomy may be required in patients with toxic megacolon, perforation, sepsis, or hemorrhage.

B. Treatment of Relapse

Up to 20% of patients have a relapse of diarrhea from *C difficile* within 1 or 2 weeks after stopping initial therapy. This may be due to reinfection or failure to eradicate the organism. Most relapses respond promptly to a second course of metronidazole therapy. Some patients have recurrent relapses that can be difficult to treat. The optimal treatment regimen for recurrent relapses is unknown. Many authorities recommend a 6-week tapering regimen of vancomycin (125 mg orally four times daily for 7 days; twice daily for 7 days; once daily for 7 days; every other day for 7 days; and every third day for 2 weeks). Controlled trials show that oral administration of a live yeast, *Saccharomyces boulardii,* 500 mg twice daily, reduces the incidence of relapse by 50%. Probiotic therapy with this agent is recommended as adjunctive therapy in patients with relapsing disease.

Bartlett JG: Clinical practice. Antibiotic-associated diarrhea. N Engl J Med 2002;346:334. [PMID: 11821511]

Bricker E et al: Antibiotic treatment for *Clostridium difficile*–associated diarrhea in adults. Cochrane Database Syst Rev 2005; (1):CD004610. [PMID: 15674956]

Loo VG et al: A predominantly clonal multi-institutional outbreak of *Clostridium difficile*–associated diarrhea with high morbidity and mortality. N Engl J Med 2005; 353:2442. [PMID: 16322602]

McDonald LC et al: An epidemic, toxin gene-variant strain of *Clostridium difficile.* N Engl J Med 2005;353:2433. [PMID: 16322603]

Morelli M et al: Clinical application of the polymerase chain reaction to diagnose *Clostridium difficile* in hospitalized patients with diarrhea. Clin Gastroenterol Hepatol 2004; 2:669. [PMID: 15290659]

Szajewska H et al: Meta-analysis: non-pathogenic yeast *Saccharomyces boulardii* in the prevention of antibiotic-associated diarrhea. Aliment Pharmacol Ther 2005;22:365. [PMID: 16128673]

INFLAMMATORY BOWEL DISEASE

The term "inflammatory bowel disease" includes ulcerative colitis and Crohn's disease. Ulcerative colitis is a chronic, recurrent disease characterized by diffuse mucosal inflammation involving only the colon. Ulcerative colitis invariably involves the rectum and may extend proximally in a continuous fashion to involve part or all of the colon. Crohn's disease is a chronic, recurrent disease characterized by patchy transmural inflammation involving any segment of the gastrointestinal tract from the mouth to the anus.

Crohn's disease and ulcerative colitis may be associated in 25% of patients with a number of extraintestinal manifestations, including oligoarticular or polyarticular nondeforming peripheral arthritis, spondylitis or sacroiliitis, episcleritis or uveitis, erythema nodosum, pyoderma gangrenosum, sclerosing cholangitis, and thromboembolic events.

Drug Therapies for Inflammatory Bowel Disease

Although ulcerative colitis and Crohn's disease appear to be distinct entities, the same pharmacologic agents are used to treat both. Despite extensive research, there are still no specific therapies for these diseases. The mainstays of therapy are 5-aminosalicylic acid derivatives, corticosteroids, immunomodulating agents (such as mercaptopurine or azathioprine), methotrexate, and infliximab.

A. 5-Aminosalicylic Acid (5-ASA)

5-ASA is a topically active agent that has a variety of anti-inflammatory effects. It is used in the active treatment of ulcerative colitis and Crohn's disease and during disease inactivity to maintain remission. It is readily absorbed from the small intestine but demonstrates minimal colonic absorption. A number of oral and topical compounds have been designed to target delivery of 5-ASA to the colon or small intestine while minimizing absorption. Commonly used formulations of 5-ASA are sulfasalazine, mesalamine, and azo compounds. Side effects of these compounds are uncommon but include nausea, rash, diarrhea, pancreatitis, and acute interstitial nephritis.

1. Oral mesalamine agents—These 5-ASA agents are coated in various pH-sensitive resins (Asacol) or packaged in timed-release capsules (Pentasa). Mesalamine tablets dissolve at pH 7.0, releasing 5-ASA in the terminal small bowel and proximal colon. Pentasa releases 5-ASA slowly throughout the small intestine and colon.

2. Azo Compounds—Sulfasalazine, balsalazide and olsalazine contain 5-ASA linked by an azo bond that requires cleavage by colonic bacterial azoreductases to release 5-ASA. Absorption of these drugs from the small intestine is negligible. After release within the colon, the 5-ASA works topically and is largely unabsorbed. Olsalazine contains two 5-ASA molecules connected by the azo bond. Balsalazide contains 5-ASA linked to an inert carrier (4-aminobenzoyl-β-alanine).

Sulfasalazine contains 5-ASA linked to a sulfapyridine moiety. It is unclear whether the sulfapyridine group has any anti-inflammatory effects. One gram of sulfasalazine contains 400 mg of 5-ASA. The sulfapyridine group, however, is absorbed and may cause side effects in 15–30% of patients—much higher than with other 5-ASA compounds. Dose-related side effects include nausea, headaches, leukopenia, oligospermia, and impaired folate metabolism. Allergic and idiosyncratic side effects are fever, rash, hemolytic anemia, neutropenia, worsened colitis, hepatitis, pancreatitis, and pneumonitis. Despite its side effects, sulfasalazine continues to be used because it is significantly less expensive than other 5-ASA agents. It should always be administered in conjunction with folate. Eighty percent of patients intolerant of sulfasalazine can tolerate mesalamine.

3. Topical mesalamine—5-ASA is provided in the form of suppositories (Canasa; 500 mg) and enemas (Rowasa; 4 g/60 mL). These formulations can deliver much higher concentrations of 5-ASA to the distal colon than oral compounds. Side effects are uncommon.

B. CORTICOSTEROIDS

A variety of intravenous, oral, and topical corticosteroid formulations have been used in inflammatory bowel disease. They have utility in the short-term treatment of moderate to severe disease. However, long-term use is associated with serious, potentially irreversible side effects and is to be avoided. The agents, route of administration, duration of use, and tapering regimens used are based more on personal bias and experience than on data from rigorous clinical trials. The most commonly used intravenous formulations have been hydrocortisone or methylprednisolone, which are given by continuous infusion or every 6 hours. Oral formulations are prednisone or methylprednisolone. Adverse events commonly occur during systemic corticosteroid therapy, including mood changes, insomnia, hypertension, weight gain, edema, elevated serum glucose levels, and moon facies. Topical preparations are provided as hydrocortisone suppositories (100 mg), foam (90 mg), and enemas (100 mg). Budesonide is an oral glucocorticoid with high topical anti-inflammatory activity but low systemic activity due to high first-pass hepatic metabolism. A controlled-release formulation is available (Entocort) that targets delivery to the terminal ileum and colon. It produces less suppression of the hypothalamic-pituitary-adrenal axis and fewer steroid-related side effects than hydrocortisone or prednisone.

C. MERCAPTOPURINE, AZATHIOPRINE, OR METHOTREXATE

Mercaptopurine and azathioprine are thiopurine drugs that are used in many patients with refractory Crohn's disease and, increasingly, in patients with ulcerative colitis. Azathioprine is converted in vivo to mercaptopurine. It is believed that the active metabolite of mercaptopurine is 6-thioguanine. Monitoring of 6-thioguanine levels is performed in some research settings but is of unproven value in the management of most patients. Allergic and nonallergic side effects of mercaptopurine and azathioprine occur in 10% of patients, including pancreatitis, bone marrow suppression, infections, hepatitis or cholestatic jaundice and, potentially, a higher risk of neoplasm.

Three competing enzymes are involved in the metabolism of mercaptopurine to its active (6-thioguanine) and inactive metabolites. About 1 person in 300 has a homozygous mutation of one of the enzymes that metabolizes thiopurine methyltransferase (TPMT), placing them at risk for profound immunosuppression; 1 person in 9 is heterozygous for TPMT, resulting in intermediate enzyme activity. Measurement of TPMT functional activity is recommended prior to initiation of therapy. Treatment should be withheld in patients with absent TPMT activity and increased slowly in those with intermediate activity. For patients with normal TPMT activity, the recommended dose of mercaptopurine is 1.5 mg/kg or of azathioprine is 2.5 mg/kg daily. Some clinicians prefer to initiate therapy with either drug at 50 mg/d for 2 weeks before increasing to the full recommended dose. For patients with intermediate activity and for patients in whom TPMT measurement is not available, both drugs should be started at 25 mg/d and increased by 25 mg every 2 weeks while monitoring for myelosuppression. For all patients, a complete blood count, liver chemistries, and amylase should be obtained every 2 weeks for 3 months, then every 3 months for the duration of therapy. If the white blood count falls below 3500–4000/mcL, the medication should be held for at least 1 week before reducing the daily dose by 25–50 mg.

Methotrexate is increasingly used in the treatment of patients with inflammatory bowel disease, especially patients with Crohn's disease who are intolerant of mercaptopurine. Methotrexate is an analog of dihydrofolic acid. Although at high doses it interferes with cell proliferation through inhibition of nucleic acid metabolism, at low doses it has anti-inflammatory properties, including inhibition of expression of tumor necrosis factor-α (TNF-α) in monocytes and macrophages. Methotrexate may be given intramuscularly, subcutaneously, or orally. Side effects of methotrexate include nausea, vomiting, diarrhea, alopecia, stomatitis, infections, bone marrow suppression, hepatitis, hepatic fibrosis, and life-threatening pneumonitis. A complete blood count and liver chemistries should be monitored every 1–3 months. Folate supplementation (1 mg/d) should be administered.

D. ANTI-TNF THERAPY

A dysregulation of the T_H1 T cell response is present in inflammatory bowel disease, especially Crohn's disease. One of the key proinflammatory cytokines in the

T$_H$1 response is TNF-α. Several antibodies to TNF currently are available or in clinical testing for the treatment of inflammatory bowel disease. Infliximab is an immunomodulating agent that represents a major advance in the treatment of patients with moderate to severe Crohn's disease and ulcerative colitis who are unresponsive to conventional therapy. Infliximab is a chimeric (human/mouse) IgG monoclonal antibody that binds with high specificity to membrane-associated TNF-α on monocytes and activated T lymphocytes, promoting apoptosis and cell death. Infliximab is administered by intravenous infusion. The half-life of infliximab after intravenous infusion is 8–10 days; however, therapeutic serum concentrations persist for approximately 8 weeks. A three-dose regimen of 5 mg/kg administered at 0, 2, and 6 weeks is recommended for acute induction, followed by infusions every 8 weeks for maintance therapy. Acute infusion reactions occur in 4–6% of infusions but occur less commonly in patients receiving concomitant immunomodulators (ie, azathioprine or methotrexate). Most are mild or moderate (nausea; headache; dizziness; urticaria; diaphoresis; or mild cardiopulmonary symptoms that include chest tightness, dyspnea, or palpitations) and can be treated by slowing the infusion rate and administering acetaminophen and diphenhydramine. Severe reactions (hypotension, severe shortness of breath, rigors, severe chest discomfort) occur in 1% and may require oxygen, diphenhydramine, hydrocortisone, and epinephrine. Delayed serum sickness-like reactions occur in 1%. With repeated, intermittent intravenous injections, antibodies to infliximab (ATI) develop in up to 40% of patients, which are associated with a shortened duration or loss of response and increased risk of acute infusion reactions. Giving infliximab in a regularly scheduled maintenance therapy (eg, every 8 weeks), concomitant use of infliximab with other immunomodulating agents (azathioprine, mercaptopurine, or methotrexate), or preinfusion treatment with corticosteroids (intravenous hydrocortisone 200 mg) significantly reduces the development of ATI.

Serious infections may occur in up to 5% of patients, including sepsis, pneumonia, abscess, and cellulitis. Patients treated with infliximab are at increased risk for the development of disseminated tuberculosis as well as other opportunistic infections (*Pneumocystis jiroveci*, listeriosis, histoplasmosis, aspergillosis, varicella). Prior to use of infliximab, patients should be screened for latent tuberculosis with PPD testing and a chest radiograph. Autoantibodies including anti-DNA antibody occur in a small number of patients; however, the development of drug-induced lupus is rare. Infliximab may cause severe hepatic reactions leading to acute hepatic failure; liver enzymes should be monitored routinely during therapy. It is speculated but unproven that infliximab may increase the risk of lymphoproliferative malignancies. Rare cases of multiple sclerosis have been reported. Infliximab may worsen congestive heart failure in patients with cardiac disease.

Although infliximab is currently the only anti-TNF agent approved in the United States for treatment of patients with inflammatory bowel disease, other agents that are commercially available or may soon be available have demonstrated efficacy in the treatment of Crohn's disease. These include adalimumab (a fully humanized IgG antibody that is approved for the treatment of rheumatoid arthritis) and certolizumab (a polyethlene glycolated Fab' fragment of humanized anti-TNF), both of which are administered by subcutaneous injection. It is unknown whether these agents will have similar efficacy to infliximab with reduced complications related to antibody formation.

Social Support for Patients with Inflammatory Bowel Disease

Inflammatory bowel disease is a lifelong illness that can have profound emotional and social impacts on the individual. Patients should be encouraged to become involved in the Crohn's and Colitis Foundation of America (CCFA). National headquarters may be contacted at 444 Park Avenue South, 11th Floor, New York, NY 10016-7374; phone 212-685-3440. Internet address: http://www.ccfa.org.

1. Crohn's Disease

ESSENTIALS OF DIAGNOSIS

- *Insidious onset.*
- *Intermittent bouts of low-grade fever, diarrhea, and right lower quadrant pain.*
- *Right lower quadrant mass and tenderness.*
- *Perianal disease with abscess, fistulas.*
- *Radiographic evidence of ulceration, stricturing, or fistulas of the small intestine or colon.*

General Considerations

One-third of cases of Crohn's disease involve the small bowel only, most commonly the terminal ileum (ileitis). Half of all cases involve the small bowel and colon, most often the terminal ileum and adjacent proximal ascending colon (ileocolitis). In 20% of cases, the colon alone is affected. One-third of patients have associated perianal disease (fistulas, fissures, abscesses). A small number of patients have involvement of the mouth (aphthous ulcers) or upper intestinal tract. Unlike ulcerative colitis, Crohn's disease is a transmural process that can result in mucosal inflammation and ulceration, stricturing, fistula development, and abscess formation. Cigarette smoking is strongly associated with the development of Crohn's disease, resistance to medical therapy, and early disease relapse.

Clinical Findings

A. Symptoms and Signs

Because of the variable location of involvement and severity of inflammation, Crohn's disease may present with a variety of symptoms and signs. In eliciting the history, the clinician should take particular note of fevers, the patient's general sense of well-being, the presence of abdominal pain, the number of liquid bowel movements per day, and prior surgical resections. Physical examination should focus on the patient's temperature, weight, and nutritional status, the presence of abdominal tenderness or an abdominal mass, rectal examination, and extraintestinal manifestations. Most commonly, there is one or a combination of the following clinical constellations.

1. Chronic inflammatory disease—This is the most common presentation and is often seen in patients with ileitis or ileocolitis. Patients report low-grade fever, malaise, weight loss, and loss of energy. There may be diarrhea, which is nonbloody and often intermittent. Cramping or steady right lower quadrant or periumbilical pain is present. Physical examination reveals focal tenderness, usually in the right lower quadrant. A palpable, tender mass that represents thickened or matted loops of inflamed intestine may be present in the lower abdomen.

2. Intestinal obstruction—Narrowing of the small bowel may occur as a result of inflammation, spasm, or fibrotic stenosis. Patients report postprandial bloating, cramping pains, and loud borborygmi. This sometimes occurs in patients with active inflammatory symptoms (as above). More commonly, however, it occurs later in the disease from chronic fibrosis without other systemic symptoms or signs of inflammation.

3. Fistulization with or without infection—A subset of patients develops sinus tracts that penetrate through the bowel and form fistulas to a number of locations. Fistulas to the mesentery are usually asymptomatic but can result in intra-abdominal or retroperitoneal abscesses manifested by fevers, chills, a tender abdominal mass, and leukocytosis. Fistulas from the colon to the small intestine or stomach can result in bacterial overgrowth with diarrhea, weight loss, and malnutrition. Fistulas to the bladder or vagina produce recurrent infections. Enterocutaneous fistulas usually occur at the site of surgical scars.

4. Perianal disease—One-third of patients with either large or small bowel involvement develop perianal disease manifested by anal fissures, perianal abscesses, and fistulas.

5. Extraintestinal manifestations—The extracolonic manifestations (described in the section on ulcerative colitis) may also be seen with Crohn's disease, particularly Crohn's colitis. Other problems may also arise. Oral aphthous lesions are common. There is an increased prevalence of gallstones due to malabsorption of bile salts from the terminal ileum. Nephrolithiasis with urate or calcium oxalate stones may occur.

B. Laboratory Findings

There is a poor correlation between laboratory studies and the patient's clinical picture. Laboratory values may reflect inflammatory activity or nutritional complications of disease. A complete blood count and serum albumin should be obtained in all patients. Anemia may reflect chronic inflammation, mucosal blood loss, iron deficiency, or vitamin B_{12} malabsorption secondary to terminal ileal inflammation or resection. Leukocytosis may reflect inflammation or abscess formation or may be secondary to corticosteroid therapy. Hypoalbuminemia may be due to intestinal protein loss (protein-losing enteropathy), malabsorption, bacterial overgrowth, or chronic inflammation. The sedimentation rate or C-reactive protein level is elevated in many patients during active inflammation. Stool specimens are sent for examination for routine pathogens, ova and parasites, leukocytes, fat, and *C difficile* toxin.

C. Special Diagnostic Studies

In most patients, the initial diagnosis of Crohn's disease is based on a compatible clinical picture with supporting endoscopic and radiographic findings. An upper gastrointestinal series with small bowel follow-through or enteroclysis is obtained in all patients with suspected small bowel involvement. Suggestive findings include ulcerations, strictures, and fistulas. Capsule imaging may help to establish a diagnosis in patients in whom the clinical suspicion for small bowel involvement is high but radiographs are normal or nondiagnostic. To evaluate the colon, a barium enema or colonoscopy is obtained. Colonoscopy offers the advantage of obtaining mucosal biopsies of the colon or terminal ileum. Typical endoscopic findings include aphthoid ulcers, linear or stellate ulcers, strictures, and segmental involvement with areas of normal-appearing mucosa adjacent to inflamed mucosa. In 10% of cases, it may be difficult to distinguish ulcerative colitis from Crohn's disease. Granulomas on biopsy are present in less than 25% of patients but are highly suggestive of Crohn's disease. When the diagnosis remains uncertain, two serologic tests may be useful in further distinguishing these two diseases. Antineutrophil cytoplasmic antibodies with perinuclear staining (p-ANCA) are found in 50–70% of patients with ulcerative colitis and 5–10% of patients with Crohn's disease. Antibodies to the yeast *Saccharomyces cerevisiae* (ASCA) are found in 60–70% of patients with Crohn's disease and 10–15% of patients with ulcerative colitis. The accuracy and predictive value of these tests in patients with indeterminate colitis remain uncertain.

Complications

A. Abscess

The presence of a tender abdominal mass with fever and leukocytosis suggests an abscess. Emergent CT of the abdomen is necessary to confirm the diagnosis. Patients should be given broad-spectrum antibiotics and, if malnourished, maintained on TPN. Percutaneous drainage or surgery is usually required.

B. OBSTRUCTION

Small bowel obstruction may develop secondary to active inflammation or chronic fibrotic stricturing and is often acutely precipitated by dietary indiscretion. Patients should be given intravenous fluids with nasogastric suction for several days. Systemic corticosteroids are indicated in patients with symptoms or signs of active inflammation but are unhelpful in patients with inactive, fixed disease. Patients unimproved on medical management require surgical resection of the stenotic area or stricturoplasty.

C. FISTULAS

The majority of enteromesenteric and enteroenteric fistulas are asymptomatic and require no specific therapy. Large abscesses associated with fistulas require percutaneous or surgical drainage. Medical therapy is effective in a subset of patients and is usually tried before surgery. Although fistulas may close temporarily in response to TPN or oral elemental diets, they recur when oral feedings are resumed. Azathioprine or mercaptopurine heals fistulas in 30–40% of patients but requires 3–6 months. Infliximab is the most effective medical therapy for chronic fistulizing Crohn's disease. Infliximab injections (5 mg/kg) given at 0, 2, and 6 weeks result in complete closure of fistulas (both perianal and abdominal) in up to 50% of patients and improvement in up to 75%. Although cyclosporine has demonstrated some value for fistulous disease, high relapse rates and the risk of toxicity have limited its use. Surgical therapy is required for symptomatic fistulas that do not respond to medical therapy. Fistulas that arise above (proximal to) areas of intestinal stricturing commonly require surgical treatment.

D. PERIANAL DISEASE

Patients with fissures, fistulas, and skin tags commonly have perianal discomfort. Severe pain should suggest a perianal abscess, which usually requires simple incision and drainage. Pelvic MRI and endoscopic ultrasonography are the best studies for evaluating perianal fistulas and abscesses. Deep abscesses require drainage with noncutting drains, which allow drainage and improve comfort while medical treatment is initiated. In small series, closure of the internal opening with a suture followed by instillation of fibrin glue into the external fistula opening achieves successful closure in two-thirds of patients. Where possible, surgical fistulotomy should be avoided in the presence of active Crohn's disease because of the risk of poor wound healing. The medical treatment of perianal fistulas can be difficult. Metronidazole, 250 mg three times daily, and ciprofloxacin, 500 mg twice daily, are commonly prescribed based on efficacy in uncontrolled studies. Aminosalicylates and corticosteroids are of no benefit. Patients unresponsive to antibiotics may be treated with mercaptopurine or azathioprine, which results in symptomatic improvement in up to two-thirds of patients but fistula closure in less than one-third. Persistent perianal fistulas are treated with intravenous infliximab, 5 mg/kg, given at 0, 2, and 6 weeks followed by either maintenance therapy with infliximab every 8 weeks or mercaptopurine or azathioprine.

E. CARCINOMA

Patients with extensive colonic Crohn's disease are at increased risk of developing colon carcinoma. Screening colonoscopy to detect dysplasia or cancer is recommended by most authorities for patients with a history of 8 or more years of Crohn's colitis. Patients with Crohn's disease have an increased risk of lymphoma and of small bowel adenocarcinoma; however, both are rare.

F. HEMORRHAGE

Unlike ulcerative colitis, severe hemorrhage is unusual in Crohn's disease.

G. MALABSORPTION

Malabsorption may arise from bacterial overgrowth in patients with enterocolonic fistulas, strictures, and stasis resulting in bacterial overgrowth, extensive jejunal inflammation, and prior surgical resections.

Differential Diagnosis

Chronic cramping abdominal pain and diarrhea are typical of both irritable bowel syndrome and Crohn's disease, but x-ray examinations are normal in the former. Acute fever and right lower quadrant pain may resemble appendicitis or *Yersinia enterocolitica* enteritis. Intestinal lymphoma causes fever, pain, weight loss, and abnormal small bowel radiographs that may mimic Crohn's disease. Patients with undiagnosed AIDS may present with fever and diarrhea. Segmental colitis may be caused by tuberculosis, *E histolytica*, *Chlamydia*, or ischemic colitis. *C difficile* or CMV infection may develop in patients with inflammatory bowel disease, mimicking disease recurrence. Diverticulitis with abscess formation may be difficult to distinguish acutely from Crohn's disease. NSAIDs may exacerbate inflammatory bowel disease and may also cause NSAID-induced colitis characterized by small bowel or colonic ulcers, erosion, or strictures that tend to be most severe in the terminal ileum and right colon.

Treatment of Active Disease

Crohn's disease is a chronic lifelong illness characterized by exacerbations and periods of remission. As no specific therapy exists, current treatment is directed toward symptomatic improvement and controlling the disease process. The treatment must address the specific problems of the individual patient. All patients with Crohn's disease should be counseled to discontinue cigarettes.

A. NUTRITION

1. Diet—Patients should eat a well-balanced diet with as few restrictions as possible. Because lactose intolerance is common, a trial off dairy products is warranted if flatulence or diarrhea is a prominent complaint. Patients with mainly colonic involvement benefit from fiber supplementation. Conversely, patients with obstructive symptoms should be placed on a low-roughage diet, ie, no raw fruits or vegetables, popcorn, nuts, etc. Resection of more than 100 cm of terminal ileum results in fat malabsorption for which a low-fat diet is recommended. Parenteral vitamin B_{12} (100 mcg intramuscularly per month) commonly is needed for patients with previous ileal resection or extensive terminal ileal disease.

2. Enteral therapy—Supplemental enteral therapy via nasogastric tube may be required for children and adolescents with poor intake and growth retardation.

3. Total parenteral nutrition—TPN is used short term in patients with active disease and progressive weight loss or those awaiting surgery who have malnutrition but cannot tolerate enteral feedings because of high-grade obstruction, high-output fistulas, severe diarrhea, or abdominal pain. It is required long term in a small subset of patients with extensive intestinal resections resulting in short bowel syndrome with malnutrition.

B. SYMPTOMATIC MEDICATIONS

There are several potential mechanisms by which diarrhea may occur in Crohn's disease in addition to active Crohn's disease. A rational empiric treatment approach often yields therapeutic improvement that may obviate the need for corticosteroids or immunosuppressive agents. Involvement of the terminal ileum with Crohn's disease or prior ileal resection may lead to reduced absorption of bile acids that may induce secretory diarrhea from the colon. This diarrhea commonly responds to cholestyramine 2–4 g or colestipol 5 g two or three times daily before meals to bind the malabsorbed bile salts. Patients with extensive ileal disease or more than 100 cm of ileal resection have such severe bile salt malabsorption that steatorrhea may arise. Such patients may benefit from a low-fat diet; bile salt-binding agents will exacerbate the diarrhea and should not be given. Patients with Crohn's disease are at risk for the development of small intestinal bacterial overgrowth due to enteral fistulas, ileal resection, and impaired motility and may benefit from a course of broad-spectrum antibiotics (see Bacterial Overgrowth, above). Other causes of diarrhea include lactase deficiency and short bowel syndrome (described in other sections). Use of antidiarrheals may provide benefit in some patients. Loperamide (2–4 mg), diphenoxylate with atropine (one tablet), or tincture of opium (5–15 drops) may be given as needed up to four times daily. Because of the risk of toxic megaco-

lon, these drugs should not be used in patients with active severe colitis.

C. SPECIFIC DRUG THERAPY

1. 5-Aminosalicylic acid agents—Mesalamine (Asacol 2.4–4.8 g/d; Pentasa 4 g/d) traditionally has been used as initial therapy for the treatment of mild to moderately active colonic and ileocolonic Crohn's disease. However, the efficacy of 5-ASA agents recently has been called into question. In early studies, remission rates of over 40% were reported in patients with mild to moderate disease compared with 20–30% in patients treated with placebo. However, recent meta-analyses of published and unpublished trial data suggest that mesalamine is of little or no value in the treatment of Crohn's disease, especially for disease involving the small intestine. Mesalamine or sulfasalazine (3–4 g/d) may be of benefit for disease confined to the colon. 5-ASA agents also appear to have little or no efficacy for maintenance of remission or for prevention of postoperative recurrences.

2. Antibiotics—Antibiotics also are widely used by clinicians for the treatment of active Crohn's disease, although meta-analyses of controlled trials suggest that they have little or no efficacy. It is hypothesized that antibiotics may reduce inflammation through alteration of gut flora, reduction of bacterial overgrowth, or treatment of microperforations. Metronidazole (10 mg/kg/d) or ciprofloxacin (500 mg twice daily) commonly are administered for 6–12 weeks.

3. Corticosteroids—Corticosteroids dramatically suppress the acute clinical symptoms or signs in most patients with both small and large bowel disease; however, they do not alter the underlying disease. An ileal-release budesonide preparation (Entocort), 9 mg once daily for 8–16 weeks, induces remission in 50–70% of patients with mild to moderate Crohn's disease involving the terminal ileum or ascending colon. After initial treatment, budesonide is tapered over 2–4 weeks in 3 mg increments. In some patients, low-dose budesonide (6 mg/d) may be used for up to 1 year to maintain remission. Budesonide is superior to mesalamine but somewhat less effective than prednisone. However, because budesonide has markedly reduced acute and chronic steroid-related adverse effects, including smaller reductions of bone mineral density, it is preferred to other systemic corticosteroids for the treatment of mild to moderate Crohn's disease involving the terminal ileum or ascending colon.

Prednisone or methylprednisolone, 40–60 mg/d, is generally administered to patients with Crohn's disease that is severe, that involves the distal colon or proximal small intestine, or that has failed treatment with budesonide. Remission or significant improvement occurs in 60–90% of patients after 8–16 weeks of therapy. After improvement at 2 weeks, tapering proceeds at 5 mg/wk until a dosage of 20 mg/d is being given. Thereafter, slow tapering by 2.5 mg/wk is recommended. Approximately 20% of patients cannot be completely withdrawn from corticosteroids without experiencing a symptomatic flare-up. Furthermore, 75% of patients who achieve initial remission on corticosteroids will experience a relapse within 1 year. Use of long-term low corticosteroid doses (2.5–10 mg/d) should be avoided, because of associated complications including aseptic necrosis of the hips, osteoporosis, cataracts, diabetes, and hypertension. Calcium and vitamin D supplementation should be administered to all patients receiving chronic corticosteroid therapy. Bone densitometry should be considered in patients with inflammatory bowel disease with other risk factors for osteoporosis and in all patients requiring long-term corticosteroids. Bisphosphonate therapy is recommended for patients with proven osteoporosis and those requiring > 3 months of corticosteroid therapy to reduce bone loss. Patients requiring long-term corticosteroid treatment should be given immunomodulatory drugs (as described below) in an effort to wean them from corticosteroids.

Patients with persisting symptoms despite oral corticosteroids or those with high fever, persistent vomiting, evidence of intestinal obstruction, severe weight loss, severe abdominal tenderness, or suspicion of an abscess should be hospitalized. In patients with a tender, palpable inflammatory abdominal mass, CT scan of the abdomen should be obtained prior to administering corticosteroids to rule out an abscess. If no abscess is identified, parenteral corticosteroids should be administered (as described for ulcerative colitis).

4. Immunomodulating drugs: Azathioprine, mercaptopurine, or methotrexate—Immunomodulating agents are used in approximately one-third of patients with Crohn's disease who have not responded to corticosteroids or who require repeated courses of long-term corticosteroids to control symptoms. These agents permit elimination or reduction of corticosteroids in over 75% and fistula closure in 30% of patients. In the United States, mercaptopurine or azathioprine are more commonly used than methotrexate. The mean time to symptomatic response is 2–4 months, so these agents are not useful for acute exacerbations. Meta-analyses of controlled trials suggest that patients with Crohn's disease treated with immunomodulating agents are three times as likely to achieve remission and 2.25 times as likely to maintain remission than those treated with corticosteroids. Once patients achieve remission, immunomodulating drugs reduce the 3-year relapse rate from over 60% to less than 25%. Methotrexate (25 mg intramuscularly or subcutaneously weekly for 12 weeks, followed by 12.5–15 mg once weekly, orally or subcutaneously) is increasingly used in patients who are unresponsive to or intolerant of mercaptopurine or azathioprine. Because oral absorption may be erratic, parenteral administration is more commonly recommended. Other immunosuppressive agents have been investigated in the treatment of Crohn's disease, including cyclosporine and thalidomide; however, efficacy has been modest and toxicity greater than with the thiopurines.

5. Immunomodulating drugs: Anti-TNF therapies—Infliximab is used for the treatment of patients with active moderate to severe Crohn's disease with an inadequate response to corticosteroids or other immunomodulators (azathioprine or mercaptopurine), symptomatic flares when corticosteroids are tapered, severe illness requiring hospitalization, or fistulizing disease. It is also used instead of corticosteroids to promote rapid initial improvement while other immunosuppressives (azathioprine, mercaptopurine) that take weeks to months to achieve therapeutic effect are being initiated. A three-dose regimen of 5 mg/kg administered at 0, 2, and 6 weeks is recommended for acute induction. Improvement occurs in two-thirds of patients and remission in one-third. After initial clinical response, symptom relapse occurs in > 80% of patients within 1 year in the absence of further maintenance therapy. Options for maintenance therapy include long-term continuation of other immunosuppressive agents (mercaptopurine, azathioprine, or methotrexate) with need for subsequent infliximab determined by the clinical course or systematic maintenance therapy with infliximab 5 mg/kg every 8 weeks (with or without concomitant immunomodulating agents). A gradual or complete loss of efficacy occurs over time in some patients, necessitating increased dosing (10 mg/kg) or decreased dosing intervals (every 6 weeks), or both, which may be partly attributable to development of ATI. Systematic maintenance therapy is associated with an increased likelihood of sustained response and a lower likelihood of developing ATI. For these reasons, maintenance therapy with infliximab is increasingly used. Concomitant therapy with low doses of other immunomodulating agents (mercaptopurine 50 mg/d, azathioprine 100 mg/d, or methotrexate 7.5 mg/wk) may also reduce development of ATI.

Adalimumab is a fully human anti-TNF monoclonal antibody that is as efficacious as infliximab for the treatment of rheumatoid arthritis. Although controlled studies of adalimumab in Crohn's disease are currently ongoing, open-label studies have demonstrated efficacy in patients who have intolerance or loss of responsiveness to infliximab.

Granulocyte-macrophage colony-stimulating factor (GM-CSF) (sargramostim) is a myeloid growth factor that may augment the innate intestinal immune system. Recent controlled studies suggest that sargramostim may have significant benefit in a subset of patients. The role of this agent, which is safer than anti-TNF therapy, in Crohn's disease is undergoing further testing.

Indications for Surgery

Over 50% of patients will require at least one surgical procedure. The main indications for surgery are intractability to medical therapy, intra-abdominal abscess, massive bleeding, symptomatic refractory internal or perianal fistulas, and intestinal obstruction. Patients with chronic obstructive symptoms due to a short segment of ileal stenosis are best treated with resection or strictureplasty (rather than chronic medical therapy), which promotes rapid return of well-being and elimination of corticosteroids. After surgery, clinical recurrence occurs in 20% of patients within 1 year and 80% within 10–15 years. Postsurgical prophylaxis with mesalamine commonly does not appear to reduce the risk of clinical recurrence. A recent randomized controlled trial reported that ornidazole (a nitroimidazole antibiotic with a superior safety profile) reduced the postoperative clinical recurrence rate at 1 year from 38% in the placebo group to 8% in the ornidazole group. Long-term immunosuppressive therapy with mercaptopurine (50 mg daily) may be effective than placebo in preventing clinical and endoscopic recurrence after ileocolic resection and is recommended for high-risk patients.

Prognosis

With proper medical and surgical treatment, the majority of patients are able to cope with this chronic disease and its complications and lead productive lives. Few patients die as a direct consequence of the disease.

Colombel JF et al: The safety profile of infliximab in patients with Crohn's disease: the Mayo Clinic experience of 500 patients. Gastroenterology 2004;126:19. [PMID: 14699483]

Hanauer S et al: Oral pentasa in the treatment of active Crohn's disease: a meta-analysis of double-blind, placebo-controlled trials. Clin Gastroenterol Hepatol 2004;2:379. [PMID: 15118975]

Hanauer S et al: Postoperative maintenance of Crohn's disease remission with 6-mercaptopurine, mesalamine, or placebo: a 2-year trial. Gastroenterology 2004;127:723. [PMID: 15362027]

Korzenik JR et al: Sargramostim for active Crohn's disease. N Engl J Med 2005;352:2193. [PMID: 15917384]

Lichtenstein GR: Infliximab: lifetime use for maintenance is appropriate in Crohn's Disease. PRO: maintenance therapy is superior to episodic therapy. Am J Gastroenterol 2005; 100:1433. [PMID: 15984959]

Loftus EV: Infliximab: lifetime use for maintenance is appropriate in Crohn's Disease. CON: "lifetime use" is an awfully long time. Am J Gastroenterol 2005;100:1435. [PMID: 15984960]

Papadakis KA et al: Safety and efficacy of adalimumab (D2E7) in Crohn's disease patients with an attenuated response to infliximab. Am J Gastroenterol 2005;100:75. [PMID: 15654784]

Rutgeerts P et al: Comparison of scheduled and episodic treatment strategies of infliximab for Crohn's disease. Gastroenterology 2004;126:402. [PMID: 14262776]

Rutgeerts P et al: Ornidazole for prophylaxis of postoperative Crohn's disease recurrence: a randomized, double-blind, placebo-controlled trial. Gastroenterology 2005;128:856. [PMID: 15825069]

Sandborn WJ et al: Budesonide for maintenance of remission in patients with Crohn's disease in medically induced remission: a predetermined pooled analysis of four randomized, double-blind, placebo-controlled trials. Am J Gastroenterol 2005;100:1780. [PMID: 16086715]

Sands B et al: Infliximab maintenance therapy for fistulizing Crohn's disease. N Engl J Med 2004;350:876. [PMID: 14985485]

Siegel CA et al: Review article: practical management of inflammatory bowel disease patients taking immunomodulators. Aliment Pharmacol Ther 2005;22:1. [PMID: 15963074]

2. Ulcerative Colitis

 ESSENTIALS OF DIAGNOSIS

- Bloody diarrhea.
- Lower abdominal cramps and fecal urgency.
- Anemia, low serum albumin.
- Negative stool cultures.
- Sigmoidoscopy is the key to diagnosis.

General Considerations

Ulcerative colitis is an idiopathic inflammatory condition that involves the mucosal surface of the colon, resulting in diffuse friability and erosions with bleeding. Approximately one-third of patients have disease confined to the rectosigmoid region (proctosigmoiditis); one-third have disease that extends to the splenic flexure (left-sided colitis); and one-third have disease that extends more proximally (extensive colitis). There is some correlation between disease extent and symptom severity. In the majority of patients, the extent of colonic involvement does not progress over time. In most patients, the disease is characterized by periods of symptomatic flare-ups and remissions. Ulcerative colitis is more common in nonsmokers and former smokers. Disease severity may be lower in active smokers and may worsen in patients who stop smoking. Appendectomy before the age of 20 years for acute appendicitis is associated with a reduced risk of developing ulcerative colitis.

Clinical Findings

A. SYMPTOMS AND SIGNS

The clinical profile in ulcerative colitis is highly variable. Bloody diarrhea is the hallmark. On the basis of several clinical and laboratory parameters, it is clinically useful to classify patients as having mild, moderate, or severe disease (Table 14–14). Patients should be asked about stool frequency, the presence and amount of rectal bleeding, cramps, abdominal pain, fecal urgency, and tenesmus. Physical examination should focus on the patient's volume status as determined by orthostatic blood pressure and pulse measurements and by nutritional status. On abdominal examination, the clinician should look for tenderness and evidence of peritoneal inflammation. Red blood may be present on digital rectal examination.

1. **Mild to moderate disease**—Patients with mild disease have a gradual onset of infrequent diarrhea (less than five movements per day) with intermittent rectal bleeding and mucus. Stools may be formed too loose in consistency. Because of rectal inflammation, there is fecal urgency and tenesmus. Left lower quad-

Table 14–14. Ulcerative colitis: Assessment of disease activity.

	Mild	Moderate	Severe
Stool frequency (per day)	< 4	4–6	> 6 (mostly bloody)
Pulse (beats/min)	< 90	90–100	> 100
Hematocrit (%)	Normal	30–40	< 30
Weight loss (%)	None	1–10	> 10
Temperature (°F)	Normal	99–100	> 100
ESR (mm/h)	< 20	20–30	> 30
Albumin (g/dL)	Normal	3–3.5	< 3

ESR = erythrocyte sedimentation rate.

rant cramps relieved by defecation are common, but there is no significant abdominal tenderness. Patients with moderate disease have more severe diarrhea with frequent bleeding. Abdominal pain and tenderness may be present but are not severe. There may be mild fever, anemia, and hypoalbuminemia.

2. Severe disease—Patients with severe disease have more than six to ten bloody bowel movements per day, resulting in severe anemia, hypovolemia, and impaired nutrition with hypoalbuminemia. Abdominal pain and tenderness are present. "Fulminant colitis" is a subset of severe disease characterized by rapidly worsening symptoms with signs of toxicity.

B. LABORATORY FINDINGS

The degree of abnormality of the hematocrit, sedimentation rate, and serum albumin reflects disease severity.

C. ENDOSCOPY

In acute colitis, the diagnosis is readily established by sigmoidoscopy. The mucosal appearance is characterized by edema, friability, mucopus, and erosions. Colonoscopy should not be performed in patients with severe disease because of the risk of perforation. After patients have demonstrated improvement on therapy, colonoscopy is sometimes performed to determine the extent of disease, which will dictate the need for subsequent cancer surveillance.

D. IMAGING

Plain abdominal radiographs are obtained in patients with severe colitis to look for significant colonic dilation. Barium enemas are of little utility in the evaluation of acute ulcerative colitis and may precipitate toxic megacolon in patients with severe disease.

Differential Diagnosis

The initial presentation of ulcerative colitis is indistinguishable from other causes of colitis, clinically as well as endoscopically. Thus, the diagnosis of idiopathic ulcerative colitis is reached after excluding other known causes of colitis. Infectious colitis should be excluded by sending stool specimens for routine bacterial cultures (to exclude *Salmonella, Shigella,* and *Campylobacter*), ova and parasites (to exclude amebiasis), and stool toxin assay for *C difficile.* Mucosal biopsy can distinguish amebic colitis from ulcerative colitis. Enteroinvasive *E coli* and *E coli* O157:H7 will not be detected on routine bacterial cultures. CMV colitis occurs in immunocompromised patients (especially those with AIDS) and is diagnosed on mucosal biopsy. Gonorrhea, chlamydial infection, herpes, and syphilis are considerations in sexually active patients with proctitis. In elderly patients with cardiovascular disease, ischemic colitis may involve the rectosigmoid. A history of radiation to the pelvic region can result in proctitis months to years later. Crohn's disease involving the colon but not the small intestine may be confused with ulcerative colitis. In 10% of patients, a distinction between Crohn's disease and ulcerative colitis may not be possible. The utility of ANCA and ASCA antibodies in these difficult patients is discussed in the section on Crohn's disease.

Treatment

There are two main treatment objectives: (1) to terminate the acute, symptomatic attack and (2) to prevent recurrence of attacks. The treatment of acute ulcerative colitis depends on the extent of colonic involvement and the severity of illness.

Patients with mild to moderate disease should eat a regular diet but limit their intake of caffeine and gas-producing vegetables. Fiber supplements decrease diarrhea and rectal symptoms (psyllium, 3.4 g twice daily; methylcellulose, 2 g twice daily; bran powder, 1 tbsp twice daily). Antidiarrheal agents should not be given in the acute phase of illness but are safe and helpful in patients with mild chronic symptoms. Loperamide (2 mg), diphenoxylate with atropine (one tablet), or tincture of opium (8–15 drops) may be given up to four times daily. Such remedies are particularly useful at nighttime and when taken prophylactically for occasions when patients may not have reliable access to toilet facilities.

A. DISTAL COLITIS

Patients with disease confined to the rectum or rectosigmoid region generally have mild but distressing symptoms. Treatment of acute disease is best approached with topical agents. Topical mesalamine is the drug of choice and is superior to topical corticosteroids. Mesalamine is administered as a suppository, 500 mg twice daily for proctitis, and as an enema, 4 g at bedtime for proctosigmoiditis, for 3–12 weeks, with 75% of patients improving (Table 14–15). Topical corticosteroids are a less expensive alternative to mesalamine but are also less effective. Hydrocortisone suppository or foam is prescribed for proctitis and hy-

Table 14–15. Treatment of ulcerative colitis.

Distal colitis
  Proctitis
    Mesalamine suppositories, 500 mg per rectum twice
      daily, or—
    Hydrocortisone foam, 90 mg per rectum daily, or—
    Hydrocortisone suppositories, 100 mg per rectum daily
  Proctosigmoiditis
    Mesalamine enema, 4 g per rectum daily, or—
    Hydrocortisone enema, 100 mg per rectum daily
Extensive colitis
  Mild to moderate
    Sulfasalazine, 1.5–3 g orally twice daily, or—
    Mesalamine tablets (delayed-release), 4.0–4.8 g/d, or—
    Balsalazide, 2.25 g three times a day
    If no response after 2–4 weeks, add prednisone, 40–60
      mg/d (taper by 5 mg/wk)
  Severe
    Methylprednisolone, 48–60 mg IV daily

---

drocortisone enema (80–100 mg) for proctosigmoiditis. Systemic effects from short-term use are very slight. For patients with distal disease who fail to improve with once daily topical therapy, the following options may be considered: (1) increase the same topical agent to twice daily, (2) combination therapy with a 5-ASA enema at bedtime and a corticosteroid enema or foam in the morning, and (3) a combination of a topical agent with an oral 5-ASA agent.

Patients whose acute symptoms resolve rapidly with acute therapy may have prolonged periods of remission that are treated successfully with intermittent courses of therapy. Patients with early or frequent relapse should be treated with maintenance therapy with mesalamine suppositories (500 mg daily) or with oral 5-ASA agents (see below).

B. MILD TO MODERATE COLITIS

1. 5-ASA Agents—Disease extending above the sigmoid colon is best treated with mesalamine or balsalazide, which result in symptomatic improvement in 50–75% of patients. Most patients improve within 3–6 weeks, though some require 2–3 months. Mesalamine, 0.8–1.6 g (Asacol) three times daily, or 1 g four times daily (Pentasa), and balsalazide, 2.25 g three times daily, are approved for active disease (Table 14–15). In a recent large multicenter study, 72% of patients treated with mesalamine 4.8 g/d achieved clinical response or remission compared with 59% treated with 2.4 g/d. Sulfasalazine is comparable in efficacy to mesalamine and because of its low cost is still commonly used as a first-line agent by many providers, though it is associated with greater side effects. To minimize side effects, sulfasalazine is begun at a dosage of 500 mg twice daily and increased gradually over 1–2 weeks to 2 g twice daily (Table 14–15). Total doses of 5–6 g/d may have greater efficacy but

are poorly tolerated. Folic acid, 1 mg/d, should be administered to all patients taking sulfasalazine.

2. Corticosteroids—Patients with mild to moderate disease who fail to improve after 2–3 weeks of 5-ASA therapy should have the addition of corticosteroid therapy. Topical therapy with hydrocortisone foam or enemas (80–100 mg once or twice daily) or 5-ASA enemas (4 g once daily) may be tried first. Patients who do not improve after 2 more weeks require systemic corticosteroid therapy. Prednisone and methylprednisolone are most commonly used. Depending on the severity of illness, the initial oral dose of prednisone is 40–60 mg daily. Rapid improvement is observed in most cases. It is usually possible to begin to taper prednisone after 2 weeks. Tapering of prednisone should proceed by no more than 5 mg/wk. After tapering to 15 mg/d, slower tapering is sometimes required. Complete tapering without symptomatic flare-ups is possible in the majority of patients.

3. Immunomodulating agents—A subset of patients either does not respond to aminosalicylates or corticosteroids or has symptomatic flares during attempts at corticosteroid tapering. Although surgical resection is traditionally recommended for patients with refractory disease, some patients may wish to avoid surgery and others have moderately severe disease for which surgery might not otherwise be warranted. Immunomodulating agents are increasingly used for the treatment of ulcerative colitis; however, the risks of these drugs from chronic immunosuppression must be weighed against the certainty of cure with surgical resection. Limited trials suggest mercaptopurine or azathioprine is of benefit in 60% of patients, allowing tapering of corticosteroids and maintenance of remission. There is less evidence that methotrexate is effective.

Based on the results of two large multicenter studies (ACT 1 and ACT 2), infliximab was recently approved in the United States for the treatment of patients with moderate to severe ulcerative colitis who have had an inadequate response to conventional therapies (oral corticosteroids, mercaptopurine or azathioprine, and mesalamine). Following a three-dose regimen of 5 mg/kg administered at 0, 2, and 6 weeks, clinical response occurred in 65% and clinical remission in 26–34%.

C. SEVERE COLITIS

About 10–15% of patients with ulcerative colitis have a more severe course. Because they may progress to fulminant colitis or toxic megacolon, hospitalization is generally required.

1. General measures—Discontinue all oral intake for 24–48 hours or until the patient demonstrates clinical improvement. TPN is indicated only in patients with poor nutritional status or if feedings cannot be reinstituted within 7–10 days. All opioid or anticholinergic agents should be discontinued. Restore circulating volume with fluids, correct electrolyte abnormalities, and consider transfusion for significant anemia (hematocrit < 25–28%). Abdominal examinations should be repeated to look for evidence of worsening distention or pain. A plain abdominal radiograph should be ordered on admission to look for evidence of colonic dilation. Send stools for bacterial (including *C difficile*) culture and examination for ova and parasites. Surgical consultation should be sought for all patients with severe disease.

2. Corticosteroid therapy—Methylprednisolone, 48–64 mg, or hydrocortisone, 300 mg, is administered in four divided doses or by continuous infusion over 24 hours. Higher or "pulse" doses are of no benefit. Hydrocortisone enemas (100 mg) may also be administered twice daily for treatment of urgency or tenesmus. In patients who have not previously received corticosteroids, administration of ACTH, 120 units/24 h, may be superior to corticosteroids. Approximately 50–75% of patients achieve remission with systemic corticosteroids within 7–10 days. Once symptomatic improvement has occurred, oral fluids are reinstituted. If fluids are well tolerated, intravenous corticosteroids are discontinued and the patient is started on oral prednisone (as described for moderate disease).

3. Anti-TNF therapies—A single infusion of infliximab, 5 mg/kg, has been shown in recent controlled and uncontrolled studies to be effective in treating severe to fulminant colitis in patients who did not improve within 4–7 days of intravenous corticosteroid therapy. In a controlled study of patients hospitalized for ulcerative colitis, colectomy was required within 3 months in 69% who received placebo therapy, compared with 47% who received infliximab. Although further studies are needed, infliximab therapy should be considered in patients with severe ulcerative colitis who have not improved with intravenous corticosteroid therapy.

4. Cyclosporine—Intravenous cyclosporine (2–4 mg/kg/d as a continuous infusion) benefits 60–75% of patients with severe colitis who have not improved after 7–10 days of corticosteroids. In patients with severe steroid-resistant colitis who are reluctant to undergo colectomy, intravenous cyclosporine may be considered as a "bridge" therapy while mercaptopurine or azathioprine therapy (which take 2–4 months for full efficacy) is initiated. Up to two-thirds of responders may be maintained in remission with a combination of oral cyclosporine for 3 months and long-term therapy with mercaptopurine or azathioprine. The relative role of infliximab versus cyclosporine in the treatment of severe colitis requires further clinical study.

4. Surgical therapy—Patients with severe disease who fail to improve after 7–10 days of corticosteroid, infliximab or cyclosporine therapy are unlikely to respond to further medical therapy, and surgery is recommended.

D. Fulminant Colitis and Toxic Megacolon

A subset of patients with severe disease has a more fulminant course with rapid progression of symptoms over 1–2 weeks and signs of severe toxicity. These patients appear quite ill, with fever, prominent hypovolemia, hemorrhage requiring transfusion, and abdominal distention with tenderness. They are at a higher risk of perforation or development of toxic megacolon and must be followed closely. Broad-spectrum antibiotics should be administered to cover anaerobes and gram-negative bacteria.

Toxic megacolon develops in less than 2% of cases of ulcerative colitis. It is characterized by colonic dilation of more than 6 cm on plain films with signs of toxicity. In addition to the therapies outlined above, nasogastric suction should be initiated. Patients should be instructed to roll from side to side and onto the abdomen in an effort to decompress the distended colon. Serial abdominal plain films should be obtained to look for worsening dilation or ischemia. Patients with fulminant disease or toxic megacolon who worsen or fail to improve within 48–72 hours should undergo surgery to prevent perforation. If the operation is performed before perforation, the mortality rate should be low.

Maintenance of Remission

Without long-term therapy, 75% of patients who initially go into remission on medical therapy will experience a symptomatic relapse within 1 year. Long-term maintenance therapy with sulfasalazine, 1–1.5 g twice daily; olsalazine, 500 mg twice daily; and mesalamine, 800 mg three times daily or 500 mg four times daily, has been shown to reduce relapse rates to less than 33%. Uncontrolled studies suggest that the immunomodulators mercaptopurine or azathioprine may be useful in patients with frequent disease relapses (more than two per year) to maintain remission. The role of long-term infliximab therapy in the maintenance of remission is unclear. In the ACT 1 and 2 studies, initial induction therapy with infliximab 0, 2, and 6 weeks, infliximab maintenance infusions were administered every 8 weeks for 30–54 weeks. At both 8 weeks and the end of the study (30 or 54 weeks), 40% of patients had a sustained clinical response and 20% were in clinical remission, a modest but impressive response in patients with more refractory disease. In considering long-term infliximab therapy, patients and providers need to weigh the long-term risks of immunosuppression against colectomy.

Risk of Colon Cancer

In patients with ulcerative colitis with disease proximal to the sigmoid colon, there is a markedly increased risk of developing colon carcinoma. In patients who have had colitis for more than 10 years, the risk of developing colon cancer increases approximately 0.5–1% per year.

Meta-analysis of observational studies suggests that the risk of colon cancer is reduced by 50% in patients treated with long-term 5-ASA therapy. Ingestion of folic acid, 1 mg/d, also is associated with a decreased risk of cancer development. Colonoscopies are recommended every 1–2 years in patients with extensive colitis, beginning 8–10 years after diagnosis. At colonoscopy, multiple (at least 32) random mucosal biopsies are taken throughout the colon at 10-cm intervals as well as biopsies of mass lesions to look for dysplasia or carcinoma. Because of the relatively high incidence of concomitant carcinoma in patients with dysplasia (either low or high grade) in flat mucosa or mass lesions, colectomy is recommended. When low-grade dysplasia is detected only in flat mucosa, some authorities recommend a repeat colonoscopy in 3–6 months to confirm the presence of dysplasia before proceeding with colectomy.

Surgery in Ulcerative Colitis

Surgery is required in 25% of patients. Severe hemorrhage, perforation, and documented carcinoma are absolute indications for surgery. Surgery is indicated also in patients with fulminant colitis or toxic megacolon that does not improve within 48–72 hours, in patients with dysplasia on surveillance colonoscopy, and in patients with refractory disease requiring long-term corticosteroids to control symptoms.

Although total proctocolectomy (with placement of an ileostomy) provides complete cure of the disease, most patients seek to avoid it out of concern for the impact it may have on their bowel function, their self-image, and their social interactions. After complete colectomy, patients may have a standard ileostomy with an external appliance, a continent ileostomy, or an internal ileal pouch that is anastomosed to the anal canal (ileal pouch-anal anastomosis). The latter maintains intestinal continuity, thereby obviating an ostomy. Under optimal circumstances, patients have five to seven loose bowel movements per day without incontinence. Endoscopic or histologic inflammation in the ileal pouch ("pouchitis") develops in over 25% of patients, resulting in increased stool frequency, fecal urgency, cramping, and bleeding, but usually resolves with a 2-week course of metronidazole (10 mg/kg/d) or ciprofloxacin (500 mg twice daily). Probiotics containing nonpathogenic strains of lactobacilli, bifidobacteria, and streptococci (VSL#3) are effective in the maintenance of remission in patients with recurrent pouchitis. Bismuth subsalicylate (Pepto Bismol, 262 mg, two tablets four times daily) has demonstrated benefit in some series. Some clinicians report that topical corticosteroids or oral budesonide 9 mg/d are of benefit. Refractory cases of proctitis can be disabling and may require conversion to a standard ileostomy.

Prognosis

Ulcerative colitis is a lifelong disease characterized by exacerbations and remissions. For most patients, the disease is readily controlled by medical therapy without need for surgery. The majority never require hospitalization. A subset of patients with more severe disease will require surgery, which results in complete cure of the disease. Properly managed, most patients with ulcerative colitis lead close to normal productive lives.

Aberra FN et al: Review article: monitoring of immunomodulators in inflammatory bowel disease. Aliment Pharmacol Ther 2005;21:307. [PMID: 15709982]

Bebb JR et al: Systematic review: how effective are the usual treatments for ulcerative colitis? Aliment Pharmacol Ther 2004; 20:143. [PMID: 15233693]

Bernstein CN: Ulcerative colitis with low-grade dysplasia. Gastroenterology 2004;127:950. [PMID: 15362049]

Gan SI et al: A new look at toxic megacolon: an update and review of incidence, etiology, pathogenesis, and management. Am J Gastroenterol 2003;98:2363. [PMID: 14638335]

Hanauer S: Medical therapy for ulcerative colitis 2004. Gastroenterology 2004;126:1582. [PMID: 15168369]

Hanauer SB et al: Delayed-release oral mesalamine at 4.8 g/day (800 mg tablet) for the treatment of moderately active ulcerative colitis: the ASCEND II Trial. Am J Gastroenterol 2005;100:2478. [PMID: 16279903]

Itzkowitz SH et al; Crohn's and Colitis Foundation of America Colon Cancer in IBD Study Group: Consensus Conference: Colorectal cancer screening and surveillance in inflammatory bowel disease. Inflam Bowel Dis 2005;11:314. [PMID: 15735438]

Jarnerot G et al: Infliximab as rescue therapy in severe to moderately severe ulcerative colitis: a randomized, placebo-controlled study. Gastroenterology 2005;128:1805. [PMID: 15940615]

Kornbluth A et al: Ulcerative colitis practice guidelines in adults (update): American College of Gastroenterology, Practice Parameters Committee. Am J Gastroenterol 2004;99:1371. [PMID: 15233681]

Probert CS et al: Infliximab in moderately severe glucocorticoid resistant ulcerative colitis: a randomized controlled trial. Gut 2003;52:998. [PMID: 12801957]

Rutgeerts P et al: Infliximab for induction and maintenance therapy for ulcerative colitis. N Engl J Med 2005;353:2462. [PMID: 16339095]

Sandborn WJ et al: Clinical management of pouchitis. Gastroenterology 2005;127:1809. [PMID: 15578518]

Sartor RB: Therapeutic manipulation of the enteric microflora in inflammatory bowel diseases: antibiotics, probiotics, and prebiotics. Gastroenterology 2004;126:1620. [PMID: 15168372]

Velayos FS et al: Effect of 5-aminosalicylate use on colorectal cancer and dysplasia risk: a systematic review and meta-analysis of observational studies. Am J Gastroenterol 2005;100: 1345. [PMID: 15929768]

3. Microscopic Colitis

Microscopic colitis is an idiopathic condition that is increasing in incidence in which patients have chronic or intermittent watery diarrhea with normal-appearing mucosa at endoscopy. A more severe illness characterized by abdominal pain, fatigue, dehydration, and weight loss may develop in a subset of patients. There appear to be two subtypes—lymphocytic colitis and collagenous colitis. In both, histologic evaluation of mucosal biopsies reveals chronic inflammation (lymphocytes, plasma cells) in the lamina propria and increased intraepithelial lymphocytes. Collagenous colitis is further characterized by the presence of a thickened band (> 10 mcm) of subepithelial collagen. Both forms occur more commonly in women, especially in the fifth to sixth decades. Symptoms tend to be chronic or recurrent but may remit in most patients after several years. Long-term NSAID therapy has been implicated as a causative factor in up to 50% of cases. Microscopic colitis occurs in up to one-third of patients with celiac sprue and should be considered in patients with continued diarrhea after institution of a gluten-free diet. Mild disease may be treated with antidiarrheal agents (loperamide, cholestyramine). NSAIDs should be discontinued. Treatment with 5-ASAs (sulfasalazine, mesalamine) is reported to be effective in uncontrolled studies. Although a controlled trial demonstrated efficacy for bismuth subsalicylate (two tablets four times daily) for 2 months, reported clinical experience has reported only modest benefit. Delayed release budesonide (Entocort) 9 mg/d for 6–8 weeks has been shown in several prospective controlled studies to induce clinical remission in more than 60–80% of patients and is well tolerated; however, clinical relapse is common after cessation of therapy. Patients who do not respond to bismuth or budesonide may be treated with systemic corticosteroids or, rarely, azathioprine. After entering remission, clinical relapse occurs in 20–30% of patients within 3 years.

Chande N et al: Interventions for treating collagenous colitis. Cochrane Database Syst Rev 2005;(4):CD003575. [PMID: 16235328]

Fernandez-Banares F et al: Collagenous and lymphocytic colitis: evaluation of clinical and histological features, response to treatment, and long-term follow up. Am J Gastroenterol 2003;98:340. [PMID: 12591052]

Feyen B et al: Meta-analysis: budesonide treatment for collagenous colitis. Aliment Pharmacol Ther 2004;20:745. [PMID: 15379834]

Miehlke S et al: Long-term follow-up of collagenous colitis after induction of clinical remission with budesonide. Aliment Pharmacol Ther 2005;22:1115. [PMID: 16305725]

DIVERTICULAR DISEASE OF THE COLON

Colonic diverticulosis increases with age, ranging from 5% in those under age 40, to 30% at age 60, to more than 50% over age 80 years in Western societies. In contrast, it is very uncommon in developing countries with much lower life expectancies. Most are asymptomatic, discovered incidentally at endoscopy or on barium enema. Complications in one-third include lower gastrointestinal bleeding and diverticulitis.

Colonic diverticula may vary in size from a few millimeters to several centimeters and in number from one to several dozen. Almost all patients with diverticulosis have involvement in the sigmoid colon; however, only 15% have proximal colonic disease.

In most patients, diverticulosis is believed to arise after many years of a diet deficient in fiber. The undistended, contracted segments of colon have higher intraluminal pressures. Over time, the contracted colonic musculature, working against greater pressures to move small, hard stools, develops hypertrophy, thickening, rigidity, and fibrosis. Diverticula may develop more commonly in the sigmoid because intraluminal pressures are highest in this region. The extent to which abnormal motility and hereditary factors contribute to diverticular disease is unknown. Patients with diffuse diverticulosis may have an inherent weakness in the colonic wall. Patients with abnormal connective tissue are also disposed to development of diverticulosis, including Ehlers-Danlos syndrome, Marfan's syndrome, and scleroderma.

1. Uncomplicated Diverticulosis

More than two-thirds of patients with diverticulosis have uncomplicated disease and no specific symptoms. In some, diverticulosis may be an incidental finding detected during colonoscopic examination or barium enema examination. Some patients have nonspecific complaints of chronic constipation, abdominal pain, or fluctuating bowel habits. It is unclear whether these symptoms are due to alterations in the colonic musculature or underlying irritable bowel syndrome. Physical examination is usually normal but may reveal mild left lower quadrant tenderness with a thickened, palpable sigmoid and descending colon. Screening laboratory studies should be normal in uncomplicated diverticulosis.

There is no reason to perform imaging studies for the purpose of diagnosing uncomplicated disease. Diverticula are best seen on barium enema. Involved segments of colon may also be narrowed and deformed. Colonoscopy is a less sensitive means of detecting diverticula.

Asymptomatic patients in whom diverticulosis is discovered and patients with a history of complicated disease (see below) should be treated with a high-fiber diet or fiber supplements (bran powder, 1–2 tbsp twice daily; psyllium or methylcellulose) (see section on constipation). Retrospective studies suggest that such treatment may decrease the likelihood of subsequent complications.

2. Diverticulitis

 ESSENTIALS OF DIAGNOSIS

- Acute abdominal pain and fever.
- Left lower abdominal tenderness and mass.
- Leukocytosis.

Clinical Findings

A. SYMPTOMS AND SIGNS

Perforation of a colonic diverticulum results in an intra-abdominal infection that may vary from microperforation (most common) with localized paracolic inflammation to macroperforation with either abscess or generalized peritonitis. Thus, there is a range from mild to severe disease. Most patients with localized inflammation or infection report mild to moderate aching abdominal pain, usually in the left lower quadrant. Constipation or loose stools may be present. Nausea and vomiting are frequent. In many cases, symptoms are so mild that the patient may not seek medical attention until several days after onset. Physical findings include a low-grade fever, left lower quadrant tenderness, and a palpable mass. Stool occult blood is common, but hematochezia is rare. Leukocytosis is mild to moderate. Patients with free perforation present with a more dramatic picture of generalized abdominal pain and peritoneal signs.

B. IMAGING

Plain abdominal films are obtained in all patients to look for evidence of free abdominal air (signifying free perforation), ileus, and small or large bowel obstruction. In patients with mild symptoms and a presumptive diagnosis of diverticulitis, empiric medical therapy is started without further imaging in the acute phase. Patients who respond to acute medical management should undergo complete colonic evaluation with colonoscopy or barium enema after resolution of clinical symptoms to corroborate the diagnosis or exclude other disorders such as colonic neoplasms. In patients who do not improve rapidly after 2–4 days of empiric therapy and in those with severe disease, CT scan of the abdomen is obtained to look for evidence of diverticulitis, including colonic diverticula and wall thickening, pericolic fat infiltration, abscess formation, or extraluminal air or contrast. Endoscopy and barium enema are contraindicated during the initial stages of an acute attack because of the risk of free perforation, though sigmoidoscopy with minimal air insufflation is sometimes required to exclude other diagnoses.

Differential Diagnosis

Localized diverticulitis must be distinguished from perforated colonic carcinoma, Crohn's disease, appendicitis, ischemic colitis, *C difficile*–associated colitis, and gynecologic disorders (ectopic pregnancy, ovarian cyst or torsion).

Complications

Fistula formation may involve the bladder, ureter, vagina, uterus, bowel, and abdominal wall. Diverticulitis may result in stricturing of the colon with partial or complete obstruction.

Treatment

A. MEDICAL MANAGEMENT

Most patients can be managed with conservative measures. Patients with mild symptoms and no peritoneal signs may be managed initially as outpatients on a clear liquid diet and broad-spectrum oral antibiotics with anaerobic activity. Reasonable regimens include amoxicillin and clavulanate potassium (875 mg/125 mg) twice daily; or metronidazole, 500 mg three times daily; plus either ciprofloxacin, 500 mg twice daily, or trimethoprim-sulfamethoxazole, 160/800 mg twice daily orally, for 7–10 days or until the patient is afebrile for 3–5 days. Symptomatic improvement usually occurs within 3 days, at which time the diet may be advanced. Patients with increasing pain, fever, or inability to tolerate oral fluids require hospitalization. Patients with severe diverticulitis (high fevers, leukocytosis, or peritoneal signs) and patients who are elderly or immunosuppressed or who have serious comorbid disease require hospitalization acutely. Patients should be given nothing by mouth and should receive intravenous fluids. If ileus is present, a nasogastric tube should be placed. Intravenous antibiotics should be given to cover anaerobic and gram-negative bacteria. Single-agent therapy with either a second-generation cephalosporin (eg, cefoxitin), piperacillin-tazobactam, or ticarcillin clavulanate appears to be as effective as combination therapy (eg, metronidazole or clindamycin plus an aminoglycoside or third-generation cephalosporin [eg, ceftazidime, cefotaxime]). Symptomatic improvement should be evident within 2–3 days. The antibiotics should be continued for 7–10 days, after which time elective evaluation with colonoscopy or barium enema should be performed.

B. SURGICAL MANAGEMENT

Approximately 20–30% of patients with diverticulitis will require surgical management. Surgical consultation should be obtained on all patients with severe disease or those who fail to improve after 72 hours of medical management. Indications for emergent surgical management include free peritonitis and large abscesses. Patients with fistulas or colonic obstruction due to chronic disease will require elective surgery.

Patients with a localized abdominal abscess can be treated acutely with a percutaneous catheter drain placed by an interventional radiologist. This permits control of the infection and resolution of the immediate infectious inflammatory process. In this manner, a subsequent single-stage elective surgical operation can be performed in which the diseased segment of colon is removed and primary colonic anastomosis performed. In patients in whom catheter drainage is not possible or helpful or in cases requiring emergency surgery, it is necessary to perform surgery in two stages. In the first stage, the diseased colon is resected and the proximal colon brought out to form a temporary colostomy. The distal colonic stump is either closed (forming a Hartmann pouch) or exteriorized as a mucous fistula. Weeks later, after inflammation and infection have completely subsided, the colon can be reconnected electively.

Prognosis

Diverticulitis recurs in one-third of patients treated with medical management. Recurrent attacks warrant elective surgical resection, which carries a lower morbidity and mortality risk than emergency surgery.

Biondo S et al: Acute colonic diverticulitis in patients under 50 years of age. Br J Surg 2002;89:1137. [PMID: 12190679]

Kircher MF et al: Frequency, sensitivity, and specificity of individual signs of diverticulitis on thin-section helical CT with colonic contrast material: experience with 312 cases. AJR Am J Roentgenol 2002;178:1313. [PMID: 12034590]

Mizuki A et al: The outpatient management of patients with acute mild-to-moderate colonic diverticulitis. Aliment Pharmacol Ther 2005;21:889. [PMID: 15801924]

Stollman N et al: Diverticular disease of the colon. Lancet 2004; 363:631. [PMID: 14987890]

3. Diverticular Bleeding

Half of all cases of acute lower gastrointestinal bleeding are attributable to diverticulosis. For a full discussion, see the section on Acute Lower Gastrointestinal Bleeding.

POLYPS OF THE COLON & SMALL INTESTINE

Polyps are discrete mass lesions that protrude into the intestinal lumen. Although most commonly sporadic, they may be inherited as part of a familial polyposis syndrome. Polyps may be divided into three major pathologic groups: mucosal neoplastic (adenomatous) polyps, mucosal nonneoplastic polyps (hyperplastic, juvenile polyps, hamartomas, inflammatory polyps), and submucosal lesions (lipomas, lymphoid aggregates, carcinoids, pneumatosis cystoides intestinalis). The nonneoplastic mucosal polyps have no malignant potential and usually are discovered incidentally at colonoscopy or barium enema. Only the adenomatous polyps have significant clinical implications and will be considered further here. Of polyps removed at colonoscopy, over 70% are adenomatous; most of the remainder are hyperplastic. Hyperplastic polyps are generally small (< 5 mm) and of no consequence. Their only importance is that they cannot be reliably distinguished from adenomatous lesions except by biopsy.

NONFAMILIAL ADENOMATOUS POLYPS

Histologically, adenomas are classified as tubular, villous, or tubulovillous. They may be flat, sessile or pedunculated (containing a stalk). They are present in 35% of adults over 50 years of age. Their significance is that over 95% of cases of adenocarcinoma of the colon are believed to arise from adenomas. It is proposed that there is an adenoma → carcinoma sequence whereby colorectal cancer develops through a continuous process from normal mucosa to adenoma to carcinoma. Most adenomas are small (< 1 cm) and have a low risk of becoming malignant; fewer than 5% of these enlarge with time. Adenomas are classified as "advanced" if they are ≥ 1 cm, or contain villous features or high-grade dysplasia. Advanced adenomas are believed to have a higher risk of harboring or progressing to malignancy. It has been estimated from longitudinal studies that it takes an average of 5 years for a medium-sized polyp to develop from normal-appearing mucosa and 10 years for a gross cancer to arise. In an asymptomatic population of male veterans over age 50 years undergoing screening with colonoscopy, invasive cancer was detected in 1%, adenomas containing high-grade dysplasia in 1.7%, and other adenomas ≥ 1 cm in size in 7.2%. The role of aspirin and NSAIDs for the chemoprevention of adenomatous polyps is discussed in the section on Colorectal Cancer.

Clinical Findings

A. SYMPTOMS AND SIGNS

Most patients with adenomatous polyps are completely asymptomatic. Chronic occult blood loss may lead to iron deficiency anemia. Large polyps may ulcerate, resulting in intermittent hematochezia.

B. FECAL OCCULT BLOOD OR MULTITARGET DNA TESTS

FOBT and, more recently, fecal DNA tests are available as part of colorectal cancer screening programs (see Colorectal Cancer: Screening for Colorectal Neoplasms). Unfortunately, both tests detect less than 20% of advanced adenomas.

C. RADIOLOGIC TESTS

Polyps are identified by means of barium enema examinations or CT colonography. Barium enema examinations (either single- or double-contrast) as currently performed detect < 50% of colorectal polyps ≥ 1 cm in size. CT colonography ("virtual colonoscopy") uses data from helical CT imaging with computer-enabled luminal image reconstruction to generate two-dimensional and three-dimensional images of the colon. Using optimal imaging software with multidetector helical CT scanners, several studies report a sensitivity of > 90% for the detection of clinically significant neoplasms (polyps > 10 mm). Other studies report sensitivities of only 50%, especially when performed for colorectal screening in asymptomatic patients. Pending further validation, CT colonography is not yet recommended for routine colorectal cancer screening, but may be best suited for patients with significant cardiac or pulmonary comorbidities—for whom colonoscopy is deemed unsafe—or in clinical settings in which endoscopic expertise is not readily available.

D. ENDOSCOPIC TESTS

Flexible sigmoidoscopy is commonly performed as part of colorectal screening programs. Approximately one-half to two-thirds of colonic adenomas are within the reach of a flexible sigmoidoscope. Polyps are seen in 10–20% of patients undergoing screening sigmoidoscopy, and polyps less than 8 mm in size should be removed by excisional biopsy. Patients with hyperplastic polyps require no further evaluation. Patients with advanced neoplasms (as defined above) have an increased risk (12%) of harboring other advanced neoplasms in the proximal colon and should undergo colonoscopy. At present, the management of patients with small adenomas without villous features or high-grade dysplasia is controversial. Opinions are conflicting about whether diminutive adenomas found on sigmoidoscopy are predictive of finding an increased prevalence of advanced neoplasms (> 1 cm or containing villous features or high-grade dysplasia) in the colon proximal to the splenic flexure during colonoscopy. In patients in whom no adenomas have been detected in the distal colon, the prevalence of advanced proximal adenomas is 2–5%; among patients with a distal adenoma less than 10 mm in size, the prevalence of advanced proximal neoplasia is 5–7%. Some physicians have not routinely performed colonoscopy in patients found to have a single small (< 5–8 mm) polyp in the distal colon on screening sigmoidoscopy. However, several professional guidelines recommend colonoscopy for all patients with adenomas found in the distal colon at sigmoidoscopy irrespective of size.

Colonoscopy allows evaluation of the entire colon and is the best means of detecting and removing adenomatous polyps. It should be performed in all patients who have positive FOBT or DNA tests or iron deficiency anemia (see Occult & Obscure Gastrointestinal Bleeding, above), as the prevalence of colonic neoplasms is increased in these patients. Colonoscopy should also be performed in patients with polyps detected on radiologic imaging studies (barium enema or CT colonography) or adenomas detected on flexible sigmoidoscopy to remove these polyps and to fully evaluate the entire colon.

Treatment

A. COLONOSCOPIC POLYPECTOMY

Most adenomatous polyps are amenable to colonoscopic removal with biopsy forceps or snare cautery. Large sessile polyps (> 2–3 cm) may be removed in piecemeal fashion or may require primary surgical resection. Complications after colonoscopic polypectomy include perforation in 0.2% and clinically significant bleeding in 0.3–1% of patients.

A malignant polyp is an adenoma that appears grossly benign at endoscopy but on histologic assessment is found to contain cancer that has penetrated through the muscularis mucosae into the submucosa. Malignant polyps may be considered to be adequately treated by polypectomy alone if (1) the polyp is completely excised and submitted for pathologic examination, (2) it is well differentiated, (3) the margin is not involved, and (4) there is no tumor budding vascular invasion. The risk of residual cancer or nodal metastasis with favorable histologic features is < 1%. The excision site of these "favorable" malignant polyps should be checked in 3 months for residual tissue. In patients with malignant polyps that have unfavorable histologic features, cancer resection is advisable if the patient is a good operative candidate.

B. POSTPOLYPECTOMY SURVEILLANCE

Adenomas can be found in 30–40% of patients when another colonoscopy is performed within 3–5 years after the initial examination. Periodic colonoscopic surveillance is therefore recommended to detect these "metachronous" adenomas, which either may be new or may have been overlooked during the initial examination. Most of these adenomas are small, without high-risk features and of little immediate clinical significance. The probability of detecting advanced neoplasms at surveillance colonoscopy is increased significantly if the polyps found on initial (index) colonoscopy were advanced (≥ 1 cm, villous features, or high-grade dysplasia) or multiple (more than two polyps) or if the patient's family includes a first-degree member with colorectal cancer. (See discussion below under Colorectal Cancer.) In these higher-risk patients, repeat or "surveillance" colonoscopy should be performed 3 years after the initial colonoscopy and polypectomy. For patients with adenomatous polyps who had low-risk features on initial colonoscopy and polypectomy (ie, one or two polyps less than 10 mm in size without villous features or high-grade dysplasia) or for higher-risk patients whose follow-up surveillance colonoscopy is negative for further polyps after 3 years, repeat colonoscopy to check for metachronous adenomas should be performed in 5 years.

Imperiale TF et al: Using risk for advanced proximal colonic neoplasia to tailor endoscopic screening for colorectal cancer. Ann Intern Med 2003;139:959. [PMID: 14678915]

Imperiale T et al: Fecal DNA versus fecal occult blood for colorectal cancer screening in an average-risk population. N Engl J Med 2004;351:2704. [PMID: 15616205]

Pickhardt P et al: Computed tomographic virtual colonoscopy to screen for colorectal neoplasia in asymptomatic adults. N Engl J Med 2003;349:2191. [PMID: 14657426]

Rockey DC et al: Analysis of air contrast barium enema, computed tomographic colonography, and colonoscopy: prospective comparison. Lancet 2005;365:305. [PMID: 15664225]

Ueno H et al: Risk factors for an adverse outcome in early invasive colorectal adenocarcinoma. Gastroenterology 2004; 127:385. [PMID: 15300569]

Van Dam J et al: AGA future trends report: CT colonography. Gastroenterology 2004;127:970. [PMID: 15362051]

HEREDITARY COLORECTAL CANCER & POLYPOSIS SYNDROMES

Up to 4% of all colorectal cancers are caused by germline genetic mutations that impose on carriers a high lifetime risk of developing colorectal cancer. Because the diagnosis of these disorders has important implications for treatment of affected members and for screening of family members, it is important to consider these disorders in patients with a family history of colorectal cancer that has affected more than one family member, those with a personal or family history of colorectal cancer developing at an early age (≤ 50 years), those with a personal or family history of multiple polyps (> 20), and those with a personal or family history of multiple extracolonic malignancies.

1. Familial Adenomatous Polyposis

Familial adenomatous polyposis (FAP) is a syndrome affecting 1:10,000 people and accounts for approximately 0.5% of colorectal cancer. The classic form of FAP is characterized by the development of hundreds to thousands of colonic adenomatous polyps and a variety of extracolonic manifestations. It is caused by an autosomally dominant inherited mutation in the adenomatous polyposis coli *(APC)* gene on chromosome 5q21 that leads to frameshifts or premature stop codons, most of which result in truncation of the *APC* gene product, a protein important in the regulation of cell adhesion and apoptosis. More than 300 different mutations have been reported. The location of the mutation affects the number of polyps formed and the type of extracolonic features seen. An attenuated variant of FAP has been recognized; an average of only 25 polyps (range of 0–500) develop in affected family members due to mutations at the 3' or 5' end of the *APC* gene. Recently, mutations in the *MYH* gene have been identified in patients with FAP who do not have mutations in the *FAP* gene. *MYH* is a recessive gene involved with base excision repair. FAP due to *MYH* mutation is inherited in an autosomal recessive fashion, hence a family history of colorectal cancer may not be evident.

Colorectal polyps develop by a mean age of 15 years and cancer at 40 years. Unless prophylactic colectomy is performed, colorectal cancer is inevitable by age 50 years. In attenuated FAP, the mean age for development of cancer is about 56 years.

Adenomatous polyps of the duodenum and periampullary area develop in over 90% of patients, resulting in a 5% lifetime risk of adenocarcinoma. Adenomas occur less frequently in the gastric antrum and small bowel and in those locations have a lower risk of malignant transformation. Gastric fundus gland polyps occur in over 50% but have an extremely low (0.6%) malignant potential.

Some patients with FAP develop a variety of other benign extraintestinal manifestations, including soft tissue tumors of the skin, desmoid tumors, osteomas, and congenital hypertrophy of the retinal pigment. They may also develop malignancies of the central nervous system (Turcot's syndrome) and tumors of the thyroid and liver (hepatoblastomas). These extraintestinal manifestations vary among families, depending in part on the type or site of mutation in the *APC* gene.

Genetic counseling and testing should be offered to patients with a diagnosis of FAP established by endoscopy and to first-degree family members of patients with the disease; testing should be done also to confirm a diagnosis of attenuated disease in patients with 20 or more adenomas. Genetic testing is best performed by sequencing the *APC* gene to identify disease-associated mutations, which are identified in approximately 90% of cases of typical FAP. Mutational assessment of *MYH* should be considered in patients with negative test results. First-degree relatives of patients with FAP should undergo genetic screening after age 10 years. A negative result can be considered to be a true negative only if an affected family member has a positive test result. If the assay cannot be done or is not informative, family members at risk should undergo yearly sigmoidoscopy beginning at 12 years of age. Once the diagnosis has been established, complete proctocolectomy with ileoanal anastomosis or colectomy with ileorectal anastomosis is recommended, usually before age 20 years. Ileorectal anastomosis affords superior bowel function but has a 10% risk of development of rectal cancer, and for that reason frequent sigmoidoscopy with fulguration of polyps is required. Sulindac and COX-2 selective agents (celecoxib) have been shown to decrease the number and size of polyps in the rectal stump but not the duodenum. Upper endoscopic evaluation of the stomach, duodenum, and periampullary area should be performed every 1–3 years to look for adenomas or carcinoma. Large (> 2 cm) periampullary adenomas require surgical resection.

Burt R et al: Genetic testing for inherited colon cancer. Gastroenterology 2005;128:1696. [PMID: 15887160]

Cruz-Correa M et al: Familial adenomatous polyposis. Gastrointest Endosc 2003;58:885. [PMID: 14652558]

Wang L et al: *MYH* mutations in patients with attenuated and classic polyposis and with young-onset colorectal cancer without polyps. Gastroenterology 2004;127:9. [PMID: 15235166]

2. Hamartomatous Polyposis Syndromes

Hamartomatous polyposis syndromes are rare and account for less than 0.1% of colorectal cancers.

Peutz-Jeghers syndrome is an autosomal dominant condition characterized by hamartomatous polyps throughout the gastrointestinal tract (most notably in the small intestine) as well as mucocutaneous pigmented macules on the lips, buccal mucosa, and skin. The hamartomas may become large, leading to bleeding, intussusception, or obstruction. Although hamartomas are not malignant, gastrointestinal malignancies (stomach, small bowel, and colon) develop in 40%, breast cancer in 50%, as well as a host of other malignancies of nonintestinal organs (gonads, pancreas). The defect has been localized to the serine threonine kinase 11 gene, and genetic testing is available.

Familial juvenile polyposis is also autosomal dominant and is characterized by several (more than ten) juvenile hamartomatous polyps located most commonly in the colon. There is an increased risk (up to 50%) of adenocarcinoma due to synchronous adenomatous polyps or mixed hamartomatous-adenomatous polyps. Genetic defects have been identified to loci on 18q and 10q (*MADH4* and *BMPR1A*). Genetic testing is available.

PTEN multiple hamartoma syndrome (Cowden disease) is characterized by hamartomatous polyps and lipomas throughout the gastrointestinal tract, trichilemmomas, and cerebellar lesions. An increased rate of malignancy is demonstrated in the thyroid, breast, and urogenital tract.

Schreibman IR et al: The hamartomatous polyposis syndromes: a clinical and molecular review. Am J Gastroenterol 2005; 100:476. [PMID: 15667510]

3. Hereditary Nonpolyposis Colorectal Cancer (HNPCC)

HNPCC is an autosomal dominant condition in which there is a markedly increased risk of developing colorectal cancer as well as a host of other cancers, including endometrial, ovarian, renal or vesical, hepatobiliary, gastric, and small intestinal cancers. It is estimated to account for up to 3% of all colorectal cancers. Affected individuals have a 60–80% lifetime risk of developing colorectal carcinoma and an over 30% lifetime risk of endometrial cancer. Unlike individuals with familial adenomatous polyposis, patients with HNPCC develop only a few adenomas, which may be flat and more often contain villous features or high-grade dysplasia. In contrast to the traditional polyp → cancer progression (which may take over 10 years), these polyps are believed to undergo rapid transformation from normal tissue → adenoma → cancer. It has been believed that HNPCC tends to develop at an earlier age than sporadic colorectal cancers (mean age: 44 years); however, in a recent study of HNPCC families, the median age at diagnosis of colorectal cancer (excluding probands) was 61 years—very similar to sporadic cancer. Compared with patients with sporadic tumors of similar pathologic stage, those with HNPCC tumors have improved survival. Synchronous or metachronous cancers occur within 10 years in up to 45% of patients.

HNPCC is caused by a defect in one of several genes that are important in the detection and repair of DNA base-pair mismatches: *MLH1, MSH2, MSH6,* and *PMS2*. Germline mutations in *MLH1* and *MSH2* account for more than 90% of the known mutations in families with HNPCC. Mutations in any of these mismatch repair genes result in a characteristic phenotypic abnormality known as microsatellite instability. In over 95% of cancers in patients with HNPCC, microsatellite instability is readily demonstrated by expansion or contraction of DNA microsatellites (short, repeated DNA sequences). Microsatellite instability also occurs in 15% of sporadic colorectal cancers, usually due to aberrant methylation of the *MLH1* promoter resulting in decreased gene expression.

A thorough family cancer history is essential to identify families that may be affected with HNPCC so that appropriate genetic and colonoscopic screening can be offered. Owing to the limitations of genetic testing for HNPCC and the medical, psychological, and social implications that such testing may have, families with suspected HNPCC should be evaluated first by a genetic counselor and should give informed consent in writing before genetic testing is performed. Patients whose families meet any of the revised "Bethesda criteria" have an increased likelihood of harboring a germline mutation in one of the mismatch repair genes and should be considered for genetic testing: (1) colorectal cancer under age 50; (2) synchronous or metachronous colorectal or HNPCC-associated tumor regardless of age (endometrial, stomach, ovary, pancreas, ureter and renal pelvis, biliary tract, brain); (3) colorectal cancer with one or more first-degree relatives with colorectal or HNPCC-related cancer, with one of the cancers occurring before age 50; (4) colorectal cancer with two or more second-degree relatives with colorectal or HNPCC cancer, regardless of age. These criteria will identify > 90% of mutation-positive HNPCC families. Tumor tissues of affected individuals or family members meeting the revised Bethesda criteria should undergo immunohistochemical staining for *MSH2, MLH1,* and *PMS2* (commercially available assays) or tested for microsatellite instability. Individuals whose tumors have normal immunohistochemical staining or do not have microsatellite instability are unlikely to have germline mutations in mismatch repair genes, do not require further genetic testing, and do not require intensive cancer surveillance. Germline testing for gene mutations is positive in > 90% of individuals whose tumors show absent histochemical staining of one of the mismatch repair genes and in 50% of those whose tumors have a high level of microsatellite instability. Germline testing is also warranted in families with a strong history consistent with HNPCC when tumors from affected members are unavailable for assessment. If a mutation is detected in a patient with cancer in one of the known mismatch genes, genetic testing of other first-degree family members is indicated.

If genetic testing documents an HNPCC gene mutation, affected relatives should be screened with colonoscopy every 1–2 years beginning at age 25 (or at age 5 years younger than the age at diagnosis of the youngest affected family member). If cancer is found, subtotal colectomy with ileorectal anastomosis (followed by annual surveillance of the rectal stump) should be performed. Upper endoscopy should be performed every 2–3 years to screen for gastric cancer. Women should undergo screening for endometrial and ovarian cancer beginning at age 25–35 years with pelvic examination, CA-125 assay, endometrial aspiration, and transvaginal ultrasound. Prophylactic hysterectomy and oophorectomy may be considered, especially in women of postchildbearing age. Similarly, consideration should be given for increased cancer surveillance in family members in proven or suspected HNPCC families who do not wish to undergo germline testing.

Hampel H et al: Screening for the Lynch syndrome (hereditary nonpolyposis colorectal cancer). N Engl J Med 2005; 352: 1851. [PMID: 15872200]

Hampel H et al: Cancer risk in hereditary nonpolyposis colorectal cancer syndrome: later age of onset. Gastroenterology 2005; 129:415. [PMID: 16083698]

Lindor NM et al: Lower cancer incidence in Amsterdam-I criteria families without mismatch repair deficiency: familial colorectal cancer type X. JAMA 2005;293:1979. [PMID: 15855431]

Terdiman JP: Colorectal cancer at a young age. Gastroenterology 2005;128:1067. [PMID: 15825087]

COLORECTAL CANCER

ESSENTIALS OF DIAGNOSIS

- Symptoms or signs depend on tumor location.
- Proximal colon: fecal occult blood, anemia.
- Distal colon: change in bowel habits, hematochezia.
- Characteristic findings on barium enema or CT colonography.
- Diagnosis established with colonoscopy.

General Considerations

Colorectal cancer is the second leading cause of death due to malignancy in the United States. Approximately 6% of Americans will develop colorectal cancer and 40% of those will die of the disease. An estimated 145,000 new cases and 55,000 deaths occur annually. Colorectal cancers are almost all adenocarcinomas, which tend to form bulky exophytic masses or annular constricting lesions. Slightly less than 50% of cancers are located distal to the splenic flexure (within the descending colon or rectosigmoid region), where they are within reach of detection by flexible sigmoidoscopy. There appears to be a gradual increase in incidence of cancers in the cecum and ascending colon, and over half of cancers now develop proximal to the splenic flexure. It is currently believed that the majority of colorectal cancers arise from malignant transformation of an adenomatous polyp. Approximately 85%

of sporadic colorectal cancers have loss of function of one or more tumor suppressor genes (eg, *p53*, *APC*, or *DCC*) due to a combination of spontaneous mutation of one allele combined with chromosomal instability that leads to deletion and loss of heterozygosity of the other allele (eg, 5q, 17q, or 18p deletion). Approximately 15% of colorectal cancers have microsatellite instability, suggesting inactivation of mismatch repair genes that is most commonly acquired but may be an indicator of unrecognized HNPCC (see above).

Risk Factors

A number of factors increase the risk of developing colorectal cancer. Recognition of these has impact on screening strategies. However, 75% of all cases occur in people with no known predisposing factors.

A. AGE

The incidence of colorectal cancer rises sharply after age 45 years, and 90% of cases occur in persons over the age of 50 years.

B. FAMILY HISTORY OF NEOPLASIA

A family history of colorectal cancer is present in 20% of patients with colon cancer. Hereditary factors are believed to contribute to 20–30% of colorectal cancers; however, the genes responsible for most of these cases have not yet been identified. Up to 5% of colorectal cancers are caused by inherited germline mutations resulting in polyposis syndromes or HNPCC (reviewed elsewhere in this chapter). Approximately 6% of the Ashkenazic Jewish population has a missense mutation in the *APC* gene *(APC I1307K)* that confers a modestly increased lifetime risk of developing colorectal cancer (OR 1.4–1.9) but phenotypically resembles sporadic colorectal cancer rather than FAP. Genetic screening is available, and patients harboring the mutation merit intensive screening.

A family history of colorectal cancer or adenomatous polyps is one of the most important risk factors for colorectal cancer. The risk of colon cancer is proportionate to the number and age of affected first-degree family members with colon cancer. People with one first-degree family member with colorectal cancer have an increased risk approximately 2 times that of the general population. However, the relative risk is 3.8 times if the family member's cancer was diagnosed at < 45 years of age, 2.2 if diagnosed at 45–59 years of age, and only 1.8 if diagnosed at > 59 years of age. Patients with two first-degree relatives have a fourfold—or 25–30% lifetime—risk of developing colon cancer. First-degree relatives of patients with adenomas also are at increased risk for colorectal neoplasia, especially if the adenoma was detected before age 60 years. Cancers arise at an earlier age in patients with a positive family history, meriting screening at an earlier age. The risk of a 40-year-old person with a positive family history is comparable to that of an average-risk 50-year-old person.

C. INFLAMMATORY BOWEL DISEASE

The risk of adenocarcinoma of the colon begins to rise 7–10 years after disease onset in patients with ulcerative colitis and Crohn's colitis. The cumulative risk approaches 5–10% after 20 years and 20% after 30 years. Chronic treatment with 5-ASA agents and folate is associated with a lower risk of cancer in patients with ulcerative colitis.

D. DIETARY FACTORS AND CHEMOPREVENTION

In epidemiologic studies, diets rich in fats and red meat are associated with an increased risk of colorectal adenomas and cancer, whereas diets high in fruits, vegetables, and fiber are associated with a decreased risk. However, two prospective, randomized controlled trials failed to demonstrate a risk reduction in the recurrence of adenomas after treatment with a diet low in fat and high in fiber, fruits, and vegetables or with fiber supplementation over a 3- to 4-year period. Both calcium carbonate (3 g/d) and folate therapy have been shown in prospective trials to yield a modest but significant reduction in the relative risk of developing colorectal neoplasia. In women, hormone replacement therapy may also be beneficial. The antioxidant vitamins A, C, and E have not been shown to be of benefit in prospective controlled studies.

Cohort and case-control studies show that prolonged regular use of aspirin (at least 325 mg twice weekly) and NSAIDs is associated with a 30–50% decrease in the incidence of colorectal cancer and adenomas. Several prospective, blinded clinical trials have shown that daily low-dose aspirin (80–325 mg) reduces the number of recurrent adenomas at 1–3 years in patients with a history of colorectal adenomas or cancer. Because chronic aspirin use is associated with a low incidence of serious complications (gastrointestinal hemorrhage, stroke), it should not be prescribed as a chemopreventive agent in people without polyps or with small adenomas unless there are other medical indications. Chronic administration of these agents may be considered in patients with a personal or family history of colorectal cancer or advanced adenomas; however, they do not obviate the need for screening and surveillance.

E. RACE

The incidence of colon adenocarcinoma is higher in blacks than in whites. It is unclear whether this is due to genetic or socioeconomic factors (eg, diet or reduced access to screening).

Clinical Findings

A. SYMPTOMS AND SIGNS

Adenocarcinomas grow slowly and may be present for several years before symptoms appear. However, asymptomatic tumors may still be detected by the presence of fecal occult blood (see Colorectal Cancer Screening, be-

low). Symptoms depend on the location of the carcinoma. Chronic blood loss from right-sided colonic cancers may cause iron deficiency anemia, manifested by fatigue and weakness. Obstruction, however, is uncommon because of the large diameter of the right colon and the liquid consistency of the fecal material. Lesions of the left colon often involve the bowel circumferentially. Because the left colon has a smaller diameter and the fecal matter is solid, obstructive symptoms may develop with colicky abdominal pain and a change in bowel habits. Constipation may alternate with periods of increased frequency and loose stools. The stool may be streaked with blood, though marked bleeding is unusual. With rectal cancers, patients note tenesmus, urgency, and recurrent hematochezia. Weight loss is uncommon. Physical examination is usually normal except in advanced disease. A mass may be palpable in the abdomen. The liver should be examined for hepatomegaly, suggesting metastatic spread. For cancers of the distal rectum, digital examination is necessary to determine whether there is extension into the anal sphincter or fixation, suggesting extension to the pelvic floor.

B. LABORATORY FINDINGS

A complete blood count is obtained to look for evidence of anemia. Elevated liver function tests are suspicious for metastatic disease. Carcinoembryonic antigen (CEA) should be measured in all patients with proved colorectal cancer. A preoperative CEA level > 5 ng/mL is a poor prognostic indicator. After complete surgical resection, CEA levels should normalize; persistently elevated levels suggest the presence of persistent disease and warrant further evaluation.

C. INSPECTION OF THE COLON

Cancers may be detected with a high degree of reliability with barium enema, CT colonography ("virtual colonoscopy"), or colonoscopy. Colonoscopy is the diagnostic procedure of choice in patients with a clinical history suggestive of colon cancer or in patients with an abnormality suspicious for cancer detected on radiographic imaging. Colonoscopy permits biopsy for pathologic confirmation of malignancy. In patients in whom colonoscopy is unable to reach the cecum (< 5% of cases) or when a nearly obstructing tumor precludes passage of the colonoscope, barium enema or CT colonography examination should be performed.

D. IMAGING

Clinicians obtain an abdominal and pelvic CT scan to assist in preoperative staging, although it is unclear that it alters surgical management in most cases. CT scans may demonstrate distal metastases but is less accurate in the determination of the level of local tumor extension (T stage) or lymphatic spread (N stage). Intraoperative assessment of the liver by direct palpation and ultrasonography is more accurate than CT scanning for the detection of hepatic metastases. For rectal cancer, pelvic MRI or endorectal ultrasonography provides important accurate in-

Table 14–16. Staging of colorectal cancer.

Joint Committee Classification	TNM			Dukes Class[1]
Stage 0				
Carcinoma in situ	Tis	N0	M0	
Stage I				
Tumor invades submucosa	T1	N0	M0	Dukes A
Tumor invades muscularis propria	T2	N0	M0	Dukes B_1
Stage II				
Tumor invades into subserosa or into nonperitonealized pericolic or perirectal tissues	T3	N0	M0	Dukes B_1 or B_2
Tumor perforates the visceral peritoneum or directly invades other organs or structures	T4	N0	M0	Dukes B_2
Stage III				
Any degree of bowel wall perforation with lymph node metastasis				
One to three pericolic or perirectal lymph nodes involved	Any T	N1	M0	Dukes C_1
Four or more pericolic or perirectal lymph nodes involved	Any T	N2	M0	Dukes C_2
Metastasis to lymph nodes along a vascular trunk	Any T	N3	M0	
Stage IV				
Presence of distant metastasis	Any T	Any N	M1	Dukes D

[1]Gastrointestinal Tumor Study Group modification of Dukes classification.

formation about the depth of penetration of the cancer through the rectal wall and pararectal lymph nodes that may guide preoperative (neoadjuvant) chemoradiotherapy and operative management. A chest CT scan should also be obtained because the systemic blood supply of the distal rectum may promote distal tumor metastasis outside the abdomen. Positron emission tomography (PET) is useful to determine recurrent colorectal cancer but currently is not used for staging of primary tumors.

Differential Diagnosis

The nonspecific symptoms of colon cancer may be confused with those of irritable bowel syndrome, diverticular disease, ischemic colitis, inflammatory bowel disease, infectious colitis, and hemorrhoids. Neoplasm must be excluded in any patient over age 40 years who reports a change in bowel habits or hematochezia or who has an unexplained iron deficiency anemia or occult blood in the stools.

Staging

Determination of the stage of colorectal cancer is important not only because it correlates with the patient's long-term survival but also because it is used to determine which patients should receive adjuvant therapy (Table 14–16). Although the Dukes classification has been widely employed in the past, the TNM system is now more commonly used.

Treatment

Resection of the primary colonic or rectal cancer is the treatment of choice for almost all patients who have

resectable lesions and can tolerate general anesthesia. Multiple studies demonstrate that minimally invasive, laparoscopically assisted colectomy results in similar outcomes and rates of recurrence to open colectomy. Regional lymph node dissection should be performed to determine staging, which guides decisions about adjuvant therapy. Even patients with extensive metastatic disease may benefit from resection of the colonic tumor to reduce the likelihood of intestinal obstruction or serious bleeding.

For rectal carcinoma, the operative approach depends on the level of the tumor above the anal verge, the size and depth of penetration, and the patient's overall condition. Clinical staging by endorectal ultrasound or MRI with endorectal coil is important in guiding the clinical approach. In carefully selected patients with small, mobile (< 4 cm), well-differentiated T1 or T2 rectal tumors that are less than 7.5 cm from the anal verge and that appear on endosonography to be localized to the rectal wall, transanal excision may be performed. This approach avoids laparotomy and spares the rectum and anal sphincter, preserving normal bowel continence. All other patients will require either a low anterior resection with a colorectal or coloanal anastomosis or an abdominoperineal resection with a colostomy, depending on how far above the anal verge the tumor is located and the extent of local tumor spread. Careful dissection of the entire mesorectum at the time of surgery has been shown to reduce local recurrence to 8%. With improvements in surgical stapling techniques, it is possible to perform low anterior resection provided there is a margin of at least 2 cm of normal tissue below the tumor. Although low resections obviate a colostomy, they are associated with increased immediate postsurgical complications (leak, dehiscence, stricture) and defecatory complaints (increased stool frequency, defecatory problems, and incontinence). With unresectable rectal cancer, the patient may be palliated with a diverting colostomy, laser fulguration, or placement of an expandable wire stent.

A. Adjuvant Therapy for Colon Cancer

Adjuvant chemotherapy and radiotherapy have been demonstrated to improve overall and tumor-free survival in selected patients with colon cancer.

1. Stage I—Because of the excellent 5-year survival rate (90–100%), no adjuvant therapy is recommended.

2. Stage II (node-negative disease)—The expected 5-year survival rate is 80%. A benefit from adjuvant chemotherapy has not been demonstrated in most controlled trials for stage II colon cancer (see discussion for Stage III disease). Patients with advanced local stage II disease (perforation, T4) may be considered for study protocols looking at the role of adjuvant chemotherapy for control of local recurrence.

3. Stage III (node-positive) disease—With surgical resection alone, the expected 5-year survival rate is 30–50%. Postoperative adjuvant chemotherapy significantly increases disease-free survival as well as overall survival and is recommended for all patients. In stage III colorectal cancer, patients treated for 6 months with intravenous 5-fluorouracil (5-FU) (bolus or continuous infusion) and leucovorin (folinic acid) who have one to three involved nodes have a 5-year survival of 65%, and those with more than three involved nodes have a 5-year survival of up to 40%. Therefore, until recently, adjuvant therapy with 5-FU and leucovorin was most widely used for stage III disease. However, in a recent multicenter trial, monotherapy with an oral 5-FU analog capecitabine yielded a similar rate of disease-free survival with a lower rate of serious side effects compared with intravenous 5-FU and leucovorin. Furthermore, a large, well-designed study (MOSAIC trial) of adjuvant therapy for stage II and III colon cancer reported at 4 years a higher rate of disease-free survival for patients treated with a combination of oxaliplatin, fluorouracil, and leucovorin (FOLFOX) (76%) than with fluorouracil and leucovorin (FL) alone (69%). Benefit was higher for stage III than stage II cancers. The addition of oxaliplatin was associated with an increased incidence of neutropenia and sensory neuropathy. Although further study is needed, combined adjuvant therapy with oxaliplatin should be considered for stage III disease in optimal candidates.

4. Stage IV (metastatic disease)—Approximately 20% of patients have metastatic disease at the time of initial diagnosis, and another 30% eventually develop metastasis. The long-term survival of these patients is only 5%, and the median survival is only 6 months in the absence of other treatment. Resection of isolated (one to three) liver or lung metastases may result in long-term (over 5 years) survival in 35–55% of cases.

For those with unresectable hepatic metastases, local ablative techniques (cryosurgery, radiofrequency or microwave coagulation, embolization, hepatic intra-arterial chemotherapy) may provide long-term tumor control. Approximately 20% of patients with metastatic disease respond to chemotherapy regimens containing intravenous 5-FU and folinic acid (leucovorin), prolonging median survival to about 11 months. The oral 5-FU agent capecitabine may be preferred in patients with advanced disease who desire the convenience of oral rather than intravenous therapy. However, the addition of either oxaliplatin (FOLFOX) or irinotecan (FOLFIRI; IFL) to 5-FU and folinic acid provides further improvement in tumor response rate (40%) and median survival (14–16 months). Currently, oxaliplatin-based regimens are commonly used as first-line therapy for metastatic disease, because irinotecan-based regimens are associated with greater toxicity (especially diarrhea and febrile neutropenia). Patients progressing with one regimen may respond to the alternative regimen, prolonging mean survival to > 20 months. Cetuximab, a monoclonal antibody to EGFR, has demonstrated improvement in tumor response rates and median survival when used in combination with irinotecan-based chemotherapeutic regimens, including tumors with resistance to irinotecan. Bevacizumab is a monoclonal antibody to vascular endothelial growth factor that is inactive as a single-agent against colorectal cancer but leads to further prolongation of mean survival by 5 months when used in combination with either irinotecan-based (IFL) or oxaliplatin-based (FOLFOX) regimens. The mean survival in patients treated with bevacizumab plus these regimens exceeds 20 months. However, bevacizumab may cause serious thromboembolic events (including stroke and myocardial infarction) in 5% of patients. Currently, the role of these effective but very expensive regimens as first-line or second-line therapy for metastatic disease is unclear.

B. Adjuvant Therapy for Rectal Cancer

Compared with colon cancer, rectal cancer has lower long-term survival rates and significantly higher rates of local tumor recurrence (25%) due to the difficulty of achieving adequate surgical resection margins. Combination therapy with fluorouracil and radiation has been shown to improve the disease-free survival rate and to decrease pelvic recurrence and is recommended for all patients with stage II and stage III rectal cancers. It has long been controversial whether chemoradiation should be administered preoperatively ("neoadjuvant") or postoperatively ("adjuvant"). Neoadjuvant therapy may decrease the size of the tumor before surgery (tumor downstaging), allowing more patients to undergo curative resection with sphincter preservation rather than abdominoperineal resection. When initial imaging studies suggest stage I disease, surgery may be performed first, followed by postoperative chemoradiation in patients found at surgery to have more advanced (stage II or III) disease. A recent, large, randomized controlled trial reported that preoperative therapy led to better patient treatment compliance, reduced local recurrence and toxicity, and a higher number of sphincter-preserving resections. Therefore, preoperative chemoradiation increasingly is recommended for patients with distal rectal cancers that are determined to be stage II or III by endorectal ultrasound or MRI.

Follow-Up after Surgery

Patients who have undergone resections for cure are followed closely to look for evidence of symptomatic or asymptomatic tumor recurrence that may be amenable to curative resection in a small number of patients. The optimal cost-effective strategy is not clear and professional guidelines provide different recommendations. Two randomized trials reported that intense follow-up with yearly colonoscopy, abdominal CT, and chest radiography did not improve overall outcome compared with most standard follow-up protocols. In the absence of consensus guidelines, the following may be recommended. Patients should be evaluated every 3–6 months for 3–5 years with history, physical examination, and CEA determinations. All patients should undergo colonoscopy either preoperatively or within 3–6 months postoperatively to exclude other synchronous colorectal neoplasms. Thereafter, surveillance colonoscopy should be performed every 3–5 years to look for metachronous polyps or cancer. Because of the high incidence of local tumor recurrence in patients with rectal cancer, sigmoidoscopy should be performed every 6–12 months for 3 years. New onset of symptoms or a rising CEA warrants investigation with chest and abdominal CT to look for recurrent or metastatic disease that may be amenable to therapy. For patients with a rising CEA with unrevealing CT imaging, a PET scan is more sensitive for the detection of occult metastatic disease.

Prognosis

The stage of disease at presentation is the most important determinant of long-term survival: stage I, > 90%; stage II, 70–80%; stage III with fewer than four positive lymph nodes, 67%; stage III with more than four positive lymph nodes, 33%; and stage IV, 5–7%. For each stage, rectal cancers have a worse prognosis. For those patients whose disease progresses despite therapy, meticulous efforts at palliative care are essential (see Chapter 5).

Screening for Colorectal Neoplasms

Colorectal cancer is ideal for screening because it is a common disease affecting 6% of men and women that is fatal in almost 50% of cases yet is curable if detected at an earlier stage. Furthermore, the vast majority of cases arise from benign adenomas that progress over many years to cancer, and removal of adenomas has

been shown to prevent the vast majority of cancers. Colorectal cancer screening has now been endorsed by the United States Preventive Services Task Force, the Agency for Health Care Policy and Research, the American Cancer Society, and every professional gastroenterology and colorectal surgery society. Although there is continued debate about the optimal cost-effective means of providing population screening, there is unanimous consent that screening *of some kind* should be offered to every patient over the age of 50 years. Several analyses suggest that the cost of screening is approximately $25,000 per year of life saved for all recommended screening strategies, which is well below the range of $40,000–$50,000 per year generally considered to be cost-effective.

A number of options for screening are available and reimbursed by third-party payers and by Medicare. The recommendations of a multidisciplinary consensus panel are listed in Table 14–17 for patients at average risk of developing colorectal cancer. Patients with first-degree relatives with colorectal cancer are at increased risk, and for these individuals more intensive screening recommendations are recommended. Recommendations for screening in families with inherited cancer syndromes or inflammatory bowel disease are provided in separate sections. (See Hereditary Colorectal Cancer and Polyposis Syndromes; Inflammatory Bowel Disease.) The advantages and disadvantages of

Table 14–17. Recommendations for colorectal cancer screening.[1]

Average-risk individuals ≥ 50 years old[2]
Annual fecal occult blood testing
Flexible sigmoidoscopy every 5 years
Annual fecal occult blood testing *and* flexible sigmoidoscopy every 5 years
Colonoscopy every 10 years
Barium enema every 5 years
Individuals with a family history of a first-degree member with colorectal neoplasia[3]
Single first-degree relative with colorectal cancer diagnosed at age ≥ **60 years:** Begin screening at age 40. Screening guidelines same as average-risk individual; however, preferred method is colonoscopy every 10 years.
Single first-degree relative with colorectal cancer diagnosed at age < **60 years,** or multiple first-degree relatives: Begin screening at age 40 or at age 10 years younger than age at diagnosis of the youngest affected relative, whichever is first in time. Recommended screening: colonoscopy every 5 years.

[1]For recommendations for families with inherited polyposis syndromes or hereditary nonpolyposis colon cancer, see separate section.
[2]Colorectal cancer screening and survelliance: clinical guidelines and rationale. Gastroenterology 2003;124:544.
[3]Screening Recommendations of American College of Gastroenterology. Am J Gastroenterol 2000;95:868.

the various options are discussed below. It is important for primary care providers to understand the relative merits of various options and to discuss them with their patients. Despite growing awareness of the importance of screening on the part of medical professionals and the public, less than 50% of patients have undergone screening of any kind. Discussion and encouragement by the primary care provider are the most important factors in achieving patient compliance with screening programs. The potential for harm from screening must be weighed against the likelihood of benefit, especially in elderly patients with comorbid illnesses and shorter life expectancy.

A. Fecal Occult Blood Test or Multitarget DNA Assay

Most colorectal cancers and some large adenomas result in increased chronic blood loss that may be detectable. A variety of tests have been developed that have varying sensitivities for fecal occult blood, some of which are in clinical testing. A guaiac-based test (Hemoccult II) has undergone the most extensive testing and has had the greatest clinical use. Two slides must be prepared from three consecutive bowel movements. To reduce the likelihood of false-positive tests, patients should abstain from aspirin (in doses greater than 325 mg/d), NSAIDs, red meat, poultry, fish, and vegetables with peroxide activity (turnips, horseradish) for 72 hours. Vitamin C may cause a false-negative test. Slides should be developed within 7 days after preparation. The World Health Organization recently endorsed another guaiac test for FOBT, Hemoccult Sensa, because it has higher sensitivity than the Hemoccult II test; however, data from large clinical trials with this test are lacking.

When FOBT is administered to the general population as part of a screening program, 1–5% of tests are positive. Patients with positive tests should undergo colonoscopy accompanied by removal of any polyps identified. If colonoscopy reveals no colorectal neoplasm, further screening for colorectal cancer can be deferred for 10 years. Of those with positive tests, 5–18% have colorectal cancer, more likely to be at an earlier stage (Dukes A or B). Adenomatous polyps are identified in 25–50% of patients with positive tests. Finding these polyps is somewhat fortuitous since most are less than 1 cm in size and unlikely to cause occult bleeding. The estimated sensitivity of a guaiac-based FOBT for colorectal cancer is only 30–50%, but 65% with immunochemical tests. Sensitivity may be increased in patients who are compliant with annual testing. In several large prospective studies, FOBT has been demonstrated to reduce mortality from colorectal cancer by 15–33%. Higher risk reductions are obtained with annual versus biennial testing.

A fecal DNA assay (Pre-Gen Plus) is commercially available for screening for colorectal neoplasia. The test analyzes fecal DNA for point mutations in the *APC*, K-*ras*, and *p53* genes, microsatellite instability, and a marker of abnormal apoptosis. In studies con-

ducted in nonscreening populations, the average sensitivity and specificity for detection of advanced adenomas and cancer are approximately 67% and 97%, respectively. However, in a recent study performed in a large asymptomatic screening population, the fecal DNA panel detected only 41% of cancers and only 18% of adenomas containing high-grade dysplasia and only 18% of all advanced neoplasms (cancers or adenomas that were ≥ 1 cm or that contained villous features or high-grade dysplasia). The FOBT (Hemoccult II) performed even worse, detecting only 14% of invasive cancers and 10% of all advanced neoplasms.

The low sensitivity of FOBT and DNA tests for advanced neoplasia makes them a less attractive choice for population-based screening than endoscopic or radiographic tests. At present, they are most suitable in settings where health care resources are limited or in patients who desire a noninvasive method of screening.

B. Flexible Sigmoidoscopy

Use of a 60-cm flexible sigmoidoscope permits visualization of the rectosigmoid and descending colon. It requires no sedation and in many centers is performed by a nurse specialist or physician's assistant. Adenomatous polyps are identified in 10–20% and colorectal cancers in 1% of patients. Polyps less than 5–8 mm in diameter should be removed by biopsy to determine the histology. All patients found to have a high-risk adenomatous polyp (> 1 cm, villous features, or high-grade dysplasia) or more than two diminutive adenomatous polyps should undergo pancolonoscopy to look for synchronous neoplasms in the proximal colon. As discussed previously, there are conflicting opinions about whether patients found to have one or two diminutive adenomas on flexible sigmoidoscopy require colonoscopy (See Adenomatous Polyps, above.) Up to 80% of cases of advanced neoplasia will be detected in flexible sigmoidoscopy screening programs provided that all patients in whom an adenoma is identified at sigmoidoscopy undergo subsequent colonoscopy. The risk of serious complications (perforation) associated with flexible sigmoidoscopy is less than 1:10,000 patients.

C. Screening Colonoscopy

Colonoscopy permits examination of the entire colon. Approximately 50% of advanced neoplasms (cancer, adenomas ≥ 1 cm, polyps with villous histology, or high-grade dysplasia) are proximal to the splenic flexure, ie, above the reach of a flexible sigmoidoscopic examination. Up to 50–60% of such patients do not have an adenomatous polyp distal to the splenic flexure at sigmoidoscopy. Therefore, screening programs that use flexible sigmoidoscopy will not identify approximately 20–30% of patients with advanced colonic neoplasia. For this reason, screening colonoscopy is the preferred screening test in patients deemed to be at higher risk due to a positive family history of colorectal cancer. Colonoscopy has been advocated by the American College of Gastroenterology as the preferred screening modality in average-risk patients as well. In a population of asymptomatic veterans between 50 and 75 years of age undergoing screening colonoscopy, the prevalence of advanced adenomas or cancer was 10.7%. To alleviate discomfort, intravenous sedation is used for most patients. The incidence of serious complications after colonoscopy (perforation, bleeding, cardiopulmonary events) is 0.3%. Although colonoscopy is believed to be the most sensitive test for detecting adenomas and cancer, it is not infallible. In several studies, the rate of colorectal cancer within 3 years of a screening colonoscopy was 0.7–0.9%, ie, 1 in 110 patients. Even skilled endoscopists may overlook polyps that are small, flat, or located behind folds. Furthermore, some precancerous polyps may undergo rapid progression to cancer.

D. DOUBLE CONTRAST BARIUM ENEMA

Like colonoscopy, barium enema permits examination of the entire colon. Barium enema has been an attractive screening technique because it was widely available, relatively inexpensive, and safe. However, it is being rapidly supplanted by colonoscopy and CT colonography. A recent multicenter trial demonstrated that the sensitivity of barium enema is only 50% for polyps ≥ 1 cm and 55–85% for early-stage cancers when compared with colonoscopy. At present, barium enema may be recommended when screening of the entire colon is desired and the patient is unable or unwilling to undergo colonoscopy, and expertise in CT colonography is unavailable.

E. CT COLONOGRAPHY (VIRTUAL COLONOSCOPY)

Using computer-assisted image reconstruction and rapid helical CT, two- and three-dimensional views can be generated of the colon lumen that simulate the view of colonoscopy. This technique is performed rapidly, requires no sedation or intravenous contrast, and has minimal risk except for radiation exposure. At this time, it requires a similar bowel cleansing regimen as colonoscopy as well as the insufflation of air into the colon through a rectal tube, which may be associated with discomfort. In several recent large studies, the accuracy of virtual colonoscopy compared with colonoscopy has been assessed for the screening of colorectal neoplasia in asymptomatic screening populations. In several studies, the sensitivity of virtual colonoscopy for the detection of polyps larger than 8–10 mm is > 90%; however, other studies report sensitivity of only 50–60%. Abnormalities identified on CT imaging require assessment by colonoscopy. Although most professional guidelines do not yet endorse virtual colonoscopy for routine colorectal screening, it is a reasonable alternative for patients in whom screening of the entire colon is desired but who are unable or unwilling to undergo colonoscopy.

Callery MP: Combined modality therapy for rectal cancer. Gastroenterology 2005;128:1516.

Colon Cancer—National Cancer Institute—Cancer Net: http://cancernet.nci.nih.gov.

Hurwitz H et al: Bevacizumab plus irinotecan, fluorouracil, and leucovorin for metastatic colorectal cancer. N Engl J Med 2004;350:2335. [PMID: 15175435]

Imperiale T et al: Fecal DNA versus fecal occult blood for colorectal cancer screening in an average-risk population. N Engl J Med 2004;351:2704. [PMID: 5616205]

Meyerhardt JA et al: Systematic therapy for colorectal cancer. N Engl J Med 2005;352:476. [PMID: 15689586]

Minsky BD: Adjuvant therapy for rectal cancer—the transatlantic view. Colorectal Dis 2003;5:416. [PMID: 12925072]

Morikawa T et al: A comparison of the immunochemical fecal occult blood test and total colonoscopy in the asymptomatic population. Gastroenterology 2005;129:422. [PMID: 16083699]

Nelson H et al: A comparison of laparoscopically assisted and open colectomy for colon cancer. N Engl J Med 2004;350:2050. [PMID: 15141043]

Nicholson FB et al: The role of CT colography in colorectal cancer screening. Am J Gastroenterol 2005;100:2316. [PMID: 16181386]

Ouyang DL et al: Noninvasive testing for colorectal cancer: a review. Am J Gastroenterol 2005;100:1393. [PMID: 15929776]

Pfister DG et al: Surveillance strategies after curative treatment of colorectal cancer. N Engl J Med 2004;350:2375. [PMID: 15175439]

Rockey DC et al: Analysis of air contrast barium enema, computed tomographic colonography, and colonoscopy: prospective comparison. Lancet 2005;365:305. [PMID: 15664225]

Schoenfeld P et al: Colonoscopic screening of average-risk women for colorectal neoplasia. N Engl J Med 2005;352:2061. [PMID: 15901859]

Twelves C et al: Capecitabine as adjuvant treatment for stage III colon cancer. N Engl J Med 2005;352:2696. [PMID: 15987918]

Van Dam J et al: AGA future trends report: CT colonography. Gastroenterology 2004;127:970. [PMID: 15362051]

Walsh JM et al: Colorectal cancer screening: clinical applications. JAMA 2003;289:1297. [PMID: 12633192]

Weitz J et al: Colorectal cancer. Lancet 2005;365:153. [PMID: 15639298]

■ ANORECTAL DISEASES

HEMORRHOIDS

ESSENTIALS OF DIAGNOSIS

- *Bright red blood per rectum.*
- *Protrusion, discomfort.*
- *Characteristic findings on external anal inspection and anoscopic examination.*

General Considerations

Internal hemorrhoids are subepithelial vascular cushions consisting of connective tissue, smooth muscle fibers, and arteriovenous communications between terminal branches of the superior rectal artery and rectal veins. They are a normal anatomic entity, occurring in all adults, that contribute to normal anal pressures and ensure a water-tight closure of the anal canal. They commonly occur in three primary locations—right anterior, right posterior, and left lateral. External hemorrhoids arise from the inferior hemorrhoidal veins located below the dentate line and are covered with squamous epithelium of the anal canal or perianal region.

Hemorrhoids may become symptomatic as a result of activities that increase venous pressure, resulting in distention and engorgement. Straining at stool, constipation, prolonged sitting, pregnancy, obesity, and low-fiber diets all may contribute. With time, redundancy and enlargement of the venous cushions may develop and result in bleeding or protrusion.

Clinical Findings

A. SYMPTOMS AND SIGNS

Patients often attribute a variety of perianal complaints to "hemorrhoids." However, the principal problems attributable to internal hemorrhoids are bleeding, prolapse, and mucoid discharge. Bleeding is manifested by bright red blood that may range from streaks of blood visible on toilet paper or stool to bright red blood that drips into the toilet bowl after a bowel movement. Rarely is bleeding severe enough to result in anemia. Initially, internal hemorrhoids are confined to the anal canal (stage I). Over time, the internal hemorrhoids may gradually enlarge and protrude from the anal opening. At first, this mucosal prolapse occurs during straining and reduces spontaneously (stage II). With progression over time, the prolapsed hemorrhoids may require manual reduction after bowel movements (stage III) or may remain chronically protruding (stage IV). Chronically prolapsed hemorrhoids may result in a sense of fullness or discomfort and mucoid perianal discharge, resulting in irritation and soiling of underclothes. Pain is unusual with internal hemorrhoids, occurring only when there is extensive inflammation and thrombosis of irreducible tissue or with thrombosis of an external hemorrhoid (see below).

B. EXAMINATION

External hemorrhoids are readily visible on perianal inspection. Nonprolapsed internal hemorrhoids are not visible but may protrude through the anus with gentle straining while the physician spreads the buttocks. Prolapsed hemorrhoids are visible as protuberant purple nodules covered by mucosa. The perianal region should also be examined for other signs of disease such as fistulas, fissures, skin tags, or dermatitis. On digital examination, uncomplicated internal hemorrhoids are neither palpable nor painful. Anoscopic evaluation, best performed in the prone jackknife position, provides optimal visualization of internal hemorrhoids.

Differential Diagnosis

Small volume rectal bleeding may be caused by anal fissure or fistula, neoplasms of the distal colon or rectum, ulcerative colitis or Crohn's colitis, infectious proctitis, or rectal ulcers. Rectal prolapse, in which a full thickness of rectum protrudes concentrically from the anus, is readily distinguished from mucosal hemorrhoidal prolapse. Proctosigmoidoscopy should be performed in all patients with hematochezia to exclude disease in the rectum or sigmoid colon that could be misinterpreted in the presence of hemorrhoidal bleeding. Patients with iron deficiency anemia should undergo colonoscopy or barium enema to exclude disease proximal to the sigmoid colon.

Treatment

A. CONSERVATIVE MEASURES

Most patients with early (stage I and stage II) disease can be managed with conservative treatment. To decrease straining with defecation, patients should be given instructions for a high-fiber diet and told to increase fluid intake with meals. Dietary fiber may be supplemented with bran powder (1–2 tbsp twice daily added to food or in 8 oz of liquid) or with commercial psyllium bulk laxatives (eg, Metamucil, Citrucel). Suppositories and rectal ointments have no demonstrated utility in the management of mild disease. Mucoid discharge may be treated effectively by the local application of a cotton ball tucked next to the anal opening after bowel movements. For edematous, prolapsed hemorrhoids, gentle manual reduction may be supplemented by suppositories (eg, Anusol with or without hydrocortisone) or topical pads containing witch hazel (eg, Tucks) that have anesthetic and astringent properties and by warm sitz baths.

B. MEDICAL TREATMENT

Patients with stage I, stage II, and stage III hemorrhoids and recurrent bleeding despite conservative measures may be treated without anesthesia with injection sclerotherapy, rubber band ligation, or application of electrocoagulation (bipolar cautery or infrared photocoagulation). The choice of therapy is dictated by operator preference, but rubber band ligation increasingly is preferred due to its ease of use and high rate of efficacy. Major complications occur in < 2%, including pelvic sepsis, pelvic abscess, urinary retention, and bleeding. Recurrence is common unless patients alter their dietary habits.

C. SURGICAL TREATMENT

Surgical excision (hemorrhoidectomy) is reserved for < 5–10% of patients with chronic severe bleeding due to stage III or stage IV hemorrhoids or patients with acute thrombosed stage IV hemorrhoids. Complications of surgical hemorrhoidectomy include postoperative pain (which may persist for 2–4 weeks) and impaired continence.

Thrombosed External Hemorrhoid

Thrombosis of the external hemorrhoidal plexus results in a perianal hematoma. It most commonly occurs in otherwise healthy young adults and may be precipitated by coughing, heavy lifting, or straining at stool. The condition is characterized by the relatively acute onset of an exquisitely painful, tense and bluish perianal nodule covered with skin that may be up to several centimeters in size. Pain is most severe within the first few hours but gradually eases over 2–3 days as edema subsides. Symptoms may be relieved with warm sitz baths, analgesics, and ointments. If the patient is evaluated in the first 24–48 hours, removal of the clot may hasten symptomatic relief. With the patient in the lateral position, the skin around and over the lump is injected subcutaneously with 1% lidocaine using a tuberculin syringe with a 30-gauge needle. An ellipse of skin is then excised and the clot evacuated. A dry gauze dressing is applied for 12–24 hours, and daily sitz baths are then begun.

Madoff RD et al: American Gastroenterological Association technical review on the diagnosis and treatment of hemorrhoids. Gastroenterology 2004;126:1463. [PMID: 15131807]

Nisar PJ et al: Managing haemorrhoids. BMJ 2003;327:847. [PMID: 14551102]

Wehrmann T et al: Hemorrhoidal elastic band ligation with flexible videoendoscopes: a prospective, randomized comparison with the conventional technique that uses rigid proctoscopes. Gastrointest Endosc 2004;60:191. [PMID: 15278043]

ANORECTAL INFECTIONS

A number of organisms can cause inflammation of the anal and rectal mucosa. Proctitis is defined as inflammation of the distal 15 cm of rectum and is characterized by anorectal discomfort, tenesmus, constipation, and discharge. Most cases of proctitis are sexually transmitted, especially by anal-receptive intercourse. Proctocolitis implies inflammation that extends above the rectum to the sigmoid colon or more proximally and is caused by entirely different organisms such as *Campylobacter, E histolytica, Shigella*, and enteroinvasive *E coli*. These organisms are discussed earlier in the section on diarrhea. Symptoms include frequent, small-volume, bloody or watery diarrhea, urgency, cramps, and tenesmus.

Etiology & Management

Several organisms may cause infectious proctitis.

A. NEISSERIA GONORRHOEAE

Gonorrhea may cause itching, burning, tenesmus, and a mucopurulent discharge. Blind swabs of the anal canal have a sensitivity of less than 60%. Swabs should be taken for Gram staining and culture during anoscopy, expressing mucopus from the anal crypts. Cultures should also be taken from the urethra and pharynx in men and from the cervix in women. Complications of untreated infections include strictures, fissures, fistulas, and perirectal abscesses.

B. TREPONEMA PALLIDUM

Anal syphilis may be asymptomatic or may lead to perianal pain and discharge. With primary syphilis, the chancre may be at the anal margin or within the

anal canal and may mimic a fissure, fistula, or ulcer. Proctitis or inguinal lymphadenopathy may be present. With secondary syphilis, condylomata lata (pale-brown, flat verrucous lesions) may be seen, with secretion of foul-smelling mucus. The diagnosis is established with dark-field microscopy of scrapings from the chancre or condylomas. The VDRL test is positive in 75% of primary cases and in 99% of secondary cases.

C. CHLAMYDIA TRACHOMATIS

Chlamydial infection may cause proctitis similar to gonorrheal proctitis or may cause lymphogranuloma venereum, characterized by proctocolitis with fever and bloody diarrhea, painful perianal ulcerations, anorectal strictures and fistulas, and inguinal adenopathy (buboes). The diagnosis is established by serology and culture of rectal discharge or rectal biopsy.

D. HERPES SIMPLEX TYPE 2

Herpes simplex virus is a common cause of anorectal infection. Symptoms occur 4–21 days after exposure and include severe pain, itching, constipation, tenesmus, urinary retention, and radicular pain from involvement of lumbar or sacral nerve roots. Small vesicles or ulcers may be seen in the perianal area or anal canal. Sigmoidoscopy is not usually necessary but may reveal vesicular or ulcerative lesions in the distal rectum. Diagnosis is established by viral culture or antigen detection assays of vesicular fluid. Symptoms resolve within 2 weeks, but viral shedding may continue for several weeks. Patients may remain asymptomatic with or without viral shedding or may have recurrent mild relapses. Treatment of acute infection with acyclovir, 400 mg orally five times daily for 5–10 days, has been shown to reduce the duration of symptoms and viral shedding. Patients with AIDS and recurrent relapses may benefit from chronic suppressive therapy (see Chapter 32).

E. CONDYLOMATA ACUMINATA

Condylomata acuminata are a significant cause of anorectal symptoms. Caused by the human papillomavirus (HPV), they are seen in up to 25% of homosexual men. HIV-positive individuals with condylomas have a higher relapse rate after therapy and a higher rate of progression to high-grade dysplasia or anal cancer. The warts are located on the perianal skin and extend within the anal canal up to 2 cm above the dentate line. Patients may have no symptoms or may report itching, bleeding, and pain. The warts may form a confluent mass that may obscure the anal opening. Treatment can be difficult. Sexual partners should also be examined and treated. Topical application of podophyllum resin, imiquimod cream 5%, or podofilox 0.5% gel is effective for small external perianal lesions. Anal canal lesions require topical application of bichloroacetic acid, cryotherapy, or electrocautery. Refractory or large lesions may be treated with local injection of interferon-α beneath the lesions or surgical excision. HIV-positive individuals with condylomas who have detectable serum HIV RNA levels should have anoscopic surveillance every 3–6 months.

Mabey D et al: Lymphogranuloma venereum. Sex Transm Infect 2002;78:90. [PMID: 12081191]

Piketty C et al: High prevalence of anal human papillomavirus infection and anal cancer precursors among HIV-infected persons in the absence of anal intercourse. Ann Intern Med 2003;138:453. [PMID: 12639077]

Vukasin P: Anal condyloma and HIV-associated anal disease. Surg Clin North Am 2002;82:1199. [PMID: 12516848]

Workowski KA et al: Sexually transmitted diseases treatment guidelines 2002. Centers for Disease Control and Prevention. MMWR Recomm Rep 2002;51(RR-6):1. (Available at http://www.cdc.gov/mmwr/preview/mmwrhtml/rr5106a1.htm.) [PMID: 12184549]

RECTAL PROLAPSE & SOLITARY RECTAL ULCER SYNDROME

Rectal prolapse is protrusion through the anus of some or all of the layers of the rectum. Hemorrhoidal (mucosal) prolapse is common (see discussion under Hemorrhoids). Full thickness is uncommon and is usually caused by surgical or traumatic injuries or from chronic, excessive straining at stool in conjunction with weakening of pelvic support structures, especially in patients who are elderly, psychotic, or paraplegic. Although prolapse initially reduces spontaneously after defecation, with time the rectal mucosa becomes chronically prolapsed, resulting in mucous discharge, bleeding, incontinence, and sphincteric damage. Patients with complete prolapse require surgical correction.

The term solitary rectal ulcer syndrome is a misnomer. The syndrome is characterized by anal pain, excessive straining at stool, and passage of mucus and blood. It is most commonly seen in young adults, especially women. Proctoscopic examination reveals either shallow ulcerations (single or multiple) or a nodular mass located anteriorly 6–10 cm above the anal verge. Biopsy is diagnostic. The disorder may be caused by rectal intussusception or prolapse with straining. Treatment is directed at decreasing straining through education of the patient, use of bulking agents, and surgical treatment of prolapse, when present.

Purkayastha S et al: A comparison of open vs. laparoscopic abdominal rectopexy for full-thickness rectal prolapse: a meta-analysis. Dis Colon Rectum 2005;48:1930. [PMID: 15981060]

Sharara AI et al: Solitary rectal ulcer syndrome: endoscopic spectrum and review of the literature. Gastrointest Endosc 2005; 62:755. [PMID: 16246692]

FECAL INCONTINENCE

There are five general requirements for bowel continence: (1) solid or semisolid stool (even healthy young adults have difficulty maintaining continence with liquid rectal contents); (2) a distensible rectal reservoir (as sigmoid contents empty into the rectum, the vault must expand to accommodate); (3) a sensation of rectal fullness (if the patient cannot sense this, overflow may occur before the patient can take appropriate action); (4) intact pelvic nerves and muscles; and (5) the ability to reach a toilet in a timely fashion.

Minor Incontinence

Many patients complain of inability to control flatus or slight soilage of undergarments that tends to occur after bowel movements or with straining or coughing. This may be due to local anal problems such as hemorrhoids and skin tags that make it difficult to form a tight anal seal, especially if stools are somewhat loose. Patients should be treated with fiber supplements to provide greater stool bulk. Coffee and other caffeinated beverages should be eliminated. The perianal skin should be cleansed with moist, lanolin-coated tissue (baby wipes) to reduce excoriation and infection. After wiping, loose application of a cotton ball near the anal opening may absorb small amounts of fecal leakage. Prolapsing hemorrhoids may be treated with band ligation or surgical hemorrhoidectomy. Control of flatus and seepage may be improved by Kegel perineal exercises. Conditions such as ulcerative proctitis that cause tenesmus and urgency, chronic diarrheal conditions, and irritable bowel syndrome may result in difficulty in maintaining complete continence, especially if a toilet is not readily available. Loperamide may be helpful to reduce urge incontinence in patients with loose stools and may be taken in anticipation of situations in which a toilet may not be readily available. The elderly may require more time or assistance to reach a toilet, which may lead to incontinence. Scheduled toileting and the availability of a bedside commode are helpful. Elderly patients with chronic constipation may develop stool impaction leading to "overflow" incontinence.

Major Incontinence

Complete uncontrolled loss of stool reflects a significant problem with central perception or neuromuscular function. Incontinence that occurs without awareness suggests a loss of central awareness (eg, dementia, cerebrovascular accident, multiple sclerosis) or peripheral nerve injury (eg, spinal cord injury, cauda equina syndrome, pudendal nerve damage due to obstetric trauma or pelvic floor prolapse, aging, or diabetes mellitus). Incontinence that occurs despite awareness and active efforts to retain stool suggests sphincteric damage, which may be caused by traumatic childbirth (especially forceps delivery), episiotomy, prolapse, prior anal surgery, and physical trauma.

Physical examination should include careful inspection of the perianal area for hemorrhoids, rectal prolapse, fissures, fistulas, and either gaping or a keyhole defect of the anal sphincter (indicating severe sphincteric injury). The perianal skin should be stimulated to confirm an intact anocutaneous reflex. Digital examination during relaxation gives valuable information about resting tone (due mainly to the internal sphincter) and contraction of the external sphincter and pelvic floor during squeezing. It also excludes fecal impaction. Anoscopy is required to evaluate for hemorrhoids, fissures, and fistulas. Proctosigmoidoscopy is useful to exclude rectal carcinoma or proctitis. Anal ultrasonography or pelvic MRI is the most reliable test for definition of anatomic defects in the external and internal anal sphincters. Anal manometry may also be useful to define the severity of weakness, to assess sensation, and to predict response to biofeedback training. In special circumstances, surface electromyography is useful to document sphincteric denervation and proctography to document perineal descent or rectal intussusception.

Patients who are incontinent only of loose or liquid stools are treated with bulking agents and antidiarrheal drugs (eg, loperamide, 2 mg before meals and prophylactically before social engagements, shopping trips, etc). Patients with incontinence of solid stool benefit from scheduled toilet use after glycerin suppositories or tap water enemas. Biofeedback training with anal sphincteric strengthening (Kegel) exercises (alternating 5-second squeeze and 10-second rest for 10 minutes twice daily) is helpful in motivated patients to lower the threshold for awareness of rectal filling—or to improve anal sphincter squeeze function—or both. Operative management is seldom needed but should be considered in patients with major incontinence due to prior injury to the anal sphincter who have failed medical therapy.

Madoff RD et al: Faecal incontinence in adults. Lancet 2004; 364:621. [PMID: 15313364]

Rao SS et al: Diagnosis and management of fecal incontinence. American College of Gastroenterology Practice Parameters Committee. Am J Gastroenterol 2004;99:1585. [PMID: 15307881]

Schnelle JF et al: Urinary and fecal incontinence in nursing homes. Gastroenterology 2004;126(1 Suppl 1):S41. [PMID: 14978637]

OTHER ANAL CONDITIONS

Anal Fissures

Anal fissures are linear or rocket-shaped ulcers that are usually less than 5 mm in length. Most fissures are believed to arise from trauma to the anal canal during defecation, perhaps caused by straining, constipation, or high internal sphincter tone. They occur most commonly in the posterior midline, but 10% occur anteriorly. Fissures that occur off the midline should raise suspicion for Crohn's disease, HIV/AIDS, tuberculosis, syphilis, or anal carcinoma. Patients complain of severe, tearing pain during defecation followed by throbbing discomfort that may lead to constipation due to fear of recurrent pain. There may be mild associated hematochezia, with blood on the stool or toilet

paper. Anal fissures are confirmed by visual inspection of the anal verge while gently separating the buttocks. Acute fissures look like cracks in the epithelium. Chronic fissures result in fibrosis and the development of a skin tag at the outermost edge (sentinel pile). Digital and anoscopic examinations may cause severe pain and may not be possible. Medical management is directed at promoting effortless, painless bowel movements. Fiber supplements and sitz baths should be prescribed. Suppositories are of no benefit. Topical 0.2–0.4% nitroglycerin ointment (1 cm of ointment) applied twice daily just inside the anus with the tip of a finger for 6–8 weeks results in healing in 50–80% of patients with chronic anal fissure; however, headaches occur in up to 40%. Injection of botulinum toxin (20 units) into the internal anal sphincter has been shown to cause healing in over 80% of patients with chronic anal fissure. Fissures may recur in up to 40% of patients treated with either nitrates or botulinum toxin. Chronic or recurrent fissures benefit from lateral internal sphincterotomy; however, minor incontinence may complicate this procedure.

Arroyo A et al: Surgical versus chemical (botulinum toxin) sphincterotomy for chronic anal fissure: long term results from a prospective randomized clinical and manometric study. Am J Surg 2005;189:429. [PMID: 15820455]

Madoff RD et al: AGA technical review on the diagnosis and care of patients with anal fissure. Gastroenterology 2003;124: 235. [PMID: 12512046]

Utzig MJ et al: Concepts in the pathogenesis and treatment of chronic anal fissure—a review of the literature. Am J Gastroenterol 2003;98:968. [PMID: 12809816]

Perianal Abscess & Fistula

The anal glands located at the base of the anal crypts at the dentate line may become infected, leading to abscess formation. Other causes of abscess include anal fissure and Crohn's disease. Abscesses may extend upward or downward through the intersphincteric plane. Symptoms of perianal abscess are throbbing, continuous perianal pain. Erythema, fluctuance, and swelling may be found in the perianal region on external examination or in the ischiorectal fossa on digital rectal examination. Perianal abscesses are treated with local incision and drainage, while ischiorectal abscesses require drainage in the operating room. After drainage of an abscess, most patients are found to have a fistula in ano.

Fistula in ano most often arises in an anal crypt and is usually preceded by an anal abscess. In patients with fistulas that connect to the rectum, other disorders such as Crohn's disease, lymphogranuloma venereum, rectal tuberculosis, and cancer should be considered. Fistulas are associated with purulent discharge that may lead to itching, tenderness, and pain. The treatment of Crohn's-related fistula is discussed elsewhere in this chapter. Treatment of idiopathic fistula in ano is by surgical incision or excision under anesthesia. Care must be taken to preserve the anal sphincters.

Pruritus Ani

Pruritus ani is characterized by perianal itching and discomfort. It may be caused by poor anal hygiene associated with fistulas, fissures, prolapsed hemorrhoids, skin tags, and minor incontinence. Conversely, overzealous cleansing with soaps may contribute to local irritation or contact dermatitis. Contact dermatitis, atopic dermatitis, bacterial infections (staphylococcus or streptococcus), parasites (pinworms, scabies), candidal infection (especially in diabetics), sexually transmitted disease (condylomata acuminata, herpes, syphilis, molluscum contagiosum), and other skin conditions (psoriasis, Paget's) must be excluded. In patients with idiopathic pruritus ani, examination may reveal erythema, excoriations, or lichenified, eczematous skin. Education is vital to successful therapy. Spicy foods, coffee, chocolate, and tomatoes may cause irritation and should be eliminated. After bowel movements, the perianal area should be cleansed with nonscented wipes premoistened with lanolin followed by gentle drying. A piece of cotton ball should be tucked next to the anal opening to absorb perspiration or fecal seepage. Anal ointments and lotions may exacerbate the condition and should be avoided. A short course of high-potency topical corticosteroid may be tried, although efficacy has not been demonstrated. Diluted capsaicin cream (0.006%) led to symptomatic relief in 75% of patients in a recent double-blind crossover study.

Oztas MO et al: Idiopathic perianal pruritus: washing compared with topical corticosteroids. Postgrad Med J 2004;80:295. [PMID: 15138322]

Weichert GE: An approach to the treatment of anogenital pruritus. Dermatol Ther 2004;17:129. [PMID: 14756897]

CARCINOMA OF THE ANUS

These tumors are relatively rare, comprising only 1–2% of all cancers of the anus and large intestine. Squamous cancers make up the majority of anal cancers. Squamous cancer involving the anal canal may be subclassified as transitional and cloacogenic carcinoma; however, these are treated similarly. Anal cancer is increased among people practicing receptive anal intercourse and those with a history of other sexually transmitted diseases. In over 80% of cases, HPV may be detected, suggesting that this virus may be a causal factor. Anal cancer is increased in HIV-infected individuals. Combined HIV and HPV infection markedly increases the risk of anal carcinoma. Bleeding, pain, and local tumor are the commonest symptoms. The lesion is often confused with hemorrhoids or other common anal disorders. These tumors tend to become annular, invade the sphincter, and spread upward via the lymphatics into the perirectal mesenteric lymphatic nodes.

Treatment depends on the tumor stage. MR scan and endoluminal ultrasound assist in determining the depth of penetration and local spread. Small (< 3 cm) superficial lesions of the perianal skin may be treated with wide local excision. Squamous cancer of the anal canal and large perianal tumors invading the sphincter or rectum are treated with combined-modality therapy that includes external radiation with simultaneous chemotherapy (fluorouracil and either mitomycin or cisplatin). Local control is achieved in 80% of patients. Radical surgery (abdominoperineal resection) is reserved for patients who fail chemotherapy and radiation therapy. The 5-year survival rate is 60–70% for localized tumors and over 25% for metastatic (stage IV) disease.

Anal Cancer (PDQ) Treatment—National Cancer Institute—Cancer Net: http://cancernet.nci.nih.gov.

Moore HG et al: Anal neoplasms. Surg Clin North Am 2002; 82:1233. [PMID: 12516851]

Welton ML et al: The etiology and epidemiology of anal cancer. Surg Oncol Clin N Am 2004;13:263. [PMID: 15137956]

Liver, Biliary Tract, & Pancreas

15

Lawrence S. Friedman, MD

JAUNDICE (Icterus)

ESSENTIALS OF DIAGNOSIS

- *Results from accumulation of bilirubin in the body tissues; cause may be hepatic or nonhepatic.*
- *Hyperbilirubinemia may be due to abnormalities in the formation, transport, metabolism, and excretion of bilirubin.*
- *Total serum bilirubin is normally 0.2–1.2 mg/dL; jaundice may not be recognizable until levels are about 3 mg/dL.*
- *Evaluation of obstructive jaundice begins with ultrasonography and is usually followed by cholangiography.*

General Considerations

Jaundice results from the accumulation of bilirubin—a reddish pigment product of heme metabolism—in the body tissues; the cause may be hepatic or nonhepatic. Hyperbilirubinemia may be due to abnormalities in the formation, transport, metabolism, and excretion of bilirubin. Total serum bilirubin is normally 0.2–1.2 mg/dL (mean levels are higher in men than women and higher in whites and hispanics than blacks), and jaundice may not be recognizable until levels are about 3 mg/dL.

Jaundice is caused by predominantly unconjugated or conjugated bilirubin in the serum (Table 15–1). Unconjugated hyperbilirubinemia may result from overproduction of bilirubin because of hemolysis; impaired hepatic uptake of bilirubin due to certain drugs; or impaired conjugation of bilirubin by glucuronide, as in Gilbert's syndrome, due to mild decreases in glucuronyl transferase, or Crigler–Najjar syndrome, caused by moderate decreases or absence of glucuronyl transferase. In the absence of liver disease, hemolysis rarely elevates the serum bilirubin level to more than 7 mg/dL. Predominantly conjugated hyperbilirubinemia may result from impaired excretion of bilirubin from the liver due to hepatocellular disease, drugs, sepsis,

hereditary disorders such as Dubin–Johnson syndrome, or extrahepatic biliary obstruction. Features of some hyperbilirubinemic syndromes are summarized in Table 15–2. The term "cholestasis" denotes retention of bile in the liver, and the term "cholestatic jaundice" is often used when conjugated hyperbilirubinemia results from impaired bile flow.

Manifestations of Diseases Associated with Jaundice

A. UNCONJUGATED HYPERBILIRUBINEMIA

Stool and urine color are normal, and there is mild jaundice and indirect (unconjugated) hyperbilirubinemia with no bilirubin in the urine. Splenomegaly occurs in hemolytic disorders except in sickle cell anemia. Abdominal or back pain may occur with acute hemolytic crises.

B. CONJUGATED HYPERBILIRUBINEMIA

1. Hereditary cholestatic syndromes or intrahepatic cholestasis—The patient may be asymptomatic; intermittent cholestasis is often accompanied by pruritus, light-colored stools, and, occasionally, malaise.

2. Hepatocellular disease—Malaise, anorexia, low-grade fever, and right upper quadrant discomfort are frequent. Dark urine, jaundice, and, in women, amenorrhea occur. An enlarged tender liver, vascular spiders, palmar erythema, ascites, gynecomastia, sparse body hair, fetor hepaticus, and asterixis may be present, depending on the cause, severity, and chronicity of liver dysfunction.

C. BILIARY OBSTRUCTION

There may be right upper quadrant pain, weight loss (suggesting carcinoma), jaundice, dark urine, and light-colored stools. Symptoms and signs may be intermittent if caused by stone, carcinoma of the ampulla, or cholangiocarcinoma. Pain may be absent early in pancreatic cancer. Occult blood in the stools suggests cancer of the ampulla. Hepatomegaly and a palpable gallbladder (Courvoisier's sign) are characteristic, but neither specific nor sensitive, of pancreatic head tumor. Fever and chills are far more common in benign obstruction and associated cholangitis.

Table 15–1. Classification of jaundice.

Type of Hyperbilirubinemia	Location and Cause
Unconjugated hyperbilirubinemia (predominant indirect-reacting bilirubin)	Increased bilirubin production (eg, hemolytic anemias, hemolytic reactions, hematoma, pulmonary infarction)
	Impaired bilirubin uptake and storage (eg, posthepatitis hyperbilirubinemia, Gilbert's syndrome, Crigler-Najjar syndrome, drug reactions)
Conjugated hyperbilirubinemia (predominant direct-reacting bilirubin)	**HEREDITARY CHOLESTATIC SYNDROMES**
	Faulty excretion of bilirubin conjugates (eg, Dubin-Johnson syndrome, Rotor's syndrome) or mutation in genes coding for bile salt transport proteins (eg, progressive familial intrahepatic cholestasis syndromes and benign recurrent intrahepatic cholestasis)
	HEPATOCELLULAR DYSFUNCTION
	Biliary epithelial damage (eg, hepatitis, hepatic cirrhosis)
	Intrahepatic cholestasis (eg, certain drugs, biliary cirrhosis, sepsis, postoperative jaundice)
	Hepatocellular damage or intrahepatic cholestasis resulting from miscellaneous causes (eg, spirochetal infections, infectious mononucleosis, cholangitis, sarcoidosis, lymphomas, industrial toxins)
	BILIARY OBSTRUCTION
	Choledocholithiasis, biliary atresia, carcinoma of biliary duct, sclerosing cholangitis, choledochal cyst, external pressure on common duct, pancreatitis, pancreatic neoplasms

Diagnostic Methods for Evaluation of Liver Disease & Jaundice (Tables 15–3, 15–4)

A. LABORATORY STUDIES

Serum alanine and aspartate aminotransferase (ALT and AST) levels vary with age and correlate with body mass index and possibly with mortality from liver disease and inversely with caffeine consumption. Normal reference values for ALT and AST may be lower than generally reported when persons with risk factors for fatty liver are excluded. Elevated ALT and AST levels result from hepatocellular necrosis or inflammation (Table 15–4). Elevated alkaline phosphatase levels are seen in cholestasis or infiltrative liver disease (such as tumor or granuloma). Alkaline phosphatase elevations of hepatic rather than bone, intestinal, or placental origin are confirmed by concomitant elevation of γ-glutamyl transpeptidase or 5'-nucleotidase levels. The differential diagnosis of any liver test elevation includes toxicity caused by drugs, herbal remedies, and toxins.

B. LIVER BIOPSY

Percutaneous liver biopsy is the definitive study for determining the cause and histologic severity of hepatocellular dysfunction or infiltrative liver disease. In patients with suspected metastatic disease or a hepatic mass, it is performed under ultrasound or CT guidance. A transjugular route can be used in patients with coagulopathy or ascites.

C. IMAGING

Demonstration of dilated bile ducts by ultrasonography or CT scan indicates biliary obstruction (90–95% sensitivity). Ultrasonography, CT scan, and MRI may also demonstrate hepatomegaly, intrahepatic tumors, and portal hypertension. Spiral arterial-phase and multislice CT scanning, in which the liver is imaged during peak hepatic enhancement while the patient holds one or two breaths, improves diagnostic accuracy. Multiphasic spiral or multislice CT, CT arterial portography, in which imaging follows intravenous contrast infusion via a catheter placed in the superior mesenteric artery, MRI with use of gadolinium or ferumoxides as contrast agents, and intraoperative ultrasonography are the most sensitive techniques for detection of individual small hepatic lesions in patients eligible for resection of metastases. Use of color Doppler ultrasound or contrast agents that produce microbubbles increases the sensitivity of transcutaneous ultrasound for detecting small neoplasms. MRI is the

Table 15–2. Hyperbilirubinemic disorders.

	Nature of Defect	Type of Hyper-bilirubinemia	Clinical and Pathologic Characteristics
Gilbert's syndrome	Reduced activity of glucuronyl transferase	Unconjugated (indirect) bilirubin	Benign, asymptomatic hereditary jaundice. Hyperbilirubinemia increased by 24- to 36-hour fast. No treatment required. Prognosis excellent.
Dubin-Johnson syndrome[1]	Faulty excretory function of hepatocytes	Conjugated (direct) bilirubin	Benign, asymptomatic hereditary jaundice. Gallbladder does not visualize on oral cholecystography. Liver darkly pigmented on gross examination. Biopsy shows centrilobular brown pigment. Prognosis excellent.
Rotor's syndrome			Similar to Dubin-Johnson syndrome, but liver is not pigmented and the gallbladder is visualized on oral cholecystography. Prognosis excellent.
Benign recurrent intrahepatic cholestasis[2]	Cholestasis, often on a familial basis	Unconjugated plus conjugated (total) bilirubin	Episodic attacks of jaundice, itching, and malaise. Onset in early life and may persist for a lifetime. Alkaline phosphatase increased. Cholestasis found on liver biopsy. (Biopsy is normal during remission.) Prognosis excellent.
Recurrent jaundice of pregnancy			Benign cholestatic jaundice of unknown cause, usually occurring in the third trimester of pregnancy. Itching, gastrointestinal symptoms, and abnormal liver excretory function tests. Cholestasis noted on liver biopsy. Prognosis excellent, but recurrence with subsequent pregnancies or use of birth control pills is characteristic.

[1]The Dubin-Johnson syndrome is caused by a point mutation in the gene coding for an organic anion transporter in bile canaliculi on chromosome 10q23–24.
[2]Mutations in genes that control hepatocellular transport systems that are involved in the formation of bile and inherited as autosomal recessive traits are on chromosomes 18q21–22, 2q24, and 7q21 in families with progressive familial intrahepatic cholestasis. Gene mutations on chromosome 18q21–22 alter a P-type ATPase expressed in the small intestine and liver and others on chromosome 2q24 alter the bile acid export pump and cause benign recurrent intrahepatic cholestasis.

most accurate technique for identifying isolated liver lesions such as hemangiomas, focal nodular hyperplasia, or focal fatty infiltration and for detecting hepatic iron overload. Because of its much lower cost (amount charged), ultrasonography ($500) is preferable to CT ($1200–$1400) or MRI ($2000) as a screening test.

Table 15–3. Liver function tests: Normal values and changes in two types of jaundice.[1]

Tests	Normal Values	Hepatocellular Jaundice	Uncomplicated Obstructive Jaundice
Bilirubin			
Direct	0.1–0.3 mg/dL	Increased	Increased
Indirect	0.2–0.7 mg/dL	Increased	Increased
Urine bilirubin	None	Increased	Increased
Serum albumin/total protein	Albumin, 3.5–5.5 g/dL	Albumin decreased Total protein, 6.5–8.4 g/dL	Unchanged
Alkaline phosphatase	30–115 units/L	Increased (+)	Increased (++++)
Prothrombin time	INR of 1.0–1.4. After vitamin K, 10% increase in 24 hours	Prolonged if damage severe and does not respond to parenteral vitamin K	Prolonged if obstruction marked, but responds to parenteral vitamin K
ALT, AST	ALT, 5–35 units/L; AST, 5–40 units/L	Increased in hepatocellular damage, viral hepatitis	Minimally increased

[1]INR, international normalized ratio; ALT, alanine aminotransferase; AST, aspartate aminotransferase.

Table 15–4. Causes of serum aminotransferase elevations.[1]

Mild Elevations[2] (< 5× normal)	Severe Elevations (> 15× normal)
Hepatic: ALT-predominant	Acute viral hepatitis
Chronic hepatitis B, C, and D	(A-E, herpes)
Acute viral hepatitis (A-E,	Medications/toxins
EBV, CMV)	Ischemic hepatitis
Steatosis/steatohepatitis	Autoimmune hepatitis
Hemochromatosis	Wilson's disease
Medications/toxins	Acute bile duct obstruc-
Autoimmune hepatitis	tion
α_1-Antitrypsin deficiency	Acute Budd-Chiari syn-
Wilson's disease	drome
Celiac disease	Hepatic artery ligation
Hepatic: AST-predominant	
Alcohol-related liver injury	
(AST:ALT > 2:1)	
Cirrhosis	
Nonhepatic	
Strenuous exercise	
Hemolysis	
Myopathy	
Thyroid disease	
Macro-AST	

Adapted from Green RM, Flamm S: AGA technical review on the evaluation of liver chemistry tests. Gastroenterology 2002;123:1367.
[1]Almost any liver disease can cause moderate aminotransferase elevations (5–15× normal).
[2]EBV, Epstein-Barr virus; CMV, cytomegalovirus; ALT, alanine aminotransferase; AST, aspartate aminotransferase.

Ultrasonography can detect gallstones with a sensitivity of 95%.

Endoscopic retrograde cholangiopancreatography (ERCP) or percutaneous transhepatic cholangiography (PTC) identifies the cause, location, and extent of biliary obstruction. Magnetic resonance cholangiopancreatography (MRCP) appears to be a sensitive, noninvasive method of detecting bile duct stones, strictures, and dilation; however, it is less reliable than ERCP for distinguishing malignant from benign strictures. ERCP requires a skilled endoscopist and may be used to demonstrate pancreatic or ampullary causes of jaundice, to carry out papillotomy and stone extraction, or to insert a stent through an obstructing lesion. Complications of ERCP include pancreatitis (5%) and, less commonly, cholangitis, bleeding, or duodenal perforation after papillotomy. Risk factors for post-ERCP pancreatitis include female gender, prior post-ERCP pancreatitis, suspected sphincter of Oddi dysfunction, and a difficult or failed cannulation. Severe complications of PTC occur in 3% and include fever, bacteremia, bile peritonitis, and intraperitoneal hemorrhage. Endoscopic ultrasonography is the most sensitive test for detecting small lesions of the ampulla or pancreatic head and for detecting portal vein invasion by pancreatic cancer. It is also accurate in detecting or excluding bile duct stones.

ASGE guideline: The role of ERCP in diseases of the biliary tract and the pancreas. Gastrointest Endosc 2005; 62:1. [PMID: 15990812]

Balistreri WF et al: Intrahepatic cholestasis: summary of an American Association for the Study of Liver Diseases Single-Topic Conference. Hepatology 2005;42:222. [PMID: 15898074]

Cheng C-L et al: Risk factors for post-ERCP pancreatitis: a prospective multicenter study. Am J Gastroenterol 2006;101: 139. [PMID: 16405547]

Elinav E et al: Correlation between serum alanine aminotransferase activity and age: an inverted U curve pattern. Am J Gastroenterol 2005;100:2201. [PMID: 16181369]

Goessling WG et al: Increased liver chemistry in an asymptomatic patient. Clin Gastroenterol Hepatol 2005;3:852. [PMID: 16234021]

Ioannou GN et al: The prevalence and predictors of elevated serum aminotransferase activity in the United States in 1999-2002. Am J Gastroenterol 2006;101:76. [PMID: 16405537]

Sheela H el al: Liver biopsy: evolving role in the new millennium. J Clin Gastroenterol 2005;39:603. [PMID: 16000929]

■ DISEASES OF THE LIVER

VIRAL HEPATITIS

 ESSENTIALS OF DIAGNOSIS

- *Prodrome of anorexia, nausea, vomiting, malaise, aversion to smoking.*
- *Fever, enlarged and tender liver, jaundice.*
- *Normal to low white cell count; abnormal liver tests, especially markedly elevated aminotransferases early in the course.*
- *Liver biopsy shows hepatocellular necrosis and mononuclear infiltrate but is rarely indicated.*

General Considerations

Hepatitis can be caused by many drugs and toxic agents as well as by numerous viruses, the clinical manifestations of which may be quite similar. Viruses causing hepatitis are (1) hepatitis A virus (HAV), (2) hepatitis B virus (HBV), (3) hepatitis C virus (HCV), (4) hepatitis D virus (HDV) (delta agent), and (5) hepatitis E virus (HEV) (an enterically transmitted hepatitis seen in epidemic form in Asia, North Africa, and Mexico). The designation hepatitis G virus (HGV) applies to a virus that rarely, if ever, causes frank hepatitis. A DNA virus designated the TT virus (TTV) has been identified in up to 7.5% of blood donors and found to be transmitted readily by blood transfusions, but an association between this virus and liver disease has not been established. A related virus known as SEN-V has been found in 2% of US blood donors, is transmitted by transfusion, and may account for some cases of transfusion-associated non-ABCDE hepatitis. In immunocompromised and rare immunocompetent persons, cytomegalovirus, Epstein–Barr virus, and herpes simplex virus should be considered in the differential diagnosis of hepatitis. Severe acute respiratory syndrome (SARS) may be associated with marked serum aminotransferase elevations. As yet unidentified pathogens account for a small percentage of cases of apparent acute viral hepatitis.

A. Hepatitis A

Figure 15–1 shows the typical course of HAV infection. HAV is a 27-nm RNA hepatovirus (in the picornavirus family) causing epidemics or sporadic cases of hepatitis. The virus is transmitted by the fecal–oral route, and its spread is favored by crowding and poor sanitation. Since introduction of the HAV vaccine in the United States in 1995, the incidence rate of HAV infection has declined by 76%. Common source outbreaks result from contaminated water or food, including inadequately cooked shellfish. A large outbreak among patrons of a restaurant in Monaca, Pennsylvania, in 2003 was traced to contaminated green onions from Mexico. The incubation period averages 30 days. HAV is excreted in feces for up to 2 weeks before clinical illness but rarely after the first week of illness. The mortality rate for hepatitis A is low, and fulminant hepatitis A is uncommon except for rare instances in which it occurs in a patient with chronic hepatitis C. Chronic hepatitis A does not occur, and there is no carrier state. Clinical illness is more severe in adults than in children, in whom it is

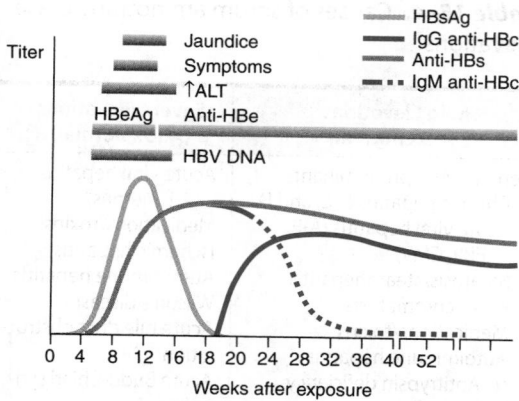

Figure 15–2. The typical course of acute type B hepatitis. (HBsAg, hepatitis B surface antigen; anti-HBs, antibody to HBsAg; HBeAg, hepatitis Be antigen; anti-HBe, antibody to HBeAg; anti-HBc, antibody to hepatitis B core antigen; ALT, alanine aminotransferase.) (Reprinted with permission from Koff RS: Acute viral hepatitis. In: *Handbook of Liver Disease.* Friedman LS, Keeffe EB [editors], 2nd ed. ©Elsevier, 2004.)

typically asymptomatic. It is the only viral hepatitis causing spiking fevers. Rare cases of acute cholecystitis during the course of acute hepatitis A have been described.

Antibody to hepatitis A (anti-HAV) appears early in the course of the illness. Both IgM and IgG anti-HAV are detectable in serum soon after the onset. Peak titers of IgM anti-HAV occur during the first week of clinical disease and disappear within 3–6 months. Detection of IgM anti-HAV is an excellent test for diagnosing acute hepatitis A but is not recommended for the evaluation of asymptomatic persons with persistently elevated serum aminotransferase levels because false-positive results occur. Titers of IgG anti-HAV rise after 1 month of the disease and may persist for years. IgG anti-HAV indicates previous exposure to HAV, noninfectivity, and immunity. In the United States, about 30% of the population have serologic evidence of previous infection.

B. Hepatitis B

Figure 15–2 shows the typical course of HBV infection. HBV is a 42-nm hepadnavirus with a partially double-stranded DNA genome, inner core protein (hepatitis B core antigen, HBcAg), and outer surface coat (hepatitis B surface antigen, HBsAg). There are eight different genotypes (A–H), which may influence the course of infection and responsiveness to antiviral therapy. HBV is usually transmitted by inoculation of infected blood or blood products or by sexual contact and is present in saliva, semen, and vaginal secretions. HBsAg-positive mothers may transmit HBV at delivery; the risk of chronic infection in the infant is as high as 90%.

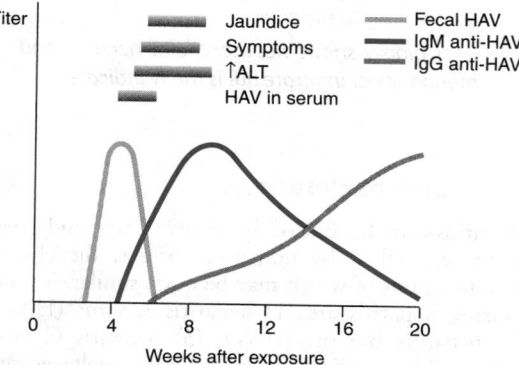

Figure 15–1. The typical course of acute type A hepatitis. (HAV, hepatitis A virus; anti-HAV, antibody to hepatitis A virus; ALT, alanine aminotransferase.) (Reprinted with permission from Koff RS: Acute viral hepatitis. In: *Handbook of Liver Disease.* Friedman LS, Keeffe EB [editors], 2nd ed. ©Elsevier, 2004.)

Table 15–5. Common serologic patterns in hepatitis B virus infection and their interpretation.

HBsAg	Anti-HBs	Anti-HBc	HBeAg	Anti-HBe	Interpretation
+	−	IgM	+	−	Acute hepatitis B
+	−	IgG[1]	+	−	Chronic hepatitis B with active viral replication
+	−	IgG	−	+	Chronic hepatitis B with low viral replication
+	+	IgG	+ or −	+ or −	Chronic hepatitis B with heterotypic anti-HBs (about 10% of cases)
−	−	IgM	+ or −	−	Acute hepatitis B
−	+	IgG	−	+ or −	Recovery from hepatitis B (immunity)
−	+	−	−	−	Vaccination (immunity)
−	−	IgG	−	−	False-positive; less commonly, infection in remote past

[1]Low levels of IgM anti-HBc may also be detected.

HBV is prevalent in men who have sex with men and in injection drug users (about 7% of human immunodeficiency virus [HIV]-infected persons are coinfected with HBV), but the greatest number of cases results from heterosexual transmission; the incidence has decreased by 75% since the 1980s. Groups at risk include patients and staff at hemodialysis centers, physicians, dentists, nurses, and personnel working in clinical and pathology laboratories and blood banks. Half of all patients with acute hepatitis B in the United States have previously been incarcerated or treated for a sexually transmitted disease. The risk of HBV infection from a blood transfusion is less than 1 in 60,000 units transfused in the United States. The incubation period of hepatitis B is 6 weeks to 6 months (average 12–14 weeks).

The onset of hepatitis B is more insidious and the aminotransferase levels are higher than in HAV infection. The risk of fulminant hepatitis is less than 1%, with a mortality rate of up to 60%. Following acute hepatitis B, HBV infection persists in 1–2% of immunocompetent adults but in a higher percentage of immunocompromised adults or children. Persons with chronic hepatitis B, particularly when HBV infection is acquired early in life and viral replication persists, are at substantial risk of cirrhosis and hepatocellular carcinoma (up to 25–40%). Men are more at risk than women. Infection caused by HBV may be associated with serum sickness, glomerulonephritis, and polyarteritis nodosa.

There are three distinct antigen–antibody systems that relate to HBV infection and circulating markers that are useful in diagnosis. Interpretation of common serologic patterns is shown in Table 15–5.

1. HBsAg—The appearance of HBsAg is the first evidence of infection, appearing before biochemical evidence of liver disease, and persists throughout the clinical illness. Persistence of HBsAg after the acute illness may be associated with clinical and laboratory evidence of chronic hepatitis for variable periods of time.

The detection of HBsAg establishes infection with HBV and implies infectivity.

2. Anti-HBs—Specific antibody to HBsAg (anti-HBs) appears in most individuals after clearance of HBsAg and after successful vaccination against hepatitis B. Disappearance of HBsAg and the appearance of anti-HBs signal recovery from HBV infection, noninfectivity, and immunity.

3. Anti-HBc—IgM anti-HBc appears shortly after HBsAg is detected. (HBcAg alone does not appear in serum.) Its presence in the setting of acute hepatitis B indicates a diagnosis of acute hepatitis B, and it fills the serologic gap in patients who have cleared HBsAg but do not yet have detectable anti-HBs. IgM anti-HBc can persist for 3–6 months or longer. IgM anti-HBc may also reappear during flares of previously inactive chronic hepatitis B. IgG anti-HBc also appears during acute hepatitis B but persists indefinitely, whether the patient recovers (with the appearance of anti-HBs in serum) or develops chronic hepatitis B (with persistence of HBsAg). In asymptomatic blood donors, an isolated anti-HBc with no other positive HBV serologic results may represent a falsely positive result or latent infection in which HBV DNA is detectable only by polymerase chain reaction testing.

4. HBeAg—HBeAg is a soluble protein found only in HBsAg-positive serum. It is a secretory form of HBcAg appearing during the incubation period shortly after the detection of HBsAg. HBeAg indicates viral replication and infectivity. Persistence of HBeAg in serum beyond 3 months indicates an increased likelihood of chronic hepatitis B. Its disappearance is often followed by the appearance of anti-HBe, signifying diminished viral replication and decreased infectivity.

5. HBV DNA—The presence of HBV DNA in serum generally parallels the presence of HBeAg, although HBV DNA is a more sensitive and precise marker of viral replication and infectivity. Very low levels of HBV DNA, detectable only by polymerase chain reaction testing, may persist in serum and liver long after a patient has recovered from acute hepatitis B, but the HBV DNA in serum is bound to IgG and is rarely infectious. In some patients with chronic hepatitis B, HBV DNA is present at high levels without HBeAg in serum because of a mutation that prevents synthesis of HBeAg in infected hepatocytes. This "pre-core mutant" appears during the course of chronic wild-type HBV infection, presumably as a result of immune pressure. When additional mutations in the core gene are present, the pre-core mutant enhances the severity of HBV and increases the risk of cirrhosis.

C. HEPATITIS D (DELTA AGENT)

HDV is a defective RNA virus that causes hepatitis only in association with hepatitis B infection and specifically only in the presence of HBsAg; it is cleared when the latter is cleared.

HDV may coinfect with HBV or may superinfect a person with chronic hepatitis B, usually by percutaneous exposure. When acute hepatitis D is coincident with acute HBV infection, the infection is generally similar in severity to acute hepatitis B alone. In chronic hepatitis B, superinfection by HDV appears to carry a worse short-term prognosis, often resulting in fulminant hepatitis or severe chronic hepatitis that progresses rapidly to cirrhosis.

In the 1970s and early 1980s, HDV was endemic in some areas, such as the Mediterranean countries, where up to 80% of HBV carriers were superinfected with it. In the United States, HDV occurred primarily among injection drug users. However, new cases of hepatitis D are now infrequent (for reasons that are not entirely clear), and cases seen today are usually from cohorts infected years ago who survived the initial impact of hepatitis D and now have inactive cirrhosis. These patients have a threefold increased risk of hepatocellular carcinoma. Diagnosis is made by detection of antibody to hepatitis D antigen (anti-HDV) or, where available, HDV RNA in serum.

D. HEPATITIS C

Figure 15–3 shows the typical course of HCV infection. HCV is a single-stranded RNA virus (hepacivirus) with properties similar to those of flavivirus. At least six major genotypes of HCV have been identified. In the past, HCV was responsible for over 90% of cases of posttransfusion hepatitis, yet only 4% of cases of hepatitis C were attributable to blood transfusions. Over 50% of cases are transmitted by injection drug use. Intranasal cocaine use, body piercing, and hemodialysis also are risk factors. The risk of sexual and maternal–neonatal transmission is low and may be greatest in a subset of patients with high circulating levels of HCV RNA. Having multiple sexual partners may increase the risk of HCV infection. Transmission via breast-feeding has not been documented. An outbreak of hepatitis C in patients with immune deficiencies occurred in some recipients of intravenous im-

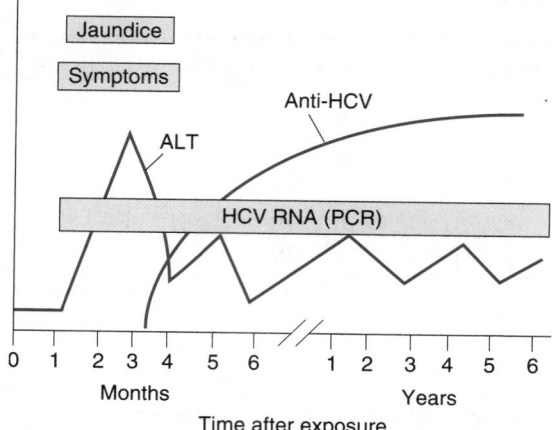

Figure 15–3. The typical course of acute and chronic hepatitis C. (ALT, alanine aminotransferase; Anti-HCV, antibody to hepatitis C virus by enzyme immunoassay; HCV RNA [PCR], hepatitis C viral RNA by polymerase chain reaction.)

mune globulin, and nosocomial transmission has occurred via multidose vials of saline used to flush Portacaths, through reuse of disposable syringes and contamination of shared saline bags, and between hospitalized patients on a liver unit. Coinfection with HCV is found in at least 30% of persons infected with HIV; HIV infection leads to an increased risk of acute hepatic failure and more rapid progression of chronic hepatitis C to cirrhosis; in addition, HCV increases the hepatotoxicity of highly active antiretroviral therapy. Covert transmission during bloody fisticuffs has even been reported. In many patients, the source of infection is unknown. There are more than 2.7 million HCV carriers in the United States and another 1.3 million previously exposed persons who have cleared the virus.

The incubation period averages 6–7 weeks, and clinical illness is often mild, usually asymptomatic, and characterized by waxing and waning aminotransferase elevations and a high rate (> 80%) of chronic hepatitis. In pregnant patients, serum aminotransferase levels frequently normalize despite persistence of viremia, only to increase again after delivery. HCV is a pathogenetic factor in mixed **cryoglobulinemia** and membranoproliferative glomerulonephritis and may be related to lichen planus, autoimmune thyroiditis, lymphocytic sialadenitis, idiopathic pulmonary fibrosis, sporadic porphyria cutanea tarda, monoclonal gammopathies, and probably lymphoma. Hepatitis C may induce insulin resistance (which in turn increases the risk of hepatic fibrosis), and the risk of type 2 diabetes mellitus is increased in persons with chronic hepatitis C. Hepatic steatosis is a particular feature of infection with HCV genotype 3 and may also occur in patients with risk factors for fatty liver (see below).

Diagnosis of hepatitis C is based on an enzyme immunoassay that detects antibodies to HCV. Anti-HCV is not protective, and in patients with acute or chronic hepatitis its presence in serum generally signifies that HCV is the cause. Limitations of the enzyme immunoassay include moderate sensitivity (false-negatives) for the diagnosis of acute hepatitis C early in the course and in healthy blood donors and low specificity (false-positives) in some persons with elevated γ-globulin levels. In these situations, a diagnosis of hepatitis C may be confirmed by using an assay for HCV RNA and, in some cases, a supplemental recombinant immunoblot assay (RIBA) for anti-HCV. Most RIBA-positive persons are potentially infectious, as confirmed by use of polymerase chain reaction-based tests to detect HCV RNA. Occasional persons are found to have anti-HCV in serum, confirmed by RIBA, without HCV RNA in serum, suggesting recovery from HCV infection in the past. Testing donated blood for HCV has helped reduce the risk of transfusion-associated hepatitis C from 10% in 1990 to about 1 case per 2 million units today.

E. HEPATITIS E

HEV is a 29- to 32-nm RNA virus similar to calicivirus and responsible for waterborne hepatitis outbreaks in India, Burma, Afghanistan, Algeria, Mexico, and recently Sudan and Iraq. It is rare in the United States but should be considered in patients with acute hepatitis after a trip to an endemic area. Illness is self-limited (no carrier state), with a high mortality rate (10–20%) in pregnant women and an increased risk of hepatic decompensation in patients with underlying chronic liver disease.

F. HEPATITIS G

The designation HGV has been applied to a flavivirus that is percutaneously transmitted and associated with chronic viremia lasting at least 10 years. HGV has been detected in 1.5% of blood donors, 50% of injection drug users, 30% of hemodialysis patients, 20% of hemophiliacs, and 15% of patients with chronic hepatitis B or C, but it does not appear to cause important liver disease or affect the response of patients with chronic hepatitis B or C to antiviral therapy. HGV coinfection may improve survival in patients with HIV infection.

Clinical Findings

The clinical picture of viral hepatitis is extremely variable, ranging from asymptomatic infection without jaundice to a fulminating disease and death in a few days.

A. SYMPTOMS

1. Prodromal phase—The onset may be abrupt or insidious, with general malaise, myalgia, arthralgia, easy fatigability, upper respiratory symptoms, and anorexia. A distaste for smoking, paralleling anorexia, may occur early. Nausea and vomiting are frequent, and diarrhea or constipation may occur. Serum sickness may be seen early in acute hepatitis B. Fever is generally present but is low-grade except in occasional cases of hepatitis A. Defervescence and a fall in pulse rate often coincide with the onset of jaundice.

Abdominal pain is usually mild and constant in the right upper quadrant or epigastrium, often aggravated by jarring or exertion, and rarely may be severe enough to simulate cholecystitis.

2. Icteric phase—Jaundice occurs after 5–10 days but may appear at the same time as the initial symptoms. In many patients, jaundice never develops. With the onset of jaundice, there is often worsening of the prodromal symptoms, followed by progressive clinical improvement.

3. Convalescent phase—There is an increasing sense of well-being, return of appetite, and disappearance of jaundice, abdominal pain and tenderness, and fatigability.

4. Course and complications—The acute illness usually subsides over 2–3 weeks with complete clinical and laboratory recovery by 9 weeks in hepatitis A and by 16 weeks in hepatitis B. In 5–10% of cases, the course may be more protracted, but less than 1% will have a fulminant course. In some cases of acute hepatitis A, clinical, biochemical, and serologic recovery may be followed by one or two relapses, but recovery is the rule. A protracted course of hepatitis A has been reported to be associated with HLA *DRB1*1301*. Hepatitis B, D, and C (and G) may become chronic (see below). Rarely, aplastic anemia may complicate the course of non-A–E hepatitis.

B. SIGNS

Hepatomegaly—rarely marked—is present in over half of cases. Liver tenderness is usually present. Splenomegaly is reported in 15% of patients, and soft, enlarged lymph nodes—especially in the cervical or epitrochlear areas—may occur. Systemic toxicity is most often encountered in hepatitis A. Slight neurocognitive impairment has been described in patients with chronic hepatitis C.

C. LABORATORY FINDINGS

The white blood cell count is normal to low, especially in the preicteric phase. Large atypical lymphocytes may occasionally be seen. Rarely, aplastic anemia follows an episode of acute hepatitis not caused by any of the known hepatitis viruses. Mild proteinuria is common, and bilirubinuria often precedes the appearance of jaundice. Acholic stools are often present during the icteric phase. Strikingly elevated AST or ALT occurs early, followed by elevations of bilirubin and alkaline phosphatase; in a minority of patients, the latter persist after aminotransferase levels have normalized. Cholestasis is occasionally marked in acute hepatitis A. Marked prolongation of the prothrombin time in severe hepatitis correlates with increased mortality.

Differential Diagnosis

The differential diagnosis includes other viral diseases such as infectious mononucleosis, cytomegalovirus infection, and herpes simplex virus infection; spirochetal diseases such as leptospirosis and secondary syphilis; brucellosis; rickettsial diseases such as Q fever; drug-induced liver disease; and shock liver (ischemic hepatitis). Occasionally, autoimmune hepatitis (see below) may have an acute onset mimicking acute viral hepatitis. Rarely, metastatic cancer of the liver may present with a hepatitis-like picture.

The prodromal phase of viral hepatitis must be distinguished from other infectious disease such as influenza, upper respiratory infections, and the prodromal stages of the exanthematous diseases. Cholestasis may mimic obstructive jaundice.

Prevention

Strict isolation of patients is not necessary, but hand washing after bowel movements is required. Thorough hand washing by medical staff who may contact contaminated utensils, bedding, or clothing is essential. Careful handling of disposable needles—including not recapping used needles—is required for medical personnel. Screening of donated blood for HBsAg, anti-HBc, and anti-HCV has reduced the risk of transfusion-associated hepatitis markedly. All pregnant women should undergo testing for HBsAg. HBV- and HCV-infected persons should practice safe sex, but there is little evidence that HCV is spread easily by sexual contact. Vaccination against HAV (after prescreening for prior immunity) and HBV is recommended for patients with chronic hepatitis C, and vaccination against HAV is recommended for patients with chronic hepatitis B.

A. HEPATITIS A

Immune globulin should be given to all *close* (eg, household) personal contacts of patients with hepatitis A and should be considered in persons who consume food prepared by an infected food handler. The recommended dose of 0.02 mL/kg intramuscularly is protective if administered during incubation. Two effective inactivated hepatitis A vaccines are available and recommended for persons living in or traveling to endemic areas (including military personnel), patients with chronic liver disease upon diagnosis, persons with clotting-factor disorders who are treated with concentrates, homosexual and bisexual men, animal handlers, illicit drug users, sewage workers, food handlers, and children and caregivers in day care centers and institutions. Routine vaccination is advised for all children in states with an incidence of hepatitis A at least twice the national average and has been recommended by the Advisory Committee on Immunization Practices

of the Centers for Disease Control and Prevention (CDC) for all children between ages 1 and 2 in the United States. HAV vaccine is also effective in the prevention of secondary spread to household contacts of primary cases. The recommended dose for adults is 1 mL (1440 ELISA units) of Havrix (GlaxoSmithKline) or 0.5 mL (50 units) of Vaqta (Merck) intramuscularly, followed by a booster dose at 6–18 months. A combined hepatitis A and B vaccine (Twinrix, GlaxoSmithKline) is available. HIV infection impairs the response to the HAV vaccine, especially in persons with a CD4 count less than 200/mcL.

B. HEPATITIS B

Hepatitis B immune globulin (HBIG) may be protective—or may attenuate the severity of illness—if given in large doses within 7 days after exposure (adult dose is 0.06 mL/kg body weight) followed by initiation of the HBV vaccine series (see below). This approach is currently recommended for persons exposed to HBsAg-contaminated material via mucous membranes or through breaks in the skin and for individuals who have had sexual contact with persons with HBV infection (irrespective of the presence or absence of HBeAg in the source). HBIG is also indicated for newborn infants of HBsAg-positive mothers followed by initiation of the vaccine series (see below).

The currently used vaccines are recombinant-derived. Initially, the vaccine was targeted to persons at high risk, including renal dialysis patients and attending personnel, patients requiring repeated transfusions, spouses of HBsAg-positive persons, men who have sex with men, injection drug users, newborns of HBsAg-positive mothers, beginning medical and nursing students, and all medical technologists. Because this strategy failed to lower the incidence of hepatitis B, the CDC recommended universal vaccination of infants and children in the United States. Over 90% of recipients of the vaccine mount protective antibody to hepatitis B; immunocompromised persons respond poorly. Reduced response to the vaccine may have a genetic basis and has also been associated with age over 40 years and celiac disease. The standard regimen for adults is 10–20 mcg initially (depending on the formulation) repeated again at 1 and 6 months, but alternative schedules have been approved, including accelerated schedules of 0, 1, 2, and 12 months and of 0, 7, and 21 days plus 12 months. For greatest reliability of absorption, the deltoid muscle is the preferred site. Vaccine formulations free of the mercury-containing preservative thimerosal are given in infants less than 6 months of age. When documentation of seroconversion is considered desirable, postimmunization anti-HBs titers may be checked. Protection appears to be excellent even if the titer wanes—at least for 15 years—and booster reimmunization is not routinely recommended but is advised for immunocompromised persons in whom anti-HBs titers fall below 10 mIU/mL. For vaccine nonresponders, three additional vaccine doses may elicit seroprotective anti-HBs levels in 30–50% of persons. Universal vaccination of neonates in countries endemic for HBV reduces the incidence of hepatocellular carcinoma.

Treatment

Bed rest is recommended only if symptoms are marked. If nausea and vomiting are pronounced or if oral intake is substantially decreased, intravenous 10% glucose is indicated. Encephalopathy or severe coagulopathy indicates impending acute hepatic failure, and hospitalization is mandatory (see below).

Dietary management consists of palatable meals as tolerated, without overfeeding; breakfast is usually best tolerated. Strenuous physical exertion, alcohol, and hepatotoxic agents are avoided. Small doses of oxazepam are safe, as metabolism is not hepatic; morphine sulfate is avoided.

Corticosteroids have no benefit in patients with viral hepatitis, including those with fulminant disease. Treatment of acute hepatitis C patients with interferon alfa or peginterferon (see later) for 6–24 weeks appreciably decreases the risk of chronic hepatitis. Because 20% of patients with acute hepatitis C clear the virus without such treatment, reserving it for patients in whom serum HCV RNA levels fail to clear after 3–4 months may be advisable. Ribavirin may be added if HCV RNA fails to clear after 3 months of interferon alfa or peginterferon. Spontaneous viral clearance is much more likely in symptomatic patients than in asymptomatic patients. Antiviral therapy is generally unnecessary in patients with acute hepatitis B. Liver transplantation should be considered in patients with acute liver failure (see below).

Prognosis

In most patients, clinical recovery is complete in 3–6 weeks. Laboratory evidence of liver dysfunction may persist for a longer period, but most patients recover completely. The overall mortality rate is less than 1%, but the rate is reportedly higher in older people.

Hepatitis A does not cause chronic liver disease, although it may persist for up to 1 year, and clinical and biochemical relapses may occur before full recovery. The mortality rate is less than 0.2%. The mortality rate for acute hepatitis B is 0.1–1%, but is higher with superimposed hepatitis D. Fulminant hepatitis C is rare in the United States. For unknown reasons, the mortality rate for hepatitis E is especially high in pregnant women (10–20%).

Chronic hepatitis, characterized by elevated aminotransferase levels for more than 6 months, develops in 1–2% of immunocompetent adults with acute hepatitis B but in as many as 90% of infected neonates and infants and a substantial proportion of immunocompromised adults. Chronic hepatitis, which progresses very slowly in many cases, develops in as many as 80% of all persons with acute hepatitis C. Ultimately, cirrhosis develops in up to 30% of those with chronic hepatitis C

and 40% of those with chronic hepatitis B; the risk of cirrhosis is even higher in patients coinfected with both viruses or with HIV. Patients with cirrhosis are at risk for hepatocellular carcinoma at a rate of 3–5% per year. Even in the absence of cirrhosis, patients with chronic hepatitis B—particularly those with active viral replication—are at increased risk.

Pearlman BL: Hepatitis C virus infection in African Americans. CID 2006;42:82. [PMID: 16323096]

Santantonio T et al: Efficacy of a 24-week course of PEG-interferon α-2b monotherapy in patients with acute hepatitis C after failure of spontaneous clearance. J Hepatol 2005;42: 329. [PMID: 15710214]

Schiff ER, guest ed: Vaccine-preventable hepatitis, a step toward elimination: reevaluating hepatitis A and B prevention. Am J Med 2005;118 (10A):1S.

Shim M et al: Susceptibility to hepatitis A in patients with chronic liver disease due to hepatitis C virus infection: missed opportunities for vaccination. Hepatology 2005;42: 688. [PMID: 16104047]

Wheeler C et al: An outbreak of hepatitis A associated with green onions. N Engl J Med 2005;353:890. [PMID: 16135833]

Zuckerman JN et al: Hepatitis A and B booster recommendations: implications for travelers. Clin Infect Dis 2005;41: 1020. [PMID: 16142669]

ACUTE HEPATIC FAILURE

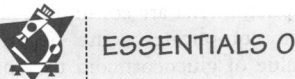 ESSENTIALS OF DIAGNOSIS

- *May be fulminant or subfulminant; both forms carry a poor prognosis.*
- *Acetaminophen and idiosyncratic drug reactions are the most common causes.*

General Considerations

Acute hepatic failure may be fulminant or subfulminant. Fulminant hepatic failure is characterized by the development of hepatic encephalopathy within 8 weeks after the onset of acute liver disease. Coagulopathy (international normalized ratio [INR] ≥ 1.5) is invariably present. Subfulminant hepatic failure occurs when these findings appear between 8 weeks and 6 months after the onset of acute liver disease and carries an equally poor prognosis.

Acetaminophen toxicity is now the most common cause of acute hepatic failure in the United States, as it has been in England for some time, accounting for 40% of cases. Suicide attempts account for 44% of cases of acetaminophen-induced hepatic failure, and unintentional overdoses account for 48%. Other causes include idiosyncratic drug reactions (now the second most common cause), viral hepatitis, poisonous mushrooms, shock, hyperthermia or hypothermia, Budd–Chiari syndrome, malignancy (most commonly lymphomas),

Wilson's disease, Reye's syndrome, fatty liver of pregnancy and other disorders of fatty acid oxidation, autoimmune hepatitis, and parvovirus B19 infection. The risk of acute hepatic failure is increased in patients with diabetes. Herbal and dietary supplements are thought to be contributory to acute hepatic failure in a substantial portion of cases, regardless of cause. Acute hepatic failure may rarely complicate grand mal seizures.

In the past, about 70% of all cases of acute hepatic failure in the United States were caused by acute viral hepatitis. Viral hepatitis now accounts for only 12% of all cases. The decline of viral hepatitis as the principal cause of acute hepatic failure is due to a decline in the contribution of hepatitis B to acute hepatic failure, possibly because of a policy of universal vaccination of infants and children. In endemic areas, hepatitis E is an important cause of acute hepatic failure. Hepatitis C appears to be a rare cause of acute hepatic failure in the United States, but acute hepatitis A or B superimposed on chronic hepatitis C is associated with a high risk of fulminant hepatitis.

Clinical Findings

In acute hepatic failure due to drug toxicity or hepatitis, extensive necrosis of large areas of the liver gives a typical pathologic picture of acute liver atrophy. A systemic inflammatory response, gastrointestinal symptoms, and hemorrhagic phenomena are common. Adrenal insufficiency often complicates acute hepatic failure. However, the value of glucocorticoid therapy is uncertain. Jaundice may be absent or minimal early, but laboratory tests show severe hepatocellular damage. In acute hepatic failure due to microvesicular steatosis (eg, Reye's syndrome), serum aminotransferase elevations may be modest (< 300 units/L).

Treatment

The treatment of acute hepatic failure is directed toward correcting metabolic abnormalities. These include coagulation defects, electrolyte and acid-base disturbances, renal failure, hypoglycemia, and encephalopathy. Prophylactic antibiotic therapy decreases the risk of infection, observed in up to 90%, but has no effect on survival and is not routinely recommended. For suspected sepsis, broad coverage is indicated. Stress gastropathy prophylaxis with an H_2-receptor blocker or proton pump inhibitor is recommended. Early administration of acetylcysteine (140 mg/kg orally followed by 70 mg/kg orally every 4 hours for an additional 17 doses or 150 mg/kg in 5% dextrose intravenously over 15 minutes followed by 50 mg/kg over 4 hours and then 100 mg/kg over 16 hours) is indicated for acetaminophen toxicity and improves cerebral blood flow and oxygenation in patients with fulminant hepatic failure due to any cause. (Acetylcysteine treatment can prolong the prothrombin time, leading to the erroneous assumption that liver failure is worsening.) Penicillin G (300,000 to 1 million units/kg/day) or silibinin (silymarin or milk

thistle), which is not licensed in the United States, is administered to patients with mushroom poisoning. Nucleoside analogs are recommended for patients with fulminant hepatitis B (see Chronic Hepatitis). Subclinical seizure activity is common in patients with acute liver failure, but the value of prophylactic phenytoin is uncertain. Early transfer to a liver transplantation center is essential. Extradural sensors may be placed to monitor intracranial pressure for impending cerebral edema.

Lactulose is administered for encephalopathy (see Cirrhosis). Mannitol, 100–200 mL of a 20% solution by intravenous infusion over 10 minutes, may decrease cerebral edema but should be used with caution in patients with renal failure. Preliminary experience suggests that intravenously administered hypertonic saline to induce hypernatremia also may reduce intracranial hypertension. Hypothermia to a temperature of 33.1°C may reduce intracranial pressure when other measures have failed and may improve survival long enough to permit liver transplantation. The value of hyperventilation and intravenous prostaglandin E_1 is uncertain. Short-acting barbiturates are considered for refractory intracranial hypertension. Hepatic-assist devices using living hepatocytes, extracorporeal whole liver perfusion, hepatocyte transplantation, and liver xenografts have shown promise experimentally and may reduce mortality in patients with acute hepatic failure superimposed on chronic liver disease. They also serve as a "bridge" to liver transplantation. However, a meta-analysis of trials (involving small numbers of patients) of the molecular adsorbent recirculating system (MARS), which is based on extracorporeal albumin dialysis, showed no significant survival benefit when compared with standard medical therapy in patients with acute liver failure.

Prognosis

The mortality rate of fulminant hepatic failure with severe encephalopathy is as high as 80%, except for acetaminophen hepatotoxicity, in which the transplant-free survival is 65% and only 8% of patients undergo liver transplantation. For patients with fulminant hepatic failure of other causes, the outlook is especially poor in patients younger than 10 and older than 40 years of age and in those with an idiosyncratic drug reaction. Spontaneous recovery is less likely for hepatitis B than for hepatitis A. Other adverse prognostic factors are a serum bilirubin level > 18 mg/dL, INR > 6.5, onset of encephalopathy more than 7 days after the onset of jaundice, and a low factor V level (< 20% of normal). For acetaminophen-induced fulminant hepatic failure, indicators of a poor outcome (which is less common than for other causes) are acidosis (pH < 7.3), INR > 6.5, and azotemia (serum creatinine ≥ 3.4 mg/dL), whereas an elevated serum α-fetoprotein level predicts a favorable outcome. An elevated blood lactate level (> 3.5 mmol/L), blood ammonia level (> 124 mcmol/L), and possibly hyperphosphatemia (> 1.2 mmol/L) also predict poor survival outcomes. Emergency liver transplantation is considered for patients with stage 2 to stage 3 encephalopathy (see later) and is associated with a 70% survival rate at 5 years.

Barshes NR et al: Support for the acutely failing liver: a comprehensive review of historic and contemporary strategies. J Am Coll Surg 2005;201:458. [PMID: 16125082]

Bhatia V et al: Predictive value of arterial ammonia for complications and outcome in acute liver failure. Gut 2006;55:98. [PMID: 16024550]

Larson AM et al: Acetaminophen-induced acute liver failure: results of a United States multicenter, prospective study. Hepatology 2005;42:1364. [PMID: 16317692]

MacQuillan GC et al: Blood lactate but not serum phosphate levels can predict patient outcome in fulminant hepatic failure. Liver Transpl 2005;11:1073. [PMID: 16123967]

Polson J et al: AASLD position paper: the management of acute liver failure. Hepatology 2005;41:1179. [PMID: 15841455]

Sass DA et al: Fulminant hepatic failure. Liver Transpl 2005;11: 594. [PMID: 15915484]

Schmidt LE et al: Alpha-fetoprotein is a predictor of outcome in acetaminophen-induced liver injury. Hepatology 2005;41: 26. [PMID: 15617097]

CHRONIC VIRAL HEPATITIS

 ESSENTIALS OF DIAGNOSIS

- *Defined by chronic infection (HBV, HCV, HDV) for greater than 6 months.*
- *Diagnosis is usually made by antibody tests and viral nucleic acid in serum.*

General Considerations

Chronic hepatitis is defined as chronic necroinflammation of the liver of more than 3–6 months' duration, demonstrated by persistently abnormal serum aminotransferase levels and characteristic histologic findings. In many cases, the diagnosis of chronic hepatitis may be made on initial presentation. The causes of chronic hepatitis include HBV, HCV, and HDV as well as autoimmune hepatitis, chronic hepatitis associated with certain medications (such as isoniazid and nitrofurantoin), Wilson's disease, and α_1-antiprotease deficiency. In the past, chronic hepatitis was categorized histologically as chronic persistent hepatitis and chronic active hepatitis. However, with improved serologic and autoimmune markers, more specific categorization became possible, based on etiology; the grade of portal, periportal, and lobular inflammation (minimal, mild, moderate, or severe); and the stage of fibrosis (none, mild, moderate, severe, cirrhosis).

Clinical Findings & Diagnosis

A. CHRONIC HEPATITIS B

Chronic hepatitis B afflicts nearly 400 million people worldwide and 1.25 million (predominantly males) in the United States. It may be noted as a continuum of acute hepatitis or diagnosed because of persistently elevated aminotransferase levels.

Early in the course, HBeAg and HBV DNA are present in serum, indicative of active viral replications and necroinflammatory activity in the liver. These persons are at risk for progression to cirrhosis (at a rate of 2–5.5% per year) and for hepatocellular carcinoma (at a rate of > 2% per year in those with cirrhosis). Low-level IgM anti-HBc is also present in about 70%. In some patients, clinical and biochemical improvement coincides with disappearance of HBeAg and reduced HBV DNA levels (< 10^5 copies/mL) in serum, appearance of anti-HBe, and integration of the HBV genome into the host genome in infected hepatocytes. If cirrhosis has not yet developed, such persons with the inactive HBsAg carrier state are at a low risk for cirrhosis and hepatocellular carcinoma. As noted, infection by a pre-core mutant of HBV or spontaneous mutation of the pre-core or pre-core promoter region of the HBV genome during the course of chronic hepatitis caused by wild-type HBV (HBeAg-negative chronic hepatitis B) may result in particularly severe chronic hepatitis with rapid progression to cirrhosis (at a rate of 8–10% per year), particularly when additional mutations in the core gene of HBV are present. HIV coinfection is also associated with an increased frequency of cirrhosis when the CD4 count is low.

B. HEPATITIS D

Acute hepatitis D infection superimposed on chronic HBV infection may result in severe chronic hepatitis, which may progress rapidly to cirrhosis and may be fatal. Patients with long-standing chronic hepatitis D and B often have inactive cirrhosis. The diagnosis is confirmed by detection of anti-HDV in serum.

C. CHRONIC HEPATITIS C

Chronic hepatitis C develops in up to 85% of patients with acute hepatitis C. It is clinically indistinguishable from chronic hepatitis due to other causes and may be the most common. Worldwide, 170 million people are infected with HCV, with 1.8% of the US population infected. In approximately 40% of cases, serum aminotransferase levels are persistently normal. The diagnosis is confirmed by detection of anti-HCV by enzyme immunoassay (EIA). In rare cases of suspected chronic hepatitis C but a negative EIA, HCV RNA is detected by polymerase chain reaction testing. Progression to cirrhosis occurs in 20% of affected patients after 20 years, with an increased risk in men, those who drink more than 50 g of alcohol daily, and possibly those who acquire HCV infection after age 40 years. African Americans have a higher rate of chronic hepatitis C but lower rates of fibrosis progression and response to therapy than whites. Immunosuppressed persons—including patients with hypogammaglobulinemia, HIV infection with a low CD4 count, or organ transplants receiving immunosuppressants—appear to progress more rapidly to cirrhosis than immunocompetent persons with chronic hepatitis C. Cannibis smoking and hepatic steatosis also appear to promote progression of fibrosis. Affected persons with persistently normal serum aminotransferase levels usually have mild chronic hepatitis with slow or absent progression to cirrhosis; however, cirrhosis is present in 10% of these patients.

Treatment (See Chapter 37)

A. CHRONIC HEPATITIS B

Patients with active viral replication (HBeAg and HBV DNA [$\geq 10^5$ copies/mL] in serum; elevated aminotransferase levels) may be treated with pegylated interferon (peginterferon) alfa-2a 180 mcg subcutaneously once weekly for 48 weeks or recombinant human interferon alfa-2b 5 million units a day or 10 million units three times a week intramuscularly for 4 months. Up to 40% of treated patients will respond with sustained normalization of aminotransferase levels, disappearance of HBeAg and HBV DNA from serum, appearance of anti-HBe, and improved survival. A response is most likely in patients with a low baseline HBV DNA level and high aminotransferase levels and is more likely in those infected with HBV genotype A (prevalent in the United States) than D (prevalent in the Middle East and South Asia). Moreover, some responders may eventually clear HBsAg from serum and liver, develop anti-HBs in serum, and thus be cured. Relapses are uncommon in such complete responders. Patients with HBeAg-negative chronic hepatitis B (pre-core mutant) have a durable sustained response rate of only 15–25% after 12 months of standard interferon alfa therapy. The response to interferon is poor in patients with HIV coinfection.

Nucleoside and nucleotide analogs may be used instead of interferon for the treatment of chronic hepatitis B and are much better tolerated. Lamivudine, 100 mg orally daily, reliably suppresses HBV DNA in serum, improves liver histology in 60% of patients, and leads to normal ALT levels in over 40% and HBeAg seroconversion in 20% of patients after 1 year of therapy. In contrast with interferon therapy, HBsAg rarely clears. However, by the end of 1 year, 15–30% of responders experience a relapse (and occasionally frank decompensation) as a result of a mutation in the polymerase gene (the YMDD motif) of HBV DNA that confers resistance to lamivudine. Moreover, hepatitis activity may recur when the drug is stopped. Therefore, despite a high rate of resistance (up to 70% by 5 years), long-term—perhaps indefinite—treatment may be required to suppress the disease when HBeAg seroconversion does not ensue. Rates of complete response increase with longer duration of therapy. In patients with advanced fibrosis or cirrhosis, continuous treatment with lamivudine reduces the risk of hepatic decompensation and hepatocellular carcinoma. A nucleotide analog, adefovir dipivoxil, has activity against wild-type and lamivudine-resistant HBV. The standard dose is 10 mg orally once a day for at least 1 year.

The drug is effective in patients who have become resistant to lamivudine. As with lamivudine, only a small number of patients achieve sustained suppression of HBV replication with adefovir, and long-term suppressive therapy is often required. Resistance to adefovir is less frequent than with lamivudine but is seen in up to 29% of patients treated for 5 years. Patients with underlying renal dysfunction are at risk of nephrotoxicity from adefovir.

Entecavir, another nucleoside analog, given in a dose of 0.5 mg daily orally or, for patients who have become resistant to lamivudine or have cirrhosis, 1 mg daily orally, was approved by the Food and Drug Administration (FDA) in 2005. The drug is more effective than lamivudine, with histologic improvement observed in 70% of treated patients and suppression of HBV DNA in serum in up to 80%, not nephrotoxic, and infrequently associated with resistance. A theoretical risk of malignancies in humans has not been confirmed.

Tenofovir, a drug used for HIV infection, also has substantial activity against HBV. Other antiviral agents such as emtricitabine, entecavir, clevudine, and telbivudine are under study, and strategies using multiple drugs are likely to be investigated.

Nucleoside and nucleotide analogs are well tolerated even in patients with decompensated cirrhosis (for whom the treatment threshold is an HBV DNA level $\geq 10^3$ copies/mL) and may be effective in patients with rapidly progressive hepatitis B ("fibrosing cholestatic hepatitis") following organ transplantation. Although therapy with these agents leads to biochemical, virologic, and histologic improvement in patients with HBeAg-negative chronic hepatitis B (pre-core mutant) and baseline HBV DNA levels $\geq 10^4$ copies/mL, relapse is frequent when therapy is stopped, and long-term treatment is often required. Resistance is most likely to develop to lamivudine and may develop to adefovir. The development of resistance occasionally results in hepatic decompensation. Sequential addition of a second antiviral agent is usually effective after resistance to the first agent has developed. Combined use of peginterferon or interferon and a nucleoside or nucleotide analog has not been shown convincingly to have a substantial advantage over the use of either type of drug alone.

Nucleoside analogs are also recommended for inactive HBV carriers prior to the initiation of immunosuppressive therapy or cancer chemotherapy to prevent reactivation. In patients infected with both HBV and HIV, antiretroviral therapy, including two drugs active against both agents (eg, lamivudine and tenovir), has been recommended when the CD4 count is less than 500/mm^3.

B. CHRONIC HEPATITIS C

Treatment of chronic hepatitis C is generally considered in patients under age 70 with more than minimal fibrosis on liver biopsy. Because of high response rates to treatment in patients infected with HCV genotype 2 or 3, treatment may be initiated in these patients without a liver biopsy. In the past, standard therapy was a combination of interferon alfa (given subcutaneously three times weekly) and ribavirin (given orally).

Pegylated interferon (peginterferon) taken only once a week is more effective than standard interferon presumably because of sustained high blood levels. Two formulations are available: Pegintron (peginterferon alfa-2b), with a 12-kDa polyethylene glycol (PEG), and Pegasys (peginterferon alfa-2a), with a 40-kDa PEG. Whether there are clinically important differences between the two formulations is unclear. With peginterferon alfa-2a administered in a dose of 180 mcg subcutaneously once per week for 48 weeks, a sustained biochemical and virologic response was achieved in 38% of patients with chronic hepatitis C compared with 17% of those treated with standard interferon. Peginterferon alfa-2b yields similar results but is given according to the patient's weight in a dose of 1.5 mcg/kg subcutaneously.

Addition of the nucleoside analog ribavirin, 1000–1200 mg daily in two divided doses, results in higher sustained response rates than interferon or peginterferon alone in previously untreated patients with chronic hepatitis C or patients who have had a relapse after an initial response to interferon alfa alone. Long-term response rates with a combination of peginterferon and ribavirin are as high as 55% (and up to 80% for HCV genotypes 2 or 3). Low levels of HCV RNA may persist in the liver, lymphocytes, and macrophages of successfully treated ("cured") patients, but the significance of this finding is uncertain. Response rates are lower in patients with advanced fibrosis, high levels of viremia, alcohol consumption, HIV coinfection, and severe steatosis and lower in blacks than in whites, in part because of a higher rate of genotype 1 among infected black patients. For prior nonresponders to standard interferon and ribavirin, sustained response rates to retreatment with peginterferon and ribavirin are only 10–15%. When used with peginterferon alfa-2b, the dose of ribavirin is also based on the patient's weight and may range from 800 mg to 1400 mg daily in two divided doses. When used with peginterferon alfa-2a, the daily ribavirin dose is 1000 mg or 1200 mg depending on whether the patient's weight is less than or greater than 75 kg. Patients infected with genotype 1a or 1b are treated for 48 weeks if there has been a decrease in the serum HCV RNA level of at least 2 logs by 12 weeks. Patients with cirrhosis or a high viral level in serum (> 800,000 IU/mL), including those infected with genotype 3, may also require 48 weeks of treatment. Those infected with genotype 2 or 3 (without cirrhosis and with low levels of viremia) are treated for 24 weeks and require a ribavirin dose of only 800 mg; preliminary findings suggest that for patients infected with these genotypes who clear the virus within 4 weeks, a total treatment duration of only 12–16 weeks may be sufficient. For patients infected with HCV genotype 1 and without any fibrosis on liver biopsy, expectant management and a repeat liver biopsy in 3–5 years are often recommended.

Peginterferon alfa with ribavirin may be beneficial in the treatment of cryoglobulinemia associated with chronic hepatitis C. "Chronic HCV carriers" with normal serum aminotransferase levels respond just as well to treatment as do patients with elevated aminotransferase levels. Patients with both HCV and HIV infections may benefit from treatment of HCV if the CD4 count is not low. Moreover, in HCV/HIV-coinfected persons, long-term liver-related mortality increases as mortality from HIV infection is reduced by highly active antiretroviral therapy.

Treatment with peginterferon alfa plus ribavirin is costly (over $12,000 for a 24-week supply), and side effects, which include flu-like symptoms, are almost universal; more serious toxicity includes psychiatric symptoms (irritability, depression), thyroid dysfunction, and bone marrow suppression. Discontinuation rates are 15–30% and higher in persons over age 60 years than in younger patients. A blood count is obtained at weeks 1, 2, and 4 after therapy is started and monthly thereafter. Interferon is contraindicated in patients with decompensated cirrhosis, profound cytopenias, severe psychiatric disorders, and autoimmune diseases. Patients taking ribavirin must be monitored for hemolysis, and, because of teratogenic effects in animals, men and women taking the drug must practice strict contraception until 6 months after conclusion of therapy. Ribavirin should be avoided in persons over age 65 years and in others in whom hemolysis could pose a risk of angina or stroke. Rash, itching, headache, cough, and shortness of breath also occur with the drug. Lactic acidosis is a concern in patients also taking highly active antiretroviral therapy for HIV infection. Erythropoietin (epoetin alfa) and granulocyte colony-stimulating factor may be used to treat therapy-induced anemia and leukopenia. Interferon is generally contraindicated in heart, lung, and renal transplant recipients because of an increased risk of organ rejection. Selected liver transplant recipients with recurrent hepatitis C may be treated with peginterferon and ribavirin, but response rates are low.

In nonresponders to interferon-based therapy, long-term "maintenance" peginterferon therapy as a strategy to prevent liver fibrosis and reduce the risk of cirrhosis and hepatocellular carcinoma is under study. "Consensus" interferon (a synthetic recombinant interferon), or alfacon, 15 mcg/day subcutaneously for 12 weeks, then 15 mcg three times a week for 36 weeks, plus ribavirin, has been reported to lead to a sustained virologic response in 37% of nonresponders to peginterferon and ribavirin. Ribavirin analogs that cause little hemolysis are also under study. New specific HCV inhibitors are under study.

C. CHRONIC HEPATITIS D

Recombinant interferon alfa-2a (9 million units three times a week for 48 weeks) may lead to normalization of serum aminotransferase levels, histologic improvement, and elimination of HDV RNA from serum in about 50% of patients with chronic hepatitis D, but relapse is common after therapy is stopped. Lamivudine and adefovir are not effective in treating chronic hepatitis D.

Prognosis

The course of chronic viral hepatitis is variable and unpredictable. The sequelae of chronic hepatitis secondary to hepatitis B include cirrhosis, liver failure, and hepatocellular carcinoma. The 5-year mortality rate is 0–2% in those without cirrhosis, 14–20% in those with compensated cirrhosis, and 70–86% following decompensation. Antiviral treatment may improve the prognosis in responders. Chronic hepatitis C is an indolent, often subclinical disease that may lead to cirrhosis and hepatocellular carcinoma after decades. Indeed, the mortality rate from transfusion-associated hepatitis C may be no different from that of an age-matched control population. Nevertheless, mortality rates clearly rise once cirrhosis develops, and mortality from cirrhosis and hepatocellular carcinoma due to hepatitis C is expected to triple in the next 10–20 years. Peginterferon plus ribavirin appears to have a beneficial effect on survival and quality of life, is cost-effective, appears to retard and even reverse fibrosis, and in responders may reduce the risk of hepatocellular carcinoma.

Alberti A et al: Short statement of the first European consensus conference on the treatment of chronic hepatitis B and C in HIV co-infected patients. J Hepatol 2005;42:615. [PMID: 15916745]

Branch AD et al, guest ed: HCV: new paradigms. Semin Liver Dis 2005;25:1.

Dienstag JL et al: American Gastroenterological Association medical position statement on the management of hepatitis C. Gastroenterology 2006;130:225. [PMID: 16401486]

Hadziyannis SJ et al: Long-term therapy with adefovir dipivoxil for HBeAg-negative chronic hepatitis B. N Engl J Med 2005;352:2673. [PMID: 15987916]

Kanwal F et al: Treatment alternatives for chronic hepatitis B infection: a cost-effectiveness analysis. Ann Intern Med 2005; 142:821. [PMID: 15897532]

Keeffe EB, guest ed: Advancing the clinical treatment of hepatitis B virus. Semin Liver Dis 2005;25(Suppl 1):1.

Keeffe EB, guest ed: Hepatitis C virus. Clin Liver Dis 2005;9: 353.

Kim AI et al: Treatment of hepatitis C. Am J Med 2005;118: 808. [PMID: 16084169]

Lau GK et al: Peginterferon alfa-2a, lamivudine, and the combination for HBeAg-positive chronic hepatitis B. N Engl J Med 2005;352:2682. [PMID: 15987917]

Management and treatment of hepatitis C virus infection in HIV-infected adults: recommendations from the Veterans Affairs Hepatitis C Resource Center Program and National Hepatitis C Program Office. Am J Gastroenterol 2005;100: 2338. [PMID: 16181388]

von Wagner M et al: Peginterferon-α-2a (40KD) and ribavirin for 16 or 24 weeks in patients with genotype 2 or 3 chronic hepatitis C. Gastroenterology 2005;129:522. [PMID: 16083709]

Wong W et al: Update on chronic hepatitis C. Clin Gastroenterol Hepatol 2005;3:507. [PMID: 15952092]

AUTOIMMUNE HEPATITIS

ESSENTIALS OF DIAGNOSIS

- *Usually young to middle-aged women.*
- *Chronic hepatitis with high serum globulins.*
- *Positive antinuclear antibody (ANA) and/or smooth muscle antibody in most common type.*
- *Responds to corticosteroids.*

Clinical Findings

A. Symptoms and Signs

Although autoimmune hepatitis is usually seen in young women, it can occur in either sex at any age. Affected younger persons are often positive for HLA-B8 and HLA-DR3; in older patients, HLA-DR4. The principal susceptibility allele among white Americans and northern Europeans is HLA *DRB1*0301;* HLA *DRB1*0401* is a secondary but independent risk factor. The onset is usually insidious, but up to 40% present with an acute attack of hepatitis and some cases follow a viral illness such as hepatitis A, Epstein-Barr infection, or measles or exposure to a drug or toxin such as nitrofurantoin. Exacerbations may occur postpartum. Twenty percent of patients are anicteric. Typically, examination reveals a healthy-appearing young woman with multiple spider nevi, cutaneous striae, acne, hirsutism, and hepatomegaly. Amenorrhea may be a presenting feature. Extrahepatic features include arthritis, Sjögren's syndrome, thyroiditis, nephritis, ulcerative colitis, and Coombs-positive hemolytic anemia.

B. Diagnostic Tests

Serum aminotransferase levels may be > 1000 units/L, and the total bilirubin is usually increased. In classic (type I) autoimmune hepatitis, ANA or smooth muscle antibody (either or both) is detected in serum. Serum γ-globulin levels are typically elevated (up to 5–6 g/dL). In patients with the latter, the EIA for antibody to HCV may be falsely positive. Other antibodies, including atypical perinuclear antineutrophil cytoplasmic antibodies (ANCA) and antibodies to histones, may be found. A second type, seen more often in Europe, is characterized by circulating antibody to liver-kidney microsomes (anti-LKM1)—directed against cytochrome P450 2D6—without anti-smooth muscle antibody or ANA. In some cases, anti-liver cytosol type 1, directed against formiminotransferase cyclodeaminase, is detected. This type of autoimmune hepatitis can be seen in patients with autoimmune polyglandular syndrome type 1. A third variant is characterized by antibodies to soluble liver antigen–liver pancreas (anti-SLA/LP) and may represent a variant of type I autoimmune hepatitis characterized by severe disease, a high relapse rate after treatment, and absence of the usual antibodies (ANA and smooth muscle antibody). Anti-SLA/LP is directed against a transfer RNA complex responsible for incorporating selenocysteine into peptide chains. Concurrent primary biliary cirrhosis or primary sclerosing cholangitis has been recognized in up to 15% of patients with autoimmune hepatitis. Liver biopsy is indicated to help establish the diagnosis, evaluate disease severity, and determine the need for treatment.

Treatment

Prednisone with or without azathioprine improves symptoms; decreases the serum bilirubin, aminotransferase, and γ-globulin levels; and reduces hepatic inflammation. Symptomatic patients with aminotransferase levels elevated tenfold (or fivefold if the serum globulins are elevated at least twofold) are optimal for therapy, and asymptomatic patients with modest enzyme elevations may be considered for therapy depending on the clinical circumstances; however, asymptomatic patients usually remain asymptomatic, have either mild hepatitis or inactive cirrhosis on liver biopsy specimens, and have a good long-term prognosis without therapy.

Prednisone or an equivalent drug is given initially in doses of 30 mg orally daily with azathioprine or mercaptopurine, 50 mg/d orally, which are generally well tolerated and permit the use of lower corticosteroid doses. Blood counts are monitored weekly for the first 2 months of therapy and monthly thereafter because of the small risk of bone marrow suppression. The dose of prednisone is lowered from 30 mg/d after 1 week to 20 mg/d and again after 2 or 3 weeks to 15 mg/d. Ultimately, a maintenance dose of 10 mg/d is achieved. While symptomatic improvement is often prompt, biochemical improvement is more gradual, with normalization of serum aminotransferase levels after several months in many cases. Histologic resolution of inflammation may require 18–24 months, the time at which repeat liver biopsy is recommended. Failure of aminotransferase levels to normalize invariably predicts lack of histologic resolution.

The response rate to therapy with prednisone and azathioprine is 80%. Fibrosis may reverse with therapy and rarely progresses after apparent biochemical and histologic remission. Once remission is achieved, therapy may be withdrawn, but the subsequent relapse rate is 50–90%. Relapses may again be treated in the same manner as the initial episode, with the same remission rate. After successful treatment of a relapse, the patient may be kept indefinitely on azathioprine (up to 2 mg/kg) and the lowest dose of prednisone needed to maintain aminotransferase levels as close to normal as possible—although another attempt at withdrawing therapy may be considered in patients remaining in remission long term (eg, ≥ 4 years). Budesonide, a corticosteroid with less toxicity than predni-

sone, does not appear to be effective in maintaining remission. Prednisone can be used to treat rare flares during pregnancy, and maintenance azathioprine does not have to be discontinued.

Nonresponders to prednisone and azathioprine (failure of serum aminotransferase levels to decrease by 50% after 6 months) may be considered for a trial of cyclosporine, tacrolimus, or methotrexate. Mycophenolate mofetil is an effective alternative to azathioprine in patients who cannot tolerate or do not respond to it. Bone density should be monitored—particularly in patients being maintained on corticosteroids—and measures undertaken to prevent or treat osteoporosis (Chapter 26). Liver transplantation may be required for treatment failures, and the disease has been recognized to recur in up to 40% of transplanted livers (and rarely to develop de novo) as immunosuppression is reduced.

Chatur N et al: Transplant immunosuppressive agents in nontransplant chronic autoimmune hepatitis: the Canadian association for the study of liver (CASL) experience with mycophenolate mofetil and tacrolimus. Liver Int 2005;25:723. [PMID: 15998421]

Feld JJ et al: Autoimmune hepatitis: effect of symptoms and cirrhosis on natural history and outcome. Hepatology 2005;42:53. [PMID: 15954109]

Krawitt EL: Autoimmune hepatitis. N Engl J Med 2006;354:54. [PMID: 16394302]

Miyake Y et al: Persistent normalization of serum alanine aminotransferase levels improves the prognosis of type 1 autoimmune hepatitis. J Hepatol 2005;43:951. [PMID: 16143423]

Tan P et al: Early treatment response predicts the need for liver transplantation in autoimmune hepatitis. Liver Int 2005;25:728. [PMID: 159984227]

ALCOHOLIC LIVER DISEASE

 ESSENTIALS OF DIAGNOSIS

- *Chronic alcohol intake usually exceeds 80 g/d in men and 30–40 g/d in women with alcoholic hepatitis or cirrhosis.*
- *Fatty liver is often asymptomatic.*
- *Alcoholic hepatitis may present as fever, right upper quadrant pain, tender hepatomegaly, and jaundice, but the patient may also be asymptomatic.*
- *AST is usually elevated but rarely above 300 units/L; AST is greater than ALT, usually by a factor of 2 or more.*
- *Often reversible but it is the most common precursor of cirrhosis in the United States.*

General Considerations

Excessive alcohol intake can lead to fatty liver, hepatitis, and cirrhosis. Alcoholic hepatitis is characterized by acute or chronic inflammation and parenchymal necrosis of the liver induced by alcohol. While alcoholic hepatitis is often a reversible disease, it is the most common precursor of cirrhosis in the United States and is associated with four to five times the number of hospitalizations and deaths as hepatitis C, which is the second most common cause of cirrhosis.

The frequency of alcoholic cirrhosis is estimated to be 10–15% among persons who consume over 50 g of alcohol (4 oz of 100-proof whiskey, 15 oz of wine, or four 12-oz cans of beer) daily for over 10 years (although the risk of cirrhosis may be lower for wine than for a comparable intake of beer or spirits). The risk of cirrhosis is lower (5%) in the absence of other cofactors such as chronic viral hepatitis. Genetic factors may also account in part for differences in susceptibility, and there are associations with polymorphisms of the genes encoding for tumor necrosis factor-α and cytochrome P450 2E1. Obesity may increase susceptibility to alcoholic liver injury. Women appear to be more susceptible than men, in part because of lower gastric mucosal alcohol dehydrogenase levels. Although alcoholic hepatitis may not develop in many patients even after several decades of alcohol abuse, it appears in a few individuals within a year after onset of excessive drinking. In general, over 80% of patients with alcoholic hepatitis have been drinking 5 years or more before any symptoms that can be attributed to liver disease develop; the longer the duration of drinking (10–15 or more years) and the larger the alcoholic consumption, the greater the probability of developing alcoholic hepatitis and cirrhosis. In individuals who drink alcohol excessively, the rate of ethanol metabolism can be sufficiently high to permit the consumption of large quantities without raising the blood alcohol level over 80 mg/dL.

The role of deficiencies in vitamins and calories in the development of alcoholic hepatitis or in the progression of this lesion to cirrhosis remains controversial but is at least contributory. Many of the adverse effects of alcohol on the liver are thought to be mediated by tumor necrosis factor α and by the oxidative metabolite acetaldehyde, which contributes to lipid peroxidation and induction of an immune response following covalent binding to proteins in the liver. Concurrent HBV or HCV infection and heterozygosity for the *HFE* gene mutation for hemochromatosis increase the severity of alcoholic liver disease.

Clinical Findings

A. SYMPTOMS AND SIGNS

The clinical presentation of alcoholic liver disease can vary from an asymptomatic patient who may have an enlarged liver to a critically ill individual who dies quickly or a patient with end-stage cirrhosis. A recent period of heavy drinking, complaints of anorexia and nausea, and the demonstration of hepatomegaly and jaundice strongly suggest the diagnosis. Abdominal

pain and tenderness, splenomegaly, ascites, fever, and encephalopathy may be present.

B. LABORATORY FINDINGS

In patients with steatosis, laboratory findings may be normal except for mild liver enzyme elevations. Anemia (usually macrocytic) may be present. Leukocytosis with shift to the left is common in patients with severe alcoholic hepatitis. Leukopenia is occasionally seen and disappears after cessation of drinking. About 10% of patients have thrombocytopenia related to a direct toxic effect of alcohol on megakaryocyte production or to hypersplenism.

AST is usually elevated but rarely above 300 units/L. AST is greater than ALT, usually by a factor of 2 or more. Serum alkaline phosphatase is generally elevated, but seldom more than three times the normal value. Serum bilirubin is increased in 60–90% of patients. Serum bilirubin levels greater than 10 mg/dL and marked prolongation of the prothrombin time ($\geq$ 6 seconds above control) indicate severe alcoholic hepatitis with a mortality rate as high as 50%. The serum albumin is depressed, and the γ-globulin level is elevated in 50–75% of individuals, even in the absence of cirrhosis. Increased transferrin saturation and hepatic iron stores are found in many alcoholic patients due to sideroblastic anemia. Folic acid deficiency may coexist.

C. LIVER BIOPSY

Liver biopsy, if done, demonstrates macrovesicular fat and, in patients with alcoholic hepatitis, polymorphonuclear infiltration with hepatic necrosis, Mallory bodies (alcoholic hyaline), and perivenular and perisinusoidal fibrosis. Micronodular cirrhosis may be present as well. The findings are identical to those of nonalcoholic steatohepatitis.

D. OTHER STUDIES

Imaging studies are used to exclude other diagnoses; they can detect moderate to severe steatosis reliably but not inflammation or fibrosis. Ultrasound helps exclude biliary obstruction and identifies subclinical ascites. CT scanning with intravenous contrast or MRI may be indicated in selected cases to evaluate patients for collateral vessels, space-occupying lesions of the liver, or concomitant disease of the pancreas.

Differential Diagnosis

Alcoholic hepatitis may be closely mimicked by cholecystitis and cholelithiasis and by drug toxicity. Other causes of hepatitis or chronic liver disease may be excluded by serologic or biochemical testing, by imaging studies, or by liver biopsy.

Treatment

A. GENERAL MEASURES

Abstinence from alcohol is essential. Fatty liver is quickly reversible with abstinence. Every effort should be made to provide sufficient amounts of carbohydrates and calories in anorectic patients to reduce endogenous protein catabolism, promote gluconeogenesis, and prevent hypoglycemia. Nutritional support (40 kcal/kg with 1.5–2 g/kg as protein) improves survival in patients with malnutrition. Use of liquid formulas rich in branched-chain amino acids does not improve survival beyond that achieved with less expensive caloric supplementation. The administration of vitamins, particularly folic acid and thiamine, is indicated, especially when deficiencies are noted; glucose administration increases the vitamin B_1 requirement and can precipitate Wernicke–Korsakoff syndrome if thiamine is not coadministered.

B. CORTICOSTEROIDS

Methylprednisolone, 32 mg/d orally for 1 month or the equivalent, may reduce short-term mortality in patients with alcoholic hepatitis and either encephalopathy or a greatly elevated bilirubin concentration and prolonged prothrombin time (specifically, when a discriminant function defined by the patient's prothrombin time minus the control prothrombin time times 4.6 plus the total bilirubin in mg/dL is > 32). Failure of the serum bilirubin level to decline after 7 days of treatment predicts nonresponse and poor long-term survival. No benefit has been demonstrated in patients with concomitant gastrointestinal bleeding.

C. OTHER THERAPIES

Pentoxifylline—an inhibitor of tumor necrosis factor—400 mg orally three times daily for 4 weeks, may reduce 1-month mortality rates in patients with severe alcoholic hepatitis, primarily by decreasing the risk of hepatorenal syndrome. Other experimental therapies include propylthiouracil, oxandrolone, S-adenosyl-L-methionine, infliximab, and extracorporeal liver support. Colchicine has been shown not to reduce mortality in patients with alcoholic cirrhosis.

Prognosis

A. SHORT-TERM

When the prothrombin time is short enough to permit liver biopsy (< 3 seconds above control), the 1-year mortality rate is 7%, rising to 20% if there is progressive prolongation of the prothrombin time during hospitalization. Individuals in whom the prothrombin time prohibits liver biopsy have a 42% mortality rate at 1 year. Other unfavorable prognostic factors are a serum bilirubin greater than 10 mg/dL, hepatic encephalopathy, azotemia, leukocytosis, lack of response to corticosteroid therapy, and possibly little steatosis on a liver biopsy specimen and reversal of portal blood flow by Doppler ultrasound. In addition to the discriminant function discussed above, the Model for End-Stage Liver Disease (MELD) score used for cirrhosis (see later) correlates with mortality from alcoholic hepatitis.

B. LONG-TERM

In the United States, the 3-year mortality rate of persons who recover from acute alcoholic hepatitis is ten times greater than that of control individuals of comparable age. Histologically severe disease is associated with continued excessive mortality rates after 3 years, whereas the death rate is not increased after the same period in those whose liver biopsies show only mild alcoholic hepatitis. Complications of portal hypertension (ascites, variceal bleeding, hepatorenal syndrome), coagulopathy, and severe jaundice following recovery from acute alcoholic hepatitis also suggest a poor long-term prognosis.

The most important prognostic consideration is continued excessive drinking. A 6-month period of abstinence is generally required before liver transplantation is considered, although this requirement has been questioned.

Dunn W et al: MELD accurately predicts mortality in patients with alcoholic hepatitis. Hepatology 2005;41:353. [PMID: 15660383]

Forrest EH et al: Analysis of factors predictive of mortality in alcoholic hepatitis and derivation and validation of the Glasgow alcoholic hepatitis score. Gut 2005;54:1174. [PMID: 16009691]

Mathurin P: Corticosteroids for alcoholic hepatitis—what's next? J Hepatol 2005;43:526. [PMID: 16026887]

Morgan TR et al: Colchicine treatment of alcoholic cirrhosis: a randomized, placebo-controlled clinical trial of patient survival. Gastroenterology 2005;128:882. [PMID: 15825072]

Srikureja W et al: MELD score is a better prognostic model than Child-Turcotte-Pugh score or Discriminant Function in patients with alcoholic hepatitis. J Hepatol 2005;42:700. [PMID: 15826720]

DRUG- & TOXIN-INDUCED LIVER DISEASE

 ESSENTIALS OF DIAGNOSIS

- Drug-induced liver disease can mimic viral hepatitis, biliary tract obstruction, or other types of liver disease.
- Clinicians must inquire about the use of many widely used therapeutic agents, including over-the-counter "natural" and "herbal" products, in any patient with liver disease.

General Considerations

The continuing synthesis, testing, and introduction of new drugs into clinical practice has resulted in an increase in toxic reactions of many types. Many widely used therapeutic agents, including over-the-counter "natural" and "herbal" products, may cause hepatic injury. The medications most commonly implicated are nonsteroidal anti-inflammatory drugs, analgesics, and antibiotics because of their widespread use. Drug-induced liver disease can mimic viral hepatitis, biliary tract obstruction, or other types of liver disease. In any patient with liver disease, the clinician must inquire carefully about the use of potentially hepatotoxic drugs or exposure to hepatotoxins. In some cases, coadministration of a second agent may increase the toxicity of the first (eg, isoniazid and rifampin, acetaminophen and alcohol). Drug toxicity may be categorized on the basis of pathogenesis or histologic appearance.

Direct Hepatotoxic Group

The liver lesion caused by this group of drugs is characterized by (1) dose-related severity, (2) a latent period following exposure, and (3) susceptibility in all individuals. Examples include acetaminophen (toxicity is enhanced by fasting and chronic alcohol use because of depletion of glutathione and induction of cytochrome P450 2E1), alcohol, carbon tetrachloride, chloroform, heavy metals, mercaptopurine, niacin, plant alkaloids, phosphorus, tetracyclines, valproic acid, and vitamin A. Statins, like all cholesterol-lowering agents, may cause serum aminotransferase elevations but rarely, if ever, cause true hepatotoxicity.

Idiosyncratic Reactions

Except for acetaminophen, most severe hepatotoxicity is idiosyncratic. Reactions of this type are (1) sporadic, (2) not related to dose, and (3) occasionally associated with features suggesting an allergic reaction, such as fever and eosinophilia. In some, toxicity results directly from a metabolite that is produced only in certain individuals on a genetic basis. Examples include amiodarone, aspirin, carbamazepine, chloramphenicol, diclofenac, flutamide, halothane, isoniazid, ketoconazole, lamotrigine, methyldopa, oxacillin, phenytoin, pyrazinamide, quinidine, streptomycin, rofecoxib and troglitazone (both withdrawn from the market in the United States), and less commonly other thiazolidinediones, and perhaps tacrine.

Cholestatic Reactions

A. Noninflammatory

The following drugs have a direct effect on bile secretory mechanisms: azathioprine, estrogens, or anabolic steroids containing an alkyl or ethinyl group at carbon 17, indinavir, mercaptopurine, methyltestosterone, and cyclosporine.

B. Inflammatory

The following drugs cause inflammation of portal areas with bile duct injury (cholangitis), often with allergic features such as eosinophilia: amoxicillin-clavulanic acid, azithromycin, chlorothiazide, chlorpromazine, chlorpropamide, erythromycin, penicillamine,

prochlorperazine, semisynthetic penicillins (eg, cloxacillin), and sulfadiazine.

Acute or Chronic Hepatitis

Medications that may result in acute or chronic hepatitis that is histologically—and in some cases clinically—indistinguishable from autoimmune hepatitis include aspirin, isoniazid (increased risk in HBV carriers), methyldopa, minocycline, nitrofurantoin, nonsteroidal anti-inflammatory drugs, and propylthiouracil. Hepatitis also can occur in patients taking cocaine, ecstasy, efavirenz, nevirapine (increased risk in HBV and HCV carriers), ritonavir (greater rate than other protease inhibitors), sulfonamides, troglitazone (withdrawn from the market in the United States), and zafirlukast as well as a variety of alternative remedies (eg, chaparral, germander, jin bu huan, skullcap, kava). In patients with jaundice due to drug-induced hepatitis, the mortality rate without liver transplantation is at least 10%.

Other Reactions

A. Fatty Liver

1. Macrovesicular—Alcohol, amiodarone, corticosteroids, methotrexate, irinotecan, oxaliplatin.

2. Microvesicular (often resulting from mitochondrial injury)—Didanosine, stavudine, tetracyclines, valproic acid, zidovudine.

B. Granulomas

Allopurinol, quinidine, quinine, phenylbutazone, phenytoin.

C. Fibrosis and Cirrhosis

Methotrexate, vitamin A.

D. Sinusoidal Obstruction Syndrome (Veno-occlusive Disease)

Antineoplastic agents (eg, pre-bone marrow transplant), pyrrolizidine alkaloids (eg, Comfrey).

E. Peliosis Hepatis (Blood-Filled Cavities)

Anabolic steroids, azathioprine, oral contraceptive steroids.

F. Neoplasms

Oral contraceptive steroids, estrogens (hepatic adenoma but not focal nodular hyperplasia); vinyl chloride (angiosarcoma).

Björnsson E et al: Outcome and prognostic markers in severe drug-induced liver disease. Hepatology 2005;42:481. [PMID: 16025496]

Chalasani N: Statins and hepatotoxicity: focus on patients with fatty liver. Hepatology 2005;41:690. [PMID: 15789367]

Charles EC et al: Evaluation of cases of severe statin-related transaminitis within a large health maintenance organization. Am J Med 2005;118:618. [PMID: 15922693]

Navarro VJ et al: Current concepts: drug-related hepatotoxicity. N Engl J Med 2006;354:731. [PMID: 16481640]

Rostom A et al: Nonsteroidal anti-inflammatory drugs and hepatic toxicity: a systematic review of randomized controlled trials in arthritis patients. Clin Gastroenterol Hepatol 2005; 3:489. [PMID: 15880319]

Stickel F et al: Herbal hepatotoxicity. J Hepatol 2005;43:901. [PMID: 16171893]

NONALCOHOLIC FATTY LIVER DISEASE

 ESSENTIALS OF DIAGNOSIS

- *Often asymptomatic.*
- *Elevated aminotransferase levels and/or hepatomegaly.*
- *Macrovesicular and/or microvesicular steatosis with or without inflammation and fibrosis on liver biopsy.*

General Considerations

Ethanol can cause hepatic steatosis (fatty liver) in the absence of malnutrition, although inadequate diets—specifically those deficient in choline, methionine, and protein—can contribute to liver damage caused by ethanol (see earlier). Causes of nonalcoholic steatosis, or nonalcoholic fatty liver disease (NAFLD), are obesity (present in ≥ 40%), diabetes mellitus (in ≥ 20%), hypertriglyceridemia (in ≥ 20%), corticosteroids, amiodarone, diltiazem, tamoxifen, irinotecan, oxaliplatin, highly active antiretroviral therapy, poisons (carbon tetrachloride and yellow phosphorus), endocrinopathies such as Cushing's syndrome and hypopituitarism, hypobetalipoproteinemia and other metabolic disorders, obstructive sleep apnea, starvation and refeeding syndrome, and total parenteral nutrition. Steatosis is nearly universal in obese alcoholic patients and is a hallmark of insulin resistance syndrome, which is characterized by obesity, diabetes, hypertriglyceridemia, and hypertension. The risk of fatty liver in persons with insulin resistance syndrome is 4 to 11 times higher than that of persons without insulin resistance. In addition to macrovesicular steatosis, histologic features may include focal infiltration by polymorphonuclear neutrophils and Mallory's hyalin, a picture indistinguishable from that of alcoholic hepatitis and referred to as nonalcoholic steatohepatitis (NASH). In patients with NAFLD, older age, obesity, and diabetes are risk factors for advanced hepatic fibrosis and cirrhosis. Cirrhosis caused by NASH appears to be uncommon in African Americans.

Microvesicular steatosis is seen with Reye's syndrome, valproic acid toxicity, high-dose tetracycline, or acute fatty liver of pregnancy and may result in fulminant hepatic failure.

Women in whom fatty liver of pregnancy develops often have a defect in fatty acid oxidation due to reduced long-chain 3-hydroxyacyl-CoA dehydrogenase activity. The exact stimulus that causes progression of steatosis to steatohepatitis and fibrosis ("second hit") is unclear. The leading possibility is lipid peroxidation and oxidative stress. Some patients with NAFLD have hepatic iron overload, and some of these patients are heterozygous for the *C282Y* gene for hemochromatosis *(HFE);* increased hepatic iron as well as severe steatosis (both attributed to insulin resistance) have been associated with hepatic fibrosis in some studies.

Clinical Findings

A. Symptoms and Signs

Most patients are asymptomatic or have mild right upper quadrant discomfort. Hepatomegaly is present in up to 75% of patients with NAFLD, but the stigmas of chronic liver disease are uncommon. Rare instances of subacute liver failure caused by previously unrecognized NASH have been described.

B. Laboratory Findings

Laboratory studies may show mildly elevated aminotransferase and alkaline phosphatase levels; however, laboratory values may be normal in up to 80% of persons with hepatic steatosis. In contrast to alcoholic liver disease, the ratio of ALT to AST is almost always greater than 1 in NAFLD, but it decreases to less than 1 as advanced fibrosis and cirrhosis develop. An AST/ALT ratio > 2.0 is highly suggestive of alcoholic liver disease. Antinuclear or smooth muscle antibodies may be detected in one-fourth of patients with nonalcoholic steatohepatitis.

C. Imaging

Macrovascular steatosis may be demonstrated on ultrasound, CT, or MRI. However, imaging does not distinguish steatosis from steatohepatitis.

D. Liver Biopsy

Percutaneous liver biopsy is diagnostic and is the only way to assess the degree of inflammation and fibrosis. The risks of the procedure must be balanced against the impact of the added information on management decisions and assessment of prognosis. The histologic spectrum includes fatty liver, isolated portal fibrosis, nonalcoholic steatohepatitis, and cirrhosis.

Treatment

Treatment consists of removing or modifying the offending factors. Weight loss, dietary fat restriction, and exercise often lead to improvement in liver tests and steatosis in obese patients with fatty liver, but the benefit of such measures is less clear in patients with steatohepatitis. Vitamin E (to reduce oxidative stress) is of uncertain benefit. Betaine (a methyl donor) may have some benefit and is under study. Metformin has been shown to reduce insulin resistance and reverse fatty liver in obese leptin-deficient mice and—in some preliminary clinical trials (but not others)—in humans. Thiazolidinediones also reverse insulin resistance and appear to improve serum aminotransferase levels and histologic features of steatohepatitis but lead to weight gain. Pentoxifylline, which inhibits tumor necrosis factor-α, improves liver biochemical test levels but is associated with a high rate of side effects, particularly nausea. Ursodeoxycholic acid, 13–15 mg/kg/d, improved liver function test results and liver histologic features in preliminary studies but not in a larger randomized trial of patients with nonalcoholic steatohepatitis. Hepatic steatosis due to total parenteral nutrition may be ameliorated—and perhaps prevented—with supplemental choline. Other agents under study include orlistat, an inhibitor of gastrointestinal lipases, recombinant human leptin, and losartan, an angiotensin II-receptor antagonist. Gastric bypass may be considered in patients with a body mass index > 35.

Prognosis

Fatty liver is readily reversible with discontinuation of alcohol or treatment of other underlying conditions. Otherwise, the course is variable. NASH may be associated with hepatic fibrosis in 40% of cases; cirrhosis develops in 10–15%; and decompensated cirrhosis occurs in 2–5% of patients. The course may be more aggressive in diabetic persons than in nondiabetic persons. Mortality is increased in patients with NAFLD and is more likely to be the result of malignancy and ischemic heart disease than liver disease. Risk factors for mortality are older age, diabetes, and cirrhosis. Steatosis is a cofactor for the progression of fibrosis in patients with other causes of chronic liver disease, such as hepatitis C. Instances of hepatocellular carcinoma in patients with cirrhosis caused by NASH have been reported. NASH accounts for a substantial percentage of cases labeled as cryptogenic cirrhosis and can recur following liver transplantation. Central obesity is an independent risk factor for death from cirrhosis.

Adams LA et al: The natural history of nonalcoholic fatty liver disease: a population-based cohort study. Gastroenterology 2005;129:113. [PMID: 16012941]

Bugianesi E et al: Insulin resistance: a metabolic pathway to chronic liver disease. Hepatology 2005;42:987. [PMID: 16250043]

Fartoux L et al: Insulin resistance is a cause of steatosis and fibrosis progression in chronic hepatitis C. Gut 2005;54:1003. [PMID: 15951550]

Hamaguchi M et al: The metabolic syndrome as a predictor of nonalcoholic fatty liver disease. Ann Intern Med 2005;143:722. [PMID: 16287793]

Kunde SS et al: Spectrum of NAFLD and diagnostic implication of the proposed new normal range for serum ALT in obese women. Hepatology 2005;42:650. [PMID: 16037946]

Sass DA et al: Nonalcoholic fatty liver disease: a clinical review. Dig Dis Sci 2005;50:171. [PMID: 15712657]

CIRRHOSIS

 ESSENTIALS OF DIAGNOSIS

- *End result of injury that leads to both fibrosis and nodular regeneration.*
- *May be reversible if cause is removed.*
- *The clinical features result from hepatic cell dysfunction, portosystemic shunting, and portal hypertension.*

General Considerations

Cirrhosis is the end result of hepatocellular injury that leads to both fibrosis and nodular regeneration throughout the liver. Cirrhosis is a serious and generally irreversible disease and is the tenth leading cause of death in the United States. In patients at increased risk of liver injury (eg, heavy alcohol use, obesity, iron overload), higher coffee and tea consumption has been reported to reduce the risk of chronic liver disease. The clinical features of cirrhosis result from hepatic cell dysfunction, portosystemic shunting, and portal hypertension.

The most common histologic classification divides cirrhosis into micronodular, macronodular, and mixed forms. These are descriptive terms rather than separate diseases, and each form may be seen in the same patient at different stages of the disease. In micronodular cirrhosis—typical of alcoholic liver disease (Laennec's cirrhosis)—the regenerating nodules are no larger than the original lobules, ie, approximately 1 mm in diameter or less.

Macronodular cirrhosis is characterized by larger nodules, which can measure several centimeters in diameter and may contain central veins. This form corresponds more or less to postnecrotic (posthepatitic) cirrhosis but does not necessarily follow episodes of massive necrosis and stromal collapse.

Clinical Findings

A. SYMPTOMS AND SIGNS

Cirrhosis may cause no symptoms for long periods. The onset of symptoms may be insidious or, less often, abrupt. Weakness, fatigability, disturbed sleep, muscle cramps, and weight loss are common. In advanced cirrhosis, anorexia is usually present and may be extreme, with associated nausea and occasional vomiting. Abdominal pain may be present and is related either to hepatic enlargement and stretching of Glisson's capsule or to the presence of ascites. Menstrual abnormalities (usually amenorrhea), impotence, loss of libido, sterility, and gynecomastia in men may occur. Hematemesis is the presenting symptom in 15–25%.

In 70% of cases, the liver is enlarged, palpable, and firm if not hard and has a sharp or nodular edge; the left lobe may predominate. Skin manifestations consist of spider nevi (invariably on the upper half of the body), palmar erythema (mottled redness of the thenar and hypothenar eminences), and Dupuytren's contractures. Evidence of vitamin deficiencies (glossitis and cheilosis) is common. Weight loss, wasting, and the appearance of chronic illness are present. Jaundice—usually not an initial sign—is mild at first, increasing in severity during the later stages of the disease. Ascites, pleural effusions, peripheral edema, and ecchymotic lesions are late findings. Encephalopathy characterized by day–night reversal, asterixis, tremor, dysarthria, delirium, drowsiness, and ultimately coma also occur late except when precipitated by an acute hepatocellular insult or an episode of gastrointestinal bleeding. Fever may be a presenting symptom in up to 35% of patients and usually reflects associated alcoholic hepatitis, spontaneous bacterial peritonitis, or intercurrent infection. Splenomegaly is present in 35–50% of cases. The superficial veins of the abdomen and thorax are dilated, reflecting the intrahepatic obstruction to portal blood flow, as do rectal varices. The veins fill from below when compressed.

B. Laboratory Findings

Laboratory abnormalities are either absent or minimal in latent or quiescent cirrhosis. Anemia, a frequent finding, is often macrocytic; causes include suppression of erythropoiesis by alcohol as well as folate deficiency, hemolysis, hypersplenism, and insidious or overt blood loss from the gastrointestinal tract. The white blood cell count may be low, reflecting hypersplenism, or high, suggesting infection; thrombocytopenia is secondary to alcoholic marrow suppression, sepsis, folate deficiency, or splenic sequestration. Prolongation of the prothrombin time may result from failure of hepatic synthesis of clotting factors.

Blood chemistries reflect hepatocellular injury and dysfunction, manifested by modest elevations of AST and alkaline phosphatase and progressive elevation of the bilirubin. Serum albumin is low; γ-globulin is increased and may be as high as in autoimmune hepatitis. The risk of diabetes mellitus is increased in patients with cirrhosis, particularly when associated with HCV infection, alcoholism, hemochromatosis, and NAFLD. Patients with alcoholic cirrhosis may have elevated serum cardiac troponin I and brain natriuretic peptide levels. Blunted cardiac inotropic and chronotropic responses to exercise, stress, and drugs, as well as reduced ventricular function and prolongation of the QT interval, are common in cirrhosis of all causes, but overt heart failure is rare in the absence of alcoholism.

Liver biopsy may show inactive cirrhosis (fibrosis with regenerative nodules) with no specific features to suggest the underlying cause. Alternatively, there may be additional features of alcoholic liver disease, chronic hepatitis, or other specific causes of cirrhosis. Combinations of routine blood tests (eg, AST, platelet count) and serum markers of hepatic fibrosis (eg, hyaluronic acid, amino-terminal propeptide of type III collagen, tissue inhibitor of matrix metalloproteinase 1) are under study as alternatives to liver biopsy for the diagnosis or exclusion of cirrhosis.

C. Imaging

Plain films of the abdomen are seldom helpful. Barium studies of the upper gastrointestinal tract may reveal the presence of esophageal or gastric varices, although endoscopy is more sensitive. Ultrasound is helpful for assessing liver size and detecting ascites or hepatic nodules, including small hepatocellular carcinomas. Together with Doppler studies, it may establish patency of the splenic, portal, and hepatic veins. Hepatic nodules are characterized further by contrast-enhanced CT scan or MRI. Nodules suspicious for malignancy may be biopsied under ultrasound or CT guidance.

D. Special Examinations

Esophagogastroduodenoscopy confirms the presence of varices and detects specific causes of bleeding in the esophagus, stomach, and proximal duodenum. Liver biopsy may be performed by laparoscopy or, in patients with coagulopathy and ascites, by a transjugular approach. In selected cases, wedged hepatic vein pressure measurement may establish the presence and cause of portal hypertension.

Differential Diagnosis

Determining the cause of cirrhosis is important prognostically and therapeutically. The most common causes of cirrhosis are chronic hepatitis C and B and alcohol. Many cases of cirrhosis are "cryptogenic," in which unrecognized NAFLD may play a role. Mutations in the keratin 8 gene have been associated with some cases of cryptogenic cirrhosis. In advanced cases, hemochromatosis may be associated with bronzing of the skin, arthritis, heart failure, and diabetes; however, most patients have no symptoms or signs. Diagnostic features include greater than 60% saturation of serum transferrin or serum ferritin level above the upper limit of normal, detection of the mutated *HFE* gene (see below), and increased staining for iron and quantitation of the iron on liver biopsy. Other metabolic diseases that may lead to cirrhosis include Wilson's disease and α_1-antiprotease (α_1-antitrypsin) deficiency. Primary biliary cirrhosis occurs more frequently in women and is associated with pruritus, significant elevation of alkaline phosphatase, elevated immunoglobulin (IgM) and hypercholesterolemia, and antimitochondrial antibody. Secondary biliary cirrhosis may result from chronic biliary obstruction due to a stone, stricture, or neoplasm and is not associated with antimitochondrial antibody. Congestive heart failure and constrictive pericarditis may lead to hepatic fibrosis ("cardiac cirrhosis") complicated by ascites and may be mistaken for other causes of cirrhosis. Hereditary hemorrhagic telangiectasia can lead to portal hypertension because of portosystemic shunting and nodular transformation of the liver.

Complications

Upper gastrointestinal tract bleeding may occur from varices, portal hypertensive gastropathy, or gastroduodenal ulcer (see Chapter 14). Hemorrhage may be massive, resulting in fatal exsanguination or encephalopathy. Varices may also result from portal vein thrombosis. Liver failure may be precipitated by alcoholism, surgery, and infection. The risk of carcinoma of the liver is increased in patients with cirrhosis. Hepatic Kupffer cell (reticuloendothelial) dysfunction and decreased opsonic activity lead to an increased risk of systemic infection.

Treatment

A. General Measures

The most important principle of treatment is abstinence from alcohol. The diet should be palatable, with adequate calories (25–35 kcal/kg body weight per day in those with compensated cirrhosis and 35–40 kcal/kg/d in those with malnutrition) and protein (1–1.2 g/kg/d in those with compensated cirrhosis and 1.5 g/kg/d in those with malnutrition) and, if there is fluid retention, sodium restriction. In the presence of hepatic encephalopathy, protein intake should be reduced to 60–80 g/d. The benefit of using specialized supplements containing branched-chain amino acids to prevent or treat hepatic encephalopathy or delay progressive liver failure is uncertain. Vitamin supplementation is desirable.

B. Treatment of Complications

1. Ascites and edema—Diagnostic paracentesis is indicated for new ascites. It is rarely associated with serious complications such as bleeding, infection, or bowel perforation even in patients with severe coagulopathy. In addition to a cell count and culture, the ascitic albumin level should be determined; a serum-ascites albumin gradient (serum albumin minus ascitic albumin) > 1.1 suggests portal hypertension. An elevated ascitic adenosine deaminase level is suggestive of tuberculous peritonitis, but the sensitivity of the test is reduced in patients with portal hypertension. Occasionally, cirrhotic ascites is chylous (rich in triglycerides); other causes of chylous ascites are malignancy, tuberculosis, and recent abdominal surgery or trauma.

Ascites in patients with cirrhosis results from portal hypertension (increased hydrostatic pressure); hypoalbuminemia (decreased oncotic pressure); peripheral vasodilation, perhaps mediated by endotoxin-induced release of nitric oxide from splanchnic and systemic vasculature, with resulting increases in renin and angiotensin levels and sodium retention by the kidneys; impaired liver inactivation of aldosterone; and increased aldosterone secretion secondary to increased renin production. Free water excretion is also impaired in cirrhosis, and hyponatremia may develop.

In all patients with cirrhotic ascites, dietary sodium intake may initially be restricted to 2000 mg/d; the intake of sodium may be liberalized slightly after diuresis ensues. In some patients, there is a rapid diminution of ascites on bed rest and dietary sodium restriction alone. In individuals with ascites, the urinary excretion of sodium is usually less than 10 mEq/L. Restriction of fluid intake (800–1000 mL/d) is required for patients with hyponatremia (serum sodium < 125 mEq/L). Treatment of severe hyponatremia with vasopressin receptor antagonists is under study.

a. Diuretics—Spironolactone, generally in combination with furosemide, should be used in patients who do not respond to salt restriction. An initial trial of furosemide 80 mg intravenously demonstrating a rise in urine sodium to 750 mmol in 8 hours may predict response to diuretic therapy. The initial dose of spironolactone is 100 mg orally daily and may be increased by 100 mg every 3–5 days (up to a maximal conventional daily dose of 400 mg/d, although higher doses have been used) until diuresis is achieved, typically preceded by a rise in the urinary sodium concentration. Monitoring for hyperkalemia is important. In patients who cannot tolerate spironolactone because of side effects, such as painful gynecomastia, amiloride (another potassium-sparing diuretic) may be used in a dose of 5–10 mg orally daily. Diuresis is augmented by the addition of a loop diuretic such as furosemide. This potent diuretic, however, will maintain its effect even with a falling glomerular filtration rate, with resultant prerenal azotemia. The dose of oral furosemide ranges from 40 mg/d to 160 mg/d, and the drug should be administered while monitoring blood pressure, urinary output, mental status, and serum electrolytes, especially potassium.

The goal of weight loss in the ascitic patient without associated peripheral edema should be no more than 1–1.5 lb/d (0.5–0.7 kg/d).

b. Large-volume paracentesis—In patients with massive ascites and respiratory compromise, ascites refractory to diuretics, or intolerable diuretic side effects, large-volume paracentesis (4–6 L) is effective. Intravenous albumin concomitantly at a dosage of 10 g/L of ascites fluid removed protects the intravascular volume, although the usefulness of this practice is debated. Moreover, use of albumin at approximately $15 per gram adds considerable expense to the procedure. Large-volume paracentesis can be repeated daily until ascites is largely resolved and may decrease the need for hospitalization. If possible, diuretics should be continued in the hope of preventing recurrent ascites.

c. Transjugular intrahepatic portosystemic shunt (TIPS)—TIPS is an effective treatment of variceal bleeding refractory to standard therapy (eg, endoscopic band ligation or sclerotherapy) and has shown benefit in the treatment of severe refractory ascites. The technique involves insertion of an expandable metal stent between a branch of the hepatic vein and portal vein over a catheter inserted via the internal jugular vein. Increased renal sodium excretion and control of ascites refractory to diuretics can be achieved in about 75% of selected cases. The success rate is lower in patients with underlying renal insufficiency. TIPS appears to be the treatment of choice for refractory hepatic hydrothorax (translocation of ascites across the diaphragm to the pleural space); video-assisted thoracoscopy with pleurodesis using talc may be effective when TIPS is contraindicated. Complications of TIPS include hepatic encephalopathy in 20–30% of cases, infection, shunt stenosis in up to 60% of cases, and shunt occlusion in up to 30% of cases. Long-term patency usually requires periodic shunt revisions. In most cases, patency can be maintained by balloon dilation, local thrombolysis, or placement of an additional stent. Because of the complications associated with TIPS and uncertainty about its long-term efficacy (reduced hepatic perfusion as a result of TIPS may conceivably shorten a patient's survival), it is currently preferred in patients who require short-term control of variceal bleeding or ascites until liver transplantation can be performed—as opposed to patients in need of definitive control of bleeding or ascites but in whom liver transplantation is not a consideration. In patients with refractory ascites, TIPS results in lower rates of ascites recurrence and hepatorenal syndrome but a higher rate of hepatic encephalopathy than occur with repeated large-volume paracentesis; a benefit in survival has been demonstrated in one study but not in others or a meta-analysis. Renal insufficiency, refractory encephalopathy, and hyperbilirubinemia are associated with mortality after TIPS.

d. Peritoneovenous shunts—In the past, peritoneovenous shunts were advocated for use in patients with refractory ascites. These shunts may be effective but carry a considerable complication rate: disseminated intravascular coagulation in 65% of patients (25% symptomatic; 5% severe), bacterial infections in 4–8%, congestive heart failure in 2–4%, and variceal bleeding from sudden expansion of intravascular volume. TIPS is now preferred for refractory ascites.

2. Spontaneous bacterial peritonitis—Spontaneous bacterial peritonitis is heralded by abdominal pain, increasing ascites, fever, and progressive encephalopathy in a patient with cirrhotic ascites; symptoms are typically mild. Paracentesis reveals an ascitic fluid with, most commonly, a total white cell count of up to 500 cells/mcL with a high percentage of polymorphonuclear cells (PMNs) (> 250/mcL) and a protein concentration of 1 g/dL or less, corresponding to decreased ascitic opsonic activity. Rapid diagnosis of bacterial peritonitis can be made with a high degree of accuracy with rapid reagent strips ("dipsticks") that detect leukocyte esterase in ascitic fluid. Cultures of ascites give the highest yield—80–90% positive—using blood culture bottles inoculated at the bedside. Common isolates are *Escherichia coli* and pneumococci. (Gram-positive cocci are the most common isolates in patients who have undergone invasive procedures such as central venous line placement.) Anaerobes are rare. Pending culture results, if there are 250 or more PMN/mcL, intravenous antibiotic therapy should be initiated with cefotaxime, 2 g every 8–12 hours for at least 5 days. Ceftriaxone and amoxicillin-clavulanic acid are alternatives. Oral ofloxacin, 400 mg twice daily, or a 2-day course of intravenous ciprofloxacin, 200 mg twice daily, followed by oral ciprofloxacin, 500 mg twice daily for 5 days, may be effective in selected patients. Supplemental administration of intravenous albumin may reduce mortality. Response to therapy can be documented, if necessary, by a decrease in the PMN count of at least 50% on repeat paracentesis 48 hours after initiation of therapy. The overall mortality rate is high—up to 30% during hospitalization and up to 70% by 1 year. In survivors, the risk of recurrent peritonitis may be decreased by long-term norfloxacin, 400 mg orally daily (although in recurrence the causative organism is often resistant to quinolones). In high-risk cirrhotic patients (eg, those with ascitic protein < 1 g/dL, serum bilirubin > 2.5 mg/dL, acute variceal bleeding), first episodes of peritonitis may be prevented by prophylactic norfloxacin, ciprofloxacin (500 mg orally twice a day), or trimethoprim-sulfamethoxazole (one double-strength tablet five times a week).

3. Hepatorenal syndrome—Hepatorenal syndrome occurs in up to 10% of patients with advanced cirrhosis and ascites and is characterized by azotemia in the absence of shock or significant proteinuria and by failure of renal function to improve following intravenous infusion of 1.5 L of isotonic saline. Oliguria, hyponatremia, and low urinary sodium are typical features. Hepatorenal syndrome is diagnosed only when other causes of renal failure (including prerenal azotemia and acute tubular necrosis) have been excluded. Type I hepatorenal syndrome is characterized by doubling of the serum creatinine to a level greater than 2.5 mg/dL or by halving of the creatinine clearance to less than 20 mL/min in less than 2 weeks. Type II hepatorenal syndrome is more slowly progressive and chronic. The cause is unknown, but the pathogenesis involves intense renal vasoconstriction, possibly because of impaired synthesis of renal vasodilators such as prostaglandin E_2 and decreased total renal blood flow; histologically, the kidneys are normal. An acute decrease in cardiac output is often the precipitating event. Treatment is often ineffective. Improvement may follow intravenous infusion of albumin in combination with one of the following: the long-acting vasoconstrictor ornipressin (but with a high rate of ischemic side effects), ornipressin and dopamine, terlipressin (a long-acting vasopressin analog not available in the United States), norepinephrine, or the somatostatin analog octreotide, subcutaneously, and midodrine, an α-adrenergic drug, orally. Prolongation of survival has been associated with use of the molecular adsorbent recirculating system (MARS), a modified dialysis method that selectively removes albumin-bound substances. Improvement and sometimes normalization of renal function may also follow placement of a TIPS. Mortality is high without liver transplantation, death being due to complicating infection or hemorrhage.

4. Hepatic encephalopathy—Hepatic encephalopathy is a state of disordered central nervous system function resulting from failure of the liver to detoxify noxious agents of gut origin because of hepatocellular dysfunction and portosystemic shunting. The clinical spectrum ranges from day–night reversal and mild intellectual impairment to coma. Patients with minimal hepatic encephalopathy have no recognizable clinical symptoms but demonstrate mild cognitive and psychomotor deficits and attention deficit on standardized tests. The stages of overt encephalopathy are (1) mild confusion, (2) drowsiness, (3) stupor, and (4) coma. Ammonia is the most readily identified and measurable toxin but is not solely responsible for the disturbed mental status. Pathogenic factors may include production of false neurotransmitters, increased sensitivity of central nervous system neurons to the inhibitory neurotransmitter γ-aminobutyric acid (GABA), an increase in circulating levels of endogenous benzodiazepines, decreased activity of urea-cycle enzymes due to zinc deficiency, decreased brain levels of myoinositol, deposition of manganese in the basal ganglia, and swelling of astrocytes in the brain. Bleeding into the intestinal tract may significantly increase the amount of protein in the bowel and precipitate rapid development of encephalopathy. Other precipitants include constipation, alkalosis, and potassium deficiency induced by diuretics, opioids, hypnotics, and sedatives; medications containing ammonium or amino compounds; paracentesis with attendant hypovolemia; hepatic or systemic infection; and portosystemic shunts (including TIPS). The diagnosis is based primarily on detection of characteristic symptoms and signs, including asterixis. The role of neuroimaging studies (eg, cerebral positron emissions tomography, magnetic resonance spectroscopy) in the diagnosis of hepatic encephalopathy is evolving.

Dietary protein should be withheld during acute episodes if the patient cannot eat. When the patient resumes oral intake, protein intake should be 60–80 g/d as tolerated; vegetable protein is better tolerated than meat protein. Gastrointestinal bleeding should be controlled and blood purged from the gastrointestinal tract. This can be accomplished with 120 mL of magnesium citrate by mouth or nasogastric tube every 3–4 hours until the stool is free of gross blood, or by administration of lactulose. The value of treating patients with minimal hepatic encephalopathy is uncertain.

Lactulose, a nonabsorbable synthetic disaccharide syrup, is digested by bacteria in the colon to short-chain fatty acids, resulting in acidification of colon contents. This acidification favors the formation of ammonium ion in the $NH_4^+ \times NH_3 + H^+$ equation; NH_4^+ is not absorbable, whereas NH_3 is absorbable and thought to be neurotoxic. Lactulose also leads to a change in bowel flora so that fewer ammonia-forming organisms are present. When given orally, the initial dose of lactulose for acute hepatic encephalopathy is 30 mL three or four times daily. The dose should then be titrated so that two or three soft stools per day are produced. When rectal use is indicated because of the patient's inability to take medicines orally, the dose is 300 mL of lactulose in 700 mL of saline or sorbitol as a retention enema for 30–60 minutes; it may be repeated every 4–6 hours. Lactilol is a less sweet disaccharide alternative available as a powder in some countries.

The ammonia-producing intestinal flora may also be controlled with neomycin sulfate, 0.5–1 g orally every 6 or 12 hours for 7 days. Side effects of neomycin include diarrhea, malabsorption, superinfection, ototoxicity, and nephrotoxicity, usually only after prolonged use. Alternative antibiotics are rifaximin 1200 mg orally daily, vancomycin, 1 g orally twice daily, or metronidazole, 250 mg orally three times daily. Patients who do not respond to lactulose alone may improve with a 1-week course of an antibiotic in addition to lactulose.

Opioids and sedatives metabolized or excreted by the liver are avoided. If agitation is marked, oxazepam, 10–30 mg, which is not metabolized by the liver, may be given cautiously by mouth or by nasogastric tube. Zinc deficiency should be corrected, if present, with oral zinc sulfate, 600 mg/d in divided doses. Eradication of *Helicobacter pylori*, which generates ammonia in the stomach, does not appear to improve encephalopathy. Sodium benzoate, 10 g orally daily, and ornithine aspartate, 9 g orally three times daily, may lower blood ammonia levels, but there is less experience with these drugs than with lactulose. The benzodiazepine competitive antagonist flumazenil is effective in about 30% of patients with severe hepatic encephalopathy, but the drug is short-acting and intravenous administration is required. Use of special dietary supplements enriched with branched-chain amino acids is usually unnecessary except in occasional patients who are intolerant of standard protein supplements. Treatment by modulating the gut flora with prebiotic and probiotic agents is under study.

5. Anemia—For iron deficiency anemia, ferrous sulfate, 0.3-g enteric-coated tablets, one tablet orally three times daily after meals, is effective. Folic acid, 1 mg/d orally, is indicated in the treatment of macrocytic anemia associated with alcoholism. Transfusions with packed red blood cells may be necessary to replace blood loss.

6. Hemorrhagic tendency—Severe hypoprothrombinemia may be treated with vitamin K (eg, phytonadione, 5 mg orally or subcutaneously daily). This treatment is ineffective when synthesis of coagulation factors is impaired because of severe hepatic disease. In such cases, correcting the prolonged prothrombin time requires large volumes of fresh frozen plasma (Chapter 13). Because the effect is transient, plasma infusions are not indicated except for active bleeding or before an invasive procedure. Use of recombinant factor VII may be an alternative.

7. Hemorrhage from esophageal varices—See Chapter 14.

8. Hepatopulmonary syndrome—Shortness of breath in patients with cirrhosis may result from pulmonary restriction and atelectasis caused by massive ascites. The hepatopulmonary syndrome is the triad of chronic liver disease, an increased alveolar–arterial gradient while the patient is breathing room air, and intrapulmonary vascular dilations or arteriovenous communications that result in a right-to-left intrapulmonary shunt and occurs in 4–29% of patients with cirrhosis. The syndrome is presumed to result from failure of the diseased liver to clear circulating pulmonary vasodilators. Patients often have dyspnea and arterial deoxygenation in the upright position (orthodeoxia) that is relieved by recumbency. The diagnosis should be suspected in a cirrhotic patient with a pulse oximetry level ≤ 97%. Contrast-enhanced echocardiography is a sensitive screening test for detecting pulmonary vascular dilations, whereas macroaggregated albumin lung perfusion scanning is more specific and is used to confirm the diagnosis. High-resolution CT may be useful for detecting dilated pulmonary vessels that may be amenable to embolization in patients who respond poorly to supplemental oxygen and is under study. Medical therapy has been disappointing; however, intravenous methylene blue and oral garlic powder may improve oxygenation in patients by inhibiting nitric oxide-induced vasodilation. The syndrome may reverse with liver transplantation, although postoperative mortality is increased in patients with a preoperative arterial oxygen tension < 60 mm Hg or with substantial intrapulmonary shunting. TIPS may provide palliation in patients with hepatopulmonary syndrome awaiting transplantation. Liver transplantation is contraindicated in patients with moderate to severe pulmonary hypertension (mean pulmonary pressure > 35 mm Hg). Pulmonary hypertension occurs in 0.7% of patients with cirrhosis and is thought to result from an excess of circulating vasoconstrictors, particularly endothelin-1. In some cases, treatment with epoprostenol or bosentan may reduce pulmonary hypertension and thereby facilitate liver transplantation; β-blockers worsen exercise capacity and are contraindicated.

C. LIVER TRANSPLANTATION

Liver transplantation is indicated in selected cases of irreversible, progressive chronic liver disease, acute hepatic failure, and certain metabolic diseases in which the metabolic defect is in the liver. Absolute contraindications include malignancy (except small hepatocellular carcinomas in a cirrhotic liver), advanced cardio-pulmonary disease (except pulmonary arteriovenous shunting due to portal hypertension and cirrhosis), and sepsis. Relative contraindications include age over 70 years, morbid obesity, portal and mesenteric vein thrombosis, active alcohol or drug abuse, HIV infection, severe malnutrition, and lack of patient understanding. With the emergence of effective antiretroviral therapy for HIV disease, a major cause of mortality in these patients has shifted to liver disease caused by HCV and HBV infection; preliminary experience suggests that the outcome of liver transplantation is comparable to that for non-HIV-infected liver transplant recipients. Alcoholics should be abstinent for 6 months. Liver transplantation should be considered in patients with worsening functional status, rising bilirubin, decreasing albumin, worsening coagulopathy, refractory ascites, recurrent variceal bleeding, or worsening encephalopathy. The major impediment to more widespread use of liver transplantation is a shortage of donor organs. Increasingly, adult living donor liver transplantation is an option for some patients. Five-year survival rates as high as 80% are now reported. Hepatocellular carcinoma, hepatitis B and C, and some cases of Budd–Chiari syndrome and autoimmune liver disease may recur in the transplanted liver. The incidence of recurrence of hepatitis B can be reduced by preoperative and postoperative treatment with lamivudine, adefovir dipivoxil, or entecavir and perioperative administration of HBIG. Immunosuppression is achieved with a combination of cyclosporine or tacrolimus, corticosteroids, azathioprine, and mycophenolate mofetil and may be complicated by infections, renal failure, neurologic disorders, and drug toxicity as well as graft rejection, vascular occlusion, or bile leaks. Patients are at risk for obesity, diabetes, and hyperlipidemia.

Prognosis

Factors determining survival include the patient's ability to stop the intake of alcohol as well as the Child-Turcotte-Pugh class (Table 15–6). The MELD score, which incorporates the serum bilirubin and creatinine levels and the INR, is also a measure of mortality risk in patients with end-stage liver disease and is particularly useful for predicting short- and intermediate-term survival and determining allocation priorities for donor livers. Hematemesis, jaundice, and ascites are unfavorable signs. In patients with a relatively low MELD score (< 21) and a low priority for liver transplantation, a low serum sodium concentration (< 130 mEq/L), an elevated hepatic venous pressure gradient, and persistent ascites appear to be independent predictors of mortality. In established cases with severe hepatic dysfunction (serum albumin < 3 g/dL, bilirubin > 3 mg/dL, ascites, encephalopathy, cachexia, and upper gastrointestinal bleeding), only 50% survive 6 months. The risk of death in this subgroup of patients with advanced cirrhosis is associated with renal insufficiency, cognitive dysfunction, ventilatory insufficiency,

Table 15–6. Modified Child-Turcotte-Pugh classification for cirrhosis.

Parameter	Numerical Score		
	1	2	3
Ascites	None	Slight	Moderate to severe
Encephalopathy	None	Slight to moderate	Moderate to severe
Bilirubin (mg/dL)	< 2.0	2–3	> 3.0
Albumin (g/dL)	> 3.5	2.8–3.5	< 2.8
Prothrombin time (seconds increased)	1–3	4–6	> 6.0

Total numerical score	Child-Turcotte-Pugh class
5–6	A
7–9	B
10–15	C

age ≥ 65 years, and prothrombin time ≥ 16 seconds. Obesity appears to be a risk factor for cirrhosis-related death or hospitalization in nonalcoholic patients. Patients with cirrhosis are at risk for the development of hepatocellular carcinoma, with rates of 3–5% per year for alcoholic and viral hepatitis-related cirrhosis (see later). Liver transplantation has markedly improved the outlook for patients who are acceptable candidates and are referred for evaluation early. In-hospital mortality from variceal bleeding in patients with cirrhosis has declined from over 40% in 1980 to 15% in 2000. Medical treatments to reverse hepatic fibrosis are under investigation.

Albillos A et al: A meta-analysis of transjugular intrahepatic portosystemic shunt versus paracentesis for refractory ascites. J Hepatol 2005;43:990. [PMID: 16139922]

Boyer TD et al: The role of transjugular portosystemic shunt in the management of portal hypertension. Hepatology 2005; 41:386. [PMID: 15660434]

Cardenas A: Hepatorenal syndrome: a dreaded complication of end-stage liver disease. Am J Gastroenterol 2005;100:460. [PMID: 15667508]

Cardenas A et al: Refractory ascites. Dig Dis 2005;23:30. [PMID: 15920323]

Córdoba J et al: Treatment of hepatic encephalopathy. Lancet 2005;365:1384. [PMID: 15836879]

D'Amico G et al: Uncovered transjugular intrahepatic portosystemic shunt for refractory ascites: a meta-analysis. Gastroenterology 2005;129:1282. [PMID: 16230081]

Murray KF et al: AASLD practice guidelines: evaluation of the patient for liver transplantation. Hepatology 2005;41: 1407. [PMID: 15880505]

Pham PT et al: Review article: current management of renal dysfunction in the cirrhotic patient. Aliment Pharmacol Ther 2005;21:949. [PMID: 15813830]

Sheer TA et al: Spontaneous bacterial peritonitis. Dig Dis 2005; 23:39. [PMID: 15920324]

Swanson KL et al: Natural history of hepatopulmonary syndrome: impact of liver transplantation. Hepatology 2005; 41:1122. [PMID: 15828054]

PRIMARY BILIARY CIRRHOSIS

 ESSENTIALS OF DIAGNOSIS

- *Occurs in middle-aged women.*
- *Often asymptomatic.*
- *Elevation of alkaline phosphatase, positive antimitochondrial antibody, elevated IgM, increased cholesterol.*
- *Characteristic liver biopsy.*
- *In later stages, can present with fatigue, jaundice, features of cirrhosis, xanthelasma, xanthoma, steatorrhea.*

General Considerations

Primary biliary cirrhosis is a chronic disease of the liver characterized by autoimmune destruction of intrahepatic bile ducts and cholestasis. It is insidious in onset, occurs usually in women aged 40–60 years, and is often detected by the chance finding of elevated alkaline phosphatase levels. Estimated incidence and prevalence rates in the United States are 4.5 and 65.4 per 100,000, respectively, in women, and 0.7 and 12.1 per 100,000, respectively, in men. The frequency of the disease among first-degree relatives of affected persons is 1.3–6%, and the concordance rate in identical twins is high. The disease is progressive and may be complicated by steatorrhea, xanthomas, xanthelasma, osteoporosis, osteomalacia, and portal hypertension. It may be associated with Sjögren's syndrome, autoimmune thyroid disease, Raynaud's syndrome, scleroderma, hypothyroidism, and celiac disease. Infection with *Novosphingobium aromaticivorans* or *Chlamydia pneumoniae* may be triggering or causative in primary biliary cirrhosis; other triggers, including viruses, such as human betaretrovirus, and xenobiotics, are also suspected. X-chromosome monosomy may be a predisposing factor. A history of urinary tract infections and smoking and use of hormone replacement therapy are risk factors.

Clinical Findings

A. SYMPTOMS AND SIGNS

Many patients are asymptomatic for years. The onset of clinical illness is insidious and is heralded by fatigue and pruritus. With progression, physical examination reveals hepatosplenomegaly. Xanthomatous lesions may occur in the skin and tendons and around the eyelids. Jaundice, steatorrhea, and signs of portal hypertension are late findings. The risk of osteopenia and osteoporosis is increased in patients with primary biliary cirrhosis (who tend to be older women) possibly due in part to polymorphisms of the vitamin D receptor.

B. LABORATORY FINDINGS

Blood counts are normal early in the disease. Liver biochemical tests reflect cholestasis with elevation of alkaline phosphatase, cholesterol (especially high-density lipoproteins), and, in later stages, bilirubin. Antimitochondrial antibodies (directed against the dihydrolipoamide acetyltransferase component of pyruvate dehydrogenase or other 2-oxo-acid enzymes in mitochondria) are present in 95% of patients, and serum IgM levels are elevated. ANAs with distinctive specificities (eg, against gp210 in the nuclear envelope or nucleoporin p62) may be detected in specialized laboratories.

Diagnosis

The diagnosis of primary biliary cirrhosis is based on the detection of cholestatic liver chemistries (often initially an isolated elevation of the alkaline phosphatase) and antimitochondrial antibodies in serum. Liver biopsy is not essential for diagnosis but permits histologic staging: I, portal inflammation with granulomas; II, bile duct proliferation, periportal inflammation; III, interlobular fibrous septa; and IV, cirrhosis.

Differential Diagnosis

The disease must be differentiated from chronic biliary tract obstruction (stone or stricture), carcinoma of the bile ducts, primary sclerosing cholangitis, sarcoidosis, cholestatic drug toxicity (eg, chlorpromazine), and in some cases chronic hepatitis. Patients with a clinical and histologic picture of primary biliary cirrhosis but no antimitochondrial antibodies are said to have "autoimmune cholangitis," which has been associated with lower serum IgM levels and a greater frequency of smooth muscle and ANAs. Many such patients are found to have antimitochondrial antibodies

by immunoblot against recombinant proteins (rather than standard immunofluorescence). Some patients have overlapping features of primary biliary cirrhosis and autoimmune hepatitis.

Treatment

Treatment is primarily symptomatic. Cholestyramine (4 g) or colestipol (5 g) in water or juice three times daily may be beneficial for the pruritus. Rifampin, 150–300 mg orally twice daily, is inconsistently beneficial. Opioid antagonists (eg, naloxone, 0.2 mcg/kg/min by intravenous infusion, or naltrexone, 50 mg/d by mouth) show promise in the treatment of pruritus. The 5-hydroxytryptamine ($5-HT_3$) serotonin receptor antagonist ondansetron may also provide some benefit. For refractory pruritus, plasmapheresis or extracorporeal albumin dialysis may be needed. Deficiencies of vitamins A, K, and D may occur if steatorrhea is present and is aggravated when cholestyramine or colestipol is administered. See Chapter 26 for discussion on prevention and treatment of osteoporosis.

Because of its lack of toxicity, ursodeoxycholic acid (12–15 mg/kg/d in one or two doses) is the preferred medical treatment (and only treatment approved by the US FDA) for primary biliary cirrhosis and has been shown to slow the progression of disease (particularly in early-stage disease), stabilize histology, improve long-term survival, reduce the risk of developing esophageal varices, and delay the need for liver transplantation. Complete normalization of liver tests occurs in 25% of treated patients, and survival is similar to that of healthy controls when the drug is given to patients with stage 1 or 2 primary biliary cirrhosis. Ursodeoxycholic acid therapy has also been reported to reduce the risk of recurrent colorectal adenomas in patients with primary biliary cirrhosis. Colchicine (0.6 mg orally twice daily) and methotrexate (15 mg/wk orally) have had some reported benefit in improving symptoms and serum levels of alkaline phosphatase and bilirubin. Methotrexate may also improve liver histology in some patients, but overall response rates have been disappointing. Penicillamine, prednisone, and azathioprine have proved to be of no benefit. Budesonide may improve liver histology but worsens osteopenia. Mycophenolate mofetil is under study. For patients with advanced disease, liver transplantation is the treatment of choice.

Prognosis

Without liver transplantation, survival averages 7–10 years once symptoms develop. Progression to liver failure is associated with the presence of anticentromere antibodies. In advanced disease, adverse prognostic markers are older age, high serum bilirubin, edema, low serum albumin, prolonged prothrombin time, and variceal hemorrhage. Among asymptomatic patients, at least one-third will become symptomatic within 15 years. The risk of hepatobiliary malignancies appears to be increased in patients with primary biliary cirrhosis. Liver transplantation for advanced primary biliary cirrhosis is associated with a 1-year survival rate of 85–90%. The disease recurs in the graft in 20% of patients by 3 years, but this does not seem to affect survival.

Combes B et al: Methotrexate (MTX) plus ursodeoxycholic acid (UDCA) in the treatment of primary biliary cirrhosis. Hepatology 2005;42:1184. [PMID: 16250039]

Corpechot C et al: The effect of ursodeoxycholic acid therapy on the natural history of primary biliary cirrhosis. Gastroenterology 2005;128:297. [PMID: 15685541]

Gershwin ME et al (eds): Primary biliary cirrhosis. Semin Liver Dis 2005;25:237.

Gershwin ME et al: USA PBC Epidemiology Group. Risk factors and comorbidities in primary biliary cirrhosis: a controlled interview-based study of 1032 patients. Hepatology 2005; 42:1194. [PMID: 16250040]

Kaplan MM et al: Primary biliary cirrhosis. N Engl J Med 2005; 353:1261. [PMID: 16177252]

HEMOCHROMATOSIS

 ESSENTIALS OF DIAGNOSIS

- *Usually diagnosed because of elevated iron saturation or serum ferritin or a family history.*
- *Most patients are asymptomatic; the disease is rarely recognized clinically before the fifth decade.*
- *Hepatic abnormalities and cirrhosis, congestive heart failure, hypogonadism, and arthritis.*
- *HFE gene mutation (usually C282Y/C282Y) is found in most cases.*

General Considerations

Hemochromatosis is an autosomal recessive disease caused in many cases by a mutation in the *HFE* gene on chromosome 6. The alteration leads to substitution of tyrosine for cysteine at position 282 *(C282Y)* in a region of the gene product involved in interaction with β_2-microglobulin. The HFE protein is thought to play an important role in the process by which duodenal crypt cells sense body iron stores. The presence of the mutation apparently reduces surface expression of an HFE–β_2-microglobulin complex on duodenal crypt cells, decreasing the affinity of the transferrin receptor for transferrin. This impairs transferrin-mediated uptake of iron from the circulation into crypt cells and results in up-regulation of duodenal metal-transporter-1 and ferroportin-1 expression on the luminal side of villous cells, leading in turn to increased iron absorption from the intestine. A decrease in the expression of hepcidin, the principal iron regulatory hormone, is also thought to lead to in-

creased ferroportin-1 expression. About 85% of persons with well-established hemochromatosis are homozygous for the *C282Y* mutation. The frequency of the gene mutation averages 7% in Northern European and North American white populations, resulting in a 0.5% frequency of homozygotes (of whom up to 88% will develop biochemical evidence of iron overload but fewer will develop clinical symptoms). By contrast, the gene mutation and hemochromatosis are uncommon in African-American and Asian-American populations. A second genetic mutation leading to substitution of aspartic acid for histidine at position 63 (H63D) of the same protein may contribute to the development of hemochromatosis in a small percentage (1.5%) of persons who are compound heterozygotes for *C282Y* and *H63D*. A third *HFE* mutation, *S65C*, appears to lead to mild to moderate hepatic iron overload without fibrosis in some cases. Rare instances of hemochromatosis result from mutations in the genes that encode transferrin receptor 2 and ferroprotein.

The disorder is characterized by increased accumulation of iron as hemosiderin in the liver, pancreas, heart, adrenals, testes, pituitary, and kidneys. Cirrhosis is more likely to develop in affected persons who drink alcohol excessively or have obesity-related steatosis than in those who do not. Eventually, hepatic and pancreatic insufficiency, congestive heart failure, and hypogonadism may develop. The disease is rarely recognized clinically before the fifth decade. Heterozygotes do not develop cirrhosis in the absence of associated disorders such as viral hepatitis or NAFLD. A juvenile-onset variant is characterized by severe iron overload, cardiac dysfunction, hypogonadotropic hypogonadism, and a high mortality rate and is infrequently associated with the *C282Y* mutation and usually linked to a mutation of a gene on chromosome 1q designated *HJV* that produces a protein called hemojuvelin or rarely to a mutation in the *HAMP* gene that encodes hepcidin.

Clinical Findings

A. SYMPTOMS AND SIGNS

The onset is usually after age 50 years—earlier in men than in women; however, because of widespread liver biochemical testing and iron screening, the diagnosis can be made long before symptoms develop. Early symptoms are nonspecific (eg, fatigue, arthralgias). Later clinical manifestations include arthropathy, hepatomegaly and evidence of hepatic insufficiency (late finding), skin pigmentation (combination of slate-gray due to iron and brown due to melanin, sometimes resulting in bronze color), cardiac enlargement with or without heart failure or conduction defects, diabetes mellitus with its complications, and impotence in men. Interestingly, population studies have shown an increased prevalence of liver disease but not of diabetes, arthritis, or heart disease in *C282Y* homozygotes. Bleeding from esophageal varices may occur, and in patients in whom cirrhosis develops, there is a 15–

20% incidence of hepatocellular carcinoma. Affected patients are at increased risk of infection with *Vibrio vulnificus, Listeria monocytogenes, Yersinia enterocolitica*, and other siderophilic organisms.

B. LABORATORY FINDINGS

Laboratory findings include mildly abnormal liver tests (AST, alkaline phosphatase), an elevated plasma iron with greater than 50% saturation of the transferrin (after an overnight fast), and an elevated serum ferritin (although a normal iron saturation and a normal ferritin do not exclude the diagnosis). Affected men are more likely than affected women to have an elevated ferritin level.

C. IMAGING

MRI and CT may show changes consistent with iron overload of the liver, and MRI can quantitate hepatic iron stores; however, these techniques are not sensitive enough for screening. Testing for *HFE* mutations is indicated in any patient with evidence of iron overload and in siblings of patients with confirmed hemochromatosis.

D. LIVER BIOPSY

In patients who are homozygous for *C282Y*, liver biopsy is often indicated to determine whether cirrhosis is present. Biopsy can be deferred, however, in patients in whom the serum ferritin level is < 1000 mcg/L, serum AST level is normal, and hepatomegaly is absent; the likelihood of cirrhosis is low in these persons. Liver biopsy is also indicated when iron overload is suspected even though the patient is not homozygous for *C282Y*. In patients with hemochromatosis, the liver biopsy characteristically shows extensive iron deposition in hepatocytes and in bile ducts and the hepatic iron index—hepatic iron content per gram of liver converted to micromoles and divided by the patient's age—is generally greater than 1.9. However, only 5% of patients with hereditary hemochromatosis identified by screening in a primary care setting have cirrhosis.

Treatment

Early diagnosis and treatment in the precirrhotic phase of hemochromatosis are of great importance. Affected patients should avoid foods rich in iron (such as red meat), alcohol, vitamin C, raw shellfish, and supplemental iron. Weekly phlebotomies of 1 or 2 units (250–500 mL) of blood (each containing about 250 mg of iron) is indicated in all symptomatic patients, those with a serum ferritin level of at least 1000 mcg/L, and those with an increased fasting iron saturation and should be continued for up to 2–3 years to achieve depletion of iron stores. This process is monitored by hematocrit and serum iron determinations. When iron store depletion is achieved (iron saturation < 50% and serum ferritin level < 50 mcg/L), maintenance phlebotomies (every 2–4 months) are continued

(although compliance has been reported to decrease with time). The chelating agent deferoxamine is indicated for patients with hemochromatosis and anemia or in those with secondary iron overload due to thalassemia who cannot tolerate phlebotomies. The drug is administered intravenously or subcutaneously in a dose of 20–40 mg/kg/d infused over 24 hours and can mobilize 30 mg of iron per day. However, treatment is painful and time-consuming. Complications of hemochromatosis—arthropathy, diabetes, heart disease, portal hypertension, and hypopituitarism—also require treatment.

The course of the disease is favorably altered by phlebotomy therapy. In precirrhotic patients, cirrhosis may be prevented. Cardiac conduction defects and insulin requirements improve with treatment. In patients with cirrhosis, varices may reverse, and the risk of variceal bleeding declines. However, cirrhotic patients must be monitored for the development of hepatocellular carcinoma. Liver transplantation for advanced cirrhosis associated with severe iron overload, including hemochromatosis, has been reported to lead to survival rates that are lower than those for other types of liver disease because of cardiac complications and an increased risk of infections.

Screening

Genetic testing is recommended for all first-degree family members of the proband; children of an affected person (*C282Y* homozygote) need to be screened only if the patient's spouse carries the *C282Y* or *H63D* mutation. Screening all white men over age 30 years or all adults over age 20 years by measurement of the transferrin saturation or perhaps the unbound iron-binding capacity has been recommended by some, but the value of screening has been questioned on the basis of recent observations that morbidity and mortality from hemochromatosis are lower than expected. Patients with otherwise unexplained chronic liver disease, arthritis, impotence, and late-onset type 1 (and possibly type 2) diabetes mellitus should be screened for iron overload.

Adams PC et al: Hemochromatosis and iron-overload screening in a racially diverse population. N Engl J Med 2005;352: 1769. [PMID: 15858186]

Bacon BR, guest ed: Iron and the liver. Semin Liver Dis 2005;25: 379.

Powell E et al: Steatosis is a cofactor in liver injury in hemochromatosis. Gastroenterology 2005;129:1937. [PMID: 16344062]

Qaseem A et al: Screening for hereditary hemochromatosis: a clinical practice guideline from the American College of Physicians. Ann Intern Med 2005;143:517. [PMID: 16204164]

Schmitt B et al: Screening primary care patients for hereditary hemochromatosis with transferrin saturation and serum ferritin levels: systematic review for the American College of Physicians. Ann Intern Med 2005;143:522. [PMID: 16204165]

Zoller H et al: Hemochromatosis: genetic testing and clinical practice. Clin Gastroenterol Hepatol 2005;3:945. [PMID: 16234038]

WILSON'S DISEASE

ESSENTIALS OF DIAGNOSIS

- *Characterized by excessive deposition of copper in the liver and brain.*
- *Rare autosomal recessive disorder that usually occurs between the first and third decades.*
- *Serum ceruloplasmin, the plasma copper-carrying protein, is low.*
- *Urinary excretion of copper and hepatic copper concentration are high.*

General Considerations

Wilson's disease (hepatolenticular degeneration) is a rare autosomal recessive disorder that usually occurs between the first and third decades. The worldwide prevalence is about 30 per million population. The condition is characterized by excessive deposition of copper in the liver and brain. The genetic defect, localized to chromosome 13, has been shown to affect a copper-transporting adenosine triphosphatase (ATP7B) in the liver and leads to copper accumulation in the liver and oxidative damage of hepatic mitochondria. Most patients are compound heterozygotes (ie, carry two different mutations). Over 200 different mutations in the Wilson disease gene have been identified, making genetic diagnosis impractical except within families in which the mutation has been identified in the index case. The *H1069Q* mutation accounts for 40% of disease alleles in populations of Northern European descent and may be associated with a neurologic presentation.

The major physiologic aberration in Wilson's disease is excessive absorption of copper from the small intestine and decreased excretion of copper by the liver, resulting in increased tissue deposition, especially in the liver, brain, cornea, and kidney. Serum ceruloplasmin, the plasma copper-carrying protein, is low. Urinary excretion of copper is high.

Clinical Findings

Wilson's disease tends to present as liver disease in adolescents and neuropsychiatric disease in young adults, but there is great variability. The diagnosis should always be considered in any child or young adult with hepatitis, splenomegaly with hypersplenism, Coombs-negative hemolytic anemia, portal hypertension, and neurologic or psychiatric abnormalities. Wilson's disease should also be considered in persons under 40 years of age with chronic or fulminant hepatitis.

Hepatic involvement may range from elevated liver tests (although the alkaline phosphatase may be low) to cirrhosis and portal hypertension. The neurologic manifestations are related to basal ganglia dysfunction and include a resting, postural, or kinetic tremor and dystonia of the bulbar musculature with resulting dysarthria and dysphagia. Psychiatric features include behavioral and personality changes and emotional lability. The pathognomonic sign of the condition is the brownish or gray-green Kayser-Fleischer ring, which represents fine pigmented granular deposits in Descemet's membrane in the cornea close to the endothelial surface. The ring is usually most marked at the superior and inferior poles of the cornea. It can frequently be seen with the naked eye and almost invariably by slit-lamp examination. It may be absent in patients with hepatic manifestations only but is usually present in those with neuropsychiatric disease. Renal calculi, the Fanconi defect, renal tubular acidosis, hypoparathyroidism, and hemolytic anemia may occur in patients with Wilson's disease.

Diagnosis

The diagnosis can be challenging and is generally based on demonstration of increased urinary copper excretion (> 100 mcg/24 h) or low serum ceruloplasmin levels (< 20 mcg/dL), and elevated hepatic copper concentration (> 250 mcg/g of dry liver). However, increased urinary copper and low serum ceruloplasmin levels are neither completely sensitive nor specific for Wilson's disease. In equivocal cases (when the serum ceruloplasmin level is normal), the diagnosis may require demonstration of low radiolabeled copper incorporation into ceruloplasmin or urinary copper determination after a penicillamine challenge. Liver biopsy may show acute or chronic hepatitis or cirrhosis. MRI of the brain may show increased basal ganglia copper even early in the course of the disease.

Treatment

Early treatment to remove excess copper is essential before it can produce neurologic or hepatic damage. Early in the treatment phase, restriction of dietary copper (shellfish, organ foods, and legumes) may be of value. Oral penicillamine (0.75–2 g/d in divided doses) is the drug of choice and enhances urinary excretion of chelated copper. Oral pyridoxine, 50 mg per week, is added, since penicillamine is an antimetabolite of this vitamin. If penicillamine treatment cannot be tolerated because of gastrointestinal, hypersensitivity, or autoimmune reactions, consider the use of trientine, 250–500 mg three times a day. Oral zinc acetate, 50 mg three times a day, interferes with intestinal absorption of copper, promotes fecal copper excretion, and may be used as maintenance therapy after decoppering with a chelating agent or as first-line therapy in presymptomatic or pregnant patients. Ammonium tetrathiomolybdate, which complexes copper in the intestinal tract, has shown promise as initial therapy for neurologic Wilson's disease.

Treatment should continue indefinitely. Supplemental vitamin E, an antioxidant, has been recommended but not rigorously studied. Once the serum nonceruloplasmin copper level is within the normal range, the dose of chelating agent can be reduced to the minimum necessary for maintaining that level. The prognosis is good in patients who are effectively treated before liver or brain damage has occurred. Liver transplantation is indicated for fulminant hepatitis (often after plasma exchange as a stabilizing measure), end-stage cirrhosis, and, in selected cases, intractable neurologic disease, although survival is lower when liver transplantation is undertaken for neurologic disease than for liver disease. Family members, especially siblings, require screening with serum ceruloplasmin, liver function tests, and slit-lamp examination or, if the causative mutation is known, with mutation analysis.

Ferenci P: Wilson's disease. Clin Gastroenterol Hepatol 2005;3: 726. [PMID: 16233999]

Ferenci P et al: Diagnostic value of quantitative hepatic copper determination in patients with Wilson's disease. Clin Gastroenterol Hepatol 2005;3:811. [PMID: 16234011]

Medici V et al: Liver transplantation for Wilson's disease: the burden of neurological and psychiatric disorders. Liver Transpl 2005;11:1056. [PMID: 16123950]

HEPATIC VEIN OBSTRUCTION (Budd–Chiari Syndrome)

 ESSENTIALS OF DIAGNOSIS

- *Right upper quadrant pain and tenderness.*
- *Ascites.*
- *Imaging studies show occlusion/absence of flow in the hepatic vein(s) or inferior vena cava.*
- *Clinical picture is similar in veno-occlusive disease but major hepatic veins are patent.*

General Considerations

Factors that predispose patients to Budd–Chiari syndrome, including hereditary and acquired hypercoagulable states, can be identified in 75% of affected patients; multiple disorders are found in 25%. Occlusion of the hepatic veins may occur from a variety of causes. Many cases are associated with polycythemia vera or other myeloproliferative diseases, which may be subclinical. In some cases, an underlying predisposition to thrombosis (eg, hyperprothrombinemia [factor II G20210A mutation], activated protein C resistance [factor V Leiden mutation], protein C or S or antithrombin deficiency, the methylenetetrahydrofolate reductase mutation, antiphospholipid antibodies) can be identified. Hepatovenous obstruction may be associated with caval webs, right-sided heart failure or constrictive pericarditis, neoplasms that cause he-

patic vein occlusion, paroxysmal nocturnal hemoglobinuria, Behçet's syndrome, blunt abdominal trauma, use of oral contraceptives, and pregnancy. Some cytotoxic agents and pyrrolizidine alkaloids ("bush teas") may cause sinusoidal obstruction syndrome (previously known as veno-occlusive disease because the terminal venules are occluded), which mimics Budd–Chiari syndrome clinically. Sinusoidal obstruction syndrome is common in patients who have undergone bone marrow transplantation, particularly those with pretransplant aminotransferase elevations or fever during cytoreductive therapy with cyclophosphamide, azathioprine, carmustine, busulfan, or etoposide or those receiving high-dose cytoreductive therapy or high-dose total body irradiation. In India, China, and South Africa, Budd–Chiari syndrome is often the result of occlusion of the hepatic portion of the inferior vena cava, presumably due to prior thrombosis, and the clinical presentation is mild but the course is frequently complicated by hepatocellular carcinoma.

Clinical Findings

A. SYMPTOMS AND SIGNS

The presentation may be fulminant, acute, subacute, or chronic. An insidious (subacute) onset is most common. Clinical manifestations generally include tender, painful hepatic enlargement, jaundice, splenomegaly, and ascites. With chronic disease, bleeding varices and hepatic coma may be evident; hepatopulmonary syndrome may occur.

B. IMAGING

Hepatic imaging studies may show a prominent caudate lobe, since its venous drainage may not be occluded. The screening test of choice is color or pulsed-Doppler ultrasonography, which has a sensitivity of 85% for detecting evidence of hepatic venous or inferior vena caval thrombosis. MRI with spin-echo and gradient-echo sequences and intravenous gadolinium injection allows visualization of the obstructed veins and collateral vessels. Direct venography can delineate caval webs and occluded hepatic veins ("spider-web" pattern) most precisely.

C. LIVER BIOPSY

Percutaneous or transjugular liver biopsy frequently shows a characteristic centrilobular congestion and fibrosis and often multiple large regenerating nodules. Liver biopsy is often contraindicated in sinusoidal obstruction syndrome because of thrombocytopenia, and the diagnosis is based on clinical findings.

Treatment

Ascites should be treated with fluid and salt restriction and diuretics. Treatable causes of Budd–Chiari syndrome should be sought. Prompt recognition and treatment of an underlying hematologic disorder may avoid the need for surgery, but the optimal anticoagulation regimen is uncertain. Infusion of a thrombolytic agent into recently occluded veins has been attempted with success. In patients with sinusoidal obstruction syndrome, defibrotide, an adenosine receptor agonist that increases endogenous tissue plasminogen activator levels, has shown promise. TIPS placement may be attempted in patients with persistent hepatic congestion or failed thrombolytic therapy, although late TIPS dysfunction is common. TIPS is now preferred over surgical decompression (side-to-side portacaval, mesocaval, or mesoatrial shunt), which has not been proven to improve long-term survival. Balloon angioplasty, in some cases with placement of an intravascular metallic stent, is preferred in patients with an inferior vena caval web and may be feasible in patients with a short segment of thrombosis in the hepatic vein. Liver transplantation is considered in patients with fulminant hepatic failure, cirrhosis and hepatocellular dysfunction, and failure of a portosystemic shunt. Patients often require lifelong anticoagulation and treatment of the underlying myeloproliferative disease; antiplatelet therapy with aspirin and hydroxyurea has been suggested as an alternative to warfarin in patients with a myeloproliferative disorder. The overall 5-year survival rate is 50–80%. Adverse prognostic factors in patients with Budd–Chiari syndrome are older age, advanced Child-Turcotte-Pugh stage, ascites, encephalopathy, elevated total bilirubin, prolonged prothrombin time, elevated serum creatinine, concomitant portal vein thrombosis, and histologic features of acute liver disease superimposed on chronic liver injury.

Bogin V et al: Budd-Chiari syndrome: in evolution. Eur J Gastroenterol Hepatol 2005;17:33. [PMID: 15647637]

Molmenti EP et al: The utility of TIPS in the management of Budd-Chiari syndrome. Ann Surg 2005;241:978. [PMID: 15912047]

Murad SD et al: Pathogenesis and treatment of Budd-Chiari syndrome combined with portal vein thrombosis. Am J Gastroenterol 2006;101:83. [PMID: 16405538]

Ruh J et al: Management of Budd-Chiari syndrome. Dig Dis Sci 2005;50:540. [PMID: 15810639]

Senzolo M et al: Update on the classification, assessment of prognosis and therapy of Budd-Chiari syndrome. Nat Clin Pract Gastroenterol Hepatol 2005;2:182. [PMID: 16265183]

THE LIVER IN HEART FAILURE

Shock liver, or ischemic hepatopathy, results from an acute fall in cardiac output due, for example, to acute myocardial infarction or arrhythmia, usually in a patient with passive congestion of the liver. Clinical hypotension may be absent (or unwitnessed). In some cases, the precipitating event is arterial hypoxemia due to respiratory failure. The hallmark is a rapid and striking elevation of serum aminotransferase levels (often > 5000 units/L); an early rapid rise in the serum lactate dehydrogenase level is also typical, but elevations of serum alkaline phosphatase and bilirubin are usually mild. The prothrombin time may be pro-longed, and encephalopathy may develop. The mortality rate due to the underlying disease is high, but in patients who recover, the aminotransferase levels return to normal quickly, usually within 1 week—in contrast to viral hepatitis.

In patients with passive congestion of the liver due to right-sided heart failure, the serum bilirubin level may be elevated, occasionally as high as 40 mg/dL, due in part to hypoxia of perivenular hepatocytes. Serum alkaline phosphatase levels are normal or slightly elevated. Hepatojugular reflux is present, and with tricuspid regurgitation the liver may be pulsatile. Ascites may be out of proportion to peripheral edema, with a high serum ascites-albumin gradient (> 1.1) and a protein content of more than 2.5 g/dL. In severe cases, signs of encephalopathy may develop.

Dichtl W et al: Cardiac hepatopathy before and after heart transplantation. Transpl Int 2005;18:697. [PMID: 15910296]

Glantzounis GK et al: The contemporary role of antioxidant therapy in attenuating liver ischemia-reperfusion injury: a review. Liver Transpl 2005;11:1031. [PMID: 16123965]

NONCIRRHOTIC PORTAL HYPERTENSION

Noncirrhotic portal hypertension must be considered in the differential diagnosis of splenomegaly or upper gastrointestinal bleeding due to esophageal or gastric varices in patients with little if any liver dysfunction. This syndrome may be due to portal vein thrombosis (with so-called cavernous transformation), splenic vein obstruction (presenting as gastric varices without esophageal varices), schistosomiasis, noncirrhotic intrahepatic portal sclerosis, nodular regenerative hyperplasia, or arterial-portal vein fistula. Aside from splenomegaly, the physical findings are not remarkable, although hepatic decompensation can follow severe gastrointestinal bleeding or a concurrent hepatic disorder, and intestinal infarction may occur when portal vein thrombosis is associated with mesenteric venous thrombosis. Endoscopy shows esophageal or gastric varices. The liver tests are usually normal, but there may be findings of hypersplenism. Color Doppler ultrasound and contrast-enhanced CT are usually the initial diagnostic tests for portal vein thrombosis. Magnetic resonance angiography (MRA) of the portal system is generally confirmatory. Endoscopic ultrasound may be helpful in some cases. In patients with jaundice, magnetic resonance cholangiography may demonstrate compression of the bile duct by a large portal cavernoma. Needle biopsy of the liver may be indicated to diagnose schistosomiasis and noncirrhotic intrahepatic portal sclerosis and may demonstrate sinusoidal dilatation. An underlying hypercoagulable state is found in many patients with portal vein thrombosis; this includes mutation G20210A of prothrombin, factor V Leiden mutation, protein C and S deficiency, antiphospholipid syndrome, mutation TT677 of methylenetetrahydrofolate reductase, elevated factor VIII levels, hyperhomocysteinemia, and myeloproliferative disorders. It is possible, however, that deficiency of protein C and S—as well as of antithrombin—is a secondary phenomenon due to portosystemic shunting and reduced hepatic blood flow. Portal vein thrombosis may occur in up to 15% of patients with cirrhosis and may be associated with hepatocellular carcinoma. Splenic vein thrombosis may complicate pancreatitis or pancreatic cancer. Pylephlebitis (septic thrombophlebitis of the portal vein) may complicate intra-abdominal inflammatory disorders such as appendicitis or diverticulitis, particularly when anaerobic organisms are involved.

If splenic vein thrombosis is the cause of variceal bleeding, splenectomy is curative. For other causes, band ligation or sclerotherapy followed by β-blockers to reduce portal pressure is initiated for variceal bleeding, and portosystemic shunting (including TIPS) is reserved for failures of endoscopic therapy; rarely progressive liver dysfunction requires liver transplantation. Anticoagulation or thrombolytic therapy may be indicated for isolated acute portal vein thrombosis if a hypercoagulable disorder is identified.

Krasinskas AM et al: Liver transplantation for severe intrahepatic noncirrhotic portal hypertension. Liver Transpl 2005;11: 627. [PMID: 15915493]

Primignani M et al: Risk factors for thrombophilia in extrahepatic portal vein obstruction. Hepatology 2005;41:603. [PMID: 15726653]

Webster GJM et al: Review article: portal vein thrombosis—new insights into aetiology and management. Aliment Pharmacol Ther 2005;21:1. [PMID: 15644039]

PYOGENIC HEPATIC ABSCESS

 ESSENTIALS OF DIAGNOSIS

- *Fever, right upper quadrant pain, jaundice.*
- *Often in setting of biliary disease but up to 40% are "cryptogenic" in origin.*
- *Detected by imaging studies.*

General Considerations

The liver can be invaded by bacteria via (1) the portal vein (pylephlebitis); (2) the common duct (ascending cholangitis); (3) the hepatic artery, secondary to bacteremia; (4) direct extension from an infectious process; and (5) traumatic implantation of bacteria through the abdominal wall. Risk factors for liver abscess include older age and male gender. Predisposing conditions include malignancy, diabetes, inflammatory bowel disease, cirrhosis, and liver transplantation.

Ascending cholangitis resulting from biliary obstruction due to a stone, stricture, or neoplasm is the most common identifiable cause of hepatic abscess in the United States. In 10% of cases, liver abscess is sec-

ondary to appendicitis or diverticulitis. At least 40% of abscesses have no demonstrable cause and are classified as cryptogenic. A dental source is identified in some cases. The most frequently encountered organisms are *E coli, Klebsiella pneumoniae, Proteus vulgaris, Enterobacter aerogenes,* and multiple microaerophilic and anaerobic species (eg, *Streptococcus milleri*). *Staphylococcus aureus* is usually the causative organism in patients with chronic granulomatous disease. Unusual causative organisms include *Salmonella, Haemophilus,* and *Yersinia.* Hepatic candidiasis, tuberculosis, and actinomycosis are seen in immunocompromised patients and those with hematologic malignancies. Rarely, hepatocellular carcinoma can present as a pyogenic abscess because of tumor necrosis, biliary obstruction, and superimposed bacterial infection. The possibility of an amebic liver abscess must always be considered (see Chapter 35).

Clinical Findings

A. SYMPTOMS AND SIGNS

The presentation is often insidious. Fever is almost always present and may antedate other symptoms or signs. Pain may be a prominent complaint and is localized to the right hypochondrium or epigastric area. Jaundice, tenderness in the right upper abdomen, and either steady or swinging fever are the chief physical findings.

B. LABORATORY FINDINGS

Laboratory examination reveals leukocytosis with a shift to the left. Liver function studies are nonspecifically abnormal. Blood cultures are positive in 50–100% of cases.

C. IMAGING

Chest roentgenograms usually reveal elevation of the diaphragm if the abscess is on the right side. Ultrasound, CT, or MRI may reveal the presence of intrahepatic defects. On MRI, characteristic findings include high signal intensity on T2-weighted images and rim enhancement. Hepatic candidiasis is seen usually in the setting of systemic candidiasis, and on CT scan the characteristic appearance is that of multiple "bullseyes," but imaging studies may be negative in neutropenic patients.

Treatment

Treatment should consist of antimicrobial agents (a third-generation cephalosporin such as cefoperazone 1–2 g intravenously every 12 hours and metronidazole 500 mg intravenously every 6 hours) that are effective against coliform organisms and anaerobes. Antibiotics are administered for 2–3 weeks, and sometimes up to 6 weeks. If the abscess is at least 5 cm in diameter or the response to antibiotic therapy is not rapid, intermittent needle aspiration or catheter or surgical (eg, laparoscopic) drainage should be done. The mortality rate is still substantial (≥ 8% in most studies) and is highest in patients with underlying biliary malignancy or severe multiorgan dysfunction. Hepatic candidiasis often responds to intravenous amphotericin B (total dose of 2–9 g). Fungal abscesses are associated with mortality rates of up to 50% and are treated with intravenous amphotericin B and drainage.

Choi D et al: Liver abscess after percutaneous radiofrequency ablation for hepatocellular carcinomas: frequency and risk factors. AJR 2005;184:1860. [PMID: 15908543]

Lederman ER et al: Pyogenic liver abscess with a focus on *Klebsiella pneumoniae* as a primary pathogen: an emerging disease with unique clinical characteristics. Am J Gastroenterol 2005;100:322. [PMID: 15667489]

Rahimian J et al: Pyogenic liver abscess: recent trends in etiology and mortality. Clin Infect Dis 2004;39:1654. [PMID: 15578367]

Tan Y-M et al: An appraisal of surgical and percutaneous drainage for pyogenic liver abscesses larger than 5 cm. Ann Surg 2005;241:485. [PMID: 15729072]

NEOPLASMS OF THE LIVER

1. Hepatocellular Carcinoma

ESSENTIALS OF DIAGNOSIS

- In Western countries, usually a complication of cirrhosis.
- Characteristic CT and MRI features and elevated serum α-fetoprotein may obviate the need for a confirmatory biopsy.

General Considerations

Malignant neoplasms of the liver that arise from parenchymal cells are called hepatocellular carcinomas; those that originate in the ductular cells are called cholangiocarcinomas.

Hepatocellular carcinomas are associated with cirrhosis in 80% of cases. Incidence rates are rising rapidly (twofold since 1978) in the United States and other Western countries, presumably because of the increasing prevalence of cirrhosis caused by chronic hepatitis C infection over the past 2–3 decades. In Western countries, risk factors for hepatocellular carcinoma in patients known to have cirrhosis are male gender, age > 55 years (although there has been an increase in the number of younger cases), nonwhite ethnicity, anti-HCV positivity, prothrombin time < 75% of control, and platelet count < 75,000/mcL. In Africa and most of Asia, hepatitis B is of major etiologic significance, whereas in Western countries and Japan, hepatitis C (sometimes in combination with "occult" HBV infection) and alcoholic cirrhosis are the most common risk factors. Other associations include hemochromatosis

(and possibly the *C282Y* carrier state), aflatoxin exposure (associated with mutation of the *P53* gene), α₁-antiprotease (α_1-antitrypsin) deficiency, and tyrosinemia. Increasingly, cirrhosis resulting from NAFLD and insulin resistance syndrome has been associated with hepatocellular carcinomas. The fibrolamellar variant of hepatocellular carcinoma occurs in young women and is characterized by a distinctive histologic picture, absence of risk factors, and indolent course.

Histologically, hepatocellular carcinoma is made up of cords or sheets of cells that roughly resemble the hepatic parenchyma. Blood vessels such as portal or hepatic veins are commonly involved by tumor.

Clinical Findings

A. Symptoms and Signs

The presence of a hepatocellular carcinoma may be unsuspected until there is deterioration in the condition of a cirrhotic patient who was formerly stable. Cachexia, weakness, and weight loss are associated symptoms. The sudden appearance of ascites, which may be bloody, suggests portal or hepatic vein thrombosis by tumor or bleeding from the necrotic tumor.

Physical examination may show tender enlargement of the liver, with an occasionally palpable mass. In Africa, the typical presentation in young patients is a rapidly expanding abdominal mass. Auscultation may reveal a bruit over the tumor or a friction rub when the process has extended to the surface of the liver.

B. Laboratory Findings

Laboratory tests may reveal leukocytosis, as opposed to the leukopenia that is frequently encountered in cirrhotic patients. Anemia is common, but a normal or elevated hematocrit may be found in up to one-third of patients owing to elaboration of erythropoietin by the tumor. Sudden and sustained elevation of the serum alkaline phosphatase in a patient who was formerly stable is a common finding. HBsAg is present in a majority of cases in endemic areas, whereas in the United States anti-HCV is found in up to 40% of cases. α-Fetoprotein levels are elevated in up to 70% of patients with hepatocellular carcinoma in Western countries (although the sensitivity is lower in blacks); however, mild elevations are also often seen in patients with chronic hepatitis. Serum levels of des-gamma-carboxy prothrombin are elevated in up to 90% of patients with hepatocellular carcinoma, but they may also be elevated in patients with vitamin K deficiency, chronic hepatitis, and metastatic cancer. Cytologic study of ascitic fluid rarely reveals malignant cells.

C. Imaging

Arterial phase helical CT scanning and MRI with contrast enhancement are the preferred imaging studies for determining the location and vascularity of the tumor. Lesions smaller than 2 cm may be difficult to characterize. Arterial phase enhancement of the lesion followed by delayed hypointensity ("washout") is most specific for hepatocellular carcinoma. Ultrasound is less sensitive and operator dependent but is used to screen for hepatic nodules in high-risk patients. Contrast-enhanced ultrasound has a sensitivity and specificity approaching those of arterial phase helical CT. Positron emission tomography is under study.

D. LIVER BIOPSY AND STAGING

Liver biopsy is diagnostic, although seeding of the needle tract by tumor is a potential risk (1–3%), and biopsy can be deferred if imaging studies and α-fetoprotein levels are diagnostic (eg, serum α-fetoprotein > 200 ng/mL and a hypervascular mass lesion > 2 cm on imaging of a cirrhotic liver) or if surgical resection is planned. Staging in the TNM classification includes the following definitions: T0: no evidence of primary tumor; T1: solitary tumor without vascular invasion; T2: solitary tumor with vascular invasion or multiple tumors none more than 5 cm; T3: multiple tumors more than 5 cm or tumor involving a major branch of the portal or hepatic vein; and T4: tumors with direct invasion of adjacent organs other than the gallbladder or with perforation of the visceral peritoneum. Alternative staging systems also incorporate liver function, tumor aggressiveness and growth rate, general health of the patient, and treatment but require refinement and validation. For example, the CLIP (Cancer of the Liver Italian Program) classification incorporates the Child-Turcotte-Pugh stage, tumor morphology (uninodular, multinodular, extensive), α-fetoprotein (less than or greater than 400 ng/mL), and vascular invasion. The BCLC (Barcelona Clinic Liver Cancer) staging system includes the Child-Turcotte-Pugh stage, tumor stage, and liver function and has the advantage of linking overall stage with preferred treatment modalities and with an estimation of life expectancy.

Treatment

Surgical resection of solitary hepatocellular carcinomas may result in cure if liver function is preserved (Child class A or possibly B). Laparoscopic liver resection has been performed in selected cases. Treatment of underlying chronic viral hepatitis, adjuvant chemotherapy, and adaptive immunotherapy may lower postsurgical recurrence rates. Liver transplantation may be appropriate for small unresectable tumors in a patient with advanced cirrhosis, with reported 5-year survival rates of up to 75%. The recurrence-free survival may be better for liver transplantation than for resection in patients with well-compensated cirrhosis and small tumors (one tumor < 5 cm or three or fewer tumors each < 3 cm in diameter [Milan criteria]). However, liver transplantation is often impractical because of the donor organ shortage and living donor liver transplantation may be considered in these cases. Chemotherapy, hormonal therapy with tamoxifen, and long-acting octreotide have not been shown to prolong life, but chemoembolization via the hepatic artery is pallia-

tive and may prolong survival in patients with a large or multifocal tumor in the absence of vascular invasion or extrahepatic spread. Injection of absolute ethanol into, radiofrequency ablation of, or cryotherapy of small tumors (< 2 cm) may prolong survival in patients who are not candidates for resection; these interventions may provide a "bridge" to liver transplantation. Radiofrequency ablation is superior to ethanol injection for tumors > 2 cm in diameter. New radiation therapy techniques and novel biologic approaches (eg, antiangiogenesis agents and inhibitors of growth-factor signaling) are under study. For patients whose disease progresses despite treatment or who present with advanced tumors, vascular invasion, or extrahepatic spread, meticulous efforts at palliative care are essential (see Chapter 5). Severe pain may develop in such patients due to expansion of the liver capsule by the tumor and requires concerted efforts at pain management, including the use of opioids (see Chapter 5).

Prognosis

In the United States, overall 1- and 5-year survival rates for patients with hepatocellular carcinoma are 23% and 5%, respectively. Five-year survival rates rise to 56% for patients with localized resectable disease (T1, T2, T3, selected T4; N0; M0) but are virtually nil for those with localized unresectable or advanced disease. The fibrolamellar variant has a better prognosis than conventional hepatocellular carcinoma, with a 5-year survival rate of 32%.

Screening & Prevention

In the patient with chronic hepatitis B or cirrhosis caused by HCV or alcohol, surveillance for the development of hepatocellular carcinoma should be considered with regular (eg, every 6 months) α-fetoprotein testing and ultrasonography. The risk of hepatocellular carcinoma in a patient with cirrhosis is 3–5% a year. The diagnosis of hepatocellular carcinoma is established (without the need for biopsy) for lesions > 2 cm when characteristic arterial hypervascularity is demonstrated on both helical CT and MRI (or on either CT or MRI if the serum α-fetoprotein level is higher than 200 mg/L). In a population of patients with cirrhosis, over 60% of nodules < 2 cm in diameter detected on a screening ultrasound prove to be hepatocellular carcinoma. Mass vaccination programs against HBV in developing countries are leading to reduced rates of hepatocellular carcinoma, whereas in the United States and western Europe the incidence of hepatocellular carcinoma is rising. Successful treatment of hepatitis C in patients with cirrhosis reduces the subsequent risk of hepatocellular carcinoma.

Bruix J et al: Management of hepatocellular carcinoma. Hepatology 2005;42:1208. [PMID: 16250051]

Chen C-J et al: Risk of hepatocellular carcinoma across a biological gradient of serum hepatitis B virus DNA level. JAMA 2006;295:65. [PMID: 16391218]

Davila JA et al: Diabetes increases the risk of hepatocellular carcinoma in the United States: a population based control study. Gut 2005;54:533. [PMID: 15753540]

El-Serag HB et al: Management of the single liver nodule in a cirrhotic patient: a decision analysis model. J Clin Gastroenterol 2005;39:152. [PMID: 15681913]

Kim WR et al: Mortality and hospital utilization for hepatocellular carcinoma in the United States. Gastroenterology 2005; 129:486. [PMID: 16083705]

Marrero JA et al: Prognosis of hepatocellular carcinoma: comparison of 7 staging systems in an American cohort. Hepatology 2005;41:707. [PMID: 15795889]

Shiina S et al: A randomized controlled trial of radiofrequency ablation with ethanol injection for small hepatocellular carcinoma. Gastroenterology 2005;129:122. [PMID: 16012942]

2. Benign Liver Neoplasms

The most common benign neoplasm of the liver is the **cavernous hemangioma,** often an incidental finding on ultrasound or CT scan. This lesion may enlarge in women who take hormonal therapy and must be differentiated from other space-occupying intrahepatic lesions, usually by MRI. Rarely, fine-needle biopsy is necessary to differentiate these lesions and does not appear to carry an increased risk of bleeding. Surgical resection of cavernous hemangiomas is rarely necessary but may be required for abdominal pain or to exclude malignancy.

In addition to rare instances of sinusoidal dilatation and peliosis hepatis, two distinct benign lesions with characteristic clinical, radiologic, and histopathologic features have been described in women taking oral contraceptives—focal nodular hyperplasia and hepatic adenoma. **Focal nodular hyperplasia** occurs at all ages but is probably not caused by oral contraceptives. It is often asymptomatic and appears as a hypervascular mass, occasionally with a central hypodense "stellate" scar on CT scan or MRI. Microscopically, focal nodular hyperplasia consists of hyperplastic units of hepatocytes with a central stellate scar containing proliferating bile ducts. It is not a true neoplasm but a nonspecific reaction to vascular abnormalities. The prevalence of hepatic hemangiomas is increased in patients with focal nodular hyperplasia. A variant termed "telangiectatic focal nodular hyperplasia" is associated with overexpression of the gene that encodes angiopoietin, a protein involved in blood vessel maturation, and appears to be a true neoplasm, like hepatic adenoma.

Hepatic adenoma occurs most commonly in the third and fourth decades of life and is usually caused by oral contraceptives; the clinical presentation is often one of acute abdominal pain due to necrosis of the tumor with hemorrhage. Hepatic adenomas occur in patients with glycogen storage disease. Rare instances of multiple hepatic adenomas in association with maturity-onset diabetes of the young occur in families with a germline mutation in hepatocyte nuclear factor 1α; this mutation may also be found in patients with sporadic adenomas. The tumor is hypovascular and reveals a cold defect on liver scan. Grossly, the cut surface appears structureless.

As seen microscopically, the hepatic adenoma consists of sheets of hepatocytes without portal tracts or central veins. The only physical finding in focal nodular hyperplasia or hepatic adenoma is a palpable abdominal mass in a minority of cases. Liver function is usually normal. Arterial phase helical CT and MRI with contrast can distinguish an adenoma from focal nodular hyperplasia in 80–90% of cases.

Cystic neoplasms of the liver, such as cystadenoma and cystadenocarcinoma, must be distinguished from simple and echinococcal cysts and von Meyenburg complexes (hamartomas).

Treatment of focal nodular hyperplasia is resection only in the symptomatic patient. The prognosis is excellent. Hepatic adenoma often undergoes necrosis and rupture, and resection is advised even in asymptomatic persons. In selected cases, laparoscopic resection or percutaneous radiofrequency ablation may be feasible. Regression of benign hepatic tumors may follow cessation of oral contraceptives.

Bioulac-Sage P et al: Clinical, morphologic, and molecular features defining so-called telangiectatic focal nodular hyperplasia of the liver. Gastroenterology 2005;128:1211. [PMID: 15887105]

Choi BY et al: The diagnosis and management of benign hepatic tumors. J Clin Gastroenterol 2005;39:401. [PMID: 15815209]

Vogt DP et al: Cystadenoma and cystadenocarcinoma of the liver: a single center experience. J Am Coll Surg 2005;200: 727. [PMID: 15848365]

■ DISEASES OF THE BILIARY TRACT

CHOLELITHIASIS (Gallstones)

ESSENTIALS OF DIAGNOSIS

- *Often asymptomatic.*
- *Classic biliary pain characterized by infrequent episodes of steady severe pain in epigastrium or right upper quadrant with radiation to right scapula.*
- *Detected on ultrasound.*

General Considerations

Gallstones are more common in women than in men and increase in incidence in both sexes and all races with aging. In the United States, over 10% of men and 20% of women have gallstones by age 65 years; the total exceeds 20 million people. Although cholesterol gallstones are less common in black people, cholelithiasis attributable to hemolysis occurs in over a third of individuals with sickle cell anemia. Native Americans of both the Northern and Southern Hemispheres have a high rate of cholesterol cholelithiasis, probably because of a predisposition resulting from "thrifty" *(LITH)* genes that promote efficient calorie utilization and fat storage. As many as 75% of Pima and other American Indian women over the age of 25 years have cholelithiasis. Other genetic mutations that predispose persons to gallstones have been identified. Obesity is a risk factor for gallstones, especially in women. Rapid weight loss also increases the risk of symptomatic gallstone formation. There is evidence that glucose intolerance and elevated serum insulin levels (insulin resistance syndrome) are risk factors for gallstones, and a high intake of carbohydrate and high dietary glycemic load increase the risk of cholecystectomy in women. A low-carbohydrate diet and physical activity may help prevent gallstones. Consumption of caffeinated coffee appears to protect against gallstones in women, and a high intake of polyunsaturated and monounsaturated fats reduces the risk of gallstones in men on an energy-balanced diet. A high-fiber diet reduces the risk of cholecystectomy in women. Hypertriglyceridemia may promote gallstone formation by impairing gallbladder motility. The incidence of gallstones is high in individuals with Crohn's disease; approximately one-third of those with inflammatory involvement of the terminal ileum have gallstones due to disruption of bile salt resorption that results in decreased solubility of the bile. The incidence of cholelithiasis is also increased in patients with diabetes mellitus, and the prevalence of gallbladder disease is increased in men (but not women) with cirrhosis and hepatitis C virus infection. Drugs such as clofibrate, octreotide, and ceftriaxone can cause gallstones. In contrast, aspirin and other nonsteroidal anti-inflammatory drugs may protect against gallstones. Prolonged fasting (over 5–10 days) can lead to formation of biliary "sludge" (microlithiasis), which usually resolves with refeeding but can lead to gallstones or biliary symptoms. Pregnancy, particularly in obese women, is associated with an increased risk of gallstones and of symptomatic gallbladder disease. Hormone replacement therapy appears to increase the risk of gallbladder disease and need for cholecystectomy.

Gallstones are classified according to their predominant chemical composition as cholesterol or calcium bilirubinate stones. The latter comprise less than 20% of the stones found in Europe or the United States but 30–40% of stones found in Japan.

Clinical Findings

Table 15–7 lists the clinical and laboratory features of several diseases of the biliary tract as well as their treatment. Cholelithiasis is frequently asymptomatic and is discovered in the course of routine radiographic study, operation, or autopsy. There is generally no need for prophylactic cholecystectomy in an asymptomatic person unless the gallbladder is calcified, gallstones are over 3 cm in diameter, or the patient is a candidate for cardiac transplantation. Ultimately, symptoms (biliary pain) develop in 10–25% of patients, and complications (such as acute cholecystitis) develop in 3% by 10 years. Occasionally, small intestinal obstruction due to "gallstone ileus" presents as the initial manifestation of cholelithiasis.

Treatment

Laparoscopic cholecystectomy is the treatment of choice for symptomatic gallbladder disease. The minimal trauma to the abdominal wall makes it possible for patients to go home within 1 day of the procedure and to return to work within 7 days (instead of weeks for those undergoing standard open cholecystectomy). In many cases, the procedure may be performed on an outpatient basis. This procedure is suitable in most patients, including those with acute cholecystitis. If problems are encountered, the surgery can be converted to a conventional open cholecystectomy. Bile duct injuries occur in 0.1% of cases done by experienced surgeons. Cholecystectomy may increase the risk of esophageal, proximal small intestinal, and colonic adenocarcinomas because of increased duodenogastric reflux and changes in intestinal exposure to bile, respectively. A conservative approach to biliary pain is advised in pregnant patients, but for patients with repeated attacks of biliary pain or acute cholecystitis, cholecystectomy can be performed—even by the laparoscopic route—preferably in the second trimester. Enterolithotomy alone is considered adequate treatment in most patients with gallstone ileus.

Persistence of symptoms after removal of the gallbladder (postcholecystectomy syndrome) implies either mistaken diagnosis, functional bowel disorder, technical error, retained or recurrent common bile duct stone, or spasm of the sphincter of Oddi (see below).

Cheno- and ursodeoxycholic acids are bile salts that when given orally for up to 2 years dissolve some cholesterol stones and may be considered in occasional, selected patients who refuse cholecystectomy. The dose is 7 mg/kg/d of each or 8–13 mg/kg of ursodeoxycholic acid in divided doses daily. They are most effective in patients with a functioning gallbladder, as determined by gallbladder visualization on oral cholecystography, and multiple small "floating" gallstones (representing not more than 15% of patients with gallstones). In half of patients, gallstones recur within 5 years after treatment is stopped. Ursodeoxycholic acid, 500–600 mg daily, reduces the risk of gallstone formation with rapid weight loss, as occurs after bariatric surgery.

Lithotripsy in combination with bile salt therapy for single radiolucent stones less than 20 mm in diameter was an option in the past but is no longer generally used in the United States.

Bini EJ et al: Prevalence of gallbladder disease among persons with hepatitis C virus infection in the United States. Hepatology 2005;41:1029. [PMID: 15770666]

Table 15–7. Diseases of the biliary tract.[1]

	Clinical Features	Laboratory Features	Diagnosis	Treatment
Gallstones	Asymptomatic	Normal	Ultrasound	None
Gallstones	Biliary pain	Normal	Ultrasound	Laparoscopic cholecystectomy
Cholesterolosis of gallbladder	Usually asymptomatic	Normal	Oral cholecystography	None
Adenomyomatosis	May cause biliary pain	Normal	Oral cholecystography	Laparoscopic cholecystectomy if symptomatic
Porcelain gallbladder	Usually asymptomatic, high risk of gallbladder cancer	Normal	X-ray or CT	Laparoscopic cholecystectomy
Acute cholecystitis	Epigastric or right upper quadrant pain, nausea, vomiting, fever, Murphy's sign	Leukocytosis	Ultrasound, HIDA scan	Antibiotics, laparoscopic cholecystectomy
Chronic cholecystitis	Biliary pain, constant epigastric or right upper quadrant pain, nausea	Normal	Ultrasound (stones), oral cholecystography (nonfunctioning gallbladder)	Laparoscopic cholecystectomy
Choledocholithiasis	Asymptomatic or biliary pain, jaundice, fever; gallstone pancreatitis	Cholestatic liver function tests; leukocytosis and positive blood cultures in cholangitis; elevated amylase and lipase in pancreatitis	Ultrasound (dilated ducts), endoscopic ultrasound, MRCP, ERCP	Endoscopic sphincterotomy and stone extraction; antibiotics for cholangitis

[1]HIDA, hepatic iminodiacetic acid; MRCP, magnetic resonance cholangiopancreatography; ERCP, endoscopic retrograde cholangiopancreatography.

Katsika D et al: Genetic and environmental influences on symptomatic gallstone disease: a Swedish study of 43,141 twin pairs. Hepatology 2005;41:1138. [PMID: 15747383]

Ko CW et al: Incidence, natural history, and risk factors for biliary sludge and stones during pregnancy. Hepatology 2005; 41:359. [PMID: 15660385]

Shao T et al: Cholecystectomy and the risk of colorectal cancer. Am J Gastroenterol 2005;100:1813. [PMID: 16086719]

Tsai C-J et al: Glycemic load, glycemic index, and carbohydrate intake in relation to risk of cholecystectomy in women. Gastroenterology 2005;129:105. [PMID: 16012940]

ACUTE CHOLECYSTITIS

ESSENTIALS OF DIAGNOSIS

- *Steady, severe pain and tenderness in the right hypochondrium or epigastrium.*
- *Nausea and vomiting.*
- *Fever and leukocytosis.*

General Considerations

Cholecystitis is associated with gallstones in over 90% of cases. It occurs when a stone becomes impacted in the cystic duct and inflammation develops behind the obstruction. Acalculous cholecystitis should be considered when unexplained fever or right upper quadrant pain occurs within 2–4 weeks of major surgery or in a critically ill patient who has had no oral intake for a prolonged period; multiorgan failure is often present. Primarily as a result of ischemic changes secondary to splanchnic vasoconstriction or intravascular coagulation, gangrene may develop, resulting in perforation. Although generalized peritonitis is possible, the leak usually remains localized and forms a chronic, well-circumscribed abscess cavity. Acute cholecystitis caused by infectious agents (eg, cytomegalovirus, cryptosporidiosis, or microsporidiosis) may occur in patients with AIDS.

Clinical Findings

A. SYMPTOMS AND SIGNS

The acute attack is often precipitated by a large or fatty meal and is characterized by the sudden appearance of steady pain localized to the epigastrium or right hypochondrium, which may gradually subside over a period of 12–18 hours. Vomiting occurs in about 75% of patients and in half of instances affords variable relief. Right upper quadrant abdominal tenderness (often with Murphy's sign, or inhibition of inspiration by pain on palpation of the right upper quadrant) is almost always present and is usually associated with muscle guarding and rebound pain. A palpable gallbladder is present in about 15% of cases. Jaundice is present in about 25% of cases and, when persistent or severe, suggests the possibility of choledocholithiasis. Fever is typical.

B. LABORATORY FINDINGS

The white blood cell count is usually high (12,000–15,000/mcL). Total serum bilirubin values of 1–4 mg/dL may be seen even in the absence of common duct obstruction. Serum aminotransferase and alkaline phosphatase are often elevated—the former as high as 300 units/mL, or even higher when associated with ascending cholangitis. Serum amylase may also be moderately elevated.

C. IMAGING

Plain films of the abdomen may show radiopaque gallstones in 15% of cases. ^{99m}Tc hepatobiliary imaging (using iminodiacetic acid compounds), also known as the hepatic iminodiacetic acid (HIDA) scan, is useful in demonstrating an obstructed cystic duct, which is the cause of acute cholecystitis in most patients. This test is reliable if the bilirubin is under 5 mg/dL (98% sensitivity and 81% specificity for acute cholecystitis). False-positive results can occur with prolonged fasting, liver disease, and chronic cholecystitis. Right upper quadrant abdominal ultrasound may show the presence of gallstones but is not sensitive for acute cholecystitis (67% sensitivity, 82% specificity); findings suggestive of acute cholecystitis are gallbladder wall thickening, pericholecystic fluid, and sonographic Murphy's sign.

Differential Diagnosis

The disorders most likely to be confused with acute cholecystitis are perforated peptic ulcer, acute pancreatitis, appendicitis in a high-lying appendix, perforated colonic carcinoma or diverticulum of the hepatic flexure, liver abscess, hepatitis, pneumonia with pleurisy on the right side, and even myocardial ischemia. Definite localization of pain and tenderness in the right hypochondrium, with radiation around to the infrascapular area, strongly favors the diagnosis of acute cholecystitis. True cholecystitis without stones suggests the rare possibility of polyarteritis nodosa affecting the cystic artery.

Complications

A. GANGRENE OF THE GALLBLADDER

Continuation or progression of right upper quadrant abdominal pain, tenderness, muscle guarding, fever,

and leukocytosis after 24–48 hours suggests severe inflammation and possible gangrene of the gallbladder. Necrosis may occasionally develop without definite signs in the obese, diabetic, elderly, or immunosuppressed patient. Other serious acute complications include gallbladder perforation (usually with formation of a pericholecystic abscess), emphysematous cholecystitis (secondary infection with a gas-forming organism), and empyema.

B. CHOLANGITIS

Cholangitis classically presents with Charcot's triad, namely, fever and chills, right upper quadrant pain, and jaundice. Although 95% of patients who present with this picture will have common duct stones, only a minority of patients with acute cholecystitis has common duct stones that will present in this manner.

C. CHRONIC CHOLECYSTITIS AND OTHER COMPLICATIONS

Chronic cholecystitis results from repeated episodes of acute cholecystitis or chronic irritation of the gallbladder wall by stones and is characterized pathologically by varying degrees of chronic inflammation of the gallbladder. Calculi are usually present. In about 4–5% of cases, the villi of the gallbladder undergo polypoid enlargement due to deposition of cholesterol that may be visible to the naked eye ("strawberry gallbladder," cholesterolosis). In other instances, adenomatous hyperplasia of all or part of the gallbladder wall may be so marked as to give the appearance of a myoma (pseudotumor). Hydrops of the gallbladder results when acute cholecystitis subsides but cystic duct obstruction persists, producing distention of the gallbladder with a clear mucoid fluid. Occasionally, a stone in the neck of the gallbladder may compress the bile duct and cause jaundice (Mirizzi's syndrome). Xanthogranulomatous cholecystitis is a rare variant of chronic cholecystitis characterized by grayish-yellow nodules or streaks, representing lipid-laden macrophages, in the wall of the gallbladder.

Cholelithiasis with chronic cholecystitis may be associated with acute exacerbations of gallbladder inflammation, common duct stone, fistulization to the bowel, pancreatitis, and, rarely, carcinoma of the gallbladder. Calcified (porcelain) gallbladder has generally been thought to have a high association with gallbladder carcinoma and to be an indication for cholecystectomy, although the risk of gallbladder cancer may be higher when calcification is mucosal rather than intramural.

Treatment

Acute cholecystitis will usually subside on a conservative regimen (withholding of oral feedings, intravenous alimentation, analgesics, and intravenous antibiotics—generally a third-generation cephalosporin such as cefoperazone 1–2 g intravenously every 12 hours with the addition of metronidazole 500 mg intravenously every 6 hours in severe cases). Meperidine may be preferable to morphine for pain because of less spasm of the sphincter of Oddi. Because of the high risk of recurrent attacks (up to 10% by 1 month and over 30% by 1 year), cholecystectomy—generally laparoscopically—should generally be performed within 2–3 days after hospitalization (and immediately if perforation or gangrene is suspected). If nonsurgical treatment has been elected, the patient (especially if diabetic or elderly) should be watched carefully for recurrent symptoms, evidence of gangrene of the gallbladder, or cholangitis. In high-risk patients, ultrasound-guided aspiration of the gallbladder, if feasible, percutaneous cholecystostomy, or endoscopic insertion of a stent into the gallbladder may postpone or even avoid the need for surgery. Cholecystectomy is mandatory when there is evidence of gangrene or perforation.

Surgical treatment of chronic cholecystitis is the same as for acute cholecystitis. If indicated, cholangiography can be performed during laparoscopic cholecystectomy. Choledocholithiasis can also be excluded by either preoperative or postoperative ERCP or MRCP.

Prognosis

The overall mortality rate of cholecystectomy is less than 1%, but hepatobiliary tract surgery is a more formidable procedure in the elderly, in whom the mortality rate is 5–10%. A technically successful surgical procedure in an appropriately selected patient is generally followed by complete resolution of symptoms.

Conway JD et al: Endoscopic stent insertion into the gallbladder for symptomatic gallbladder disease in patients with end-stage liver disease. Gastrointest Endosc 2005;61:32. [PMID: 15672053]

Lau H et al: Early versus delayed-interval laparoscopic cholecystectomy for acute cholecystitis: a meta-analysis. Surg Endosc 2006;20:82. [PMID: 16247580]

Makela JT et al: Acute cholecystitis in the elderly. Hepatogastroenterology 2005;52:999. [PMID: 16001616]

PRE- & POSTCHOLECYSTECTOMY SYNDROMES

Precholecystectomy

In a small group of patients (mostly women) with biliary pain, conventional radiographic studies of the upper gastrointestinal tract and gallbladder—including cholangiography—are unremarkable. In some such cases, emptying of the gallbladder is markedly reduced on gallbladder scintigraphy following injection of cholecystokinin; cholecystectomy may be curative. In some cases, histologic examination of the resected gallbladder shows chronic cholecystitis or microlithiasis. An additional diagnostic consideration is sphincter of Oddi dysfunction (see below).

Postcholecystectomy

Following cholecystectomy, some patients complain of continuing symptoms, ie, right upper quadrant pain, flatulence, and fatty food intolerance. The persistence of symptoms in this group of patients suggests the possibility of an incorrect diagnosis prior to cholecystectomy, eg, esophagitis, pancreatitis, radiculopathy, or functional bowel disease. It is important to rule out the possibility of choledocholithiasis or common duct stricture as a cause of persistent symptoms. Pain may also be associated with dilation of the cystic duct remnant, neuroma formation in the ductal wall, foreign body granuloma, or traction on the common duct by a long cystic duct.

The clinical presentation of right upper quadrant pain, chills, fever, or jaundice should suggest biliary tract disease. Endoscopic ultrasonography or retrograde cholangiography may be necessary to demonstrate or exclude biliary tract disease. Biliary pain associated with elevated liver tests and a dilated bile duct suggests sphincter of Oddi dysfunction or stenosis. Biliary manometry may be useful for documenting elevated baseline sphincter of Oddi pressures typical of sphincter dysfunction when biliary pain is associated with elevated liver tests (twofold) or a dilated bile duct (> 12 mm) (sphincter of Oddi dysfunction type II) but is not necessary when both are present (sphincter of Oddi dysfunction type I) and is associated with a high risk of pancreatitis. (Analogous criteria have been developed for pancreatic sphincter dysfunction.) Biliary scintigraphy and MRCP following intravenous administration of secretin show promise as screening tests for sphincter dysfunction. Endoscopic sphincterotomy is most likely to relieve symptoms when they are associated with elevated liver chemistry tests, a dilated common duct, or an elevated sphincter of Oddi pressure, although many patients continue to have some pain. In some cases, treatment with calcium channel blockers, long-acting nitrates, or possibly injection of the sphincter with botulinum toxin may be beneficial. In refractory cases, surgical sphincteroplasty or removal of the cystic duct remnant may be considered.

Baillie J: Sphincter of Oddi dysfunction: overdue for an overhaul. Am J Gastroenterol 2005;100:1217. [PMID: 15929746]

Fogel EL et al: Abdominal pain with fluctuating elevation of amylase and AST. Clin Gastroenterol Hepatol 2005;3:538. [PMID: 15952095]

Madura JA et al: Surgical sphincteroplasty in 446 patients. Arch Surg 2005;140:504. [PMID: 15897447]

Rastogi A et al: Controversies concerning pathophysiology and management of acalculous biliary-type abdominal pain. Dig Dis Sci 2005;50:1391. [PMID: 16110827]

CHOLEDOCHOLITHIASIS & CHOLANGITIS

 ESSENTIALS OF DIAGNOSIS

- *Often a history of biliary pain or jaundice.*
- *Sudden onset of severe right upper quadrant or epigastric pain, which may radiate to the right scapula or shoulder.*
- *Occasional patients present with painless jaundice.*
- *Nausea and vomiting.*
- *Fever, which may be followed by hypothermia and gram-negative shock, jaundice, and leukocytosis.*
- *Stones in bile duct most reliably detected by ERCP or endoscopic ultrasound.*

General Considerations

About 15% of patients with gallstones have choledocholithiasis (common bile duct stones). The percentage rises with age, and the frequency in elderly people with gallstones may be as high as 50%. Common duct stones usually originate in the gallbladder but may also form spontaneously in the common duct after cholecystectomy. The risk is increased twofold in persons with a juxtapapillary duodenal diverticulum. The stones are frequently "silent" as no symptoms result unless there is obstruction.

Clinical Findings

A. SYMPTOMS AND SIGNS

A history of biliary pain or prior jaundice may be obtained. Biliary pain results from rapid increases in common bile duct pressure due to obstructed bile flow. The features that suggest the presence of a common duct stone are (1) frequently recurring attacks of right upper abdominal pain that is severe and persists for hours, (2) chills and fever associated with severe pain, and (3) a history of jaundice associated with episodes of abdominal pain. The combination of pain, fever (and chills), and jaundice represents **Charcot's triad** and denotes the classic picture of cholangitis. The addition of altered sensorium and hypotension (Reynold's pentad) connotes acute suppurative cholangitis and represents an endoscopic emergency.

Hepatomegaly may be present in calculous biliary obstruction, and tenderness is usually present in the right upper quadrant and epigastrium. Common duct obstruction lasting longer than 30 days results in liver damage leading to cirrhosis. Hepatic failure with portal hypertension occurs in untreated cases.

B. LABORATORY FINDINGS

Acute obstruction of the bile duct typically produces a transient albeit striking increase in serum aminotransferase levels (> 1000 units/L). Bilirubinuria and elevation of serum bilirubin are present if the common duct remains obstructed; levels commonly fluctuate. Serum alkaline phosphatase levels rise more slowly and are suggestive of obstructive jaundice. Not uncommonly, serum amylase elevations are present because of secondary pancreatitis. When extrahepatic obstruction persists for more than a few weeks, differentiation of obstruction from chronic cholestatic liver disease becomes more difficult. Leukocytosis is present in patients with cholangitis. Prolongation of the prothrombin time can result from the obstructed flow of bile to the intestine. In contrast to hepatocellular dysfunction, hypoprothrombinemia due to obstructive jaundice will respond to 10 mg of parenteral vitamin K or water-soluble oral vitamin K (phytonadione, 5 mg) within 24–36 hours.

C. IMAGING

Ultrasonography and CT scan may demonstrate dilated bile ducts. and radionuclide imaging may show impaired bile flow. Endoscopic ultrasonography, helical CT, and magnetic resonance cholangiography have been found to be accurate in demonstrating common duct stones and may be used in patients thought to be at low or intermediate risk for choledocholithiasis. ERCP (occasionally with intraductal ultrasound) or percutaneous transhepatic cholangiography provides the most direct and accurate means of determining the cause, location, and extent of obstruction. If the likelihood that obstruction is caused by a stone or that cholangitis is present is high, ERCP is the procedure of choice because it permits sphincterotomy with stone extraction or stent placement. Endoscopic balloon dilation of the sphincter of Oddi is associated with a higher rate of pancreatitis than endoscopic sphincterotomy and is generally reserved for patients with coagulopathy, in whom the risk of bleeding is lower with balloon dilation than with sphincterotomy.

Differential Diagnosis

The most common cause of obstructive jaundice is common duct stone. Next in frequency are neoplasms of the pancreas, ampulla of Vater, or common duct. Extrinsic compression of the common duct may result from metastatic carcinoma (usually from the gastrointestinal tract or breast) involving porta hepatis lymph nodes or, rarely, from a large duodenal diverticulum. Gallbladder cancer extending into the common duct often presents as obstructive jaundice. Chronic cholestatic liver diseases (primarily biliary cirrhosis, sclerosing cholangitis, drug-induced) must be considered. Hepatocellular jaundice can usually be differentiated by the history, clinical findings, and liver tests, but liver biopsy is necessary on occasion. Recurrent pyogenic cholangitis should be considered in persons from Asia (and occasionally elsewhere) with intrahepatic biliary stones (particularly in the left ductal system) and with recurrent cholangitis.

Treatment

Common duct stone in a patient with cholelithiasis or cholecystitis is usually treated by endoscopic sphincterotomy and stone extraction followed by laparoscopic cholecystectomy. For the poor-risk patient with cholelithiasis and choledocholithiasis, however, cholecystectomy may be deferred after endoscopic sphincterotomy because the risk of subsequent cholecystitis is low. ERCP with sphincterotomy should be performed before cholecystectomy in patients with gallstones and jaundice (serum total bilirubin > 5 mg/dL), a dilated common bile duct (> 7 mm), or stones in the bile duct seen on ultrasound or CT scans. (Stones may ultimately recur in up to 12% of patients, particularly when the bile duct diameter is ≥ 15 mm or there are brown pigment stones at time of the initial sphincterotomy.) In patients with biliary pancreatitis that resolves rapidly, the stone usually passes into the intestine, and ERCP prior to cholecystectomy is not necessary if an intraoperative cholangiogram is done.

Choledocholithiasis discovered at laparoscopic cholecystectomy may be managed via laparoscopic common duct exploration or, if necessary, conversion to open surgery or by postoperative endoscopic sphincterotomy. Operative findings of choledocholithiasis are palpable stones in the common duct, dilation or thickening of the wall of the common duct, or stones in the gallbladder small enough to pass through the cystic duct. Laparoscopic intraoperative cholangiography should be done at the time of cholecystectomy in patients with liver enzyme elevations but a common duct diameter of less than 5 mm; if a ductal stone is found, the duct is explored. In the postcholecystectomy patient with choledocholithiasis, endoscopic sphincterotomy with stone extraction is preferable to transabdominal surgery. Lithotripsy (endoscopic or external), direct cholangioscopy, or biliary stenting may be a therapeutic consideration for large stones. For the patient with a T tube and common duct stone, the stone may be extracted via the T tube. A properly placed T tube should drain bile at the operating table and continuously thereafter; otherwise, it should be considered blocked or dislocated. The volume of bile drainage varies from 100 mL to 1000 mL daily (average, 200–400 mL). Above-average drainage may be due to obstruction at the ampulla (usually by edema).

Postoperative antibiotics are not administered routinely after biliary tract surgery. Cultures of the bile are always taken at operation. If biliary tract infection was present preoperatively or is apparent at operation, ampicillin (500 mg every 6 hours intravenously) with gentamicin (1.5 mg/kg intravenously every 8 hours) and metronidazole (500 mg intravenously every 6 hours) or ciprofloxacin (250 mg intravenously every 12 hours) or a third-generation cephalosporin (eg, cefoperazone, 1–2 g intravenous every 12 hours) is administered postoperatively until the results of sensitivity tests on culture specimens are available. A T-tube cholangiogram should be done before the tube is removed, usually about 3 weeks after surgery. A small amount of bile frequently leaks from the tube site for a few days.

Urgent ERCP, sphincterotomy, and stone extraction are generally indicated for choledocholithiasis complicated by ascending cholangitis and are preferred to surgery. Before ERCP, liver function should be evaluated thoroughly. Prothrombin time should be restored to normal by parenteral administration of vitamin K (see above). Ciprofloxacin, 250 mg intravenously every 12 hours, penetrates well into bile and is effective treatment for cholangitis. An alternative regimen in severely ill patients is mezlocillin, 3 g intravenously every 4 hours, plus either metronidazole or gentamicin (or both). The dose of metronidazole is 500 mg intravenously every 6 hours (if there has been no prior manipulation of the duct); the dose of gentamicin is 2 mg/kg intravenously as loading dose, plus 1.5 mg/kg every 8 hours adjusted for renal function. Aminoglycosides should not be given for more than a few days because the risk of aminoglycoside nephrotoxicity is increased in patients with cholestasis. Emergent decompression of the bile duct, generally by ERCP, is required for patients who are septic or fail to improve on antibiotics within 12–24 hours. Medical therapy alone is most likely to fail in patients with tachycardia, serum albumin < 3 g/dL, marked hyperbilirubinemia, and prothrombin time > 14 seconds on admission. If sphincterotomy cannot be performed, decompression by a biliary stent or nasobiliary catheter can be done. Once decompression is achieved, antibiotics are generally continued for at least another three days. Elective cholecystectomy can be undertaken after resolution of cholangitis, unless the patient remains unfit for surgery.

Baron TH et al: Endoscopic balloon dilation of the biliary sphincter compared to endoscopic biliary sphincterotomy for removal of common bile duct stones during ERCP: a metaanalysis of randomized, controlled trials. Am J Gastroenterol 2004;99: 1455.

Kim Y-J et al: Preoperative evaluation of common bile duct stones in patients with gallstone disease. AJR 2005;184: 1854. [PMID: 15908542]

Kondo S et al: Detection of common bile duct stones: comparison between endoscopic ultrasonography, magnetic resonance cholangiography, and helical-computed-tomographic cholangiography. Eur J Radiol 2005;54:271. [PMID: 15837409]

Nathanson LK et al: Preoperative ERCP versus laparoscopic choledochotomy for clearance of select bile duct calculi. Ann Surg 2005;242:188. [PMID: 16041208]

Sharma BC et al: Endoscopic biliary drainage by nasobiliary drain or by stent placement in patients with acute cholangitis. Endoscopy 2005;37:439. [PMID: 15844022]

BILIARY STRICTURE

Benign biliary strictures are the result of surgical anastomosis or injury in about 95% of cases. The remainder of cases are caused by blunt external injury to the abdomen, pancreatitis, erosion of the duct by a gallstone, or prior endoscopic sphincterotomy.

Signs of injury to the duct may or may not be recognized in the immediate postoperative period. If complete occlusion has occurred, jaundice will develop rapidly; more often, however, a tear has been accidentally made in the duct, and the earliest manifestation of injury may be excessive or prolonged loss of bile from the surgical drains. Bile leakage may predispose to localized infection, which in turn accentuates scar formation and the ultimate development of a fibrous stricture.

Cholangitis is the most common complication of stricture. Typically, the patient experiences episodes of pain, fever, chills, and jaundice within a few weeks to months after cholecystectomy. Physical findings may include jaundice during an attack of cholangitis and right upper quadrant abdominal tenderness.

Serum alkaline phosphatase is usually elevated. Hyperbilirubinemia is variable, fluctuating during exacerbations and usually remaining in the range of 5–10 mg/dL. Blood cultures may be positive during an episode of cholangitis. MRCP can be valuable in demonstrating the stricture, whereas ERCP and PTC permit biopsy and cytologic specimens and allow dilation and stent placement, thereby avoiding surgical repair in some cases. Placement of multiple plastic stents appears to be more effective than placement of a single stent. Metal stents, which often cannot be removed endoscopically, are generally avoided in benign strictures unless life expectancy is less than 2 years. The use of covered metal stents, which are more easily removed endoscopically than uncovered metal stents, as well as bioabsorbable stents, is under study. When malignancy cannot be excluded with certainty, additional endoscopic diagnostic approaches may be considered—if available—including endoscopic ultrasonography, intraductal ultrasound, and choledochoscopy (cholangioscopy).

Differentiation from cholangiocarcinoma may ultimately require surgical exploration. Significant hepatocellular disease due to secondary biliary cirrhosis will inevitably occur if a biliary stricture is not treated. Operative treatment of a stricture frequently necessitates performance of an end-to-end ductal repair, choledochojejunostomy, or hepaticojejunostomy to reestablish bile flow into the intestine.

Matlock J et al: Endoscopic therapy of benign biliary strictures. Rev Gastrointest Disord 2005;5:206. [PMID: 16369216]

Siriwardana HPP et al: Systematic appraisal of the role of metallic endobiliary stents in the treatment of benign bile duct stricture. Ann Surg 2005;242:10. [PMID: 15973096]

Zoepf T et al: Balloon dilatation vs. balloon dilatation plus bile duct endoprostheses for treatment of anastomotic biliary strictures after liver transplantation. Liver Transpl 2006;12:88. [PMID: 16382450]

PRIMARY SCLEROSING CHOLANGITIS

 ESSENTIALS OF DIAGNOSIS

- *Most common in men aged 20–50 years.*
- *Often associated with ulcerative colitis.*
- *Progressive jaundice, itching, and other features of cholestasis.*
- *Diagnosis based on characteristic cholangiographic findings.*
- *10% risk of cholangiocarcinoma.*

General Considerations

Primary sclerosing cholangitis is an uncommon disease characterized by a diffuse inflammation of the biliary tract leading to fibrosis and strictures of the biliary system. The disease is most common in men aged 20–40 years, with a prevalence rate in the United States of 21 per 100,000 men and 6 per 100,000 women, and is closely associated with ulcerative colitis (and occasionally Crohn's colitis), which is present in approximately two-thirds of patients with primary sclerosing cholangitis; however, clinically significant sclerosing cholangitis develops in only 1–4% of patients with ulcerative colitis. As in ulcerative colitis, smoking is associated with a decreased risk of primary sclerosing cholangitis. Primary sclerosing cholangitis is associated with the histocompatible antigens HLA-B8 and -DR3 or -DR4, suggesting that genetic factors may play an etiologic role. ANCA, with fluorescent staining characteristics and target antigens distinct from those found in patients with Wegener's granulomatosis or vasculitis, are found in 30–80% of patients. In patients with AIDS, sclerosing cholangitis may result from infections caused by cytomegalovirus, cryptosporidium, or microsporidium. Rarely, a clinical and radiologic picture of sclerosing cholangitis can follow an episode of septic shock.

Clinical Findings

A. SYMPTOMS AND SIGNS

Primary sclerosing cholangitis presents as progressive obstructive jaundice, frequently associated with fatigue, pruritus, anorexia, and indigestion. Patients may be diagnosed in the presymptomatic phase because of an elevated alkaline phosphatase level. Complications of chronic cholestasis, such as osteoporosis and malabsorption of fat-soluble vitamins, may occur late in the course. Esophageal varices are most likely in patients with a platelet count below 150,000/mcL, low serum albumin, and advanced histologic stage. In patients with primary sclerosing cholangitis, ulcerative colitis is frequently characterized by rectal sparing and backwash ileitis.

B. DIAGNOSTIC FINDINGS

The diagnosis of primary sclerosing cholangitis is increasingly made by magnetic resonance cholangiography, the sensitivity of which approaches that of ERCP. Characteristic cholangiographic findings are segmental fibrosis of bile ducts with saccular dilatations between strictures. Biliary obstruction by a stone or tumor should be excluded. The disease may be confined to small intrahepatic bile ducts, in which case MRCP and ERCP are normal and the diagnosis is suggested by liver biopsy. These patients have a longer survival and lower rate of cholangiocarcinoma than patients with involvement of the large ducts. Liver biopsy also allows staging, which is based on the degree of fibrosis. In addition to ANCA, patients may have serum antinuclear, anticardiolipin, antithyroperoxidase, and anti-*Saccharomyces cerevisiae* antibodies and rheumatoid factor. Occasional patients have clinical and histologic features of both sclerosing cholangitis and autoimmune hepatitis. Even more rarely, an association with chronic pancreatitis (sclerosing pancreaticocholangitis) is seen, and this entity is often responsive to corticosteroids. In general, the diagnosis of primary sclerosing cholangitis is difficult to make after biliary surgery or intrahepatic artery chemotherapy, which may result in bile duct injury and secondary sclerosing cholangitis. Primary sclerosing cholangitis must be distinguished from idiopathic adulthood ductopenia, a rare disorder affecting young to middle-aged adults who manifest cholestasis resulting from loss of interlobular and septal bile ducts yet who have a normal cholangiogram.

Complications

Cholangiocarcinoma may complicate the course of primary sclerosing cholangitis in at least 10% of cases and may be difficult to diagnose by cytologic examination or biopsy because of false-negative results. A serum CA 19-9 level > 100 units/mL is suggestive but not diagnostic of cholangiocarcinoma. Patients with ulcerative colitis and primary sclerosing cholangitis are at high risk for colorectal neoplasia.

Treatment

Treatment with corticosteroids and broad-spectrum antimicrobial agents has been used with inconsistent and unpredictable results. Episodes of acute bacterial cholangitis may be treated with ciprofloxacin (750 mg twice daily orally or intravenously). Ursodeoxycholic acid in standard doses (10–15 mg/kg/d orally) may improve liver function test results but does not appear to alter the natural history. However, recent experience suggests that high-dose ursodeoxycholic acid (22–25 mg/kg/d) may reduce cholangiographic progression and liver fibrosis but does not appear to improve survival or prevent cholangiocarcinoma. Other drugs such as cyclosporine and tacrolimus are under study. Careful endoscopic evaluation of the biliary tree may permit balloon dilation of localized strictures. If there is a major stricture, short-term placement of a stent may relieve symptoms and improve biochemical abnormalities with sustained improvement after the stent is removed. Repeated balloon dilation of a recurrent dominant bile duct stricture may improve survival. However, long-term stenting may increase the rate of complications such as cholangitis. In patients without cirrhosis, surgical resection of a dominant bile duct stricture may lead to longer survival than endoscopic therapy by decreasing the subsequent risk of cholangiocarcinoma. In patients with ulcerative colitis, primary sclerosing cholangitis is an independent risk factor for the development of colorectal dysplasia and cancer, and strict adherence to a colonoscopic surveillance program is advisable. Treatment with ursodeoxycholic acid has been reported to reduce the risk of colorectal dysplasia and carcinoma in patients with ulcerative colitis and primary sclerosing cholangitis. For patients with cirrhosis and clinical decompensation, liver transplantation is the procedure of choice.

Prognosis

Survival of patients with primary sclerosing cholangitis averages 10 years once symptoms appear. Adverse prognostic markers are older age, higher serum bilirubin and AST levels, lower albumin levels, and a history of variceal bleeding. Variceal bleeding is also a risk factor for cholangiocarinoma. Actuarial survival rates with liver transplantation are as high as 85% at 3 years, but rates are much lower once cholangiocarcinoma has developed. Following transplantation, patients have an increased risk of nonanastomotic biliary strictures and—in those with ulcerative colitis—colon cancer. The retransplantation rate is higher than that for primary biliary cirrhosis. Those patients who are unable to undergo liver transplantation will ultimately require high-quality palliative care (see Chapter 5).

Cullen SN et al: Review article: current management of primary sclerosing cholangitis. Aliment Pharmacol Ther 2005;21: 933. [PMID: 15813829]

Loftus EV Jr et al: PSC-IBD: a unique form of inflammatory bowel disease associated with primary sclerosing cholangitis. Gut 2005;54:91. [PMID: 15591511]

Olsson R et al: High-dose ursodeoxycholic acid in primary sclerosing cholangitis: a 5-year multicenter, randomized, controlled study. Gastroenterology 2005;129:1464. [PMID: 16285948]

Talwalkar JA et al: Primary sclerosing cholangitis. Inflamm Bowel Dis 2005;11:62. [PMID: 15674115]

CARCINOMA OF THE BILIARY TRACT

ESSENTIALS OF DIAGNOSIS

- *Presents with obstructive jaundice, usually painless, often with dilated biliary tree.*
- *Pain is more common in gallbladder carcinoma than cholangiocarcinoma.*

- *A Courvoisier (dilated) gallbladder may be detected.*
- *Diagnosis by cholangiography with biopsy and brushings for cytology.*

General Considerations

Carcinoma of the gallbladder occurs in approximately 2% of all people operated on for biliary tract disease. It is notoriously insidious, and the diagnosis is often made unexpectedly at surgery. Cholelithiasis (often large, symptomatic stones) is usually present. Other risk factors are chronic infection of the gallbladder with *Salmonella typhi*, gallbladder polyps over 1 cm in diameter, mucosal calcification of the gallbladder (porcelain gallbladder), and anomalous pancreaticobiliary ductal junction. Genetic factors include K-*ras* and *TP53* mutations. Spread of the cancer—by direct extension into the liver or to the peritoneal surface—may be the initial manifestation. The TNM classification includes the following stages: Tis, carcinoma in situ; T1a, tumor invades lamina propria, and T1b, tumor invades muscle layer; T2, tumor invades perimuscular connective tissue, no extension beyond serosa (visceral peritoneum) or into liver; T3, tumor perforates the serosa or directly invades the liver or adjacent organ or structure; T4, tumor invades the main portal vein or hepatic artery or invades multiple extrahepatic organs or structures; N1, regional lymph node metastasis; and M1, distant metastasis.

Carcinoma of the bile ducts (cholangiocarcinoma) accounts for 3% of all cancer deaths in the United States, and the incidence and mortality rates have increased dramatically in the past two decades. It is more prevalent in persons aged 50–70, with a slight male predominance. Two-thirds arise at the confluence of the hepatic ducts (Klatskin tumors), and one-fourth arise in the distal extrahepatic bile duct; the remainder are intrahepatic (peripheral), the incidence of which is continuing to rise. Staging is similar to that for carcinoma of the gallbladder. The frequency of carcinoma in persons with choledochal cysts has been reported to be over 14% at 20 years, and surgical excision is recommended. There is an increased incidence in patients with Caroli's disease, a biliary-enteric anastomosis, and ulcerative colitis, especially those with primary sclerosing cholangitis, cirrhosis, and past exposure to thorotrast, a contrast agent. In southeast Asia, hepatolithiasis and infection of the bile ducts with helminths (*Clonorchis sinensis, Opisthorchis viverrini*) are associated with chronic cholangitis and an increased risk of cholangiocarcinoma. Hepatitis C virus infection, HIV infection, diabetes mellitus, and tobacco smoking are additional risk factors for intrahepatic cholangiocarcinoma.

Clinical Findings

A. SYMPTOMS AND SIGNS

Progressive jaundice is the most common and usually the first sign of obstruction of the extrahepatic biliary system.

Pain in the right upper abdomen with radiation into the back is usually present early in the course of gallbladder carcinoma, but this occurs later in the course of bile duct carcinoma. Anorexia and weight loss are common and often associated with fever and chills due to cholangitis. Rarely, hematemesis or melena results from erosion of tumor into a blood vessel (hemobilia). Fistula formation between the biliary system and adjacent organs may also occur. The course is usually one of rapid deterioration, with death occurring within a few months.

Physical examination reveals profound jaundice. A palpable gallbladder with obstructive jaundice usually is said to signify malignant disease (Courvoisier's law); however, this clinical generalization has been proved to be accurate only about 50% of the time. Hepatomegaly is usually present and is associated with liver tenderness. Ascites may occur with peritoneal implants. Pruritus and skin excoriations are common.

B. LABORATORY FINDINGS

Laboratory examination reveals predominantly conjugated hyperbilirubinemia, with total serum bilirubin values ranging from 5 to 30 mg/dL. There is usually concomitant elevation of the alkaline phosphatase and serum cholesterol. AST is normal or minimally elevated. An elevated CA 19-9 level may help distinguish cholangiocarcinoma from a benign biliary stricture (in the absence of cholangitis).

C. IMAGING

Ultrasonography and contrast-enhanced, triple-phase, helical CT may show a gallbladder mass in gallbladder carcinoma and intrahepatic mass or biliary dilation in carcinoma of the bile ducts. CT may also show involved regional lymph nodes and atrophy of a hepatic lobe because of vascular encasement with compensatory hypertrophy of the unaffected lobe. MRI with MRCP and gadolinium enhancement permits visualization of the entire biliary tree and detection of vascular invasion and obviates the need for angiography and, in some cases, direct cholangiography; it has become the imaging procedure of choice but may understage malignant hilar strictures. Preliminary observations suggest that positron emission tomography can detect cholangiocarcinomas as small as 1 cm, but false-positive results occur. The most helpful diagnostic studies before surgery are either percutaneous transhepatic or endoscopic retrograde cholangiography with biopsy and cytologic specimens, although false-negative biopsy and cytology results are common. Endoscopic ultrasound with fine-needle aspiration of tumors, choledochoscopy, and intraductal ultrasonography also have roles in the diagnosis of cholangiocarcinoma.

Treatment

In young and fit patients, curative surgery may be attempted if the tumor is well localized. The 5-year survival rate for localized carcinoma of the gallbladder (stage 1, T1a, N0, M0) is as high as 80% with laparoscopic cholecystectomy but drops to 15%, even with a more extended open resection, if there is muscular invasion (T1b). If the tumor is unresectable at laparotomy, biliary-enteric bypass (eg, Roux-en-Y hepaticojejunostomy) can be performed. Carcinoma of the bile ducts is curable by surgery in less than 10% of cases. If resection margins are negative, the 5-year survival rate may be as high as 47% for intrahepatic cholangiocarcinomas and 54% for distal cholangiocarcinomas, but the perioperative mortality rate may be as high as 10%. Palliation can be achieved by placement of a self-expandable metal stent via an endoscopic or percutaneous transhepatic route. Covered metal stents may be more cost-effective than uncovered metal stents because of a lower risk of stent occlusion, but they are not associated with longer survival. For hilar tumors, there is controversy as to whether unilateral or bilateral stents should be inserted. Plastic stents are less expensive but more prone to occlude than metal ones; they are suitable for patients expected to survive only a few months. Preliminary experience suggests that photodynamic therapy in combination with stent placement prolongs survival when compared with stent placement alone in patients with nonresectable cholangiocarcinoma. Radiotherapy may relieve pain and contribute to biliary decompression. There is limited response to chemotherapy such as with gemcitabine. In general, the prognosis is poor, with few patients surviving for more than 12 months after surgery. Although cholangiocarcinoma is generally considered to be a contraindication to liver transplantation because of rapid tumor recurrence, an 80% 5-year survival rate has been reported in patients with stage I and II cholangiocarcinoma undergoing chemoradiation and exploratory laparotomy followed by liver transplantation.

For those patients whose disease progresses despite treatment, meticulous efforts at palliative care are essential (see Chapter 5).

Brugge WR: Endoscopic techniques to diagnose and manage biliary tumors. J Clin Oncol 2005;23:4561. [PMID: 16002848]

Khan SA et al: Cholangiocarcinoma. Lancet 2005;366:1303. [PMID: 16214602]

Lazaridis KN et al: Cholangiocarcinoma. Gastroenterology 2005; 128:1655. [PMID: 15887157]

Shaib YH et al: Risk factors of intrahepatic cholangiocarcinoma in the United States: a case-control study. Gastroenterology 2005;128:620. [PMID: 15765398]

■ DISEASES OF THE PANCREAS

ACUTE PANCREATITIS

ESSENTIALS OF DIAGNOSIS

- *Abrupt onset of deep epigastric pain, often with radiation to the back.*
- *History of previous episodes, often related to alcohol intake.*

- *Nausea, vomiting, sweating, weakness.*
- *Abdominal tenderness and distention and fever.*
- *Leukocytosis, elevated serum amylase, elevated serum lipase.*

General Considerations

Acute pancreatitis is thought to result from "escape" of activated pancreatic enzymes from acinar cells into surrounding tissues. Most cases are related to biliary tract disease (a passed gallstone, usually < 5 mm in diameter) or heavy alcohol intake. The exact pathogenesis is not known but may include edema or obstruction of the ampulla of Vater, resulting in reflux of bile into pancreatic ducts, or direct injury to the acinar cells. Among the numerous other causes or associations are hypercalcemia, hyperlipidemias (chylomicronemia, hypertriglyceridemia, or both), abdominal trauma (including surgery), drugs (including azathioprine, mercaptopurine, asparaginase, pentamidine, didanosine, valproic acid, tetracyclines, estrogen and tamoxifen [by raising serum triglycerides], sulfonamides, mesalamine, thiazides, and possibly glucocorticoids), vasculitis, infections (eg, mumps, cytomegalovirus, *Mycobacterium avium* complex), peritoneal dialysis, cardiopulmonary bypass, ERCP, and genetic mutations that also predispose to chronic pancreatitis (see below). In patients with pancreas divisum, a congenital anomaly in which the dorsal and ventral pancreatic ducts fail to fuse, acute pancreatitis may result from stenosis of the minor papilla with obstruction to flow from the accessory pancreatic duct, although concomitant mutations in the cystic fibrosis transmembrane conductance regulator *(CFTR)* gene have also been reported to account for acute pancreatitis in some patients with pancreas divisum. Acute pancreatitis may also result from anomalous union of the pancreaticobiliary duct. Rarely, acute pancreatitis may be the presenting manifestation of a pancreatic or ampullary neoplasm. Apparently "idiopathic" acute pancreatitis is often caused by occult biliary microlithiasis and may be caused by sphincter of Oddi dysfunction involving the pancreatic duct. No more than 20% of cases are truly idiopathic. Smoking may increase the risk of alcoholic and idiopathic pancreatitis.

Pathologic changes in acute pancreatitis vary from acute edema and cellular infiltration to necrosis of the acinar cells, hemorrhage from necrotic blood vessels, and intra- and extrapancreatic fat necrosis. All or part of the pancreas may be involved.

Clinical Findings

A. SYMPTOMS AND SIGNS

Epigastric abdominal pain, generally abrupt in onset, is steady, boring, and severe and often made worse by walking and lying supine and better by sitting and leaning forward. The pain usually radiates into the back but may radiate to the right or left. Nausea and vomiting are usually present. Weakness, sweating, and anxiety are noted in severe attacks. There may be a history of alcohol intake or a heavy meal immediately preceding the attack, or a history of milder similar episodes or biliary colic in the past.

The abdomen is tender mainly in the upper part, most often without guarding, rigidity, or rebound. The abdomen may be distended, and bowel sounds may be absent with associated ileus. Fever of 38.4–39°C, tachycardia, hypotension (even true shock), pallor, and cool clammy skin are often present. Mild jaundice is common. Occasionally, an upper abdominal mass due to the inflamed pancreas or a pseudocyst may be palpated. Acute renal failure (usually prerenal) may occur early in the course of acute pancreatitis.

B. Assessment of Severity

Ranson's criteria are generally used in assessing the severity of acute alcoholic pancreatitis on presentation (pancreatitis due to other causes is assessed by similar criteria).

1. When three or more of the following are present on admission, a severe course complicated by pancreatic necrosis can be predicted with a sensitivity of 60–80%:

   Age over 55 years.

   White blood cell count over 16,000/mcL.

   Blood glucose over 200 mg/dL.

   Serum LDH over 350 units/L.

   AST over 250 units/L.

2. Development of the following in the first 48 hours indicates a worsening prognosis:

   Hematocrit drop of more than 10 percentage points.

   Blood urea nitrogen (BUN) rise greater than 5 mg/dL.

   Arterial P_{O_2} of less than 60 mm Hg.

   Serum calcium of less than 8 mg/dL.

   Base deficit over 4 mEq/L.

   Estimated fluid sequestration of more than 6 L.

3. Mortality rates correlate with the number of criteria present:

Number of criteria	Mortality rate
0–2	1%
3–4	16%
5–6	40%
7–8	100%

An APACHE II score ≥ 8 also correlates with mortality.

C. Laboratory Findings

Serum amylase and lipase are elevated—usually more than three times the upper limit of normal—within 24 hours in 90% of cases; their return to normal is variable depending on the severity of disease; lipase remains elevated longer than amylase and is slightly more accurate for the diagnosis of acute pancreatitis. Leukocytosis (10,000–30,000/mcL), proteinuria, granular casts, glycosuria (10–20% of cases), hyperglycemia, and elevated serum bilirubin may be present. Blood urea nitrogen and serum alkaline phosphatase may be elevated and coagulation tests abnormal. In patients with clear evidence of acute pancreatitis, a serum ALT level of more than 150 units/L suggests biliary pancreatitis. Decrease in serum calcium may reflect saponification and correlates well with severity of disease. Levels lower than 7 mg/dL (when serum albumin is normal) are associated with tetany and an unfavorable prognosis. Patients with acute pancreatitis caused by hypertriglyceridemia generally have fasting triglyceride levels above 1000 mg/dL. An early rise in the hematocrit value above 47% suggests hemoconcentration and is thought to predict severe disease. An elevated C-reactive protein (> 150 mg/L) concentration after 48 hours also suggests the development of pancreatic necrosis.

Other tests that offer the possibility of simplicity, rapidity, ease of use, and low cost—including urinary trypsinogen-2, trypsinogen activation peptide, and carboxypeptidase B—are under study, and a urinary dipstick for trypsinogen activation peptide is nearing commercial release. In patients in whom ascites or left pleural effusions develop, fluid amylase content is high. Electrocardiography may show ST–T wave changes.

D. Imaging

Plain radiographs of the abdomen may show gallstones, a "sentinel loop" (a segment of air-filled small intestine most commonly in the left upper quadrant), the "colon cutoff sign"—a gas-filled segment of transverse colon abruptly ending at the area of pancreatic inflammation—or linear focal atelectasis of the lower lobe of the lungs with or without pleural effusion. Ultrasound is often not helpful in diagnosing acute pancreatitis because of intervening bowel gas but may identify gallstones in the gallbladder. CT scan is useful in demonstrating an enlarged pancreas when the diagnosis of pancreatitis is uncertain, in detecting pseudocysts, and in differentiating pancreatitis from other possible intra-abdominal catastrophes. Intravenous contrast-enhanced CT following aggressive volume resuscitation is of particular value after the first 3 days of severe acute pancreatitis to identify areas of necrotizing pancreatitis and to assess prognosis (Table 15–8), although the use of intravenous contrast may increase the risk of complications of pancreatitis and of renal failure and should be avoided when the serum creatinine level is greater than 1.5 mg/dL. MRI appears to be a suitable alternative to CT. The presence of a fluid collection in the pancreas correlates with an increased mortality rate. CT-guided needle aspiration of areas of necrotizing pancreatitis after the third day may disclose infection, usually by enteric organisms, which invariably leads to death unless surgical debridement is ultimately performed. The presence of gas bubbles on CT scan implies that infection by gas-

Table 15–8. Severity index for acute pancreatitis.

CT Grade		Points	Necrosis		Severity Index	Mortality Rate (%)
			%	Additional Points		
A	Normal pancreas	0	0	0	0	0
B	Pancreatic enlargement	1	0	0	1	0
C	Pancreatic inflammation and/or peripancreatic fat	2	< 30	2	4	< 3
D	Single peripancreatic fluid collection	3	30–50	4	7	6
E	Two or more fluid collections or retroperitoneal air	4	> 50	6	10	> 17

Adapted from Balthazar EJ: Acute pancreatitis: assessment of severity with clinical and CT evaluation. Radiology 2002;223:603.

forming organisms is present. Endoscopic ultrasonography is useful in identifying occult biliary disease (eg, small stones, sludge), which, including microlithiasis, is present in a majority of patients with apparently idiopathic acute pancreatitis. ERCP is generally not indicated after a first attack of acute pancreatitis unless there is associated cholangitis or jaundice, but MRCP or endoscopic ultrasonography can be considered. After repeated attacks of idiopathic acute pancreatitis, aspiration of bile for crystal analysis may confirm the suspicion of microlithiasis, and manometry of the pancreatic duct sphincter may detect sphincter of Oddi dysfunction as a cause of pancreatitis.

Differential Diagnosis

Acute pancreatitis must be differentiated from an acutely perforated duodenal ulcer, acute cholecystitis, acute intestinal obstruction, leaking aortic aneurysm, renal colic, and acute mesenteric vascular insufficiency or thrombosis. Serum amylase may also be elevated in high intestinal obstruction, in gastroenteritis, in mumps not involving the pancreas (salivary amylase), in ectopic pregnancy, after administration of opioids, and after abdominal surgery. Serum lipase may also be elevated in many of these conditions.

Complications

Intravascular volume depletion secondary to leakage of fluids in the pancreatic bed and ileus with fluid-filled loops of bowel may result in prerenal azotemia and even acute tubular necrosis without overt shock. This usually occurs within 24 hours of the onset of acute pancreatitis and lasts 8–9 days. Some patients require peritoneal dialysis or hemodialysis.

As mentioned above, sterile or infected necrotizing pancreatitis may complicate the course of 5–10% of cases and accounts for most of the deaths. The risk of infection does not correlate with the extent of necrosis. Pancreatic necrosis is often associated with fever, leukocytosis, and, in some cases, shock and is associated with organ failure (eg, pulmonary, renal, gastrointestinal bleeding) in 50% of cases. Because infected pancreatic necrosis is almost always an indication for operative treatment, fine-needle aspiration of necrotic tissue under CT guidance should be performed (if necessary, repeatedly) for Gram stain and culture.

A serious complication of acute pancreatitis is acute respiratory distress syndrome (ARDS); cardiac dysfunction may be superimposed. It usually occurs 3–7 days after the onset of pancreatitis in patients who have required large volumes of fluid and colloid to maintain blood pressure and urinary output. Most patients with ARDS require assisted respiration with positive end-expiratory pressure.

Pancreatic abscess is a suppurative process characterized by rising fever, leukocytosis, and localized tenderness and epigastric mass usually 6 or more weeks into the course of acute pancreatitis. This may be associated with a left-sided pleural effusion or an enlarging spleen secondary to splenic vein thrombosis. In contrast to infected necrosis, the mortality rate is low following drainage.

Pseudocysts, encapsulated fluid collections with high enzyme content, commonly appear in pancreatitis when CT scans are used to monitor the evolution of an acute attack. Pseudocysts that are smaller than 6 cm in diameter often resolve spontaneously. They most commonly are within or adjacent to the pancreas but can present anywhere (eg, mediastinal, retrorectal), by extension along anatomic planes. Pseudocysts are multiple in 14% of cases. Pseudocysts may become secondarily infected, necessitating drainage as for an abscess. Erosion of the inflammatory process into a blood vessel can result in a major hemorrhage into the cyst.

Pancreatic ascites may present after recovery from acute pancreatitis as a gradual increase in abdominal girth and persistent elevation of the serum amylase level in the absence of frank abdominal pain. Marked elevations in the ascitic protein (> 3 g/dL) and amylase (> 1000 units/L) concentrations are typical. The condition results from rupture of the pancreatic duct or drainage of a pseudocyst into the peritoneal cavity.

Rare complications of acute pancreatitis include hemorrhage caused by erosion of a blood vessel to form a pseudoaneurysm and colonic necrosis. Chronic pancreatitis develops in about 10% of cases. Permanent diabetes mellitus and exocrine pancreatic insufficiency occur uncommonly after a single acute episode.

Treatment

A. MANAGEMENT OF ACUTE DISEASE

In most patients, acute pancreatitis is a mild disease that subsides spontaneously within several days. The pancreas is "rested" by a regimen of withholding food and liquids by mouth, bed rest, and, in patients with moderately severe pain or ileus and abdominal distention or vomiting, nasogastric suction. Pain is controlled with meperidine, up to 100–150 mg intramuscularly every 3–4 hours as necessary. In those with severe hepatic or renal dysfunction, the dose may need to be reduced. (Morphine has been thought to cause sphincter of Oddi spasm but is probably an acceptable alternative.) Oral intake of fluid and foods can be resumed when the patient is largely free of pain and has bowel sounds (even if the serum amylase is still elevated). Clear liquids are then given first, and gradual advancement to a low-fat diet is prescribed, guided by the patient's tolerance and by the absence of pain. Following recovery from acute biliary pancreatitis, laparoscopic cholecystectomy is generally performed, although in selected cases endoscopic sphincterotomy alone may be done. In patients with recurrent pancreatitis associated with pancreas divisum, insertion of a stent in the minor papilla (or minor papilla sphincterotomy) may reduce the frequency of subsequent attacks, although complications of such therapy are frequent.

In more severe pancreatitis—particularly necrotizing pancreatitis—there may be considerable leakage of fluids, necessitating large amounts of intravenous fluids to maintain intravascular volume. The importance of aggressive intravenous hydration cannot be overemphasized. Calcium gluconate must be given intravenously if there is evidence of hypocalcemia with tetany. Infusions of fresh frozen plasma or serum albumin may be necessary in patients with coagulopathy or hypoalbuminemia. With colloid solutions, there may be an increased risk of developing ARDS. If shock persists after adequate volume replacement (including packed red cells), pressors may be required. For the patient requiring a large volume of parenteral fluids, central venous pressure and blood gases should be monitored at regular intervals. Total parenteral nutrition (including lipids) should be considered in patients who have severe pancreatitis and ileus and will be without oral nutrition for at least 7–10 days. Enteral nutrition via a nasogastric or nasojejunal feeding tube is preferable but may not be tolerated in some patients with an ileus. Imipenem (500 mg every 8 hours intravenously) and possibly cefuroxime (1.5 g intravenously three times daily, then 250 mg orally twice daily) administered for up to 14 days to patients with sterile pancreatic necrosis appear to reduce the risk of pancreatic infection and mortality and the combination of ciprofloxacin and metronidazole may reduce the frequency of infected necrosis and multiorgan failure (but not mortality), but the routine use of antibiotics in patients with < 30% pancreatic necrosis is not indicated. The role of intravenous somatostatin in severe acute pancreatitis is uncertain, but octreotide is thought to have no benefit. There is conflicting evidence as to whether the risk of pancreatitis after ERCP can be reduced by the administration of somatostatin or gabexate mesilate, a protease inhibitor. Allopurinol and ulinastatin, another protease inhibitor, have been reported to reduce the frequency of post-ERCP pancreatitis. Lexipafant, an antagonist of platelet-activating factor, appears to be of no benefit.

The patient with severe pancreatitis requires attention in an intensive care unit. Close follow-up of white blood count, hematocrit, serum electrolytes, serum calcium, serum creatinine, BUN, serum AST and lactate dehydrogenase, and arterial blood gases is mandatory. Cultures of blood, urine, sputum, and pleural effusion (if present) and needle aspirations of areas of pancreatic necrosis (with CT guidance) should be obtained.

B. TREATMENT OF COMPLICATIONS AND FOLLOW-UP

A surgeon should be consulted in all cases of severe acute pancreatitis. If the diagnosis is in doubt and investigations indicate a strong possibility of a serious surgically correctable lesion (eg, perforated peptic ulcer), exploration is indicated. When acute pancreatitis is unexpectedly found on exploratory laparotomy, it is usually wise to close without intervention. If the pancreatitis appears mild and cholelithiasis is present, cholecystectomy or cholecystostomy may be justified. When severe pancreatitis results from choledocholithiasis—particularly if jaundice (serum total bilirubin > 5 mg/dL) or cholangitis is present—ERCP with endoscopic sphincterotomy and stone extraction is indicated. MRCP may be useful in selecting patients for therapeutic ERCP.

Operation may improve survival in patients with necrotizing pancreatitis and clinical deterioration with multiorgan failure or lack of resolution by 4–6 weeks. Surgery is nearly always indicated for infected necrosis. The goal of surgery is to debride necrotic pancreas and surrounding tissue and establish adequate drainage. Outcomes are best if surgery is delayed until the necrosis has organized, usually about 4 weeks after disease onset. In selected cases, nonsurgical drainage of necrotizing pancreatitis under radiologic or endoscopic guidance may be feasible, at least as a temporizing measure, depending on local expertise. Peritoneal lavage has not been shown to improve survival in severe acute pancreatitis, in part because the risk of late septic complications is not reduced.

The development of a pancreatic abscess is an indication for prompt percutaneous or surgical drainage. Chronic pseudocysts require endoscopic, percutaneous catheter, or surgical drainage when infected or associated with persisting pain, pancreatitis, or common duct obstruction. For pancreatic infections, imipenem, 500 mg every 8 hours intravenously, is a good choice of antibiotic because it achieves bactericidal levels in pancreatic tissue for most causative organisms.

Prognosis

Mortality rates for acute pancreatitis have declined from at least 10% to around 5% since the 1980s, but the mortality rate for severe acute pancreatitis (more than three Ranson criteria) remains at least 20%. Half of the deaths occur within the first 2 weeks, usually from multiorgan failure. Multiorgan failure that persists beyond the first 48 hours is associated with a mortality rate of over 50%. Later deaths occur because of complications of infected necrosis. Recurrences are common in alcoholic pancreatitis.

Draganov P et al: "Idiopathic" pancreatitis. Gastroenterology 2005;128:756. [PMID: 15765410]

Eatock FC et al: A randomized study of early nasogastric versus nasojejunal feeding in severe acute pancreatitis. Am J Gastroenterol 2005;100:432. [PMID: 15667504]

Garg PK et al: Association of extent and infection of pancreatic necrosis with organ failure and death in acute necrotizing pancreatitis. Clin Gastroenterol Hepatol 2005;3:159. [PMID: 15704050]

Lankisch PG et al: The role of antibiotic prophylaxis in the treatment of acute pancreatitis. J Clin Gastroenterol 2006;40:149. [PMID: 16394877]

Trivedi CD et al: Drug-induced pancreatitis: an update. J Clin Gastroenterol 2005;39:709. [PMID: 16082282]

UK Working Party on Acute Pancreatitis: UK guidelines for the management of acute pancreatitis. Gut 2005;54(suppl iii):1. [PMID: 15831893]

Vege SS et al: Management of pancreatic necrosis in severe acute pancreatitis. Clin Gastroenterol Hepatol 2005;3:192. [PMID: 15704054]

Werner J et al: Management of acute pancreatitis: from surgery to interventional intensive care. Gut 2005;54:426. [PMID: 15710995]

CHRONIC PANCREATITIS

ESSENTIALS OF DIAGNOSIS

- *Chronic or intermittent epigastric pain, steatorrhea, weight loss, abnormal pancreatic imaging.*
- *A mnemonic for the predisposing factors of chronic pancreatitis is TIGAR-O: toxic-metabolic, idiopathic, genetic; autoimmune, recurrent and severe acute pancreatitis, or obstructive.*

General Considerations

Chronic pancreatitis occurs most often in patients with alcoholism (70–80% of all cases). The risk of chronic pancreatitis increases with the duration and amount of alcohol consumed, but pancreatitis devel-

ops in only 5–10% of heavy drinkers. Ethanol is thought to cause secretion of insoluble pancreatic proteins that calcify and occlude the pancreatic duct. Progressive fibrosis and destruction of functioning glandular tissue then occur, perhaps as a result of repeated episodes of necroinflammation and activation of pancreatic stellate cells. Tobacco smoking has been reported to accelerate progression of alcoholic chronic pancreatitis. About 2% of patients with hyperparathyroidism develop pancreatitis. In tropical Africa and Asia, tropical pancreatitis, related in part to malnutrition, is the most common cause of chronic pancreatitis. A stricture, stone, or tumor obstructing the pancreas can lead to obstructive chronic pancreatitis. Autoimmune chronic pancreatitis is associated with hypergammaglobulinemia (IgG_4 in particular) and often with ANA and antibodies to carbonic anhydrase IV and is responsive to corticosteroids. About 10–20% of cases are idiopathic. Genetic factors may predispose to chronic pancreatitis in some of these cases. For example, a mutant trypsinogen gene *(PRSS1)* for hereditary pancreatitis, transmitted as an autosomal dominant trait with variable penetrance, has been identified on chromosome 7. Furthermore, mutations of the cystic fibrosis transmembrane conductance regulator *(CFTR)* gene have been identified in as many as 50% of patients with idiopathic chronic pancreatitis and no other clinical features of cystic fibrosis. Mutations of the pancreatic secretory trypsin inhibitory gene *(PSTI,* serine protease inhibitor, *SPINK1)* and possibly the gene for uridine 5'-diphosphate glucuronosyltransferase have also been associated with idiopathic chronic pancreatitis. A useful mnemonic for the predisposing factors to chronic pancreatitis is TIGAR-O: toxic-metabolic, idiopathic, genetic; autoimmune, recurrent and severe acute pancreatitis, or obstructive.

The pathogenesis of chronic pancreatitis may be explained by the SAPE (sentinel acute pancreatitis event) hypothesis by which the first (sentinel) acute pancreatitis event initiates an inflammatory process that results in both injury and later fibrosis. In many cases, chronic pancreatitis is a self-perpetuating disease characterized by chronic pain or recurrent episodes of acute pancreatitis and ultimately by pancreatic exocrine or endocrine insufficiency. After many years, chronic pain may resolve spontaneously or as a result of surgery tailored to the cause of pain. Over 80% of adults develop diabetes 25 years after the clinical onset of chronic pancreatitis.

Clinical Findings

A. SYMPTOMS AND SIGNS

Persistent or recurrent episodes of epigastric and left upper quadrant pain with referral to the upper left lumbar region are typical. Anorexia, nausea, vomiting, constipation, flatulence, and weight loss are common. Abdominal signs during attacks consist chiefly of tenderness over the pancreas, mild muscle guarding, and ileus. Attacks may last only a few hours or as long as 2 weeks; pain may eventually be almost continuous. Steatorrhea (as indicated by bulky, foul, fatty stools) may occur late in the course.

B. LABORATORY FINDINGS

Serum amylase and lipase may be elevated during acute attacks; however, a normal amylase does not exclude the diagnosis. Serum alkaline phosphatase and bilirubin may be elevated owing to compression of the common duct. Glycosuria may be present. Excess fecal fat may be demonstrated on chemical analysis of the stool; pancreatic insufficiency generally is confirmed by response to therapy with pancreatic enzyme supplements; the secretin stimulation test can be used if available, as can detection of decreased fecal chymotrypsin or elastase levels, although the latter tests lack sensitivity and specificity. Vitamin B_{12} malabsorption is detectable in about 40% of patients, but clinical deficiency of vitamin B_{12} and fat-soluble vitamins is rare. Accurate diagnostic tests are available for the major trypsinogen gene mutations, but because of uncertainty about the mechanisms linking heterozygous *CFTR* and *PSTI* mutations with pancreatitis, genetic testing for mutations in these two genes is not currently recommended.

C. IMAGING

Plain films show calcifications due to pancreaticolithiasis in 30% of affected patients. CT may show calcifications not seen on plain films as well as ductal dilation and heterogeneity or atrophy of the gland. Occasionally, the findings raise suspicion of pancreatic cancer ("tumefactive chronic pancreatitis"). ERCP is the most sensitive imaging study for chronic pancreatitis and may show dilated ducts, intraductal stones, strictures, or pseudocyst, but the results may be normal in patients with so-called minimal change pancreatitis. MRCP and endoscopic ultrasonography (with pancreatic tissue sampling) are less invasive alternatives to ERCP. Characteristic imaging features of autoimmune chronic pancreatitis include diffuse enlargement of the pancreas and irregular narrowing of the main pancreatic duct.

Complications

Opioid addiction is common. Other frequent complications include often brittle diabetes mellitus, pancreatic pseudocyst or abscess, cholestatic liver enzymes with or without jaundice, common bile duct stricture, steatorrhea, malnutrition, and peptic ulcer. Pancreatic cancer develops in 4% of patients after 20 years; the risk may relate to tobacco and alcohol use. In patients with hereditary pancreatitis, the risk of pancreatic cancer rises after age 50 years and reaches 19% by age 70 years.

Treatment

Correctable coexistent biliary tract disease should be treated surgically.

Table 15–9. Selected pancreatic enzyme preparations.

Product	Enzyme Content Per Unit Dose		
	Lipase	Amylase	Protease
Conventional preparations			
Viokase	8000	30,000	30,000
Pancrelipase	8000	30,000	30,000
Enteric-coated microencapsulated preparations			
Creon 10	10,000	33,200	37,500
Creon 20	20,000	66,400	75,000
Lipram CR 10	10,000	33,200	37,500
Lipram UL 12	12,000	39,000	39,000
Lipram PM 16	16,000	48,000	48,000
Lipram UL 18	18,000	58,500	58,500
Lipram CR 20	20,000	66,400	75,000
Pancrease	4500	20,000	25,000
Pancrease MT10	10,000	30,000	30,000
Pancrease MT16	16,000	48,000	48,000
Pancrease MT20	20,000	56,000	44,000
Ultrase MT12	12,000	39,000	39,000
Ultrase MT20	20,000	65,000	65,000

Modified from *Drug Facts and Comparisons*, 2005.

A. MEDICAL MEASURES

A low-fat diet should be prescribed. Alcohol is forbidden because it frequently precipitates attacks. Narcotics should be avoided if possible. Steatorrhea is treated with pancreatic supplements that are selected on the basis of their high lipase activity. A total dose of 30,000 units of lipase in capsules is given with meals (Table 15–9). Higher doses may be required in some cases. The tablets should be taken at the start of, during, and at the end of a meal. Concurrent administration of H_2-receptor antagonists (eg, ranitidine, 150 mg orally twice daily), a proton pump inhibitor (eg, omeprazole, 20–60 mg orally daily), or sodium bicarbonate, 650 mg orally before and after meals, decreases the inactivation of lipase by acid and may thereby further decrease steatorrhea. In selected cases of alcoholic pancreatitis and in cystic fibrosis, enteric-coated microencapsulated preparations may offer an advantage. However, in patients with cystic fibrosis, high-dose pancreatic enzyme therapy has been associated with strictures of the ascending colon. Pain secondary to idiopathic chronic pancreatitis may be alleviated in some cases by the use of pancreatic enzymes (not enteric-coated) or octreotide, 200 mcg subcutaneously three times daily. Associated diabetes should be treated (see Chapter 27). Autoimmune chronic pancreatitis is treated with prednisone 40 mg/d orally for 1–2 months, followed by a taper of 5 mg every 2–4 weeks.

B. SURGICAL AND ENDOSCOPIC TREATMENT

Endoscopic therapy or surgery may be indicated in chronic pancreatitis to drain persistent pseudocysts, relieve biliary obstruction, treat other complications, attempt to relieve pain, or exclude pancreatic cancer. The objectives of such interventions are to eradicate biliary tract disease, ensure a free flow of bile into the duodenum, and eliminate obstruction of the pancreatic duct. Liver fibrosis may regress after biliary drainage. Distal common bile duct obstruction may be relieved by endoscopic placement of multiple bile duct stents. When obstruction of the duodenal end of the pancreatic duct can be demonstrated by ERCP, dilation or placement of a stent in the duct or resection of the tail of the pancreas with implantation of the distal end of the duct by pancreaticojejunostomy may be successful. When the pancreatic duct is diffusely dilated, anastomosis between the duct after it is split longitudinally and a defunctionalized limb of jejunum (modified Puestow procedure), in some cases combined with resection of the head of the pancreas, is associated with relief of pain in 80% of cases. In advanced cases, subtotal or total pancreatectomy may be considered as a last resort but has variable efficacy and is associated with a high rate of pancreatic insufficiency and diabetes. Perioperative administration of somatostatin or octreotide may reduce the risk of postoperative pancreatic fistulas. Endoscopic or surgical drainage is indicated for symptomatic pseudocysts and, in many cases, those over 6 cm in diameter. Endoscopic ultrasound may facilitate selection of an optimal site for endoscopic drainage. Pancreatic ascites or pancreaticopleural fistulas due to a disrupted pancreatic duct can be managed by endoscopic placement of a stent across the disrupted duct. Fragmentation of stones in the pancreatic duct by lithotripsy and endoscopic removal of stones from the duct, pancreatic sphincterotomy, or pseudocyst drainage may relieve pain in selected patients. For patients with chronic pain and nondilated ducts, a percutaneous celiac plexus nerve block may be considered under either CT or endoscopic ultrasound guidance, with pain relief (albeit often short-lived) in approximately 50% of patients.

Prognosis

Chronic pancreatitis is a serious disease that often leads to chronic disability. The prognosis is best in patients with recurrent acute pancreatitis caused by a remediable condition such as cholelithiasis, choledocholithiasis, stenosis of the sphincter of Oddi, or hyperparathyroidism. Medical management of the hyperlipidemia frequently associated with the condition may also prevent recurrent attacks of pancreatitis. In alcoholic pancreatitis, pain relief is most likely when a dilated pancreatic duct can be decompressed. In patients with disease not amenable to decompressive surgery, addiction to narcotics is a frequent outcome of treatment.

Aparisi L et al: Antibodies to carbonic anhydrase and IgG4 levels in idiopathic chronic pancreatitis: relevance for diagnosis of autoimmune pancreatitis. Gut 2005;54:703. [PMID: 15831920]

Gabbrielli A et al: Efficacy of main pancreatic-duct endoscopic drainage in patients with chronic pancreatitis, continuous pain, and dilated duct. Gastrointest Endosc 2005;61:576. [PMID: 15812411]

Maisonneuve P et al: Cigarette smoking accelerates progression of alcoholic chronic pancreatitis. Gut 2005;54:510. [PMID: 15753536]

Nahon Uzan K et al: Is idiopathic chronic pancreatitis an autoimmune disease? Clin Gastroenterol Hepatol 2005;3:903. [PMID: 16234029]

Tadenuma H et al: Long-term results of extracorporeal shock-wave lithotripsy and endoscopic therapy for pancreatic stones. Clin Gastroenterol Hepatol 2005;3:1128. [PMID: 16271345]

CARCINOMA OF THE PANCREAS & THE PERIAMPULLARY AREA

ESSENTIALS OF DIAGNOSIS

- *Obstructive jaundice (may be painless).*
- *Enlarged gallbladder (may be painful).*
- *Upper abdominal pain with radiation to back, weight loss, and thrombophlebitis are usually late manifestations.*

General Considerations

Carcinoma is the most common neoplasm of the pancreas. About 75% are in the head and 25% in the body and tail of the organ. Carcinomas involving the head of the pancreas, the ampulla of Vater, the distal common bile duct, and the duodenum are considered together, because they are usually indistinguishable clinically; of these, carcinomas of the pancreas constitute over 90%. They comprise 2% of all cancers and 5% of cancer deaths. Risk factors include age, obesity, tobacco use, chronic pancreatitis, prior abdominal radiation, and family history. New-onset diabetes mellitus after age 50 years should raise the possibility of early pancreatic cancer. About 7–8% of patients with pancreatic cancer have a family history of pancreatic cancer in a first-degree relative, compared with 0.6% of control subjects. Pancreatic cancer can also occur as part of several hereditary syndromes, including hereditary pancreatitis, familial atypical multiple mole melanoma, Peutz–Jeghers syndrome, ataxia-telangiectasia, familial breast cancer (*BRCA-2*), and hereditary nonpolyposis colorectal cancer. Polymorphisms of the genes for methylene tetrahydrofolate reductase and thymidylate synthase have been reported to be associated with pancreatic cancer. Neuroendocrine tumors account for 2–5% of pancreatic neoplasms. Cystic neoplasms account for only 1% of pancreatic cancers, but they are important because they are often mistaken for pseudocysts. A cystic neoplasm should be suspected when a cystic lesion in the pancreas is found in the absence of a history of pancreatitis. Whereas serous cystadenomas (which account for 32–39% of cystic pancreatic neoplasms and also occur in patients with von Hippel–Lindau disease) are benign, mucinous cystic neoplasms (defined by the presence of ovarian stroma) (10–45%), intraductal papillary mucinous neoplasms (21–33%), solid pseudopapillary neoplasms (< 5%), and cystic islet cell tumors (3–5%) are premalignant, although their prognoses are better than the prognosis of adenocarcinoma of the pancreas, unless the neoplasm is locally advanced.

Clinical Findings

A. SYMPTOMS AND SIGNS

Pain is present in over 70% of cases and is often vague, diffuse, and located in the epigastrium or left upper quadrant when the lesion is in the tail. Radiation of pain into the back is common and sometimes predominates. Sitting up and leaning forward may afford some relief, and this usually indicates that the lesion has spread beyond the pancreas and is inoperable. Diarrhea, perhaps due to maldigestion, is an occasional early symptom. Migratory thrombophlebitis is a rare sign. Weight loss is a common but late finding and may be associated with depression. Occasionally a patient presents with acute pancreatitis in the absence of an alternative cause. Jaundice is usually due to biliary obstruction by a cancer in the pancreatic head. A palpable gallbladder is also indicative of obstruction by neoplasm (Courvoisier's law), but there are frequent exceptions. A hard, fixed, occasionally tender mass may be present. In advanced cases, a hard periumbilical (Sister Joseph's) nodule may be palpable.

B. LABORATORY FINDINGS

There may be mild anemia. Glycosuria, hyperglycemia, and impaired glucose tolerance or true diabetes mellitus are found in 10–20% of cases. The serum amylase or lipase level is occasionally elevated. Liver function tests may suggest obstructive jaundice. Steatorrhea in the absence of jaundice is uncommon. Occult blood in the stool is suggestive of carcinoma of the ampulla of Vater (the combination of biliary obstruction and bleeding may give the stools a distinctive silver appearance). CA 19-9, with a sensitivity of 70% and a specificity of 87%, has not proved sensitive enough for early detection of pancreatic cancer; increased values are also found in acute and chronic pancreatitis and cholangitis. Point mutations in codon 12 of the K-*ras* oncogene are found in 70–100%, and inactivation of the tumor suppressor genes *P16* on chromosome 9, *TP53* on chromosome 17, and *MADH4* on chromosome 18 is found in 95%, 75%, and 55% of pancreatic cancers, respectively.

C. IMAGING

With carcinoma of the head of the pancreas, the upper gastrointestinal series may show a widening of the duodenal loop, mucosal abnormalities in the duodenum ranging from edema to invasion or ulceration, spasm, or compression. Ultrasound is not reliable because of interference by intestinal gas. Multiphase

thin-cut spiral CT scanning is generally the initial diagnostic procedure and detects a mass in over 80% of cases. CT scanning identifies metastases, delineates the extent of the tumor, and allows for percutaneous fine-needle aspiration for cytologic studies and tumor markers. MRI is an alternative to CT scanning. Preliminary experience suggests that positron emission tomography is a sensitive technique for detecting pancreatic cancer and metastases. Selective celiac and superior mesenteric arteriography may demonstrate vessel invasion by tumor, a finding that would interdict attempts at surgical resection, but it is less widely used since the advent of multiphase spiral CT. Endoscopic ultrasonography is more sensitive than CT scanning for detecting pancreatic cancer and equivalent to CT scanning for determining nodal involvement and resectability. A normal endoscopic ultrasound excludes pancreatic cancer. Endoscopic ultrasonography may also be used to guide fine-needle aspiration for tissue diagnosis and tumor markers. ERCP may clarify an ambiguous CT scan or MRI study by delineating the pancreatic duct system or confirming an ampullary or biliary neoplasm. In patients with bile duct obstruction, preoperative endoscopic placement of a biliary stent does not appear to reduce operative mortality or morbidity. MRCP appears to be at least as sensitive as ERCP in diagnosing pancreatic cancer. In some centers, pancreatoscopy or intraductal ultrasonography can be used to evaluate filling defects in the pancreatic duct and assess resectability of intraductal papillary mucinous tumors. With obstruction of the splenic vein, splenomegaly or gastric varices are present, the latter delineated by endoscopy, endoscopic ultrasonography, or angiography.

Cystic neoplasms can be distinguished by their appearance on CT, endoscopic ultrasonography, and ERCP and features of the cyst fluid on gross and cytologic analysis. For example, serious cystadenomas may have a central scar or honeycomb appearance; mucinous cystadenomas are unilocular or multilocular and contain mucin-rich fluid with high carcinoembryonic antigen levels; and intraductal papillary mucinous neoplasms are associated with a dilated pancreatic duct and extrusion of gelatinous material from the ampulla.

Staging of pancreatic cancer by the TNM classification includes the following definitions: Tis: carcinoma in situ; T1: tumor limited to the pancreas, 2 cm or less in greatest dimension; T2: tumor limited to the pancreas, more than 2 cm in greatest dimension; T3: tumor extends beyond the pancreas but without involvement of the celiac axis or the superior mesenteric artery; T4, tumor involves the celiac axis or the superior mesenteric artery (unresectable primary tumor).

Treatment

Abdominal exploration is usually necessary when cytologic diagnosis cannot be made or if resection is to be attempted, which includes about 30% of patients. In a patient with a localized mass in the head of the pancreas and without jaundice, laparoscopy may detect tiny peritoneal or liver metastases and thereby avoid resection in 4–13% of patients. Radical pancreaticoduodenal (Whipple) resection is indicated for lesions strictly limited to the head of the pancreas, periampullary zone, and duodenum (T1, N0, M0). Five-year survival rates are 20–25% in this group and as high as 40% in those with negative resection margins and without lymph node involvement. Preoperative endoscopic decompression of an obstructed bile duct may not be necessary but is often achieved with a plastic stent or short metal stent. The best surgical results are achieved at centers that specialize in the multidisciplinary treatment of pancreatic cancer. Adjuvant or neoadjuvant chemotherapy with gemcitabine and fluorouracil, possibly combined with irradiation, appears to be of benefit. When resection is not feasible, endoscopic stenting of the bile duct is performed to relieve jaundice. A plastic stent is generally placed if the patient's anticipated survival is less than 6 months (or surgery is planned). A metal stent is preferred when anticipated survival is 6 months or greater. Surgical biliary bypass may be considered in patients expected to survive at least 6 months. Surgical duodenal bypass may be considered in patients in whom duodenal obstruction is expected to develop later; alternatively, endoscopic placement of a self-expandable duodenal stent may be feasible. Chemoradiation may be used for palliation of unresectable cancer confined to the pancreas. Chemotherapy has been disappointing in metastatic pancreatic cancer, although improved response rates have been reported with gemcitabine. Novel small molecules, including fluoropyrimidines, nucleoside cytidine analogues, and topoisomerase inhibitors, are under study. Celiac plexus nerve block or thoracoscopic splanchnicectomy may improve pain control. Photodynamic therapy is under study.

Surgical resection is indicated for all mucinous cystic neoplasms, symptomatic serous cystadenomas, and cystic tumors that remain undefined after spiral CT, endoscopic ultrasound, and diagnostic aspiration. In the absence of locally advanced disease, survival is higher than for adenocarcinoma. Endoscopic resection or ablation, with temporary placement of a pancreatic duct stent, may be feasible for ampullary adenomas, but patients must be followed for recurrence.

Prognosis

Carcinoma of the pancreas, especially in the body or tail, has a poor prognosis. Reported 5-year survival rates range from 2% to 5%. Lesions of the ampulla have a better prognosis, with reported 5-year survival rates of 20–40% after resection; jaundice and lymph node involvement are adverse prognostic factors. In carefully selected patients, resection of cancer of the pancreatic head is feasible and results in reasonable survival. In persons with a family history of pancreatic cancer, screening with spiral CT and endoscopic ultrasonography should be considered beginning 10 years before the age at which pancreatic cancer was diagnosed in a family member.

For those patients whose disease progresses despite treatment, meticulous efforts at palliative care are essential (see Chapter 5).

Chari ST et al: Probability of pancreatic cancer following diabetes: a population-based study. Gastroenterology 2005;129: 504. [PMID: 16083707]

Guidelines for the management of patients with pancreatic cancer periampullary and ampullary carcinomas. Gut 2005;54(Suppl V):v1. [PMID: 15888770]

Hammarström LE: Endobiliary stents for palliation in patients with malignant obstructive jaundice. J Clin Gastroenterol 2005;39:413. [PMID: 15815210]

Klapman JB et al: Negative predictive value of endoscopic ultrasound in a large series of patients with a clinical suspicion of pancreatic cancer. Am J Gastroenterol 2005;100:2658. [PMID: 16393216]

Lockhart AC et al: Treatment for pancreatic cancer: current therapy and continued progress. Gastroenterology 2005; 128:1642. [PMID: 15887156]

Ryan DP et al: Case 20-2005: a 58-year-old man with locally advanced pancreatic cancer. N Engl J Med 2005;352:2734. [PMID: 15987923]

Scheiman JM: Cystic lesion of the pancreas. Gastroenterology 2005;128:463. [PMID: 15685556]

Breast

16

Armando E. Giuliano, MD

■ BENIGN BREAST DISORDERS

FIBROCYSTIC CONDITION

ESSENTIALS OF DIAGNOSIS

- *Painful, often multiple, usually bilateral masses in the breast.*
- *Rapid fluctuation in the size of the masses is common.*
- *Frequently, pain occurs or worsens and size increases during premenstrual phase of cycle.*
- *Most common age is 30–50. Rare in postmenopausal women not receiving hormonal replacement.*

General Considerations

Fibrocystic condition is the most frequent lesion of the breast. Although commonly referred to as "fibrocystic disease," it does not, in fact, represent a pathologic or anatomic disorder. It is common in women 30–50 years of age but rare in postmenopausal women who are not taking hormonal replacement medications. Estrogen is considered a causative factor. There may be an increased risk in women who drink alcohol, especially women between 18 and 22 years of age. Fibrocystic condition encompasses a wide variety of histologic changes. These lesions are always associated with benign changes in the breast epithelium, some of which are found so commonly in normal breasts that they are probably variants of normal breast histology but have nonetheless been termed a "condition" or "disease."

The microscopic findings of fibrocystic condition include cysts (gross and microscopic), papillomatosis, adenosis, fibrosis, and ductal epithelial hyperplasia. Although fibrocystic condition has generally been considered to increase the risk of subsequent breast cancer, only the variants in which proliferation (especially with atypia) of epithelial components is demonstrated represent true risk factors.

Clinical Findings

A. SYMPTOMS AND SIGNS

Fibrocystic condition may produce an asymptomatic lump in the breast that is discovered by accident, but pain or tenderness often calls attention to the mass. There may be discharge from the nipple. In many cases, discomfort occurs or worsens during the premenstrual phase of the cycle, at which time the cysts tend to enlarge. Fluctuation in size and rapid appearance or disappearance of a breast mass are common with this condition. Multiple or bilateral masses are common, and many patients will give a history of a transient lump in the breast or cyclic breast pain.

B. DIAGNOSTIC TESTS

Because a mass due to fibrocystic condition is frequently indistinguishable from carcinoma on the basis of clinical findings, suspicious lesions should be biopsied. Fine-needle aspiration cytology may be used, but if a suspicious mass that is nonmalignant on cytologic examination does not resolve over several months, it should be excised. Surgery should be conservative, since the primary objective is to exclude cancer. Occasionally, core needle biopsy will suffice. Simple mastectomy or extensive removal of breast tissue is rarely, if ever, indicated for fibrocystic condition.

Differential Diagnosis

Pain, fluctuation in size, and multiplicity of lesions are the features most helpful in differentiating fibrocystic condition from carcinoma. If a dominant mass is present, the diagnosis of cancer should be assumed until disproved by biopsy. Final diagnosis depends on pathologic analysis of the excisional biopsy specimen. Mammography may be helpful, but the breast tissue in these young women is usually too radiodense to permit a worthwhile study. Sonography is useful in differentiating a cystic mass from a solid mass.

Treatment

When the diagnosis of fibrocystic condition has been established by previous biopsy or is likely because the history is classic, aspiration of a discrete mass suggestive of a cyst is indicated to alleviate pain and, more importantly, to confirm the cystic nature of the mass. The patient is reexamined at intervals thereafter. If no fluid is obtained by aspiration, if fluid is bloody, if a mass persists after aspiration, or if at any time during follow-up a persistent or recurrent lump is noted, biopsy is performed.

Breast pain associated with generalized fibrocystic condition is best treated by avoiding trauma and by wearing a good supportive brassiere during the night and day. Hormone therapy is not advisable, because it does not cure the condition and has undesirable side effects. Danazol (100–200 mg orally twice daily), a synthetic androgen, has been used for patients with severe pain. This treatment suppresses pituitary gonadotropins, but androgenic effects (acne, edema, hirsutism) usually make this treatment intolerable; in practice, it is rarely used. Similarly, tamoxifen reduces some symptoms of fibrocystic condition, but because of its side effects it is not useful for young women unless it is given to reduce the risk of cancer. Postmenopausal women receiving hormone replacement therapy may stop hormones to reduce pain. The use of evening primrose oil (a natural form of gamolenic acid) has been shown in studies to decrease pain in 44–58% of users and should be considered for treatment. The dose of gamolenic acid is six capsules of 500 mg orally twice daily. Studies have also demonstrated a low-fat diet or decreasing dietary fat intake may reduce the painful symptoms associated with fibrocystic condition.

The role of caffeine consumption in the development and treatment of fibrocystic condition is controversial. Some studies suggest that eliminating caffeine from the diet is associated with improvement while other studies refute the benefit entirely. Many patients are aware of these studies and report relief of symptoms after giving up coffee, tea, and chocolate. Similarly, many women find vitamin E (400 IU daily) helpful. However, these observations remain anecdotal.

Prognosis

Exacerbations of pain, tenderness, and cyst formation may occur at any time until the menopause, when symptoms usually subside, except in patients receiving hormonal replacement therapy. The patient should be advised to examine her own breasts each month just after menstruation and to inform her practitioner if a mass appears. The risk of breast cancer developing in women with fibrocystic condition showing proliferative or atypical changes in the epithelium is higher than that of the general population. These women should be monitored carefully with physical examinations and imaging studies, such as mammography.

Lucas JH et al: Breast cyst aspiration. Am Fam Physician 2003; 68:1983. [PMID: 14655807]

Marchant DJ: Benign breast disease. Obstet Gynecol Clin North Am 2002;29:1. [PMID: 11892859]

Morrow M: The evaluation of common breast problems. Am Fam Physician 2000;61:2371. [PMID: 10794579]

Norlock FE: Benign breast pain in women: a practical approach to evaluation and treatment. J Am Med Womens Assoc 2002;57:85. [PMID: 11991427]

Terry MB et al: Lifetime alcohol intake and breast cancer risk. Ann Epidemiol 2006;16:230. [PMID: 16230024]

FIBROADENOMA OF THE BREAST

This common benign neoplasm occurs most frequently in young women, usually within 20 years after puberty. It is somewhat more frequent and tends to occur at an earlier age in black women. Multiple tumors are found in 10–15% of patients.

The typical fibroadenoma is a round or ovoid, rubbery, discrete, relatively movable, nontender mass 1–5 cm in diameter. It is usually discovered accidentally. Clinical diagnosis in young patients is generally not difficult. In women over 30 years, fibrocystic condition of the breast and carcinoma of the breast must be considered. Cysts can be identified by aspiration or ultrasonography. Fibroadenoma does not normally occur after the menopause but may occasionally develop after administration of hormones.

No treatment is usually necessary if the diagnosis can be made by needle biopsy or cytologic examination. Excision or vacuum-assisted core needle removal with pathologic examination of the specimen is performed if the diagnosis is uncertain. In a 2005 study, cryoablation, or freezing of the fibroadenoma, appears to be a safe procedure if the lesion is consistent with fibroadenoma on histology prior to ablation. Cryoablation is not appropriate for all fibroadenomas because some are too large to freeze. The advantages of cryoablation over observation are not clear. It is usually not possible to distinguish a large fibroadenoma from a phyllodes tumor on the basis of needle biopsy results.

Phyllodes tumor is a fibroadenoma-like tumor with cellular stroma that grows rapidly. It may reach a large size and, if inadequately excised, will recur locally. The lesion can be benign or malignant. If benign, phyllodes tumor is treated by local excision with a margin of surrounding breast tissue. The treatment of malignant phyllodes tumor is more controversial, but complete removal of the tumor with a rim of normal tissue avoids recurrence. Because these tumors may be large, simple mastectomy is sometimes necessary. Lymph node dissection is not performed, since the sarcomatous portion of the tumor metastasizes to the lungs and not the lymph nodes.

Grady I et al: Ultrasound-guided, vacuum-assisted, percutaneous excision of breast lesions: an accurate technique in the diagnosis of atypical ductal hyperplasia. J Am Coll Surg 2005;201:14. [PMID: 15978438]

Hartmann LC et al: Benign breast disease and the risk of breast cancer. N Engl J Med 2005;353:229. [PMID: 16034008]

Jacklin RK et al: Optimising preoperative diagnosis in phyllodes tumour of the breast. J Clin Pathol 2006 [Epub ahead of print]. [PMID: 16461806]

Kaufman CS et al: Office based cryoablation of breast fibroadenomas with long-term follow-up. Breast J 2005;11:344. [PMID: 16174156]

NIPPLE DISCHARGE

In order of decreasing frequency, the following are the most common causes of nipple discharge in the nonlactating breast: duct ectasia, intraductal papilloma, and carcinoma. The important characteristics of the discharge and some other factors to be evaluated by history and physical examination are as follows:

1. Nature of the discharge (serous, bloody, or other).
2. Association with a mass.
3. Unilateral or bilateral.
4. Single or multiple duct discharge.
5. Discharge is spontaneous (persistent or intermittent) or must be expressed.
6. Discharge is produced by pressure at a single site or by general pressure on the breast.
7. Relation to menses.
8. Premenopausal or postmenopausal.
9. Patient is taking contraceptive pills or estrogen.

Spontaneous, unilateral, serous or serosanguineous discharge from a single duct is usually caused by an intraductal papilloma or, rarely, by an intraductal cancer. A mass may not be palpable. The involved duct may be identified by pressure at different sites around the nipple at the margin of the areola. Bloody discharge is suggestive of cancer but is more often caused by a benign papilloma in the duct. Cytologic examination may identify malignant cells, but negative findings do not rule out cancer, which is more likely in women over age 50 years. In any case, the involved duct—and a mass if present—should be excised. A ductogram (a mammogram of a duct after radiopaque dye has been injected) is of limited value since excision of the suspicious ductal system is indicated regardless of findings. Ductoscopy, evaluation of the ductal system with a small scope inserted through the nipple is being studied as a means of identifying intraductal lesions but is not yet practical in the clinical setting.

In premenopausal women, spontaneous multiple duct discharge, unilateral or bilateral, most noticeable just before menstruation, is often due to fibrocystic condition. Discharge may be green or brownish. Papillomatosis and ductal ectasia are usually detected only by biopsy. If a mass is present, it should be removed.

A milky discharge from multiple ducts in the nonlactating breast occurs from hyperprolactinemia. Serum prolactin levels should be obtained to search for a pituitary tumor. Thyroid-stimulating hormone (TSH) helps exclude causative hypothyroidism. Numerous antipsychotic drugs and other drugs may also cause a milky discharge that ceases on discontinuance of the medication.

Oral contraceptive agents or estrogen replacement therapy may cause clear, serous, or milky discharge from a single duct, but multiple duct discharge is more common. In the premenopausal woman, the discharge is more evident just before menstruation and disappears on stopping the medication. If it does not stop and is from a single duct, exploration may be considered.

A purulent discharge may originate in a subareolar abscess and require removal of the abscess and the related lactiferous sinus.

When localization is not possible, no mass is palpable, and the discharge is nonbloody, the patient should be reexamined every 3 or 4 months for a year, and mammography should be done. Although most discharge is from a benign process, patients may find it annoying or disconcerting. To eliminate the discharge, proximal duct excision can be considered both for treatment and diagnosis. Cytologic examination of the nipple discharge for exfoliated cancer cells may rarely be helpful in determining a diagnosis. In addition, the duct may be catheterized and washed out with an isotonic solution (ductal lavage) to evaluate cells for atypia. Regardless of the method of analysis, ductal excision is both therapeutic as well as diagnostic.

Dietz JR et al: Directed duct excision by using mammary ductoscopy in patients with pathologic nipple discharge. Surgery 2002;132:582. [PMID: 12407341]

Dooley WC et al: Office-based breast ductoscopy for diagnosis. Am J Surg 2004;188:415. [PMID: 15474438]

Escobar PF et al: The clinical applications of mammary ductoscopy. Am J Surg 2006;191:211. [PMID: 16442948]

Pritt B et al: Diagnostic value of nipple cytology: study of 466 cases. Cancer 2004;102:233. [PMID: 15368315]

Sauter ER et al: Fiberoptic ductoscopy findings in women with and without spontaneous nipple discharge. Cancer 2005; 103:914. [PMID: 15666326]

Sauter ER et al: The association of bloody nipple discharge with breast pathology. Surgery 2004;136:780. [PMID: 15467662]

Simmons R et al: Nonsurgical evaluation of pathologic nipple discharge. Ann Surg Oncol 2003;10:113. [PMID: 12620904]

FAT NECROSIS

Fat necrosis is a rare lesion of the breast but is of clinical importance because it produces a mass (often accompanied by skin or nipple retraction) that is indistinguishable from carcinoma. Trauma is presumed to be the cause, though only about 50% of patients give a history of injury. Ecchymosis is occasionally present. If untreated, the mass effect gradually disappears. The safest course is to obtain a biopsy. Needle biopsy is often adequate, but frequently the entire mass must be excised, primarily to exclude carcinoma. Fat necrosis is common after segmental resection, radiation therapy, or flap reconstruction after mastectomy.

Tan PH et al: Fat necrosis of the breast—A review. Breast 2006; 15:313. [PMID: 16198567]

BREAST ABSCESS

During nursing, an area of redness, tenderness, and induration may develop in the breast. The organism most commonly found in these abscesses is *Staphylococcus aureus*. In the early stages, the infection can often be treated while nursing is continued from that breast by administering an antibiotic such as dicloxacillin or oxacillin, 250 mg orally four times daily for 7–10 days (see Puerperal Mastitis, Chapter 18). If the lesion progresses to form a localized mass with local and systemic signs of infection, surgical drainage is performed and nursing is discontinued. Often needle or catheter drainage is adequate, but surgical incision and drainage may be necessary.

A subareolar abscess may develop (rarely) in young or middle-aged women who are not lactating. These infections tend to recur after incision and drainage unless the area is explored during a quiescent interval, with excision of the involved lactiferous duct or ducts at the base of the nipple. Otherwise, infection in the nonlactating breast is very rare. In the nonlactating breast, inflammatory carcinoma must always be considered. Thus, findings suggestive of abscess or cellulitis in the nonlactating breast are an indication for incision and biopsy of any indurated tissue that does not resolve promptly with antibiotics. If the abscess can be percutaneously drained and completely resolves, the patient may be monitored conservatively.

Berna-Serna JD et al: Percutaneous management of breast abscesses. An experience of 39 cases. Ultrasound Med Biol 2004;30:1. [PMID: 14962601]

Dener C et al: Breast abscesses in lactating women. World J Surg 2003;27:130. [PMID: 12616423]

DISORDERS OF THE AUGMENTED BREAST

At least 4 million American women have had breast implants. Breast augmentation is performed by placing implants under the pectoralis muscle or, less desirably, in the subcutaneous tissue of the breast. Most implants are made of an outer silicone shell filled with a silicone gel, saline, or some combination of the two. Capsule contraction or scarring around the implant develops in about 15–25% of patients, leading to a firmness and distortion of the breast that can be painful. Some require removal of the implant and capsule.

Implant rupture may occur in as many as 5–10% of women, and bleeding of gel through the capsule is noted even more commonly. Although silicone gel may be an immunologic stimulant, there is no increase in autoimmune disorders in patients with such implants. The Food and Drug Administration (FDA) has advised symptomatic women with ruptured implants to discuss possible surgical removal with their physicians. However, women who are asymptomatic and have no evidence of rupture of a silicone gel prosthesis should probably not undergo removal of the implant. Women with symptoms of autoimmune illnesses should address the possibility of removal with their practitioner.

Studies have failed to show any association between implants and an increased incidence of breast cancer. However, breast cancer may develop in a patient with a silicone gel prosthesis, as it does in women without them. Detection in patients with implants is more difficult because mammography is less able to detect early lesions. However, after a woman who had mastectomy undergoes breast reconstruction with implants, local recurrence of cancer is usually cutaneous or subcutaneous and is easily detected by palpation.

If a cancer develops in a patient with implants, it should be treated in the same manner as in women without implants. Such women should be offered the option of mastectomy or breast-conserving therapy, which may require removal or replacement of the implant. Radiotherapy of the augmented breast often results in marked capsular contracture. Adjuvant treatments should be given for the same indications as for women who have no implants.

Adams WP et al: Decision and management algorithms to address patient and food and drug administration concerns regarding breast augmentation and implants. Plast Reconstr Surg 2004;114:1252. [PMID: 15457045]

Brinton LA et al: Risk of connective tissue disorders among breast implant patients. Am J Epidemiol 2004;160:619. [PMID: 15383405]

Englert H et al: Augmentation mammoplasty and "silicone-osis." Intern Med J 2004;34:668. [PMID: 15610211]

Fryzek JP et al: Silicone breast implants. J Rheumatol 2005;32:201. [PMID: 15700387]

■ CARCINOMA OF THE FEMALE BREAST

 ESSENTIALS OF DIAGNOSIS

- *Risk factors include delayed childbearing, positive family history of breast cancer or genetic mutations (BRCA1, BRCA2), and personal history of breast cancer or some types of fibrocystic condition.*

- *Most women with breast cancer do not have identifiable risk factors.*

- *Early findings: Single, nontender, firm to hard mass with ill-defined margins; mammographic abnormalities and no palpable mass.*

- *Later findings: Skin or nipple retraction; axillary lymphadenopathy; breast enlargement, erythema, edema, pain; fixation of mass to skin or chest wall.*

INCIDENCE & RISK FACTORS

Next to skin cancer, breast cancer is the most common type of cancer in women, second only to lung cancer as a cause of death. The probability of developing breast cancer increases throughout life. The mean and the median age of women with breast cancer is between 60 and 61 years.

There will be about 214,640 new cases of breast cancer and about 41,430 deaths from this disease in women in the United States in 2006. An additional

61,980 cases of ductal carcinoma in situ will be detected, principally by screening mammography. Breast cancer will develop in one of every eight or nine American women during her lifetime. The incidence of breast cancer continues to increase, but recently mortality has appeared to decrease slightly. This reflects both early detection and increased use of systemic therapy. Breast cancer is three to four times more likely to develop in women whose mothers or sisters had breast cancer than in those without this family history. Risk is further increased in patients whose mothers' or sisters' breast cancers occurred before menopause or were bilateral and in those with a family history of breast cancer in two or more first-degree relatives as well as in women of Ashkenazi Jewish descent. However, there is no history of breast cancer among female relatives in over 75% of patients. Nulliparous women and women whose first full-term pregnancy was after age 35 have a 1.5 times higher incidence of breast cancer than multiparous women. Late menarche and artificial menopause are associated with a lower incidence, whereas early menarche (under age 12) and late natural menopause (after age 50) are associated with a slight increase in risk. Fibrocystic condition, when accompanied by proliferative changes, papillomatosis, or atypical epithelial hyperplasia, is associated with an increased incidence. A woman who had cancer in one breast is at increased risk for cancer developing in the other breast. In these women, a contralateral cancer develops at the rate of 1% or 2% per year. Women with cancer of the uterine corpus have a risk of breast cancer significantly higher than that of the general population, and women with breast cancer have a comparably increased risk for endometrial cancer. In the United States, breast cancer is more common in whites. The incidence of the disease among nonwhites (mostly blacks) is increasing, especially in younger women. In general, rates reported from developing countries are low, whereas rates are high in developed countries, with the notable exception of Japan. Some of the variability may be due to underreporting in the developing countries, but a real difference probably exists. Dietary factors, particularly increased fat consumption, may account for some differences in incidence. Oral contraceptives do not appear to increase the risk of breast cancer. There is evidence that administration of estrogens to postmenopausal women may result in a slightly increased risk of breast cancer, but only with higher, long-term doses of estrogens. Concomitant administration of progesterone and estrogen may markedly increase the incidence of breast cancer compared with the use of estrogen alone. The Women's Health Initiative prospective randomized study of hormone replacement therapy stopped treatment with estrogen and progesterone early because of an increased risk of breast cancer compared with untreated controls or women treated with estrogen alone. Alcohol consumption increases the risk slightly. Some inherited breast cancers have been found to be associated with a gene on chromosome 17. This gene, BRCA1, is mutated in families with early-onset breast cancer and ovarian cancer. Breast cancer will develop in as many as 85% of women with BRCA1 gene mutations during their lifetime. Other genes are associated with increased risk of breast and other cancers, such as BRCA2 (associated with a gene on chromosome 13); ataxia-telangiectasia mutation; and mutation of p53, the tumor suppressor gene. Mutations to p53 have been found in approximately 1% of breast cancers in women under 40 years of age. Genetic testing is commercially available for women at high risk for breast cancer. Women with genetic mutations in whom breast cancer develops may be treated in the same way as women who do not have mutations (ie, lumpectomy), though data are emerging to suggest an increased recurrence rate for these women. Such women with mutations often elect bilateral mastectomy as treatment. Some states have enacted legislation to prevent insurance companies from considering mutations as "preexisting conditions," preventing insurability.

Women at greater than normal risk for developing breast cancer (Table 16–1) should be identified by their practitioners, taught the techniques of breast self-examination (BSE), and followed carefully. Those with an exceptional family history should be counseled and given the option of genetic testing. Some of these high-risk women may consider prophylactic mastectomy or tamoxifen.

The National Surgical Adjuvant Breast Project (NS-ABP) conducted the Breast Cancer Prevention Trial (BCPT), which studied the efficacy of tamoxifen as a preventive agent in women who never had breast cancer but were at high risk for developing the disease. Women who received tamoxifen for 5 years had about a 50% reduction in noninvasive and invasive cancers compared with women taking placebo. However, women above the age of 50 who received the drug had an increased incidence of endometrial cancer and deep venous

Table 16–1. Factors associated with increased risk of breast cancer.[1]

Race	White
Age	Older
Family history	Breast cancer in mother, sister, or daughter (especially bilateral or premenopausal)
Genetics	BRCA1 or BRCA2 mutation
Previous medical history	Endometrial cancer Proliferative forms of fibrocystic disease Cancer in other breast
Menstrual history	Early menarche (under age 12) Late menopause (after age 50)
Reproductive history	Nulliparous or late first pregnancy

[1]Normal lifetime risk in white women = 1 in 8 or 9.

thrombosis. Unfortunately, no survival data will be produced from this trial because it was stopped.

The selective estrogen receptor modulator (SERM) raloxifene, effective in preventing osteoporosis, has also shown some promise in preventing breast cancer. The Multiple Outcomes of Raloxifene Evaluations (MORE) trial demonstrated that raloxifene reduced breast cancer risk in women being treated with the drug for osteoporosis. The MORE trial, whose principal aim was to determine the effect of raloxifene on bone, was extended by 4 years (Continuing Outcomes Relevant to Evista (CORE) trial) to better evaluate the effect of raloxifene on breast cancer risk. After 8 years of treatment, raloxifene demonstrated an overall reduction of invasive breast cancer of 66%. Although, it appears that raloxifene is more effective than tamoxifen in reducing the risk of breast cancer, the studies are not comparable since the tamoxifen trial was observing women at increased risk for breast cancer while the MORE/CORE trial was observing women with low bone density and with a lower risk of breast cancer. While it does appear that older women with osteopenia will benefit from the bone effects and breast cancer risk reduction of raloxifene, its efficacy compared with tamoxifen still requires study.

The Study of Tamoxifen and Raloxifene (STAR) trial is ongoing with early results expected in 2007. Similar to tamoxifen, aromatase inhibitors (AI) have shown great success in treating breast cancer with fewer side effects, although bone loss is a significant side effect of this long-term treatment.

Several large multicenter studies (eg, International Breast Cancer Intervention Study II [IBIS-II] and National Cancer Institute of Canada Clinical Trials Group [NCIC CTG]) are underway to determine whether AIs have a role in preventing breast cancer.

In addition to pharmaceutical therapy, patients continue to seek a way to prevent breast cancer. There has been considerable research on incorporating diet and exercise into the lifestyle of women who may be at risk for cancer. The Women's Health Initiative Randomized Controlled Dietary Modification Trial was conducted to determine whether decreasing dietary fat intake would reduce the incidence of breast cancer recurrence after initial treatment. Although the trial demonstrated a decrease in recurrence in the follow-up period, it did not reach statistical significance.

Andrews L et al: Psychological impact of genetic testing for breast cancer susceptibility in women of Ashkenazi Jewish background: a prospective study. Genet Test 2004;8:240. [PMID: 15727246]

Cauley JA et al: Continued breast cancer risk reduction in postmenopausal women treated with raloxifene: 4-year results from the MORE trial. Multiple outcomes of raloxifene evaluation. Breast Cancer Res Treat 2001;65:125. [PMID: 11261828]

Colditz GA: Estrogen, estrogen plus progestin therapy, and risk of breast cancer. Clin Cancer Res 2005;11(2 Pt 2):909s. [PMID: 15701886]

Cuzick J: Aromatase inhibitors for breast cancer prevention. J Clin Oncol 2005;23:1636. [PMID: 15755971]

Ettinger B et al: Reduction of vertebral fracture risk in postmenopausal women with osteoporosis treated with raloxifene: results from a 3-year randomized clinical trial. Multiple Outcomes of Raloxifene Evaluation (MORE) Investigators. JAMA 1999;282:637. [PMID: 10517716]

Fabian CJ et al: Selective estrogen-receptor modulators for primary prevention of breast cancer. J Clin Oncol 2005;23:1644. [PMID: 15755972]

Fisher B et al: Tamoxifen for the prevention of breast cancer: current status of the National Surgical Adjuvant Breast and Bowel Project P-1 study. J Natl Cancer Inst 2005;97:1652. [PMID: 16288118]

Jemal A et al: Cancer Statistics, 2006. CA Cancer J Clin 2006; 56:106. [PMID: 16514137]

Kalidas M et al: Aromatase inhibitors for the treatment and prevention of breast cancer. Clin Breast Cancer 2005;6:27. [PMID: 15899070]

Martino S et al; CORE Investigators: Continuing outcomes relevant to Evista: breast cancer incidence in postmenopausal osteoporotic women in a randomized trial of raloxifene. J Natl Cancer Inst 2004;96:1751. [PMID: 15572757]

Miller WR: Aromatase inhibitors and breast cancer. Minerva Endocrinol 2006;31:27. [PMID: 16498362]

Narod SA et al: Prevention and management of hereditary breast cancer. J Clin Oncol 2005;23:1656. [PMID: 15755973]

Palma M et al: BRCA1 and BRCA2: the genetic testing and the current management options for mutation carriers. Crit Rev Oncol Hematol 2006;57:1. [PMID: 16337408]

Prentice RL et al: Low-fat dietary pattern and risk of invasive breast cancer: the Women's Health Initiative Randomized Controlled Dietary Modification Trial. JAMA 2006;295: 629. [PMID: 16467232]

Rebbeck TR et al: Bilateral prophylactic mastectomy reduces breast cancer risk in BRCA1 and BRCA2 mutation carriers: the PROSE Study Group. J Clin Oncol 2004;22:1055. [PMID: 14981104]

Rossouw JE et al: Risks and benefits of estrogen plus progestin in healthy postmenopausal women: principal results from the Women's Health Initiative randomized controlled trial. JAMA 2002;288:321. [PMID: 12117397]

U.S. Preventive Services Task Force. Genetic risk assessment and BRCA mutation testing for breast and ovarian cancer susceptibility: recommendation statement. Ann Intern Med 2005;143:355. [PMID: 16144894]

Vogel VG et al: The study of tamoxifen and raloxifene: preliminary enrollment data from a randomized breast cancer risk reduction trial. Clin Breast Cancer 2002;3:153. [PMID: 12123540]

Wrensch MR et al: Breast cancer risk in women with abnormal cytology in nipple aspirates of breast fluid. J Natl Cancer Inst 2001;93:1791. [PMID: 11734595]

EARLY DETECTION OF BREAST CANCER

Screening Programs

A number of mass screening programs consisting of physical and mammographic examination of the breasts of asymptomatic women have been conducted. Such programs frequently identify about 10 cancers per 1000 women older than age 50 years and about two cancers per 1000 women younger than age 50 years. About 80% of these women have negative axillary lymph nodes at the time of surgery, whereas only 50% of nonscreened women found in the course of usual medical practice have uninvolved axillary nodes. Detecting breast cancer before it has spread to the axillary nodes greatly increases the chance of survival, and about 85% of such women will survive at least 5 years.

Both physical examination and mammography are necessary for maximum yield in screening programs, since about 35–50% of early breast cancers can be discovered only by mammography and another 40% can be detected only by palpation by clinician. About one-third of the abnormalities detected on screening mammograms will be found to be malignant when biopsy is performed. The probability of cancer on a screening mammogram is directly related to the Breast Imaging and Reporting Data System (BIRADS) assessment, and work-up should be performed based on this classification. Women 20–40 years of age should have a breast examination as part of routine medical care every 2–3 years. Women over age 40 years should have annual breast examinations. The sensitivity of mammography varies from approximately 60% to 90%. This sensitivity depends on several factors, including patient age (breast density) and tumor size, location, and mammographic appearance. In young women with dense breasts, mammography is less sensitive than in older women with fatty breasts, in whom mammography can detect at least 90% of malignancies. Smaller tumors, particularly those without calcifications, are more difficult to detect, especially in dense breasts. The lack of sensitivity and the low incidence of breast cancer in young women have led to questions concerning the value of mammography for screening in women 40–50 years of age. The specificity of mammography in women under 50 years varies from about 30% to 40% for nonpalpable mammographic abnormalities to 85% to 90% for clinically evident malignancies.

Screening recommendations for women in their 40s are based, in part, on trials from Sweden. Two trials showed a statistical advantage for screening women in their 40s, and a meta-analysis similarly revealed a statistical survival advantage for screened women with longer follow-up. In March 1997, the National Cancer Advisory Board recommended that women in their 40s with average risk factors should have screening mammography every 1–2 years and that women at higher risk should seek medical advice on when to begin screening. Studies continue to support the value of screening mammography in women over 40 years. Such women should have annual mammography and physical examination.

The beneficial effect of screening in women aged 50–69 years is undisputed and has been confirmed by all clinical trials. The efficacy of screening in older women—those older than 70 years—is inconclusive and is difficult to determine because few women were screened.

Self-Examination

BSE has not been shown to improve survival. Despite this and despite possible increased biopsy rates, it is a useful technique since many patients do detect their own cancer, and women often feel more in control and proactive by performing BSE. Because of the absence of strong evidence supporting the value of BSE, the American Cancer Society no longer recommends monthly BSE beginning at age 20 years. The recommendation is that patients be made aware of the potential benefits, limitations, and harms (increased biopsies or false-positive results) associated with BSE. Women who chose to perform BSE should be advised regarding the proper technique. Premenopausal women should perform the examination 7–8 days after the menstrual period. The breasts should be inspected initially while standing before a mirror with the hands at the sides, overhead, and pressed firmly on the hips to contract the pectoralis muscles. Masses, asymmetry of breasts, and slight dimpling of the skin may become apparent as a result of these maneuvers. Next, in a supine position, each breast should be carefully palpated with the fingers of the opposite hand. Some women discover small breast lumps more readily when their skin is moist while bathing or showering. Physicians should instruct women in the technique of self-examination and advise them to report a mass or other abnormality. While BSE is not a recommended practice, patients should recognize and report any breast changes to their practitioners as it remains an important facet of proactive care.

Imaging

Mammography is the most reliable means of detecting breast cancer before a mass can be palpated. Slowly growing cancers can be identified by mammography at least 2 years before reaching a size detectable by palpation. Film screen mammography delivers less than 0.4 cGy to the mid breast per view and has largely replaced the older xeromammographic technique, which delivers more radiation. Although full-field digital mammography provides an easier method to maintain and review mammograms, it has not been proven that it provides better images or increases detection rates more than film mammography. A large study of 50,000 women comparing film screen to digital mammography showed no difference in overall cancer detection. However, in subset analysis, digital mammography seems slightly superior in young women with dense breasts. Computer-assisted detection (CAD) has not shown any increase in detection of cancers and is not routinely performed at centers with experienced mammographers.

Calcifications are the most easily recognized mammographic abnormality. The most common findings associated with carcinoma of the breast are clustered polymorphic microcalcifications. Such calcifications are usually at least five to eight in number, aggregated in one part of the breast and differing from each other in size and shape, often including branched or V- or Y-shaped configurations. There may be an associated mammographic mass density or, at times, only a mass density with no calcifications. Such a density usually has irregular or ill-defined borders and may lead to architectural distortion within the breast. A small mass or architectural distortion, particularly in a dense breast, may be subtle and difficult to detect.

Indications for mammography are as follows: (1) to screen at regular intervals women at high risk for developing breast cancer (see above); (2) to evaluate each breast when a diagnosis of potentially curable breast cancer has been made, and at yearly intervals thereafter; (3) to evaluate a questionable or ill-defined breast mass or other suspicious change in the breast; (4) to search for an occult breast cancer in a woman with metastatic disease in axillary nodes or elsewhere from an unknown primary; (5) to screen women prior to cosmetic operations or prior to biopsy of a mass, to examine for an unsuspected cancer; (6) to monitor those women with breast cancer who have been treated with breast-conserving surgery and radiation; and (7) to monitor the contralateral breast in those women with breast cancer treated with mastectomy.

Patients with a dominant or suspicious mass must undergo biopsy despite mammographic findings. The mammogram should be obtained prior to biopsy so that other suspicious areas can be noted and the contralateral breast can be checked. Mammography is never a substitute for biopsy because it may not reveal clinical cancer in a very dense breast, as may be seen in young women with fibrocystic changes, and may not reveal medullary cancers.

Communication and documentation among the patient, the referring practitioner, and the interpreting physician are critical for high-quality screening and diagnostic mammography. The patient should be told about *how* she will receive timely results of her mammogram; that mammography does not "rule out" cancer; and that she may receive a correlative examination such as ultrasound at the mammography facility if referred for a suspicious lesion. She should also be aware of the technique and need for breast compression and that this may be uncomfortable. The mammography facility should be informed *in writing* of abnormal physical examination findings. It is strongly recommended in the Agency for Health Care Policy and Research (AHCPR) Clinical Practice Guidelines that all mammography reports be communicated with the patient as well as the health care provider in writing. Additional phone communication about any abnormal findings should take place between the interpreting and referring practitioners. MRI and ultrasound may be useful screening modalities in women who are at high risk for breast cancer, but not for the general population. The sensitivity of MRI is much higher than mammography; however, the specificity is significantly lower and this results in multiple unnecessary biopsies. The increased sensitivity despite decreased specificity may be considered a reasonable trade-off for those at increased risk for developing breast cancer, but not for normal-risk population. MRI is useful in women with breast implants to determine the character of a lesion present in the breast and to search for

implant rupture. In addition, positron emission tomography (PET) may play a role in imaging atypical lesions but only after diagnostic mammography has been performed. PET has demonstrated the ability to improve breast cancer diagnosis in small pilot studies, but the primary role remains evaluation of metastatic deposits.

Baxter N: Canadian Task Force on Preventive Health Care: Preventive health care, 2001 update: should women be routinely taught breast self-examination to screen for breast cancer? CMAJ 2001;164:1837. [PMID: 11450279]

Byrne AM et al: Positron emission tomography in the staging and management of breast cancer. Br J Surg 2004;91:1398. [PMID: 15499650]

Elmore JG et al: Screening for breast cancer. JAMA 2005; 293:1245. [PMID: 15755947]

Humphrey LL et al: Breast cancer screening: a summary of the evidence for the U.S. Preventive Services Task Force. Ann Intern Med 2002;137(5 Part 1):347. [PMID: 12204020]

Kosters JP et al: Regular self-examination or clinical examination for early detection of breast cancer. Cochrane Database Syst Rev 2003;(2):CD003373. [PMID: 12804462]

Kriege M et al: The Magnetic Resonance Imaging Screening Study Group: Efficacy of magnetic resonance imaging and mammography for breast cancer screening in women with a familial or genetic predisposition. Obstet Gynecol Surv 2005;60:107. [PMID: 15671899]

Kumar R et al: Potential of dual-time-point imaging to improve breast cancer diagnosis with (18)F-FDG PET. J Nucl Med 2005;46:1819. [PMID: 16269595]

Nystrom L et al: Long-term effects of mammography screening: updated overview of the Swedish randomised trials. Lancet 2001;359:909. [PMID: 11918907]

Pisano ED et al; Digital Mammographic Imaging Screening Trial (DMIST) Investigators Group: Diagnostic performance of digital versus film mammography for breast cancer screening. N Engl J Med 2005;353:1773. [PMID: 16169887]

Reddy DH et al: Incorporating new imaging models in breast cancer management. Curr Treat Options Oncol 2005;6:135. [PMID: 15717995]

Smith RA et al: American Cancer Society guidelines for the early detection of cancer, 2005. CA Cancer J Clin 2005;55:31. [PMID: 15661685]

Taylor P et al: Impact of computer-aided detection prompts on the sensitivity and specificity of screening mammography. Health Technol Assess 2005;9:1. [PMID: 15717938]

Weaver DL et al: Pathologic findings from the Breast Cancer Surveillance Consortium: population-based outcomes in women undergoing biopsy after screening mammography. Cancer 2006;106:732. [PMID: 16411214]

Clinical Clues to Early Detection of Breast Cancer

A. SYMPTOMS AND SIGNS

The presenting complaint in about 70% of patients with breast cancer is a lump (usually painless) in the breast. About 90% of breast masses are discovered by the patient herself. Less frequent symptoms are breast pain; nipple discharge; erosion, retraction, enlargement, or itching of the nipple; and redness, generalized hardness, enlargement, or shrinking of the breast. Rarely, an axil-

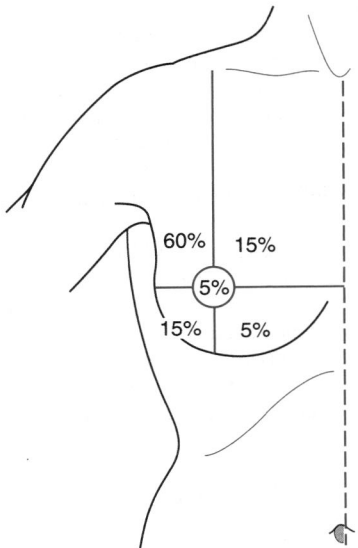

Figure 16–1. Frequency of breast carcinoma at various anatomic sites.

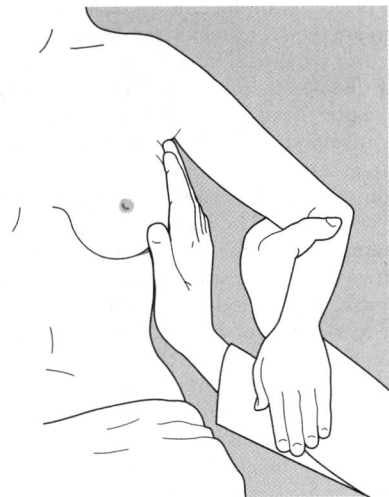

Figure 16–2. Palpation of axillary region for enlarged lymph nodes.

lary mass or swelling of the arm may be the first symptom. Back or bone pain, jaundice, or weight loss may be the result of systemic metastases, but these symptoms are rarely seen on initial presentation.

The relative frequency of carcinoma in various anatomic sites in the breast is shown in Figure 16–1.

Inspection of the breast is the first step in physical examination and should be carried out with the patient sitting, arms at her sides and then overhead. Abnormal variations in breast size and contour, minimal nipple retraction, and slight edema, redness, or retraction of the skin can be identified. Asymmetry of the breasts and retraction or dimpling of the skin can often be accentuated by having the patient raise her arms overhead or press her hands on her hips to contract the pectoralis muscles. Axillary and supraclavicular areas should be thoroughly palpated for enlarged nodes with the patient sitting (Figure 16–2). Palpation of the breast for masses or other changes should be performed with the patient both seated and supine with the arm abducted (Figure 16–3). Palpation with a rotary motion of the examiner's fingers as well as a horizontal stripping motion has been recommended.

Breast cancer usually consists of a nontender, firm or hard mass with poorly delineated margins (caused by local infiltration). Slight skin or nipple retraction is an important sign. Minimal asymmetry of the breast may be noted. Very small (1–2 mm) erosions of the nipple epithelium may be the only manifestation of Paget's carcinoma. Watery, serous, or bloody discharge from the nipple is an occasional early sign but is more often associated with benign disease.

A lesion smaller than 1 cm in diameter may be difficult or impossible for the examiner to feel and yet may be discovered by the patient. She should always be

asked to demonstrate the location of the mass; if the practitioner fails to confirm the patient's suspicions, the examination should be repeated in 2–3 months, preferably 1–2 weeks after the onset of menses. During the premenstrual phase of the cycle, increased innocuous nodularity may suggest neoplasm or may obscure an underlying lesion. If there is any question regarding the nature of an abnormality under these circumstances, the patient should be asked to return after her period. Ultrasound is often valuable and mammography essential when an area is felt by the patient to be abnormal but the physician feels no mass. MRI may be considered, but the lack of specificity should be discussed by the practitioner and the patient.

Metastases tend to involve regional lymph nodes, which may be palpable. One or two movable, nontender, not particularly firm axillary lymph nodes 5 mm or less in diameter are frequently present and are

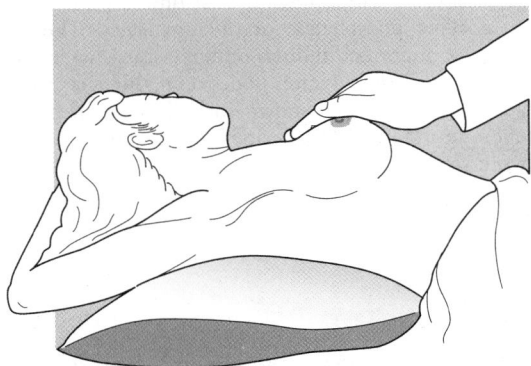

Figure 16–3. Palpation of breasts. Palpation is performed with the patient supine and arm abducted.

generally of no significance. Firm or hard nodes larger than 1 cm are typical of metastases. Axillary nodes that are matted or fixed to skin or deep structures indicate advanced disease (at least stage III). Microscopic metastases are present in about 30% of patients with clinically negative nodes. On the other hand, if the examiner thinks that the axillary nodes are involved, that impression will be borne out by histologic section in about 85% of cases. The incidence of positive axillary nodes increases with the size of the primary tumor. Noninvasive cancers (in situ) do not metastasize.

In most cases, no nodes are palpable in the supraclavicular fossa. Firm or hard nodes of any size in this location or just beneath the clavicle are suggestive of metastatic cancer and should be biopsied. Ipsilateral supraclavicular or infraclavicular nodes containing cancer indicate that the tumor is in an advanced stage (stage III or IV). Edema of the ipsilateral arm, commonly caused by metastatic infiltration of regional lymphatics, is also a sign of advanced cancer.

B. LABORATORY FINDINGS

A consistently elevated sedimentation rate may be the result of disseminated cancer. Liver or bone metastases may be associated with elevation of serum alkaline phosphatase. Hypercalcemia is an occasional important finding in advanced cancer of the breast. Carcinoembryonic antigen (CEA) and CA 15-3 or CA 27-29 may be used as markers for recurrent breast cancer but are not helpful in diagnosing early lesions. Many scientists are further investigating breast cancer markers through proteomics and hormone assays. These studies are ongoing and may prove to be helpful in early detection or evaluation of prognosis.

C. IMAGING FOR METASTASES

Chest radiographs may show pulmonary metastases. CT scanning of the liver and brain is of value only when metastases are suspected in these areas. Bone scans utilizing ^{99m}Tc-labeled phosphates or phosphonates are more sensitive than skeletal radiographs in detecting metastatic breast cancer. Bone scanning has not proved to be of clinical value as a routine preoperative test in the absence of symptoms, physical findings, or abnormal alkaline phosphatase or calcium levels. The frequency of abnormal findings on bone scan parallels the status of the axillary lymph nodes on pathologic examination. PET has been shown to be less useful than a bone scan to identify metastatic bone lesions. It is effective in soft tissue or visceral metastases in patients with signs or symptoms of metastatic disease. PET scanning combined with CT (PET-CT) is an effective screening method for detecting soft tissue metastases and is replacing CT scans.

D. DIAGNOSTIC TESTS

1. Biopsy—The diagnosis of breast cancer depends ultimately on examination of tissue or cells removed by biopsy. Treatment should never be undertaken without an unequivocal histologic or cytologic diagnosis of cancer. The safest course is biopsy examination of all suspicious masses found on physical examination and of suspicious lesions demonstrated by mammography. About 60% of lesions clinically thought to be cancer prove on biopsy to be benign, and about 30% of lesions believed to be benign are found to be malignant. These findings demonstrate the fallibility of clinical judgment and the necessity for biopsy.

All breast masses require a histologic diagnosis with one probable exception, that being a nonsuspicious, presumably fibrocystic mass, in a premenopausal woman. Rather, these masses can be observed through one or two menstrual cycles. However, if the mass does not completely resolve during this time, it must be biopsied. Figures 16–4 and 16–5 present algorithms for management of breast masses in premenopausal and postmenopausal patients.

The simplest biopsy method is needle biopsy, either by aspiration of tumor cells (fine-needle aspiration cytology) or by obtaining a small core of tissue with a hollow needle (core biopsy).

Fine-needle aspiration cytology is a useful technique whereby cells are aspirated with a small needle and examined cytologically. This technique can be performed easily with no morbidity and is much less expensive than excisional or open biopsy. The main disadvantages are that it requires a pathologist skilled in the cytologic diagnosis of breast cancer and that it is subject to sampling problems, particularly because deep lesions may be missed. Furthermore, noninvasive cancers usually cannot be distinguished from invasive cancers. The incidence of false-positive diagnoses is extremely low, perhaps 1–2%. The false-negative rate is as high as 10%. Most experienced clinicians would not leave a suspicious dominant mass in the breast even when fine-needle aspiration cytology is negative unless the clinical diagnosis, breast imaging studies, and cytologic studies were all in agreement, such as a fibrocystic lesion or fibroadenoma.

Large-needle (core needle) biopsy removes a core of tissue with a large cutting needle. Hand-held biopsy devices make large-core needle biopsy of a palpable mass easy and cost effective in the office with local anesthesia. As in the case of any needle biopsy, the main problem is sampling error due to improper positioning of the needle, giving rise to a false-negative test result.

Open biopsy under local anesthesia as a separate procedure prior to deciding upon definitive treatment is the most reliable means of diagnosis. Needle biopsy or aspiration, when positive, offers a more rapid approach with less expense and morbidity, but when nondiagnostic it must be followed by open biopsy. Open biopsy consists of either an incisional biopsy or an excisional biopsy. An incisional biopsy is one in which an incision is made and only a portion of the breast abnormality is removed for histologic evaluation. An excisional biopsy is also done through an incision in the skin, but with the intent to remove the entire abnormality, not simply a sample. Incisional biopsies are rarely performed.

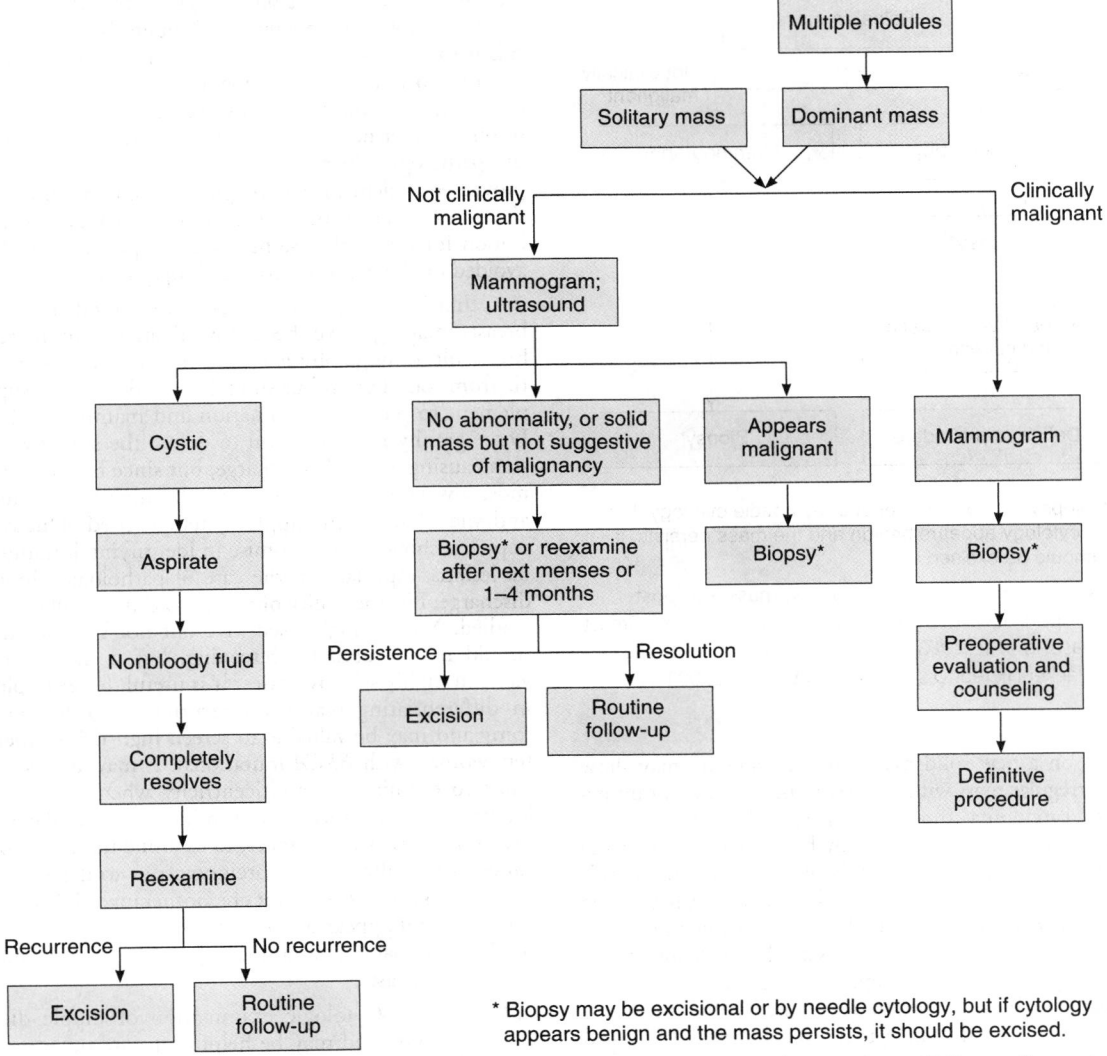

Figure 16–4. Evaluation of breast masses in premenopausal women. (Modified from Giuliano AE: Breast disease. In: *Practical Gynecologic Oncology*, 3rd ed. Berek JS, Hacker NF [editors]. Williams & Wilkins, 2000.)

Additional evaluation for metastatic disease and therapeutic options can be discussed with the patient after the histologic or cytologic diagnosis of cancer has been established. This approach has the advantage of avoiding unnecessary procedures, since cancer is found in the minority of patients biopsied for a breast lump. In situ cancers are not easily diagnosed cytologically and usually require excisional biopsy.

As an alternative in highly suspicious circumstances, the patient may be admitted to the hospital, where the diagnosis is made on frozen section of tissue obtained by open biopsy under general anesthesia. If the frozen section is positive, the surgeon can proceed immediately with operation. This one-step method is rarely used today except when a cytologic study has suggested cancer but is not diagnostic and there is a high clinical suspicion of malignancy in a patient well prepared for the diagnosis of cancer and its treatment options.

In general, the two-step approach—outpatient biopsy followed by definitive operation at a later date—is preferred in the diagnosis and treatment of breast cancer, because patients can be given time to adjust to the diagnosis of cancer, can consider alternative forms of therapy, and can seek a second opinion if they wish. There is no adverse effect from the short delay of the two-step procedure, and this is the recommendation of the NCI.

2. Ultrasonography—Ultrasonography is performed primarily to differentiate cystic from solid lesions. Though not diagnostic, ultrasound may reveal features highly suggestive of malignancy such as irregular mar-

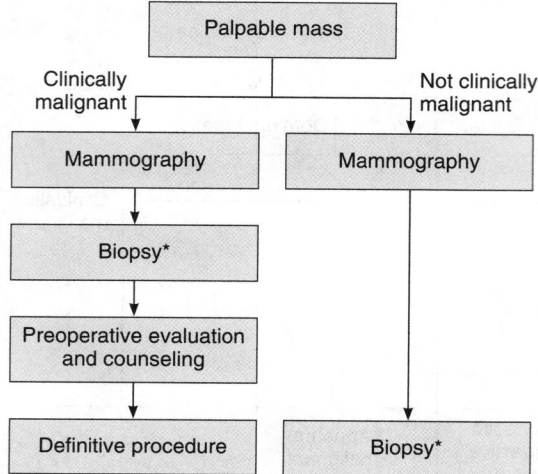

```
                    ┌─────────────────┐
                    │  Palpable mass  │
                    └─────────────────┘
       Clinically                    Not clinically
       malignant                       malignant
          ┌──────────────┐         ┌──────────────┐
          │ Mammography  │         │ Mammography  │
          └──────────────┘         └──────────────┘
          ┌──────────────┐
          │   Biopsy*    │
          └──────────────┘
      ┌──────────────────────┐
      │ Preoperative evaluation │
      │    and counseling       │
      └──────────────────────┘
      ┌──────────────────────┐   ┌──────────────┐
      │ Definitive procedure │   │   Biopsy*    │
      └──────────────────────┘   └──────────────┘
```

* Biopsy may be excisional or by needle cytology, but if cytology appears benign and the mass persists, it should be excised.

Figure 16–5. Evaluation of breast masses in postmenopausal women. (Modified from Giuliano AE: Breast disease. In: *Practical Gynecologic Oncology*, 3rd ed. Berek JS, Hacker NF [editors]. Williams & Wilkins, 2000.)

gins on a new solid mass. Ultrasonography may show an irregular mass within a cyst in the rare case of intracystic carcinoma. If a tumor is palpable and feels like a cyst, an 18-gauge needle can be used to aspirate the fluid and make the diagnosis of cyst. If a cyst is aspirated and the fluid is nonbloody, it does not have to be examined cytologically. If the mass does not recur, no further diagnostic test is necessary. Nonpalpable mammographic densities that appear benign should be investigated with ultrasound to determine whether the lesion is cystic or solid. These may even be needle biopsied with ultrasound guidance.

3. Mammography—When a suspicious abnormality is identified by mammography alone and cannot be palpated by the clinician, the lesion should be biopsied by a **computerized stereotactic guided core needle** technique. Under mammographic guidance, a biopsy needle can be inserted into the lesion by the mammographer, and a core of tissue for histologic examination or cells for cytology can then be examined. Vacuum assistance increases the amount of tissue obtained and improves diagnosis.

Mammographic localization biopsy is performed by obtaining a mammogram in two perpendicular views and placing a needle or hook-wire near the abnormality so that the surgeon can use the metal needle or wire as a guide during operation to locate the lesion. After mammography confirms the position of the needle in relation to the lesion, an incision is made and the subcutaneous tissue is dissected until the needle is identified. Using the films as a guide, the abnormality can then be localized and excised. It often happens that the abnormality cannot even be palpated through the incision—this is the case with microcalcifications—and thus it is essential to obtain a mammogram of the specimen to document that the lesion was excised. At that time, a second marker needle can further localize the lesion for the pathologist. Stereotactic core needle biopsies have proved equivalent to mammographic localization biopsies. Core biopsy is preferable to mammographic localization for accessible lesions since an operation can be avoided by the use of stereotactic biopsy techniques.

4. Other imaging modalities—Other modalities of breast imaging have been investigated. Automated breast ultrasonography is useful in distinguishing cystic from solid lesions but should be used only as a supplement to physical examination and mammography. Ductography may be useful to define the site of a lesion causing a bloody discharge, but since biopsy is almost always indicated, ductography may be omitted and the blood-filled nipple system excised. Ductoscopy has shown some promise in identifying intraductal lesions, especially in the case of pathologic nipple discharge, but the utility of this procedure is still being studied. MRI is highly sensitive but not specific and should not be used for screening, but it may be of value in highly selective cases. It is useful, for example, in differentiating scar from recurrence postlumpectomy and may be valuable to screen high-risk women (eg, women with *BRCA* mutations). It may also be of value to examine for multicentricity when there is a known primary cancer; to examine the contralateral breast in women with cancer; to examine the extent of cancer, especially lobular carcinomas; or to determine the response to neoadjuvant chemotherapy. PET scanning does not appear useful in evaluating the breast itself but is valuable to examine regional lymphatics and distant metastases.

5. Cytology—Cytologic examination of nipple discharge or cyst fluid may be helpful on rare occasions. As a rule, mammography (or ductography) and breast biopsy are required when nipple discharge or cyst fluid is bloody or cytologically questionable. Ductal lavage, a technique that washes individual duct systems with saline and loosens epithelial cells for cytologic evaluation, is being evaluated as a risk assessment tool but appears to be of little value.

Baker JA et al: Breast US: assessment of technical quality and image interpretation. Radiology 2002;223:229. [PMID: 11930071]

Dooley WC: Routine operative breast endoscopy for bloody nipple discharge. Ann Surg Oncol 2002;9:920. [PMID: 12417516]

Eubank WB et al: Evolving role of positron emission tomography in breast cancer imaging. Semin Nucl Med 2005;35:84. [PMID: 15765372]

Hollingsworth AB: Perspectives on preoperative staging with breast MRI. J Am Coll Surg 2004;199:173. [PMID: 15217651]

Lenahan C et al: The role of tumor markers in breast cancer management. Curr Surg 2004;61:532. [PMID: 15590016]

Ljung BM et al: Cytology of ductal lavage fluid of the breast. Diagn Cytopathol 2004;30:143. [PMID: 14986293]

DIFFERENTIAL DIAGNOSIS

The lesions to be considered most often in the differential diagnosis of breast cancer are the following, in descending order of frequency: fibrocystic condition of the breast, fibroadenoma, intraductal papilloma, lipoma, and fat necrosis.

STAGING

Currently, the American Joint Committee on Cancer and the International Union Against Cancer have agreed on a TNM (tumor, regional lymph nodes, distant metastases) staging system for breast cancer. The use of this uniform TNM staging system enhances communication between investigators and clinicians. Table 16–2 sets forth the TNM classification.

PATHOLOGIC TYPES

Numerous pathologic subtypes of breast cancer can be identified histologically (Table 16–3). These types are distinguished by the histologic appearance and growth pattern of the tumor. In general, breast cancer arises either from the epithelial lining of the large or intermediate-sized ducts (ductal) or from the epithelium of the terminal ducts of the lobules (lobular). The cancer may be invasive or in situ. Most breast cancers arise from the intermediate ducts and are invasive (invasive ductal, infiltrating ductal), and most histologic types are merely subtypes of invasive ductal cancer with unusual growth patterns (colloid, medullary, scirrhous, mucinous, etc). Ductal carcinoma that has not invaded the extraductal tissue is intraductal or in situ ductal. Lobular carcinoma may be either invasive or in situ. In situ lobular carcinoma is primarily a risk factor for the development of invasive ductal cancer.

Except for the in situ cancers, the histologic subtypes have only a slight bearing on prognosis when outcomes are compared after accurate staging. Various histologic parameters, such as invasion of blood vessels, tumor differentiation, invasion of breast lymphatics, and tumor necrosis have been examined, but they too seem to have little prognostic value.

The noninvasive cancers by definition are confined by the basement membrane of the ducts and lack the ability to spread. However, in patients whose biopsies show noninvasive intraductal cancer, associated invasive ductal cancers metastasize to lymph nodes in about 1–3% of cases.

SPECIAL CLINICAL FORMS OF BREAST CANCER

Paget's Carcinoma

The basic lesion is usually an infiltrating ductal carcinoma, usually well differentiated, or a ductal carcinoma in situ (DCIS). The ducts of the nipple epithelium are infiltrated, but gross nipple changes are often minimal, and a tumor mass may not be palpable. The first symptom is often itching or burning of the nipple, with superficial erosion or ulceration. The diagnosis is established by biopsy of the erosion.

Paget's carcinoma is not common (about 1% of all breast cancers), but it is important because the nipple changes appear innocuous and the diagnosis frequently is missed. The nipple changes are often diagnosed and treated as dermatitis or bacterial infection, leading to delay in detection. When the lesion consists of nipple changes only, the incidence of axillary metastases is less than 5%, and the prognosis is excellent. When a breast mass is also present, the incidence of axillary metastases rises, with an associated marked decrease in prospects for cure by surgical or other treatment.

Inflammatory Carcinoma

This is the most malignant form of breast cancer and constitutes less than 3% of all cases. The clinical findings consist of a rapidly growing, sometimes painful mass that enlarges the breast. The overlying skin becomes erythematous, edematous, and warm. Often there is no distinct mass, since the tumor infiltrates the involved breast diffusely. The diagnosis should be made when the redness involves more than one-third of the skin over the breast and biopsy shows infiltrating carcinoma with invasion of the subdermal lymphatics. The inflammatory changes, often mistaken for an infection, are caused by carcinomatous invasion of the subdermal lymphatics, with resulting edema and hyperemia. If the practitioner suspects infection but the lesion does not respond rapidly (1–2 weeks) to antibiotics, biopsy should be performed. Metastases tend to occur early and widely, and for this reason inflammatory carcinoma is rarely curable. Mastectomy is seldom indicated unless chemotherapy and radiation have resulted in clinical remission with no evidence of distant metastases. In these cases, residual disease in the breast may be eradicated. Radiation, hormone therapy, and chemotherapy are the measures most likely to be of value rather than operation.

Breast Cancer Occurring during Pregnancy or Lactation

Breast cancer complicates approximately one in 3000 pregnancies. The diagnosis is frequently delayed, because physiologic changes in the breast may obscure the lesion. This results in a tendency of both patients and practitioners to misinterpret findings and to delay biopsy. When the cancer is confined to the breast, the 5-year survival rate after mastectomy is about 70%. Axillary metastases are already present in 60–70% of patients, and for them the 5-year survival rate after mastectomy is only 30–40%. Pregnancy (or lactation) is not a contraindication to operation, and treatment should be based on the stage of the disease as in the nonpregnant (or nonlactating) woman. Overall survival rates have improved, since cancers are now diagnosed in pregnant women earlier than in the past. Breast-conserving surgery may be performed—and radiation and chemotherapy given—even during the pregnancy.

Table 16–2. TNM staging for breast cancer.

Primary tumor (T)	
Definitions for classifying the primary tumor (T) are the same for clinical and for pathologic classification. If the measurement is made by physical examination, the examiner will use the major headings (T1, T2, or T3). If other measurements, such as mammographic or pathologic measurements, are used, the subsets of T1 can be used. Tumors should be measured to the nearest 0.1 cm increment.	
TX	Primary tumor cannot be assessed
T0	No evidence of primary tumor
Tis	Carcinoma in situ
Tis (DCIS)	Ductal carcinoma in situ
Tis (LCIS)	Lobular carcinoma in situ
Tis (Paget's)	Paget's disease of the nipple with no tumor

Note: Paget's disease associated with a tumor is classified according to the size of the tumor.

T1	Tumor 2 cm or less in greatest dimension
T1mic	Microinvasion 0.1 cm or less in greatest dimension
T1a	Tumor more than 0.1 cm but not more than 0.5 cm in greatest dimension
T1b	Tumor more than 0.5 cm but not more than 1 cm in greatest dimension
T1c	Tumor more than 1 cm but not more than 2 cm in greatest dimension
T2	Tumor more than 2 cm but not more than 5 cm in greatest dimension
T3	Tumor more than 5 cm in greatest dimension
T4	Tumor of any size with direct extension to (a) chest wall or (b) skin, only as described below
T4a	Extension to chest wall, not including pectoralis muscle
T4b	Edema (including peau d'orange) or ulceration of the skin of the breast, or satellite skin nodules confined to the same breast
T4c	Both T4a and T4b
T4d	Inflammatory carcinoma

Regional lymph nodes (N)	
Clinical	
NX	Regional lymph nodes cannot be assessed (eg, previously removed)
N0	No regional lymph node metastasis
N1	Metastasis to movable ipsilateral axillary lymph node(s)
N2	Metastases in ipsilateral axillary lymph nodes fixed or matted, or in clinically apparent[1] ipsilateral internal mammary nodes in the *absence* of clinically evident axillary lymph node metastasis
N2a	Metastasis in ipsilateral axillary lymph nodes fixed to one another (matted) or to other structures
N2b	Metastasis only in clinically apparent[1] ipsilateral internal mammary nodes and in the *absence* of clinically evident axillary lymph node metastasis

N3	Metastasis in ipsilateral infraclavicular lymph node(s) with or without axillary lymph node involvement, or in clinically apparent[1] ipsilateral internal mammary lymph node(s) and in the *presence* of clinically evident axillary lymph node metastasis; or metastasis in ipsilateral supraclavicular lymph node(s) with or without axillary or internal mammary lymph node involvement
N3a	Metastasis in ipsilateral infraclavicular lymph node(s)
N3b	Metastasis in ipsilateral internal mammary lymph node(s) and axillary lymph node(s)
N3c	Metastasis in ipsilateral supraclavicular lymph node(s)

Pathologic (pN)[2]

pNX	Regional lymph nodes cannot be assessed (eg, previously removed, or not removed for pathologic study)
pN0	No regional lymph node metastasis histologically, no additional examination for isolated tumor cells

Note: Isolated tumor cells (ITC) are defined as single tumor cells or small cell clusters not greater than 0.2 mm, usually detected only by immunohistochemical (IHC) or molecular methods but which may be verified on hematoxylin and eosin stains. ITCs do not usually show evidence of malignant activity, eg, proliferation or stromal reaction.

pN0(i–)	No regional lymph node metastasis histologically, negative IHC
pN0(i+)	No regional lymph node metastasis histologically, positive IHC, no IHC cluster greater than 0.2 mm
pN0(mol–)	No regional lymph node metastasis histologically, negative molecular findings (RT-PCR)[3]
pN0(mol+)	No regional lymph node metastasis histologically, positive molecular findings (RT-PCR)[3]
pN1	Metastasis in one to three axillary lymph nodes, and/or in internal mammary nodes with microscopic disease detected by sentinel lymph node dissection but not clinically apparent[4]
pN1mi	Micrometastasis (greater than 0.2 mm, none greater than 2.0 mm)
pN1a	Metastasis in one to three axillary lymph nodes
pN1b	Metastasis in internal mammary nodes with microscopic disease detected by sentinel lymph node dissection but not clinically apparent[4]
pN1c	Metastasis in one to three axillary lymph nodes and in internal mammary lymph nodes with microscopic disease detected by sentinel lymph node dissection but not clinically apparent.[4] (If associated with greater than three positive axillary lymph nodes, the internal mammary nodes are classified as pN3b to reflect increased tumor burden)

Table 16–2. TNM staging for breast cancer. (continued)

		Distant metastasis (M)	
pN2	Metastasis in four to nine axillary lymph nodes, or in clinically apparent[4] internal mammary lymph nodes in the *absence* of axillary lymph node metastasis	MX	Distant metastasis cannot be assessed
		M0	No distant metastasis
		M1	Distant metastasis
pN2a	Metastasis in four to nine axillary lymph nodes (at least one tumor deposit greater than 2.0 mm)		

			Stage grouping		
pN2b	Metastasis in clinically apparent[4] internal mammary lymph nodes in the *absence* of axillary lymph node metastasis				
pN3	Metastasis in 10 or more axillary lymph nodes, or in infraclavicular lymph nodes, or in clinically apparent[4] ipsilateral internal mammary lymph nodes in the *presence* of one or more positive axillary lymph nodes; or in more than three axillary lymph nodes with clinically negative microscopic metastasis in internal mammary lymph nodes; or in ipsilateral supraclavicular lymph nodes	Stage 0	Tis	N0	M0
		Stage I	T1[5]	N0	M0
		Stage IIA	T0	N1	M0
			T1[5]	N1	M0
			T2	N0	M0
		Stage IIB	T2	N1	M0
			T3	N0	M0
		Stage IIIA	T0	N2	M0
			T1[5]	N2	M0
			T2	N2	M0
pN3a	Metastasis in 10 or more axillary lymph nodes (at least one tumor deposit greater than 2.0 mm), or metastasis to the infraclavicular lymph nodes	T3	N1	M0	
		T3	N2	M0	
		Stage IIIB	T4	N0	M0
			T4	N1	M0
pN3b	Metastasis in clinically apparent[4] ipsilateral internal mammary lymph nodes in the *presence* of one or more positive axillary lymph nodes; or in more than three axillary lymph nodes and in internal mammary lymph nodes with microscopic disease detected by sentinel lymph node dissection but not clinically apparent[4]		T4	N2	M0
		Stage IIIC	Any T	N3	M0
		Stage IV	Any T	Any N	M1
pN3c	Metastasis in ipsilateral supraclavicular lymph nodes				

Note: Stage designation may be changed if postsurgical imaging studies reveal the presence of distant metastases, provided that the studies are carried out within 4 months of diagnosis in the absence of disease progression and provided that the patient has not received neoadjuvant therapy.

[1]*Clinically apparent* is defined as detected by imaging studies (excluding lymphoscintigraphy) or by clinical examination or grossly visible pathologically.
[2]Classification is based on axillary lymph node dissection with or without sentinal lymph node dissection. Classification based solely on sentinel lymph node dissection without subsequent axillary lymph node dissection is designated (sn) for "sentinal node," eg, pN0(i+)(sn).
[3]RT-PCR: reverse transcriptase/polymerase chain reaction.
[4]*Clinically apparent* is defined as detected by imaging studies (excluding lymphoscintigraphy) or by clinical examination. *Not clinically apparent* is defined as not detected by imaging studies (excluding lymphoscintigraphy) or by clinical examination.
[5]T1 includes T1mic.
Reproduced from *AJCC Cancer Staging Manual*, 6th edition. Springer, 2002.

Bilateral Breast Cancer

Clinically evident simultaneous bilateral breast cancer occurs in less than 5% of cases, but there is as high as a 20–25% incidence of later occurrence of cancer in the second breast. Bilaterality occurs more often in familial breast cancer, in women under age 50 years, and when the tumor in the primary breast is lobular. The incidence of second breast cancers increases directly with the length of time the patient is alive after her first cancer—about 1–2% per year.

In patients with breast cancer, mammography should be performed before primary treatment and at regular intervals thereafter, to search for occult cancer in the opposite breast or conserved ipsilateral breast. Routine biopsy of the opposite breast is usually not warranted even for lobular cancer.

Noninvasive Cancer

Noninvasive cancer can occur within the ducts (ductal carcinoma in situ, DCIS) or lobules (lobular carcinoma in situ, LCIS). LCIS, although thought to be a premalignant lesion or a risk factor for breast cancer, in fact may behave like DCIS. In a 2004 analysis of multiple NSABP studies, invasive lobular breast cancer not only developed in patients with LCIS but it developed in the same breast and indexed location as the original LCIS. Although more research needs to be done in this area, the invasive potential of LCIS is

Table 16–3. Histologic types of breast cancer.

Type	Frequency of Occurrence
Infiltrating ductal (not otherwise specified)	80–90%
Medullary	5–8%
Colloid (mucinous)	2–4%
Tubular	1–2%
Papillary	1–2%
Invasive lobular	6–8%
Noninvasive	4–6%
Intraductal	2–3%
Lobular in situ	2–3%
Rare cancers	< 1%
Juvenile (secretory)	
Adenoid cystic	
Epidermoid	
Sudoriferous	

being reconsidered. DCIS tends to be unilateral and most often progresses to invasive cancer if untreated. In approximately 40–60% of women who have DCIS treated with biopsy alone, invasive cancer develops within the same breast.

The treatment of intraductal lesions is controversial. DCIS can be treated by wide excision with or without radiation therapy or with total mastectomy. Conservative management is advised in this patient population with small lesions amenable to lumpectomy until further data are developed. Although research is defining the malignant potential of LCIS, it may be well managed with observation, but patients unwilling to accept the increased risk of breast cancer may be offered surgical excision of the area in question or even bilateral total mastectomy. Currently, accepted standards of care offer the alternative of chemoprevention, using agents such as tamoxifen, which is effective in preventing invasive breast cancer from developing in both LCIS and intraductal carcinoma in situ that has been completely excised. Axillary metastases from in situ cancers should not occur unless there is an occult invasive cancer. Sentinel node biopsy may be indicated in large DCIS treated with mastectomy.

Barni S et al: Locally advanced breast cancer. Curr Opin Obstet Gynecol 2006;18:47. [PMID: 16493260]

Fisher ER et al: Pathologic findings from the National Surgical Adjuvant Breast and Bowel Project: twelve-year observations concerning lobular carcinoma in situ. Cancer 2004; 100:238. [PMID: 14716756]

Kawase K et al: Paget's disease of the breast: there is a role for breast-conserving therapy. Ann Surg Oncol 2005;12:391. [PMID: 15915373]

Khan A et al: Diagnosis and management of ductal carcinoma in situ. Curr Treat Options Oncol 2004;5:131. [PMID: 14990207]

Lerebours F et al: Update on inflammatory breast cancer. Breast Cancer Res 2005;7:52. [PMID: 15743511]

Ring AE et al: Breast cancer and pregnancy. Ann Oncol 2005; 16: 1855. [PMID: 16030024]

Tai P et al: Short- and long-term cause-specific survival of patients with inflammatory breast cancer. BMC Cancer 2005; 5:137. [PMID: 16242046]

BIOMARKERS

The presence or absence of estrogen receptors (ER) and progesterone receptors (PR) in the cytoplasm of tumor cells is of paramount importance in managing patients with breast cancer. Patients whose primary tumors are receptor-positive have a more favorable course than those whose tumors are receptor-negative. Receptors are of value in determining adjuvant therapy and for treatment of advanced disease. Up to 60% of patients with metastatic breast cancer will respond to hormonal manipulation if their tumors contain estrogen receptors. Fewer than 5% of patients with metastatic, ER-negative tumors can be treated successfully in this fashion.

Receptor status is valuable not only in managing metastatic disease but also in helping select patients for adjuvant therapy. Adjuvant hormonal therapy (tamoxifen) or AIs with receptor-positive tumors and adjuvant chemotherapy with receptor-negative tumors improve survival rates even in the absence of lymph node metastases (see Adjuvant Therapy, below).

PR status may be a more sensitive indicator than ER status of patients who may respond to hormonal manipulation. Up to 80% of patients with metastatic PR-positive tumors improve with hormonal manipulation. Receptors have no relationship to response to chemotherapy.

In addition to ER status and PR status, the rate at which tumor divides and the differentiation of the cells (proliferative indices) are important. In order to establish the rate of growth and differentiation, the amount and type of DNA is measured with flow cytometry.

The ER status, PR status, proliferative indices, and HER-2/*neu* status of the tumor should be determined at the time of initial biopsy. This is performed on paraffin-fixed tissue by immunohistochemistry. HER-2/*neu* overexpression is scored using a numerical system: 1+ is not an overexpressor, 2+ is borderline, and 3+ is an overexpressor. In the case of 2+ expression, fluorescence in situ hybridization (FISH) is recommended to more accurately assess HER-2/*neu* amplification and provide better prognostic information. It is critical to understand the receptor status prior to initiating any adjuvant therapy because it may change after hormonal therapy or chemotherapy as well as aid in the assessment of prognosis. While individually these biomarkers provide insight to appropriate adjuvant therapy, when combined they provide a great deal of information regarding risk of recurrence. A new test, Oncotype DX, combines 21 genetic markers, including estrogen receptor, progesterone receptor, and HER-2/*neu* expression in a tumor specimen. The researchers were able to categorize risk of recurrence into three groups: high risk, intermediate risk, and low risk. In addition, the test is able to identify that the high-risk group was more likely to benefit from chemotherapy in addition to tamoxifen while the low risk group did not. This type of test is quite helpful when the survival advantage of therapy is difficult to determine but is only appropriate for ER-positive node-negative tumors. Its applicability is limited by its experience and lack of prospective corroboration.

Another promising biomarker being studied is vascular endothelial growth factor (VEGF), a protein that stimulates the growth of blood vessels. Elevated levels of VEGF may be a marker for a tumor that is more aggressive since it has the ability to develop blood vessels and grow. While researchers look for more specific markers to determine the presence of breast cancer, these markers also provide insight to targeted methods of treatment. Other markers being evaluated are *p53, nm23*, DNA 5c exceeding rate (DNA 5cER), G-actin, urokinase-type plasminogen activator (u-PA), and its type-1 inhibitor (PAI-1).

Konecny G et al: Quantitative association between HER-2/*neu* and steroid hormone receptors in hormone receptor-positive primary breast cancer. J Natl Cancer Inst 2003;95:142. [PMID: 12529347]

Paik S et al: A multigene assay to predict recurrence of tamoxifen treated, node-negative breast cancer. N Eng J Med 2004; 351:2817. [PMID: 15591335]

Winston JS et al: HER-2/*neu* evaluation in breast cancer are we there yet? Am J Clin Pathol 2004;121:S33. [PMID: 15298149]

Zhang W et al: Biomarker analysis on breast ductal lavage cells in women with and without breast cancer. Int J Cancer 2006 [Epub ahead of print]. [PMID: 16477639]

CURATIVE TREATMENT

Treatment may be curative or palliative. Curative treatment is advised for clinical stage I, II, and III disease (Table 16–2). Patients with locally advanced (T3, T4) and even inflammatory tumors may be cured with multimodality therapy, but in most palliation is all that can be expected. Palliative treatment is appropriate for all patients with stage IV disease and for previously treated patients in whom distant metastases develop or who have unresectable local cancers.

The growth potential of tumors and host resistance factors vary widely from patient to patient and may be altered during the course of the disease. The doubling time of breast cancer cells ranges from several weeks in a rapidly growing lesion to years in slowly growing ones. Assuming that the rate of doubling is constant and that the neoplasm originates in one cell, a carcinoma with a doubling time of 100 days may not reach clinically detectable size (1 cm) for about 8 years. Rapidly growing cancers have a much shorter preclinical course and a greater tendency to metastasize by the time a breast mass is discovered.

The long preclinical growth phase and the tendency of breast cancers to metastasize have led clinicians to believe that most breast cancer is a systemic disease at the time of diagnosis. Although it may be true that breast cancer cells are released from the tumor prior to diagnosis, variations in the host–tumor relationship prohibit the growth of disseminated disease in many patients. Clearly, not all breast cancer is systemic at the time of diagnosis. For this reason, a pessimistic attitude concerning the management of breast cancer is unwarranted. Most patients can be cured.

Controversy surrounds the timing of surgery with respect to the menstrual cycle. Some suggest that operation during the time of unopposed estrogen adversely affects survival, but most studies support no such effect. Several randomized trials are currently examining this question.

Choice of Primary Therapy

The extent of disease and its biologic aggressiveness are the principal determinants of the outcome of primary therapy. Clinical and pathologic staging help in assessing extent of disease (Table 16–2), but each is to some extent imprecise. Other factors such as DNA flow cytometry, tumor grade, hormone receptor assays, and oncogene amplification may be of prognostic value but are not important in determining the type of local therapy.

Controversy surrounds the choice of primary therapy of stage I, II, and III breast carcinoma. A number of states require physicians to inform patients of alternative treatment methods in the management of breast cancer. Currently, the standard of care for stage I, stage II, and most stage III cancer is surgical resection followed by adjuvant radiation or systemic therapy when indicated.

Breast-Conserving Therapy

Many nonrandomized trials, the randomized Milan trial, and a large randomized trial conducted by the NSABP in the United States show that disease-free survival rates are similar for patients treated by partial mastectomy plus axillary dissection followed by radiation therapy and for those treated by modified radical mastectomy (total mastectomy plus axillary dissection). All patients whose axillary nodes contained tumor received adjuvant chemotherapy.

In the NSABP trial, patients were randomized to three treatment types: (1) "lumpectomy" (removal of the tumor with *confirmed* tumor-free margins) plus whole breast irradiation, (2) lumpectomy alone, and (3) total mastectomy. All patients underwent axillary lymph node dissection, and some had tumors as large as 4 cm with (or without) palpable axillary lymph nodes. With 20 years of follow-up, the lowest local recurrence rate was among patients treated with lumpectomy and postoperative irradiation, approximately 14%; the highest—nearly 40%—was among patients treated with lumpectomy alone. However, the overall survival as well as the distant disease-free survival were similar among the three treatment groups. This study shows that lumpectomy and axillary dissection with postoperative radiation therapy are as effective as modified radical mastectomy for the management of patients with stage I and stage II breast cancer.

The results of these and other trials have demonstrated that much less aggressive surgical treatment of the primary lesion than has previously been thought necessary gives equivalent therapeutic results and may preserve an acceptable cosmetic appearance.

Tumor size is a major consideration in determining the feasibility of breast conservation. The lumpectomy trial of the NSABP randomized patients with tumors as large as 4 cm. To achieve an acceptable cosmetic result, the patient must have a breast of sufficient size to enable excision of a 4-cm tumor without considerable deformity. Therefore, large size is only a relative contraindication. Subareolar tumors, also difficult to excise without deformity, are not contraindications to breast conservation. Clinically detectable multifocality is a relative contraindication to breast-conserving surgery, as is fixation to the chest wall or skin or involvement of the nipple or overlying skin. The patient—not the surgeon—should be the judge of what is cosmetically acceptable.

Axillary dissection is valuable in preventing axillary recurrences, in staging cancer, and in planning therapy. Intraoperative lymphatic mapping and sentinel node dissection identify lymph nodes most likely to harbor metastases if present in the axillary nodes. A trial from Milan with very short follow-up showed no survival difference between axillary dissection and sentinel node biopsy in **node-negative** women. Results suggest that sentinel node biopsy can safely replace axillary dissection for staging and treatment in histopathologically node-negative women at experienced centers. At an international consensus conference in Philadelphia in 2001, participants recommended sentinel node biopsy as an alternative to axillary dissection in selected patients with invasive cancer. Bone marrow biopsy with examination by immunocytochemistry to detect early metastases may be as sensitive a staging procedure as axillary dissection and may identify patients at high risk for disseminating disease.

Recommendations

Earlier consensus held that breast-conserving surgery with radiation was the preferred form of treatment for patients with early-stage breast cancer. Despite the numerous randomized trials showing no survival benefit of mastectomy over breast-conserving partial mastectomy and irradiation, breast-conserving surgery appears underutilized and mastectomy remains the more common treatment. About 25% of patients in the United States with stage I or stage II breast cancer are treated with breast-conserving surgery and radiation therapy, compared with 75% treated with mastectomy. Use of breast-conserving surgery and radiation

therapy varies by region of the country, ranging from 15% in the South Central United States to 30% in the Pacific Region.

Modified radical mastectomy (total mastectomy plus axillary lymph node dissection) has been the standard therapy for most patients with breast cancer. This operation removes the entire breast, overlying skin, nipple, and areolar complex as well as the underlying pectoralis fascia with the axillary lymph nodes in continuity. The major advantage of modified radical mastectomy is that radiation therapy may not be necessary. The disadvantage, of course, is the psychological impact associated with breast loss. Radical mastectomy, which removes the underlying pectoralis muscle, should be performed rarely, if at all. Axillary node dissection is not indicated for noninfiltrating cancers, because nodal metastases are rarely present. Skin-sparing mastectomy is currently gaining favor but is appropriate in only a small subgroup of patients.

Radiotherapy after partial mastectomy consists of 5–6 weeks of five daily fractions to a total dose of 5000–6000 cGy. Most radiation oncologists use a boost dose. Currently, several studies are underway examining the utility and recurrence rates after intraoperative radiation or dose dense radiation in which the time course of radiation is shortened. Current studies suggest that radiotherapy after mastectomy may improve survival in a subset of patients and meta-analyses suggest radiation after lumpectomy may improve survival. The use of radiation in mastectomy patients is being further researched in a large cooperative trial to better identify which subgroups will benefit. Researchers are also examining the utility of axillary irradiation as an alternative to axillary dissection in the clinically node-negative patient with sentinel node metastases.

Preoperatively, full discussion with the patient regarding the rationale for operation and various alternative forms of treatment is essential. Breast-conserving surgery and radiation should be offered whenever possible, since most patients would prefer to save the breast. Breast reconstruction, immediate or delayed, should be discussed with patients who choose or require mastectomy. Patients should have an interview with a reconstructive plastic surgeon to discuss options prior to making a decision regarding reconstruction. Time is well spent preoperatively in educating the patient and family about these matters.

Adjuvant Systemic Therapy

Following surgery and radiation therapy, chemotherapy or hormonal therapy is advocated for most patients with curable breast cancer. The objective of adjuvant systemic therapy is to eliminate the occult metastases responsible for late recurrences while they are microscopic and most vulnerable to anticancer agents. In addition, adjuvant chemotherapy may decrease local recurrence in patients treated with breast conservation, whereas adjuvant hormonal manipulation decreases contralateral breast cancer occurrence.

Even the earliest studies comparing placebo with chemotherapy drugs having minimal activity such as L-phenylalanine mustard showed an improvement in both disease-free and overall survival for women disease free postoperatively. The landmark study from Milan, Italy evaluating the effect of 1 year of adjuvant cyclophosphamide, methotrexate, and fluorouracil (CMF) given on days 1 and 8 of each month for 12 months, showed a significant improvement in survival for premenopausal women with node-positive disease. After 20 years of follow-up, significant improvement in survival persisted among those receiving chemotherapy. CMF rapidly became the standard management for premenopausal women with node-positive breast cancer. Subsequently, the use of chemotherapy for postmenopausal women and those at less risk than node-positive women was evaluated. Systemic chemotherapy improves survival in all groups of women treated. The improvement in survival appears to be about 30% of the patients' risk of death; that is, a woman with a 30% chance of recurrence and death derives about a 10% overall improvement in survival. This risk reduction analysis has been confirmed in numerous studies and meta-analyses.

On the basis of the superiority of anthracycline-containing regimens in metastatic breast cancer, both doxorubicin and epirubicin have been studied extensively in the adjuvant setting and have been compared to CMF regimens. Studies comparing Adriamycin (doxorubicin) and cyclophosphamide (AC) or epirubicin and cyclophosphamide (EC) with CMF have shown that treatment with anthracycline-containing regimens are at least as effective, and perhaps more effective, as treatment with CMF. The NSABP B-23 compared four cycles of AC with six cycles of CMF and demonstrated the equivalence of these two regimens in node-negative, ER-negative disease. Whereas four cycles of AC or EC have not demonstrated improved survival compared with CMF, the use of six cycles of fluorouracil plus AC (FAC) or fluorouracil plus EC (FEC) has shown improved survival compared with CMF alone. For node-negative patients, most oncologists offer four cycles of AC or six cycles of CMF in the adjuvant setting.

For node-positive patients, taxanes are now frequently combined with anthracycline-based regimens. The Cancer and Leukemia Group B (CALGB) study comparing four cycles of AC to four cycles of AC followed by four cycles of paclitaxel showed about a 20% proportional reduction in recurrence and a 4% absolute improvement in disease-free survival with the use of paclitaxel. Paclitaxel is FDA-approved for and increasingly used as adjuvant therapy in node-positive breast cancer. Unfortunately, a subsequent study by the NSABP failed to show any benefits of the use of paclitaxel except in ER-negative patients with positive nodes as did later results of the CALGB study. A 2002 National Institutes of Health (NIH) consensus panel felt that firm conclusions about the use of taxanes could not be drawn and recommended that patients receive adjuvant taxanes only in the context of a clinical trial. However, based on trends in improved survival, most oncologists add a taxane to AC for node-positive women. A trial comparing six cycles of FAC to six cycles of docetaxel, doxorubicin, and cyclophosphamide (TAC) showed an improvement in disease-free survival for patients receiving the addition of paclitaxel. This benefit was most marked for patients with positive nodes and was seen in both ER-negative and ER-positive tumors. Until more information is obtained, the role of taxanes in the adjuvant setting remains unclear.

Controversy exists as to whether patients whose tumors overexpress the HER-2/*neu* oncogene benefit more from anthracycline regimens than from CMF regimens. Retrospective analysis of randomized trials suggests that patients with HER-2/*neu* overexpression may benefit more from doxorubicin than patients with HER-2/*neu*-negative disease. These retrospective studies have numerous problems including the analysis of HER-2/*neu* on paraffin tissue blocks. Trastuzumab (Herceptin), when studied in the metastatic setting, has proved effective in combination with chemotherapy in patients with HER-2/*neu* overexpression. Published in early 2006, a multicenter trial from Finland by the Fin-Her collaborative group, studied the use of trastuzumab in combination with docetaxel or vinorelbine for patients with early breast cancer that demonstrated HER-2/*neu* overexpression. The 3-year recurrence-free survival was better in those who took trastuzumab than in those who did not receive the antibody, 89% versus 78%, respectively. In another study from Brussels, the HERA trial, a similar disease-free survival at interim analysis was demonstrated when giving trastuzumab subsequent to adjuvant chemotherapy in early breast cancer. While both these studies require additional follow-up, the ability to reduce recurrence in the adjuvant setting is promising and many medical oncologists are adding trastuzumab to their adjuvant chemotherapy regimens in early breast cancer with HER-2/*neu* overexpression.

The overall duration of adjuvant chemotherapy still remains uncertain. However, based on the meta-analysis performed in the Oxford Overview (Early Breast Cancer Trialists' Collaborative Group), the current recommendation is for 3–6 months of the commonly used regimens. The addition of taxanes required an additional duration of therapy of up to 6 months. Increasing the frequency of chemotherapy administration (dose dense chemotherapy) has been shown to be superior to standard dosing. It is often used when there is a greater risk of recurrence or in the younger patient, since it is a difficult regimen to tolerate physically.

Adjuvant hormonal therapy is also highly effective in decreasing recurrence and mortality in women with ER-positive tumors. The standard regimen has been tamoxifen for 5 years. Hormonal therapy decreases the risk of breast cancer mortality by approximately 25%. This appears to be effective regardless of age and may be used in both premenopausal and postmenopausal women. More recently, the AIs have been shown to be effective in the adjuvant setting. The large Arimidex, Tamoxifen, Alone or in Combination (ATAC) trial in postmenopausal women with ER-positive disease showed improved disease-free survival in patients treated with anastrozole compared with those treated with tamoxifen alone or even with the combination of tamoxifen and anastrozole. In addition, anastrozole showed a decrease of over 50% in the recurrence of contralateral breast tumors and fewer side effects such as endometrial cancers, hot flushes, and thromboembolic events. However, anastrozole did have an increase in fractures related to bone loss and the use of the drug. Anastrozole is increasingly being used in the adjuvant setting in postmenopausal women. Because of the extensive long-term data supporting the use of tamoxifen, the American Society of Clinical Oncology, continues to recommend the use of tamoxifen for adjuvant hormonal therapy in the absence of significant contraindications; anastrozole is recommended when there are contraindications to tamoxifen. In addition, anastrozole is being used after patients complete tamoxifen therapy or prior to completing therapy (year 2 or 3) to further decrease recurrences.

Use of high-dose chemotherapy with stem cell support has not demonstrated a consistent, favorable impact on survival and should not be used outside of clinical trials. Although it is clear that dose intensity to a specific threshold is essential, there is no clear benefit to high-dose therapy with stem cell support.

An NIH consensus conference has reexamined the standards for adjuvant therapy of breast cancer. Since the last conference on this topic in 2000, the long-term advantage of systemic therapy has been further established. No new prognostic factors have been validated to aid in the selection of patients for adjuvant treatment. Its use should be based on the patient's age; on the size, histopathologic grade, and hormone receptor status of the breast tumor; and on the status of the regional lymph nodes. The value of HER-2/*neu*, *p53*, angiogenesis factors, and vascular invasion is being investigated, but they remain to be proven prognostic factors. Studies are being conducted evaluating trastuzumab in the adjuvant and neoadjuvant setting in a group of patients with newly diagnosed disease in which the tumors overexpress HER-2/*neu*. The NIH panel concluded that regardless of other factors, adjuvant systemic chemotherapy with drug combinations improves survival and should be used for most women who have potentially curable breast cancer. The use of anthracyclines is superior to combinations without anthracyclines. Tamoxifen should be used as a systemic agent in all women whose tumors are hormone receptor positive—regardless of age, menopausal status, or other prognostic factors. HER-2/*neu* status should not affect the choice of agents or the use of hormone therapy. Ovarian ablation in premenopausal patients with ER-positive tumors may produce a benefit similar to that of adjuvant systemic chemotherapy. Taxanes have

demonstrated benefit in patients with metastatic cancer and are being used in node-negative patients as is trastuzumab. Adjuvant systemic therapy should not be given to women who have small node-negative breast cancers with favorable histologic findings and tumor markers such as mucinous or tubular carcinoma, ER-positive, low grade.

In practice, most medical oncologists are currently using systemic adjuvant therapy for patients with either node-negative or node-positive breast cancer. Prognostic factors other than nodal status being used to determine the patient's risks are tumor size, ER and PR status, nuclear grade, histologic type, proliferative rate, and oncogene expression (Table 16–4). The assumption is made that all patients with node-negative aggressive tumors should receive adjuvant therapy except those who have serious coexistent medical problems. In general, systemic chemotherapy decreases the chance of recurrence by about 30%. Most patients tolerate at least tamoxifen. The use of chemotherapy or hormonal therapy prior to resection of the primary tumor (neoadjuvant) is gaining popularity. This enables the assessment of in vivo chemosensitivity. A complete tumor response in vivo prior to operation appears to be associated with improvement in survival. Neoadjuvant chemotherapy also permits breast conservation by shrinking the primary tumor in women who would otherwise need mastectomy for local control. There was considerable concern as to the timing of sentinel lymph node biopsy (SLNB), since the chemotherapy may affect any cancer present in the lymph nodes. After several studies, it is still unclear as to the appropriate timing of the procedure. A large multi-center study, NSABP B-27, studied this question as an adjunct to a neoadjuvant efficacy trial. The false-nega-

Table 16–4. Prognostic factors in node-negative breast cancer.

Prognostic Factor	Increased Recurrence	Decreased Recurrence
Size	T3, T2	T1, T0
Hormone receptors	Negative	Positive
DNA flow cytometry	Aneuploid	Diploid
Histologic grade	High	Low
Tumor labeling index	< 3%	> 3%
S phase fraction	> 5%	< 5%
Lymphatic or vascular invasion	Present	Absent
Cathepsin D	High	Low
HER-2/*neu* oncogene	High	Low
Epidermal growth factor receptor	High	Low

tive rate was as high as 10.7%, which is well above the false-negative rate outside the neoadjuvant setting (< 1–5%). Many physicians recommend performing SLNB prior to administering the chemotherapy in order to avoid a false-negative result. If a complete dissection is necessary, this can be completed at the time of the definitive surgery. While SLNB is critical to staging, the timing remains physician dependent and its role with neoadjuvant therapy is unclear.

Important questions remaining to be answered are the timing and duration of adjuvant and neoadjuvant chemotherapy, which chemotherapeutic agents should be applied for which subgroups of patients, the use of combinations of hormonal therapy and chemotherapy, and the value of prognostic factors other than hormone receptors in predicting response to therapy. Adjuvant systemic therapy is not generally used in patients with small tumors and those with negative lymph nodes who have favorable tumor markers. However, a small disease-free survival benefit, even in patients with small favorable tumors, has been suggested. It appears that adjuvant systemic therapy benefits all breast cancer patients, but the clinician and patient must decide if the benefits outweigh the risks, complications, and expense.

Delaney G: Recent advances in the use of radiotherapy to treat early breast cancer. Curr Opin Obstet Gynecol 2005;17:27. [PMID: 15711408]

Early Breast Cancer Trialists' Collaborative Group: Favourable and unfavourable effects on long-term survival of radiotherapy for early breast cancer: an overview of the randomised trials. Lancet 2000;355:1757. [PMID: 10832826]

Fisher B et al: Twenty-year follow-up of a randomized trial comparing total mastectomy, lumpectomy, and lumpectomy plus irradiation for the treatment of invasive breast cancer. N Engl J Med 2002;347:1233. [PMID: 12393820]

Fisher B et al: Treatment of axillary lymph node-negative, estrogen receptor-negative breast cancer: updated findings from National Surgical Adjuvant Breast and Bowel Project clinical trials. J Natl Cancer Inst 2004;96:1823. [PMID: 15601638]

Fisher B et al: Sentinel node biopsy after neoadjuvant chemotherapy in breast cancer: results from National Surgical Adjuvant Breast and Bowel Project Protocol B-27. J Clin Oncol 2005;23:2694. [PMID: 15837984]

Howell A et al: ATAC Trialists' Group: Results of the ATAC (Arimidex, Tamoxifen, Alone or in Combination) trial after completion of 5 years' adjuvant treatment for breast cancer. Lancet 2005;365:60. [PMID: 15639680]

Joensuu H et al; FinHer Study Investigators: Adjuvant docetaxel or vinorelbine with or without trastuzumab for breast cancer. N Engl J Med 2006;354:809. [PMID: 16495393]

Keshtgar MR et al: New approaches in breast cancer management: sentinel node biopsy and intraoperative radiotherapy. Int J Fertil Womens Med 2005;50(5 Pt 1):218. [PMID: 16468472]

Lemanski C et al: Intraoperative radiotherapy given as a boost for early breast cancer: Long-term clinical and cosmetic results. Int J Radiat Oncol Biol Phys 2006;64:1410. [PMID: 16442241]

Love RR: Meeting highlights: international consensus panel on the treatment of primary breast cancer. J Clin Oncol 2002; 20:1955. [PMID: 11919263]

Mamounas EP et al: Paclitaxel after doxorubicin plus cyclophosphamide as adjuvant chemotherapy for node-positive breast cancer: results from NSABP B-28. J Clin Oncol 2005;23: 3686. [PMID: 15897552]

Muller V et al: Bone marrow micrometastases and circulating tumor cells: current aspects and future perspectives. Breast Cancer Res 2004;6:258. [PMID: 15535856]

Piccart-Gebhart MJ et al; Herceptin Adjuvant (HERA) Trial Study Team: Trastuzumab after adjuvant chemotherapy in HER2-positive breast cancer. N Engl J Med 2005;353:1659. [PMID: 16236737]

Posther KE et al: Sentinel node skills verification and surgeon performance: data from a multicenter clinical trial for early-stage breast cancer. Ann Surg 2005;242:593. [PMID: 16192820]

Sokolowicz LE et al: Hormonal therapy for primary breast cancer: scientific rationale and status of clinical research. Curr Oncol Rep 2005;7:31. [PMID: 15610684]

Stolier AJ et al: Postlumpectomy insertion of the MammoSite brachytherapy device using the scar entry technique: initial experience and technical considerations. Breast J 2005;11: 199. [PMID: 15871706]

The National Institutes of Health Consensus Development Conference: Adjuvant Therapy for Breast Cancer. Bethesda, Maryland, USA. November 1-3, 2000. Proceedings. J Natl Cancer Inst Monogr 2001;(30):1. [PMID: 12083020]

Veronesi U et al: Twenty-year follow-up of randomized study comparing breast-conserving surgery with radical mastectomy for early breast cancer. N Engl J Med 2002;347:1227. [PMID: 12393819]

Vinh-Hung V et al: Breast-conserving surgery with or without radiotherapy: pooled-analysis for risks of ipsilateral breast tumor recurrence and mortality. J Natl Cancer Inst 2004;96: 115. [PMID: 14734701]

Vogel C et al: Efficacy and safety of trastuzumab as a single agent in first-line treatment of HER2-overexpressing metastatic breast cancer. J Clin Oncol 2002;3:719. [PMID: 11821453]

PALLIATIVE TREATMENT

This section covers palliative therapy of disseminated disease incurable by surgery (stage IV).

Radiotherapy

Palliative radiotherapy may be advised for primary treatment of locally advanced cancers with distant metastases to control ulceration, pain, and other manifestations in the breast and regional nodes. Irradiation of the breast and chest wall and the axillary, internal mammary, and supraclavicular nodes should be undertaken in an attempt to cure locally advanced and inoperable lesions when there is no evidence of distant metastases. A small number of patients in this group are cured in spite of extensive breast and regional node involvement.

Palliative irradiation is of value also in the treatment of certain bone or soft tissue metastases to control pain or avoid fracture. Radiotherapy is especially useful in the treatment of isolated bony metastasis, chest wall recurrences, brain metastases, and acute spinal cord compression.

Hormone & Targeted Therapy

Disseminated disease may shrink—or grow less rapidly—after endocrine therapy such as administration of

Table 16–5. Agents commonly used for hormonal management of metastatic breast cancer.

Drug	Action	Dose, Route, Frequency	Major Side Effects
Tamoxifen citrate (Nolvadex)	Selective estrogen receptor modulator	20 mg by mouth daily	Hot flushes, uterine bleeding, thrombophlebitis, rash
Fulvestrant (Faslodex)	Steroidal estrogen receptor antagonist	250 mg intramuscularly monthly	Gastrointestinal upset, headache, back pain, hot flushes, pharyngitis
Toremifene citrate (Fareston)	Selective estrogen receptor modulator	40 mg by mouth daily	Hot flushes, sweating, nausea, vaginal discharge, dry eyes, dizziness
Diethylstilbestrol (DES)	Estrogen	5 mg by mouth three times daily	Fluid retention, uterine bleeding, thrombophlebitis, nausea
Goserelin (Zoladex)	Synthetic leutinizing hormone releasing analogue	3.6 mg subcutaneously monthly	Arthralgias, blood pressure changes, hot flushes, headaches, vaginal dryness
Megestrol acetate (Megace)	Progestin	40 mg by mouth four times daily	Fluid retention
Letrozole (Femara)	Aromatase inhibitor	2.5 mg by mouth daily	Hot flushes, arthralgia/arthritis, myalgia
Anastrozole (Arimidex)	Aromatase inhibitor	1 mg by mouth daily	Hot flushes, skin rashes, nausea and vomiting
Exemestane (Aromasin)	Aromatase inhibitor	25 mg by mouth daily	Hot flushes, increased arthralgia/arthritis, myalgia, and alopecia

hormones (eg, estrogens, androgens, progestins; see Table 16–5); ablation of the ovaries, adrenals, or pituitary; or administration of drugs that block hormone receptor sites (eg, antiestrogens) or drugs that block the synthesis of hormones (eg, AIs). Hormonal manipulation is usually more successful in postmenopausal women even if they have received estrogen replacement therapy. Treatment should be based on the presence of ER protein in the primary tumor or metastases. The rate of response is nearly equal in premenopausal and postmenopausal women with ER-positive tumors. A favorable response to hormonal manipulation occurs in about one-third of patients with metastatic breast cancer. Of those whose tumors contain ERs, the response is about 60% and perhaps as high as 80% for patients whose tumors contain PRs as well. Because only 5–10% of women whose tumors do not contain ERs respond, they should not receive hormonal therapy except in unusual circumstances, eg, in an older patient who cannot tolerate chemotherapy. Because the quality of life during a remission induced by endocrine manipulation is often superior to a remission following cytotoxic chemotherapy, it is usually best to try endocrine manipulation first in cases in which the ER status is unknown. In addition, women with ER-positive tumors who do not respond to hormone therapy or experience progression should be placed on a different form of hormonal manipulation. Women whose tumor has failed to respond to tamoxifen and gone on to a third-generation AI have shown equal if not better response than those who respond to tamoxifen. However, when receptor status is unknown and the disease is progressing rapidly or involves visceral organs, endocrine ther-

apy is rarely successful, and introducing it may waste valuable time.

In addition to radiotherapy, bisphosphonate therapy has shown excellent results in delaying and reducing skeletal events in women with bony metastases. Bisphosphonates are also sometimes used in conjunction with AIs to decrease the potential bony events associated with those drugs. Further research examining the utility of bisphosphonates in conjunction with other therapies and in early breast cancer treatment is being conducted.

In general, only one type of therapy should be given at a time unless it is necessary to irradiate a destructive lesion of weight-bearing bone while the patient is receiving another regimen. The regimen should be changed only if the disease is clearly progressing. This is especially important for patients with destructive bone metastases, since changes in the status of these lesions are difficult to determine radiographically. A plan of therapy that would simultaneously minimize toxicity and maximize benefits is often best achieved by hormonal manipulation.

The choice of endocrine therapy depends on the menopausal status of the patient. Women within 1 year of their last menstrual period are arbitrarily considered to be premenopausal, whereas women whose menstruation ceased more than a year ago are postmenopausal. If endocrine therapy is the initial choice, it is referred to as primary hormonal manipulation; subsequent endocrine treatment is called secondary or tertiary hormonal manipulation.

Trastuzumab is a monoclonal antibody that binds to HER-2/*neu* receptors on the cancer cell and has been shown to be highly effective in HER-2/*neu*-expressive cancers. In metastatic disease, for patients with HER-2/*neu* oncogene overexpression, trastuzumab has been shown to increase survival when combined with AC or paclitaxel. Ongoing studies are evaluating trastuzumab in combination with other agents for adjuvant chemotherapy regimens in newly diagnosed cases.

In addition, compelling data have been reported regarding the use of an antiangiogenesis drug bevacizumab (Avastin) in the treatment of metastatic disease. Based on the amount of VEGF detected in the primary tumor, bevacizumab can increase overall survival and disease-free survival when used in combination with chemotherapy when metastases are present. Studies are ongoing and hold a great deal of promise.

A. THE PREMENOPAUSAL PATIENT

1. Primary hormonal therapy—The potent antiestrogen tamoxifen is by far the most common and preferred method of hormonal manipulation in the premenopausal patient. Tamoxifen is usually given orally in a dose of 20 mg daily. There is no significant difference in survival or response between tamoxifen therapy and bilateral oophorectomy. The average remission is about 12 months. Tamoxifen can be given with little morbidity and few side effects. Toremifene, a tamoxifen analog, has similar side effects but is less likely to cause uterine cancer. Controversy continues about whether a response to tamoxifen is predictive of probable success with other forms of endocrine manipulation.

Bilateral oophorectomy is less desirable than primary hormonal manipulation in premenopausal women because tamoxifen is so well tolerated. However, oophorectomy can be achieved rapidly and safely by surgery, or if the patient is a poor operative risk, by irradiation of the ovaries. Chemical ovarian ablation using a gonadotropin-releasing hormone (GnRH) analog can also be utilized. Oophorectomy presumably works by eliminating estrogens, progestins, and androgens, which stimulate growth of the tumor. AIs should not be used in a patient with functioning ovaries.

2. Secondary or tertiary hormonal therapy— Although patients who do not respond to tamoxifen or oophorectomy should be treated with cytotoxic drugs, those who respond and then relapse may subsequently respond to another form of endocrine treatment (Table 16–5). The initial choice for secondary endocrine manipulation has not been clearly defined.

Patients who improve after oophorectomy but subsequently relapse should receive tamoxifen or an AI. If one fails, the other may be tried but is not likely to succeed. Megestrol acetate, a progesterone agent, may be considered. Both drugs cause less morbidity and mortality than surgical adrenalectomy, can be discontinued once the patient improves, and are not associated with the many problems of postsurgical hypoadrenalism, so that patients who require chemotherapy are more easily managed. Adrenalectomy or hypophysectomy induced regression in 30–50% of patients who previously re-

sponded to oophorectomy, but these procedures are rarely done today. Pharmacologic hormonal manipulation has replaced these invasive procedures. Toremifene has shown no added value when tumors no longer respond to tamoxifen. AIs are of value when a tumor had responded to tamoxifen or oophorectomy but then progresses.

B. THE POSTMENOPAUSAL PATIENT

1. Primary hormonal therapy—Tamoxifen, 20 mg orally daily, or anastrozole, 1 mg orally daily, is the initial therapy of choice for postmenopausal women with metastatic breast cancer amenable to endocrine manipulation. Anastrozole (an AI) has fewer side effects than tamoxifen, the former therapy of choice, and is at least equally as effective. The main side effects of tamoxifen are nausea, vomiting, skin rash, and hot flushes. Rarely, it may induce hypercalcemia in patients with bony metastases. The main side effects of anastrozole are similar but lower in incidence; however, osteoporosis and bone fractures are significant. Other AIs are letrozole or exemestane. They have similar efficacy and side effect profiles.

2. Secondary or tertiary hormonal therapy—AIs have achieved the status of primary hormonal therapy in postmenopausal women since trials comparing an AI, anastrozole, with tamoxifen suggest that the former is just as effective and has fewer side effects. AIs are also available for the treatment of advanced breast cancer in postmenopausal women after tamoxifen treatment. In the event that the patient responds to AI, but then has progression of disease, an antiestrogen, fulvestrant (Faslodex) has shown a great deal of promise with about 20–30% of women benefiting from use. Postmenopausal patients who do not respond to SERM or AI should be given cytotoxic drugs such as CMF or AC. Postmenopausal women who respond initially to a SERM or AI but later manifest progressive disease may be crossed over to cytotoxic drugs. Androgens have many toxicities and should rarely be used. As in premenopausal patients, neither hypophysectomy nor adrenalectomy is being performed.

Chemotherapy

Cytotoxic drugs should be considered for the treatment of metastatic breast cancer (1) if visceral metastases are present (especially brain or lymphangitic pulmonary), (2) if hormonal treatment is unsuccessful or the disease has progressed after an initial response to hormonal manipulation, or (3) if the tumor is ER-negative. The most useful single chemotherapeutic agent to date is doxorubicin (Adriamycin), with a response rate of 40–50%. Single agents are rarely used but rather are given in combination with other cytotoxic drugs.

Combination chemotherapy using multiple agents has proved to be more effective, with objectively observed favorable responses achieved in 60–80% of patients with stage IV disease. Various combinations of drugs have been used, and clinical trials are always ongoing to identify a combination to increase survival and reduce undesirable side effects. Doxorubicin (40 mg/m^2 intravenously on day 1) and cyclophosphamide (200 mg/m^2 orally on days 3–6) produce an objective response in about 85% of patients so treated. Other chemotherapeutic regimens have consisted of various combinations of drugs, including cyclophosphamide, vincristine, methotrexate, fluorouracil, and taxanes with response rates ranging up to 60–70%. Prior adjuvant chemotherapy does not seem to alter response rates in patients who relapse. Researchers continue to study new drugs and combinations of chemotherapy agents such as capecitabine, mitoxantrone, vinorelbine, gemcitabine, irinotecan, cisplatin, and carboplatin. Many of these agents or combinations are available to patients in a clinical trial setting or by physician's choice. For patients whose tumors have progressed after many therapies and who are considering additional therapy, clinical trial participation with experimental drugs in phase II or III testing should be encouraged.

Nausea and vomiting are well controlled with drugs that directly affect the central nervous system, such as ondansetron and granisetron. These drugs are selective antagonists of serotonin receptors in the central nervous system and block nausea caused by cytotoxic chemotherapy. Growth factors such as erythropoietin (epoetin alfa), which stimulates red blood cell production and mimics the effect of erythropoietin, and filgrastim (granulocyte colony-stimulating factor; G-CSF), which stimulates proliferation and differentiation of hematopoietic cells, prevent life-threatening anemia and neutropenia seen commonly with high doses of chemotherapy. These agents greatly diminish the incidence of infections that may complicate the use of myelosuppressive chemotherapy.

The taxanes (paclitaxel and docetaxel) have been shown to be very effective for patients with metastatic breast cancer. They have usually been given after failure of combination chemotherapy for metastatic disease or relapse shortly after completion of adjuvant chemotherapy. However, they are becoming more important in both the management of metastatic disease and even adjuvant therapy. These drugs have response rates of 30–40% in patients with metastatic disease. They may be especially valuable in treating anthracycline-resistant tumors. Both agents are being used after treatment with anthracyclines in patients with advanced disease as well as in adjuvant and neoadjuvant settings. High-dose chemotherapy and autologous bone marrow or stem cell transplantation aroused widespread interest for the treatment of metastatic breast cancer. With this technique, the patient receives high doses of cytotoxic agents, eradicating the marrow, for which the patient subsequently undergoes autologous bone marrow or stem cell transplantation. Complete response rates are as high as 30–35%—considerably better than what can be achieved with conventional chemotherapy. Most randomized trials, however, comparing high-dose chemotherapy with stem cell support show no improvement in survival over conventional chemotherapy. A study purporting to show a survival advantage to high-dose chemotherapy in South Africa was found to be falsified and

discredited. Enthusiasm for high-dose chemotherapy with stem cell support has waned, but additional studies continue and recently showed a beneficial effect in some high-risk women. The technique is extremely costly, and the treatment itself is associated with a mortality rate of about 3–7%.

Bernard-Marty C et al: Facts and controversies in systemic treatment of metastatic breast cancer. Oncologist 2004;9: 617. [PMID: 15561806]

Bhatnagar AS: Review of the development of letrozole and its use in advanced breast cancer and in the neoadjuvant setting. Breast 2006;15(1 Suppl):3. [PMID: 16500235]

Fricker J: Letrozole better than tamoxifen in postmenopausal women. Lancet Oncol 2005;6:137. [PMID: 15759362]

Harvey HA: Optimizing bisphosphonate therapy in patients with breast cancer on endocrine therapy. Semin Oncol 2004;31 (6 Suppl 12):23. [PMID: 15719598]

Gould RE et al: Update on aromatase inhibitors in breast cancer. Curr Opin Obstet Gynecol 2006;18:41. [PMID: 16493259]

Hussain SA et al: Endocrine therapy and other targeted therapies for metastatic breast cancer. Expert Rev Anticancer Ther 2004;4:1179. [PMID: 15606341]

Ingle JN et al; North Central Cancer Treatment Group Trial N0032: Fulvestrant in women with advanced breast cancer after progression on prior aromatase inhibitor therapy: North Central Cancer Treatment Group Trial N0032. J Clin Oncol 2006;24:1052. [PMID: 16505423]

Mouridsen HT: Aromatase inhibitors in advanced breast cancer. Semin Oncol 2004;31(6 Suppl 12):3. [PMID: 15719595]

Pandit-Taskar N et al: Radiopharmaceutical therapy for palliation of bone pain from osseous metastases. J Nucl Med 2004; 45:1358. [PMID: 15299062]

Slamon DJ et al: Use of chemotherapy plus a monoclonal antibody against HER2 for metastatic breast cancer that overexpresses HER2. N Engl J Med 2001;344:783. [PMID: 11248153]

Smith I: Goals of treatment for patients with metastatic breast cancer. Semin Oncol 2006;33(1 Suppl 2):2. [PMID: 16472711]

Stadtmauer EA et al: Conventional-dose chemotherapy compared with high-dose chemotherapy plus autologous hematopoietic stem-cell transplantation for metastatic breast cancer. N Engl J Med 2000;342:1069. [PMID: 10760307]

PROGNOSIS

Stage of breast cancer is the most reliable indicator of prognosis (Table 16–6). Patients with disease localized to the breast and no evidence of regional spread after microscopic examination of the lymph nodes have by far the most favorable prognosis. Axillary lymph node status is the best-analyzed prognostic factor and correlates with survival at all tumor sizes. In addition, increased number of axillary nodes involved correlates directly with lower survival rates. Biologic markers of tumor aggressiveness such as estrogen, PRs, grade, and others are important prognostic variables because patients with aggressive tumors and no evidence of metastases to the axillary lymph nodes have a much higher recurrence rate than do patients with hormone receptor-positive tumors and no regional metastases. The histologic subtype of breast cancer (eg, medullary, lobular, colloid) seems to have little significance in prognosis once these tumors are truly invasive. Flow cy-

Table 16–6. Approximate survival (%) of patients with breast cancer by TNM stage.

TNM Stage	Five Years	Ten Years
0	95	90
I	85	70
IIA	70	50
IIB	60	40
IIIA	55	30
IIIB	30	20
IV	5–10	2
All	65	30

tometry of tumor cells to analyze DNA index and S-phase frequency aid in prognosis. Tumors with marked aneuploidy have a poor prognosis (see Table 16–4). HER-2/*neu* oncogene amplification, epidermal growth factor receptors, and cathepsin D may have some prognostic value, but no markers are as significant as lymph node metastases in predicting outcome.

The mortality rate of breast cancer patients exceeds that of age-matched normal controls for nearly 20 years. Thereafter, the mortality rates are equal, though deaths that occur among breast cancer patients are often directly the result of tumor. Five-year statistics do not accurately reflect the final outcome of therapy.

When cancer is localized to the breast, with no evidence of regional spread after pathologic examination, the clinical cure rate with most accepted methods of therapy is 75% to greater than 90%. Variations to this generalization may be related to the hormonal receptor content of the tumor, tumor size, host resistance, or associated illness. Patients with small mammographically detected biologically favorable tumors and no evidence of axillary spread have a 5-year survival rate greater than 95%. When the axillary lymph nodes are involved with tumor, the survival rate drops to 50–70% at 5 years and probably around 25–40% at 10 years. In general, breast cancer appears to be somewhat more malignant in younger than in older women, and this may be related to the fact that fewer younger women have ER-positive tumors.

For those patients whose disease progresses despite treatment, studies suggest supportive group therapy may improve survival. As they approach the end of life, such patients will require meticulous efforts at palliative care (see Chapter 5).

Hayes DF: Prognostic and predictive factors for breast cancer: translating technology to oncology. J Clin Oncol 2005;23: 1596. [PMID: 15755959]

FOLLOW-UP CARE

After primary therapy, patients with breast cancer should be monitored for life for at least two reasons: to detect recurrences and to observe the opposite breast for a second primary carcinoma. Local and distant recurrences occur most frequently within the first 2–5 years. During this period, the patient should be examined more frequently. Thereafter, examination is done annually. Special attention is paid to the contralateral breast because a new primary breast malignancy will develop in 20–25% of patients. The patient should examine her own breast monthly, and a mammogram should be obtained annually. In some cases, metastases are dormant for long periods and may appear 10–15 years or longer after removal of the primary tumor. Estrogen and progestational agents are rarely used for a patient free of disease after treatment of primary breast cancer, particularly if the tumor was hormone receptor positive. Studies nevertheless have failed to show an adverse effect of hormonal agents in patients who are free of disease. Even pregnancy has not been clearly associated with shortened survival of patients rendered disease free—yet most oncologists are reluctant to advise a young patient with breast cancer that she may become pregnant, and most are less than enthusiastic about prescribing hormone replacement therapy for the postmenopausal breast cancer patient. The use of estrogen replacement therapy may be considered for a woman with a history of breast cancer after discussion of the benefits and risks of such therapy for conditions such as osteoporosis and hot flushes, but it is not recommended.

Local Recurrence

The incidence of local recurrence correlates with tumor size, the presence and number of involved axillary nodes, the histologic type of tumor, the presence of skin edema or skin and fascia fixation with the primary tumor, and the type of initial local (breast) therapy. Local recurrence on the chest wall after total mastectomy and axillary dissection develops in as many as 8% of patients. When the axillary nodes are not involved, the local recurrence rate is less than 5%, but the rate is as high as 25% when they are heavily involved. A similar difference in local recurrence rate was noted between small and large tumors. Factors such as multifocal cancer, in situ tumors, positive resection margins, chemotherapy, and radiotherapy have an effect on local recurrence in patients treated with breast-conserving surgery.

Chest wall recurrences usually appear within the first several years but may occur as late as 15 or more years after mastectomy. All suspicious nodules and skin lesions should be biopsied. Local excision or localized radiotherapy may be feasible if an isolated nodule is present. If lesions are multiple or accompanied by evidence of regional involvement in the internal mammary or supraclavicular nodes, the disease is best managed by radiation treatment of the entire chest wall including the parasternal, supraclavicular, and axillary areas and usually by systemic therapy.

Local recurrence after mastectomy usually signals the presence of widespread disease and is an indication for studies to search for evidence of metastases. Distant metastases will develop within 2 years in most patients with locally recurrent tumor after mastectomy. When there is no evidence of metastases beyond the chest wall and regional nodes, irradiation for cure or complete local excision should be attempted. Patients with local recurrence may be cured with local resection and radiation. After partial mastectomy, local recurrence may not have as serious a prognostic significance as after mastectomy. However, those patients in whom a recurrence develops have a worse prognosis than those who do not. It is speculated that the ability of a cancer to recur locally after radiotherapy is a sign of aggressiveness and resistance to therapy. Completion of the mastectomy should be done for local recurrence after partial mastectomy; some of these patients will survive for prolonged periods, especially if the breast recurrence is DCIS or more than 5 years after initial treatment. Systemic chemotherapy or hormonal treatment should be used for women in whom disseminated disease develops or those in whom local recurrence occurs.

Edema of the Arm

Significant edema of the arm occurs in about 10–30% of patients after axillary dissection with or without mastectomy. It occurs more commonly if radiotherapy has been given or if there was postoperative infection. Partial mastectomy with radiation to the axillary lymph nodes is followed by chronic edema of the arm in 10–20% of patients. In the past, it was routine to perform an axillary dissection as it is more accurate for staging than axillary sampling. In an axillary dissection, it is recommended that at least level I and II lymph nodes (approximately 15–20 lymph nodes) be removed, in combination with partial mastectomy or as part of the mastectomy. After considerable research in the last decade, sentinel lymph node dissection has proved to be a more accurate form of axillary staging with less morbidity. Because a sentinel lymph node dissection usually only removes the first one to three lymph nodes that would be affected by carcinoma if it had spread to the axilla, it can provide accurate staging without the side effects of edema or infection. It does not replace axillary dissection if the sentinel lymph nodes are involved with metastases, although this is still being studied. Judicious use of radiotherapy, with treatment fields carefully planned to spare the axilla as much as possible, can greatly diminish the incidence of edema, which will occur in only 5% of patients if no radiotherapy is given to the axilla after a partial mastectomy and lymph node dissection.

Late or secondary edema of the arm may develop years after treatment, as a result of axillary recurrence or of infection in the hand or arm, with obliteration of lymphatic channels. Infection in the arm or hand on the dissected side should be treated with antibiotics, rest, and elevation. When edema develops, careful examination of the axilla for recurrence should be done. If there is no sign of recurrence, the swollen extremity should be treated with rest and elevation. A mild diuretic may be helpful. If there is no improvement, a compressor pump or manual decompression decreases the swelling, and the patient is then fitted with an elastic glove or sleeve. Most patients are not bothered enough by mild edema to wear an uncomfortable glove or sleeve and will treat themselves with elevation or manual decompression alone. Benzopyrones have been reported to decrease lymphedema but are not approved for this use in the United States. Rarely, edema may be severe enough to interfere with use of the limb.

Breast Reconstruction

Breast reconstruction is usually feasible after standard or modified radical mastectomy. Reconstruction should be discussed with patients prior to mastectomy, because it offers an important psychological focal point for recovery. Reconstruction is not an obstacle to the diagnosis of recurrent cancer. The most common breast reconstruction has been implantation of a silicone gel prosthesis in the subpectoral plane between the pectoralis minor and pectoralis major muscles. Although the FDA has placed a moratorium on the purely cosmetic use of silicone gel implants because of possible leakage of silicone and possible associated autoimmune phenomena, they can be used in breast reconstruction after mastectomy with appropriate prior patient consent. Most plastic surgeons currently would place a saline-filled prosthesis rather than a silicone gel implant. Alternatively, autologous tissue can be used for reconstruction.

Autologous tissue flaps are aesthetically superior to implant reconstruction in most patients. They also have the advantage of not feeling like a foreign body to the patient. The most popular autologous technique currently is the trans-rectus abdominis muscle flap (TRAM flap), which is done by rotating the rectus abdominis muscle with attached fat and skin cephalad to make a breast mound. The free TRAM flap is done by completely removing the rectus with overlying fat and skin and using microvascular surgical techniques to reconstruct the vascular supply on the chest wall. A latissimus dorsi flap can be swung from the back but offers less fullness than the TRAM flap and is therefore less acceptable cosmetically. Reconstruction may be performed immediately (at the time of initial mastectomy) or may be delayed until later, usually when the patient has completed adjuvant therapy. When considering reconstructive options, concomitant illnesses should be considered, since the ability of an autologous flap to survive depends on medical comorbidities. In addition, the need for radiotherapy may affect the choice of reconstruction as radiation may increase fibrosis around an implant or decrease the volume of a flap.

Risks of Pregnancy

Data are insufficient to determine whether interruption of pregnancy improves the prognosis of patients who are identified to have potentially curable breast cancer and who receive definitive treatment during pregnancy. Theoretically, the increasingly high levels of estrogen produced by the placenta as the pregnancy progresses could be detrimental to the patient with occult metastases of hormone-sensitive breast cancer. Moreover, occult metastases are present in most patients with positive axillary nodes, and treatment by adjuvant chemotherapy could be potentially harmful to the fetus early in gestation, although chemotherapy may be given to pregnant women later. Under these circumstances, interruption of early pregnancy seems reasonable, with progressively less rationale for the procedure as term approaches. The decision is affected by many factors, including the patient's desire to have the baby and the prognosis especially when axillary nodes are involved.

Equally important is the advice regarding future pregnancy (or abortion in case of pregnancy) to be given to women of child-bearing age who have had definitive treatment for breast cancer. It is assumed that pregnancy will be harmful if occult metastases are present, though this has not been demonstrated. Patients whose tumors are ER negative (most younger women) may not be affected by pregnancy. To date, no adverse effect of pregnancy on survival of pregnant women who have had breast cancer has been demonstrated, though most oncologists advise against it.

In patients with inoperable or metastatic cancer (stage IV disease), induced abortion is usually advisable because of the possible adverse effects of hormonal treatment, radiotherapy, or chemotherapy upon the fetus.

Ascherman JA et al: Implant reconstruction in breast cancer patients treated with radiation therapy. Plast Reconstr Surg 2006;117:359. [PMID: 16462313]

Cocquyt VF et al: Better cosmetic results and comparable quality of life after skin-sparing mastectomy and immediate autologous breast reconstruction compared to breast conservative treatment. Br J Plast Surg 2003;56:462. [PMID: 12890459]

Ducic I et al: Safety and risk factors for breast reconstruction with pedicled transverse rectus abdominis musculocutaneous flaps: a 10-year analysis. Ann Plast Surg 2005;55:559. [PMID: 16327450]

Langer S et al: Lymphatic mapping improves staging and reduces morbidity in women undergoing total mastectomy for breast carcinoma. Am Surg 2004;70:881. [PMID: 15529842]

Salhab M et al: Skin-sparing mastectomy and immediate breast reconstruction: patient satisfaction and clinical outcome. Int J Clin Oncol 2006;11:51. [PMID: 16508729]

van der Veen P et al: Lymphedema development following breast cancer surgery with full axillary resection. Lymphology 2004; 37:206. [PMID: 15693539]

■ CARCINOMA OF THE MALE BREAST

ESSENTIALS OF DIAGNOSIS

- *A painless lump beneath the areola in a man usually over 50 years of age.*

- *Nipple discharge, retraction, or ulceration may be present.*

GENERAL CONSIDERATIONS

Breast cancer in men is a rare disease; the incidence is only about 1% of that in women. The average age at occurrence is about 60—somewhat older than the most common presenting age in women. There may be an increased incidence of breast cancer in men with prostate cancer. The prognosis, even in stage I cases, is worse in men than in women. Blood-borne metastases are commonly present when the male patient appears for initial treatment. These metastases may be latent and may not become manifest for many years. As in women, hormonal influences are probably related to the development of male breast cancer. There is a high incidence of both breast cancer and gynecomastia in Bantu men, theoretically owing to failure of estrogen inactivation by a liver damaged by associated liver disease. It is important to note that first-degree relatives of men with breast cancer are considered to be at high risk. This risk should be taken into account when discussing options with the patient and family. In addition, *BRCA2* mutations are common in men with breast cancer. Men with breast cancer, especially with a history of prostate cancer, should receive genetic counseling.

Clinical Findings

A painless lump, occasionally associated with nipple discharge, retraction, erosion, or ulceration, is the primary complaint. Examination usually shows a hard, ill-defined, nontender mass beneath the nipple or areola. Gynecomastia not uncommonly precedes or accompanies breast cancer in men. Nipple discharge is an uncommon presentation for breast cancer in men but is an ominous finding associated with carcinoma in nearly 75% of cases.

Breast cancer staging is the same in men as in women. Gynecomastia and metastatic cancer from another site (eg, prostate) must be considered in the differential diagnosis. Benign tumors are rare, and biopsy should be performed on all males with a defined breast mass.

Treatment

Treatment consists of modified radical mastectomy in operable patients, who should be chosen by the same criteria as women with the disease. Breast conserving therapy is rarely performed. Irradiation is the first step in treating localized metastases in the skin, lymph nodes, or skeleton that are causing symptoms. Examination of the cancer for hormone receptor proteins is of value in predicting response to endocrine ablation. Men commonly have ER-positive tumors. Adjuvant chemotherapy is used for the same indications as in breast cancer in women.

Because breast cancer in men is frequently a disseminated disease, endocrine therapy is of considerable importance in its management. Tamoxifen is the main drug for management of advanced breast cancer in men. Tamoxifen (20 mg orally daily) should be the initial treatment. There is little experience with AIs though they should be effective. Castration in advanced breast cancer is a successful measure and more beneficial than the same procedure in women but is rarely used. Objective evidence of regression may be seen in 60–70% of men with hormonal therapy for metastatic disease—approximately twice the proportion in women. The average duration of tumor growth remission is about 30 months, and life is prolonged. Bone is the most frequent site of metastases from breast cancer in men (as in women), and hormonal therapy relieves bone pain in most patients so treated. The longer the interval between mastectomy and recurrence, the longer the remission following treatment. As in women, there is correlation between ERs of the tumor and the likelihood of remission following hormonal therapy.

AIs should replace adrenalectomy in men as it has in women. Corticosteroid therapy alone has been considered to be efficacious but probably has no value when compared with major endocrine ablation. Either tamoxifen or AIs may be primary or secondary hormonal manipulation.

Estrogen therapy—5 mg of diethylstilbestrol three times daily orally—may be effective hormonal manipulation after others have been successful and failed, just as in women. Androgen therapy may exacerbate bone pain. Chemotherapy should be administered for the same indications and using the same dosage schedules as for women with metastatic disease or for adjuvant treatment.

Prognosis

The prognosis of breast cancer is poorer in men than in women. The crude 5- and 10-year survival rates for clinical stage I breast cancer in men are about 58% and 38%, respectively. For clinical stage II disease, the 5- and 10-year survival rates are approximately 38% and 10%. The survival rates for all stages at 5 and 10 years are 36% and 17%. For those patients whose disease progresses despite treatment, meticulous efforts at palliative care are essential (see Chapter 5).

Fentiman IS et al: Male breast cancer. Lancet 2006;367:595. [PMID: 16488803]

Kwiatkowska E et al: Somatic mutations in the *BRCA2* gene and high frequency of allelic loss of *BRCA2* in sporadic male breast cancer. Int J Cancer 2002;98:943. [PMID: 11948477]

Loerzel VW et al: Male breast cancer. Clin J Oncol Nurs 2004; 8: 191. [PMID: 15108421]

Weiss JR et al: Epidemiology of male breast cancer. Cancer Epidemiol Biomarkers Prev 2005;14:20. [PMID: 15668471]

Gynecology

17

H. Trent MacKay, MD, MPH

ABNORMAL PREMENOPAUSAL BLEEDING

 ESSENTIALS OF DIAGNOSIS

- *Blood loss of over 80 mL per cycle.*
- *Excessive bleeding, often with the passage of clots, may occur at regular menstrual intervals (menorrhagia) or irregular intervals (dysfunctional uterine bleeding).*
- *Etiology most commonly dysfunctional uterine bleeding on a hormonal basis.*

General Considerations

Normal menstrual bleeding lasts an average of 4 days (range, 2–7 days), with a mean blood loss of 40 mL. Blood loss of over 80 mL per cycle is abnormal and frequently produces anemia. Excessive bleeding, often with the passage of clots, may occur at regular menstrual intervals (menorrhagia) or irregular intervals (dysfunctional uterine bleeding). When there are fewer than 21 days between the onset of bleeding episodes, the cycles are likely to be anovular. Ovulation bleeding, a single episode of spotting between regular menses, is quite common. Heavier or irregular intermenstrual bleeding warrants investigation.

Dysfunctional uterine bleeding is usually caused by overgrowth of endometrium due to estrogen stimulation without adequate progesterone to stabilize growth; this occurs in anovular cycles. Anovulation commonly occurs in teenagers, in women aged late 30s to late 40s, and in extremely obese women or those with polycystic ovary syndrome.

Clinical Findings

A. SYMPTOMS AND SIGNS

The diagnosis of the disorders underlying the bleeding usually depends on the following: (1) A careful description of the duration and amount of flow, related pain, and relationship to the last menstrual period (LMP). The presence of blood clots or the degree of inconvenience caused by the bleeding may be more useful indicators. (2) A history of pertinent illnesses or weight change. (3) A history of all medications the patient has taken in the past month. (4) A history of coagulation disorders in the patient or family members. (5) A careful pelvic examination to look for pregnancy, uterine myomas, adnexal masses, or infection.

B. LABORATORY STUDIES

Cervical smears should be obtained as needed for cytologic and culture studies. Blood studies should include a complete blood count, sedimentation rate, and glucose levels to rule out diabetes. Diabetes may occasionally initially present with abnormal bleeding. A test for pregnancy and studies of thyroid function and coagulation disorders should be considered in the clinical evaluation. Up to 18% of women with severe menorrhagia may have a coagulopathy. Tests for ovulation in cyclic menorrhagia include basal body temperature records, serum progesterone measured 1 week before the expected onset of menses, and analysis of an endometrial biopsy specimen for secretory activity shortly before the onset of menstruation.

C. IMAGING

Ultrasound may be useful to evaluate endometrial thickness or to diagnose intrauterine or ectopic pregnancy or adnexal masses. Endovaginal ultrasound with saline infusion sonohysterography may be used to diagnose endometrial polyps or subserous myomas. MRI can definitively diagnose submucous myomas and adenomyosis.

D. CERVICAL BIOPSY AND ENDOMETRIAL CURETTAGE

Biopsy, curettage, or aspiration of the endometrium and curettage of the endocervix may be necessary to diagnose the cause of bleeding. These and other invasive gynecologic diagnostic procedures are described in Table 17–1. Polyps, endometrial hyperplasia, and submucous myomas are commonly identified in this way. If cancer of the cervix is suspected, colposcopically directed biopsies and endocervical curettage are indicated as first steps.

E. HYSTEROSCOPY

Hysteroscopy can visualize endometrial polyps, submucous myomas, and exophytic endometrial cancers,

Table 17–1. Common gynecologic diagnostic procedures.

Colposcopy

Visualization of cervical, vaginal, or vulvar epithelium under 5–50× magnification with and without dilute acetic acid to identify abnormal areas requiring biopsy. An office procedure.

D&C

Dilation of the cervix and curettage of the entire endometrial cavity, using a metal curette or suction cannula and often using forceps for the removal of endometrial polyps. Can usually be done in the office under local anesthesia.

Endometrial biopsy

Removal of one or more areas of the endometrium by means of a curette or small aspiration device without cervical dilation. Diagnostic accuracy similar to D&C. An office procedure performed under local anesthesia.

Endocervical curettage

Removal of endocervical epithelium with a small curette for diagnosis of cervical dysplasia and cancer. An office procedure performed under local anesthesia.

Hysteroscopy

Visual examination of the uterine cavity with a small fiberoptic endoscope passed through the cervix. Biopsies, and excision of myomas can be performed. Can be done in the office under local anesthesia or in the operating room under general anesthesia.

Saline infusion sonohysterography

Introduction of saline solution into endometrial cavity with catheter to visualize submucous myomas or endometrial polyps by transvaginal ultrasound. May be performed in the office with oral analgesia.

Hysterosalpingography

Injection of radiopaque dye through the cervix to visualize the uterine cavity and oviducts. Mainly used in investigation of infertility.

Laparoscopy

Visualization of the abdominal and pelvic cavity through a small fiberoptic endoscope passed through a subumbilical incision. Permits diagnosis, tubal sterilization, and treatment of many conditions previously requiring laparotomy. General anesthesia is usually used.

---

and the procedure can be followed immediately by dilatation and curettage (D&C).

Treatment

Premenopausal patients with abnormal uterine bleeding include those with submucous myomas, infection, early abortion, or pelvic neoplasms. The history, physical examination, and laboratory findings should identify such patients, who require definitive therapy depending on the cause of the bleeding. A large group of patients remains, most of whom have dysfunctional uterine bleeding on a hormonal basis.

Dysfunctional uterine bleeding can usually be treated hormonally. Women over the age of 35 should have endometrial sampling to rule out endometrial hyperplasia or carcinoma prior to initiation of hormonal therapy. Progestins, which limit and stabilize endometrial growth, are generally effective. Medroxyprogesterone acetate, 10 mg/d, or norethindrone acetate, 5 mg/d, should be given for 10–14 days starting on day 15 of the cycle, following which withdrawal bleeding (so-called medical curettage) will occur. The treatment is repeated for several cycles; it can be reinstituted if amenorrhea or dysfunctional bleeding recurs. In women who are bleeding actively, any of the combination oral contraceptives can be given four times daily for 1 or 2 days followed by two pills daily through day 5 and then one pill daily through day 20; after withdrawal bleeding occurs, pills are taken in the usual dosage for three cycles. In cases of intractable heavy bleeding, danazol, 200 mg four times daily, is sometimes used to create an atrophic endometrium. Alternatively, a GnRH agonist such as depot leuprolide, 3.75 mg intramuscularly monthly, or nafarelin, 0.2–0.4 mg intranasally twice daily, can be used for up to 6 months to create a temporary cessation of menstruation by ovarian suppression.

In cases of heavy bleeding, intravenous conjugated estrogens, 25 mg every 4 hours for three or four doses, can be used, followed by oral conjugated estrogens, 2.5 mg daily, or ethinyl estradiol, 20 mcg daily, for 3 weeks, with the addition of medroxyprogesterone acetate, 10 mg daily for the last 10 days of treatment, or a combination oral contraceptive daily for 3 weeks. This will thicken the endometrium and control the bleeding. If the abnormal bleeding is not controlled by hormonal treatment, hysteroscopy, saline infusion sonohysterography, or a D&C is necessary to check for polyps, submucous myomas, or endometrial cancer.

Endometrial ablation through the hysteroscope with laser photocoagulation or electrocautery—or blindly with hyperthermia or cryotherapy—is an option; these techniques are designed to reduce or prevent any future menstrual flow.

Nonsteroidal anti-inflammatory drugs (NSAIDs) such as naproxen or mefenamic acid in the usual anti-inflammatory doses will often reduce blood loss in menorrhagia—even that associated with a copper intrauterine device (IUD). The levonorgestrel-releasing IUD will markedly reduce menstrual blood loss and may be a good alternative to other medical or surgical therapies.

Prolonged use of a progestin, as in a minipill, in injectable contraceptives, or in the therapy of endometriosis, can also lead to intermittent bleeding, sometimes severe. In this instance, the endometrium is atrophic and fragile. If bleeding occurs, it should be treated with estrogen as follows: ethinyl estradiol, 20 mcg/d for 7 days, or conjugated estrogens, 1.25 mg/d for 7 days.

It is useful for the patient and the clinician to discuss stressful situations or lifestyles that may contribute to anovulation and dysfunctional bleeding, such as prolonged emotional turmoil or excessive use of drugs or alcohol.

Albers JR et al: Abnormal uterine bleeding. Am Fam Physician 2004;69:1915. [PMID: 15117012]

Hurskainen R et al: Levonorgestrel-releasing intrauterine system in the treatment of heavy menstrual bleeding. Curr Opin Obstet Gynecol 2004;16:487. [PMID: 15534445]

Tabor A et al: Endometrial thickness as a test for endometrial cancer in women with postmenopausal vaginal bleeding. Obstet Gynecol 2002;99:663. [PMID: 12039131]

POSTMENOPAUSAL VAGINAL BLEEDING

 ESSENTIALS OF DIAGNOSIS

- *Vaginal bleeding that occurs 6 months or more following cessation of menstrual function.*
- *Bleeding is usually painless.*
- *Bleeding may be a single episode of spotting or profuse bleeding for days or months.*

General Considerations

Vaginal bleeding that occurs 6 months or more following cessation of menstrual function should be investigated. The most common causes are atrophic endometrium, endometrial proliferation or hyperplasia, endometrial or cervical cancer, and administration of estrogens with or without added progestin. Other causes include atrophic vaginitis, trauma, endometrial polyps, friction ulcers of the cervix associated with prolapse of the uterus, and blood dyscrasias. Uterine bleeding is usually painless, but pain will be present if the cervix is stenotic, if bleeding is severe and rapid, or if infection or torsion or extrusion of a tumor is present. The patient may report a single episode of spotting or profuse bleeding for days or months.

Diagnosis

The vulva and vagina should be inspected for areas of bleeding, ulcers, or neoplasms. A cytologic smear of the cervix and vaginal pool should be taken. If available, transvaginal sonography (TVS) should be used to measure endometrial thickness. A measurement of 5 mm or less indicates a low likelihood of hyperplasia or endometrial cancer, although up to 4% of endometrial cancers may be missed with sonography. If the thickness is greater than 5 mm or there is a heterogeneous appearance to the endometrium, endocervical curettage and endometrial biopsy or D&C preferably with hysteroscopy should be performed.

Treatment

Endometrial biopsy or D&C may be curative. Simple endometrial hyperplasia calls for cyclic progestin therapy (medroxyprogesterone acetate, 10 mg/d, or norethindrone acetate, 5 mg/d) for 21 days of each month for 3 months. A repeat endometrial biopsy should be performed. If endometrial hyperplasia with atypical cells or carcinoma of the endometrium is found, hysterectomy is necessary.

PREMENSTRUAL SYNDROME (Premenstrual Tension)

The premenstrual syndrome is a recurrent, variable cluster of troublesome physical and emotional symptoms that develop during the 7–14 days before the onset of menses and subside when menstruation occurs. The syndrome intermittently affects about 40% of all premenopausal women, primarily those 25–40 years of age. In about 10–15% of affected women, the syndrome may be severe. Although not every woman experiences all the symptoms or signs at one time, many describe bloating, breast pain, ankle swelling, a sense of increased weight, skin disorders, irritability, aggressiveness, depression, inability to concentrate, libido change, lethargy, and food cravings. The pathogenesis of premenstrual syndrome is still uncertain. Psychosocial factors may play a role.

Current treatment methods are mainly empiric. The clinician should provide the best support possible for the patient's emotional and physical distress. This includes the following:

1. Careful evaluation of the patient, with understanding, explanation, and reassurance, is of first importance.

2. Advise the patient to keep a daily diary of all symptoms for 2–3 months, to help in evaluating the timing and characteristics of the syndrome. If her symptoms occur throughout the month rather than in the 2 weeks before menses, she may be depressed or may have other emotional problems in addition to premenstrual syndrome.

3. For mild to moderate symptoms, a program of aerobic exercise; reduction of caffeine, salt, and alcohol intake; and an increase in complex carbohydrates in the diet may be helpful.

4. When physical symptoms predominate, spironolactone, 100 mg daily during the luteal phase, is effective for reduction of bloating and breast tenderness. Oral contraceptives or injectable progestin medroxyprogesterone acetate (DMPA) will decrease breast pain and cramping. NSAIDs, such as 500 mg of mefenamic acid three times a day, will reduce a number of symptoms but not breast pain.

5. When mood disorders predominate, serotonin reuptake inhibitors such as 20 mg/d of fluoxetine, either daily or only on symptom days, are effective in relieving tension, irritability, and dysphoria with few side effects.

6. When the above regimens are not effective, ovarian function can be suppressed with continuous high-dose progestin (20–30 mg/d of oral medroxyprogesterone acetate [MPA] or 150 mg of DMPA every 3 months or GnRH agonist with add-back therapy if continued for more than 6 months).

Johnson SR: Premenstrual syndrome, premenstrual dysphoric disorder, and beyond: a clinical primer for practitioners. Obstet Gynecol 2004;104:845. [PMID: 15458909]

DYSMENORRHEA

1. Primary Dysmenorrhea

Primary dysmenorrhea is menstrual pain associated with ovulatory cycles in the absence of pathologic findings. The pain usually begins within 1–2 years after the menarche and may become more severe with time. The frequency of cases increases up to age 20 and then decreases with age and markedly with parity. Fifty to 75 percent of women are affected at some time and 5–6% have incapacitating pain.

Primary dysmenorrhea is low, midline, wave-like, cramping pelvic pain often radiating to the back or inner thighs. Cramps may last for 1 or more days and may be associated with nausea, diarrhea, headache, and flushing. The pain is produced by uterine vasoconstriction, anoxia, and sustained contractions mediated by prostaglandins.

Clinical Findings

The pelvic examination is normal between menses; examination during menses may produce discomfort, but there are no pathologic findings.

Treatment

NSAIDs (ibuprofen, ketoprofen, mefenamic acid, naproxen) are generally helpful. Drugs should be started at the onset of bleeding to avoid inadvertent drug use during early pregnancy. Medication should be continued on a regular basis for 2–3 days. Ovulation can be suppressed and dysmenorrhea usually prevented by oral contraceptives or depot-medroxyprogesterone acetate. For women who do not wish to use hormonal contraception, other therapies that have shown at least some benefit include local heat; thiamine, 100 mg/d orally; vitamin E, 200 units/d orally from 2 days prior to and for the first 3 days of menses; the Japanese herbal remedy toki-shakuyaku-san, 2.5 g 3 times daily; and high-frequency transcutaneous electrical nerve stimulation.

2. Secondary Dysmenorrhea

Secondary dysmenorrhea is menstrual pain for which an organic cause exists. It usually begins well after menarche, sometimes even as late as the third or fourth decade of life.

Clinical Findings

The history and physical examination commonly suggest endometriosis or pelvic inflammatory disease (PID). Other causes may be submucous myoma, IUD use, cervical stenosis with obstruction, or blind uterine horn (rare).

Diagnosis

Laparoscopy is often needed to differentiate endometriosis from PID. Submucous myomas can be detected most reliably by MRI but also by hysterogram, by hysteroscopy, or by passing a sound or curette over the uterine cavity during D&C. Cervical stenosis may result from induced abortion, creating crampy pain at the time of expected menses with no blood flow; this is easily cured by passing a sound into the uterine cavity after administering a paracervical block.

Treatment

A. SPECIFIC MEASURES

Periodic use of analgesics, including the NSAIDs given for primary dysmenorrhea, may be beneficial, and oral contraceptives may give relief, particularly in endometriosis. Danazol and GnRH agonists are effective in the treatment of endometriosis (see below).

B. SURGICAL MEASURES

If disability is marked or prolonged, laparoscopy or exploratory laparotomy is usually warranted. Definitive surgery depends on the degree of disability and the findings at operation.

French L: Dysmenorrhea. Am Fam Physician 2005;71:285. [PMID: 15686299]

Proctor M et al: Dysmenorrhea. Clin Evid 2004;12:2524. [PMID: 1565806]

VAGINITIS

ESSENTIALS OF DIAGNOSIS

- *Vaginal irritation.*
- *Pruritus.*
- *Pain.*
- *Unusual discharge.*

General Considerations

Inflammation and infection of the vagina are common gynecologic problems, resulting from a variety of pathogens, allergic reactions to vaginal contraceptives or other products, or the friction of coitus. The normal vaginal pH is 4.5 or less, and *Lactobacillus* is the predominant organism. At the time of the midcycle estrogen surge, clear, elastic, mucoid secretions from the cervical os are often profuse. In the luteal phase and during pregnancy, vaginal secretions are thicker, white, and sometimes adherent to the vaginal walls. These normal secretions can be confused with vaginitis by concerned women.

Clinical Findings

When the patient complains of vaginal irritation, pain, or unusual discharge, a careful history should be taken, noting the onset of the LMP; recent sexual activity; use of contraceptives, tampons, or douches; and the presence of vaginal burning, pain, pruritus, or unusually profuse or malodorous discharge. The physical examination should include careful inspection of the vulva and speculum examination of the vagina and cervix. The cervix is cultured for *Gonococcus* or *Chlamydia* if applicable. A specimen of vaginal discharge is examined under the microscope in a drop of 0.9% saline solution to look for trichomonads or clue cells and in a drop of 10% potassium hydroxide to search for *Candida*. The vaginal pH should be tested; it is frequently greater than 4.5 in infections due to trichomonads and bacterial vaginosis. A bimanual examination to look for evidence of pelvic infection should follow.

A. Vulvovaginal Candidiasis

Pregnancy, diabetes, and use of broad-spectrum antibiotics or corticosteroids predispose patients to *Candida* infections. Heat, moisture, and occlusive clothing also contribute to the risk. Pruritus, vulvovaginal erythema, and a white curd-like discharge that is not malodorous are found. Microscopic examination with 10% potassium hydroxide reveals filaments and spores. Cultures with Nickerson's medium may be used if *Candida* is suspected but not demonstrated.

B. Trichomonas vaginalis Vaginitis

This protozoal flagellate infects the vagina, Skene's ducts, and lower urinary tract in women and the lower genitourinary tract in men. It is transmitted through coitus. Pruritus and a malodorous frothy, yellow-green discharge occur, along with diffuse vaginal erythema and red macular lesions on the cervix in severe cases. Motile organisms with flagella are seen by microscopic examination of a wet mount with saline solution.

C. Bacterial Vaginosis

This condition is considered to be a polymicrobial disease that is not sexually transmitted. An overgrowth of *Gardnerella* and other anaerobes is often associated with increased malodorous discharge without obvious vulvitis or vaginitis. The discharge is grayish and sometimes frothy, with a pH of 5.0–5.5. An amine-like ("fishy") odor is present if a drop of discharge is alkalinized with 10% potassium hydroxide. On wet mount in saline, epithelial cells are covered with bacteria to such an extent that cell borders are obscured (clue cells). Vaginal cultures are generally not useful in diagnosis.

D. Condylomata Acuminata (Genital Warts)

Warty growths on the vulva, perianal area, vaginal walls, or cervix are caused by various types of the human papillomavirus (HPV). They are sexually transmitted. Pregnancy and immunosuppression favor growth. Vulvar lesions may be obviously wart-like or may be diagnosed only after application of 4% acetic acid (vinegar) and colposcopy, when they appear whitish, with prominent papillae. Fissures may be present at the fourchette. Vaginal lesions may show diffuse hypertrophy or a cobblestone appearance. Cervical lesions may be visible only by colposcopy after pretreatment with 4% acetic acid. These lesions may be related to dysplasia and cervical cancer. Vulvar cancer is also currently considered to be associated with HPV infection.

Treatment

A. Vulvovaginal Candidiasis

A variety of regimens are available to treat vulvovaginal candidiasis. Women with uncomplicated vulvovaginal candidiasis will usually respond to a 1- to 3-day regimen of a topical azole. Women with complicated infection (including four or more episodes in 1 year, severe signs and symptoms, non-albicans species, uncontrolled diabetes, HIV infection, corticosteroid treatment, or pregnancy) should receive 7–14 days of a topical regimen or two doses of fluconazole 3 days apart. (Pregnant women should use only topical azoles.)

1. Single-dose regimens—Miconazole, 200-mg vaginal suppository; tioconazole, 6.5%, 5 g; or sustained-release butoconazole, 2% cream, 5 g.

2. Three-day regimens—Butoconazole (2% cream, 5 g once daily), clotrimazole (two 100-mg vaginal tablets once daily), teraconazole (0.8% cream, 5 g, or 80-mg suppository once daily), or miconazole (200 mg vaginal suppository once daily).

3. Seven-day regimens—The following regimens are given once daily: clotrimazole (1% cream or 100-mg vaginal tablet), miconazole (2% cream, 5 g, or 100-mg vaginal suppository), or teraconazole (0.4% cream, 5 g).

4. Fourteen-day regimen—Nystatin (100,000-unit vaginal tablet once daily).

5. Recurrent vulvovaginitis (maintenance therapy)—Clotrimazole (500-mg vaginal suppository once weekly or 200 mg cream twice weekly) or fluconazole (100, 150, or 200 mg orally once weekly) are effective regimens for maintenance therapy for up to 6 months.

B. Trichomonas vaginalis Vaginitis

Treatment of both partners simultaneously is recommended; metronidazole, 2 g orally as a single dose or 500 mg orally twice a day for 7 days, is usually used. In the case of treatment failure in the absence of reexposure, the patient should be re-treated with metronidazole, 500 mg orally twice a day for 7 days. If treatment failure occurs again, give metronidazole, 2 g orally once daily for 3–5 days. If this is not effective in eradicating the organisms, metronidazole susceptibility testing can be arranged with the CDC at 770-488-4115.

C. Bacterial Vaginosis

The recommended regimens are metronidazole, 500 mg orally twice daily for 7 days, clindamycin vaginal cream

(2%, 5 g), once daily for 7 days, or metronidazole gel (0.75%, 5 g), twice daily for 5 days. Alternative regimens include metronidazole, 2 g orally as a single dose, clindamycin, 300 mg orally twice daily for 7 days, or clindamycin ovules, 100 g intravaginally at bedtime for 3 days.

D. CONDYLOMATA ACUMINATA

Recommended treatments for vulvar warts include podophyllum resin 10–25% in tincture of benzoin (do not use during pregnancy or on bleeding lesions) or 80–90% trichloroacetic or bichloroacetic acid, carefully applied to avoid the surrounding skin. The pain of bichloroacetic or trichloroacetic acid application can be lessened by a sodium bicarbonate paste applied immediately after treatment. Podophyllum resin must be washed off after 2–4 hours. Freezing with liquid nitrogen or a cryoprobe and electrocautery are also effective. Patient-applied regimens include podofilox 0.5% solution or gel and imiquimod 5% cream. Vaginal warts may be treated with cryotherapy with liquid nitrogen, trichloroacetic acid, or podophyllum resin. Extensive warts may require treatment with CO_2 laser under local or general anesthesia. Interferon is not recommended for routine use because it is very expensive, associated with systemic side effects, and no more effective than other therapies. Routine examination of sex partners is not necessary for the management of genital warts since the risk of reinfection is probably minimal and curative therapy to prevent transmission is not available. However, partners may wish to be examined for detection and treatment of genital warts and other sexually transmitted diseases. While condom use does not appear to prevent HPV transmission, it may result in accelerated regression of associated lesions, including untreated cervical intraepithelial neoplasia (CIN) and in accelerated clearance of genital HPV infection in women.

Anderson MR et al: Evaluation of vaginal complaints. JAMA 2004;291:1368. [PMID: 15026404]

Holmes KK et al: Effectiveness of condoms in preventing sexually transmitted infections. Bull World Health Organ 2004;82: 454. [PMID: 15356939]

Sexually transmitted disease treatment guidelines 2006. Centers for Disease Control and Prevention. MMWR Recomm Rep 2006;55(RR11):1. [PMID: 16888612]

CERVICITIS

Infection of the cervix must be distinguished from physiologic ectopy of columnar epithelium, which is common in young women. Mucopurulent cervicitis is characterized by a red edematous cervix with a purulent yellow discharge. The infection may result from a sexually transmitted pathogen such as *Neisseria gonorrhoeae, Chlamydia,* or herpesvirus (which presents with vesicles and ulcers on the cervix during a primary herpetic infection), although in most cases none of these organisms can be isolated.

Mucopurulent cervicitis is an insensitive predictor of either gonorrheal or chlamydial infection and in ad-

dition has a low positive predictive value. Treatment should be based on microbiologic testing. Presumptive antibiotic treatment of mucopurulent cervicitis is not indicated unless there is a high prevalence of either *N gonorrhoeae* or *Chlamydia* in the population or if the patient is unlikely to return for treatment. (See Chapter 33 for discussion.)

CERVICAL POLYPS

Cervical polyps commonly occur after menarche and are occasionally noted in postmenopausal women. The cause is not known, but inflammation may play an etiologic role. The principal symptoms are discharge and abnormal vaginal bleeding. However, abnormal bleeding should not be ascribed to a cervical polyp without sampling the endocervix and endometrium. The polyps are visible in the cervical os on speculum examination.

Cervical polyps must be differentiated from polypoid neoplastic disease of the endometrium, small submucous pedunculated myomas, and endometrial polyps. Cervical polyps rarely contain malignant foci.

Treatment

Cervical polyps can generally be removed in the office by avulsion with a uterine packing forceps or ring forceps. If the cervix is soft, patulous, or definitely dilated and the polyp is large, surgical D&C is required (especially if the pedicle is not readily visible). Hysteroscopy may aid removal and lead to identification of concomitant endometrial disease. Because of the possibility of endometrial disease, cervical polypectomy should routinely be accompanied by endometrial sampling.

Spiewankiewicz B et al: Hysteroscopy in cases of endocervical polyps. Eur J Gynaecol Oncol 2003;24:67. [PMID: 12691321]

CYST & ABSCESS OF BARTHOLIN'S DUCT

Trauma or infection may involve Bartholin's duct, causing obstruction of the gland. Drainage of secretions is prevented, leading to pain, swelling, and abscess formation. The infection usually resolves and pain disappears, but stenosis of the duct outlet with distention often persists. Reinfection causes recurrent tenderness and further enlargement of the duct.

The principal symptoms are periodic painful swelling on either side of the introitus and dyspareunia. A fluctuant swelling 1–4 cm in diameter in the inferior portion of either labium minus is a sign of occlusion of Bartholin's duct. Tenderness is evidence of active infection.

Pus or secretions from the gland should be cultured for gonococci, chlamydiae, and other pathogens and treated accordingly (see Chapter 33); frequent warm soaks may be helpful. If an abscess develops, aspiration or incision and drainage are the simplest forms of therapy, but the problem may recur. Marsupialization (in the absence of an abscess), incision and drainage with the insertion of an indwelling Word catheter, or laser treatment will establish a new duct opening. Antibiotics are unnecessary unless cellulitis is present. An asymptomatic cyst does not require therapy.

Omole F et al: Management of Bartholin's duct cyst and gland abscess. Am Fam Physician 2003;68:135. [PMID: 12887119]

EFFECTS OF EXPOSURE TO DIETHYLSTILBESTROL IN UTERO

Between 1947 and 1971, diethylstilbestrol (DES) was widely used in the United States for diabetic women during pregnancy and to treat threatened abortion. It is estimated that at least 2–3 million fetuses were exposed. A relationship between fetal DES exposure and clear cell carcinoma of the vagina was later discovered, and a number of other related anomalies have since been noted. In one-third of all exposed women, there are changes in the vagina (adenosis, septa), cervix (deformities and hypoplasia of the vaginal portion of the cervix), or uterus (T-shaped cavity).

All women known to be exposed prenatally are advised to have an initial colposcopic examination to outline vaginal and cervical areas of abnormal epithelium, followed by cytologic examination of the vagina (all four quadrants of the upper half of the vagina) and cervix at yearly intervals. Lugol's iodine stain of the vagina and cervix will also outline areas of metaplastic squamous epithelium.

Many women are not aware of having been exposed to DES. Therefore, in the age groups at risk (35–59 years), examiners should pay attention to structural changes of the vagina and cervix that may signal the possibility of DES exposure and indicate the need for follow-up.

The incidence of clear cell carcinoma is approximately 1 in 1000 exposed women, and the incidence of cervical and vaginal intraepithelial neoplasia (dysplasia and carcinoma in situ) is twice as high as in unexposed women. DES daughters have more difficulty conceiving and have an increased incidence of early abortion, ectopic pregnancy, and premature births. In addition, mothers treated with DES in pregnancy appear to have a small increase in the incidence of breast cancer, beginning 20 years after exposure.

Schrager S et al: Diethylstilbesterol exposure. Am Fam Physician 2004;69:2395. [PMID: 15168959]

CERVICAL INTRAEPITHELIAL NEOPLASIA (Dysplasia of the Cervix)

ESSENTIALS OF DIAGNOSIS

- *The presumptive diagnosis is made by an abnormal Pap smear of an asymptomatic woman with no grossly visible cervical changes.*
- *Diagnose by colposcopically directed biopsy.*
- *Increased in women with HIV.*

General Considerations

The squamocolumnar junction of the cervix is an area of active squamous cell proliferation. In childhood, this junction is located on the exposed vaginal portion of the cervix. At puberty, because of hormonal influence and possibly because of changes in the vaginal pH, the squamous margin begins to encroach on the single-layered, mucus-secreting epithelium, creating an area of metaplasia (transformation zone). Factors associated with coitus (see Prevention, below) may lead to cellular abnormalities, which over a period of time can result in the development of squamous cell dysplasia or cancer. There are varying degrees of dysplasia (Table 17–2), defined by the degree of cellular atypia; all types must be observed and treated if they persist or become more severe.

Clinical Findings

There are no specific symptoms or signs of CIN. The presumptive diagnosis is made by cytologic screening of an asymptomatic population with no grossly visible cervical changes. All visibly abnormal cervical lesions should be biopsied.

Diagnosis

A. CYTOLOGIC EXAMINATION (PAPANICOLAOU SMEAR)

Screening should begin within 3 years of the onset of sexually activity or at age 21. Testing should be done an-

Table 17–2. Classification systems for Papanicolaou smears.

Numerical	Dysplasia	CIN	Bethesda System
1	Benign	Benign	Normal
2	Benign with inflammation	Benign with inflammation	Normal, ASC-US
3	Mild dysplasia	CIN I	Low-grade SIL
3	Moderate dysplasia	CIN II	High-grade SIL
3	Severe dysplasia	CIN III	
4	Carcinoma in situ		
5	Invasive cancer	Invasive cancer	Invasive cancer

CIN = cervical intraepithelial neoplasia; ASC-US = atypical squamous cells of undetermined significance; SIL = squamous intraepithelial lesion.

nually for 3 years and then at least every 3 years if no ab-normality is detected. After age 65 or 70, if there have been no abnormalities on the last 3 cytologic tests, screening may be discontinued. With liquid-based cytol-ogy (LCB), the initial interval may be increased to every 2 years. Specimens should be taken from a nonmenstru-ating patient, spread on a single slide, and fixed or rinsed directly into preservative solution if LCB is to be used. A specimen should be obtained from the squamocolumnar junction with a wooden or plastic spatula and from the endocervix with a cotton swab or nylon brush.

Cytologic reports from the laboratory may describe findings in one of several ways (see Table 17–2). While use of class 1–5 is now rare, the CIN classification contin-ues to be used along with a description of abnormal cells, including evidence of HPV. The Bethesda System uses the terminology "squamous intraepithelial lesions (SIL)," low-grade or high-grade. Cytopathologists consider a Pap smear to be a medical consultation and will recommend further diagnostic procedures, treatment for infection, and comments on factors preventing adequate evaluation of the specimen. Reflex testing for high-risk HPV types with thin layer cytologic smears is useful for triage of atypia (atypical squamous cells of unknown significance; ASC-US). The routine use of combined cytologic screening and high-risk HPV testing is appropriate in women over the age of 30 who are being screened no more frequently than every 3 years. Women who have undergone hyster-ectomy for benign disease do not need to be screened.

B. COLPOSCOPY

Women with ASC-US and a negative HPV screening may be followed-up in 1 year. If the HPV screen is posi-tive, colposcopy should be performed. If HPV screening is unavailable, repeat cytology may be done at 4- to 6-month intervals until two consecutive normal results, or the patient may be referred directly for colposcopy. All patients with SIL or atypical glandular cells should un-dergo colposcopy. Viewing the cervix with 10–20× mag-nification allows for assessment of the size and margins of an abnormal transformation zone and determination of extension into the endocervical canal. The application of 3–5% acetic acid (vinegar) dissolves mucus, and the acid's desiccating action sharpens the contrast between normal and actively proliferating squamous epithelium. Abnormal changes include white patches and vascular atypia, which indicate areas of greatest cellular activity. Paint the cervix with Lugol's solution (strong iodine solu-tion [Schiller's test]). Normal squamous epithelium will take the stain; nonstaining squamous epithelium should be biopsied. (The single-layered, mucus-secreting en-docervical tissue will not stain either but can readily be distinguished by its darker pink, shinier appearance.)

C. BIOPSY

Colposcopically directed punch biopsy and endocervical curettage are office procedures. If colposcopy is not available, the normal-appearing cervix shedding atypical cells can be evaluated by endocervical curettage and multiple punch biopsies of nonstaining squamous epi-thelium or biopsies from each quadrant of the cervix. Data from both cervical biopsy and endocervical curet-tage are important in deciding on treatment.

Prevention

Cervical infection with the HPV is associated with a high percentage of all cervical dysplasias and cancers. There are over 70 recognized HPV subtypes, of which types 6 and 11 tend to cause genital warts and mild dysplasia, while types 16, 18, 31, and others cause higher-grade cellular changes. In 2006, the FDA approved a vaccine to prevent cervical cancer and vaginal and vulvar pre-cancers caused by HPV types 16 and 18, and to protect against low-grade and pre-cancerous lesions and genital warts caused by HPV types 6, 11, 16, and 18. The vaccine, Gardisil, is rec-ommended for all girls and women aged 11 to 26. Girls as young as nine should receive the vaccine at the judgement of the practitioner. A therapeutic vaccine to treat existing HPV infections is in earlier stages of development.

Cervical cancer is epidemiologically related to the number of sexual partners a woman has had and the number of other female partners a male partner has had. Use of the diaphragm or condom has some protective ef-fect. Long-term oral contraceptive users develop more dysplasias and cancers of the cervix than users of other forms of birth control, and smokers, as well as women exposed to second-hand smoke, are also at increased risk. Preventive measures include regular cytologic screening to detect abnormalities, limiting the number of sexual partners, using a diaphragm or condom for coitus, and stopping smoking or exposure to second-hand smoke.

Women with HIV infection appear to be at in-creased risk for the disease and of recurrent disease after treatment. Women with HIV infection should receive regular cytologic screening and should be fol-lowed closely after treatment for CIN.

Treatment

Treatment varies depending on the degree and extent of CIN. Biopsies should always precede treatment.

A. CAUTERIZATION OR CRYOSURGERY

The use of either hot cauterization or freezing (cryosur-gery) is effective for noninvasive small lesions visible on the cervix without endocervical extension.

B. CO₂ LASER

This well-controlled method minimizes tissue destruc-tion. It is colposcopically directed and requires special training. It may be used with large visible lesions. In current practice, it involves the vaporization of the transformation zone on the cervix and the distal 5–7 mm of endocervical canal.

C. LOOP RESECTION

When the CIN is clearly visible in its entirety, a wire loop can be used for excisional biopsy. Cutting and hemostasis are effected with a low-voltage electrosurgical machine (Bovie). This office procedure with local anesthesia is quick and uncomplicated.

D. CONIZATION OF THE CERVIX

Conization is surgical removal of the entire transformation zone and endocervical canal. It should be reserved for cases of severe dysplasia or cancer in situ (CIN III), particularly those with endocervical extension. The procedure can be performed with the scalpel, the CO_2 laser, the needle electrode, or by large-loop excision.

E. FOLLOW-UP

Because recurrence is possible—especially in the first 2 years after treatment—and because the false-negative rate of a single cervical cytologic test is 20%, close follow-up is imperative. Vaginal cytologic examination should be repeated at 3-month intervals for at least 1 year.

Bundrick JB et al: Screening for cervical cancer and initial treatment of patients with abnormal results from Papanicolaou testing. Mayo Clin Proc 2005;80:1063. [PMID: 16092586]

Franco EL et al: Vaccination against human Papillomavirus infection: a new paradigm in cervical cancer control. Vaccine 2005;23:2388. [PMID: 15755633]

Wright TC Jr et al: 2001 Consensus guidelines for the management of women with cervical cytological abnormalities. JAMA 2002;287:2120. [PMID: 11966387]

CARCINOMA OF THE CERVIX

ESSENTIALS OF DIAGNOSIS

- *Abnormal uterine bleeding and vaginal discharge.*
- *Cervical lesion may be visible on inspection as a tumor or ulceration.*
- *Vaginal cytology usually positive; must be confirmed by biopsy.*

General Considerations

Cancer appears first in the intraepithelial layers (the preinvasive stage, or carcinoma in situ). Preinvasive cancer (CIN III) is a common diagnosis in women 25–40 years of age and is etiologically related to infection with HPV. Two to 10 years are required for carcinoma to penetrate the basement membrane and invade the tissues. After invasion, death usually occurs within 3–5 years in untreated or unresponsive patients.

Clinical Findings

A. SYMPTOMS AND SIGNS

The most common signs are metrorrhagia, postcoital spotting, and cervical ulceration. Bloody or purulent, odorous, nonpruritic discharge may appear after invasion. Bladder and rectal dysfunction or fistulas and pain are late symptoms.

B. CERVICAL BIOPSY AND ENDOCERVICAL CURETTAGE, OR CONIZATION

These procedures are necessary steps after a positive Papanicolaou smear to determine the extent and depth of invasion of the cancer. Even if the smear is positive, treatment is never justified until definitive diagnosis has been established through biopsy.

C. "STAGING," OR ESTIMATE OF GROSS SPREAD OF CANCER OF THE CERVIX

The depth of penetration of the malignant cells beyond the basement membrane is a reliable clinical guide to the extent of primary cancer within the cervix and the likelihood of metastases. It is customary to stage cancers of the cervix under anesthesia as shown in Table 17–3. Further assessment may be carried out by abdominal and pelvic CT scanning or MRI.

Complications

Metastases to regional lymph nodes occur with increasing frequency from stage I to stage IV. Paracervical extension occurs in all directions from the cervix. The ureters are often obstructed lateral to the cervix, causing hydroureter and hydronephrosis and consequently impaired kidney function. Almost two-thirds of patients with untreated carcinoma of the cervix die of uremia when ureteral obstruction is bilateral. Pain in the back, in the distribution of the lumbosacral plexus, is often indicative of neurologic involvement. Gross edema of the legs may be indicative of vascular and lymphatic stasis due to tumor.

Vaginal fistulas to the rectum and urinary tract are severe late complications. Hemorrhage is the cause of death in 10–20% of patients with extensive invasive carcinoma.

Prevention

In 2006, the FDA approved a vaccine to prevent cervical cancer caused by HPV types 16, and 18, and to protect against low-grade and precancerous lesions and genital warts caused by HPV types 6, 11, 16, and 18. The vaccine, Gardisil is recommended for all girls and women aged 11 to 26. Girls as young as nine should receive the vaccine if clinically indicated.

Treatment

A. EMERGENCY MEASURES

Vaginal hemorrhage originates from gross ulceration and cavitation in stage II–IV cervical carcinoma. Ligation and suturing of the cervix are usually not feasible, but ligation of the uterine or hypogastric arteries may be lifesaving when other measures fail. Styptics such as Monsel's solution or acetone are effective, although delayed sloughing may result in further bleeding. Wet vaginal packing is helpful. Emergency irradiation usually controls bleeding.

Table 17–3. FIGO[1] staging of cancer of the cervix.

Preinvasive carcinoma	
Stage 0	Carcinoma in situ.
Invasive carcinoma	
Stage I	Carcinoma strictly confined to the cervix.
IA	Invasive cancer diagnosed only by microscopy.
	IA1 Measured invasion of stroma no greater than 3 mm in depth and no wider than 7 mm.
	IA2 Measured invasion of stroma greater than 3 mm in depth and no greater than 5 mm in depth and no wider than 7 mm.
IB	Clinical lesions confined to the cervix or pre-clinical lesions greater than 1A. All gross lesions, even with superficial invasion, are stage IB.
	IB1 Clinical lesions no greater than 4 cm.
	IB2 Clinical lesions greater than 4 cm.
Stage II	Carcinoma extends beyond the cervix but has not extended to the pelvic wall. The carcinoma involves the vagina but not as far as the lower third.
IIA	No obvious parametrial involvement.
IIB	Obvious parametrial involvement.
Stage III	Carcinoma has extended either to the lower-third of the vagina or to the pelvic side-wall. All cases of hydronephrosis.
IIIA	Involvement of lower third of vagina. No extension to pelvic sidewall.
IIIB	Extension onto the pelvic wall and/or hydronephrosis or nonfunctioning kidney.
Stage IV	Carcinoma extended beyond the true pelvis or clinically involving the mucosa of the bladder or rectum.
IVA	Spread of growth to adjacent organs.
IVB	Spread of growth to distant organs.

[1]International Federation of Gynecology and Obstetrics

B. SPECIFIC MEASURES

1. Carcinoma in situ (stage 0)—In women who have completed childbearing, total hysterectomy is the treatment of choice. In women who wish to retain the uterus, acceptable alternatives include cervical conization or ablation of the lesion with cryotherapy or laser. Close follow-up with Papanicolaou smears every 3 months for 1 year and every 6 months for another year is necessary after cryotherapy or laser.

2. Invasive carcinoma—Microinvasive carcinoma (stage IA) is treated with simple, extrafascial hysterectomy. Stage IB and stage IIA cancers may be treated with either radical hysterectomy or radiation therapy. Stage IIB and stage III and IV cancers are treated with

radiation therapy plus concurrent cisplatin-based chemotherapy. Because radical surgery results in fewer long-term complications than irradiation and may allow preservation of ovarian function, it may be the preferred mode of therapy in younger women without contraindications to major surgery.

Prognosis

The overall 5-year relative survival rate for carcinoma of the cervix is 68% in white women and 55% in black women in the United States. Survival rates are inversely proportionate to the stage of cancer: stage 0, 99–100%; stage IA, > 95%; stage IB–IIA, 80–90%; stage IIB, 65%; stage III, 40%; and stage IV, < 20%.

ACOG Practice Bulletin. Diagnosis and treatment of cervical carcinomas, Number 35, May 2002. Obstet Gynecol 2002; 99 (5 Pt 1):855. [PMID: 11978302]

Lonky NM: Reducing death from cervical cancer: examining the prevention paradigms. Obstet Gynecol Clin North Am 2002;29:599. [PMID: 12509087]

LEIOMYOMA OF THE UTERUS (Fibroid Tumor)

 ESSENTIALS OF DIAGNOSIS

- *Irregular enlargement of the uterus (may be asymptomatic).*
- *Heavy or irregular vaginal bleeding, dysmenorrhea.*
- *Acute and recurrent pelvic pain if the tumor becomes twisted on its pedicle or infarcted.*
- *Symptoms due to pressure on neighboring organs (large tumors).*

General Considerations

Uterine leiomyoma is the most common benign neoplasm of the female genital tract. It is a discrete, round, firm, often multiple uterine tumor composed of smooth muscle and connective tissue. The most convenient classification is by anatomic location: (1) intramural, (2) submucous, (3) subserous, (4) intraligamentous, (5) parasitic (ie, deriving its blood supply from an organ to which it becomes attached), and (6) cervical. A submucous myoma may become pedunculated and descend through the cervix into the vagina.

Clinical Findings

A. SYMPTOMS AND SIGNS

In nonpregnant women, myomas are frequently asymptomatic. However, they can cause urinary frequency, dysmenorrhea, heavy bleeding (often with anemia), or other complications due to the presence of an abdominal mass.

Occasionally, degeneration occurs, causing intense pain. Infertility may be due to a myoma that significantly distorts the uterine cavity.

B. Laboratory Findings

Hemoglobin levels may be decreased as a result of blood loss, but in rare cases polycythemia is present, presumably as a result of the production of erythropoietin by the myomas.

C. Imaging

Ultrasonography will confirm the presence of uterine myomas and can be used sequentially to monitor growth. When multiple subserous or pedunculated myomas are being followed, ultrasonography is important to exclude ovarian masses. MRI can delineate intramural and submucous myomas accurately. Hysterography or hysteroscopy can also confirm cervical or submucous myomas.

Differential Diagnosis

Irregular myomatous enlargement of the uterus must be differentiated from the similar but symmetric enlargement that may occur with pregnancy or adenomyosis (the presence of endometrial glands and stroma in the myometrium). Subserous myomas must be distinguished from ovarian tumors. Leiomyosarcoma is an unusual tumor occurring in 0.5% of women operated on for symptomatic myoma. It is very rare under the age of 40 and increases in incidence thereafter.

Treatment

A. Emergency Measures

If the patient is markedly anemic as a result of long, heavy menstrual periods, preoperative treatment with depot medroxyprogesterone acetate, 150 mg intramuscularly every 28 days, or danazol, 400–800 mg orally daily, will slow or stop bleeding, and medical treatment of anemia can be given prior to surgery. Emergency surgery is required for acute torsion of a pedunculated myoma. The only emergency indication for myomectomy during pregnancy is torsion; abortion is not an inevitable result.

B. Specific Measures

Women who have small asymptomatic myomas should be examined at 6-month intervals. If necessary, elective myomectomy can be done to preserve the uterus. Myomas do not require surgery on an urgent basis unless they cause significant pressure on the ureters, bladder, or bowel or severe bleeding leading to anemia or unless they are undergoing rapid growth. Cervical myomas larger than 3–4 cm in diameter or pedunculated myomas that protrude through the cervix must be removed. Submucous myomas can be removed using a hysteroscope and laser or resection instruments.

Because the risk of surgical complications increases with the increasing size of the myoma, preoperative re-

duction of myoma size is desirable. GnRH analogs such as depot leuprolide, 3.75 mg intramuscularly monthly, or nafarelin, 0.2–0.4 mg intranasally twice a day, are used preoperatively for 3- to 4-month periods to induce reversible hypogonadism, which temporarily reduces the size of myomas, suppresses their further growth, and reduces surrounding vascularity.

C. Surgical Measures

Surgical measures available for the treatment of myoma are laparoscopic or abdominal myomectomy and total or subtotal abdominal, vaginal, or laparoscopy-assisted vaginal hysterectomy. Myomectomy is the treatment of choice during the childbearing years. Recent developments include transcatheter bilateral uterine artery embolization, myolysis with MRI-guided high frequency focused ultrasound, or laser cauterization. While these approaches are promising and potentially cost-effective alternatives, randomized clinical trials to compare long-term outcomes of these new methods with conventional therapy are needed.

Prognosis

Surgical therapy is curative. Future pregnancies are not endangered by myomectomy, although cesarean delivery may be necessary after wide dissection with entry into the uterine cavity.

Beinfeld MT et al: Cost-effectiveness of uterine artery embolization and hysterectomy for uterine fibroids. Radiology 2004; 230:207. [PMID: 14695395]

Wallach EE et al: Uterine myomas: An overview of development, clinical features, and management. Obstet Gynecol 2004;104: 393. [PMID: 15292018]

CARCINOMA OF THE ENDOMETRIUM

 ESSENTIALS OF DIAGNOSIS

- *Abnormal bleeding is the presenting sign in 80% of cases.*
- *Pap smear is frequently negative.*
- *After a negative pregnancy test, endometrial tissue is required to confirm the diagnosis.*

General Considerations

Adenocarcinoma of the endometrium is the second most common cancer of the female genital tract. It occurs most often in women 50–70 years of age. Some patients will have taken unopposed estrogen in the past; their increased risk appears to persist for 10 or more years after stopping the drug. Obesity, nulliparity, diabetes, and polycystic ovaries with prolonged anovulation and the extended use of tamoxifen for the treatment of breast cancer are also risk factors.

Abnormal bleeding is the presenting sign in 80% of cases. Endometrial carcinoma may cause obstruction of the cervix with collection of pus (pyometra) or blood (hematometra) causing lower abdominal pain. However, pain generally occurs late in the disease, with metastases or infection.

Papanicolaou smears of the cervix occasionally show atypical endometrial cells but are an insensitive diagnostic tool. Endocervical and endometrial sampling is the only reliable means of diagnosis. Adequate specimens of each can usually be obtained during an office procedure performed following local anesthesia (paracervical block). Simultaneous hysteroscopy can be a valuable addition in order to localize polyps or other lesions within the uterine cavity. Vaginal ultrasonography may be used to determine the thickness of the endometrium as an indication of hypertrophy and possible neoplastic change.

Pathologic assessment is important in differentiating hyperplasias, which often can be treated with cyclic oral progestins.

Prevention

Prompt endometrial sampling for patients who report abnormal menstrual bleeding or postmenopausal uterine bleeding will reveal many incipient as well as clinical cases of endometrial cancer. Younger women with chronic anovulation are at risk for endometrial hyperplasia and subsequent endometrial cancer. They can reduce the risk of hyperplasia almost completely with the use of oral contraceptives or cyclic progestin therapy.

Staging

Examination under anesthesia, endometrial and endocervical sampling, chest radiography, intravenous urography, cystoscopy, sigmoidoscopy, TVS, and MRI will help determine the extent of the disease and its appropriate treatment. The staging is based on the surgical and pathologic evaluation.

Treatment

Treatment consists of total hysterectomy and bilateral salpingo-oophorectomy. Peritoneal material for cytologic examination is routinely taken and lymph node sampling may be done. If invasion deep into the myometrium has occurred or if sampled lymph nodes are positive for tumor, postoperative irradiation is indicated. The role of adjuvant chemotherapy alone or with irradiation is currently under investigation. Palliation of advanced or metastatic endometrial adenocarcinoma may be accomplished with large doses of progestins, eg, medroxyprogesterone, 400 mg intramuscularly weekly, or megestrol acetate, 80–160 mg daily orally.

Prognosis

With early diagnosis and treatment, the overall 5-year survival is 80–85%. With stage I disease, the depth of myometrial invasion is the strongest predictor of survival,

with a 98% 5-year survival with less than 66% depth of invasion and 78% survival with 66% or greater invasion.

Amant F et al: Endometrial cancer. Lancet 2005;366:491. [PMID: 16084259]

Mariani A et al: Surgical stage I endometrial cancer: predictors of distant failure and death. Gynecol Oncol 2002;87:274. [PMID: 12468325]

CARCINOMA OF THE VULVA

ESSENTIALS OF DIAGNOSIS

- *History of genital warts.*
- *History of prolonged vulvar irritation, with pruritus, local discomfort, or slight bloody discharge.*
- *Early lesions may suggest or include nonneoplastic epithelial disorders.*
- *Late lesions appear as a mass, an exophytic growth, or a firm, ulcerated area in the vulva.*
- *Biopsy is necessary to make the diagnosis.*

General Considerations

The majority of cancers of the vulva are squamous lesions that classically have occurred in women over 50 years of age. Several subtypes (particularly 16, 18, and 31) of the HPV have been identified in some but not all vulvar cancers. As with squamous cell lesions of the cervix, a grading system of vulvar intraepithelial neoplasia (VIN) from mild dysplasia to carcinoma in situ has been established.

Differential Diagnosis

Biopsy is essential for the diagnosis of VIN and vulvar cancer and should be performed with any localized atypical vulvar lesion, including white patches. Multiple skin-punch specimens can be taken in the office under local anesthesia, with care to include tissue from the edges of each lesion sampled.

Benign vulvar disorders that must be excluded in the diagnosis of carcinoma of the vulva include chronic granulomatous lesions (eg, lymphogranuloma venereum, syphilis), condylomas, hidradenoma, or neurofibroma. Lichen sclerosus and other associated leukoplakic changes in the skin should be biopsied. The likelihood that a superimposed vulvar cancer will develop in a woman with a nonneoplastic epithelial disorder (vulvar dystrophy) ranges from 1% to 5%.

Treatment

A. GENERAL MEASURES

Early diagnosis and treatment of irritative or other predisposing causes, such as lichen sclerosis and VIN, should be pursued. A 7:3 combination of betamethasone and crotamiton is particularly effective for itching. After an initial response, fluorinated steroids should be replaced with hydrocortisone because of their skin atrophying effect. For lichen sclerosus, recommended treatment is clobetasol propionate cream 0.05% twice daily for 2–3 weeks, then once daily until symptoms resolve. Application one to three times a week can be used for long-term maintenance therapy.

B. SURGICAL MEASURES

High-grade VIN may be treated with a variety of approaches including topical chemotherapy, laser ablation, wide local excision, skinning vulvectomy, and simple vulvectomy. Small, invasive basal cell carcinoma of the vulva should be excised with a wide margin. If the VIN is extensive or multicentric, laser therapy or superficial surgical removal of vulvar skin may be required. In this way, the clitoris and uninvolved portions of the vulva may be spared.

Invasive carcinoma confined to the vulva without evidence of spread to adjacent organs or to the regional lymph nodes is treated with wide local excision and inguinal lymphadenectomy or wide local excision alone if invasion is less than 1 mm. Patients with more advanced disease may receive preoperative radiation, chemotherapy, or both.

Prognosis

Basal cell carcinomas very seldom metastasize, and carcinoma in situ by definition has not metastasized. With adequate excision, the prognosis for both lesions is excellent. Patients with invasive vulvar squamous cell carcinoma 2 cm in diameter or less, without inguinal lymph node metastases, have an 85–90% chance of a 5-year survival. If the lesion is greater than 2 cm and lymph node involvement is present, the likelihood of 5-year survival is approximately 40%.

de Hullu JA et al: Modern management of vulvar cancer. Curr Opin Obstet Gynecol 2004;16:65. [PMID: 15128010]

Montana GS: Carcinoma of the vulva: combined modality treatment. Curr Treat Options Oncol 2004;5:85. [PMID: 14990203]

ENDOMETRIOSIS

 ESSENTIALS OF DIAGNOSIS

- Pelvic pain related to menstrual cycle.
- Dysmenorrhea.
- Dyspareunia.
- Increased frequency among infertile women.

General Considerations

Endometriosis is an aberrant growth of endometrium outside the uterus, particularly in the dependent parts of the pelvis and in the ovaries and is the most common cause of secondary dysmenorrhea. While retrograde menstruation is the most widely accepted cause, its pathogenesis and natural course are not fully understood. The overall prevalence in the United States is 6–10% and is fourfold to fivefold greater among infertile women.

Clinical Findings

Women with endometriosis will complain of pelvic pain, which may be associated with infertility, dyspareunia, or rectal pain with bleeding. Initially, pain tends to start 2–7 days before the onset of menses and becomes increasingly severe until flow slackens. With increasing duration of disease, pain may become continuous. Pelvic examination may disclose tender nodules in the cul-de-sac or rectovaginal septum, uterine retroversion with decreased uterine mobility, cervical motion tenderness, or an adnexal mass or tenderness. However, most women with endometriosis have a normal pelvic examination.

Endometriosis must be distinguished from PID, ovarian neoplasms, and uterine myomas. Bowel invasion by endometrial tissue may produce blood in the stool that must be distinguished from bowel neoplasm. Paradoxically, the severity of pain associated with endometriosis may be inversely related to the anatomic extent of the disease.

Imaging is of limited value. Ultrasound examination will often reveal complex fluid-filled masses that cannot be distinguished from neoplasms. MRI is more sensitive and specific than ultrasound, particularly in the diagnosis of adnexal masses. However, the clinical diagnosis of endometriosis is presumptive and usually confirmed by laparoscopy.

Treatment

A. MEDICAL TREATMENT

Medical treatment, using a variety of hormonal therapies, is effective in the amelioration of pain associated with endometriosis. However, there is no evidence that any of these agents increase the likelihood of pregnancy. Their preoperative use is of questionable value in reducing the difficulty of surgery. Most of these regimens are designed to inhibit ovulation over 4–9 months and lower hormone levels, thus preventing cyclic stimulation of endometriotic implants and decreasing their size. The optimum duration of therapy is not clear, and the relative merits in terms of side effects and long-term risks and benefits show insignificant differences when compared with each other and, in mild cases, with placebo.

1. The GnRH analogs such as nafarelin nasal spray, 0.2–0.4 mg twice daily, or long-acting injectable leuprolide acetate, 3.75 mg intramuscularly monthly, used for 6 months, suppress ovulation. Side effects of vasomotor symptoms and bone demineralization may be relieved by "add-back" therapy with norethindrone, 5–10 mg daily.

2. Danazol is used for 4–6 months in the lowest dose necessary to suppress menstruation, usually 200–400 mg twice daily. Danazol has a high incidence of androgenic side effects, including decreased breast size, weight gain, acne, and hirsutism.

3. Any of the combination oral contraceptives, the contraceptive patch, or vaginal ring may be used continuously for 6–12 months. Breakthrough bleeding can be treated with conjugated estrogens, 1.25 mg daily for 1 week, or estradiol, 2 mg daily for 1 week.

4. Medroxyprogesterone acetate, 100 mg intramuscularly every 2 weeks for four doses and then 100 mg every 4 weeks; add oral estrogen or estradiol valerate, 30 mg intramuscularly, for breakthrough bleeding. Use for 6–9 months.

5. Low-dose oral contraceptives can also be given cyclically; prolonged suppression of ovulation will often inhibit further stimulation of residual endometriosis, especially if taken after one of the therapies mentioned above.

6. Analgesics, with or without codeine, may be needed during menses. NSAIDs may be helpful.

B. SURGICAL MEASURES

Surgical treatment of endometriosis—particularly extensive disease—is effective both in reducing pain and in promoting fertility. Laparoscopic ablation of endometrial implants along with uterine nerve ablation significantly reduces pain. Ablation of implants and, if necessary, removal of ovarian endometriomas enhance fertility, although subsequent pregnancy rates are related to the severity of disease. Women with disabling pain who no longer desire childbearing can be treated definitively with total abdominal hysterectomy and bilateral salpingo-oophorectomy (TAH-BSO).

Prognosis

The prognosis for reproductive function in early or moderately advanced endometriosis is good with conservative therapy. TAH-BSO is curative for patients with severe and extensive endometriosis with pain.

Giudice LC et al: Endometriosis. Lancet 2004;364:1789. [PMID: 15541453]

Winkel CA: Evaluation and management of women with endometriosis. Obstet Gynecol 2003;102:397. [PMID: 12907119]

PELVIC ORGAN PROLAPSE

Cystocele, rectocele, and enterocele are vaginal hernias commonly seen in multiparous women. Cystocele is a hernia of the bladder wall into the vagina, causing a soft anterior fullness. Cystocele may be accompanied by urethrocele, which is not a hernia but a sagging of the urethra following its detachment from the pubic symphysis during childbirth. Rectocele is a herniation of the terminal rectum into the posterior vagina, caus-

ing a collapsible pouch-like fullness. Enterocele is a vaginal vault hernia containing small intestine, usually in the posterior vagina and resulting from a deepening of the pouch of Douglas. Two or all three types of hernia may occur in combination. Pelvic organ prolapse is often associated with symptoms of pelvic pressure or a dragging sensation as well as bowel or lower urinary tract dysfunction. Stress urinary incontinence is a frequent symptom.

Supportive measures include a high-fiber diet. Weight reduction in obese patients and limitation of straining and lifting are helpful. Pessaries may reduce cystocele, rectocele, or enterocele temporarily and are helpful in women who do not wish surgery or are chronically ill. The only cure for symptomatic cystocele, rectocele, enterocele, or stress urinary Incontinence is corrective surgery.

UTERINE PROLAPSE

Uterine prolapse most commonly occurs as a delayed result of childbirth injury to the pelvic floor (particularly the transverse cervical and uterosacral ligaments). Unrepaired obstetric lacerations of the levator musculature and perineal body augment the weakness. Attenuation of the pelvic structures with aging and congenital weakness can accelerate the development of prolapse.

In slight prolapse, the uterus descends only part way down the vagina; in moderate prolapse, the corpus descends to the introitus and the cervix protrudes slightly beyond; and in marked prolapse (procidentia), the entire cervix and uterus protrude beyond the introitus and the vagina is inverted. Inability to walk comfortably because of protrusion or discomfort from the presence of a vaginal mass is an indication that surgical treatment should be considered.

Treatment

The type of surgery depends on the extent of prolapse and the patient's age and her desire for menstruation, pregnancy, and coitus. The simplest, most effective procedure is vaginal hysterectomy with appropriate repair of the cystocele and rectocele. If the patient desires pregnancy, a partial resection of the cervix with plication of the cardinal ligaments can be attempted. For elderly women who do not desire coitus, partial obliteration of the vagina is surgically simple and effective. Uterine suspension with sacrospinous cervicocolpopexy may be an effective approach in older women who wish to avoid hysterectomy but preserve coital function. A well-fitted vaginal pessary (eg, inflatable doughnut type, Gellhorn pessary) may give relief if surgery is refused or contraindicated.

Clemons JL et al: Risk factors associated with an unsuccessful pessary fitting trial in women with pelvic organ prolapse. Am J Obstet Gynecol 2004;190:345. [PMID: 14981372]

Novara G et al: Surgery for pelvic organ prolapse: current status and future perspectives. Curr Opin Urol 2005;15:256. [PMID: 15928515]

PELVIC INFLAMMATORY DISEASE
(Salpingitis, Endometritis)

ESSENTIALS OF DIAGNOSIS

- *Uterine, adnexal, or cervical motion tenderness.*
- *Absence of a competing diagnosis.*

General Considerations

PID is a polymicrobial infection of the upper genital tract associated with the sexually transmitted organisms *N gonorrhoeae* and *Chlamydia trachomatis* as well as endogenous organisms, including anaerobes, *Haemophilus influenzae*, enteric gram-negative rods, and streptococci. It is most common in young, nulliparous, sexually active women with multiple partners. Other risk markers include nonwhite race, douching, and smoking. The use of oral contraceptives or barrier methods of contraception may provide significant protection.

Tuberculous salpingitis is rare in the United States but more common in developing countries; it is characterized by pelvic pain and irregular pelvic masses not responsive to antibiotic therapy. It is not sexually transmitted.

Clinical Findings

A. SYMPTOMS AND SIGNS

Patients with PID may have lower abdominal pain, chills and fever, menstrual disturbances, purulent cervical discharge, and cervical and adnexal tenderness. Right upper quadrant pain (Fitz-Hugh and Curtis syndrome) may indicate an associated perihepatitis. However, diagnosis of PID is complicated by the fact that many women may have subtle or mild symptoms that are not readily recognized as PID.

B. MINIMUM DIAGNOSTIC CRITERIA

Women with uterine adnexal or cervical motion tenderness should be considered to have PID and be treated with antibiotics unless there is a competing diagnosis such as ectopic pregnancy or appendicitis.

C. ADDITIONAL CRITERIA

The following criteria may be used to enhance the specificity of the diagnosis: (1) oral temperature greater than 38.3 °C, (2) abnormal cervical or vaginal discharge with white cells on saline microscopy, (3) elevated erythrocyte sedimentation rate, (4) elevated C-reactive protein, and (5) laboratory documentation of cervical infection with *N gonorrhoeae* or *C trachomatis*. Endocervical culture should be performed routinely, but treatment should not be delayed while awaiting results.

D. DEFINITIVE CRITERIA

In selected cases where the diagnosis based on clinical or laboratory evidence is uncertain, the following criteria may be used: (1) histopathologic evidence of endometritis on endometrial biopsy, (2) TVS or MRI showing thickened fluid-filled tubes with or without free pelvic fluid or tubo-ovarian complex, and (3) laparoscopic abnormalities consistent with PID.

Differential Diagnosis

Appendicitis, ectopic pregnancy, septic abortion, hemorrhagic or ruptured ovarian cysts or tumors, twisted ovarian cyst, degeneration of a myoma, and acute enteritis must be considered. PID is more likely to occur when there is a history of PID, recent sexual contact, recent onset of menses, or an IUD in place or if the partner has a sexually transmitted disease. Acute PID is highly unlikely when recent intercourse has not taken place or an IUD is not being used. A sensitive serum pregnancy test should be obtained to rule out ectopic pregnancy. Culdocentesis will differentiate hemoperitoneum (ruptured ectopic pregnancy or hemorrhagic cyst) from pelvic sepsis (salpingitis, ruptured pelvic abscess, or ruptured appendix). Pelvic and vaginal ultrasonography is helpful in the differential diagnosis of ectopic pregnancy of over 6 weeks. Laparoscopy is often used to diagnose PID, and it is imperative if the diagnosis is not certain or if the patient has not responded to antibiotic therapy after 48 hours. The appendix should be visualized at laparoscopy to rule out appendicitis. Cultures obtained at the time of laparoscopy are often specific and helpful.

Treatment

A. HOSPITALIZATION

Patients with acute PID should be admitted for intravenous antibiotic therapy if (1) surgical emergencies such as appendicitis cannot be ruled out, (2) the patient has a tubo-ovarian abscess, (3) the patient is pregnant, (4) the patient is unable to follow or tolerate an outpatient regimen, (5) the patient has not responded clinically to outpatient therapy, or (6) the patient has severe illness, nausea and vomiting, or high fever. In the past, many experts recommended that all patients with PID be hospitalized for bed rest and supervised treatment with parenteral antibiotics. However, a recent large, randomized clinical trial suggests that in women with mild to moderate PID, there is no difference between inpatient and outpatient therapy in short-term clinical outcomes or in long-term reproductive outcomes. Patients with tubo-ovarian abscesses should have direct inpatient observation for at least 24 hours before switching to outpatient parenteral therapy.

B. ANTIBIOTICS

Early treatment with appropriate antibiotics effective against *N gonorrhoeae*, *C trachomatis*, and the endogenous organisms listed above is essential to prevent long-term sequelae. The sexual partner should be examined and treated appropriately.

Two inpatient regimens have been shown to be effective in the treatment of acute PID: (1) Cefoxitin, 2 g intravenously every 6 hours, or cefotetan, 2 g every 12 hours, plus doxycycline, 100 mg intravenously or orally every 12 hours. This regimen is continued for at least 24 hours after the patient shows significant clinical improvement. Doxycycline, 100 mg twice daily, should be continued to complete a total of 14 days therapy. If a tubo-ovarian abscess is present, it is advisable to add oral clindamycin or metronidazole to the doxycycline to provide more effective anaerobic coverage. (2) Clindamycin, 900 mg intravenously every 8 hours, plus gentamicin intravenously in a loading dose of 2 mg/kg followed by 1.5 mg/kg every 8 hours. This regimen is continued for at least 24 hours after the patient shows significant clinical improvement and is followed by either clindamycin, 450 mg four times daily, or doxycycline, 100 mg twice daily, to complete a total of 14 days of therapy.

Limited data exist on other parenteral regimens. Two regimens providing broad-spectrum coverage have been investigated in at least one clinical trial: (1) ofloxacin, 400 mg intravenously every 12 hours, or levofloxacin, 500 mg intravenously once daily, plus metronidazole, 500 mg intravenously every 8 hours; and (2) ampicillin-sulbactam, 3 g intravenously every 6 hours, plus doxycycline, 100 mg intravenously or orally every 12 hours.

Two outpatient regimens are recommended: (1) ofloxacin, 400 mg orally twice daily for 14 days, or levofloxacin, 500 mg orally once daily for 14 days, plus metronidazole, 500 mg orally twice daily, for 14 days; and (2) either a single dose of cefoxitin, 2 g intramuscularly, with probenecid, 1 g orally, or ceftriaxone, 250 mg intramuscularly, plus doxycycline, 100 mg orally twice daily, for 14 days.

C. SURGICAL MEASURES

Tubo-ovarian abscesses may require surgical excision or transcutaneous or transvaginal aspiration. Unless rupture is suspected, institute high-dose antibiotic therapy in the hospital, and monitor therapy with ultrasound. In 70% of cases, antibiotics are effective; in 30%, there is inadequate response in 48–72 hours, and intervention is required. Unilateral adnexectomy is acceptable for unilateral abscess. Hysterectomy and bilateral salpingo-oophorectomy may be necessary for overwhelming infection or in cases of chronic disease with intractable pelvic pain.

Prognosis

In spite of treatment, long-term sequelae, including repeated episodes of infection, chronic pelvic pain, dyspareunia, ectopic pregnancy, or infertility, develop in one-fourth of women with acute disease. The risk of infertility increases with repeated episodes of salpingitis: it is estimated at 10% after the first episode, 25% after a second episode, and 50% after a third episode.

Banikarim C et al: Pelvic inflammatory disease in adolescents. Semin Pediatr Infect Dis 2005;16:175. [PMID: 16044391]

Sexually transmitted disease treatment guidelines 2006. Centers for Disease Control and Prevention. MMWR Recomm Rep 2006;55(RR11):1. [PMID: 16888612]

OVARIAN TUMORS

ESSENTIALS OF DIAGNOSIS

- *Vague gastrointestinal discomfort.*
- *Pelvic pressure and pain.*
- *Many cases of early-stage cancer are asymptomatic.*
- *Pelvic examination, CA 125, and ultrasound are mainstays of diagnosis.*

General Considerations

Ovarian tumors are common. Most are benign, but malignant ovarian tumors are the leading cause of death from reproductive tract cancer. The wide range of types and patterns of ovarian tumors is due to the complexity of ovarian embryology and differences in tissues of origin (Table 17–4).

In women with no family history of ovarian cancer, the lifetime risk is 1.6%, whereas a woman with one affected first-degree relative has a 5% lifetime risk. With two or more affected first-degree relatives, the risk is 7%. Approximately 3% of women with two or more affected first-degree relatives will have a hereditary ovarian cancer syndrome with a lifetime risk of 40%. Women with a BRCA1 gene mutation have a 45% lifetime risk of ovarian cancer and those with a BRAC2 mutation a 25% risk. These women should be screened annually with TVS and CA 125 testing, and prophylactic oophorectomy is recommended by age 35 or whenever childbearing is completed because of the high risk of disease. The benefits of such screening for women with one or no affected first-degree relatives are unproved, and the risks associated with unnecessary surgical procedures may outweigh the benefits in low-risk women.

Clinical Findings

A. SYMPTOMS AND SIGNS

Unfortunately, most women with both benign and malignant ovarian neoplasms are either asymptomatic or experience only mild nonspecific gastrointestinal symptoms or pelvic pressure. Women with early disease are typically detected on routine pelvic examination. Women with advanced malignant disease may experience abdominal pain and bloating, and a palpable abdominal mass with ascites is often present.

Table 17–4. Ovarian functional and neoplastic tumors.

Tumor	Incidence	Size	Consistency	Menstrual Irregularities	Endocrine Effects	Potential for Malignancy	Special Remarks
Follicle cysts	Rare in childhood; frequent in menstrual years; never in postmenopausal years.	< 6 cm, often bilateral.	Moderate	Occasional	Occasional anovulation with persistently proliferative endometrium	None	Usually disappear spontaneously within 2–3 months.
Corpus luteum cysts	Occasional, in menstrual years.	4–6 cm, unilateral.	Moderate	Occasional delayed period	Prolonged secretory phase	None	Functional cysts. Intraperitoneal bleeding occasionally.
Theca lutein cysts	Occurs with hydatidiform mole, choriocarcinoma; also with gonadotropin or clomiphene therapy.	To 4–5 cm, multiple, bilateral. (Ovaries may be ≥ 20 cm in diameter.)	Tense	Amenorrhea	hCG elevated as a result of trophoblastic proliferation	None	Functional cysts. Hematoperitoneum or torsion of ovary may occur. Surgery is to be avoided.
Inflammatory (tubo-ovarian abscess)	Concomitant with acute salpingitis.	To 15–20 cm, often bilateral.	Variable, painful	Menometrorrhagia	Anovulation usual	None	Unilateral removal indicated if possible.
Endometriotic cysts	Never in preadolescent or postmenopausal years. Most common in women aged 20–40 years.	To 10–12 cm, occasionally bilateral.	Moderate to softened	Rare	None	Very rare	Associated pelvic endometriosis. Medical treatment or conservative surgery recommended.
Teratoid tumors: Benign teratomas (dermoid cysts)	Childhood to postmenopause.	< 15 cm; 15% are bilateral.	Moderate to softened	None	None	Rare	Torsion can occur. Partial oophorectomy recommended.
Malignant teratomas	< 1% of ovarian tumors. Usually in infants and young adults.	> 20 cm, unilateral.	Irregularly firm	None	Occasionally, hCG elevated	All	Surgery alone may be curative.
Cystadenoma, cystadenocarcinoma	Common in reproductive years.	Serous: < 25 cm, 33% bilateral; mucinous: up to 1 cm, 10% bilateral.	Moderate to softened	None	None	> 50% for serous, about 5% for mucinous	Peritoneal implants often occur with serous, rarely with mucinous. If mucinous tumor is ruptured, pseudomyxoma peritonei may occur.

(continued)

763

Table 17–4. Ovarian functional and neoplastic tumors. (continued)

Tumor	Incidence	Size	Consistency	Menstrual Irregularities	Endocrine Effects	Potential for Malignancy	Special Remarks
Endometrioid carcinoma	15% of ovarian carcinomas.	Moderate, 13% bilateral.	Firm	None	None	All	Adenocarcinoma of endometrium coexists in 15–30% of cases.
Fibroma	< 5% of ovarian tumors.	Usually < 15 cm.	Very firm	None	None	Rare	Ascites in 20% (rarely, pleural fluid).
Arrhenoblastoma	Rare. Average age 30 years or more.	Often small (< 10 cm), unilateral.	Firm to softened	Amenorrhea	Androgens elevated	< 20%	Recurrences are moderately sensitive to irradiation.
Theca cell tumor (thecoma)	Uncommon.	< 10 cm, unilateral.	Firm	Occasional irregularity	Estrogens or androgens elevated	< 1%	
Granulosa cell tumor	Uncommon. Usually in prepubertal girls or women older than 50 years.	May be very small.	Firm to softened	Menometrorrhagia	Estrogens elevated	15–20%	Recurrences are moderately sensitive to irradiation.
Dysgerminoma	About 1–2% of ovarian tumors.	< 30 cm, bilateral in 33%.	Moderate to softened	None	—	All	Very radiosensitive.
Brenner tumor	About 1% of ovarian tumors.	< 30 cm, unilateral.	Firm	None	—	Very rare	> 50% occur in postmenopausal years.
Secondary ovarian tumors	10% of fatal malignant disease in women.	Varies; often bilateral.	Firm to softened	Occasional	Very rare (thyroid, adrenocortical origin)	All	Bowel or breast metastases to ovary common.

B. LABORATORY FINDINGS

An elevated serum CA 125 (> 35 units) indicates a greater likelihood that an ovarian tumor is malignant. CA 125 is elevated in 80% of women with epithelial ovarian cancer overall but in only 50% of women with early disease. Furthermore, serum CA 125 may be elevated in premenopausal women with benign disease such as endometriosis.

C. IMAGING STUDIES

TVS is useful for screening high-risk women but has inadequate sensitivity for screening low-risk women. Ultrasound is helpful in differentiating ovarian masses that are benign and likely to resolve spontaneously from those with malignant potential. Color Doppler imaging may further enhance the specificity of ultrasound diagnosis.

Differential Diagnosis

Once an ovarian mass has been detected, it must be categorized as functional, benign neoplastic, or potentially malignant. Predictive factors include age, size of the mass, ultrasound configuration, CA 125 levels, the presence of symptoms, and whether the mass is unilateral or bilateral. In a premenopausal woman, an asymptomatic, mobile, unilateral, simple cystic mass less than 7.5 cm may be observed for 4–6 weeks. Most will resolve spontaneously. If the mass is larger or unchanged on repeat pelvic examination and TVS, surgical evaluation is required.

Most ovarian masses in postmenopausal women require surgical evaluation. However, a postmenopausal woman with an asymptomatic unilateral simple cyst less than 5 cm in diameter and a normal CA 125 level may be followed closely with TVS. All others require surgical evaluation.

Laparoscopy may be used when an ovarian mass is small enough to be removed with a laparoscopic approach. If malignancy is suspected, preoperative workup should include chest radiograph, evaluation of liver and kidney function, and hematologic indices.

Treatment

If a malignant ovarian mass is suspected, surgical evaluation should be performed by a gynecologic oncologist. For benign neoplasms, tumor removal or unilateral oophorectomy is usually performed. For ovarian cancer in an early stage, the standard therapy is complete surgical staging followed by abdominal hysterectomy and bilateral salpingo-oophorectomy with omentectomy and selective lymphadenectomy. With more advanced disease, aggressive removal of all visible tumor improves survival. Except for women with low-grade ovarian cancer in an early stage, postoperative chemotherapy is indicated. Several chemotherapy regimens are effective, such as the combination of cisplatin or carboplatin with paclitaxel, with clinical response rates of up to 60–70%.

Prognosis

Unfortunately, approximately 75% of women with ovarian cancer are diagnosed with advanced disease after regional or distant metastases have become established. The overall 5-year survival is approximately 17% with distant metastases, 36% with local spread, and 89% with early disease.

Cannistra SA: Cancer of the ovary. N Engl J Med 2004;351: 2519. [PMID: 15590954]

Guppy AE et al: Epithelial ovarian cancer: a review of current management. Clin Oncol 2005;17:399. [PMID: 16149282]

POLYCYSTIC OVARY SYNDROME

 ESSENTIALS OF DIAGNOSIS

- *Clinical or biochemical evidence of hyperandrogenism.*
- *Oligoovulation or anovulation.*
- *Polycystic ovaries on ultrasonography.*

General Considerations

Polycystic ovary syndrome (PCOS) is a common endocrine disorder affecting 5–10% of women of reproductive age and is a common source of chronic anovulation. The underlying etiology is unknown, although most of these women have an aberration of gonadotropin stimulation. This is manifested by an increased release of luteinizing hormone (LH) relative to follicle-stimulating hormone (FSH), resulting in an increased production of androstenedione and testosterone by ovarian theca cells. The androstenedione undergoes aromatization to estrone and converted to estradiol in the ovarian granulosa cells. The high estrone levels are believed to cause suppression of pituitary FSH and constant LH stimulation of the ovary results in anovulation, multiple cysts, and theca cell hyperplasia with excess androgen output.

Women with Cushing's syndrome, congenital adrenal hyperplasia, and androgen-secreting adrenal tumors also tend to have high circulating androgen levels and anovulation with polycystic ovaries; these disorders must be ruled out in women with presumed PCOS.

Clinical Findings

PCOS is manifested by hirsutism (50% of cases), obesity (40%), and virilization (20%). Fifty percent of patients have amenorrhea, 30% have abnormal uterine bleeding, and 20% have normal menstruation. In addition, they show insulin resistance and hyperinsulinemia, and these women are at increased risk for early-onset type 2 diabetes. The patients are generally infertile, although they may ovulate occasionally. They have an increased long-term risk of cancer of the breast and endometrium because of unopposed estrogen secretion.

Differential Diagnosis

Anovulation in the reproductive years may also be due to (1) premature menopause (high FSH and LH levels); (2) rapid weight loss, extreme physical exertion (normal FSH and LH levels for age), or obesity; (3) discontinuation of hormonal contraceptives (anovulation for 6 months or more occasionally occurs); (4) pituitary adenoma with elevated prolactin (galactorrhea may or may not be present); and (5) hyperthyroidism or hypothyroidism. When amenorrhea has persisted for 6 months or more without a diagnosis, FSH, LH, prolactin, and TSH should be checked. Women with clinical evidence of androgen excess should have total testosterone, DHEA-S, and 17-hydroxyprogesterone measured. A 10-day course of progestin (eg, medroxyprogesterone acetate, 10 mg/d) will cause withdrawal bleeding if estrogen levels are high. This will aid in the diagnosis and prevent endometrial hyperplasia. Because of the high risk of insulin resistance and dyslipidemia, all women with PCOS should have a 2-hour glucose determination after a 75-g glucose load and a lipoprotein profile.

Treatment

In obese patients with PCOS, weight reduction is often effective. If the patient wishes to become pregnant, clomiphene or other drugs can be used for ovulatory stimulation. (See Infertility, this chapter.) The addition of dexamethasone, 0.5 mg at bedtime, to a clomiphene regimen may increase the likelihood of ovulation by suppression of ACTH and any circulating adrenal androgens. For women who are unresponsive to clomiphene, 3- to 6-month courses of the oral hypoglycemic agents metformin, 500 mg three times daily, rosiglitazone 4 mg daily, or pioglitazone 30–45 mg daily may bring resumption of regular cycles and ovulation. These agents reduce the hyperinsulinemia and hyperandrogenemia in PCOS.

If the patient does not desire pregnancy, medroxyprogesterone acetate, 10 mg/d for the first 10 days of each month, should be given. This will ensure regular shedding of the endometrium so that hyperplasia will not occur. If contraception is desired, a low-dose combination oral contraceptive can be used; this is also useful in controlling hirsutism, for which treatment must be continued for 6–12 months before results are seen.

Hirsutism may be managed with epilation and electrolysis. Dexamethasone, 0.5 mg each night, is helpful in women with excess adrenal androgen secretion. If hirsutism is severe, some patients will elect to have a hysterectomy and bilateral oophorectomy followed by estrogen replacement therapy. Spironolactone, an aldosterone antagonist, is also useful for hirsutism in doses of 25 mg three or four times daily. Flutamide, 250 mg

daily, and finasteride, 5 mg daily, are also effective for treating hirsutism. Because these three agents are potentially teratogenic, they should be used only in conjunction with secure contraception.

Ehrmann DA: Polycystic ovarian syndrome. N Engl J Med 2005; 352:1223. [PMID: 15788499]

PAINFUL INTERCOURSE (Dyspareunia)

Questions related to sexual functioning should be asked as part of the reproductive history. Two helpful questions are, "Are you sexually active?" and "Are you having any sexual difficulties at this time?"

During the pelvic examination, the patient should be placed in a half-sitting position and given a handheld mirror and then asked to point out the site of pain and describe the type of pain.

Etiology

A. VULVOVAGINITIS

Vulvovaginitis is inflammation or infection of the vagina. Areas of marked tenderness in the vulvar vestibule without visible inflammation occasionally show lesions resembling small condylomas on colposcopy (see Vaginitis, this chapter).

B. VAGINISMUS

Vaginismus is voluntary or involuntary contraction of muscles around the introitus. It results from fear, pain, sexual trauma, or having learned negative attitudes toward sex during childhood.

C. REMNANTS OF THE HYMEN

The hymen is usually adequately stretched during initial intercourse, so that pain does not occur subsequently. In some women, the pain of initial intercourse may produce vaginismus. In others, a thin or thickened rim or partial rim of hymen remains after several episodes of intercourse, causing pain.

D. INSUFFICIENT LUBRICATION OF THE VAGINA

See vaginal atrophy in the section on Menopausal Syndrome, this chapter.

E. INFECTION, ENDOMETRIOSIS, TUMORS, OR OTHER PATHOLOGIC CONDITIONS

Pain occurring with deep thrusting during coitus is usually due to acute or chronic infection of the cervix, uterus, or adnexa; endometriosis; adnexal tumors; or adhesions resulting from prior pelvic disease or operation. Careful history taking and a pelvic examination will generally help in the differential diagnosis.

F. VULVODYNIA

This is the most frequent cause of dyspareunia in premenopausal women. It is characterized by a sensation of burning along with other symptoms including pain, itching, stinging, irritation, and rawness. The discomfort may be constant or intermittent, focal or diffuse, and experienced as either deep or superficial. There are generally no physical findings except minimal erythema that may be associated with a subset of vulvodynia, vulvar vestibulitis. Vulvar vestibulitis is normally asymptomatic, but the pain is associated with touching or pressure on the vestibule such as with vaginal entry or insertion of a tampon.

Treatment

A. VULVOVAGINITIS

Lesions resembling warts on colposcopy or biopsy should be treated in the appropriate way (see Vaginitis). Irritation from spermicides may be a factor. The couple may be helped by a discussion of noncoital techniques to achieve orgasm until the infection subsides.

B. VAGINISMUS

Sexual counseling and education on anatomy and sexual functioning may be appropriate. The patient can be instructed in self-dilation, using a lubricated finger or test tubes of graduated sizes. Before coitus (with adequate lubrication) is attempted, the patient—and then her partner—should be able to easily and painlessly introduce two fingers into the vagina. Penetration should never be forced, and the woman should always be the one to control the depth of insertion during dilation or intercourse. Injection of botulinum toxin has been used successfully in refractory cases.

C. REMNANTS OF THE HYMEN

In rare situations, manual dilation of a remaining hymen under general anesthesia is necessary. Surgery should be avoided.

D. INSUFFICIENT LUBRICATION OF THE VAGINA

If inadequate sexual arousal is the cause, sexual counseling is helpful. Lubricants may be used during sexual foreplay. For women with low plasma estrogen levels, use of a lubricant during coitus is sometimes sufficient. If not, estrogen vaginal cream or an estradiol vaginal ring may be used. The ring may be worn continuously and replaced every 3 months. Concomitant progestin therapy is not needed with the ring.

E. INFECTION, ENDOMETRIOSIS, TUMORS, OR OTHER PATHOLOGIC CONDITIONS

Medical treatment of acute cervicitis, endometritis, or salpingitis and temporary abstention from coitus usually relieve pain. Hormonal or surgical treatment of endometriosis may be helpful. Dyspareunia resulting from chronic PID or any condition causing extensive adhesions or fixation of pelvic organs is difficult to treat without extirpative surgery. Couples can be advised to try coital positions that limit deep thrusting and to use manual and oral sexual techniques.

F. VULVODYNIA

Since the cause of vulvodynia is unknown, management is difficult. Few treatment approaches have been subjected to methodologically rigorous trials. A variety of topical agents have been tried, although only topical anesthetics (eg, estrogen cream and a compounded mixture of topical amitriptyline 2% and baclofen 2% in a water washable base) have been useful in relieving vulvodynia. Useful oral medications include tricyclic antidepressants, such as amitriptyline in gradually increasing doses from 10 mg/d to 75–100 mg/d; various selective serotonin reuptake inhibitors; and anticonvulsants, such as gabapentin starting with 300 mg three times a day and increasing to 1200 mg three times a day. Biofeedback and physical therapy, with a physical therapist experienced with the treatment of vulvar pain, have been shown to be helpful. Surgery—usually consisting of vestibulectomy—has been useful for women with introital dyspareunia.

Haefner HK et al: The vulvodynia guideline. J Low Genit Tract Dis 2005;9:40. [PMID: 15870521]

INFERTILITY

A couple is said to be infertile if pregnancy does not result after 1 year of normal sexual activity without contraceptives. About 25% of couples experience infertility at some point in their reproductive lives; the incidence of infertility increases with age. The male partner contributes to about 40% of cases of infertility, and a combination of factors is common.

Diagnostic Survey

During the initial interview, the clinician can present an overview of infertility and discuss a plan of study. Separate private consultations are then conducted, allowing appraisal of psychosexual adjustment without embarrassment or criticism. Pertinent details (eg, sexually transmitted disease or prior pregnancies) must be obtained. The ill effects of cigarettes, alcohol, and other recreational drugs on male fertility should be discussed. Prescription drugs that impair male potency should be discussed as well. The gynecologic history should include queries regarding the menstrual pattern. The present history includes use and types of contraceptives, douches, libido, sex techniques, frequency and success of coitus, and correlation of intercourse with time of ovulation. Family history includes repeated abortions and maternal DES use.

General physical and genital examinations are performed on both partners. Basic laboratory studies include complete blood count, urinalysis, cervical culture for *Chlamydia,* serologic test for syphilis, rubella antibody determination, and thyroid function tests. Tay-Sachs screening should be offered if both parents are Ashkenazi Jews as well as couples of French-Canadian or Cajun ancestry; sickle cell screening should be offered if both parents are black.

The patient is instructed to chart her basal body temperature orally daily on arising and to record on a graph episodes of coitus and days of menstruation. Self-performed urine tests for the midcycle LH surge enhance temperature observations relating to ovulation. Couples should be advised that coitus resulting in conception occurs during the 6-day period ending with the day of ovulation.

The male partner is instructed to bring a complete ejaculate for analysis. Men must abstain from sexual activity for at least 3 days before the semen is obtained. A clean, dry, wide-mouthed bottle for collection is preferred. Condoms should not be used, as the protective powder or lubricant may be spermicidal. Semen should be examined within 1–2 hours after collection. Semen is considered normal with the following minimum values: volume, 1.5–5 mL; concentration, 20 million sperm per milliliter; motility, 60%; and normal forms, 35%. If the sperm count is abnormal, further evaluation includes a search for exposure to environmental and workplace toxins, alcohol or drug abuse, and hypogonadism.

A. First Testing Cycle

While the contribution of cervical factors to infertility is controversial, most gynecologists include a postcoital test in their workup. The test is scheduled for just before ovulation (eg, day 12 or 13 in an expected 28-day cycle). Preovulation timing can be enhanced by serial urinary LH tests. The patient is examined within 6 hours after coitus. The cervical mucus should be clear, elastic, and copious owing to the influence of the preovular estrogen surge. (The mucus is scantier and more viscid before and after ovulation.) A good spinnbarkeit (stretching to a fine thread 4 cm or more in length) is desirable. A small drop of cervical mucus should be obtained from within the cervical os and examined under the microscope. The presence of five or more active sperm per high-power field constitutes a satisfactory postcoital test. If no spermatozoa are found, the test should be repeated (assuming that active spermatozoa were present in the semen analysis). Sperm agglutination and sperm immobilization tests should be considered if the sperm are immotile or show ineffective tail motility.

The presence of more than three white blood cells per high-power field in the postcoital test suggests cervicitis in the woman or prostatitis in the man. When estrogen levels are normal, the cervical mucus dried on the slide will form a fern-like pattern when viewed with a low-power microscope. This type of mucus is necessary for normal sperm transport.

The serum progesterone level should be measured at the midpoint of the secretory phase (21st day); a level of > 3 ng/mL confirms ovulation.

B. Second Testing Cycle

Hysterosalpingography using an oil dye is performed within 3 days following the menstrual period. This x-ray study will demonstrate uterine abnormalities (septa, polyps, submucous myomas) and tubal obstruction. A repeat x-ray film 24 hours later will confirm tubal patency if there is wide pelvic dispersion of the dye. This test has been associated with an increased pregnancy rate by some observers. If the woman has had prior pelvic inflammation, one should give doxycycline, 100 mg twice daily, beginning immediately before and for 7 days after the x-ray study.

C. Further Testing

1. Gross deficiencies of sperm (number, motility, or appearance) require repeat analysis. Zona-free hamster egg penetration tests are available to evaluate the ability of human sperm to fertilize an egg.

2. Obvious obstruction of the uterine tubes requires assessment for microsurgery or in vitro fertilization.

3. Absent or infrequent ovulation requires additional laboratory evaluation. Elevated FSH and LH levels indicate ovarian failure causing premature menopause. Elevated LH levels in the presence of normal FSH levels confirm the presence of polycystic ovaries. Elevation of blood prolactin (PRL) levels suggests pituitary microadenoma.

4. Ultrasound monitoring of folliculogenesis may reveal the occurrence of unruptured luteinized follicles.

5. Endometrial biopsy in the luteal phase associated with simultaneous serum progesterone levels will rule out luteal phase deficiency.

D. Laparoscopy

Approximately 25% of women whose basic evaluation is normal will have findings on laparoscopy explaining their infertility (eg, peritubal adhesions, endometriotic implants).

Treatment

A. Medical Measures

Fertility may be restored by appropriate treatment in many patients with endocrine imbalance, particularly those with hypothyroidism or hyperthyroidism. Antibiotic treatment of cervicitis is of value. In women with abnormal postcoital tests and demonstrated antisperm antibodies causing sperm agglutination or immobilization, condom use for up to 6 months may result in lower antibody levels and improved pregnancy rates.

Women who engage in vigorous athletic training often have low sex hormone levels; fertility improves with reduced exercise and some weight gain.

B. Surgical Measures

Excision of ovarian tumors or ovarian foci of endometriosis can improve fertility. Microsurgical relief of tubal obstruction due to salpingitis or tubal ligation will reestablish fertility in a significant number of cases. In special instances of cornual or fimbrial block, the prognosis with newer surgical techniques has become much better. Peritubal adhesions or endometriotic implants often can be treated via laparoscopy or via laparotomy immediately following laparoscopic examination if prior consent has been obtained.

With varicocele in the male, sperm characteristics are often improved following surgical treatment.

C. INDUCTION OF OVULATION

1. Clomiphene citrate—Clomiphene citrate stimulates gonadotropin release, especially LH. Consequently, plasma estrone (E_1) and estradiol (E_2) also rise, reflecting ovarian follicle maturation. If E_2 rises sufficiently, an LH surge occurs to trigger ovulation.

After a normal menstrual period or induction of withdrawal bleeding with progestin, one should give 50 mg of clomiphene orally daily for 5 days. If ovulation does not occur, the dosage is increased to 100 mg orally daily for 5 days. If ovulation still does not occur, the course is repeated with 150 mg daily and then 200 mg daily for 5 days, with the addition of chorionic gonadotropin, 10,000 units intramuscularly, 7 days after clomiphene.

The rate of ovulation following this treatment is 90% in the absence of other infertility factors. The pregnancy rate is high. Twinning occurs in 5% of these patients, and three or more fetuses are found in rare instances (< 0.5% of cases). An increased incidence of congenital anomalies has not been reported. Painful ovarian cyst formation occurs in 8% of patients and may warrant discontinuation of therapy. Several studies have suggested a twofold to threefold increased risk of ovarian cancer with the use of clomiphene for more than 1 year.

In the presence of increased androgen production (DHEA-S > 200 mcg/dL), the addition of dexamethasone, 0.5 mg, or prednisone, 5 mg, at bedtime, improves the response to clomiphene. Dexamethasone should be discontinued after pregnancy is confirmed.

2. Bromocriptine—Bromocriptine is used only if PRL levels are elevated and there is no withdrawal bleeding following progesterone administration (otherwise, clomiphene is used). To minimize side effects (nausea, diarrhea, dizziness, headache, fatigue), bromocriptine should be taken with meals. The initial dosage is 2.5 mg once daily, increased to two or three times daily in increments of 1.25 mg. The drug is discontinued once pregnancy has occurred.

3. Human menopausal gonadotropins (hMG)—hMG or recombinant FSH is indicated in cases of hypogonadotropism and most other types of anovulation (exclusive of ovarian failure). Because of the complexities, laboratory tests, and expense associated with this treatment, these patients should be referred to a specialist.

4. Gonadotropin-releasing hormone (GnRH)—Hypothalamic amenorrhea unresponsive to clomiphene will be reliably and successfully treated with subcutaneous pulsatile GnRH. Use of this substance will avoid the dangerous ovarian complications and the 25% incidence of multiple pregnancy associated with hMG, although the overall rate of ovulation and pregnancy is lower than when hMG is used.

D. TREATMENT OF ENDOMETRIOSIS

See above.

E. TREATMENT OF INADEQUATE TRANSPORT OF SPERM

Intrauterine insemination of concentrated washed sperm has been used to bypass a poor cervical environment associated with scant or hostile cervical mucus. The sperm must be handled by sterile methods, washed in sterile saline or tissue culture solutions, and centrifuged. A small amount of fluid (0.5 mL) containing the sperm is then instilled into the uterus.

F. ARTIFICIAL INSEMINATION IN AZOOSPERMIA

If azoospermia is present, artificial insemination by a donor usually results in pregnancy, assuming female function is normal. The use of frozen sperm is currently preferable to fresh sperm because the frozen specimen can be held pending cultures and blood test results for sexually transmitted diseases, including HIV infection.

G. ASSISTED REPRODUCTIVE TECHNOLOGIES (ART)

Couples who have not responded to traditional infertility treatments, including those with tubal disease, severe endometriosis, oligospermia, and immunologic or unexplained infertility, may benefit from in vitro fertilization (IVF), gamete intrafallopian transfer (GIFT), and zygote intrafallopian transfer (ZIFT). These techniques are complex and require a highly organized team of specialists. All of the procedures involve ovarian stimulation to produce multiple oocytes, oocyte retrieval by TVS-guided needle aspiration, and handling of the oocytes outside the body. With IVF, the eggs are fertilized in vitro and the embryos transferred to the uterine fundus. Intracytoplasmic sperm injection (ICSI) allows fertilization with a single sperm. It was originally intended for couples with male factor infertility, but it is now used in approximately half of all IVF procedures in the United States.

GIFT involves the placement of sperm and eggs in the uterine tube by laparoscopy or minilaparotomy. With ZIFT, fertilization occurs in vitro, and the early development of the embryo occurs in the uterine tube after transfer by laparoscopy or minilaparotomy. The later two procedures are used infrequently. In ART cycles using fresh, nondonor eggs, the overall rate of live births per cycle for the 399 programs reporting results in the United States in 2003 was 28.3%. Age is an important determinant of success—for couples under the age of 35, the average rate of live birth was 43% per cycle, while the rate for women over 42 was 5.9%. In 2003, 34.2% of pregnancies were multiple.

Prognosis

The prognosis for conception and normal pregnancy is good if minor (even multiple) disorders can be identified and treated; it is poor if the causes of infertility are severe, untreatable, or of prolonged duration (over 3 years).

It is important to remember that in the absence of identifiable causes of infertility, 60% of couples will achieve a pregnancy within 3 years. Couples with unexplained infertility who do not achieve pregnancy within 3 years should be offered ovulation induction or assisted reproductive technology. Also, offering appropriately timed information about adoption is considered part of a complete infertility regimen.

Centers for Disease Control and Prevention, American Society for Reproductive Medicine: 2003 Assisted Reproductive Technology Success Rates. 2005, Atlanta, GA. http://www.cdc.gov/ART/ART2003/index.htm

Frey KA et al: Initial evaluation and management of infertility by the primary care physician. Mayo Clin Proc 2004;79:1439. [PMID: 15544024]

CONTRACEPTION

Voluntary control of childbearing benefits women, men, and their children. Contraception should be available to all women and men of reproductive ages. Education about contraception and access to contraceptive pills or devices are especially important for sexually active teenagers and for women following childbirth or abortion.

1. Oral Contraceptives

Combined Oral Contraceptives

A. EFFICACY AND METHODS OF USE

Oral contraceptives have a perfect use failure rate of 0.3% and a typical use failure rate of 8%. Their primary mode of action is suppression of ovulation. The pills can be initially started on the first day of the menstrual cycle, the first Sunday after the onset of the cycle or on any day of the cycle. If started on any day other than the first day of the cycle, a backup method should be used. There are also pills packaged to be taken continuously for 84 days, followed by 7 days of placebos. If an active pill is missed at any time, and no intercourse occurred in the past 5 days, two pills should be taken immediately and a backup method should be used for 7 days. If intercourse occurred in the previous 5 days, emergency contraception should be used immediately, and the pills restarted the following day. A backup method should be used for 5 days.

B. BENEFITS OF ORAL CONTRACEPTIVES

Noncontraceptive benefits of oral contraceptives include lighter menses, reducing the likelihood of anemia. Dysmenorrhea is relieved for most women. Functional ovarian cysts are less likely with oral contraceptive use. The risk of ovarian and endometrial cancer is decreased. The risks of salpingitis and ectopic pregnancy may be diminished. Acne is usually improved. The frequency of developing myomas is lower in long-term users (> 4 years). There is a beneficial effect on bone mass.

C. SELECTION OF AN ORAL CONTRACEPTIVE

Any of the combination oral contraceptives containing 35 mcg or less of estrogen are suitable for most women. There is some variation in potency of the various progestins in the pills, but there are essentially no clinically significant differences for most women among the progestins in the low-dose pills. Women who have acne or hirsutism may benefit from use of one of the pills containing the third-generation progestins, desogestrel, drospirenone, or norgestimate, as they are the least androgenic. A combination regimen with 84 active and 7 inert pills that results in only four menses per year is available. The low-dose oral contraceptives commonly used in the United States are listed in Table 17–5.

Table 17–5. Commonly used low-dose oral contraceptives.

Name	Progestin	Estrogen (Ethinyl Estradiol)	Cost per Month[1]
COMBINATION			
Alesse	0.1 mg levonorgestrel	20 mcg	$35.32
Loestrin 1/20 Microgestin 1/20	1 mg norethindrone acetate	20 mcg	$50.33 $28.66
Mircette	0.15 mg desogestrel	20 mcg	$41.30
Loestrin 1.5/30 Microgestin 1.5/30	1.5 mg norethindrone acetate	30 mcg	$50.33 $28.94
Lo-Ovral Low-ogestrel	0.3 mg norgestrel	30 mcg	$37.54 $30.52
Nordette Levlen Levora	0.15 mg levonorgestrel	30 mcg	$50.33 $36.50 $30.93
Ortho-Cept Desogen	0.15 mg desogestrel	30 mcg	$48.33 $34.02

(continued)

Table 17–5. Commonly used low-dose oral contraceptives. (continued)

Name	Progestin	Estrogen (Ethinyl Estradiol)	Cost per Month[1]
Yasmin	3 mg drospirenone	30 mcg	$43.94
Brevicon Modicon Necon 0.5/35	0.5 mg norethindrone	35 mcg	$45.83 $52.71 $32.14
Demulen 1/35 Zovia 1/35E	1 mg ethynodiol diacetate	35 mcg	$37.07 $29.88
Norinyl 1/35 Ortho-Novum 1/35 Necon 1/35	1 mg norethindrone	35 mcg	$46.19 $48.33 $29.47
Ortho-Cyclen	0.25 mg norgestimate	35 mcg	$46.13
Ovcon 35	0.4 mg norethindrone	35 mcg	$42.92
COMBINATION: OTHER			
Seasonale	0.15 mg levonorgestrel	30 mcg	$51.13
TRIPHASIC			
Estrostep	1.0 mg norethindrone acetate (days 1–5) 1.0 mg norethindrone acetate (days 6–12) 1.0 mg norethindrone acetate (days 13–21)	20 mcg 30 mcg 35 mcg	$42.92
Cyclessa	0.1 mg desogestrel (days 1–7) 0.125 mg desogestrel (days 8–14) 0.15 mg desogestrel (days 15–21)	25 mcg	$39.52
Ortho-Tri-Cyclen Lo	0.18 norgestimate (days 1–7) 0.21 norgestimate (days 8–14) 0.25 norgestimate (days 15–21)	25 mcg	$44.07
Triphasil Trivora Tri-Levlen	0.05 mg levonorgestrel (days 1–6) 0.075 mg levonorgestrel (days 7–11) 0.125 mg levonorgestrel (days 12–21)	30 mcg 40 mcg 30 mcg	$31.90 $27.49 $34.88
Ortho-Novum 7/7/7	0.5 mg norethindrone (days 1–7) 0.75 mg norethindrone (days 8–14) 1 mg norethindrone (days 15–21)	35 mcg	$46.13
Ortho-Tri-Cyclen	0.15 mg norgestimate (days 1–7) 0.215 mg norgestimate (days 8–14) 0.25 mg norgestimate (days 15–21)	35 mcg	$41.99
Tri-Norinyl	0.5 mg norethindrone (days 1–7) 1 mg norethindrone (days 8–16) 0.5 mg norethindrone (days 17–21)	35 mcg	$44.08
PROGESTIN-ONLY MINIPILL			
Ortho Micronor Nor-QD	0.35 mg norethindrone to be taken continuously	(None)	$56.13 $48.80
Ovrette	0.075 mg norgestrel to be taken continuously	(None)	$35.34

[1]Average wholesale price (AWP, for AB-rated generic when available) for quantity listed. Source: *Red Book Update*, Vol. 25, No. 1, January 2006. AWP may not accurately represent the actual pharmacy cost because wide contractual variations exist among institutions.

D. DRUG INTERACTIONS

Several drugs interact with oral contraceptives to decrease their efficacy by causing induction of microsomal enzymes in the liver, by increasing sex hormone-binding globulin, and by other mechanisms. Some commonly prescribed drugs in this category are phenytoin, phenobarbital (and other barbiturates), primidone, carbamazepine, and rifampin. Women taking these drugs should use another means of contraception for maximum safety.

E. CONTRAINDICATIONS AND ADVERSE EFFECTS

Oral contraceptives have been associated with many adverse effects; they are contraindicated in some situations and should be used with caution in others (Table 17–6).

1. Myocardial infarction—The risk of heart attack is higher with use of oral contraceptives, particularly with pills containing 50 mcg of estrogen or more. Cigarette smoking, obesity, hypertension, diabetes, or hypercholesterolemia increases the risk. Young nonsmoking women have minimal increased risk. Smokers over age 35 and women with other cardiovascular risk factors should use other methods of birth control.

2. Thromboembolic disease—An increased rate of venous thromboembolism is found in oral contracep-

Table 17–6. Contraindications to use of oral contraceptives.

Absolute contraindications
Pregnancy
Thrombophlebitis or thromboembolic disorders (past or present)
Stroke or coronary artery disease (past or present)
Cancer of the breast (known or suspected)
Undiagnosed abnormal vaginal bleeding
Estrogen-dependent cancer (known or suspected)
Benign or malignant tumor of the liver (past or present)
Uncontrolled hypertension
Diabetes with vascular disease
Age over 35 and smoking > 15 cigarettes daily
Known thrombophilia
Migraine with aura
Active hepatitis
Surgery or orthopedic injury requiring prolonged immobilization
Relative contraindications
Migraine without aura
Hypertension
Cardiac or renal disease
Diabetes
Gallbladder disease
Cholestasis during pregnancy
Sickle cell disease (S/S or S/C type)
Lactation

---

tive users, especially if the dose of estrogen is 50 mcg or more. While the overall risk is very low (15 per 100,000 woman-years), several studies have reported a twofold increased risk in women using oral contraceptives containing the progestins gestodene (not available in the United States) or desogestrel compared with women using oral contraceptives with levonorgestrel and norethindrone. Women in whom thrombophlebitis develops should stop using this method, as should those at risk for thrombophlebitis because of surgery, fracture, serious injury, or immobilization. Women with a known thrombophilia should not use oral contraceptives.

3. Cerebrovascular disease—Overall, a small increased risk of hemorrhagic stroke and subarachnoid hemorrhage and a somewhat greater increased risk of thrombotic stroke has been found; smoking, hypertension, and age over 35 years are associated with increased risk. Women should stop using contraceptives if such warning symptoms as severe headache, blurred or lost vision, or other transient neurologic disorders develop.

4. Carcinoma—A relationship between long-term (3–4 years) oral contraceptive use and occurrence of cervical dysplasia and cancer has been found in various studies. A 2002 study showed that there is no increased risk of breast cancer in women aged 35–64 who are current or former users of oral contraceptives. Women with a family history of breast cancer or women who started oral contraceptive use at a young age are not at increased risk. Combination oral contraceptives reduce the risk of endometrial carcinoma by 40% after 2 years of use and 60% after 4 or more years of use. The risk of ovarian cancer is reduced by 30% with pill use for less than 4 years, by 60% with use for 5–11 years, and by 80% after 12 or more years. Rarely, oral contraceptives have been associated with the development of benign or malignant hepatic tumors; this may lead to rupture of the liver, hemorrhage, and death. The risk increases with higher dosage, longer duration of use, and older age.

5. Hypertension—Oral contraceptives may cause hypertension in some women; the risk is increased with longer duration of use and older age. Women in whom hypertension develops while using oral contraceptives should use other contraceptive methods. However, with regular blood pressure monitoring, nonsmoking women under the age of 40 with well-controlled mild hypertension may use oral contraceptives.

6. Headache—Migraine or other vascular headaches may occur or worsen with pill use. If severe or frequent headaches develop while using this method, it should be discontinued. Women with migraine headaches with an aura should not use oral contraceptives.

7. Lactation—Combined oral contraceptives can impair the quantity and quality of breast milk. While it is preferable to avoid the use of combination oral contraceptives during lactation, the effects on milk quality are small and are not associated with developmental abnormalities in infants. Combination oral contraceptives should be started no earlier than 6 weeks postpartum to allow for establishment of lactation. Progestin-only pills, levonorgestrel implants, and depot medroxyprogesterone acetate are alternatives with no adverse effects on milk quality.

8. Other disorders—Depression may occur or be worsened with oral contraceptive use. Fluid retention may occur. Patients who had cholestatic jaundice during pregnancy may develop it while taking birth control pills.

F. MINOR SIDE EFFECTS

Nausea and dizziness may occur in the first few months of pill use. A weight gain of 2–5 lb commonly occurs. Spotting or breakthrough bleeding between menstrual periods may occur, especially if a pill is skipped or taken late; this may be helped by switching to a pill of slightly greater potency (see section C, above). Missed menstrual periods may occur, especially with low-dose pills. A pregnancy test should be performed if pills have been skipped or if two or more menstrual periods are missed. Depression, fatigue, and decreased libido can occur. Chloasma may occur, as in pregnancy, and is increased by exposure to sunlight.

Progestin Minipill

A. EFFICACY AND METHODS OF USE

Formulations containing 0.35 mg of norethindrone or 0.075 mg of norgestrel are available in the United States. Their efficacy is similar to that of combined oral contraceptives. The minipill is believed to prevent conception by causing thickening of the cervical mucus to make it hostile to sperm, alteration of ovum transport (which may account for the higher rate of ectopic pregnancy with these pills), and inhibition of implantation. Ovulation is inhibited inconsistently with this method. The minipill is begun on the first day of a menstrual cycle and then taken continuously for as long as contraception is desired.

B. ADVANTAGES

The low dose and absence of estrogen make the minipill safe during lactation; it may increase the flow of milk. It is often tried by women who want minimal doses of hormones and by patients who are over age 35. They lack the cardiovascular side effects of combination pills. The minipill can be safely used by women with sickle cell disease (S/S or S/C).

C. COMPLICATIONS AND CONTRAINDICATIONS

Minipill users often have bleeding irregularities (eg, prolonged flow, spotting, or amenorrhea); such patients may need regular pregnancy tests. Ectopic pregnancies are more frequent, and complaints of abdominal pain should be investigated with this in mind. The absolute contraindications and many of the relative contraindications listed in Table 17–6 apply to the minipill. Minor

side effects of combination oral contraceptives such as weight gain and mild headache may also occur with the minipill.

Hatcher RA et al: Contraceptive Technology 18th edition 2004. Ardent Media, New York.

Reproductive Health and Research; World Health Organization: Medical Eligibilty Criteria for Contraceptive Use. WHO/RHR 2004, Geneva. http://www.who.int/reproductive-health/publications/mec/index.htm

Reproductive Health and Research; World Health Organization: Selected Practice Recommendations for Contraceptive Use. WHO/RHR 2004, Geneva. http://www.who.int/reproductive-health/publications/spr/index.htm

Seibert C et al: Prescribing oral contraceptives for women older than 35 years of age. Ann Intern Med 2003;138:54. [PMID: 12513046]

2. Contraceptive Injections & Implants (Long-Acting Progestins)

The injectable progestin medroxyprogesterone acetate (DMPA) is approved for contraceptive use in the United States. There is extensive worldwide experience with this method over the past 3 decades. The medication is given as a deep intramuscular injection of 150 mg every 3 months and has a contraceptive efficacy of 99.7%. A subcutaneous preparation, containing 104 mg of DMPA is available in the United States. Common side effects include irregular bleeding, amenorrhea, weight gain, and headache. It is associated with bone mineral loss that is usually reversible after discontinuation of the method. Users commonly have irregular bleeding initially and subsequently develop amenorrhea. Ovulation may be delayed after the last injection. Contraindications are similar to those for the minipill.

A monthly injectable containing both depot medroxyprogesterone acetate and an estrogen, estradiol cypionate (Lunelle), has been available in the United States, although it is not being marketed currently. It is highly effective, with a first-year pregnancy rate of 0.2% and a side effect profile similar to that of oral contraceptives.

The other long-acting progestin contraceptive is the Norplant system, a contraceptive implant containing levonorgestrel that is no longer available in the United States. The system consists of six small Silastic capsules that are inserted subcutaneously in the inner aspect of the upper arm. They release daily and provide highly effective contraception for 5 years. In the first year of use, Norplant is 99.8% effective. Contraceptive effectiveness drops slightly in succeeding years, but even in the fifth year it is more effective than the combination pill. The most common side effects include irregular bleeding and spotting, amenorrhea, headache, acne, and weight gain. Irregular bleeding is the most common reason for discontinuation. Hormone levels drop rapidly after removal of the implants, and there is no delay in the return of fertility. Contraindications are similar to those for the minipill. Insertion of the implants requires a minor surgical procedure under local anesthesia. Removal is also done under local anesthesia and may be more difficult than insertion. Removal may be facilitated by the "U" technique, involving use of a modified vasectomy clamp through a 4-mm incision parallel to the implants between implants three and four.

Berenson AB et al: Effects of hormonal contraception on bone mineral density after 24 months of use. Obstet Gynecol 2004; 103:899. [PMID: 15121563]

Kaunitz AM: Beyond the pill: new data and options in hormonal and intrauterine contraception. Am J Obstet Gynecol 2005; 192:998. [PMID: 15846172]

World Health Organization: WHO Statement on Hormonal Contraception and Bone Health 2005 http://www.who.nt/reproductive-health/family_planning/docs/hormonal_contraception_bone_health.pdf

3. Other Hormonal Methods

A transdermal contraceptive patch containing 150 mcg norelgestromin and 20 mcg ethinyl estradiol and measuring 20 cm^2 is available. The patch is applied to the lower abdomen, upper torso, or buttock once a week for 3 consecutive weeks, followed by 1 week without the patch. It appears that the average steady-state concentration of ethinyl estradiol with the patch is approximately 60% higher than with a 35 mcg pill. However, there is currently no evidence for an increased incidence of estrogen-related side effects. The mechanism of action, side effects, and efficacy are similar to those associated with oral contraceptives, although compliance may be better.

A contraceptive vaginal ring that measures 54 mm in diameter and releases 120 mcg of etonogestrel and 15 mcg of ethinyl estradiol daily is available. The ring is soft and flexible and is placed in the upper vagina for 3 weeks, removed, and replaced 1 week later. The efficacy, mechanism of action, and systemic side effects are similar to those associated with oral contraceptives. In addition, users may experience an increased incidence of vaginal discharge.

Veres S et al: A comparison between the vaginal ring and oral contraceptives. Obstet Gynecol 2004;104:555. [PMID: 15339769]

4. Intrauterine Devices

IUDs available in the United States include the Mirena (which releases levonorgestrel) and the copper-bearing TCu380A. The mechanism of action of IUDs is thought to involve either spermicidal or inhibitory effects on sperm capacitation and transport. IUDs are not abortifacients.

The Mirena is effective for 5 years, and the TCu380A for 10 years. The hormone-containing IUDs have the advantage of reducing cramping and menstrual flow.

The IUD is an excellent contraceptive method for most women. The devices are highly effective, with failure rates similar to those achieved with surgical sterilization. Nulliparity is not a contraindication to IUD use.

Women who are not in mutually monogamous relationships should use condoms for protection from sexually transmitted diseases. The Mirena may have a protective effect against upper tract infection similar to that of the oral contraceptives.

Insertion

Insertion can be performed during or after the menses, at midcycle to prevent implantation, or later in the cycle if the patient has not become pregnant. Most clinicians wait for 6–8 weeks postpartum before inserting an IUD. When insertion is performed during lactation, there is greater risk of uterine perforation or embedding of the IUD. Insertion immediately following abortion is acceptable if there is no sepsis and if follow-up insertion a month later will not be possible; otherwise, it is wise to wait until 4 weeks postabortion.

Contraindications & Complications

Contraindications to use of IUDs are outlined in Table 17–7.

A. PREGNANCY

A copper-containing IUD can be inserted within 5 days following a single episode of unprotected mid-cycle coitus as a postcoital contraceptive. An IUD should not be inserted into a pregnant uterus. If pregnancy occurs as an IUD failure, there is a greater chance of spontaneous abortion if the IUD is left in situ (50%) than if it is removed (25%). Spontaneous abortion with an IUD in place is associated with a high risk of severe sepsis, and death can occur rapidly. Women using an IUD who become pregnant should have the IUD removed if the string is visible. It can be removed at the time of abortion if this is desired. If the string is not visible and the patient wants to continue the pregnancy, she should be informed of the serious risk of sepsis and, occasionally, death with such pregnancies. She should be informed that any flu-

Table 17–7. Contraindications to IUD use.

Absolute contraindications
Pregnancy
Acute or subacute pelvic inflammatory disease or purulent cervicitis
Significant anatomic abnormality of uterus
Unexplained uterine bleeding
Active liver disease (Mirena only)
Relative contraindications
History of pelvic inflammatory disease since the last pregnancy
Lack of available follow-up care
Menorrhagia or severe dysmenorrhea (copper IUD)
Cervical or uterine neoplasia

IUD = intrauterine device.

like symptoms such as fever, myalgia, headache, or nausea warrant immediate medical attention for possible septic abortion.

Since the ratio of ectopic to intrauterine pregnancies is increased among IUD wearers, clinicians should search for adnexal masses in early pregnancy and should always check the products of conception for placental tissue following abortion.

B. PELVIC INFECTION

There is an increased risk of pelvic infection during the first month following insertion. The subsequent risk of pelvic infection appears to be primarily related to the risk of acquiring sexually transmitted infections. Infertility rates do not appear to be increased among women who have previously used the currently available IUDs. At the time of insertion, women with an increased risk of sexually transmitted diseases should be screened for gonorrhea and *Chlamydia*. Women with a history of recent or recurrent pelvic infection are not good candidates for IUD use.

C. MENORRHAGIA OR SEVERE DYSMENORRHEA

The copper IUD can cause heavier menstrual periods, bleeding between periods, and more cramping, so it is generally not suitable for women who already suffer from these problems. However, hormone-releasing IUDs can be tried in these cases, as they often cause decreased bleeding and cramping with menses. NSAIDs are also helpful in decreasing bleeding and pain in IUD users.

D. COMPLETE OR PARTIAL EXPULSION

Spontaneous expulsion of the IUD occurs in 10–20% of cases during the first year of use. Any IUD should be removed if the body of the device can be seen or felt in the cervical os.

E. MISSING IUD STRINGS

If the transcervical tail cannot be seen, this may signify unnoticed expulsion, perforation of the uterus with abdominal migration of the IUD, or simply retraction of the string into the cervical canal or uterus owing to movement of the IUD or uterine growth with pregnancy. Once pregnancy is ruled out, one should probe for the IUD with a sterile sound or forceps designed for IUD removal, after administering a paracervical block. If the IUD cannot be detected, pelvic ultrasound will demonstrate the IUD if it is in the uterus. Alternatively, obtain anteroposterior and lateral x-rays of the pelvis with another IUD or a sound in the uterus as a marker, to confirm an extrauterine IUD. If the IUD is in the abdominal cavity, it should generally be removed by laparoscopy or laparotomy. Open-looped all-plastic IUDs such as the Lippes Loop can be left in the pelvis without danger, but ring-shaped IUDs may strangulate a loop of bowel and copper-bearing IUDs may cause tissue reaction and adhesions.

Perforations of the uterus are less likely if insertion is performed slowly, with meticulous care taken to follow directions applicable to each type of IUD.

ACOG Committee on Practice Bulletins-Gynecology: ACOG practice bulletin. Clinical Management Guidelines for Obstetrician-Gynecologists. Number 59, January 2005. Intrauterine device. Obstet Gynecol 2005;105:223. [PMID: 15625179]

5. Diaphragm & Cervical Cap

The diaphragm (with contraceptive jelly) is a safe and effective contraceptive method with features that make it acceptable to some women and not others. Failure rates range from 6% to 16%, depending on the motivation of the woman and the care with which the diaphragm is used. The advantages of this method are that it has no systemic side effects and gives significant protection against pelvic infection and cervical dysplasia as well as pregnancy. The disadvantages are that it must be inserted near the time of coitus and that pressure from the rim predisposes some women to cystitis after intercourse.

The cervical cap (with contraceptive jelly) is similar to the diaphragm but fits snugly over the cervix only (the diaphragm stretches from behind the cervix to behind the pubic symphysis). The cervical cap is more difficult to insert and remove than the diaphragm. The main advantages are that it can be used by women who cannot be fitted for a diaphragm because of a relaxed anterior vaginal wall or by women who have discomfort or develop repeated bladder infections with the diaphragm. However, failure rates are 16% (typical use) and 9% (perfect use) in nulliparous women and 32% (typical use) and 26% (perfect use) in parous women.

Because of the small risk of toxic shock syndrome, a cervical cap or diaphragm should not be left in the vagina for over 12–18 hours, nor should these devices be used during the menstrual period.

6. Contraceptive Foam, Cream, Film, Sponge, Jelly, & Suppository

These products are available without prescription, are easy to use, and are fairly effective, with typical failure rates of 10–22%. All contain the spermicide nonoxynol-9, which also has some virucidal and bactericidal activity. Nonoxynol-9 does not appear to adversely affect the vaginal colonization of hydrogen peroxide-producing lactobacilli. A 2002 study suggests that nonoxynol-9 is not protective against HIV infection, particularly in women who have frequent intercourse.

Raymond EG et al: Contraceptive effectiveness and safety of five nonoxynol-9 spermicides: a randomized trial. Obstet Gynecol 2004;103;430. [PMID: 14990402]

Van Damme L et al: Effectiveness of COL-1492, a nonoxynol-9 vaginal gel, on HIV-1 transmission in female sex workers: a randomised controlled trial. Lancet 2002;360:971. [PMID: 12383665]

7. Condom

The male condom of latex or animal membrane affords good protection against pregnancy—equivalent to that of a diaphragm and spermicidal jelly; latex (but not animal membrane) condoms also offer protection against many sexually transmitted diseases, including HIV. When a spermicide, such as vaginal foam, is used with the condom, the failure rate approaches that of oral contraceptives. The disadvantages of condoms are dulling of sensation and spillage of semen due to tearing, slipping, or leakage with detumescence of the penis.

A female condom made of polyurethane is available in the United States. The reported failure rates range from 5% to 21%; the efficacy is comparable to that of the diaphragm. This is the only female-controlled method that offers significant protection from both pregnancy and sexually transmitted diseases.

Holmes KK et al: Effectiveness of condoms in preventing sexually transmitted infections. Bull World Health Organ 2004;82: 454. [PMID: 15356939]

8. Contraception Based on Awareness of Fertile Periods

These methods are most effective when the couple restricts intercourse to the postovular phase of the cycle or uses a barrier method at other times. Well-instructed, motivated couples may be able to achieve low pregnancy rates with fertility awareness methods. However, properly done randomized clinical trials comparing the efficacy of most of these methods with other contraceptive methods do not exist.

Grimes DA et al: Fertility awareness-based methods for contraception: systematic review of randomized controlled trials. Contraception 2005;72:85. [PMID: 16022845]

"Symptothermal" Natural Family Planning

The basis for this approach is patient-observed increase in clear elastic cervical mucus, brief abdominal midcycle discomfort ("mittelschmerz"), and a sustained rise of the basal body temperature about 2 weeks after onset of menstruation. Unprotected intercourse is avoided from shortly after the menstrual period, when fertile mucus is first identified, until 48 hours after ovulation, as identified by a sustained rise in temperature and the disappearance of clear elastic mucus.

Calendar Method

After the length of the menstrual cycle has been observed for at least 8 months, the following calculations are made: (1) The first fertile day is determined by subtracting 18 days from the shortest cycle, and (2) the last fertile day is determined by subtracting 11 days from the longest cycle. For example, if the observed cycles run from 24 to 28 days, the fertile period would extend from the sixth day of the cycle (24 minus 18) through the 17th day (28 minus 11). Day 1 of the cycle is the first day of menses.

Basal Body Temperature Method

This method indicates the safe time for intercourse after ovulation has passed. The temperature must be taken immediately upon awakening, before any activity. A slight drop in temperature often occurs 12–24 hours before ovulation, and a rise of about 0.4°C occurs 1–2 days after ovulation. The elevated temperature continues throughout the remainder of the cycle. Data suggest that the risk of pregnancy increases starting 5 days prior to the day of ovulation, peaks on the day of ovulation, and then rapidly decreases to zero by the day after ovulation.

Standard Days Method

This fertility awareness method requires the use of a set of beads that reminds the couple to avoid intercourse (or use a barrier method of contraception) during days 8 through 19 of the menstrual cycle. The beads are in a circle and color-coded to show the days when a woman is likely to become pregnant and the days that are "safe" during the cycle. A movable ring is repositioned to a new bead each day starting on the first day of menses. In a small multicenter trial, the perfect use failure rate was 5% and the typical use failure rate was 12%. The method is applicable to women with a history of menstrual cycles between 29 and 32 days.

Arevalo M et al: Efficacy of a new method of family planning: the Standard Days Method. Contraception 2002;65:333. [PMID: 12057784]

TwoDay Method

The TwoDay method requires that women be able to identify cervical secretions by observation or touching them in underwear or toilet paper, by touching the genitals, or by the sensation of wetness in the genital area or on underwear. The woman then uses a two-question algorithm to determine whether she is fertile. She asks herself: 1) Did I note secretions today? and 2) Did I note secretions yesterday? If the answer to either of these questions is "yes," she should consider herself fertile. In a multicenter study of 450 women, effectiveness with perfect use was 96.5% and with typical use 76.3%.

Arevelo M et al: Efficacy of the new TwoDay Method of family planning. Fertil Steril 2004;82:885. [PMID: 15482764]

9. Emergency Contraception

If unprotected intercourse occurs in midcycle and the woman is certain she has not inadvertently become pregnant earlier in the cycle, the following regimens are effective in preventing implantation. These methods should be started as soon as possible and within 120 hours after unprotected coitus. (1) Levonorgestrel, 0.75 mg given in two doses 12 hours apart (available in the United States prepackaged as Plan B), has a 1% failure rate, when taken within 72 hours, and is associated with less nausea and vomiting than the following combination regimen. A recent study has demonstrated that levonorgestrel, 1.5 mg as a single dose, given within 72 hours after intercourse, is slightly more effective than the two-dose regimen. It remains efficacious up to 120 hours after intercourse, though less so compared with earlier use. (2) Ethinyl estradiol, 50 mcg, with 0.5 mg norgestrel (available in the United States prepackaged as Preven), given in a regimen of two tablets initially followed by two tablets 12 hours later. A comparable regimen includes four pills 12 hours apart of Lo/Ovral, Nordette, or Levlen, or the same regimen with the yellow pills of Triphasil or Tri-Levlen. The failure rate is approximately 3%, and antinausea medication should be provided. Mifepristone, 10 mg as a single dose, has been shown to have the same failure rate as the levonorgestrel regimen. It is not currently available at this dose in the United States.

IUD insertion within 5 days after one episode of unprotected midcycle coitus will also prevent pregnancy; copper-bearing IUDs have been tested for this purpose. Information on clinics or individual clinicians providing emergency contraception in the United States may be obtained by calling 1-888-668-2528.

American College of Obstetricians and Gynecologists: ACOG Practice Bulletin. Clinical Management Guidelines for Obstetrician-Gynecologists, Number 69, December 2005. Emergency contraception. Obstet Gynecol 2005;106:1443. [PMID: 16319278]

von Hertzen H et al: Low dose mifepristone and two regimens of levonorgestrel for emergency contraception: a WHO multicentre randomized trial. Lancet 2002;360:1803. [PMID: 12480356]

10. Abortion

Since the legalization of abortion in the United States in 1973, the related maternal mortality rate has fallen markedly, because illegal and self-induced abortions have been replaced by safer medical procedures. Abortions in the first trimester of pregnancy are performed by vacuum aspiration under local anesthesia or with medical regimens. Dilation and evacuation, a variation of vacuum aspiration is generally used in the second trimester. Techniques utilizing intra-amniotic instillation of hypertonic saline solution or various prostaglandins regimens, along with medical or osmotic dilators are occasionally used after 18 weeks. Overall, legal abortion in the United States has a mortality rate of less than 1:100,000. Rates of morbidity and mortality rise with length of gestation. Currently in the United States, 87% of abortions are performed before 13 weeks' gestation and only 1.4% are performed after 20 weeks. If abortion is chosen, every effort should be made to encourage the patient to seek an early procedure. While numerous state laws limiting access to abortion and a federal law banning a rarely-used variation of dilation and evacuation have been enacted,

abortion remains legal and available until fetal viability under Roe v. Wade.

Complications resulting from abortion include retained products of conception (often associated with infection and heavy bleeding) and unrecognized ectopic pregnancy. Immediate analysis of the removed tissue for placenta can exclude or corroborate the diagnosis of ectopic pregnancy. Women who have fever, bleeding, or abdominal pain after abortion should be examined; use of broad-spectrum antibiotics and reaspiration of the uterus are frequently necessary. Hospitalization is advisable if acute salpingitis requires intravenous administration of antibiotics. Complications following illegal abortion often need emergency care for hemorrhage, septic shock, or uterine perforation.

Rh immune globulin should be given to all Rh-negative women following abortion. Contraception should be thoroughly discussed and contraceptive supplies or pills provided at the time of abortion. Prophylactic antibiotics are indicated; for example a one-dose regimen of doxycycline, 200 mg orally 1 hour before the procedure. Many clinics prescribe tetracycline, 500 mg four times daily for 5 days after the procedure, as presumptive treatment for *Chlamydia*.

Long-term sequelae of repeated induced abortions have been studied, but as yet there is no consensus on whether there are increased rates of fetal loss or premature labor. It is felt that such adverse sequelae can be minimized by performing early abortion with minimal cervical dilation or by the use of osmotic dilators to induce gradual cervical dilation. A population-based study showed no evidence of an increased risk of breast cancer in women who had undergone an induced abortion.

Mifepristone (RU 486) is approved by the FDA as an oral abortifacient; the dose is 600 mg orally on day 1. It is followed by 400 mcg orally of misoprostol (a prostaglandin) on day 3. This combination is 95% successful in terminating pregnancies of up to 9 weeks' duration with minimum complications. Although not approved by the FDA for this indication, a combination of intramuscular methotrexate, 50 mg/m^2 of body surface area, followed 7 days later by vaginal misoprostol, 800 mcg, was 98% successful in terminating pregnancy at 8 weeks or less. Minor side effects, such as nausea, vomiting, and diarrhea, are common with these regimens. There is a 5–10% incidence of hemorrhage or incomplete abortion requiring curettage. There is a recent report of four deaths occurring within 1 week of medical abortion, associated with endometritis and toxic shock caused by *Clostridium sordellii*. To improve diagnosis and treatment of this entity, clinicians should be aware of the constellation of presenting symptoms of tachycardia, hypotension, edema, hemoconcentration, profound leukocytosis, and absence of fever.

ACOG: ACOG practice bulletin: Clinical management guidelines of Obstetrician-Gynecologists. Number 67, October 2005. Medical management of abortion. Obstet Gynecol 2005;106:871. [PMID: 16199653]

Fischer M et al: Fatal toxic shock syndrome associated with *Clostridium sordellii* after medical abortion. N Engl J Med 2005;353:2352. [PMID: 16319384]

Grimes DA et al: Induced abortion: an overview for internists. Ann Intern Med 2004;140:620. [PMID: 15096333]

11. Sterilization

In the United States, sterilization is the most popular method of birth control for couples who want no more children. Although sterilization is reversible in some instances, reversal surgery in both men and women is costly, complicated, and not always successful. Therefore, patients should be counseled carefully before sterilization and should view the procedure as final.

Vasectomy is a safe, simple procedure in which the vas deferens is severed and sealed through a scrotal incision under local anesthesia. Long-term follow-up studies on vasectomized men show no excess risk of cardiovascular disease. Several studies have shown a possible association with prostate cancer, but the evidence is weak and inconsistent.

Female sterilization procedures include laparoscopic bipolar electrocoagulation, or plastic ring application on the uterine tubes, or minilaparotomy with Pomeroy tubal resection. The advantages of laparoscopy are minimal postoperative pain, small incisions, and rapid recovery. The advantages of minilaparotomy are that it can be performed with standard surgical instruments under local or general anesthesia. However, there is more postoperative pain and a longer recovery period. The cumulative 10-year failure rate for all methods combined is 1.85%, varying from 0.75% for postpartum partial salpingectomy and laparoscopic unipolar coagulation to 3.65% for spring clips; this fact should be discussed with women preoperatively. Some studies have found an increased risk of menstrual irregularities as a long-term complication of tubal ligation, but findings in different studies have been inconsistent. A new method of transcervical sterilization, Essure, is approved by the FDA. The method involves the placement of an expanding microcoil of titanium into the proximal uterine tube under hysteroscopic guidance. The efficacy rate at 1 year is 99.8%.

Magos A et al: Hysteroscopic tubal sterilization. Obstet Gynecol Clin North Am 2004;31:705. [PMID: 15450329]

Pollack A et al: ACOG practice bulletin. Benefits and risks of sterilization. Obstet Gynecol 2003;102:647. [PMID: 12962966]

RAPE

ESSENTIALS OF DIAGNOSIS

- *Women neither secretly want to be raped nor do they expect, encourage, or enjoy rape.*
- *Rape is always a terrifying experience in which most victims fear for their lives.*

- *The rapist is usually a hostile man who uses sexual intercourse to terrorize and humiliate a woman.*

General Considerations

Rape, or sexual assault, is legally defined in different ways in various jurisdictions. Clinicians and emergency department personnel who deal with rape victims should be familiar with the laws pertaining to sexual assault in their own state. From a medical and psychological viewpoint, it is essential that persons treating rape victims recognize the nonconsensual and violent nature of the crime. About 95% of reported rape victims are women. Penetration may be vaginal, anal, or oral and may be by the penis, hand, or a foreign object. The absence of genital injury does not imply consent by the victim. The assailant may be unknown to the victim or, more frequently, may be an acquaintance or even the spouse.

"Unlawful sexual intercourse," or statutory rape, is intercourse with a female before the age of majority even with her consent.

Rape represents an expression of anger, power, and sexuality on the part of the rapist. The rapist is usually a hostile man who uses sexual intercourse to terrorize and humiliate a woman. Women neither secretly want to be raped nor do they expect, encourage, or enjoy rape.

Rape involves severe physical injury in 5–10% of cases and is always a terrifying experience in which most victims fear for their lives. Consequently, all victims suffer some psychological aftermath. Moreover, some rape victims may acquire sexually transmissible disease or become pregnant.

Because rape is a personal crisis, each patient will react differently. The rape trauma syndrome comprises two principal phases. (1) Immediate or acute: Shaking, sobbing, and restless activity may last from a few days to a few weeks. The patient may experience anger, guilt, or shame or may repress these emotions. Reactions vary depending on the victim's personality and the circumstances of the attack. (2) Late or chronic: Problems related to the attack may develop weeks or months later. The lifestyle and work patterns of the individual may change. Sleep disorders or phobias often develop. Loss of self-esteem can rarely lead to suicide.

Clinicians and emergency department personnel who deal with rape victims should work with community rape crisis centers whenever possible to provide ongoing support and counseling.

General Office Procedures

The clinician who first sees the alleged rape victim should be empathetic. Begin with a statement such as, "This is a terrible thing that has happened to you. I want to help."

1. Secure written consent from the patient, guardian, or next of kin for gynecologic examination and for photographs if they are likely to be useful as evidence. If police are to be notified, do so, and obtain advice on the preservation and transfer of evidence.

2. Obtain and record the history in the patient's own words. The sequence of events, ie, the time, place, and circumstances, must be included. Note the date of the LMP, whether or not the woman is pregnant, and the time of the most recent coitus prior to the sexual assault. Note the details of the assault such as body cavities penetrated, use of foreign objects, and number of assailants. Note whether the victim is calm, agitated, or confused (drugs or alcohol may be involved). Record whether the patient came directly to the hospital or whether she bathed or changed her clothing. Record findings but do not issue even a tentative diagnosis lest it be erroneous or incomplete.

3. Have the patient disrobe while standing on a white sheet. Hair, dirt, and leaves, underclothing, and any torn or stained clothing should be kept as evidence. Scrape material from beneath fingernails and comb pubic hair for evidence. Place all evidence in separate clean paper bags or envelopes and label carefully.

4. Examine the patient, noting any traumatized areas that should be photographed. Examine the body and genitals with a Wood light to identify semen, which fluoresces; positive areas should be swabbed with a premoistened swab and air-dried in order to identify acid phosphatase. Colposcopy can be used to identify small areas of trauma from forced entry especially at the posterior fourchette.

5. Perform a pelvic examination, explaining all procedures and obtaining the patient's consent before proceeding gently with the examination. Use a narrow speculum lubricated with water only. Collect material with sterile cotton swabs from the vaginal walls and cervix and make two air-dried smears on clean glass slides. Wet and dry swabs of vaginal secretions should be collected and refrigerated for subsequent acid phosphatase and DNA evaluation. Swab the mouth (around molars and cheeks) and anus in the same way, if appropriate. Label all slides carefully. Collect secretions from the vagina, anus, or mouth with a premoistened cotton swab, place at once on a slide with a drop of saline, and cover with a coverslip. Look for motile or nonmotile sperm under high, dry magnification, and record the percentage of motile forms.

6. Perform appropriate laboratory tests as follows. Culture the vagina, anus, or mouth (as appropriate) for *N gonorrhoeae* and *Chlamydia*. Perform a Papanicolaou smear of the cervix, a wet mount for *Trichomonas vaginalis*, a baseline pregnancy test, and VDRL test. A confidential test for HIV antibody can be obtained if desired by the patient and repeated in 2–4 months if initially negative. Repeat the pregnancy test if the next menses is missed, and repeat the VDRL test in 6 weeks. Obtain blood (10 mL without anticoagulant) and urine (100 mL) specimens if there is a history of forced ingestion or injection of drugs or alcohol.

7. Transfer clearly labeled evidence, eg, laboratory specimens, directly to the clinical pathologist in charge or to the responsible laboratory technician, in the presence of witnesses (never via messenger), so that the rules of evidence will not be breached.

Treatment

Give analgesics or sedatives if indicated. Administer tetanus toxoid if deep lacerations contain soil or dirt particles.

Give ceftriaxone, 125 mg intramuscularly, to prevent gonorrhea. In addition, give metronidazole, 2 g as a single dose, and azithromycin 1 g orally or doxycycline, 100 mg twice daily for 7 days to treat chlamydial infection. Incubating syphilis will probably be prevented by these medications, but the VDRL test should be repeated 6 weeks after the assault.

Prevent pregnancy by using one of the methods discussed under Emergency Contraception, if necessary (this chapter).

Vaccinate against hepatitis B. Consider HIV prophylaxis (see Chapter 31).

Make sure the patient and her family and friends have a source of ongoing psychological support.

Cantu M et al: Evaluation and management of the sexually assaulted woman. Emerg Med Clin North Am 2003;21:737. [PMID: 12962356]

MENOPAUSAL SYNDROME

 ESSENTIALS OF DIAGNOSIS

- *Cessation of menses due to aging or to bilateral oophorectomy.*
- *Elevation of FSH and LH levels.*
- *Hot flushes and night sweats (in 80% of women).*
- *Decreased vaginal lubrication; thinned vaginal mucosa with or without dyspareunia.*

General Considerations

The term "menopause" denotes the final cessation of menstruation, either as a normal part of aging or as the result of surgical removal of both ovaries. In a broader sense, as the term is commonly used, it denotes a 1- to 3-year period during which a woman adjusts to a diminishing and then absent menstrual flow and the physiologic changes that may be associated—hot flushes, night sweats, and vaginal dryness.

The average age at menopause in Western societies today is 51 years. Premature menopause is defined as ovarian failure and menstrual cessation before age 40;

this often has a genetic or autoimmune basis. Surgical menopause due to bilateral oophorectomy is common and can cause more severe symptoms owing to the sudden rapid drop in sex hormone levels.

There is no objective evidence that cessation of ovarian function is associated with severe emotional disturbance or personality changes. However, mood changes toward depression and anxiety can occur at this time. Furthermore, the time of menopause often coincides with other major life changes, such as departure of children from the home, a midlife identity crisis, or divorce. These events, coupled with a sense of the loss of youth, may exacerbate the symptoms of menopause and cause psychological distress.

Clinical Findings

A. SYMPTOMS AND SIGNS

1. Cessation of menstruation—Menstrual cycles generally become irregular as menopause approaches. Anovular cycles occur more often, with irregular cycle length and occasional menorrhagia. Menstrual flow usually diminishes in amount owing to decreased estrogen secretion, resulting in less abundant endometrial growth. Finally, cycles become longer, with missed periods or episodes of spotting only. When no bleeding has occurred for 1 year, the menopausal transition can be said to have occurred. Any bleeding after this time warrants investigation by endometrial curettage or aspiration to rule out endometrial cancer.

2. Hot flushes—Hot flushes (feelings of intense heat over the trunk and face, with flushing of the skin and sweating) occur in 80% of women as a result of the decrease in ovarian hormones. Hot flushes can begin before the cessation of menses. An increase in pulsatile release of GnRH from the hypothalamus is believed to trigger the hot flushes by affecting the adjacent temperature-regulating area of the brain. Hot flushes are more severe in women who undergo surgical menopause. Flushing is more pronounced late in the day, during hot weather, after ingestion of hot foods or drinks, or during periods of tension. Occurring at night, they often cause sweating and insomnia and result in fatigue on the following day.

3. Vaginal atrophy—With decreased estrogen secretion, thinning of the vaginal mucosa and decreased vaginal lubrication occur and may lead to dyspareunia. The introitus decreases in diameter. Pelvic examination reveals pale, smooth vaginal mucosa and a small cervix and uterus. The ovaries are not normally palpable after the menopause. Continued sexual activity will help prevent tissue shrinkage.

4. Osteoporosis—Osteoporosis may occur as a late sequela of menopause.

B. LABORATORY FINDINGS

Serum FSH and LH levels are elevated. Vaginal cytologic examination will show a low estrogen effect with predominantly parabasal cells, indicating lack of epithelial maturation due to hypoestrinism.

Treatment

A. NATURAL MENOPAUSE

Education and support from health providers, midlife discussion groups, and reading material will help most women having difficulty adjusting to the menopause. Physiologic symptoms can be treated as follows.

1. Vasomotor symptoms—Oral conjugated estrogens, 0.3 mg or 0.625 mg, estradiol, 0.5 or 1 mg, or estrone sulfate, 0.625 mg; or estradiol can be given transdermally as skin patches that are changed once or twice weekly and secrete 0.05–0.1 mg of hormone daily. When either form of estrogen is used, add a progestin (medroxyprogesterone acetate) to prevent endometrial hyperplasia or cancer. The hormones can be given in several differing regimens. Give estrogen on days 1–25 of each calendar month, with 5–10 mg of medroxyprogesterone acetate added on days 14–25. Withhold hormones from day 26 until the end of the month, when the endometrium will be shed, producing a light, generally painless monthly period. Alternatively, give the estrogen along with 2.5 mg of medroxyprogesterone acetate daily, without stopping. This regimen causes some initial bleeding or spotting, but within a few months it produces an atrophic endometrium that will not bleed. If the patient has had a hysterectomy, a progestin need not be used.

Data from the Women's Health Initiative (WHI) study suggest that women should not use combination progestin-estrogen therapy for more than 3 or 4 years. In this study, the increased risk of cardiovascular disease, cerebrovascular disease, and breast cancer with this regimen outweighed the benefits. Women who cannot find relief with alternative approaches may wish to consider continuing use of combination therapy after a thorough discussion of the risks and benefits. Alternatives to hormone therapy for vasomotor symptoms include selective serotonin reuptake inhibitors such as paroxetine 12.5 mg or 25 mg/d, venlafaxine 75 mg/d. Gabapentin, an antiseizure medication, is also effective at 900 mg/d. Clonidine given orally or transdermally, 100–150 mcg daily, may also reduce the frequency of hot flushes, but its use is limited by side effects, including dry mouth, drowsiness, and hypotension.

2. Vaginal atrophy—An estradiol vaginal ring that can be left in place for 3 months and is suitable for long-term use provides effective relief of vaginal atrophy. There is minimal systemic absorption of estradiol with the ring, and progestin therapy to protect the endometrium is unnecessary. Short-term use of estrogen vaginal cream will relieve symptoms of atrophy, but because of variable absorption, therapy with either the vaginal ring or systemic hormone replacement is preferable. Testosterone propionate 1–2%, 0.5–1 g, in a vanishing cream base used in the same manner is also effective if estrogen is contraindicated. A bland lubricant such as unscented cold cream or water-soluble gel can be helpful at the time of coitus.

3. Osteoporosis—(See also discussion in Chapter 26.) Women should ingest at least 800 mg of calcium daily throughout life. Nonfat or low-fat milk products, calcium-fortified orange juice, green leafy vegetables, corn tortillas, and canned sardines or salmon consumed with the bones are good dietary sources. In addition, 1 g of elemental calcium should be taken as a daily supplement at the time of the menopause and thereafter; calcium supplements should be taken with meals to increase their absorption. Vitamin D, 400 units/d from food, sunlight, or supplements, is necessary to enhance calcium absorption. A daily program of energetic walking and exercise to strengthen the arms and upper body helps maintain bone mass.

Women most at risk for osteoporotic fractures should consider bisphosphonates, raloxifene, or hormone replacement therapy. This includes white and Asian women, especially if they have a family history of osteoporosis; are thin, short, cigarette smokers, and physically inactive; or have had a low calcium intake in adult life.

B. RISKS OF HORMONE THERAPY

Double-blinded randomized, controlled trials have shown no overall cardiovascular benefit with estrogen-progestin replacement therapy in a group of postmenopausal women with or without established coronary disease. Both in the WHI trial and the Heart and Estrogen/Progestin Replacement Study (HERS), the overall health risks (increased risk of coronary heart events, strokes, thromboembolic disease, breast cancers, gallstones) exceeded the benefits from the use of combination estrogen and progesterone. Progestins counteract some but not all favorable effects of estrogen. Women who have been receiving long-term estrogen-progestin hormone replacement therapy (HRT), even in the absence of complications should be encouraged to stop, especially if they do not have menopausal symptoms. An ancillary study of the WHI study showed that not only did estrogen-progestin HRT not benefit cognitive

function but there was a small increased risk of cognitive decline in that group compared with women in the placebo group. The unopposed estrogen arm of the WHI trial demonstrated a decrease in the risk of hip fracture, a small but nonsignificant decrease in breast cancer, but an increased risk of stroke and no evidence of protection from coronary heart disease. The study also showed a small increase in the combined risk of mild cognitive impairment and dementia with estrogen use compared with placebo, similar to the estrogen-progestin arm. (See also discussions of estrogen and progestin replacement therapy in Chapter 26.)

C. SURGICAL MENOPAUSE

The abrupt hormonal decrease resulting from oophorectomy generally results in severe vasomotor symptoms and rapid onset of dyspareunia and osteoporosis unless treated. Estrogen replacement is generally started immediately after surgery. Conjugated estrogens 1.25 mg, estrone sulfate 1.25 mg, or estradiol 2 mg is given for 25 days of each month. After age 45–50 years, this dose can be tapered to 0.625 mg of conjugated estrogens or equivalent.

Anderson GL: Effects of conjugated equine estrogen in postmenopausal women with hysterectomy: the Women's Health Initiative randomized controlled trial. JAMA 2004;291:1701. [PMID: 15082697]

National Institutes of Health: National Institutes of Health State-of-the-Science Conference statement: management of menopause-related symptoms. Ann Intern Med 2005;142:1003. [PMID: 15968015]

Rapp SR et al: Effect of estrogen plus progestin on global cognitive function in postmenopausal women: the Women's Health Initiative Memory Study: a randomized controlled trial. JAMA 2003;289:2663. [PMID: 12771113]

Rossouw JE et al: Risks and benefits of estrogen plus progestin in healthy postmenopausal women: principal results from the Women's Health Initiative randomized controlled trial. JAMA 2002;288:321. [PMID: 12117397]

Shumaker SA et al: Conjugated equine estrogens and incidence of probable dementia and mild cognitive impairment in postmenopausal women: Women's Health Initiative Memory Study. JAMA 2004;291:2947. [PMID: 15213206]

Obstetrics

William R. Crombleholme, MD

18

DIAGNOSIS & DIFFERENTIAL DIAGNOSIS OF PREGNANCY

It is advantageous to diagnose pregnancy as promptly as possible when a sexually active woman misses a menstrual period or has symptoms suggestive of pregnancy. In the event of a desired pregnancy, prenatal care can begin early, and potentially harmful medications and activities such as drug and alcohol use, smoking, and occupational chemical exposure can be halted. In the event of an unwanted pregnancy, counseling about adoption or termination of the pregnancy can be provided at an early stage.

Pregnancy Tests

All urine or blood pregnancy tests rely on the detection of human chorionic gonadotropin (hCG) produced by the placenta. hCG levels increase shortly after implantation, approximately double every 48 hours, reach a peak at 50–75 days, and fall to lower levels in the second and third trimesters. Laboratory and home pregnancy tests use monoclonal antibodies specific for hCG. These tests are performed on serum or urine and are accurate at the time of the missed period or shortly after it.

Compared with intrauterine pregnancies, ectopic pregnancies may show lower levels of hCG that level off or fall in serial determinations. Quantitative assays of hCG repeated at 48- to 72-hour intervals are used in the diagnosis of ectopic pregnancy as well as in cases of molar pregnancy, threatened abortion, and missed abortion. Comparison of hCG levels between laboratories may be misleading in a given patient because different international standards may produce results that vary by as much as twofold.

Manifestations of Pregnancy

The following symptoms and signs are usually due to pregnancy, but none are diagnostic. A record of the time and frequency of coitus is helpful for diagnosing and dating a pregnancy.

A. SYMPTOMS

Amenorrhea, nausea and vomiting, breast tenderness and tingling, urinary frequency and urgency, "quickening" (perception of first movement noted at about the 18th week), weight gain.

B. SIGNS (IN WEEKS FROM LAST MENSTRUAL PERIOD)

Breast changes (enlargement, vascular engorgement, colostrum), abdominal enlargement, cyanosis of vagina and cervical portio (about the seventh week), softening of the cervix (seventh week), softening of the cervicouterine junction (eighth week), generalized enlargement and diffuse softening of the corpus (after eighth week).

The uterine fundus is palpable above the pubic symphysis by 12–15 weeks from the last menstrual period (LMP) and reaches the umbilicus by 20–22 weeks. Fetal heart tones can be heard by Doppler at 10–12 weeks of gestation and at 20 weeks with an ordinary fetoscope.

Differential Diagnosis

The nonpregnant uterus enlarged by myomas can be confused with the gravid uterus, but it is usually very firm and irregular. An ovarian tumor may be found midline, displacing the nonpregnant uterus to the side or posteriorly. Ultrasonography and a pregnancy test will provide accurate diagnosis in these circumstances.

ESSENTIALS OF PRENATAL CARE

The first prenatal visit should occur as early as possible after the diagnosis of pregnancy and should include the following: history, physical examination, laboratory tests, advice to patients, and tests and procedures.

History

Ask the patient's age, ethnic background, and occupation. Gather information about onset of LMP and its normality, possible conception dates, bleeding after LMP, medical history, all prior pregnancies (duration, outcome, and complications), and symptoms of present pregnancy. Discuss with the patient her nutritional habits as well as any use of caffeine, tobacco, alcohol, or drugs (Table 18–1). Determine whether there is any family history of congenital anomalies and heritable diseases, a personal history of childhood varicella, or prior sexually transmitted diseases (STDs) or risk factors for HIV infection.

Physical Examination

Height, weight, and blood pressure should be measured, and a general physical examination should be done. Abdominal and pelvic examination should in-

Table 18–1. Common drugs that are teratogenic or fetotoxic.[1]

ACE inhibitors	Griseofulvin
Alcohol	Hypoglycemics, oral
Amantadine	(older drugs)
Androgens	Isotretinoin
Anticonvulsants	Lithium
Aminoglutethimide	Methotrexate
Carbamazepine	Misoprostol
Phenytoin	NSAIDs (third trimester)
Valproic acid	Opioids (prolonged use)
Aspirin and other salicylates	Progestins
(third trimester)	Radioiodine (antithyroid)
Benzodiazepines	Reserpine
Carbarsone (amebicide)	Ribavirin
Chloramphenicol (third	Sulfonamides (third trimester)
trimester)	Tetracycline (third trimester)
Cyclophosphamide	Thalidomide
Diazoxide	Tobacco smoking
Diethylstilbestrol	Trimethoprim (third
Disulfiram	trimester)
Ergotamine	Warfarin and other cou-
Estrogens	marin anticoagulants

[1]Many other drugs are also contraindicated during pregnancy. Evaluate any drug for its need versus its potential adverse effects. Further information can be obtained from the manufacturer or from any of several teratogenic registries around the country.
ACE = angiotensin-converting enzyme; NSAIDs = nonsteroidal anti-inflammatory drugs.

clude the following: (1) estimate of uterine size or measure fundal height; (2) evaluation of bony pelvis for symmetry and adequacy; (3) evaluation of cervix for structural anatomy, infection, effacement, dilation; (4) detection of fetal heart sounds by Doppler device after 10 weeks or fetoscope after 18 weeks.

Laboratory Tests

Urinalysis, culture of a clean-voided midstream urine sample, complete blood count with red cell indices, serologic test for syphilis, rubella antibody titer, history of varicella infection, blood group, Rh type, atypical antibody screening, and hepatitis B surface antigen (HBsAg) evaluation. HIV screening should be offered to all pregnant women. Cervical cultures are usually obtained for *Neisseria gonorrhoeae* and chlamydia, along with a Papanicolaou smear of the cervix. All black women should have sickle cell screening. Women of African, Asian, or Mediterranean ancestry with anemia or low mean corpuscular volume (MCV) values should have hemoglobin electrophoresis performed to identify abnormal hemoglobins (Hb S, C, F, α-thalassemia, β-thalassemia). Tuberculosis skin testing is indicated for high-risk

immigrant and local populations. Genetic counseling with the option of chorionic villus sampling or genetic amniocentesis should be offered to all women who will be 35 years of age or older at delivery and those who have had prior offspring with chromosomal abnormalities. Noninvasive first trimester screening for nuchal translucency and serum levels of PAPP-A (pregnancy-associated plasma protein A) and free β subunit of hCG can also be offered. Blood screening for Tay-Sachs and Canavan disease is offered to Jewish women with Jewish partners (especially those of Ashkenazi descent), and couples of French-Canadian or Cajun ancestry should also be screened as possible Tay-Sachs carriers. Screening for cystic fibrosis is offered to all pregnant women. Hepatitis C antibody screening should be offered to pregnant women who are at high risk for infection.

Pregnant women who work in medical-dental health care or the police and fire departments and those who are household contacts of a hepatitis B virus carrier or a hemodialysis patient and are HBsAg-negative at prenatal screening are at high risk for acquiring hepatitis B. They should be vaccinated during pregnancy.

Advice to Patients

A. Prenatal Visits

Prenatal care should begin early and maintain a schedule of regular prenatal visits: 0–28 weeks, every 4 weeks; 28–36 weeks, every 2 weeks; 36 weeks on, weekly.

B. Diet

1. Eat a balanced diet containing the major food groups.
2. Take prenatal vitamins with iron and folic acid.
3. Expect to gain 20–40 lb. Do not diet to lose weight during pregnancy.
4. Decrease caffeine intake to 0–1 cup of coffee, tea, or caffeinated cola daily.
5. Avoid eating raw or rare meat or fish suspected of elevated levels of mercury.
6. Eat fresh fruits and vegetables and wash them before eating.

C. Medications

Do not take medications unless prescribed or authorized by your provider.

D. Alcohol and Other Drugs

Abstain from alcohol, tobacco, and all recreational ("street") drugs. No safe level of alcohol intake has been established for pregnancy. Fetal effects are manifest in the **fetal alcohol syndrome**, which includes growth restriction, facial abnormalities, and serious central nervous system dysfunction. These effects are thought to result from direct toxicity of ethanol itself as well as of its metabolites such as acetaldehyde. Characteristic findings include shortened palpebral fissures, low-set ears, midfacial hypoplasia, a smooth philtrum, a thin upper lip, microcephaly, mental retardation, and attention deficit disorder. Skeletal and cardiac abnormalities may also be seen.

Cigarette smoking results in fetal exposure to carbon monoxide and nicotine, and this is thought to eventuate in a number of adverse pregnancy outcomes. An increased risk of abruptio placentae, placenta previa, and premature rupture of the membranes is documented among women who smoke. Premature delivery occurs 20% more frequently among smoking pregnant women, and the birth weights of their infants are on average 200 g lower than infants of nonsmokers. Women who smoke should quit smoking or at least reduce the number of cigarettes smoked per day to as few as possible. Pregnant women should also avoid exposure to environmental smoke ("passive smoking").

Sometimes compounding the above effects on pregnancy outcome are the independent adverse effects of illicit drugs. Cocaine use in pregnancy is associated with an increased risk of premature rupture of membranes, preterm delivery, placental abruption, intrauterine growth restriction, neurobehavioral deficits, and sudden infant death syndrome. Similar adverse pregnancy effects are associated with amphetamine use, perhaps reflecting the vasoconstrictive potential of both amphetamines and cocaine. Adverse effects associated with opioid use include intrauterine growth restriction, prematurity, and fetal death.

E. X-Rays and Noxious Exposures

Avoid x-rays unless essential and approved by a physician and with shielding. Inform your dentist and your providers that you are pregnant. Avoid chemical or radiation hazards. Avoid excessive heat in hot tubs or saunas. Avoid handling cat feces or cat litter. Wear gloves when gardening.

F. Rest and Activity

Obtain adequate rest each day. Abstain from strenuous physical work or activities, particularly when heavy lifting or weight bearing is required. Exercise regularly at a mild to moderate level. Avoid exhausting or hazardous exercises or new athletic training programs during pregnancy. Heart rate should be kept below 140 beats/min during exercise.

G. Birth Classes

Enroll with your partner in a childbirth preparation class well before your due date.

Tests & Procedures

A. Each Visit

Weight, blood pressure, fundal height, fetal heart rate are measured, and a urine specimen is obtained and tested for protein and glucose. Review any concerns the patient may have about pregnancy, health, and nutrition.

B. 6–12 Weeks

Confirm uterine size and growth by pelvic examination. Document fetal heart tones (audible at 10–12 weeks of gestation by Doppler). Perform transvaginal chorionic villus sampling between 10 and 12 weeks when indicated or screening for trisomy 18, 21, and cardiac defects using nuchal translucency measurement on sonography, free β-hCG, and PAPP-A at 11–13 weeks.

C. 12–18 Weeks

Genetic counseling should be offered for women age 35 years or older at delivery and for those with a family history of congenital anomalies or a previous child with a chromosomal abnormality, metabolic disease, or neural tube defect. Amniocentesis is performed as indicated and requested by the patient.

D. 12–24 Weeks

Fetal ultrasound examination to determine pregnancy dating and evaluate fetal anatomy is done. An earlier examination provides the most accurate dating, and a later examination demonstrates fetal anatomy in greater detail. The best compromise is at 18–20 weeks of gestation.

E. 16–20 Weeks

Maternal serum alpha-fetoprotein testing is offered to all women to screen for neural tube defects. In some states, such testing is mandatory. Serum alpha-fetoprotein is combined with measurement of estriol and hCG (triple screen) or inhibin A (quad screen) for the detection of fetal Down syndrome.

F. 20–24 Weeks

Instruct patient in symptoms and signs of preterm labor and rupture of membranes. Consider cervical length measurement by ultrasound after 18 weeks with history of prior preterm delivery (> 2.5 cm is normal).

G. 24 Weeks to Delivery

Ultrasound examination is performed as indicated. Typically, fetal size and growth are evaluated when fundal height is 3 cm less than or more than expected for gestational age. In multiple pregnancies, ultrasound should be performed every 4 weeks to evaluate for discordant growth.

H. 26–28 Weeks

Screening for gestational diabetes by a 50-g glucose load (Glucola) and a 1-hour post-Glucola blood glucose determination. Abnormal values should be followed up with a 3-hour glucose tolerance test (see Table 18–3).

I. 28 Weeks

If initial antibody screen is negative, repeat antibody testing for Rh-negative patients, but result is not required before $Rh_o(D)$ immune globulin is administered.

J. 28–32 Weeks

Repeat the complete blood count to evaluate for anemia of pregnancy.

K. 28 WEEKS TO DELIVERY

Determine fetal position and presentation. Question the patient at each visit for symptoms or signs of preterm labor or rupture of membranes. Assess maternal perception of fetal movement at each visit. Antepartum fetal testing is performed as medically indicated.

L. 36 WEEKS TO DELIVERY

Repeat syphilis and HIV testing, cervical cultures for *N gonorrhoeae*, and *Chlamydia trachomatis* in at-risk patients. Discuss with the patient the indicators of onset of labor, admission to hospital, management of labor and delivery, and options for analgesia and anesthesia. Weekly cervical examinations are not necessary unless indicated to assess a specific clinical situation. Elective delivery (whether by induction or cesarean section) prior to 39 weeks of gestation requires confirmation of fetal lung maturity.

The CDC has recommended universal prenatal culture-based screening for group B streptococcal colonization in pregnancy. A single standard culture of the distal vagina and anorectum is collected at 35–37 weeks. No prophylaxis is needed if the screening culture is negative. Patients whose cultures are positive receive intrapartum penicillin prophylaxis with labor. Patients with risk factors such as a previous infant with invasive group B streptococcal disease, or group B streptococcal bacteriuria during the pregnancy, or delivery at less than 37 weeks of gestation also receive intrapartum prophylaxis. Patients whose cultures at 35–37 weeks were not done or whose results are not known receive prophylaxis only with the risk factors of intrapartum temperature greater than 38 °C or membrane rupture greater than 18 hours.

The routine recommended regimen for prophylaxis is penicillin G, 5 million units intravenously as a loading dose and then 2.5 million units intravenously every 4 hours until delivery. In penicillin-allergic patients not at high risk for anaphylaxis, 2 g of cefazolin can be given intravenously as an initial dose and then 1 g intravenously every 8 hours until delivery. In patients at high risk for anaphylaxis, use vancomycin 1 g intravenously every 12 hours until delivery or, after confirmed susceptibility testing of group B streptococcal isolate, clindamycin 900 mg intravenously every 8 hours or erythromycin 500 mg intravenously every 6 hours until delivery.

M. 41 WEEKS AND BEYOND

Examine the cervix to determine the probability of successful induction of labor. Based on this, induction of labor is undertaken if the cervix is favorable (generally, cervix ≥ 2 cm dilated ≥ 50% effaced, vertex at −1 station, soft cervix, and midposition); if unfavorable, antepartum fetal testing is begun.

Kirkham C et al: Evidence-based prenatal care: Part I. General prenatal care and counseling issues. Am Fam Physician 2005;71:1307. [PMID: 15832534]

Schrag S et al: Prevention of perinatal group B streptococcal disease. Revised guidelines from CDC. MMWR Recomm Rep 2002;51(RR-11):1. [PMID: 12211284]

NUTRITION IN PREGNANCY

Nutrition in pregnancy can affect maternal health and infant size and well-being. Pregnant women should have nutrition counseling early in prenatal care and access to supplementary food programs if necessary. Counseling should stress abstention from alcohol, smoking, and recreational drugs. Caffeine and artificial sweeteners should be used only in small amounts. "Empty calories" should be avoided, and the diet should contain the following foods: protein foods of animal and vegetable origin, milk and milk products, whole-grain cereals and breads, and fruits and vegetables—especially green leafy vegetables.

Weight gain in pregnancy should be 20–40 lb, which includes the added weight of the fetus, placenta, and amniotic fluid and of maternal reproductive tissues, fluid, blood, increased fat stores, and increased lean body mass. Maternal fat stores are a caloric reserve for pregnancy and lactation; weight restriction in pregnancy to avoid developing such fat stores may affect the development of other fetal and maternal tissues and is not advisable. Obese women can have normal infants with less weight gain (15–20 lb) but should be encouraged to eat high-quality foods. Normally, a pregnant woman gains 2–5 lb in the first trimester and slightly less than 1 lb/wk thereafter. She needs approximately an extra 200–300 kcal/d (depending on energy output) and 30 g/d of additional protein for a total protein intake of about 75 g/d. Appropriate caloric intake in pregnancy helps prevent the problems associated with low birth weight.

Rigid salt restriction is not necessary. While consumption of highly salted snack foods and prepared foods is not desirable, 2–3 g/d of sodium is permissible. The increased calcium needs of pregnancy (1200 mg/d) can be met with milk, milk products, green vegetables, soybean products, corn tortillas, and calcium carbonate supplements.

The increased need for iron and folic acid should be met from foods as well as vitamin and mineral supplements. (See section on anemia in pregnancy.) Megavitamins should not be taken in pregnancy, as they may result in fetal malformation or disturbed metabolism. However, a balanced prenatal supplement containing 30–60 mg of elemental iron, 0.5–0.8 mg of folate, and the recommended daily allowances of various vitamins and minerals is widely used in the United States and is probably beneficial to many women with marginal diets. There is evidence that periconceptional folic acid supplements can decrease the risk of neural tube defects in the fetus. For this reason, the United States Public Health Service recommends the consumption of 0.4 mg of folic acid per day for all pregnant and reproductive age women. Women with a prior pregnancy complicated by neural tube defect may require higher supplemental doses as determined by their providers. Lactovegetarians and ovolactovegetarians do well in pregnancy; vegetarian women who eat neither eggs nor milk products should have their diets assessed for adequate calories and protein and should take oral vitamin B_{12} supplements during pregnancy and lactation.

Picciano MF: Pregnancy and lactation: physiological adjustments, nutritional requirements and the role of dietary supplements. J Nutr 2003;133:1997S. [PMID: 12771353]

Rosello-Soberon ME et al: Twin pregnancies: eating for three? Maternal nutrition update. Nutr Rev 2005;63:295. [PMID: 16220640]

TRAVEL & IMMUNIZATIONS DURING PREGNANCY

During an otherwise normal low-risk pregnancy, travel can be planned most safely between the 18th and 32nd weeks. Commercial flying in pressurized cabins does not pose a threat to the fetus. An aisle seat will allow frequent walks. Adequate fluids should be taken during the flight.

It is not advisable to travel to endemic areas of yellow fever in Africa or Latin America; similarly, it is inadvisable to travel to areas of Africa or Asia where chloroquine-resistant falciparum malaria is a hazard, since complications of malaria are more common in pregnancy.

Ideally, all immunizations should precede pregnancy. Live virus products are contraindicated (measles, rubella, yellow fever), including smallpox. Inactivated poliovaccine (Salk) can be used instead of the oral vaccine. Vaccines against pneumococcal pneumonia, meningococcal meningitis, and hepatitis A can be used as indicated. Influenza vaccine is indicated in all pregnant women who will be in their second or third trimester during "flu season." The CDC lists pregnant women in the high-risk group even with vaccine shortages.

Pooled immune globulin to prevent hepatitis A is safe and does not carry a risk of HIV transmission. Hepatitis A vaccine contains formalin-inactivated virus but can be given in pregnancy when needed. Chloroquine can be used for malaria prophylaxis in pregnancy, and proguanil is also safe.

Water should be purified by boiling, since iodine purification may provide more iodine than is safe during pregnancy.

Do not use prophylactic antibiotics or bismuth subsalicylate during pregnancy to prevent diarrhea. Use oral rehydration fluids, and treat bacterial diarrhea with erythromycin or ampicillin if necessary.

VOMITING OF PREGNANCY (Morning Sickness) & HYPEREMESIS GRAVIDARUM (Pernicious Vomiting of Pregnancy)

 ESSENTIALS OF DIAGNOSIS

- *Morning or evening nausea and vomiting.*
- *Persistent vomiting severe enough to result in weight loss, dehydration, starvation ketosis, hypochloremic alkalosis, hypokalemia.*
- *May have transient elevation of liver enzymes.*
- *Appears related to high or rising serum hCG.*
- *More common with multiple gestation or hydatidiform mole.*

General Considerations

Nausea and vomiting begin soon after the first missed period and cease by the fifth month of gestation. Up to three-fourths of women complain of nausea and vomiting during early pregnancy, with the vast majority noting nausea throughout the day. This problem exerts no adverse effects on the pregnancy and does not presage other complications.

Persistent, severe vomiting during pregnancy—hyperemesis gravidarum—can be disabling and require hospitalization. Thyroid dysfunction can be associated with hyperemesis gravidarum, so it is advisable to determine thyroid-stimulating hormone (TSH) and free T_4 values in these patients.

Treatment

A. MILD NAUSEA AND VOMITING OF PREGNANCY

Reassurance and dietary advice are all that is required in most instances. Because of possible teratogenicity, drugs used during the first half of pregnancy should be restricted to those of major importance to life and health. Antiemetics, antihistamines, and antispasmodics are generally unnecessary to treat nausea of pregnancy. Vitamin B_6 (pyridoxine), 50–100 mg/d orally, is nontoxic and may be helpful in some patients.

B. HYPEREMESIS GRAVIDARUM

Hospitalize the patient in a private room at bed rest. Give nothing by mouth for 48 hours, and maintain hydration and electrolyte balance by giving appropriate parenteral fluids and vitamin supplements as indicated. Rarely, total parenteral nutrition may become necessary. As soon as possible, place the patient on a dry diet consisting of six small feedings daily plus clear liquids 1 hour after eating. Prochlorperazine rectal suppositories may be useful. After in-patient stabilization, the patient can be maintained at home even if she requires intravenous fluids in addition to her oral intake.

Jewell D et al: Interventions for nausea and vomiting in early pregnancy. Cochrane Database Syst Rev 2003;(4):CD000145. [PMID: 14583914]

Verberg MF et al: Hyperemesis gravidarum, a literature review. Hum Reprod Update 2005;11:527. [PMID: 16006438]

SPONTANEOUS ABORTION

 ESSENTIALS OF DIAGNOSIS

- *Intrauterine pregnancy at less than 20 weeks.*
- *Low or falling levels of hCG.*

- *Bleeding, midline cramping pain.*
- *Open cervical os.*
- *Complete or partial expulsion of products of conception.*

General Considerations

About three-fourths of spontaneous abortions occur before the 16th week; of these, three-fourths occur before the eighth week. Almost 20% of all clinically recognized pregnancies terminate in spontaneous abortion.

More than 60% of spontaneous abortions result from chromosomal defects due to maternal or paternal factors; about 15% appear to be associated with maternal trauma, infections, dietary deficiencies, diabetes mellitus, hypothyroidism, the lupus anticoagulant-anticardiolipin-antiphospholipid antibody syndrome or anatomic malformations. There is no reliable evidence that abortion may be induced by psychic stimuli such as severe fright, grief, anger, or anxiety. In about one-fourth of cases, the cause of abortion cannot be determined. There is no evidence that video display terminals or associated electromagnetic fields are related to an increased risk of spontaneous abortion.

It is important to distinguish women with a history of incompetent cervix from those with more typical early abortion and those with premature labor or rupture of the membranes. Characteristically, incompetent cervix presents as "silent" cervical dilation (ie, with minimal uterine contractions) between 16 and 28 weeks of gestation. Women with incompetent cervix often present with significant cervical dilation (2 cm or more) and minimal symptoms. When the cervix reaches 4 cm or more, active uterine contractions or rupture of the membranes may occur secondary to the degree of cervical dilation. This does not change the primary diagnosis. Factors that predispose to incompetent cervix are a history of incompetent cervix with a previous pregnancy, cervical conization or surgery, cervical injury, diethylstilbestrol (DES) exposure, and anatomic abnormalities of the cervix. Prior to pregnancy or during the first trimester, there are no methods for determining whether the cervix will eventually be incompetent. After 14–16 weeks, ultrasound may be used to evaluate the internal anatomy of the lower uterine segment and cervix for the funneling and shortening abnormalities consistent with cervical incompetence.

Clinical Findings

A. Symptoms and Signs

1. Threatened abortion—Bleeding or cramping occurs, but the pregnancy continues. The cervix is not dilated.

2. Inevitable abortion—The cervix is dilated and the membranes may be ruptured, but passage of the products of conception has not occurred. Bleeding and cramping persist, and passage of the products of conception is considered inevitable.

3. Complete abortion—The fetus and placenta are completely expelled. Pain ceases, but spotting may persist.

4. Incomplete abortion—Some portion of the products of conception (usually placental) remain in the uterus. Only mild cramps are reported, but bleeding is persistent and often excessive.

5. Missed abortion—The pregnancy has ceased to develop, but the conceptus has not been expelled. Symptoms of pregnancy disappear. There is a brownish vaginal discharge but no free bleeding. Pain does not develop. The cervix is semifirm and slightly patulous; the uterus becomes smaller and irregularly softened; the adnexa are normal.

B. Laboratory Findings

Pregnancy tests show low or falling levels of hCG. A complete blood count should be obtained if bleeding is heavy. Determine Rh type, and give $Rh_o(D)$ immune globulin if the type is Rh-negative. All tissue recovered should be assessed by a pathologist and may be sent for genetic analysis in selected cases.

C. Ultrasonographic Findings

The gestational sac can be identified at 5–6 weeks from the LMP, a fetal pole at 6 weeks, and fetal cardiac activity at 6–7 weeks. Serial observations are often required to evaluate changes in size of the embryo. A small, irregular sac without a fetal pole with accurate dating is diagnostic of an abnormal pregnancy.

Differential Diagnosis

The bleeding that occurs in abortion of a uterine pregnancy must be differentiated from the abnormal bleeding of an ectopic pregnancy and anovular bleeding in a nonpregnant woman. The passage of hydropic villi in the bloody discharge is diagnostic of hydatidiform mole.

Treatment

A. General Measures

1. Threatened abortion—Place the patient at bed rest for 24–48 hours followed by gradual resumption of usual activities, with abstinence from coitus and douching. Hormonal treatment is contraindicated. Antibiotics should be used only if there are signs of infection.

2. Missed abortion—This calls for counseling regarding the fate of the pregnancy and planning for its elective termination at a time chosen by the patient and physician. Insertion of a laminaria to dilate the cervix followed by aspiration is the method of choice for a missed abortion. Prostaglandin vaginal tablets (misoprostol) are an effective alternative.

B. SURGICAL MEASURES

1. Incomplete or inevitable abortion—Prompt removal of any products of conception remaining within the uterus is required to stop bleeding and prevent infection. Analgesia and a paracervical block are useful, followed by uterine exploration with ovum forceps or uterine aspiration.

2. Cerclage and restriction of activities—These are the treatments of choice for incompetent cervix. A variety of suture materials including a 5-mm Mersilene band can be used to create a purse-string type of stitch around the cervix, using either the McDonald or Shirodkar method. Cerclage should be undertaken with caution when there is advanced cervical dilation or when the membranes are prolapsed into the vagina. Rupture of the membranes and infection are specific contraindications to cerclage. Cervical cultures for *N gonorrhoeae*, chlamydia, and group B streptococci should be obtained before or at the time of cerclage.

Aleman A et al: Bed rest during pregnancy for preventing miscarriage. Cochrane Database Syst Rev 2005;(2):CD003576. [PMID: 15846669]

RECURRENT (Habitual) ABORTION

Recurrent abortion has been defined as the loss of three or more previable (< 500 g) pregnancies in succession. Recurrent abortion occurs in about 0.4–0.8% of all pregnancies. Abnormalities related to recurrent abortion can be identified in approximately half of the couples. If a woman has lost three previous pregnancies without identifiable cause, she still has a 70–80% chance of carrying a fetus to viability. If she has aborted four or five times, the likelihood of a successful pregnancy is 65–70%.

Recurrent abortion is a clinical rather than pathologic diagnosis. The clinical findings are similar to those observed in other types of abortion (see above).

Treatment

A. PRECONCEPTION THERAPY

Preconception therapy is aimed at detection of maternal or paternal defects that may contribute to abortion. A thorough general and gynecologic examination is essential. Polycystic ovaries should be ruled out. A random blood glucose test and thyroid function studies (including thyroid antibodies) should be done. Detection of lupus anticoagulant and other hemostatic abnormalities (proteins S and C and antithrombin III deficiency, hyperhomocysteinemia, anticardiolipin antibody, factor V Leiden mutations) and an antinuclear antibody test may be indicated with second trimester losses. Endometrial tissue should be examined in the postovulation stage of the cycle to determine the adequacy of the response of the endometrium to hormones. The competency of the cervix must be determined and hysteroscopy or hysterography used to exclude submucous myomas and congenital anoma-

lies. Chromosomal (karyotype) analysis of both partners rules out balanced translocations (found in 5% of infertile couples).

Studies have focused on the major histocompatibility complex of chromosome 6, which carries HLA loci and other genes that may influence reproductive success. Some women demonstrate a lack of maternal antibody response to paternal lymphocytes, which is customarily found in normal women after successful childbearing. However, several randomized controlled trials have found no benefit of intravenous immunoglobulin therapy for recurrent spontaneous abortion.

B. POSTCONCEPTION THERAPY

Provide early prenatal care and schedule frequent office visits. Complete bed rest is justified only for bleeding or pain. Empiric sex steroid hormone therapy is contraindicated.

Prognosis

The prognosis is excellent if the cause of abortion can be corrected.

Christiansen OB et al: Evidence-based investigations and treatments of recurrent pregnancy loss. Fertil Steril 2005;83: 821. [PMID: 15820784]

ECTOPIC PREGNANCY

 ESSENTIALS OF DIAGNOSIS

- *Amenorrhea or irregular bleeding and spotting.*
- *Pelvic pain, usually adnexal.*
- *Adnexal mass by clinical examination or ultrasound.*
- *Failure of serum level of hCG to double every 48 hours.*
- *No intrauterine pregnancy on transvaginal ultrasound with serum β-hCG of > 2000 mU/mL.*

General Considerations

Ectopic implantation occurs in about one out of 150 live births. About 98% of ectopic pregnancies are tubal. Other sites of ectopic implantation are the peritoneum or abdominal viscera, the ovary, and the cervix. Any condition that prevents or retards migration of the fertilized ovum to the uterus can predispose to an ectopic pregnancy, including a history of infertility, pelvic inflammatory disease, ruptured appendix, and prior tubal surgery. Combined intrauterine and extrauterine pregnancy (heterotopic) may occur rarely. In the United States, undiagnosed or undetected ectopic pregnancy is currently the most common cause of maternal death during the first trimester.

Clinical Findings

A. SYMPTOMS AND SIGNS

They may be acute or chronic.

1. Acute (40%)—Severe lower quadrant pain occurs in almost every case. It is sudden in onset, lancinating, intermittent, and does not radiate. Backache is present during attacks. Shock occurs in about 10%, often after pelvic examination. At least two-thirds of patients give a history of abnormal menstruation; many have been infertile.

2. Chronic (60%)—Blood leaks from the tubal ampulla over a period of days, and considerable blood may accumulate in the peritoneum. Slight but persistent vaginal spotting is reported, and a pelvic mass can be palpated. Abdominal distention and mild paralytic ileus are often present.

B. LABORATORY FINDINGS

Blood studies may show anemia and slight leukocytosis. Quantitative serum pregnancy tests will show levels generally lower than expected for normal pregnancies of the same duration. If pregnancy tests are followed over a few days, there may be a slow rise or a plateau rather than the near doubling every 2 days associated with normal early intrauterine pregnancy or the falling levels that occur with spontaneous abortion.

C. IMAGING

Ultrasonography can reliably demonstrate a gestational sac 6 weeks from the LMP and a fetal pole at 7 weeks if located in the uterus. An empty uterine cavity raises a strong suspicion of extrauterine pregnancy, which can occasionally be revealed by endovaginal ultrasound. Specified levels of serum hCG have been reliably correlated with ultrasound findings of an intrauterine pregnancy. For example, an hCG level of 6500 mU/mL with an empty uterine cavity by transabdominal ultrasound is virtually diagnostic of an ectopic pregnancy. Similarly, an hCG value of 2000 mU/mL or more can be indicative of an ectopic pregnancy if no products of conception are detected within the uterine cavity by transvaginal ultrasound.

D. SPECIAL EXAMINATIONS

With the advent of high-resolution transvaginal ultrasound, culdocentesis is rarely used in evaluation of possible ectopic pregnancy. Laparoscopy is the surgical procedure of choice both to confirm an ectopic pregnancy and in most cases to permit pelviscopic removal of the ectopic pregnancy without the need for exploratory laparotomy.

Differential Diagnosis

Clinical and laboratory findings suggestive or diagnostic of pregnancy will distinguish ectopic pregnancy from many acute abdominal illnesses such as acute appendicitis, acute pelvic inflammatory disease, ruptured corpus luteum cyst or ovarian follicle, and urinary calculi. Uterine enlargement with clinical findings similar to those found in ectopic pregnancy is also characteristic of an aborting uterine pregnancy or hydatidiform mole. Ectopic pregnancy should be suspected when postabortal tissue examination fails to reveal placenta. Steps must be taken for immediate diagnosis, including prompt microscopic tissue examination, ultrasonography, and serial hCG titers every 48 hours. Patients must be warned of possible ectopic pregnancy problems and monitored very closely.

Treatment

When a patient with an ectopic pregnancy is unstable or when surgical therapy is planned, the patient is hospitalized. Blood is typed and cross-matched. Ideally, diagnosis and operative treatment should precede frank rupture of the tube and intra-abdominal hemorrhage.

Surgical treatment is definitive. In a stable patient, diagnostic laparoscopy is the initial surgical procedure performed. Depending on the size of the ectopic pregnancy and whether or not it has ruptured, salpingostomy with removal of the ectopic or a partial or complete salpingectomy can usually be performed pelviscopically. Clinical conditions permitting, patency of the contralateral tube can be established by injection of indigo carmine into the uterine cavity and flow through the contralateral tube confirmed visually by the surgeon.

In a stable patient, methotrexate (50 mg/m²) intramuscularly—given as single or multiple doses—is acceptable medical therapy for early ectopic pregnancy. Favorable criteria are that the pregnancy should be less than 3.5 cm in largest dimension and unruptured, with no active bleeding.

Iron therapy for anemia may be necessary during convalescence. Give Rh_o(D) immune globulin (300 mcg) to Rh-negative patients.

Prognosis

Repeat tubal pregnancy occurs in about 12% of cases. This should not be regarded as a contraindication to future pregnancy, but the patient requires careful observation and early ultrasound confirmation of an intrauterine pregnancy.

Bickell NA et al: Time and risk of ruptured tubal pregnancy. Obstet Gynecol 2004;104:789. [PMID: 15458903]

Lipscomb GH et al: Comparison of multidose and single-dose methotrexate protocols for the treatment of ectopic pregnancy. Am J Obstet Gynecol 2005;192:1844. [PMID: 15970826]

PREECLAMPSIA-ECLAMPSIA

 ESSENTIALS OF DIAGNOSIS

Preeclampsia

- *Blood pressure of ≥ 140 mm Hg systolic or ≥ 90 mm Hg diastolic after 20 weeks of gestation.*

- Proteinuria of ≥ 0.3 g in 24 hours.

Severe Preeclampsia

- Blood pressure of ≥ 160 mm Hg systolic or ≥ 110 mm Hg diastolic.
- Proteinuria ≥ 5 g in 24 hours or 4+ on dipstick.
- Oliguria of < 500 mL in 24 hours.
- Thrombocytopenia.
- Hemolysis, elevated liver enzymes, low platelets (HELLP).
- Pulmonary edema.
- Fetal growth restriction.

General Considerations

Preeclampsia is defined as the presence of elevated blood pressure and proteinuria during pregnancy. Eclampsia occurs with the addition of seizures. Classically, the presence of three elements was required for the diagnosis of preeclampsia-eclampsia: hypertension, proteinuria, and edema. Edema was difficult to objectively quantify and is no longer a required element.

Preeclampsia-eclampsia can occur any time after 20 weeks of gestation and up to 6 weeks postpartum. It is a disease unique to pregnancy, with the only cure being delivery of the fetus and placenta. Preeclampsia-eclampsia develops in approximately 7% of pregnant women in the United States. Primiparas are most frequently affected; however, the incidence of preeclampsia-eclampsia is increased with multiple pregnancies, chronic hypertension, diabetes, renal disease, collagen-vascular and autoimmune disorders, and gestational trophoblastic disease. Five percent of women with preeclampsia progress to eclampsia. Uncontrolled eclampsia is a significant cause of maternal death.

The basic cause of preeclampsia-eclampsia is not known. Epidemiologic studies suggest an immunologic cause for preeclampsia, since it occurs predominantly in women who have had minimal exposure to sperm (having used barrier methods of contraception) or have new consorts, in primigravidas, and in women both of whose parents have similar HLA antigens. Preeclampsia is an endothelial disorder resulting from poor placental perfusion, which releases a factor that injures the endothelium, causing activation of coagulation and an increased sensitivity to pressors. Before the syndrome becomes clinically manifest in the second half of pregnancy, there has been vasospasm in various small vessel beds, accounting for the pathologic changes in maternal organs and the placenta with consequent adverse effects on the fetus.

The use of diuretics, dietary restriction or enhancement, sodium restriction, aspirin, and vitamin-mineral supplements such as calcium or vitamin C and E have not yet been confirmed to be useful in clinical studies. The only cure is termination of the pregnancy at a time as favorable as possible for fetal survival.

Clinical Findings

Clinically, the severity of preeclampsia-eclampsia can be measured with reference to the six major sites in which it exerts its effects: the central nervous system, the kidneys, the liver, the hematologic and vascular systems, and the fetal-placental unit. By evaluating each of these areas for the presence of mild to moderate versus severe preeclampsia-eclampsia, the degree of involvement can be assessed, and an appropriate management plan can be formulated that is integrated with gestational age assessment (Table 18–2).

A. PREECLAMPSIA

1. Mild to moderate—Precise differentiation between mild and moderate preeclampsia is difficult because the abnormalities that define the disease are quite variable and fail to accurately predict progression to more severe

Table 18–2. Indicators of mild to moderate versus severe preeclampsia-eclampsia.

Site	Indicator	Mild to Moderate	Severe
Central nervous system	Symptoms and signs	Hyperreflexia Headache	Seizures Blurred vision Scotomas Headache Clonus Irritability
Kidney	Proteinuria	0.3–5 g/24 h	> 5 g/24 h or catheterized urine with 4+ protein
	Uric acid	↑ > 4.5 mg/dL	↑↑ > 4.5 mg/dL
	Urinary output	> 20–30 mL/h	< 20–30 mL/h
Liver	AST, ALT, LDH	Normal	Elevated LFTs Epigastric pain Ruptured liver
Hematologic	Platelets Hemoglobin	> 100,000/mcL Normal range	< 100,000/mcL Elevated
Vascular	Blood pressure	< 160/110 mm Hg	> 160/110 mm Hg
	Retina	Arteriolar spasm	Retinal hemorrhages
Fetal-placental unit	Growth restriction	Absent	Present
	Oligohydramnios	May be present	Present
	Fetal distress	Absent	Present

AST = aspartate aminotransferase; ALT = alanine aminotransferase; LDH = lactate dehydrogenase; LFTs = liver function tests.

disease. Symptoms are generally minimal or mild. With mild preeclampsia, patients usually have few complaints, and the diastolic blood pressure is less than 90–100 mm Hg. Edema is usually more pronounced with moderate disease, and diastolic blood pressures are in the range of 90–110 mm Hg. The platelet count is over 100,000/mcL, antepartum fetal testing is reassuring, central nervous system irritability is minimal, epigastric pain is not present, and liver enzymes are not elevated.

2. Severe—Symptoms are more dramatic and persistent. The blood pressure is often quite high, with readings over 160/110 mm Hg. Thrombocytopenia (platelet counts < 100,000/mcL) may be present and progress to disseminated intravascular coagulation. Severe epigastric pain may be present from hepatic subcapsular hemorrhage with significant stretch or rupture of the liver capsule. The HELLP syndrome (hemolysis, elevated liver enzymes, low platelets) is a form of severe preeclampsia.

B. ECLAMPSIA

The occurrence of seizures defines eclampsia. It is a manifestation of severe central nervous system involvement. The other abnormal findings of severe preeclampsia are also observed with eclampsia.

Differential Diagnosis

Preeclampsia-eclampsia can mimic and be confused with many other diseases, including chronic hypertension, chronic renal disease, primary seizure disorders, gallbladder and pancreatic disease, immune or thrombotic thrombocytopenic purpura, and hemolytic-uremic syndrome. It must always be considered a possibility in any pregnant woman beyond 20 weeks of gestation. It is particularly difficult to diagnose when preexisting disease such as hypertension is present. Uric acid values can be quite helpful in such situations, since hyperuricemia is uncommon in pregnancy except with gout, renal failure, or preeclampsia-eclampsia.

Treatment

A. PREECLAMPSIA

Early recognition is the key to treatment. This requires careful attention to the details of prenatal care—especially subtle changes in blood pressure and weight. The objectives are to prolong pregnancy if possible, to allow fetal lung maturity while preventing progression to severe disease and eclampsia. The critical factors are the gestational age of the fetus, fetal pulmonary maturity status, and the severity of maternal disease. Preeclampsia-eclampsia at 36 weeks or more of gestation is managed by delivery regardless of how mild the disease is judged to be. Prior to 36 weeks, severe preeclampsia-eclampsia requires delivery except in unusual circumstances associated with extreme fetal prematurity, in which case prolongation of pregnancy may be attempted. Epigastric pain, thrombocytopenia, and visual disturbances are strong indications for de-

livery of the fetus. For mild to moderate preeclampsia-eclampsia, bed rest is the cornerstone of therapy. This increases central blood flow to the kidneys, heart, brain, liver, and placenta and may stabilize or even improve the degree of preeclampsia-eclampsia for a period of time.

Bed rest may be attempted at home or in the hospital. Prior to making this decision, the provider should evaluate the six sites of involvement listed in Table 18–2 and make an assessment about the severity of disease.

1. Home management—Home management with bed rest may be attempted for patients with mild preeclampsia and a stable home situation. This requires homemaking assistance, rapid access to the hospital, a reliable patient, and the ability to obtain frequent blood pressure readings. A home health nurse can often provide frequent home visits and assessment.

2. Hospital care—Hospitalization is required for women with moderate or severe preeclampsia or those with unreliable home situations. Regular assessment of blood pressure, reflexes, urine protein, and fetal heart tones and activity are required. A complete blood count, platelet count, and electrolyte panel including liver enzymes should be checked every 1 or 2 days. A 24-hour urine collection for creatinine clearance and total protein should be obtained on admission and repeated as indicated. Sedatives and opioids should be avoided because the fetal central nervous system depressant effects interfere with fetal testing. Magnesium sulfate is not used until the diagnosis of severe preeclampsia-eclampsia is made or until labor occurs.

Fetal evaluation should be obtained as part of the workup. If the patient is being admitted to the hospital, fetal testing must be performed on the same day to make certain that the fetus is safe. This may be done by fetal heart rate testing with nonstress or stress testing or by biophysical profile. A regular schedule of fetal surveillance must then be followed. Daily fetal kick counts can be recorded by the patient herself. Consideration should be given to amniocentesis to evaluate fetal lung maturity status if hospitalization occurs at 30–37 weeks of gestation. If immaturity is present, corticosteroids (betamethasone 12 mg or dexamethasone 16 mg, two doses intramuscularly 12–24 hours apart) can be administered to the mother. Fetuses between 26 and 30 weeks of gestation can be presumed to be immature, and corticosteroids should be given.

The method of delivery is determined by the maternal and fetal status. Cesarean section is reserved for the usual fetal indications.

B. ECLAMPSIA

1. Emergency care—If the patient is convulsing, she is turned on her side to prevent aspiration and to improve blood flow to the placenta. Fluid or food is aspirated from the glottis or trachea. The seizure may be stopped by giving an intravenous bolus of either magnesium sulfate, 4 g, or diazepam, 5–10 mg, over 4 minutes or until the seizure stops. A continuous intravenous infusion of magnesium sulfate is then started at a rate of 2–3 g/h unless the patient is known to have significantly reduced renal function. Magnesium blood levels are then checked every 4–6 hours and the infusion rate adjusted to maintain a therapeutic blood level (4–6 mEq/L). Urinary output is checked hourly and the patient assessed for signs of possible magnesium toxicity such as loss of deep tendon reflexes or decrease in respiratory rate and depth, which can be reversed with calcium gluconate.

2. General care—The occurrence of eclampsia necessitates delivery once the patient is stabilized. It is important, however, that assessment of the status of the patient and fetus take place first. Continuous fetal monitoring must be performed and blood typed and cross-matched quickly. A urinary catheter is inserted to monitor urinary output, and blood is sent for complete blood count, platelets, liver enzymes, uric acid, creatinine or urea nitrogen, and electrolytes. If hypertension is present with diastolic values over 110 mm Hg, antihypertensive medications should be administered to reduce the diastolic blood pressure to 90–100 mm Hg. Lower blood pressures than this may induce placental insufficiency through reduced perfusion. Hydralazine given in 5- to 10-mg increments intravenously every 20 minutes is frequently used to lower blood pressure. Nifedipine, 10 mg sublingually or orally, or labetalol, 10–20 mg intravenously, both every 20 minutes, can also be used.

3. Delivery—Except in unusual circumstances, delivery is mandated once eclampsia has occurred. Vaginal delivery may be attempted if the patient has already been in active labor or the cervix is quite favorable *and* the patient is clinically stable. The rapidity with which delivery must be achieved depends on the fetal and maternal status following the seizure and the availability of laboratory data on the patient. Oxytocin may be used to induce or augment labor. Regional analgesia or anesthesia is acceptable. Cesarean section is used for the usual obstetric indications or when rapid delivery is necessary for maternal or fetal indications.

4. Postpartum—Magnesium sulfate infusion (2–3 g/h) should be continued until preeclampsia-eclampsia has begun to resolve postpartum (which may take 1–7 days), but in any case for at least 24 hours. The most reliable indicator of this resolution is the onset of diuresis with urinary output of over 100–200 mL/h. When this occurs, magnesium sulfate can be discontinued. Late-onset preeclampsia-eclampsia can occur during the postpartum period. It is usually manifested by either hypertension or seizures. Treatment is the same as prior to delivery—ie, with magnesium sulfate—although other antiseizure medications can be used since the fetus is no longer present.

Lain KY et al: Contemporary concepts of the pathogenesis and management of preeclampsia. JAMA 2002;287:3183. [PMID: 12076198]

Sibai BM: Diagnosis, prevention, and management of eclampsia. Obstet Gynecol 2005;105:402. [PMID: 15684172]

GESTATIONAL TROPHOBLASTIC DISEASE (Hydatidiform Mole & Choriocarcinoma)

 ESSENTIALS OF DIAGNOSIS

Hydatidiform Mole

- *Amenorrhea.*
- *Irregular uterine bleeding.*
- *Serum hCG β-subunit > 40,000 mU/mL.*
- *Passage of grape-like clusters of enlarged edematous villi per vagina.*
- *Ultrasound of uterus with characteristic heterogeneous echogenic image and no fetus or placenta.*
- *Cytogenetic composition is 46,XX (85%), completely of paternal origin.*

General Considerations

Gestational trophoblastic disease is a spectrum of disorders that includes hydatidiform mole, invasive mole, and choriocarcinoma. Partial moles generally show evidence of an embryo or gestational sac; are polyploid, slower-growing, and less symptomatic; and often present clinically as a missed abortion. Partial moles tend to follow a benign course, while complete moles have a greater tendency to become choriocarcinomas.

The highest rates of gestational trophoblastic disease occur in some developing countries, with rates of 1:125 pregnancies in certain areas of Asia. In the United States, the frequency is 1:1500 pregnancies. Risk factors include low socioeconomic status, a history of mole, and age below 18 or above 40. Approximately 10% of women require further treatment after evacuation of the mole; 5% develop choriocarcinoma.

Clinical Findings

A. SYMPTOMS AND SIGNS

Excessive nausea and vomiting occur in over one-third of patients with hydatidiform mole. Uterine bleeding, beginning at 6–8 weeks, is observed in virtually all instances. In about one-fifth of cases, the uterus is larger than would be expected in a normal pregnancy of the same duration. Bilaterally enlarged cystic ovaries are sometimes palpable. They are the result of ovarian hyperstimulation due to excess of hCG.

Preeclampsia-eclampsia, frequently of the fulminating type, may develop during the second trimester of pregnancy, but this is unusual.

Choriocarcinoma may be manifested by continued or recurrent uterine bleeding after evacuation of a mole or following delivery, abortion, or ectopic pregnancy. The presence of an ulcerative vaginal tumor, pelvic mass, or evidence of distant metastatic tumor may be the presenting observation. The diagnosis is established by pathologic examination of curettings or by biopsy.

B. LABORATORY FINDINGS

A serum hCG β-subunit value above 40,000 mU/mL or a urinary hCG value in excess of 100,000 units/24 h increases the likelihood of hydatidiform mole.

C. IMAGING

Ultrasound has virtually replaced all other means of preoperative diagnosis of hydatidiform mole. A preoperative chest film is indicated to rule out pulmonary metastases of trophoblast.

Treatment

A. SPECIFIC (SURGICAL) MEASURES

The uterus should be emptied as soon as the diagnosis of hydatidiform mole is established, preferably by suction. Ovarian cysts should not be resected nor ovaries removed; spontaneous regression of theca lutein cysts will occur with elimination of the mole.

If malignant tissue is discovered at surgery or during the follow-up examination, chemotherapy is indicated.

Thyrotoxicosis indistinguishable clinically from that of thyroid origin may occur. While hCG usually has minimal TSH-like activity, the very high hCG levels associated with moles result in the release of T_3 and T_4 and cause hyperthyroidism. Patients thyrotoxic on this basis should be stabilized with β-blockers prior to induction of anesthesia for their surgical evacuation. Surgical removal of the mole promptly corrects the thyroid overactivity.

B. FOLLOW-UP MEASURES

Effective contraception (preferably birth control pills) should be prescribed. Weekly quantitative hCG level measurements are initially required. Following successful surgical evacuation, moles show a progressive decline in hCG. After two negative weekly tests (< 5 mU/mL), the interval may be increased to monthly for 6 months and then to every 2 months for a total of 1 year. If levels plateau or begin to rise, the patient should be evaluated by repeat chest film and dilatation and curettage (D&C) before the initiation of chemotherapy.

C. ANTITUMOR CHEMOTHERAPY

For low-risk patients with a good prognosis, methotrexate, 0.4 mg/kg intramuscularly over a 5-day period, or dactinomycin, 10–12 mcg/kg/d intravenously over a 5-day period, is used (see Table 40–3). The side effects—anorexia, nausea and vomiting, stomatitis, rash, diarrhea, and bone marrow depression—usually are revers-

ible in about 3 weeks and can be ameliorated by the administration of leucovorin (0.1 mg/kg) intramuscularly. Repeated courses of methotrexate 2 weeks apart generally are required to destroy the trophoblast and maintain a zero chorionic gonadotropin titer, as indicated by β-hCG determination. Patients with a poor prognosis should be referred to a cancer center, where multiple-agent chemotherapy probably will be given.

D. SUPPORTIVE MEASURES

Oral contraceptives (if acceptable) or another reliable birth control method should be prescribed to avoid the hazard and confusion of elevated hCG from a new pregnancy. The hCG levels should be negative for 6 months to 1 year before pregnancy is again attempted. In the pregnancy following a mole, the hCG level should be checked 6 weeks postpartum.

Prognosis

Five years survival after courses of chemotherapy, even when metastases have been demonstrated, can be expected in at least 85% of cases of choriocarcinoma.

Fulop V et al: Molecular biology of gestational trophoblastic neoplasia: a review. J Reprod Med 2004;49:415. [PMID: 15283047]

Smith HO et al: Choriocarcinoma and gestational trophoblastic disease. Obstet Gynecol Clin North Am 2005;32:661. [PMID: 16310678]

THIRD-TRIMESTER BLEEDING

Five to 10 percent of women have vaginal bleeding in late pregnancy. The clinician must distinguish between placental causes (placenta previa, placental abruption, vasa previa) and nonplacental causes (infection, disorders of the lower genital tract, systemic disease). The approach to bleeding in late pregnancy should be conservative and expectant unless fetal distress or risk of maternal hemorrhage occurs.

The patient should be hospitalized and placed at bed rest with continuous fetal monitoring. A complete blood count (including platelets) should be obtained and two to four units of blood typed and cross-matched. Coagulation studies should be ordered as clinically indicated. Ultrasound examination should be performed to determine placental location. Speculum and digital pelvic examinations are done only after ultrasound study has ruled out placenta previa. Continuous electronic fetal monitoring is required to exclude fetal distress. While uterine contractions, pain, or tenderness often indicate associated abruptio placentae, an ultrasound negative for retroplacental clot does not exclude it.

If the patient is at less than 36 weeks of gestation, continued hospitalization and bed rest may be necessary, especially with placenta previa during the initial 7–10 days following vaginal bleeding. If the patient has close proximity to the hospital and immediate access, can be on strict bed rest, and has complete resolution of bleeding and uterine contractions, home management may be considered. She must be well instructed and counseled regarding the risks. Patients with vaginal bleeding at less than 36 weeks of gestation should also be considered for amniocentesis to test for fetal lung maturity. Corticosteroid therapy (betamethasone 12 mg intramuscularly, two doses 12–24 hours apart) is indicated if fetal lung immaturity is present.

Usta IM et al: Placenta previa-accreta: risk factors and complications. Am J Obstet Gynecol 2005;193(3 Pt 2):1045. [PMID: 16157109]

MEDICAL CONDITIONS COMPLICATING PREGNANCY

Anemia

Plasma volume increases 50% during pregnancy, while red cell volume increases 25%, causing lower hemoglobin and hematocrit values, which are maximally changed around the 24th to 28th weeks. Anemia in pregnancy is often defined as a hemoglobin measurement below 10 g/dL or hematocrit below 30%. Anemia is very common in pregnancy, causing fatigue, anorexia, dyspnea, and edema. Prevention through optimal nutrition and iron and folic acid supplementation is desirable.

A. IRON DEFICIENCY ANEMIA

Many women enter pregnancy with low iron stores resulting from heavy menstrual periods, previous pregnancies, breast-feeding, or poor nutrition. It is difficult to meet the increased requirement for iron through diet, and anemia often develops unless iron supplements are given. Red cells may not become hypochromic and microcytic until the hematocrit has fallen significantly. When this occurs, a serum iron level below 40 mcg/dL and a transferrin saturation less than 10% are consistent with iron deficiency anemia (see Chapter 13). Treatment consists of a diet containing iron-rich foods and 60 mg of oral elemental iron (eg, 300 mg of ferrous sulfate) three times a day with meals. Iron is best absorbed if taken with a source of vitamin C (raw fruits and vegetables, lightly cooked greens). All pregnant women should take daily iron supplements.

B. FOLIC ACID DEFICIENCY ANEMIA

Folic acid deficiency anemia is the main cause of macrocytic anemia in pregnancy, since vitamin B_{12} deficiency anemia is rare in the childbearing years. The daily requirement of folic acid doubles from 0.4 mg to 0.8 mg in pregnancy. Twin pregnancies, infections, malabsorption, and use of anticonvulsant drugs such as phenytoin can precipitate folic acid deficiency. The anemia may first be seen in the puerperium owing to the increased need for folate during lactation.

The diagnosis is made by finding macrocytic red cells and hypersegmented neutrophils in a blood smear (see Chapter 13). However, blood smears in pregnancy may be difficult to interpret, since they frequently show iron deficiency changes as well. Because the deficiency is hard to diagnose and folate intake is inadequate in some socioeconomic groups, 0.8–1 mg of oral folic acid is given as a supplement in pregnancy; the dose in established deficiency is 1–5 mg/d.

Good sources of folate in food are leafy green vegetables, orange juice, peanuts, and beans. Cooking and storage of food destroy folic acid. Strict vegetarians who eat no eggs or milk products should take vitamin B_{12} supplements during pregnancy and lactation.

C. SICKLE CELL ANEMIA

Women with sickle cell anemia are subject to serious complications in pregnancy. The anemia becomes more severe, and crises may occur more frequently. Complications include infections, bone pain, pulmonary infarction, congestive heart failure, and preeclampsia. There is an increased rate of spontaneous abortion and higher maternal and perinatal mortality rates. Intensive medical treatment may improve the outcome for mother and fetus. Frequent indicated transfusions of packed cells or leukocyte-poor washed red cells lower the level of hemoglobin S and elevate the level of hemoglobin A; this minimizes the severity of anemia and the risk of sickle cell crises.

Genetic counseling should be offered to patients with sickle cell disease or sickle trait. They may wish to undergo first-trimester chorionic villus biopsy or second-trimester amniocentesis to determine whether the abnormality has been passed on to the fetus. Intrauterine devices and oral contraceptives are relatively contraindicated, but progestin-only contraceptives may be used. Women with sickle cell trait alone usually have an uncomplicated gestation except for an increased risk of urinary tract infection. Sickle cell-hemoglobin C disease in pregnancy is similar to sickle cell anemia and is treated similarly.

Bodnar LM et al: Predictors of pregnancy and postpartum haemoglobin concentrations in low-income women. Public Health Nutr 2004;7:701. [PMID: 15369607]

Lupus Anticoagulant-Anticardiolipin-Antiphospholipid Antibody Syndrome

The presence of antibodies to phospholipids and a variety of clinical symptoms, including vascular thromboses, thrombocytopenia, and recurrent pregnancy loss, characterize the lupus anticoagulant-anticardiolipin-antiphospholipid antibody syndrome. Many of these patients have systemic lupus erythematosus–like symptoms but do not meet specific diagnostic criteria for that disease. The lupus anticoagulant and anticardiolipin antibody may occur in these patients, and both may cause arterial and venous thromboses. Detection of these antiphospholipid antibodies may require a combination of laboratory tests. The lupus anticoagulant will prolong both the partial thromboplastin time and the Russell viper venom time. The latter is a more sensitive predictor of disease. Such patients should also be screened for the presence of the factor V Leiden mutation. Anticardiolipin antibody may be detected with enzyme-linked immunosorbent assay (ELISA) testing. Either antibody may cause false-positive serologic tests for syphilis.

This syndrome may require treatment with anticoagulant medications. In a small number of patients with recurrent pregnancy loss and a diagnosis of lupus anticoagulant syndrome, improved outcomes have been reported following treatment with heparin anticoagulation (8000–20,000 units in two or three doses daily) or low-molecular-weight heparin (1 mg/kg twice daily) and low-dose aspirin begun before or early in pregnancy and continued until the postpartum period. The addition of monthly infusions of intravenous immunoglobulin to this regimen did not improve outcomes in such patients.

Empson M et al: Prevention of recurrent miscarriage for women with antiphospholipid antibody or lupus anticoagulant. Cochrane Database Syst Rev 2005;(2):CD002859. [PMID: 15846641]

Levine JS et al: The antiphospholipid syndrome. N Engl J Med 2002;346:752. [PMID: 11882732]

Asthma

The effect of pregnancy on asthma is unpredictable. About 50% of patients have no change, 25% improve, and 25% get worse. Management of acute and chronic asthma during pregnancy does not differ significantly from that of nonpregnant women. The goal is to maintain maternal $PO_2 > 80$ mm Hg to sustain normal fetal oxygenation (see Chapter 9).

Blaiss MS: Management of asthma during pregnancy. Allergy Asthma Proc 2004;25:375. [PMID: 15709447]

AIDS during Pregnancy

Heterosexual acquisition (45%) and injection drug use (17%) are the principal identified modes of HIV infection in women. Asymptomatic infection is associated with a normal pregnancy rate and no increased risk of adverse pregnancy outcomes. There is no evidence that pregnancy causes AIDS progression.

Although some fetuses appear to acquire HIV infection antenatally by transplacental transmission, approximately two-thirds are infected close to or during the time of delivery. Zidovudine (500 mg/d orally) given to the mother antenatally starting at 14 weeks of gestation and during labor (1 mg/kg/h intravenously) and then to the infant (2 mg/kg orally four times daily) for the first 6 weeks of life reduces the transmission rate from 25% to 8%. HIV-positive pregnant women should be assessed by CD4 count, plasma RNA levels, and prior or current antiretroviral use. In general, pregnant HIV-positive women should receive at least zidovudine but also highly active antiretroviral therapy (HAART) appropriate for their HIV disease status after counseling regarding the potential impact of therapy on the fetus and infant after delivery. Although information is limited, zidovudine has been associated with mild anemia in infants at birth but only efavirenz has been clearly linked with anomalies (myelomeningocele). The use of prophylactic elective cesarean section before the onset of labor or rupture of the membranes to prevent vertical transmission of HIV infection from mother to fetus has been shown to reduce the transmission rate to 2% in infants of mothers taking zidovudine. There is limited information on the impact of elective cesarean section on transmission rates in infants of mothers on HAART or with viral loads less than 1000 copies/mL. However, with HAART therapy and undetectable viral loads (< 50 copies/mL), there may be no additional benefit of cesarean delivery. HIV-infected women should be advised not to breast-feed their infants.

Abrams EJ: Prevention of mother-to-child transmission of HIV— successes, controversies and critical questions. AIDS Rev 2004;6:131. [PMID: 15595430]

Public Health Service Task Force Recommendations for Use of Antiretroviral Drugs in Pregnant HIV-1 Infected Women for Maternal Health and Interventions to Reduce Perinatal HIV-1 Transmission in the United States. http://www.hivatis.org.

Watts DH: Management of human immunodeficiency virus in pregnancy. N Engl J Med 2002;346:1879. [PMID: 12063373]

Diabetes Mellitus

Pregnancy is associated with increased tissue resistance to insulin, resulting in increased levels of blood insulin as well as glucose and triglycerides. These changes are due to placental lactogen and elevated circulating estrogens and progesterone. Although pregnancy does not appear to alter the long-term consequences of diabetes, retinopathy and nephropathy may first appear or become worse during pregnancy. Debate continues over whether gestational diabetics are women whose glucose intolerance is solely a function of their pregnancy compared with their nonpregnant state. Alternatively, pregnancy may merely serve to unmask an underlying propensity for glucose intolerance, which will be evident even in the nonpregnant state at some time in the future if not in the immediate postpartum period. However, goals for glycemic control during pregnancy are the same whether the diagnosis is made before or during the pregnancy.

Prepregnancy counseling and evaluation of diabetic women should include a complete chemistry panel, HbA_{1c} determination, 24-hour urine collection for total protein and creatinine clearance, funduscopic examination, and an ECG. Any medical problems should be addressed, and HbA_{1c} levels of 6% should be achieved before pregnancy. Euglycemia should be established before conception and maintained during pregnancy with daily home glucose monitoring by the patient. A well-planned dietary program is a key component, with an intake of 1800–2200 kcal/d divided into three meals and three snacks. Insulin is given subcutaneously in a split-dose regimen with frequent dosage adjustments. Patients taking some oral agents prior to pregnancy should be switched to insulin. However, limited information suggests that agents such as glyburide may be safe and effective in pregnancy. The use of continuous insulin pump therapy has been found to be very useful during pregnancy in women with type 1 diabetes mellitus.

Congenital anomalies result from hyperglycemia during the first 4–8 weeks of pregnancy. They occur in 4–10% of diabetic pregnancies (two to three times the rate in nondiabetic pregnancies). Euglycemia in the early weeks of pregnancy, when organogenesis is occurring, reduces the rate of anomalies to near-normal levels. Even so, because few women with diabetes begin a rigorous program to achieve euglycemia until well after they have become pregnant, congenital anomalies are the principal cause of perinatal fetal deaths in diabetic pregnancies. All women with diabetes should receive counseling about pregnancy and, when the decision has been made to start a family, should receive prepregnancy management by providers experienced in diabetic pregnancies.

Fasting and preprandial glucose values are lower during pregnancy in both diabetic and nondiabetic women. Euglycemia is considered to be 60–80 mg/dL while fasting and 30–45 minutes before meals and < 120 mg/dL 2 hours after meals. This is the target for good diabetic control during pregnancy. Glycated hemoglobin levels help determine the quality of glucose control both before and during pregnancy.

While perinatal problems for mother and baby are decreased by fastidious diabetic control, the incidence of hydramnios, preeclampsia-eclampsia, infections, and prematurity is increased even in carefully managed diabetic pregnancies. Diabetes is an inherently unstable disease characterized by fluctuations of blood glucose levels, particularly late in pregnancy. The risk of fetal demise in the third trimester (stillbirth) and neonatal death increases with the level of hyperglycemia. Consequently, pregnant women with diabetes must receive regular antepartum fetal testing (nonstress testing, contraction stress testing, biophysical profile) during the third trimester. The timing of delivery is dictated by the quality of diabetic control, the presence or absence of medical complications, and fetal status. The goal is to reach 39 weeks (38 completed weeks) and then proceed with delivery. Confirmation of lung maturity is necessary only for delivery prior to 39 weeks. Cesarean sections are performed for obstetric indications.

Because 15% of patients with gestational diabetes require insulin during pregnancy and because the infants of gestational diabetics have some risks similar to those of infants of diabetic mothers (particularly macrosomia), screening of women for glucose intolerance has been recommended between the 24th and 28th weeks of pregnancy (Table 18–3). Patients with gestational diabetes should be evaluated 6–8 weeks postpar-

Table 18–3. Screening and diagnostic criteria for gestational diabetes mellitus.

Screening for gestational diabetes mellitus
1. 50-g oral glucose load, administered between the 24th and 28th weeks, without regard to time of day or time of last meal. Universal blood glucose screening is indicated for patients who are of Hispanic, African, Native American, South or East Asian, Pacific Island, or Indigenous Australian ancestry. Other patients who have no known diabetes in first-degree relatives, are under 25 years of age, have normal weight before pregnancy, and have no history of abnormal glucose metabolism or poor obstetric outcome do not require routine screening.
2. Venous plasma glucose measure 1 hour later.
3. Value of 130 mg/dL (7.2 mmol/L) or above in venous plasma indicates the need for a full diagnostic glucose tolerance test.

Diagnosis of gestational diabetes mellitus
1. 100-g oral glucose load, administered in the morning after overnight fast lasting at least 8 hours but not more than 14 hours, and following at least 3 days of unrestricted diet (> 150 g carbohydrate) and physical activity.
2. Venous plasma glucose is measured fasting and at 1, 2, and 3 hours. Subject should remain seated and should not smoke throughout the test.
3. Two or more of the following venous plasma concentrations must be equaled or exceeded for a diagnosis of gestational diabetes: fasting, 95 mg/dL (5.3 mmol/L); 1 hour, 180 mg/dL (10 mmol/L); 2 hours, 155 mg/dL (8.6 mmol/L); 3 hours, 140 mg/dL (7.8 mmol/L).

tum by a 2-hour oral glucose tolerance test (75 g glucose load).

ACOG Practice Bulletin. Clinical Management Guidelines for Obstetrician-Gynecologists. Number 60, March 2005. Pregestational diabetes mellitus. Obstet Gynecol 2005; 105:675. [PMID: 15738045]

Blayo A et al: Screening and diagnosis of gestational diabetes. Diabetes Metab 2004;30:575. [PMID: 15671929]

Langer O et al: A comparison of glyburide and insulin in women with gestational diabetes mellitus. N Engl J Med 2000;343: 1134. [PMID: 11036118]

Heart Disease

Overall, 5% of maternal deaths are due to heart disease. Most heart disease complicating pregnancy in the United States is congenital heart disease. Normal pregnancy causes a faster pulse, an increase of cardiac output of more than 30%, and a rise in plasma volume greater than red cell mass with relative hemodilution. Vital capacity and oxygen consumption rise only slightly.

For practical purposes, the functional capacity of the heart is the best single measurement of cardiopulmonary status.

FUNCTIONAL CARDIAC ASSESSMENT

Class I	Ordinary physical activity causes no discomfort (perinatal mortality rate about 5%).
Class II	Ordinary activity causes discomfort and slight disability (perinatal mortality rate 10–15%).
Class III	Less than ordinary activity causes discomfort or disability; patient is barely compensated (perinatal mortality rate about 35%).
Class IV	Patient decompensated; any physical activity causes acute distress (perinatal mortality rate over 50%).

In general, patients with class I or class II functional disability (80% of pregnant women with heart disease) do well obstetrically, with four-fifths of maternal deaths due to heart disease occurring in women with class III or class IV disability. Congestive failure is the usual cause of death. Most deaths occur in the early puerperium. Pregnancy is contraindicated in Eisenmenger's complex, in primary pulmonary hypertension, in severe mitral stenosis with secondary pulmonary hypertension, and in Marfan's syndrome, in which the aorta is prone to dissection and rupture. In addition, pregnancy is poorly tolerated in patients with aortic stenosis, aortic coarctation, tetralogy of Fallot, and active rheumatic carditis.

Therapeutic abortion and elective sterilization should be offered to patients with significant cardiac disease. Cesarean section should be performed only for obstetric indications. Women with valvular heart disease, mitral valve prolapse associated with mitral insufficiency, or idiopathic hypertrophic cardiomyopathy should receive appropriate antibiotic prophylaxis against infective endocarditis during labor and delivery or termination of pregnancy.

Earing MG et al: Congenital heart disease and pregnancy: maternal and fetal risks. Clin Perinatol 2005;32:913. [PMID: 16325669]

Peripartum Cardiomyopathy

Cardiac failure that develops during pregnancy or during the first 6 months postpartum in a woman without a history of heart disease and with no cause for heart failure other than pregnancy is termed peripartum cardiomyopathy. The incidence varies from 1:4000 to 1:1000. It is higher in Africa. It occurs more often in older women, those with twins, and in patients with pregnancy-induced hypertension. The cause of peripartum cardiomyopathy is unknown. In patients who continue to have symptoms and signs of disease for more than 6 months postpartum, the mortality rate is high, and subsequent pregnancy is especially dangerous.

Symptoms of peripartum cardiomyopathy are those of congestive heart failure. An ECG may reveal tachycardia and atrial or ventricular arrhythmias. Death may occur as a result of arrhythmia or embolism. Autopsy usually reveals an enlarged, dilated heart, and mural thrombi (the source of pulmonary and systemic emboli) are often found.

The treatment of peripartum cardiomyopathy is that of congestive cardiomyopathy (see Chapter 10). Patients with persistent cardiomegaly or mural thrombi shown by echocardiography require anticoagulant therapy. The long-term prognosis in these patients depends on whether cardiomegaly resolves within 6 months after the onset of symptoms. If it does not resolve, the 5-year mortality rate is 6%. If cardiomegaly does not resolve and another pregnancy intervenes, cardiomyopathy recurs in 50% of cases, with a 19% mortality rate.

Phillips SD et al: Peripartum cardiomyopathy: current therapeutic perspective. Curr Treat Options Cardiovasc Med 2004; 6:481. [PMID: 15496265]

Herpes Genitalis (See also Chapter 6)

Infection of the lower genital tract by herpes simplex virus type 2 (HSV-2) is a common STD of potential seriousness to pregnant women and their newborn infants. Although up to 20% of women in an obstetric practice may have antibodies to HSV-2, a history of the infection is unreliable and the incidence of neonatal infection is low (1:20,000–1:3000 live births). Most infected neonates are born to women with no symptoms, signs, or history of infection.

Women who have had *primary* herpes infection late in pregnancy are at high risk for shedding virus at delivery. Some authors suggest use of prophylactic acyclovir, 400 mg orally twice daily, to decrease the likelihood of active lesions at the time of labor and delivery.

Women with a history of *recurrent* genital herpes have a neonatal attack rate of 5% and should be followed by clinical observation and culture of any suspicious lesions. Since asymptomatic viral shedding is not predictable by antepartum cultures, current recommendations do not include routine cultures in individuals with a history of herpes without active disease. However, when labor begins, vulvar and cervical inspection and cultures should be performed, with prompt treatment of a newborn after a positive culture.

For treatment, see Chapter 32. The use of acyclovir in pregnancy is acceptable when there is significant fetal or neonatal risk.

Cesarean section is indicated at the time of labor if there are prodromal symptoms, active genital lesions, or a positive cervical culture obtained within the preceding week.

Brown ZA et al: Genital herpes complicating pregnancy. Obstet Gynecol 2005;106:845. [PMID: 16199646]

Hypertensive Disease

Hypertensive disease in women of childbearing age is usually essential hypertension, but secondary causes should be considered: coarctation of the aorta, pheochromocytoma, hyperaldosteronism, and renovascular and renal hypertension.

Preeclampsia is superimposed on 20% of pregnancies in hypertensive women and appears earlier, is more severe, and is more often associated with intrauterine growth restriction. It may be difficult to determine whether or not hypertension in a pregnant woman precedes or derives from the pregnancy if she is not examined until after the 20th week. Serum uric acid can help differentiate, since it is elevated with preeclampsia and generally normal in chronic hypertension unless the patient is receiving diuretics. If hypertension persists for 6–8 weeks postpartum, essential hypertension is likely.

Pregnant women with chronic hypertension require medication only if the diastolic pressure is sustained at or above 100 mm Hg. For initiation of treatment, methyldopa has the longest record of safety in a starting dosage of 250 mg orally twice daily. Therapy with β-blockers or calcium channel blockers is also acceptable (see Tables 11–7, 11–9). The goal is to keep the diastolic pressure between 80 mm Hg and 100 mm Hg.

If a hypertensive woman is being managed successfully by medical treatment when she registers for antenatal care, one may generally continue the antihypertensive medication. Diuretics may be continued in pregnancy. Angiotensin-converting enzyme inhibitors should be replaced with a drug of another class because of reports of fetal and neonatal renal failure with these compounds.

Use of antihypertensive medications in preeclampsia remains controversial. This should be attempted only with significant fetal prematurity, absence of fetal compromise, and close supervision of the patient.

Therapeutic abortion may be indicated in cases of severe hypertension during pregnancy. If pregnancy is allowed to continue, the risk to the fetus must be assessed periodically in anticipation of early delivery. An early second-trimester ultrasound examination will confirm the duration of pregnancy, and follow-up examinations after 28 weeks will evaluate intrauterine growth restriction.

James PR et al: Management of hypertension before, during, and after pregnancy. Heart 2004;90:1499. [PMID: 15547046]

Maternal Hepatitis B & C Carrier State

There are an estimated 200 million chronic carriers of hepatitis B virus worldwide. Among these people there is an increased incidence of chronic active hepatitis, cirrhosis, and hepatocellular carcinoma. The frequency of the hepatitis B carrier state varies from 1% in the United States and Western Europe to 35% in parts of Africa and Asia. All pregnant women should be screened for HBsAg. Transmission of the virus to the baby after delivery is likely if both surface antigen and e antigen are positive. Vertical transmission can be blocked by the immediate postdelivery administration to the newborn of 0.5 mL of hepatitis B immunoglobulin and hepatitis B vaccine intramuscularly. The vaccine dose is repeated at 1 and 6 months of age.

Hepatitis C virus infection is the most common chronic blood-borne infection in the United States. Risk factors for transmission include blood transfusion, injection drug use, employment in patient care or clinical laboratory work, exposure to a sex partner or household member who has had a history of hepatitis, exposure to multiple sex partners, and low socioeconomic level. The average rate of hepatitis C virus (HCV) infection among infants born to HCV-positive, HIV-negative women is 5–6%. However, the average infection rate increases to 14% when mothers are coinfected with HCV and HIV. The principal factor associated with transmission is the presence of HCV RNA in the mother at the time of birth.

Ranger-Rogez S et al: Hepatitis B mother-to-child transmission. Expert Rev Anti Infect Ther 2004;2:133. [PMID: 15482178]

Acute Fatty Liver of Pregnancy

Acute fatty liver of pregnancy is a disorder limited to the gravid state. It occurs in the third trimester of pregnancy and involves acute hepatic failure. With improved recognition and immediate delivery, the mortality range is now 20–30%. The disorder is usually seen after the 35th week of gestation and is more common in primigravidas and those with twins. The incidence is about 1:14,000 deliveries.

The cause of acute fatty liver of pregnancy is not known. However, as many as 20% of cases may be due to a homozygous fetal deficiency of long-chain 3-hydroxyacyl-coenzyme A dehydrogenase (LCHAD) deficiency in a heterozygous mother. Pathologic findings are unique to the disorder, with fatty engorgement of hepatocytes. Clinical onset is gradual, with flu-like symptoms that progress to the development of abdominal pain, jaundice, encephalopathy, disseminated intravascular coagulation, and death. On examination, the patient shows signs of hepatic failure.

Laboratory findings show marked elevation of alkaline phosphatase but only moderate elevations of alanine aminotransferase (ALT) and aspartate aminotransferase (AST). Prothrombin time and bilirubin are also elevated. The white blood cell count is elevated, and the platelet count is depressed. Hypoglycemia may be extreme.

The differential diagnosis is that of fulminant hepatitis. However, liver aminotransferases for fulminant hepatitis are higher (> 1000 units/mL) than those for acute fatty liver of pregnancy (usually < 500 units/mL). It is also important to review the appropriate history and perform the appropriate tests for toxins that cause liver failure. Preeclampsia may involve the liver but typically does not cause jaundice. The elevations in liver function tests in patients with preeclampsia usually do not reach the levels seen in patients with acute fatty liver of pregnancy.

Diagnosis of acute fatty liver of pregnancy mandates immediate delivery. Supportive care during labor includes administration of glucose, platelets, and fresh frozen plasma as needed. Vaginal delivery is preferred. Resolution of encephalopathy occurs over days, and supportive care with a low-protein diet is needed.

Recurrence rates for this liver disorder are unclear but probably increased in families with proven LCHAD deficiency. Most authorities advise against subsequent pregnancy, but there have been reported cases of successful outcomes in later pregnancies.

Steingrub JS: Pregnancy-associated severe liver dysfunction. Crit Care Clin 2004;20:763. [PMID: 15388201]

Seizure Disorders

Epileptic women contemplating pregnancy who have not had a seizure for 5 years should consider a prepregnancy trial of withdrawal from treatment. Those with recurrent epilepsy should use a single drug with blood level monitoring. Trimethadione and valproate are contraindicated during pregnancy; phenytoin and carbamazepine may be teratogenic in the first trimester and should not be used unless absolutely necessary. There is limited information available on the safety of newer antiepilepsy drugs (eg, lamotrigine), and they should only be used if unavoidable.

Phenobarbital is considered the drug of choice. Serum levels should be measured in each trimester and dosage adjustments made to keep serum levels in the low normal therapeutic range. Pregnant women taking phenobarbital and phenytoin should receive vitamin supplements, including folic acid and vitamin D, throughout pregnancy. Oral vitamin K, 10–20 mg/d, is administered during the last month to help prevent bleeding problems in the newborn, who is at risk of bleeding tendencies due to decreased levels of clotting factors. Such infants should receive an injection of vitamin K_1, 1 mg subcutaneously immediately after delivery, and should have clotting studies 2–4 hours later. Breast-feeding is not contraindicated for infants of mothers taking antiseizure medications.

Syphilis, Gonorrhea, & *Chlamydia trachomatis* Infection
(See also Chapters 33 and 34)

These STDs have significant consequences for mother and child. Untreated syphilis in pregnancy will cause late abortion, stillbirth, transplacental infection, and congenital syphilis. Gonorrhea will produce large-joint arthritis by hematogenous spread as well as ophthalmia neonatorum. Maternal chlamydial infections are largely asymptomatic but are manifested in the newborn by inclusion conjunctivitis and, at age 2–4 months, by pneumonia. The diagnosis of each can be reliably made by appropriate laboratory tests, which should be included in all prenatal care. The sexual partners of women with STDs should be identified and treated also if that can be done.

Berman SM: Maternal syphilis: pathophysiology and treatment. Bull World Health Organ 2004;82:433. [PMID: 15356936]

Group B Streptococcal Infection

Group B streptococci frequently colonize the lower female genital tract, with an asymptomatic carriage rate in pregnancy of 5–30%. This rate depends on maternal age, gravidity, and geographic variation. Vaginal carriage is asymptomatic and intermittent, with spontaneous clearing in approximately 30% and recolonization in about 10% of women. Adverse perinatal outcomes associated with group B streptococcal colonization include urinary tract infection, intrauterine infection, premature rupture of membranes, preterm delivery, and postpartum endometritis.

Women with postpartum endometritis due to infection with group B streptococci, especially after cesarean section, develop fever, tachycardia, and abdominal distention, usually within 24 hours after delivery. Approximately 35% of these women are bacteremic.

Group B streptococcal infection is a common cause of neonatal sepsis. Transmission rates are high, yet the rate of neonatal sepsis is surprisingly low at less than 4:1000 live births. Unfortunately, the mortality rate associated with early-onset disease can be as high as 50% in premature infants and approaches 25% even in those at term. Moreover, these infections can contribute markedly to chronic morbidity, including mental retardation and neurologic disabilities. Late-onset disease develops through contact with hospital nursery personnel. Up to 45% of these health care workers can carry the bacteria on their skin and transmit the infection to newborns.

CDC recommendations for screening for and prophylaxis of group B streptococcal colonization are set forth in this chapter in the section on tests and procedures.

Akker-van Marle ME et al: Cost-effectiveness of different treatment strategies with intrapartum antibiotic prophylaxis to prevent early-onset group B streptococcal disease. BJOG 2005;112:820. [PMID: 15924544]

Davies HD et al: Multicenter study of a rapid molecular-based assay for the diagnosis of group B *Streptococcus* colonization in pregnant women. Clin Infect Dis 2004;39:1129. [PMID: 15486835]

Varicella

Commonly known as chickenpox, varicella-zoster virus (VZV) infection has a fairly benign course when incurred during childhood but may result in serious illness in adults, particularly during pregnancy. Infection results in lifelong immunity. Approximately 95% of women born in the United States have VZV antibodies by the time they reach reproductive age. The incidence of VZV infection during pregnancy has been reported as up to 7:10,000.

The incubation period for this infection is 10–20 days. A primary infection follows and is characterized by a flu-like syndrome with malaise, fever, and development of a pruritic maculopapular rash on the trunk which becomes vesicular and then crusts. Pregnant women are prone to the development of VZV pneumonia, often a fulminant infection sometimes requiring respiratory support. After primary infection, the virus becomes latent, ascending to dorsal root ganglia. Subsequent reactivation can occur as zoster, often under circumstances of immunocompromise, although this is rare during pregnancy.

Two types of fetal infection have been documented. The first is congenital VZV syndrome, which typically occurs in 0.4–2% of fetuses exposed to primary VZV infection during the first trimester. Anomalies include limb and digit abnormalities, microphthalmos, and microcephaly.

Infection during the second and third trimesters is less threatening. Maternal IgG crosses the placenta, protecting the fetus. The only infants at risk for severe infection are those born after maternal viremia but before development of maternal protective antibody. Maternal infection manifesting 5 days before or after delivery is the time period arbitrarily determined to be most hazardous for transmission to the fetus.

Diagnosis is commonly made on clinical grounds. Laboratory verification of recent infection is made most often by antibody detection techniques, including ELISA, fluorescent antibody, and hemagglutination inhibition. Serum obtained by cordocentesis may be tested for VZV IgM to document fetal infection.

Varicella-zoster immune globulin (VZIG) has been shown to prevent or modify the symptoms of infection in some women. Treatment success depends on identification of susceptible women at or just following exposure. Women with a questionable or negative history of chickenpox should be checked for antibody, since the overwhelming majority will have been exposed previously. If the antibody is negative, VZIG (625 units intramuscularly) should be given within 96 hours after exposure. There are no known adverse effects of VZIG administration during pregnancy. Infants born within 5 days after onset of maternal infection should also receive VZIG (125 units).

Infected pregnant women should be closely observed and hospitalized at the earliest signs of pulmonary involvement. Intravenous acyclovir (10–15 mg/kg every 8 hours for 7–10 days) is recommended in the treatment of VZV pneumonia.

Tan MP et al: Chickenpox in pregnancy: Revisited. Reprod Toxicol 2006;21:410. [PMID: 15979274]

Thyroid Disease

Thyrotoxicosis during pregnancy may result in fetal anomalies, late abortion, or preterm labor and fetal hyperthyroidism with goiter. Thyroid storm in late pregnancy or labor is a life-threatening emergency.

Radioactive isotope therapy must never be given during pregnancy. The thyroid inhibitor of choice is propylthiouracil, which acts to prevent further thyroxine formation by blocking iodination of tyrosine. There is a 2- to 3-week delay before the pretreatment hormone level begins to fall. The initial dose of propylthiouracil is 100–150 mg orally three times a day; the dose is lowered as the euthyroid state is approached. It is desirable to keep free T_4 in the high normal range during pregnancy. A maintenance dose of 100 mg/d minimizes the chance of fetal hypothyroidism and goiter.

Recurrent postpartum thyroiditis occurs 3–6 months after delivery. A hyperthyroid state of 1–3 months' duration is followed by hypothyroidism, sometimes misdiagnosed as depression. Thyroperoxidase antibodies and thyroglobulin antibodies are present. Recovery is spontaneous in over 90% of cases after 3–6 months.

Maternal hypothyroidism—even subclinical hypothyroidism manifested only by elevated levels of TSH—may adversely affect subsequent neuropsychological development of the child. Mothers with known or suspected hypothyroidism should have the TSH level measured at the first prenatal visit. Replacement therapy with levothyroxine should be adjusted to maintain levels of TSH in the normal range.

Lafranchi SH et al: Is thyroid inadequacy during gestation a risk factor for adverse pregnancy and developmental outcomes? Thyroid 2005;15:60. [PMID: 15687825]

Tuberculosis

The diagnosis of tuberculosis in pregnancy is made by history taking, physical examination, and skin testing, with special attention to women from ethnic groups with a high prevalence of the disease (such as women from southeast Asia). Chest films should not be obtained as a routine screening measure in pregnancy but should be used only in patients with a skin test conversion or with suggestive findings in the history and physical examination. Abdominal shielding must be used if a chest film is obtained.

If adequately treated, tuberculosis in pregnancy has an excellent prognosis. There is no increase in spontaneous abortion, fetal problems, or congenital anomalies.

Treatment is with isoniazid and ethambutol or isoniazid and rifampin (see Chapters 9 and 33). Because isoniazid therapy may result in vitamin B_6 deficiency, a supplement of 50 mg/d of vitamin B_6 should be given simultaneously. Streptomycin, ethionamide, and most other antituberculous drugs should be avoided in pregnancy.

Urinary Tract Infection

The urinary tract is especially vulnerable to infections during pregnancy because the altered secretions of steroid sex hormones and the pressure exerted by the gravid uterus upon the ureters and bladder cause hypotonia and congestion and predispose to urinary stasis. Labor and delivery and urinary retention postpartum also may initiate or aggravate infection. *Escherichia coli* is the offending organism in over two-thirds of cases.

From 2% to 8% of pregnant women have asymptomatic bacteriuria, which some believe to be associated with an increased risk of prematurity. It is estimated that pyelonephritis will develop in 20–40% of these women if untreated.

A first-trimester urine culture is indicated in women with a history of recurrent or recent episodes of urinary tract infection. If the culture is positive, treatment should be initiated as a prophylactic measure. Nitrofurantoin (100 mg orally twice daily), ampicillin (500 mg orally four times daily), and cephalexin (500 mg orally four times daily) are acceptable medications for 3–7 days. Sulfonamides should not be given in the third trimester because they may interfere with bilirubin binding and thus impose a risk of neonatal hyperbilirubinemia and kernicterus. Fluoroquinolones are also contraindicated because of their potential teratogenic effects on fetal cartilage and bone. If bacteriuria returns, suppressive medication (one daily dose of an appropriate antibiotic) for the remainder of the pregnancy is indicated. Acute pyelonephritis requires hospitalization for intravenous administration of antibiotics until the patient is afebrile; this is followed by a full course of oral antibiotics.

Le J et al: Urinary tract infections during pregnancy. Ann Pharmacother 2004;38:1692. [PMID: 15340129]

SURGICAL COMPLICATIONS DURING PREGNANCY

Elective major surgery should be avoided during pregnancy. Normal uncomplicated pregnancy does not alter operative risk except as it may interfere with the diagnosis of abdominal disorders and increase the technical problems of intra-abdominal surgery. Abortion is not a serious hazard after operation unless peritoneal sepsis or other significant complications occur. During the first trimester, congenital anomalies may theoretically be induced in the developing fetus by hypoxia. Thus, the second trimester is usually the optimal time for operative procedures.

Appendicitis

Appendicitis occurs in about 1 of 1500 pregnancies. Diagnosis may be difficult, since the appendix is often carried high and to the right, away from McBurney's point, as the uterus enlarges, and localization of pain does not always occur. Nausea, vomiting, fever, and leukocytosis occur regularly. Any right-sided abdominal pain associated with these symptoms should arouse suspicion. In at least 20% of obstetric patients, the diagnosis of appendicitis is not made until rupture oc-

curs and peritonitis has become established. Such a delay may lead to premature labor or abortion. With early diagnosis and appendectomy, the prognosis is good for mother and baby.

Cohen-Kerem R et al: Pregnancy outcome following non-obstetric surgical intervention. Am J Surg 2005;190:467. [PMID: 16105538]

Carcinoma of the Breast

Cancer of the breast (see also Chapter 16) is diagnosed approximately once in 3500 pregnancies. Pregnancy may accelerate the growth of cancer of the breast, and delay in diagnosis affects the outcome of treatment. Inflammatory carcinoma is an extremely virulent type of breast cancer that occurs most commonly during lactation. Prepregnancy mammography should be encouraged for women over age 35 who are anticipating a pregnancy.

Breast enlargement during pregnancy obscures parenchymal masses, and breast tissue hyperplasia decreases the accuracy of mammography. Any discrete mass should be evaluated by aspiration to verify its cystic structure, with fine-needle biopsy if it is solid. A definitive diagnosis may require excisional biopsy under local anesthesia. If breast biopsy confirms the diagnosis of cancer, surgery should be done regardless of the stage of the pregnancy. If spread to the regional glands has occurred, irradiation or chemotherapy should be considered. Under these circumstances, the alternatives are termination of an early pregnancy or delay of therapy for fetal maturation.

Choledocholithiasis, Cholecystitis, & Idiopathic Cholestasis of Pregnancy

Severe choledocholithiasis and cholecystitis are not uncommon during pregnancy. When they do occur, it is usually in late pregnancy or in the puerperium. About 90% of patients with cholecystitis have gallstones; 90% of stones will be visualized by ultrasonography. Symptomatic relief may be all that is required.

Conventional gallbladder surgery in pregnant women should be attempted only in complicated cases (eg, obstruction), because it may increase the perinatal mortality rate to about 15%. Cholecystostomy and lithotomy may be all that is feasible during advanced pregnancy, cholecystectomy being deferred until after delivery. On the other hand, withholding surgery may result in necrosis and perforation of the gallbladder and peritonitis. Cholangitis due to impacted common duct stone requires surgical removal of gallstones and establishment of biliary drainage. Endoscopic retrograde cholangiopancreatography and endoscopic retrograde sphincterotomy can be performed safely in pregnant women if precautions are taken to minimize exposure to radiation. In the early to mid second trimester, laparoscopic cholecystectomy can be performed with minimal maternal morbidity and no fetal mortality.

Idiopathic cholestasis of pregnancy is due to a hereditary metabolic (hepatic) deficiency aggravated by the high estrogen levels of pregnancy. It causes intrahepatic biliary obstruction of varying degrees. The rise in bile acids is sufficient in the third trimester to cause severe, intractable, generalized itching and sometimes clinical jaundice. There may be mild elevations in blood bilirubin and alkaline phosphatase levels. The fetus is also threatened by this condition. An increased incidence of preterm delivery has been reported as well as unexplained intrauterine fetal demise. For this reason, antenatal surveillance of the fetus is mandatory in patients with this diagnosis. Resins such as cholestyramine (4 g orally three times a day) absorb bile acids in the large bowel and relieve pruritus but are difficult to take and may cause constipation. Their use requires vitamin K supplementation. Limited but very encouraging experience has been reported with ursodeoxycholic acid, 16 mg/kg/d orally for 3 weeks, or dexamethasone, 12 mg/d orally for 7 days. The disorder is relieved once the infant has been delivered, but it recurs in subsequent pregnancies and sometimes with the use of oral contraceptives.

Ovarian Tumors

The most common adnexal mass in early pregnancy is the corpus luteum, which may become cystic and enlarge to 6 cm in diameter. Any persistent mass over 6 cm should be evaluated by ultrasound examination; unilocular cysts are likely to be corpus luteum cysts, whereas septated or semisolid tumors are likely to be neoplasms. The incidence of malignancy in ovarian masses over 6 cm in diameter is 2.5%. Ovarian tumors may undergo torsion and cause abdominal pain and nausea and vomiting and must be differentiated from appendicitis, other bowel disease, and ectopic pregnancy. Patients with suspected ovarian cancer should be referred to a tertiary perinatal center to determine whether the pregnancy can progress to fetal viability or whether treatment should be instituted without delay.

PREVENTION OF HEMOLYTIC DISEASE OF THE NEWBORN (Erythroblastosis Fetalis)

The antibody anti-$Rh_o(D)$ is responsible for most severe instances of hemolytic disease of the newborn (erythroblastosis fetalis). About 15% of whites and much lower proportions of blacks and Asians are $Rh_o(D)$-negative. If an $Rh_o(D)$-negative woman carries an $Rh_o(D)$-positive fetus, she may develop antibodies against $Rh_o(D)$ when fetal red cells enter her circulation during small fetomaternal bleeding episodes in the early third trimester or during delivery, abortion, ectopic pregnancy, abruptio placentae, or other antepartum bleeding problems. This antibody, once produced, remains in the woman's circulation and poses the threat of hemolytic disease for subsequent Rh-positive fetuses.

Passive immunization against hemolytic disease of the newborn is achieved with $Rh_o(D)$ immune globulin, a purified concentrate of antibodies against $Rh_o(D)$ an-

tigen. The $Rh_o(D)$ immune globulin (one vial of 300 mcg intramuscularly) is given to the mother within 72 hours after delivery (or spontaneous or induced abortion or ectopic pregnancy). The antibodies in the immune globulin destroy fetal Rh-positive cells so that the mother will not produce anti-$Rh_o(D)$. During her next Rh-positive gestation, erythroblastosis will be prevented. An additional safety measure is the routine administration of the immune globulin at the 28th week of pregnancy. The passive antibody titer that results is too low to significantly affect an Rh-positive fetus. The maternal clearance of the globulin is slow enough that protection will continue for 12 weeks.

Hemolytic disease of varying degrees, from mild to serious, continues to occur in association with Rh subgroups (C, c, or E) or Kell, Kidd, and other factors. Therefore, the presence of atypical antibodies should be checked in the third trimester of all pregnancies.

Matijevic R et al: Diagnosis and management of Rh alloimmunization. Fetal Diagn Ther 2005;20:393. [PMID: 16113560]

PREVENTION OF PRETERM (Premature) LABOR

Preterm (premature) labor is labor that begins before the 37th week of pregnancy; it is responsible for 85% of neonatal illnesses and deaths. The onset of labor is a result of a complex sequence of biologic events involving regulatory factors that are still poorly understood. Significant risk factors for the onset of preterm labor are a past history of preterm delivery, premature rupture of the membranes, urinary tract infection, exposure to DES, multiple gestation, and abdominal or cervical surgery. In high-risk women (prior preterm birth), ultrasound measurement of cervical length (< 25 mm) in the second trimester may also identify a significant risk.

Low rates of preterm delivery are associated with success in educating patients to identify regular, frequent uterine contractions and in alerting medical and nursing staff to evaluate these patients early and initiate treatment if cervical changes can be identified. Distinguishing true from false labor in patients with a history of previous preterm births can be facilitated by the use of fetal fibronectin measurement in cervicovaginal specimens. This ubiquitous protein can be released by several different stimuli. Its absence (< 50 ng/mL) in the face of uterine contractions in a patient with a previous preterm birth has a negative predictive value of 93–97% for delivery within 7–14 days. Despite initial promising findings, several prospective randomized controlled trials have failed to demonstrate a benefit of home uterine activity monitoring in preventing preterm birth. On the other hand, a recent study has suggested that weekly injections of 17α-hydroxyprogesterone caproate from 16 to 36 weeks of gestation in women with a history of preterm delivery can substantially reduce the rate of recurrent preterm birth.

In more acute situations, intravenous magnesium sulfate is effective, as are intravenous β-adrenergic drugs. Magnesium sulfate is given as a 4- or 6-g bolus followed by a continuous infusion of 2–3 g/h. The rate may be increased by 1 g/h every 30 minutes to 2 hours until contractions cease or a blood magnesium concentration of 6–8 mg/dL is reached. Magnesium levels are determined every 4–6 hours to monitor the therapeutic blood level. After contractions have ceased for 12–24 hours, magnesium can be stopped and the situation reassessed.

Uterine smooth muscle is largely under sympathetic nervous system control, and stimulation of β$_2$-adrenergic receptors relaxes the myometrium. Consequently, inhibition of uterine contractility often can be accomplished by the administration of β-adrenergic drugs such as terbutaline. Alternatively, use of an oxytocin receptor antagonist might also be expected to inhibit uterine contractility. However, trials of one such antagonist, atosiban, have shown only minimal efficacy.

Terbutaline can be given as an intravenous infusion starting at 2.5 mcg/min and increased by 2.5 mcg/min every 20 minutes until contractions cease or to a maximum dose of 20 mcg/min. Terbutaline can also be administered as subcutaneous injections of 250 mcg every 3 hours. Oral terbutaline therapy following parenteral treatment is often elected and consists of giving 2.5–5 mg every 4–6 hours. With terbutaline, a dose-related elevation of heart rate of 20–40 beats/min may occur. An increase of systolic blood pressure up to 10 mm Hg is likely, and the diastolic pressure may fall 10–15 mm Hg during the infusion. Nifedipine has also been used in doses of 10–20 mg orally every 4–6 hours. Blood pressure may fall with nifedipine, but cardiac output increases considerably. Transient elevation of blood glucose, insulin, and fatty acids together with slight reduction of serum potassium have been reported with β-adrenergic drugs. Fetal tachycardia may be slight or absent. No drug-related perinatal deaths have been reported with β-agonists. Maternal side effects requiring dose limitation are tachycardia (≥ 120 beats/min), palpitations, and nervousness. Fluids should be limited to 2500 mL/24 h. Serious side effects (pulmonary edema, chest pain with or without electrocardiographic changes) are often idiosyncratic, not dose-related, and warrant termination of therapy.

One must identify cases in which untimely delivery is the sole threat to the life or health of the infant. An effort should be made to eliminate (1) maternal conditions that compromise the intrauterine environment and make premature birth the lesser risk, eg, preeclampsia-eclampsia; (2) fetal conditions that either are helped by early delivery or render attempts to stop premature labor meaningless, eg, severe erythroblastosis fetalis; and (3) clinical situations in which it is likely that an attempt to stop labor will be futile, eg, ruptured membranes with chorioamnionitis, cervix fully effaced and dilated more than 3 cm, or strong labor in progress.

In pregnancies of less than 34 weeks' duration, betamethasone, 12 mg intramuscularly, or dexamethasone, 16 mg intramuscularly, repeated in 12–24 hours, is administered to hasten fetal lung maturation and permit delivery 48 hours after initial treatment when further prolongation of pregnancy is contraindicated.

Goldenberg RL: The management of preterm labor. Obstet Gynecol 2002;100(5 Part 1):1020. [PMID: 12423870]

Klein LL et al: Infection and preterm birth. Obstet Gynecol Clin North Am 2005;32:397. [PMID: 16125040]

Meis PJ et al: Prevention of recurrent preterm delivery by 17 alpha-hydroxyprogesterone caproate. N Engl J Med 2003; 348:2379. [PMID: 12802023]

LACTATION

Breast-feeding should be encouraged by education throughout pregnancy and the puerperium. Mothers should be told the benefits of breast-feeding—it is emotionally satisfying, promotes mother-infant bonding, is economical, and gives significant immunity to the infant. The period of amenorrhea associated with frequent and consistent breast-feeding provides some (although not completely reliable) birth control until menstruation begins at 6–12 months postpartum or the intensity of breast-feeding diminishes. If the mother must return to work, even a brief period of nursing is beneficial. Transfer of immunoglobulins in colostrum and breast milk protects the infant against many systemic and enteric infections. Macrophages and lymphocytes transferred to the infant from breast milk play an immunoprotective role. The intestinal flora of breast-fed infants inhibits the growth of pathogens. Breast-fed infants have fewer bacterial and viral infections, less severe diarrhea, and fewer allergy problems than bottle-fed infants and are less apt to be obese as children and in adult life.

Frequent breast-feeding on an infant-demand schedule enhances milk flow and successful breast-feeding. Mothers breast-feeding for the first time need help and encouragement from providers, nurses, and other nursing mothers. Milk supply can be increased by increased suckling and increased rest.

Nursing mothers should have a fluid intake of over 2 L/d. The United States RDA calls for 21 g of extra protein (over the 44 g/d baseline for an adult woman) and 550 extra kcal/d in the first 6 months of nursing. Calcium intake should be 1200 mg/d. Continuation of a prenatal vitamin and mineral supplement is wise. Strict vegetarians who eschew both milk and eggs should always take vitamin B$_{12}$ supplements during pregnancy and lactation.

Effects of Drugs in a Nursing Mother

Drugs taken by a nursing mother may accumulate in milk and be transmitted to the infant (Table 18–4). The amount of drug entering the milk depends on the drug's lipid solubility, mechanism of transport, and degree of ionization.

Table 18–4. Drugs and substances that require a careful assessment of risk before they are prescribed for breast-feeding women.[1]

Category	Specific Drugs or Compounds	Management Plan and Rationale
Analgesic drugs	Meperidine, oxycodone	Use alternatives to meperidine and oxycodone. Breast-fed infants whose mothers were receiving meperidine had a higher risk of neurobehavioral depression than breast-fed infants whose mothers were receiving morphine. In breast-fed infants, the level of exposure to oxycodone may reach 10% of the therapeutic dose. For potent analgesia, morphine may be given cautiously. Acetaminophen and nonsteroidal anti-inflammatory drugs are safe.
Antiarthritis drugs	Gold salts, methotrexate, high-dose aspirin	Consider alternatives to gold therapy. Although the bioavailability of elemental gold is unknown, a small amount is excreted in breast milk for a prolonged period. Therefore, the total amount of elemental gold that an infant could ingest may be substantial. No toxicity has been reported. Consider alternatives to methotrexate therapy, although low-dose methotrexate therapy for breast-feeding women with rheumatic diseases had lower risks of adverse effects in their infants than did anticancer chemotherapy. High-dose aspirin should be used with caution, since there is a case report of metabolic acidosis in a breast-fed infant whose mother was receiving high-dose therapy. Although the risk seems small, the infant's condition should be monitored clinically if the mother is receiving long-term therapy with high-dose aspirin.
Anticoagulant drugs	Phenindione[2]	Use alternatives to phenindione. Currently available vitamin K antagonists such as warfarin and acenocoumarol are considered safe, as is heparin.
Antidepressant drugs and lithium	Fluoxetine, doxepin, lithium[2]	Use fluoxetine, doxepin, and lithium with caution. Although the concentrations of these drugs in breast milk are low, colic (with fluoxetine) and sedation (with doxepin) have been reported in exposed infants. Near-therapeutic plasma concentrations of lithium were reported in an infant exposed to the drug in utero and through breast-feeding. The incidence of these adverse events is unknown.
Antiepileptic drugs	Phenobarbital, ethosuximide, primidone	In breast-fed infants, the level of exposure to phenobarbital, ethosuximide, and primidone may exceed 10% of the weight-adjusted therapeutic dose. Consider alternatives such as carbamazepine, phenytoin, and valproic acid.
Antimicrobial drugs	Chloramphenicol, tetracycline	Use alternatives to chloramphenicol and tetracycline. Idiosyncratic aplastic anemia is a possibility among breast-fed infants whose mothers are receiving chloramphenicol. Although tetracycline-induced discoloration of the teeth of breast-fed infants has not been reported, the potential risk of this event needs to be clearly communicated to lactating women.
Anticancer drugs	All (eg, cyclophosphamide,[2] methotrexate,[2] doxorubicin[2])	Because of their potent pharmacologic effects, cytotoxic drugs should not be given to breast-feeding women.
Anxiolytic drugs	Diazepam, alprazolam	Avoid long-term use of diazepam and alprazolam in breast-feeding women. Intermittent use poses little risk to their infants, but regular use may result in the accumulation of the drug and its metabolites in the infants. Lethargy and poor weight gain have been reported in an infant exposed to diazepam in breast milk, and the withdrawal syndrome was reported in a breast-fed infant after the mother discontinued alprazolam.
Cardiovascular and antihypertensive drugs	Acebutolol, amiodarone, atenolol, nadolol, sotalol	The use of acebutolol, amiodarone, atenolol, nadolol, and sotalol by breast-feeding women may cause relatively high levels of exposure among their infants, and these agents should therefore be used with caution. The two β-adrenergic antagonists propranolol and labetalol are considered safe.
Endocrine drugs and hormones	Estrogens, bromocriptine[2]	Estrogens and bromocriptine may suppress milk production. Oral contraceptives containing little or no estrogen have smaller risk than formulations with higher concentrations of estrogen. Nevertheless, caution should be exercised in their use.

(continued)

Table 18–4. Drugs and substances that require a careful assessment of risk before they are prescribed for breast-feeding women.[1] (continued)

Category	Specific Drugs or Compounds	Management Plan and Rationale
Immunosuppressive drugs	Cyclosporine,[2] azathioprine	Maternal plasma concentrations of cyclosporine and azathioprine should be monitored. In nine reported cases in breast-fed infants who were exposed to azathioprine in breast milk, no obvious adverse effects were noted.
Respiratory drugs	Theophylline	Theophylline should be used with caution. When the mother's doses are high, the levels of exposure in the infant may be substantial (ie, 20% of the therapeutic dose).
Radioactive compounds	All	Breast-feeding should be stopped until the level of radioactivity in milk has returned to the background level.
Drugs of abuse	All	The use of drugs of abuse precludes breast-feeding; cocaine-induced toxicity has been reported among breast-fed infants whose mothers abused cocaine. Methadone, used for the treatment of addiction, is safe for infants of breast-feeding women, at doses of up to 80 mg/d. Buprenorphine may be a safer alternative to methadone.
Nonmedicinal substances	Ethanol, caffeine, nicotine	In order to avoid exposure of the infant to ethanol, the mother should not consume alcohol or should consume no more than one drink 2 to 3 hours before breast-feeding. The ingestion of moderate amounts of caffeine should be safe. Because of the effects of second-hand smoke and the fact that nicotine is excreted in breast milk, smoking is contraindicated in breast-feeding women.
Miscellaneous compounds	Iodides and iodine, ergotamine,[2] ergonovine	Use alternatives to iodine-containing antiseptic agents. Ergotamine and ergonovine may suppress prolactin secretion in breast-feeding women. However, the use of methylergonovine to stimulate uterine involution is considered safe in breast-feeding women.

[1]Data modified from Ito S: Drug therapy for breast-feeding women. N Engl J Med 2000;343:120. Drugs for which there is no information are not included, although a careful risk assessment is necessary before such drugs are prescribed.
[2]The use of this drug or these drugs by breast-feeding women is contraindicated according to the American Academy of Pediatrics.

Suppression of Lactation

A. MECHANICAL SUPPRESSION

The simplest and safest method of suppressing lactation after it has started is to gradually transfer the baby to a bottle or a cup over a 3-week period. Milk supply will decrease with decreased demand, and minimal discomfort ensues. If nursing must be stopped abruptly, the mother should avoid nipple stimulation, refrain from expressing milk, and use a snug brassiere. Ice packs and analgesics can be helpful. If suppression is desired before nursing has begun, use this same technique. Engorgement will gradually recede over a 2- to 3-day period.

B. HORMONAL SUPPRESSION

Oral and long-acting injections of hormonal preparations were used at one time to suppress lactation. Because of their questionable efficacy and particularly because of associated side effects such as thromboembolic episodes and hair growth, their use for this purpose has been abandoned. Similarly, lactation suppression with bromocriptine is to be avoided because

of reports of severe hypertension, seizures, strokes, and myocardial infarctions associated with its use.

Dyson L et al: Interventions for promoting the initiation of breast-feeding. Cochrane Database Syst Rev 2005;(2):CD001688. [PMID: 15846621]

Ito S: Drug therapy for breast-feeding women. N Engl J Med 2000;343:118. [PMID: 10891521]

PUERPERAL MASTITIS (See also Chapter 16)

Postpartum mastitis occurs sporadically in nursing mothers shortly after they return home, or it may occur in epidemic form in the hospital. *Staphylococcus aureus* is usually the causative agent. Inflammation is generally unilateral, and women nursing for the first time are more often affected. Rarely, inflammatory carcinoma of the breast can be mistaken for puerperal mastitis.

Mastitis frequently begins within 3 months after delivery and may start with a sore or fissured nipple. There is obvious cellulitis in an area of breast tissue, with redness, tenderness, local warmth, and fever. Treatment consists of antibiotics effective against penicillin-resistant staphylococci (dicloxacillin or a cephalosporin, 500 mg orally every 6 hours for 5–7 days) and regular emptying of the breast by nursing followed by expression of any remaining milk by hand or with a mechanical suction device. Failure to respond to usual antibiotics within 3 days should prompt consideration of resistant staphylococci.

If the mother begins antibiotic therapy before suppuration begins, infection can usually be controlled in 24 hours. If delay is permitted, breast abscess can result. Incision and drainage are required for abscess formation. Despite puerperal mastitis, the baby usually thrives without prophylactic antimicrobial therapy.

Allergic & Immunologic Disorders

19

Jeffrey L. Kishiyama, MD, & Daniel C. Adelman, MD

■ ATOPIC DISEASE

ALLERGIC RHINITIS

 ESSENTIALS OF DIAGNOSIS

- *Seasonal or perennial occurrence of nasal pruritus, congestion, rhinorrhea, or paroxysms of sneezing, which may be associated with lower respiratory symptoms, eye erythema, pruritus, irritation, tearing, or eczematous dermatitis.*
- *Environmental aeroallergen exposure.*
- *Presence of specific-IgE antibody to tested aeroallergens.*

Clinical Findings

In addition to the symptoms listed above, up to 40% of patients with allergic rhinitis also manifest lower respiratory symptoms: cough, wheezing, chest tightness, or dyspnea. The physical examination may reveal edematous or inflamed nasal mucosa. In severe cases, the affected mucosa may be pale, boggy, or blue-tinged from vascular engorgement and venous congestion. Nasal symptoms can be nonspecific, however, and the differential diagnosis can include viral rhinitis, bacterial sinusitis, vasomotor rhinitis, nasal polyposis, drug-induced rhinitis, hormonal rhinitis, rhinitis medicamentosa, atrophic rhinitis, gastroesophageal reflux, and systemic disorders such as thyroid disease or Wegener's granulomatosis. Even a basic understanding of regional aeroallergen patterns and seasons can aid the clinician during the evaluation of patients presenting with acute or chronic rhinitis.

Patients with moderate to severe disease, those who are potential candidates for allergen immunotherapy, and those with strong predisposing factors for atopic diatheses (eg, a strong family history of atopy or ongoing exposure to potential sources of allergen) should undergo testing. Since the development of rhinitis precedes the presentation of asthma in over 50% of cases,

early intervention may decrease the risk of more severe clinical allergic disease. Patients with comorbidities or associated complications such as allergic asthma, allergic conjunctivitis, chronic cough, sinusitis, polyposis, eczema, or otitis media may also benefit from evaluation by a subspecialist.

Treatment

The three basic principles of allergy management are avoidance of the allergen, symptomatic pharmacologic therapy, and specific allergen immunotherapy. Patients with suboptimal responses to reasonable therapeutic interventions benefit from diagnostic allergy skin testing.

A. AVOIDANCE THERAPY

Avoidance is the most effective treatment for any allergic condition but may be limited in its applicability. It cures the clinical manifestations but does not reduce the sensitivity to the allergen.

1. Pollens—Airborne allergens can travel significant distances, but concentrations are highest near their source. Pollen release occurs in the early morning, and airborne levels depend on temperature and wind velocity. Closing windows and remaining in air-conditioned environments can decrease exposure when pollen counts are high.

2. Animal danders—If the allergy is slight, the patient may benefit from merely keeping the animal out of the bedroom; usually, however, it is necessary to remove the animal from the home altogether. Hypersensitivity to animal dander can be exquisite, and passively transferred dander can accumulate to significant levels in "off-limits" areas. Washing or otherwise treating the fur of a live animal has not been proved to reduce allergenicity.

3. House dust and dust mites—The mattress and pillows should be encased in dust mite-proof material, and all other bedding should be washed weekly and dried at high temperature. The bedroom floor should be uncarpeted. The room should be dusted frequently. Electronic air purifiers are of unproved effectiveness for dust mite reduction since the primary source of exposure is the bed. Acaricides are not recommended. Dust mite reduction interventions can be successful adjunctive measures to medical therapy, can signifi-

Table 19–1. Effectiveness of agents used in treatment of allergic disorders.

Drug Class	Sneezing	Pruritus	Rhinorrhea	Congestion	Inflammation	Onset of Action
Antihistamines	++++	++++	+++	+	−	Rapid
Sympathomimetics	−	−	+	++++	−	Rapid
Corticosteroids	+++	+++	+++	++++	++++	Slow (days)
Cromolyn-nedocromil sodium	++	+	+	+	++	Slow (weeks)
Anticholinergics	−	−	++++	−	−	Rapid
Immunotherapy	++++	++++	++++	++++	++++	Slow (months)

cantly reduce symptoms, and can reduce bronchial hyperreactivity and medication requirements in sensitized patients.

4. Mold spores—Out of doors, mold spores are unavoidable during certain seasons. Nevertheless, activities such as gardening and farming can be associated with acute high levels of exposure and should be avoided. Indoor mold contamination can be controlled by repairing leaks, by preventing mold buildup in bathrooms and around windows, and by replacement of mold-contaminated carpeting.

B. DRUG THERAPY

Three classes of pharmacotherapy are useful for IgE-mediated diseases, based on (1) inhibition of release of mediators from mast cells, (2) inhibition of the action of mediators on their target cells, and (3) reversal of the vascular and inflammatory responses in the target tissues (Table 19–1).

1. Antihistamines—Antihistamine drugs competitively inhibit the binding of histamine to H_1 receptors and are useful for the treatment of IgE-mediated allergy. There are a number of such drugs, but the use of first-generation antihistamines (chlorpheniramine, brompheniramine, diphenhydramine, clemastine, hydroxyzine) are limited by sedation, neurocognitive impairment, and dry mucous membranes. Rare complications include seizures and tachyarrhythmias. Second-generation nonsedating histamine H_1-receptor-blocking drugs, loratadine, fexofenadine, and desloratadine appear not to be associated with arrhythmias and, along with cetirizine, are the systemic drugs of choice. Cetirizine is mildly sedating, but the incidence of side effects is markedly lower than that of its parent compound, hydroxyzine. Azelastine is a topical antihistamine preparation that is applied intranasally to decrease its systemic side effects. Because of methodologic issues, publication bias, and inability to generalize findings, providing a rank order of potency and clinical efficacy for the available antihistamines is difficult. Clinical tolerance or tachyphylaxis does not occur at prescribed dosages but *an incomplete response to antihistamine therapy often indicates the need for combined treatment with a corticosteroid nasal spray.* This highlights the necessity to con-

trol both the early phase and late phase of the allergic response for optimal symptom control.

Antihistamine therapy only rarely alleviates symptoms of asthma, although it is not contraindicated when used to treat concomitant rhinitis or pruritus. The antipruritic effect of antihistamines may be a useful adjunct in treatment of eczematous diseases.

2. Sympathomimetic drugs—Adrenergic agonists are used for both α-adrenergic (vasoconstricting) and β-adrenergic (bronchodilating) properties. α-Adrenergic agonists can be used orally (pseudoephedrine) or topically (phenylephrine, naphazoline, oxymetazoline) as nasal decongestants and topically as conjunctival vasoconstrictors. Daily use of topical preparations can lead to rapid development of rebound vasodilation (rhinitis medicamentosa). The main side effects of oral decongestants are insomnia, tremor, and tachycardia.

3. Corticosteroids—These drugs have a therapeutic role in virtually all types of allergic diseases because of their anti-inflammatory action rather than by their immunosuppressive effects. Systemic use for the treatment of allergic disease, however, requires close attention to toxicity. Corticosteroids are available in oral, intramuscular, intravenous, intranasal, and bronchial inhalation forms; as eye drops; and in topical formulations for dermatologic use. Short-term systemic burst therapy can be used for treatment of severe asthma, marked allergic rhinitis, allergic fungal sinusitis, and allergic bronchopulmonary aspergillosis. Because of complications, including cataracts, corneal ulceration, keratitis, and glaucoma, the prescription of corticosteroid eye drops should be reserved for ophthalmologists.

Topical corticosteroid nasal sprays are effective and appear safe for long-term use, but epistaxis can occur and nasal septum perforation is a rare complication. Although the dosages and formulations available for the treatment of asthma vary greatly in terms of dosage and clinical potency, intranasal preparations of flunisolide, fluticasone, beclomethasone, mometasone, budesonide, and triamcinolone are similarly efficacious for the treatment of allergic rhinitis. *Long-term topical corticosteroid therapy for allergic rhinitis is an essential aspect of management of the inflammatory phase of the disease.* It may take several days of consistent use before optimal responses are seen, but these compounds have consistently proved superior to antihistamine monotherapy for control of nasal pruritus, sneezing, and nasal congestion. Surprisingly, they may also provide some relief from concomitant eye pruritus and have shown positive effects on sleep, which can be adversely affected in patients with allergic rhinitis. Topical corticosteroids may also be effective for treatment of vasomotor rhinitis and may be used as adjunctive treatment for sinusitis in combination with antibiotic therapy.

4. Cromolyn sodium and sodium nedocromil— Pretreatment with these drugs prevents the response to allergen by stabilizing the mast cell, although the specific molecular mechanisms of action are unknown. Although unrelated, they have similar effects and, because of poor bioavailability, are effective only when applied directly to the involved organ. Their action is short-lived, so that they must be given three or four times a day. Cromolyn is available as a bronchial inhaler, nasal spray, and ophthalmologic preparation; nedocromil is available in metered-dose inhalers. In comparison with topical corticosteroids they appear to be much less potent, but the drugs have very few side effects and wide margins of safety.

5. Anticholinergic agents—Ipratropium bromide is effective as a nasal topical agent for use in rhinitis. Mucous membrane glandular secretion is under cholinergic control and can be inhibited by anticholinergic agents. First-generation antihistamines have systemic anticholinergic activity, but ipratropium is preferred as adjunctive treatment of allergic rhinitis or as primary treatment for many types of nonallergic rhinitis. Ipratropium does not alleviate sneezing, pruritus, or nasal congestion but can be useful for treatment of postnasal drip and rhinorrhea.

6. Leukotriene antagonists—Montelukast is an effective drug for the treatment of asthma. To a much more limited degree, leukotriene antagonists can be efficacious for the treatment of allergic rhinitis, either as monotherapy or combined with an antihistamine. By inhibiting leukotriene-mediated vasodilation vascular permeability and by potentially reducing eosinophilic inflammation, orally administered montelukast can provide symptomatic relief, especially for nasal congestion. It is less effective than intranasal corticosteroids, however.

C. IMMUNOTHERAPY

Treatment of atopy—especially allergic rhinitis—by the repeated long-term injection of allergen has been shown in many controlled clinical trials to be an effective method for reducing or eliminating symptoms and signs of the allergic disorder.

1. Indications—The severity and duration of a patient's symptoms should be considered when selecting candidates for allergen immunotherapy. This treatment is recommended for patients with severe allergic rhinoconjunctivitis who respond poorly to drug ther-

apy, those seeking to lower their long-term medication requirements, and for those whose allergens are not avoidable. Immunotherapy is unequivocally effective in patients with allergic rhinitis and allergic conjunctivitis who react to pollens, mold, and house dust mites. It reduces immunologic hypersensitivity, symptoms, and medication requirements. In children with documented allergic rhinitis, immunotherapy may reduce the risk of subsequent development of asthma. The efficacy of immunotherapy in allergic asthma is still debated, but a meta-analysis of 20 randomized, controlled trials done by Abramson showed a positive benefit in patients with allergic asthma. The lower clinical response rates observed in asthma have been attributed to the multifactorial nature of the disease. Immunotherapy is of no value in atopic dermatitis.

2. Immunologic effects—"Allergen immunotherapy" is preferable to "desensitization" because the immunologic basis for this treatment has not been clearly elucidated. Nevertheless, certain immunologic changes can be induced by these injections. Circulating levels of IgE antibodies specific to the injected allergens increase slightly during the first few months, then decrease, eventually to substantially lower levels than before treatment. Seasonal rises in IgE antibodies to pollens are blunted or eliminated. IgG blocking antibody is produced. Changes in regulatory T cells favoring suppression of IgE antibody production and apoptosis of antigen-specific T cell clones have been noted. TH2 cytokine responses may be shifted toward TH1 responses in peripheral blood mononuclear cells. Higher thresholds for release of inflammatory mediators and decreases in late-phase allergic reactions might also be related to the reduction in biologic sensitivity of end-organ systems (eyes, nose, bronchi, and skin).

3. Clinical effects—Most patients with allergic rhinitis caused by aeroallergens become more tolerant to natural pollen exposure during successive seasons while receiving immunotherapy. A small minority becomes completely asymptomatic, but most patients enjoy a significant decrease in symptoms and medication usage. Only high-dose injected immunotherapy has been demonstrated to be effective. A beneficial response may persist for years after treatment is stopped. The clinical effects and immunologic responses are antigen-specific, but the treatment may also decrease the risk of developing new environmental sensitivities.

4. Procedure—A sterile aqueous solution of the allergen or allergens responsible for the patient's disease is administered by subcutaneous injection in increasing doses once or twice a week until a maintenance dose is reached, at which time the interval is advanced to every 4 weeks. The maintenance dose is typically one to ten thousand times the starting dose. Ascending doses are used to minimize the risk of systemic allergic reactions during initial stages of immunotherapy. Three to 5 years is a typical course of therapy. Oral immunotherapy remains experimental in the United States, and sublingual or low-dose immunotherapy is unconventional and of unproved efficacy.

5. Adverse effects—Reactions to treatment may be local or systemic. Localized immediate and late-phase skin reactions occur at injection sites. These are not harmful, but the dose must be adjusted to avoid excessively large or prolonged local reactions. Immediate systemic reactions or anaphylaxis is a potential problem with each injection and must be prevented by monitoring of dosage. The patient remains at the treatment facility for at least 20 minutes after each injection so that drugs and equipment for treating anaphylaxis will be available if needed. No long-term adverse consequences of aqueous allergen extract immunotherapy are known to have occurred in immunocompetent individuals.

Abramson MJ et al: Allergen immunotherapy for asthma. Cochrane Database Syst Rev 2000; CD001186. [PMID: 10796617]

Meltzer EO et al: Rhinosinusitis: Establishing definitions for clinical research and patient care. J Allergy Clin Immunol 2004; 114(6 Suppl):155. [PMID: 15577865]

Moller C et al: Pollen immunotherapy reduces the development of asthma in children with seasonal rhinoconjunctivitis (the PAT-study). J Allergy Clin Immunol 2002;109:251. [PMID: 11842293]

Norman PS: Immunotherapy: 1999–2004. J Allergy Clin Immunol 2004;113:1013. [PMID: 15208577]

Togias A: Rhinitis and asthma: Evidence for respiratory system integration. J Allergy Clin Immunol 2003;111:1171. [PMID: 12789212]

ANAPHYLAXIS, URTICARIA, & ANGIOEDEMA

ESSENTIALS OF DIAGNOSIS

- *Anaphylaxis is a systemic reaction with cutaneous symptoms, associated with dyspnea, visceral edema, and hypotension.*
- *Urticaria is characterized by large, irregularly shaped, pruritic, erythematous wheals.*
- *Angioedema is painless, deep, subcutaneous swelling, often involving periorbital, circumoral, and facial regions.*
- *These disorders may be diagnosed clinically, especially in the context of allergen exposure; detection of specific IgE or elevated serum tryptase can confirm the diagnosis.*

General Considerations

Certain allergens—especially drugs, insect venoms, and foods—may induce an IgE antibody response, causing a generalized release of mediators from mast cells and resulting in systemic anaphylaxis. This potentially fatal condition affects both nonatopic and atopic persons. Isolated urticaria and angioedema are more common cutaneous forms of anaphylaxis with a better prognosis.

Food allergies cause an estimated 150 fatalities per year in the United States, most cases being due to ingestion of peanuts, tree nuts, shellfish, and fish. Common childhood food allergies such as milk, soy, wheat, and egg are often outgrown over time if strict avoidance is practiced. β-Lactam antibiotics may be involved in 400–800 fatalities per year, and stinging insect venom causes about 50 fatalities per year. Chronic relapsing urticaria, angioedema, and, less commonly, anaphylaxis, however, are not always due to IgE-mediated hypersensitivity. In a minority of cases—perhaps 10% or less—underlying systemic disorders such as systemic mastocytosis or subclinical infection or inflammatory disorders may be manifested by episodic urticaria or angioedema. Idiopathic causes are commonly responsible for chronic or relapsing symptoms, suggesting that some cases may be associated with autoimmune processes including the production of histamine-liberating autoantibodies directed against Fcε mast cell membrane receptors. A review of 593 patients with recurrent episodes of anaphylaxis seeking medical attention at a university medical center revealed that most (70%) anaphylactic episodes in adults were classified as idiopathic in nature. In contrast, the bulk (35–55%) of anaphylactic reactions in children are caused by food allergies. Twenty percent of the population will experience urticaria or angioedema during their lifetime, and the estimated prevalence of idiopathic anaphylaxis is 34,000 patients in the United States.

Clinical Findings

A. SYMPTOMS AND SIGNS

The manifestations are (1) hypotension or shock from widespread vasodilation or dysrhythmia, (2) respiratory distress from bronchospasm or laryngeal edema, (3) gastrointestinal and uterine muscle contraction, and (4) flushing, pruritus, urticaria, and angioedema.

B. LABORATORY FINDINGS

In vivo allergy skin testing and in vitro RAST testing can detect allergen-specific IgE for a variety of foods, hymenoptera (bee, wasp, hornet, fire ant) venom, latex, and some medicines. Skin testing for food allergy is appropriate only if the patient has symptoms consistent with IgE-mediated allergy (eg, urticaria, angioedema, or anaphylaxis) within 2 hours after eating the suspect food.

Determination of serum tryptase can be used to identify recent anaphylactic reactions or other reactions due to systemic mast cell activation. Tryptase is a mast cell-derived neutral protease with a half-life of 60–90 minutes. Elevated tryptase levels have been associated with anaphylaxis, systemic mastocytosis, and non-IgE-mediated diseases characterized by mast cell degranulation ("anaphylactoid reactions"). Histamine is released during these disorders and has a very short serum half-life but may be briefly detectable during symptomatic periods.

If IgE-mediated hypersensitivity is not found and symptoms become relapsing or chronic (over 6 weeks in duration), a screening battery of laboratory tests may be done after a thorough history and physical examination. Appropriate diagnostic testing should follow any positive findings on examination or review of systems. Patients suffering from recurrent angioedema should also be tested for C1-esterase inhibitor deficiency. Measuring a serum C4 level is an easy screening test for C1-esterase inhibitor deficiency/hereditary angioedema because it will be low in most cases.

Treatment

A. TREATMENT OF ANAPHYLAXIS

At the first suspicion of anaphylaxis, airway, breathing, and circulation are assessed. If systemic anaphylaxis is suspected, aqueous epinephrine 1:1000 in a dose of 0.2–0.5 mL (0.2–0.5 mg) is injected intramuscularly. Repeated injections can be given every 5–15 minutes as necessary. Between 40% and 70% of patients suffering from severe anaphylaxis will require more than one injection of epinephrine. Injection in the anterolateral thigh may lead to more predictable and rapid absorption compared with sites in the arm. Epinephrine can stabilize hemodynamics, cause bronchodilation, and prevent further mast cell degranulation. Rapid intravenous infusion of large volumes of fluids (saline, lactated Ringer's injection, plasma, colloid solutions, or plasma expanders) is essential to replace loss of intravascular plasma into tissues in patients with hypotension caused by marked vasodilation. Other vasopressor drugs (high-dose dopamine, norepinephrine, phenylephrine) may be necessary if the patient remains hypotensive.

Airway obstruction is caused by edema of the larynx and hypopharynx or by bronchospasm. The former is treated by maintenance of an airway with endotracheal intubation or tracheostomy. Inhalation of selective β_2-adrenergic agonists such as albuterol or terbutaline and intravenous administration of aminophylline (0.5 mg/kg/h IV with 6 mg/kg loading dose over 30 minutes) are effective for bronchospasm.

Antihistamines (H_1- and H_2-receptor antagonists such as diphenhydramine (25–50 mg orally, intramuscularly, or intravenously every 4–6 hours) and ranitidine (150 mg orally every 12 hours or 50 mg intramuscularly or intravenously every 6–8 hours) may be useful adjuvant therapies for alleviating the cutaneous manifestations of urticaria or angioedema and pruritus and for the gastrointestinal and uterine smooth muscle spasms. Corticosteroids will not reverse respiratory obstruction or shock but may reduce prolonged reactions or relapses. Long-term combined oral antihistamine and prednisone therapy reduces the number and severity of attacks in patients with frequent life-threatening episodes of idiopathic anaphylaxis. Medical therapy does not reliably prevent true IgE-mediated hypersensitivity reactions.

There may be a clinical biphasic or late-phase response in anaphylaxis, causing a recrudescence of symptoms hours (most commonly 6–12 hours) after exposure to the allergen. The incidence of late phase reactions is estimated to be between 1% and 20%. Since this may occur after subsidence of the immediate-phase response, all patients with anaphylaxis should be monitored for up to 24 hours, discharged with injectable epinephrine, and educated about the possible recurrence of symptoms.

Anaphylaxis in a patient being treated with β-adrenergic blocker drugs is a special problem because of refractoriness to epinephrine and selective β-adrenergic agonists. Higher doses of adrenergic drugs are required for the desired effect; glucagon (0.5–1 mg intravenously, intramuscularly, or subcutaneously may be repeated 30 minutes later) in patients taking β-blockers may be beneficial. Patients being treated with angiotensin-converting enzyme inhibitors may suffer from more severe hypotension due to blockade of renin-angiotensin-dependent compensatory mechanisms.

B. TREATMENT OF URTICARIA AND ANGIOEDEMA

These disorders are discussed fully in Chapter 6. If urticaria or angioedema is found to be secondary to underlying inflammatory or infectious processes, treatment of the primary disorder can lead to remission of cutaneous symptoms.

C. VENOM IMMUNOTHERAPY

Patients demonstrating immediate hypersensitivity reactions to stinging insects (honey bees, wasps, hornets, yellow jackets, and imported fire ants) with documented venom-specific IgE on allergy skin testing should receive venom immunotherapy for prevention of anaphylaxis. A 5-year course of venom-specific immunotherapy is indicated for persons suffering from generalized urticaria, angioedema, bronchospasm, or hypotension after insect venom exposure. Large isolated local reactions to insect stings are not a predisposing factor for systemic anaphylaxis. Untreated individuals have a 50–60% risk of anaphylactic response to subsequent stings. Venom immunotherapy is highly protective, affording 98% protection from life-threatening reactions on rechallenge. Rarely, anaphylaxis has been associated with other biting insects, including *Triatoma* and mosquito, but diagnostic reagents and therapeutic extracts are not consistently available for these other species.

Charous BL et al: Natural rubber latex allergy after 12 years: recommendations and perspectives. J Allergy Clin Immunol 2002;109:31. [PMID: 11799362]

Kaplan AP: Diagnostic tests for urticaria and angioedema. Clin Allergy Immunol 2000;15:111. [PMID: 10943290]

Kemp SF et al: Anaphylaxis: a review of causes and mechanisms. J Allergy Clin Immunol 2002;110:341. [PMID: 12209078]

Lieberman P: Anaphylaxis. Med Clin North Am 2006;90:77. [PMID: 16310525]

Moffitt JE et al: Stinging insect hypersensitivity: A practice parameter update. J Allergy Clin Immunol 2004;113:1204. [PMID: 15480329]

DRUG & FOOD ALLERGY

General Considerations

Some drugs are clearly more immunogenic than others, and this can be reflected in the incidence of drug hypersensitivity. A partial list of drugs frequently implicated in drug reactions includes β-lactam antibiotics, sulfonamides, phenytoin, carbamazepine, allopurinol, muscle relaxants used for general anesthesia, nonsteroidal anti-inflammatory drugs, antisera, and antiarrhythmic agents. Many drugs can be associated with recognizable known toxicities, drug interactions, or idiosyncratic reactions that are not immune-mediated. These must be distinguished from true hypersensitivity reactions because the prognosis and management differ. Some estimate that only 10% or less of adverse reactions to drugs are true hypersensitivity reactions. Patients with multidrug hypersensitivity are quite rare, and those reporting "allergies" to more than three distinct classes of drugs should be carefully evaluated since intolerance to many of these drug classes may not be immunologic.

Four foods account for 90% of food allergy in adults: peanuts, tree nuts, fish, and shellfish. Food hypersensitivity must be distinguished from food intolerance, which is more common and more variable in terms of underlying mechanism. An example of food intolerance would be lactose intolerance, which is due to an enzyme deficiency rather than an IgE-mediated hypersensitivity.

Clinical Findings

A. SYMPTOMS AND SIGNS

The development of symptoms and the nature of the adverse drug reaction can suggest whether an immunologic process is responsible for symptoms. Factors to consider include type of symptoms, history of previous drug exposure, time of onset after starting the drug, presence of other systemic involvement, coexisting illness, and concurrent drug use. In previously sensitized individuals, immediate hypersensitivity is manifested by rapid development of urticaria, angioedema, or anaphylaxis. Delayed onset of urticaria accompanied by fever, arthralgias, and nephritis may indicate the development of an immune complex-mediated disorder. Drug fever and Stevens-Johnson syndrome probably act by immune hypersensitivity mechanisms. In genetically slow acetylators and in AIDS patients with depleted hepatic glutathione levels, drugs such as sulfamethoxazole are not rapidly excreted during drug metabolism. This altered drug metabolism favors the generation of haptenated immunoreactive metabolites as well as drug reactions, such as delayed morbilliform eruptions. Other types of immune-mediated dermatologic drug reactions include lupus-like syndromes caused by procainamide, isoniazid, phenytoin, or hydralazine. Drugs that have been associated with the development of systemic or cutaneous vasculitis include leukotriene receptor antagonists, allopurinol, phenytoin, thiazides, nonsteroidal anti-inflammatory drugs, furosemide, cimetidine, gold, hydralazine, and many antibiotics (eg, penicillin, sulfonamides, quinolones, and tetracycline). Cutaneous vasculitides are usually associated with fixed lesions, with histologically-proven immune-complex involvement.

Food hypersensitivity is manifest by immediate hypersensitivity reactions or, more rarely, atopic dermatitis. Onset of allergic food reactions is rapid, usually within minutes to a couple of hours of ingestion, and the reaction is usually quite reproducible. Oral allergy syndrome is a self-limited form of fruit and vegetable hypersensitivity, where symptoms are confined to the oropharynx. Due to cross-reactivity between certain fruit and vegetable allergens and certain seasonal pollens, ingestion of these foods causes pruritus of lips, tongue and palate without systemic anaphylaxis. The most common cross-reacting foods and pollens are apples and carrots, which cross-react with birch pollen; melons and bananas, which cross-react with ragweed pollen. Many of these antigens involved in oral allergy syndrome are heat labile and denature during cooking.

B. LABORATORY FINDINGS

1. Allergy testing—Allergy skin testing is only available for a limited number of drugs (penicillin, insulin, streptokinase, chymopapain, heterologous serum), since patients may react to the native drug as well as any metabolite that covalently binds to native protein and becomes immunoreactive. Skin testing is available for patients with suspected immediate hypersensitivity to penicillin or β-lactam antibiotics (see Chapter 37). The degree of cross-reactivity between the cephalosporin antibiotics and penicillins is uncertain. The incidence of IgE-mediated hypersensitivity appears to be less than 5%. There appears to be no allergic cross-reactivity between the monobactam antibiotics (aztreonam) and penicillin or other β-lactam antibiotics. A high degree of cross-reactivity exists between penicillin and the carbapenem, imipenem, so this drug should be given to the penicillin-allergic patient with the same degree of caution as if the patient were to receive penicillin.

If the likelihood of immunologic reaction is low—based on the history and the assessment of likely offending agents—and if no allergy testing is available, judicious test dose challenges may be considered in a monitored setting. If the likelihood of IgE-mediated reaction is significant, these challenges are risky and rapid drug desensitization is indicated.

The gold standard for allergy food testing is skin-prick testing with actual food items, but due to the inconvenience and potential risk for systemic reactions, this form of testing is usually preceded by IgE RAST testing or skin prick testing with commercially available extracts or both.

2. Provocation tests—Occasionally, direct allergen challenge of the target organ or tissue under controlled conditions is required for definitive diagnosis. Such challenges may be bronchial, nasal, conjunctival, oral, or cutaneous. A positive test confirms that the test substance can cause the reaction, but it does not prove that an immunologic mechanism is responsible.

a. Bronchoprovocation testing—Natural provocation field testing can be done by having the patient make serial determinations of peak expiratory flow rate using a portable peak flowmeter during periods of natural exposure to a suspected airborne allergen. Bronchoprovocation is not necessary in the routine diagnosis of allergic asthma, but it may be helpful in some cases of occupational asthma. Bronchial provocation with exercise or with inhalation of methacholine, histamine, or cold air can document the presence of nonspecific bronchial hyperreactivity during the diagnostic workup for respiratory symptoms but does not detect allergic sensitivities.

b. Oral provocation—In most cases of suspected allergy to a food or drug, placebo-controlled oral challenge is the definitive test. To be considered a positive result, the reported clinical findings must be reproduced during provocation testing. A blinded provocation test may be preceded by an open challenge (no placebo control), which, if negative, negates the necessity for logistically difficult blinded challenge. Freeze-dried foods in large opaque capsules provide a sufficient dose of allergen for testing. This should not be done in patients with suspected food- or drug-induced anaphylaxis.

Treatment

For IgE-mediated drug hypersensitivity, acute rapid desensitization may allow administration of a drug if there is no suitable alternative treatment regimen. This procedure carries a significant risk and should be undertaken in an intensively monitored setting. This is accomplished by a course of oral or parenteral doses starting with extremely low doses (dilutions of 1×10^{-6} or 1×10^{-5} units) and increasing to the full dose over a period of hours. IgE-mediated reactivity diminishes during the course of this desensitization, creating a temporary drug-specific refractory state. During the refractory period, skin histamine responsiveness is maintained, and mast cells may be activated by other stimuli but the patient may receive the desired drug with a very low risk of anaphylaxis. Acute rapid desensitization may work through cellular mechanisms different from those involved in standard injection immunotherapy, and the refractory period is maintained only throughout the course of uninterrupted therapy.

Various slow desensitization protocols have been developed for patients suffering from late-appearing morbilliform eruptions (eg, AIDS patients with sulfamethoxazole-induced dermatitis). These eruptions are not IgE-mediated, and the slow reintroduction of drug allows for less haptenation during sulfonamide metabolism with generation of less immunoreactive drug metabolites. This form of desensitization is distinct from rapid desensitization of IgE-mediated drug allergy. Desensitization for non–IgE-mediated drug reactions has been successful for aspirin, nonsteroidal anti-inflammatory drugs, and allopurinol.

Any history or finding consistent with toxic epidermal necrolysis or Stevens-Johnson syndrome would be an absolute contraindication for drug readministration.

For any proven food hypersensitivity, strict avoidance is the only rational recommendation. Patients should also be provided with an epinephrine autoinjector (Epi-pen) if indicated.

Clark S et al: Multicenter study of emergency department visits for food allergies. J Allergy Clin Immunol 2004;113: 347. [PMID: 14767453]

Grammer LC et al: Drug allergy and protocols for management of drug allergies, 3rd edition. Part II. General principles of prevention of allergic drug reactions. Allergy Asthma Proc 2004; 25:267. [PMID: 15510589]

Gruchalla R: Understanding drug allergies. J Allergy Clin Immunol 2000;105(6 Pt 2):S637. [PMID: 10856171]

IMMUNE COMPLEX DISEASE (Serum Sickness)

 ESSENTIALS OF DIAGNOSIS

- *Fever, pruritus, and arthropathy.*
- *Reaction is delayed in onset, usually 7–10 days, when specific IgG antibodies are generated against the allergen.*
- *Immune complexes found circulating in serum or deposited in affected tissues.*

General Considerations

Serum sickness reactions occur when immune complexes are formed by the binding of antigens (eg, drugs, heterologous serum) to antibodies. Deposition of these complexes in tissues or in vascular endothelium can produce immune complex-mediated tissue injury by activation of complement, generation of anaphylatoxins, chemoattraction of polymorphonuclear leukocytes, and tissue injury. The commonly affected organs include skin (urticaria, vasculitis), joints (arthritis), and kidney (nephritis).

Clinical Findings

A. SYMPTOMS AND SIGNS

Constitutional symptoms, such as drug fever, are common.

B. LABORATORY FINDINGS

The specific IgG antibody may be present in sufficient quantity in serum to be detected by the precipitin-in-gel method. Detection of these precipitating antibodies by gel diffusion can be useful in the diagnosis of allergic bronchopulmonary aspergillosis or hypersensitivity pneumonitis. Enzyme-linked immunosorbent assay (ELISA) will detect antibodies present in lesser amounts.

Circulating antigen-nonspecific immune complexes can be detected in a variety of malignancies and in autoimmune, hypersensitivity, and infectious diseases. Immunohistochemical techniques can identify immune complexes or complement fragments deposited in tissue biopsy specimens. Depressed serum levels of C3, C4, or CH50 may be sought as nonspecific evidence of immune complex disease with consumption of soluble factors.

The erythrocyte sedimentation rate is increased, and other nonspecific laboratory findings may include elevated hepatic aminotransferases or reduced complement levels. Circulating immune complexes may be found, but current assays are limited in sensitivity. Evidence of nephritis may be found by observing red cell casts at urinalysis.

Treatment

This disease is self-limited, so treatment is usually conservative. Aspirin will relieve the arthralgias. Antihistamines and topical corticosteroids will control the dermatitis. Corticosteroid therapy may be necessary for serious reactions—especially glomerulonephritis, neuropathy, and other manifestations of vasculitis.

PSEUDOALLERGIC REACTIONS

These reactions resemble immediate hypersensitivity reactions but are not mediated by allergen-IgE interaction. Instead, direct mast cell activation occurs. Examples of pseudoallergic or "anaphylactoid" reactions include the now rare "red man syndrome" from rapid infusion of vancomycin, direct mast cell activation by opioids, and radiocontrast reactions. In contrast to IgE-mediated reactions, these can often be prevented by prophylactic medical regimens.

Radiocontrast Media Reactions

Reactions to radiocontrast media do not appear to be mediated by IgE antibodies, yet clinically they are similar to anaphylaxis. If a patient has had an anaphylactoid reaction to conventional radiocontrast media, the risk for a second reaction upon reexposure may be as high as 30%. Patients with asthma or those being treated with β-adrenergic blocking medications may be at increased risk. The management of patients at risk for radiocontrast medium reactions includes use of the low-osmolality contrast preparations and prophylactic administration of prednisone (50 mg orally every 6 hours beginning 18 hours before the procedure) and diphenhydramine (25–50 mg intramuscularly 60 minutes before the procedure). The use of the lower-osmolality radiocontrast media in combination

with the pretreatment regimen decreases the incidence of reactions to less than 1%.

■ IMMUNODEFICIENCY DISORDERS

The primary immunologic deficiency diseases include congenital and acquired disorders of humoral immunity (B cell function) or cell-mediated immunity (T cell function). Most of these diseases are rare, and since they are genetically determined, are seen primarily in children. Several immunodeficiency disorders affect adults and are discussed below. The WHO classification of immunodeficiency disorders more often affecting adults is set forth in the accompanying box.

WHO CLASSIFICATION

- Primary Immunodeficiency Disorders:
  Selective IgA deficiency.
  Common variable immunodeficiency.
  X-linked agammaglobulinemia.
  Immunodeficiency with normal serum globulins or hyperimmunoglobulinemia.
  Immunodeficiency with thymoma.
- Secondary Immunodeficiency Disorders (for example, AIDS)

Bonilla FA et al: Primary immunodeficiency diseases. J Allergy Clin Immunol 2003;111:S571. [PMID: 12592303]

Buckley RH: Advances in immunology: primary immunodeficiency diseases due to defects in lymphocytes. N Engl J Med 2000;343:1313. [PMID: 11058677]

Cooper MA et al: Primary immunodeficiencies. Am Fam Physician 2003;68:2001. [PMID: 14655810]

Fischer A: Human primary immunodeficiency diseases: a perspective. Nat Immunol 2004;5:23. [PMID: 14699405]

SELECTIVE IMMUNOGLOBULIN A DEFICIENCY

Selective IgA deficiency is the most common primary immunodeficiency disorder and is characterized by the absence of serum IgA with normal levels of IgG and IgM; its prevalence is about 1:500 individuals. Most persons are asymptomatic because of compensatory increases in secreted IgG and IgM. Some affected patients have frequent and recurrent infections such as sinusitis, otitis, and bronchitis. Some cases of IgA deficiency may spontaneously remit. When IgG$_2$ subclass deficiency occurs in combination with IgA deficiency, affected patients are more susceptible to encapsulated bacteria and the degree of immune impairment can be more severe. Patients with a combined IgA and IgG subclass deficiency should be assessed for functional antibody responses to glycoprotein antigen immunization.

Atopic disease and autoimmune disorders can be associated with IgA deficiency. Occasionally, a sprue-like syndrome with steatorrhea has been associated with an isolated IgA deficit. Treatment with commercial immune globulin is ineffective, since IgA and IgM are present only in trace quantities in these preparations. Frequent infusions of plasma (containing IgA) or unwashed blood transfusions are hazardous, since anti-IgA antibodies may develop, resulting in systemic anaphylaxis or serum sickness.

Cunningham-Rundles C: Physiology of IgA and IgA deficiency. J Clin Immunol 2001;21:303. [PMID: 11720003]

COMMON VARIABLE IMMUNODEFICIENCY

 ESSENTIALS OF DIAGNOSIS

- *Defect in terminal differentiation of B cells, with absent plasma cells and deficient synthesis of secreted antibody.*
- *Frequent sinopulmonary infections secondary to humoral immune deficiency.*
- *Confirmation by evaluation of serum immunoglobulin levels and deficient functional antibody responses.*

General Considerations

The most common cause of panhypogammaglobulinemia in adults is common variable immunodeficiency, a heterogeneous immunodeficiency disorder clinically characterized by an increased incidence of recurrent infections, autoimmune phenomena, and neoplastic diseases. The onset generally is during adolescence or early adulthood but can occur at any age. The prevalence of common variable immunodeficiency is about 1:80,000 in the United States.

Clinical Findings

A. SYMPTOMS AND SIGNS

The pattern of immunoglobulin isotype deficiency is variable. Most patients present with significantly depressed IgG levels, but over time all antibody classes (IgG, IgA, and IgM) may be affected. Increased susceptibility to pyogenic infections is the hallmark of the disease. Virtually all patients suffer from recurrent si-

nusitis, with bronchitis, otitis, pharyngitis, and pneumonia also being common infections. Infections may be prolonged or associated with unusual complications such as meningitis or sepsis.

Gastrointestinal disorders are commonly associated with common variable immunodeficiency, and a sprue-like syndrome, with diarrhea, steatorrhea, malabsorption, protein-losing enteropathy, and hepatosplenomegaly, may develop in patients. Paradoxically, there is an increased incidence of autoimmune disease (20%), although patients may not display the usual serologic markers. Autoimmune cytopenias are most common, but autoimmune endocrinopathies, seronegative rheumatic disease, and gastrointestinal disorders are also commonly seen. Lymph nodes may be enlarged in these patients, yet biopsies show marked reduction in plasma cells. Noncaseating granulomas are frequently found in the spleen, liver, lungs, or skin. There is an increased propensity for the development of B cell neoplasms (50- to 400-fold increase risk of lymphoma), gastric carcinomas, and skin cancers.

B. LABORATORY FINDINGS

Diagnosis is confirmed in patients with recurrent infections by demonstration of functional or quantitative defects in antibody production. Serum IgG levels are usually less than 250 mg/dL; serum IgA and IgM levels are also subnormal. Decreased to absent functional antibody responses to protein antigen immunizations establish the diagnosis.

The cause of the panhypogammaglobulinemia in the majority of common variable immunodeficiency patients is an intrinsic B cell defect preventing terminal maturation into antibody-secreting plasma cells. In a small number, excessive suppressor T cell activity that inhibits B cells—or helper T cell activity inadequate to assist B cells to make antibody—has been identified. The absolute B cell count in the peripheral blood in most patients, despite the underlying cellular defect, is normal. A subset of these patients have concomitant T cell immunodeficiency with increased numbers of activated CD8 cells, splenomegaly, and decreased delayed-type hypersensitivity.

Treatment

Patients may be treated aggressively with antibiotics at the first sign of infection. Since antibody deficiency predisposes patients to high-risk pyogenic infections, antibiotic coverage should be sure to cover encapsulated bacteria. Only after the development of bronchiectasis or after sinus surgery do patients become significantly affected by more virulent organisms such as *Staphylococcus aureus* or *Pseudomonas aeruginosa*. Maintenance intravenous immune globulin (IGIV) therapy is indicated, with infusions of 300–500 mg/kg of IGIV given at about monthly intervals. Adjustment of dosage or of the infusion interval is made on the basis of clinical responses and steady-state trough serum IgG levels. Such therapy is effective in decreasing the incidence of potentially life-threatening infections and increasing quality of life. The yearly cost of monthly infusions can be in excess of $20,000–$30,000.

Cunningham-Rundles C: Immune deficiency: office evaluation and treatment. Allergy Asthma Proc 2003;24:409. [PMID: 14763242]

Kokron CM et al: Clinical and laboratory aspects of common variable immunodeficiency. An Acad Bras Cienc 2004;76: 707. [PMID: 15558152]

Sneller MC: Common variable immunodeficiency. Am J Med Sci 2001;321:42. [PMID: 11202479]

DISEASES OF IMMUNOGLOBULIN OVERPRODUCTION (Gammopathies)

The monoclonal gammopathies include those diseases in which there is a proliferation of a single clone of immunoglobulin-forming cells that produce a homogeneous heavy chain, light chain, or complete molecule. The amino acid sequence of the variable (V) regions is fixed, and only one type (κ or λ) of light chain is produced. Polyclonal gammopathies result from proliferation of many B cell clones, resulting in a diffuse increase of immunoglobulins.

1. Monoclonal Gammopathy of Uncertain Significance

ESSENTIALS OF DIAGNOSIS

- M protein in the serum without symptoms or signs of multiple myeloma, macroglobulinemia, amyloidosis, or lymphoma.
- Less than 10% plasma cells in the bone marrow.

General Considerations

The incidence of monoclonal gammopathy of uncertain significance (MGUS) increases with age and may approach 3% in persons 70 years of age or older. Lymphoid malignancies, amyloidosis, or multiple myeloma will develop in as many as one-third of patients with apparently benign monoclonal gammopathies. No specific therapy is necessary, but close observation is required. MGUS patients should be periodically monitored for changes in serum M proteins, urinary Bence Jones proteins, evidence of renal failure, anemia, hypercalcemia, lytic bone lesions, or bone marrow plasmacytoses. Risk of developing a malignant disorder is 12% at 10 years, 25% at 20 years, and 30% at 25 years. Parameters that suggest a favorable prognosis include (1) concentrations of homogeneous immunoglobulin less than 2 g/dL, (2) no increase in concentration of the immunoglobulin from the time of diagnosis, (3) no decrease in the concentration of normal immunoglobulins, (4) absence of a homogeneous

light chain in the urine, and (5) normal hematocrit and serum albumin.

Clinical Findings

A. SYMPTOMS AND SIGNS

No clinical symptoms are associated with MGUS. In patients with MGUS, the quantity of M protein is stable, and the lymphadenopathy, splenomegaly, or bony lesions seen with multiple myeloma are absent.

B. LABORATORY FINDINGS

The diagnosis of MGUS is made upon finding of a monoclonal spike on serum protein electrophoresis, confirmed by immunoelectrophoresis to be a homogeneous immunoglobulin with either κ or γ light chains.

Kyle RA et al: A long-term study of prognosis in monoclonal gammopathy of undetermined significance. N Engl J Med 2002;346:564. [PMID: 11856795]

Rajkumar SV: MGUS and smoldering multiple myeloma: update on pathogenesis, natural history, and management. Hematology (Am Soc Hematol Educ Program) 2005;340. [PMID: 16304401]

2. Multiple Myeloma (See Chapter 13)

3. Waldenström's Macroglobulinemia (See Chapter 13)

4. Amyloidosis

ESSENTIALS OF DIAGNOSIS

- The diagnosis is based on clinical suspicion, family history, and preexisting long-standing infection or debilitating illness.
- Microscopic examination of biopsy (eg, gingival, renal, rectal) or surgical specimens is diagnostic.
- Fine-needle biopsy of subcutaneous abdominal fat is a simple and reliable method for diagnosing secondary systemic amyloidosis.

General Considerations

Amyloidosis is a group of disorders manifested by impaired organ function due to infiltration with insoluble protein fibrils. Different fibrils can be correlated with the clinical syndromes. In primary amyloidosis (AL), the protein fibrils are monoclonal immunoglobulin light chains, whereas in secondary amyloidosis (AA), protein deposits are derived from acute phase reactant apolipoprotein precursors. Familial amyloidosis syndromes commonly cause infiltrative neuropathies. Other types of amyloidosis may also be hereditary. Over 20 types of fibrils have been identified in amyloid deposits. Amyloidosis due to deposition of β_2-microglobulin in carpal ligaments occurs in long-term hemodialysis patients.

Clinical Findings

A. SYMPTOMS AND SIGNS

The symptoms and signs of primary amyloidosis are due to amyloid infiltration and subsequent malfunction of the infiltrated organ (eg, nephritic syndrome and renal failure, cardiomyopathy and cardiac conduction defects, Alzheimer's disease, intestinal malabsorption and pseudo-obstruction, carpal tunnel syndrome, macroglossia, peripheral neuropathy, end-organ insufficiency of endocrine glands, respiratory failure, capillary damage with ecchymosis). Secondary amyloidosis is more often limited to the liver, spleen, and adrenals. Familial syndromes commonly cause infiltrative neuropathies.

B. LABORATORY TESTS

The diagnosis of primary amyloidosis is based on clinical suspicion with corroboration provided by detection of a monoclonal gammopathy on serum protein electrophoresis and microscopic examination of abdominal fat pad aspirates; rectal or gingival biopsies reveal amyloid protein (green birefringence under polarizing microscope after Congo red staining). In systemic disease, rectal or gingival biopsies show a sensitivity of about 80%, bone-marrow biopsy about 50%, and abdominal fat aspiration between 70% and 80%. The latter is a simple and reliable method for diagnosing systemic amyloidosis.

Differential Diagnosis

When evaluating a patient with suspected primary amyloidosis, it is important to consider other causes of the presenting symptoms and signs, including multiple myeloma, hemochromatosis, sarcoidosis, Waldenström's macroglobulinemia, metastatic tumors, and other cause of nephrotic syndrome, such as lupus nephritis.

Treatment

Treatment of localized amyloid tumors is by surgical excision. There is no effective treatment of systemic amyloidosis, and death usually occurs within 1–3 years. Care is generally supportive, although hemodialysis and immunosuppressive therapy may be useful. When concomitant multiple myeloma is found, it is treated in the standard way (see Chapter 13). Secondary disease is usually approached by aggressively treating the predisposing disease, but remission of fibril deposition does not occur. Bone marrow transplant after chemotherapy has been used in selected patients.

5. Heavy Chain Disease (α, γ, μ)

These are rare disorders in which the abnormal serum and urine protein is a part of a homogeneous α, γ, or μ heavy chain. The clinical presentation is more typical of lymphoma than multiple myeloma, and there are no destructive bone lesions. γ Chain disease presents as a lymphoproliferative disorder with autoimmune features. α Chain disease is frequently associated with severe diarrhea and infiltration of the lamina propria of the small intestine with abnormal plasma cells. μ Chain disease is associated with chronic lymphocytic leukemia.

Ando Y et al: A novel tool for detecting amyloid deposits in systemic amyloidosis in vitro and in vivo. Lab Invest 2003;83:1751. [PMID: 14691293]

Gahrton G: New therapeutic targets in multiple myeloma. Lancet 2004;364:1648. [PMID: 15530610]

Merlini G et al: Molecular mechanisms of amyloidosis. N Engl J Med 2003;349:583. [PMID: 12904524]

■ AUTOIMMUNITY

Autoimmune diseases cannot be explained by a solitary cause or mechanism. Small amounts of autoantibodies are normally produced and may have physiologic roles in cellular interactions. Positive serologic findings may be found years before the development of pathogenic autoimmunity or clinical illness, and in some cases, they represent normal immunity or "benign autoimmunity" without disease. The major theories regarding the development of autoimmune disease are (1) release of normally sequestered antigens; (2) escape from anergy or defective apoptosis (programmed cell death) leading to abnormal autoreactive cellular clones; (3) shared antigens between the host and microorganisms, ie, "molecular mimicry"; and (4) defects in helper or suppressor T cell function. A genetic susceptibility is also a likely determinant of autoimmune disease. In nearly all autoimmune diseases, multiple mechanisms of autoimmunity are operative.

Cell-Mediated Autoimmunity

Certain autoimmune diseases are mediated by T cells that have become specifically immunized to autologous tissues. Cytotoxic or killer T cells generated by this aberrant immune response injure specific organs in the absence of serum autoantibodies. Diminished suppressor T cell activity or loss of clonal anergy results in disordered regulation of immune function and consequent autoreactivity. The immune damage in systemic (non-organ-specific) diseases such as systemic lupus erythematosus may be due to such a mechanism.

Antibody-Mediated Autoimmunity

Several autoimmune diseases have been shown to be caused by autoantibodies in the absence of cell-mediated autoimmunity. The autoimmune hemolytic anemias, idiopathic thrombocytopenia, and Goodpasture's syndrome appear to be mediated solely by autoantibodies directed against autologous cell membrane constituents. In these diseases, antibody attaches to cell membranes and fixes complement; the ensuing inflammatory reaction injures the cells.

Anti-receptor antibodies that compete with or mimic physiologic agonists for cellular receptors cause several diseases. In Graves' disease, antibodies are present that bind to thyroid cells' thyroid-stimulating hormone receptors and thereby stimulate thyroid hormone production. In rare instances of type 1 diabetes mellitus, anti-insulin receptor antibodies cause insulin resistance in peripheral target tissues. Antibodies to acetylcholine receptors of the myoneural junction in myasthenia gravis block neuromuscular transmission and produce muscle weakness.

Immune Complex Disease

In this group of diseases (systemic lupus erythematosus, lupus nephritis, rheumatoid arthritis, some drug-induced hemolytic anemias, and thrombocytopenias), autologous tissues are injured as "innocent bystanders." Autoantibodies are not directed against cellular components of the target organ but rather against autologous or heterologous antigens in the serum. The resultant antigen-antibody complexes bind nonspecifically to autologous membranes (eg, glomerular basement membrane) and fix complement. Fixation and subsequent activation of complement components produce a local inflammatory response resulting in tissue injury.

AUTOIMMUNE DISEASES
(See also Chapter 20)

The diagnosis and treatment of specific autoimmune diseases are described elsewhere in this book. Autoantibodies associated with certain autoimmune diseases may not be pathogenetic but are thought to be markers or by-products of the injury (eg, autoimmune thyroiditis and antithyroglobulin antibody). See Table 19–2 for autoantibody patterns in connective tissue diseases.

TESTS FOR AUTOANTIBODIES ASSOCIATED WITH AUTOIMMUNE DISEASE

Agglutination Assays

Red cells are incubated with purified specific antigen (eg, thyroglobulin), which is adsorbed to the cell surface. The antigen-coated cells are suspended in the patient's serum, and antibody is detected by red cell agglutination. Antigen-coated latex particles are substituted for red cells in latex fixation tests.

Enzyme-Linked Immunosorbent Assay

Antibodies to various tissue antigens can be readily detected by these tests. Extracted and purified antigens are fixed to a plastic microtiter well or beads. The patient's serum is added, and excess proteins are removed by washing and centrifugation. Adherent immunoglobulin is then detected when a second antibody coupled to an enzyme (eg, alkaline phosphatase) is added. Finally, the enzyme's substrate is added; color forms and is measured in a spectrophotometer. This test can also be adapted for antigen detection by placing the antibody on the plastic surface. ELISA is very sensitive and less cumbersome than radioimmunoassay techniques.

Immunofluorescence Microscopy

This technique is most frequently used for detection of antinuclear antibody (ANA). Frozen sections of mouse liver or other substrates are cut and placed on glass slides or, alternatively, monolayers of cultured cell lines may be used. A patient's serum is placed over the sections and incubated. Fluorescein-conjugated rabbit anti-human immunoglobulin is then applied and washed. ANA specifically binds to the nucleus, and the fluorescein conjugate binds to the human antibody. Fluorescence of the cell nucleus on microscopy indicates a positive test.

Complement Fixation

Specific antigen, unknown serum, and complement are combined. Sheep red blood cells coated with antisheep cell antibody are added for 30 minutes at 37 °C. If antigen-specific antibody is present in the patient's serum, complement is bound and consumed, preventing lysis of sheep red cells.

Arbuckle MR: Development of autoantibodies before the clinical onset of systemic lupus erythematosus. N Engl J Med 2003; 349:1526. [PMID: 14561795]

Benito-Garcia E et al: Guidelines for immunologic laboratory testing in the rheumatic diseases: anti-Sm and anti-RNP antibody tests. Arthritis Rheum 2004;51:1030. [PMID: 15593352]

D'Cruz D: Testing for autoimmunity in humans. Toxicol Lett 2002;127:93. [PMID: 12052646]

Newkirk MM: Rheumatoid factors: host resistance or autoimmunity? Clin Immunol 2002;104:1. [PMID: 12139942]

■ IMMUNOGENETICS & TRANSPLANTATION

ASSOCIATIONS BETWEEN HLA ANTIGENS & SPECIFIC DISEASES

In humans, very striking associations are observed between particular HLA antigens and specific diseases. Some of these are listed in Table 19–3. In some diseases, the HLA molecule may be implicated in the pathogenesis. In others, the specific HLA allele may be linked to a gene determining immune responsiveness to a particular antigen.

Table 19–2. Autoantibodies: Associations with connective tissue diseases.

Suspected Disease State	Test	Primary Disease Association (Sensitivity, Specificity)	Other Disease Associations	Comments
CREST syndrome	Anticentromere antibody	CREST (70–90%, high)	Scleroderma (10–15%), Raynaud's disease (10–30%).	Predictive value of a positive test is > 95% for scleroderma or related disease (CREST, Raynaud's). Diagnosis of CREST is made clinically.
Systemic lupus erythematosus (SLE)	Antinuclear antibody (ANA)	SLE (> 95%, low)	Rheumatoid arthritis (30–50%), discoid lupus, scleroderma (60%), drug-induced lupus (100%), Sjögren's syndrome (80%), miscellaneous inflammatory disorders.	Often used as a screening test; a negative test virtually excludes SLE; a positive test, while nonspecific, increases posttest probability of SLE. Titer does not correlate with disease activity.
	Anti-double-stranded-DNA (anti-ds-DNA)	SLE (60–70%, high)	Lupus nephritis, rarely rheumatoid arthritis, other connective tissue disease, usually in low titer.	Predictive value of a positive test is > 90% for SLE if present in high titer; a decreasing titer may correlate with worsening renal disease. Titer generally correlates with disease activity.
	Anti-Smith antibody (anti-Sm)	SLE (30–40%, high)		SLE-specific. A positive test substantially increases posttest probability of SLE. Test rarely indicated.
Mixed connective tissue disease (MCTD)	Anti-ribonucleoprotein antibody (RNP)	Scleroderma (20–30%, low), MCTD (95–100%, low)	SLE (30%), Sjögren's syndrome, rheumatoid arthritis (10%), discoid lupus (20–30%).	A negative test essentially excludes MCTD; a positive test in high titer, while nonspecific, increases posttest probability of MCTD.
Rheumatoid arthritis	Rheumatoid factor (RF)	Rheumatoid arthritis (50–90%)	Other rheumatic diseases, chronic infections, some malignances, some healthy individuals, elderly patients.	Titer does not correlate with disease activity.
Scleroderma	Anti-Scl-70 antibody	Scleroderma (15–20%, low)		Predictive value of a positive test is > 95% for scleroderma.
Sjögren's syndrome	Anti-SS-A/Ro antibody	Sjögren's (60–70%, low)	SLE (30–40%), rheumatoid arthritis (10%), subacute cutaneous lupus, vasculitis.	Useful in counseling women of childbearing age with known connective tissue disease, since a positive test is associated with a small but real risk of neonatal SLE and congenital heart block.
Wegener's granulomatosis	Antineutrophil cytoplasmic antibody (ANCA)	Wegener's granulomatosis (systemic necrotizing vasculitis) (56–96%, high)	Crescentic glomerulonephritis or other systemic vasculitis (eg, polyarteritis nodosa).	Ability of this assay to reflect disease activity remains unclear.

CREST = calcinosis, Raynaud's phenomenon, esophageal dysmotility, sclerodactyly, and telangiectasia.
Modified, with permission, from Harvey AM et al (editors): The Principles and Practice of Medicine, 22nd ed. Appleton & Lange, 1988; White RH, Robbins DL: Clinical significance and interpretation of antinuclear antibodies. West J Med 1987;147:210; and Tan EM: Autoantibodies to nuclear antigens (ANA): their immunobiology and medicine. Adv Immunol 1982;33:167.

The standard method for detecting HLA-A, -B, and -C antigens is that of lymphocyte microcytotoxicity. Lymphocytes isolated from peripheral blood or lymph nodes are added to each well of a typing tray filled with sera containing the appropriate cytotoxic alloantibody. When complement is added, cells to which antibody has been specifically bound will have complement activated at the cell surface, resulting in cell death or lysis. It is thus possible to type for all of the known HLA-A, -B, and -C specificities. An appre-

Table 19–3. Association between the presence of various HLA markers and selected autoimmune diseases.

Disease	Associated HLA Marker[1]	Relative Risk of Disease[2]
Ankylosing spondylitis	B27	87.4
Reactive arthropathy, including Reiter's syndrome	B27	37.0
Rheumatoid arthritis	DR4	4.2
Behçet's syndrome	B51	3.8
Systemic lupus erythematosus	DR3	5.8
Insulin-dependent (type 1) diabetes mellitus	DR3	3.3
	DQB1*0201	2.4
	DR4	6.4
	DQB1*0302	9.5
	DR2	0.19
	DRB*1501[3]	
	DRB*0101[3]	
	DQB1*0602[3]	0.15
Idiopathic Addison's disease	DR3	6.3
Graves' disease	DR3	3.7
Hashimoto's disease	DR11	3.2
Postpartum thyroiditis	DR4	5.3
Celiac disease	DR3	10.8
	DQB1*0201[3]	
	DQA1*0501[3]	
	DR7,11	6.0–10.00
	DR7, DQB1*0201[3]	
	DR11, DQA1*0501[3]	
Dermatitis herpetiformis	DR3	15.9
Sicca syndrome	DR3	9.7
Myasthenia gravis	DR3	2.5
	B8	3.4
Idiopathic membranous glomerulonephritis	DR3	12.0
Goodpasture's syndrome	DR2	15.9
Multiple sclerosis	DR2	4.1
	DRB1*1501[3]	
	DRB5*0101[3]	
	DQB1*0602[3]	
Pemphigus vulgaris (among Ashkenazi Jews)	DR4	14.4
Psoriasis vulgaris	Cw6	13.3
Birdshot retinochoroidopathy	A29	109.0

[1]Symbols with asterisks indicate alleles, and symbols without asterisks indicate serologically defined antigens. For each disease, the marker or markers with the strongest associations are given. In many cases in which it is difficult to decide whether HLA-DR or -DQ markers are responsible for association, both markers are given.

[2]The relative risk indicates the frequency of a disease in persons with the HLA marker as compared with persons without the marker. A positive association (ie, when the HLA marker is more frequent in persons with the disease than in those without it) is indicated by a relative risk of more than 1.0, a negative association by a relative risk of less than 1.0, and no association by a relative risk of 1.0.

[3]The risk has not been assessed separately for this allele.

Reproduced, with permission, from Svejgaard A: MHC and disease associations. In: Herzenberg LA et al (editors). *Weir's Handbook of Experimental Immunology*, 5th ed. Blackwell Science, 1996.

ciable majority of typing serum samples are obtained from multiparous women since they form antibodies to fetal alloantigens.

Typing for the class II antigens HLA-DR and -DQ by serologic methods is technically more difficult. Antigens of the HLA-D, -DR, -DQ, and -DP series may also be detected by in vitro mixed lymphocyte culture. Lymphocytes of one individual (responder cells) will undergo proliferation upon encountering lymphocytes from another individual possessing foreign HLA-DR and -DQ antigens (stimulator cells). Lymphocyte proliferation can be readily measured by DNA incorporation of tritiated thymidine. Responders possessing matching -DR and -DQ antigens will remain nonreactive.

Increasingly, HLA class II typing is being performed by molecular technology. The DNA sequences for the HLA genes and their flanking sequences are known. Selected primers that amplify the gene of interest using the polymerase chain reaction technique are known as sequence-specific primers. HLA typing by PCR provides better resolution than serologic identification because typing is done at the genetic level.

Gonzalez S et al: Immunogenetics, HLA-B27 and spondyloarthropathies. Curr Opin Rheumatol 1999;11:257. [PMID: 10411379]

McCurdy D: Genetic susceptibility to the connective tissue diseases. Curr Opin Rheumatol 1999;11:399. [PMID: 10503661]

Shiina T et al: An update of the HLA genomic region, locus information and disease associations: 2004. Tissue Antigens 2004;64:631. [PMID: 15546336]

CLINICAL TRANSPLANTATION

Organ transplants are in widespread use. Limitations include the scarcity of donor organs and expense. Failure to achieve successful grafts is primarily due to histoincompatibility and lack of safe and effective immunosuppressive regimens to halt rejection. Avoiding transmission of infectious agents (eg, HIV, hepatitis B virus, hepatitis C virus, cytomegalovirus) from donor to recipient requires extensive pretransplant serologic testing.

Kidney Transplantation

End-stage renal disease is the indication for kidney transplantation. Factors that determine outcome include antigenic disparity (ABO blood groups and major histocompatibility or HLA) between donor and recipient, the type of immunologic response mounted by the host, and the immunosuppressive regimen used to prevent graft rejection. Nonimmunologic factors that affect the risk of chronic rejection include age and race of recipient; donor age; length of time on dialysis; and coexisting hyperlipidemia, hypertension, or cytomegalovirus infection.

Kidneys from living related donors who are HLA-identical and also red cell ABO-matched grafts have 90% survival at 1 year; grafts from less-well matched relatives and from living unrelated donors have lower

rates. Antigens are matched for HLA-A, -B and -DR loci, with -DR compatibility most important for long-term graft survival. Grafts from cadaver donors with zero HLA mismatches have a half-life of 11.3 years. Those with six mismatches have a half-life of 6.8 years, compared with those from HLA-identical siblings, which have a half-life of 23.6 years.

Some donors are highly sensitized to HLA antigens from previous transfusions, ie, possess high panel reactive antibody levels. It may be difficult to find a suitable donor, since a positive cross-match by cytotoxicity testing is likely and would be a contraindication to transplant. Donor screening is performed in all cases to assess suitability, rule out hypertension or anatomic anomalies, and avoid transmission of hepatitis viruses, HIV, and other infectious agents. Owing to the scarcity of related donors, living unrelated donors may be used in certain circumstances. Pretreatment of recipients with blood transfusions from the donor appears to extend graft survival even longer.

Delayed allograft function can be due to hyperacute graft rejection, postischemic acute tubular necrosis, cyclosporine toxicity, or obstructive nephropathy. If conservative measures do not improve function or patients are at high risk for allograft rejection, renal biopsy should be performed for definitive diagnostic purposes. Renal allograft rejection may be due to hyperacute rejection from binding of cytotoxic antibodies and complement activation, acute rejection from cellular immune responses, or chronic rejection. A form of interstitial nephritis secondary to polyomavirus infection is associated with aggressive immunosuppression. Noninvasive methods to diagnose rejection are being developed. To replace the need for renal biopsy, studies of mRNA reveal that the levels of FOXP3 in urinary cells may serve as a mechanistically informative biomarker of acute rejection.

Chronic allograft nephropathy is characterized by vasculopathy and immune-mediated graft obliteration. Previous acute rejection is strongly linked with later chronic rejection, and severity of those episodes has prognostic implications. Cyclosporine-induced nephrotoxicity and recurrent or de novo renal disease are also significant factors affecting long-term survival.

High-Dose Chemotherapy with Hematopoietic Progenitor Cell (Stem Cell) Transplantation

Transient myelosuppression after cancer chemotherapy is a well-established adverse effect of such treatments. For most regimens, it is rapidly reversible and requires no intervention. Some malignancies (eg, many leukemias, lymphomas, and chemotherapy-sensitive breast and small-cell lung carcinomas) may demonstrate a higher cure rate with higher-dose therapy; however, associated with this approach is an increase in hematologic toxicity. Administering the maximal tolerated chemotherapy dose and restoring all hematopoietic functions as rapidly as possible has led to evolution of the concept of hematopoietic progenitor cell (HPC) or "stem cell" transplant. HPC transplants have also expanded somewhat into the therapy of certain nonmalignant disorders of hematopoiesis and hematologic function; examples are aplastic anemia, sickle cell anemia, thalassemia, myelodysplasia, amyloidosis, and paroxysmal nocturnal hemoglobinuria.

The sources of HPC are the bone marrow, peripheral blood, and cord blood. They comprise less than 0.5–1% of all nucleated bone marrow cells. Although HPCs are "rare" cells, they can be obtained from the peripheral blood by apheresis. As the peripheral blood has approximately one-fortieth the number of circulating HPCs as the bone marrow, these cells must be "mobilized" by the administration of cytotoxic chemotherapy (with the harvest being performed during the recovery phase) or enriched by the administration of hematopoietic growth factors. The cells are frozen and administered at a later date. Transplantation of HPC from umbilical cord blood can be used in unrelated donors, with a potentially lower rate of graftversus-host disease, or may be autologous, from frozen stored blood.

Because syngeneic transplants between identical (monozygotic) twins are rare, the two predominant transplants are autologous, where the HPCs are harvested from and returned to the patient; or allogeneic, where the source is an HLA-matched donor, ideally a sibling. The goals of the two procedures—and their associated adverse effects—are frequently different. Allogeneic transplants are most commonly offered to patients with malignant and nonmalignant disorders involving the bone marrow. Chemotherapy is given to ablate the marrow, resulting in maximal suppression or eradication of the recipient's native immune system. The bone marrow is repopulated by infusion of donor cells containing not only HPCs but also functional donor T lymphocytes. These T cells can cause graft-versus-host disease, in which the recipient's tissues are recognized as nonself. While this is occasionally desirable, as in the "graft-versus-leukemia" effect, it is the cause of considerable morbidity and can be fatal. There are two separate phases of graft-versus-host disease: acute, secondary to cytokine-mediated cytotoxicity against the cells of the liver, the mucosa of the gastrointestinal tract, and skin; and chronic, characterized by fibrosis and collagen deposition and resembling autoimmune disease such as scleroderma. The incidence of graft-versus-host disease can be decreased by depleting the donor marrow of T cells, but this is associated with a higher incidence of graft failure and, in the case of leukemia, a higher relapse rate. Allogeneic peripheral HPC transplants have been attempted, and graft-versus-host disease in such cases does not appear to be as severe.

Autologous HPC transplants are performed solely for the treatment of malignancies. In these cases the chemotherapy is intensively myelosuppressive although not necessarily myeloablative. One prominent exception is patients with chronic myelogenous leukemia in blast crisis, who receive their autologous HPC in an effort to return their disease to the chronic phase. Since patients usually have some residual immune function and are receiving their own HPC—and thus do not require posttransplant immunosuppression—the risk of opportunistic infections and immunosuppression-related neoplasia is markedly reduced.

The success rates of HPC transplantation depend mostly on the underlying disease and the associated risk of relapse (in cases of leukemia), the level of matching between donor and recipient (and thus the likelihood of graft-versus-host disease), the age of the recipient, and the complications associated with conditioning (venoocclusive liver disease and infection). Overall, the survival rates at 1 year are about 60–70% in aplastic anemia and 40–75% in various forms of leukemia and other neoplasms such as non-Hodgkin's lymphomas; results in breast carcinoma are less well defined.

Horwitz ME et al: Chronic graft-versus-host disease. Blood Rev 2006;20:15. [PMID 16426941]

Muthukumar T et al: Messenger RNA for FOXP3 in the urine of renal allograft recipients. N Engl J Med 2005;353:2342. [PMID: 16319383]

Nankivell BJ et al: The natural history of chronic allograft nephropathy. N Engl J Med 2003;349:2288. [PMID: 14668458]

Sankari BR et al: Immunosuppression after kidney transplantation: current strategies and drug interactions. J Med Liban 2004;52:234. [PMID: 16432988]

Shizura JA et al: Hematopoietic stem and progenitor cells. Clinical and preclinical regeneration of the hematolymphoid system. Ann Rev Med 2005;56:509. [PMID: 15660525]

Strom TB: Rejection—More than the eye can see. N Engl J Med 2005;353:2394. [PMID: 16319390]

Valcarcel D et al: Conventional versus reduced-intensity conditioning regimen for allogeneic stem cell transplantation in patients with hematologic malignancies. Eur J Haematol 2005;74:144. [PMID: 15654906]

MECHANISM OF ACTION OF IMMUNOSUPPRESSIVE DRUGS

The most frequently used immunosuppressive drugs and their modes of action are briefly summarized below.

Corticosteroids

This group of drugs has potent and direct anti-inflammatory effects on immunocompetent cells. Corticosteroids inhibit lymphocyte proliferation and cell-mediated immune responses more severely than they inhibit antibody responses. T helper cells, eosinophils, and monocytes are reduced in peripheral blood. Corticosteroids down-regulate cytokine gene expression through interference with transcription regulation. By inhibition of phospholipase A_2, synthesis of inflammatory arachidonic acid metabolites (prostaglandins and leukotrienes) is suppressed. Corticosteroids have been shown to block the activation of T cells by interleukin-1 (IL-1) derived from macrophages. They also inhibit the expression of class II histocompatibility antigens on the macrophage surface, thereby interfering with presentation of antigen to T cells. Cumulatively, these cellular changes result in reduced inflammatory responses.

Cytotoxic Drugs

The most frequently used cytotoxic drugs are the antimetabolites (see below) and cyclophosphamide. Cyclophosphamide is an alkylating agent that damages cells by cross-linking DNA. Although this cycle-specific drug is most effective in killing cells going through the mitotic cycle, it can also cause intermitotic cell injury and death. Cyclophosphamide can inhibit both T and B cell immunity as well as inflammation. Azathioprine and cyclophosphamide are effective inhibitors of the production of serum antibodies.

Antimetabolites

Antimetabolites used for immune modulation include methotrexate, an inhibitor of folic acid synthesis, azathioprine, a structural analog of mercaptopurine and an antagonist of purine synthesis; and leflunomide, an inhibitor of de novo pyrimidine synthesis. Azathioprine is a phase-specific drug that kills rapidly replicating cells. It inhibits proliferation of both T and B cells as well as macrophages. Methotrexate inhibits rapidly proliferating cells in S phase and suppresses both cell-mediated and humoral immunity as well as inflammation. Without immunosuppression, the incidence of graft-versus-host disease after allogeneic HPC transplant is almost 100%; this can be reduced to 20–30% with immunosuppressive therapy, especially the combination of methotrexate and cyclosporine, in addition to corticosteroids. Cyclosporine prevents T cell activation, while methotrexate inhibits the function of T cells that are already activated. When leflunomide is combined with methotrexate for the treatment of rheumatoid arthritis, it is more effective than methotrexate alone but the risk of hepatic toxicity is also increased. As monotherapy, it appears to be comparable to methotrexate or sulfasalazine.

Cyclosporine

This cyclic polypeptide derived from a fungus is used as an immunosuppressive drug in organ transplant recipients. Cyclosporine binds to cyclophilin, a cytoplasmic protein, thereby interfering with calcium-dependent events including secretion of interleukin-2 (IL-2) by T lymphocytes. Since IL-2 is necessary for T cell replication, this drug is a potent inhibitor of T cell proliferation and thereby inhibits T cell-mediated immune responses. Little effect has been shown on direct B cell immune responses or on inflammation. Its toxic effects are primarily on renal and, to a lesser extent, hepatic function. In addition to methotrexate, methylprednisolone has also been used with cyclosporine to treat graft-versus-host disease, although T cell-directed immunotoxins have not proved to be of any benefit. A recently developed microemulsion formulation offers improved oral bioavailability, safety, and efficacy.

Tacrolimus/Sirolimus/Everolimus

Like cyclosporine, tacrolimus also inhibits calcineurin-dependent phosphorylation of nuclear transcription factors, thereby inhibiting T cell activation and subsequent production of IL-2 and interferon-γ. Tacrolimus is approximately 100 times more potent than cyclosporine and, in many cases, is now preferred over cyclosporine. Rates of graft-versus-host disease are lower for tacrolimus-based regimens. Tacrolimus appears to be at least as effective as cyclosporine and possibly better as prophylaxis of acute rejection. The major toxicities include hyperglycemia, nephrotoxicity, and neurotoxicity. Topical formulations are well tolerated and have shown efficacy in the treatment of atopic dermatitis and allergic contact dermatitis.

Sirolimus, a macrocyclic immunosuppressive agent and product of *Streptomyces hygroscopicus,* inhibits cellular proliferation stimulated by growth factor driven signal transduction in response to alloantigens. It binds to FK506 binding protein 12 (FKBP12), which in turn binds FKBP12-rapamycin associated protein, arresting the cell cycle in the G1 phase. This allows sirolimus to act synergistically with cyclosporine. In particular, sirolimus added to other calcineurin antagonists appears to be less commonly associated with immunosuppression-induced neoplasms or lymphoproliferative diseases. Everolimus, a derivative of sirolimus, has a similar mechanism of action.

Tacrolimus and sirolimus are approved for use in kidney and liver transplantation as primary immunosuppressive agents and as rescue therapy but may also be used to prevent graft-versus-host disease. Everolimus is not approved by the US Food and Drug Administration.

Mycophenolate Mofetil

Mycophenolate mofetil is a prodrug used primarily as an adjunctive agent in kidney transplantation. By blocking lymphocyte production of guanine nucleotides, it inhibits T and B lymphocyte proliferation. Its use in combination with cyclosporine or tacrolimus has led to a lower incidence of acute allograft rejection, reducing the need for high-dose corticosteroids or OKT3 (muromonab-CD3).

Humanized Anti-Interleukin-2 Receptor Antibody

Several humanized monoclonal antibodies directed to the low-affinity IL-2 receptor are approved for use in kidney transplantation. Daclizumab and basiliximab target CD25, the IL-2 receptor, which is expressed on activated T cells. When combined with calcineurin inhibitors, they can be used for induction during transplantation. These antibodies, administered during the first 4–8 weeks following the transplant, result in a reduction of the incidence of acute graft rejection to about 25% when added to standard immunosuppressive therapy. Although the incidence of acute rejection is not substantially lower than that of other combinations of immunosuppressive agents, there appears to be a lower incidence and severity of side effects compared with antilymphocyte alternatives.

Muromonab-CD3

A murine monoclonal antibody, muromonab-CD3, is directed against human CD3, the T cell receptor. Indicated for acute graft rejection refractory to corticosteroids, large doses of the drug purge T cells from the systemic circulation. The drug has numerous side effects related to the release of cytokines, including fever, myalgias, dyspnea, and aseptic meningitis, and has also been associated with increased susceptibility to cytomegalovirus infection. Most patients are limited to a single course of therapy since recurrent courses may be associated with the production of neutralizing antibodies or posttransplant lymphoproliferative disease.

Other Monoclonal Antibodies

Rituximab specifically binds to CD20, a pan-B cell marker. Initially approved for use in B cell lymphoma, it is also used for posttransplant lymphoproliferative disease. It is being investigated for other B cell-mediated disorders but does suppress humoral immunity.

IMMUNOMODULATING THERAPIES

Co-Stimulatory Blockade

Abatacept is the first medication in a new class of drugs for the treatment of rheumatoid arthritis that selectively modulate the CD80 or CD86-CD28 co-stimulatory signal required for full T-cell activation. CD80 or CD86 on the surface of an antigen-presenting cell binds to CD28 on the T-cell, facilitating T cell activation. The naturally occurring inhibitory molecule known as cytotoxic T-lymphocyte antigen 4 (CTLA4) is induced on the surface of the T cell. CTLA4 has a markedly greater affinity for CD80 or CD86 than does CD28, thus out competing CD28 for CD80 or CD86 binding. Abatacept is a recombinant fusion protein comprising the extracellular domain of human CTLA4 and a fragment of the Fc domain of human IgG_1, which has been modified to prevent complement fixation.

Belatacept differs from abatacept by two specific amino acid substitutions conferring greater binding avidity to CD80 andCD86. In combination with mycophenolate mofetil and corticosteroids after an induction phase with basiliximab, belatacept was found to be noninferior to a cyclosporine-based regimen in kidney transplantation.

Cytokine Therapy

The experimental and clinical applications of cytokines, as biologic response modifiers and therapeutic agents, have been greatly expanded in recent years. Some cytokines, such as tumor necrosis factor and interferon alfa,

have direct antitumor activity. Other cytokines affect tumor immune responses by lymphokine-activated killer cells, tumor-infiltrating lymphocytes, and activated natural killer cells. Cytokines have been used to activate immune cells ex vivo prior to adoptive transfer or have been given concurrently with activated effector cells. Clinical trials of cellular adoptive therapy, with IL-2 activated killer cells, for the treatment of renal cell carcinoma and melanoma have demonstrated feasibility and regression of metastasis in some patients. Modest results, significant morbidity, and high cost have hampered widespread adoption of these techniques.

Interferon alfa is used in hairy cell leukemia, chronic myelogenous leukemia, Kaposi's sarcoma, and chronic active hepatitis B and C. Interferon beta is used for multiple sclerosis and interferon gamma for the treatment of chronic granulomatous disease. Constitutional symptoms are common with cytokine therapy, and in some instances toxicity is considerable.

Tumor Necrosis Factor Antagonists

Several approaches are available to mitigate the biologic effects of tumor necrosis factor (TNF), a cytokine produced by macrophages and other antigen-presenting cells. Three molecules have been designed to inhibit binding of TNF to its cellular receptor and thereby reduce its cellular and biologic effects. Etanercept is a dimeric construct—containing the soluble TNF receptor—joined to the Fc domain of a human IgG molecule. Infliximab is a chimeric antibody molecule containing a human Fc domain and a murine variable region. Adalimumab is a recombinant human monoclonal antibody that binds to TNF-α and impairs cytokine receptor binding. All are disease-modifying antirheumatic drugs that have been shown to slow joint destruction and markedly decrease symptoms of rheumatoid arthritis. Etanercept has shown efficacy in ankylosing spondylitis. It must be administered by subcutaneous injection twice weekly; infliximab is given intravenously every 2 months. These TNF antagonists should not be administered to patients with active infection, and the full scope of associated adverse effects is still not clear. Possible association without proven causation has been cited between TNF antagonists and lymphoma, demyelinating syndromes, and hematologic abnormalities. The incidence of ANAs is increased in patients receiving these drugs but frank drug-induced lupus appears rare.

Soluble IL-1 Receptor Antagonist

Anakinra, a recombinant, nonglycosylated soluble IL-1 receptor antagonist, competitively inhibits the binding of IL-1 to its cellular receptor. IL-1 is a major immunomodulatory cytokine, proinflammatory agent, and endogenous pyrogen. Through receptor blockade, anakinra has proved to be anti-inflammatory and efficacious in the treatment of rheumatoid arthritis for patients who have not responded or are unable to tolerate antimetabolites or TNF antagonists. There does appear to be an increased incidence of infections in patients receiving anakinra, and hypersensitivity reactions may also occur.

Anti-IgE

Omalizumab is a recombinant, humanized, murine monoclonal antibody with affinity for human IgE. By binding to the Fc-binding domain of circulating serum IgE, omalizumab prevents IgE binding to Fc-receptors on human mast cells. With ongoing subcutaneously injected treatment, tissue mast cells are effectively "disarmed" and less capable of activation through allergen-IgE interactions. Both early and late phase allergic reactions can be suppressed, and omalizumab has shown to be effective for control of symptoms, improvement in pulmonary function, and improvement in quality of life for patients with allergic asthma and allergic rhinitis. Improvement is not sustained after cessation of therapy, and chronic treatment is necessary for long-term disease control.

Intravenous Gamma Globulin

IGIV has numerous immunomodulatory and anti-inflammatory activities and is the standard of care for immunologically mediated disorders such as Kawasaki's syndrome and for antibody replacement in humoral immunodeficiency. When used in humoral immunodeficiency, serum IgG levels can become normal but the IGIV contains virtually no IgM and only traces of IgA.

Each lot of IGIV produced from donated serum contains millions of antibody specificities, reflecting the humoral immune repertoire from thousands of normal blood donors. Most current products undergo numerous purification and viral inactivation steps, including solvent-detergent treatment or pasteurization. The antibody reactivities can be directed against a wide range of foreign and self antigens. In addition to the above disorders, IGIV is effective in Guillain-Barré syndrome, immune-mediated neuropathies, idiopathic thrombocytopenic purpura, pediatric HIV infection, and after bone marrow transplantation. Many other potential indications have been supported only by anecdotal reports or uncontrolled trials.

Cobbold SP: New trends in immunosuppression. Int Immunopharmacol 2005;5:1. [PMID: 15589453]

Eisen HJ et al; RAD B253 Study Group: Everolimus for the prevention of allograft rejection and vasculopathy in cardiac transplant recipients. N Engl J Med 2003;349:847. [PMID: 12944570]

First MR: Immunosuppressive agents and their actions. Transplant Proc 2002;34:1369. [PMID: 12176401]

Genovese MC et al: Abatacept for rheumatoid arthritis refractory to tumor necrosis factor alpha inhibition. N Engl J Med 2005;353:1114. [PMID: 16162882]

Halloran PF: Immunosuppressive drugs for kidney transplantation. N Engl J Med 2004;351:2715. [PMID: 15616206]

John Looney R et al: Use of intravenous immunoglobulin G (IVIG). Best Pract Res Clin Haematol 2006;19:3. [PMID: 16377538]

Kahan BD: Sirolimus-based immunosuppression: present state of the art. J Nephrol 2004;17(Suppl 8):S32. [PMID: 15599884]

Olsen NJ et al: New drugs for rheumatoid arthritis. N Engl J Med 2004; 350:2167. [PMID: 15152062]

Vincenti F et al; Belatacept Study Group: Co-stimulation blockade with belatacept in renal transplantation. N Engl J Med 2005;353:770. [PMID: 16120857]

Arthritis & Musculoskeletal Disorders

20

David B. Hellmann, MD, MACP, & John H. Stone, MD, MPH

■ DIAGNOSIS & EVALUATION

Examination of the Patient

In the patient with arthritis, the two clinical clues most helpful for diagnosis are the joint pattern and the presence or absence of extra-articular manifestations. The joint pattern is defined by the answers to three questions: (1) Is inflammation present? (2) How many joints are involved? and (3) What joints are affected? Joint inflammation is manifested by redness, warmth, swelling, and morning stiffness of at least 30 minutes' duration. Both the number of affected joints and the specific sites of involvement affect the differential diagnosis (Table 20–1). Some diseases—gout, for example—are characteristically monarticular, whereas other diseases, such as rheumatoid arthritis, are chiefly polyarticular. The location of joint involvement can also be distinctive. Only two diseases frequently cause prominent involvement of the distal interphalangeal (DIP) joint: osteoarthritis and psoriatic arthritis. Extra-articular manifestations such as fever, rash, nodules, or neuropathy narrow the differential diagnosis further (see Table 20–1).

Arthrocentesis & Examination of Joint Fluid

Synovial fluid examination (Table 20–2) may provide specific diagnostic information in joint disease. Contraindications to arthrocentesis include infection of the overlying skin, bleeding disorder, or inability of the patient to cooperate. For patients who are receiving long-term anticoagulation therapy with warfarin, joints can be aspirated if the international normalized ratio (INR) is less than 3.0. In such patients, use of a small-gauge needle (eg, 22F or 25F) and application of firm pressure to the aspiration site are prudent measures. Most large joints are easily aspirated (Figure 20–1).

A. Types of Studies

1. Gross examination—If fluid is opaque, a Gram stain is indicated. If bloody, a bleeding disorder, trauma, or traumatic tap is most likely.

2. Microscopic examination—Compensated polarized light microscopy identifies and distinguishes monosodium urate (gout, negatively birefringent) and calcium pyrophosphate (pseudogout, positive birefringent) crystals.

3. Culture—Bacterial cultures as well as special studies for gonococci, tubercle bacilli, or fungi are ordered as appropriate.

B. Interpretation

Although synovial fluid analysis is diagnostic in infectious or microcrystalline arthritis, there is considerable overlap in the cytologic and biochemical values obtained in these and other diseases (Table 20–3). These studies do make possible, however, a differentiation according to severity of inflammation. Inflammatory joint fluids have more than 3000 white blood cells per microliter, of which 50% or more are polymorphonuclear neutrophils (Table 20–2). Noninflammatory fluids usually have less than 3000/mcL white cells and less than 25% polymorphonuclear neutrophils. Synovial fluid glucose and protein levels add little information.

■ DEGENERATIVE & CRYSTAL-INDUCED ARTHRITIS

DEGENERATIVE JOINT DISEASE (Osteoarthritis)

ESSENTIALS OF DIAGNOSIS

- *A degenerative disorder without systemic manifestations.*
- *Commonly secondary to other articular disease.*
- *Pain relieved by rest; morning stiffness brief; articular inflammation minimal.*
- *X-ray findings: narrowed joint space, osteophytes, increased density of subchondral bone, bony cysts.*

Table 20–1. Diagnostic value of the joint pattern.

Character-istic	Status	Representative Disease
Inflammation	Present	Rheumatoid arthritis, systemic lupus erythematosus, gout
	Absent	Osteoarthritis
Number of involved joints	Monarticular	Gout, trauma, septic arthritis, Lyme disease, osteoarthritis
	Oligoarticular (2–4 joints)	Reiter's disease, psoriatic arthritis, inflammatory bowel disease
	Polyarticular (≥ 5 joints)	Rheumatoid arthritis, systemic lupus erythematosus
Site of joint involvement	Distal interphalangeal	Osteoarthritis, psoriatic arthritis (not rheumatoid arthritis)
	Metacarpophalangeal, wrists	Rheumatoid arthritis, systemic lupus erythematosus (not osteoarthritis)
	First metatarsal phalangeal	Gout, osteoarthritis

General Considerations

Osteoarthritis, the most common form of joint disease, is chiefly a disease of aging. Ninety percent of all people have radiographic features of osteoarthritis in weight-bearing joints by age 40. Symptomatic disease also increases with age.

This arthropathy is characterized by degeneration of cartilage and by hypertrophy of bone at the articular margins. Inflammation is usually minimal. Hereditary and mechanical factors may be involved in the pathogenesis.

Degenerative joint disease is divided into two types: (1) primary, which most commonly affects some or all of the following: the terminal interphalangeal joints (Heberden's nodes) and less commonly the proximal interphalangeal (PIP) joints (Bouchard's nodes), the metacarpophalangeal (MCP) and carpometacarpal joints of the thumb, the hip, the knee, the metatarsophalangeal (MTP) joint of the big toe, and the cervical and lumbar spine; and (2) secondary, which may occur in any joint as a sequela to articular injury resulting from either intra-articular (including rheumatoid arthritis) or extra-articular causes. The injury may be acute, as in a fracture; or chronic, as that due to occupational overuse of a joint, metabolic disease (eg, hyperparathyroidism, hemochromatosis, ochronosis), or neurologic disorders (tabes dorsalis; see below). Obesity is a risk factor for knee osteoarthritis and probably for the hip. Recreational running does not increase the incidence of osteoarthritis, but participation in competitive contact sports does. Jobs requiring frequent bending and carrying increase the risk of knee osteoarthritis.

Clinical Findings

A. Symptoms and Signs

The onset is insidious. Initially, there is articular stiffness, seldom lasting more than 15 minutes; this develops later into pain on motion of the affected joint and is made worse by activity or weight bearing and relieved by rest. Deformity may be absent or minimal; however, bony enlargement of the interphalangeal joints is occasionally prominent, and flexion contracture or varus deformity of the knee is not unusual. There is no ankylosis, but limitation of motion of the affected joint or joints is common. Crepitus may often

Table 20–2. Examination of joint fluid.

Measure	(Normal)	Group I (Noninflammatory)	Group II (Inflammatory)	Group III (Purulent)
Volume (mL) (knee)	< 3.5	Often > 3.5	Often > 3.5	Often > 3.5
Clarity	Transparent	Transparent	Translucent to opaque	Opaque
Color	Clear	Yellow	Yellow to opalescent	Yellow to green
WBC (per mcL)	< 200	200–300	3000–50,000	> 50,000[1]
Polymorphonuclear leukocytes	< 25%	< 25%	50% or more	75% or more[1]
Culture	Negative	Negative	Negative	Usually positive
Glucose (mg/dL)	Nearly equal to serum	Nearly equal to serum	> 25, lower than serum	< 25, much lower than serum

[1]Counts are lower with infections caused by organisms of low virulence or if antibiotic therapy has been started.

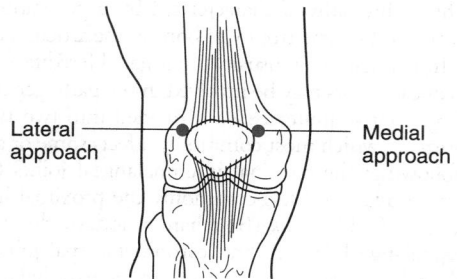

Figure 20–1. Aspiration of the knee joint. The knee joint—the most commonly aspirated joint—can be entered either medially or laterally. The patient should be supine, with the leg fully extended. Apply pressure on the side of the joint opposite to the puncture site to assist in directing the needle toward the bulging synovium. From the lateral approach, the needle (held parallel to the examining table) is directed medially, just beneath the patella, into the suprapatellar space. From the medial approach, the needle (held parallel to the examining table) is introduced between the patella and the medial condyle and advanced upward and laterally, beneath the patella and into the joint space. (Reproduced, with permission, from Nicoll D et al: *Pocket Guide to Diagnostic Tests.* McGraw-Hill, 1997.)

be felt in the joint. Joint effusion and other articular signs of inflammation are mild. There are no systemic manifestations.

B. LABORATORY FINDINGS

Osteoarthritis does not cause elevation of the erythrocyte sedimentation rate (ESR) or other laboratory signs of inflammation.

C. IMAGING

Radiographs may reveal narrowing of the joint space; sharpened articular margins; osteophyte formation and lipping of marginal bone; and thickened, dense subchondral bone. Bone cysts may also be present.

Differential Diagnosis

Because articular inflammation is minimal and systemic manifestations are absent, degenerative joint disease should seldom be confused with other arthritides. The distribution of joint involvement in the hands also helps distinguish osteoarthritis from rheumatoid arthritis. Osteoarthritis chiefly affects the DIP and PIP joints and spares the wrist and MCP joints (except at the thumb); rheumatoid arthritis involves the wrists and MCP joints and spares the DIP joints. Furthermore, the joint enlargement is bony-hard and cool in osteoarthritis but spongy and warm in rheumatoid arthritis. Skeletal symptoms due to degenerative changes in joints—especially in the spine—may cause coexistent metastatic neoplasia, osteoporosis, multiple myeloma, or other bone disease to be overlooked.

Prevention

Weight reduction reduces the risk of developing symptomatic knee osteoarthritis. Maintaining normal

Table 20–3. Differential diagnosis by joint fluid groups.

Group I (Noninflammatory)	Group II (Inflammatory)	Group III (Purulent)	Hemorrhagic
Degenerative joint disease	Rheumatoid arthritis	Pyogenic bacterial infections	Hemophilia or other hemorrhagic diathesis
Trauma[1]	Acute crystal-induced synovitis (gout and pseudogout)		Trauma with or without fracture
Osteochondritis dissecans	Reiter's syndrome		Neuropathic arthropathy
Osteochondromatosis	Ankylosing spondylitis		Pigmented villonodular synovitis
Neuropathic arthropathy[1]	Psoriatic arthritis		Synovioma
Subsiding or early inflammation	Arthritis accompanying ulcerative colitis and regional enteritis		Hemangioma and other benign neoplasms
Hypertrophic osteoarthropathy[2]	Rheumatic fever[2]		
Pigmented villonodular synovitis[1]	Systemic lupus erythematosus[2]		
	Progressive systemic sclerosis (scleroderma)[2]		
	Tuberculosis		
	Mycotic infections		

[1]May be hemorrhagic.
[2]Noninflammatory or inflammatory group.
Reproduced from Rodnan GP (editor): Primer on the rheumatic diseases, 7th ed. JAMA 1973;224(Suppl):662.

vitamin D levels may reduce the occurrence and progression of osteoarthritis, in addition to being important for bone health.

Treatment

A. GENERAL MEASURES

For patients with mild to moderate osteoarthritis of weight-bearing joints, a supervised walking program may result in clinical improvement of functional status without aggravating the joint pain. Weight loss can also improve the symptoms.

B. ANALGESIC AND ANTI-INFLAMMATORY DRUGS

Nonsteroidal anti-inflammatory drugs (NSAIDs) (see Table 5-5) are more effective (and more toxic) than acetaminophen for osteoarthritis of the knee or hip. Their superiority is most convincing in those with severe disease. Patients with mild disease should start with acetaminophen (2.6-4 g/d). Glucosamine and chondroitin sulfate are also effective and safe for knee osteoarthritis; glucosamine may even reduce progression of knee osteoarthritis. NSAIDs should be considered for patients who do not respond to acetaminophen, chondroitin sulfate, and glucosamine. (See discussion of NSAID toxicity in the section on treatment of rheumatoid arthritis.) High doses of NSAIDs, as used in more inflammatory arthritides, are unnecessary.

For many patients, it is possible eventually to reduce the dosage or limit use of drugs to periods of exacerbation. For patients with knee osteoarthritis and effusion, intra-articular injection of triamcinolone (20-40 mg) may obviate the need for analgesics or NSAIDs. Corticosteroid injections up to four times a year appear to be safe. Intra-articular injections of sodium hyaluronate reduce symptoms moderately in some patients. Capsaicin cream 0.025% applied twice daily can also reduce knee pain without NSAIDs. Doxycycline, though not FDA approved for treating osteoarthritis, has shown promise in reducing the progression of knee osteoarthritis.

C. SURGICAL MEASURES

Total hip replacement provides excellent symptomatic and functional improvement when that joint is seriously afflicted, as indicated by severely restricted walking and pain at rest, particularly at night. Knee replacement is also effective. Arthroscopic surgery for knee osteoarthritis is ineffective. Experimental techniques to repair focal cartilage loss in the knee by autologous chondrocyte transplantation are promising. However, the indications for and limitations of this procedure require further definition.

Prognosis

Marked disability is less common in patients with osteoarthritis than in those with rheumatoid arthritis, but symptoms may be quite severe and limit activity

considerably (especially with involvement of the hips, knees, and cervical spine).

Bjordal JM et al: Non-steroidal anti-inflammatory drugs, including cyclo-oxygenase-2 inhibitors in osteoarthritis knee pain: meta-analysis of randomised placebo controlled trials. BMJ 2004;329:1317. [PMID: 15561731]

Brandt KD et al: Effects of doxycycline on progression of osteoarthritis: results of a randomized, placebo-controlled, double-blind trial. Arthritis Rheum 2005;52:2015. [PMID: 15986343]

Felson DT: Clinical practice. Osteoarthritis of the knee. N Engl J Med 2006;354:841. [PMID: 16495396]

Fransen M: Dietary weight loss and exercise for obese adults with knee osteoarthritis: modest weight loss targets, mild exercise, modest effects. Arthritis Rheum 2004;50:1366. [PMID: 15146405]

Schumacher HR et al: Injectable corticosteroids in treatment of arthritis of the knee. Am J Med 2005;118:1208. [PMID: 16271901]

Witt C et al: Acupuncture in patients with osteoarthritis of the knee: a randomised trial. Lancet 2005;366:136. [PMID: 16005336]

CRYSTAL DEPOSITION ARTHRITIS

1. Gouty Arthritis

 ESSENTIALS OF DIAGNOSIS

- Acute onset, typically nocturnal and usually monarticular, often involving the first MTP joint.
- Polyarticular involvement more common in patients with longstanding disease.
- Identification of urate crystals in joint fluid or tophi is diagnostic.
- Dramatic therapeutic response to NSAIDs.
- With chronicity, urate deposits in subcutaneous tissue, bone, cartilage, joints, and other tissues.

General Considerations

Gout is a metabolic disease of heterogeneous nature, often familial, associated with abnormal amounts of urates in the body and characterized early by a recurring acute arthritis, usually monarticular, and later by chronic deforming arthritis. The associated hyperuricemia is due to overproduction or underexcretion of uric acid—sometimes both. The disease is especially common in Pacific islanders, eg, Filipinos and Samoans. It is rarely caused by a specifically determined genetic aberration (eg, Lesch-Nyhan syndrome). Secondary gout, which may have a heritable component, is related to acquired causes of hyperuricemia, eg, medication use (especially diuretics, cyclosporine, low-dose aspirin, and niacin), myeloproliferative disorders, multiple myeloma, hemoglobinopathies, chronic renal disease, hypothyroidism, psoriasis, sarcoidosis, and lead poisoning (Table 20-4). Alcohol ingestion promotes hyperuricemia by in-

Table 20–4. Origin of hyperuricemia.

Primary hyperuricemia
  A. Increased production of purine
    1. Idiopathic
    2. Specific enzyme defects (eg, Lesch-Nyhan syndrome, glycogen storage diseases)
  B. Decreased renal clearance of uric acid (idiopathic)
Secondary hyperuricemia
  A. Increased catabolism and turnover of purine
    1. Myeloproliferative disorders
    2. Lymphoproliferative disorders
    3. Carcinoma and sarcoma (disseminated)
    4. Chronic hemolytic anemias
    5. Cytotoxic drugs
    6. Psoriasis
  B. Decreased renal clearance of uric acid
    1. Intrinsic kidney disease
    2. Functional impairment of tubular transport
      a. Drug-induced (eg, thiazides, probenecid)
      b. Hyperlacticacidemia (eg, lactic acidosis, alcoholism)
      c. Hyperketoacidemia (eg, diabetic ketoacidosis, starvation)
      d. Diabetes insipidus (vasopressin-resistant)
      e. Bartter's syndrome

Modified from Rodnan GP: Gout and other crystalline forms of arthritis. Postgrad Med (Oct) 1975;58:6.

creasing urate production and decreasing the renal excretion of uric acid. Finally, hospitalized patients frequently suffer attacks of gout because of changes in diet, fluid intake, or medications that lead either to rapid reductions or increases in the serum urate level.

About 90% of patients with primary gout are men, usually over 30 years of age. In women, the onset is typically postmenopausal. The characteristic lesion is the tophus, a nodular deposit of monosodium urate monohydrate crystals, with an associated foreign body reaction. These are found in cartilage, subcutaneous and periarticular tissues, tendon, bone, the kidneys, and elsewhere. Urates have been demonstrated in the synovial tissues (and fluid) during acute arthritis; indeed, the acute inflammation of gout is believed to be activated by the phagocytosis by polymorphonuclear cells of urate crystals with the ensuing release from the neutrophils of chemotactic and other substances capable of mediating inflammation. The precise relationship of hyperuricemia to gouty arthritis is still obscure, since chronic hyperuricemia is found in people who never develop gout or uric acid stones. Rapid fluctuations in serum urate levels, either increasing or decreasing, are important factors in precipitating acute gout. The mechanism of the late, chronic stage of gouty arthritis is better understood. This is characterized pathologically by tophaceous in-

vasion of the articular and periarticular tissues, with structural derangement and secondary degeneration (osteoarthritis).

Uric acid kidney stones are present in 5–10% of patients with gouty arthritis. Hyperuricemia correlates highly with the likelihood of developing stones, with the risk of stone formation reaching 50% in patients with a serum urate level above 13 mg/dL. Chronic urate nephropathy is caused by the deposition of monosodium urate crystals in the renal medulla and pyramids. Although progressive renal failure occurs in a substantial percentage of patients with chronic gout, the role of hyperuricemia in causing this outcome is controversial, because many patients with gout have numerous confounding risk factors for renal failure (eg, hypertension, alcohol use, lead exposure, and other risk factors for vascular disease).

Unless there is a rapid breakdown of cellular nucleic acid following aggressive treatment of leukemia or lymphoma, uric acid-lowering drugs need not be instituted until arthritis, renal calculi, or tophi become apparent. Asymptomatic hyperuricemia should not be treated.

Clinical Findings

A. SYMPTOMS AND SIGNS

The acute arthritis is characterized by its sudden onset, frequently nocturnal, either without apparent precipitating cause or following rapid fluctuations in serum urate levels. Either increases or decreases in the serum urate level can precipitate a gout attack. Common precipitants are alcohol excess (particularly beer), changes in medications that affect urate metabolism, and in the hospitalized patient fasting before medical procedures. The MTP joint of the great toe is the most susceptible joint ("podagra"), although others, especially those of the feet, ankles, and knees, are commonly affected. Gouty attacks may develop in periarticular soft tissues such as the arch of the foot. Hips and shoulders are rarely affected. More than one joint may occasionally be affected during the same attack; in such cases, the distribution of the arthritis is usually asymmetric. As the attack progresses, the pain becomes intense. The involved joints are swollen and exquisitely tender and the overlying skin tense, warm, and dusky red. Fever is common and may reach 39 °C. Local desquamation and pruritus during recovery from the acute arthritis are characteristic of gout but are not always present. Tophi may be found in the external ears, hands, feet, olecranon, and prepatellar bursas. They usually develop years after the initial attack of gout.

Asymptomatic periods of months or years commonly follow the initial acute attack. After years of recurrent severe monarthritis attacks of the lower extremities and untreated hyperuricemia, gout can evolve into a chronic, deforming polyarthritis of upper and lower extremities that mimics rheumatoid arthritis.

B. Laboratory Findings

The serum uric acid is elevated (> 7.5 mg/dL) in 95% of patients who have serial measurements during the course of an attack. However, a single uric acid determination is normal in up to 25% of cases, so it does not exclude gout, especially in patients taking uricopenic drugs. During an acute attack, the ESR and white cell count are frequently elevated. Material aspirated from a tophus shows the typical crystals of sodium urate and confirms the diagnosis. Further confirmation is obtained by identification of sodium urate crystals by compensated polariscopic examination of wet smears prepared from joint fluid aspirates. Such crystals are negatively birefringent and needle-like and may be found free or in neutrophils.

C. Imaging

Early in the disease, radiographs show no changes. Later, punched-out erosions with an overhanging rim of cortical bone ("rat bite") develop. When these are adjacent to a soft tissue tophus, they are diagnostic of gout.

Differential Diagnosis

Acute gout is often confused with cellulitis. Bacteriologic studies usually exclude acute pyogenic arthritis. Pseudogout is distinguished by the identification of calcium pyrophosphate crystals (strong positive birefringence) in the joint fluid, usually normal serum uric acid, the x-ray appearance of chondrocalcinosis, and the relative therapeutic ineffectiveness of colchicine.

Chronic tophaceous arthritis may resemble chronic rheumatoid arthritis; gout is suggested by an earlier history of monarthritis and is established by the demonstration of urate crystals in a suspected tophus. Likewise, hips and shoulders are generally spared in tophaceous gout. Biopsy may be necessary to distinguish tophi from rheumatoid nodules. An x-ray appearance similar to that of gout may be found in rheumatoid arthritis, sarcoidosis, multiple myeloma, hyperparathyroidism, or Hand-Schüller-Christian disease. Chronic lead intoxication may result in attacks of gouty arthritis (saturnine gout); abdominal pain, peripheral neuropathy, renal insufficiency, and basophilic stippling of red cells are clues to the diagnosis.

Treatment

A. Acute Attack

Arthritis is treated first and hyperuricemia weeks or months later, if at all. Sudden reduction of serum uric acid often precipitates further episodes of gouty arthritis.

1. NSAIDs—These drugs (see Table 5–5) are the treatment of choice for acute gout. Traditionally, indomethacin has been the most frequently used agent, but all of the other newer NSAIDs are probably equally effective. Indomethacin is initiated at a dosage of 25–50 mg orally every 8 hours and continued until the symptoms have resolved (usually 5–10 days). Active peptic ulcer disease, impaired renal function, and a history of allergic reaction to NSAIDs are contraindications. For patients at high risk for upper gastrointestinal bleeding, a cyclooxygenase type 2 (COX-2) inhibitor may be an appropriate first choice for management of an acute gout attack. Long-term use of COX-2 inhibitors is not advised because of the association with increased risk of cardiovascular events, which has led to the removal of some drugs from the US market (eg, rofecoxib and valdecoxib).

2. Colchicine—Colchicine is no longer recommended for the treatment of acute gout flares. Its use during the intercritical period to prevent gout attacks is discussed below.

3. Corticosteroids—Corticosteroids often give dramatic symptomatic relief in acute episodes of gout and will control most attacks. They are most useful in patients with contraindications to the use of NSAIDs. If the patient's gout is monarticular, intra-articular administration (eg, triamcinolone, 10–40 mg depending on the size of the joint) is most effective. For polyarticular gout, corticosteroids may be given intravenously (eg, methylprednisolone, 40 mg/d tapered over 7 days) or orally (eg, prednisone, 40–60 mg/d tapered over 7 days). Gouty and septic arthritis can coexist, albeit rarely. Therefore, joint aspiration and Gram stain with culture of synovial fluid should be performed before corticosteroids are given.

B. Management Between Attacks

Treatment during symptom-free periods is intended to minimize urate deposition in tissues, which causes chronic tophaceous arthritis, and to reduce the frequency and severity of recurrences.

1. Diet—Potentially reversible causes of hyperuricemia are a high-purine diet, obesity, alcohol consumption, and use of certain medications (see below). Beer consumption appears to confer a higher risk of gout than does whiskey or wine. Higher levels of meat and seafood consumption are associated with increased risks of gout, whereas a higher level of dairy products consumption is associated with a decreased risk. Although dietary purines usually contribute only 1 mg/dL to the serum uric acid level, moderation in eating foods with high purine content is advisable (Table 20–5). A high liquid intake and, more importantly, a daily urinary output of 2 L or more will aid urate excretion and minimize urate precipitation in the urinary tract.

2. Avoidance of hyperuricemic medications—Thiazide and loop diuretics inhibit renal excretion of uric acid and should be avoided in patients with gout. Similarly, low doses of aspirin (< 3 g daily) aggravate hyperuricemia, as does niacin.

3. Colchicine—Patients with a single episode of gout who are willing to lose weight and stop drinking alcohol are at low risk for another attack and unlikely to benefit from chronic medical therapy. In contrast, older individ-

Table 20–5. The purine content of foods.[1]

Low-purine foods

Refined cereals and cereal products, cornflakes, white bread, pasta, flour, arrowroot, sago, tapioca, cakes

Milk, milk products, and eggs

Sugar, sweets, and gelatin

Butter, polyunsaturated margarine, and all other fats

Fruit, nuts, and peanut butter

Lettuce, tomatoes, and green vegetables (except those listed below)

Cream soups made with low-purine vegetables but without meat or meat stock

Water, fruit juice, cordials, and carbonated drinks

High-purine foods

All meats, including organ meats, and seafood

Meat extracts and gravies

Yeast and yeast extracts, beer, and other alcoholic beverages

Beans, peas, lentils, oatmeal, spinach, asparagus, cauliflower, and mushrooms

[1]The purine content of a food reflects its nucleoprotein content and turnover. Foods containing many nuclei (eg, liver) have many purines, as do rapidly growing foods such as asparagus. The consumption of large amounts of a food containing a small concentration of purines may provide a greater purine load than consumption of a small amount of a food containing a large concentration of purines.

Reproduced, with permission, from Emmerson BT: The management of gout. N Engl J Med 1996;334:445.

uals with mild chronic renal failure who require diuretic use and have a history of multiple attacks of gout are more likely to benefit from pharmacologic treatment. In general, the higher the uric acid level and the more frequent the attacks, the more likely that chronic medical therapy will be beneficial.

There are two indications for daily colchicine administration. First, colchicine can be used to prevent future attacks. For the person who has mild hyperuricemia and occasional attacks of gouty arthritis, chronic colchicine prophylaxis may be all that is needed. The usual dose is 0.6 mg either once or twice a day. Patients who have coexisting moderate renal insufficiency or heart failure should take colchicine only once a day in order to avoid the peripheral neuromyopathy that can complicate the use of higher doses. Second, colchicine can also be used when uricosuric drugs or allopurinol (see below) are started, to suppress attacks precipitated by abrupt changes in the serum uric acid level.

4. Reduction of serum uric acid—Indications for a urate lowering intervention include frequent acute arthritis not controlled by colchicine prophylaxis, tophaceous deposits, or renal damage. Hyperuricemia with infrequent attacks of arthritis may not require treatment; asymptomatic hyperuricemia should not be treated. If instituted, the goal of medical treatment is to maintain the serum uric acid at or below 5 mg/dL, which should prevent crystallization of urate.

Two classes of agents may be used to lower the serum uric acid—the uricosuric drugs and allopurinol (neither is of value in the treatment of acute gout). The choice of one or the other depends on the result of a 24-hour urine uric acid determination. A value under 800 mg/d indicates undersecretion of uric acid, which is amenable to uricosuric agents if renal function is preserved. Patients with more than 800 mg of uric acid in a 24-hour urine collection are overproducers and require allopurinol.

a. Uricosuric drugs—These drugs, which block the tubular reabsorption of filtered urate thereby reducing the metabolic urate pool, prevent the formation of new tophi and reduce the size of those already present. When administered concomitantly with colchicine, they may lessen the frequency of recurrences of acute gout. The indication for uricosuric treatment is the increasing frequency or severity of acute attacks. Uricosuric agents are ineffective in patients with renal insufficiency, with a serum creatinine of more than 2 mg/dL.

The following uricosuric drugs may be used: (1) Probenecid, 0.5 g orally daily initially, with gradual increase to 1–2 g daily; or (2) sulfinpyrazone, 50–100 mg orally twice daily initially, with gradual increase to 200–400 mg twice daily. Hypersensitivity to either with fever and rash occurs in 5% of cases; gastrointestinal complaints are observed in 10%. Probenecid also inhibits the excretion of penicillin, indomethacin, dapsone, and acetazolamide.

Precautions with uricosuric drugs. It is important to maintain a daily urinary output of 2000 mL or more in order to minimize the precipitation of uric acid in the urinary tract. This can be further prevented by giving alkalinizing agents (eg, potassium citrate, 30–80 mEq/d orally) to maintain a urine pH of above 6.0. Uricosuric drugs are avoided in patients with a history of uric acid nephrolithiasis. Aspirin in moderate doses antagonizes the action of uricosuric agents, but low doses (325 mg or less per day) do not; doses greater than 3 g daily are themselves uricosuric.

b. Allopurinol—The xanthine oxidase inhibitor allopurinol promptly lowers plasma urate and urinary uric acid concentrations and facilitates tophus mobilization. The drug is of special value in uric acid overproducers; in tophaceous gout; in patients unresponsive to the uricosuric regimen; and in gouty patients with uric acid renal stones. It should be used in low doses in patients with renal insufficiency and is not indicated in asymptomatic hyperuricemia. The most frequent adverse effect is the precipitation of an acute gouty attack. However, the most common sign of hypersensitivity to allopurinol (occurring in 2% of cases) is a pruritic rash that may progress to toxic epidermal necrolysis. Vasculitis and hepatitis are other rare complications.

The initial daily dose of allopurinol is 300 mg/d for patients who have normal renal function and who are taking prophylactic colchicine. In the absence of prophylactic colchicine, the initial dose should be 100 mg/d orally. The dose of allopurinol can be increased in a week if needed to achieve the desired serum uric acid level of ≤ 5.0 mg/dL. Successful treatment usually requires a dose of 300–400 mg of allopurinol daily. The maximum daily dose is 800 mg. Allopurinol can be used in renal disease, but the dose must be reduced to decrease the chance of side effects.

Allopurinol interacts with other drugs. The combined use of allopurinol and ampicillin causes a drug rash in 20% of patients. Allopurinol can increase the half-life of probenecid, while probenecid increases the excretion of allopurinol. Thus, a patient taking both drugs may need to use slightly higher than usual doses of allopurinol and lower doses of probenecid. Allopurinol potentiates the effect of azathioprine. If allopurinol cannot be avoided, the dose of azathioprine should be reduced by 75% before allopurinol is started.

Febuxostat, a new xanthine oxidase inhibitor, is being evaluated in phase three trials. Patients who have had hypersensitivity reactions to allopurinol, the only xanthine oxidase inhibitor now on the market, appear to tolerate febuxostat.

C. CHRONIC TOPHACEOUS ARTHRITIS

With rigorous medical compliance, allopurinol shrinks tophi and in time can lead to their disappearance. Resorption of extensive tophi requires maintaining a serum uric acid below 5 mg/dL, which may be achievable only with concomitant use of allopurinol and a uricosuric agent. Surgical excision of large tophi offers mechanical improvement in selected deformities.

D. GOUT IN THE TRANSPLANT PATIENT

Hyperuricemia and gout commonly develop in many transplant patients because they have decreased renal function and require drugs that inhibit uric acid excretion (especially cyclosporine and diuretics). Treating these patients is challenging: NSAIDs are usually contraindicated because of renal impairment; intravenous colchicine is generally avoided for acute gout because of its narrow therapeutic index (particularly in renal dysfunction); and corticosteroids are already being used. Often the best approach for monarticular gout—after excluding infection—is injecting corticosteroids into the joint (see above). For polyarticular gout, increasing the dose of systemic corticosteroid may be the only alternative. Since transplant patients often have multiple attacks of gout, long-term relief requires lowering the serum uric acid with allopurinol. (Renal impairment seen in many transplant patients makes uricosuric agents ineffective.) Allopurinol doses should be lowered in patients with renal dysfunction and adjusted according to their effect on the serum uric acid level.

Prognosis

Without treatment, the acute attack may last from a few days to several weeks. The intervals between acute at-

tacks vary up to years, but the asymptomatic periods often become shorter if the disease progresses. Chronic gouty arthritis occurs after repeated attacks of acute gout, but only after inadequate treatment. The younger the patient at the onset of disease, the greater the tendency to a progressive course. Destructive arthropathy is rarely seen in patients whose first attack is after age 50.

Patients with gout are anecdotally thought to have an increased incidence of hypertension, renal disease (eg, nephrosclerosis, interstitial nephritis, pyelonephritis), diabetes mellitus, hypertriglyceridemia, and atherosclerosis.

Becker MA et al: Febuxostat compared with allopurinol in patients with hyperuricemia and gout. N Engl J Med 2005; 353:2450. [PMID: 16339094]

Choi HK et al: Alcohol intake and risk of incident gout in men: a prospective study. Lancet 2004;363:1277. [PMID: 15094272]

Choi HK et al: Pathogenesis of gout. Ann Intern Med 2005;143: 499. [PMID: 16204163]

Terkeltaub RA: Clinical practice. Gout. N Engl J Med 2003;349: 1647. [PMID: 14573737]

2. Chondrocalcinosis & Pseudogout

Chondrocalcinosis is the presence of calcium-containing salts in articular cartilage. Diagnosed radiologically, it may be familial and is commonly associated with a wide variety of metabolic disorders, eg, hemochromatosis, hyperparathyroidism, ochronosis, diabetes mellitus, hypothyroidism, Wilson's disease, and gout. Pseudogout (also called calcium pyrophosphate dihydrate [CPPD] deposition disease) is most often seen in persons age 60 or older, is characterized by acute, recurrent and rarely chronic arthritis involving large joints (most commonly the knees and the wrists) and is almost always accompanied by chondrocalcinosis of the affected joints. Other joints frequently affected are the MCPs, hips, shoulders, elbows, and ankles. Involvement of the DIP and PIP joints is no more common in CPPD deposition disease than in other age-matched controls. Pseudogout, like gout, frequently develops 24–48 hours after major surgery. Identification of calcium pyrophosphate crystals in joint aspirates is diagnostic of pseudogout. With light microscopy, the rhomboid-shaped crystals differ from the needle-shaped gout crystals. A red compensator is used for positive identification, since pseudogout crystals are blue when parallel and yellow when perpendicular to the axis of the compensator. Urate crystals give the opposite pattern. X-ray examination shows not only calcification (usually symmetric) of cartilaginous structures but also signs of degenerative joint disease (osteoarthritis). Unlike gout, pseudogout is usually associated with normal serum urate levels and is not dramatically improved by colchicine.

Treatment of chondrocalcinosis is directed at the primary disease, if present. Some of the NSAIDs (salicylates, indomethacin, naproxen, and other drugs) are helpful in the treatment of acute episodes. Patients at increased risk for upper gastrointestinal bleeding may use a COX-2 inhibitor to treat acute attacks of pseudogout. Long-term use of COX-2 inhibitors is not advised because of the association with increased risk of cardiovascular events, which has led to the removal of some drugs from the US market (eg, rofecoxib and valdecoxib). Colchicine, 0.6 mg orally twice daily, is more effective for prophylaxis than for acute attacks. Aspiration of the inflamed joint and intra-articular injection of triamcinolone, 10–40 mg, depending on the size of the joint, are also of value in resistant cases.

Wise CM: Crystal-associated arthritis in the elderly. Clin Geriatr Med 2005;21:491. [PMID: 15911203]

■ PAIN SYNDROMES

NECK PAIN

ESSENTIALS OF DIAGNOSIS

- *Most chronic neck pain is caused by degenerative joint disease and responds to conservative approaches.*
- *Whiplash, the most common type of traumatic injury to the neck, responds to early mobilization.*
- *Serious erosive disease of joints in the neck that may lead to neurologic complications sometimes occurs in rheumatoid arthritis and occasionally in ankylosing spondylitis; the usual joint involved in these disorders is the atlantoaxial joint (C1–2).*

General Considerations

At any point in time, about 15% of adults are experiencing neck pain. The prevalence of neck pain peaks at age 50 and develops more commonly in women than in men. A large group of articular and extra-articular disorders are characterized by pain that may involve simultaneously the neck, shoulder girdle, and upper extremity. Diagnostic differentiation may be difficult. Some represent primary disorders of the cervicobrachial region; others are local manifestations of systemic disease. It is frequently not possible to make a specific diagnosis.

Clinical Findings

A. SYMPTOMS AND SIGNS

Neck pain may be limited to the posterior region or, depending on the level of the symptomatic joint, may radiate segmentally to the occiput, anterior chest, shoulder girdle, arm, forearm, and hand. It may be intensified by active or passive neck motions. The general distribution of pain and paresthesias corresponds roughly to the involved dermatome in the upper extremity. Radiating pain in the upper extremity is often intensified by hyperextension of the neck and deviation of the head to the involved side. Limitation of cervical movements is the most common objective finding. Neurologic signs depend on the extent of compression of nerve roots or the spinal cord. Compression of the spinal cord may cause paraparesis or paraplegia.

B. IMAGING

The radiographic findings depend on the cause of the pain; many plain radiographs are completely normal in patients who have suffered an acute cervical strain. Loss of cervical lordosis is often seen but is nonspecific. In osteoarthritis, comparative reduction in height of the involved disk space is a frequent finding. The most common late radiographic finding is osteophyte formation anteriorly, adjacent to the disk; other chronic abnormalities occur around the apophysial joint clefts, chiefly in the lower cervical spine.

Use of advanced imaging techniques is indicated in the patient who has severe pain of unknown cause that fails to respond to conservative therapy or in the patient who has evidence of myelopathy. MRI is more sensitive than CT in detecting disk disease, extradural compression, and intramedullary cord disease. CT is preferable for demonstration of fractures.

Differential Diagnosis & Treatment

The causes of neck pain include acute and chronic cervical strain or sprains, herniated nucleus pulposus, osteoarthritis, ankylosing spondylitis, rheumatoid arthritis, fibromyalgia, osteomyelitis, neoplasms, polymyalgia rheumatica, compression fractures, and functional disorders.

A. NONSPECIFIC NECK PAIN

In the absence of trauma or evidence of infection, malignancy, neurologic findings, or systemic inflammation, the patient can be treated conservatively. Conservative therapy can include rest, analgesics, or physical therapy.

B. ACUTE CERVICAL MUSCULOTENDINOUS STRAIN

Cervical strain is generally caused by mechanical postural disorders, overexertion, or injury (eg, whiplash). Acute episodes are associated with pain, decreased cervical spine motion, and paraspinal muscle spasm, resulting in stiffness of the neck and loss of motion. Muscle trigger points can often be localized. After whiplash injury, patients often experience not only neck pain but also shoulder girdle discomfort and headache. Management includes administration of analgesics. Soft cervical collars are commonly recommended, but evidence suggests they may delay recovery. Acupuncture, manipulation, or physical therapy can help some patients, but the precise role of these treatments is not well established. Corticosteroid injection into cervical facet joints is ineffective. Gradual return to full activity is encouraged.

C. HERNIATED NUCLEUS PULPOSUS

Rupture or prolapse of the nucleus pulposus of the cervical disks into the spinal canal causes pain radiating at a C6–7 level. When intra-abdominal pressure is increased by coughing, sneezing, or other movements, symptoms are aggravated, and cervical muscle spasm may occur. Neurologic abnormalities include decreased reflexes of the deep tendons of the biceps and triceps and decreased sensation and muscle atrophy or weakness in the forearm or hand. Cervical traction, bed rest, and other conservative measures are usually successful. Radicular symptoms usually respond to conservative therapy, including NSAIDs, activity modification, intermittent cervical traction, and neck immobilization. Cervical epidural corticosteroid injections may help those who fail conservative therapy. Surgery is indicated for unremitting pain and progressive weakness despite a full trial of conservative therapy and if a surgically correctable abnormality is identified by MRI or CT myelography. Surgical decompression achieves excellent results in 70–80% of such patients.

D. ARTHRITIC DISORDERS

Cervical spondylosis (degenerative arthritis) is a collective term describing degenerative changes that occur in the apophysial joints and intervertebral disk joints, with or without neurologic signs. Osteoarthritis of the articular facets is characterized by progressive thinning of the cartilage, subchondral osteoporosis, and osteophytic proliferation around the joint margins. Degeneration of cervical disks and joints may occur in adolescents but is more common after age 40. Degeneration is progressive and is marked by gradual narrowing of the disk space, as demonstrated by x-ray. Osteocartilaginous proliferation occurs around the margin of the vertebral body and gives rise to osteophytic ridges that may encroach upon the intervertebral foramina and spinal canal, causing compression of the neurovascular contents.

Osteoarthritis of the cervical spine is often asymptomatic but may cause diffuse neck pain. A minority of patients with neck pain also suffer from radicular pain or myelopathy. Myelopathy develops insidiously and is manifested by sensory dysfunction and clumsy hands. Some patients also complain of unsteady walking, urinary frequency and urgency, or electrical shock sensations with neck flexion or extension (Lhermitte's sign). Weakness, sensory loss, and spasticity with exaggerated reflexes develop below the level of spinal cord compression. Amyotrophic lateral sclerosis, multiple sclerosis, syringomyelia, spinal cord tumors, and tropical spastic paresis from HTLV-1 infection can mimic myelopathy from cervical arthritis. The mainstay of conservative therapy is immobilizing the cervical spine

with a collar. With moderate to severe neurologic symptoms, surgical treatment is indicated.

Atlantoaxial subluxation may occur in patients with either rheumatoid arthritis or ankylosing spondylitis. Inflammation of the synovial structures resulting from erosion and laxity of the transverse ligament can lead to neurologic signs of spinal cord compression. Treatment may vary from use of a cervical collar or more rigid bracing to operative treatment, depending on the degree of subluxation and neurologic progression. Surgical treatment for stabilization of the cervical spine is a last resort.

E. OTHER DISORDERS

Osteomyelitis and neoplasms are discussed below. Osteoporosis is discussed in Chapter 26.

Hendriks EJ et al: Prognostic factors for poor recovery in acute whiplash patients. Pain 2005;114:408. [PMID: 15777866]

Hoving JL et al: Manual therapy, physical therapy, or continued care by a general practitioner for patients with neck pain. A randomized, controlled trial. Ann Intern Med 2002;136: 713. [PMID: 12020139]

White P et al: Acupuncture versus placebo for the treatment of chronic mechanical neck pain: a randomized, controlled trial. Ann Intern Med 2004;141:911. [PMID: 15611488]

THORACIC OUTLET SYNDROMES

Thoracic outlet syndromes result from compression of the neurovascular structures supplying the upper extremity. Symptoms and signs arise from intermittent or continuous pressure on elements of the brachial plexus and the subclavian or axillary vessels (veins or arteries) by a variety of anatomic structures of the shoulder girdle region. The neurovascular bundle can be compressed between the anterior or middle scalene muscles and a normal first thoracic rib or a cervical rib. Most commonly thoracic outlet obstruction is caused by sagging of the shoulder girdle resulting from aging, obesity, or pendulous breasts. Faulty posture, occupation, or thoracic muscle hypertrophy from physical activity (eg, weight-lifting, baseball pitching) may be other predisposing factors.

Thoracic outlet obstruction presents in most patients with some combination of four symptoms involving the upper extremity, namely pain, numbness, weakness, and swelling. The predominant symptoms depend on whether the obstruction chiefly affects neural or vascular structures. The onset of symptoms is usually gradual but can be sudden. Some patients spontaneously notice aggravation of symptoms with specific positioning of the arm. Pain radiates from the point of compression to the base of the neck, the axilla, the shoulder girdle region, arm, forearm, and hand. Paresthesias are common and distributed to the volar aspect of the fourth and fifth digits. Sensory symptoms may be aggravated at night or by prolonged use of the extremities. Weakness and muscle atrophy are the principal motor abnormalities. Vascular symptoms consist of arterial ischemia characterized by pallor of the fingers on elevation of the extremity, sensitivity to cold, and, rarely, gangrene of the digits or venous obstruction marked by edema, cyanosis, and engorgement.

Reflexes are usually not altered. When the site of compression is between the upper rib and clavicle, partial obliteration of subclavian artery pulsation may be demonstrated by abduction of the arm to a right angle with the elbow simultaneously flexed and rotated externally at the shoulder so that the entire extremity lies in the coronal plane. Neck or arm position has no effect on the diminished pulse, which remains constant in the subclavian steal syndrome.

Chest radiography will identify patients with cervical rib (although most patients with cervical ribs are asymptomatic). MRI with the arms held in different positions is useful in identifying sites of impaired blood flow. Intra-arterial or venous obstruction is confirmed by angiography. Determination of conduction velocities of the ulnar and other peripheral nerves of the upper extremity may help localize the site of their compression.

Thoracic outlet syndrome must be differentiated from osteoarthritis of the cervical spine, tumors of the superior pulmonary sulcus, cervical spinal cord, or nerve roots, and periarthritis of the shoulder.

Treatment is directed toward relief of compression of the neurovascular bundle. Greater than 95% of patients can be treated successfully with conservative therapy consisting of physical therapy and avoiding postures or activities that compress the neurovascular bundle. Some women will benefit from a support bra. Operative treatment, required by less than 5% of patients, is more likely to relieve the neurologic rather than the vascular component that causes symptoms.

Brantigan CO et al: Diagnosing thoracic outlet syndrome. Hand Clin 2004;20:27. [PMID: 15005381]

Divi V et al: Thoracic outlet decompression for subclavian vein thrombosis: experience in 71 patients. Arch Surg 2005;140: 54. [PMID: 15655206]

LOW BACK PAIN

Low back pain is experienced at some time by up to 80% of the population. The differential diagnosis is broad and includes muscular strain, primary spine disease (eg, disk herniation, degenerative arthritis), systemic diseases (eg, metastatic cancer), and regional diseases (eg, aortic aneurysm). A precise diagnosis cannot be made in the majority of cases. Even when anatomic defects—such as vertebral osteophytes or a narrowed disk space—are present, clinical disease cannot be assumed since such defects are common in asymptomatic patients. The majority of patients will improve in 1–4 weeks and need no evaluation beyond the initial history and physical examination. The diagnostic challenge is to identify those patients who require more extensive or urgent evaluation.

In practice, this means identifying those patients with pain caused by (1) infection, (2) cancer, (3) in-flammatory back disease such as ankylosing spondylitis, (4) or nonrheumatologic conditions, especially expanding aortic aneurysm. Significant or progressive neurologic deficits also require identification. If there is no evidence of these problems, conservative therapy is called for.

1. Clinical Approach to Diagnosis

General History & Physical Examination

Low back pain is a final common pathway of many processes; the pain of vertebral osteomyelitis, for example, is not very different in quality and intensity from that due to back strain of the weekend gardener. Historical factors of importance include smoking, weight loss, age over 50, and cancer, all of which are risk factors for vertebral body metastasis. Osteomyelitis most frequently occurs in adults with a history of recurrent urinary tract infections and is especially common in diabetics.

Previous peptic ulcer disease suggests that a patient's back pain is due to a penetrating ulcer. A history of a cardiac murmur should raise concern about endocarditis, since back pain is a not uncommon manifestation. A background of renal stones might indicate another cause of referred back pain.

History of the Back Pain

Certain qualities of a patient's pain can indicate a specific diagnosis. Low back pain radiating down the buttock and below the knee suggests a herniated disk causing nerve root irritation. Other conditions—including sacroiliitis, facet joint degenerative arthritis, spinal stenosis, or irritation of the sciatic nerve from a wallet—also cause this pattern.

The diagnosis of disk herniation is further suggested by physical examination (see below) and confirmed by imaging techniques. Disk herniation can be asymptomatic, so its presence does not invariably link it to the symptom.

Low back pain at night, unrelieved by rest or the supine position, suggests the possibility of malignancy, either vertebral body metastasis (chiefly from prostate, breast, lung, multiple myeloma, or lymphoma) or a cauda equina tumor. Similar pain can also be caused by compression fractures (from osteoporosis or myeloma).

Symptoms of large or rapidly evolving neurologic deficits identify patients who need urgent evaluation for possible cauda equina tumor, epidural abscess or, rarely, massive disk herniation. Even with a herniated disk and nerve root impingement, pain is the most prominent symptom; numbness and weakness are less commonly reported and when present are of the magnitude consistent with compression of a single nerve root. Thus, symptoms of bilateral leg weakness (from multiple lumbar nerve root compressions) or of saddle area anesthesia, bowel or bladder incontinence, or impotence (indicating multiple sacral nerve root compressions) indicate a cauda equina process.

Low back pain that worsens with rest and improves with activity is characteristic of ankylosing spondylitis or other seronegative spondyloarthropathies, especially when the onset is insidious and begins before age 40. Most degenerative back diseases produce precisely the opposite pattern, with rest alleviating and activity aggravating the pain. Low back pain causing the patient to writhe occurs in renal colic but can also indicate a leaking aneurysm. The pain associated with pseudoclaudication from lumbar spinal stenosis is discussed below.

Physical Examination of the Back

Several physical findings should be sought because they help identify those few patients who need more than conservative management.

Neurologic examination of the lower extremities will detect the small deficits produced by disk disease and the large deficits complicating such problems as cauda equina tumors. A positive straight leg raising test indicates nerve root irritation. The examiner performs the test on the supine patient by passively raising the patient's ipsilateral leg. The test is positive if radicular pain is produced with the leg raised 60 degrees or less. It has a specificity of 40% but is 95% sensitive in patients with herniation at the L4–5 or L5–S1 level (the sites of 95% of disk herniations). It can be falsely negative, especially in patients with herniation above the L4–5 level. The crossed straight leg sign is positive when raising the contralateral leg reproduces the sciatica. It has a sensitivity of 25% but is 90% specific for disk herniation.

Detailed examination of the sacral and lumbar nerve roots, especially L5 and S1, is essential for detecting neurologic deficits associated with back pain. Disk herniation produces deficits predictable for the site involved (Table 20–6). Deficits of multiple nerve roots suggest a cauda equina tumor or an epidural abscess, both requiring urgent evaluation and treatment.

Measurement of spinal motion in the patient with acute pain is rarely of diagnostic utility and usually simply confirms that pain limits motion. An exception is the decreased range of motion in multiple regions of the spine (cervical, thoracic, and lumbar) in a diffuse spinal disease such as ankylosing spondylitis. By the time the patient has such limits, however, the diagnosis is usually straightforward.

If back pain is not severe and does not itself limit motion, Schober's test of lumbar motion is helpful in early diagnosis of ankylosing spondylitis. To perform this test, two marks are made, one 10 cm above S1 and another 5 cm below. The patient then bends forward as far as possible, and the distance between the points is measured. Normally, the distance increases at least 5 cm. Anything less indicates reduced lumbar motion, which in the absence of severe pain is most commonly due to ankylosing spondylitis or other seronegative spondyloarthropathies.

Palpation of the spine usually does not yield diagnostic information. Point tenderness over a vertebral body is reported to suggest osteomyelitis, but this association is uncommon. A step-off noted between the spinous process of adjacent vertebral bodies may indicate spondylolisthesis, but the sensitivity of this finding is extremely low. Tenderness of the soft tissues overlying the greater trochanter of the hip is a manifestation of trochanteric bursitis.

Inspection of the spine is not often of value in identifying serious causes of low back pain. The classic posture of ankylosing spondylitis is a late finding. Scoliosis of mild degree is not associated with an increased risk of clinical back disease. Cutaneous neurofibromas can identify the rare patient with nerve root encasement.

Examination of the hips should be part of the complete examination. While hip arthritis usually produces groin pain, some patients have buttock or low back symptoms.

Further Examination

If the history and physical examination do not suggest the presence of infection, cancer, inflammatory back disease, major neurologic deficits, or pain referred from abdominal or pelvic disease, further evaluation can be eliminated or deferred while conservative therapy is tried. The great majority of patients will improve with conservative care over 1–4 weeks.

Regular radiographs of the lumbosacral spine give 20 times the radiation dose of a chest radiograph and provide limited, albeit important, information. Oblique films double the radiation dose and are not routinely needed. Radiographs can provide evidence of vertebral body osteomyelitis, cancer, fractures, or ankylosing spondylitis. Degenerative changes in the lumbar spine are ubiquitous in patients over 40 and do not prove clinical disease. Plain radiographs have very low sensitivity or specificity for disk disease. Thus, plain radiographs are warranted promptly for patients suspected of having infection, cancer, or fractures; selected other patients who do not improve after 2–4 weeks of conservative therapy are also candidates. The Agency for Health Care Policy and Research guidelines for obtaining lumbar radiographs are summarized in Table 20–7.

Table 20–6. Neurologic testing of lumbosacral nerve disorders.

Nerve Root	Motor	Reflex	Sensory Area
L4	Dorsiflexion of foot	Knee jerk	Medial calf
L5	Dorsiflexion of great toe	None	Medial forefoot
S1	Eversion of foot	Ankle jerk	Lateral foot

Table 20–7. AHRQ criteria for lumbar radiographs in patients with acute low back pain.

Possible fracture
Major trauma
Minor trauma in patients > 50 years
Long-term corticosteroid use
Osteoporosis
> 70 years
Possible tumor or infection
> 50 years
< 20 years
History of cancer
Constitutional symptoms
Recent bacterial infection
Injection drug use
Immunosuppression
Supine pain
Nocturnal pain

Agency for Healthcare Research and Quality (modified from JAMA 1997;277:1784).

MRI provides exquisite anatomic detail but is reserved for patients who are considering surgery or have evidence of a systemic disease. For example, MRI is needed urgently for any patient in whom an epidural mass or cauda equina tumor is suspected but not for a patient believed to have a routine disk herniation, since most will improve over 4–6 weeks of conservative therapy. Noncontrast CT does not image cauda equina tumors or other intradural lesions, and if used instead of MRI it must include intrathecal contrast.

Radionuclide bone scanning has limited usefulness. It is most useful for early detection of vertebral body osteomyelitis or osteoblastic metastases. The bone scan is normal in multiple myeloma because lytic lesions do not take up isotope.

2. Management

While any management plan must be individualized, key elements of most conservative treatments for back pain include analgesia and education. Analgesia can usually be provided with NSAIDs (see Table 5–5), but severe pain may require opioids (see Table 5–6). Rarely does the need for opioids extend beyond 1–2 weeks.

Diazepam, cyclobenzaprine, carisoprodol, and methocarbamol have been prescribed as muscle relaxants, though their sedative effects may limit their use. They should be reserved for patients who do not respond to NSAIDs and should also be limited to courses of 1–2 weeks. Their use should be avoided in older patients, who are at risk for falling. All patients should be taught how to protect the back in daily activities—ie, not to lift heavy objects, to use the legs rather than the back when lifting, to use a chair with arm rests, and to rise from bed by first rolling to one side and then using the arms to push to an upright position. Back manipulation for benign, mechanical low back pain appears safe and as effective as therapies provided by physicians.

Rest and back exercises, once thought to be cornerstones of conservative therapy, are now known to be ineffective for acute back pain. Advice to rest in bed is less effective than advice to remain active. No bed rest with continuation of ordinary activities as tolerated is superior to 2 days of bed rest, 7 days of bedrest, and back mobilizing exercises. Similarly, for acute back pain, exercise therapy is not effective. The value of corsets or traction is dubious. Epidural corticosteroid injections can provide short-term relief of sciatica but do not improve functional status or reduce the need for surgery. In double-blind studies, repeated injections have been no more effective than a single injection. For chronic low back pain, yoga is as effective as a back exercise program and more effective than a self-care book. Corticosteroid injections into facet joints are ineffective for chronic low back pain.

Surgical consultation is needed urgently for any patient with a major or evolving neurologic deficit. Surgery for disk disease is indicated when there is documentation of herniation by imaging, persistent pain, and a consistent neurologic deficit that has failed to respond to 4–6 weeks of conservative therapy. Percutaneous lumbar discectomy, performed under local anesthesia, is a safe and effective (up to 75%) alternative to laminectomy. The percutaneous procedure is contraindicated in the presence of tumor, infection, spondylolisthesis, foraminal stenosis, loose disk fragments, or severe facet joint arthritis.

Complaints without objective findings suggest a psychological role in symptom formation. Treatment includes reassurance and nonopioid analgesics.

Arden NK et al: A multicentre randomized controlled trial of epidural corticosteroid injections for sciatica: the WEST study. Rheumatology 2005;44:1399. [PMID: 16030082]

Cherkin DC et al: A review of the evidence for the effectiveness, safety, and cost of acupuncture, massage therapy, and spinal manipulation for back pain. Ann Intern Med 2003;138:898. [PMID: 12779300]

Hagen K et al: Bed rest for acute low-back pain and sciatica. Cochrane Database Syst Rev 2004:(4);CD001254. [PMID: 15495012]

Manheimer E et al: Meta-analysis: acupuncture for low back pain. Ann Intern Med 2005;142:651. [PMID: 15838072]

Sherman KJ et al: Comparing yoga, exercise, and a self-care book for chronic low back pain: a randomized, controlled trial. Ann Intern Med 2005;143:849. [PMID: 16365466]

Speed C: Low back pain. BMJ 2004;328:1119. [PMID: 15130982]

van Poppel MN et al: An update of a systematic review of controlled clinical trials on the primary prevention of back pain at the workplace. Occup Med (Lond) 2004;54:345. [PMID: 15289592]

LUMBAR SPINAL STENOSIS

ESSENTIALS OF DIAGNOSIS

- *Most patients are older than 60 years.*

- *Presenting symptom is often back pain radiating to the buttocks and thighs.*
- *Pain often interferes with walking and worsened by lumbar extension.*
- *Back and leg pain often associated with numbness and paresthesia.*
- *Preservation of pedal pulses helps exclude vascular claudication.*
- *Diagnosis best confirmed by MRI.*

General Considerations

Lumbar spinal stenosis, defined as narrowing of the spinal canal with compression of the nerve roots, may be congenital or (more commonly) acquired. It most frequently results from enlarging osteophytes at the facet joints, hypertrophy of the ligamentum flavum, and protrusion or bulging of intervertebral disks. Lumbar spinal stenosis may produce symptoms by directly compressing nerve roots or by compressing nutrient arterioles that supply the nerve roots.

Clinical Findings

A. Symptoms and Signs

Since age is the greatest risk factor for spinal degenerative changes, most patients with lumbar spinal stenosis are over 60 years old. Patients typically complain of either leg pain or trouble walking. The pain may originate in the low back but will extend below the buttock into the thigh in nearly 90% of patients. In approximately 50% of patients, the pain will extend below the knee. The pain is often a combination of aching and numbness, which characteristically worsens with walking. The pain can also be brought on by prolonged standing. Not infrequently the symptoms are bilateral. Many patients are more troubled by poor balance, unsteadiness of gait, or leg weakness that develops as they walk. Some describe these neuroclaudication symptoms as developing "spaghetti legs" or "walking like a drunk sailor." Because the lumbar spinal canal volume increases with back flexion and decreases with extension, some patients observe that they have fewer symptoms walking uphill than down. The back and lower extremity examination in patients with lumbar spinal stenosis is often unimpressive. Fewer than 10% have a positive straight leg raise sign, 25% have diminished deep tendon reflexes, and 60% have slight proximal weakness. Walking with the patient may reveal unsteadiness, although usually the patient's perception of gait disturbance is greater than that of an observer.

B. Imaging

The diagnosis of spinal stenosis in a patient with symptoms is best confirmed by MRI.

Differential Diagnosis

The onset of symptoms with standing, the location of the maximal discomfort to the thighs, and the preservation of pedal pulses help distinguish the "pseudo-claudication" of spinal stenosis from true claudication caused by vascular insufficiency. Distinguishing spinal stenosis from disk herniation can be challenging since both conditions can produce pain radiating down the back of the leg. Features that favor spinal stenosis are the gradual onset of symptoms, the marked exacerbation with walking, and the amelioration of symptoms with sitting or lumbar flexion. Complaints of bilateral aching in the buttocks associated with stiffness may make some practitioners consider the diagnosis of polymyalgia rheumatica. However, patients with lumbar spinal stenosis do not have the shoulder or neck symptoms characteristic of polymyalgia rheumatica.

Treatment

Weight loss and exercises aimed at reducing lumbar lordosis, which aggravates symptoms of spinal stenosis, can help. Lumbar epidural corticosteroid injections provide some immediate relief for about 50% of patients and more sustained relief for approximately 25%. When disabling symptoms persist, decompressive laminectomy provides at least short-term relief in approximately 80%.

Chang Y et al: The effect of surgical and nonsurgical treatment on longitudinal outcomes of lumbar spinal stenosis over 10 years. J Am Geriatr Soc 2005;53:785. [PMID: 15877553]

Sengupta DK et al: Lumbar spinal stenosis. Treatment strategies and indications for surgery. Orthop Clin North Am 2003; 34:281. [PMID: 12914268]

FIBROMYALGIA

 ESSENTIALS OF DIAGNOSIS

- *Most frequent in women aged 20–50.*
- *Chronic widespread musculoskeletal pain syndrome with multiple tender points.*
- *Fatigue, headaches, numbness common.*
- *Objective signs of inflammation absent; laboratory studies normal.*
- *Partially responsive to exercise, tricyclic antidepressants.*

General Considerations

Fibromyalgia is one of the most common rheumatic syndromes in ambulatory general medicine affecting 3–10% of the general population. It shares many features with the chronic fatigue syndrome, namely, an increased frequency among women aged 20–50, absence of objective findings, and absence of diagnostic laboratory test results. While many of the clinical features of the two conditions overlap, musculoskeletal pain predominates in fibromyalgia whereas lassitude dominates the chronic fatigue syndrome.

The cause is unknown, but sleep disorders, depression, viral infections, and aberrant perception of painful stimuli have all been proposed. Fibromyalgia can be a rare complication of hypothyroidism, rheumatoid arthritis or, in men, sleep apnea.

Clinical Findings

The patient complains of chronic aching pain and stiffness, frequently involving the entire body but with prominence of pain around the neck, shoulders, low back, and hips. Fatigue, sleep disorders, subjective numbness, chronic headaches, and irritable bowel symptoms are common. Even minor exertion aggravates pain and increases fatigue. Physical examination is normal except for "trigger points" of pain produced by palpation of various areas such as the trapezius, the medial fat pad of the knee, and the lateral epicondyle of the elbow.

Differential Diagnosis

Fibromyalgia is a diagnosis of exclusion. A detailed history and repeated physical examination can obviate the need for extensive laboratory testing. Rheumatoid arthritis and systemic lupus erythematosus (SLE) present with objective physical findings or abnormalities on routine testing, including the ESR and C-reactive protein. Thyroid function tests are useful, since hypothyroidism can produce a secondary fibromyalgia syndrome. Polymyositis produces weakness rather than pain. The diagnosis of fibromyalgia probably should be made hesitantly in a patient over age 50 and should never be invoked to explain fever, weight loss, or any other objective signs. Polymyalgia rheumatica produces shoulder and pelvic girdle pain, is associated with anemia and an elevated ESR, and occurs after age 50. Hypophosphatemic states, such as oncogenic osteomalacia, should also be included in the differential diagnosis of musculoskeletal pain unassociated with physical findings. In contrast to fibromyalgia, oncogenic osteomalacia usually produces pain in only a few areas and is associated with a low serum phosphate level.

Treatment

Patient education is essential. Patients can be comforted that they have a diagnosable syndrome treatable by specific though imperfect therapies and that the course is not progressive. There is modest efficacy of amitriptyline, fluoxetine, chlorpromazine, or cyclobenzaprine. Amitriptyline is initiated at a dosage of 10 mg orally at bedtime and gradually increased to 40–50 mg depending on efficacy and toxicity. Fewer than 50% of the pa-

tients experience a sustained improvement. Exercise programs are also beneficial. NSAIDs are generally ineffective. Tramadol and acetaminophen combinations have ameliorated symptoms modestly in short-term trials. Opioids and corticosteroids are ineffective and should not be used to treat fibromyalgia. Acupuncture is also ineffective.

Prognosis

All patients have chronic symptoms. With treatment, however, many do eventually resume increased activities. Progressive or objective findings do not develop.

Assefi NP et al: A randomized clinical trial of acupuncture compared with sham acupuncture in fibromyalgia. Ann Intern Med 2005;143:10. [PMID: 15998750]

Bennett RM et al: Tramadol and acetaminophen combination tablets in the treatment of fibromyalgia pain: a double-blind, randomized, placebo-controlled study. Am J Med 2003;114:537. [PMID: 12753877]

Goldenberg DL et al: Management of fibromyalgia syndrome. JAMA 2004;292:2388. [PMID: 15547167]

CARPAL TUNNEL SYNDROME

An entrapment neuropathy, carpal tunnel syndrome is a painful disorder caused by compression of the median nerve between the carpal ligament and other structures within the carpal tunnel. The contents of the tunnel can be increased by organic lesions such as synovitis of the tendon sheaths or carpal joints, recent or malhealed fractures, tumors, and occasionally congenital anomalies. Even though no anatomic lesion is apparent, flattening or even circumferential constriction of the median nerve may be observed during operative section of the ligament. The disorder may occur in pregnancy, is seen in individuals with a history of repetitive use of the hands, and may follow injuries of the wrists. There is a familial type of carpal tunnel syndrome in which no etiologic factor can be identified.

Carpal tunnel syndrome can also be a feature of many systemic diseases: rheumatoid arthritis and other rheumatic disorders (inflammatory tenosynovitis); myxedema, localized amyloidosis in chronic renal failure, sarcoidosis, and leukemia (tissue infiltration); acromegaly; and hyperparathyroidism.

Clinical Findings

Pain, burning, and tingling in the distribution of the median nerve (the palmar surface of the thumb and first two and a half fingers) is the initial symptom. Aching pain may radiate proximally into the forearm and occasionally proximally to the shoulder and over the neck and chest. Pain is exacerbated by manual activity, particularly by extremes of volar flexion or dorsiflexion of the wrist. It is most bothersome at night. Impairment of sensation in the median nerve distribution may or may not be demonstrable. Subtle disparity between the affected and opposite sides can be shown by testing for two-point discrimination or by requiring the patient to identify different textures of cloth by rubbing them between the tips of the thumb and the index finger. Tinel's or Phalen's sign may be positive. (Tinel's sign is tingling or shock-like pain on volar wrist percussion; Phalen's sign is pain or paresthesia in the distribution of the median nerve when the patient flexes both wrists to 90 degrees with the dorsal aspects of the hands held in apposition for 60 seconds.) The carpal compression test, in which numbness and tingling are induced by the direct application of pressure over the carpal tunnel, may be more sensitive and specific than the Tinel and Phalen tests. Muscle weakness or atrophy, especially of the thenar eminence, appears later than sensory disturbances. Specific examinations include electromyography and determinations of segmental sensory and motor conduction delay. Sensory conduction delay is evident before motor delay.

Differential Diagnosis

This syndrome should be differentiated from other cervicobrachial pain syndromes, from compression syndromes of the median nerve in the forearm or arm, and from mononeuritis multiplex. When left-sided, it may be confused with angina pectoris.

Treatment

Treatment is directed toward relief of pressure on the median nerve. When a causative lesion is discovered, it is treated appropriately. Otherwise, patients in whom causative carpal tunnel syndrome is suspected should modify their hand activities and have the affected wrist splinted for 2–6 weeks. NSAIDs can also be added. Patients should be referred to a specialist for injection of corticosteroid into the carpal tunnel or for operation when they do not improve or when thenar muscle atrophy or weakness develops. Muscle strength returns gradually, but complete recovery cannot be expected when atrophy is pronounced.

Katz JN et al: Clinical practice. Carpal tunnel syndrome. N Engl J Med 2002;346:1807. [PMID: 12050342]

Ly-Pen D et al: Surgical decompression versus local steroid injection in carpal tunnel syndrome: a one-year, prospective, randomized, open, controlled clinical trial. Arthritis Rheum 2005;52:612. [PMID: 15692981]

MacDermid JC et al: Clinical diagnosis of carpal tunnel syndrome: a systematic review. J Hand Ther 2004;17:309. [PMID: 15162113]

DUPUYTREN'S CONTRACTURE

This relatively common disorder is characterized by hyperplasia of the palmar fascia and related structures, with nodule formation and contracture of the palmar fascia. The cause is unknown, but the condition has a genetic predisposition and occurs primarily in white men over 50 years of age. The incidence is higher among alcoholic patients and those with chronic systemic disorders (especially cirrhosis). It is also associated with systemic fibrosing syndrome, which includes Peyronie's disease, mediastinal and retroperitoneal fibrosis, and Riedel's struma. The onset may be acute, but slowly progressive chronic disease is more common.

Dupuytren's contracture manifests itself by nodular or cord-like thickening of one or both hands, with the fourth and fifth fingers most commonly affected. The patient may complain of tightness of the involved digits, with inability to satisfactorily extend the fingers, and on occasion there is tenderness. The resulting cosmetic problems may be unappealing, but in general the contracture is well tolerated since it exaggerates the normal position of function of the hand. Fasciitis involving other areas of the body may lead to plantar fibromatosis (10% of patients) or Peyronie's disease (1–2%).

If the palmar nodule is growing rapidly, injections of triamcinolone into the nodule may be of benefit. Surgical intervention is indicated in patients with significant flexion contractures, depending on the location, but recurrence is not uncommon.

Hart MG et al: Clinical associations of Dupuytren's disease. Postgrad Med J 2005;81:425. [PMID: 15998816]

COMPLEX REGIONAL PAIN SYNDROME (Reflex Sympathetic Dystrophy)

Complex regional pain syndrome is a rare disorder of the extremities characterized by autonomic and vasomotor instability. The cardinal symptoms and signs are diffuse pain (characteristically localized to an arm or hand, leg or foot), swelling of the involved extremity, disturbances of color and temperature in the affected limb, dystrophic changes in the overlying skin and nails, and limited range of motion. Use of the former name of this entity, reflex sympathetic dystrophy, is now discouraged because the precise role of the sympathetic nervous system is unclear and dystrophy is not an inevitable sequela of the syndrome. Most cases are preceded by direct physical trauma, often of relatively minor nature, to the soft tissues, bone, or nerve. Any extremity can be involved, but the syndrome most commonly occurs in the hand and is associated with ipsilateral restriction of shoulder motion (shoulder-hand syndrome). The syndrome proceeds through phases: pain, swelling, and skin color and temperature changes develop early and, if untreated, lead to atrophy and dystrophy. The swelling in complex regional pain syndrome is diffuse ("catcher's mitt hand") and not restricted to joints. Pain is often burning in quality, intense, and often greatly worsened by minimal stimuli such as light touch. The shoulder-hand variant of this disorder sometimes complicates myocardial infarction or injuries to the neck or shoulder. Complex regional pain syndrome may occur after a knee injury or after arthroscopic knee surgery. There are no systemic symptoms. In the early phases of the syndrome, bone scans are sensitive, showing diffuse increased uptake in the affected extremity. X-rays eventually reveal severe generalized osteopenia. In the post-traumatic variant, this is known as Sudeck's atrophy. Symptoms and findings are bilateral in some. This syndrome should be differentiated from other cervicobrachial pain syndromes, rheumatoid arthritis, thoracic outlet obstruction, and scleroderma, among others.

Early mobilization after injury, surgery, or myocardial infarction reduces the likelihood of developing the syndrome. In addition to addressing the underlying disorder, treatment is directed toward restoration of function. Physical therapy is the cornerstone of treatment. Many patients will also benefit from drug therapies, especially antidepressant agents (eg, nortriptyline initiated at a dosage of 10 mg orally at bedtime and gradually increased to 40–75 mg at bedtime). In resistant cases, prednisone, 30–40 mg/d orally for 2 weeks and then tapered over 2 weeks, may be effective. Regional nerve blocks and dorsal-column stimulation have also been demonstrated to be helpful. Patients who have restricted shoulder motion may benefit from the treatment described for scapulohumeral periarthritis. The prognosis partly depends on the stage in which the lesions are encountered and the extent and severity of associated organic disease. Early treatment offers the best prognosis for recovery.

Birklein F: Complex regional pain syndrome. J Neurol 2005; 252:131. [PMID: 15729516]

Mailis A et al: Sympathectomy for neuropathic pain. Cochrane Database Syst Rev 2003;(2):CD002918. [PMID: 12804444]

Mailis-Gagnon A et al: Spinal cord stimulation for chronic pain. Cochrane Database Syst Rev 2004;(3):CD003783. [PMID: 15266501]

BURSITIS

Inflammation of the synovium-like cellular membrane overlying bony prominences may be secondary to trauma, infection, or arthritic conditions such as gout, rheumatoid arthritis, or osteoarthritis. The most common locations are the subdeltoid, olecranon, ischial, trochanteric, semi-membranous-gastrocnemius (Baker's cyst), and prepatellar bursae.

There are several ways to distinguish bursitis from arthritis. Bursitis is more likely than arthritis to begin abruptly and cause focal tenderness and swelling. Olecranon bursitis, for example, causes an oval (or, if chronic, bulbous) swelling at the tip of the elbow, whereas elbow joint inflammation produces more diffuse swelling. Similarly, a patient with prepatellar bursitis has a small focus of swelling over the kneecap but no distention of the knee joint itself. Active and passive ranges of motion are usually much more limited in arthritis than in bursitis. A patient with trochanteric bursitis will have normal internal rotation of the hip, whereas a patient with hip arthritis will not. Bursitis caused by trauma responds to local heat, rest, NSAIDs, and local corticosteroid injections.

Bursitis can result from infection. The two most common sites are the olecranon and prepatellar bursae. Acute swelling and redness at either of these two sites calls for aspiration to rule out infection. The absence of fever does not exclude infection; and one-third of those with septic olecranon bursitis are afebrile. A bursal fluid white blood cell count of greater than 1000/mcL indicates inflammation from infection, rheumatoid arthritis, or gout. In septic bursitis, the white cell count averages over 50,000/mcL. Most cases are caused by *Staphylococcus aureus;* the Gram stain is positive in two-thirds. Treatment involves antibiotics and repeated aspiration for tense effusions.

Chronic, stable olecranon bursa swelling unaccompanied by erythema or other signs of inflammation does not suggest infection and does not require aspiration. Aspiration of the olecranon bursa in rheumatoid arthritis and in gout runs the risk of creating a chronic drainage site, which can be reduced by using a small needle (25-gauge if possible) and pulling the skin over the bursa before introducing it. Applying a pressure bandage may also help prevent chronic drainage. Surgical removal of the bursa is indicated only for cases in which repeated infections occur. Repetitive minor trauma to the olecranon bursa should be eliminated by avoiding resting the elbow on a hard surface or by wearing an elbow pad.

A bursa can also become symptomatic when it ruptures. This is particularly true for Baker's cyst, whose rupture can cause calf pain and swelling that mimic thrombophlebitis. Ruptured Baker's cysts are imaged easily by sonography or MRI. In most cases, imaging is unnecessary because the cyst and an associated knee effusion are detectable on physical examination. It may be important to exclude a deep venous thrombosis, which can be mimicked by a ruptured Baker's cyst. Treatment of a ruptured cyst includes rest, leg elevation, and injection of triamcinolone, 20–40 mg into the knee (which communicates with the cyst). Rarely, Baker's cyst can compress vascular structures and cause leg edema and true thrombophlebitis.

Cohen SP et al: Corticosteroid injections for trochanteric bursitis: is fluoroscopy necessary? A pilot study. Br J Anaesth 2005; 94:100. [PMID: 15516348]

SPORTS MEDICINE INJURIES

Musculoskeletal problems commonly occur as a result of both serious athletic pursuits and activities of daily living. For most such disorders, the diagnosis is made easily. Physical therapy is an increasingly important adjunct to the management of these disorders.

1. Rotator Cuff Disorders

A substantial majority of shoulder problems stem from disorders of the rotator cuff. The tendons of the rotator cuff form a musculotendinous unit near their insertions into the proximal humerus. As a result of years of cumulative irritation, attenuation of these tendons occurs. Among the relevant muscles, the supraspinatus is most often affected. Distinguishing between the various soft tissue disorders that cause shoulder pain is difficult. Rotator cuff tendinitis, subacromial bursitis, partial and complete rotator cuff tears, and calcific tendinitis frequently cause similar symptoms. In addition, these disorders often occur together, although precise distinction is frequently unimportant for purposes of therapy.

Clinical Findings

Patients usually present with nonspecific pain localized to the shoulder, often noticed more at night when lying on the affected side. Locking sensations occur with motion of the shoulder, particularly through abduction. Because of the shared innervation, symptoms are frequently referred down the proximal lateral arm. With rotator cuff tears, the patient may be unable to abduct or flex the shoulder, depending on the site of the tear.

The rotator cuff may be palpated just lateral to the head of the acromion. Maximum tenderness is usually noted over the supraspinatus insertion. The acromioclavicular joint may also be tender if there is accompanying degenerative arthritis in that joint. There may be prominent crepitus. Pain with range of motion is most pronounced between 60 and 120 degrees of abduction, the site of greatest impingement of the rotator cuff tissues between the humerus and coracoacromial arch.

For patients with partial rotator cuff tendon ruptures, the findings are identical to those of chronic tendinitis and bursitis. Patients with partial ruptures often demonstrate mild abduction weakness. With complete ruptures, weakness of abduction (and, to a lesser extent, flexion) is substantial, even though full range of motion may be maintained by the shoulder's accessory rotator muscles. Patients with complete tears usually have positive "drop arm" signs: inability to sustain passive abduction of the arm to 90 degrees.

Treatment

For most rotator cuff disorders, the central tenets of therapy are rest and abstention from inciting activities. Temporary use of a sling is helpful in enforcing rest. NSAIDs and moist heat afford some relief. For patients with symptoms persisting after 2 weeks of conservative management, injections of a corticosteroid preparation (eg, 1 mL of triamcinolone, 40 mg/mL) mixed with 2–3 mL of lidocaine hydrochloride (1–2%) may be useful. Tears or partial tears of the rotator cuff tendons that are believed to be chronic do not preclude a corticosteroid injection. Most patients obtain significant relief with one injection, but the procedure—along with continued rest—may be repeated after 2–3 weeks. Physical therapy is valuable for refractory cases—if the patient does not maintain the shoul-

der's normal range of motion, stiffness and impaired function from a "frozen shoulder" may ensue.

Aside from patients with complete rotator cuff tears, only those who do not improve after months of conservative therapy are candidates for operation. Persistent symptoms may be a sign of complete tear, which may be diagnosed by MRI. Patients with symptoms that continue in the absence of a complete tear, however, sometimes require surgery to excise the inferolateral portion of the acromion, release obstructed soft tissue, and repair partial tendon tears. Depending on the patient's symptoms and functional status, complete tears may not always require surgical repair. Patients over 75 years of age rarely have symptoms or limitations that necessitate surgery. Moreover, surgical repairs are frequently less successful because of the attrition of the rotator cuff that occurs with aging.

Gerdesmeyer L et al: Extracorporeal shock wave therapy for the treatment of chronic calcifying tendonitis of the rotator cuff: a randomized controlled trial. JAMA 2003;290:2573. [PMID: 14625334]

Grant HJ et al: Evaluation of interventions for rotator cuff pathology: a systematic review. J Hand Ther 2004;17:274. [PMID: 15162111]

Haahr JP et al: Exercises versus arthroscopic decompression in patients with subacromial impingement: a randomised, controlled study in 90 cases with a one year follow up. Ann Rheum Dis 2005;64:760. [PMID: 15834056]

Luime JJ et al: Does this patient have an instability of the shoulder or a labrum lesion? JAMA 2004;292:1989. [PMID: 15507585]

2. Lateral & Medial Epicondylitis

These disorders are better known by their sports associations: "tennis elbow" and "golf elbow," respectively. Lateral epicondylitis is the more common of the two. The conditions are caused by overuse, and the pain results from minor tears in the tendons of the forearm's extensor and flexor muscles.

Clinical Findings

The patient presents with pain at the site of tendon insertion. Tasks that require grasping and squeezing, such as shaking hands or opening jars, cause pain.

The diagnoses are easily confirmed on physical examination by elicitation of point tenderness over the involved site. The characteristic pain may also be reproduced by extension or flexion of the wrist against pressure. Clenching the fist and extending the wrist against the pressure of the examiner's palm is a useful maneuver for localizing lateral epicondylitis. Medial epicondylitis may be demonstrated by performing the same maneuver in flexion.

Treatment

The use of "counterforce" straps (bands worn distal to the elbow, over the bulk of the forearm musculature), intended to decrease the forces transmitted to the elbow during activity, are inadequate substitutes for rest. NSAIDs are effective in mild cases. Symptoms that persist after 2 weeks of conservative therapy usually respond either to infiltration of triamcinolone, 10–20 mg mixed with 1–2 mL of 1% lidocaine, around the involved epicondyle—or to physiotherapy. Results are quicker with corticosteroid injections but longer-lasting with physiotherapy. Botulinum toxin injection can also ameliorate lateral epicondylitis symptoms but runs the risk of causing digital paresis. After the pain and tenderness have subsided, patients may begin a physical therapy program involving daily stretching of the flexor and extensor tendons.

Smidt N et al: Corticosteroid injections, physiotherapy, or a wait-and-see policy for lateral epicondylitis: a randomised controlled trial. Lancet 2002;359:657. [PMID: 11879861]

Trudel D et al: Rehabilitation for patients with lateral epicondylitis: a systematic review. J Hand Ther 2004;17:243. [PMID: 15162109]

Wong SM et al: Treatment of lateral epicondylitis with botulinum toxin: a randomized, double-blind, placebo-controlled trial. Ann Intern Med 2005;143:793. [PMID: 16330790]

3. Patellofemoral Syndrome

Patellofemoral syndrome is among the most common causes of knee complaints in primary care medicine, particularly among adolescent and young adult patients. The syndrome frequently gives rise to the chief complaint of anterior knee pain. A variety of injuries or anatomic abnormalities predispose patients to irregular patellar movements, leading to the patellofemoral syndrome. Such predisposing conditions include imbalance of quadriceps strength, patella alta, recurrent patellar subluxation, direct trauma to the patella, and meniscal injuries. For most of these causes, the therapeutic approach is similar.

Clinical Findings

Patients frequently have difficulty localizing the source of their complaint but generally confirm that the pain is in the front of the knee, around or underneath the patella. Questions regarding specific precipitants of the pain may be useful in establishing the diagnosis. For example, because of the flexion load, patients have difficulty going up or down staircases (down is usually associated with greater symptoms). Another characteristic symptom is the positive "theater" sign: after remaining seated for a prolonged period, patients describe extreme discomfort with their first few steps after rising. The symptoms improve with further walking. Finally, patients with patellofemoral syndrome often complain of crepitus, joint locking, or sensations of joint instability, all of which lack readily confirmed anatomic explanations.

The physical examination is less useful than the history in establishing the diagnosis, but a significant number of patients have characteristic physical findings. In particular, when the knee is held in slight flexion, gentle pressure against the patella as the patient contracts the quadriceps muscles may reproduce the symptoms. In some cases, with the knee extended and the quadriceps relaxed, the typical pain may be reproduced by digital pressure under the medial or lateral border of the patella, with side-to-side movement of the bone. Inflammatory findings on examination are incompatible with the diagnosis of patellofemoral syndrome and suggest other disorders.

Treatment

Therapy includes avoidance of flexion loads and strengthening of the quadriceps. Referral to a physical therapist is helpful in educating the patient about home exercises. Many patients learn that the most effective therapy is bicycling, with the seat high enough to permit nearly full knee extension with each cycle. Although most cases respond to these interventions and even resolve altogether, some persist for years. Even in the latter, conservative therapy remains the rule; operation is rarely indicated. There is only limited evidence for the effectiveness of NSAIDs in short-term pain reduction associated with the patellofemoral pain syndrome. The evidence supporting the use of glycosaminoglycan polysulfate is conflicting. Bracing is no more effective than a home exercise program.

Heintjes E et al: Pharmacotherapy for patellofemoral pain syndrome. Cochrane Database Syst Rev 2004;(3):CD003470. [PMID: 15266488]

Lun VM et al: Effectiveness of patellar bracing for treatment of patellofemoral pain syndrome. Clin J Sport Med 2005;15:235. [PMID: 16003037]

4. Overuse Syndromes of the Knee

Runners—particularly those who overtrain, fail to stretch prior to running, or do not attain the proper level of conditioning before starting a running program—may develop a variety of painful overuse syndromes of the knee. Most of these conditions are forms of tendinitis or bursitis that can be diagnosed on examination. The most common conditions include anserine bursitis, the iliotibial band syndrome, and popliteal and patellar tendinitis.

Clinical Findings

Symptoms resulting from all of these conditions worsen as the patient continues to run and often require cessation of the activity. Anserine bursitis results in pain medial and inferior to the knee joint over the medial tibia. The iliotibial band syndrome and popliteal tenosynovitis may be difficult to differentiate, because the popliteus tendon inserts into the lateral femoral condyle underneath the iliotibial band. Both conditions result in pain on the lateral side of the knee. Patellar tendinitis, a cause of anterior knee discomfort, typically occurs at the tendon's insertion into the patella rather than at its more inferior insertion.

All of these diagnoses are confirmed by palpation at the relevant sites around the knee. None is associated with joint effusions or other signs of synovitis.

Treatment

Rest and abstention from the associated physical activities for a period of days to weeks are essential. Once pain has subsided, a program of gentle stretching (particularly prior to resuming exercise) may prevent recurrence. Corticosteroid injections with lidocaine may be useful when intense discomfort is present, but caution must be used when injecting corticosteroids into the region of a tendon to avoid rupture.

5. Medial Meniscus Injuries

Tears of the medial meniscus are the most common knee injuries encountered in primary care. Because the medial meniscus is tethered firmly to the underlying tibia, injuries to the medial meniscus occur ten times more commonly than injuries to the lateral meniscus. Both result from a twisting action exerted on the knee joint while the foot is in a weight-bearing position.

Clinical Findings

The injury is heralded by a tearing or popping sensation followed by severe pain. Occasionally, meniscal tears result from seemingly minor trauma. In contrast to ligamentous injuries, in which hemorrhage causes immediate swelling, effusions associated with meniscal injuries accumulate over hours and are typically worse the day after the injury. Several days after resolution (full or partial), the patient may experience joint locking or instability, recurrent swelling with activity, and pain. The sensation of locking, which may result from mechanical blockage by a fragment of torn meniscus, more commonly results from "pseudolocking" caused by muscle spasm and swelling.

Joint effusion is usually present, frequently accompanied by a ballottable patella. Tenderness may be localized to the medial joint line, and range of motion in the knee may be restricted. In patients without an acutely painful, swollen knee, McMurray's test may suggest the diagnosis. This test is performed with the patient supine and the hip and knee in full flexion. The examiner has one hand on the involved knee and the other on the ipsilateral foot. As the foot is externally rotated, the examiner extends the patient's knee. The presence of a "snap" (palpable or audible) suggests a medial meniscus lesion. MRI is the optimal test for confirming the diagnosis if plain films exclude other conditions.

Treatment

Initial management is conservative, with elevation of the joint and application of a compression dressing and ice. Weight bearing should be minimized for the first few days after the injury but may be resumed slowly thereafter. The patient should perform quadriceps-strengthening exercises under the instruction of a physical therapist. Surgery is reserved for patients with symptoms that recur upon resumption of normal activities or for patients with irreducible locking caused by mechanical problems.

Jackson JL et al: Evaluation of acute knee pain in primary care. Ann Intern Med 2003;139:575. [PMID: 14530229]

6. Ankle Sprains

Ankle sprains are among the most common of all sports injuries. Most sprains involve the lateral ligament complex, particularly the anterior talofibular ligament. In more severe injuries, the calcaneofibular ligament may also be involved. If both of these ligaments are ruptured, the injury results in significant joint instability and is classified as a grade III (severe) sprain. (Grades I and II correspond to mild and moderate injuries, respectively.) This section reviews only the type of ankle sprain resulting from inversion (varus) injuries, which account for 85% of all sprains.

Clinical Findings

Varus sprains include a spectrum of severity, ranging from slight loss of function to injuries in which the swelling is prompt, the pain prominent, and weight bearing impossible. A history of hearing a "pop" at the time of injury is frequently associated with the latter.

Hemorrhage resulting from torn ligaments and damaged peroneal muscle tendons may cause substantial ecchymosis. Tenderness is typically present at the site of injury, and the associated swelling may be considerable. Stability of the anterior talofibular and calcaneofibular ligaments should be assessed with the "anterior drawer" sign: With the foot held in slight plantar flexion, the examiner cups the patient's heel with one hand and the patient's shin with the other. The examiner then applies gentle anterior force in the plane of the patient's foot. Excessive anterior motion of the foot constitutes a positive test (grade III sprain). Plain radiographs exclude associated bony injury.

Treatment

Most ankle sprains—even grade III—are treated identically. The acronym "RICE" (rest, ice, compression, elevation) applies more accurately to ankle sprains than to any other injury. Early application of a compression dressing is essential to control swelling and provide stability to the traumatized joint. An Aircast ankle brace may be more effective than an elastic support bandage. Weight bearing should be minimal, with liberal use of crutches. Elevation of the ankle for several days hastens functional recovery by diminishing pain and swelling, and ice is also helpful (alternating 30 minutes on, 30 minutes off). The ice should be applied on top of the compression dressing and not against the skin both because close apposition of the dressing to the skin is critical to control swelling and because direct application of ice is uncomfortable and even deleterious to the skin. Referral to a physical therapist may expedite recovery. Patients should be informed that symptoms from lateral ankle sprains may take weeks or months to resolve, and that this period will be prolonged by premature attempts to bear weight on the injured ankle. Surgical repairs of ruptured lateral ligaments provide excellent outcomes but are usually necessary only in cases of chronically unstable joints.

Boyce SH et al: Management of ankle sprains: a randomised controlled trial of the treatment of inversion injuries using an elastic support bandage or an Aircast ankle brace. Br J Sports Med 2005;39:91. [PMID: 15665204]

7. Plantar Fasciitis

The most common cause of foot pain in outpatient medicine is plantar fasciitis, which results from constant strain on the plantar fascia at its insertion into the medial tubercle of the calcaneus. Although certain inflammatory disorders such as the seronegative spondyloarthropathies predispose patients to enthesopathies, the majority of cases occur in patients with no associated disease. Most occur as the result of excessive standing and improper footwear.

Clinical Findings

Patients with plantar fasciitis report severe pain on the bottoms of their feet in the morning—the first steps out of bed in particular—but the pain subsides after a few minutes of ambulation.

The diagnosis may be confirmed by palpation over the plantar fascia's insertion on the medial heel. Radiographs have no role in the diagnosis of this condition—heel spurs frequently exist in patients without plantar fasciitis, and most symptomatic patients do not have heel spurs.

Treatment

Treatment consists of imposing an interval of days without prolonged standing and the use of arch supports. Arch supports give relief by requiring the arches to bear more of the patient's weight, thus unloading the plantar enthesis. NSAIDs may provide some relief. In severe cases, a corticosteroid with lidocaine injection (small volume—no more than a total of 1.5 mL) directly into the most tender area on the sole of the foot is helpful. Rare patients require release of the plantar fascia from its attachment site at the os calcis.

■ AUTOIMMUNE DISEASES

The autoimmune disorders are a protean group of acquired diseases in which genetic factors also play a role. They have in common widespread immunologic alterations and often share features of generalized inflammation.

Because of overlapping clinical features, differentiation among autoimmune diseases may be challenging, particularly in their early stages. These illnesses share certain clinical features, and differentiation among them is often difficult because of this. Common findings include synovitis, pleuritis, myocarditis, endocarditis, pericarditis, peritonitis, vasculitis, myositis, skin rash, and nephritis. Laboratory tests may reveal Coombs-positive hemolytic anemia, thrombocytopenia, leukopenia, immunoglobulin excesses or deficiencies, antinuclear antibodies (which include antibodies to many nuclear constituents, including DNA and extractable nuclear antigen), rheumatoid factors, cryoglobulins, false-positive serologic tests for syphilis, other antiphospholipid antibodies, elevated muscle enzymes, and hypocomplementemia.

Some of the laboratory abnormalities found in autoimmune diseases (eg, false-positive serologic tests for syphilis, rheumatoid factor) occur in asymptomatic individuals. These changes may also be demonstrated in certain asymptomatic relatives of patients with connective tissue diseases, in older persons, in patients using certain medications, and in patients with chronic infectious diseases.

RHEUMATOID ARTHRITIS

ESSENTIALS OF DIAGNOSIS

- *Prodromal systemic symptoms of malaise, fever, weight loss, and morning stiffness.*
- *Onset usually insidious and in small joints; progression is centripetal and symmetric; deformities common.*
- *Radiographic findings: juxta-articular osteoporosis, joint erosions, and narrowing of the joint spaces.*
- *Rheumatoid factor usually present. The anticyclic citrullinated peptide (CCP) test also has a high sensitivity and specificity for rheumatoid arthritis.*
- *Extra-articular manifestations: subcutaneous nodules, pleural effusion, pericarditis, lymphadenopathy, splenomegaly with leukopenia, and vasculitis.*

General Considerations

Rheumatoid arthritis is a chronic systemic inflammatory disease of unknown cause, chiefly affecting synovial membranes of multiple joints. The disease has a wide clinical spectrum with considerable variability in joint and extra-articular manifestations. The prevalence in the general population is 1–2%; female patients outnumber males almost 3:1. The usual age at onset is 20–40 years, although rheumatoid arthritis may begin at any age. Susceptibility to rheumatoid arthritis is genetically determined. Many patients have a class II HLA epitope with an identical five-amino-acid sequence; this is known as the "shared epitope." If not treated appropriately, rheumatoid arthritis has a strong tendency to shorten life and cause severe disability. Consequently, early, aggressive treatment is now the standard of care.

The pathologic findings in the joint include chronic synovitis with pannus formation. The pannus erodes cartilage, bone, ligaments, and tendons. In the acute phase, effusion and other manifestations of inflammation are common. In the late stage, organization may result in fibrous ankylosis; true bony ankylosis is rare. In both acute and chronic phases, inflammation of soft tissues around the joints may be prominent and is a significant factor in joint damage.

The microscopic findings most characteristic of rheumatoid arthritis are those of the subcutaneous nodule. This is a granuloma with a central zone of fibrinoid necrosis, a surrounding palisade of radially arranged elongated connective tissue cells, and a periphery of chronic granulation tissue. Pathologic alterations indistinguishable from those of the subcutaneous nodule are occasionally seen in the myocardium, pericardium, endocardium, heart valves, visceral pleura, lungs, sclera, dura mater, spleen, larynx, and other tissues. In the era of more effective treatment, secondary amyloidosis is now very rare.

Clinical Findings

A. SYMPTOMS AND SIGNS

The clinical manifestations of rheumatoid disease are highly variable. Although acute presentations may occur, the onset of articular signs of inflammation is usually insidious, with prodromal symptoms of malaise, weight loss, and vague periarticular pain or stiffness. Symmetric joint swelling with stiffness, warmth, tenderness, and pain are characteristic. Stiffness persisting for more than 30 minutes (and usually many hours) is prominent in the morning, subsiding later in the day. The duration of morning stiffness is a useful indicator of disease activity. Stiffness may recur after daytime inactivity and be much more severe after strenuous activity. Although any joint may be affected, the PIP and MCP joints of the fingers as well as the wrists, knees, ankles, and toes are most often involved. Monarticular disease is occasionally seen early. Synovial cysts and rupture of tendons may occur. Entrapment syndromes are not unusual—particularly of the median nerve at the carpal tunnel of the wrist. Palmar erythema is noted occasionally, as are tiny hemorrhagic infarcts in the nail folds or finger pulps. Twenty percent of patients have subcutaneous nodules, most commonly situated over bony prominences but also observed in the bursas and tendon sheaths. Nodules correlate with the presence of rheumatoid factor in serum ("seropositivity"), as do most other extra-articular manifestations. Dryness of the eyes, mouth, and other mucous membranes is found especially in advanced disease (see Sjögren's Syndrome). Other ocular manifestations include episcleritis and scleromalacia, the latter due to scleral nodules and capable of causing retinal detachment. Pericarditis and pleural disease, when present, are frequently silent clinically. Nonspecific pericarditis and pleuritis are found in 25–40% of patients at autopsy. Additional nonspecific lesions associated with rheumatoid arthritis include inflammation of small arteries, pulmonary fibrosis, mononuclear cell infiltration of skeletal muscle and perineurium, and hyperplasia of lymph nodes. Aortitis is a rare late complication that can result in aortic regurgitation or rupture and is usually associated with evidence of rheumatoid vasculitis elsewhere in the body.

After months or years, deformities may occur; the most common are ulnar deviation of the fingers, boutonnière deformity (hyperextension of the DIP joint with flexion of the PIP joint), "swan-neck" deformity (flexion of the DIP joint with extension of the PIP joint), and valgus deformity of the knee. Atrophy of skin or muscle is common, caused by the combined effects of disease and treatment (particularly prednisone). A small number of patients have splenomegaly and lymph node enlargement. A small subset of patients with rheumatoid arthritis have Felty's syndrome, the occurrence of splenomegaly and neutropenia, usually in the setting of severe, destructive arthritis. Felty's syndrome must be distinguished from the large granular lymphocyte syndrome, with which it shares many features.

B. LABORATORY FINDINGS

Serum protein abnormalities are often present. The most specific blood test for rheumatoid arthritis is antibody to cyclic citrullinated peptide (specificity ~95%). However, in early disease the CCP antibody has a sensitivity of only 50%. Rheumatoid factor, an IgM antibody directed against the Fc fragment of IgG, is present in the sera of more than 75% of patients and has a specificity of approximately 90%. High titers of rheumatoid factor are commonly associated with severe rheumatoid disease. Titers may also be significantly elevated in a number of diverse conditions, including syphilis, sarcoidosis, infective endocarditis, tuberculosis, leprosy, and parasitic infections. The prevalence of seropositivity also rises with age in healthy individuals. Asymptomatic relatives of patients with autoimmune diseases are more likely to be rheumatoid factor positive as well. Antinuclear antibodies are demonstrable in 20% of patients, although their titers are lower than in SLE.

During both the acute and chronic phases, the ESR and the immune globulins (most commonly IgM and IgG) are typically elevated. A moderate hypochromic normocytic anemia is common. The white cell count is normal or slightly elevated, but leukopenia may occur, often in the presence of splenomegaly (eg, Felty's syndrome). The platelet count is often elevated, roughly in proportion to the severity of overall joint inflammation. Joint fluid examination is valuable, reflecting abnormalities that are associated with varying degrees of inflammation. (See Tables 20–1 and 20–2.)

C. IMAGING

Of all the laboratory tests, x-ray changes are the most specific for rheumatoid arthritis. X-rays performed during the first 6 months of symptoms, however, are usually normal. The earliest changes occur in the wrists or feet and consist of soft tissue swelling and juxta-articular demineralization. Later, diagnostic changes of uniform joint space narrowing and erosions develop. The erosions are often first evident at the ulnar styloid and at the juxta-articular margin, where the bony surface is not protected by cartilage. Diagnostic changes also occur in the cervical spine, with C1–2 subluxation, but these changes usually take many years to develop. Both MRI and ultrasonography are more sensitive than radiographs in detecting bony and soft tissue changes in rheumatoid arthritis. However, the value of MRI and ultrasound in early diagnosis relative to that of plain radiographs, particularly given cost considerations, has not been established.

Differential Diagnosis

The differentiation of rheumatoid arthritis from other joint conditions and immune-mediated disorders can be difficult. However, certain clinical features are helpful. Osteoarthritis, for example, spares the wrist and the MCP joints, in contrast to rheumatoid arthritis. Degenerative joint disease (osteoarthritis) is not associated with constitutional manifestations and the joint pain is characteristically relieved by rest, unlike the morning stiffness of rheumatoid arthritis. Signs of articular inflammation, prominent in rheumatoid arthritis, are usually minimal in degenerative joint disease. Although gouty arthritis is almost always intermittent and monarticular in the early years, it may evolve with time into a chronic polyarticular process that mimics rheumatoid arthritis. Gouty tophi resemble rheumatoid nodules both in typical location and appearance. The early history of intermittent monarthritis and the presence of synovial urate crystals are distinctive features of gout. Septic arthritis can be distinguished by chills and fever, demonstration of the causative organism in joint fluid, and the frequent presence of a primary focus elsewhere, eg, gonococcal arthritis. Septic arthritis can complicate rheumatoid arthritis and should be considered whenever a patient with rheumatoid arthritis has one joint inflamed out of proportion to the rest. Lyme disease typically involves only one joint, most commonly the knee, and is associated with positive serologic tests (see Chapter 34). Human parvovirus B19 infection in adults can occasionally mimic rheumatoid arthritis. The mean age at onset is approximately 35 years. Arthralgias are much more prominent than arthritis, and rash—on the cheeks, torso, or extremities—is common. The patients are rheumatoid factor–negative, do not have erosions, and have IgM antibodies to human parvovirus B19 infection.

Malar rash, photosensitivity, discoid skin lesions, alopecia, high titer antibodies to double-stranded DNA, glomerulonephritis, and central nervous system abnormalities point to the diagnosis of SLE. Polymyalgia rheumatica occasionally causes polyarthralgias in patients over age 50, but these patients remain rheumatoid factor–negative and have chiefly proximal muscle pain and stiffness, centered on the shoulder and hip girdles. Rheumatic fever is characterized by the migratory nature of the arthritis, an elevated antistreptolysin titer, and a more dramatic and prompt response to aspirin; carditis and erythema marginatum may occur in adults, but chorea and subcutaneous nodules virtually never do. Finally, a variety of cancers produce paraneoplastic syndromes, including polyarthritis. One form is hypertrophic pulmonary osteoarthropathy most often produced by lung and gastrointestinal carcinomas, characterized by a rheumatoid-like arthritis associated with clubbing, periosteal new bone formation, and a negative rheumatoid factor. Diffuse swelling of the hands with palmar fasciitis occurs in a variety of cancers, especially ovarian carcinoma.

Treatment

A. BASIC PROGRAM (NONPHARMACOLOGIC MANAGEMENT)

The primary objectives in treating rheumatoid arthritis are reduction of inflammation and pain, preservation of function, and prevention of deformity. Patient satisfaction and the success of therapy depend on how effectively the clinician utilizes the nonpharmacologic measures outlined in the following paragraphs.

1. Education and emotional factors—The clinician should explain the disease, describe its fluctuations, and involve the patient and family in decisions about therapy.

2. Physical and occupational therapies—Physical and occupational therapists understand nonpharmacologic treatments of arthritis (described below) and can effectively teach them. The therapist can develop a program the patient can follow at home, with only periodic monitoring.

3. Systemic rest—The amount of systemic rest required depends on the presence and severity of inflammation. With mild inflammation, 2 hours of rest each day may suffice. In general, rest should be continued until significant improvement is sustained for at least 2 weeks; thereafter, the program may be liberalized. However, the increase of physical activity must proceed gradually and with appropriate support for any involved weight-bearing joints.

4. Articular rest—Decrease of articular inflammation may be expedited by joint rest. Relaxation and stretching of the hip and knee muscles, to prevent flexion contractures, can be accomplished by having the patient lie in the prone position for 15 minutes several times daily. Sitting in a flexed position for prolonged periods is a poor form of joint rest. Appropriate adjustable supports provide rest for inflamed weight-bearing joints, relieve spasm, and may reduce deformities, soft tissue contracture, or instability of the ligaments. The supports must be removable to permit daily range of motion and exercise of the affected extremities (see below).

5. Exercise—Exercises are designed to preserve joint motion, muscular strength, and endurance. Initially, for inflammatory disease, passive range of motion and isometric exercises (such as straight leg raising) are best tolerated. In hydrotherapy, the buoyancy of water permits maximum isotonic and isometric exercise with no more stress on joints than active range of motion exercises. As tolerance for exercise increases and the activity of the disease subsides, progressive resistance exercises may be introduced. Patients should follow the general rule of eliminating any exercise that produces increased pain 1 hour after the exercise has ended.

6. Heat and cold—These are used primarily for their muscle-relaxing and analgesic effects. Radiant or moist heat is generally most satisfactory. Exercise may be better performed after exposure to heat. Some patients derive more relief of joint pain from local application of cold.

7. Assistive devices—Patients with significant hip or knee arthritis may benefit from having an elevated toilet, a gripping bar, or a cane. Patients hold the cane in the hand opposite to the affected knee or hip, thus leaning away from the affected joint. Crutches or walkers may be needed for patients with more extensive disease.

8. Splints—Splints may provide joint rest, reduce pain, and prevent contracture, but their use should be guided by certain principles.

a. Night splints of the hands or wrists (or both) should maintain the extremity in the position of optimum function. The elbow and shoulder lose motion so rapidly that other local measures and corticosteroid injections are usually preferable to splints.

b. The best "splint" for the hip is prone-lying for several hours a day on a firm bed. For the knee, pronelying may suffice, but splints in maximum tolerated extension are frequently needed. Ankle splints are of the simple right-angle type.

c. Splints should be applied for the shortest period needed, should be made of lightweight materials for comfort, and should be easily removable for range-of-motion exercises once or twice daily to prevent loss of motion.

d. Corrective splints, such as those for overcoming knee flexion contractures, should be used under the guidance of a clinician familiar with their proper use.

Note: Avoidance of prolonged sitting or knee pillows may decrease the need for splints.

9. Weight loss—For overweight patients, achieving ideal body weight will reduce the wear and tear placed on arthritic joints of the lower extremities.

B. NONSTEROIDAL ANTI-INFLAMMATORY DRUGS

The first drug used to treat rheumatoid arthritis is an NSAID. These agents have analgesic and anti-inflammatory effects but do not prevent erosions or alter disease progression. A number of NSAIDs are available, including aspirin, ibuprofen, naproxen, sulindac, diclofenac, nabumetone, etodolac, ketoprofen, celecoxib, and others.

NSAIDs work in arthritis by the same mechanism that causes side effects: inhibition of COX, the enzyme that converts arachidonic acid to prostaglandins. Although prostaglandins play important roles in promoting inflammation and pain, they also help maintain homeostasis in several organs—especially the stomach, where prostaglandin E serves as a local hormone responsible for gastric mucosal cytoprotection. The discovery that COX exists in two isomers—COX-1 (which is expressed continuously in many cells and is responsible for the salutary effects of prostaglandins) and COX-2 (which is induced by cytokines and expressed in inflammatory tissues)—was initially of little practical consequence since all traditional NSAIDs inhibit both isomers.

However, selective COX-2 inhibitors (eg, celecoxib) are FDA-approved for the treatment of osteoarthritis and rheumatoid arthritis. Compared with traditional NSAIDs, COX-2 inhibitors are as effective for treating rheumatoid arthritis but less likely in some circumstances to cause upper gastrointestinal tract adverse events (eg, obstruction, perforation, hemorrhage, or ulceration). Long-term use of COX-2 inhibitors, particularly in the absence of concomitant aspirin use, has been associated with an increased risk of cardiovascular events, leading to the removal of some COX-2 inhibitors from the market and intense scrutiny of all drugs in that class.

1. Gastrointestinal side effects—In terms of efficacy, all NSAIDs appear equivalent. Anecdotes suggest that indomethacin is more effective than other NSAIDs for ankylosing spondylitis (see below). For rheumatoid arthritis, no NSAID is convincingly more effective than another.

For traditional NSAIDs that inhibit both COX-1 and COX-2, gastrointestinal side effects, such as gastric ulceration, perforation, and gastrointestinal hemorrhage, are the most common serious side effects. The overall rate of bleeding with NSAID use in the general population is low (1:6000 users or less) but is increased by long-term use, higher NSAID dose, concomitant corticosteroids or anticoagulants, the presence of rheumatoid arthritis, history of peptic ulcer disease or alcoholism, and age over 70. Twenty-five percent of all hospitalizations and deaths from peptic ulcer disease result from traditional NSAID therapy. Each year, 1:1000 patients with rheumatoid arthritis will require hospitalization for NSAID-related gastrointestinal bleeding or perforation. Although all traditional NSAIDs can cause massive gastrointestinal bleeding, the risk may be higher with indomethacin and piroxicam, probably because these drugs preferentially inhibit COX-1 in the stomach.

There are two approaches to reducing the gastrointestinal toxicity of NSAIDs. One approach is to use a traditional NSAID and add either a proton pump inhibitor (eg, omeprazole 20 mg orally daily), famotidine 40 mg orally twice daily, or misoprostol. The efficacy of misoprostol is limited by its poor tolerability; 20% of patients discontinue the medication because of diarrhea and bloating associated with full doses (200 mcg orally four times daily). Giving smaller amounts of misoprostol (eg, 100 mcg four times daily) or using less frequent dosing (eg, 200 mcg twice daily) improves tolerance while reducing efficacy only modestly. Misoprostol is an abortifacient and is contraindicated in patients who are or might become pregnant. Sucralfate, antacids, and ranitidine either do not work or do not work as well as proton pump inhibitors. The expense of proton pump inhibitors and misoprostol dictates that their use should be reserved for patients with risk factors for NSAID-induced gastrointestinal toxicity (noted above). Patients who have recently recovered from an NSAID-induced bleeding gastric ulcer appear to be at high risk for rebleeding (about 5% in 6 months) when an NSAID is reintroduced, even if prophylactic measures such as proton pump inhibitors are used. NSAIDs can also affect the lower intestinal tract, causing perforation or aggravating inflammatory bowel disease.

Acute liver injury from NSAIDs is rare, occurring in about 1 of every 25,000 patients using these agents. Having rheumatoid arthritis or taking sulindac may increase the risk.

2. Renal side effects—All of the NSAIDs, including aspirin and the COX-2 inhibitors, can produce renal toxicity, including interstitial nephritis, nephrotic syndrome, prerenal azotemia, and aggravation of hypertension. Hyperkalemia due to hyporeninemic hypoaldosteronism may also be seen. The risk of renal toxicity is low but is increased by age over 60, a history of renal disease, congestive heart failure, ascites, and diuretic use. COX-2 inhibitors appear to cause as much nephrotoxicity as traditional NSAIDs.

3. Platelet effects—All NSAIDs except the nonacetylated salicylates and the COX-2 inhibitors interfere with platelet function and prolong bleeding time. For all older NSAIDs except aspirin, the effect on bleeding time resolves as the drug is cleared. Aspirin irreversibly inhibits platelet function, so the bleeding time effect resolves only as new platelets are made. COX-2 inhibitors, which differ from other NSAIDs in not inhibiting platelet function, do not increase the risk of bleeding with surgical procedures as most NSAIDs do. Unfortunately, this failure to inhibit platelets is now known to lead to increased risks of myocardial infarc-

tion and stroke, particularly when the medications are used in high doses for prolonged periods of time. Patients requiring low-dose aspirin who are not compliant have a greater risk of developing a thrombotic event while taking a "coxib" than while taking a traditional NSAID. Whether combination therapy with low-dose aspirin and a coxib maintains the gastrointestinal advantage of selective COX-2 inhibitors is not yet known.

Although groups of patients with rheumatoid arthritis respond similarly to NSAIDs, individuals may respond differently—an NSAID that works for one patient may not work for another. Thus, if the first NSAID chosen is not effective after 2–3 weeks of use, another should be tried.

C. ADDITIONAL DRUGS

Disease-modifying antirheumatic drugs (DMARDs) should be started as soon as the diagnosis of rheumatoid disease is certain.

1. Methotrexate—Methotrexate is usually the treatment of choice for patients with rheumatoid arthritis who do not respond to NSAIDs. Methotrexate is generally well tolerated and often produces a beneficial effect in 2–6 weeks—compared with the 2- to 6-month onset of action for drugs such as gold, penicillamine, and antimalarials. The usual initial dose is 7.5 mg of methotrexate orally once weekly. If the patient has tolerated methotrexate but has not responded in 1 month, the dose can be increased to 15 mg orally once per week. The maximal dose is approximately 25 mg/wk. The most frequent side effects are gastric irritation and stomatitis. If needed to minimize gastrointestinal toxicity, methotrexate can be administered by subcutaneous or intramuscular injection. A severe, potentially life-threatening interstitial pneumonitis occurs rarely and usually responds to cessation of the drug and institution of corticosteroids. Hepatotoxicity with fibrosis and cirrhosis is another important toxic effect that appears to be very rare, with a risk of approximately 1:1000 after 5 years of methotrexate therapy. Still, methotrexate is contraindicated in a patient with any form of chronic hepatitis. Diabetes, obesity, and renal disease increase the risk of hepatotoxicity. Liver function tests should be monitored every 4–8 weeks, along with the complete blood count, serum creatinine, and serum albumin. Heavy alcohol use increases the hepatotoxicity, so patients should be advised to drink alcohol in extreme moderation, if at all. In a patient with no risk factors for hepatotoxicity, liver biopsy is not needed initially but is performed if aminotransferase levels are elevated, despite dosage reduction, in 6 out of 12 monthly determinations or if the serum albumin falls below normal. Cytopenia due to bone marrow suppression and infection are other important potential problems. The risk of developing cytopenia is much higher in patients with a serum creatinine of 2 mg/dL or higher. Side effects, including hepatotoxicity, may be reduced by prescribing either daily folate (1 mg) or weekly leucovorin calcium (2.5–5 mg taken 24 hours after the dose of methotrexate). Methotrexate is associated with an increased risk of B cell lymphomas, some of which resolve following the discontinuation of the medication. The combination of methotrexate and other folate antagonists, such as trimethoprim-sulfamethoxazole, should be used cautiously, since pancytopenia can result. Probenecid should also be avoided since it increases methotrexate drug levels and toxicity.

2. Tumor necrosis factor inhibitors—Inhibitors of tumor necrosis factor (TNF) are fulfilling the aim of targeted therapy for rheumatoid arthritis. These medications are frequently added to the treatment of patients who have not responded adequately to methotrexate, and increasingly are added simultaneously with methotrexate for patients with poor prognostic factors. TNF—a cytokine central to the inflammatory cascade in rheumatoid arthritis—activates lymphocytes and leukocytes, stimulates the elaboration of other cytokines, and is found in elevated concentrations in rheumatoid synovium. Three inhibitors are in use: etanercept, infliximab, and adalimumab. Etanercept, a soluble recombinant TNF receptor:Fc fusion protein, is administered at a dosage of 25 mg subcutaneously twice weekly or 50 mg once per week. Infliximab, a chimeric monoclonal antibody, is administered at a dosage of 3–10 mg/kg intravenously initially and then repeated after 2, 6, 10, and 14 weeks. Adalimumab, a recombinant monoclonal antibody that binds to TNF receptor sites, and is given at a dosage of 40 mg subcutaneously every other week. Each drug produces substantial improvement in more than 60% of patients. Each is usually very well tolerated. Minor irritation at injection sites is the most common side effect of etanercept and adalimumab. Rarely, nonrecurrent leukopenia develops in patients. The use of TNF blockers reduces the need for prednisone, thereby avoiding or attenuating some of the major side effects of corticosteroids. TNF plays a physiologic role in combating many types of infection; TNF inhibitors have been associated with an increased risk of certain opportunistic infections, such as tuberculosis. Screening for latent tuberculosis (see Chapter 9) is now recommended before the initiation of TNF blockers. It is prudent to suspend TNF blockers when a fever or other manifestations of a clinically important infection develops in a patient. Demyelinating neurologic complications that resemble multiple sclerosis have been reported rarely in patients taking TNF inhibitors, but the true magnitude of this risk—likely quite small—has not been determined with precision. Contrary to expectation, TNF inhibitors were not effective in the treatment of congestive heart failure. The use of infliximab, in fact, was associated with increased morbidity in a congestive heart failure trial. Consequently, TNF inhibitors should be used with extreme caution in patients with congestive heart failure. Infliximab can rarely cause anaphylaxis and induce anti-DNA antibodies (but rarely clinically evident SLE). A final concern about TNF inhibitors is the expense, which is more than $10,000 per year.

3. Antimalarials—Hydroxychloroquine sulfate is the antimalarial agent most often used against rheumatoid arthritis. Monotherapy with hydroxychloroquine should be reserved for patients with mild disease because only 25–50% will respond and in some of those cases only after 3–6 months of therapy. Hydroxychloroquine is often used in combination with other conventional DMARDs, particularly methotrexate and sulfasalazine. The advantage of hydroxychloroquine is its comparatively low toxicity, especially at a dosage of 200–400 mg/d orally (not to exceed 6.5 mg/kg/d). The most important reaction, pigmentary retinitis causing visual loss, is rare at this dose. Ophthalmologic examinations every 6–12 months are required when this drug is used for long-term therapy. Other reactions include neuropathies and myopathies of both skeletal and cardiac muscle, which usually improve when the drug is withdrawn.

4. Corticosteroids—These drugs usually produce an immediate and dramatic anti-inflammatory effect in rheumatoid arthritis, and they may be able to slow the rate of bony destruction. However, their multitudinous side effects greatly limit their long-term use, particularly in doses > 5.0–7.5 mg/d orally of prednisone.

Corticosteroids may be used on a short-term basis to tide patients over acute disabling episodes, to facilitate other treatment measures (eg, physical therapy), or to manage serious extra-articular manifestations (eg, pericarditis, necrotizing scleritis). They may also be indicated for active and progressive disease that does not respond favorably to conservative management and when there are contraindications to or therapeutic failure of methotrexate, gold salts, or other disease-modifying agents.

No more than 10 mg of prednisone or equivalent per day is appropriate for articular disease. Many patients do reasonably well on 5–7.5 mg daily. (The use of 1 mg tablets, to facilitate doses of < 5 mg/d, is encouraged.) When the corticosteroids are to be discontinued, they should be tapered gradually on a planned schedule appropriate to the duration of treatment. All patients receiving long-term corticosteroid therapy should take measures to prevent osteoporosis.

Intra-articular corticosteroids may be helpful if one or two joints are the chief source of difficulty. Intra-articular triamcinolone, 10–40 mg depending on the size of the joint to be injected, may be given for symptomatic relief, but not more than four times a year.

5. Sulfasalazine—This drug is a second-line agent for rheumatoid arthritis. It is usually introduced at a dosage of 0.5 g orally twice daily and then increased each week by 0.5 g until the patient improves or the daily dose reaches 3 g. Side effects, particularly neutropenia and thrombocytopenia, occur in 10–25% and are serious in 2–5%. Sulfasalazine also causes hemolysis in patients with glucose-6-phosphate dehydrogenase (G6PD) deficiency, so a G6PD level should be checked before initiating sulfasalazine. Patients taking sulfasalazine should have complete blood counts monitored every 2–4 weeks for the first 3 months, then every 3 months.

6. Leflunomide—Leflunomide, a pyrimidine synthesis inhibitor, is also FDA-approved for treatment of rheumatoid arthritis. It can be used alone or combined with methotrexate. Administration is started at a dosage of 100 mg/d orally for 3 days followed by a maintenance dosage of 20 mg daily. The most frequent side effects are diarrhea, rash, reversible alopecia, and hepatotoxicity. Some patients experience dramatic unexplained weight loss. The drug is carcinogenic, teratogenic, and has a half-life of 2 weeks. Thus, it is contraindicated in premenopausal women or in men who wish to father children.

7. Minocycline—Minocycline is more effective than placebo for rheumatoid arthritis. It is reserved for early, mild cases, since its efficacy is modest, and it works better during the first year of rheumatoid arthritis. The mechanism of action is not clear, but tetracyclines do have anti-inflammatory properties, including the ability to inhibit destructive enzymes such as collagenase. The dosage of minocycline is 200 mg daily. Adverse effects are uncommon except for dizziness, which occurs in about 10%.

8. Combination therapy—Certain combinations of two or more DMARDs have been shown to be effective in treating rheumatoid arthritis. The most common combination therapy has been methotrexate with one of the anti-TNF agents. Combination therapy has been traditionally reserved for patients who have not responded adequately to individual agents. Recent studies suggest that combination therapy produces superior results to sequential monotherapy. If the benefits of combination therapy and the long-term safety of biologic agents are confirmed, then combination therapy will become the initial treatment of choice for patients with rheumatoid arthritis.

D. Other Therapies

Anakinra, a recombinant form of human IL-1 receptor antagonist, may be given to adult patients who have failed one or more DMARDs. Anakinra can be used alone or in combination with DMARDs other than TNF-blocking agents. This drug must be administered daily by subcutaneous injection. The efficacy of anakinra is generally less than that of TNF inhibitors. Because anakinra has been associated with an increased incidence of serious infection, it should be discontinued whenever suggestive symptoms develop.

Experiments have documented the efficacy of blocking T cell activation with proteins that prevent the interaction of T cells and antigen presenting cells. Abatacept, a recombinant protein made by fusing a fragment of the Fc domain of human IgG with the extracellular domain of a T cell inhibitory molecule (CTLA4), is a new medication based on this approach that has received FDA approval for use in rheumatoid arthritis. Finally, clinical trials of therapies designed to deplete B cells in rheumatoid arthritis are under way.

E. Surgical Measures

See section on Some Orthopedic Procedures for Arthritic Joints at the end of this chapter.

Course & Prognosis

Determining the best initial treatment is difficult because patients in whom rheumatoid arthritis is suspected can follow two widely divergent courses. Of all patients who present with polyarthritis that appears to be (but probably is not) rheumatoid arthritis, 50–75% experience remission within 2 years. These patients are often negative for antibody to cyclic citrullinated peptide or rheumatoid factor, have good functional status even during disease activity, and are commonly seen in community practices but rarely in academic centers. Clearly, conservative therapy makes good sense for this patient population.

For patients whose joint symptoms persist beyond 2 years, the outcome is not so favorable. Patients in this group are known to have shorter longevity, dying on average 10–15 years earlier than people without rheumatoid arthritis. The impact of more effective therapies, such as the combination of methotrexate and biologic agents, on these data is not clear. The most common causes of death are infection, respiratory or renal failure, and gastrointestinal disease, many of which can be attributed in large part to complications of conventional DMARD use. In recent years, there has been a growing appreciation of the impact of cardiovascular mortality in rheumatoid arthritis, a complication likely associated with the disease process itself as well as the adverse effects of treatment. Factors that identify those at particular risk for early death include positive rheumatoid factor, poor functional status, more than 30 inflamed joints, and extra-articular manifestations (eg, rheumatoid lung disease). These patients, then, need aggressive therapy early, since extensive bone damage can occur during the first 2 years.

Since some patients with polyarthritis will remit and others will sustain substantial damage within the first 2 years, a guidepost for early decisions about aggressive treatment is needed. Patients who have polyarthritis lasting more than 12 weeks and who are seropositive for rheumatoid factor and cyclic citrullinated peptide are those at greatest risk for having persistent disease and are appropriate candidates for aggressive therapy. Although genetic risk factors for developing rheumatoid arthritis have been identified, it has not been possible in this way to consistently identify those patients needing aggressive therapy.

Edwards JC et al: Efficacy of B cell-targeted therapy with rituximab in patients with rheumatoid arthritis. N Engl J Med 2004;350:2572. [PMID: 15201414]

Genovese MC et al: Abatacept for rheumatoid arthritis refractory to tumor necrosis factor alpha inhibition. N Engl J Med 2005;353:1114. [PMID: 16162882]

Goekoop-Ruiterman YPM et al: Clinical and radiographic outcomes of four different treatment strategies in patients with early rheumatoid arthritis (the BeSt study): a randomized, controlled trial. Arthritis Rheum 2005;52:3381. [PMID: 16258899]

O'Dell JR: Therapeutic strategies for rheumatoid arthritis. N Engl J Med 2004;350:2591. [PMID: 15201416]

Quinn MA et al: Very early treatment with infliximab in addition to methotrexate in early, poor-prognosis rheumatoid arthritis. Arthritis Rheum 2005;52:27. [PMID: 15641102]

Raza K et al: Predictive value of antibodies to cyclic citrullinated peptide in patients with very early inflammatory arthritis. J Rheumatol 2005;32:231. [PMID: 15693082]

Wassenberg S et al: Very low-dose prednisolone in early rheumatoid arthritis retards radiographic progression over two years: a multicenter, double-blind, placebo-controlled trial. Arthritis Rheum 2005;52:3371. [PMID: 16255011]

ADULT STILL'S DISEASE

Still's disease is considered a variant of rheumatoid arthritis in which high spiking fevers are much more prominent, especially at the outset, than arthritis. This syndrome also occurs in adults. Most adults are in their 20s or 30s; onset after age 60 is rare. The fever is dramatic, often spiking to 40 °C, associated with sweats and chills, and then plunging to several degrees below normal. Many patients initially complain of sore throat. An evanescent salmon-colored nonpruritic rash, chiefly on the chest and abdomen, is a characteristic feature. However, the rash can easily be missed since it often appears only with the fever spike. Many patients also have lymphadenopathy and pericardial effusions. Joint symptoms are mild or absent in the beginning, but a destructive arthritis, especially of the wrists, may develop months later. Anemia and leukocytosis, with white blood counts sometimes exceeding 40,000/mcL, are the rule. Ferritin levels are exceptionally high (> 3000 mg/mL) in more than 70% of cases of adult Still's disease—for reasons that are not clear. A low percentage (< 20%) of serum ferritin that is glycosylated may be even more specific for adult Still's disease. Although the diagnosis requires exclusion of other causes of fever, the diagnosis of adult Still's disease is strongly suggested by the fever pattern, sore throat, and the classic rash. About half of the patients respond to high-dose aspirin (eg, 1 g three times orally daily) or other NSAIDs, and half require prednisone, sometimes in doses greater than 60 mg/d orally. TNF inhibitors may be helpful for some patients with refractory adult Still's disease, but most patients treated with these agents achieve only partial remissions. More complete and dramatic responses have been achieved with the IL-1 receptor antagonist anakinra.

Fautrel B et al: Tumor necrosis factor-alpha blocking agents in refractory adult Still's disease: An observational study of 20 cases. Ann Rheum Dis 2005;64:262. [PMID: 15184196]

Fitzgerald AA et al: Rapid responses to anakinra in patients with refractory adult-onset Still's disease. Arthritis Rheum 2005; 52:1794. [PMID: 15934079]

SYSTEMIC LUPUS ERYTHEMATOSUS

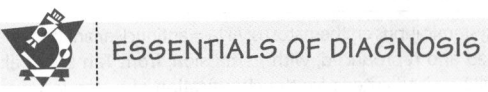

ESSENTIALS OF DIAGNOSIS

- *Occurs mainly in young women.*
- *Rash over areas exposed to sunlight.*
- *Joint symptoms in 90% of patients. Multiple system involvement.*
- *Depression of hemoglobin, white blood cells, platelets.*
- *Glomerulonephritis, central nervous system disease, and complications of antiphospholipid antibodies are major sources of disease morbidity.*
- *Serologic findings: antinuclear antibodies (100%), anti-native DNA antibodies (approximately two-thirds), and low serum complement levels (particularly during disease flares).*

General Considerations

SLE is an inflammatory autoimmune disorder that may affect multiple organ systems. Many of its clinical manifestations are secondary to the trapping of antigen-antibody complexes in capillaries of visceral structures or to autoantibody-mediated destruction of host cells (eg, thrombocytopenia). The clinical course is marked by spontaneous remission and relapses. The severity may vary from a mild episodic disorder to a rapidly fulminant, life-threatening illness.

The prevalence of SLE is influenced by many factors, including gender, race, and genetic inheritance. About 85% of patients are women. Sex hormones appear to play some role; most cases develop after menarche and before menopause. Among older individuals, the gender distribution is more equal. Race is also a factor, as SLE occurs in 1:1000 white women but in 1:250 black women. Familial occurrence of SLE has been repeatedly documented, and the disorder is concordant in 25–70% of identical twins. If a mother has SLE, her daughters' risks of developing the disease are 1:40 and her sons' risks are 1:250. Aggregation of serologic abnormalities (positive antinuclear antibody) is seen in asymptomatic family members, and the prevalence of other rheumatic diseases is increased among close relatives of patients. The importance of specific genes in SLE is emphasized by the high frequency of certain HLA haplotypes, especially DR2 and DR3, and null complement alleles. Genes that regulate programmed cell death (apoptosis) also appear to be important in the pathogenesis of SLE.

Before making a diagnosis of SLE, it is imperative to ascertain that the condition has not been induced by a drug. A host of pharmacologic agents have been implicated as causing a lupus-like syndrome, but only a few cause the disorder with appreciable frequency (Table 20–8). Procainamide, hydralazine, and isoniazid are the best-studied drugs. While antinuclear antibody tests and other serologic findings become positive in many persons receiving these agents, clinical manifestations occur in only a few.

Four features of drug-induced lupus separate it from SLE: (1) the sex ratio is nearly equal; (2) nephritis and central nervous system features are not ordinarily

Table 20–8. Drugs associated with lupus erythematosus.

Definite association	
Chlorpromazine	Methyldopa
Hydralazine	Procainamide
Isoniazid	Quinidine
Possible association	
β-Blockers	Nitrofurantoin
Captopril	Penicillamine
Carbamazepine	Phenytoin
Cimetidine	Propylthiouracil
Ethosuximide	Sulfasalazine
Levodopa	Sulfonamides
Lithium	Trimethadione
Methimazole	
Unlikely association	
Allopurinol	Penicillin
Chlorthalidone	Phenylbutazone
Gold salts	Reserpine
Griseofulvin	Streptomycin
Methysergide	Tetracyclines
Oral contraceptives	

Modified and reproduced, with permission, from Hess EV, Mongey AB: Drug-related lupus. Bull Rheum Dis 1991;40:1.

present; (3) hypocomplementemia and antibodies to native DNA are absent; and (4) the clinical features and most laboratory abnormalities often revert toward normal when the offending drug is withdrawn.

The diagnosis of SLE should be suspected in patients having a multisystem disease with serologic positivity (eg, antinuclear antibody, false-positive serologic test for syphilis). Differential diagnosis includes rheumatoid arthritis, systemic vasculitis, scleroderma, inflammatory myopathies, viral hepatitis, sarcoidosis, acute drug reactions, and drug-induced lupus.

The diagnosis of SLE can be made with reasonable probability if 4 of the 11 criteria set forth in Table 20–9 are met. These criteria, developed as guidelines for the inclusion of patients in research studies, do not supplant clinical judgment in the diagnosis of SLE.

Clinical Findings

A. SYMPTOMS AND SIGNS

The systemic features include fever, anorexia, malaise, and weight loss. Most patients have skin lesions at some time; the characteristic "butterfly" (malar) rash affects fewer than half of patients. Other cutaneous manifestations are discoid lupus, typical fingertip lesions, periungual erythema, nail fold infarcts, and splinter hemorrhages. Alopecia is common. Mucous membrane lesions tend to occur during periods of exacerbation. Raynaud's phenomenon, present in about 20% of patients, often antedates other features of the disease.

Joint symptoms, with or without active synovitis, occur in over 90% of patients and are often the earliest manifestation. The arthritis is seldom deforming; erosive changes are almost never noted on radiographs. Subcutaneous nodules are rare.

Ocular manifestations include conjunctivitis, photophobia, transient or permanent monocular blindness, and blurring of vision. Cotton-wool spots on the retina (cytoid bodies) represent degeneration of nerve fibers due to occlusion of retinal blood vessels.

Pleurisy, pleural effusion, bronchopneumonia, and pneumonitis are frequent. Restrictive lung disease is often demonstrated. Alveolar hemorrhage is rare, but potentially life-threatening.

The pericardium is affected in the majority of patients. Cardiac failure may result from myocarditis and hypertension. Cardiac arrhythmias are common. Atypical verrucous endocarditis of Libman-Sacks is usually clinically silent but occasionally can produce acute or chronic valvular incompetence—most commonly mitral regurgitation—and can serve as a source of emboli.

Mesenteric vasculitis occasionally occurs in SLE and may closely resemble polyarteritis nodosa, includ-

Table 20–9. Criteria for the classification of SLE. (A patient is classified as having SLE if any 4 or more of 11 criteria are met.)

1. Malar rash
2. Discoid rash
3. Photosensitivity
4. Oral ulcers
5. Arthritis
6. Serositis
7. Renal disease
   a. > 0.5 g/d proteinuria, or—
   b. ≥ 3+ dipstick proteinuria, or—
   c. Cellular casts
8. Neurologic disease
   a. Seizures, or—
   b. Psychosis (without other cause)
9. Hematologic disorders
   a. Hemolytic anemia, or—
   b. Leukopenia (< 4000/mcL), or—
   c. Lymphopenia (< 1500/mcL), or—
   d. Thrombocytopenia (< 100,000/mcL)
10. Immunologic abnormalities
    a. Positive LE cell preparation, or—
    b. Antibody to native DNA, or—
    c. Antibody to Sm, or—
    d. False-positive serologic test for syphilis
11. Positive ANA

SLE = systemic lupus erythematosus; ANA = antinuclear antibody. Modified and reproduced, with permission, from Tan EM et al: The 1982 revised criteria for the classification of systemic lupus erythematosus. Arthritis Rheum 1982;25:1271.

Table 20–10. Frequency (%) of autoantibodies in rheumatic diseases.

	ANA	Anti-Native DNA	Rheu-matoid Factor	Anti-Sm	Anti-SS-A	Anti-SS-B	Anti-SCL-70	Anti-Centro-mere	Anti-Jo-1	ANCA
Rheumatoid arthritis	30–60	0–5	80	0	0–5	0–2	0	0	0	0
Systemic lupus erythematosus	95–100	60	20	10–25	15–20	5–20	0	0	0	0–1
Sjögren's syndrome	95	0	75	0	65	65	0	0	0	0
Diffuse scleroderma	80–95	0	30	0	0	0	33	1	0	0
Limited sclero-derma (CREST syndrome)	80–95	0	30	0	0	0	20	50	0	0
Polymyositis/der-matomyositis	80–95	0	33	0	0	0	0	0	20–30	0
Wegener's granulomatosis	0–15	0	50	0	0	0	0	0	0	93–96[1]

[1]Frequency for generalized, active disease.
ANA = antinuclear antibodies; Anti-Sm = anti-Smith antibody; anti-SCHL-70 = anti-scleroderma antibody; ANCA = antineutrophil cytoplasmic antibody; CREST = calcinosis cutis, Raynaud's phenomenon, esophageal motility disorder, sclerodactyly, and telangiectasia.

ing the presence of aneurysms in medium-sized blood vessels. Abdominal pain (particularly postprandial), ileus, peritonitis, and perforation may result.

Neurologic complications of SLE include psychosis, organic brain syndrome, seizures, peripheral and cranial neuropathies, transverse myelitis, and strokes. Severe depression and psychosis are sometimes exacerbated by the administration of large doses of corticosteroids. Several forms of glomerulonephritis may occur, including mesangial, focal proliferative, diffuse proliferative, and membranous (see Chapter 22). Some patients may also have interstitial nephritis. With appropriate therapy, the survival rate even for patients with serious renal disease (proliferative glomerulonephritis) is favorable, albeit a substantial portion of patients with severe lupus nephritis still eventually require renal replacement therapy.

B. LABORATORY FINDINGS

(Tables 20–10, 20–11, and 19–2.) SLE is characterized by the production of many different autoantibodies, some of which produce specific laboratory abnormalities (eg, hemolytic anemia). Antinuclear antibody tests are sensitive but not specific for SLE—ie, they are positive in virtually all patients with lupus but are positive also in many patients with nonlupus conditions such as rheumatoid arthritis, various forms of hepatitis, and interstitial lung disease. Antibodies to double-stranded DNA and to Sm are specific for SLE but not sensitive, since they are present in only 60% and 30% of patients, respectively. Depressed serum complement—a finding suggestive of disease activity—often

returns toward normal in remission. Anti-double-stranded DNA antibody levels also correlate with disease activity in some patients; anti-Sm levels do not.

Three types of antiphospholipid antibodies occur (Table 20–11). The first causes the biologic false-posi-

Table 20–11. Frequency of laboratory abnormalities in systemic lupus erythematosus.

Anemia	60%
Leukopenia	45%
Thrombocytopenia	30%
Biologic false-positive tests for syphilis	25%
Antiphospholipid antibodies	
Lupus anticoagulant	7%
Anti-cardiolipin antibody	25%
Direct Coombs-positive	30%
Proteinuria	30%
Hematuria	30%
Hypocomplementemia	60%
ANA	95–100%
Anti-native DNA	50%
Anti-Sm	20%

ANA = antinuclear antibody; Anti-Sm = anti-Smith antibody.
Modified and reproduced, with permission, from Hochberg MC et al: Systemic lupus erythematosus: a review of clinicolaboratory features and immunologic matches in 150 patients with emphasis on demographic subsets. Medicine 1985;64:285.

tive tests for syphilis; the second is the lupus anticoagulant, which despite its name is a risk factor for venous and arterial thrombosis and miscarriage. It is most commonly identified by prolongation of the activated partial thromboplastin time, an in vitro phenomenon related to antibody reacting to phospholipid in the test materials. Anticardiolipin antibodies are the third type of antiphospholipid antibodies. In many cases, the "anticardiolipin antibody" appears to be directed at a serum cofactor (β_2-glycoprotein-I) rather than at phospholipid itself. Abnormality of urinary sediment is almost always found in association with renal lesions. Showers of red blood cells, with or without casts, and proteinuria (varying from mild to nephrotic range) are frequent during exacerbation of the disease; these usually abate with remission.

Treatment

Patient education and emotional support, as described for rheumatoid arthritis, are especially important for patients with lupus. Patients with drug-induced SLE usually respond to withdrawal of the offending agent. Since the various manifestations of idiopathic SLE affect prognosis differently and since SLE activity often waxes and wanes, drug therapy—both the choice of agents and the intensity of their use—must be tailored to match disease severity. Patients with photosensitivity should be cautioned against sun exposure and should apply a protective lotion to the skin while out of doors. Skin lesions often respond to the local administration of corticosteroids. Minor joint symptoms can usually be alleviated by rest and NSAIDs.

Antimalarials (hydroxychloroquine) may be helpful in treating lupus rashes or joint symptoms that do not respond to NSAIDs. When these are used, the dose should not exceed 400 mg/d (≤ 6.5 mg/kg/d), and biannual monitoring for retinal changes is recommended. Drug-induced neuropathy and myopathy may be erroneously ascribed to the underlying disease. The androgenic corticosteroid danazol may be effective therapy for thrombocytopenia not responsive to corticosteroids. Dehydroepiandrosterone (DHEA) has a therapeutic role comparable to that of the antimalarial agents in the treatment of SLE, but its side effects (particularly acne) are troubling to some patients.

Corticosteroids are required for the control of certain complications. (Systemic corticosteroids are not usually given for minor arthritis, skin rash, leukopenia, or the anemia associated with chronic disease.) Glomerulonephritis, hemolytic anemia, pericarditis or myocarditis, alveolar hemorrhage, central nervous system involvement, and thrombotic thrombocytopenic purpura all require corticosteroid treatment and often other interventions as well. Forty to 60 mg of oral prednisone is often needed initially; however, the lowest dose of corticosteroid that controls the condition should be used. Central nervous system lupus may require higher doses of corticosteroids than are usually given; however, corticosteroid psychosis may mimic

lupus cerebritis, in which case reduced doses are appropriate. Immunosuppressive agents such as cyclophosphamide, mycophenolate mofetil, and azathioprine are used in cases resistant to corticosteroids. Treatment of severe lupus nephritis includes an induction phase and a maintenance phase. Cyclophosphamide, which improves renal survival but not patient survival, was for many years the standard treatment for both phases of lupus nephritis. More recently, mycophenolate mofetil, which appears to be more effective and less toxic than cyclophosphamide, is emerging as the treatment of choice for many patients with lupus nephritis. Very close follow-up is needed to watch for potential side effects when immunosuppressants are given; these agents should be administered by physicians experienced in their use. When cyclophosphamide is required, gonadotropin-releasing hormone analogs can be given to protect a woman against the risk of premature ovarian failure. For patients with the antiphospholipid syndrome—the presence of antiphospholipid antibodies and compatible clinical events—anticoagulation is the treatment of choice. Moderate intensive anticoagulation with warfarin to achieve an INR of 2.0–3.0 is as effective as more intensive regimens. Pregnant patients with recurrent fetal loss associated with antiphospholipid antibodies should be treated with low-molecular-weight heparin plus aspirin.

Course & Prognosis

The prognosis for patients with systemic lupus appears to be considerably better than older reports implied. From both community settings and university centers, 10-year survival rates exceeding 85% are routine. In most patients, the illness pursues a relapsing and remitting course. Corticosteroids, often needed in doses of 40 mg/d or more during severe flares, can usually be tapered to low doses (5–10 mg/d) when the disease is inactive. However, there are some in whom the disease pursues a virulent course, leading to serious impairment of vital structures such as lung, heart, brain, or kidneys, and the disease may lead to death. With improved control of lupus activity and with increasing use of corticosteroids and immunosuppressive drugs, the mortality and morbidity patterns in lupus have changed. Mortality in SLE shows a bimodal pattern. In the early years after diagnosis, infections—especially with opportunistic organisms—are the leading cause of death, followed by active SLE, chiefly due to renal or central nervous system disease. In later years, accelerated atherosclerosis, attributed in part to corticosteroid use, becomes a major cause of death. Indeed, the incidence of myocardial infarction is five times higher in persons with SLE than in the general population. Therefore, it is especially important for SLE patients to avoid smoking and to minimize other conventional risk factors for atherosclerosis (eg, hypercholesterolemia, hypertension, obesity, and inactivity). Patients with SLE should receive influenza vaccination every year and pneumococcal vaccination every 5 years. Since some reports indicate that SLE patients have a higher risk of developing malignancy, preventive cancer screening recommendations should be followed assiduously. With more patients living longer, it has become evident that avascular necrosis of bone, affecting most commonly the hips and knees, is responsible for substantial morbidity. Still, the outlook for most patients with SLE has become increasingly favorable.

Arbuckle MR et al: Development of autoantibodies before the clinical onset of systemic lupus erythematosus. N Engl J Med 2003;349:1499. [PMID: 14561795]

Asanuma Y et al: Premature coronary-artery atherosclerosis in systemic lupus erythematosus. N Engl J Med 2003;349:2407. [PMID: 14681506]

Ginzler EM: Mycophenolate mofetil or intravenous cyclophosphamide for lupus nephritis. N Engl J Med 2005;353:2219. [PMID: 16306519]

Petri M et al: Combined oral contraceptives in women with systemic lupus erythematosus. N Engl J Med 2005;353:2550. [PMID: 16354891]

Somers EC et al: Use of a gonadotropin-releasing hormone analog for protection against premature ovarian failure during cyclophosphamide therapy in women with severe lupus. Arthritis Rheum 2005;52:2761. [PMID: 16142702]

ANTIPHOSPHOLIPID SYNDROME

ESSENTIALS OF DIAGNOSIS

- *Hypercoagulability, with recurrent thromboses in either the venous or arterial circulation.*
- *Thrombocytopenia is common.*
- *Pregnancy complications, specifically pregnancy losses after the first trimester.*
- *Lifelong anticoagulation with warfarin is recommended currently for patients with serious complications of this syndrome, as recurrent events are common.*

General Considerations

A primary **antiphospholipid antibody syndrome** (APS) is diagnosed in patients who have recurrent venous or arterial occlusions, recurrent fetal loss, or thrombocytopenia in the presence of antiphospholipid antibodies but not other features of SLE. In fewer than 1% of patients with antiphospholipid antibodies, a potentially devastating syndrome known as the "catastrophic antiphospholipid syndrome" occurs, leading to diffuse thromboses, thrombotic microangiopathy, and multiorgan system failure.

Clinical Findings

A. SYMPTOMS AND SIGNS

Patients are often asymptomatic until suffering a thrombotic complication of this syndrome. Thrombotic events may occur in either the arterial or venous circulations. Thus, deep venous thromboses, pulmonary emboli, cerebrovascular accidents are typical clinical events among patients with the APS. Budd-Chiari syndrome, cerebral sinus vein thrombosis, myocardial or digital infarctions, and other thrombotic events also occur. A variety of other symptoms and signs are often attributed to the APS, including mental status changes, livedo reticularis, skin ulcers, microangiopathic nephropathy, and cardiac valvular dysfunction—typically mitral regurgitation that may mimic Libman-Sacks endocarditis. Livedo reticularis is strongly associated with the subset of patients with APS in whom arterial ischemic events develop.

B. LABORATORY FINDINGS

As noted in the discussion of SLE, three types of antiphospholipid antibody are believed to contribute to this syndrome: (1) anti-cardiolipin antibodies; (2) a "lupus anticoagulant" that prolongs certain coagulation tests (see below); and (3) an antibody associated with a biologic false-positive test for syphilis (see Table 10–11). Anti-cardiolipin antibodies are typically measured with enzyme immunoassays for either IgG or IgM. In general, IgG anti-cardiolipin antibodies are believed to be more pathologic than IgM. A clue to the presence of a lupus anticoagulant, which may occur in individuals who do not have SLE, may be detected by a prolongation of the partial thromboplastin time (which, paradoxically, is associated with a thrombotic tendency rather than a bleeding risk). A finding more sensitive for a lupus anticoagulant, however, is prolongation of a specialized coagulation assay known as the Russell viper venom time (RVVT). In the presence of a lupus anticoagulant, the RVVT is prolonged and does not correct with mixing studies. With the last type of antiphospholipid antibody, the patient has a positive rapid plasma reagin (RPR), but negative specific anti-treponemal assays.

Differential Diagnosis

The exclusion of other autoimmune disorders, particularly those in the SLE spectrum, is essential, as such disorders may be associated with additional complications requiring alternative treatments. Other genetic or acquired conditions associated with hypercoagulability such as protein C, protein S, factor V Leiden, and antithrombin III deficiency should be excluded. The thrombocytopenia associated with APS must be distinguished from immune thrombocytopenic purpura. Catastrophic APS has a broad differential, including sepsis, pulmonary-renal syndromes, systemic vasculitis, disseminated intravascular coagulation, and thrombotic thrombocytopenic purpura.

Treatment

Present recommendations for anticoagulation are to treat patients with warfarin to maintain an INR of 2.0–3.0. Patients who have recurrent thrombotic events on this level of anticoagulation may require higher INRs (> 3.0), but the bleeding risk increases substantially with this degree of anticoagulation. Guidelines indicate that patients with APS should be treated with anticoagulation for life. Because of the teratogenic effects of warfarin, subcutaneous heparin and baby aspirin is the usual approach to prevent pregnancy complications in women with APS. In patients with catastrophic APS, a three-pronged approach is taken in the acute setting: intravenous heparin, high doses of corticosteroids, and either intravenous immune globulin or plasmapheresis.

Finazzi G et al: A randomized clinical trial of high-intensity warfarin vs. conventional antithrombotic therapy for the prevention of recurrent thrombosis in patients with the antiphospholipid syndrome (WAPS). J Thromb Haemost 2005;3:848. [PMID: 15869575]

Frances C et al: Dermatologic manifestations of the antiphospholipid syndrome: two hundred consecutive cases. Arthritis Rheum 2005;52:1785. [PMID: 15934071]

Trilolo G et al: Randomized study of subcutaneous low molecular weight heparin plus aspirin versus intravenous immunoglobulin in the treatment of recurrent fetal loss associated with antiphospholipid antibodies. Arthritis Rheum 2003;48:728. [PMID: 12632426]

Turiel M et al: Five-year follow-up by transesophageal echocardiographic studies in primary antiphospholipid syndrome. Am J Cardiol 2005;96:574. [PMID: 16098314]

SYSTEMIC SCLEROSIS (Scleroderma)

ESSENTIALS OF DIAGNOSIS

- *Widespread thickening of skin in diffuse systemic sclerosis, including truncal involvement, with areas of increased pigmentation and depigmentation.*
- *Thickening confined to the face and neck, distal arms, feet and hands in limited systemic sclerosis.*
- *Raynaud's phenomenon and antinuclear antibodies are present in virtually all patients.*
- *Systemic features of dysphagia, hypomotility of gastrointestinal tract, pulmonary fibrosis, and cardiac and renal involvement.*

General Considerations

Systemic sclerosis is a chronic disorder characterized by diffuse fibrosis of the skin and internal organs. The causes of systemic sclerosis are not known, but autoimmunity, fibroblast dysregulation, graft-versus-host disease from fetal lymphocytes retained in the maternal circulation, and occupational exposure to silica have been implicated. Symptoms usually appear in the third to fifth decades, and women are affected two to three times as frequently as men.

Two forms of systemic sclerosis are generally recognized: limited (80% of patients) and diffuse (20%).

Two bedside clues help distinguish the two subsets. First, in the CREST syndrome (representing calcinosis cutis, Raynaud's phenomenon, esophageal motility disorder, sclerodactyly, and telangiestasia), hardening of the skin (scleroderma) is limited to the face and hands. In contrast, in diffuse scleroderma, the skin changes also involve the trunk and proximal extremities. Second, tendon friction rubs, especially frequent over the wrists, ankles, and knees, occur uniquely (but not universally) in diffuse scleroderma. In general, patients with CREST syndrome have better outcomes than those with diffuse disease, largely because renal failure or interstitial lung disease rarely develops in patients with limited disease. Cardiac disease is also more characteristic of diffuse systemic sclerosis. Curiously, however, patients with limited disease are more susceptible to digital ischemia, leading to finger loss and to life-threatening pulmonary hypertension. Gastrointestinal involvement (gut hypomotility) may occur in both forms of systemic sclerosis, leading to such potentially serious complications as pseudoobstruction.

Clinical Findings

A. SYMPTOMS AND SIGNS

Most frequently, the disease makes its appearance in the skin, although visceral involvement may precede the cutaneous features. Polyarthralgia and Raynaud's phenomenon (present in 90% of patients) are early manifestations. Subcutaneous edema, fever, and malaise are common. With time the skin becomes thickened and hidebound, with loss of normal folds. Telangiectasia, pigmentation, and depigmentation are characteristic. Ulceration about the fingertips and subcutaneous calcification are seen. Dysphagia due to esophageal dysfunction is common and results from abnormalities in motility and later from fibrosis. Fibrosis and atrophy of the gastrointestinal tract cause hypomotility, and malabsorption results from bacterial overgrowth. Large-mouthed diverticuli occur in the jejunum, ileum, and colon. Diffuse pulmonary fibrosis and pulmonary vascular disease are reflected in restrictive lung physiology and low diffusing capacities. Cardiac abnormalities include pericarditis, heart block, myocardial fibrosis, and right heart failure secondary to pulmonary hypertension. Scleroderma renal crisis, resulting from obstruction of smaller renal blood vessels, is a marker for a poor outcome even though many cases can now be treated effectively with angiotensin-converting enzyme inhibitors.

B. LABORATORY FINDINGS

Mild anemia is often present. Among patients with severe renal disease, the peripheral blood smear can show findings consistent with a microangiopathic hemolytic anemia (because of mechanical damage to red cells from diseased small vessels). Elevation of the ESR is unusual. Proteinuria and cylindruria appear in association with renal involvement. Antinuclear antibody tests are nearly always positive, frequently in high titers (Tables 20–10 and 19–2). The scleroderma antibody (SCL-70) directed against topoisomerase III is found in one-third of patients with diffuse systemic sclerosis and in 20% of those with CREST syndrome; an anticentromere antibody is seen in 50% of those with CREST syndrome and in 1% of individuals with diffuse systemic sclerosis (Tables 20–10 and 19–2). Although present in only a minority of patients with diffuse systemic sclerosis, anti-Scl-70 antibodies may portend a poor prognosis, with a high likelihood of serious internal organ involvement (eg, interstitial lung disease). Anticentromere antibodies are highly specific for limited systemic sclerosis, but they also occur occasionally in overlap syndromes. Other scleroderma autoantibodies are those directed against RNA polymerases (anti-RNAP I, II, III) and B23. Anti-RNAP antibodies are associated with diffuse skin changes, cardiac and renal involvement, and increased mortality. Antibodies to B23 are associated with pulmonary hypertension.

Differential Diagnosis

Several diseases with principally cutaneous manifestations may mimic systemic sclerosis in their skin findings. These disorders include morphea and limited systemic sclerosis, two diseases often categorized as forms of "localized" scleroderma. These disorders are generally limited to circumscribed areas of the skin and usually have excellent outcomes. Morphea is associated with lavender plaques, typically located over the trunk. Linear scleroderma may be associated with atrophy of underlying muscle and bone and may cause deformities that are both cosmetically and functionally disabling.

Eosinophilic fasciitis is a rare disorder presenting with skin changes that resemble diffuse systemic sclerosis. The inflammatory abnormalities, however, are limited to the fascia rather than the dermis and epidermis. Moreover, patients with eosinophilic fasciitis are distinguished from those with systemic scleroderma by the presence of peripheral blood eosinophilia, the absence of Raynaud's phenomenon, the good response to prednisone, and an association (in some cases) with paraproteinemias.

The eosinophilia-myalgia syndrome was first noted in patients who ingested L-tryptophan, an essential amino acid once sold as an over-the-counter remedy for insomnia and premenstrual symptoms (before removal from the market). Since banning of L-tryptophan sales, the eosinophilia-myalgia syndrome has essentially disappeared.

Treatment

Treatment of systemic sclerosis is symptomatic and supportive. There is no medication that is known to alter the underlying disease process. However, interventions for management of specific organ manifestations of this disease have improved substantially. Severe Raynaud's syndrome may respond to calcium channel blockers, eg, long-acting nifedipine, 30–120 mg/d orally, or to losartan, 50 mg/d orally. Intravenous iloprost, a prostacyclin analog that causes vasodilation and platelet inhibition, is moderately effective in healing digital ulcers. Patients with esophageal disease should take medications in liquid or crushed form. Esophageal reflux can be reduced and the risk of scarring diminished by avoidance of late-night meals and elevation of the head of the bed. In addition, proton pump inhibitors (eg, omeprazole, 20–40 mg/d orally), the only drugs that achieve near-complete inhibition of gastric acid production, are remarkably effective for refractory esophagitis. Patients with delayed gastric emptying maintain their weight better if they eat small, frequent meals and remain upright for at least 2 hours after eating. Octreotide, a somatostatin analog, helps some patients with bacterial overgrowth and pseudoobstruction. Malabsorption due to bacterial overgrowth also responds to antibiotics, eg, tetracycline, 500 mg four times orally daily. The hypertensive crises associated with systemic sclerosis renal crisis must be treated early and aggressively (in the hospital) with angiotensin-converting enzyme inhibitors, eg, captopril, 37.5–75 mg/d orally in three divided doses. Prednisone has little or no role in the treatment of scleroderma. Cyclophosphamide, a drug with many important side effects, may improve severe interstitial lung disease. Bosentan, an endothelin receptor antagonist, improves exercise capacity and cardiopulmonary hemodynamics in patients with pulmonary hypertension and helps prevent digital ulceration.

The 9-year survival rate in scleroderma averages approximately 40%. The prognosis tends to be worse in those with diffuse scleroderma, in blacks, in males, and in older patients. In most cases, death results from renal, cardiac, or pulmonary failure. Those persons in whom severe internal organ involvement does not develop in the first 3 years have a substantially better prognosis, with 72% surviving at least 9 years. Breast and lung cancer may be more common in patients with scleroderma.

Girgis RE et al: Long-term outcome of bosentan treatment in idiopathic pulmonary arterial hypertension and pulmonary arterial hypertension associated with the scleroderma spectrum of diseases. J Heart Lung Transplant 2005;24:1626. [PMID: 16210140]

Herrick AL: Pathogenesis of Raynaud's phenomenon. Rheumatology (Oxford) 2005;44:587. [PMID: 15741200]

Ioannidis JP et al: Mortality in systemic sclerosis: an international meta-analysis of individual patient data. Am J Med 2005;118: 2. [PMID: 1563920]

Jimenez SA et al: Microchimerism and systemic sclerosis. Curr Opin Rheumatol 2005;17:86. [PMID: 15604910]

Korn JH et al: Digital ulcers in systemic sclerosis: prevention by treatment with bosentan, an oral endothelin receptor antagonist. Arthritis Rheum 2004;50:3985. [PMID: 15593188]

Steen VD: Autoantibodies in systemic sclerosis. Semin Arthritis Rheum 2005;35:35. [PMID: 16084222]

Steen V et al: Predictors of isolated pulmonary hypertension in patients with systemic sclerosis and limited cutaneous involvement. Arthritis Rheum 2003;48:516. [PMID: 12571862]

IDIOPATHIC INFLAMMATORY MYOPATHIES (Polymyositis & Dermatomyositis)

ESSENTIALS OF DIAGNOSIS

- Bilateral proximal muscle weakness.
- Characteristic cutaneous manifestations in dermatomyositis (Gottron's papules, heliotrope rash).
- Diagnostic tests: elevated creatine kinase and other muscle enzymes, muscle biopsy, electromyography.
- Increased risk of malignancy, particularly in adult dermatomyositis.
- Inclusion body myositis can mimic polymyositis but is less responsive to treatment.

General Considerations

Polymyositis and dermatomyositis are systemic disorders of unknown cause whose principal manifestation is muscle weakness. Although their clinical presentations (aside from the presence of certain skin findings in dermatomyositis, some of which are pathognomonic) and treatments are similar, the two diseases are pathologically quite distinct. They affect persons of any age group, but the peak incidence is in the fifth and sixth decades of life. Women are affected twice as commonly as men, and the diseases (particularly polymyositis) also occur more often among blacks than whites. There is an increased risk of malignancy, especially in adult patients with dermatomyositis. Indeed, up to one patient in four with dermatomyositis has an occult malignancy. Malignancies may be evident at the time of presentation with the muscle disease but may not be detected until months afterward in some cases. Rare patients with dermatomyositis have skin disease without overt muscle involvement, a condition termed "dermatomyositis sine myositis."

Clinical Findings

A. SYMPTOMS AND SIGNS

Polymyositis may begin abruptly, but the usual presentation is one of gradual and progressive muscle weakness. The weakness chiefly involves proximal muscle groups of the upper and lower extremities as well as the neck. Leg weakness (eg, difficulty in rising from a chair or climbing stairs) typically precedes arm symptoms. In contrast to myasthenia gravis, polymyositis and dermatomyositis do not cause facial or ocular muscle weakness. Pain and tenderness of affected muscles occur in one-fourth of cases, but these are rarely the chief complaints. About one-fourth of patients have dysphagia. In contrast to scleroderma, which affects the smooth muscle of the lower esophagus and can cause a "sticking" sensation below the sternum, polymyositis or dermatomyositis involves the striated muscles of the upper pharynx and can make initiation of deglutition difficult. Muscle atrophy and contractures occur as late complications of advanced disease. Clinically significant myocarditis is uncommon even though there is often creatine kinase-MB elevation. Patients who are bed-bound from myositis should be screened for respiratory muscle weakness that can be severe enough to cause CO_2 retention and to require mechanical ventilation.

In dermatomyositis, the characteristic rash is dusky red and may appear in a malar distribution mimicking the classic rash of SLE. Facial erythema beyond the malar distribution is also characteristic of dermatomyositis. Erythema also occurs over other areas of the face, neck, shoulders, and upper chest and back ("shawl sign"). Periorbital edema and a purplish (heliotrope) suffusion over the eyelids are typical signs. Periungual erythema, dilations of nailbed capillaries, and scaly patches over the dorsum of PIP and MCP joints (Gottron's sign) are highly suggestive. Scalp involvement by dermatomyositis may mimic psoriasis. Infrequently, the cutaneous findings of this disease precede the muscle inflammation by weeks or months. Diagnosing polymyositis in patients over age 70 years can be difficult because weakness may be overlooked or attributed erroneously to idiopathic frailty. Polymyositis can remain undiagnosed or will be misdiagnosed as hepatitis because of elevations in alanine aminotransferase (ALT) and aspartate aminotransferase (AST) levels. A subset of patients with polymyositis and dermatomyositis develop the "antisynthetase syndrome," a group of findings including inflammatory arthritis, Raynaud's phenomenon, interstitial lung disease, and often severe muscle disease associated with certain autoantibodies (eg, anti-Jo1 antibodies).

B. LABORATORY FINDINGS

Measurement of serum levels of muscle enzymes, especially creatine kinase and aldolase, is most useful in diagnosis and in assessment of disease activity. Anemia is uncommon. The ESR is not appreciably elevated in half of the patients. Rheumatoid factor is found in a minority of patients. Antinuclear antibodies are present in many patients, and anti-Jo-1 antibodies are seen in the subset of patients who have associated interstitial lung disease (Tables 20–10 and 19–2). Chest radiographs are usually normal, although interstitial fibrosis is occasionally seen. Electromyographic abnormalities consisting of polyphasic potentials, fibrillations, and high-frequency action potentials are helpful in establishing the diagnosis. None of the studies are specific. The search for an occult malignancy should begin with a history and physical examination, supplemented with a complete blood count, comprehensive biochemical panel, serum protein electrophoresis, and urinalysis, and should include age- and risk-appropriate cancer screening tests. If these evaluations are unrevealing, more invasive or extensive laboratory evaluations are probably not cost-effective. No matter how extensive the initial screening, some malignancies will not become evident for months after the initial presentation.

C. MUSCLE BIOPSY

Biopsy of clinically involved muscle is the only specific diagnostic test. The pathology findings in polymyositis and dermatomyositis are distinct. Although both include lymphoid inflammatory infiltrates, the findings in dermatomyositis are localized to perivascular regions and there is evidence of humoral and complement-mediated destruction of microvasculature associated with the muscle. In addition to its vascular orientation, the inflammatory infiltrate in dermatomyositis centers on the interfascicular septa and is located around, rather than in, muscle fascicles. A pathological hallmark of dermatomyositis is perifascicular atrophy. In contrast, the pathology of polymyositis characteristically includes endomysial infiltration of the inflammatory infiltrate. Owing to the sometimes patchy distribution of pathologic abnormalities, however, false-negative biopsies sometimes occur in both disorders.

Differential Diagnosis

Muscle inflammation may occur as a component of SLE, systemic sclerosis, Sjögren's syndrome, and overlap syndromes. In those cases, associated findings usually permit the precise diagnosis of the primary condition.

Inclusion body myositis, because of its tendency to mimic polymyositis, is a common cause of "treatment-resistant polymyositis." In contrast to the epidemiologic features of polymyositis, however, the typical inclusion body myositis patient is white, male, and over the age of 50. The onset of inclusion body myositis is even more insidious than that of polymyositis or dermatomyositis (eg, occurring over years rather than months), and asymmetric distal motor weakness is common in inclusion body myositis. Creatine phosphokinase (CPK) levels in inclusion body myositis are often minimally elevated and are normal in 25%. Muscle biopsy shows characteristic intracellular vacuoles by light microscopy either tubular or filamentous inclusions in the nucleus or cytoplasm by electron microscopy. Inclusion body myositis is less likely to respond to therapy and is associated with characteristic pathologic findings evident on frozen section or electron microscopy.

Hyperthyroidism and hypothyroidism may both be associated with proximal muscle weakness. Hypothyroidism is associated also with elevations of CPK. Patients with polymyalgia rheumatica are over the age of 50 and—in contrast to patients with polymyositis—have pain but no objective weakness. Disorders of the peripheral and central nervous systems (eg, chronic inflammatory polyneuropathy, multiple sclerosis, myasthenia gravis, Eaton-Lambert disease, and amyotrophic lateral sclerosis) can produce weakness but are distinguished by characteristic symptoms and neurologic signs and often by distinctive electromyographic abnormalities. A number of systemic vasculitides (polyarteritis nodosa, microscopic polyangiitis, the Churg-Strauss syndrome, Wegener's granulomatosis, and mixed cryoglobulinemia) can produce profound weakness through vasculitic neuropathy. The muscle weakness associated with these disorders, however, is typically distal and asymmetric, at least in the early stages.

Many drugs, including corticosteroids, alcohol, clofibrate, penicillamine, tryptophan, and hydroxychloroquine, can produce proximal muscle weakness. Chronic use of colchicine at doses as low as 0.6 mg twice a day in patients with moderate renal insufficiency can produce a mixed neuropathy-myopathy that mimics polymyositis. The weakness and muscle enzyme elevation reverse with cessation of the drug. HMG-CoA reductase inhibitors, which are frequently used to treat hypercholesterolemia, can cause myopathy and rhabdomyolysis. Although only about 0.1% of patients taking a statin drug alone develop myopathy, concomitant administration of other drugs (especially gemfibrozil, cyclosporine, niacin, macrolide antibiotics, azole antifungals, and protease inhibitors) increases the risk. Statin-induced muscle inflammation resolves after cessation of these medications. Polymyositis can occur as a complication of HIV or HTLV-I infection and with zidovudine therapy as well.

Treatment

Most patients respond to corticosteroids. Often a daily dose of 40–60 mg or more of oral prednisone is required initially. The dose is then adjusted downward according to the response of sequentially observed serum levels of muscle enzymes. Long-term use of corticosteroids is often needed, and the disease may recur or reemerge when they are withdrawn. Patients with an associated neoplasm have a poor prognosis, although remission may follow treatment of the tumor; corticosteroids may or may not be effective in these patients. In patients resistant or intolerant to corticosteroids, therapy with methotrexate or azathioprine may be helpful. Intravenous immune globulin has also been shown to be effective for dermatomyositis resistant to prednisone. TNFs do not appear to be effective in the inflammatory myopathies. Mycophenolate mofetil (1.0–1.5 g twice daily) may be useful as a steroid-sparing agent. B cell depletion therapies—eg, rituximab (either 375 mg/m^2 administered intravenously once weekly for 4 weeks, or 1 g/wk intravenously for 2 weeks)—are a promising avenue of current investigation.

Danko K et al: Long-term survival of patients with idiopathic inflammatory myopathies according to clinical features: a longitudinal study of 162 cases. Medicine 2004;83:35. [PMID: 14747766]

Edge JC et al: Mycophenolate mofetil as an effective corticosteroid-sparing therapy for recalcitrant dermatomyositis. Arch Dermatol 2006;142:65. [PMID: 16415388]

Troyanov Y et al: Novel classification of idiopathic inflammatory myopathies based on overlap syndrome features and autoantibodies: analysis of 100 French Canadian patients. Medicine (Baltimore) 2005;84:231. [PMID: 16010208]

OVERLAP (or Mixed) CONNECTIVE TISSUE DISEASE

Many patients with symptoms and signs compatible with a connective tissue disease have features consistent with more than one type of rheumatic disease. Special attention has been drawn to patients who have overlapping features of SLE, systemic sclerosis, and inflammatory myopathy. Initially, these patients were thought to have a distinct entity ("mixed connective tissue disease") defined by a specific autoantibody to ribonuclear protein (RNP). In many patients, the manifestations evolve to one predominant disease in time, such as scleroderma, and many patients with antibodies to RNP develop unequivocal SLE. Therefore, "overlap connective tissue disease" is the preferred designation for patients having features of different rheumatic diseases. Treatments are guided more by the distribution and severity of patients' organ system involvement than by therapies specific to these diverse syndromes.

Bodolay E et al: Five-year follow-up of 665 Hungarian patients with undifferentiated connective tissue disease (UCTD). Clin Exp Rheumatol 2003;21:313. [PMID: 12846049]

Wigley FM et al: The prevalence of undiagnosed pulmonary arterial hypertension in subjects with connective tissue disease at the secondary health care level of community-based rheumatologists (the UNCOVER study). Arthritis Rheum 2005;52:2125. [PMID: 15986394]

SJÖGREN'S SYNDROME

ESSENTIALS OF DIAGNOSIS

- *Ninety percent of patients are women; the average age is 50 years.*
- *Dryness of eyes and dry mouth (sicca components) are the most common features; they occur alone or in association with rheumatoid arthritis or other connective tissue disease.*
- *Rheumatoid factor and other autoantibodies common.*
- *Increased incidence of lymphoma.*

General Considerations

Sjögren's syndrome, an autoimmune disorder, is the result of chronic dysfunction of exocrine glands in many areas of the body. It is characterized by dryness of the eyes, mouth, and other areas covered by mucous membranes and is frequently associated with a rheumatic disease, most often rheumatoid arthritis. The disorder is predominantly a disease of women, in a ratio of 9:1, with greatest incidence between age 40 and 60 years.

Disorders with which Sjögren's syndrome is frequently associated include rheumatoid arthritis, SLE, primary biliary cirrhosis, scleroderma, polymyositis, Hashimoto's thyroiditis, polyarteritis, and interstitial pulmonary fibrosis. When Sjögren's syndrome occurs without rheumatoid arthritis, HLA-DR2 and -DR3 antigens are present with increased frequency.

Clinical Findings

A. SYMPTOMS AND SIGNS

Keratoconjunctivitis sicca results from inadequate tear production caused by lymphocyte and plasma cell infiltration of the lacrimal glands. Ocular symptoms are usually mild. Burning, itching, and the sensation of having a foreign body or a grain of sand in the eye occur commonly. For some patients, the initial manifestation is the inability to tolerate wearing contact lenses. Many patients with more severe ocular dryness notice ropy secretions across their eyes, especially in the morning. Photophobia may signal corneal ulceration resulting from severe dryness. For most patients, symptoms of dryness of the mouth (xerostomia) dominate those of dry eyes. Patients frequently complain of a "cotton mouth" sensation and difficulty swallowing foods, especially dry foods like crackers, unless they are washed down with liquids. The persistent oral dryness causes most patients to carry water bottles or other liquid dispensers from which they sip constantly. A few patients have such severe xerostomia that they have difficulty speaking. Persistent xerostomia results often in rampant dental carries; carries at the gum line strongly suggest Sjögren's syndrome. Some patients are most troubled by loss of taste and smell. Parotid enlargement, which may be chronic or relapsing, develops in one-third of patients. Desiccation may involve the nose, throat, larynx, bronchi, vagina, and skin.

Systemic manifestations include dysphagia, vasculitis, pleuritis, obstructive lung disease (in the absence of smoking), neuropsychiatric dysfunction (most commonly peripheral neuropathies), and pancreatitis; they may be related to the associated diseases noted above. Renal tubular acidosis (type I, distal) occurs in 20% of patients. Chronic interstitial nephritis, which may result in impaired renal function, may be seen. A glomerular lesion is rarely observed but may occur secondary to associated cryoglobulinemia.

B. LABORATORY FINDINGS

Laboratory findings include mild anemia, leukopenia, and eosinophilia. Polyclonal hypergammaglobulinemia, rheumatoid factor positivity (70%), and antinuclear antibodies (95%) are all common findings.

Antibodies against the cytoplasmic antigens SS-A and SS-B (also called Ro and La, respectively) are often present in Sjögren's syndrome and tend to correlate with the presence of extraglandular manifestations (Tables 20–10 and 19–2). Thyroid-associated autoimmunity is a common finding among patients with Sjögren's syndrome.

Useful ocular diagnostic tests include the Schirmer test, which measures the quantity of tears secreted. Lip biopsy, a simple procedure, is the only specific diagnostic technique and has minimal risk; if lymphoid foci are seen in accessory salivary glands, the diagnosis is confirmed. Biopsy of the parotid gland should be reserved for patients with atypical presentations such as unilateral gland enlargement.

Treatment & Prognosis

Treatment is symptomatic and supportive. Artificial tears applied frequently will relieve ocular symptoms and avert further desiccation. The mouth should be kept well lubricated. Sipping water frequently or using sugar-free gums and hard candies usually relieves dry mouth symptoms. Pilocarpine (5 mg orally four times daily) and the acetylcholine derivative cevimeline (30 mg orally three times daily) may improve xerostomia symptoms. Atropinic drugs and decongestants decrease salivary secretions and should be avoided. A program of oral hygiene, including fluoride treatment, is essential in order to preserve dentition. If there is an associated rheumatic disease, its systemic treatment is not altered by the presence of Sjögren's syndrome.

Although Sjögren's syndrome may compromise patients' quality of life significantly, the disease is usually consistent with a normal life span. Poor prognoses are influenced mainly by the presence of systemic features associated with underlying disorders, the development in some patients of lymphocytic vasculitis, the occurrence of a painful peripheral neuropathy, and the complication (in a minority of patients) of lymphoma. The patients (3–10% of the total Sjögren's population) at greatest risk for developing lymphoma are those with severe exocrine dysfunction, marked parotid gland enlargement, splenomegaly, vasculitis, peripheral neuropathy, anemia, and mixed monoclonal cryoglobulinemia.

Brito-Zeron P et al: Circulating monoclonal immunoglobulins in Sjögren syndrome: prevalence and clinical significance in 237 patients. Medicine (Baltimore) 2005;84:90. [PMID: 15758838]

Garcia-Carrasco M et al: Primary Sjögren syndrome: clinical and immunologic disease patterns in a cohort of 400 patients. Medicine (Baltimore) 2002;81:270. [PMID: 12169882]

Ono M et al: Therapeutic effect of cevimeline on dry eye in patients with Sjögren's syndrome: a randomized, double-blind clinical study. Am J Ophthalmol 2004;138:6. [PMID: 15234277]

Ramos-Casals M et al: Cutaneous vasculitis in primary Sjogren syndrome: classification and clinical significance of 52 patients. Medicine (Baltimore) 2004;83:96. [PMID: 15028963]

RHABDOMYOLYSIS

 ESSENTIALS OF DIAGNOSIS

- Associated with crush injuries to muscle, prolonged immobility, drug toxicities, hypothermia, and other causes.
- Massive acute elevations of muscle enzymes that peak quickly and usually resolve within days once the inciting injury has been identified and removed.

General Considerations

Defined strictly, rhabdomyolysis is necrosis of skeletal muscle and may be encountered in a wide variety of clinical settings, alone or in concert with other disorders of muscle. When the term "rhabdomyolysis" is used without being otherwise defined, healthcare providers ordinarily think of the syndrome of crush injury to muscle, associated with myoglobinuria, renal insufficiency, markedly elevated creatine kinase levels and, frequently, multiorgan failure as a consequence of other complications of the trauma. Renal insufficiency in myoglobinuria is caused by tubular injury resulting from excessive quantities of filtered myoglobin. This complication is nearly always associated with hypovolemia. Experimental models of severe rhabdomyolysis in which blood volume and pressure are maintained ordinarily are not associated with acute tubular necrosis. From a practical point of view, however, many patients who suffer crush injuries are indeed volume-contracted, and oliguric renal failure is encountered routinely.

In addition to crush injuries, prolonged immobility, particularly after drug overdose or intoxication and commonly associated with exposure hypothermia, may be associated with rhabdomyolysis. Often there is little evidence for muscle injury on external examination of these patients—and specifically, neither myalgia nor myopathy presents. The clue to muscle necrosis in such individuals may be a urinary dipstick testing positive for blood in the absence of red cells in the sediment. This false-positive finding is due to myoglobinuria, which results in a positive reading for blood. Such an abnormality is investigated by serum creatine kinase determination. Other studies elevated in rhabdomyolysis include ALT and lactate dehydrogenase (LDH)—and once again, these studies may be obtained for other reasons, such as suspected liver disease or hemolysis. When disproportionately elevated, it is prudent to establish that they are not of muscle origin by confirming them with creatine kinase determination.

A number of other causes of rhabdomyolysis are encountered. Statins, agents used commonly to treat hyperlipidemia, are common offenders (see above). The presence of compromised renal and hepatic function, diabetes, and hypothyroidism as well as concomitant use of other medications all increase the risk of rhabdomyolysis in those patients taking statins. Both acute alcohol intoxication and even intramuscular injections may cause some elevation of creatine kinase.

Treatment

Vigorous fluid resuscitation (4–6 L/d, with careful monitoring for fluid overload), mannitol (100 mg/d), and urine alkalinization are suggested early in the course, but definitive evidence for the efficacy of these measures is lacking. On occasion, oliguric tubular necrosis may be converted to a nonoliguric variety, and—though the prognosis for recovery of renal function and mortality is the same—many clinicians believe it is easier to care for nonoliguric disease because hyperkalemia and pulmonary edema are less important concerns. Myopathic complications of statins usually resolve within several weeks of discontinuing the drug.

Allison RC et al: The other medical causes of rhabdomyolysis. Am J Med Sci 2003;326:79. [PMID: 12920439]

Thompson PD et al: Statin-associated myopathy. JAMA 2003; 289:1681. [PMID: 12672737]

■ VASCULITIS SYNDROMES

"Vasculitis" is a heterogeneous group of disorders characterized by the pathologic features of inflammation within the walls of affected blood vessels. The major forms of primary systemic vasculitis are listed in Table 20–12. The first consideration in classifying cases of vasculitis is the size of the major vessels involved: large, medium, or small. The presence of the clinical signs and symptoms shown in Table 20–13 help distinguish among these three groups. After determining the size of the major vessels involved, other issues that contribute to the classification include the following:

- Does the process involve arteries, veins, or both?
- What are the patient's demographic characteristics (age, gender, ethnicity, smoking status)?
- Which organs are involved?
- Is there evidence of immune complex deposition?
- Is there granulomatous inflammation on tissue biopsy?
- Are antineutrophil cytoplasmic antibodies (ANCA) present?

In addition to the disorders considered to be primary vasculitides, there are also multiple forms of vasculitis that are associated with other known underlying conditions.

Table 20–12. Classification scheme of vasculitides according to size of predominant blood vessels involved.

Primary vasculitides
  Predominantly large-vessel vasculitides
    Takayasu's arteritis
    Giant cell arteritis (temporal arteritis)
    Behçet's disease[1]
  Predominantly medium-vessel vasculitides
    Polyarteritis nodosa
    Buerger's disease
  Predominantly small-vessel vasculitides
    Immune-complex mediated
      Cutaneous leukocytoclastic angiitis ("hypersensitivity vasculitis")
      Henoch-Schönlein purpura
      Essential cryoglobulinemia[2]
      "ANCA-associated" disorders[3]
      Wegener's granulomatosis[2]
      Microscopic polyangiitis[2]
      Churg-Strauss syndrome[2]

[1]May involve small, medium, and large-sized blood vessels.
[2]Frequent overlap of small and medium-sized blood vessel involvement.
[3]Not all forms of these disorders are always associated with ANCA.
ANCA = antineutrophil cytoplasmic antibodies.

These "secondary" forms of vasculitis occur in the setting of infections (eg, hepatitis B or C), connective tissue disorders, inflammatory bowel disease, malignancies, and reactions to medications. Only the major primary forms of vasculitis are discussed here.

POLYARTERITIS NODOSA

ESSENTIALS OF DIAGNOSIS

- *Classic polyarteritis nodosa involves only medium-sized vessels (specifically arteries), but involvement of smaller arterioles is sometimes observed.*
- *Clinical findings depend on the arteries involved.*
- *Common symptoms and signs include fever and other constitutional symptoms, abdominal pain, livedo reticularis, mononeuritis multiplex, anemia, and elevated acute phase reactants (ESR or C-reactive protein or both).*
- *Classic polyarteritis nodosa is often associated with a renin-mediated hypertension caused by kidney involvement but spares the lung.*
- *Ten percent of cases are associated with hepatitis B.*

Table 20–13. Typical clinical manifestations of large-, medium-, and small-vessel involvement by vasculitis.

Large	Medium	Small
Constitutional symptoms: fever, weight loss, malaise, arthralgias/arthritis		
Limb claudication	Cutaneous nodules	Purpura
Asymmetric blood pressures	Ulcers	Vesiculobullous lesions
	Livedo reticularis	Urticaria
Absence of pulses	Digital gangrene	Glomerulonephritis
Bruits	Mononeuritis multiplex	Alveolar hemorrhage
Aortic dilation	Microaneurysms	Cutaneous extravascular necrotizing granulomas
		Splinter hemorrhages
		Uveitis
		Episcleritis
		Scleritis

General Considerations

Polyarteritis nodosa, described in 1866, is acknowledged widely as the first form of vasculitis reported in the medical literature. For many years, all forms of inflammatory vascular disease were termed "polyarteritis nodosa." In recent decades, numerous subtypes of vasculitis have been recognized, greatly narrowing the spectrum of vasculitis called polyarteritis nodosa. Although the term is reserved currently for necrotizing arteritis of medium-sized vessels that has a predilection for involving the skin, peripheral nerves, mesenteric vessels (including renal arteries), heart, and brain, the disease can involve most organs. Polyarteritis nodosa is relatively rare, with a prevalence of about 30 per 1 million people. Approximately 10% of cases of polyarteritis nodosa are caused by hepatitis B. Most cases of hepatitis B–associated disease occur within 6 months of hepatitis B infection.

Clinical Findings

A. SYMPTOMS AND SIGNS

The clinical onset is usually insidious, with fever, malaise, weight loss, and other symptoms developing over weeks to months. Pain in the extremities is often a prominent early feature caused by arthralgia, myalgia (particularly affecting the calves), or neuropathy. The combination of mononeuritis multiplex (with the most common finding being foot-drop) and features of a systemic illness is one of the earliest specific clues to the presence of an underlying vasculitis. Polyarteritis nodosa is among the forms of vasculitis most commonly associated with vasculitic neuropathy.

In polyarteritis nodosa, the typical skin findings—livedo reticularis, subcutaneous nodules, and skin ulcers—reflect the involvement of deeper, medium-sized blood vessels. Digital gangrene is not an unusual occurrence. The most common cutaneous presentation is lower extremity ulcerations, usually occurring near the malleoli. Involvement of the renal arteries leads to a renin-mediated hypertension (much less characteristic of vasculitides involving smaller blood vessels). For unclear reasons, classic polyarteritis nodosa seldom (if ever) involves the lung, with the occasional exception of the bronchial arteries.

Abdominal pain—particularly diffuse periumbilical pain precipitated by eating—is common but often difficult to attribute to mesenteric vasculitis in the early stages. Nausea and vomiting are common symptoms. Infarction compromises the function of major viscera and may lead to acalculous cholecystitis or appendicitis. Some patients present dramatically with an acute abdomen caused by mesenteric vasculitis and gut perforation or with hypotension resulting from rupture of a microaneurysm in the liver, kidney, or bowel.

Subclinical cardiac involvement is common in polyarteritis nodosa, and overt cardiac dysfunction occasionally occurs (eg, myocardial infarction secondary to coronary vasculitis, or myocarditis).

B. LABORATORY FINDINGS

Most patients with polyarteritis nodosa have a slight anemia, and leukocytosis is common. Acute phase reactants are often (but not always) strikingly elevated. A major challenge in making the diagnosis of polyarteritis nodosa, however, is the absence of a disease-specific serologic test (eg, an autoantibody). Patients with classic polyarteritis nodosa are ANCA-negative and may have low titers of rheumatoid factor or antinuclear antibodies, both of which are nonspecific findings. In patients with polyarteritis nodosa, appropriate serologic tests for active hepatitis B infection must be performed.

C. BIOPSY AND ANGIOGRAPHY

The diagnosis of polyarteritis nodosa requires confirmation with either a tissue biopsy or an angiogram. Biopsies of symptomatic sites such as skin (from the edge of an ulcer or the center of a nodule), nerve, or muscle have reasonably high (albeit imperfect) sensitivities. The least invasive tests should usually be obtained first, but biopsy of an involved organ is essential. If performed by experienced physicians, tissue biopsies normally have high benefit-risk ratios because of the importance of establishing the diagnosis. Patients in whom polyarteritis nodosa is suspected—eg, on the basis of mesenteric ischemia or new-onset hypertension occurring in the setting of a systemic illness—may be diagnosed by the angiographic finding of aneurysmal dilations in the renal, mesenteric, or hepatic arteries. Angiography must be performed cautiously in patients with baseline renal dysfunction.

Treatment

For polyarteritis nodosa, corticosteroids in high doses (up to 60 mg of oral prednisone daily) may control fever and constitutional symptoms and heal vascular lesions. Pulse methylprednisolone (eg, 1 g intravenously daily for 3 days) may be necessary for patients who are critically ill at presentation. Immunosuppressive agents, especially cyclophosphamide, lower the risk of disease-related death and morbidity among patients who have severe disease. For patients with polyarteritis nodosa associated with hepatitis B, the preferred treatment regimen is a short course of prednisone accompanied by lamivudine (100 mg/d orally) and plasmapheresis (three times a week for up to 6 weeks).

Prognosis

Without treatment, the 5-year survival rate in these disorders is poor—on the order of 20%. With appropriate therapy, remissions are possible in many cases and the 5-year survival rate has improved to 60–90%. Poor prognostic factors are renal insufficiency, proteinuria, gastrointestinal ischemia, central nervous system disease, and cardiac involvement. Substantial morbidity and even death may result from adverse effects of cyclophosphamide and corticosteroids. Consequently, these therapies require careful monitoring and expert management. In contrast to many other forms of systemic vasculitis, disease relapses in polyarteritis following the successful induction of remission are the exception rather than the rule, occurring in only about 10% of cases.

Bourgarit A et al: Deaths occurring during the first year after treatment onset for polyarteritis nodosa, microscopic polyangiitis, and Churg-Strauss syndrome: a retrospective analysis of causes and factors predictive of mortality based on 595 patients. Medicine (Baltimore) 2005;84:323. [PMID: 16148732]

Guillevin L et al: Hepatitis B virus-associated polyarteritis nodosa: clinical characteristics, outcome, and impact of treatment in 115 patients. Medicine (Baltimore) 2005;84:313. [PMID: 16148731]

POLYMYALGIA RHEUMATICA & GIANT CELL ARTERITIS

ESSENTIALS OF DIAGNOSIS

- *Giant cell (temporal) arteritis is characterized by headache, jaw claudication, polymyalgia rheumatica, visual abnormalities, and a markedly elevated ESR.*
- *The hallmark of polymyalgia rheumatica is pain and stiffness in shoulders and hips lasting for several weeks without other explanation.*

General Considerations

Polymyalgia rheumatica and giant cell arteritis probably represent a spectrum of one disease: Both affect the same population (patients over the age of 50), show preference for the same HLA haplotypes, and show similar patterns of cytokines in blood and arteries. Polymyalgia rheumatica and giant cell arteritis also frequently coexist. The important differences between the two conditions are that polymyalgia rheumatica alone does not cause blindness and responds to low-dose (10–20 mg/d) prednisone therapy, whereas giant cell arteritis can cause blindness and large artery complications and requires high-dose therapy (40–60 mg/d).

Clinical Findings

A. POLYMYALGIA RHEUMATICA

Polymyalgia rheumatica is a clinical diagnosis based on pain and stiffness of the shoulder and pelvic girdle areas, frequently in association with fever, malaise, and weight loss. In approximately two-thirds of cases, polymyalgia occurs in the absence of giant cell arteritis. Because of the stiffness and pain in the shoulders, hips, and lower back, patients have trouble combing their hair, putting on a coat, or rising from a chair. In contrast to polymyositis and polyarteritis nodosa, polymyalgia rheumatica does not cause muscular weakness either through primary muscle inflammation or secondary to nerve infarction. A few patients have joint swelling, particularly of the knees, wrists, and sternoclavicular joints. Anemia and elevated acute phase reactants (often markedly elevated ESRs, for example) are present in the most cases, but cases of polymyalgia rheumatica occurring with normal acute phase reactants are well-documented. The differential diagnosis of malaise, anemia, and striking acute phase reactant elevations includes rheumatic diseases such as rheumatoid arthritis, systemic vasculitis, multiple myeloma and other malignant disorders, and chronic infections such as bacterial endocarditis and osteomyelitis.

B. GIANT CELL ARTERITIS

Giant cell arteritis is a systemic panarteritis affecting medium-sized and large vessels in patients over the age of 50. The incidence of this disease increases with each decade of life. The mean age at onset is approximately 72 years. Giant cell arteritis is also called temporal arteritis because that artery is frequently involved, as are other extracranial branches of the carotid artery. About 50% of patients with giant cell arteritis also have polymyalgia rheumatica. The classic symptoms suggesting that a patient has arteritis are headache, scalp tenderness, visual symptoms (particularly amaurosis fugax or diplopia), jaw claudication, or throat pain. The temporal artery is usually normal on physical examination but may be nodular, enlarged, tender, or pulseless. Blindness usually results from the syndrome of anterior ischemic optic neuropathy, caused by occlusive arteritis of the posterior ciliary branch of the ophthalmic artery.

The ischemic optic neuropathy of giant cell arteritis may produce no funduscopic findings for the first 24–48 hours after the onset of blindness.

Asymmetry of pulses in the arms, a murmur of aortic regurgitation, or bruits heard near the clavicle resulting from subclavian artery stenoses identify patients in whom giant cell arteritis has affected the aorta or its major branches. Large vessel involvement—characterized chiefly by aneurysm of the thoracic aortic or stenosis of the subclavian, vertebral, carotid, and basilar arteries—occurs in approximately 25% of patients with giant cell arteritis, sometimes years after the diagnosis. Forty percent of patients with giant cell arteritis have nonclassic symptoms at presentation, chiefly respiratory tract problems (most frequently dry cough), mononeuritis multiplex (most frequently with painful paralysis of a shoulder), or fever of unknown origin. Giant cell arteritis accounts for 15% of all cases of fever of unknown origin in patients over the age of 65. The fever can be as high as 40 °C and is frequently associated with rigors and sweats. In contrast to patients with infection, patients with giant cell arteritis and fever usually have normal white blood cell counts (before prednisone is started). Thus, in an older patient with fever of unknown origin, marked elevations of acute phase reactants, and a normal white blood count, giant cell arteritis must be considered even in the absence of specific features such as headache or jaw claudication. In some cases, instead of having the well-known symptom of jaw claudication, patients complain of vague pain affecting other locations, including the tongue, nose, or ears. Indeed, unexplained head or neck pain in an older patient may signal the presence of giant cell arteritis.

C. LABORATORY FINDINGS

Nearly 90% of patients with giant cell arteritis have ESRs > 50 mm/h. The ESR in this disorder is often > 100 mm/h, but cases in which the ESR is low or even normal do occur. In one series, 5% of patients with biopsy-proven giant cell arteritis had ESRs < 40 mm/h. Patients with biopsy-proven giant cell arteritis with normal C-reactive proteins have also been described. Most patients also have a mild normochromic, normocytic anemia and thrombocytosis. The alkaline phosphatase (liver source) is elevated in 20% of patients with giant cell arteritis.

Treatment

A. POLYMYALGIA RHEUMATICA

Patients with isolated polymyalgia rheumatica (ie, those not having "above the neck" symptoms of headache, jaw claudication, scalp tenderness, or visual symptoms) are treated with prednisone, 10–20 mg/d orally. If the patient does not experience a dramatic improvement within 72 hours, the diagnosis should be revisited. Usually after 2–4 weeks of treatment, slow tapering of the prednisone can be attempted. Most patients require some dose of prednisone for a minimum of approximately 1 year; 6 months is too short in most cases. Disease flares are common (50% or more) as prednisone is tapered. The addition of weekly methotrexate may increase the chance of successfully tapering prednisone in some patients.

B. GIANT CELL ARTERITIS

The urgency of early diagnosis and treatment in giant cell arteritis relates to the prevention of blindness. Once blindness develops, it is usually permanent. Therefore, when a patient has symptoms and findings suggestive of temporal arteritis, therapy with prednisone (60 mg/d orally) should be initiated immediately and a temporal artery biopsy performed promptly. Retrospective studies suggest that low-dose aspirin (~ 81 mg/d orally) may reduce the chance of visual loss or stroke in patients with giant cell arteritis and should be added to prednisone in the initial treatment. Although it is prudent to obtain a temporal artery biopsy as soon as possible after instituting treatment, diagnostic findings of giant cell arteritis may still be present 2 weeks (or even considerably longer) after starting corticosteroids. Typically, a positive biopsy shows inflammatory infiltrate in the media and adventitia with lymphocytes, histiocytes, plasma cells, and giant cells. An adequate biopsy specimen is essential (at least 2 cm in length is ideal), because the disease may be segmental. Unilateral temporal artery biopsies are positive in approximately 80–85% of patients, but bilateral biopsies add incrementally to the yield (10–15% in some studies, less in others). Prednisone should be continued in a dosage of 60 mg/d for about 1 month before tapering. When only the symptoms of polymyalgia rheumatica are present, temporal artery biopsy is not necessary.

In adjusting the dosage of corticosteroid, the ESR is a useful but not absolute guide to disease activity. A common error is treating the ESR rather than the patient. The ESR often rises slightly as the prednisone is tapered, even as the disease remains quiescent. Because elderly individuals often have baseline ESRs that are above the normal range, mild ESR elevations should not be an occasion for renewed treatment with prednisone in patients who are asymptomatic. Thoracic aortic aneurysms occur 17 times more frequently in patients with giant cell arteritis than in normal individuals. The aneurysms can develop at any time but typically occur 7 years after the diagnosis of giant cell arteritis is made.

Bongartz T et al: Large-vessel involvement in giant cell arteritis. Curr Opin Rheumatol 2006;18:10. [PMID: 16344614]

Gonzalez-Gay MA et al: Giant cell arteritis: disease patterns of clinical presentation in a series of 240 patients. Medicine (Baltimore) 2005;84:269. [PMID: 16148727]

Gonzalez-Gay MA et al: Giant cell arteritis: laboratory tests at the time of diagnosis in a series of 240 patients. Medicine (Baltimore) 2005;84:277. [PMID: 16148728]

Nesher G et al: Low-dose aspirin and prevention of cranial ischemic complications in giant cell arteritis. Arthritis Rheum 2004;50:1332. [PMID: 15077317]

Seo P et al: Large-vessel vasculitis. Arthritis Care Res 2004;51: 128. [PMID: 14872466]

WEGENER'S GRANULOMATOSIS

 ESSENTIALS OF DIAGNOSIS

- Originally defined by the triad of upper respiratory tract disease, lower respiratory disease, and glomerulonephritis.
- Suspect if mild respiratory symptoms (eg, nasal congestion, sinusitis) are refractory to usual treatment.
- Pathology defined by the triad of small vessel vasculitis, granulomatous inflammation, and necrosis.
- Ninety percent of patients with severe, active disease have ANCAs, usually directed against proteinase-3 (less commonly against myeloperoxidase).
- Renal disease often rapidly progressive without treatment.

General Considerations

Wegener's granulomatosis, which has an estimated incidence of approximately 12 cases per million individuals per year, is the prototype of diseases associated with antineutrophil cytoplasmic antibodies (ANCA). (Other "ANCA-associated vasculitides" include microscopic polyangiitis and the Churg-Strauss syndrome.) Wegener's granulomatosis is characterized in its full expression by vasculitis of small arteries, arterioles, and capillaries, necrotizing granulomatous lesions of both upper and lower respiratory tract, glomerulonephritis, and other organ manifestations. Without treatment, generalized disease is invariably fatal, with most patients surviving less than 1 year after diagnosis. It occurs most commonly in the fourth and fifth decades of life and affects men and women with equal frequency.

Clinical Findings

A. SYMPTOMS AND SIGNS

The disorder usually develops over 4–12 months, with 90% of patients presenting with upper or lower respiratory tract symptoms or both. Upper respiratory tract symptoms can include nasal congestion, sinusitis, otitis media, mastoiditis, inflammation of the gums, or stridor due to subglottic stenosis. Since many of these symptoms are common, the underlying disease is not often suspected until the patient develops systemic symptoms or the original problem is refractory to treatment. The lungs are affected initially in 40% and eventually in 80%, with symptoms including cough, dyspnea, and hemoptysis. Other early symptoms can include a migratory oligoarthritis with a predilection

for large joints; a variety of symptoms related to ocular disease (unilateral proptosis from orbital pseudotumor; red eye from scleritis, episcleritis, anterior uveitis, or peripheral ulcerative keratitis); purpura or other skin lesions; and dysesthesia due to neuropathy. Renal involvement, which develops in three-fourths of the cases, may be subclinical until renal insufficiency is advanced. Fever, malaise, and weight loss are common.

Physical examination can be remarkable for congestion, crusting, ulceration, bleeding, and even perforation of the nasal septum. Destruction of the nasal cartilage with "saddle nose" deformity occurs late. Otitis media, proptosis, scleritis, episcleritis, and conjunctivitis are other common findings. Newly acquired hypertension, a frequent feature of polyarteritis nodosa, is rare in Wegener's granulomatosis. Venous thrombotic events (eg, deep venous thrombosis and pulmonary embolism) are now recognized to be a common occurrence in Wegener's granulomatosis, at least in part because of the tendency of the disease to involve veins as well as arteries. Vigilance must be maintained for venous thrombotic events.

Although limited forms of Wegener's granulomatosis have been described in which the kidney is spared initially, renal disease will develop in the majority of untreated patients. In such cases, the urinary sediment invariably contains red cells, with or without white cells, and red cell casts. Renal biopsy discloses a segmental necrotizing glomerulonephritis with multiple crescents; this is characteristic but not diagnostic. Pathologists characterize the renal lesion of Wegener's granulomatosis (and other forms of "ANCA-associated vasculitis") as a pauci-immune glomerulonephritis because of the relative absence (compared with immune complex–mediated disorders) of immunoreactants—IgG, IgM, IgA, and complement proteins—within glomeruli.

B. LABORATORY FINDINGS

Most patients have slight anemia, mild leukocytosis, and elevated acute phase reactants. Chest CT is more sensitive than chest radiography; lesions include infiltrates, nodules, masses, and cavities. Often the radiographs prompt concern about lung cancer. Hilar adenopathy is unusual in Wegener's granulomatosis; if present, sarcoidosis, tumor, or infection is more likely. Other common laboratory or radiographic abnormalities include hematuria, red blood cell casts, extensive sinusitis, and even bony sinus erosions.

Histologic features of Wegener's granulomatosis include vasculitis, granulomatous inflammation, geographic necrosis, and acute and chronic inflammation. The full range of pathologic changes are usually evident only on thoracoscopic lung biopsy. Granulomas, observed only rarely in renal biopsy specimens, are found much more commonly on lung biopsy specimens. Nasal biopsies often do not show vasculitis but may show chronic inflammation and other changes which, interpreted by an experienced pathologist, can serve as convincing evidence of the diagnosis.

Serum tests for ANCA help in the diagnosis of Wegener's granulomatosis and related forms of vasculitis (Tables 20–10 and 19–2). Several different types of ANCA are recognized, but the two subtypes relevant to systemic vasculitis are those directed against proteinase-3 (PR3) and myeloperoxidase (MPO). Antibodies to these two antigens are termed, respectively, PR3-ANCA and MPO-ANCA. The cytoplasmic pattern of immunofluorescence (C-ANCA) caused by PR3-ANCA has a high specificity (> 90%) for either Wegener's granulomatosis or a closely related disease, microscopic polyangiitis (or, less commonly, the Churg-Strauss syndrome). In the setting of active disease, particularly cases in which the disease is severe and generalized to multiple organ systems, the sensitivity of PR3-ANCA is > 95%. A substantial percentage of patients with "limited" Wegener's granulomatosis—disease that does not pose an immediate threat to life and is often confined to the respiratory tract—are ANCA-negative. Although ANCA testing may be very helpful when used properly, it does not eliminate the need in most cases for confirmation of the diagnosis by tissue biopsy. Furthermore, ANCA levels correlate erratically with disease activity, and changes in titer should not dictate changes in therapy in the absence of supporting clinical data. The perinuclear (P-ANCA) pattern, caused by MPO-ANCA, is more likely to occur in microscopic polyangiitis or Churg-Strauss but may also be found in Wegener's granulomatosis. Approximately 10–25% of patients with classic Wegener's granulomatosis have MPO-ANCA. Owing to involvement of the same types of blood vessels, similar patterns of organ involvement, and the possibility of failing to identify granulomatous pathology on tissue biopsies because of sampling error, Wegener's granulomatosis is often difficult to differentiate from microscopic polyangiitis. The crucial distinctions between the two disorders are the tendencies for Wegener's granulomatosis to involve the upper respiratory tract (including the ears) and to cause granulomatous inflammation.

All positive immunofluorescence assays for ANCA should be confirmed by enzyme immunoassays for the specific autoantibodies directed against PR3 or MPO.

Treatment

Early treatment is crucial in preventing the devastating end-organ complications of this disease, and often in preserving life. While Wegener's granulomatosis may involve the sinuses or lung for months, once proteinuria or hematuria develops, progression to renal failure can be rapid (over several weeks). Remissions of at least a temporary nature have been induced in more than 90% of patients treated with conventional approaches to therapy, but disease relapses occur in a substantial proportion of those patients who achieve remission. For patients with severe Wegener's granulomatosis, cyclophosphamide remains the standard of care for remission induction. Cyclophosphamide is best given daily by mouth; intermittent high-dose intravenous cyclophosphamide is less effective. Unfortunately, the traditional therapy of oral cyclophosphamide continued for 12 months after the patient achieves remission has resulted in severe toxicity, including a 2.4 times increased risk of all malignancies, a 33-fold increase in bladder cancer, and a 60% chance of ovarian failure. Consequently, the current approach to remission induction in severe cases is to use cyclophosphamide for 3–6 months, followed by a switch to a regimen more likely to be tolerated well. In patients with remission induced by 3–6 months of cyclophosphamide and corticosteroids, azathioprine (up to 2 mg/kg/d orally) has been shown to be as effective as cyclophosphamide in maintaining disease remissions (at least for up to 12–15 months). Before the institution of azathioprine, patients should be tested (through a commercially available blood test) for deficiencies in the level of thiopurine methyltransferase, an enzyme essential to the metabolism of azathioprine. Another current option for remission maintenance is methotrexate, 20–25 mg/wk (administered either PO or IM). Because of its superior side-effect profile, methotrexate is viewed as an appropriate substitute for cyclophosphamide in patients who do not have significant renal dysfunction (of any cause) or immediately life-threatening disease. Treatment with TNF inhibitors, particularly etanercept, does not appear to be effective.

Goek ON et al: Randomized controlled trials in vasculitis associated with anti-neutrophil cytoplasmic antibodies. Curr Opin Rheumatol 2005;17:257. [PMID: 15838233]

Merkel PA et al: High incidence of venous thrombotic events among patients with Wegener granulomatosis: the Wegener's Clinical Occurrence of Thrombosis (WeCLOT) Study. Ann Intern Med 2005;142:620. [PMID: 15838068]

Seo P et al: Damage caused by Wegener's granulomatosis and its treatment: prospective data from the Wegener's Granulomatosis Etanercept Trial (WGET). Arthritis Rheum 2005; 52:2168. [PMID: 15986348]

Wegener's Granulomatosis Etanercept Trial (WGET) Research Group: Etanercept plus standard therapy for Wegener's granulomatosis. N Engl J Med 2005;352:351. [PMID: 15673801]

MICROSCOPIC POLYANGIITIS

 ESSENTIALS OF DIAGNOSIS

- *Necrotizing vasculitis of small- and medium-sized vessels in both the arterial and venous circulations.*
- *Frequently involves the lung and kidneys with typical complications of alveolar hemorrhage and glomerulonephritis.*
- *Associated with ANCA in three-fourths of all cases, usually anti-myeloperoxidase antibodies (MPO-ANCA) that cause a P-ANCA pattern on immunofluorescence testing. ANCA directed against pro-*

teinase-3 (PR3-ANCA) can also be observed in microscopic polyangiitis.

General Considerations

Microscopic polyangiitis, as its name implies, is the term given to nongranulomatous vasculitis involving small blood vessels. It is often associated with ANCAs that produce a P-ANCA pattern on immunofluorescence testing and are directed against MPO, a constituent of neutrophil granules. Because microscopic polyangiitis may involve medium-sized as well as small blood vessels and because it tends to affect capillaries within the lungs and kidneys, its spectrum overlaps those of both polyarteritis nodosa and Wegener's granulomatosis.

In a minority of cases, microscopic polyangiitis appears to be induced by reactions to medications, particularly propylthiouracil, hydralazine, allopurinol, penicillamine, and sulfasalazine. In rare instances, these drugs induce a systemic vasculitis associated with MPO-ANCA. Such syndromes usually resolve with discontinuation of the offending drug.

Clinical Findings

A. Symptoms and Signs

A wide variety of findings suggesting vasculitis of small blood vessels may develop in microscopic polyangiitis. These include palpable purpura and numerous other signs of cutaneous vasculitis; hematuria, proteinuria, and red blood cell casts in the urine; and pulmonary hemorrhage. The renal lesion is a segmental, necrotizing glomerulonephritis, often with localized intravascular coagulation and the observation of intraglomerular thrombi upon renal biopsy. The pathologic findings in the lung are typically those of capillaritis. Vasculitic neuropathy (mononeuritis multiplex) is also common in microscopic polyangiitis.

Microscopic polyangiitis is the most common cause of pulmonary-renal syndromes, being several times more common than Goodpasture's (antiglomerular basement membrane) syndrome. In a subset of patients with microscopic polyangiitis, interstitial lung fibrosis that mimics usual interstitial pneumonitis is the presenting condition. Microscopic polyangiitis is defined as a pauci-immune necrotizing vasculitis with few or no immune deposits that (1) affects small blood vessels (capillaries, venules, or arterioles); (2) often includes glomerulonephritis and pulmonary capillaritis; and, (3) is often associated with ANCA (antimyeloperoxidase > antiproteinase-3). Distinguishing this disease from Wegener's granulomatosis may be challenging in some cases. Microscopic polyangiitis is not associated with the chronic destructive upper respiratory tract disease often found in Wegener's granulomatosis. Moreover, as noted, a critical difference between the two diseases is the absence of granulomatous inflammation in micro-

scopic polyangiitis. Because their treatments may differ, microscopic polyangiitis must also be differentiated from polyarteritis nodosa. Microscopic polyangiitis usually requires treatment with both cyclophosphamide and corticosteroids.

B. Laboratory Findings

As noted, three-fourths of patients with microscopic polyangiitis are ANCA-positive. Elevated acute phase reactants are also typical of active disease. Careful scrutiny of the urine sediment is essential to excluding active renal disease.

Treatment

In microscopic polyangiitis, patients are likely to require cyclophosphamide because of the urgency in treating pulmonary hemorrhage and glomerulonephritis. Cyclophosphamide may be administered either in an oral daily regimen or via intermittent (usually monthly) intravenous pulses. The typical oral dose is 2 mg/kg/d, but this may need to be decreased substantially for patients with significant renal dysfunction (for example, the dose for patients receiving dialysis is 0.8–1.0 mg/kg/d). For intermittent administration, cyclophosphamide is usually dosed at 750 mg/m^2 (500 mg/m^2 for those with renal failure). Whenever cyclophosphamide is used, *Pneumocystis jiroveci* prophylaxis with either single-strength trimethoprim-sulfamethoxazole or dapsone 100 mg daily is essential. Following the induction of remission, azathioprine is a reasonable choice to replace cyclophosphamide.

Prognosis

The key to effecting good outcomes is early diagnosis. Compared with patients who have Wegener's granulomatosis, those who have microscopic polyangiitis are more likely to have significant fibrosis on renal biopsy because of later diagnosis. The likelihood of disease recurrence following remission in microscopic polyangiitis is about 33%.

Bonaci-Nikolic B et al: Antineutrophil cytoplasmic antibody (ANCA)-associated autoimmune diseases induced by antithyroid drugs: comparison with idiopathic ANCA vasculitides. Arthritis Res Ther 2005;7:R1072. [PMID: 16207324]

Hogan SL et al: Predictors of relapse and treatment resistance in antineutrophil cytoplasmic antibody-associated small-vessel vasculitis. Ann Intern Med 2005;143:621. [PMID: 16263884]

Seo P et al: The antineutrophil cytoplasmic antibody-associated vasculitides. Am J Med 2004;117:39. [PMID: 15210387]

CRYOGLOBULINEMIA

Vasculitis secondary to cryoglobulinemia occurs in only a small minority of patients with cryoglobulins in their serum, but this diagnosis should be considered when patients present with palpable purpura, especially when recurrent, and peripheral neuropathy. A proliferative glomerulonephritis that strongly resembles lupus nephritis may complicate cryoglobulinemia. Abnormal liver function tests, abdominal pain, and pulmonary disease may also occur. The diagnosis is based on a compatible clinical picture and a positive serum test for cryoglobulins. Type I cryoglobulins (monoclonal proteins that lack rheumatoid factor activity) are more commonly seen in lymphoproliferative disease. (Type I cryoglobulins usually cause hyperviscosity syndromes rather than vasculitis.) The diseases most commonly associated with cryoglobulinemic vasculitis are hepatitis C and connective tissues diseases, especially Sjögren's syndrome. Type II (monoclonal antibody with rheumatoid factor activity) and Type III (polyclonal antibody with rheumatoid factor activity) cryoglobulins cause vasculitis. Because 90% of cryoglobulinemia cases are associated with hepatitis C infections, the optimal approach to treatment is viral suppression with interferon-α with or without ribavirin. Pegylated forms of interferon-α are now the standard of care for mixed cryoglobulinemia because this form of the drug requires less frequent administration. Because immunosuppressive agents may facilitate viral replication, corticosteroids, cyclophosphamide, and other interventions (including plasmapheresis) should be reserved for organ-threatening complications. B cell depletion using agents such as rituximab appears to be a promising avenue of therapy.

Cacoub P et al: PEGylated interferon alfa-2b and ribavirin treatment in patients with hepatitis C virus-related systemic vasculitis. Arthritis Rheum 2005;52:911. [PMID: 15751068]

Ferri C et al: Mixed cryoglobulinemia: demographic, clinical, and serologic features and survival in 231 patients. Semin Arthritis Rheum 2004;33:355. [PMID: 15190522]

Quartuccio L: Rituximab treatment for glomerulonephritis in HCV-associated mixed cryoglobulinaemia: efficacy and safety in the absence of steroids. Rheumatology (Oxford) 2006; 45:842. [PMID: 16418196]

HENOCH-SCHÖNLEIN PURPURA

Henoch-Schönlein purpura, the most common systemic vasculitis in children, occurs in adults as well. Typical features are palpable purpura, abdominal pain, arthritis, and hematuria. Pathologic features include leukocytoclastic vasculitis with IgA deposition. The cause is not known.

The purpuric skin lesions are typically located on the lower extremities but may also be seen on the hands, arms, trunk, and buttocks. Joint symptoms are present in the majority of patients, the knees and ankles being most commonly involved. Abdominal pain secondary to vasculitis of the intestinal tract is often associated with gastrointestinal bleeding. Hematuria signals the presence of a renal lesion that is usually reversible, although it occasionally may progress to renal insufficiency. Children tend to have more frequent and more serious gastrointestinal vasculitis, whereas adults more often suffer from renal disease. Biopsy of

the kidney reveals segmental glomerulonephritis with crescents and mesangial deposition of IgA.

The disease is usually self-limited, lasting 1–6 weeks, and subsides without sequelae if renal involvement is not severe. Chronic courses with persistent or intermittent skin disease are more likely to occur in adults than in children. Corticosteroids (eg, prednisone 20–40 mg/d orally) are effective in treating some disease manifestations of Henoch-Schönlein purpura but are not universally effective. Some patients with persistent disease appear to benefit from pulse doses of methylprednisolone (1 g/day IV for 3 days). The incremental efficacy of steroid-sparing drugs such as azathioprine and mycophenolate mofetil—often used in the setting of renal disease—is not known.

Halling SF et al: Henoch Schönlein nephritis: clinical findings related to renal function and morphology. Pediatr Nephrol 2005;20:46. [PMID: 15503170]

Nadrous HF et al: Pulmonary involvement in Henoch-Schönlein purpura. Mayo Clin Proc 2004;79:1151. [PMID: 15357037]

RELAPSING POLYCHONDRITIS

This disease is characterized by inflammatory destructive lesions of cartilaginous structures, principally the ears, nose, trachea, and larynx. Nearly 40% of cases are associated with another disease, especially either other immunologic disorders (such as SLE, rheumatoid arthritis, or Hashimoto's thyroiditis) or cancers (such as multiple myeloma). The disease, which is usually episodic, affects males and females equally. The cartilage is painful, swollen, and tender during an attack and subsequently becomes atrophic, resulting in permanent deformity. Biopsy of the involved cartilage shows inflammation and chondrolysis. Noncartilaginous manifestations of the disease include fever, episcleritis, uveitis, deafness, aortic insufficiency, and rarely glomerulonephritis. In 85% of patients, a migratory, asymmetric, and seronegative arthropathy occurs, affecting both large and small joints and the costochondral junctions.

Prednisone, 0.5–1 mg/kg/d orally, is often effective. Dapsone (100–200 mg/d orally) may also be effective, sparing the need for chronic high-dose corticosteroid treatment. Involvement of the tracheobronchial tree, leading to tracheomalacia, may lead to difficult management issues.

Kent PD et al: Relapsing polychondritis. Curr Opin Rheumatol 2004;16:56. [PMID: 14673390]

BEHÇET'S SYNDROME

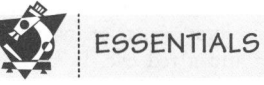 ESSENTIALS OF DIAGNOSIS

- *Most commonly occurs among persons of Asian, Turkish, or Middle Eastern background, but may affect persons of any demographic profile.*

- Recurrent, painful aphthous ulcers of the mouth and genitals.

- Additional cutaneous findings include erythema nodosum–like lesions, a follicular rash, and the "pathergy" phenomenon (formation of a sterile pustule at the site of a needle stick).

- Either anterior or posterior uveitis. Posterior uveitis may be asymptomatic until significant damage to the retina has occurred.

- Variety of neurologic lesions that can mimic multiple sclerosis, particularly through involvement of the white matter of the brainstem.

General Considerations

Named after the Turkish dermatologist who first described it, this disease is of unknown cause. Essentially all of its protean manifestations, however, are believed to result from vasculitis that may involve all types of blood vessels: small, medium, and large, on both the arterial and venous side of the circulation.

Clinical Findings

A. SYMPTOMS AND SIGNS

The hallmark of Behçet's disease is painful aphthous ulceration in the mouth. These lesions, which usually occur multiply, may be found on the tongue, gums, and inner surfaces of the oral cavity. Genital lesions, similar in appearance, are also common but do not occur in all patients. Other cutaneous lesions of Behçet's disease include tender, erythematous, papular lesions that resemble erythema nodosum. (On biopsy, however, many of these lesions are shown to be secondary to vasculitis rather than septal panniculitis.) These erythema nodosum–like lesions have a tendency to ulcerate, a major difference between the lesions of Behçet's disease and the erythema nodosum seen in cases of sarcoidosis and inflammatory bowel disease. An erythematous follicular rash that occurs frequently on the upper extremities may be a subtle feature of the disease. The pathergy phenomenon is frequently underappreciated (unless the patient is asked); in this phenomenon, sterile pustules develop at sites where needles have been inserted into the skin (eg, for phlebotomy) in some patients.

A nonerosive arthritis occurs in about two-thirds of patients, most commonly affecting the knees and ankles. Eye involvement may be one of the most devastating complications of Behçet's disease. Posterior uveitis, in essence a retinal venulitis, may lead to the insidious destruction of large areas of the retina before the patient becomes aware of visual problems. Anterior uveitis, associated with photophobia and a red eye, is intensely symptomatic. This complication may lead to a hypopyon, the accumulation of pus in the anterior chamber. If not treated properly with mydriatic agents to dilate the pupil and corticosteroid eyedrops to diminish inflammation, the anterior uveitis of Behçet's may lead to synechial formation between the iris and lens, resulting in permanent pupillary distortion.

Central nervous system involvement is another cause of major potential morbidity in Behçet's disease. The central nervous system lesions that may mimic multiple sclerosis radiologically often result in serious disability or death. Findings include sterile meningitis (recurrent meningeal headaches associated with a lymphocytic pleocytosis), cranial nerve palsies, seizures, encephalitis, mental disturbances, and spinal cord lesions. Finally, patients with Behçet's disease have a hypercoagulable tendency that may lead to complicated venous thrombotic events, particularly multiple deep venous thrombosis, pulmonary emboli, cerebral sinus thrombosis, and other problems associated with clotting.

The clinical course may be chronic but is often characterized by remissions and exacerbations.

B. LABORATORY FINDINGS

There are no pathognomonic laboratory features of Behçet's disease. Although patients with Behçet's disease often have elevated acute phase reactants, there is no autoantibody or other assay that is distinctive. No markers of hypercoagulability specific to Behçet's have been identified. Behçet's disease is known to have a genetic risk factor (HLA B51), but this gene is neither necessary nor sufficient to cause the disease and is of little help in making the diagnosis or determining prognosis.

Treatment

Corticosteroids (1 mg/kg/d of oral prednisone) are a mainstay of therapy for severe disease manifestations. Azathioprine (2 mg/kg/d orally) may be an effective steroid-sparing agent. Cyclophosphamide (2 mg/kg/d orally) is indicated for severe ocular and central nervous system complications of Behçet's. Both colchicine (0.6 mg once to three times daily orally) and thalidomide (100 mg/d orally) help ameliorate the mucocutaneous findings of Behçet's. TNF inhibition demonstrates some promise as a therapeutic approach, but large studies are lacking to date.

Calamia KT et al: Major vessel involvement in Behçet disease. Curr Opin Rheumatol 2005;17:1. [PMID: 15604898]

Kural-Seyahi E et al: The long-term mortality and morbidity of Behçet syndrome: a 2-decade outcome survey of 387 patients followed at a dedicated center. Medicine (Baltimore) 2003;82:60. [PMID: 12544711]

Melikoglu M et al: Short-term trial of etanercept in Behçet's disease: a double blind, placebo controlled study. J Rheumatol 2005;32:98. [PMID: 15630733]

PRIMARY ANGIITIS OF THE CENTRAL NERVOUS SYSTEM

Primary angiitis of the central nervous system is a syndrome with several possible causes that produces small and medium-sized vasculitis limited to the brain and spinal cord. Biopsy-proved cases have predominated in men who present with a history of weeks to months of headaches, encephalopathy, and multifocal strokes. Systemic signs and symptoms are absent, and routine laboratory tests are usually normal. MRI of the brain is almost always abnormal, and the spinal fluid often reveals a mild lymphocytosis and a modest increase in protein level. Angiograms classically reveal a "string of beads" pattern produced by alternating segments of arterial narrowing and dilation. However, neither the MRI nor the angiogram appearance is specific for vasculitis. Many conditions, including vasospasm, can produce the same angiographic pattern as vasculitis. Definitive diagnosis requires a compatible clinical picture; exclusion of infection, neoplasm, or metabolic disorder or drug exposure (eg, cocaine) that can mimic primary angiitis of the central nervous system; and a positive brain biopsy. When a patient meeting the above criteria has a positive angiogram without a confirming biopsy, the diagnosis should be considered possible. Angiographically defined cases of central nervous system vasculopathy differ from biopsy-proved cases chiefly involving women who have had an abrupt onset of headaches and stroke (often in the absence of encephalopathy) with normal spinal fluid findings. Many patients who fit this clinical profile and have disease diagnosed by angiography (but not biopsy) may have vasospasm rather than true vasculitis. Such cases may require shorter and less intensive courses of immunosuppression—or none at all—as opposed to those with biopsy-proved cases. The latter usually improve with prednisone therapy and may require cyclophosphamide. In recent years, cases of central nervous system vasculitis associated with cerebral amyloid angiopathy have been reported. These cases often respond well to corticosteroids, albeit the long-term natural history remains poorly defined.

Scolding NJ et al: Abeta-related angiitis: primary angiitis of the central nervous system associated with cerebral amyloid angiopathy. Brain 2005;128:500. [PMID: 15659428]

■ SERONEGATIVE SPONDYLOARTHROPATHIES

The seronegative spondyloarthropathies are ankylosing spondylitis, psoriatic arthritis, Reiter's syndrome (also called reactive arthritis), and the arthritis associated with inflammatory bowel disease. These disorders are noted for male predominance, onset usually before age 40, inflammatory arthritis of the spine or the large peripheral joints (or both), uveitis in a significant minority, the absence of autoantibodies in the serum, and a striking association with HLA-B27. Present in only 8% of normal whites and 4% of normal blacks, HLA-B27 is positive

in 90% of patients with ankylosing spondylitis and 75% with Reiter's syndrome. HLA-B27 also occurs in 50% of the psoriatic and inflammatory bowel disease patients who have sacroiliitis. Patients with only peripheral arthritis in these latter two syndromes do not show an increase in HLA-B27.

That HLA-B27 itself (and not some other gene) confers susceptibility to these diseases has been demonstrated by experiments with transgenic rats. When the human HLA-B27 gene is expressed in rats, the animals develop a spinal and peripheral arthritis, psoriasiform nail and skin changes, and bowel inflammation. Thus, HLA-B27 is an important risk factor for the spondyloarthropathies. However, some patients with these disorders are HLA-B27-negative, and the great majority of HLA-B27-positive individuals do not develop spondyloarthropathies. The gene is therefore neither necessary nor sufficient to cause spondyloarthropathies.

Infection also appears to play a key role in some of the spondyloarthropathies, especially Reiter's syndrome, which characteristically develops days to weeks after bacterial dysentery or a nongonococcal sexually transmitted infection (see below). The interplay of susceptibility genes and environmental infections is demonstrated by the fact that the risk of developing Reiter's syndrome is 0.2% in the general population, 2% in the HLA-B27 individuals, and 20% in patients with HLA-B27 who become infected with *Salmonella, Shigella,* or enteric organisms. Despite these gains in our understanding of the importance of HLA-B27 and infection, the precise mechanism by which genes and infection cause spondyloarthropathy is not yet known.

ANKYLOSING SPONDYLITIS

 ESSENTIALS OF DIAGNOSIS

- *Chronic low backache in young adults, generally worst in the morning.*
- *Progressive limitation of back motion and of chest expansion.*
- *Transient (50%) or permanent (25%) peripheral arthritis.*
- *Anterior uveitis in 20–25%.*
- *Diagnostic radiographic changes in sacroiliac joints.*
- *Elevated ESR and negative serologic tests for rheumatoid factor.*
- *HLA-B27 testing is most helpful when there is an indeterminate probability of disease.*

General Considerations

Ankylosing spondylitis is a chronic inflammatory disease of the joints of the axial skeleton, manifested clinically by pain and progressive stiffening of the spine. The age at onset is usually in the late teens or early 20s. The incidence is greater in males than in females, and symptoms are more prominent in men, with ascending involvement of the spine more likely to occur.

Clinical Findings

A. SYMPTOMS AND SIGNS

The onset is usually gradual, with intermittent bouts of back pain that may radiate down the thighs. As the disease advances, symptoms progress in a cephalad direction and back motion becomes limited, with the normal lumbar curve flattened and the thoracic curvature exaggerated. Chest expansion is often limited as a consequence of costovertebral joint involvement. Radicular symptoms due to cauda equina fibrosis may occur years after onset of the disease. In advanced cases, the entire spine becomes fused, allowing no motion in any direction. Transient acute arthritis of the peripheral joints occurs in about 50% of cases, and permanent changes in the peripheral joints—most commonly the hips, shoulders, and knees—are seen in about 25%.

Spondylitic heart disease, characterized chiefly by atrioventricular conduction defects and aortic insufficiency, occurs in 3–5% of patients with longstanding severe disease. Anterior uveitis is associated in as many as 25% of cases and may be a presenting feature. Pulmonary fibrosis of the upper lobes, with progression to cavitation and bronchiectasis mimicking tuberculosis, may occur, characteristically long after the onset of skeletal symptoms. Constitutional symptoms similar to those of rheumatoid arthritis are absent in most patients.

B. LABORATORY FINDINGS

The ESR is elevated in 85% of cases, but serologic tests for rheumatoid factor are characteristically negative. Anemia may be present but is often mild. HLA-B27 is found in 90% of white patients and 50% of black patients with ankylosing spondylitis. Because this antigen occurs in 8% of the healthy white population (and 4% of healthy blacks), it is not a specific diagnostic test.

C. IMAGING

The earliest radiographic changes are usually in the sacroiliac joints. In the first few months of the disease process, the sacroiliac changes may be detectable only by CT scanning. Later, erosion and sclerosis of these joints are evident on plain radiographs. Involvement of the apophysial joints of the spine, ossification of the annulus fibrosus, calcification of the anterior and lateral spinal ligaments, and squaring and generalized demineralization of the vertebral bodies may occur in more advanced stages. The term "bamboo spine" has been used to describe the late radiographic appearance of the spinal column.

Additional radiographic findings include periosteal new bone formation on the iliac crest, ischial tuberosi-

ties and calcanei, and alterations of the pubic symphysis and sternomanubrial joint similar to those of the sacroiliacs. Radiologic changes in peripheral joints, when present, tend to be asymmetric and lack the demineralization and erosions seen in rheumatoid arthritis.

Differential Diagnosis

In contrast to ankylosing spondylitis, rheumatoid arthritis predominantly affects multiple, small, peripheral joints of the hands and feet. Rheumatoid arthritis also spares the sacroiliac joints, and has little effect on the rest of the spine except for C1–C2. Finally, rheumatoid arthritis is often associated with rheumatoid nodules and with rheumatoid factor, not with HLA-B27. The history and physical findings of ankylosing spondylitis serve to distinguish this disorder from other causes of low back pain such as disk disease, osteoporosis, soft tissue trauma, and tumors. The most valuable distinguishing radiologic sign of ankylosing spondylitis is the appearance of the sacroiliac joints, although a similar pattern may be seen in Reiter's syndrome and in the arthritis associated with inflammatory intestinal diseases and psoriasis. In ankylosing hyperostosis (diffuse idiopathic skeletal hyperostosis [DISH], Forestier's disease), there is exuberant osteophyte formation. The osteophytes are thicker and more anterior than the syndesmophytes of ankylosing spondylitis, and the sacroiliac joints are not affected. The x-ray appearance of the sacroiliac joints in spondylitis should be distinguished from that in osteitis condensans ilii.

Treatment

A. BASIC PROGRAM

The general principles of managing chronic arthritis (see above) apply equally well to ankylosing spondylitis. The importance of postural and breathing exercises should be stressed.

B. DRUG THERAPY

The NSAIDs are used in the treatment of this disorder. Of these, indomethacin appears to be the most effective, though it can be quite toxic. The dosage of indomethacin is usually 25–50 mg orally three times a day, but the smallest effective dose should be used. Indomethacin may produce a variety of untoward reactions, including headache, giddiness, nausea and vomiting, peptic ulcer, renal insufficiency, depression, and psychosis. Other NSAIDs are valuable alternatives and may be used as primary therapy. Sulfasalazine (1000 mg twice daily) is sometimes useful for the peripheral arthritis in patients with spondyloarthropathies but has little symptomatic effect on spinal and sacroiliac joint disease. Curiously, corticosteroids have minimal impact on the arthritis—particularly the spondylitis—of ankylosing spondylitis. Studies with TNF inhibitors demonstrate that these agents are highly effective in both the spinal and peripheral arthritis of ankylosing spondylitis. Either etanercept (25 mg subcutaneously twice a week) or infliximab (5 mg/kg every other month by IV infusion) is reasonable for patients whose symptoms are refractory to physical therapy and other interventions.

Prognosis

Almost all patients have persistent symptoms over decades; rare individuals experience long-term remissions. The severity of disease varies greatly, with about 10% of patients having work disability after 10 years. Developing hip disease within the first 2 years of disease onset presages a worse prognosis. The availability of TNF inhibitors has improved the outlook dramatically for many patients with ankylosing spondylitis, and the early use of these therapies may attenuate many of the long-term disabilities otherwise characteristic of this disease.

Baraliakos X et al: Magnetic resonance imaging examinations of the spine in patients with ankylosing spondylitis before and after therapy with the tumor necrosis factor alpha receptor fusion protein etanercept. Arthritis Rheum 2005;52:1216. [PMID: 15818694]

Braun J et al: Persistent clinical response to the anti-TNF-alpha antibody infliximab in patients with ankylosing spondylitis over 3 years. Rheumatology (Oxford) 2005;44:670. [PMID: 15757965]

van der Heijde D et al: Efficacy and safety of infliximab in patients with ankylosing spondylitis: Results of a randomized, placebo-controlled trial (ASSERT). Arthritis Rheum 2005; 52:582. [PMID: 15692973]

Wanders A et al: Nonsteroidal antiinflammatory drugs reduce radiographic progression in patients with ankylosing spondylitis: A randomized clinical trial. Arthritis Rheum 2005;52: 1756. [PMID: 15934081]

Ward MM: Prospects for disease modification in ankylosing spondylitis: Do nonsteroidal antiinflammatory drugs do more than treat symptoms? Arthritis Rheum 2005;52:1634. [PMID: 15934065]

PSORIATIC ARTHRITIS

ESSENTIALS OF DIAGNOSIS

- *Psoriasis precedes onset of arthritis in 80% of cases.*
- *Arthritis usually asymmetric, with "sausage" appearance of fingers and toes; resembles rheumatoid arthritis; rheumatoid factor is negative.*
- *Sacroiliac joint involvement common; ankylosis of the sacroiliac joints may occur.*
- *Radiographic findings: osteolysis; pencil-in-cup deformity; relative lack of osteoporosis; bony ankylosis; asymmetric sacroiliitis and atypical syndesmophytes.*

General Considerations

In 15–20% of patients with psoriasis, arthritis coexists. The patterns or subsets of arthritis that may accompany psoriasis include the following:

1. Joint disease that resembles rheumatoid arthritis in which polyarthritis is symmetric. Usually, fewer joints are involved than in rheumatoid arthritis.

2. An oligoarticular form that may lead to considerable destruction of the affected joints.

3. A pattern of disease in which the DIP joints are primarily affected. Early, this may be monarticular, and often the joint involvement is asymmetric. Pitting of the nails and onycholysis are frequently associated.

4. A severe deforming arthritis (arthritis mutilans) in which osteolysis is marked.

5. A spondylitic form in which sacroiliitis and spinal involvement predominate; 50% of these patients are HLA-B27-positive.

Clinical Findings

A. SYMPTOMS AND SIGNS

Although psoriasis usually precedes the onset of arthritis, arthritis precedes or occurs simultaneously with the skin disease in approximately 20% of cases. Arthritis is at least five times more common in patients with severe skin disease than in those with only mild skin findings. Occasionally, however, patients may have a single patch of psoriasis (typically hidden in the scalp, gluteal cleft, or umbilicus) and are unaware of its connection to the arthritis. Thus, a detailed search for cutaneous lesions is essential in patients with arthritis of new onset. Also, the psoriatic lesions may have cleared when arthritis appears—in such cases, the history is most useful in diagnosing previously unexplained cases of mono- or oligoarthritis. Nail pitting, a residue of previous psoriasis, is sometimes the only clue.

B. LABORATORY FINDINGS

Laboratory studies show an elevation of the ESR, but rheumatoid factor is not present. Uric acid levels may be high, reflecting the active turnover of skin affected by psoriasis. There is a correlation between the extent of psoriatic involvement and the level of uric acid, but gout is no more common than in patients without psoriasis. Desquamation of the skin may also reduce iron stores.

C. IMAGING

Radiographic findings are most helpful in distinguishing the disease from other forms of arthritis. There are marginal erosions of bone and irregular destruction of joint and bone, which, in the phalanx, may give the appearance of a sharpened pencil. Fluffy periosteal new bone may be marked, especially at the insertion of muscles and ligaments into bone. Such changes will also be seen along the shafts of metacarpals, metatarsals, and phalanges. Paravertebral ossification occurs, which may be distinguished from ankylosing spondylitis by the absence of ossification in the anterior aspect of the spine.

Treatment

Treatment regimens are symptomatic. NSAIDs are usually sufficient for mild cases. Corticosteroids are less effective in psoriatic arthritis than in other forms of inflammatory arthritis. In addition, they may exacerbate the skin disease during tapers. Antimalarials may also exacerbate psoriasis. In resistant cases, methotrexate may be helpful. For cases with disease that is refractory to methotrexate, etanercept or infliximab is usually effective for both arthritis and psoriatic skin disease. Successful treatment of the skin lesions (eg, by PUVA therapy) commonly—though not invariably—is accompanied by an improvement in peripheral articular symptoms. Both the cutaneous and the articular findings associated with psoriasis respond dramatically in most cases to TNF inhibitors. Alefacept, a biologic agent that is administered by subcutaneous injection, blocks the activation and proliferation of memory effector T cells by binding to CD2. This drug is a promising new treatment for psoriatic arthritis as well as cutaneous disease.

Antoni CE et al: Sustained benefits of infliximab therapy for dermatologic and articular manifestations of psoriatic arthritis: results from the infliximab multinational psoriatic arthritis controlled trial (IMPACT). Arthritis Rheum 2005;52:1227. [PMID: 15818699]

Gottlieb AB: Alefacept for psoriasis and psoriatic arthritis. Ann Rheum Dis 2005;64(Suppl 4):iv58. [PMID: 16239390]

REACTIVE ARTHRITIS

ESSENTIALS OF DIAGNOSIS

- Fifty to 80 percent of patients are HLA-B27-positive.
- Oligoarthritis, conjunctivitis, urethritis, and mouth ulcers most common features.
- Usually follows dysentery or a sexually transmitted infection.

General Considerations

Reactive arthritis (formerly called Reiter's syndrome) is a clinical tetrad of urethritis, conjunctivitis (or, less commonly, uveitis), mucocutaneous lesions, and aseptic arthritis. It occurs most commonly in young men, is associated with HLA-B27 in 80% of white patients and 50–60% of blacks, and often follows infection (see above).

Clinical Findings

A. SYMPTOMS AND SIGNS

Most cases of reactive arthritis develop within days or weeks after either a dysenteric infection (with *Shigella, Salmonella, Yersinia, Campylobacter*) or a sexually transmitted infection (with *Chlamydia trachomatis* or perhaps *Ureaplasma urealyticum*). Whether the inciting infection is sexually transmitted or dysenteric does not affect the subsequent manifestations but does influence the gender ratio: The ratio is 1:1 after enteric infections but 9:1 with male predominance after sexually transmitted infections.

Although affected joints are culture-negative, fragments of putative organisms have been identified by polymerase chain reaction studies on synovial fluid. The exact role of infection remains unclear.

The arthritis is most commonly asymmetric and frequently involves the large weight-bearing joints (chiefly the knee and ankle); sacroiliitis or ankylosing spondylitis is observed in at least 20% of patients, especially after frequent recurrences. Systemic symptoms including fever and weight loss are common at the onset of disease. The mucocutaneous lesions may include balanitis, stomatitis, and keratoderma blennorrhagicum, indistinguishable from pustular psoriasis. Involvement of the fingernails in Reiter's syndrome may also mimic psoriatic changes. Carditis and aortic regurgitation may occur. While most signs of the disease disappear within days or weeks, the arthritis may persist for several months or even years. Recurrences involving any combination of the clinical manifestations are common and are sometimes followed by permanent sequelae, especially in the joints.

B. IMAGING

Radiographic signs of permanent or progressive joint disease may be seen in the sacroiliac as well as the peripheral joints.

Differential Diagnosis

Gonococcal arthritis can initially mimic reactive arthritis, but the marked improvement after 24–48 hours of antibiotic administration and the culture results distinguish the two disorders. Rheumatoid arthritis, ankylosing spondylitis, and psoriatic arthritis must also be considered. By causing similar oral, ocular, and joint lesions, Behçet's disease may also mimic reactive arthritis. The oral lesions of reactive arthritis, however, are typically painless, in contrast to those of Behçet's.

The association of reactive arthritis and HIV has been debated, but evidence now indicates that it is equally common in sexually active men regardless of HIV status.

Treatment

NSAIDs have been the mainstay of therapy. Antibiotics given at the time of a nongonococcal sexually transmitted infection reduce the chance that the individual will develop this disorder. Unfortunately, once reactive arthritis has developed, antibiotics do not alleviate symptoms. Patients who fail NSAIDs and tetracycline may respond to sulfasalazine, 1000 mg orally twice daily, or to methotrexate, 7.5–20 mg orally per week. Anti-TNF agents (etanercept, infliximab, adalimumab) are effective options in most patients with disease that is refractory to more conventional therapies.

Colmegna I et al: Recent advances in reactive arthritis. Curr Rheumatol Rep 2005;7:201. [PMID: 15918996]

ARTHRITIS & INFLAMMATORY INTESTINAL DISEASES

One-fifth of patients with inflammatory bowel disease have arthritis, making it second only to anemia as the most common extraintestinal manifestation. Arthritis complicates Crohn's disease somewhat more frequently than it does ulcerative colitis. In both diseases, two distinct forms of arthritis occur. The first is peripheral arthritis—usually a nondeforming asymmetric oligoarthritis of large joints—in which the activity of the joint disease parallels that of the bowel disease. The arthritis usually begins months to years after the bowel disease, but occasionally the joint symptoms develop earlier and may be prominent enough to cause the patient to overlook intestinal symptoms. The second form of arthritis is a spondylitis that is indistinguishable by symptoms or x-ray from ankylosing spondylitis and follows a course independent of the bowel disease. About 50% of these patients are HLA-B27-positive.

Controlling the intestinal inflammation usually eliminates the peripheral arthritis. The spondylitis often requires NSAIDs, which need to be used cautiously since these agents may activate the bowel disease in a few patients. Range-of-motion exercises as prescribed for ankylosing spondylitis can be helpful.

About two-thirds of patients with Whipple's disease experience arthralgia or arthritis, most often an episodic, large-joint polyarthritis. The arthritis usually precedes the gastrointestinal manifestations by years. In fact, the arthritis resolves as the diarrhea develops. Thus, Whipple's disease should be considered in the differential diagnosis of unexplained episodic arthritis.

■ INFECTIOUS ARTHRITIS*

NONGONOCOCCAL ACUTE BACTERIAL (Septic) ARTHRITIS

 ESSENTIALS OF DIAGNOSIS

- Sudden onset of acute arthritis, usually monar-

*Lyme disease is discussed in Chapter 34.

ticular, most often in large weight-bearing joints and wrists.
- Previous joint damage or injection drug abuse common risk factors.
- Infection with causative organisms commonly found elsewhere in body.
- Joint effusions are usually large, with white blood counts commonly > 50,000/mcL.

General Considerations

Nongonococcal acute bacterial arthritis is a disease of an abnormal host. The key risk factors are persistent bacteremia (eg, injection drug use, endocarditis) and damaged joints (eg, rheumatoid arthritis). *S aureus* is the most common cause of nongonococcal septic arthritis, followed by group A and group B streptococci. Gram-negative septic arthritis, once rare, has become more common, especially in injection drug users and in other immunocompromised hosts. *Escherichia coli* and *Pseudomonas aeruginosa* are the most common gram-negative isolates in adults.

The widespread use of arthroscopy and prosthetic joint surgery has also increased the frequency of septic arthritis. In the latter conditions, *Staphylococcus epidermidis* is the usual offending organism. Pathologic changes include varying degrees of acute inflammation, with synovitis, effusion, abscess formation in synovial or subchondral tissues, and, if treatment is not adequate, articular destruction.

Clinical Findings

A. SYMPTOMS AND SIGNS

The onset is usually sudden, with acute pain, swelling, and heat of one joint—most frequently the knee. Other commonly affected sites are the hip, wrist, shoulder, and ankle. Unusual sites, such as the sternoclavicular or sacroiliac joint, can be involved in injection drug users. Chills and fever are common but are absent in up to 20% of patients. Infection of the hip usually does not produce apparent swelling but results in groin pain greatly aggravated by walking.

B. LABORATORY FINDINGS

Blood cultures are positive in approximately 50% of patients. The leukocyte count of the synovial fluid exceeds 50,000/mcL and often 100,000/mcL, with 90% or more polymorphonuclear cells. Synovial fluid glucose is usually low. Gram stain of the synovial fluid is positive in 75% of staphylococcal infections and in 50% of gram-negative infections.

C. IMAGING

Radiographs are usually normal early in the disease, but evidence of demineralization may be present within days of onset. Bony erosions and narrowing of the joint space followed by osteomyelitis and periostitis may be seen within 2 weeks.

Differential Diagnosis

The septic course with chills and fever, the acute systemic reaction, the joint fluid findings, evidence of infection elsewhere in the body, and the evidence of response to appropriate antibiotics are diagnostic of bacterial arthritis. Gout and pseudogout are excluded by the failure to find crystals on synovial fluid analysis. Acute rheumatic fever and rheumatoid arthritis commonly involve many joints; Still's disease may mimic septic arthritis, but laboratory evidence of infection is absent. Pyogenic arthritis may be superimposed on other types of joint disease, notably rheumatoid arthritis. Indeed, septic arthritis must be excluded (by joint fluid examination) in any patient with rheumatoid arthritis who has a joint strikingly more inflamed than the other joints.

Treatment

Prompt systemic antibiotic therapy of any septic arthritis should be based on the best clinical judgment of the causative organism and the results of smear and culture of joint fluid, blood, urine, or other specific sites of potential infection. If the organism cannot be determined clinically, treatment should be started with bactericidal antibiotics effective against staphylococci, pneumococci, and gram-negative organisms.

Frequent (even daily) local aspiration is indicated when synovial fluid rapidly reaccumulates and causes symptoms. Immediate surgical drainage is reserved for septic arthritis of the hip, because that site is inaccessible to repeated aspiration. For most other joints, surgical drainage by arthroscopy or open technique is used only if medical therapy fails over 2–4 days to improve the fever and the synovial fluid volume, white blood count, and culture results. Pain can be relieved with local hot compresses and by immobilizing the joint with a splint or traction. Rest, immobilization, and elevation are used at the onset of treatment. Early active motion exercises within the limits of tolerance will hasten recovery.

Prognosis

The outcome of septic arthritis depends largely on the antecedent health of the patient, the causative organism (eg, *S aureus* bacterial arthritis is associated with a poor functional outcome in about 40% of cases), and the promptness of treatment. Five to 10 percent of patients with an infected joint die of respiratory complications of sepsis. The mortality rate is 30% for patients with polyarticular sepsis. Bony ankylosis and articular destruction commonly also occur if treatment is delayed or inadequate.

Nolla JM et al: Group B streptococcus (*Streptococcus agalactiae*) pyogenic arthritis in nonpregnant adults. Medicine (Baltimore) 2003;82:119. [PMID: 12640188]

Ross JJ et al: Sternoclavicular septic arthritis: review of 180 cases. Medicine (Baltimore) 2004;83:139. [PMID: 15118542]

Zimmerli W et al: Prosthetic-joint infections. N Engl J Med 2004;351:1645. [PMID: 15483283]

GONOCOCCAL ARTHRITIS

 ESSENTIALS OF DIAGNOSIS

- *Prodromal migratory polyarthralgias.*
- *Tenosynovitis most common sign.*
- *Purulent monarthritis in 50%.*
- *Characteristic skin rash.*
- *Most common in young women during menses or pregnancy.*
- *Symptoms of urethritis frequently absent.*
- *Dramatic response to antibiotics.*

General Considerations

In contrast to nongonococcal bacterial arthritis, gonococcal arthritis usually occurs in otherwise healthy individuals. Host factors, however, influence the expression of the disease: Gonococcal arthritis is two to three times more common in women than in men, is especially common during menses and pregnancy, and is rare after age 40. Gonococcal arthritis is also common in male homosexuals, whose high incidence of asymptomatic gonococcal pharyngitis and proctitis predisposes them to disseminated gonococcal infection. Some of the signs of disseminated gonococcal infection may result from an immunologic reaction to nonviable fragments of the organism's cell wall; this may explain the frequent inability to culture organisms from skin and joint lesions. Recurrent disseminated gonococcal infection should prompt testing of the patient's CH50 level to evaluate for a congenital deficiency of the terminal complement components C7 and C8.

Clinical Findings

A. SYMPTOMS AND SIGNS

One to 4 days of migratory polyarthralgias involving the wrist, knee, ankle, or elbow is the most common initial course. Thereafter, two patterns emerge, one (60% of patients) characterized by tenosynovitis and the other (40%) by purulent monarthritis, most frequently involving the knee. Less than half of patients have fever, and less than one-fourth have any genitourinary symptoms. Most patients will have asymptomatic but highly characteristic skin lesions that usually consist of two to ten small necrotic pustules distributed over the extremities, especially the palms and soles.

B. LABORATORY FINDINGS

The peripheral blood leukocyte count averages about 10,000 cells/mcL and is elevated in less than one-third of patients. The synovial fluid white blood cell count, however, is typically over 50,000 cells/mcL. The synovial fluid Gram stain is positive in one-fourth of cases and culture in less than half. Positive blood cultures are seen in 40% of patients with tenosynovitis and virtually never in patients with suppurative arthritis. Urethral, throat, and rectal cultures should be done in all patients, since they are often positive in the absence of local symptoms. Culturing *Neisseria gonorrhoeae* is facilitated by rapid transport to the microbiology laboratory, inoculation on appropriate media, and incubation in carbon dioxide.

C. IMAGING

Radiographs are usually normal or show only soft tissue swelling.

Differential Diagnosis

Reactive arthritis can produce acute monarthritis in a young person but is distinguished by negative cultures, sacroiliitis, and failure to respond to antibiotics. Lyme disease involving the knee is less acute, does not show positive cultures, and may be preceded by known tick exposure and characteristic rash. The synovial fluid analysis will exclude gout, pseudogout, and nongonococcal bacterial arthritis. Rheumatic fever and sarcoidosis can produce migratory tenosynovitis but have other distinguishing features. Infective endocarditis with septic arthritis can mimic disseminated gonococcal infection.

Treatment

In most cases, patients in whom gonococcal arthritis is suspected should be admitted to the hospital to confirm the diagnosis, to exclude endocarditis, and to start treatment. While outpatient treatment has been recommended in the past, the rapid rise in gonococci resistant to penicillin makes initial inpatient treatment advisable. Approximately 4–5% of all gonococcal isolates produce a β-lactamase that confers penicillin resistance. An additional 15–20% of gonococcal species have chromosomal mutations that result in relative resistance to penicillin. Therefore, the recommendations for initial treatment of gonococcal arthritis are to give ceftriaxone, 1 g intravenously daily (or cefotaxime, 1 g intravenously every 8 hours); spectinomycin, 2 g intramuscularly every 12 hours, may be used for patients with β-lactam allergies). Once improvement from parenteral antibiotics has been achieved for 24–48 hours, patients can be switched to oral cefixime, 400 mg orally twice daily, or, in regions with low rates of quinolone resistance, levofloxacin 500 mg orally daily or ciprofloxacin 500 mg orally twice daily, to complete a 7- to 10-day course.

Prognosis

Generally, gonococcal arthritis responds dramatically in 24–48 hours after initiation of antibiotics so that daily joint aspirations are rarely needed. Complete recovery is the rule.

Bardin T: Gonococcal arthritis. Best Pract Res Clin Rheumatol 2003;17:201. [PMID: 12787521]

RHEUMATIC MANIFESTATIONS OF HIV INFECTION

Infection with HIV has been associated with various rheumatic disorders, most commonly arthralgias or reactive arthritis. More rarely myositis, psoriatic arthritis, Sjögren's syndrome, or vasculitis has been reported to occur (see Chapter 31). It is possible that these disorders stem directly from HIV infection itself or from the many other infections that occur in immunodeficient patients. The rheumatic syndromes may follow the diagnosis of AIDS or may precede it by several months. Thus, coexistent HIV infection must be considered in patients presenting with reactive arthritis. The lower extremity joints, especially the knees and ankles, are most commonly affected. Often, as in classic Reiter's syndrome (reactive arthritis), Achilles tendon inflammation (enthesopathy) or knee periarthritis is a prominent and distinguishing feature. Many patients respond to NSAIDs, though a few are unresponsive and develop progressive deformities. In the era of highly active antiretroviral therapies, immunosuppressive medications can be used if necessary in HIV patients, though with reluctance and great caution. Finally, medications used to treat HIV, particularly the protease inhibitors, may be associated with musculoskeletal side effects, chiefly arthralgias.

Calabrese LH et al: Rheumatic complications of human immunodeficiency virus infection in the era of highly active antiretroviral therapy: emergence of a new syndrome of immune reconstitution and changing patterns of disease. Semin Arthritis Rheum 2005;35:166. [PMID: 16325657]

VIRAL ARTHRITIS

Arthritis may be a manifestation of many viral infections. It is generally mild and of short duration, terminating without lasting ill effects. Mumps arthritis may occur in the absence of parotitis. Rubella arthritis, which occurs more commonly in adults than in children, may appear immediately before, during, or soon after the disappearance of the rash. Its usual polyarticular and symmetric distribution mimics that of rheumatoid arthritis. However, the seronegative tests for rheumatoid factor and the rising rubella titers in convalescent serum help confirm the diagnosis. Postrubella vaccination arthritis may have its onset as long as 6 weeks following vaccination and occurs in all age groups. In adults, arthritis may follow infection with human parvovirus B19 and sometimes mimics rheumatoid arthritis.

Transient polyarthritis may be associated with type B hepatitis and typically occurs before the onset of jaundice; it may occur in anicteric hepatitis as well. Urticaria or other types of skin rash may be present. Indeed, the clinical picture may be indistinguishable from that of serum sickness. Serum transaminase levels are elevated, and hepatitis B surface antigen is most often present. Serum complement levels are usually low during active arthritis and become normal after remission of arthritis. False-positive tests for rheumatoid factor, when present, disappear within several weeks. The arthritis is mild; it rarely lasts more than a few weeks and is self-limiting and without deformity. Hepatitis C infection may be associated with chronic polyarthralgia or polyarthritis that mimics rheumatoid arthritis, both in the distribution of involved joints and the fact that many patients infected with hepatitis C are rheumatoid factor positive in at least low titers.

Mariette X: Hepatitis C virus, arthritides, and arthromyalgia. Joint Bone Spine 2003;70:246. [PMID: 12951305]

Masuko-Hongo K et al: Virus-associated arthritis. Best Pract Res Clin Rheumatol 2003;17:309. [PMID: 12787527]

■ INFECTIONS OF BONES

Direct microbial contamination of bones results from open fracture, surgical procedures, gunshot wounds, diagnostic needle aspirations, and therapeutic or self-administered drug injections.

Indirect or secondary infections are first noticed in other areas of the body and extend to bones by hematogenous routes.

ACUTE PYOGENIC OSTEOMYELITIS

ESSENTIALS OF DIAGNOSIS

- Fever and chills associated with pain and tenderness of involved bone.
- Aspiration of involved bone is usually diagnostic.
- Culture of blood or lesion tissue is essential for precise diagnosis.
- ESR often extremely high (eg, > 100 mm/h).
- Radiographs early in the course are typically negative.

General Considerations

Osteomyelitis is a serious infection that is often difficult to diagnose and treat. Infection of bone occurs as a consequence of (1) hematogenous dissemination of bacteria, (2) invasion from a contiguous focus of infection, and (3) skin breakdown in the setting of vascular insufficiency.

Clinical Findings

A. SYMPTOMS AND SIGNS

1. Hematogenous osteomyelitis—Osteomyelitis resulting from bacteremia is a disease associated with sickle cell disease, injection drug users, or the elderly. Patients with this form of osteomyelitis often present with sudden onset of high fever, chills, and pain and tenderness of the involved bone. The site of osteomyelitis and the causative organism depend on the host. Among patients with hemoglobinopathies such as sickle cell anemia, osteomyelitis is caused by salmonellae ten times as often as by other bacteria. Osteomyelitis in injection drug users develops most commonly in the spine. Although in this setting S aureus is most common, gram-negative infections, especially P aeruginosa and Serratia species, are also frequent pathogens. Rapid progression to epidural abscess causing fever, pain, and sensory and motor loss is not uncommon. In older patients with hematogenous osteomyelitis, the most common sites are the thoracic and lumbar vertebral bodies. Risk factors for these patients include diabetes, intravenous catheters, and indwelling urinary catheters. These patients often have more subtle presentations, with low-grade fever and gradually increasing bone pain.

2. Osteomyelitis from a contiguous focus of infection—Prosthetic joint replacement, decubitus ulcer, neurosurgery, and trauma most frequently cause soft tissue infections that can spread to bone. S aureus and S epidermidis are the most common organisms. Localized signs of inflammation are usually evident, but high fever and other signs of toxicity are usually absent.

3. Osteomyelitis associated with vascular insufficiency—Patients with diabetes and vascular insufficiency are susceptible to developing a very challenging form of osteomyelitis. The foot and ankle are the most commonly affected sites. Infection originates from an ulcer or other break in the skin that is usually still present when the patient presents but may appear disarmingly unimpressive. Bone pain is often absent or muted by the associated neuropathy. Fever is also commonly absent. One of the best bedside clues that the patient has osteomyelitis is the ability to easily advance a sterile probe through a skin ulcer to bone.

B. IMAGING AND LABORATORY FINDINGS

The plain film is the most readily available imaging procedure to establish the diagnosis of osteomyelitis, but it can be falsely negative early. Early radiographic findings may include soft tissue swelling, loss of tissue planes, and periarticular demineralization of bone. About 2 weeks after onset of symptoms, erosion of bone and alteration of cancellous bone appear, followed by periostitis.

MRI, CT, and nuclear medicine bone scanning are more sensitive than conventional radiography. MRI is the most sensitive and is particularly helpful in demonstrating the extent of soft tissue involvement. Radionuclide bone scanning is most valuable when osteomyelitis is suspected but no site is obvious. Nuclear medicine studies may also detect multifocal sites of infection. Ultrasound is useful in diagnosing the presence of effusions within joints and extra-articular soft tissue fluid collections but not in detecting bone infections.

Identifying the offending organism is a crucial step in selection of antibiotic therapy. Bone biopsy for culture is required except in those with hematogenous osteomyelitis, who have positive blood cultures. Cultures from overlying ulcers, wounds, or fistulas are unreliable.

Differential Diagnosis

Acute hematogenous osteomyelitis should be distinguished from suppurative arthritis, rheumatic fever, and cellulitis. More subacute forms must be differentiated from tuberculosis or mycotic infections of bone and Ewing's sarcoma or, in the case of vertebral osteomyelitis, from metastatic tumor. When osteomyelitis involves the vertebrae, it commonly traverses the disk—a finding not observed in tumor.

Complications

Inadequate treatment of bone infections results in chronicity of infection, and this possibility is increased by delaying diagnosis and treatment. Extension to adjacent bone or joints may complicate acute osteomyelitis. Recurrence of bone infections often results in anemia, a markedly elevated ESR, weight loss, weakness and, rarely, amyloidosis or nephrotic syndrome. Pseudoepitheliomatous hyperplasia, squamous cell carcinoma, or fibrosarcoma may occasionally arise in persistently infected tissues.

Treatment

Most patients require both debridement of necrotic bone and prolonged administration of antibiotics. Patients with vertebral body osteomyelitis and epidural abscess require urgent neurosurgical decompression. Depending on the site and extent of debridement, surgical procedures to stabilize, fill in, cover, or revascularize may be needed. Traditionally, antibiotics have been administered parenterally for at least 4–6 weeks. Oral therapy with quinolones (eg, ciprofloxacin, 750 mg twice daily) for 6–8 weeks has been shown to be as effective as standard parenteral antibiotic therapy for chronic osteomyelitis with susceptible organisms. When treating osteomyelitis caused by *S aureus*, quinolones are usually combined with rifampin, 300 mg orally twice daily.

Prognosis

If sterility of the lesion is achieved within 2–4 days, a good result can be expected in most cases if there is no compromise of the patient's immune system. However, progression of the disease to a chronic form may occur. It is especially common in the lower extremities and in patients in whom circulation is impaired (eg, diabetics).

Lew D et al: Osteomyelitis. Lancet 2004:24;364:369. [PMID: 15276398]

MYCOTIC INFECTIONS OF BONES & JOINTS

Fungal infections of the skeletal system are usually secondary to a primary infection in another organ, frequently the lungs (see Chapter 36). Although skeletal lesions have a predilection for the cancellous portions of long bones and vertebral bodies, the predominant lesion—a granuloma with varying degrees of necrosis and abscess formation—does not produce a characteristic clinical picture.

Differentiation from other chronic focal infections depends on culture studies of synovial fluid or tissue obtained from the local lesion. Serologic tests provide presumptive support of the diagnosis.

1. Candidiasis

Candidal osteomyelitis most commonly develops in debilitated, malnourished patients undergoing prolonged hospitalization for cancer, neutropenia, trauma, complicated abdominal surgical procedures, or injection drug use. Infected intravenous catheters frequently serve as a hematogenous source. Prosthetic joints can also be infected by *Candida*.

For susceptible *Candida* species, fluconazole, 200 mg orally twice daily, is probably as effective as amphotericin B.

Garbino J et al: An unusual cause of vertebral osteomyelitis: Candida species. Scand J Infect Dis 2003;35:288. [PMID: 12839165]

2. Coccidioidomycosis

Coccidioidomycosis of bones and joints is usually secondary to primary pulmonary infection. Arthralgia with periarticular swelling, especially in the knees and ankles, occurring as a nonspecific manifestation of systemic coccidioidomycosis, should be distinguished from actual bone or joint infection. Osseous lesions commonly occur in cancellous bone of the vertebrae or near the ends of long bones at tendinous insertions. These lesions are initially osteolytic and thus may mimic metastatic tumor or myeloma.

The precise diagnosis depends on recovery of *Coccidioides immitis* from the lesion or histologic examination of tissue obtained by open biopsy. Rising titers of complement-fixing antibodies also provide evidence of the disseminated nature of the disease.

Oral azole antifungal agents (fluconazole 200–400 mg daily, or itraconazole 200 mg twice daily) have become the treatment of choice for bone and joint coc-cidioidomycosis. Chronic infection is rarely cured with antifungal agents and may require operative exci-sion of infected bone and soft tissue; amputation may be the only solution for stubbornly progressive infec-tions. Immobilization of joints by plaster casts and avoidance of weight bearing provide benefit. Synovec-tomy, joint debridement, and arthrodesis are reserved for more advanced joint infections.

3. Histoplasmosis

Focal skeletal or joint involvement in histoplasmosis is rare and generally represents dissemination from a pri-mary focus in the lungs. Skeletal lesions may be single or multiple and are not characteristic.

Steinbach WJ et al: Review of newer antifungal and immuno-modulatory strategies for invasive aspergillosis. Clin Infect Dis 2003;37(Suppl 3):S157. [PMID: 12975751]

Stratov I: Management of Aspergillus osteomyelitis: report of failure of liposomal amphotericin B and response to vori-conazole in an immunocompetent host and literature re-view. Eur J Clin Microbiol Infect Dis 2003;22:277. [PMID: 12734721]

Wheat LJ et al: Histoplasmosis. Infect Dis Clin North Am 2003; 17:1. [PMID: 12751258]

TUBERCULOSIS OF BONES & JOINTS

ESSENTIALS OF DIAGNOSIS

- *A disease of children, the elderly, or those with HIV infection.*
- *In most cases, a single site of bone or joint is in-fected.*
- *Spine—especially lower thoracic—or knee most common sites.*
- *Chest radiographs abnormal in less than half.*

General Considerations

Most tuberculous infections in the United States are caused by the human strain of *Mycobacterium tubercu-losis* (see Chapter 9). Infection of the musculoskeletal system is caused by hematogenous spread from a pri-mary lesion of the respiratory tract; it may occur shortly after primary infection or may be seen years later as a disease reactivation. Tuberculosis of the tho-racic or lumbar spine (Pott's disease) usually occurs in the absence of extraspinal infection. It is a disease of children in developing nations and of the elderly in the United States. Tuberculosis of peripheral joints is almost always monarticular, with the knee the most common site. Extra-articular tuberculosis occurs in only 20%.

Clinical Findings

A. SYMPTOMS AND SIGNS

The onset of symptoms is generally insidious and not accompanied by general manifestations of fever, sweat-ing, toxicity, or prostration. Pain may be mild at on-set, is usually worse at night, and may be accompanied by stiffness. As the disease process progresses, limita-tion of joint motion becomes prominent because of muscle contractures and joint destruction. The knee is the most commonly involved peripheral joint. Symp-toms of pulmonary tuberculosis may also be present.

Local findings during the early stages may be lim-ited to tenderness, soft tissue swelling, joint effusion, and increase in skin temperature about the involved area. As the disease progresses without treatment, muscle atrophy and deformity become apparent. Ab-scess formation with spontaneous drainage externally leads to sinus formation. Progressive destruction of bone in the spine may cause a hump spine or gibbus deformity, especially in the thoracolumbar region.

B. LABORATORY FINDINGS

The precise diagnosis rests on recovery of the acid-fast organism from joint fluid, pus, or tissue specimens. Biopsy of the bony lesion, synovium, or a regional lymph node may demonstrate the characteristic histo-pathologic picture of caseating necrosis and giant cells.

C. IMAGING

There is a latent period between the onset of symp-toms and the initial positive radiographic finding. The earliest changes of tuberculous arthritis are those of soft tissue swelling and distention of the capsule by ef-fusion. Subsequently, bone atrophy causes thinning of the trabecular pattern, narrowing of the cortex, and enlargement of the medullary canal. As joint disease progresses, destruction of cartilage, both in the spine and in peripheral joints, is manifested by narrowing of the joint cleft and focal erosion of the articular surface, especially at the margins. Where the lesion is limited to bone, especially in the cancellous portion of the me-taphysis, radiography may demonstrate single or mul-tilocular cysts surrounded by sclerotic bone. With spinal tuberculosis, CT scanning is helpful in demonstrating paraspinal soft tissue extensions of the infection (eg, psoas abscess, epidural extension).

Differential Diagnosis

Tuberculosis of the musculoskeletal system must be dif-ferentiated from all subacute and chronic infections, rheumatoid arthritis, gout, and, occasionally, osseous dys-plasia. In the spine, metastatic tumor may be suggested.

Complications

Destruction of bones or joints may occur in a few weeks or months if adequate treatment is not provided. Deformity due to joint destruction, abscess formation with spread into adjacent soft tissues, and sinus formation are common. Paraplegia is the most serious complication of spinal tuberculosis. As healing of severe joint lesions takes place, spontaneous fibrous or bony ankylosis follows.

Treatment (See also Chapter 9)

A. GENERAL MEASURES

General care is especially important when prolonged recumbency is necessary; skillful nursing care must be provided.

B. CHEMOTHERAPY

See Chapter 9. Cure with chemotherapy without need for operation may be achieved in most cases, even with extensive disease.

C. SURGICAL MEASURES

In acute infections where synovitis is the predominant feature, treatment can be conservative, at least initially. Immobilization by splint or plaster, aspiration, and chemotherapy may suffice to control the infection. Synovectomy may be valuable for less acute hypertrophic lesions that involve tendon sheaths, bursae, or joints.

Wardle N et al: Orthopaedic manifestations of tuberculosis. Hosp Med 2004;65:228. [PMID: 15127678]

ARTHRITIS IN SARCOIDOSIS

The frequency of arthritis among patients with sarcoidosis is variously reported between 10% and 35%. It is usually acute in onset, but articular symptoms may appear insidiously and often antedate other manifestations of the disease. Knees and ankles are most commonly involved, but any joint may be affected. Distribution of joint involvement is usually polyarticular and symmetric. The arthritis is commonly self-limited, resolving after several weeks or months and rarely resulting in chronic arthritis, joint destruction, or significant deformity. Sarcoid arthropathy is often associated with erythema nodosum, but the diagnosis is contingent on the demonstration of other extra-articular manifestations of sarcoidosis and, notably, biopsy evidence of noncaseating granulomas. In chronic arthritis, radiographs show typical changes in the bones of the extremities with intact cortex and cystic changes.

Treatment of arthritis in sarcoidosis is usually symptomatic and supportive. Colchicine may be of value. A short course of corticosteroids may be effective in patients with severe and progressive joint disease.

Abril A et al: Rheumatologic manifestations of sarcoidosis. Curr Opin Rheumatol 2004;16:51. [PMID: 14673389]

Torralba KD et al: Sarcoid arthritis: a review of clinical features, pathology, and therapy. Sarcoidosis Vasc Diffuse Lung Dis 2003;20:95. [PMID: 12870718]

■ TUMORS & TUMOR-LIKE LESIONS OF BONE

ESSENTIALS OF DIAGNOSIS

- *Persistent pain, swelling, or tenderness of a skeletal part.*
- *Pathologic ("spontaneous") fractures.*
- *Suspicious areas of bony enlargement, deformity, radiodensity, or radiolucency on x-ray.*
- *Histologic evidence of bone neoplasm on biopsy specimen.*

General Considerations

Primary tumors of bone are relatively uncommon in comparison with secondary or metastatic neoplasms. They are, however, of great clinical significance because some grow rapidly and metastasize widely.

Although tumors of bone have been categorized classically as primary or secondary, there is some disagreement about which tumors are primary to the skeleton. Tumors of mesenchymal origin that reflect skeletal tissues (eg, bone, cartilage, and connective tissue) and tumors developing in bones that are of hematopoietic, nerve, vascular, fat cell, and notochordal origin should be differentiated from secondary malignant tumors that involve bone by direct extension or hematogenous spread. Because of the great variety of bone tumors, it is difficult to establish a satisfactory simple classification of bone neoplasms.

Clinical Findings

Persistent skeletal pain and swelling, with or without limitation of motion of adjacent joints or spontaneous fracture, are indications for prompt clinical, radiographic, laboratory, and possibly biopsy examination. Radiographs may reveal the location and extent of the lesion and certain characteristics that may suggest the specific diagnosis. The so-called classic radiographic findings of certain tumors (eg, punched-out areas of the skull in multiple myeloma, "sun ray" appearance of osteogenic sarcoma, and "onion peel" effect of Ewing's sarcoma), although suggestive, are not pathognomonic. Even a bone tumor's histologic characteristics, considered in isolation, provide incomplete information about the nature of the disease. The age of the patient, the duration of complaints, the site of involvement and the number of bones involved, and the presence or absence of associated systemic disease—as well as the histologic characteristics—must all be considered for proper management.

The possibility of benign developmental skeletal abnormalities, metastatic neoplastic disease, infections (eg, osteomyelitis), posttraumatic bone lesions, or metabolic disease of bone must always be kept in mind. If bone tumors occur in or near the joints, they may be confused with the various types of arthritis, especially monarticular arthritis.

Specific Bone Tumors

Tumors arising from osteoblastic connective tissue include osteoid osteoma and osteosarcoma. Osteoid osteomas are benign tumors seen in children and adolescents. Interstitial laser photocoagulation is the treatment of choice. Osteosarcoma, the most common malignancy of bone, typically occurs in an adolescent who presents with pain or swelling in a bone or joint (especially in or around the knee). Since the symptoms often appear to begin following a sports-related injury, accurate diagnosis may be delayed. Osteosarcoma can also develop in patients with Paget's disease of bone, enchondromatosis, fibrous dysplasia, or hereditary multiple exostoses. Osteosarcomas are treated by resection and chemotherapy, with 5-year survival rates improving from 15% in 1965 to 60% at this time. Fibrosarcomas, which are derived from nonosteoblastic connective tissue, have a prognosis similar to that of the osteogenic sarcomas. Tumors derived from cartilage include enchondromas, chondromyxoid fibromas, and chondrosarcomas. Histologic examination is confirmatory in this group, and the prognosis with appropriate curettement or surgery is generally good.

Other bone tumors include giant cell tumors (osteoclastomas), chondroblastomas, and Ewing's sarcoma. Of these, chondroblastomas are almost always benign. About 50% of giant cell tumors are benign, while the rest may be frankly malignant or recur after excision. Ewing's sarcoma, which affects children, adolescents, and young adults, has a 50% mortality rate in spite of chemotherapy, irradiation, and surgery.

Treatment

Although prompt action is essential for optimal treatment of certain bone tumors, accurate diagnosis is required because of the great potential for harm that may result from temporization, radical or ablative operations, or unnecessary irradiation.

Westhovens R et al: Musculoskeletal manifestations of benign and malignant tumors of bone. Curr Opin Rheumatol 2003;15: 70. [PMID: 12496513]

NEUROGENIC ARTHROPATHY (Charcot's Joint)

Neurogenic arthropathy is joint destruction resulting from loss or diminution of proprioception, pain, and temperature perception. Although traditionally associated with tabes dorsalis, it is more frequently seen in diabetic neuropathy, syringomyelia, spinal cord injury, pernicious anemia, leprosy, and peripheral nerve injury. Prolonged administration of hydrocortisone by the intra-articular route may also cause Charcot's joint. As normal muscle tone and protective reflexes are lost, secondary degenerative joint disease ensues, resulting in an enlarged, boggy, painless joint with extensive cartilage erosion, osteophyte formation, and multiple loose joint bodies. Radiographic changes may be degenerative or hypertrophic in the same patient.

Treatment is directed against the primary disease; mechanical devices are used to assist in weight bearing and prevention of further trauma. In some instances, amputation becomes unavoidable.

Anderson JJ et al: Bisphosphonates for the treatment of Charcot neuroarthropathy. J Foot Ankle Surg 2004;43:285. [PMID: 15480402]

■ OTHER RHEUMATIC DISORDERS

RHEUMATIC MANIFESTATIONS OF CANCER

Rheumatologic syndromes may be the presenting manifestations for a variety of cancers. Dermatomyositis in adults, for example, is associated with cancer. In middle-aged or older patients with polyarthritis that mimics rheumatoid arthritis but is associated with new onset of clubbing and periosteal new bone formation, hypertrophic pulmonary osteoarthropathy, a disorder commonly associated with both malignant diseases (eg, lung and intrathoracic cancers) and nonmalignant ones (eg, cyanotic heart disease, cirrhosis, and lung abscess), should be suspected. Palmar fasciitis is characterized by bilateral palmar swelling and finger contraction and may be the first indication of cancer, particularly ovarian carcinoma. Palpable purpura due to leukocytoclastic vasculitis may be the presenting complaint in myeloproliferative disorders. Hairy cell leukemia can be associated with medium-sized vessel vasculitis such as polyarteritis nodosa. Acute leukemia can produce joint pains that are disproportionately severe in comparison to the minimal swelling and heat that are present. Leukemic arthritis complicates approximately 5% of cases. Rheumatic manifestations of myelodysplastic syndromes include cutaneous vasculitis, lupus-like syndromes, neuropathy, and episodic intense arthritis. Erythromelalgia, a painful warmth and redness of the extremities that (unlike Raynaud's) improves with cold exposure or with elevation of the extremity, is often associated with myeloproliferative diseases.

Chakravarty E et al: Rheumatic syndromes associated with malignancy. Curr Opin Rheumatol 2003;15:35. [PMID: 12496508]

PALINDROMIC RHEUMATISM

Palindromic rheumatism is a disease of unknown cause characterized by frequent recurring attacks (at irregular intervals) of acutely inflamed joints. Periarticular pain with swelling and transient subcutaneous nodules may also occur. The attacks cease within several hours to several days. The knee and finger joints are most commonly affected, but any peripheral joint may be involved. Systemic manifestations other than fever do not occur. Although hundreds of attacks may take place over a period of years, there is no permanent articular damage. Laboratory findings are usually normal. Palindromic rheumatism must be distinguished from acute gouty arthritis and an atypical acute onset of rheumatoid arthritis. In some patients, palindromic rheumatism is a prodrome of rheumatoid arthritis.

Symptomatic treatment with NSAIDs is usually all that is required during the attacks. Hydroxychloroquine may be of value in preventing recurrences.

AVASCULAR NECROSIS OF BONE

Avascular necrosis of bone is a complication of corticosteroid use, trauma, SLE, pancreatitis, alcoholism, gout, sickle cell disease, and infiltrative diseases (eg, Gaucher's disease). The most commonly affected sites are the proximal and distal femoral heads, leading to hip or knee pain. Many patients with hip disease actually first present with pain referred to the knee. Physical examination will reveal that it is internal rotation of the hip—not movement of the knee—that is painful. Other commonly affected sites include the ankle, shoulder, and elbow. Initially, radiographs are often normal; MRI, CT scan, and bone scan are all more sensitive techniques. Treatment involves avoidance of weight bearing on the affected joint for at least several weeks. The value of surgical core decompression is controversial. For osteonecrosis of the hip, a variety of procedures designed to preserve the femoral head have been developed for early disease, including vascularized and nonvascularized bone grafting procedures. These procedures are most effective in avoiding or forestalling the need for total hip arthroplasty in young patients who do not have advanced disease. Without a successful intervention of this nature, the natural history of avascular necrosis is usually progression of the bony infarction to cortical collapse, resulting in significant joint dysfunction. Total hip replacement is the usual outcome for all patients who are candidates for that procedure.

Mont MA et al: Outcome of non-vascularized bone grafting for osteonecrosis of the femoral head. Clin Orthop 2003;417: 84. [PMID: 14646705]

Shannon BD et al: Femoral osteotomies for avascular necrosis of the femoral head. Clin Orthop Relat Res 2004;418:34. [PMID: 15043090]

■ SOME ORTHOPEDIC PROCEDURES FOR ARTHRITIC JOINTS

Synovectomy

This procedure attempts to eliminate inflammation at a joint by surgically removing as much of the synovium as possible. The procedure has been performed most commonly in patients with rheumatoid arthritis who, despite medical therapy, have a persistent pannus of inflamed synovium (usually around a wrist or a knee). Patients with degenerative diseases do not have marked synovial inflammation and are not candidates for this procedure.

Unfortunately, synovium can regrow. Even in patients with rheumatoid arthritis, the long-term benefits of synovectomy remain unproved.

Arthroplasty

Realigning arthritic joints (arthroplasty) generally does not work as well as complete joint replacement, but it can defer the need for joint replacement. The typical candidate is an adult under 50 years of age who has severe osteoarthritis of one compartment of the knee (typically the medial compartment). Excising a wedge of femur will realign the patient's knee so as to shift weight to the compartment with normal cartilage and thereby eliminate or reduce the patient's pain.

Tendon Rupture

This is a fairly common complication in rheumatoid arthritis and requires immediate orthopedic referral. The most common sites are the finger flexors and extensors, the patellar tendon, and the Achilles tendon.

Arthrodesis

Arthrodesis (fusion) is being used less now than formerly, but a chronically infected, painful joint may be an indication for this surgical procedure.

Total Joint Arthroplasty

In the last 3 decades, remarkable progress has been made in the replacement of severely damaged joints with prosthetic materials. Although many different joints can be replaced, the largest experience and greatest success have been with hip and knee replacement. Indication for total joint arthroplasty is severe pain (usually including pain at rest) accompanied by loss of function and severe destruction of the joint on x-ray. Age is also a consideration, as the durability of artificial joints beyond 10–15 years is limited with older surgical techniques and unproved with newer techniques. Thus, patients over 65 are less likely than younger ones to face the challenge of revision.

Whatever the patient's age, success of the replacement depends on the amount of physical stress to which the prosthetic components are subjected. Vigorous impact activity, even with the most advanced biomaterials and design, will result in failure of the prosthesis with time. Revision operations are technically more difficult, and the results may not be as good as with the primary procedure. The patient, therefore, must understand the limitations of joint replacement and the consequences of unrestrained joint usage.

A. TOTAL HIP ARTHROPLASTY

Hip replacement was originally designed for use in patients over 65 years of age with severe osteoarthritis. In these patients—usually less active physically—the prosthesis not only functioned well but outlasted the patients. Severe arthritis that fails to respond to conservative measures remains the principal indication for hip arthroplasty. Hip arthroplasty may also be indicated in younger patients severely disabled by painful hip disease (eg, rheumatoid arthritis). Contraindications to the operation include active infection and neurotrophic joint disease. Obesity is a relative contraindication. Serious complications may occur in about 1% of patients and include thrombophlebitis, pulmonary embolization, infection, and dislocation of the joint. Extensive experience has now been accumulated, and the short-term results are highly successful in properly selected patients. The long-term success has been limited by loosening of the prosthesis, a complication seen in 30–50% of patients 10 years after replacement with "first generation" techniques. Although loosening and periprosthetic osteolysis were blamed on the cement, second-generation cementing techniques for prosthetic hips have proved more durable than cementless hips in one out of four cases.

B. TOTAL KNEE ARTHROPLASTY

The indications and contraindications for total knee arthroplasty are similar to those for hip arthroplasty. Results are slightly better in osteoarthritis patients than in those with rheumatoid arthritis. Complications are similar to those with hip arthroplasty. The failure rate of knee arthroplasty is slightly higher than that of hip arthroplasty.

Huo MH: What's new in hip arthroplasty. J Bone Joint Surg Am 2003;85-A:1852. [PMID: 12954856]

Salvati EA et al: Thromboembolism following total hip replacement. J Long Term Eff Med Implants 2003;13:325. [PMID: 14649571]

Sutton PM et al: Treatment of anaemia after joint replacement. A double-blind, randomised, controlled trial of ferrous sulphate versus placebo. J Bone Joint Surg Br 2004;86:31. [PMID: 14765861]

Fluid & Electrolyte Disorders

21

Masafumi Fukagawa, MD, PhD, Kiyoshi Kurokawa, MD, MACP, &
Maxine A. Papadakis, MD

APPROACH TO THE PATIENT

History, Physical Examination, & Basic Laboratory Tests

In many instances, electrolyte disorders are asymptomatic, thus the clinician should never overlook abnormal values in routine laboratory studies. Nevertheless, symptoms such as lethargy, weakness, confusion, delirium, and seizures may develop, especially in the presence of an abnormal serum sodium concentration. Often these symptoms are mistaken for primary neurologic or metabolic disorders. Muscle weakness occurs in patients with severe hypokalemia, hyperkalemia, and hypophosphatemia; confusion, seizures, and coma may develop in those with severe hypercalcemia. Measurement of electrolytes (sodium, potassium, chloride, bicarbonate, calcium, magnesium, and phosphorus) is indicated for any patient with even vague neuromuscular symptoms.

In addition to taking a careful history, the diagnosis and treatment of fluid and electrolyte disorders are based on (1) assessment of total body water and its distribution, (2) serum electrolyte concentrations, (3) urine electrolyte concentrations, and (4) serum osmolality.

A. BODY WATER

Changes of total body water content are best evaluated by documenting changes in body weight. Table 21–1 shows the sex difference in total body water and the decrease in total body water that occurs with aging. Two-thirds of total body water (40% of body weight) is intracellular fluid (ICF), while one-third (20% of body weight) is extracellular fluid (ECF). Water may be lost from either or both of the fluid compartments. Circulatory and neurologic symptoms, physical examination, and laboratory tests (serum and urine sodium, serum urea nitrogen, serum creatinine) can identify the compartment from which fluid is lost.

One-fourth of extracellular fluid (5% of body weight) is retained within the blood vessels as plasma (effective circulating volume). Effective circulating volume may be assessed by physical examination (blood pressure, pulse rate, jugular vein dilation). In addition to the invasive measurement of central venous pressure or pulmonary wedge pressure, noninvasive measurement of the diameter of the inferior vena cava by ultra-

sonography may be useful for assessment of effective circulating volume.

B. SERUM ELECTROLYTES

Table 21–2 shows the normal values for serum electrolytes. Electrolyte disorders may be suspected by considering the history and underlying disease and the medications the patient is taking.

C. EVALUATION OF URINE

Urinalysis provides information about underlying renal disorders. Samples also should be obtained for analysis of urine electrolyte abnormalities. An electrolyte concentration in urine is a useful indicator of renal handling of water and the electrolyte, ie, whether the kidney loses or preserves the electrolyte.

In addition to the total urine per day, a spot urine may be used. Simple concentration, or concentration per gram creatinine excretion, is usually sufficient for initial analysis. More precisely, fractional excretion is used. Fractional excretion (FE) of an electrolyte X (FE$_X$) is calculated using a random urine sample with simultaneously obtained serum samples for X and creatinine (Cr).

$$FE_X(\%) = \frac{Urine\ X/Serum\ X}{Urine\ Cr/Serum\ Cr} \times 100$$

D. SERUM OSMOLALITY

Serum osmolality (normally 285–295 mosm/kg) can be calculated from the following formula:

$$Osmolality = 2(Na^+\ mEq/L) + \frac{Glucose\ mg/dL}{18} + \frac{BUN\ mg/dL}{2.8}$$

(1 mosm of glucose equals 180 mg/L and 1 mosm of urea nitrogen equals 28 mg/L). Solute concentration is usually expressed in terms of osmolality. The number of particles in solution (ie, osmolytes; either molecules or ions) determines the number of milliosmoles. Each particle has a unit value of 1, so if a substance ionizes, each ion contributes the same amount as a nonionizable molecule. More importantly, permeability of the particle across the cell membrane determines whether it

887

Table 21–1. Total body water (as percentage of body weight) in relation to age and sex.

Age	Male	Female
18–40	60%	50%
41–60	60–50%	50–40%
Over 60	50%	40%

acts as a physiologically active osmolyte. Tonicity refers to osmolytes that are impermeable to the cell wall. Since osmolytes do not equilibrate on either side of the cell wall, it is tonicity that leads to osmosis, fluid shifts, stimulation of thirst, and secretion of antidiuretic hormone (ADH). Substances that easily permeate cell membranes (eg, urea, ethanol) are not effective osmolytes and therefore do not cause shifting of fluid in body fluid compartments. For example, glucose in solution is nonionizable. Therefore, 1 mmol of glucose has an osmole concentration of 1 mosm/kg H_2O. One millimole of NaCl, however, forms two ions in water (one Na^+ and one Cl^-) and has an osmole concentration of roughly 2 mosm/kg H_2O. "Osmoles per kilogram of water" is *osmolality;* "osmoles per liter of solution" is *osmolarity.* At the solute concentration of body fluids, the two measurements correspond so closely that they are interchangeable. A discrepancy between actual and calculated osmolality suggests the accumulation of unmeasured osmoles (osmolar gap).

Riggs JE: Neurologic manifestations of electrolyte disturbances. Neurol Clin 2002;20:157. [PMID: 11754308]

■ DISORDERS OF SODIUM CONCENTRATION

An abnormal serum sodium concentration does not necessarily imply abnormal sodium balance but rather implies abnormal water balance. Thus, most instances of abnormal sodium concentration are associated with abnormal serum osmolality and shifts of water across the cell membrane. By contrast, abnormal sodium balance results in an edematous state or in volume depletion.

HYPONATREMIA

ESSENTIALS OF DIAGNOSIS

- *Extracellular fluid volume and serum osmolality are important determinants of etiology.*
- *Most cases of hyponatremia result from water imbalance, not sodium imbalance.*
- *Hospitalized patients treated with hypotonic fluid are at increased risk for the development of hyponatremia.*
- *Treatment strategy should be based not only on pathophysiology but on the severity and speed of development.*

General Considerations

Hyponatremia (defined as a serum sodium concentration less than 130 mEq/L) is the most common electrolyte abnormality observed in a general hospitalized population, seen in about 2% of patients.

The initial approach to its investigation is the determination of serum osmolality (Figure 21–1).

The Urine Sodium

Although most cases of hyponatremia result from water imbalance, not sodium imbalance, measurement of urine sodium helps distinguish renal from nonrenal causes of hyponatremia. Urine sodium exceeding 20 mEq/L is consistent with renal salt wasting (diuretics, angiotensin-converting enzyme (ACE) inhibitors, mineralocorticoid deficiency, salt-losing nephropathy). Urine sodium less than 10 mEq/L or fractional excretion of sodium less than 1% (unless diuretics have been given) implies avid sodium retention by the kidney to compensate for extrarenal fluid losses from vomiting, diarrhea, sweating, or third-spacing, as with ascites.

Isotonic & Hypertonic Hyponatremia

Isotonic and hypertonic hyponatremia should be initially ruled out by determining serum osmolality, blood lipids, and blood glucose.

Table 21–2. Normal values and mass conversion factors.[1]

	Normal Plasma Values	Mass Conversion
Na^+	135–145 mEq/L	23 mg = 1 mEq
K^+	3.5–5 mEq/L	39 mg = 1 mEq
Cl^-	98–107 mEq/L	35 mg = 1 mEq
HCO_3^-	22–28 mEq/L	61 mg = 1 mEq
Ca	8.5–10.5 mg/dL	40 mg = 1 mmol
Phosphorus	2.5–4.5 mg/dL	31 mg = 1 mmol
Mg	1.6–3 mg/dL	24 mg = 1 mmol
Osmolality	280–295 mosm/kg	…

[1]Ca and Mg are measured as their total concentration. Ca ion concentration is about half the total calcium concentration, while Mg ion concentration is about two-thirds the total magnesium concentration.
Modified and reproduced, with permission, from Cogan MG: *Fluid and Electrolytes: Physiology and Pathophysiology.* McGraw-Hill, 1991.

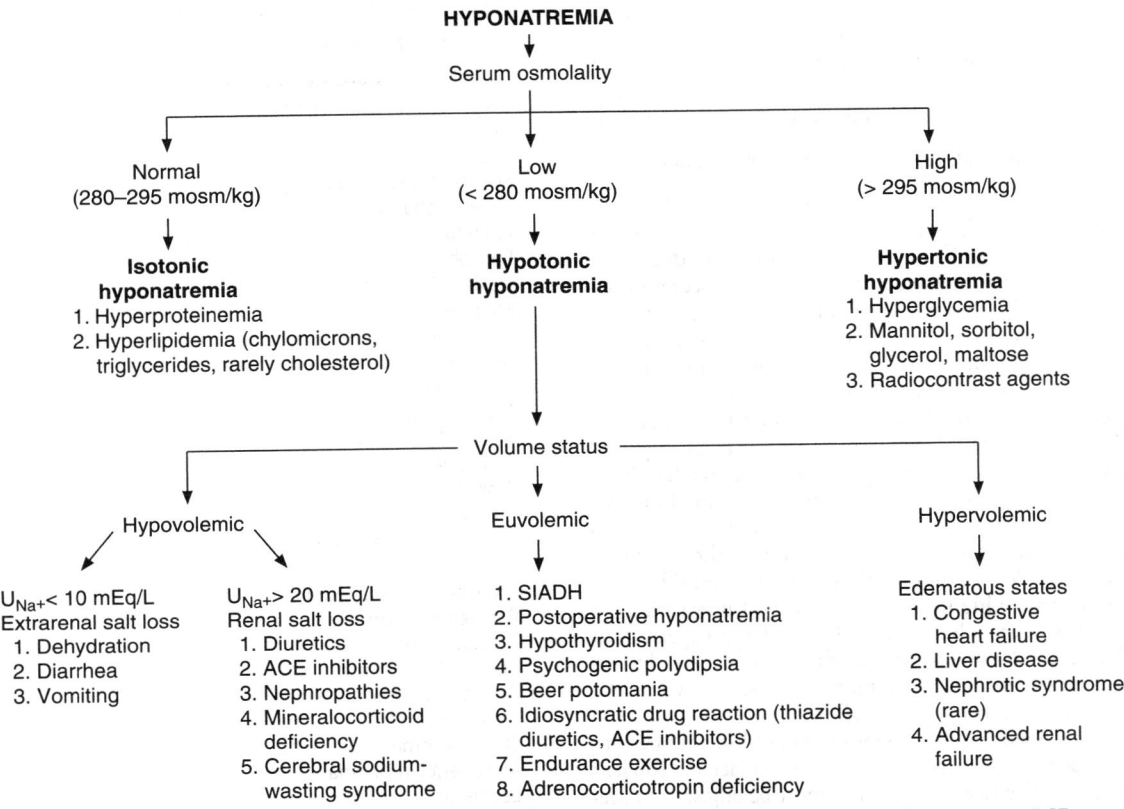

HYPONATREMIA

Serum osmolality

| Normal (280–295 mosm/kg) | Low (< 280 mosm/kg) | High (> 295 mosm/kg) |

Isotonic hyponatremia
1. Hyperproteinemia
2. Hyperlipidemia (chylomicrons, triglycerides, rarely cholesterol)

Hypotonic hyponatremia

Hypertonic hyponatremia
1. Hyperglycemia
2. Mannitol, sorbitol, glycerol, maltose
3. Radiocontrast agents

Volume status

| Hypovolemic | Euvolemic | Hypervolemic |

$U_{Na^+} < 10$ mEq/L
Extrarenal salt loss
1. Dehydration
2. Diarrhea
3. Vomiting

$U_{Na^+} > 20$ mEq/L
Renal salt loss
1. Diuretics
2. ACE inhibitors
3. Nephropathies
4. Mineralocorticoid deficiency
5. Cerebral sodium-wasting syndrome

1. SIADH
2. Postoperative hyponatremia
3. Hypothyroidism
4. Psychogenic polydipsia
5. Beer potomania
6. Idiosyncratic drug reaction (thiazide diuretics, ACE inhibitors)
7. Endurance exercise
8. Adrenocorticotropin deficiency

Edematous states
1. Congestive heart failure
2. Liver disease
3. Nephrotic syndrome (rare)
4. Advanced renal failure

Figure 21–1. Evaluation of hyponatremia using serum osmolality and extracellular fluid volume status. ACE = angiotensin-converting enzyme; SIADH = syndrome of inappropriate antidiuretic hormone. (Adapted, with permission, from Narins RG et al: Diagnostic strategies in disorders of fluid, electrolyte and acid-base homeostasis. Am J Med 1982;72:496.)

Isotonic hyponatremia can be seen with hyperlipidemia and hyperproteinemia. Because of marked increases, lipids (chylomicrons; triglycerides, which make the blood visibly lipemic; and very occasionally cholesterol, which may not make the blood visibly lipemic) and proteins (> 10 g/dL, eg, intravenous immunoglobulin therapy) occupy a disproportionately large portion of the plasma volume. Plasma osmolality remains normal because its measurement is unaffected by the lipids or proteins. A decreased volume of water results, so that the sodium concentration in total plasma volume is decreased. Because the sodium concentration in the plasma water is actually normal, hyperlipidemia and hyperproteinemia cause so-called "pseudohyponatremia." Most laboratories measure serum electrolytes using ion-specific electrodes and thus avoid misdiagnosis unless dilution of samples is needed before direct measurement.

Hypertonic hyponatremia is most commonly seen with hyperglycemia. When blood glucose becomes acutely elevated, water is drawn from the cells into the extracellular space, diluting the serum sodium. The plasma sodium level falls 2 mEq/L for every 100 mg/dL rise when the glucose concentration is be-

tween 200 and 400 mg/dL. If the glucose concentration is above 400 mg/dL, the plasma sodium concentration falls 4 mEq/L for every 100 mg/dL rise in glucose. This "dilutional or translocational hyponatremia" is not "pseudohyponatremia," since the sodium concentration does indeed fall. Infusion of hypertonic solutions containing osmotically active osmoles (eg, mannitol) may also cause hypertonic hyponatremia by drawing water to the extracellular space.

Hypotonic Hyponatremia

Hypotonic hyponatremia is true hyponatremia in a physiologic sense. In this abnormality, water shifts into the cell, usually resulting in increased ICF.

Because the capacity of the kidney to excrete electrolyte-free water is potentially great—up to 20–30 L/d—in the presence of a normal glomerular filtration rate (GFR) (100 L/d), electrolyte-free water intake must theoretically exceed 30 L/d for hyponatremia to develop. Instead, in hypotonic hyponatremia, retention of electrolyte-free water nearly always occurs because of impaired excretion (renal failure, inappropriate ADH excess, etc).

Determinations of the urine osmolality and urine sodium are useful diagnostic tools.

Once a diagnosis of hypotonic hyponatremia has been made, an accurate determination of the patient's volume status is essential in directing further evaluation.

A. HYPOVOLEMIC HYPOTONIC HYPONATREMIA

Hyponatremia with decreased extracellular fluid volume occurs in the setting of renal or extrarenal volume loss (Figure 21–1). Total body sodium is decreased. To maintain intravascular volume, ADH secretion increases, and free water is retained. The drive to replenish intravascular volume overrides the need to sustain normal osmolality; losses of salt and water are replaced by water alone. The combination of low fractional excretion of sodium (< 0.5%) and low fractional urea clearance (< 55%) is the best way to predict improvement with saline therapy. Hyponatremia has been shown to develop in patients with intracranial diseases through renal sodium wasting. Unlike those with syndrome of inappropriate ADH secretion, these patients are hypovolemic, though plasma levels of ADH are inappropriately high for the osmolality. Observations in patients with subarachnoid hemorrhage suggest that the cerebral salt-wasting syndrome is caused by increased secretion of brain natriuretic peptide with suppression of aldosterone secretion.

Treatment consists of replacement of lost volume with isotonic or half-normal (0.45%) saline or lactated Ringer's infusion. The rate of correction must be adjusted to prevent permanent cerebral damage (see below).

B. EUVOLEMIC HYPOTONIC HYPONATREMIA

1. Clinical syndromes—
a. Syndrome of inappropriate antidiuretic hormone secretion (SIADH)—(Table 21–3.) Hypovolemia physiologically stimulates ADH secretion, so the diagnosis of SIADH is made only if the patient is euvolemic. In SIADH, increased ADH release occurs without osmolality-dependent or volume-dependent physiologic stimulation. Normal regulation of ADH release occurs from both the central nervous system and the chest via baroreceptors and neural input. It follows that the causes of SIADH are disorders affecting the central nervous system—structural, metabolic, psychiatric, or pharmacologic—or the lungs. Furthermore, some carcinomas, such as small cell lung carcinoma, synthesize ADH. Other states associated with SIADH include administration of drugs that either increase ADH secretion or potentiate its action.

(1) Patterns of abnormal antidiuretic hormone secretion—

*(a) Random secretion—*ADH release is unrelated to osmoregulation. This pattern is seen in carcinomas and central nervous system diseases.

*(b) Reset osmostat—*This variant is characterized by ADH secretion appropriately suppressed at very low serum osmolalities but with ADH osmoregulation downset to a lower level of "normal." Therefore,

Table 21–3. Causes of syndrome of inappropriate secretion of ADH (SIADH).

Central nervous system disorders
  Head trauma
  Stroke
  Subarachnoid hemorrhage
  Hydrocephalus
  Brain tumor
  Encephalitis
  Guillain-Barré syndrome
  Meningitis
  Acute psychosis
  Acute intermittent porphyria
Pulmonary lesions
  Tuberculosis
  Bacterial pneumonia
  Aspergillosis
  Bronchiectasis
  Neoplasms
  Positive pressure ventilation
Malignancies
  Bronchogenic carcinoma
  Pancreatic carcinoma
  Prostatic carcinoma
  Renal cell carcinoma
  Adenocarcinoma of colon
  Thymoma
  Osteosarcoma
  Malignant lymphoma
  Leukemia
Drugs
  Increased ADH production
    Antidepressants: tricyclics, monoamine oxidase inhibitors, SSRIs
    Antineoplastics: cyclophosphamide, vincristine
    Carbamazepine
    Methylenedioxymethylamphetamine (MDMA; Ecstasy)
    Clofibrate
    Neuroleptics: thiothixene, thioridazine, fluphenazine, haloperidol, trifluoperazine
  Potentiated ADH action
    Carbamazepine
    Chlorpropamide, tolbutamide
    Cyclophosphamide
    NSAIDs
    Somatostatin and analogs
    Amiodarone
Others
  Postoperative
  Pain
  Stress
  AIDS
  Pregnancy (physiologic)
  Hypokalemia

ADH = antidiuretic hormone; SSRIs = selective serotonin reuptake inhibitors; NSAIDs = nonsteroidal anti-inflammatory drugs.

ADH is secreted at a subnormal serum osmolality threshold (< 280 mosm/kg). Appropriate urinary dilution can be attained but at low serum osmolalities. This pattern is seen in the elderly, and in patients with pulmonary processes, tuberculosis, or malnutrition. During pregnancy, the physiologic reset osmostat may suppress osmolality by about 10 mmol/kg of water.

(c) *Leak of antidiuretic hormone*—In conditions such as basilar skull fractures, low levels of ADH are "leaked" into the circulation despite hypo-osmolality. If serum osmolality rises to normal, ADH secretion increases appropriately and then continues to respond normally if osmolality further increases.

(2) *Clinical features*—SIADH is characterized by (1) hyponatremia; (2) decreased osmolality (< 280 mosm/kg) with inappropriately increased urine osmolality (> 150 mosm/kg); (3) absence of cardiac, renal, or liver disease; (4) normal thyroid and adrenal function (see Chapter 26 for thyroid function tests and cosyntropin stimulation test); and (5) urine sodium usually over 20 mEq/L. Natriuresis compensates for the slight increase in volume from ADH secretion. The mechanisms that regulate sodium excretion in response to increases in extracellular volume, such as suppression of the sympathetic nervous and renin–angiotensin systems and increased secretion of atrial natriuretic factor, are preserved and account for the increase in urinary sodium. The expansion of extracellular volume is not large enough to cause clinical hypervolemia, hypertension, or edema. Other changes frequently seen in SIADH include low blood urea nitrogen (BUN) (< 10 mg/dL) and hypouricemia (< 4 mg/dL), which are not only dilutional but result from increased urea and uric acid clearances in response to the volume-expanded state. A high BUN suggests a volume-contracted state, which excludes a diagnosis of SIADH.

b. Hyponatremia after a surgery or procedure— Severe postoperative hyponatremia can develop in 2 days or less after elective surgery in healthy patients, especially premenopausal women. Most have received excessive postoperative hypotonic fluid in the setting of elevated ADH levels related to pain of surgery with continuing excretion of hypertonic urine. Patients awake normally from general anesthesia, but within 2 days develop nausea, headache, seizures, and even respiratory arrest.

Similar mechanisms have been suspected for hyponatremia after colonoscopy. This is not a direct effect of the large volume of liquid-cleansing agents such as polyethylene glycol solution but is due to the diarrhea, nausea, vomiting, and potential volume depletion sometimes produced by these agents. Increased oral water intake or hypotonic fluid administration after colonoscopy (in the presence of elevated ADH) may then result in hyponatremia; occasionally, if thirst is impaired, hypernatremia results.

c. Hypothyroidism—Hyponatremia is not commonly caused by hypothyroidism, but it can occur on oc-

casion with serum sodium levels as low as 105 mEq/L. Water retention is the cause, probably both from inappropriately elevated ADH levels and from alterations in the handling of water by the kidneys.

d. Psychogenic polydipsia and beer potomania— Marked excess free water intake (generally > 10 L/d) may produce hyponatremia. Euvolemia is maintained through the renal excretion of sodium. Urine sodium is therefore generally elevated (> 20 mEq/L), but unlike SIADH, levels of ADH are suppressed. Urine osmolality is appropriately low (< 300 mosm/kg) as the increased free water is excreted. Hyponatremia from bursts of ADH occurs in manic-depressive patients with excess free water intake. Psychogenic polydipsia is observed in patients with psychological problems, and these patients frequently take drugs interfering with water excretion. Similarly, excessive intake of beer, which contains very small amounts of sodium (< 5 mEq/L), can cause severe hyponatremia in cirrhotic patients, who have elevated ADH and often a decreased GFR.

e. Idiosyncratic diuretic reaction—In addition to hyponatremia developing from volume contraction due to diuretic therapy (see above), a less common diuretic-induced hyponatremia can occur in euvolemic patients, typically from thiazides. This syndrome is most often seen in healthy older women (over 70 years of age) often after a few days of therapy. The mechanism for the hyponatremia appears to be a combination of excessive renal sodium loss and water retention.

f. Idiosyncratic ACE inhibitor reactions— ACE inhibitors can cause central polydipsia and increased ADH secretion, both of which result in severe, symptomatic hyponatremia. ACE does not block the conversion of angiotensin I to angiotensin II in the brain. Thus, angiotensin II converted in the brain stimulates thirst and ADH secretion.

g. Endurance exercise hyponatremia—Hyponatremia after endurance exercise (eg, triathlon events) may be caused by a combination of excessive hypotonic fluid intake and continued ADH secretion. Reperfusion of the exercise-induced ischemic splanchnic bed causes delayed absorption of excessive quantities of hypotonic fluid ingested during exercise. Sustained elevation of ADH prevents water excretion in this setting. The retention of hypotonic fluid may be further exacerbated by nonsteroidal anti-inflammatory drugs (NSAIDs) frequently used by athletes. New guidelines encourage runners to drink between 400 mL/h and 800 mL/h as opposed to the previous "as much as possible" advice. However, the clinical relevance of this new recommendation remains to be determined.

h. Mineralocorticoid-responsive hyponatremia in the elderly—In a subgroup of elderly patients, hyponatremia does not resolve in response to water restriction even though they are euvolemic with high ADH levels. These patients may respond to fludrocortisone treatment.

i. Adrenal deficiency—This is an important but often overlooked cause of euvolemic hyponatremia. The adrenal insufficiency may be either primary or secondary, due to adrenocorticotropin (ACTH) deficiency. Routine laboratory data may not easily distinguish hyponatremia due to ACTH deficiency from that of SIADH. However, low plasma bicarbonate (or total CO_2) levels suggest ACTH deficiency.

j. Methylenedioxymethylamphetamine ("Ecstasy") abuse—Abuse of 3,4-methylenedioxymethylamphetamine (MDMA), also known as "Ecstasy," can lead to severe neurologic symptoms, including seizures, brain edema, and herniation from severe hyponatremia. MDMA and its metabolites have been shown to induce enhanced ADH release from the hypothalamus.

k. Selective serotonin reuptake inhibitors (SSRIs)—SIADH induced by selective serotonin (or epinephrine) reuptake inhibitors, such as fluoxetine, paroxetine, and rofloxacin, is fairly common in geriatric patients. Enhanced secretion or action of ADH may result from increased serotonergic tone.

l. Amiodarone—SIADH during amiodarone-loading has been reported. Hyponatremia usually improves with dose reduction.

m. Hyponatremia in HIV-infected patients—Hyponatremia is seen in up to 50% of patients hospitalized for HIV infection and in 20% of ambulatory AIDS patients, often associated with pneumonia and central nervous system processes. If hyponatremia is present at the time of hospital admission, it is just as likely to be due to hypovolemic gastrointestinal loss as to euvolemic SIADH. However, if hyponatremia develops after hospital admission, most patients have euvolemic SIADH. Infrequently, hypovolemic hyponatremia is due to adrenal insufficiency—from infections or ketoconazole toxicity, isolated mineralocorticoid deficiency with hyporeninemic hypoaldosteronism, or an HIV-specific impairment in renal sodium conservation.

2. Treatment—

a. Symptomatic hyponatremia—Symptomatic hyponatremia is usually seen in patients with serum sodium levels less than 120 mEq/L. If there are central nervous system symptoms, hyponatremia should be rapidly treated at any level of serum sodium concentration.

(1) Rate and degree of correction—Central pontine myelinolysis may occur from osmotically induced demyelination due to overly rapid correction of serum sodium (an increase of more than 1 mEq/L/h, or 25 mEq/L within the first day of therapy). Hypoxic–anoxic episodes during hyponatremia may contribute to the demyelination. Premenopausal women in whom hyponatremic encephalopathy develops are about 25 times more likely than menopausal women to die or suffer permanent brain damage, suggesting a hormonal role in the pathophysiology of this disorder.

A reasonable approach is to increase the serum sodium concentration by no more than 1–2 mEq/L/h and not more than 25–30 mEq/L in the first 2 days; the rate should be reduced to 0.5–1 mEq/L/h as soon as neurologic symptoms improve. The initial goal is to achieve a serum sodium concentration of 125–130 mEq/L, guarding against overcorrection.

(2) Saline plus furosemide—Hypertonic (eg, 3%) saline with furosemide is indicated for symptomatic hyponatremic patients. If 3% saline without a diuretic is administered to a patient with SIADH, the serum sodium concentration increases temporarily, but euvolemic patients excrete the excess sodium. If furosemide (0.5–1 mg/kg intravenously) is added, however, the kidney cannot concentrate urine even in the presence of high levels of ADH. Infusion of 3% saline is accompanied by excretion of isotonic urine with a net loss of free water. The sodium concentration of 3% saline is 513 mEq/L. To determine how much 3% saline to administer, a spot urinary Na^+ is determined after a furosemide diuresis has begun. The excreted Na^+ is replaced with 3% saline, empirically begun at 1–2 mL/kg/h and then adjusted based on urinary output and urinary sodium. For example, after administration of furosemide, urine volume may be 400 mL/h and sodium plus potassium excretion 100 mEq/L. The excreted Na^+ plus K^+ is 40 mEq/h, which is replaced with 78 mL/h of 3% saline (40 mEq/h divided by 513 mEq/L). Free water loss is about 1% of total body water. Therefore, an approximately 1% rise in plasma sodium concentration (1–1.5 mEq/L/h) can be expected. Measurements of plasma sodium should be done approximately every 4 hours and the patient observed closely.

b. Asymptomatic hyponatremia—In asymptomatic hyponatremia, the correction rate of hyponatremia need be no more than 0.5 mEq/L/h. No specific treatment is needed for patients with reset osmostats.

(1) Water restriction—Water intake should be restricted to 0.5–1 L/d. A gradual increase of serum sodium will occur over days.

(2) 0.9% saline—0.9% saline with furosemide may be used in asymptomatic patients whose serum sodium is less than 120 mEq/L. Urinary sodium and potassium losses are replaced as above.

(3) Demeclocycline—Demeclocycline (300–600 mg twice daily) is useful for patients who cannot adhere to water restriction or need additional therapy; it inhibits the effect of ADH on the distal tubule. Onset of action may require 1 week, and concentrating may be permanently impaired. Therapy with demeclocycline in cirrhosis appears to increase the risk of renal failure.

(4) Fludrocortisone—Hyponatremia occurring as part of the cerebral salt-wasting syndrome can be treated with fludrocortisone.

(5) Selective vasopressin V2 antagonist—The renal effect of ADH on water excretion is mediated by the V2 receptor. Oral selective V2 antagonists have been in clinical trials and should become available for treatment of SIADH in the near future.

C. Hypervolemic Hypotonic Hyponatremia

Hyponatremia with increased extracellular fluid volume is seen when hyponatremia is accompanied by edema-associated disorders such as congestive heart failure, cirrhosis, nephrotic syndrome, and advanced renal disease (Figure 21–1). In congestive heart failure, total body sodium is increased, yet effective circulating volume is sensed as inadequate by baroreceptors. Increased ADH and aldosterone results, with retention of water and sodium.

The urine sodium concentration is generally less than 10 mEq/L unless the patient has been taking diuretics.

Treatment

A. Water Restriction

The treatment of hyponatremia is that of the underlying condition (eg, improving cardiac output in congestive heart failure) and water restriction (to < 1–2 L of water daily).

B. Diuretics and V2 Antagonists

To hasten excretion of water and salt, use of diuretics may be indicated. Because diuretics may worsen hyponatremia, the patient must be cautioned not to increase free water intake. A potential role for V2 antagonists for the treatment of hyponatremia in congestive heart failure is under investigation.

C. Hypertonic (3%) Saline

Hypertonic saline administration is dangerous in volume-overloaded states and is not routinely recommended. In patients with severe hyponatremia (serum sodium < 110 mEq/L) and central nervous system symptoms, judicious administration of small amounts (100–200 mL) of 3% saline with diuretics may be necessary. Emergency dialysis should also be considered.

Adrogue HJ et al: Hyponatremia. N Engl J Med 2000;342:1581. [PMID: 0844078]

Castello L et al: Hyponatremia in liver cirrhosis: pathophysiological principles of management. Dig Liver Dis 2005;37:73. [PMID: 15733516]

Decaux G et al: Treatment of symptomatic hyponatremia. Am J Med Sci 2003;326:25. [PMID: 11320492]

Goh KP: Management of hyponatremia. Am Fam Physician 2004;69:2387. [PMID: 15168958]

Goldsmith SR: Current treatments and novel pharmacologic treatments for hyponatremia in congestive heart failure. Am J Cardiol 2005;95(9A):14B. [PMID: 15847853]

Hoorn EJ et al: Diagnostic approach to a patient with hyponatremia: traditional versus physiology-based options. QJM 2005; 98:529. [PMID: 15955797]

Milionis HJ et al: The hyponatremic patient: a systematic approach to laboratory diagnosis. CMAJ 2002;166:1056. [PMID: 12002984]

Moritz ML et al: The pathophysiology and treatment of hyponatremic encephalopathy: an update. Nephrol Dial Transplant 2003;18:2486. [PMID: 14605269]

HYPERNATREMIA

 ESSENTIALS OF DIAGNOSIS

- *Occurs most commonly when water intake or water supplementation is inadequate, as in patients with altered mental status.*
- *Urine osmolality helps differentiate renal from nonrenal water loss.*

General Considerations

An intact thirst mechanism usually prevents hypernatremia (> 145 mEq/L). Thus, whatever the underlying disorder (eg, dehydration, lactulose or mannitol therapy, central and nephrogenic diabetes insipidus), excess water loss can cause hypernatremia only when adequate water intake is not possible, as with unconscious patients.

Rarely, excessive sodium intake may cause hypernatremia. Hypernatremia in primary aldosteronism is mild and usually does not cause symptoms. Hypernatremia in the presence of salt and water overload is uncommon but has been reported in very ill patients in the course of therapy.

Clinical Findings

A. Symptoms and Signs

When dehydration exists, orthostatic hypotension and oliguria are typical findings. Because water shifts from the cells to the intravascular space to protect volume status, these symptoms may be delayed. Hyperthermia, delirium, and coma may be seen with severe hyperosmolality.

B. Laboratory Findings

1. Urine osmolality > 400 mosm/kg—Renal water-conserving ability is functioning.

 a. Nonrenal losses—Hypernatremia will develop if water ingestion fails to keep up with hypotonic losses from excessive sweating, exertional losses from the respiratory tract, or through stool water. Lactulose causes an osmotic diarrhea with loss of free water.

 b. Renal losses—Whereas diabetic hyperglycemia can cause pseudohyponatremia (see above), progressive volume depletion from the osmotic diuresis of glycosuria can result in true hypernatremia. Osmotic diuresis can occur with the use of mannitol or urea.

2. Urine osmolality < 250 mosm/kg—A dilute urine with osmolality less than 250 mosm/kg with hypernatremia is characteristic of central and nephrogenic diabetes insipidus. Nephrogenic diabetes insipidus, seen with lithium or demeclocycline therapy, after relief of prolonged urinary tract obstruction, or with interstitial nephritis, results from renal insensitivity to ADH. Hypercalcemia and hypokalemia may be contributing factors when present.

Treatment

Treatment of hypernatremia is directed toward correcting the cause of the fluid loss and replacing water and, as needed, electrolytes. In response to increases in plasma osmolality, brain cells synthesize solutes—or idiogenic osmoles—which increase osmotic flow of water back into the brain cells to regulate their volume. This begins 4–6 hours after dehydration and takes several days to reach a steady state. If hypernatremia is too rapidly corrected, the osmotic imbalance may cause water to preferentially enter brain cells, causing cerebral edema and potentially severe neurologic impairment. Fluid therapy should be administered over a 48-hour period, aiming for a decrease in serum sodium of 1 mEq/L/h (1 mmol/L/h). Potassium and phosphate may be added as indicated by serum levels; other electrolytes are also monitored frequently.

A. Choice of Type of Fluid for Replacement

1. Hypernatremia with hypovolemia—Severe hypovolemia should be treated with isotonic (0.9%) saline to restore the volume deficit and to treat the hyperosmolality, since the osmolality of isotonic saline (308 mosm/kg) is often lower than that of the plasma. This should be followed by 0.45% saline to replace any remaining free water deficit. Milder volume deficit may be treated with 0.45% saline and 5% dextrose in water.

2. Hypernatremia with euvolemia—Water drinking or 5% dextrose and water intravenously will result in excretion of excess sodium in the urine. If the GFR is decreased, diuretics will increase urinary sodium excretion but may impair renal concentrating ability, increasing the quantity of water that needs to be replaced.

3. Hypernatremia with hypervolemia—Treatment consists of providing water as 5% dextrose in water to reduce hyperosmolality, but this will expand vascular volume. Thus, loop diuretics such as furosemide (0.5–1 mg/kg) should be administered intravenously to remove the excess sodium. In severe renal insufficiency, hemodialysis may be necessary.

B. Calculation of Water Deficit

When calculating fluid replacement, both the deficit and the maintenance requirements should be added to each 24-hour replacement regimen.

1. Acute hypernatremia—In acute dehydration without much solute loss, free water loss is similar to the weight loss. Initially, 5% dextrose in water may be used. As correction of water deficit progresses, therapy should continue with 0.45% saline with dextrose.

2. Chronic hypernatremia—Water deficit is calculated to restore normal osmolality for total body water. Total body water (TBW) (Table 21–1) correlates with

muscle mass and therefore decreases with advancing age, cachexia, and dehydration and is lower in women than in men. Current TBW equals 0.4–0.6 % current body weight.

$$\text{Volume (in L)} \atop \text{to be replaced} = \text{Current TBW} \times \frac{\left[Na^+\right] - 140}{140}$$

Adrogue HJ et al: Hypernatremia. N Engl J Med 2000;342:1493. [PMID: 10816188]

Fall PJ: Hyponatremia and hypernatremia. A systematic approach to causes and their correction. Postgrad Med 2000;107:75. [PMID: 10844943]

Kugler JP et al: Hyponatremia and hypernatremia in the elderly. Am Fam Physician 2000;61:3623. [PMID: 10892634]

Lin M et al: Disorders of water imbalance. Emerg Med Clin North Am 2005;23:749. [PMID: 15982544]

■ HYPEROSMOLAR DISORDERS & OSMOLAR GAPS

HYPEROSMOLALITY WITH TRANSIENT OR NO SIGNIFICANT SHIFT IN WATER

Urea and alcohol are two substances that readily cross cell membranes and can produce hyperosmolality. Because of its permeant nature, urea has little effect on the shift of water across the cell membrane. Alcohol quickly equilibrates between intracellular and extracellular water, adding 22 mosm/L for every 1000 mg/L of ethanol. This measured hyperosmolality does not produce symptoms by itself because of the equilibrium described, but in any case of stupor or coma in which measured osmolality exceeds that calculated from values of serum Na^+ and glucose and BUN, ethanol intoxication should be considered as a possible explanation of the discrepancy (osmolar gap). Toxic alcohol ingestion, particularly methanol or ethylene glycol, also causes an osmolar gap characterized by anion gap metabolic acidosis (see Chapter 39).

The combination of anion gap metabolic acidosis and an osmolar gap exceeding 10 mosm/kg is not specific for toxic alcohol ingestion. Nearly 50% of patients with alcoholic ketoacidosis or lactic acidosis have similar findings, caused in part by elevations of endogenous glycerol, acetone, and acetone metabolites (see Metabolic Acidosis).

HYPEROSMOLALITY ASSOCIATED WITH SIGNIFICANT SHIFTS IN WATER

Increased concentrations of solutes that do not readily enter cells produce a shift of water from the intracellular space to effect a true intracellular dehydration. Sodium and glucose are the solutes commonly involved.

In these instances, the hyperosmolality does produce symptoms.

Clinical symptoms are mainly referred to the central nervous system. The severity of symptoms depends on the degree of hyperosmolality and rapidity of development. In acute hyperosmolality, symptoms of somnolence and confusion can appear when the osmolality exceeds 320–330 mosm/L, and coma, respiratory arrest, and death can result when it exceeds 340–350 mosm/L.

Chiasson JL et al: Diagnosis and treatment of diabetic ketoacidosis and the hyperglycemic hyperosmolar state. CMAJ 2003; 168:859. [PMID: 12668546]

Delaney MF et al: Diabetic ketoacidosis and hyperglycemic hyperosmolar nonketotic syndrome. Endocrinol Metab Clin North Am 2000;29:683. [PMID: 11149157]

Stoner GD: Hyperosmolar hyperglycemic state. Am Fam Physician 2005;71:1723. [PMID: 15887451]

■ DISORDERS OF POTASSIUM CONCENTRATION

HYPOKALEMIA

 ESSENTIALS OF DIAGNOSIS

- *Severe hypokalemia may induce dangerous arrhythmias and even rhabdomyolysis.*
- *Rule out intracellular potassium shifts.*
- *Assess urinary potassium excretion to rule out renal loss.*
- *When renal loss is suspected, evaluate mineralocorticoid action by urinary sodium and potassium excretion, transtubular [K⁺] gradient, and plasma aldosterone level.*

General Considerations

The total potassium content of the body is 50 mEq/kg, more than 95% of which is intracellular. The plasma potassium concentration is maintained in a narrow range through two main regulating mechanisms: potassium shift between intracellular and extracellular compartments and modulation of renal potassium excretion. A deficit of 4–5 mEq/kg exists for each 1 mEq/L decrement in serum potassium concentration below a level of 4 mEq/L.

Clinical Findings

A. SYMPTOMS AND SIGNS

Muscular weakness, fatigue, and muscle cramps are frequent complaints in mild to moderate hypokale-

mia. Smooth muscle involvement may result in constipation or ileus. Flaccid paralysis, hyporeflexia, hypercapnia, tetany, and rhabdomyolysis may be seen with severe hypokalemia (< 2.5 mEq/L).

B. LABORATORY FINDINGS

The electrocardiogram (ECG) shows decreased amplitude and broadening of T waves, prominent U waves, premature ventricular contractions, and depressed ST segments. Hypokalemia also increases the likelihood of digitalis toxicity. Thus, in patients with heart disease, hypokalemia induced by certain drugs such as β₂-adrenergic agonists and diuretics may impose a substantial risk.

Pathophysiology & Diagnosis

Hypokalemia can occur as a result of shifting of potassium intracellularly from the extracellular space, extrarenal potassium loss (or insufficient potassium intake), or renal potassium loss (Table 21–4). Potassium uptake by

Table 21–4. Causes of hypokalemia.

Decreased potassium intake
Potassium shift into the cell
  Increased postprandial secretion of insulin
  Alkalosis
  Trauma (via β-adrenergic stimulation?)
  Periodic paralysis (hypokalemic)
  Barium intoxication
Renal potassium loss
  Increased aldosterone (mineralocorticoid) effects
    Primary hyperaldosteronism
    Secondary aldosteronism (dehydration, heart failure)
    Renovascular hypertension
    Malignant hypertension
    Ectopic ACTH-producing tumor
    Gitelman's syndrome
    Bartter's syndrome
    Cushing's syndrome
    Licorice (European)
    Renin-producing tumor
    Congenital abnormality of steroid metabolism (eg, adrenogenital syndrome, 17α-hydroxylase defect, apparent mineralocorticoid excess, 11β-hydroxylase deficiency)
  Increased flow of distal nephron
    Diuretics (furosemide, thiazides)
    Salt-losing nephropathy
  Hypomagnesemia
    Unreabsorbable anion
    Carbenicillin, penicillin
  Renal tubular acidosis (type I or II)
    Fanconi's syndrome
    Interstitial nephritis
    Metabolic alkalosis (bicarbonaturia)
  Congenital defect of distal nephron
    Liddle's syndrome
Extrarenal potassium loss
  Vomiting, diarrhea, laxative abuse
  Villous adenoma, Zollinger-Ellison syndrome

Table 21–5. Genetic disorders associated with electrolyte metabolism disturbances.

Disease	Site of Mutation
Potassium	
Hypokalemia	
Hypokalemic periodic paralysis	Dihydropyridine-sensitive skeletal muscle voltage-gated calcium channel
Bartter's syndrome	Na⁺-K⁺-2Cl⁻ cotransporter, K⁺ channel (ROMK), or Cl⁻ channel of thick ascending limb of Henle (hypofunction), barttin
Gitelman's syndrome	Thiazide-sensitive Na⁺-Cl⁻ cotransporter
Liddle's syndrome	β or γ subunit of amiloride-sensitive Na⁺ channel (hyperfunction)
Apparent mineralocorticoid excess	11β-hydroxysteroid dehydrogenase (failure to inactivate cortisol)
Glucocorticoid-remediable hyperaldosteronism	Regulatory sequence of 11β-hydroxylase controls aldosterone synthase inappropriately
Hyperkalemia	
Hyperkalemic periodic paralysis	α subunit of calcium channel
Pseudohypoaldosteronism type I	β or γ subunit of amiloride-sensitive Na⁺ channel (hypofunction)
Pseudohypoaldosteronism type II (Gordon syndrome)	HNK2, HNK4
Calcium	
Familial hypocalciuric hypercalcemia	Ca²⁺-sensing protein (hypofunction)
Familial hypocalcemia	Ca²⁺-sensing protein (hyperfunction)
Phosphate	
Hypophosphatemic rickets	*PEX* gene, FGF-23
Magnesium	
Hypomagnesemia-hypercalciuria syndrome	Paracellin-1
Water	
Nephrogenic diabetes insipidus	Vasopressin receptor-2 (Type 1), aquaporin-2
Acid-base	
Proximal RTA	Na⁺ HCO₃⁻ cotransporter
Distal RTA	Cl⁻ HCO₃⁻ exchanger H⁺-ATPase
Proximal and distal RTA	Carbonic anhydrase II

FGF-23 = fibroblast growth factor 23; RTA = renal tubular acidosis.

the cell is stimulated by insulin in the presence of glucose. It is also facilitated by β-adrenergic stimulation, whereas α-adrenergic stimulation blocks it. All of these effects are transient. Self-limited hypokalemia occurs in 50–60% of trauma patients, perhaps related to enhanced release of epinephrine. Profound hypokalemia due to barium or cesium intoxication has been reported that may also be the result of transport of potassium into cells. Hypokalemia in the presence of acidosis suggests profound potassium depletion and requires urgent treatment.

The most common cause of hypokalemia, especially in developing countries, is gastrointestinal loss due to infectious diarrhea. The potassium concentration in intestinal secretion is 10 times higher (80 mEq/L) than in gastric juice. Aldosterone, which facilitates urinary potassium excretion through enhanced potassium secretion at the distal renal tubules, is the most important regulator of body potassium content. Urinary potassium concentration is low (< 20 mEq/L) as a result of extrarenal fluid loss (eg, diarrhea, vomiting) and inappropriately high (> 40 mEq/L) with urinary losses (eg, mineralocorticoid excess, Bartter's syndrome, Liddle's syndrome). Various genetic mutations that affect fluid and electrolyte metabolism, including disorders of potassium metabolism, have been reported recently, for which the presence or absence of hypertension may serve as a clue to the diagnosis (Table 21–5). Licorice-induced hypokalemia results from inhibition of 11β-hydroxysteroid dehydrogenase, which inactivates cortisol. Cortisol thus escapes degradation, binds to aldosterone receptors, and exerts aldosterone-like effects. It has been shown that homozygous mutations of the related gene lead to apparent mineralocorticoid excess. For an example, a mutation of a mineralocorticoid receptor increases its affinity to progesterone. In affected patients, hypertension and hypokalemia develop during pregnancy.

The transtubular [K⁺] gradient (TTKG) is a simple and rapid evaluation of net potassium secretion. TTKG is calculated as follows:

$$TTKG = \frac{Urine\ K^+/Plasma\ K^+}{Urine\ osm/Plasma\ osm}$$

Hypokalemia with a TTKG > 4 suggests renal potassium loss with increased distal K⁺ secretion. In such cases, plasma renin and aldosterone levels are helpful in differential diagnosis. The presence of nonabsorbed anions, including bicarbonate, also increases TTKG.

Magnesium is an important cofactor for potassium uptake and for maintenance of intracellular potassium levels. Loop diuretics (eg, furosemide) cause substantial renal potassium and magnesium losses. Magnesium depletion should be suspected in refractory hypokalemia despite potassium repletion.

Treatment

The safest way to treat mild to moderate deficiency is with oral potassium, and all potassium formulations are easily absorbed. Dietary potassium is almost entirely coupled to phosphate—rather than chloride—and is therefore not effective in correcting potassium loss associated with chloride depletion, such as from diuretics or vomiting. In the setting of abnormal renal function and mild to moderate diuretic dosage, 20 mEq/d of oral potassium is generally sufficient to prevent hypokalemia, but 40–100 mEq/d over a period of days to weeks is needed to treat hypokalemia and fully replete potassium stores.

Intravenous potassium replacement is indicated for patients with severe hypokalemia and for those who cannot take oral supplementation. For severe deficiency, potassium may be given through a peripheral intravenous line in a concentration that should not exceed 40 mEq/L at rates of up to 40 mEq/L/h. Continuous ECG monitoring is indicated, and the serum potassium level should be checked every 3–6 hours. For the initial administration, avoid glucose-containing fluid to prevent further shifts of potassium into the cells. Magnesium deficiency also needs to be corrected at the same time, particularly in refractory hypokalemia.

Coca SG et al: The cardiovascular implications of hypokalemia. Am J Kidney Dis 2005;45:233. [PMID: 15685500]

Cohn JN et al: New guidelines for potassium replacement in clinical practice. Arch Intern Med 2000;160:2429. [PMID: 10979053]

Groeneveld JH et al: An approach to the patient with severe hypokalemia: the potassium quiz. QJM 2005;98:305. [PMID: 15760922]

Schaefer TJ et al: Disorders of potassium. Emerg Med Clin North Am 2005;23:723. [PMID: 15982543]

Welfare W et al: Challenges in managing profound hypokalemia. BMJ 2002;324:269. [PMID: 11823358]

HYPERKALEMIA

 ESSENTIALS OF DIAGNOSIS

- Hyperkalemia may develop in patients taking ACE inhibitors, angiotensin receptor blockers, potassium-sparing diuretics, or their combination, even with no or only mild renal dysfunction.

- The ECG may show peaked T waves, widened QRS and biphasic QRS–T complexes, or may be normal despite life-threatening hyperkalemia.

- Measurement of plasma potassium level differentiates potassium leak from blood cells in cases of clotting, leukocytosis, and thrombocytosis from elevated serum potassium.

- Rule out extracellular potassium shift from the cells in acidosis and assess renal potassium excretion.

General Considerations

Hyperkalemia usually develops in patients with advanced renal dysfunction but can also develop with no or only mild renal dysfunction. Many cases of hyper-

kalemia are spurious or associated with acidosis (Table 21–6). The common practice of repeatedly clenching and unclenching a fist during venipuncture may raise the potassium concentration by 1–2 mEq/L by causing acidosis and consequent potassium loss from cells.

Intracellular potassium shifts to the extracellular fluid in hyperkalemia associated with acidosis. Serum potassium concentration rises about 0.7 mEq/L for every decrease of 0.1 pH unit during acidosis. Potassium movement out of cells occurs primarily in metabolic acidosis due to the accumulation of minerals such as NH_4Cl or HCl. The inability of the chloride anion to permeate the cell membrane results in the transcellular exchange of H^+ for K^+. Metabolic acidosis from organic acids (keto acids and lactic acid) does not induce hyperkalemia. Unlike the minerals, these organic acids easily permeate cell membranes and retard $Na^+–K^+$-ATPase. The hyperkalemia frequently observed

Table 21–6. Causes of hyperkalemia.

Spurious
  Leakage from erythrocytes when separation of serum from clot is delayed (plasma K^+ normal)
  Marked thrombocytosis or leukocytosis with release of K^+ (plasma K^+ normal)
  Repeated fist clenching during phlebotomy, with release of K^+ from forearm muscles
  Specimen drawn from arm with K^+ infusion
Decreased excretion
  Renal failure, acute and chronic
  Renal secretory defects (may or may not have frank renal failure): renal transplant, interstitial nephritis, systemic lupus erythematosus, sickle cell disease, amyloidosis, obstructive uropathy
  Hyporeninemic hypoaldosteronism (often in diabetic patients with mild to moderate nephropathy) or selective hypoaldosteronism (some patients with AIDS)
  Heparin (regardless of molecular size; suppresses aldosterone secretion)
  Drugs that inhibit potassium excretion (spironolactone, eplerenone, triamterene, ACE inhibitors, angiotensin II receptor blockers, trimethoprim, NSAIDs, cyclosporine, tacrolimus)
Shift of K^+ from within the cell
  Massive release of intracellular K^+ in burns, rhabdomyolysis, hemolysis, severe infection, internal bleeding, vigorous exercise
  Metabolic acidosis (in the case of organic acid accumulation—eg, lactic acidosis—a shift of K^+ does not occur since organic acid can easily move across the cell membrane)
  Hypertonicity (solvent drag)
  Insulin deficiency (metabolic acidosis may not be apparent)
  Hyperkalemic periodic paralysis
  Drugs: succinylcholine, arginine, digitalis toxicity, β-adrenergic antagonists
  α-Adrenergic stimulation?
Excessive intake of K^+

ACE = angiotensin-converting enzyme; NSAIDs = nonsteroidal anti-inflammatory drugs.

in diabetic ketoacidosis is not due to the acidosis but to a combination of the hyperosmolality (the intracellular K^+ concentration of the dehydrated cell increases and K^+ diffuses extracellularly) and deficiencies of insulin, catecholamines, and aldosterone. Aminocaproic acid, a synthetic amino acid structurally related to lysine and arginine used for the prevention of operative blood loss, may induce shift of potassium. In the absence of acidosis, serum potassium concentration rises about 1 mEq/L when there is a total body potassium excess of 1–4 mEq/kg. However, the higher the serum potassium concentration, the smaller the excess necessary to raise the potassium levels further.

Mineralocorticoid deficiency from Addison's disease (high renin) or chronic kidney disease (low renin) is another cause of hyperkalemia with decreased renal excretion of potassium. Mineralocorticoid resistance due to genetic disorders, interstitial renal disease, or urinary tract obstruction also leads to hypokalemia.

ACE inhibitors or angiotensin receptor blockers, commonly used in patients with congestive heart failure or renal insufficiency, may cause hyperkalemia. Recent trends involving simultaneous use of spironolactone or eplerenone, or β-blockers further increases the risk of hyperkalemia. Thiazide or loop diuretics and sodium bicarbonate may be effective in minimizing hyperkalemia. Mild hyperkalemia that recurs often in patients in the absence of ACE inhibitor drug therapy is usually due to type IV renal tubular acidosis (RTA). Heparin inhibits aldosterone production by inhibiting the final enzymatic step in its manufacture in the adrenal glands, and thus can be a cause of hyperkalemia.

Trimethoprim is structurally related to amiloride and triamterene, and all three drugs inhibit renal potassium excretion through suppression of sodium channels in the distal nephron. Serum potassium levels rise progressively over 4–5 days in patients treated with standard or high-dose trimethoprim (combined with sulfamethoxazole or dapsone), especially if there is concurrent renal insufficiency. Over 50% of inpatients taking this drug have potassium levels over 5 mEq/L, and 20% have marked hyperkalemia (> 5.5 mEq/L). The potassium concentration returns to baseline after drug discontinuation.

In addition, it is of note that immunosuppressive drugs such as cyclosporine and tacrolimus can induce hyperkalemia in organ transplant recipients—and especially in kidney transplant patients. This is partly due to the suppression of basolateral Na^+–K^+-ATPase in principal cells. Furthermore, five cases have been recently reported of severe hyperkalemia and cardiovascular disturbances caused by the use of drugs with K_{ATP} channel-opening properties (K-channel syndrome), such as nicorandil, cyclosporine, or isoflurane. The hyperkalemia was successfully reversed by the administration of glibenclamide.

Hyperkalemia is commonly seen in HIV-infected patients and has been attributed to impaired renal excretion of potassium due to the use of pentamidine or trimethoprim-sulfamethoxazole or to hyporeninemic hypoaldosteronism.

Clinical Findings

An elevated K^+ concentration interferes with normal neuromuscular function to produce muscle weakness and, rarely, flaccid paralysis; abdominal distention and diarrhea may occur. Electrocardiography is not a sensitive method for detecting hyperkalemia, since nearly half of patients with a serum potassium level greater than 6.5 mEq/L will not manifest ECG changes. ECG changes in hyperkalemia include peaked T waves of increased amplitude, widening of the QRS, and biphasic QRS–T complexes. Inhibition of atrial depolarization despite normal conduction through usual pathways may occur. This sinoventricular rhythm resembles a junctional mechanism and occurs because of greater sensitivity of atrial myocytes to hyperkalemia than is the case for ventricular muscle cells. The heart rate may be slow; ventricular fibrillation and cardiac arrest are terminal events.

Treatment

First confirm that the elevated level of serum K^+ is genuine. Potassium concentration can be measured in plasma rather than in serum to avoid leakage of potassium out of cells into the serum of the blood sample in the course of clotting, which may be observed in thrombocytosis. Renal dysfunction should be ruled out at the initial assessment.

Treatment consists of withholding potassium and giving cation exchange resins by mouth or enema. Sodium polystyrene sulfonate, 40–80 g/d in divided doses, is usually effective. Emergent treatment of hyperkalemia is indicated if cardiac toxicity or muscular paralysis is present or if the hyperkalemia is severe (serum potassium > 6.5–7 mEq/L) even in the absence of ECG changes. Insulin plus 10–50% glucose (5–10 g of glucose per unit of insulin) may be given to deposit K^+ with glycogen in the liver (Table 21–7). Calcium may be given intravenously as an antagonist ion—but not when digoxin toxicity is suspected, since calcium may augment the deleterious effects of digoxin on the heart. Transcellular shifts of potassium can also be mediated by β_2-adrenergic stimulation. Thus, one or two standard doses of nebulized albuterol can reduce serum K^+ 0.5–1 mEq/L within 30 minutes after administration in dialysis patients, and this effect is sustained for at least 2 hours. Sodium bicarbonate can be given intravenously as an emergency measure in severe hyperkalemia; the increase in blood pH results in a shift of K^+ into cells. Hemodialysis or peritoneal dialysis may be required to remove K^+ in the presence of protracted renal insufficiency. Therapy of the precipitating event proceeds concurrently.

Gross P et al: Hyperkalemia: again. Nephrol Dial Transplant 2004;19:2163. [PMID: 15299094]

Halperin ML et al: Potassium. Lancet 1998;352:135. [PMID: 9672294]

Kamel KS et al: Controversial issues in the treatment of hyperkalemia. Nephrol Dial Transplant 2003;18:2215. [PMID: 14551344]

Palmer BF: Managing hyperkalemia caused by inhibitors of the renin-angiotensin-aldosterone system. N Engl J Med 2004; 351:585. [PMID: 15295051]

Table 21–7. Treatment of hyperkalemia.

EMERGENCY					
Modality	**Mechanism of Action**	**Onset**	**Duration**	**Prescription**	**K+ Removed from Body**
Calcium	Antagonizes cardiac conduction abnormalities	0–5 minutes	1 hour	Calcium gluconate 10%, 5–30 mL intravenously; or calcium chloride 5%, 5–30 mL intravenously	0
Bicarbonate	Distributes K+ into cells	15–30 minutes	1–2 hours	NaHCO$_3$, 44–88 mEq (1–2 ampules) intravenously	0
Insulin	Distributes K+ into cells	15–60 minutes	4–6 hours	Regular insulin, 5–10 units intravenously, plus glucose 50%, 25 g (1 ampule) intravenously	0
Albuterol	Distributes K+ into cells	15–30 minutes	2–4 hours	Nebulized albuterol, 10–20 mg in 4 mL normal saline, inhaled over 10 minutes	0

NONEMERGENCY				
Modality	**Mechanism of Action**	**Duration of Treatment**	**Prescription**	**K+ Removed from Body**
Loop diuretic	↑ Renal K+ excretion	0.5–2 hours	Furosemide, 40–160 mg intravenously or orally with or without NaHCO3, 0.5–3 mEq/kg daily	Variable
Sodium polystyrene sulfonate (Kayexalate)	Ion-exchange resin binds K+	1–3 hours	Oral: 15–30 g in 20% sorbitol (50–100 mL) Rectal: 50 g in 20% sorbitol	0.5–1 mEq/g
Hemodialysis	Extracorporeal K+ removal	48 hours	Blood flow ≥ 200–300 mL/min Dialysate [K+] ~ 0	200–300 mEq
Peritoneal dialysis	Peritoneal K+ removal	48 hours	Fast exchange, 3–4 L/h	200–300 mEq

Modified and reproduced, with permission, from Cogan MG: *Fluid and Electrolytes: Physiology and Pathophysiology.* McGraw-Hill, 1991.

Singer M et al: Reversal of life-threatening, drug-related potassium-channel syndrome by glibenclamide. Lancet 2005; 365:1873. [PMID: 15924984]

Tamirisa KP et al: Spironolactone-induced renal insufficiency and hyperkalemia in patients with heart failure. Am Heart J 2004;148:971. [PMID: 15632880]

■ DISORDERS OF CALCIUM CONCENTRATION

The normal total plasma (or serum) calcium concentration is 9–10.3 mg/dL. It is ionized calcium (normal: 4.7–5.3 mg/dL) that is physiologically active and is necessary for muscle contraction and nerve function.

Calcium-sensing protein, a receptor-like protein with the special function of detecting extracellular calcium ion concentrations, has been identified in parathyroid cells and in the kidney. Some diseases (eg, familial hypocalcemia and familial hypocalciuric hypercalcemia) associated with disturbed calcium me-

tabolism are due to functional defects of this protein (Table 21–5).

HYPOCALCEMIA

 ESSENTIALS OF DIAGNOSIS

- *Often mistaken as a neurologic disorder.*
- *Check for decreased parathyroid hormone (PTH), vitamin D, or magnesium depletion.*
- *If the ionized calcium level is normal despite a low total serum calcium, calcium metabolism is usually normal.*

General Considerations

Development of true hypocalcemia (decreased ionized calcium) implies insufficient action of PTH or active vitamin D. The most common cause of low total serum calcium is hypoalbuminemia; correction of serum calcium concentration is needed to accurately reflect the ionized calcium concentration. When albumin is low, serum Ca^{2+} concentration is depressed in a ratio of 0.8–1 mg of Ca^{2+} to 1 g of albumin. Thus,

$$\text{Corrected calcium}^{2+} \text{ (mg/dL)} =$$
$$Ca^{2+} \text{ (mg/dL)} + 0.8 \sim 1.0 \times (4 - \text{albumin [g/dL])}$$

Important causes of hypocalcemia are listed in Table 21–8.

The most common cause of hypocalcemia is renal failure, in which decreased production of active vitamin D_3 and hyperphosphatemia both play a role (see Chapter 22). Some cases of primary hypoparathyroidism are due to mutation of calcium-sensing protein in which inappropriate suppression of PTH release leads to hypocalcemia (see Chapter 15). Hypocalcemia in pancreatitis is also a marker for severe disease. Elderly hospitalized patients with low ionized serum calcium and hypophosphatemia, with or without an elevated parathyroid level, are likely deficient in vitamin D.

Clinical Findings

A. SYMPTOMS AND SIGNS

Hypocalcemia increases excitation of nerve and muscle cells, primarily affecting the neuromuscular and cardiovascular systems. Extensive spasm of skeletal muscle causes cramps and tetany. Laryngospasm with stridor can obstruct the airway. Convulsions can occur as well as paresthesias of lips and extremities and abdominal pain. Chvostek's sign (contraction of the facial muscle in response to tapping the facial nerve anterior to the ear) and Trousseau's sign (carpal spasm occurring after occlusion of the brachial artery with a blood pressure cuff for 3 minutes) are usually readily elicited. Prolongation of the QT interval (due to lengthened ST segment) predisposes to the development of ventricular arrhythmias. In chronic hypoparathyroidism, cataracts and calcification of basal ganglia of the brain may appear (see Hypoparathyroidism, Chapter 26).

B. LABORATORY FINDINGS

Serum calcium concentration is low (< 9 mg/dL). In true hypocalcemia, the ionized serum calcium concentration is also low (< 4.7 mg/dL). Serum phosphate is usually elevated in hypoparathyroidism or end-stage renal failure, whereas it is suppressed in early-stage renal failure or vitamin D deficiency.

Serum magnesium concentration is commonly low, and hypomagnesemia reduces both PTH release and tissue responsiveness to PTH, causing hypocalcemia. In respiratory alkalosis, total serum calcium is normal but ionized calcium is low. The ECG shows a prolonged QT interval.

Treatment[1]

A. SEVERE, SYMPTOMATIC HYPOCALCEMIA

In the presence of tetany, arrhythmias, or seizures, calcium gluconate 10% (10–20 mL) administered intravenously over 10–15 minutes is indicated. Because of the short duration of action, calcium infusion is usually required. Ten to 15 milligrams of calcium per kilogram body weight, or six to eight 10-mL vials of 10% calcium gluconate (558–744 mg of calcium), is added to 1 L of D_5W and infused over 4–6 hours. By monitoring the serum calcium level frequently (every 4–6 hours), the infusion rate is adjusted to maintain the serum calcium level at 7–8.5 mg/dL.

B. ASYMPTOMATIC HYPOCALCEMIA

Oral calcium (1–2 g) and vitamin D preparations are used. Calcium carbonate is well tolerated and less expensive than many other calcium tablets. The low serum Ca^{2+} associated with low serum albumin concentration does not require replacement therapy. If serum Mg^{2+} is low, therapy must include replacement of magnesium, which by itself will usually correct hypocalcemia.

Table 21–8. Causes of hypocalcemia.

Decreased intake or absorption
  Malabsorption
  Small bowel bypass, short bowel
  Vitamin D deficit (decreased absorption, decreased production of 25-hydroxyvitamin D or 1,25-dihydroxyvitamin D)
Increased loss
  Alcoholism
  Chronic renal insufficiency
  Diuretic therapy
Endocrine disease
  Hypoparathyroidism (genetic, acquired; including hypomagnesemia and hypermagnesemia)
  Sepsis
  Pseudohypoparathyroidism
  Calcitonin secretion with medullary carcinoma of the thyroid
  Familial hypocalcemia
Physiologic causes
  Associated with decreased serum albumin[1]
  Decreased end-organ response to vitamin D
  Hyperphosphatemia
  Induced by aminoglycoside antibiotics, plicamycin, loop diuretics, foscarnet

[1]Ionized calcium concentration is normal.

Ariyan CE et al: Assessment and management of patients with abnormal calcium. Crit Care Med 2004;32(4 Suppl):S146. [PMID: 15064673]

Diercks DB et al: Electrocardiographic manifestations: electrolyte abnormalities. J Emerg Med 2004;27:153. [PMID: 15261358]

---

[1]See also Chapter 26 for discussion of the treatment of hypoparathyroidism.

Lyman D: Undiagnosed vitamin D deficiency in the hospitalized patient. Am Fam Physician 2005;71:299. [PMID: 15686300]

HYPERCALCEMIA

 ESSENTIALS OF DIAGNOSIS

- *Primary hyperparathyroidism and malignancy-associated hypercalcemia are the most common causes.*
- *Hypercalciuria usually precedes hypercalcemia.*
- *Most often, asymptomatic, mild hypercalcemia (≤ 11 mg/dL) is due to primary hyperparathyroidism, whereas the symptomatic, severe hypercalcemia (≥ 14 mg/dL) is due to hypercalcemia of malignancy.*

General Considerations

Important causes of hypercalcemia are listed in Table 21–9. Primary hyperparathyroidism and malignancy account for 90% of all cases of hypercalcemia. Primary hyperparathyroidism is the most common cause of hypercalcemia (usually mild) in ambulatory patients.

Table 21–9. Causes of hypercalcemia.

Increased intake or absorption
    Milk-alkali syndrome
    Vitamin D or vitamin A excess
Endocrine disorders
    Primary hyperparathyroidism
    Tertiary hyperparathyroidism (renal insufficiency, malabsorption)
    Acromegaly
    Adrenal insufficiency
    Pheochromocytoma
    Hyperparathyroidism
Neoplastic diseases
    Tumors producing PTH-related proteins (ovary, kidney, lung)
    Multiple myeloma (elaboration of osteoclast-activating factor)
    Lymphoma (occasionally from production of calcitriol)
Miscellaneous causes
    Thiazide diuretic use
    Sarcoidosis and other granulomatous diseases (production of calcitriol)
    Paget's disease of bone
    Hypophosphatasia
    Immobilization
    Familial hypocalciuric hypercalcemia
    Complications of renal transplantation
    Lithium intake

PTH = parathyroid hormone.

Chronic hypercalcemia (over 6 months) or some manifestation such as nephrolithiasis also suggests a benign cause. Tumor production of PTH-related proteins (PTHrP) is the most common paraneoplastic endocrine syndrome, accounting for most cases of hypercalcemia in inpatients (see Table 40–6). The neoplasm is clinically apparent in nearly all cases when the hypercalcemia is detected, and the prognosis is poor.

Milk-alkali syndrome, which had become rare with the advent of nonabsorbable antacid therapy for ulcer disease, has had a resurgence related to calcium ingestion for prevention of osteoporosis. In the milk-alkali syndrome, massive calcium and vitamin D ingestion can cause hypercalcemic nephropathy. Because of the decreased GFR, retention of the alkali in the calcium antacid occurs and causes metabolic alkalosis, which can be worsened by the vomiting associated with this disorder.

Hypercalcemia also causes nephrogenic diabetes insipidus. Development of polyuria is mediated through activation of calcium-sensing receptors in collecting ducts. Volume depletion further worsens hypercalcemia.

Clinical Findings

A. Symptoms and Signs

Hypercalcemia may affect gastrointestinal, renal, and neurologic function. The focus of the history and physical examination should be on the duration of the process of hypercalcemia and evidence for a neoplasm. Mild hypercalcemia is often asymptomatic. Symptoms usually occur if the serum calcium is above 12 mg/dL and tend to be more severe if hypercalcemia develops acutely. Symptoms irrespective of cause are constipation and polyuria, except in hypocalciuric hypercalcemia, in which polyuria is absent. Other gastrointestinal symptoms may include nausea, vomiting, anorexia, and peptic ulcer disease. Renal colic or hematuria from nephrolithiasis may be present. Polyuria from hypercalciuria-induced nephrogenic diabetes insipidus can result in volume depletion and azotemia. Neurologic manifestations may range from mild drowsiness to weakness, depression, lethargy, stupor, and coma in severe hypercalcemia. Ventricular extrasystoles and idioventricular rhythm occur and can be accentuated by digitalis.

B. Laboratory Findings

A significant elevation of serum calcium is seen; the level must be interpreted in relation to the serum albumin level (see Hypocalcemia, above). A high serum chloride concentration and a low serum phosphate concentration in a ratio > 33 to 1 is suggestive of primary hyperparathyroidism where PTH decreases proximal tubular phosphate reabsorption. A low serum chloride concentration with a high serum bicarbonate concentration, along with elevations of BUN and creatinine, suggests milk-alkali syndrome. The highest serum calcium levels (> 15 mg/dL) generally occur in malignancy. More than 200 mg/d of urinary calcium excretion suggests hypercalciuria; less than 100 mg/d suggests hypocalciuria. Hypercalciuric patients—such as those with malignancy or those receiving oral active vitamin D therapy—may easily develop hypercalcemia in case of volume depletion. Serum phosphate may or may not be low, depending on the cause. Hypocalciuric hypercalcemia occurs in milk-alkali syndrome, thiazide diuretic use, and familial hypocalciuric hypercalcemia.

The chest radiograph may reveal a malignancy or granulomatous disease. The ECG shows a shortened QT interval. Measurements of PTH and PTHrP help distinguish between malignancy-associated hypercalcemia (suppressed PTH, elevated PTHrP) and hyperparathyroidism (elevated PTH).

Treatment

Until the primary disease can be brought under control, renal excretion of calcium with resultant decrease in serum calcium concentration is promoted. Excretion of Na^+ is accompanied by excretion of Ca^{2+}.

The tendency in hypercalcemia is toward volume depletion from nephrogenic diabetes insipidus. Therefore, establishing euvolemia and inducing natriuresis by giving saline with furosemide is the emergency treatment of choice. In dehydrated patients with normal cardiac and renal function, 0.45% saline or 0.9% saline can be given rapidly (250–500 mL/h). Intravenous furosemide (20–40 mg every 2 hours) prevents volume overload and enhances Ca^{2+} excretion. Thiazides can actually worsen hypercalcemia (as can furosemide if inadequate saline is given).

Bisphosphonates are the mainstay of treatment of hypercalcemia of malignancy. They are safe, effective, and normalize calcium in more than 70% of patients, although it may require up to 48–72 hours before their full therapeutic effect is achieved. In emergency cases, dialysis with low or no calcium dialysate may be needed. A calcimimetic agent, cinacalcet hydrochloride, that suppresses PTH secretion and decreases serum calcium concentration holds promise as a future treatment option. See Chapter 40 for a discussion of the treatment of hypercalcemia of malignancy and Chapter 26 for a discussion of the treatment of hypercalcemia of hyperparathyroidism.

Typically, patients with end-stage renal disease who receive long-term dialysis develop hypocalcemia and hyperphosphatemia if they do not receive proper supplementation of calcium and active vitamin D. On the other hand, hypercalcemia can sometimes develop, particularly in the setting of severe secondary hyperparathyroidism, characterized by high levels of PTH and subsequent release of calcium from bone. Therapy may include intravenous vitamin D, which further increases the serum calcium concentration. Another type of hypercalcemia occurs when the PTH levels are low. In this setting, bone turnover is decreased, which results in a low buffering capacity for calcium. When calcium is administered in calcium-containing phosphate binders or in the dialysate, or when vitamin D is administered, hypercalcemia results. Hypercalcemia in dialysis patients usually occurs in the presence of hyperphosphatemia, and severe metastatic calcification, eg, involving blood vessels, may occur. Malignancy should also be considered as a cause of the hypercalcemia.

Bilezikian JP et al: Clinical practice. Asymptomatic primary hyperparathyroidism. N Engl J Med 2004;350:1746. [PMID: 15103001]

Caroll MF et al: A practical approach to hypercalcemia. Am Fam Physician 2003;67:1959. [PMID: 12751658]

Inzucchi SE: Management of hypercalcemia. Diagnostic workup, therapeutic options for hyperparathyroidism and other common causes. Postgrad Med 2004;115:27. [PMID: 15171076]

Sarko J: Bone and mineral metabolism. Emerg Med Clin North Am 2005;23:703. [PMID: 15982542]

Schwartz SR et al: Hypercalcemic hypocalciuria: a critical differential diagnosis for hyperparathyroidism. Otolaryngol Clin North Am 2004;37:887. [PMID: 15262523]

■ DISORDERS OF PHOSPHORUS CONCENTRATION

In plasma, phosphate is mainly present as inorganic phosphate, and this fraction is very small (< 0.2% of total phosphate). However, body phosphate metabolism is regulated through plasma inorganic phosphate.

Important determinants of plasma inorganic phosphate concentration are its renal excretion, intestinal absorption, and shift between the intracellular and extracellular spaces. In general, the kidney is the most important regulator of the serum phosphate level. PTH decreases the absorption of phosphate in the proximal tubule while 1–25 dihydroxy-vitamin D3 increases tubular phosphate reabsorption. Renal proximal tubular reabsorption of phosphate is decreased by volume expansion, corticosteroid administration, and proximal tubular dysfunction, such as occurs in Fanconi's syndrome due to myeloma or other diseases. Fibroblast growth factor 23 (FGF-23) is an additional phosphaturic hormone. Intestinal absorption of phosphate is facilitated by active vitamin D. PTH, which both stimulates phosphate release from bone and is phosphaturic, can lead to hypophosphatemia and to depletion of bone phosphate store if hypersecretion continues.

Growth hormone, on the other hand, augments proximal tubular reabsorption of phosphate. Cellular phosphate uptake is stimulated by various factors and conditions, including alkalemia, insulin, epinephrine, feeding, hungry bone syndrome, and accelerated cell proliferation.

Phosphorus metabolism and homeostasis are intimately related to calcium metabolism. See sections on metabolic bone disease in Chapter 26.

HYPOPHOSPHATEMIA

ESSENTIALS OF DIAGNOSIS

• *Severe hypophosphatemia may cause tissue hypooxygenation and even rhabdomyolysis.*

- *Renal loss of phosphate can be diagnosed by measuring urinary phosphate excretion and by calculating maximal tubular phosphate reabsorption rate (TmP/GFR).*
- *PTH is one of the major factors that decrease TmP/GFR, leading to renal loss of phosphate.*

General Considerations

Hypophosphatemia may occur in the presence of normal phosphate stores. Serious depletion of body phosphate stores may exist with low, normal, or high concentrations of phosphorus in serum. Leading causes of hypophosphatemia are listed in Table 21–10.

In the presence of **severe** hypophosphatemia (1 mg/dL or less), affinity of hemoglobin for oxygen is

Table 21–10. Causes of hypophosphatemia.

Diminished supply or absorption
Starvation
Parenteral alimentation with inadequate phosphate content
Malabsorption syndrome, small bowel bypass
Absorption blocked by oral aluminum hydroxide or bicarbonate
Vitamin D–deficient and vitamin D–resistant osteomalacia
Increased loss
Phosphaturic drugs: theophylline, diuretics, bronchodilators, corticosteroids
Hyperparathyroidism (primary or secondary)
Hyperthyroidism
Renal tubular defects permitting excessive phosphaturia (congenital, induced by monoclonal gammopathy, heavy metal poisoning), alcoholism
Hypokalemic nephropathy
Inadequately controlled diabetes mellitus
Hypophosphatemic rickets
Phosphatonins of oncogenic osteomalacia (eg, FGF-23 production)
Intracellular shift of phosphorus
Administration of glucose
Anabolic steroids, estrogen, oral contraceptives, β-adrenergic agonists, xanthine derivatives
Respiratory alkalosis
Salicylate poisoning
Electrolyte abnormalities
Hypercalcemia
Hypomagnesemia
Metabolic alkalosis
Abnormal losses followed by inadequate repletion
Diabetes mellitus with acidosis, particularly during aggressive therapy
Recovery from starvation or prolonged catabolic state
Chronic alcoholism, particularly during restoration of nutrition; associated with hypomagnesemia
Recovery from severe burns

FGF-23 = fibroblast growth factor-23.

increased through a decrease in the erythrocyte 2,3-diphosphoglycerate concentration. This impairs tissue oxygenation and thus cell metabolism, which underlies the effects of hypophosphatemia such as muscle weakness or even rhabdomyolysis.

Severe hypophosphatemia is common and multifactorial in alcoholic patients. In acute alcohol withdrawal, increased plasma insulin and epinephrine along with respiratory alkalosis promote intracellular shift of phosphate. Vomiting, diarrhea, and poor dietary intake contribute to hypophosphatemia. Chronic alcohol use results in a decrease in the renal threshold of phosphate excretion. This renal tubular dysfunction reverses after a month of abstinence. Patients with chronic obstructive pulmonary disease and asthma commonly have hypophosphatemia, attributed to xanthine derivatives causing shifts of phosphate intracellularly and the phosphaturic effects of β-adrenergic agonists, loop diuretics, xanthine derivatives, and corticosteroids. The metabolic syndrome, a major contributor to coronary heart disease risk, is associated with low phosphate (and magnesium) levels but the clinical significance of these disturbances is unclear. Refeeding or glucose administration to phosphate-depleted patients may cause fatal hypophosphatemia.

Moderate hypophosphatemia (1.0–2.5 mg/dL) occurs commonly in hospitalized patients and may not reflect decreased phosphate stores. Hypophosphatemia is a potent stimulator of 1α-hydroxylation of vitamin D in the kidney to form active vitamin D. However, in oncogenic osteomalacia, which accompanies various mesenchymal tumors, activation of vitamin D is suppressed in spite of hypophosphatemia. This suppression may be due to overproduction of phosphatonins, such as FGF-23. Serum phosphate levels also decrease transiently after food intake, thus fasting samples are recommended for an accurate analysis.

Clinical Findings

A. Symptoms and Signs

Acute, severe hypophosphatemia (0.1–0.2 mg/dL) can lead to rhabdomyolysis, paresthesias, and encephalopathy (irritability, confusion, dysarthria, seizures, and coma). Respiratory failure or failure to wean from a respirator may occur. Arrhythmias and heart failure are uncommon but serious manifestations. Acute hemolytic anemia has been reported with increased erythrocyte fragility and platelet dysfunction with petechial hemorrhages. There is increased susceptibility to gram-negative sepsis from impaired chemotaxis of leukocytes.

Chronic severe depletion may be manifested by anorexia, pain in muscles and bones, and fractures.

B. Laboratory Findings

Evaluation of urinary phosphate excretion is a useful clue to the diagnosis of hypophosphatemia. A spot urine with > 20 mg/dL of phosphate suggests renal phosphate loss. Tubular phosphate reabsorption can be assessed by TmP/GFR.

$$\frac{TmP}{GFR} = \frac{Serum\ Pi - (UPi \times UV)}{GFR}$$

where serum Pi = serum phosphate concentration
UPi = urine phosphate concentration
UV = urine volume

The normal range of TmP/GFR is 2.5–4.5 mg/dL; lower values indicate urinary phosphate loss. The main factors regulating TmP/GFR are PTH and phosphate intake. Increase of PTH or phosphate intake decreases TmP/GFR, so that more phosphate is excreted into the urine.

Measurement of plasma PTH or PTHrP levels may be helpful. Serum FGF-23 levels can also be measured; however, the clinical usefulness of doing so remains to be established.

Other clinical features may be suggestive of specific causes of hypophosphatemia. Evidence of anemia due to hemolysis may be present (eg, elevated serum lactate dehydrogenase). Rhabdomyolysis results in elevated serum creatine kinase (which contains mostly the MM fraction but also some MB fraction) and, in many cases, myoglobin in the urine. Other values vary according to the cause. Renal glycosuria and hypouricemia together with hypophosphatemia indicate Fanconi's syndrome. In chronic depletion, radiographs and biopsies of bones show changes resembling those of osteomalacia.

Treatment

Treatment is best directed toward prophylaxis by including phosphate in repletion and maintenance fluids. A rapid decline in calcium levels can occur with parenteral administration of phosphate; therefore, when possible, oral replacement of phosphate is preferable. Moderate hypophosphatemia (1.0–2.5 mg/dL) is usually asymptomatic and does not require treatment. The hypophosphatemia in patients with diabetic ketoacidosis will usually correct with normal dietary intake. Chronic hypophosphatemia can be treated with oral phosphate repletion. Phosphate salts are available in skim milk (approximately 1 g [33 mmol]/L). Tablets or capsules of mixtures of sodium and potassium phosphate may be given to provide 0.5–1 g (18–32 mmol) per day. For severe, symptomatic hypophosphatemia (serum phosphorus 1 mg/ dL), an infusion should provide 279–310 mg (9–10 mmol)/12 h until the serum phosphorus exceeds 1 mg/dL and the patient can be switched to oral therapy. The infusion rate should be decreased if hypotension occurs. Because the response to phosphate supplementation is not predictable, monitoring of plasma phosphate, calcium, and potassium every 6 hours is necessary. A magnesium deficit often coexists and should be treated simultaneously.

Contraindications to therapy with phosphate salts include hypoparathyroidism, renal insufficiency, tissue damage and necrosis, and hypercalcemia. When hyperglycemia due to any cause is treated, phosphate accompanies glucose into cells, and hypophosphatemia may ensue.

Gaasbeek A et al: Hypophosphatemia: an update on its etiology and treatment. Am J Med 2005;118:1094. [PMID: 16194637]

Shiber JR et al: Serum phosphate abnormalities in the emergency department. J Emerg Med 2002;23:395. [PMID: 12480022]

Taylor BE et al: Treatment of hypophosphatemia using a protocol based on patient weight and serum phosphorus level in a surgical intensive care unit. J Am Coll Surg 2004;198:198. [PMID: 14759775]

HYPERPHOSPHATEMIA

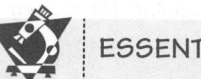 ESSENTIALS OF DIAGNOSIS

- *Renal failure is the most common cause.*
- *Hyperphosphatemia in the presence of hypercalcemia imposes a high risk of metastatic calcification.*

General Considerations

Chronic renal insufficiency from decreased excretion of phosphorus and decreased renal hydroxylation of 25-hydroxyvitamin D to 1,25-dihydroxyvitamin D is the main cause of hyperphosphatemia. Other causes are listed in Table 21–11. Children normally have higher serum phosphate levels than adults.

Clinical Findings

A. SYMPTOMS AND SIGNS

The clinical manifestations are those of the underlying disorder (eg, chronic renal failure) of hypocalcemia. Inadequately treated hyperphosphatemia in chronic renal failure leads to secondary hyperparathyroidism, renal osteodystrophy, and extraosseous calcification of soft tissues.

B. LABORATORY FINDINGS

In addition to elevated phosphate, blood chemistry abnormalities are those of the underlying disease.

Treatment

In acute and chronic renal failure, dialysis will reduce serum phosphate. Absorption of phosphate can be reduced by administration of calcium carbonate, 0.5– 1.5 g three times daily with meals (500 mg tablets). Another phosphate binder is sevelamer hydrochloride, which can be titrated to target phosphorus levels using 800–1600 mg three times daily with meals (400 and

Table 21–11. Causes of hyperphosphatemia.

Massive load of phosphate into the extracellular fluid
  Exogenous sources
    Hypervitaminosis D
    Laxatives or enemas containing phosphate
    Intravenous phosphate supplement
  Endogenous sources
    Rhabdomyolysis (especially if renal insufficiency coexists)
    Cell destruction by chemotherapy of malignancy, particularly lymphoproliferative diseases
    Metabolic acidosis (lactic acidosis, ketoacidosis)
    Respiratory acidosis (phosphate incorporation into cells is disturbed)
Decreased excretion into urine
  Renal failure (acute, chronic)
  Hypoparathyroidism
  Pseudohypoparathyroidism
  Excessive growth hormone (acromegaly)
Pseudohyperphosphatemia
  Multiple myeloma
  Hypertriglyceridemia
  Cell lysis

800 mg tablets and 403 mg capsules). Because this agent does not contain calcium or aluminum, it may be especially useful for patients with hypercalcemia or uremia. Despite its usefulness, it has been suspected of producing mild hyperchloremic metabolic acidosis in patients with chronic kidney disease. The 2004 Calcium Acetate Renagel Evaluation (CARE) study on the treatment of hyperphosphatemia in hemodialysis patients concluded that in the absence of hypercalcemia, calcium therapy is more effective than sevelamer in the control of serum phosphorus and the calcium-phosphate product.

Akizawa T et al: New strategies for the treatment of secondary hyperparathyroidism. Am J Kidney Dis 2003;41(3 Suppl 1): S100. [PMID: 12612963]

Friedman EA: Consequences and management of hyperphosphatemia in patients with renal insufficiency. Kidney Int Suppl 2005;(95):S1. [PMID: 15882307]

Qunibi WY et al: Treatment of hyperphosphatemia in hemodialysis patients: The Calcium Acetate Renagel Evaluation (CARE Study). Kidney Int 2004;65:1914. [PMID: 15086935]

Shiber JR et al: Serum phosphate abnormalities in the emergency department. J Emerg Med 2002;23:39. [PMID: 12480022]

■ DISORDERS OF MAGNESIUM CONCENTRATION

The normal plasma concentration is 1.5–2.5 mEq/L, with about one-third bound to protein and two-thirds existing as free cation. Excretion of magnesium ion is via the kidney. Normally, about 3% of magnesium filtered by the glomerulus is excreted in urine. Magnesium exerts physiologic effects on the nervous system resembling those of calcium. Magnesium acts directly upon the myoneural junction.

Altered concentration of Mg^{2+} in the plasma usually provokes an associated alteration of Ca^{2+}. Hypermagnesemia suppresses secretion of PTH with consequent hypocalcemia. Severe and prolonged magnesium depletion impairs secretion of PTH with consequent hypocalcemia. Hypomagnesemia may impair end-organ response to PTH as well.

HYPOMAGNESEMIA

 ESSENTIALS OF DIAGNOSIS

- *Serum concentration of magnesium may not be decreased even in the presence of magnesium depletion. Check urinary magnesium excretion if renal magnesium wasting is suspected.*
- *Causes neurologic symptoms and arrhythmias.*
- *Impairs release of PTH.*

General Considerations

Causes of hypomagnesemia are listed in Table 21–12. Normomagnesemia does not exclude magnesium depletion because only 1% of total body magnesium is in the

Table 21–12. Causes of hypomagnesemia.

Diminished absorption or intake
  Malabsorption, chronic diarrhea, laxative abuse
  Prolonged gastrointestinal suction
  Small bowel bypass
  Malnutrition
  Alcoholism
  Total parenteral alimentation with inadequate Mg^{2+} content
Increased renal loss
  Diuretic therapy (loop diuretics, thiazide diuretics)
  Hyperaldosteronism, Gitelman's syndrome (a variant of Bartter's syndrome)
  Hyperparathyroidism, hyperthyroidism
  Hypercalcemia
  Volume expansion
  Tubulointerstitial diseases
  Transplant kidney
  Drugs (aminoglycoside, cetuximab, cisplatin, amphotericin B, pentamidine)
Others
  Diabetes mellitus
  Post parathyroidectomy (hungry bone syndrome)
  Respiratory alkalosis
  Pregnancy

extracellular fluid. Nearly 50% of hospitalized patients in whom serum electrolytes are ordered have unrecognized hypomagnesemia. Up to 40% of patients with hypomagnesemia have hypokalemia, and up to 50% have hypocalcemia. Hypomagnesemia and hypokalemia share many etiologies, including diuretics, diarrhea, alcoholism, aminoglycosides, and amphotericin B. Renal potassium wasting also occurs from hypomagnesemia, and is refractory to potassium replacement until magnesium is repleted. Hypomagnesemia also suppresses PTH release and causes end-organ resistance to it and to low 1,25-vitamin D levels. This hypocalcemia is also refractory to calcium replacement until the magnesium is repleted. In addition, molecular mechanisms of magnesium wasting have been revealed in some hereditary disorders.

Clinical Findings

A. SYMPTOMS AND SIGNS

Common symptoms are those of hypokalemia and hypocalcemia, with weakness and muscle cramps. There is marked neuromuscular and central nervous system hyperirritability, with tremors, athetoid movements, jerking, nystagmus, and a positive Babinski response. There may be hypertension, tachycardia, and ventricular arrhythmias. Confusion and disorientation may be prominent features.

B. LABORATORY FINDINGS

Urinary excretion of magnesium exceeding 10–30 mg/d or a fractional excretion more than 2% indicates renal magnesium wasting. In calculating fractional excretion of magnesium, since only 30% is protein bound, it follows that 70% of circulating magnesium is filtered by the glomerulus. In addition to hypomagnesemia, hypocalcemia and hypokalemia are often present. The ECG shows a prolonged QT interval, due to lengthening of the ST segment. PTH secretion is often suppressed (see Hypocalcemia, above).

Treatment

Magnesium oxide, 250–500 mg by mouth once or twice daily, is useful for repleting stores in patients with chronic hypomagnesemia. Treatment of symptomatic hypomagnesemia can include an infusion of 1–2 g of magnesium sulfate, followed by an infusion of 6 g magnesium sulfate in at least 1 L of fluids over 24 hours, repeated for up to 7 days to replete magnesium stores. Magnesium sulfate may also be given intramuscularly in a dosage of 200–800 mg/d (8–33 mmol/d) in four divided doses. Serum levels must be monitored daily and dosage adjusted to keep the concentration from rising above 2.5 mmol/L. Tendon reflexes may also be checked, since hypermagnesemia causes hyporeflexia. K^+ and Ca^{2+} replacement may be required as well, but patients with hypokalemia and hypocalcemia of hypomagnesemia do not recover without magnesium supplementation.

Patients with normal renal function can excrete excess magnesium and hypermagnesemia should not develop with replacement dosages. In patients with renal insufficiency, replacement of magnesium should be done cautiously to avoid hypermagnesemia. Reduced doses (50–75% dose reduction) and more frequent monitoring (at least twice daily) are indicated.

Tong GM et al: Magnesium deficiency in critical illness. J Intensive Care Med 2005;20:3. [PMID: 15665255]

Topf JM et al: Hypomagnesemia and hypermagnesemia. Rev Endocr Metab Disord 2003;4:195. [PMID: 127P66548]

Touyz RM: Magnesium in clinical medicine. Front Biosci 2004; 9:1278. [PMID: 14977544]

HYPERMAGNESEMIA

 ESSENTIALS OF DIAGNOSIS

- *Almost always associated with renal insufficiency and a history of chronic intake of magnesium-containing drugs.*

General Considerations

Magnesium excess is almost always the result of renal insufficiency and the inability to excrete what has been taken in from food or drugs, especially the long-term use of antacids and laxatives. Magnesium replacement should be done cautiously in patients with renal insufficiency, and dose reductions up to 75% may be needed to avoid hypermagnesemia.

Clinical Findings

A. SYMPTOMS AND SIGNS

Muscle weakness, decreased deep tendon reflexes, mental obtundation, and confusion are characteristic manifestations. Weakness—even flaccid paralysis—ileus, urinary retention, and hypotension are noted. There may be respiratory muscle paralysis or cardiac arrest.

B. LABORATORY FINDINGS

Serum Mg^{2+} is elevated. In the common setting of renal insufficiency, concentrations of BUN and of serum creatinine, phosphate, and uric acid are elevated; serum K^+ may be elevated. Serum Ca^{2+} is often low. The ECG shows increased PR interval, broadened QRS complexes, and peaked T waves, probably related to associated hyperkalemia.

Treatment

Treatment is directed toward alleviating renal insufficiency. Calcium acts as an antagonist to Mg^{2+} and may be given intravenously as calcium chloride, 500 mg or more at a rate of 100 mg (4.5 mmol)/min. Hemodialysis or peritoneal dialysis may be necessary to remove the magnesium, particularly when there is severe renal failure.

Long-term use of magnesium-containing drugs, such as magnesium hydroxylate and magnesium sulfate, should be avoided in patients with renal insufficiency.

Topf JM et al: Hypomagnesemia and hypermagnesemia. Rev Endocr Metab Disord 2003;4:195. [PMID: 12766548]

■ ACID–BASE DISORDERS

To assess a patient's acid–base status, measurement of arterial pH, P_{CO_2}, and plasma bicarbonate (HCO_3^-) is needed. Blood gas analyzers directly measure pH and P_{CO_2}, and the HCO_3^- value is calculated from the Henderson–Hasselbalch equation:

$$pH = 6.1 + \log \frac{HCO_3^-}{0.3 \times P_{CO_2}}$$

The total venous CO_2 measurement is a more direct determination of HCO_3^-. Because of the dissociation characteristics of carbonic acid (H_2CO_3) at body pH, dissolved CO_2 is almost exclusively in the form of HCO_3^-, and for clinical purposes the total carbon dioxide content is equivalent ($\pm$ 3 mEq/L) to the HCO_3^- concentration:

$$H^+ + HCO_3^- \leftrightarrow H_2CO_3 \leftrightarrow CO_2 + H_2O$$

If precise measurements of oxygenation are not needed or if oxygen saturation obtained from the pulse oximeter is adequate, venous blood gases generally provide useful information for assessment of acid–base balance and can be used interchangeably with arterial blood gases since the arteriovenous differences in pH and P_{CO_2} are small and relatively constant. Venous blood pH is usually 0.03–0.04 units lower than that of arterial blood, and venous blood P_{CO_2} is 7 or 8 mm Hg higher. Calculated HCO_3^- concentration in venous blood is at most 2 mEq/L higher than that of arterial blood. Serum HCO_3^- measurement also provides equivalent information to the arterial base deficit in surgical intensive care unit patients. An important exception to the rule of interchangeability between arterial and venous blood gases for determination of acid–base balance is during cardiopulmonary arrest. In this setting, arterial pH may be 7.41 and venous pH 7.15, and arterial blood P_{CO_2} can be 32 mm Hg with a venous blood P_{CO_2} of 74 mm Hg.

Types of Acid–Base Disorders

There are two types of acid–base disorders: respiratory and metabolic. Primary respiratory disorders affect blood acidity by causing changes in P_{CO_2}, and primary metabolic disorders are caused by disturbances in the HCO_3^- concentration. The primary disturbances are usually accompanied by compensatory changes; however, even though these changes attenuate a pH shift from the normal value (7.40), they do not fully compensate for the primary acid–base disorders even if the disorders are chronic. Therefore, if the pH is less than 7.40, the primary process is acidosis (either respiratory or metabolic). If the pH is higher than 7.40, the primary process is either respiratory or metabolic alkalosis. The presence of one disorder with its appropriate compensatory change is a simple disorder.

Mixed Acid–Base Disorders

The presence of more than one simple disorder (not compensatory) is a mixed disorder. Double or triple disorders can coexist but not quadruple ones, because simultaneous respiratory acidosis and alkalosis are not possible.

Clinicians frequently find it difficult to decide if a mixed disorder is present. One useful scheme is to determine if the degree of compensation for the primary disorder is appropriate (Table 21–13). In respiratory disorders, if the magnitude of compensation in HCO_3^- level differs from what is predicted, the patient has a mixed disorder. Therefore, superimposed metabolic acidosis will decrease HCO_3^- to lower than the predicted level, and a metabolic alkalosis will increase HCO_3^- over the predicted value. For example, a patient with chronic respiratory acidosis and P_{CO_2} of 60 mm Hg should have a HCO_3^- of 31 mEq/L (assuming that normal HCO_3^- is 24 mEq/L). If the HCO_3^- is 25 mEq/L, a superimposed metabolic acidosis exists, and if the HCO_3^- is 45 mEq/L, there is a superimposed metabolic alkalosis. Using data from Table 21–13, similar calculations can be made for primary metabolic disorders.

Furthermore, corrected bicarbonate ($cHCO_3^-$), calculated from measured HCO_3^- plus the increase in anion gap (see box), is useful to assess the superimposed metabolic alkalosis or normal anion gap metabolic acidosis. In increased anion gap acidosis, there must be a mole for mole decrease in HCO_3^- as anion gap increases. Therefore, an HCO_3^- value higher or lower than normal (24 mEq/L) indicates the concomitant presence of metabolic alkalosis or normal anion gap acidosis, respectively.

**STEP-BY-STEP ANALYSIS OF
ACID-BASE STATUS**

Step 1: Determine the primary (or main) disorder—whether it is metabolic or respiratory—from blood, pH, HCO_3^-, and P_{CO_2} values.

Step 2: Determine the presence of mixed acid-base disorders by calculating the range of compensatory responses (Table 21–13).

Step 3: Calculate the anion gap (Table 21–14).

Step 4: Calculate the corrected HCO_3^- concentration if the anion gap is increased (see above).

Step 5: Examine the patient to determine whether the clinical signs are compatible with the acid-base analysis thus obtained.

Table 21–13. Primary acid-base disorders and expected compensation.

Disorder	Primary Defect	Compensatory Response	Magnitude of Compensation
Respiratory acidosis			
Acute	$\uparrow P_{CO_2}$	$\uparrow HCO_3^-$	$\uparrow HCO_3^-$ 1 mEq/L per 10 mm Hg $\uparrow P_{CO_2}$
Chronic	$\uparrow P_{CO_2}$	$\uparrow HCO_3^-$	$\uparrow HCO_3^-$ 3.5 mEq/L per 10 mm Hg $\uparrow P_{CO_2}$
Respiratory alkalosis			
Acute	$\downarrow P_{CO_2}$	$\downarrow HCO_3^-$	$\downarrow HCO_3^-$ 2 mEq/L per 10 mm Hg $\downarrow P_{CO_2}$
Chronic	$\downarrow P_{CO_2}$	$\downarrow HCO_3^-$	$\downarrow HCO_3^-$ 5 mEq/L per 10 mm Hg $\downarrow P_{CO_2}$
Metabolic acidosis	$\downarrow HCO_3^-$	$\downarrow P_{CO_2}$	$\downarrow P_{CO_2}$ 1.3 mm Hg per 1 mEq/L $\downarrow HCO_3^-$
Metabolic alkalosis	$\uparrow HCO_3^-$	$\uparrow P_{CO_2}$	$\uparrow P_{CO_2}$ 0.7 mm Hg per 1 mEq/L $\uparrow HCO_3^-$

Haber RJ: A practical approach to acid-base disorders. West J Med 1991;155:146. [PMID: 1843849]

Herd AM: An approach to complex acid-base problems: keeping it simple. Can Fam Physician 2005;51:226. [PMID: 15751566]

Kellum JA: Determinants of plasma acid-base balance. Crit Care Clin 2005;21:329. [PMID: 15781166]

Williamson JC: Acid-base disorders: classification and management strategies. Am Fam Physician 1995;52:584. [PMID: 7625331]

METABOLIC ACIDOSIS

ESSENTIALS OF DIAGNOSIS

- *Decreased HCO_3^- with acidemia.*
- *Classified into high anion gap acidosis and normal anion gap acidosis.*
- *The highest anion gap acidoses are seen in lactic acidosis, ketoacidosis, or toxins.*
- *Normal anion gap acidosis is mainly caused by gastrointestinal HCO_3^- loss or RTA. Urinary anion gap may help distinguish between these causes.*

General Considerations

The hallmark of metabolic acidosis is decreased HCO_3^-, seen also in respiratory alkalosis (see above), but the pH distinguishes between the two disorders. Calculation of the anion gap is useful in determining the cause of the metabolic acidosis (Table 21–14). The anion gap represents the difference between readily measured anions and cations.

In plasma,

$$Na^+ + \frac{Unmeasured}{cations} = HCO_3^- + Cl^- + \frac{Unmeasured}{anions}$$

$$Anion\ gap = Na^+ - (HCO_3^- + Cl^-)$$

The major unmeasured cations are calcium (1 mEq/L), magnesium (2 mEq/L), γ-globulins, and potassium (4 mEq/L). The major unmeasured anions are negatively charged albumin (2 mEq/L per g/dL), phosphate (2 mEq/L), sulfate (1 mEq/L), lactate (1–2 mEq/L), and other organic anions (3–4 mEq/L). Traditionally, the normal anion gap has been 12 ± 4 mEq/L.

Table 21–14. Abnormal anion gap.[1]

Decreased (< 6 mEq)
  Hypoalbuminemia (decreased unmeasured anion)
  Plasma cell dyscrasias
    Monoclonal protein (cationic paraprotein) (accompanied by chloride and bicarbonate)
  Bromide intoxication
Increased (>12 mEq)
  Metabolic anion
    Diabetic ketoacidosis
    Alcoholic ketoacidosis
    Lactic acidosis
    Renal insufficiency (PO_4^{3-}, SO_4^{2-})
    Starvation
    Metabolic alkalosis (increased number of negative charges on protein)
  Drug or chemical anion
    Salicylate intoxication
    Sodium carbenicillin therapy
    Methanol (formic acid)
    Ethylene glycol (oxalic acid)
Normal (6–12 mEq)
  Loss of HCO_3^-
    Diarrhea
    Recovery from diabetic ketoacidosis
    Pancreatic fluid loss ileostomy (unadapted)
    Carbonic anhydrase inhibitors
  Chloride retention
    Renal tubular acidosis
    Ileal loop bladder
  Administration of HCl equivalent or NH_4Cl
    Arginine and lysine in parenteral nutrition

[1]Reference ranges for anion gap may vary based on differing laboratory methods.

With the current generation of autoanalyzers, the reference range may be lower (6 ± 1 mEq/L), primarily from an increase in Cl^- values. Despite its usefulness, the serum anion gap can be misleading. Non-acid–base disorders that may contribute to an error in anion gap interpretation include hypoalbuminemia (see below), antibiotic administration (eg, carbenicillin is an unmeasured anion; polymyxin is an unmeasured cation), hypernatremia, or hyponatremia.

Decreased Anion Gap

A decreased anion gap can occur because of a reduction in unmeasured anions or an increase in unmeasured cations.

A. DECREASED UNMEASURED ANIONS

If the sodium concentration remains normal but HCO_3^- and Cl^- increase, the anion gap will decrease. This is seen when there are decreased unmeasured anions, especially in hypoalbuminemia, which explains the low anion gap that frequently occurs in patients with hepatic cirrhosis. For every 1 g/dL decline in serum albumin, a 2 mEq/L decrease in anion gap will occur. Thus, without such a correction, the presence of an increased anion gap acidosis may be overlooked in patients who have marked hypoalbuminemia.

B. INCREASED UNMEASURED CATIONS

If the sodium concentration falls because of addition of unmeasured cations but HCO_3^- and Cl^- remain unchanged, the anion gap will decrease. This is seen in (1) severe hypercalcemia, hypermagnesemia, or hyperkalemia; (2) IgG myeloma, where the immunoglobulin is cationic in 70% of cases; and (3) lithium toxicity.

Jurado RL et al: Low anion gap. South Med J 1998;91:624. [PMID: 9671832]

Increased Anion Gap Acidosis (Increased Unmeasured Anions)

The hallmark of this disorder is that metabolic acidosis (thus low HCO_3^-) is associated with normal serum Cl^-, so that the anion gap increases. Normochloremic metabolic acidosis generally results from addition to the blood of nonchloride acids such as lactate, acetoacetate, β-hydroxybutyrate, and exogenous toxins. Unmeasured anions such as isocitrate, alpha-ketoglutarate, malate and D-lactate, may further contribute to the anion gap of lactic acidosis, diabetic ketoacidosis, and acidosis of unknown etiology. An exception is uremia, with underexcretion of organic acids and anions.

A. LACTIC ACIDOSIS

Lactic acid is formed from pyruvate in anaerobic glycolysis. Therefore, most of the lactate is produced in tissues with high rates of glycolysis, such as gut (responsible for over 50% of lactate production), skeletal muscle, brain, skin, and erythrocytes. Normally, lactate levels remain low (1 mEq/L) because of metabolism of lactate principally by the liver through gluconeogenesis or oxidation via the Krebs cycle. Furthermore, the kidneys metabolize about 30% of lactate.

In lactic acidosis, lactate levels are at least 4–5 mEq/ L but commonly 10–30 mEq/L. The mortality rate exceeds 50%. There are two basic types of lactic acidosis, both associated with increased lactate production and decreased lactate utilization. Type A is characterized by hypoxia or decreased tissue perfusion, whereas in type B there is no clinical evidence of hypoxia.

Type A (hypoxic) lactic acidosis is the more common type, resulting from poor tissue perfusion; cardiogenic, septic, or hemorrhagic shock; and carbon monoxide or cyanide poisoning. These conditions not only cause lactic acid production to increase peripherally but, more importantly, hepatic metabolism of lactate to decrease as liver perfusion declines. In addition, severe acidosis impairs the ability of the liver to extract the perfused lactate.

Type B lactic acidosis may be due to metabolic causes, such as diabetes, ketoacidosis, liver disease, renal failure, infection, leukemia, or lymphoma, or it may occur as a result of toxicity from ethanol, methanol, salicylates, isoniazid, or metformin. Propylene glycol, used as a vehicle for intravenous agents such as nitroglycerin, etomidate, and high-dose diazepam, may cause lactic acidosis from liver metabolism. Nutritional problems are important causes of lactic acidosis. Parenteral nutrition without thiamin causes severe refractory lactic acidosis from the deranged metabolism of pyruvate. Patients with short bowel syndrome may develop D-lactic acidosis with encephalopathy due to carbohydrate malabsorption in the intestine and subsequent fermentation by colonic bacteria.

AIDS without AIDS-related lymphoma is associated with type B lactic acidosis. Treatment of HIV patients with nucleoside analog reverse transcriptase inhibitors may cause lactic acidosis due to mitochondrial toxicity.

Idiopathic lactic acidosis, usually in debilitated patients, has an extremely high mortality rate. (For treatment of lactic acidosis, see below and Chapter 27.)

B. DIABETIC KETOACIDOSIS

This metabolic abnormality is characterized by hyperglycemia and metabolic acidosis (pH < 7.25 or plasma bicarbonate < 16 mEq/L). Anion gap metabolic acidosis is the acid–base disturbance generally ascribed to diabetic ketoacidosis:

$$H^+ + B^- + NaHCO_3 \leftrightarrow CO_2 + NaB + H_2O$$

where B^- is β-hydroxybutyrate or acetoacetate. The anion gap should be calculated from the serum electrolytes as measured, since correction of the serum sodium for the dilutional effect of hyperglycemia will incorrectly exaggerate the anion gap. The increased anion gap is due to hyperketonemia (acetoacetate and β-hydroxybutyrate) and at times to an increase in serum lactate secondary to reduced tissue perfusion and increased anaerobic metabolism. If a rise in anion gap from normal is equal to a fall in HCO_3^-, a diagnosis of simple metabolic acidosis can be made. However, the presence of concurrent metabolic alkalosis or normal anion gap metabolic acidosis is suggested if the value of the measured HCO_3^- plus the increase in anion gap ($cHCO_3^-$) is higher or lower than the normal value for HCO_3^-, respectively.

During the recovery phase of diabetic ketoacidosis, anion gap acidosis can be transformed into hyperchloremic non-anion gap acidosis. The mechanism for this is as follows: As GFR increases from NaCl therapy of diabetic ketoacidosis, the retention of Cl^- causes a mild decrease in the anion gap from dilution. More importantly, the increased GFR causes the urinary excretion of ketone salts (NaB), which are formed as bicarbonate is consumed:

$$HB + NaHCO_3 \rightarrow NaB + H_2CO_3$$

The kidney reabsorbs ketone anions poorly but can compensate for the loss of anions (and therefore Na^+) by increasing the reabsorption of Cl^-. Conversely, even on presentation, patients with diabetic ketoacidosis and normal renal perfusion may have marked ketonuria, severe metabolic acidosis, and only a mildly increased anion gap. Again, the variable relationship between the rise in the anion gap and the fall in the HCO_3^- can occur with the urinary loss of Na^+ or K^+ salts of β-hydroxybutyrate, which will lower the anion gap without altering the H^+ excretion or the severity of the acidosis. Because Ketostix reacts to acetoacetate, less to acetone, and not at all to the predominant keto acid, β-hydroxybutyrate, the test may become more positive even as the patient improves owing to the metabolism of hydroxybutyrate. Thus, the patient's clinical status and the reduction of the anion gap are better markers of improvement than monitoring the serum acetone test. Conversely, in the presence of concomitant lactic acidosis, a shift in the redox state can increase β-hydroxybutyrate and decrease the readily detectable acetoacetate, thus lowering the nitroprusside reaction.

C. ALCOHOLIC KETOACIDOSIS

This is a common disorder of chronically malnourished patients who consume large quantities of alcohol daily. Most of these patients have mixed acid–base disorders (10% have a triple acid–base disorder). Although decreased HCO_3^- is usual, 50% of the patients may have normal or alkalemic pH. Three types of metabolic acidosis are seen in alcoholic ketoacidosis: (1) Ketoacidosis is due to β-hydroxybutyrate and acetoacetate excess. (2) Lactic acidosis: Alcohol metabolism increases the NADH:NAD ratio, causing increased production and decreased utilization of lactate. Accompanying thiamin deficiency, which inhibits pyruvate carboxylase, further enhances lactic acid production in many cases. Moderate to severe elevations of lactate (> 6 mmol/L) are seen with concomitant disorders such as sepsis, pancreatitis, or hypoglycemia. (3) Hyperchloremic acidosis from bicarbonate loss in the urine is associated with ketonuria (see above). Metabolic alkalosis occurs from volume contraction and vomiting. Respiratory alkalosis results from alcohol withdrawal, pain, or associated disorders such as sepsis or liver disease. Half of the patients have either hypoglycemia or hyperglycemia. When serum glucose levels are greater than 250 mg/dL, the distinction from diabetic ketoacidosis is difficult. The diagnosis of alcoholic ketoacidosis is supported by the absence of a diabetic history and by no evidence of glucose intolerance after initial therapy.

D. TOXINS

(See also Chapter 39.) Multiple toxins and drugs can increase the anion gap by increasing endogenous acid production. Examples include methanol (metabolized to formic acid), ethylene glycol (glycolic and oxalic acid), and salicylates (salicylic acid and lactic acid), which can cause a mixed disorder of metabolic acidosis with respiratory alkalosis. In toluene poisoning, a metabolite hippurate is rapidly excreted by the kidney and may present as a normal anion gap acidosis. Isopropyl alcohol, which is metabolized to acetone, increases the osmolar gap, but not the anion gap.

E. UREMIC ACIDOSIS

At GFRs below 20 mL/min, the inability to excrete H^+ with retention of acid anions such as PO_4^{3-} and SO_4^{2-} results in an increased anion gap acidosis, which rarely is severe. The unmeasured anions "replace" HCO_3^- (which is consumed as a buffer). Hyperchloremic normal anion gap acidosis develops in milder cases of renal insufficiency.

Normal Anion Gap Acidosis (Table 21–15)

The hallmark of this disorder is that the low HCO_3^- of metabolic acidosis is associated with hyperchloremia, so that the anion gap remains normal. The most common causes are gastrointestinal HCO_3^- loss and defects in renal acidification (renal tubular acidoses). The urinary anion gap can differentiate between these two common causes (see below).

A. GASTROINTESTINAL HCO_3^- LOSS

Bicarbonate is secreted in multiple areas in the gastrointestinal tract. Small bowel and pancreatic secretions contain large amounts of HCO_3^-. Therefore, massive diarrhea or pancreatic drainage can result in HCO_3^- loss because of increased HCO_3^- secretion and decreased absorption. Hyperchloremia occurs because the ileum and colon secrete HCO_3^- in a one-to-one exchange for Cl^- by countertransport. The resultant volume contraction causes further increased Cl^- retention by the kidney in the setting of decreased anion,

Table 21–15. Hyperchloremic, normal anion gap metabolic acidoses.

| | Renal Defect | Serum [K⁺] | Distal H⁺ Secretion | | | Urinary Anion Gap | Treatment |
			Urinary NH₄⁺ Plus Minimal Urine pH	Titratable Acid			
Gastrointestinal HCO₃⁻ loss	None	↓	< 5.5	↑↑		Negative	Na⁺, K⁺, and HCO₃⁻ as required
Renal tubular acidosis							
I. Classic distal	Distal H⁺ secretion	↓	> 5.5	↓		Positive	NaHCO₃ (1–3 mEq/kg/d)
II. Proximal secretion	Proximal H⁺	↓	< 5.5	Normal		Positive	NaHCO₃ or KHCO₃ (10–15 mEq/kg/d), thiazide
IV. Hyporeninemic hypoaldosteronism	Distal Na⁺ reabsorption, K⁺ secretion, and H⁺ secretion	↑	< 5.5	↓		Positive	Fludrocortisone (0.1–0.5 mg/d), dietary K⁺ restriction, furosemide (40–160 mg/d), NaHCO₃ (1–3 mEq/kg/d)

Modified and reproduced, with permission, from Cogan MG: *Fluid and Electrolytes: Physiology and Pathophysiology.* McGraw-Hill, 1991.

HCO_3^-. Patients with ureterosigmoidostomies can develop hyperchloremic metabolic acidosis because the colon secretes HCO_3^- in the urine in exchange for Cl^-.

B. Renal Tubular Acidosis (RTA)

Hyperchloremic acidosis with a normal anion gap and normal (or near normal) GFR , and in the absence of diarrhea, defines RTA. The defect is either inability to excrete H^+ (inadequate generation of new HCO_3^-) or inappropriate reabsorption of HCO_3^-. Three major types can be differentiated by the clinical setting, urinary pH, urinary anion gap (see below), and serum K^+ level. (The term "type III renal tubular acidosis" is no longer used because of the controversies surrounding its definition.) Recently, the mechanisms of each abnormality have been better elucidated by identifying the responsible molecules and their gene mutations.

1. Classic distal RTA (type I)—This disorder is characterized by hypokalemic hyperchloremic metabolic acidosis and is due to selective deficiency in H^+ secretion in α intercalated cells in the collecting tubule. Despite acidosis, urinary pH cannot be acidified and is above 5.5, which retards the binding of H^+ to phosphate (H^+ + $HPO_4^{2-} \rightarrow H_2PO_4$), and thus inhibits titratable acid excretion. Furthermore, urinary excretion of $NH_4^+Cl^-$ is decreased, and the urinary anion gap is positive (see below). Enhanced K^+ excretion occurs probably because there is less competition from H^+ in the distal nephron transport system. Furthermore, as a response to renal salt wasting, hyperaldosteronism occurs. Nephrocalcinosis and nephrolithiasis frequently accompany this disorder since chronic acidosis decreases tubular calcium reabsorption. The hypercalciuria, alkaline urine, and lowered level of urinary citrate cause calcium phosphate stones and nephrocalcinosis.

Distal RTA develops as a consequence of dysproteinemic syndromes, autoimmune disease, and drugs and toxins such as amphotericin B.

2. Proximal RTA (type II)—Proximal RTA is a hypokalemic hyperchloremic metabolic acidosis due to a selective defect in the proximal tubule's ability to adequately reabsorb filtered HCO_3^-. Carbonic anhydrase inhibitors (acetazolamide) can cause proximal RTA. About 90% of filtered HCO_3^- is absorbed by the proximal tubule. The distal nephron has a limited ability to absorb HCO_3^- but becomes overwhelmed and does not function adequately when there is increased delivery. Eventually, distal delivery of filtered HCO_3^- declines because the plasma HCO_3^- level has dropped as a result of progressive urinary HCO_3^- wastage. When the plasma HCO_3^- level drops to 15–18 mEq/L, delivery of HCO_3^- drops to the point where the distal nephron is no longer overwhelmed and can regain function. At that point, bicarbonaturia disappears, and urinary pH can be acidic. Thiazide-induced volume contraction can be used to enhance proximal HCO_3^- reabsorption, leading to the decrease in distal HCO_3^- delivery and improvement of bicarbonaturia and renal acidification. The increased delivery of HCO_3^- to the distal nephron also increases K^+ secretion, and hypokalemia results if a patient is loaded with excess HCO_3^- and K^+ is not adequately supplemented. Proximal RTA often exists with other defects of absorption in the proximal tubule, resulting in glucosuria, aminoaciduria, phosphaturia, and uricaciduria. Causes include multiple myeloma with Fanconi's syndrome and nephrotoxic drugs.

3. Hyporeninemic hypoaldosteronemic RTA (type IV)—Type IV is the most common form of RTA in clinical practice. This is the only type characterized by hyperkalemic, hyperchloremic acidosis. The defect is aldosterone deficiency or antagonism, which impairs distal nephron Na^+ reabsorption and K^+ and H^+ excretion. Renal salt wasting is frequently present. Relative hypoaldosteronism from hyporeninemia is most commonly found in diabetic nephropathy, tubulointerstitial renal diseases, hypertensive nephrosclerosis, and AIDS. In patients with these disorders, caution must be taken when using drugs that can exacerbate the hyperkalemia, such as ACE inhibitors (which will further reduce aldosterone levels), aldosterone receptor blockers such as spironolactone, and NSAIDs.

C. DILUTIONAL ACIDOSIS

Rapid dilution of plasma volume by 0.9% NaCl may cause a mild hyperchloremic acidosis.

D. RECOVERY FROM DIABETIC KETOACIDOSIS

See earlier section, Increased Anion Gap Acidosis (Increased Unmeasured Anion).

E. POSTHYPOCAPNIA

In prolonged respiratory alkalosis, HCO_3^- decreases and Cl^- increases from decreased renal $NH_4^+Cl^-$ excretion. If the respiratory alkalosis is corrected quickly, PCO_2 will increase acutely but HCO_3^- will remain low until the kidneys can generate new HCO_3^-, which generally takes several days. In the meantime, the increased PCO_2 with low HCO_3^- causes metabolic acidosis.

F. HYPERALIMENTATION

Hyperalimentation fluids may contain amino acid solutions that acidify when metabolized, such as arginine hydrochloride and lysine hydrochloride.

Urinary Anion Gap to Assess Hyperchloremic Metabolic Acidosis

Increased renal $NH_4^+Cl^-$ excretion to enhance H^+ removal is a normal physiologic response to metabolic acidosis. NH_3 reacts with H^+ to form NH_4^+, which is accompanied by the anion Cl^- for excretion. The normal daily urinary excretion of NH_4Cl of about 30 mEq can be increased up to 200 mEq in response to acid load.

Urinary anion gap from a random urine sample ($[Na^+ + K^+] - Cl^-$) reflects the ability of the kidney to excrete NH_4Cl as in the following equation:

$$Na^+ + K^+ + NH^{4+} = Cl^- + 80$$

where 80 is the average value for the difference in the urinary anions and cations other than Na^+, K^+, NH_4^+, and Cl. Therefore, urinary anion gap is equal to ($80 - NH_4^+$), and thus aids in the distinction between gastrointestinal and renal causes of hyperchloremic acidosis. If the cause of the metabolic acidosis is gastrointestinal HCO_3^- loss (diarrhea), the renal acidification ability remains normal and NH_4Cl excretion increases

in response to the acidosis. The urinary anion gap is negative (eg, –30 mEq/L). If the cause is distal RTA, the urinary anion gap is positive (eg, +25 mEq/L), since the basic lesion in the disorder is the inability of the kidney to excrete H^+ and thus the inability to increase NH_4Cl excretion. In proximal (type II) RTA, the kidney has defective HCO_3^- reabsorption, leading to increased HCO_3^- excretion rather than decreased NH_4Cl excretion. Thus, the urinary anion gap is often negative in proximal (type II) RTA.

Urinary pH may not as readily differentiate between the two causes. Despite acidosis, if volume depletion from diarrhea causes inadequate Na^+ delivery to the distal nephron and therefore decreased exchange with H^+, urinary pH may not be lower than 5.3. In the presence of this relatively high urine pH, however, H^+ excretion continues due to buffering of NH_3 to NH_4^+, since the pK of this reaction is as high as 9.1. Potassium depletion, which can accompany diarrhea (and surreptitious laxative abuse), may also impair renal acidification. Thus, when volume depletion is present, the urinary anion gap is a better measurement of ability to acidify the urine than urinary pH.

When large amounts of other anions are present in the urine, the urinary anion gap may not be reliable. In such a situation, NH_4^+ excretion can be estimated using the urinary osmolar gap.

$$NH_4^+ \text{ excretion (mmol/L)} =$$
$$0.5 \times \text{Urinary osmolar gap} =$$
$$0.5 \text{ [U osm} - 2(\text{U Na}^+ + \text{U K}^+) + \text{U urea} + \text{U glucose]}$$

where urinary (U) concentrations and osmolality are in millimoles per liter.

Clinical Findings

A. SYMPTOMS AND SIGNS

Symptoms of metabolic acidosis are mainly those of the underlying disorder. Compensatory hyperventilation is an important clinical sign and may be misinterpreted as a primary respiratory disorder; when severe, Kussmaul respirations (deep, regular, sighing respirations) are seen.

B. LABORATORY FINDINGS

Blood pH, serum HCO_3^-, and PCO_2 are decreased. Anion gap may be normal (hyperchloremic) or increased (normochloremic). Hyperkalemia may be seen (see above).

Treatment

A. INCREASED ANION GAP ACIDOSIS

Treatment is aimed at the underlying disorder, such as insulin and fluid therapy for diabetes and appropriate volume resuscitation to restore tissue perfusion. The metabolism of lactate will produce HCO_3^- and increase pH. The use of supplemental HCO_3^- is indicated for treatment of hyperkalemia (Table 21–7) and some forms of normal anion gap acidosis but has been controversial for treatment of increased anion gap metabolic acidosis.

Controversy remains about the efficacy and safety of alkali therapy for severe metabolic acidosis. Administration of large amounts of HCO_3^- may have deleterious effects, including hypernatremia and hyperosmolality. Furthermore, intracellular pH may decrease because administered HCO_3^- is converted to CO_2, which easily diffuses into cells. There, it combines with water to create additional hydrogen ions and worsening of intracellular acidosis. Theoretically, this could impair cellular function, but the clinical significance of this phenomenon is uncertain.

In addition, alkali administration is known to stimulate phosphofructokinase activity, thus exacerbating lactic acidosis via enhanced lactate production. Ketogenesis is also augmented by alkali therapy.

In salicylate intoxication, however, alkali therapy must be started unless blood pH is already alkalinized by respiratory alkalosis, since the increment in pH converts salicylate to more impermeable salicylic acid and thus prevents central nervous system damage. In alcoholic ketoacidosis, thiamin should be given together with glucose to avoid the development of Wernicke's encephalopathy. The amount of HCO_3^- deficit can be calculated as follows:

$$\text{Amount of } HCO_3^- \text{ deficit} = 0.5 \times \text{body weight} \times (24 - HCO_3^-)$$

Half of the calculated deficit should be administered within the first 3–4 hours to avoid overcorrection and volume overload. In methanol intoxication, ethanol has been used as a competitive substrate for alcohol dehydrogenase, which metabolizes methanol to formaldehyde. Recently, direct inhibition of alcohol dehydrogenase by fomepizole has been reported. Fomepizole may be used in methanol intoxication in the near future.

B. NORMAL ANION GAP ACIDOSIS

Treatment of RTA is mainly achieved by administration of alkali (either as bicarbonate or citrate) to correct metabolic abnormalities and prevent nephrocalcinosis and renal failure.

Large amounts of alkali (10–15 mEq/kg/d) may be required to treat proximal RTA because most of the alkali is excreted into the urine, which exacerbates hypokalemia. Thus, a mixture of sodium and potassium salts, such as K-Shohl solution, is preferred. The addition of thiazides may reduce the amount of alkali required, but hypokalemia may develop. Correction of type 1 distal RTA requires a smaller amount of alkali (1–3 mEq/kg/d) and potassium supplementation as needed.

For the treatment of type IV RTA, dietary potassium restriction may be needed and potassium-retaining drugs should be withdrawn. Fludrocortisone may be effective in cases with hypoaldosteronism, but

should be used with care, preferably in combination with loop diuretics. In some cases, alkali supplementation (1–3 mEq/kg/d) may be required.

Casaletto JJ: Differential diagnosis of metabolic acidosis. Emerg Med Clin North Am 2005;23:771. [PMID: 15982545]

Forni LG et al: Circulating anions usually associated with the Krebs cycle in patients with metabolic acidosis. Crit Care 2005;9:R591. [PMID: 16277723]

Hassan H et al: Evaluation of serum anion gap in patients with liver cirrhosis of diverse etiologies. Mt Sinai J Med 2004; 71:281. [PMID: 15365595]

Levraut J et al: Treatment of metabolic acidosis. Curr Opin Crit Care 2003;9:260. [PMID: 11576874]

Matin MJ et al: Use of serum bicarbonate measurement in place of arterial base deficit in the surgical intensive care unit. Arch Surg 2005;140:745. [PMID: 16103283]

Soriano JR: Renal tubular acidosis: the clinical entity. J Am Soc Nephrol 2002;13:2160. [PMID: 12138150]

METABOLIC ALKALOSIS

 ESSENTIALS OF DIAGNOSIS

- High HCO_3^- with alkalemia.
- Evaluate effective circulating volume by physical examination and check urinary chloride concentration. This will help differentiate saline-responsive metabolic alkalosis from saline-unresponsive alkalosis.

Classification

Metabolic alkalosis is characterized by high HCO_3^-. The high HCO_3^- is also seen in chronic respiratory acidosis (see below), but pH differentiates the two disorders. Abnormalities that generate HCO_3^- within the body are called "initiation factors" of metabolic alkalosis, whereas abnormalities that promote renal conservation of HCO_3^- are called "maintenance factors." Metabolic alkalosis may remain even after the initiation factors have disappeared.

It is useful to classify the causes of metabolic alkalosis into two groups based on "saline responsiveness" or urinary Cl^-, which are markers for volume status (Table 21–16). Saline-responsive metabolic alkalosis is a sign of extracellular volume contraction, and saline-unresponsive alkalosis implies a volume-expanded state. It is rare for a compensatory increase in PCO_2 to exceed 55 mm Hg. A higher value implies a superimposed respiratory acidosis.

A. SALINE-RESPONSIVE METABOLIC ALKALOSIS

Saline-responsive metabolic alkalosis is by far the more common disorder. It is characterized by normotensive extracellular volume contraction and hypokalemia. Less frequently, hypotension or orthostatic hypoten-

Table 21–16. Metabolic alkalosis.

Saline-Responsive ($U_{Cl} < 10$ mEq/d)	Saline-Unresponsive ($U_{Cl} > 10$ mEq/d)
Excessive body bicarbonate content	**Excessive body bicarbonate content**
Renal alkalosis	Renal alkalosis
Diuretic therapy	Normotensive
Poorly reabsorbable anion therapy: carbenicil- lin, sulfate, phosphate	Bartter's syndrome (renal salt wasting and secon- dary hyperaldosteronism)
Posthypercapnia	Severe potassium depletion
Gastrointestinal alkalosis	Refeeding alkalosis
Loss of HCl from vomiting or nasogastric suction	Hypercalcemia and hypoparathyroidism
Intestinal alkalosis: chloride diarrhea	Hypertensive
Exogenous alkali	Endogenous mineralocorticoids
$NaHCO_3$ (baking soda)	Primary aldosteronism
Sodium citrate, lactate, gluconate, acetate	Hyperreninism
Transfusions	Adrenal enzyme deficiency: 11- and 17-hydroxylase
Antacids	Liddle's syndrome
Normal body bicarbonate content	Exogenous mineralocorticoids
"Contraction alkalosis"	Licorice

Modified and reproduced, with permission, from Narins RG et al: Diagnostic strategies in disorders of fluid, electrolyte and acid-base homeostasis. Am J Med 1982;72:496.

sion may be seen. In vomiting or nasogastric suction, for example, loss of acid (HCl) initiates the alkalosis, but volume contraction from loss of Cl^- sustains the alkalosis because the decline in GFR causes avid renal Na^+ and HCO_3^- reabsorption. Because there is Cl^- depletion from loss of HCl, NaCl, and KCl from the stomach, the available anion is HCO_3^-, whose reabsorption is increased proximally, and urine pH may remain acidic despite alkalemia (paradoxic aciduria). Renal Cl^- reabsorption (as well as Na^+ reabsorption) is high, and the urinary Cl^- is therefore low (< 10–20 mEq/L). In alkalosis, bicarbonaturia may force Na^+ excretion as the accompanying cation even if volume depletion is present. Therefore, urinary Cl^- is preferred to urinary Na^+ as a measure of extracellular volume. An exception to the usefulness of urinary Cl^- is in patients who have recently received diuretics. Their urine may contain high Na^+ and Cl^- despite extracellular volume contraction. If diuretics are discontinued, the urinary Cl^- will decrease.

Metabolic alkalosis is generally associated with hypokalemia. This is due partly to the direct effect of alkalosis per se on renal potassium excretion and partly to secondary hyperaldosteronism from volume depletion. Hypokalemia induced in this fashion further worsens the metabolic alkalosis by increasing bicarbonate reabsorption in the proximal tubule and hydrogen ion secretion in the distal tubule. Administration of KCl will correct the disorder. Repletion of KCl is important to reverse the disorder.

1. Contraction alkalosis—Diuretics can acutely decrease extracellular volume from urinary loss of NaCl and water. There is no associated bicarbonaturia, so that body HCO_3^- content remains normal. However,

plasma HCO_3^- increases because of extracellular fluid contraction—the reverse of what occurs in dilutional acidosis.

2. Posthypercapnia alkalosis—In chronic respiratory acidosis, compensatory increases in HCO_3^- occur (Table 21–13). Hypercapnia also directly affects the proximal tubule to decrease NaCl reabsorption, which can cause extracellular volume depletion. If PCO_2 is corrected rapidly, as with mechanical ventilation, metabolic alkalosis will ensue until adequate bicarbonaturia occurs. Hypovolemia will inhibit bicarbonaturia until Cl^- is repleted. Many patients with chronic respiratory acidosis receive diuretics, which further exacerbates the metabolic alkalosis.

B. SALINE-UNRESPONSIVE ALKALOSIS

1. Hyperaldosteronism—Primary hyperaldosteronism causes expansion of extracellular volume with hypertension. Metabolic alkalosis with hypokalemia results from the renal mineralocorticoid effect. In an attempt to decrease extracellular volume, high levels of NaCl are excreted, and for that reason the urinary Cl^- is high (> 20 mEq/L, often higher). Therapy with NaCl will only increase volume expansion and hypertension and will not treat the underlying problem of mineralocorticoid excess.

2. Alkali administration with decreased GFR—Despite large ingestions of HCO_3^-, enhanced bicarbonaturia almost always prevents a patient with normal renal function from developing metabolic alkalosis. However, with renal insufficiency, urinary excretion of bicarbonate is inadequate. If large amounts of HCO_3^- or metabolizable salts of organic acids such as sodium lactate, sodium citrate, or sodium gluconate are consumed, as with intensive antacid therapy, metabolic alkalosis will occur. In milk-alkali syndrome, large and sustained ingestion of absorbable antacids and milk causes renal insufficiency from hypercalcemia. Decreased GFR prevents appropriate bicarbonaturia from the ingested alkali, and metabolic alkalosis occurs. Volume contraction from renal hypercalcemic effects further exacerbates the alkalosis.

Clinical Findings

A. SYMPTOMS AND SIGNS

There are no characteristic symptoms or signs. Orthostatic hypotension may be encountered. Weakness and hyporeflexia occur if serum K^+ is markedly low. Tetany and neuromuscular irritability occur rarely.

B. LABORATORY FINDINGS

The arterial blood pH and bicarbonate are elevated. The arterial P_{CO_2} is increased. Serum potassium and chloride are decreased. There may be an increased anion gap.

Treatment

Mild alkalosis is generally well tolerated. Severe or symptomatic alkalosis (pH > 7.60) requires urgent treatment.

A. SALINE-RESPONSIVE METABOLIC ALKALOSIS

Therapy for saline-responsive metabolic alkalosis is aimed at correction of extracellular volume deficit. Depending on the degree of hypovolemia, adequate amounts of 0.9% NaCl and KCl should be administered. Discontinuation of diuretics and administration of H_2-blockers in patients whose alkalosis is due to nasogastric suction can be useful. If impaired pulmonary or cardiovascular status prohibits adequate volume repletion, acetazolamide, 250–500 mg intravenously every 4–6 hours, can be used. One must be alert to the possible development of hypokalemia, since potassium depletion can be induced by forced kaliuresis via bicarbonaturia. Administration of acid can be used as emergency therapy. HCl, 0.1 mol/L, is infused via a central vein (the solution is sclerosing). Dosage is calculated to decrease the HCO_3^- level by 50% over 2–4 hours, assuming an HCO_3^- volume of distribution (L) of 0.5 % body weight (kg). Patients with marked renal insufficiency may require dialysis.

B. SALINE-UNRESPONSIVE METABOLIC ALKALOSIS

Therapy for saline-unresponsive metabolic alkalosis includes surgical removal of a mineralocorticoid-producing tumor and blockage of aldosterone effect with an ACE inhibitor or with spironolactone. Metabolic alkalosis in primary aldosteronism can be treated only with potassium repletion.

Bartholow C et al: Hypokalemia and metabolic alkalosis: algorithms for combined clinical problem solving. Compr Ther 2000;26:114. [PMID: 10822791]

Galla JH: Metabolic alkalosis. J Am Soc Nephrol 2000;11:369. [PMID: 10665945]

RESPIRATORY ACIDOSIS (Hypercapnia)

Respiratory acidosis results from decreased alveolar ventilation and subsequent hypercapnia. Pulmonary as well as nonpulmonary disorders can cause hypoventilation. The clinician must be mindful of readily reversible causes of respiratory acidosis, especially opioid-induced central nervous system depression.

Acute respiratory failure is associated with severe acidosis and only a small increase in the plasma bicarbonate. After 6–12 hours, the primary increase in P_{CO_2} evokes a renal compensatory response to generate more HCO_3^-, which tends to ameliorate the respiratory acidosis. This usually takes several days to complete.

Chronic respiratory acidosis is generally seen in patients with underlying lung disease, such as chronic obstructive pulmonary disease. Urinary excretion of acid in the form of NH_4^+ and Cl^- ions results in the characteristic hypochloremia of chronic respiratory acidosis. When chronic respiratory acidosis is corrected suddenly, especially in patients who receive mechanical ventilation, there is a 2- to 3-day lag in renal bicarbonate excretion, resulting in posthypercapnic metabolic alkalosis.

Clinical Findings

A. SYMPTOMS AND SIGNS

With acute onset, there is somnolence and confusion, and myoclonus with asterixis may be seen. Coma from CO_2 narcosis ensues. Severe hypercapnia increases cerebral blood flow and cerebrospinal fluid pressure. Signs of increased intracranial pressure (papilledema, pseudotumor cerebri) may be seen.

B. LABORATORY FINDINGS

Arterial pH is low and P_{CO_2} is increased. Serum HCO_3^- is elevated, but not enough to completely compensate for the hypercapnia. If the disorder is chronic, hypochloremia is seen.

Treatment

Because opioid drug overdose is an important reversible cause of acute respiratory acidosis, naloxone, 0.04–2 mg intravenously (see Chapter 39), is administered to all such patients if no obvious cause for respiratory depression is present. In all forms of respiratory acidosis, treatment is directed at the underlying disorder to improve ventilation.

Epstein SK et al: Respiratory acidosis. Respir Care 2001;46:366. [PMID: 11262556]

Madias NE et al: Cross-talk between two organs: how the kidney responds to disruption of acid–base balance by the lung. Nephron Physiol 2003;93:61. [PMID: 12660492]

RESPIRATORY ALKALOSIS (Hypocapnia)

Respiratory alkalosis, or hypocapnia, occurs when hyperventilation reduces the P_{CO_2}, which increases the pH. The most common cause of respiratory alkalosis is hyperventilation syndrome (Table 21–17), but bacterial septicemia and cirrhosis are other common causes. Symptoms in acute respiratory alkalosis are related to decreased cerebral blood flow induced by the disorder. Pregnancy is another cause of chronic respiratory alkalosis, probably from progesterone stimulation of the respiratory center, producing an average P_{CO_2} of 30 mm Hg.

Determination of appropriate compensatory changes in the HCO_3^- is useful to sort out the presence of an associated metabolic disorder (see above under Mixed Acid–Base Disorders).

As in respiratory acidosis, the changes in HCO_3^- values are greater if the respiratory alkalosis is chronic (Table 21–13). Although serum HCO_3^- is frequently below 15 mEq/L in metabolic acidosis, it is unusual to see such a low level in respiratory alkalosis, and its presence would imply a superimposed (noncompensatory) metabolic acidosis.

Clinical Findings

A. SYMPTOMS AND SIGNS

In acute cases (hyperventilation), there is light-headedness, anxiety, paresthesias, numbness about the mouth, and a tingling sensation in the hands and feet. Tetany occurs in more severe alkalosis from a fall in ionized calcium. In chronic cases, findings are those of the responsible condition.

B. LABORATORY FINDINGS

Arterial blood pH is elevated, and P_{CO_2} is low. Serum bicarbonate is decreased in chronic respiratory alkalosis.

Treatment

Treatment is directed toward the underlying cause. In acute hyperventilation syndrome from anxiety, rebreathing into a paper bag will increase the P_{CO_2}. The processes are usually self-limited since muscle weakness caused by hyperventilation-induced alkalemia will suppress ventilation. Sedation may be necessary if the process persists. Rapid correction of chronic respiratory alkalosis may result in metabolic acidosis as P_{CO_2} is increased in the setting of a previous compensatory decrease in HCO_3^-.

Foster GT et al: Respiratory alkalosis. Respir Care 2001;46:384. [PMID: 11262557]

Laffey JG et al: Hypocapnia. N Engl J Med 2002;347:43. [PMID: 12097540]

Table 21–17. Causes of respiratory alkalosis.

Hypoxia
    Decreased inspired oxygen tension
    High altitude
    Ventilation/perfusion inequality
    Hypotension
    Severe anemia
CNS-mediated disorders
    Voluntary hyperventilation
        Anxiety-hyperventilation syndrome
    Neurologic disease
    Cerebrovascular accident (infarction, hemorrhage)
    Infection
    Trauma
    Tumor
    Pharmacologic and hormonal stimulation
        Salicylates
        Nicotine
        Xanthines
        Pregnancy (progesterone)
    Hepatic failure
    Gram-negative septicemia
    Recovery from metabolic acidosis
    Heat exposure
Pulmonary disease
    Interstitial lung disease
    Pneumonia
    Pulmonary embolism
    Pulmonary edema
Mechanical overventilation

Adapted from Gennari FJ: Respiratory acidosis and alkalosis. In: *Maxwell and Kleeman's Clinical Disorders of Fluid and Electrolyte Metabolism,* 5th ed. Narins RG (editor). McGraw-Hill, 1994.

■ FLUID MANAGEMENT

An average adult whose entire intake is parenteral would require for maintenance 2500–3000 mL of 5% dextrose in 0.2% saline solution (34 mEq Na^+ plus 34 mEq Cl^-/L). To each liter, 30 mEq of KCl could be added. In 3 L, the total chloride intake would be 192 mEq, which is easily tolerated. Guidelines for gastrointestinal fluid losses are shown in Table 21–18.

Weight loss or gain is the best indication of water balance. Insensible water loss should be further considered in febrile patients. Water loss increases by 100–150 mL/d for each degree of body temperature over 37 °C.

In situations requiring maintenance or maintenance plus replacement of fluid and electrolyte by parenteral infusion, the total daily ration should be administered continuously over the 24-hour period to ensure the best utilization by the patient.

If parenteral fluids are the only source of water, electrolytes, and calories for longer than a week, more complex fluids containing amino acids, lipids, trace

Table 21–18. Replacement guidelines for sweat and gastrointestinal fluid losses.

	Average Electrolyte Composition				Replacement Guidelines per Liter Lost				
	Na^+ (mEq/L)	K^+ (mEq/L)	Cl^- (mEq/L)	HCO_3^- (mEq/L)	0.9% Saline (mL)	0.45% Saline (mL)	D_5W (mL)	KCl (mEq/L)	7.5% NaHCO$_3$ (45 mEq HCO$_3^-$/amp)
Sweat	30–50	5	50			500	500	5	
Gastric secretions	20	10	10			300	700	20	
Pancreatic juice	130	5	35	115		400	600	5	2 amps
Bile	145	5	100	25	600			400	5	0.5 amp
Duodenal fluid	60	15	100	10		1000		15	0.25 amp
Ileal fluid	100	10	60	60		600	400	10	1 amp
Colonic diarrhea	140[1]	10	85	60		1000		10	1 amp

[1]In the absence of diarrhea, colonic fluid Na^+ levels are low (40 mEq/L).

metals, and vitamins may be indicated. (See Total Parenteral Nutrition, Chapter 29.)

For parenteral alimentation, 620 mg (20 mmol) of phosphorus is required for every 1000 nonprotein kcal to maintain phosphate balance and to ensure anabolic function. For prolonged parenteral fluid maintenance, a daily ration is 620–1240 mg (20–40 mmol) of phosphorus.

Kidney

22

Suzanne Watnick, MD, & Gail Morrison, MD

▪ APPROACH TO RENAL DISEASE

Renal disease presents in one of two ways: discovered incidentally during a routine medical evaluation or with evidence of renal dysfunction such as hypertension, edema, nausea, and hematuria. The initial approach in both situations should be to assess the cause and severity of renal abnormalities. In all cases this evaluation includes (1) an estimation of disease duration, (2) a careful urinalysis, and (3) an assessment of the glomerular filtration rate (GFR). The history and physical examination, though equally important, are variable among renal syndromes—thus, specific symptoms and signs are discussed under each disease entity. Further diagnostic categorization is according to anatomic distribution: prerenal disease, postrenal disease, and intrinsic renal disease. Intrinsic renal disease can further be divided into glomerular, tubular, interstitial, and vascular abnormalities.

DISEASE DURATION

Renal disease may be acute or chronic. Acute renal failure is worsening of renal function over hours to days, resulting in the retention of nitrogenous wastes (such as urea nitrogen) and creatinine in the blood. Retention of these substances is called azotemia. Chronic renal failure (chronic kidney disease) results from an abnormal loss of renal function over months to years. Differentiating between the two is important for diagnosis, treatment, and outcome. Oliguria is unusual in chronic renal insufficiency. Anemia (from low renal erythropoietin production) is rare in the initial period of acute renal failure. Small kidneys are most consistent with chronic kidney disease, whereas normal to large-size kidneys can be seen with both chronic and acute disease.

URINALYSIS

A urinalysis has been likened to "a poor man's renal biopsy." The urine is collected in midstream or, if that is not feasible, by bladder catheterization. The urine should be examined within 1 hour after collection to avoid destruction of formed elements. Urinalysis includes a dipstick examination followed by microscopic assessment if the dipstick has positive findings. The dipstick examination measures urinary specific gravity, pH, protein, hemoglobin, glucose, ketones, bilirubin, nitrites, and leukocyte esterase. Microscopy searches for all formed elements—crystals, cells, casts, and infecting organisms.

Various findings on the urinalysis are indicative of certain patterns of renal disease. A bland urinary sediment is common, especially in chronic kidney disease and prerenal and postrenal disorders. The presence of hematuria with dysmorphic red blood cells, red blood cell casts, and proteinuria is indicative of glomerulonephritis. Red blood cells are misshapen during passage from the capillary through the glomerular basement membrane into the urinary space of Bowman's capsule.

Casts are composed of Tamm-Horsfall urinary mucoprotein in the shape of the nephron segment where they were formed. Heavy proteinuria and lipiduria are consistent with the nephrotic syndrome. Pigmented granular casts and renal tubular epithelial cells alone or in casts suggest acute tubular necrosis. White blood cells, including neutrophils and eosinophils, white blood cell casts, red blood cells, and small amounts of protein can be found in interstitial nephritis and pyelonephritis (Table 22–1); Wright's stain can detect eosinophiluria. Pyuria alone can indicate a urinary tract infection. Hematuria and proteinuria are discussed more thoroughly below.

Proteinuria

Proteinuria is defined as excessive protein excretion in the urine, generally greater than 150–160 mg/24 h in adults. Significant proteinuria is a sign of an underlying renal abnormality, usually glomerular in origin when greater than 1 g/d. It is typically accompanied by other clinical abnormalities—elevated blood urea nitrogen (BUN) and serum creatinine levels, abnormal urinary sediment, or evidence of systemic illness (eg, fever, rash, vasculitis).

There are four primary reasons for development of proteinuria: (1) Functional proteinuria is a benign process stemming from stressors such as acute illness, exercise, and "orthostatic proteinuria." The latter condition, generally found in people under age 30 years, results in the excretion of abnormal amounts of urinary protein, typically less than 1 g/d. The orthostatic nature of the proteinuria is confirmed by measuring

Table 22–1. Significance of specific urinary casts.

Type	Significance
Hyaline casts	Concentrated urine, febrile disease, after strenuous exercise, in the course of diuretic therapy (not indicative of renal disease)
Red cell casts	Glomerulonephritis
White cell casts	Pyelonephritis, interstitial nephritis (indicative of infection or inflammation)
Renal tubular cell casts	Acute tubular necrosis, interstitial nephritis
Coarse, granular casts	Nonspecific; can represent acute tubular necrosis
Broad, waxy casts	Chronic renal failure (indicative of stasis in enlarged collecting tubules)

an 8-hour overnight supine urinary protein excretion, which should be less than 50 mg. (2) Overload proteinuria can result from overproduction of circulating, filterable plasma proteins (monoclonal gammopathies), such as Bence Jones proteins associated with multiple myeloma. Urinary protein electrophoresis will exhibit a discrete protein peak. Other examples of overload proteinuria include myoglobinuria in rhabdomyolysis and hemoglobinuria in hemolysis. (3) Glomerular proteinuria results from effacement of epithelial cell foot processes and altered glomerular permeability with an increased filtration fraction of normal plasma proteins. Glomerular diseases exhibit some degree of proteinuria. The urinary electrophoresis will have a pattern exhibiting a large albumin spike indicative of increased permeability of albumin across a damaged glomerular basement membrane (GBM). (4) Tubular proteinuria occurs as a result of faulty reabsorption of normally filtered proteins in the proximal tubule, such as β_2-microglobulin and immunoglobulin light chains. Causes include acute tubular necrosis, toxic injury (lead, aminoglycosides), drug-induced interstitial nephritis, and hereditary metabolic disorders (Wilson's disease and Fanconi's syndrome).

Evaluation of proteinuria by urinary dipstick primarily detects albumin and intact globulins, while overlooking positively charged light chains of immunoglobulins. These proteins can be detected by the addition of sulfosalicylic acid to the urine specimen. Precipitation indicates the presence of paraproteins.

The next step—and the most reliable way to quantify proteinuria—is a 24-hour urine collection. A finding of greater than 150 mg/24 h is abnormal, and greater than 3.5 g/24 h is consistent with nephrotic-range proteinuria. A simpler but less accurate method is to collect a random urine sample. The ratio of urinary protein concentration to urinary creatinine concentration ($U_{protein}/U_{creatinine}$) correlates with 24-hour urine protein collection (< 0.2 is normal and corresponds to excretion of less than 200 mg/24 h). If a patient has proteinuria with loss of renal function, renal biopsy may be indicated, particularly if the renal insufficiency is acute in onset. The clinical consequences of proteinuria are discussed in the section on the nephrotic syndrome. The benefit of a urine protein-to-creatinine ratio is the ease of collection and the lack of error from overcollection or undercollection.

In both diabetics and nondiabetics, therapy aimed at reducing proteinuria may also reduce progression of renal disease. Angiotensin-converting enzyme (ACE) inhibitors are effective by lowering efferent arteriolar resistance out of proportion to afferent arteriolar resistance, thereby reducing glomerular capillary pressure and lowering urinary protein excretion. Other effects include alterations of glomerular mesangial proliferation. ACE inhibitors can be used in patients despite compromised GFR as long as significant hyperkalemia does not occur and serum creatinine rises less than 30% and stabilizes over 2 months. Large randomized controlled trials (ie, the RENAAL and IDNT studies) have also proved the benefit of angiotensin II receptor blockers in reducing proteinuria and preventing progression of renal disease in diabetic nephropathy. Recently, "head-to-head" comparisons of an ACE-I and an angiotensin receptor blocker (ARB) have shown the ARB to be no better than the ACE-I in preventing progression of renal disease in diabetic persons with proteinuria. The consequences of dietary restrictions in patients with proteinuria are discussed in the section on chronic kidney disease.

Hematuria

Hematuria is significant if there are more than three red cells per high-power field. It is usually detected incidentally by the urine dipstick examination or clinically following an episode of macroscopic hematuria. The diagnosis must be confirmed via microscopic examination, as false-positive dipstick tests can be caused by vitamin C, beets and rhubarb, bacteria, and myoglobin. Transient hematuria is common, but in patients under 40 years it is less often of clinical significance.

Hematuria may be due to renal or extrarenal causes. Extrarenal causes are addressed in Chapter 23; most worrisome are urologic malignancies. Renal causes account for approximately 10% of cases and are best considered anatomically as glomerular or nonglomerular. The most common extraglomerular sources include cysts, calculi, interstitial nephritis, and renal neoplasia. Glomerular causes include immunoglobulin A (IgA) nephropathy, thin GBM disease, postinfectious glomerulonephritis, membranoproliferative glomerulonephritis, and systemic nephritic syndromes.

Currently, the United States Health Preventive Services Task Force does not recommend screening for hematuria. See Chapter 23 for evaluation of hematuria.

ESTIMATION OF GFR

The GFR provides a useful index of overall renal function; however, patients with renal disease can actually have a normal or increased GFR. The GFR measures the amount of plasma ultrafiltered across the glomerular capillaries and correlates with the ability of the kidneys to filter fluids and various substances. Daily GFR in normal individuals is variable, with a range of 150–250 L/24 h or 100–120 mL/min/1.73 m² of body surface area. GFR can be measured indirectly by determining the renal clearance of plasma substances that are not bound to plasma proteins, are freely filterable across the glomerulus, and are neither secreted nor reabsorbed along the renal tubules.

The formula used to determine the renal clearance of a substance is

$$C = \frac{U \times V}{P}$$

where C is the clearance, U and P are the urine and plasma concentrations of the substance (mg/dL), and V is the urine flow rate (mL/min). Inulin and creatinine clearance are used as markers of GFR. Inulin clearance following a continuous infusion is one of the most accurate methods for measurement of GFR. The cost and the complexity of the administration and analysis of inulin preclude its routine use. In clinical practice, the clearance rate of endogenous creatinine, the creatinine clearance, is the usual means of estimating GFR. Creatinine is a product of muscle metabolism produced at a relatively constant rate and cleared by renal excretion. It is freely filterable by the glomerulus and not reabsorbed by the renal tubules. With stable renal function, creatinine production and excretion are equal; thus, plasma creatinine concentrations remain constant. However, it is not a perfect indicator of GFR for the following reasons: (1) A small amount is normally eliminated by tubular secretion, and the fraction secreted progressively increases as GFR declines (overestimating GFR); (2) with severe renal failure, gut microorganisms degrade creatinine; (3) an individual's meat intake and muscle mass affect baseline plasma creatinine levels; (4) commonly used drugs such as aspirin, cimetidine, probenecid, and trimethoprim reduce tubular secretion of creatinine, increasing the plasma creatinine concentration and falsely indicating renal dysfunction; and (5) the accuracy of the measurement necessitates a stable plasma creatinine concentration over a 24-hour period, so that during the development of and recovery from acute renal failure, the creatinine clearance is of questionable value (Table 22–2).

To measure creatinine clearance, collect a 24-hour urine sample and determine the plasma creatinine level on the same day. An incomplete or prolonged urine collection is a common source of error. One way of estimating the completeness of the collection is to calculate a 24-hour creatinine excretion; the amount should be constant:

Table 22–2. Conditions affecting serum creatinine independently of glomerular filtration rate.

Condition	Mechanism
Conditions causing elevation	
Ketoacidosis	Noncreatinine chromogen
Cephalothin, cefoxitin	Noncreatinine chromogen
Flucytosine	Noncreatinine chromogen
Other drugs: aspirin, cimetidine, probenecid, trimethoprim	Inhibition of tubular creatinine secretion
Conditions causing decrease	
Advanced age	Physiologic decrease in muscle mass
Cachexia	Pathologic decrease in muscle mass
Liver disease	Decreased hepatic creatine synthesis and cachexia

$U_{cr} \times V = 15\text{–}20$ mg/kg for healthy young women

$U_{cr} \times V = 20\text{–}25$ mg/kg for healthy young men

The creatinine clearance (C_{cr}) is approximately 100 mL/min/1.73 m² in healthy young women and 120 mL/min/1.73 m² in healthy young men. The C_{cr} declines by an average of 0.8 mL/min/yr after age 40 years as part of the aging process, but 35% of subjects in one study had no decline in renal function over 10 years. Because urine collection may be difficult, C_{cr} can be estimated from the formula of Cockcroft and Gault, which incorporates age, sex, and weight to estimate C_{cr} from plasma creatinine levels without any urinary measurements:

$$C_{cr} = \frac{(140 - \text{Age}) \times \text{Weight (kg)}}{P_{cr} \times 72}$$

For women, the estimated GFR is multiplied by 0.85 because muscle mass is less. This formula overestimates GFR in patients who are obese or edematous, and is most accurate when normalized for body surface area of 1.73 m². A more complicated but more accurate assessment can be obtained via the 4-variable Modification of Diet in Renal Disease (MDRD) formula. This requires SCr, gender, race, and age; the formula can be found at www.nephron.com under the heading "MDRD GFR."

Urea is another index helpful in assessing renal function. It is synthesized mainly in the liver and is the end product of protein catabolism. Urea is freely filtered by the glomerulus, and about 30–70% is reabsorbed in the nephron. Unlike creatinine clearance, which overestimates GFR, urea clearance underestimates GFR. Urea reabsorption may be decreased in well-hydrated patients, whereas dehydration causes increased reabsorption, increasing BUN. A normal BUN:creatinine ratio

Table 22–3. Conditions affecting BUN independently of GFR.

Increased BUN
Reduced effective circulating blood volume (prerenal azotemia)
Catabolic states (gastrointestinal bleeding, corticosteroid use)
High-protein diets
Tetracycline
Decreased BUN
Liver disease
Malnutrition
Sickle cell anemia
SIADH

BUN = blood urea nitrogen; GFR = glomerular filtration rate; SIADH = syndrome of inappropriate antidiuretic hormone.

is 10:1. With dehydration, the ratio can increase to 20:1 or higher. Other causes of increased BUN include increased catabolism (gastrointestinal bleeding, cell lysis, and corticosteroid usage), increased dietary protein, and decreased renal perfusion (congestive heart failure, renal artery stenosis) (Table 22–3). Reduced BUN is seen in liver disease and in the syndrome of inappropriate antidiuretic hormone (SIADH) secretion.

As patients approach end-stage renal disease (ESRD), a more accurate measure of GFR than creatinine clearance is the average of the creatinine and urea clearances. The creatinine clearance overestimates GFR, as mentioned above, while the urea clearance underestimates GFR. Therefore, an average of the two more accurately approximates the true GFR.

IMAGING STUDIES

Radionuclide Studies

Radionuclide studies can measure renal function. [^{125}I]Iothalamate gives a surprisingly accurate measurement of GFR. It is injected intravenously, excreted renally, and sampled from the venous circulation over time. Technetium-labeled diethylenetriamine pentaacetic acid (^{99m}Tc-DTPA) is freely filtered by the glomerulus and not reabsorbed and is used to estimate GFR. Technetium-labeled dimercaptosuccinic acid (^{99m}Tc-DMSA) is bound to the tubules and provides an assessment of functional renal mass. [^{131}I]Orthoiodohippurate is secreted into the renal tubules and assesses renal plasma flow (RPF). The indications for nuclear renography are to measure function and flow, to determine the contribution of each kidney to overall renal function, to demonstrate the presence or absence of functioning renal tissue in mass lesions, to detect obstruction, and to evaluate renovascular disease.

Poor flow along with poor function is consistent with acute tubular necrosis or ESRD. Decreased flow to one kidney suggests arterial occlusion of that kidney. To further investigate renal artery stenosis, the test is done both with and without captopril (see Chapter 11).

Ultrasonography

Ultrasonography can identify the thickness and echogenicity of the renal cortex, medulla, and pyramids, and a distended urinary collecting system. Kidney size can be determined; a kidney less than 9 cm in length in an adult indicates significant irreversible renal disease. A difference in size of more than 1.5 cm between the two kidneys is observed in unilateral renal disease. Renal ultrasound is also performed to search for hydronephrosis and obstruction, to characterize renal mass lesions, to screen for autosomal dominant polycystic kidney disease, to evaluate the perirenal space, to localize the kidney for a percutaneous invasive procedure, and to assess postvoiding residual urine volume of the bladder.

Intravenous Urography

The intravenous pyelogram (IVP) had been the standard imaging procedure for evaluating the urinary tract since it provides an assessment of the kidneys, ureters, and bladder. An IVP necessitates the injection of contrast and is relatively contraindicated in patients at increased risk for acute renal failure (eg, diabetes mellitus with serum creatinine greater than 2 mg/dL, severe volume contraction, or prerenal azotemia), chronic kidney disease with serum creatinine greater than 5 mg/dL, and multiple myeloma. IVP is performed to obtain a detailed view of the pelvicaliceal system, assess renal size and shape, detect and localize renal stones, and assess renal function. It is particularly useful in diagnosing certain disorders such as medullary sponge kidney and papillary necrosis. Ultrasonography is replacing IVP to avoid dye administration, and helical CT scanning is replacing IVP for stone evaluation.

CT Scanning

CT scanning is required for further investigation of abnormalities detected by ultrasound or IVP. Although routine CT requires radiographic contrast administration, no contrast is necessary if the reason for the study is to demonstrate hemorrhage or calcifications in the kidneys such as suspected stone disease. Noncontrast helical CT scanning to detect renal stones is 95% sensitive and 98% specific in patients with acute flank pain. Because contrast is filtered by the glomeruli and concentrated in the tubules, there is enhancement of parenchymal tissue, making abnormalities such as cysts or neoplasms easily identified and allowing good visualization of renal vessels and ureters. CT scanning is especially useful for evaluation of solid or cystic lesions in the kidney or the retroperitoneal space, particularly if the ultrasound results are suboptimal.

MRI Scanning

MRI can easily distinguish renal cortex from medulla. Loss of corticomedullary function in a variety of disorders (eg, glomerulonephritis, hydronephrosis, renal vascular occlusion, and renal failure) will be evident on MRI. Renal cysts can also be identified by MRI. For some solid lesions, MRI may be superior to CT scans. MRI is indicated as an addition or alternative to CT scanning for staging renal cell cancer and as a substitute for CT scanning in the evaluation of a renal mass, especially for patients in whom contrast is contraindicated; in addition, the adrenals are well imaged. MRI is nearly 100% sensitive and 96–98% specific for the diagnosis of renal artery stenosis.

Arteriography & Venography

Renal arteriography is useful in the evaluation of atherosclerotic or fibrodysplastic stenotic lesions, aneurysms, vasculitis, and renal mass lesions. Venography is the best test for diagnosis of renal vein thrombosis, though CT scanning and MRI are less invasive for this purpose.

RENAL BIOPSY

Indications for percutaneous needle biopsy include (1) unexplained acute renal failure or chronic kidney disease; (2) acute nephritic syndromes; (3) unexplained proteinuria and hematuria; (4) previously identified and treated lesions to plan future therapy; (5) systemic diseases associated with kidney dysfunction, such as systemic lupus erythematosus, Goodpasture's syndrome, and Wegener's granulomatosis, to confirm the extent of renal involvement and to guide management; (6) suspected transplant rejection, to differentiate it from other causes of acute renal failure; and (7) to guide treatment. If a patient is unwilling to accept therapy based on biopsy findings, the risk of biopsy may outweigh its benefit. Relative contraindications include a solitary or ectopic kidney (exception: transplant allografts), horseshoe kidney, uncorrected bleeding disorder, severe uncontrolled hypertension, renal infection, renal neoplasm, hydronephrosis, ESRD, congenital anomalies, multiple cysts, or an uncooperative patient.

Prior to biopsy, patients should have well-controlled blood pressure; blood work should include a hematocrit, platelet count, prothrombin time, and partial thromboplastin time. After biopsy, hematuria occurs in nearly all patients. Fewer than 10% will have macroscopic hematuria. Patients should remain supine for 4–6 hours postbiopsy. A patient with a 6-hour postbiopsy hematocrit more than 3% lower than baseline should be closely monitored.

Percutaneous kidney biopsies are generally safe. One percent of patients will experience significant bleeding and 0.1–0.3% will require blood transfusions. More than half of patients will have at least a small hematoma. Risk of major bleeding persists up to 72 hours after the biopsy. Any type of anticoagulation therapy should be held for 5–7 days postbiopsy if possible. The risks of nephrectomy and mortality are about 0.06–0.08%. When a percutaneous needle biopsy is technically not feasible and renal tissue is deemed clinically essential, a closed renal biopsy via

interventional radiologic techniques or open renal biopsy under general anesthesia can be done.

Barnett AH et al: Diabetics Exposed to Telmisartan and Enalapril Study Group: Angiotensin-receptor blockade versus converting-enzyme inhibition in type 2 diabetes and nephropathy. N Engl J Med 2004;351:1952. [PMID: 15516696]

Carman TL et al: Noninvasive imaging of the renal arteries. Urol Clin North Am 2001;28:815. [PMID: 11791497]

Cohen RA et al: Clinical practice. Microscopic hematuria. N Engl J Med 2003;348:2330. [PMID: 12788998]

Johnson CA et al: Clinical practice guidelines for chronic kidney disease in adults: Part II. Glomerular filtration rate, proteinuria, and other markers. Am Fam Physician 2004;70:1091. [PMID: 15456118]

Manjunath G et al: Estimating the glomerular filtration rate. Postgrad Med 2001;110:55. [PMID: 11787409]

Whittier WL et al: Timing of complications in percutaneous renal biopsy. J Am Soc Nephrol 2004;15:142. [PMID: 14694166]

■ ACUTE RENAL FAILURE

ESSENTIALS OF DIAGNOSIS

- Sudden increase in BUN or serum creatinine.
- Oliguria often associated.
- Symptoms and signs depend on cause.

General Considerations

Five percent of hospital admissions and 30% of intensive care unit (ICU) admissions carry a diagnosis of acute renal failure, and it will develop in 25% of hospitalized patients. Acute renal failure is defined as a sudden decrease in renal function, resulting in an inability to maintain fluid and electrolyte balance and to excrete nitrogenous wastes. Serum creatinine is a convenient marker. In the absence of functioning kidneys, serum creatinine concentration will typically increase by 1–1.5 mg/dL daily—although with certain conditions, such as rhabdomyolysis, serum creatinine can increase more rapidly. Acute renal failure is now also being termed "acute kidney injury" since it may be a more appropriately descriptive term.

Clinical Findings

A. SYMPTOMS AND SIGNS

The uremic milieu of acute renal failure can cause nonspecific symptoms. When present, they are often due to azotemia or its underlying cause. Azotemia can cause nausea, vomiting, malaise, and altered sensorium. Hypertension is rare, but fluid homeostasis is often altered. Hypovolemia can cause prerenal disease, whereas hyper-

Table 22-4. Classification and differential diagnosis of acute renal failure.

	Prerenal Azotemia	Postrenal Azotemia	Intrinsic Renal Disease		
			Acute Tubular Necrosis (Oliguric or Polyuric)	Acute Glomerulonephritis	Acute Interstitial Nephritis
Etiology	Poor renal perfusion	Obstruction of the urinary tract	Ischemia, nephrotoxins	Poststreptococcal; collagen-vascular disease	Allergic reaction; drug reaction
Urinary indices Serum BUN:Cr ratio	> 20:1	> 20:1	< 20:1	> 20:1	< 20:1
U_{Na} (mEq/L)	< 20	Variable	> 20	< 20	Variable
FE_{Na} (%)	< 1	Variable	> 1	< 1	< 1; > 1
Urine osmolality (mosm/kg)	> 500	< 400	250–300	Variable	Variable
Urinary sediment	Benign or hyaline casts	Normal or red cells, white cells, or crystals	Granular (muddy brown) casts, renal tubular casts	Dysmorphic red cells and red cell casts	White cells, white cell casts, with or without eosinophils

BUN:Cr = blood urea nitrogen:creatinine ratio; U_{Na} = urinary concentration of sodium; FE_{Na} = fractional excretion of sodium.

volemia can result from intrinsic or postrenal disease. Pericardial effusions can occur with azotemia, and a pericardial friction rub can be present. Effusions may result in cardiac tamponade. Arrhythmias occur especially with hyperkalemia. The lung examination may show rales in the presence of hypervolemia. Acute renal failure can cause nonspecific diffuse abdominal pain and ileus as well as platelet dysfunction; thus, bleeding is more common in these patients. The neurologic examination reveals encephalopathic changes with asterixis and confusion; seizures may ensue.

B. LABORATORY FINDINGS

Elevated BUN and creatinine are present, though these elevations do not in themselves distinguish acute from chronic renal failure. Hyperkalemia often occurs from impaired renal potassium excretion. The ECG can reveal peaked T waves, PR prolongation, and QRS widening. A long QT segment can occur with hypocalcemia. Anion gap metabolic acidosis (due to decreased organic acid clearance) is often noted. Hyperphosphatemia occurs when phosphorus cannot be secreted by damaged tubules either with or without increased cell catabolism. Hypocalcemia with metastatic calcium phosphate deposition may be observed when the product of calcium and phosphorus exceeds 70 mg/dL. Anemia can occur as a result of decreased erythropoietin production over weeks, and associated platelet dysfunction is typical.

Classification & Etiology

Acute renal failure can be divided into three categories: prerenal azotemia, intrinsic renal disease, and post-renal azotemia. Identifying the cause is the first step toward treating the patient (Table 22–4).

A. PRERENAL AZOTEMIA

Prerenal azotemia is the most common cause of acute renal failure, accounting for 40–80% of cases, depending on the population studied. It is due to renal hypoperfusion. This is an appropriate physiologic change. If it can be immediately reversed with restoration of renal blood flow, renal parenchymal damage does not occur. If hypoperfusion persists, ischemia can result, causing intrinsic renal failure.

Decreased renal perfusion can occur in one of three ways: a decrease in intravascular volume, a change in vascular resistance, or low cardiac output. Causes of volume depletion include hemorrhage, gastrointestinal losses, dehydration, excessive diuresis, extravascular space sequestration, pancreatitis, burns, trauma, and peritonitis.

Changes in vascular resistance can occur systemically with sepsis, anaphylaxis, anesthesia, and afterload-reducing drugs. ACE inhibitors prevent efferent renal arteriolar constriction out of proportion to the afferent arteriole; thus, GFR will decrease. Nonsteroidal anti-inflammatory drugs (NSAIDs) prevent afferent arteriolar vasodilation by inhibiting prostaglandin-mediated signals. Thus, in cirrhosis and congestive heart failure, when prostaglandins are recruited to increase renal blood flow, NSAIDs will have particularly deleterious effects. Epinephrine, norepinephrine, high-dose dopamine, anesthetic agents, and cyclosporine also can cause renal vasoconstriction. Renal artery stenosis causes increased resistance and decreased perfusion.

Low cardiac output is a state of low effective renal arterial blood flow. This occurs in states of cardiogenic shock, congestive heart failure, pulmonary embolism, and pericardial tamponade. Arrhythmias and valvular disorders can also reduce cardiac output. In the ICU setting, positive pressure ventilation will decrease venous return, also decreasing cardiac output.

When GFR falls acutely, it is important to determine whether acute renal failure is due to prerenal or intrinsic renal causes. The history and physical examination are important, and urinalysis can be helpful. The BUN:creatinine ratio will typically exceed 20:1 due to increased urea reabsorption. In an oliguric patient, another useful index is the fractional excretion of sodium (FE_{Na}). With decreased GFR, the kidney will reabsorb salt and water avidly if there is no intrinsic tubular dysfunction. Thus, patients with prerenal failure should have a low fractional excretion percent of sodium (< 1%). The FE_{Na} is calculated as follows: FE_{Na} = clearance of Na^+/GFR = clearance of Na^+/creatinine clearance:

$$FE_{Na} = \frac{Urine_{sodium}/Plasma_{sodium}}{Urine_{creatinine}/Plasma_{creatinine}} \times 100\%$$

Oliguric states are more accurately assessed with this formula than nonoliguric states because the kidneys do not avidly reabsorb water and sodium in nonoliguric states. (Oliguria is defined as urinary output < 400–500 mL/d.) Diuretics can cause increased sodium excretion. Thus, if the FE_{Na} is high within 12–24 hours after diuretic administration, the cause of acute renal failure may not be accurately predicted. Acute renal failure due to glomerulonephritis can have a low FE_{Na} because sodium reabsorption and tubular function may not be compromised.

Treatment of prerenal azotemia depends entirely on its cause, but maintenance of euvolemia, attention to serum potassium, and avoidance of nephrotoxic drugs are the benchmarks of therapy. This involves careful assessment of volume status, drug usage, and cardiac function.

B. POSTRENAL AZOTEMIA

Postrenal azotemia is the least common cause of acute renal failure, accounting for approximately 5–10% of cases, but is important to detect because of its reversibility. It occurs when urinary flow from both kidneys, or a single functioning kidney, is obstructed. Each nephron has an elevated intraluminal pressure, causing a decrease in GFR.

Causes include urethral obstruction, bladder dysfunction or obstruction, and obstruction of both ureters or renal pelvises. In men, benign prostatic hyperplasia is the most common cause. Patients taking anticholinergic drugs are particularly at risk. Bladder, prostate, and cervical cancers as well as retroperitoneal processes and neurogenic bladder can also cause obstruction. Less common causes are blood clots, bilateral ureteral stones, urethral stones or stricture, and bilateral papillary necrosis. In patients with a single

functioning kidney, obstruction of a solitary ureter can cause postrenal azotemia.

Patients may be anuric or polyuric and may complain of lower abdominal pain. Obstruction can be constant or intermittent and partial or complete. On examination, the patient may have an enlarged prostate, distended bladder, or mass detected on pelvic examination.

Laboratory examination may initially reveal high urine osmolality, low urine sodium, high BUN:creatinine ratio, and low FE_{Na}. These indices are similar to a prerenal picture because extensive intrinsic renal damage has not occurred. After several days, the urine sodium increases as the kidneys fail and are unable to concentrate the urine—thus, isosthenuria is present. The urine sediment is generally benign.

Patients with acute renal failure and suspected postrenal azotemia should undergo bladder ultrasonography and bladder catheterization if hydroureter and hydronephrosis are present along with an enlarged bladder. These patients often undergo a postobstructive diuresis, and care should be taken to avoid dehydration. Rarely, obstruction is not diagnosed by ultrasonography. For example, patients with retroperitoneal fibrosis from tumor or radiation may not show dilation of the urinary tract. If suspicion does exist, a CT scan or MRI can establish the diagnosis. Prompt treatment of obstruction within days by catheters, stents, or other surgical procedures can result in complete reversal of the acute process.

C. INTRINSIC RENAL FAILURE

Intrinsic renal disorders account for up to 50% of all cases of acute renal failure. Intrinsic (or parenchymal) dysfunction is considered after prerenal and postrenal causes have been excluded. The sites of injury are the tubules, interstitium, vasculature, and glomeruli.

ACUTE TUBULAR NECROSIS

ESSENTIALS OF DIAGNOSIS

- *Acute renal insufficiency.*
- *Clinical scenario consistent with diagnosis (ischemic or toxic insult).*
- *Urine sediment with pigmented granular casts and renal tubular epithelial cells.*

General Considerations

Acute renal failure due to tubular damage is termed acute tubular necrosis and accounts for 85% of intrinsic acute renal failure. The two major causes of acute tubular necrosis are ischemia and toxin exposure. Ischemia causes tubular damage from states of low perfusion and is often preceded by a state of prerenal azotemia. Ischemic acute renal failure is characterized not only by inadequate GFR but also by renal blood flow inadequate to maintain parenchymal cellular formation. This occurs in the setting of prolonged hypotension or hypoxemia, such as dehydration, shock, and sepsis. Major surgical procedures can involve prolonged periods of hypoperfusion, which are exacerbated by vasodilating anesthetic agents.

The other major cause of acute tubular necrosis is nephrotoxin exposure. Exogenous nephrotoxins more commonly cause damage than endogenous nephrotoxins.

A. EXOGENOUS NEPHROTOXINS

Up to 25% of hospitalized patients receiving therapeutic levels of aminoglycosides sustain some degree of acute tubular necrosis. Nonoliguric renal failure typically occurs after 5–10 days of exposure. Predisposing factors include underlying renal damage, dehydration, and advanced age. Aminoglycosides can remain in renal tissues for up to a month, so renal function may not recover for some time after stopping the medication. Monitoring of peak and trough levels is important, but trough levels are more helpful in predicting renal toxicity. Gentamicin is as nephrotoxic as tobramycin; streptomycin is the least nephrotoxic of the aminoglycosides, likely due to the number of cationic amino side chains present on each molecule. Amphotericin B is typically nephrotoxic after a dose of 2–3 g. This causes severe vasoconstriction with distal tubular damage and can lead to distal renal tubular acidosis with hypokalemia and nephrogenic diabetes insipidus. Vancomycin, acyclovir, and several cephalosporins have been known to cause acute tubular necrosis.

Radiographic contrast media can be directly nephrotoxic. Contrast nephropathy is the third leading cause of new acute renal failure in hospitalized patients. It probably results from the synergistic combination of direct renal tubular epithelial cell toxicity and renal medullary ischemia. Predisposing factors include advanced age, preexisting renal disease (serum creatinine > 2 mg/dL), volume depletion, diabetic nephropathy, congestive heart failure, multiple myeloma, repeated doses of contrast, and recent exposure to other nephrotoxic agents, including NSAIDs and ACE inhibitors. The combination of diabetes mellitus and renal dysfunction poses the greatest risk (15–50%) for contrast nephropathy. Lower volumes of contrast with lower osmolality are recommended in high-risk patients. Toxicity usually occurs 24–48 hours after the radiocontrast study. Nonionic contrast media may be less toxic, but this has never been proved. Prevention should be the goal when using these agents. Patients should be hydrated with 1 L of 0.45% saline over 12 hours both before and after the contrast administration—cautiously in patients with preexisting cardiac dysfunction. Neither mannitol nor furosemide offers benefit over saline hydration. In fact, furosemide may lead to increased rates of renal dysfunction in this setting. In some but not all studies, N-acetylcysteine given before and after contrast decreased the incidence of dye-induced nephrotoxicity. Its benefit

seems more pronounced in subjects with a lower GFR. Acetylcysteine is a thiol-containing antioxidant with little toxicity whose mechanism of action is unclear. With little harm and possible benefit, administering acetylcysteine 600 mg orally every 12 hours twice, before and after a dye load, for patients at risk for acute renal failure, is a reasonable strategy. Investigators have shown a benefit using sodium bicarbonate rather than normal saline as the isotonic volume expander. Other nephrotoxic agents should be avoided during the day before and after dye administration.

Cyclosporine toxicity is usually dose dependent. It causes distal tubular dysfunction from severe vasoconstriction. Regular blood level monitoring is important to prevent nephrotoxicity. With patients who are taking cyclosporine for renal transplant rejection, kidney biopsy is often necessary to distinguish transplant rejection from cyclosporine toxicity. Renal function usually improves after reducing the dose or stopping the drug.

Other exogenous nephrotoxins include antineoplastics, such as cisplatin and organic solvents, and heavy metals such as mercury, cadmium, and arsenic.

B. ENDOGENOUS NEPHROTOXINS

Endogenous nephrotoxins include heme-containing products, uric acid, and paraproteins. Myoglobinuria as a consequence of rhabdomyolysis leads to acute tubular necrosis. Necrotic muscle releases large amounts of myoglobin, which is freely filtered across the glomerulus. The myoglobin is reabsorbed by the renal tubules, and direct damage can occur. Distal tubular obstruction from pigmented casts and intrarenal vasoconstriction can also cause damage. This type of renal failure occurs in the setting of crush injury, or muscle necrosis from prolonged unconsciousness, seizures, cocaine, and alcohol abuse. Dehydration and acidosis predispose to the development of myoglobinuric acute renal failure. Patients may complain of muscular pain and often have signs of muscle injury. Rhabdomyolysis of clinical importance commonly occurs with a serum creatine kinase (CK) greater than 20,000–50,000 IU/L. One study showed that 58% of patients with acute renal failure from rhabdomyolysis had CK levels greater than 16,000 IU/L. Only 11% of patients without renal failure had CK values greater than 16,000 IU/L. The globin moiety of myoglobin will cause the urine dipstick to read falsely positive for hemoglobin: the urine appears dark brown, but no red cells are present. With lysis of muscle cells, patients also become hyperkalemic, hyperphosphatemic, and hyperuricemic. The mainstay of treatment is hydration. Other adjunctive treatments include mannitol for free radical clearance and diuresis as well as alkalinization of the urine. These modalities have not been proved to change outcomes in human trials.

Hemoglobin can cause a similar form of acute renal tubular necrosis. Massive intravascular hemolysis is seen in transfusion reactions and in certain hemolytic anemias. Reversal of the underlying disorder and hydration are the mainstays of treatment.

Hyperuricemia can occur in the setting of rapid cell turnover and lysis. Chemotherapy for germ cell neoplasms and leukemia and lymphoma are the primary causes. Acute renal failure occurs with intratubular deposition of uric acid crystals; serum uric acid levels are often greater than 20 mg/dL and urine uric acid levels greater than 600 mg/24 h. A urine uric acid to urine creatinine ratio greater than 1.0 indicates risk of acute renal failure.

Bence Jones protein seen in conjunction with multiple myeloma can cause direct tubular toxicity and tubular obstruction. Other renal complications from multiple myeloma include hypercalcemia and proximal renal tubular acidosis.

Clinical Findings

A. Symptoms and Signs

See Acute Renal Failure.

B. Laboratory Findings

Urinalysis may show evidence of acute tubular damage. The urine may be brown. On microscopic examination, an active sediment may show pigmented granular casts or "muddy brown" casts. Renal tubular epithelial cells and epithelial cell casts are often present as well (see Table 22–1). Hyperkalemia and hyperphosphatemia are commonly encountered.

Treatment

Treatment is aimed at hastening recovery and avoiding complications. Preventive measures should be taken to avoid volume overload and hyperkalemia. Loop-blocking diuretics have been used in large doses (eg, furosemide in doses ranging from 20 mg to 160 mg orally or intravenously twice daily) to effect adequate diuresis and may help convert oliguric to nonoliguric renal failure. Such a conversion has never been shown to affect outcomes such as mortality, though. One recent retrospective study has shown potentially worse outcomes in patients who receive doses of furosemide, including nonrecovery of renal function and an increased risk of death. A more recent prospective randomized controlled trial has shown no difference between the administration of large doses of diuretics versus placebo on either recovery from acute renal failure or death. Widespread use of diuretics in critically ill patients with acute renal failure should be discouraged. Side effects of supranormal dosing include deafness. This is mainly due to peak furosemide levels and can be avoided by the use of a furosemide drip. A starting dose of 0.2–0.6 mg/kg/h is appropriate, increasing to a maximum of 1 mg/kg/h. A bolus of the hourly dose should be administered at the beginning of treatment. Intravenous thiazide diuretics can be used to augment urinary output; chlorothiazide, 500 mg intravenously every 8–12 hours, is a reasonable choice. Short-term effects also include activation of

the renin–angiotensin system. Nutritional support should maintain adequate intake while preventing excessive catabolism. Dietary protein restriction of 0.6 g/kg/d helps prevent metabolic acidosis. Hypocalcemia and hyperphosphatemia can be improved with diet and phosphate-binding agents, such as aluminum hydroxide (500 mg orally with meals) over the short term, calcium carbonate (500–1500 mg orally three times daily), calcium acetate (667 mg, two or three tablets, orally before meals), or sevelamer (800–1600 mg orally three times daily). Hypocalcemia should not be treated in patients with rhabdomyolysis unless they are symptomatic. Hypermagnesemia can occur because of reduced magnesium excretion by the renal tubules, so magnesium-containing antacids and laxatives should be avoided in these patients. Dosages must be adjusted according to the estimated degree of renal impairment for drugs eliminated by the kidney.

Indications for dialysis in acute renal failure from acute tubular necrosis or other intrinsic disorders are as follows: life-threatening electrolyte disturbances (such as hyperkalemia), volume overload unresponsive to diuresis, worsening acidosis, and uremic complications (eg, encephalopathy, pericarditis, and seizures). In gravely ill patients, less severe but worsening abnormalities may also be indications for dialytic support.

Course & Prognosis

The clinical course of acute tubular necrosis is often divided into three phases: initial injury, maintenance, and recovery. The maintenance phase is expressed as either oliguric (urinary output < 500 mL/d) or nonoliguric. Nonoliguric acute tubular necrosis has a better outcome. Conversion from oliguric to nonoliguric states may be attempted but has not been shown to change the prognosis. Drugs such as dopamine and diuretics are sometimes used for this purpose but have not been shown to improve outcomes. "Renal dose" dopamine (1–3 mcg/kg/min) can increase renal blood flow but can also potentiate arrhythmias and myocardial ischemia. In numerous studies, dopamine use in this setting has been shown to have no benefit. Average duration of the maintenance phase is 1–3 weeks but may be several months. Cellular repair and removal of tubular debris occur during this period. The recovery phase is heralded by diuresis. GFR begins to rise; BUN and serum creatinine fall. Other treatments for acute tubular necrosis, such as atrial natriuretic peptide use, have not proven beneficial. Ongoing randomized controlled studies are looking at the usefulness of intensive versus conventional renal replacement therapy for a survival benefit.

The mortality rate from acute renal failure is 20–50% in medical illness and up to 70% in a surgical setting. Increased mortality is associated with advanced age, severe underlying disease, and multisystem organ failure. Leading causes of death are infections, fluid and electrolyte disturbances, and worsening of underlying disease. Mortality rates have not changed significantly over 20 years, making prevention of acute renal failure a high priority.

INTERSTITIAL NEPHRITIS

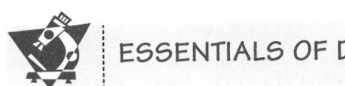 ESSENTIALS OF DIAGNOSIS

- Fever.
- Transient maculopapular rash.
- Acute renal insufficiency.
- Pyuria (including eosinophiluria), white blood cell casts, and hematuria.

General Considerations

Acute interstitial nephritis accounts for 10–15% of cases of intrinsic renal failure. An interstitial inflammatory response with edema and possible tubular cell damage is the typical pathologic finding. Cell-mediated immune reactions prevail over humoral responses. T lymphocytes can cause direct cytotoxicity or release lymphokines that recruit monocytes and inflammatory cells.

Although drugs account for over 70% of cases, acute interstitial nephritis also occurs in infectious diseases, immunologic disorders, or as an idiopathic condition. The most common drugs are penicillins and cephalosporins, sulfonamides and sulfonamide-containing diuretics, NSAIDs, rifampin, phenytoin, and allopurinol. Infectious causes include streptococcal infections, leptospirosis, cytomegalovirus, histoplasmosis, and Rocky Mountain spotted fever. Immunologic entities are more commonly associated with glomerulonephritis, but systemic lupus erythematosus, Sjögren's syndrome, sarcoidosis, and cryoglobulinemia can cause interstitial nephritis.

Clinical Findings

Clinical features can include fever (> 80%), rash (25–50%), arthralgias, and peripheral blood eosinophilia (80%). The urine often contains red cells (95%), white cells, and white cell casts. Proteinuria can be a feature, particularly in NSAID-induced interstitial nephritis, but is usually modest. Eosinophiluria can be detected by Wright's or Hansel's stain.

Treatment & Prognosis

Acute interstitial nephritis often carries a good prognosis. Recovery occurs over weeks to months, but acute dialytic therapy may be necessary in up to one-third of all patients before resolution. Patients rarely progress to ESRD. Those with prolonged courses of oliguric failure and advanced age have a worse prognosis. Treatment consists of supportive measures and re-moval of the inciting agent. If renal failure persists after these steps, a short course of corticosteroids can be given. Short-term, high-dose methylprednisolone (0.5–1 g/d for 1–4 days) or prednisone (60 mg/d for 1–2 weeks) followed by a prednisone taper can be used in these more severe cases of drug-induced interstitial nephritis.

GLOMERULONEPHRITIS

 ESSENTIALS OF DIAGNOSIS

- Hematuria, dysmorphic red cells, red cell casts, and mild proteinuria.
- Dependent edema and hypertension.
- Acute renal insufficiency.

General Considerations

Acute glomerulonephritis is a relatively uncommon cause of acute renal failure, accounting for about 5% of cases of intrinsic renal failure. Pathologically, inflammatory glomerular lesions are seen. These include mesangioproliferative, focal and diffuse proliferative, and crescentic lesions. The larger the percentage of glomeruli involved and the more severe the lesion, the more likely it is that the patient will have a poor clinical outcome.

Categorization of acute glomerulonephritis can be done by serologic analysis. Markers include antineutrophil cytoplasmic antibodies (ANCA), anti-GBM antibodies, and other immune markers of disease.

Immune complex deposition usually occurs when moderate antigen excess over antibody production occurs. Complexes formed with marked antigen excess tend to remain in the circulation. Antibody excess with large antigen–antibody aggregates usually results in phagocytosis and clearance of the precipitates by the mononuclear phagocytic system in the liver and spleen. Causes include IgA nephropathy (Berger's disease), peri-infectious or postinfectious glomerulonephritis, endocarditis, lupus nephritis, cryoglobulinemic glomerulonephritis (often associated with hepatitis C virus), and membranoproliferative glomerulonephritis.

Anti-GBM–associated acute glomerulonephritis is either confined to the kidney or associated with pulmonary hemorrhage. The latter is termed "Goodpasture's syndrome." Injury is related to autoantibodies aimed against type IV collagen in the GBM rather than to immune complex deposition.

Pauci-immune acute glomerulonephritis is a form of small-vessel vasculitis associated with ANCA, causing primary and secondary renal diseases that do not have direct immune complex deposition or antibody binding. Tissue injury is believed to be due to cell-mediated immune processes. An example is Wegener's granulomatosis, a systemic necrotizing vasculitis of small arteries and veins associated with intravascular and extravascular granuloma formation. In addition to glomerulonephritis, these patients can have upper airway, pulmonary, and skin manifestations of disease. Cytoplasmic ANCA (C-ANCA) is both specific (88%) and sensitive (95%) for this entity. Microscopic polyangiitis is another pauci-immune vasculitis causing acute glomerulonephritis. Perinuclear staining (P-ANCA) is the common pattern. ANCA-associated and anti-GBM-associated acute glomerulonephritis can evolve to crescentic glomerulonephritis and often have poor outcomes unless treatment is started early. Both are described more fully below.

Other vascular causes of acute glomerulonephritis include malignant hypertension and the thrombotic microangiopathies such as hemolytic-uremic syndrome (see Chapter 11) and thrombotic thrombocytopenic purpura (see Chapter 13).

Clinical Findings

A. SYMPTOMS AND SIGNS

Patients with acute glomerulonephritis are often hypertensive and edematous, and have an abnormal urinary sediment. The edema is found first in body parts with low tissue tension, such as the periorbital and scrotal regions.

B. LABORATORY FINDINGS

Dipstick and microscopic evaluation will reveal evidence of hematuria, moderate proteinuria (usually < 2 g/d), and cellular elements such as red cells, red cell casts, and white cells. Red cell casts are specific for glomerulonephritis, and a detailed search is warranted. Twenty-four hour urine for protein excretion and creatinine clearance quantifies the amount of proteinuria and documents the degree of renal dysfunction. However, in cases of rapidly changing serum creatinine values, the urinary creatinine clearance is an unreliable marker of GFR. FE_{Na} is usually low unless renal dysfunction is marked.

Further tests include complement levels (C3, C4, CH50), ASO titer, anti-GBM antibody levels, ANCAs, antinuclear antibody titers, cryoglobulins, hepatitis serologies, blood cultures, renal ultrasound, and occasionally renal biopsy.

Treatment

Depending on the nature and severity of disease, treatment can consist of high-dose corticosteroids and cytotoxic agents such as cyclophosphamide. Plasma exchange can be used in Goodpasture's disease as a temporizing measure until chemotherapy can take effect. Treatment and prognosis for specific diseases are discussed more fully below.

Albright RC Jr: Acute renal failure: a practical update. Mayo Clin Proc 2001;76:67. [PMID: 11155415]

Briguori C et al: Contrast agent-associated nephrotoxicity. Prog Cardiovasc Dis 2003;45:493. [PMID: 12800130]

Cantarovich F et al: High-dose furosemide for established ARF: a prospective, randomized, double-blind, placebo-controlled, multicenter trial. Am J Kidn Dis 2004;44:402. [PMID: 15332212]

Edwards BF: Postoperative renal insufficiency. Med Clin North Am 2001;85:1241. [PMID: 11565497]

Esson ML et al: Diagnosis and treatment of acute tubular necrosis. Ann Intern Med 2002;137:744. [PMID: 12416948]

Kodner CM et al: Diagnosis and management of acute interstitial nephritis. Am Fam Physician 2003;67:2527. [PMID: 12825841]

Malinoski DJ et al: Crush injury and rhabdomyolysis. Crit Care Clin 2004;20:171. [PMID: 14979336]

Mehta R et al: Diuretics, mortality, and nonrecovery of renal function in acute renal failure. JAMA 2002;288:2547. [PMID: 12444861]

Merten GJ et al: Prevention of contrast-induced nephropathy with sodium bicarbonate: a randomized controlled trial. JAMA 2004;291:2328. [PMID: 15150204]

Parmet S et al: JAMA patient page. Acute renal failure. JAMA 2002;288:2634. [PMID: 12444873]

Perazella MA: Drug-induced renal failure: update on new medications and unique mechanisms of nephrotoxicity. Am J Med Sci 2003;325:349. [PMID: 12811231]

Sauret JM et al: Rhabdomyolysis. Am Fam Physician 2002;65:907. [PMID: 11898964]

Singri N et al: Acute renal failure. JAMA 2003;289:747. [PMID: 12585954]

Vinen CS et al: Acute glomerulonephritis. Postgrad Med J 2003;79:206. [PMID: 12743337]

Warnock DG: Towards a definition and classification of acute kidney injury. J Am Soc Nephrol 2005;16:3149. [PMID: 16207828]

■ CHRONIC KIDNEY DISEASE

ESSENTIALS OF DIAGNOSIS

- *Progressive azotemia over months to years.*
- *Symptoms and signs of uremia when nearing end-stage disease.*
- *Hypertension in the majority.*
- *Isosthenuria and broad casts in urinary sediment are common.*
- *Bilateral small kidneys on ultrasound are diagnostic.*

General Considerations

Chronic kidney disease affects up to 20 million Americans, or one in nine adults. Most are unaware of the condition because they remain asymptomatic until the disease has significantly progressed. The National Kid-

Table 22–5. Stages of chronic kidney disease: a clinical action plan.[1,2]

Stage	Description	GFR (mL/min/ 1.73 m^2)	Action[3]
1	Kidney damage with normal or ↑ GFR	≥ 90	Diagnosis and treatment. Treatment of comorbid conditions. Slowing of progression. Cardiovascular disease risk reduction.
2	Kidney damage with mildly ↓	60–89	Estimating progression.
3	Moderately ↓	30–59	Evaluating and treating complications.
4	Severely ↓	15–29	Preparation for kidney replacement therapy.
5	Kidney failure	< 15 (or dialysis)	Replacement (if uremia is present).

[1]From National Kidney Foundation, KDOQI, chronic kidney disease guidelines.
[2]Chronic kidney disease is defined as either kidney damage or GFR < 60 mL/min/1.73 m^2 for 3 or more months. Kidney damage is defined as pathologic abnormalities or markers of damage, including abnormalities in blood or urine tests or imaging studies.
[3]Includes actions from preceding stages.
GFR = glomerular filtration rate.

ney Foundation has developed a new staging system that helps clinicians formulate practice plans (Table 22–5). Over 70% of cases of late-stage chronic kidney disease are due to diabetes mellitus or hypertension. Glomerulonephritis, cystic diseases, and other urologic diseases account for another 12%, and 15% of patients have other or unknown causes. The major causes of chronic renal failure are listed in Table 22–6.

Chronic kidney disease is rarely reversible and leads to a progressive decline in renal function. This occurs even after an inciting event has been removed. Reduction in renal mass leads to hypertrophy of the remaining nephrons with hyperfiltration, and the GFR in these nephrons is transiently at supranormal levels. These adaptations place a burden on the remaining nephrons and lead to progressive glomerular sclerosis and interstitial fibrosis, suggesting that hyperfiltration may worsen renal function. However, decreased renal mass in kidney donors is not associated with chronic renal failure.

Clinical Findings

A. SYMPTOMS AND SIGNS

The symptoms of chronic kidney disease often develop slowly and are nonspecific (Table 22–7). Individuals can remain asymptomatic until renal failure is far advanced (GFR < 10–15 mL/min). Manifestations include fatigue, weakness, and malaise. Gastrointestinal complaints, such as anorexia, nausea, vomiting, a metallic taste in the mouth, and hiccups, are common. Neurologic problems include irritability, difficulty in concentrating, insomnia, subtle memory defects, restless legs, and twitching. Pruritus is common and difficult to treat. As uremia progresses, decreased libido, menstrual irregularities, chest pain from pericarditis, and paresthesias can develop. Symptoms of drug toxicity—especially for drugs eliminated by the kidney—increase as renal clearance worsens.

On physical examination, the patient appears chronically ill. Hypertension is common. The skin may be yellow, with signs of easy bruisability. Rarely seen in the dialysis era is uremic frost, a cutaneous re-

Table 22–6. Major causes of chronic renal failure.

Glomerulopathies
  Primary glomerular diseases:
    1. Focal and segmental glomerulosclerosis
    2. Membranoproliferative glomerulonephritis
    3. IgA nephropathy
    4. Membranous nephropathy
  Secondary glomerular diseases:
    1. Diabetic nephropathy
    2. Amyloidosis
    3. Postinfectious glomerulonephritis
    4. HIV-associated nephropathy
    5. Collagen-vascular diseases
    6. Sickle cell nephropathy
    7. HIV-associated membranoproliferative glomerulonephritis
Tubulointerstitial nephritis
  Drug hypersensitivity
  Heavy metals
  Analgesic nephropathy
  Reflux/chronic pyelonephritis
  Idiopathic
Hereditary diseases
  Polycystic kidney disease
  Medullary cystic disease
  Alport's syndrome
Obstructive nephropathies
  Prostatic disease
  Nephrolithiasis
  Retroperitoneal fibrosis/tumor
  Congenital
Vascular diseases
  Hypertensive nephrosclerosis
  Renal artery stenosis

Table 22–7. Symptoms and signs of uremia.

Organ System	Symptoms	Signs
General	Fatigue, weakness	Sallow-appearing, chronically ill
Skin	Pruritus, easy bruisability	Pallor, ecchymoses, excoriations, edema, xerosis
ENT	Metallic taste in mouth, epistaxis	Urinous breath
Eye		Pale conjunctiva
Pulmonary	Shortness of breath	Rales, pleural effusion
Cardiovascular	Dyspnea on exertion, retrosternal pain on inspiration (pericarditis)	Hypertension, cardiomegaly, friction rub
Gastrointestinal	Anorexia, nausea, vomiting, hiccups	
Genitourinary	Nocturia, impotence	Isosthenuria
Neuromuscular	Restless legs, numbness and cramps in legs	
Neurologic	Generalized irritability and inability to concentrate, decreased libido	Stupor, asterixis, myoclonus, peripheral neuropathy

flection of ESRD. Uremic fetor is the characteristic fishy odor of the breath. Cardiopulmonary signs may include rales, cardiomegaly, edema, and a pericardial friction rub. Mental status can vary from decreased concentration to confusion, stupor, and coma. Myoclonus and asterixis are additional signs of uremic effects on the central nervous system.

The term "uremia" is used for this clinical syndrome, but the exact cause remains unknown. BUN and serum creatinine are considered markers for unknown toxins, with parathyroid hormone (PTH) believed to be one such toxin.

In any patient with renal failure, it is important to identify and correct all possibly reversible causes. Urinary tract infections, obstruction, extracellular fluid volume depletion, nephrotoxins, hypertension, and congestive heart failure should be excluded (Table 22–8). Any of the above can worsen underlying chronic renal failure.

B. LABORATORY FINDINGS

The diagnosis of renal failure is made by documenting elevations of the BUN and serum creatinine concentrations. Further evaluation is needed to differentiate between acute and chronic renal failure. Evidence of previously elevated BUN and creatinine, abnormal prior urinalyses, and stable but abnormal serum creatinine on successive days is most consistent with a chronic process. It is helpful to plot the inverse of serum creatinine ($1/S_{Cr}$) versus time if three or more prior measurements are available; this estimates time to ESRD (Figure 22–1). If the slope of the line acutely declines, new causes of renal failure should be excluded as outlined above. Anemia, metabolic acidosis, hyperphosphatemia, hypocalcemia, and hyperkalemia can occur with both acute and chronic renal failure. The urinalysis shows isosthenuria if tubular concentrating and diluting ability are impaired. The urinary sediment can show broad waxy casts as a result of dilated, hypertrophic nephrons.

C. IMAGING

The finding of small echogenic kidneys bilaterally (< 10 cm) by ultrasonography supports a diagnosis of chronic renal failure, though normal or even large kidneys can be seen with chronic renal failure caused by adult polycystic kidney disease, diabetic nephropathy, HIV-associated nephropathy, multiple myeloma, amyloidosis, and obstructive uropathy. Radiologic evidence of renal osteodystrophy is another helpful finding, since x-ray changes of secondary hyperparathyroidism do not appear unless parathyroid levels have been elevated for at least 1 year. Evidence of subperiosteal reabsorption along the radial sides of the digital bones of the hand confirms hyperparathyroidism.

Complications

A. HYPERKALEMIA

Potassium balance generally remains intact in chronic renal failure until the GFR is less than 10–20 mL/min.

Table 22–8. Reversible causes of renal failure.

Reversible Factors	Diagnostic Clues
Infection	Urine culture and sensitivity tests
Obstruction	Bladder catheterization, then renal ultrasound
Extracellular fluid volume depletion	Orthostatic blood pressure and pulse: ↓ blood pressure and ↑ pulse upon sitting up from a supine position
Hypokalemia, hypercalcemia, and hyperuricemia (usually > 15 mg/dL)	Serum electrolytes, calcium, phosphate, uric acid
Nephrotoxic agents	Drug history
Hypertension	Blood pressure, chest x-ray
Congestive heart failure	Physical examination, chest x-ray

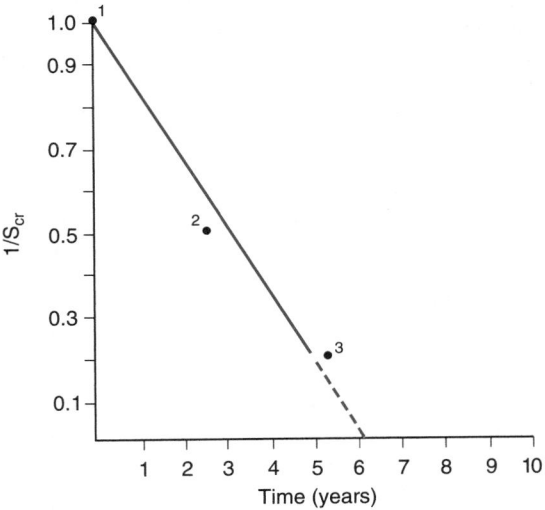

Figure 22–1. Decline in renal function plotted against time to end-stage renal disease (ESRD). The solid line indicates the linear decline in renal function over time. The dotted line indicates the approximate time to ESRD.

[1] Value of serum creatinine level = 1.0 mg/dL
[2] Value of serum creatinine level = 2.0 mg/dL
[3] Value of serum creatinine level = 5.0 mg/dL

However, certain states pose an increased risk of hyperkalemia at higher GFRs. Endogenous causes include any type of cellular destruction such as hemolysis and trauma, hyporeninemic hypoaldosteronism (type IV renal tubular acidosis, seen particularly in diabetes mellitus), and acidemic states (0.6 mEq/L elevation in K^+ for each 0.1 unit decrease in pH). Exogenous causes include diet (eg, citrus fruits and salt substitutes containing potassium) and drugs that decrease K^+ secretion (amiloride, triamterene, spironolactone, NSAIDs, ACE inhibitors) or block cellular uptake (β-blockers).

Treatment of acute hyperkalemia involves cardiac monitoring, intravenous calcium chloride or gluconate, insulin administration with glucose, bicarbonate, and an orally or rectally administered ion exchange resin (sodium polystyrene sulfonate). The resin exchanges sodium for potassium and can administer a significant sodium load to a patient. β-Agonists, such as albuterol, may also be used in acute cases. Chronic hyperkalemia is best treated with dietary potassium restriction (2 g/d) and sodium polystyrene sulfonate when necessary. The usual dose is 15–30 g once a day in juice or sorbitol.

B. ACID–BASE DISORDERS

Damaged kidneys are unable to excrete the 1 mEq/kg/d of acid generated by metabolism of dietary proteins. The resultant metabolic acidosis is primarily due to loss of renal mass. This limits production of ammonia (NH_3) and limits buffering of H^+ in the urine. (Other causes include decreased filtration of titratable acids such as sulfates and phosphates, decreased proximal tubular bicarbonate resorption, and decreased renal tubular hydrogen ion secretion.) Although patients with chronic renal failure are in positive hydrogen ion balance, the arterial blood pH is maintained at 7.33–7.37 and serum bicarbonate concentration rarely falls below 15 mEq/L. The excess hydrogen ions are buffered by the large calcium carbonate and calcium phosphate stores in bone. This contributes to the renal osteodystrophy of chronic renal failure described below.

The serum bicarbonate level should be maintained at greater than 21 mEq/L according to recently published national guidelines. Alkali supplements include sodium bicarbonate, calcium bicarbonate, and sodium citrate. Citrate salts increase the absorption of dietary aluminum and should be avoided in patients exposed to aluminum. Administration should begin with 20–30 mmol/d of alkali divided into two doses per day and titrated as needed.

C. CARDIOVASCULAR COMPLICATIONS

Long-term complications of chronic kidney disease include a high risk of morbidity and mortality of cardiovascular disease in comparison to the general population. Mortality due to a cardiovascular cause accounts for 45% of all deaths of patients receiving dialysis. The precise biologic mechanisms for this are unclear but may have to do with the uremic milieu, underlying coexistent comorbidities, and a hesitancy to perform investigative procedures in patients with chronic kidney disease.

1. Hypertension—As renal failure progresses, hypertension due to salt and water retention usually develops. Hyperreninemic states and exogenous erythropoietin administration can also exacerbate hypertension. Hypertension is the most common complication of ESRD and must be meticulously controlled. Failure to do so can accelerate the progression of renal damage.

Control of hypertension can be achieved with salt and water restriction, weight loss if indicated, and pharmacologic therapy. The ability of the kidney to adjust to variations in sodium and water intake becomes limited as renal failure progresses. An elevated sodium chloride intake leads to congestive heart failure, edema, and hypertension, whereas low salt intake leads to volume contraction and hypotension. A mildly decreased salt diet (4 g/d) can be started, and salt intake should be reduced to 2 g/d if hypertension persists. Initial drug therapy can include ACE inhibitors or angiotensin II receptor blockers (if serum potassium and GFR permit), calcium channel-blocking agents, diuretics, and β-blocking agents. The adjunctive drugs that are often needed (eg, clonidine, hydralazine, minoxidil) reflect the difficulty of achieving and maintaining hypertensive control in these patients. Goal blood pressure for patients with chronic kidney disease is less than 130/80 mm Hg.

2. Pericarditis—With uremia, pericarditis may develop. The cause is believed to be retention of metabolic toxins. Symptoms include chest pain and fever. Pulsus paradoxus can be present. A friction rub may be auscultated, but the lack of a rub does not rule out a significant pericardial effusion. Chest radiography will show an enlarged cardiac silhouette, and an ECG will show characteristic findings as explained in Chapter 10. Cardiac tamponade can occur; these patients have signs of poor cardiac output, with jugular venous distention and lungs clear to auscultation. Pericarditis is an absolute indication for initiation of hemodialysis.

3. Congestive heart failure—Patients with ESRD tend toward a high cardiac output. They often have extracellular fluid overload, shunting of blood through an arteriovenous fistula for dialysis, and anemia. In addition to hypertension, these abnormalities cause increased myocardial work and oxygen demand. Patients with chronic kidney disease may also have accelerated rates of atherosclerosis. All of these factors contribute to left ventricular hypertrophy and dilation, present in 75% of patients starting dialysis. PTH may also play a role in the pathogenesis of the cardiomyopathy of renal failure.

Water and salt intake should be controlled in patients who are oliguric or anuric. Diuretics are of value, though certain thiazides are ineffective when the GFR is less than 10–15 mL/min. Loop diuretics are commonly used, and higher doses are required as renal function declines. Digoxin should be used with caution since it is excreted by the kidney. The proved efficacy of ACE inhibitors in congestive heart failure holds true for patients with chronic renal failure. Despite the risks of hyperkalemia and worsening renal function, ACE inhibitors can be used for patients with a serum creatinine greater than 3 mg/dL with close supervision. Along with angiotensin II receptor blockers, ACE inhibitors have been shown to slow the progression to ESRD, even for patients with advanced chronic kidney disease. (See above section regarding treatment of proteinuria.) Once a patient is receiving dialysis, these risks become less relevant. When an ACE inhibitor or ARB drug is initiated, patients should have serum creatinine and potassium checked within 5–14 days.

D. HEMATOLOGIC COMPLICATIONS

1. Anemia—The anemia of chronic renal failure is characteristically normochromic and normocytic. It is due primarily to decreased erythropoietin production, which becomes clinically significant when GFR falls below 20–25 mL/min. Many patients are iron deficient as well. Low-grade hemolysis and blood loss from platelet dysfunction or hemodialysis play an additional role.

Recombinant erythropoietin (epoetin alfa) is used in patients whose hematocrits are less than 33%. The effective dose can vary; the starting dose is 50 units/kg (3000–4000 units/dose) once or twice a week. It can be given intravenously (eg, in the hemodialysis patient) or subcutaneously (eg, in any predialysis or dialysis patient). Subcutaneous administration is preferable to intravenous administration because it requires a 33% lower dose for the same effect. Recombinant darbepoietin is also now available. Its administration is less frequent, and intravenous and subcutaneous doses have equivalent effects. Iron stores must be adequate to ensure response. Hemodialysis patients typically require 50–200 mg intravenous iron each month due to expected blood loss at dialysis. Other patients with serum ferritin less than 100 ng/mL or iron saturation less than 20% should also receive iron supplementation. Depending on the clinical situation, iron therapy should be withheld if the serum ferritin is greater than 800 ng/mL. Oral therapy with ferrous sulfate, 325 mg once daily to three times daily, is adequate but not always well tolerated, and gut absorption of iron is impaired in uremic patients. Ferrous fumarate is the best-accepted formulation, and intravenous iron may be used in dialysis patients. Hypertension is a complication of epoetin alfa therapy in about 20% of patients. It develops more abruptly in the patients with the lowest hematocrit values at initiation of therapy, and in those with the greatest rate of rise in hemoglobin. The dosage may require adjustment, or antihypertensive drugs may need to given. Hemoglobin levels should rise no more than 1 g/dL every 3–4 weeks.

2. Coagulopathy—The coagulopathy of chronic kidney disease is mainly caused by platelet dysfunction. Platelet counts are only mildly decreased, but the bleeding time is prolonged. Platelets show abnormal adhesiveness and aggregation. Clinically, patients can have petechiae, purpura, and an increased tendency for bleeding during surgery.

Treatment is required only in patients who are symptomatic. Raising the hematocrit to 30% can reduce bleeding time in many patients. Desmopressin (25 mcg intravenously every 8–12 hours for two doses) is effective and often used in preparation for surgery. It causes release of factor VIII bound to von Willebrand's factor from endothelial cells. Conjugated estrogens, 0.6 mg/kg diluted in 50 mL of 0.9% sodium chloride infused over 30–40 minutes daily, or 2.5–5 mg orally for 5–7 days, have an effect for several weeks. Dialysis improves the bleeding time but does not normalize it. Peritoneal dialysis is preferable to hemodialysis because the latter requires heparin to prevent clotting in the dialyzer. Cryoprecipitate (10–15 bags) is rarely used and lasts less than 24 hours.

E. NEUROLOGIC COMPLICATIONS

Uremic encephalopathy does not occur until GFR falls below 10–15 mL/min. Encephalopathy may be due to tertiary hyperparathyroidism, where an elevated PTH level or, rarely, hypercalcemia, can be the culprit. PTH may be one of the uremic toxins. Symptoms begin with difficulty in concentrating and can progress to lethargy, confusion, and coma. Physical findings include nystagmus, weakness, asterixis, and hyperreflexia. These symptoms and signs may improve after initiation of dialysis.

Neuropathy is found in 65% of patients who receive dialysis or who will need it soon but not until GFR is 10% of normal. Peripheral neuropathies manifest themselves as sensorimotor polyneuropathies (stocking and glove distribution) and isolated or multiple isolated mononeuropathies. Patients can have restless legs, loss of deep tendon reflexes, and distal pain. The earlier initiation of dialysis may prevent peripheral neuropathies, and the response to dialysis is variable. Other neuropathies result in impotence and autonomic dysfunction.

F. DISORDERS OF MINERAL METABOLISM

The disorders of calcium, phosphorus, and bone are referred to as renal osteodystrophy. The most common disorder is osteitis fibrosa cystica—the bony changes of secondary hyperparathyroidism. This affects ~ 50% of patients nearing ESRD. As GFR decreases below 25% of normal, phosphorus excretion is impaired. Hyperphosphatemia leads to hypocalcemia, stimulating secretion of PTH, which has a phosphaturic effect and normalizes serum phosphorus. This continuous process leads to markedly elevated PTH levels and high bone turnover with osteoclastic bone resorption and subperiosteal lesions. Metastatic calcifications, such as tumoral calcinosis, can occur. Radiographically, lesions are most prominent in the phalanges and lateral ends of the clavicles.

Osteomalacia is a form of renal osteodystrophy with low bone turnover (affecting ~ 10% of patients nearing ESRD). With worsening renal function, there is decreased renal conversion of 25-hydroxycholecalciferol to the 1,25-dihydroxy form. Gut absorption of calcium is diminished, leading to hypocalcemia and abnormal bone mineralization. Deposition of aluminum in bone can also lead to osteomalacia. Elevated aluminum levels are seen in patients after years of chronic aluminum hydroxide administration for phosphorus binding. This entity is seen with decreasing frequency because aluminum-based binders are used less in the chronic setting and water used for hemodialysis is now cleared of aluminum.

Adynamic bone disease is a disorder of low bone turnover. More than 25% of patients nearing ESRD show evidence of minimal osteoid and decreased or absent bone remodeling. Its frequency is increasing because of increased use of active vitamin D analogs, which suppress PTH production.

All of the above entities can cause bony pain and proximal muscle weakness. Spontaneous bone fractures can occur that are slow to heal. When the calcium-phosphorus product (serum calcium [mg/dL] × serum phosphate [mg/dL]) is above 60–70, metastatic calcifications are commonly seen in blood vessels, soft tissues, lungs, and myocardium. Treatment should begin with dietary phosphorus restriction to 1000 mg/d. Oral phosphorus-binding agents, such as calcium carbonate or calcium acetate, act in the gut and are given in divided doses three or four times daily with meals. These should be titrated to a serum calcium of less than 10 mg/dL (preventing hypercalcemia) and serum phosphorus of 2.7–4.6 mg/dL in patients with a GFR of 15–59 mL/min/1.73 m^2 and serum phosphorus of 3.5–5.5 mg/dL in patients with a GFR of less than 15 mL/min/1.73 m^2. Sevelemer and lanthanum carbonate are other phosphorus-binding agents that do not contain calcium; they are particularly useful in patients with hypercalcemia, although long-term effects are unknown. Aluminum hydroxide is an effective phosphorus binder but can cause osteomalacia and neurologic complications. It can be used in the acute setting for serum phosphorus greater than 7 mg/dL, but long-term use should be avoided. If aluminum levels are high, chelation with deferoxamine can be effective. Vitamin D or vitamin D analogs should be given with secondary hyperparathyroidism (iPTH more than two to three times normal) if phosphorus levels are less than 5.5 mg/dL and calcium less than 10 mg/dL. Vitamin D suppresses PTH and increases serum calcium and phosphorus levels; both need to be monitored closely to prevent hypercalcemia and hyperphosphatemia. If calcitriol is used, the dosage should be 0.25–0.5 mcg daily or every other day initially. Cinacalcet can be used if elevated serum phosphorus or calcium levels prohibit the use of vitamin D analogs. Cinacalcet is a calcimimetic agent that targets the calcium-sensing receptor on the chief cells of the parathyroid gland.

G. ENDOCRINE DISORDERS

Circulating insulin levels are higher because of decreased renal insulin clearance. Glucose intolerance can occur in chronic renal failure when GFR is less than 10–20 mL/min. Primarily, this is due to peripheral insulin resistance. Fasting glucose levels are usually normal or only slightly elevated. Therefore, patients can be either hyperglycemic or hypoglycemic depending on the predominant disturbance. Most commonly, diabetic patients require decreased doses of hypoglycemic agents.

Decreased libido and impotence are common in chronic renal failure. Men have decreased testosterone levels; women are often anovulatory. Despite a high degree of infertility, pregnancy can occur—particularly in women who are well dialyzed and well nourished. Therefore, contraception is advisable for women who wish to become pregnant.

Treatment

A. DIETARY MANAGEMENT

Every patient with chronic renal failure should be evaluated by a renal nutritionist. Specific recommendations should be made concerning protein, salt, water, potassium, and phosphorus intake.

1. Protein restriction—Experimental models have shown that protein restriction slows the progression to ESRD; however, this has not been consistently proved in clinical trials. The MDRD Study was meant to clarify the issue, but the results were inconclusive. A subsequent meta-analysis of five clinical trials did show a significant benefit but did not control for certain effects such as ACE inhibitor therapy. The benefits of protein restriction in slowing the rate of decline of GFR must be weighed against the risk of cachexia upon the institution of dialysis. Low serum albumin at the start of dialysis is one of the strongest predictors of mortality in this population. In general, protein intake should not exceed 1 g/kg/d, and if protein restriction proves to be beneficial, the level of restriction may be increased to 0.6–0.8 g/kg/d.

2. Salt and water restriction—In advanced renal failure, the kidney is unable to adapt to large changes in sodium intake. Intake greater than 3–4 g/d can lead to edema, hypertension, and congestive heart failure, whereas intake of less than 1 g/d can lead to volume depletion and hypotension. For the nondialysis patient approaching ESRD, 2 g/d of sodium is an initial recommendation. A daily intake of 1–2 L of fluid maintains water balance.

3. Potassium restriction—Restriction is needed once the GFR has fallen below 10–20 mL/min. Patients should receive detailed lists concerning potassium content of foods and should limit their intake to less than 60–70 mEq/d. Normal intake is about 100 mEq/d.

4. Phosphorus restriction—The phosphorus level should be kept below 4.6 mg/dL, with a dietary restriction of 800–1000 mg/d. Foods rich in phosphorus such as cola beverages, eggs, dairy products, and meat should be limited. Below a GFR of 20–30 mL/min, phosphorus binders are usually required. The treatment of hyperphosphatemia is discussed in the section on disorders of mineral metabolism.

5. Magnesium restriction—Magnesium is excreted primarily by the kidneys. Dangerous hypermagnesemia is rare unless the patient ingests medications high in magnesium or receives it parenterally. All magnesium-containing laxatives and antacids are relatively contraindicated in renal failure.

B. Dialysis

When conservative management of ESRD is inadequate, hemodialysis, peritoneal dialysis, and kidney transplantation are alternatives (see below). According to the Kidney Disease Outcomes Quality Initiative (KDOQI) guidelines, dialysis should be started when a patient has a GFR of 10 mL/min or serum creatinine of 8 mg/dL. Diabetic patient should start when the GFR reaches 15 mL/min or serum creatinine is 6 mg/dL. Other indications for dialysis include (1) uremic symptoms, such as pericarditis, encephalopathy, or coagulopathy; (2) fluid overload unresponsive to diuresis; (3) refractory hyperkalemia; (4) severe metabolic acidosis (pH < 7.20); and (5) neurologic symptoms, such as seizures or neuropathy. Preparation for dialysis requires a team approach. Dietitians, social workers, psychiatrists, and transplant surgeons should be involved as well as primary care physicians and nephrol-

ogists. The patient and family need early counseling regarding the risks and benefits of therapy. The options of not starting or withdrawing dialysis should be discussed openly.

1. Hemodialysis—Hemodialysis requires a constant flow of blood along one side of a semipermeable membrane with a cleansing solution, or dialysate, along the other. Diffusion and convection allow the dialysate to remove unwanted substances from the blood while adding back needed components. Vascular access for hemodialysis can be accomplished by an arteriovenous fistula (the preferred method) or prosthetic graft. Indwelling catheters should be considered temporary measures. Native fistulas typically last longer than prosthetic shunts but require longer time (6–8 weeks or more after surgical construction) before they can be used. Infection, thrombosis, and aneurysm formation are complications seen more often in grafts than fistulas. *Staphylococcus aureus* is the most common infecting agent.

Patients typically require hemodialysis three times a week. Sessions last 3–5 hours depending on patient size, type of dialyzer used, and other factors. Periodic measurement of dialysis adequacy should determine the duration of treatment. Home hemodialysis is an option that is becoming less popular because of the need for a trained helper, large equipment, and costs. Nocturnal and daily hemodialysis are other forms of hemodialysis that offer improved outcomes in certain populations. Unfamiliarity with home hemodialysis and the financial impact with most current reimbursement schemes are currently limiting the availability of these modalities.

2. Peritoneal dialysis—With peritoneal dialysis, the peritoneal membrane is the "dialyzer." Fluids and solutes move across the capillary bed that lies between the visceral and parietal layers of the membrane into the dialysate. Dialysate enters the peritoneal cavity through a catheter. The most common kind of peritoneal dialysis is continuous ambulatory peritoneal dialysis (CAPD). Patients exchange the dialysate four to six times a day. Continuous cyclic peritoneal dialysis (CCPD) utilizes a cycler machine to automatically perform exchanges at night. The dialysate remains in the peritoneal cavity between exchanges. As with hemodialysis, actual peritoneal dialysis prescriptions are guided by adequacy measurements.

The percentage of dialysis patients using peritoneal dialysis has been decreasing over the past several years. Peritoneal dialysis permits greater patient autonomy; its continuous nature minimizes the symptomatic swings observed in hemodialysis patients; and poorly dialyzable compounds such as phosphates are better cleared, which permits less dietary restriction. The dialysate removes large amounts of albumin, and nutritional status must be closely watched.

The most common complication of peritoneal dialysis is peritonitis. Rates are as high as 0.8 episodes per patient-year. The patient can experience nausea and vomiting, abdominal pain, diarrhea or constipation, and fever. The dialysate can be cloudy and contain greater than 100 white cells/mcL of which over 50% are polymorphonuclear neutrophils. *S aureus* is the most common infecting organism.

The total costs of peritoneal dialysis and hemodialysis are approximately the same. Equipment expenses are less for peritoneal dialysis, but the costs of peritonitis are high. Patients treated with both modalities more often prefer peritoneal dialysis to hemodialysis.

Survival rates on dialysis depend on the underlying disease process. Five-year Kaplan-Meier survival rates vary from 21% for patients with diabetes to 47% for patients with glomerulonephritis. Overall 5-year survival is currently estimated at 36%. Patients undergoing dialysis have an average life expectancy of 3–4 years, but survival for as long as 25 years is seen depending on the disease entity. Studies are conflicting regarding the survival advantage associated with either peritoneal dialysis or hemodialysis.

C. Kidney Transplantation

Up to 50% of all patients with ESRD are suitable for transplantation. Age is becoming less of a barrier. Two-thirds of kidney transplants come from deceased donors, with the remainder from living related or unrelated donors. Immunosuppressive drugs include corticosteroids, azathioprine, mycophenolate mofetil, tacrolimus, cyclosporine, and rapamycin. A patient with a deceased-donor renal transplant typically requires stronger immunosuppression than patients with living related kidney donor transplants. However, this depends to a great extent on the degree of HLA-type matching. The 1- and 5-year kidney graft survival rates are approximately 94% and 76%, respectively, for living related and living unrelated donor transplants and 88% and 65%, respectively, for deceased donor transplants. The average wait for a cadaveric transplant is 2–4 years; this is becoming progressively longer as more people are going onto waiting lists while the deceased donor pool is not expanding. Aside from medication use, the life of a transplanted patient can return to nearly normal.

Prognosis

Mortality is higher for patients undergoing dialysis than for age-matched controls. Yearly mortality is 21.2 deaths per 100 patient-years. The expected remaining lifetime for the age group 55–64 is 22 years, whereas that of the ESRD population is 5 years. The most common cause of death is cardiac dysfunction (45%). Other causes include infection (14%), cerebrovascular disease (6%), and malignancy (4%). Diabetes, age, a low serum albumin, lower socioeconomic status, and inadequate dialysis are all significant predictors of mortality.

For those who require dialysis to sustain life but elect not to undergo dialysis, death ensues within days to weeks. In general, uremia develops and patients lose consciousness prior to death. Arrhythmias can occur as a result of electrolyte imbalance. Volume overload and dyspnea can be managed by volume restriction and opioids as described in Chapter 5. Meticulous efforts at palliative care are essential.

Barry JM: Current status of renal transplantation. Patient evaluations and outcomes. Urol Clin North Am 2001;28: 677. [PMID: 11791486]

Block GA et al: Cinacalcet for secondary hyperparathyroidism in patients receiving hemodialysis. N Engl J Med 2004;350: 1516. [PMID: 15071126]

Bolton WK et al: Preparing the patient for renal replacement therapy. Teamwork optimizes outcomes. Postgrad Med 2002; 111:97. [PMID: 12082923]

Collins AJ et al: Cardiovascular disease in end-stage renal disease patients. Am J Kidney Dis 2001;38(4 Suppl 1):S26. [PMID: 11576917]

Fan SL et al: Bisphosphonates in renal osteodystrophy. Curr Opin Nephrol Hypertens 2001;10:581. [PMID: 11496050]

Go AS et al: Chronic kidney disease and the risks of death, cardiovascular events, and hospitalization. N Engl J Med 2004; 351:1296. [PMID: 15385656]

JAMA patient page. Kidney failure. JAMA 2001;286:2898. [PMID: 11767735]

Jardine AG et al: Cardiovascular complications of renal disease. Heart 2001;86:459. [PMID: 11559693]

Levey AS et al: National Kidney Foundation: National Kidney Foundation practice guidelines for chronic kidney disease: evaluation, classification, and stratification. Ann Intern Med 2003;139:137. Erratum in Ann Intern Med 2003;139:605. [PMID: 12859163]

Mathur RV et al: Calciphylaxis. Postgrad Med J 2001;77:557. [PMID: 11524512]

Ramanathan V et al: Renal transplantation. Semin Nephrol 2001; 21:213. [PMID: 11245782]

Ruggenenti P et al: Progression, remission, regression of chronic renal diseases. Lancet 2001;357:1601. [PMID: 11377666]

Smogorzewski MJ: Central nervous dysfunction in uremia. Am J Kidney Dis 2001;38(4 Suppl 1):S122. [PMID: 11576937]

RENAL ARTERY STENOSIS

The two most common forms of renal artery stenosis are atherosclerotic ischemic renal disease and fibromuscular dysplasia. The prevalence of this condition has been estimated only by autopsy and angiographic studies. Approximately 5% of Americans with hypertension suffer from renal artery stenosis.

Atherosclerotic ischemic renal disease accounts for 67–95% of all cases of renal artery stenosis. It occurs most commonly in those over 45 years of age with a history of atherosclerotic disease. Other risk factors include renal insufficiency, diabetes mellitus, tobacco use, and hypertension.

Clues to diagnosis include refractory hypertension, new-onset hypertension in an older patient, pulmonary edema with poorly controlled blood pressure, and acute renal failure upon starting an ACE inhibitor. In addition to hypertension, physical examination may reveal an audible abdominal bruit on the affected side. Laboratory values can show elevated BUN and serum creatinine levels in the setting of significant renal ischemia, and abdominal ultrasound discloses asymmetric kidney size when one renal artery is affected out of proportion to the other.

Three prevailing methods used for screening are Doppler ultrasonography, captopril renography, and magnetic resonance angiography (MRA). Doppler ultrasonography is highly sensitive and specific (> 90% with an experienced ultrasonographer) and relatively inexpensive. However, this method is extremely operator and patient dependent. Measurements of blood flow must be made at the aorta and along each third of the renal artery in order to assess the disease. This test is a poor choice for patients who are obese, unable to lie supine, or have interfering bowel gas patterns.

Captopril renography capitalizes on the difference in renal perfusion with and without ACE inhibitors. A kidney distal to a significant stenosis requires high angiotensin II levels to maintain adequate perfusion. With an ACE inhibitor, perfusion is markedly diminished. The affected kidney enhances less, whereas the unaffected one enhances more in the setting of a captopril challenge. Sensitivity ranges from 75% to 100% and specificity from 60% to 90%. This procedure is not as accurate in moderate to severe renal insufficiency.

MRA is an excellent but expensive way to screen for renal artery stenosis. Sensitivity is 99–100%. Specificity ranges from 71% to 96%. Turbulent blood flow can cause false-positive results.

Renal angiography is the gold standard for diagnosis. CO_2 subtraction angiography can be used in place of dye when the risk of dye nephropathy exists—eg, in diabetic patients with renal insufficiency. Lesions are most commonly found in the proximal third or ostial region of the renal artery. The risk of atheroembolic phenomena after angiography is not trivial in this population, ranging from 5% to 10%.

Treatment is controversial. Options include medical management, angioplasty with or without stenting, and surgical bypass. Angioplasty might reduce the number of antihypertensive medications but does not significantly change outcome in comparison to patients medically managed. Stenting produces significantly better angioplastic results. However, blood pressure is equally improved, and serum creatinines are similar at 6 months of observation. Angioplasty is equally as effective as, and safer than, surgical revision.

Fibromuscular dysplasia primarily affects young women. Unexplained hypertension in a young woman is reason to screen for this disorder. The noninvasive tests mentioned above should be used for detection. This disorder has a characteristic "beads-on-a-string" appearance on angiography. Treatment with percutaneous transluminal angioplasty is often curative.

Bloch MJ et al: Clinical insights into the diagnosis and management of renovascular disease. An evidence-based review. Minerva Med 2004;95:357. [PMID: 15467512]

Kalra PA et al: Atherosclerotic renovascular disease in United States patients aged 67 years or older: risk factors, revascularization, and prognosis. Kidney Int 2005;68:293. [PMID: 15954920]

Korsakas S et al: Delay of dialysis in end-stage renal failure: prospective study on percutaneous renal artery interventions. Kidney Int 2004;65:251. [PMID: 14675057]

Nordmann AJ et al: Balloon angioplasty versus medical therapy for hypertensive patients with renal artery obstruction. Cochrane Database Syst Rev 2003;(3):CD002944. [PMID: 12917937]

Safian RD et al: Renal artery stenosis. N Engl J Med 2001;8:344. [PMID: 11172181]

■ GLOMERULONEPHROPATHIES

Abnormalities of glomerular function can be caused by damage to the major components of the glomerulus: the epithelium (podocytes), basement membrane, capillary endothelium, or mesangium. The damage is often manifested as an inflammatory process. A specific histologic pattern of glomerular injury can be seen on renal biopsy, one of the most helpful techniques available for defining the cause of glomerular disease. Clinically, hematuria, proteinuria, hypertension, and a reduced GFR are typical findings of glomerular diseases presenting as *nephritic* syndromes; heavy proteinuria (> 3.5 g/24 h), hypoalbuminemia, hyperlipidemia, and edema are typical findings of glomerular diseases presenting as *nephrotic* syndromes.

Classification

Glomerular diseases generally can be classified into one of three major syndromes: nephritic syndrome, nephrotic syndrome, and asymptomatic renal disease. Specific glomerular diseases usually exhibit characteristics of one of the above syndromes, though some can have varying components of all three.

Glomerular diseases can also be classified according to whether they cause only renal abnormalities (primary renal disease) or whether the renal abnormalities result from a systemic disease (secondary renal disease).

NEPHRITIC SYNDROME

ESSENTIALS OF DIAGNOSIS

- *Edema.*
- *Hypertension.*
- *Hematuria (with or without dysmorphic red cells, red blood cell casts).*

General Considerations

Acute glomerulonephritis usually signifies an inflammatory process causing renal dysfunction over days to weeks that may or may not resolve. If the inflammatory process is severe, the glomerulonephritis may lead to a greater than 50% loss of nephron function over the course of just weeks to months. Such a process, called rapidly progressive acute glomerulonephritis, can cause permanent damage to glomeruli if not identified and treated rapidly. Prolonged inflammatory changes can result in chronic glomerulonephritis with persistent renal abnormalities that progress to ESRD.

Clinical Findings

A. SYMPTOMS AND SIGNS

Edema is first seen in regions of low tissue pressure such as the periorbital and scrotal areas. Hypertension, if present, is due to volume overload rather than vasoactive substances such as angiotensin II, whose levels are low.

B. LABORATORY FINDINGS

1. Serum chemistries—There are no serum chemistries characteristic of nephritic syndrome, but certain special tests are often performed depending on the history and the results of the preliminary evaluation. These include complement levels, antinuclear antibodies (ANA), cryoglobulins, hepatitis serologies, ANCA, anti-GBM antibodies, antistreptolysin O (ASO) titers, and C3 nephritic factor (Figure 22–2).

2. Urinalysis—The urinalysis shows red blood cells. These may be misshapen from traversing a damaged capillary membrane—so-called dysmorphic red blood cells. Red blood cell casts and moderate degrees of proteinuria are also characteristic of the urinary sediment. Placing the patient in a lordotic position for an hour increases sensitivity for finding red cell casts in the next urine specimen.

3. Biopsy—Renal biopsy should be considered if there are no other contraindications to biopsy (eg, bleeding disorders, thrombocytopenia, uncontrolled hypertension). Rapidly progressive glomerulonephritis is likely when over 50% of glomeruli contain crescents. The type of disease can be categorized according to the immunofluorescent pattern and appearance on electron microscopy (Table 22–9).

Treatment

Treatment includes aggressive reduction of hypertension and fluid overload and specific therapeutic maneuvers aimed at the underlying cause. Salt and water restriction, diuretic therapy, and possibly dialysis are needed. The inflammatory glomerular injury may require corticosteroids and cytotoxic agents. (See specific diseases discussed below.)

POSTINFECTIOUS GLOMERULONEPHRITIS

Postinfectious glomerulonephritis is most often due to infection with nephritogenic group A β-hemolytic streptococci, especially type 12. It can occur sporadically or in clusters and during epidemics can account for up to 10% of known streptococcal infections. It commonly appears after pharyngitis or impetigo. Onset occurs within 1–3 weeks after infection (average, 7–10 days).

Other causes of postinfectious glomerulonephritis include bacteremic states such as systemic *S aureus* infection. Infective endocarditis and shunt infections cause similar lesions.

These are referred to as peri-infectious glomerulonephritides. Viral, fungal, and parasitic causes include hepatitis B or C, cytomegalovirus infection, infectious mononucleosis, coccidioidomycosis, malaria, and toxoplasmosis.

Clinical Findings

A. SYMPTOMS AND SIGNS

The patient is oliguric, edematous, and variably hypertensive.

B. LABORATORY FINDINGS

Serum complement levels are low; in postinfectious glomerulonephritis due to group A streptococcal infection, ASO titers can be high unless the immune response has been blunted with previous antibiotic treatment. Classically, the urine is described as cola-colored. Urinary red blood cells, red cell casts, and proteinuria under 3.5 g/d are present. On microscopy, this entity appears as a diffuse proliferative glomerulonephritis. Immunofluorescence shows IgG and C3 in a granular pattern in the mesangium and along the capillary basement membrane. Electron microscopy shows large, dense subepithelial deposits or "humps."

Treatment

Treatment for this entity is supportive. Appropriate antibiotics should be used. Antihypertensives, salt restriction, and diuretics should be used if needed. Corticosteroids have not been shown to improve outcome. Prognosis in children is very favorable, but adults are more prone to crescent formation and chronic renal insufficiency. A rapidly progressive glomerulonephritis will develop in less than 5% of adults, and a smaller percentage of adults will progress to ESRD.

IGA NEPHROPATHY & HENOCH-SCHÖNLEIN PURPURA

IgA Nephropathy

IgA nephropathy (Berger's disease) is a primary renal disease of IgA deposition in the glomerular mesangium. The inciting cause is unknown, but the same lesion is seen in Henoch-Schönlein purpura. IgA nephropathy is also associated with hepatic cirrhosis, celiac disease, and infections such as with HIV and cytomegalovirus.

IgA nephropathy is the most common form of acute glomerulonephritis in the United States and is even more prevalent worldwide, particularly in Asia. It

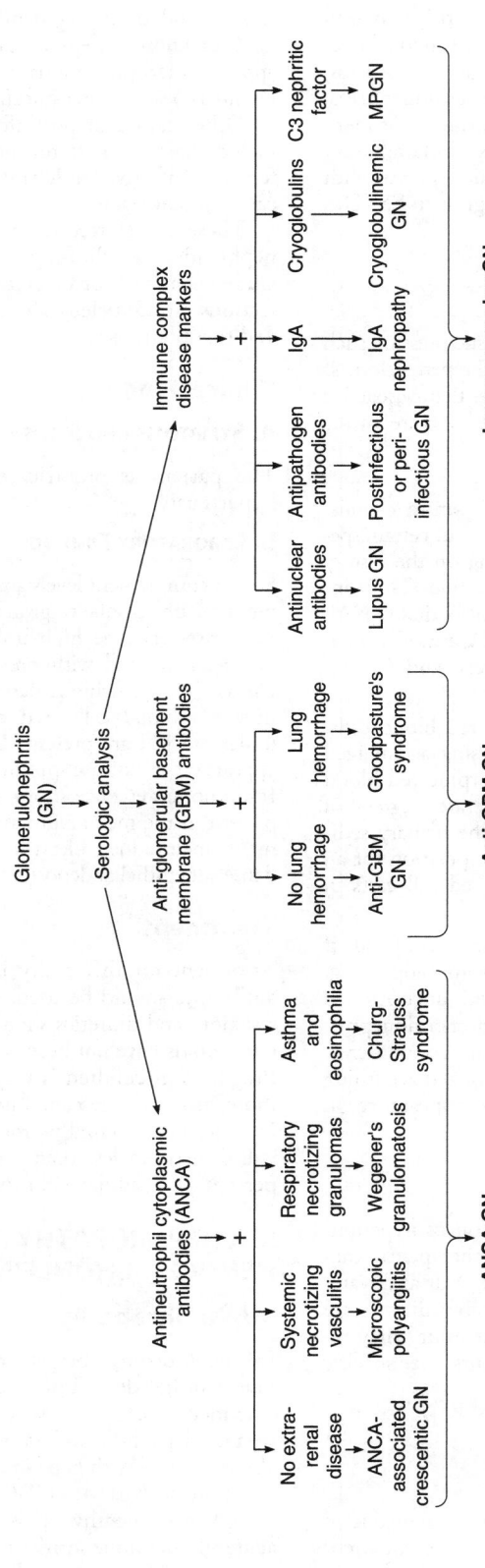

Figure 22–2. **Serologic analysis of patients with glomerulonephritis.** (Reproduced, with permission, from Jennette JC et al: *Primer on Kidney Diseases.* Academic Press, 1994.)

Table 22–9. Classification and findings in glomerulonephritis: nephritic syndromes.

	Etiology	Histopathology	Pathogenesis
Acute (postinfectious) glomerulonephritis	Streptococci, other bacteria	Light: Diffuse proliferative glomerulonephritis Immunofluorescence: IgG; C3, granular pattern Electron microscopy: Subepithelial deposits or "humps"	Trapped immune complexes
IgA nephropathy (Berger's disease and Henoch-Schönlein purpura)	In association with viral upper respiratory tract infections; gastrointestinal infection or flu-like syndrome	Light: Mesangioproliferative glomerulonephritis Immunofluorescence: IgA (with or without IgG, C3) Electron microscopy: Mesangial deposits	Unknown
Rapidly progressive glomerulonephritis	Lupus erythematosus, mixed cryoglobulinemia, subacute infective endocarditis, shunt infections	Light: Crescentic glomerulonephritis Immunofluorescence: IgG, IgA; C3, granular pattern Electron microscopy: Deposits in subepithelium, subendothelium, or mesangium	Trapped immune complexes
	Goodpasture's syndrome or idiopathic	Light: Crescentic glomerulonephritis Immunofluorescence: IgG; C3, linear pattern Electron microscopy: Widening of GBM	Anti-GBM antibodies
	Wegener's granulomatosis, polyarteritis, idiopathic	Light: Crescentic glomerulonephritis Immunofluorescence: No immunoglobulins Electron microscopy: No deposits	Unknown

GBM = glomerular basement membrane.

is most commonly seen in children and young adults, with males affected two to three times more commonly than females.

An episode of gross hematuria is the most common presenting complaint. Frequently, this is associated with an upper respiratory infection (50%), gastrointestinal symptoms (10%), or a flu-like illness (15%). The urine becomes red or cola-colored 1–2 days after onset. In contrast to postinfectious glomerulonephritis, this feature has been called "synpharyngitic hematuria" since there is no significant latent period. Other findings include asymptomatic microscopic hematuria as an incidental finding and the nephrotic syndrome (see below). Approximately one-third of patients will experience a clinical remission. Forty to 50 percent of patients will have progressive renal insufficiency. The remainder will show chronic microscopic hematuria and a stable serum creatinine. The most unfavorable prognostic indicator is proteinuria greater than 1 g/d; others include hypertension, persistent microscopic hematuria and proteinuria, glomerulosclerosis, and abnormal renal function.

The serum IgA level is increased in up to 50% of patients, and for that reason a normal serum IgA does not rule out the disease. Serum complement levels are usually normal, and renal biopsy is the standard for diagnosis. Glomeruli show a focal glomerulonephritis with diffuse mesangial IgA deposits and proliferation of mesangial cells. IgG and C3 can also be seen in the mesangium of all glomeruli. Skin biopsy often reveals granular deposits of IgA in dermal capillaries of affected patients.

In patients with significant proteinuria (> 1 g/d), ACE inhibitors or ARB drugs should be used to reduce proteinuria and hypertension. The target blood pressure is less than 130/80 mm Hg. In patients with proteinuria of 1.0–3.5 g/d, corticosteroid therapy has proven beneficial. A recent regimen showed a 2% doubling of creatinine after 6 years in the treatment group versus a 21% doubling of creatinine in the control group. The regimen consisted of giving methylprednisolone, 1 g/d intravenously, for 3 days during months 1, 3, and 5, plus prednisone in a dosage of 0.5 mg/kg every other day for 6 months. This was aimed at patients with creatinine clearances greater than 70 mL/min. Other treatments have included fish oil, with variable results in clinical trials. Recent studies that have shown a benefit also show that low doses (2–5 g/d) are just as efficacious as high doses (9–12 g/d). A recent meta-analysis has showed no benefit from fish oil, but there was a trend toward benefit in patients with more proteinuria. There are very few side effects of long-term fish oil administration aside from fishy breath and eructations. Renal transplantation is an excellent option for patients with ESRD, but recurrent disease has been documented in 30% of patients 5–10 years posttransplant. Fortunately, recurrent disease rarely leads to failure of the allograft.

Henoch-Schönlein Purpura (Anaphylactoid Purpura)

This disease is a leukocytoclastic vasculitis of unknown cause. It is most common in children and has a male predominance. It classically presents with palpable purpura, arthralgias, and abdominal symptoms such as nausea, colic, and melena. Purpuric skin lesions are most often found on the lower extremities. Renal insufficiency is common with a nephritic presentation. The renal lesions are identical to those found in IgA nephropathy. Most patients will recover fully over several weeks.

Further details about Henoch-Schönlein purpura are provided in Chapter 20.

David JC et al: What is the difference between IgA nephropathy and Henoch-Schönlein purpura nephritis? Kidney Int 2001; 59:823. [PMID: 11231337]

Donadio JV et al: IgA nephropathy. N Engl J Med 2002; 347:738. [PMID: 12213946]

Gedalia A: Henoch-Schönlein purpura. Curr Rheumatol Rep 2004;6:195. [PMID: 15134598]

Julian BA et al: IgA nephropathy: an update. Curr Opin Nephrol Hypertens 2004;13:171. [PMID: 15202611]

Lang MM et al: Identifying poststreptococcal glomerulonephritis. Nurse Pract 2001;26:34. [PMID: 11521409]

PAUCI-IMMUNE GLOMERULONEPHRITIS (ANCA-Associated)

Pauci-immune glomerular lesions are seen with Wegener's granulomatosis, Churg-Strauss disease, and microscopic polyangiitis. All are small-vessel vasculitides. Wegener's granulomatosis also involves granulomatous inflammation of the respiratory tract with a necrotizing vasculitis of small and medium-sized vessels. Microscopic polyangiitis (polyarteritis) is similar to Wegener's granulomatosis without granulomatous inflammation, but both commonly exhibit a necrotizing glomerulonephritis. ANCA-associated glomerulonephritis can also present as a primary renal lesion. The pathogenesis of these entities is unknown, but more than 80% of pauci-immune glomerulonephritis is associated with antineutrophil cytoplasmic antibodies.

Clinical Findings

A. SYMPTOMS AND SIGNS

Symptoms of a systemic inflammatory disease, including fever, malaise, and weight loss, may be present. In addition to hematuria and proteinuria from glomerular inflammation, some patients exhibit purpura from dermal capillary involvement and mononeuritis multiplex from nerve arteriolar involvement. Ninety percent of patients with Wegener's granulomatosis will have upper or lower respiratory tract symptoms with nodular lesions that can cavitate and bleed.

B. LABORATORY FINDINGS

Serologically, ANCA subtype analysis can be done. A cytoplasmic pattern (C-ANCA) is specific for antiproteinase-3 antibodies, while a perinuclear pattern (P-ANCA) is specific for antimyeloperoxidase antibodies. Over 90%

of patients with Wegener's syndrome will have C-ANCA; the remainder can have a P-ANCA pattern. Microscopic angiitis will have either a P-ANCA or C-ANCA pattern about 80% of the time. Pathologically, the small vessels and glomeruli will lack immune deposits (pauci-immune); however, a cell-mediated immune response is often seen. Necrotizing lesions and crescents signify a rapidly progressive glomerulonephritis.

Treatment

Treatment should be instituted early if aggressive disease is suspected. High doses of corticosteroids (methylprednisolone, 1–2 g/d for 3 days, followed by prednisone, 1 mg/kg for 1 month, with a slow taper over the next 6 months) and cytotoxic agents (cyclophosphamide, 0.5–1.0 g/m^2 intravenously or 1.5–2 mg/kg orally for 3–6 months tapered over 1 year) are recommended for controlling end-organ damage. Intravenous cyclophosphamide is likely associated with fewer side effects and is just as efficacious as corticosteroids. Without treatment, prognosis is extremely poor, but with the above regimen, complete remission can be achieved in about 75% of patients. The addition of plasmapheresis does not seem to improve outcomes. Prognosis depends mainly on the extent of glomerular involvement before treatment is started. ANCA levels can be monitored to help determine the efficacy of treatment.

ANTI-GLOMERULAR BASEMENT MEMBRANE GLOMERULONEPHRITIS & GOODPASTURE'S SYNDROME

Goodpasture's syndrome is defined by the clinical constellation of glomerulonephritis and pulmonary hemorrhage; injury to both is mediated by anti-GBM antibodies. Up to one-third of patients with anti-GBM glomerulonephritis have no evidence of lung injury. Anti-GBM-associated glomerulonephritis accounts for about 10% of patients with rapidly progressive acute glomerulonephritis. The incidence in males is approximately six times that in females, and the disease occurs most commonly in the second and third decades but has a wide range. It has been associated with influenza A infection, hydrocarbon solvent exposure, and HLA-DR2 and -B7 antigens.

Clinical Findings

A. SYMPTOMS AND SIGNS

The onset of disease is preceded by an upper respiratory tract infection in 20–60% of cases. Patients experience hemoptysis, dyspnea, and possible respiratory failure. Hypertension and edema are seen as components of the nephritic syndrome.

B. LABORATORY FINDINGS

Laboratory evaluation can show iron deficiency anemia, and complement levels are normal. Sputum contains hemosiderin-laden macrophages. Chest radiographs can show shifting pulmonary infiltrates due to pulmonary hemorrhage. The diffusion capacity of carbon monoxide is markedly increased. Diagnosis is confirmed by finding circulating anti-GBM antibodies, which are positive in over 90% of patients.

Treatment

The treatment of choice is a combination of plasma exchange therapy to remove circulating antibodies and administration of immunosuppressive drugs to prevent formation of new antibodies and control the inflammatory response. Corticosteroids are given initially in pulse doses of prednisone or methylprednisolone, 1–2 g/d for 3 days, then 1 mg/kg/d. Cyclophosphamide is administered intravenously at a dose of 0.5–1.0 g/m² or orally at a dosage of 2–3 mg/kg/d. Daily plasmapheresis is performed for up to 2 weeks. A poorer prognosis exists in patients with oliguria and a serum creatinine greater than 6–7 mg/dL. Anti-GBM antibody levels should decrease as the clinical course improves.

CRYOGLOBULIN-ASSOCIATED GLOMERULONEPHRITIS

Essential (mixed) cryoglobulinemia is a disorder associated with cold-precipitable immunoglobulins (cryoglobulins). Glomerular disease results from the precipitation of cryoglobulins in glomerular capillaries. The cause is typically an underlying infection such as hepatitis B and C or other occult viral, bacterial, and fungal infections.

Patients exhibit necrotizing skin lesions in dependent areas, arthralgias, fever, and hepatosplenomegaly. Serum complement levels are depressed. Rheumatoid factor is often elevated when cryoglobulins are present. Rapidly progressive glomerulonephritis is seen on pathologic examination with the presence of crescents.

Treatment consists of aggressively treating the underlying infection. Pulse corticosteroids, plasma exchange, and cytotoxic agents can be used. Interferon-α (IFN-α) has been shown to benefit patients with hepatitis C–related cryoglobulinemia.

Booth AD et al: Pan-Thames Renal Research Group: Outcome of ANCA-associated renal vasculitis: a 5-year retrospective study. Am J Kidney Dis 2003;41:776. [PMID: 12666064]

Gaskin G et al: Plasmapheresis in antineutrophil cytoplasmic antibody-associated systemic vasculitis. Ther Apher 2001;5:176. [PMID: 11467753]

Harper L et al: ANCA-associated renal vasculitis at the end of the twentieth century--a disease of older patients. Rheumatology (Oxford) 2005;44:495. [PMID: 15613403]

Hudson BG et al: Alport's syndrome, Goodpasture's syndrome, and type IV collagen. N Engl J Med 2003;348:2543. [PMID: 12815141]

Jara LJ et al: Pulmonary-renal vasculitic disorders: differential diagnosis and management. Curr Rheumatol Rep 2003;5:107. [PMID: 12628041]

Jennett JC et al: Microscopic polyangiitis (microscopic polyarteritis). Semin Diagn Pathol 2001;18:3. [PMID: 11296991]

Levy JB et al: Long-term outcome of anti-glomerular basement membrane antibody disease treated with plasma exchange and immunosuppression. Ann Intern Med 2001;134:1033. [PMID: 11388816]

Madaio MP et al: The diagnosis of glomerular diseases: acute glomerulonephritis and the nephrotic syndrome. Arch Intern Med 2001;161:25. [PMID: 11146695]

Vinen CS et al: Acute glomerulonephritis. Postgrad Med J 2003; 79:206. [PMID: 12743337]

NEPHROTIC SYNDROME

ESSENTIALS OF DIAGNOSIS

- Urine protein excretion > 3.5 g/1.73 m² per 24 hours.
- Hypoalbuminemia (albumin < 3 g/dL).
- Peripheral edema.

General Considerations

In adults, about one-third of patients with nephrotic syndrome have a systemic renal disease such as diabetes mellitus, amyloidosis, or systemic lupus erythematosus. With the current epidemic of type 2 diabetes mellitus, this proportion is slowly increasing. The remainder have idiopathic nephrotic syndrome. The four most common are minimal change disease, focal glomerular sclerosis, membranous nephropathy, and membranoproliferative glomerulonephritis.

Clinical Findings

A. SYMPTOMS AND SIGNS

Peripheral edema is a hallmark of the nephrotic syndrome, occurring when the serum albumin concentration is less than 3 g/dL. Edema is most likely due to sodium retention (from renal disease) rather than arterial underfilling from low plasma oncotic pressure. Initially this presents in the dependent areas of the body such as the lower extremities; however, such edema can become generalized. Patients can experience dyspnea due to pulmonary edema, pleural effusions, and diaphragmatic compromise with ascites. Complaints of abdominal fullness may also be present in patients with ascites.

Patients may show symptoms and signs of infection more frequently than the general population owing to loss of immunoglobulins and certain complement moieties in the urine.

B. LABORATORY FINDINGS

1. Urinalysis—Proteinuria occurs as a result of an alteration of the negative charge in the GBM. The screening test for proteinuria is the urinary dipstick analysis; however, this test indicates albumin only. The addition of sulfosalicylic acid to the urine sedi-

Table 22–10. Classification and findings in glomerulonephritis: nephrotic syndromes.

	Etiology	Histopathology	Pathogenesis
Minimal change disease (nil disease; lipoid nephrosis)	Associated with allergy, Hodgkin's disease, NSAIDs	Light: Normal (with or without mesangial proliferation) Immunofluorescence: No immunoglobulins Electron microscopy: Fusion foot processes	Unknown
Focal and segmental glomerulosclerosis	Associated with heroin abuse, HIV infection, reflux nephropathy, obesity	Light: Focal segmental sclerosis Immunofluorescence: IgM and C3 in sclerotic segments Electron microscopy: Fusion foot processes	Unknown
Membranous nephropathy	Associated with non-Hodgkin's lymphoma, carcinoma (gastrointestinal, renal, bronchogenic, thyroid), gold therapy, penicillamine, lupus erythematosus	Light: Thickened GBM and spikes Immunofluorescence: Granular IgG and C3 along capillary loops Electron microscopy: Dense deposits in subepithelial area	In situ immune complex formation
Membranoproliferative glomerulonephropathy	Type I associated with upper respiratory infection	Light: Increased mesangial cells and matrix with splitting of GBM Immunofluorescence: Granular C3, C1q, C4 with IgG and IgM Electron microscopy: Dense deposits in subendothelium	Unknown
	Type II	Light: Same as type I Immunofluorescence: C3 only Electron microscopy: Dense material in GBM	Unknown

NSAIDs = nonsteroidal anti-inflammatory drugs; GBM = glomerular basement membrane.

ment allows abnormal paraproteins to be detected. Urine dipstick testing can detect as little as 15 mg/dL of protein, but the results must be interpreted along with the urine specific gravity. Trace protein seen on highly concentrated specimens may be insignificant, while trace protein on dilute specimens may indicate true renal disease.

Microscopically, the urinary sediment has relatively few cellular elements or casts. However, if marked hyperlipidemia is present, patients can have oval fat bodies in the urine. These represent lipid deposits in sloughed renal tubular epithelial cells. They appear as "grape clusters" under light microscopy and "Maltese crosses" under polarized light.

2. Blood chemistries—Characteristic blood chemistries include a decreased serum albumin (< 3 g/dL) and total serum protein less than 6 g/dL. Hyperlipidemia occurs in over 50% of those with early nephrotic syndrome. As patients excrete larger amounts of protein per day, the frequency of hyperlipidemia increases. There is increased hepatic production of lipids (cholesterol and apolipoprotein B), owing to a fall in oncotic pressure. There is also decreased clearance of very low-density lipoproteins, causing hypertriglyceridemia. Patients can also have an elevated erythrocyte sedimentation rate as a result of alterations in some plasma components such as increased levels of fibrinogen.

Other less common tests may be necessary depending on the patient's clinical presentation, including complement levels, serum and urine protein electrophoresis, ANA, and serologic tests for hepatitis. Patients may become deficient in vitamin D, zinc, and copper from loss of binding proteins in the urine; they are prone to infection, in part from urinary losses of immunoglobulins.

3. Renal biopsy—Specific classification and findings are shown in Table 22–10. Specimens are examined by light microscopy, with immunofluorescent stains, and by electron microscopy. Renal biopsy is often performed in adults with new-onset idiopathic nephrotic syndrome if a primary renal disease that may require drug therapy (eg, corticosteroids, cytotoxic agents) is suspected. Significantly elevated creatinine levels may indicate irreversible renal disease mitigating the usefulness of renal biopsy. Disease due to amyloid or diabetes mellitus often does not need to be biopsied, since nephrotic range proteinuria in these diseases represents irreversible damage, although bone marrow transplant with high-dose chemotherapy can be considered in some patients with amyloid. The role of biopsy for other systemic renal diseases is debated. However, it can be useful for prognosis and treatment. An occasional unexpected diagnosis is made, such as membranous nephropathy due to lupus erythematosus without serologic evidence of that illness.

Management of Nephrotic Syndrome

A. PROTEIN LOSS

The daily total dietary protein intake should replace the daily urinary protein losses so as to avoid negative nitrogen balance. Protein malnutrition often occurs with urinary protein losses greater than 10 g/d. In the past, protein restriction was suggested for patients with renal insufficiency because experimental animal models had demonstrated a decrease in glomerulosclerosis among those animals fed low-protein diets. The largest human trial to date (the MDRD Study) did not show a significant benefit, but two recent meta-analyses have shown a mild renal benefit. For this reason, the KDOQI recommends protein restriction to 0.6 g/kg/d in patients with a GFR less than 25 mL/min prior to starting dialysis.

B. EDEMA

Dietary salt restriction is essential for managing edema; most patients also require diuretic therapy. Commonly used diuretics include thiazide and loop diuretics. Both are highly protein bound. With hypoalbuminemia, diuretic delivery to the kidney is reduced, and patients often require large doses. The combination of loop and thiazide diuretics can potentiate the diuretic effect. This may be needed for patients with refractory fluid retention associated with pleural effusions and ascites.

C. HYPERLIPIDEMIA

Hypercholesterolemia and hypertriglyceridemia occur as outlined above. Dietary management in patients with nephrotic syndrome is of little value; however, dietary modification and exercise should be advocated. Aggressive pharmacologic treatment should be pursued. This is discussed in Chapter 27.

D. HYPERCOAGULABLE STATE

Patients with serum albumin less than 2 g/dL can become hypercoagulable. Nephrotic patients have urinary losses of antithrombin III, protein C, and protein S and increased platelet activation. Patients are prone to renal vein thrombosis and other venous thromboemboli, particularly with membranous glomerulopathy. Anticoagulation therapy is warranted for at least 3–6 months in patients with evidence of thrombosis. Patients with renal vein thrombosis and recurrent thromboemboli require indefinite anticoagulation.

■ NEPHROTIC DISEASE IN PRIMARY RENAL DISORDERS

MINIMAL CHANGE DISEASE

Minimal change disease is most commonly seen in children but is occasionally present in adults. In patients over 40 years with primary nephrotic syndrome, the incidence of minimal change disease is 20–25%, with equal distribution between men and women. In younger patients, there is a male predominance. Minimal change disease can be idiopathic but also occurs following viral upper respiratory infections, in association with tumors such as Hodgkin's disease, with drugs (gold and lithium), and with hypersensitivity reactions (especially to NSAIDs and bee stings).

Clinical Findings

A. SYMPTOMS AND SIGNS

Patients can exhibit the manifestations of nephrotic syndrome. They are more susceptible to infection, especially with gram-positive organisms, have a tendency toward thromboembolic events, develop severe hyperlipidemia, and experience protein malnutrition. Minimal change disease can rarely cause acute renal failure due to tubular changes and interstitial edema.

B. HISTOLOGIC FINDINGS

Glomeruli show no changes on light microscopy or immunofluorescence. On electron microscopy, there is a characteristic fusion of epithelial foot processes. A subgroup of patients also shows mesangial cell proliferation. These people have more hematuria and hypertension and respond poorly to corticosteroid treatment.

Treatment

Treatment is with prednisone, 1 mg/kg/d. In children, the response is excellent, but about 10% of patients become corticosteroid resistant after 4–6 weeks. Adults often require longer therapy. It can take up to 16 weeks to achieve a response to corticosteroids. Treatment should be continued for several weeks after complete remission of proteinuria. A significant number of patients will relapse and require further corticosteroid treatment. Patients with frequent relapses and corticosteroid resistance may need cyclophosphamide or chlorambucil to induce subsequent remissions. Progression to ESRD is rare. Complications most often arise from prolonged corticosteroid use.

MEMBRANOUS NEPHROPATHY

Membranous nephropathy is the most common cause of primary nephrotic syndrome in adults. It is an immune-mediated disease characterized by immune complex deposition in the subepithelial portion of glomerular capillary walls. The antigens in primary disease are not known. Secondary disease is associated with infections, such as hepatitis B, endocarditis, and syphilis; autoimmune disease, such as systemic lupus erythematosus, mixed connective tissue disease, and thyroiditis; carcinoma; and certain drugs, such as gold, penicillamine, and captopril. Membranous nephropathy occurs most commonly in adults in their fifth and sixth decades and almost always after age 30 years.

Clinical Findings

A. SYMPTOMS AND SIGNS

Patients exhibit the signs of nephrotic syndrome and have a higher incidence of renal vein thrombosis than most nephrotic patients. A higher incidence of occult neoplasms of lung, stomach, and colon is found in people over 50 years of age. The course of disease is variable, with about 50% of patients progressing to ESRD over 3–10 years. Poorer outcome is associated with concomitant tubulointerstitial fibrosis, male gender, elevated serum creatinine, hypertension, and heavy proteinuria (> 10 g/d).

B. LABORATORY FINDINGS

By light microscopy, capillary wall thickness is increased without inflammatory changes or cellular proliferation. When stained with silver methenamine, a "spike and dome" pattern may be observed owing to projections of excess GBM between the subepithelial deposits. Immunofluorescence shows IgG and C3 uniformly along capillary loops. Electron microscopy shows a discontinuous pattern of dense deposits along the subepithelial surface of the basement membrane.

Treatment

Treatment is controversial. After underlying causes are excluded, treatment depends on the risk of renal disease progression. One algorithm is based on the degree of proteinuria. In patients with proteinuria less than 3.5 g/d, the risk of progression is low. These individuals should be closely monitored with a low-salt diet, strict blood pressure control, and an ACE inhibitor for reduction of proteinuria. Patients with proteinuria of 3.5–8 g/d but normal renal function are at medium risk. They should follow the above suggestions and can elect immunosuppressive regimens with corticosteroids and chlorambucil or cyclophosphamide for 6 months, although 65% of these patients experience partial or complete remission within 3–4 years. Cyclosporine is a second choice. The highest-risk patients—those with greater than 8 g/d of proteinuria and possible renal dysfunction—might receive corticosteroids with a cytotoxic agent as first-line immunosuppressant therapy, though the choice of cyclosporine is also reasonable. These treatments should be carefully chosen in consultation with a nephrologist. Patients with membranous nephropathy are excellent candidates for transplant.

FOCAL SEGMENTAL GLOMERULAR SCLEROSIS

This lesion can present as idiopathic disease or secondary to such conditions as heroin use, morbid obesity, and HIV infection. Clinically, patients show evidence of nephrotic syndrome, but they also have more nephritic features than membranous nephropathy or min-imal change disease. Eighty percent of patients have microscopic hematuria at presentation, and many are hypertensive. Decreased renal function is present in 25–50% at time of diagnosis. Patients with focal segmental glomerular sclerosis and nephrotic syndrome typically progress to ESRD in 6–8 years.

Diagnosis requires renal biopsy. Light microscopy shows the lesions of focal segmental glomerular sclerosis. It is thought that these lesions occur first in the juxtamedullary glomeruli and are then seen in the superficial renal cortex. IgM and C3 are seen in the sclerotic lesions on immunofluorescence. Electron microscopy shows fusion of epithelial foot processes as seen in minimal change disease (Table 22–10).

Treatment is controversial, though supportive care for nephrotic patients is indicated. Longer courses of corticosteroids are now being used because a higher percentage of patients enter remission. High-dose oral prednisone (1–1.5 mg/kg/d) for 2–3 months followed by a slow taper can induce remission in over half of patients. Most patients achieve remission within 5–9 months. Other cytotoxic drug therapy can be considered but is disappointing (< 20% remission in most series).

Cattran DC: Idiopathic membranous glomerulonephritis. Kidney Int 2001;59:1983. [PMID: 11318974]

Chun MJ et al: Focal segmental glomerulosclerosis in nephrotic adults: presentation, prognosis, and response to therapy of the histologic variants. J Am Soc Nephrol 2004; 15:2169. [PMID: 15284302]

DeSanto NG et al: Nephrotic edema. Semin Nephrol 2001;21: 262. [PMID: 11320491]

Fogo AB: Minimal change disease and focal segmental glomerulosclerosis. Nephrol Dial Transplant 2001;16(Suppl 6):74. [PMID: 11568250]

Madaio MP et al: The diagnosis of glomerular diseases: acute glomerulonephritis and the nephrotic syndrome. Arch Intern Med 2001;161:25. [PMID: 11146695]

Ponticelli C et al: Treatment of membranous nephropathy. Nephrol Dial Transplant 2001;16(Suppl 5):8. [PMID: 11509678]

Schwarz A: New aspects of the treatment of nephrotic syndrome. J Am Soc Nephrol 2001;12(Suppl 17):S44. [PMID: 11251031]

■ NEPHROTIC DISEASE FROM SYSTEMIC DISORDERS

AMYLOIDOSIS

Amyloidosis consists of extracellular deposition of the fibrous protein amyloid in one or more sites in the body. The amyloid fibrils are composed of proteins that have formed β-pleated sheets, a definitive characteristic. Primary renal amyloidosis (AL amyloidosis) may occur in the absence of systemic disease or associated with multiple myeloma; indeed, both are plasma cell dyscrasias. Secondary amyloidosis (AA amyloidosis) is due to a chronic inflammatory disease, such as rheumatoid arthritis, inflammatory bowel disease, or chronic infection. The acute phase reactant serum amyloid A is synthesized in the liver and deposited in the tissues. Primary amyloidosis usually occurs in older age groups and displays a benign urinary sediment; the amyloid is derived from immunoglobulin light chain. The degree of proteinuria is not associated with the extent of renal lesions. Kidneys can be enlarged as a result of amyloid deposition. Pathologically, glomeruli are filled with amorphous deposits that stain positive with Congo red and show green birefringence.

Treatment options are few. Remissions can occur in secondary amyloidosis if the inciting agent is removed. Primary amyloidosis of the kidney progresses to ESRD in an average of 2–3 years. Five-year overall survival is less than 20%, with death occurring from ESRD and heart disease. The use of alkylating agents and corticosteroids—eg, melphalan and prednisone—can reduce proteinuria and improve renal function in a small percentage of patients. Melphalan and stem cell transplantation are associated with high toxicity (45% mortality) but induce remission in 80% of the remaining patients. Renal transplant is an option in patients with secondary amyloid.

DIABETIC NEPHROPATHY

Diabetic nephropathy is the most common cause of ESRD in the United States (about 4000 cases a year). Type 1 diabetes mellitus carries a 30–40% chance of nephropathy after 20 years, whereas type 2 has a 15–20% chance after 20 years. ESRD is much more likely to develop in persons with type 1 diabetes mellitus, probably because of fewer comorbidities and deaths before ESRD ensues. With the current epidemic of type 2 diabetes mellitus, rates of diabetic nephropathy are projected to continue to increase over at least the next 2 decades. Patients at higher risk include males, African Americans, and Native Americans.

The nephrotic syndrome develops in patients at risk for nephropathy. Diabetic retinopathy is often present in these patients. Initial screening of diabetics should always include urine examination for microalbuminuria. Dipstick examination may not be sensitive enough; a 24-hour urine collection is the accepted standard measure. (An albumin excretion of > 30 mg/d is abnormal.) However, an early morning spot urine albumin or albumin-creatinine ratio is adequate. (More than 30 mg of albumin per gram of creatinine is considered abnormal.) In patients prone to nephropathy, microalbuminuria will develop within 10–15 years after onset of diabetes and progress over the next 3–7 years to overt proteinuria. During the onset of subclinical proteinuria, aggressive treatment is necessary. Strict glycemic control and treatment of hypertension have been proven to slow progression of disease. In particular, ACE inhibitors and ARBs lower the rate of progression to clinical proteinuria and slow progression to ESRD. They may reduce intraglomerular pressure as well

as treat hypertension. Even in the subset of patients with markedly diminished renal function, ARBs seem to provide renal benefit if patients can tolerate the medication from the perspective of hyperkalemia and the acute decrease in GFR.

The most common lesion in diabetic nephropathy is diffuse glomerulosclerosis, but nodular glomerulosclerosis (Kimmelstiel-Wilson nodules) is pathognomonic. The kidneys in these patients are usually enlarged as a result of cellular hypertrophy and proliferation. At the onset of diabetic nephropathy, glomerular disease will cause an increase in GFR. As the nephropathy progresses, with the development of macroalbuminuria, the GFR returns to normal and continues to decrease.

Patients with diabetes are prone to other renal disease. These include papillary necrosis, chronic interstitial nephritis, and type IV (hyporeninemic hypoaldosteronemic) renal tubular acidosis. Patients are more susceptible to acute renal failure from contrast material and have a poor prognosis once dialysis is begun.

HIV-ASSOCIATED NEPHROPATHY

HIV-associated nephropathy can present as the nephrotic syndrome in patients with HIV infection. Most patients are young black men. In these patients, the more common mode of acquisition of HIV is through injection drug use.

Patients can have a nephrotic picture with normal complement levels. Light microscopy shows focal segmental glomerulosclerosis as described above. Lesions can be of the collapsing variety and often exhibit severe tubulointerstitial damage.

Small, uncontrolled studies have shown that highly active antiretroviral therapy (HAART) for a prolonged course can slow progression of disease. Despite this minimal evidence, HAART has been recommended for use in these patients given the therapy's other beneficial effects and reasonable toxicity profile. Corticosteroid treatment has been used with variable success at a dosage of 1 mg/kg/d along with cyclosporine and ACE inhibitors.

Barnett AH et al; Diabetics Exposed to Telmisartan and Enalapril Study Group: Angiotensin-receptor blockade versus converting-enzyme inhibition in type 2 diabetes and nephropathy. N Engl J Med 2004;351:1952. [PMID: 15516696]

Finne P et al: Incidence of end-stage renal disease in patients with type 1 diabetes. JAMA 2005;294:1782. [PMID: 16219881]

Merlini G et al: Molecular mechanisms of amyloidosis. N Engl J Med 2003;349:583. [PMID: 12904524]

Remuzzi G et al: Clinical practice. Nephropathy in patients with type 2 diabetes. N Engl J Med 2002;346:1145. [PMID: 11948275]

Ruggenenti P et al; Bergamo Nephrologic Diabetes Complications Trial (BENEDICT) Investigators: Preventing microalbuminuria in type 2 diabetes. N Engl J Med 2004;351: 1941. [PMID: 15516697]

Strippoli GF et al: Effects of angiotensin converting enzyme inhibitors and angiotensin II receptor antagonists on mortality and renal outcomes in diabetic nephropathy: systematic review. BMJ 2004;329:828. [PMID: 15459003]

Szczech LA et al: The clinical epidemiology and course of the spectrum of renal diseases associated with HIV infection. Kidney Int 2004;66:1145. [PMID: 15327410]

■ DISEASES DEMONSTRATING NEPHRITIC & NEPHROTIC COMPONENTS

SYSTEMIC LUPUS ERYTHEMATOSUS

Systemic lupus erythematosus is a systemic autoimmune disease in which renal involvement is common. In various series, clinical renal involvement ranges from 35% to 90%.

Patients present with glomerular syndromes such as nephritic or nephrotic syndromes and asymptomatic renal disease. Nonglomerular syndromes include tubulo-interstitial nephritis and vasculitis. All patients with systemic lupus erythematosus should have routine urinalyses to monitor for the appearance of hematuria or proteinuria. If urinary abnormalities are detected, renal biopsy is often performed. The type of glomerular injury depends on the site of immune complex deposition. The World Health Organization (WHO) classifies the renal glomerular lesions as follows: type I, normal; type II, mesangial proliferative; type III, focal and segmental proliferative; type IV, diffuse proliferative; and type V, membranous nephropathy.

Individuals with type I and type II patterns require no treatment. Transformation of these types to a more active lesion is usually accompanied by an increase in lupus serologic activity and evidence of deteriorating renal function (eg, rising serum creatinine, increasing proteinuria). Repeat biopsy to confirm the transformation in these patients is standard. Patients with extensive type III lesions and all type IV lesions should receive aggressive immunosuppressive therapy. Poorest prognostic features in patients with type IV lesions are an elevated serum creatinine, hematocrit less than 26%, and black race. Indications for treatment of type V disease are unclear; however, if superimposed proliferative lesions exist, aggressive therapy should be instituted.

Corticosteroids are the mainstay of treatment (methylprednisolone 1 g intravenously daily for 3 days followed by prednisone, 60 mg orally daily for 4–6 weeks) but are associated with many side effects and may not prevent progression of chronic lesions. Cytotoxic agents, such as cyclophosphamide, are almost always added because they improve long-term renal survival in patients with aggressive type III and type IV nephritis. However, a recent study has shown the potential benefit of mycophenolate mofetil as an alternative form of induction therapy. In a recent randomized noninferiority study, patients using mycophenolate mofetil had similar rates of full remission at 24 weeks in comparison to those using cyclophosphamide. These agents are typically used for 18–24 months

(eg, cyclophosphamide intravenously every month for six doses and then every 3 months for six doses). Studies suggest that mycophenolate mofetil is less toxic than cyclophosphamide, does not cause ovarian failure, and may be more acceptable to patients, although long-term follow-up needs to be examined. Ongoing trials of other therapies include cyclosporine and azathioprine as longer-term options, too. The return of serologic measurements to normal can be useful in monitoring treatment. Markers include double-stranded DNA (dsDNA) antibodies, C3, C4, CH50, and serum creatinine. Urinary protein and sediment are also helpful markers. Patients with systemic lupus erythematosus who undergo dialysis have a favorable prospect for long-term survival. Patients with kidney transplants have recurrent renal disease in 8% of cases.

HEPATITIS C VIRUS INFECTION

Renal disease in the setting of hepatitis C viral infection was not well-recognized until 1993. Now it accounts for approximately 8% of patients with ESRD. Three clinicopathologic glomerular syndromes associated with hepatitis C are secondary membranoproliferative glomerulonephritis, cryoglobulinemic glomerulonephritis, and membranous nephropathy. A type I membranoproliferative glomerulonephritis (MPGN) is the most common lesion in patients requiring renal biopsy. These patients typically have hematuria and proteinuria, hypertension, and anemia. Occasionally, they exhibit the nephrotic syndrome. Many have elevated serum transaminases and an elevated rheumatoid factor. Of patients studied in one series, 50% had hepatomegaly. Hypocomplementemia is very common, with C4 typically more reduced than C3. Cryoglobulinemic disease is discussed above. Membranous glomerulopathy is the least common of the three and presents with a typical nephrotic picture. Neither cryoglobulins nor rheumatoid factor is present.

In patients with MPGN not receiving treatment for liver disease, the question arises whether to initiate therapy for renal disease. The main indications for therapy are poor renal function, nephrotic syndrome, new or worsening hypertension, fibrosis or tubulointerstitial disease on biopsy, and progressive disease. IFN-α may result in suppression of viremia and improvement in hepatic function. Renal function rarely improves unless viral suppression occurs; however, renal function often worsens when therapy is abated. Ribavirin is relatively contraindicated in renal disease because of the dose-related hemolysis that occurs with renal dysfunction. Despite this, some case series have shown benefit with combined IFN-α and ribavirin in closely monitored settings.

IDIOPATHIC MEMBRANOPROLIFERATIVE GLOMERULONEPHRITIS

MPGN in its primary form is an idiopathic syndrome that can present with nephritic or nephrotic features. (The secondary form can be seen in the immune complex, paraprotein deposition, and thrombotic microangiopathic glomerulonephritides discussed above.) Most patients are under 30 years of age. At least two major subgroups are recognized: type I and type II.

Patients with type I MPGN have a history of recent upper respiratory tract infection about a third of the time. Patients typically have a nephrotic picture, and complement levels are low. Histologically, the GBM is thickened because of immune complex deposition and abnormal mesangial cell proliferation between the GBM and the endothelial cells. This gives a characteristic "splitting" appearance to the capillary wall. Immunofluorescence shows IgG, IgM, and granular deposits of C3, C1q, and C4 (Table 22–10).

Type II MPGN often presents with a nephritic picture and is less common than type I. Light microscopy is similar to type I. Serologically, type II is associated with C3 nephritic factor, which is a circulating IgG antibody. Electron microscopy shows a characteristic dense deposit of homogeneous material that replaces part of the GBM.

Treatment of this disorder is controversial. After ruling out secondary causes, it consists of corticosteroid therapy (there is no standard dosage for adults) and antiplatelet drugs (aspirin, 500–975 mg/d, plus dipyridamole 225 mg/d). The rationale for antiplatelet therapy is that platelet consumption is increased in MPGN and may play a role in glomerular injury. Fifty percent of patients used to progress to ESRD in 10 years; these rates may now be slightly lower with the introduction of more aggressive therapy. Less favorable prognostic findings include type II disease, early renal insufficiency, hypertension, and persistent nephrotic syndrome. Both types of MPGN will recur after renal transplantation; however, type II recurs more commonly.

Contreras G et al: Sequential therapies for proliferative lupus nephritis. N Engl J Med 2004;350:971. [PMID: 14999109]

Fine DM: Pharmacological therapy of lupus nephritis. JAMA 2005;293:3053. [PMID: 15972568]

Flanc RS et al: Treatment for lupus nephritis. Cochrane Database Syst Rev 2004;(1):CD002922. [PMID: 14973998]

Ginzler EM et al: Mycophenolate mofetil or intravenous cyclophosphamide for lupus nephritis. N Engl J Med 2005;353: 2219. [PMID: 16306519]

Meyers CM et al: Hepatitis C and renal disease: an update. Am J Kidney Dis 2003;42:631. [PMID: 14520615]

Moroni G et al: Antiphospholipid antibodies are associated with an increased risk for chronic renal insufficiency in patients with lupus nephritis. Am J Kidney Dis 2004;43:28. [PMID: 14712424]

Nakopoulou L: Membranoproliferative glomerulonephritis. Nephrol Dial Transplant 2001;16(Suppl 6):71. [PMID: 11568249]

■ TUBULOINTERSTITIAL DISEASES

Tubulointerstitial disease may be acute or chronic. Acute disease is most commonly associated with toxins and ischemia. Interstitial edema, infiltration with polymorphonuclear neutrophils, and tubular cell necrosis

Table 22–11. Causes of acute tubulointerstitial nephritis.

Drug reactions
  Antibiotics
    β-Lactam antibiotics: methicillin, penicillin, ampicillin, cephalosporins
    Ciprofloxacin
    Erythromycin
    Sulfonamides
    Tetracycline
    Vancomycin
    Trimethoprim-sulfamethoxazole
    Ethambutol
    Rifampin
  Nonsteroidal anti-inflammatory drugs
  Diuretics
    Thiazides
    Furosemide
  Miscellaneous
    Allopurinol
    Cimetidine
    Phenytoin
Systemic infections
  Bacteria
    Streptococcus
    Corynebacterium diphtheriae
    Legionella
  Viruses
    Epstein-Barr virus
  Others
    Mycoplasma
    Rickettsia rickettsii
    Leptospira icterohaemorrhagiae
    Toxoplasma
Idiopathic
  Tubulointerstitial nephritis-uveitis (TIN–U)

can be seen. (See Acute Renal Failure, above, and Table 22–11.) Chronic disease is associated with insult from an acute factor or progressive insult without any obvious acute cause. Interstitial fibrosis and tubular atrophy are present, with a mononuclear cell predominance. The chronic disorders are described below.

CHRONIC TUBULOINTERSTITIAL DISEASES

ESSENTIALS OF DIAGNOSIS

- *Kidney size: small and contracted.*
- *Decreased urinary concentrating ability.*
- *Hyperchloremic metabolic acidosis.*
- *Hyperkalemia.*
- *Reduced GFR.*

General Considerations

There are four main causes of chronic tubulointerstitial disease. These are discussed below. Other causes include multiple myeloma and gout, which are discussed in the section on multisystem disease with variable kidney involvement (below).

A. OBSTRUCTIVE UROPATHY

The most common cause of chronic tubulointerstitial disease is prolonged obstruction of the urinary tract. In partial obstruction, urinary output alternates between polyuria (due to vasopressin insensitivity) and oliguria (due to decreased GFR). Azotemia and hypertension (due to increased renin-angiotensin production) are usually present. The major causes are prostatic disease in men; ureteral calculus in a single functioning kidney; bilateral ureteral calculi; carcinoma of the cervix, colon, and bladder; and retroperitoneal tumors or fibrosis.

Abdominal, rectal, and genitourinary examinations are helpful. Urinalysis can show hematuria, pyuria, and bacteriuria but is often benign. Abdominal ultrasound may detect mass lesions, hydroureter, and hydronephrosis. CT scanning and MRI provide more detailed information.

B. VESICOURETERAL REFLUX

Reflux nephropathy is primarily a disorder of childhood and occurs when urine passes retrograde from the bladder to the kidneys during voiding. It is the second most common cause of chronic tubulointerstitial disease. It occurs as a result of an incompetent vesicoureteral sphincter. Urine can extravasate into the interstitium; an inflammatory response develops, and fibrosis occurs. The inflammatory response is due to either bacteria or normal urinary components.

Patients are adolescents or young adults with hypertension, renal insufficiency, and a history of urinary tract infections as a child. Focal glomerulosclerosis is often seen. This is a cause of substantial proteinuria, unusual in most tubular diseases. Renal ultrasound or IVP can show renal scarring and hydronephrosis. Although most damage occurs before age 5 years, progressive renal deterioration to ESRD continues as a result of the early insults.

C. ANALGESICS

Analgesic nephropathy is most commonly seen in patients who ingest large quantities of analgesic combinations. The drugs of concern are phenacetin, paracetamol, aspirin, and NSAIDs. Chronic ingestion of 1 g/ d for 3 years is the typical amount needed for renal dysfunction. This disorder occurs most frequently in individuals who are using analgesics for chronic headaches, muscular pains, and arthritis. Most patients grossly underestimate their analgesic use.

Tubulointerstitial inflammation and papillary necrosis are seen on pathologic examination. Papillary tip and inner medullary concentrations of some analgesics are tenfold higher than in the renal cortex. Phenacetin— once a common cause of this disorder and now rarely available—is metabolized in the papillae by the prostaglandin hydroperoxidase pathway to reactive intermediates that bind covalently to interstitial cell macromolecules, causing necrosis. Aspirin and other NSAIDs may worsen the damage by decreasing medullary blood flow (via inhibition of prostaglandin synthesis) and decreasing glutathione levels (which are necessary for detoxification).

Patients can exhibit hematuria, mild proteinuria, polyuria (from tubular damage), anemia (from gastrointestinal bleeding), and sterile pyuria. As a result of papillary necrosis, sloughed papillae can be found in the urine. An IVP may be helpful for detecting these—contrast will fill the area of the sloughed papillae, leaving a "ring shadow" sign at the papillary tip.

D. HEAVY METALS

Environmental exposure to heavy metals—such as lead and cadmium—is seen infrequently now in the United States. Chronic lead exposure can lead to tubulointerstitial disease. Individuals at risk are those with occupational exposure (eg, welders who work with lead-based paint) and drinkers of alcohol distilled in automobile radiators (moonshine users). Lead is filtered by the glomerulus and is transported across the proximal convoluted tubules, where it accumulates and causes cell damage. Fibrosed arterioles and cortical scarring also lead to damaged kidneys. Proximal tubular damage leads to decreased secretion of uric acid, resulting in hyperuricemia and saturnine gout. Patients commonly are hypertensive. Diagnosis is most reliably performed with a calcium disodium edetate (EDTA) chelation test. Urinary excretion of more than 600 mg of lead in 24 hours following 1 g of EDTA indicates excessive lead exposure.

Occupational exposure to cadmium also causes proximal tubular dysfunction. Hypercalciuria and nephrolithiasis can be seen. Other heavy metals that can cause tubulointerstitial disease include mercury and bismuth.

Clinical Findings

A. SYMPTOMS AND SIGNS

Polyuria is common because tubular damage leads to inability to concentrate the urine. Dehydration can also occur as a result of a salt-wasting defect in some individuals.

B. LABORATORY FINDINGS

Patients are hyperkalemic because the distal tubules become aldosterone resistant. A hyperchloremic renal tubular acidosis is characteristic. The cause of the renal tubular acidosis is threefold: (1) reduced ammonia production, (2) inability to acidify the distal tubules, and (3) proximal tubular bicarbonate wasting. The urinalysis is nonspecific, as opposed to that seen in acute interstitial nephritis. Proteinuria is typically less than 2 g/d (owing to inability of the proximal tubule to reabsorb freely filterable proteins); a few cells may be seen; and broad waxy casts are often present.

Treatment

Treatment depends first upon identifying the disorder responsible for renal dysfunction. The degree of interstitial fibrosis that has developed can help predict recovery of renal function. Once there is evidence for loss of parenchyma (small shrunken kidneys or interstitial fibrosis on biopsy), nothing can prevent the progression toward ESRD. Treatment is then directed at medical management. Tubular dysfunction may require potassium and phosphorus restriction and sodium, calcium, or bicarbonate supplements.

If hydronephrosis is present, relief of obstruction should be accomplished promptly. Prolonged obstruction leads to further tubular damage—particularly in the distal nephron—which may be irreversible despite relief of obstruction. Neither surgical correction of reflux nor medical therapy with antibiotics can prevent deterioration toward ESRD once renal scarring has occurred.

Patients in whom lead nephropathy is suspected should continue chelation therapy with EDTA if there is no evidence of irreversible renal damage (eg, renal scarring or small kidneys). Continued exposure should be avoided.

Treatment of analgesic nephropathy requires withdrawal of all analgesics. Stabilization or improvement of renal function may occur if significant interstitial fibrosis is not present. Hydration during exposure to analgesics may also have some beneficial effects.

Harris DC: Tubulointerstitial renal disease. Curr Opin Nephrol Hypertens 2001;10:303. [PMID: 11342791]

Huerta C et al: Nonsteroidal anti-inflammatory drugs and risk of ARF in the general population. Am J Kidney Dis 2005;45: 531. [PMID: 15754275]

Kodner CM et al: Diagnosis and management of acute interstitial nephritis. Am Fam Physician 2003;67:2527. [PMID: 12825841]

■ CYSTIC DISEASES OF THE KIDNEY

Renal cysts are epithelium-lined cavities filled with fluid or semisolid material. They develop primarily from renal tubular elements. One or more simple cysts are found in 50% of individuals over the age of 50 years. They are rarely symptomatic and have little clinical significance. In contrast, generalized cystic diseases are associated with cysts scattered throughout the cortex and medulla of both kidneys and can progress to ESRD (Table 22–12).

SIMPLE OR SOLITARY CYSTS

Simple cysts account for 65–70% of all renal masses. They are generally found at the outer cortex and contain fluid that is consistent with an ultrafiltrate of plasma. Most are found incidentally on ultrasonographic examination. Simple cysts are typically asymptomatic but can become infected.

The main concern with simple cysts is to differentiate them from malignancy, abscess, or polycystic kidney disease. Renal cystic disease can develop in dialysis patients. These cysts have a potential for progression to malignancy. Ultrasound and CT scanning are the recommended procedures for evaluating these masses. Simple cysts must meet three sonographic criteria to be considered benign: (1) echo free, (2) sharply demarcated mass with smooth walls, and (3) an enhanced back wall (indicating good transmission through the cyst). Complex cysts can have thick walls, calcifications, solid components, and mixed echogenicity. On CT scan, the simple

Table 22–12. Clinical features of renal cystic disease.

	Simple Renal Cysts	Acquired Renal Cysts	Autosomal Dominant Polycystic Kidney Disease	Medullary Sponge Kidney	Medullary Cystic Kidney
Prevalence	Common	Dialysis patients	1:1000	1:5000	Rare
Inheritance	None	None	Autosomal dominant	None	Autosomal dominant
Age at onset	...	...	20–40	40–60	Adulthood
Kidney size	Normal	Small	Large	Normal	Small
Cyst location	Cortex and medulla	Cortex and medulla	Cortex and medulla	Collecting ducts	Corticomedullary junction
Hematuria	Occasional	Occasional	Common	Rare	Rare
Hypertension	None	Variable	Common	None	None
Associated complications	None	Adenocarcinoma in cysts	Urinary tract infections, renal stones, cerebral aneurysms 10–15%, hepatic cysts 40–60%	Renal stones, urinary tract infections	Polyuria, salt wasting
Renal failure	Never	Always	Frequently	Never	Always

cyst should have a smooth thin wall that is sharply de-marcated. It should not enhance with contrast media. A renal cell carcinoma will enhance but typically is of lower density than the rest of the parenchyma. Arteriography can also be used to evaluate a mass preoperatively. A renal cell carcinoma is hypervascular in 80%, hypovascular in 15%, and avascular in 5% of cases.

If a cyst meets the criteria for being benign, peri-odic reevaluation is the standard of care. If the lesion is not consistent with a simple cyst, surgical exploration is recommended.

AUTOSOMAL DOMINANT POLYCYSTIC KIDNEY DISEASE

This disorder is among the most common hereditary diseases in the United States, affecting 500,000 indi-viduals, or 1 in 800 live births. Fifty percent of pa-tients will have ESRD by age 60 years. The disease has variable penetrance but accounts for 10% of dialysis patients in the United States. At least two genes ac-count for this disorder: *ADPKD1* on the short arm of chromosome 16 (85–90% of patients) and *ADPKD2* on chromosome 4 (10–15%). Patients with the *PKD2* mutation have slower progression of disease and longer life expectancy than those with *PKD1*. Other sporadic cases without these mutations have also been recognized.

Clinical Findings

Abdominal or flank pain and microscopic or gross he-maturia are present in most patients. A history of uri-nary tract infections and nephrolithiasis is common. A family history is positive in 75% of cases, and more than 50% of patients have hypertension (see below) that may antedate the clinical manifestations of the disease. Patients have large kidneys that may be palpa-ble on abdominal examination. The combination of hypertension and an abdominal mass should suggest the disease. Forty to 50 percent have concurrent he-patic cysts. Pancreatic and splenic cysts occur also. He-moglobin and hematocrit tend to be maintained as a result of erythropoietin production by the cysts. The urinalysis may show hematuria and mild proteinuria. In patients with *PKD1*, ultrasonography confirms the diagnosis—two or more cysts in patients under age 30 years (sensitivity of 88.5%), two or more cysts in each kidney in patients age 30–59 years (sensitivity of 100%), and four or more cysts in each kidney in patients age 60 years or older are diagnostic for autosomal domi-nant polycystic kidney disease. If sonographic results are unclear, CT scan is recommended and highly sensitive.

Complications & Treatment

A. Pain

Abdominal or flank pain is caused by infection, bleed-ing into cysts, and nephrolithiasis. Bed rest and anal-gesics are recommended. Cyst decompression can help with chronic pain.

B. Hematuria

Gross hematuria is most commonly due to rupture of a cyst into the renal pelvis, but it can also be caused by a renal stone or urinary tract infection. Hematuria typically resolves within 7 days with bed rest and hy-dration. Recurrent bleeding should suggest the possi-bility of underlying renal cell carcinoma, particularly in men over age 50 years.

C. Renal Infection

An infected renal cyst should be suspected in patients who have flank pain, fever, and leukocytosis. Blood cul-tures may be positive, and urinalysis may be normal be-cause the cyst does not communicate directly with the urinary tract. CT scans can be helpful because an in-fected cyst may have an increased wall thickness. Bacte-rial cyst infections are difficult to treat. Antibiotics with cystic penetration should be used, eg, fluoroquin-olones, trimethoprim-sulfamethoxazole, and chloram-phenicol. Treatment may require 2 weeks of parenteral therapy followed by long-term oral therapy.

D. Nephrolithiasis

Up to 20% of patients have kidney stones, primarily calcium oxalate. Hydration (2–3 L/d) is recommended.

E. Hypertension

Fifty percent of patients have hypertension at time of presentation, and it will develop in most patients dur-ing the course of the disease. Cyst-induced ischemia appears to cause activation of the renin–angiotensin system, and cyst decompression can lower blood pres-sure temporarily. Hypertension should be treated ag-gressively, as this may prolong the time to ESRD. (Di-uretics should be used cautiously since the effect on renal cyst formation is unknown.)

F. Cerebral Aneurysms

About 10–15% of these patients have arterial aneu-rysms in the circle of Willis. Screening arteriography is not recommended unless the patient has a family his-tory of aneurysms or is undergoing elective surgery with a high risk of developing hypertension.

G. Other Complications

Vascular problems include mitral valve prolapse in up to 25% of patients, aortic aneurysms, and aortic valve abnormalities. Colonic diverticula are more common in patients with polycystic kidneys.

Prognosis

No medical therapy has been shown to prevent the de-velopment of renal failure, though treatment of hyper-tension and a low-protein diet may slow the progres-sion of disease.

MEDULLARY SPONGE KIDNEY

This disease is a relatively common and benign disorder that is present at birth and not usually diagnosed until the fourth or fifth decade. It is caused by autosomal dominant mutations in the *MCKD1* or *MCKD2* genes on chromosomes 1 and 16, respectively. Kidneys have a marked irregular enlargement of the medullary and interpapillary collecting ducts. This is associated with medullary cysts that are diffuse, giving a "Swiss cheese" appearance in these regions.

Clinical Findings

Medullary sponge kidney presents with gross or microscopic hematuria, recurrent urinary tract infections, or nephrolithiasis. Common abnormalities are a decreased urinary concentrating ability and nephrocalcinosis; less common is incomplete type I distal renal tubular acidosis. The diagnosis is confirmed with IVP, which shows striations in the papillary portions of the kidney produced by the accumulation of contrast in dilated collecting ducts.

Treatment

There is no known therapy. Adequate fluid intake (2 L/d) helps prevent stone formation. If hypercalciuria is present, thiazide diuretics are recommended because they decrease calcium excretion. Alkali therapy is recommended if renal tubular acidosis is present.

Prognosis

Renal function is well maintained unless there are complications from recurrent urinary tract infections and nephrolithiasis.

JUVENILE NEPHRONOPHTHISIS-MEDULLARY CYSTIC DISEASE

This is a rare disorder associated with almost universal progression to ESRD. The childhood type—juvenile nephronophthisis—is an autosomal recessive disorder caused by mutations in the *NPH1*, *NPH2*, and *NPH3* genes; the type appearing in adulthood—medullary cystic disease—is autosomal dominant. Both types are manifested by multiple small renal cysts at the corticomedullary junction and medulla. The cortex becomes fibrotic, and as the disease progresses, interstitial inflammation and glomerular sclerosis appear.

Clinical Findings

Patients with both forms exhibit polyuria, pallor, and lethargy. Hypertension occurs at the later stages of disease. The juvenile form causes growth retardation and ESRD before age 20 years. Patients require large amounts of salt and water as a result of renal salt wasting. Ultrasound and CT scan show small, scarred kidneys, and an open renal biopsy may be necessary to recover tissue from the corticomedullary junction.

Treatment & Prognosis

There is no current medical therapy that will prevent progression to renal failure. Adequate salt and water intake are essential to replenish renal losses.

Peters DJ et al: Autosomal-dominant polycystic kidney disease: modification of disease progression. Lancet 2001;358:1439. [PMID: 11705510]

Rizk D et al: Cystic and inherited kidney diseases. Am J Kidney Dis 2003;42:1305. [PMID: 14655206]

Terada N et al: Risk factors for renal cysts. BJU Int 2004;93: 1300. [PMID: 15180627]

Torres VE et al: Autosomal dominant polycystic kidney disease. Nefrologia 2003;23(Suppl 1):14. [PMID: 12708359]

Wilson PD: Polycystic kidney disease. N Engl J Med 2004;350: 151. [PMID: 11568249]

■ MULTISYSTEM DISEASES WITH VARIABLE KIDNEY INVOLVEMENT[1]

MULTIPLE MYELOMA

Multiple myeloma is a malignancy of plasma cells (see Chapter 13). Renal involvement occurs in about 25% of all patients. "Myeloma kidney" is the presence of light chain immunoglobulins (Bence Jones protein) in the urine causing renal toxicity. Bence Jones protein causes direct renal tubular toxicity and results in tubular obstruction by precipitating in the tubules. The earliest tubular damage results in Fanconi's syndrome (a type II proximal renal tubular acidosis). The proteinuria seen with multiple myeloma is primarily due to light chains that are not detected on urine dipstick, which mainly detects albumin. Glomerular amyloidosis can develop in patients with multiple myeloma; in these patients, dipstick protein determinations are positive. Hypercalcemia and hyperuricemia are frequently seen. Other conditions resulting in renal dysfunction include plasma cell infiltration of the renal parenchyma and a hyperviscosity syndrome compromising renal blood flow. Therapy for acute renal failure attributed to multiple myeloma includes correction of hypercalcemia, volume repletion, and chemotherapy for the underlying malignancy. Previously, plasmapheresis had been con-

---

[1]Other diseases with variable involvement described elsewhere in this chapter include systemic lupus erythematosus, diabetes mellitus, and the vasculitides such as Wegener's granulomatosis and Goodpasture's disease.

sidered appropriate to decrease the burden of existing monoclonal proteins while awaiting chemotherapeutic regimens to take effect. Recently, however, in the largest randomized prospective trial to date, plasmapheresis did not provide any renal benefit to these patients.

SICKLE CELL DISEASE

Renal dysfunction associated with sickle cell disease is most commonly due to sickling of red blood cells in the renal medulla because of low oxygen tension and hypertonicity. Congestion and stasis lead to hemorrhage, interstitial inflammation, and papillary infarcts. Clinically, hematuria is common. Damage to renal capillaries also leads to diminished concentrating ability. Isosthenuria (urine osmolality equal to that of serum) is routine, and patients can easily become dehydrated. Papillary necrosis occurs as well. These abnormalities are commonly encountered in sickle cell trait. Sickle cell glomerulopathy is less common but will inexorably progress to ESRD. Its primary clinical manifestation is proteinuria. Optimal treatment requires adequate hydration and control of the sickle cell disease.

TUBERCULOSIS

The classic renal manifestation of tuberculosis is the presence of microscopic pyuria with a sterile urine culture—or "sterile pyuria." More often, other bacteria are present in addition. Microscopic hematuria is often present with pyuria. Urine cultures are the gold standard for diagnosis. Three to six first morning midstream specimens should be performed to improve sensitivity. Papillary necrosis and cavitation of the renal parenchyma occur less frequently, as do ureteral strictures and calcifications. Adequate drug therapy can result in resolution of renal involvement.

GOUT & THE KIDNEY

The kidney is the primary organ for excretion of uric acid. Patients with proximal tubular dysfunction have decreased excretion of uric acid and are more prone to gouty attacks. Depending on the pH and uric acid concentration, deposition can occur in the tubules, the interstitium, or the urinary tract. The more alkaline pH of the interstitium causes urate salt deposition, whereas the acidic environment of the tubules and urinary tract causes uric acid crystal deposition at high concentrations.

Three disorders are commonly seen: (1) uric acid nephrolithiasis, (2) acute uric acid nephropathy, and (3) chronic urate nephropathy. Renal dysfunction with uric acid nephrolithiasis stems from obstructive nephropathy. Acute uric acid nephropathy presents similarly to acute tubulointerstitial nephritis with di-

rect toxicity from uric acid crystals. Chronic urate nephropathy is caused by deposition of urate crystals in the alkaline medium of the interstitium; this can lead to fibrosis and atrophy.

Treatment between gouty attacks involves avoidance of food and drugs causing hyperuricemia, aggressive hydration, and pharmacotherapy aimed at reducing serum uric acid levels. These disorders are seen in both "overproducers" and "underexcretors" of uric acid. The latter situation may seem counterintuitive; however, these patients have hyperacidic urine, which explains the deposition of relatively insoluble uric acid crystals.

■ THE KIDNEY & AGING

Renal mass declines progressively after the fourth decade. The renal medulla is spared in comparison to the cortex. Renal blood flow decreases with a resultant increase in arteriolar resistance. This allows for an increased filtration fraction and a relative sparing of the GFR. After the age of 40 years, GFR declines at a rate of approximately 0.8 mL/min/1.73 m^2/yr (though some older patients show little or no change). Serum creatinine values remain relatively constant because of decreased muscle mass along with the decrease in GFR. GFR impairment is partially due to thickening of the GBM, leading to glomerulosclerosis.

Renal tubular changes include impaired sodium handling, decreased concentration and dilutional ability, and impaired acidification. Thus, older patients are more prone to volume overload, hyponatremia and hypernatremia, and acidosis. Decreased renin synthesis and 1α-hydroxylase activity are also observed. These abnormalities can result in hyperkalemia, hypocalcemia, and elevated PTH activity.

More adverse drug reactions occur in older patients. Three main pharmacokinetic changes occur: (1) altered volume of distribution, (2) altered drug half-life, and (3) altered elimination. The latter two are directly related to impaired renal clearance of drug.

The average age of patients starting dialysis is 61 years; the average age of patients receiving dialysis is 65 years. Both are increasing steadily. Hemodialysis is the modality of choice for those with functional impairment. Peritoneal dialysis is tolerated much better in those with cardiovascular disease. Sudden fluid and electrolyte shifts can cause hypotension, ischemia, and arrhythmias.

Renal transplantation is being offered to older individuals more often as it seems to benefit even those over 65 years. The main complications in this population are infection and cardiovascular disease. A reduced corticosteroid requirement with the introduction of steroid-sparing agents, such as cyclosporine, has diminished infection rates.

Clark WF et al; Canadian Apheresis Group: Plasma exchange when myeloma presents as acute renal failure: a randomized, controlled trial. Ann Intern Med 2005;143:777. [PMID: 16330788]

Corso A et al: Urinary proteins in multiple myeloma: correlation with clinical parameters and diagnostic implications. Ann Hematol 2003;82:487. [PMID: 12838370]

Kapoor M et al: Malignancy and renal disease. Crit Care Clin 2001;17:571. [PMID: 11525049]

Kramer HJ et al: The association between gout and nephrolithiasis in men: The Health Professionals' Follow-Up Study. Kidney Int 2003;64:1022. [PMID: 12911552]

Pandit SR et al: Management of renal dysfunction in multiple myeloma. Curr Treat Options Oncol 2003;4:239. [PMID: 12718801]

Scheinman JI: Sickle cell disease and the kidney. Semin Nephrol 2003;23:66. [PMID: 12563602]

Wise GJ et al: Genitourinary manifestations of tuberculosis. Urol Clin North Am 2003;30:111. [PMID: 12580563]

Urology

23

Marshall L. Stoller, MD, Christopher J. Kane, MD, FACS, & Peter R. Carroll, MD, FACS

■ UROLOGIC EVALUATION

HISTORY

Pain

Pain in the genitourinary tract is usually associated with distention of a hollow viscus (ureteral obstruction, urinary retention) or the capsule of an organ (acute prostatitis, acute pyelonephritis). Pain may be local or referred. Pain associated with malignancy is usually a late manifestation and indicative of advanced disease.

A. RENAL PAIN

Pain of renal origin is usually located in the ipsilateral costovertebral angle. It may radiate to the umbilicus and may be referred to the ipsilateral testicle in men or the labium in women. In infection, the pain is typically constant, whereas in obstruction it may come and go. Nausea and vomiting may result from reflex stimulation of the celiac ganglion. Patients with intraperitoneal pathology will typically lie motionless to avoid pain, while patients with renal disease will move about to try to find a more comfortable position.

B. URETERAL PAIN

Ureteral pain is usually acute and a result of obstruction. Distention of the ureter along with hyperperistalsis and spasm of the smooth muscle of the ureter may result in two different pain patterns. Distention may cause a constant dull ache, while the spasms result in colic. The site of obstruction is often predicted by the site of pain. Upper ureteral obstruction may result in pain referred to the scrotum in males or to the labium in females. Midureteral obstruction may cause pain in the lower quadrant and thus may be confused with appendicitis in right-sided ureteral obstruction or diverticulitis in left-sided ureteral obstruction. Lower ureteral obstruction may cause inflammation of the ureteral orifice and thus be associated with symptoms of vesical irritability.

C. VESICAL PAIN

Acute urinary retention results in severe suprapubic discomfort. Chronic urinary retention is usually pain-less despite tremendous vesical distention. Suprapubic pain not related to the act of micturition is rarely vesical in origin. Acute cystitis pain is usually referred to the distal urethra and is associated with micturition.

D. PROSTATIC PAIN

Prostatic pain is associated with inflammation and is located in the perineum. Pain radiates to the lumbosacral spine, inguinal canals, or lower extremities. Because of its location near the bladder neck, inflammatory processes of the prostate result in irritative voiding complaints.

E. PENILE PAIN

Pain in the flaccid penis is secondary to inflammatory processes caused by sexually transmitted diseases or paraphimosis, a condition of the uncircumcised male in which the retracted foreskin is trapped behind the glans penis, resulting in vascular congestion and painful swelling of the glans. Pain in the erect penis may be due to Peyronie's disease (fibrous plaque of the tunica albuginea, resulting in painful curvature of the erect penis) or to priapism (prolonged painful erection).

F. TESTICULAR PAIN

Acute conditions such as trauma, torsion of the testis or one of its appendices, or epididymo-orchitis cause acute pain within the scrotum with radiation to the ipsilateral groin. Chronic pain may persist for months following successful treatment of acute epididymitis. Chronic pain produced by a varicocele or hydrocele results in "heaviness" without radiation. Disorders of the kidney, retroperitoneal structures, or inguinal canal may result in pain referred to the testis.

Hematuria

Gross hematuria in adults is considered a sign of malignancy until proved otherwise.

The character of the hematuria may provide a clue to the site of origin. **Initial hematuria**, the presence of blood at the beginning of the urinary stream that clears during the stream, implies an anterior (penile) urethral source. **Terminal hematuria**, the presence of blood at the end of the urinary stream, implies a bladder neck or prostatic urethral source. **Total hematuria**, the presence of blood throughout the urinary stream, implies a bladder or upper tract source.

954

Associated symptoms provide clues to the cause. Hematuria associated with renal colic suggests ureteral stone, but the passage of blood clots from a bleeding tumor mimics this scenario. Irritative voiding symptoms in a young woman may suggest acute bacterial infection and associated hemorrhagic cystitis, yet the same picture in an older woman or in any male raises concerns about neoplasm. In any situation, if cultures are negative or hematuria persists after therapy, further evaluation is warranted. In the absence of other symptoms, gross hematuria may be more indicative of tumor, but staghorn calculi, glomerulonephropathies, and polycystic kidney disease are in the differential.

Irritative Voiding Symptoms

Urgency is the sudden desire to void. It is observed in inflammatory conditions such as cystitis or in hyperreflexic neuropathic conditions such as neurogenic bladders resulting from upper motor neuron lesions. **Dysuria** (painful urination) is usually associated with inflammation. The pain is typically referred to the tip of the penis in men or to the urethra in women. **Frequency** is the increased number of voids during the daytime, and **nocturia** is nocturnal frequency. Adults normally void five or six times a day and once at most during the nighttime hours. Increased numbers of voidings may result from increased urinary output or decreased functional bladder capacity. Diabetes mellitus, diabetes insipidus, excess fluid ingestion, and diuretics (including caffeine and alcohol) are a few of the causes of increased urinary output. Decreased functional bladder capacities may result from bladder outlet obstruction (increased residual urine volume results in a lower functional capacity), neurogenic bladder disorders (spasticity and reduced compliance), extrinsic bladder compression (uterine fibroids, radiation-induced fibrosis, pelvic neoplasms), or psychological factors (anxiety).

Obstructive Voiding Symptoms

Hesitancy is a delay in the initiation of micturition. It results from the increased time required for the bladder to attain the high pressure necessary to exceed that of the urethra in the obstructed setting. **Decreased force of stream** results from the high resistance the bladder faces and is often associated with a decrease in caliber of the stream. **Intermittency** and **postvoid dribbling** are interruption of the urinary stream and the uncontrolled release of the terminal few drops of urine, respectively. Obstructive symptoms are most commonly due to benign prostatic hyperplasia, urethral stricture, or neurogenic bladder disorders. Prostatic or urethral carcinoma and foreign body are other causes.

Incontinence

Urinary incontinence is the involuntary loss of urine. The history permits subclassification into one of four categories of incontinence. Such a distinction is necessary, as the evaluation and treatment vary with each of the categories. With **total incontinence**, patients lose urine at all times and in all positions. **Stress incontinence** is the loss of urine associated with activities that result in an increase in intra-abdominal pressure (coughing, sneezing, lifting, exercising). Uncontrolled loss of urine preceded by a strong urge to void is known as **urge incontinence**. Chronic urinary retention may result in **overflow incontinence**.

Systemic Manifestations

Fever, when associated with other symptoms of a urinary tract infection (see below), helps localize the site of infection. In women, high fevers occur in acute pyelonephritis. Fevers are not typical of uncomplicated cystitis. In men, a febrile urinary tract infection implies acute pyelonephritis, acute prostatitis, or acute epididymitis. Fever may also be associated with malignancy of the kidney, bladder, or testis.

Weight loss and malaise may also be associated with tumor or disease states associated with chronic renal failure.

Other Symptoms

Hematospermia, the presence of blood in the ejaculate, results from inflammation of the prostate or seminal vesicles. Blood in the initial portion of the ejaculate implicates the prostate, whereas terminal hematospermia implies a seminal vesicle origin. Workup should include urinalysis, digital rectal examination (DRE) with prostate massage, and microscopic evaluation of the expressed prostatic secretions. More invasive procedures such as cystoscopy or transrectal ultrasound with prostate biopsy are reserved for patients with hematuria or abnormal rectal examinations, respectively. Persistent hematospermia warrants similar testing. The risk of malignancy with isolated hematospermia, normal urinalysis, and normal DRE is low.

Pneumaturia, the presence of gas in the urine, is usually secondary to a fistula between the bladder and the gastrointestinal tract. Diverticulitis is the most common cause, followed by colonic carcinoma, Crohn's disease, and radiation enteritis. The patient reports bubbles or particulate matter in the urine. On occasion, pneumaturia may be due to infection by gas-producing organisms.

Urethral discharge is the most common symptom of sexually transmitted diseases. Dysuria and urethral itching are seen in association with the discharge. A bloody urethral discharge, especially in an elderly patient, suggests urethral carcinoma.

Cloudy urine may be secondary to a urinary tract infection, yet in the absence of infection it can be a result of an alkaline urinary pH. Such conditions result in phosphate crystal precipitation. Chyluria, the presence of lymph in the urine, results from a fistula between the urinary tract and the lymphatic system. Filariasis, tuberculosis, and retroperitoneal tumors are some of the possible causes of this rare symptom.

PHYSICAL EXAMINATION

General Examination

The pallor of anemia and cachexia may be seen in malignancy. Gynecomastia may occur with testicular carcinomas or as a complication of hormonal therapy in prostatic cancer. Hypertension can be a result of renovascular disease or adrenal cancer.

Detailed Examination

A. KIDNEY

Because of the liver, the right kidney is lower than the left. The lower pole of the right kidney may be palpable in thin patients, yet the left kidney is usually not palpable unless abnormally enlarged. To palpate the kidney, one hand is placed posteriorly over the costovertebral angle to push the kidney anteriorly, while the second hand is placed anteriorly under the costal margin. With inspiration, the kidney may be palpated between the two hands.

Auscultation of the upper abdominal quadrants in hypertensive patients may reveal a systolic bruit associated with renal artery stenosis or an arteriovenous malformation; however, aortic bruits or transmitted heart murmurs may give similar findings.

Patients with flank pain should be tested for hyperesthesia of the overlying skin by pin testing, as this may be secondary to nerve root irritation and radiculitis rather than being of renal origin.

B. BLADDER

The normal adult bladder is not palpable unless filled with at least 150 mL of urine. Percussion is better than palpation in diagnosing the distended bladder. Dullness is appreciated over the full bladder and changes to tympany if the air-filled bowel is anterior to the bladder.

Bimanual examination under anesthesia is helpful in the evaluation of patients with suspected bladder neoplasms. In the male, the bladder is palpated between the abdominal wall and the rectum while in the female it is palpated between the abdominal wall and the vagina. This is the best means of assessing vesical mobility and thus resectability.

C. PENIS

The foreskin must be retracted in the uncircumcised male to permit inspection of the urethral meatus and glans. The position of the urethral meatus and the presence of urethral discharge, inflammation, penile tumor, and skin lesions must be noted. In **phimosis**, the foreskin cannot be retracted over the glans. In **paraphimosis**, the foreskin has been left retracted behind the glans, resulting in painful engorgement and edema of the glans. If not attended to, this may result in glandu-

lar ischemia. Congenital anomalies of position of the urethral meatus are called **hypospadias** when the meatus is located on the ventral aspect of the penis, scrotum, or perineum and **epispadias** when it is located on the dorsal aspect of the penis. A thick yellow urethral discharge is seen in gonococcal urethritis, whereas a thin clear or white discharge is noted in nongonococcal urethritis. Palpation of the dorsal penile shaft for plaques of Peyronie's disease and of the ventral surface for urethral tumors should be performed.

D. SCROTUM AND ITS CONTENTS

The most common referral to the urologist concerning the scrotum is for evaluation of a mass. It is important to determine whether the lesion resides within the testicle or is related to the epididymis or cord structures. The testes are palpated between the fingertips of both hands. Normal testes measure 4.5×2.5 cm and are rubbery in consistency. The epididymis rests posterolateral to the testis and varies in its degree of testicular attachment. Masses arising from within the testes are usually malignant; those from the epididymis and spermatic cord structures are usually benign. Transillumination will frequently distinguish solid and cystic lesions.

The history and physical examination can determine the diagnosis in the majority of cases. Tumors of the testis are usually painless, firm, solid lesions within the substance of the testis. These lesions do not transilluminate.

Acute epididymitis is an acute infectious process and is associated with painful enlargement of the epididymis. Fever and irritative voiding symptoms are common. In advanced states, the infection can spread to the testis, making the distinction between the epididymis and the testicle difficult on physical examination. The entire scrotal contents may be painful on palpation, yet relief may be offered to the supine patient by elevation of the scrotum above the pubic symphysis (Prehn's sign).

A **hydrocele** is a collection of fluid between the two layers of the tunica vaginalis. The diagnosis is readily made by transillumination. Evaluation of the testis is necessary, as approximately 10% of testicular tumors may have an associated hydrocele.

A **varicocele** is engorgement of the internal spermatic veins above the testis. These almost always occur on the left side as the left spermatic vein empties into the left renal vein while the right empties into the inferior vena cava below the level of the renal vein. Varicoceles should diminish in size or disappear with the patient in the supine position. The sudden onset of a right varicocele should raise the question of a retroperitoneal malignancy resulting in obstruction of the right spermatic vein.

Torsion of the testis typically occurs in the 10- to 20-year age group and presents with acute onset of pain and swelling within the testis. Examination reveals a painful testis that may have a "high lie" in relation to the other testis. The acute onset, lack of voiding symptoms, and the different age distribution may help distinguish it from epididymitis.

Torsion of the appendices of the testis or epididymis may be indistinguishable from torsion of the testis and affects a similar age group as torsion of the testis. On occasion a small palpable lump on the superior pole of the testis or epididymis is discernible that may appear blue when the skin is pulled tautly over it ("blue dot sign").

E. RECTAL EXAMINATION IN THE MALE

Inspection for anal pathology (fissures, warts, carcinoma, hemorrhoids) should be performed first. Upon insertion of the finger, anal tone can be estimated and a bulbocavernosus reflex can be elicited. As the anal and urinary sphincter derive from a common innervation, clues to neurogenic disorders may be obtained. The entire prostate is then examined, with attention being directed toward size and consistency. The normal prostate is approximately 4×4 cm and weighs 25 g. Normal consistency is that of the contracted thenar eminence with the thumb opposed to the little finger. Rubbery enlargement of the prostate is noted in benign prostatic hyperplasia. Induration may be perceived with carcinoma but also with chronic inflammation. The remainder of the rectum is then examined to exclude primary rectal disease.

F. PELVIC EXAMINATION IN THE FEMALE

Examination of the introitus should include inspection for atrophic changes, ulcers, discharge, and warts. The urethral meatus can be inspected for caruncles (more commonly seen in postmenopausal patients, and as a reddened area at the inferior margin of the meatus) and palpated for tumors or diverticula. Bimanual examination of the bladder, uterus, and adnexa should be performed with two fingers in the vagina and one hand on the abdomen, and attention is directed toward abnormal masses.

URINALYSIS

Collection of Specimens

In the male, a clean-catch urine specimen is obtained in separate aliquots. Such a scheme may permit localization of disease. The first 5–10 mL is collected and represents the urethral specimen; a midstream specimen reflects conditions in the bladder and upper urinary tracts. If necessary, the prostate is then massaged and the expressed secretions collected. If no fluid is obtained, the next 2–3 mL of urine is collected, which reflects prostatic pathology. (See also Hematuria.)

Dipstick Urinalysis

A. PH

There is no role for dipstick urinalysis screening for urinary tract disorders in asymptomatic adults except for pregnant women. Urinary pH (range 5.0–8.0) may be helpful in the diagnosis and treatment of some uro-

logic conditions. Alkaline urine in a patient with a urinary tract infection suggests the presence of a urea-splitting organism, most commonly *Proteus mirabilis*, though some strains of *Klebsiella*, *Pseudomonas*, *Providencia*, and *Staphylococcus* may also produce urease. Acidic urine in a patient with urolithiasis suggests uric acid or cystine stones. Failure to acidify the urine below a pH of 5.5 despite a metabolic acidosis suggests a distal renal tubular acidosis.

B. PROTEIN

Dipsticks using bromphenol blue can detect protein in concentrations exceeding 10 mg/dL. It measures albumin and is not sensitive for the light chain of immunoglobulins (Bence Jones proteins). False-positive results are seen in urine containing numerous leukocytes or epithelial cells. (See Proteinuria in Chapter 22.)

C. UROBILINOGEN AND BILIRUBIN

Urobilinogen is formed from the catabolism of conjugated bilirubin in the gut by bacteria, and the majority is cleared by the liver. Normally, only 1–4 mg of urobilinogen is excreted in the urine per day. Hemolytic processes or hepatocellular disease can lead to increased urinary levels, while complete biliary obstruction or broad-spectrum antibiotics that alter the gut bacterial flora may result in absent urinary urobilinogen. Unconjugated bilirubin is not filtered by the glomerulus, while only 1% of conjugated bilirubin is filtered. Normally no bilirubin is detected by urinary dipstick, since only concentrations greater than 0.4 mg/dL are detectable. Conditions manifesting elevated conjugated bilirubin in the serum will result in higher urinary levels. Ascorbic acid may cause false-negative results, while phenazopyridine may cause false-positive results.

D. GLUCOSE AND KETONES

Only small amounts of glucose are normally excreted in the urine, and these levels are below the sensitivity of the dipstick. Any positive finding requires evaluation for diabetes. The test is specific for glucose and does not cross-react with any other sugars. Ascorbic acid or elevated ketones may result in false-negative results.

Ketones are not normally found in the urine, but fasting, postexercise states, and pregnancy may result in elevated urinary ketones. Diabetics often demonstrate elevated urinary ketone levels prior to an elevation in serum levels. False-positive results occur in dehydration or in the presence of levodopa metabolites, mesna (sodium mercaptoethanesulfonate), and other sulfhydryl-containing compounds.

E. NITRITES

Normally, the urine does not contain nitrites. Many gram-negative bacteria can reduce nitrate to nitrite, which is thus an indicator of bacteriuria. However, the low sensitivity of the test requires clarification. Adequate numbers of bacteria must be present (10^5 organisms/mL), nitrates must be available in the urine, and the bacteria must be in contact with the urine for a sufficient time (usually 4 hours). Therefore, the first morning voided sample is preferable. False-negative results may be due to non–nitrate-reducing organisms, frequent urination, dilute or acidic urine (pH < 6.0), and the presence of urobilinogen. False-positive results are usually secondary to contaminated specimens, so that bacteria are indeed present in the sample yet not present in the urinary tract.

F. LEUKOCYTE ESTERASE

Leukocyte esterase is an enzyme produced by white cells. The dipstick detects leukocytes in the urine, which is thus suggestive but not diagnostic for bacteria. False-positive tests result from specimen contamination. False-negative tests result from high specific gravity, glycosuria, the presence of urobilinogen, and medications, including rifampin, phenazopyridine, and ascorbic acid.

G. BLOOD

The urinary dipstick for blood measures intact erythrocytes, free hemoglobin, and myoglobin. False-positive results in women may occur as a result of contamination at collection with menstrual blood. Concentrated urine may also cause a false-positive result, as patients normally excrete 1000 erythrocytes per milliliter of urine. Vigorous exercise and vitamins or foods associated with high oxidant levels may also give a false-positive result. High ascorbic acid levels may give a false-negative result.

Microscopic Urinalysis

A. LEUKOCYTES

The presence of more than five leukocytes per high-power field is considered significant pyuria. Leukocytes in the urine are indicative of injury to the urinary tract, which may or may not be due to infection. Other causes of pyuria include calculous disease, strictures, neoplasm, genitourinary tuberculosis, glomerulonephropathy, or interstitial cystitis. Leukocyte counts will vary by the state of hydration, method of collection, and degree of injury to the urinary tract.

B. ERYTHROCYTES

The presence of more than five erythrocytes per high-power field on a single occasion or more than three erythrocytes per high-power field on multiple examinations is considered significant and warrants further investigation. (See Evaluation of Hematuria, below.) The appearance of the red cells sometimes provides a clue to their origin within the urinary tract. Dysmorphic (irregularly shaped) cells have an uneven distribution of hemoglobin and cytoplasm, and usually indicate glomerular disease. Red cells that are round, with evenly distributed hemoglobin, suggest disease along the epithelial lining of the urinary tract. All patients with hematuria (even with concurrent anticoagulants) require further diagnostic workup (see below); mor-

phology, though of interest, is not of sufficient accuracy to allow firm diagnostic conclusions.

C. EPITHELIAL CELLS

The presence of squamous epithelial cells in the urinary sediment is indicative of contamination and thus requires a repeat collection. Transitional epithelial cells are occasionally noted in normal urinary sediment, but if present in large numbers or clumps they cause concern about possible neoplasm. Cytologic examination may be necessary to confirm the finding.

D. BACTERIA AND YEASTS

The identification of organisms in an uncontaminated specimen implies infection, which must be confirmed by culture. The presence of several organisms per high-power field usually correlates with a culture count of 10^5 organisms per milliliter. Gram staining may further aid in characterizing the organism. *Candida albicans* is the most common yeast seen in the urine, and characteristic budding and clumps are typically observed. For yeast, colony count per milliliter does not necessarily correlate with the severity of infection.

E. CASTS

Casts are formed in the distal tubules and collecting ducts as a result of Tamm–Horsfall mucoprotein precipitation (the most common excreted protein in urine). They congregate near the edges of the coverslip and are detected best in a fresh specimen viewed under low power. If the urine is devoid of cells, hyaline casts are formed. Casts with entrapped red cells are indicative of glomerulonephritis or vasculitis. Leukocyte casts are suggestive of pyelonephritis. Epithelial casts in small numbers are normal, but in large numbers they suggest intrinsic renal disease. Granular casts result from degeneration of other cellular casts and also suggest intrinsic renal disease.

F. CRYSTALS

Uric acid, oxalate, and cystine crystals are more often precipitated in acid urine, while phosphate crystals are more commonly seen in alkaline urine. The presence of uric acid, phosphate, and oxalate crystals can be seen in normal patients as well as in stone-formers. Cystine crystals, with a characteristic hexagonal benzene ring shape, are seen only in patients with cystinuria and are thus pathologic.

■ EVALUATION OF HEMATURIA

If gross hematuria occurs, a description of the timing (initial, terminal, total) may provide a clue to the localization of disease. Associated symptoms (ie, renal colic, irritative voiding symptoms, constitutional symptoms) should be investigated. Drug ingestion and associated medical problems may also provide diagnostic clues. Anticoagulants, analgesic abuse (papillary necrosis), cyclophosphamide (chemical cystitis), antibiotics (interstitial nephritis), diabetes mellitus, sickle cell trait or disease (papillary necrosis), a history of stone disease, or malignancy should all be investigated. The presence of hematuria in patients receiving anticoagulation therapy warrants a complete evaluation consisting of upper tract imaging, cystoscopy, and urine cytology.

Physical examination should emphasize signs of systemic disease (fever, rash, lymphadenopathy, abdominal or pelvic masses) as well as signs of medical renal disease (hypertension, volume overload). Urologic evaluation may demonstrate an enlarged prostate, flank mass, or urethral disease.

Initial laboratory investigations include a urinalysis and urine culture. Proteinuria and casts suggest renal origin. Irritative voiding symptoms, bacteriuria, and a positive urine culture in the female suggest urinary tract infection, but follow-up urinalysis is important after treatment to ensure resolution of the hematuria.

Further evaluation includes urinary cytology, upper tract imaging, and cystoscopy. Cytology especially assists in the diagnosis of bladder neoplasm, and three voided samples are recommended to maximize sensitivity. Upper tract imaging (usually abdominal and pelvic CT scanning with and without contrast) may identify neoplasms of the kidney or ureter as well as identifying benign conditions such as urolithiasis, obstructive uropathy, papillary necrosis, medullary sponge kidney, or polycystic kidney disease. CT urography and MRI have replaced intravenous pyelography (IVP) when imaging the upper tracts for sources of hematuria. The role of ultrasonographic evaluation of the urinary tract for hematuria is unclear. Although it may provide adequate information for the kidney, its sensitivity in detecting ureteral disease is lower. In addition, its higher degree of operator dependence may further confound the issue. Cystoscopy can be used to assess for bladder or urethral neoplasm, benign prostatic enlargement, and radiation or chemical cystitis. For gross hematuria, cystoscopy is ideally performed while the patient is actively bleeding to allow better localization (ie, lateralize to one side of the upper tracts, bladder, or urethra).

In patients with gross or microscopic hematuria, an upper tract source (kidneys and ureters) can be identified in 10% of cases. For upper tract sources, stone disease accounts for 40%, medical renal disease (medullary sponge kidney, glomerulonephritis, papillary necrosis) for 20%, renal cell carcinoma for 10%, and transitional cell carcinoma of the ureter or renal pelvis for 5%. In the absence of infection, gross hematuria from a lower tract source is most commonly from transitional cell carcinoma of the bladder. Microscopic hematuria in the male is most commonly from benign prostatic hyperplasia. In patients with negative evaluations, repeat evaluations are warranted to avoid a missed malignancy; however, the ideal frequency of such evaluations is not defined. Urinary cytology can

be repeated in 3–6 months, and cystoscopy and upper tract imaging after a year.

Avidor Y et al: Clinical significance of gross hematuria and its evaluation in patients receiving anticoagulant and aspirin treatment. Urology 2000;55:22. [PMID: 10654888]

Chow KM et al: Asymptomatic isolated microscopic haematuria: long-term follow-up. QJM 2004;97:739. [PMID: 15496530]

Grossfeld G et al: Evaluation of asymptomatic microscopic hematuria in adults: the American Urological Association best practice policy—part I: definition, detection, prevalence, and etiology. Urology 2001;57:599. [PMID: 11306356]

Ripley TL et al: Early evaluation of hematuria in a patient receiving anticoagulant therapy and detection of malignancy. Pharmacotherapy 2004;24:1638. [PMID: 15537566]

Rosenstein D et al: Urologic emergencies. Med Clin North Am 2004;88:495. [PMID: 15049590]

Yun EJ et al: Evaluation of the patient with hematuria. Med Clin North Am 2004;88:329. [PMID: 15049581]

■ GENITOURINARY TRACT INFECTIONS

Urinary tract infections are among the most common entities encountered in medical practice. In acute infections, a single pathogen is usually found, whereas two or more pathogens are often seen in chronic infections. Coliform bacteria are responsible for most non-nosocomial, uncomplicated urinary tract infections, with *Escherichia coli* being the most common. Such infections typically are sensitive to a wide variety of orally administered antibiotics and respond quickly. Nosocomial infections often are due to more resistant pathogens and may require parenteral antibiotics. Renal infections are of particular concern because if they are inadequately treated, loss of renal function may result. Previously, a colony count $> 10^5$/mL was considered the criterion for urinary tract infection. However, it is now recognized that up to 50% of women with symptomatic infections have lower counts. In addition, the presence of pyuria correlates poorly with the diagnosis of urinary tract infection, and thus urinalysis alone is not adequate for diagnosis. With respect to treatment, soft-tissue infections (pyelonephritis, prostatitis) require intensive therapy for 1–2 weeks, while mucosal infections (cystitis) may require 1–3 days of therapy.

Classification & Pathogenesis

First infections—ie, first documented infections—in young women tend to be uncomplicated. **Unresolved bacteriuria** occurs when the urinary tract is never sterilized during therapy. This may result from bacterial resistance to therapy, noncompliance, mixed infections with organisms having different susceptibilities, renal insufficiency, or the rapid emergence of resistance from an initially sensitive organism. **Persistent bacteriuria** occurs when the urinary tract is initially sterilized during therapy but a persistent source of infection in contact with the urinary tract remains. This may result from infected stones, chronic pyelonephritis or prostatitis, vesicoenteric or vesicovaginal fistulas, obstructive uropathy, foreign bodies, or urethral diverticula. **Reinfections** occur when new infections with new pathogens occur following successful treatment.

Ascending infection from the urethra is the most common route. Women are particularly at risk for urinary tract infections because the female urethra is short and the vagina becomes colonized with bacteria. Sexual intercourse is a major precipitating factor in young women, and the use of diaphragms and spermicidal creams (alters normal vaginal bacterial flora) further increases the risk for cystitis. Pyelonephritis most commonly results from ascent of infection up the ureter. **Hematogenous spread** to the urinary tract is uncommon, the exceptions being tuberculosis and cortical renal abscesses. **Lymphogenous spread** is rare. **Direct extension** from other organs may occur, especially from intraperitoneal abscesses in inflammatory bowel disease or pelvic inflammatory disease.

Susceptibility Factors

A. BACTERIAL VIRULENCE FACTORS

Over 90% of first infections are caused by *E coli*. Although there are over 150 strains of *E coli*, most infections are caused by only five serogroups (O1, O4, O6, O18, and O75). It appears that strains implicated in infection have a higher degree of bacterial adherence, which is mediated by the bacterial fimbriae or pili. A relationship between the type of fimbriae and the type of infection exists. P-fimbriated strains of *E coli* are associated with pyelonephritis in normal urinary tracts, whereas strains without P fimbriae are associated with pyelonephritis only when vesicoureteral reflux is present.

B. HOST SUSCEPTIBILITY FACTORS

1. Bladder and upper tract factors—Intrinsic defense mechanisms in the bladder include efficient emptying of the bladder with voiding, which decreases colony counts; a protective glycosaminoglycan layer, which interferes with bacterial adherence; and the antimicrobial properties of urine (high osmolality and extremes of pH). The presence of vesicoureteral reflux, diminished renal blood flow, or intrinsic renal disease may increase the likelihood of upper tract involvement.

2. Female-specific factors—The anatomically short female urethra facilitates the ascent of organisms from the introitus into the bladder. Women with recurrent urinary tract infections have more adhesive receptors on their genitourinary mucosa and therefore have more binding sites for pathogens. Women whose mucosal secretions lack fucosyltransferase activity ("nonsecretors") are more prone to urinary tract infections. The lack of this enzyme results in lack of expression of the A, B, and H blood group antigens that normally may mask some of the bacterial adhesin receptors, making these receptors more available for pathogen binding.

3. Male-specific factors—A higher incidence of urinary tract infections in the uncircumcised male in comparison to the circumcised male has been observed. The mucosal surface of the foreskin has a propensity for colonization with P-fimbriated bacteria in a fashion analogous to that of the female introitus. The prostate in normal males secretes zinc, which is a potent antibacterial agent and thus prevents ascending infection. Lower zinc levels are seen in prostatic secretions of men with bacterial prostatitis.

Prevention of Reinfections

Prophylactic antibiotic therapy is given to prevent recurrence after treatment of urinary tract infection. Women who have more than three episodes of cystitis per year are considered candidates for prophylaxis. Prior to institution of therapy, a thorough urologic evaluation is warranted to exclude any anatomic abnormality (stones, reflux, fistula, etc). Only selected antimicrobial agents are effective in prophylaxis. To be successful, the agent must eliminate pathogenic bacteria from the fecal or introital reservoirs and not cause bacterial resistance. Single dosing at bedtime or at the time of intercourse is the recommended schedule. The three most commonly used agents for prophylaxis are trimethoprim-sulfamethoxazole (40 mg/200 mg), nitrofurantoin (100 mg), and cephalexin (250 mg).

Deville WL et al: The urine dipstick test useful to rule out infections. A meta-analysis of the accuracy. BMC Urol 2004;4:4. [PMID: 15175113]

Hooton TM et al: Acute uncomplicated cystitis in an era of increasing antibiotic resistance: a proposed approach to empirical therapy. Clin Infect Dis 2004;39:75. [PMID: 15206056]

Johnson JR: Laboratory diagnosis of urinary tract infections in adult patients. Clin Infect Dis 2004;39:873. [PMID: 15472825]

Liu H et al: Appropriate antibiotic treatment of genitourinary infections in hospitalized patients. Am J Med 2005;118(Suppl 7A):14S. [PMID: 15993673]

Miller LG et al: Treatment of uncomplicated urinary tract infections in an era of increasing antimicrobial resistance. Mayo Clin Proc 2004;79:1048. [PMID: 15301333]

Tambyah PA: Catheter-associated urinary tract infections: diagnosis and prophylaxis. Int J Antimicrob Agents 2004;24(Suppl 1):44. [PMID: 15364306]

ACUTE CYSTITIS

 ESSENTIALS OF DIAGNOSIS

- *Irritative voiding symptoms.*
- *Patient usually afebrile.*
- *Positive urine culture; blood cultures may also be positive.*

General Considerations

Acute cystitis is an infection of the bladder most commonly due to the coliform bacteria (especially *E coli*) and occasionally gram-positive bacteria (enterococci). The route of infection is typically ascending from the urethra. Viral cystitis due to adenovirus is sometimes seen in children but is rare in adults.

Clinical Findings

A. SYMPTOMS AND SIGNS

Irritative voiding symptoms (frequency, urgency, dysuria) and suprapubic discomfort are common. Women may experience gross hematuria, and symptoms in women may often appear following sexual intercourse. Physical examination may elicit suprapubic tenderness, but examination is often unremarkable. Systemic toxicity is absent.

B. LABORATORY FINDINGS

Urinalysis shows pyuria and bacteriuria and varying degrees of hematuria. The degree of pyuria and bacteriuria does not necessarily correlate with the severity of symptoms. Urine culture is positive for the offending organism, but colony counts exceeding 10^5/mL are not essential for the diagnosis.

C. IMAGING

Follow-up imaging is warranted only if pyelonephritis, recurrent infections, or anatomic abnormalities are suspected.

Differential Diagnosis

In women, infectious processes such as vulvovaginitis and pelvic inflammatory disease can usually be distinguished by pelvic examination and urinalysis. In men, urethritis and prostatitis may be distinguished by physical examination (urethral discharge or prostatic tenderness). Cystitis in men is rare and implies a pathologic process such as infected stones, prostatitis, or chronic urinary retention requiring further investigation.

Noninfectious causes of cystitis-like symptoms include pelvic irradiation, chemotherapy (cyclophosphamide), bladder carcinoma, interstitial cystitis, voiding dysfunction disorders, and psychosomatic disorders.

Treatment

Uncomplicated cystitis in women can be treated with short-term antimicrobial therapy, which consists of single-dose therapy or 1–3 days of therapy. Trimethoprim-sulfamethoxazole can be ineffective in significant numbers of patients because of the emergence of resistant organisms. Fluoroquinolones and nitrofurantoin are now the drugs of choice for uncomplicated cystitis (Table 23–1). Because uncomplicated cystitis is rare in men, elucidation of the underlying problem with ap-

propriate investigations is warranted. Hot sitz baths or urinary analgesics (phenazopyridine, 200 mg orally three times daily) may provide symptomatic relief.

Prognosis

Infections typically respond rapidly to therapy, and failure to respond suggests resistance to the selected drug or anatomic abnormalities requiring further investigation.

Fihn SD: Clinical practice. Acute uncomplicated urinary tract infection in women. N Engl J Med 2003;349:259. [PMID: 12867610]

Gupta K: Addressing antibiotic resistance. Dis Mon 2003;49:99. [PMID: 12601340]

Nicolle LE: Urinary tract infection: traditional pharmacologic therapies. Am J Med 2002;113(Suppl 1A):35S. [PMID: 12113870]

ACUTE PYELONEPHRITIS

 ESSENTIALS OF DIAGNOSIS

- *Fever.*
- *Flank pain.*
- *Irritative voiding symptoms.*
- *Positive urine culture.*

General Considerations

Acute pyelonephritis is an infectious inflammatory disease involving the kidney parenchyma and renal pelvis. Gram-negative bacteria are the most common causative agents including *E coli*, *Proteus*, *Klebsiella*, *Enterobacter*, and *Pseudomonas*. Gram-positive bacteria are less commonly seen but include *Enterococcus faecalis* and *Staphylococcus aureus*. The infection usually ascends from the lower urinary tract—with the exception of *S aureus*, which usually is spread by a hematogenous route.

Clinical Findings

A. SYMPTOMS AND SIGNS

Symptoms include fever, flank pain, shaking chills, and irritative voiding symptoms (urgency, frequency, dysuria). Associated nausea and vomiting, and diarrhea are common. Signs include fever and tachycardia. Costovertebral angle tenderness is usually pronounced.

B. LABORATORY FINDINGS

Complete blood count shows leukocytosis and a left shift. Urinalysis shows pyuria, bacteriuria, and varying degrees of hematuria. White cell casts may be seen. Urine culture demonstrates heavy growth of the offending agent, and blood culture may also be positive.

Table 23–1. Empirical therapy for urinary tract infections.

Diagnosis	Antibiotic	Route	Duration	Cost per Duration Noted[1]
Acute pyelonephritis	Ampicillin, 1 g every 6 hours, and gentamicin, 1 mg/kg every 8 hours	Intravenously	21 days	$780.00 not including intravenous supplies
	Ciprofloxacin, 750 mg every 12 hours	Orally	21 days	$229.00
	Ofloxacin, 200–300 mg every 12 hours	Orally	21 days	$270.00
	Trimethoprim-sulfamethoxazole, 160/800 mg every 12 hours[2]	Orally	21 days	$46.00
Chronic pyelonephritis	Same as for acute pyelonephritis, but duration of therapy is 3–6 months			
Acute cystitis	Cephalexin, 250–500 mg every 6 hours	Orally	1–3 days	$16.00/3 days (500 mg)
	Ciprofloxacin, 250–500 mg every 12 hours	Orally	1–3 days	$31.00/3 days (500 mg)
	Nitrofurantoin (macrocrystals), 100 mg every 12 hours	Orally	7 days	$26.00
	Norfloxacin, 400 mg every 12 hours	Orally	1–3 days	$24.00/3 days
	Ofloxacin, 200 mg every 12 hours	Orally	1–3 days	$32.00/3 days
	Trimethoprim-sulfamethoxazole, 160/800 mg, two tablets[2]	Orally	Single dose	$2.00
Acute bacterial prostatitis	Same as for acute pyelonephritis		21 days	
Chronic bacterial prostatitis	Ciprofloxacin, 250–500 mg every 12 hours	Orally	1–3 months	$311.00/1 month (500 mg)
	Ofloxacin, 200–400 mg every 12 hours	Orally	1–3 months	$407.00/1 month (400 mg)
	Trimethoprim-sulfamethoxazole, 160/800 mg every 12 hours[2]	Orally	1–3 months	$69.00/1 month
Acute epididymitis				
Sexually transmitted	Ceftriaxone, 250 mg as single dose, plus: Doxycycline, 100 mg every 12 hours	Intramuscularly Orally	10 days	$17.00/250 mg $27.00
Non-sexually transmitted	Same as for chronic bacterial prostatitis	Orally	3 weeks	

[1]Average wholesale price, (AWP, for AB-rated generic when available) for quantity listed. Source: *Red Book Update,* Vol. 25, No. 5, May 2006. AWP may not accurately represent the actual pharmacy cost because wide contractual variations exist among institutions.
[2]Increasing resistance noted (up to 20%).

C. IMAGING

In complicated pyelonephritis, renal ultrasound may show hydronephrosis from a stone or other source of obstruction.

Differential Diagnosis

Acute intra-abdominal disease such as appendicitis, cholecystitis, pancreatitis, or diverticulitis must be distinguished from pyelonephritis. A normal urinalysis is usually seen in gastrointestinal disorders; however, on occasion, inflammation from adjacent bowel (appendicitis or diverticulitis) may result in hematuria or pyuria. Abnormal liver function tests or elevated amy-lase levels may assist in the differentiation. Lower lobe pneumonia is distinguishable by the abnormal chest radiograph.

In males, the main differential diagnosis for acute pyelonephritis includes acute epididymitis, acute prostatitis, and acute cystitis. Physical examination and the location of the pain should permit this distinction.

Complications

Sepsis with shock can occur with acute pyelonephritis. In diabetics, emphysematous pyelonephritis resulting from gas-producing organisms may be life-threatening if not adequately treated. Healthy adults usually recover complete renal function, yet if coexistent renal disease is present, scarring or chronic pyelonephritis may result. Inadequate therapy could result in abscess formation.

Treatment

Severe infections or complicating factors require hospital admission. Urine and blood cultures are obtained to identify the causative agent and to determine antimicrobial sensitivity. Intravenous ampicillin and an aminoglycoside are initiated prior to obtaining sensitivity results (Table 23–1). In the outpatient setting, quinolones or nitrofurantoin may be initiated (Table 23–1). Antibiotics are adjusted according to sensitivities. Fevers may persist for up to 72 hours; failure to respond warrants radiographic imaging (ultrasound) to exclude complicating factors that may require intervention. Catheter drainage may be necessary in the face of urinary retention and nephrostomy drainage if there is ureteral obstruction. In inpatients, intravenous antibiotics are maintained for 24 hours after the fever resolves, and oral antibiotics are then given to complete a 7-day course of therapy. Follow-up urine cultures are mandatory several weeks following the completion of treatment.

Prognosis

With prompt diagnosis and appropriate treatment, acute pyelonephritis carries a good prognosis. Complicating factors, underlying renal disease, and increasing patient age may lead to a less favorable outcome.

Miller O 2nd et al: Urinary tract infection and pyelonephritis. Emerg Med Clin North Am 2001;19:655. [PMID: 11554280]

ACUTE BACTERIAL PROSTATITIS

ESSENTIALS OF DIAGNOSIS

- *Fever.*
- *Irritative voiding symptoms.*
- *Perineal or suprapubic pain; exquisite tenderness common on rectal examination.*
- *Positive urine culture.*

General Considerations

Acute bacterial prostatitis is usually caused by gram-negative rods, especially *E coli* and *Pseudomonas* species and less commonly by gram-positive organisms (eg, enterococci). The most likely routes of infection include ascent up the urethra and reflux of infected urine into the prostatic ducts. Lymphatic and hematogenous routes are probably rare.

Clinical Findings

A. SYMPTOMS AND SIGNS

Perineal, sacral, or suprapubic pain, fever, and irritative voiding complaints are common. Varying degrees of obstructive symptoms may occur as the acutely inflamed prostate swells, which may lead to urinary retention. High fevers and a warm and often exquisitely tender prostate are detected on examination. Care should be taken in performing a gentle rectal examination, as vigorous manipulations may result in septicemia. Prostatic massage is contraindicated.

B. LABORATORY FINDINGS

Complete blood count shows leukocytosis and a left shift. Urinalysis shows pyuria, bacteriuria, and varying degrees of hematuria. Urine cultures will demonstrate the offending pathogen.

Differential Diagnosis

Acute pyelonephritis or acute epididymitis should be distinguishable by the location of pain as well as by physical examination. Acute diverticulitis is occasionally confused with acute prostatitis; however, the history and urinalysis should permit clear distinction. Urinary retention from benign or malignant prostatic enlargement is distinguishable by initial or follow-up rectal examination.

Treatment

Hospitalization may be required, and parenteral antibiotics (ampicillin and aminoglycoside) should be initiated until organism sensitivities are available (Table 23–1). After the patient is afebrile for 24–48 hours, oral antibiotics (eg, quinolones) are used to complete 4–6 weeks of therapy. If urinary retention develops, urethral catheterization or instrumentation is contraindicated, and a percutaneous suprapubic tube is required. Follow-up urine culture and examination of prostatic secretions should be performed after the completion of therapy to ensure eradication.

Prognosis

With effective treatment, chronic bacterial prostatitis is rare.

Hua VN et al: Acute and chronic prostatitis. Med Clin North Am 2004;88:483. [PMID: 15049589]

CHRONIC BACTERIAL PROSTATITIS

ESSENTIALS OF DIAGNOSIS

- *Irritative voiding symptoms.*
- *Perineal or suprapubic discomfort, often dull and poorly localized.*

- *Positive expressed prostatic secretions and culture.*

General Considerations

Although chronic bacterial prostatitis may evolve from acute bacterial prostatitis, many men have no history of acute infection. Gram-negative rods are the most common etiologic agents, but only one gram-positive organism (*Enterococcus*) is associated with chronic infection. Routes of infection are the same as discussed for acute infection.

Clinical Findings

A. SYMPTOMS AND SIGNS

Clinical manifestations are variable. Some patients are asymptomatic, but most have varying degrees of irritative voiding symptoms. Low back and perineal pain are not uncommon. Many patients report a history of urinary tract infections. Physical examination is often unremarkable, though the prostate may feel normal, boggy, or indurated.

B. LABORATORY FINDINGS

Urinalysis is normal unless a secondary cystitis is present. Expressed prostatic secretions demonstrate increased numbers of leukocytes (> 10 per high-power field), especially lipid-laden macrophages. Leukocyte and bacterial counts from expressed prostatic secretions do not correlate with severity of symptoms. However, this finding is consistent with inflammation and is not diagnostic of bacterial prostatitis. Culture of the secretions or the postprostatic massage urine specimen is necessary to make the diagnosis.

C. IMAGING

Imaging tests are not necessary, though pelvic radiographs or transrectal ultrasound may demonstrate prostatic calculi.

Differential Diagnosis

Chronic urethritis may mimic chronic prostatitis, though cultures of the fractionated urine may localize the source of infection. Cystitis may be secondary to prostatitis, but fractionated urine samples should localize the infection. Anal disease may share some of the symptoms of prostatitis, but physical examination should permit a distinction between the two.

Treatment

Few antimicrobial agents attain therapeutic intraprostatic levels in the absence of acute inflammation. Trimethoprim does diffuse into the prostate, and trimethoprim-sulfamethoxazole is associated with the best cure rates (Table 23–1). Other effective agents include carbenicillin, erythromycin, cephalexin, and the quinolones. The optimal duration of therapy remains controversial, ranging from 6 to 12 weeks. Symptomatic relief may be provided by anti-inflammatory agents (indomethacin, ibuprofen) and hot sitz baths.

Prognosis

Chronic bacterial prostatitis is difficult to cure, but its symptoms and tendency to cause recurrent urinary tract infections can be controlled by suppressive antibiotic therapy.

NONBACTERIAL PROSTATITIS

 ESSENTIALS OF DIAGNOSIS

- *Irritative voiding symptoms.*
- *Perineal or suprapubic discomfort, similar to that of chronic bacterial prostatitis.*
- *Positive expressed prostatic secretions, but culture is negative.*

General Considerations

Nonbacterial prostatitis is the most common of the prostatitis syndromes, and its cause is unknown. Speculation implicates chlamydiae, mycoplasmas, ureaplasmas, and viruses, but no substantial proof exists. In some cases, nonbacterial prostatitis may represent a noninfectious inflammatory disorder. Some investigators have postulated an autoimmune origin. Because the cause of nonbacterial prostatitis remains unknown, the diagnosis is usually one of exclusion.

Clinical Findings

A. SYMPTOMS AND SIGNS

The clinical presentation is identical to that of chronic bacterial prostatitis; however, no history of urinary tract infections is present. The National Institutes of Health Chronic Prostatitis Symptom Index (NIH-CPSI) has been validated to quantify symptoms of chronic nonbacterial prostatitis or chronic pelvic pain syndrome (CPPS).

B. LABORATORY FINDINGS

Increased numbers of leukocytes are seen on expressed prostatic secretions, but all cultures are negative.

Differential Diagnosis

The major distinction is from chronic bacterial prostatitis. The absence of a history of urinary tract infection and of positive cultures makes the distinction (Table 23–2). In older men with irritative voiding symptoms and negative cultures, the possibility of bladder cancer

Table 23–2. Clinical characteristics of prostatitis and prostatodynia syndromes.

Findings	Acute Bacterial Prostatitis	Chronic Bacterial Prostatitis	Nonbacterial Prostatitis	Prostatodynia
Fever	+	–	–	–
Urinalysis	+	–	–	–
Expressed prostatic secretions	Contraindicated	+	+	–
Bacterial culture	+	+	–	–

must be excluded. Urinary cytologic examination and cystoscopy are warranted.

Treatment

Because of the uncertainty regarding the etiology of nonbacterial prostatitis, a trial of antimicrobial therapy directed against *Ureaplasma*, *Mycoplasma*, or *Chlamydia* is warranted. Erythromycin (250 mg orally four times daily) can be initiated for 14 days yet should be continued (for 3–6 weeks) only if a favorable clinical response ensues. Some symptomatic relief may be obtained with anti-inflammatory agents or sitz baths. Dietary restrictions are not necessary unless the patient relates a history of symptom exacerbation by certain substances such as alcohol, caffeine, and perhaps certain foods.

Prognosis

Annoying, recurrent symptoms are common, but serious sequelae have not been identified.

Krieger JN et al: Does the chronic prostatitis/pelvic pain syndrome differ from nonbacterial prostatitis and prostatodynia? J Urol 2000;164:1554. [PMID: 11025703]

Litwin MS: A review of the development and validation of the National Institutes of Health Chronic Prostatitis Symptom Index. Urology 2002;60(6 Suppl):14. [PMID: 12521581]

Nickel JC et al: Prevalence, diagnosis, characterization, and treatment of prostatitis, interstitial cystitis, and epididymitis in outpatient urological practice: the Canadian PIE Study. Urology 2005;66:935. [PMID: 16286098]

PROSTATODYNIA

Prostatodynia is a noninflammatory disorder that affects young and middle-aged men and has variable causes, including voiding dysfunction and pelvic floor musculature dysfunction. The term "prostatodynia" is a misnomer, as the prostate is actually normal.

Clinical Findings

A. SYMPTOMS AND SIGNS

Symptoms are the same as those seen with chronic prostatitis, yet there is no history of urinary tract infection. Additional symptoms may include hesitancy and interruption of flow. Patients may relate a lifelong his-

tory of voiding difficulty. Physical examination is unremarkable, but increased anal sphincter tone and periprostatic tenderness may be observed.

B. LABORATORY FINDINGS

Urinalysis is normal. Expressed prostatic secretions show normal numbers of leukocytes. Urodynamic testing may show signs of dysfunctional voiding (detrusor contraction without urethral relaxation, high urethral pressures, spasms of the urinary sphincter) and is indicated in patients failing empiric trials of α-blockers or anticholinergics.

Differential Diagnosis

Normal urinalysis will distinguish it from acute infectious processes. Examination of expressed prostatic secretions will distinguish this entity from prostatitis syndromes (Table 23–2).

Treatment

Bladder neck and urethral spasms can be treated by α-blocking agents (terazosin, 1–10 mg orally once a day, or doxazosin, 1–8 mg orally once a day). Pelvic floor muscle dysfunction may respond to diazepam and biofeedback techniques. Sitz baths may contribute to symptomatic relief.

Prognosis

Prognosis is variable depending upon the specific cause.

Krieger JN: The problem with prostatitis. What do we know? What do we need to know? J Urol 2004;172:432. [PMID: 15247696]

Schaeffer A et al: Chronic prostatitis. Clin Evid 2003;(10): 994. [PMID: 15555133]

Zvara P et al: Minimally invasive therapies for prostatitis. Curr Urol Rep 2004;5:320. [PMID: 15260937]

ACUTE EPIDIDYMITIS

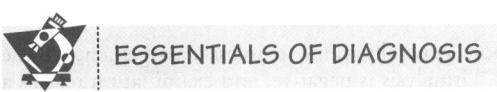 ESSENTIALS OF DIAGNOSIS

- *Fever.*
- *Irritative voiding symptoms.*

• *Painful enlargement of epididymis.*

General Considerations

Most cases of acute epididymitis are infectious and can be divided into one of two categories that have different age distributions and etiologic agents. Sexually transmitted forms typically occur in men under age 40 years, are associated with urethritis, and result from *Chlamydia trachomatis* or *Neisseria gonorrhoeae*. Non-sexually transmitted forms typically occur in older men, are associated with urinary tract infections and prostatitis, and are caused by gram-negative rods. The route of infection is probably via the urethra to the ejaculatory duct and then down the vas deferens to the epididymis. Amiodarone has been associated with self-limited epididymitis.

Clinical Findings

A. SYMPTOMS AND SIGNS

Symptoms may follow acute physical strain (heavy lifting), trauma, or sexual activity. Associated symptoms of urethritis (pain at the tip of the penis and urethral discharge) or cystitis (irritative voiding symptoms) may occur. Pain develops in the scrotum and may radiate along the spermatic cord or to the flank. Fever and scrotal swelling are usually apparent. Early in the course, the epididymis may be distinguishable from the testis; however, later the two may appear as one enlarged, tender mass. The prostate may be tender on rectal examination.

B. LABORATORY FINDINGS

Complete blood count shows leukocytosis and a left shift. In the sexually transmitted variety, Gram staining of a smear of urethral discharge may be diagnostic of gram-negative intracellular diplococci (*N gonorrhoeae*). White cells without visible organisms on urethral smear represent nongonococcal urethritis, and *C trachomatis* is the most likely pathogen. In the non-sexually transmitted variety, urinalysis shows pyuria, bacteriuria, and varying degrees of hematuria. Urine cultures will demonstrate the offending pathogen.

C. IMAGING

Scrotal ultrasound may aid in the diagnosis if examination is difficult because of the presence of a large hydrocele or because questions exist regarding the diagnosis.

Differential Diagnosis

Tumors generally cause painless enlargement of the testis. Urinalysis is negative, and examination reveals a normal epididymis. Scrotal ultrasound is helpful to define the pathology. Testicular torsion usually occurs in prepubertal males but is occasionally seen in young adults. Acute onset of symptoms and a negative urinalysis favor testicular torsion or torsion of one of the testicular or epididymal appendages. Prehn's sign (elevation of the scrotum above the pubic symphysis improves pain from epididymitis) may be helpful but is not reliable.

Treatment

Bed rest with scrotal elevation is important in the acute phase. Treatment is directed toward the identified pathogen (Table 23–1). The sexually transmitted variety is treated with 10–21 days of antibiotics, and the sexual partner must be treated as well. Non-sexually transmitted forms are treated for 21–28 days with appropriate antibiotics, at which time evaluation of the urinary tract is warranted to identify underlying disease.

Prognosis

Prompt treatment usually results in a favorable outcome. Delayed or inadequate treatment may result in epididymo-orchitis, decreased fertility, or abscess formation.

Chan PT et al: Inflammatory conditions of the male excurrent ductal system. Part I. J Androl 2002;23:453. [PMID: 12065446]

Hagley M: Epididymo-orchitis and epididymitis: a review of causes and management of unusual forms. Int J STD AIDS 2003;14:372. [PMID: 12816663]

■ URINARY STONE DISEASE

Urinary stone disease is exceeded in frequency as a urinary tract disorder only by infections and prostatic disease and is estimated to afflict 240,000–720,000 Americans per year. Men are more frequently affected by urolithiasis than women, with a ratio of 3:1. Initial presentation predominates in the third and fourth decades. The ratio of men to women approaches parity in the sixth and seventh decades.

Urinary calculi are polycrystalline aggregates composed of varying amounts of crystalloid and a small amount of organic matrix. Stone formation requires saturated urine that is dependent upon pH, ionic strength, solute concentration, and complexation. There are five major types of urinary stones: calcium oxalate, calcium phosphate, struvite, uric acid, and cystine. The most common types are composed of calcium, and for that reason most urinary stones (85%) are radiopaque. Uric acid stones can be radiolucent yet frequently are composed of a combination of uric acid and calcium oxalate and thus are radiopaque. Cystine stones frequently have a smooth-edged ground-glass appearance.

Geographic factors contribute to the development of stones. Areas of high humidity and elevated temperatures appear to be contributing factors, and the incidence of symptomatic ureteral stones is greatest during hot summer months.

Diet and fluid intake may be important factors in the development of urinary stones. Those afflicted with recurrent urinary stone disease are encouraged to maintain a diet restricted in sodium and protein intake. Sodium should be restricted to 100 mEq/d. Increased sodium intake will increase sodium and calcium excretion, increase monosodium urate saturation (that can act as a nidus for stone growth), increase the relative saturation of calcium phosphate, and decrease urinary citrate excretion. All of these factors encourage stone growth. Protein intake should be limited to 1 g/kg/d. An increased protein load can also increase calcium, oxalate, and uric acid excretion and decrease urinary citrate excretion.

Carbohydrates and fats have not been proved to have any impact on urinary stone disease. Bran can significantly decrease urinary calcium by increasing bowel transit time and mechanically binding to calcium. Excess intake of oxalate and purines can increase the incidence of stones in predisposed individuals. Although a reduction in dietary calcium results in reduced urinary calcium, the concurrent increase in urinary oxalate may promote stone formation. Only type II absorptive hypercalciuric patients (see below) benefit from a low-calcium diet. Persons in sedentary occupations have a higher incidence of stones than manual laborers.

Genetic factors may contribute to urinary stone formation. Cystinuria is an autosomal recessive disorder. Homozygous individuals have markedly increased excretion of cystine and frequently have numerous recurrent episodes of urinary stones despite attempts to optimize medical treatment. Distal renal tubular acidosis may be transmitted as a hereditary trait, and urolithiasis occurs in up to 75% of patients affected with this disorder.

Clinical Findings

A. SYMPTOMS AND SIGNS

Obstructing urinary stones usually present with colic. Pain usually occurs suddenly and may awaken patients from sleep. It is localized to the flank, is usually severe, and may be associated with nausea and vomiting. Patients are constantly moving—in sharp contrast to those with an acute abdomen. The pain may occur episodically and may radiate anteriorly over the abdomen. As the stone progresses down the ureter, the pain may be referred into the ipsilateral testis or labium. If the stone becomes lodged at the ureterovesicular junction, patients will complain of marked urinary urgency and frequency. Stone size does not correlate with the severity of the symptoms.

B. METABOLIC EVALUATION

Stone analysis should be performed on recovered stones. Controversy exists in deciding which patients need a thorough metabolic evaluation for stone disease. Uncomplicated first-time stone-formers should probably undergo blood screening for abnormalities of serum calcium, phosphate, electrolytes, and uric acid as a baseline.

More extensive evaluation is required in recurrent stone-formers or patients with a family history of stone disease. A 24-hour urine collection on a random diet should ascertain volume, urinary pH, and calcium, uric acid, oxalate, phosphate, sodium, and citrate excretion. A second collection on a restricted calcium (400 mg/d) and sodium (100 mEq/d) diet is undertaken to subcategorize patients, if necessary. Serum parathyroid hormone (PTH) and calcium load tests can be performed at a third visit. A calcium load test is performed as follows: After a patient has been on a restricted calcium diet for at least 1 week, the patient is told to fast from 9 PM. The patient discards the early morning voided specimen (7 AM). While still fasting, the patient voids at 9 AM, which is the fasting sample. The patient then ingests 1 g of calcium gluconate, and all urine is collected from 9 AM to 1 PM, the calcium load sample. Table 23–3 demonstrates the di-

Table 23–3. Diagnostic criteria of different types of hypercalciuria.

	Absorptive Type I	Absorptive Type II	Absorptive Type III	Resorptive	Renal
Serum					
Calcium	N	N	N	↑	N
Phosphorus	N	N	↓	↓	N
PTH	N	N	N	↑	↑
Vitamin D	N	N	↑	↑	↑
Urinary calcium					
Fasting	N	N	↑	↑	↑
Restricted	↑	N	↑	↑	↑
After calcium load	↑	↑	↑	↑	↑

PTH = parathyroid hormone; ↑ = elevated; ↓ = low; N = normal.

agnostic criteria for the hypercalciuric states. (See discussion below.)

C. LABORATORY FINDINGS

Urinalysis usually reveals microscopic or gross hematuria (~90%). However, the absence of microhematuria does not exclude urinary stones. Infection must be excluded, because the combination of infection and urinary tract obstruction requires prompt intervention as described below. Urinary pH is a valuable clue to the cause of the possible stone. Normal urine pH is 5.85. There is a normal postprandial urinary alkaline tide. Numerous dipstick measurements are valuable in the complete workup of a stone patient. Persistent urinary pH below 5.5 is suggestive of uric acid or cystine stones, both relatively radiolucent as seen on plain films of the abdomen. In contrast, a persistent pH above 7.2 is suggestive of a struvite infection stone, radiopaque on plain films.

D. IMAGING

A plain film of the abdomen and renal ultrasound examination will diagnose most stones. Spiral CT has emerged as a first-line tool in evaluating flank pain. All stones whether radiopaque or radiolucent on plain abdominal radiographs will be visible on noncontrast CT except the rare calculi due to the protease inhibitor indinivir. Stones suspected of being located at the ureterovesicular junction can be imaged with abdominal ultrasonography with the aid of the acoustic window of a full bladder. Alternatively, transvaginal or transrectal ultrasonography will help identify calculi near the ureterovesicular junction.

Medical Treatment & Prevention

To reduce the recurrence rate of urinary stones, one must attempt to achieve a stone-free status. Small stone fragments may serve as a nidus for future stone development. Selected patients must be thoroughly evaluated to reduce stone recurrence rates. Uric acid stone-formers may have recurrences within months if appropriate therapy is not initiated. If no medical treatment is provided after surgical stone removal, stones will generally recur in 50% of patients within 5 years. Of greatest importance in reducing stone recurrence is an increased fluid intake. Absolute volumes are not established, but doubling previous fluid intake is recommended. Patients are encouraged to ingest fluids during meals, 2 hours after each meal (when the body is most dehydrated), and prior to going to sleep in the evening—enough to awaken the patient to void—and to ingest additional fluids during the night. Increasing fluids only during daylight hours may not dilute a supersaturated urine overnight and thus initiate a new stone.

A. CALCIUM NEPHROLITHIASIS

1. Hypercalciuric—Hypercalciuric calcium nephrolithiasis (> 200 mg/24 h; > 4 mg/kg/24 h) can be caused by absorptive, resorptive, and renal disorders.

Absorptive hypercalciuria is secondary to increased absorption of calcium at the level of the small bowel, predominantly in the jejunum, and can be further subdivided into types I, II, and III. Type I absorptive hypercalciuria is independent of calcium intake. There is increased urinary calcium on a regular or even a calcium-restricted diet. Treatment is centered upon decreasing bowel absorption of calcium. Cellulose phosphate, a chelating agent, is an effective form of therapy. An average dose is 10–15 g in three divided doses. It binds to the calcium and impedes small bowel absorption due to its increased bulk. Cellulose phosphate does not change the intestinal transport mechanism. It should be given with meals so it will be available to bind to the calcium. Taking this chelating agent prior to bedtime is ineffective. Postmenopausal women should be treated with caution. It is interesting, however, that there is no enhanced decline in bone density after long-term use. Inappropriate use without an initial metabolic evaluation (see above) may result in a negative calcium balance and a secondary parathyroid stimulation. Long-term use without follow-up metabolic surveillance may result in hypomagnesuria and secondary hyperoxaluria and recurrent calculi. Routine follow-up every 6–8 months will help encourage medical compliance and permit adjustments in medical therapy based upon repeat metabolic studies.

Thiazide therapy is an alternative to cellulose phosphate in the treatment of type I absorptive hypercalciuria. Thiazides decrease renal calcium excretion but have no impact on intestinal absorption. This therapy results in increased bone density of approximately 1% per year. Thiazides have limited long-term utility (< 5 years) since they may lose their hypocalciuric effect with continued therapy.

Type II absorptive hypercalciuria is diet dependent. Decreasing calcium intake by 50% (approximately 400 mg/d) will decrease the hypercalciuria to normal values (150–200 mg/24 h). There is no specific medical therapy.

Type III absorptive hypercalciuria is secondary to a renal phosphate leak. This results in increased vitamin D synthesis and secondarily increased small bowel absorption of calcium. This can be readily reversed by orthophosphates (250 mg three to four times per day). Orthophosphates do not change intestinal absorption but rather inhibit vitamin D synthesis.

Resorptive hypercalciuria is secondary to hyperparathyroidism. Hypercalcemia, hypophosphatemia, hypercalciuria, and an elevated PTH value are found. Appropriate surgical resection of the parathyroid adenoma cures the disease and the urinary stones. Medical management is invariably a failure.

Renal hypercalciuria occurs when the renal tubules are unable to efficiently reabsorb filtered calcium, and hypercalciuria results. Spilling calcium in the urine results in secondary hyperparathyroidism. Serum calcium typically is normal. Thiazides are effective long-term therapy in patients with this disorder.

2. Hyperuricosuric—Hyperuricosuric calcium nephrolithiasis is secondary to dietary excesses or uric acid metabolic defects. Both disorders can be treated with purine dietary restrictions or allopurinol therapy (or both). In contrast to uric acid nephrolithiasis, patients with hyperuricosuric calcium stones typically maintain a urinary pH greater than 5.5. Monosodium urates absorb and adsorb inhibitors and promote heterogeneous nucleation. Hyperuricosuric calcium nephrolithiasis is probably secondary to epitaxy, or heterogeneous nucleation. In such situations, similar crystal structures (ie, uric acid and calcium oxalate) can grow together with the aid of a protein matrix infrastructure.

3. Hyperoxaluric—Hyperoxaluric calcium nephrolithiasis is usually due to primary intestinal disorders. Patients usually present with a history of chronic diarrhea frequently associated with inflammatory bowel disease or steatorrhea. Increased bowel fat combines with intraluminal calcium to form a soap-like product. Calcium is therefore unavailable to bind to oxalate, which is then freely and rapidly absorbed. A small increase in oxalate absorption will significantly increase stone formation. If the diarrhea or steatorrhea cannot be effectively curtailed, oral calcium supplements should be given with meals. More than 2 g/d of ascorbic acid will increase urinary oxalate levels. Emphasis on encouraging increased fluid intake is required for these patients as for all stone-formers.

4. Hypocitraturic—Hypocitraturic calcium nephrolithiasis may be secondary to chronic diarrhea, type I (distal) renal tubular acidosis, chronic hydrochlorothiazide treatment, and, in rare cases, is idiopathic. Any condition that results in metabolic acidosis (including prolonged fasting, hypomagnesemia, and hypokalemia) will decrease urinary citrate excretion, since it will be consumed by the citric acid cycle within the mitochondria of proximal tubular cells. Hypocitraturia is frequently associated with other forms of calcium stone formation. Citrate appears to bind to calcium in solution, thereby decreasing available calcium for stone formation. Potassium citrate supplements are usually effective. Urinary citrate is decreased in acidosis and is increased during alkalosis. The potassium will supplement the frequently associated hypokalemic states, and citrate will help to correct the acidosis. A typical dose is 20 mEq three times a day (available in solution and in 10-mEq waxed tablets), or 30 mEq of crystal formulations twice a day.

B. URIC ACID CALCULI

The average urinary pH is 5.85. Uric acid stone-formers typically have urinary pH values less than 5.5. The pK of uric acid is 5.75, at which point half of the uric acid is ionized as a urate salt and is soluble, while the other half is insoluble. Increasing the pH above 6.5 dramatically increases solubility and can effectively dissolve large calculi. Potassium citrate is the most frequently used medication to increase urinary pH. It can

be given in liquid preparation, as crystals that need to be taken with fluids, or as tablets (10 mEq), two by mouth three or four times daily. Compliant urinary alkalinization may dissolve uric acid calculi at a rate of 1 cm (as measured on plain abdominal radiograph) of stone per month. Patients with uric acid calculi should be given Nitrazine pH paper with which to monitor the effectiveness of their urinary alkalinization. Other contributing factors include hyperuricemia, myeloproliferative disorders, malignancy with increased uric acid production, abrupt and dramatic weight loss, and uricosuric medications. If hyperuricemia is present, allopurinol (300 mg/d) may be given. Although pure uric acid stones are relatively radiolucent, most have some calcium components and can be visualized on plain abdominal radiographs. Renal ultrasonography is a helpful adjunct for appropriate diagnosis and long-term management.

C. STRUVITE CALCULI

Struvite stones are synonymous with magnesium-ammonium-phosphate stones. They are commonly seen in women with recurrent urinary tract infections recalcitrant to appropriate antibiotics. They rarely form as ureteral stones without prior upper tract endourologic intervention. Frequently, a struvite stone is discovered as a large staghorn calculus forming a cast of the renal collecting system. Struvite stones are radiodense. Urinary pH is high, usually above 7.2. These stones are formed secondary to urease-producing organisms, including *Proteus, Pseudomonas, Providencia*, and, less commonly, *Klebsiella, Staphylococcus*, and *Mycoplasma*. An *E coli* urinary tract infection is not consistent with an infectious reservoir originating from a struvite calculus. These frequently large stones are relatively soft and amenable to percutaneous nephrolithotomy. Appropriate perioperative antibiotics are required. They can recur rapidly, and efforts should be taken to render the patient stone-free. Postoperative irrigation through nephrostomy tubes can eliminate small fragments. Acetohydroxamic acid is an effective urease inhibitor, but it is poorly tolerated by most patients because of its gastrointestinal toxicity.

D. CYSTINE CALCULI

Cystine stones are a result of abnormal excretion of cystine, ornithine, lysine, and arginine. Cystine is the only amino acid that becomes insoluble in urine. These stones are particularly difficult to manage medically. Prevention is centered around increased fluid intake, alkalinization of the urine above pH 7.5 (monitored with Nitrazine pH paper), and a variety of medications including penicillamine and tiopronin (α-mercaptoproprionylglycine). There are no known inhibitors of cystine calculi.

Surgical Treatment

Forced intravenous fluids will not push stones down the ureter. Effective peristalsis directing a bolus of urine down the ureter requires opposing ureteral walls to approach each other and touch, which large dilated systems cannot do. In fact, diuresis is counterproductive and will exacerbate the pain. Associated fever may represent infection, a medical emergency requiring prompt drainage by a ureteral catheter or a percutaneous nephrostomy tube. Antibiotics alone are inadequate unless obstruction is drained.

A. URETERAL STONES

Impediment to urine flow by ureteral stones usually occurs at three sites: (1) at the ureteropelvic junction, (2) at the crossing of the ureter over the iliac vessels, and finally (3) as the ureter enters the bladder at the ureterovesicular junction. Prediction of spontaneous stone passage is difficult. Stones less than 6 mm in diameter as seen on a plain abdominal radiograph will usually pass spontaneously. Conservative observation with appropriate pain medications is appropriate for the first 6 weeks. There is new evidence that oral corticosteroids, α-blockers, and calcium channel blockers may enhance stone passage of observed ureteral stones. α-Blockers are safe and well tolerated. Typical agents and dosages are tamsulosin, 0.4 mg orally once daily; terazosin, 5 mg orally once daily; or doxazosin, 4 mg orally once daily. If spontaneous stone passage has failed, either because of lack of progression of the stone or intolerance of the pain, therapeutic intervention is required. Distal ureteral stones are best managed either with ureteroscopic stone extraction or in situ extracorporeal shock wave lithotripsy (SWL). Ureteroscopic stone extraction involves placement of a small endoscope through the urethra and into the ureter. Under direct vision, basket extraction or fragmentation followed by extraction is performed. Complications during endoscopic retrieval increase as the duration of conservative observation increases beyond 6 weeks. Indications for earlier intervention include severe pain unresponsive to medications, fever, persistent nausea and vomiting requiring intravenous hydration, social requirements requiring return to work, or anticipated travel. Most upper tract stones that enter the bladder can exit the urethra with minimal discomfort.

In situ SWL, an alternative, utilizes an external energy source that is focused upon the stone. This focused energy is additive, resulting in minimal tissue insult except at the focus where the stone is positioned with the aid of fluoroscopy or ultrasonography. This can be performed under anesthesia as an outpatient procedure and usually results in stone fragmentation. Most stone fragments will pass uneventfully within 2 weeks, but those that have not passed within 3 months are unlikely to pass without intervention. Women of childbearing age are best not treated with SWL for a stone in the lower ureter, as the impact upon the ovary is unknown.

Proximal and midureteral stones—those above the inferior margin of the sacroiliac joint—can be treated with SWL or ureteroscopy. SWL is delivered directly to the stone (in situ) without the need to push the stone back

into the renal pelvis. To help ensure adequate drainage after SWL, a double J ureteral stent is frequently placed. Double J stents do not ensure passage of stone fragments after SWL. Occasionally, stone fragments will obstruct the ureter after SWL. Conservative management will usually result in spontaneous resolution with eventual passage of the stone fragments. If this is unsuccessful, adequate proximal drainage through a percutaneous nephrostomy tube will facilitate passage. In rare instances, ureteroscopic extraction will be required.

B. RENAL STONES

Patients with renal calculi presenting without pain, urinary tract infections, or obstruction need not be treated. They should be followed with serial abdominal radiographs or renal ultrasonographic examinations. If calculi are growing or become symptomatic, intervention should be undertaken. Renal stones less than 2 cm in diameter are best treated with SWL. Stones located in the inferior calix frequently result in suboptimal stone-free rates as measured at 3 months by x-ray. Such stones and others of larger diameter are best treated via percutaneous nephrolithotomy. Perioperative antibiotic coverage should be given on the basis of preoperative urine cultures.

Dellabella M et al: Randomized trial of the efficacy of tamsulosin, nifedipine and phloroglucinol in medical expulsive therapy for distal ureteral calculi. J Urol 2005;174:167. [PMID: 15947613]

Heneghan JP et al: Helical CT for nephrolithiasis and ureterolithiasis: comparison of conventional and reduced radiation-dose techniques. Radiology 2003;229:575. [PMID: 14526095]

Maalouf NM et al: Novel insights into the pathogenesis of uric acid nephrolithiasis. Curr Opin Nephrol Hypertens 2004; 13:181. [PMID: 15202612]

Pak CY: Medical management of urinary stone disease. Nephron Clin Pract 2004;98:c49. [PMID: 15499203]

Pak CY et al: Predictive value of kidney stone composition in the detection of metabolic abnormalities. Am J Med 2003;115: 26. [PMID: 12867231]

Parmar MS: Kidney stones. BMJ 2004;328:1420. [PMID: 15191979]

Stoller ML et al: The primary stone event: a new hypothesis involving a vascular etiology. J Urol 2004;171:1920. [PMID: 15076312]

Tiselius HG: Epidemiology and medical management of stone disease. BJU Int 2003;91:758. [PMID: 12709088]

■ URINARY INCONTINENCE

Urinary incontinence is most common in older patients. Its prevalence varies from 5% to 15% in the community to perhaps more than 50% in long-term care facilities. The normal urinary bladder can store relatively large volumes of urine at low pressures. Continence is dependent upon a compliant reservoir and sphincteric efficiency that has two components: the involuntary smooth muscle of the bladder neck and the voluntary skeletal muscle of the external sphincter. (See also discussion in Chapter 4.)

Classification

Urinary incontinence occurs when urine leaks involuntarily and can be classified into one of four categories.

A. TOTAL INCONTINENCE

With total incontinence, patients lose urine at all times and in all positions. This results when sphincteric efficiency is lost (previous surgery, nerve damage, cancerous infiltration) or when an abnormal connection between the urinary tract and the skin exists that bypasses the urinary sphincter (vesicovaginal or ureterovaginal fistulas).

B. STRESS INCONTINENCE

Stress incontinence is the loss of urine associated with activities that result in an increase in intra-abdominal pressure (coughing, sneezing, lifting, exercising). Patients do not leak in the supine position. Laxity of the pelvic floor musculature—most commonly seen in the multiparous woman or in patients who have undergone pelvic surgery—results in urethral sphincteric insufficiency.

C. URGE INCONTINENCE

The uncontrolled loss of urine that is preceded by a strong, unexpected urge to void is known as urge incontinence. It is unrelated to position or activity and is indicative of detrusor hyperreflexia or sphincter dysfunction. Inflammatory conditions or neurogenic disorders of the bladder are commonly associated with urge incontinence.

D. OVERFLOW INCONTINENCE

Chronic urinary retention may result in overflow incontinence. Incontinence results from the chronically distended bladder receiving an additional increment of urine, so that intravesical pressure just exceeds the outlet resistance, allowing a small amount of urine to dribble out.

Clinical Findings

A. SYMPTOMS AND SIGNS

The history is the most important step in the evaluation of urinary incontinence. It may be supplemented with a voiding diary prepared by the patient. Physical examination is important to exclude fistula for cases of total incontinence, neurologic abnormalities in cases of urge incontinence (spasticity, flaccidity, rectal sphincter tone), or the distended bladder in cases of overflow incontinence. Rectal examination will reveal the general function of the pelvic floor. Normal anal tone suggests an intact external sphincter. A tender levator ani suggests an overfacilitated pelvic floor. A lax sphincter suggests a lower motor neuron lesion. The bulbocavernosus reflex further confirms the integrity of the lower motor neurons. This reflex is confirmed by feeling an anal contraction in response to pressure on the glans penis or the clitoris.

B. LABORATORY FINDINGS

Urinalysis and urine culture are important to exclude urinary tract infection in cases of urge incontinence. Abnormal renal function may be detected in cases of overflow incontinence. Patients in whom overflow incontinence is suspected can have postvoid residual urine volume assessed by urethral catheterization or ultrasonography.

C. SPECIAL TESTS

Urinary continence depends upon both bladder and sphincteric mechanisms; dysfunction of either component may result in incontinence. Urodynamic evaluation can assess both bladder and sphincteric function. Such testing is indicated in patients with moderate to severe incontinence, those suspected of having neurologic disease, and those with urge incontinence when infection and neoplasm have been excluded.

Bladder capacity, accommodation, sensation, voluntary control, contractility, and response to pharmacologic intervention can be assessed by cystometry. Cystometry is performed by filling the bladder with water and simultaneously recording intravesical pressure.

During filling, the normal bladder has the ability to maintain a low pressure. As volume increases, compliance increases. Normal sensation is first appreciated with volumes less than 150 mL. There is a strong sensation prior to micturition. Normal capacity in an adult bladder is 350–500 mL. Micturition is consciously initiated starting with pelvic floor relaxation followed by a sustained bladder contraction. Normal bladder function will empty the bladder completely. Uninhibited contractions during the normal filling phase are abnormal and are usually associated with a strong urge to void. Causes of decreased urinary capacity include incontinence, infections, interstitial cystitis, radiation damage, upper motor neuron lesions, and postoperative changes. Increased bladder capacity is seen with chronic urinary tract obstruction, lower motor neuron lesions, and sensory neuropathies.

Responses to routine medications during cystometry will help confirm a diagnosis and facilitate appropriate therapy. Lack of an appropriate detrusor contraction may be secondary to poor bladder muscle function or inadequate filling.

Sphincteric function assessment is necessary in the evaluation of urinary incontinence. More formal evaluation of the urinary sphincter may be performed using urethral profilometry, electromyography, or combined video studies.

Treatment

A. TOTAL INCONTINENCE

True incontinence is due to anatomic abnormalities, either congenital or acquired. Congenital defects, including bladder exstrophy, ectopic ureteral orifices, and urethral diverticula, and acquired lesions such as vesicovaginal fistulas require surgical correction. Sphincter injuries following prostatectomy may be managed by periurethral bulking agents, a urethral sling, or placement of an artificial urinary sphincter.

B. STRESS INCONTINENCE

In patients with stress urinary incontinence, the bladder neck will descend below the midportion of the pubic symphysis when viewed on a lateral stress cystogram. Urodynamic investigations usually reveal a shortened functional urethral length, decreased urethral closure pressure, minimal augmentation of closure pressure with stress activities, decreased urethral pressure and length when assuming an upright position, and decreased closure pressure with bladder filling.

If hypoestrogenism of the vagina or urethra is discovered, topical estrogen creams applied locally are indicated. Surgical treatment is centered upon placing the bladder neck into an appropriate anatomic location, allowing increased intra-abdominal pressure to be transmitted to both the bladder and the bladder neck. These procedures also lengthen the urethra. Transvaginal sling suspension or suprapubic (culpocystourethropexy) approaches can pull the bladder neck into proper position. Less invasive procedures include periurethral injectables to increase outlet resistance and insertion of tension-free vaginal tape. Surgery is usually corrective in the short- to intermediate-term. Long-term outcomes are variable and depend on patient factors and the procedure.

C. URGE INCONTINENCE

The etiology of urge urinary incontinence includes urethral or detrusor instability or a combination of these mechanisms. Treatment is medical rather than surgical. Effective agents include anticholinergic medications (oxybutinin, 5–15 mg/d, or tolterodine, 2–4 mg/d) or tricyclic antidepressants (imipramine, 25–75 mg orally at bedtime). Sacral nerve stimulation can be effective in treating refractory urinary urge incontinence.

D. OVERFLOW INCONTINENCE

Placement of a urethral catheter is both diagnostic and therapeutic in the acute setting. Further treatment must address the underlying disease. Men with benign prostatic hyperplasia can be treated with medical therapy, prostatectomy, or newer less invasive procedures (see below). Patients with urethral strictures can be treated with a direct internal urethrotomy or open urethroplasty. Neurogenic causes (external sphincteric spasticity) may be managed with intermittent catheterization regimens with or without pharmacotherapy.

Assessment and treatment of urinary incontinence. Scientific Committee of the First International Consultation on Incontinence. Lancet 2000;355:2153. [PMID: 2035843]

Khullar V et al: Treatment of urge-predominant mixed urinary incontinence with tolterodine extended release: a randomized, placebo-controlled trial. Urology 2004;64:269. [PMID: 15302476]

Moore K: Duloxetine: a new approach for treating stress urinary incontinence. Int J Gynaecol Obstet 2004;86(Suppl 1):S53. [PMID: 15302567]

Nygaard IE et al: Stress urinary incontinence. Obstet Gynecol 2004;104:607. [PMID: 15339776]

Parmet S et al: JAMA patient page. Stress incontinence. JAMA 2003;290:426. [PMID: 12865384]

Schuessler B et al: Pharmacologic treatment of stress urinary incontinence: expectations for outcome. Urology 2003;62(4 Suppl 1):31. [PMID: 14550835]

Teleman PM et al: WHILA study group: overactive bladder: prevalence, risk factors and relation to stress incontinence in middle-aged women. BJOG 2004;111:600. [PMID: 15198789]

Watson NM: Use of the Agency for Health Care Policy and Research Urinary Incontinence Guideline in nursing homes. J Am Geriatr Soc 2003;51:1779. [PMID: 14687358]

INTERSTITIAL CYSTITIS

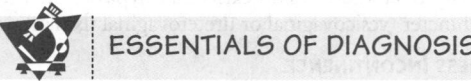

ESSENTIALS OF DIAGNOSIS

- *Pain with a full bladder or urinary urgency.*
- *Submucosal petechiae on cystoscopic examination.*
- *Diagnosis of exclusion.*

General Considerations

Interstitial cystitis is characterized by pain with bladder filling that is relieved by emptying and is often associated with urgency and frequency. This is a diagnosis of exclusion, and patients must have a negative urine culture and cytology and no other obvious cause such as radiation cystitis, chemical cystitis (cyclophosphamide), vaginitis, urethral diverticulum, or genital herpes. Up to 40% of patients referred to urologists for interstitial cystitis may actually be found to have a different diagnosis after careful evaluation.

Population-based studies have demonstrated a prevalence of between 18 and 40 per 100,000 people. Both sexes are involved, but most patients are women, with a mean age of 40 years at onset. Patients with interstitial cystitis are more likely to report bladder problems in childhood, and there appears to be a higher prevalence in Jewish women. Up to 50% of patients may experience spontaneous remission of symptoms, with a mean duration of 8 months without treatment.

The etiology of interstitial cystitis is unknown, and it is most likely not a single disease but rather several diseases with similar symptoms. Associated diseases include severe allergies, irritable bowel syndrome, or inflammatory bowel disease. Theories regarding the cause of interstitial cystitis include increased epithelial permeability, neurogenic causes (sensory nervous system abnormalities), and autoimmunity.

Clinical Findings

A. SYMPTOMS AND SIGNS

Pain with bladder filling that is relieved with urination or urgency, frequency, and nocturia are the most common symptoms. Exposures such as pelvic radiation or prior cyclophosphamide should be inquired about. Examination should exclude genital herpes, vaginitis, or a urethral diverticulum.

B. LABORATORY FINDINGS

Urinalysis and urine culture are obtained to exclude infectious causes. Urinary cytology is obtained to exclude bladder malignancy. Urodynamic testing assesses bladder sensation and compliance and excludes detrusor instability.

C. CYSTOSCOPY

The bladder is distended with fluid (hydrodistention) to detect glomerulations (submucosal hemorrhage), which may or may not be present. Biopsy should be performed to exclude other causes such as carcinoma, eosinophilic cystitis, and tuberculous cystitis. The presence of submucosal mast cells is not needed to make the diagnosis of interstitial cystitis.

Differential Diagnosis

Exposures to radiation or cyclophosphamide are obtained by the history. Bacterial cystitis, genital herpes, or vaginitis can be excluded by urinalysis, culture, and physical examination. A urethral diverticulum may be suspected if palpation of the urethra demonstrates an indurated mass that results in the expression of pus from the urethral meatus. Urethral carcinoma presents as a firm mass on palpation.

Treatment

There is no cure for interstitial cystitis, but most patients achieve symptomatic relief from one of several approaches, including hydrodistention, which is usually done as part of the diagnostic evaluation. Approximately 20–30% of patients will notice symptomatic improvement following this maneuver. Also of importance is the measurement of bladder capacity during hydrodistention, since patients with very small bladder capacities (< 200 mL) are unlikely to respond to medical therapy.

Amitriptyline is often used as first-line medical therapy in patients with interstitial cystitis. Both central and peripheral mechanisms may contribute to its activity. Nifedipine and other calcium channel blockers have also demonstrated some activity in patients with interstitial cystitis. Pentosan polysulfate sodium (Elmiron) is an oral synthetic sulfated polysaccharide that helps restore integrity to the epithelium of the bladder in a subset of patients and has been evaluated in a placebo-controlled trial. Other options include intravesical instillation of dimethyl sulfoxide (DMSO), heparin, or bacillus Calmette-Guérin (BCG), the latter achieving up to 60% response rates. A group of investigators and the Interstitial Cystitis Clinical Trials Group performed a randomized controlled trial that showed no statistically significant improvement with intravesical BCG over placebo.

Other treatment modalities include transcutaneous electric nerve stimulation (TENS) and acupuncture. Surgical therapy for interstitial cystitis should be considered only as a last resort and may require cystourethrectomy with urinary diversion.

Chancellor MB et al: Treatment of interstitial cystitis. Urology 2004;63(3 Suppl 1):85. [PMID: 15013658]

Comiter CV: Sacral neuromodulation for the symptomatic treatment of refractory interstitial cystitis: a prospective study. J Urol 2003;169:1369. [PMID: 12629364]

Irwin P et al: Reinvestigation of patients with a diagnosis of interstitial cystitis: common things are sometimes common. J Urol 2005;174:584. [PMID: 16006903]

Mayer R et al; Interstitial Cystitis Clinical Trials Group: A randomized controlled trial of intravesical bacillus Calmette-Guerin for treatment refractory interstitial cystitis. J Urol 2005;173:1186. [PMID: 15758738]

Propert KJ et al: A prospective study of interstitial cystitis: results of longitudinal followup of the interstitial cystitis data base cohort. The Interstitial Cystitis Data Base Study Group. J Urol 2000;163:1434. [PMID: 10751852]

Selo-Ojeme DO et al: Interstitial cystitis. J Obstet Gynaecol 2004;24:216. [PMID: 15203611]

van Ophoven A et al: A prospective, randomized, placebo controlled, double-blind study of amitriptyline for the treatment of interstitial cystitis. J Urol 2004;172:533. [PMID: 15247722]

■ MALE ERECTILE DYSFUNCTION & SEXUAL DYSFUNCTION

Erectile dysfunction is defined as the consistent inability to maintain an erect penis with sufficient rigidity to allow sexual intercourse. This condition is thought to affect 10 million American men, and its incidence is age related. Approximately 25% of all men older than age 65 years suffer from this disorder. Most cases of male erectile disorders have an organic rather than a psychogenic cause. Normal male erection is a neurovascular phenomenon relying on an intact autonomic and somatic nerve supply to the penis, smooth and striated musculature of the corpora cavernosa and pelvic floor, and arterial inflow supplied by the paired pudendal arteries. Erection is precipitated and maintained by an increase in arterial flow, active relaxation of the smooth muscle elements of the sinusoids within the corporal bodies of the penis, and an increase in venous resistance. Contraction of the bulbocavernosus and ischiocavernosus muscles results in further rigidity of the penis. The neurotransmitters that initiate and contribute to male erection include nitric oxide, vasoactive intestinal peptide, acetylcholine, and prostaglandins.

Male sexual dysfunction may be manifested in a variety of ways, and the history is critical to the proper classification and subsequent treatment. Androgens have a strong influence on the sexual desire of men. A **loss of libido** may indicate androgen deficiency on the basis of either hypothalamic, pituitary, or testicular disease. Serum testosterone and gonadotropin levels may help localize the site of disease. **Loss of erections** may result from arterial, venous, neurogenic, or psychogenic causes. Concurrent medical problems may damage one or more of the mechanisms. In addition, many medications, especially antihypertensives, are associated with erectile dysfunction. Centrally acting sympatholytics (methyldopa, clonidine, reserpine) can result in loss of erection, while vasodilators, α-blockers, and diuretics rarely alter erections. β-Blockers and spironolactone may result in loss of libido. It is important to determine whether the patient ever has any normal erections in the early morning or during sleep. If normal erections do occur, an organic cause is unlikely. The gradual loss of erections over a period of time is more suggestive of an organic cause. The **loss of emission** (lack of antegrade seminal fluid during ejaculation) may result from several underlying disorders. **Retrograde ejaculation** may occur as a result of mechanical disruption of the bladder neck, especially following transurethral resection of the prostate or sympathetic denervation as a result of medications (α-blockers), diabetes mellitus, or radical pelvic or retroperitoneal surgery. Androgen deficiency may also result in lack of emission by decreasing the amount of prostatic and seminal vesicle secretions. If libido and erection are intact, the **loss of orgasm** is usually of psychological origin. **Premature ejaculation** is usually an anxiety-related disorder and rarely has an organic cause. The history may elucidate the presence of a new partner, unreasonable expectations about performance, or emotional disorders. Pharmacologic therapy with clomipramine 25 mg prior to intercourse has been effective in delaying ejaculation.

Clinical Findings

A. SYMPTOMS AND SIGNS

Erectile dysfunction should be clearly distinguished from problems of ejaculation, libido, and orgasm. The degree of the dysfunction (whether chronic, occasional, or situational) as well as its timing should be noted. The history should include inquiries about hyperlipidemia, hypertension, depression, neurologic disease, diabetes mellitus, renal failure, and adrenal and thyroid disorders. Trauma to the pelvis or pelvic or peripheral vascular surgery also identifies patients at increased risk of impotence. A complete recording of drug use should be made, since about 25% of all cases of sexual dysfunction may be drug related. The excessive use of alcohol and recreational drugs should be recorded as well, since each is associated with an increased risk of sexual dysfunction. Depression is a risk factor for erectile dysfunction.

During the physical examination, secondary sexual characteristics should be assessed. Neurologic and pe-

ripheral vascular examination should be performed. Motor and sensory examination should be performed as well as palpation and quantification of lower extremity vascular pulsations. The genitalia should be examined, noting the presence of penile scarring or plaque formation (Peyronie's disease) and any abnormalities in size or consistency of either testicle. Examination of the prostate is essential.

B. LABORATORY FINDINGS

Laboratory evaluation is limited and should consist of a complete blood count, urinalysis, lipid profile, determination of serum testosterone, glucose, and prolactin. Patients with abnormalities of testosterone or prolactin require further evaluation with measurement of serum follicle-stimulating hormone (FSH) and luteinizing hormone (LH), and endocrinologic consultation is advised.

C. SPECIAL TESTS

Further testing is based on the patient's goals. Patients who will accept only noninvasive forms of therapy may be offered medical therapy or a vacuum constriction device, as described below. Most patients undergo further evaluation with direct injection of vasoactive substances into the penis. Such substances (prostaglandin E_1, papaverine, or a combination of drugs) will induce erections in men with intact vascular systems. Patients who respond with a rigid erection require no further vascular evaluation. However, organic and psychogenic impotence can be differentiated by use of nocturnal penile tumescence testing, where the frequency as well as the rigidity of erections are recorded by a simple device attached to the penis before sleep. Patients with psychogenic impotence will have nocturnal erections of adequate frequency and rigidity.

Additional vascular testing is indicated in patients who fail to achieve an erection with injection of vasoactive substances on serial attempts using increasing doses or combination of drugs and who would consider vascular reconstructive surgery. Diagnostic tests, such as duplex ultrasound, penile cavernosography, and pudendal arteriography, can separate arterial from venous erectile dysfunction and help predict which patients may benefit from vascular surgery.

Treatment

The vast majority of men suffering from erectile dysfunction can be treated successfully with one of the approaches outlined below. Men who do not suffer from organic dysfunction will probably benefit from behaviorally oriented sex therapy.

A. HORMONAL REPLACEMENT

Testosterone injections (200 mg intramuscularly every 3 weeks) or topical patches (2.5–6 mg/d) are offered to men with documented androgen deficiency who have undergone endocrinologic evaluation as described and in whom prostatic cancer has been excluded by prostate-specific antigen (PSA) screening and DRE.

B. VACUUM CONSTRICTION DEVICE

The vacuum constriction device is a cylindric device that draws the penis into an erect state by inducing a vacuum within the cylinder. Once adequate tumescence has been achieved, a rubber constriction device or band is placed around the proximal penis to prevent loss of erection, and the cylinder is removed. Such devices are suitable for patients with venous disorders of the penis and those who fail to achieve an adequate erection with injection of vasoactive substances. Complications are rare.

C. VASOACTIVE THERAPY

Direct injection of vasoactive prostaglandins into the penis is an acceptable form of treatment for most men with impotence. These injections are performed using a tuberculin syringe. The base and lateral aspect of the penis is used as the injection site to avoid injury to the superficial blood supply located anteriorly. Complications are rare and include dizziness, local pain, fibrosis, and infection. A prolonged erection requiring aspiration of blood and injection of epinephrine and phenylephrine to achieve detumescence occurs very rarely. A mechanism of delivering vasoactive prostaglandins (alprostadil) via a urethral suppository has been developed, and results are good. Pellet sizes are 125, 250, 500, and 1000 mcg.

Sexual stimulation with subsequent nitric oxide neural release will initiate penile erections. Decreasing the breakdown of cyclic guanosine monophosphate (cGMP) has revolutionized the treatment of erectile dysfunction. Sildenafil (Viagra) inhibits phosphodiesterase 5 (PDE-5)—itself an inhibitor of erection—and allows cGMP to function unopposed. Ordinarily, nitric oxide-mediated release from parasympathetic nerves and endothelium generates this compound, and prolongation of its half-life results in sustained inflow of blood into the erect penis. Fifty milligrams taken 1 hour prior to anticipated sexual activity is recommended, with peak action at 2 hours. There is no effect on libido, nor is priapism a problem, but the additive effect on nitrates may lead to exaggerated cardiac preload reduction and hypotension. Thus, the drug is contraindicated in patients taking nitroglycerin. All patients being evaluated for acute chest pain should be asked if they are taking sildenafil before administering nitroglycerin. Fixed atherosclerotic disease in the aortoiliac system is associated with diminished efficacy. Newer PDE-5 inhibitors, including vardenafil (Levitra) and tadalafil (Cialis), have a longer half-life and are similarly effective. Some patients who do not respond to one PDE-5 inhibitor may respond to one of the other agents. Apomorphine SL is a dopamine D_1 and D_2 agonist and is now approved for use in Europe.

D. PENILE PROSTHESES

Prosthetic devices may be implanted directly into the paired corporal bodies. Such prostheses may be rigid, malleable, hinged, or inflatable. Each is manufactured in a variety of sizes and diameters. Inflatable models may result in a more cosmetic appearance but may be associated with a greater likelihood of mechanical failure.

E. VASCULAR RECONSTRUCTION

Patients with disorders of the arterial system are candidates for various forms of arterial reconstruction, including endarterectomy and balloon dilation for proximal arterial occlusion and arterial bypass procedures utilizing arterial (epigastric) or venous (deep dorsal vein) segments for distal occlusion. Patients with venous disorders may be managed with ligation of certain veins (deep dorsal or emissary veins) or the crura of the corpora cavernosa. Experience with vascular reconstructive procedures is still limited, and many patients so treated still fail to achieve a rigid erection.

Carson CC et al; Patient Response with Vardenafil in Sildenafil Non-Responders (PROVEN) Study Group: Erectile response with vardenafil in sildenafil nonresponders: a multicentre, double-blind, 12-week, flexible-dose, placebo-controlled erectile dysfunction clinical trial. BJU Int 2004;94: 1301. [PMID: 15610110]

Gonzalgo ML et al: Clinical efficacy of sildenafil citrate and predictors of long-term response. J Urol 2003;170:503. [PMID: 12853809]

Lue TF: Erectile dysfunction. N Engl J Med 2000;342:1802. [PMID: 10853004]

Montague DK et al: Contemporary aspects of penile prosthesis implantation. Urol Int 2003;70:141. [PMID: 12592043]

Morales A: Erectile dysfunction: an overview. Clin Geriatr Med 2003;19:529. [PMID: 14567005]

Mulhall JP: Deciphering erectile dysfunction drug trials. J Urol 2003;170(2 Pt 1):353. [PMID: 12853774]

Nehra A et al: Vardenafil improved patient satisfaction with erectile hardness, orgasmic function and sexual experience in men with erectile dysfunction following nerve sparing radical prostatectomy. J Urol 2005;173:2067. [PMID: 15879836]

Seftel AD: Erectile dysfunction in the elderly: epidemiology, etiology and approaches to treatment. J Urol 2003;169:1999. [PMID: 12771705]

Seidman SN: The aging male: androgens, erectile dysfunction, and depression. J Clin Psychiatry 2003;64(Suppl 10):31. [PMID: 12971814]

Waldinger MD: On-demand treatment of premature ejaculation with clomipramine and paroxetine: a randomized, double-blind fixed-dose study with stopwatch assessment. Eur Urol 2004;46(4):510. [PMID: 15363569]

MALE INFERTILITY

Primary infertility affects 15–20% of married couples. Approximately one-third of cases result from male factors, one-third from female factors, and one-third from combined factors. It is thus critical to have simultaneous evaluation of both partners. Clinical evaluation is warranted following 6 months of unprotected intercourse. Endocrinologic profiles and detailed semen analyses are the cornerstones of laboratory investigations after the history and physical examination (see Figure 23–1). **Oligospermia** is the presence of less than 20 million sperm/

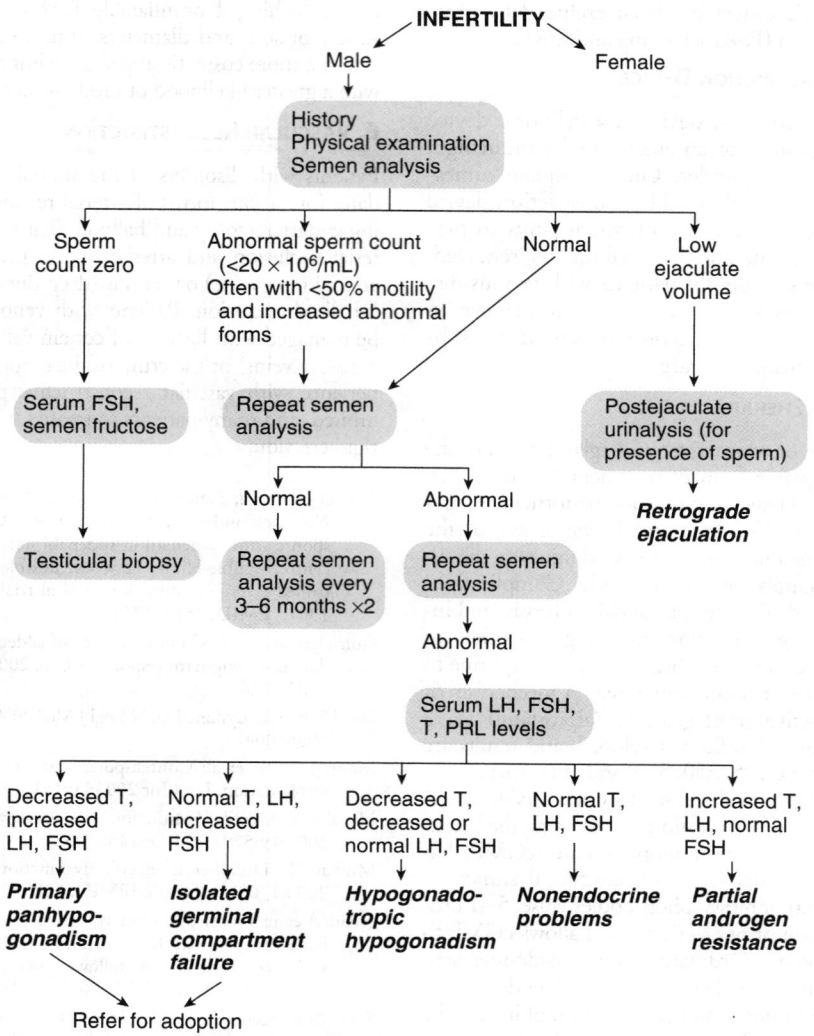

Figure 23–1. Male infertility: evaluation of male factor infertility. FSH = follicle-stimulating hormone; LH = luteinizing hormone; PRL = prolactin; T = testosterone. (From Nicoll D et al [editors]: *Pocket Guide to Diagnostic Tests.* McGraw-Hill, 2004. Adapted, with permission, from Swerdloff RS, Boyers SM: evaluation of the male partner of an infertile couple: an algorithmic approach. JAMA 1982;247:2418. Copyright © 1982 by The American Medical Association.)

mL in the ejaculate; **azoospermia** is the absence of sperm. As spermatogenesis takes approximately 74 days, it is thus important to review events from the past 3 months.

Clinical Findings

A. SYMPTOMS AND SIGNS

The history should include prior testicular insults (torsion, cryptorchidism, trauma), infections (mumps orchitis, epididymitis), environmental factors (excessive heat, radiation, chemotherapy), medications (anabolic

steroids, cimetidine, and spironolactone may affect spermatogenesis; phenytoin may lower FSH; sulfasalazine and nitrofurantoin affect sperm motility), and drugs (alcohol, marijuana). Sexual habits, frequency and timing of intercourse, use of lubricants, and each partner's previous fertility experiences are important. Loss of libido and headaches or visual disturbances may indicate a pituitary tumor. The past medical or surgical history may reveal thyroid or liver disease (abnormalities of spermatogenesis), diabetic neuropathy (retrograde ejaculation), radical pelvic or retroperitoneal surgery (absent seminal emission secondary to sympathetic nerve injury), or hernia repair (damage to the vas deferens or testicular blood supply).

Physical examination should pay particular attention to features of hypogonadism: underdeveloped secondary sexual characteristics, diminished male pattern hair distribution (axillary, body, facial, pubic), eunuchoid skeletal proportions (arm span 2 inches > height; upper to lower body ratio < 1.0), and gynecomastia. The scrotal contents should be carefully evaluated. Testicular size should be noted (normal size approximately 4.5 × 2.5 cm, volume 18 mL). Varicoceles should be looked for in the standing position and on occasion may be appreciated only with the Valsalva maneuver. The vas deferens, epididymis, and prostate should be palpated.

B. LABORATORY FINDINGS

Semen analysis should be performed after 72 hours of abstinence. The specimen should be analyzed within 1 hour after collection. Abnormal sperm concentrations are less than 20 million/mL. Normal semen volumes range between 1.5 and 5 mL (volumes < 1.5 mL may result in inadequate buffering of the vaginal acidity and may be due to retrograde ejaculation or androgen insufficiency). Normal sperm motility and morphology demonstrate 50–60% motile cells and more than 60% normal morphology. Abnormal motility may result from antisperm antibodies or infection. Abnormal morphology may result from a varicocele, infection, or exposure history.

Endocrinologic evaluation is warranted if sperm counts are low or if there is a clinical basis (from the history and physical examination) for suspecting an endocrinologic origin. Testing should include serum FSH, LH, and testosterone. Elevated FSH and LH and low testosterone (hypergonadotropic hypogonadism) are associated with primary testicular failure, which is usually irreversible. Low FSH and LH associated with low testosterone occur in secondary testicular failure (hypogonadotropic hypogonadism) and may be of hypothalamic or pituitary origin. Such defects may be correctable. In such cases, serum prolactin should be checked to exclude pituitary prolactinoma.

C. IMAGING

Scrotal ultrasound may detect a subclinical varicocele. Vasography may be required in patients with suspected ductal obstruction.

D. SPECIAL TESTS

Azoospermic patients should have postmasturbation urine samples centrifuged and analyzed for sperm to exclude retrograde ejaculation. Azoospermic patients and patients with ejaculate volumes less than 1 mL should have fructose levels determined on the ejaculate. Fructose is produced in the seminal vesicles and if absent in the ejaculate implies obstruction of the ejaculatory ducts.

Treatment

A. GENERAL MEASURES

Education with respect to the proper timing for intercourse in relation to the female's ovulatory cycle as well as the avoidance of spermicidal lubricants should be discussed. In cases of toxic exposure or medication-related factors, the offending agent should be removed. Patients with active genitourinary tract infections should be treated with appropriate antibiotics.

B. ENDOCRINE THERAPY

Hypogonadotropic hypogonadism may be treated with chorionic gonadotropin once primary pituitary disease has been excluded or treated. Dosage is usually 2000 international units intramuscularly three times a week. If sperm counts fail to rise after 12 months, FSH therapy should be initiated. Menotropins (Pergonal) is available as a premixed vial of 75 international units of FSH and 75 international units of LH. The usual dosage ranges from one-half to one vial intramuscularly three times per week.

C. RETROGRADE EJACULATION THERAPY

Oligospermic patients with retrograde ejaculation may benefit from α-adrenergic agonists (pseudoephedrine, 60 mg orally three times a day) or imipramine (25 mg orally three times a day). Medical failures may require the collection of postmasturbation urine for intrauterine insemination or electroejaculation in the case of absent emission.

D. VARICOCELE

Surgical approaches to varicoceles may be accomplished via a scrotal, inguinal, or laparoscopic approach. More recently, percutaneous venographic approaches have been developed, obviating the need for an anesthetic.

E. DUCTAL OBSTRUCTION

The level of obstruction must be delineated via a vasogram prior to operative treatment. Mechanical obstruction of the ejaculatory duct may be corrected by transurethral resection and unroofing of the ducts in the prostatic urethra. Obstruction of the vas deferens is best managed by a microsurgical approach, and a vasovasostomy or vasoepididymostomy may be required.

F. ASSISTED REPRODUCTIVE TECHNIQUES

Advances in reproductive technology may provide alternatives to patients who have failed other means of treating reduced sperm counts and motility. Such measures include intrauterine insemination, in vitro fertilization, and gamete intrafallopian transfer.

Brugh VM 3rd et al: Male factor infertility: evaluation and management. Med Clin North Am 2004;88:367. [PMID: 15049583]
Hirsh A: Male subfertility. BMJ 2003;327:669. [PMID: 14500443]

Makar RS et al: The evaluation of infertility. Am J Clin Pathol 2002;117(Suppl):S95. [PMID: 14569805]

■ BENIGN PROSTATIC HYPERPLASIA

 ESSENTIALS OF DIAGNOSIS

- *Obstructive or irritative voiding symptoms.*
- *May have enlarged prostate on rectal examination.*
- *Absence of urinary tract infection, neurologic disorder, stricture disease, prostatic or bladder malignancy.*

General Considerations

Benign prostatic hyperplasia is the most common benign tumor in men, and its incidence is age related. The prevalence of histologic benign prostatic hyperplasia in autopsy studies rises from approximately 20% in men aged 41–50 years, to 50% in men aged 51–60, and to over 90% in men over 80 years of age. Although clinical evidence of disease occurs less commonly, symptoms of prostatic obstruction are also age related. At age 55 years, approximately 25% of men report obstructive voiding symptoms. At age 75 years, 50% of men report a decrease in the force and caliber of the urinary stream.

Risk factors for the development of benign prostatic hyperplasia are poorly understood. Some studies have suggested a genetic predisposition and some have noted racial differences. Approximately 50% of men under age 60 years who undergo surgery for benign prostatic hyperplasia may have a heritable form of the disease. This form is most likely an autosomal dominant trait, and first-degree male relatives of such patients carry an increased relative risk of approximately fourfold.

Etiology

The etiology is not completely understood, but the disorder seems to be multifactorial and under endocrine control. The prostate is composed of both stromal and epithelial elements, and each, either alone or in combination, can give rise to hyperplastic nodules and the symptoms associated with benign prostatic hyperplasia. Each element may be targeted in medical management schemes.

Laboratory and clinical studies have identified two factors necessary for the development of benign prostatic hyperplasia: dihydrotestosterone (DHT) and aging. Animal studies have demonstrated that the aging prostate becomes more sensitive to androgens. Prostatic growth in aging dogs appears to be related more to a decrease in cell death than to an increase in cell proliferation. Laboratory studies have suggested several theories in this area: (1) stromal-epithelial interactions (stroma cell may regulate growth of epithelial cell or other stromal cells via a paracrine or autocrine mechanism by secreting growth factors such as basic fibroblast growth factor or transforming growth factor-β), and (2) aging may result in stem cells undergoing a block in the maturation process, preventing them from entering into programmed cell death (apoptosis). The impact of aging in animal studies appears to be mediated via estrogen synergism. In canines, estrogens induce the androgen receptor; alter steroid metabolism, resulting in higher levels of intraprostatic DHT; inhibit cell death when given in the presence of androgens; and stimulate stroma collagen production.

Studies have demonstrated that benign prostatic hyperplasia is under endocrine control. Castration results in the regression of established disease and improvement in urinary symptoms. Administration of a luteinizing hormone-releasing hormone (LHRH) analog in men reversibly shrinks established benign prostatic hyperplasia, resulting in objective improvement in flow rate and subjective improvement in symptoms. Further investigations have demonstrated a positive correlation between levels of free testosterone and estrogen and the volume of the gland. The latter may suggest that the association between aging and benign prostatic hyperplasia might reflect increasing estrogen levels of aging, resulting in induction of the androgen receptor and thus sensitizing the prostate to free testosterone. However, no studies to date have been able to demonstrate elevated estrogen receptor levels in humans with the disease.

Pathology

Benign prostatic hyperplasia is truly a hyperplastic process, resulting from an increase in cell numbers. Microscopic evaluation reveals a nodular growth pattern consisting of varying amounts of stroma or epithelium. Stroma is composed of varying amounts of collagen and smooth muscle. The differential representation of various histologic components of benign prostatic hyperplasia in part explains the potential responsiveness to medical therapy. Thus, α-blocker therapy may result in excellent responses in patients with benign prostatic hyperplasia when there is a significant component of smooth muscle, while hyperplasia composed predominantly of epithelium might respond better to 5α-reductase inhibitors. Patients with significant components of collagen in the stroma may not respond to either form of medical therapy. Responsiveness to specific therapy cannot reliably be predicted (see below).

As benign prostatic hyperplasia nodules in the transition zone enlarge, they compress the outer zones of the prostate, resulting in the formation of a "surgical capsule." This boundary separates the transition zone from the peripheral zone of the gland and serves as a cleavage plane for open enucleation of the prostate during simple prostatectomy (surgery that removes the zone of the prostate around the urethra leaving the peripheral portion of the prostate and prostate capsule).

Pathophysiology

The symptoms of benign prostatic hyperplasia can be related either to the obstructive component of the prostate or to the secondary response of the bladder to the outlet resistance. The obstructive component can be subdivided into mechanical obstruction and dynamic obstruction.

As prostatic enlargement occurs, mechanical obstruction may result from intrusion into the urethral lumen or bladder neck, resulting in a higher bladder outlet resistance. Prostatic size on DRE correlates poorly with symptoms.

The dynamic component of prostatic obstruction explains the variable nature of the symptoms. The prostatic stroma is composed of smooth muscle and collagen and is rich in adrenergic nerve supply. The level of autonomic stimulation thus sets a "tone" to the prostatic urethra. α-Blocker therapy decreases this tone, resulting in a decrease in outlet resistance.

The irritative voiding complaints (see below) of benign prostatic hyperplasia result from the secondary response of the bladder to the increased outlet resistance. Bladder outlet obstruction results in detrusor muscle hypertrophy and hyperplasia as well as collagen deposition. The latter is most likely responsible for a decrease in bladder compliance, but detrusor instability also occurs. On gross inspection, thickened detrusor muscle bundles are seen as trabeculations on cystoscopic examination. If left unchecked, mucosal herniation between detrusor muscle bundles ensues, resulting in diverticulum formation ("false" diverticula composed of mucosa and serosa only).

Clinical Findings

A. SYMPTOMS

The symptoms of benign prostatic hyperplasia can be divided into obstructive and irritative complaints. Obstructive symptoms include hesitancy, decreased force and caliber of the stream, sensation of incomplete bladder emptying, double voiding (urinating a second time within 2 hours), straining to urinate, and postvoid dribbling. Irritative symptoms include urgency, frequency, and nocturia.

The American Urological Association (AUA) has developed a self-administered questionnaire that is reliable in identifying patients who need therapy and in monitoring the response to therapy. The AUA symptom index (Table 23–4) is perhaps the single most important tool used in the evaluation of patients with this disorder and

should be calculated for all patients before starting therapy. The answers to seven questions quantitate the severity of obstructive or irritative complaints on a scale of 0–5. Thus, the score can range from 0 to 35, in increasing severity of symptoms.

A detailed history focusing on the urinary tract should be obtained to exclude other possible causes of symptoms such as prostate cancer or disorders unrelated to the prostate such as urinary tract infection, neurogenic bladder, or urethral stricture.

B. SIGNS

A physical examination, DRE, and a focused neurologic examination should be performed on all patients. The size and consistency of the prostate should be noted, but prostate size does not correlate with the severity of symptoms or the degree of obstruction. Benign prostatic hyperplasia usually results in a smooth, firm, elastic enlargement of the prostate. Induration, if detected, must alert the physician to the possibility of cancer, and further evaluation is needed (ie, PSA, transrectal ultrasound, and biopsy). Examination of the lower abdomen should be performed to assess for a distended bladder.

C. LABORATORY FINDINGS

Urinalysis should be performed to exclude infection or hematuria, and serum creatinine should be measured to assess renal function. Renal insufficiency from benign prostatic hyperplasia is fairly rare, occurring in only about 2% of patients with lower urinary tract symptoms on initial presentation. If renal insufficiency is detected, upper urinary tract imaging is warranted. Patients with renal insufficiency are at an increased risk for complications following operative treatment for benign prostatic hyperplasia. A serum PSA is considered optional, yet most physicians will include it in the initial evaluation. PSA certainly increases the ability to detect prostate cancer over DRE alone; however, because there is much overlap between levels seen in benign prostatic hyperplasia and prostate cancer, its use remains controversial (see below in the section on screening for prostate cancer).

D. IMAGING

Upper tract imaging (IVP, CT, or renal ultrasound) is recommended only in the presence of concomitant urinary tract disease or complications from benign prostatic hyperplasia (ie, hematuria, urinary tract infection, renal insufficiency, history of stone disease).

E. CYSTOSCOPY

Cystoscopy is not recommended to determine the need for treatment but may assist in determining the surgical approach in patients opting for invasive therapy.

F. ADDITIONAL TESTS

Cystometrograms and urodynamic profiles should be reserved for patients with suspected neurologic disease or those who have failed prostate surgery. Flow rates,

Table 23–4. American Urological Association symptom index for benign prostatic hyperplasia.[1]

Questions to Be Answered	Not at All	Less Than One Time in Five	Less Than Half the Time	About Half the Time	More Than Half the Time	Almost Always
1. Over the past month, how often have you had a sensation of not emptying your bladder completely after you finish urinating?	0	1	2	3	4	5
2. Over the past month, how often have you had to urinate again less than 2 hours after you finished urinating?	0	1	2	3	4	5
3. Over the past month, how often have you found you stopped and started again several times when you urinated?	0	1	2	3	4	5
4. Over the past month, how often have you found it difficult to postpone urination?	0	1	2	3	4	5
5. Over the past month, how often have you had a weak urinary stream?	0	1	2	3	4	5
6. Over the past month, how often have you had to push or strain to begin urination?	0	1	2	3	4	5
7. Over the past month, how many times did you most typically get up to urinate from the time you went to bed at night until the time you got up in the morning?	0 (None)	1 (1 time)	2 (2 times)	3 (3 times)	4 (4 times)	5 (5 times)

[1]Sum of seven circled numbers equals the symptom score. See text for explanation.
Reproduced, with permission, from Barry MJ et al: The American Urological Association symptoms index for benign prostatic hyperplasia. J Urol 1992;148:1549.

postvoid residual urine determination, and pressure-flow studies are considered optional.

Differential Diagnosis

Other obstructive conditions of the lower urinary tract such as urethral stricture, bladder neck contracture, bladder stone, or carcinoma of the prostate must be considered when evaluating men with presumptive benign prostatic hyperplasia. A history of prior urethral instrumentation, urethritis, or trauma should be elucidated to exclude urethral stricture or bladder neck contracture. Hematuria and pain are commonly associated with bladder stones. Carcinoma of the prostate may be detected by abnormalities on the DRE or an elevated PSA (see below). A urinary tract infection can mimic the irritative symptoms of benign prostatic hyperplasia and can be readily identified by urinalysis and culture; however, a urinary tract infection can also be a complication of benign prostatic hyperplasia. Carcinoma of the bladder, especially carcinoma in situ, may also present with irritative voiding complaints; however, urinalysis usually shows evidence of hematuria. Patients with a neurogenic bladder may also have many of the same symptoms and signs as those with benign prostatic hyperplasia; however, a history of neurologic disease, stroke,

diabetes mellitus, or back injury may be obtained, and diminished perineal or lower extremity sensation or alterations in rectal sphincter tone or the bulbocavernosus reflex might be observed on examination. Simultaneous alterations in bowel function (constipation) might also suggest the possibility of a neurologic disorder.

Treatment

Clinical practice guidelines exist for the evaluation and treatment of patients with benign prostatic hyperplasia (Figure 23–2). Following evaluation as outlined above, patients should be offered various forms of therapy for benign prostatic hyperplasia. Patients are advised to consult with their primary care physicians and make an educated decision on the basis of the relative efficacy and side effects of the treatment options (Table 23–5).

Patients with mild symptoms (AUA scores 0–7) should be managed by watchful waiting only. Absolute surgical indications are refractory urinary retention (failing at least one attempt at catheter removal), large bladder diverticula, or any of the following sequelae of benign prostatic hyperplasia: recurrent urinary tract infection, recurrent gross hematuria, bladder stones, or renal insufficiency.

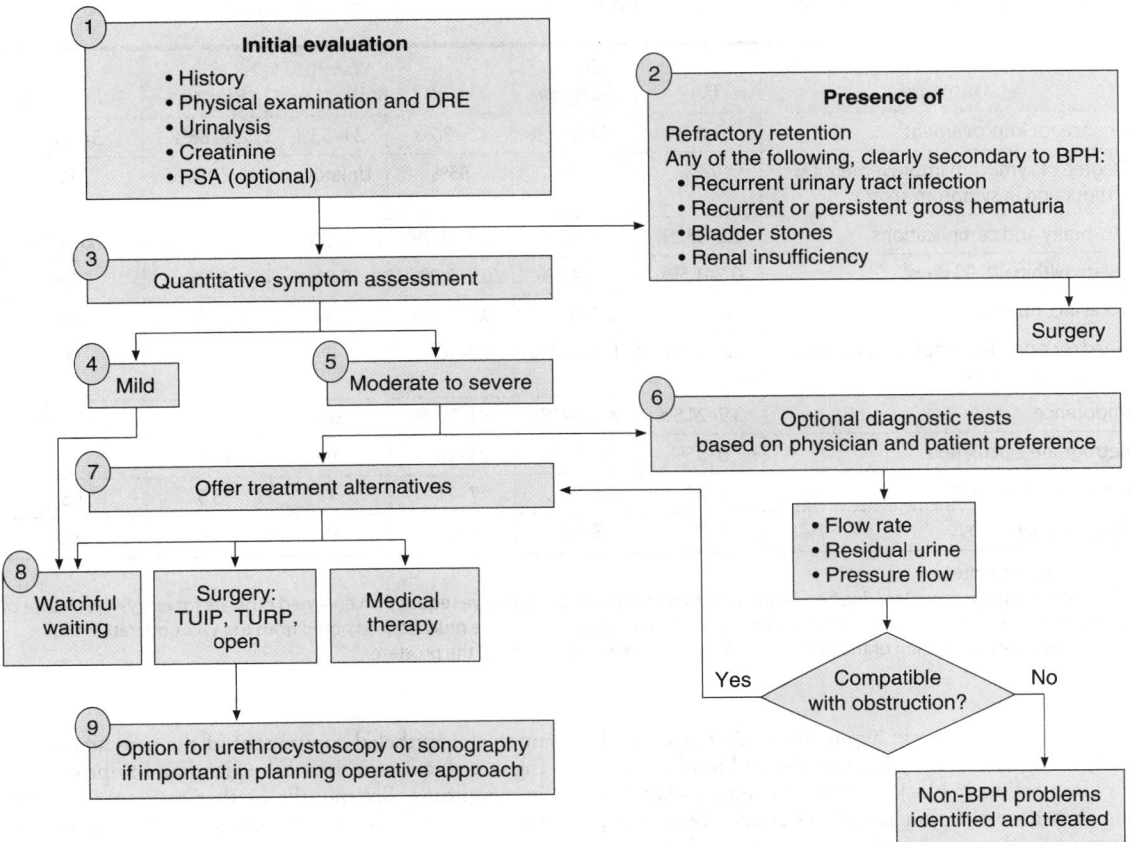

Figure 23–2. Benign prostatic hyperplasia decision diagram. DRE = digital rectal examination; PSA = prostate-specific antigen; BPH = benign prostatic hyperplasia; TUIP = transurethral incision of the prostate; TURP = transurethral resection of the prostate.

A. WATCHFUL WAITING

The risk of progression or complications is uncertain. However, in men with symptomatic disease, it is clear that progression is not inevitable and that some men undergo spontaneous improvement or resolution of their symptoms.

Retrospective studies on the natural history of benign prostatic hyperplasia are inherently subject to bias, relating in part to patient selection and also to the type and extent of follow-up. Very few prospective studies addressing the natural history have been reported. One small series demonstrated that approximately 10% of symptomatic men may progress to urinary retention while 50% of patients demonstrate marked improvement or resolution of symptoms. Recently, a large randomized study was reported comparing finasteride with placebo in men with moderate to severely symptomatic disease and enlarged prostates on DRE. Patients in the placebo arm demonstrated a 7% risk of developing urinary retention over 4 years.

Men with moderate or severe symptoms can also be managed in this fashion if they so choose. The opti-

mal interval for follow-up is not defined, nor are the specific end points for intervention.

B. MEDICAL THERAPY

1. α-Blockers—The human prostate and bladder base contains α_1-adrenoceptors, and the prostate will show a contractile response to such agonists. The contractile properties of the prostate and bladder neck seem to be mediated primarily by α_{1a}-receptors. α-Blockade has been shown to result in both objective and subjective degrees of improvement in the symptoms and signs of benign prostatic hyperplasia in some patients. α-Blockers can be classified according to their receptor selectivity as well as their half-life (Table 23–6).

The efficacies of phenoxybenzamine and prazosin are comparable with respect to symptomatic relief; however, the higher side-effect profile of phenoxybenzamine, resulting from its lack of α-receptor specificity, precludes its use in patients with benign prostatic hyperplasia. Prazosin is effective; however, it requires dose titration and twice daily dosing. Typical side ef-

Table 23–5. Balance sheet for benign prostatic hyperplasia treatment outcomes.[1]

Outcome	TUIP	Open Surgery	TURP	Watchful Waiting	α-Blockers	Finasteride[2]
Chance for improvement[1]	78–83%	94–99.8%	75–96%	31–55%	59–86%	54–78%
Degree of symptom improvement (% reduction in symptom score)	73%	79%	85%	Unknown	51%	31%
Morbidity and complications[1]	2.2–33.3%	7–42.7%	5.2–30.7%	1–5%	2.9–43.3%	13.6–8.8%
Death within 30–90 days[1]	0.2–1.5%	1–4.6%	0.5–3.3%	0.8%	0.8%	0.8%
Total incontinence[1]	0.1–1.1%	0.3–0.7%	0.7–1.4%	2%	2%	2%
Need for operative treatment for surgical complications[1]	1.3–2.7%	0.6–14.1%	0.7–10.1%	0	0	0
Impotence[1]	3.9–24.5%	4.7–39.2%	3.3–34.8%	3%	3%	2.5–5.3%
Retrograde ejaculation	6–55%	36–95%	25–99%	0	4–11%	0
Loss of work in days	7–21	21–28	7–21	1	3.5	1.5
Hospital stay in days	1–3	5–10	3–5	0	0	0

[1]90% confidence interval.

[2]Most of the data reviewed for finasteride are derived from three trials that have required an enlarged prostate for entry. The chance of improvement in men with symptoms yet minimally enlarged prostates may be much less, as noted from the VA Cooperative Trial. TUIP = transurethral incision of the prostate; TURP = transurethral resection of the prostate.

fects include orthostatic hypotension, dizziness, tiredness, retrograde ejaculation, rhinitis, and headache.

Long-acting α-blockers allow for once-a-day dosing, but dose titration is still necessary. Terazosin is started at a dosage of 1 mg orally daily for 3 days, increased to 2 mg orally daily for 11 days, then 5 mg orally daily. Additional dose escalation to 10 mg orally daily can be performed if necessary. Doxazosin is started at a dosage of 1 mg orally daily for 7 days, increased to 2 mg orally daily for 7 days, then 4 mg orally daily. Additional dose escalation to 8 mg orally daily can be performed if necessary. Side effects are similar to those described above for prazosin. Terazosin improves symptoms and in numerous studies is superior to placebo or finasteride. Alfuzosin is a long-acting α-blocker; its dose is 10 mg orally once daily and does not require titration.

The most recent advance in α-blocker therapy has been the identification of subtypes of α_1-receptors. The α_{1a}-receptors are localized to the prostate and bladder neck, and selective blockade results in fewer systemic side effects (orthostatic hypotension, dizziness, tiredness, rhinitis, and headache), thus obviating the need for dose titration. The dose of tamsulosin is 0.4 mg orally daily taken 30 minutes after a meal. Several randomized, double-blind, placebo-controlled trials have been performed comparing terazosin, doxazosin, tamsulosin, and alfuzosin with placebo. All agents have demonstrated safety and efficacy.

2. 5α-Reductase inhibitors—Finasteride is a 5α-reductase inhibitor that blocks the conversion of testosterone to dihydrotestosterone. This drug impacts upon the epithelial component of the prostate, resulting in reduction in size of the gland and improvement in symptoms. Six months of therapy is required for maximum effects on prostate size (20% reduction) and symptomatic improvement.

Several randomized, double-blind, placebo-controlled trials have been performed comparing finasteride with placebo. Efficacy, safety, and durability are well established. However, symptomatic improvement is seen only in men with enlarged prostates (> 40 mL). Side effects include decreased libido, decrease in volume of ejaculate, and impotence. Serum PSA is reduced by approximately 50% in patients receiving finasteride therapy. Therefore, in order to compare with pre-finasteride levels, the serum PSA of a patient taking finasteride should be doubled.

Table 23–6. α-Blockade for benign prostatic hyperplasia.

Agent	Action	Dose
Phenoxybenzamine	α_1- and α_2-Blockade	5–10 mg twice daily
Prazosin	α_1-Blockade	1–5 mg twice daily
Terazosin	α_1-Blockade	1–10 mg daily
Doxazosin	α_1-Blockade	1–8 mg daily
Alfuzosin	α_1-Blockade	10 mg daily
Tamsulosin	α_{1a}-Blockade	0.4 or 0.8 mg daily

A recent report suggests that finasteride therapy may decrease the incidence of urinary retention and the need for operative treatment in men with enlarged prostates and moderate to severe symptoms. The larger the prostate over 40 mL, the greater the apparent relative-risk reduction. However, optimal identification of appropriate patients for prophylactic therapy remains to be determined. Dutasteride is a well-tolerated 5α-reductase inhibitor that appears to be similar to finasteride in its effectiveness; its dose is 0.5 mg orally daily.

3. Combination therapy—The four-arm Veterans Administration Cooperative Trial compared placebo, finasteride alone, terazosin alone, and combination of finasteride and terazosin. Over 1200 patients participated, and significant decreases in symptom scores and increases in urinary flow rates were seen only in the arms containing terazosin. However, enlarged prostates were not an entry criterion; in fact, prostate size in this study was much smaller than in previous controlled trials using finasteride (32 versus 52 mL). Other randomized, placebo-controlled trials comparing finasteride with placebo in men with lower urinary tract symptoms and large prostates showed finasteride to be beneficial for reducing symptoms, increasing urinary flow rate, and reducing the risk of complications due to benign prostatic hyperplasia as well as reducing the number of men who required surgery for benign prostatic hyperplasia. The Medical Therapy of Prostatic Symptoms (MTOPs) trial is a large, randomized, placebo-controlled trial comparing finasteride, doxazosin, the combination of the two, and placebo in 3047 men observed for a mean of 4.5 years. Long-term combination therapy with doxazosin and finasteride was safe and reduced the risk of overall clinical progression of benign prostatic hyperplasia significantly more than did treatment with either drug alone. Combination therapy and finasteride alone reduced the long-term risk of acute urinary retention and the need for invasive therapy. Combination therapy had the risks of additional side effects and the cost of two medications.

4. Phytotherapy—Phytotherapy is the use of plants or plant extracts for medicinal purposes. Its use in benign prostatic hyperplasia has been popular in Europe for years, and its use in the United States is growing as a result of patient-driven enthusiasm. Several plant extracts have been popularized, including the saw palmetto berry, the bark of *Pygeum africanum*, the roots of *Echinacea purpurea* and *Hypoxis rooperi*, pollen extract, and the leaves of the trembling poplar. The mechanisms of action of these agents are unknown. A recent, prospective, randomized, double-blind, placebo-controlled trial revealed no improvement in symptoms, urinary flow rate, or quality of life for men with benign prostatic hyperplasia with saw palmetto treatment compared with placebo.

C. CONVENTIONAL SURGICAL THERAPY

1. Transurethral resection of the prostate (TURP)— Ninety-five percent of simple prostatectomies can be performed endoscopically. Most of these procedures are per-formed under a spinal anesthetic and require a 1- to 2-day hospital stay. Symptom scores and flow rate improvement are superior following TURP relative to any minimally invasive therapy; however, the length of the hospital stay is greater. Much controversy revolves around possible higher rates of morbidity and mortality associated with TURP in comparison with open surgery, but the higher rates observed in one study probably related to more significant comorbidities in the TURP patients compared with the patients who received open surgical treatment. Several other studies could not confirm the difference in mortality when controlling for age and comorbidities. The risks of TURP include retrograde ejaculation (75%), impotence (5–10%), and urinary incontinence (< 1%). Complications include bleeding, urethral stricture or bladder neck contracture, perforation of the prostate capsule with extravasation, and, if severe, transurethral resection syndrome, a hypervolemic, hyponatremic state resulting from absorption of the hypotonic irrigating solution. Clinical manifestations of the syndrome include nausea, vomiting, confusion, hypertension, bradycardia, and visual disturbances. The risk of transurethral resection syndrome increases with resection times over 90 minutes. Treatment includes diuresis and, in severe cases, hypertonic saline administration.

2. Transurethral incision of the prostate (TUIP)— Men with moderate to severe symptoms and small prostates often have posterior commissure hyperplasia or an "elevated bladder neck." These patients will often benefit from incision of the prostate. The procedure is more rapid and less morbid than TURP. Outcomes in well-selected patients are comparable, though a lower rate of retrograde ejaculation has been reported (25%). The technique involves two incisions using the Collins knife at the 5 and 7 o'clock positions. The incisions are started just distal to the ureteral orifices and extended outward to the verumontanum.

3. Open simple prostatectomy—When the prostate is too large to remove endoscopically, open enucleation is necessary. What size is "too large" depends upon the surgeon's experience with TURP. Glands over 100 g are usually considered for open enucleation. In addition to size, other relative indications for open prostatectomy include concomitant bladder diverticulum or bladder stone and whether dorsal lithotomy positioning is or is not possible.

Open prostatectomies can be performed with either a suprapubic or retropubic approach. Simple suprapubic prostatectomy is performed transvesically and is the operation of choice if there is concomitant bladder pathology. After the bladder is opened, a semicircular incision is made in the bladder mucosa distal to the trigone. The dissection plane is initiated sharply, and blunt dissection with the finger is then performed to deliver the adenoma. The apical dissection should be performed sharply to avoid injury to the distal sphincteric mechanism. After the adenoma is removed, hemostasis is attained with suture ligatures and both a urethral and a suprapubic catheter are inserted prior to closure.

In simple retropubic prostatectomy, the bladder is not entered but rather a transverse incision is made in the surgical capsule of the prostate and the adenoma is enucleated as described above. Only a urethral catheter is needed at the end of the case.

D. MINIMALLY INVASIVE THERAPY

1. Laser therapy—Many techniques of laser surgery for the prostate have been described. Two main energy sources of lasers have been utilized—neodymium:yttrium-aluminum-garnet (Nd:YAG) and holmium-YAG.

Several different coagulation necrosis techniques have been described. Transurethral laser-induced prostatectomy (TULIP) is performed under transrectal ultrasound guidance. The instrument is placed in the urethra and transrectal ultrasound is used to direct the device as it is slowly pulled from the bladder neck to the apex. The depth of treatment is monitored with ultrasound.

Most urologists prefer to use visually directed laser techniques. Visual coagulative necrosis is performed under cystoscopic control, and the laser fiber is pulled through the prostate at several designated areas depending upon the size and configuration of the gland. Four-quadrant and sextant approaches have been described for lateral lobes, with additional treatments directed at enlarged median lobes. Coagulative techniques do not create an immediate visual defect in the prostatic urethra—tissue is sloughed over the course of several weeks up to 3 months following the procedure.

Visual contact ablative techniques take longer in the operating room because the fiber is placed in direct contact with the prostate tissue, which is vaporized. A new laser technique that is gaining popularity is photovaporization of the prostate (PVP) using a high-power KTP laser. An immediate defect is obtained in the prostatic urethra, similar to that seen during TURP.

Interstitial laser therapy places fibers directly into the prostate, usually under cystoscopic control. At each puncture, the laser is fired, resulting in submucosal coagulative necrosis. Irritative voiding symptoms may be less in these patients as the urethral mucosa is spared and prostate tissue is resorbed by the body rather than sloughed.

Advantages to laser surgery include minimal blood loss, rare occurrence of transurethral resection syndrome, the ability to treat patients while on anticoagulation therapy, and outpatient surgery. Disadvantages are the lack of tissue for pathologic examination, the longer postoperative catheterization time, the more frequent irritative voiding complaints, and the expense of laser fibers and generators.

Large multicenter, randomized studies with long-term follow-up are needed in comparing laser prostate surgery with TURP and other forms of minimally invasive surgery.

2. Transurethral needle ablation of the prostate (TUNA)—This procedure uses a specially designed urethral catheter that is passed into the urethra. Interstitial radiofrequency needles are then deployed from the tip of the catheter, piercing the mucosa of the prostatic urethra. Radiofrequencies are then used to heat the tissue, resulting in coagulative necrosis. Bladder neck and median lobe enlargement are not well treated by TUNA. Subjective and objective improvement in voiding occurs. In randomized trials comparing TUNA to TURP, similar improvement was seen when comparing life scores, peak urinary flow rates, and postvoid residual urine.

3. Transurethral electrovaporization of the prostate—This technique uses the standard resectoscope but replaces a conventional loop with a variation of a grooved rollerball. High current densities result in heat vaporization of tissue, creating a cavity in the prostatic urethra. Because the device requires slower sweeping speeds over the prostatic urethra and the depth of vaporization is approximately one-third of a standard loop, this procedure usually takes longer than a standard TURP. Long-term comparative data are needed.

4. Hyperthermia—Microwave hyperthermia is most commonly delivered with a transurethral catheter. Some devices cool the urethral mucosa to decrease the risk of injury. However, if temperatures do not go above 45 °C, cooling is unnecessary. Symptom score and flow rate improvement are obtained, but (as with laser surgery) large randomized studies with long-term follow-up are needed to assess durability and cost-effectiveness.

5. High-intensity focused ultrasound (HIFU)—HIFU is another means of performing thermal tissue ablation. A specially designed dual-function ultrasound probe is placed in the rectum. This probe allows transrectal imaging of the prostate and also delivers short bursts of high-intensity focused ultrasound energy, which heats the prostate tissue and causes coagulative necrosis. Bladder neck and median lobe enlargement are not well treated by HIFU. Ongoing clinical trials demonstrate some improvement in symptom score and flow rate, but the durability of the response is not known.

6. Intraurethral stents—Intraurethral stents are placed endoscopically in the prostatic fossa to keep the prostatic urethra patent. They are usually covered by urothelium within 4–6 months following insertion. These devices are typically used for patients with limited life expectancies who are not deemed good surgical or anesthetic candidates; however, with the advent of other minimally invasive techniques requiring minimal anesthesia (conscious sedation, or prostatic blocks), their application has become more limited.

7. Transurethral balloon dilation of the prostate—Balloon dilation of the prostate is performed with specially designed catheters that permit dilation of the prostatic fossa alone or dilation of the prostatic fossa and bladder neck. The technique is most effective in small prostates (< 40 mL), and although it may result in improvement in symptom score and flow rates, the effects are transient. This technique is rarely used today.

Andriole GL et al: Safety and tolerability of the dual 5-alpha-reductase inhibitor dutasteride in the treatment of benign prostatic hyperplasia. Eur Urol 2003;44:82. [PMID: 12814679]

Bent S et al: Saw palmetto for benign prostatic hyperplasia. N Engl J Med 2006;354:557. [PMID: 16467543]

Bhargava S et al: A rational approach to benign prostatic hyperplasia evaluation: recent advances. Curr Opin Urol 2004; 14:1. [PMID: 15091041]

Djavan B et al: Benign prostatic hyperplasia progression and its impact on treatment. Curr Opin Urol 2004;14:45. [PMID: 15091050]

Dutkiewicz S: Long-term treatment with doxazosin in men with benign prostatic hyperplasia: 10-year follow-up. Int Urol Nephrol 2004;36:169. [PMID: 15368687]

Kaplan SA: Use of alpha-adrenergic inhibitors in treatment of benign prostatic hyperplasia and implications on sexual function. Urology 2004;63:428. [PMID: 15028431]

Kortmann BB et al: Urodynamic effects of alpha-adrenoceptor blockers: a review of clinical trials. Urology 2003;62:1. [PMID: 12837408]

McConnell JD et al; Medical Therapy of Prostatic Symptoms (MTOPS) Research Group: The long-term effect of doxazosin, finasteride, and combination therapy on the clinical progression of benign prostatic hyperplasia. N Engl J Med 2003;349:2387. [PMID: 14681504]

O'Leary MP: Lower urinary tract symptoms/benign prostatic hyperplasia: maintaining symptom control and reducing complications. Urology 2003;62(3 Suppl 1):15. [PMID: 12957196]

Schulman CC: Lower urinary tract symptoms/benign prostatic hyperplasia: minimizing morbidity caused by treatment. Urology 2003;62(3 Suppl 1):24. [PMID: 12957197]

Thorpe A et al: Benign prostatic hyperplasia. Lancet 2003;361:1359. [PMID: 12711484]

Wilt TJ et al: Tamsulosin for benign prostatic hyperplasia. Cochrane Database Syst Rev 2003;(1):CD002081. [PMID: 12535426]

■ MALIGNANT GENITOURINARY TRACT DISORDERS

PROSTATE CANCER

ESSENTIALS OF DIAGNOSIS

- *Prostatic induration on DRE or elevation of PSA.*
- *Most often asymptomatic.*
- *Rarely: systemic symptoms (weight loss, bone pain).*

General Considerations

Prostatic cancer is the most common cancer detected in American men and the second leading cause of cancer-related death. In the United States in 2005, over 232,000 new cases of prostate cancer were diagnosed, and about 30,300 deaths resulted. However, the clinical incidence of the disease does not match the prevalence noted at autopsy, where more than 40% of men over 50 years of age are found to have prostatic carcinoma. Most such occult cancers are small and contained within the prostate gland. Few are associated with regional or distant disease. The incidence of prostatic cancer increases with age. Whereas 30% of men aged 60–69 years will have the disease, autopsy incidence increases to 67% in men aged 80–89 years. Although the prevalence of prostatic cancer in autopsy specimens around the world varies little, the clinical incidence is considerably different (high in North America and European countries, intermediate in South America, and low in the Far East), suggesting that environmental or dietary differences among populations may be important for prostatic cancer growth. A 50-year-old American man has a lifetime risk of 40% for latent cancer, 9.5% for developing clinically apparent cancer, and a 2.9% risk of death due to prostatic cancer. Blacks, men with a family history of prostatic cancer, and those with a history of high dietary fat intake are at increased risk of developing it.

Clinical Findings

A. SYMPTOMS AND SIGNS

Prostate cancer may be manifested as focal nodules or areas of induration within the prostate at the time of DRE. However, a large number of prostate cancers are associated with palpably normal prostates and are detected on the basis of elevations in serum PSA.

Rarely, patients present with signs of urinary retention (palpable bladder) or neurologic symptoms as a result of epidural metastases and cord compression. Obstructive voiding symptoms are most often due to benign prostatic hyperplasia, which occurs in the same age group. However, large or locally extensive prostatic cancers can cause obstructive voiding symptoms. Lymph node metastases can lead to lower extremity lymphedema. As the axial skeleton is the most common site of metastases, patients may present with back pain or pathologic fractures.

B. LABORATORY FINDINGS

1. Serum tumor markers—PSA is a glycoprotein produced only in the cytoplasm of benign and malignant prostate cells. The serum level correlates with the volume of both benign and malignant prostatic tissue. Measurement of PSA may be useful in detecting and staging prostatic cancer, monitoring response to treatment, and detecting recurrence before it becomes obvious clinically. As a first-line screening test, PSA will be elevated in approximately 10–15% of men self-referred for screening. Approximately 18–30% of men with intermediate degrees of elevation (4.1–10 ng/mL; normal < 4 ng/mL) will be found to have prostatic cancer. Between 50% and 70% of those with elevations greater than 10 ng/mL will have prostatic cancer. (See age-specific PSA reference ranges under Screening for Prostatic Cancer, below.) Patients with intermediate levels of PSA will usually have localized and therefore potentially curable cancers. However, it should be remembered that approximately 20% of patients who undergo radical prostatectomy for localized prostatic cancer will have normal levels of PSA.

In untreated patients with prostatic cancer, the level of PSA correlates with the volume and stage of the disease. Whereas most organ-confined cancers are associated with PSA levels less than 10 ng/mL, more advanced disease (seminal vesicle invasion, lymph node involvement, or occult distant metastases) is more common in patients with PSA levels in excess of 40 ng/mL. Approximately 98% of patients with metastatic prostatic cancer will have elevated PSA. However, there are occasional cancers that are localized despite substantial elevations in PSA. Therefore, treatment decisions in patients with untreated cancers cannot be made on the basis of PSA testing alone. A rising level of PSA after treatment is usually consistent with progressive disease whether it is locally recurrent or metastatic.

2. Miscellaneous laboratory testing—Patients in urinary retention or those with ureteral obstruction due to locally or regionally advanced prostatic cancers may present with elevations in serum urea nitrogen or creatinine. Patients with bony metastases may have elevations in alkaline phosphatase or hypercalcemia. Laboratory and clinical evidence of disseminated intravascular coagulation can occur in patients with advanced prostatic cancers.

3. Prostatic biopsy—Transrectal ultrasound-guided biopsy is a better method for detection of prostatic cancer than finger-guided biopsy. The use of a spring-loaded, 18-gauge biopsy needle has allowed transrectal biopsy to be performed with little patient discomfort and low attendant morbidity. Local anesthesia is commonly used and increases the tolerability of the procedure. The specimen preserves glandular architecture and allows for accurate grading as described below. Transrectal ultrasound-guided biopsy specimens are taken from the apex, mid portion, and base of the prostate in men who have an abnormal DRE or an elevated serum PSA. Extended-pattern biopsies, including a total of at least ten biopsies, are associated with improved cancer detection and risk stratification of patients with newly diagnosed disease. Patients with abnormalities of the seminal vesicles can have guided biopsies of these structures performed to allow for detection of local tumor invasion.

C. IMAGING

Modern transrectal ultrasound instrumentation provides high-definition images of the prostate. Transrectal ultrasonography has been used largely for the staging of prostatic carcinomas. In addition, transrectal ultrasound-guided—rather than digitally guided—biopsy of the prostate is a more accurate way to investigate suspicious lesions. Most prostatic cancers are hypoechoic.

MRI of the prostate allows for evaluation of the prostatic lesion as well as regional lymph nodes. The positive predictive value for detection of both capsular penetration and seminal vesicle invasion is similar for both transrectal ultrasound and MRI. CT scanning plays little role in evaluation because of its inability to accurately identify or stage prostatic cancers.

Radionuclide bone scan is superior to conventional plain skeletal x-rays in detecting bony metastases. Most prostatic cancer metastases are multiple and are most commonly localized to the axial skeleton. Because of the high frequency of abnormal scans in patients in this age group resulting from degenerative joint disease, plain films are often useful in evaluating patients with indeterminate radionuclide findings. Intravenous urography and cystoscopy are not routinely used to evaluate patients with prostatic cancer.

Imaging can be tailored to the likelihood of advanced disease in newly diagnosed patients. Asymptomatic patients with well to moderately well differentiated cancers—thought to be localized to the prostate on DRE and transurethral ultrasound and associated with normal or only modest elevations of PSA (ie, < 10 ng/mL)—need no further evaluation.

Those with more advanced local lesions, symptoms of metastases (ie, bone pain), high-grade prostate cancer, and elevations in PSA greater than 20 ng/mL should undergo radionuclide bone scan. Cross-sectional imaging of the prostate is usually indicated only in those patients in the latter group who have negative bone scans in an attempt to detect lymph node metastases. Patients found to have enlarged pelvic lymph nodes are candidates for fine-needle aspiration. Despite application of modern and sophisticated imaging, understaging of prostatic cancer occurs in at least 20% of patients.

Screening for Prostatic Cancer

The reported incidence of prostate cancer rose significantly in the United States when early detection techniques (PSA testing and transrectal ultrasound) became widely available. The goal of a screening effort should be to detect and effectively treat only those prostatic carcinomas most likely to cause morbidity or mortality if left untreated. Detection of latent, nonprogressive cancers would expose patients to unnecessary treatment and its attendant complications and costs. Whether screening for prostatic cancer will result in a decrease in yearly mortality rates due to the disease is the subject of much current debate.

The screening tests currently available include DRE, PSA testing, and transrectal ultrasound. Depending on the patient population being evaluated, detection rates using DRE alone will vary from 1.5% to 7%. Unfortunately, most cancers detected in this way are advanced (stages T3 or greater). Transrectal ultrasound should not be used as a first-line screening tool because of its expense, its low specificity (and therefore high biopsy rate), and the fact that it increases the detection rate very little when compared with the combined use of DRE and PSA testing.

PSA testing will increase the detection rate of prostatic cancers compared with DRE. Approximately 2–2.5% of men older than 50 years of age will be found to have prostatic cancer using PSA testing compared with a rate of approximately 1.5% using DRE alone. PSA is not specific for cancer, and there is considerable overlap of values between men with benign prostatic hyperplasia and those with prostatic cancers. The sensitivity, specificity, and positive predictive value of PSA and DRE are listed in Table 23–7. PSA-detected cancers are more likely to be localized compared with those detected with DRE alone.

To improve the performance of PSA as a screening test, several investigators have developed alternative methods for its use. The serial measurement of PSA (PSA velocity) may increase specificity for cancer detection with little loss in sensitivity. A rate of change in PSA greater than 0.75 ng/mL per year is associated with an increased likelihood of cancer detection. In a patient with a normal DRE, an elevated PSA, and a normal transrectal ultrasound, the indications for prostate biopsy may be refined by calculating PSA density (serum PSA/volume of the prostate as measured by ultrasound). Patients with high PSA density are more likely to have disease in spite of a normal DRE and normal transrectal ultrasound. Some have found measurement of PSA transition zone density (the zone of the prostate that undergoes enlargement during development of benign prostatic hyperplasia) to be more predictive of the presence or absence of cancer than PSA density calculated using the entire prostate volume. As PSA concentration is directly related to patient age, establishment of age-specific reference ranges would increase specificity (fewer older men with benign prostatic hyperplasia would undergo evaluation) and increase sensitivity (more younger men with cancer would undergo evaluation). Age-specific reference ranges have been established: men 40–49, < 2.5 ng/mL; men 50–59, < 3.5 ng/mL; men 60–69, < 4.5 ng/mL; and men 70–79, < 6.5 ng/mL (based on a previously normal serum PSA of < 4 ng/mL). Black men have lower age-specific reference ranges (age 40–49, < 2 ng/mL; age 50–59, < 4 ng/mL; age 60–69, < 4.5 ng/mL; age 70–79, < 5.5 ng/mL). The most recent attempt at refining PSA has been the measurement of free serum and protein-bound levels (cancer patients have a lower percentage of free serum PSA). Numerous centers are analyzing this assay to define an optimal cutoff level. Generally, men with free fractions exceeding 25% are unlikely to have prostate cancer, whereas those with free fractions less than 10% have an approximately 50% chance of having prostate cancer. Early reports using cutoffs of 18–20% of free PSA resulted in 5–10% lost sensitivity for 15–40% gains in specificity. The frequency of PSA testing remains a matter of some debate. In men with a normal DRE and a PSA > 2.5 ng/mL, PSA testing should be performed yearly because approximately 50% of these patients convert to having a PSA > 4 ng/mL. It can be performed biennially in those with a normal DRE and serum PSA < 2.5 ng/mL. Conversion in this group is much less likely.

Pathology & Staging

The majority of prostatic cancers are adenocarcinomas. Most arise in the periphery of the prostate (peripheral zone), though a small percentage arise in the central (5–10%) and transition zones (20%) of the gland. Most pathologists employ the Gleason grading system whereby a "primary" grade is applied to the architectural pattern of cancerous glands occupying the largest area of the specimen and a "secondary" pattern is assigned to the next largest area of cancerous growth. Grading is based on architectural (rather than histologic) criteria, and five possible "grades" are possible. Adding the score of the primary and secondary patterns gives a Gleason score. Grade correlates well with tumor volume, stage, and prognosis. The TNM classification of the American Joint Cancer Committee for prostatic cancer is shown in Table 23–8.

The likelihood of success of surveillance or treatment can be predicted using risk assessment tools that combine stage, grade, PSA level, and number and extent of positive prostate biopsies among other information. Several tools are available on the Internet for private use (eg, http://mskcc.org/mskcc/html/5794.cfm). One of the most widely used risk prediction tools is the Kattan nomogram; it uses serum PSA to predict the likelihood that a patient will be disease-free at 5 years after radical prostatectomy or radiation therapy, depending on the tumor stage, grade, and PSA level.

The patterns of prostatic cancer progression have been well defined. The likelihood of both local invasion and metastases is greater in larger or less well-differentiated cancers. Small and well-differentiated cancers (grades 1 and 2) are usually confined within the prostate, whereas large-volume (> 4 mL) or poorly differentiated (grades 4 and 5) cancers are more com-

Table 23–7. Screening for prostatic cancer: Test performance.

Test	Sensitivity	Specificity	Positive Predictive Value
Abnormal PSA (> 4 ng/mL)	0.67	0.97	0.43
Abnormal DRE	0.50	0.94	0.24
Abnormal PSA or DRE	0.84	0.92	0.28
Abnormal PSA *and* DRE	0.34	0.995	0.49

DRE = digital rectal examination; PSA = prostate-specific antigen.
Modified from Kramer BS et al: Prostate cancer screening: what we know and what we need to know. Ann Intern Med 1993;119:914.

Table 23–8. TNM staging system for prostate cancer.

T: Primary tumor	
Tx	Cannot be assessed
T0	No evidence of primary tumor
T1a	Carcinoma in 5% or less of tissue resected; normal DRE
T1b	Carcinoma in more than 5% of tissue resected; normal DRE
T1c	Detected from elevated PSA alone; normal DRE
T2a	Tumor in ≤1/2 of one lobe
T2b	Tumor in >1/2 of one lobe
T2c	Tumor in both lobes
T3a	Extracapsular extension
T3b	Seminal vesicle involvement
T4	Adjacent organ involvement
N: Regional lymph nodes	
Nx	Cannot be assessed
N0	No regional lymph node metastasis
N1	Metastasis in one or more regional lymph nodes
M: Distant metastasis	
Mx	Cannot be assessed
M0	No distant metastasis
M1a	Metastasis to nonregional lymph node(s)
M1b	Metastasis to bone(s)
M1c	Metastasis to other site(s) with or without bone disease

DRE = digital rectal examination; PSA = prostate-specific antigen.

monly locally extensive or metastatic to regional lymph nodes or bone. Penetration of the prostatic capsule by cancer is common and often occurs along perineural spaces. Seminal vesicle invasion is associated with a high likelihood of regional or distant disease. Lymphatic metastases are most often identified in the obturator lymph node chain. The axial skeleton, as mentioned previously, is the most common site of distant metastases.

Treatment

A. LOCALIZED DISEASE

What constitutes the optimal form of treatment for patients with clinically localized cancers remains controversial. Treatment decisions are at present made on the basis of tumor grade and stage and the age and health of the patient. Although selected patients may be candidates for surveillance based on age or health and the presence of small-volume or well-differentiated cancers, most patients with an anticipated survival in excess of 10 years should be considered for treatment. Both radiation therapy and radical prostatectomy allow for acceptable levels of local control. The first large, prospective, randomized trial of watchful waiting compared with radical prostatectomy was reported recently. Six hundred ninety-five men were

randomized and monitored for a median of 8.2 years. Radical prostatectomy reduced disease-specific mortality, overall mortality, and risks of metastasis and local progression. The absolute reduction in the risk of death after 10 years was small, but the reductions in the risks of metastasis and local tumor progression were substantial. This trial accrued patients in Sweden between 1989 and 1999, so the patients enrolled likely had a greater burden of disease than is average for patients who are newly diagnosed in areas where PSA screening is common. Patients need to be advised of all treatment options (including surveillance) along with the particular benefits, risks, and limitations.

B. RADICAL PROSTATECTOMY

In radical prostatectomy, the seminal vesicles, prostate, and ampullae of the vas deferens are removed. Refinements in technique have allowed maintenance of urinary continence in most patients and erectile function in selected patients. Radical prostatectomy can be performed via open retropubic surgery, transperineally, or laparoscopically, with or without the assistance of surgical robotics. Local recurrence is uncommon after radical prostatectomy, and its incidence is related to pathologic stage. Organ-confined cancers rarely recur. However, cancers found to be locally extensive (capsular penetration, seminal vesicle invasion) are associated with higher local (10–25%) and distant (20–50%) relapse rates.

Ideal candidates for the procedure include healthy patients with stages T1 and T2 prostatic cancers. Patients with advanced local tumors (T3 and T4) and those with lymph node metastases are rarely candidates for this procedure, although surgery is sometimes used in combination with hormonal therapy and postoperative radiation therapy for select high-risk patients.

Patients with advanced pathologic stage or positive surgical margins are at an increased risk for local and distant tumor relapse. Such patients are often considered candidates for adjuvant therapy (radiation for positive margins or androgen deprivation for lymph node metastases). Although adjuvant radiation seems to be associated with fewer local recurrences (0–5% with radiation versus 15–30% without), it has little or no impact on distant failure rates (30–35% with radiation versus 30–45% without).

C. RADIATION THERAPY

Radiation can be delivered by a variety of techniques including use of external beam radiotherapy and transperineal implantation of radioisotopes. Morbidity is limited, and the survival of patients with localized cancers (T1, T2, and selected T3) approaches 65% at 10 years. As with surgery, the likelihood of local failure correlates with technique and tumor stage. The likelihood of a positive prostatic biopsy more than 18 months after radiation varies between 20% and 60% in selected series. Patients with local recurrence are at an increased risk of cancer progression and cancer death compared with those who have negative biopsies. Ambiguous target definitions, inadequate radiation doses, and understaging of patients may be responsible for the failure noted in some series. Newer techniques of radiation (implantation, conformal therapy using three-dimensional reconstruction of CT-based tumor volumes, heavy particle, charged particle, and heavy charged particle) may improve local control rates. Three-dimensional conformal radiation delivers a higher dose because of improved targeting and appears to be associated with improved efficacy and a lower likelihood of adverse side effects compared with previous radiation techniques. As a result of improvements in imaging—most notably transrectal ultrasound—there has been a resurgence of interest in brachytherapy, the implantation of permanent or temporary radioactive sources (palladium, iodine, or iridium) into the prostate. Brachytherapy can be combined with external beam radiation in patients with higher-grade or higher-volume disease or as monotherapy in those with low-grade or low-volume malignancies.

D. Surveillance

A positive impact of localized prostatic cancer treatment with regard to survival has not been conclusively demonstrated. Surveillance alone may be an appropriate form of management for selected patients with prostatic cancer. However, many patients in such series are older and have very small and well-differentiated cancers. Because of profound stage migration due to the widespread use of serum PSA screening, patients with prostate cancer in heavily screened societies have cancers that are lower stage and grade and with lower serum PSA at diagnosis. Depending on the age and health of the patient, many of these very low-volume, low-grade cancers may never progress to clinical significance. So, careful surveillance of low-risk patients with serial PSA levels, rectal examination, and periodic repeat prostate biopsies to assess grade and extent of tumor is reasonable. The goal of surveillance is to recognize and treat patients with early evidence of progression effectively and to avoid treatment in patients who may never experience progression. End points for intervention in patients on surveillance regimens have not been clearly defined and surveillance regimens remain investigational.

E. Cryosurgery

Cryosurgery is a technique whereby liquid nitrogen is circulated through small hollow-core needles inserted into the prostate under ultrasound guidance. The freezing process results in tissue destruction. There has been a resurgence of interest in less invasive forms of therapy for localized prostate cancer as well as several recent technical innovations, including improved percutaneous techniques, expertise in transrectal ultrasound, improved cryotechnology, and better understanding of cryobiology. The positive biopsy rate after cryoablation ranges between 7% and 23%.

F. Locally and Regionally Advanced Disease

Prostatic cancers associated with minimal degrees of capsular penetration are candidates for standard irradiation or surgery. Those with locally extensive cancers, including those with seminal vesicle and bladder neck invasion, are at increased risk for both local and distant relapse despite conventional therapy. Currently, a variety of investigational regimens are being tested in an effort to improve local and distant relapse rates in such patients. Combination therapy (androgen deprivation combined with surgery or irradiation), newer forms of irradiation, and hormonal therapy alone are being tested in such patients, as are neoadjuvant and adjuvant chemotherapy. Neoadjuvant and adjuvant androgen deprivation therapy combined with external beam radiation therapy have demonstrated improved survival over external beam radiation therapy alone.

G. Metastatic Disease

Since death due to prostatic carcinoma is almost invariably a result of failure to control metastatic disease, research has emphasized efforts to improve control of distant disease. It is well known that most prostatic carcinomas are hormone dependent, and approximately 70–80% of men with metastatic prostatic carcinoma will respond to various forms of androgen deprivation. Testosterone, the major circulating androgen, is produced by Leydig cells in the testes (95%), with a smaller amount being produced by peripheral conversion of other steroids. Although 98% of serum testosterone is protein bound, free testosterone enters prostate cells and is converted to DHT, the major intracellular androgen. DHT binds a cytoplasmic receptor protein, and the complex moves to the cell nucleus, where it modulates transcription. Androgen deprivation may be induced at several levels along the pituitary–gonadal axis using a variety of methods or agents (Table 23–9). Use of LHRH agonists (leuprolide, goserelin)—drugs delivered in monthly or 3-monthly depot—has allowed induction of androgen deprivation without orchiectomy or administration of diethylstilbestrol. Presently, administration of LHRH agonists and orchiectomy are the most common forms of primary androgen blockade used. Because of its rapid onset of action, ketoconazole should be considered in patients with advanced prostatic cancer who present with spinal cord compression, bilateral ureteral obstruction, or disseminated intravascular coagulation. Although testosterone is the major circulating androgen, the adrenal gland secretes the androgens dehydroepiandrosterone, dehydroepiandrosterone sulfate, and androstenedione. Some investigators believe that suppressing both testicular and adrenal androgens will allow for a better initial and longer response than methods that inhibit production of only testicular androgens. Complete androgen blockade can be achieved by combining an antiandrogen with use of an LHRH agonist or orchiectomy. Nonsteroidal antiandrogen agents appear to act by competitively binding the receptor for DHT, the intracellular androgen responsible

Table 23–9. Androgen ablation for prostatic cancer.

Level	Agent	Dose	Sequelae
Pituitary, hypothalamus	Estrogens	1–3 mg daily	Gynecomastia, hot flushes, thromboembolic disease, erectile dysfunction
	LHRH agonists	Monthly or 3-monthly depot injection	Erectile dysfunction, hot flushes, gynecomastia, rarely anemia
Adrenal	Ketoconazole	400 mg three times daily	Adrenal insufficiency, nausea, rash, ataxia
	Aminoglutethimide	250 mg four times daily	Adrenal insufficiency, nausea, rash, ataxia
	Corticosteroids	Prednisone: 20–40 mg daily	Gastrointestinal bleeding, fluid retention
Testis	Orchiectomy		Gynecomastia, hot flushes, erectile dysfunction
Prostate cell	Antiandrogens	Flutamide: 250 mg three times daily Bicalutamide: 50 mg daily	No erectile dysfunction when used alone; nausea, diarrhea

LHRH = luteinizing hormone-releasing hormone.

for prostatic cell growth and development. A meta-analysis of trials comparing the use of either an LHRH agonist or orchiectomy alone with the use of either in combination with an antiandrogen agent shows marginal (if any) benefit to the use of combination therapy. However, patients at risk of disease-related symptoms (bone pain, obstructive voiding symptoms) due to the initial elevation of serum testosterone that accompanies the use of an LHRH agonist should receive antiandrogens initially. Bisphosphonates are increasingly being used with metastatic bone disease.

Docetaxel has recently been shown to improve survival in men with hormone-refractory prostate cancer. Docetaxel is the first cytotoxic chemotherapy agent to improve survival in patients with prostate cancer. Current research is underway combining docetaxel with hormonal therapy, radiation therapy, and surgery to find effective combinations for high-risk patients. Immune therapies are also under intense investigation and have shown promise for patients with advanced prostate cancer.

Bill-Axelson A et al: Radical prostatectomy versus watchful waiting in early prostate cancer. N Engl J Med 2005;352:1977. [PMID: 15888698]

Carroll PR et al: Third international conference on innovations and challenges in prostate cancer: prevention, detection and treatment. J Urol 2003;170:S3. [PMID: 14610403]

Guise TA et al: Role of bisphosphonates in prostate cancer bone metastases. Semin Oncol 2003;30:717. [PMID: 14571419]

Han M et al: Prostate-specific antigen and screening for prostate cancer. Med Clin North Am 2004;88:245. [PMID: 15049577]

Hernandez J et al: Diagnosis and treatment of prostate cancer. Med Clin North Am 2004;88:267. [PMID: 15049578]

Hernandez J et al: Prostate-specific antigen: a review of the validation of the most commonly used cancer biomarker. Cancer 2004;101:894. [PMID: 15329895]

Higgins B et al: The Prostate Cancer Prevention Trial: current status. J Urol 2004;171(2 Pt 2):S15. [PMID: 14713747]

Hittelman AB et al: Update of staging and risk assessment for prostate cancer patients. Curr Opin Urol 2004;14:163. [PMID: 15069307]

Kattan MW et al: Algorithms for prostate-specific antigen recurrence after treatment of localized prostate cancer. Clin Prostate Cancer 2003;1:221. [PMID: 15040880]

Klotz LH et al: Active surveillance with selective delayed intervention for favorable risk prostate cancer: clinical experience and a 'number needed to treat' analysis. Can J Urol 2006; 13(Suppl 1):48. [PMID: 16526983]

Meng MV et al: Treatment of patients with high risk localized prostate cancer: results from cancer of the prostate strategic urological research endeavor (CaPSURE). J Urol 2005;173:1557. [PMID: 15821485]

Nelson JB et al: Prostate cancer: radical prostatectomy. Urol Clin North Am 2003;30:703. [PMID: 14680309]

Parnes HL et al: Prostate cancer chemoprevention agent development: the National Cancer Institute, Division of Cancer Prevention portfolio. J Urol 2004;171:S68. [PMID: 14713758]

Petrylak DP et al: Docetaxel and estramustine compared with mitoxantrone and prednisone for advanced refractory prostate cancer. N Engl J Med 2004;351:1513. [PMID: 15470214]

Shinohara K: Prostate cancer: cryotherapy. Urol Clin North Am 2003;30:725. [PMID: 14680310]

Wilson SS et al: Screening for prostate cancer: current recommendations. Urol Clin North Am 2004;31:219. [PMID: 15123402]

BLADDER CANCER

ESSENTIALS OF DIAGNOSIS

- *Irritative voiding symptoms.*
- *Gross or microscopic hematuria.*
- *Positive urinary cytology in most patients.*
- *Filling defect within bladder noted on imaging.*

General Considerations

Bladder cancer is the second most common urologic cancer; it occurs more commonly in men than women (2.7:1), and the mean age of patients at diagnosis is 65 years. Cigarette smoking and exposure to industrial dyes or solvents are risk factors for the disease and account for approximately 60% and 15% of new cases, respectively.

Clinical Findings

A. SYMPTOMS AND SIGNS

Hematuria—gross or microscopic, chronic or intermittent—is the presenting symptom in 85–90% of patients with bladder cancer. Irritative voiding symptoms (urinary frequency and urgency) will occur in a small percentage of patients as a result of the location or size of the cancer. Most patients with bladder cancer will fail to have signs of the disease because of its superficial nature. Masses detected on bimanual examination may be present in patients with large-volume or deeply infiltrating cancers. Hepatomegaly or supraclavicular lymphadenopathy may be present in patients with metastatic disease, and lymphedema of the lower extremities may be present as a result of locally advanced cancers or metastases to pelvic lymph nodes.

B. LABORATORY FINDINGS

Urinalysis will reveal hematuria in the majority of cases. On occasion, it may be accompanied by pyuria. Azotemia may be present in a small number of cases associated with ureteral obstruction. Anemia may occasionally be due to chronic blood loss or to bone marrow metastases. Exfoliated cells from normal and abnormal urothelium can be readily detected in voided urine specimens. Cytology may be useful in detecting the disease at the time of initial presentation or to detect recurrence. Cytology is very sensitive in detecting cancers of higher grade and stage (80–90%) but less so in detecting superficial or well-differentiated lesions (50%). Sensitivity of detection using exfoliated cells may be enhanced by flow cytometry.

C. IMAGING

Bladder cancers may be detected using intravenous urography, ultrasound, CT, or MRI where filling defects within the bladder are noted. However, the presence of cancer is confirmed by cystoscopy and biopsy, so imaging is useful primarily for evaluating the upper urinary tract and in staging the more advanced lesions.

D. CYSTOURETHROSCOPY AND BIOPSY

The diagnosis and staging of bladder cancers are made by cystoscopy and transurethral resection. If cystoscopy—performed usually under local anesthesia—confirms the presence of bladder cancer, the patient is scheduled for transurethral resection under general or regional anesthesia. A careful bimanual examination is performed initially and at the end of the procedure, noting the size, position, and degree of fixation of a mass, if present. Any suspicious lesions are resected using electrocautery. Resection is carried down to the muscular elements of the bladder wall so as to allow complete staging. Random bladder and, on occasion, prostatic urethral biopsies are performed to detect occult disease elsewhere in the bladder and, therefore, identify patients at high risk of recurrence and progression.

Pathology & Selection of Treatment

Ninety-eight percent of primary bladder cancers are epithelial malignancies, with the majority being transitional cell carcinomas (90%). These latter cancers most often appear as papillary growths, but higher-grade lesions are often sessile and ulcerated. Grading is based on histologic appearance: size, pleomorphism, mitotic rate, and hyperchromatism. The frequency of recurrence and progression are strongly correlated with grade. Whereas progression may be noted in few grade I cancers (19–37%), it is common with poorly differentiated lesions (33–67%). Carcinoma in situ is recognizable as a flat, nonpapillary, anaplastic epithelium and may occur focally or diffusely, but it is most often found in association with papillary bladder cancers. Its presence identifies a patient at increased risk of recurrence and progression.

Adenocarcinomas and squamous cell cancers account for approximately 2% and 7%, respectively, of all bladder cancers detected in the United States. The latter is often associated with schistosomiasis, vesical calculi, or chronic catheter use.

Bladder cancer staging is based on the extent of bladder wall penetration and the presence of either regional or distant metastases. The TNM classification of the American Joint Cancer Committee for bladder cancer is shown in Table 23–10.

The natural history of bladder cancer is based on two separate but related processes: tumor recurrence and progression to higher-stage disease. Both are related to tumor grade and stage. At initial presentation, approximately 50–80% of bladder cancers will be superficial: Ta, Tis, or T1. Lymph node metastases and progression are uncommon in such patients when they are properly treated, and survival is excellent at 81%. Patients with superficial cancers (Ta, T1) are treated with complete transurethral resection and the selective use of intravesical chemotherapy. The latter is used to prevent or delay recurrence. Patients who present with large, high-grade, recurrent Ta lesions or T1 cancers and those with carcinoma in situ are good candidates for intravesical chemotherapy. Patients with more invasive (T2, T3) but still localized cancers are at risk of both nodal metastases and progression, and they require more aggressive surgery, irradiation, or the combination of chemotherapy and selective surgery or irradiation due to the much higher risk of progression compared to patients with lower-stage lesions. Patients with evidence of lymph node or distant metastases should undergo systemic chemotherapy initially.

Table 23–10. TNM staging system for bladder cancer.

T: Primary tumor

Tx	Cannot be assessed
T0	No evidence of primary tumor
Tis	Carcinoma in situ (CIS)
Ta	Noninvasive papillary carcinoma
T1	Invasion into lamina propria
T2a	Invasion into superficial layer of muscularis propria
T2b	Invasion into deep layer of muscularis propria
T3a	Microscopic invasion into perivesical tissue
T3b	Macroscopic invasion into perivesical tissue
T4a	Invasion into adjacent organs
T4b	Invasion into pelvic sidewall

N: Regional lymph nodes

Nx	Cannot be assessed
N0	No regional lymph node metastasis
N1	Metastasis in a single lymph node 2 cm or less
N2	Metastasis in a single lymph node > 2 cm and < 5 cm or multiple nodes none > 5 cm
N3	Metastasis in lymph node > 5 cm

M: Distant metastasis

Mx	Cannot be assessed
M0	No distant metastasis
M1	Distant metastasis present

Treatment

A. INTRAVESICAL CHEMOTHERAPY

Immunotherapeutic or chemotherapeutic agents can be delivered directly into the bladder by a urethral catheter. They can be used to eradicate existing disease or to reduce the likelihood of recurrence in those who have undergone complete transurethral resection. Such therapy is more effective in the latter situation. Most agents are administered weekly for 6–12 weeks. The use of maintenance therapy after the initial induction regimen may be beneficial. Efficacy may be increased by prolonging contact time to 2 hours. Common agents include thiotepa, mitomycin, doxorubicin, and BCG, the latter being the most effective agent when compared with the others. BCG and mitomycin have similar efficacy in retarding disease progression and patient survival. Side effects of intravesical chemotherapy include irritative voiding symptoms and hemorrhagic cystitis. Systemic effects are rare. Patients who develop symptoms from BCG may require antituberculous therapy.

B. SURGICAL TREATMENT

Although transurethral resection is the initial form of treatment for all bladder cancers as it is diagnostic, allows for proper staging, and will control superficial cancers, muscle infiltrating cancers will require more aggressive treatment. Partial cystectomy may be indicated in patients with solitary lesions and those with cancers in a bladder diverticulum. Radical cystectomy entails re-

moval of the bladder, prostate, seminal vesicles, and surrounding fat and peritoneal attachments in men and in women also the uterus, cervix, urethra, anterior vaginal vault, and usually the ovaries. Bilateral pelvic lymph node dissection is performed simultaneously.

Urinary diversion can be performed using a conduit of small or large bowel. However, continent forms of diversion have been developed that avoid the necessity of an external appliance and significantly improve quality of life for patients who are candidates.

C. RADIOTHERAPY

External beam radiotherapy delivered in fractions over a 6- to 8-week period is generally well tolerated, but approximately 10–15% of patients will develop bladder, bowel, or rectal complications. Unfortunately, local recurrence is common after radiotherapy (30–70%). Increasingly, radiotherapy is being combined with systemic chemotherapy in an effort to improve local and distant relapse rates.

D. CHEMOTHERAPY

Fifteen percent of patients with newly diagnosed bladder cancer will present with metastatic disease, and 40% of those thought to have localized disease at the time of cystectomy or definitive radiotherapy will develop metastases usually within 2 years after the start of treatment. Cisplatin-based combination chemotherapy will result in partial or complete responses in 15–35% and 15–45% of patients, respectively.

Combination chemotherapy has been integrated into trials of surgery and radiotherapy. It has been used to decrease recurrence rates with either modality and in an attempt to preserve the bladder in those treated with radiation. Chemotherapy should be considered before surgery in those with bulky lesions or those suspected of having regional disease. Chemoradiation may be best suited for those with T2 or limited T3 disease without hydronephrosis. Alternatively, chemotherapy has been employed postoperatively in patients who have undergone cystectomy and have been found to be at high risk of recurrence. In current practice, adjuvant chemotherapy when indicated—ie, when the primary tumor invades perivesical fat or adjacent organs or when lymph nodes are found to have metastatic disease—is being offered mainly to patients being treated with radical cystectomy.

Carroll PR: Urothelial carcinoma: cancers of the bladder, ureter and renal pelvis. In: *Smith's General Urology,* 16th ed. Tanagho EA, McAninch JW (editors). McGraw-Hill, 2003.

Droller MJ: Primary care update on kidney and bladder cancer: a urologic perspective. Med Clin North Am 2004;88:309. [PMID: 15049580]

Kim HL et al: The current status of bladder preservation in the treatment of muscle invasive bladder cancer. J Urol 2000; 164(3 Part 1):627. [PMID: 10953112]

Krejci KG et al: Immunotherapy for urological malignancies. J Urol 2004;171(2 Pt 1):870. [PMID: 14713844]

Shelley MD et al: Intravesical bacillus Calmette-Guérin versus mitomycin C for Ta and T1 bladder cancer. Cochrane Database Syst Rev 2003;(3):CD003231. [PMID: 12917955]

CANCERS OF THE URETER & RENAL PELVIS

Cancers of the renal pelvis and ureter are rare and occur more commonly in smokers, in those with Balkan nephropathy, in those exposed to Thorotrast (a contrast agent with radioactive thorium in use until the 1960s), or in those with a long history of analgesic abuse. The majority are transitional cell carcinomas. Gross or microscopic hematuria occurs in most patients, and flank pain secondary to bleeding and obstruction occurs less commonly. Like primary bladder cancers, urinary cytology is often positive. The most common signs identified at the time of IVP or CT include an intraluminal filling defect, unilateral nonvisualization of the collecting system, and hydronephrosis. Ureteral and renal pelvic tumors must be differentiated from calculi, blood clots, papillary necrosis, or inflammatory or infectious lesions. On occasion, such lesions are accessible to direct biopsy, fulguration, or resection using a ureteroscope. Treatment is based on the site, size, depth of penetration, and number of tumors present. Most such cancers are excised with laparoscopic or open nephroureterectomy (renal pelvic and upper ureteral lesions) or segmental excision of the ureter (distal ureteral lesions). Endoscopic resection may be indicated in patients with limited renal function and in the management of focal, low-grade, upper tract cancers.

PRIMARY TUMORS OF THE KIDNEY

1. Renal Cell Carcinoma

 ESSENTIALS OF DIAGNOSIS

- Gross or microscopic hematuria.
- Flank pain or mass in some patients.
- Systemic symptoms such as fever, weight loss may be prominent.
- Solid renal mass on imaging.

General Considerations

Renal cell carcinoma accounts for 2.6% of all adult cancers. In the United States in 2005, approximately 36,160 cases of renal cell carcinoma were diagnosed and 12,660 deaths resulted. Renal cell carcinoma has a peak incidence in the sixth decade of life and a male-to-female ratio of 2:1.

The cause is unknown. Cigarette smoking is the only significant environmental risk factor that has been identified. Familial settings for renal cell carcinoma have been identified (von Hippel–Lindau syndrome) as well as an association with dialysis-related acquired cystic disease, but sporadic tumors are far more common.

Table 23–11. TNM staging system for kidney cancer.

T: Primary tumor	
Tx	Cannot be assessed
T0	No evidence of primary tumor
T1	Tumor 7 cm or less limited to kidney
T1a	Tumor 4 cm or less limited to kidney
T1b	Tumor more than 4 cm but not more than 7 cm limited to kidney
T2	Tumor > 7 cm limited to kidney
T3a	Tumor invades adrenal gland or perinephric tissue
T3b	Tumor extends into renal vein or vena cava
T3c	Tumor extends into renal vein or vena cava above diaphragm
T4	Tumor invades outside of Gerota's fascia
N: Regional lymph nodes	
Nx	Cannot be assessed
N0	No regional lymph node metastasis
N1	Metastasis in a single lymph node
N2	Metastasis in multiple nodes
M: Distant metastasis	
Mx	Cannot be assessed
M0	No distant metastasis
M1	Distant metastasis present

Renal cell carcinoma originates from the proximal tubule cells. Various cell types (clear, granular, spindle) and histologic patterns (acinar, papillary, solid) are observed. However, cell type and histologic pattern do not affect treatment. The TNM classification of the American Joint Cancer Committee for kidney cancer is shown in Table 23–11.

Clinical Findings

A. SYMPTOMS AND SIGNS

Historically, 60% of patients presented with gross or microscopic hematuria. Flank pain or an abdominal mass was detected in approximately 30% of cases. The triad of flank pain, hematuria, and mass was found in only 10–15% of patients and is often a sign of advanced disease. Symptoms of metastatic disease (cough, bone pain) occur in 20–30% of patients at presentation. Because of the more widespread use of ultrasound and CT scanning for diverse indications, renal tumors are being detected incidentally in patients with no urologic symptoms.

B. LABORATORY FINDINGS

Hematuria is present in 60% of patients. Paraneoplastic syndromes are not uncommon in renal cell carcinoma. Erythrocytosis from increased erythropoietin production occurs in 5%, though anemia is far more common; hypercalcemia may be present in up to 10% of patients. Stauffer's syndrome is a reversible syndrome of hepatic dysfunction in the absence of metastatic disease.

C. IMAGING

Renal masses are often first detected by intravenous urography or CT scans. Further evaluation requires ultrasound to determine whether it is solid or cystic. CT scanning is the most valuable imaging test for renal cell carcinoma. It confirms the character of the mass and further stages the lesion with respect to regional lymph nodes, renal vein, or hepatic involvement. It also provides valuable information regarding the contralateral kidney (function, bilaterality of neoplasm). Chest radiographs exclude pulmonary metastases, and bone scans should be performed for large tumors and in patients with bone pain or elevated alkaline phosphatase levels. MRI and duplex Doppler ultrasonography are excellent methods of assessing for the presence and extent of tumor thrombus within the renal vein or vena cava in selected patients.

Differential Diagnosis

Solid lesions of the kidney are renal cell carcinoma until proved otherwise. Other solid masses include angiomyolipomas (fat density usually visible by CT), transitional cell cancers of the renal pelvis (more centrally located, involvement of the collecting system, positive urinary cytology reports), adrenal tumors (superoanterior to the kidney) and oncocytomas (indistinguishable from renal cell carcinoma preoperatively), and renal abscesses.

Treatment & Prognosis

Radical nephrectomy is the primary treatment for localized renal cell carcinoma. Patients with a single kidney, bilateral lesions, or significant medical renal disease should be considered for laparoscopic or open partial nephrectomy. Patients with a normal contralateral kidney and good renal function but a small cancer may be good candidates for partial nephrectomy as well. The use of radiofrequency or cryosurgical ablation is being studied. Tumors confined to the renal capsule (T1–T2) demonstrate 5-year disease-free survivals of 90–100%. Tumors extending beyond the renal capsule (T3 or T4) and node-positive tumors have 50–60% and 0–15% 5-year disease-free survivals, respectively.

No effective chemotherapy is available for metastatic renal cell carcinoma. Vinblastine is the single most effective agent, with short-term partial response rates of 15%. Bevacizumab can prolong time to progression in those with metastatic disease. Biologic response modifiers have received much attention, including interferon-α and interleukin-2. Partial response rates of 15–20% and 15–35%, respectively, have been reported. Responders tend to have lower tumor burdens, metastatic disease confined to the lung, and a high performance status. Patients with metastatic kidney cancer and good performance status who have resectable primary tumors should undergo cytoreductive nephrectomy if possible. Two randomized trials have shown a benefit to surgery followed by the use of systemic therapy—specifically, biologic response modifiers—compared with the use of systemic therapy alone.

Several new drugs, specifically, vascular endothelial growth factor (VEGF) and Raf-kinase inhibitors, have recently demonstrated effectiveness in patients with advanced kidney cancer. The drugs are oral agents, well tolerated, and active especially against clear cell carcinoma with ~40% response rates. The sequencing and combination of these agents, with and without cytokine therapy, is an active area of investigation.

One subgroup of metastatic patients has demonstrated long-term survival, namely, those with solitary resectable metastases. In this setting, radical nephrectomy with resection of the metastasis has resulted in 5-year disease-free survival rates of 15–30%. Bisphosphonates can be effective for metastatic bone disease.

Dhote R et al: Risk factors for adult renal cell carcinoma. Urol Clin North Am 2004;31:237. [PMID: 15123404]

Flanigan RC et al: Nephrectomy followed by interferon alfa-2b compared with interferon alfa-2b alone for metastatic renal-cell cancer. N Engl J Med 2001;345:1655. [PMID: 11759643]

Mickisch GH et al: Radical nephrectomy plus interferon-alfa-based immunotherapy compared with interferon alfa alone in metastatic renal-cell carcinoma: a randomised trial. Lancet 2001;358:966. [PMID: 11583750]

Motzer RJ et al: Activity of SU11248, a multitargeted inhibitor of vascular endothelial growth factor receptor and platelet-derived growth factor receptor, in patients with metastatic renal cell carcinoma. J Clin Oncol 2006;24:16. [PMID: 16330672]

Motzer RJ et al: Prognostic factors for survival in previously treated patients with metastatic renal cell carcinoma. J Clin Oncol 2004;22:454. [PMID: 14752067]

Rini BI: New approaches in advanced renal cell carcinoma. Urol Oncol 2005;23:65. [PMID: 15885585]

Saika T et al: Long-term outcome of laparoscopic radical nephrectomy for pathologic T1 renal cell carcinoma. Urology 2003; 62:1018. [PMID: 14665347]

2. Other Primary Tumors of the Kidney

Oncocytomas account for 3–5% of renal tumors and are indistinguishable from renal cell carcinoma by all imaging modalities. The biologic potential of these lesions is not well defined. These tumors are seen in other organs, including the adrenals, the salivary glands, and the thyroid and parathyroid glands.

Angiomyolipomas are rare benign tumors composed of fat, smooth muscle, and blood vessels. They are most commonly seen in patients with tuberous sclerosis (often multiple and bilateral) or in young to middle-aged women. CT scanning may identify the fat component, which is diagnostic for angiomyolipoma. Asymptomatic lesions less than 5 cm in diameter usually do not require intervention.

SECONDARY TUMORS OF THE KIDNEY

The kidney is not an infrequent site for metastatic disease. Of the solid tumors, the lung is the most common (20%), followed by breast (10%), stomach (10%), and the contralateral kidney (10%). Lymphoma, both Hodgkin's and non-Hodgkin's, may also involve the kidney, though it tends to be a diffusely infiltrative process resulting in renal enlargement rather than a discrete mass.

PRIMARY TUMORS OF THE TESTIS

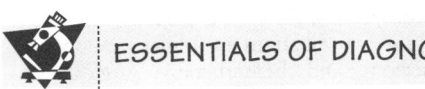

ESSENTIALS OF DIAGNOSIS

- *Commonest neoplasm in men aged 20–35 years.*
- *Typical presentation as a patient-identified painless nodule.*
- *Orchiectomy necessary for diagnosis.*

General Considerations

Malignant tumors of the testis are rare, with approximately two to three new cases per 100,000 males being reported in the United States each year. Ninety to 95 percent of all primary testicular tumors are germ cell tumors (seminoma and nonseminoma), while the remainder are nongerminal neoplasms (Leydig cell, Sertoli cell, gonadoblastoma). The lifetime probability of developing testicular cancer is 0.2% for an American white male. For the purposes of this review, we will consider only germ cell tumors. Survival in testicular cancer has improved dramatically in recent years as a result of the development and application of effective combination chemotherapy.

Testicular cancer is slightly more common on the right than on the left, which parallels the increased incidence of cryptorchism on the right side. One to 2 percent of primary testicular tumors are bilateral, and up to 50% of these men have a history of unilateral or bilateral cryptorchism. Primary bilateral testicular tumors may occur synchronously or asynchronously but tend to be of the same histology. Seminoma is the most common histologic finding in bilateral *primary* testicular tumors, while malignant lymphoma is the most common bilateral testicular tumor.

Although the cause of testicular cancer is unknown, both congenital and acquired factors have been associated with tumor development. Approximately 5% of testicular tumors develop in a patient with a history of cryptorchism, with seminoma being the most common. However, 5–10% of these tumors occur in the contralateral, normally descended testis. The relative risk of development of malignancy is highest for the intra-abdominal testis (1:20) and lower for the inguinal testis (1:80). Placement of the cryptorchid testis into the scrotum (orchiopexy) does not alter the malignant potential of the cryptorchid testis; however, it does facilitate examination and tumor detection.

In animal models, exogenous estrogen administration during pregnancy has been associated with an in-creased relative risk for testicular tumors ranging from 2.8 to 5.3. Other acquired factors such as trauma and infection-related testicular atrophy have been associated with testicular tumors; however, a causal relationship has not been established.

Histopathology & Clinical Staging

From a treatment standpoint, testicular carcinoma can be divided into two major categories: (1) nonseminomas, which include embryonal cell carcinomas (20%), teratomas (5%), choriocarcinomas (< 1%), and mixed cell types (40%), and (2) seminomas (35%). In a commonly used staging system for nonseminoma germ cell tumors, a stage A lesion is confined to the testis; stage B demonstrates regional lymph node involvement in the retroperitoneum; and stage C indicates distant metastasis. For seminoma, the M.D. Anderson system is commonly used. In this system, a stage I lesion is confined to the testis, a stage II lesion has spread to the retroperitoneal lymph nodes, and a stage III lesion has supradiaphragmatic nodal or visceral involvement. The TNM classification of the American Joint Cancer Committee for testis cancer is shown in Table 23–12.

Clinical Findings

A. SYMPTOMS AND SIGNS

The most common symptom of testicular cancer is painless enlargement of the testis. Sensations of heaviness are not unusual. Patients are usually the first to recognize an abnormality, yet the typical delay in seeking

Table 23–12. TNM staging system for testicular cancer.

T: Primary tumor	
Tx	Cannot be assessed
T0	No evidence of primary tumor
Tis	Intratubular cancer (carcinoma in situ)
T1	Limited to testis without vascular invasion
T2	Invades beyond tunica albuginea or into epididymis, or limited to testis with vascular invasion
T3	Invades spermatic cord
T4	Invades scrotum
N: Regional lymph nodes	
Nx	Cannot be assessed
N0	No regional lymph node metastasis
N1	Metastasis in a single lymph node 2 cm or less
N2	Metastasis in a single lymph node > 2 cm and < 5 cm or multiple nodes none > 5 cm
N3	Metastasis in lymph node > 5 cm
M: Distant metastasis	
Mx	Cannot be assessed
M0	No distant metastasis
M1a	Metastasis to nonregional lymph node(s) or lung(s)
M1b	Distant metastasis to sites other than nonregional lymph node(s) or lung(s)

medical attention ranges from 3 to 6 months. Acute testicular pain resulting from intratesticular hemorrhage occurs in approximately 10% of cases. Ten percent of patients are asymptomatic at presentation, and 10% manifest symptoms relating to metastatic disease such as back pain (retroperitoneal metastases), cough (pulmonary metastases), or lower extremity edema (vena cava obstruction).

A testicular mass or diffuse enlargement of the testis is found in the majority of cases on physical examination. Secondary hydroceles may be present in 5–10% of cases. In advanced disease, supraclavicular adenopathy may be detected, and abdominal examination may palpate a retroperitoneal mass. Gynecomastia is seen in 5% of germ cell tumors.

B. LABORATORY FINDINGS

Several biochemical markers are important in the diagnosis and treatment of testicular carcinoma, including human chorionic gonadotropin (hCG), α-fetoprotein, and lactate dehydrogenase (LDH). α-Fetoprotein is never elevated in seminomas, and while hCG is occasionally elevated in seminomas, levels tend to be lower than those seen in nonseminomas. LDH may be elevated in either type of tumor. Liver function tests may be elevated in the presence of hepatic metastases, and anemia may be present in advanced disease. In patients with advanced disease who will receive chemotherapy, renal function is assessed with a 24-hour urine creatinine clearance.

C. IMAGING

Scrotal ultrasound can readily determine whether the mass is intratesticular or extratesticular in origin. Once the diagnosis of testicular cancer has been established by inguinal orchiectomy, clinical staging of the disease is accomplished by chest, abdominal, and pelvic CT scanning.

Differential Diagnosis

An incorrect diagnosis is made at the initial examination in up to 25% of patients with testicular tumors. The differential diagnosis of scrotal masses has been discussed previously in this chapter. Scrotal ultrasonography should be performed if any uncertainty exists with respect to the diagnosis. Although most intratesticular masses are malignant, one benign lesion, an epidermoid cyst, may rarely be seen. Epidermoid cysts are usually very small benign nodules located just underneath the tunica albuginea; on occasion, however, they can be large.

Treatment

Inguinal exploration with early vascular control of the spermatic cord structures is the initial intervention to exclude neoplasm. If cancer cannot be excluded by examination of the testis, radical orchiectomy is warranted. Scrotal approaches and open testicular biopsies should be avoided. Further therapy is dependent upon the histology of the tumor as well as the clinical stage.

The 5-year disease-free survival rates for stage I and IIa (retroperitoneal disease < 10 cm in diameter) seminomas treated by radical orchiectomy and retroperitoneal irradiation are 98% and 92–94%, respectively. High-stage seminomas of stage IIb (> 10 cm retroperitoneal involvement) and stage III receive primary chemotherapy (etoposide and cisplatin or cisplatin, etoposide, and bleomycin). Ninety-five percent of patients with stage III disease will attain a complete response following orchiectomy and chemotherapy. Surgical resection of residual retroperitoneal masses is warranted only if the mass is larger than 3 cm in diameter, under which circumstances 40% will harbor residual carcinoma.

Up to 75% of stage A nonseminomas are cured by orchiectomy alone. Currently, such patients may be treated by modified retroperitoneal lymph node dissections designed to preserve the sympathetic innervation for ejaculation. Selected patients who meet specific criteria may be offered surveillance. These criteria are as follows: (1) tumor is confined within the tunica albuginea; (2) tumor does not demonstrate vascular invasion; (3) tumor markers normalize after orchiectomy; (4) radiographic imaging shows no evidence of disease (chest x-ray and CT); and (5) the patient is reliable. Patients most likely to experience relapse on a surveillance regimen include those with predominantly embryonal cancer and those with vascular or lymphatic invasion identified in the orchiectomy specimen. Surveillance should be considered an active process both by the physician and by the patient. Patients are followed monthly for the first 2 years and bimonthly in the third year. Tumor markers are obtained at each visit, and chest x-ray and CT scans are obtained every 3–4 months. Follow-up continues beyond the initial 3 years; however, the majority of relapses will occur within the first 8–10 months. With rare exceptions, patients who relapse can be cured by chemotherapy or surgery. The 5-year disease-free survival rate for patients with stage A disease ranges from 96% to 100%. For low-volume stage B disease, 90% 5-year disease-free survival is attainable.

Patients with bulky retroperitoneal disease (> 3 cm nodes) or metastatic nonseminomas are treated with primary cisplatin-based combination chemotherapy following orchiectomy (etoposide and cisplatin or cisplatin, etoposide, and bleomycin). If tumor markers normalize and a residual mass greater than 3 cm is apparent on imaging studies, resection of that mass is mandatory because 20% of the time it will harbor residual cancer and 40% of the time it will be teratoma. Even if patients have a complete response to chemotherapy, retroperitoneal lymphadenectomy is advocated by some as 10% of patients may harbor residual carcinoma and 10% may have teratoma in the retroperitoneum. If tumor markers fail to normalize following primary chemotherapy, salvage chemotherapy is required (cisplatin, etoposide, bleomycin, ifosfamide).

Prognosis

Patients with bulky retroperitoneal or disseminated disease treated with primary chemotherapy followed by surgery have a 5-year disease-free survival rate of 55–80%.

Heidenreich A et al: Organ-sparing surgery for malignant germ cell tumor of the testis. J Urol 2001;166:2161. [PMID: 11696727]

Huyghe E et al: Increasing incidence of testicular cancer worldwide: a review. J Urol 2003;170:5. [PMID: 12796635]

Jewett MA et al: Management of recurrence and follow-up strategies for patients with nonseminoma testis cancer. Urol Clin North Am 2003;30:819. [PMID: 14680317]

Patel MI et al: Management of recurrence and follow-up strategies for patients with seminoma and selected high-risk groups. Urol Clin North Am 2003;30:803. [PMID: 14680316]

SECONDARY TUMORS OF THE TESTIS

Secondary tumors of the testis are rare. Lymphoma is the most common testis tumor in a patient over the age of 50 years and is the most common secondary neoplasm of the testis, accounting for 5% of all testicular tumors. It may be seen in three clinical settings: (1) as a late manifestation of widespread lymphoma, (2) as the initial presentation of clinically occult disease, and (3) as primary extranodal disease. Radical orchiectomy is indicated to make the diagnosis. Prognosis is related to the stage of disease.

Metastasis to the testis is rare. The most common primary site is the prostate, followed by the lung, gastrointestinal tract, melanoma, and kidney.

Nervous System

24

Michael J. Aminoff, MD, DSc, FRCP

HEADACHE

Headache is such a common complaint and can occur for so many different reasons that its proper evaluation may be difficult. Headaches of acute onset are discussed in Chapter 2. Chronic headaches are commonly due to migraine, tension, or depression, but they may be related to intracranial lesions, head injury, cervical spondylosis, dental or ocular disease, temporomandibular joint dysfunction, sinusitis, hypertension, and a wide variety of general medical disorders. Although underlying structural lesions are not present in most patients presenting with headache, it is nevertheless important to bear this possibility in mind. About one-third of patients with brain tumors, for example, present with a primary complaint of headache.

The intensity, quality, and site of pain—and especially the duration of the headache and the presence of associated neurologic symptoms—may provide clues to the underlying cause. Migraine or tension headaches are often described as pulsating or throbbing; a sense of tightness or pressure is also common with tension headache. Sharp lancinating pain suggests a neuritic cause; ocular or periorbital icepick-like pains occur with migraine or cluster headache; and a dull or steady headache is typical of an intracranial mass lesion. Ocular or periocular pain suggests an ophthalmologic disorder; band-like pain is common with tension headaches; and lateralized headache is common with migraine or cluster headache. In patients with sinusitis, there may be tenderness of overlying skin and bone. With intracranial mass lesions, headache may be focal or generalized; in patients with trigeminal or glossopharyngeal neuralgia, the pain is localized to one of the divisions of the trigeminal nerve or to the pharynx and external auditory meatus, respectively.

Inquiry should be made of precipitating factors. Recent sinusitis or hay fever, dental surgery, head injury, or symptoms suggestive of a systemic viral infection may suggest the underlying cause. Migraine may be exacerbated by emotional stress, fatigue, foods containing nitrite or tyramine, or the menstrual period. Alcohol may precipitate cluster headache. Temporomandibular joint dysfunction causes headache or facial pain that comes on with chewing; trigeminal or glossopharyngeal neuralgia may also be precipitated by chewing, and masticatory claudication sometimes occurs with giant cell arteritis. Cough-induced headache occurs with structural lesions of the posterior fossa, but in many instances no specific cause can be found.

The timing of symptoms is important. Headaches are typically worse on awakening in patients with sinusitis or an intracranial mass. Cluster headaches tend to occur at the same time each day or night. Tension headaches are worse with stress or at the end of the day.

The onset of severe headache in a previously well patient is more likely than chronic headache to relate to an intracranial disorder such as subarachnoid hemorrhage or meningitis. The need for further investigation is determined by the initial clinical impression.

A progressive headache disorder, new onset of headache in middle or later life, headaches that disturb sleep or are related to exertion, and headaches that are associated with neurologic symptoms or a focal neurologic deficit usually require cranial MRI or CT scan to exclude an intracranial mass lesion. Signs of meningeal irritation and impairment of consciousness also indicate the need for further investigation (cranial CT scan or MRI and examination of the cerebrospinal fluid) to exclude subarachnoid hemorrhage or meningeal infection. The diagnosis and treatment of primary neurologic disorders associated with headache are considered separately under these disorders.

1. Tension Headache

Patients frequently complain of poor concentration and other vague nonspecific symptoms, in addition to constant daily headaches that are often vise-like or tight in quality and may be exacerbated by emotional stress, fatigue, noise, or glare. The headaches are usually generalized, may be most intense about the neck or back of the head, and are not associated with focal neurologic symptoms.

When treatment with simple analgesics is not effective, a trial of antimigrainous agents (see Migraine, below) is worthwhile. Techniques to induce relaxation are also useful and include massage, hot baths, and biofeedback. Exploration of underlying causes of chronic anxiety is often rewarding. Local injection of botulinum toxin type A is sometimes helpful, has few systemic adverse effects, and requires only infrequent administration.

2. Depression Headache

Depression headaches are frequently worse on arising in the morning and may be accompanied by other symptoms of depression. Headaches are occasionally the focus of a somatic delusional system. Antidepressant drugs are often helpful, as may be psychiatric consultation.

3. Migraine

ESSENTIALS OF DIAGNOSIS

- *Headache, usually pulsatile.*
- *Nausea, vomiting, photophobia, and phono-phobia are common accompaniments.*
- *May be transient neurologic symptoms (commonly visual) preceding headache of classic migraine.*
- *No preceding aura is common.*

General Considerations

The pathophysiology of migraine probably relates to the neurotransmitter serotonin. Headache may result from release of neuropeptides acting as neurotransmitters at trigeminal nerve branches, leading to an inflammatory process; another possible mechanism involves activation of the dorsal raphe nucleus.

Clinical Findings

Classic migrainous headache is a lateralized throbbing headache that occurs episodically following its onset in adolescence or early adult life, although not all headaches that are throbbing in character are of migrainous origin. Moreover, in many cases the headaches do not conform to this pattern, although their associated features and response to antimigrainous preparations nevertheless suggest that they have a similar basis. In this broader sense, migrainous headaches may be lateralized or generalized, may be dull or throbbing, and are sometimes associated with anorexia, nausea, vomiting, photophobia, phonophobia, and blurring of vision. They usually build up gradually and may last for several hours or longer. They have been related to dilation and excessive pulsation of branches of the external carotid artery. Focal disturbances of neurologic function may precede or accompany the headaches and have been attributed to constriction of branches of the internal carotid artery. Visual disturbances occur quite commonly and may consist of field defects; of luminous visual hallucinations such as stars, sparks, unformed light flashes (photopsia), geometric patterns, or zigzags of light; or of some combination of field defects and luminous hallucinations (scintillating scotomas). Other focal disturbances such as aphasia or numbness, tingling, clumsiness, or weakness in a circumscribed distribution may also occur.

Patients often give a family history of migraine. Attacks may be triggered by emotional or physical stress, lack or excess of sleep, missed meals, specific foods (eg, chocolate), alcoholic beverages, menstruation, or use of oral contraceptives.

An uncommon variant is **basilar artery migraine**, in which blindness or visual disturbances throughout both visual fields are initially accompanied or followed by dysarthria, disequilibrium, tinnitus, and perioral and distal paresthesias and are sometimes followed by transient loss or impairment of consciousness or by a confusional state. This, in turn, is followed by a throbbing (usually occipital) headache, often with nausea and vomiting.

In **ophthalmoplegic migraine**, lateralized pain—often about the eye—is accompanied by nausea, vomiting, and diplopia due to transient external ophthalmoplegia. The ophthalmoplegia is due to third nerve palsy, sometimes with accompanying sixth nerve involvement, and may outlast the orbital pain by several days or even weeks. The ophthalmic division of the fifth nerve has also been affected in some patients. Ophthalmoplegic migraine is rare; more common causes of a painful ophthalmoplegia are internal carotid artery aneurysms and diabetes.

In rare instances, the neurologic or somatic disturbance accompanying typical migrainous headaches becomes the sole manifestation of an attack ("migraine equivalent"). Very rarely, the patient may be left with a permanent neurologic deficit following a migrainous attack.

Treatment

Management of migraine consists of avoidance of any precipitating factors, together with prophylactic or symptomatic pharmacologic treatment if necessary.

A. SYMPTOMATIC THERAPY

During acute attacks, many patients find it helpful to rest in a quiet, darkened room until symptoms subside. A simple analgesic (eg, aspirin, acetaminophen, ibuprofen, or naproxen) taken right away often provides relief, but treatment with extracranial vasoconstrictors or other drugs is sometimes necessary. Cafergot, a combination of ergotamine tartrate (1 mg) and caffeine (100 mg), is often particularly helpful; one or two tablets are taken at the onset of headache or warning symptoms, followed by one tablet every 30 minutes, if necessary, up to six tablets per attack and ten tablets per week. Because of impaired absorption or vomiting during acute attacks, oral medication sometimes fails to help. Cafergot given rectally as suppositories (one-half to one suppository containing 2 mg of ergotamine) or dihydroergotamine mesylate (0.5–1 mg intravenously or 1–2 mg subcutaneously or intramuscularly) may be useful in such cases. Alternatively, prochlorperazine administered rectally (25 mg suppository) or intravenously (10 mg) may be prescribed. Ergotamine-containing preparations may affect the gravid uterus and thus should be avoided during pregnancy. Sumatriptan, which has a high affinity for serotonin₁ receptors, is a rapidly effective agent for aborting attacks when given subcutaneously by an autoinjection device. It can also be taken in a nasal form, but absorption is limited, and an oral preparation is available. Zolmitriptan, another selective serotonin$_1$ receptor agonist, has high bioavailability after oral administration and is also effective for the acute treatment of migraine. The optimal initial dose is 5 mg, and relief usually occurs within 1 hour. A newly developed nasal formulation has a rapid onset of action. A number of other triptans are available, including rizatriptan, naratriptan, almotriptan, frovatriptan, and eletriptan. Eletriptan (up to 80 mg over 24 hours) is useful for acute therapy and frovatriptan, which has a longer half-life, may be worthwhile for patients with prolonged attacks (up to 7.5 mg over 24 hours). Triptans should probably be avoided in pregnancy, are contraindicated in patients with coronary or peripheral vascular disease, and may cause nausea or vomiting. The neuroleptic droperidol is also helpful in aborting acute attacks. Metoclopramide given intravenously may be helpful and is being studied. Narcotic analgesics are needed in rare instances, such as meperidine (100 mg intramuscularly) or butorphanol tartrate by nasal spray (1 mg/spray in one nostril, repeated after 3 or 4 hours if necessary). Intravenous propofol in subanesthetic doses may help in intractable cases.

B. PROPHYLACTIC THERAPY

Prophylactic treatment may be necessary if migrainous headaches occur more frequently than two or three times a month. Some of the more common drugs used for this purpose are listed in Table 24–1. Their mode of action is unclear and may involve both an effect on extracerebral vasculature and a cerebral effect, eg, by stabilizing serotonergic neurotransmission. Several drugs

may have to be tried in turn before the headaches are brought under control. Once a drug has been found to help, it should be continued for several months. If the patient remains headache-free, the dose can then be tapered and the drug eventually withdrawn. Botulinum toxin type A is also effective for migraine prevention in some patients; it has few systemic side effects and need only be given at intervals of several months. Although acupuncture has been widely used in the prophylaxis of migraine, a randomized controlled trial failed to show any difference between it and sham acupuncture.

Calcium channel antagonist drugs may decrease the frequency of attacks after an interval of several weeks, but the severity and duration of attacks are not influenced. They should not be used with β-blockers. The angiotensin-converting enzyme receptor blocker, candesartan, may also be effective and is undergoing evaluation.

4. Cluster Headache (Migrainous Neuralgia)

Cluster headache affects predominantly middle-aged men. Its cause is unclear but may relate to a vascular headache disorder or a disturbance of serotonergic mechanisms. Activation of cells in the ipsilateral hypothalamus has been shown to occur. There is often no family history of headache or migraine. Episodes of severe unilateral periorbital pain occur daily for several weeks and are often accompanied by one or more of the following: ipsilateral nasal congestion, rhinorrhea, lacrimation, redness of the eye, and Horner's syndrome. Episodes often occur at night, awaken the patient, and last for less than 2 hours. Spontaneous remission then occurs, and the patient remains well for

Table 24–1. Prophylactic treatment of migraine.

Drug	Usual Adult Daily Dose	Common Side Effects
Propranolol[1]	80–240 mg	Fatigue, lassitude, depression, insomnia, nausea, vomiting, constipation.
Amitriptyline	10–150 mg	Sedation, dry mouth, constipation, weight gain, blurred vision, edema, hypotension, urinary retention.
Imipramine	10–150 mg	Similar to those of amitriptyline (above).
Sertraline	50–200 mg	Anxiety, insomnia, sweating, tremor, gastrointestinal disturbances.
Fluoxetine	20–60 mg	Similar to those of sertraline (above).
Cyproheptadine	12–20 mg	Sedation, dry mouth, epigastric discomfort, gastrointestinal disturbances.
Clonidine	0.2–0.6 mg	Dry mouth, drowsiness, sedation, headache, constipation.
Verapamil[2]	80–160 mg	Headache, hypotension, flushing, edema, constipation. May aggravate atrioventricular nodal heart block and congestive heart failure.

[1]Other β-blockers have also been used (eg, timolol and metoprolol).
[2]Other calcium channel antagonists (eg, nimodipine, nicardipine, and diltiazem) have also been used.
Botulinum toxin type A injected locally into the scalp is effective for prophylaxis in some patients. The antiseizure agents valproic acid (500–1500 mg), gabapentin (900–2400 mg), and topiramate (50–200 mg) are also effective and are detailed in Table 24–3. Valproic acid should be avoided during pregnancy.

weeks or months before another bout of closely spaced attacks occurs. During a bout, many patients report that alcohol triggers an attack; others report that stress, glare, or ingestion of specific foods occasionally precipitates attacks. In occasional patients, typical attacks of pain and associated symptoms recur at intervals without remission. This variant has been referred to as chronic cluster headache.

Examination reveals no abnormality apart from Horner's syndrome that either occurs transiently during an attack or, in longstanding cases, remains as a residual deficit between attacks.

Treatment of an individual attack with oral drugs is generally unsatisfactory, but subcutaneous sumatriptan (6 mg) or dihydroergotamine (1–2 mg) or inhalation of 100% oxygen (7 L/min for 15 minutes) may be effective. Butorphanol tartrate, a synthetic opioid agonist-antagonist, may also be helpful when administered by nasal spray. The dose is 1 mg (one spray in one nostril), repeated after 60–90 minutes if necessary. Ergotamine tartrate is an effective prophylactic and can be given as rectal suppositories (0.5–1 mg at night or twice daily), by mouth (2 mg daily), or by subcutaneous injection (0.25 mg three times daily for 5 days per week). Various prophylactic agents that have been found to be effective in individual patients are valproate, cyproheptadine, lithium carbonate (monitored by plasma lithium determination), prednisone (20–40 mg daily or on alternate days for 2 weeks, followed by gradual withdrawal), and verapamil (240–480 mg daily).

5. Posttraumatic Headache

A variety of nonspecific symptoms may follow closed head injury, regardless of whether consciousness is lost. Headache is often a conspicuous feature. Some authorities believe that psychological factors may be important because there is no correlation of severity of the injury with neurologic signs.

The headache itself usually appears within a day or so following injury, may worsen over the ensuing weeks, and then gradually subsides. It is usually a constant dull ache, with superimposed throbbing that may be localized, lateralized, or generalized. It is sometimes accompanied by nausea, vomiting, or scintillating scotomas.

Disequilibrium, sometimes with a rotatory component, may also occur and is often enhanced by postural change or head movement. Impaired memory, poor concentration, emotional instability, and increased irritability are other common complaints and occasionally are the sole manifestations of the syndrome. The duration of symptoms relates in part to the severity of the original injury, but even trivial injuries are sometimes followed by symptoms that persist for months.

Special investigations are usually not helpful. The electroencephalogram may show minor nonspecific changes, while the electronystagmogram sometimes suggests either peripheral or central vestibulopathy. CT scans or MRI of the head usually show no abnormal findings.

Treatment is difficult, but optimistic encouragement and graduated rehabilitation, depending on the occupational circumstances, are advised. Headaches often respond to simple analgesics, but severe headaches may necessitate treatment with amitriptyline, propranolol, or ergot derivatives.

6. Cough Headache

Severe head pain may be produced by coughing (and by straining, sneezing, and laughing) but, fortunately, usually lasts for only a few minutes or less. The pathophysiologic basis of the complaint is not known, and often there is no underlying structural lesion. However, intracranial lesions, usually in the posterior fossa (eg, Arnold-Chiari malformation), are present in about 10% of cases, and brain tumors or other space-occupying lesions may certainly present in this way. Accordingly, CT scanning or MRI should be undertaken in all patients and repeated annually for several years, since a small structural lesion may not show up initially.

The disorder is usually self-limited, although it may persist for several years. For unknown reasons, symptoms sometimes clear completely after lumbar puncture. Indomethacin (75–150 mg daily) may provide relief.

7. Headache Due to Giant Cell (Temporal or Cranial) Arteritis

The superficial temporal, vertebral, ophthalmic, and posterior ciliary arteries are often the most severely affected pathologically. Most patients are elderly. The major symptom is headache, often associated with or preceded by myalgia, malaise, anorexia, weight loss, and other nonspecific complaints. Loss of vision is the most feared manifestation and occurs quite commonly. Clinical examination often reveals tenderness of the scalp and over the temporal arteries. Further details, including approaches to treatment, are given in Chapter 20.

8. Headache Due to Intracranial Mass Lesions

Intracranial mass lesions of all types may cause headache owing to displacement of vascular structures. Posterior fossa tumors often cause occipital pain, and supratentorial lesions lead to bifrontal headache, but such findings are too inconsistent to be of value in attempts at localizing a pathologic process. The headaches are nonspecific in character and may vary in severity from mild to severe. They may be worsened by exertion or postural change and may be associated with nausea and vomiting, but this is true of migraine also. Headaches are also a feature of pseudotumor cerebri (see below). Signs of focal or diffuse cerebral dysfunction or of increased intracranial pressure will indicate the need for further investigation. Similarly, a progressive headache disorder or the new onset of headaches in middle or later life merits investigation if no cause is apparent.

9. Headache Due to Other Neurologic Causes

Cerebrovascular disease may be associated with headache, but the mechanism is unclear. Headache may occur with internal carotid artery occlusion or carotid dissection and after carotid endarterectomy. Diagnosis is facilitated by the clinical accompaniments and the circumstances in which the headache developed.

Acute severe headache accompanies subarachnoid hemorrhage and meningeal infections; accompanying signs of meningeal irritation and impairment of consciousness indicate the need for further investigations.

Dull or throbbing headache is a frequent sequela of lumbar puncture and may last for several days. It is aggravated by the erect posture and alleviated by recumbency. The exact mechanism is unclear, but it is commonly attributed to leakage of cerebrospinal fluid through the dural puncture site. Its incidence may be reduced if a small-diameter needle is used for the spinal tap, and perhaps also if the patient lies prone or supine after the procedure.

Ashkenazi A et al: The evolving management of migraine. Curr Opin Neurol 2003;16:341. [PMID: 12858071]

Friedman BW et al: A trial of metoclopramide vs. sumatriptan for the emergency department treatment of migraines. Neurology 2005;64:463. [PMID: 15699376]

Kaniecki R: Headache assessment and management. JAMA 2003; 289:1430. [PMID: 12636467]

Linde K et al: Acupuncture for patients with migraine: a randomized controlled trial. JAMA 2005;293:2118. [PMID: 15870415]

May A: Cluster headache: pathogenesis, diagnosis, and management. Lancet 2005;366:843. [PMID: 16139660]

Parmet S et al: JAMA patient page. Headaches. JAMA 2003;289: 1462. [PMID: 12636471]

Schoenen J et al: Headache with focal neurological signs or symptoms: a complicated differential diagnosis. Lancet Neurol 2004;3:237. [PMID: 15039036]

FACIAL PAIN

1. Trigeminal Neuralgia

 ESSENTIALS OF DIAGNOSIS

- *Brief episodes of stabbing facial pain.*
- *Pain is in the territory of the second and third division of the trigeminal nerve.*
- *Pain exacerbated by touch.*

General Considerations

Trigeminal neuralgia ("tic douloureux") is most common in middle and later life. It affects women more frequently than men.

Clinical Findings

Momentary episodes of sudden lancinating facial pain occur and commonly arise near one side of the mouth and shoot toward the ear, eye, or nostril on that side. The pain may be triggered or precipitated by such factors as touch, movement, drafts, and eating. Indeed, in order to lessen the likelihood of triggering further attacks, many patients try to hold the face still while talking. Spontaneous remissions for several months or longer may occur. As the disorder progresses, however, the episodes of pain become more frequent, remissions become shorter and less common, and a dull ache may persist between the episodes of stabbing pain. Symptoms remain confined to the distribution of the trigeminal nerve (usually the second or third division) on one side only.

Differential Diagnosis

The characteristic features of the pain in trigeminal neuralgia usually distinguish it from other causes of facial pain. Neurologic examination shows no abnormality except in a few patients in whom trigeminal neuralgia is symptomatic of some underlying lesion, such as multiple sclerosis or a brainstem neoplasm, in which case the finding will depend on the nature and site of the lesion. Similarly, CT scans and radiologic contrast studies are normal in patients with classic trigeminal neuralgia.

In a young patient presenting with trigeminal neuralgia, multiple sclerosis must be suspected even if there are no other neurologic signs. In such circumstances, findings on evoked potential testing and examination of cerebrospinal fluid may be corroborative. When the facial pain is due to a posterior fossa tumor, CT scanning and MRI generally reveal the lesion.

Treatment

The drugs most helpful for treatment are oxcarbazepine (although not approved by the US Food and Drug Administration [FDA] for this indication) or carbamazepine, with monitoring by serial blood counts and liver function tests. If these medications are ineffective or cannot be tolerated, phenytoin should be tried. (Doses and side effects of these drugs are shown in Table 24–3). Baclofen (10–20 mg three or four times daily) may also be helpful, either alone or in combination with one of these other agents. Gabapentin may also relieve pain, especially in patients who do not respond to conventional medical therapy and those with multiple sclerosis. Depending on response and tolerance, up to 2400 mg/d is given in divided doses.

In the past, alcohol injection of the affected nerve, rhizotomy, or tractotomy was recommended if pharmacologic treatment was unsuccessful. More recently, however, posterior fossa exploration has frequently revealed some structural cause for the neuralgia (despite normal findings on CT scans, MRI, or arteriograms), such as an anomalous artery or vein impinging on the trigeminal nerve root. In such cases, simple decompression and separation of the anomalous vessel from the nerve root produce lasting relief of symptoms. In elderly patients with a limited life expectancy, radiofrequency rhizotomy is sometimes preferred because it is easy to perform, has few complications, and provides symptomatic relief for a period of time. Gamma radiosurgery to the trigeminal root is another noninvasive approach that appears to be successful in 80% of patients, with essentially no side effects other than facial paresthesias in a few instances. Surgical exploration generally reveals no abnormality and is inappropriate in patients with trigeminal neuralgia due to multiple sclerosis.

Liu JK et al: Treatment of trigeminal neuralgia. Neurosurg Clin North Am 2004;15:319. [PMID: 15246340]

Rozen TD: Trigeminal neuralgia and glossopharyngeal neuralgia. Neurol Clin 2004;22:185. [PMID: 15062534]

2. Atypical Facial Pain

Facial pain without the typical features of trigeminal neuralgia is generally a constant, often burning pain that may have a restricted distribution at its onset but soon spreads to the rest of the face on the affected side and sometimes involves the other side, the neck, or the back of the head as well. The disorder is especially common in middle-aged women, many of them depressed, but it is not clear whether depression is the cause of or a reaction to the pain. Simple analgesics should be given a trial, as should tricyclic antidepressants, carbamazepine, oxcarbazepine, and phenytoin; the response is often disappointing. Opioid analgesics pose a danger of addiction in patients with this disorder. Attempts at surgical treatment are not indicated.

3. Glossopharyngeal Neuralgia

Glossopharyngeal neuralgia is an uncommon disorder in which pain similar in quality to that in trigeminal neuralgia occurs in the throat, about the tonsillar fossa, and sometimes deep in the ear and at the back of the tongue. The pain may be precipitated by swallowing, chewing, talking, or yawning and is sometimes accompanied by syncope. In most instances, no underlying structural abnormality is present; multiple sclerosis is sometimes responsible. Oxcarbazepine and carbamazepine (see Table 24–3) are the treatments of choice and should be tried before any surgical procedures are considered. Microvascular decompression is generally preferred over destructive surgical procedures such as partial rhizotomy in medically refractory cases and is often effective without causing severe complications.

4. Postherpetic Neuralgia

Herpes zoster (shingles) is due to infection of the nervous system by varicella-zoster virus. About 15% of patients who develop shingles suffer from postherpetic neuralgia. This complication seems especially likely to occur in the elderly, when the rash is severe, and when the first division of the trigeminal nerve is affected. A history of shingles and the presence of cutaneous scarring resulting from shingles aid in the diagnosis. Severe pain with shingles correlates with the intensity of postherpetic symptoms.

The incidence of postherpetic neuralgia may be reduced by the treatment of shingles with oral acyclovir or famciclovir, but this is disputed; systemic corticosteroids do not help. Zoster vaccine markedly reduces morbidity from herpes zoster and postherpetic neuralgia among older adults. Management of the established complication is essentially medical. If simple analgesics fail to help, a trial of a tricyclic antidepressant (eg, amitriptyline, up to 100–150 mg/d) in conjunction with a phenothiazine (eg, perphenazine, 2–8 mg/d) is often effective. Other patients respond to carbamazepine (up to 1200 mg/d), phenytoin (300 mg/d), gabapentin (up to 3600 mg/d), or pregabalin (up to 300 mg/d). A combination of gabapentin and morphine taken orally may provide better analgesia at lower doses of each agent than either taken alone. Topical application of capsaicin cream (eg, Zostrix, 0.025%) is sometimes helpful, perhaps because of depletion of pain-mediating peptides from peripheral sensory neurons, and topical lidocaine (5%) is also worthy of trial.

Gilron I et al: Morphine, gabapentin, or their combination for neuropathic pain. N Engl J Med 2005;352:1324. [PMID: 15800228]

Johnson RW et al: Treatment of herpes zoster and postherpetic neuralgia. BMJ 2003;326:748. [PMID: 12676845]

5. Facial Pain Due to Other Causes

Facial pain may be caused by temporomandibular joint dysfunction in patients with malocclusion, abnormal bite, or faulty dentures. There may be tenderness of the masticatory muscles, and an association between pain onset and jaw movement is sometimes noted. This pattern differs from that of jaw (masticatory) claudication, a symptom of giant cell arteritis, in which pain develops progressively with mastication. Treatment of the underlying joint dysfunction relieves symptoms.

A relationship of facial pain to chewing or temperature changes may suggest a dental disturbance. The cause is sometimes not obvious, and diagnosis requires careful dental examination and x-rays. Sinusitis and ear infections causing facial pain are usually recognized by the history of respiratory tract infection, fever, and, in some instances, aural discharge. There may be localized tenderness. Radiologic evidence of sinus infection or mastoiditis is confirmatory.

Glaucoma is an important ocular cause of facial pain, usually localized to the periorbital region.

On occasion, pain in the jaw may be the principal manifestation of angina pectoris. Precipitation by exertion and radiation to more typical areas establish the cardiac origin.

EPILEPSY

ESSENTIALS OF DIAGNOSIS

- *Recurrent seizures.*
- *Characteristic electroencephalographic changes accompany seizures.*
- *Mental status abnormalities or focal neurologic symptoms may persist for hours postictally.*

General Considerations

The term "epilepsy" denotes any disorder characterized by recurrent seizures. A seizure is a transient disturbance of cerebral function due to an abnormal paroxysmal neuronal discharge in the brain. Epilepsy is common, affecting approximately 0.5% of the population in the United States.

Etiology

Epilepsy has several causes. Its most likely cause in individual patients relates to the age at onset.

A. IDIOPATHIC OR CONSTITUTIONAL EPILEPSY

Seizures usually begin between 5 and 20 years of age but may start later in life. No specific cause can be identified, and there is no other neurologic abnormality.

B. SYMPTOMATIC EPILEPSY

There are many causes for recurrent seizures.

1. Pediatric age groups—Congenital abnormalities and perinatal injuries may result in seizures presenting in infancy or childhood.

2. Metabolic disorders—Withdrawal from alcohol or drugs is a common cause of recurrent seizures, and other metabolic disorders such as uremia and hypoglycemia or hyperglycemia may also be responsible.

3. Trauma—Trauma is an important cause of seizures at any age, but especially in young adults. Posttraumatic epilepsy is more likely to develop if the dura mater was penetrated and generally becomes manifest within 2 years following the injury. However, seizures developing in the first week after head injury do not necessarily imply that future attacks will occur. There is no clear evidence that prophylactic anticonvulsant drug treatment reduces the incidence of posttraumatic epilepsy.

4. Tumors and other space-occupying lesions—Neoplasms may lead to seizures at any age, but they are an especially important cause of seizures in middle and later life, when the incidence of neoplastic disease increases. The seizures are commonly the initial symptoms of the tumor and often are partial (focal) in character. They are most likely to occur with structural lesions involving the frontal, parietal, or temporal regions. Tumors must be excluded by appropriate imaging studies in all patients with onset of seizures after 30 years of age, focal seizures or signs, or a progressive seizure disorder.

5. Vascular diseases—Vascular diseases become increasingly frequent causes of seizures with advancing age and are the most common cause of seizures with onset at age 60 years or older.

6. Degenerative disorders—Alzheimer's disease and other degenerative disorders are a cause of seizures in later life.

7. Infectious diseases—Infectious diseases must be considered in all age groups as potentially reversible causes of seizures. Seizures may occur with an acute infective or inflammatory illness, such as bacterial meningitis or herpes encephalitis, or in patients with more longstanding or chronic disorders such as neurosyphilis or cerebral cysticercosis. In patients with AIDS, they may result from central nervous system toxoplasmosis, cryptococcal meningitis, secondary viral encephalitis, or other infective complications. Seizures are a common sequela of supratentorial brain abscess, developing most frequently in the first year after treatment.

Classification of Seizures

Seizures can be categorized in various ways, but the descriptive classification proposed by the International League Against Epilepsy is clinically the most useful. Seizures are divided into those that are generalized and those affecting only part of the brain (partial seizures) (Table 24–2).

A. PARTIAL SEIZURES

The initial clinical and electroencephalographic manifestations of partial seizures indicate that only a restricted part of one cerebral hemisphere has been activated. The ictal manifestations depend on the area of the brain involved. Partial seizures are subdivided into simple seizures, in which consciousness is preserved, and complex seizures, in which it is impaired. Partial seizures of either type sometimes become secondarily generalized, leading to a tonic, clonic, or tonic-clonic attack.

1. Simple partial seizures—Simple seizures may be manifested by focal motor symptoms (convulsive jerking) or somatosensory symptoms (eg, paresthesias or tingling) that spread (or "march") to different parts of the limb or body depending on their cortical representation. In other instances, special sensory symptoms (eg, light flashes or buzzing) indicate involvement of visual, auditory, olfactory, or gustatory regions of the brain, or there may be autonomic symptoms or signs (eg, abnormal epigastric sensations, sweating, flushing,

Table 24–2. Seizure classification.

Seizure Type	Key Features	Other Associated Features
Partial seizures	Involvement of only restricted part of brain; may become secondarily generalized	
Simple partial	Consciousness preserved	May be manifested by focal motor, sensory, or autonomic symptoms
Complex partial	Consciousness impaired	Above symptoms may precede, accompany, or follow
Generalized seizures	Diffuse involvement of brain at onset	
Absence (petit mal)	Consciousness impaired briefly; patient often unaware of attacks	May be clonic, tonic, or atonic components (ie, loss of postural tone); autonomic components (eg, enuresis); or accompanying automatisms Almost always begin in childhood and frequently cease by age 20
Atypical absences	May be more gradual onset and termination than typical absence	More marked changes in tone may occur
Myoclonic seizures	Single or multiple myoclonic jerks	
Tonic-clonic (grand mal)	Tonic phase: Sudden loss of consciousness, with rigidity and arrest of respiration, lasting < 1 minute Clonic phase: Jerking occurs, usually for < 2–3 minutes Flaccid coma: Variable duration	May be accompanied by tongue biting, incontinence, or aspiration; commonly followed by postictal confusion variable in duration
Status epilepticus	Repeated seizures without recovery between them; a fixed and enduring epileptic condition lasting 30 minutes	

pupillary dilation). The sole manifestations of some seizures are phenomena such as dysphasia, dysmnesic symptoms (eg, déjà vu, jamais vu), affective disturbances, illusions, or structured hallucinations, but such symptoms are usually accompanied by impairment of consciousness.

2. Complex partial seizures—Impaired consciousness may be preceded, accompanied, or followed by the psychic symptoms mentioned above, and automatisms may occur. Such seizures may also begin with some of the other simple symptoms mentioned above.

B. GENERALIZED SEIZURES

There are several different varieties of generalized seizures, as outlined below. In some circumstances, seizures cannot be classified because of incomplete information or because they do not fit into any category.

1. Absence (petit mal) seizures—These are characterized by impairment of consciousness, sometimes with mild clonic, tonic, or atonic components (ie, reduction or loss of postural tone), autonomic components (eg, enuresis), or accompanying automatisms. Onset and termination of attacks are abrupt. If attacks occur during conversation, the patient may miss a few words or may break off in mid sentence for a few sec-

onds. The impairment of external awareness is so brief that the patient is unaware of it. Absence seizures almost always begin in childhood and frequently cease by the age of 20 years, although occasionally they are then replaced by other forms of generalized seizure. Electroencephalographically, such attacks are associated with bursts of bilaterally synchronous and symmetric 3-Hz spike-and-wave activity. A normal background in the electroencephalogram and normal or above-normal intelligence imply a good prognosis for the ultimate cessation of these seizures.

2. Atypical absences—There may be more marked changes in tone, or attacks may have a more gradual onset and termination than in typical absences.

3. Myoclonic seizures—Myoclonic seizures consist of single or multiple myoclonic jerks.

4. Tonic-clonic (grand mal) seizures—In these seizures, which are characterized by sudden loss of consciousness, the patient becomes rigid and falls to the ground, and respiration is arrested. This tonic phase, which usually lasts for less than a minute, is followed by a clonic phase in which there is jerking of the body musculature that may last for 2 or 3 minutes and is then followed by a stage of flaccid coma. During the seizure, the tongue or lips may be bitten, urinary or fecal incontinence may occur, and the patient may be injured. Immediately after the seizure, the patient may either recover consciousness, drift into sleep, have a further convulsion without recovery of consciousness between the attacks (**status epilepticus**), or after recovering consciousness have a further convulsion (**serial seizures**). In other cases, patients will behave in an abnormal fashion in the immediate postictal period, without subsequent awareness or memory of events (**postepileptic automatism**). Headache, disorientation, confusion, drowsiness, nausea, soreness of the muscles, or some combination of these symptoms commonly occurs postictally.

5. Tonic, clonic, or atonic seizures—Loss of consciousness may occur with either the tonic or clonic accompaniments described above, especially in children. Atonic seizures (**epileptic drop attacks**) have also been described.

Clinical Findings

A. SYMPTOMS AND SIGNS

Nonspecific changes such as headache, mood alterations, lethargy, and myoclonic jerking alert some patients to an impending seizure hours before it occurs. These prodromal symptoms are distinct from the aura which may precede a generalized seizure by a few seconds or minutes and which is itself a part of the attack, arising locally from a restricted region of the brain.

In most patients, seizures occur unpredictably at any time and without any relationship to posture or ongoing activities. Occasionally, however, they occur at a particular time (eg, during sleep) or in relation to external precipitants such as lack of sleep, missed meals, emotional stress, menstruation, alcohol ingestion (or alcohol withdrawal; see below), or use of certain drugs. Fever and nonspecific infections may also precipitate seizures in known epileptics. In a few patients, seizures are provoked by specific stimuli such as flashing lights or a flickering television set (**photosensitive epilepsy**), music, or reading.

Clinical examination between seizures shows no abnormality in patients with idiopathic epilepsy, but in the immediate postictal period, extensor plantar responses may be seen. The presence of lateralized or focal signs postictally suggests that seizures may have a focal origin. In patients with symptomatic epilepsy, the findings on examination will reflect the underlying cause.

B. IMAGING

MRI is indicated for patients with focal neurologic symptoms or signs, focal seizures, or electroencephalographic findings of a focal disturbance; some clinicians routinely order imaging studies for all patients with new-onset seizure disorders. Such studies should certainly be performed in patients with clinical evidence of a progressive disorder and in those presenting with new onset of seizures after the age of 20 years, because of the possibility of an underlying neoplasm. A chest radiograph should also be obtained in such patients, since the lungs are a common site for primary or secondary neoplasms.

C. LABORATORY AND OTHER STUDIES

Initial investigations should always include a full blood count, blood glucose determination, liver and renal function tests, and serologic tests for syphilis. The hematologic and biochemical screening tests are important both in excluding various causes of seizures and in providing a baseline for subsequent monitoring of long-term effects of treatment.

Electroencephalography may support the clinical diagnosis of epilepsy (by demonstrating paroxysmal abnormalities containing spikes or sharp waves), may provide a guide to prognosis, and may help classify the seizure disorder. Classification of the disorder is important for determining the most appropriate anticonvulsant drug with which to start treatment. For example, absence (petit mal) and complex partial seizures may be difficult to distinguish clinically, but the electroencephalographic findings and treatment of choice differ in these two conditions. Finally, by localizing the epileptogenic source, the electroencephalographic findings are important in evaluating candidates for surgical treatment.

Differential Diagnosis

The distinction between the various disorders likely to be confused with generalized seizures is usually made on the basis of the history. The importance of obtaining an eyewitness account of the attacks cannot be overemphasized.

A. DIFFERENTIAL DIAGNOSIS OF PARTIAL SEIZURES

1. Transient ischemic attacks—These attacks are distinguished from seizures by their longer duration, lack of spread, and symptoms. Level of consciousness, which is unaltered, does not distinguish them. There is a loss of motor or sensory function (eg, weakness or numbness) with transient ischemic attacks, whereas positive symptoms (eg, convulsive jerking or paresthesias) characterizes seizures.

2. Rage attacks—Rage attacks are usually situational and lead to goal-directed aggressive behavior.

3. Panic attacks—These may be hard to distinguish from simple or complex partial seizures unless there is evidence of psychopathologic disturbances between attacks and the attacks have a clear relationship to external circumstances.

B. DIFFERENTIAL DIAGNOSIS OF GENERALIZED SEIZURES

1. Syncope—Syncopal episodes usually occur in relation to postural change, emotional stress, instrumentation, pain, or straining. They are typically preceded by pallor, sweating, nausea, and malaise and lead to loss of consciousness accompanied by flaccidity; recovery occurs rapidly with recumbency, and there is no post-ictal headache or confusion. In some instances, however, motor accompaniments may simulate a seizure. Serum creatine kinase measured about 3 hours after the event is generally normal after syncopal episodes but markedly elevated after tonic-clonic seizures.

2. Cardiac dysrhythmias—Cerebral hypoperfusion due to a disturbance of cardiac rhythm should be suspected in patients with known cardiac or vascular disease or in elderly patients who present with episodic loss of consciousness. Prodromal symptoms are typically absent. A relationship of attacks to physical activity and the finding of a systolic murmur is suggestive of aortic stenosis. Repeated Holter monitoring may be necessary to establish the diagnosis; monitoring initiated by the patient ("event monitor") may be valuable if the disturbances of consciousness are rare.

3. Brainstem ischemia—Loss of consciousness is preceded or accompanied by other brainstem signs. Basilar artery migraine and vertebrobasilar vascular disease are discussed elsewhere in this chapter.

4. Pseudoseizures—The term "pseudoseizures" is used to denote both hysterical conversion reactions and attacks due to malingering when these simulate epileptic seizures. Many patients with pseudoseizures also have true seizures or a family history of epilepsy. Although pseudoseizures tend to occur at times of emotional stress, this may also be the case with true seizures.

Clinically, the attacks superficially resemble tonic-clonic seizures, but there may be obvious preparation before pseudoseizures occur. Moreover, there is usually no tonic phase; instead, there is an asynchronous thrashing of the limbs, which increases if restraints are imposed and which rarely leads to injury. Consciousness may be normal or "lost," but in the latter context the occurrence of goal-directed behavior or of shouting, swearing, etc, indicates that it is feigned. Postictally, there are no changes in behavior or neurologic findings.

Laboratory studies may aid in recognition of pseudoseizures. There are no electrocerebral changes, whereas the electroencephalogram changes during organic seizures accompanied by loss of consciousness. The serum level of prolactin has been found to increase dramatically between 15 and 30 minutes after a tonic-clonic convulsion in most patients, whereas it is unchanged after a pseudoseizure. Serum creatine kinase levels also increase after convulsions but not pseudoseizures.

Treatment

A. GENERAL MEASURES

For patients with recurrent seizures, drug treatment is prescribed with the goal of preventing further attacks and is usually continued until there have been no seizures for at least 3 years. Epileptic patients should be advised to avoid situations that could be dangerous or life-threatening if further seizures should occur. State legislation may require clinicians to report to the state department of public health any patients with seizures or other episodic disturbances of consciousness.

1. Choice of medication—The drug with which treatment is best initiated depends on the type of seizures to be treated (Table 24–3). The dose of the selected drug is gradually increased until seizures are controlled or side effects prevent further increases. If seizures continue despite treatment at the maximal tolerated dose, a second drug is added and the dose increased depending on tolerance; the first drug is then gradually withdrawn. In treatment of partial and secondarily generalized tonic-clonic seizures, the success rate is higher with carbamazepine, phenytoin, or valproic acid than with phenobarbital or primidone. Gabapentin, topiramate, lamotrigine, oxcarbazepine, levetiracetam, and zonisamide are newer antiepileptic drugs that are effective for partial or secondarily generalized seizures. Felbamate is also effective for such seizures but, because it may cause aplastic anemia or fulminant hepatic failure, should be used only in selected patients unresponsive to other measures. Tiagabine is another adjunctive agent for partial seizures. In most patients with seizures of a single type, satisfactory control can be achieved with a single anticonvulsant drug. Treatment with two drugs may further reduce seizure frequency or severity, but usually only at the cost of greater toxicity. Treatment with more than two drugs is almost always unhelpful unless the patient is having seizures of different types.

2. Monitoring—Monitoring serum drug levels has led to major advances in the management of seizure disorders. The same daily dose of a particular drug leads to markedly different blood concentrations in different patients, and this will affect the therapeutic response. In general, the dose of an antiepileptic agent is increased depending on the clinical response regardless of the serum drug level. The trough drug level is then measured to provide a reference point for the maximum tolerated dose. Dosing should not be based simply on serum levels because many patients require levels that exceed the therapeutic range ("toxic levels") but tolerate these without ill effect. Steady-state drug levels in the blood should be measured after treatment is initiated, dosage is changed, or another drug is added to the therapeutic regimen and when seizures are poorly controlled. Dose adjustments are then guided by the laboratory findings. The most common cause of a lower concentration of drug than expected for the prescribed dose is poor patient compliance. Compliance can be improved by limiting to a minimum the number of daily doses. Recurrent seizures or status epilepticus may result if drugs are taken erratically, and in some circumstances noncompliant patients may be better off without any medication.

All anticonvulsant drugs have side effects, and some of these are shown in Table 24–3.

Table 24–3. Drug treatment for seizures.

Drug	Usual Adult Daily Dose	Minimum No. of Daily Doses	Time to Steady-State Drug Levels	Optimal Drug Level	Selected Side Effects and Idiosyncratic Reactions
Generalized tonic-clonic (grand mal) or partial (focal) seizures					
Phenytoin	200–400 mg	1	5–10 days	10–20 mcg/mL	Nystagmus, ataxia, dysarthria, sedation, confusion, gingival hyperplasia, hirsutism, megaloblastic anemia, blood dyscrasias, skin rashes, fever, systemic lupus erythematosus, lymphadenopathy, peripheral neuropathy, dyskinesias.
Carbamazepine (extended-release formulation)	600–1200 mg	2–3 (2)	3–4 days	4–8 mcg/mL	Nystagmus, dysarthria, diplopia, ataxia, drowsiness, nausea, blood dyscrasias, hepatotoxicity, hyponatremia. May exacerbate myoclonic seizures.
Valproic acid	1500–2000 mg	3	2–4 days	50–100 mcg/mL	Nausea, vomiting, diarrhea, drowsiness, alopecia, weight gain, hepatotoxicity, thrombocytopenia, tremor, pancreatitis.
Phenobarbital	100–200 mg	1	14–21 days	10–40 mcg/mL	Drowsiness, nystagmus, ataxia, skin rashes, learning difficulties, hyperactivity.
Primidone	750–1500 mg	3	4–7 days	5–15 mcg/mL	Sedation, nystagmus, ataxia, vertigo, nausea, skin rashes, megaloblastic anemia, irritability.
Felbamate[1,2]	1200–3600 mg	3	4–5 days	?	Anorexia, nausea, vomiting, headache, insomnia, weight loss, dizziness, hepatotoxicity, aplastic anemia.
Gabapentin[2]	900–1800 mg	3	1 day	?	Sedation, fatigue, ataxia, nystagmus, weight loss.
Lamotrigine[2,4]	100–500 mg	2	4–5 days	?	Sedation, skin rash, visual disturbances, dyspepsia, ataxia.
Topiramate[2,4]	200–400 mg	2	4 days	?	Somnolence, nausea, dyspepsia, irritability, dizziness, ataxia, nystagmus, diplopia, renal calculi, weight loss, hypohidrosis, hyperthermia.
Oxcarbazepine[4]	900–1800 mg	2	2–3 days	?	As for carbamazepine.
Levetiracetam[2]	1000–3000 mg	2	2 days	?	Somnolence, ataxia, headache, behavioral changes.
Zonisamide[2]	200–600 mg	1–2	10 days	?	Somnolence, ataxia, anorexia, nausea, vomiting, rash, confusion, renal calculi. Do not use in patients with sulfonamide allergy.
Tiagabine[3]	32–56 mg	2	2 days	?	Somnolence, anxiety, dizziness, poor concentration, tremor, diarrhea.
Pregabalin	150–160 mg	2	2–4 days	?	Somnolence, dizziness, poor concentration, weight gain, thrombocytopenia, skin rashes, anaphylactoid reactions

Table 24–3. Drug treatment for seizures. (continued)

Drug	Usual Adult Daily Dose	Minimum No. of Daily Doses	Time to Steady-State Drug Levels	Optimal Drug Level	Selected Side Effects and Idiosyncratic Reactions
Absence (petit mal) seizures					
Ethosuximide	100–1500 mg	2	5–10 days	40–100 mcg/mL	Nausea, vomiting, anorexia, headache, lethargy, unsteadiness, blood dyscrasias, systemic lupus erythematosus, urticaria, pruritus.
Valproic acid	1500–2000 mg	3	2–4 days	50–100 mcg/mL	See above.
Clonazepam	0.04–0.2 mg/kg	2	?	20–80 ng/mL	Drowsiness, ataxia, irritability, behavioral changes, exacerbation of tonic-clonic seizures.
Myoclonic seizures					
Valproic acid	1500–2000 mg	3	2–4 days	50–100 mcg/mL	See above.
Clonazepam	0.04–0.2 mg/kg	2	?	20–80 ng/mL	See above.

[1]Not to be used as a first-line drug; when used, blood counts should be performed regularly (every 2–4 weeks). Should be used only in selected patients because of risk of aplastic anemia and hepatic failure.
[2]Approved as adjunctive therapy for partial and secondarily generalized seizures.
[3]Approved as adjunctive therapy for partial seizures.
[4]Approved as monotherapy for partial seizures.

In most patients, a complete blood count should be performed at least annually because of the risk of anemia or blood dyscrasia. Treatment with certain drugs may require more frequent monitoring or use of additional screening tests. For example, periodic tests of hepatic function are necessary if valproic acid, carbamazepine, or felbamate is used, and serial blood counts are important with carbamazepine, ethosuximide, or felbamate.

3. Discontinuance of medication—Only when patients have been seizure-free for several (at least 3) years should withdrawal of medication be considered. Unfortunately, there is no way of predicting which patients can be managed successfully without treatment, although seizure recurrence is more likely in patients who initially failed to respond to therapy, those with seizures having focal features or of multiple types, and those with continuing electroencephalographic abnormalities. Dose reduction should be gradual over a period of weeks or months, and drugs should be withdrawn one at a time. If seizures recur, treatment is reinstituted with the same drugs used previously. Seizures are no more difficult to control after a recurrence than before.

4. Surgical treatment—Patients with surgically remediable epilepsy or seizures refractory to pharmacologic management may be candidates for operative treatment, which is best undertaken in specialized centers.

5. Vagal nerve stimulation—Treatment by chronic vagal nerve stimulation for adults and adolescents with medically refractory partial-onset seizures is approved in the United States and provides an alternative approach for patients who are not optimal candidates for surgical treatment. The mechanism of therapeutic action is unknown. Adverse effects consist mainly of transient hoarseness during stimulus delivery.

B. SPECIAL CIRCUMSTANCES

1. Solitary seizures—In patients who have had only one seizure, investigation as outlined above should exclude an underlying cause requiring specific treatment. An EEG should also be performed, preferably within 24 hours after the seizure, because the findings may influence management—especially when focal abnormalities are present. Prophylactic anticonvulsant drug treatment is generally not required unless further attacks occur or investigations reveal some underlying pathology that itself is untreatable. The risk of seizure recurrence varies in different series between about 30% and 70%. Epilepsy should not be diagnosed on the basis of a solitary seizure. If seizures occur in the context of transient, nonrecurrent systemic disorders such as acute cerebral anoxia, the diagnosis of epilepsy is inaccurate, and long-term prophylactic anticonvulsant drug treatment is unnecessary.

2. Alcohol withdrawal seizures—One or more generalized tonic-clonic seizures may occur within 48 hours or so of withdrawal from alcohol after a period of high or chronic intake. Patients should be hospitalized for at least 24 hours for observation and to follow the severity of withdrawal symptoms. If the seizures have consistently focal features, the possibility of an associated structural abnormality, often traumatic in origin, must be considered. Head CT scan or MRI should be performed in patients with new onset of generalized seizures and whenever there are focal features associated with any seizures. Treatment with anticonvulsant drugs is generally not required for alcohol withdrawal seizures, since they are self-limited. Benzodiazepines (diazepam or lorazepam) are effective and safe for preventing further seizures. Status epilepticus may rarely follow alcohol withdrawal and is managed along conventional lines (see below). Further attacks will not occur if the patient abstains from alcohol.

3. Tonic-clonic status epilepticus—Poor compliance with the anticonvulsant drug regimen is the most common cause; others include alcohol withdrawal, intracranial infection or neoplasms, metabolic disorders, and drug overdose. The mortality rate may be as high as 20%, and among survivors the incidence of neurologic and mental sequelae may be high. The prognosis relates to the length of time between onset of status epilepticus and the start of effective treatment.

Status epilepticus is a medical emergency. Initial management includes maintenance of the airway and 50% dextrose (25–50 mL) intravenously in case hypoglycemia is responsible. If seizures continue, 10 mg of diazepam is given intravenously over the course of 2 minutes, and the dose is repeated after 10 minutes if necessary. Alternatively, a 4-mg intravenous bolus of lorazepam, repeated once after 10 minutes if necessary, is given in place of diazepam. This is usually effective in halting seizures for a brief period but occasionally causes respiratory depression.

Regardless of the response to diazepam or lorazepam, phenytoin (18–20 mg/kg) is given intravenously at a rate of 50 mg/min; this provides initiation of long-term seizure control. The drug is best injected directly but can also be given in saline; it precipitates, however, if injected into glucose-containing solutions. Because arrhythmias may develop during rapid administration of phenytoin, electrocardiographic monitoring is prudent. Hypotension may complicate phenytoin administration, especially if diazepam has also been given. In the United States, injectable phenytoin has been replaced by fosphenytoin, which is rapidly and completely converted to phenytoin following intravenous administration. No dosing adjustments are necessary because fosphenytoin is expressed in terms of phenytoin equivalents (PE); fosphenytoin is less likely to cause reactions at the infusion site, can be given with all common intravenous solutions, and may be administered at a faster rate (150 mg PE/min). It is also more expensive.

If seizures continue, phenobarbital is then given in a loading dose of 10–20 mg/kg intravenously by slow or intermittent injection (50 mg/min). Respiratory depression and hypotension are common complications and should be anticipated; they may occur also with diazepam alone, although less commonly. If these measures fail, general anesthesia with ventilatory assistance and neuromuscular junction blockade may be required. Alternatively, intravenous midazolam may provide control of refractory status epilepticus; the suggested loading dose is 0.2 mg/kg, followed by 0.05–0.2 mg/kg/h.

After status epilepticus is controlled, an oral drug program for the long-term management of seizures is started, and investigations into the cause of the disorder are pursued.

4. Nonconvulsive status epilepticus—Absence (petit mal) and complex partial status epilepticus are characterized by fluctuating abnormal mental status, confusion, impaired responsiveness, and automatism. Electroencephalography is helpful both in establishing the diagnosis and in distinguishing the two varieties. Initial treatment with intravenous diazepam is usually helpful regardless of the type of status epilepticus, but phenytoin, phenobarbital, carbamazepine, and other drugs may also be needed to obtain and maintain control in complex partial status epilepticus.

Brathen G et al: EFNS guidelines on the diagnosis and management of alcohol-related seizures: report of a EFNS task force. Eur J Neurol 2005;12:816. [PMID: 16053464]

Chang BS et al: Epilepsy. N Engl J Med 2003;349:1257. [PMID: 14507951]

Kelso AR et al: Advances in epilepsy. Br Med Bull 2005;72:135. [PMID: 15845748]

Schachter SC: Epilepsy: major advances in treatment. Lancet Neurol 2004;3:11. [PMID: 14693100]

Vazquez B: Monotherapy in epilepsy: role of the newer antiepileptic drugs. Arch Neurol 2004;61:1361. [PMID: 15364680]

DYSAUTONOMIA

 ESSENTIALS OF DIAGNOSIS

- *Abnormalities of blood pressure, heart rate, sweating, intestinal motility, sphincter control, sexual function, respiration, or ocular function, occurring in isolation or any combination.*

General Considerations

Dysautonomia may occur as a result of central or peripheral pathologic processes. It is manifested by a variety of symptoms that may occur in isolation or in various combinations and relate to abnormalities of blood pressure regulation, thermoregulatory sweating, gastrointestinal function, sphincter control, sexual function, respiration, and ocular function. Syncope, a symptom of dysautonomia, is characterized by a transient loss of consciousness, usually accompanied by hypotension and bradycardia. It may occur in response to emotional stress, postural hypotension, vigorous exercise in a hot environment, obstructed venous return to the heart, acute pain or its anticipation, fluid loss, and a variety of other circumstances.

A. CENTRAL NEUROLOGIC CAUSES

Disease at certain sites in the central nervous system, regardless of its nature, may lead to dysautonomic symptoms. Postural hypotension, which is usually the most troublesome and disabling symptom, may result from spinal cord transection and other myelopathies (eg, due to tumor or syringomyelia) above the T6 level or from brainstem lesions such as syringobulbia and posterior fossa tumors. Sphincter or sexual disturbances may result from cord lesions below T6. Certain primary degenerative disorders are responsible for dysautonomia occurring in isolation (**pure autonomic failure**) or in association with more widespread abnormalities (**multisystem atrophy** or **Shy-Drager syndrome**) that may include parkinsonian, pyramidal symptoms, and cerebellar deficits.

B. PERIPHERAL NEUROLOGIC CAUSES

A pure autonomic neuropathy may occur acutely or subacutely after a viral infection or as a paraneoplastic disorder related usually to small cell lung cancer, particularly in association with certain antibodies, such as anti-Hu or those directed at neuronal nicotinic acetylcholine receptors. Typically, presenting symptoms include postural hypotension, impaired thermoregulatory sweating, xerostomia or xerophthalmia, abnormal gastrointestinal motility, dilated pupils, or acute urinary retention. Dysautonomia is often conspicuous in patients with Guillain-Barré syndrome, manifesting with marked hypotension or hypertension or cardiac arrhythmias that may have a fatal outcome. It may also occur with diabetic, uremic, amyloidotic, and various other metabolic or toxic neuropathies; in association with leprosy or Chagas' disease; and as a feature of certain hereditary neuropathies with autosomal dominant or recessive inheritance or an X-linked pattern. Autonomic symptoms are prominent in the crises of hepatic porphyria. Patients with botulism or the Lambert-Eaton myasthenic syndrome may have constipation, urinary retention, and a sicca syndrome as a result of impaired cholinergic function.

Clinical Findings

A. SYMPTOMS AND SIGNS

Dysautonomic symptoms include syncope, postural hypotension, paroxysmal hypertension, persistent tachycardia without other cause, facial flushing, hypohidrosis or hyperhidrosis, vomiting, constipation, diarrhea, dysphagia, abdominal distention, disturbances of micturition or defecation, apneic episodes, and declining night vision. In syncope, prodromal malaise, nausea, headache, diaphoresis, pallor, visual disturbance, loss of postural tone, and a sense of weakness and impending loss of consciousness are followed by actual loss of consciousness. Although the patient is usually flaccid, some motor activity is not uncommon, and urinary (and rarely fecal) incontinence may also occur, thereby

simulating a seizure. Recovery is rapid once the patient becomes recumbent, but headache, nausea, and fatigue are common postictally.

B. EVALUATION OF THE PATIENT

Clinical evaluation is important to exclude reversible, nonneurologic causes of symptoms. Postural hypotension and syncope, for example, may relate to a reduced cardiac output (eg, from aortic stenosis or cardiomyopathy), paroxysmal cardiac dysrhythmias, volume depletion, various medications, and endocrine and metabolic disorders such as Addison's disease, hypothyroidism or hyperthyroidism, pheochromocytoma, and carcinoid syndrome. Testing of autonomic function helps establish the diagnosis of dysautonomia, to exclude other causes of symptoms, to assess the severity of involvement, and to guide prognostication. Such testing includes evaluating the cardiovascular response to the Valsalva maneuver, startle, mental stress, postural change, and deep respiration, and the sudomotor (sweating) responses to warming or a deep inspiratory gasp. Tilt-table testing may reproduce syncopal or presyncopal symptoms. Pharmacologic studies to evaluate the pupillary responses, radiologic studies of the bladder or gastrointestinal tract, uroflowmetry and urethral pressure profiles, and recording of nocturnal penile tumescence may also be necessary in selected cases. Further investigation depends on the presence of other associated neurologic abnormalities. In patients with a peripheral cause, work-up for peripheral neuropathy may be required as discussed below. For those with evidence of a central lesion, imaging studies will exclude a treatable structural cause.

Treatment

The most disabling symptom of dysautonomia is usually postural hypotension and syncope. Abrupt postural change, prolonged recumbency, and other precipitants should be avoided. Medications associated with postural hypotension should be discontinued or reduced in dose. Treatment may include wearing waist-high elastic hosiery, salt supplementation, sleeping in a semierect position (which minimizes the natriuresis and diuresis that occur during recumbency), and fludrocortisone (0.1–0.2 mg daily). Vasoconstrictor agents may be helpful and include midodrine (2.5–10 mg three times daily) and ephedrine (15–30 mg three times daily). Other agents that have been used occasionally or experimentally are dihydroergotamine, yohimbine, and clonidine; refractory cases may respond to erythropoietin (epoetin alfa) or desmopressin. Patients must be monitored for recumbent hypertension. Postprandial hypotension is helped by caffeine. There is no satisfactory treatment for disturbances of sweating, but an air-conditioned environment is helpful in avoiding extreme swings in body temperature.

Chen-Scarabelli C et al: Neurocardiogenic syncope. BMJ 2004; 329:336. [PMID: 15297344]

Freeman R: Autonomic peripheral neuropathy. Lancet 2005;365: 1259. [PMID: 15811460]

SENSORY DISTURBANCES

Patients may complain of either lost or abnormal sensations. The term "numbness" is often used by patients to denote loss of feeling, but the word also has other meanings and the patient's intention must be clarified. Abnormal spontaneous sensations are generally called paresthesias, and unpleasant or painful sensations produced by a stimulus that is usually painless are called dysesthesias.

Sensory symptoms may be due to disease located anywhere along the peripheral or central sensory pathways. The character, site, mode of onset, spread, and temporal profile of sensory symptoms must be established and any precipitating or relieving factors identified. These features—and the presence of any associated symptoms—help identify the origin of sensory disturbances, as do the physical signs as well. Sensory symptoms or signs may conform to the territory of individual peripheral nerves or nerve roots. Involvement of one side of the body—or of one limb in its entirety—suggests a central lesion. Distal involvement of all four extremities suggests polyneuropathy, a cervical cord or brainstem lesion, or—when symptoms are transient—a metabolic disturbance such as hyperventilation syndrome. Short-lived sensory complaints may be indicative of sensory seizures or cerebral ischemic phenomena as well as metabolic disturbances. In patients with cord lesions, there may be a transverse sensory level. "Dissociated sensory loss" is characterized by loss of some sensory modalities with preservation of others. Such findings may be encountered in patients with either peripheral or central disease and must therefore be interpreted in the clinical context in which they are found.

The absence of sensory signs in patients with sensory symptoms does not mean that symptoms have a nonorganic basis. Symptoms are often troublesome before signs of sensory dysfunction have had time to develop.

WEAKNESS & PARALYSIS

Loss of muscle power may result from central disease involving the upper or lower motor neurons; from peripheral disease involving the roots, plexus, or peripheral nerves; from disorders of neuromuscular transmission; or from primary disorders of muscle. The clinical findings help localize the lesion and thus reduce the number of diagnostic possibilities.

Weakness due to upper motor neuron lesions is characterized by selective involvement of certain muscle groups and is associated with spasticity, increased tendon reflexes, and extensor plantar responses. The site of upper motor neuron (pyramidal) involvement may be indicated by the presence of other clinical signs or by the distribution of the motor deficit. Lower motor neuron lesions lead to muscle wasting as well as weakness, with flaccidity and loss of tendon reflexes, but no change in the plantar responses unless the neurons subserving them are directly involved. Fasciculations may be evident over affected muscles. In distinguishing between a root, plexus, or peripheral nerve lesion, the distribution of the motor deficit and of any sensory changes is of particular importance. In patients with disturbances of neuromuscular transmission, weakness is patchy in distribution, often fluctuates over short periods of time, and is not associated with sensory changes. In myopathic disorders, weakness is usually most marked proximally in the limbs, is not associated with sensory loss or sphincter disturbance, and is not accompanied by muscle wasting or loss of tendon reflexes—at least not until an advanced stage.

TRANSIENT ISCHEMIC ATTACKS

 ESSENTIALS OF DIAGNOSIS

- *Focal neurologic deficit of acute onset.*
- *Clinical deficit resolves completely within 24 hours.*
- *Risk factors for vascular disease often present.*

General Considerations

Transient ischemic attacks are characterized by focal ischemic cerebral neurologic deficits that last for less than 24 hours (usually less than 1–2 hours). About 30% of patients with stroke have a history of transient ischemic attacks, and proper treatment of the attacks is an important means of prevention. The incidence of stroke does not relate to either the number or the duration of individual attacks but is increased in patients with hypertension or diabetes. The risk of stroke is highest in the month after a transient ischemic attack (particularly in the first 48 hours) and progressively declines thereafter.

Etiology

An important cause of transient cerebral ischemia is embolization. In many patients with these attacks, a source is readily apparent in the heart or a major extracranial artery to the head, and emboli sometimes are visible in the retinal arteries. Moreover, an embolic phenomenon explains why separate attacks may affect different parts of the territory supplied by the same major vessel. Cardiac causes of embolic ischemic attacks include atrial fibrillation, rheumatic heart disease, mitral valve disease, infective endocarditis, atrial myxoma, and mural thrombi complicating myocardial infarction. Atrial septal defects and patent foramen ovale may permit emboli from the veins to reach the brain ("paradoxical emboli"). An ulcerated plaque on a major artery to the brain may serve as a source of emboli. In the anterior circulation, atherosclerotic changes occur most commonly in the region of the carotid bifurcation extracranially, and these changes may cause a bruit. In some patients with transient ischemic attacks or strokes, an acute or recent hemorrhage is found to have occurred into this atherosclerotic plaque, and this finding may have pathologic significance. Patients with AIDS have an increased risk of developing transient ischemic deficits or strokes.

Less common abnormalities of blood vessels that may cause transient ischemic attacks include fibromuscular dysplasia, which affects particularly the cervical internal carotid artery; atherosclerosis of the aortic arch; inflammatory arterial disorders such as giant cell arteritis, systemic lupus erythematosus, polyarteritis, and granulomatous angiitis; and meningovascular syphilis. Hypotension may cause a reduction of cerebral blood flow if a major extracranial artery to the brain is markedly stenosed, but this is a rare cause of transient ischemic attack.

Hematologic causes of ischemic attacks include polycythemia, sickle cell disease, and hyperviscosity syndromes. Severe anemia may also lead to transient focal neurologic deficits in patients with preexisting cerebral arterial disease.

The **subclavian steal syndrome** may lead to transient vertebrobasilar ischemia. Symptoms develop when there is localized stenosis or occlusion of one subclavian artery proximal to the source of the vertebral artery, so that blood is "stolen" from this artery. A bruit in the supraclavicular fossa, unequal radial pulses, and a difference of 20 mm Hg or more between the systolic blood pressures in the arms should suggest the diagnosis in patients with vertebrobasilar transient ischemic attacks.

Clinical Findings

A. SYMPTOMS AND SIGNS

The symptoms of transient ischemic attacks vary markedly among patients; however, the symptoms in a given individual tend to be constant in type. Onset is abrupt and without warning, and recovery usually occurs rapidly, often within a few minutes.

If the ischemia is in the carotid territory, common symptoms are weakness and heaviness of the contralateral arm, leg, or face, singly or in any combination. Numbness or paresthesias may also occur either as the sole manifestation of the attack or in combination with the motor deficit. There may be slowness of movement, dysphasia, or monocular visual loss in the eye contralateral to affected limbs. During an attack, examination may reveal flaccid weakness with pyramidal distribution, sensory changes, hyperreflexia or an extensor plantar response on the affected side, dysphasia, or any combination of these findings. Subsequently, examination

reveals no neurologic abnormality, but the presence of a carotid bruit or cardiac abnormality may provide a clue to the cause of symptoms.

Vertebrobasilar ischemic attacks may be characterized by vertigo, ataxia, diplopia, dysarthria, dimness or blurring of vision, perioral numbness and paresthesias, and weakness or sensory complaints on one, both, or alternating sides of the body. These symptoms may occur singly or in any combination. Drop attacks due to bilateral leg weakness, without headache or loss of consciousness, may occur, sometimes in relation to head movements.

The natural history of attacks is variable. Some patients will have a major stroke after only a few attacks, whereas others may have frequent attacks for weeks or months without having a stroke. Attacks may occur intermittently over a long period of time, or they may stop spontaneously. In general, carotid ischemic attacks are more liable than vertebrobasilar ischemic attacks to be followed by stroke. The stroke risk is greater in patients older than 60 years, in diabetics, or after transient ischemic attacks that last longer than 10 minutes and with symptoms or signs of weakness, speech impairment, or gait disturbance.

B. IMAGING

CT scan of the head will exclude the possibility of a small cerebral hemorrhage or a cerebral tumor masquerading as a transient ischemic attack. A number of noninvasive techniques, such as ultrasonography, have been developed for studying the cerebral circulation and imaging the major vessels to the head. Carotid duplex ultrasonography is useful for detecting significant stenosis of the internal carotid artery, but arteriography remains important for demonstrating the status of the cerebrovascular system. MR angiography may reveal stenotic lesions of large vessels but is less sensitive than conventional arteriography. Accordingly, if findings on CT scan are normal, if there is no cardiac source of embolization, and if age and general condition indicate that the patient is a good operative risk, bilateral carotid arteriography should be considered in the further evaluation of carotid ischemic attacks, although the ultrasound findings may help in selecting patients for study.

C. LABORATORY AND OTHER STUDIES

Clinical and laboratory evaluation must include assessment for hypertension, heart disease, hematologic disorders, diabetes mellitus, hyperlipidemia, and peripheral vascular disease. It should include complete blood count, fasting blood glucose and serum cholesterol and homocysteine determinations, serologic tests for syphilis, and an ECG and chest x-ray. Echocardiography with bubble contrast is performed if a cardiac source is likely, and blood cultures are obtained if endocarditis is suspected. Holter monitoring is indicated if a transient, paroxysmal disturbance of cardiac rhythm is suspected.

Differential Diagnosis

Focal seizures usually cause abnormal motor or sensory phenomena such as clonic limb movements, paresthesias, or tingling, rather than weakness or loss of feeling. Symptoms generally spread ("march") up the limb and may lead to a generalized tonic-clonic seizure.

Classic migraine is easily recognized by the visual premonitory symptoms, followed by nausea, headache, and photophobia, but less typical cases may be hard to distinguish. The patient's age and medical history (including family history) may be helpful in this regard. Patients with migraine commonly have a history of episodes since adolescence and report that other family members have a similar disorder.

Focal neurologic deficits may occur during periods of hypoglycemia in diabetic patients receiving insulin or oral hypoglycemic agent therapy.

Treatment

When arteriography reveals a surgically accessible high-grade stenosis (70–99% in luminal diameter) on the side appropriate to carotid ischemic attacks and there is relatively little atherosclerosis elsewhere in the cerebrovascular system, operative treatment (carotid thromboendarterectomy) reduces the risk of ipsilateral carotid stroke, especially when transient ischemic attacks are of recent onset (< 1 month). Surgery is not indicated for mild stenosis (< 30%); its benefits are unclear with severe stenosis plus diffuse intracranial atherosclerotic disease. See Chapter 12 for additional discussion.

In patients with carotid ischemic attacks who are poor operative candidates (and thus have not undergone arteriography) or who are found to have extensive vascular disease, medical treatment should be instituted. Similarly, patients with vertebrobasilar ischemic attacks are treated medically and are not subjected to arteriography unless there is clinical evidence of stenosis or occlusion in the carotid or subclavian arteries.

Medical treatment is aimed at preventing further attacks and stroke. Cigarette smoking should be stopped, and cardiac sources of embolization, hypertension, diabetes, hyperlipidemia, arteritis, or hematologic disorders should be treated appropriately.

A. Embolization from the Heart

If anticoagulants are indicated for the treatment of embolism from the heart, they should be started immediately, provided there is no contraindication to their use. There is no advantage in delay, and the common fear of causing hemorrhage into a previously infarcted area is misplaced, since there is a far greater risk of further embolism to the cerebral circulation if treatment is withheld. Treatment is initiated with intravenous heparin (in a loading dose of 5000–10,000 units of standard-molecular-weight heparin, and maintenance infusion of 1000–2000 units per hour depending on the partial thromboplastin time), while warfarin sodium is introduced in a daily dose of 5–15 mg orally, depending on the international normalized ratio (INR). Warfarin is more effective than aspirin in reducing the incidence of cardioembolic events, but when its use is contraindicated, aspirin (325 mg daily) may be used in patients with nonrheumatic atrial fibrillation to reduce the risk of stroke.

B. Embolization from the Cerebrovascular System

In patients with presumed or angiographically verified atherosclerotic changes in the extracranial or intracranial cerebrovascular circulation, antithrombotic medication is prescribed. The evidence supporting a therapeutic role for aspirin to suppress platelet aggregation is convincing. Platelets adhere to and aggregate around an atherosclerotic plaque and release various substances including thromboxane A_2. Treatment with aspirin significantly reduces the frequency of transient ischemic attacks and the incidence of stroke or myocardial infarcts in high-risk patients. A daily dose of 325 mg is adequate; higher doses may provide added benefit but are associated with a higher incidence of gastrointestinal side effects. Dipyridamole is not as effective; it is unclear whether it offers any advantage over aspirin alone when added to aspirin for stroke prevention. In patients intolerant of aspirin, clopidogrel (75 mg) can be used instead. Some physicians use anticoagulant drugs (eg, warfarin, with temporary heparinization until the dose of warfarin is adequate) unless they are medically contraindicated, continuing them for 3–6 months before they are tapered and ultimately replaced with aspirin, which is continued for another year. However, a recent study concluded that warfarin was associated with higher rates of adverse effects without providing benefit over aspirin.

Surgical extracranial-intracranial arterial anastomosis is generally not helpful in patients with transient ischemic attacks associated with stenotic lesions of the distal internal carotid or the proximal middle cerebral arteries.

Chimowitz MI et al: Comparison of warfarin and aspirin for symptomatic intracranial arterial stenosis. N Engl J Med 2005;352:1305. [PMID: 15800226]

Elkind MS: Secondary stroke prevention: review of clinical trials. Clin Cardiol 2004;27(Suppl 2):II25. [PMID: 15188933]

Nguyen-Huynh MN et al: Transient ischemic attack: a neurologic emergency. Curr Neurol Neurosci Rep 2005;5:13. [PMID: 15676103]

STROKE

 ESSENTIALS OF DIAGNOSIS

- Sudden onset of characteristic neurologic deficit.
- Patient often has history of hypertension, diabetes mellitus, valvular heart disease, or atherosclerosis.

- *Distinctive neurologic signs reflect the region of the brain involved.*

General Considerations

In the United States, stroke remains the third leading cause of death, despite a general decline in the incidence of stroke in the last 30 years. The precise reasons for this decline are uncertain, but increased awareness of risk factors (hypertension, diabetes, hyperlipidemia, cigarette smoking, cardiac disease, AIDS, recreational drug abuse, heavy alcohol consumption, family history of stroke) and improved prophylactic measures and surveillance of those at increased risk have been contributory. Elevation of the blood homocysteine level is also a risk factor for stroke, but it is unclear whether this risk is reduced by treatment to lower the level. A previous stroke makes individual patients more susceptible to additional strokes.

For years, strokes have been subdivided pathologically into infarcts (thrombotic or embolic) and hemorrhages, and clinical criteria for distinguishing between these possibilities have been emphasized. However, it is often difficult to determine on clinical grounds the pathologic basis for stroke (Table 24–4).

1. Lacunar Infarction

Lacunar infarcts are small lesions (usually < 5 mm in diameter) that occur in the distribution of short penetrating arterioles in the basal ganglia, pons, cerebellum, anterior limb of the internal capsule, and, less commonly, the deep cerebral white matter. Lacunar infarcts are associated with poorly controlled hypertension or diabetes and have been found in several clinical syndromes, including contralateral pure motor or pure sensory deficit, ipsilateral ataxia with crural paresis, and dysarthria with clumsiness of the hand. The neurologic deficit may progress over 24–36 hours before stabilizing.

Lacunar infarcts are sometimes visible on CT scans as small, punched-out, hypodense areas, but in other patients no abnormality is seen. In some instances, patients with a clinical syndrome suggestive of lacunar infarction are found on CT scanning to have a severe hemispheric infarct.

The prognosis for recovery from the deficit produced by a lacunar infarct is usually good, with partial or complete resolution occurring over the following 4–6 weeks in many instances.

Norrving B: Long-term prognosis after lacunar infarction. Lancet Neurology 2003;2:238. [PMID: 12849212]

2. Cerebral Infarction

Thrombotic or embolic occlusion of a major vessel leads to cerebral infarction. Causes include the disorders predisposing to transient ischemic attacks (see above) and atherosclerosis of cerebral arteries. The resulting deficit depends on the particular vessel involved and the extent of any collateral circulation. Cerebral ischemia leads to release of excitatory and other neuropeptides that may augment calcium flux into neurons, thereby leading to cell death and increasing the neurologic deficit.

Clinical Findings

A. SYMPTOMS AND SIGNS

Onset is usually abrupt, and there may then be very little progression except that due to brain swelling. Clinical evaluation should always include examination of the heart and auscultation over the subclavian and carotid vessels to determine whether there are any bruits.

1. Obstruction of carotid circulation—Occlusion of the ophthalmic artery is probably symptomless in most cases because of the rich orbital collaterals, but its transient embolic obstruction can lead to amaurosis fugax—sudden and brief loss of vision in one eye.

Occlusion of the anterior cerebral artery distal to its junction with the **anterior communicating artery** causes weakness and cortical sensory loss in the contralateral leg and sometimes mild weakness of the arm, especially proximally. There may be a contralateral grasp reflex, paratonic rigidity, and abulia (lack of initiative) or frank confusion. Urinary incontinence is not uncommon, particularly if behavioral disturbances are conspicuous. Bilateral anterior cerebral infarction is especially likely to cause marked behavioral changes and memory disturbances. Unilateral anterior cerebral artery occlusion proximal to the junction with the anterior communicating artery is generally well tolerated because of the collateral supply from the other side.

Middle cerebral artery occlusion leads to contralateral hemiplegia, hemisensory loss, and homonymous hemianopia (ie, bilaterally symmetric loss of vision in half of the visual fields), with the eyes deviated to the side of the lesion. If the dominant hemisphere is involved, global aphasia is also present. It may be impossible to distinguish this clinically from occlusion of the internal carotid artery. With occlusion of either of these arteries, there may also be considerable swelling of the hemisphere, leading to drowsiness, stupor, and coma in extreme cases. Occlusions of different branches of the middle cerebral artery cause more limited findings. For example, involvement of the anterior main division leads to a predominantly expressive dysphasia and to contralateral paralysis and loss of sensations in the arm, the face, and, to a lesser extent, the leg. Posterior branch occlusion produces a receptive (Wernicke's) aphasia and a homonymous visual field defect. With involvement of the nondominant hemisphere, speech and comprehension are preserved, but there may be a confusional state, dressing apraxia, and constructional and spatial deficits.

2. Obstruction of vertebrobasilar circulation—Occlusion of the **posterior cerebral artery** may lead to a thalamic syndrome in which contralateral he-

Table 24–4. Features of the major stroke subtypes.

Stroke Type and Subtype	Clinical Features	Diagnosis	Treatment
Ischemic stroke			
Lacunar infarct	Small (< 5 mm) lesions in the basal ganglia, pons, cerebellum, or internal capsule; less often in deep cerebral white matter; prognosis generally good; clinical features depend on location, but may worsen over first 24–36 hours.	CT may reveal small hypodensity but is often normal.	Aspirin; long-term management is to control risk factors (hypertension and diabetes).
Carotid circulation obstruction	See text—signs vary depending on occluded vessel.	Noncontrast CT to exclude hemorrhage; CT may be normal during first 6–24 hours of an ischemic stroke, whereas diffusion-weighted MRI is more sensitive; electrocardiography, blood glucose, complete blood count, and tests for hypercoagulable states, hyperlipidemia are indicated; echocardiography or Holter monitoring in selected instances.	Select patients for intravenous thrombolytics (see text); aspirin (325 mg/d orally) is first-line therapy; if stroke occurs during aspirin therapy, clopidogrel may be substituted for aspirin; anticoagulation with heparin for cardioembolic strokes, and sometimes for evolving stroke when no contraindications exist.
Vertebrobasilar occlusion	See text—signs vary based on location of occluded vessel	As for carotid circulation obstruction	As for carotid circulation obstruction
Hemorrhagic stroke			
Spontaneous intracerebral hemorrhage	Commonly associated with hypertension; also with bleeding disorders, amyloid angiopathy. Location: basal ganglia more common than pons, thalamus, cerebellum, or cerebral white matter.	Noncontrast CT is superior to MRI for detecting bleeds of < 48 hours duration; laboratory tests to identify bleeding disorder; angiography may be indicated to exclude aneurysm or AVM. Do not perform lumbar puncture.	Most managed supportively, but cerebellar bleeds or hematomas with gross mass effect benefit from urgent surgical evacuation.
Subarachnoid hemorrhage	Present with sudden onset of worst headache of life, may lead rapidly to loss of consciousness; signs of meningeal irritation often present; etiology usually aneurysm or AVM, but 20% have no source identified.	CT to confirm diagnosis, but may be normal in rare instances; if CT negative and suspicion high, perform lumbar puncture to look for red blood cells or xanthochromia; angiography to determine source of bleed in candidates for treatment.	See sections on AVM and aneurysm.
Intracranial aneurysm	Most located in the anterior circle of Willis and are typically asymptomatic until subarachnoid bleed occurs; 20% rebleed in first 2 weeks.	CT indicates subarachnoid hemorrhage, and angiography then demonstrates aneurysms; angiography may not reveal aneurysm if vasospasm present.	Prevent further bleeding by clipping aneurysm or coil embolization; nimodipine helps prevent vasospasm; reverse vasospasm by intravenous fluids and induced hypertension after aneurysm has been obliterated, if no other aneurysms are present; angioplasty may also reverse symptomatic vasospasm.
AVMs	Focal deficit from hematoma or AVM itself.	CT reveals bleed, and may reveal the AVM; may be seen by MRI. Angiography demonstrates feeding vessels and vascular anatomy.	Surgery indicated if AVM has bled or to prevent further progression of neurologic deficit; other modalities to treat nonoperable AVMs are available at specialized centers.

AVMs = arteriovenous malformations.

misensory disturbance occurs, followed by the development of spontaneous pain and hyperpathia. There is often a macular-sparing homonymous hemianopia and sometimes a mild, usually temporary, hemiparesis. Depending on the site of the lesion and the collateral circulation, the severity of these deficits varies and other deficits may also occur, including involuntary movements and alexia. Occlusion of the main artery beyond the origin of its penetrating branches may lead solely to a macular-sparing hemianopia.

Vertebral artery occlusion distally, below the origin of the anterior spinal and posterior inferior cerebellar arteries, may be clinically silent because the circulation is maintained by the other vertebral artery. If the remaining vertebral artery is congenitally small or severely atherosclerotic, however, a deficit similar to that of basilar artery occlusion is seen unless there is good collateral circulation from the anterior circulation through the circle of Willis. When the small paramedian arteries arising from the vertebral artery are occluded, contralateral hemiplegia and sensory deficit occur in association with an ipsilateral cranial nerve palsy at the level of the lesion. An obstruction of the **posterior inferior cerebellar artery** or an obstruction of the vertebral artery just before it branches to this vessel leads ipsilaterally to spinothalamic sensory loss involving the face, ninth and tenth cranial nerve lesions, limb ataxia and numbness, and Horner's syndrome, combined with contralateral spinothalamic sensory loss involving the limbs.

Occlusion of both **vertebral arteries** or the **basilar artery** leads to coma with pinpoint pupils, flaccid quadriplegia and sensory loss, and variable cranial nerve abnormalities. With partial basilar artery occlusion, there may be diplopia, visual loss, vertigo, dysarthria, ataxia, weakness or sensory disturbances in some or all of the limbs, and discrete cranial nerve palsies. In patients with hemiplegia of pontine origin, the eyes are often deviated to the paralyzed side, whereas in patients with a hemispheric lesion, the eyes commonly deviate from the hemiplegic side.

Occlusion of any of the major **cerebellar arteries** produces vertigo, nausea, vomiting, nystagmus, ipsilateral limb ataxia, and contralateral spinothalamic sensory loss in the limbs. If the superior cerebellar artery is involved, the contralateral spinothalamic loss also involves the face; with occlusion of the anterior inferior cerebellar artery, there is ipsilateral spinothalamic sensory loss involving the face, usually in conjunction with ipsilateral facial weakness and deafness. Massive cerebellar infarction may lead to coma, tonsillar herniation, and death.

3. Coma—Infarction in either the carotid or vertebrobasilar territory may lead to loss of consciousness. For example, an infarct involving one cerebral hemisphere may lead to such swelling that the function of the other hemisphere or the rostral brainstem is disturbed and coma results. Similarly, coma occurs with bilateral brainstem infarction when this involves the reticular formation, and it occurs with brainstem compression after cerebellar infarction.

B. IMAGING

Radiography of the chest may reveal cardiomegaly or valvular calcification; the presence of a neoplasm would suggest that the neurologic deficit is due to metastasis rather than stroke, or rarely to nonbacterial thrombotic endocarditis. A CT scan of the head (without contrast) is important in excluding cerebral hemorrhage, but it may not permit distinction between a cerebral infarct and tumor. CT scanning is preferable to MRI in the acute stage because it is quicker and because intracranial hemorrhage is not easily detected by MRI within the first 48 hours after a bleeding episode. In selected patients, carotid duplex studies, MRI and MR angiography, and conventional angiography may also be necessary. Diffusion-weighted MRI is more sensitive than standard MRI in detecting cerebral ischemia.

C. LABORATORY AND OTHER STUDIES

Investigations should include a complete blood count, sedimentation rate, blood glucose determination, and serologic tests for syphilis. Antiphospholipid antibodies (lupus anticoagulants and anticardiolipin antibodies) promote thrombosis and are associated with an increased incidence of stroke. Similarly, elevated serum cholesterol and lipids and serum homocysteine may indicate an increased risk of thrombotic stroke. Electrocardiography will help exclude a cardiac arrhythmia or recent myocardial infarction that might be serving as a source of embolization. Blood cultures should be performed if endocarditis is suspected, echocardiography if heart disease is suspected, and Holter monitoring if paroxysmal cardiac arrhythmia requires exclusion. Examination of the cerebrospinal fluid is not always necessary but may be helpful if there is diagnostic uncertainty; it should be delayed until after CT scanning.

Treatment

If the neurologic deficit progresses over the following minutes or hours, administering heparin may limit or arrest further deterioration. Since the signs of progressing stroke may be simulated by an intracerebral hematoma, the latter must be excluded by immediate CT scanning or angiography before the patient is heparinized.

Intravenous thrombolytic therapy with recombinant tissue plasminogen activator (0.9 mg/kg to a maximum of 90 mg, with 10% given as a bolus over 1 minute and the remainder over 1 hour) is effective in reducing the neurologic deficit in selected patients without CT evidence of intracranial hemorrhage when administered within 3 hours after onset of ischemic stroke, but later administration has not been proved effective or safe. Recent hemorrhage, increased risk of hemorrhage (eg, treatment with anticoagulants), arterial puncture at a noncompressible site, and systolic pressure above 185 mm Hg or diastolic pressure above 110 mm Hg are among the contraindications to this treatment. Early management of a completed stroke otherwise consists of attention to general supportive measures. During the acute stage, there may be marked brain swelling and edema, with symptoms and signs of increasing intracranial pressure, an increasing neurologic deficit, or herniation syndrome. Prednisone (up to 100 mg/d) or dexamethasone (16 mg/d) has been used in an attempt to reduce vasogenic cerebral edema, but the evidence that corticosteroids are of any benefit is conflicting. Dehydrating hyperosmolar agents have also been prescribed in efforts to reduce brain swelling, but there is little evidence of any lasting benefit. Likewise, clinical benefit from treatment with vasodilators such as papaverine is minimal. Neither hypercapnia nor hypocapnia has been shown to have any benefit. Barbiturates are known to decrease neuronal metabolism and energy requirements and have been reported to improve functional recovery in experimental stroke models; their use in humans, however, is experimental. Attempts to lower the blood pressure of hypertensive patients during the acute phase (ie, within 2 weeks) of a stroke should generally be avoided, as there is loss of cerebral autoregulation and lowering the blood pressure may further compromise ischemic areas. However, if the systolic pressure exceeds 200 mm Hg, it can be lowered with continuous monitoring to 170–200 mm Hg and then, after 2 weeks, it can be reduced further to less than 140/90 mm Hg.

Anticoagulant drugs should be started when there is a cardiac source of embolization. Treatment is with intravenous heparin while warfarin is introduced. The target is an INR of 2.0–3.0 for the prothrombin time. If the CT scan shows no evidence of hemorrhage and the cerebrospinal fluid is clear, anticoagulant treatment may be started without delay. Some physicians prefer to wait for 2 or 3 days before initiating anticoagulant treatment; the CT scan is then repeated and anticoagulant therapy is initiated if it again shows no evidence of hemorrhagic transformation.

Physical therapy has an important role in the management of patients with impaired motor function. Passive movements at an early stage will help prevent contractures. As cooperation increases and some recovery begins, active movements will improve strength and coordination. In all cases, early mobilization and active rehabilitation are important. Occupational therapy may improve morale and motor skills, while speech therapy may be beneficial in patients with expressive dysphasia or dysarthria. When there is a severe and persisting motor deficit, a device such as a leg brace, toe spring, frame, or cane may help the patient move about, and the provision of other aids to daily living may improve the quality of life.

Prognosis

The prognosis for survival after cerebral infarction is better than after cerebral or subarachnoid hemorrhage. The only proved effective therapy for acute stroke re-

quires initiation within 3 hours after stroke onset, and the prognosis therefore depends on the time that elapses before arrival at the hospital. Patients receiving such treatment with tissue plasminogen activator are at least 30% more likely to have minimal or no disability at 3 months than those not treated by this means. Loss of consciousness after a cerebral infarct implies a poorer prognosis than otherwise. The extent of the infarct governs the potential for rehabilitation. Patients who have had a cerebral infarct are at risk for additional strokes and for myocardial infarcts. Statin therapy to lower serum lipid levels may reduce this risk. Antiplatelet therapy reduces the recurrence rate by 30% among patients without a cardiac cause for the stroke who are not candidates for carotid endarterectomy. Nevertheless, the cumulative risk of recurrence of noncardioembolic stroke is still 3–7% annually. A 2-year comparison did not show benefit of warfarin (INR 1.4–2.8) over aspirin (325 mg daily), and higher doses of warfarin should be avoided as they lead to an increased incidence of major bleeding. Patients with massive strokes from which meaningful recovery is unlikely should receive palliative care (see Chapter 5).

Anticoagulants and antiplatelet agents in acute ischemic stroke: report of the Joint Stroke Guideline Development Committee of the American Academy of Neurology and the American Stroke Association (a division of the American Heart Association). Stroke 2002;33:1934. [PMID: 12105379]

Bath P: Anticoagulants and antiplatelet agents in acute ischaemic stroke. Lancet Neurol 2002;1:405. [PMID: 12849358]

Caplan LR: Treatment of patients with stroke. Arch Neurol 2002; 59:703. [PMID: 12020249]

Hart RG et al: Lessons from the Stroke Prevention in Atrial Fibrillation trials. Ann Intern Med 2003;138:831. [PMID: 12755555]

Straus SE et al: New evidence for stroke prevention: scientific review. JAMA 2002;288:1388. [PMID: 12234233]

Subramaniam S et al: Massive cerebral infarction. Neurologist 2005;11:150. [PMID: 15860137]

3. Intracerebral Hemorrhage

Spontaneous intracerebral hemorrhage in patients with no angiographic evidence of an associated vascular anomaly (eg, aneurysm or angioma) is usually due to hypertension. The pathologic basis for hemorrhage is probably the presence of microaneurysms that develop on perforating vessels of 100–300 mcm in diameter in hypertensive patients. Hypertensive intracerebral hemorrhage occurs most frequently in the basal ganglia and less commonly in the pons, thalamus, cerebellum, and cerebral white matter. Hemorrhage may extend into the ventricular system or subarachnoid space, and signs of meningeal irritation are then found. Hemorrhages usually occur suddenly and without warning, often during activity.

In addition to its association with hypertension, nontraumatic intracerebral hemorrhage may occur with hematologic and bleeding disorders (eg, leukemia, thrombocytopenia, hemophilia, or disseminated intravascular coagulation), anticoagulant therapy, liver disease, cerebral amyloid angiopathy, high alcohol intake, and primary or secondary brain tumors. There is also an association with advancing age and male sex. Bleeding is primarily into the subarachnoid space when it occurs from an intracranial aneurysm or arteriovenous malformation (see below), but it may be partly intraparenchymal as well. In some cases, no specific cause for cerebral hemorrhage can be identified.

Clinical Findings

A. SYMPTOMS AND SIGNS

With hemorrhage into the cerebral hemisphere, consciousness is initially lost or impaired in about one-half of patients. Vomiting occurs very frequently at the onset of bleeding, and headache is sometimes present. Focal symptoms and signs then develop, depending on the site of the hemorrhage. With hypertensive hemorrhage, there is generally a rapidly evolving neurologic deficit with hemiplegia or hemiparesis. A hemisensory disturbance is also present with more deeply placed lesions. With lesions of the putamen, loss of conjugate lateral gaze may be conspicuous. With thalamic hemorrhage, there may be a loss of upward gaze, downward or skew deviation of the eyes, lateral gaze palsies, and pupillary inequalities.

Cerebellar hemorrhage may present with sudden onset of nausea and vomiting, disequilibrium, headache, and loss of consciousness that may terminate fatally within 48 hours. Less commonly, the onset is gradual and the course episodic or slowly progressive—clinical features suggesting an expanding cerebellar lesion. In yet other cases, however, the onset and course are intermediate, and examination shows lateral conjugate gaze palsies to the side of the lesion; small reactive pupils; contralateral hemiplegia; peripheral facial weakness; ataxia of gait, limbs, or trunk; periodic respiration; or some combination of these findings.

B. IMAGING

CT scanning (without contrast) is important not only in confirming that hemorrhage has occurred but also in determining the size and site of the hematoma. It is superior to MRI for detecting intracranial hemorrhage of less than 48 hours duration. If the patient's condition permits further intervention, cerebral angiography may be undertaken thereafter to determine whether an aneurysm or arteriovenous malformation is present (see below).

C. LABORATORY AND OTHER STUDIES

A complete blood count, platelet count, bleeding time, prothrombin and partial thromboplastin times, and liver and renal function tests may reveal a predisposing cause for the hemorrhage. Lumbar puncture is contraindicated because it may precipitate a herniation syndrome in patients with a large hematoma, and CT scanning is superior in detecting intracerebral hemorrhage.

Treatment

Neurologic management is generally conservative and supportive, regardless of whether the patient has a profound deficit with associated brainstem compression, in which case the prognosis is grim, or a more localized deficit not causing increased intracranial pressure or brainstem involvement. Such therapy may include ventilatory support, blood pressure regulation, seizure prophylaxis, control of fever, osmotherapy, and nutritional supplementation. Intracranial pressure may require monitoring. Ventricular drainage may be required in patients with intraventricular hemorrhage and acute hydrocephalus. Decompression may be helpful when a superficial hematoma in cerebral white matter is exerting a mass effect and causing incipient herniation. In patients with cerebellar hemorrhage, prompt surgical evacuation of the hematoma is appropriate, because spontaneous unpredictable deterioration may otherwise lead to a fatal outcome and because operative treatment may lead to complete resolution of the clinical deficit. The treatment of underlying structural lesions or bleeding disorders depends on their nature. Randomized trials of recombinant activated factor VII given within a few hours of onset are in progress, and preliminary reports are encouraging.

Mayer SA et al: Treatment of intracerebral haemorrhage. Lancet Neurol 2005;4:662. [PMID: 16168935]

4. Subarachnoid Hemorrhage

 ESSENTIALS OF DIAGNOSIS

- Sudden severe headache.
- Signs of meningeal irritation usually present.
- Obtundation is common.
- Focal deficits frequently absent.

General Considerations

Between 5% and 10% of strokes are due to subarachnoid hemorrhage. Although hemorrhage is usually from rupture of an aneurysm or arteriovenous malformation, no specific cause can be found in 20% of cases.

Clinical Findings

A. SYMPTOMS AND SIGNS

Subarachnoid hemorrhage has a characteristic clinical picture. Its onset is with sudden headache of a severity never experienced previously by the patient. This may be followed by nausea and vomiting and by a loss or impairment of consciousness that can either be transient or progress inexorably to deepening coma and death. If consciousness is regained, the patient is often confused and irritable and may show other symptoms of an altered mental status. Neurologic examination generally reveals nuchal rigidity and other signs of meningeal irritation, except in deeply comatose patients. A focal neurologic deficit is occasionally present and may suggest the site of the underlying lesion.

B. Imaging

A CT scan should be performed immediately to confirm that hemorrhage has occurred and to search for clues regarding its source. It is preferable to MRI because it is faster and more sensitive in detecting hemorrhage in the first 24 hours. CT findings sometimes are normal in patients with suspected hemorrhage, and the cerebrospinal fluid must then be examined for the presence of blood or xanthochromia before the possibility of subarachnoid hemorrhage is discounted.

Cerebral arteriography may be undertaken to determine the source of bleeding; it is not performed unless or until the patient's condition has stabilized and is good enough so that operative treatment is feasible. In general, bilateral carotid and vertebral arteriography are necessary because aneurysms are often multiple, while arteriovenous malformations may be supplied from several sources. MR angiography may also permit these vascular anomalies to be visualized but is less sensitive than conventional arteriography.

Treatment

The measures outlined below in the section on stupor and coma are applied to comatose patients. Conscious patients are confined to bed, advised against any exertion or straining, treated symptomatically for headache and anxiety, and given laxatives or stool softeners. If there is severe hypertension, the blood pressure can be lowered gradually, but not below a diastolic level of 100 mm Hg. Phenytoin is generally prescribed routinely to prevent seizures. Further comment concerning the specific operative management of arteriovenous malformations and aneurysms follows.

5. Intracranial Aneurysm

ESSENTIALS OF DIAGNOSIS

- Subarachnoid hemorrhage or focal deficit.
- Abnormal imaging studies.

General Considerations

Saccular aneurysms ("berry" aneurysms) tend to occur at arterial bifurcations, are frequently multiple (20% of cases), and are usually asymptomatic. They may be associated with polycystic kidney disease and coarctation of the aorta. Risk factors for aneurysm formation include smoking, hypertension, and hypercholesterolemia. Most aneurysms are located on the anterior part of the circle of Willis—particularly on the anterior or posterior communicating arteries, at the bifurcation of the middle cerebral artery, and at the bifurcation of the internal carotid artery.

Clinical Findings

A. Symptoms and Signs

Aneurysms may cause a focal neurologic deficit by compressing adjacent structures. However, most are asymptomatic or produce only nonspecific symptoms until they rupture, at which time subarachnoid hemorrhage results. There is often a paucity of focal neurologic signs in patients with subarachnoid hemorrhage, but when present, such signs may relate either to a focal hematoma or to ischemia in the territory of the vessel with the ruptured aneurysm. Hemiplegia or other focal deficit sometimes occurs after a delay of 4–14 days and is due to focal arterial spasm in the vicinity of the ruptured aneurysm. This spasm is of uncertain, probably multifactorial, cause, but it sometimes leads to significant cerebral ischemia or infarction, and it may further aggravate any existing increase in intracranial pressure. Subacute hydrocephalus due to interference with the flow of cerebrospinal fluid may occur after 2 or more weeks, and this leads to a delayed clinical deterioration that is relieved by shunting.

In some patients, "warning leaks" of a small amount of blood from the aneurysm precede the major hemorrhage by a few hours or days. They lead to headaches, sometimes accompanied by nausea and neck stiffness, but the true cause of these symptoms is often not appreciated until massive hemorrhage occurs.

B. Imaging

The CT scan generally confirms that subarachnoid hemorrhage has occurred, but occasionally it is normal. Angiography (bilateral carotid and vertebral studies) generally indicates the size and site of the lesion, sometimes reveals multiple aneurysms, and may show arterial spasm. If subarachnoid hemorrhage is confirmed by lumbar puncture or CT scanning but arteriograms show no abnormality, the examination should be repeated after 2 weeks, because vasospasm may have prevented detection of an aneurysm during the initial study.

C. Laboratory and Other Studies

The cerebrospinal fluid is bloodstained. The electroencephalogram sometimes indicates the side or site of hemorrhage but frequently shows only a diffuse abnormality. Electrocardiographic evidence of arrhythmias or myocardial ischemia has been well described and probably relates to excessive sympathetic activity. Peripheral leukocytosis and transient glycosuria are also common findings.

Treatment

The major aim of treatment is to prevent further hemorrhages. Definitive treatment requires surgical clipping of the aneurysm base or endovascular treatment (coil embolization) by interventional radiologists; the latter is sometimes feasible even for inoperable aneurysms. Otherwise, medical management as outlined above for subarachnoid hemorrhage is continued for about 6 weeks and is followed by gradual mobilization.

The risk of further hemorrhage is greatest within a few days of the first hemorrhage; approximately 20% of patients will have further bleeding within 2 weeks and 40% within 6 months. Attempts have been made to reduce this risk pharmacologically. Treatment with an antifibrinolytic agent such as aminocaproic acid during the first 14 days reduces the risk of recurrent hemorrhage but is associated with such an increase in cerebral ischemic complications that the mortality rate and the degree of disability among survivors are unchanged. Thus, early operation (ie, within about 2 days of hemorrhage) is preferred for good operative candidates.

Calcium channel-blocking agents have helped reduce or reverse experimental vasospasm, and nimodipine has been shown to reduce, in neurologically normal patients, the incidence of ischemic deficits from arterial spasm without producing any side effects. The dose of nimodipine is 60 mg every 4 hours orally for 21 days. After surgical obliteration of any aneurysms, symptomatic vasospasm may also be treated by intravascular volume expansion, induced hypertension, or transluminal balloon angioplasty of involved intracranial vessels.

With regard to unruptured aneurysms, those that are symptomatic merit prompt treatment, either surgically or by endovascular coil embolization, whereas small asymptomatic ones discovered incidentally are often monitored arteriographically and corrected surgically only if they increase in size to over 10 mm.

Doerfler A et al: Endovascular treatment of cerebrovascular disease. Curr Opin Neurol 2004;17:481. [PMID: 15247546]

Molyneux AJ et al: International Subarachnoid Aneurysm Trial (ISAT) of neurosurgical clipping versus endovascular coiling in 2143 patients with ruptured intracranial aneurysms: a randomised comparison of effects on survival, dependency, seizures, rebleeding, subgroups, and aneurysm occlusion. Lancet 2005;366:809. [PMID: 16139655]

Roos Y et al: Antifibrinolytic therapy for aneurysmal subarachnoid hemorrhage: a major update of a Cochrane review. Stroke 2003;34:2308. [PMID: 12933970]

Wiebers DO et al: Unruptured intracranial aneurysms: natural history, clinical outcome, and risks of surgical and endovascular treatment. Lancet 2003;362:103. [PMID: 12867109]

6. Arteriovenous Malformations

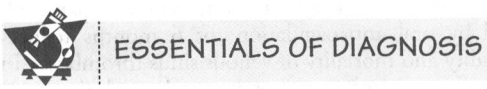

ESSENTIALS OF DIAGNOSIS

- Sudden onset of subarachnoid and intracerebral hemorrhage.

- Distinctive neurologic signs reflect the region of the brain involved.
- Signs of meningeal irritation in patients presenting with subarachnoid hemorrhage.
- Seizures or focal deficits may occur.

General Considerations

Arteriovenous malformations are congenital vascular malformations that result from a localized maldevelopment of part of the primitive vascular plexus and consist of abnormal arteriovenous communications without intervening capillaries. They vary in size, ranging from massive lesions that are fed by multiple vessels and involve a large part of the brain to lesions so small that they are hard to identify at arteriography, surgery, or autopsy. In approximately 10% of cases, there is an associated arterial aneurysm, while 1–2% of patients presenting with aneurysms have associated arteriovenous malformations. Clinical presentation may relate to hemorrhage from the malformation or an associated aneurysm or may relate to cerebral ischemia due to diversion of blood by the anomalous arteriovenous shunt or due to venous stagnation. Regional maldevelopment of the brain, compression or distortion of adjacent cerebral tissue by enlarged anomalous vessels, and progressive gliosis due to mechanical and ischemic factors may also be contributory. In addition, communicating or obstructive hydrocephalus may occur and lead to symptoms.

Clinical Findings

A. Symptoms and Signs

1. Supratentorial lesions—Most cerebral arteriovenous malformations are supratentorial, usually lying in the territory of the middle cerebral artery. Initial symptoms consist of hemorrhage in 30–60% of cases, recurrent seizures in 20–40%, headache in 5–25%, and miscellaneous complaints (including focal deficits) in 10–15%. Up to 70% of arteriovenous malformations bleed at some point in their natural history, most commonly before the patient reaches the age of 40 years. This tendency to bleed is unrelated to the lesion site or to the patient's sex, but small arteriovenous malformations are more likely to bleed than large ones. Arteriovenous malformations that have bled once are more likely to bleed again. Hemorrhage is commonly intracerebral as well as into the subarachnoid space, and it has a fatal outcome in about 10% of cases. Focal or generalized seizures may accompany or follow hemorrhage, or they may be the initial presentation, especially with frontal or parietal arteriovenous malformations. Headaches are especially likely when the external carotid arteries are involved in the malformation. These sometimes simulate migraine but more commonly are nonspecific in character, with nothing about them to suggest an underlying structural lesion.

In patients presenting with subarachnoid hemorrhage, examination may reveal an abnormal mental status and signs of meningeal irritation. Additional findings may help localize the lesion and sometimes indicate that intracranial pressure is increased. A cranial bruit always suggests the possibility of a cerebral arteriovenous malformation, but bruits may also be found with aneurysms, meningiomas, acquired arteriovenous fistulas, and arteriovenous malformations involving the scalp, calvarium, or orbit. Bruits are best heard over the ipsilateral eye or mastoid region and are of some help in lateralization but of no help in localization. Absence of a bruit in no way excludes the possibility of arteriovenous malformation.

2. Infratentorial lesions—Brainstem arteriovenous malformations are often clinically silent, but they may hemorrhage, cause obstructive hydrocephalus, or lead to progressive or relapsing brainstem deficits. Cerebellar arteriovenous malformations may also be clinically inconspicuous but sometimes lead to cerebellar hemorrhage.

B. IMAGING

In patients presenting with suspected hemorrhage, CT scanning indicates whether subarachnoid or intracerebral bleeding has recently occurred, helps localize its source, and may reveal the arteriovenous malformation. If the CT scan shows no evidence of bleeding but subarachnoid hemorrhage is diagnosed clinically, the cerebrospinal fluid should be examined.

When intracranial hemorrhage is confirmed but the source of hemorrhage is not evident on the CT scan, arteriography is necessary to exclude aneurysm or arteriovenous malformation. MR angiography is not sensitive enough for this purpose. Even if the findings on CT scan suggest arteriovenous malformation, arteriography is required to establish the nature of the lesion with certainty and to determine its anatomic features so that treatment can be planned. The examination must generally include bilateral opacification of the internal and external carotid arteries and the vertebral arteries. Arteriovenous malformations typically appear as a tangled vascular mass with distended tortuous afferent and efferent vessels, a rapid circulation time, and arteriovenous shunting. Findings on plain radiographs of the skull are often normal unless an intracerebral hematoma is present, in which case there may be changes suggestive of raised intracranial pressure and displacement of a calcified pineal gland.

In patients presenting without hemorrhage, CT scan or MRI usually reveals the underlying abnormality, and MRI frequently also shows evidence of old or recent hemorrhage that may have been asymptomatic. The nature and detailed anatomy of any focal lesion identified by these means are delineated by angiography, especially if operative treatment is under consideration.

C. LABORATORY AND OTHER STUDIES

Electroencephalography is usually indicated in patients presenting with seizures and may show consistently focal or lateralized abnormalities resulting from the underlying cerebral arteriovenous malformation. This should be followed by CT scanning.

Treatment

Surgical treatment to prevent further hemorrhage is justified in patients with arteriovenous malformations that have bled, provided that the lesion is accessible and the patient has a reasonable life expectancy. Surgical treatment is also appropriate if intracranial pressure is increased and to prevent further progression of a focal neurologic deficit. In patients presenting solely with seizures, anticonvulsant drug treatment is usually sufficient, and operative treatment is unnecessary unless there are further developments.

Definitive operative treatment consists of excision of the arteriovenous malformation if it is surgically accessible. Arteriovenous malformations that are inoperable because of their location are sometimes treated solely by embolization; although the risk of hemorrhage is not reduced, neurologic deficits may be stabilized or even reversed by this procedure. Two other techniques for the treatment of intracerebral arteriovenous malformations are injection of a vascular occlusive polymer through a flow-guided microcatheter and permanent occlusion of feeding vessels by positioning detachable balloon catheters in the desired sites and then inflating them with quickly solidifying contrast material. Stereotactic radiosurgery with the gamma knife is also useful in the management of inoperable cerebral arteriovenous malformations.

Choi JH et al: Brain arteriovenous malformations in adults. Lancet Neurol 2005;4:299. [PMID: 15847843]

Fleetwood IG et al: Arteriovenous malformations. Lancet 2002; 359:863. [PMID: 11897302]

7. Intracranial Venous Thrombosis

Intracranial venous thrombosis may occur in association with intracranial or maxillofacial infections, hypercoagulable states, polycythemia, sickle cell disease, and cyanotic congenital heart disease and in pregnancy or during the puerperium. It is characterized by headache, focal or generalized convulsions, drowsiness, confusion, increased intracranial pressure, and focal neurologic deficits—and sometimes by evidence of meningeal irritation. The diagnosis is confirmed by CT scanning, MRI, MR venography, or angiography.

Treatment includes anticonvulsant drugs if seizures have occurred and antiedema agents (eg, dexamethasone, 4 mg four times daily and continued as necessary) or other measures to reduce intracranial pressure. Anticoagulation with dose-adjusted intravenous heparin followed by oral anticoagulation for 6 months reduces morbidity and mortality of venous sinus thrombosis. In cases refractory to heparin, endovascular techniques including catheter-directed thrombolytic therapy (urokinase) and thrombectomy, are sometimes helpful.

Biousse V et al: Cerebral venous thrombosis. Curr Treat Options Neurol 2003;5:409. [PMID: 12895403]

Cakmak S et al: Cerebral venous thrombosis: clinical outcome and systematic screening of prothrombotic factors. Neurology 2003;60:1175. [PMID: 12682328]

8. Spinal Cord Vascular Diseases

ESSENTIALS OF DIAGNOSIS

- *Sudden onset of back or limb pain and neurologic deficit in limbs.*
- *Motor, sensory, or reflex changes in limbs depending on level of lesion.*
- *Imaging studies distinguish between infarct and hematoma.*

Infarction of the Spinal Cord

Infarction of the spinal cord is rare. It occurs only in the territory of the anterior spinal artery because this vessel, which supplies the anterior two-thirds of the cord, is itself supplied by only a limited number of feeders. Infarction usually results from interrupted flow in one or more of these feeders, eg, with aortic dissection, aortography, polyarteritis, or severe hypotension, or after surgical resection of the thoracic aorta. The paired posterior spinal arteries, by contrast, are supplied by numerous arteries at different levels of the cord.

Since the anterior spinal artery receives numerous feeders in the cervical region, infarcts almost always occur caudally. Clinical presentation is characterized by acute onset of flaccid, areflexive paraplegia that evolves after a few days or weeks into a spastic paraplegia with extensor plantar responses. There is an accompanying dissociated sensory loss, with impairment of appreciation of pain and temperature but preservation of sensations of vibration and position. Treatment is symptomatic.

Goodin DS: Neurological complications of aortic disease and surgery. In: *Neurology and General Medicine,* 3rd ed. Aminoff MJ (editor). Churchill Livingstone, 2001.

Epidural or Subdural Hemorrhage

Epidural or subdural hemorrhage may lead to sudden severe back pain followed by an acute compressive myelopathy necessitating urgent spinal MRI or myelography and surgical evacuation. It may occur in patients with bleeding disorders or those who are taking anticoagulant drugs, sometimes following trauma or lumbar puncture. Epidural hemorrhage may also be related to a vascular malformation or tumor deposit.

Arteriovenous Malformation of the Spinal Cord

Arteriovenous malformations of the cord are congenital lesions that present with spinal subarachnoid hemorrhage or myeloradiculopathy. Since most of these malformations are located in the thoracolumbar region, they lead to motor and sensory disturbances in the legs and to sphincter disorders. Pain in the legs or back is often severe. Examination reveals an upper, lower, or mixed motor deficit in the legs; sensory deficits are also present and are usually extensive, although occasionally they are confined to radicular distribution. Cervical arteriovenous malformations lead also to symptoms and signs in the arms. Spinal MRI may not detect the arteriovenous malformation, and negative findings do not exclude the diagnosis. In general, the diagnosis is suggested at myelography (performed with the patient prone and supine) when serpiginous filling defects due to enlarged vessels are found. Selective spinal arteriography confirms the diagnosis. Most lesions are extramedullary, are posterior to the cord (lying either intra- or extradurally), and can easily be treated by ligation of feeding vessels and excision of the fistulous anomaly or by embolization procedures. Delay in treatment may lead to increased and irreversible disability or to death from recurrent subarachnoid hemorrhage.

INTRACRANIAL & SPINAL SPACE-OCCUPYING LESIONS

1. Primary Intracranial Tumors

ESSENTIALS OF DIAGNOSIS

- *Generalized or focal disturbance of cerebral function, or both.*
- *Increased intracranial pressure in some patients.*
- *Neuroradiologic evidence of space-occupying lesion.*

General Considerations

Half of all primary intracranial neoplasms (Table 24–5) are gliomas and the remainder meningiomas, pituitary adenomas, neurofibromas, and other tumors. Certain tumors, especially neurofibromas, hemangioblastomas, and retinoblastomas, may have a familial basis, and congenital factors bear on the development of craniopharyngiomas. Tumors may occur at any age, but certain gliomas show particular age predilections (Table 24–5).

Clinical Findings

A. SYMPTOMS AND SIGNS

Intracranial tumors may lead to a generalized disturbance of cerebral function and to symptoms and signs of increased intracranial pressure. In consequence, there may be personality changes, intellectual decline, emotional lability, seizures, headaches, nausea, and malaise.

Table 24–5. Primary intracranial tumors.

Tumor	Clinical Features	Treatment and Prognosis
Glioblastoma multiforme	Presents commonly with nonspecific complaints and increased intracranial pressure. As it grows, focal deficits develop.	Course is rapidly progressive, with poor prognosis. Total surgical removal is usually not possible. Radiation therapy and chemotherapy may prolong survival.
Astrocytoma	Presentation similar to glioblastoma multiforme but course more protracted, often over several years. Cerebellar astrocytoma may have a more benign course.	Prognosis is variable. By the time of diagnosis, total excision is usually impossible; tumor often is not radiosensitive. In cerebellar astrocytoma, total surgical removal is often possible.
Medulloblastoma	Seen most frequently in children. Generally arises from roof of fourth ventricle and leads to increased intracranial pressure accompanied by brainstem and cerebellar signs. May seed subarachnoid space.	Treatment consists of surgery combined with radiation therapy and chemotherapy.
Ependymoma	Glioma arising from the ependyma of a ventricle, especially the fourth ventricle; leads to early signs of increased intracranial pressure. Arises also from central canal of cord.	Tumor is not radiosensitive and is best treated surgically if possible.
Oligodendroglioma	Slow-growing. Usually arises in cerebral hemisphere in adults. Calcification may be visible on skull x-ray.	Treatment is surgical and usually successful.
Brainstem glioma	Presents during childhood with cranial nerve palsies and then with long tract signs in the limbs. Signs of increased intracranial pressure occur late.	Tumor is inoperable; treatment is by irradiation and shunt for increased intracranial pressure.
Cerebellar hemangioblastoma	Presents with disequilibrium, ataxia of trunk or limbs, and signs of increased intracranial pressure. Sometimes familial. May be associated with retinal and spinal vascular lesions, polycythemia, and renal cell carcinoma.	Treatment is surgical.
Pineal tumor	Presents with increased intracranial pressure, sometimes associated with impaired upward gaze (Parinaud's syndrome) and other deficits indicative of midbrain lesion.	Ventricular decompression by shunting is followed by surgical approach to tumor; irradiation is indicated if tumor is malignant. Prognosis depends on histopathologic findings and extent of tumor.
Craniopharyngioma	Originates from remnants of Rathke's pouch above the sella, depressing the optic chiasm. May present at any age but usually in childhood, with endocrine dysfunction and bitemporal field defects.	Treatment is surgical, but total removal may not be possible.
Acoustic neurinoma	Ipsilateral hearing loss is most common initial symptom. Subsequent symptoms may include tinnitus, headache, vertigo, facial weakness or numbness, and long tract signs. (May be familial and bilateral when related to neurofibromatosis.) Most sensitive screening tests are MRI and brainstem auditory evoked potential.	Treatment is excision by translabyrinthine surgery, craniectomy, or a combined approach. Outcome is usually good.
Meningioma	Originates from the dura mater or arachnoid; compresses rather than invades adjacent neural structures. Increasingly common with advancing age. Tumor size varies greatly. Symptoms vary with tumor site—eg, unilateral proptosis (sphenoidal ridge); anosmia and optic nerve compression (olfactory groove). Tumor is usually benign and readily detected by CT scanning; may lead to calcification and bone erosion visible on plain x-rays of skull.	Treatment is surgical. Tumor may recur if removal is incomplete.
Primary cerebral lymphoma	Associated with AIDS and other immunodeficient states. Presentation may be with focal deficits or with disturbances of cognition and consciousness. May be indistinguishable from cerebral toxoplasmosis.	Treatment is high-dose methotrexate followed by radiation therapy. Prognosis depends on CD4 count at diagnosis.

If the pressure is increased in a particular cranial compartment, brain tissue may herniate into a compartment with lower pressure. The most familiar syndrome is herniation of the temporal lobe uncus through the tentorial hiatus, which causes compression of the third cranial nerve, midbrain, and posterior cerebral artery. The earliest sign of this is ipsilateral pupillary dilation, followed by stupor, coma, decerebrate posturing, and respiratory arrest. Another important herniation syndrome consists of displacement of the cerebellar tonsils through the foramen magnum, which causes medullary compression leading to apnea, circulatory collapse, and death. Other herniation syndromes are less common and of less clear clinical importance.

Intracranial tumors also lead to focal deficits depending on their location.

1. Frontal lobe lesions—Tumors of the frontal lobe often lead to progressive intellectual decline, slowing of mental activity, personality changes, and contralateral grasp reflexes. They may lead to expressive aphasia if the posterior part of the left inferior frontal gyrus is involved. Anosmia may also occur as a consequence of pressure on the olfactory nerve. Precentral lesions may cause focal motor seizures or contralateral pyramidal deficits.

2. Temporal lobe lesions—Tumors of the uncinate region may be manifested by seizures with olfactory or gustatory hallucinations, motor phenomena such as licking or smacking of the lips, and some impairment of external awareness without actual loss of consciousness. Temporal lobe lesions also lead to depersonalization, emotional changes, behavioral disturbances, sensations of déjà vu or jamais vu, micropsia or macropsia (objects appear smaller or larger than they are), visual field defects (crossed upper quadrantanopia), and auditory illusions or hallucinations. Left-sided lesions may lead to dysnomia and receptive aphasia, while right-sided involvement sometimes disturbs the perception of musical notes and melodies.

3. Parietal lobe lesions—Tumors in this location characteristically cause contralateral disturbances of sensation and may cause sensory seizures, sensory loss or inattention, or some combination of these symptoms. The sensory loss is cortical in type and involves postural sensibility and tactile discrimination, so that the appreciation of shape, size, weight, and texture is impaired. Objects placed in the hand may not be recognized (astereognosis). Extensive parietal lobe lesions may produce contralateral hyperpathia and spontaneous pain (thalamic syndrome). Involvement of the optic radiation leads to a contralateral homonymous field defect that sometimes consists solely of lower quadrantanopia. Lesions of the left angular gyrus cause Gerstmann's syndrome (a combination of alexia, agraphia, acalculia, right-left confusion, and finger agnosia), whereas involvement of the left submarginal gyrus causes ideational apraxia. Anosognosia (the denial, neglect, or rejection of a paralyzed limb) is seen in patients with lesions of the nondominant (right)

hemisphere. Constructional apraxia and dressing apraxia may also occur with right-sided lesions.

4. Occipital lobe lesions—Tumors of the occipital lobe characteristically produce crossed homonymous hemianopia or a partial field defect. With left-sided or bilateral lesions, there may be visual agnosia both for objects and for colors, while irritative lesions on either side can cause unformed visual hallucinations. Bilateral occipital lobe involvement causes cortical blindness in which there is preservation of pupillary responses to light and lack of awareness of the defect by the patient. There may also be loss of color perception, prosopagnosia (inability to identify a familiar face), simultagnosia (inability to integrate and interpret a composite scene as opposed to its individual elements), and Balint's syndrome (failure to turn the eyes to a particular point in space, despite preservation of spontaneous and reflex eye movements). The denial of blindness or a field defect constitutes Anton's syndrome.

5. Brainstem and cerebellar lesions—Brainstem lesions lead to cranial nerve palsies, ataxia, incoordination, nystagmus, and pyramidal and sensory deficits in the limbs on one or both sides. Intrinsic brainstem tumors, such as gliomas, tend to produce an increase in intracranial pressure only late in their course. Cerebellar tumors produce marked ataxia of the trunk if the vermis cerebelli is involved and ipsilateral appendicular deficits (ataxia, incoordination and hypotonia of the limbs) if the cerebellar hemispheres are affected.

6. False localizing signs—Tumors may lead to neurologic signs other than by direct compression or infiltration, thereby leading to errors of clinical localization. These false localizing signs include third or sixth nerve palsy and bilateral extensor plantar responses produced by herniation syndromes, and an extensor plantar response occurring ipsilateral to a hemispheric tumor as a result of compression of the opposite cerebral peduncle against the tentorium.

B. IMAGING

CT scanning or MRI with gadolinium enhancement may detect the lesion and may also define its location, shape, and size; the extent to which normal anatomy is distorted; and the degree of any associated cerebral edema or mass effect. CT scanning is less helpful with tumors in the posterior fossa, but MRI is of particular value there. The characteristic appearance of meningiomas on CT scanning is virtually diagnostic, ie, a lesion in a typical site (parasagittal and sylvian regions, olfactory groove, sphenoidal ridge, tuberculum sellae) that appears as a homogeneous area of increased density in noncontrast CT scans and enhances uniformly with contrast.

Arteriography may show stretching or displacement of normal cerebral vessels by the tumor and the presence of tumor vascularity. The presence of an avascular mass is a nonspecific finding that could be due to tumor, hematoma, abscess, or any space-occupying lesion. In patients with normal hormone levels and an intrasellar mass, angiography is necessary to distinguish with confidence between a pituitary adenoma and an arterial aneurysm.

C. LABORATORY AND OTHER STUDIES

The electroencephalogram provides supporting information concerning cerebral function and may show either a focal disturbance due to the neoplasm or a more diffuse change reflecting altered mental status. Lumbar puncture is rarely necessary; the findings are seldom diagnostic, and the procedure carries the risk of causing a herniation syndrome.

Treatment

Treatment depends on the type and site of the tumor (Table 24–5) and the condition of the patient. Complete surgical removal may be possible if the tumor is extra-axial (eg, meningioma, acoustic neuroma) or is not in a critical or inaccessible region of the brain (eg, cerebellar hemangioblastoma). Surgery also permits the diagnosis to be verified and may be beneficial in reducing intracranial pressure and relieving symptoms even if the neoplasm cannot be completely removed. Clinical deficits are sometimes due in part to obstructive hydrocephalus, in which case simple surgical shunting procedures often produce dramatic benefit. In patients with malignant gliomas, radiation therapy increases median survival rates regardless of any preceding surgery, and its combination with chemotherapy provides additional benefit. Indications for irradiation in the treatment of patients with other primary intracranial neoplasms depend on tumor type and accessibility and the feasibility of complete surgical removal. Corticosteroids help reduce cerebral edema and are usually started before surgery. Herniation is treated with intravenous dexamethasone (10–20 mg as a bolus, followed by 4 mg every 6 hours) and intravenous mannitol (20% solution given in a dose of 1.5 g/kg over about 30 minutes). Anticonvulsants are also commonly administered in standard doses (see Table 24–3) but are not indicated for prophylaxis in patients who have no history of seizures. For those patients whose disease deteriorates despite treatment, palliative care is important (see Chapter 5).

Behin A et al: Primary brain tumours in adults. Lancet 2003; 361:323. [PMID: 12559880]

Sarin R et al: Medical decompressive therapy for primary and metastatic intracranial tumours. Lancet Neurol 2003;2: 357. [PMID: 12849152]

Sirven JI et al: Seizure prophylaxis in patients with brain tumors: a meta-analysis. Mayo Clin Proc 2004;79:1489. [PMID: 15595331]

Taillibert S et al: Palliative care in patients with primary brain tumors. Curr Opin Oncol 2004;16:587. [PMID: 15627022]

Wen PY et al: Malignant gliomas. Curr Neurol Neurosci Rep 2004;4:218. [PMID: 15102348]

Whittle IR: Surgery for gliomas. Curr Opin Neurol 2002;15:663. [PMID: 12447103]

Wrensch M et al: Epidemiology of primary brain tumors: current concepts and review of the literature. Neuro-oncol 2002;4:278. [PMID: 12356358]

2. Metastatic Intracranial Tumors

Cerebral Metastases

Metastatic brain tumors present in the same way as other cerebral neoplasms, ie, with increased intracranial pressure, with focal or diffuse disturbance of cerebral function, or with both of these manifestations. Indeed, in patients with a single cerebral lesion, the metastatic nature of the lesion may only become evident on histopathologic examination. In other patients, there is evidence of widespread metastatic disease, or an isolated cerebral metastasis develops during treatment of the primary neoplasm.

The most common source of intracranial metastasis is carcinoma of the lung; other primary sites are the breast, kidney, and gastrointestinal tract. Most cerebral metastases are located supratentorially. Laboratory and radiologic studies used to evaluate patients with metastases are those described for primary neoplasms. They include MRI and CT scanning performed both with and without contrast material. Lumbar puncture is necessary only in patients with suspected carcinomatous meningitis (see below). In patients with verified cerebral metastasis from an unknown primary, investigation is guided by symptoms and signs. In women, mammography is indicated; in men under 50, germ cell origin is sought since both have therapeutic implications.

In patients with only a single cerebral metastasis who are otherwise well, it may be possible to remove the lesion and then treat with irradiation; the latter may also be selected as the sole treatment. In patients with multiple metastases or widespread systemic disease, the prognosis is poor; stereotactic radiotherapy may help in some instances, but in others treatment is palliative only.

Kaal EC et al: Therapeutic management of brain metastases. Lancet Neurol 2005;4:289. [PMID: 15847842]

Leptomeningeal Metastases (Carcinomatous Meningitis)

The neoplasms metastasizing most commonly to the leptomeninges are carcinoma of the breast, lymphomas, and leukemia. Leptomeningeal metastases lead to multifocal neurologic deficits, which may be associated with infiltration of cranial and spinal nerve roots, direct invasion of the brain or spinal cord, obstructive hydrocephalus, or some combination of these factors.

The diagnosis is confirmed by examination of the cerebrospinal fluid. Findings may include elevated cerebrospinal fluid pressure, pleocytosis, increased protein concentration, and decreased glucose concentration. Cytologic studies may indicate that malignant cells are present; if not, spinal tap should be repeated at least twice to obtain further samples for analysis.

CT scans showing contrast enhancement in the basal cisterns or showing hydrocephalus without any evidence of a mass lesion support the diagnosis. Gadolinium-enhanced MRI frequently shows enhancing foci in the leptomeninges. Myelography may show deposits on multiple nerve roots.

Treatment is by irradiation to symptomatic areas, combined with intrathecal methotrexate. The long-term prognosis is poor—only about 10% of patients survive for 1 year—and palliative care is therefore important (see Chapter 5).

3. Intracranial Mass Lesions in AIDS Patients

Primary cerebral lymphoma is a common complication in patients with AIDS. This leads to disturbances in cognition or consciousness, focal motor or sensory deficits, aphasia, seizures, and cranial neuropathies. Similar clinical disturbances may result from **cerebral toxoplasmosis**, which is also a common complication in patients with AIDS (see Chapters 31 and 35). Neither CT nor MRI findings distinguish these two disorders, and serologic tests for toxoplasmosis are unreliable in AIDS patients. Accordingly, for neurologically stable patients, a trial of treatment for toxoplasmosis with sulfadiazine (100 mg/kg/d up to 8 g/d in four divided doses) and pyrimethamine (75 mg/d for 3 days, then 25 mg/d) is recommended for 3 weeks; the imaging studies are then repeated, and if any lesion has improved, the regimen is continued indefinitely. If any lesion does not improve, cerebral biopsy is necessary. Primary cerebral lymphoma is treated with whole-brain irradiation.

Cryptococcal meningitis is a common opportunistic infection in AIDS patients. Clinically, it may resemble cerebral toxoplasmosis or lymphoma, but cranial CT scans are usually normal. The diagnosis is made on the basis of cerebrospinal fluid studies, with positive India ink staining in 75–80% and cryptococcal antigen tests in 95% of cases. Treatment is with amphotericin B plus flucytosine, as set forth in Table 36–1, followed by fluconazole.

Bicanic T et al: Cryptococcal meningitis. Br Med Bull 2005; 72:99. [PMID: 15838017]

4. Primary & Metastatic Spinal Tumors

Approximately 10% of spinal tumors are intramedullary. Ependymoma is the most common type of intramedullary tumor; the remainder are other types of glioma. Extramedullary tumors may be extradural or intradural in location. Among the primary extramedullary tumors, neurofibromas and meningiomas are relatively common, are benign, and may be intradural or extradural. Carcinomatous metastases, lymphomatous or leukemic deposits, and myeloma are usually extradural; in the case of metastases, the prostate, breast, lung, and kidney are common primary sites.

Tumors may lead to spinal cord dysfunction by direct compression, by ischemia secondary to arterial or venous obstruction, and, in the case of intramedullary lesions, by invasive infiltration.

Clinical Findings

A. SYMPTOMS AND SIGNS

Symptoms usually develop insidiously. Pain is often conspicuous with extradural lesions; is characteristically aggravated by coughing or straining; may be radicular, localized to the back, or felt diffusely in an extremity; and may be accompanied by motor deficits, paresthesias, or numbness, especially in the legs. When sphincter disturbances occur, they are usually particularly disabling. Pain, however, often precedes specific neurologic symptoms from epidural metastases.

Examination may reveal localized spinal tenderness. A segmental lower motor neuron deficit or dermatomal sensory changes (or both) are sometimes found at the level of the lesion, while an upper motor neuron deficit and sensory disturbance are found below it.

B. IMAGING

Findings on plain radiography of the spine may be normal but are commonly abnormal when there are metastatic deposits. CT myelography or MRI may be necessary to identify and localize the site of cord compression. The combination of known tumor elsewhere in the body, back pain, and either abnormal plain films of the spine or neurologic signs of cord compression is an indication to perform these studies on an urgent basis. Some clinicians proceed to myelography based solely on new back pain in a cancer patient. If a complete block is present at lumbar myelography, a cisternal myelogram is performed to determine the upper level of the block and to investigate the possibility of block higher in the cord.

C. LABORATORY FINDINGS

The cerebrospinal fluid removed at myelography is often xanthochromic and contains a greatly increased protein concentration with normal cell content and glucose concentration.

Treatment

Intramedullary tumors are treated by decompression and surgical excision (when feasible) and by irradiation. The prognosis depends on the cause and severity of cord compression before it is relieved.

Treatment of epidural spinal metastases consists of irradiation, irrespective of cell type. Dexamethasone is also given in a high dosage (eg, 25 mg four times daily for 3 days, followed by rapid tapering of the dosage, depending on response) to reduce cord swelling and relieve pain. Surgical decompression is reserved for patients with tumors that are unresponsive to irradiation or have previously been irradiated and for cases in which there is some uncertainty about the diagnosis. The long-term outlook is poor, but radiation treatment may at least delay the onset of major disability.

5. Brain Abscess

ESSENTIALS OF DIAGNOSIS

- Symptoms and signs of expanding intracranial mass.
- May be signs of primary infection or congenital heart disease.
- Fever may be absent.

General Considerations

Brain abscess presents as an intracranial space-occupying lesion and arises as a sequela of disease of the ear or nose, may be a complication of infection elsewhere in the body, or may result from infection introduced intracranially by trauma or surgical procedures. The most common infective organisms are streptococci, staphylococci, and anaerobes; mixed infections are not uncommon.

Clinical Findings

A. SYMPTOMS AND SIGNS

Headache, drowsiness, inattention, confusion, and seizures are early symptoms, followed by signs of increasing intracranial pressure and then a focal neurologic deficit. There may be little or no systemic evidence of infection.

B. IMAGING

A CT scan of the head characteristically shows an area of contrast enhancement surrounding a low-density core. Similar abnormalities may be found in patients with metastatic neoplasms. MRI findings often permit earlier recognition of focal cerebritis or an abscess. Arteriography indicates the presence of a space-occupying lesion, which appears as an avascular mass with displacement of normal cerebral vessels, but this procedure provides no clue to the nature of the lesion. Examination of the cerebrospinal fluid does not help in diagnosis and may precipitate a herniation syndrome.

C. TREATMENT

Treatment consists of intravenous antibiotics, combined with surgical drainage (aspiration or excision) if necessary to reduce the mass effect, or sometimes to establish the diagnosis. Abscesses smaller than 2 cm can often be cured medically. Broad-spectrum antibiotics are used if the infecting organism is unknown. A common regimen is penicillin G (2 million units every 2 hours intravenously) plus either chloramphenicol (1–2 g intravenously every 6 hours), metronidazole (750 mg intravenously every 6 hours), or both. Nafcillin is added if *Staphylococcus aureus* infection is suspected. Antimicrobial treatment is usually continued parenterally for 6–8 weeks, followed by orally for a further 2–3 weeks. The patient should be monitored by serial CT scans or MRI every 2 weeks and at deterioration. Dexamethasone (4–25 mg four times daily, depending on severity, followed by tapering of dose, depending on response) may reduce any associated edema, but intravenous mannitol is sometimes required.

Kastrup O et al: Neuroimaging of infections. NeuroRx 2005;2: 324. [PMID: 15897953]

NONMETASTATIC NEUROLOGIC COMPLICATIONS OF MALIGNANT DISEASE

A variety of nonmetastatic neurologic complications of malignant disease (see Table 40–6) can be recognized. Metabolic encephalopathy due to electrolyte abnormalities, infections, drug overdose, or the failure of some vital organ may be reflected by drowsiness, lethargy, restlessness, insomnia, agitation, confusion, stupor, or coma. The mental changes are usually associated with tremor, asterixis, and multifocal myoclonus. The electroencephalogram is generally diffusely slowed. Laboratory studies are necessary to detect the cause of the encephalopathy, which must then be treated appropriately.

Immune suppression resulting from either the malignant disease or its treatment (eg, by chemotherapy) predisposes patients to brain abscess, progressive multifocal leukoencephalopathy, meningitis, herpes zoster infection, and other opportunistic infectious diseases. Moreover, an overt or occult cerebrospinal fluid fistula, as occurs with some tumors, may also increase the risk of infection. CT scanning aids in the early recognition of a brain abscess, but metastatic brain tumors may have a similar appearance. Examination of the cerebrospinal fluid is essential in the evaluation of patients with meningitis but is of no help in the diagnosis of brain abscess.

Table 24–6. Some anticholinergic antiparkinsonian drugs.

Drug	Usual Daily Dose
Benztropine mesylate (Cogentin)	1–6 mg
Biperiden (Akineton)	2–12 mg
Orphenadrine (Disipal, Norflex)	150–400 mg
Procyclidine (Kemadrin)	7.5–30 mg
Trihexyphenidyl (Artane)	6–20 mg

Modified, with permission, from Aminoff MJ: Pharmacologic management of parkinsonism and other movement disorders. In: *Basic & Clinical Pharmacology*, 8th ed. Katzung BG (editor). McGraw-Hill, 2001.

Cerebrovascular disorders that cause neurologic complications in patients with systemic cancer include nonbacterial thrombotic endocarditis and septic embolization. Cerebral, subarachnoid, or subdural hemorrhages may occur in patients with myelogenous leukemia and may be found in association with metastatic tumors, especially malignant melanoma. Spinal subdural hemorrhage sometimes occurs after lumbar puncture in patients with marked thrombocytopenia.

Disseminated intravascular coagulation occurs most commonly in patients with acute promyelocytic leukemia or with some adenocarcinomas and is characterized by a fluctuating encephalopathy, often with associated seizures, that frequently progresses to coma or death. There may be few accompanying neurologic signs. Venous sinus thrombosis, which usually presents with convulsions and headaches, may also occur in patients with leukemia or lymphoma. Examination commonly reveals papilledema and focal or diffuse neurologic signs. Anticonvulsants, anticoagulants, and drugs to lower the intracranial pressure may be of value.

Paraneoplastic cerebellar degeneration occurs most commonly in association with carcinoma of the lung. Symptoms may precede those due to the neoplasm itself, which may be undetected for several months or even longer. Typically, there is a pancerebellar syndrome causing dysarthria, nystagmus, and ataxia of the trunk and limbs. The disorder probably has an autoimmune basis. Treatment is of the underlying malignant disease.

Encephalopathy, characterized by impaired recent memory, disturbed affect, hallucinations, and seizures, occurs in some patients with carcinomas. The cerebrospinal fluid is often abnormal. EEGs may show diffuse slow-wave activity, especially over the temporal regions. Pathologic changes are most marked in the inferomedian portions of the temporal lobes. There is no specific treatment.

Malignant disease may be associated with sensorimotor polyneuropathy and less commonly with pure sensory neuropathy (ie, dorsal root ganglionitis) or autonomic neuropathy. A subacute motor neuronopathy may be associated with lymphomas.

Dermatomyositis or a myasthenic syndrome may be seen in patients with underlying carcinoma (see Chapter 20). The myasthenic syndrome may have an autoimmune basis and differs clinically from myasthenia gravis.

Bataller L et al: Paraneoplastic neurologic syndromes. Neurol Clin 2003;21:221. [PMID: 12690651]

PSEUDOTUMOR CEREBRI (Benign Intracranial Hypertension)

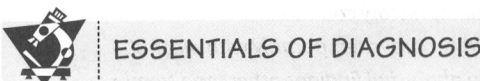

ESSENTIALS OF DIAGNOSIS

- *Headache, worse on straining.*
- *Visual obscurations or diplopia may occur.*
- *Level of consciousness may be impaired.*
- *Other deficits depend on cause of intracranial hypertension or on herniation syndrome.*
- *Examination reveals papilledema.*

General Considerations

There are many causes of pseudotumor cerebri. Thrombosis of the transverse venous sinus as a noninfectious complication of otitis media or chronic mastoiditis is one cause, and sagittal sinus thrombosis may lead to a clinically similar picture. Other causes include chronic pulmonary disease, endocrine disturbances such as hypoparathyroidism or Addison's disease, vitamin A toxicity, and the use of tetracycline or oral contraceptives. Cases have also followed withdrawal of corticosteroids after long-term use. In many instances, however, no specific cause can be found, and the disorder remits spontaneously after several months.

Clinical Findings

A. Symptoms and Signs

Symptoms of pseudotumor cerebri consist of headache, diplopia, and other visual disturbances due to papilledema and abducens nerve dysfunction. Examination reveals the papilledema and some enlargement of the blind spots, but patients otherwise look well.

B. Imaging

Investigations reveal no evidence of a space-occupying lesion, and the CT scan shows small or normal ventricles. MR venography is helpful in screening for thrombosis of the intracranial venous sinuses.

C. Laboratory Findings

Lumbar puncture confirms the presence of intracranial hypertension, but the cerebrospinal fluid is normal. Laboratory studies help exclude some of the other causes mentioned earlier.

Treatment

Untreated pseudotumor cerebri leads to secondary optic atrophy and permanent visual loss. Acetazolamide (250 mg orally three times daily) reduces formation of cerebrospinal fluid and can be used to start treatment. Oral corticosteroids (eg, prednisone, 60–80 mg daily) may also be necessary. Obese patients should be advised to lose weight. Repeated lumbar puncture to lower the intracranial pressure by removal of cerebrospinal fluid is effective, but pharmacologic approaches to treatment are now more satisfactory. Treatment is monitored by checking visual acuity and visual fields, funduscopic appearance, and pressure of the cerebrospinal fluid.

If medical treatment fails to control the intracranial pressure, surgical placement of a lumboperitoneal or other shunt—or subtemporal decompression or optic nerve sheath fenestration—should be undertaken to preserve vision.

In addition to the above measures, any specific cause of pseudotumor cerebri requires appropriate treatment. Thus, hormone therapy should be initiated if there is an underlying endocrine disturbance. Discontinuing the use of tetracycline, oral contraceptives, or vitamin A will allow for resolution of pseudotumor cerebri due to these agents. If corticosteroid withdrawal is responsible, the medication should be reintroduced and then tapered more gradually.

Friedman DI: Pseudotumor cerebri. Neurol Clin 2004;22:99. [PMID: 15062530]

SELECTED NEUROCUTANEOUS DISEASES

Tuberous Sclerosis

Tuberous sclerosis may occur sporadically or on a familial basis with autosomal dominant inheritance. The responsible gene is located on the long arm of chromosome 9 in at least some cases. Its pathogenesis is unknown. Neurologic presentation is with seizures and progressive psychomotor retardation beginning in early childhood. The cutaneous abnormality, adenoma sebaceum, becomes manifest usually between 5 and 10 years of age and typically consists of reddened nodules on the face (cheeks, nasolabial folds, sides of the nose, and chin) and sometimes on the forehead and neck. Other typical cutaneous lesions include subungual fibromas, shagreen patches (leathery plaques of subepidermal fibrosis, situated usually on the trunk), and leaf-shaped hypopigmented spots. Associated abnormalities include retinal lesions and tumors, benign rhabdomyomas of the heart, lung cysts, benign tumors in the viscera, and bone cysts.

The disease is slowly progressive and leads to increasing mental deterioration. There is no specific treatment, but anticonvulsant drugs may help in controlling seizures.

Neurofibromatosis

Neurofibromatosis may occur either sporadically or on a familial basis with autosomal dominant inheritance. Two distinct forms are recognized: Type 1 (**Recklinghausen's disease**) is characterized by multiple hyperpigmented macules and neurofibromas and type 2 by **eighth nerve tumors**, often accompanied by other intracranial or intraspinal tumors. Among familial cases, the gene for type 1 is located on chromosome 17 and that for type 2 on chromosome 22.

Neurologic presentation is usually with symptoms and signs of tumor. Multiple neurofibromas characteristically are present and may involve spinal or cranial nerves, especially the eighth nerve. Examination of the superficial cutaneous nerves usually reveals palpable mobile nodules. In some cases, there is an associated marked overgrowth of subcutaneous tissues (plexiform neuromas), sometimes with an underlying bony abnormality. Associated cutaneous lesions include axillary freckling and patches of cutaneous pigmentation (café au lait spots). Malignant degeneration of neurofibromas occasionally occurs and may lead to peripheral sarcomas. Meningiomas, gliomas (especially optic nerve gliomas), bone cysts, pheochromocytomas, scoliosis, and obstructive hydrocephalus may also occur.

It may be possible to correct disfigurement by plastic surgery. Intraspinal or intracranial tumors and tumors of peripheral nerves should be treated surgically if they are producing symptoms.

Neff BA et al: Current concepts in the evaluation and treatment of neurofibromatosis type ll. Otolaryngol Clin North Am 2005;38:671. [PMID: 16012314]

Reynolds RM et al: Von Recklinghausen's neurofibromatosis: neurofibromatosis type 1. Lancet 2003;361:1552. [PMID: 12737880]

Sturge-Weber Syndrome

Sturge-Weber syndrome consists of a congenital, usually unilateral, cutaneous capillary angioma involving the upper face, leptomeningeal angiomatosis, and, in many patients, choroidal angioma. It has no sex predilection and usually occurs sporadically. The cutaneous angioma sometimes has a more extensive distribution over the head and neck and is often quite disfiguring, especially if there is associated overgrowth of connective tissue. Focal or generalized seizures are the usual neurologic presentation and may commence at any age. There may be contralateral homonymous hemianopia, hemiparesis and hemisensory disturbance, ipsilateral glaucoma, and mental subnormality. Skull x-rays taken after the first 2 years of life usually reveal gyriform ("tramline") intracranial calcification, especially in the parieto-occipital region, due to mineral deposition in the cortex beneath the intracranial angioma.

Treatment is aimed at controlling seizures pharmacologically. Ophthalmologic advice should be sought concerning the management of choroidal angioma and of increased intraocular pressure.

MOVEMENT DISORDERS

1. Benign Essential (Familial) Tremor

 ESSENTIALS OF DIAGNOSIS

- Postural tremor of hands, head, or voice.
- Family history common.
- May improve temporarily with alcohol.
- No abnormal findings other than tremor.

General Considerations

The cause of benign essential tremor is uncertain, but it is sometimes inherited in an autosomal dominant manner. Responsible genes have been identified at 3q13 and 2p22-p25.

Clinical Findings

A. SYMPTOMS AND SIGNS

Tremor may begin at any age and is enhanced by emotional stress. The tremor usually involves one or both hands, the head, or the hands and head, while the legs tend to be spared. Examination reveals no other abnormalities. Ingestion of a small quantity of alcohol commonly provides remarkable but short-lived relief by an unknown mechanism.

Although the tremor may become more conspicuous with time, it generally leads to little disability. Occasionally, it interferes with manual skills and leads to impairment of handwriting. Speech may also be affected if the laryngeal muscles are involved.

B. TREATMENT

Treatment is often unnecessary. When it is required because of disability, propranolol may be helpful but will need to be continued indefinitely in daily doses of 60–240 mg. However, intermittent therapy is sometimes useful in patients whose tremor becomes exacerbated in specific predictable situations. Primidone may be helpful when propranolol is ineffective, but patients with essential tremor are often very sensitive to it. Therefore, the starting dose is 50 mg daily, and the daily dose is increased by 50 mg every 2 weeks depending on the patient's response; a maintenance dose of 125 mg three times daily is commonly effective. Occasional patients do not respond to these measures but are helped by alprazolam (up to 3 mg daily in divided doses), clozapine (30–50 mg twice daily), or mirtazapine (15 or 30 mg at night). Benefit has been reported with topiramate titrated up to a dose of 400 mg daily over about 8 weeks.

Disabling tremor unresponsive to medical treatment may be helped by contralateral thalamotomy. Unilateral high-frequency thalamic stimulation is an alternative approach that is equally effective, is associated with only mild and transient side effects, and is therefore preferred. Bilateral thalamotomy has significant morbidity, whereas the risks of bilateral stimulation are appreciably lower.

Louis ED: Essential tremor. Lancet Neurol 2005;4:100. [PMID: 15664542]

Pathwa R et al: Essential tremor: differential diagnosis and current therapy. Am J Med 2003;115:134. [PMID: 12893400]

Sydow O et al: Multicentre European study of thalamic stimulation in essential tremor: a six year follow up. J Neurol Neurosurg Psychiatry 2003;74:1387. [PMID: 14570831]

2. Parkinsonism

 ESSENTIALS OF DIAGNOSIS

- *Any combination of tremor, rigidity, bradykinesia, progressive postural instability.*
- *Seborrhea of skin quite common.*
- *Mild intellectual deterioration may occur.*

General Considerations

Parkinsonism is a relatively common disorder that occurs in all ethnic groups, with an approximately equal sex distribution. The most common variety, idiopathic Parkinson's disease (paralysis agitans), begins most often between 45 and 65 years of age.

Etiology

Parkinsonism may rarely occur on a familial basis, and the parkinsonian phenotype may result from mutations of several different genes. Postencephalitic parkinsonism is becoming increasingly rare. Exposure to certain toxins (eg, manganese dust, carbon disulfide) and severe carbon monoxide poisoning may lead to parkinsonism. Typical parkinsonism has occurred in individuals who have taken 1-methyl-4-phenyl-1,2,5,6-tetrahydropyridine (MPTP) for recreational purposes. This compound is converted in the body to a neurotoxin that selectively destroys dopaminergic neurons in the substantia nigra. Reversible parkinsonism may develop in patients receiving neuroleptic drugs (see Chapter 25), reserpine, or metoclopramide. Only rarely is hemiparkinsonism the presenting feature of a progressive space-occupying lesion.

In idiopathic parkinsonism, dopamine depletion due to degeneration of the dopaminergic nigrostriatal system leads to an imbalance of dopamine and acetylcholine, which are neurotransmitters normally present in the corpus striatum. Treatment is directed at redressing this imbalance by blocking the effect of acetylcholine with anticholinergic drugs or by the administration of levodopa, the precursor of dopamine.

Clinical Findings

Tremor, rigidity, bradykinesia, and postural instability are the cardinal features of parkinsonism and may be present in any combination. There may also be a mild decline in intellectual function. The tremor of about four to six cycles per second is most conspicuous at rest, is enhanced by emotional stress, and is often less severe during voluntary activity. Although it may ultimately be present in all limbs, the tremor is commonly confined to one limb or to the limbs on one side for months or years before it becomes more generalized. In some patients, tremor is absent.

Rigidity (an increase in resistance to passive movement) is responsible for the characteristically flexed posture seen in many patients, but the most disabling symptoms of parkinsonism are due to bradykinesia, manifested as a slowness of voluntary movement and a reduction in automatic movements such as swinging of the arms while walking. Curiously, however, effective voluntary activity may briefly be regained during an emergency (eg, the patient is able to leap aside to avoid an oncoming motor vehicle).

Clinical diagnosis of the well-developed syndrome is usually simple. The patient has a relatively immobile face with widened palpebral fissures, infrequent blinking, and a certain fixity of facial expression. Seborrhea of the scalp and face is common. There is often mild blepharoclonus, and a tremor may be present about the mouth and lips. Repetitive tapping (about twice per second) over the bridge of the nose produces a sustained blink response (Myerson's sign). Other findings may include saliva drooling from the mouth, perhaps due to impairment of swallowing; soft and poorly modulated voice; a variable rest tremor and rigidity in some or all of the limbs; slowness of voluntary movements; impairment of fine or rapidly alternating movements; and micrographia. There is typically no muscle weakness (provided that sufficient time is allowed for power to be developed) and no alteration in the tendon reflexes or plantar responses. It is difficult for the patient to arise from a sitting position and begin walking. The gait itself is characterized by small shuffling steps and a loss of the normal automatic arm swing; there may be unsteadiness on turning, difficulty in stopping, and a tendency to fall.

Differential Diagnosis

Diagnostic problems may occur in mild cases, especially if tremor is minimal or absent. For example, mild hypokinesia or slight tremor is commonly attributed to old age. Depression, with its associated expressionless face, poorly modulated voice, and reduction in voluntary activity, can be difficult to distinguish from mild parkinsonism, especially since the two disorders may coexist; in some cases, a trial of antidepressant drug therapy is necessary. The family history, the character of the tremor, and lack of other neurologic signs should distinguish essential tremor from parkinsonism. Wilson's disease can be distinguished by its early age at onset, the presence of other abnormal movements, Kayser-Fleischer rings, and chronic hepatitis, and by increased concentrations of copper in the tissues. Huntington's disease presenting with rigidity and bradykinesia may be mistaken for parkinsonism unless the family history and accompanying dementia are recognized. In Shy-Drager syndrome (also called multisystem atrophy), the clinical features of parkinsonism are accompanied by autonomic insufficiency (leading to postural hypotension, anhidrosis, disturbances of sphincter control, impotence, etc) and more widespread neurologic deficits (pyramidal, lower motor neuron, or cerebellar signs). In progressive supranuclear palsy, bradykinesia and rigidity are accompanied by a supranuclear disorder of eye movements, pseudobulbar palsy, and axial dystonia. Creutzfeldt-Jakob disease may be accompanied by features of parkinsonism, but dementia is usual, myoclonic jerking is common, ataxia and pyramidal signs may be conspicuous, and the electroencephalographic findings are usually characteristic. In cortical-basal ganglionic degeneration, parkinsonism is accompanied by conspicuous signs of cortical dysfunction (eg, apraxia, sensory inattention, dementia, aphasia).

Treatment

Treatment is symptomatic. No therapy has been shown to slow disease progression, but trials of several putative neuroprotective agents are in progress, as are various trials of gene therapy.

A. MEDICAL MEASURES

Drug treatment is not required early in the course of parkinsonism, but the nature of the disorder and the availability of medical treatment for use when necessary should be discussed with the patient.

1. Amantadine—Patients with mild symptoms but no disability may be helped by amantadine. This drug improves all of the clinical features of parkinsonism, but its mode of action is unclear. Side effects include restlessness, confusion, depression, skin rashes, edema, nausea, constipation, anorexia, postural hypotension, and disturbances of cardiac rhythm. However, these are relatively uncommon with the usual dose (100 mg twice daily).

2. Anticholinergic drugs—Anticholinergics are more helpful in alleviating tremor and rigidity than bradykinesia. Treatment is started with a small dose (Table 24–6) and gradually increased until benefit occurs or side effects limit further increments. If treatment is ineffective, the drug is gradually withdrawn and another preparation then tried.

Common side effects include dryness of the mouth, nausea, constipation, palpitations, cardiac arrhythmias, urinary retention, confusion, agitation, restlessness, drowsiness, mydriasis, increased intraocular pressure, and defective accommodation.

Anticholinergic drugs are contraindicated in patients with prostatic hyperplasia, narrow-angle glaucoma, or obstructive gastrointestinal disease and are often tolerated poorly by the elderly.

3. Levodopa—Levodopa, which is converted in the body to dopamine, improves all of the major features of parkinsonism, including bradykinesia, but does not stop progression of the disorder. The most common early side effects of levodopa are nausea, vomiting, and hypotension, but cardiac arrhythmias may also occur. Dyskinesias, restlessness, confusion, and other behavioral changes tend to occur somewhat later and become more common with time. Levodopa-induced dyskinesias may take any conceivable form, including chorea, athetosis, dystonia, tremor, tics, and myoclonus. An even later complication is the "on-off phenomenon," in which abrupt but transient fluctuations in the severity of parkinsonism occur unpredictably but frequently during the day. The "off" period of marked bradykinesia has been shown to relate in some instances to falling plasma levels of levodopa. During the "on" phase, dyskinesias are often conspicuous but mobility is increased.

Carbidopa, which inhibits the enzyme responsible for the breakdown of levodopa to dopamine, does not cross the blood-brain barrier. When levodopa is given in combination with carbidopa, the extracerebral breakdown of levodopa is diminished. This reduces the amount of levodopa required daily for beneficial effects, and it lowers the incidence of nausea, vomiting, hypotension, and cardiac irregularities. Such a combination does not prevent the development of the "on-off phenomenon," and the incidence of other side effects (dyskinesias or psychiatric complications) may actually be increased.

Sinemet, a commercially available preparation that contains carbidopa and levodopa in a fixed ratio (1:10 or 1:4), is generally used. Treatment is started with a small dose—eg, one tablet of Sinemet 25/100 (containing 25 mg of carbidopa and 100 mg of levodopa) three times daily—and gradually increased depending on the response. Sinemet CR is a controlled-release formulation (containing 25 or 50 mg of carbidopa and 100 or 200 mg of levodopa). It is sometimes helpful in reducing fluctuations in clinical response to treatment and in reducing the frequency with which medication must be taken. The commercially available combination of levodopa with both carbidopa and entacapone (Stalevo) may also be helpful in this context and is discussed in the following section on COMT inhibitors. Response fluctuations are also reduced by keeping the daily intake of protein at the recommended minimum and taking the main protein meal as the last meal of the day.

The dyskinesias and behavioral side effects of levodopa are dose-related, but reduction in dose may eliminate any therapeutic benefit.

Levodopa therapy is contraindicated in patients with psychotic illness or narrow-angle glaucoma. It should not be given to patients taking monoamine oxidase A inhibitors or within 2 weeks of their withdrawal, because hypertensive crises may result. Levodopa should be used with care in patients with suspected malignant melanomas or with active peptic ulcers because of concerns that it may exacerbate these disorders.

4. Dopamine agonists—Dopamine agonists act directly on dopamine receptors, and their use in parkinsonism is associated with a lower incidence of the response fluctuations and dyskinesias that occur with long-term levodopa therapy. They were previously reserved for patients who had either become refractory to levodopa or developed the "on-off phenomenon."

However, they are now best given either before the introduction of levodopa or with a low dose of Sinemet 25/100 (carbidopa 25 mg and levodopa 100 mg), one tablet three times daily when dopaminergic therapy is first introduced; the dose of Sinemet is kept constant, while the dose of the agonist is gradually increased. Two agonists, bromocriptine and pergolide, are ergot derivatives. The initial dosage of bromocriptine is 1.25 mg twice daily; this is increased by 2.5 mg at 2-week intervals until benefit occurs or side effects limit further increments. The usual daily maintenance dose in patients with parkinsonism is between 10 and 30 mg. Pergolide is similarly started in a low dose (eg, 0.05 mg daily) and built up gradually depending on the response and tolerance.

Side effects include anorexia, nausea, vomiting, constipation, postural hypotension, digital vasospasm, cardiac arrhythmias, various dyskinesias and mental disturbances, headache, nasal congestion, erythromelalgia, and pulmonary infiltrates. There are rare reports of pericardial, pleural, or pulmonary fibrosis; cardiac valvopathy has also been associated with pergolide therapy (in as many as 30% of patients). Bromocriptine and pergolide have largely been replaced with other agents because of these side effects.

Pramipexole and ropinirole are two newer dopamine agonists that are not ergot derivatives. They are effective in early Parkinson's disease as well as in advanced stages of the disease. In each case, the daily dose is built up gradually. Pramipexole is started at a dosage of 0.125 mg three times daily, and the dose is doubled after 1 week and again after another week; the daily dose is then increased by 0.75 mg at weekly intervals depending on response and tolerance. Most patients require between 0.5 and 1.5 mg three times daily. Ropinirole is begun in a dosage of 0.25 mg three times daily, and the total daily dose is increased at weekly intervals by 0.75 mg until the fourth week and by 1.5 mg thereafter. Most patients require between 2 and 8 mg three times daily for benefit. Adverse effects include fatigue, somnolence, nausea, peripheral edema, dyskinesias, confusion, and postural hypotension. Less commonly, an irresistible urge to sleep may occur, sometimes in inappropriate and hazardous circumstances.

5. Selegiline—Selegiline is a monoamine oxidase B inhibitor that is sometimes used as adjunctive treatment for parkinsonism in patients receiving levodopa. By inhibiting the metabolic breakdown of dopamine, selegiline has been used to improve fluctuations or declining response to levodopa. In general, however, the response to treatment with it has been disappointing. The drug is taken in a standard dose of 5 mg with breakfast and 5 mg with lunch. It may increase any adverse effects of levodopa.

There are reasons to believe that selegiline may arrest the progression of Parkinson's disease. Studies have failed to establish this conclusively, but this remains an important consideration for patients who are young or have mild disease.

6. COMT inhibitors—Catecholamine-*O*-methyltransferase inhibitors reduce the metabolism of levodopa to 3-*O*-methyldopa and thereby alter the plasma pharmacokinetics of levodopa, leading to more sustained plasma levels and more constant dopaminergic stimulation of the brain. Two such agents, tolcapone and entacapone, are currently available and may be used as an adjunct to levodopa-carbidopa in patients with response fluctuations or an otherwise inadequate response and who either have failed with other adjunctive therapies or are not candidates for such therapies. Treatment results in reduced response fluctuations, with a greater period of responsiveness to administered levodopa. Tolcapone is given in a dosage of 100 mg or 200 mg three times daily, and entacapone is given as 200 mg with each dose of Sinemet (levodopa-carbidopa). With either preparation, the dose of Sinemet taken concurrently may have to be reduced by up to one-third to avoid side effects such as dyskinesias, confusion, hypotension, and syncope. Diarrhea is sometimes troublesome. Because rare cases of fulminant hepatic failure have followed its use, tolcapone should be avoided in patients with preexisting liver disease. Serial liver function tests should be performed at 2-week intervals for the first year and at longer intervals thereafter in patients receiving the drug—as recommended by the manufacturer. Hepatotoxicity has not been reported with entacapone, which is therefore the preferred agent, and serial liver function tests are not required.

Stalevo is the commercial preparation of levodopa combined with both carbidopa and entacapone. It is best used in patients already stabilized on equivalent doses of carbidopa/levodopa and entacapone. It is priced at or below the price of the individual ingredients (ie, carbidopa/levodopa and entacapone) and has the added convenience of requiring fewer tablets to be taken daily. It is available in three strengths: Stalevo 50 (12.5 mg of carbidopa, 50 mg of levodopa, and 200 mg of entacapone), Stalevo 100 (25 mg of carbidopa, 100 mg of levodopa, and 200 mg of entacapone), and Stalevo 150 (37.5 mg of carbidopa, 150 mg of levodopa, and 200 mg of entacapone).

7. Atypical antipsychotics—Confusion and psychotic symptoms, which may be iatrogenic, often respond to atypical antipsychotic agents, which have few extrapyramidal side effects and do not block the effects of dopaminergic medication. Olanzapine, quetiapine, and risperidone may be tried, but the most effective of these agents is clozapine, a dibenzodiazepine derivative. Clozapine may rarely cause marrow suppression, and weekly blood counts are therefore necessary for patients taking it. The patient is started on 6.25 mg at bedtime and the dosage increased to 25–100 mg/d as needed. In low doses, it may also improve iatrogenic dyskinesias.

B. GENERAL MEASURES

Physical therapy or speech therapy helps many patients. The quality of life can often be improved by the provision of simple aids to daily living, eg, rails or banisters placed strategically about the home, special table

cutlery with large handles, nonslip rubber table mats, and devices to amplify the voice.

C. SURGICAL MEASURES

Thalamotomy or pallidotomy may be helpful for patients who become unresponsive to medical treatment or have intolerable side effects from antiparkinsonian agents, especially if they have no evidence of diffuse vascular disease or significant cognitive decline. Surgery should generally be confined to one side because the morbidity is considerably greater after bilateral procedures. Because of their morbidity, ablative procedures have generally been supplanted by deep brain stimulation, discussed in the following section. Surgical implantation of adrenal medullary or fetal substantia nigra tissue into the caudate nucleus has been reported to benefit some patients, but other investigators have failed to substantiate such claims or have found only modest benefits or major adverse effects. Such procedures are therefore best regarded as experimental, and further studies are required to define the role of cellular therapies.

D. BRAIN STIMULATION

High-frequency thalamic stimulation is effective in suppressing the rest tremor of Parkinson's disease, and chronic bilateral stimulation of the subthalamic nuclei or globus pallidus internus may benefit all the major features of the disease. Electrical stimulation of the brain has the advantage over ablative procedures of being reversible and of causing minimal or no damage to the brain, and is therefore the preferred surgical approach to treatment. There is no evidence that the natural history of Parkinson's disease is affected.

Bjorklund A et al: Neural transplantation for the treatment of Parkinson's disease. Lancet Neurology 2003;2:437. [PMID: 12849125]

Christine CW et al: Clinical differentiation of parkinsonian syndromes: prognostic and therapeutic relevance. Am J Med 2004;117:412. [PMID: 15380498]

Krack P et al: Five-year follow-up of bilateral stimulation of the subthalamic nucleus in advanced Parkinson's disease. N Engl J Med 2003;349:1925. [PMID: 14614167]

Samii A et al: Parkinson's disease. Lancet 2004;363:1783. [PMID: 15172778]

Wu SS et al: Treatment of Parkinson's disease: what's on the horizon? CNS Drugs 2005;19:723. [PMID: 16142989]

3. Huntington's Disease

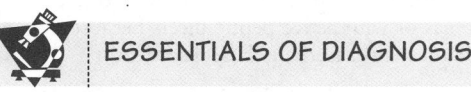

ESSENTIALS OF DIAGNOSIS

- *Gradual onset and progression of chorea and dementia or behavioral change.*
- *Family history of the disorder.*
- *Responsible gene identified on chromosome 4.*

General Considerations

Huntington's disease is characterized by chorea and dementia. It is inherited in an autosomal dominant manner and occurs throughout the world, in all ethnic groups, with a prevalence rate of about 5 per 100,000. The gene responsible for the disease is on the short arm of chromosome No. 4. At 4p16.3 there is an expanded and unstable CAG trinucleotide repeat.

Clinical Findings

A. SYMPTOMS AND SIGNS

Clinical onset is usually between 30 and 50 years of age. The disease is progressive and usually leads to a fatal outcome within 15–20 years. The initial symptoms may consist of either abnormal movements or intellectual changes, but ultimately both occur. The earliest mental changes are often behavioral, with irritability, moodiness, antisocial behavior, or a psychiatric disturbance, but a more obvious dementia subsequently develops. The dyskinesia may initially be no more than an apparent fidgetiness or restlessness, but eventually choreiform movements and some dystonic posturing occur. Progressive rigidity and akinesia (rather than chorea) sometimes occur in association with dementia, especially in cases with childhood onset.

B. IMAGING

CT scanning usually demonstrates cerebral atrophy and atrophy of the caudate nucleus in established cases. MRI and positron emission tomography (PET) have shown reduced glucose utilization in an anatomically normal caudate nucleus.

Differential Diagnosis

Chorea developing with no family history of choreoathetosis should not be attributed to Huntington's disease, at least not until other causes of chorea have been excluded clinically and by appropriate laboratory studies. Nongenetic causes of chorea include stroke, systemic lupus erythematosus and related disorders, paraneoplastic syndromes, infection with HIV, and various medications. In younger patients, self-limiting Sydenham's chorea develops after group A streptococcal infections on rare occasions. If a patient presents solely with progressive intellectual failure, it may not be possible to distinguish Huntington's disease from other causes of dementia unless there is a characteristic family history or a dyskinesia develops.

A clinically similar autosomal dominant disorder (**dentatorubral-pallidoluysian atrophy**), manifested by chorea, dementia, ataxia, and myoclonic epilepsy, is uncommon except in persons of Japanese ancestry. It is due to a mutant gene mapping to 12p13.31. Treatment is as for Huntington's disease.

Treatment

There is no cure for Huntington's disease; progression cannot be halted; and treatment is purely symptomatic. The reported biochemical changes suggest a relative underactivity of neurons containing gamma-aminobutyric acid (GABA) and acetylcholine or a relative overactivity of dopaminergic neurons. Treatment with drugs blocking dopamine receptors, such as phenothiazines or haloperidol, may control the dyskinesia and any behavioral disturbances. Haloperidol treatment is usually begun with a dose of 1 mg once or twice daily, which is then increased every 3 or 4 days depending on the response. Tetrabenazine, a drug that depletes central monoamines, is widely used in Europe to treat dyskinesia but is not available in the United States. Reserpine is similar in its actions to tetrabenazine and may be helpful; the daily dose is built up gradually to between 2 and 5 mg, depending on the response. Behavioral disturbances may respond to clozapine. Attempts to compensate for the relative GABA deficiency by enhancing central GABA activity or to compensate for the relative cholinergic underactivity by giving choline chloride have not been therapeutically helpful. High levels of somatostatin (a neuropeptide) have recently been reported in certain areas of the brain in patients with Huntington's disease, and the therapeutic response to cysteamine (a selective depleter of somatostatin in the brain) is currently under study. Neuroprotective strategies are also being explored.

Offspring should be offered genetic counseling. Genetic testing permits presymptomatic detection and definitive diagnosis of the disease.

Cardosi F: Chorea: non-genetic causes. Curr Opin Neurol 2004;17:433. [PMID: 15247538]

MacDonald ME et al: Huntington's disease. Neuromolecular Med 2003;4:7. [PMID: 14528049]

Rosenblatt A et al: Predictors of neuropathological severity in 100 patients with Huntington's disease. Ann Neurol 2003;54:488. [PMID: 14520661]

4. Idiopathic Torsion Dystonia

 ESSENTIALS OF DIAGNOSIS

- *Dystonic movements and postures.*
- *Normal birth and developmental history. No other neurologic signs.*
- *Investigations (including CT scan or MRI) reveal no cause of dystonia.*

General Considerations

Idiopathic torsion dystonia may occur sporadically or on a hereditary basis, with autosomal dominant, autosomal recessive, and X-linked recessive modes of transmission. One responsible gene is located at 9q34 (and has been named *DYT1*) and involves a unique mutation consisting of a GAG deletion in the dominantly inherited disorder, and maps to the long arm of the X chromosome in the X-linked recessive form; the responsible gene in the autosomal recessive disorder is unknown. Other autosomal dominant forms have also been recognized, with different or unidentified genetic loci. Symptoms may begin in childhood or later and persist throughout life.

Clinical Findings

The disorder is characterized by the onset of abnormal movements and postures in a patient with a normal birth and developmental history, no relevant past medical illness, and no other neurologic signs. Investigations (including CT scan) reveal no cause for the abnormal movements. Dystonic movements of the head and neck may take the form of torticollis, blepharospasm, facial grimacing, or forced opening or closing of the mouth. The limbs may also adopt abnormal but characteristic postures. The age at onset influences both the clinical findings and the prognosis. With onset in childhood, there is usually a family history of the disorder, symptoms commonly commence in the legs, and progression is likely until there is severe disability from generalized dystonia. In contrast, when onset is later, a positive family history is unlikely, initial symptoms are often in the arms or axial structures, and severe disability does not usually occur, although generalized dystonia may ultimately develop in some patients. If all cases are considered together, about one-third of patients eventually become so severely disabled that they are confined to chair or bed, while another one-third are affected only mildly.

Differential Diagnosis

Before a diagnosis of idiopathic torsion dystonia is made, it is imperative to exclude other causes of dystonia. Perinatal anoxia, birth trauma, and kernicterus are common causes of dystonia, but abnormal movements usually then develop before the age of 5, the early development of the patient is usually abnormal, and a history of seizures is not unusual. Moreover, examination may reveal signs of mental retardation or pyramidal deficit in addition to the movement disorder. Dystonic posturing may also occur in Wilson's disease, Huntington's disease, or parkinsonism; as a sequela of encephalitis lethargica or previous neuroleptic drug therapy; and in certain other disorders. In these cases, diagnosis is based on the history and accompanying clinical manifestations.

Treatment

Idiopathic torsion dystonia usually responds poorly to drugs. Levodopa, diazepam, baclofen, carbamazepine, amantadine, or anticholinergic medication (in high dosage) is occasionally helpful; if not, a trial of treatment with phenothiazines or haloperidol may be worthwhile.

In each case, the dose has to be individualized, depending on response and tolerance. However, the doses of these latter drugs that are required for benefit lead usually to mild parkinsonism. Stereotactic thalamotomy is sometimes helpful in patients with predominantly unilateral dystonia, especially when this involves the limbs. The usefulness of deep brain stimulation is under study.

A distinct variety of dominantly inherited dystonia, mapping to a genetic locus on chromosome 14q, is remarkably responsive to levodopa.

Bressman SB et al: Dystonia: phenotypes and genotypes. Rev Neurol (Paris) 2003;159:849. [PMID: 14628853]

Defazio G et al: Epidemiology of primary dystonia. Lancet Neurol 2004;3:673. [PMID: 15488460]

Kanovsky P: Dystonia: a disorder of motor programming or motor execution? Mov Disord 2002;17:1143. [PMID: 12465050]

Nemeth AH: The genetics of primary dystonias and related disorders. Brain 2002;125:695. [PMID: 11912106]

5. Focal Torsion Dystonia

A number of the dystonic manifestations that occur in idiopathic torsion dystonia may also occur as isolated phenomena. They are best regarded as focal dystonias that either occur as formes frustes of idiopathic torsion dystonia in patients with a positive family history or represent a focal manifestation of the adult-onset form of that disorder when there is no family history. Mapping of responsible genes to chromosome 8 *(DYT6)* and chromosome 18 *(DYT7)* has been reported in some instances of cervical or cranial dystonia. Medical treatment is generally unsatisfactory. A trial of the drugs used in idiopathic torsion dystonia is worthwhile, however, since a few patients do show some response. In addition, with restricted dystonias such as blepharospasm or torticollis, local injection of botulinum A toxin into the overactive muscles may produce worthwhile benefit for several weeks or months and can be repeated as needed.

Both blepharospasm and oromandibular dystonia may occur as an isolated focal dystonia. The former is characterized by spontaneous involuntary forced closure of the eyelids for a variable interval. Oromandibular dystonia is manifested by involuntary contraction of the muscles about the mouth causing, for example, involuntary opening or closing of the mouth, roving or protruding tongue movements, and retraction of the platysma.

Spasmodic torticollis, usually with onset between 25 and 50 years of age, is characterized by a tendency for the neck to twist to one side. This initially occurs episodically, but eventually the neck is held to the side. Spontaneous resolution may occur in the first year or so. The disorder is otherwise usually lifelong. Selective section of the spinal accessory nerve and the upper cervical nerve roots is sometimes helpful if medical treatment is unsuccessful. Local injection of botulinum A toxin provides benefit in most cases.

Writer's cramp is characterized by dystonic posturing of the hand and forearm when the hand is used for writing and sometimes when it is used for other tasks, eg, playing the piano or using a screwdriver or eating utensils. Drug treatment is usually unrewarding, and patients are often best advised to learn to use the other hand for activities requiring manual dexterity. Injections of botulinum A toxin are helpful in some instances.

6. Myoclonus

Occasional myoclonic jerks may occur in anyone, especially when drifting into sleep. General or multifocal myoclonus is common in patients with idiopathic epilepsy and is especially prominent in certain hereditary disorders characterized by seizures and progressive intellectual decline, such as the lipid storage diseases. It is also a feature of various rare degenerative disorders, notably Ramsay Hunt syndrome, and is common in subacute sclerosing panencephalitis and Creutzfeldt-Jakob disease. Generalized myoclonic jerking may accompany uremic and other metabolic encephalopathies, result from therapy with levodopa or cyclic antidepressants, occur in alcohol or drug withdrawal states, or follow anoxic brain damage. It also occurs on a hereditary or sporadic basis as an isolated phenomenon in otherwise healthy subjects.

Segmental myoclonus is a rare manifestation of a focal spinal cord lesion. It may also be the clinical expression of **epilepsia partialis continua**, a disorder in which a repetitive focal epileptic discharge arises in the contralateral sensorimotor cortex, sometimes from an underlying structural lesion. An electroencephalogram is often helpful in clarifying the epileptic nature of the disorder, and CT or MRI scan may reveal the causal lesion.

Myoclonus may respond to certain anticonvulsant drugs, especially valproic acid, or to one of the benzodiazepines, particularly clonazepam (see Table 24–3). It may also respond to piracetam (up to 16.8 g daily). Myoclonus following anoxic brain damage is often responsive to oxitriptan (5-hydroxytryptophan), an investigational agent that is the precursor of serotonin, and sometimes to clonazepam. Oxitriptan is given in gradually increasing doses up to 1–1.5 mg daily. In patients with segmental myoclonus, a localized lesion should be searched for and treated appropriately.

Caviness JN et al: Myoclonus: current concepts and recent advances. Lancet Neurol 2004;3:598. [PMID: 15380156]

Jimenez-Jimenez FJ et al: Drug-induced myoclonus: frequency, mechanisms and management. CNS Drugs 2004;18:93. [PMID: 14728056]

7. Wilson's Disease

In this metabolic disorder, abnormal movement and posture may occur with or without coexisting signs of liver involvement. It is discussed in Chapter 15.

8. Drug-Induced Abnormal Movements

Phenothiazines and butyrophenones may produce a wide variety of abnormal movements, including par-

kinsonism, akathisia (ie, motor restlessness), acute dystonia, chorea, and tardive dyskinesia. These complications are discussed in Chapter 25. Chorea may also develop in patients receiving levodopa, bromocriptine, anticholinergic drugs, phenytoin, carbamazepine, lithium, amphetamines, or oral contraceptives, and it resolves with withdrawal of the offending substance. Similarly, dystonia may be produced by levodopa, bromocriptine, lithium, metoclopramide, or carbamazepine; and parkinsonism by reserpine, tetrabenazine, and metoclopramide. Postural tremor may occur with a variety of drugs, including epinephrine, isoproterenol, theophylline, caffeine, lithium, thyroid hormone, tricyclic antidepressants, and valproic acid.

9. Restless Legs Syndrome

This disorder may occur as a primary (idiopathic) disorder or in relation to pregnancy, iron-deficiency anemia, peripheral neuropathy, or periodic leg movements of sleep. It may have a hereditary basis. Restlessness and curious sensory disturbances lead to an irresistible urge to move the limbs, especially during periods of relaxation. Disturbed nocturnal sleep and excessive daytime somnolences may result. Therapy is with long-acting dopamine agonists or with benzodiazepines such as clonazepam. Levodopa is also helpful but may lead to an augmentation of symptoms, so that its use is generally reserved for those who fail other measures. In some instances, opiates are required to control symptoms.

Schapira AH: Restless legs syndrome: an update on treatment options. Drugs 2004;64:149. [PMID: 14717617]

10. Gilles de la Tourette's Syndrome

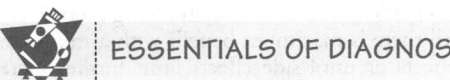

ESSENTIALS OF DIAGNOSIS

- *Multiple motor and phonic tics.*
- *Symptoms begin before age 21 years.*
- *Tics occur frequently for at least 1 year.*
- *Tics vary in number, frequency, and nature over time.*

Clinical Findings

Motor tics are the initial manifestation in 80% of cases and most commonly involve the face, whereas in the remaining 20%, the initial symptoms are phonic tics; ultimately a combination of different motor and phonic tics develop in all patients. These are noted first in childhood, generally between the ages of 2 and 15. Motor tics occur especially about the face, head, and shoulders (eg, sniffing, blinking, frowning, shoulder shrugging, head thrusting, etc). Phonic tics commonly consist of grunts, barks, hisses, throat-clearing, coughs, etc, but sometimes also of verbal utterances including coprolalia (obscene speech). There may also be echolalia (repetition of the speech of others), echopraxia (imitation of others' movements), and palilalia (repetition of words or phrases). Some tics may be self-mutilating in nature, such as nail-biting, hair-pulling, or biting of the lips or tongue. The disorder is chronic, but the course may be punctuated by relapses and remissions. Obsessive-compulsive behaviors are commonly associated and may be more disabling than the tics themselves. A family history is sometimes obtained and inheritance has been attributed to an autosomal dominant gene with variable penetrance; linkage to 18q22.1 has been noted in some instances.

Examination usually reveals no abnormalities other than the tics. In addition to obsessive-compulsive behavior disorders, psychiatric disturbances may occur because of the associated cosmetic and social embarrassment. Electroencephalography may show minor nonspecific abnormalities of no diagnostic relevance.

The diagnosis of the disorder is often delayed for years, the tics being interpreted as psychiatric illness or some other form of abnormal movement. Patients are thus often subjected to unnecessary treatment before the disorder is recognized. The tic-like character of the abnormal movements and the absence of other neurologic signs should differentiate this disorder from other movement disorders presenting in childhood. Wilson's disease, however, can simulate the condition and should be excluded.

Treatment

Treatment is symptomatic and may need to be continued indefinitely. Haloperidol is generally regarded as the drug of choice. It is started in a low daily dose (0.25 mg) that is gradually increased (by 0.25 mg every 4 or 5 days) until there is maximum benefit with a minimum of side effects or until side effects limit further increments. A total daily dose of between 2 and 8 mg is usually optimal, but higher doses are sometimes necessary. Treatment with clonazepam (in a dose that depends on response and tolerance) or clonidine (2–5 mcg/kg/d) may also be helpful, and it seems sensible to begin with one of these drugs in order to avoid some of the long-term extrapyramidal side effects of haloperidol. Phenothiazines, such as fluphenazine (2–15 mg daily), have been used, but patients unresponsive to haloperidol are usually unresponsive to these as well.

Pimozide, an oral dopamine-blocking drug related to haloperidol, may be helpful in patients who cannot tolerate or have not responded to haloperidol. Treatment is started with 1 mg daily and the daily dose increased by 1–2 mg every 10 days; the average dose is between 7 and 16 mg daily. Injection of botulinum toxin type A at the site of the most distressing tics is sometimes worthwhile.

Treatment with risperidone, calcium channel blockers, tetrabenazine, clomipramine, metoclopramide, or

pergolide has yielded mixed results or encouraging findings in preliminary studies that require confirmation. Bilateral high-frequency thalamic stimulation has been helpful in some, otherwise intractable, cases and is currently under study.

Singer HS: Tourette's syndrome: from behaviour to biology. Lancet Neurol 2005;4:149. [PMID: 15721825]

DEMENTIA

Dementia, the symptom complex of progressive global impairment of intellectual function, is a major medical, social, and economic problem that is worsening as the number of elderly people in the general population increases. It is discussed in Chapter 4, and the only point to be reiterated here is the importance of recognizing early any treatable or reversible causes of dementia, such as normal-pressure hydrocephalus, intracranial mass lesions, vascular disease, hypothyroidism, thiamine or vitamin B_{12} deficiency, Wilson's disease, hepatic or renal failure, neurosyphilis, and the chronic meningitides.

MULTIPLE SCLEROSIS

ESSENTIALS OF DIAGNOSIS

- *Episodic neurologic symptoms.*
- *Patient usually under 55 years of age at onset.*
- *Single pathologic lesion cannot explain clinical findings.*
- *Multiple foci best visualized by MRI.*

General Considerations

This common neurologic disorder, which probably has an autoimmune basis, has its greatest incidence in young adults. Epidemiologic studies indicate that multiple sclerosis is much more common in persons of western European lineage who live in temperate zones. No population with a high risk for multiple sclerosis exists between latitudes 40° N and 40° S. Genetic, dietary, and climatic factors cannot account for these differences. Nevertheless, a genetic susceptibility to the disease is likely, based on twin studies, familial cases, and an association with specific HLA antigens (HLA-DR2). Pathologically, focal—often perivenular—areas of demyelination with reactive gliosis are found scattered in the white matter of brain and spinal cord and in the optic nerves.

Clinical Findings

A. SYMPTOMS AND SIGNS

The common initial presentation is weakness, numbness, tingling, or unsteadiness in a limb; spastic paraparesis; retrobulbar neuritis; diplopia; disequilibrium; or a sphincter disturbance such as urinary urgency or hesitancy. Symptoms may disappear after a few days or weeks, although examination often reveals a residual deficit.

Several forms of the disease are recognized. In most patients, there is an interval of months or years after the initial episode before new symptoms develop or the original ones recur (**relapsing-remitting disease**). Eventually, however, relapses and usually incomplete remissions lead to increasing disability, with weakness, spasticity, and ataxia of the limbs, impaired vision, and urinary incontinence. The findings on examination at this stage commonly include optic atrophy, nystagmus, dysarthria, and pyramidal, sensory, or cerebellar deficits in some or all of the limbs. In some of these patients, the clinical course changes so that a steady deterioration occurs, unrelated to acute relapses (**secondary progressive disease**).

Less commonly, symptoms are steadily progressive from their onset, and disability develops at a relatively early stage (**primary progressive disease**). The diagnosis cannot be made with confidence unless the total clinical picture indicates involvement of different parts of the central nervous system at different times.

A number of factors (eg, infection, trauma) may precipitate or trigger exacerbations. Relapses are also more likely during the 2 or 3 months following pregnancy, possibly because of the increased demands and stresses that occur in the postpartum period.

B. IMAGING

MRI of the brain or cervical cord is often helpful in demonstrating the presence of a multiplicity of lesions. CT scans are less helpful.

In patients presenting with myelopathy alone and in whom there is no clinical or laboratory evidence of more widespread disease, myelography or MRI may be necessary to exclude a congenital or acquired surgically treatable lesion. The foramen magnum region must be visualized to exclude the possibility of Arnold-Chiari malformation, in which parts of the cerebellum and the lower brainstem are displaced into the cervical canal and produce mixed pyramidal and cerebellar deficits in the limbs.

C. LABORATORY AND OTHER STUDIES

A definitive diagnosis can never be based solely on the laboratory findings. If there is clinical evidence of only a single lesion in the central nervous system, multiple sclerosis cannot properly be diagnosed unless it can be shown that other regions are affected subclinically. The electrocerebral responses evoked by monocular visual stimulation with a checkerboard pattern stimulus, by monaural click stimulation, and by electrical stimulation of a sensory or mixed peripheral nerve have been used to detect subclinical involvement of the visual, brainstem auditory, and somatosensory pathways, respectively. Other disorders may also be characterized by multifocal electrophysiologic abnormalities.

There may be mild lymphocytosis or a slightly increased protein concentration in the cerebrospinal fluid, especially soon after an acute relapse. Elevated IgG in cerebrospinal fluid and discrete bands of IgG (oligoclonal bands) are present in many patients. The presence of such bands is not specific, however, since they have been found in a variety of inflammatory neurologic disorders and occasionally in patients with vascular or neoplastic disorders of the nervous system.

D. DIAGNOSIS

Multiple sclerosis should not be diagnosed unless there is evidence that two or more different regions of the central white matter have been affected at different times. A diagnosis of clinically definite disease can be made in patients with a relapsing-remitting course and evidence on examination of at least two lesions involving different regions of the central white matter. The diagnosis is probable in patients with multifocal white matter disease but only one clinical attack, or with a history of at least two clinical attacks but signs of only a single lesion.

Treatment

At least partial recovery from acute exacerbations can reasonably be expected, but further relapses may occur without warning, and there is no means of preventing progression of the disorder. Some disability is likely to result eventually, but about half of all patients are without significant disability even 10 years after onset of symptoms.

Recovery from acute relapses may be hastened by treatment with corticosteroids, but the extent of recovery is unchanged. A high dose (eg, prednisone, 60 or 80 mg) is given daily for 1 week, after which medication is tapered over the following 2 or 3 weeks. Such a regimen is often preceded by methylprednisolone, 1 g intravenously for 3 days. Long-term treatment with corticosteroids provides no benefit and does not prevent further relapses. In patients with relapsing-remitting or secondary progressive disease, treatment with β-interferon or with daily subcutaneous administration of glatiramer acetate reduces the frequency of exacerbations. Natalizumab, an alpha4 integrin antagonist that reduces the development of brain lesions in experimental models, reduces the relapse rate; however, its use in multiple sclerosis has been suspended after progressive multifocal leukoencephalopathy developed in two patients. Several studies have suggested that immunosuppressive therapy with cyclophosphamide, azathioprine, methotrexate, cladribine, or mitoxantrone may help arrest the course of secondary progressive multiple sclerosis. The evidence of benefit is incomplete, however. There is little evidence that plasmapheresis is helpful in multiple sclerosis. Intravenous immunoglobulins may reduce the clinical attack rate in relapsing-remitting disease, but the available studies are inadequate to permit treatment recommendations. Statins may have immunomodulatory effects, and their possible role in the treatment of multiple sclerosis is being studied.

Treatment for spasticity (see below) and for neurogenic bladder may be needed in advanced cases. Excessive fatigue must be avoided, and patients should rest during periods of acute relapse.

Compston A et al: Multiple sclerosis. Lancet 2002;359:1221. [PMID: 11955556]

Filippini G et al: Interferons in relapsing remitting multiple sclerosis: a systematic review. Lancet 2003;361:545. [PMID: 12598138]

Goodin DS et al: Disease modifying therapies in multiple sclerosis: subcommittee of the American Academy of Neurology and the MS Council for Clinical Practice Guidelines. Neurology 2002;58;169. [PMID: 11805241]

Neuhaus O et al: Are statins a treatment option for multiple sclerosis? Lancet Neurol 2004;3:369. [PMID: 15157852]

VITAMIN E DEFICIENCY

Vitamin E deficiency may produce a disorder somewhat similar to Friedreich's ataxia (see below). There is spinocerebellar degeneration involving particularly the posterior columns of the spinal cord and leading to limb ataxia, sensory loss, absent tendon reflexes, slurring of speech, and, in some cases, pigmentary retinal degeneration. The disorder may occur as a consequence of malabsorption or on a hereditary basis. Treatment is with α-tocopheryl acetate (eg, Aquasol E capsules or drops) as discussed in Chapter 29.

SPASTICITY

The term "spasticity" is commonly used for an upper motor neuron deficit, but it properly refers to a velocity-dependent increase in resistance to passive movement that affects different muscles to a different extent, is not uniform in degree throughout the range of a particular movement, and is commonly associated with other features of pyramidal deficit. It is often a major complication of stroke, cerebral or spinal injury, static perinatal encephalopathy, and multiple sclerosis.

Physical therapy with appropriate stretching programs is important during rehabilitation after the development of an upper motor neuron lesion and in subsequent management of the patient. The aim is to prevent joint and muscle contractures and perhaps to modulate spasticity.

Drug management is important also, but treatment may increase functional disability when increased extensor tone is providing additional support for patients with weak legs. Dantrolene weakens muscle contraction by interfering with the role of calcium. It is best avoided in patients with poor respiratory function or severe myocardial disease. Treatment is begun with 25 mg once daily, and the daily dose is built up by 25 mg increments every 3 days, depending on tolerance, to a maximum of 100 mg four times daily. Side effects include diarrhea, nausea, weakness, hepatic dysfunction (that may rarely be fatal, especially in women older than 35), drowsiness, light-headedness, and hallucinations.

Lioresal is an effective drug for treating spasticity of spinal origin and painful flexor (or extensor) spasms. The maximum recommended daily dose is 80 mg; treatment is started with a dose of 5 or 10 mg twice daily and then built up gradually. Side effects include gastrointestinal disturbances, lassitude, fatigue, sedation, unsteadiness, confusion, and hallucinations. Diazepam may modify spasticity by its action on spinal interneurons and perhaps also by influencing supraspinal centers, but effective doses often cause intolerable drowsiness and vary with different patients. Tizanidine, a centrally acting α_2-adrenergic agonist, is as effective as these other agents but is probably better tolerated. The daily dose is built up gradually, usually to 8 mg taken three times daily. Side effects include sedation, lassitude, hypotension, and dryness of the mouth.

Motor-point blocks by intramuscular phenol have been used to reduce spasticity selectively in one or a few important muscles and may permit return of function in patients with incomplete myelopathies. Intramuscular administration of botulinum toxin may also be helpful. Intrathecal injection of phenol or absolute alcohol may be helpful in more severe cases, but greater selectivity can be achieved by nerve root or peripheral nerve neurolysis. These procedures should not be undertaken until the spasticity syndrome is fully evolved, ie, only after about 1 year or so, and only if long-term drug treatment either has been unhelpful or carries a significant risk to the patient.

In patients with severe spasticity and limited use of the legs, a surgically implanted lioresal pump may provide significant relief and improve hygiene. Repeated transcutaneous electrical nerve stimulation may supplement medical treatment. A number of surgical procedures, eg, adductor or heel cord tenotomy, may also help in the management of spasticity and facilitate patient management. For example, obturator neurectomy is helpful in patients with marked adductor spasms that interfere with personal hygiene or cause gait disturbances. Posterior rhizotomy reduces spasticity, but its effect may be short-lived, whereas anterior rhizotomy produces permanent wasting and weakness in the muscles that are denervated.

Spasticity may be exacerbated by decubitus ulcers, urinary or other infections, and nociceptive stimuli.

Gordon MF et al: Repeated dosing of botulinum toxin type A for upper limb spasticity following stroke. Neurology 2004;63: 1971. [PMID: 15557529]

Gracies JM: Pathophysiology of spastic paresis. I: Paresis and soft tissue changes. Muscle Nerve 2005;31:535. [PMID: 15714510]

Gracies JM: Pathophysiology of spastic paresis. II: Emergence of muscle overactivity. Muscle Nerve 2005;31:552. [PMID: 15714511]

MYELOPATHIES IN AIDS

A variety of myelopathies may occur in patients with AIDS. These are discussed in Chapter 31.

MYELOPATHY OF HUMAN T CELL LEUKEMIA VIRUS INFECTION

Human T cell leukemia virus (HTLV-1), a human retrovirus, is transmitted by breast-feeding, sexual contact, blood transfusion, and contaminated needles. Most patients are asymptomatic, but after a variable latent period (which may be as long as several years) a myelopathy develops in some instances. The MRI, electrophysiologic, and cerebrospinal fluid findings are similar to those of multiple sclerosis, but HTLV-1 antibodies are present in serum and spinal fluid. There is no specific treatment.

Nagai M et al: Human T-cell lymphotropic virus type I and neurological diseases. J Neurovirol 2003;9:228. [PMID: 12707853]

SUBACUTE COMBINED DEGENERATION OF THE SPINAL CORD

Subacute combined degeneration of the spinal cord is due to vitamin B_{12} deficiency, such as occurs in pernicious anemia. It is characterized by myelopathy with predominant pyramidal and posterior column deficits, sometimes in association with polyneuropathy, mental changes, or optic neuropathy. Megaloblastic anemia may also occur, but this does not parallel the neurologic disorder, and the former may be obscured if folic acid supplements have been taken. Treatment is with vitamin B_{12}. For pernicious anemia, a convenient therapeutic regimen is 100 mg cyanocobalamin intramuscularly daily for 1 week, then weekly for 1 month, and then monthly for the remainder of the patient's life.

WERNICKE'S ENCEPHALOPATHY

Wernicke's encephalopathy is characterized by confusion, ataxia, and nystagmus leading to ophthalmoplegia (lateral rectus muscle weakness, conjugate gaze palsies); peripheral neuropathy may also be present. It is due to thiamine deficiency and in the United States occurs most commonly in alcoholics. It may also occur in patients with AIDS. In suspected cases, thiamine (50 mg) is given intravenously immediately and then intramuscularly on a daily basis until a satisfactory diet can be ensured. Intravenous glucose given before thiamine may precipitate the syndrome or worsen the symptoms. The diagnosis is confirmed by the response in 1 or 2 days to treatment, which must not be delayed while laboratory confirmation is obtained.

McIntosh C et al: Alcohol and the nervous system. J Neurol Neurosurg Psychiatry 2004;75 (Suppl 3):iii16. [PMID: 15316040]

STUPOR & COMA

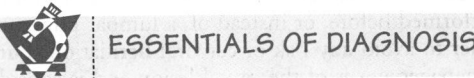

ESSENTIALS OF DIAGNOSIS

- *Level of consciousness is depressed.*

- *Stuporous patients respond only to repeated vigorous stimuli.*
- *Comatose patients are unarousable and unresponsive.*

General Considerations

The patient who is stuporous is unresponsive except when subjected to repeated vigorous stimuli, while the comatose patient is unarousable and unable to respond to external events or inner needs, although reflex movements and posturing may be present.

Coma is a major complication of serious central nervous system disorders. It can result from seizures, hypothermia, metabolic disturbances, or structural lesions causing bilateral cerebral hemispheric dysfunction or a disturbance of the brainstem reticular activating system. A mass lesion involving one cerebral hemisphere may cause coma by compression of the brainstem.

Assessment & Emergency Measures

The diagnostic workup of the comatose patient must proceed concomitantly with management. Supportive therapy for respiration or blood pressure is initiated; in hypothermia, all vital signs may be absent and all such patients should be rewarmed before the prognosis is assessed.

The patient can be positioned on one side with the neck partly extended, dentures removed, and secretions cleared by suction; if necessary, the patency of the airways is maintained with an oropharyngeal airway. Blood is drawn for serum glucose, electrolyte, and calcium levels; arterial blood gases; liver and renal function tests; and toxicologic studies as indicated. Dextrose 50% (25 g), naloxone (0.4–1.2 mg), and thiamine (50 mg) are given intravenously.

Further details are then obtained from attendants of the patient's medical history, the circumstances surrounding the onset of coma, and the time course of subsequent events. Abrupt onset of coma suggests subarachnoid hemorrhage, brainstem stroke, or intracerebral hemorrhage, whereas a slower onset and progression occur with other structural or mass lesions. A metabolic cause is likely with a preceding intoxicated state or agitated delirium. On examination, attention is paid to the behavioral response to painful stimuli, the pupils and their response to light, the position of the eyes and their movement in response to passive movement of the head and ice-water caloric stimulation, and the respiratory pattern.

A. RESPONSE TO PAINFUL STIMULI

Purposive limb withdrawal from painful stimuli implies that sensory pathways from and motor pathways to the stimulated limb are functionally intact. Unilateral absence of responses despite application of stimuli to both sides of the body in turn implies a corticospinal lesion; bilateral absence of responsiveness suggests brainstem involvement, bilateral pyramidal tract lesions, or psychogenic unresponsiveness. Inappropriate responses may also occur. Decorticate posturing may occur with lesions of the internal capsule and rostral cerebral peduncle, decerebrate posturing with dysfunction or destruction of the midbrain and rostral pons, and decerebrate posturing in the arms accompanied by flaccidity or slight flexor responses in the legs in patients with extensive brainstem damage extending down to the pons at the trigeminal level.

B. Ocular Findings

1. Pupils—Hypothalamic disease processes may lead to unilateral Horner's syndrome, while bilateral diencephalic involvement or destructive pontine lesions may lead to small but reactive pupils. Ipsilateral pupillary dilation with no direct or consensual response to light occurs with compression of the third cranial nerve, eg, with uncal herniation. The pupils are slightly smaller than normal but responsive to light in many metabolic encephalopathies; however, they may be fixed and dilated following overdosage with atropine, scopolamine, or glutethimide, and pinpoint (but responsive) with opiates. Pupillary dilation for several hours following cardiopulmonary arrest implies a poor prognosis.

2. Eye movements—Conjugate deviation of the eyes to the side suggests the presence of an ipsilateral hemispheric lesion or a contralateral pontine lesion. A mesencephalic lesion leads to downward conjugate deviation. Dysconjugate ocular deviation in coma implies a structural brainstem lesion unless there was preexisting strabismus.

The oculomotor responses to passive head turning and to caloric stimulation relate to each other and provide complementary information. In response to brisk rotation of the head from side to side and to flexion and extension of the head, normally conscious patients with open eyes do not exhibit contraversive conjugate eye deviation (doll's-head eye response) unless there is voluntary visual fixation or bilateral frontal pathology. With cortical depression in lightly comatose patients, a brisk doll's-head eye response is seen. With brainstem lesions, this oculocephalic reflex becomes impaired or lost, depending on the site of the lesion.

The oculovestibular reflex is tested by caloric stimulation using irrigation with ice water. In normal subjects, jerk nystagmus is elicited for about 2 or 3 minutes, with the slow component toward the irrigated ear. In unconscious patients with an intact brainstem, the fast component of the nystagmus disappears, so that the eyes tonically deviate toward the irrigated side for 2–3 minutes before returning to their original position. With impairment of brainstem function, the response becomes perverted and finally disappears. In metabolic coma, oculocephalic and oculovestibular reflex responses are preserved, at least initially.

C. Respiratory Patterns

Diseases causing coma may lead to respiratory abnormalities. Cheyne-Stokes respiration may occur with bihemispheric or diencephalic disease or in metabolic disorders. Central neurogenic hyperventilation occurs with lesions of the brainstem tegmentum; apneustic breathing (in which there are prominent end-inspiratory pauses) suggests damage at the pontine level (eg, due to basilar artery occlusion); and atactic breathing (a completely irregular pattern of breathing with deep and shallow breaths occurring randomly) is associated with lesions of the lower pontine tegmentum and medulla.

1. Stupor & Coma Due to Structural Lesions

Supratentorial mass lesions tend to affect brain function in an orderly way. There may initially be signs of hemispheric dysfunction, such as hemiparesis. As coma develops and deepens, cerebral function becomes progressively disturbed, producing a predictable progression of neurologic signs that suggest rostrocaudal deterioration.

Thus, as a supratentorial mass lesion begins to impair the diencephalon, the patient becomes drowsy, then stuporous, and finally comatose. There may be Cheyne-Stokes respiration; small but reactive pupils; doll's-head eye responses with side-to-side head movements but sometimes an impairment of reflex upward gaze with brisk flexion of the head; tonic ipsilateral deviation of the eyes in response to vestibular stimulation with cold water; and initially a positive response to pain but subsequently only decorticate posturing. With further progression, midbrain failure occurs. Motor dysfunction progresses from decorticate to bilateral decerebrate posturing in response to painful stimuli; Cheyne-Stokes respiration is gradually replaced by sustained central hyperventilation; the pupils become middle-sized and fixed; and the oculocephalic and oculovestibular reflex responses become impaired, perverted, or lost. As the pons and then the medulla fail, the pupils remain unresponsive; oculovestibular responses are unobtainable; respiration is rapid and shallow; and painful stimuli may lead only to flexor responses in the legs. Finally, respiration becomes irregular and stops, the pupils often then dilating widely.

In contrast, a subtentorial (ie, brainstem) lesion may lead to an early, sometimes abrupt disturbance of consciousness without any orderly rostrocaudal progression of neurologic signs. Compressive lesions of the brainstem, especially cerebellar hemorrhage, may be clinically indistinguishable from intraparenchymal processes.

A structural lesion is suspected if the findings suggest focality. In such circumstances, a CT scan should be performed before, or instead of, a lumbar puncture in order to avoid any risk of cerebral herniation. Further management is of the causal lesion and is considered separately under the individual disorders.

2. Stupor & Coma Due to Metabolic Disturbances

Patients with a metabolic cause of coma generally have signs of patchy, diffuse, and symmetric neurologic involvement that cannot be explained by loss of function at any single level or in a sequential manner, although focal or lateralized deficits may occur in hypoglycemia. Moreover, pupillary reactivity is usually preserved, while other brainstem functions are often grossly impaired. Comatose patients with meningitis, encephalitis, or subarachnoid hemorrhage may also exhibit little in the way of focal neurologic signs, however, and clinical evidence of meningeal irritation is sometimes very subtle in comatose patients. Examination of the cerebrospinal fluid in such patients is essential to establish the correct diagnosis.

In patients with coma due to cerebral ischemia and hypoxia, the absence of pupillary light reflexes at the time of initial examination indicates that there is little chance of regaining independence; by contrast, preserved pupillary light responses, the development of spontaneous eye movements (roving, conjugate, or better), and extensor, flexor, or withdrawal responses to pain at this early stage imply a relatively good prognosis.

Treatment of metabolic encephalopathy is of the underlying disturbance and is considered in other chapters. If the cause of the encephalopathy is obscure, all drugs except essential ones may have to be withdrawn in case they are responsible for the altered mental status.

Laureys S et al: Brain function in coma, vegetative state, and related disorders. Lancet Neurol 2004;3:537. [PMID: 15324722]

Malik K et al: Evaluating the comatose patient. Rapid neurologic assessment is key to appropriate management. Postgrad Med 2002;111:38. [PMID: 11868313]

3. Brain Death

The definition of brain death is controversial, and diagnostic criteria have been published by many different professional organizations. In order to establish brain death, the irreversibly comatose patient must be shown to have lost all brainstem reflex responses, including the pupillary, corneal, oculovestibular, oculocephalic, oropharyngeal, and respiratory reflexes, and should have been in this condition for at least 6 hours. Spinal reflex movements do not exclude the diagnosis, but ongoing seizure activity or decerebrate or decorticate posturing is not consistent with brain death. The apnea test (presence or absence of spontaneous respiratory activity at a $PaCO_2$ of at least 60 mm Hg) serves to determine whether the patient is capable of respiratory activity.

Reversible coma simulating brain death may be seen with hypothermia (temperature < 32°C) and overdosage with central nervous system depressant drugs, and these conditions must be excluded. Certain ancillary tests may assist the determination of brain death but are not essen-

tial. An isoelectric electroencephalogram, when the recording is made according to the recommendations of the American Electroencephalographic Society, may help in confirming the diagnosis. Alternatively, the demonstration of an absent cerebral circulation by intravenous radioisotope cerebral angiography or by four-vessel contrast cerebral angiography is confirmatory.

Booth CM et al: Is this patient dead, vegetative, or severely neurologically impaired? Assessing outcome for comatose survivors of cardiac arrest. JAMA 2004;291:870. [PMID: 14970067]

Young GB et al: A critique of ancillary tests for brain death. Neurocrit Care 2004;1:499. [PMID: 16174956]

4. Persistent Vegetative State

Patients with severe bilateral hemispheric disease may show some improvement from an initially comatose state, so that, after a variable interval, they appear to be awake but lie motionless and without evidence of awareness or higher mental activity. This persistent vegetative state has been variously referred to as akinetic mutism, apallic state, or coma vigil. Most patients in this persistent vegetative state will die in months or years, but partial recovery has occasionally occurred and in rare instances has been sufficient to permit communication or even independent living.

5. Locked-In Syndrome (De-efferented State)

Acute destructive lesions (eg, infarction, hemorrhage, demyelination, encephalitis) involving the ventral pons and sparing the tegmentum may lead to a mute, quadriparetic but conscious state in which the patient is capable of blinking and of voluntary eye movement in the vertical plane, with preserved pupillary responses to light. Such a patient can mistakenly be regarded as comatose. Physicians should recognize that "locked-in" individuals are fully aware of their surroundings. The prognosis is variable, but recovery has occasionally been reported—in some cases including resumption of independent daily life, though this may take up to 2 or 3 years.

HEAD INJURY

Trauma is the most common cause of death in young people, and head injury accounts for almost half of these trauma-related deaths. The prognosis following head injury depends on the site and severity of brain damage. Some guide to prognosis is provided by the mental status, since loss of consciousness for more than 1 or 2 minutes implies a worse prognosis than otherwise. Similarly, the degree of retrograde and posttraumatic amnesia provides an indication of the severity of injury and thus of the prognosis. Absence of skull fracture does not exclude the possibility of severe head injury. During the physical examination, special attention should be given to the level of consciousness and extent of any brainstem dysfunction.

Table 24–7. Acute cerebral sequelae of head injury.

Sequelae	Clinical Features	Pathology
Concussion	Transient loss of consciousness with bradycardia, hypotension, and respiratory arrest for a few seconds followed by retrograde and posttraumatic amnesia. Occasionally followed by transient neurologic deficit.	Bruising on side of impact (coup injury) or contralaterally (contrecoup injury).
Cerebral contusion or laceration	Loss of consciousness longer than with concussion. May lead to death or severe residual neurologic deficit.	Cerebral contusion, edema, hemorrhage, and necrosis. May have subarachnoid bleeding.
Acute epidural hemorrhage	Headache, confusion, somnolence, seizures, and focal deficits occur several hours after injury and lead to coma, respiratory depression, and death unless treated by surgical evacuation.	Tear in meningeal artery, vein, or dural sinus, leading to hematoma visible on CT scan.
Acute subdural hemorrhage	Similar to epidural hemorrhage, but interval before onset of symptoms is longer. Treatment is by surgical evacuation.	Hematoma from tear in veins from cortex to superior sagittal sinus or from cerebral laceration, visible on CT scan.
Cerebral hemorrhage	Generally develops immediately after injury. Clinically resembles hypertensive hemorrhage. Surgical evacuation is sometimes helpful.	Hematoma, visible on CT scan.

Note: Patients who have lost consciousness for 2 minutes or more following head injury should be admitted to the hospital for observation, as should patients with focal neurologic deficits, lethargy, or skull fractures. If admission is declined, responsible family members should be given clear instructions about the need for, and manner of, checking on them at regular (hourly) intervals and for obtaining additional medical help if necessary.

Skull radiographs or CT scans may provide evidence of fractures. Because injury to the spine may have accompanied head trauma, cervical spine radiographs (especially in the lateral projection) should always be obtained in comatose patients and in patients with severe neck pain or a deficit possibly related to cord compression.

CT scanning has an important role in demonstrating intracranial hemorrhage and may also provide evidence of cerebral edema and displacement of midline structures.

Cerebral Injuries

These are summarized in Table 24–7 along with comments about treatment. Increased intracranial pressure may result from ventilatory obstruction, abnormal neck position, seizures, dilutional hyponatremia, or cerebral edema; an intracranial hematoma requiring surgical evacuation may also be responsible. Other measures that may be necessary to reduce intracranial pressure include induced hyperventilation, intravenous mannitol infusion, and intravenous furosemide; corticosteroids provide no benefit in this context.

Scalp Injuries & Skull Fractures

Scalp lacerations and depressed or compound depressed skull fractures should be treated surgically as appropriate. Simple skull fractures require no specific treatment.

The clinical signs of basilar skull fracture include bruising about the orbit (raccoon sign), blood in the external auditory meatus (Battle's sign), and leakage of cerebrospinal fluid (which can be identified by its glucose content) from the ear or nose. Cranial nerve palsies (involving especially the first, second, third, fourth, fifth, seventh, and eighth nerves in any combination) may also occur. If there is any leakage of cerebrospinal fluid, conservative treatment, with elevation of the head, restriction of fluids, and administration of acetazolamide (250 mg four times daily), is often helpful; but if the leak continues for more than a few days, lumbar subarachnoid drainage may be necessary. Antibiotics are given if infection occurs, based on culture and sensitivity studies. Only very occasional patients require intracranial repair of the dural defect because of persistence of the leak or recurrent meningitis.

Late Complications of Head Injury

The relationship of chronic subdural hemorrhage to head injury is not always clear. In many elderly persons there is no history of trauma, but in other cases a head injury, often trivial, precedes the onset of symptoms by several weeks. The clinical presentation is usually with mental changes such as slowness, drowsiness, headache, confusion, memory disturbances, personality change, or even dementia. Focal neurologic deficits such as hemiparesis or hemisensory disturbance may also occur but are less common. CT scan is an important means of detecting the hematoma, which is sometimes bilateral. Treatment is by surgical evacuation to prevent cerebral compression and tentorial herniation. There is no clear evidence that prophylactic anticonvulsant therapy reduces the incidence of posttraumatic seizures.

Normal-pressure hydrocephalus may follow head injury, subarachnoid hemorrhage, or meningoencephalitis.

Other late complications of head injury include posttraumatic seizure disorder and posttraumatic headache.

Dutton RP et al: Traumatic brain injury. Curr Opin Crit Care 2003;9:503. [PMID: 14639070]

Vincent JL et al: Primer on medical management of severe brain injury. Crit Care Med 2005;33:1392. [PMID: 15942361]

Winter CD et al: A review of the current management of severe traumatic brain injury. Surgeon 2005;3:329. [PMID: 16245652]

SPINAL TRAUMA

ESSENTIALS OF DIAGNOSIS

- History of preceding trauma.
- Development of acute neurologic deficit.
- Signs of myelopathy on examination.

General Considerations

While spinal cord damage may result from whiplash injury, severe injury usually relates to fracture-dislocation causing compression or angular deformity of the cord either cervically or in the lower thoracic and upper lumbar regions. Extreme hypotension following injury may also lead to cord infarction.

Clinical Findings

Total cord transection results in immediate flaccid paralysis and loss of sensation below the level of the lesion. Reflex activity is lost for a variable period, and there is urinary and fecal retention. As reflex function returns over the following days and weeks, spastic paraplegia or quadriplegia develops, with hyperreflexia and extensor plantar responses, but a flaccid atrophic (lower motor neuron) paralysis may be found depending on the segments of the cord that are affected. The bladder and bowels also regain some reflex function, permitting urine and feces to be expelled at intervals. As spasticity increases, flexor or extensor spasms (or both) of the legs become troublesome, especially if the patient develops bed sores or a urinary tract infection. Paraplegia with the legs in flexion or extension may eventually result.

With lesser degrees of injury, patients may be left with mild limb weakness, distal sensory disturbance, or both. Sphincter function may also be impaired, urinary urgency and urgency incontinence being especially common. More particularly, a unilateral cord lesion leads to an ipsilateral motor disturbance with accompanying impairment of proprioception and con-

tralateral loss of pain and temperature appreciation below the lesion (Brown-Séquard syndrome). A central cord syndrome may lead to a lower motor neuron deficit and loss of pain and temperature appreciation, with sparing of posterior column functions. A radicular deficit may occur at the level of the injury—or, if the cauda equina is involved, there may be evidence of disturbed function in several lumbosacral roots.

Treatment

Treatment of the injury consists of immobilization and—if there is cord compression—decompressive laminectomy and fusion. Early treatment with high doses of corticosteroids (eg, methylprednisolone, 30 mg/kg by intravenous bolus, followed by 5.4 mg/kg/h for 23 hours) has been shown to improve neurologic recovery if commenced within 8 hours after injury. Treatment with G_{M1} ganglioside for 3 or 4 weeks is an experimental approach that has also been helpful. Anatomic realignment of the spinal cord by traction and other orthopedic procedures is also important. Subsequent care of the residual neurologic deficit—paraplegia or quadriplegia—requires treatment of spasticity and care of the skin, bladder, and bowels.

McDonald JW et al: Spinal-cord injury. Lancet 2002;359:417. [PMID: 11844532]

SYRINGOMYELIA

Destruction or degeneration of gray and white matter adjacent to the central canal of the cervical spinal cord leads to cavitation and accumulation of fluid within the spinal cord. The precise pathogenesis is unclear, but many cases are associated with Arnold-Chiari malformation, in which there is displacement of the cerebellar tonsils, medulla, and fourth ventricle into the spinal canal, sometimes with accompanying meningomyelocele. In such circumstances, the cord cavity connects with and may merely represent a dilated central canal. In other cases, the cause of cavitation is less clear. There is a characteristic clinical picture, with segmental atrophy and areflexia and loss of pain and temperature appreciation in a "cape" distribution owing to the destruction of fibers crossing in front of the central canal. Thoracic kyphoscoliosis is usually present. With progression, involvement of the long motor and sensory tracts occurs as well, so that a pyramidal and sensory deficit develops in the legs. Upward extension of the cavitation (syringobulbia) leads to dysfunction of the lower brainstem and thus to bulbar palsy, nystagmus, and sensory impairment over one or both sides of the face.

Syringomyelia, ie, cord cavitation, may also occur in association with an intramedullary tumor or following severe cord injury, and the cavity then does not communicate with the central canal.

In patients with Arnold-Chiari malformation, there are commonly skeletal abnormalities on plain x-rays of the skull and cervical spine. CT scans show caudal displacement of the fourth ventricle. MRI or positive contrast myelography may demonstrate the malformation itself. Focal cord enlargement is found at myelography or by MRI in patients with cavitation related to past injury or intramedullary neoplasms.

Treatment of Arnold-Chiari malformation with associated syringomyelia is by suboccipital craniectomy and upper cervical laminectomy, with the aim of decompressing the malformation at the foramen magnum. The cord cavity should be drained, and if necessary an outlet for the fourth ventricle can be made. In cavitation associated with intramedullary tumor, treatment is surgical, but radiation therapy may be necessary if complete removal is not possible. Posttraumatic syringomyelia is also treated surgically if it leads to increasing neurologic deficits or to intolerable pain.

Arnett B: Arnold-Chiari malformation. Arch Neurol 2003;60: 898. [PMID: 12810499]

Levine DN: The pathogenesis of syringomyelia associated with lesions at the foramen magnum: a critical review of existing theories and proposal of a new hypothesis. J Neurol Sci 2004;220:3. [PMID: 15140600]

DEGENERATIVE MOTOR NEURON DISEASES

ESSENTIALS OF DIAGNOSIS

- Weakness.
- No sensory loss or sphincter disturbance.
- Progressive course.
- No identifiable underlying cause other than genetic basis in familial cases.

General Considerations

This group of degenerative disorders is characterized clinically by weakness and variable wasting of affected muscles, without accompanying sensory changes.

Motor neuron disease in adults generally commences between 30 and 60 years of age. There is degeneration of the anterior horn cells in the spinal cord, the motor nuclei of the lower cranial nerves, and the corticospinal and corticobulbar pathways. The disorder is usually sporadic, but familial cases may occur and several genetic mutations or loci have been identified.

Classification

Five varieties have been distinguished on clinical grounds.

A. PROGRESSIVE BULBAR PALSY

Bulbar involvement predominates owing to disease processes affecting primarily the motor nuclei of the cranial nerves.

B. PSEUDOBULBAR PALSY

Bulbar involvement predominates in this variety also, but it is due to bilateral corticobulbar disease and thus reflects upper motor neuron dysfunction.

C. PROGRESSIVE SPINAL MUSCULAR ATROPHY

This is characterized primarily by a lower motor neuron deficit in the limbs due to degeneration of the anterior horn cells in the spinal cord.

D. PRIMARY LATERAL SCLEROSIS

There is a purely upper motor neuron deficit in the limbs.

E. AMYOTROPHIC LATERAL SCLEROSIS

A mixed upper and lower motor neuron deficit is found in the limbs. This disorder is sometimes associated with dementia or parkinsonism.

Clinical Findings

A. SYMPTOMS AND SIGNS

Difficulty in swallowing, chewing, coughing, breathing, and talking (dysarthria) occur with bulbar involvement. In progressive bulbar palsy, there is drooping of the palate; a depressed gag reflex; pooling of saliva in the pharynx; a weak cough; and a wasted, fasciculating tongue. In pseudobulbar palsy, the tongue is contracted and spastic and cannot be moved rapidly from side to side. Limb involvement is characterized by motor disturbances (weakness, stiffness, wasting, fasciculations) reflecting lower or upper motor neuron dysfunction; there are no objective changes on sensory examination, although there may be vague sensory complaints. The sphincters are generally spared.

The disorder is progressive, and amyotrophic lateral sclerosis is usually fatal within 3–5 years; death usually results from pulmonary infections. Patients with bulbar involvement generally have the poorest prognosis.

B. LABORATORY AND OTHER STUDIES

Electromyography may show changes of chronic partial denervation, with abnormal spontaneous activity in the resting muscle and a reduction in the number of motor units under voluntary control. In patients with suspected spinal muscular atrophy or amyotrophic lateral sclerosis, the diagnosis should not be made with confidence unless such changes are found in at least three spinal regions (cervical, thoracic, lumbosacral) or two spinal regions and the bulbar musculature. Motor conduction velocity is usually normal but may be slightly reduced, and sensory conduction studies are also normal. Biopsy of a wasted muscle shows the histologic changes of denervation. The serum creatine kinase may be slightly elevated but never reaches the extremely high values seen in some of the muscular dystrophies. The cerebrospinal fluid is normal.

A familial form of amyotrophic lateral sclerosis has been described with autosomal dominant inheritance, related to mutations in the copper-zinc superoxide dismutase gene on the long arm of chromosome 21. Other familial forms with dominant or recessive inheritance have also been identified and mapped to other genetic loci. X-linked bulbospinal neuronopathy is associated with an expanded trinucleotide repeat sequence on the androgen receptor gene and carries a more benign prognosis than other forms of motor neuron disease. There have been recent reports of juvenile spinal muscular atrophy due to hexosaminidase deficiency, with abnormal findings on rectal biopsy and reduced hexosaminidase A in serum and leukocytes. Pure motor syndromes resembling motor neuron disease may also occur in association with monoclonal gammopathy or multifocal motor neuropathies with conduction block. A motor neuronopathy may also develop in Hodgkin's disease and has a relatively benign prognosis. Infective anterior horn cell diseases (polio virus or West Nile virus infection) can generally be distinguished by the acute onset and monophasic course of the illness, as discussed elsewhere in this book.

Treatment

Riluzole, 50 mg orally twice daily, which reduces the presynaptic release of glutamate, may slow progression of amyotrophic lateral sclerosis. There is otherwise no specific treatment except in patients with gammopathy, in whom plasmapheresis and immunosuppression may lead to improvement. Therapeutic trials of various neurotrophic factors to slow disease progression have yielded generally disappointing results. Symptomatic and supportive measures may include prescription of anticholinergic drugs (such as trihexyphenidyl, amitriptyline, or atropine) or use of a portable suction machine if drooling is troublesome, braces or a walker to improve mobility, and physical therapy to prevent contractures. Behavioral modification (eg, exercising facial muscles and encouraging frequent swallowing) or over-the-counter decongestants may also help mild drooling. Spasticity may be helped by baclofen or diazepam. A semiliquid diet or nasogastric tube feeding may be needed if dysphagia is severe. Gastrostomy or cricopharyngomyotomy is sometimes resorted to in extreme cases of predominant bulbar involvement, and tracheostomy may be necessary if respiratory muscles are severely affected; however, in the terminal stages of these disorders, the aim of treatment should be to keep patients as comfortable as possible. Information on palliative care is provided in Chapter 5.

McGeer EG et al: Pharmacologic approaches to the treatment of amyotrophic lateral sclerosis. BioDrugs 2005;19:31. [PMID: 15691215]

Winhammar JM et al: Assessment of disease progression in motor neuron disease. Lancet Neurol 2005;4:229. [PMID: 15778102]

PERIPHERAL NEUROPATHIES

Peripheral neuropathies can be categorized on the basis of the structure primarily affected. The predominant pathologic feature may be axonal degeneration (axonal or neuronal neuropathies) or paranodal or segmental demyelination. The distinction may be possible on the basis of neurophysiologic findings. Motor and sensory conduction velocity can be measured in accessible segments of peripheral nerves. In axonal neuropathies, conduction velocity is normal or reduced only mildly and needle electromyography provides evidence of denervation in affected muscles. In demyelinating neuropathies, conduction may be slowed considerably in affected fibers, and in more severe cases, conduction is blocked completely, without accompanying electromyographic signs of denervation.

Nerves may be injured or compressed by neighboring anatomic structures at any point along their course. Common **mononeuropathies** of this sort are considered below. They lead to a sensory, motor, or mixed deficit that is restricted to the territory of the affected nerve. A similar clinical disturbance is produced by peripheral nerve tumors, but these are rare except in patients with Recklinghausen's disease. Multiple mononeuropathies suggest a patchy multifocal disease process such as vasculopathy (eg, diabetes, arteritis), an infiltrative process (eg, leprosy, sarcoidosis), radiation damage, or an immunologic disorder (eg, brachial plexopathy). Diffuse **polyneuropathies** lead to a symmetric sensory, motor, or mixed deficit, often most marked distally. They include the hereditary, metabolic, and toxic disorders; idiopathic inflammatory polyneuropathy (Guillain-Barré syndrome); and the peripheral neuropathies that may occur as a nonmetastatic complication of malignant diseases. Involvement of motor fibers leads to flaccid weakness that is most marked distally; dysfunction of sensory fibers causes impaired sensory perception. Tendon reflexes are depressed or absent. Paresthesias, pain, and muscle tenderness may also occur.

1. Polyneuropathies & Mononeuritis Multiplex

 ESSENTIALS OF DIAGNOSIS

- *Weakness, sensory disturbances, or both in the extremities.*
- *Pain sometimes common.*
- *Depressed or absent tendon reflexes.*
- *May be family history of neuropathy.*
- *May be history of systemic illness or toxic exposure.*

The cause of polyneuropathy or mononeuritis multiplex is suggested by the history, mode of onset, and predominant clinical manifestations. Laboratory workup includes a complete blood count and sedimentation rate, serum protein electrophoresis, and immunophoresis, determination of plasma urea and electrolytes, liver and thyroid function tests, tests for rheumatoid factor and antinuclear antibody, HBsAg determination, a serologic test for syphilis, fasting blood glucose level, urinary heavy metal levels, cerebrospinal fluid examination, and chest radiography. These tests should be ordered selectively, as guided by symptoms and signs. Measurement of nerve conduction velocity is important in confirming the peripheral nerve origin of symptoms and providing a means of following clinical changes, as well as indicating the likely disease process (ie, axonal or demyelinating neuropathy). Cutaneous nerve biopsy may help establish a precise diagnosis (eg, polyarteritis, amyloidosis). In about half of cases, no specific cause can be established; of these, slightly less than half are subsequently found to be heredofamilial.

Treatment is of the underlying cause, when feasible, and is discussed below under the individual disorders. Physical therapy helps prevent contractures, and splints can maintain a weak extremity in a position of useful function. Anesthetic extremities must be protected from injury. To guard against burns, patients should check the temperature of water and hot surfaces with a portion of skin having normal sensation, measure water temperature with a thermometer, and use cold water for washing or lower the temperature setting of their hot-water heaters. Shoes should be examined frequently during the day for grit or foreign objects in order to prevent pressure lesions.

Patients with polyneuropathies or mononeuritis multiplex are subject to additional nerve injury at pressure points and should therefore avoid such behavior as leaning on elbows or sitting with crossed legs for lengthy periods.

Neuropathic pain is sometimes troublesome and may respond to simple analgesics such as aspirin. Narcotics or narcotic substitutes may be necessary for severe hyperpathia or pain induced by minimal stimuli, but their use should be avoided as much as possible. The use of a frame or cradle to reduce contact with bedclothes may be helpful. Many patients experience episodic stabbing pains, which may respond to phenytoin, carbamazepine, gabapentin, pregabalin, or tricyclic antidepressants.

Symptoms of autonomic dysfunction are occasionally troublesome. Postural hypotension is often helped by wearing waist-high elastic stockings and sleeping in a semierect position at night. Fludrocortisone reduces postural hypotension, but doses as high as 1 mg/d are sometimes necessary in diabetics and may lead to recumbent hypertension. Midodrine, an α-agonist, is sometimes helpful in a dose of 2.5–10 mg three times daily. Impotence and diarrhea are difficult to treat; a flaccid neuropathic bladder may respond to parasympathomimetic drugs such as bethanechol chloride, 10–50 mg three or four times daily.

Inherited Neuropathies

A. CHARCOT-MARIE-TOOTH DISEASE (HMSN TYPE I, II)

Several distinct varieties of Charcot-Marie-Tooth disease can be recognized. There is usually an autosomal dominant mode of inheritance, but occasional cases occur on a sporadic, recessive, or X-linked basis. The responsible gene is commonly located on the short arm of chromosome 17 and less often shows linkage to chromosome 1 or the X chromosome. It has also been linked to several other chromosomes, emphasizing the genetic heterogeneity of the disorder. Clinical presentation may be with foot deformities or gait disturbances in childhood or early adult life. Slow progression leads to the typical features of polyneuropathy, with distal weakness and wasting that begin in the legs, a variable amount of distal sensory loss, and depressed or absent tendon reflexes. Tremor is a conspicuous feature in some instances. Electrodiagnostic studies show a marked reduction in motor and sensory conduction velocity (hereditary motor and sensory neuropathy [HMSN] type I).

In other instances (HMSN type II), motor conduction velocity is normal or only slightly reduced, sensory nerve action potentials may be absent, and signs of chronic partial denervation are found in affected muscles electromyographically. The predominant pathologic change is axonal loss rather than segmental demyelination.

A similar disorder may occur in patients with progressive distal spinal muscular atrophy, but there is no sensory loss; electrophysiologic investigation reveals that motor conduction velocity is normal or only slightly reduced, and nerve action potentials are normal.

B. DEJERINE-SOTTAS DISEASE (HMSN TYPE III)

The disorder may occur on a sporadic, autosomal dominant or, less commonly, autosomal recessive basis. Onset in infancy or childhood leads to a progressive motor and sensory polyneuropathy with weakness, ataxia, sensory loss, and depressed or absent tendon reflexes. The peripheral nerves may be palpably enlarged and are characterized pathologically by segmental demyelination, Schwann cell hyperplasia, and thin myelin sheaths. Electrophysiologically, there is slowing of conduction, and sensory action potentials may be unrecordable.

C. FRIEDREICH'S ATAXIA

Patients generally present in childhood or early adult life with this autosomal recessive disorder, which has been related to an unstable mutation of the *X25* gene on chromosome 9q13–q21.1. The gait becomes atactic, the hands become clumsy, and other signs of cerebellar dysfunction develop accompanied by weakness of the legs and extensor plantar responses. Involvement of peripheral sensory fibers leads to sensory disturbances in the limbs and depressed tendon reflexes.

There is bilateral pes cavus. Pathologically, there is a marked loss of cells in the posterior root ganglia and degeneration of peripheral sensory fibers. In the central nervous system, changes are conspicuous in the posterior and lateral columns of the cord. Electrophysiologically, conduction velocity in motor fibers is normal or only mildly reduced, but sensory action potentials are small or absent.

D. REFSUM'S DISEASE (HMSN TYPE IV)

This autosomal recessive disorder is due to a disturbance in phytanic acid metabolism. Clinically, pigmentary retinal degeneration is accompanied by progressive sensorimotor polyneuropathy and cerebellar signs. Auditory dysfunction, cardiomyopathy, and cutaneous manifestations may also occur. Motor and sensory conduction velocity are reduced, often markedly, and there may be electromyographic evidence of denervation in affected muscles. Dietary restriction of phytanic acid and its precursors may be helpful therapeutically. Plasmapheresis to reduce stored phytanic acid may help at the initiation of treatment.

E. PORPHYRIA

Peripheral nerve involvement may occur during acute attacks in both variegate porphyria and acute intermittent porphyria. Motor symptoms usually occur first, and weakness is often most marked proximally and in the upper limbs rather than the lower. Sensory symptoms and signs may be proximal or distal in distribution. Autonomic involvement is sometimes pronounced. The electrophysiologic findings are in keeping with the results of neuropathologic studies suggesting that the neuropathy is axonal in type. Hematin (4 mg/kg intravenously over 15 minutes once or twice daily) may lead to rapid improvement. A high-carbohydrate diet and, in severe cases, intravenous glucose or levulose may also be helpful. Propranolol (up to 100 mg every 4 hours) may control tachycardia and hypertension in acute attacks. Porphyria is discussed further in Chapter 40.

Neuropathies Associated with Systemic & Metabolic Disorders

A. DIABETES MELLITUS

In this disorder, involvement of the peripheral nervous system may lead to symmetric sensory or mixed polyneuropathy, asymmetric motor radiculoneuropathy or plexopathy (diabetic amyotrophy), thoracoabdominal radiculopathy, autonomic neuropathy, or isolated lesions of individual nerves. These may occur singly or in any combination and are discussed in Chapter 27.

B. UREMIA

Uremia may lead to a symmetric sensorimotor polyneuropathy that tends to affect the lower limbs more than the upper limbs and is more marked distally than proximally (see Chapter 22). The diagnosis can be confirmed electrophysiologically, for motor and sensory conduction velocity is moderately reduced. The neuropathy improves both clinically and electrophysiologically with renal transplantation and to a lesser extent with chronic dialysis.

C. ALCOHOLISM AND NUTRITIONAL DEFICIENCY

Many alcoholics have an axonal distal sensorimotor polyneuropathy that is frequently accompanied by painful cramps, muscle tenderness, and painful paresthesias and is often more marked in the legs than in the arms. Symptoms of autonomic dysfunction may also be conspicuous. Motor and sensory conduction velocity may be slightly reduced, even in subclinical cases, but gross slowing of conduction is uncommon. A similar distal sensorimotor polyneuropathy is a well-recognized feature of beriberi (thiamine deficiency). In vitamin B_{12} deficiency, distal sensory polyneuropathy may develop but is usually overshadowed by central nervous system manifestations (eg, myelopathy, optic neuropathy, or intellectual changes).

D. PARAPROTEINEMIAS

A symmetric sensorimotor polyneuropathy that is gradual in onset, progressive in course, and often accompanied by pain and dysesthesias in the limbs may occur in patients (especially men) with multiple myeloma. The neuropathy is of the axonal type in classic lytic myeloma, but segmental demyelination (primary or secondary) and axonal loss may occur in sclerotic myeloma and lead to predominantly motor clinical manifestations. Both demyelinating and axonal neuropathies are also observed in patients with paraproteinemias without myeloma. A small fraction will develop myeloma if serially followed. The demyelinating neuropathy in these patients may be due to the monoclonal protein's reacting to a component of the nerve myelin. The neuropathy of classic multiple myeloma is poorly responsive to therapy. The polyneuropathy of benign monoclonal gammopathy may respond to immunosuppressant drugs and plasmapheresis.

Polyneuropathy may also occur in association with macroglobulinemia and cryoglobulinemia and sometimes responds to plasmapheresis. Entrapment neuropathy, such as carpal tunnel syndrome, is more common than polyneuropathy in patients with (nonhereditary) generalized amyloidosis. With polyneuropathy due to amyloidosis, sensory and autonomic symptoms are especially conspicuous, whereas distal wasting and weakness occur later; there is no specific treatment.

Neuropathies Associated with Infectious & Inflammatory Diseases

A. LEPROSY

Leprosy is an important cause of peripheral neuropathy in certain parts of the world. Sensory disturbances are mainly due to involvement of intracutaneous nerves. In tuberculoid leprosy, they develop at the same time and in the same distribution as the skin lesion but may be more extensive if nerve trunks lying beneath the lesion are also involved. In lepromatous leprosy, there is more extensive sensory loss, and this develops earlier and to a greater extent in the coolest regions of the body, such as the dorsal surfaces of the hands and feet, where the bacilli proliferate most actively. Motor deficits result from involvement of superficial nerves where their temperature is lowest, eg, the ulnar nerve in the region proximal to the olecranon groove, the median nerve as it emerges from beneath the forearm flexor muscle to run toward the carpal tunnel, the peroneal nerve at the head of the fibula, and the posterior tibial nerve in the lower part of the leg; patchy facial muscular weakness may also occur owing to involvement of the superficial branches of the seventh cranial nerve.

Motor disturbances in leprosy are suggestive of multiple mononeuropathy, whereas sensory changes resemble those of distal polyneuropathy. Examination, however, relates the distribution of sensory deficits to the temperature of the tissues; in the legs, for example, sparing frequently occurs between the toes and in the popliteal fossae, where the temperature is higher. Treatment is with antileprotic agents (see Chapter 33).

B. AIDS

A variety of neuropathies occur in HIV-infected patients (see Chapter 31). Patients with AIDS may develop a chronic symmetric sensorimotor axonal **polyneuropathy** associated usually with no abnormal cerebrospinal fluid findings. Treatment is symptomatic. AIDS patients may also develop progressive **polyradiculopathy** or radiculomyelopathy that leads to leg weakness and urinary retention; sensory loss is less conspicuous than in polyneuropathy. The cerebrospinal fluid may show mononuclear pleocytosis and increased protein and low glucose concentrations. Cytomegalovirus is responsible in at least some cases. The prognosis is generally poor, but some patients respond to intravenous ganciclovir (2.5 mg/kg every 8 hours for 10 days, then 7.5 mg/kg daily 5 days per week).

An inflammatory **demyelinating polyradiculoneuropathy** sometimes occurs in HIV-seropositive patients without AIDS and may follow an acute, subacute, or chronic course. Weakness is usually more conspicuous distally than proximally and tends to overshadow sensory symptoms. Tendon reflexes are depressed or absent. The cerebrospinal fluid shows an increased cell count and protein concentration. Treatment with plasmapheresis has helped some patients. Spontaneous improvement may also occur. Seropositive patients without AIDS may also develop a **mononeuropathy multiplex** that sometimes responds to treatment with plasmapheresis.

C. Lyme Borreliosis

The neurologic manifestations of Lyme disease include meningitis, meningoencephalitis, polyradiculo-

neuropathy, mononeuropathy multiplex, and cranial neuropathy. Serologic tests establish the underlying disorder. Treatment is described in Chapter 34.

D. Sarcoidosis

Cranial nerve palsies (especially facial palsy), multiple mononeuropathy and, less commonly, symmetric polyneuropathy may all occur, the latter sometimes preferentially affecting either motor or sensory fibers. Improvement may occur with use of corticosteroids.

E. Polyarteritis

Involvement of the vasa nervorum by the vasculitic process may result in infarction of the nerve. Clinically, one encounters an asymmetric sensorimotor polyneuropathy (mononeuritis multiplex) that pursues a waxing and waning course. Corticosteroids and cytotoxic agents—especially cyclophosphamide—may be of benefit in severe cases.

F. Rheumatoid Arthritis

Compressive or entrapment neuropathies, ischemic neuropathies, mild distal sensory polyneuropathy, and severe progressive sensorimotor polyneuropathy can occur in rheumatoid arthritis.

Neuropathy Associated with Critical Illness

Patients in intensive care units with sepsis and multiorgan failure sometimes develop polyneuropathies. This may be manifested initially by unexpected difficulty in weaning patients from a mechanical ventilator and in more advanced cases by wasting and weakness of the extremities and loss of tendon reflexes. Sensory abnormalities are relatively inconspicuous. The neuropathy is axonal in type. Its pathogenesis is obscure, and treatment is supportive. The prognosis is good provided patients recover from the underlying critical illness.

Toxic Neuropathies

Axonal polyneuropathy may follow exposure to industrial agents or pesticides such as acrylamide, organophosphorus compounds, hexacarbon solvents, methyl bromide, and carbon disulfide; metals such as arsenic, thallium, mercury, and lead; and drugs such as phenytoin, perhexiline, isoniazid, nitrofurantoin, vincristine, and pyridoxine in high doses. Detailed occupational, environmental, and medical histories and recognition of clusters of cases are important in suggesting the diagnosis. Treatment is by preventing further exposure to the causal agent. Isoniazid neuropathy is prevented by pyridoxine supplementation.

Diphtheritic neuropathy results from a neurotoxin released by the causative organism and is common in many areas. Palatal weakness may develop 2–4 weeks after infection of the throat, and infection of the skin may similarly be followed by focal weakness of neighboring muscles. Disturbances of accommodation may occur about 4–5 weeks after infection and distal sensorimotor demyelinating polyneuropathy after 1–3 months.

Neuropathies Associated with Malignant Diseases

Both a sensorimotor and a purely sensory polyneuropathy may occur as a nonmetastatic complication of malignant diseases (see Table 40–6). The sensorimotor polyneuropathy may be mild and occur in the course of known malignant disease, or it may have an acute or subacute onset, lead to severe disability, and occur before there is any clinical evidence of the cancer, occasionally following a remitting course.

Acute Idiopathic Polyneuropathy (Guillain-Barré Syndrome)

 ESSENTIALS OF DIAGNOSIS

- Acute or subacute progressive polyradiculoneuropathy.
- Usually ascending, symmetric weakness.
- Paresthesias are more variable.
- Acute dysautonomia may be life-threatening.

A. GENERAL CONSIDERATIONS

This acute or subacute polyradiculoneuropathy sometimes follows infective illness, inoculations, or surgical procedures. There is an association with preceding *Campylobacter jejuni* enteritis. The disorder probably has an immunologic basis, but the precise mechanism is unclear.

B. CLINICAL FINDINGS

1. Symptoms and signs—The main complaint is of weakness that varies widely in severity in different patients and often has a proximal emphasis and symmetric distribution. It usually begins in the legs, spreading to a variable extent but frequently involving the arms and often one or both sides of the face. The muscles of respiration or deglutition may also be affected. Sensory symptoms are usually less conspicuous than motor ones, but distal paresthesias and dysesthesias are common, and neuropathic or radicular pain is present in many patients. Autonomic disturbances are also common, may be severe, and are sometimes life-threatening; they include tachycardia, cardiac irregularities, hypotension or hypertension, facial flushing, abnormalities of sweating, pulmonary dysfunction, and impaired sphincter control.

2. Laboratory findings—The cerebrospinal fluid characteristically contains a high protein concentration with a normal cell content, but these changes may take 2 or 3 weeks to develop. Electrophysiologic studies may reveal marked abnormalities, which do not necessarily parallel the clinical disorder in their temporal course. Pathologic examination has shown primary demyelination or, less commonly, axonal degeneration.

C. DIFFERENTIAL DIAGNOSIS

When the diagnosis is made, the history and appropriate laboratory studies should exclude the possibility of porphyric, diphtheritic, or toxic (heavy metal, hexacarbon, organophosphate) neuropathies. The temporal course excludes other peripheral neuropathies. Poliomyelitis, botulism, and tick paralysis must also be considered as they cause weakness of acute onset. The presence of pyramidal signs, a markedly asymmetric motor deficit, a sharp sensory level, or early sphincter involvement should suggest a focal cord lesion.

D. PROGNOSIS

Most patients eventually make a good recovery, but this may take many months, and 10–20% patients of are left with persisting disability.

E. TREATMENT

Treatment with prednisone is ineffective and may prolong recovery time. Plasmapheresis is of value; it is best performed within the first few days of illness and is best reserved for clinically severe or rapidly progressive cases or those with ventilatory impairment. Intravenous immunoglobulin (400 mg/kg/d for 5 days) is also helpful and imposes less stress on the cardiovascular system than plasmapheresis. Patients should be admitted to intensive care units if their forced vital capacity is declining, and intubation is considered if the forced vital capacity reaches 15 mL/kg, dyspnea becomes evident, or the oxygen saturation declines. Respiratory toilet and chest physical therapy help prevent atelectasis. Marked hypotension may respond to volume replacement or pressor agents. Low-dose heparin to prevent pulmonary embolism should be considered.

Approximately 3% of patients with acute idiopathic polyneuropathy have one or more clinically similar relapses, sometimes several years after the initial illness. Plasma exchange therapy may produce improvement in chronic and relapsing inflammatory polyneuropathy.

Chronic Inflammatory Polyneuropathy

Chronic inflammatory demyelinating polyneuropathy, an acquired immunologically mediated disorder, is clinically similar to Guillain-Barré syndrome except that it has a relapsing or steadily progressive course over months or years. In the relapsing form, partial recovery may occur after some relapses, but in other instances there is no recovery between exacerbations. Although remission may occur spontaneously with time, the disorder frequently follows a progressive downhill course leading to severe functional disability.

Electrodiagnostic studies show marked slowing of motor and sensory conduction, and focal conduction block. Signs of partial denervation may also be present owing to secondary axonal degeneration. Nerve biopsy may show chronic perivascular inflammatory infiltrates in the endoneurium and epineurium, without accompanying evidence of vasculitis. However, a normal nerve biopsy result or the presence of nonspecific abnormalities does not exclude the diagnosis.

Corticosteroids may be effective in arresting or reversing the downhill course. Treatment is usually begun with prednisone, 60 mg daily, continued for 2–3 months or until a definite response has occurred. If no response has occurred despite 3 months of treatment, a higher dose may be tried. In responsive cases, the dose is gradually tapered, but most patients become corticosteroid-dependent, often requiring prednisone, 20 mg daily on alternate days, on a long-term basis. Patients unresponsive to corticosteroids may benefit instead from treatment with a cytotoxic drug such as azathioprine. There are increasing anecdotal reports of short-term benefit with plasmapheresis; high-dose intravenous immunoglobulin treatment (eg, 400 mg/kg/d) may produce clinical improvement lasting for weeks to months.

Briemberg HR et al: Inflammatory neuropathies. Curr Neurol Neurosci Rep 2005;5:66. [PMID: 15676111]

Donofrio PD: Immunotherapy of idiopathic inflammatory neuropathies. Muscle Nerve 2003;28:273. [PMID: 12929187]

Kieseier BC et al: Advances in understanding and treatment of immune-mediated disorders of the peripheral nervous system. Muscle Nerve 2004;30:131. [PMID: 15266629]

Mendell JR et al: Clinical practice. Painful sensory neuropathy. N Engl J Med 2003;348:1243. [PMID: 12660389]

Polydefkis M et al: New insights into diabetic polyneuropathy. JAMA 2003;290:1371. [PMID: 12966130]

Wolfe GI et al: Painful peripheral neuropathy and its nonsurgical treatment. Muscle Nerve 2004;30:3. [PMID: 15221874]

2. Mononeuropathies

ESSENTIALS OF DIAGNOSIS

- Focal motor or sensory deficit.
- Deficit is in territory of an individual peripheral nerve.

An individual nerve may be injured along its course or may be compressed, angulated, or stretched by neighboring anatomic structures, especially at a point where it passes through a narrow space (entrapment neuropathy). The relative contributions of mechanical factors and ischemia to the local damage are not clear. With involvement of a sensory or mixed nerve, pain is commonly felt distal to the lesion. Symptoms never develop

with some entrapment neuropathies, resolve rapidly and spontaneously in others, and become progressively more disabling and distressing in yet other cases. The precise neurologic deficit depends on the nerve involved. Percussion of the nerve at the site of the lesion may lead to paresthesias in its distal distribution.

Entrapment neuropathy may be the sole manifestation of subclinical polyneuropathy, and this must be borne in mind and excluded by nerve conduction studies. Such studies are also indispensable for the accurate localization of the focal lesion.

In patients with acute compression neuropathy such as may occur in intoxicated individuals ("Saturday night palsy"), no treatment is necessary. Complete recovery generally occurs, usually within 2 months, presumably because the underlying pathology is demyelination. However, axonal degeneration can occur in severe cases, and recovery then takes longer and may never be complete.

In chronic compressive or entrapment neuropathies, avoidance of aggravating factors and correction of any underlying systemic conditions are important. Local infiltration of the region about the nerve with corticosteroids may be of value; in addition, surgical decompression may help if there is a progressively increasing neurologic deficit or if electrodiagnostic studies show evidence of partial denervation in weak muscles.

Peripheral nerve tumors are uncommon, except in Recklinghausen's disease, but also give rise to mononeuropathy. This may be distinguishable from entrapment neuropathy only by noting the presence of a mass along the course of the nerve and by demonstrating the precise site of the lesion with appropriate electrophysiologic studies. Treatment of symptomatic lesions is by surgical removal if possible.

Carpal Tunnel Syndrome

See Chapter 20.

Pronator Teres or Anterior Interosseous Syndrome

The median nerve gives off its motor branch, the anterior interosseous nerve, below the elbow as it descends between the two heads of the pronator teres muscle. A lesion of either nerve may occur in this region, sometimes after trauma or owing to compression from, for example, a fibrous band. With anterior interosseous nerve involvement, there is no sensory loss, and weakness is confined to the pronator quadratus, flexor pollicis longus, and the flexor digitorum profundus to the second and third digits. Weakness is more widespread and sensory changes occur in an appropriate distribution when the median nerve itself is affected. The prognosis is variable. If improvement does not occur spontaneously, decompressive surgery may be helpful.

Ulnar Nerve Lesions

Ulnar nerve lesions are likely to occur in the elbow region as the nerve runs behind the medial epicondyle and descends into the cubital tunnel. In the condylar groove, the ulnar nerve is exposed to pressure or trauma. Moreover, any increase in the carrying angle of the elbow, whether congenital, degenerative, or traumatic, may cause excessive stretching of the nerve when the elbow is flexed. Ulnar nerve lesions may also result from thickening or distortion of the anatomic structures forming the cubital tunnel, and the resulting symptoms may also be aggravated by flexion of the elbow, because the tunnel is then narrowed by tightening of its roof or inward bulging of its floor. A severe lesion at either site causes sensory changes in the medial $1^1/_2$ digits and along the medial border of the hand. There is weakness of the ulnar-innervated muscles in the forearm and hand. With a cubital tunnel lesion, however, there may be relative sparing of the flexor carpi ulnaris muscle. Electrophysiologic evaluation using nerve stimulation techniques allows more precise localization of the lesion.

If conservative measures are unsuccessful in relieving symptoms and preventing further progression, surgical treatment may be necessary. This consists of nerve transposition if the lesion is in the condylar groove, or a release procedure if it is in the cubital tunnel.

Ulnar nerve lesions may also develop at the wrist or in the palm of the hand, usually owing to repetitive trauma or to compression from ganglia or benign tumors. They can be subdivided depending on their presumed site. Compressive lesions are treated surgically. If repetitive mechanical trauma is responsible, this is avoided by occupational adjustment or job retraining.

Radial Nerve Lesions

The radial nerve is particularly liable to compression or injury in the axilla (eg, by crutches or by pressure when the arm hangs over the back of a chair). This leads to weakness or paralysis of all the muscles supplied by the nerve, including the triceps. Sensory changes may also occur but are often surprisingly inconspicuous, being marked only in a small area on the back of the hand between the thumb and index finger. Injuries to the radial nerve in the spiral groove occur characteristically during deep sleep, as in intoxicated individuals (Saturday night palsy), and there is then sparing of the triceps muscle, which is supplied more proximally. The nerve may also be injured at or above the elbow; its purely motor posterior interosseous branch, supplying the extensors of the wrist and fingers, may be involved immediately below the elbow, but then there is sparing of the extensor carpi radialis longus, so that the wrist can still be extended. The superficial radial nerve may be compressed by handcuffs or a tight watch strap.

Femoral Neuropathy

The clinical features of femoral nerve palsy consist of weakness and wasting of the quadriceps muscle, with sensory impairment over the anteromedian aspect of the thigh and sometimes also of the leg to the medial malleolus, and a depressed or absent knee jerk. Isolated femoral neuropathy may occur in diabetics or from compression by retroperitoneal neoplasms or hematomas (eg, expanding aortic aneurysm). Femoral neuropathy may also result from pressure from the inguinal ligament when the thighs are markedly flexed and abducted, as in the lithotomy position.

Meralgia Paresthetica

The lateral femoral cutaneous nerve, a sensory nerve arising from the L2 and L3 roots, may be compressed or stretched in obese or diabetic patients and during pregnancy. The nerve usually runs under the outer portion of the inguinal ligament to reach the thigh, but the ligament sometimes splits to enclose it. Hyperextension of the hip or increased lumbar lordosis—such as occurs during pregnancy—leads to nerve compression by the posterior fascicle of the ligament. However, entrapment of the nerve at any point along its course may cause similar symptoms, and several other anatomic variations predispose the nerve to damage when it is stretched. Pain, paresthesia, or numbness occurs about the outer aspect of the thigh, usually unilaterally, and is sometimes relieved by sitting. Examination shows no abnormalities except in severe cases when cutaneous sensation is impaired in the affected area. Symptoms are usually mild and commonly settle spontaneously. Hydrocortisone injections medial to the anterosuperior iliac spine often relieve symptoms temporarily, while nerve decompression by transposition may provide more lasting relief.

Sciatic & Common Peroneal Nerve Palsies

Misplaced deep intramuscular injections are probably still the most common cause of sciatic nerve palsy. Trauma to the buttock, hip, or thigh may also be responsible. The resulting clinical deficit depends on whether the whole nerve has been affected or only certain fibers. In general, the peroneal fibers of the sciatic nerve are more susceptible to damage than those destined for the tibial nerve. A sciatic nerve lesion may therefore be difficult to distinguish from peroneal neuropathy unless there is electromyographic evidence of involvement of the short head of the biceps femoris muscle. The common peroneal nerve itself may be compressed or injured in the region of the head and neck of the fibula, eg, by sitting with crossed legs or wearing high boots. There is weakness of dorsiflexion and eversion of the foot, accompanied by numbness or blunted sensation of the anterolateral aspect of the calf and dorsum of the foot.

Tarsal Tunnel Syndrome

The tibial nerve, the other branch of the sciatic, supplies several muscles in the lower extremity, gives origin to the sural nerve, and then continues as the posterior tibial nerve to supply the plantar flexors of the foot and toes. It passes through the tarsal tunnel behind and below the medial malleolus, giving off calcaneal branches and the medial and lateral plantar nerves that supply small muscles of the foot and the skin on the plantar aspect of the foot and toes. Compression of the posterior tibial nerve or its branches between the bony floor and ligamentous roof of the tarsal tunnel leads to pain, paresthesias, and numbness over the bottom of the foot, especially at night, with sparing of the heel. Muscle weakness may be hard to recognize clinically. Compressive lesions of the individual plantar nerves may also occur more distally, with clinical features similar to those of the tarsal tunnel syndrome. Treatment is surgical decompression.

Brown WF, Bolton CF, Aminoff MJ (eds): Neuromuscular Function and Disease, 2 vols. Saunders, 2002.

Katz JN et al: Clinical practice. Carpal tunnel syndrome. N Engl J Med 2002; 346:1807. [PMID: 12050342]

Facial Neuropathy

An isolated facial palsy may occur in patients with HIV seropositivity, sarcoidosis, or Lyme disease (see Chapter 34), but most often it is idiopathic (Bell's palsy).

3. Bell's Palsy

ESSENTIALS OF DIAGNOSIS

- *Sudden onset of lower motor neuron facial palsy.*
- *Hyperacusis or impaired taste may occur.*
- *No other neurologic abnormalities.*

General Considerations

Bell's palsy is an idiopathic facial paresis of lower motor neuron type that has been attributed to an inflammatory reaction involving the facial nerve near the stylomastoid foramen or in the bony facial canal. Increasing evidence incriminates reactivation of herpes simplex virus infection in the geniculate ganglion at least in some instances. The disorder is more common in pregnant women or in persons with diabetes.

Clinical Findings

The facial paresis generally comes on abruptly, but it may worsen over the following day or so. Pain about the ear precedes or accompanies the weakness in many cases but usually lasts for only a few days. The face itself feels stiff and pulled to one side. There may be ipsilateral restriction of eye closure and difficulty with eating and fine facial movements. A disturbance of taste is common, owing to involvement of chorda tympani fibers, and hyperacusis due to involvement of fibers to the stapedius occurs occasionally.

Treatment

Other disorders that can produce a facial palsy and require specific treatment, such as tumors, Lyme disease, AIDS, sarcoidosis, and herpes zoster infection of the geniculate ganglion, must be excluded. The management of Bell's palsy is controversial. Approximately 60% of cases recover completely without treatment, presumably because the lesion is so mild that it leads merely to conduction block. Considerable improvement occurs in most other cases, and only about 10% of all patients have permanent disfigurement or other long-term sequelae. Treatment is unnecessary in most cases but is indicated for patients in whom an unsatisfactory outcome can be predicted. The best clinical guide to progress is the severity of the palsy during the first few days after presentation. Patients with clinically complete palsy when first seen are less likely to make a full recovery than those with an incomplete one. A poor prognosis for recovery is also associated with advanced age, hyperacusis, and severe initial pain. Electromyography and nerve excitability or conduction studies provide a guide to prognosis but not early enough to aid in the selection of patients for treatment.

The only medical treatment that may influence the outcome is administration of corticosteroids, but this is unclear. Many clinicians nevertheless routinely prescribe corticosteroids for patients with Bell's palsy seen within 5 days of onset. The author prescribes them only when the palsy is clinically complete or there is severe pain. Treatment with prednisone, 60 or 80 mg daily in divided doses for 4 or 5 days, followed by tapering of the dose over the next 7–10 days, is a satisfactory regimen. It is helpful to protect the eye with lubricating drops (or lubricating ointment at night) and a patch if eye closure is not possible. It is unclear whether acyclovir or other antiviral agents confer any benefit. There is no evidence that surgical procedures to decompress the facial nerve are of benefit.

Gilden DH: Clinical practice. Bell's palsy. N Engl J Med 2004; 351:1323. [PMID: 15385659]

Holland NJ et al: Recent developments in Bell's palsy. BMJ 2004; 329:553. [PMID: 15345630]

DISCOGENIC NECK PAIN

ESSENTIALS OF DIAGNOSIS

- *Neck pain, sometimes radiating to arms.*
- *Restricted neck movements.*
- *Motor, sensory, or reflex changes in arms with root involvement.*
- *Neurologic deficit in legs, gait disorder, or sphincter disturbance with cord involvement.*

General Considerations

A variety of congenital abnormalities may involve the cervical spine and lead to neck pain; these include hemivertebrae, fused vertebrae, basilar impression, and instability of the atlantoaxial joint. Traumatic, degenerative, infective, and neoplastic disorders may also lead to pain in the neck. When rheumatoid arthritis involves the spine, it tends to affect especially the cervical region, leading to pain, stiffness, and reduced mobility; displacement of vertebrae or atlantoaxial subluxation may lead to cord compression that can be life-threatening if not treated by fixation. Further details are given in Chapter 20 (including a discussion on low back pain), and discussion here is restricted to disk disease.

Acute Cervical Disk Protrusion

Acute cervical disk protrusion leads to pain in the neck and radicular pain in the arm, exacerbated by head movement. With lateral herniation of the disk, motor, sensory, or reflex changes may be found in a radicular (usually C6 or C7) distribution on the affected side (Figure 24–1); with more centrally directed herniations, the spinal cord may also be involved, leading to spastic paraparesis and sensory disturbances in the legs, sometimes accompanied by impaired sphincter function. The diagnosis is confirmed by MRI or CT myelography. In mild cases, bed rest or intermittent neck traction may help, followed by immobilization of the neck in a collar for several weeks. If these measures are unsuccessful or the patient has a significant neurologic deficit, surgical removal of the protruding disk may be necessary.

Cervical Spondylosis

Cervical spondylosis results from chronic cervical disk degeneration, with herniation of disk material, secondary calcification, and associated osteophytic outgrowths. One or more of the cervical nerve roots may be compressed, stretched, or angulated; and myelopathy may also develop as a result of compression, vascular insufficiency, or recurrent minor trauma to the cord. Patients present with neck pain and restricted head movement, occipital headaches, radicular pain and other sensory disturbances in the arms, weakness of the arms or legs, or some combination of these symptoms. Examination generally reveals that lateral flexion and rotation of the neck are limited. A segmental pattern of weakness or dermatomal sensory loss (or both) may be found unilaterally or bilaterally in the upper limbs, and tendon reflexes mediated by the affected root or roots are depressed. The C5 and C6 nerve roots are most commonly involved, and examination frequently then reveals weakness of muscles supplied by these roots (eg, deltoids, supraspinatus and infraspinatus, biceps, brachioradialis), pain or sensory loss about the shoulder and outer border of the arm and forearm, and depressed biceps and brachioradialis reflexes. Spastic paraparesis may also be present if there is an associated myelopathy, sometimes accompanied by posterior column or spinothalamic sensory deficits in the legs.

Plain radiographs of the cervical spine show osteophyte formation, narrowing of disk spaces, and encroachment on the intervertebral foramina, but such changes are common in middle-aged persons and may be unrelated to the presenting complaint. CT or MRI helps confirm the diagnosis and exclude other structural causes of the myelopathy.

Restriction of neck movements by a cervical collar may relieve pain. Operative treatment may be necessary to prevent further progression if there is a significant neurologic deficit or if root pain is severe, persistent, and unresponsive to conservative measures.

BRACHIAL & LUMBAR PLEXUS LESIONS

Brachial Plexus Neuropathy

Brachial plexus neuropathy may be idiopathic, sometimes occurring in relationship to a number of different nonspecific illnesses or factors. In other instances, brachial plexus lesions follow trauma or result from congenital anomalies, neoplastic involvement, or injury by various physical agents. In rare instances, the disorder occurs on a familial basis.

Idiopathic brachial plexus neuropathy (neuralgic amyotrophy) characteristically begins with severe pain about the shoulder, followed within a few days by weakness, reflex changes, and sensory disturbances involving especially the C5 and C6 segments. Symptoms and signs are usually unilateral but may be bilateral. Wasting of affected muscles is sometimes profound. The disorder relates to disturbed function of cervical roots or part of the brachial plexus, but its precise cause is unknown. Recovery occurs over the ensuing months but may be incomplete. Treatment is purely symptomatic.

Cervical Rib Syndrome

Compression of the C8 and T1 roots or the lower trunk of the brachial plexus by a cervical rib or band arising from the seventh cervical vertebra leads to weakness and wasting of intrinsic hand muscles, especially those in the thenar eminence, accompanied by pain and numbness in the medial two fingers and the ulnar border of the hand and forearm. The subclavian artery may also be compressed, and this forms the basis of Adson's test for diagnosing the disorder; the radial pulse is diminished or obliterated on the affected side when the seated patient inhales deeply and turns the head to one side or the other. Electromyography, nerve conduction studies, and somatosensory evoked potential studies may help confirm the diagnosis. X-rays sometimes show the cervical rib or a large transverse process of the seventh cervical vertebra, but normal findings do not exclude the possibility of a cervical band. Treatment of the disorder is by surgical excision of the rib or band.

Peripheral nerve

Nerve root

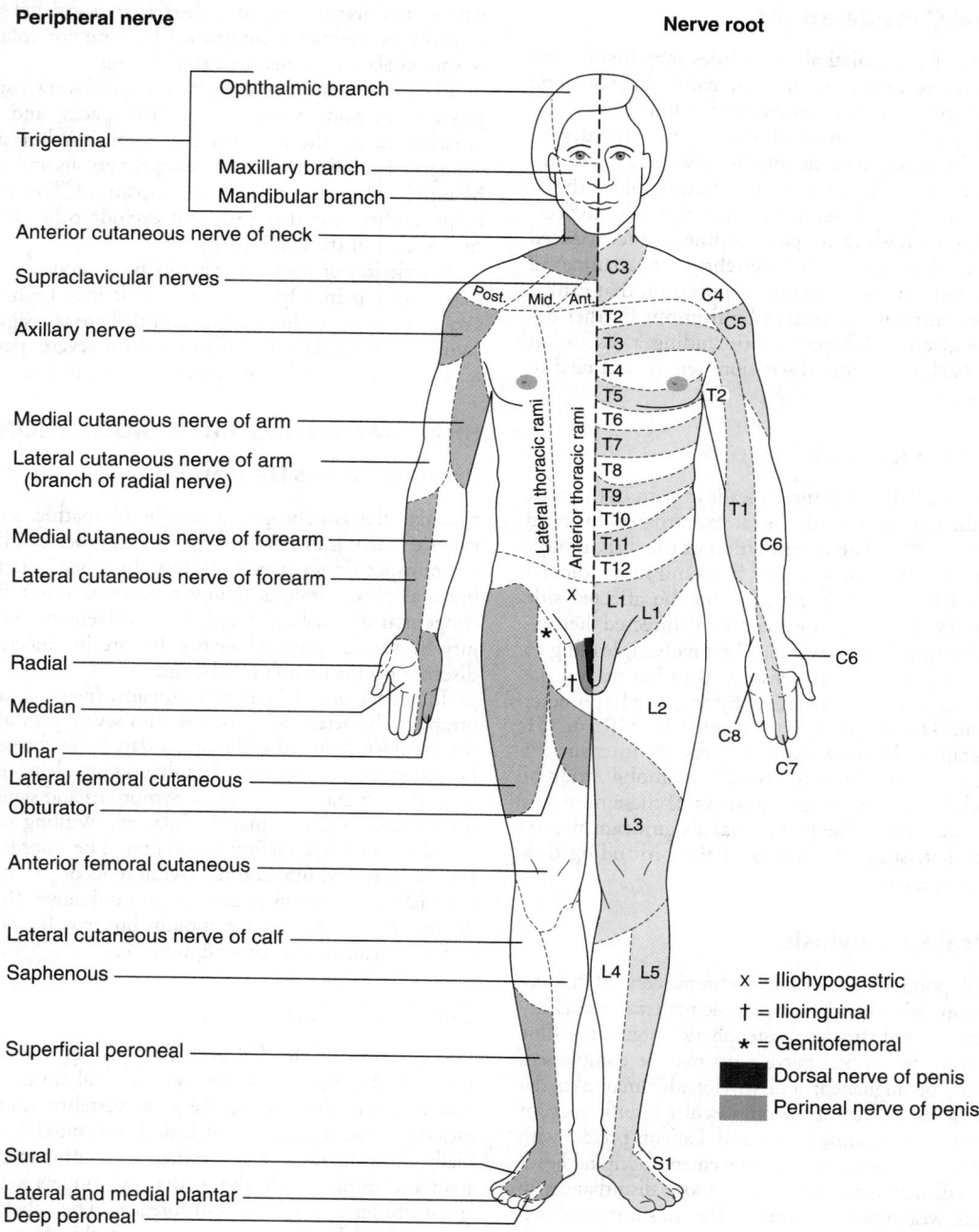

Figure 24–1. Cutaneous innervation. The segmental or radicular (root) distribution is shown on the left side of the body and the peripheral nerve distribution on the right side. **Above:** anterior view; **facing page:** posterior view. (Reproduced, with permission, from Simon RP et al: Clinical Neurology, 4th ed. McGraw-Hill, 1999.)

Lumbosacral Plexus Lesions

A lumbosacral plexus lesion may develop in association with diseases such as diabetes, cancer, or bleeding disorders or in relation to injury. It occasionally occurs as an isolated phenomenon similar to idiopathic brachial plexopathy, and pain and weakness then tend to be more conspicuous than sensory symptoms. The distribution of symptoms and signs depends on the level and pattern of neurologic involvement.

Nerve root

Peripheral nerve

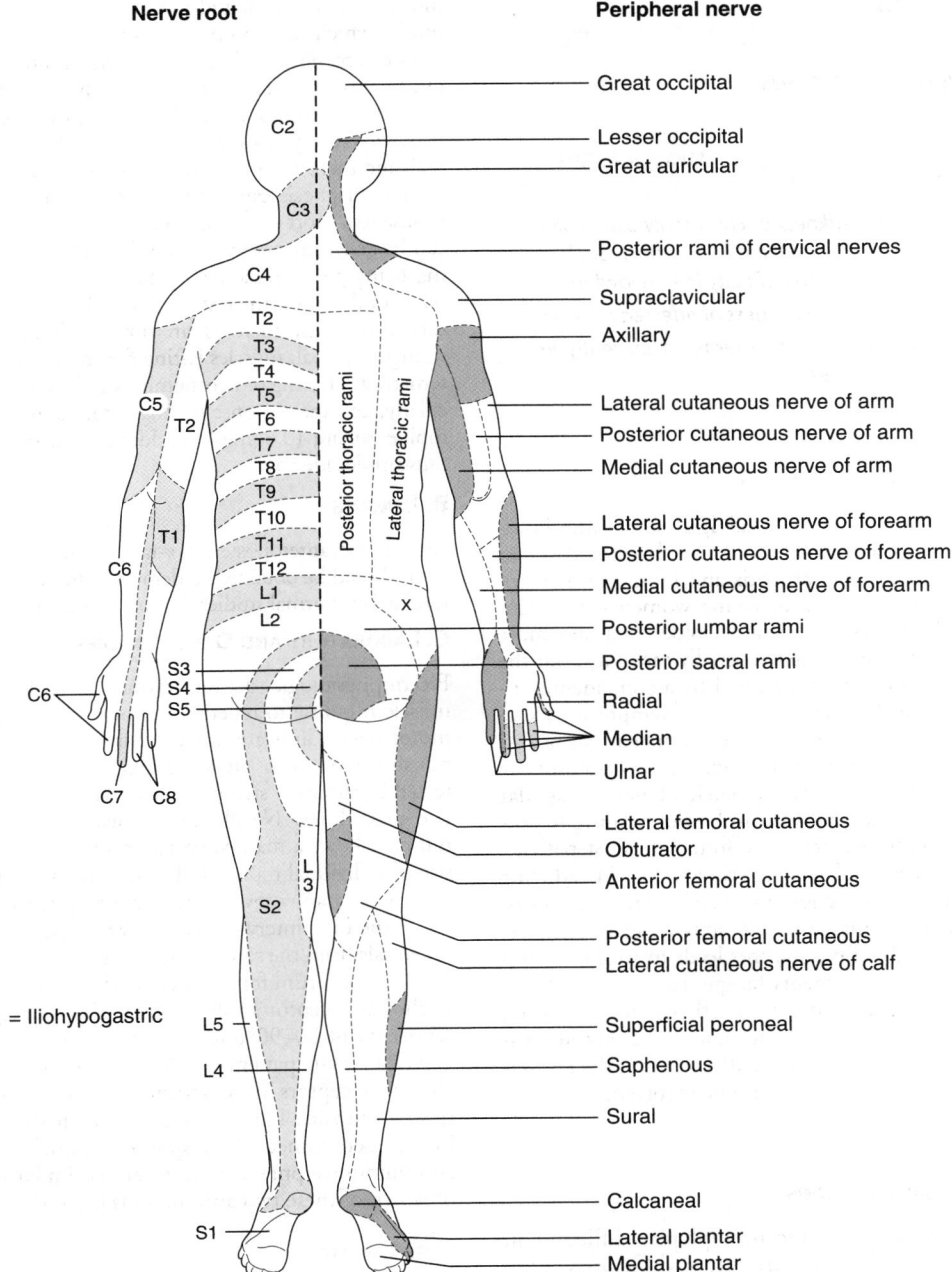

- Great occipital
- Lesser occipital
- Great auricular
- Posterior rami of cervical nerves
- Supraclavicular
- Axillary
- Lateral cutaneous nerve of arm
- Posterior cutaneous nerve of arm
- Medial cutaneous nerve of arm
- Lateral cutaneous nerve of forearm
- Posterior cutaneous nerve of forearm
- Medial cutaneous nerve of forearm
- Posterior lumbar rami
- Posterior sacral rami
- Radial
- Median
- Ulnar
- Lateral femoral cutaneous
- Obturator
- Anterior femoral cutaneous
- Posterior femoral cutaneous
- Lateral cutaneous nerve of calf
- Superficial peroneal
- Saphenous
- Sural
- Calcaneal
- Lateral plantar
- Medial plantar

Posterior thoracic rami

Lateral thoracic rami

x = Iliohypogastric

Figure 24–1. Continued

DISORDERS OF NEUROMUSCULAR TRANSMISSION

1. Myasthenia Gravis

ESSENTIALS OF DIAGNOSIS

- *Fluctuating weakness of commonly used voluntary muscles, producing symptoms such as diplopia, ptosis, and difficulty in swallowing.*
- *Activity increases weakness of affected muscles.*
- *Short-acting anticholinesterases transiently improve the weakness.*

General Considerations

Myasthenia gravis occurs at all ages, sometimes in association with a thymic tumor or thyrotoxicosis, as well as in rheumatoid arthritis and lupus erythematosus. It is most common in young women with HLA-DR3; if thymoma is associated, older men are more commonly affected. Onset is usually insidious, but the disorder is sometimes unmasked by a coincidental infection that leads to exacerbation of symptoms. Exacerbations may also occur before the menstrual period and during or shortly after pregnancy. Symptoms are due to a variable degree of block of neuromuscular transmission caused by autoantibodies binding to acetylcholine receptors; these are found in most patients with the disease and have a primary role in reducing the number of functioning acetylcholine receptors. Additionally, cellular immune activity against the receptor is found. Clinically, this leads to weakness; initially powerful movements fatigue readily. The external ocular muscles and certain other cranial muscles, including the masticatory, facial, and pharyngeal muscles, are especially likely to be affected, and the respiratory and limb muscles may also be involved.

Clinical Findings

A. SYMPTOMS AND SIGNS

Patients present with ptosis, diplopia, difficulty in chewing or swallowing, respiratory difficulties, limb weakness, or some combination of these problems. Weakness may remain localized to a few muscle groups, especially the ocular muscles, or may become generalized. Symptoms often fluctuate in intensity during the day, and this diurnal variation is superimposed on a tendency to longer-term spontaneous relapses and remissions that may last for weeks. Nevertheless, the disorder follows a slowly progressive course and may have a fatal outcome owing to respiratory complications such as aspiration pneumonia.

Clinical examination confirms the weakness and fatigability of affected muscles. In most cases, the extraocular muscles are involved, and this leads to ocular palsies and ptosis, which are commonly asymmetric. Pupillary responses are normal. The bulbar and limb muscles are often weak, but the pattern of involvement is variable. Sustained activity of affected muscles increases the weakness, which improves after a brief rest. Sensation is normal, and there are usually no reflex changes.

The diagnosis can generally be confirmed by the response to a short-acting anticholinesterase. Edrophonium can be given intravenously in a dose of 10 mg (1 mL), 2 mg being given initially and the remaining 8 mg about 30 seconds later if the test dose is well tolerated; in myasthenic patients, there is an obvious improvement in strength of weak muscles lasting for about 5 minutes. Alternatively, 1.5 mg of neostigmine can be given intramuscularly, and the response then lasts for about 2 hours; atropine sulfate (0.6 mg) should be available to reverse muscarinic side effects.

B. IMAGING

Lateral and anteroposterior x-rays of the chest and CT scans should be obtained to demonstrate a coexisting thymoma, but normal studies do not exclude this possibility.

C. LABORATORY AND OTHER STUDIES

Electrophysiologic demonstration of a decrementing muscle response to repetitive 2- or 3-Hz stimulation of motor nerves indicates a disturbance of neuromuscular transmission. Such an abnormality may even be detected in clinically strong muscles with certain provocative procedures. Needle electromyography of affected muscles shows a marked variation in configuration and size of individual motor unit potentials, and single-fiber electromyography reveals an increased jitter, or variability, in the time interval between two muscle fiber action potentials from the same motor unit.

Assay of serum for elevated levels of circulating acetylcholine receptor antibodies is useful because it has a sensitivity of 80–90% for the diagnosis of myasthenia gravis. Certain patients without antibodies to acetylcholine receptors have serum antibodies to muscle-specific tyrosine kinase (MuSK), which should therefore be determined; the response to anticholinesterase and immunosuppressive treatment is similar regardless of which of these two antibodies is present.

Treatment

Medication such as aminoglycosides that may exacerbate myasthenia gravis should be avoided. Anticholinesterase drugs provide symptomatic benefit without influencing the course of the disease. Neostigmine, pyridostigmine, or both can be used, the dose being determined on an individual basis. The usual dose of neostigmine is 7.5–30 mg (average, 15 mg) taken four times daily; of pyridostigmine, 30–180 mg (average, 60 mg) four times daily. Overmedication may temporarily increase weakness, which is then unaffected or enhanced by intravenous edrophonium.

Thymectomy usually leads to symptomatic benefit or remission and should be considered in all patients younger than age 60, unless weakness is restricted to the extraocular muscles. If the disease is of recent onset and only slowly progressive, operation is sometimes delayed for a year or so, in the hope that spontaneous remission will occur.

Treatment with corticosteroids is indicated for patients who have responded poorly to anticholinesterase drugs and have already undergone thymectomy. It is often introduced with the patient in the hospital, since weakness may initially be aggravated. Once weakness has stabilized after 2–3 weeks or any improvement is sustained, further management can be on an outpatient basis. Alternate-day treatment is usually well tolerated, but if weakness is enhanced on the nontreatment day it may be necessary for medication to be taken daily. The dose of corticosteroids is determined on an individual basis, but an initial high daily dose (eg, prednisone, 60–100 mg) can gradually be tapered to a relatively low maintenance level as improvement occurs; total withdrawal is difficult, however. Treatment with azathioprine may also be effective. The usual dose is 2–3 mg/kg orally daily after a lower initial dose.

In patients with major disability in whom conventional treatment is either unhelpful or contraindicated, plasmapheresis or intravenous immunoglobulin therapy may be beneficial. It may also be useful for stabilizing patients before thymectomy and for managing acute crisis. Mycophenolate mofetil, an immunosuppressant, has also been used, and preliminary studies indicate that it may provide symptomatic benefit and allow the corticosteroid dose to be reduced.

Keesey JC: Clinical evaluation and management of myasthenia gravis. Muscle Nerve 2004;29:484. [PMID: 15052614]

Zhou L et al: Clinical comparison of muscle-specific tyrosine kinase (MuSK) antibody-positive and -negative myasthenic patients. Muscle Nerve 2004;30:55. [PMID: 15221879]

2. Myasthenic Syndrome (Lambert-Eaton Syndrome)

 ESSENTIALS OF DIAGNOSIS

- *Variable weakness, typically improving with activity.*
- *Dysautonomic symptoms may also be present.*
- *A history of malignant disease may be obtained.*

General Considerations

Myasthenic syndrome (see Table 40–6) may be associated with small-cell carcinoma, sometimes developing before the tumor is diagnosed, and occasionally occurs with certain autoimmune diseases. There is defective release of acetylcholine in response to a nerve impulse, and this leads to weakness, especially of the proximal muscles of the limbs.

As is not the case in myasthenia gravis, however, power steadily increases with sustained contraction. The diagnosis can be confirmed electrophysiologically, because the muscle response to stimulation of its motor nerve increases remarkably if the nerve is stimulated repetitively at high rates, even in muscles that are not clinically weak.

Treatment with plasmapheresis and immunosuppressive drug therapy (prednisone and azathioprine) may lead to clinical and electrophysiologic improvement, in addition to therapy aimed at tumor when present. Prednisone is usually initiated in a daily dose of 60–80 mg and azathioprine in a daily dose of 2 mg/kg. Guanidine hydrochloride (25–50 mg/kg/d in divided doses) is occasionally helpful in seriously disabled patients, but adverse effects of the drug include marrow suppression. The response to treatment with anticholinesterase drugs such as pyridostigmine or neostigmine, either alone or in combination with guanidine, is variable.

3. Botulism

The toxin of *Clostridium botulinum* prevents the release of acetylcholine at neuromuscular junctions and autonomic synapses. Botulism occurs most commonly following the ingestion of contaminated home-canned food and should be suggested by the development of sudden, fluctuating, severe weakness in a previously healthy person. Symptoms begin within 72 hours following ingestion of the toxin and may progress for several days. Typically, there is diplopia, ptosis, facial weakness, dysphagia, and nasal speech, followed by respiratory difficulty and finally by weakness that appears last in the limbs. Blurring of vision (with unreactive dilated pupils) is characteristic, and there may be dryness of the mouth, constipation (paralytic ileus), and postural hypotension. Sensation is preserved, and the tendon reflexes are not affected unless the involved muscles are very weak. If the diagnosis is suspected, the local health authority should be notified and a sample of serum and contaminated food (if available) sent to be assayed for toxin. Support for the diagnosis may be obtained by electrophysiologic studies; with repetitive stimulation of motor nerves at fast rates, the muscle response increases in size progressively.

Patients should be hospitalized in case respiratory assistance becomes necessary. Treatment is with trivalent antitoxin, once it is established that the patient is not allergic to horse serum. Guanidine hydrochloride (25–50 mg/kg/d in divided doses) to facilitate release of acetylcholine from nerve endings sometimes helps to increase muscle strength. Anticholinesterase drugs are of no value. Respiratory assistance and other supportive measures should be provided as necessary. Further details are provided in Chapter 33.

4. Disorders Associated with Use of Aminoglycosides

Aminoglycoside antibiotics, eg, gentamicin, may produce a clinical disturbance similar to botulism by preventing the release of acetylcholine from nerve endings, but symptoms subside rapidly as the responsible drug is eliminated from the body. These antibiotics are particularly dangerous in patients with preexisting disturbances of neuromuscular transmission and are therefore best avoided in patients with myasthenia gravis.

MYOPATHIC DISORDERS

1. Muscular Dystrophies

ESSENTIALS OF DIAGNOSIS

- Muscle weakness, often in a characteristic distribution.
- Age at onset and inheritance pattern depend on the specific dystrophy.

General Considerations

These inherited myopathic disorders are characterized by progressive muscle weakness and wasting. They are subdivided by mode of inheritance, age at onset, and clinical features, as shown in Table 24–8. In the Duchenne type, pseudohypertrophy of muscles frequently occurs at some stage; intellectual retardation is common; and there may be skeletal deformities, muscle contractures, and cardiac involvement. The serum creatine kinase level is increased, especially in the Duchenne and Becker varieties, and mildly increased also in limb-girdle dystrophy. Electromyography may help confirm that weakness is myopathic rather than neurogenic. Similarly, histopathologic examination of a muscle biopsy specimen may help confirm that weakness is due to a primary disorder of muscle and to distinguish between various muscle diseases.

A genetic defect on the short arm of the X chromosome has been identified in Duchenne dystrophy. The affected gene codes for the protein dystrophin, which is markedly reduced or absent from the muscle of patients with the disease. Dystrophin levels are generally normal in the Becker variety, but the protein is qualitatively altered.

Duchenne muscular dystrophy can now be recognized early in pregnancy in about 95% of women by genetic studies; in late pregnancy, DNA probes can be used on fetal tissue obtained for this purpose by am-

Table 24–8. The muscular dystrophies.

Disorder	Inheritance	Age at Onset (years)	Distribution	Prognosis	Genetic Locus
Duchenne type	X-linked recessive	1–5	Pelvic, then shoulder girdle; later, limb and respiratory muscles.	Rapid progression. Death within about 15 years after onset.	Xp21
Becker's	X-linked recessive	5–25	Pelvic, then shoulder girdle.	Slow progression. May have normal life span.	Xp21
Limb-girdle (Erb's)	Autosomal recessive, dominant or sporadic	10–30	Pelvic or shoulder girdle initially, with later spread to the other.	Variable severity and rate of progression. Possible severe disability in middle life.	Multiple
Facioscapulo-humeral	Autosomal dominant	Any age	Face and shoulder girdle initially; later, pelvic girdle and legs.	Slow progression. Minor disability. Usually normal life span.	4q35
Emery-Dreifuss	X-linked recessive or autosomal dominant	5–10	Humeroperoneal or scapuloperoneal.	Variable.	Xq28, 1q11, 1q21.2
Distal	Autosomal dominant or recessive	40–60	Onset distally in extremities; proximal involvement later.	Slow progression.	2q13, 2p13
Ocular	Autosomal dominant (may be recessive)	Any age (usually 5–30)	External ocular muscles; may also be mild weakness of face, neck, and arms.		
Oculopharyngeal	Autosomal dominant	Any age	As in the ocular form but with dysphagia		14q11.2–q13
Myotonic dystrophy	Autosomal dominant	Any age (usually 20–40)	Face, neck, distal limbs.	Slow progression.	19q13.2–q13.3; 3q21.3

niocentesis. The genes causing some of the other muscular dystrophies are listed in Table 24–8.

There is no specific treatment for the muscular dystrophies, but it is important to encourage patients to lead as normal lives as possible. Prednisone (0.75 mg/kg daily) improves muscle strength and function in boys with Duchenne dystrophy, but side effects need to be monitored. Prolonged bed rest must be avoided, as inactivity often leads to worsening of the underlying muscle disease. Physical therapy and orthopedic procedures may help counteract deformities or contractures.

Kirschner J et al: The congenital and limb-girdle muscular dystrophies. Arch Neurol 2004;61:189. [PMID: 14967765]

Moxley RT 3rd et al: Practice parameter: corticosteroid treatment of Duchenne dystrophy: report of the Quality Standards Subcommittee of the American Academy of Neurology and the Practice Committee of the Child Neurology Society. Neurology 2005;64:13. [PMID: 15642897]

2. Myotonic Dystrophy

Myotonic dystrophy, a slowly progressive, dominantly inherited disorder, usually manifests itself in the third or fourth decade but occasionally appears early in childhood. The genetic defect has been localized to the long arm of chromosome 19 in the type 1 disorder. Myotonia leads to complaints of muscle stiffness and is evidenced by the marked delay that occurs before affected muscles can relax after a contraction. This can often be demonstrated clinically by delayed relaxation of the hand after sustained grip or by percussion of the belly of a muscle. In addition, there is weakness and wasting of the facial, sternocleidomastoid, and distal limb muscles. Associated clinical features include cataracts, frontal baldness, testicular atrophy, diabetes mellitus, cardiac abnormalities, and intellectual changes. In myotonic dystrophy type 2, the clinical features are similar but a different gene is involved (3q21.3). Electromyographic sampling of affected muscles reveals myotonic discharges in addition to changes suggestive of myopathy.

Myotonia can be treated with phenytoin (100 mg three times daily), quinine sulfate (300–400 mg three times daily), or procainamide (0.5–1 g four times daily). More recently, tocainide and mexiletine have been used. Phenytoin is preferred, since the other drugs may have undesirable effects on cardiac conduction. Neither the weakness nor the course of the disorder is influenced by treatment.

Machuca-Tzili L et al: Clinical and molecular aspects of the myotonic dystrophies: a review. Muscle Nerve 2005;32:1. [PMID: 15770660]

3. Myotonia Congenita

Myotonia congenita is commonly inherited as a dominant trait. The responsible gene may be on the long arm of chromosome 7. Generalized myotonia without weakness is usually present from birth, but symptoms may not appear until early childhood. Patients complain of muscle stiffness that is enhanced by cold and inactivity and relieved by exercise. Muscle hypertrophy, at times pronounced, is also a feature. A recessive form with later onset is associated with slight weakness and atrophy of distal muscles. Treatment with quinine sulfate, procainamide, tocainide, mexiletine, or phenytoin may help the myotonia, as in myotonic dystrophy.

4. Polymyositis & Dermatomyositis

See Chapter 20.

5. Inclusion Body Myositis

This disorder, of unknown cause, begins insidiously, usually after middle age, with progressive proximal weakness of first the lower and then the upper extremities. Distal weakness is usually mild. Serum creatine kinase levels may be normal or increased. The diagnosis is confirmed by muscle biopsy. In contrast to polymyositis, corticosteroid therapy is usually ineffective. The role of intravenous immunoglobulin therapy is unclear.

Mastaglia FL et al: Inflammatory myopathies: clinical, diagnostic and therapeutic aspects. Muscle Nerve 2003;27:407. [PMID: 12661042]

6. Mitochondrial Myopathies

The mitochondrial myopathies are a clinically diverse group of disorders that on pathologic examination of skeletal muscle with the modified Gomori stain show characteristic "ragged red fibers" containing accumulations of abnormal mitochondria. Patients may present with progressive external ophthalmoplegia or with limb weakness that is exacerbated or induced by activity. Other patients present with central neurologic dysfunction, eg, myoclonic epilepsy (myoclonic epilepsy, ragged red fiber syndrome, or MERRF), or the combination of myopathy, encephalopathy, lactic acidosis, and stroke-like episodes (MELAS). These disorders result from separate abnormalities of mitochondrial DNA. (See also Chapter 20.)

7. Myopathies Associated with Other Disorders

Myopathy may occur in association with chronic hypokalemia, any endocrinopathy, and in patients taking corticosteroids, chloroquine, colchicine, clofibrate, emetine, aminocaproic acid, lovastatin, bretylium tosylate, or drugs causing potassium depletion. Weakness is mainly proximal, and serum creatine kinase is typically normal, except in hypothyroidism and some of the toxic myopathies. Treatment is of the underlying cause. Myopathy also occurs with chronic alcoholism, whereas acute reversible muscle necrosis may occur shortly after acute alcohol intoxication. Inflammatory myopathy may occur in patients taking penicillamine; myotonia may be induced by clofibrate, and preexisting myotonia may be exacerbated or unmasked by depolarizing muscle relaxants (eg, suxamethonium), β-blockers (eg, propranolol), fenoterol, ritodrine and, possibly, certain diuretics.

PERIODIC PARALYSIS SYNDROME

Periodic paralysis may have a familial (dominant inheritance) basis. Episodes of flaccid weakness or paralysis occur, sometimes in association with abnormalities of the plasma potassium level. Strength is normal between attacks. **Hypokalemic periodic paralysis** is characterized by attacks that tend to occur on awakening, after exercise, or after a heavy meal and may last for several days. Patients should avoid excessive exertion. A low-carbohydrate and low-salt diet may help prevent attacks, as may acetazolamide, 250–750 mg/d. An ongoing attack may be aborted by potassium chloride given orally or by intravenous drip, provided the ECG can be monitored and renal function is satisfactory. In young Asian men, it is commonly associated with hyperthyroidism; treatment of the endocrine disorder then prevents recurrences. In **hyperkalemic periodic paralysis**, attacks also tend to occur after exercise but usually last for less than an hour. They may be terminated by intravenous calcium gluconate (1–2 g) or by intravenous diuretics (furosemide, 20–40 mg), glucose, or glucose and insulin; daily acetazolamide or chlorothiazide may prevent recurrences. Genetic linkage studies suggest that many families with this disorder have a defect in the sodium channel gene on the long arm of chromosome 17. **Normokalemic periodic paralysis** is similar clinically to the hyperkalemic variety, but the plasma potassium level remains normal during attacks; treatment is with acetazolamide.

Renner DR et al: Periodic paralyses and nondystrophic myotonias. Adv Neurol 2002;88:235. [PMID: 11908229]

Psychiatric Disorders

25

Stuart J. Eisendrath, MD, & Jonathan E. Lichtmacher, MD

■ PSYCHIATRIC ASSESSMENT

Psychiatric diagnosis rests upon the established principles of a thorough history and examination. All of the forces contributing to the individual's life situation must be identified, and this can be done only if the examination includes the history, mental status, medical conditions (including drugs), and pertinent social, cultural, and environmental factors impinging on the individual.

The examination of a psychiatric patient must include a complete medical history and physical examination (with emphasis on the neurologic examination) as well as all necessary laboratory and other special studies. Physical illness may frequently present as psychiatric disease, and vice versa. In many instances, the physical examination is completed by the primary care provider who is working with a psychiatrist.

Interview

Every psychiatric history should cover the following points: (1) complaint, from the patient's viewpoint; (2) the present illness, or the evolution of the symptoms; (3) neurovegetative signs such as libido, appetite, and sleep; (4) previous disorders and the nature and extent of their treatment; (5) the family history—important for genetic aspects and family influences; (6) the personal history—childhood development, adolescent adjustment, level of education, and adult coping patterns; (7) current life functioning, with attention to vocational, social, educational, and avocational areas; and (8) present or past use of alcohol and other drugs.

It is often essential to obtain additional information from the family. Observing interactions of the patient with significant others in the context of a family interview may give important diagnostic information and may even underscore the nature of the problem and suggest a therapeutic approach.

The formal mental status examination should be particularly detailed when there is any evidence or high risk of cognitive dysfunction. The mental status examination includes the following: (1) Appearance: Note unusual modes of dress, use of makeup, etc. (2) Activity and behavior: Gait, gestures, coordination of bodily movements, etc. (3) Affect: Outward manifestation of emotions such as depression, anger, elation, fear, resentment, or lack of emotional response. (4) Mood: The patient's report of feelings and observable emotional manifestations. (5) Speech: Coherence, spontaneity, articulation, hesitancy in answering, and duration of response. (6) Content of thought: Associations, preoccupations, obsessions, depersonalization, delusions, hallucinations, paranoid ideation, anger, fear, or unusual experiences; suicidal and homicidal ideation. (7) Thought process: Loose associations, flight of ideas, thought blocking, tangentiality, circumstantiality, perseveration, racing thought. (8) Cognition: (a) orientation to person, place, time, and circumstances; (b) remote and recent memory and recall; (c) calculations, digit retention (six forward is normal), serial sevens or threes; (d) general fund of knowledge (presidents, states, distances, events); (e) abstracting ability, often tested with common proverbs or with analogies and differences (eg, "How are a lie and a mistake the same, and how are they different?"); (f) ability to identify by naming, reading, and writing specified test names and objects; (g) ideomotor function, which combines understanding and the ability to perform a task (eg, "Show me how to throw a ball"); (h) ability to reproduce geometric constructions (eg, parallelogram, intersecting squares); and (i) right-left differentiation. (9) Judgment regarding commonsense problems such as what to do when one runs out of medicine. (10) Insight into the nature and extent of the current difficulty and its ramifications in the patient's daily life.

Formal cognitive screens can quantify impairments and point to the need for further evaluation. The Mini-Mental State Examination produces a numerical score with up to 30 points given for correct answers to questions (likely organic < 27 points) (Figure 25–1). Specific cognitive assessment must be performed, since many patients are able to cover a deficit in routine conversation.

Special Diagnostic Aids

Many tests and evaluation procedures are available that can be used to support and clarify initial diagnostic impressions.

A. PSYCHOLOGICAL TESTING

Testing by a psychologist may measure intelligence and cognitive functioning; provide information about personality, feelings, psychodynamics, and psychopathology; and help differentiate psychic problems from

COMPLETE IF INDICATED CLINICALLY
(Ask general question and then ask specific questions to the right.)

Orientation *(Score 1 for each correct; max = 10)*
Where are you?
    Name this place (building or hospital)
    What floor are you on now?
    What state are you in?
    What country are you in?
    (If not in a country, score correct if city is correct.)
    What city are you in (or near) now?
What is the date today?
    What year is it?
    What season is it?
    What month is it?
    What is the day of the week?
    What is the date today?

Registration *(Score 1 for each object correctly repeated; max = 3)*
    Name three objects (ball, flag, and tree) and have the patient repeat them.
(Say objects at about 1 word per second. If patient misses object, ask patient to repeat them after you until he/she learns them. Stop at 6 repeats.)

Attention and calculation *(Score 1 for each correct to 65; max = 5)*
    Subtract 7s from 100 in a serial fashion to 65
(Alternatively, subtract serial 3s from 20 or spell WORLD backwards.)

Recall *(Score 1 for each object recalled; max = 3)*
    Do you recall the names of the three objects?

Language (max = 8)
    Ask the patient to provide names of a watch and pen as you show them to him/her
        (Score 1 for each object correct; max = 2)
    Repeat "No ifs, ands, or buts."
        (Only one trial. Score 1 if correct; max = 1)
    Give the patient a piece of plain blank paper and say, "Take the paper in your right hand (1), fold it in half (2), and put it on the floor (3)."
        (Score 1 for each part done correctly; max = 3)
    Ask the patient to read and perform the following task written on paper: Close your eyes.
        (Score 1 if patient closes eyes; max = 1)
    Ask the patient to write a sentence on a piece of paper.
        (Score total of 1 if sentence has a subject, object and verb; max = 1)

Construction
    Ask patient to copy the two interlocking pentagons.
        (Score total of 1, if all 10 angles are present and the two angles intersect. Ignore tremor and rotation; max = 1)

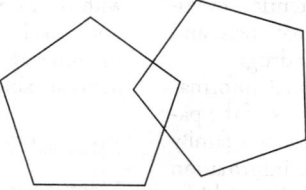

Total Score *(Maximum = 30, likely organic < 27)*

Figure 25–1. Mini-Mental State Exam. (Adapted from Folstein MF et al: Mini-mental state: a practical method for grading the cognitive state of patients for the clinician. J Psychiatr Res 1975;12:189.)

organic ones. The place of such tests is similar to that of other tests in medicine—helpful in diagnostic problems but may be an unnecessary expense if the diagnosis is clear.

1. Objective tests—These tests provide quantitative evaluation compared to standard norms.

a. Intelligence tests—The test most frequently used is the Wechsler Adult Intelligence Scale–Revised (WAIS-R). Intelligence tests often reveal more than IQ. The results, given expert interpretation, can quantify intellectual deterioration that has occurred.

b. Minnesota Multiphasic Personality Inventory (MMPI-2)—The MMPI-2 is an empirically based test of personality assessment. The patient's scores are interpreted in comparison with data about others with the same response pattern to assess psychopathologic changes.

c. Screening instruments—These tests include the Beck Depression Inventory, which quantifies degrees of dysphoria, and the Patient Health Questionnaire, which is a broad measure of the patient's concerns and assists with differential diagnosis.

d. Neuropsychological assessment—Such an assessment is made when an organic deficit is present but information on anatomic location and extent of dysfunction is required.

2. Projective tests—These tests are unstructured, so that the patient is forced to respond in ways that reflect fantasies and individual modes of adaptation. They are particularly useful in identifying psychotic disorders and unconscious motivations.

a. Rorschach Psychodiagnostics—This test utilizes ten inkblots to provide important information on psychodynamic themes and aberrations.

b. Thematic Apperception Test (TAT)—This test uses 20 pictures of people in different situations to assess areas of interpersonal conflicts.

B. NEUROLOGIC EVALUATION

Consultation is often necessary and may include specialized tests. Brain imaging is useful for detecting structural abnormalities in the patient who presents with a nondefinitive history and examination (eg, dissociative episodes, unusual psychotic episodes not explained by drug abuse, or an acute change in mental status). MRI is particularly useful in delineating lesions and identifying demyelinating and degenerative diseases (eg, Huntington's disease). Electroencephalography is particularly useful for the diagnosis of seizure disorders and in differentiating delirium from depression or dementia. Typically, delirium is associated with generalized electroencephalographic slowing, while depression and dementia do not have this change. Single photon emission computed tomography (SPECT), functional MRI (fMRI), and positron emission tomography (PET) provide tomographic images of brain activity. These imaging modalities are opening new understanding of brain functioning.

Formulation of the Diagnosis

A psychiatric diagnosis must be based on positive evidence accumulated by the above techniques. It must not be based simply on the exclusion of organic findings.

A thorough psychiatric evaluation has therapeutic as well as diagnostic value and should be expressed in ways best understood by the patient, family, and other clinicians.

Crum RM et al: Population-based norms for the Mini-Mental State Examination by age and educational level. JAMA 1993;269:2386. [PMID: 8479064]

Lowe B et al: Comparative validity of three screening questionnaires for DSM IV depressive disorders and physicians' diagnoses. J Affect Disord 2004;78:131. [PMID: 14706723]

■ TREATMENT APPROACHES

The approaches to treatment of psychiatric patients are, in a broad sense, similar to those in other branches of medicine. For example, the internist treating a patient with heart disease uses not only **medical** measures such as drugs and pacemakers but also **psychological** techniques to change attitudes and behaviors, **social** and **environmental** manipulation to mitigate deleterious influences, and **behavioral** techniques to change behavior patterns.

Regardless of the methods used, treatment must be directed toward an objective, ie, it must be **goal-oriented**. This usually involves (1) obtaining active cooperation on the part of the patient, (2) establishing reasonable goals and modifying the goal if failure occurs, (3) emphasizing positive behavior (goals) instead of symptom behavior (problems), (4) delineating the method, and (5) setting a time frame (which can be modified later).

The clinician must resist pressures for instantaneous results. In almost all cases, psychiatric treatment involves the active participation of the significant people in the patient's life. Time must be spent with the patient, but the frequency and duration of appointments are highly variable and should be adjusted to meet both the patient's psychological needs and financial restrictions. Adherence (collaboration) is the end product of many factors, the most important being clear communication, attention to cost, and simple dosage regimens when drugs are prescribed. The clinician can unwittingly promote chronic illness by prescribing medication inappropriately. The patient may come to believe that problems respond only to medication, and the more drugs prescribed, the stronger the misconception becomes.

Psychiatric Consultation

All clinicians are in an excellent position to meet their patients' emotional needs in an organized and competent way, referring to psychiatrists for consultation or for ongoing treatment of patients whose problems are considered beyond the expertise of the referring clinician. The most pressing problems involve evaluation of suicidal or assaultive potential and diagnostic differentiation in mood disorders and psychoses. Psychiatric problems associated with unusual psychopharmacologic therapy and with medications used in other branches of medicine may require pharmacologic consultation. When a psychiatric referral is made, it should be conducted like any other referral: in an open manner, with full explanation of the problem to the patient.

Hospitalization

Hospital care may be indicated when patients are too sick to care for themselves or when they present serious threats to themselves or others, when observation and diagnostic procedures are necessary, or when specific kinds of treatment such as complex medication trials or a hospital environment ("milieu therapy") are required. Symptoms calling for hospitalization include self-neglect, violent or bizarre behavior, suicidal risk, paranoid ideation or delusions, marked intellectual impairment, and poor judgment. The trend over recent years has been to admit patients to hospitals and treat them aggressively with the expectation of prompt discharge to the next appropriate level of care—day hospital, halfway house, outpatient therapy, etc. The decision to propose involuntary hospitalization should be taken only after weighing the potential benefits to the patient and the community against the individual's loss of autonomy.

The disadvantages of psychiatric hospitalization include decreased self-confidence as a result of needing hospitalization, the stigma of being a "psychiatric patient," possible increased dependency and regression, and the expense. Generally, there is no advantage to prolonged hospital stays for most psychiatric disorders. Partial hospitalization or "day" programs are providing many of the benefits of hospitalization without some of the disadvantages; in these programs, the patient attends daytime treatment but sleeps at home.

Bateman A et al: Health service utilization costs for borderline personality disorder patients treated with psychoanalytically oriented partial hospitalization versus general psychiatric care. Am J Psychiatry 2003;160:169. [PMID: 12505818]

Hedrick SC et al: Effectiveness of collaborative care depression treatment in Veterans' Affairs primary care. J Gen Intern Med 2003;18:9. [PMID: 12534758]

■ COMMON PSYCHIATRIC DISORDERS

STRESS & ADJUSTMENT DISORDERS (Situational Disorders)

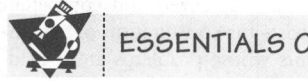

ESSENTIALS OF DIAGNOSIS

- Anxiety or depression clearly secondary to an identifiable stress.

- Subsequent symptoms of anxiety or depression commonly elicited by similar stress of lesser magnitude.

- Alcohol and other drugs are commonly used in self-treatment.

General Considerations

Stress exists when the adaptive capacity of the individual is overwhelmed by events. The event may be an insignificant one objectively considered, and even favorable changes (eg, promotion and transfer) requiring adaptive behavior can produce stress. For each individual, stress is subjectively defined, and the response to stress is a function of each person's personality and physiologic endowment.

Classification & Clinical Findings

Opinion differs about what events are most apt to produce stress reactions. The causes of stress are different at different ages—eg, in young adulthood, the sources of stress are found in the marriage or parent-child relationship, the employment relationship, and the struggle to achieve financial stability; in the middle years, the focus shifts to changing spousal relationships, problems with aging parents, and problems associated with having young adult offspring who themselves are encountering stressful situations; in old age, the principal concerns are apt to be retirement, loss of physical capacity, major personal losses, and thoughts of death.

An individual may react to stress by becoming anxious or depressed, by developing a physical symptom, by running away, having a drink, starting an affair, or in limitless other ways. Common subjective responses are fear (of repetition of the stress-inducing event), rage (at frustration), guilt (over aggressive impulses), and shame (over helplessness). Acute and reactivated stress may be manifested by restlessness, irritability, fatigue, increased startle reaction, and a feeling of tension. Inability to concentrate, sleep disturbances (insomnia, bad dreams), and somatic preoccupations often lead to self-medication, most commonly with alcohol or other central nervous system depressants. Maladaptive behavior in response to stress is called adjustment disorder, with the major symptom specified (eg, "adjustment disorder with depressed mood").

Posttraumatic stress disorder (PTSD)—included among the anxiety disorders in *DSM-IV*—is a syndrome characterized by "reexperiencing" a traumatic event (eg, rape, severe burns, military combat) and decreased responsiveness and avoidance of current events associated with the trauma. Patients with PTSD experience physiologic hyperarousal, including startle reactions, intrusive thoughts, illusions, overgeneralized associations, sleep problems, nightmares, dreams about the precipitating event, impulsivity, difficulties in concentration, and hyperalertness. The symptoms may be precipitated or exacerbated by events that are a reminder of the original stress. Symptoms frequently arise after a long latency period (eg, child abuse can result in later-onset posttraumatic stress syndrome). The sooner therapy is initiated after the trauma, the better the prognosis. Therapy at that time should be brief and simple (once in a safe environment), expecting quick recovery and promoting a sense of mastery over the traumatic event.

Treatment initiated later, when symptoms have crystallized, includes programs for cessation of alcohol and other drug abuse, group and individual psychotherapy, and improved social support systems. The therapeutic approach is to facilitate the normal recovery that was blocked at the time of the trauma.

Differential Diagnosis

Adjustment disorders must be distinguished from anxiety disorders, affective disorders, and personality disorders exacerbated by stress and from somatic disorders with psychic overlay.

Treatment

A. BEHAVIORAL

Stress reduction techniques include immediate symptom reduction (eg, rebreathing in a bag for hyperventilation) or early recognition and removal from a stress source before full-blown symptoms appear. It is often helpful for the patient to keep a daily log of stress precipitators, responses, and alleviators. Relaxation and exercise techniques are also helpful in reducing the reaction to stressful events.

B. SOCIAL

The stress reactions of life crisis problems are—more than any other category—a function of psychosocial upheaval, and patients frequently present with somatic symptoms. While it is not easy for the patient to make necessary changes (or they would have been made long ago), it is important for the therapist to establish the framework of the problem, since the patient's denial system may obscure the issues. Clarifying the problem allows the patient to begin viewing it within the proper context and facilitates the sometimes difficult decisions the patient eventually must make (eg, change of job or relocation of adult-dependent offspring).

C. PSYCHOLOGICAL

Prolonged in-depth psychotherapy is seldom necessary in cases of isolated stress response or adjustment disorder. Supportive psychotherapy (see above) with an emphasis on the here and now and strengthening of existing defenses is a helpful approach so that time and the patient's own resiliency can restore the previous level of function. In posttraumatic stress syndromes, psychological debriefing in a single session, once a mainstay in prevention of PTSD, is now considered to be ineffective and possibly harmful. Posttraumatic stress syndromes respond to interventions that help patients integrate the event in an adaptive way with some sense of mastery in having survived the trauma. Early cognitive behavioral therapy has been shown to speed recovery. Marital problems are a major area of concern, and it is important that the clinician have available a dependable referral source when marriage counseling is indicated.

D. MEDICAL

Judicious use of sedatives (eg, lorazepam, 1–2 mg orally daily) for a limited time and as part of an overall treatment plan can provide relief from acute anxiety symptoms. Problems arise when the situation becomes chronic through inappropriate treatment or when the treatment approach supports the development of chronicity.

In PTSD, early treatment of anxious arousal with β-blockers (eg, propranolol, 80–160 mg daily) may lessen the peripheral symptoms of anxiety (eg, tremors, palpitations) and help prevent development of the disorder; however, research in this area is preliminary. Antidepressant drugs—particularly selective serotonin reuptake inhibitors (SSRIs)—in full dosage are helpful in ameliorating depression, panic attacks, sleep disruption, and startle responses in chronic PTSD. Sertraline and paroxetine are approved by the US Food and Drug Administration (FDA) for this purpose. Antiseizure medications such as carbamazepine (400–800 mg daily) will often mitigate impulsivity and difficulty with anger management. Benzodiazepines such as clonazepam (1–4 mg daily) will reduce anxiety and panic attacks when used in adequate dosage, but dependency problems are a concern, particularly when the patient has had such problems in the past.

Prognosis

Return to satisfactory function after a short period is part of the clinical picture of this syndrome. Resolution may be delayed if others' responses to the patient's difficulties are thoughtlessly harmful or if the secondary gains outweigh the advantages of recovery. The longer the symptoms persist, the worse the prognosis.

Ehlers A et al: Early psychological interventions for survivors of trauma: a review. Biol Psychiatry 2003;53:817. [PMID: 12725974]

Schoenfeld FB et al: Current concepts in pharmacotherapy for posttraumatic stress disorder. Psychiatr Serv 2004;55:519. [PMID: 15128960]

Vaiva G et al: Immediate treatment with propranolol decreases posttraumatic stress disorder two months after trauma. Biol Psychiatry 2003;54:947. [PMID: 14573324]

ANXIETY DISORDERS & DISSOCIATIVE DISORDERS

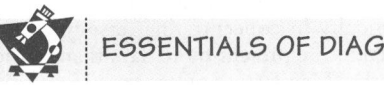 ESSENTIALS OF DIAGNOSIS

- *Overt anxiety or an overt manifestation of a defense mechanism (such as a phobia), or both.*

- Not limited to an adjustment disorder.
- Somatic symptoms referable to the autonomic nervous system or to a specific organ system (eg, dyspnea, palpitations, paresthesias).
- Not a result of physical disorders, psychiatric conditions (eg, schizophrenia), or drug abuse (eg, cocaine).

General Considerations

Stress, fear, and anxiety all tend to be interactive. The principal components of anxiety are **psychological** (tension, fears, difficulty in concentration, apprehension) and **somatic** (tachycardia, hyperventilation, palpitations, tremor, sweating). Other organ systems (eg, gastrointestinal) may be involved in multiple-system complaints. Fatigue and sleep disturbances are common. Sympathomimetic symptoms of anxiety are both a response to a central nervous system state and a reinforcement of further anxiety. Anxiety can become self-generating, since the symptoms reinforce the reaction, causing it to spiral. This is often the case when the anxiety is an epiphenomenon of other medical or psychiatric disorders.

Anxiety may be free-floating, resulting in acute anxiety attacks, occasionally becoming chronic. When one or several defense mechanisms (see above) are functioning, the consequences are well-known problems such as phobias, conversion reactions, dissociative states, obsessions, and compulsions. Lack of structure is frequently a contributing factor, as noted in those people who have "Sunday neuroses." They do well during the week with a planned work schedule but cannot tolerate the unstructured weekend. Planned-time activities tend to bind anxiety, and many people have increased difficulties when this is lost, as in retirement.

Some believe that various manifestations of anxiety are not a result of unconscious conflicts but are "habits"—persistent patterns of nonadaptive behavior acquired by learning. The "habits," being nonadaptive, are unsatisfactory ways of dealing with life's problems—hence the resultant anxiety. Help is sought only when the anxiety becomes too painful. Exogenous factors such as stimulants (eg, caffeine, cocaine) must be considered as a contributing factor.

Clinical Findings

A. GENERALIZED ANXIETY DISORDER

This is the most common of the clinically significant anxiety disorders. Initial manifestations appear at age 20–35 years, and there is a slight predominance in women. The anxiety symptoms of apprehension, worry, irritability, difficulty in concentrating, insomnia, and somatic complaints are present more days than not for at least 6 months. Manifestations can include cardiac (eg, tachycardia, increased blood pressure), gastrointes-

tinal (eg, increased acidity, nausea, epigastric pain), and neurologic (eg, headache, near-syncope) systems. The focus of the anxiety may be a number of everyday activities.

B. PANIC DISORDER

This is characterized by short-lived, recurrent, unpredictable episodes of intense anxiety accompanied by marked physiologic manifestations. Agoraphobia, fear of being in places where escape is difficult, such as open spaces or public places, may be present. Distressing symptoms and signs such as dyspnea, tachycardia, palpitations, headaches, dizziness, paresthesias, choking, smothering feelings, nausea, and bloating are associated with feelings of impending doom (alarm response). Recurrent sleep panic attacks (not nightmares) occur in about 30% of panic disorders. Anticipatory anxiety develops in all these patients and further constricts their daily lives. Panic disorder tends to be familial, with onset usually under age 25; it affects 3–5% of the population, and the female-to-male ratio is 2:1. The premenstrual period is one of heightened vulnerability. Patients frequently undergo emergency medical evaluations (eg, for "heart attacks" or "hypoglycemia") before the correct diagnosis is made. Gastrointestinal symptoms are especially common, occurring in about one-third of cases. Myocardial infarction, pheochromocytoma, hyperthyroidism, and various recreational drug reactions can mimic panic disorder. Mitral valve prolapse may be present but is not usually a significant factor. Patients who have recurrent panic disorder often become **demoralized, hypochondriacal, agoraphobic**, and **depressed**. These individuals are at increased risk for major depression and the suicide attempts associated with that disorder. Alcohol abuse (about 20%) results from self-treatment and is not infrequently combined with dependence on sedatives. Some patients have atypical panic attacks associated with seizure-like symptoms that often include psychosensory phenomena (a history of stimulant abuse often emerges). About 25% of panic disorder patients also have obsessive-compulsive disorder (OCD).

C. OBSESSIVE-COMPULSIVE DISORDER

In the obsessive-compulsive reaction, the irrational idea or the impulse persistently intrudes into awareness. Obsessions (constantly recurring thoughts such as fears of exposure to germs) and compulsions (repetitive actions such as washing the hands many times) are recognized by the individual as absurd and are resisted, but anxiety is alleviated only by ritualistic performance of the action or by deliberate contemplation of the intruding idea or emotion. Many patients do not mention the symptoms and must be asked about them. These patients are usually predictable, orderly, conscientious, and intelligent—traits that are seen in many compulsive behaviors such as food binging and purging and compulsive running. There is an overlapping of OCD and other behaviors ("OCD spectrum"), including tics, trichotillomania (hair pulling), onychophagia (nail biting), hypochondriasis, Tourette's syndrome, and eating disorders (see Chapter 29). The 2–3% incidence of OCD in the general population is much higher than was previously recognized. In addition, there is a high comorbidity of OCD and major depression; two-thirds of OCD patients will develop major depression during their lifetime. Male to female ratios are similar, with the highest rates occurring in the young, divorced, separated, and unemployed (all high-stress categories). Neurologic abnormalities of fine motor coordination and involuntary movements are common. Under extreme stress, these patients sometimes exhibit paranoid and delusional behaviors, often associated with depression, and can mimic schizophrenia.

D. Phobic Disorder

Phobic ideation can be considered a mechanism of "displacement" in which patients transfer feelings of anxiety from their true object to one that can be avoided. However, since phobias are ineffective defense mechanisms, there tends to be an increase in their scope, intensity, and number. Social phobias are global or specific; in the former, all social situations are poorly tolerated, while the latter group includes performance anxiety or well-delineated phobias. Agoraphobia (fear of open places and public areas) is frequently associated with severe panic attacks, and it often develops in early adult life, making a normal lifestyle difficult.

E. Dissociative Disorder

Fugue (the sudden, unexpected travel away from one's home with inability to recall one's past), amnesia, somnambulism, dissociative identity disorder (multiple personality disorder), and depersonalization are all dissociative states. The reaction is precipitated by emotional crisis. The symptom produces anxiety reduction and a temporary solution of the crisis. Mechanisms include repression and isolation as well as particularly limited concentration as seen in hypnotic states. Dissociative symptoms are similar in many ways to symptoms seen in patients with temporal lobe dysfunction.

Treatment

In all cases, underlying medical disorders must be ruled out (eg, cardiovascular, endocrine, respiratory, and neurologic disorders and substance-related syndromes, both intoxication and withdrawal states). These and other disorders can coexist with panic disorder.

A. Medical

1. Generalized anxiety—Benzodiazepines are the anxiolytics of choice in the acute management of generalized anxiety (Table 25–1). They are almost immediately effective. Antidepressants can be efficacious for the long-term treatment of generalized anxiety disorder, panic disorder, social phobia, and OCD.

All of the benzodiazepines may be given orally, and several are available in parenteral formulations. Benzo-

diazepines such as lorazepam are absorbed rapidly when given intramuscularly. In psychiatric disorders, the benzodiazepines are usually given orally; in controlled medical environments (eg, the ICU), where the rapid onset of respiratory depression can be assessed, they are often given intravenously. Onset of action is a function of the rate of absorption (related to lipophilic property) and varies, with diazepam and clorazepate being the most rapidly absorbed. This characteristic, along with high lipid solubility, may explain the popularity of diazepam. In the average case of anxiety, diazepam, 5–10 mg orally every 6–8 hours as needed, is a reasonable starting regimen.

The duration of action of the benzodiazepines varies as a function of the active metabolites they produce. Benzodiazepines such as lorazepam do not produce active metabolites and have intermediate half-lives of 10–20 hours, characteristics useful in treating elderly patients. Ultra-short-acting agents such as triazolam have half-lives of 1–3 hours and may lead to rebound withdrawal anxiety. Longer-acting benzodiazepines such as flurazepam and diazepam produce active metabolites, have half-lives of 20–120 hours, and should be avoided in the elderly. Since people vary widely in their response and since the drugs are long-lasting, the dosage must be individualized. Once this is established, an adequate dose early in the course of symptom development will obviate the need for "pill popping," which contributes to dependency problems. Panic disorder does not usually respond to benzodiazepines other than clonazepam and alprazolam. Those high-potency benzodiazepines and the antidepressants are most commonly used for panic disorder. Notably, alprazolam has a relatively short half-life and over time can lead to interdose rebound anxiety, although the extended release form is available and obviates some of this difficulty.

Whether the indications for benzodiazepines are anxiety or insomnia, the drugs should be used judiciously. The longer-acting benzodiazepines are used for the treatment of alcohol withdrawal and anxiety symptoms; the intermediate drugs are useful as sedatives for insomnia (eg, lorazepam), while short-acting agents (eg, midazolam) are used for medical procedures such as endoscopy.

The side effects of all the benzodiazepine antianxiety agents are patient and dose dependent. As the dosage exceeds the levels necessary for sedation, the side effects include disinhibition, ataxia, dysarthria, nystagmus, and errors of commission. (The patient should be told not to operate machinery until he or she is well stabilized without side effects.)

Paradoxical agitation, anxiety, psychosis, confusion, mood lability, and anterograde amnesia have been reported, particularly with the shorter-acting benzodiazepines. These agents produce cumulative clinical effects with repeated dosage (especially if the patient has not had time to metabolize the previous dose), additive effects when given with other classes of sedatives or alcohol (many apparently "accidental" deaths are the result of concomitant use of sedatives and alcohol), and resid-

Table 25–1. Commonly used antianxiety and hypnotic agents.

Drug	Usual Daily Oral Dose	Usual Daily Maximum Dose	Cost for 30 Days Treatment Based on Maximum Dosage[1]
Benzodiazepines (used for anxiety)			
Alprazolam (Xanax)[2]	0.5 mg	4 mg	$117.60
Chlordiazepoxide (Librium)[3]	10–20 mg	100 mg	$40.80
Clonazepam (Klonopin)[3]	1–2 mg	10 mg	$177.00
Clorazepate (Tranxene)[3]	15–30 mg	60 mg	$260.40
Diazepam (Valium)[3]	5–15 mg	30 mg	$27.90
Lorazepam (Ativan)[2]	2–4 mg	4 mg	$76.80
Oxazepam (Serax)[2]	10–30 mg	60 mg	$98.40
Benzodiazepines (used for sleep)			
Estazolam (Prosom)[2]	1 mg	2 mg	$29.70
Flurazepam (Dalmane)[3]	15 mg	30 mg	$10.50
Midazolam (Versed IV)[4]	5 mg IV		$3.58/dose
Quazepam (Doral)[3]	7.5 mg	15 mg	$117.90
Temazepam (Restoril)[2]	15 mg	30 mg	$26.40
Triazolam (Halcion)[5]	0.125 mg	0.25 mg	$20.24
Miscellaneous (used for anxiety)			
Buspirone (Buspar)[2]	10–30 mg	60 mg	$218.10
Phenobarbital[3]	15–30 mg	90 mg	$2.10
Miscellaneous (used for sleep)			
Chloral hydrate (Noctec)[2]	500	1000 mg	$8.39
Eszopiclone (Lunesta)[5]	2–3 mg	3 mg	$111.00
Hydroxyzine (Vistaril)[2]	50 mg	100 mg	$66.60
Zolpidem (Ambien)[5]	5–10 mg	10 mg	$111.90
Zaleplon (Sonata)[6]	5–10 mg	10 mg	$91.50

[1]Average wholesale price (AWP, for AB-rated generic when available) for quantity listed. Source: *Red Book Update*, Vol. 25, No. 5, May 2006. AWP may not accurately represent the actual pharmacy cost because wide contractual variations exist among institutions.
[2]Intermediate physical half-life (10–20 hours).
[3]Long physical half-life (> 20 hours).
[4]Intravenously for procedures.
[5]Short physical half-life (1–6 hours).
[6]Short physical half-life (about 1 hour).

ual effects after termination of treatment (particularly in the case of drugs that undergo slow biotransformation).

Overdosage results in respiratory depression, hypotension, shock syndrome, coma, and death. Flumazenil, a benzodiazepine antagonist, is effective in overdosage. Overdosage (see Chapter 39) and withdrawal states are medical emergencies. Serious side effects of chronic excessive dosage are development of tolerance, resulting in increasing dose requirements, and physiologic dependence, resulting in withdrawal symptoms similar in appearance to alcohol and barbiturate withdrawal (withdrawal effects must be distinguished from reemergent anxiety). Abrupt withdrawal of sedative drugs may cause serious and even fatal convulsive seizures. Psychosis, delirium, and autonomic dysfunction have also been described. Both duration of action and duration of exposure are major factors.

Common withdrawal symptoms after low to moderate daily use of benzodiazepines are classified as somatic (disturbed sleep, tremor, nausea, muscle aches), psychological (anxiety, poor concentration, irritability, mild depression), or perceptual (poor coordination, mild paranoia, mild confusion). The presentation of symptoms will vary depending on the half-life of the drug. There are no significant side effects on organ systems other than the brain, and the drugs are safe in most medical conditions. Benzodiazepine interactions with other drugs are listed in Table 25–2.

Antidepressants are the first-line medications for sustained treatment of generalized anxiety disorder, having the advantage of not causing serious physiologic dependency problems. At initiation of treatment, antidepressants can themselves be anxiogenic—thus, an initial dose, in conjunction with short-term treatment with a benzo-

Table 25–2. Benzodiazepine interactions with other drugs.

Drug	Effects
Antacids	Decreased absorption of benzodiazepines
Cimetidine	Increased half-life of diazepam and triazolam
Contraceptives	Increased levels of diazepam and triazolam
Digoxin	Alprazolam and diazepam raise digoxin level
Disulfiram	Increased duration of action of sedatives
Isoniazid	Increased plasma diazepam
Levodopa	Inhibition of antiparkinsonism effect
Propoxyphene	Impaired clearance of diazepam
Rifampin	Decreased plasma diazepam
Warfarin	Decreased prothrombin time

diazepine, is often indicated. Venlafaxine (a sustained-release serotonin and norepinephrine reuptake inhibitor) is FDA-approved for the treatment of generalized anxiety disorder in usual antidepressant doses (75–225 mg). Initial daily dosing should start low (37.5–75 mg) and be titrated upward as needed. SSRIs, such as paroxetine, are also used. Similarly, buspirone, sometimes used as an augmenting agent in the treatment of depression and compulsive behaviors, is also effective for generalized anxiety. Buspirone is usually given in a dosage of 15–60 mg/d in three divided doses. Higher doses tend to be counterproductive and produce gastrointestinal symptoms and dizziness. There is a 2- to 4-week delay before antidepressants and buspirone take effect, and patients require education regarding this lag. Sleep is sometimes negatively affected. β-Blockers such as propranolol may help reduce peripheral somatic symptoms. Alcohol is the most frequently self-administered drug and should be interdicted. The highly addicting drugs with a narrow margin of safety such as glutethimide, ethchlorvynol, methprylon, meprobamate, and the barbiturates (with the exception of phenobarbital) should be avoided. Phenobarbital, in addition to its anticonvulsant properties, is a reasonably safe and very inexpensive sedative but has the disadvantage of causing hepatic microsomal enzyme stimulation (not the case with benzodiazepines), which markedly reduces its usefulness if any other relevant medications are being used by the patient.

2. Panic attacks—Panic attacks may be treated in several ways. A sublingual dose of lorazepam (0.5–2 mg) or alprazolam (0.5–1 mg) is often effective for urgent treatment. For sustained treatment, SSRIs are the initial drugs of choice (adequate blood levels will require dosages similar to those used in the treatment of depression). For example, sertraline starting at 25 mg/d and increased after 1 week to 50 mg/d may be effective. Because of initial agitation in response to antidepressants, doses should start low and be very gradually increased. High-potency benzodiazepines may be used

for symptomatic treatment as the antidepressant dose is titrated upward. Clonazepam (1–6 mg/d orally) and alprazolam (0.5–6 mg/d orally) are effective alternatives to antidepressants. Both drugs may produce marked withdrawal if stopped abruptly and should always be tapered. Because of chronicity of the disorders and the problem of dependency with benzodiazepine drugs, it is generally desirable to use antidepressant drugs as the principal pharmacologic approach. Antidepressants have been used in conjunction with β-blockers in resistant cases. Propranolol (40–160 mg/d orally) can mute the peripheral symptoms of anxiety without significantly affecting motor and cognitive performance. They block symptoms mediated by sympathetic stimulation (eg, palpitations, tremulousness) but not nonadrenergic symptoms (eg, diarrhea, muscle tension). Contrary to current belief, they usually do not cause depression as a side effect and can be used cautiously in patients with depression. Valproate has been found to be as effective in panic disorder as the antidepressants and is another useful alternative.

3. Phobic disorder—Phobic disorder may be part of the panic disorder and is treated within that framework. Global social phobias may be treated with SSRIs, such as paroxetine, sertraline, and fluvoxamine, or monoamine oxidase (MAO) inhibitors in the same dosage as used for depression. Gabapentin, an anticonvulsant with anxiolytic properties, may be an alternative to antidepressants in the treatment of social phobia in a dosage of 300–3600 mg/d, depending on response versus sedation. Specific phobias such as performance anxiety may respond to moderate doses of β-blockers, such as propranolol, 20–40 mg 1 hour prior to exposure. A sustained effect is often not obtained with drugs alone; a combination of drugs, behavioral techniques, and cognitive psychotherapy is most effective. If there is any indication of seizure-like phenomena, carbamazepine or valproic acid should be considered.

4. Obsessive-compulsive disorder—OCD responds to serotonergic drugs in about 60% of cases and usually requires a longer response time than for depression (up to 12 weeks). Clomipramine has proved effective in doses equivalent to those used for depression. Fluoxetine (an SSRI drug) has been widely used in this disorder but in doses higher than those used in depression (up to 60–80 mg/d). The other SSRI drugs such as sertraline, paroxetine, and fluvoxamine are being used with comparable efficacy, each with its own side-effect profile. Buspirone in doses of 15–60 mg/d appears to be effective primarily as an anti-obsessional augmenting agent for the SSRI drugs. Psychosurgery has a limited place in selected cases of severe unremitting OCD. The stereotactic techniques now being used, including modified cingulotomy, are great improvements over the crude methods of the past.

B. BEHAVIORAL

Behavioral approaches are widely used in various anxiety disorders, often in conjunction with medication. Any of the behavioral techniques (see above) can be used beneficially in altering the contingencies (precipitating factors or rewards) supporting any anxiety-provoking behavior. Relaxation techniques can sometimes be helpful in reducing anxiety. Desensitization, by exposing the patient to graded doses of a phobic object or situation, is an effective technique and one that the patient can practice outside the therapy session. Emotive imagery, wherein the patient imagines the anxiety-provoking situation while at the same time learning to relax, helps decrease the anxiety when the patient faces the real-life situation. Physiologic symptoms in panic attacks respond well to relaxation training. Exposure techniques with response prevention are useful for OCD.

C. PSYCHOLOGICAL

Cognitive behavioral approaches have been effective in treatment of panic disorders, phobias, and OCD when erroneous beliefs need correction. These approaches share a common technique of exposing the individual to the feared object or situation. The combination of medical and cognitive behavioral therapy is more effective than either alone. Group therapy is the treatment of choice when the anxiety is clearly a function of the patient's difficulties in dealing with others, and if these other people are part of the family, it is appropriate to include them and initiate family or couples therapy.

D. SOCIAL

Peer support groups for panic disorder and agoraphobia have been particularly helpful. Social modification may require measures such as family counseling to aid acceptance of the patient's symptoms and avoid counterproductive behavior in behavioral training. Any help in maintaining the social structure is anxiety-alleviating, and work, school, and social activities should be maintained. School and vocational counseling may be provided by professionals, who often need help from the clinician in defining the patient's limitations.

Prognosis

Anxiety disorders are usually of longstanding and may be quite difficult to treat. All can be relieved to varying degrees with medications and behavioral techniques. The prognosis is much better if the commonly observed anxiety-panic-phobia-depression cycle can be broken with a combination of the therapeutic interventions discussed above.

Kaplan A et al: A review of pharmacologic treatments for obsessive-compulsive disorder. Psychiatr Serv 2003;54:1111. [PMID: 12883138]

Leopola U et al: Sertraline versus imipramine treatment of comorbid panic disorder and major depressive disorder. J Clin Psychiatry 2003;64:654. [PMID: 12823079]

Rickels K et al: Paroxetine treatment of generalized anxiety disorder: a double blind, placebo controlled study. Am J Psychiatry 2003;160:749. [PMID: 12668365]

SOMATOFORM DISORDERS (Abnormal Illness Behaviors)

 ESSENTIALS OF DIAGNOSIS

- Physical symptoms may involve one or more organ systems and are not intentional.
- Subjective complaints exceed objective findings.
- Correlations of symptom development and psychosocial stresses.
- Combination of biogenetic and developmental patterns.

General Considerations

A major source of diagnostic confusion in medicine has been to assume cause-and-effect relationships when parallel conditions exist. This problem is particularly vexing in situations where the individual exhibits psychosocial distress that could well be secondary to a chronic illness but has been assumed to be primary and causative. An example is the person with a chronic bowel disease who becomes querulous and demanding. Is this behavior a result of problems of coping with a chronic disease, or is it a personality pattern that causes the gastrointestinal problem?

Vulnerability in one or more organ systems and exposure to family members with somatization problems play a major role in the development of particular symptoms, and the "functional" versus "organic" dichotomy is a hindrance to good treatment. Clinicians should suspect psychiatric disorders in a number of conditions. For example, 45% of patients complaining of palpitations had lifetime psychiatric diagnoses including generalized anxiety, depression, panic, and somatization disorders. Similarly, 33–44% of patients who undergo coronary angiography for chest pain but have negative results have been found to have panic disorder.

In any patient presenting with a condition judged to be somatoform, depression must be considered in the diagnosis.

Clinical Findings

A. CONVERSION DISORDER

"Conversion" (formerly "hysterical conversion") of psychic conflict into physical symptoms in parts of the body innervated by the sensorimotor system (eg, paralysis, aphonia) is a disorder that is more common in individuals from lower socioeconomic classes and certain cultures. The defense mechanisms used in this condition are repression (a barring from consciousness) and isolation (a splitting of the affect from the idea). The somatic manifestation that takes the place of anxiety is typically paralysis, and in some instances the organ dysfunction may have symbolic meaning (eg, arm paralysis in marked anger). Pseudoepileptic ("hysterical") seizures are often difficult to differentiate from intoxication states or panic attacks. Retention of consciousness, random flailing with asynchronous movements of the right and left sides, and resistance to having the nose and mouth pinched closed during the attack all point toward a pseudoepileptic event. Electroencephalography, particularly in a video-EEG assessment unit, during the attack is the most helpful diagnostic aid in excluding genuine seizure states. Serum prolactin levels rise abruptly in the postictal state only in true epilepsy. La belle indifférence (an unconcerned affect) is not a significant identifying characteristic, as commonly believed. Important criteria in diagnosis include a history of conversion or somatization disorder, modeling the symptom after someone else who had a similar presentation, a serious precipitating emotional event, associated psychopathology (eg, depression, schizophrenia, personality disorders), a temporal correlation between the precipitating event and the symptom, and a temporary "solving of the problem" by the conversion. It is important to identify physical disorders with unusual presentations (eg, multiple sclerosis).

B. SOMATIZATION DISORDER (BRIQUET'S SYNDROME, HYSTERIA)

This is characterized by multiple physical complaints referable to several organ systems. Anxiety, panic disorder, and depression are often present, and **major depression** is an important consideration in the differential diagnosis. There is a significant relationship (20%) to a lifetime history of panic-agoraphobia-depression. It usually occurs before age 30 and is ten times more common in women. Polysurgery is often a feature of the history. Preoccupation with medical and surgical therapy becomes a lifestyle that excludes most other activities. The symptoms are a reflection of maladaptive coping techniques and reactivity of the particular organ system. There is often evidence of longstanding somatic symptoms (particularly dysmenorrhea, a lump in the throat, vomiting, shortness of breath, burning in the sex organs, painful extremities, and amnesia), often with a history of similar organ system involvement in other family members. Multiple symptoms that constantly change and inability of more than three doctors to make a diagnosis are strong clues to the problem.

C. PAIN DISORDER ASSOCIATED WITH PSYCHOLOGICAL FACTORS (FORMERLY SOMATOFORM PAIN DISORDER)

This involves a long history of complaints of severe pain not consonant with anatomic and clinical signs. This diagnosis must not be one of exclusion and should be made only after extended evaluation has established a clear correlation of psychogenic factors with exacerbations and remissions of complaints.

D. HYPOCHONDRIASIS

This is a fear of disease and preoccupation with the body, with perceptual amplification and heightened re-

sponsiveness. A process of social learning is usually involved, frequently with a role model who was a member of the family and may be a part of the underlying psychodynamic causation. It is common in panic disorders.

E. FACTITIOUS DISORDERS

These disorders, in which symptom production is intentional, are not somatoform conditions in that symptoms are produced consciously, in contrast to the unconscious process of the above conditions. They are characterized by self-induced symptoms or false physical and laboratory findings for the purpose of deceiving clinicians or other hospital personnel. The deceptions may involve self-mutilation, fever, hemorrhage, hypoglycemia, seizures, and an almost endless variety of manifestations—often presented in an exaggerated and dramatic fashion (Munchausen syndrome). "Munchausen by proxy" is the term used when a parent creates an illness in a child so the adult (usually the mother) can maintain a relationship with clinicians. The duplicity may be either simple or extremely complex and difficult to recognize. The patients are frequently connected in some way with the health professions; they are often migratory; and there is no apparent external motivation other than achieving the patient role.

Complications

A poor doctor-patient relationship, with iatrogenic disorders and "doctor shopping," tends to exacerbate the problem. Sedative and analgesic dependency is the most common iatrogenic complication.

Treatment

A. MEDICAL

Medical support with careful attention to building a therapeutic practitioner-patient relationship is the mainstay of treatment. It must be accepted that the patient's distress is real. Every problem not found to have an organic basis is not necessarily a mental disease. Diligent attempts should be made to relate symptoms to adverse developments in the patient's life. It may be useful to have the patient keep a meticulous diary, paying particular attention to various pertinent factors evident in the history. Regular, frequent, short appointments that are not symptom-contingent may be helpful. Drugs (frequently abused) should not be prescribed to replace appointments. One person should be the primary clinician, and consultants should be used mainly for evaluation. An empathic, realistic, optimistic approach must be maintained in the face of the expected ups and downs. Ongoing reevaluation is necessary, since somatization can coexist with a concurrent physical illness.

B. PSYCHOLOGICAL

Psychological approaches can be used by the primary clinician when it is clear that the patient is ready to make some changes in lifestyle in order to achieve symptomatic relief. This is often best approached on a here-and-now basis and oriented toward pragmatic changes rather than an exploration of early experiences that the patient frequently fails to relate to current distress. Group therapy with other individuals who have similar problems is sometimes of value to improve coping, allow ventilation, and focus on interpersonal adjustment. Hypnosis or lorazepam interviews used early are helpful in resolving conversion disorders. If the primary clinician has been working with the patient on psychological problems related to the physical illness, the groundwork is often laid for successful psychiatric referral.

For patients who have been identified as having a factitious disorder, early psychiatric consultation is indicated. There are two main treatment strategies for these patients. One consists of a conjoint confrontation of the patient by both the primary clinician and the psychiatrist. The patient's disorder is portrayed as a cry for help, and psychiatric treatment is recommended. The second approach avoids direct confrontation and attempts to provide a face-saving way to relinquish the symptom without overt disclosure of the disorder's origin. Techniques such as biofeedback and self-hypnosis may foster recovery using this strategy. Another face-saving approach is to use a double bind with the patient. For example, the patient is told there are two possible diagnoses: (1) an organic disease that should respond to the next medical intervention (usually modest and noninvasive), or (2) factitious disorder for which the patient will need psychiatric treatment. Given these options, many patients will choose to recover and not have to admit the origin of their problem.

C. BEHAVIORAL

Behavioral therapy is probably best exemplified by biofeedback techniques. In biofeedback, the particular abnormality (eg, increased peristalsis) must be recognized and monitored by the patient and therapist (eg, by an electronic stethoscope to amplify the sounds). This is immediate feedback, and after learning to recognize it, the patient can then learn to identify any change thus produced (eg, a decrease in bowel sounds) and so become a conscious originator of the feedback instead of a passive recipient. Relief of the symptom operantly conditions the patient to utilize the maneuver that relieves symptoms (eg, relaxation causing a decrease in bowel sounds). With emphasis on this type of learning, the patient is able to identify symptoms early and initiate the countermaneuvers, thus decreasing the symptomatic problem. Migrainoid and tension headaches have been particularly responsive to biofeedback methods.

D. SOCIAL

Social endeavors include family, work, and other interpersonal activity. Family members should come for some appointments with the patient so they can learn how best to live with the patient. This is particularly important in treatment of somatization and pain dis-

orders. Peer support groups provide a climate for encouraging the patient to accept and live with the problem. Ongoing communication with the employer may be necessary to encourage long-term continued interest in the employee. Employers can become just as discouraged as clinicians in dealing with employees who have chronic problems.

Prognosis

The prognosis is much better if the primary clinician is able to intervene early before the situation has deteriorated. After the problem has crystallized into chronicity, it is very difficult to effect change.

Krahn LE et al: Patients who strive to be ill: factitious disorder with physical symptoms. Am J Psychiatry 2003;160:1163. [PMID: 12777276]

Yeung A et al: Somatoform disorders. West J Med 2002;176:253. [PMID: 12208832]

CHRONIC PAIN DISORDERS

ESSENTIALS OF DIAGNOSIS

- *Chronic complaints of pain.*
- *Symptoms frequently exceed signs.*
- *Minimal relief with standard treatment.*
- *History of having seen many clinicians.*
- *Frequent use of several nonspecific medications.*

General Considerations

A problem in the management of pain is the lack of distinction between acute and chronic pain syndromes. Most clinicians are adept at dealing with acute pain problems but have difficulty handling the patient with a chronic pain disorder. This type of patient frequently takes too many medications, stays in bed a great deal, has seen many clinicians, has lost skills, and experiences little joy in either work or play. All relationships suffer (including those with clinicians), and life becomes a constant search for succor. The search results in complex clinician-patient relationships that usually include many drug trials, particularly sedatives, with adverse consequences (eg, irritability, depressed mood) related to long-term use. Treatment failures provoke angry responses and depression from both the patient and the clinician, and the pain syndrome is exacerbated. When frustration becomes too great, a new clinician is found, and the cycle is repeated. The longer the existence of the pain disorder, the more important become the psychological factors of anxiety and depression. As with all other conditions, it is counterproductive to speculate about whether the pain is "real." It is real to the patient, and

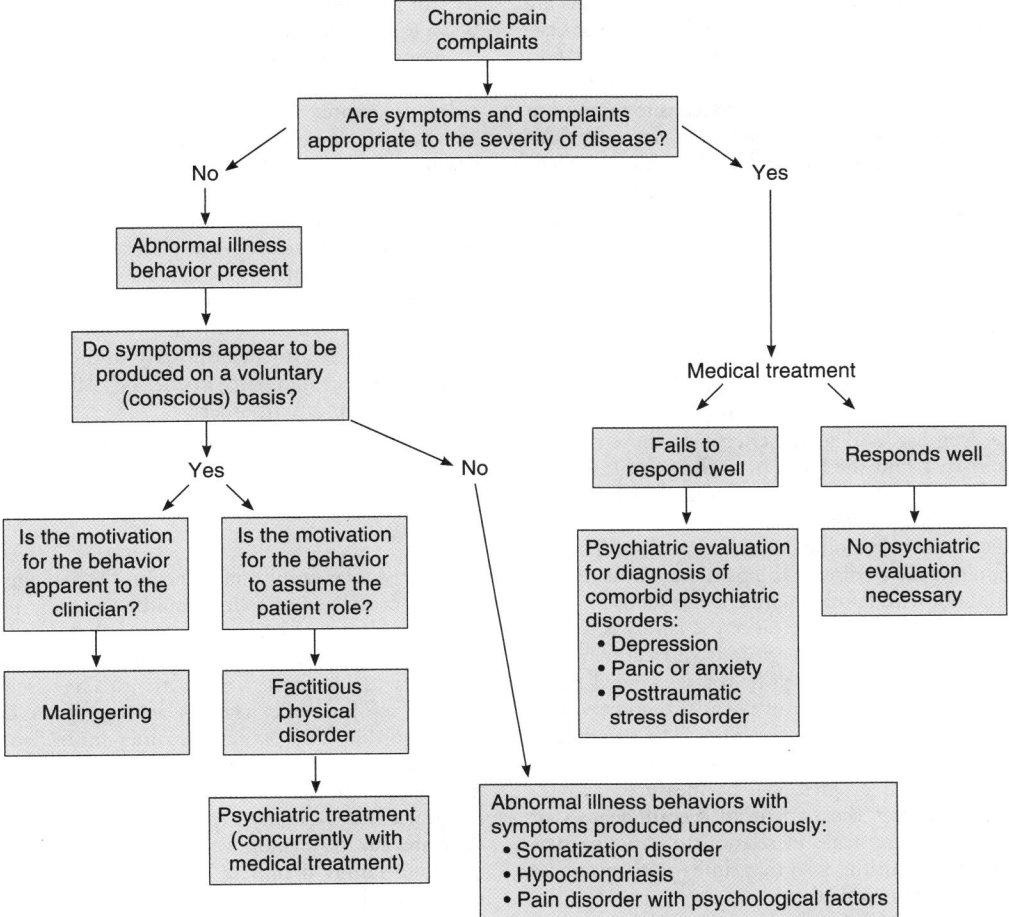

Figure 25–2. Algorithm for assessing psychiatric component of chronic pain. (Modified and reproduced, with permission, from Eisendrath SJ: Psychiatric aspects of chronic pain. Neurology 1995;45[Suppl 9]:S26.)

acceptance of the problem must precede a mutual endeavor to alleviate the disturbance.

Clinical Findings

Components of the chronic pain syndrome consist of anatomic changes, chronic anxiety and depression, anger, and changed lifestyle. Usually, the anatomic problem is irreversible, since it has already been subjected to many interventions with increasingly unsatisfactory results. An algorithm for assessing chronic pain and differentiating it from other psychiatric conditions is illustrated in Figure 25–2.

Chronic anxiety and depression produce heightened irritability and overreaction to stimuli. A marked decrease in pain threshold is apparent. This pattern develops into a hypochondriacal preoccupation with the body and a constant need for reassurance. The pressure on the clinician becomes wearing and often leads to covert rejection devices, such as not being available or making referrals to other clinicians. This is perceived by the patient, who then intensifies the effort to find help, and the typical cycle is repeated. Anxiety and depression are seldom discussed, almost as if there is a tacit agreement not to deal with these issues.

Changes in lifestyle involve some of the pain behaviors. These usually take the form of a family script in which the patient accepts the role of being sick, and this role then becomes the focus of most family interactions and may become important in maintaining the family, so that neither the patient nor the family wants the patient's role to change. Demands for attention and efforts to control the behavior of others revolve around the central issue of control of other people (including clinicians). Cultural factors frequently play a role in the behavior of the patient and how the significant people around the patient cope with the problem. Some cultures encourage demonstrative behavior, while others value the stoic role.

Another secondary gain that frequently maintains the patient in the sick role is financial compensation or other benefits ("green poultice"). Frequently, such systems are structured so that they reinforce the maintenance of sickness and discourage any attempts to give up the role. Clinicians unwittingly reinforce this role because of the very nature of the practice of medicine, which is to respond to complaints of illness. Helpful suggestions from the clinician are often met with responses like, "Yes, but…." Medications then become the principal approach, and drug dependency problems may develop.

Treatment

A. BEHAVIORAL

The cornerstone of a unified approach to chronic pain syndromes is a comprehensive behavioral program. This is necessary to identify and eliminate pain reinforcers, to decrease drug use, and to use effectively those positive reinforcers that shift the focus from the pain. It is critical that the patient be made a partner in the effort to alleviate pain. The clinician must shift from the idea of biomedical cure to ongoing care of the patient. The patient should agree to discuss the pain only with the clinician and not with family members; this tends to stabilize the patient's personal life, since the family is usually tired of the subject. At the beginning of treatment, the patient should be assigned self-help tasks graded up to maximal activity as a means of positive reinforcement. The tasks should not exceed capability. The patient can also be asked to keep a self-rating chart to log accomplishments, so that progress can be measured and remembered. Instruct the patient to record degrees of pain on a self-rating scale in relation to various situations and mental attitudes so that similar circumstances can be avoided or modified.

Avoid positive reinforcers for pain such as marked sympathy and attention to pain. Emphasize a positive response to productive activities, which remove the focus of attention from the pain. Activity is also desensitizing, since the patient learns to tolerate increasing activity levels.

Biofeedback techniques (see Somatoform Disorders, above) and hypnosis have been successful in ameliorating some pain syndromes. Hypnosis tends to be most effective in patients with a high level of denial, who are more responsive to suggestion. Hypnosis can be used to lessen anxiety, alter perception of the length of time that pain is experienced, and encourage relaxation.

B. MEDICAL

A *single clinician* in charge of the comprehensive treatment approach is the highest priority. Consultations as indicated and technical procedures done by others are appropriate, but the care of the patient should remain in the hands of the primary clinician. Referrals should not be allowed to raise the patient's hopes unrealistically or to become a way for the clinician to reject the case. The attitude of the doctor should be one of honesty, interest, and hopefulness—not for a cure but for control of pain and improved function. If the

patient manifests opioid addiction, detoxification may be an early treatment goal.

Nonsteroidal anti-inflammatory drugs are often the first-line of treatment for pain. If opioid analgesics or sedatives are prescribed, they should not be given on an "as-needed" schedule (see Chapter 5). A fixed schedule lessens the conditioning effects of these drugs. Tricyclic antidepressants (TCAs) (eg, nortriptyline) and venlafaxine in doses up to those used in depression may be helpful, particularly in neuropathic pain syndromes. In other conditions, their effects on pain may be less clear, but ameliorating depression is usually important nonetheless. Gabapentin, an anticonvulsant with possible applications in the treatment of anxiety disorders, has been shown to be useful in postherpetic and diabetic neuropathy and somatoform disorders.

In addition to medications, a variety of alternative strategies may be offered, including physical therapy and acupuncture.

C. SOCIAL

Involvement of family members and other significant persons in the patient's life should be an early priority. The best efforts of both patient and therapists can be unwittingly sabotaged by other persons who may feel that they are "helping" the patient. They frequently tend to reinforce the negative aspects of the chronic pain disorder. The patient becomes more dependent and less active, and the pain syndrome becomes an immutable way of life. The more destructive pain behaviors described by many experts in chronic pain disorders are the results of well-meaning but misguided efforts of family members. Ongoing therapy with the family can be helpful in the early identification and elimination of these behavior patterns.

D. PSYCHOLOGICAL

In addition to group therapy with family members and others, groups of patients can be helpful if properly led. The major goal, whether of individual or group therapy, is to gain patient involvement. A group can be a powerful instrument for achieving this goal, with the development of group loyalties and cooperation. People will frequently make efforts with group encouragement that they would never make alone. Individual therapy should be directed toward strengthening existing defenses and improving self-esteem. For example, teaching patients to challenge expectations induced by chronic pain may lead to improved functioning. As an illustration, many chronic pain patients, making assumptions more derived from acute injuries, incorrectly believe they will damage themselves by attempting to function. The rapport between patient and clinician, as in all psychotherapeutic efforts, is the major factor in therapeutic success.

Ciaramella A et al: When pain is not fully explained by organic lesion: a psychiatric perspective on chronic pain patients. Eur J Pain 2004;8:3. [PMID: 14690670]

Evers AW et al: Tailored cognitive-behavioral therapy in early rheumatoid arthritis for patients at risk: a randomized controlled trial. Pain 2002;100:141. [PMID: 12435467]

Lin EH et al: Effect of improving depression care on pain and functional outcomes among older adults with arthritis: a randomized controlled trial. JAMA 2003;290:2428. [PMID: 14612479]

PSYCHOSEXUAL DISORDERS

The stages of sexual activity include **excitement** (arousal), **orgasm**, and **resolution**. The precipitating excitement or arousal is psychologically determined. Arousal response leading to plateau is a physiologic and psychological phenomenon of vasocongestion, a parasympathetic reaction causing erection in men and labial-clitoral congestion in women. The orgasmic response includes emission in men and clonic contractions of the analogous striated perineal muscles of both men and women. Resolution is a gradual return to normal physiologic status.

While the arousal stimuli—vasocongestive and orgasmic responses—constitute a single response in a well-adjusted person, they can be considered as separate stages that can produce different syndromes responding to different treatment procedures.

Clinical Findings

There are three major groups of sexual disorders.

A. PARAPHILIAS (SEXUAL AROUSAL DISORDERS)

In these conditions, formerly called "deviations" or "variations," the excitement stage of sexual activity is associated with sexual objects or orientations different from those usually associated with adult sexual stimulation. The stimulus may be a woman's shoe, a child, animals, instruments of torture, or incidents of aggression. The pattern of sexual stimulation is usually one that has early psychological roots. Poor experiences with sexual activity frequently reinforce this pattern over time.

Exhibitionism is the impulsive behavior of exposing the genitalia to unsuspecting strangers in order to achieve sexual excitation. It is a childhood sexual behavior carried into adult life.

Transvestism consists of recurrent cross-dressing behavior in a heterosexual man for the purpose of sexual excitation. Such fetishistic behavior can be part of masturbation foreplay. Transvestism in homosexuality and transsexualism is not for the purpose of sexual excitement but is a function of preference or gender identity disorder.

Voyeurism involves the achievement of sexual arousal by watching the activities of an unsuspecting person, usually in various stages of undress or sexual activity. In both exhibitionism and voyeurism, excitation leads to masturbation as a replacement for sexual activity.

Pedophilia is the use of a child of either sex to achieve sexual arousal and, in many cases, gratification. Contact is frequently oral, with either participant being dominant, but pedophilia includes intercourse

of any type. Adults of both sexes engage in this behavior, but because of social and cultural factors it is more commonly identified with men. The pedophile has difficulty in adult sexual relationships, and men who perform this act are frequently impotent.

Incest involves a sexual relationship with a person in the immediate family, most frequently a child. In many ways it is similar to pedophilia (intrafamilial pedophilia). Incestuous feelings are fairly common, but cultural mores are usually sufficiently strong to act as a barrier to the expression of sexual feelings.

Sexual sadism is the attainment of sexual arousal by inflicting pain upon the sexual object. Much sexual activity has aggressive components (eg, biting, scratching). However, forced sexual acquiescence (eg, rape) is considered to be primarily an act of aggression.

Sexual masochism is the achievement of erotic pleasure by being humiliated, enslaved, physically bound, and restrained. It is life-threatening, since neck binding or partial asphyxiation usually forms part of the ritual. The practice is much more common in men than in women.

Necrophilia is sexual intercourse with a dead body or the use of parts of a dead body for sexual excitation, often with masturbation.

B. GENDER IDENTITY DISORDER

Core gender identity reflects a biologic self-image—the conviction that "I am a boy" or "I am a girl" that is usually well developed by age 3 or 4. Gender dysphoria refers to the development of a sexual identity that is the opposite of the biologic one.

Transsexualism is an attempt to deny and reverse biologic sex by maintaining sexual identity with the opposite gender. Transsexuals do not alternate between gender roles; rather, they assume a fixed role of attitudes, feelings, fantasies, and choices consonant with those of the opposite sex, all of which clearly date back to early development. For example, male to female transsexuals in early childhood behave, talk, and fantasize as if they were girls. They do not grow out of feminine patterns; they do not work in professions traditionally considered to be masculine; and they have no interest in their own penises either as evidence of maleness or as organs for erotic behavior. The desire for sex change starts early and may culminate in assumption of a feminine lifestyle, hormonal treatment, and use of surgical procedures, eg, castration and vaginoplasty.

C. PSYCHOSEXUAL DYSFUNCTION

This category includes a large group of vasocongestive and orgasmic disorders. Often, they involve problems of sexual adaptation, education, and technique that are often initially discussed with, diagnosed by, and treated by the primary care provider.

There are two conditions common in men: erectile dysfunction and ejaculation disturbances.

Erectile dysfunction (impotence) is inability to achieve or maintain an erection firm enough for satisfactory intercourse; patients sometimes use the term to mean premature ejaculation. Careful questioning is necessary, since causes of this vasocongestive disorder can be psychological, physiologic, or both. The majority are pathophysiologic and, to varying degrees, treatable. After onset of the problem, a history of occasional erections—especially nocturnal penile tumescence, which may be evaluated by a simple monitoring device, or a sleep study in the sleep laboratory—is usually evidence that the dysfunction is psychological in origin, with the caveat that decreased nocturnal penile tumescence occurs in some depressed patients. **Psychological erectile dysfunction** is caused by interpersonal or intrapsychic factors (eg, marital disharmony, depression). **Organic factors** are discussed in Chapter 23.

Ejaculation disturbances include premature ejaculation, inability to ejaculate, and retrograde ejaculation. (One may ejaculate even though impotent.) Ejaculation is usually connected with orgasm, and ejaculatory control is an acquired behavior that is minimal in adolescence and increases with experience. Pathogenic factors are those that interfere with learning control, most frequently sexual ignorance. Intrapsychic factors (anxiety, guilt, depression) and interpersonal maladaptation (marital problems, unresponsiveness of mate, power struggles) are also common. Organic causes include interference with sympathetic nerve distribution (often due to surgery or trauma) and the effects of pharmacologic agents (eg, SSRIs or sympatholytics).

In women, the two most common forms of sexual dysfunction are vaginismus and frigidity.

Vaginismus is a conditioned response in which a spasm of the perineal muscles occurs if there is any stimulation of the area. The desire is to avoid penetration. Sexual responsiveness and vasocongestion may be present, and orgasm can result from clitoral stimulation.

Frigidity is a complex condition in which there is a general lack of sexual responsiveness. The woman has difficulty in experiencing erotic sensation and does not have the vasocongestive response. Sexual activity varies from active avoidance of sex to an occasional orgasm. Orgasmic dysfunction—in which a woman has a vasocongestive response but varying degrees of difficulty in reaching orgasm—is sometimes differentiated from frigidity. Causes for the dysfunctions include poor sexual techniques, early traumatic sexual experiences, interpersonal disharmony (marital struggles, use of sex as a means of control), and intrapsychic problems (anxiety, fear, guilt). Organic causes include any conditions that might cause pain in intercourse, pelvic pathology, mechanical obstruction, and neurologic deficits.

Disorders of sexual desire consist of diminished or absent libido in either sex and may be a function of organic or psychological difficulties (eg, anxiety, phobic avoidance). Any chronic illness can sap desire. Hormonal disorders, including hypogonadism or use of antiandrogen compounds such as cyproterone acetate, and chronic renal failure contribute to deterioration in sexual activity. Although menopause may lead to diminution of sexual desire in some women, the relationship between menopause and libido is compli-

cated and may be influenced by sociocultural factors. Alcohol, sedatives, opioids, marijuana, and some medications may affect sexual drive and performance.

Treatment

A. PARAPHILIAS AND GENDER IDENTITY DISORDERS

1. Psychological—Sexual arousal disorders involving variant sexual activity (paraphilia), particularly those of a more superficial nature (eg, voyeurism) and those of recent onset, are responsive to psychotherapy in a moderate percentage of cases. The prognosis is much better if the motivation comes from the individual rather than the legal system; unfortunately, however, judicial intervention is frequently the only stimulus to treatment, because the condition persists and is reinforced until conflict with the law occurs. Therapies frequently focus on barriers to normal arousal response; the expectation is that the variant behavior will decrease as normal behavior increases.

2. Behavioral—Aversive and operant conditioning techniques have been tried frequently in gender role disorders but have only occasionally been successful. In some cases, the sexual arousal disorders improve with modeling, role-playing, and conditioning procedures. Emotive imagery is occasionally helpful in lessening anxiety in fetish problems.

3. Social—Although they do not produce a change in sexual arousal patterns or gender role, self-help groups have facilitated adjustment to an often hostile society. Attention to the family is particularly important in helping persons in such groups to accept their situation and alleviate their guilt about the role they think they had in creating the problem.

4. Medical—Medroxyprogesterone acetate, a suppressor of libidinal drive, is used to mute disruptive sexual behavior in men of all ages. Onset of action is usually within 3 weeks, and the effects are generally reversible. Fluoxetine or other SSRIs at depression doses (see Table 25–8) may reduce some of the compulsive sexual behaviors including the paraphilias. A recent focus of study in the treatment of severe paraphilia has been agonists of luteinizing hormone–releasing hormone. Although some transsexuals are treated with genital reconstructive surgery, many others are screened out by trial periods of living as the other sex prior to operation.

B. PSYCHOSEXUAL DYSFUNCTION

1. Medical—Identification of a contributory reversible cause is most important. Even if the condition is not reversible, identification of the specific cause helps the patient to accept the condition. Marital disharmony, with its exacerbating effects, may thus be avoided. Of all the sexual dysfunctions, erectile dysfunction is the condition most likely to have an organic basis. Sildenafil citrate, a phosphodiesterase type 5 inhibitor, is an effective oral agent for the treatment of penile erectile dysfunction in the recommended dose of 25–100 mg 1 hour prior to intercourse. Sildenafil is effective for SSRI-induced erectile dysfunction in men and in some cases for SSRI-associated sexual dysfunction in women. Use of the medication in conjunction with any nitrates, particularly in individuals with coronary artery disease, can have significant hypotensive effects leading to death in some cases. The medication, which does not appear to impact sexual desire, should be used only once a day. The newer phosphodiesterase type 5 inhibitors tadalafil and vardenafil have similar efficacy. Because of their common effect in delaying ejaculation, the SSRIs have been effective in premature ejaculation.

2. Behavioral—Syndromes resulting from conditioned responses have been treated by conditioning techniques, with excellent results. Vaginismus responds well to desensitization with graduated Hegar dilators along with relaxation techniques. Masters and Johnson have used behavioral approaches in all of the sexual dysfunctions, with concomitant supportive psychotherapy and with improvement of the communication patterns of the couple.

3. Psychological—The use of psychotherapy by itself is best suited for those cases in which interpersonal difficulties or intrapsychic problems predominate. Anxiety and guilt about parental injunctions against sex may contribute to sexual dysfunction. Even in these cases, however, a combined behavioral-psychological approach usually produces results most quickly.

4. Social—The proximity of other people (eg, a mother-in-law) in a household is frequently an inhibiting factor in sexual relationships. In such cases, some social engineering may alleviate the problem.

Kostis JB et al: Sexual dysfunction and cardiac risk (The Second Princeton Consensus Conference). Am J Cardiol 2005;96: 313. [PMID: 16018863]

Shiri R et al: Effect of chronic diseases on incidence of erectile dysfunction. Urology 2003;62:1097. [PMID: 14665363]

Worthington JJ et al: Treatment of antidepressant-induced sexual dysfunction. Drugs Today 2003;39:887. [PMID: 14702134]

PERSONALITY DISORDERS

 ESSENTIALS OF DIAGNOSIS

- *Long history dating back to childhood.*
- *Recurrent maladaptive behavior.*
- *Low self-esteem and lack of confidence.*
- *Minimal introspective ability with a tendency to blame others for all problems.*
- *Major difficulties with interpersonal relationships or society.*
- *Depression with anxiety when maladaptive behavior fails.*

General Considerations

An individual's personality structure, or character, is an integral part of self-image. It reflects genetics, interpersonal influences, and recurring patterns of behavior adopted in order to cope with the environment. The classification of subtypes of personality disorders depends on the predominant symptoms and their severity. The most severe disorders—those that bring the patient into greatest conflict with society—tend to be classified as antisocial (psychopathic) or borderline.

Personality disorders can be considered a matrix for some of the more severe psychiatric problems (eg, schizotypal, relating to schizophrenia, and avoidance types, relating to some anxiety disorders).

Classification & Clinical Findings

See Table 25–3.

Differential Diagnosis

Patients with personality disorders tend to show anxiety and depression when pathologic coping mechanisms fail, and their symptoms can be similar to those occurring with anxiety disorders. Occasionally, the more severe cases may decompensate into psychosis under stress and mimic other psychotic disorders.

Treatment

A. SOCIAL

Social and therapeutic environments such as day hospitals, halfway houses, and self-help communities utilize peer pressures to modify the self-destructive behavior. The patient with a personality disorder often has failed to profit from experience, and difficulties with authority impair the learning experience. The use of peer relationships and the repetition possible in a structured setting of a helpful community enhance the behavioral treatment opportunities and increase learning. When problems are detected early, both the school and the home can serve as foci of intensified social pressure to change the behavior, particularly with the use of behavioral techniques.

B. BEHAVIORAL

The behavioral techniques used are principally operant conditioning and aversive conditioning. The former simply emphasizes the recognition of acceptable behavior and its reinforcement with praise or other tangible rewards. Aversive responses usually mean punishment, although this can range from a mild rebuke to some specific punitive responses such as deprivation of privileges. Extinction plays a role in that an attempt is made not to respond to inappropriate behavior, and the lack of response eventually causes the person to abandon that type of behavior. Pouting and tantrums, for example, dimin-

Table 25–3. Personality disorders: Classification and clinical findings.

Personality Disorder	Clinical Findings
Paranoid	Defensive, oversensitive, secretive, suspicious, hyperalert, with limited emotional response.
Schizoid	Shy, introverted, withdrawn, avoids close relationships.
Obsessive-compulsive	Perfectionist, egocentric, indecisive, with rigid thought patterns and need for control.
Histrionic (hysterical)	Dependent, immature, seductive, egocentric, vain, emotionally labile.
Schizotypal	Superstitious, socially isolated, suspicious, with limited interpersonal ability, eccentric behaviors, and odd speech.
Narcissistic	Exhibitionist, grandiose, preoccupied with power, lacks interest in others, with excessive demands for attention.
Avoidant	Fears rejection, hyperreacts to rejection and failure, with poor social endeavors and low self-esteem.
Dependent	Passive, overaccepting, unable to make decisions, lacks confidence, with poor self-esteem.
Antisocial	Selfish, callous, promiscuous, impulsive, unable to learn from experience, has legal problems.
Borderline	Impulsive; has unstable and intense interpersonal relationships; is suffused with anger, fear, and guilt; lacks self-control and self-fulfillment; has identity problems and affective instability; is suicidal (a serious problem—up to 80% of hospitalized borderline patients make an attempt at some time during treatment, and the incidence of completed suicide is as high as 5%); aggressive behavior, feelings of emptiness, and occasional psychotic decompensation. This group has a high drug abuse rate, which plays a role in symptoms. There is extensive overlap with other diagnostic categories, particularly mood disorders and posttraumatic stress disorder.

ish quickly when such behavior elicits no reaction. Dialectical behavioral therapy is a program of individual and group therapy specifically designed for patients with chronic suicidality and borderline personality disorder. It blends mindfulness and a cognitive-behavioral model to address self-awareness, interpersonal functioning, affective lability, and reactions to stress.

C. PSYCHOLOGICAL

Psychological intervention is best conducted in group settings. Group therapy is helpful when specific interpersonal behavior needs to be improved. This mode of treatment also has a place with so-called acting-out patients, ie, those who frequently act in an impulsive and inappropriate way. The peer pressure in the group tends to impose restraints on rash behavior. The group also quickly identifies the patient's types of behavior and helps improve the validity of the patient's self-assessment, so that the antecedents of the unacceptable behavior can be effectively handled, thus decreasing its frequency. Individual therapy should initially be supportive, ie, helping the patient to restabilize and mobilize defenses. If the individual has the ability to observe his or her own behavior, a longer-term and more introspective therapy may be warranted. The therapist must be able to handle countertransference feelings (which are frequently negative), maintain appropriate boundaries in the relationship (no physical contacts, however well-meaning), and refrain from premature confrontations and interpretations.

D. MEDICAL

Hospitalization is indicated in the case of serious suicidal or homicidal danger. In most cases, treatment can be accomplished in the day treatment center or self-help community. Antipsychotics may be required for short periods in conditions that have temporarily decompensated into transient psychoses (eg, haloperidol, 2–5 mg orally every 3–4 hours until the patient has quieted down and is regaining contact with reality). Olanzapine (2.5–10 mg/d) or risperidone (0.5–2 mg/d) may be given with lorazepam (1–2 mg orally every 4 hours as needed). In some cases, these drugs are required only for several days and can be discontinued after the patient has regained a previously established level of adjustment; they can also provide ongoing support. Carbamazepine, 400–800 mg orally daily in divided doses, decreases the severity of behavioral dyscontrol. Antidepressants have improved anxiety, depression, and sensitivity to rejection in some borderline patients. SSRIs may have a role in reducing aggressive behavior in impulsive aggressive patients.

Prognosis

Antisocial and borderline categories generally have a guarded prognosis. Those patients with poor outcomes are more likely to have a history of parental abuse and a family history of mood disorder, whereas persons with mild schizoid or passive-aggressive tendencies have a better prognosis with appropriate treatment.

Rocca P et al: Treatment of borderline personality disorder with risperidone. J Clin Psychiatry 2002;63:241. [PMID: 11926724]

Swenson CR et al: Implementing dialectical behavior therapy. Psychiat Ser 2002;53:171. [PMID: 11821547]

SCHIZOPHRENIC & OTHER PSYCHOTIC DISORDERS

ESSENTIALS OF DIAGNOSIS

- *Social withdrawal, usually slowly progressive, often with deterioration in personal care.*
- *Loss of ego boundaries, with inability to perceive oneself as a separate entity.*
- *Loose thought associations, often with slowed thinking or overinclusive and rapid shifting from topic to topic.*
- *Autistic absorption in inner thoughts and frequent sexual or religious preoccupations.*
- *Auditory hallucinations, often of a derogatory nature.*
- *Delusions, frequently of a grandiose or persecutory nature.*
- *Symptoms of at least 6 months' duration.*

Frequent additional signs:

- *Flat affect and rapidly alternating mood shifts irrespective of circumstances.*
- *Hypersensitivity to environmental stimuli, with a feeling of enhanced sensory awareness.*
- *Variability or changeable behavior incongruent with the external environment.*
- *Concrete thinking with inability to abstract; inappropriate symbolism.*
- *Impaired concentration worsened by hallucinations and delusions.*
- *Depersonalization, wherein one behaves like a detached observer of one's own actions.*

General Considerations

The schizophrenic disorders are a group of syndromes manifested by massive disruption of thinking, mood, and overall behavior as well as poor filtering of stimuli. The characterization and nomenclature of the disorders are quite arbitrary and are influenced by sociocultural factors and schools of psychiatric thought.

It is currently believed that the schizophrenic disorders are of multifactorial cause, with genetic, environmental, and neurotransmitter pathophysiologic components. At present, there is no laboratory method for confirming the diagnosis of schizophrenia. There may or may not be a history of a major disruption in the individual's life (failure, loss, physical illness) before gross psychotic deterioration is evident.

Schizophrenic symptoms have been classified into positive and negative categories. Positive symptoms include hallucinations, delusions, and formal thought disorders; these symptoms appear to be related to increased dopaminergic (D_2) activity in the mesolimbic region. Negative symptoms include diminished sociability, restricted affect, and poverty of speech; these symptoms appear to be related to decreased D_2 activity in the mesocortical system.

"Other psychotic disorders" are conditions that are similar to schizophrenic disorders in their acute symptoms but have a less pervasive influence over the long term. The patient usually attains higher levels of functioning. The acute psychotic episodes tend to be less disruptive of the person's lifestyle, with a fairly quick return to previous levels of functioning.

Classification

A. SCHIZOPHRENIC DISORDERS

Schizophrenic disorders are subdivided on the basis of certain prominent phenomena that are frequently present. **Disorganized (hebephrenic) schizophrenia** is characterized by marked incoherence and an incongruous or silly affect. **Catatonic schizophrenia** is distinguished by a marked psychomotor disturbance of either excitement (purposeless and stereotyped) or rigidity with mutism. Infrequently, there may be rapid alternation between excitement and stupor (see under catatonic syndrome, below). **Paranoid schizophrenia** includes marked persecutory or grandiose delusions often consonant with hallucinations of similar content and with less marked disorganization of speech and behavior. **Undifferentiated schizophrenia** denotes a category in which symptoms are not specific enough to warrant inclusion of the illness in the other subtypes. **Residual schizophrenia** is a classification that includes persons who have clearly had an episode warranting a diagnosis of schizophrenia but who at present have no overt psychotic symptoms, although they show milder signs such as social withdrawal, flat affect, and eccentric behaviors.

B. DELUSIONAL DISORDERS

Delusional disorders are psychoses in which the predominant symptoms are persistent, nonbizarre delusions with minimal impairment of daily functioning. (The schizophrenic disorders show significant impairment.) Intellectual and occupational activities are little affected, whereas social and marital functioning tend to be markedly involved. Hallucinations are not usually present. Common delusional themes include paranoid delusions of persecution, delusions of being related to or loved by a well-known person, and delusions that one's partner is unfaithful.

C. SCHIZOAFFECTIVE DISORDERS

Schizoaffective disorders are those cases that fail to fit comfortably either in the schizophrenic or in the affective categories. They are usually cases with affective symptoms that precede or develop concurrently with psychotic manifestations. There has been increasing interest in studying prodromal schizophrenia with a goal to early treatment.

D. SCHIZOPHRENIFORM DISORDERS

Schizophreniform disorders are similar in their symptoms to schizophrenic disorders except that the duration of prodromal, acute, and residual symptoms is more than 1 week but less than 6 months.

E. BRIEF PSYCHOTIC DISORDERS

These disorders last less than 1 week. They are the result of psychological stress. The shorter duration is significant and correlates with a more acute onset and resolution as well as a much better prognosis.

F. LATE LIFE PSYCHOSIS

Brain abnormalities occur in 40% of patients who develop psychotic symptoms after age 60. The psychotic symptoms are typical, and there are other findings such as low IQ scores and diminished cognitive function.

G. ATYPICAL PSYCHOSES

This group includes a wide range of conditions with psychotic symptoms. The cause is often not clear, but later events (eg, new symptoms) may clarify the diagnosis. The most common example is chronic psychosis developing either during periods of heavy abuse of drugs or at some time after the drug use has ceased. Other conditions include temporal lobe dysfunction, HIV infection, and a number of the conditions noted in the differential diagnosis (see below). They often have a good premorbid history, a precipitous onset, and an episodic course with symptom-free intervals.

Clinical Findings

A. SYMPTOMS AND SIGNS

The symptoms and signs of schizophrenia vary markedly among individuals as well as in the same person at different times. The patient's **appearance** may be bizarre, although the usual finding is a mild to moderate unkempt blandness. **Motor activity** is generally reduced, although extremes ranging from catatonic stupor to frenzied excitement occur. **Social behavior** is characterized by marked withdrawal coupled with disturbed interpersonal relationships and a reduced ability to experience pleasure. Dependency and a poor self-image are common. **Verbal utterances** are variable, the language being concrete yet symbolic, with unassociated rambling statements (at times interspersed with mutism) during an acute episode. Neologisms (made-up words or phrases), echolalia (repetition of words spoken by others), and verbigeration (repetition of senseless words or phrases) are occasionally present. **Affect** is usually flattened, with occasional inappropriateness. **Depression** is present in almost all cases but may be less apparent during the acute psychotic episode and more obvious during recovery. Depression is sometimes confused with akinetic side ef-

fects of antipsychotic drugs. It is also related to **boredom**, which increases symptoms and decreases the response to treatment. Work is generally unavailable and time unfilled, providing opportunities for counterproductive activities such as drug abuse, withdrawal, and increased psychotic symptoms.

Thought content may vary from a paucity of ideas to a rich complex of delusional fantasy with archaic thinking. One frequently notes after a period of conversation that little if any information has actually been conveyed. Incoming stimuli produce varied responses. In some cases a simple question may trigger explosive outbursts, whereas at other times there may be no overt response whatsoever (catatonia). When paranoid ideation is present, the patient is often irritable and less cooperative. **Delusions** (false beliefs) are characteristic of paranoid thinking, and they usually take the form of a preoccupation with the supposedly threatening behavior exhibited by other individuals. This ideation may cause the patient to adopt active countermeasures such as locking doors and windows, taking up weapons, covering the ceiling with aluminum foil to counteract radar waves, and other bizarre efforts. Somatic delusions revolve around issues of bodily decay or infestation. **Perceptual distortions** usually include auditory hallucinations—visual hallucinations are more commonly associated with organic mental states—and may include illusions (distortions of reality) such as figures changing in size or lights varying in intensity. Cenesthetic hallucinations (eg, a burning sensation in the brain, feeling blood flowing in blood vessels) occasionally occur. Lack of humor, feelings of dread, depersonalization (a feeling of being apart from the self), and fears of annihilation may be present. Any of the above symptoms generate higher anxiety levels, with heightened arousal and occasional panic and suicidal ideation, as the individual fails to cope.

The development of the acute episode in schizophrenia frequently is the end product of a gradual decompensation. Frustration and anxiety appear early, followed by depression and alienation, along with decreased effectiveness in day-to-day coping. This often leads to feelings of panic and increasing disorganization, with loss of the ability to test and evaluate the reality of perceptions. The stage of so-called psychotic resolution includes delusions, autistic preoccupations, and psychotic insight, with acceptance of the decompensated state. The process is frequently complicated by the use of caffeine, alcohol, and other recreational drugs. Life expectancy of schizophrenics is as much as 20% shorter than that of cohorts in the general population (usually because of a higher mortality rate in younger people).

Polydipsia may produce water intoxication with hyponatremia—characterized by symptoms of confusion, lethargy, psychosis, seizures, and occasionally death—in any psychiatric disorder, but most commonly in schizophrenia. These problems exacerbate the schizophrenic symptoms. Possible pathogenetic factors in polydipsia include a hypothalamic defect, inappropriate antidiuretic hormone (ADH) secretion, neuroleptic medications (anticholinergic effects, stimulation of hypothalamic thirst center, effect on ADH), smoking (nicotine and syndrome of inappropriate antidiuretic hormone [SIADH]), psychotic thought processes (delusions), and other medications (eg, diuretics, antidepressants, lithium, alcohol). Other causes of polydipsia must be ruled out (eg, diabetes mellitus, diabetes insipidus, renal disease).

B. IMAGING

Ventricular enlargement and cortical atrophy, as seen on CT scan, have been correlated with chronic course, severe cognitive impairment, and nonresponsiveness to neuroleptic medications. Decreased frontal lobe activity seen on PET scan has been associated with negative symptoms.

Differential Diagnosis

One should not hesitate to reconsider the diagnosis of schizophrenia in any person who has received that diagnosis in the past, particularly when the clinical course has been atypical. A number of these patients have been found to actually have atypical episodic affective disorders that have responded well to lithium. Manic episodes often mimic schizophrenia. Furthermore, schizophrenia has been diagnosed in many individuals because of inadequacies in psychiatric nomenclature. Thus, schizophrenia was often inappropriately diagnosed in persons with brief reactive psychoses, OCD, paranoid disorders, and schizophreniform disorders.

Psychotic depressions, psychotic organic mental states, and any illness with psychotic ideation tend to be confused with schizophrenia, partly because of the regrettable tendency to use the terms interchangeably. Adolescent phases of growth and counterculture behaviors constitute another area of diagnostic confusion. It is particularly important to avoid a misdiagnosis in these groups, because of the long-term implications arising from having such a serious diagnosis made in a formative stage of life.

Medical disorders such as thyroid dysfunction, adrenal and pituitary disorders, reactions to toxic materials (eg, mercury, PCBs), and almost all of the organic mental states in the early stages must be ruled out. Postpartum psychosis is discussed under Mood Disorders. **Complex partial seizures**, especially when psychosensory phenomena are present, are an important differential consideration. Toxic drug states arising from prescription, over-the-counter, herbal and street drugs may mimic all of the psychotic disorders. The chronic use of amphetamines, cocaine, and other stimulants frequently produces a psychosis that is almost identical to the acute paranoid schizophrenic episode. The presence of formication and stereotypy suggests the possibility of stimulant abuse. Phencyclidine (see below), a very common street drug, may cause a reaction that is difficult to distinguish from other psychotic disorders. Cerebellar signs, excessive salivation, dilated pupils, and increased deep tendon reflexes should alert the clinician to the possibility of a toxic psychosis. Industrial chemical toxicity (both organic and metallic), degenerative disorders, and metabolic deficiencies must be considered in the differential diagnosis.

Catatonic syndrome, frequently assumed to exist solely as a component of schizophrenic disorders, is actually the end product of a number of illnesses, including various organic conditions. Neoplasms, viral and bacterial encephalopathies, central nervous system hemorrhage, metabolic derangements such as diabetic ketoacidosis, sedative withdrawal, and hepatic and renal malfunction have all been implicated. It is particularly important to realize that drug toxicity (eg, overdoses of antipsychotic medications such as fluphenazine or haloperidol) can cause catatonic syndrome, which may be misdiagnosed as a catatonic schizophrenic disorder and inappropriately treated with more antipsychotic medication.

Treatment

A. MEDICAL

Hospitalization is often necessary, particularly when the patient's behavior shows gross disorganization. The presence of competent family members lessens the need for hospitalization, and each case should be judged individually. The major considerations are to prevent self-inflicted harm or harm to others and to provide the patient's basic needs. A full medical evaluation and CT scan or MRI should be considered in first episodes of schizophreniform disorder and other psychotic episodes of unknown cause.

Antipsychotic medications (see below) are the treatment of choice. They block the response to stimulation. The relapse rate can be reduced by 50% with proper maintenance neuroleptic therapy. Long-acting, injectable depot neuroleptics are used in noncompliant patients or nonresponders to oral medication.

Antipsychotic drugs include the "typical" neuroleptics **phenothiazines, thioxanthenes** (both similar in structure), **butyrophenones, dihydroindolones, dibenzoxazepines**, and **benzisoxazoles**, and the newer "atypical" neuroleptics clozapine, risperidone, olanzapine, quetiapine, and ziprasidone (Table 25–4). Generally, increasing milligram potency of the typical neuroleptics is associated with decreasing anticholinergic and adrenergic side effects and increasing extrapyramidal symptoms (Table 25–5). For example, chlorpromazine has lower potency and more severe anticholinergic and adrenergic side effects. The increased anticholinergic effect of chlorpromazine, however, lowers the risk of extrapyramidal symptoms.

The Clinical Antipsychotic Trials of Intervention Effectiveness (CATIE) study was a complex investigation that compared "atypical" and "typical" neuroleptic drugs. Although it was not definitive, it suggested similar antipsychotic efficacy for both classes and a tendency for the atypicals, particularly olanzapine, to be better tolerated leading to enhanced compliance.

The phenothiazines comprise the bulk of the currently used "typical" neuroleptic drugs. The only butyrophenone

Table 25–4. Commonly used antipsychotics.

Drug	Usual Daily Oral Dose	Usual Daily Maximum Dose[1]	Cost per Unit	Cost for 30 Days Treatment Based on Maximum Dosage[2]
Phenothiazines				
Chlorpromazine (Thorazine; others)	100–400 mg	1 g	$1.05/200 mg	$157.50
Thioridazine (Mellaril)	100–400 mg	600 mg	$1.10/200 mg	$99.00
Mesoridazine (Serentil)	50–200 mg	400 mg		Not available in USA
Perphenazine (Trilafon)[3]	16–32 mg	64 mg	$1.54/16 mg	$184.80
Trifluoperazine (Stelazine)	5–15 mg	60 mg	$1.58/10 mg	$284.40
Fluphenazine (Permitil, Prolixin)[3]	2–10 mg	60 mg	$1.15/10 mg	$207.00
Thioxanthenes				
Thiothixene (Navane)[3]	5–10 mg	80 mg	$0.65/10 mg	$156.00
Dihydroindolone				
Molindone (Moban)	30–100 mg	225 mg	$4.05/50 mg	$546.75
Dibenzoxazepine				
Loxapine (Loxitane)	20–60 mg	200 mg	$2.57/50 mg	$308.40
Dibenzodiazepine				
Clozapine (Clozaril)	300–450 mg	900 mg	$3.33/100 mg	$899.10
Butyrophenone				
Haloperidol (Haldol)	2–5 mg	60 mg	$3.12/20 mg	$280.80
Benzisoxazole				
Risperidone[4] (Risperdal)	2–6 mg	10 mg	$6.70/2 mg	$835.78
Thienbenzodiazepine				
Olanzapine (Zyprexa)	5–10 mg	10 mg	$11.76/10 mg	$352.80
Dibenzothiazepine				
Quetiapine (Seroquel)	200–400 mg	800 mg	$6.62/200 mg	$612.00
Benzisothiazolyl piperazine				
Ziprasidone (Geodon)	40–160 mg	160 mg	$5.72/80 mg	$343.02
Dipiperazine				
Aripiprazole (Abilify)	10–15 mg	30 mg	$16.33/30 mg	$489.97

[1]Can be higher in some cases.
[2]Average wholesale price (AWP, for AB-rated generic when available) for quantity listed. Source: *Red Book Update*, Vol. 25, No. 5, May 2006. AWP may not accurately represent the actual pharmacy cost because wide contractual variations exist among institutions.
[3]Indicates piperazine structure.
[4]For risperidone, daily doses above 6 mg increase the risk of extrapyramidal syndrome. Risperidone 6 mg is approximately equivalent to haloperidol 20 mg.

commonly used in psychiatry is haloperidol, which is totally different in structure but very similar in action and side effects to the piperazine phenothiazines such as fluphenazine, perphenazine, and trifluoperazine. These drugs and haloperidol (dopamine [D_2] receptor blockers) have high potency and a paucity of autonomic side effects and act to markedly lower arousal levels. Molindone and loxapine, while less potent, are similar in action, side effects, and safety to the piperazine phenothiazines.

The first "atypical" (novel) antipsychotic drug developed, clozapine, a dibenzodiazepine derivative, has dopamine (D_4) receptor-blocking activity as well as central se-

rotonergic, histaminergic, and α-noradrenergic receptor-blocking activity. It is effective in the treatment of about 30% of psychoses resistant to other neuroleptic drugs. Research suggests that clozapine may have specific efficacy in decreasing suicidality in patients with schizophrenia. It is associated with a 1% risk of agranulocytosis, which requires weekly white blood cell count monitoring for the first 6 months followed by monitoring every other week. Weekly monitoring for 1 month after discontinuation of the medication is recommended. Because of an association between clozapine and myocarditis, the drug is contraindicated in patients with severe heart disease.

Table 25–5. Relative potency and side effects of antipsychotics.

Drug	Chlorpromazine:Drug Potency Ratio	Anticholinergic Effects[1]	Extrapyramidal Effect[1]
Phenothiazines			
Chlorpromazine	1:1	4	1
Thioridazine	1:1	4	1
Mesoridazine	1:2	3	2
Perphenazine	1:10	2	3
Trifluoperazine	1:20	1	4
Fluphenazine	1:50	1	4
Thioxanthene			
Thiothixene	1:20	1	4
Dihydroindolone			
Molindone	1:10	2	3
Dibenzoxazepine			
Loxapine	1:10	2	3
Butyrophenone			
Haloperidol	1:50	1	4
Dibenzodiazepine			
Clozapine	1:1	4	—
Benzisoxazole			
Risperidone	1:50	1	1
Thienbenzodiazepine			
Olanzapine	1:20	1	1
Dibenzothiazepine			
Quetiapine	1:1	1	—
Benzisothiazolyl piperazine			
Ziprasidone	1:1	1	1
Dipiperazine			
Aripiprazole	1:20	1	0

[1]4 = strong effect; 1 = weak effect.

Risperidone is an antipsychotic that blocks some serotonin receptors (5-HT$_2$) and dopamine receptors (D$_2$). Risperidone causes fewer extrapyramidal side effects than the typical antipsychotics at doses less than 6 mg. It appears to be as effective as haloperidol and possibly as effective as clozapine in treatment-resistant patients without requiring weekly white cell counts. Risperidone-induced hyperprolactinemia, even on low doses, has been reported, and that effect is thought to be more common with risperidone than with other atypical antipsychotics. Risperidone is available in a long-acting injectable preparation.

Olanzapine is a potent blocker of muscarinic, anticholinergic, 5-HT$_2$, and dopamine D$_1$, D$_2$, and D$_4$ receptors. High doses of olanzapine (12.5–17.5 mg daily) appear to be more effective than lower doses. The drug appears to be more effective than haloperidol in the treatment of negative symptoms. It is available in an orally disintegrating form for patients who are unable to tolerate standard oral dosing and in an injectable form for the management of acute agitation associated with schizophrenia and bipolar disorder. Serum alanine aminotransferase is more elevated in patients taking olanzapine than in those taking haloperidol. Olanzapine is associated with a much lower incidence of dystonic reaction than haloperidol and is perhaps less likely to induce tardive dyskinesia. Its most common side effects include somnolence, agitation, nervousness, headache, insomnia, dizziness, and significant weight gain. Multiple case reports have linked olanzapine and clozapine to new-onset type 2 diabetes. Further investigation is ongoing to clarify the risk, risk factors, and pathophysiology. The manufacturer has alerted physicians to an association between olanzapine and a significantly higher risk of stroke and death in elderly patients.

Quetiapine is a neuroleptic with greater 5-HT$_2$ relative to D$_2$ receptor blockade as well as a relatively high affinity for α_1- and α_2-adrenergic receptors. It appears to be as efficacious as haloperidol in treating positive and negative symptoms of schizophrenia, with less extrapyramidal side effects even at high doses. More common side effects include somnolence, dizziness, and postural hypotension. Because of an association with lens changes seen in patients on long-term treatment, an eye examination to detect cataract formation is recommended at initiation of treatment and then at 6-month intervals during treatment.

Ziprasidone has both anti-dopamine receptor and anti-serotonin receptor effects, with good efficacy for both positive and negative symptoms of schizophrenia. Ziprasidone is not associated with significant weight gain, hyperlipidemia, or new-onset diabetes and offers a good alternative for some patients. It has been implicated in QTc interval delay of > 500 ms in some patients, although in several cases of overdose there were no incidents of torsades de pointes or sudden death. Patients taking ziprasidone should be screened for cardiac risk factors. A pretreatment ECG is indicated for patients at risk for cardiac sequelae (including patients taking other medications that might prolong the QTc interval).

Aripiprazole is the first neuroleptic that is a dopamine stabilizer. A partial agonist at the dopamine D_2 and serotonin 5-HT$_1$ receptors and an antagonist at 5-HT$_2$ receptors, it is effective against positive and negative symptoms of schizophrenia. It functions as an antagonist or agonist, depending on the dopaminergic activity at the dopamine receptors. This may help decrease side effects. More activating than sedating, aripiprazole is thought to impose a low risk of extrapyramidal symptoms, weight gain, hyperprolactinemia, and delayed QT interval.

None of the antipsychotics produce true physical dependency. All decrease adrenergic responses. Despite higher costs, atypical neuroleptics are often considered preferable to traditional antipsychotics because they are thought to be associated with reduced extrapyramidal symptoms and a lesser risk of tardive dyskinesia.

Clinical Indications

The antipsychotics are used to treat all forms of the schizophrenias as well as psychotic ideation in organic brain psychoses, delirium and dementia, drug-induced psychoses, psychotic depression, and mania. They are also effective in Tourette's disorder. They quickly lower the arousal (activity) level and, perhaps indirectly, gradually improve socialization and thinking. The improvement rate is about 80%. Patients whose behavioral symptoms worsen with use of antipsychotic drugs may have an undiagnosed organic condition such as anticholinergic toxicity.

Symptoms that are ameliorated by these drugs include hyperactivity, hostility, aggression, delusions, hallucinations, irritability, and poor sleep. Individuals with acute psychosis and good premorbid function respond quite well. The most common cause of failure in the treatment of acute psychosis is inadequate dosage, and the most common cause of relapse is noncompliance.

Although typical antipsychotics are efficacious in the treatment of so-called positive symptoms of schizophrenia such as hallucinations and delusions, atypical antipsychotics are thought to have efficacy in reducing both positive symptoms and negative symptoms such as withdrawal, psychomotor retardation, and poor interpersonal relationships. Antidepressant drugs may be used in conjunction with neuroleptics if significant depression is present. Resistant cases may require concomitant use of lithium, carbamazepine, or valproic acid. The addition of a benzodiazepine drug to the neuroleptic regimen may prove helpful in treating the agitated or catatonic psychotic patient who has not responded to neuroleptics alone—lorazepam, 1–2 mg orally, can produce a rapid resolution of catatonic symptoms and may allow maintenance with a lower neuroleptic dose. Electroconvulsive therapy (ECT) has also been effective in treating catatonia.

Dosage Forms & Patterns

The dosage range is quite broad. For example, risperidone, 0.5–1 mg orally at bedtime, may be sufficient for the elderly person with mild dementia, whereas up to 6 mg/d may be used in a young patient with acute schizophrenia. For quick response, an atypical antipsychotic may be started in combination with a benzodiazepine (eg, risperidone oral solution, 2 mg, or olanzapine, 10 mg orally, and lorazepam, 2 mg orally, every 2–4 hours as needed). In an acutely distressed, psychotic patient one might use haloperidol, 10 mg intramuscularly, which is absorbed rapidly and achieves an initial tenfold plasma level advantage over equal oral doses. Psychomotor agitation, racing thoughts, and general arousal are quickly reduced. The dose can be repeated every 3–4 hours; when the patient is less symptomatic, oral doses can replace parenteral administration in most cases. In the elderly, both atypical (eg, risperidone 0.25 mg–0.5 mg daily or olanzapine 1.25 mg daily) and conventional (eg haloperidol 0,5 mg daily or perphenazine 2 mg daily) antipsychotics, often used effectively in small doses for behavioral control, have been linked to premature death in some cases.

Various factors play a role in the absorption of oral medications. Of particular importance are previous gastrointestinal surgery and concomitant administration of other drugs. There are racial differences in metabolizing the neuroleptic drugs—eg, many Asians require only about half the usual dosage. Bioavailability is influenced by other factors such as smoking or hepatic microsomal enzyme stimulation with alcohol or barbiturates and enzyme-altering drugs such as carbamazepine or methylphenidate. Neuroleptic plasma drug level determinations are not currently of major clinical assistance.

Divided daily doses are not necessary after a maintenance dose has been established, and most patients can then be maintained on a single daily dose, usually taken at bedtime. This is particularly appropriate in a case where the sedative effect of the drug is desired for nighttime sleep, and undesirable sedative effects can be avoided during the day. Risperidone is an exception, being given twice daily. First-episode patients especially should be tapered off medications after about 6 months of stability and carefully monitored; their rate of relapse is lower than that of multiple-episode patients.

Psychiatric patients—particularly paranoid individuals—often neglect to take their medication. In these cases and in nonresponders to oral medication, the enanthate and decanoate (the latter is slightly longer-lasting and has fewer extrapyramidal side effects) forms of fluphenazine or the decanoate form of haloperidol may be given by deep subcutaneous injection or intramuscularly to achieve an effect that will usually last 7–28 days. A patient who cannot be depended on to take oral medication (or who overdoses on minimal provocation) will generally agree to come to the clinician's office for a "shot." The usual dose of the fluphenazine long-acting preparations is 25 mg every 2 weeks. Dosage and frequency of administration vary from about 100 mg weekly to 12.5 mg monthly. Use the smallest effective amount as infrequently as possible. A monthly injection of 25 mg of fluphenazine decanoate is equivalent to about 15–20 mg of oral fluphenazine daily. Risperidone is the first atypical neuroleptic now available in a long-acting injectable form (25–50 mg intramuscularly every 2 weeks). Concomitant use of a benzodiazepine (eg, lorazepam, 2 mg orally twice daily) may permit reduction of the required dosage of oral or parenteral antipsychotic drug.

Intravenous haloperidol, the neuroleptic most commonly used by this route, is often used in critical care units in the management of agitated, delirious patients. Intravenous haloperidol should be given no faster than 1 mg/min to reduce cardiovascular side effects, such as torsades de pointes, and is associated with a lower risk of extrapyramidal side effects.

Side Effects

For both typical and atypical neuroleptic agents, a range of side effects has been reported. The most common anticholinergic side effects include dry mouth (which can lead to ingestion of caloric liquids and weight gain or hyponatremia), blurred near vision, urinary retention (particularly in elderly men with enlarged prostates), delayed gastric emptying, esophageal reflux, ileus, delirium, and precipitation of acute glaucoma in patients with narrow anterior chamber angles. Other autonomic effects include orthostatic hypotension and sexual dysfunction—problems in achieving erection, ejaculation (including retrograde ejaculation), and orgasm in men (approximately 50% of cases) and women (approximately 30%). Delay in achieving orgasm is often a factor in medication noncompliance. Electrocardiographic changes occur frequently, but clinically significant arrhythmias are much less common. Elderly patients and those with preexisting cardiac disease are at greater risk. The most frequently seen electrocardiographic changes include diminution of the T wave amplitude, appearance of prominent U waves, depression of the ST segment, and prolongation of the QT interval. Thioridazine has been given an FDA warning for dose-related QTc delay and risk of fatal cardiac arrhythmias. As noted above, ziprasidone can produce QTc prolongation. An ECG prior to treatment in some patients may be indicated. In some critical care patients, torsades de pointes has been associated with the use of high-dose intravenous haloperidol (usually > 30 mg/24 h).

Associations have been suggested between the atypical neuroleptics and new-onset diabetes, hyperlipidemia, QTc prolongation, and weight gain (Table 25–6). The FDA has particularly noted the risk of hyperglycemia and new-onset diabetes in this class of medication that is not related to weight gain. Monitoring of weight, fasting blood sugar and lipids prior to initiation of treatment and at regular intervals thereafter is an important part of medication monitoring. Neuroleptic medications in general may have metabolic and endocrine effects, including weight gain, hyperglycemia, infrequent temperature irregularities (particularly in hot weather), and water intoxication, that may be due to inappropri-

Table 25–6. Adverse factors associated with atypical antipsychotics.

	Weight Gain	Hyperlipidemia	New–Onset Diabetes	QTc Prolongation[1]
Clozapine	+++	+	+	+/–
Olanzapine	+++	+	+	+/–
Risperidone	++	Unclear data	Unclear data	+
Quetiapine	++	Unclear data	Unclear data	++
Ziprasidone	+/–	–	–	+++

[1]QTc prolongation is a side effect of many medications and suggests a possible risk for arrhythmia. Among atypical neuroleptics, only ziprasidone carries a special warning regarding the risk of QTc prolongation.
Adapted from Consensus Development Conference on Antipsychotic Drugs and Obesity and Diabetes. Diabetes Care 2004;27:596.

ate ADH secretion. Lactation and menstrual irregularities are common (antipsychotic drugs should be avoided, if possible, in breast cancer patients because of potential trophic effects of elevated prolactin levels on the breast). Both antipsychotic and antidepressant drugs inhibit sperm motility. Bone marrow depression and cholestatic jaundice occur rarely; these are hypersensitivity reactions, and they usually appear in the first 2 months of treatment. They subside on discontinuance of the drug. There is cross-sensitivity among all of the phenothiazines, and a drug from a different group should be used when allergic reactions occur.

Clozapine is associated with a 1.6% risk of **agranulocytosis** (higher in persons of Ashkenazi Jewish ancestry), and its use must be strictly monitored with weekly blood counts during the first 6 months of treatment, with monitoring every other week thereafter. Discontinuation of the medication requires weekly monitoring of the white blood cell count for 1 month. Recently, clozapine has been associated with fatal myocarditis and is contraindicated in patients with severe heart disease. In addition, clozapine lowers the seizure threshold and has many side effects, including sedation, hypotension, increased liver enzyme levels, hypersalivation, respiratory arrest, weight gain, and changes in both the ECG and the EEG.

Photosensitivity, retinopathy, and hyperpigmentation are associated with use of fairly high dosages of chlorpromazine and thioridazine. The appearance of particulate melanin deposits in the lens of the eye is related to the total dose given, and patients on long-term medication should have periodic eye examinations. Teratogenicity has not been causally related to these drugs, but prudence is indicated particularly in the first trimester of pregnancy. The seizure threshold is lowered, but it is safe to use these medications in epileptics who take anticonvulsants.

The **neuroleptic malignant syndrome (NMS)** is a catatonia-like state manifested by extrapyramidal signs, blood pressure changes, altered consciousness, and hyperpyrexia; it is an uncommon but serious complication of neuroleptic treatment. Muscle rigidity, involuntary movements, confusion, dysarthria, and dysphagia are accompanied by pallor, cardiovascular instability, fever, pulmonary congestion, and diaphoresis and may result in stupor, coma, and death. The cause may be related to a number of factors, including poor dosage control of neuroleptic medication, affective illness, decreased serum iron, dehydration, and increased sensitivity of dopamine receptor sites. Lithium in combination with a neuroleptic drug may increase vulnerability, which is already increased in patients with an affective disorder. In most cases, the symptoms develop within the first 2 weeks of antipsychotic drug treatment. The syndrome may occur with small doses of the drugs. Intramuscular administration is a risk factor. Elevated creatine kinase and leukocytosis with a shift to the left are present early in about half of cases. Treatment includes controlling fever and providing fluid support. Dopamine agonists such as bromocriptine, 2.5–10 mg orally three times a

day, and amantadine, 100–200 mg orally twice a day, have also been useful. Dantrolene, 50 mg intravenously as needed, is used to alleviate rigidity (do not exceed 10 mg/kg/d due to hepatotoxicity risk). There is ongoing controversy about the efficacy of these three agents as well as the use of calcium channel blockers and benzodiazepines. ECT has been used effectively in resistant cases. Clozapine has been used with relative safety and fair success as an antipsychotic drug for patients who have had NMS. The syndrome must be differentiated from acute lethal catatonia, malignant hyperthermia, neurotoxic syndromes (including AIDS), and a variety of other conditions such as viral encephalitis, Wilson's disease, central anticholinergic syndrome, and hypertonic states (eg, tetany, strychnine poisoning).

Akathisia is the most common (about 20%) so-called **extrapyramidal symptom**. It usually occurs early in treatment (but may persist after neuroleptics are discontinued) and is frequently mistaken for anxiety or exacerbation of psychosis. It is characterized by a subjective desire to be in constant motion followed by an inability to sit or stand still and consequent pacing. It may include suicidality or feelings of fright, rage, terror, or sexual torment. Insomnia is often present. In all cases, reevaluate the dosage requirement or the type of neuroleptic drug. One should inquire also about cigarette smoking, which in women has been associated with an increased incidence of akathisia. Antiparkinsonism drugs such as trihexyphenidyl, 2–5 mg orally three times daily, or benztropine mesylate, 1–2 mg twice daily, may be helpful. In resistant cases, symptoms may be alleviated by propranolol, 30–80 mg/d orally, diazepam, 5 mg three times daily, or amantadine, 100 mg orally three times daily.

Acute dystonias usually occur early, although a late (tardive) occurrence is reported in patients (mostly men after several years of therapy) who previously had early severe dystonic reactions and a mood disorder (see below). Younger patients are at higher risk for acute dystonias. The most common signs are bizarre muscle spasms of the head, neck, and tongue. Frequently present are torticollis, oculogyric crises, swallowing or chewing difficulties, and masseter spasms. Laryngospasm is particularly dangerous. Back, arm, or leg muscle spasms are occasionally reported. Diphenhydramine, 50 mg intramuscularly, is effective for the acute crisis; one should then give benztropine mesylate, 2 mg orally twice daily, for several weeks, and then discontinue gradually, since few of the extrapyramidal symptoms require long-term use of the antiparkinsonism drugs (all of which are about equally efficacious—though trihexyphenidyl tends to be mildly stimulating and benztropine mildly sedating).

Drug-induced parkinsonism is indistinguishable from idiopathic parkinsonism, but it is reversible, occurs later in treatment than the preceding extrapyramidal symptoms, and in some cases appears after neuroleptic withdrawal. The condition includes the typical signs of apathy and reduction of facial and arm movements (akinesia, which can mimic depression), festinating gait, rigidity, loss of postural reflexes, and pill-rolling tremor. AIDS patients seem particularly vulnerable to extrapyramidal side effects. High-potency neuroleptics often require antiparkinsonism drugs (see Table 24–6). The neuroleptic dosage should be reduced, and immediate relief can be achieved with antiparkinsonism drugs in the same dosages as above. After 4–6 weeks, these antiparkinsonism drugs can often be discontinued with no recurrent symptoms. In any of the extrapyramidal symptoms, amantadine, 100–400 mg daily, may be used instead of the antiparkinsonism drugs. Neuroleptic-induced catatonia is similar to catatonic stupor with rigidity, drooling, urinary incontinence, and cogwheeling. It usually responds slowly to withdrawal of the offending medication and use of antiparkinsonism agents.

Tardive dyskinesia is a syndrome of abnormal involuntary stereotyped movements of the face, mouth, tongue, trunk, and limbs that may occur after months or (usually) years of treatment with neuroleptic agents. The syndrome affects 20–35% of patients who have undergone long-term neuroleptic therapy. Predisposing factors include older age, many years of treatment, cigarette smoking, and diabetes mellitus. Pineal calcification is higher in this condition by a margin of 3:1. There are no known differences among any of the antipsychotic drugs in the development of this syndrome. Although the atypical antipsychotics appear to offer lower risk, the CATIE study did not address the long-term effects of these drugs.

Early manifestations include fine worm-like movements of the tongue at rest, difficulty in sticking out the tongue, facial tics, increased blink frequency, or jaw movements of recent onset. Later manifestations may include bucco-linguo-masticatory movements, lip smacking, chewing motions, mouth opening and closing, disturbed gag reflex, puffing of the cheeks, disrupted speech, respiratory distress, or choreoathetoid movements of the extremities (the last being more prevalent in younger patients). The symptoms do not necessarily worsen and in rare cases may lessen even though neuroleptic drugs are continued. The dyskinesias do not occur during sleep and can be voluntarily suppressed for short periods. Stress and movements in other parts of the body will often aggravate the condition.

Early signs of dyskinesia must be differentiated from those reversible signs produced by ill-fitting dentures or nonneuroleptic drugs such as levodopa, TCAs, antiparkinsonism agents, anticonvulsants, and antihistamines. Other neurologic conditions such as Huntington's chorea can be differentiated by history and examination.

The emphasis should be on prevention. Use the least amount of neuroleptic drug necessary to mute the psychotic symptoms; atypical drugs appear to offer less risk as first line agents. Detect early manifestations of dyskinesias. When these occur, stop anticholinergic drugs and gradually discontinue neuroleptic drugs. Weight loss and cachexia sometimes appear on withdrawal of neuroleptics. In an indeterminate number of cases, the dyskinesias will remit. Keep the patient off the drugs until re-

emergent psychotic symptoms dictate their resumption, at which point they are restarted in low doses and gradually increased until there is clinical improvement. If neuroleptic drugs are restarted, clozapine and olanzapine appear to offer less risk of recurrence. The use of adjunctive agents such as benzodiazepines or lithium may help directly or indirectly by allowing control of psychotic symptoms with a low dosage of neuroleptics. If the dyskinesic syndrome recurs and it is necessary to continue neuroleptic drugs to control psychotic symptoms, informed consent should be obtained. Benzodiazepines, buspirone (in doses of 15–60 mg/d), phosphatidylcholine, clonidine, calcium channel blockers, vitamin E, and propranolol all have had limited usefulness in treating the dyskinetic side effects.

B. SOCIAL

Environmental considerations are most important in the individual with a chronic illness, who usually has a history of repeated hospitalizations, a continued low level of functioning, and symptoms that never completely remit. Family rejection and work failure are common. In these cases, board and care homes staffed by personnel experienced in caring for psychiatric patients are most important. There is frequently an inverse relationship between stability of the living situation and the amounts of required antipsychotic drugs, since the most salutary environment is one that reduces stimuli. Nonresidential self-help groups such as Recovery, Inc., should be utilized whenever possible. They provide a setting for sharing, learning, and mutual support and are frequently the only social involvement with which this type of patient is comfortable. Vocational rehabilitation and work agencies (eg, Goodwill Industries, Inc.) provide assessment, training, and job opportunities at a level commensurate with the person's clinical condition.

C. PSYCHOLOGICAL

The need for psychotherapy varies markedly depending on the patient's current status and history. In a person with a single psychotic episode and a previously good level of adjustment, supportive psychotherapy may help the patient reintegrate the experience, gain some insight into antecedent problems, and become a more self-observant individual who can recognize early signs of stress. Insight-oriented psychotherapy is often counterproductive in this type of disorder. Research suggests that cognitive behavioral therapy—in conjunction with medication management—may have some efficacy in the treatment of symptoms of schizophrenia. Cognitive behavioral therapy for schizophrenia involves helping the individual challenge their psychotic thinking and alter their response to hallucinations. Family therapy should be given concomitantly to help alleviate the patient's stress and to assist relatives in coping with the patient.

D. BEHAVIORAL

Behavioral techniques (see above) are most frequently used in therapeutic settings such as day treatment centers, but there is no reason why they cannot be incorporated into family situations or any therapeutic setting. Many behavioral techniques are used unwittingly (eg, positive reinforcement—whether it be a word of praise or an approving nod—after some positive behavior), and with some careful thought this approach can be a powerful instrument for helping a person learn behaviors that will facilitate social acceptance. Music from portable cassette players with earphones is one of many ways to divert the patient's attention from auditory hallucinations.

Prognosis

In any psychosis, in the large majority of patients the prognosis is excellent for alleviation of positive symptoms such as hallucinations or delusions treated with medication. Negative symptoms such as diminished affect and sociability are much more difficult to treat but appear responsive to atypical antipsychotics. Unavailability of structured work situations and lack of family therapy are two other reasons why the prognosis is so guarded in such a large percentage of schizophrenic patients. Psychosis connected with a history of serious drug abuse has a guarded prognosis because of the central nervous system damage, usually from the drugs themselves and associated medical illnesses.

Chandran GJ et al: Neuroleptic malignant syndrome: case report and discussion. CMAJ 2003;169:439. [PMID: 12952806]

Eisendrath SJ, Chamberlain J: Psychiatric problems. In: *Current Diagnosis and Treatment in Critical Care*, 2nd ed. Bongard FS, Sue DY (editors). McGraw-Hill, 2002.

Freedman R: Schizophrenia. N Engl J Med 2003;349:1738. [PMID: 14585943]

Koro CE et al: Assessment of independent effect of olanzapine and risperidone on risk of diabetes among patients with schizophrenia: population-based nested case-control study. BMJ 2002;325:243. [PMID: 12153919]

Lieberman JA et al: Clinical Antipsychotic Trials of Intervention Effectiveness (CATIE) Investigators: Effectiveness of antipsychotic drugs in patients with chronic schizophrenia. N Engl J Med 2005;353:1286. [PMID: 16172203]

Wang PS et al: Risk of death in elderly users of conventional vs. atypical antipsychotic medications. N Engl J Med 2005; 353:2335. [PMID: 16319382]

MOOD DISORDERS
(Depression & Mania)

 ESSENTIALS OF DIAGNOSIS

Present in most depressions:

- *Lowered mood, varying from mild sadness to intense feelings of guilt, worthlessness, and hopelessness.*
- *Difficulty in thinking, including inability to concentrate, ruminations, and lack of decisiveness.*
- *Loss of interest, with diminished involvement in work and recreation.*

- *Somatic complaints such as headache; disrupted, lessened, or excessive sleep; loss of energy; change in appetite; decreased sexual drive.*
- *Anxiety.*

Present in some severe depressions:

- *Psychomotor retardation or agitation.*
- *Delusions of a hypochondriacal or persecutory nature.*
- *Withdrawal from activities.*
- *Physical symptoms of major severity, eg, anorexia, insomnia, reduced sexual drive, weight loss, and various somatic complaints.*
- *Suicidal ideation.*

Present in mania:

- *Mood ranging from euphoria to irritability.*
- *Sleep disruption.*
- *Hyperactivity.*
- *Racing thoughts.*
- *Grandiosity.*
- *Variable psychotic symptoms.*

General Considerations

Depression is extremely common, with up to 30% of primary care patients having depressive symptoms. Depression may be the final expression of (1) genetic factors (neurotransmitter dysfunction), (2) developmental problems (personality problems, childhood events), or (3) psychosocial stresses (divorce, unemployment). It frequently presents in the form of somatic complaints with negative medical workups. Although sadness and grief are normal responses to loss, depression is not. Patients experiencing normal grief tend to produce sympathy and sadness in the clinician caregiver; depression often produces frustration and irritation in the clinician. Grief is usually accompanied by intact self-esteem, whereas depression is marked by a sense of guilt and worthlessness.

Mania is often combined with depression and may occur alone, together with mania in a mixed episode, or in cyclic fashion with depression.

Clinical Findings

In general, there are four major types of depressions, with similar symptoms in each group.

A. Adjustment Disorder with Depressed Mood

Depression may occur in reaction to some identifiable stressor or adverse life situation, usually loss of a person by death (grief reaction), divorce, etc; financial reversal (crisis); or loss of an established role, such as being needed. Anger is frequently associated with the loss, and this in turn often produces a feeling of guilt. The disorder occurs within 3 months of the stressor and causes significant impairment in social or occupational functioning. The symptoms range from mild sadness, anxiety, irritability, worry, lack of concentration, discouragement, and somatic complaints to the more severe symptoms of the next group.

B. Depressive Disorders

The subclassifications include major depressive disorder and dysthymia.

1. Major depressive disorder—A major depressive disorder (eg, "endogenous" unipolar disorder, melancholia) consists of at least one episode of serious mood depression that occurs at any time of life. Many consider a physiologic or metabolic aberration to be causative. Complaints vary widely but most frequently include a loss of interest and pleasure (anhedonia), withdrawal from activities, and feelings of guilt. Also included are inability to concentrate, some cognitive dysfunction, anxiety, chronic fatigue, feelings of worthlessness, somatic complaints (unidentifiable somatic complaints frequently indicate depression), loss of sexual drive, and thoughts of death. Diurnal variation with improvement as the day progresses is common. Vegetative signs that frequently occur are insomnia, anorexia with weight loss, and constipation. Occasionally, severe agitation and psychotic ideation (paranoid thinking, somatic delusions) are present. These symptoms are more common in depressed persons who are older than 50 years. Paranoid symptoms may range from general suspiciousness to ideas of reference with delusions. The somatic delusions frequently revolve around feelings of impending annihilation or hypochondriacal beliefs (eg, that the body is rotting away with cancer). Hallucinations are uncommon.

Subcategories include **major depression with atypical features** characterized by hypersomnia, overeating, lethargy, and rejection sensitivity. **Major depression with a seasonal onset (seasonal affective disorder)** is a dysfunction of circadian rhythms that occurs more commonly in the winter months and is believed to be due to decreased exposure to full-spectrum light. Common symptoms include carbohydrate craving, lethargy, hyperphagia, and hypersomnia. **Major depression with postpartum onset** usually occurs 2 weeks to 6 months postpartum.

Most women (up to 80%) experience some mild letdown of mood in the postpartum period. For some of these (10–15%), the symptoms are more severe and similar to those usually seen in serious depression, with an increased emphasis on concerns related to the baby (obsessive thoughts about harming it or inability to care for it). When psychotic symptoms occur, there is frequently associated sleep deprivation, volatility of behavior, and manic-like symptoms. Postpartum psychosis is much less common (< 2%), often occurs within the first 2 weeks, and requires early and aggressive management. Biologic vulnerability with hormonal changes and psychosocial stressors all play a role. The chances of a second episode are about 25% and may be reduced with prophylactic treatment.

2. Dysthymia—Dysthymia is a chronic depressive disturbance. Sadness, loss of interest, and withdrawal from activities over a period of 2 or more years with a relatively persistent course is necessary for this diagnosis. Generally, the symptoms are milder but longer-lasting than those in a major depressive episode.

3. Premenstrual dysphoric disorder—Depressive symptoms during the late luteal phase of the menstrual cycles may occur throughout the year.

C. Bipolar Disorders

Bipolar disorders consist of episodic mood shifts into mania, major depression, hypomania, and mixed mood states. The ability of bipolar disorder to mimic aspects of many other Axis I disorders and a high comorbidity with substance abuse can make the initial diagnosis of bipolar disorder difficult.

1. Mania—A manic episode is a mood change characterized by elation with hyperactivity, over involvement in life activities, increased irritability, flight of ideas, easy distractibility, and little need for sleep. The overenthusiastic quality of the mood and the expansive behavior initially attract others, but the irritability, mood lability with swings into depression, aggressive behavior, and grandiosity usually lead to marked interpersonal difficulties. Activities may occur that are later regretted, eg, excessive spending, resignation from a job, a hasty marriage, sexual acting out, and exhibitionistic behavior, with alienation of friends and family. Atypical manic episodes can include gross delusions, paranoid ideation of severe proportions, and auditory hallucinations usually related to some grandiose perception. The episodes begin abruptly (sometimes precipitated by life stresses) and may last from several days to months. Spring and summer tend to be the peak periods. Generally, the manic episodes are of shorter duration than the depressive episodes. In almost all cases, the manic episode is part of a broader bipolar (manic-depressive) disorder. Patients with four or more discrete episodes of a mood disturbance in 1 year are called "rapid cyclers." (Substance abuse, particularly cocaine, can mimic rapid cycling.) These patients have a higher incidence of hypothyroidism. Manic patients differ from patients with schizophrenia in that the former use more effective interpersonal maneuvers, are more sensitive to the social maneuvers of others, and are more able to utilize weakness and vulnerability in others to their own advantage. Creativity has been positively correlated with mood disorders, but the best work done is between episodes of mania and depression.

2. Cyclothymic disorders—These are chronic mood disturbances with episodes of depression and hypomania. The symptoms must have at least a 2-year duration and are milder than those that occur in depressive or manic episodes. Occasionally, the symptoms will escalate into a full-blown manic or depressive episode, in which case reclassification as bipolar I or bipolar II disorder would be warranted.

D. Mood Disorders Secondary to Illness and Drugs

Any illness, severe or mild, can cause significant depression. Conditions such as rheumatoid arthritis, multiple sclerosis, and chronic heart disease are particularly likely to be associated with depression, as are other chronic illnesses. Hormonal variations clearly play a role in some depressions. Varying degrees of depression occur at various times in schizophrenic disorders, central nervous system disease, and organic mental states. **Alcohol dependency** frequently coexists with serious depression.

The classic model of drug-induced depression occurs with the use of reserpine, both in a clinical and a neurochemical sense. Corticosteroids and oral contraceptives are commonly associated with affective changes. Antihypertensive medications such as methyldopa, guanethidine, and clonidine have been associated with the development of depressive syndromes, as have digitalis and antiparkinsonism drugs (eg, levodopa). It is unusual for β-blockers to produce depression when given for short periods, such as in the treatment of performance anxiety. Sustained use of β-blockers for medical conditions such as hypertension may produce depression in some patients, although the literature is unclear on this subject. It is also unclear whether non–lipid-soluble β-blockers are less likely to be associated with depression than lipid-soluble ones. Infrequently, disulfiram and anticholinesterase drugs may be associated with symptoms of depression. All stimulant use results in a depressive syndrome when the drug is withdrawn. Alcohol, sedatives, opiates, and most of the psychedelic drugs are depressants and, paradoxically, are often used in self-treatment of depression.

Differential Diagnosis

Since depression may be a part of any illness—either reactively or as a secondary symptom—careful attention must be given to personal life adjustment problems and the role of medications (eg, reserpine, corticosteroids, levodopa). Schizophrenia, partial complex seizures, organic brain syndromes, panic disorders, and anxiety disorders must be differentiated. Subtle thyroid dysfunction must be ruled out.

Complications

The longer the depression continues, the more crystallized it becomes—particularly when there is an element of secondary reinforcement. The most important complication is suicide, which often includes some elements of aggression. Suicide rates in the general population vary from 9 per 100,000 in Spain to 20 per 100,000 in the United States to 58 per 100,000 in Hungary. In individuals with depression, the lifetime risk rises to 10–15%. Men tend toward successful suicide, particularly in older age groups, whereas women make more attempts with lower mortality rates. An increased suicide rate is being observed in the younger population, ages 15–35. Patients with cancer, respiratory illnesses, AIDS, and those being maintained on hemodialysis have higher suicide rates. Alcohol is a significant factor in many suicide attempts.

There are four major groups of people who make suicide attempts. By far the greatest number fall into the category of **situational problems** (the despair of ordinary people). There is often great ambivalence—they don't really want to die, but they don't want to go on as before either. A suicide attempt in such cases may be an impulsive or aggressive act not associated with significant depression. In other cases a suicide attempt is clearly a stratagem for **controlling or hurting others**.

The high-risk groups are those with severe depressions or psychotic illnesses. **Severe depression** may be due to exogenous conditions (eg, AIDS, whose victims have a suicide rate over 30 times that of the general population) or endogenous conditions (eg, panic disorders). This group also includes those who may not be diagnosed as having depression but who are overwhelmed by a serious stressful situation (eg, the man charged with child molestation who hangs himself in his cell). Anxiety, panic, and fear are major findings in suicidal behavior. A patient may seem to make a dramatic improvement, but the lifting of depression may be due to the patient's decision to commit suicide. Those with **psychotic illness** tend not to verbalize their concerns, are unpredictable, and are often successful but make up only a small percentage of the total.

Suicide is ten times more prevalent in patients with schizophrenia than in the general population, and jumping from bridges is a more common means of attempted suicide by schizophrenics than by others. In one study of 100 jumpers, 47% had schizophrenia.

The immediate goal of psychiatric evaluation is to assess the current suicidal risk and the need for hospitalization versus outpatient management. The intent is less likely to be truly suicidal, for example, if small amounts of poison or drugs were ingested or scratching of wrists was superficial, if the act was performed in the vicinity of others or with early notification of others, or if the attempt was arranged so that early detection would be anticipated. Alcohol, hopelessness, delusional thoughts, and complete or nearly complete loss of interest in life or ability to experience pleasure are all positively correlated with suicide attempts. Other risk factors are previous attempts, a family history of suicide, medical or psychiatric illness (eg, anxiety, depression, psychosis), male sex, older age, contemplation of violent methods, a humiliating social stressor, and drug use (including long-term sedative or alcohol use), which contributes to impulsiveness or mood swings. Successful treatment of the patient at risk for suicide cannot be achieved if the patient continues to abuse drugs.

The patient's current mood status is best evaluated by direct evaluation of plans and concerns about the future, personal reactions to the attempt, and thoughts about the reactions of others. The patient's immediate resources should be assessed—people who can be significantly involved (most important), family support, job situation, financial resources, etc.

If hospitalization is not indicated (eg, gestures, impulsive attempts; see above), the clinician must formulate and institute a treatment plan or make an adequate referral. Medication should be dispensed in small amounts to at-risk patients. Although TCAs and SSRIs are associated with an equal incidence of suicide attempts, the risk of successful suicide is higher with TCA overdose. Guns and drugs should be removed from the patient's household. Driving should be interdicted until the patient improves. The problem is often worsened by the long-term complications of the suicide attempt, eg, brain damage due to hypoxia, peripheral neuropathies caused by staying for long periods in one position causing nerve compressions, and medical or surgical problems such as esophageal strictures and tendon dysfunctions.

The reasons for self-mutilation, most commonly wrist cutting (but also autocastration, autoamputation, and autoenucleation, which are associated with psychoses), may be very different from the reasons for a suicide attempt. The initial treatment plan, however, should presume suicidal ideation, and conservative treatment should be initiated.

Sleep disturbances in the depressions are discussed below.

Treatment of Depression

A. MEDICAL

Depression associated with reactive disorders usually does not call for drug therapy and can be managed by psychotherapy and the passage of time. In severe cases—particularly when vegetative signs are significant and symptoms have persisted for more than a few weeks—antidepressant drug therapy is often effective. Drug therapy is also suggested by a family history of major depression in first-degree relatives or a past history of prior episodes.

The antidepressant drugs may be conveniently classified into three groups: (1) the newer antidepressants, including the SSRIs and bupropion, venlafaxine, nefazodone, and mirtazapine, (2) the TCAs and clinically similar drugs, and (3) the MAO inhibitors (see Table 25–8). These groups are described in greater detail below. ECT is effective in all types of depression and will also rapidly resolve a manic episode. It is also very effective for postpartum depression. Megavitamin treatment, acupuncture, and electrosleep are of unproved usefulness for any psychiatric condition.

Hospitalization is necessary if suicide is a major consideration or if complex treatment modalities are required.

Drug selection is influenced by the history of previous responses if that information is available. If a relative has responded to a particular drug, this suggests that the patient may respond similarly. If no background information is available, a drug such as sertraline, 50 mg daily, or desipramine, starting with 50 mg and gradually increasing to 150 mg daily, can be selected and a *full trial* insti-

tuted. The medication trial should be monitored with patient assessments every 1–2 weeks until week 6. If successful, the medication should be continued for 6–12 months at the full therapeutic dose before tapering is considered. Antidepressants should usually be continued indefinitely at full dosage in individuals with more than two episodes after age 40 or one episode after age 50. If the response is inadequate despite a diagnosis supported by review and adequate drug levels, a second drug (eg, citalopram) should be substituted and given a trial. If the second drug fails, augmentation with lithium (eg, 600–900 mg/d) or thyroid medication (eg, liothyronine, 25 mcg/d) should be considered. Dysthymia is also treated in this way. The Agency for Health Care Policy and Research has produced clinical practice guidelines that outline one algorithm of treatment decisions (Figure 25–3).

Psychotic depression can be treated with a combination of an antipsychotic such as olanzapine and an antidepressant such as an SSRI at their usual doses. Mifepristone may have specific and early activity against psychotic depression.

Major depression with atypical features or seasonal onset can be treated with an MAO inhibitor or an SSRI with good results.

Stimulants such as dextroamphetamine (5–30 mg/d) and methylphenidate (10–45 mg/d) have enjoyed a resurgence of interest for the short-term treatment of depression in medically ill and geriatric patients. Their 50–60% efficacy rate is slightly below that of other agents. The stimulants are notable for rapid onset of action (hours) and a paucity of side effects (tachycardia, agitation) in most patients. They are usually given in two divided doses early in the day (eg, 7 AM and noon) so as to avoid interfering with sleep. These agents may also be useful as adjunctive agents in refractory depression.

Caution: Depressed patients may have suicidal thoughts, and the amount of drug dispensed should be appropriately controlled. The older TCAs have a narrow therapeutic index, and one advantage of the newer drugs is their wider margin of safety. Nonetheless, even with newer agents, because of the possibility of suicidality early in antidepressant treatment, close follow-up is indicated. This is particularly true in the treatment of children and adolescents where suicide risk has received special scrutiny. In all cases of pharmacologic management of depressed states, caution is indicated until the risk of suicide is considered minimal.

1. SSRIs and atypical antidepressants—The chief advantages of these agents are that they do not generally cause significant cardiovascular or anticholinergic side effects, as do the TCAs. The SSRIs include fluoxetine, sertraline, paroxetine, fluvoxamine, citalopram and its enantiomer escitalopram. The atypical antidepressants are bupropion, which appears to exert its effect through the dopamine neurotransmitter system; venlafaxine and duloxetine, both of which inhibit the reuptake of both serotonin and norepinephrine; nefazodone, which blocks the reuptake of serotonin but also inhibits the 5-HT$_2$ postsynaptic receptors; and

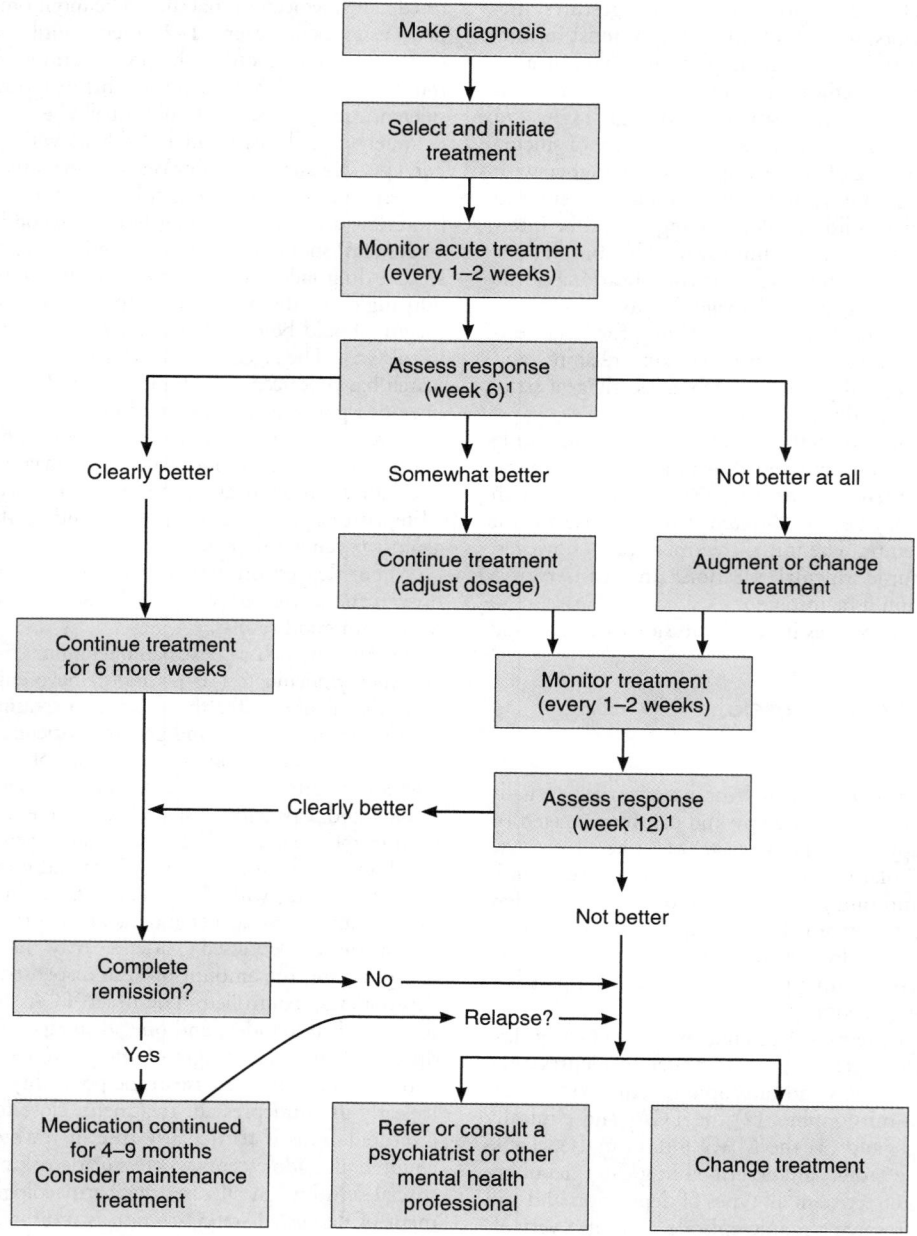

Figure 25–3. Overview of treatment for depression. (Reproduced, with permission, from Agency for Health Care Policy and Research: Depression in Primary Care. Vol. 2: Treatment of Major Depression. United States Department of Health and Human Services, 1993.)

[Footnote within figure:]
[1]Times of assessment (weeks 6 and 12) rest on very modest data. It may be necessary to revise the treatment plan earlier for patients not responding at all.

mirtazapine, which selectively blocks presynaptic α_2-adrenergic receptors and enhances both noradrenergic and serotonergic transmission. All of these antidepressants are effective in the treatment of depression, both typical and atypical. The SSRI drugs have been effective in the treatment of panic attacks, bulimia, generalized anxiety disorder, OCD, and PTSD. They do not seem to be as clearly effective in some pain syndromes as the TCAs, although venlafaxine may have some efficacy in the treatment of neuropathic pain, and duloxetine is FDA-approved for the treatment of diabetic peripheral neuropathy.

Most of the drugs in this group tend to be activating and are given in the morning so as not to interfere with sleep. Some patients, however, may have sedation, requiring that the drug be given at bedtime. This reaction occurs most commonly with paroxetine, fluvoxamine, and mirtazapine. The SSRIs can be given in once-daily dosage. Nefazodone and venlafaxine are usually given twice daily. Bupropion and venlafaxine are available in extended-release formulations and can be given once daily. There is usually some delay in response; fluoxetine, for example, requires 2–6 weeks to act in depression, 4–8 weeks to be effective in panic disorder, and 6–12 weeks in treatment of OCD. The starting dose (10–20 mg) is the usual daily dose for depression, while OCD may require up to 80 mg daily. Some patients, particularly the elderly, may tolerate and benefit from as little as 10 mg/d or every other day. The other SSRIs have shorter half-lives and a lesser effect on hepatic enzymes, which reduces their impact on the metabolism of other drugs (thus not increasing significantly the serum concentrations of other drugs as much as fluoxetine). The shorter half-lives also allow for more rapid clearing if adverse side effects appear. Venlafaxine appears to be more effective with doses greater than 200 mg/d, although some individuals respond to doses as low as 75 mg/d.

The side effects common to all of these drugs are headache, nausea, tinnitus, insomnia, and nervousness. Akathisia has been common with the SSRIs; other extrapyramidal symptoms (eg, dystonias) have occurred infrequently but particularly in withdrawal states. Sexual side effects of erectile dysfunction, retrograde ejaculation, and dysorgasmia are very common with the SSRIs. Antidotes to SSRI-induced sexual dysfunction are occasionally helpful. Sildenafil, 25–50 mg 1 hour prior to sexual activity, can improve erectile dysfunction in some patients. Cyproheptadine, 4 mg orally prior to sexual activity, may be helpful in countering drug-induced anorgasmia. Adjunctive bupropion (75–150 mg daily) may also help with restoring erectile function. The SSRIs are strong serotonin uptake blockers and may in high dosage or in combination with MAO inhibitors, including the antiparkinsonian drug selegiline, cause a "**serotonin syndrome**." This syndrome is manifested by rigidity, hyperthermia, autonomic instability, myoclonus, confusion, delirium, and coma. This syndrome can be a particularly troublesome problem in the elderly. Several cases of angina have been reported in association with SSRIs. However, current research indicates that SSRIs are safer agents to use than TCAs in patients with cardiac disease. A study has found that sertraline is a safe and effective antidepressant treatment in patients with acute myocardial infarction or unstable angina.

Withdrawal syndromes have been reported for the SSRIs and venlafaxine. These include dysphoric mood, agitation, and a flu-like state. These medications should be discontinued gradually over a period of weeks or months to reduce the risk of withdrawal phenomena.

Fluoxetine, fluvoxamine, sertraline, venlafaxine, and citalopram in customary antidepressant doses do not appear to increase the risk of major fetal malformation when used during pregnancy. Recent evidence, however, has suggested that paroxetine may be associated with a twofold increased risk of cardiac abnormalities. Postpartum developmental effects are thought to be minimal, but this question calls for ongoing investigation. Peripartum effects may be a of concern and are documented anecdotally in the literature. The risk of depression to the mother and fetus needs to be part of the discussion with the patient about treatment options. The decision to use SSRIs and other psychotropic agents during pregnancy and postpartum must be based on a thorough risk-benefit analysis for each individual. A recent review of the literature on antidepressants levels in breast-feeding mothers and their infants suggests that nortriptyline, paroxetine, and sertraline are least likely to lead to detectable levels in infants.

Venlafaxine is reported to be well-tolerated without significant anticholinergic or cardiovascular side effects. Nausea, nervousness, and profuse sweating appear to be the major side effects. Venlafaxine appears to have few drug-drug interactions. It does require monitoring of blood pressure because dose-related hypertension may develop in some individuals. Nefazodone appears to lack the anticholinergic effects of the TCAs and the agitation sometimes induced by SSRIs. Nefazodone should not be given with terfenadine, astemizole, or cisapride. (Terfenadine and astemizole are not commercially available in the United States.) Because nefazodone inhibits the liver's cytochrome P450 3A4 isoenzymes, concurrent use of these medications can lead to serious QT prolongation, ventricular tachycardia, or death. Through the same mechanism of enzyme inhibition, nefazodone can elevate cyclosporine levels sixfold to tenfold. Nefazodone has been given an FDA warning because it has been implicated in liver failure in rare cases. Pretreatment and ongoing monitoring of liver enzymes are indicated.

Mirtazapine is thought to enhance central noradrenergic and serotonergic activity with minimal sexual side effects compared with the SSRIs. Its action as a potent antagonist of histaminergic receptors may make it a useful agent for patients with depression and insomnia. Its most common adverse side effects include somnolence, increased appetite, weight gain, lipid abnormalities, and dizziness. There are reports of agranulocytosis in 2 of 2796 patients. Although it is metabolized by P450 isoenzymes, it is not an inhibitor of this system. It is given in a single dose at bedtime starting at 15 mg and increasing in 15-mg increments every week or every other week up to 45 mg.

Duloxetine may also result in small increases in blood pressure. Common side effects include dry mouth, dizziness, and fatigue. Inhibitors of 1A2 and 2D6 may increase duloxetine levels with a risk of toxicity.

2. Tricyclic antidepressants and clinically similar drugs—These drugs were the mainstay of drug therapy for depression for many years. They have also been effective in panic disorders, pain syndromes, and anxiety states. Specific ones have been effective in OCD (clomipramine), enuresis (imipramine), psychotic depression (amoxapine), and reduction of craving in cocaine withdrawal (desipramine).

TCAs are characterized more by their similarities than by their differences. There is a lag in clinical response for up to several weeks, partly as a result of side effects that prevent rapid increase in dosage and partly because of their neurotransmitter effects. They tend to affect both serotonin and norepinephrine reuptake; some drugs act mainly on the former and others principally on the latter neurotransmitter system. Individuals receiving the same dosages vary markedly in therapeutic drug levels achieved (elderly patients require smaller doses), and determination of plasma drug levels is helpful when clinical response has been disappointing. Nortriptyline is usually effective when plasma levels are between 50 and 150 ng/mL; imipramine at plasma levels of 200–250 ng/mL; and desipramine at plasma levels of 100–250 ng/mL. High blood levels are not more effective than moderate levels and may be counterproductive (eg, delirium, seizures). Patients with gastrointestinal side effects benefit from plasma level monitoring to assess absorption of the drug. Most TCAs can be given in a single dose at bedtime, starting at fairly low doses (eg, nortriptyline 25 mg orally) and increasing by 25 mg every several days as tolerated until the therapeutic response is achieved (eg, nortriptyline, 100–150 mg) or to maximum dose if necessary (eg, nortriptyline, 150 mg). The most common cause of treatment failure is an inadequate trial. A full trial consists of giving maximum daily dosage for at least 6 weeks. To reach maximum dosage, the trial encompasses a total of about 8 weeks. Because of marked anticholinergic and sedating side effects, clomipramine is started at a low dose (25 mg/d orally) and increased slowly in divided doses up to 100 mg/d, held at that level for several days, and then gradually increased as necessary up to 250 mg/d. Any of the TCA-like drugs should be started at very low doses (eg, 10–25 mg/d) and increased slowly in the treatment of panic disorder.

The TCAs have anticholinergic side effects to varying degrees (amitriptyline 100 mg is equivalent to atropine 5 mg). One must be particularly wary of the effect in elderly men with prostatic hyperplasia. The anticholinergic effects also predispose to other medical problems such as heat stroke or dental problems from xerostomia. Orthostatic hypotension is fairly common, may not remit with time, and may predispose to falls and hip fractures in the elderly. Cardiac effects of the TCAs are functions of the anticholinergic effect, direct myocardial depression (quinidine-like effect), and interference with adrenergic neurons. These factors may produce altered rate, rhythm, and contractility, particularly in patients with preexisting cardiac

disease, such as bundle-branch or bifascicular block. Electrocardiographic changes range from benign ST segment and T wave changes and sinus tachycardia to a variety of complex and serious arrhythmias, the latter requiring a change in medication. Because TCAs have class I antiarrhythmic effects, they should be used with caution in patients with ischemic heart disease, arrhythmias, or conduction disturbances. SSRIs or the atypical antidepressants may be better initial choices for this population. TCAs lower the seizure threshold so this is of particular concern in patients with a propensity for seizures (eg, previous head injury, alcohol withdrawal). Loss of libido and erectile, ejaculatory, and orgasmic dysfunction are fairly common and can compromise compliance. Trazodone rarely causes priapism, which requires treatment within 12 hours (epinephrine 1:1000 injected into the corpus cavernosum). Delirium, agitation, and mania are infrequent complications. Sudden discontinuation of some of these drugs can produce "cholinergic rebound," manifested by headaches and nausea with abdominal cramps. Overdoses of TCAs are often serious because of the narrow therapeutic index and quinidine-like effects (see Chapter 39).

3. Monoamine oxidase inhibitors—The MAO inhibitors are generally used as third-line drugs for depression (after a failure of SSRIs, TCAs, or the atypical antidepressants) because of the dietary and other restrictions required (see below and Table 25–7). They should be considered third-line drugs for refractory panic disorder and depression. This may change in the future, as MAO inhibitor skin patches are expected to become available. They bypass the gastrointestinal tract so that dietary restrictions will not be necessary.

MAO inhibitors are administered in gradual stepwise dosage and may be given in the morning or evening, depending upon their effect on sleep. They tend to take effect in a fairly low dosage range (Table 25–8). Blood levels are not congruent with therapeutic response.

The MAO inhibitors commonly cause symptoms of orthostatic hypotension (which may persist) and sympathomimetic effects of tachycardia, sweating, and tremor. Nausea, insomnia (often associated with intense afternoon drowsiness), and sexual dysfunction

Table 25–7. Principal dietary restrictions in MAOI use.

1. Cheese, except cream cheese and cottage cheese and fresh yogurt
2. Fermented or aged meats such as bologna, salami
3. Broad bean pods such as Chinese bean pods
4. Liver of all types
5. Meat and yeast extracts
6. Red wine, sherry, vermouth, cognac, beer, ale
7. Soy sauce, shrimp paste, sauerkraut

MAOI = monoamine oxidase inhibitor.

Table 25–8. Commonly used antidepressants.

Drug	Usual Daily Oral Dose (mg)	Usual Daily Maximum Dose (mg)	Sedative Effects[1]	Anticho-linergic Effects[1]	Cost per Unit	Cost for 30 Days Treatment Based on Maximum Dosage[2]
SSRIs						
Fluoxetine (Prozac, Sarafem)	5–40	80	< 1	< 1	$2.67/20 mg	$320.40
Fluvoxamine (Luvox)	100–300	300	1	< 1	$2.64/100 mg	$237.60
Nefazodone (Serzone)	300–600	600	2	< 1	$1.60/200 mg	$144.00
Paroxetine (Paxil)	20–30	50	1	1	$2.73/20 mg	$163.80
Sertraline (Zoloft)	50–150	200	< 1	< 1	$2.90/100 mg	$174.00
Citalopram (Celexa)	20	40	< 1	1	$2.53/40 mg	$75.90
Escitalopram (Lexapro)	10	20	< 1	1	$2.81/20 mg	$84.30
TRICYCLIC AND CLINICALLY SIMILAR COMPOUNDS						
Amitriptyline (Elavil)	150–250	300	4	4	$1.16/150 mg	$69.60
Amoxapine (Asendin)	150–200	400	2	2	$1.67/100 mg	$200.40
Clomipramine (Anafranil)	100	250	3	3	$1.47/75 mg	$157.20
Desipramine (Norpramin)	100–250	300	1	1	$1.50/100 mg	$135.00
Doxepin (Sinequan)	150–200	300	4	3	$1.00/100 mg	$90.00
Imipramine (Tofranil)	150–200	300	3	3	$1.22/50 mg	$219.60
Maprotiline (Ludiomil)	100–200	300	4	2	$0.93/75 mg	$111.60
Nortriptyline (Aventyl, Pamelor)	100–150	150	2	2	$1.62/50 mg	$148.20
Protriptyline (Vivactil)	15–40	60	1	3	$1.58/10 mg	$248.40
MONOAMINE OXIDASE INHIBITORS						
Phenelzine (Nardil)	45–60	90	...	...	$0.60/15 mg	$108.00
Tranylcypromine (Parnate)	20–30	50	...	...	$0.80/10 mg	$120.00
OTHER COMPOUNDS						
Venlafaxine XR (Effexor)	150–225	225	1	< 1	$3.52/75 mg	$316.80
Duloxetine (Cymbalta)	40	60	2	3	$3.84/60 mg	$115.30
Mirtazapine (Remeron)	15–45	45	4	2	$2.80/30 mg	$165.46
Bupropion XL (Wellbutrin XL)	300[3]	450[3]		< 1	$4.65/300 mg	$245.21
Bupropion SR (Wellbutrin SR)	300	400[4]		< 1	$3.76/200 mg	$226.12
Trazodone (Desyrel)	100–300	400	4	< 1	$0.73/100 mg	$87.60
Trimipramine (Surmontil)	75–200	200	4	4	$2.96/100 mg	$177.60

[1]4 = strong effect; 1 = weak effect.

[2]Average wholesale price (AWP, for AB-rated generic when available) for quantity listed. Source: *Red Book Update*, Vol. 25, No. 5, May 2006. AWP may not accurately represent the actual pharmacy cost because wide contractual variations exist among institutions.

[3]Wellbutrin XL is a once-daily form of bupropion. Bupropion is still available as immediate release, and, if used, no single dose should exceed 150 mg.

[4]200 mg twice daily.

SSRIs = serotonin selective reuptake inhibitors.

are common. Trazodone, 25–75 mg orally at bedtime, may ameliorate the MAO-induced insomnia. Central nervous system effects include agitation and toxic psychoses. Dietary limitations (Table 25–7) and abstinence from drug products containing phenylpropanolamine, phenylephrine, meperidine, dextromethorphan, and pseudoephedrine are mandatory for MAO-A type inhibitors (those marketed for treatment of depression), since the reduction of available monoamine oxidase leaves the patient vulnerable to exogenous amines (eg, tyramine in foodstuffs).

Treatment for a resultant hypertensive crisis has been the same as for pheochromocytoma (see Chapter 26), but there have been reports of success with nifedipine, 10 mg chewed and placed under the tongue, normalizing blood pressure in 1–5 minutes. The restrictions on the proscribed foodstuffs and sympathomimetic drugs are in effect during treatment and for 2–3 weeks after cessation of therapy. Termination of therapy with MAO inhibitors may be associated with anxiety, agitation, cognitive slowing, and headache. Very gradual withdrawal and short-term benzodiazepine therapy will ameliorate symptoms.

4. Switching and combination therapy—If the therapeutic response has been poor after an adequate trial with the chosen drug, the diagnosis should be reassessed. Assuming that the trial has been adequate and the diagnosis is correct, a trial with a drug from another group is appropriate. In switching from one group to another, an adequate "washout time" must be allowed. This is critical in certain situations—eg, in switching from an MAO inhibitor to a TCA, allow 2–3 weeks between stopping one drug and starting another; in switching from an SSRI to an MAO inhibitor, allow 4–5 weeks. In switching within groups—eg, from one TCA to another (amitriptyline to desipramine, etc)—no washout time is needed, and one can rapidly decrease the dosage of one drug while increasing the other. Combining two antidepressants requires caution and is usually reserved for refractory patients after psychiatric consultation.

However, in any of the three groups, one can augment the antidepressant drug if the therapeutic response has been less than satisfactory. Psychiatric consultation may be helpful in selecting the augmenting agent. Lithium is an excellent augmentation agent for the 25–40% of depressed patients who do not respond to an adequate trial of an antidepressant. Half of these patients will respond to the addition of lithium (600–900 mg/d) with an enhanced antidepressant effect.

5. Maintenance and tapering—When clinical relief of symptoms is obtained, medication is continued for 12 months in the effective maintenance dosage, which is the dosage required in the acute stage. The full dosage should be continued indefinitely when the individual has a first episode before age 20 or after age 50, is over age 40 with two episodes, or has had three episodes at any age. Major depression should often be considered as a chronic disease. If the medication is being tapered, it should be done gradually over several months, monitoring closely for relapse.

6. Drug interactions—Interactions with other drugs are listed in Table 25–9.

7. Electroconvulsive therapy—ECT causes a generalized central nervous system seizure (peripheral convulsion is not necessary) by means of electric current. The key objective is to exceed the seizure threshold, which can be accomplished by a variety of means. Electrical stimulation is more reliable and simpler than the use of chemical convulsants. The mechanism of action is not known, but it is thought to involve major neurotransmitter responses at the cell membrane. Current insufficient to cause a seizure produces no therapeutic benefit.

ECT is the most effective (about 70–85%) treatment of severe depression—particularly the delusions and agitation commonly seen with depression in the elderly. It is indicated when medical conditions preclude the use of antidepressants or in cases of nonresponsiveness to these medications. Comparative controlled studies of ECT in severe depression show that it is more effective than chemotherapy. It is also effective in the manic disorders and psychoses during pregnancy (when drugs may be contraindicated). It has not been shown to be helpful in chronic schizophrenic disorders, and it is generally not used in acute schizophrenic episodes unless drugs are not effective and it is urgent that the psychosis be controlled (eg, a catatonic stupor complicating an acute medical condition).

The most common side effects are memory disturbance and headache. Memory loss or confusion is usually related to the number and frequency of ECT treatments and proper oxygenation during treatment. Unilateral ECT is associated with less memory loss than bilateral ECT. Some memory loss is occasionally permanent, but most memory faculties return to full capacity within several weeks. There have been reports that lithium administration concurrent with ECT resulted in greater memory loss. Before anesthesia was used, spinal compression fractures and severe anticipatory anxiety were common.

Increased intracranial pressure is a serious contraindication. Other problems such as cardiac disorders, aortic aneurysms, bronchopulmonary disease, and venous thrombosis are relative contraindications and must be evaluated in light of the severity of the medical problem versus the need for ECT. Serious complications arising from ECT occur in less than 1 in 1000 cases. Most of these problems are cardiovascular or respiratory in nature (eg, aspiration of gastric contents). Poor patient understanding and lack of acceptance of the technique by the public are the biggest obstacles to the use of ECT.

8. Phototherapy—Phototherapy is used in major depression with seasonal onset. It consists of exposure (at a 3-foot distance) to a light source of 2500 lux for 2 hours daily. Light visors are an adaptation that provides greater mobility and an adjustable light intensity. The price of these full-spectrum light sources ranges

Table 25–9. Antidepressant drug interactions with other drugs.

Drug	Effects
Tricyclic and other non-MAOI antidepressants	
Antacids	Decreased absorption of antidepressants
Anticoagulants	Increased hypoprothrombinemic effect
Cimetidine	Increased antidepressant blood levels and psychosis
Clonidine	Decreased antihypertensive effect
Digitalis	Increased incidence of heart block
Disulfiram	Increased antidepressant blood levels
Guanethidine	Decreased antihypertensive effect
Haloperidol	Increased clomipramine levels
Insulin	Decreased blood sugar
Lithium	Increased lithium levels with fluoxetine
Methyldopa	Decreased antihypertensive effect
Other anticholinergic drugs	Marked anticholinergic responses
Phenytoin	Increased blood levels
Procainamide	Decreased ventricular conduction
Procarbazine	Hypertensive crisis
Propranolol	Increased hypotension
Quinidine	Decreased ventricular conduction
Rauwolfia derivatives	Increased stimulation
Sedatives	Increased sedation
Sympathomimetic drugs	Increased pressor effect
Terfenadine,[1] astemizole,[1] cisapride	Torsades de pointes
MAOIs	
Antihistamines	Increased sedation
Belladonna-like drugs	Increased blood pressure
Dextromethorphan	Same as meperidine
Guanethidine	Decreased blood pressure
Insulin	Decreased blood sugar
Levodopa	Increased blood pressure
Meperidine	Increased agitation, seizures, coma, death
Methyldopa	Decreased blood pressure
Pseudoephedrine	Hypertensive crisis (increased blood pressure)
Reserpine	Increased blood pressure and temperature
Succinylcholine	Increased neuromuscular blockade
Sulfonylureas	Decreased blood sugar
Sympathomimetic drugs	Increased blood pressure

[1]Terfenadine and astemizole are not commercially available in the United States.
MAOIs = monoamine oxidase inhibitors.

between $300 and $400. The dosage varies, with some patients requiring morning and night exposure. One effect is alteration of biorhythm through melatonin mechanisms.

9. Experimental treatments—In preliminary studies, transcranial magnetic stimulation appears to be effective in nonpsychotic depression. Vagal nerve stimulation has shown promise in extremely refractory cases and has recently been approved by the FDA.

B. PSYCHOLOGICAL

It is seldom possible to engage an individual in penetrating psychotherapeutic endeavors during the acute stage of a severe depression. While medications may be taking effect, a supportive approach to strengthen existing defenses and appropriate consideration of the patient's continuing need to function at work, to engage in recreational activities, etc, are necessary as the severity of the depression lessens. If the patient is not seriously depressed, it is often quite appropriate to initiate intensive psychotherapeutic efforts, since flux periods are a good time to effect change. A catharsis of repressed anger and guilt may be beneficial. Therapy during or just after the acute stage may focus on coping techniques, with some practice of alternative choices. When lack of self-confidence and identity problems are factors in the depression, individual psychotherapy can be oriented to ways of improving self-esteem, increasing assertiveness, and lessening dependency. Interpersonal psychotherapy for depression has shown efficacy in the treatment of acute depression, helping patients master interpersonal stresses and develop new coping strategies. Cognitive behavioral therapy for depression addresses patients' patterns of negative thoughts, called cognitive distortions, that lead to feelings of depression and anxiety. Treatment usually includes homework assignments such as keeping a journal of cognitive distortions and of positive responses to them. As previously noted, numerous studies have shown that the combination of drug therapy plus interpersonal psychotherapy or cognitive behavioral therapy is more effective than either modality alone. It is usually helpful to involve the spouse or other significant family members early in treatment. Mindfulness based cognitive therapy is a new form of therapy showing promise in reducing depression recurrence. This therapy incorporates meditation and teaches patients to distance themselves from depressive thinking.

C. SOCIAL

Flexible use of appropriate social services can be of major importance in the treatment of depression. Since alcohol is often associated with depression, early involvement in alcohol treatment programs such as Alcoholics Anonymous can be important to future success (see Alcohol Dependency and Abuse, below). The structuring of daily activities during severe depression is often quite difficult for the patient, and loneliness is often a major factor. The help of family, employer, or friends is often necessary to mobilize the patient who experiences no joy in daily activities and tends to remain uninvolved and to deteriorate. Insistence on sharing activities will help involve the patient in simple but important daily functions. In some severe cases, the use of day treatment centers or support groups of a specific type (eg, mastectomy groups) is indicated. It is not unusual for a patient to have multiple legal, financial, and vocational problems requiring legal and vocational assistance.

D. BEHAVIORAL

When depression is a function of self-defeating coping techniques such as passivity, the role-playing approach can be useful. Behavioral techniques, including desensitization, may be used in problems such as phobias where depression is a by-product. When depression is a regularly used interpersonal style, behavioral counseling to family members or others can help in extinguishing the behavior in the patient.

Treatment of Mania

Acute manic or hypomanic symptoms will respond to lithium or valproic acid after several days of treatment, but it is increasingly common to use atypical neuroleptics as adjunctive treatment or monotherapy. High-potency benzodiazepines (eg, clonazepam) may also be useful adjuncts in managing acute cases. Some schizoaffective disorders and some cases of so-called schizophrenia are probably atypical bipolar affective disorder, for which lithium treatment may be effective.

A. NEUROLEPTICS

Acute manic symptoms of agitation and psychosis may be treated initially with the atypical antipsychotic olanzapine, (eg, 5–20 mg orally), risperidone (2–3 mg orally), or aripiprazole (15–30 mg) in conjunction with a benzodiazepine if indicated. Alternatively, when behavioral control is immediately necessary, olanzapine in an injectable form (2.5–10 mg intramuscularly) or haloperidol, 5–10 mg orally or intramuscularly repeated as needed until symptoms subside, may be used. The dosage of the neuroleptic may be gradually reduced after lithium or another mood stabilizer is started (see below). Olanzapine is approved as a maintenance treatment for bipolar disorder.

B. CLONAZEPAM

Clonazepam can be an alternative or adjunct to a neuroleptic in controlling acute behavioral symptoms. Clonazepam has the advantage of causing no extrapyramidal side effects. Although 1–2 mg orally every 4–6 hours may be effective, up to 16 mg/d may be necessary.

C. LITHIUM

As a prophylactic drug for bipolar affective disorder, lithium significantly decreases the frequency and severity of both manic and depressive attacks in about 70% of patients. A positive response is more predictable if the patient has a low frequency of episodes (no more than two per year with intervals free of psychopathology). A positive response occurs more frequently in individuals who have blood relatives with a diagnosis of manic or hypomanic attacks. Patients who swing rapidly back and forth between manic and depressive attacks (at least four cycles per year) usually respond poorly to lithium prophylaxis initially, but some improve with continued long-term treatment. Carbamazepine (see below) has been used with success in this group.

In addition to its use in manic states, lithium is sometimes useful in the prophylaxis of recurrent unipolar depressions (perhaps undiagnosed bipolar disorder). Lithium may ameliorate nonspecific aggressive behaviors and dyscontrol syndromes. The dosages are the same as used in bipolar disorder. Most patients with bipolar disease can be managed long-term with lithium alone, although some will require continued or intermittent use of a neuroleptic, antidepressant, or carbamazepine. An excellent resource for information pertaining to lithium is the Information Centers, Madison Institute of Medicine, 7617 Mineral Point Road, Suite 300, Madison, WI 53717-1914.

Before treatment, the clinical workup should include a medical history and physical examination; complete blood count; T_4, thyroid-stimulating hormone, blood urea nitrogen (BUN), serum creatinine, and serum electrolyte determinations; urinalysis; and electrocardiography in patients over age 45 or with a history of cardiac disease.

1. Dosage—Lithium carbonate is generally prescribed in the 300 mg unit. In a small minority of patients, a slow release form or units of different dosage may be required. Lithium citrate is available as a syrup. The dosage is that required to maintain blood levels in the therapeutic range. For acute attacks, this ranges from 1 to 1.5 mEq/L. Although there is controversy about the optimal long-term maintenance dose, many clinicians reduce the acute level to 0.6–1 mEq/L in order to reduce side effects. The dose required to meet this need will vary in different individuals. For acute mania, doses of 1200–1800 mg/d are generally recommended. Augmentation of antidepressants is usually achieved with half of these doses. Once-a-day dosage is acceptable, but most patients have less nausea when they take the drug in divided doses with meals.

Lithium is readily absorbed, with peak serum levels occurring within 1–3 hours and complete absorption in 8 hours. Half of the total body lithium is excreted in 18–24 hours (95% in the urine). Blood for lithium levels should be drawn 12 hours after the last dose. Serum levels should be measured 5–7 days after initiation of treatment and changes in dose. For maintenance treatment, lithium levels should be monitored initially every 1–2 months but may be measured every 6–12 months in stable, long-term patients. Levels should be monitored more closely when there is any condition that causes volume depletion (eg, diarrhea, dehydration, use of diuretics).

2. Side effects—Mild gastrointestinal symptoms (take lithium with food), fine tremors (treat with propranolol, 20–60 mg/d orally, only if persistent), slight muscle weakness, and some degree of somnolence are early side effects that are usually transient. Moderate polyuria (reduced renal responsiveness to ADH) and polydipsia (associated with increased plasma renin concentration) are often present. Potassium administration can blunt this effect, as may once-daily dosing of lithium. Weight gain (often a result of calories in fluids taken for polydipsia) and leukocytosis not due to infection are fairly common.

Other side effects include goiter (3%; often euthyroid), hypothyroidism (10%; concomitant administration of lithium and iodide or lithium and carbamazepine enhances the hypothyroid and goitrogenic effect of either drug), changes in the glucose tolerance test toward a diabetes-like curve, nephrogenic diabetes insipidus (usually resolving about 8 weeks after cessation of lithium therapy), nephrotic syndrome, edema, folate deficiency, and pseudotumor cerebri (ophthalmoscopy is indicated if there are complaints of headache or blurred vision). A metallic taste, hair loss, and Raynaud's phenomenon have been reported in a few cases. Thyroid and kidney function should be checked at 3- to 4-month intervals. Most of these side effects subside when lithium is discontinued; when residual side effects exist, they are usually not serious. Most clinicians treat lithium-induced hypothyroidism (more common in women) with thyroid hormone while continuing lithium therapy. Hypercalcemia and elevated parathyroid hormone levels occur in some patients. Electrocardiographic abnormalities (principally T wave flattening or inversion) may occur during lithium administration but are not of major clinical significance. Sinoatrial block may occur, particularly in the elderly. Other drugs that prolong intraventricular conduction, such as TCAs, must be used cautiously in conjunction with lithium. Lithium impairs ventilatory function in patients with airway obstruction. Lithium alone does not have a significant effect on sexual function, but when combined with benzodiazepines (clonazepam in most symptomatic patients) it causes sexual dysfunction in about 50% of men. Lithium may precipitate or exacerbate psoriasis in some patients.

Patients receiving long-term lithium therapy may have cogwheel rigidity and, occasionally, other extrapyramidal signs. Lithium potentiates the parkinsonian effects of haloperidol. Long-term lithium therapy has also been associated with a relative lowering of the level of memory and perceptual processing (affecting compliance in some cases). Some impairment of attention and emotional reactivity has also been noted. Lithium-induced delirium with therapeutic lithium levels is an infrequent complication usually occurring in the elderly and may persist for several days after serum levels have become negligible. Encephalopathy has occurred in patients receiving combined lithium and neuroleptic therapy and in those who have cerebrovascular disease, thus requiring careful evaluation of patients who develop neurotoxic signs at subtoxic blood levels.

Some reports have suggested that the long-term use of lithium may have adverse effects on renal function (with interstitial fibrosis or tubular atrophy). A rise in serum creatinine levels is an indication for in-depth evaluation of renal function and consideration of alternative treatments if the individual can tolerate a change. Incontinence has been reported in women, apparently related to changes in bladder cholinergic-adrenergic balance.

Prospective studies suggest that the overall risk imposed by lithium in pregnancy may be overemphasized. However, lithium exposure in early pregnancy does increase the frequency of congenital anomalies, especially Ebstein's and other major cardiovascular anomalies. For women who take psychotropic medications who become pregnant, the decision to make a change in medication is complex and requires informed consent regarding the relative risks to the patient and fetus. Indeed, the risk of untreated bipolar disorder carries its own risks for pregnancy. Formula feeding should be considered in mothers taking lithium, since concentration in breast milk is one-third to half that in serum.

Frank toxicity usually occurs at blood lithium levels above 2 mEq/L. Because sodium and lithium are reabsorbed at the same loci in the proximal renal tubules, any sodium loss (diarrhea, use of diuretics, or excessive perspiration) results in increased lithium levels. Symptoms and signs include vomiting and diarrhea, the latter exacerbating the problem since more sodium is lost and more lithium is absorbed. Other symptoms and signs, some of which may not be reversible, include tremors, marked muscle weakness, confusion, dysarthria, vertigo, choreoathetosis, ataxia, hyperreflexia, rigidity, lack of coordination, myoclonus, seizures, opisthotonos, and coma. Toxicity is more severe in the elderly, who should be maintained on slightly lower serum levels. Lithium overdosage may be accidental or intentional or may occur as a result of poor monitoring.

Patients with massive ingestions of lithium or blood lithium levels above 2.5 mEq/L should be treated with induced emesis and gastric lavage. If renal function is normal, osmotic and saline diuresis increases renal lithium clearance. Urinary alkalinization is also helpful, since sodium bicarbonate decreases lithium reabsorption in the proximal tubule, as does acetazolamide as well. Aminophylline potentiates the diuretic effect by increasing the clearance of lithium. Drugs affecting the distal loop have no effect on lithium reabsorption. Blood lithium levels above 2.5 mEq/L (confirmed by cerebrospinal fluid lithium levels) should be considered an indication for hemodialysis.

Compliance with lithium therapy is adversely affected by the loss of some hypomanic experiences valued by the patient. These include social extroversion and a sense of heightened enjoyment in many activities such as sex and business dealings, often with increased productivity in the latter.

3. Drug interactions—Patients receiving lithium should use diuretics with caution and only under close medical supervision. The thiazide diuretics cause in-

Table 25–10. Lithium interactions with other drugs.

Drug	Effects
ACE inhibitors	↑ Lithium levels
Fluoxetine	↑ Lithium levels
Ibuprofen	↑ Lithium levels
Indomethacin	↑ Lithium levels
Methyldopa	Rigidity, mutism, fascicular twitching
Osmotic diuretics (urea, mannitol)	↑ Lithium excretion
Phenylbutazone	↑ Lithium levels
Potassium-sparing diuretics (spironolactone, amiloride, triamterene)	↑ Lithium levels
Sodium bicarbonate	↑ Lithium excretion
Succinylcholine	↑ Duration of action of succinylcholine
Theophylline, aminophylline	↑ Lithium excretion
Thiazide diuretics	↑ Lithium levels
Valproic acid	↓ Lithium levels
COX-2 inhibitors	↑ Lithium levels

ACE = angiotensin-converting enzyme; COX-2 = cyclooxygenase-2.

creased lithium reabsorption from the proximal renal tubules, resulting in increased serum lithium levels (Table 25–10), and adjustment of lithium intake must be made to compensate for this. Reduce lithium dosage by 25–40% when the patient is receiving 50 mg of hydrochlorothiazide daily. Potassium-sparing diuretics (spironolactone, amiloride, triamterene) may also increase serum lithium levels and require careful monitoring of lithium levels. Loop diuretics (furosemide, ethacrynic acid, bumetanide) do not appear to alter serum lithium levels. Concurrent use of lithium and angiotensin-converting enzyme inhibitors requires a 50–75% reduction in lithium intake to achieve therapeutic lithium levels.

D. Valproic Acid

Valproic acid (divalproex) is an antiseizure drug whose activity is at least partially related to GABA neurotransmission. It is a first-line treatment for mania because it has a broader index of safety than lithium. This issue is particularly important in AIDS or other medically ill patients prone to dehydration or malabsorption with wide swings in serum lithium levels. Valproic acid has also been used effectively in panic disorder and migraine headache. Treatment is often started at a dose of 750 mg/d

orally in divided doses, and dosage is then titrated to achieve therapeutic serum levels. Oral loading in acutely manic bipolar patients in an inpatient setting (initiated at a dosage of 20 mg/kg/d) can safely achieve serum therapeutic levels in 2–3 days. Concomitant use of aspirin, carbamazepine, warfarin, or phenytoin may affect serum levels. Gastrointestinal symptoms are the main side effects. Liver function tests, complete blood counts, glucose levels, and weight should be monitored, and teratogenic effects are a concern.

E. Carbamazepine

Carbamazepine, an antiseizure drug that stabilizes the activity of cell membranes, has been used with increasing frequency in the treatment of bipolar patients who cannot be satisfactorily treated with lithium (nonresponsive, excessive side effects, or rapid cycling). It is often effective at 800–1600 mg/d orally. It has also been used in the treatment of resistant depressions, alcohol withdrawal, and hallucinations (in conjunction with neuroleptics) and in patients with behavioral dyscontrol or panic attacks. It suppresses some phases of kindling (see Stimulants) and has been used to treat residual symptoms in previous stimulant abusers (eg, PTSD with impulse control problems). Dose-related side effects include sedation and ataxia. Dosages start at 400–600 mg orally daily and are increased slowly to therapeutic levels. Skin rashes and a mild reduction in white count are common. SIADH occurs rarely. Nonsteroidal antiinflammatory drugs (except aspirin), the antibiotics erythromycin and isoniazid, the calcium channel blockers verapamil and diltiazem (but not nifedipine), fluoxetine, propoxyphene, and cimetidine all increase carbamazepine levels. Carbamazepine can be effective in conjunction with lithium, although there have been reports of reversible neurotoxicity with the combination. Carbamazepine stimulates hepatic microsomal enzymes and so tends to decrease levels of haloperidol and oral contraceptives. It also lowers T_4, free T_4, and T_3 levels. Cases of fetal malformation (particularly spina bifida) have been reported along with growth deficiency and developmental delay. Liver tests and complete blood counts should be monitored in patients taking carbamazepine. **Oxcarbazepine**, a derivative of carbamazepine, does not appear to induce its own metabolism and is associated with fewer drug interactions, although it may impose a higher risk of hyponatremia. FDA-approved for partial seizures, oxcarbazepine may have efficacy in acute mania. It appears to be a safer alternative to carbamazepine due to its lower risk of hepatotoxicity.

F. Newer Anticonvulsants

Lamotrigine is thought to inhibit neuronal sodium channels and the release of the excitatory amino acids, glutamate and aspartate. It is FDA approved for long-term maintenance of bipolar disorder. Two double-blind studies support its efficacy in the treatment of acute bipolar depression as adjunctive therapy or as monotherapy. Its metabolism is inhibited by coadministration of valproic acid—doubling its half-life—and accelerated by hepatic enzyme-inducing agents such as carbamazepine. More frequent mild side effects include headache, dizziness, nausea, and diplopia. Rash occurring in 10% of patients is an indication for immediate cessation of dosing, since lamotrigine has been associated with Stevens-Johnson syndrome (1:1000) and, rarely, toxic epidermal necrolysis. Dosing starts at 25–50 mg/d and is titrated upward slowly to decrease the likelihood of rash. Slower titration and a lower total dose are indicated for patients taking valproic acid. **Topiramate**, which has been labeled for use as an anticonvulsant, has been found to be effective in the adjunctive treatment of bipolar disorder in a series of open-label studies. It has the unique feature of promoting weight loss as a side effect. Other common side effects include somnolence, difficulty with memory, dizziness, and anxiety.

G. CALCIUM CHANNEL BLOCKERS

Calcium channel blockers (eg, verapamil) have been used in bipolar states that have failed to respond to lithium, carbamazepine, or valproic acid. This has come about with the realization that a number of drugs used in psychiatry (eg, lithium, antidepressants, neuroleptics, and carbamazepine) have calcium channel–blocking activity. There is also preliminary evidence that these drugs may be useful in the treatment of tardive dyskinesia and panic attacks. Verapamil may be safer than lithium or carbamazepine during pregnancy, although it decreases uterine contractility and must be discontinued before delivery.

Prognosis

Reactive depressions are usually time-limited, and the prognosis with treatment is good if a pathologic pattern of adjustment does not intervene. Major affective disorders frequently respond well to a full trial of drug treatment.

Mania and bipolar disorder have a good prognosis with adequate treatment.

Glassman AH et al: Sertraline treatment of major depression in patients with acute MI or unstable angina. JAMA 2002; 288:701. [PMID: 12169073]

Nulman I et al: Child development following exposure to tricyclic antidepressants or fluoxetine throughout fetal life: a prospective, controlled study. Am J Psychiatry 2002;159:1889. [PMID: 12411224]

Nurnberg HG et al: Treatment of antidepressant-associated sexual dysfunction with sildenafil: a randomized controlled trial. JAMA 2003;289:56. [PMID: 12503977]

Segal ZV et al: Challenges in preventing relapse in major depression. A report of a National Institute of Mental Health Workshop on state of the science of relapse prevention in major depression. J Affect Disord 2003;77:97. [PMID: 14607387]

Swartz HA et al: A pilot study of brief interpersonal psychotherapy for depression among women. Psychiatr Serv 2004;55:448. [PMID: 15067162]

Williams M et al: Paroxetine (Paxil) and congenital malformations. CMAJ 2005;173:1320. [PMID: 16272192]

SLEEP DISORDERS

Sleep consists of two distinct states as shown by electroencephalographic studies: (1) REM (rapid eye movement) sleep, also called dream sleep, D state sleep, paradoxic sleep, and (2) NREM (non-REM) sleep, also called S stage sleep, which is divided into stages 1, 2, 3, and 4 and is recognizable by different electroencephalographic patterns. Stages 3 and 4 are "delta" sleep. Dreaming occurs mostly in REM and to a lesser extent in NREM sleep.

Sleep is a cyclic phenomenon, with four or five REM periods during the night accounting for about one-fourth of the total night's sleep (1.5–2 hours). The first REM period occurs about 80–120 minutes after onset of sleep and lasts about 10 minutes. Later REM periods are longer (15–40 minutes) and occur mostly in the last several hours of sleep. Most stage 4 (deepest) sleep occurs in the first several hours.

Age-related changes in normal sleep include an unchanging percentage of REM sleep and a marked decrease in stage 3 and stage 4 sleep, with an increase in wakeful periods during the night. These normal changes, early bedtimes, and daytime naps play a role in the increased complaints of insomnia in older people. Variations in sleep patterns may be due to circumstances (eg, "jet lag") or to idiosyncratic patterns ("night owls") in persons who perhaps because of different "biologic rhythms" habitually go to bed late and sleep late in the morning. Creativity and rapidity of response to unfamiliar situations are impaired by loss of sleep. There are also rare individuals who have chronic difficulty in adapting to a 24-hour sleep-wake cycle (desynchronization sleep disorder), which can be resynchronized by altering exposure to light.

The three major sleep disorders are discussed below.

1. Dyssomnias (Insomnia)

Classification & Clinical Findings

Patients may complain of difficulty getting to sleep or staying asleep, intermittent wakefulness during the night, early morning awakening, or combinations of any of these. Transient episodes are usually of little significance. Stress, caffeine, physical discomfort, daytime napping, and early bedtimes are common factors.

Psychiatric disorders are often associated with persistent insomnia. **Depression** is usually associated with fragmented sleep, decreased total sleep time, earlier onset of REM sleep, a shift of REM activity to the first half of the night, and a loss of slow wave sleep—all of which are nonspecific findings. In **manic disorders**, sleeplessness is a cardinal feature and an important early sign of impending mania in bipolar cases. Total sleep time is decreased, with shortened REM latency and increased REM activity. Sleep-related panic attacks occur in the transition from stage 2 to stage 3 sleep in some patients with a longer REM latency in the sleep pattern preceding the attacks.

Abuse of alcohol may cause or be secondary to the sleep disturbance. There is a tendency to use alcohol as a means of getting to sleep without realizing that it disrupts the normal sleep cycle. Acute alcohol intake produces a decreased sleep latency with reduced REM sleep during the first half of the night. REM sleep is increased in the second half of the night, with an increase in total amount of slow wave sleep (stages 3 and 4). Vivid dreams and frequent awakenings are common. Chronic alcohol abuse increases stage 1 and decreases REM sleep (most drugs delay or block REM sleep), with symptoms persisting for many months after the individual has stopped drinking. Acute alcohol or other sedative withdrawal causes delayed onset of sleep and REM rebound with intermittent awakening during the night.

Heavy smoking (more than a pack a day) causes difficulty falling asleep—apparently independently of the often associated increase in coffee drinking. Excess intake near bedtime of caffeine, cocaine, and other stimulants (eg, over-the-counter cold remedies) causes decreased total sleep time—mostly NREM sleep—with some increased sleep latency.

Sedative-hypnotics—specifically, the benzodiazepines, which are the most commonly prescribed drugs to promote sleep—tend to increase total sleep time, decrease sleep latency, and decrease nocturnal awakening, with variable effects on NREM sleep. Withdrawal causes just the opposite effects and results in continued use of the drug for the purpose of preventing withdrawal symptoms. Antidepressants decrease REM sleep (with marked rebound on withdrawal in the form of nightmares) and have varying effects on NREM sleep. The effect on REM sleep correlates with reports that REM sleep deprivation produces improvement in some depressions.

Persistent insomnias are also related to a wide variety of medical conditions, particularly delirium, pain, respiratory distress syndromes, uremia, asthma, and thyroid disorders. Adequate analgesia and proper treatment of medical disorders will reduce symptoms and decrease the need for sedatives.

Treatment

In general, there are two broad classes of treatment for insomnia, and the two may be combined: psychological (cognitive-behavioral) and pharmacologic. In situations of acute distress, such as a grief reaction, pharmacologic measures may be most appropriate. With primary insomnia, however, initial efforts should be psychologically based. This is particularly true in the elderly to avoid the potential adverse reactions of medications. The elderly population is at risk for complaints of insomnia because sleep becomes lighter and more easily disrupted with aging. Medical disorders that become more common with age may also predispose to insomnia.

A. PSYCHOLOGICAL

Psychological strategies should include educating the patient regarding good sleep hygiene: (1) Go to bed only when sleepy. (2) Use the bed and bedroom only for sleeping and sex. (3) If still awake after 20 minutes, leave the bedroom and only return when sleepy. (4) Get up at the same time every morning regardless of the amount of sleep during the night. (5) Discontinue caffeine and nicotine, at least in the evening if not completely. (6) Establish a daily exercise regimen. (7) Avoid alcohol as it may disrupt continuity of sleep. (8) Limit fluids in the evening. (9) Learn and practice relaxation techniques. A recent study suggests that cognitive behavioral therapy for insomnia was as effective as zolpidem with benefits sustained 1 year after treatment.

The clinician should also discuss any myths or misconceptions about sleep that the patient may hold.

B. MEDICAL

When the above measures are insufficient, medications may be useful. Pharmacologic measures currently rely primarily on safe hypnotic medications that are difficult to overdose with. Lorazepam (0.5 mg orally nightly), temazepam (7.5–15 mg orally nightly) and the nonbenzodiazepine hypnotics, zolpidem (5–10 mg orally nightly), and zaleplon (5–10 mg orally nightly), are often effective for the elderly population and can be given in larger doses—twice what is prescribed for the elderly—in younger patients. A new nonbenzodiazepine hypnotic, eszopiclone (2–3 mg), is similar in action to zolpidem and zaleplon but dissimilar in that it is not restricted to short-term use. A lower dose of 1 mg is indicated in the elderly or those with hepatic impairment. It is important to note that short-acting agents like triazolam or zolpidem may lead to amnestic episodes if used on a daily ongoing basis. Longer-acting agents such as flurazepam (half-life of > 48 hours) may accumulate in the elderly and lead to cognitive slowing, ataxia, falls, and somnolence. In general, it is appropriate to use medications for short courses of 1–2 weeks. The medications described above have largely replaced barbiturates as hypnotic agents because of their greater safety in overdose and their lesser hepatic enzyme induction effects. Antihistamines such as diphenhydramine (25 mg nightly) or hydroxyzine (25 mg nightly) may also be useful for sleep, as they produce no pharmacologic dependency; their anticholinergic effects may, however, produce confusion or urinary symptoms in the elderly. Trazodone, an atypical antidepressant, is a non–habit-forming, effective sleep medication in lower than antidepressant doses (25–150 mg at bedtime). Priapism is a rare side effect requiring emergent treatment.

Triazolam has achieved popularity as a hypnotic drug because of its very short duration of action. Because it has been associated with dependency, transient psychotic reactions, anterograde amnesia, and rebound anxiety, it has been removed from the market in several European countries. If used, it must be prescribed only for short periods of time.

2. Hypersomnias (Disorders of Excessive Sleepiness)

The hypersomnias are a more severe problem than insomnia.

Classification & Clinical Findings

A. SLEEP APNEA

This disorder is characterized by cessation of breathing for at least 30 episodes (each lasting about 10 seconds) during the night. There are two types: obstructive and central. (See Chapter 9.)

B. NARCOLEPSY

Narcolepsy consists of a tetrad of symptoms: (1) Sudden, brief (about 15 minutes) sleep attacks that may occur during any type of activity; (2) cataplexy—sudden loss of muscle tone involving specific small muscle groups or generalized muscle weakness that may cause the person to slump to the floor, unable to move, often associated with emotional reactions and sometimes confused with seizure disorder; (3) sleep paralysis—a generalized flaccidity of muscles with full consciousness in the transition zone between sleep and waking; and (4) hypnagogic hallucinations, visual or auditory, which may precede sleep or occur during the sleep attack. The attacks are characterized by an abrupt transition into REM sleep—a necessary criterion for diagnosis. The disorder begins in early adult life, affects both sexes equally, and usually levels off in severity at about 30 years of age.

REM sleep behavior disorder, characterized by motor dyscontrol and often violent dreams during REM sleep, may be related to narcolepsy.

C. KLEINE-LEVIN SYNDROME

This syndrome, which occurs mostly in young men, is characterized by hypersomnic attacks three or four times a year lasting up to 2 days, with hyperphagia, hypersexuality, irritability, and confusion on awakening. It has often been associated with antecedent neurologic insults. It usually remits after age 40.

D. NOCTURNAL MYOCLONUS

Periodic lower leg movements occur during sleep with subsequent daytime sleepiness, anxiety, depression, and cognitive impairment.

Treatment

Narcolepsy can be managed by daily administration of a stimulant such as dextroamphetamine sulfate, 10 mg in the morning, with increased dosage as necessary. Modafinil is a schedule IV medication FDA-approved for treating the excessive daytime fatigue of narcolepsy. Usual dosing is 200 mg each morning. Its mechanism of action is unknown, yet it is thought to be less of an abuse risk than stimulants that are primarily dopaminergic.

Common side effects include headache and anxiety; however, modafinil appears to be generally well tolerated. Modafinil may reduce the efficacy of cyclosporine, oral contraceptives, and other medications by inducing their hepatic metabolism. Imipramine, 75–100 mg daily, has been effective in treatment of cataplexy but not narcolepsy.

Nocturnal myoclonus and REM sleep behavior disorder can be treated with clonazepam with variable results. There is no treatment for Kleine-Levin syndrome.

Treatment of sleep apnea is discussed in Chapter 9.

3. Parasomnias (Abnormal Behaviors during Sleep)

These disorders are fairly common in children and less so in adults.

Classification & Clinical Findings

A. SLEEP TERROR

Sleep terror (pavor nocturnus) is an abrupt, terrifying arousal from sleep, usually in preadolescent boys although it may occur in adults as well. It is distinct from sleep panic attacks. Symptoms are fear, sweating, tachycardia, and confusion for several minutes, with amnesia for the event.

B. NIGHTMARES

Nightmares occur during REM sleep; sleep terrors in stage 3 or stage 4 sleep.

C. SLEEPWALKING

Sleepwalking (somnambulism) includes ambulation or other intricate behaviors while still asleep, with amnesia for the event. It affects mostly children aged 6–12 years, and episodes occur during stage 3 or stage 4 sleep in the first third of the night and in REM sleep in the later sleep hours. Sleepwalking in elderly people may be a feature of dementia. Idiosyncratic reactions to drugs (eg, marijuana, alcohol) and medical conditions (eg, partial complex seizures) may be causative factors in adults.

D. ENURESIS

Enuresis is involuntary micturition during sleep in a person who usually has voluntary control. Like other parasomnias, it is more common in children, usually in the 3–4 hours after bedtime, but is not limited to a specific stage of sleep. Confusion during the episode and amnesia for the event are common.

Treatment

Treatment for sleep terrors is with benzodiazepines (eg, diazepam, 5–20 mg at bedtime), since it will suppress stage 3 and stage 4 sleep. Somnambulism responds to the same treatment for the same reason, but simple safety measures should not be neglected. Enuresis may respond to imipramine, 50–100 mg at bedtime, although desmopressin nasal spray (an ADH preparation) has increasingly become the treatment of choice for nocturnal enuresis. Behavioral approaches (eg, bells that ring when the pad gets wet) have also been successful.

Brielmaier BD: Eszopiclone (Lunesta): a new nonbenzodiazepine hypnotic. Proc (Bayl Univ Med Cent) 2006;19:54. [PMID: 16424933]

Jacobs GD et al: Cognitive behavioral therapy and pharmacotherapy for insomnia: a randomized controlled trial and direct comparison. Arch Intern Med 2004;164:1888. [PMID: 15463047]

Jindal RD et al: Maintenance treatment of insomnia: what can we learn from the depression literature? Am J Psychiatry 2004; 161:19. [PMID: 14702243]

DISORDERS OF AGGRESSION

Acts performed with the deliberate intent of causing physical harm to persons or property have a wide variety of causative features. Aggression and violence are symptoms rather than diseases, and most frequently they are not associated with an underlying medical condition. Clinicians are unable to predict dangerous behavior with greater than chance accuracy. Depression, schizophrenia, personality disorders, mania, paranoia, temporal lobe dysfunction, and organic mental states may be associated with acts of aggression. Impulse control disorders are characterized by physical abuse (usually of the aggressor's domestic partner or children), by pathologic intoxication, by impulsive sexual activities, and by reckless driving. Anabolic steroid usage by athletes has been associated with increased tendencies toward violent behavior.

In the United States, a significant proportion of all violent deaths are alcohol-related. The ingestion of even small amounts of alcohol can result in pathologic intoxication that resembles an acute organic mental condition. Amphetamines, crack cocaine, and other stimulants are frequently associated with aggressive behavior. Phencyclidine is a drug commonly associated with violent behavior that is occasionally of a bizarre nature, partly due to lowering of the pain threshold. Domestic violence and rape are much more widespread than previously recognized. Awareness of the problem is to some degree due to increasing recognition of the rights of women and the understanding by women that they do not have to accept abuse. Acceptance of this kind of aggressive behavior inevitably leads to more, with the ultimate aggression being murder—20–50% of murders in the United States occur within the family. Police are called in more domestic disputes than all other criminal incidents combined. Children living in such family situations frequently become victims of abuse.

Features of individuals who have been subjected to long-term physical or sexual abuse are as follows: trouble expressing anger, staying angry longer, general passivity in relationships, feeling "marked for life" with an accompanying feeling of deserving to be victimized, lack of trust, and dissociation of affect from experiences. They are prone to express their psychological distress with somatization symptoms, often pain complaints. They may also have symptoms related to posttraumatic stress, as discussed above. The clinician should be suspicious about the origin of any injuries not fully explained, particularly if such incidents recur.

Treatment

A. PSYCHOLOGICAL

Management of any violent individual includes appropriate psychological maneuvers. Move slowly, talk slowly with clarity and reassurance, and evaluate the situation. Strive to create a setting that is minimally disturbing, and eliminate people or things threatening to the violent individual. Do not threaten or abuse, and do not touch or crowd the person. Allow no weapons in the area (an increasing problem in hospital emergency departments). Proximity to a door is comforting to both the patient and the examiner. Use a negotiator the violent person can relate to comfortably. Food and drink are helpful in defusing the situation (as are cigarettes for those who smoke). Honesty is important. Make no false promises, bolster the patient's self-esteem, and continue to engage the subject verbally until the situation is under control. This type of individual does better with strong external controls to replace the lack of inner controls over the long term. Close probationary supervision and judicially mandated restrictions can be most helpful. There should be a major effort to help the individual avoid drug use (eg, Alcoholics Anonymous). Victims of abuse are essentially treated as any victim of trauma and, not infrequently, have evidence of PTSD.

B. PHARMACOLOGIC

Pharmacologic means are often necessary whether or not psychological approaches have been successful. This is particularly true in the agitated or psychotic patient. The drug of choice in psychotic aggressive states is haloperidol, 5–10 mg intramuscularly every hour until symptoms are alleviated. Benzodiazepine sedatives (eg, diazepam, 5 mg orally or intravenously every several hours) can be used for mild to moderate agitation, but an antipsychotic drug is preferred for management of the seriously violent and psychotic patient. Chronic aggressive states, particularly in retardation and brain damage (rule out causative organic conditions and medications such as anticholinergic drugs in amounts sufficient to cause confusion), have been ameliorated with propranolol, 40–240 mg/d orally, or pindolol, 5 mg twice daily orally (pindolol causes less bradycardia and hypotension). Carbamazepine and valproic acid are effective in the treatment of aggression and explosive disorders, particularly when associated with known or suspected brain lesions. Lithium and SSRIs are also effective for some intermittent explosive outbursts. Buspirone (10–45 mg/d orally) is helpful for aggression, particularly in mentally retarded patients.

C. PHYSICAL

Physical management is necessary if psychological and pharmacologic means are not sufficient. It requires the active and visible presence of an adequate number of personnel (five or six) to reinforce the idea that the situation is under control despite the patient's lack of inner controls. Such an approach often precludes the need for actual physical restraint. When adequate personnel are not available, however, two people shielded by a mattress (single-bed size) can usually corner and subdue the patient without injury to anyone. Seclusion rooms and restraints should be used only when necessary (ambulatory restraints are an alternative), and the patient must then be observed at frequent intervals. Design of corridors and seclusion rooms is important. Narrow corridors, small spaces, and crowded areas exacerbate the potential for violence in an anxious patient.

D. OTHER

The treatment of victims (eg, battered women) is challenging and often complicated by their reluctance to leave the situation. Reasons for staying vary, but common themes include the fear of more violence because of leaving, the hope that the situation may ameliorate (in spite of steady worsening), and the financial aspects of the situation, which are seldom to the woman's advantage. Concerns for the children often finally compel the woman to seek help. An early step is to get the woman into a therapeutic situation that provides the support of others in similar straits. Al-Anon is frequently a valuable asset and quite appropriate when alcohol is a factor. The group can support the victim while she gathers strength to consider alternatives without being paralyzed by fear. Many cities now offer temporary emergency centers and counseling. Use the available resources, attend to any medical or psychiatric problems, and maintain a compassionate interest. Some states now require physicians to report injuries caused by abuse to police authorities.

Jonassen JA et al: Identification of physician and patient attributes that influence the likelihood of screening for intimate partner violence. Acad Med 2003;78(10 Suppl):S20. [PMID: 14557085]

McFarlane J et al: Abuse during pregnancy and femicide: urgent implications for women's health. Obstet Gynecol 2002;100: 27. [PMID: 12100800]

Walthan CN et al: Interventions for violence against women: scientific review. JAMA 2003;327:708. [PMID: 12578492]

■ SUBSTANCE USE DISORDERS (Drug Dependency, Drug Abuse)

The term "drug dependency" is used in a broad sense here to include both addictions and habituations. It involves the triad of compulsive drug use referred to as drug addiction, which includes: (1) a **psychological dependence** or craving and the behavior involved in procurement of the drug; (2) **physiologic dependence**, with withdrawal symptoms on discontinuance of the drug; and (3) **tolerance**, ie, the need to increase the dose to obtain the desired effects. Drug dependency is a function of the amount of drug used and the duration of usage. The amount needed to produce dependency varies with the nature of the drug and the idiosyncratic nature of the user. The frequency of use is usually daily, and the duration is inevitably greater than 2–3 weeks. Polydrug abuse is very common. Transgenerational continuity of drug abuse is also common.

There is accumulating evidence that an impairment syndrome exists in many former (and current) drug users. It is believed that drug use produces damaged neurotransmitter receptor sites and that the consequent imbalance produces symptoms that may mimic other psychiatric illnesses. "Kindling"—repeated stimulation of the brain—renders the individual more susceptible to focal brain activity with minimal stimulation. Stimulants and depressants can produce kindling, leading to relatively spontaneous effects no longer dependent on the original stimulus. These effects may be manifested as mood swings, panic, psychosis, and occasionally overt seizure activity. The imbalance also results in personal nonproductivity: frequent job changes, marital problems, and generally erratic behavior. Patients with PTSD frequently have treated themselves with a variety of drugs. Chronic abusers of a wide variety of drugs exhibit cerebral atrophy on CT scans, a finding that may relate to the above symptoms. Early recognition is important, mainly to establish realistic treatment programs that are chiefly symptom-directed.

The clinician faces three problems with substance abuse: (1) the prescribing of substances such as sedatives, stimulants, or opioids that might produce dependency; (2) the treatment of individuals who have already abused drugs, most commonly alcohol; and (3) the detection of illicit drug use in patients presenting with psychiatric symptoms. The usefulness of urinalysis for detection of drugs varies markedly with different drugs and under different circumstances (pharmacokinetics is a major factor). Water-soluble drugs (eg, alcohol, stimulants, opioids) are eliminated in a day or so. Lipophilic substances (eg, barbiturates, tetrahydrocannabinol) appear in the urine over longer periods of time: several days in most cases, 1–2 months in chronic marijuana users. Sedative drug determinations are quite variable, amount of drug and duration of use being important determinants. False-positives can be a problem related to ingestion of some legitimate drugs (eg, phenytoin for barbiturates, phenylpropanolamine for amphetamines, chlorpromazine for opioids) and some foods (eg, poppy seeds for opioids, coca leaf tea for cocaine). Manipulations can alter the legitimacy of the testing. Dilution, either in vivo or in vitro, can be detected by checking urine specific gravity. Addition of ammonia, vinegar, or salt may invalidate the test, but odor and pH determinations are simple. Hair analysis can determine drug use over longer periods, particularly sequential drug-taking patterns. The sensitivity and reliability of such tests are considered good, and the method may be complementary to urinalysis.

Kosten TR et al: Management of drug and alcohol withdrawal. N Engl J Med 2003;348:1786. [PMID: 12724485]

Rigotti NA: Treatment of tobacco use and dependence. N Engl J Med 2002;346:506. [PMID: 12088292]

Thom B: From alcoholism treatment to the alcohol harm reduction strategy for England: an overview of alcohol policy since 1950. Am J Addict 2005;14:416. [PMID: 16257879]

ALCOHOL DEPENDENCY & ABUSE (Alcoholism)

 ESSENTIALS OF DIAGNOSIS

Major criteria:

- Physiologic dependence as manifested by evidence of withdrawal when intake is interrupted.
- Tolerance to the effects of alcohol.
- Evidence of alcohol-associated illnesses, such as alcoholic liver disease, cerebellar degeneration.
- Continued drinking despite strong medical and social contraindications and life disruptions.
- Impairment in social and occupational functioning.
- Depression.
- Blackouts.

Other signs:

- Alcohol stigmas: alcohol odor on breath, alcoholic facies, flushed face, scleral injection, tremor, ecchymoses, peripheral neuropathy.
- Surreptitious drinking.
- Unexplained work absences.
- Frequent accidents, falls, or injuries of vague origin; in smokers, cigarette burns on hands or chest.
- Laboratory tests: elevated values of liver function tests, mean corpuscular volume, serum uric acid, and triglycerides.

General Considerations

Alcoholism is a syndrome consisting of two phases: problem drinking and alcohol addiction. Problem drinking is the repetitive use of alcohol, often to alleviate anxiety or solve other emotional problems. Alcohol addiction is a true addiction similar to that which occurs following the repeated use of other sedative-hypnotics. Alcohol and other drug abuse patients have a much higher prevalence of lifetime psychiatric disorders. While male-to-female ratios in alcoholic treatment agencies remain at 4:1, there is evidence that the rates are converging. Women delay seeking help, and when they do they tend to seek it in medical or mental health settings. Adoption and twin studies indicate some genetic influence. Ethnic distinctions are important—eg, 40% of Japanese have aldehyde dehydrogenase deficiency and are more susceptible to the effects of alcohol. Depression is often present and should be evaluated carefully. The majority of suicides and intrafamily homicides involve alcohol. Alcohol is a major factor in rapes and other assaults.

There are several screening instruments that may help identify alcoholism. One of the most useful is the CAGE questionnaire (see Table 1–10).

Clinical Findings

A. ACUTE INTOXICATION

The signs of alcoholic intoxication are the same as those of overdosage with any other central nervous system depressant: drowsiness, errors of commission, psychomotor dysfunction, disinhibition, dysarthria, ataxia, and nystagmus. For a 70-kg person, an ounce of whiskey, a 4- to 6-oz glass of wine, or a 12-oz bottle of beer (roughly 15, 11, and 13 grams of alcohol, respectively) may raise the level of alcohol in the blood by 25 mg/dL. For a 50-kg person, the blood alcohol level would rise even higher (35 mg/dL) with the same consumption. Blood alcohol levels below 50 mg/dL rarely cause significant motor dysfunction. Intoxication as manifested by ataxia, dysarthria, and nausea and vomiting indicates a blood level above 150 mg/dL, and lethal blood levels range from 350 to 900 mg/dL. In severe cases, overdosage is marked by respiratory depression, stupor, seizures, shock syndrome, coma, and death. Serious overdoses are frequently due to a combination of alcohol with other sedatives.

B. WITHDRAWAL

There is a wide spectrum of manifestations of alcoholic withdrawal, ranging from anxiety, decreased cognition, and tremulousness through increasing irritability and hyperreactivity to full-blown **delirium tremens**. Symptoms of mild withdrawal, including tremor, elevated vital signs, and anxiety, begin within about 8 hours after the last drink and usually have passed by day 3. Generalized seizures occur within the first 24–38 hours and are more prevalent in persons who have a history of withdrawal syndromes. Delirium tremens is an acute organic psychosis that is usually manifest within 24–72 hours after the last drink (but may occur up to 7–10 days later). It is characterized by mental confusion, tremor, sensory hyperacuity, visual hallucinations (often of snakes, bugs, etc), autonomic hyperactivity, diaphoresis, dehydration, electrolyte disturbances (hypokalemia, hypomagnesemia), seizures, and cardiovascular abnormalities. The acute withdrawal syndrome is often completely unexpected and occurs when the patient has been hospitalized for some unrelated problem and presents as a diagnostic problem. Suspect alcohol withdrawal in every unexplained delirium. The mortality rate from delirium tremens has steadily decreased with early diagnosis and improved treatment.

In addition to the immediate withdrawal symptoms, there is evidence of persistent longer-term ones, including sleep disturbances, anxiety, depression, excitability, fatigue, and emotional volatility. These symptoms may persist for 3–12 months, and in some cases they become chronic.

C. ALCOHOLIC (ORGANIC) HALLUCINOSIS

This syndrome occurs either during heavy drinking or on withdrawal and is characterized by a paranoid psychosis without the tremulousness, confusion, and clouded sensorium seen in withdrawal syndromes. The patient appears normal except for the auditory hallucinations, which are frequently persecutory and may cause the patient to behave aggressively and in a paranoid fashion.

D. CHRONIC ALCOHOLIC BRAIN SYNDROMES

These encephalopathies are characterized by increasing erratic behavior, memory and recall problems, and emotional instability—the usual signs of organic brain injury due to any cause. Wernicke-Korsakoff syndrome due to thiamine deficiency may develop with a series of episodes. Wernicke's encephalopathy consists of the triad of confusion, ataxia, and ophthalmoplegia (typically sixth nerve). Early recognition and treatment with thiamine can minimize damage. One of the possible sequelae is Korsakoff's psychosis, characterized by both anterograde and retrograde amnesia, with confabulation early in the course. Early recognition and treatment of the alcoholic with intravenous thiamine and B complex vitamins can minimize damage.

Differential Diagnosis

The differential diagnosis of problem drinking is essentially between primary alcoholism (when no other major psychiatric diagnosis exists) and secondary alcoholism, when alcohol is used as self-medication for major underlying psychiatric problems such as schizophrenia or affective disorder. The differentiation is important, since the latter group requires treatment for the specific psychiatric problem.

The differential diagnosis of alcohol withdrawal includes other sedative withdrawals and other causes of delirium. Acute alcoholic hallucinosis must be differentiated from other acute paranoid states such as amphetamine psychosis or paranoid schizophrenia. An accurate history is the most important differentiating factor. The history and laboratory test results (elevated liver function tests, increased mean corpuscular volume, increased serum uric acid and triglycerides, decreased serum potassium and magnesium) are the

most important features in differentiating chronic organic brain syndromes due to alcohol from those due to other causes. The form of the brain syndrome is of little help—eg, chronic brain syndromes from lupus erythematosus may be associated with confabulation similar to that resulting from longstanding alcoholism.

Complications

The medical, economic, and psychosocial problems of alcoholism are staggering. The central and peripheral nervous system complications include chronic brain syndromes, cerebellar degeneration, cardiomyopathy, and peripheral neuropathies. Direct effects on the liver include cirrhosis, esophageal varices, and eventual hepatic failure. Indirect effects include protein abnormalities, coagulation defects, hormone deficiencies, and an increased incidence of liver neoplasms.

Fetal alcohol syndrome includes one or more of the following developmental defects in the offspring of alcoholic women: (1) low birth weight and small size with failure to catch up in size or weight (2) mental retardation, with an average IQ in the 60s, and (3) a variety of birth defects, with a large percentage of facial and cardiac abnormalities. The fetuses are very quiet in utero, and there is an increased frequency of breech presentations. There is a higher incidence of delayed postnatal growth and behavior development. The risk is appreciably higher the more alcohol ingested by the mother each day. Cigarette and marijuana smoking as well as cocaine use can produce similar effects on the fetus.

Treatment of Problem Drinking

A. PSYCHOLOGICAL

The most important consideration for the clinician is to suspect the problem early and take a nonjudgmental attitude, although this does not mean a passive one. The problem of **denial** must be faced, preferably with significant family members at the first meeting. This means dealing from the beginning with any enabling behavior of the spouse or other significant people. Enabling behavior allows the alcoholic to avoid facing the consequences of his or her behavior.

There must be an emphasis on the things that can be done. This approach emphasizes the fact that the clinician cares and strikes a positive and hopeful note early in treatment. Valuable time should not be wasted trying to find out why the patient drinks; come to grips early with the immediate problem of how to stop the drinking. Although total abstinence should be the ultimate goal, a harm reduction model indicates that gradual progress toward abstinence can be a useful treatment stratagem.

B. SOCIAL

Get the patient into Alcoholics Anonymous and the spouse into Al-Anon. Success is usually proportionate to the utilization of Alcoholics Anonymous, religious counseling, and other resources. The patient should be seen frequently for short periods and charged an appropriate fee.

Do not underestimate the importance of religion, particularly since the alcoholic is often a dependent person who needs a great deal of support. Early enlistment of the help of a concerned religious adviser can often provide the turning point for a personal conversion to sobriety.

One of the most important considerations is the patient's job—fear of losing a job is one of the most powerful motivations for giving up drink. The business community has become painfully aware of the problem, with the result that about 70% of the Fortune 500 companies offer programs to their employees to help with the problem of alcoholism. In the latter case, some specific recommendations to employers can be offered: (1) Avoid placement in jobs where the alcoholic must be alone, eg, as a traveling buyer or sales executive. (2) Use supervision but not surveillance. (3) Keep competition with others to a minimum. (4) Avoid positions that require quick decision making on important matters (high-stress situations). In general, commitment to abstinence and avoidance of situations that might be conducive to drinking are most predictive of a good outcome.

C. MEDICAL

Hospitalization is not usually necessary. It is sometimes used to dramatize a situation and force the patient to face the problem of alcoholism, but generally it should be used on medical indications.

Because of the many medical complications of alcoholism, a complete physical examination with appropriate laboratory tests is mandatory, with special attention to the liver and nervous system. The most definitive biologic marker for chronic alcoholism is carbohydrate deficient transferrin, which can detect heavy use (60 mg/d over 7–10 days) with high specificity. Two other tests that may provide clues to an alcohol problem are γ-glutamyl transpeptidase measurement (levels above 30 units/L are suggestive of heavy drinking) and mean corpuscular volume (> 95 fL in men and > 100 fL in women). If both are elevated, a serious drinking problem is likely. Use of other recreational drugs with alcohol skews and negates the significance of these tests. High-density lipoprotein cholesterol elevations combined with elevated γ-glutamyl transpeptidase concentrations also can help identify heavy drinkers.

Use of sedatives as a replacement for alcohol is not desirable. The usual result is concomitant use of sedatives and alcohol and worsening of the problem. Lithium is not helpful in the treatment of alcoholism.

Disulfiram (250–500 mg/d orally) has been used for many years as an aversive drug to discourage alcohol use. Disulfiram inhibits alcohol dehydrogenase, causing toxic reactions when alcohol is consumed. The results have generally been of limited effectiveness and depend on the motivation of the individual to be compliant.

Naltrexone, an opiate antagonist, in a dosage of 50 mg daily, has been helpful in lowering relapse rates over the 3–6 months after cessation of drinking, apparently by lessening the pleasurable effects of alcohol. One study suggests that naltrexone is most effective when given during periods of drinking in combination with therapy that supports abstinence but accepts the fact that relapses occur. Naltrexone is FDA-approved for maintenance therapy. Studies indicate that it reduces alcohol craving when used as part of a comprehensive treatment program. Acamprosate (333–666 mg orally three times daily) has recently become available for maintenance of abstinence and can be continued even during periods of relapse.

Topiramate, an anticonvulsant, may have efficacy in reducing alcohol consumption and craving in patients with alcohol dependence by blunting mesolimbic dopamine.

D. BEHAVIORAL

Conditioning approaches have been used in some settings in the treatment of alcoholism, most commonly as a type of aversion therapy. For example, the patient is given a drink of whiskey and then a shot of apomorphine, and proceeds to vomit. In this way a strong association is built up between the vomiting and the drinking. Although this kind of treatment has been successful in some cases, many people do not sustain the learned aversive response.

Treatment of Hallucinosis & Withdrawal

A. MEDICAL

1. Alcoholic hallucinosis—Alcoholic hallucinosis, which can occur either during or on cessation of a prolonged drinking period, is not a typical withdrawal syndrome and is handled differently. Since the symptoms are primarily those of a psychosis in the presence of a clear sensorium, they are handled like any other psychosis: hospitalization (when indicated) and adequate amounts of antipsychotic drugs. Haloperidol, 5 mg orally twice a day for the first day or so, usually ameliorates symptoms quickly, and the drug can be decreased and discontinued over several days as the patient improves. It then becomes necessary to deal with the chronic alcohol abuse, which has been discussed.

2. Withdrawal symptoms—The onset of withdrawal symptoms is usually 8–12 hours and the peak intensity of symptoms is 48–72 hours after alcohol consumption is stopped. Providing adequate central nervous system depressants (eg, benzodiazepines) is important to counteract the excitability resulting from sudden cessation of alcohol intake. The choice of a specific sedative is less important than using adequate doses to bring the patient to a level of moderate sedation, and this will vary from person to person. Mild dependency requires "drying out." In some instances for outpatients, a short course of tapering benzodiazepines—eg, 20 mg of diazepam initially, decreasing by 5 mg daily—may be a useful adjunct. In moderate to severe withdrawal, hospitalize the patient and use diazepam orally in a dosage of 5–10 mg hourly depending on the clinical need as judged by withdrawal symptoms, including nausea, tremor, autonomic hyperactivity, agitation; tactile, visual, and auditory hallucinations; and disorientation. This type of symptom-driven medication regimen for withdrawal appears to reduce total benzodiazepine usage over fixed-dose schedules. Antipsychotic drugs should not be used. Monitoring of vital signs and fluid and electrolyte levels is essential for the severely ill patient.

In very severe withdrawal, intravenous administration is necessary. After stabilization, the amount of diazepam required to maintain a sedated state may be given orally every 8–12 hours. If restlessness, tremulousness, and other signs of withdrawal persist, the dosage is increased until moderate sedation occurs. The dosage is then gradually reduced by 20% every 24 hours until withdrawal is complete. This usually requires a week or so of treatment. Clonidine, 5 mcg/kg orally every 2 hours, or the patch formulation of appropriate dosage strength, suppresses cardiovascular signs of withdrawal and has some anxiolytic effect. Carbamazepine, 400–800 mg daily orally, compares favorably with benzodiazepines for alcohol withdrawal.

Atenolol, as an adjunct to benzodiazepines, can reduce symptoms of alcohol withdrawal. The daily oral atenolol dose is 100 mg when the heart rate is above 80 beats per minute and 50 mg for a heart rate between 50 and 80 beats per minute. Atenolol should not be used when bradycardia is present.

Meticulous examination for other medical problems is necessary. Alcoholic hypoglycemia can occur with low blood alcohol levels (see Chapter 27). Alcoholics commonly have liver disease and associated clotting problems and are also prone to injury—and the combination all too frequently leads to undiagnosed subdural hematoma.

Phenytoin does not appear to be useful in managing alcohol withdrawal seizures per se. Sedating doses of benzodiazepines are effective in treating alcohol withdrawal seizures. Thus, other anticonvulsants are not usually needed unless there is a preexisting seizure disorder.

A general diet should be given, and vitamins in high doses: thiamine, 50 mg intravenously initially, then intramuscularly on a daily basis; pyridoxine, 100 mg/d; folic acid, 1 mg/d; and ascorbic acid, 100 mg twice a day. Intravenous glucose solutions should not be given prior to thiamine for fear of precipitation of Wernicke's syndrome. Thiamine is necessary as a ketolase enzyme cofactor. Concurrent administration is satisfactory, and hydration should be meticulously assessed on an ongoing basis.

Chronic brain syndromes secondary to a long history of alcohol intake are not clearly responsive to thiamine and vitamin replenishment. Attention to the social and environmental care of this type of patient is paramount.

B. PSYCHOLOGICAL AND BEHAVIORAL

The comments in the section on problem drinking apply here also; these methods of treatment become the primary consideration after successful treatment of withdrawal or alcoholic hallucinosis. Psychological and social measures should be initiated in the hospital shortly before discharge. This increases the possibility of continued post-hospitalization treatment.

Dongier M: What are the treatment options for comorbid alcohol abuse and depressive disorders? J Psychiatry Neurosci 2005; 30:224. [PMID: 16262111]

Johnson BA et al: Oral topiramate for the treatment of alcohol dependence: a randomized controlled trial. Lancet 2003; 361:1677. [PMID: 12767733]

Mayo-Smith MF et al: Management of alcohol withdrawal delirium. An evidence-based practice guideline. Arch Intern Med 2004;164:1405. Erratum in: Arch Intern Med 2004; 164:2068. dosage error in text. [PMID: 15249349]

Moore AA et al: Beyond alcoholism: identifying older, at risk drinkers in primary care. J Stud Alcohol 2002;63:316. [PMID: 12086132]

Morgenstern J et al: Examining mechanisms of action in 12-step treatment. J Stud Alcohol 2002;63:665. [PMID: 14643940]

Williams SH: Medications for treating alcohol dependence. Am Fam Physician 2005;72:1775. [PMID: 16300039]

OTHER DRUG & SUBSTANCE DEPENDENCIES

Opioids

The terms "opioids" and "narcotics" are used interchangeably and include a group of drugs with actions that mimic those of morphine. The group includes natural derivatives of opium (opiates), synthetic surrogates (opioids), and a number of polypeptides, some of which have been discovered to be natural neurotransmitters. The principal narcotic of abuse is heroin (metabolized to morphine), which is not used as a legitimate medication. The other common opioids are prescription drugs that differ in milligram potency, duration of action, and agonist and antagonist capabilities (see Chapter 1). All of the opioid analgesics can be reversed by the opioid antagonist naloxone.

The clinical symptoms and signs of mild narcotic intoxication include changes in mood, with feelings of euphoria; drowsiness; nausea with occasional emesis; needle tracks; and miosis. The incidence of snorting and inhaling heroin ("smoking") is increasing, particularly among cocaine users. This coincides with a decrease in the availability of methaqualone (no longer marketed) and other sedatives used to temper the cocaine "high" (see discussion of cocaine under Stimulants, below). Overdosage causes respiratory depression, peripheral vasodilation, pinpoint pupils, pulmonary edema, coma, and death.

Dependency is a major concern when continued use of narcotics occurs, although withdrawal causes only moderate morbidity (similar in severity to a bout of "flu"). Addicted patients sometimes consider themselves more addicted than they really are and may not require a withdrawal program. Grades of withdrawal are categorized from 0 to 4: grade 0 includes craving and anxiety;

grade 1, yawning, lacrimation, rhinorrhea, and perspiration; grade 2, previous symptoms plus mydriasis, piloerection, anorexia, tremors, and hot and cold flashes with generalized aching; grades 3 and 4, increased intensity of previous symptoms and signs, with increased temperature, blood pressure, pulse, and respiratory rate and depth. In withdrawal from the most severe addiction, vomiting, diarrhea, weight loss, hemoconcentration, and spontaneous ejaculation or orgasm commonly occur. Complications of heroin administration include infections (eg, pneumonia, septic emboli, hepatitis, and HIV infection from using nonsterile needles), traumatic insults (eg, arterial spasm due to drug injection, gangrene), and pulmonary edema.

Treatment for overdosage (or suspected overdosage) is naloxone, 2 mg intravenously. If an overdose has been taken, the results are dramatic and occur within 2 minutes. Since the duration of action of naloxone is much shorter than that of the narcotics, the patient must be under close observation. Hospitalization, supportive care, repeated naloxone administration, and observation for withdrawal from other drugs should be maintained for as long as necessary.

Treatment for withdrawal begins if grade 2 signs develop. If a withdrawal program is necessary, use methadone, 10 mg orally (use parenteral administration if the patient is vomiting), and observe. If signs (piloerection, mydriasis, cardiovascular changes) persist for more than 4–6 hours, give another 10 mg; continue to administer methadone at 4- to 6-hour intervals until signs are not present (rarely more than 40 mg of methadone in 24 hours). Divide the total amount of drug required over the first 24-hour period by 2 and give that amount every 12 hours. Each day, reduce the total 24-hour dose by 5–10 mg. Thus, a moderately addicted patient initially requiring 30–40 mg of methadone could be withdrawn over a 4- to 8-day period. Clonidine, 0.1 mg several times daily over a 10- to 14-day period, is both an alternative and an adjunct to methadone detoxification; it is not necessary to taper the dose. Clonidine is helpful in alleviating cardiovascular symptoms but does not significantly relieve anxiety, insomnia, or generalized aching. There is a protracted abstinence syndrome of metabolic, respiratory, and blood pressure changes over a period of 3–6 months.

Narcotic antagonists (eg, naltrexone) can also be used successfully for treatment of the patient who has been free of opioids for 7–10 days. Naltrexone blocks the narcotic "high" of heroin when 50 mg is given orally every 24 hours initially for several days and then 100 mg is given every 48–72 hours. Liver disorders are a major contraindication. Compliance tends to be poor, partly because of the dysphoria that can persist long after opioid discontinuance. Buprenorphine, a partial agonist, is approved for office-based management of opiate addiction. Its use requires special training.

Alternative strategies for the treatment of opioid withdrawal have included rapid and ultrarapid detoxification techniques. In rapid detoxification, withdrawal is precipitated by opioid antagonists followed by naltrexone maintenance. Ultrarapid detoxification precipitates withdrawal with opioid antagonists under general anesthesia in a hospital. However, recent data do not support the use of either method. Methadone maintenance programs are of some value in chronic recidivism. Under carefully controlled supervision, the narcotic addict is maintained on fairly high doses of methadone (40–120 mg/d) that satisfy craving and block the effects of heroin to a great degree.

Sedatives (Anxiolytics)

See Anxiety Disorders, this chapter.

Psychedelics

About 6000 species of plants have psychoactive properties. All of the common psychedelics (LSD, mescaline, psilocybin, dimethyltryptamine, and other derivatives of phenylalanine and tryptophan) can produce similar behavioral and physiologic effects. An initial feeling of tension is followed by emotional release such as crying or laughing (1–2 hours). Later, perceptual distortions occur, with visual illusions and hallucinations, and occasionally there is fear of ego disintegration (2–3 hours). Major changes in time sense and mood lability then occur (3–4 hours). A feeling of detachment and a sense of destiny and control occur (4–6 hours). Of course, reactions vary among individuals, and some of the drugs produce markedly different time frames. Occasionally, the acute episode is terrifying (a "bad trip"), which may include panic, depression, confusion, or psychotic symptoms. Preexisting emotional problems, the attitude of the user, and the setting where the drug is used affect the experience.

Treatment of the acute episode primarily involves protection of the individual from erratic behavior that may lead to injury or death. A structured environment is usually sufficient until the drug is metabolized. In severe cases, antipsychotic drugs with minimal side effects (eg, haloperidol, 5 mg intramuscularly) may be given every several hours until the individual has regained control. In cases where "flashbacks" occur (mental imagery from a "bad trip" that is later triggered by mild stimuli such as marijuana, alcohol, or psychic trauma), a short course of an antipsychotic drug—eg, olanzapine, 5–10 mg/d, or risperidone, 2 mg/d, initially, and up to 20 mg/d and 6 mg/d, respectively—is usually sufficient. Lorazepam, 1–2 mg orally or intramuscularly every 2 hours as needed for acute agitation, may be a useful adjunct. An occasional patient may have "flashbacks" for much longer periods and require small doses of neuroleptic drugs over the longer term.

Phencyclidine

Phencyclidine (PCP, angel dust, peace pill, hog), developed as an anesthetic agent, first appeared as a street drug deceptively sold as tetrahydrocannabinol (THC). Because it is simple to produce and mimics to some degree the traditional psychedelic drugs, PCP has become a common deceptive substitute for LSD, THC, and mescaline. It is available in crystals, capsules, and tablets to be inhaled, injected, swallowed, or smoked (it is commonly sprinkled on marijuana).

Absorption after smoking is rapid, with onset of symptoms in several minutes and peak symptoms in 15–30 minutes. Mild intoxication produces euphoria accompanied by a feeling of numbness. Moderate intoxication (5–10 mg) results in disorientation, detachment from surroundings, distortion of body image, combativeness, unusual feats of strength (partly due to its anesthetic activity), and loss of ability to integrate sensory input, especially touch and proprioception. Physical symptoms include dizziness, ataxia, dysarthria, nystagmus, retracted upper eyelid with blank stare, hyperreflexia, and tachycardia. There are increases in blood pressure, respiration, muscle tone, and urine production. Usage in the first trimester of pregnancy is associated with an increase in spontaneous abortion and congenital defects. Severe intoxication (20 mg or more) produces an increase in degree of moderate symptoms, with the addition of seizures, deepening coma, hypertensive crisis, and severe psychotic ideation. The drug is particularly long-lasting (several days to several weeks) owing to high lipid solubility, gastroenteric recycling, and the production of active metabolites. Overdosage may be fatal, with the major causes of death being hypertensive crisis, respiratory arrest, and convulsions. Acute rhabdomyolysis has been reported and can result in myoglobinuric renal failure.

Differential diagnosis involves the whole spectrum of street drugs, since in some ways phencyclidine mimics sedatives, psychedelics, and marijuana in its effects. Blood and urine testing can detect the acute problem.

Treatment is discussed in Chapter 39.

Marijuana

Cannabis *sativa*, a hemp plant, is the source of marijuana. The parts of the plant vary in potency. The resinous exudate of the flowering tops of the female plant (hashish, charas) is the most potent, followed by the dried leaves and flowering shoots of the female plant (bhang) and the resinous mass from small leaves of inflorescence (ganja). The least potent parts are the lower branches and the leaves of the female plant and all parts of the male plant. Mercury may be a contaminant in marijuana grown in volcanic soil. The drug is usually inhaled by smoking. Effects occur in 10–20 minutes and last 2–3 hours. "Joints" of good quality contain about 500 mg of marijuana (which contains approximately 5–15 mg of tetrahydrocannabinol with a half-life of 7 days). Marijuana soaked in formaldehyde and dried ("AMP") has produced unusual effects, including autonomic discharge and severe though transient cognitive impairment.

With moderate dosage, marijuana produces two phases: mild euphoria followed by sleepiness. In the acute state, the user has an altered time perception, less inhibited emotions, psychomotor problems, impaired immediate memory, and conjunctival injection. High doses produce transient psychotomimetic effects. No specific treatment is necessary except in the case of the occasional "bad trip," in which case the person is treated in the same way as for psychedelic usage. Marijuana frequently aggravates existing mental illness and adversely affects motor performance.

Studies of long-term effects have conclusively shown abnormalities in the pulmonary tree. Laryngitis and rhinitis are related to prolonged use, along with chronic obstructive pulmonary disease. Electrocardiographic abnormalities are common, but no long-term cardiac disease has been linked to marijuana use. Chronic usage has resulted in depression of plasma testosterone levels and reduced sperm counts. Abnormal menstruation and failure to ovulate have occurred in some women. Cognitive impairments are common. Health care utilization for a variety of health problems is increased in chronic marijuana smokers. Sudden withdrawal produces insomnia, nausea, myalgia, and irritability. Psychological effects of chronic marijuana usage are still unclear. Urine testing is reliable if samples are carefully collected and tested. Detection periods span 4–6 days in acute users and 20–50 days in chronic users.

Stimulants: Amphetamines & Cocaine

Stimulant abuse is quite common, either alone or in combination with abuse of other drugs. The **amphetamines**, including Methedrine ("speed")—one variant is a smokable form called "ice," which gives an intense and fairly long-lasting high—methylphenidate, and phenmetrazine, are under prescription control, but street availability remains high. Moderate usage of any of the stimulants produces hyperactivity, a sense of enhanced physical and mental capacity, and sympathomimetic effects. The clinical picture of acute stimulant intoxication includes sweating, tachycardia, elevated blood pressure, mydriasis, hyperactivity, and an acute brain syndrome with confusion and disorientation. Tolerance develops quickly, and, as the dosage is increased, hypervigilance, paranoid ideation (with delusions of parasitosis), stereotypy, bruxism, tactile hallucinations of insect infestation, and full-blown psychoses occur, often with persecutory ideation and aggressive responses. Stimulant withdrawal is characterized by depression with symptoms of hyperphagia and hypersomnia.

People who have used stimulants chronically (eg, anorexigenics) occasionally become sensitized (**"kindling"**) to future use of stimulants. In these individuals, even small amounts of mild stimulants such as caffeine can cause symptoms of paranoia and auditory hallucinations.

Cocaine is a stimulant. It is a product of the coca plant. The derivatives include seeds, leaves, coca paste, cocaine hydrochloride, and the free base of cocaine. Coca paste is a crude extract that contains 40–80% cocaine sulfate and other impurities. Cocaine hydrochloride is the salt and the most commonly used form. Free base, a purer (and stronger) derivative called "crack," is prepared by simple extraction from cocaine hydrochloride.

There are various modes of use. Coca leaf chewing involves toasting the leaves and chewing with alkaline material (eg, the ash of other burned leaves) to enhance buccal absorption. One achieves a mild high, with onset in 5–10 minutes and lasting for about an hour. Intranasal use is simply snorting cocaine through a straw. Absorption is slowed somewhat by vasoconstriction (which may eventually cause tissue necrosis and septal perforation); the onset of action is in 2–3 minutes, with a moderate high (euphoria, excitement, increased energy) lasting about 30 minutes. The purity of the cocaine is a major determinant of the high. Intravenous use of cocaine hydrochloride or "freebase" is effective in 30 seconds and produces a short-lasting, fairly intense high of about 15 minutes' duration. The combined use of cocaine and ethanol results in the metabolic production of cocaethylene by the liver. This substance produces more intense and long-lasting cocaine-like effects. Smoking freebase (volatilized cocaine because of the lower boiling point) acts in seconds and results in an intense high lasting several minutes. The intensity of the reaction is related to the marked lipid solubility of the freebase form and produces by far the most severe medical and psychiatric symptoms.

Cardiovascular collapse, arrhythmias, myocardial infarction, and transient ischemic attacks have been reported. Seizures, strokes, migraine symptoms, hyperthermia, and lung damage may occur, and there are several obstetric complications, including spontaneous abortion, abruptio placentae, teratogenic effects, delayed fetal growth, and prematurity. Cocaine can cause anxiety, mood swings, and delirium, and chronic use can cause the same problems as other stimulants (see above).

Clinicians should be alert to cocaine use in patients presenting with unexplained nasal bleeding, headaches, fatigue, insomnia, anxiety, depression, and chronic hoarseness. Sudden withdrawal of the drug is not life-threatening but usually produces craving, sleep disturbances, hyperphagia, lassitude, and severe depression (sometimes with suicidal ideation) lasting days to weeks.

Treatment is imprecise and difficult. Since the high is related to blockage of dopamine reuptake, the dopamine agonist bromocriptine, 1.5 mg orally three times a day, alleviates some of the symptoms of craving associated with acute cocaine withdrawal. Other dopamine agonists such as apomorphine, levodopa, and amantadine are under study for this purpose. Carbamazepine may be a useful adjunct in treating symptoms of alcohol withdrawal, and desipramine in moderate doses has been useful in helping maintain abstinence in the early stages of treatment. Treatment of psychosis is the same as that of any psychosis: antipsychotic drugs in dosages sufficient to alleviate the symptoms. Any medical symptoms (eg, hyperthermia, seizures, hypertension) are treated specifically. These approaches should be used in conjunction with a structured program, most often based on the Alcoholics Anonymous model. Hospitalization may be required if self-harm or violence toward others is a perceived threat (usually indicated by paranoid delusions).

Caffeine

Caffeine, along with nicotine and alcohol, is one of the most commonly used drugs worldwide. About 10 billion pounds of coffee (the richest source of caffeine) are consumed yearly throughout the world. Tea, cocoa, and cola drinks also contribute to an intake of caffeine that is often astoundingly high in a large number of people. Low to moderate doses (30–200 mg/d) tend to improve some aspects of performance (eg, vigilance). The approximate content of caffeine in a (180-mL) cup of beverage is as follows: brewed coffee, 80–140 mg; instant coffee, 60–100 mg; decaffeinated coffee, 1–6 mg; black leaf tea, 30–80 mg; tea bags, 25–75 mg; instant tea, 30–60 mg; cocoa, 10–50 mg; and 12-oz cola drinks, 30–65 mg. A 2-oz chocolate candy bar has about 20 mg. Some herbal teas (eg, "morning thunder") contain caffeine. Caffeine-containing analgesics usually contain approximately 30 mg per unit. Symptoms of caffeinism (usually associated with ingestion of over 500 mg/d) include anxiety, agitation, restlessness, insomnia, a feeling of being "wired," and somatic symptoms referable to the heart and gastrointestinal tract. It is common for a case of caffeinism to present as an anxiety disorder. It is also common for caffeine and other stimulants to precipitate severe symptoms in compensated schizophrenic and manic-depressive patients. Chronically depressed patients often use caffeine drinks as self-medication. This diagnostic clue may help distinguish some major affective disorders. Withdrawal from caffeine (> 250 mg/d) can produce headaches, irritability, lethargy, and occasional nausea.

Miscellaneous Drugs, Solvents

The principal over-the-counter drugs of concern have been phenylpropanolamine and an assortment of antihistaminic agents, frequently in combination with a mild analgesic promoted as cold remedies. Medications containing phenylpropanolamine have been removed from sale in the United States due to an FDA ban. The major problem in use of phenylpropanolamine relates to its side effects as a stimulant, including precipitation of anxiety states, increased pressure effects, auditory and visual hallucinations, paranoid ideation, and occasionally delirium. Aggressiveness and some loss of impulse control were reported as well as sleep disturbances even with small doses.

Antihistamines usually produce some central nervous system depression—thus their use as over-the-counter sedatives. Practically all of the so-called sleep aids are antihistamines. Drowsiness may be a problem. The mixture of antihistamines with alcohol usually exacerbates the central nervous system effects. Scopolamine and bromides have generally been removed from over-the-counter products.

The abuse of laxatives sometimes can lead to electrolyte disturbances that may contribute to the manifestations of a delirium. The greatest use of laxatives tends to be in the elderly and in those with eating disorders, both of whom are the most vulnerable to physiologic changes.

Anabolic steroids are being abused by people who wish to increase muscle mass for cosmetic reasons or for greater strength. In addition to the medical problems, the practice is associated with significant mood swings, aggressiveness, and paranoid delusions. Alcohol and stimulant use is higher in these individuals. Withdrawal symptoms of steroid dependency include fatigue, depressed mood, restlessness, and insomnia.

Amyl nitrite has been used as an "orgasm expander." The changes in time perception, "rush," and mild euphoria caused by the drug prompted its nonmedical use, and popular lore concerning the effects of inhalation just prior to orgasm has led to increased use. Subjective effects last from 5 seconds to 15 minutes. Tolerance develops readily, but there are no known withdrawal symptoms. Abstinence for several days reestablishes the previous level of responsiveness. Long-term effects may include damage to the immune system and respiratory difficulties.

Sniffing of solvents and inhaling of gases (including aerosols) produce a form of inebriation similar to that of the volatile anesthetics. Agents include gasoline, toluene, petroleum ether, lighter fluids, cleaning fluids, paint thinners, and solvents that are present in many household products (eg, nail polish, typewriter correction fluid). Typical intoxication states include euphoria, slurred speech, hallucinations, and confusion, and with high doses, acute manifestations are unconsciousness and cardiorespiratory depression or failure; chronic exposure produces a variety of symptoms related to the liver, kidney, bone marrow, or heart. Lead encephalopathy can be associated with sniffing leaded gasoline. In addition, studies of workers chronically exposed to jet fuel showed significant increases in neurasthenic symptoms, including fatigue, anxiety, mood changes, memory difficulties, and somatic complaints. These same problems have been noted in long-term solvent abuse.

The so-called designer drugs are synthetic substitutes for commonly used recreational drugs and are produced in small, clandestine laboratories. The most common designer drugs have been methyl analogues of fentanyl and have been used as heroin substitutes. MDMA (methylenedioxymethamphetamine), an amphetamine derivative sometimes called "ecstasy," is also a designer drug with high abuse potential and neurotoxicity. Often not detected by standard toxicology screens, these substances can present a vexing problem for clinicians faced with symptoms from a totally unknown cause.

Collins ED et al: Anesthesia-assisted vs buprenorphine- or clonidine-assisted heroin detoxification and naltrexone induction: a randomized trial. JAMA 2005;294:903. [PMID: 16118380]

Fudala PJ et al: Office-based treatment of opiate addiction with sublingual-tablet formulation of buprenorphine and naloxone. N Engl J Med 2003;349:949. [PMID: 12954743]

Khalsa JH et al: Clinical consequences of marijuana. J Clin Pharmacol 2002;42 (11 Suppl):7S. [PMID: 12412830]

■ DELIRIUM, DEMENTIA, & OTHER COGNITIVE DISORDERS (Formerly: Organic Brain Syndrome)

ESSENTIALS OF DIAGNOSIS

- *Transient or permanent brain dysfunction.*
- *Cognitive impairment to varying degrees: may include impaired recall and recent memory, inability to focus attention, random psychomotor activity such as stereotypy, and problems in perceptual processing, often with psychotic ideation.*
- *Emotional disorders frequently present: depression, anxiety, irritability.*
- *Behavioral disturbances may include problems of impulse control, sexual acting-out, attention deficits, aggression, and exhibitionism.*

General Considerations

The organic problem may be a primary brain disease or a secondary manifestation of some general disorder. All of the cognitive disorders show some degree of impaired thinking depending on the site of involvement, the rate of onset and progression, and the duration of the underlying brain lesion. Emotional disturbances (eg, depression) are often present as significant comorbidities. The behavioral disturbances tend to be more common with chronicity, more directly related to the underlying personality or central nervous system vulnerability to drug side effects, and not necessarily correlated with cognitive dysfunction.

The causes of cognitive disorders are listed in Table 25–11.

Clinical Findings

The manifestations are many and varied and include problems with orientation, short or fluctuating attention span, loss of recent memory and recall, impaired judgment, emotional lability, lack of initiative, impaired impulse control, inability to reason through problems, depression (worse in mild to moderate types), confabulation (not limited to alcohol organic brain syndrome), constriction of intellectual functions, visual and auditory hallucinations, and delusions. Physical findings will

Table 25–11. Etiology of delirium and other cognitive disorders.

Disorder	Possible Causes
Intoxication	Alcohol, sedatives, bromides, analgesics (eg, pentazocine), psychedelic drugs, stimulants, and household solvents.
Drug withdrawal	Withdrawal from alcohol, sedative-hypnotics, corticosteroids.
Long-term effects of alcohol	Wernicke-Korsakoff syndrome.
Infections	Septicemia; meningitis and encephalitis due to bacterial, viral, fungal, parasitic, or tuberculous organisms or to central nervous system syphilis; acute and chronic infections due to the entire range of microbiologic pathogens.
Endocrine disorders	Thyrotoxicosis, hypothyroidism, adrenocortical dysfunction (including Addison's disease and Cushing's syndrome), pheochromocytoma, insulinoma, hypoglycemia, hyperparathyroidism, hypoparathyroidism, panhypopituitarism, diabetic ketoacidosis.
Respiratory disorders	Hypoxia, hypercapnia.
Metabolic disturbances	Fluid and electrolyte disturbances (especially hyponatremia, hypomagnesemia, and hypercalcemia), acid-base disorders, hepatic disease (hepatic encephalopathy), renal failure, porphyria.
Nutritional deficiencies	Deficiency of vitamin B_1 (beriberi), vitamin B_{12} (pernicious anemia), folic acid, nicotinic acid (pellagra); protein-calorie malnutrition.
Trauma	Subdural hematoma, subarachnoid hemorrhage, intracerebral bleeding, concussion syndrome.
Cardiovascular disorders	Myocardial infarctions, cardiac arrhythmias, cerebrovascular spasms, hypertensive encephalopathy, hemorrhages, embolisms, and occlusions indirectly cause decreased cognitive function.
Neoplasms	Primary or metastatic lesions of the central nervous system, cancer-induced hypercalcemia.
Seizure disorders	Ictal, interictal, and postictal dysfunction.
Collagen-vascular and immunologic disorders	Autoimmune disorders, including systemic lupus erythematosus, Sjögren's syndrome, and AIDS.
Degenerative diseases	Alzheimer's disease, Pick's disease, multiple sclerosis, parkinsonism, Huntington's chorea, normal pressure hydrocephalus.
Medications	Anticholinergic drugs, antidepressants, H_2-blocking agents, digoxin, salicylates (chronic use), and a wide variety of other over-the-counter and prescribed drugs.

naturally vary according to the cause. The EEG usually shows generalized slowing in delirium.

A. DELIRIUM

Delirium (acute confusional state) is a transient global disorder of attention, with clouding of consciousness, usually a result of systemic problems (eg, drugs, hypoxemia). Onset is usually rapid. The mental status fluctuates (impairment is usually least in the morning), with varying inability to concentrate, maintain attention, and sustain purposeful behavior. ("Sundowning"—mild to moderate delirium at night—is more common in patients with preexisting dementia and may be precipitated by hospitalization, drugs, and sensory deprivation.) There is a marked deficit of short-term memory and recall. Anxiety and irritability are common. Amnesia is retrograde (impaired recall of past memories) and anterograde (inability to recall events after the onset of the delirium). Orientation problems follow the inability to retain information. Perceptual disturbances (often visual hallucinations) and psychomotor restlessness with insomnia are com-

mon. Autonomic changes include tachycardia, dilated pupils, and sweating. The average duration is about 1 week, with full recovery in most cases. Delirium can coexist with dementia.

B. DEMENTIA

(See also Chapter 4.) Dementia is characterized by chronicity and deterioration of selective mental functions. Onset is insidious over months to years in most cases. Dementia is usually progressive, more common in the elderly, and rarely reversible even if underlying disease can be corrected. Dementia can be classified as cortical or subcortical.

There are three types of cortical dementia: (1) primary degenerative dementia (eg, Alzheimer's), accounting for about 50–60% of cases; (2) atherosclerotic (multi-infarct) dementia, 15–20% of cases (this figure is probably low because of the tendency to overuse the diagnosis of Alzheimer's dementia); and (3) mixtures of the first two types or dementia due to miscellaneous causes, 15–20% of cases (see also Chapter 4). Examples of primary degenerative dementia are Alzheimer's dementia (most common) and Pick, Creutzfeldt-Jakob, and Huntington dementias (less common).

In all types, loss of impulse control (sexual and language) is common. The tenuous level of functioning makes the individual most susceptible to minor physical and psychological stresses. The course depends on the underlying cause, and the general trend is steady deterioration.

HIV infection can produce a primary neurogenic disorder (partially due to neuronal loss) and secondary effects due to opportunistic infections, neoplasias, or the effects of drug therapy. At present there has been a reduction in dementia symptoms in both early and late stages, perhaps due to earlier use of zidovudine. The general trend is variable, and patients require ongoing monitoring of neuropsychiatric status.

Pseudodementia is a term applied to depressed patients who appear to be demented. These patients are often identifiable by their tendency to complain about memory problems vociferously rather than try to cover them up. They usually say they can't complete cognitive tasks but with encouragement can often do so. In some reports, they can be considered to have depression-induced reversible dementia that remits when the depression resolves.

C. AMNESTIC SYNDROME

This is a memory disturbance without delirium or dementia. It is usually associated with thiamine deficiency and chronic alcohol use (eg, Korsakoff's syndrome). There is an impairment in the ability to learn new information or recall previously learned information.

D. SUBSTANCE-INDUCED HALLUCINOSIS

This condition is characterized by persistent or recurrent hallucinations (usually auditory) without the other symptoms usually found in delirium or dementia. Alcohol or hallucinogens are often the cause. There does not have to be any other mental disorder, and there may be complete spontaneous resolution.

E. PERSONALITY CHANGES DUE TO A GENERAL MEDICAL CONDITION (FORMERLY ORGANIC PERSONALITY SYNDROME)

This syndrome is characterized by emotional lability and loss of impulse control along with a general change in personality. Cognitive functions are preserved. Social inappropriateness is common. Loss of interest and lack of concern with the consequences of one's actions are often present. The course depends on the underlying cause (eg, frontal lobe contusion may resolve completely).

Differential Diagnosis

The differential diagnosis consists mainly of schizophrenia and the other psychoses, which are sometimes confused with cognitive disorders are often accompanied by psychotic symptoms.

Complications

Chronicity may result from delayed correction of the defect, eg, subdural hematoma, low-pressure hydrocephalus. Accidents secondary to impulsive behavior and poor judgment are a major consideration. Secondary depression and impulsive behavior not infrequently lead to suicide attempts. Drugs—particularly sedatives—may worsen thinking abilities and contribute to the overall problems.

Treatment

(See also Chapter 4.)

A. MEDICAL

Delirium should be considered a syndrome of acute brain dysfunction analogous to acute renal failure. The first aim of treatment is to identify and correct the etiologic medical problem. Evaluation should consist of a comprehensive physical examination including a search for neurologic abnormalities, infection, or hypoxia. Routine laboratory tests may include serum electrolytes, serum glucose, BUN, serum creatinine, liver function tests, thyroid function tests, arterial blood gases, complete blood count, serum calcium, phosphorus, magnesium, vitamin B_{12}, folate, blood cultures, urinalysis, and cerebrospinal fluid analysis. Discontinue drugs that may be contributing to the problem (eg, analgesics, corticosteroids, cimetidine, lidocaine, anticholinergic drugs, central nervous system depressants, mefloquine). Do not overlook any possibility of reversible organic disease. Electroencephalography, CT, MRI, PET, and SPECT evaluations may be helpful in diagnosis. Ideally, the patient should be monitored without further medications while the evaluation is carried out. There are, however, two indications for medication in delirious states: behavioral control (eg, pulling out lines) and subjective distress (eg, pronounced fear due to hallucinations). If these indications are present, medications may be used. If there is any hint of alcohol or substance withdrawal (the most common cause of delirium in the general hospital), a benzodiazepine such as lorazepam (1–2 mg every hour) can be given parenterally. If there is little likelihood of withdrawal syndrome, haloperidol is often used in doses of 1–10 mg every hour. Given intravenously, it appears to impose slight risk of extrapyramidal side effects. In addition to the medication, a pleasant, comfortable, nonthreatening, and physically safe environment with adequate nursing or attendant services should be provided. Once the underlying condition has been identified and treated, adjunctive medications can be tapered.

Treatment of dementia syndrome usually involves symptomatic management with one exception. Since there is a cholinergic deficiency in Alzheimer's disease, research has focused on drugs to increase cholinergic activity by inhibiting cholinesterase. Tacrine was the first reversible cholinesterase inhibitor approved by the FDA.

Three better-tolerated FDA-approved cholinesterase inhibitors are donepezil (5–10 mg at night), rivastigmine (3–6 mg twice daily), and galantamine (8–12 mg twice daily). Donepezil and galantamine doses need adjustment for liver disease, and the galantamine dose should be adjusted for renal failure. They are thought to be efficacious in the short-term preservation of cognitive function and activities of daily living in mild to moderate dementia and, unlike tacrine, are not thought to be hepatotoxic. Gastrointestinal side effects are common but may be least frequent with donepezil. Further research continues to clarify the long-term efficacy of these medications on cognition and behavior. None of the cholinesterase inhibitors to date are thought to slow disease progression. An *N*-methyl-D-aspartate (NMDA) receptor antagonist, memantine, is the first medication approved by the FDA for the treatment of moderate to severe Alzheimer's disease. Memantine may improve performance and cognition in some patients and has been used as an augmenting agent with the cholinesterase inhibitors.

Aggressiveness and rage states in central nervous system disease can be reduced with lipophilic β-blockers (eg, propranolol, metoprolol) in moderate doses. Since the serotonergic system has been implicated in arousal conditions, drugs that affect serotonin have been found to be of some benefit in aggression and agitation. Included in this group are lithium, trazodone, buspirone, and clonazepam. Dopamine blockers (eg, the neuroleptic drugs such as haloperidol) have been used for many years to attenuate aggression. Atypical neuroleptics may have a role in selected geriatric patients; however, there are reports of increased mortality in some studies related to the use of atypical neuroleptics in this population. There are also recent reports of reduced agitation in Alzheimer's disease from carbamazepine, 100–400 mg/d orally (with slow increase as needed). Emotional lability in some cases responds to small doses of imipramine (25 mg orally one to three times per day) or fluoxetine (5–20 mg/d orally); depression, which often occurs early in the course of Alzheimer's dementia, responds to the usual doses of antidepressant drugs, preferably those with the least anticholinergic side effects (eg, SSRIs and MAO inhibitors).

Cerebral vasodilators were originally used on the assumption that cerebral arteriosclerosis and ischemia were the principal causes of the dementias. Although there is a slight reduction of blood flow in primary degenerative dementia (probably as a result of the basic disorder), there is no evidence that this is a major factor in this group of disorders or that vasodilators are of value. Ergotoxine alkaloids (ergoloid mesylates: Hydergine, others) have been studied with mixed results; improvement in ambulatory self-care and depressed mood has been noted, but there has been no improvement of cognitive functioning on any standardized tests. Hyperbaric oxygen treatment has not produced significant improvement. Stimulant drugs (eg, methylphenidate) do not change cognitive function but can improve affect and mood, which helps the caretakers cope with the problem.

Failing sensory functions should be supported as necessary, with hearing aids, cataract surgery, etc.

B. Social

Substitute home care, board and care, or convalescent home care may be most useful when the family is unable to care for the patient. The setting should include familiar people and objects, lights at night, and a simple schedule. Counseling may help the family to cope with problems and may help keep the patient at home as long as possible. Information about local groups can be obtained from the Alzheimer's Disease and Related Disorders Association, 70 East Lake Street, Suite 600, Chicago, IL 60601. Volunteer services, including homemakers, visiting nurses, and adult protective services, may be helpful in maintaining the patient at home.

C. Behavioral

Behavioral techniques include operant responses that can be used to induce positive behaviors, eg, paying attention to the patient who is trying to communicate appropriately, and extinction by ignoring inappropriate responses. Alzheimer's patients can learn skills and retain them but do not recall the circumstances in which they were learned.

D. Psychological

Formal psychological therapies are not usually helpful and may make things worse by taxing the patient's limited cognitive resources.

Prognosis

The prognosis is good for recovery of mental functioning in delirium when the underlying condition is reversible. For most dementia syndromes, the prognosis is for gradual deterioration, although new drug treatments may prove helpful.

Clegg A et al: Clinical and cost-effectiveness of donepezil, rivastigmine, and galantamine for Alzheimer's disease. Int J Technol Assess Health Care 2002;18:497. [PMID: 12391943]

Reisberg B et al: Memantine in moderate-to-severe Alzheimer's disease. N Engl J Med 2003;348:1333. [PMID: 12672860]

Trinh N et al: Efficacy of cholinesterase inhibitors in the treatment of neuropsychiatric symptoms and functional impairment in Alzheimer disease, a meta-analysis. JAMA 2003; 289:210. [PMID: 12517232]

■ GERIATRIC PSYCHIATRIC DISORDERS (See also Chapter 4)

There are three basic factors in the process of aging: biologic, sociologic, and psychological.

The complex **biologic** changes depend on inherited characteristics (the best chance of long life is to have long-lived parents), nutrition, declining sensory functions such as hearing or vision, disease, trauma, and lifestyle. A definite correlation between hearing loss and paranoid ideation exists in the elderly. (See Dementia, above.) As a person ages, relatively minor disorders or combinations of disorders may cause deficits in cognition and affective response. Hypochondriasis is frequently a mechanism of compensating for decreased function (eg, preoccupation with bowel function).

The **sociologic** factors derive from stresses connected with occupation, family, and community. Any or all of these areas may be disrupted in a general phenomenon of "disengagement" and lack of intimacy that older people experience as friends die, the children move away, and the surroundings become less familiar. Retirement commonly precipitates a major disruption in a well-established life structure. This is particularly stressful in the person whose compulsive devotion to a job has inhibited the development of other interests, so that sudden loss of this outlet leaves a void that is not easily filled. New duties, such as caring for a spouse with dementia, may also lead to depression.

The **psychological** withdrawal of the elderly person is frequently related to a loss of self-esteem, which is based on the economic insecurity of older age with its congruent loss of independence, the recognition of decreasing physical and mental ability, loneliness, and the fear of approaching death. The process of aging is often poorly accepted, and the real or imagined loss of physical attractiveness may have a traumatic impact that the plastic surgeon can only soften for a time. In a culture that stresses physical and sexual attractiveness, it is difficult for some people to accept the change.

Clinical Findings & Complications

The most common psychiatric syndrome in the elderly is dementia of varying degrees. Psychotic ideation (usually paranoid) may coexist with dementia. Frequently, in milder cases, the individual is aware of the deficiency in cognition and becomes depressed about actual or threatened loss of function. Depression may then amplify the apparent cognitive decline.

Overt depression, often presenting as a somatic complaint, is often related to life changes (80% of people over age 65 have some kind of medical problem). Alcoholism is present in approximately 15% of older patients presenting with psychiatric symptoms. The incidence of suicide is higher in elderly people— loneliness, age, and medical problems being directly related. Deprivation of full-spectrum light may be a factor in some patients (eg, nursing home residents). Anxiety, often associated with organic illness, heightens preexisting confusion in the patient with cognitive dysfunction.

Abuse of the elderly—both physical neglect (passive) and physical injury (active)—demands early recognition. Bruises, welts, fractures, and debilitation should alert the clinician. The battered elderly are probably just as numerous as battered children, but less reported, and require the same diligence in clinician recognition.

Polypharmacy (with both prescription and over-the-counter drugs) is a major cause of accidents (often with resultant hip fracture) and illness in the elderly. Cognitive impairment increases as the number of drugs used increases; sedatives and anticholinergic drugs are the major culprits (eg, overuse in sleep problems). The increased and varied complaints are often an attempt to compensate and divert attention from decreased mental function.

Treatment

A. SOCIAL

Socialization, a structured schedule of activities, familiar surroundings, continued achievement, and avoidance of loneliness (probably the most important factor) are some of the major considerations in prevention and amelioration of the psychiatric problems of old age. The patient can be supported in the primary environment by various agencies that can help avoid a premature change of habits. For patients with disabilities that make it difficult to cope with the problems of living alone, homemaker services can assist in continuing the day-to-day activities of the household; visiting nurses can administer medications and monitor the physical condition of the patient; and geriatric social groups can help maintain socialization and human contacts. In the hospital or nursing home, attention to the kinds of people placed in the same room is most important (mix active and inactive patients).

B. MEDICAL

Treatment of any reversible components of a dementia syndrome is obviously the major medical consideration. One commonly overlooked factor is self-medication, frequently with nonprescription drugs or herbal remedies that further impair the patient's already precarious functioning. Common culprits are antihistamines and anticholinergic drugs, sometimes mixed with alcohol abuse.

Any signs of psychosis, such as paranoid ideation, agitation, and delusions, respond very well to *small doses* of antipsychotics. Risperidone, 0.25–1 mg orally daily, or olanzapine, 1.25–5 mg orally once a day, will usually decrease psychotic ideation markedly; monitoring for significant orthostatic hypotension (resulting in dizziness, falls, fractures) is mandatory with these agents.

Antidepressants (in one-third to half the doses given to young adults) are used when indicated for depression. Occasionally, a stimulant in small doses (eg, methylphenidate, 5–30 mg orally usually given in two doses at 7 AM and noon) can be used to treat apathy. The stimulant may help increase the patient's energy for social involvement and help the patient to maintain life activities.

The appropriate use of wine and beer for mild sedative effects is quite rewarding in the hospital and other care facilities as well as at home.

C. BEHAVIORAL

The impaired cognitive abilities of the geriatric patient necessitate simple behavioral techniques. Positive responses to appropriate behavior encourage the patient to repeat desirable kinds of behavior, and frequent repetition offsets to some degree the defects in recent memory and recall. It also results in participation—a most important element, since there is a tendency in the older population to withdraw, thus increasing isolation and functional decline.

One must be careful not to reinforce and encourage obstreperous behavior by responding to it; in this way, extinction or at least gradual reduction of inappropriate behavior will occur. At the same time, the obstreperous behavior often represents a nondirective response to frustration and inability to function, and a structured program of activity is necessary.

D. PSYCHOLOGICAL

Patients may require help in adjusting to changing roles and commitments and in finding new goals and viewpoints. The older person steadily loses an important commodity—the future—and may attempt to compensate by preoccupation with the past. Involvement with the present and psychotherapy on a here-and-now basis can help make the adjustment easier.

Lane HY et al: Shifting from haloperidol to risperidone for behavioral disturbances in dementia: safety, response predictors, and mood effects. J Clin Psychopharmacol 2002;22:4. [PMID: 11799336]

Unutzer J et al: Collaborative care management of late-life depression in the primary care setting: a randomized controlled trial. JAMA 2002;288:2836. [PMID: 12472325]

■ PSYCHIATRIC PROBLEMS ASSOCIATED WITH HOSPITALIZATION & MEDICAL & SURGICAL DISORDERS

Diagnostic Categories

A. ACUTE PROBLEMS

1. Delirium with psychotic features secondary to the medical or surgical problem, or compounded by effect of treatment.
2. Acute anxiety, often related to ignorance and fear of the immediate problem as well as uncertainty about the future.

3. Anxiety as an intrinsic aspect of the medical problem (eg, hyperthyroidism).
4. Denial of illness, which may present during acute or intermediate phases of illness.

B. INTERMEDIATE PROBLEMS

1. Depression as a function of the illness or acceptance of the illness, often associated with realistic or fantasied hopelessness about the future.
2. Behavioral problems, often related to denial of illness and, in extreme cases, causing the patient to leave the hospital against medical advice.

C. RECUPERATIVE PROBLEMS

1. Decreasing cooperation as the patient sees improvement and compliance are not compelled.
2. Readjustment problems with family, job, and society.

General Considerations

A. ACUTE PROBLEMS

1. "Intensive care unit psychosis"—The stressful ICU environment may be a cause of delirium. Critical care unit factors include sleep deprivation, increased arousal, mechanical ventilation, and social isolation. Other causes include those common to delirium and require vigorous investigation (see Delirium, above).

2. Pre- and postsurgical anxiety states—Such problems are common and commonly ignored. Presurgical anxiety is very common and is principally a fear of death (many surgical patients make out their wills). Patients may be fearful of anesthesia (improved by the preoperative anesthesia interview), the mysterious operating room, and the disease processes that might be uncovered by the surgeon. Such fears frequently cause people to delay examinations that might result in earlier surgery and a greater chance of cure.

The opposite of this is **surgery proneness**, the quest for surgery to escape from overwhelming life stresses. Polysurgery patients may be classified as "factitious" ones. Dynamic motivations include narcissism, societal pressures (eg, breast implants), unconscious guilt, a masochistic need to suffer, an attempt to deal with another family member's illness, and somatoform disorders and body dysmorphic disorder (an obsession that a body part is disfigured). More apparent reasons may include an attempt to get relief from pain and a lifestyle that has become almost exclusively medically oriented, with all of the risks entailed in such an endeavor.

Postsurgical anxiety states are usually related to pain, procedures, and loss of body image. Acute pain problems are quite different from chronic pain disorders (see Chronic Pain Disorders, this chapter); the former are readily handled with adequate analgesic medication (see Chapter 5). Alterations in body image, as with amputations, ostomies, and mastectomies, often raise concerns about relationships with others.

3. Iatrogenic problems—These usually pertain to medications, complications of diagnostic and treatment procedures, and impersonal and unsympathetic staff behavior. Polypharmacy is often a factor. Patients with unsolved diagnostic problems are at higher risk. They are desirous of relief, and the quest engenders more diagnostic procedures with a higher incidence of complications. The upset patient and family may be very demanding. Excessive demands usually result from anxiety. Such behavior is best handled with calm and measured responses.

B. Intermediate Problems

1. Prolonged hospitalization—Prolonged hospitalization presents unique problems in certain hospital services, eg, burn units, orthopedic services, and tuberculosis wards. The acute problems of the severely burned patient are discussed in Chapter 38. The problems often are behavioral difficulties related to length of hospitalization and necessary procedures. For example, in burn units, pain is a major problem in addition to anxiety about procedures. Disputes with staff are common and often concern pain medication or ward privileges. Some patients regress to infantile behavior and dependency. Staff members must agree about their approach to the patient in order to ensure the smooth functioning of the unit.

Denial of illness may present in the patient with acute myocardial infarction. Intervention by an authority figure (eg, immediate work supervisor) may help the patient accept treatment and eventually abandon the defense of denial.

2. Depression—Depression frequently occurs during this period. Therapeutic drugs (eg, corticosteroids) may be a factor. Depression can contribute to irritability and overt anger. Severe depression can lead to anorexia, which further complicates healing and metabolic balance. It is during this period that the issue of disfigurement arises—relief at survival gives way to concern about future function and appearance.

C. Recuperative Problems

1. Anxiety—Anxiety about return to the posthospital environment can cause regression to a dependent position. Complications increase, and staff forbearance again is tested. Anxiety occurring at this stage usually is handled more easily than previous behavior problems.

2. Posthospital adjustment—Adjustment difficulties after discharge are related to the severity of the deficits and the use of outpatient facilities (eg, physical therapy, rehabilitation programs, psychiatric outpatient treatment). Some patients may experience posttraumatic stress symptoms (eg, from traumatic injuries or even from necessary medical treatments). Lack of appropriate follow-up can contribute to depression in the patient, who may feel that he or she is making

poor progress and may have thoughts of "giving up." Reintegration into work, educational, and social endeavors may be slow. Life is simply much more difficult when one is disfigured, disabled, or disfranchised.

Clinical Findings

The symptoms that occur in these patients are similar to those discussed in previous sections of this chapter, eg, delirium, stress and adjustment disorders, anxiety, and depression. Behavior problems may include lack of cooperation, increased complaints, demands for medication, sexual approaches to nurses, threats to leave the hospital, and actual signing out against medical recommendations. The underlying personality structure of the individual is a major factor in coping styles (eg, the compulsive individual increases indecision, the hysterical individual increases dramatic behavior).

Differential Diagnosis

Delirium and dementia (including cases associated with HIV infection and drug abuse) must always be ruled out, since they often present with symptoms resembling anxiety, depression, or psychosis. Personality disorders existing prior to hospitalization often underlie the various behavior problems, but particularly the management problems.

Complications

Prolongation of hospitalization causes increased expense, deterioration of patient-staff relationships, and increased probabilities of iatrogenic and legal problems. The possibility of increasing posthospital treatment problems is enhanced.

Treatment

A. Medical

The most important consideration by far is to have one clinician in charge, a clinician whom the patient trusts and who is able to oversee multiple treatment approaches (see Somatoform Disorders, above). In acute problems, attention must be paid to metabolic imbalance, alcohol withdrawal, and previous drug use—prescribed, recreational, or over-the-counter. Adequate sleep and analgesia are important in the prevention of delirium. When absolute behavioral control is urgently needed, agents such as propofol, dexmedetomidine, opioids, and midazolam have been used.

Most clinicians are attuned to the early detection of the surgery-prone patient. Plastic and orthopedic surgeons are at particular risk. Appropriate consultations may help detect some problems and mitigate future ones.

Postsurgical anxiety states can be alleviated by personal attention from the surgeon. Anxiety is not so effectively lessened by ancillary medical personnel, whom the patient perceives as lesser authorities, until after the physician has reassured the patient. Inappropriate use of "as needed" analgesia places an unfair burden on the nurse. "Patient-controlled analgesia" can improve pain control, decrease anxiety, and minimize side effects.

Depression should be recognized early. If severe, it may be treated by antidepressant medications (see Antidepressant Drugs, above). High levels of anxiety can be lowered with judicious use of anxiolytic agents. Unnecessary medications tend to reinforce the patient's impression that there must be a serious illness or medication would not be required.

B. Psychological

Prepare the patient and family for what is to come. This includes the types of units where the patient will be quartered, the procedures that will be performed, and any disfigurements that will result from surgery. Repetition improves understanding. The nursing staff can be helpful, since patients frequently confide a lack of understanding to a nurse but are reluctant to do so to the physician.

Denial of illness is frequently a block to acceptance of treatment. This too should be handled with family members present (to help the patient face the reality of the situation) in a series of short interviews (for reinforcement). Dependency problems resulting from long hospitalization are best handled by focusing on the changes to come as the patient makes the transition to the outside world. Key figures are teachers, vocational counselors, and physical therapists. Challenges should be realistic and practical and handled in small steps.

Depression is usually related to the loss of familiar hospital supports, and the outpatient therapists and counselors help to lessen the impact of the loss. Some of the impact can be alleviated by anticipating, with the patient and family, the signal features of the common depression to help prevent the patient from assuming a permanent sick role (invalidism).

Suicide is always a concern when a patient is faced with despair. An honest, compassionate, and supportive approach will help sustain the patient during this trying period.

C. Behavioral

Prior desensitization can significantly allay anxiety about medical procedures. A "dry run" can be done to reinforce the oral description. Cooperation during acute problem periods can be enhanced by the use of appropriate reinforcers such as a favorite nurse or helpful family member. People who are positive reinforcers are even more helpful during the intermediate phases when the patient becomes resistant to the seemingly endless procedures (eg, debridement of burned areas).

Specific situations (eg, psychological dependency on the respirator) can be corrected by weaning with appropriate reinforcers (eg, watching a favorite movie on a videorecorder when disconnected from the ventilator). Behavioral approaches should be used in a positive and optimistic way for maximal reinforcement.

Relaxation techniques and attentional distraction can be used to block side effects of a necessary treatment (eg, nausea in cancer chemotherapy).

D. Social

A change in environment requires adaptation. Because of the illness, admission and hospitalization may be more easily handled than discharge. Reintegration into society can be difficult. In some cases, the family is a negative influence. A predischarge evaluation must be made to determine whether the family will be able to cope with the physical or mental changes in the patient. Working with the family while the patient is in the acute stage may presage a successful transition later on.

Development of a new social life can be facilitated by various self-help organizations (eg, the stoma club). Sharing problems with others in similar circumstances eases the return to a social life, which may be quite different from that prior to the illness.

Prognosis

The prognosis is good in all patients who have reversible medical and surgical conditions. It is guarded when there is serious functional loss that impairs vocational, educational, or societal possibilities—especially in the case of progressive and ultimately life-threatening illness.

Blumenthal JA et al: Depression as a risk factor for mortality after coronary artery bypass surgery. Lancet 2003;362:604. [PMID: 12944059]

Ciechanowski P et al: Influence of patient attachment style on self-care and outcomes in diabetes. Psychosom Med 2004; 66:720. [PMID: 15385697]

Hogarth DK et al: Management of sedation in mechanically ventilated patients. Curr Opin Crit Care 2004;10:40. [PMID: 15166848]

Endocrinology

26

Paul A. Fitzgerald, MD

Hormones exert their effects by interacting with receptors on the cell surface (catecholamines and peptide hormones) or in the cytoplasm and nucleus (thyroid and steroid hormones). Endocrine disorders result from an excess or deficiency of hormonal effects.

■ COMMON PRESENTATIONS IN ENDOCRINOLOGY

UNINTENDED WEIGHT LOSS

Uncontrolled diabetes mellitus may be associated with weight loss, polyphagia, polydipsia, and polyuria. Anorexia and nausea may be seen with diabetic ketoacidosis and with adrenal insufficiency (due either to pituitary adrenocorticotropic hormone [ACTH] deficiency or to Addison's disease). Patients with severe diabetes insipidus may also lose weight. Patients with hyperthyroidism typically lose weight despite increased appetite; some patients with hypothyroidism lose weight because of diminished appetite. About 15% of patients with pheochromocytoma lose over 10% of their basal weight. Some patients with Cushing's syndrome lose weight as a result of muscle wasting.

A great variety of nonendocrine conditions enter into the differential diagnosis of unintended weight loss (see Chapter 2). Anorexia is frequently a side effect of medications or radiation therapy and is also seen with azotemia, AIDS, and many gastrointestinal conditions. Malignancies typically produce diminished appetite and cachexia. Tuberculosis may cause weight loss even when occult. Chronic respiratory insufficiency is often associated with weight loss. Psychiatric illnesses producing diminished appetite include depressed or agitated affective disorder, catatonia, and anorexia nervosa.

ABNORMAL SKIN PIGMENTATION

Increased skin pigmentation can be caused by excessive ACTH secretion in Addison's disease and can occur after bilateral adrenalectomy for Cushing's disease (Nelson's syndrome). Pigmentation can be generalized or may be localized to palmar creases, extensor joint surfaces, tongue, nails, belt or bra lines, freckles, or new scars.

Pigmentation of the upper lip, forehead, or malar eminences, known as **chloasma**, can be caused by pregnancy ("mask of pregnancy"), oral contraceptives, or estrogen replacement therapy.

Acanthosis nigricans presents as velvety brown thickened skin of the neck and axillae. It may be associated with syndromes of severe insulin resistance type A (ovarian dysfunction and hirsutism) or type B (autoimmune). It may also be familial or associated with obesity, acromegaly, or thyroid disease. Acanthosis presenting after age 35 years is often a sign of an underlying malignancy, such as hepatocellular carcinoma.

Pretibial areas of pigmentation are common in diabetes ("diabetic shin spots") as a result of minor trauma or following necrobiosis lipoidica diabeticorum.

Prominent lentigines can be a sign of Carney's complex, an autosomal dominant condition associated with atrial myxomas, schwannomas, and endocrine overactivity (eg, tumors of the thyroid, gonads, or pigmented adrenal nodular hyperplasia). Similar skin pigmentation is seen in Peutz–Jeghers syndrome with an increased risk of intestinal polyposis, adenocarcinoma, breast cancer, and tumors of the gonads and thyroid.

Diffuse hyperpigmentation is seen in POEMS (polyneuropathy, organomegaly, endocrinopathy, monoclonal gammopathy, skin changes) syndrome; adrenal insufficiency, hypoparathyroidism, diabetes, osteosclerotic bone lesions, or thiamine deficiency may occur.

Gray-brown ("bronze") hyperpigmentation is caused by hemochromatosis, which can cause endocrine deficiencies such as diabetes mellitus. An orange skin discoloration is characteristic of jaundice and carotenodermia (caused by ingestion of large amounts of carotene in vegetables, seaweed, or vitamin preparations).

Patchy hypopigmentation can be due to vitiligo, a condition sometimes associated with Addison's disease and with other endocrine deficiencies as part of the polyglandular autoimmune syndrome. Hypopigmentation can also be a manifestation of cobalamin deficiency, trisomy 13, and various dermatologic conditions.

Patients undergoing chronic hemodialysis frequently become hyperpigmented, and hypopigmentation has also been reported. Other causes of hyperpigmentation include sprue, malnutrition, HIV infection, and porphyria. Hyperpigmentation may be caused by certain drugs: amiodarone, arsenic, bleomycin, busulfan, clofazimine, hydroxychloroquine, chlorpromazine, doxorubicin (nail beds), imipramine, methimazole, minocycline, niacin, primaquine, propylthiouracil, topical tretinoin, and zidovudine (nails).

OBESITY

See Nutrition, Chapter 29.

GYNECOMASTIA

ESSENTIALS OF DIAGNOSIS

- *Enlargement of the male breast, often asymmetric or unilateral.*
- *Glandular gynecomastia characterized by tenderness.*
- *Fatty gynecomastia typically nontender.*
- *Must be distinguished from tumors or mastitis.*

General Considerations

Gynecomastia refers to a female-appearing male breast. Pubertal gynecomastia is common and the swelling usually subsides spontaneously within a year. Gynecomastia is particularly common in teenagers who are very tall or overweight. Gynecomastia develops in about 50% of athletes who abuse androgens and anabolic steroids. It is seen in Klinefelter's syndrome, which affects 1:500 men. (See section on Klinefelter's syndrome.) Gynecomastia can develop in HIV-infected patients treated with highly active antiretroviral therapy (HAART), especially in men receiving efavirenz or didanosine; breast enlargement resolves spontaneously in 73% of patients within 9 months. Gynecomastia is common among elderly men, particularly when there is associated weight gain. However, it can be the first sign of a serious disorder. Patients with Peutz–Jeghers syndrome are prone to development of gynecomastia caused by testicular tumors.

The causes of gynecomastia are multiple and diverse (Table 26–1).

Clinical Findings

A. SYMPTOMS AND SIGNS

Gynecomastia is graded according to severity: I, mild; II, moderate; III, severe. Fatty gynecomastia is usually diffuse and nontender. Glandular enlargement beneath the areola may be tender. Pubertal gynecomastia is characterized by tender discoid enlargement of breast tissue 2–3 cm in diameter beneath the areola.

B. LABORATORY FINDINGS

Laboratory measurements of plasma levels of prolactin (PRL) (see Hyperprolactinemia) and the β-subunit of human chorionic gonadotropin (β-hCG). Detectable

Table 26–1. Causes of gynecomastia.

Idiopathic	Bicalutamide
	Busulfan
Physiologic causes	Chorionic gonadotropin
Neonatal period	Cimetidine
Puberty	Clomiphene
Aging	Cyclophosphamide
Obesity	Diazepam
	Diethylstilbestrol
Endocrine diseases	Digitalis preparations
Androgen resistance syndromes	Estrogens (oral or topical)
	Ethionamide
Aromatase excess syndrome (sporadic or familial)	Finasteride
	Flutamide
	Goserelin
Diabetic lymphocytic mastitis	HAART (highly active antiretroviral therapy)
Hyperprolactinemia	Haloperidol
Hyperthyroidism	Hydroxyzine
Klinefelter's syndrome	Isoniazid
Male hypogonadism	Ketoconazole
Partial 17-ketosteroid reductase deficiency	Leuprolide
	Marijuana
	Meprobamate
Systemic diseases	Methadone
Chronic liver disease	Methyldopa
Chronic renal disease	Metoclopramide
Neurologic disorders	Mirtazapine
Refeeding after starvation	Molindone
Spinal cord injury	Nilutamide
	Omeprazole
	Opioids
Neoplasms	Penicillamine
Adrenal tumors	Phenothiazines
Bronchogenic carcinoma	Progestins
Carcinoma of the breast	Protease inhibitors
Hepatocellular carcinoma (rare)	Reserpine
	Risperidone
Testicular tumors	Somatropin (growth hormone)
Drugs (partial list)	Spironolactone
Alcohol	Testosterone
Alkylating agents	Thioridazine
Amiodarone	Tricyclic antidepressants
Anabolic steroids	
Androgens	

levels of β-hCG implicate a testicular tumor (germ cell or Sertoli cell) or other malignancy (usually lung or liver). Detectable low levels of serum β-hCG (< 5 mU/mL) may be reported in men with primary hypogonadism and high serum luteinizing hormone (LH) levels if the assay for β-hCG cross-reacts with LH. Measurements of plasma testosterone and LH are valuable in the diagnosis of primary or secondary hypogonadism. A low testosterone and high LH are seen in primary hypogonadism. High testosterone levels plus high LH levels characterize partial androgen resistance. Serum estradiol is determined but is usually normal; increased levels may result from testicular tumors, increased β-hCG, liver disease, obesity, adrenal tumors (rare), true hermaphroditism (rare), or gain of function mutations affecting the aromatase gene (rare). Many estrogens and substances with estrogenic activity are not detected by estradiol assays. Serum thyroid-stimulating hormone (TSH) (sensitive) and free thyroxine (FT$_4$) levels are also determined. A karyotype (for Klinefelter's syndrome) is obtained in men with persistent gynecomastia without obvious cause.

Investigation of unclear cases should include a chest radiograph to search for metastatic or bronchogenic carcinoma. Needle biopsy with cytologic examination may be performed on suspicious areas of male breast enlargement (especially when unilateral or asymmetric) to distinguish gynecomastia from tumor or mastitis.

Treatment

Pubertal gynecomastia often resolves spontaneously within 1–2 years. Drug-induced gynecomastia resolves after the offending drug is removed. Spironolactone can be stopped, with substitution of a selective aldosterone antagonist such as eplerenone. Patients with painful or persistent (> 12 months) gynecomastia may be treated with a 3- to 9-month course of a selective estrogen receptor modulator (SERM; eg, raloxifene or tamoxifen). SERM therapy is much more effective for glandular ("lumpy") gynecomastia than for diffuse fatty gynecomastia. There is some evidence that raloxifene, taken orally in a dose of 60 mg daily, may be the more effective drug. Aromatase inhibitors (eg, letrozole, anastrozole, or exemestane) are marginally effective and should not ordinarily be used for adolescent boys, since long-term therapy may prevent epiphyseal fusion. Surgical correction is reserved for patients with persistent or severe gynecomastia, since results are often disappointing. Endoscopically assisted transaxillary liposuction and subcutaneous mastectomy may produce acceptable results. Generally, it is prudent to treat patients for gynecomastia only when it becomes a troubling and continuing problem for them.

Lawrence SE et al: Beneficial effects of tamoxifen and raloxifene in the treatment of pubertal gynecomastia. J Pediatr 2004; 145:71. [PMID: 15238910]

Mira JA et al: Gynaecomastia in HIV-infected men on highly active antiretroviral therapy: association with efavirenz and didanosine treatment. Antivir Ther 2004;9:511. [PMID: 15456082]

Ramon Y et al: Multimodality gynecomastia repair by cross-chest power-assisted superficial liposuction combined with endoscopic-assisted pull-through excision. Ann Plast Surg 2005; 55:591. [PMID: 16327457]

Rhoden EL et al: Treatment of testosterone-induced gynecomastia with the aromatase inhibitor, anastrozole. Int J Impot Res 2004;16:95. [PMID: 14963480]

ERECTILE DYSFUNCTION & DIMINISHED LIBIDO IN MEN

Erectile dysfunction is a frequent problem. Psychogenic factors as well as endocrine, vascular, or neurologic abnormalities may be important. Hypogonadism of whatever origin is associated with lack of libido and erectile dysfunction. These can also be the first clinical manifestations of a hyperprolactinemic disorder. Other endocrine causes include hyperthyroidism, Addison's disease, and acromegaly. Impotence in men with diabetes may be related to inadequate penile blood flow or autonomic neuropathy. Vascular disease is a frequent factor in impotence in elderly men. Vascular claudication of the legs along with related impotence is known as **Leriche's syndrome.**

Many pharmacologic agents are known to cause varying degrees of impotence (Table 26–2). Selective serotonin reuptake inhibitors (SSRIs, eg, fluoxetine) cause reduced libido. SSRIs and clomipramine cause delayed ejaculation.

Evaluation and treatment of erectile dysfunction are covered in Chapters 23 and 25.

CRYPTORCHISM

One or both testes may be absent from the scrotum at birth in about 20% of premature or low-birth-weight male infants and in 3–6% at full term infants. Cryptorchism is found in 1–2% of males after 1 year of age but must be distinguished from retractile testes, which require no treatment. Cryptorchism should be corrected before age 12–24 months in an attempt to reduce the risk of infertility, which occurs in up to 75% of men with bilateral cryptorchism and in 50% of men with unilateral cryptorchism. It is not clear, however, whether such early orchiopexy improves ultimate fertility. Some patients have underlying hypogonadism.

The ultimate incidence of significant testicular neoplasia is about 0.002% in normal males, 0.06% in cryptorchid males, and up to 5% in patients with intra-abdominal testes.

Table 26–2. Drugs causing erectile dysfunction.

Alcohol	Marijuana
Amphetamines	Methadone
Antihistamines	Methyldopa
Barbiturates	Metoclopramide
β-Blockers	Monoamine oxidase inhibitors
Butyrophenones	Opioids
Carbamazepine	Phenothiazines
Cimetidine	Sedatives
Clonidine	Spironolactone
Cocaine	Selective serotonin reuptake inhibitors
Guanethidine	Thiazides
Ketoconazole	Tricyclic antidepressants
Leuprolide	

If the testes are not palpable, ultrasound or MRI can be used to locate them. Alternatively, hCG, 1500 units intramuscularly daily for 3 days, causes a significant rise in testosterone if the testes are present. Therapy with hCG results in a testicular descent rate of about 25%.

Orchiopexy decreases the risk of neoplasia when performed before 10 years of age. Orchiectomy after puberty is an option for intra-abdominal testes.

Henna MR et al: Hormonal cryptorchidism therapy: systematic review with metanalysis of randomized clinical trials. Pediatr Surg Int 2004;20:357. [PMID: 15221359]

Kolon TF et al: Cryptorchidism: diagnosis, treatment, and long-term prognosis. Urol Clin North Am 2004;31:469. [PMID: 15313056]

BONE PAIN & PATHOLOGIC FRACTURES

Onset of pathologic fractures at an early age is seen in osteogenesis imperfecta (blue scleras may be present). Painful bowing of the bones and pseudofractures suggest rickets or osteomalacia. Vitamin D deficiency is a common cause of bone pain, and all patients with non-traumatic bone pain (or reduced bone density) should have a serum 25-hydroxyvitamin D determination. Any serum 25-hydroxyvitamin D level under 20 ng/mL (50 nmol/L) is considered low and an indication for vitamin D supplementation, although being considered in the "normal range" by many laboratories. Hyperparathyroidism or malignancy is suspected in patients with bone pain and hypercalcemia. Back pain or pathologic fractures in hypogonadal men and women implicate osteoporosis; such pain may be relieved with calcitonin. In cases of osteopenia of unknown cause, hyperthyroidism and Cushing's syndrome should also be considered. Bone pain may also occur as a result of primary or metastatic tumors, multiple myeloma, and Paget's disease; such pain may be relieved with bisphosphonates, such as intravenous zoledronic acid or oral alendronate. However, bisphosphonates themselves commonly cause bone pain.

MUSCLE CRAMPS & TETANY

Muscle cramps are usually caused by sports or occupational muscle injury. Nocturnal leg cramps are commonly idiopathic but are associated with diabetes mellitus, Parkinson's disease, central nervous system or spinal cord lesions, peripheral neuropathy, hemodialysis, peripheral vascular disease, and cisplatin or vincristine. Various other drugs can cause myalgias that patients describe as cramps (eg, cimetidine, cholestyramine). Alkalosis due to any cause (eg, severe vomiting or hyperventilation) may decrease ionized calcium and cause muscle cramping and paresthesias. Leg cramps during walking may be due to vascular insufficiency, hyperthyroidism, or hypothyroidism. A common cause for muscle pain, though not usually with cramping, is 3-hydroxy-3-methylglutaryl coenzyme A (HMG-CoA) reductase inhibitor (statin) therapy for hyperlipidemia; serum creatine kinase (CK) levels may

be elevated in the presence of rhabdomyolysis, but are usually normal with statin-associated myopathy. Other medications can cause muscle cramping, including cholinesterase inhibitors, bisphosphonates, and chemotherapeutic agents (eg, imatinib). Acute arsenic intoxication can cause muscle cramps along with dysphagia, nausea, vomiting, and thirst. Muscle pain may be caused by dermatomyositis; CK levels are elevated. Diffuse muscle tenderness, especially with "trigger points" and normal serum CK levels, may indicate, fibromyalgia (see Chapter 20).

McArdle's disease is caused by muscle phosphorylase deficiency; patients present with muscle fatigue, cramping, and high serum CK levels; vitamin B_6 (pyridoxine) supplementation reduces muscle cramps. Carnitine palmitoyltransferase II deficiency is a genetic disorder of lipid metabolism; presenting symptoms and signs include myalgia, cramping, myoglobinuria, and elevated serum CK levels. Other conditions that may cause muscle cramping include stiff man syndrome (abdominal and back cramping), Brody's disease, phosphoglycerate kinase deficiency (myoglobinuria), muscle phosphofructokinase deficiency (Tarui's disease), and neuromyotonia (Isaac's syndrome).

Diffuse, recurrent, or severe muscle cramping requires evaluation for hypocalcemia (see Table 21–8). Treatment of hypocalcemia is discussed in Chapter 21. Magnesium deficiency must be considered in tetany unresponsive to calcium.

For patients with recurrent, severe, or prolonged muscle cramping, gabapentin, 600–1200 mg/d orally, appears to be effective. Adverse effects of gabapentin may include leukopenia and central nervous system toxicities. Quinine, long used to prevent nocturnal muscle cramps, can cause arrhythmias, dizziness, hemolytic-uremic syndrome, and agranulocytosis. The US Food and Drug Administration has prohibited the marketing of quinine for leg cramps because of these side effects. Leg cramps, usually nocturnal, affect 45% of women during pregnancy; oral calcium or magnesium citrate supplementation twice daily may also improve cramping.

Exertional claudication caused by peripheral artery disease may be treated with oral pentoxifylline, cilostazol, angioplasty, or arterial bypass; the differential diagnosis includes neurogenic claudication, usually caused by spinal stenosis.

Recurrent cervicofacial and laryngeal dystonias, as well as hand cramps, have been successfully treated with injections of botulinum toxin.

de Carvalho M et al: Cramps, muscle pain, and fasciculations: not always benign? Neurology 2004;63:721. [PMID: 15326252]

Schwellnus MP et al: Serum electrolyte concentrations and hydration status are not associated with exercise associated muscle cramping (EAMC) in distance runners. Br J Sports Med 2004;38:488. [PMID: 15273192]

MENTAL CHANGES

Disturbances of mentation may be important indications of underlying endocrine disorders. Nervousness, irritability, apathy, and depression can be seen in both men and women with hypogonadism. Postpartum depression occurs in 10–15% of women. Premenstrual dysphoric disorder is common and may be due in part to an adverse reaction to progesterone. Oral or transdermal progestins also cause a similar syndrome. Anxiety and extreme irritability can be seen in patients with hyperthyroidism. Adult cretinism is the result of prolonged hypothyroidism in infancy. In adults, hypothyroidism is accompanied by mental slowness, depression, and lethargy. Occasionally, it may be manifested by delusional psychosis ("myxedema madness"). Pheochromocytoma may cause anxiety, confusion, or psychosis. Prolonged hypocalcemia from untreated hypoparathyroidism may be associated with intellectual deterioration. Hypoglycemia of any origin may cause confusion, abnormal speech, and behavioral or personality changes as well as sudden loss of consciousness, somnolence and prolonged lethargy, or coma; frank psychosis can occur but is rare. Mild hypercalcemia causes fatigue and emotional irritability. Severe hypercalcemia can cause confusion, psychosis, and coma. Confusion may occur in hypopituitarism or Addison's disease. Confusion, lethargy, and nausea may be the presenting symptoms of hyponatremia. Insomnia, mood changes, anxiety, and psychosis can be associated with Cushing's syndrome or high-dose corticosteroid administration. Rapid changes in corticosteroid status (either a sudden increase or a sudden decrease) may be associated with acute psychosis. Porphyria may cause affective and thought disorders, particularly during acute attacks.

Mental changes may result from vitamin deficiencies caused by malnutrition, malabsorption, and other conditions. Deficiency in vitamin B_1 (thiamine) is usually seen in alcoholism and can cause Korsakoff's syndrome with typical memory loss and confabulation. Deficiency in vitamin B_2 (riboflavin) may cause personality deterioration and occurs commonly with psychotropic and antimalarial drugs and with diabetes and other diseases. Vitamin B_3 (niacin) deficiency is seen with poor nutrition, alcoholism, mercaptopurine toxicity, and malignant carcinoid syndrome and can cause irritability, dementia, dermatitis, and diarrhea. Vitamin B_6 (pyridoxine) deficiency is frequently seen in alcoholics or during treatment with isoniazid or levodopa and can cause irritability, depression, and neuropathy. Deficiency of vitamin B_{12} (cobalamin) is caused by insufficient gastric intrinsic factor and may be seen at any age; however, it is more common in the elderly, affecting about 10% of people over age 70 years. Vitamin B_{12} deficiency may cause depression, irritability, paranoia, mania, psychotic symptoms, cognitive impairment, obsessive–compulsive disorder, and dementia. Although vitamin B_{12} deficiency is usually associated with other neurologic symptoms such as paresthesias and leg weakness, mental changes may occur in the absence of neurologic symptoms and without megaloblastic anemia. When serum vitamin B_{12} levels are borderline low, an elevated serum level of methylmalonic acid is an additional indication of vitamin B_{12} deficiency.

Disturbance in mentation is always an indication to evaluate for the endocrine and metabolic disorders discussed above. However, cognitive changes are more typically caused by organic brain or cerebrovascular disease, psychiatric problems, alcoholism, or drug abuse.

■ DISEASES OF THE HYPOTHALAMUS & PITUITARY GLAND

Anterior pituitary gland function is controlled by hypothalamic hormones and by direct feedback inhibition. The **posterior pituitary** receives antidiuretic hormone and oxytocin from the hypothalamus, secreting them under central nervous system control (Table 26–3). Hypothalamic hormones generally stimulate the anterior pituitary except for dopamine, which inhibits the pituitary from spontaneously secreting PRL.

ANTERIOR HYPOPITUITARISM

ESSENTIALS OF DIAGNOSIS

- Loss of one, all, or any combination of anterior pituitary hormones.
- ACTH deficiency reduces adrenal secretion of cortisol, testosterone, and epinephrine; aldosterone secretion remains intact.
- Growth hormone (GH) deficiency causes short stature in children; adults experience asthenia, obesity, and increased cardiac mortality.
- PRL deficiency inhibits postpartum lactation.
- TSH deficiency causes secondary hypothyroidism.
- LH and follicle-stimulating hormone (FSH) deficiency cause hypogonadism and infertility in men and women.

General Considerations

Hypopituitarism can be caused by either hypothalamic or pituitary dysfunction. Patients with hypopituitarism may have single or multiple hormonal deficiencies. When one hormonal deficiency is discovered, others must be sought.

Mass lesions causing hypopituitarism include pituitary adenomas, granulomas, Rathke's cleft cysts, apoplexy, metastatic carcinomas, aneurysms, and brain tumors such as craniopharyngioma, meningioma, germinoma, glioma, chondrosarcoma, and chordoma of the clivus. Langerhans cell histiocytosis usually presents in youth with diabetes

Table 26–3. Pituitary hormones.

Anterior pituitary
  Growth hormone (GH)[1]
  Prolactin (PRL)
  Adrenocorticotropic hormone (ACTH)
  Thyroid-stimulating hormone (TSH)
  Luteinizing hormone (LH)[2]
  Follicle-stimulating hormone (FSH)
Posterior pituitary
  Arginine vasopressin (AVP)[3]
  Oxytocin

[1]GH closely resembles human placental lactogen (hPL).
[2]LH closely resembles human chorionic gonadotropin (hCG).
[3]AVP is identical with antidiuretic hormone (ADH).

insipidus or hypopituitarism. Osteolytic bone lesions are noted on skeletal x-rays. Autoimmune hypophysitis, postpartum pituitary necrosis (Sheehan's syndrome), eclampsia–preeclampsia, sickle cell disease, and African trypanosomiasis are rare causes.

A pituitary tumor may be part of the syndrome of multiple endocrine neoplasia type 1 (MEN 1), with tumors of the parathyroid glands and pancreatic islets.

Hypopituitarism without mass lesions may be genetic or idiopathic, or may be caused by trauma, cranial radiation, surgery, encephalitis, hemochromatosis, autoimmunity, or stroke. It may also occur after coronary artery bypass grafting. About 25–30% of survivors of moderate to severe traumatic brain injury (Glasgow coma scale ≤ 13/15) have at least one anterior pituitary hormone deficiency. Following aneurysmal subarachnoid hemorrhage, at least one pituitary hormone deficiency develops in about 55% of survivors.

Physiologic isolated hypogonadotrophic hypogonadism is common, occurring with severe illness, malnutrition, and extreme prolonged exercise (in women). It is also commonly found among obese patients with type 2 diabetes mellitus. Long-term intrathecal administration of opioids causes hypogonadotropic hypogonadism in the overwhelming majority of patients; GH deficiency and secondary adrenal insufficiency each occurs in about 15% of such patients. High-dose oral methadone can also cause hypogonadotropic hypogonadism that may persist after stopping the drug.

Congenital combined pituitary hormone deficiency occurs in about 1:8000 births. Depending on the genetic defect, it may be transmitted as an autosomal recessive, autosomal dominant, or X-linked recessive trait. Mutations have been found in genes that encode transcription factors necessary for pituitary development. Mutations in the *PROP1* gene are found in about 50% of patients with genetic combined pituitary hormone deficiency. Mutations in other genes, such as *POU1F1*, *LHX3*, *LHX4*, and *HESX1*, can also cause hypopituitarism. Some of these patients exhibit benign pituitary enlargement that may regress spontaneously.

Kallmann's syndrome is the most common cause of congenital isolated gonadotropin deficiency. It is usually sporadic but may be familial. Three different genetic inheritance patterns can occur: X-linked recessive (Kal 1), autosomal dominant (Kal 2), or autosomal recessive (Kal 3). Kallmann's syndrome has an incidence of 1:10,000 males and 1:50,000 females. It is associated with hyposmia caused by hypoplasia of the olfactory bulbs. In Kallmann's syndrome, about 50% of patients have unilateral renal agenesis; some patients may also exhibit cryptorchidism, sensorineural deafness, cerebellar dysfunction, bilateral synkinesis, nystagmus, cleft lip, or high-arched palate.

Clinical Findings

Manifestations of hypopituitarism vary depending on which specific hormones are lacking and whether their deficiency is partial or complete.

A. SYMPTOMS AND SIGNS

Gonadotropin deficiency includes loss of LH and FSH, which causes hypogonadism and infertility. Patients with isolated gonadotropin deficiency may present as delayed adolescence. (See also discussion of primary amenorrhea.) Congenital gonadotropin deficiency in males may be associated with congenital micropenis or cryptorchism.

Hypogonadotropic hypogonadism is also seen in patients with congenital adrenal hypoplasia, a rare X-linked disorder caused by a mutation in the *DAX-1* gene. Boys with *DAX-1* gene mutations usually present during infancy or childhood with adrenal insufficiency caused by failure to form the permanent zone of the adrenal cortex. Boys who survive beyond childhood usually fail to enter puberty as a result of hypogonadotropic hypogonadism. However, those with partial loss-of-function mutations in *DAX-1* can present in adulthood with hypogonadotropic hypogonadism and subtle signs of adrenal failure.

In acquired gonadotropin deficiency, both men and women lose axillary, pubic, and body hair gradually, particularly if they are also hypoadrenal. Men may note diminished beard growth. Libido is diminished. Women have amenorrhea; men note decreased erections. Most patients are infertile. Androgen deficiency predisposes patients to osteopenia and muscle atrophy. (See section on secondary amenorrhea.)

TSH deficiency causes hypothyroidism with manifestations such as fatigue, weakness, weight change, and hyperlipidemia. (See Hypothyroidism and Myxedema.)

ACTH deficiency results in diminished cortisol secretion (see Adrenocortical Hypofunction). Symptoms may include weakness, fatigue, weight loss, and hypotension. Patients with partial ACTH deficiency continue to have some cortisol secretion and may not have symptoms until stressed by illness or surgery. Adrenal mineralocorticoid secretion continues, so manifestations of adrenal insufficiency in hypopituitarism are usually less striking than in bilateral adrenal gland destruction

(Addison's disease); hyponatremia may occur, especially when ACTH and TSH deficiencies are both present.

GH deficiency in adulthood tends to cause mild to moderate central obesity, increased systolic blood pressure, and relative increases in low-density lipoprotein (LDL) cholesterol. GH deficiency also results in a small heart with reduced cardiac output, asthenia, and feelings of social isolation.

Panhypopituitarism is the absence of all anterior pituitary hormones. Combined pituitary hormone deficiency (CPHD) refers to a deficiency of several anterior pituitary hormones. Patients with *PROP1* gene mutations gradually develop CPHD, usually presenting with short stature and growth failure due to GH and TSH deficiency; lack of pubertal development occurs due to deficiencies in FSH and LH. Patients with *PROP1* gene mutations gradually develop ACTH-cortisol deficiency, and typically require corticosteroid replacement therapy by age 18 years. In addition to the manifestations noted above, patients with long-standing hypopituitarism tend to have dry, pale, finely textured skin. The face has fine wrinkles and an apathetic countenance.

B. LABORATORY FINDINGS

The fasting blood glucose may be low. Hyponatremia is often present. Hyperkalemia usually does not occur, since aldosterone production is not affected.

The free tetraiodothyronine (thyroxine, T_4) level is low, and TSH is not elevated. Plasma levels of sex steroids (testosterone and estradiol) are low or low normal, as are the serum gonadotropins as well. Elevated PRL levels are found in patients with prolactinomas, acromegaly, and hypothalamic disease.

ACTH deficiency causes functional atrophy of the adrenal cortex within 2 weeks of pituitary damage. Therefore, the diagnosis of secondary hypoadrenalism may be confirmed by holding any corticosteroid medication on the day of the test and by administering cosyntropin (synthetic $ACTH_{1-24}$), 0.25 mg (intramuscularly or intravenously); blood is drawn 30–60 minutes after the injection. A serum cortisol of ≥ 20 mcg/dL (550 nmol/mL), random or stimulated, rules out the diagnosis. A baseline ACTH level is low or normal in secondary hypoadrenalism, distinguishing it from primary adrenal disease.

Deficiency of epinephrine occurs with secondary adrenal insufficiency, since high local concentrations of cortisol are required to induce the production of the enzyme phenylethanolamine *N*-methyltransferase (PNMT) that catalyzes the conversion of norepinephrine to epinephrine in the adrenal medulla.

The diagnosis of GH deficiency is made difficult by the pulsatile nature of GH secretion and individual variability. GH deficiency is present in 96% of patients with three or more other pituitary hormone deficiencies. The insulin hypoglycemia test, long considered the "gold standard," is actually unreliable, cumbersome, and uncomfortable; it is contraindicated in the elderly, in patients

with cardiovascular or cerebrovascular disease, and in patients with any history of seizures, an abnormal electroencephalogram (EEG), or recent brain surgery. Other GH stimulation tests require the administration of intravenous arginine and oral carbidopa and levodopa (combination) in patients pretreated with propranolol or estrogen. However, these tests do not discriminate well between normal individuals and patients with presumed GH deficiency (patients with three or more other pituitary hormone deficiencies). Serum insulin-like growth factor (IGF-I) levels are in the normal range in about 50% of adults with GH deficiency. However, very low levels of IGF-I (< 84 mcg/L) are indicative of GH deficiency except in conditions that naturally suppress serum IGF-I (eg, malnutrition, prolonged fasting, oral estrogen, hypothyroidism, uncontrolled diabetes mellitus, liver failure). In GH deficiency, exercise-stimulated serum GH levels usually fail to rise and remain at < 5 ng/mL; however, by age 40 years, most normal adults have lost their GH response to exercise.

Because hemochromatosis can cause hypopituitarism, in patients with hypopituitarism without an established etiology, it is prudent to screen for hemochromatosis with a serum iron and transferrin saturation or ferritin.

C. IMAGING

MRI provides the best visualization of parasellar lesions. In hemochromatosis, MRI shows a very hypointense anterior lobe on T1-weighted images, which is surrounded by hyperintense cerebrospinal fluid on T2-weighted images. The posterior pituitary usually has a high-intensity signal on sagittal T1-weighted MRI that is lacking in central diabetes insipidus. In Langerhans cell histiocytosis, MRI may reveal a mass lesion, thickening of the pituitary stalk, or be normal.

Differential Diagnosis

Reversible hypogonadotropic hypogonadism may occur with serious illness, malnutrition, or anorexia nervosa. The clinical situation and the presence of normal adrenal and thyroid function allow ready distinction from hypopituitarism. Profound hypogonadotropic hypogonadism develops in men who receive gonadotropin-releasing hormone (GnRH) therapy for prostate cancer; it usually persists following cessation of therapy. Hypogonadotropic hypogonadism usually develops in patients receiving high-dose methadone or chronic intrathecal infusion of opioids; both GH deficiency and secondary adrenal insufficiency occur in 15% of such patients. Secondary adrenal insufficiency may persist for many months following high-dose corticosteroid therapy.

Severe illness causes functional suppression of TSH and T_4. Hyperthyroxinemia reversibly suppresses TSH. Administration of triiodothyronine (Cytomel) suppresses TSH and T_4. Bexarotene, used to treat cutaneous T cell lymphoma, suppresses TSH secretion, resulting in temporary central hypothyroidism. Corticosteroids or meges-trol treatment reversibly suppresses endogenous ACTH and cortisol secretion.

Complications

Patients with destructive lesions (eg, tumors) may develop complications related to them or to surgery or radiation therapy. Among patients with craniopharyngiomas, diabetes insipidus is found in 16% preoperatively and in 60% postoperatively. Hyponatremia often presents abruptly during the first 2 weeks following pituitary surgery. Visual field impairment may occur. Hypothalamic damage may result in morbid obesity as well as cognitive and emotional problems. Conventional radiation therapy results in an increased incidence of small vessel ischemic strokes and second tumors.

Patients with untreated hypoadrenalism and a stressful illness may become febrile and die in shock and coma.

Adults with GH deficiency have experienced an increased cardiovascular morbidity. Rarely, acute hemorrhage may occur in large pituitary tumors, manifested by rapid loss of vision, headache, and evidence of acute pituitary failure (pituitary apoplexy) requiring emergency decompression of the sella.

Treatment

Transsphenoidal removal of pituitary tumors will sometimes reverse hypopituitarism. Postoperative hyponatremia often occurs; serum sodium must be checked frequently for 2 weeks after pituitary surgery. Hypogonadism due to PRL excess usually resolves during treatment with dopamine agonists. Endocrine substitution therapy must be used before, during, and often permanently after such procedures.

GH-secreting tumors may respond to octreotide (see section on acromegaly). Radiation therapy with x-ray, gamma knife, or heavy particles may be necessary but increases the likelihood of hypopituitarism.

The mainstay of substitution therapy for pituitary insufficiency remains lifetime hormone replacement.

A. Corticosteroids

Hydrocortisone tablets, 15–30 mg/d orally in divided doses, should be given. Most patients do well with 15 mg in the morning and 5–10 mg in the late afternoon. Patients with partial ACTH deficiency (basal morning serum cortisol above 8 mg/dL [220 mmol/L]) require hydrocortisone replacement in lower doses of about 5 mg orally twice daily. Some patients feel better taking prednisone, 3–7.5 mg/d orally. A mineralocorticoid is rarely needed. To determine the optimal corticosteroid replacement dosage, it is necessary to monitor patients carefully for manifestations of overreplacement (Cushing's syndrome) or underreplacement. A serum white blood cell count (WBC) with a relative differential can be useful, since a relative neutrophilia and lymphopenia

can indicate overreplacement with corticosteroid, and vice versa. Additional corticosteroids must be given during states of stress, eg, during infection, trauma, or surgical procedures. For mild illness, corticosteroid doses are doubled or tripled. For trauma or surgical stress, hydrocortisone is given in doses of 50 mg intramuscularly or intravenously every 6 hours and then reduced to normal doses as the stress subsides. Patients with adrenal insufficiency are advised to wear a medical alert bracelet describing their condition and treatment.

Patients with secondary adrenal insufficiency due to treatment with corticosteroids at supraphysiologic doses require their usual daily dose of corticosteroid during surgery and acute illness; supplemental hydrocortisone is not usually required.

B. Thyroid

Levothyroxine is given to correct hypothyroidism only after the patient is assessed for cortisol deficiency or is already receiving corticosteroids. (See Hypothyroidism.) The typical maintenance dose is about 1.6 mcg/kg body weight. However, dosage requirements vary widely, averaging 0.125 mg daily with a range of 0.025–0.3 mg daily. The optimal replacement dose of thyroxine for each patient must be carefully assessed clinically on an individual basis. Serum FT_4 levels usually need to be in the high-normal range for adequate replacement. Assessment of serum TSH is useless for monitoring patients, since levels are always low with TSH deficiency.

C. Sex Hormones

Hypogonadotropic hypogonadism often develops in patients with hyperprolactinemia; it may be reversed with treatment of the hyperprolactinemia. (See Hyperprolactinemia.)

Androgen replacement is discussed in the section on male hypogonadism. Estrogen replacement is discussed in the section on female hypogonadism. Women with hypopituitarism and androgen deficiency may be treated with compounded dehydroepiandrosterone (DHEA) in doses of about 30 mg/d orally. DHEA therapy tends to increase pubic and axillary hair and improve libido, alertness, and stamina.

To improve spermatogenesis, hCG (equivalent to LH) may be given at a dosage of 2000–3000 units intramuscularly three times weekly and testosterone replacement is discontinued. The dose of hCG is adjusted to normalize serum testosterone levels. After 6–12 months of hCG treatment, if the sperm count remains low, hCG injections are continued along with injections of FSH: follitropin-β (synthetic recombinant FSH) or urofollitropins (urine-derived FSH). An alternative for patients with an intact pituitary (eg, Kallmann's syndrome) is the use of leuprolide (GnRH analog) by intermittent subcutaneous infusion. With either treatment, testicular volumes double within 5–12 months, and spermatogenesis occurs in most cases. With persistent treatment and the help of intracytoplasmic sperm injection for some cases, the total pregnancy success rate is about 70%. Clomiphene, 25–50 mg orally daily, can sometimes stimulate a man's own pituitary gonadotropins (when his pituitary is intact), thereby increasing testosterone and sperm production.

For fertility induction in females, ovulation may be induced with clomiphene, 50 mg daily for 5 days every 2 months. Follitropins and hCG can induce multiple births and should be used only by those experienced with their administration. (See Hypogonadism and Chapter 17.)

D. HUMAN GROWTH HORMONE (hGH)

Recombinant human growth hormone (rhGH) has been synthesized as a 191-amino acid sequence (somatropin) identical to hGH; an rhGH of 192 amino acids (somatrem) is also available and is of equal potency. Symptomatic adults with severe GH deficiency (serum IGF-I below 85 mcg/L) may be treated with a subcutaneous rhGH injection starting at a dosage of about 0.2 mg (0.6 IU)/day, administered three or four times weekly. The dosage of rhGH is increased every 2–4 weeks by increments of 0.1 mg (0.3 IU) until side effects occur or a sufficient salutary response and a normal serum IGF-I level are achieved. A sustained-release injectable suspension of GH has been developed (somatropin depot). It can be given once monthly and is therefore more convenient than standard rhGH preparations; however, its safety and dosing in adults remain to be established. If the desired effects (eg, improved energy and mentation, reduction in visceral adiposity) are not seen within 3–6 months at maximum tolerated dosage, rhGH therapy is discontinued.

During pregnancy, rhGH may be safely administered to women with hypopituitarism at their usual pregestational dose during the first trimester, tapering the dose during the second trimester, and discontinuing rhGH during the third trimester.

Oral estrogen replacement reduces hepatic IGF-I production. Therefore, prior to commencing rhGH therapy, oral estrogen is changed to a transdermal or transvaginal estradiol.

Side effects of rhGH therapy may include peripheral edema, hand stiffness, arthralgias, myalgias, headache, pseudotumor cerebri, gynecomastia, carpal tunnel syndrome, tarsal tunnel syndrome, hypertension, and proliferative retinopathy. Side effects are more common in older patients, those with greater weight and higher body mass index (BMI), and those with adult-onset GH deficiency. Such symptoms usually remit promptly after a sufficient reduction in dosage. Excessive doses of rhGH could cause acromegaly; patients receiving long-term therapy require careful clinical monitoring. Serum IGF-I levels should be kept in the normal range and periodic determinations of serum IGF-I levels are helpful in guiding therapeutic dosing.

GH should not be administered during critical illness since, in one study, administration of very high doses of rhGH to patients in an intensive care unit was shown to increase overall mortality. There is no role for GH replacement in the somatopause of aging.

E. OTHER TREATMENT

Selective transsphenoidal resection of pituitary adenomas can often restore normal pituitary function. Cabergoline, bromocriptine, or quinagolide may reverse the hypogonadism seen in hyperprolactinomas. (See Disorders of Prolactin Secretion.) Disseminated Langerhans cell histiocytosis may be treated with bisphosphonates to improve bone pain; treatment with 2-chlorodeoxyadenosine has been reported to produce complete remission.

Prognosis

The prognosis depends on the primary cause. Hypopituitarism resulting from a pituitary tumor may be reversible with dopamine agonists or with careful selective resection of the tumor. Spontaneous recovery from hypopituitarism associated with pituitary stalk thickening has been reported. Patients can also recover from functional hypopituitarism, eg, hypogonadism due to starvation or severe illness, suppression of ACTH by corticosteroids, or suppression of TSH by hyperthyroidism.

Functionally, most patients with hypopituitarism do very well with hormone replacement. Men with infertility who are treated with hCG/FSH or GnRH are likely to resume spermatogenesis if they have a history of sexual maturation, descended testicles, and a baseline serum inhibin level over 60 pg/mL. Women under age 40 years, with infertility due to hypogonadotropic hypogonadism, can usually have successful induction of ovulation.

Agha A et al: Conventional glucocorticoid replacement overtreats adult hypopituitary patients with partial ACTH deficiency. Clin Endocrinol (Oxf) 2004;60:688. [PMID: 15163331]

Böttner A et al: *PROP1* mutations cause progressive deterioration of anterior pituitary function including adrenal insufficiency: a longitudinal analysis. J Clin Endocrinol Metab 2004;89:5256. [PMID: 15472232]

Kreitschmann-Andermahr I et al: Prevalence of pituitary deficiency in patients after aneurysmal subarachnoid hemorrhage. J Clin Endocrinol Metab 2004;89:4986. [PMID: 15472195]

Leal-Cerro A et al: Prevalence of hypopituitarism and growth hormone deficiency in adults long-term after severe traumatic brain injury. Clin Endocrinol (Oxf) 2005;62:525. [PMID: 15853820]

Maison P et al: Impact of growth hormone (GH) treatment of cardiovascular risk factors in GH-deficient adults: a meta-analysis of blinded, randomized, placebo-controlled trials. J Clin Endocrinol Metab 2004;89:2192. [PMID: 15126541]

Smith JC: Hormone replacement therapy in hypopituitarism. Expert Opin Pharmacother 2004;5:1023. [PMID: 15155105]

Verrees M et al: Pituitary tumor apoplexy: characteristics, treatment, and outcomes. Neurosurg Focus 2004;16:E6. [PMID: 15191335]

POSTERIOR HYPOPITUITARISM

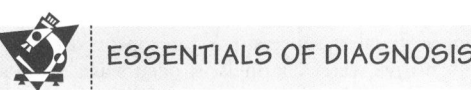

ESSENTIALS OF DIAGNOSIS

- *Antidiuretic hormone (ADH) deficiency causes central diabetes insipidus with polyuria (2–20 L/d)* and polydipsia; hypernatremia occurs if fluid intake is inadequate.

- Oxytocin deficiency causes lactation failure in postpartum women.

General Considerations

Diabetes insipidus is an uncommon disease characterized by an increase in thirst and the passage of large quantities of urine of low specific gravity (usually < 1.006 with ad libitum fluid intake). The urine is otherwise normal. It is caused by a deficiency of vasopressin or resistance to vasopressin.

Primary central diabetes insipidus (without an identifiable organic lesion noted on MRI of the pituitary and hypothalamus) accounts for about one-third of all cases. Many such cases appear to be due to autoimmunity against hypothalamic arginine vasopressin (AVP)-secreting cells; pituitary stalk thickening can often be detected on pituitary MRI scanning. The cause may also be genetic. Familial diabetes insipidus occurs as a dominant genetic trait with symptoms developing at about 2 years of age. Diabetes insipidus also occurs in Wolfram syndrome, a rare autosomal recessive disorder that is also known by the acronym DIDMOAD (diabetes insipidus, type 1 diabetes mellitus, optic atrophy, and deafness). DIDMOAD manifestations usually present in childhood but may not occur until adulthood, along with depression and cognitive problems. **Secondary central diabetes insipidus** is due to damage to the hypothalamus or pituitary stalk by tumor, hypophysitis, anoxic encephalopathy, surgical or accidental trauma, infection (eg, encephalitis, tuberculosis, syphilis), sarcoidosis, or multifocal Langerhans cell (eosinophilic) granulomatosis ("histiocytosis X"). Metastases to the pituitary are more likely to cause diabetes insipidus (33%) than are pituitary adenomas (1%).

Vasopressinase-induced diabetes insipidus may be seen in the last trimester of pregnancy and in the puerperium; it is often associated with oligohydramnios, preeclampsia, or hepatic dysfunction. A circulating enzyme destroys native vasopressin; however, synthetic desmopressin is unaffected. The condition usually responds to desmopressin therapy (see below) and subsides spontaneously.

Nephrogenic diabetes insipidus is a disorder caused by a defect in the kidney tubules that interferes with water reabsorption. The polyuria is unresponsive to vasopressin. These patients have normal secretion of vasopressin. Congenital nephrogenic diabetes insipidus is present from birth and is due to defective expression of renal vasopressin V2 receptors or vasopressin-sensitive water channels. It occurs as a familial X-linked trait; adults often have hyperuricemia as well.

Acquired forms of vasopressin-resistant diabetes insipidus are usually less severe and are seen in pyelo-nephritis, renal amyloidosis, myeloma, potassium depletion, Sjögren's syndrome, sickle cell anemia, or chronic hypercalcemia. The disorder may occur also as a corticosteroid effect or as an acute side effect of diuretics. Certain drugs (eg, demeclocycline, lithium, foscarnet, or methicillin) may induce nephrogenic diabetes insipidus. The recovery from acute tubular necrosis may also be associated with transient nephrogenic diabetes insipidus. (See Kidney Disorders.)

Clinical Findings

A. SYMPTOMS AND SIGNS

The symptoms of the disease are intense thirst, especially with a craving for ice water, and polyuria, the volume of ingested fluid varying from 2 L to 20 L daily, with correspondingly large urine volumes. Partial diabetes insipidus presents with less intense symptoms and should be suspected in patients with unremitting enuresis. Most patients with diabetes insipidus are able to maintain fluid balance by continuing to ingest large volumes of water. However, diabetes insipidus may present with hypernatremia and dehydration in patients without free access to water, or with a damaged hypothalamic thirst center and altered thirst sensation. Diabetes insipidus is aggravated by administration of high-dose corticosteroids, which increases renal free water clearance.

B. LABORATORY FINDINGS

The diagnosis of diabetes insipidus as a cause of polyuria or hypernatremia requires clinical judgment. There is no single diagnostic laboratory test. Evaluation for diabetes insipidus should include an accurate 24-hour urine collection that is measured for volume and creatinine. A urine volume of < 2 L/24 h (in the absence of hypernatremia) essentially rules out diabetes insipidus. Serum is assayed for glucose, urea nitrogen, calcium, potassium, sodium, and uric acid. Hyperuricemia occurs in many patients with diabetes insipidus, since reduced vasopressin stimulation of the renal V1 receptor causes a reduction in the renal tubular clearance of urate.

If the clinical situation implicates central diabetes insipidus (and no other causes for polyuria are present; see Differential Diagnosis, below), a supervised "vasopressin challenge test" may be given: Desmopressin acetate is given in an initial dose of 0.05–0.1 mL (5–10 mcg) intranasally (or 1 mcg subcutaneously or intravenously), with measurement of urine volume for 12 hours prior to and 12 hours after administration. Serum sodium must be obtained immediately in the event of symptoms of hyponatremia. The dosage of desmopressin is doubled if the response is marginal. Patients with central diabetes insipidus notice a distinct reduction in thirst and polyuria; serum sodium stays normal except in some salt-losing conditions.

In nonfamilial central diabetes insipidus, MRI of the pituitary and hypothalamus and of the skull is done to look for mass lesions. The pituitary stalk may be thickened, which may be a manifestation of Langerhans cell histiocytosis, sarcoidosis, or lymphocytic hypophysitis. Absence of a posterior pituitary "bright spot" on T1-weighted MRI is suggestive of central diabetes insipidus.

When nephrogenic diabetes insipidus is a diagnostic consideration, measurement of serum vasopressin is done during modest fluid restriction; typically, the vasopressin level is high.

Differential Diagnosis

Central diabetes insipidus must be distinguished from polyuria caused by diabetes mellitus, Cushing's syndrome or corticosteroid treatment, lithium, hypercalcemia, hypokalemia, and the nocturnal polyuria of Parkinson's disease. It must also be distinguished from nephrogenic diabetes insipidus (see above), the excessive fluid intake seen in psychogenic polydipsia, central nervous system sarcoidosis, and intravenous fluid administration.

Complications

If water is not readily available, the excessive output of urine will lead to severe dehydration. Patients with an impaired thirst mechanism are very prone to hypernatremia, particularly since they usually also have impaired mentation and forget to take their desmopressin. All the complications of the primary disease may eventually become evident. In patients who are receiving desmopressin acetate therapy, there is a danger of induced water intoxication.

Treatment

A. DIABETES INSIPIDUS

Desmopressin acetate is the treatment of choice for central diabetes insipidus. It is also useful in diabetes insipidus associated with pregnancy or the puerperium, since desmopressin is resistant to degradation by the circulating vasopressinase.

Desmopressin is available as an oral preparation (0.1 or 0.2 mg tablets) that is given in a starting dose of 0.05 mg twice daily and increased to a maximum of 0.4 mg every 8 hours, if required. Oral desmopressin is particularly useful for patients with sinusitis from the nasal preparation. Mild increases in hepatic enzymes can occur with the oral preparation. Gastrointestinal symptoms and asthenia may also occur.

The nasal preparation (100 mcg/mL solution) is given every 12–24 hours as needed for thirst and polyuria. It may be administered via metered-dose nasal inhaler containing 0.1 mL/spray or via a plastic calibrated tube. Patients are started with 0.05–0.1 mL every 12–24 hours, and the dose is then individualized according to response.

Desmopressin is also available as a parenteral preparation containing 4 mcg/mL. For central diabetes insipidus, it is given intravenously, intramuscularly, or subcutaneously in doses of 1–4 mcg every 12–24 hours as needed to treat thirst or hypernatremia.

Adverse reactions to desmopressin have included nasal irritation, occasional agitation, and erythromelalgia. Hyponatremia is uncommon if minimum effective doses are used and the patient allows thirst to occur periodically.

Mild cases of diabetes insipidus require no treatment other than adequate fluid intake. Reduction of aggravating factors (eg, corticosteroids, which directly increase renal free water clearance) will improve polyuria. Both central and nephrogenic diabetes insipidus respond partially to hydrochlorothiazide, 50–100 mg/d orally (with potassium supplement or amiloride). Nephrogenic diabetes insipidus may respond to combined treatments of indomethacin-hydrochlorothiazide, indomethacin-desmopressin, or indomethacin-amiloride. Indomethacin, 50 mg orally every 8 hours, is effective in acute cases.

Psychotherapy is required for most patients with compulsive water drinking. Thioridazine and lithium are best avoided if drug therapy is needed, since they cause polyuria.

B. OXYTOCIN DEFICIENCY

Women lacking oxytocin are unable to nurse their infants. Oxytocin induces the contraction of myoepithelial cells surrounding the mammary alveoli, which leads to the ejection of milk. Both oxytocin and milk removal are required for postpartum alveolar proliferation and successful lactation.

Nasal oxytocin (Syntocinon) is not available in the United States. It is used to promote milk let-down in normal postpartum women and with variable success in women with hypopituitarism. The dosage is one puff into each nostril in the sitting position 2–3 minutes before nursing.

Prognosis

Central diabetes insipidus appearing after pituitary surgery usually remits after days to weeks but may be permanent if the upper pituitary stalk is cut.

Chronic central diabetes insipidus is ordinarily more an inconvenience than a dire medical condition. Treatment with desmopressin allows normal sleep and activity. Hypernatremia can occur, especially when the thirst center is damaged, but diabetes insipidus does not otherwise reduce life expectancy, and the prognosis is that of the underlying disorder.

Oxytocin deficiency is a permanent condition. It does not affect life expectancy.

Smith CJA et al: Phenotype-genotype correlations in a series of Wolfram syndrome families. Diabetes Care 2004;27:2003. [PMID: 15277431]

Verbalis JG: Disorders of body water homeostasis. Best Pract Res Clin Endocrinol Metab 2003;17:471. [PMID: 14687585]

ACROMEGALY & GIGANTISM

ESSENTIALS OF DIAGNOSIS

- *Excessive growth of hands, feet, jaw, and internal organs; or gigantism before closure of epiphyses.*
- *Amenorrhea, headaches, visual field loss, weakness.*
- *Soft, doughy, sweaty handshake.*
- *Elevated IGF-I.*
- *Serum GH not suppressed following oral glucose.*

General Considerations

GH exerts much of its growth-promoting effects through the release of IGF-I produced in the liver and other tissues.

Acromegaly is nearly always caused by a pituitary adenoma. These tumors may be locally invasive, particularly into the cavernous sinus. Less than 1% are malignant. Most are macroadenomas (over 1 cm in diameter). Acromegaly is usually sporadic but may rarely be familial. The disease may be associated with endocrine tumors of the parathyroids or pancreas (MEN 1). Acromegaly may also be seen in McCune–Albright syndrome and as part of Carney's complex (atrial myxoma, acoustic neuroma, and spotty skin pigmentation). Acromegaly is rarely caused by ectopic growth hormone-releasing hormone (GHRH) or GH secreted by a lymphoma, hypothalamic tumor, bronchial carcinoid, or pancreatic tumor.

Clinical Findings

A. SYMPTOMS AND SIGNS

Excessive GH causes tall stature and gigantism if it occurs before closure of epiphyses. Afterward, acromegaly develops. The term "acromegaly," meaning extremity enlargement, seriously understates the manifestations. The hands enlarge and a doughy, moist handshake is characteristic. The fingers widen, causing patients to enlarge their rings. Carpal tunnel syndrome is common. The feet also grow, particularly in shoe width. Facial features coarsen since the bones and sinuses of the skull enlarge; hat size increases. The mandible becomes more prominent, causing prognathism and malocclusion. Tooth spacing widens.

Macroglossia occurs, as does hypertrophy of pharyngeal and laryngeal tissue; this causes a deep, coarse voice and sometimes makes intubation difficult. Obstructive sleep apnea may occur. A goiter may be noted. Hypertension (50%) and cardiomegaly are common. At diagnosis, about 10% of acromegalic patients have overt heart failure, with a dilated left ventricle and a reduced ejection fraction. Weight gain is typical, particularly of muscle and bone. Insulin resistance is usually present and frequently causes diabetes mellitus (30%). Arthralgias and degenerative arthritis occur. Overgrowth of vertebral bone can cause spinal stenosis. Colon polyps are common, especially in patients with skin papillomas. The skin may also manifest hyperhidrosis, thickening, cystic acne, and areas of acanthosis nigricans.

GH-secreting pituitary tumors usually cause some degree of hypogonadism, either by cosecretion of PRL or by direct pressure upon normal pituitary tissue. Decreased libido and impotence are common, as are irregular menses or amenorrhea. Secondary hypothyroidism sometimes occurs; hypoadrenalism is unusual. Headaches are frequent. Temporal hemianopia may occur as a result of the optic chiasm being impinged by a suprasellar growth of the tumor.

B. LABORATORY FINDINGS

The patient should be fasting for at least 8 hours (except for water), not acutely ill, and should not have exercised on the day of testing. A serum specimen is obtained and assayed for the following: IGF-I (increased to over five times normal in most acromegalics), PRL (cosecreted by many GH-secreting tumors), glucose (diabetes is common in acromegaly), liver enzymes and blood urea nitrogen (BUN) (hepatic or renal failure can misleadingly elevate GH), serum calcium (to screen for hyperparathyroidism), serum inorganic phosphorus (frequently elevated), serum free T_4, and TSH (secondary hypothyroidism is common in acromegaly; primary hypothyroidism may increase PRL, and hyperthyroidism may occur as a result of excess TSH).

Glucose syrup (75 g) is then administered orally, and serum GH is measured 60 minutes afterward; acromegaly is excluded if the serum GH is less than 1 ng/mL (immunoradiometric assay [IRMA] or chemiluminescent assays) or less than 2 ng/mL (older radioimmunoassays) after glucose syrup, and if the serum IGF-I is normal.

C. IMAGING

MRI shows a pituitary tumor in 90% of acromegalics. MRI is generally superior to CT scanning, especially in the postoperative setting. Radiographs of the skull may show an enlarged sella and thickened skull. Radiographs may also show tufting of the terminal phalanges of the fingers and toes. A lateral view of the foot shows increased thickness of the heel pad.

Differential Diagnosis

Active acromegaly must be distinguished from familial coarse features, large hands and feet, and isolated prognathism and from inactive ("burned-out") acromegaly in which there has been a spontaneous remission due to infarction of the pituitary adenoma. GH-induced gigantism must be differentiated from familial tall stature and from aromatase deficiency. (See Osteoporosis.)

Misleadingly high serum GH levels can be caused by exercise or eating just prior to the test; acute illness or agitation; hepatic or renal failure; malnourishment; diabetes mellitus; or concurrent treatment with estrogens, β-blockers, or clonidine.

Complications

Complications include hypopituitarism, hypertension, glucose intolerance or frank diabetes mellitus, cardiac enlargement, and cardiac failure. Carpal tunnel syndrome may cause thumb weakness and thenar atrophy. Arthritis of hips, knees, and spine can be troublesome. Cord compression may be seen. Visual field defects may be severe and progressive. Acute loss of vision or cranial nerve palsy may occur if the tumor undergoes spontaneous hemorrhage and necrosis (pituitary apoplexy). Patients with acromegaly are more likely to develop colon polyps.

Treatment

Endoscopic transnasal, transsphenoidal pituitary microsurgery removes the adenoma while preserving anterior pituitary function in most patients. Surgical remission is achieved in about 70% of patients followed over 3 years. GH levels fall immediately; diaphoresis and carpal tunnel syndrome often improve within a day after surgery. Transsphenoidal surgery is usually well tolerated, but complications occur in about 10% of patients, including infection, cerebrospinal fluid leak, and hypopituitarism. Hyponatremia can occur 4–13 days postoperatively and is manifested by nausea, vomiting, headache, malaise, or seizure. It is prudent to monitor serum sodium levels postoperatively. Dietary salt supplements for 2 weeks postoperatively may prevent this complication.

Patients who do not have a clinical or biochemical remission after surgery are treated with a dopamine agonist (eg, cabergoline), somatostatin analogs, pegvisomant, or a combination of these medications. **Cabergoline** may be used first, since it is an oral medication. Cabergoline therapy is most successful for tumors that secrete both PRL and GH, but can also be effective for patients with normal serum PRL levels. Therapy with cabergoline will shrink one-third of such tumors by more than 50%. The initial dose is 0.25 mg orally twice weekly, which is gradually increased to a maximum dosage of 1 mg twice weekly, if tolerated by the patient based upon serum GH and IGF-I levels. Side effects of cabergoline include nausea, fatigue, constipation, abdominal pain, and dizziness. Cabergoline is expensive.

Octreotide and **lanreotide** are somatostatin analogs that are given by subcutaneous injection. Short-acting octreotide acetate in doses of 50 mcg is injected three times daily. Responders who tolerate the drug are switched to long-acting octreotide acetate injectable suspension in a dosage of 20 mg intragluteally per month. The dosage may be adjusted—up to a maximum of 40 mg monthly—to maintain the serum GH between 1 and 2.5 ng/mL, keeping IGF-I levels normal. Lanreotide SR (not available in the United States) is given by subcutaneous injection at a dosage of 30 mg every 7–14 days. Lanreotide Autogel (not available in the United States) is a newer formulation that is administered by deep subcutaneous injection in doses of 60–120 mg every 28 days; this preparation is better tolerated than lanreotide SR. All somatostatin analogs are expensive and must be continued indefinitely or until other treatment has been effective. Octreotide long-acting release (LAR) preparations (Sandostatin LAR depot) are superior to shorter-acting octreotide, ultimately achieving serum GH levels under 2 ng/mL in 79% of patients and normal serum IGF-I levels in 53% of patients. Headaches often improve, and tumor shrinkage of about 30% may be expected. Acromegalic patients with pretreatment serum GH levels exceeding 20 ng/mL are less likely to respond to octreotide therapy. Side effects are experienced by about one-third of patients and include injection site pain, loose acholic stools, abdominal discomfort, or cholelithiasis.

Pegvisomant is a GH receptor antagonist that blocks the effects of GH. Pegvisomant therapy produces symptomatic relief and normalizes serum IGF-I levels in over 90% of acromegalic patients. The starting dosage is 10 mg subcutaneously daily. The maintenance dosage can be increased by 5–10 mg every 4–6 weeks, based on serum IGF-I levels and liver transaminase levels; the maximum dosage is 30 mg subcutaneously daily. Pegvisomant does not shrink GH-secreting tumors. Patients need to be monitored carefully with visual field examinations, GH levels, and MRI scanning of the pituitary. Side effects of pegvisomant can include injection site reactions, hepatitis, edema, flu-like syndrome, nausea, and hypertension. In acromegalic diabetics, hypoglycemic drugs are reduced to avoid hypoglycemia during pegvisomant therapy. The effectiveness of pegvisomant is reduced by coadministration of opioids or propoxyphene. Pegvisomant is extraordinarily expensive.

Acromegalic patients who have not had a complete remission with transsphenoidal surgery or medical therapy may be treated with **stereotactic radiosurgery** administered by gamma knife, heavy particle radiation, or adapted linear accelerator. Some medical centers are using pituitary gamma knife radiosurgery as the initial treatment with reported success rates of 20–90%. Radiosurgery precisely radiates the pituitary tumor in a single session and reduces radiation to the normal brain. However, it cannot be used for pituitary tumors with suprasellar extension due to the risk of damaging the optic chiasm. Radiosurgery can be used for pituitary tumors invading the cavernous sinus, since cranial nerves III, IV, V, and VI are less susceptible to radiation damage. Radiosurgery can also be used for patients who have not responded to conventional radiation therapy.

Prognosis

Patients with acromegaly have increased morbidity and mortality from cardiovascular disorders; those who are treated and have a glucose-suppressed serum GH level less than 2.5 ng/mL (radioimmunoassay) or under 1 ng/mL (immunofluorometric assay) and normal age-adjusted serum IGF-I levels have reduced morbidity and mortality. Patients with untreated or persistent acromegaly tend to have premature cardiovascular disease and progressive acromegalic symptoms. Transsphenoidal pituitary surgery is successful in 80–90% of patients with tumors less than 2 cm in diameter and GH levels less than 50 ng/mL. Extrasellar extension of the pituitary tumor, particularly cavernous sinus invasion, reduces the likelihood of surgical cure. Adjuvant medical therapy has been quite successful in treating patients who are not cured by pituitary surgery. Postoperatively, normal pituitary function is usually preserved. Soft tissue swelling regresses but bone enlargement is permanent. Hypertension frequently persists despite successful surgery. Conventional radiation therapy (alone) produces a remission in about 40% of patients by 2 years and 75% of patients by 5 years after treatment. Gamma knife or cyberknife radiosurgery reduces GH levels an average of 77%, with 20% of patients having a full remission after 12 months. Patients with pituitary adenomas that abut the optic chiasm can be treated with cyberknife radiosurgery, controlling tumor growth and preserving vision in most patients. Heavy particle pituitary radiation produces a remission in about 70% of patients by 2 years and 80% of patients by 5 years. Radiation therapy eventually produces some degree of hypopituitarism in most patients. Conventional radiation therapy may cause some degree of organic brain syndrome and predisposes to small strokes. Patients must receive lifelong follow-up, with regular monitoring of serum GH and IGF-I levels. Serum GH levels over 5 ng/mL and rising IGF-I levels usually indicate a recurrent tumor.

Hypopituitarism may occur, due to the tumor itself, pituitary surgery, or radiation therapy. Hypopituitarism may develop years following radiation therapy, so patients must have regular clinical monitoring of their pituitary function.

Castinetti F et al: Outcome of gamma knife radiosurgery in 82 patients with acromegaly: correlation with initial hypersecretion. J Clin Endocrinol Metab 2005;90:4483. [PMID: 15899958]

Cozzi R et al: Cabergoline addition to depot somatostatin analogues in resistant acromegalic patients: efficacy and lack of predictive value of prolactin status. Clin Endocrinol (Oxf) 2004;61:209. [PMID: 15272916]

Feenstra J et al: Combined therapy with somatostatin analogues and weekly pegvisomant in active acromegaly. Lancet 2005; 365:1644. [PMID: 15885297]

Ferone D et al: Current diagnostic guidelines for biochemical diagnosis of acromegaly. Minerva Endocrinol 2004;29: 207. [PMID: 15765030]

Serri O et al: Long-term biochemical status and disease-related morbidity in 53 postoperative patients with acromegaly. J Clin Endocrinol Metab 2004;89:658. [PMID: 14764777]

HYPERPROLACTINEMIA

 ESSENTIALS OF DIAGNOSIS

- Women: Menstrual cycle disturbances (oligomenorrhea, amenorrhea); galactorrhea; infertility.
- Men: Hypogonadism; decreased libido and erectile dysfunction; infertility.
- Elevated serum PRL.
- CT scan or MRI often demonstrates pituitary adenoma.

General Considerations

Elevated serum PRL can be caused by numerous conditions (Table 26–4). PRL-secreting pituitary tumors are more common in women than in men and are usually sporadic but may rarely be familial as part of MEN 1. Most are microadenomas (< 1 cm in diameter) that do not grow even with pregnancy or oral contraceptives. However, some giant prolactinomas can spread into the cavernous sinuses and suprasellar areas; rarely, they may erode the floor of the sella to invade the sinuses.

Clinical Findings

A. Symptoms and Signs

Hyperprolactinemia due to any cause may result in hypogonadotropic hypogonadism and reduced fertility. Men usually have erectile dysfunction and diminished libido; gynecomastia sometimes occurs, but rarely with galactorrhea. Women may note oligomenorrhea or amenorrhea, though some women continue to menstruate normally. Galactorrhea, defined as lactation in the absence of nursing, is common. Of women with secondary amenorrhea and galactorrhea, about 70% have hyperprolactinemia. Untreated hypogonadism ultimately increases the risk for developing osteoporosis.

Pituitary prolactinomas may cosecrete growth hormone and cause acromegaly (see above). Large tumors may cause headaches, visual symptoms, and pituitary insufficiency.

B. Laboratory Findings

Evaluate for conditions known to cause hyperprolactinemia, particularly pregnancy (serum hCG), hypothyroidism (serum FT_4 and TSH), renal failure (BUN and serum creatinine), cirrhosis (clinical evaluation and serum bilirubin and liver enzymes) and hyperparathyroidism (serum calcium). Men are evaluated for hypogonadism with determinations of serum total and free testosterone, LH, and FSH. Women who have amenorrhea are assessed for hypogonadism with determinations of serum

Table 26–4. Causes of hyperprolactinemia.

Physiologic Causes	Pharmacologic Causes	Pathologic Causes
Exercise	Amoxapine	Acromegaly
Idiopathic	Amphetamines	Chronic chest wall stimulation (postthora-
Macroprolactinemia ("big prolactin")	Anesthetic agents	cotomy, postmastectomy, herpes zos-
Pregnancy	Antipsychotics (conventional and	ter, breast problems, chest acupuncture,
Puerperium	atypical)	nipple rings, etc)
Sleep (REM phase)	Butyrophenones	Cirrhosis
Stress (trauma, surgery)	Cimetidine and ranitidine (not famoti-	Hypothalamic disease
Suckling	dine or nizatidine)	Hypothyroidism
	Estrogens	Multiple sclerosis
	Hydroxyzine	Optic neuromyelitis
	Methyldopa	Pituitary stalk section
	Metoclopramide	Prolactin-secreting tumors
	Opioids	Pseudocyesis (false pregnancy)
	Nicotine	Renal failure (especially with zinc deficiency)
	Phenothiazines	Spinal cord lesions
	Protease inhibitors	Systemic lupus erythematosus
	Progestins	
	Reserpine	
	Risperidone	
	Selective serotonin reuptake inhibitors	
	Tricyclic antidepressants	
	Verapamil	

estradiol, LH, and FSH. An assay for macroprolactinemia should be considered for patients with hyperprolactinemia who are relatively asymptomatic and have no apparent cause for hyperprolactinemia. Patients with pituitary macroadenomas (> 3 cm in diameter) should have PRL measured on serial dilutions of serum, since IRMA assays may otherwise report falsely low titers, the "high-dose hook effect." Patients with macroprolactinomas or manifestations of possible hypopituitarism should be evaluated for hypopituitarism as described above.

C. IMAGING

When hyperprolactinemia persists without obvious cause, MRI of the pituitary and hypothalamus is indicated. Small prolactinomas may thus be demonstrated, but clear differentiation from normal variants is not always possible.

Differential Diagnosis

The causes of hyperprolactinemia are shown in Table 26–4. Chronic nipple stimulation, nipple piercing, augmentation or reduction mammoplasty, and mastectomy may stimulate PRL secretion. The pituitary tumor of acromegaly can cosecrete GH and PRL. Hyperprolactinemia may also be idiopathic. Increased pituitary size is a normal variant in young women. About 10% of hyperprolactinemic patients are found to be secreting macroprolactin, a relatively inactive "big prolactin"; pituitary MRI is normal in 78% of cases.

The differential diagnosis for galactorrhea includes the small amount of breast milk that can be expressed from

the nipple in many parous women that is not cause for concern. Nipple stimulation from nipple rings, chest surgery, or acupuncture can cause galactorrhea; serum PRL levels may be normal or minimally elevated. Some women can have galactorrhea with normal serum PRL levels and no discernible cause (idiopathic). Normal breast milk may be various colors besides white. Bloody galactorrhea requires an evaluation for breast malignancy.

Treatment

Medications known to increase PRL should be stopped if possible. Hyperprolactinemia due to hypothyroidism is corrected by thyroxine. Patients with hyperprolactinemia not induced by drugs, hypothyroidism, or pregnancy should be examined by pituitary MRI.

Women with microprolactinomas who have amenorrhea or are desirous of contraception may safely take oral contraceptives or estrogen replacement—there is minimal risk of stimulating enlargement of the microadenoma. Patients with infertility and hyperprolactinemia may be treated with a dopamine agonist in an effort to improve fertility. Women who elect to receive no treatment have an increased risk of developing osteoporosis; such women require periodic bone densitometry.

Pituitary macroprolactinomas (> 10 mm in diameter) have a higher risk of progressive growth, particularly during treatment with estrogen or testosterone replacement therapy or during pregnancy. Therefore, patients with macroprolactinomas should not be treated with sex hormone replacement therapy unless they are in remission with dopamine agonist medication or surgery. Pregnant women with macroprolactinomas should continue to receive treatment with dopamine agonists throughout the pregnancy to prevent tumor growth.

A. DOPAMINE AGONISTS

Dopamine agonists are the initial treatment of choice for patients with giant prolactinomas and those with hyperprolactinemia desiring restoration of normal sexual function and fertility. Of the ergot-derived dopamine agonists, cabergoline is usually the best tolerated and is prescribed beginning with a dosage of 0.25 mg orally once weekly for 1 week, then 0.25 mg twice weekly for the next week, then 0.5 mg twice weekly. Further dosage increases may be required monthly, based on serum PRL levels, up to a maximum of 1.5 mg twice weekly. Higher doses of cabergoline, (≥ 2 mg daily, have been reported to cause mitral valve regurgitation. Alternative drugs include bromocriptine (1.25–20 mg/d orally) and pergolide (0.125–2 mg/d orally). Women who experience nausea with oral preparations may find relief with deep vaginal insertion of cabergoline or bromocriptine tablets; vaginal irritation sometimes occurs. Quinagolide (Norprolac; not available in the United States) is a non-ergot-derived dopamine agonist for patients intolerant or resistant to ergot-derived medications; the starting dosage is 0.075 mg/d orally, increasing as needed and tolerated to a maximum of 0.6 mg/d.

Dopamine agonists are given at bedtime to minimize side effects of fatigue, nausea, dizziness, and orthostatic hypotension. These symptoms usually improve with dosage reduction and continued use. Erythromelalgia is rare. Dopamine agonists can cause a variety of psychiatric side effects that are not dose related and may take weeks to resolve once the dopamine agonist is discontinued. Therefore, dopamine agonists should be used judiciously in psychiatric patients whose antipsychotic medications have caused hyperprolactinemia.

With dopamine agonist treatment, 90% of patients with prolactinomas experience a fall in serum PRL to 10% or less of pretreatment levels; about 80% of treated patients achieve a normal serum PRL level. Shrinkage of a pituitary adenoma occurs early, but the maximum effect may take up to a year. Nearly half of prolactinomas—even massive tumors—shrink more than 50%. Such shrinkage of giant prolactinomas can result in spinal fluid rhinorrhea. Discontinuing therapy after months or years usually results in the reappearance of hyperprolactinemia and galactorrhea-amenorrhea, but some patients with microadenomas remain in remission.

Because dopamine agonists usually restore fertility promptly, many pregnancies have resulted; no teratogenicity has been noted with any of the dopamine agonists. However, women with microadenomas may have treatment safely withdrawn during pregnancy. Macroadenomas may enlarge significantly during pregnancy; if therapy is withdrawn, such patients must be monitored clinically with serum PRL determinations and with computer-assisted visual field perimetry. Women with macroprolactinomas who have responded to dopamine agonists may safely receive oral contraceptive agents as long as they continue receiving therapy.

B. SURGICAL TREATMENT

For most patients with prolactinomas, therapy with dopamine agonists is overwhelmingly preferable to surgery, particularly for giant prolactinomas that distort surgical fields. Transsphenoidal pituitary surgery may be urgently required for large tumors undergoing apoplexy or those severely compromising visual fields. It is also used electively for patients who do not tolerate or respond to dopamine agonists. Craniotomy is rarely indicated, since even large tumors can usually be decompressed via the transsphenoidal approach.

C. RADIATION THERAPY

Radiation therapy is reserved for patients with macroadenomas that are growing despite treatment with dopamine agonists. A single gamma knife or cyberknife treatment is preferable for certain patients whose optic chiasm is clear of tumor, since it is generally safer and more convenient than conventional radiation therapy. Conventional radiation therapy must be given over 5 weeks and carries a high risk of eventual hypopituitarism. Other possible side effects include some degree of memory impairment and an increased long-term risk of second tumors and small vessel ischemic strokes. After radiation therapy, patients are advised to take low-dose aspirin to reduce their stroke risk.

Colao A et al: Outcome of cabergoline treatment in men with prolactinoma: effects of a 24-month treatment on prolactin levels, tumor mass, recovery of pituitary function, and semen analysis. J Clin Endocrinol Metab 2004;89:1704. [PMID: 15070934]

Delgrange E: Cabergoline and mitral regurgitation. N Engl J Med 2006;354:420. [PMID: 16436779]

Gibney J et al: The impact on clinical practice of routine screening for macroprolactin. J Clin Endocrinol Metab 2005;90: 3927. [PMID: 15811931]

Haddad PM et al: Antipsychotic-induced hyperprolactinaemia: mechanisms, clinical features and management. Drugs 2004; 64:2291. [PMID: 15456328]

Molitch ME: Medication-induced hyperprolactinemia. Mayo Clin Proc 2005;80:1050. [PMID: 16092584]

Sodi R et al: Testosterone replacement-induced hyperprolactinaemia: case report and review of the literature. Ann Clin Biochem 2005;42(Pt 2):153. [PMID: 15829128]

■ DISEASES OF THE THYROID GLAND

TESTS OF THYROID FUNCTION (Table 26–5)

The thyroid tests discussed in this section are ordinarily very helpful in the evaluation of thyroid disor-

Table 26–5. Appropriate use of thyroid tests.

	Test	Comment
Screening	Serum thyroid-stimulating hormone (TSH) (sensitive assay)	Most sensitive test for primary hypothyroidism and hyperthyroidism
	Free thyroxine (FT$_4$)	Excellent test
For hypothyroidism	Serum TSH	High in primary and low in secondary hypothyroidism
	Antithyroglobulin and antithyroperoxidase antibodies	Elevated in Hashimoto's thyroiditis
For hyperthyroidism	Serum TSH (sensitive assay)	Suppressed except in TSH-secreting pituitary tumor or pituitary hyperplasia (rare)
	Triiodothyronine (T$_3$) (radioiodine)	Elevated
	^{123}I uptake and scan	Increased uptake; diffuse versus "hot" areas on scan
	Antithyroglobulin and antimicrosomal antibodies	Elevated in Graves' disease
	Thyroid-stimulating immunoglobulin (TSI); TSH receptor antibody (TSH-R Ab [stim])	Usually (65%) positive in Graves' disease
For nodules	Fine-needle aspiration biopsy (FNAB)	Best diagnostic method for thyroid cancer
	^{123}I uptake and scan	Cancer is usually "cold"; less reliable than FNA[1] biopsy
	^{99m}Tc scan	Vascular versus avascular
	Ultrasonography	Useful to assist FNA[1] biopsy. Useful in assessing the risk of malignancy (multinodular goiter or pure cysts are less likely to be malignant). Useful to monitor nodules and patients after thyroid surgery for carcinoma.

[1]Fine-needle aspiration.

ders. However, many conditions and drugs alter serum T$_4$ levels without affecting clinical status (Table 26–6).

The tests most widely used in clinical practice are serum immunoassays for TSH and FT$_4$. Assays for FT$_4$ have largely supplanted measurements of total T$_4$, resin T$_3$ uptake (RT$_3$U), and free thyroxine index (FT$_4$I).

1. Serum Thyroid Tests

TSH Immunoassay

There is considerable debate about what constitutes a normal range for serum TSH levels. The normal range for ultrasensitive TSH levels is generally stated to be 0.4–5.5 mU/L. However, over 95% of normal individuals have serum TSH concentrations under 3.0 mU/L. There is a high risk of finding antithyroid antibodies in patients with serum TSH in the upper range of normal (3.0–5.5 mU/L), but most such patients are asymptomatic. The serum TSH level varies during the day, usually within the normal range, being higher in the early morning and after strenuous exercise, sleep deprivation, or working night shifts.

TSH levels as low as 0.01 mU/L can be detected by ultrasensitive "third-generation" assays. To diagnose hyperthyroidism, an assay sensitive to at least 0.1 mU/

L (sensitive "second-generation" assay) should be used. Because of discrepancies between different TSH assay methods, it is prudent to recheck unexpected results with a different assay.

TSH levels are **decreased** in patients with primary hyperthyroidism (eg, Graves' disease, toxic multinodular goiter, toxic nodule, subacute thyroiditis, or release of stored hormone in Hashimoto's thyroiditis). They may also be suppressed in some clinically euthyroid individuals with autonomous thyroid secretion (eg, euthyroid Graves' ophthalmopathy). TSH can also be suppressed by metformin and by thyroid hormone administration in either excessive or adequate replacement amounts. TSH is also frequently low during severe nonthyroidal illness; distinction from hypopituitarism can usually be made clinically.

Dopamine and dopamine agonists (levodopa, bromocriptine) can cause suppression of TSH and may cause true secondary hypothyroidism during prolonged administration. Other conditions associated with decreased TSH include pregnancy (especially with morning sickness), hCG-secreting trophoblastic tumors, acute psychiatric illness (1% incidence), and urgent administration of corticosteroids. Certain drugs cause mild suppression of TSH without clinical hyperthyroidism; these include nonsteroidal anti-inflamma-

Table 26–6. Factors causing misleading serum thyroxine (T_4) measurements without affecting clinical status.[1]

Factors Increasing T_4	Factors Decreasing T_4
Laboratory error	Laboratory error
AIDS (increased thyroid-binding globulin)	Severe illness (eg, chronic renal failure, major surgery, caloric deprivation)
Autoimmunity	Acute psychiatric problems
Acute illness (eg, viral hepatitis, chronic active hep- atitis; primary biliary cirrhosis; acute intermittent porphyria; AIDS)	Cirrhosis
	Nephrotic syndrome
	Hereditary thyroid-binding globulin deficiency
High-estrogen states (may also increase total T_3)	Drugs
Oral estrogen-containing contraceptives	Androgens
Pregnancy	Asparaginase
Estrogen replacement therapy	Carbamazepine
Tamoxifen	Chloral hydrate
Acute psychiatric problems	Fenclofenac
Hyperemesis gravidarum and morning sickness	Fluorouracil
(may also increase T_3)	Corticosteroids
Familial thyroid-binding abnormalities	Halofenate (lowers triglycerides and uric acid; not marketed in the United States)
Generalized resistance to thyroid hormone	Mitotane
Drugs	Nicotinic acid
Amiodarone	Oxcarbazepine
Amphetamines	Phenobarbital
Clofibrate	Phenylbutazone
Heparin (dialysis method)	Phenytoin (T_4 may be as low as 2 mcg/dL)
Heroin	Salicylates (large doses)
Levothyroxine (T_4) replacement therapy	Sertraline
Methadone (may also increase T_3)	Triiodothyronine (T_3) therapy
Perphenazine	

[1]Symptomatic hyperthyroidism or hypothyroidism may also be present incidentally.

tory drugs, amphetamine, octreotide, opioids, and certain calcium channel blockers (especially nifedipine; also verapamil, but not diltiazem).

In clinically euthyroid persons age 60 years or older, the TSH is very low (≤ 0.1 mU/L) in 3% and mildly low (0.1–0.4 mU/L) in 9%. The chance of developing atrial fibrillation is higher with very low TSH (2.8% yearly) than with normal TSH (1.1% yearly). Asymptomatic patients with very low TSH are followed closely but not treated unless atrial fibrillation or other manifestations of hyperthyroidism develop.

TSH levels are **elevated** in primary hypothyroidism, either clinical or subclinical. They may also be elevated or inappropriately normal in the very rare cases of hyperthyroidism due to pituitary neoplastic or nonneoplastic inappropriate secretion of thyrotropin. Autoimmune disease may also falsely elevate serum TSH levels by interfering with the assay. Assay interference can cause spuriously high serum TSH levels in patients with heterophile antibodies or anti-mouse antibodies. TSH may be elevated after strenuous exercise or in the morning after sleep deprivation. TSH may be transiently elevated during recovery from nonthyroidal illness and in about 14% of patients with acute psychiatric admissions; the TSH re-turns to normal in the great majority of these patients. TSH may be mildly elevated in some individuals, especially elderly women (10% incidence). Such patients with normal T_4 levels must be carefully evaluated for subtle signs of hypothyroidism (eg, fatigue, depression, hyperlipidemia). About 18% later become definitely hypothyroid.

Free Thyroxine Immunoassay

FT_4 is a direct measurement of the serum concentration of free (unbound) T_4. FT_4 represents only about 0.025% of the serum concentration of the total T_4. It is the only metabolically active fraction of T_4 that freely enters cells to produce its effects.

When performed properly, this assay is superior to the total T_4 assay and FT_4I, since it is not affected by variations in protein binding. It is the procedure of choice for following the thyroid's changing secretion of T_4 during treatment for hyperthyroidism. Serum FT_4 levels may be suppressed in patients with severe nonthyroid illness. In patients receiving heparin, measured levels of FT_4 may be falsely high, particularly when a dialysis assay is used. Serum FT_4 levels rise transiently in acute nonthyroidal illness, when thyroid-binding protein frequently falls.

Thyroxine Immunoassay

This test measures the total serum concentration of T_4 (bound and free). An increased serum T_4 confirms a clinical diagnosis of hyperthyroidism, while a decreased serum T_4 confirms a clinical diagnosis of hypothyroidism. It is affected by altered states of T_4 binding (see Table 26–6). Therefore, this test is usually run with a resin T_3 uptake to provide an FT_4I (see below).

Resin T_3 (or T_4) Uptake (RT$_3$U or RT$_4$U)

This is an indirect inverse test of serum thyroid-binding proteins (TBPs)—ie, it is high when TBPs are low. The assay involves adding labeled T_3 or T_4 to the serum sample; it competes with the patient's T_4 for binding to TBP. This mixture is then added to a thyroid hormone-binding resin. The resin is then assayed for its uptake of the label. A high resin uptake indicates that the patient's serum contains relatively low amounts of TBP or high levels of T_4.

This test corrects a total serum T_4 measurement for the effect of increased or decreased binding, creating a free T_4 index (see below). A low resin uptake (high TBP) is seen with estrogen therapy, pregnancy, acute hepatitis, genetic TBP increase, and hypothyroidism. A low resin uptake with low TBP may be seen in severe illness. A high resin uptake (low TBP) is seen with hyperthyroidism and with chronic liver disease, nephrotic syndrome, anabolic steroid administration, and high-dose corticosteroid administration.

Free Thyroxine Index

The product of T_4 and resin T_3 uptake ($T_4 \times T_3$ uptake) helps correct for abnormalities of T_4 binding. A good FT_4 assay is more accurate.

The FT_4I, when calculated using the RT_3U, may be elevated in euthyroid patients with familial dysalbuminemic hyperthyroxinemia. This is a benign autosomal dominant trait in which an abnormal albumin molecule binds T_4 with much greater affinity than T_3. The RT_3U is not decreased (failing to compensate for the increased binding, as it would for thyroxine binding globulin [TBG] excess), because the T_3 used in the RT_3U assay is not significantly affected. Serum levels of FT_4 and TSH are normal.

Total Triiodothyronine

This test is of value in the diagnosis of thyrotoxicosis with normal T_4 values (T_3 thyrotoxicosis). Determination of serum total triiodothyronine (TT_3) can also be useful, along with serum TSH, to screen for excessive thyroxine replacement. TT_3 levels are not useful for the diagnosis of hypothyroidism. Serum TT_3 levels can be misleadingly elevated in women who are pregnant or who take oral estrogen, due to the high serum levels of TBG in these conditions. **Note:** When blood is collected in tubes using a gel barrier, certain immunoassays (eg, Immulite but not Axsym analyzers) report serum TT_3 levels that are falsely elevated in 24% of normal patients.

Free Triiodothyronine

Free triiodothyronine (FT_3) measures the very tiny amount of T_3 that circulates unbound. It is useful in looking for hyperthyroidism or thyroxine overreplacement in women who are pregnant or taking oral estrogen.

2. Thyroid Radioactive Iodine Uptake & Scan

Radioiodine (^{123}I or ^{131}I) Uptake of Thyroid Gland

A. ELEVATED

Graves' disease, dietary iodine deficiency, toxic nodular goiter, pregnancy, early Hashimoto's thyroiditis, some thyroid enzyme deficiencies, nephrotic syndrome, recovery from subacute thyroiditis, and recovery from thyroid hormone suppression.

B. LOW

Administration of iodides or iodine in any form (drugs, radiology contrast dyes, etc), antithyroid drugs, subacute thyroiditis, thyroid hormone administration, thyroid gland damage (from thyroiditis, surgery, or radioiodine), hypopituitarism, ectopic functioning thyroid tissue, azotemia, severe (high-turnover) Graves' disease, heart failure, and some thyroid enzyme abnormalities.

Radioiodine Scans

A rectilinear scan over the neck may be obtained after radioiodine administration, thereby obtaining a life-sized picture of thyroid uptake. Radioactive iodine (RAI) scans are useful also for detecting metastatic thyroid cancer. (See Thyroid Cancer.) Following administration of a treatment dose of ^{131}I for thyroid cancer, a whole-body scan is useful for detecting metastases.

3. Other Thyroid Tests

Thyroid Antibodies

Antibodies against several thyroid constituents (thyroglobulin and thyroperoxidase) are most commonly found in Hashimoto's thyroiditis and Graves' disease. Antithyroid antibodies are found in about 5–10% of normal subjects. There is an increasing incidence with age. About 20% of hospitalized patients have detectable antithyroid antibodies. In the latter, the titers tend to be low, and they increase with age. Thyroid-stimulating antibody (TSAb, TSH-R Ab[stim]) serum titers are elevated in approximately 80% of patients with Graves' disease and in about 14% of patients with Hashitoxicosis. These titers—and those of antithyroglobulin and antithyroperoxidase antibodies—often decrease during pregnancy and during treatment of Graves' disease with antithyroid drugs. TSAb titers have been used with variable results to predict the rate of relapse of Graves' disease after long-term thiourea therapy.

Serum Thyroglobulin

The level of serum thyroglobulin rises in autoimmune thyroid disease, thyroid injury or inflammation, and thyroid cancer. Levels are of little value in diagnosing or distinguishing among these conditions, but they provide a useful marker in thyroid cancer to indicate recurrence of disease and the need for further studies and therapy. (See Thyroid Cancer.) Serum thyroglobulin is to be distinguished from serum TBG (see above).

Calcitonin Assay

This test is elevated in medullary thyroid carcinoma, azotemia, hypercalcemia, pernicious anemia, thyroiditis, and pregnancy. High levels are also seen in many other malignancies such as carcinomas of the lung (45%), pancreas, breast (38%), and colon (24%).

Fine-Needle Thyroid Biopsy

Aspiration of thyroid tissue with a fine needle (25 gauge) is helpful in the diagnosis of thyroid disorders, especially nodular lesions. This technique has become the preferred approach to the diagnosis of thyroid masses. (See Nodular Thyroid.)

4. Effect of Nonthyroidal Illness & Drugs on Thyroid Function Tests

Many factors affect thyroid function tests, causing misleading laboratory evidence of hypothyroidism or hyperthyroidism in patients who are clinically euthyroid. (See Table 26–6.)

Serum T_4 is frequently low in patients with severe illness, caloric deprivation, or major surgery who have accelerated peripheral metabolism of serum T_4 to reverse T_3 (rT_3). Furthermore, in most patients who are critically ill, there is a circulating inhibitor of thyroid hormone binding to serum TBPs. This causes the RT_3U to be misleadingly low, causing the computed FT_4I to be very low. The presence of a very low serum T_4 in severe nonthyroidal illness indicates a poor prognosis.

Direct assays of FT_4 often show low levels of FT_4 in severe illness. Because studies of giving replacement T_4 to such patients have shown no improvement in survival, they are considered "euthyroid." Serum TSH tends to be suppressed in severe nonthyroidal illness, making the diagnosis of concurrent primary hypothyroidism quite difficult, although the presence of a goiter suggests the diagnosis.

The clinician must decide whether such severely ill patients (with a low serum T_4 but nonelevated TSH) might have hypothyroidism due to pituitary insufficiency. Patients without symptoms of prior brain le-

sion or hypopituitarism are very unlikely to suddenly develop hypopituitarism during an unrelated illness. Patients with diabetes insipidus, hypopituitarism, or other signs of a central nervous system lesion may have T_4 given empirically. Patients receiving prolonged dopamine infusions may develop true secondary hypothyroidism due to direct dopamine suppression of TSH-secreting cells.

Certain antiseizure medications cause low serum FT_4 levels by accelerating hepatic conversion of T_4 to T_3; serum TSH levels are normal.

Ando T et al: Thyrotropin receptor antibodies: new insights into their actions and clinical relevance. Best Pract Res Clin Endocrinol Metab 2005;19:33. [PMID: 15826921]

Bowen RA et al: Effect of blood collection tubes on total triiodothyronine and other laboratory assays. Clin Chem 2005;51:424. [PMID: 15576427]

Helfand M; U.S. Preventive Services Task Force: Screening for subclinical thyroid dysfunction in nonpregnant adults: a summary of the evidence for the U.S. Preventive Services Task Force. Ann Intern Med 2004;140:128. [PMID: 14734337]

THYROID NODULES & MULTINODULAR GOITER

 ESSENTIALS OF DIAGNOSIS

- Single or multiple thyroid nodules are commonly found with careful thyroid examinations.
- Thyroid function tests mandatory.
- Thyroid biopsy for single or dominant nodules or for a history of prior head–neck or chest–shoulder radiation.
- Ultrasound examination useful for biopsy and follow-up.
- Clinical follow-up required.

General Considerations

Palpable enlargement of the thyroid (goiter) may be diffuse or nodular and is detectable in 4% of North American adults. The incidence of goiter is higher in iodine-deficient geographic areas (see Endemic Goiter, below). The presence of a goiter warrants further testing and follow-up. Most patients with goiter are euthyroid, but there is a high incidence of hypothyroidism or hyperthyroidism. Diffuse and multinodular goiters are ordinarily benign and may be caused by numerous conditions, eg, benign multinodular goiter, iodine deficiency, pregnancy (in areas of iodine deficiency), Graves' disease, Hashimoto's thyroiditis, subacute thyroiditis, or infections. A solitary thyroid nodule is most often a benign adenoma, colloid nodule, or cyst but may sometimes be a primary thyroid malignancy or (less frequently) a metastatic neoplasm. The risk of a palpable nodule being malignant is higher among patients with a history of head–neck radiation, a family history of thyroid cancer, or a personal history of another malignancy. The risk of malignancy is higher if a thyroid nodule is large, adherent to the trachea or strap muscles, or associated with lymphadenopathy.

Thyroid nodules are often discovered incidentally during radiologic procedures performed for other reasons. Nonpalpable thyroid nodules < 1 cm in diameter are benign in 98.4% of cases. Nodules that are palpable or ≥ 1 cm in diameter have a higher chance of being malignant. In patients with Hashimoto's thyroiditis, a palpable solitary thyroid nodule of ≥ 1 cm diameter has about an 8% chance of being malignant.

Clinical Findings (Table 26–7)

A. SYMPTOMS AND SIGNS

The thyroid is best examined in a well-lighted room. The seated patient is given water to drink and the anterior neck is observed during swallowing. The thyroid moves upward during swallowing and may be visible in a thin neck; enlargement or asymmetry of the thyroid may be noted. Palpation of the thyroid is best done from behind a seated patient using the second and third fingers of both hands. As the patient swallows water, thyroid nodules may be perceived moving beneath the fingers. The location of any nodules should be noted, along with their size, firmness, and tenderness. The neck should be examined for lymphadenopathy. An enlarged thyroid should be auscultated for bruits.

Most small thyroid nodules are asymptomatic and are discovered incidentally on routine neck inspection or palpation; some are discovered as an incidental finding during radiologic imaging of the neck. Graves' disease, toxic multinodular goiter, hyperfunctioning nodules, and subacute thyroiditis can cause hyperthyroidism. Hashimoto's thyroiditis may cause goiter and hypothyroidism.

A thyroid nodule or multinodular goiter can grow to become visible and of concern to the patient. Particularly large nodular goiters can become a cosmetic embarrassment. Nodules can grow large enough to cause discomfort, hoarseness, or dysphagia. Retrosternal large multinodular goiters can cause dyspnea due to tracheal compression. Large substernal goiters may cause superior vena cava syndrome, manifested by facial erythema and jugular vein distention that progress to cyanosis and facial edema when both arms are kept raised over the head (Pemberton's sign).

B. LABORATORY FINDINGS

Thyroid nodules are an indication for thyroid function testing. Serum determinations for TSH (sensitive assay) and FT_4 are preferred. Tests for antithyroperoxidase antibodies and antithyroglobulin antibodies may also be helpful. Very high antibody levels are found in Hashimoto's thyroiditis. However, thyroiditis frequently coexists with malignancy, so suspicious nodules should always be biopsied.

Fine-needle aspiration (FNA) biopsy is the best way to assess a nodule for malignancy. A 25-gauge needle is used to biopsy suspicious nodules. The needle is attached to a syringe and special syringe holder. The bi-

Table 26–7. Clinical evaluation of thyroid nodules.[1]

Clinical Evidence	Low Index of Suspicion	High Index of Suspicion
History	Family history of goiter; residence in area of endemic goiter	Previous therapeutic radiation of head, neck, or chest; hoarseness
Physical characteristics	Older women; soft nodule; multinodular goiter	Young adults, men; solitary, firm nodule; vocal cord paralysis; enlarged lymph nodes; distant metastatic lesions
Serum factors	High titer of antithyroid antibody; hypothyroidism; hyperthyroidism	
Fine-needle aspiration biopsy	Colloid nodule or adenoma	Papillary carcinoma, follicular neoplasm, medullary or anaplastic carcinoma
Scanning techniques		
Uptake of [123]I	"Hot" nodule	"Cold" nodule
Ultrasonogram	Cystic lesion	Solid lesion
Roentgenogram	Shell-like calcification	Punctate calcification
Thyroxine therapy	Regression after 0.05–0.1 mg/d for 6 months or more	Increase in size

[1]Clinically suspicious nodules should be evaluated with fine-needle aspiration biopsy.

opsy is done without local anesthesia. The success rate of FNA biopsy is increased by ultrasound guidance. Care must be taken to avoid bloody dilution of the specimens. Material obtained is placed on a slide and a thin smear is obtained by laying a second slide over the material and then drawing the slides apart. One slide is air dried while the other is preserved in 95% alcohol. Two or more biopsies may be obtained. Reading by an experienced cytopathologist is mandatory.

In one review of thyroid FNA biopsies, about 70% were benign, 5% malignant, 15% nondiagnostic, and 10% indeterminate or "suspicious." With indeterminate "suspicious" FNA cytology, the risk of malignancy has been reported to be 15% for follicular neoplasms, 20% for Hurthle cell neoplasms, and 82% for papillary carcinoma. The risk of a nodule (with indeterminate FNA cytology) being malignant is even higher in young patients and those with nodules that are fixed or over 2 cm in diameter. Therefore, most patients with indeterminate FNA cytology undergo thyroid surgery. However, a subgroup of elderly patients with "suspicious" cytology (nodules < 4 cm in diameter) has a malignancy rate of just 5%; such patients may elect to be monitored every 4–6 months with palpation and ultrasound.

Cystic nodules yielding serous fluid are usually benign, but fluid should be submitted for cytologic testing. Cystic nodules yielding bloody fluid have a higher chance of being malignant. Repeat FNA biopsy is done if the cytology is nondiagnostic (eg, diluted with blood or hypocellular) and the lesion remains palpable.

False-positive thyroid FNA biopsies occur at a rate of about 4%. False-negative thyroid FNA biopsies also occur at an overall rate of about 4%, less commonly when performed under ultrasound and interpreted by cytopathologists at major university centers. False-negative thyroid FNAs delay surgical excision and lead to an increased risk of vascular and capsular invasion by the malignancy. Patients who have a negative thyroid FNA should have observational follow-up, ideally with both palpation and ultrasound; nodules that continue to grow should be rebiopsied or excised.

C. IMAGING

Neck ultrasound should be performed on most patients with thyroid nodules, since it frequently adds important information. Ultrasound is more accurate than palpation in measuring the size of a nodule and can help determine whether a palpable nodule is part of a multinodular goiter, thus having less chance of being malignant. Ultrasound is also helpful in evaluating thyroid nodules. The following ultrasound characteristics of thyroid nodules increase the likelihood of malignancy: irregular margins, intranodular vascular spots, or microcalcifications. FNA biopsy is performed on such nodules—even if they are nonpalpable—if they are over 8 mm in diameter. Ultrasound-guided FNA biopsy is helpful in obtaining representative and adequate specimens, especially from complex thyroid nodules. Ultrasonography is generally preferred over CT and MRI because of its accuracy, ease of use, and lower cost.

RAI (^{123}I or ^{131}I) scans have limited utility in the evaluation of thyroid nodules. Hypofunctioning (cold) nodules have a somewhat increased risk of being malignant, but most are benign. Hyperfunctioning (hot) nodules are ordinarily benign but may sometimes be malignant. RAI scanning and uptake are helpful if a patient is found to have evidence of hyperthyroidism. (See Hyperthyroidism, below.)

Treatment

All thyroid nodules, including those with benign cytology, need to be followed by regular periodic palpation and rebiopsied if growth occurs. Thyroid ultrasound is useful for following nodules that are difficult to palpate. Patients with elevated levels of serum TSH are treated with T_4 replacement. Otherwise, for small nodules, T_4 is not required. For larger nodules (> 2 cm), if TSH levels are elevated or normal, "suppression" with levothyroxine sodium (0.05–0.1 mg daily) can be considered. Levothyroxine should not be administered if the baseline TSH is low, since that is an indication of autonomous thyroid secretion, such that levothyroxine treatment will be ineffective and liable to cause clinical thyrotoxicosis. Long-term levothyroxine suppression of TSH tends to keep nodules from enlarging, but only a few will actually shrink. Additional nodules develop in fewer treated patients. Suppressive levothyroxine therapy is most suitable for younger patients. All patients require regular careful clinical evaluation and thyroid palpation or ultrasound examinations. Levothyroxine suppression therapy should usually not be given to patients with cardiovascular problems since it may increase the risk for angina and arrhythmia. Levothyroxine suppression causes a small loss of bone density in many postmenopausal women. Bisphosphonate or other therapy for osteoporosis may be indicated. Patients at risk for osteoporosis are advised to have periodic bone density testing.

A. SOLITARY THYROID NODULES

Palpable solitary thyroid nodules call for FNA biopsy. A solitary thyroid nodule in a patient with a remote history of radiation therapy to the head or neck (or exposure to nuclear fallout) is considered at high risk for malignancy and the nodule is resected. Cystic nodules can be managed by removal of fluid for cytologic examination, which may deflate the cyst. However, cysts tend to recur, requiring repeated aspirations. Solitary nodules in a patient with hyperthyroidism are an indication for RAI scan, which generally distinguishes toxic adenoma from Graves' disease. However, Graves' disease may occasionally be unilateral owing to agenesis of the contralateral lobe, so additional studies with antithyroid antibodies may be helpful. A "hot" nodule is usually benign but is resected to cure the hyperthyroidism.

B. MULTINODULAR GOITERS

A thyroid containing multiple nodules is likely to be a benign multinodular goiter. Nevertheless, FNA biopsy is performed on any nodule that is growing or is particularly dominant or hard. Large retrosternal goiters rarely harbor a malignancy but can be followed by CT scan or MRI. Continued growth or compressive symptoms are reasons for surgical excision. Patients found to be hyperthyroid may have a radioactive iodine scan and uptake for additional evaluation, especially if ^{131}I is a therapeutic consideration.

C. NONPALPABLE THYROID NODULES

Nonpalpable small thyroid nodules are incidentally discovered in about 25–50% of scans of the neck (MRI, CT, ultrasound) done for other reasons. Such nodules are sometimes referred to as "thyroid incidentalomas." In one series, only 2% of such thyroids were found to have a significant malignancy after surgical resection. However, other series have found a higher risk of malignancy in nonpalpable thyroid nodules. Therefore, ultrasound-guided FNA biopsy should be considered for nonpalpable thyroid nodules 1.5 cm in diameter. For nodules < 1.5 cm diameter, ultrasound-guided FNA biopsy should be considered for patients with a history of head–neck irradiation or a family history of thyroid cancer. Smaller thyroid nodules with a suspicious appearance on ultrasound (calcified, solitary, or irregular) should also be considered for ultrasound-guided FNA biopsy. For incidentally discovered thyroid nodules of borderline concern, follow-up thyroid ultrasound in 3–4 months may be helpful; growing lesions may be biopsied or resected.

Microscopic "micropapillary" carcinoma is a variant of normal, being found in 24% of thyroidectomies performed for benign thyroid disease when 2-mm sections were carefully examined. It thus appears that the overwhelming majority of these microscopic foci never become clinically significant. The surgical pathology report of such a tiny papillary carcinoma that is otherwise benign does not justify aggressive follow-up or treatment because a cancer diagnosis is unwarranted and harmful. All that may be required is yearly follow-up with palpation of the neck and mild TSH suppression by thyroxine.

Prognosis

The great majority of thyroid nodules are benign. Benign thyroid nodules may involute but usually persist or grow slowly. About 89% of thyroid nodules will increase their volume by ≥ 15% over 5 years; cystic nodules are less likely to grow. Cytologically benign nodules that grow are unlikely to be malignant; in one series, only 1 of 78 rebiopsied nodules was found to be malignant. The prognosis for patients with thyroid nodules that prove to be malignant is determined by the histologic type and other factors (see below). Overall, differentiated thyroid carcinoma has an excellent prognosis, but metastases do occur. Multinodular goiters tend to persist or grow slowly, even in iodine-deficient areas where iodine repletion usually does not shrink estab-

lished goiters. Patients with small incidentally discovered nonpalpable thyroid nodules are at very low risk for malignancy, and even those that are malignant have a minor effect on morbidity and mortality.

Hegedüs L: Clinical practice. The thyroid nodule. N Engl J Med 2004;351:1764. [PMID: 15496625]

Kang HW et al: Prevalence, clinical and ultrasonographic characteristics of thyroid incidentalomas. Thyroid 2004;14:29. [PMID: 15009911]

Kessler A et al: Accuracy and consistency of fine-needle aspiration biopsy in the diagnosis and management of solitary thyroid nodules. Isr Med Assoc J 2005;7:371. [PMID: 15984379]

Liebeskind A et al: Rates of malignancy in incidentally discovered thyroid nodules evaluated with sonography and fine-needle aspiration. J Ultrasound Med 2005;24:629. [PMID: 15840794]

Nam-Goong IS et al: Ultrasonography-guided fine-needle aspiration of thyroid incidentaloma: correlation with pathological findings. Clin Endocrinol (Oxf) 2004;60:21. [PMID: 14678283]

THYROID CANCER
(Table 26–8)

 ESSENTIALS OF DIAGNOSIS

- Painless swelling in region of thyroid.
- Thyroid function tests usually normal.
- Past history of irradiation to head and neck region may be present.
- Positive thyroid needle aspiration.

General Considerations

The incidence of papillary and follicular (differentiated) thyroid carcinomas increases with age. The female:male ratio is 3:1. In the United States, thyroid cancer is diagnosed in nearly 26,000 people yearly, and about 1 in every 250 people eventually receives this diagnosis. About 13% of persons in the United States are found to have microscopic thyroid cancer at autopsy. Clearly, most thyroid cancers remain microscopic and indolent. However, larger thyroid cancers (palpable or ≥ 1 cm in diameter) are more malignant and require treatment.

Papillary thyroid carcinoma is the most common thyroid malignancy. Pure papillary or mixed papillary-follicular carcinoma represents about 81% of all thyroid cancers. It usually presents as a single nodule, but it can arise out of a multinodular goiter. Papillary thyroid carcinoma is commonly multifocal within the gland, with other foci usually arising de novo rather than representing intraglandular metastases.

Papillary thyroid carcinoma is caused by certain genetic mutations or translocations. Activating mutations of the *ras* oncogene can cause benign thyroid adenomas or nodular goiter. Additional activating mutations in *BRAF*

Table 26–8. Some characteristics of thyroid cancer.

	Papillary	Follicular	Medullary	Anaplastic
Incidence	Most common	Common	Uncommon	Uncommon
Average age	42	50	50	57
Females	70%	72%	56%	56%
Deaths due to thyroid cancer	6%	24%	33%	98%
Invasion				
Juxtanodal	+++++	+	++++++	+++
Blood vessels	+	+++	+++	+++++
Distant sites	+	+++	++	++++
Resemblance to normal thyroid	+	+++	+	±
^{123}I uptake	+	++++	0	0
Degree of malignancy	+	++ to +++	+ to ++++	++++++++

or *TRK* genes can lead to papillary carcinoma. About 45% of papillary thyroid carcinomas are caused by over-expression of the *ret* oncogene by the translocation of certain gene promoters to it, producing *retPTC-1*, *retPTC-2*, or *retPTC-3*. Radiation treatments to the head and neck region tend to cause *retPTC-1*. Nuclear fallout exposure tends to cause *retPTC-3*, resulting in more aggressive papillary thyroid carcinomas. Additional loss of the *p53* tumor suppressor gene can cause progression of papillary thyroid carcinoma to anaplastic thyroid carcinoma.

Exposure to radiation therapy to the head and neck poses a particular threat to children who then have an increased lifetime risk of developing thyroid pathology, including papillary thyroid carcinoma; thyroid malignancy may emerge between 10 and 40 years after exposure, with a peak occurrence 20–25 years later. Following the Chernobyl explosion, the risk for developing papillary thyroid carcinoma was highest among children who were under 5 years old at the time of exposure; emergence of more aggressive papillary thyroid carcinoma occurred within 6–7 years after exposure.

Papillary thyroid carcinoma can occur in rare familial syndromes as an autosomal dominant trait, caused by loss of various tumor suppressor genes. Such syndromes (with associated features) include familial papillary carcinoma (with papillary renal carcinoma); familial nonmedullary thyroid carcinoma; familial polyposis (with large intestine polyps and gastrointestinal tumors); Gardner's syndrome (with small and large intestine polyps, fibromas, lipomas, osteomas); and Turcot's syndrome (with large intestine polyps and brain tumors).

Generally speaking, papillary carcinoma is the least aggressive thyroid malignancy. However, the tumor spreads via lymphatics within the thyroid, becoming multifocal in 60% of patients and involving both lobes in 30% of patients. About 80% of patients have microscopic metastases to cervical lymph nodes; palpable lymph node involvement is present in 15% of adults and 60% of youths. Unlike other forms of can-

cer, patients with papillary thyroid carcinoma who have palpable lymph node metastases do not have a particularly increased mortality rate; however, their risk of local recurrence is increased.

Occult metastases to the lung occur in 10–15% of differentiated thyroid cancer; such lung metastases may be first noted on the whole-body scan following ^{131}I therapy. About 70% of small lung metastases resolve following ^{131}I therapy; however, larger pulmonary metastases have only a 10% remission rate.

Chronic low-grade papillary carcinoma can sometimes undergo a late anaplastic transformation into an aggressive carcinoma.

Follicular thyroid carcinoma results from certain gene mutations or translocations. Aberrant DNA methylation, activation of the *ras* oncogene, and mutations of the *MEN1* gene can result in benign follicular adenomas. Loss of function of *PPARg* or the *3P* tumor suppressor gene can lead to follicular carcinoma, and additional loss of the *p53* tumor suppressor gene can produce anaplastic carcinoma.

Follicular thyroid carcinoma and adenomas develop in patients with Cowden's disease, a rare autosomal dominant familial syndrome caused by loss of a tumor suppressor gene; such patients tend to have macrocephaly, multiple hamartomas, early-onset breast cancer, intestinal polyps, facial papules, and other skin and mucosal lesions.

Follicular and Hürthle cell carcinoma accounts for about 14% of thyroid malignancies and is generally more aggressive than papillary carcinoma. Rarely, some follicular carcinomas secrete enough T_4 to cause thyrotoxicosis if the tumor load becomes significant. Metastases commonly are found in neck nodes, bone, and lungs. Most follicular thyroid carcinomas avidly absorb iodine, making possible diagnostic scanning and treatment with ^{131}I after total thyroidectomy. Certain follicular histopathologic features are associated with a high risk of metastasis and recurrence: poorly differentiated and Hürthle cell (oncocytic) variants. The latter variants do not take up RAI.

Medullary thyroid carcinoma is often caused by an activating mutation of the *ret* oncogene on chromosome 10. Mutation analysis of the *ret* oncogene's exons 10, 11, 13, and 14 detects 95% of the mutations causing MEN 2A and 90% of the mutations causing familial medullary thyroid carcinoma. Patients with MEN 2B have activating mutations in exon 16 of the *ret* oncogene. These germline mutations can be detected by DNA analysis of peripheral white blood cells, allowing identification of gene carriers within the family. When a family with MEN 2A or familial medullary thyroid carcinoma does not have an identifiable *ret* oncogene mutation, gene carriers may still be identified using family linkage analysis. Somatic mutations of the *ret* oncogene can be identified in the tumors of 30% of patients with sporadic (nonfamilial) medullary thyroid carcinoma. (See Multiple Endocrine Neoplasia.)

Medullary thyroid carcinoma represents about 3% of thyroid cancers. About one-third of cases are sporadic, one-third are familial, and one-third are associated with MEN type 2. Therefore, discovery of a medullary thyroid carcinoma makes genetic analysis mandatory, as noted above. If a gene defect is discovered, related family members must have genetic screening for that specific gene defect. Even when no gene defect is detectable, family members should have regular thyroid surveillance. Medullary thyroid carcinoma arises from parafollicular thyroid cells that can secrete calcitonin, prostaglandins, serotonin, ACTH, corticotropin-releasing hormone (CRH), and other peptides. These peptides can cause symptoms and can be used as tumor markers. Early local metastases are usually present, usually to adjacent muscle and trachea as well as to local and mediastinal lymph nodes. Eventually, late metastases may appear in the bones, lungs, adrenals, or liver. Metastases to the neck may be detected by ultrasound. Metastases are best detected using [18F]fluorodeoxyglucose positron emission tomography (18FDG-PET) whole-body scanning. Medullary thyroid carcinoma does not concentrate iodine.

Anaplastic thyroid carcinoma is caused by certain gene mutations, including inactivating mutations of the *p53* tumor suppressor gene, as described above for papillary and follicular thyroid carcinomas. Anaplastic thyroid carcinoma represents about 2% of thyroid cancers. It usually presents in an older patient as a rapidly enlarging mass in a multinodular goiter. It is the most aggressive thyroid carcinoma and metastasizes early to surrounding nodes and distant sites. Local pressure symptoms include dysphagia or vocal cord paralysis. This tumor does not concentrate iodine.

Other thyroid malignancies together represent about 3% of thyroid cancers. **Lymphoma** of the thyroid is more common in older women. It usually presents as a rapidly enlarging, painful mass arising out of a multinodular or diffuse goiter affected by autoimmune thyroiditis, with which it may be confused microscopically. About 20% of cases have concomitant hypothyroidism. Thyroid lymphomas are most commonly B cell lymphomas (50%) or mucosa-associated lymphoid tissue (MALT; 23%); other types include follicular, small lymphocytic, and Burkitt's lymphoma and Hodgkin's disease. Thyroidectomy is rarely required. **Metastatic cancers** may sometimes involve the thyroid, particularly bronchogenic, breast, and renal carcinomas and malignant melanoma.

Clinical Findings

A. SYMPTOMS AND SIGNS

Thyroid carcinoma usually presents as a palpable, firm, nontender nodule in the thyroid. Most thyroid carcinomas are asymptomatic, but large thyroid cancers can cause neck discomfort, dysphagia, or hoarseness (due to pressure on the recurrent laryngeal nerve). About 3% of thyroid malignancies present with a metastasis, usually to local lymph nodes but sometimes to distant sites such as bone or lung. Metastatic functioning differentiated thyroid carcinoma can sometimes secrete enough thyroid hormone to produce thyrotoxicosis.

Medullary thyroid carcinoma frequently causes flushing and persistent diarrhea (30%), which may be the initial clinical feature. Patients with metastases often experience fatigue as well as other symptoms. Cushing's syndrome develops in about 5% of patients from secretion of ACTH or CRH. Signs of pressure or invasion of surrounding tissues are present in anaplastic or large tumors; recurrent laryngeal nerve palsy can occur.

B. LABORATORY FINDINGS

(FNA is discussed above in the section on nodular thyroid.) Thyroid function tests are generally normal unless there is concomitant thyroiditis. Follicular carcinoma may secrete enough T_4 to suppress TSH and cause clinical hyperthyroidism.

Serum thyroglobulin is high in most metastatic papillary and follicular tumors, making this a useful marker for recurrent or metastatic disease. Caution must be exercised for the following reasons: (1) Circulating antithyroglobulin antibodies can cause erroneous thyroglobulin determinations. (2) Thyroglobulin levels may be misleadingly elevated in thyroiditis, which often coexists with carcinoma. (3) Certain thyroglobulin assays falsely report the continued presence of thyroglobulin after total thyroidectomy and tumor resection, causing undue concern about possible metastases. Therefore, unexpected thyroglobulin levels should prompt a repeat assay in another reference laboratory.

Serum calcitonin levels are usually elevated in medullary thyroid carcinoma, making this a marker for metastatic disease. However, serum calcitonin may be elevated in many other conditions such as thyroiditis, pregnancy, azotemia, hypercalcemia, and other malignancies, including pheochromocytomas, carcinoid tumors, and carcinomas of the lung, pancreas, breast, and colon.

Serum calcitonin and carcinoembryonic antigen (CEA) determinations should be obtained before surgery for medullary carcinoma, then regularly in postoperative follow-up: every 4 months for 5 years, then every 6 months for life. Calcitonin levels remain elevated in patients with persistent tumor but also in some patients with apparent cure or indolent disease. Therefore, rising levels of calcitonin (or CEA) are the best indication for recurrence. Serum calcitonin levels > 250 pg/mL are also an indication for recurrent or metastatic medullary thyroid carcinoma. Serum CEA levels are usually elevated with medullary carcinoma, making this a useful second marker; however, it is not specific for this carcinoma.

Because up to two-thirds of medullary thyroid carcinoma cases are familial or MEN 2 (both autosomal dominant), siblings and children of patients with medullary carcinoma are advised to have genetic testing to detect *ret* oncogene mutations. (See discussion of medullary thyroid carcinoma, above.)

C. IMAGING

1. Radioactive iodine scanning—RAI (^{131}I or ^{123}I) thyroid and whole-body scanning are not usually helpful in the initial diagnosis of thyroid cancer. In the past, RAI scanning was performed in patients with thyroid nodules to determine whether they were "cold," a sign of malignancy. However, this did not provide sufficient sensitivity and has been supplanted by FNA biopsy. Prior to thyroidectomy, whole-body RAI scanning is not very sensitive for metastatic disease, since the normal thyroid competes for RAI with metastases, which are less avid for RAI. Consequently, RAI scanning is used after thyroidectomy for surveillance as described below.

2. Ultrasound of the neck—Ultrasound of the neck is useful in determining the size and location of the malignancy as well as the location of any neck metastases. Neck ultrasound is a simple and useful procedure and should be performed routinely on all patients with thyroid cancer for the initial diagnosis and for follow-up.

3. CT scanning—CT scanning may demonstrate metastases and is particularly useful for localizing and following lung metastases. However, CT scanning is less sensitive than ultrasound for detecting metastases within the neck. Iodinated contrast should never be given prior to RAI scanning or RAI therapy, since the large amounts of iodine in contrast media competitively inhibit the uptake of RAI by the thyroid, greatly reducing the effectiveness of subsequent RAI scanning and therapy. Medullary carcinoma in the thyroid, nodes, and liver may calcify, but lung metastases rarely do so.

4. MRI—MRI is particularly useful for imaging bone metastases.

5. PET scanning—PET scanning is particularly useful for detecting thyroid cancer metastases that do not have sufficient iodine uptake to be visible on RAI scans. ^{18}FDG-PET is quite sensitive and allows tumor volumetric determinations. The sensitivity of ^{18}FDG-PET scanning for differentiated thyroid cancer is enhanced if the

patient is hypothyroid or receiving thyrotropin, which increases the metabolic activity of differentiated thyroid cancer. Disadvantages of PET scanning include its lack of specificity for thyroid cancer as well as its expense and lack of availability in many locations.

Differential Diagnosis

Lymphocytic thyroiditis, multinodular goiter, and colloid nodules can be distinguished from malignancies by FNA biopsy. However, FNA cannot distinguish benign follicular adenoma from follicular carcinoma. Overall, in such "suspicious" cases, the risk of malignancy is about 20% higher in fixed lesions over 4 cm in diameter. The risk of malignancy is 5% for nodules in elderly patients with lesions under 4 cm in diameter having "suspicious" cytology.

Neuroendocrine carcinomas may metastasize to the thyroid and be confused with medullary thyroid carcinoma.

False-positive ^{131}I scans are common with normal residual thyroid tissue and have been reported with Zenker's diverticulum, struma ovarii, pleuropericardial cyst, gastric pull-up, and ^{131}I-contaminated bodily secretions. False-negative ^{131}I scans are common in early metastatic differentiated thyroid carcinoma but occur also in more advanced disease, including 14% of bone metastases.

Complications

The complications vary with the type of carcinoma. Differentiated thyroid carcinomas may have local or distant metastases. One-third of medullary carcinomas may secrete serotonin and prostaglandins, producing flushing and diarrhea, and may be complicated by the coexistence of pheochromocytomas or hyperparathyroidism. The risks of radical neck surgery include permanent hypoparathyroidism and vocal cord palsy due to recurrent laryngeal nerve damage; permanent hypothyroidism is expected after thyroidectomy and should always be treated adequately.

Treatment of Differentiated Thyroid Carcinoma

A. SURGICAL TREATMENT

Surgical removal is the treatment of choice for thyroid carcinomas. Neck ultrasound is useful both preoperatively and in follow-up. For differentiated papillary and follicular carcinoma, thyroidectomy with limited removal of cervical lymph nodes is adequate. However, for patients with Hürthle cell carcinoma or medullary thyroid carcinoma who have metastases to lymph nodes, modified radical neck dissection is recommended. Highly skilled surgeons can perform neartotal thyroidectomies with a less than 1% rate of serious complications (hypoparathyroidism or recurrent laryngeal nerve damage). Other series have reported up to an 11% incidence of permanent hypoparathyroidism after total thyroidectomy.

Thyroidectomy requires at least an overnight hospital admission, since late bleeding, airway problems, and tetany can occur. Ambulatory thyroidectomy is potentially dangerous and should not be done.

The incidence of hypoparathyroidism may be reduced if accidentally resected parathyroids are immediately autotransplanted into the neck muscles. The advantage of near-total thyroidectomy for differentiated thyroid carcinoma is that multicentric foci of carcinoma are more apt to be resected and there is then less normal thyroid tissue to compete with cancer for ^{131}I administered later for scans or treatment. Subtotal thyroidectomy is acceptable for adults under age 45 years who have a single small tumor (≤ 1 cm in diameter). Neck muscle dissections are usually avoided for differentiated thyroid carcinoma. T_4 is prescribed in doses of 0.05–0.1 mg/d immediately postoperatively. The dosage is adjusted to keep the serum TSH slightly suppressed during long-term follow-up of differentiated thyroid carcinoma.

About 2–4 months after surgery, a whole-body ^{131}I scan is performed. T_4 is stopped for 6 weeks prior to the scan, thereby causing hypothyroidism; TSH then rises and stimulates iodide uptake and thyroglobulin release from residual tumor or normal thyroid. Iodine-containing foods and contrast media are avoided.

Metastases to the brain are best treated surgically, since treatment with radiation or RAI is ineffective. Patients with bulky recurrent tumor in the neck region also benefit from surgery.

B. MEDICAL TREATMENT AND CHEMOTHERAPY

Patients who have had a thyroidectomy for differentiated thyroid cancer must take thyroid hormone replacement for life. Serum TSH levels must be monitored. Patients with differentiated thyroid carcinoma, including Hürthle cell carcinoma, should be given oral thyroxine in doses that suppress serum TSH without causing clinical thyrotoxicosis. An ultrasensitive TSH assay should be used; serum TSH should be suppressed below 0.1 mU/L for patients with stage II disease and below 0.05 mU/L for patients with stage III–IV disease. Patients receiving T_4 suppression therapy have been reported, as a group, to have slightly lower bone density than age-matched controls. However, for patients who are clinically euthyroid, T_4 suppression therapy has a minimal effect upon bone and fracture risk. Nevertheless, patients receiving T_4 suppression therapy are advised to have periodic bone densitometry.

Thyroid carcinomas are extraordinarily resistant to chemotherapy. Zoledronic acid, an intravenous bisphosphonate, has proven useful for osseous metastases from other solid tumors and has been used for patients with thyroid bone metastases, but its effectiveness is unknown.

C. RADIOACTIVE IODINE THERAPY

Following total or near-total thyroidectomy, patients with differentiated thyroid carcinoma receive an RAI neck and whole-body scan, either while hypothyroid, or after thyrotropin administration. In patients with visible RAI uptake, those with stage II–IV cancer should be treated with adjuvant ^{131}I therapy, when possible. The use of RAI therapy for patients with stage I differentiated thyroid cancer (with residual thyroid bed RAI uptake) is controversial; there has been no demonstrable improvement in survival in this group of patients following RAI therapy, although RAI therapy reduces the risk of local recurrence. Some groups advocate RAI therapy for patients with stage I disease whose primary tumor was over 1 cm in diameter. Patients must have demonstrated uptake of RAI on diagnostic scanning to warrant RAI therapy. For patients who have ^{131}I therapy, the dose of ^{131}I for thyroid "remnant ablation" (residual normal thyroid with perhaps thyroid cancer in the thyroid bed) in those with no nodal involvement is 30–100 mCi, with the higher doses given to patients with large primary tumors or tumors at the surgical margin. Patients with local lymph node involvement typically receive 100 mCi of ^{131}I; patients with more extensive neck node involvement or distant metastases receive 150–200 mCi of ^{131}I.

Prior to ^{131}I therapy, patients must be allowed to become hypothyroid, since high TSH levels stimulate thyroid cancer cells to actively absorb more iodine, and hypothyroidism reduces the renal clearance of iodine. Being hypothyroid is uncomfortable for most patients. Because levothyroxine (T_4) has a much longer half-life than T_3, the following protocol is suggested to prepare patients for ^{131}I therapy: 8 weeks prior to ^{131}I therapy, levothyroxine replacement therapy is stopped and T_3 (Cytomel) is substituted at a dose of 12.5 mcg orally twice daily; 6 weeks prior to ^{131}I therapy, the Cytomel is increased to 25 mcg orally twice daily; 16 days prior to ^{131}I therapy, the Cytomel is discontinued.

Recombinant human thyrotropin (rhTSH) injections do not stimulate RAI uptake sufficiently to prepare patients with stage II–IV cancer for ^{131}I ablative therapy of thyroid cancer. Also, patients receiving thyrotropin injections are euthyroid and have a high renal clearance of RAI, reducing the effectiveness of ^{131}I therapy. However, many centers are using rhTSH to stimulate ^{131}I uptake for thyroid remnant ablation in patients with stage I cancer. Such patients can also have their T_4 withdrawn for 1 week before the rhTSH and ^{131}I therapy to allow endogenous TSH levels to rise and provide additional stimulation of RAI uptake. Thyrotropin stimulation is also useful for patients with functional metastases whose serum TSH is always suppressed.

Patients must follow a low-iodine diet for 2 weeks before ^{131}I therapy. Just before therapy, serum is obtained for measurement of TSH (to make certain it is > 30 mcU/mL), thyroglobulin, and hCG (in all reproductive-age women). Pregnant women may not receive RAI therapy. Women are advised to avoid pregnancy for at least 4 months following ^{131}I therapy. Men have been found to have abnormal spermatozoa for up to 6 months following ^{131}I therapy and are advised to use contraceptive methods during that time.

Sodium ^{131}I, 30–50 mCi (1110–1850 MBq), is administered orally to patients with an original papillary or follicular carcinoma ≥ 1.5 cm in diameter and also to patients having persistent RAI uptake in the thyroid bed following near-total thyroidectomy. Patients with extrathyroidal uptake from metastatic disease are given larger doses of about 125–150 mCi (5550 MBq) ^{131}I orally in the hospital. A posttherapy whole-body scan performed 1 week after ^{131}I treatment will often detect metastases that were not visible on pretreatment scans.

Four days following ^{131}I therapy, Cytomel is resumed at a dose of 25 mcg orally twice daily for 1 week, reduced to 12.5 mcg twice daily for the next week. At the same time, T$_4$ is resumed and continued at a full thyroid replacement dose.

About 35% of patients with metastatic differentiated thyroid carcinoma have poor uptake of RAI into metastases. Lithium inhibits the release of ^{131}I from differentiated thyroid cancer and may increase the absorbed radiation dose; however, prospective treatment trials are lacking.

^{131}I therapy in doses over 100 mCi (3799 MBq) can cause gastritis, temporary oligospermia, sialadenitis, and xerostomia. RAI therapy can cause neurologic decompensation in patients with brain metastases; it is advisable to treat such patients with prednisone 30–40 mg orally daily for several days before and after ^{131}I therapy. Cumulative doses of ^{131}I over 500 mCi can cause infertility, pancytopenia (4%), and leukemia (0.3%). The kidneys excrete RAI. To reduce the risk of radiation-induced side effects, patients receiving dialysis for renal failure require a dosage reduction to only 20% of the usual dose of ^{131}I.

D. Treatment of Other Thyroid Malignancies

Patients with anaplastic thyroid carcinoma are treated with local resection and radiation. Lovastatin, an HMG-CoA inhibitor, has been demonstrated to cause differentiation and apoptosis of anaplastic thyroid carcinoma cells in vitro; however, clinical studies have not been performed. Anaplastic thyroid carcinoma does not respond to ^{131}I therapy and is resistant to chemotherapy.

Patients with thyroid MALT lymphomas have a low risk of recurrence after simple thyroidectomy. Patients with other thyroid lymphomas are best treated with external radiation therapy; chemotherapy is added for extensive lymphoma. Patients with systemic lymphomas involving the thyroid are usually treated with chemotherapy.

Patients with medullary thyroid carcinoma are treated surgically; repeated neck dissections are often required over time.

Patients with medullary thyroid carcinoma are advised to have genetic testing for *ret* protooncogene mutations. Patients who are discovered to have a germline mutation may require surveillance for other manifestations of MEN; genetic testing of first-degree relatives is also advisable. It is advisable that children with a *ret* protooncogene mutation have a prophylactic total thyroidectomy, ideally by age 6 years (MEN 2A) or at age 6 months (MEN 2B). Medullary thyroid carcinoma does not take up ^{131}I.

E. External Radiation Therapy

External radiation may be delivered to bone metastases. Brain metastases do not usually respond to ^{131}I and are best resected or treated with gamma knife radiosurgery.

F. Surveillance

Patients with differentiated thyroid carcinoma must be observed long term for recurrent or metastatic disease. Follow-up must include physical examinations and laboratory testing to ensure that patients remain clinically euthyroid with a suppressed TSH. To achieve suppression of serum TSH, the required dose of thyroxine may be such that serum FT$_4$ levels may be slightly elevated; in that case, measurement of serum T$_3$ or free T$_3$ (women who are pregnant or receiving oral estrogens) can be useful to ensure the patient is not frankly hyperthyroid. Thyrotoxicosis can be caused by overreplacement with thyroxine or by the growth of functioning metastases.

Neck palpation has a sensitivity of only 16% for detecting cervical lymph node metastases. Therefore, a combination of surveillance techniques must be used to detect recurrent or metastatic thyroid cancer.

1. Neck ultrasound—Neck ultrasound should be used in all patients with thyroid carcinoma to supplement neck palpation. It is prudent to perform a thyroid/neck ultrasound in all patients with thyroid cancer preoperatively, 3 months postoperatively, and regularly thereafter. Ultrasound is more sensitive for lymph node metastases than either CT or MRI scanning. Small inflammatory nodes may be detected postoperatively and do not necessarily indicate metastatic disease, but follow-up is necessary. Ultrasound-guided FNA biopsy should be performed on suspicious lesions.

2. Serum thyroglobulin (Tg)—Thyroglobulin is produced by normal thyroid tissue and by most differentiated thyroid carcinomas. It is only after a total or near-total thyroidectomy and ^{131}I remnant ablation that serum thyroglobulin (Tg) becomes a useful tumor marker for patients with differentiated papillary or follicular thyroid cancer. The usefulness of serum Tg is negated by the presence of anti-thyroglobulin antibodies. Anti-Tg antibodies tend to persist but may become less evident several years after total thyroidectomy and during the last trimester of pregnancy. For patients without serum anti-Tg antibodies, Tg measurement is a useful tumor marker.

Detectable levels of thyroglobulin are commonly encountered in patients who have had incomplete thyroidectomies and ^{131}I remnant ablations and do not necessarily indicate the presence of residual or metastatic thyroid cancer. However, baseline or stimulated serum Tg levels ≥ 2 ng/mL indicate the need for a repeat neck ultrasound and further scanning. If serum Tg levels remain ≥ 2 ng/mL in the presence of normal scanning, it is prudent to repeat the serum Tg in a national reference laboratory. Rising serum levels of thyroglobulin are particularly worrisome.

In one series of patients with differentiated thyroid cancer following thyroidectomy, there was a 21% incidence of metastases in patients with serum Tg < 1 ng/mL (while receiving thyroxine for TSH suppression). Therefore, *stimulated* serum Tg measurements should be used and *always* with neck ultrasound. The usefulness of routinely doing a radioiodine scan (see below) in low-risk patients is controversial but continues to be done in most centers during stimulation following either rhTSH or thyroid hormone withdrawal, according to the protocols described below.

3. Radioactive iodine (RAI: ^{131}I or ^{123}I) whole-body scanning—Despite its limitations, RAI has traditionally been used to detect metastatic differentiated thyroid cancer and to determine whether the cancer is amenable to treatment with ^{131}I. RAI scanning is particularly useful for high-risk patients and those with anti-thyroglobulin antibodies that make serum thyroglobulin determinations unreliable.

The ^{131}I isotope may be used in scanning doses of < 3 mCi (111 MBq) or given within 2 weeks of RAI treatment to avoid "stunning" metastases such that they take up less of the RAI therapy dose. The radioisotope ^{123}I may be used in scanning doses of 5 mCi (185 MBq), does not stun tumors, and allows single-photon emission computed tomography (SPECT) to better localize metastases. Initial RAI scanning is typically performed about 2–4 months following surgery for differentiated thyroid carcinoma. Whole-body scanning should be performed for at least 30 minutes for at least 140,000 counts and spot views of the neck should be obtained for at least 35,000 counts.

About 65% of metastases are detectable by RAI scanning, but only after optimal preparation: Patients should ideally have a total or near-total thyroidectomy, since any residual normal thyroid competes for RAI with metastases, which are less avid for iodine. To avoid nonradioactive iodine competitive inhibition of RAI uptake, intravenous iodinated contrast must be avoided for at least 2 months before scanning; patients must follow a low-iodine diet for at least 2 weeks before scanning and continue to limit iodine consumption until the scan is complete or until after ^{131}I therapy. In addition, patients must have high levels of TSH to stimulate metastases to take up more RAI, making them visible on scanning. This can be accomplished by allowing the patient to become hypothyroid or by administering synthetic rhTSH. The use of rhTSH has become more widespread for surveillance scanning and stimulated thyroglobulin determinations following thyroidectomy for differentiated thyroid carcinoma, due to its convenience for the patient. However, rhTSH-stimulated scanning is slightly less sensitive than hypothyroid-stimulated scanning. For stage I–II patients, it is reasonable to perform a thyroid-withdrawal scan once; if it is negative and the serum thyroglobulin is < 2 ng/mL, an rhTSH scan can be performed 1 and 3 years thereafter.

a. Thyrotropin-stimulated serum Tg and radioiodine scanning—The use of recombinant human thyrotropin-α (Thyrogen; rhTSH) injections can replace thyroid withdrawal with much less discomfort for most patients. Thyrotropin stimulates uptake of RAI and production of thyroglobulin by differentiated thyroid cancer or residual thyroid. The use of rhTSH is particularly suited to "low-risk" patients: those with a small papillary thyroid carcinoma who have had a total or near-total thyroidectomy and have no known local or distal metastases and a serum thyroglobulin < 1 mcg/L during thyroxine suppression of serum TSH. In about 21% of such "low-risk" patients, rhTSH stimulates serum thyroglobulin to above 2 mcg/L; such patients have a 23% risk of local neck metastases and a 13% risk of distant metastases. Stimulated radioiodine neck and whole-body scanning can detect only about half of these metastases because they are small or not avid for iodine.

Thyrotropin must be kept refrigerated and may be administered according to the following protocol: Thyroxine replacement is held for 2 days before rhTSH and for 3 days afterward. On Monday and Tuesday, thyrotropin 0.9 mg is administered intragluteally (not intravenously). On Wednesday, serum is drawn for TSH and thyroglobulin determinations. Immediately thereafter, RAI is administered in a scanning dose (see above). On Friday, serum is drawn for thyroglobulin and the whole-body scan is performed.

Side effects of thyrotropin injections include nausea (11%) and headache (7%). Hyperthyroidism can occur in patients with significant metastases or residual normal thyroid. Thyrotropin has caused neurologic deterioration in 7% of patients with central nervous system metastases.

The combination of thyrotropin-stimulated scanning and thyroglobulin levels detects a thyroid remnant or cancer with a sensitivity of 84%. However, the presence of anti-thyroglobulin antibodies renders the serum thyroglobulin determination uninterpretable. Thyrotropin stimulation does not prepare patients for ^{131}I treatment; they must be prepared for treatment by becoming hypothyroid as described below.

b. Thyroid withdrawal-stimulated serum Tg and radioiodine scanning—Patients are allowed to become hypothyroid; high levels of endogenous TSH stimulate the uptake of RAI and production of thyroglobulin by thyroid cancer or residual thyroid. Being hypothyroid is uncomfortable for most patients. Because T_4 has a much longer half-life than T_3, the following protocol is suggested to prepare patients for RAI scanning: Eight weeks prior to RAI scanning, levothyroxine replacement therapy is stopped and T_3 (Cytomel) is substituted at a dose of 12.5 mcg orally twice daily. Six weeks prior to RAI scanning, the Cytomel is increased to 25 mcg twice daily. Seventeen days prior to RAI scanning, the Cytomel is discontinued. Prior to scanning, serum TSH is assayed to confirm that it is > 30 mcU/mL; serum hCG is assayed to screen for pregnancy; serum thyroglobulin titers are also determined. Following radioisotope scanning, or 4 days after ^{131}I therapy (see above), Cytomel is resumed at a dose of 25 mcg twice daily for 1 week, reduced to 12.5 mcg twice daily for the next week. At the same time, T_4 is resumed and continued at a full thyroid replacement dose.

Patients with **papillary carcinoma** should have at least two annual consecutively negative stimulated serum thyroglobulin determinations < 1mcg/L and normal RAI scans (if done) before they are considered to be in remission. Patients with persistent RAI uptake restricted to the thyroid bed need not have repeated ^{131}I therapies if neck ultrasound appears benign and serum thyroglobulin is < 5 ng/mL. Further radioiodine or other scans may be required for patients with more aggressive papillary-follicular, follicular, or medullary thyroid carcinomas, prior metastases, rising serum thyroglobulin levels, or other evidence of metastases.

Patients often have a negative whole-body radioiodine scan but have serum thyroglobulin levels that are > 2 ng/mL. In such cases, another thyroglobulin assay should be sent to a different reference laboratory to confirm the accuracy of the thyroglobulin determination. Patients with serum Tg levels > 2 ng/mL require close continued monitoring. Those with progressively rising Tg levels are at high risk for occult thyroid cancer metastases. Other scanning methods may be used in an effort to detect such metastases. (See below.)

4. Positron emission tomography scanning— PET whole-body scanning using [18]FDG-PET is a relatively sensitive method for detecting thyroid cancer metastases—particularly those that are not revealed on RAI scanning. PET scanning is particularly useful for detecting thyroid cancer metastases in patients with a detectable serum thyroglobulin (especially serum thyroglobulin levels > 10 ng/mL and rising) who have a normal whole-body RAI scan and an unrevealing neck ultrasound. PET scanning can be combined with a CT scan; the resultant PET/CT fusion scan is 60% sensitive for detecting metastases that are not visible by other methods. This scan is less sensitive for small brain metastases. [18]FDG-PET scanning detects the metabolic activity of tumor tissue; for differentiated thyroid carcinoma, this scan is more sensitive when the patient is hypothyroid or pretreated with thyrotropin as described above. One problem with [18]FDG-PET scanning is its lack of specificity. For example, false-positives can occur with benign hepatic tumors, sarcoidosis, radiation therapy, suture granulomas, reactive lymph nodes, or inflammation at surgical sites that can persist for months. False-positive uptake can also occur in muscles and brown fat in the neck and shoulders, axillae, mediastinum, perinephric regions, intercostal paravertebral spaces, and paravertebral muscles. A fusion [18]FDG-PET/CT (no contrast) scan improves specificity but cannot distinguish thyroid carcinoma from other unrelated malignancies that may be present concurrently. Smaller metastases are often present on PET scanning before becoming visible on CT or even MRI scanning.

[18]FDG-PET scanning is particularly sensitive for detecting medullary thyroid carcinoma (MTC) metastases, and prescan thyrotropin does not improve the PET scan sensitivity for MTC.

5. Other scanning—Thallium-201 (^{201}Tl) scans may be useful for detecting metastatic differentiated thyroid carcinoma when the ^{131}I scan is normal but serum thyroglobulin is elevated. MRI scanning is particularly useful for imaging metastases in the brain, mediastinum, or bones. CT scanning is useful for imaging and monitoring pulmonary metastases.

Prognosis

Differentiated thyroid carcinoma carries a generally good prognosis, particularly for adults under age 45 years, despite the fact that about 15% of these patients are subsequently found to have metastases. The following characteristics imply a worse prognosis: older age, male sex, bone or brain metastases, large pulmonary metastases, and lack of ^{131}I uptake into metastases. Certain papillary histologic types are associated with a higher risk of recurrence: tall cell, columnar cell, and diffuse sclerosing types. Staging and survival rates are presented in Table 26–9. Brain metastases are detected in 1%; they reduce median survival to 12 months, but their prognosis is improved by surgical resection. Patients with follicular carcinoma have a cancer mortality rate that is 3.4 times higher than patients with papillary carcinoma. The Hürthle cell variant of follicular carcinoma is more aggressive. Patients with primary tumors over 1 cm in diameter who undergo limited thyroid surgery (subtotal thyroidectomy or lobectomy) have a 2.2-fold increased mortality over those having total or near-total thyroidectomies. Patients who have not received ^{131}I ablation have mortality rates that are increased twofold by 10 years and threefold by 25 years (over those who have received ablation). The risk of cancer recurrence is twofold higher in men than in women and 1.7-fold higher in multifocal than in unifocal tumors.

Medullary thyroid carcinoma is typically fairly indolent but more aggressive than differentiated thyroid cancer. The overall 10-year survival rate is 90% when the tumor is confined to the thyroid, 70% for those with metastases to cervical lymph nodes, and 20% for those with distant metastases. Patients with sporadic disease usually have lymph node involvement at the time of diagnosis, whereas distal metastases may not be noted for years. Familial cases or those associated with MEN 2A tend to be less aggressive; the 10-year survival rate is higher, in part due to earlier detection. Medullary thyroid carcinoma that is seen in MEN 2B is more aggressive, arises earlier in life, and carries a worse overall prognosis. Women with medullary thyroid carcinoma who are under age 40 years also have a better prognosis. A better prognosis is also obtained in patients undergoing total thyroidectomy and neck dissection; radiation therapy reduces recurrence in patients with metastases to neck nodes. The mortality rate is increased 4.5-fold when primary or metastatic tumor tissue stains heavily for myelomonocytic antigen M-1. Conversely, tumors with heavy immunoperoxidase staining for calcitonin are associated

Table 26–9. Pathologic tumor-node-metastasis (pTNM) staging and tumor-related survival rates for adults with appropriately treated differentiated (papillary) thyroid carcinoma based upon patient age, primary tumor size and invasiveness (T), lymph node involvement (N), and distant metastases (M).[1]

Stage	Description	Five-Year Survival	Ten-Year Survival
1	Under 45: any T, any N, no M Over 45: T ≤1 cm, no N, no M	99%	98%
2	Under 45: any T, any N, any M Over 45: T >1 cm limited to thyroid, no N, no M	99%	85%
3	Over 45: T beyond thyroid capsule, no N, no M; or any T, regional N, no M	95%	70%
4	Over 45: any T, any N, any M	80%	61%

From Alsanea O et al: Surgery 2000;128:1043; Loh KC et al: J Endocrinol Metab 1997;82:3553; and Hay ID: Endocrinol Metabol Clin North Am 1990;19:545.
[1]Patients having a relatively worse prognosis include those with follicular thyroid carcinoma and those with familial differentiated thyroid carcinoma.

with prolonged survival even in the presence of significant metastases.

Anaplastic thyroid carcinoma has a 1-year survival rate of about 10% and a 5-year survival rate of about 5%. Patients with fully localized tumors on MRI have a better prognosis.

Patients with localized lymphoma have nearly 100% 5-year survival. Those with disease outside the thyroid have a 63% 5-year survival. However, the prognosis is better for those with the MALT type. Patients presenting with stridor, pain, laryngeal nerve palsy, or mediastinal extension tend to fare worse.

Driedger AA et al: Two cases of thyroid carcinoma that were not stimulated by recombinant human thyrotropin. J Clin Endocrinol Metab 2004;89:589. [PMID: 14764766]

Fernandes JK et al: Overview of the management of differentiated thyroid cancer. Curr Treat Options Oncol 2005;6: 47. [PMID: 15610714]

Giles Y et al: The advantage of total thyroidectomy to avoid reoperation for incidental thyroid cancer in multinodular goiter. Arch Surg 2004;139:179. [PMID: 14769577]

Hamady ZZ et al: Surgical pathological second opinion in thyroid malignancy: impact on patients' management and prognosis. Eur J Surg Oncol 2005;31:74. [PMID: 15642429]

Kim TY et al: Metastasis to the thyroid diagnosed by fine-needle aspiration biopsy. Clin Endocrinol (Oxf) 2005;62:236. [PMID: 15670202]

Lin JD et al: Papillary thyroid carcinomas with lung metastases. Thyroid 2004;14:1091. [PMID: 15650364]

Mazzaferri EL et al: A consensus report of the role of serum thyroglobulin as a monitoring method for low-risk patients with papillary thyroid carcinoma. J Clin Endocrinol Metab 2003;88:1433. [PMID: 12679418]

Robbins RJ et al: Real-time prognosis for metastatic thyroid carcinoma based on 2-[18F]fluoro-2-deoxy-D-glucose-positron emission tomography scanning. J Clin Endocrinol Metab 2006;91:498. [PMID: 16303836]

Sawka AM et al: A systematic review and metaanalysis of the effectiveness of radioactive iodine remnant ablation for well-differentiated thyroid cancer. J Clin Endocrinol Metab 2004;89:3668. [PMID: 15292285]

ENDEMIC GOITER

 ESSENTIALS OF DIAGNOSIS

- *Common in regions of the world with low-iodine diets.*
- *High rate of congenital hypothyroidism and cretinism.*
- *Goiters may become multinodular and grow to great size.*
- *Most adults with endemic goiter are found to be euthyroid; however, some are hypothyroid or hyperthyroid.*
- *Impaired cognition and hearing may be subtle or severe in congenital hypothyroidism.*

General Considerations

Approximately 5% of the world's population have goiters. Of these, about 75% are in persons dwelling in areas of iodine deficiency. Such areas are found in 115 countries, mostly in developing areas but also in Europe. In iodine-deficient patients, smoking or pregnancy can induce goiter growth.

In Pescopagano, Italy, 60% of adults have goiters. Hyperthyroidism (present or past) occurred in 2.9%; hypothyroidism was overt in 0.2% and subclinical in 3.8%. The incidence of thyroid cancer was less than 0.1%. Up to 0.5% of iodine-deficient populations have full-blown cretinism, with less severe manifestations of congenital hypothyroidism being even more common (eg, isolated deafness, short stature, or impaired mentation). Intelligence quotients in iodine-deficient adults are an average of 13 points lower than expected. Although iodine deficiency is the most common cause of endemic goiter, certain foods (eg, sorghum, millet, maize, cassava), mineral deficiencies (selenium, iron), and water pollutants can themselves cause goiter or aggravate a goiter proclivity caused by iodine deficiency. Pregnancy is associated with an increase in size of thyroid nodules and the emergence of new nodules. Some individuals are particularly susceptible to goiter owing to congenital partial defects in thyroid enzyme activity.

Clinical Findings

A. SYMPTOMS AND SIGNS

Endemic goiters may become multinodular and very large. Growth often occurs during pregnancy and may cause compressive symptoms.

Substernal goiters are usually asymptomatic but can cause tracheal compression, respiratory distress and failure, dysphagia, superior vena cava syndrome, gastrointestinal bleeding from esophageal varices, palsies of the phrenic or recurrent laryngeal nerves, or Horner's syndrome. Cerebral ischemia and stroke can result from arterial compression or thyrocervical steal syndrome. Substernal goiters can rarely cause pleural or pericardial effusions. The incidence of significant malignancy is less than 1%.

Some patients with endemic goiter may become hypothyroid. Others may become thyrotoxic as the goiter grows and becomes more autonomous, especially if iodine is added to the diet.

B. LABORATORY FINDINGS

The serum T_4 is usually normal. Serum TSH is generally normal. TSH falls in the presence of hyperthyroidism if a multinodular goiter has become autonomous in the presence of sufficient amounts of iodine for thyroid hormone synthesis. TSH rises with hypothyroidism. Thyroid RAI uptake is usually elevated, but it may be normal if iodine intake has improved. Serum levels of antithyroid antibodies are usually either undetectable or in low titers. Serum thyroglobulin is often elevated.

Differential Diagnosis

Endemic goiter must be distinguished from all other forms of nodular goiter that may coexist in an endemic region (see above).

Prevention

Iodine supplementation was started in Switzerland in 1922, initially by adding 5 mg of potassium iodide per kilogram of salt, with later increases to the current level of 20 mg/kg salt. Iodized salt has greatly reduced the incidence of endemic goiter. Unfortunately, many iodine-deficient countries have inadequate programs for iodine supplementation. The minimum dietary requirement for iodine is about 50 mcg daily, with optimal iodine intake being 150–300 mcg daily. Iodine sufficiency is assessed by measurement of urinary iodide excretion, the target being more than 10 mcg/dL.

Initiating iodine supplementation in a geographic area causes an increased frequency of hyperthyroidism in the first year, followed by greatly reduced rates of toxic nodular goiter and Graves' disease thereafter.

Treatment

The addition of potassium iodide to table salt greatly reduces the prevalence of endemic goiter and cretinism but is less effective in shrinking established goiter. Concurrent deficiencies in both vitamin A and iodine increase the risk of endemic goiter and concurrent repletion of both iodide and vitamin A reduces goiter in endemic goiter regions. Dietary iodine supplementation increases the risk of autoimmune thyroid dysfunction, which may result in hypothyroidism or thyrotoxicosis. Excessive iodine intake may increase the risk of goiter. T_4 supplementation can shrink goiters and reduce the risk of further goiter growth, but such treatment likewise carries a risk of inducing hyperthyroidism in individuals with autonomous multinodular goiters; therefore, T_4 suppression should not be started in patients with suppressed TSH levels.

Adults with large multinodular goiter may require thyroidectomy for cosmesis, compressive symptoms, or thyrotoxicosis. Following partial thyroidectomy in iodine-deficient geographic areas, there is a high goiter recurrence rate, so total thyroidectomy is preferred when surgery is indicated. Certain patients may be treated with ^{131}I for large compressive goiters. Such patients may rarely develop Graves' disease 3–10 months after treatment.

Bellantone R et al: Predictive factors for recurrence after thyroid lobectomy for unilateral non-toxic goiter in an endemic area: results of a multivariate analysis. Surgery 2004;136: 1247. [PMID: 15657583]

Valentino R et al: Screening a coastal population in Southern Italy: iodine deficiency and prevalence of goitre, nutritional aspects and cardiovascular risk factors. Nutr Metab Cardiovasc Dis 2004;14:15. [PMID: 15053159]

HYPOTHYROIDISM & MYXEDEMA

ESSENTIALS OF DIAGNOSIS

- *Weakness, fatigue, cold intolerance, constipation, weight change, depression, menorrhagia, hoarseness.*
- *Dry skin, bradycardia, delayed return of deep tendon reflexes.*
- *Anemia, hyponatremia.*
- T_4 *and RAI uptake usually low.*
- *TSH elevated in primary hypothyroidism.*

General Considerations

Thyroid hormone deficiency may affect almost all body functions. The degree of severity ranges from mild and unrecognized hypothyroid states to striking myxedema. The fluid retention seen in myxedema is caused by the interstitial accumulation of hydrophilic mucopolysaccharides, which leads to lymphedema. Hyponatremia is the result of impaired renal tubular sodium reabsorption due to reductions in Na^+–K^+-ATPase. Cellular proteins are also affected in myxedema.

Hypothyroidism may be due to primary disease of the thyroid gland itself or lack of pituitary TSH. Florid hypothyroidism, ie, myxedema and cretinism, is readily recognized on clinical grounds alone, but mild hypothyroidism often escapes detection without screening (ie, serum TSH). Maternal hypothyroidism during pregnancy results in offspring with IQ scores that are an average 7 points lower than those of euthyroid mothers.

Goiter may be noted when hypothyroidism is due to Hashimoto's thyroiditis, iodide deficiency, genetic thyroid enzyme defects, drug goitrogens (lithium, iodide, propylthiouracil or methimazole, phenylbutazone, sulfonamides, amiodarone, interferon-α, interferon-β, interleukin-2), food goitrogens in iodide-deficient areas (eg, turnips, cassavas), or, rarely, peripheral resistance to thyroid hormone or infiltrating diseases (eg, cancer, sarcoidosis). A hypothyroid phase occurs in subacute (de Quervain's) viral thyroiditis following initial hyperthyroidism.

Goiter is usually absent when hypothyroidism is due to deficient pituitary TSH secretion, or destruction of the gland by surgery, external radiation, or ^{131}I. Patients who have received central nervous system radiation for leukemia have a 15% chance of developing hypothyroidism years later. Patients with primary pulmonary hypertension have a 22% incidence of hypothyroidism.

Amiodarone, because of its high iodine content, causes clinically significant hypothyroidism in about 8% of patients. The T_4 level is normal or low, and the TSH is elevated, usually over 20 ng/dL. Another 17% of patients develop milder elevations of TSH and are asymptomatic. Low-dose amiodarone is less likely to cause hypothyroidism. Cardiac patients with amiodarone-induced symptomatic hypothyroidism are treated with just enough T_4 to relieve symptoms. Hypothyroidism usually resolves if amiodarone is discontinued. Patients with a high iodine intake from other sources may also develop hypothyroidism, especially if they have underlying lymphocytic thyroiditis.

Patients with chronic hepatitis C have an increased risk of autoimmune thyroiditis, with 21% having antithyroid antibodies and 13% having hypothyroidism. The risk of thyroid dysfunction is even higher when patients are treated with interferon. Interferon-α and interferon-β treatment can induce thyroid dysfunction (usually hypothyroidism, sometimes hyperthyroidism) in 6% of patients. Spontaneous resolution occurs in over 50% of cases once interferon is discontinued.

Clinical Findings

These may vary from the rather rare full-blown myxedema to mild states of hypothyroidism, which are far

more common. Hypothyroidism is a common disorder; therefore, a clinician should request thyroid function tests for any patient with the nonspecific symptoms and signs of hypothyroidism.

A. Symptoms and Signs

1. Early—Frequent symptoms are fatigue, lethargy, weakness, arthralgias or myalgias, muscle cramps, cold intolerance, constipation, dry skin, headache, and menorrhagia. Physical findings may be few or absent. Features may include thin, brittle nails, thinning of hair, and pallor. Delayed relaxation of deep tendon reflexes and bradycardia are sometimes noted.

2. Late—The symptoms are variable but may include slow speech, absence of sweating, constipation, peripheral edema, pallor, hoarseness, decreased sense of taste and smell, muscle cramps, aches and pains, dyspnea, weight changes (usually gain, but weight loss is not rare), and diminished auditory acuity. Some women have amenorrhea; others have menorrhagia. Galactorrhea may also be present. Physical findings may include goiter, puffiness of the face and eyelids, typical carotenemic skin color, thinning of the outer halves of the eyebrows, thickening of the tongue, hard pitting edema, and effusions into the pleural, peritoneal, and pericardial cavities, as well as into joints. Cardiac enlargement ("myxedema heart") is often due to pericardial effusion. The heart rate is slow; the blood pressure is more often normal than low, and reversible diastolic hypertension may be found. Hypothermia may be present. Pituitary enlargement due to hyperplasia of TSH-secreting cells, which is reversible following thyroid therapy, may be seen in long-standing hypothyroidism. Hypothyroidism rarely causes true obesity.

B. Laboratory Findings

The FT_4 may be low or low normal. TSH is increased with primary hypothyroidism but is low or normal with pituitary insufficiency. Other laboratory abnormalities may often be seen: increased serum cholesterol, liver enzymes, and creatine kinase; increased serum PRL; and hyponatremia, hypoglycemia, and anemia (with normal or increased mean corpuscular volume). Titers of antibodies against thyroperoxidase and thyroglobulin are high in patients with Hashimoto's thyroiditis. Serum T_3 is not a good test for hypothyroidism.

Some clinically euthyroid patients have mildly elevated levels of serum TSH (5–10 mIU/L) without any other manifestations of hypothyroidism; serum FT_4 levels are normal. Such patients are said to have "subclinical hypothyroidism."

Differential Diagnosis

Hypothyroidism can be mistaken for other conditions that cause states of asthenia, unexplained menstrual disorders, myalgias, constipation, weight change, hyperlipidemia, and anemia. Myxedema enters into the differential diagnosis of unexplained heart failure that does not respond to digitalis or diuretics, and unexplained ascites. The protein content of myxedematous effusions is high. The thick tongue may be confused with that seen in primary amyloidosis. Pernicious anemia may be suggested by the pallor and the macrocytic anemia sometimes seen in myxedema; the two disorders may even coexist. Some cases of depression, primary psychosis, and structural diseases of the brain have been confused with myxedema. The pituitary is often quite enlarged in primary hypothyroidism due to reversible hyperplasia of TSH-secreting cells; the concomitant hyperprolactinemia seen in hypothyroidism can lead to the mistaken diagnosis of a TSH-secreting or PRL-secreting pituitary adenoma.

A number of factors can lower serum T_4 levels without causing true hypothyroidism (see Table 26–6). Autoimmune disease can cause false elevations of TSH by interfering with the assay. Serum TSH may be elevated transiently in acute psychiatric illness and during recovery from nonthyroidal illness. A high TSH can also be caused by thyrotropin-secreting pituitary tumors. Patients with TSH resistance, caused by a mutation in the gene encoding the TSH receptor, have high serum TSH levels despite usually being clinically and biochemically euthyroid.

Complications

Complications are mostly cardiac in nature, occurring as a result of advanced coronary artery disease and congestive failure, which may be precipitated by overly vigorous thyroid therapy. There is an increased susceptibility to infection. Megacolon has been described in long-standing hypothyroidism. Organic psychoses with paranoid delusions may occur ("myxedema madness"). Rarely, adrenal crisis may be precipitated by thyroid therapy. Hypothyroidism is a rare cause of infertility, which may respond to thyroid medication. Pregnancy in a woman with untreated hypothyroidism often results in miscarriage. On the other hand, if the hypothyroidism is due to autoimmune disease, it may improve during pregnancy. Sellar enlargement and even well-defined TSH-secreting tumors may develop in untreated cases. These tumors decrease in size after replacement therapy is instituted.

A rare complication of severe hypothyroidism is deep stupor, at times progressing to **myxedema coma**, with severe hypothermia, hypoventilation, hyponatremia, hypoxia, hypercapnia, and hypotension. Convulsions and abnormal central nervous system signs may occur. Myxedema coma is often induced by an underlying infection; cardiac, respiratory, or central nervous system illness; cold exposure; or drug use. It is most often seen in elderly women. The mortality rate from myxedema coma is high. Myxedematous patients are unusually sensitive to opioids and may die from average doses.

Refractory hyponatremia is often seen in severe myxedema. Inappropriate secretion of ADH has been observed in some patients, but a defect in distal tubular reabsorption of sodium and water has been demonstrated in many others.

Treatment

Levothyroxine (thyroxine; T_4) is the treatment of choice. It is partially converted in the body to T_3, the more active thyroid hormone. Hypothyroid patients who are taking thyroxine replacement typically have serum T_3 levels that are lower than normal, owing to their lack of thyroidal T_3 secretion. Oral administration of T_3 causes abnormal peaks in serum T_3 and the usefulness of T_3 for hypothyroidism is controversial; a sustained-release T_3 preparation is not commercially available.

In patients taking a certain daily dose of levothyroxine, significant increases in serum T_4 levels are seen within 1–2 weeks, and near-peak levels are seen within 3–4 weeks. It is best taken in the morning with water, avoiding concomitant intake of foods and drugs that may interfere with its absorption (see below). Brand preparations of levothyroxine in the United States appear to be bioequivalent to each other and certain generics. Before therapy with thyroid hormone is commenced, the hypothyroid patient requires at least a clinical assessment for adrenal insufficiency, which would require concurrent treatment.

A. BEGINNING TREATMENT FOR HYPOTHYROIDISM

Patients without coronary insufficiency who are under age 60 years may receive starting doses of oral levothyroxine of 50–100 mcg/daily up to a maximum of 1.6 mcg/kg body weight daily. Women who are pregnant and significantly hypothyroid may begin therapy with levothyroxine at doses of 100–150 mcg orally daily. Patients with coronary disease or those who are over age 60 years are treated with smaller initial doses of levothyroxine, 25–50 mcg daily; higher initial doses may be used if such patients are severely hypothyroid. The dose can be increased by 25 mcg every 1–3 weeks until the patient is euthyroid. Hypothyroid patients with ischemic heart disease may begin thyroxine therapy following coronary artery angioplasty or bypass.

Patients with severe hypothyroidism require larger initial doses of levothyroxine, particularly since myxedema itself can interfere with the intestinal absorption of T_4.

Myxedema coma is a medical emergency with a high mortality rate. It is caused by hypothyroidism but is usually precipitated by an acute illness or trauma. Patients have the manifestations of hypothyroidism as well as impaired mentation. Hyponatremia and hypoglycemia are often present. Levothyroxine sodium 400 mcg is given intravenously as a loading dose, followed by 100 mcg intravenously daily. The hypothermic patient is warmed only with blankets, since faster warming can precipitate cardiovascular collapse. Patients with hypercapnia require intubation and assisted mechanical ventilation. Infections must be detected and treated aggressively. Patients in whom concomitant adrenal insufficiency is suspected are treated with hydrocortisone, 100 mg intravenously, followed by 25–50 mg every 8 hours.

B. Long-Term Treatment of Hypothyroidism

It is important to stress to the patient that levothyroxine therapy must be continued long-term and that regular clinical reassessments will be required for life. Most patients ultimately require levothyroxine in doses of 75–250 mcg orally daily.

For most hypothyroid patients, a stable maintenance dose can usually be found. However, the dosage requirement can rise, due to increased hepatic metabolism of thyroxine induced by certain medications: carbamazepine, phenobarbitol, phenytoin, rifabutin, rifampin, and the antitumor drug imatinib (Gleevec). Amiodarone can cause changes in thyroxine dose requirements by various mechanisms. Malabsorption of thyroxine can be caused by coadministration of thyroxine with certain medications: antacids, bile acid binding resins, calcium, didanosine, magnesium, and iron salts (including iron found in multivitamins with minerals).

Women with hypothyroidism typically require increased doses of T_4 during pregnancy and during therapy with oral estrogen. Conversely, T_4 dosage requirements for women often decrease with delivery, cessation of oral estrogen, and menopause.

There is no standardized optimal dose of levothyroxine, so each patient's dose must be based on careful clinical assessment. Although serum TSH levels can be helpful in determining optimal dosing, it is important not to rely entirely on this test alone.

During pregnancy, it is critical to administer adequate levothyroxine to a hypothyroid woman. Although the fetal thyroid begins secreting thyroid hormone at about 18 weeks of gestation, fetal thyroid development is not complete until term. Maternal T_4 crosses the placenta, and the fetus is at least partially dependent upon maternal T_4 for central nervous system development—particularly in the second trimester. Maternal hypothyroidism after the first trimester appears to cause some developmental delay in offspring. It is therefore important to carefully follow women with hypothyroidism during their pregnancies with serum TSH (FT_4 concentrations in hypopituitarism) determinations every 4–6 weeks and to increase T_4 replacement progressively as required.

There is considerable individual variation in the requirement for additional T_4 replacement during pregnancy. For women receiving replacement thyroxine, it is prudent to increase thyroxine dosages by 30% as soon as pregnancy is confirmed.

The increased T_4 dosage requirements during pregnancy are believed to be due to several factors: (1) Rising estrogen levels during pregnancy increase TBG serum concentrations, reducing FT_4 levels. (2) Placental deiodinase promotes the turnover of T_4. (3) Supplemental iron and prenatal multivitamins containing iron can bind to oral T_4 and reduce its intestinal absorption. Similarly, supplemental calcium can also reduce T_4 absorption. Therefore, it is important that patients take their T_4 replacement at least 4 hours before or after such dietary supplements. Postpartum, T_4 replacement requirements ordinarily return to prepregnancy levels.

Elevated serum TSH levels usually indicate underreplacement with levothyroxine. However, before increasing the T_4 dosage, it is wise to (1) confirm that the patient is receiving the prescribed dosage of thyroxine replacement and (2) question the patient about compliance and the presence of angina. It is also important to consider the following: A high TSH in a patient receiving standard replacement doses of T_4 may indicate malabsorption of levothyroxine due to concurrent administration with binding substances, particularly iron preparations, sucralfate, aluminum hydroxide antacids, calcium supplements, and soy milk or soy protein supplements. Bile acid-binding resins such as cholestyramine can bind T_4 and impair its absorption even when administered 5 hours before the T_4. Malabsorption of T_4 can also occur in short bowel syndrome; therapy with medium chain triglyceride oil may improve absorption. Impaired absorption of T_4 can also be caused by diarrhea of any cause or malabsorption due to sprue, regional enteritis, liver disease, or pancreatic exocrine insufficiency. Serum TSH may be elevated transiently in acute psychiatric illness and during recovery from nonthyroidal illness. Autoimmune disease can cause false elevations of TSH by interfering with the assay. A high TSH can also be caused by thyrotropin-secreting pituitary tumors. TSH may be increased by phenothiazines and atypical antipsychotics.

Suppressed serum TSH levels < 0.1 mU/L (using a sensitive assay) may indicate overreplacement with levothyroxine; if such a patient has manifestations of hyperthyroidism, the dosage of levothyroxine is reduced. However, some patients with suppressed serum TSH levels exhibit no symptoms of hyperthyroidism. For such patients, it is important to determine whether hypopituitarism or severe nonthyroidal illness is present, which can result in low serum TSH levels without hyperthyroidism. TSH can also be suppressed by certain medications, such as nonsteroidal anti-inflammatory drugs, opioids, nifedipine, verapamil, and urgent administration of corticosteroids. Absent such conditions, a clinically euthyroid patient with a low serum TSH should be given a lower dosage of levothyroxine. Patients who exhibit hypothyroid symptoms on the reduced dosage of levothyroxine may have their higher dosage resumed, unless they have coronary insufficiency.

Some hypothyroid patients treated with levothyroxine complain of hypothyroid-type symptoms, particularly fatigue, despite having normal or suppressed levels of TSH and normal levels of FT_4. Such patients require careful assessment for other concurrent illnesses such as adrenal insufficiency, hypogonadism, anemia, or depression. If such conditions are treated and hypothyroid-type symptoms persist despite normal or low TSH levels, a serum T_3 level (FT_3 in pregnancy and women receiving oral estrogens) may help make the difficult decision about whether to increase the levothyroxine dose. If the serum T_3 level is low or low normal, such a patient may benefit from a careful increase in T_4 dosage; if a definite clinical benefit is achieved, the higher dose is continued. However, long-term monitoring for atrial arrhythmias and for osteoporosis is recommended for such patients, though such complications are uncommon in those who are clinically euthyroid. The malaise felt by some hypothyroid patients despite apparent optimal replacement therapy with T_4 may be caused by a low concentration of T_3 in certain tissues. Studies adding T_3 to T_4 therapy have not typically shown objective improvement, but patients tend to lose weight and to subjectively prefer combined T_4/T_3 mixtures to T_4 alone. A Dutch double-blind study of 141 hypothyroid patients found that most patients subjectively preferred not T_4 but a combined T_4/T_3 preparation in 5:1 or 10:1 ratios, such that TSH was often suppressed; satisfaction correlated with weight loss.

Prognosis

With early treatment, striking transformations take place both in appearance and mental function. Return to a normal state is usually the rule, but relapses will occur if treatment is interrupted. On the whole, response to thyroid treatment is most satisfactory. However, untreated hypothyroid patients in whom myxedema coma develops have a high mortality rate.

Hypothyroidism caused by interferon-α resolves within 17 months of stopping the drug in 50% of patients. Long-term maintenance therapy with unduly large doses of thyroid hormone can cause symptomatic hyperthyroidism.

Alexander EK et al: Timing and magnitude of increases in levothyroxine requirements during pregnancy in women with hypothyroidism. N Engl J Med 2004;351:241. [PMID: 15254282]

Antonelli A et al: Thyroid disorders in chronic hepatitis C. Am J Med 2004;117:10. [PMID: 15210382]

Appelhof BC et al: Combined therapy with levothyroxine and liothyronine in two ratios, compared with levothyroxine monotherapy in primary hypothyroidism: a double-blind, randomized, controlled clinical trial. J Clin Endocrinol Metab 2005;90:2666. [PMID: 15705921]

Casey BM et al: Subclinical hypothyroidism and pregnancy outcomes. Obstet Gynecol 2005;105:239. [PMID: 15684146]

Danzi S et al: Potential uses of T3 in the treatment of human disease. Clin Cornerstone 2005;(7 Suppl 2):S9. [PMID: 16399246]

Escobar-Morreale HF et al: Treatment of hypothyroidism with combinations of levothyroxine plus liothyronine. J Clin Endocrinol Metab 2005;90:4946. [PMID: 15928247]

Rodriguez I et al: Factors associated with mortality of patients with myxoedema coma: prospective study in 11 cases treated in a single institution. J Endocrinol 2004;180:347. [PMID: 14765987]

Roos A et al: The starting dose of levothyroxine in primary hypothyroidism treatment: a prospective, randomized, double-blind trial. Arch Intern Med 2005;165:1714. [PMID: 16087818]

Tell R et al: Long-term incidence of hypothyroidism after radiotherapy in patients with head-and-neck cancer. Int J Radiat Oncol Biol Phys 2004;60:395. [PMID: 15380571]

Wekking EM et al: Cognitive functioning and well-being in euthyroid patients on thyroxine replacement therapy for primary hypothyroidism. Eur J Endocrinol 2005;153:747. [PMID: 16322379]

HYPERTHYROIDISM (Thyrotoxicosis)

 ESSENTIALS OF DIAGNOSIS

- *Sweating, weight loss or gain, anxiety, loose stools, heat intolerance, irritability, fatigue, weakness, menstrual irregularity.*
- *Tachycardia; warm, moist skin; stare; tremor.*
- *In Graves' disease: goiter (often with bruit); ophthalmopathy.*
- *Suppressed TSH in primary hyperthyroidism; increased T_4, FT_4, T_3, FT_3.*

General Considerations

The term "thyrotoxicosis" refers to the clinical manifestations associated with serum levels of T_4 or T_3 that are excessive for the individual (hyperthyroidism). The causes are many and diverse, as described below.

A. GRAVES' DISEASE

Graves' disease (known as Basedow's disease in Europe) is the most common cause of thyrotoxicosis. It is an autoimmune disorder affecting the thyroid gland, characterized by an increase in synthesis and release of thyroid hormones; the thyroid gland is typically enlarged. Graves' disease is much more common in women than in men (8:1), and its onset is usually between the ages of 20 and 40 years. It may be accompanied by infiltrative ophthalmopathy (Graves' exophthalmos) and, less commonly, by infiltrative dermopathy (pretibial myxedema). The thymus gland is typically hyperplastic and enlarged. Graves' disease may also be associated with other systemic autoimmune disorders such as pernicious anemia, myasthenia gravis, and diabetes mellitus. It has a familial tendency, and histocompatibility studies have shown an association with group HLA-B8 and HLA-DR3. The pathogenesis of the hyperthyroidism of Graves' disease involves the formation of autoantibodies that bind to the TSH receptor in thyroid cell membranes and stimulate the gland to hyperfunction. TSH-R Ab[stim] are demonstrable in the plasma of about 80% of patients with Graves' disease. Other antibodies such as antinuclear antibody (ANA) are generated in Graves' disease, with antithyroperoxidase or antithyroglobulin antibodies being increased in most patients. Patients with Graves' disease have an increased risk of developing Addison's disease, alopecia areata, celiac disease, diabetes mellitus type 1, myasthenia gravis, cardiomyopathy, and hypokalemic periodic paralysis.

B. TOXIC ADENOMAS

Autonomous toxic adenomas of the thyroid may be single (Plummer's disease) or multiple (toxic multinodular goiter). These adenomas are not accompanied by infiltrative ophthalmopathy or dermopathy. Antithyroid antibodies are usually not present in the plasma, and tests for TSH-R Ab[stim] are negative.

C. SUBACUTE THYROIDITIS

Subacute thyroiditis typically presents with a moderately enlarged, tender thyroid, and hyperthyroidism. It is thought to be due to a viral infection. If the gland is nontender, the disorder is called "silent thyroiditis." Hyperthyroidism is followed by hypothyroidism. During thyrotoxicosis, thyroid RAI uptake is low. A similar problem is seen with interleukin-2 therapy and after neck surgery for hyperparathyroidism. Patients taking lithium may rarely experience thyrotoxicosis due to silent thyroiditis. Symptoms mimic a manic episode such that the diagnosis is often missed.

D. JODBASEDOW DISEASE

Jodbasedow disease, or iodine-induced hyperthyroidism, may occur in patients with multinodular goiters after intake of large amounts of iodine in the diet or in the form of radiographic contrast materials or drugs, especially amiodarone.

E. THYROTOXICOSIS FACTITIA

Thyrotoxicosis factitia is due to ingestion of excessive amounts of exogenous thyroid hormone. Isolated epidemics of thyrotoxicosis have been caused by consumption of ground beef contaminated with bovine thyroid gland.

F. STRUMA OVARII

Thyroid tissue is contained in about 3% of ovarian dermoid tumors and teratomas. This thyroid tissue may autonomously secrete thyroid hormone due to a toxic nodule or in concert with the woman's thyroid gland in Graves' disease or toxic multinodular goiter.

G. PITUITARY TUMOR

TSH hypersecretion by the pituitary may be caused by a tumor and is a rare cause of hyperthyroidism. Serum TSH is elevated or normal (determined by a sensitive TSH assay) in the presence of true thyrotoxicosis. No ophthalmopathy is present. Antithyroid antibodies and TSH-R Ab[stim] are usually normal. TSH hypersecretion may be caused by a pituitary adenoma, in which case it is known as "neoplastic inappropriate secretion of thyrotropin." The tumor may present as a mass lesion following treatment of hyperthyroidism. The pituitary adenoma is usually removed by transsphenoidal surgery. Larger tumors may require radiation therapy; treatment with a somatostatin analog (octreotide, lanreotide) is also usually effective.

Hyperthyroidism is treated symptomatically with propranolol. This condition may also be due to pituitary hyperplasia, in which case it is known as "nonneoplastic inappropriate secretion of thyrotropin." Pituitary hyperplasia may be detected on MRI scan as pituitary enlargement without a discrete adenoma being visible. This condition appears to be due to a diminished feedback effect of T_4 upon the pituitary. It may be familial, but it can also be caused by prolonged untreated hypothyroidism, especially in youth. Hyperthyroid symptoms are treated with propranolol. Definitive treatment is with radioactive iodine or thyroid surgery.

H. HASHIMOTO'S THYROIDITIS

Hashimoto's thyroiditis may cause transient hyperthyroidism during the initial destructive phase. This is also seen in some patients receiving interferon-α, interferon-β, and interleukin-2.

I. PREGNANCY AND TROPHOBLASTIC TUMORS

Postpartum thyroiditis is common, occurring in 5–9% of women in the first 6 months after delivery. Transient hyperthyroidism results from the release of stored thyroid hormone following damage to the thyroid by thyroperoxidase antibodies whose IgG subclasses activate the complement cascade. The damaged thyroid is then unable to produce thyroid hormone, and hypothyroidism ensues. Most of these women eventually return to a euthyroid state, but one-third of them remain hypothyroid. Therapy is with propranolol during the hyperthyroid phase, followed by T_4 during hypothyroidism. Women with postpartum thyroiditis may experience depression. About 75% of women experience recurrence after a subsequent pregnancy.

Although hCG generally has a low affinity for the thyroid's TSH receptors, very high serum levels of hCG may cause sufficient receptor activation to cause thyrotoxicosis. Mild gestational hyperthyroidism may occur during the first 4 months of pregnancy, when hCG levels are very high. Pregnant women are more likely to have thyrotoxicosis and hyperemesis gravidarum if they have high serum levels of asialo-hCG, a subfraction of hCG with greater affinity for TSH receptors.

Thyrotoxicosis may also be caused by the high serum levels of hCG seen in molar pregnancy, choriocarcinoma, and testicular malignancies.

J. THYROID CARCINOMA

Metastatic functioning thyroid carcinoma is a rare cause of thyrotoxicosis.

K. AMIODARONE-INDUCED THYROTOXICOSIS

Amiodarone is used to treat cardiac arrhythmias. The drug is concentrated in thyroid, adipose tissue, heart, and skeletal muscle and is 38% iodine by weight; its elimination half-life can be as long as 100 days. Among patients in the United States taking amiodarone, hyperthyroidism develops in about 3%; the incidence of hyperthyroidism is higher in Europe and in iodine-deficient geographic areas. Hyperthyroidism can occur 4 months to 3 years after initiation of amiodarone and may develop many months after amiodarone has been discontinued. Thyrotoxicosis may cause angina or a relapse of the cardiac arrhythmia. Since high levels of T_4 and FT_4 are normally seen in patients taking amiodarone, suppressed TSH (sensitive assay) must be present along with a greatly elevated T_4 (> 20 mcg/dL) or T_3 (> 200 ng/dL). (**Note:** *Hypo*thyroidism occurs in an additional 6% of patients receiving amiodarone after 2–39 weeks of therapy.) Amiodarone-induced thyrotoxicosis can occur by various mechanisms.

Type I amiodarone-induced thyrotoxicosis is caused by active elaboration of excessive thyroid hormone and may occur by either of two mechanisms: (1) Free iodine may cause toxic multinodular goiter in iodine-deficient patients with preexisting autonomous thyroid nodules (jodbasedow phenomenon). This is infrequently encountered in iodine-sufficient countries such as the United States. Thyroid RAI uptake ranges from low to high. (2) Excessive free iodine can trigger an immunologic attack on the thyroid; this may cause Graves' disease, commonly with diffuse thyroid enlargement and antithyroid peroxidase antibodies (70%). The presence of proptosis, TSH-R Ab[stim], or thyrotropin-binding inhibitory immunoglobulin (TBII) is diagnostic. Thyroid RAI uptake is usually negligible in the United States; however, up to 80% of such patients in Europe have detectable or normal RAI uptake.

Treatment of type I amiodarone-induced thyrotoxicosis usually requires a prolonged course of methimazole. After two doses of methimazole, iopanoic acid or sodium ipodate may be added to the regimen to further block conversion of T_4 to T_3; the recommended dosage for each is 500 mg orally twice daily for 3 days, followed by 500 mg once daily until thyrotoxicosis is resolved. β-Blockers may be required. Withdrawal of amiodarone does not have a significant therapeutic effect for several months. Therapy with ^{131}I may be successful in some patients with adequate RAI uptake. Thyroidectomy is reserved for resistant cases.

Type II amiodarone-induced thyrotoxicosis is caused by destructive thyroiditis, which releases stored thyroid hormone from damaged cells; hyperthyroidism can last 1–3 months and may be followed by hypothyroidism. Thyroid RAI uptake is very low. Serum levels of interleukin-6 (IL-6) are usually quite elevated. Treatment consists of prednisone plus either iopanoic acid or ipodate sodium (see above). β-Blockers may be required. Withdrawal of amiodarone is not usually necessary. Because the condition is transient, thyroidectomy is rarely required.

Patients are likely to have type I amiodarone-induced thyrotoxicosis if they have a pretreatment history of multinodular goiter or autoimmune thyroid disease, if they have proptosis, or if they have elevated serum levels of antithyroperoxidase or antithyroglobulin antibodies or TSH-R Ab[stim]. A thyroid RAI uptake is not usually obtained in the United States but may be useful elsewhere. It may be necessary to obtain a thyroid ultrasound with color flow Doppler sonography. Ultrasound can usually detect thyroid nodularity characteristic of toxic multinodular goiter. In Graves' disease blood flow is normal or increased, whereas in destructive thyroiditis blood flow is decreased. In practice, the accuracy of this test depends on the proficiency of the ultrasonographer.

Patients in atrial fibrillation usually require anticoagulation with warfarin; close monitoring of the international normalized ratio (INR) is required, since both methimazole and hyperthyroidism potentiate the hypoprothrombinemia of anticoagulants. Hyperthyroidism increases the catabolism of vitamin K-dependent clotting factors, and methimazole potentiates anti-vitamin K activity. Changing thyroid levels also modify the coagulation profile.

Clinical Findings

A. SYMPTOMS AND SIGNS

Thyrotoxicosis due to any cause produces many different manifestations of variable intensity among different individuals. Patients may complain of nervousness, restlessness, heat intolerance, increased sweating, fatigue, weakness, muscle cramps, frequent bowel movements, or weight change (usually loss). There may be palpitations or angina pectoris. Women frequently report menstrual irregularities.

Hypokalemic periodic paralysis occurs in about 15% of Asian or Native American men with thyrotoxicosis. It usually presents abruptly with paralysis (and few thyrotoxic symptoms), often after intravenous dextrose, oral carbohydrate, or vigorous exercise. Attacks last 7–72 hours.

Signs of thyrotoxicosis may include stare and lid lag, fine resting finger tremors, moist warm skin, hyperreflexia, fine hair, and onycholysis. Chronic thyrotoxicosis may cause osteoporosis. A minority of patients develop clubbing and swelling of the fingers (acropachy). Graves' disease usually presents with additional findings of goiter (often with a bruit), but some patients have no palpable thyroid enlargement.

Cardiac manifestations of thyrotoxicosis commonly include a forceful heart beat, premature atrial contractions, and sinus tachycardia. Atrial fibrillation or atrial tachycardia occurs in about 8% of patients with thyrotoxicosis, more commonly in men, the elderly, and those with ischemic or valvular heart disease. Thyrotoxicosis itself can cause a thyrotoxic cardiomyopathy, and the onset of atrial fibrillation can precipitate congestive heart failure.

Ophthalmopathy is clinically apparent in 20–40% of patients with Graves' disease, but in no other condition causing hyperthyroidism. It usually consists of chemosis, conjunctivitis, and mild exophthalmos (proptosis). More severe lymphocytic infiltration of the eye muscles occurs in 5–10%, pushing the eye forward, producing clinical exophthalmos and sometimes diplopia due to extraocular muscle entrapment. The optic nerve may be compressed in severe cases, causing progressive loss of color vision, visual fields, and visual acuity. Corneal drying may occur with inadequate lid closure. Eye changes may sometimes be asymmetric or unilateral. The severity of the eye disease is not closely correlated with the severity of the thyrotoxicosis. Some patients with Graves' ophthalmopathy are clinically euthyroid.

Exophthalmometry should be performed on all patients with Graves' disease to document their degree of exophthalmos and detect progression of orbitopathy. The protrusion of the eye beyond the orbital rim is measured with a prism instrument (Hertel exophthalmometer). Maximum normal eye protrusion varies between kindreds and races, being about 22 mm for blacks, 20 mm for whites, and 18 mm for Asians.

Diplopia can also be caused by coexistent ocular **myasthenia gravis**, which is more common in Graves' disease and is usually mild, often with selective eye involvement. Acetylcholinesterase receptor antibody (AChR Ab) levels are elevated in only 36% of such patients, and a thymoma is present in 9%.

Graves' dermopathy (pretibial myxedema) occurs in about 3% of patients with Graves' disease, usually in the pretibial region. Glycosaminoglycan accumulation and lymphoid infiltration occur in affected skin, which becomes erythematous with a thickened, rough texture.

Thyroid acropachy is an extreme and unusual manifestation of Graves' disease. It presents with digital clubbing, swelling of fingers and toes, and a periosteal reaction of extremity bones. It is ordinarily associated with ophthalmopathy and thyroid dermopathy. Most patients are smokers. The presence of thyroid acropachy is an indication of the severity of the autoimmunity; most patients have high serum titers of thyroid-stimulating immunoglobulin. Patients with thyroid acropachy are at greater risk for having concurrent Graves' dermopathy and severe ophthalmopathy. However, acropachy itself does not usually cause clinical complaints.

B. LABORATORY FINDINGS

Serum T_3, T_4, thyroid resin uptake, and FT_4 are usually all increased. Sometimes the T_4 level may be normal but the serum T_3 is elevated. Blood that is to be assayed for serum T_3 should be collected in tubes without a gel barrier, which can cause false elevations in serum T_3 in certain assays. A reliable sensitive TSH assay is the best test for thyrotoxicosis; it is suppressed except in the very rare cases of pituitary inappropriate secretion of thyrotropin. Other laboratory abnormalities may include hypercalcemia, increased alkaline phosphatase, anemia, and decreased granulocytes.

TSH-R Ab[stim] levels are usually high (75%). Second-generation TSH-R Ab assays using human recombinant TSH-R are more sensitive for Graves' disease. Antithyroglobulin or antithyroperoxidase antibodies are usually elevated in Graves' disease but are nonspecific. Serum ANA and anti-double-stranded DNA antibodies are also usually elevated without any evidence of lupus erythematosus or other collagen-vascular disease.

Patients with subacute thyroiditis often have an increased erythrocyte sedimentation rate.

Thyroid RAI uptake and scan is usually performed on patients with an established diagnosis of thyrotoxicosis. A high RAI uptake is seen in Graves' disease and toxic nodular goiter but can be seen in other conditions as well. A low radioactive iodine uptake is characteristic of subacute thyroiditis but can also be seen in other conditions. (For conditions affecting radioactive iodine uptake, see section on tests of thyroid function.)

C. IMAGING

MRI of the orbits is the imaging method of choice to visualize Graves' ophthalmopathy affecting the extraocular muscles. CT scanning and ultrasound can also be used. Imaging is required only in severe cases or in euthyroid exophthalmos that must be distinguished from orbital tumors or other disorders.

Differential Diagnosis

True thyrotoxicosis must be distinguished from those conditions elevating serum T_4 without affecting clinical status (see Table 26–6). Serum T_3 can be misleadingly elevated when blood is collected in tubes using a gel barrier, which causes certain immunoassays (eg, Immulite but not Axsym analyzers) to report serum total T_3 levels that are falsely elevated in 24% of normal patients.

Hyperthyroidism may be confused with anxiety neurosis or mania, but in the latter, the thyroid is not enlarged and thyroid function tests are usually normal. Problems of diagnosis occur in patients with acute psychiatric disorders, about 30% of whom have hyperthyroxinemia without thyrotoxicosis. The TSH is not suppressed, distinguishing psychiatric disorder from true hyperthyroidism. T_4 levels return to normal gradually.

Exogenous thyroid administration will present the same laboratory features as thyroiditis. A rare pituitary tumor may resemble thyrotoxicosis with high levels of TSH.

Some states of hypermetabolism without thyrotoxicosis—notably severe anemia, leukemia, polycythemia, and cancer—rarely cause confusion. Pheochromocytoma is often associated with hypermetabolism, tachycardia, weight loss, and profuse sweating. Acromegaly may also produce tachycardia, sweating, and thyroid enlargement. Appropriate laboratory tests will easily distinguish these entities.

Cardiac disease (eg, atrial fibrillation, angina) refractory to treatment suggests the possibility of underlying ("apathetic") hyperthyroidism. Other causes of ophthalmoplegia (eg, myasthenia gravis) and exophthalmos (eg, orbital tumor, pseudotumor) must be considered. Thyrotoxicosis must also be considered in the differential diagnosis of muscle weakness and osteoporosis. Diabetes mellitus and Addison's disease may coexist with thyrotoxicosis.

Complications

Cardiac complications of thyrotoxicosis include atrial fibrillation with a ventricular response that is difficult to control. Episodes of periodic paralysis induced by exercise or heavy carbohydrate ingestion and accompanied by hypokalemia may complicate thyrotoxicosis in Asian or Native American men. Hypercalcemia, osteoporosis, and nephrocalcinosis may occur. Decreased libido, impotence, decreased sperm count, and gynecomastia may be noted in men with hyperthyroidism.

Patients who have "subclinical hyperthyroidism" (suppressed TSH but normal FT_4 and clinically euthyroid) generally do well without treatment. In most such patients, serum TSH reverts to normal within 2 years. No accelerated bone loss has been noted. In one series, one of seven patients with subclinical hyperthyroidism developed clinical hyperthyroidism after about 2 years.

Treatment

The methods used to treat thyrotoxicosis will vary according to the cause and severity of the hyperthyroidism, the patient's age, the clinical situation, and the desires of the patient.

A. Graves' Disease

The treatment of Graves' disease involves a choice of methods rather than a method of choice.

1. Propranolol—Propranolol is generally used for symptomatic relief until the hyperthyroidism is resolved. It effectively relieves the tachycardia, tremor, diaphoresis, and anxiety that occur with hyperthyroidism due to any cause. It is the initial treatment of choice for thyroid storm. The periodic paralysis seen in association with thyrotoxicosis is also effectively treated with β-blockade. It has no effect on thyroid hormone secretion. Treatment is usually begun with propranolol 20 mg orally, which is increased progressively until an adequate response is achieved, usually 20–40 mg four times daily. Doses as high as 80 mg four times daily are occasionally required. A long-acting (LA) propranolol formulation is available that provides more consistent relief; doses are 60, 80, 120, and 160 mg. Propranolol LA is initially given every 12 hours for patients with severe hyperthyroidism, due to accelerated metabolism of the propranolol; it may be given once daily as hyperthyroidism improves.

2. Thiourea drugs—Methimazole or propylthiouracil is generally used for young adults or patients with mild thyrotoxicosis, small goiters, or fear of isotopes. Carbimazole is another thiourea, available outside the United States, that is converted to methimazole in vivo. Aged patients usually respond particularly well. They may be administered long-term. These drugs are also useful for preparing hyperthyroid patients for surgery and elderly patients for radioactive iodide treatment. The drugs do not permanently damage the thyroid and are associated with a lower chance of posttreatment hypothyroidism (compared with radioactive iodide or surgery). Thioureas are usually continued for 12–24 months before being discontinued. When thiourea therapy is discontinued, there is a high recurrence rate for hyperthyroidism (about 50%). A better likelihood of long-term remission is seen in patients with small goiters or mild hyperthyroidism and those requiring small doses of thiourea. Patients whose

thyroperoxidase and thyroglobulin antibodies remain high after 2 years of therapy have been reported to have only a 10% rate of relapse. Thiourea therapy may be continued long-term for patients who are tolerating it well.

Agranulocytosis occurs in about 0.3% of patients taking methimazole and about 0.4% of patients taking propylthiouracil. Agranulocytosis usually occurs in the first 60 days of therapy, and it develops in a few patients after 5 months of therapy. There is a genetic tendency to develop agranulocytosis with thiourea therapy; if a close relative has had this adverse reaction, other therapies should be considered for the patient. Patients are warned that if a sore throat or febrile illness develops, they should stop the drug while a WBC is rechecked. The agranulocytosis is generally reversible; recovery is not improved by filgrastim (granulocyte colony-stimulating factor [G-CSF]). Periodic surveillance of the WBC during treatment has been advocated, but the onset of agranulocytosis is generally abrupt.

Other side effects common to thiourea drugs include pruritus, allergic dermatitis, nausea, and dyspepsia. Antihistamines may control mild pruritus without discontinuation of the drug. Since the two thiourea drugs are similar, patients who have had a major allergic reaction from one should not be given the other.

Primary hypothyroidism may occur. The patient may become clinically hypothyroid for 2 weeks or more before TSH levels rise, having been suppressed by the preceding hyperthyroidism. Therefore, the patient's changing thyroid status is best monitored clinically and with serum levels of FT_4. Rapid growth of the goiter usually occurs if prolonged hypothyroidism is allowed to develop; the goiter may sometimes become massive but usually regresses rapidly with thyroid hormone replacement.

a. Methimazole—Methimazole has the advantage of requiring less frequent dosing and fewer pills than propylthiouracil. Patients treated with methimazole (compared with those taking propylthiouracil) have a lower risk of developing fulminant hepatic necrosis; methimazole therapy is also less likely to cause ^{131}I treatment failure. Rare complications peculiar to methimazole include serum sickness, cholestatic jaundice, loss of taste, alopecia, nephrotic syndrome, and hypoglycemia. Methimazole is given orally in initial doses of 30–60 mg once daily; it may also be administered twice daily to reduce the likelihood of gastrointestinal upset. The dosage is reduced as manifestations of hyperthyroidism resolve and as the FT_4 level falls toward normal. Methimazole is discontinued 4 days prior to ^{131}I therapy for Graves' disease and resumed at a lower dose 3 days after ^{131}I therapy to avoid recurrence of hyperthyroidism. About 4 weeks after ^{131}I therapy, methimazole may be discontinued if the patient is euthyroid.

b. Propylthiouracil—Propylthiouracil is the drug of choice during breast-feeding or pregnancy, possibly causing fewer problems in the newborn. Rare complications peculiar to propylthiouracil include arthritis, lupus erythematosus, aplastic anemia, thrombocytopenia, and hypoprothrombinemia. Acute hepatitis occurs rarely and is treated with prednisone but may progress to liver failure. Propylthiouracil is given orally in initial doses of 300–600 mg daily in four divided doses. The dosage and frequency of administration are reduced as symptoms of hyperthyroidism resolve and the FT_4 level approaches normal. During pregnancy, the dose of propylthiouracil is kept below 200 mg/d to avoid goitrous hypothyroidism in the infant.

3. Iodinated contrast agents—These agents provide effective temporary treatment for thyrotoxicosis of any cause. Iopanoic acid (Telepaque) or ipodate sodium (Bilivist, Oragrafin) is given orally in a dosage of 500 mg twice daily for 3 days, then 500 mg once daily. These agents inhibit peripheral 5′-monodeiodination of T_4, thereby blocking its conversion to active T_3. Within 24 hours, serum T_3 levels fall an average of 62%. For patients with Graves' disease, methimazole is begun first to block iodine organification; the next day, ipodate sodium or iopanoic acid may be added. The iodinated contrast agents are particularly useful for patients who are very symptomatically thyrotoxic (see Thyroid Storm, below). They offer a therapeutic option for patients with T_4 overdosage, subacute thyroiditis, and amiodarone-induced thyrotoxicosis and for those intolerant to thioureas and for newborns with thyrotoxicosis (due to maternal Graves' disease). Treatment periods of 8 months or more are possible, but efficacy tends to wane with time. In Graves' disease, thyroid RAI uptake may be suppressed during treatment but typically returns to pretreatment uptake by 7 days after discontinuation of the drug, allowing ^{131}I treatment.

4. Radioactive iodine (^{131}I)—The administration of RAI is an excellent method of destroying overactive thyroid tissue (either diffuse or toxic nodular goiter). The RAI damages the cells that concentrate it. There are ample data to conclude that patients who are treated with RAI in adulthood do not have an increased risk of subsequent thyroid cancer, leukemia, or other malignancies. Similarly, individuals who were treated with RAI as teenagers have not shown any increased risk of malignancy in a 36-year retrospective study. Children born to parents previously treated with ^{131}I show normal rates of congenital abnormalities.

Because fetal radiation is harmful, *RAI should not be given to pregnant women.* It is prudent to obtain a sensitive pregnancy test (serum β-hCG) on all women of reproductive age prior to ^{131}I therapy.

Most patients may receive ^{131}I while being symptomatically treated with just propranolol, which is then reduced in dosage as hyperthyroxinemia resolves. However, some patients (those with coronary diseases, the elderly, or those with severe hyperthyroidism) are usually rendered euthyroid with a thiouracil drug (see above) while the dosage of propranolol is reduced. Treatment with methimazole is discontinued for about 1 week prior to ^{131}I therapy. A higher rate of ^{131}I treatment failure has been reported in patients with Graves' disease who have been receiving methimazole or propylthioura-cil. However, therapy with ^{131}I will usually be effective if the methimazole is discontinued about 6 days before RAI therapy and if the therapeutic dosage of ^{131}I is adjusted (upward) according to ^{123}I uptake on the pretherapy scan.

Following ^{131}I treatment for hyperthyroidism, Graves' ophthalmopathy appears or worsens in 15% of patients and improves in none, whereas during treatment with methimazole, ophthalmopathy worsens in 3% and improves in 2% of patients. Among patients receiving 3 months of prednisone following ^{131}I treatment, preexistent ophthalmopathy worsens in none and improves in 67%.

Smoking increases the risk of having a flare in ophthalmopathy following ^{131}I treatment and also reduces the effectiveness of prednisone treatment. Therefore, patients who smoke are strongly encouraged to quit prior to ^{131}I treatment.

FT_4 levels may sometimes drop within 2 months after ^{131}I treatment, but then rise again to thyrotoxic levels, at which time thyroid RAI uptake is low. This phenomenon is caused by a release of stored thyroid hormone from injured thyroid cells and does not indicate a treatment failure. In fact, serum FT_4 then falls abruptly to hypothyroid levels.

There is a high incidence of hypothyroidism several years after ^{131}I even when small doses are given. However, hypothyroidism also occurs quite frequently years after surgical or medical treatment of Graves' disease, and eventual hypothyroidism may be part of the natural history of this condition. Lifelong clinical follow-up is mandatory, with measurements of FT_4 and TSH when indicated.

5. Thyroid surgery—Thyroid surgery for Graves' disease and toxic nodular goiter has been performed less frequently as RAI treatment has become more widely accepted. Thyroidectomy may be performed for pregnant women whose thyrotoxicosis is not controlled with low doses of thioureas, and for women who desire to become pregnant in the very near future. Children with Graves' disease usually undergo thyroidectomy. Surgery is also an option for nodular goiters, when there is a suspicion for malignancy. The Hartley–Dunhill operation is the surgical procedure of choice for patients with Graves' disease; this operation consists of a total resection of one lobe and a subtotal resection of the other lobe, leaving about 4 g of thyroid tissue. Subtotal thyroidectomy of both lobes is often used, but ultimately results in a 9% recurrence rate for hyperthyroidism. Total thyroidectomy of both lobes poses an increased risk for hypoparathyroidism and damage to the recurrent laryngeal nerve.

Patients are ordinarily rendered euthyroid preoperatively with a thiourea drug. Ipodate sodium or iopanoic acid (500 mg orally twice daily) may be used in addition to a thiourea to accelerate the decline in serum T_3. Propranolol is given until the serum T_3 (or free T_3) is normal preoperatively. Thyroid vascularity is reduced by preoperative treatment with either ipodate sodium or iopanoic acid (500 mg twice daily for 3 days) or iodine (eg, Lugol's solution, two or three drops orally daily for several days). If a patient undergoes surgery while thyrotoxic, larger doses of propranolol are given perioperatively to reduce the likelihood of thyroid crisis.

Morbidity includes possible damage to the recurrent laryngeal nerve, with resultant vocal cord paralysis. Hypoparathyroidism also occurs, which means that calcium levels must be checked postoperatively. When a thyroidectomy is performed by a competent, experienced neck surgeon, surgical complications are uncommon. Thyroid surgery should be performed as an inpatient, with at least an overnight observational period.

B. Toxic Solitary Thyroid Nodules

Hyperthyroidism caused by a single hyperfunctioning thyroid nodule may be treated symptomatically with propranolol as in Graves' disease. Definitive treatment is with surgery or RAI. For patients under age 40 years, surgery is usually recommended; patients are made euthyroid with a thiourea preoperatively and given several days of iodine, ipodate sodium, or iopanoic acid before surgery as in Graves' disease (see above). Transient postoperative hypothyroidism resolves spontaneously. Permanent hypothyroidism occurs in about 14% of patients by 6 years after surgery. Patients over age 40 years with a toxic solitary nodule are offered RAI. Permanent hypothyroidism occurs in about one-third of patients by 8 years after RAI. The nodule remains palpable in 50% and may grow in 10% of patients after RAI.

C. Toxic Multinodular Goiter

Hyperthyroidism caused by a toxic multinodular goiter may also be treated symptomatically with propranolol as in Graves' disease. This disorder usually affects older individuals, so RAI is ordinarily selected over surgery as the definitive treatment. Thioureas do reverse hyperthyroidism, but there is a 95% recurrence rate after they are stopped. Older patients who are quite thyrotoxic are rendered nearly euthyroid with methimazole, which is stopped at least 3 days before RAI treatment. Meanwhile, the patient follows a low-iodine diet; this is done to enhance the thyroid gland's uptake of RAI, which may be relatively low in this condition (compared to Graves' disease). Relatively high doses of RAI are usually required; recurrent thyrotoxicosis and hypothyroidism are common, so patients must be followed closely. Surgery is generally reserved for pressure symptoms or cosmetic indications. Patients are prepared for surgery as in Graves' disease (see above).

D. Subacute (de Quervain's) Thyroiditis

Patients with hyperthyroidism due to subacute thyroiditis are treated symptomatically with propranolol. Ipodate sodium or iopanoic acid, 500 mg orally daily, promptly corrects elevated T_3 levels and is continued for 15–60 days until the serum FT_4 level normalizes. The condition sub-

sides spontaneously within weeks to months. Thioureas are ineffective, since thyroid hormone production is actually low in this condition. RAI is ineffective, since the thyroid's iodine uptake is low. Since periods of hypothyroidism may occur following the initial inflammatory episode, patients should have close clinical follow-up, with serum FT_4 measurement when necessary. Prompt treatment of the transient hypothyroidism may reduce the incidence of recurrent thyroiditis. Pain can usually be managed with aspirin or other nonsteroidal anti-inflammatory drugs.

E. Hashimoto's Thyroiditis

Rarely, hyperthyroidism develops as a result of release of stored thyroid hormone during severe Hashimoto's thyroiditis. The thyroperoxidase or thyroglobulin antibodies are usually high, but RAI uptake is low, thus distinguishing it from Graves' disease. This is especially common in postpartum women, in whom it may be transient. Treatment is with propranolol. Patients are monitored carefully for the development of hypothyroidism and treated according to their thyroid status.

F. Treatment of Complications

1. Graves' ophthalmopathy—The risk of having a "flare" of ophthalmopathy following ^{131}I treatment for hyperthyroidism is about 6% for nonsmokers and 23% for smokers. For acute, progressive exophthalmos, intravenous methylprednisolone, begun promptly, is superior to oral prednisone, possibly due to improved compliance. Methylprednisolone is given intravenously, 500 mg weekly for 6 weeks, then 250 mg weekly for 6 weeks. If oral prednisone is chosen for treatment, it must be given promptly in daily doses of 40–60 mg/d orally, with dosage reduction over several weeks. Higher initial prednisone doses of 80–120 mg/d are used when there is optic nerve compression. Prednisone alleviates eye symptoms in 64% of nonsmokers, but only 14% of smokers respond well. Thiazolidinediones (pioglitazone, rosiglitazone) may aggravate ophthalmopathy and should be avoided.

Progressive active exophthalmos may be treated with retrobulbar radiation therapy using a supervoltage linear accelerator (4–6 MeV) to deliver 20 Gy over 2 weeks to the extraocular muscles, avoiding the cornea and lens. Prednisone in high doses is given concurrently. Patients who respond well to orbital radiation include those with signs of acute inflammation, recent exophthalmos (< 6 months), or optic nerve compression. Patients with chronic proptosis and orbital muscle restriction respond less well. Retrobulbar radiation does not cause cataracts or tumors; however, it can cause radiation-induced retinopathy (usually subclinical) in about 5% of patients overall, mostly in diabetics.

For severe cases, orbital decompression surgery may save vision, though diplopia often persists postoperatively. General eye protective measures include wearing glasses to protect the protruding eye and taping the lids shut during sleep if corneal drying is a problem. Methylcellulose drops and gels ("artificial tears") may also help. Tarsorrhaphy or canthoplasty can frequently help protect the cornea and provide improved appearance. Hypothyroidism and hyperthyroidism must be treated promptly.

2. Cardiac complications—

a. Sinus tachycardia—Sinus tachycardia or heart pounding is usually present in thyrotoxicosis. Treatment consists of treating the thyrotoxicosis. A β-blocker (as described above) such as propranolol is used in the interim unless there is an associated cardiomyopathy.

b. Atrial fibrillation—Atrial fibrillation may be the presenting manifestation of hyperthyroidism and may precipitate heart failure. Persistent atrial fibrillation is present in 2.9% of men and 1.4% of women when hyperthyroidism is diagnosed. The incidence of atrial fibrillation in hyperthyroidism increases with age, reaching 8% in patients over age 70 years. Electrical cardioversion is unlikely to convert atrial fibrillation to normal sinus rhythm while the patient is thyrotoxic. Spontaneous conversion to normal sinus rhythm tends to occur in about 56% of patients with achievement of euthyroidism, but that likelihood decreases with age. Elective cardioversion may be used for those patients in whom atrial fibrillation persists for 4 months after resolution of hyperthyroidism. Hyperthyroidism must be treated immediately (see above). Other drugs, including digoxin, β-blockers, anticoagulants, may be required.

*(1) Digoxin—*Digoxin is used to slow a fast ventricular response to thyrotoxic atrial fibrillation; it must be used in larger than normal doses because of increased clearance and an increased number of cardiac cellular sodium pumps requiring inhibition. Digoxin doses are reduced as hyperthyroidism is corrected.

*(2) β-Blockers—*β-Blockers may also reduce the ventricular rate, but they must be used with caution—particularly in patients with cardiomegaly or signs of heart failure—since their negative inotropic effect may precipitate congestive heart failure. Therefore, an initial trial of a short-duration β-blocker should be considered, such as esmolol intravenously. If a β-blocker is used, doses of digoxin must be reduced.

*(3) Anticoagulants—*Anticoagulation is indicated to prevent arterial thromboembolism in thyrotoxicosis-induced atrial fibrillation in the following situations: left atrial enlargement on echocardiogram, global left ventricular dysfunction, recent congestive heart failure, hypertension, recurrent atrial fibrillation, or a history of previous thromboembolism. The doses of warfarin required in thyrotoxicosis are smaller than normal because of an accelerated plasma clearance of vitamin K-dependent clotting factors. Higher warfarin doses are usually required as hyperthyroidism subsides.

c. Heart failure—Heart failure due to thyrotoxicosis may be caused by extreme tachycardia, cardiomyopathy, or both. Very aggressive treatment of the hyperthyroidism is required in either case (see Thyroid Crisis, below). The tachycardia from atrial fibrillation is treated with digoxin as above. Intravenous furosemide is typically required. If tachycardia appears to be the main cause of the failure, β-blockers are administered cautiously as described above.

Congestive heart failure may occur as a result of low-output dilated cardiomyopathy in the setting of hyperthyroidism. It is uncommon and may be caused by an idiosyncratic severe toxic effect of hyperthyroidism upon certain hearts. Cardiomyopathy may occur at any age and without preexisting cardiac disease. β-Blockers and calcium channel blockers are avoided. Emergency treatment may include afterload reduction, diuretics, digoxin, and other inotropic agents while the patient is being rendered euthyroid. Heart failure usually persists despite correction of hyperthyroidism.

d. Apathetic hyperthyroidism—Apathetic hyperthyroidism may present with angina pectoris. Treatment is directed at reversing the hyperthyroidism as well as providing standard antianginal therapy. Coronary angioplasty or bypass grafting can often be avoided by prompt diagnosis and treatment.

3. Thyroid crisis or "storm"—This disorder, rarely seen today, is an extreme form of thyrotoxicosis that may occur with stressful illness, thyroid surgery, or RAI administration and is manifested by marked delirium, severe tachycardia, vomiting, diarrhea, dehydration, and, in many cases, very high fever. The mortality rate is high.

A thiourea drug is given (eg, methimazole, 15–25 mg orally every 6 hours or propylthiouracil, 150–250 mg orally every 6 hours). Ipodate sodium (500 mg/d orally) can be helpful if begun 1 hour after the first dose of thiourea. Iodide is given 1 hour later as Lugol's solution (10 drops three times daily orally) or as sodium iodide (1 g intravenously slowly). Propranolol is given (cautiously in the presence of heart failure; see above) in a dosage of 0.5–2 mg intravenously every 4 hours or 20–120 mg orally every 6 hours. Hydrocortisone is usually given in doses of 50 mg orally every 6 hours, with rapid dosage reduction as the clinical situation improves. Aspirin is avoided since it displaces T_4 from TBG, raising FT_4 serum levels. Definitive treatment with ^{131}I or surgery is delayed until the patient is euthyroid.

4. Hyperthyroidism and pregnancy—The prevalence of hyperthyroidism in pregnancy—most commonly due to Graves' disease—is about 0.2%. Struma ovarii is rare. Diagnosis may be difficult, since normal pregnancy may be accompanied by tachycardia, warm skin, heat intolerance, increased sweating, and a palpable thyroid. Laboratory tests are helpful: The FT_4 is clearly elevated, while the TSH is suppressed. However, apparent lack of full TSH suppression can be seen due to misidentification of hCG as TSH in certain assays. Although the total T_4 is elevated in most pregnant women, values over 20 mcg/dL are encountered only in hyperthyroidism. The T_3 resin uptake, which is low in normal pregnancy because of high TBG concentration, is normal or high in thyrotoxic subjects. Pregnancy can have a beneficial effect upon the thyrotoxicosis of Graves' disease, with decreasing antibody titers and decreasing FT_4 levels as the pregnancy advances. However, there is an increased risk of thyroid storm, preeclampsia–eclampsia, congestive heart failure, premature delivery, and abruptio placentae. Newborns have an increased risk of intrauterine growth retardation, prematurity, and transient thyrotoxicosis from transplacental transfer of TSH-R Ab[stim]. Pregnant women with hyperthyroidism are treated with methimazole or propylthiouracil in the smallest dose possible, permitting mild hyperthyroidism to occur since it is usually well tolerated. The drug does cross the placenta and rarely may induce TSH hypersecretion and fetal goiter. Thyroid hormone administration to the mother does not prevent hypothyroidism in the fetus, since T_4 and T_3 do not freely cross the placenta. Fetal hypothyroidism is rare if the mother's hyperthyroidism is controlled with small daily doses of propylthiouracil (50–150 mg/d orally) or methimazole (5–15 mg/d orally). Thyroidectomy is reserved for women who are allergic or resistant to antithyroid drugs (usually due to noncompliance) or who have very large goiters.

During lactation, women treated with propylthiouracil secrete very little of it into breast milk. Methimazole is secreted in somewhat higher concentrations in breast milk. However, the use of either propylthiouracil or methimazole during breast-feeding does not significantly affect the infant's thyroid hormone levels, and both drugs are approved for nursing mothers by the American Academy of Pediatrics. No adverse reactions to these drugs (eg, rash, hepatic dysfunction, leukopenia) have been reported in breast-fed infants. Recommended doses are 20 mg or less daily for methimazole and 450 mg or less daily for propylthiouracil. It is recommended that the medication be taken just after breast-feeding.

5. Graves' dermopathy—An uncommon complication of Graves' disease, dermopathy is an abnormal thickening of the skin due to deposition of glycosaminoglycans. It is known as "pretibial myxedema" since it usually occurs in the anterior lower leg, sometimes also including the dorsum of the foot. Treatment involves application of a topical corticosteroid (eg, fluocinolone) with nocturnal plastic occlusive dressings.

6. Thyrotoxic hypokalemic periodic paralysis—Thyrotoxicosis must always be suspected in Asian or Native American men with sudden symmetric flaccid paralysis, hypokalemia, and hypophosphatemia, especially since classic signs of thyrotoxicosis may be lacking. Therapy with oral propranolol, 3 mg/kg, normalizes the serum potassium and phosphate levels and reverses the paralysis within 2–3 hours. No intravenous potassium or phosphate is ordinarily required. Intravenous dextrose and oral carbohydrate aggravate the condition and are to be avoided. Therapy is continued with propranolol, 60–80 mg every 8 hours (or sustained-action propranolol daily at equivalent daily dosage), along with a thiourea drug such as methimazole to treat the hyperthyroidism.

Prognosis

Graves' disease may rarely subside spontaneously and may even result in spontaneous hypothyroidism. However, it usually persists. The ocular, cardiac, and psychological complications can become very serious and persistent even after treatment. Patients with atrial fibrillation experience a spontaneous remission rate of 56% as thyroid levels decline with treatment. Permanent hypoparathyroidism and vocal cord palsy are risks of surgical thyroidectomy. Recurrences are common following thiourea therapy but also occur after low-dose ^{131}I therapy or subtotal thyroidectomy. With adequate treatment and long-term follow-up, the results are usually good. However, despite treatment for their hyperthyroidism, women experience an increased long-term risk of death from thyroid disease, cardiovascular disease, stroke, and fracture of the femur. Posttreatment hypothyroidism is common. It may occur within a few months or up to several years after RAI therapy or subtotal thyroidectomy. Malignant exophthalmos has a poor prognosis unless treated aggressively.

Subclinical hyperthyroidism refers to asymptomatic individuals with a low serum TSH and normal FT_4 and T_3. Such patients generally do not progress to overt thyrotoxicosis. However, they may be at some increased risk for bone loss, so bone densitometry is performed periodically. In persons over age 60 years, serum TSH is very low (< 0.1 mU/L) in 3% and mildly low (0.1–0.4 mU/L) in 9%. The chance of developing atrial fibrillation is 2.8% yearly in elderly patients with very low TSH and 1.1% yearly in those with mildly low TSH. Asymptomatic persons with very low TSH are followed closely but are not treated unless they develop atrial fibrillation or other manifestations of hyperthyroidism.

Azizi F et al: Effect of long-term continuous methimazole treatment of hyperthyroidism: comparison with radioiodine. Eur J Endocrinol 2005;152:695. [PMID: 15879354]

Chi SY et al: A prospective, randomized comparison of bilateral subtotal thyroidectomy versus unilateral total and contralateral subtotal thyroidectomy for Graves' disease. World J Surg 2005;29:160. [PMID: 15650802]

Cooper DS: Antithyroid drugs. N Engl J Med 2005;352:905. [PMID: 15745981]

Diez JJ: Goiter in adult patients aged 55 years and older: etiology and clinical features in 634 patients. J Gerontol A Biol Sci Med Sci 2005;60:920. [PMID: 16079218]

He CT et al: Comparison of single daily dose of methimazole and propylthiouracil in the treatment of Graves' hyperthyroidism. Clin Endocrinol (Oxf) 2004;60:676. [PMID: 15163329]

Holm IA et al: Smoking and other lifestyle factors and the risk of Graves' hyperthyroidism. Arch Intern Med 2005;165:1606. [PMID: 16043678]

Kahaly GJ et al: Randomized, single blind trial of intravenous versus oral steroid monotherapy in Graves' orbitopathy. J Clin Endocrinol Metab 2005;90:5234. [PMID: 15998777]

McKeown NJ et al: Hyperthyroidism. Emerg Med Clin North Am 2005;23:669. [PMID: 15982540]

Migneco A et al: Management of thyrotoxic crisis. Eur Rev Med Pharmacol Sci 2005;9:69. [PMID: 15850146]

Panzer C et al: Rapid preparation for severe hyperthyroid Graves' disease. J Clin Endocrinol Metab 2004;89:2142. [PMID: 15126532]

Wakelkamp IM et al: Orbital irradiation for Graves' ophthalmopathy: is it safe? A long-term follow-up study. Ophthalmology 2004;111:1557. [PMID: 15288988]

Woeber KA: Observations concerning the natural history of subclinical hyperthyroidism. Thyroid 2005;15:687. [PMID: 16053385]

THYROIDITIS

ESSENTIALS OF DIAGNOSIS

- Swelling of thyroid gland, sometimes causing pressure symptoms in acute and subacute forms; painless enlargement and rubbery firmness in chronic form.
- Thyroid function tests variable.
- Serum antithyroperoxidase and antithyroglobulin antibody levels usually elevated in Hashimoto's thyroiditis.

General Considerations

Thyroiditis may be classified as follows: (1) chronic lymphocytic ("Hashimoto's") thyroiditis due to autoimmunity, (2) subacute thyroiditis, (3) suppurative thyroiditis, and (4) Riedel's thyroiditis.

Hashimoto's thyroiditis (also known as chronic lymphocytic or autoimmune thyroiditis) is an autoimmune condition and the most common thyroid disorder in the United States. Elevated serum levels of antithyroid antibodies are found in 3% of men and 13% of women. Women over the age of 60 years have a 25% incidence of elevated serum levels of antithyroid antibodies. The incidence of Hashimoto's thyroiditis varies by kindred and by race; in persons older than 12 years of age in the United States, elevated levels of antithyroid antibodies are found in 14.3% of whites, 10.9% of Mexican-Americans, and 5.3% of blacks. Subclinical thyroiditis is extremely common, as evidenced in autopsy series that have found focal thyroiditis in about 40% of women and 20% of men. However, only 1% of the population has serum antithyroid antibody titers greater than 1:6400.

Hashimoto's thyroiditis tends to be familial and is six times more common in women than in men. Its frequency is increased by dietary iodine supplementation. Certain drugs (amiodarone, interferon-α, interferon-β, interleukin-2, G-CSF) frequently induce thyroid autoantibodies. Childhood or occupational exposure to head–neck external beam radiation increases the lifetime risk of Hashimoto's thyroiditis.

Hashimoto's thyroiditis often progresses to hypothyroidism, which is usually permanent, remitting in fewer than 5% of cases. The development of hypothyroidism may be linked to thyrotropin receptor–blocking antibodies, which are detected in 10% of patients with Hashimoto's thyroiditis. Among patients with Hashimoto's thyroiditis, hypothyroidism is more likely to develop in smokers than in nonsmokers, possibly due to the thiocyanates found in cigarette smoke. High serum levels of thyroid peroxidase antibody also predict progression from subclinical hypothyroidism to symptomatic hypothyroidism.

Uncommonly, Hashimoto's thyroiditis causes acute destruction of thyroid tissue and release of stored thyroid hormone, causing transient thyrotoxicosis. Rarely, a hypofunctioning gland may become hyperfunctioning with the onset of coexistent Graves' disease; in patients with Graves' disease, Hashimoto's thyroiditis is usually present concurrently.

Clinical Findings

A. SYMPTOMS AND SIGNS

1. Hashimoto's thyroiditis—The thyroid gland is usually diffusely enlarged, firm, and finely nodular. One thyroid lobe may be asymmetrically enlarged, raising concerns about neoplasm. Patients with Hashimoto's thyroiditis who have a thyroid nodule should have an ultrasound-guided FNA biopsy, since the risk of concurrent papillary thyroid cancer is about 8% in such patients. Although patients may complain of neck tightness, pain and tenderness are not usually present. About 10% of cases are atrophic, the gland being fibrotic, particularly in elderly women.

Systemic manifestations of Hashimoto's thyroiditis are mostly related to ambient levels of thyroid hormone. However, depression and chronic fatigue are more common in such patients, even after correction of hypothyroidism. About one-third of patients with Hashimoto's thyroiditis have mild dry mouth (xerostomia) or dry eyes (keratoconjunctivitis sicca) of an autoimmune nature related to Sjögren's syndrome. It may be associated with myasthenia gravis, which is usually of mild severity, mainly affecting the extraocular muscles and having a relatively low incidence of detectable AChR Ab or thymic disease.

Hashimoto's thyroiditis is sometimes associated with adrenal insufficiency (Schmidt's syndrome) and other endocrine deficiencies as part of polyglandular autoimmunity. Thyroiditis is also more common in patients with other autoimmune conditions, such as inflammatory bowel disease or celiac disease (10%). Hashimoto's thyroiditis is very rarely associated with myocarditis, encephalopathy, or membranous nephropathy. Women with gonadal dysgenesis (Turner's syndrome) have a 15% incidence of significant thyroid dysfunction by age 40 years. Thyroiditis is also commonly seen in patients with hepatitis C. Women with Hashimoto's thyroiditis have an increased risk of miscarriage in the first trimester of pregnancy.

Painless postpartum thyroiditis refers to autoimmune thyroiditis that occurs soon after delivery in 7.2%

of women. Women in whom postpartum thyroiditis develops have a 70% chance of recurrence after subsequent pregnancies. It occurs most commonly in women who have high levels of thyroid peroxidase antibody in the first trimester of pregnancy or immediately after delivery. It is also more common in women with other autoimmunity or a family history of Hashimoto's thyroiditis. There is some evidence that the autoimmunity may be triggered by the accumulation of fetal cells in the maternal thyroid during pregnancy, a condition known as microchimerism. Postpartum thyroiditis is typically accompanied by hyperthyroidism that begins 1–6 months after delivery and persists for only 1–2 months. Then, hypothyroidism tends to develop in affected women beginning 4–8 months after delivery. Although 80% of affected women subsequently recover normal thyroid function, permanent hypothyroidism eventually develops in about 50% within 7 years. Permanent hypothyroidism is more common in women who are multiparous or who have had a spontaneous abortion.

Painless sporadic thyroiditis is thought to be a subacute form of Hashimoto's thyroiditis that is similar to painless postpartum thyroiditis except that it is not related to pregnancy. It accounts for about 1% of cases of thyrotoxicosis. Thyrotoxic symptoms are usually mild; a small, nontender goiter may be palpated in about 50% of such patients. High serum thyroid peroxidase antibody concentrations are found in only 50% of such patients. The course is similar to painless postpartum thyroiditis.

2. Subacute thyroiditis—Subacute thyroiditis—also called de Quervain's thyroiditis, granulomatous thyroiditis, and giant cell thyroiditis—is relatively common, accounting for about 5% of clinical thyroid disease. It usually presents as an acute, usually painful enlargement of the thyroid gland, often with dysphagia. The pain may radiate to the ears. Patients usually manifest a low-grade fever and fatigue. The manifestations may persist for weeks or months and may be associated with malaise. In patients who experience pain, it is called "painful subacute thyroiditis." If there is no pain, it is called "silent thyroiditis." Subacute thyroiditis often follows an upper respiratory infection and its incidence peaks in the summer. A viral etiology has been proposed but not firmly established. Thyrotoxicosis develops in 50% of affected patients and tends to last for several weeks. Subsequently, hypothyroidism develops that lasts 4–6 months. Normal thyroid function typically returns within 12 months, but 5% of patients develop persistent hypothyroidism. Young and middle-aged women are most commonly affected.

3. Suppurative thyroiditis—Suppurative thyroiditis is caused by an infection of the thyroid gland, usually bacterial. However, low-grade mycobacterial, fungal, and parasitic (eg, *Pneumocystis jiroveci*) infections have been described, frequently in patients with AIDS. Suppurative thyroiditis is quite rare, since the thyroid is re-sistant to infection, largely due to its high iodine content. Affected patients usually are febrile and have severe pain, tenderness, redness, and fluctuation in the region of the thyroid gland. It tends to affect patients with pre-existent thyroid disease. It is also more likely to affect patients who are immunosuppressed or infirm.

4. Riedel's thyroiditis—Riedel's thyroiditis is also called invasive fibrous thyroiditis, Riedel's struma, woody thyroiditis, ligneous thyroiditis, and invasive thyroiditis. It usually causes hypothyroidism and may cause hypoparathyroidism as well. It is the rarest form of thyroiditis and is found most frequently in middle-aged or elderly women. Enlargement is often asymmetric; the gland is stony hard and adherent to the neck structures, causing signs of compression and invasion, including dysphagia, dyspnea, pain, and hoarseness. It is usually a manifestation of a multifocal systemic fibrosis syndrome, with anterior neck symptoms predominating. Related conditions include retroperitoneal fibrosis, fibrosing mediastinitis, sclerosing cervicitis, subretinal fibrosis, and biliary tract sclerosis. It may respond to therapy with tamoxifen (see Treatment, below).

B. LABORATORY FINDINGS

With hyperthyroidism due to subacute thyroiditis or Hashimoto's thyroiditis, serum FT_4 levels tend to be proportionally higher than T_3 levels, since the hyperthyroidism is due to the passive release of stored thyroid hormone, which is predominantly T_4; this is in contrast to Graves' disease and toxic nodular goiter, where T_3 is relatively more elevated. Because T_4 is less active than T_3, the hyperthyroidism seen in thyroiditis is usually less severe. Serum levels of TSH are suppressed in hyperthyroidism due to thyroiditis.

Thyroid autoantibodies are most commonly demonstrable in Hashimoto's thyroiditis but may also be present in the other types of thyroiditis. Patients with Hashimoto's thyroiditis and clinically evident disease usually have increased circulating levels of antithyroid peroxidase (90%) or antithyroglobulin (40%) antibodies. Antithyroid antibodies decline during pregnancy and are often undetectable in the third trimester. Once Hashimoto's thyroiditis has been diagnosed, monitoring of these antibody levels is not necessary. The serum TSH level is elevated if thyroid hormone is not elaborated in adequate amounts by the thyroid gland.

The erythrocyte sedimentation rate (ESR) is markedly elevated, and antithyroid antibodies are low, which helps differentiate this form of thyroiditis from others. Aspiration biopsy is usually not required but shows characteristic giant multinucleated cells.

In **suppurative thyroiditis,** the leukocyte count and ESR are usually elevated; when suspected, an FNA biopsy with Gram stain and culture is required.

C. IMAGING

Ultrasound in cases of Hashimoto's thyroiditis typically shows a gland with characteristic diffuse heterogeneous density and hypoechogenicity. Ultrasound of the thyroid helps distinguish thyroiditis from multinodular goiter or thyroid nodules that are suspicious for malignancy. Ultrasound is also helpful in guiding FNA biopsy of small suspicious thyroid nodules. Color-flow Doppler ultrasonography can help distinguish thyroiditis from Graves' disease, since patients with Graves' disease have a hypervascular thyroid gland, whereas in thyroiditis there is normal or reduced vascularity.

RAI scan and uptake may be helpful in determining the cause of hyperthyroidism, distinguishing thyroiditis from Graves' disease, since patients with subacute thyroiditis exhibit a very low RAI uptake. In patients with chronic Hashimoto's thyroiditis (euthyroid or hypothyroid), RAI uptake may be normal or high with uneven uptake on the scan; scanning is not useful in making the diagnosis.

Complications

In the suppurative forms of thyroiditis, any of the complications of infection may occur; the subacute and chronic forms of the disease are complicated by the effects of pressure on the neck structures: dyspnea and, in Riedel's struma, vocal cord palsy. Hashimoto's thyroiditis may lead to hypothyroidism or transient thyrotoxicosis. Perimenopausal women with high serum levels of antithyroperoxidase antibodies have a higher relative risk of depression independently of ambient thyroid hormone levels. Graves' disease may sometimes develop. Papillary thyroid carcinoma or thyroid lymphoma may rarely be associated with chronic thyroiditis and must be considered in the diagnosis of uneven painless enlargements that continue in spite of treatment; such patients require FNA biopsy. Hashimoto's thyroiditis may be associated with Addison's disease, hypoparathyroidism, diabetes, pernicious anemia, biliary cirrhosis, vitiligo, and other autoimmune conditions.

Differential Diagnosis

Thyroiditis must be considered in the differential diagnosis of all types of goiters, especially if enlargement is rapid. The very low RAI uptake in subacute thyroiditis with elevated T_4 and T_3 is helpful. Chronic thyroiditis, especially if the enlargement is uneven and if there is pressure on surrounding structures, may resemble carcinoma, and both disorders may be present in the same gland. The subacute and suppurative forms of thyroiditis may resemble any infectious process in or near the neck structures. Thyroid autoantibody tests have been of help in the diagnosis of chronic lymphocytic (Hashimoto's) thyroiditis, but the tests are not specific and may also be positive in patients with multinodular goiters, malignancy (eg, thyroid carcinoma, lymphoma), and concurrent Graves' disease.

Treatment

A. Suppurative Thyroiditis

Treatment is with antibiotics and with surgical drainage when fluctuation is marked.

B. Subacute Thyroiditis

All treatment is empiric and must be continued for several weeks. Recurrence is common. The drug of choice is aspirin, which relieves pain and inflammation. Thyrotoxic symptoms are treated with propranolol, 10–40 mg orally every 6 hours. Iodinated contrast agents cause a prompt fall in serum T_3 levels and a dramatic improvement in thyrotoxic symptoms. Sodium ipodate (Oragrafin, Bilivist) or iopanoic acid (Telepaque) is given orally in doses of 500 mg orally daily until serum FT_4 levels return to normal. Transient hypothyroidism is treated with T_4 (0.05–0.1 mg/d orally) if symptomatic.

C. Hashimoto's Thyroiditis

If hypothyroidism is present, levothyroxine should be given in the usual replacement doses (0.05–0.2 mg orally daily). In patients with a large goiter and normal or elevated serum TSH, T_4 may be given in doses sufficient to suppress serum TSH in an effort to shrink the thyroid. Suppressive doses of T_4 tend to shrink the goiter an average of 30% over 6 months. If the goiter does not regress, lower replacement doses of T_4 may be given. If the thyroid gland is only minimally enlarged and the patient is euthyroid (with normal TSH levels), regular observation is in order, since hypothyroidism may develop subsequently—often years later. (See Hypothyroidism section.)

In one study involving 21 patients with Hashimoto's thyroiditis and subclinical hypothyroidism, simvastatin (20 mg orally daily) improved thyroid function over 8 weeks, possibly by stimulating apoptosis of certain types of lymphocytes. In another study, selenium selenite (200 mcg daily orally for 3 months) reduced the serum levels of antithyroperoxidase antibodies by 49% versus a 10% reduction in the placebo arm. The long-term effectiveness of statins or selenium therapy on the course of Hashimoto's thyroiditis is unknown.

Hyperthyroidism may develop in patients with Hashimoto's thyroiditis due to the release of stored hormone by the thyroid, which is caused by inflammation. This condition has variably been termed "hashitoxicosis" or "painless sporadic thyroiditis;" it is known as postpartum painless thyroiditis when it occurs in women after delivery. Such patients may have only mild thyrotoxicosis and may not require therapy. Patients who are more symptomatic may be treated with propranolol (see Subacute Thyroiditis); they should have a 24-hour ^{123}I thyroid uptake and scan to determine whether Graves' disease may be present. In patients with low RAI uptake, propranolol is continued; sodium ipodate or iopanoic acid may also be given in doses of 500 mg daily orally until the patient is euthyroid to block the peripheral conversion of T_4 to T_3. Patients having low RAI uptake do not respond to thiourea medication. Because RAI is excreted in breast milk, nursing mothers having RAI scanning should always be scanned with ^{123}I, since it is less toxic than ^{131}I; breast milk must be pumped and discarded for 2 days after ^{123}I scanning.

D. RIEDEL'S STRUMA

The treatment of choice for invasive fibrous thyroiditis, like that of its related conditions, is tamoxifen, 20 mg orally twice daily. Tamoxifen can induce partial to complete remissions in most patients within 3–6 months. Tamoxifen treatment must be continued for years. Its mode of action appears to be unrelated to its antiestrogen activity. Short-term corticosteroid treatment may be added for partial alleviation of pain and compression symptoms. Surgical decompression usually fails to permanently alleviate compression symptoms; such surgery is difficult due to dense fibrous adhesions, making surgical complications more likely.

Prognosis

In subacute thyroiditis, spontaneous remissions and exacerbations are common, and therapy is supportive; the disease process may smolder for months. Hashimoto's thyroiditis is occasionally associated with other autoimmune disorders (diabetes mellitus, Addison's disease, pernicious anemia, etc). In general, however, patients with Hashimoto's thyroiditis have an excellent prognosis, since the condition either remains stable for years or progresses slowly to hypothyroidism, which is easily treated. Women with postpartum thyroiditis usually regain normal thyroid function. Papillary thyroid carcinoma carries a relatively good prognosis when it occurs in patients with Hashimoto's thyroiditis.

Gullu S et al: In vivo and in vitro effects of statins on lymphocytes in patients with Hashimoto's thyroiditis. Eur J Endocrinol 2005;153:41. [PMID: 15994744]

Jung YJ et al: A case of Riedel's thyroiditis treated with tamoxifen: another successful outcome. Endocr Pract 2004;10:483. [PMID: 16033720]

Pearce EN et al: Thyroiditis. N Engl J Med 2003;348:2646. [PMID: 12826640]

Smyth PP et al: Sequential studies on thyroid antibodies during pregnancy. Thyroid 2005;15:474. [PMID: 15929669]

Stagnaro-Green A: Postpartum thyroiditis. Best Pract Res Clin Endocrinol Metab 2004;18:303. [PMID: 15157842]

■ THE PARATHYROIDS

The main physiologic effects of parathyroid hormone (PTH) are as follows: (1) It increases the osteoclastic activity in bone, with increased delivery of calcium and phosphorus to the circulation; (2) it increases the renal tubular reabsorption of calcium in the glomerular filtrate; (3) it inhibits the net absorption of phosphate and bicarbonate by the renal tubule; and (4) it stimulates the synthesis of 1,25-dihydroxycholecalciferol by the kidney. All of these steps result in a net increase in the amount of serum ionized calcium. Serum calcium is largely bound to albumin. Therefore, ionized calcium should be determined, or the serum calcium level should be corrected for serum albumin level as follows:

$$\text{"Corrected" serum Ca}^{2+} = \text{Serum Ca}^{2+} \text{ mg/dL} + (0.8 \times [4.0 - \text{Albumin g/dL}])$$

HYPOPARATHYROIDISM & PSEUDOHYPOPARATHYROIDISM

ESSENTIALS OF DIAGNOSIS

- Tetany, carpopedal spasms, tingling of lips and hands, muscle and abdominal cramps, psychological changes.
- Positive Chvostek's sign and Trousseau's phenomenon.
- Serum calcium low; serum phosphate high; alkaline phosphatase normal; urine calcium excretion reduced.
- Serum magnesium may be low.

General Considerations

Hypoparathyroidism is most commonly seen following thyroidectomy, when it is usually transient but may be permanent. It may also occur after surgical removal of a parathyroid adenoma for primary hyperparathyroidism due to suppression of the remaining normal parathyroids and accelerated remineralization of the skeleton (hungry bone syndrome).

Calcium-sensing receptors (CaSR) on parathyroid gland cells sense the serum calcium concentration and alter PTH hormone secretion by way of G-protein-coupled mechanisms. Gain-of-function (constitutive activation) mutations of the *CaSR* gene essentially "fool" the parathyroid glands, resulting in hypocalcemia without elevations in serum PTH hormone levels. Such mutations cause "autosomal dominant hypocalcemia with hypercalciuria" (ADHH) from deficient secretion of PTH hormone. The prevalence of ADHH in the population is about 1 in 70,000 and it typically presents in infancy with hypocalcemic seizures.

Hypoparathyroidism, deafness, and renal dysplasia (HDR or Barakat) syndrome is an autosomal dominant condition caused by haploinsufficiency or mutations of the gene *GATA3*. The hypocalcemia is present from birth but may not be detected until the occurrence of mental retardation or hypocalcemic tetany. The mostly high-frequency deafness is present at birth. Various renal and vesicoureteral anomalies occur.

Hypoparathyroidism may also be seen in DiGeorge's syndrome, along with congenital cardiac and facial anomalies; hypocalcemia usually presents with tetany in infancy, but some cases are not detected until adulthood.

Parathyroid deficiency may also be the result of damage from heavy metals such as copper (Wilson's disease) or iron (hemochromatosis, transfusion hemosiderosis), granulomas, sporadic autoimmunity, Riedel's thyroiditis, tumors, or infection.

Functional hypoparathyroidism may also occur as a result of magnesium deficiency (malabsorption, chronic alcoholism), which prevents the secretion of PTH. Correction of hypomagnesemia results in rapid disappearance of the condition. Hypoparathyroidism may rarely occur after neck irradiation.

Polyglandular autoimmunity type I (PGA-1) is also known as autoimmune polyendocrinopathy-candidiasis-ectodermal dystrophy (APECED). PGA-1 presents in childhood with at least two of the following manifestations: candidiasis, hypoparathyroidism, or Addison's disease. Cataracts, uveitis, alopecia, vitiligo, or autoimmune thyroid disease may also develop.

Fat malabsorption occurs in 20% of patients with PGA-1 and may present as weight loss, diarrhea, or malabsorption of vitamin D, a fat-soluble vitamin used to treat the hypoparathyroidism. The fat malabsorption may be due to a deficiency in the jejunal enteroendocrine cells that produce cholecystokinin, causing a reduction in bile acid secretion.

Pseudohypoparathyroidism is a group of disorders characterized by hypocalcemia due to renal resistance to PTH. There are several subtypes caused by different mutations involving the PTH receptor or its G protein or adenylyl cyclase. PTH levels are high and the PTH receptors in bone are typically not involved, such that bony changes of hyperparathyroidism may be evident. Various phenotypic abnormalities may be associated—classically, short stature, round face, obesity, short fourth metacarpals, ectopic bone formation, and mental retardation. Patients without hypocalcemia but sharing the phenotypic abnormalities are said to have "pseudopseudohypoparathyroidism."

Clinical Findings

A. SYMPTOMS AND SIGNS

Acute hypoparathyroidism causes tetany, with muscle cramps, irritability, carpopedal spasm, and convulsions; tingling of the circumoral area, hands, and feet is almost always present. Symptoms of the chronic disease are lethargy, personality changes, anxiety state, blurring of vision due to cataracts, parkinsonism, and mental retardation.

Chvostek's sign (facial muscle contraction on tapping the facial nerve in front of the ear) is positive, and Trousseau's phenomenon (carpal spasm after application of a cuff) is present. Cataracts may occur; the nails may be thin and brittle; the skin is dry and scaly, at times with fungus infection (candidiasis), and there may be loss of hair (eyebrows); and deep tendon reflexes may be hyperactive. Papilledema and elevated

cerebrospinal fluid pressure are occasionally seen. Teeth may be defective if the onset of the disease occurs in childhood.

B. LABORATORY FINDINGS

Serum calcium is low, serum phosphate high, urinary calcium low, and alkaline phosphatase normal. PTH levels are low. Serum magnesium should be determined since hypomagnesemia frequently accompanies hypocalcemia and may exacerbate symptoms and decrease parathyroid function.

C. IMAGING

Radiographs or CT scans of the skull may show basal ganglia calcifications; the bones may be denser than normal. Cutaneous calcification may occur.

D. OTHER EXAMINATIONS

Slit-lamp examination may show early posterior lenticular cataract formation. The electrocardiogram (ECG) shows prolonged QT intervals and T wave abnormalities. Patients with chronic hypoparathyroidism tend to have increased bone mineral density, particularly in the lumbar spine.

Complications

Acute tetany with stridor, especially if associated with vocal cord palsy, may lead to respiratory obstruction requiring tracheostomy. The complications of chronic hypoparathyroidism largely depend on the duration of the disease. There may be associated autoimmunity causing sprue syndrome, pernicious anemia, or Addison's disease. In long-standing cases, cataract formation and calcification of the basal ganglia are seen. Occasionally, parkinsonian symptoms or choreoathetosis develop. Ossification of the paravertebral ligaments may occur with nerve root compression; surgical decompression may be required. Seizures are common in untreated patients. Overtreatment with vitamin D and calcium may produce nephrocalcinosis and impairment of renal function.

Differential Diagnosis

The symptoms of hypocalcemic tetany may be confused with paresthesias, muscle cramps, or tetany due to respiratory alkalosis, in which the serum calcium is normal. In fact, hyperventilation tends to accentuate hypocalcemic symptoms. Chronic hypocalcemia can cause heart failure and be confused with myocardial infarction and ischemic cardiomyopathy.

At times hypoparathyroidism is misdiagnosed as idiopathic epilepsy, choreoathetosis, or brain tumor (on the basis of brain calcifications, convulsions, choked disks) or, more rarely, as "asthma" (on the basis of stridor and dyspnea). Hypocalcemia is frequently seen in patients with hypoalbuminemia; serum levels of ionized calcium are normal.

Hypocalcemia may also be due to malabsorption of calcium, magnesium, or vitamin D; patients do not always have diarrhea. Hypocalcemia may also be caused by certain drugs: loop diuretics, plicamycin, phenytoin, alendronate, and foscarnet. In addition, hypocalcemia may be seen in cases of rapid intravascular volume expansion or due to chelation from transfusions of large volumes of citrated blood. Hypocalcemia is also frequently seen following parathyroidectomy for hyperparathyroidism. It is also observed in patients with acute pancreatitis. Hypocalcemia may develop in some patients with certain osteoblastic metastatic carcinomas (especially breast, prostate) instead of the expected hypercalcemia. Hypocalcemia with hyperphosphatemia (simulating hypoparathyroidism) is seen in azotemia but may also be caused by large doses of intravenous, oral, or rectal phosphate preparations and by chemotherapy of responsive lymphomas or leukemias.

Hypocalcemia with hypercalciuria may be due to a familial syndrome involving a mutation in the calcium-sensing receptor; such patients have levels of serum PTH that are in the normal range, distinguishing it from hypoparathyroidism. It is transmitted as an autosomal dominant disorder. Such patients are hypercalciuric; treatment with calcium and vitamin D may cause nephrocalcinosis.

Treatment

A. EMERGENCY TREATMENT FOR ACUTE ATTACK (HYPOPARATHYROID TETANY)

This usually occurs after surgery and requires immediate treatment.

1. Airway—Be sure an adequate airway is present.

2. Intravenous calcium gluconate—Calcium gluconate, 10–20 mL of 10% solution intravenously, may be given *slowly* until tetany ceases. Ten to 50 mL of 10% calcium gluconate may be added to 1 L of 5% glucose in water or saline and administered by slow intravenous drip. The rate should be adjusted so that the serum calcium is maintained between 8 mg/dL and 9 mg/dL.

3. Oral calcium—Calcium salts should be given orally as soon as possible to supply 1–2 g of calcium daily. Liquid calcium carbonate (Titralac Plus), 500 mg/5

mL, may be especially useful. The dosage is 1–3 g calcium daily. Calcium citrate contains 21% calcium, but a higher proportion is absorbed with less gastrointestinal intolerance.

4. Vitamin D preparations—(Table 26–10.) Therapy should be started as soon as oral calcium is begun. The active metabolite of vitamin D, 1,25-dihydroxycholecalciferol (calcitriol), has a very rapid onset of action, and if toxicity develops it is not long-lasting. It is of great use in the treatment of acute hypocalcemia. Therapy is commenced at a dosage of 0.25 mcg orally each morning with upward dosage titration to near normocalcemia. Ultimately, doses of 0.5–2 mcg/d are usually required.

Calcifediol (25-hydroxyvitamin D_3), another option for treatment, has an intermediate onset and duration of action; the usual starting dose is 20 mcg/d orally.

Dihydrotachysterol is faster in onset of action and is three times more potent than ergocalciferol. The usual daily maintenance dose is 0.125–1 mg/d orally. It is more expensive than vitamin D_2.

5. Magnesium—If hypomagnesemia is present (chronic alcoholism, malnutrition, renal loss, drugs such as cisplatin, etc), it must be corrected to treat the resulting hypocalcemia. Acutely, magnesium sulfate is given intravenously, 1–2 g every 6 hours. Chronic magnesium replacement may be given as magnesium oxide tablets (600 mg), one or two per day, or as a combined magnesium and calcium preparation (Dolomite, others).

6. Transplantation of cryopreserved parathyroid tissue removed during prior surgery—Transplantation restores normocalcemia in about 23%.

B. MAINTENANCE TREATMENT

The goal should be to maintain the serum calcium in a slightly low but asymptomatic range (8–8.6 mg/dL). This will minimize the hypercalciuria that would otherwise occur and provides a margin of safety against overdosage and hypercalcemia, which may produce permanent damage to renal function. Calcium supplementation (1–2 g/d) is given, along with a vitamin D preparation. Patients with chronic hypoparathyroidism may be treated with vitamin D_2 (ergocalciferol). The usual dose ranges from 25,000 to 150,000 units/d. It is a slow-acting preparation, and if toxicity devel-

Table 26–10. Vitamin D preparations used in the treatment of hypoparathyroidism.

	Available Preparations	Daily Dose	Duration of Action
Ergocalciferol ergosterol, (vitamin D_2, calciferol)	Capsules of 50,000 IU; 8000 IU/mL oral solution	25,000–200,000 units	6–18 weeks
Dihydrotachysterol (DHT)	Tablets and capsules of 0.125, 0.2, and 0.4 mg; 0.2 mg/mL oral solution	0.2–1 mg	1–3 weeks
Calcitriol (Rocaltrol)	Capsules of 0.25 and 0.5 mcg; 1 mcg/mL oral solution; 1 mcg/mL for injection	0.25–4 mcg	$^1/_2$–2 weeks

ops, hypercalcemia—treatable with hydration and prednisone—may persist for weeks after it is discontinued. Ergocalciferol usually produces a more stable serum calcium level than do the shorter-acting preparations. Despite its high cost, calcitriol is being used with increasing frequency for the treatment of chronic hypoparathyroidism; the maintenance dosage of calcitriol ranges from 0.25 mcg/d to 2.0 mcg/d. Monitoring of serum calcium at regular intervals (at least every 3 months) is mandatory.

PTH acts upon the kidney to increase tubular reabsorption of calcium. Therefore, patients with hypoparathyroidism are prone to hypercalciuria and calcium nephrolithiasis during treatment. Target serum calcium levels should be 8–8.6 mg/dL, keeping it mildly low to avoid hypercalciuria. It is prudent to monitor urine calcium with "spot" urine determinations and keep the level below 30 mg/dL if possible. Hypercalciuria may respond to oral hydrochlorothiazide, usually given with a potassium supplement.

Caution: Phenothiazine drugs should be administered with caution to hypocalcemic patients, since they may precipitate extrapyramidal symptoms. Furosemide should be avoided, since it may worsen hypocalcemia.

Prognosis

The outlook is good if the diagnosis is made promptly and treatment instituted. Any dental changes, cataracts, and brain calcifications are permanent. Periodic blood chemical evaluation is required, since changes in calcium levels may call for modification of the treatment schedule. Hypercalcemia that develops in patients with seemingly stable, treated hypoparathyroidism may be a presenting sign of Addison's disease.

Tartaglia F et al: Randomized study on oral administration of calcitriol to prevent symptomatic hypocalcemia after total thyroidectomy. Am J Surg 2005;190:424. [PMID: 16105530]

Tfelt-Hansen J et al: The calcium-sensing receptor in normal physiology and pathophysiology: a review. Crit Rev Clin Lab Sci 2005;42:35. [PMID: 15697170]

HYPERPARATHYROIDISM

ESSENTIALS OF DIAGNOSIS

- *Patients frequently asymptomatic, detected by screening.*
- *Renal stones, polyuria, hypertension, constipation, fatigue, mental changes.*
- *Bone pain; rarely, cystic lesions and pathologic fractures.*
- *Serum and urine calcium elevated; urine phosphate high with low to normal serum phosphate; alkaline phosphatase normal to elevated.*
- *Elevated PTH.*

General Considerations

Primary hyperparathyroidism is characterized by chronic poorly regulated excessive secretion of PTH by one or more parathyroid glands that results in hypercalcemia. It is an increasingly recognized disorder, present in up to 0.1% of adult patients examined. It can be seen at any age but is more frequent in persons over the age of 50 years and is three times more common in women than in men.

The disease is caused by hypersecretion of PTH, usually by a single parathyroid adenoma (80%), and less commonly by hyperplasia by two or more parathyroid glands (20%), or carcinoma (≤ 1%). However, when hyperparathyroidism presents before age 30 years, there is a higher incidence of multiglandular disease (36%) and carcinoma (5%). The size of the parathyroid adenoma correlates with the serum PTH level.

Parathyroid adenomas or hyperplasia can be familial (about 5%) and may be part of MEN types 1, 2A, and 2B. In MEN 1, multiglandular hyperparathyroidism is usually the initial manifestation and ultimately occurs in 90% of affected individuals. Hyperparathyroidism in MEN 2A is less frequent that in MEN 1 and is usually milder. Familial hyperparathyroidism can occur without multiple endocrine neoplasia. It can also occur in the hyperparathyroidism-jaw tumor syndrome, a rare autosomal dominant familial condition in which parathyroid cystic adenomas or carcinomas are associated with ossifying fibromas of the mandible and maxilla as well as renal lesions (cysts, hamartomas, Wilms tumors) (Table 26–11).

Hyperparathyroidism results in the excessive excretion of calcium and phosphate by the kidneys. PTH stimulates renal tubular reabsorption of calcium; however, hyperparathyroidism causes hypercalcemia and an increase in calcium in the glomerular filtrate that overwhelms tubular reabsorption capacity, resulting in hypercalciuria. At least 5% of renal stones are associated with this disease. Diffuse parenchymal calcification (nephrocalcinosis) is seen less commonly. Chronic bone resorption induced by excessive PTH in the circulation may produce diffuse demineralization, pathologic fractures, or cystic bone lesions throughout the skeleton ("osteitis fibrosa cystica").

In chronic renal failure, hyperphosphatemia and decreased renal production of 1,25-dihydroxycholecalciferol $(1,25[OH]_2D_3)$ initially produce a decrease in ionized calcium. The parathyroid glands are stimulated (secondary hyperparathyroidism) and may enlarge, becoming autonomous (tertiary hyperparathyroidism). The bone disease seen in this setting is known as "renal osteodystrophy." Diabetics seem somewhat less prone to develop this syndrome. Hypercalcemia often occurs after renal transplant but usually subsides spontaneously.

Parathyroid carcinoma is a rare cause of hyperparathyroidism but is more common in patients with se-

Table 26–11. Multiple endocrine neoplasia (MEN) syndromes: incidence of tumor types.

Tumor Type	MEN 1 (Wermer's Syndrome)	MEN 2A (Sipple's Syndrome)	MEN 2B
Parathyroid	95%	20–50%	Rare
Pancreatic	54%		
Pituitary	42%		
Medullary thyroid carcinoma		> 90%	80%
Pheochromocytoma		20–35%	60%
Mucosal and gastrointestinal ganglioneuromas		Rare	> 90%
Subcutaneous lipoma	30%		
Adrenocortical adenoma	30%		
Thoracic carcinoid	15%		
Thyroid adenoma	Occasional		
Facial angiofibromas and collagenomas	85%		

vere hypercalcemia. About 50% of parathyroid carcinomas are palpable.

Clinical Findings

A. SYMPTOMS AND SIGNS

Hypercalcemia is typically discovered accidentally by routine chemistry panels. Most patients are asymptomatic. Parathyroid adenomas are usually so small and deeply located in the neck that they are almost never palpable; when a mass is palpated, it usually turns out to be an incidental thyroid nodule.

Although many patients with mild hypercalcemia offer no complaints, symptomatic patients are said to have problems with "bones, stones, abdominal groans, psychic moans, with fatigue overtones." The manifestations are categorized as skeletal, urinary tract, and those associated with hypercalcemia.

1. Skeletal manifestations—Hyperparathyroidism causes a loss of cortical bone and a gain of trabecular bone. Bone mineral concentration tends to be decreased in the distal radius and in the midshaft of the femur but not in the femoral neck. Similarly, bone mineral is decreased in vertebral posterior processes but increased in the vertebral bodies. Significant bone demineralization is uncommon in mild hyperparathyroidism, but osteitis fibrosa cystica may present as pathologic fractures or as "brown tumors" or cysts of the jaw. More commonly, patients have bone pain and arthralgias.

2. Urinary tract manifestations—Polyuria and polydipsia may be present and are due to hypercalcemia-induced nephrogenic diabetes insipidus. Calcium-containing kidney stones are reported in about 18% of those with newly discovered primary hyperparathyroidism. Nephrocalcinosis and renal failure can occur.

3. Manifestations of hypercalcemia—Mild hypercalcemia is often asymptomatic. In more severe cases, thirst, anorexia, nausea, and vomiting are present. Constipation, fatigue, anemia, weight loss, and hypertension are commonly found. Pancreatitis occurs in 3%. Some patients have neuromuscular disorders such as muscle weakness, easy fatigability, or paresthesias. Depression, intellectual weariness, and increased sleep requirement are common. Pruritus and psychosis or even coma may accompany severe hypercalcemia. Calcium may precipitate in the corneas ("band keratopathy") or soft tissue (calciphylaxis).

4. Hyperparathyroidism during pregnancy—About 67% of women with primary hyperparathyroidism during pregnancy experience complications such as nephrolithiasis, hyperemesis, pancreatitis, muscle weakness, cognitive changes, and hypercalcemic crisis. About 80% of fetuses experience complications of maternal hyperparathyroidism, including fetal demise, preterm delivery, low birth weight, postpartum neonatal tetany, and permanent hypoparathyroidism.

B. LABORATORY FINDINGS

The hallmark of primary hyperparathyroidism is hypercalcemia: serum calcium > 10.5 mg/dL or ionized calcium. In hyperproteinemic states, the total serum calcium may be elevated but the ionized fraction is normal, whereas in primary hyperparathyroidism, the ionized calcium is almost always over 5.4 mg/dL (1.4 mmol/L). In practice, serum ionized calcium determinations have not proved to be very helpful clinically. The serum phosphate is often low (< 2.5 mg/dL). The urine calcium excretion may be high or normal (averaging 250 mg/g creatinine) but it is usually low for the degree of hypercalcemia. There is an excessive loss of phosphate in the urine in the presence of hypophosphatemia (25% of cases) to low-normal serum phosphate. (In secondary hyperparathyroidism due to renal failure, the serum phosphate is high.) The alkaline phosphatase is elevated only if bone disease is present. The plasma chloride and uric acid levels may be elevated. Vitamin D deficiency is common in patients with hyperparathyroidism, and it is prudent to screen for vitamin D deficiency with a serum 25-OH vitamin D determination. Low serum 25-OH vitamin D levels (< 20 mcg/L; < 50 nmol/L) can aggravate hyperparathyroidism and its bone manifestations; vitamin D replacement may be helpful in treating patients with hyperparathyroidism. (See below.)

Elevated serum levels of PTH confirm the diagnosis of hyperparathyroidism. The best immunoassay recognizes the intact molecule at two different sites—the amino terminal and the carboxyl terminal ends—with two different antibodies. This assay, known as IRMA, is specific and sensitive, making it easier to distinguish primary hyperparathyroidism from other causes of hypercalcemia.

All patients with apparent hyperparathyroidism should be screened for familial benign hypocalciuric hypercalcemia with a 24-hour urine for calcium and creatinine. Patients should discontinue thiazide diuretics prior to this test. Calcium excretion of < 50 mg/24 hours (or < 5 mg/dL on a random urine) is not typical for primary hyperparathyroidism and indicates possible familial benign hypocalciuric hypercalcemia. (See below.)

C. IMAGING

Preoperative sestamibi-iodine subtraction scanning and neck ultrasonography have been used to locate parathyroid adenomas in patients with hyperparathyroidism, in an effort to improve the outcome and limit the invasiveness of neck surgery. Parathyroid imaging is crucial for patients who have had prior neck surgery. However, the usefulness of preoperative parathyroid localizing imaging studies for first neck explorations remains controversial. Imaging is not useful for the diagnosis of hyperparathyroidism, which must be made by serum calcium and PTH determinations. Preoperative scanning does not improve the outcome of initial bilateral neck explorations performed by a surgeon with special expertise in parathyroid surgery. Therefore, preoperative imaging has been used mainly to improve the outcome for limited neck exploration, with only modest success. See Surgery, below. Small benign thyroid nodules are discovered incidentally in nearly 50% of patients with hyperparathyroidism who have imaging with ultrasound or MRI.

CT and MRI scanning are not ordinarily required or useful for initial preoperative parathyroid localizing studies, since these scanning techniques are less sensitive for identifying tiny parathyroid adenomas. However, for repeat neck operations and when ectopic parathyroids are suspected, MRI is preferred since it offers better soft tissue contrast than CT scanning and is less adversely affected by postoperative changes in the neck. Three-dimensional technetium-99m sestamibi scanning can also help localize ectopic parathyroid glands.

Bone radiographs are usually normal and are not required to make the diagnosis of hyperparathyroidism. There may be demineralization, subperiosteal resorption of bone (especially in the radial aspects of the fingers), or loss of the lamina dura of the teeth. There may be cysts throughout the skeleton, mottling of the skull ("salt-and-pepper appearance"), or pathologic fractures. Articular cartilage calcification (chondrocalcinosis) is sometimes found.

Patients with renal osteodystrophy may have ectopic calcifications around joints or in soft tissue. Such patients may exhibit radiographic changes of osteopenia, osteitis fibrosa, or osteosclerosis, alone or in combination. Osteosclerosis of the vertebral bodies is known as "rugger jersey spine."

Complications

Pathologic fractures are more common in patients with hyperparathyroidism than in the general population. Urinary tract infection due to stone and obstruction may lead to renal failure and uremia. If the serum calcium level rises rapidly, clouding of sensorium, renal failure, and rapid precipitation of calcium throughout the soft tissues may occur. Peptic ulcer and pancreatitis may be intractable before surgery. Insulinomas or gastrinomas may be associated, as well as pituitary tumors (MEN type 1). Pseudogout may complicate hyperparathyroidism both before and after surgical removal of tumors. Hypercalcemia during gestation produces neonatal hypocalcemia.

In secondary hyperparathyroidism due to renal failure, high serum calcium and phosphate levels may cause disseminated calcification in the skin, soft tissues, and arteries (calciphylaxis); this can result in painful ischemic necrosis of skin and gangrene, cardiac arrhythmias, and respiratory failure. The actual serum levels of calcium and phosphate have not correlated well with calciphylaxis, but a calcium (mg/dL) × phosphate (mg/dL) product over 70 is usually present.

Differential Diagnosis

A. ARTIFACT

A report of hypercalcemia may be due to laboratory error or excess tourniquet time and should always be repeated. Hypercalcemia may be due to high serum protein concentrations; in the presence of high or low serum albumin concentrations, a serum ionized calcium is more dependable than the total serum calcium concentration. Hypercalcemia may also be seen with dehydration; spurious elevations in serum calcium have been reported with severe hypertriglyceridemia, when the calcium assay uses spectophotometry.

B. HYPERCALCEMIA OF MALIGNANCY

Many malignant tumors (breast, lung, pancreas, uterus, hypernephroma, etc) can produce hypercalcemia. In some cases (breast carcinoma especially), bony metastases are present. In others, no metastases to bone can be demonstrated. Most of these tumors secrete PTH-related protein (PTHrP), which has tertiary structural homologies to PTH and causes bone resorption and hypercalcemia similar to those of PTH. The clinical features of the hypercalcemia of cancer can closely simulate hyperparathyroidism. Serum phosphate is often low, but the plasma level of PTH by IRMA is *low*. Serum PTHrP may be elevated.

Multiple myeloma is a common cause of hypercalcemia in the older population. Many other hematologic cancers such as monocytic leukemia, T cell leukemia and lymphoma, Burkitt's lymphoma, etc, have also been associated with hypercalcemia. Multiple myeloma causes renal dysfunction; resultant increased levels of carboxyl terminal PTH may cause it to be confused with hyperparathyroidism if a carboxyl terminal PTH assay is used. Serum protein and urine electrophoresis and bone marrow biopsy establish the diagnosis.

C. SARCOIDOSIS AND OTHER GRANULOMATOUS DISORDERS

Macrophages and perhaps other cells present in granulomatous tissue have the ability to synthesize $1,25(OH)_2D_3$. Hypercalcemia has been reported in patients with sarcoidosis, tuberculosis, berylliosis, histoplasmosis, coccidioidomycosis, leprosy, and even foreign-body granuloma. Increased intestinal calcium absorption and hypercalciuria are more common than hypercalcemia. Serum levels of $1,25(OH)_2D_3$ are elevated. In patients with sarcoidosis, serum levels of angiotensin-converting enzyme (ACE) are usually elevated. [18]FDG-PET scanning may localize hypermetabolic foci of active disease. Ketoconazole is an antifungal agent that inhibits macrophage 1-hydroxylation of 25-hydroxyvitamin D, thereby improving the hypercalcemia of sarcoidosis and tuberculosis. In all conditions, treatment is directed at the underlying disorder.

D. CALCIUM OR VITAMIN D INGESTION

Ingestion of large amounts of calcium (usually as an antacid) or vitamin D can cause hypercalcemia, which is reversible following its cessation. If it persists, the possibility of associated hyperparathyroidism should be strongly considered.

In vitamin D intoxication, patients may take large amounts of vitamin D for unclear reasons, so a check of all medications is important. Hypercalcemia may persist for several weeks. Serum levels of 25-hydroxycholecalciferol ($25[OH]D_3$) are helpful to confirm the diagnosis. A brief course of corticosteroid therapy may be necessary if hypercalcemia is severe.

E. FAMILIAL BENIGN HYPOCALCIURIC HYPERCALCEMIA

Familial benign hypocalciuric hypercalcemia can be easily mistaken for mild hyperparathyroidism. It is a common autosomal dominant inherited disorder (prevalence: 1 in 16,000) caused by a loss-of-function mutation in the gene encoding the CaSR. CaSRs are found on the surface of the parathyroid glands and allow the parathyroid glands to vary PTH hormone secretion according to serum PTH levels. Reduced function of the CaSR causes the parathy-

roid glands to falsely "sense" hypocalcemia and inappropriately release slightly excessive amounts of PTH. At the same time, the renal tubule CaSRs are also affected, causing hypocalciuria. Familial benign hypocalciuric hypercalcemia is characterized by hypercalcemia, hypocalciuria (usually < 50 mg/24 h), variable hypermagnesemia, and normal or minimally elevated levels of PTH. These patients do not normalize their hypercalcemia after subtotal parathyroid removal and should not be subjected to surgery. The condition has an excellent prognosis and is easily diagnosed with a family history and urinary calcium clearance determination.

F. ADRENAL INSUFFICIENCY

Hypercalcemia is common in untreated Addison's disease. This is partly due to disinhibition of calcium uptake by the renal tubule and gut. Additionally, Addison's disease can cause dehydration and hyperproteinemia, resulting in higher levels of nonionized calcium.

G. HYPERTHYROIDISM

Increased bone turnover is a feature of thyrotoxicosis. Mild hypercalcemia may also be present.

H. OTHER CAUSES

Other causes of hypercalcemia are shown in Table 21–9. Modest hypercalcemia is also occasionally seen in patients taking thiazide diuretics or lithium; such patients may have an inappropriately nonsuppressed PTH level with hypercalcemia. Prolonged immobilization at bed rest may also cause hypercalcemia, especially in adolescents and patients with extensive Paget's disease of bone. Hypercalcemia is noted in up to one-third of acutely ill patients being treated in intensive care units, particularly patients with acute renal failure. Serum PTH levels are usually slightly elevated, consistent with mild hyperparathyroidism. Bisphosphonates can increase serum calcium in 20% and serum PTH becomes high in 10%, mimicking hyperparathyroidism.

Treatment

A. SURGICAL PARATHYROIDECTOMY

Parathyroidectomy is recommended for patients with symptomatic hyperparathyroidism, kidney stones, bone disease, and pregnancy.

Some patients with seemingly asymptomatic hyperparathyroidism may be surgical candidates for other reasons such as (1) serum calcium 1 mg/dL above the upper limit of normal with urine calcium excretion > 50 mg/24 h (off thiazide diuretics), (2) urine calcium excretion over 400 mg/24 h, (3) cortical bone density (wrist, hip) ≥ 2 SD below normal, (4) relative youth (under age 50–60 years), (5) difficulty ensuring medical follow-up, or (6) pregnancy. During pregnancy, parathyroidectomy is performed in the second trimester.

Patients who undergo surgery for "asymptomatic" hyperparathyroidism have been reported to have modest benefits in social and emotional function, with improvements in anxiety and phobias being reported in comparison to similar patients who are monitored without surgery.

An intraoperative "quick" serum PTH determination is advisable to document the removal of the correct gland; if the serum PTH does not drop to < 50% of the highest preremoval value 10 minutes after removal of an abnormal-looking parathyroid gland, cure is unlikely and the excision is expanded to a bilateral neck exploration. Intraoperative PTH determinations are less helpful at predicting cure in patients with multiple abnormal parathyroid glands when abnormal glands remain in the neck.

Preoperative parathyroid imaging has been used in an attempt to allow unilateral minimally invasive neck surgery. The usefulness of preoperative parathyroid imaging was evaluated in a series of 350 patients with sporadic primary hyperparathyroidism. A single gland was predicted by sestamibi in 83%, by ultrasound in 85%, and by concordance of both in 59% of patients. Unilateral neck exploration, directed by these studies, resulted in success rate of only 73%, 77%, and 82%, respectively, despite the intraoperative quick PTH assay predicting success. Even in patients with concordant sestamibi and ultrasound scans, and an intraoperative PTH drop of > 50%, at least one additional abnormal parathyroid gland is left behind in the contralateral neck in 15% of patients.

Bilateral neck exploration is usually advisable for all patients without preoperative localization studies for the following: (1) patients with a family history of hyperparathyroidism, (2) patients with a personal or family history of MEN, and (3) patients wanting an optimal chance of success with a single surgery. Patients undergoing unilateral neck exploration can have the incision widened for bilateral neck exploration if two abnormal glands are found or if the serum quick PTH falls by < 50%. Parathyroid glands are not uncommonly supernumerary (five or more) or ectopic (eg, intrathyroidal, carotid sheath, mediastinum).

Parathyroid hyperplasia is commonly seen with chronic renal failure. When surgery is performed, a subtotal parathyroidectomy is optimally treated surgically; three and one-half glands are usually removed, and a metal clip is left to mark the location of residual parathyroid tissue.

Parathyroid carcinoma can cause severe hypercalcemia associated with very high serum levels of PTH. Preoperative localizing studies usually detect a large invasive tumor. Therapy consists of en bloc resection of the tumor and the ipsilateral thyroid lobe. Metastases to local and to distant sites occur in about 50% of patients. Reoperation for neck recurrence is usually necessary. Adjuvant treatment includes radiation therapy. Intravenous bisphosphonate (zoledronic acid) and calcimimetic agents (NPS R-568) are used for treatment of hypercalcemia.

Complications: Serum PTH levels fall below normal in 70% of patients within hours after successful surgery, commonly causing hypocalcemic paresthesias or even tetany. Hypocalcemia tends to occur the evening after surgery or on the next day. Therefore, frequent postoperative monitoring of serum ionized calcium (or serum calcium plus albumin) is advisable beginning the evening after surgery. Once hypercalcemia has resolved, liquid or chewable calcium carbonate is given orally to reduce the likelihood of hypocalcemia. Symptomatic hypocalcemia is treated with larger doses of calcium; calcitriol (0.25–1 mcg daily orally) may be added, with the dosage depending on symptom severity. Magnesium salts are sometimes required postoperatively, since adequate magnesium is required for functional recovery of the remaining suppressed parathyroid glands.

In about 12% of patients having successful parathyroid surgery, PTH levels rise above normal (while serum calcium is normal or low) by 1 week postoperatively. This secondary hyperparathyroidism is probably due to "hungry bones" and is treated with calcium and vitamin D preparations. Such therapy is usually needed only for 3–6 months but is required chronically by some patients.

Hyperthyroidism commonly occurs immediately following parathyroid surgery. It is caused by release of stored thyroid hormone during surgical manipulation of the thyroid. Short-term treatment with propranolol may be required for several days.

B. MEDICAL MEASURES

1. Fluids—Hypercalcemia is treated with a large fluid intake unless contraindicated. Severe hypercalcemia requires hospitalization and intensive hydration with intravenous saline. (See Chapter 21.)

2. Bisphosphonates—Intravenous bisphosphonates are potent inhibitors of bone resorption and can temporarily treat the hypercalcemia of hyperparathyroidism, malignancy, or immobilization. They may relieve bone pain as with patients with metastatic breast or prostate cancer. Pamidronate in doses of 30–90 mg (in 0.9% saline) is administered intravenously over 2–4 hours. Zoledronic acid 2–4 mg is administered intravenously over 15 to 20 minutes; it is quite effective but also very expensive. These drugs cause a gradual decline in serum calcium over several days that may last for weeks to months. Such intravenous bisphosphonates are used generally for patients with severe hyperparathyroidism in preparation for surgery. Oral bisphosphonates, such as alendronate, are not effective for treating the hypercalcemia or hypercalciuria of hyperparathyroidism. However, oral alendronate has been shown to improve bone mineral density in the lumbar spine and hip (not distal radius) and may be used for asymptomatic patients with hyperparathyroidism who have a low bone mineral density.

3. Calcimimetics—Cinacalcet hydrochloride is a calcimimetic agent that binds to sites of the parathyroid glands' extracellular calcium-sensing receptors (CaSR) to increase their affinity for extracellular calcium, thereby decreasing PTH secretion. Cinacalcet may be administered orally in doses of 30–250 mg daily. Patients with primary hyperparathyroidism have also been treated successfully with cinacalcet in oral doses of 30–50 mg twice daily, with 73% of patients achieving normocalcemia. Administering cinacalcet for secondary parathyroidism of renal failure causes a drop of serum PTH levels to < 250 pg/mL in 41% of patients receiving dialysis. Cinacalcet is given to patients with severe hypercalcemia due to parathyroid carcinoma at initial doses of 30 mg orally twice daily and increased progressively to 60 mg twice daily, then 90 mg twice daily to a maximum of 90 mg every 6–8 hours. Cinacalcet is usually well-tolerated but may cause nausea and vomiting, which are usually transient. It is very expensive.

4. Vitamin D and vitamin D analogs—

a. Primary hyperparathyroidism—For patients with vitamin D deficiency, careful vitamin D replacement may be beneficial to patients with hyperparathyroidism. Aggravation of hypercalcemia does not ordinarily occur. Serum PTH levels may fall with vitamin D replacement in doses of 400 to 1200 units daily. Occasionally, larger doses are required to achieve normal 25-OH vitamin D levels.

b. Secondary and tertiary hyperparathyroidism associated with renal failure—*Calcitriol,* given orally or intravenously after dialysis, suppresses parathyroid hyperplasia of renal failure. Certain vitamin D analogs suppress PTH secretion but cause less hypercalcemia than calcitriol. *Doxercalciferol* (Hectorol) is administered three times weekly orally with hemodialysis to patients with azotemic secondary hyperparathyroidism in the following doses according to serum immunoradiometric PTH (iPTH) levels: give 10 mcg three times weekly for iPTH > 400 pg/mL and increase the dose by 2.5 mcg every 8 weeks if iPTH remains > 300 pg/mL, to a maximum dose of 20 mcg three times weekly. If iPTH drops to < 100 pg/mL, doxercalciferol is held for 1 week and the dose is reduced by at least 2.5 mcg. *Paricalcitol* (Zemplar) is administered intravenously during dialysis three times weekly in starting doses of 0.04–0.1 mcg/kg body weight; the dosage is increased for iPTH levels > 300 pg/mL to a maximum dose of 0.24 mcg/kg three times weekly; paricalcitol is held if iPTH levels drop to < 100 pg/mL.

5. Other measures—Patients with mild, asymptomatic hyperparathyroidism may be monitored closely medically. Such patients are advised to keep active, avoid immobilization, and drink adequate fluids. They need to avoid thiazide diuretics, large doses of vitamins A, and calcium-containing antacids or supplements. Serum calcium and albumin are checked about twice yearly, renal function and urine calcium once yearly, and three-site bone density (distal radius, hip, and spine) every 2 years.

Estrogen replacement, given to postmenopausal women, reduces hypercalcemia slightly. Similarly, raloxifene (a selective estrogen receptor modulator) also reduces the hypercalcemia of hyperparathyroidism, reducing serum calcium levels an average of 0.4 mg/dL.

Digitalis preparations are avoided, since patients with hypercalcemia are sensitive to its toxic effects. Propranolol may be useful for preventing the adverse cardiac effects of hypercalcemia. Corticosteroid therapy is ineffective for treating hypercalcemia in hyperparathyroidism.

Renal osteodystrophy is caused by secondary hyperthyroidism during renal failure. It can be prevented or delayed by avoiding hyperphosphatemia by dietary avoidance of phosphate and with phosphate binding medication.

C. MONITORING PATIENTS WITH ASYMPTOMATIC PRIMARY HYPERPARATHYROIDISM

Patients with mild asymptomatic hyperparathyroidism may not need therapy. However, they should be monitored closely for the development of symptoms of hypercalcemia and worsening hypercalcemia. Patients should be evaluated every 6 months with determination of blood pressure and serum calcium. Rising serum calcium should prompt further evaluation and determination of PTH levels. Serum creatinine should be measured yearly. A bone density should ideally be determined every 1 to 2 years at 3 points: wrist, hip, and vertebrae.

Prognosis

Completely asymptomatic patients with mild hypercalcemia may be observed and treated medically without compromising survival. There can be unexplained exacerbations and partial remissions. Surgical removal of sporadic parathyroid adenomas generally results in a permanent cure. Patients with MEN 1 undergoing subtotal parathyroidectomy may experience long remissions, but hyperparathyroidism usually recurs.

Spontaneous cure due to necrosis of the tumor has been reported but is exceedingly rare. The bones, in spite of severe cyst formation, deformity, and fracture, will heal if a parathyroid tumor is successfully removed. The presence of pancreatitis increases the mortality rate. Acute pancreatitis usually resolves with correction of hypercalcemia, whereas subacute or chronic pancreatitis tends to persist. Significant renal damage may progress even after removal of an adenoma. Parathyroid carcinoma tends to invade local structures and may sometimes metastasize; repeat surgical resections and radiation therapy can prolong life. Aggressive surgical and medical management of parathyroid carcinoma can result in an 85% 5-year survival rate and a 57% 10-year survival rate.

Block GA et al: Cinacalcet for secondary hyperparathyroidism in patients receiving hemodialysis. N Engl J Med 2004;350:1516. [PMID: 15071126]

Coburn JW et al: Doxercalciferol safely suppresses PTH levels in patients with secondary hyperparathyroidism associated with chronic kidney disease stages 3 and 4. Am J Kidney Dis 2004;43:877. [PMID: 15112179]

Grey A et al: Vitamin D repletion in patients with primary hyperparathyroidism and coexistent vitamin D insufficiency. N Engl J Med 2005;90:2122. [PMID: 15644400]

Lambert LA et al: Surgical treatment of hyperparathyroidism in patients with multiple endocrine neoplasia type 1. Arch Surg 2005;140:374. [PMID: 15841561]

Peacock M et al: Cinacalcet hydrochloride maintains long-term normocalcemia in patients with primary hyperparathyroidism. J Clin Endocrinol Metab 2005;90:135. [PMID: 15522938]

Rao DS et al: Randomized controlled clinical trial of surgery versus no surgery in patients with mild asymptomatic primary hyperparathyroidism. J Clin Endocrinol Metab 2004;89:5415. [PMID: 15531491]

Siperstein A et al: Prospective evaluation of sestamibi scan, ultrasonography, and rapid PTH to predict the success of limited exploration for sporadic primary hyperparathyroidism. Surgery 2004;136:872. [PMID: 15467674]

Skinner MA et al: Prophylactic thyroidectomy in multiple endocrine neoplasia type 2A. N Engl J Med 2005;353:1105. [PMID: 16162881]

■ METABOLIC BONE DISEASE

The term "metabolic bone disease" denotes those conditions producing diffusely decreased bone density (osteopenia) and diminished bone strength. It is categorized by histologic appearance: osteoporosis (common; bone matrix and mineral both decreased) and osteomalacia (unusual; bone matrix intact, mineral decreased).

OSTEOPOROSIS

ESSENTIALS OF DIAGNOSIS

- Asymptomatic to severe backache from vertebral fractures.
- Spontaneous fractures often discovered incidentally on radiography; loss of height.
- Serum PTH, calcium, phosphorus, and alkaline phosphatase usually normal.
- Serum 25-hydroxyvitamin D levels often low as a comorbid condition.
- Demineralization, especially of spine, hip, pelvis, and wrist.

General Considerations

Osteoporosis is the most common metabolic bone disease. Osteoporosis is caused by a reduction and disarray of bone's microarchitectural organic collagenous matrix, which normally accounts for about 40% of bone mass and provides bone's tensile strength. Inorganic calcium and phosphate compounds, largely calcium hydroxyapetite, mineralize the available collagenous bone matrix and normally provide about 60% of bone mass and most of bone's compressive strength.

Osteoporosis is estimated to cause 1.5 million fractures annually in the United States—mainly of the spine and hip. The morbidity and indirect mortality rates are very high. Since the usual form of the disease is clinically evident in middle life and beyond and since women are more frequently affected than men, it is often referred to as "postmenopausal" osteoporosis. It is characterized by a decrease in the amount of bone present to a level below which it is capable of maintaining the structural integrity of the skeleton. The rate of bone formation is often normal, whereas the rate of bone resorption is increased. There is a greater loss of trabecular bone than compact bone, accounting for the primary features of the disease, ie, crush fractures of vertebrae, fractures of the neck of the femur, and fractures of the distal end of the radius. Whatever bone is present is normally mineralized.

Osteogenesis imperfecta is caused by a major mutation in the gene encoding for type I collagen, the major collagen constituent of bone. This causes severe osteoporosis; spontaneous fractures occur in utero or during childhood. Certain polymorphisms in the genes encoding type I collagen are common, particularly in whites, resulting in collagen disarray and predisposing to hypogonadal (eg, menopausal) or idiopathic osteoporosis.

Etiology

The causes of osteoporosis are listed in Table 26–12.

Clinical Findings

A. SYMPTOMS AND SIGNS

Osteoporosis is usually asymptomatic until fractures occur. It may present as backache of varying degrees of severity or as a spontaneous fracture or collapse of a vertebra. Loss of height is common. Once osteoporosis is identified, a carefully directed history and physical examination must be performed to determine its cause (see Table 26–12).

B. LABORATORY FINDINGS

Serum calcium, phosphate, and PTH are normal. The alkaline phosphatase is usually normal but may be slightly elevated, especially following a fracture. Once osteoporosis is identified, further testing for thyrotoxicosis, hypogonadism, and vitamin D deficiency may be required. Celiac disease should be screened for with serum immunoglobulin A (IgA) endomysial antibody and tissue transglutaminase antibody determinations. Vitamin D deficiency is very common and serum determination of 25-hydroxyvitamin D should be obtained for every individual with low bone density. Serum 25-hydroxyvitamin D levels below 20 ng/mL are considered frank vitamin D deficiency. Lesser degrees of vitamin D deficiency (serum 25-hydroxyvitamin D levels between 20 ng/mL and 30 ng/mL) may also increase the risk for hip fracture. (See Osteomalacia, below.)

Table 26–12. Etiologic classification of osteoporosis.[1]

Hormone deficiency	**Genetic disorders**
Estrogen (women)	Aromatase deficiency
Androgen (men)	Type I collagen mutations
Hormone excess	Osteogenesis imperfecta
Cushing's syndrome or corticosteroid administration	Idiopathic juvenile and adult osteoporosis
Thyrotoxicosis	Ehlers-Danlos syndrome
Hyperparathyroidism	Marfan's syndrome
Immobilization and microgravity	Homocystinuria
Tobacco	**Miscellaneous**
Alcoholism	Celiac disease
Malignancy, especially multiple myeloma	Anorexia nervosa
Medications	Protein-calorie malnutrition
Excessive vitamin D intake	Vitamin C deficiency
Excessive vitamin A intake	Copper deficiency
Heparin therapy	Liver disease
	Rheumatoid arthritis
	Uncontrolled diabetes mellitus
	Systemic mastocytosis

[1]See Table 26–14 for causes of osteomalacia.

C. BONE DENSITOMETRY

Dual energy x-ray absorptiometry (DXA) can determine the bone mineral density of the hip or spine. Peripheral DXA (pDXA) can measure the bone density of the forearm, finger, and heel. Single-energy x-ray absorptiometry (SXA) measures bone density in the wrist or heel. These tests deliver negligible radiation, and the measurements are quite accurate. Typically, DXA is used to determine the bone density of the lumbar spine and hip. Bone densitometry should be performed on all patients who are at risk for osteoporosis or osteomalacia (Table 26–13). Bone densitometry cannot distinguish osteoporosis from osteomalacia; in fact, both are often present. Also, the bone mineral density does not directly measure bone quality and is only fairly successful at predicting fractures. Vertebral bone mineral density may be misleadingly high in compressed vertebrae and in patients with extensive arthritis. DXA also overestimates the bone mineral density of taller persons and underestimates the bone mineral density of smaller persons. Quantitative computed tomography (QCT) delivers more radiation but is more accurate in the latter situations.

Bone mineral density in typically expressed in gm/cm^2, for which there are different normal ranges for each bone and for each type of DXA-measuring machine. The "T score" is a simplified way of reporting bone density in which the patient's bone mineral density is compared to the young normal mean and expressed as a standard deviation score. The World Health Organization has established criteria for defining osteoporosis in postmenopausal white women, based on T score:

T score ≥ –1.0: Normal.

T score –1.0 to –2.5: Osteopenia ("low bone density").

T score < –2.5: Osteoporosis.

T score < –2.5 with a fracture: Severe osteoporosis.

This classification is somewhat arbitrary and there really is no bone mineral density fracture threshold; instead, the fracture risk increases about twofold for each standard deviation drop in bone mineral density. In fact, most women with fragility fractures have bone densities above –2.5. Surveillance DXA bone densitometry is recommended for postmenopausal women with a frequency according to their T scores: obtain DXA every 5 years for T scores –1.0 to –1.5, every 3–5 years for scores –1.5 to –2.0, and every 1–2 years for scores under –2.0.

The "Z score" is used to express bone density in premenopausal women, younger men, and children, The Z score is a statistical term that is used for expressing an individual's bone density as standard deviation from age-matched, race-matched, and sex-matched means.

Differential Diagnosis

Osteoporosis has many causes (see Table 26–12). Additionally, osteopenia and fractures can be caused by osteomalacia (see below) and bone marrow neoplasia such as myeloma or metastatic bone disease. These conditions coexist in many patients.

Treatment

A. SPECIFIC MEASURES

Several treatment options are available, so a regimen is tailored to each patient. Generally, treatment is indicated for all women with osteoporosis (T scores below

Table 26–13. Indications for measuring bone density.

Chronic (> 1 month) corticosteroid (> 6 mg prednisone)
  therapy
Chronic diseases associated with osteoporosis
Alcoholism
Anorexia nervosa
Hypogonadism of any cause: women or men
Hyperparathyroidism
Hyperthyroidism
Liver disease
Low body mass index (BMI < 19 kg/m^2)
Immobilization (eg, paraplegia)
Inflammatory bowel disease
Protein–calorie malnutrition
Renal failure
Chronic disorders associated with osteomalacia
Hypocalcemia
Hypophosphatemia
Malabsorption
Nephrotic syndrome
Renal failure
Vitamin D deficiency
Family history of osteoporosis or hip fracture
Fracture following minimal or no trauma
Fracture following minimal trauma
Loss of height or thoracic kyphosis (dowager's hump)
Radiologic suspicion for low bone density
Radiologic diagnosis of vertebral crush deformity

−2.5) and for all patients who have had fragility fractures. Prophylactic treatment should also be considered for patients with advanced osteopenia (T scores between −2.0 and −2.5).

1. Bisphosphonates—Bisphosphonates work similarly, inhibiting osteoclast-induced bone resorption. They increase bone density significantly and reduce the incidence of both vertebral and nonvertebral fractures. Bisphosphonates have also been effective in preventing corticosteroid-induced osteoporosis. To ensure intestinal absorption, oral bisphosphonates must be taken in the morning with at least 8 oz of plain water at least 30 minutes before consumption of anything else. The patient must remain upright after taking bisphosphonates to reduce the risk of esophagitis. These medications are excreted in the urine. However, no dosage adjustments are required for patients with creatinine clearances above 35 mL/min. There has been little experience giving bisphosphonates to patients with severe renal insufficiency; if given, the dose would need to be greatly reduced and serum phosphate levels monitored.

Bisphosphonates may be given orally once monthly or weekly; which is more convenient than daily therapy and equally effective. Available oral preparations include **alendronate**, 70 mg orally once weekly (tablet or solution), and **risedronate**, 35 mg orally once weekly. Both these medications reduce the risk of both vertebral and nonver-

tebral fractures. Studies sponsored by the manufacturer of alendronate found that alendronate was significantly more potent than risedronate and equally well tolerated. Another bisphosphonate, **ibandronate sodium**, is taken once monthly in a dose of 150 mg orally. Once-monthly ibandronate is convenient and reduces the risk of vertebral fractures but not nonvertebral fractures; its effectiveness has not been directly compared with other bisphosphonates. Oral bisphosphonates can cause esophagitis, especially in patients with hiatal hernia and gastroesophageal reflux.

For patients who cannot tolerate oral bisphosphonates or for whom oral bisphosphonates are contraindicated, intravenous bisphosphonates are available. **Zoledronic acid** is a third-generation bisphosphonate and a potent osteoclast inhibitor. It can be given every 6–12 months in doses of 2–4 mg intravenously over 15–30 minutes. **Pamidronate** is an older parenteral bisphosphonate that can be given in doses of 30–60 mg by slow intravenous infusion in normal saline solution every 3–6 months. Transient postinfusion fever occurs fairly commonly (26%). Osteonecrosis of the jaw has been reported in patients receiving intravenous zoledronic acid and pamidronate for treatment of hypercalcemia and bone metastases, for which the drugs had been administered more frequently than for osteoporosis.

Both oral and parenteral bisphosphonates can cause bone, joint, or muscle pains as well as fatigue. Pains can be migratory or diffuse and can vary in severity from mild to incapacitating. The onset of pain is variable and may occur anytime from 1 day to 1 year after therapy is initiated, with a mean of 14 days. The pain can be transient, lasting several days and usually resolving spontaneously but typically recurring with subsequent doses. When the bisphosphonate is discontinued, most patients experience gradual relief of pain. Some women taking alendronate or risedronate for osteoporosis have experienced painful, necrotic, nonhealing lesions of the jaw after tooth extraction. For patients with painful exposed bone, treatment is 90% effective (without resolution of the exposed bone) using antibiotics along with 0.12% chlorohexidine antiseptic mouth wash. Patients receiving bisphosphonates must receive regular dental care and try to avoid dental extraction. Another reported adverse effect reported with bisphosphonates is ocular inflammation, manifested by blurred vision, eye pain, uveitis, conjunctivitis, and scleritis, which remits after discontinuation of the drug. Other side effects can include nausea, anemia, dyspnea, and leg edema. In patients taking bisphosphonates, hypercalcemia is seen in 20% and serum PTH levels increase above normal in 10%, mimicking primary hyperparathyroidism.

All bisphosphonates inhibit osteoclastic bone resorption by binding to active bone remodeling sites and inhibiting osteoclasts; the half-life of alendronate in bone is 10 years. The effects of long-term bisphosphonate therapy on bone strength are unknown.

2. Sex hormones—Hypogonadal women who take estrogen replacement therapy have a lower risk of developing osteoporosis. Postmenopausal estrogen replacement is valuable as an osteoporosis prevention measure and this should be one factor in the complex decision about whether to take hormone replacement therapy. Low doses of estrogen appear to be adequate to prevent postmenopausal osteoporosis. (see Hormone Replacement Therapy, HRT). Once osteoporosis has developed, estrogen replacement is not an effective treatment. Although HRT does increase bone mineral density in postmenopausal women with osteoporosis, it has not been demonstrated to significantly reduce fracture rates. Treatment with a selective estrogen receptor modulator should also be considered (see raloxifene below). Men with hypogonadism may be treated with testosterone (see Male Hypogonadism).

3. Selective estrogen receptor modulators—Raloxifene, 60 mg/d orally, can be used by postmenopausal women in place of estrogen for prevention of osteoporosis. Bone density increases about 1% over 2 years in postmenopausal women versus 2% increases with estrogen replacement. It reduces the risk of vertebral fractures by about 40% but does not appear to reduce the risk of nonvertebral fractures. Raloxifene produces a reduction in LDL cholesterol but not the rise in HDL cholesterol seen with estrogen. It has no direct effect on coronary plaque. Unlike estrogen, raloxifene does not reduce hot flushes; in fact, it often intensifies them. It does not relieve vaginal dryness. Unlike estrogen, raloxifene does not cause endometrial hyperplasia, uterine bleeding, or cancer, nor does it cause breast soreness. The risk of breast cancer is reduced 76% in women taking raloxifene for 3 years. Since it is a potential teratogen, it is contraindicated in premenopausal women.

Raloxifene increases the risk for thromboembolism and should not be used by women with such a history. Leg cramps can also occur.

4. Calcitonin—A nasal spray of calcitonin-salmon (Miacalcin) is available that contains 2200 units/mL in 2-mL metered-dose bottles. The usual dose is one puff (0.09 mL, 200 IU) once daily, alternating nostrils. Nasal administration causes significantly less nausea and flushing than the parenteral route. However, nasal symptoms such as rhinitis and epistaxis occur commonly; other less common adverse reactions include flu-like symptoms, allergy, arthralgias, back pain, and headache. Five years of therapy increases bone 2–3% and reduces the number of new vertebral fractures. Both nasal and parenteral calcitonin have analgesic effects on bone pain; reduction of pain may be noted within 2–4 weeks after commencing therapy. Calcitonin reduces the incidence of vertebral fractures, but its effect upon nonvertebral fractures has not been established.

5. Vitamin D and calcium—Adequate dietary intakes of vitamin D and calcium are required throughout life to maintain peak bone mass and reduce the risk of subsequent osteoporosis and osteomalacia.

Vitamin D supplementation is useful for the prevention of osteomalacia and postmenopausal osteoporosis. It reduces the incidence of vertebral fractures by

37% and may slightly reduce the incidence of nonvertebral fractures. Oral vitamin D is given in doses of 400–1000 IU daily. Higher doses of vitamin D may be required for patients with serum levels of 25-hydroxyvitamin D below 20 ng/mL and those with intestinal malabsorption.

Calcium supplementation alone has only a minor effect on the prevention of osteoporosis and such supplementation has not been established to reduce fracture risk significantly. Nevertheless, it is recommended for patients at high risk for osteoporosis (see above) and for those with established osteoporosis. Calcium supplements may reduce the risk of colon cancer. Calcium supplementation may be given as calcium citrate (0.4–0.7 g elemental calcium per day) or calcium carbonate (1–1.5 g elemental calcium per day).

6. Teriparatide—Teriparatide (Forteo, Parathar) is an analog of PTH. Teriparatide stimulates the production of new collagenous bone matrix that must be mineralized. Patients receiving teriparatide must have sufficient intake of vitamin D and calcium. When administered to patients with osteoporosis in doses of 20 mcg/d subcutaneously for 2 years, teriparatide dramatically improves bone density in most bones except the distal radius. The recommended dose should not be exceeded, since teriparatide has caused osteosarcoma in rats when administered in very high doses. The drug should not be used by patients with Paget's disease of bone or by patients with open epiphyses or hypercalcemia. Patients with a past history of osteosarcoma or chondrosarcoma should not use this medication. Side effects may include dizziness and leg cramps. Teriparatide is approved only for a 2-year course of treatment.

Precautions: Hypercalcemia may develop in patients who are taking teriparatide if they also take corticosteroids and thiazide diuretics along with oral calcium supplementation.

Following a course of teriparitide, a course of bisphosphonates should be considered in order to retain the improved bone density.

B. GENERAL MEASURES

For prevention and treatment of osteoporosis, the diet should be adequate in protein, total calories, calcium, and vitamin D. Pharmacologic corticosteroid doses should be reduced or discontinued if possible. Thiazides may be useful if hypercalciuria is present. High-impact physical activity (eg, jogging) significantly increases bone density in men and women. Stair-climbing increases bone density in women. Patients who cannot exercise vigorously should be encouraged to engage in other exercise regularly, thereby increasing strength and reducing the risk of falling. Weight training is also helpful to increase muscle strength as well as bone density. Measures should be taken to avoid falls at home (eg, adequate lighting, handrails on stairs, handholds in bathrooms). Patients who have weakness or balance problems must use a cane or a walker; rolling walkers should have a brake mechanism. Balance exercises (eg, tai chi) can reduce the risk of falls. Patients should be kept active; bedridden patients should be given active or passive exercises. The spine may be adequately supported (though braces or corsets are usually not well tolerated), but rigid or excessive immobilization must be avoided. Alcohol and smoking should be avoided.

Prognosis

The prognosis is good for preventing postmenopausal osteoporosis in women if estrogen or raloxifene is started early in menopause and maintained for years. However, the adverse effects of oral combined HRT are now known, reducing its use. Hypogonadal women, especially those not receiving HRT, must assure sufficient intake of vitamin D and calcium to prevent osteomalacia; but this does not prevent osteoporosis. Bone mineral density densitometries can detect whether progressive osteopenia or frank osteoporosis is developing. Bisphosphonates can reverse progressive osteopenia and osteoporosis and decrease fracture risk.

Hypogonadal men are also at risk for developing osteoporosis. Testosterone administration can prevent osteoporosis. Men with prostate cancer may not receive testosterone replacement and should be monitored with bone densitometries. Bisphosphonate therapy can reverse progressive osteopenia and osteoporosis in men.

Black DM et al: One year of alendronate after one year of parathyroid hormone (1–84) for osteoporosis. N Engl J Med 2005;353:555. [PMID: 16093464]

Bone HG et al: Ten years' experience with alendronate for osteoporosis in postmenopausal women. N Engl J Med 2004;18:1189. [PMID: 15028823]

Cosman F et al: Daily and cyclic parathyroid hormone in women receiving alendronate. N Engl J Med 2005;353:566. [PMID: 16093465]

Genant HK et al: Treatment with raloxifene for 2 years increases vertebral bone mineral density as measured by volumetric quantitative computed tomography. Bone 2004;35:1164. [PMID: 15542042]

Grant AM et al; RECORD Trial Group: Oral vitamin D$_3$ and calcium for secondary prevention of low-trauma fractures in elderly people (Randomised Evaluation of Calcium Or vitamin D, RECORD): a randomised placebo-controlled trial. Lancet 2005;365:1621. [PMID: 15885294]

Jackson RD et al; Women's Health Initiative Investigators: Calcium plus vitamin D supplementation and the risk of fractures. N Engl J Med 2006;354:669. [PMID: 16481635]

Johnell O et al: Raloxifene reduces risk of vertebral fractures and breast cancer in postmenopausal women regardless of prior hormone therapy. J Fam Pract 2004;53:789. [PMID: 15469774]

McClung MR et al: Opposite bone remodeling effects of teriparatide and alendronate in increasing bone mass. Arch Intern Med 2005;165:1762. [PMID: 16087825]

Stenson WF et al: Increased prevalence of celiac disease and need for routine screening among patients with osteoporosis. Arch Intern Med 2005;165:393. [PMID: 15738367]

OSTEOMALACIA

 ESSENTIALS OF DIAGNOSIS

- *Painful proximal muscle weakness (especially pelvic girdle); bone pain and tenderness.*
- *Decreased bone density from diminished mineralization of osteoid.*
- *Laboratory abnormalities may include increases in alkaline phosphatase, decreased 25-hydroxyvitamin D, or hypocalcemia, hypocalciuria, hypophosphatemia, secondary hyperparathyroidism.*
- *Classic radiologic features may be present.*

General Considerations

Defective mineralization of the growing skeleton in childhood causes permanent bone deformities (rickets). Defective skeletal mineralization in adults is known as osteomalacia.

Osteomalacia is commonly caused by a deficiency in vitamin D. Ergocalciferol (vitamin D$_2$) is derived from plants and is used in most pharmaceutical preparations of vitamin D. Cholecalciferol (vitamin D$_3$) is synthesized in the skin, under the influence of ultraviolet radiation, from 7-dehydrocholesterol. Both vitamin D$_2$ and vitamin D$_3$ are used to fortify foods and have equivalent potency. Two sequential hydroxylations are necessary for full biologic activity: The first one takes place in the liver—to 25(OH)D$_3$—and the second one in the kidney, resulting in the formation of the most potent biologic metabolite of vitamin D, 1,25(OH)$_2$D$_3$. The main action of vitamin D is to increase the absorption of calcium and phosphate from the intestine. However, vitamin D appears to have other systemic effects, since 1,25(OH)$_2$D receptors are also found in other tissues, including the parathyroids, bones, kidneys, skin, brain, pituitary, activated lymphocytes, and various tumors.

Etiology (Table 26–14)

Osteomalacia is a common disorder and is caused by any condition that results in inadequate calcium or phosphate mineralization of bone osteoid.

A. VITAMIN D DEFICIENCY AND RESISTANCE

Vitamin D deficiency impairs the intestinal absorption of calcium and is the most common cause of osteomalacia. Vitamin D deficiency (serum 25[OH]D < 50 nmol/L or < 20 ng/mL) was found in 24.3% of postmenopausal women from 25 countries in the MORE study. The incidence varied: < 1% in Southeast Asia, 29.3% in the United States, and 36% in Italy. Severe vitamin D deficiency (serum 25[OH]D < 25 nmol/L or

Table 26–14. Causes of osteomalacia.[1]

Vitamin disorders
 Decreased availability of vitamin D
 Insufficient sunlight exposure
 Nutritional deficiency of vitamin D
 Malabsorption
 Nephrotic syndrome
 Vitamin D-dependent rickets type I
 Liver disease
 Chronic renal failure
 Phenytoin, carbamazepine, or barbiturate therapy
Dietary calcium deficiency
Phosphate deficiency
 Decreased intestinal absorption
 Nutritional deficiency of phosphorus
 Malabsorption
 Phosphate-binding antacid therapy
 Increased renal loss
 X-linked hypophosphatemic rickets
 Tumoral hypophosphatemic osteomalacia
 Association with other disorders, including parapro-
  teinemias, glycogen storage diseases, neurofibroma-
  tosis, Wilson's disease, and Fanconi's syndrome
Disorders of bone matrix
 Hypophosphatasia
 Fibrogenesis imperfecta
 Axial osteomalacia
Inhibitors of mineralization
 Aluminum
 Bisphosphonates

[1]See Table 26–12 for causes of osteoporosis.

< 10 ng/mL) was found in 4.1% of these women; 3.5% in the United States and 12.5% in Italy. Vitamin D deficiency is particularly common in the institutionalized elderly, with the incidence exceeding 60% in some groups not receiving vitamin D supplementation. In one study of elderly individuals age 98 years or older, 95% had undetectable levels of vitamin D. Deficiency of vitamin D may arise from insufficient sun exposure, malnutrition, or malabsorption (due to pancreatic insufficiency, cholestatic liver disease, sprue, inflammatory bowel disease, jejunoileal bypass, Billroth type II gastrectomy, etc). Cholestyramine binds bile acids necessary for vitamin D absorption. Patients with severe nephrotic syndrome lose large amounts of vitamin D-binding protein in the urine, and osteomalacia may also develop.

Vitamin D-dependent rickets type I is caused by a rare autosomal recessive defect in renal synthesis of $1,25(OH)_2D$. It presents in childhood with rickets; osteomalacia develops in adults unless treated with oral calcitriol in doses of 0.5–1 mcg daily. Vitamin D-dependent rickets type II (now better known as hereditary $1,25[OH]_2D$-resistant rickets) is caused by a ge-

netic defect in the $1,25(OH)_2D$ receptor. It presents in childhood with rickets and alopecia. Adults respond variably to oral calcitriol in very large doses (2–6 mcg daily).

Anticonvulsants (eg, phenytoin, carbamazepine, valproate, phenobarbital) inhibit the hepatic production of $25(OH)D$ and sometimes cause osteomalacia. Phenytoin can also directly inhibit bone mineralization. Serum levels of $1,25(OH)_2D$ are usually normal.

B. DEFICIENT CALCIUM INTAKE

Rickets and osteomalacia continue to be common problems in many tropical countries despite adequate exposure to sunlight. A nutritional deficiency of calcium can occur in any severely malnourished patient. Some degree of calcium deficiency is common in the elderly, since intestinal calcium absorption declines with age. Ingestion of excessive wheat bran also causes calcium malabsorption.

C. PHOSPHATE DEFICIENCY

Phosphatonin is a circulating peptide that inhibits sodium-dependent phosphate transport in the renal tubule; high levels of this peptide cause excessive phosphaturia, resulting in hypophosphatemia. X-linked hypophosphatemic rickets is associated with high levels of phosphatonin, probably caused by familial or sporadic mutations in PHEX endopeptidase, which fails to cleave phosphatonin.

Oncogenic osteomalacia is caused by excessive production of phosphatonin by a wide variety of soft tissue tumors (87% benign). The condition is characterized by hypophosphatemia, excessive phosphaturia, reduced serum $1,25(OH)_2D$ concentrations, and osteomalacia. Excessive renal phosphate losses are also seen in proximal renal tubular acidosis and Fanconi's syndrome. Some cases of hyperphosphaturia are idiopathic.

Other causes of hypophosphatemic osteomalacia include poor nutrition, alcoholism, or chelation of phosphate in the gut by aluminum hydroxide antacids, calcium acetate (Phos-Lo), or sevelamer hydrochloride (Renagel).

D. ALUMINUM TOXICITY

Bone mineralization is inhibited by aluminum. Osteomalacia may occur in patients receiving long-term renal hemodialysis with tap water dialysate or from aluminum-containing antacids used to reduce phosphate levels. Osteomalacia may develop in patients being maintained on long-term total parenteral nutrition if the casein hydrolysate used for amino acids contains high levels of aluminum.

E. HYPOPHOSPHATASIA

Skeletal alkaline phosphatase is an enzyme that is necessary to form normal bone. Alkaline phosphatase cleaves pyrophosphate, an inhibitor of mineralization, thereby allowing normal mineralization of the bone matrix. There are four distinct alkaline phosphatase isomers;

only one is found in bone and it is also in liver and kidney and is therefore known as tissue-nonspecific alkaline phosphatase ("bone" alkaline phosphatase).

Hypophosphatasia, a deficiency of tissue-nonspecific alkaline phosphatase effect, is a rare genetic cause of osteomalacia that is commonly misdiagnosed as osteoporosis. The incidence in the United States is about 1 in 100,000 live births; about 1 in 300 adults is a carrier. More than 60 different mutations in the gene encoding tissue-nonspecific alkaline phosphatase (designated *ALPL*) have been described, and transmission can be autosomal recessive or autosomal dominant. The phenotypic presentation of hypophosphatasia is extremely variable. At its worst extreme, it can present as a stillborn without dentition or calcified bones. At its mildest, hypophosphatasia can present in middle age with premature loss of teeth, foot pain (due to metatarsal stress fractures), thigh pain (due to femoral pseudofractures), or arthritis (due to chondrocalcinosis). Serum alkaline phosphatase (collected in a non-EDTA tube) is low for age in patients with hypophosphatasia. To confirm the diagnosis, a 24-hour urine should be assayed for phosphoethanolamine, a substrate for tissue-nonspecific alkaline phosphatase, whose excretion is always elevated in patients with hypophosphatasia. Prenatal genetic testing, by way of chorionic villus biopsy, is available for the infantile form of hypophosphatasia. There is no proven therapy for hypophosphatasia, except for supportive care. Teriparatide, a useful therapy for osteoporosis, has been administered to some patients with hypophosphatasia, but its long-term efficacy is unknown.

F. Fibrogenesis Imperfecta Ossium

This rare condition sporadically affects middle-aged patients, who present with progressive bone pain and pathologic fractures. Bones have a dense "fishnet" appearance on x-ray. MRI of unfractured bone shows low signal intensity on both T1- and T2-weighted imaging. Serum alkaline phosphatase levels are elevated. Some patients have a monoclonal gammopathy, indicating a possible plasma cell dyscrasia causing an impairment in osteoblast function and collagen disarray. Remission has been reported after repeated courses of melphalan, corticosteroids, and vitamin D analog over 3 years.

Clinical Findings

The clinical manifestations of defective bone mineralization depend on the age at onset and the severity. In adults, osteomalacia is typically asymptomatic at first. Eventually, bone pain occurs, along with muscle weakness due to calcium deficiency. Fractures may occur with little or no trauma.

Diagnostic Tests

Serum is obtained for calcium, albumin, phosphate, alkaline phosphatase, PTH, and 25[OH]D₃ determina-

tions. Bone densitometry helps document the degree of osteopenia. X-rays may show diagnostic features.

In one series of biopsy-proved osteomalacia, alkaline phosphatase was elevated in 94% of patients; the calcium or phosphorus was low in 47% of patients; 25(OH)D₃ was low in 29% of patients; pseudofractures were seen in 18% of patients; and urinary calcium was low in 18% of patients. $1,25(OH)_2D_3$ may be low even when 25(OH)D₂ levels are normal.

Bone biopsy is not usually necessary but is diagnostic of osteomalacia if there is significant unmineralized osteoid.

Differential Diagnosis

Osteomalacia usually can be distinguished from osteoporosis by the relative absence of biochemical abnormalities in the latter. Phosphate deficiency must be distinguished from hypophosphatemia seen in hyperparathyroidism.

Prevention & Treatment

Prevention of vitamin D deficiency may be achieved with adequate sunlight exposure and vitamin D supplements. In the United States, the current recommended daily allowance (RDA) of vitamin D is at least 10 mcg (400 IU) daily. However, in sunlight-deprived individuals (eg, veiled women, confined patients, or residents of higher latitudes during winter), the RDA should be 1000 IU daily. In such individuals, vitamin D supplements should be given prophylactically. Patients receiving long-term phenytoin therapy may be treated prophylactically with vitamin D, 50,000 IU orally every 2–4 weeks.

Vitamin D deficiency is treated with ergocalciferol (D₂), 50,000 IU orally once or twice weekly for 6–12 months, followed by at least 1000 IU daily. Ergocalciferol has a long duration of action and may also be given orally every 2 months in doses of 50,000 IU. In patients with intestinal malabsorption, oral doses of 25,000–100,000 IU of vitamin D₂ daily may be required. Some patients with steatorrhea respond better to oral 25(OH)D₃ (calcifediol), 50–100 mcg/d. All patients receive supplemental oral calcium salts (eg, calcium citrate or calcium carbonate), which are given with meals. Recommended doses of calcium are as follows: calcium citrate (eg, Citracal), 0.4–0.6 g elemental calcium per day, or calcium carbonate (eg, OsCal, Tums), 1–1.5 g elemental calcium per day.

In hypophosphatemic osteomalacia, nutritional deficiencies are corrected, aluminum-containing antacids are discontinued, and patients with renal tubular acidosis are given bicarbonate therapy. In patients with sporadic adult-onset hypophosphatemia, hyperphosphaturia, and low serum $1,25(OH)_2D$ levels, a search is conducted for occult tumors that may be resected; whole-body MRI scanning may be required.

For those with X-linked or idiopathic hypophosphatemia and hyperphosphaturia, oral phosphate supplements must be given long-term; calcitriol, 0.25–0.5 mcg/d, is given also to improve the impaired calcium absorption caused by the oral phosphate. Human recombinant growth hormone reduces phosphaturia and may be added to the above regimen.

Bielesz B et al: Renal phosphate loss in hereditary and acquired disorders of bone mineralization. Bone 2004;35:1229. [PMID: 15589204]

Hanley DA et al: Vitamin D insufficiency in North America. J Nutr 2005;135:332. [PMID: 15671237]

Jan de Beur SM: Tumor-induced osteomalacia. JAMA 2005;294:1260. [PMID: 16160135]

Lyman D: Undiagnosed vitamin D deficiency in the hospitalized patient. Am Fam Physician 2005;71:299. [PMID: 15686300]

Pelger RC et al: Severe hypophosphatemic osteomalacia in hormone-refractory prostate cancer metastatic to the skeleton: natural history and pitfalls in management. Bone 2005;36:1. [PMID: 15663996]

PAGET'S DISEASE OF BONE (Osteitis Deformans)

 ESSENTIALS OF DIAGNOSIS

- Often asymptomatic.
- Bone pain may be the first symptom.
- Kyphosis, bowed tibias, large head, deafness, and frequent fractures that vary with location of process.
- Serum calcium and phosphate normal; alkaline phosphatase elevated; urinary hydroxyproline elevated.
- Dense, expanded bones on x-ray.

General Considerations

Paget's disease of bone is a common condition manifested by one or more bony lesions having high bone turnover and disorganized osteoid formation. Involved bones become vascular, weak, and deformed. Paget's disease is present in 1–2% of the population of the United States, with a higher prevalence in the elderly and in the Northeast. It is usually discovered incidentally during radiology imaging or because of incidentally discovered elevations in serum alkaline phosphatase. Only 27% of affected individuals are symptomatic at the time of diagnosis. Familial Paget's disease is unusual but is generally more severe than sporadic cases. A rare form occurs in young people.

Clinical Findings

A. SYMPTOMS AND SIGNS

Paget's disease is usually diagnosed in patients over 40 years of age and is often mild and asymptomatic. It can involve just one bone (monostotic) or multiple bones (polyostotic), particularly the skull, femur, tibia, pelvis, and humerus. Pain is the usual first symptom. The bones become soft, leading to bowed tibias, kyphosis, and frequent fractures with slight trauma. If the skull is involved, the patient may report headaches and an increased hat size. Deafness may occur. Increased vascularity over the involved bones causes increased warmth.

B. LABORATORY FINDINGS

Serum calcium and phosphorus are normal, but serum alkaline phosphatase is markedly elevated. Urinary hydroxyproline is also elevated in active disease. Serum calcium may be elevated, particularly if the patient is at bed rest.

C. IMAGING

The involved bones are expanded and denser than normal on radiographs. Multiple fissure fractures may be seen in the long bones. The initial lesion may be destructive and radiolucent, especially in the skull ("osteoporosis circumscripta"). Technetium pyrophosphate bone scans are helpful in delineating activity of bone lesions even before any radiologic changes are apparent.

Differential Diagnosis

Paget's disease must be differentiated from primary bone lesions such as osteogenic sarcoma, multiple myeloma, and fibrous dysplasia and from secondary bone lesions such as metastatic carcinoma and osteitis fibrosa cystica. Fibrogenesis imperfecta ossium is a rare symmetric disorder that can mimic the features of Paget's disease; alkaline phosphate is likewise elevated. If serum calcium is elevated, hyperparathyroidism may be present in some patients as well.

Complications

Fractures are frequent and occur with minimal trauma. If immobilization takes place and there is an excessive calcium intake, hypercalcemia and kidney stones may develop. Vertebral collapse may lead to spinal cord compression. Osteosarcoma may develop in long-standing lesions. Sarcomatous change is suggested by a marked increase in bone pain, sudden rise in alkaline phosphatase, and appearance of a new lytic lesion. The increased vascularity may give rise to high-output cardiac failure. Arthritis frequently develops in joints adjacent to involved bone.

Extensive skull involvement may cause cranial nerve palsies from impingement of the neural foramina. Ischemic neurologic events may occur as a result of a vascular "steal" phenomenon. Involvement of the auditory region frequently causes hearing loss (mixed sensorineural and conductive) and occasionally tinnitus or vertigo.

Treatment

Asymptomatic patients require no treatment except for those with extensive skull involvement, in whom prophylactic treatment may prevent deafness and stroke.

A. BISPHOSPHONATES

Bisphosphonates have become the treatment of choice for Paget's disease. The oral compounds should all be taken with 8 oz of plain water only. Bisphosphonates are usually given cyclically. Therapy is given until a therapeutic response occurs, as evidenced by normalization of the serum alkaline phosphatase. Patients are then given a break from therapy for about 3 months or until the serum alkaline phosphatase becomes elevated again; another cycle is then commenced.

Alendronate, 20–40 mg orally daily (or 70 mg orally once weekly) for 3-month cycles, is also effective. It must be taken in the morning, at least 30–60 minutes before breakfast. Its main side effect is esophagitis, so recumbency after dosing is prohibited, and the drug is contraindicated in patients with a history of esophagitis, esophageal stricture, dysphagia, hiatal hernia, or achalasia.

Tiludronate, 400 mg orally daily for 3 months, is very effective in reducing the activity of bone lesions. It should not be taken within 2 hours of meals, aspirin, indomethacin, calcium, magnesium, or aluminum-containing antacids. Esophagitis is uncommon, so recumbency after dosing is not restricted, and the drug may be taken in the evening as well as during the day. The most common side effects have been gastrointestinal, including abdominal pain in 13% and nausea in 9%.

Risedronate, 30 mg orally daily for 3-month cycles, has been effective in normalizing alkaline phosphatase and eliminating bone pain in the majority of patients. It has been generally well tolerated, but arthralgias and gastrointestinal side effects do occur.

Parenteral bisphosphonates are particularly useful for patients who cannot tolerate oral bisphosphonates. **Pamidronate**, 60–120 mg intravenously over 2–4 hours, may produce improvements lasting several months. Alkaline phosphatase may continue to drop for 6 months after treatment. (See Treatment of Hypercalcemia.) **Zoledronic acid** can be given every 6–12 months in doses of 2–4 mg intravenously over 20 minutes. Six months following a single infusion of zoledronic acid, patients had a clinical response rate of 96%, compared with 74% in patients receiving daily oral risedronate. Intravenous zoledronic acid has been demonstrated to be significantly more effective than daily risedronate. Postinfusion fever, fatigue, myalgia, bone pain, and ocular problems occur commonly and may sometimes be severe. Nonhealing jaw ulcers after tooth extraction may occur.

B. NASAL CALCITONIN-SALMON

Miacalcin, 200 IU/unit dose spray, is administered as one spray daily, alternating nostrils. It is just as effective as the parenteral preparation and is associated with fewer side effects. Nasal irritation may occur, as may occasional epistaxis. Calcitonin has been used for many years to treat Paget's disease. However, its use has declined dramatically with the introduction of more potent bisphosphonates.

Prognosis

The prognosis in general is good, but sarcomatous changes (in 1–3%) can alter it unfavorably. In general, the prognosis is worse the earlier in life the disease starts. Fractures usually heal well. In the severe forms, marked deformity, intractable pain, and cardiac failure are found. These complications should become rare with prompt bisphosphonate treatment.

Cundy T et al: Recombinant osteoprotegerin for juvenile Paget's disease. N Engl J Med 2005;353:918. [PMID: 16135836]

Langston AL et al: Management of Paget's disease of bone. Rheumatology (Oxford) 2004;43:955. [PMID: 15187244]

Reid IR et al: Comparison of a single infusion of zoledronic acid with risedronate for Paget's disease. N Engl J Med 2005; 353:898. [PMID: 16135834]

Walsh JP et al: A randomized clinical trial comparing oral alendronate and intravenous pamidronate for the treatment of Paget's disease of bone. Bone 2004;34:747. [PMID: 15050907]

■ DISEASES OF THE ADRENAL CORTEX

ACUTE ADRENOCORTICAL INSUFFICIENCY (Adrenal Crisis)

ESSENTIALS OF DIAGNOSIS

- *Weakness, abdominal pain, fever, confusion, nausea, vomiting, and diarrhea.*
- *Low blood pressure, dehydration; skin pigmentation may be increased.*
- *Serum potassium high, sodium low, BUN high.*
- *Cosyntropin (ACTH$_{1-24}$) unable to stimulate a normal increase in serum cortisol.*

General Considerations

Acute adrenal insufficiency is an emergency caused by insufficient cortisol. Crisis may occur in the course of treatment of chronic insufficiency, or it may be the presenting manifestation of adrenal insufficiency. Acute adrenal crisis is more commonly seen in primary adrenal insufficiency (Addison's disease) than in disorders of the pituitary gland causing secondary adrenocortical hypofunction.

Adrenal crisis may occur in the following situations: (1) following stress, eg, trauma, surgery, infection, or prolonged fasting in a patient with latent insufficiency; (2) following sudden withdrawal of adrenocortical hormone in a patient with chronic insufficiency or in a patient with temporary insufficiency due to suppression by exogenous corticosteroidsor megestrol; (3) following bilateral adrenalectomy or removal of a functioning adrenal tumor that had suppressed the other adrenal; (4) following sudden destruction of the pituitary gland (pituitary necrosis), or when thyroid hormone is given to a patient with hypoadrenalism; and (5) following injury to both adrenals by trauma, hemorrhage, anticoagulant therapy, thrombosis, infection or, rarely, metastatic carcinoma.

Clinical Findings

A. SYMPTOMS AND SIGNS

The patient complains of headache, lassitude, nausea and vomiting, abdominal pain, and often diarrhea. Confusion or coma may be present. Fever may be 40.6 °C or more. The blood pressure is low. Patients with preexisting type 1 diabetes may present with recurrent hypoglycemia and reduced insulin requirements. Other signs may include cyanosis, dehydration, skin hyperpigmentation, and sparse axillary hair (if hypogonadism is also present). Meningococcemia may be associated with purpura and adrenal insufficiency secondary to adrenal infarction (Waterhouse–Friderichsen syndrome).

B. LABORATORY FINDINGS

The eosinophil count may be high. Hyponatremia or hyperkalemia (or both) are usually present. Hypoglycemia is frequent. Hypercalcemia may be present. Blood, sputum, or urine culture may be positive if bacterial infection is the precipitating cause of the crisis.

The diagnosis is made by a simplified cosyntropin stimulation test, which is performed as follows: (1) Synthetic $ACTH_{1-24}$ (cosyntropin), 0.25 mg, is given parenterally. (2) Serum is obtained for cortisol between 30 and 60 minutes after cosyntropin is administered. Normally, serum cortisol rises to at least 20 mcg/dL. For patients receiving corticosteroid treatment, hydrocortisone must not be given for at least 8 hours before the test. Other corticosteroids (eg, prednisone, dexamethasone) do not interfere with specific assays for cortisol.

Plasma ACTH is markedly elevated if the patient has primary adrenal disease (generally > 200 pg/mL).

Differential Diagnosis

Acute adrenal insufficiency must be distinguished from other causes of shock (eg, septic, hemorrhagic, cardiogenic). Hyperkalemia is also seen with gastrointestinal bleeding, rhabdomyolysis, hyperkalemic paralysis, and certain drugs (eg, ACE inhibitors, spironolactone). Hyponatremia is seen in many other conditions (eg, hypothyroidism, diuretic use, heart failure, cirrhosis, vomiting, diarrhea, severe illness, or major surgery). Acute adrenal insufficiency must be distinguished from an acute abdomen in which neutrophilia is the rule, whereas adrenal insufficiency is characterized by a relative lymphocytosis and eosinophilia.

More than 90% of serum cortisol is protein bound and low serum levels of binding proteins result in misleadingly low serum cortisol determinations by most assays. Nearly 40% of critically ill patients, with serum albumin < 2.5 g/dL, have low serum total cortisol levels but normal serum free cortisol levels and normal adrenal function.

Treatment

A. ACUTE PHASE

If the diagnosis is suspected, draw a blood sample for cortisol determination and treat with hydrocortisone, 100–300 mg intravenously, and saline *immediately*, without waiting for the results. Thereafter, give hydrocortisone phosphate or hydrocortisone sodium succinate, 100 mg intravenously immediately, and continue intravenous infusions of 50–100 mg every 6 hours for the first day. Give the same amount every 8 hours on the second day and then adjust the dosage in view of the clinical picture.

Since bacterial infection frequently precipitates acute adrenal crisis, broad-spectrum antibiotics should be administered empirically while waiting for the results of initial cultures. Hypoglycemia should be vigorously treated while serum electrolytes, BUN, and creatinine are monitored.

B. CONVALESCENT PHASE

When the patient is able to take food by mouth, give oral hydrocortisone, 10–20 mg every 6 hours, and reduce dosage to maintenance levels as needed. Most patients ultimately require hydrocortisone twice daily (AM, 10–20 mg; PM, 5–10 mg). Mineralocorticoid therapy is not needed when large amounts of hydrocortisone are being given, but as the dose is reduced it is usually necessary to add fludrocortisone acetate, 0.05–0.2 mg daily. Some patients never require fludrocortisone or become edematous at doses of more than 0.05 mg once or twice weekly. Once the crisis has passed, the patient must be evaluated to assess the degree of permanent adrenal insufficiency and to establish the cause if possible.

Prognosis

Rapid treatment will usually be life-saving. However, acute adrenal insufficiency is frequently unrecognized and untreated since its manifestations mimic more common conditions; lack of treatment leads to shock that is unresponsive to volume replacement and vasopressors, resulting in death.

Hamrahian AH et al: Measurements of serum free cortisol in critically ill patients. N Engl J Med 2004;350:1629. [PMID: 15084695]

Jahangir-Hekmat M et al: Adrenal insufficiency attributable to adrenal hemorrhage: long-term follow-up with reference to glucocorticoid and mineralocorticoid function and replacement. Endocr Pract 2004;10:55. [PMID: 15251623]

CHRONIC ADRENOCORTICAL INSUFFICIENCY (Addison's Disease)

 ESSENTIALS OF DIAGNOSIS

- *Weakness, easy fatigability, anorexia, weight loss; nausea and vomiting, diarrhea; abdominal pain, muscle and joint pains; amenorrhea.*
- *Sparse axillary hair; increased skin pigmentation, especially of creases, pressure areas, and nipples.*
- *Hypotension, small heart.*
- *Serum sodium may be low; potassium, calcium, and BUN may be elevated; neutropenia, mild anemia, eosinophilia, and relative lymphocytosis may be present.*
- *Plasma cortisol levels are low or fail to rise after administration of corticotropin.*
- *Plasma ACTH level is elevated.*

General Considerations

Addison's disease is an uncommon disorder caused by destruction or dysfunction of the adrenal cortices. It is characterized by chronic deficiency of cortisol, aldosterone, and adrenal androgens and causes skin pigmentation that can be subtle or strikingly dark. Volume and sodium depletion and potassium excess eventually occur in primary adrenal failure. In contrast, if chronic adrenal insufficiency is secondary to pituitary failure (atrophy, necrosis, tumor), mineralocorticoid production (controlled by the renin–angiotensin system) persists and hyperkalemia is not present. Furthermore, if ACTH is not elevated, skin pigmentary changes are not encountered.

Etiology

Autoimmune destruction of the adrenals is the most common cause of Addison's disease in the United States (accounting for about 80% of spontaneous cases). It may occur alone or as part of a polyglandular autoimmune (PGA) syndrome. Type 1 PGA is also known as autoimmune polyendocrinopathy-candidiasis-ectodermal dystrophy (APCED) syndrome and is caused by a defect in T cell-mediated immunity inherited as an autosomal recessive trait. It usually presents in early childhood with mucocutaneous candidiasis, followed by hypoparathyroidism and dystrophy of the teeth and nails; Addison's disease usually appears by age 15 years. Partial or late expression of the syndrome is common. A varied spectrum of associated diseases may be seen in adulthood, including hypogonadism, hypothyroidism, pernicious anemia, alopecia, vitiligo, hepatitis, malabsorption, and Sjögren's syndrome.

Type 2 PGA usually presents in adulthood with autoimmune adrenal insufficiency (no hypoparathyroidism) that is HLA related. It is associated with autoimmune thyroid disease (usually hypothyroidism, sometimes hyperthyroidism), vitiligo, type 1 diabetes, alopecia areata, or celiac sprue. Autoimmune Addison's disease can also be associated with primary ovarian failure (40% of women before age 50 years), testicular failure (5%), and pernicious anemia (4%). The combination of Addison's disease and hypothyroidism is known as Schmidt's syndrome.

Tuberculosis was formerly a leading cause of Addison's disease. The association is now relatively rare in the United States but common where tuberculosis is more prevalent.

Bilateral adrenal hemorrhage may occur during sepsis, heparin-associated thrombocytopenia or anticoagulation, or with antiphospholipid antibody syndrome. It may occur in association with major surgery or trauma, presenting about 1 week later with pain, fever, and shock. It may also occur spontaneously.

Adrenoleukodystrophy is an X-linked peroxisomal disorder causing accumulation of very long-chain fatty acids in the adrenal cortex, testes, brain, and spinal cord. It may present at any age and accounts for one-third of cases of Addison's disease in boys. Aldosterone deficiency occurs in 9%. Hypogonadism is common. Psychiatric symptoms often include mania, psychosis, or cognitive impairment. Neurologic deterioration may be severe or mild (particularly in heterozygote women), mimics symptoms of multiple sclerosis, and can occur years after the onset of adrenal insufficiency.

Rare causes of adrenal insufficiency include lymphoma, metastatic carcinoma, coccidioidomycosis, histoplasmosis, cytomegalovirus infection (more frequent in patients with AIDS), syphilitic gummas, scleroderma, amyloid disease, and hemochromatosis.

Familial glucocorticoid deficiency is caused by a mutation in the gene encoding the adrenal ACTH receptor. Triple A (Allgrove's) syndrome is characterized by variable expression of the following: adrenal ACTH resistance with cortisol deficiency, achalasia, alacrima, nasal voice, and neuromuscular disease of varying severity (hyperreflexia to spastic paraplegia). Cortisol deficiency usually presents in infancy but may not occur until the third decade of life. Congenital adrenal hypoplasia causes adrenal insufficiency due to absence of the adrenal cortex; patients may also have hypogonadotropic hypogonadism, myopathy, and high-frequency hearing loss. Patients with hereditary defects in adrenal enzymes for cortisol synthesis develop **congenital adrenal hyperplasia** due to ACTH stimulation. The most common enzyme defect is P-450c21 (21-hydroxylase). Patients with severely defective P-450c21 enzymes manifest deficiency of mineralocorticoids (salt wasting) in addition to deficient cortisol and excessive androgens. Women with milder enzyme defects have adequate cortisol but develop hirsutism in adolescence or adulthood and are said to have "late-onset" congenital adrenal hyperplasia. (See Hirsutism section.)

Isolated hypoaldosteronism can be caused by various conditions. Hyporeninemic hypoaldosteronism can be caused by renal tubular acidosis type IV and is commonly seen with diabetic nephropathy, hypertensive nephrosclerosis, tubulointerstitial diseases, and AIDS; patients present with hyperkalemia, hyperchloremia, and metabolic acidosis (see Chapter 21). Hyperreninemic hypoaldosteronism can be seen in patients with myotonic dystrophy, aldosterone synthase deficiency, and congenital adrenal hyperplasia. Some patients with congenital adrenal hyperplasia (CYP17 deficiency) may present in adulthood with hyperkalemia, hypertension, and hypogonadism; cortisol deficiency is also usually present but may not be clinically evident.

Clinical Findings

A. SYMPTOMS AND SIGNS

The symptoms may include weakness and fatigability, weight loss, myalgias, arthralgias, fever, anorexia, nausea and vomiting, anxiety, and mental irritability. Some of these symptoms may be due to high serum levels of IL-6. Pigmentary changes consist of diffuse tanning over non-exposed as well as exposed parts or multiple freckles; hyperpigmentation is especially prominent over the knuckles, elbows, knees, and posterior neck and in palmar creases and nail beds. Nipples and areolas tend to darken. The skin in pressure areas such as the belt or brassiere lines and the buttocks also darkens. New scars are pigmented. Some patients have associated vitiligo (10%). Emotional changes are common. Hypoglycemia, when present, may worsen the patient's weakness and mental functioning, rarely leading to coma. Manifestations of other autoimmune disease (see above) may be present. Patients tend to be hypotensive and orthostatic; about 90% have systolic blood pressures under 110 mm Hg; blood pressure over 130 mm Hg is rare. Other findings may include a small heart, hyperplasia of lymphoid tissues, and scant axillary and pubic hair (especially in women).

Patients with adult-onset adrenoleukodystrophy may present with neuropsychiatric symptoms, sometimes without adrenal insufficiency.

B. LABORATORY FINDINGS

The white count usually shows moderate neutropenia, lymphocytosis, and a total eosinophil count over 300/mcL. Among patients with *chronic* Addison's disease, the serum sodium is usually low (90%) while the potassium is elevated (65%). Patients with diarrhea may not be hyperkalemic. Fasting blood glucose may be low. Hypercalcemia may be present. Young men with idiopathic Addison's disease are screened for adrenoleukodystrophy by determining plasma very long-chain fatty acid levels; affected patients have high levels.

Low plasma cortisol (< 3 mcg/dL) at 8 AM is diagnostic, especially if accompanied by simultaneous elevation of the plasma ACTH level (usually > 200 pg/mL). The diagnosis is made by a simplified cosyntropin stimulation test, which is performed as follows: (1) Synthetic ACTH$_{1-24}$ (cosyntropin), 0.25 mg, is given parenterally. (2) Serum is obtained for cortisol between 30 and 60 minutes after cosyntropin is administered. Normally, serum cortisol rises to at least 20 mcg/dL. For patients receiving corticosteroid treatment, hydrocortisone must not be given for at least 8 hours before the test. Other corticosteroids (eg, prednisone, dexamethasone) do not interfere with specific assays for cortisol.

Serum DHEA levels are under 1000 ng/mL in 100% of patients with Addison's disease and a serum DHEA above 1000 ng/mL excludes the diagnosis However, serum DHEA levels below 1000 ng/mL are not helpful, since about 15% of the general population have such low DHEA levels, particularly children and elderly individuals. Antiadrenal antibodies are found in the serum in about 50% of cases of autoimmune Addison's disease. Antibodies to thyroid (45%) and other tissues may be present.

Elevated plasma renin activity indicates the presence of depleted intravascular volume and the need for higher doses of fludrocortisone replacement.

C. IMAGING

When Addison's disease is not clearly autoimmune, a chest radiograph is obtained to look for tuberculosis, fungal infection, or cancer as possible causes. CT scan of the abdomen will show small noncalcified adrenals in autoimmune Addison's disease. The adrenals are enlarged in about 85% of cases due to metastatic or granulomatous disease. Calcification is noted in about 50% of cases of tuberculous Addison's disease but is also seen with hemorrhage, fungal infection, pheochromocytoma, and melanoma.

Differential Diagnosis

Addison's disease should be considered in any patient with hypotension or hyperkalemia. Unexplained weight loss, weakness, and anorexia may be mistaken for occult cancer. Nausea, vomiting, diarrhea, and abdominal pain may be misdiagnosed as intrinsic gastrointestinal disease. The hyperpigmentation may be confused with that due to ethnic or racial factors. Weight loss may simulate anorexia nervosa. The neurologic manifestations of Allgrove's syndrome and adrenoleukodystrophy (especially in women) often mimic multiple sclerosis. Hemochromatosis also enters the differential diagnosis of skin hyperpigmentation, but it should be remembered that it may truly be a cause of Addison's disease as well as diabetes mellitus and hypoparathyroidism. Serum ferritin is increased in most cases of hemochromatosis and is a useful screening test. About 17% of patients with AIDS have symptoms of cortisol resistance. AIDS can also cause frank adrenal insufficiency.

Complications

Any of the complications of the underlying disease (eg, tuberculosis) are more likely to occur, and the patient is susceptible to intercurrent infections that may precipitate crisis. Associated autoimmune diseases are common (see above).

Treatment

A. SPECIFIC THERAPY

Replacement therapy should include a combination of corticosteroids and mineralocorticoids. In mild cases, hydrocortisone alone may be adequate.

Hydrocortisone is the drug of choice. Most addisonian patients are well maintained on 15–25 mg of hydrocortisone orally daily in two divided doses, two-thirds in the morning and one-third in the late afternoon or early evening. Some patients respond better to prednisone in a dosage of about 2–3 mg in the morning and 1–2 mg in the evening. Adjustments in dosage are made according to the clinical response. A proper dose usually results in a normal differential white count. Many patients, however, do not obtain sufficient salt-retaining effect and require fludrocortisone supplementation or extra dietary salt.

Fludrocortisone acetate has a potent sodium-retaining effect. The dosage is 0.05–0.3 mg orally daily or every other day. In the presence of postural hypotension, hyponatremia, or hyperkalemia, the dosage is increased. Similarly, in patients with fatigue, elevated plasma renin activity indicates the need for a higher replacement dose of fludrocortisone. If edema, hypokalemia, or hypertension ensues, the dose is decreased.

DHEA is given to some women with adrenal insufficiency. Women taking DHEA 50 mg orally each morning have experienced an improvement in their overall sense of well-being, mood, and sexuality. Because over-the-counter preparations of DHEA have variable potencies, it is best to have the pharmacy formulate this with pharmaceutical-grade DHEA.

B. GENERAL MEASURES

All infections should be treated immediately and vigorously, and the dose of hydrocortisone should be raised appropriately. The dose of corticosteroid should also be raised in case of trauma, surgery, stressful diagnostic procedures, or other forms of stress. The maximum hydrocortisone dose for severe stress is 50 mg intravenously or intramuscularly every 6 hours. Lower doses, oral or parenteral, are used for less severe stress. The dose is reduced back to normal as the stress subsides. Patients are advised to wear a medical alert bracelet or medal reading, "Adrenal insufficiency—takes hydrocortisone."

For patients with adrenoleukodystrophy, therapy with "Lorenzo's oil" normalizes serum very long-chain fatty acid concentrations but is ineffective clinically. Neurologic manifestations may improve following hematopoietic stem cell transplantation from normal donors.

Prognosis

Patients with Addison's disease can expect a normal life expectancy if their adrenal insufficiency is diag-nosed and treated with appropriate replacement doses of corticosteroids and (if required) mineralocorticoids. However, associated conditions can pose additional health risks. For example, patients with adrenoleukodystrophy or Allgrove syndrome may suffer from neurologic disease. Patients with adrenal tuberculosis may have a serious systemic infection that requires treatment. Adrenal crisis can occur in patients who stop their medication or who experience stress such as infection, trauma, or surgery without appropriately higher doses of corticosteroids. Patients who take excessive doses of corticosteroid replacement can develop Cushing's syndrome, which imposes its own risks. Many patients with treated Addison's disease complain of chronic low-grade fatigue. Such fatigue may be due to epinephrine deficiency, which can result from adrenal destruction. Fatigue may also be an indication of suboptimal dosing of medication, electrolyte imbalance, or concurrent problems such as hypothyroidism or diabetes mellitus. However, most patients with Addison's disease are able to live fully active lives.

Alonso N et al: Evaluation of two replacement regimens in primary adrenal insufficiency patients. Effect on clinical symptoms, health-related quality of life and biochemical parameters. J Endocrinol Invest 2004;27:449. [PMID: 15279078]

Betterle C et al: Autoimmune polyglandular syndrome Type 2: the tip of an iceberg? Clin Exp Immunol 2004;137:225. [PMID: 15270837]

Libe R et al: Effects of dehydroepiandrosterone (DHEA) supplementation on hormonal, metabolic and behavioral status in patients with hypoadrenalism. J Endocrinol Invest 2004;27:736. [PMID: 15636426]

CUSHING'S SYNDROME (Hypercortisolism)

 ESSENTIALS OF DIAGNOSIS

- *Central obesity, muscle wasting, thin skin, easy bruisability, psychological changes, hirsutism, purple striae.*
- *Osteoporosis, hypertension, poor wound healing.*
- *Hyperglycemia, glycosuria, leukocytosis, lymphocytopenia, hypokalemia.*
- *Elevated serum cortisol and urinary free cortisol. Lack of normal suppression by dexamethasone.*

General Considerations

The term Cushing's "syndrome" refers to the manifestations of excessive corticosteroids, commonly due to supraphysiologic doses of corticosteroid drugs and rarely due to spontaneous production of excessive corticosteroids by the adrenal cortex. Cases of spontaneous Cushing's syndrome are rare (2.6 new cases yearly per million population) and have several possible causes.

About 40% of cases are due to Cushing's "disease," by which is meant the manifestations of hypercortisolism due to ACTH hypersecretion by the pituitary. Cushing's disease is caused by a benign pituitary adenoma that is typically very small (< 5 mm). It is at least three times more frequent in women than men.

About 10% of cases are due to nonpituitary neoplasms (eg, small cell lung carcinoma), which produce excessive amounts of ectopic ACTH. Hypokalemia and hyperpigmentation are commonly found in this group.

About 15% of cases are due to ACTH from a source that cannot be initially located.

About 30% of cases are due to excessive autonomous secretion of cortisol by the adrenals—independently of ACTH, serum levels of which are usually low. Most such cases are due to a unilateral adrenal tumor: Benign adrenal adenomas are generally small and produce mostly cortisol; adrenal carcinomas are usually large when discovered and can produce excessive cortisol as well as androgens, with resultant hirsutism and virilization. ACTH-independent macronodular adrenal hyperplasia can also produce hypercortisolism due to the adrenal cortex cells' abnormal stimulation by hormones such as catecholamines, arginine vasopressin, serotonin, hCG/LH, or gastric inhibitory polypeptide; in the latter case, hypercortisolism may be intermittent and food dependent and serum ACTH may not be completely suppressed. Pigmented bilateral adrenal macronodular adrenal hyperplasia is a rare cause of Cushing's syndrome in children and young adults; it may be an isolated condition or part of the Carney complex.

Clinical Findings

A. SYMPTOMS AND SIGNS

Patients with Cushing's syndrome usually have central obesity with a plethoric "moon face," "buffalo hump," supraclavicular fat pads, protuberant abdomen, and thin extremities; oligomenorrhea or amenorrhea (or impotence in the male); weakness, backache, and headache; hypertension; osteoporosis; avascular bone necrosis; and acne and superficial skin infections. Patients may have thirst and polyuria (with or without glycosuria), renal calculi, glaucoma, purple striae (especially around the thighs, breasts, and abdomen), and easy bruisability. Wound healing is impaired. Mental symptoms may range from diminished ability to concentrate to increased lability of mood to frank psychosis. Patients are susceptible to opportunistic infections.

B. LABORATORY FINDINGS

Glucose tolerance is impaired as a result of insulin resistance. Polyuria is present as a result of increased free water clearance; diabetes mellitus with glycosuria may worsen it. Patients with Cushing's syndrome often have leukocytosis with relative granulocytosis and lymphope-

nia. Hypokalemia (but not hypernatremia) may be present, particularly in cases of ectopic ACTH secretion.

Tests for Hypercortisolism

The easiest screening test for hypercortisolism involves giving dexamethasone, 1 mg orally, at 11 PM and collecting serum for cortisol determination at about 8 AM the next morning; a cortisol level under 5 mcg/dL (fluorometric assay) or under 2 mcg/dL (high-performance liquid chromatography [HPLC] assay) excludes Cushing's syndrome with 98% certainty. Antiseizure drugs (eg, phenytoin, phenobarbital, primidone) and rifampin accelerate the metabolism of dexamethasone, in that way causing a false-positive dexamethasone suppression test. Estrogens—during pregnancy or as oral contraceptives or estrogen replacement therapy—may also cause lack of dexamethasone suppressibility.

Patients with an abnormal dexamethasone suppression test require further investigation, which includes a 24-hour urine collection for free cortisol and creatinine. An abnormally high 24-hour urine free cortisol (or free cortisol to creatinine ratio of > 95 mcg cortisol/g creatinine) helps confirm hypercortisolism. A misleadingly high urine free cortisol excretion occurs with high fluid intake. In pregnancy, urine free cortisol is increased, while 17-hydroxycorticosteroids remain normal and diurnal variability of serum cortisol is normal. Carbamazepine and fenofibrate cause false elevations of urine free cortisol when determined by HPLC.

In cases of blatant Cushing's syndrome, no further confirmation of hypercortisolism is necessary. In less certain cases, a 2-day dexamethasone suppression test can also be done by giving dexamethasone, 0.5 mg orally every 6 hours for 48 hours: urine is collected on the second day. Urine free cortisol over 20 mcg/d or urine 17-hydroxycorticosteroid over 4.5 mg/d also helps confirm hypercortisolism.

A midnight serum cortisol level > 7.5 mcg/dL is indicative of Cushing's syndrome and distinguishes it from other conditions associated with a high urine free cortisol (pseudo-Cushing states; see Differential Diagnosis, below). Requirements for this test include being in the same time zone for at least 3 days, being without food for at least 3 hours, and having an indwelling intravenous line established in advance for the blood draw.

Due to the inconvenience of obtaining a midnight blood specimen for serum cortisol, salivary cortisol assays have proved useful. However, the saliva must be collected in special tubes and analyzed only in laboratories that have demonstrated expertise with the assay. Using an enzyme-linked immunosorbent assay, midnight salivary cortisol levels are normally < 0.15 mcg/dL (4.0 nmol/L). Midnight salivary cortisol levels that are consistently > 0.25 mcg/dL (7.0 nmol/L) are nearly diagnostic of endogenous Cushing's syndrome.

Interestingly, hypercortisolism without Cushing's syndrome can occur in several conditions: severe depression, anorexia nervosa, alcoholism, and familial cortisol resistance. (See Differential Diagnosis, below.)

Finding the Cause of Hypercortisolism

Once hypercortisolism is confirmed, aplasma ACTH is obtained. It must be collected properly in a plastic tube on ice and processed quickly by a laboratory with a reliable, sensitive assay. A level of ACTH below the normal range (below about 20 pg/mL) indicates a probable adrenal tumor, whereas higher levels are produced by pituitary or ectopic ACTH-secreting tumors.

Localizing Techniques

In ACTH-dependent Cushing's syndrome, MRI of the pituitary demonstrates a pituitary lesion in about 50% of cases. Premature cerebral atrophy is often noted. When the pituitary MRI is normal or shows a tiny irregularity that may be incidental, selective catheterization of the inferior petrosal sinus veins draining the pituitary is performed. ACTH levels in the inferior petrosal sinus that are more than twice the simultaneous peripheral venous ACTH levels are indicative of pituitary Cushing's disease. Inferior petrosal sinus sampling is also done during CRH administration, which ordinarily causes the ACTH levels in the inferior petrosal sinus to be over three times the peripheral ACTH level when the pituitary is the source of ACTH.

When inferior petrosal sinus ACTH concentrations are not above the requisite levels, a search for an ectopic source of ACTH is undertaken.

Location of ectopic sources of ACTH commences with CT scanning of the chest and abdomen, with special attention to the lungs (for carcinoid or small cell carcinomas), the thymus, the pancreas, and the adrenals. In patients with ACTH-dependent Cushing's syndrome, chest masses should not be assumed to be the source of ACTH, since opportunistic infections are common, so it is prudent to biopsy a chest mass to confirm the pathologic diagnosis prior to resection.

CT scanning fails to detect the source of ACTH in about 40% of patients with ectopic ACTH secretion. ^{111}In-octreotide scanning is also useful in detecting occult tumors, but [18]FDG-PET scanning is not usually helpful. Some ectopic ACTH-secreting tumors elude discovery, necessitating bilateral adrenalectomy.

In non-ACTH-dependent Cushing's syndrome, a CT scan of the adrenals can localize the adrenal tumor in most cases.

Differential Diagnosis

Alcoholic patients can have hypercortisolism and many clinical manifestations of Cushing's syndrome. Depressed patients also have hypercortisolism that can be nearly impossible to distinguish biochemically from Cushing's syndrome but without clinical signs of Cushing's syndrome. Some adolescents develop violaceous striae on the abdomen, back, and breasts; these

are known as "striae distensae" and are not indicative of Cushing's syndrome. Cushing's syndrome can be misdiagnosed as anorexia nervosa (and vice versa) owing to the muscle wasting and extraordinarily high urine free cortisol levels found in anorexia. Patients with severe obesity frequently have an abnormal dexamethasone suppression test, but the urine free cortisol is usually normal, as is diurnal variation of serum cortisol. Patients with familial cortisol resistance have hyperandrogenism, hypertension, and hypercortisolism without actual Cushing's syndrome. In patients with familial partial lipodystrophy type I, central obesity and a moon facies develop, along with thin extremities due to atrophy of subcutaneous fat. However, these patients' muscles are strong and may be hypertrophic, distinguishing this condition from Cushing's syndrome. Patients receiving antiretroviral therapy for HIV-1 infection frequently develop partial lipodystrophy with thin extremities and central obesity with a dorsocervical fat pad ("buffalo hump") that may mimic Cushing's syndrome.

Complications

Cushing's syndrome, if untreated, produces serious morbidity and even death. The patient may suffer from any of the complications of hypertension or of diabetes. Susceptibility to infections is increased. Compression fractures of the osteoporotic spine and aseptic necrosis of the femoral head may cause marked disability. Nephrolithiasis and psychosis may occur. Following bilateral adrenalectomy for Cushing's disease, a pituitary adenoma may enlarge progressively, causing local destruction (eg, visual field impairment) and hyperpigmentation; this complication is known as Nelson's syndrome.

Treatment

Cushing's disease is best treated by transsphenoidal selective resection of the pituitary adenoma. After pituitary surgery, the rest of the pituitary usually returns to normal function; however, the pituitary corticotrophs remain suppressed and require 6–36 months to recover normal function. Hydrocortisone or prednisone replacement therapy is necessary in the meantime. Patients who do not have a remission (or who have a recurrence) should be treated by bilateral laparoscopic adrenalectomy. Another treatment option for patients with ACTH-secreting pituitary tumors is stereotactic pituitary radiosurgery (gamma knife or cyberknife), which normalizes urine free cortisol in two-thirds of patients within 12 months. Conventional radiation therapy results in a 23% cure rate.

Pituitary radiosurgery can also be used to treat Nelson's syndrome, the progressive enlargement of ACTH-secreting pituitary tumors following bilateral adrenalectomy. Patients who are not surgical candidates may be given a trial of ketoconazole in doses of about 200 mg every 6 hours; liver enzymes must be monitored for progressive elevation.

Adrenal neoplasms secreting cortisol are resected laparoscopically. The contralateral adrenal is suppressed, so postoperative hydrocortisone replacement is required until recovery occurs. Metastatic adrenal carcinomas may be treated with mitotane; ketoconazole or metyrapone can help suppress hypercortisolism in unresectable adrenal carcinoma.

Ectopic ACTH-secreting tumors should be located, when possible, and surgically resected. If that cannot be done, laparascopic bilateral adrenalectomy is recommended. Medical treatment with ketoconazole or metyrapone (or both) may partially suppress the hypercortisolism; however, metyrapone may exacerbate female virilization. The somatostatin analog octreotide, given parenterally, suppresses ACTH secretion in about one-third of such cases.

Prognosis

Patients with Cushing's syndrome from a benign adrenal adenoma experience a 5-year survival of 95% and a 10-year survival of 90%, following a successful adrenalectomy. Patients with Cushing's disease from a pituitary adenoma experience a similar survival if their pituitary surgery is successful. However, transsphenoidal surgery incurs a failure rate of about 10–20%, often due to the adenoma's ectopic position or invasion of the cavernous sinus. Those patients who have a complete remission after transsphenoidal surgery have about a 15–20% chance of recurrence over the next 10 years. Patients with failed pituitary surgery may require pituitary radiation therapy, which has its own morbidity. Bilateral adrenalectomy is often complicated by infection; recurrence of hypercortisolism may occur as a result of growth of an adrenal remnant stimulated by high levels of ACTH. The prognosis for patients with ectopic ACTH-producing tumors is dependent upon the aggressiveness and stage of the particular tumor. Patients with ACTH of unknown source have a 5-year survival rate of 65% and a 10-year survival rate of 55%. Patients with adrenal carcinoma have a median survival of 7 months.

Findling JW et al: The low-dose dexamethasone suppression test: a reevaluation in patients with Cushing's syndrome. J Clin Endocrinol Metab 2004;89:1222. [PMID: 15001614]

Hammer GD et al: Transsphenoidal microsurgery for Cushing's disease: initial outcome and long-term results. J Clin Endocrinol Metab 2004;89:6348. [PMID: 15579802]

Ilias I et al: Cushing's syndrome due to ectopic corticotropin secretion: twenty years' experience at the National Institutes of Health. J Clin Endocrinol Metab 2005;90:4955. [PMID: 15914534]

Liu C et al: Cavernous and inferior petrosal sinus sampling in the evaluation of ACTH-dependent Cushing's syndrome. Clin Endocrinol (Oxf) 2004;61:478. [PMID: 15473881]

Pacak K et al: The role of [¹⁸F]fluordeoxyglucose positron emission tomography and [¹¹¹In]-diethylenetriaminepentaacetate-D-Phe-pentetreotide scintigraphy in the localization of ectopic adrenocorticotropin-secreting tumors causing Cushing's syndrome. J Clin Endocrinol Metab 2004;89:2214. [PMID: 15126544]

Viardot A et al: Reproducibility of nighttime salivary cortisol and its use in the diagnosis of hypercortisolism compared with urinary free cortisol and overnight dexamethasone suppression test. J Clin Endocrinol Metab 2005;90:5730. [PMID: 16014408]

Woo YS et al: Clinical and biochemical characteristics of adrenocorticotropin-secreting macroadenomas. J Clin Endocrinol Metab 2005;90:4963. [PMID: 15886242]

HIRSUTISM & VIRILIZATION

 ESSENTIALS OF DIAGNOSIS

- *Hirsutism, acne, menstrual disorders.*
- *Virilization may occur: increased muscularity, androgenic alopecia, deepening of the voice, enlargement of the clitoris.*
- *Rarely, a palpable pelvic tumor.*
- *Urinary 17-ketosteroids and serum DHEAS and androstenedione elevated in adrenal disorders; variable in others.*
- *Serum testosterone is often elevated.*

General Considerations

Hirsutism is defined as excessive terminal hair growth that appears in a male pattern in women. Hirsutism is frequently quantitated according to the Ferriman-Gallwey scale, which grades the presence of androgen sensitive hair from 0 (no hair) to 4 (virile) in 9 areas of the body (maximum score = 36). About 5% of reproductive age women are hisute, with Ferriman-Gallwey scores ≥ 8.

Major androgens include testosterone, androstenedione, and DHEAS. In women, circulating testosterone is derived from direct ovarian secretion (60%) and from peripheral conversion from androstenedione (40%). Androstenedione is secreted in about equal amounts by the adrenals and ovaries. DHEAS is secreted exclusively by the adrenals.

Testosterone is the most potent androgen, but 98% circulates in a bound state: About 65% is strongly bound to sex hormone-binding globulin (SHBG), while 33% is weakly bound to albumin. Only free testosterone and a portion of the weakly bound testosterone can enter target cells to exert an androgenic effect. Assays have therefore been devised to measure "total," "free," or "free and weakly bound" testosterone.

Testosterone is converted in the skin to dihydrotestosterone, which actually stimulates the hair follicle. Dihydrotestosterone is metabolized to androstanediol glucuronide, which can be measured and is elevated in most cases of hirsutism.

Etiology

Hirsutism may be caused by the following disorders.

A. Idiopathic or Familial

Most women with hirsutism or androgenic alopecia have no detectable hyperandrogenism. Patients often have a strong familial predisposition to hirsutism that may be considered normal in the context of their genetic background. Such patients may have elevated serum levels of androstenediol glucuronide, a metabolite of dihydrotestosterone that is produced by skin in cosmetically unacceptable amounts.

B. Polycystic Ovary Syndrome (Hyperthecosis, Stein–Leventhal Syndrome)

Polycystic ovary syndrome (PCOS) is a common functional disorder of the ovaries, affecting about 4–6% of premenopausal women in the United States. It accounts for at least 50% of all cases of clinical hirsutism. Patients frequently have amenorrhea or oligomenorrhea with anovulation and obesity. The serum LH:FSH ratio is often greater than 2.0. Both adrenal and ovarian androgen hypersecretion are commonly present. Insulin resistance and obesity are common; fasting insulin levels are elevated in 70% of cases. Women with PCOS have a 35% risk of depression, compared with 10.7% in age-matched controls. Diabetes mellitus is present in about 13% of cases. Hypertension and hyperlipidemia are often present, increasing the risk of cardiovascular disease. Women frequently regain normal menstrual cycles with aging.

C. Steroidogenic Enzyme Defects

Baby girls with "classic" 21-hydroxylase deficiency have ambiguous genitalia and may become virilized unless treated with corticosteroid replacement; about 50% of such patients have clinically evident mineralocorticoid deficiency (salt-wasting) as well.

About 2% of patients with adult-onset hirsutism have been found to have a partial defect in adrenal 21-hydroxylase, whose phenotypic expression is delayed until adolescence or adulthood; such patients do not have salt-wasting. These women are more likely to develop polycystic ovaries and adrenal adenomas.

Some rare patients with hyperandrogenism and hypertension have 11-hydroxylase deficiency. This is distinguished from cortisol resistance by high cortisol serum levels in the latter and by high serum 11-deoxycortisol levels in the former.

Patients with an XY karyotype and a deficiency in 17β-hydroxysteroid dehydrogenase-3 or a deficiency in 5α-reductase-2 may present as phenotypic girls in whom virilization develops at puberty.

D. Neoplastic Disorders

Ovarian tumors are very uncommon causes of hirsutism (0.8%) and include arrhenoblastomas, Sertoli-Leydig cell tumors, dysgerminomas, and hilar cell tumors. Adrenal carcinoma is a rare cause of Cushing's syndrome and hyperandrogenism that can be quite virilizing. Pure androgen-secreting adrenal tumors occur very rarely; about 50% are malignant.

E. Other Rare Causes of Hirsutism

Other rare causes of hirsutism include acromegaly and ACTH-induced Cushing's syndrome. Maternal virilization during pregnancy may occur as a result of a luteoma of pregnancy, hyperreactio luteinalis, or polycystic ovaries. In postmenopausal women, diffuse stromal Leydig cell hyperplasia is a rare cause of hyperandrogenism. Pharmacologic causes include minoxidil, cyclosporine, phenytoin, anabolic steroids, diazoxide, and certain progestins.

Clinical Findings

A. Symptoms and Signs

Modest androgen excess from any source increases sexual hair (chin, upper lip, abdomen, and chest) and increases sebaceous gland activity, producing acne. Menstrual irregularities, anovulation, and amenorrhea are common. If androgen excess is pronounced, defeminization (decrease in breast size, loss of feminine adipose tissue) and virilization (frontal balding, muscularity, clitoromegaly, and deepening of the voice) occur. Virilization implicates the presence of an androgen-producing neoplasm.

Hypertension may be seen in rare patients with Cushing's syndrome, adrenal 11-hydroxylase deficiency, or cortisol resistance syndrome.

A pelvic examination may disclose clitoromegaly or ovarian enlargement that may be cystic or neoplastic.

B. Laboratory Testing and Imaging

Serum androgen testing is mainly useful to screen for rare occult adrenal or ovarian neoplasms. Some general guidelines are presented here, though exceptions are common.

Serum is assayed for total testosterone and free testosterone. Certain assays for free testosterone are not reliable, including the free androgen index, the analog free testosterone assay, and the electrochemical luminescence assay. It is best to specify the assay desired, eg, free testosterone by equilibrium dialysis, calculated free testosterone, or non-sex-hormone-bound testosterone assay.

A serum testosterone level greater than 200 ng/dL or free testosterone greater than 40 ng/dL indicates the need for pelvic examination and ultrasound. If that is negative, an adrenal CT scan is performed.

A serum androstenedione level greater than 1000 ng/dL also implicates an ovarian or adrenal neoplasm.

Patients with milder elevations of serum testosterone or androstenedione usually are treated with an oral contraceptive.

Patients with very elevated serum DHEAS (> 700 mcg/dL) have an adrenal source of androgen. This usually is due to adrenal hyperplasia and rarely to adrenal carcinoma. An adrenal CT scan is performed.

No firm guidelines exist as to which patients (if any) with hyperandrogenism should be screened for "late-onset" 21-hydroxylase deficiency. The evaluation requires levels of serum 17-hydroxyprogesterone to be drawn at baseline and at 30–60 minutes after the intramuscular injection of 0.25 mg of cosyntropin (ACTH$_{1-24}$). This test should ideally be done during the follicular phase of a woman's menstrual cycle. Patients with congenital adrenal hyperplasia will usually have a baseline 17-hydroxyprogesterone level over 300 ng/dL or a stimulated level over 1000 ng/dL. The diagnosis, once made, is interesting academically but not helpful to the patient since corticosteroid treatment is not particularly more effective in this condition than are other treatment modalities (see below).

Patients with any clinical signs of Cushing's syndrome should receive a screening test. (See Cushing's Syndrome.)

Serum levels of FSH and LH are elevated if amenorrhea is due to ovarian failure. An LH:FSH ratio greater than 2.0 is common in patients with PCOS. On abdominal ultrasound, about 33% of normal young women have polycystic ovaries, so the appearance of ovarian cysts on ultrasound is not helpful.

Virilizing tumors of the ovary can usually be detected by pelvic ultrasound or MRI. However, small virilizing ovarian tumors may not be detectable on imaging studies; selective venous sampling for testosterone may be used for diagnosis in such patients.

Treatment

Any underlying cause of hyperandrogenism must be detected and treated if possible. Postmenopausal women with severe hyperandrogenism should undergo laparoscopic bilateral oophorectomy (if CT scan of the adrenals and ovaries is normal), since small hilar cell tumors of the ovary may not be visible on scans. Girls with hyperandrogenism due to classic salt-wasting congenital adrenal hyperplasia may be treated with laparoscopic bilateral adrenalectomy. Any drugs causing hirsutism are stopped. Treatment options for other cases are summarized in the following.

Spironolactone may be taken in doses of 50–100 mg twice daily orally on days 5–25 of the menstrual cycle or daily if used concomitantly with an oral contraceptive. Hyperkalemia or hyponatremia is uncommon.

Cyproterone acetate is a potent antiandrogen with progestational activity. A dose of 2 mg orally is effective. An oral contraceptive is usually prescribed also. Cyproterone is not available in the United States but is available elsewhere as the progestin element in an oral contraceptive (Diane-35: ethinyl estradiol 35 mcg with cyproterone acetate 2 mg). Side effects may include fatigue, nausea, or depression.

Finasteride inhibits 5α-reductase, the enzyme that converts testosterone to active dihydrotestosterone in the skin. Given as 2.5-mg doses orally daily, it provides modest reduction in hirsutism over 6 months—somewhat less than that achieved with spironolactone. Finasteride is ineffective for androgenic alopecia in women. Side effects are rare.

Flutamide inhibits androgen reception uptake and also suppresses serum androgen. It is given orally in a dosage of 250 mg/d for the first year and then 125 mg/d for maintenance. Used with an oral contraceptive, it appears to be more effective than spironolactone in improving hirsutism, acne, and male pattern baldness. Women with congenital adrenal hyperplasia, who take replacement hydrocortisone, experience decreased renal cortisol clearance when treated with flutamide, resulting in lower hydrocortisone dosage requirements; corticosteroid replacement doses should be reduced when flutamide is added for treatment of hirsutism. Hepatotoxicity has been reported but is rare.

Oral contraceptives stimulate menses (if that is desired) and reduce acne vulgaris, but are less effective for hirsutism. Contraceptives containing ethinyl estradiol 0.3 mg with either desogestrel 0.15 mg or levonorgestrel 0.15 mg appear to be equally effective.

Metformin, 500 mg orally three times daily with meals, given to women with PCOS and amenorrhea, tends to restore normal menses and reduce hirsutism. It is contraindicated in renal disease. Gastrointestinal side effects are usually tolerable. Metformin can be taken by nondiabetics without causing hypoglycemia.

Simvastatin, a "statin," when added to oral contraceptive therapy, has been reported to further decrease serum free testosterone by 16%, besides improving patients' serum lipid profiles.

Local treatment by shaving or depilatories, waxing, electrolysis, or bleaching should be encouraged. Eflornithine (Vaniqua 13.9%) topical cream retards hair growth when applied twice daily to unwanted facial hair; improvement is noted within 4–8 weeks. However, local skin irritation may occur. Hirsutism returns with discontinuation. Laser therapy is an effective treatment for facial hirsutism, particularly for women with dark hair and light skin; complications include skin hypopigmentation (rare) and hyperpigmentation, which occurs in 20% but usually resolves.

Women with androgenic alopecia may be effectively treated with topical minoxidil 2% solution applied twice daily to a dry scalp. Hypertrichosis is an unwanted side effect of topical minoxidil, occurring in 3–5% of treated women; it may affect the forehead, cheeks, upper lip, or chin. Hypertrichosis resolves within 1–6 months after the drug is stopped.

Note: Antiandrogen treatments must be given only to nonpregnant women. Women must be counseled to take oral contraceptives, when indicated, and avoid pregnancy, since use during pregnancy causes malformations and pseudohermaphroditism in male infants.

Azziz R et al: Androgen excess in women: experience with over 1000 consecutive patients. J Clin Endocrinol Metab 2004; 89:453. [PMID: 14764747]

Chang RJ: A practical approach to the diagnosis of polycystic ovary syndrome. Am J Obstet Gynecol 2004;191:713. [PMID: 15467530]

Ganic MA et al: Comparison of efficacy of spironolactone with metformin in the management of polycystic ovary syndrome: an open-label study. J Clin Endocrinol Metab 2004; 89:2756. [PMID: 15181054]

Ortega-Gonzalez C et al: Responses of serum androgen and insulin resistance to metformin and pioglitazone in obese, insulin-resistant women with polycystic ovary syndrome. J Clin Endocrinol Metab 2005;90:1360. [PMID: 15598674]

Palomba S et al: Prospective parallel randomized, double-blind, double-dummy controlled clinical trial comparing clomiphene citrate and metformin as the first-line treatment for ovulation induction in nonobese anovulatory women with polycystic ovary syndrome. J Clin Endocrinol Metab 2005; 90:4068. [PMID: 15840746]

Rosenfield RL: Clinical practice. Hirsutism. N Engl J Med 2005; 353:2578. [PMID: 16354894]

Souter I et al: The prevalence of androgen excess among patients with minimal unwanted hair growth. Am J Obstet Gynecol 2004;191:1914. [PMID: 15592272]

PRIMARY HYPERALDOSTERONISM

 ESSENTIALS OF DIAGNOSIS

- *Hypertension, polyuria, polydipsia, muscular weakness.*
- *Hypokalemia, alkalosis.*
- *Elevated plasma and urine aldosterone levels and low plasma renin level.*

General Considerations

Classic hyperaldosteronism (with hypokalemia) accounts for about 0.7% of cases of hypertension. Milder hyperaldosteronism, without hypokalemia, is more common, with a prevalence of 5–14% among hypertensives. The disorder is more common in women. Primary hyperaldosteronism may be due to unilateral adrenocortical adenoma (Conn's syndrome, 73%) or bilateral cortical hyperplasia (27%), which may be corticosteroid suppressible due to an autosomal-dominant genetic defect allowing ACTH stimulation of aldosterone production.

Clinical Findings

A. Symptoms and Signs

Hypertension, muscular weakness (at times with paralysis simulating periodic paralysis), paresthesias with frank tetany, headache, polyuria, and polydipsia are the main complaints. Hypertension is typically moderate. Some patients have only diastolic hypertension, without other symptoms and signs. Malignant hypertension is rare. Edema is rarely seen in primary hyperaldosteronism.

B. Laboratory Findings

For a patient to be properly tested for hyperaldosteronism, all antihypertensive medications must be dis-

continued. Calcium channel blockers can normalize aldosterone secretion, thus interfering with the diagnosis. β-Blockers suppress plasma renin activity in patients with essential hypertension. The patient must have a high sodium intake (> 120 mEq/d) during the entire evaluation period; plasma potassium may be low. A 24-hour urine collection is assayed for aldosterone, free cortisol, and creatinine. A low plasma renin activity (< 5 mcg/dL) with 24-hour urine aldosterone over 20 mcg indicates hyperaldosteronism. A urine aldosterone of less than 20 mcg/24 h is seen with rare adrenal or gonadal enzyme defects in the activity of 17α-hydroxylase (associated with ambiguous genitalia or primary amenorrhea) or 11β-hydroxylase (associated with virilization).

The ratio of plasma aldosterone concentration to plasma renin activity has been used to screen for hyperaldosteronism. Unfortunately, this test lacks sensitivity and specificity.

Once hyperaldosteronism is diagnosed, plasma is assayed for 18-hydroxycorticosterone; a level over 85 ng/dL is seen with adrenal neoplasms, whereas levels under 85 ng/dL are nondiagnostic. Additionally, plasma can be assayed for aldosterone at 8 AM while the patient is supine after overnight recumbency and again after 4 hours upright. Patients with an adrenal adenoma usually have a baseline plasma aldosterone level greater than 20 mcg/dL that does not rise. In one study, serum aldosterone levels fell (after 4 hours upright) in 63% of patients with a unilateral aldosteronoma and in no patients with bilateral adrenal hyperplasia. Patients with hyperplasia typically have a baseline plasma aldosterone level less than 20 mcg/dL that rises during upright posture. Exceptions occur.

C. Imaging

If biochemical testing implicates an adrenal aldosterone-secreting adenoma, a thin-section CT scan of the adrenals is obtained. A discrete adrenal adenoma (> 1 cm in diameter with normal contralateral adrenal) is found is 60–80% of such patients. However, about 20% of such "adenomas" are found to be hyperplasia at surgery. A dexamethasone-suppressed ^{131}I-labeled 6β-iodomethyl-19-norcholesterol scan (adrenal scintigraphy) can identify an aldosteronoma but may yield misleading results. Therefore, it is often prudent to supplement CT localization with adrenal vein catheterization for aldosterone.

Differential Diagnosis

The differential diagnosis of hyperaldosteronism includes other causes of hypokalemia (see Chapter 21) in patients with essential hypertension. For example, many hypertensive patients taking diuretics develop hypokalemia even while taking potassium-sparing diuretics or potassium supplements. Chronic depletion of intravascular volume stimulates renin secretion and secondary hyperaldosteronism. Thus, it is important to discontinue diuretics and ensure adequate hydration and sodium intake when assessing a patient for primary hyperaldosteronism (see above).

Excessive ingestion of real licorice (black and derived from anise) may produce hypertension and hypokalemia caused by a derivative of its glycyrrhizinic acid inhibiting 11β-hydroxysteroid dehydrogenase, thereby enhancing cortisol's mineralocorticoid effect. Oral contraceptives may increase aldosterone secretion in some patients. Renal vascular disease can cause severe hypertension with hypokalemia; plasma renin activity is high, distinguishing it from primary hyperaldosteronism.

Excessive adrenal secretion of other corticosteroids (besides aldosterone) may also cause hypertension with hypokalemia. This occurs with certain congenital adrenal enzyme disorders such as P-450c11 deficiency (increased deoxycorticosterone with virilization and deficient cortisol) or P-450c17 deficiency (increased deoxycorticosterone, corticosterone, and progesterone but deficient estradiol and testosterone). Primary cortisol resistance can cause hypertension and hypokalemia; renin and aldosterone are suppressed, while plasma levels of cortisol, ACTH, and deoxycorticosterone are high. Liddle's syndrome is an autosomal dominant cause of hypertension and hypokalemia resulting from excessive sodium absorption from the renal tubule; renin and aldosterone levels are low. Thyrotoxicosis and familial periodic paralysis may also present with hypokalemia. Hyperaldosteronism may rarely be due to a malignant ovarian tumor.

Complications

All of the complications of chronic hypertension are encountered in primary hyperaldosteronism. Progressive renal damage is less reversible than hypertension. Following unilateral adrenalectomy for Conn's syndrome, suppression of the contralateral adrenal may result in temporary postoperative hypoaldosteronism, characterized by hyperkalemia and hypotension.

Treatment

Conn's syndrome (unilateral adrenal adenoma secreting aldosterone) is treated by laparoscopic adrenalectomy, though lifelong spironolactone therapy is an option. Bilateral adrenal hyperplasia is best treated with spironolactone; bilateral adrenalectomy corrects the hypokalemia but not the hypertension and should *not* be performed. Antihypertensive agents may also be necessary. Hyperplasia sometimes responds well to dexamethasone suppression.

Prognosis

The hypertension is reversible in about two-thirds of cases but persists or returns in spite of surgery in the remainder. The prognosis is much improved by early diagnosis and treatment. Only 2% of aldosterone-secreting adrenal tumors are malignant.

The low renin levels found in this condition (and in about 25% of cases of essential hypertension) also imply a relatively good prognosis.

Al Fehaily M et al: Clinical manifestations of aldosteronoma. Surg Clin North Am 2004;84:887. [PMID: 15145241]

Seiler L et al: Diagnosis of primary aldosteronism: value of different screening parameters, and influence of antihypertensive medication. Eur J Endocrinol 2004;150:329. [PMID: 15012618]

Tiu SC et al: The use of aldosterone-renin ratio as a diagnostic test for primary hyperaldosteronism and its test characteristics under different conditions of blood sampling. J Clin Endocrinol Metab 2005;90:72. [PMID: 15483077]

Vasan RS et al: Serum aldosterone and the incidence of hypertension in nonhypertensive persons. N Engl J Med 2004;351:33. [PMID: 15229305]

Young WF et al: Role for adrenal venous sampling in primary aldosteronism. Surgery 2004;136:1227. [PMID: 15657580]

■ DISEASES OF THE ADRENAL MEDULLA

PHEOCHROMOCYTOMA

ESSENTIALS OF DIAGNOSIS

- *"Attacks" of headache, perspiration, palpitations.*
- *Hypertension, frequently sustained but often paroxysmal, especially during surgery or delivery.*
- *Attacks of nausea, abdominal pain, chest pain, weakness, dyspnea, tremor, visual disturbance.*
- *Anxiety, tremor, or weight loss.*
- *Elevated urinary catecholamines or their metabolites. Normal serum T_4 and TSH.*

General Considerations

Pheochromocytomas are rare, being found in less than 0.3% of hypertensive individuals. The incidence is higher in patients with moderate to severe hypertension. About two new cases per million population are diagnosed annually. However, in autopsy cases, the incidence of pheochromocytoma is 250–1300 cases per million, indicating that most cases are not diagnosed during life. The hypertension is caused by excessive plasma levels of norepinephrine or neuropeptide Y. Patients have disease characterized by paroxysmal or sustained hypertension due to a tumor located in either or both adrenals or anywhere along the sympathetic nervous chain, and rarely in such aberrant locations as the thorax, bladder, or brain. Primary extra-adrenal pheochromocytomas are known as "paragangliomas." Pheochromocytomas are characterized by a rough "rule of tens": About 10% of cases are not associated with hypertension; 10% of cases are extra-adrenal, and of those about 10% of cases are extra-abdominal (paraganglioma); 10% of cases occur in children. In about 10% of cases, the tumor involves both adrenal glands (bilateral adrenal tumors tend to occur more frequently in familial cases); and about 10% of cases have metastatic disease noted around the time of diagnosis. Initially occult metastases are later discovered in another 5% of cases.

Familial pheochromocytomas are usually bilateral (70% of cases) and may be associated with the following: calcitonin-secreting medullary thyroid carcinoma and hyperparathyroidism (MEN type 2), medullary thyroid carcinoma and the syndrome of multiple mucosal neuromas (MEN type 2B), neurofibromatosis (Recklinghausen's disease), and islet cell tumors (rare).

Pheochromocytomas develop in about 20% of patients with von Hippel–Lindau disease (hemangiomas of the retina, cerebellum, brainstem, and spinal cord; pancreatic cysts; renal cysts, adenomas, and carcinomas); inheritance is autosomal dominant.

Familial paragangliomas arise in patients harboring pathologic sequence variants in the succinate dehydrogenase gene subunits: SDHB, SDHC, and SDHD. Multiple paragangliomas typically arise at an early age and are often malignant.

Only about 10% of affected patients have a family history of pheochromocytoma or paraganglioma. However, family histories are unreliable and phenotypic penetrance is variable. About 20–30% of these patients harbor germline mutations, making such patients prone to development of additional tumors.

Clinical Findings

A. SYMPTOMS AND SIGNS

Pheochromocytomas can be lethal unless they are diagnosed and treated appropriately. They typically cause attacks of severe headache (80% of patients), perspiration (70% of patients), and palpitations (60% of patients); other symptoms may include anxiety (50% of patients), a sense of impending doom, or tremor (40% of patients). Vasomotor changes during an attack cause mottled cyanosis and facial pallor; as the attack subsides, facial flushing may occur as a result of reflex vasodilation. Other findings may include tachycardia, precordial or abdominal pain, vomiting, increasing nervousness and irritability, increased appetite, and loss of weight. Anginal attacks may occur. Physical findings usually include hypertension (90% of patients), which may be sustained (20% of patients), sustained with paroxysms (50% of patients), or paroxysmal only (25% of patients). There may be cardiac enlargement and cardiomyopathy, postural tachycardia (change of more than 20 beats/min) and postural hypotension, and mild elevation of basal body temper-

ature. Retinal hemorrhage or cerebrovascular hemorrhage occurs occasionally.

Catastrophic hypertensive crisis and fatal cardiac arrhythmias can occur spontaneously or may be triggered by intravenous contrast dye or glucagon injection, needle biopsy of the mass, anesthesia, and surgical procedures.

The manifestations of pheochromocytoma are quite varied and mimic other conditions. Some patients are normotensive and asymptomatic. In addition to the above symptoms, some patients can present with psychosis or confusion, seizures, hyperglycemia, bradycardia, hypotension, constipation, paresthesias, or Raynaud's phenomenon. Other patients may have pulmonary edema and heart failure due to cardiomyopathy. Epinephrine secretion may cause episodic tachyarrhythmias, hypotension, or syncope. Some patients may be entirely asymptomatic despite high serum levels of catecholamines. Others may present with abdominal discomfort from a large hemorrhagic pheochromocytoma, or with pain from metastatic disease.

In addition to catecholamines and their metabolites, pheochromocytomas secrete a wide range of other peptides that can sometimes cause symptoms of Cushing's syndrome (ACTH), erythrocytosis (erythropoietin), or hypercalcemia (PTHrP).

B. LABORATORY FINDINGS

Hypermetabolism is present; thyroid function tests are normal, including serum T_4, FT_4, T_3, and TSH. Hyperglycemia is present in about 35% of patients but is usually mild. Leukocytosis is common. The ESR is sometimes elevated. Plasma renin activity may be increased by catecholamines.

C. SPECIAL TESTS

The most sensitive test for secretory pheochromocytoma is plasma fractionated free metanephrines; false-positive results are fairly common. Assay of urinary catecholamines and metanephrines (total and fractionated) and creatinine detects most pheochromocytomas, especially when samples are obtained during or immediately following an episodic attack. A 24-hour urine specimen is usually obtained, although an overnight or shorter collection may be used; patients with pheochromocytomas generally have more that 2.2 mcg of total metanephrine per milligram of creatinine, and more than 135 mcg total catecholamines per gram creatinine. Urinary assay for total metanephrines is about 97% sensitive for detecting functioning pheochromocytomas. Urinary assay for vanillylmandelic acid (VMA) is about 89% sensitive and is not usually required.

Testing for catecholamines and metanephrines should be done using high-performance liquid chromatography with electrochemical detection (HPLC-ECD); this minimizes false test results. Nevertheless, some drugs and foods can interfere with certain assays, and stresses can also cause misleading elevations in catecholamine excretion (Table 26–15). About 10% of

Table 26–15. Factors potentially causing misleading catecholamine or metanephrine results: high-performance liquid chromatography with electrochemical detection (HPLC-ECD).

Drugs	Foods	Conditions
Acetaminophen[2]	Bananas[1]	Amyotrophic lateral
Aldomet[2]	Caffeine[1]	sclerosis[1]
Amphetamines[1]	Coffee[2]	Brain lesions[1]
Bronchodilators[1]	Peppers[2]	Carcinoid[1]
Buspirone[2]		Eclampsia[1]
Captopril[2]		Emotion, severe[1]
Cocaine[1]		Exercise, vigorous[1]
Cimetidine[2]		Guillain-Barré
Codeine[2]		syndrome[1]
Decongestants[1]		Hypoglycemia[1]
Ephedrine[1]		Lead poisoning[1]
Fenfluramine[3]		Myocardial infarct,
Isoproterenol[1]		acute[1]
Levodopa[2]		Pain, severe[1]
Labetalol[1,2]		Porphyria, acute[1]
Mandelamine[2]		Psychosis, acute[1]
Metoclopramide[2]		Quadriplegia[1]
Nitroglycerin[1]		Renal failure[3]
Viloxazine[2]		

[1]Increases catecholamine excretion.
[2]May cause confounding peaks on HPLC chromatograms.
[3]Decreases catecholamine excretion.

hypertensive patients have a misleadingly elevated level of one or more tests.

Direct assay of epinephrine and norepinephrine in blood and urine during or following an attack is a sensitive test for pheochromocytoma associated with paroxysmal hypertension. Plasma free metanephrine concentrations may also be used. Proper, quiet collection of plasma specimens is essential.

Serum chromogranin A is elevated in 90% of patients with pheochromocytoma and the levels correlate with tumor size, being higher in patients with metastatic disease. Serum chromogranin A levels can be misleadingly elevated in patients with azotemia or hypergastrinemia, and in those treated with corticosteroids or proton pump inhibitors. Serum may also be assayed for neuron-specific enolase; high levels implicate a malignant pheochromocytoma, while normal levels are nonspecific.

Pharmacologic provocative and suppressive tests that evaluate the rise or fall in blood pressure are usually not required or recommended.

Genetic testing should ideally be performed on all patients with pheochromocytoma or paraganglioma. Testing for VHL, *ret* protooncogene, and SDHB/SDHD mutations is advisable. Family members may then be screened for the specific gene mutation.

D. Imaging

1. CT and MRI scanning—Imaging should not usually replace biochemical testing, since incidental adrenal adenomas are common (2–4% of scans) and can be misleading. When a pheochromocytoma is suspected because of biochemical testing or a genetic condition predisposing to pheochromocytoma, a CT scan of the abdomen is performed, with thin sections through the adrenals. A noncontrast CT should be followed by a CT scan using nonionic contrast, which reduces the risk catecholamine release from a pheochromocytoma. Glucagon should not be used during scanning, since it can provoke hypertensive crisis; similarly, intravenous contrast can precipitate hypertensive crisis, particularly in patients whose hypertension is uncontrolled.

MRI scanning has the advantage of not requiring intravenous contrast dye; its lack of radiation makes it the imaging of choice during pregnancy and childhood. On T2-weighted MRI, adrenal tumors that are hyperintense relative to liver have an increased likelihood of being pheochromocytomas. Both CT and MRI scanning have a sensitivity of about 90% for adrenal pheochromocytoma and a sensitivity of 95% for adrenal tumors over 0.5 cm in diameter. However, both CT and MRI are less sensitive for detecting recurrent tumors, metastases, and extra-adrenal paragangliomas. If no adrenal tumor is found, the scan is extended to include the entire abdomen, pelvis, and chest.

2. Nuclear imaging—A whole-body [123I]*m*-Iodobenzylguanidine ([123I]mIBG) scan can localize tumors with a sensitivity of 85% and a specificity of 99%. It is less sensitive for MEN 2A- or MEN 2B-related pheochromocytomas. Preoperative [123I]mIBG scanning is not usually required to confirm that a unilateral adrenal mass is a pheochromocytoma in a patient with classic clinical and biochemical presentation. Preoperative whole-body [123I]mIBG scanning can be useful when the CT scan cannot locate a suspected pheochromocytoma, making a paraganglioma more likely; it can also be useful when the CT scan is ambiguous for pheochromocytoma. It is prudent to perform a whole-body [123I]mIBG scan about 3 months postoperatively to determine if metastatic or recurrent tumor is present. Drugs that reduce [123I]mIBG uptake should be avoided, including tricyclic antidepressants and cyclobenzaprine (6 weeks), amphetamines, nasal decongestants, phenothiazines, haloperidol, diet pills, labetalol, and cocaine (2 weeks).

Somatostatin receptor imaging using ^{111}In-labeled octreotide is only 25% sensitive for detecting an adrenal pheochromocytoma. However, ^{111}In-labeled octreotide scanning is quite sensitive for detecting extra-adrenal pheochromocytomas (paragangliomas) and metastatic pheochromocytomas, sometimes locating tumors that were missed by [123I]mIBG scanning.

PET scanning usually detects tumors using ^{18}F-labeled deoxyglucose or ^{18}F-labeled dopamine, and may demonstrate tumors that are not visible on [123I]mIBG scanning. Combining PET scan with noncontrast CT produces a PET/CT fusion scan with exceptional sensitivity.

Differential Diagnosis

Tachycardia, tremor, palpitation, and hypermetabolism may give rise to confusion with thyrotoxicosis. Pheochromocytoma may also be misdiagnosed as essential hypertension, myocarditis, glomerulonephritis or other renal lesions, toxemia of pregnancy, eclampsia, and psychoneurosis (anxiety attack). It can sometimes be mistaken for an acute abdomen.

Other conditions that have manifestations similar to those of pheochromocytoma include acute intermittent porphyria, hypogonadal vascular instability (hot flushes), cocaine or amphetamine use, clonidine withdrawal, hypertensive crisis caused by foods containing tyramine (eg, cheeses) in patients taking monoamine oxidase inhibitor antidepressants, labile hypertension, and unstable angina. Patients with erythromelalgia can have hypertensive crises; their episodic painful flushing and leg swelling are relieved by cold, distinguishing this condition from pheochromocytoma. Pheochromocytomas can cause chest pain and electrocardiographic changes that mimic acute cardiac ischemia. Renal artery stenosis can cause severe hypertension and may coexist with pheochromocytoma.

False-positive testing for catecholamines and metabolites occurs in about 10% of hypertensives, but levels are usually less than 50% above normal and typically normalize with repeat testing.

Complications

All of the complications of severe hypertension may be encountered. Additionally, a catecholamine-induced cardiomyopathy may develop. Sudden death may occur due to cardiac arrhythmia. Acute respiratory distress syndrome has been reported. Hypertensive crises with sudden blindness or cerebrovascular accidents are not uncommon. Paroxysms may be precipitated by sudden movement, by manipulation during or after pregnancy, by emotional stress or trauma, or during surgical removal of the tumor. Decongestant medications, fluoxetine, and other SSRIs may induce hypertensive paroxysms. Cardiomyopathy may develop. Occasionally, the initial manifestation of pheochromocytoma may be hypotension or even shock.

After removal of the tumor, a state of severe hypotension and shock (resistant to epinephrine and norepinephrine) may ensue with precipitation of renal failure or myocardial infarction. Hypotension and shock may occur from spontaneous infarction or hemorrhage of the tumor.

On rare occasions, a patient dies as a result of the complications of diagnostic tests or during surgery. During surgery, pheochromocytoma cells may be seeded within the peritoneum, resulting in multifocal recurrent tumors.

Treatment

Laparoscopic removal of the tumor or tumors is the treatment of choice. Very large and invasive tumors are treated with open laparotomy. Patients with small familial or bilateral pheochromocytomas may undergo selective resection of the tumors, sparing the adrenal cortex; however, there is a recurrence rate of 10% over 10 years. Preoperative administration of α-adrenergic-blocking drugs has made pheochromocytoma surgery much safer in recent years. Phenoxybenzamine is given initially in a dosage of 10 mg orally every 12 hours, increasing gradually—about every 3 days—until hypertension is controlled. The usual maintenance dose is 40–120 mg daily. Optimal α-blockade is achieved when supine arterial pressure is below 160/90 mm Hg and standing arterial pressure is above 80/45 mm Hg. Calcium channel blockers such as sustained-release nifedipine or nicardipine are also effective, are better tolerated than α-blockers, and may be coadministered with α-blockers. Labetalol therapy is avoided, since it has been associated with more postoperative hypotension, causes interference in some urinary catecholamine assays, and reduces [^{123}I]mIBG scanning sensitivity.

After appropriate antihypertensive therapy, propranolol (10–40 mg four times orally daily), can be used to control tachycardia and other arrhythmias. Blood pressure control should be maintained for a minimum of 4–7 days or until optimal cardiac status is established. The ECG should be monitored until it becomes stable. (It may take a week or even months to correct electrocardiographic changes in patients with catecholamine myocarditis, and it may be prudent to defer surgery until then in such cases.) Patients must be very closely monitored during surgery to promptly detect sudden changes in blood pressure or cardiac arrhythmias.

Hypertensive crisis can be managed initially with oral nifedipine 10 mg (chewed pierced capsule). Intraoperative severe hypertension is managed with continuous intravenous nicardipine (a short-acting calcium channel blocker), 2–6 mcg/kg/min, or nitroprusside, 0.5–10 mcg/kg/min. Prolonged nitroprusside administration can cause cyanide toxicity. Tachyarrhythmia is treated with intravenous atenolol (1 mg boluses), esmolol, or lidocaine.

Autotransfusion of 1–2 units of blood at 12 hours preoperatively plus generous intraoperative volume replacement reduces the risk of postresection hypotension caused by desensitization of the vascular α_1-receptors. Shock may therefore occur following removal of the pheochromocytoma. It is treated with intravenous saline or colloid and high doses of intravenous norepinephrine. Intravenous 5% dextrose is infused postoperatively to prevent hypoglycemia.

Because there may be multiple or metastatic tumors, it is essential to recheck urinary catecholamine levels postoperatively (at least 2 weeks after surgery). It is also prudent to perform a whole-body [^{123}I]mIBG scan about 3 months postoperatively, since previously undetected metastases may become visible. Thereafter, blood pressure and symptoms must be rechecked regularly for life; urinary catecholamines and metanephrines are also rechecked regularly, at least every 6 months for 5 years, and immediately if hypertension or symptoms recur or if metastases are evident.

For inoperable or metastatic tumors, metyrosine may be added to reduce catecholamine synthesis. Metyrosine is a competitive blocker in the synthesis of catecholamines that is also useful; the initial dosage is 250 mg four times daily, increased daily by increments of 250–500 mg to a maximum of 4 g/d. Metyrosine causes central nervous system side effects and crystalluria; hydration must be ensured. Metastatic pheochromocytomas may be treated with combination chemotherapy (eg, cyclophosphamide, vincristine, and dacarbazine) or with high doses of [^{131}I]mIBG.

Prognosis

The prognosis depends on how early the diagnosis is made. The malignancy of a pheochromocytoma cannot be determined by histologic examination. A tumor is considered malignant if metastases are present; this may take many years to become clinically evident. Therefore, lifetime surveillance is required. Malignancy is more likely for paragangliomas and for large pheochromocytomas (> 7 cm in diameter). The prognosis is good for patients with smaller, benign pheochromocytomas that are resected before causing cardiovascular damage. Hypertension usually resolves after successful surgery, but may persist or return in 25% of patients despite successful surgery. Although this may be essential hypertension, biochemical reevaluation is then required, looking for a second or metastatic pheochromocytoma.

Before the advent of blocking agents, the surgical mortality rate was as high as 30%, but this has rapidly decreased. A team approach—endocrinologist, anesthesiologist, and surgeon—is critically important. With optimal management, the surgical mortality rate is less than 3%.

Patients with metastatic pheochromocytoma and paraganglioma have a 5-year survival rate of 44% after surgery; patients who have their primary tumor resected and subsequently receive high-dose [^{131}I]mIBG therapy have been reported to have a 5-year survival rate of 75%. Patients with a heavy and increasing tumor burden and distant metastases have a worse prognosis; patients with multiple pulmonary metastases have limited survival. Those with metastases limited to the abdomen have a better prognosis. Some patients have an indolent malignancy and experience a prolonged survival.

Ilias I et al: Current approaches and recommended algorithm for the diagnostic localization of pheochromocytoma. J Clin Endocrinol Metab 2004;89:479. [PMID: 14764749]

Kercher KW et al: Laparoscopic curative resection of pheochromocytomas. Ann Surg 2005;241:919. [PMID: 15912041]

Khorram-Manesh A et al: Mortality associated with pheochromocytoma in a large Swedish cohort. Eur J Surg Oncol 2004; 30:556. [PMID: 15135486]

Lenders JW et al: Phaeochromocytoma. Lancet 2005;366:665. [PMID: 16112304]

Neumann HP et al: Distinct clinical features of paraganglioma syndromes associated with SDHB and SDHD gene mutations. JAMA 2004;292:943. [PMID: 15328326]

Rose B et al: High-dose 131I-metaiodobenzylguanadine therapy for 12 patients with malignant pheochromocytoma. Cancer 2003;98:239. [PMID: 12872341]

■ PANCREATIC & DUODENAL NEUROENDOCRINE TUMORS*

ISLET CELL TUMORS

 ESSENTIALS OF DIAGNOSIS

- *Half the tumors are nonsecretory; weight loss, abdominal pain, or jaundice may be presenting signs.*
- *Secretory tumors cause a variety of manifestations depending upon the hormones secreted.*

General Considerations

The pancreatic islets are composed of several types of cells, each with distinct chemical and microscopic features: the A cells (20%) secrete glucagon, the B cells (70%) secrete insulin, and the D cells (5%) secrete somatostatin or gastrin. F cells secrete "pancreatic polypeptide." Each type of cell may give rise to benign or malignant neoplasms that may be multiple and usually present with a clinical syndrome related to hypersecretion of a native or ectopic hormonal product. The endocrine diagnosis of a particular pancreatic islet neoplasm depends on first suspecting it from its clinical manifestations. Many tumors secrete two or more different hormones.

Insulinomas are usually (about 82%) benign and secrete excessive amounts of insulin (as well as proinsulin and C-peptide), which causes hypoglycemia. The tumors may be multiple, especially in familial MEN 1—about 12% of cases (see Chapter 27).

Gastrinomas secrete excessive quantities of the hormone gastrin (as well as "big" gastrin), which stimulates the stomach to hypersecrete acid, thereby causing hyperplastic gastric rugae and peptic ulceration (Zollinger–Ellison syndrome). Most gastrinomas are benign, but some are malignant and metastasize to the liver. Gastrinomas are typically found in the duodenum (49%), pancreas (24%), or lymph nodes (11%).

---

*Diabetes mellitus and hyperglycemia are discussed in Chapter 27.

Presenting symptoms and signs include abdominal pain (75%), diarrhea (73%), heartburn (44%), bleeding (25%), or weight loss (17%). Endoscopy usually discovers prominent gastric folds (94%). Sporadic Zollinger–Ellison syndrome is rarely suspected at the onset of symptoms; typically, there is a 5-year delay in diagnosis. About 22% of patients have MEN 1. MEN 1 usually presents in patients who are younger; hyperparathyroidism may occur from 14 years preceding the Zollinger–Ellison diagnosis to 38 years afterward. (See Multiple Endocrine Neoplasia, below.) Therapy with high doses of proton pump inhibitors (quadruple usual doses) is usually effective. Surgery is not usually performed because of the low cure rates, particularly in patients with MEN 1. Note that serum gastrin levels tend to be high in any patient who is taking a proton pump inhibitor; hypercalcemia also stimulates gastrin release.

The 5-, 10-, and 20-year survival rates with MEN 1 are 94%, 75%, and 58%, respectively, while the survival rates for sporadic Zollinger–Ellison syndrome are 62%, 50%, and 31%, respectively. (See Chapter 14.)

Glucagonomas are usually malignant; weight loss and liver metastases are ordinarily present by the time of diagnosis. They usually secrete other hormones besides glucagon, often gastrin. Other initial symptoms often include diarrhea, nausea, peptic ulcer, or necrolytic migratory erythema. About 35% of patients ultimately develop diabetes. The median survival is 2.8 years after diagnosis.

Somatostatinomas are very rare and are associated with weight loss, diabetes mellitus, malabsorption, and hypochlorhydria.

Other rare tumors secrete excessive amounts of **vasoactive intestinal polypeptide (VIP)**, a substance that causes profuse watery diarrhea (Verner–Morrison syndrome). Treatment with octreotide improves the symptoms but does not halt tumor growth. Symptomatic improvement with calcitonin treatment has also been reported.

Islet cell tumors can secrete ectopic hormones in addition to native hormones, often in combinations producing a variety of clinical syndromes. They may secrete ACTH, producing Cushing's syndrome. Secretion of serotonin can produce an atypical carcinoid syndrome manifested by pain, diarrhea, and weight loss; skin flushing occurs in only 39% of patients. Pancreatic carcinoid tumors grow slowly but usually metastasize to local and distant sites, particularly to other endocrine organs.

Islet cell tumors may be part of the syndrome of multiple endocrine adenomatosis type I (with pituitary and parathyroid adenomas).

Localization of noninsulinoma pancreatic islet cell tumors and their metastases is best done with somatostatin receptor scintigraphy (SRS); SRS detects about 75% of noninsulinomas. CT and MRI are also useful. Insulinomas can usually be located preoperatively by endoscopic ultrasonography. For insulinomas, preoperative localization studies are less successful and have the following sensitivities: ultrasonography 25%, CT 25%, endoscopic ultrasonography 27%, transhepatic portal vein sampling 40%, arteriography 45%, intraoperative palpation 55%, and intraoperative pancreatic ultrasound 75%. Nearly all insulinomas can be successfully located at surgery by intraoperative palpation and ultrasound. An abdominal CT scan is usually obtained, but extensive preoperative localization procedures, especially with invasive methods, are not required. Tumors may be located in the pancreatic head or neck (57%), body (15%), or tail (19%) or in the duodenum (9%).

Direct resection of the tumor (or tumors), which often spreads locally, is the primary form of therapy for all types of islet cell neoplasm except Zollinger–Ellison syndrome, where use of high doses of a proton pump inhibitor is the therapy of choice. Insulinomas are resected. However, in MEN 1, insulinomas are rarely cured, so surgery is reserved for dominant masses in such cases. Palliation of functioning malignant disease often requires both antihormonal and anticancer chemotherapy. The use of streptozocin, doxorubicin, and asparaginase, especially for malignant insulinoma, has produced some encouraging results, though these drugs are quite toxic. The hypoglycemia of insulinoma may be counteracted by verapamil or diazoxide. Octreotide LAR is useful in the therapy of islet cell tumors with the exception of insulinoma; monthly subcutaneous injections of 20–30 mg are required.

The prognosis in these neoplasms is variable. The surgical complication rate is about 40%, with patients commonly developing fistulas and infections. Extensive pancreatic resection may cause diabetes mellitus. The overall 5-year survival is higher with functional tumors (77%) than with nonfunctional ones (55%) and higher with benign tumors (91%) than with malignant ones (55%).

Finlayson E et al: Surgical treatment of insulinomas. Surg Clin North Am 2004;84:775. [PMID: 15145234]

Hirshberg B et al: Malignant insulinoma: spectrum of unusual clinical features. Cancer 2005;104:264. [PMID: 15937909]

Norton JA et al: Resolved and unresolved controversies in the surgical management of patients with Zollinger-Ellison syndrome. Ann Surg 2004;240:757. [PMID: 15492556]

Warner RR: Enteroendocrine tumors other than carcinoid: a review of clinically significant advances. Gastroenterology 2005;128:1668. [PMID: 15887158]

■ DISEASES OF THE TESTES

MALE HYPOGONADISM

 ESSENTIALS OF DIAGNOSIS

- *Diminished libido and erections.*
- *Decreased growth of body hair.*

- *Testes may be small or normal in size. Serum testosterone is usually decreased.*

- *Serum gonadotropins (LH and FSH) are decreased in hypogonadotropic hypogonadism; they are increased in testicular failure (hypergonadotropic hypogonadism).*

General Considerations

Male hypogonadism is caused by deficient testosterone secretion by the testes. It may be classified according to whether it is due to (1) insufficient gonadotropin secretion by the pituitary (hypogonadotropic) or (2) pathology in the testes themselves (hypergonadotropic) (Table 26–16). The evaluation for hypogonadism begins with a serum testosterone or free testosterone measurement. A low serum testosterone is evaluated with serum LH and FSH levels. Patients with low gonadotropins are further evaluated for other pituitary abnormalities, including hyperprolactinemia.

Etiology

A. Hypogonadotropic Hypogonadism

A deficiency in FSH and LH may be isolated or associated with other pituitary hormonal abnormalities. (See

Table 26–16. Causes of male hypogonadism.

Hypogonadotropic (Low or Normal LH)	Hypergonadotropic (High LH)
Alcohol	Antitumor chemotherapy
Chronic illness	Bilateral anorchia
Congenital syndromes	Idiopathic
Constitutional delay	Klinefelter's syndrome
Cushing's syndrome	Leprosy
Drugs	Lymphoma
Estrogen-secreting tumors (testicular, adrenal)	Male climacteric
	Mumps
GnRH agonist (leuprolide)	Myotonic dystrophy
Hemochromatosis	Noonan's syndrome
Hypopituitarism	Orchitis
Hypothyroidism	Radiation therapy
Idiopathic	Sertoli cell-only syndrome
Kallmann's syndrome	Testicular trauma
Ketoconazole	Tuberculosis
17-Ketosteroid reductase deficiency	Uremia
Malnourishment	
Marijuana	
Obesity (BMI > 40)	
Prader-Willi syndrome	
Prior androgens	
Spironolactone	

GnRH = gonadotropin-releasing hormone; BMI = body mass index.

Hypopituitarism.) Patients must be evaluated for signs of Cushing's syndrome or adrenal insufficiency, growth hormone excess or deficiency, and thyroid hormone excess or deficiency.

Acquired hypogonadotropic hypogonadism may be due to pituitary or hypothalamic factors but may be idiopathic. Hyperprolactinemia (see Table 26–4) may also induce hypogonadism.

Hypogonadotropic hypogonadism can develop in men receiving GnRH agonist therapy for prostate cancer and can persist following cessation of therapy.

B. Hypergonadotropic Hypogonadism

A failure in testicular secretion of testosterone causes a rise in LH. If testicular Sertoli cell function is deficient, FSH will be elevated. Conditions that can cause testicular failure include viral infection (eg, mumps), irradiation, cancer chemotherapy, autoimmunity, myotonic dystrophy, uremia, XY gonadal dysgenesis, partial 17-ketosteroid reductase deficiency, Klinefelter's syndrome, and male climacteric.

Klinefelter's syndrome (seminiferous tubule dysgenesis) is a common cause of male hypogonadism that is due to the expression of an abnormal karyotype, classically 47,XXY. Other forms are common, eg, 46,XY/47,XXY mosaicism, 48,XXYY, 48,XXXY, or 46,XX males.

The manifestations of Klinefelter's syndrome are variable. Testes feel normal during childhood, but during adolescence they usually become firm, fibrotic, small, and nontender to palpation. Although puberty occurs at the normal time, the degree of virilization is variable. About 85% of patients have some gynecomastia at puberty.

Other common findings include tall stature and abnormal body proportions that are unusual for hypogonadal men (height greater than arm span; crown-pubis length greater than pubis-floor). Patients with multiple X or Y chromosomes are more apt to have mental deficiency and other abnormalities such as clinodactyly or synostosis. They may also exhibit problems with coordination and social skills. Other problems include a higher incidence of breast cancer, chronic pulmonary disease, varicosities of the legs, and diabetes mellitus (8% of patients); impaired glucose tolerance occurs in an additional 19% of patients.

Most men (about 95%) have azoospermia, but men with 46,XY/47,XXY mosaicism may be fertile. The diagnosis is confirmed by karyotyping or by determining the presence of RNA for X-inactive-specific transcriptase (XIST) in peripheral blood leukocytes by polymerase chain reaction.

The serum testosterone is low, and FSH and LH are elevated. Sometimes the serum testosterone is normal, but serum free testosterone is usually low.

All causes of gynecomastia (see Table 26–1) must be differentiated from Klinefelter's syndrome.

C. Androgen Insensitivity

Partial resistance to testosterone is a rare condition in which phenotypic males have variable degrees of apparent hypogonadism, hypospadias, cryptorchism, and gynecomastia. Serum testosterone levels are normal.

Clinical Findings

A. Symptoms and Signs

Hypogonadism that is congenital or acquired during childhood presents as delayed puberty. Men with acquired hypogonadism have variable manifestations. Most men experience decreased libido. Others complain of erectile dysfunction, hot sweats, fatigue, or depression. Their presenting complaint may also be infertility, gynecomastia, headache, fracture, or other symptoms related to the cause or result of the hypogonadism. The patient's history often gives a clue to the cause (Table 26–16).

Physical signs associated with hypogonadism may include decreased body, axillary, beard, or pubic hair; such diminished sexual hair growth is not reliably present except after years of severe hypogonadism. Men in whom hypogonadism develops tend to lose muscle mass and gain weight due to an increase in subcutaneous fat. Examination should include measurements of arm span and height. Testicular size should be assessed with an orchidometer (normal volume is about 10–25 mL; normal length is usually over 6 cm). Testicular size may decrease but usually remains within the normal range in men with postpubertal hypogonadotropic hypogonadism, but it may be diminished with testicular injury or Klinefelter's syndrome. The testes must also be carefully palpated for masses, since Leydig cell tumors may secrete estrogen and present with hypogonadism. The testicles must be carefully examined for evidence of trauma, infiltrative lesions (eg, lymphoma), or ongoing infection (eg, leprosy, tuberculosis).

B. Laboratory Findings

The hemoglobin and hematocrit may be slightly below the male range due to hypogonadism.

To evaluate a man for hypogonadism, the morning serum total testosterone concentration is determined. Normal ranges for serum testosterone have been derived from nonfasting morning blood specimens, which tend to be the highest of the day. Later in the day, serum testosterone levels can be 25–50% lower. Therefore, a serum testosterone drawn fasting or late in the day may be misleadingly below the "normal range." Serum testosterone levels in men are highest at age 20–30 years and slightly lower at age 30–40 years; testosterone falls gradually but progressively after age 40 years. Elderly men have higher levels of SHBG, with consequently lower levels of free testosterone. Newer automated chemiluminescent assays measure serum total testosterone less accurately than older radioimmunoassays. Chemiluminescent kit assays tend to suffer interference from hyperlipidemia and also generally underestimate serum testosterone levels. Very low serum testosterone levels, measured by chemiluminescent assay, accurately diagnose severe male hypogo-

nadism; however, mildly low serum testosterone levels should be viewed skeptically and repeated, along with an assay for free testosterone (see below).

Only about 2% of serum testosterone circulates free from protein binding. About 98% of serum testosterone is bound to either SHBG or albumin. Serum testosterone is tightly bound to SHBG and not available to tissues, whereas testosterone is weakly bound to albumin and is bioavailable to tissues. Assays that measure both free testosterone and non-SHBG testosterone are described as assays for "free and weakly bound testosterone." Testing for serum free testosterone is especially important for detecting hypogonadism in elderly men, who generally have high levels of SHBG. Different assay methodologies for free testosterone are in use. Assays using equilibrium dialysis, calculated free testosterone, and non-SHBG-bound testosterone are reasonably accurate. However, the free androgen index, direct radioimmunoassay, and analog free testosterone assays are inaccurate.

In patients with low or borderline-low serum testosterone levels, serum LH and FSH should be measured. LH and FSH tend to be high in patients with hypergonadotropic hypogonadism but low or inappropriately normal in men with hypogonadotropic hypogonadism. Testosterone stimulates erythropoiesis in men, causing the normal red blood count range to be higher in men than in women; mild anemia is common in men with hypogonadism, with red blood counts below the normal male range. For men with long-standing male hypogonadism, bone densitometry is recommended. Men with severe osteoporosis may require treatment with bisphosphonates and vitamin D, in addition to testosterone replacement therapy. (See Osteoporosis section.)

1. Hypogonadotropic hypogonadism—Men with hypogonadotropic hypogonadism have low serum testosterone levels without a compensatory increase in gonadotropins. A serum PRL determination is obtained but may be elevated for many reasons (see Table 26–4). Men with gynecomastia may be screened for partial 17-ketosteroid reductase deficiency with serum determinations for androstenedione and estrone, which are elevated in this condition. X-linked congenital adrenal hypoplasia is a rare condition in which a *DAX-1* gene mutation causes hypogonadotropic hypogonadism and azoospermia, which usually presents in adolescence; the associated primary adrenal insufficiency usually presents in childhood, but it may remain undiagnosed into adulthood. The serum estradiol level may be elevated in patients with cirrhosis and in rare cases of estrogen-secreting tumors (testicular Leydig cell tumor or adrenal carcinoma). Men with no discernible definite cause for hypogonadotropic hypogonadism should be screened for hemochromatosis and have an MRI of the pituitary and hypothalamic region to look for a tumor or other lesion. (See Hypopituitarism.)

2. Hypergonadotropic hypogonadism—Men with hypergonadotropic hypogonadism have low serum testosterone levels with a compensatory increase in gonadotropins. Klinefelter's syndrome can be confirmed by karyotyping or by measurement of leukocyte XIST. Testicular biopsy is usually reserved for younger patients in whom the reason for primary hypogonadism is unclear.

Treatment

Testosterone replacement is ordinarily commenced once the diagnosis of hypogonadism is confirmed and the cause determined. It is prudent to screen older men for prostate cancer before testosterone therapy is begun. Testosterone helps reverse sexual dysfunction and muscle atrophy. Men with Klinefelter's syndrome have a reduced risk of developing verbal fluency problems if testosterone therapy is begun at the time of normal puberty.

Topical testosterone gel has become the preferred method for administering testosterone. Topical 1% testosterone gel is commercially available as Androgel or Testim (2.5-g and 5-g packets); Androgel is odorless, while Testim has a musky odor. The starting dose is 5 g (50 mg testosterone) applied once daily to clean, dry skin of the shoulders, upper arms, or abdomen. The skin serves as a reservoir that slowly releases about 10% of the testosterone into the blood; serum testosterone levels reach a steady state in 1–3 days. The gel should not be applied to the genitals. The entire contents of a packet are squeezed onto the palm and then immediately applied. The hands should be washed and the application site allowed to dry for 3–5 minutes before dressing. A shirt must be worn during contact with women or children to prevent transfer of testosterone to them. The serum testosterone level should be determined about 14 days after starting therapy; if the level remains below normal or the clinical response is inadequate, the dose may be increased to 7.5 g or 10 g.

Testosterone transdermal systems (skin patches) are available in two formulations for application to nongenital skin. The testosterone may be mixed with the adhesive (eg, Testoderm II, 5 mg/d) with a new patch applied daily to a different site; this system leaves a sticky residue but causes little skin irritation. A different patch uses testosterone in a reservoir system applied to skin (eg, Androderm); this system adheres more tightly to the skin but may cause more skin irritation. Both produce reliable serum levels of testosterone that are somewhat lower that those achieved with injections. The patch systems also suffer from being rather inconvenient and expensive.

Hypogonadism may also be treated with parenteral testosterone (enanthate or cypionate). The usual dose is about 300 mg intramuscularly every 3 weeks or 200 mg every 2 weeks. The preparation is oil based and is usually given in the gluteal area. The dose is adjusted according to the patient's response.

Oral androgen preparations include methyltestosterone and fluoxymesterone. These oral preparations have rarely caused liver tumors or peliosis hepatis with long-term use. Cholestatic jaundice occurs in 1–2% of patients but usually remits after the medication is discontinued. The oral androgens are not as effective as parenteral testosterone.

Men with mosaic Klinefelter's syndrome (eg, 46,XY/47,XXY) may be fertile. However, men with nonmosaic Klinefelter's syndrome (eg, 47,XXY) are usually azoospermic; fertility may be achieved by testicular sperm retrieval and in vitro intracytoplasmic sperm injection (ICSI) into an ovum.

Men with hypogonadotropic hypogonadism must receive further evaluation and specific treatment (see Hypopituitarism).

Testosterone replacement therapy may cause a minimal reduction in serum HDL levels and has no effect on LDL levels; testosterone therapy has never been demonstrated to increase the incidence of cardiovascular disease, myocardial infarction, or stroke.

Testosterone therapy can aggravate benign prostatic hypertrophy (BPH). However, aggravation of voiding problems is uncommon. In men with BPH, finasteride may be coadministered with testosterone to reduce prostate size. The incidence of prostate cancer does not appear to be increased by testosterone therapy. However, testosterone therapy is contraindicated in the presence of active prostate cancer. It is prudent to monitor serum prostate-specific antigen (PSA) levels before and during testosterone therapy. Hypogonadal men who have had a prostatectomy for low-grade prostate cancer, and who have remained in complete remission for several years, may have testosterone therapy given cautiously while monitoring sensitive serum PSA levels.

Erythrocytosis develops in some men who are treated with testosterone. Erythrocytosis is more common with intramuscular injections of testosterone enanthate than with transcutaneous testosterone. It is particularly common in men receiving intramuscular testosterone enanthate in doses of 200 mg intramuscularly every 2 weeks. However, no increase in the incidence of thromboembolic events has been reported.

Testosterone therapy tends to aggravate sleep apnea in older men, likely through central nervous system effects. Surveillance for sleep apnea is recommended during testosterone therapy and a formal evaluation with nocturnal pulse oximetry recording is recommended for all high-risk patients. A man's risk for sleep apnea may be approximated by determining an "adjusted neck circumference" with the following algorithm: Measure the neck circumference in centimeters; add 4 cm if the patient is hypertensive; add 3 cm if the patient snores; add 3 cm if the patient chokes or gasps most nights. Adjusted neck circumference: < 43 = low risk; 43–48 = moderate risk; > 48 = high risk.

Men who are treated with testosterone frequently experience some increase in acne, which is usually mild and tolerated; topical antiacne therapy or a reduction in testosterone replacement dosage may be required. During the initiation of testosterone replacement therapy, gynecomastia develops in some men, which usually is mild and tends to resolve spontaneously; switching from testosterone injections to testosterone transdermal gel may help this condition.

Prognosis of Male Hypogonadism

If hypogonadism is due to a pituitary lesion, the prognosis is that of the primary disease (eg, tumor, necrosis). The prognosis for restoration of virility is good if testosterone is given.

Bojesen A et al: Increased mortality in Klinefelter syndrome. J Clin Endocrinol Metab 2004;89:3830. [PMID: 15292313]

Greenstein A et al: Does sildenafil combined with testosterone gel improve erectile dysfunction in hypogonadal men in whom testosterone supplement therapy alone failed? J Urol 2005; 173:530. [PMID: 15643239]

Lanfranco F et al: Klinefelter's syndrome. Lancet 2004;364:273. [PMID: 15262106]

Matsumoto AM et al: Serum testosterone assays—accuracy matters. J Clin Endocrinol Metab 2004;89:529. [PMID: 14764756]

Rhoden EL et al: Risks of testosterone-replacement therapy and recommendations for monitoring. N Engl J Med 2004;350: 482. [PMID: 14749457]

Wang C et al: Measurement of total serum testosterone in adult men: comparison of current laboratory methods versus liquid chromatography-tandem mass spectrometry. J Clin Endocrinol Metab 2004;89:534. [PMID: 14764758]

TESTICULAR TUMORS IN ADULTS
(See also Chapter 23)

About 95% of testicular tumors are germ cell tumors (seminomas or nonseminomas). Seminomas do not produce α-fetoprotein, but about 5–10% produce some hCG. Nonseminomas, on the other hand, produce increased serum levels of one or both of these markers in about 90% of cases. Men with liver disease may have misleadingly high levels of α-fetoprotein. Most germ cell tumors are sensitive to cisplatin-based combined chemotherapy. Sperm banking is advised.

About 5% of testicular tumors are Leydig or Sertoli cell tumors. Leydig cell tumors tend to produce estrogen (75%) and cause gynecomastia and impotence on that basis; they may sometimes produce androgens that can cause pseudoprecocious puberty in boys. Sertoli cell tumors may also produce estrogen (30%) with feminization; gynecomastia may be due to hCG secretion (25%).

Some testicular tumors may be small and nonpalpable yet may secrete sufficient amounts of hCG or estrogen to cause gynecomastia or impotence. Testicular ultrasound may help reveal small tumors.

After unilateral orchiectomy for testicular cancer, an elevated FSH level prior to further treatment indicates a patient at higher risk for cancer in the remaining testis.

Garner MJ et al: Epidemiology of testicular cancer: an overview. Int J Cancer 2005;116:331. [PMID: 15818625]

Hussain A: Germ cell tumors. Curr Opin Oncol 2005;17:268. [PMID: 15818173]

Huyghe E et al: Fertility after testicular cancer treatments: results of a large multicenter study. Cancer 2004;100:732. [PMID: 14770428]

Oosterhuis JW et al: Testicular germ-cell tumours in a broader perspective. Nat Rev Cancer 2005;5:210. [PMID: 15738984]

■ AMENORRHEA & MENOPAUSE
(See also Chapter 17)

PRIMARY AMENORRHEA

Menarche ordinarily occurs between ages 11 and 15 years (average in the United States: 12.7 years). The failure of any menses to appear is termed primary amenorrhea, and evaluation is commenced (1) at age 14 years if neither menarche nor breast development has occurred or if height is in the lowest 3%, or (2) at age 16 years if menarche has not occurred.

Etiology of Primary Amenorrhea

The causes of primary amenorrhea include hypothalamic-pituitary causes, hyperandrogenism, ovarian causes, pseudohermaphroditism, uterine causes, and pregnancy.

A. HYPOTHALAMIC-PITUITARY CAUSES (WITH LOW OR NORMAL FSH)

A genetic deficiency of GnRH and gonadotropins may be isolated or associated with other pituitary deficiencies or diminished olfaction (Kallmann's syndrome). Hypothalamic lesions, particularly craniopharyngioma, may be present. Pituitary tumors may be nonsecreting or may secrete PRL or GH. Cushing's syndrome may be caused by corticosteroid treatment, a cortisol-secreting adrenal tumor, or an ACTH-secreting pituitary tumor. Hypothyroidism can delay adolescence. Head trauma or encephalitis can cause gonadotropin deficiency. Primary amenorrhea may also be caused by constitutional delay of adolescence, organic illness, vigorous exercise (eg, ballet dancing, running), stressful life events, dieting, or anorexia nervosa; however, these conditions should not be assumed to account for amenorrhea without a full physical and endocrinologic evaluation. (See section on Hypopituitarism.)

B. HYPERANDROGENISM (WITH LOW OR NORMAL FSH)

Excess testosterone may be secreted by adrenal tumors or by adrenal hyperplasia caused by steroidogenic enzyme defects such as P-450c21 deficiency (salt-wasting) or P-450c11 deficiency (hypertension). Ovarian tumors or polycystic ovaries may also secrete excess testosterone. Androgenic steroids may also cause this syndrome.

C. Ovarian Causes (with High FSH)

Gonadal dysgenesis (Turner's syndrome and variants; see below) is a frequent cause of primary amenorrhea. Ovarian failure due to autoimmunity is a common cause. Rare deficiencies in certain ovarian steroidogenic enzymes are causes of primary hypogonadism without virilization: 3β-hydroxysteroid dehydrogenase deficiency (adrenal insufficiency with low serum 17-hydroxyprogesterone) and P-450c17 deficiency (hypertension and hypokalemia with high serum 17-hydroxyprogesterone). A whole-body deficiency in P-450 aromatase (P-450arom) activity produces female hypogonadism associated with polycystic ovaries, tall stature, osteoporosis, and virilization.

D. Pseudohermaphroditism (with High LH)

An enzymatic defect in testosterone synthesis may present as a sexually immature phenotypic girl with primary amenorrhea. Complete androgen resistance (testicular feminization) presents as a phenotypic young woman without sexual hair but with normal breast development and primary amenorrhea. In both cases, the uterus is absent and testes are intra-abdominal or cryptorchid. Intra-abdominal testes are surgically resected. Such patients are treated as normal but infertile, hypogonadal women.

E. Uterine Causes (with Normal FSH)

Congenital absence or malformation of the uterus may be responsible for primary amenorrhea, as may an unresponsive or atrophic endometrium. An imperforate hymen is occasionally the reason for the absence of visible menses.

F. Pregnancy (with High hCG)

Pregnancy may be the cause of primary amenorrhea even when the patient denies ever having had sexual intercourse.

Clinical Findings

A. Symptoms and Signs

Patients with primary amenorrhea require a thorough history and physical examination to look for signs of the conditions noted above. Headaches or visual field abnormalities implicate a hypothalamic or pituitary tumor. Signs of pregnancy may be present. Blood pressure abnormalities, acne, and hirsutism should be noted. Short stature may be seen with an associated growth hormone or thyroid hormone deficiency. Short stature with manifestations of gonadal dysgenesis indicates Turner's syndrome (see below). Olfaction testing screens for Kallmann's syndrome. Obesity and short stature may be signs of Cushing's syndrome. Tall stature may be due to eunuchoidism or gigantism. Hirsutism or virilization suggests excessive testosterone.

An external pelvic examination plus a rectal examination should be performed to assess hymenal patency and the presence of a uterus.

B. Laboratory Findings

The initial endocrine evaluation should include serum determinations of FSH, LH, PRL, testosterone, TSH, FT_4, and hCG (pregnancy test). Patients who are virilized or hypertensive require serum electrolyte determinations and further hormonal evaluation. Girls with low-normal FSH and LH—especially those with high PRL levels—are evaluated by MRI of the hypothalamus and pituitary. Girls who have a normal uterus and high FSH without the classic features of Turner's syndrome may require a karyotype to diagnose X chromosome mosaicism.

Treatment

Treatment of primary amenorrhea is directed at the underlying cause. Girls with permanent hypogonadism are treated with estrogen replacement therapy (see below).

Torstveit MK et al: Participation in leanness sports but not training volume is associated with menstrual dysfunction: a national survey of 1276 elite athletes and controls. Br J Sports Med 2005;39:141. [PMID: 15728691]

Warren MP et al: The genetics, diagnosis and treatment of amenorrhea. Minerva Ginecol 2004;56:437. [PMID: 15531861]

SECONDARY AMENORRHEA & MENOPAUSE

Secondary amenorrhea is defined as the absence of menses for 3 consecutive months in women who have passed menarche. Menopause is defined as the terminal episode of naturally occurring menses; it is a retrospective diagnosis, usually made after 6 months of amenorrhea.

Etiology

The causes of secondary amenorrhea include pregnancy, hypothalamic-pituitary causes, hyperandrogenism, uterine causes, premature ovarian failure, and menopause.

A. Pregnancy (High hCG)

Pregnancy is the most common cause for secondary amenorrhea in women of childbearing age. The differential diagnosis includes rare ectopic secretion of hCG by a choriocarcinoma or bronchogenic carcinoma.

B. Hypothalamic-Pituitary Causes (with Low or Normal FSH)

The hypothalamus must release GnRH in a pulsatile manner for the pituitary to secrete gonadotropins. GnRH pulses occurring more than once per hour favor LH secretion, while less frequent pulses favor FSH secretion. In normal ovulatory cycles, GnRH pulses in the follicular phase are rapid and favor LH synthesis and ovulation; ovarian luteal progesterone is then secreted that slows GnRH pulses, causing FSH secretion during the luteal phase. Most women with hypothalamic amenorrhea have a persistently low frequency of GnRH pulses.

Secondary "hypothalamic" amenorrhea may be caused by stressful life events such as school examinations or leaving home. Such women usually have a history of normal sexual development and irregular menses since menarche. Amenorrhea may also be the result of strict dieting, vigorous exercise, organic illness, or anorexia nervosa. Intrathecal infusion of opioids causes amenorrhea in most women. These conditions should not be assumed to account for amenorrhea without a full physical and endocrinologic evaluation. Young women in whom the results of evaluation and progestin withdrawal test are normal have noncyclic secretion of gonadotropins resulting in anovulation. Such women typically recover spontaneously but should have regular evaluations and a progestin withdrawal test about every 3 months to detect loss of estrogen effect.

PRL elevation due to any cause (see section on hyperprolactinemia) may cause amenorrhea. Pituitary tumors or other lesions may cause hypopituitarism. Corticosteroid excess of any cause suppresses gonadotropins.

C. HYPERANDROGENISM (WITH LOW-NORMAL FSH)

Elevated serum levels of testosterone can cause hirsutism, virilization, and amenorrhea. In PCOS, GnRH pulses are persistently rapid, favoring LH synthesis with excessive androgen secretion; reduced FSH secretion impairs follicular maturation. Progesterone administration can slow the GnRH pulses, thus favoring FSH secretion that induces follicular maturation. Rare causes include adrenal P-450c21 deficiency, ovarian or adrenal malignancies, ectopic ACTH secretion by a malignancy, and Cushing's disease. Anabolic steroids also cause amenorrhea.

D. UTERINE CAUSES (WITH NORMAL FSH)

Infection of the uterus commonly occurs following delivery or D&C but may occur spontaneously. Endometritis due to tuberculosis or schistosomiasis should be suspected in endemic areas. Endometrial scarring may result, causing amenorrhea (Asherman's syndrome). Such women typically continue to have monthly premenstrual symptoms. The vaginal estrogen effect is normal. Diagnosis and treatment are best done by direct hysteroscopic inspection of the endometrium and lysis of adhesions. A small Foley catheter is left in the uterus for 1 week while antibiotics are given. The catheter is then replaced by an intrauterine device (IUD) for about 2 months. Cyclic estrogen and progestin are given to build up the endometrial lining. After such treatment, menses usually resume and fertility is possible, but spontaneous abortions and other pregnancy complications occur commonly.

E. PREMATURE OVARIAN FAILURE (WITH HIGH FSH)

This refers to primary hypogonadism that occurs before age 40 years. It affects about 1% of women. About 30%

of such cases are due to autoimmunity against the ovary. About 8% of cases are due to X chromosome mosaicism. Other causes include surgical bilateral oophorectomy, radiation therapy for pelvic malignancy, and chemotherapy. Women who have undergone hysterectomy are prone to premature ovarian failure even though the ovaries were left intact. Myotonic dystrophy, galactosemia, and mumps oophoritis are additional causes. Other cases may be familial or idiopathic. Ovarian failure is usually irreversible. Treatment consists of estrogen replacement therapy plus a progestin if the uterus is present.

F. MENOPAUSE (WITH HIGH FSH)

"Climacteric" is defined as the period of natural physiologic decline in ovarian function, generally occurring over about 10 years. By about age 40 years, the remaining ovarian follicles are those that are the least sensitive to gonadotropins. Increasing titers of FSH are required to stimulate estradiol secretion. Estradiol levels may actually rise during early climacteric. Frequent anovulation tends to cause menometrorrhagia (dysfunctional uterine bleeding). Fertility declines progressively. Psychological symptoms may include depression and irritability. Women may experience fatigue, insomnia, headache, diminished libido, or rheumatologic symptoms. Vasomotor instability (hot flushes) is experienced by 80% of women, lasting seconds to many minutes. Hot flushes with drenching sweats may be most severe at night or may be triggered by emotional stress. Some women continue to menstruate for many months despite symptoms of estrogen deficiency. Estrogen supplementation provides symptomatic relief.

The normal age for menopause in the United States ranges between 48 and 55 years, with an average of about 51.5 years. Serum estradiol levels fall and the remaining estrogen after menopause is estrone, derived mainly from peripheral aromatization of adrenal androstenedione. Such peripheral production of estrone is enhanced by obesity and liver disease. Individual differences in estrone levels partly explain why the symptoms noted above may be minimal in some women but severe in others. The acute symptoms of estrogen deficiency noted above tend to decline in severity within several years after menopause. However, about 35% of women have symptoms for more than 5 years. The late manifestations of estrogen deficiency include urogenital atrophy with vaginal dryness and dyspareunia; dysuria, frequency, and incontinence may occur. Increased bone osteoclastic activity increases the risk for osteoporosis and fractures. The skin becomes more wrinkled. Increases in the LDL:HDL cholesterol ratio cause an increased risk for arteriosclerosis.

Clinical Findings

A. SYMPTOMS AND SIGNS

All women with amenorrhea require a complete history and physical examination. Nausea and breast engorgement are typical signs of early pregnancy. Hot flushes are common in ovarian failure. Headache or visual field abnormalities are seen with pituitary or hypothalamic tumors. Complaints of thirst and polyuria require evaluation; diabetes insipidus implicates a hypothalamic lesion. Goiter may be due to hyperthyroidism. Weight loss, diarrhea, or skin darkening may indicate adrenal insufficiency. Weight loss with a distorted body image implicates anorexia nervosa. The breasts are examined carefully for galactorrhea, a common sign of hyperprolactinemia. Hirsutism or virilization may be a sign of hyperandrogenism. Manifestations of hypercortisolism (eg, weakness, psychiatric changes, hypertension, central obesity, hirsutism, thin skin, ecchymoses) may indicate alcoholism or Cushing's syndrome. Signs of acromegaly or gigantism may also indicate a pituitary tumor. Signs of systemic illness (eg, cirrhosis, renal failure) should be appreciated. Various drugs may elevate PRL and cause amenorrhea (see section on Hyperprolactinemia). Needle tracks may indicate heroin or amphetamine abuse.

A careful pelvic examination is always required to check for uterine or adnexal enlargement and to obtain a Papanicolaou smear and a vaginal smear for assessment of estrogen effect. Various life stresses, vigorous exercise, and "crash" dieting all predispose to amenorrhea; however, such factors should not be assumed to account for amenorrhea without a complete workup to screen for other causes.

B. Laboratory Findings

Since pregnancy is the most common cause of amenorrhea, women of childbearing age are immediately screened with a serum or urine hCG (pregnancy test). An elevated hCG overwhelmingly indicates pregnancy; false-positive testing may occur very rarely with ectopic hCG secretion (eg, choriocarcinoma or bronchogenic carcinoma). Women without an elevated hCG receive further laboratory evaluation including serum PRL, FSH, LH, TSH, and plasma potassium. Hyperprolactinemia or hypopituitarism (without obvious cause; see section on Hypopituitarism) should prompt an MRI study of the pituitary region. Routine testing for renal and hepatic function (eg, BUN, serum creatinine, bilirubin, alkaline phosphatase, and alanine aminotransferase) is also performed. A serum testosterone level is obtained in hirsute or virilized women. Patients with manifestations of hypercortisolism receive a 1-mg overnight dexamethasone suppression test for initial screening (see section on Cushing's syndrome). Nonpregnant women without any laboratory abnormality may receive a 10-day course of a progestin (eg, medroxyprogesterone acetate, 10 mg/d); absence of withdrawal menses typically indicates a lack of estrogen or a uterine abnormality.

Treatment

Therapy of hypogonadism generally consists of hormone replacement therapy (see below). The doses of estrogen required for symptomatic relief from vasomotor symptoms are sometimes higher than typical physiologic replacement doses. Slow, deep breathing can also ameliorate hot flushes. Tamoxifen and raloxifene offer bone protection but aggravate hot flushes. Treatment or prevention of postmenopausal osteoporosis with bisphosphonates such as alendronate, risedronate, or intravenous zoledronic acid (see section on Osteoporosis) is another therapeutic option. Women with low serum testosterone levels may experience hypoactive sexual desire disorder (HSDD) that may respond to low-dose testosterone replacement.

Estrogen Replacement Therapy

The Women's Health Initiative (WHI) monitored 16,606 postmenopausal women in the United States in a prospective, double-blinded, placebo-controlled study of postmenopausal HRT. A control group of women taking a daily placebo was compared to (1) women receiving daily conventional-dose oral combined HRT (conjugated equine estrogens [CEE] 0.625 mg/d with medroxyprogesterone acetate [MPA] 2.5 mg/d) and (2) women, having had a hysterectomy, receiving only CEE 0.625 mg/d.

The WHI risk–benefit findings (described below) have dramatically changed postmenopausal HRT. To reduce the risks of HRT, lower-dose estrogen regimens are now preferred over conventional-dose therapy. Estrogen preparations other than CEE are increasingly favored. Transdermal and vaginal estrogen preparations are now widely preferred over oral estrogen replacement. Also, the potential adverse effects of progestins are now recognized, such that women taking very low-dose estrogen replacement may receive progestin therapy only periodically, if at all. For moderate to high-dose estrogen therapy, progestins are being used in lower doses. Also, clinicians are now tending to prescribe progestins other than MPA. A progestin-eluting intrauterine device prevents endometrial hyperplasia while avoiding systemic progestin exposure.

Oral estrogen preparations include CEEs (0.3, 0.45, 0.625, 0.9, and 1.25 mg), ethinyl estradiol (20 and 50 mcg), estradiol (0.5, 1, 1.5, and 2 mg), estropipate (0.75, 1.5, 3, and 6 mg), plant-derived esterified estrogens (eg, Menest, Estratab, 0.3, 0.625, and 2.5 mg), and synthetic estrogens (eg, Cenestin, 0.3, 0.625, 0.9, and 1.25 mg).

Oral estrogen plus progestin preparations include CEE with MPA (Prempro 0.3/1.5, 0.45/1.5, 0.625/2.5, and 0.625/5), CEE for 14 days cycled with CEE plus MPA for 14 days (Premphase 0.625, 0.625/5), estradiol with norethindrone acetate (Activella 1/0.5), ethinyl estradiol with norethindrone acetate (Femhrt 1/5, 5 mcg/1 mg/tablet), and estradiol with norgestimate (Ortho-Prefest, sequences of estradiol 1 mg/d for 3 days, alternating with a combination of 1 mg estradiol/0.09 mg norgestimate daily for 3 days). Oral contraceptives can also be used for combined HRT.

Transdermal estradiol: Estradiol can be delivered systemically with different transdermal systems.

1. Transdermal systems with estradiol mixed with adhesive: These systems tend to cause minimal skin irritation. Of the following preparations, the Vivelle-Dot patches are the smallest and least obtrusive. Available preparations include Esclim, Vivelle, and Vivelle-Dot (0.025, 0.0375, 0.05, 0.075, or 0.1 mg/d), replaced twice weekly; Alora (0.025, 0.05, 0.075, or 0.1 mg/d), replaced twice weekly; Climara (0.025, 0.0375, 0.05, 0.06, 0.075, or 0.1 mg/d), replaced weekly; FemPatch (0.025 mg/d), replaced weekly; and Menostar (0.014 mg/d), replaced weekly. This type of estradiol skin patch can be cut in half and applied to the skin without proportionately greater loss of potency.

2. Transdermal systems with estradiol in a drug reservoir: These systems cause significant skin irritation in some women. Available preparations include Estraderm (0.05 or 0.1 mg/d), replaced twice weekly.

3. Transdermal systems with estradiol (E) and norethindrone acetate (NA) mixed with adhesive: Available preparations include Combipatch (0.05 mg/d E and 0.14 mg/d NA or 0.05 mg/d E and 0.25 mg/d NA), replaced twice weekly. The addition of a progestin increases the likelihood of side effects compared with therapy with estrogen alone.

4. Transdermal estradiol gel (EstroGel, 0.6%) is available in a metered-dose dispenser that delivers 1.25 g estradiol per actuation. The gel is applied to one arm from the wrist to the shoulder daily after bathing. To avoid spreading the estradiol to others, the hands should be washed and precautions taken to avoid prolonged skin contact with children.

Vaginal estrogen: Urogenital atrophy commonly develops in postmenopausal women and can cause dryness of the vagina, genital itching, burning, and dyspareunia. Urinary symptoms can include urgency and dysuria. Vaginal estrogen is intended to deliver estrogen directly to local tissues in an effort to reduce these symptoms, while minimizing systemic estrogen exposure. Some estrogen is absorbed systemically and can relieve menopausal symptoms. Systemically absorbed estrogen avoids first-pass liver metabolism, causing less hypertriglyceridemia and prothrombotic effects than oral estrogen. Manufacturers recommend that these preparations be used for only 3–6 months in women with an intact uterus, since vaginal estrogen can cause endometrial proliferation. However, most clinicians use them for longer periods. Vaginal estrogen can be administered in three different ways:

1. Estrogen vaginal creams: These creams are administered intravaginally with a measured-dose applicator daily for 2 weeks for atrophic vaginitis, then administered one to three times weekly. Available preparations include conjugated equine estrogens (Premarin, 0.626 mg/g cream), 0.25–0.5 g cream vaginally; dienestrol (Ortho Dienestrol, 10 mg/g cream), 0.25–0.5 g cream vaginally; estradiol (Estrace, 0.1 mg/g cream), 1 g cream vaginally; and estropipate (Ogen, 1.5 mg/g cream), 0.25–0.5 g vaginally.

2. Estradiol vaginal tablets: These tablets are sold prepackaged in a disposable applicator and can be administered deep intravaginally daily for 2 weeks for atrophic vaginitis, then twice weekly. The tablets dissolve into a gel that gradually releases estradiol. Available preparations include vaginal estradiol tablets (Vagifem, 25 mcg/tablet).

3. Estradiol vaginal rings: These rings are inserted manually into the upper third of the vagina, worn continuously, and replaced every 90 days. Only a small amount of the released estradiol enters the systemic circulation. Vaginal rings do not usually interfere with sexual intercourse. If a ring is removed or descends into the introitus, it may be washed in warm water and reinserted. Available preparations include Estring (2 mg estradiol/ring, releasing 0.0075 mg/d) and Femring (12.4 mg estradiol/ring, releasing 0.05 mg/d, or 24.8 mg estradiol/ring, releasing 0.10 mg/d).

Oral progestins: For a woman with an intact uterus, long-term conventional-dose unopposed systemic estrogen therapy can cause endometrial hyperplasia, which typically results in dysfunctional uterine bleeding (DUB) and can rarely lead to endometrial cancer. Progestin therapy transforms proliferative into secretory endometrium, causing a menses when given intermittently or no bleeding when given continuously.

The type of progestin preparation, its dosage, and the timing of administration may be tailored to the given situation. Progestins may be given daily, monthly, or at longer intervals. When given episodically, progestins are usually administered for 7–14 day periods. Progestins are available in different formulations: Micronized progesterone (Prometrium, 100 mg/capsule), medroxyprogesterone acetate (Provera, Amen, Cycrin; 2.5, 5.0, and 10 mg/scored tablet), norethindrone acetate (Aygestin, 5 mg/tablet), and norethindrone (Micronor, Nor-QD; 0.35 mg/tablet).

Topical progesterone (20–50 mg/d) may reduce hot flushes in women who are intolerant to oral hormone replacement therapy. It may be applied to the upper arms, thighs, or inner wrists daily. It may be compounded as micronized progesterone 250 mg/mL in a transdermal gel. Its effects upon the breast and endometrium are unknown.

Progesterone-releasing IUDs: Progesterone-releasing intrauterine devices can be useful for women receiving estrogen replacement therapy, since they can reduce the incidence of DUB and endometrial carcinoma without exposing women to the significant risks of systemic progestins.

Benefits of estrogen replacement therapy: Estrogen replacement without progestin (unopposed): Surprisingly, the WHI study found that postmenopausal women who received conventional-dose estrogen-only therapy had a reduced risk for breast cancer (seven fewer cases/year per 10,000 women) compared with a placebo group. The WHI study also found that women who received estrogen therapy experienced a reduced number of hip fractures (six fewer fractures/year per 10,000 women) compared with placebo. Unopposed estrogen therapy had no discernible effect upon the risk for heart attacks, colorectal cancer, or overall mortality.

Women receiving unopposed conventional-dose daily conjugated estrogen and medroxyprogesterone acetate (0.625 mg and 2.5 mg, respectively), for an average of 5.6 years, experienced a lower risk of developing diabetes (3.5%) versus those taking a placebo (4.2%).

Serum levels of atherogenic lipoprotein(a) are reduced by estrogen replacement with or without daily or cycled progestins. Improvement in serum HDL cholesterol is greatest with unopposed estrogen but is also seen with the addition of a progestin.

Estrogen replacement improves or eliminates postmenopausal hot flushes and diaphoretic episodes. Vaginal moisture is improved. Libido is enhanced in some women. Sleep disturbances are common in menopause and can be reversed with estrogen replacement. Sex hormone replacement may also improve the body pain and reduced physical function experienced by some women at the time of menopause.

Perimenopause-related depression is improved by unopposed estrogen replacement; the addition of a progestin may negate this effect. Estrogen replacement, when initiated at the time of menopause or oophorectomy, has been reported to help protect cognitive function, particularly verbal memory, whereas estrogen replacement that is begun many years after menopause confers little or no benefit on cognition. Estrogen therapy does not appear to reduce the risk of Alzheimer's dementia.

Unopposed estrogen replacement improves glycemic control in women with type 2 diabetes mellitus. Estrogen replacement does not prevent facial skin wrinkling; however, it may improve facial skin moisture and thickness, reducing seborrhea and atrophy.

Risks of estrogen replacement therapy: The risks of estrogen replacement depend on the dose. Conventional doses (eg, oral conjugated estrogens ≥ 0.625 mg/d or transdermal estradiol ≥ 0.05 mg/d) carry higher risks than lower doses (eg, oral conjugated estrogens, ≤ 0.3 mg/d or transdermal estradiol ≤ 0.025 mg/d). Route of administration also affects risks, since oral estrogens pass through the liver and increase hepatic production of clotting factors (thereby increasing the risks of thrombotic stroke), whereas transdermal or vaginal administration of estrogen does not significantly increase clotting proclivity. The risks for HRT also depend on whether estrogen is administered alone (unopposed HRT) or with a progestin (combined HRT).

Estrogen replacement without progestin (unopposed HRT): Conventional-dose unopposed estrogen replacement increases the risk of endometrial hyperplasia and DUB, which often prompts patients to stop the estrogen. Lower-dose unopposed estrogen has a much lower risk of DUB. Recurrent dysfunctional bleeding necessitates a pelvic examination and possibly an endometrial biopsy.

Unopposed estrogen in conventional doses may increase the risk for endometrial carcinoma, although the absolute risk remains low. A Cochrane Database Review found no increased risk of endometrial carcinoma in a review of 30 randomized controlled trials. Therefore, lower-dose unopposed estrogen replacement confers a negligible risk for endometrial cancer.

Long-term conventional-dose unopposed estrogen increases the mortality risk from ovarian cancer, although the absolute risk is small. The annual age-adjusted ovarian cancer death rates for women taking estrogen replacement for ≥ 10 years are 64:100,000 for current users, 38:100,000 for former users, and 26:100,000 for women who had never taken estrogen. Lower-dose estrogen replacement is believed to confer a negligible increased risk for ovarian cancer.

The WHI study has reported that conventional doses of unopposed oral estrogen do not increase the risk of breast cancer; in fact, somewhat fewer breast cancers were found in women taking estrogen alone, compared with placebo. However, the WHI trial was stopped in 2002 because of an increased risk of stroke among women taking conjugated oral estrogens in doses of 0.625 mg daily; the risk was about 44 strokes per 10,000 person-years versus about 32 per 10,000 person-years in women taking placebo. Transdermal or transvaginal estrogen is not expected to increase the risk of stroke.

Conventional-dose oral estrogen replacement increases the risk of deep venous thrombosis. It can cause hypertriglyceridemia, particularly in women with preexistent hyperlipidemia, rarely resulting in pancreatitis. Postmenopausal estrogen therapy also slightly increases the risk of gallstones and cholecystitis. Oral estrogens reduce the effectiveness of growth hormone replacement. These side effects can be reduced or avoided by using nonoral estrogen replacement.

Elderly women, receiving long-term conventional-dose estrogen replacement, experience an increased risk of urinary incontinence. Some women complain of estrogen-induced edema or mastalgia. Estrogen replacement has been reported to lower the seizure threshold in some women with epilepsy. Untreated large pituitary prolactinomas may enlarge if exposed to estrogen.

Estrogen replacement with a progestin (combined HRT): The WHI study found that women who received long-term conventional oral doses of combined HRT (conjugated estrogens 0.625 mg/d plus medroxyprogesterone acetate 2.5 mg/d) had an increased risk of deep venous thrombosis (3.5 per 1000 person-years) compared with women receiving placebo (1.7 per 1000 person-years).

Conventional-dose oral combined HRT results in an increased risk for myocardial infarction (24% or six additional heart attacks per 10,000 women), mostly in women with high-risk LDL levels or preexistent coronary disease. Most of the risk for myocardial infarction occurs in the first year of therapy. This increased risk is attributable to the progestin component, since the estrogen-only arm of the WHI study found no increased risk of myocardial infarction.

Long-term conventional-dose oral combined HRT increases breast density and increases the risk for abnormal mammograms (9.4% versus 5.4% for placebo). There is also a higher risk for breast cancer (8 cases per 10,000 women/year versus 6.5 cases per 10,000 women/year for placebo); no increased risk of breast cancer has been found with estrogen-only HRT. This increased risk for breast cancer appears to mostly affect relatively thin women with a BMI < 24.4. The Iowa Women's Health Study reported an increase in breast cancer with HRT only in women consuming more than 1 oz of alcohol weekly. No accelerated risk of breast cancer has been seen in users of HRT who have benign breast disease or a family history of breast cancer.

The Women's Health Initiative Mental Study (WHIMS) followed the effect of combined conventional-dose oral HRT on cognitive function in women 65–79 years old. HRT did not protect these older women from cognitive decline. In fact, they experienced an increased risk for severe dementia at a rate of 23 more cases/year for every 10,000 women over age 65 years.

In the WHI study, women receiving conventional-dose combined oral HRT experienced an increased risk of stroke (31 strokes per 10,000 women/year versus 26 strokes per 10,000 women/year for placebo). Stroke risk was also increased by hypertension, diabetes, and smoking.

Women taking combined estrogen–progestin replacement do not experience an increased risk of ovarian cancer. They do experience an increased risk of developing asthma.

Progestins may cause moodiness, particularly in women with a history of premenstrual dysphoric disorder. Cycled progestins may trigger migraines in certain women. Many other adverse reactions have been reported, including breast tenderness, alopecia, and fluid retention. Contraindications to the use of progestins include thromboembolic disorders, liver disease, breast cancer, and pregnancy.

Androgen replacement: Women who have undergone a bilateral oophorectomy almost invariably have low serum androgens. Women with panhypopituitarism tend to have particularly low androgen levels. However, after natural menopause, the ovaries and adrenals continue to secrete testosterone, such that postmenopausal women are not always androgen deficient. Androgen deficiency contributes to hot flushes, loss of libido and sexual hair, muscle atrophy, and osteoporosis. Selected women may be treated with low-dose methyltestosterone, which is available in combination with conjugated estrogens (eg, Estratest). Tablets contain either 1.25 mg conjugated estrogens with 2.5 mg methyltestosterone or 0.625 mg conjugated estrogens with 1.25 mg methyltestosterone. Estratest is usually started at the lowest strength every 2 days, alternating days with standard estrogen replacement (see above). It should be given cyclically at the lowest dose that controls symptoms. At small doses, side effects of

androgens are usually minimal but may include nausea, polycythemia, emotional changes, paresthesias, electrolyte disturbances, and potentiation of anticoagulant therapy. Reduction in HDL cholesterol may negate the beneficial effect on cardiovascular mortality conferred by estrogen replacement therapy. Cholestatic jaundice and elevation of liver enzymes occur rarely. Hepatocellular neoplasms and peliosis hepatis, rare complications of oral androgens at higher doses, have not been reported with lower doses. Side effects of excess androgen treatment include hirsutism and virilization. Androgens should not be given to women with liver disease or during pregnancy or breast-feeding.

Selective estrogen receptor modulators (SERMs) (eg, raloxifene; Evista) are an alternative to estrogen replacement for hypogonadal women at risk for osteoporosis who prefer not to take estrogens because of their contraindications (eg, breast or uterine cancer) or side effects. Raloxifene does not reduce hot flushes, vaginal dryness, skin wrinkling, or breast atrophy; it does not improve cognition. However, in doses of 60 mg/d orally, it inhibits bone loss without stimulating effects upon the breasts or endometrium. Because raloxifene may slightly increase the risk of venous thromboembolism, it should not be used by women at prolonged bed rest or by those prone to thrombosis. In contrast with the use of estrogen replacement therapy, concomitant progesterone therapy is not needed, and raloxifene does not increase the risk of development of breast cancer. Tibolone (Livial) is an SERM whose metabolites have mixed estrogenic, progestogenic, and weak androgenic activity. It is comparable to HRT for the treatment of climacteric-related complaints. It does not appear to significantly stimulate proliferation of breast or endometrial tissue. It depresses both serum triglycerides and HDL cholesterol. Long-term studies are lacking. It is not available in the United States.

Phytoestrogens are substances found in plants that bind to estrogen receptors. Phytoestrogens, found in soy and red clover extracts, do not appear to significantly improve menopausal hot flushes, cognitive function, bone density, or plasma lipids.

Testosterone replacement therapy in women: Low serum testosterone levels develop in women following bilateral oophorectomy and also later in menopause. Serum testosterone levels are extremely low in women with panhypopituitarism. Low serum testosterone levels are a major cause of HSDD and may also cause fatigue, a diminished sense of well-being, and a dulled enthusiasm for life. Testosterone replacement may increase sexual activity and desire in women with HSDD.

Testosterone replacement may be given orally as methyltestosterone, compounded in capsules and taken orally in doses of 1.25–2.5 mg daily. At these doses, methyltestosterone has not been associated with peliosis hepatis. Testosterone can also be compounded as a cream containing 1 mg/mL, with 1 mL applied to the low abdomen daily. A testosterone skin patch is being developed for women that will deliver testosterone transdermally 0.3 mg/d and will be changed twice weekly. Women receiving testosterone therapy must be monitored for the appearance of any acne or hirsutism, and serum testosterone levels are determined periodically if women feel that they are benefitting and long-term testosterone therapy is instituted.

Anderson GL et al: Effects of conjugated equine estrogen in postmenopausal women with hysterectomy: the Women's Health Initiative randomized controlled trial. JAMA 2004;291:701. [PMID: 15082697]

Barnabei VM et al; Women's Health Initiative Investigators: Menopausal symptoms and treatment-related effects of estrogen and progestin in the Women's Health Initiative. Obstet Gynecol 2005;105(5 Pt 1):1063. [PMID: 15863546]

Cushman M et al; Women's Health Initiative Investigators: Estrogen plus progestin and risk of venous thrombosis. JAMA 2004;292:1573. [PMID: 15467059]

Evans ML et al: Management of postmenopausal hot flushes with venlafaxine hydrochloride: a randomized, controlled trial. Obstet Gynecol 2005;105:161. [PMID: 15625158]

Johnson SR et al: Uterine and vaginal effects of unopposed ultralow-dose transdermal estradiol. Obstet Gynecol 2005; 105:779. [PMID: 15802405]

Lethaby A et al: Hormone replacement therapy in postmenopausal women: endometrial hyperplasia and irregular bleeding. Cochrane Database Syst Rev 2004;(3):CD000402. [PMID: 15266429]

Reed SD et al: Dose of progestin in postmenopausal-combined hormone therapy and risk of endometrial cancer. Am J Obstet Gynecol 2004;191:1146. [PMID: 15507934]

Sherwin BB: Estrogen and memory in women: how can we reconcile the findings? Horm Behav 2005;47:371. [PMID: 15708768]

Simon J et al: Testosterone patch increases sexual activity and desire in surgically menopausal women with hypoactive sexual desire disorder. J Clin Endocrinol Metab 2005;90:5226. [PMID: 16014407]

Wise PM et al: Are estrogens protective or risk factors in brain injury and neurodegeneration? Reevaluation after the Women's health initiative. Endocr Rev 2005;26:308. [PMID: 15851820]

TURNER'S SYNDROME
(Gonadal Dysgenesis)

Turner's syndrome is a chromosomal disorder associated with primary hypogonadism, short stature, and other phenotypic anomalies. It is a common cause of primary amenorrhea and early ovarian failure. Patients with the classic syndrome lack one of the two X chromosomes and have a 45,XO karyotype.

Typical Turner's Syndrome
(45,XO Gonadal Dysgenesis)

Features of Turner's syndrome (Table 26–17) are variable and may be subtle in girls with mosaicism. Typical manifestations in adulthood include short stature, hypogonadism, webbed neck, high-arched palate, wide-spaced nipples, hypertension, and renal abnormalities. Emotional disorders are common. 45,XO accounts for about 50% of cases. Less than 3% of these zygotes survive to term, with the incidence of Turner's syndrome being about 2:10,000 female newborns.

Table 26–17. Manifestations of Turner's syndrome.

Short stature
Distinctive facial features
   Ptosis
   Micrognathia
   Low-set ears
   Epicanthal folds
Sexual infantilism due to gonadal dysgenesis with primary amenorrhea (80%)
Early ovarian failure with secondary amenorrhea (20%)
Webbed neck (40%)
Low hairline
High-arched palate
Cubitus valgus
Short fourth metacarpals (50%)
Lymphedema of hands and feet (30%)
Hypoplastic widely spaced nipples
Hyperconvex nails
Pigmented nevi
Keloid formation (eg, surgical scars or after ear piercing)
Recurrent otitis media
Renal abnormalities (60%)
   Horseshoe kidney
   Hydronephrosis
Hypertension (idiopathic or due to coarctation or renal disease)
Gastrointestinal bleeding from intestinal telangiectases (rare)
Impaired space-form recognition, direction sense, and mathematical reasoning
Cardiovascular anomalies
   Coarctation of the aorta (10–20%)
   Aortic stenosis
   Bicuspid aortic valve
   Aortic dissection due to coarctation and cystic medial necrosis of the aorta
Associated conditions
   Obesity
   Diabetes mellitus (types 1 and 2)
   Dyslipidemia
   Hyperuricemia
   Hashimoto's thyroiditis
   Achlorhydria
   Cataracts, corneal opacities
   Neuroblastoma (1%)
   Rheumatoid arthritis
   Inflammatory bowel disease

Girls with Turner's syndrome may be diagnosed at birth, since they tend to be small and may exhibit severe lymphedema. Evaluation for childhood short stature often leads to the diagnosis. Growth hormone and somatomedin levels are normal. Hypogonadism presents as "delayed adolescence" (primary amenorrhea, 80%) or early ovarian failure (20%); girls with 45,XO

Turner (blood karyotyping) who enter puberty are typically found to have mosaicism if other tissues are karyotyped. Hypogonadism is confirmed in girls who have high serum levels of FSH and LH. A blood karyotype showing 45,XO (or X chromosome abnormalities or mosaicism) establishes the diagnosis.

Treatment of short stature with daily injections of growth hormone (0.1 unit/kg/d) plus an androgen (eg, oxandrolone) for at least 4 years before epiphysial fusion increases final height by a mean of about 10.3 cm over the mean predicted height of 144.2 cm. Such growth hormone treatment rarely causes pseudotumor cerebri. After age 12 years, estrogen therapy is begun with low doses of conjugated estrogens (0.3 mg) or ethinyl estradiol (5 mcg) given on days 1–21 per month. When growth stops, HRT is begun with estrogen and progestin; transdermal estrogen may be used to initiate pubertal development.

Women with Turner's syndrome have a reduced life expectancy due in part to their increased risk for diabetes mellitus (types 1 and 2), hypertension, dyslipidemia, and osteoporosis. Diagnostic vigilance and aggressive treatment of these conditions reduce the risk of aortic aneurysm dissection, ischemic heart disease, stroke, and fracture. Patients are prone to keloid formation after surgery or ear piercing. Yearly ocular examinations and periodic thyroid evaluations are recommended. It is advisable to evaluate all patients with Turner's syndrome with an ultrasound, CT, or MRI examination of the chest and abdomen, looking for cardiac, aortic, and renal abnormalities. Patients with a prominent webbed neck also tend to have a bicuspid aortic valve and aortic coarctation. Aortic aneurysms are common, as are cases of unilateral renal agenesis.

Turner's Syndrome Variants

A. 46,X (ABNORMAL X) KARYOTYPE

An abnormality or deletion of certain genes on the short arm of the X chromosome causes short stature and other signs of Turner's syndrome; some gonadal function and even fertility are possible. Transmission of Turner's syndrome from mother to daughter can occur. There may be an increased risk of trisomy 21 in the conceptuses of women with Turner's syndrome. Abnormalities or deletions of other genes located on both the long and short arms of the X chromosome can produce gonadal dysgenesis with few other somatic features.

B. 45,XO/46,XX MOSAICISM

This karyotype results in a modified form of Turner's syndrome. Such girls tend to be taller and may have more gonadal function and fewer other manifestations of Turner's syndrome.

C. OTHER VARIANTS

45,XO/46,XY mosaicism can produce some manifestations of Turner's syndrome. Patients may have ambiguous genitalia or male infertility with an otherwise normal phenotype. Germ cell tumors, such as gonadoblastomas and seminomas, develop in about 10% of patients with 45,XO/46,XY mosaicism; most such tumors are benign.

El-Mansoury M et al: Hypothyroidism is common in Turner syndrome: results of a five-year follow-up. J Clin Endocrinol Metab 2005;90:2131. [PMID: 15623818]

Cardoso G et al: Current and lifetime psychiatric illness in women with Turner syndrome. Gynecol Endocrinol 2004;19:313. [PMID: 15726728]

Gravholt CH: Epidemiological, endocrine and metabolic features of Turner syndrome. Eur J Endocrinol 2004;151:657. [PMID: 15588233]

Ho VB et al: Major vascular anomalies in Turner syndrome: prevalence and magnetic resonance angiographic features. Circulation 2004;110:1694. [PMID: 15353492]

Hogler W et al: Importance of estrogen on bone health in Turner syndrome: a cross-sectional and longitudinal study using dual-energy X-ray absorptiometry. J Clin Endocrinol Metab 2004;89:193. [PMID: 14715849]

Ostberg JE et al: A comparison of echocardiography and magnetic resonance imaging in cardiovascular screening of adults with Turner syndrome. J Clin Endocrinol Metab 2004;89:5966. [PMID: 15579745]

Soriano-Guillen L et al: Adult height and pubertal growth in Turner syndrome after treatment with recombinant growth hormone. J Clin Endocrinol Metab 2005;90:5197. [PMID: 15998771]

Sybert VP et al: Turner's syndrome. N Engl J Med 2004;351:1227. [PMID: 15371589]

■ MULTIPLE ENDOCRINE NEOPLASIA

Syndromes of MEN are inherited as autosomal dominant traits and cause a predisposition to the development of tumors in different tissues, particularly involving endocrine glands (see Table 26–11).

MEN 1 (Wermer's Syndrome)

MEN 1 is a familial autosomal dominant multiglandular syndrome, with a prevalence of 2–10 per 100,000 people. The presentation of MEN 1 is quite variable, even in the same kindred. Parathyroid, enteropancreatic, and pituitary tumors can be present in one individual, though not necessarily at the same time. Nonendocrine tumors also occur, such as subcutaneous lipomas, facial angiofibromas, and collagenomas. In some affected individuals, tumors may start developing in childhood, whereas in others, tumors develop late in adult life.

About 90% of patients with MEN 1 gave germline mutations that are inherited as an autosomal dominant trait. Patients with MEN 1 usually have detectable mutations in the 10 exons of the *menin* gene, located on the long arm of chromosome 11 (11q13). MEN 1 gene testing is available at a few centers and is able to detect the specific mutation in 60–95% of cases. If no mutation is detected, genetic linkage analysis can be done if there are several affected members in the kindred. Gene testing permits the rest of the kindred to be tested for the specific gene defect and allows informed genetic counseling.

With close endocrine surveillance of affected individuals, the initial biochemical manifestations (usually hypercalcemia) can often be detected as early as age 14–18 years in patients with a MEN 1 gene mutation, although clinical manifestations do not usually present until the third or fourth decade.

Hyperparathyroidism is the first clinical manifestation of MEN 1 in two-thirds of affected patients, but it may present at any time of life. Patients with the MEN 1 mutation have a > 90% lifetime risk of developing hyperparathyroidism. Hyperparathyroidism presents with hypercalcemia, caused by hyperplasia or adenomas of several parathyroid glands. The hyperparathyroidism of MEN 1 is notoriously difficult to treat surgically, due to multiple gland involvement and the frequency of supernumerary glands and ectopic parathyroid tissue. Typically, three and one-half glands are resected, leaving one-half of the most normal-appearing gland intact. Also, during neck surgery, a thymectomy is performed to resect any intrathymic parathyroid glands or occult thymic carcinoid tumors. Nevertheless, the surgical failure rate is about 38%, and there is a recurrence rate of about 16%, with hypercalcemia often recurring many years after neck surgery. Aggressive parathyroid resection can cause permanent hypoparathyroidism. Patients with persistent or recurrent hyperparathyroidism should avoid oral calcium supplements and thiazide diuretics; oral therapy with calcimimetic drug, such as cinacalcet, is effective but expensive. The diagnosis and treatment of hyperparathyroidism is described earlier in this chapter.

Enteropancreatic tumors occur in about 75% of patients with MEN 1. **Nonsecretory neuroendocrine tumors** occur and do not secrete hormones; they tend to be large and very aggressive. **Gastrinomas** occur in about 35% of patients with MEN 1; they secrete gastrin, thereby causing severe gastric hyperacidity (Zollinger–Ellison syndrome) with peptic ulcer disease or diarrhea. Concurrent hypercalcemia, due to hyperparathyroidism (see above), stimulates gastrin and gastric acid secretion; control of the hypercalcemia often reduces gastric acid secretion and serum gastrin levels. These gastrinomas tend to be small, multiple, and ectopic; they are frequently found outside the pancreas, usually in the duodenum. Gastrinomas of MEN 1 can metastasize to the liver; but in patients with MEN 1, depending upon the kindred, hepatic metastases tend to be less aggressive than those from sporadic gastrinomas. Treatment of patients with gastrinomas in MEN 1 is usually conservative, utilizing long-term high-dose proton pump inhibitor therapy and control of hypercalcemia; surgery is palliative and usually reserved for aggressive gastrinomas and those tumors arising in the

duodenum. Zollinger–Ellison syndrome is also discussed in Chapter 14.

Insulinomas cause hyperinsulinism and fasting hypoglycemia. They occur in about 15% of patients with MEN 1. Surgery is usually attempted, but the tumors can be small, multiple, and difficult to detect. The diagnosis and treatment of insulinomas are described in Chapter 27. Glucagonomas (1.6%) secrete glucagon and cause diabetes and migratory necrolytic erythema. VIPomas (1%) secrete VIP and cause profuse watery diarrhea, hypokalemia, and achlorhydria (WDHA, Verner–Morrison syndrome). Somatostatinomas (0.7%) can cause diabetes mellitus, steatorrhea, and cholelithiasis.

Pituitary adenomas occur in about 42% of patients with MEN 1. They are more common in women (50%) than men (31%) and are the presenting tumor in 17% of patients with MEN 1. These tumors tend to be more aggressive macroadenomas (> 1 cm diameter, 85%) compared to sporadic pituitary tumors (42%). Of MEN 1-associated pituitary tumors, about 62% secrete PRL, 8% secrete GH, 13% secrete both PRL and GH, and 13% are nonsecretory; only 4% secrete ACTH and cause Cushing's disease. The diagnosis and treatment of pituitary tumors and Cushing's disease were described earlier in this chapter. These pituitary tumors can produce local pressure effects and hypopituitarism.

Adrenal adenomas or **hyperplasia** occurs in about 37% of patients with MEN 1 and 50% are bilateral. They are generally benign and nonfunctional. In one series, one out of 12 of these patients developed a feminizing adrenal carcinoma. These adrenal lesions are pituitary independent.

Nonendocrine tumors occur commonly in MEN 1. Small facial angiofibromas and subcutaneous lipomas are common. Collagenomas can present as firm dermal nodules. Malignant melanomas have been reported.

The differential diagnosis of MEN 1 includes sporadic or familial tumors of the pituitary, parathyroids, or pancreatic islets. Hypercalcemia (from any cause) may cause gastrointestinal symptoms and increased gastrin levels, simulating a gastrinoma. Routine suppression of gastric acid secretion with H_2-blockers or proton pump inhibitors causes a physiologic increase in serum gastrin that can be mistaken for a gastrinoma. H_2-blockers and metoclopramide cause hyperprolactinemia, simulating a pituitary prolactinoma.

Variants of MEN 1 also occur. Kindreds with MEN 1 Burin variant have a high prevalence of prolactinomas, late-onset hyperparathyroidism, and carcinoid tumors, but rarely enteropancreatic tumors.

MEN 2A (Sipple's Syndrome)

MEN 2A is a rare familial multiglandular syndrome that is inherited as an autosomal dominant trait. Patients with MEN 2A should have genetic testing for a *ret* protooncogene (RET) mutation. Their first-degree relatives may then be tested for the specific RET mutation. Patients with MEN 2A may have **medullary thyroid carcinoma** (> 90%); hyperparathyroidism

(20–50%), due to hyperplasia or multiple adenomas in over 70% of cases; **pheochromocytomas** (20–35%), which are often bilateral; or **Hirschsprung's disease**. The medullary thyroid carcinoma is of mild to moderate aggressiveness. Children harboring an MEN 2A RET gene mutation are advised to have a prophylactic total thyroidectomy by age 6 years.

Siblings or children of patients with MEN 2A should have genetic testing to determine if they have a mutation of the *ret* protooncogene (RET) on chromosome 10cen-10q11.2; this identifies about 95% of affected individuals. Each kindred has a certain *ret* codon mutation that correlates with the particular variation in the MEN 2 syndrome, such as the age of onset and aggressiveness of medullary thyroid cancer. The specific mutation as well as case histories of family members should guide the timing for prophylactic thyroidectomy. Before any surgical procedure, MEN 2 carriers should be screened for pheochromocytoma. There is incomplete penetrance, and about 30% of those with such mutations never manifest endocrine tumors.

Patients may be screened for medullary thyroid carcinoma with a serum calcitonin drawn after 3 days of omeprazole, 20 mg orally twice daily; calcitonin levels rise in the presence of medullary thyroid carcinoma to above 80 pg/mL in women or above 190 pg/mL in men.

MEN 2B

MEN 2B is a familial, autosomal dominant multiglandular syndrome that is caused by a mutation of the *ret* protooncogene (RET) on chromosome 10. MEN 2B is characterized by mucosal neuromas (> 90%) with bumpy and enlarged lips and tongue, Marfan-like habitus (75%), adrenal pheochromocytomas (60%) that are rarely malignant and often bilateral, and medullary thyroid carcinoma (80%). Patients also have intestinal abnormalities (75%) such as intestinal ganglioneuromas, skeletal abnormalities (87%), and delayed puberty (43%). Medullary thyroid carcinoma is aggressive and presents early in life. Therefore, infants having a parent with MEN 2B receive genetic screening; those carrying the RET mutation undergo a prophylactic total thyroidectomy by age 6 months.

Gertner ME et al: Multiple endocrine neoplasia type 2. Curr Treat Options Oncol 2004;5:315. [PMID: 15233908]

Lairmore TC et al: Clinical genetic testing and early surgical intervention in patients with multiple endocrine neoplasia type 1 (MEN 1). Ann Surg 2004;239:637. [PMID: 15082967]

Lambert LA et al: Surgical treatment of hyperparathyroidism in patients with multiple endocrine neoplasia type 1. Arch Surg 2005;140:374. [PMID: 15841561]

Levy-Bohbot N et al; Groupe des Tumeurs Endocrines: Prevalence, characteristics and prognosis of MEN 1-associated glucagonomas, VIPomas, and somatostatinomas: study from the GTE (Groupe des Tumeurs Endocrines) registry. Gastroenterol Clin Biol 2004;28:1075. [PMID: 15657529]

Malone JP et al: Hyperparathyroidism and multiple endocrine neoplasia. Otolaryngol Clin North Am 2004;37:715. [PMID: 15262511]

Skinner MA et al: Prophylactic thyroidectomy in multiple endocrine neoplasia type 2A. N Engl J Med 2005;353:1105. [PMID: 16162881]

■ CLINICAL USE OF CORTICOSTEROIDS

Mechanisms of Action

Cortisol is a steroid hormone that is normally secreted by the adrenal cortex in response to ACTH. It exerts its action by binding to nuclear receptors, which then act upon chromatin to regulate gene expression, producing effects throughout the body.

Relative Potencies

Hydrocortisone and cortisone acetate, like cortisol, have mineralocorticoid effects that become excessive at higher doses. Other synthetic corticosteroids such as prednisone, dexamethasone, and deflazacort (an oxazoline derivative of prednisolone) have minimal mineralocorticoid activity. The potencies relative to hydrocortisone are listed in Table 26–18. Anticonvulsant drugs (eg, phenytoin, carbamazepine, phenobarbital) accelerate the metabolism of corticosteroids other than hydrocortisone, making them significantly less potent. Megestrol, a synthetic progestin, has slight corticosteroid activity that becomes significant when administered in high doses for appetite stimulation.

Table 26–18. Systemic versus topical activity of corticosteroids.[1]

	Systemic Activity	Topical Activity
Prednisone	4–5	1–2
Fluprednisolone	8–10	10
Triamcinolone	5	1
Triamcinolone acetonide	5	40
Dexamethasone	30–120	10
Betamethasone	30	5–10
Betamethasone valerate	—	50–150
Methylprednisolone	5	5
Fluocinolone acetonide	—	40–100
Flurandrenolone acetonide	—	20–50
Fluorometholone	1–2	40
Deflazacort	3–4	—

[1]Hydrocortisone = 1 in potency.

Table 26–19. Management of patients receiving systemic corticosteroids.

- Do not administer corticosteroids unless absolutely indicated or more conservative measures have failed.
- Keep dosage and duration of administration to the minimum required for adequate treatment.
- Screen for tuberculosis before treatment with a purified protein derivative (PPD) test or chest x-ray.
- Screen for diabetes mellitus before treatment and at each physician visit. Teach the patient about the symptoms of hyperglycemia and to test urine weekly for glucose.
- Screen for hypertension before treatment and at each physician visit.
- Screen for glaucoma and cataracts before treatment, 3 months into treatment, and then at least yearly.
- Prepare the patient and family for possible adverse effects on mood, memory, and cognitive function. Inform them about other possible side effects, particularly weight gain, osteoporosis, and aseptic necrosis of bone.
- Institute a vigorous physical exercise and isometric regimen tailored to each patient's disabilities.
- Administer calcium (1 g elemental calcium) and vitamin D₃, 400–800 IU orally daily. Check spot morning urines, and alter dosage to keep urine calcium concentration below 30 mg/dL. If the patient is receiving thiazide diuretics, check for hypercalcemia, and administer only 500 mg elemental calcium daily. Consider a bisphosphonate such as alendronate (5–10 mg orally daily or 70 mg orally weekly) or periodic intravenous infusions of pamidronate or zoledronic acid.
- Avoid prolonged bed rest that will accelerate muscle weakness and bone mineral loss. Ambulate early after fractures.

- Treat hypogonadism in women or men.
- Avoid elective surgery, if possible. Vitamin A in a daily dose of 20,000 units orally for 1 week may improve wound healing, but it is not prescribed in pregnancy.
- Avoid activities that could cause falls or other trauma.
- Watch for fungal or yeast infections of skin, nails, mouth, vagina, and rectum, and treat appropriately.
- Ulcer prophylaxis: Administer oral corticosteroids with meals. If administered with nonsteroidals, consider prophylaxis with omeprazole, 20–40 mg/d. Corticosteroids alone do not need prophylaxis with H₂-blockers or omeprazole. Avoid large doses of antacids containing aluminum hydroxide (many popular brands); aluminum hydroxide binds phosphate and may cause a hypophosphatemic osteomalacia that can compound corticosteroid osteoporosis.
- Treat infections aggressively. Consider unusual pathogens.
- Weigh daily. Use dietary measures to avoid obesity and optimize nutrition.
- Measure height frequently. This serves to document the degree of axial spine demineralization and compression.
- Treat edema as indicated.
- Monitor plasma potassium for hypokalemia. Treat as indicated.
- Obtain bone densitometry before treatment and then periodically. Treat osteoporosis.
- Counsel to avoid smoking and excessive ethanol consumption.
- With dosage reduction, watch for signs of adrenal insufficiency or corticosteroid withdrawal syndrome.

Adverse Effects

Prolonged treatment with systemic corticosteroids causes a variety of adverse effects that can be life-threatening. Patients should be thoroughly informed of the major possible side effects of treatment such as insomnia, personality change, weight gain, muscle weakness, polyuria, kidney stones, diabetes mellitus, sex hormone suppression, occasional amenorrhea in women, candidiasis and opportunistic infections, osteoporosis with fractures, or aseptic necrosis of bones, particularly of the hips, which may become manifest many months after even brief treatment (see section on Cushing's syndrome). Alendronate, 5–10 mg orally daily, prevents the development of osteoporosis among patients receiving prolonged courses of corticosteroids. For convenience, alendronate (70 mg) or risedronate (35 mg) may be taken orally once weekly. Ibandronate, 150 mg orally, may be taken once monthly. For patients who are unable to tolerate oral bisphosphonates (due to esophagitis, hiatal hernia, or gastritis), periodic intravenous infusions of pamidronate, 60–90 mg, or zoledronic acid, 2–4 mg, should also be effective. It is wise to follow an organized treatment plan such as the one outlined in Table 26–19.

Buttgereit F et al: Optimised glucocorticoid therapy: the sharpening of an old spear. Lancet 2005;365:801. [PMID: 15733723]

Gluck O et al: Recognizing and treating glucocorticoid-induced osteoporosis in patients with pulmonary diseases. Chest 2004;125:1859. [PMID: 15136401]

Rhen T et al: Antiinflammatory action of glucocorticoids—new mechanisms for old drugs. N Engl J Med 2005;353:1711. [PMID: 16236742]

Diabetes Mellitus & Hypoglycemia 27

Umesh Masharani, MB, BS, MRCP(UK)

■ DIABETES MELLITUS

 ESSENTIALS OF DIAGNOSIS

Type 1 diabetes:
- *Polyuria, polydipsia, and weight loss associated with random plasma glucose ≥ 200 mg/dL.*
- *Plasma glucose of 126 mg/dL or higher after an overnight fast, documented on more than one occasion.*
- *Ketonemia, ketonuria, or both.*
- *Islet autoantibodies are frequently present.*

Type 2 diabetes:
- *Most patients are over 40 years of age and obese.*
- *Polyuria and polydipsia. Ketonuria and weight loss generally are uncommon at time of diagnosis. Candidal vaginitis in women may be an initial manifestation. Many patients have few or no symptoms.*
- *Plasma glucose of 126 mg/dL or higher after an overnight fast on more than one occasion. After 75 g oral glucose, diagnostic values are 200 mg/dL or more 2 hours after the oral glucose.*
- *Hypertension, dyslipidemia, and atherosclerosis are often associated.*

Epidemiologic Considerations

In 2002, an estimated 18.2 million people in the United States had diabetes mellitus, of which approximately 1 million have type 1 diabetes and the rest mostly have type 2 diabetes. A third group that was designated as "other specific types" by the American Diabetes Association (ADA) (Table 27–1) number only in the thousands. Among these are the rare monogenic defects of either B cell function or of insulin action, primary diseases of the exocrine pancreas, endocrinopathies, and drug-induced diabetes. Updated information about the prevalence of

diabetes in the United States is available from the Centers for Disease Control and Prevention (http://www.cdc.gov/diabetes/pubs/estimates.htm).

Classification & Pathogenesis

Diabetes mellitus is a syndrome with disordered metabolism and inappropriate hyperglycemia due to either a deficiency of insulin secretion or to a combination of insulin resistance and inadequate insulin secretion to compensate. Type 1 diabetes is due to pancreatic islet B cell destruction predominantly by an autoimmune process, and these patients are prone to ketoacidosis. Type 2 diabetes is the more prevalent form and results from insulin resistance with a defect in compensatory insulin secretion (Table 27–2).

A. TYPE 1 DIABETES MELLITUS

This form of diabetes is immune-mediated in over 90% of cases and idiopathic in less than 10%. The rate of pancreatic B cell destruction is quite variable, being rapid in some individuals and slow in others. Type 1 diabetes is usually associated with ketosis in its untreated state. It occurs at any age but most commonly arises in children and young adults with a peak incidence before school age and again at around puberty. It is a catabolic disorder in which circulating insulin is virtually absent, plasma glucagon is elevated, and the pancreatic B cells fail to respond to all insulinogenic stimuli. Exogenous insulin is therefore required to reverse the catabolic state, prevent ketosis, reduce the hyperglucagonemia, and reduce blood glucose.

The highest incidence of immune-mediated type 1 diabetes is in Scandinavia and northern Europe, where the yearly incidence per 100,000 youngsters 14 years of age or less is as high as 37 in Finland, 27 in Sweden, 22 in Norway, and 19 in the United Kingdom. The incidence of type 1 diabetes generally decreases across the rest of Europe to 10 in Greece and 8 in France. Surprisingly, the island of Sardinia has as high an incidence as Finland (37) even though in the rest of Italy, including the island of Sicily, it is only 10 per 100,000 per year. The United States averages 15 per 100,000, with higher incidences in states more densely populated with persons of Scandinavian descent such as Minnesota. The lowest incidence of type 1 diabetes worldwide was found to be less than 1 per 100,000

Table 27–1. Other specific types of diabetes mellitus.

Genetic defects of pancreatic B cell function
    MODY 1 (HNF-4α); rare
    MODY 2 (glucokinase); less rare
    MODY 3 (HNF-1α); accounts for two-thirds of all MODY
    MODY 4 (IPF-1); very rare
    MODY 5 (HNF-1β); very rare
    MODY 6 (neuroD1); very rare
    Mitochondrial DNA
Genetic defects in insulin action
    Type A insulin resistance
    Leprechaunism
    Rabson-Mendenhall syndrome
    Lipoatrophic diabetes
Diseases of the exocrine pancreas
Endocrinopathies
Drug- or chemical-induced diabetes
Other genetic syndromes (Down's, Klinefelter's, Turner's, others) sometimes associated with diabetes

---

MODY = maturity-onset diabetes of the young.

per year in China and parts of South America. The global incidence of type 1 diabetes is increasing (approximately 3% each year).

Certain HLAs are strongly associated with the development of type 1 diabetes. About 95% of patients with type 1 diabetes possess either HLA-DR3 or HLA-DR4, compared with 45–50% of white controls. HLA-DQ genes are even more specific markers of type 1 susceptibility, since a particular variety *(HLA-DQB1*0302)* is found in the DR4 patients with type 1, while a "protective" gene *(HLA-DQB1*0602)* is often present in the DR4 controls. In addition, most patients with type 1 diabetes at diagnosis have circulating antibodies to islets (islet cell antibodies, ICA), insulin (IAA), glutamic acid decarboxylase (GAD65), and to tyrosine phosphatases (IA-2 and IA2-β). These antibodies facilitate screening

of siblings of affected children as well as adults with atypical features of type 2 for an autoimmune cause of their diabetes (Table 27–3). The antibody levels decline with increasing duration of the disease. Also, once patients are treated with insulin, low levels of anti-insulin antibodies develop.

Family members of diabetic probands are at increased lifetime risk for developing type 1 diabetes. The offspring of a mother with type 1 diabetes has a risk of 3%, whereas the risk is 6% if the father is affected. The risk in siblings is related to the number of HLA haplotypes that the sibling shares with the diabetic proband. If one haplotype is shared, the risk is 6% and if two haplotypes are shared, the risk increases to 12–25%. The highest risk is for identical twins, where the concordance rate is 25–50%.

Certain unrecognized patients with a milder expression of type 1 diabetes initially retain enough B cell function to avoid ketosis but as their B cell mass diminishes later in life, dependence on insulin therapy develops. Islet cell antibody surveys among northern Europeans indicate that up to 15% of "type 2" patients may actually have this mild form of type 1 diabetes (latent autoimmune diabetes of adulthood; LADA).

1. Immune-mediated type 1 diabetes mellitus— Immune-mediated type 1 diabetes is believed to result from an infectious or toxic insult to persons whose immune system is genetically predisposed to develop a vigorous autoimmune response either against altered pancreatic B cell antigens or against molecules of the B cell resembling the viral protein (molecular mimicry). Extrinsic factors that affect B cell function include damage caused by viruses such as mumps or coxsackie B4 virus, by toxic chemical agents, or by destructive cytotoxins and antibodies released from sensitized immunocytes. Specific HLA immune response genes are believed to predispose patients to a destructive autoimmune response against their own islet cells (autoaggression), which is mediated primarily by cytotoxic T cells. Amelioration of hyperglycemia in patients given an immunosuppressive agent (eg, cyclosporine)

Table 27–2. Clinical classification of common diabetes mellitus syndromes.

Type	Ketosis	Islet Cell Antibodies	HLA Association	Treatment
Type 1				
(A) Immune-mediated	Present	Present at onset	Positive	Eucaloric healthy diet and preprandial rapid-acting insulin, plus basal insulin replacement with intermediate-acting or long-acting insulin
(B) Idiopathic	Present	Absent	Absent	
Type 2				
(A) Nonobese	Absent	Absent	Negative	(1) Eucaloric diet alone (2) Diet plus insulin or oral agents
(B) Obese	Absent	Absent	Negative	(1) Weight reduction (2) Hypocaloric diet, plus oral agents or insulin

Table 27–3. Diagnostic sensitivity and specificity of autoimmune markers in patients with newly diagnosed type 1 diabetes mellitus.

	Sensitivity	Specificity
Glutamic acid decarboxylase (GAD65)	70–90%	99%
Insulin (IAA)	40–70%	99%
Tyrosine phosphatase (IA-2)	50–70%	99%

shortly after onset of type 1 diabetes lends further support to the pathogenetic role of autoimmunity.

2. Idiopathic type 1 diabetes mellitus—Fewer than 10% of subjects have no evidence of pancreatic B cell autoimmunity to explain their insulinopenia and ketoacidosis. This subgroup has been classified as "idiopathic type 1 diabetes" and designated as "type 1B." Although only a minority of patients with type 1 diabetes fall into this group, most of these are of Asian or African origin. It was recently reported that about 4% of the West Africans with ketosis-prone diabetes are homozygous for a mutation in PAX-4 (Arg133Trp)—a gene that is essential for the development of pancreatic islets.

B. Type 2 Diabetes Mellitus

This represents a heterogeneous group of conditions that used to occur predominantly in adults, but it is now more frequently encountered in children and adolescents. More than 90% of all diabetic persons in the United States are included under this classification. Circulating endogenous insulin is sufficient to prevent ketoacidosis but is inadequate to prevent hyperglycemia in the face of increased needs owing to tissue insensitivity. In most cases of this type of diabetes, the cause is unknown.

Tissue insensitivity to insulin has been noted in most type 2 patients irrespective of weight and has been attributed to several interrelated factors. These include a putative (and as yet undefined) genetic factor, which is aggravated in time by additional enhancers of insulin resistance such as aging, a sedentary lifestyle, and abdominal-visceral obesity. In addition, there is an accompanying deficiency in the response of pancreatic B cells to glucose. Both the tissue resistance to insulin and the impaired B cell response to glucose appear to be further aggravated by increased hyperglycemia (glucose toxicity), and both defects are ameliorated by treatment that reduces the hyperglycemia toward normal. Most epidemiologic data indicate strong genetic influences, since in monozygotic twins over 40 years of age, concordance develops in over 70% of cases within a year whenever type 2 diabetes develops in one twin. Attempts to identify genetic markers for type 2 have as yet been unsuccessful, although linkage to a gene on chromosome 2 encoding a cysteine protease, calpain-10, has been reported in a Mexican-

American population. However, its association with other ethnic populations and any role it plays in the pathogenesis of type 2 diabetes remain to be clarified.

The degree and prevalence of obesity varies among different racial groups with type 2 diabetes. While obesity is apparent in no more than 30% of Chinese and Japanese patients with type 2, it is found in 60–70% of North Americans, Europeans, or Africans with type 2 and approaches 100% of patients with type 2 among Pima Indians or Pacific Islanders from Nauru or Samoa.

Patients with this most common form of diabetes have an insensitivity to endogenous insulin. When an associated defect of insulin production prevents adequate compensation for this insulin resistance, nonketotic mild diabetes occurs. Hyperplasia of pancreatic B cells is often present and probably accounts for the fasting hyperinsulinism and exaggerated insulin and proinsulin responses to glucose and other stimuli seen early in the disease. After several years' duration of diabetes, chronic deposition of amyloid in the islets may combine with inherited genetic defects to progressively impair B cell function.

The mechanisms underlying the insulin resistance of type 2 diabetes are poorly understood. Obesity is generally associated with abdominal distribution of fat, producing an abnormally high waist-to-hip ratio. This "visceral" obesity, due to accumulation of fat in the omental and mesenteric regions, correlates with insulin resistance; subcutaneous abdominal fat seems to have less of an association with insulin insensitivity. Exercise may affect the deposition of visceral fat as suggested by CT scans of Japanese wrestlers, whose extreme obesity is predominantly subcutaneous. Their daily vigorous exercise program prevents accumulation of visceral fat, and they have normal serum lipids and euglycemia despite daily intakes of 5000–7000 kcal and development of massive subcutaneous obesity. Several **adipokines**, secreted by fat cells, can affect insulin action in obesity. Two of these, **leptin** and **adiponectin**, seem to increase sensitivity to insulin, presumably by increasing hepatic responsiveness. Two others—**tumor necrosis factor-α**, which inactivates insulin receptors, and the newly discovered peptide **resistin**—interfere with insulin action on glucose metabolism and have been reported to be elevated in obese animal models. Mutations or abnormal levels of these adipokines may contribute to the development of insulin resistance in human obesity.

Hyperglycemia per se can impair insulin action by causing accumulation of hexosamines in muscle and fat tissue and inhibiting glucose transport (acquired glucose toxicity). Correction of hyperglycemia reverses this acquired insulin resistance.

C. Other Specific Types of Diabetes Mellitus

1. Maturity-onset diabetes of the young (MODY)—This subgroup is a relatively rare monogenic disorder characterized by non–insulin-dependent diabetes with autosomal dominant inheritance and an age at onset of

25 years or younger. Patients are nonobese, and their hyperglycemia is due to impaired glucose-induced secretion of insulin. Six types of MODY have been described. Except for MODY 2, in which a glucokinase gene is defective, all other types involve mutations of a nuclear transcription factor that regulates islet gene expression.

MODY 2 is quite mild, associated with only slight fasting hyperglycemia and few if any microvascular diabetic complications. It generally responds well to hygienic measures or low doses of oral hypoglycemic agents. MODY 3—the most common form—accounts for two-thirds of all MODY cases. The clinical course is similar to that of idiopathic type 2 diabetes in terms of microangiopathy and failure to respond to oral agents with time.

2. Diabetes due to mutant insulins—This is a very rare subtype of nonobese type 2 diabetes, with no more than ten families having been described. Since affected individuals were heterozygous and possessed one normal insulin gene, diabetes was mild, did not appear until middle age, and showed autosomal dominant genetic transmission. There is generally no evidence of clinical insulin resistance, and these patients respond well to standard therapy.

3. Diabetes due to mutant insulin receptors—Defects in one of their insulin receptor genes have been found in more than 40 people with diabetes, and most have extreme insulin resistance associated with acanthosis nigricans. In very rare instances when both insulin receptor genes are abnormal, newborns present with a leprechaun-like phenotype and seldom live through infancy.

4. Diabetes mellitus associated with a mutation of mitochondrial DNA—Since sperm do not contain mitochondria, only the mother transmits mitochondrial genes to her offspring. Diabetes due to a mutation of mitochondrial DNA that impairs the transfer of leucine or lysine into mitochondrial proteins has been described. Most patients have a mild form of diabetes that responds to oral hypoglycemic agents; some have a nonimmune form of type 1 diabetes. Two-thirds of patients with this subtype of diabetes have a hearing loss, and a smaller proportion (15%) had a syndrome of myopathy, encephalopathy, lactic acidosis, and stroke-like episodes (MELAS).

5. Wolfram's syndrome—Wolfram's syndrome is an autosomal recessive neurodegenerative disorder first evident in childhood. It consists of diabetes insipidus, diabetes mellitus, optic atrophy, and deafness, hence the acronym DIDMOAD. It is due to mutations in a gene named *WFS1*, which encodes a 100.3 KDa transmembrane protein localized in the endoplasmic reticulum. The function of the protein is not known. The diabetes mellitus, which is nonimmune and not linked to specific HLA antigens, usually presents in the first decade together with the optic atrophy. Cranial diabetes insipidus and sensorineural deafness develop during the second decade in 60–75% of patients. Ureterohydronephrosis, neurogenic bladder, cerebellar ataxia, peripheral neuropathy, and psychiatric illness develop later in many patients.

Insulin Resistance Syndrome (Syndrome X; Metabolic Syndrome)

Twenty-five percent of the general nonobese nondiabetic population has insulin resistance of a magnitude similar to that seen in type 2 diabetes. These insulin-resistant nondiabetic individuals are at much higher risk for developing type 2 diabetes than insulin-sensitive persons. In addition to diabetes, these individuals have increased risk for elevated plasma triglycerides, lower high-density lipoproteins (HDLs), and higher blood pressure—a cluster of abnormalities termed syndrome X. These associations have now been expanded to include small, dense, low-density lipoprotein (LDL), hyperuricemia, abdominal obesity, prothrombotic state with increased levels of plasminogen activator inhibitor type 1 (PAI-1), and proinflammatory state. These clusters of abnormalities significantly increase the risk of atherosclerotic disease.

It has been postulated that hyperinsulinemia and insulin resistance play a direct role in these metabolic abnormalities, but supportive evidence is inconclusive. Although hyperinsulinism and hypertension often coexist in whites, that is not the case in blacks or Pima Indians. Moreover, patients with hyperinsulinism due to insulinoma are not hypertensive, and there is no fall in blood pressure after surgical removal of the insulinoma restores normal insulin levels. The main value of grouping these disorders as a syndrome, however, is to remind clinicians that the therapeutic goals are not only to correct hyperglycemia but also to manage the elevated blood pressure and dyslipidemia that result in increased cerebrovascular and cardiac morbidity and mortality in these patients. Clinicians aware of this syndrome are more cautious in prescribing therapies that correct hypertension but may raise lipids (diuretics, β-blockers) or that correct hyperlipidemia but increase insulin resistance, with aggravation of diabetes (niacin). Finally, the use of long-acting insulins and sulfonylureas that promote sustained hyperinsulinism may have to be moderated, with insulin-sparing drugs such as metformin or a thiazolidinedione being preferable, if the hypothesis behind the insulin resistance syndrome is ever substantiated.

Clinical Findings

The principal clinical features of the two major types of diabetes mellitus are listed for comparison in Table 27–4.

Patients with type 1 diabetes have a characteristic symptom complex. An absolute deficiency of insulin results in accumulation of circulating glucose and fatty acids, with consequent hyperosmolality and hyperketonemia.

Patients with type 2 diabetes may or may not have characteristic features. The presence of obesity or a

Table 27–4. Clinical features of diabetes at diagnosis.

	Type 1 Diabetes	Type 2 Diabetes
Polyuria and thirst	++	+
Weakness or fatigue	++	+
Polyphagia with weight loss	++	–
Recurrent blurred vision	+	++
Vulvovaginitis or pruritus	+	++
Peripheral neuropathy	+	++
Nocturnal enuresis	++	–
Often asymptomatic	–	++

strongly positive family history for mild diabetes suggests a high risk for the development of type 2 diabetes.

A. SYMPTOMS AND SIGNS

1. Type 1 diabetes—Increased urination is a consequence of osmotic diuresis secondary to sustained hyperglycemia. This results in a loss of glucose as well as free water and electrolytes in the urine. Thirst is a consequence of the hyperosmolar state, as is blurred vision, which often develops as the lenses are exposed to hyperosmolar fluids.

Weight loss despite normal or increased appetite is a common feature of type 1 when it develops subacutely. The weight loss is initially due to depletion of water, glycogen, and triglycerides; thereafter, reduced muscle mass occurs as amino acids are diverted to form glucose and ketone bodies.

Lowered plasma volume produces symptoms of postural hypotension. Total body potassium loss and the general catabolism of muscle protein contribute to the weakness.

Paresthesias may be present at the time of diagnosis, particularly when the onset is subacute. They reflect a temporary dysfunction of peripheral sensory nerves, which clears as insulin replacement restores glycemic levels closer to normal, suggesting neurotoxicity from sustained hyperglycemia.

When absolute insulin deficiency is of acute onset, the above symptoms develop abruptly. Ketoacidosis exacerbates the dehydration and hyperosmolality by producing anorexia and nausea and vomiting, interfering with oral fluid replacement.

The patient's level of consciousness can vary depending on the degree of hyperosmolality. When insulin deficiency develops relatively slowly and sufficient water intake is maintained, patients remain relatively alert and physical findings may be minimal. When vomiting occurs in response to worsening ketoacidosis, dehydration progresses and compensatory mechanisms become inadequate to keep serum osmolality below 320–330 mosm/L. Under these circumstances, stupor or even coma may occur. The fruity breath odor of acetone further suggests the diagnosis of diabetic ketoacidosis.

Hypotension in the recumbent position is a serious prognostic sign. Loss of subcutaneous fat and muscle wasting are features of more slowly developing insulin deficiency. In occasional patients with slow, insidious onset of insulin deficiency, subcutaneous fat may be considerably depleted.

2. Type 2 diabetes—While many patients with type 2 diabetes present with increased urination and thirst, many others have an insidious onset of hyperglycemia and are asymptomatic initially. This is particularly true in obese patients, whose diabetes may be detected only after glycosuria or hyperglycemia is noted during routine laboratory studies. Occasionally, type 2 patients may present with evidence of neuropathic or cardiovascular complications because of occult disease present for some time prior to diagnosis. Chronic skin infections are common. Generalized pruritus and symptoms of vaginitis are frequently the initial complaints of women. Diabetes should be suspected in women with chronic candidal vulvovaginitis as well as in those who have delivered large babies (> 9 lb, or 4.1 kg) or have had polyhydramnios, preeclampsia, or unexplained fetal losses.

Obese diabetics may have any variety of fat distribution; however, diabetes seems to be more often associated in both men and women with localization of fat deposits on the upper segment of the body (particularly the abdomen, chest, neck, and face) and relatively less fat on the appendages, which may be quite muscular. Standardized tables of waist-to-hip ratio indicate that ratios of "greater than 0.9" in men and "greater than 0.8" in women are associated with an increased risk of diabetes in obese subjects. Mild hypertension is often present in obese diabetics. Eruptive xanthomas on the flexor surface of the limbs and on the buttocks and lipemia retinalis due to hyperchylomicronemia can occur in patients with uncontrolled type 2 diabetes who also have a familial form of hypertriglyceridemia.

B. LABORATORY FINDINGS

1. Urinalysis—

a. Glucosuria—A specific and convenient method to detect glucosuria is the paper strip impregnated with glucose oxidase and a chromogen system (Clinistix, Diastix), which is sensitive to as little as 0.1% glucose in urine. Diastix can be directly applied to the urinary stream, and differing color responses of the indicator strip reflect glucose concentration.

A normal renal threshold for glucose as well as reliable bladder emptying is essential for interpretation.

b. Ketonuria—Qualitative detection of ketone bodies can be accomplished by nitroprusside tests (Acetest or Ketostix). Although these tests do not detect β-hydroxybutyric acid, which lacks a ketone group, the semiquantitative estimation of ketonuria thus obtained is nonetheless usually adequate for clinical purposes.

2. Blood testing procedures—

a. Glucose tolerance test—

(1) Methodology and normal fasting glucose— Plasma or serum from venous blood samples has the advantage over whole blood of providing values for glucose that are independent of hematocrit and that reflect the glucose concentration to which body tissues are exposed. For these reasons, and because plasma and serum are more readily measured on automated equipment, they are used in most laboratories. If serum is used or if plasma is collected from tubes that lack an agent to block glucose metabolism (such as fluoride), samples should be refrigerated and separated within 1 hour after collection. The glucose concentration is 10–15% higher in plasma or serum than in whole blood because structural components of blood cells are absent.

(2) Criteria for laboratory confirmation of diabetes mellitus— If the fasting plasma glucose level is 126 mg/dL or higher on more than one occasion, further evaluation of the patient with a glucose challenge is unnecessary. However, when fasting plasma glucose is less than 126 mg/dL in suspected cases, a standardized oral glucose tolerance test may be done (Table 27–5).

For proper evaluation of the test, the subjects should be normally active and free from acute illness. Medications that may impair glucose tolerance include diuretics, contraceptive drugs, glucocorticoids, niacin, and phenytoin.

Because of difficulties in interpreting oral glucose tolerance tests and the lack of standards related to aging, these tests are being replaced by documentation of fasting hyperglycemia.

b. Glycated hemoglobin (hemoglobin A₁) measurements—

b. Glycated hemoglobin (hemoglobin A_1) measurements— Hemoglobin becomes glycated by ketoamine reactions between glucose and other sugars and the free amino groups on the α and β chains. Only glycation of the N-terminal valine of the beta chain imparts sufficient negative charge to the hemoglobin molecule to allow separation by charge dependent techniques. These charge separated hemoglobins are collectively referred to as hemoglobin A_1 (HbA_1). The major form of HbA_1 is hemoglobin A_{1c} (HbA_{1c}) where glucose is the carbohydrate. HbA_{1c} comprises 4–6% of total hemoglobin A_1. The remaining HbA_1 species contain fructose-1,6 diphosphate (HbA_{1a1}); glucose-6-phosphate (HbA_{1a2}); and unknown carbohydrate moiety (HbA_{1b}). The hemoglobin A_{1c} fraction is abnormally elevated in diabetic persons with chronic hyperglycemia. Methods for measuring HbA_{1c} include electrophoresis, cation-exchange chromatography, boronate affinity chromatography, and immunoassays. Office-based immunoassays using capillary blood give a result in about 9 minutes and this allows for immediate feedback to the patients regarding their glycemic control.

Since glycohemoglobins circulate within red blood cells whose life span lasts up to 120 days, they generally reflect the state of glycemia over the preceding 8–12 weeks, thereby providing an improved method of assessing diabetic control. The HbA_{1c} value, however, is weighted to more recent glucose levels (previous month) and this explains why significant changes in HbA_{1c} are observed with short-term (1 month) changes in mean plasma glucose levels. Measurements should be made in patients with either type of diabetes mellitus at 3- to 4-month intervals so that adjustments in therapy can be made if HbA_{1c} is either subnormal or if it is more than 2% above the upper limits of normal for a particular laboratory. In patients monitoring their own blood glucose levels, HbA_{1c} values provide a valuable check on the accuracy of monitoring. In patients who do not monitor their own blood glucose levels, HbA_{1c} values are essential for adjusting therapy. Data from the Diabetes Control and Complications Trial (DCCT) showed that there is a linear relationship between the HbA_{1c} and the mean of seven-point capillary blood glucose profiles (preprandial, postprandial, and bedtime). Thus, mean plasma glucose levels of 170, 205, 240, and 275 mg/dL approximately correlate with HbA_{1c} values of 7%, 8%, 9%, and 10%, respectively. Use of HbA_{1c} for screening is controversial. Sensitivity in detecting known diabetes cases by HbA_{1c} measurements is only 85%, indicating that diabetes cannot be excluded by a normal value. On the other hand, elevated HbA_{1c} assays are fairly specific (91%) in identifying the presence of diabetes.

The accuracy of HbA_{1c} values can be affected by hemoglobin variants or derivatives; the effect depends on the specific hemoglobin variant or derivative and the specific assay used. Immunoassays that use an antibody to the glycated amino terminus of β globin do not recognize the terminus of the γ globin of hemoglobin F. Thus, in patients with high levels of hemoglobin F, immunoassays give falsely low values of HbA_{1c}. Cation-exchange chromatography separates hemoglobin species by charge differences. Hemoglobin variants that co-

Table 27–5. The Diabetes Expert Committee criteria for evaluating the standard oral glucose tolerance test.[1]

	Normal Glucose Tolerance	Impaired Glucose Tolerance	Diabetes Mellitus[2]
Fasting plasma glucose (mg/dL)	< 100	100–125	≥ 126
Two hours after glucose load (mg/dL)	< 140	≥ 140–199	≥ 200

[1] Give 75 g of glucose dissolved in 300 mL of water after an overnight fast in persons who have been receiving at least 150–200 g of carbohydrate daily for 3 days before the test.

[2] A fasting plasma glucose ≥ 126 mg/dL is diagnostic of diabetes if confirmed on a subsequent day.

elute with HbA_{1c} can lead to an overestimation of the HbA_{1c} value. Chemically modified derivatives of hemoglobin such as carbamoylation (in renal failure) or acetylation (high-dose aspirin therapy) can similarly co-elute with HbA_{1c} by some assay methods.

Any condition that shortens erythrocyte survival or decreases mean erythrocyte age (eg, recovery from acute blood loss, hemolytic anemia) will falsely lower HbA_{1c} irrespective of the assay method used. Alternative methods such as fructosamine (see below) should be considered for these patients. Vitamins C and E are reported to falsely lower test results possibly by inhibiting glycation of hemoglobin.

c. Serum fructosamine—Serum fructosamine is formed by nonenzymatic glycosylation of serum proteins (predominantly albumin). Since serum albumin has a much shorter half-life than hemoglobin, serum fructosamine generally reflects the state of glycemic control for only the preceding 1–2 weeks. Reductions in serum albumin (eg, nephrotic state or hepatic disease) will lower the serum fructosamine value. When abnormal hemoglobins or hemolytic states affect the interpretation of glycohemoglobin or when a narrower time frame is required, such as for ascertaining glycemic control at the time of conception in a diabetic woman who has recently become pregnant, serum fructosamine assays offer some advantage. Normal values vary in relation to the serum albumin concentration and are 1.5–2.4 mmol/L when the serum albumin level is 5 g/dL.

d. Self-monitoring of blood glucose—Capillary blood glucose measurements performed by patients themselves, as outpatients, are extremely useful. In type 1 patients in whom "tight" metabolic control is attempted, they are indispensable. There are several paper strip (glucose oxidase, glucose dehydrogenase, or hexokinase) methods for measuring glucose on capillary blood samples. A reflectance photometer or an amperometric system is then used to measure the reaction that takes place on the reagent strip. A large number of blood glucose meters are now available. All are accurate, but they vary with regard to speed, convenience, size of blood samples required, and cost. Popular models include those manufactured by LifeScan (One Touch), Bayer Corporation (Glucometer Elite, DEX), Roche Diagnostics (Accu-Chek), Abbott Laboratories (ExacTech, Precision, FreeStyle), and Home Diagnostics (Prestige). A Freestyle Flash meter, for example, requires only 0.3 mL of blood and gives a result in 7 seconds—and illustrates how there has been continued progress in this technologic area. Various glucometers appeal to a particular consumer need and are relatively inexpensive, ranging from $50.00 to $100.00 each. The more expensive models compute blood glucose averages and can be attached to printers for data records and graph production. Test strips remain a major expense, costing 50–75 cents apiece. In self-monitoring of blood glucose, patients must prick a finger with a 28 to 30 gauge lancets, which can be facilitated by a small plastic trigger device such as an Autolet (Ames Co.), SoftClix (Boehringer-Mannheim), or Penlet (Lifescan, Inc.). When used for multiple patients, as in a clinic, physician's office, or hospital ward, disposable finger-rest platforms are required to avoid inadvertent transmission of blood-borne viral diseases. Some meters such as the FreeStyle (Abbott Laboratories) have been approved for measuring glucose in blood samples obtained at alternative sites such as the forearm and thigh. There is, however, a 5- to 20-minute lag in the glucose response on the arm with respect to the glucose response on the finger. Forearm blood glucose measurements could therefore result in a delay in detection of rapidly developing hypoglycemia.

The clinician should be aware of the limitations of the self-monitoring glucose systems. First, a few of the older meters (such as the One Touch Profile) are calibrated against whole blood glucose concentrations even though the test strip measures the glucose in the plasma fraction. This means the displayed values are 10% to 15% *lower* than the laboratory glucose result. Second, increases or decreases in hematocrit can decrease or increase the measured glucose values. The mechanism underlying this effect is not known but presumably it is due to the impact of red cells on the diffusion of plasma into the reagent layer. Third, the meters and the test strips are calibrated over the glucose concentrations ranging from 60 mg/dL to 160 mg/dL, and the accuracy is not as good for higher and lower glucose levels. When the glucose is less than 60 mg/dL, the difference between the meter and the laboratory value may be as much as 20%. Fourth, glucose oxidase–based amperometric systems underestimate glucose levels in the presence of high oxygen tension. This may be important in the critically ill who are receiving supplemental oxygen; under these circumstances, a glucose dehydrogenase–based system may be preferable. The accuracy of data obtained by glucose monitoring requires education of the patient in sampling and measuring procedures as well as in proper calibration of the instruments. Bedside glucose monitoring in a hospital setting requires rigorous quality control programs and certification of personnel to avoid errors.

e. Continuous glucose monitoring systems—Two continuous glucose monitoring systems are currently available for clinical use. The system manufactured by Medtronic Minimed involves inserting a subcutaneous sensor (rather like an insulin pump cannula) that measures glucose concentrations in the interstitial fluid for 72 hours. In the newest version of the system (Guardian RT), the glucose values are available for review by the patient at the time of measurement. There are also options to set alarms for dangerously low or high glucose values. The other system ("Glucowatch") measures glucose in interstitial fluid extracted through intact skin by applying a low electric current (reverse iontophoresis). This process can cause local skin irritation, and sweating distorts the glucose measurement. Both systems require calibration with finger blood glucose measurements. The main value of these systems appears to be in identifying episodes of asymptomatic hypoglycemia, especially at night.

3. Lipoprotein abnormalities in diabetes—Circulating lipoproteins are just as dependent on insulin as is the plasma glucose. In type 1 diabetes, moderately deficient control of hyperglycemia is associated with only a slight elevation of LDL cholesterol and serum triglycerides and little if any change in HDL cholesterol. Once the hyperglycemia is corrected, lipoprotein levels are generally normal. However, in obese patients with type 2 diabetes, a distinct "diabetic dyslipidemia" is characteristic of the insulin resistance syndrome. Its features are a high serum triglyceride level (300–400 mg/dL), a low HDL cholesterol (less than 30 mg/dL), and a qualitative change in LDL particles, producing a smaller dense particle whose membrane carries supranormal amounts of free cholesterol. These smaller dense LDL particles are more susceptible to oxidation, which renders them more atherogenic. Since a low HDL cholesterol is a major feature predisposing to macrovascular disease, the term "dyslipidemia" has preempted the term "hyperlipidemia," which mainly denoted the elevated triglycerides. Measures designed to correct the obesity and hyperglycemia, such as exercise, diet, and hypoglycemic therapy, are the treatment of choice for diabetic dyslipidemia, and in occasional patients in whom normal weight was achieved, all features of the lipoprotein abnormalities cleared. Since primary disorders of lipid metabolism may coexist with diabetes, persistence of lipid abnormalities after restoration of normal weight and blood glucose should prompt a diagnostic workup and possible pharmacotherapy of the lipid disorder. Chapter 28 discusses these matters in detail.

Differential Diagnosis

A. HYPERGLYCEMIA SECONDARY TO OTHER CAUSES

Secondary hyperglycemia has been associated with various disorders of insulin target tissues (liver, muscle, and adipose tissue) (Table 27–6). Other secondary causes of carbohydrate intolerance include endocrine disorders—often specific endocrine tumors—associated with excess production of growth hormone, glucocorticoids, catecholamines, glucagon, or somatostatin. In the first four situations, peripheral responsiveness to insulin is impaired. With excess of glucocorticoids, catecholamines, or glucagon, increased hepatic output of glucose is a contributory factor; in the case of catecholamines, decreased insulin release is an additional factor in producing carbohydrate intolerance, and with excess somatostatin production it is the major factor.

A rare syndrome of extreme insulin resistance associated with acanthosis nigricans afflicts either young women with androgenic features as well as insulin receptor mutations or older people, mostly women, in whom a circulating immunoglobulin binds to insulin receptors and reduces their affinity to insulin.

Table 27–6. Secondary causes of hyperglycemia.

Hyperglycemia due to tissue insensitivity to insulin
  Hormonal tumors (acromegaly, Cushing's syndrome, glucagonoma, pheochromocytoma)
  Pharmacologic agents (corticosteroids, sympathomimetic drugs, niacin)
  Liver disease (cirrhosis, hemochromatosis)
  Muscle disorders (myotonic dystrophy)
  Adipose tissue disorders (lipodystrophy, truncal obesity)
  Insulin receptor disorders (acanthosis nigricans syndromes, leprechaunism)
Hyperglycemia due to reduced insulin secretion
  Hormonal tumors (somatostatinoma, pheochromocytoma)
  Pancreatic disorders (pancreatitis, hemosiderosis, hemochromatosis)
  Pharmacologic agents (thiazide diuretics, phenytoin, pentamidine)

Medications such as diuretics, phenytoin, niacin, and high-dose corticosteroids can produce hyperglycemia that is reversible once the drugs are discontinued or when diuretic-induced hypokalemia is corrected. Chronic pancreatitis or subtotal pancreatectomy reduces the number of functioning B cells and can result in a metabolic derangement very similar to that of genetic type 1 diabetes except that a concomitant reduction in pancreatic A cells may reduce glucagon secretion so that relatively lower doses of insulin replacement are needed. Insulin-dependent diabetes is occasionally associated with Addison's disease and autoimmune thyroiditis (**Schmidt's syndrome,** or **polyglandular failure syndrome**). This occurs more commonly in women and represents an autoimmune disorder in which there are circulating antibodies to adrenocortical and thyroid tissue, thyroglobulin, and gastric parietal cells.

B. NONDIABETIC GLYCOSURIA

Nondiabetic glycosuria (renal glycosuria) is a benign asymptomatic condition wherein glucose appears in the urine despite a normal amount of glucose in the blood, either basally or during a glucose tolerance test. Its cause may vary from an autosomally transmitted genetic disorder to one associated with dysfunction of the proximal renal tubule (Fanconi's syndrome, chronic renal failure), or it may merely be a consequence of the increased load of glucose presented to the tubules by the elevated glomerular filtration rate during pregnancy. As many as 50% of pregnant women normally have demonstrable sugar in the urine, especially during the third and fourth months. This sugar is practically always glucose except during the late weeks of pregnancy, when lactose may be present.

Clinical Trials in Diabetes

A fundamental controversy regarding whether diabetic microangiopathy is related exclusively to the existence and duration of hyperglycemia or whether it reflects a separate genetic disorder have been resolved by the findings of the DCCT and of the United Kingdom Prospective Diabetes Study (UKPDS), which confirmed the beneficial effects of improved glycemic control in both type 1 and type 2 diabetes, respectively (see below). In addition, with increased understanding of the pathophysiology of both type 1 and type 2 diabetes, large prospective studies have been initiated in attempts to prevent onset of these disorders. Investigators with the Diabetes Prevention Trial 1 (DPT-1) and the Diabetes Prevention Program (DPP) have recently reported their findings (see below).

A. CLINICAL TRIALS IN TYPE 1 DIABETES

1. Diabetes Prevention Trial-1 —This multicenter study sponsored by the National Institutes of Health was designed to determine whether the development of type 1 diabetes mellitus could be prevented or delayed by immune intervention therapy. Daily low-dose insulin injections were administered for up to 8 years in first-degree relatives of type 1 diabetic patients who were selected as being at high risk for development of type 1 diabetes because of detectable islet cell antibodies and reduced early-insulin release. Unfortunately, this immune intervention failed to affect the onset of type 1 diabetes compared with a randomized untreated group. A related study using oral insulin in lower risk first-degree relatives who have islet cell antibodies but whose early insulin release remains intact also failed to show an effect on the onset of type 1 diabetes. After an average of 4.3 years of observation, type 1 diabetes developed in about 35% of persons in both the oral insulin and the placebo groups.

2. The Diabetes Control and Complications Trial —A long-term therapeutic study involving 1441 patients with type 1 diabetes mellitus reported that "near" normalization of blood glucose resulted in a delay in the onset and a major slowing of the progression of established microvascular and neuropathic complications of diabetes during a follow-up period of up to 10 years. Multiple insulin injections (66%) or insulin pumps (34%) were used in the intensively treated group, who were trained to modify their therapy in response to frequent glucose monitoring. The conventionally treated groups used no more than two insulin injections, and clinical well-being was the goal with no attempt to modify management based on HbA_{1c} determinations or the glucose results.

In half of the patients, a mean hemoglobin A_{1c} of 7.2% (normal: < 6%) and a mean blood glucose of 155 mg/dL were achieved using intensive therapy, while in the conventionally treated group HbA_{1c} averaged 8.9% with an average blood glucose of 225 mg/dL. Over the study period, which averaged 7 years, there was an approximately 60% reduction in risk between the two groups in regard to diabetic retinopathy, nephropathy, and neuropathy. Intensively treated patients had a threefold greater risk of serious hypoglycemia as well as

a greater tendency toward weight gain. However, there were no deaths definitely attributable to hypoglycemia in any persons in the DCCT study, and no evidence of posthypoglycemic cognitive damage was detected.

The general consensus of the ADA is that intensive insulin therapy associated with comprehensive self-management training should become standard therapy in patients with type 1 diabetes mellitus after the age of puberty. Exceptions include those with advanced renal disease and the elderly, since in these groups the detrimental risks of hypoglycemia outweigh the benefits of tight glycemic control.

3. Immune Intervention Trials in New-Onset Type 1 Diabetes—At the time of diagnosis of type 1 diabetes, patients still have significant B cell function. This explains why soon after diagnosis patients go into a partial clinical remission ("honeymoon") requiring little or no insulin. This clinical remission is short-lived, however, and eventually patients lose all B cell function and have more labile glucose control. Attempts have been made to prolong this partial clinical remission using drugs such as cyclosporine, azathioprine, prednisone, and antithymocyte globulin. These drugs have had limited efficacy, and there are concerns about toxicity and the need for continuous treatment.

Newer agents that may induce immune tolerance and appear to have few side effects have been used in new-onset type 1 patients. Three small studies, one with a heat shock protein peptide (DiaPep277) and two with anti-CD3 antibodies, have demonstrated that these agents can preserve endogenous insulin production. Larger phase 2 clinical trials are currently in progress.

B. CLINICAL TRIALS IN TYPE 2 DIABETES

While patients with type 2 were not studied in the DCCT, the eye, kidney, and nerve abnormalities are quite similar in both types of diabetes, and it is likely that similar underlying mechanisms apply. Several important differences, however, must be considered. Since patients with type 2 diabetes are generally older with a high incidence of macrovascular disease, an episode of severe hypoglycemia entails much greater risk than it would in a younger patient with type 1 diabetes. Moreover, weight gain may be much greater in obese persons with type 2 diabetes in whom intensive insulin therapy is attempted. These risks take on a greater relevance in older patients with type 2 diabetes because the prevalence of microangiopathy is relatively lower than in those patients with type 1 diabetes; preventing microvascular disease in patients with type 2 diabetes is much less likely to influence morbidity and mortality because of the greater consequences of their macrovascular disease.

To address the issues raised by the DCCT findings as well as a previous concern that sulfonylureas may *increase* cardiovascular deaths, as reported in 1970 by the University Group Diabetes Program, randomized clinical trials of intensive therapy have been conducted in patients with type 2 diabetes.

1. The Diabetes Prevention Program—This study was aimed at discovering whether treatment with either diet and exercise or metformin could prevent the onset of type 2 diabetes in people with impaired glucose tolerance; 3234 overweight men and women aged 25–85 years with impaired glucose tolerance participated in the study. Intervention with a low-fat diet and 150 minutes of moderate exercise (equivalent to a brisk walk) per week reduced the risk of progression to type 2 diabetes by 71% compared with a matched control group. Participants taking 80 mg of metformin twice a day reduced their risk of developing type 2 diabetes by 31%, but this intervention was relatively ineffective in those who were either less obese or in the older age group.

With the demonstration that intervention can be successful in preventing progression to diabetes in these subjects, a recommendation has been made to change the terminology from the less comprehensible "impaired glucose tolerance" to "prediabetes." The latter is a term that the public can better understand and thus respond to by implementing healthier diet and exercise habits.

2. Kumamoto Study—The Kumamoto study involved a relatively small number of patients with type 2 diabetes (n = 110) who were nonobese and only slightly insulin-resistant, requiring less than 30 units of insulin per day for intensive therapy. Over a 6-year period, it was shown that intensive insulin therapy, achieving a mean HbA_{1c} of 7.1%, significantly reduced microvascular end points compared with conventional insulin therapy achieving a mean HbA_{1c} of 9.4%. Cardiovascular events were neither worsened nor improved by intensive therapy, and weight changes were likewise not influenced by either form of treatment.

3. The Veterans Administration Cooperative Study—This investigation involved 153 obese men who were moderately insulin-resistant and who were monitored for only 27 months. Intensive insulin treatment resulted in mean HbA_{1c} differences from conventional insulin treatment (7.2% versus 9.5%) that were comparable to those reported from the Kumamoto Study. However, a difference in cardiovascular outcome in this study has prompted some concern. While conventional insulin therapy resulted in 26 total cardiovascular events, there were 35 total cardiovascular events in the intensively treated group. This difference in the relatively small population was not statistically significant, but when the total events were broken down to *major* events (myocardial infarction, stroke, cardiovascular death, congestive heart failure, or amputation), the 18 major events in the group treated intensively with insulin were reported to be statistically greater (P = .04) than the ten major events occurring with conventional treatment. While this difference may be a chance consequence of studying too few patients for too short a time, it raises the possibility that insulin-resistant patients with visceral obesity and long-standing type 2 diabetes may develop a greater risk of serious cardiovascular mis-

hap when intensively treated with high doses of insulin. At the end of the study, 64% of the intensively treated group were either receiving (1) an average of 113 units of insulin per day when only two injections per day were used or (2) a mean dosage of 133 units per day when multiple injections were used. Unfortunately, the UKPDS (see below), which did not discern any effect of intensive therapy on cardiovascular outcomes, does not resolve the concern generated by the Veterans Administration Study since their patient population consisted of newly diagnosed diabetic patients in whom the obese subgroup seemed to be less insulin-resistant, requiring a median insulin dose for intensive therapy of only 60 units per day by the twelfth year of the study.

4. The United Kingdom Prospective Diabetes Study—This multicenter study was designed to establish, in type 2 diabetic patients, whether the risk of macrovascular or microvascular complications could be reduced by intensive blood glucose control with oral hypoglycemic agents or insulin and whether any particular therapy was of advantage. A total of 3867 patients aged 25–65 years with newly diagnosed diabetes were recruited between 1977 and 1991, and studied over 10 years. The median age at baseline was 54 years; 44% were overweight (> 120% over ideal weight); and baseline HbA_{1c} was 9.1%. Therapies were randomized to include a control group on diet alone and separate groups intensively treated with either insulin or sulfonylurea (chlorpropamide, glyburide, or glipizide). Metformin was included as a randomization option in a subgroup of 342 overweight patients, and much later in the study an additional subgroup of both normal-weight and overweight patients who were responding unsatisfactorily to sulfonylurea therapy were randomized to either continue on their sulfonylurea therapy alone or to have metformin combined with it.

In 1987, an additional modification was made to evaluate whether tight control of blood pressure with stepwise antihypertensive therapy would prevent macrovascular and microvascular complications in 758 hypertensive patients among this UKPDS population compared with 390 of them whose blood pressure was treated less intensively. The tight control group was randomly assigned to treatment with either an angiotensin-converting enzyme (ACE) inhibitor (captopril) or a β-blocker (atenolol). Both drugs were stepped up to maximum dosages of 100 mg/d and then, if blood pressure remained higher than the target level of < 150/85 mm Hg, more drugs were added in the following stepwise sequence: a diuretic, slow-release nifedipine, methyldopa, and prazosin—until the target level of tight control was achieved. In the control group, hypertension was conventionally treated to achieve target levels < 180/105 mm Hg, but these patients were not prescribed either ACE inhibitors or β-blockers.

a. Results of the UKPDS—Intensive treatment with either sulfonylureas, metformin, combinations of those two, or insulin achieved mean HbA_{1c} levels of

7%. This level of glycemic control decreases the risk of microvascular complications (retinopathy and nephropathy) in comparison with conventional therapy (mostly diet alone), which achieved mean levels of HbA_{1c} of 7.9%. Weight gain occurred in intensively treated patients except when metformin was used as monotherapy. No cardiovascular benefit and no adverse cardiovascular outcomes were noted regardless of the therapeutic agent. Hypoglycemic reactions occurred in the intensive treatment groups, but only one death from hypoglycemia was documented during 27,000 patient-years of intensive therapy.

When therapeutic subgroups were analyzed, some unexpected and paradoxical results were noted. Among the obese patients, intensive treatment with insulin or sulfonylureas did not reduce microvascular complications compared with diet therapy alone. This was in contrast to the significant benefit of intensive therapy with these drugs in the total group. Furthermore, intensive therapy with metformin was more beneficial in obese persons than diet alone with regard to fewer myocardial infarctions, strokes, and diabetes-related deaths, but there was no significant reduction by metformin of diabetic microvascular complications as compared with the diet group. Moreover, in the subgroup of obese and nonobese patients in whom metformin was added to sulfonylurea failures, rather than showing a benefit, there was a 96% *increase* in diabetes-related deaths compared with the matched cohort of patients with unsatisfactory glycemic control on sulfonylureas who remained on their sulfonylurea therapy. Chlorpropamide also came out poorly on subgroup analysis in that those receiving it as intensive therapy did less well regarding progression to retinopathy than those conventionally treated with diet.

Intensive antihypertensive therapy to a mean of 144/82 mm Hg had beneficial effects on microvascular disease as well as on all diabetes-related end points, including virtually all cardiovascular outcomes, in comparison with looser control at a mean of 154/87 mm Hg. In fact, the advantage of reducing hypertension by this amount was substantially more impressive than the benefit achieved by improving the degree of glycemic control from a mean HbA_{1c} of 7.9% to 7%. More than half of the patients needed two or more drugs for adequate therapy of their hypertension, and there was no demonstrable advantage of ACE inhibitor therapy over therapy with β-blockers with regard to diabetes end points. Use of a calcium channel blocker added to both treatment groups appeared to be safe over the long term in this diabetic population despite some controversy in the recent literature about its safety in diabetics.

b. Implications of the UKPDS—It appears that glycemic control to levels of HbA_{1c} to 7% shows benefit in reducing total diabetes end points, including a 25% reduction in microvascular disease as compared with HbA_{1c} levels of 7.9%. This reassures those who have questioned whether the value of intensive ther-

apy, so convincingly shown by the DCCT in type 1 diabetes, can safely be extrapolated to older patients with type 2 diabetes. It also argues against the concept of a "threshold" of glycemic control since in this group there was a benefit from this modest reduction of HbA_{1c} below 7.9% whereas in the DCCT a threshold was suggested in that further benefit was less apparent at HbA_{1c} levels below 8%.

Because of the complexity of the overall design in which many of the original therapy groups received additional medications to achieve glycemic goals but remained assigned to their group, statistical analysis may have been compromised by these multiple crossovers. For instance, in the diet group that was used as a control for all the drug treatment groups, only 58% of their total "patient-years" were actually drug-free while the remainder consisted of nonintensive therapy with various hypoglycemic drug regimens to avoid unacceptable hyperglycemia. This probably partly explains why the mean HbA_{1c} for this group was only 7.9% on "diet alone" therapy for over 10 years. In view of these crossovers within treatment groups, caution is suggested regarding several subgroup analyses that are controversial. These include the implication that metformin was superior to insulin or sulfonylureas in reducing diabetes-related end points in obese patients compared with diet therapy even though all three treatment groups achieved the same degree of glycemic control. Conversely, the finding of excess mortality in the subgroup of patients receiving combination therapy with metformin and sulfonylureas need not necessarily preclude this combination in patients doing poorly on sulfonylureas alone, although it certainly indicates a need for clarification of this important question.

Probably the most striking implication of the UKPDS is the benefit to the *hypertensive* type 2 diabetic patient of intensive control of blood pressure. There was no demonstrable advantage of ACE inhibitor therapy on outcome despite a number of short-term reports in smaller populations, implying that these drugs have special efficacy in reducing glomerular pressure beyond their general antihypertensive effects. Moreover, slow-release nifedipine showed no evidence of cardiac toxicity in this study despite some previous reports claiming that calcium channel blockers may be hazardous in patients with diabetes. Finally, the greater benefit in diabetes end points from antihypertensive than from antihyperglycemic treatments may be that the difference between the mean blood pressures achieved (144/82 mm Hg versus 154/87 mm Hg) is therapeutically more influential than the slight difference in HbA_{1c} (7% versus 7.9%). Greater hyperglycemia in the control group would most likely have rectified this discrepancy in outcomes.

5. The STENO-2 Study—The Steno-2 study was designed in 1990 to validate the efficacy of targeting multiple concomitant risk factors for both microvascular and macrovascular disorders in type 2 diabetes. A prospective, randomized, open, blinded end point design was used where 160 patients with type 2 diabetes and microalbuminuria were assigned to conventional therapy with their general practitioner or to intensive care at the Steno Diabetes Center. The intensively treated group had step-wise introduction of lifestyle and pharmacologic interventions aimed at keeping glycated hemoglobin less than 6.5%, blood pressure less than 130/80 mm Hg; total cholesterol < 175 mg/dL, and triglycerides < 150 mg/dL. All the intensively treated group received ACE inhibitors and if intolerant, an angiotensin II-receptor blocker. The lifestyle component of intensive intervention included reduction in dietary fat intake to less than 30% of total calories; smoking cessation program; light to moderate exercise; daily vitamin-mineral supplement of vitamin C, E, and chromium picolinate. Initially aspirin was only given as secondary prevention to patients with a history of ischemic cardiovascular disease; later all patients received aspirin. After a mean follow-up of 7.8 years, cardiovascular events (eg, myocardial infarction, angioplasties, coronary bypass grafts, strokes, amputations, vascular surgical interventions) developed in 44% of patients in the conventional arm and only in 24% in the intensive multifactorial arm—about a 50% reduction. Rates of nephropathy, retinopathy, and autonomic neuropathy were also lower in the multifactorial intervention arm by 62% and 63%, respectively.

The data from the UKPDS and this study provide support for guidelines recommending vigorous treatment of concomitant microvascular and cardiovascular risk factors in patients with type 2 diabetes.

Treatment Regimens

A. DIET

A well-balanced, nutritious diet remains a fundamental element of therapy. However, in more than half of cases, diabetic patients fail to follow their diet. In prescribing a diet, it is important to relate dietary objectives to the type of diabetes. In obese patients with mild hyperglycemia, the major goal of diet therapy is weight reduction by caloric restriction. Thus, there is less need for exchange lists, emphasis on timing of meals, or periodic snacks, all of which are so essential in the treatment of insulin-requiring nonobese diabetics. This type of patient represents the most frequent challenge for the clinician. Weight reduction is an elusive goal that can only be achieved by close supervision and education of the obese patient. See Chapter 29 for dietary management of obesity.

1. American Diabetes Association recommendations—The ADA releases an annual position statement on medical nutrition therapy that replaces the calculated ADA diet formula of the past with suggestions for an individually tailored dietary prescription based on metabolic, nutritional, and lifestyle requirements. They contend that the concept of one diet for "diabetes" and the prescription of an "ADA diet" no longer can apply to both major types of diabetes. In

their recommendations for persons with type 2 diabetes, the 55–60% carbohydrate content of previous diets has been reduced considerably because of the tendency of high carbohydrate intake to cause hyperglycemia, hypertriglyceridemia, and a lowered HDL cholesterol. In obese type 2 patients, glucose and lipid goals join weight loss as the focus of therapy. These patients are advised to limit their carbohydrate content by substituting noncholesterologenic monounsaturated oils such as olive oil, rapeseed (canola) oil, or the oils in nuts and avocados. This maneuver is also indicated in type 1 patients on intensive insulin regimens in whom near-normoglycemic control is less achievable on higher carbohydrate diets. They should be taught "carbohydrate counting" so they can administer 1 unit of regular insulin or short-acting insulin analog for each 10 or 15 g of carbohydrate eaten at a meal. In these patients, the ratio of carbohydrate to fat will vary among individuals in relation to their glycemic responses, insulin regimens, and exercise pattern.

The current recommendations for both types of diabetes continue to limit cholesterol to 300 mg daily and advise a daily protein intake of 10–20% of total calories. They suggest that saturated fat be no higher than 8–9% of total calories with a similar proportion of polyunsaturated fat and that the remainder of caloric needs be made up of an individualized ratio of monounsaturated fat and of carbohydrate containing 20–35 g of dietary fiber. Poultry, veal, and fish continue to be recommended as a substitute for red meats for keeping saturated fat content low. The present ADA position statement proffers no evidence that reducing protein intake below 10% of intake (about 0.8 g/kg/d) is of any benefit in patients with nephropathy and renal impairment, and doing so may be detrimental.

Exchange lists for meal planning can be obtained from the American Diabetes Association and its affiliate associations or from the American Dietetic Association, 216 W. Jackson Blvd., Chicago, IL 60606 (312-899-0040). Their Internet address is http://www.eatright.org.

2. Dietary fiber—Plant components such as cellulose, gum, and pectin are indigestible by humans and are termed dietary "fiber." Insoluble fibers such as cellulose or hemicellulose, as found in bran, tend to increase intestinal transit and may have beneficial effects on colonic function. In contrast, soluble fibers such as gums and pectins, as found in beans, oatmeal, or apple skin, tend to retard nutrient absorption rates so that glucose absorption is slower and hyperglycemia may be slightly diminished. Although its recommendations do not include insoluble fiber supplements such as added bran, the ADA recommends food such as oatmeal, cereals, and beans with relatively high soluble fiber content as staple components of the diet in diabetics. High soluble fiber content in the diet may also have a favorable effect on blood cholesterol levels.

3. Artificial sweeteners—Aspartame (NutraSweet) has proved to be a popular sweetener for diabetic patients. It consists of two amino acids (aspartic acid and phenylalanine) that combine to produce a nutritive sweetener 180 times as sweet as sucrose. A major limitation is that it cannot be used in baking or cooking because of its lability to heat.

The nonnutritive sweetener saccharin continues to be available in certain foods and beverages despite warnings by the Food and Drug Administration (FDA) about its potential long-term carcinogenicity to the bladder. The latest position statement of the ADA concludes that all nonnutritive sweeteners that have been approved by the FDA (such as aspartame and saccharin) are safe for consumption by all people with diabetes. Two other nonnutritive sweeteners have been approved by the FDA as safe for general use: sucralose (Splenda) and acesulfame potassium (Sunett, Sweet One, DiabetiSweet). These are both highly stable and, in contrast to aspartame, can be used in cooking and baking.

Nutritive sweeteners such as sorbitol and fructose have increased in popularity. Except for acute diarrhea induced by ingestion of large amounts of sorbitol-containing foods, their relative risk has yet to be established. Fructose represents a "natural" sugar substance that is a highly effective sweetener and induces only slight increases in plasma glucose levels. However, because of potential adverse effects of large amounts of fructose (up to 20% of total calories) on raising serum cholesterol and LDL cholesterol, the ADA feels it may have no overall advantage as a sweetening agent in the diabetic diet. This does not preclude, however, ingestion of fructose-containing fruits and vegetables or fructose-sweetened foods in moderation.

B. Drugs for Treating Hyperglycemia

(Table 27–7.) The drugs for treating type 2 diabetes fall into several categories: (1) Drugs that primarily stimulate insulin secretion by binding to the sulfonylurea receptor. Sulfonylureas remain the most widely prescribed drugs for treating hyperglycemia. The meglitinide analog repaglinide and the D-phenylalanine derivative nateglinide also bind the sulfonylurea receptor and stimulate insulin secretion. (2) Drugs that alter insulin action: Metformin works in the liver. The thiazolidinediones appear to have their main effect on skeletal muscle and adipose tissue. (3) Drugs that principally affect absorption of glucose: The α-glucosidase inhibitors acarbose and miglitol are such currently available drugs. (4) Drugs that mimic incretin effect or prolong incretin action: Exenatide and DPP 1V inhibitors fall into this category. (5) Other: Pramlintide lowers glucose by suppressing glucagon and slowing gastric emptying.

1. Drugs that primarily stimulate insulin secretion by binding to the sulfonylurea receptor on the beta cell—

a. Sulfonylureas—The primary mechanism of action of the sulfonylureas is to stimulate insulin release from pancreatic B cells. Specific receptors on the surface of pancreatic B cells bind sulfonylureas in the rank order of their insulinotropic potency (glyburide with the greatest affinity and tolbutamide with the least affinity). It has been shown that activation of these receptors closes potassium channels, resulting in depolarization of the B cell. This depolarized state permits calcium to enter the cell and actively promote insulin release.

Sulfonylureas are not indicated for use in type 1 diabetes patients since these drugs require functioning pancreatic B cells to produce their effect on blood glucose. These drugs are used in patients with type 2 diabetes, in whom acute administration improves the early phase of insulin release that is refractory to acute glucose stimulation. Sulfonylureas are metabolized by the liver and apart from acetohexamide, whose metabolite is more active than the parent compound, the metabolites of all the other sulfonylureas are weakly active or inactive. The metabolites are excreted by the kidney and, in the case of the second-generation sulfonylureas, partly excreted in the bile. Sulfonylureas are generally contraindicated in patients with severe hepatic or renal impairment. Idiosyncratic reactions are rare, with skin rashes or hematologic toxicity (leukopenia, thrombocytopenia) occurring in less than 0.1% of users.

(1) First-generation sulfonylureas (tolbutamide, tolazamide, acetohexamide, chlorpropamide)—**Tolbutamide** is supplied as 500-mg tablets. It is rapidly oxidized in the liver to inactive metabolites, and its approximate duration of effect is relatively short (6–10 hours). Tolbutamide is probably best administered in divided doses (eg, 500 mg before each meal and at bedtime); however, some patients require only one or two tablets daily with a maximum dose of 3000 mg/d. Because of its short duration of action, which is independent of renal function, tolbutamide is probably the safest sulfonylurea to use if liver function is normal. Prolonged hypoglycemia has been reported rarely with tolbutamide, mostly in patients receiving certain antibacterial sulfonamides (sulfisoxazole), phenylbutazone for arthralgias, or the oral azole antifungal drugs to treat candidiasis. These drugs apparently compete with tolbutamide for oxidative enzyme systems in the liver, resulting in maintenance of high levels of unmetabolized, active sulfonylurea in the circulation.

Tolazamide is supplied in tablets of 100, 250, and 500 mg. It has a longer duration of action than tolbutamide, lasting up to 20 hours, with maximal hypoglycemic effect occurring between the fourth and fourteenth hours. It is often effective, as are other longer-acting sulfonylureas also, when tolbutamide fails to correct prebreakfast hyperglycemia. Tolazamide is metabolized to several compounds that retain hypoglycemic effects. If more than 500 mg/d is required, the dose should be divided and given twice daily. Doses larger than 1000 mg daily do not improve the degree of glycemic control.

Acetohexamide and chlorpropamide are now rarely used. Chlorpropamide has a prolonged biologic effect, and severe hypoglycemia can occur especially in the el-

Table 27–7. Drugs for treatment of type 2 diabetes mellitus.

Drug	Tablet Size	Daily Dose	Duration of Action
Sulfonylureas			
Tolbutamide (Orinase)	500 mg	0.5–2 g in two or three divided doses	6–12 hours
Tolazamide (Tolinase)	100, 250, and 500 mg	0.1–1 g as single dose or in two divided doses	Up to 24 hours
Acetohexamide (Dymelor)[2]	250 and 500 mg	0.25–1.5 g as single dose or in two divided doses	8–24 hours
Chlorpropamide (Diabinese)[2]	100 and 250 mg	0.1–0.5 g as single dose	24–72 hours
Glyburide			
(Diaβeta, Micronase)	1.25, 2.5, and 5 mg	1.25–20 mg as single dose or in two divided doses	Up to 24 hours
(Glynase)	1.5, 3, and 6 mg	1.5–18 mg as single dose or in two divided doses	Up to 24 hours
Glipizide			
(Glucotrol)	5 and 10 mg	2.5–40 mg as single dose or in two divided doses on an empty stomach	6–12 hours
(Glucotrol XL)	5 and 10 mg	Up to 20 or 30 mg daily as a single dose	Up to 24 hours
Gliclazide (not available in US)	80 mg	40–80 mg as single dose; 160–320 mg as divided dose	12 hours
Glimepiride (Amaryl)	1, 2, and 4 mg	1–4 mg as single dose	Up to 24 hours
Meglitinide analogs			
Repaglinide (Prandin)	0.5, 1, and 2 mg	4 mg in two divided doses given 15 minutes before breakfast and dinner	3 hours
D-Phenylalanine derivative			
Nateglinide (Starlix)	60 and 120 mg	60 or 120 mg twice daily before meals	1.5 hours
Biguanides			
Metformin (Glucophage)	500, 850, and 1000 mg	1–2.5 g; 1 tablet with meals two or three times daily	7–12 hours
Extended-release metformin (Glucophage XR)	500 mg	500–2000 mg once a day	Up to 24 hours
Thiazolidinediones			
Rosiglitazone (Avandia)	2, 4, and 8 mg	4–8 mg daily (can be divided)	Up to 24 hours
Pioglitazone (Actos)	15, 30, and 45 mg	15–45 mg daily	Up to 24 hours
α-Glucosidase inhibitors			
Acarbose (Precose)	50 and 100 mg	75–300 mg in three divided doses with first bite of food	4 hours
Miglitol (Glyset)	25, 50, and 100 mg	75–300 mg in three divided doses with first bite of food	4 hours
Incretins			
Exenatide (Byetta)	5 mcg and 10 mcg	5 mcg within 1 hour of breakfast and dinner. Increase to 10 mcg twice a day after about a month Refrigerate between use	6 hours
Others			
Pramlintide (Symlin)	5 mL vial containing 0.6 mg/mL	For insulin-treated type 2 patients, start at 60 mcg dose three times a day (10 units on U100 insulin syringe). Increase to 120 mcg three times a day (20 units on U100 insulin syringe) if no nausea for 3–7 days. Give immediately before meal. For type 1 patients, start at 15 mcg three times a day (2.5 units on U100 insulin syringe) and increase by increments of 15 mcg to a maximum of 60 mcg three times a day, as tolerated. To avoid hypoglycemia, lower insulin dose by 50% on initiation of therapy.	

derly as their renal clearance declines with aging. Its other side effects include alcohol-induced flushing and hyponatremia due to its effect on vasopressin secretion and action.

(2) Second-generation sulfonylureas (glyburide, glipizide, gliclazide, glimepiride)—Glyburide, glipizide, gliclazide, and glimepiride are 100–200 times more potent than tolbutamide. These drugs should be used with caution in patients with cardiovascular disease or in elderly patients, in whom prolonged hypoglycemia would be especially dangerous.

Glyburide is available in 1.25-mg, 2.5-mg, and 5-mg tablets. The usual starting dose is 2.5 mg/d, and the average maintenance dose is 5–10 mg/d given as a single morning dose; maintenance doses higher than 20 mg/d are not recommended. Some reports suggest that 10 mg is a maximum daily therapeutic dose, with 15–20 mg having no additional benefit in poor responders and doses over 20 mg actually worsening hyperglycemia. Glyburide is metabolized in the liver into products with hypoglycemic activity, which probably explains why assays specific for the unmetabolized compound suggest a plasma half-life of only 1–2 hours, yet the biologic effects of glyburide are clearly persistent 24 hours after a single morning dose in diabetic patients. Glyburide is unique among sulfonylureas in that it not only binds to the pancreatic B cell membrane sulfonylurea receptor but also becomes sequestered within the B cell. This may also contribute to its prolonged biologic effect despite its relatively short circulating half-life. A "Press Tab" formulation of "micronized" glyburide—easy to divide in half with slight pressure if necessary—is available in tablet sizes of 1.5 mg, 3 mg, and 6 mg.

Glyburide has few adverse effects other than its potential for causing hypoglycemia, which at times can be prolonged. Flushing has rarely been reported after ethanol ingestion. It does not cause water retention, as chlorpropamide does, but rather slightly enhances free water clearance. Glyburide is absolutely contraindicated in the presence of hepatic impairment and should not be used in patients with renal insufficiency, in elderly patients, or in those who would be put at serious risk from an episode of hypoglycemia.

Glipizide is available in 5-mg and 10-mg tablets. For maximum effect in reducing postprandial hyperglycemia, this agent should be ingested 30 minutes before meals, since rapid absorption is delayed when the drug is taken with food. The recommended starting dose is 5 mg/d, with up to 15 mg/d given as a single daily dose before breakfast. When higher daily doses are required, they should be divided and given before meals. The maximum dose recommended by the manufacturer is 40 mg/d, although doses above 10–15 mg probably provide little additional benefit in poor responders and may even be *less* effective than smaller doses.

At least 90% of glipizide is metabolized in the liver to inactive products, and 10% is excreted unchanged in the urine. Glipizide therapy is therefore contraindicated in patients with hepatic or renal impairment,

who would be at high risk for hypoglycemia; but because of its lower potency and shorter duration of action, it is preferable to glyburide in elderly patients. Glipizide has also been marketed as Glucotrol-XL in 5-mg and 10-mg tablets. It provides extended release during transit through the gastrointestinal tract with greater effectiveness in lowering prebreakfast hyperglycemia than the shorter-duration immediate-release standard glipizide tablets. However, this formulation appears to have sacrificed its lower propensity for severe hypoglycemia compared with longer-acting glyburide without showing any demonstrable therapeutic advantages over glyburide.

Gliclazide (not available in the United States) is another intermediate duration sulfonylurea with a duration of action of about 12 hours. It is available as 80 mg tablets. The recommended starting dose is 40–80 mg/d with a maximum dose of 320 mg. Doses of 160 mg and above are given as divided doses before breakfast and dinner. The drug is metabolized by the liver; the metabolites and conjugates have no hypoglycemic effect. An extended release preparation is available.

Glimepiride is given once daily as monotherapy or in combination with insulin to lower blood glucose in diabetes patients who cannot control their glucose level through diet and exercise. Glimepiride achieves blood glucose lowering with the lowest dose of any sulfonylurea compound, and this tends to increase its cost-effectiveness. A single daily dose of 1 mg/d has been shown to be effective, and the maximal recommended dose is 8 mg. It has a long duration of action with a pharmacodynamic half-life of 5 hours, allowing once-daily administration, which improves compliance. It is completely metabolized by the liver to relatively inactive metabolic products.

b. Meglitinide analogs—Repaglinide is structurally similar to glyburide but lacks the sulfonic acid-urea moiety. It acts by binding to the sulfonylurea receptor and closing the ATP-sensitive potassium channel. It is rapidly absorbed from the intestine and then undergoes complete metabolism in the liver to inactive biliary products, giving it a plasma half-life of less than 1 hour. The drug therefore causes a brief but rapid pulse of insulin. The starting dose is 0.5 mg three times a day 15 minutes before each meal. The dose can be titrated to a maximal daily dose of 16 mg. Like the sulfonylureas, repaglinide can be used in combination with metformin. Hypoglycemia is the main side effect. In clinical trials, when the drug was compared with a long-duration sulfonylurea (glyburide), there was a trend toward less hypoglycemia. Like the sulfonylureas also, repaglinide causes weight gain. Metabolism is by cytochrome P450 3A4 isoenzyme, and other drugs that induce or inhibit this isoenzyme may increase or inhibit (respectively) the metabolism of repaglinide. The drug may be useful in patients with renal impairment or in the elderly. It remains to be shown that this drug has significant advantages over short-acting sulfonylureas.

c. D-Phenylalanine derivative—Nateglinide stimulates insulin secretion by binding to the sulfonylurea receptor and closing the ATP-sensitive potassium channel. This compound is rapidly absorbed from the intestine, reaching peak plasma levels within 1 hour. It is metabolized in the liver and has a plasma half-life of about 1.5 hours. Like repaglinide, it causes a brief rapid pulse of insulin, and when given before a meal it reduces the postprandial rise in blood glucose. The drug is available as 60-mg and 120-mg tablets. The 60-mg dose is used in patients who have mild elevations in HbA_{1c}. For most patients, the recommended starting and maintenance dose is 120 mg three times a day before meals. Like the other insulin secretagogues, its main side effects are hypoglycemia and weight gain. This drug has been approved for use either alone or in combination with metformin.

2. Drugs that alter insulin action—

a. Metformin—Metformin (1,1-dimethylbiguanide hydrochloride) is used, either alone or in conjunction with other oral agents or insulin, in the treatment of patients with type 2 diabetes.

Metformin's primary action is on the liver, reducing hepatic gluconeogenesis by activating adenosine monophosphate-activated protein kinase (AMPK), which acts as an intracellular energy sensor, and has a critical role regulating gluconeogenesis. LKB1 is a protein threonine kinase that phosphorylates and activates AMPK; it was recently reported that deletion of LKB1 function in the liver results in hyperglycemia with increased gluconeogenic and lipogenic gene expression. The deletion of LKB1 also eliminated the glucose lowering effect of metformin, providing genetic proof for the hypothesis that metformin lowers glucose levels by AMP kinase activation.

Metformin has a half-life of 1.5–3 hours, is not bound to plasma proteins, and is not metabolized in humans, being excreted unchanged by the kidneys.

Metformin may be used as an adjunct to diet for the control of hyperglycemia and its associated symptoms in patients with type 2 diabetes, particularly those who are obese or are not responding optimally to maximal doses of sulfonylureas. A side benefit of metformin therapy is its tendency to improve both fasting and postprandial hyperglycemia and hypertriglyceridemia in obese diabetics without the weight gain associated with insulin or sulfonylurea therapy. Metformin is not indicated for patients with type 1 diabetes and is contraindicated in diabetics with serum creatinine levels of 1.5 mg/dL or higher, hepatic insufficiency, alcoholism, or a propensity to develop tissue hypoxia.

Metformin is dispensed as 500 mg, 850 mg, and 1000 mg tablets. A 500 mg extended-release preparation is also available. Although the maximal dosage is 2.55 g, little benefit is seen above a total dose of 2000 mg. It is important to begin with a low dose and increase the dosage very gradually in divided doses—taken with meals—to reduce minor gastrointestinal upsets. A common schedule would be one 500 mg tablet three times a day with meals or one 850 mg or 1000 mg tablet twice daily at breakfast and dinner. One to four tablets of the extended-release preparation can be given once a day.

The most frequent side effects of metformin are gastrointestinal symptoms (anorexia, nausea, vomiting, abdominal discomfort, diarrhea), which occur in up to 20% of patients. These effects are dose-related, tend to occur at onset of therapy, and often are transient. However, in 3–5% of patients, therapy may have to be discontinued because of persistent diarrheal discomfort.

Hypoglycemia does not occur with therapeutic doses of metformin, which permits its description as a "euglycemic" or "antihyperglycemic" drug rather than an oral hypoglycemic agent. Dermatologic or hematologic toxicity is rare.

Lactic acidosis has been reported as a side effect but is uncommon with metformin in contrast to phenformin. While therapeutic doses of metformin reduce lactate uptake by the liver, serum lactate levels rise only minimally if at all, since other organs such as the kidney can remove the slight excess. However, if tissue hypoxia occurs, the metformin-treated patient is at higher risk for lactic acidosis due to compromised lactate removal. Similarly, when renal function deteriorates, affecting not only lactate removal by the kidney but also metformin excretion, plasma levels of metformin rise far above the therapeutic range and block hepatic uptake enough to provoke lactic acidosis without associated increases in lactic acid production. Almost all reported cases have involved subjects with associated risk factors that should have contraindicated its use (renal, hepatic, or cardiorespiratory insufficiency, alcoholism, advanced age). Acute renal failure can occur rarely in certain patients receiving radiocontrast agents. Metformin therapy should therefore be temporarily halted on the day of the test and for 2 days following injection of radiocontrast agents to avoid potential lactic acidosis if renal failure occurs.

b. Thiazolidinediones—Drugs of this class of antihyperglycemic agents sensitize peripheral tissues to insulin. They bind a nuclear receptor called peroxisome proliferator-activated receptor gamma (PPAR-γ) and affect the expression of a number of genes and regulate the release of the adipokines—resistin and adiponectin—from adipocytes. Adiponectin secretion is stimulated, which sensitizes tissues to the effects of insulin, and resistin secretion is inhibited, which reduces insulin resistance. Observed effects of thiazolidinediones include increased glucose transporter expression (GLUT 1 and GLUT 4), decreased free fatty acid levels, decreased hepatic glucose output, and increased differentiation of preadipocytes into adipocytes. Like the biguanides, this class of drugs does not cause hypoglycemia. Troglitazone, the first drug in this class to go into widespread clinical use, has been withdrawn from clinical use because of drug-associated fatal liver failure.

Two other drugs in the same class are available for clinical use: rosiglitazone and pioglitazone. Both are effective as monotherapy and in combination with sulfonylureas or metformin or insulin. When used as monotherapy, these drugs lower HbA_{1c} by about 1 or 2 percentage points. When used in combination with insulin, they can result in a 30–50% reduction in insulin dosage, and some patients can come off insulin completely. The combination of a thiazolidinedione and metformin has the advantage of not causing hypoglycemia. Patients inadequately managed on sulfonylureas can do well on a combination of sulfonylurea and rosiglitazone or pioglitazone. About 25% of patients in clinical trials fail to respond to these drugs, presumably because they are significantly insulinopenic.

The thiazolidinediones not only lower glucose but also have effects on lipids and other cardiovascular risk factors. Rosiglitazone therapy is associated with increases in total cholesterol, LDL-cholesterol (15%), and HDL-cholesterol (10%). There is a reduction in free fatty acids of about 8–15%. The changes in triglycerides were generally not different from placebo. The increase in the LDL-cholesterol need not necessarily be detrimental—studies with troglitazone showed that there is a shift from the atherogenic small dense LDL particles to larger, less dense LDL particles. Pioglitazone in clinical trials lowered triglycerides (9%) and increased HDL-cholesterol (15%) but did not cause a consistent change in total cholesterol and LDL-cholesterol levels. A prospective randomized comparison of the metabolic effects of pioglitazone and rosiglitazone on patients who had previously taken troglitazone showed similar effects on HbA1c and weight gain. Pioglitazone-treated subjects, however, had lower total cholesterol, LDL-cholesterol, and triglycerides when compared with rosiglitazone. The thiazolidinediones have also been demonstrated to decrease levels of plasminogen activator inhibitor type 1, matrix metalloproteinase 9, C-reactive protein, and interleukin 6. Small prospective studies have also demonstrated that treatment with these drugs lead to improvements in the biochemical and histologic features of nonalcoholic fatty liver disease. These effects make these drugs particularly beneficial for patients with the metabolic syndrome. The thiazolidinediones also may limit vascular smooth muscle proliferation after injury, and there are reports that troglitazone and pioglitazone reduce neointimal proliferation after coronary stent placement. Also, in one double-blind, placebo-controlled study, rosiglitazone was shown to be associated with a decrease in the ratio of urinary albumin to creatinine excretion.

Anemia occurs in 4% of patients treated with these drugs, but this effect may be due to a dilutional effect of increased plasma volume rather than a reduction in red cell mass. Weight gain occurs especially when the drug is combined with a sulfonylurea or insulin. Edema occurs in about 3–4% of patients receiving monotherapy with rosiglitazone or pioglitazone. The edema occurs more frequently (10–15%) in patients receiving concomitant insulin therapy and may result in congestive heart failure. The drugs are contraindicated in diabetic individuals with New York Heart Association class III and IV cardiac status. Rosiglitazone has recently been reported as being associated with new onset or worsening macular edema. Apparently, this is a rare side effect

and most of these patients also had peripheral edema. The macular edema resolved or improved once the drug was discontinued. The dosage of rosiglitazone is 4–8 mg daily and of pioglitazone 15–45 mg daily, and the drugs do not have to be taken with food. Rosiglitazone is primarily metabolized by the CYP 2C8 isoenzyme and pioglitazone is metabolized by CYP 2C8 and CYP 3A4.

These two agents have so far not (unlike troglitazone) caused drug-induced hepatotoxicity. The FDA has, however, recommended that patients should not initiate drug therapy if there is clinical evidence of active liver disease or the alanine aminotransferase (ALT) level is 2.5 times greater than the upper limit of normal. Obviously, caution should be used in initiation of therapy in patients with even mild ALT elevations. Liver function tests should be performed prior to initiation of treatment and periodically thereafter.

3. Drugs that affect absorption of glucose—α-Glucosidase inhibitors competitively inhibit the α-glucosidase enzymes in the gut that digest dietary starch and sucrose. Two of these drugs—acarbose and miglitol—are available for clinical use. Both are potent inhibitors of glucoamylase, α-amylase, and sucrase but have less effect on isomaltase and hardly any on trehalase and lactase. Acarbose binds 1000 times more avidly to the intestinal disaccharidases than do products of carbohydrate digestion or sucrose. A fundamental difference between acarbose and miglitol is in their absorption. Acarbose has the molecular mass and structural features of a tetrasaccharide, and very little (about 2%) crosses the microvillar membrane. Miglitol, however, has a structural similarity with glucose and is absorbable. Both drugs delay the absorption of carbohydrate and lower postprandial glycemic excursion.

a. Acarbose—Acarbose is available as 50-mg and 100-mg tablets. The recommended starting dose of acarbose is 50 mg twice daily, gradually increasing to 100 mg three times daily. For maximal benefit on postprandial hyperglycemia, acarbose should be given with the first mouthful of food ingested. In diabetic patients, it reduces postprandial hyperglycemia by 30–50%, and its overall effect is to lower the HbA_{1c} by 0.5–1%.

The principal adverse effect, seen in 20–30% of patients, is flatulence. This is caused by undigested carbohydrate reaching the lower bowel, where gases are produced by bacterial flora. In 3% of cases, troublesome diarrhea occurs. This gastrointestinal discomfort tends to discourage excessive carbohydrate consumption and promotes improved compliance of type 2 patients with their diet prescriptions. When acarbose is given alone, there is no risk of hypoglycemia. However, if combined with insulin or sulfonylureas, it might increase the risk of hypoglycemia from these agents. A slight rise in hepatic aminotransferases has been noted in clinical trials with acarbose (5% versus 2% in placebo controls, and particularly with doses > 300 mg/d). The levels generally return to normal on stopping the drug.

In the UKPDS, approximately 2000 patients on diet, sulfonylurea, metformin, or insulin therapy were randomized to acarbose or placebo therapy. By 3 years, 60% of the patients had discontinued the drug, mostly because of gastrointestinal symptoms. If one looked only at the 40% who remained on the drug, they had an 0.5% lower HbA_{1c} compared with placebo.

b. Miglitol—Miglitol is similar to acarbose in terms of its clinical effects. It is indicated for use in diet- or sulfonylurea-treated patients with type 2 diabetes. Therapy is initiated at the lowest effective dosage of 25 mg three times a day. The usual maintenance dose is 50 mg three times a day, although some patients may benefit from increasing the dose to 100 mg three times a day. Gastrointestinal side effects occur as with acarbose. The drug is not metabolized and is excreted unchanged by the kidney. Theoretically, absorbable α-glucosidase inhibitors could induce a deficiency of one or more of the α-glucosidases involved in cellular glycogen metabolism and biosynthesis of glycoproteins. This does not occur in practice because, unlike the intestinal mucosa, which sees a high concentration of the drug, the blood level is 200-fold to 1000-fold lower than the concentration needed to inhibit intracellular α-glucosidases. Miglitol should not be used in renal failure, when its clearance would be impaired.

4. Incretins—Oral glucose provokes a threefold to fourfold higher insulin response than an equivalent dose of glucose given intravenously. This is because the oral glucose causes a release of gut hormones, principally glucagon-like peptide 1 (GLP-1) and glucose dependent insulinotropic polypeptide (GIP1), that amplify the glucose-induced insulin release. This "incretin effect" is reduced in patients with type 2 diabetes. GLP-1 secretion (but not GIP1 secretion) is impaired in patients with type 2 diabetes and when GLP-1 is infused in patients with type 2 diabetes, it stimulates insulin secretion and lowers glucose levels. GLP-1, unlike the sulfonylureas, has only a modest insulin stimulatory effect at normoglycemic concentrations. This means that GLP-1 has a lower risk for hypoglycemia than the sulfonylureas.

In addition to its insulin stimulatory effect, GLP-1 also has a number of other pancreatic and extrapancreatic effects. It suppresses glucagon secretion and so may ameliorate the hyperglucagonemia that is present in people with diabetes and improve postprandial hyperglycemia. GLP-1 preserves islet integrity and reduces apoptotic cell death of human islet cells in culture. In mice, streptozotocin-induced apoptosis is significantly reduced by coadministration of exendin-4 or exenatide, a GLP-1 receptor agonist. GLP-1 acts on the stomach delaying gastric emptying; the importance of this effect on glucose lowering is illustrated by the observation that antagonizing the deceleration of gastric emptying markedly reduces the glucose lowering effect of GLP-1. GLP-1 receptors are present in the central nervous system, and intracerebroventricular administration of GLP-1 in wild type mice, but not in GLP-1 receptor knockout mice, inhibits feeding. Type 2 diabetic patients undergoing GLP-1 infusion are less hungry; it is unclear whether this is mainly due to a deceleration of gastric emptying or whether there is a central nervous system effect as well.

a. Exenatide— GLP-1 is rapidly proteolysed by dipeptidyl peptidase IV (DPP IV), and therefore for clinical effect would need to be administered as a continuous infusion. Exendin 4 or exenatide is a GLP-1 receptor agonist isolated from the saliva of the Gila Monster (a venomous lizard) that is more resistant to DPP IV action and, when given to type 2 diabetics by subcutaneous injection twice a day, lowers blood glucose and HbA_{1c} levels. Exenatide appears to have the same effects as GLP-1 on glucagon suppression and gastric emptying. In clinical trials, adding exenatide therapy to patients with type 2 diabetes already taking metformin or a sulfonylurea, or both, further lowered the HbA_{1c} value by 0.4% to 0.6% over a 30-week period. These patients also experienced a weight loss of 3–6 pounds. In an open label extension study up to 80 weeks, the HbA_{1c} reduction was sustained and there was further weight loss (to a total loss of about 10 pounds). The main side effect was nausea, affecting over 40% of the patients. The nausea was dose-dependent and declined with time. The risk of hypoglycemia was higher in persons taking sulfonylureas. Exenatide is dispensed as two fixed-dose pens (5 mcg and 10 mcg). It is injected 60 minutes before breakfast and before dinner. Patients should be prescribed the 5 mcg pen for the first month and, if tolerated, the dose can then be increased to 10 mcg twice a day. The drug is less stable than insulin and needs to be refrigerated between injections.

b. Oral DPP IV inhibitors—These agents, which work by prolonging the action of endogenously released GLP-1, are in clinical trials for use in type 2 diabetes.

5. Others—Pramlintide is a synthetic analog of islet amyloid polypeptide (IAPP or amylin). When given subcutaneously, it delays gastric emptying, suppresses glucagon secretion, and decreases appetite. It is approved for use both in type 1 diabetes and in insulin-treated type 2 diabetes. In 6-month clinical studies with type 1 and insulin-treated type 2 patients, those on the drug had an approximately 0.4% reduction in HbA_{1c} and about 1.7 kg weight loss compared with placebo. The HbA_{1c} reduction was sustained for 2 years but some of the weight was regained. The drug is given by injection immediately before the meal. Hypoglycemia can occur, and it is recommended that the short-acting or premixed insulin doses be reduced by 50% when the drug is started. Nausea was the other main side effect, affecting 30–50% of persons but tended to improve with time. In patients with type 1 diabetes, the initial dose of pramlintide is 15 mcg before each meal and titrated up by 15 mcg increments to a maintenance dose of 30 mcg or 60 mcg before each meal. In patients with type 2 diabetes, the starting dose is 60 mcg premeals increased to 120 mcg in 3 to 7 days if no significant nausea occurs.

6. Drug combinations—Several drug combinations are available in different dose sizes, including glyburide and metformin (Glucovance); glipizide and metformin (Metaglip); rosiglitazone and metformin (Avandamet); pioglitazone and metformin (ACTOplus Met); and rosiglitazone and glimepiride (Avandaryl). These drug combinations, however, limit the clinician's ability to optimally adjust dosage of the individual drugs and for that reason are not recommended.

7. Safety of the antihyperglycemic agents—The UKPDS has put to rest previous concerns regarding the safety of sulfonylureas. It did not confirm any cardiovascular hazard among over 1500 patients treated intensively with sulfonylureas for over 10 years, compared with a comparable number who received either insulin or diet therapy. Analysis of a subgroup of obese patients receiving metformin also showed no hazard and even a slight reduction in cardiovascular deaths compared with conventional therapy.

The currently available thiazolidinediones have not to date exhibited the idiosyncratic hepatotoxicity seen with troglitazone. However, these drugs can precipitate congestive heart failure and should not be used in patients with New York Heart Association class III and IV cardiac status. Lactic acidosis from metformin (see above) is quite rare and probably not a major problem with its use in the absence of major risk factors such as impaired renal or hepatic disease or conditions predisposing to hypoxia.

D. INSULIN

Insulin is indicated for type 1 diabetes as well as for type 2 diabetic patients with insulinopenia whose hyperglycemia does not respond to diet therapy either alone or combined with other hypoglycemic drugs.

With the development of highly purified human insulin preparations, immunogenicity has been markedly reduced, thereby decreasing the incidence of therapeutic complications such as insulin allergy, immune insulin resistance, and localized lipoatrophy at the injection site. However, the problem of achieving optimal insulin delivery remains unsolved with the present state of technology. It has not been possible to reproduce the physiologic patterns of intraportal insulin secretion with subcutaneous injections of short-acting or longer-acting insulin preparations.

Even so, with the help of appropriate modifications of diet and exercise and careful monitoring of capillary blood glucose levels at home, it has often been possible to achieve acceptable control of blood glucose by using various mixtures of short- and longer-acting insulins injected at least twice daily or portable insulin infusion pumps.

1. Characteristics of available insulin preparations—Commercial insulin preparations differ with respect to the time of onset and duration of their biologic action (Table 27–8).

a. Species of insulin—Human insulin is produced by recombinant DNA techniques (biosynthetic human insulin) as Humulin (Eli Lilly) and as Novolin (Novo Nordisk). It is dispensed as either regular (R) or NPH (N) formulations. Five analogs of human insulin—three rapidly acting (insulin lispro, insulin aspart, insulin glulisine) and two long-acting (insulin glargine and insulin detemir)—have been approved by the FDA for clinical use (see below) (Table 27–9). Animal insulins are no longer available in the United States.

b. Purity of insulin—"Purified" insulin is defined by FDA regulations as the degree of purity wherein proinsulin contamination is less than 10 ppm. All insulins presently available contain less than 10 ppm of proinsulin and are labeled as "purified." These purified insulins seem to preserve their potency quite well, so that refrigeration is recommended but not crucial. During travel, reserve supplies of insulin can thus be readily transported for weeks without losing potency if protected from extremes of heat or cold.

c. Concentration of insulin—At present, insulins in the United States are available in a concentration of 100 units/mL (U100), and all are dispensed in 10-mL vials. With the popularity of "low-dose" (0.5- or 0.3-mL) disposable insulin syringes, U100 can be measured with acceptable accuracy in doses as low as 1–2 units. For use in rare cases of severe insulin resistance in which large quantities of insulin are required, U500 regular human insulin (Humulin R) is available from Eli Lilly.

2. Insulin preparations—Four principal types of insulins are available: (1) rapid-acting insulin analogs with more rapid onset and a shorter duration of action than regular insulin after subcutaneous injection;

Table 27–8. Summary of bioavailability characteristics of the insulins.

Insulin Preparations	Onset of Action	Peak Action	Effective Duration
Insulins lispro, aspart, glulisine	5–15 minutes	1–1.5 hours	3–4 hours
Human regular	30–60 minutes	2 hours	6–8 hours
Human NPH	2–4 hours	6–7 hours	10–20 hours
Insulin glargine	1.5 hours	Flat	~24 hours
Insulin detemir	1 hour	Flat	17 hours

Table 27–9. Insulin preparations available in the United States.[1]

Rapid-acting human insulin analogs
  Insulin lispro (Humalog, Lilly)
  Insulin aspart (Novolog, Novo Nordisk)
  Insulin glulisine (Apidra, Sanofi Aventis)
Short-acting regular insulin
  Regular insulin (Lilly, Novo Nordisk)
Intermediate-acting insulins
  NPH insulin (Lilly, Novo Nordisk)
Premixed insulins
  70% NPH/30% regular (70/30 insulin - Lilly, Novo Nordisk)
  50% NPH/50% regular (50/50 insulin - Lilly)
  70% NPL /30% insulin lispro (Humalog Mix 75/25 - Lilly)
  50% NPL/50% insulin lispro (Humalog Mix 50/50 - Lilly)
  70% insulin aspart protamine/30% insulin aspart (Novolog Mix 70/30 - Novo Nordisk)
Long-acting human insulin analogs
  Insulin glargine (Lantus, Sanofi Aventis)
  Insulin detemir (Levemir, Novo Nordisk)

[1]All insulins available in the United States are recombinant human or human insulin analog origin. All the insulins are dispensed at U100 concentration. There is an additional U500 preparation of regular insulin.
NPH = neutral protamine Hagedorn.

(2) short-acting regular insulin; (3) intermediate-acting; and (4) long-acting, with slow onset of action (Table 27–9 and Figure 27–1). Rapid-acting insulin analogs and regular insulin are dispensed as clear solutions at neutral pH and contain small amounts of zinc to improve their stability and shelf life. The long-acting insulin analogs are also dispensed as clear solutions; insulin glargine is at acidic pH and insulin detemir is at neutral pH. NPH insulin is dispensed as a turbid suspension at neutral pH with protamine in phosphate buffer. The Lente series of insulin (ultralente and lente) are no longer available in the United States. The rapid-acting insulin analogs, intermediate-acting, and long-acting insulins are designed for subcutaneous administration, while regular insulin can also be given intravenously. Insulin aspart has been approved for intravenous use, but there is no advantage in using this insulin over regular for this purpose.

a. Rapid-acting insulin analogs—Insulin lispro (Humalog) is an insulin analog produced by recombinant technology, wherein two amino acids near the carboxyl terminal of the B chain have been reversed in position: Proline at position B28 has been moved to B29 and lysine has been moved from B29 to B28. Insulin aspart (Novolog) is a single substitution of proline by aspartic acid at position B28. Insulin glulisine (Apidra) differs from human insulin in that the amino acid asparagine at position B3 is replaced by lysine and the lysine in position B29 by glutamic acid. These changes result in these three analogs having less tendency to form hexamers, in contrast to human insulin. When injected subcutaneously, the analogs quickly dissociate into monomers and are absorbed very rapidly, reaching peak serum values in as soon as 1 hour—in contrast to regular human insulin, whose hexamers require considerably more time to dissociate and become absorbed. The amino acid changes in these analogs do not interfere with their binding to the insulin receptor, with the circulating half-life, or with their immunogenicity, which are all identical with those of human regular insulin.

Clinical trials have demonstrated that the optimal times of preprandial subcutaneous injection of comparable doses of the rapid-acting insulin analogs and of regular human insulin are 20 minutes and 60 minutes, respectively, before the meal. While this more rapid onset of action has been welcomed as a great convenience by diabetic patients who object to waiting as long as 60 minutes after injecting regular human insulin before they can begin their meal, patients must be taught to ingest adequate absorbable carbohydrate early in the meal to avoid hypoglycemia during the meal. Another desirable feature of insulin lispro is that its duration of action remains at about 4 hours irrespective of dosage. This contrasts with regular insulin, whose duration of action is prolonged when larger doses are used.

The rapid-acting analogs are also commonly used in pumps. In a double-blind crossover study comparing insulin lispro with regular insulin in insulin pumps, persons using insulin lispro had lower HbA$_{1c}$ values and improved postprandial glucose control with the same frequency of hypoglycemia. The concern remains that in the event of pump failure, users of the rapid-acting insulin analogs will have more rapid onset of hyperglycemia and ketosis.

b. Short-acting regular insulin—Regular insulin is a short-acting soluble crystalline zinc insulin whose effect appears within 30 minutes after subcutaneous injection and lasts 5–7 hours when usual quantities are administered. Intravenous infusions of regular insulin are particularly useful in the treatment of diabetic ketoacidosis and during the perioperative management of insulin-requiring diabetics. When intravenous insulin is needed for hyperglycemic emergencies, the rapid-acting insulin analogs have no advantage over regular human insulin, which is instantly converted to the monomeric form when given intravenously. Regular insulin is indicated when the subcutaneous insulin requirement is changing rapidly, such as after surgery or during acute infections—although the rapid-acting insulin analogs may be preferable in these situations.

For markedly insulin-resistant persons who would otherwise require large volumes of insulin solution, a U500 preparation of human regular insulin is available. Since a U500 syringe is not available, a U100 insulin syringe or tuberculin syringe is used to measure doses. The physician should carefully note dosages in both units and volume to avoid overdosage.

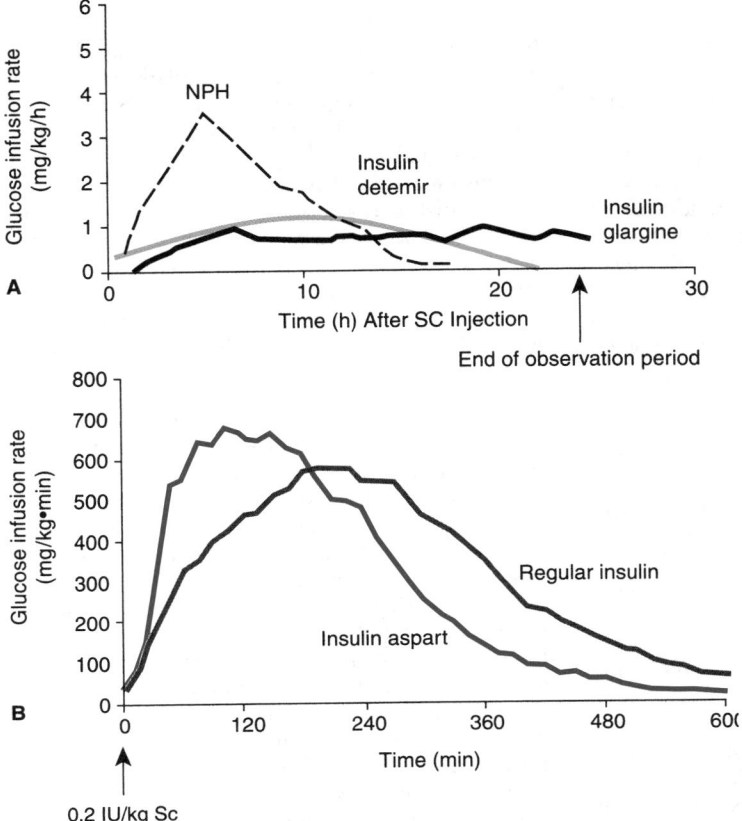

Figure 27–1. Extent and duration of action of various types of insulin–euglycemic hyperinsulinemic clamps in normal volunteers. **A:** Intermediate neutral protamine Hagedorn (NPH) insulin and long-acting insulin analogs. **B:** Regular insulin and rapid-acting insulin analogs.

c. Intermediate-acting neutral protamine Hagedorn (NPH) insulin—NPH (**neutral protamine Hagedorn or isophane) insulin** is an intermediate-acting insulin whose onset of action is delayed by combining 2 parts soluble crystalline zinc insulin with 1 part protamine zinc insulin. This produces equivalent amounts of insulin and protamine, so that neither is present in an uncomplexed form ("isophane").

Its onset of action is delayed to 2–4 hours, and its peak response is generally reached in about 8–10 hours. Because its duration of action is often less than 24 hours (with a range of 10–20 hours), most patients require at least two injections daily to maintain a sustained insulin effect. Occasional vials of NPH insulin have tended to show unusual clumping of their contents or "frosting" of the container, with considerable loss of bioactivity. This instability is rare and occurs less frequently if NPH human insulin is refrigerated when not in use and if bottles are discarded after 1 month of use.

d. Long-acting insulins—

(1) Insulin glargine—This agent is an insulin analog in which the asparagine at position 21 of the A chain of the human insulin molecule is replaced by glycine and two arginines are added to the carboxyl terminal of the B chain. The arginines raise the iso-electric point of the molecule closer to neutral, making it more soluble in an acidic environment. In contrast, human insulin has an isoelectric point of pH 5.4. Insulin glargine is a clear insulin which, when injected into the neutral pH environment of the subcutaneous tissue, forms microprecipitates that slowly release the insulin into the circulation. It lasts for about 24 hours without any pronounced peaks and is given once a day to provide basal coverage. This insulin cannot be mixed with the other human insulins because of its acidic pH. When this insulin was given as a single injection at bedtime to type 1 patients, fasting hyperglycemia was better controlled when compared with bedtime NPH insulin. The clinical trials also suggest that there may be less nocturnal hypoglycemia with this insulin when compared with NPH insulin.

In one clinical trial involving type 2 patients, insulin glargine was associated with a slightly higher progression of retinopathy when compared with NPH insulin. The frequency was 7.5% with the analog and 2.7% with the NPH. This finding, however, was not seen in other clinical trials with this analog. Insulin glargine does have a sixfold greater affinity for IGF-1 receptor compared with the human insulin. There has also been a report that insulin glargine had increased mitogenicity compared with human insulin in a human osteosarcoma cell line. The significance of these observations is not yet clear. Because of lack of safety data, use of insulin glargine during pregnancy is not recommended.

(2) Insulin detemir—This agent is an insulin analog in which the tyrosine at position 30 of the β chain has been removed and a 14-C fatty acid chain (tetradecanoic acid) is attached to the lysine at position 29 by acylation. The fatty acid chain makes the molecule more lipophilic than native insulin and the addition of zinc stabilizes the molecule and leads to formation of hexamers. After injection, self-association at the injection site and albumin binding in the circulation via the fatty acid side chain, leads to slower distribution to peripheral target tissues and prolonged duration of action. The affinity of insulin determir is fourfold to fivefold lower than that of human soluble insulin and therefore the U100 formulation of insulin detemir has an insulin concentration of 2400 nmol/mL compared with 600 nmol/mL for NPH. The duration of action for insulin detemir is about 17 hours at therapeutically relevant doses. It is recommended that the insulin be injected once or twice a day to achieve a stable basal coverage. This insulin has been reported to have lower within-subject pharmacodynamic variability compared with NPH insulin and insulin glargine. In vitro studies do not suggest any clinically relevant albumin binding interactions between insulin detemir and fatty acids or protein-bound drugs. Since there is a vast excess (~400,000) of albumin binding sites available in plasma per insulin detemir molecule, it is unlikely that hypoalbuminemic disease states will affect the ratio of bound to free insulin detemir.

e. Mixtures of insulin—Since intermediate insulins require several hours to reach adequate therapeutic levels, their use in patients with type 1 diabetes requires supplements of regular or rapid-acting insulin analogs preprandially. For convenience, regular or rapid-acting insulin analogs and NPH insulin may be mixed together in the same syringe and injected subcutaneously in split dosage before breakfast and supper. It is recommended that the regular insulin or rapid-acting insulin analog be withdrawn first, then the NPH insulin and that the injection be given immediately after loading the syringe. Stable premixed insulins (70% NPH and 30% regular or 50% of each) are available as a convenience to patients who have difficulty mixing insulin because of visual problems or impairment of manual dexterity. Premixed preparations of insulin lispro and NPH insulins are unstable because of exchange of insulin lispro with the human insulin in the protamine complex. Consequently, the soluble component becomes over time a mixture of regular and insulin lispro at varying ratios. In an attempt to remedy this, an intermediate insulin composed of isophane complexes of protamine with insulin lispro was developed called NPL (neutral protamine lispro). This insulin has the same duration of action as NPH insulin. Premixed combinations of NPL and insulin lispro (eg, 75:25, 50:50, and 25:75 of NPL:insu-

lin lispro) have been tested. Both 75% NPL/25% insulin lispro mixture (Humalog Mix 75/25) and 50% NPL/50% insulin lispro mixture (Humalog Mix 50/50) are available for clinical use. Similarly, a 70% insulin aspart protamine/30% insulin aspart (NovoLogMix 70/30) is available. The main advantages of these mixtures is that they can be given within 15 minutes of starting a meal and they are superior in controlling the postprandial glucose rise after a carbohydrate rich meal. These benefits have not translated into improvements in HbA_{1c} levels when compared with the usual 70% NPH/30% regular mixture.

The longer-acting insulin analogs cannot be mixed with either regular insulin or the rapid-acting insulin analogs.

3. Methods of insulin administration—

a. Insulin syringes and needles—Plastic disposable syringes are available in 1-mL, 0.5-mL, and 0.3-mL sizes. The "low-dose" 0.3-mL syringes have become increasingly popular, because many diabetics do not take more than 30 units of insulin in a single injection except in rare instances of extreme insulin resistance. Two lengths of needles are available: short (8 mm) and long (12.7 mm). Long needles are preferable in obese patients to reduce variability of insulin absorption. Ultrafine needles as small as 31 gauge reduce the pain of injections. "Disposable" syringes may be reused until blunting of the needle occurs (usually after three to five injections). Sterility adequate to avoid infection with reuse appears to be maintained by recapping syringes between uses. Cleansing the needle with alcohol may not be desirable since it can dissolve the silicone coating and can increase the pain of skin puncturing.

Any part of the body covered by loose skin can be used, such as the abdomen, thighs, upper arms, flanks, and upper buttocks. Preparation with alcohol is no longer required prior to injection as long as the skin is clean. Rotation of sites continues to be recommended to avoid delayed absorption when fibrosis or lipohypertrophy occurs from repeated use of a single site. However, considerable variability of absorption rates from different sites, particularly with exercise, may contribute to the instability of glycemic control in certain type 1 patients if injection sites are rotated too frequently in different areas of the body. Consequently, it is best to limit injection sites to a single region of the body and rotate sites within that region. The abdomen is recommended for subcutaneous injections, since regular insulin has been shown to absorb more rapidly from there than from other subcutaneous sites. The effect of anatomic regions appears to be much less pronounced with the analog insulins.

b. Insulin pen injector devices—Insulin pens eliminate the need for carrying insulin vials and syringes. Cartridges of insulin lispro, insulin aspart, insulin glargine, regular insulin, NPH insulin, and 70% NPH/30% regular insulin are available for reusable pens (Novo Nordisk,

Becton Dickinson, and Sanofi Aventis pens). Disposable prefilled pens are also available for insulin lispro, NPH, 70% NPH/30% regular, 75% NPL/25% insulin lispro, 50% NPL/50% insulin lispro, and 70% insulin aspart protamine/30% insulin aspart. Thirty-one gauge needles (5, 6, and 8 mm long) for these pens make injections almost painless.

c. Insulin pumps—In the United States, Medtronic Mini-Med, Animas, and Deltec Cozmo insulin infusion pumps are available for subcutaneous delivery of insulin. These pumps are small (about the size of a pager) and very easy to program. They offer many features, including the ability to set a number of different basal rates throughout the 24 hours and to adjust the time over which bolus doses are given. They also are able to detect pressure build-up if the catheter is kinked. Improvements have also been made in the infusion sets. The catheter connecting the insulin reservoir to the subcutaneous cannula can be disconnected, allowing the patient to remove the pump temporarily (eg, for bathing). The great advantage of continuous subcutaneous insulin infusion (CSII) is that it allows for establishment of a basal profile tailored to the patient. The patient therefore is able to eat with less regard to timing because the basal insulin infusion should maintain constant blood glucose between meals. Also the ability to adjust the basal insulin infusion makes it easier for the patient to manage glycemic excursions that occur with exercise.

CSII therapy is appropriate for patients who are motivated, mechanically inclined, educated about diabetes (diet, insulin action, treatment of hypoglycemia and hyperglycemia), and willing to monitor their blood glucose four to six times a day. Known complications of CSII include ketoacidosis, which can occur when insulin delivery is interrupted, and skin infections. Another disadvantage is its cost and the time demanded of physicians and staff in initiating therapy.

d. Inhaled insulin—A novel method for delivering a preprandial powdered form of insulin by inhalation (Exubera) has been approved by the FDA. In the clinical trials that led to the approval of this preparation, approximately 2500 adult patients with type 1 and type 2 diabetes were studied. The inhaled insulin was as effective as subcutaneous regular insulin in controlling postprandial glucose excursions, but the studies did not compare inhaled insulin with the short-acting insulin analogs.

Pharmacokinetic studies of the inhaled preparation show that it is rapidly absorbed and its onset of action is 32 minutes, compared with 48 and 41 minutes for regular insulin and insulin lispro, respectively. However, the metabolic effect is slower, and the duration of action is longer than insulin lispro and comparable to regular insulin. The bioavailability of inhaled insulin is about 10%, and so patients would need to inhale about 300–400 units of insulin a day. Inhaled insulin is administered 10 minutes prior to meals using a combination of 1- and 3-mg unit doses; 1 mg of inhaled insulin is equivalent to 3 units subcutaneous insulin injection.

Because consecutive inhalation of three 1-mg blisters is associated with a 30–40% greater insulin exposure than one 3-mg dose blister, the two regimens are not interchangeable. A small decrease in pulmonary function (forced expiratory volume in 1 second [FEV_1] and single-breath diffusing capacity for carbon monoxide [$D_{L_{CO}}$]) was seen in the first few months of use, but in the phase 3 studies lasting 2 years, patients did not experience clinically significant effects on pulmonary function. The clinical trials excluded patients with pulmonary disorders. Inhaled insulin does result in higher insulin antibody titers than subcutaneous insulin, but the studies so far have not shown any clinical impact on dosage or control. Other side effects associated with Exubera therapy include cough, shortness of breath, sore throat, and dry mouth. Smokers have higher insulin levels than nonsmokers, so this insulin preparation is contraindicated in patients who smoke or who have discontinued smoking for less than 6 months. The FDA has recommended pulmonary function tests at baseline, after 6 months of treatment and every year thereafter, even if there are no pulmonary symptoms.

E. TRANSPLANTATION

Pancreas **transplantation** at the time of renal transplantation is becoming more widely accepted. Patients undergoing simultaneous pancreas and kidney transplantation have an 85% chance of pancreatic graft survival and a 92% chance of renal graft survival after 1 year. Solitary pancreatic transplantation in the absence of a need for renal transplantation should be considered only in those rare patients who fail all other insulin therapeutic approaches and who have frequent severe hypoglycemia or who have life-threatening complications related to their lack of metabolic control.

Islet cell transplantation is a minimally invasive procedure, and investigators in Edmonton, Canada, have reported initial insulin independence in a small number of patients with type 1 diabetes who underwent this procedure. Using islets from multiple donors and corticosteroid-free immunosuppression, percutaneous transhepatic portal vein transplantation of islets was achieved in over 20 subjects. Although all of the initial cohort was able to achieve insulin independence posttransplantation (some for more than 2 years of follow-up), a decline in insulin secretion has occurred over time and the subjects have again required supplemental insulin. All patients had complete correction of severe hypoglycemic reactions, leading to a marked improvement in overall quality of life. Even if long-term insulin independence is demonstrated, wide application of this procedure for the treatment of type 1 diabetes is limited by the dependence on multiple donors and the requirement for potent long-term immunotherapy.

General Considerations in Treatment of Diabetes

Insulin-treated patients with diabetes can have a full and satisfying life. However, "free" diets and unrestricted activity are still not advised. Until new methods of insulin replacement are developed that provide more normal patterns of insulin delivery in response to metabolic demands, multiple feedings with carbohydrate counting will continue to be recommended, and certain occupations potentially hazardous to the patient or others will continue to be prohibited because of risks due to hypoglycemia. The American Diabetic Association can act as a patient advocate in case of employment questions.

Exercise increases the effectiveness of insulin, and moderate exercise is an excellent means of improving utilization of fat and carbohydrate in diabetic patients. A judicious balance of the size and frequency of meals with moderate regular exercise can often stabilize the insulin dosage in diabetics who tend to slip out of control easily. Strenuous exercise can precipitate hypoglycemia in an unprepared patient, and diabetics must therefore be taught to reduce their insulin dosage in anticipation of strenuous activity or to take supplemental carbohydrate. Injection of insulin into a site farthest away from the muscles most involved in exercise may help ameliorate exercise-induced hypoglycemia, since insulin injected in the proximity of exercising muscle may be more rapidly mobilized.

All diabetic patients must receive adequate instruction on personal hygiene, especially with regard to care of the feet, skin, and teeth. All infections (especially pyogenic ones) provoke the release of high levels of insulin antagonists such as catecholamines or glucagon and thus bring about a marked increase in insulin requirements. Supplemental regular insulin is often required to correct hyperglycemia during infection.

Steps in the Management of the Diabetic Patient

A. Diagnostic Examination

Any features of the clinical picture that suggest end-organ insensitivity to insulin, such as visceral obesity, must be identified. The family history should document not only the incidence of diabetes in other members of the family but also the age at onset, whether it was associated with obesity, and whether insulin was required. An attempt should be made to characterize the diabetes as type 1 or type 2, based on the clinical features present and on whether or not ketonuria accompanies the glycosuria. For the occasional patient, measurement of islet cell, glutamic acid decarboxylase (GAD65), insulin antibodies, and ICA 512 antibodies can help distinguish between type 1 and type 2 diabetes. Many patients in whom type 1 diabetes is newly diagnosed still have significant endogenous insulin production, and C peptide levels may not reliably distinguish between type 1 and type 2 diabetes. Other factors that increase cardiac risk, such as smoking history, presence of hypertension or hyperlipidemia, or oral contraceptive pill use, should be recorded.

Laboratory diagnosis should document fasting plasma glucose levels above 126 mg/dL or postprandial values consistently above 200 mg/dL and whether ketonuria accompanies the glycosuria. A glycohemoglobin measurement is useful for assessing the effectiveness of future therapy. Some flexibility of clinical judgment is appropriate when diagnosing diabetes mellitus in the elderly patient with borderline hyperglycemia.

Baseline values include fasting plasma triglycerides, total cholesterol and HDL-cholesterol, electrocardiography, renal function studies, peripheral pulses, and neurologic, podiatric, and ophthalmologic examinations to help guide future assessments.

B. Patient Education (Self-Management Training)

Since diabetes is a lifelong disorder, education of the patient and the family is probably the most important obligation of the clinician who provides initial care. The best persons to manage a disease that is affected so markedly by daily fluctuations in environmental stress, exercise, diet, and infections are the patients themselves and their families. The "teaching curriculum" should include explanations by the physician or nurse of the nature of diabetes and its potential acute and chronic hazards and how they can be recognized early and prevented or treated. Self-monitoring of blood glucose should be emphasized, especially in insulin-requiring diabetic patients, and instructions must be given on proper testing and recording of data. Patients should be provided with algorithms they can use to adjust the timing and quantity of their insulin dose, food, and exercise in response to measured blood glucose values. The targets for blood glucose control should be elevated appropriately in elderly patients since they have the greatest risk if subjected to hypoglycemia and the least long-term benefit from more rigid glycemic control. Advice on personal hygiene, including detailed instructions on foot care as well as individual instruction on diet and specific hypoglycemic therapy, should be provided. Patients should be told about community agencies, such as Diabetes Association chapters, that can serve as a continuing source of instruction. Finally, vigorous efforts should be made to persuade new diabetics who smoke to give up the habit, since large vessel peripheral vascular disease and debilitating retinopathy are less common in nonsmoking diabetic patients.

C. Therapy

Treatment must be individualized on the basis of the type of diabetes and specific needs of each patient. However, certain general principles of management can be outlined for hyperglycemic states of different types.

1. Type 2 diabetes—

a. The obese patient with type 2 diabetes—The most common type of diabetic patient is obese, is non–insulin-dependent, and has hyperglycemia because of insensitivity to normal or elevated circulating levels of insulin.

(1) Weight reduction—Treatment is directed toward achieving weight reduction, and prescribing a diet is only one means to this end. Behavior modification to achieve adherence to the diet—as well as increased physical activity to expend energy—is also required. Cure can be achieved by reducing adipose stores, with consequent restoration of tissue sensitivity to insulin, but weight reduction is hard to achieve and even more difficult to maintain with our current therapies. The presence of diabetes with its added risk factors may motivate the obese diabetic to greater efforts to lose weight. (See also Chapter 29.)

(2) Hypoglycemic agents—If the patient is not able to achieve target glycemic control with weight management and exercise, then pharmacologic therapy is indicated. The choice of initial agent depends on a number of factors, including comorbid conditions, adverse reactions to the medications, ability of the patient to monitor for hypoglycemia, drug cost, and patient and physician preferences. **Metformin** is advantageous because apart from lowering glucose without the risk of hypoglycemia, it also lowers triglycerides and promotes some modest weight loss. The drug, however, cannot be used in patients with renal failure, and gastrointestinal side effects develop in some patients at even the lowest doses. **Thiazolidinediones** improve peripheral insulin resistance and lower glucose without causing hypoglycemia. They also have been reported to improve nonalcoholic fatty liver disease, have beneficial effects on the lipid profile and some other cardiovascular risk factors, decrease microalbuminuria, and reduce neointimal tissue hyperplasia after coronary artery stent placement. These drugs, however, can cause fluid retention and are contraindicated in patients with heart failure. They also very commonly increase weight, which patients find distressing, affecting adherence. The drugs are also contraindicated in patients with active liver disease and in patients with liver enzymes ≥ 2.5 times the upper limit of normal. **Sulfonylureas** have been available for many years and their use in combination with metformin is well established. They do, however, have the propensity of causing hypoglycemia and weight gain. The α-**glucosidase inhibitors** have modest glucose lowering effects and have gastrointestinal side effects. **Exenatide** has a lower risk of hypoglycemia than the sulfonylureas and promotes weight loss. However, it needs to be given by injection, causes nausea, and is contraindicated in patients with gastroparesis. Exenatide is also expensive and lacks long-term safety data.

For most obese patients with mild type 2 diabetes, metformin is the first-line agent. If it proves to be inadequate, then a second agent should be added. In those patients where the problem is hyperglycemia after a carbohydrate rich meal (such as dinner), then a short-acting secretagogue before meals may suffice to get the glucose levels into the target range. Patients with nonalcoholic fatty liver disease or microalbuminuria may be candidates for one of the thiazolidinediones. Subjects who are very concerned about weight gain may benefit from a trial of exenatide. If two agents are inadequate, then a third agent is added, although data regarding efficacy of such combined therapy are limited. Experienced clinicians have found that instead of maximizing the dose of each agent before adding another agent, some patients are more tolerant of submaximal combinations of drugs. Insulin therapy should be instituted if combination of oral agents (and exenatide) fail to restore euglycemia. Weight-reducing interventions should continue and may allow for simplification of this regimen in the future.

When the combination of oral agents (and exenatide) fail to achieve euglycemia in patients with type 2 diabetes, various insulin regimens may be effective. There is no consensus about how insulin therapy should be instituted. One proposed regimen is to continue the oral combination therapy and then simply add a bedtime dose of NPH or long-acting insulin analog (insulin glargine or insulin detemir) to reduce excessive nocturnal hepatic glucose output and improve fasting glucose levels. If the patient does not achieve target glucose levels during the day, then daytime insulin treatment can be initiated. A convenient insulin regimen under these circumstances is a split dose of 70/30 NPH/regular mixture (or Humalog Mix 75/25 or NovoLogMix 70/30) before breakfast and before dinner. If this regimen fails to achieve satisfactory glycemic goals or is associated with unacceptable frequency of hypoglycemic episodes, then a more intensive regimen of multiple insulin injections can be instituted as in patients with type 1 diabetes. Metformin principally reduces hepatic glucose output and the thiazolidinediones improve peripheral insulin resistance, so it is a reasonable option to continue these drugs when insulin therapy is instituted. The sulfonylureas also have been shown to be of continued benefit. Thus, the continued use of the oral drugs may permit the use of lower doses of insulin and simpler regimens. There is no data on the continued administration of exenatide under these circumstances.

b. The nonobese patient with type 2 diabetes— Nonobese patients with type 2 diabetes frequently have increased visceral adiposity—the so-called metabolically obese normal weight patient—and the treatment algorithm is much the same as in the obese patient except there is not as much emphasis on weight loss. However, exercise remains an important aspect of treatment. Persons who do not have central obesity or insulin resistance should be evaluated for other types of diabetes such as latent autoimmune diabetes of adulthood (LADA) or maturity onset diabetes of the young (MODY). Patients with LADA can initially be treated with oral agents but require insulin within a few years, so experienced clinicians often prescribe insulin for these patients when the diagnosis is made.

2. Type 1 diabetes—Traditional once- or twice-daily insulin regimens are usually ineffective in type 1 patients without residual endogenous insulin. In these patients, information and counseling based on the findings of the DCCT (see above) should be provided

Table 27–10. Examples of intensive insulin regimens using rapid-acting insulin analogs (insulin lispro, aspart, or glulisine) and NPH, or insulin glargine in a 70-kg man with type 1 diabetes.[1-3]

	Pre-Breakfast	Pre-Lunch	Pre-Dinner	At Bedtime
Rapid-acting insulin analog	5 units	4 units	6 units	—
NPH insulin	3 units	3 units	2 units	8–9 units
		OR		
Rapid-acting insulin analog	5 units	4 units	6 units	—
Insulin glargine	—	—	—	15–16 units

[1]Assumes that patient is consuming approximately 75 g carbohydrate at breakfast, 60 g at lunch, and 90 g at dinner.
[2]The dose of rapid-acting insulin can be raised by 1 or 2 units if extra carbohydrate (15–30 g) is ingested or if premeal blood glucose is > 170 mg/dL. Rapid-acting insulin can be mixed in the same syringe with NPH insulin.
[3]Insulin glargine (or insulin detemir) cannot be mixed with any of the available insulins and must be given as a separate injection.
NPH = neutral protamine Hagedorn.

about the advantages of taking multiple injections of insulin in conjunction with self-blood glucose monitoring. If near-normalization of blood glucose is attempted, at least three or four measurements of capillary blood glucose and three or four insulin injections are necessary.

A combination of rapid-acting insulin analogs and long-acting insulin analogs allows for more physiologic insulin replacement. The rapid-acting insulin analogs have been advocated as a safer and much more convenient alternative to regular human insulin for preprandial use. In a study comparing regular insulin with insulin lispro, daily insulin doses and hemoglobin A_{1c} levels were similar, but insulin lispro improved postprandial control, reduced hypoglycemic episodes, and improved patient convenience compared with regular insulin. However, because of their relatively short duration (no more than 3–4 hours), the rapid-acting insulin analogs need to be combined with longer-acting insulins to provide basal coverage and avoid hyperglycemia prior to the next meal. In addition to carbohydrate content of the meal, the effect of simultaneous fat ingestion must also be considered a factor in determining the rapid-acting insulin analog dosage required to control the glycemic increment during and just after the meal. With low-carbohydrate content and high-fat intake, there is an increased risk of hypoglycemia from insulin lispro within 2 hours after the meal. Table 27–10 illustrates some regimens that might be appropriate for a 70-kg person with type 1 diabetes eating meals providing standard carbohydrate intake and moderate to low fat content.

Multiple injections of NPH insulin can be mixed in the same syringe as the insulin lispro, insulin aspart, and insulin glulisine. Insulin glargine is usually given once in the evening to provide 24-hour coverage. This insulin *cannot be mixed* with any of the other insulins and must be given as a separate injection. There are occasional patients in whom insulin glargine does not seem to last for

24 hours, and in such cases it needs to be given twice a day. Insulin detemir may also need to be given twice a day to get adequate 24-hour basal coverage.

Continuous subcutaneous insulin infusion (CSII) by portable battery-operated "open loop" devices currently provides the most flexible approach, allowing the setting of different basal rates throughout the 24 hours and permitting patients to delay or skip meals and vary meal size and composition. The dosage is usually based on providing 50% of the estimated insulin dose as basal and the remainder as intermittent boluses prior to meals. For example, a 70-kg man requiring 35 units of insulin per day may require a basal rate of 0.7 units per hour throughout the 24 hours with the exception of 3 AM to 8 AM, when 0.8 units per hour might be appropriate (for the dawn phenomenon). The meal bolus would depend on the carbohydrate content of the meal and the premeal blood glucose value. One unit per 15 g of carbohydrate plus 1 unit for 50 mg/dL of blood glucose above a target value (eg, 120 mg/dL) is a common starting point. Further adjustments to basal and bolus dosages would depend on the results of blood glucose monitoring. The majority of patients use the rapid-acting insulin analogs in the pumps. One of the more difficult therapeutic problems in managing patients with type 1 diabetes is determining the proper adjustment of insulin dose when the prebreakfast blood glucose level is high. Occasionally, the prebreakfast hyperglycemia is due to the Somogyi effect, in which nocturnal hypoglycemia leads to a surge of counterregulatory hormones to produce high blood glucose levels by 7 AM. However, a more common cause for prebreakfast hyperglycemia is the waning of circulating insulin levels by the morning. Also, the "dawn phenomenon"—reduced tissue sensitivity to insulin between 5 AM and 8 AM—is present in as many as 75% of type 1 patients and can aggravate the hyperglycemia.

Table 27–11. Prebreakfast hyperglycemia: Classification by blood glucose and insulin levels.

	Blood Glucose (mg/dL)			Free Immunoreactive Insulin (microunit/mL)		
	10:00 PM	3:00 AM	7:00 AM	10:00 PM	3:00 AM	7:00 AM
Somogyi effect	90	40	200	High	Slightly high	Normal
Dawn phenomenon	110	110	150	Normal	Normal	Normal
Waning of insulin dose plus dawn phenomenon	110	190	220	Normal	Low	Low
Waning of insulin dose plus dawn phenomenon plus Somogyi effect	110	40	380	High	Normal	Low

Table 27–11 shows that diagnosis of the cause of pre-breakfast hyperglycemia can be facilitated by self-monitoring of blood glucose at 3 AM in addition to the usual bedtime and 7 AM measurements. This is required for only a few nights, and when a particular pattern emerges from monitoring blood glucose levels overnight, appropriate therapeutic measures can be taken. The Somogyi effect can be treated by eliminating the dose of intermediate insulin at dinnertime and giving it at a lower dosage at bedtime or by supplying more food at bedtime. When a waning insulin level is the cause, then either increasing the evening dose or shifting it from dinnertime to bedtime (or both) can be effective. A bedtime dose either of insulin glargine or insulin detemir provides more sustained overnight insulin levels than human NPH and may be effective in managing refractory prebreakfast hyperglycemia. If this fails, insulin pump therapy may be required. When the dawn phenomenon alone is present, the dosage of intermediate insulin can be divided between dinnertime and bedtime; when insulin pumps are used, the basal infusion rate can be increased (eg, from 0.8 unit/h to 0.9 unit/h from 6 AM until breakfast).

Acceptable Levels of Glycemic Control

See above for a discussion of the DCCT and the UKPDS and their implications for diabetes therapy. A reasonable aim of therapy is to approach normal glycemic excursions without provoking severe or frequent hypoglycemia. What has been considered "acceptable" control includes blood glucose levels of 90–130 mg/dL before meals and after an overnight fast, and levels no higher than 180 mg/dL 1 hour after meals and 150 mg/dL 2 hours after meals. Glycohemoglobin levels should be no higher than 1% above the upper limit of the normal range for any particular laboratory. It should be emphasized that the value of blood pressure control was as great as or greater than glycemic control in type 2 patients as regards microvascular as well as macrovascular complications.

Complications of Insulin Therapy

A. HYPOGLYCEMIA

Hypoglycemic reactions, the most common complication of insulin therapy, may result from delay in taking a meal or unusual physical exertion. With more type 1 patients attempting "tight" control, this complication has become even more frequent. In older diabetics, in those taking only longer-acting insulins, and often in those attempting to maintain euglycemia on infusion pumps, autonomic counterregulatory responses are less readily elicited during hypoglycemia, and central nervous system dysfunction may occur, ie, mental confusion, bizarre behavior, and ultimately coma. Even focal neurologic deficits mimicking stroke may be observed. More rapid development of hypoglycemia from the effects of regular insulin causes signs of autonomic hyperactivity, both sympathetic (tachycardia, palpitations, sweating, tremulousness) and parasympathetic (nausea, hunger), that may progress to coma and convulsions. Except for sweating, most of the sympathetic symptoms of hypoglycemia are blunted in patients receiving β-blocking agents for angina or hypertension. Though not absolutely contraindicated, these drugs must be used with caution in insulin-requiring diabetics, and β_1-selective blocking agents are preferred.

1. Altered awareness of hypoglycemia—Since autonomic responses correlate strongly with "awareness" of hypoglycemia, many poorly controlled diabetics—whose nervous systems have adapted to chronic hyperglycemia—may trigger adrenergic alarms at levels of blood glucose above the usual hypoglycemic range. Conversely, type 1 patients overtreated with insulin may be unaware of critically low levels of blood glucose because of an adaptive blunting of their alarm systems owing to repeated episodes of hypoglycemia. This has been shown to be reversible if higher average blood glucose levels are maintained in these patients to avoid recurrent hypoglycemia over a period of several weeks.

As evidenced by results of the DCCT, the risk of frequent severe hypoglycemic episodes is greatly increased when "normalization" of the blood glucose is attempted with presently available methods of insulin delivery, and this is independent of the species of insulin used. "Near normalization" is therefore a safer target for therapy to avoid hypoglycemic unawareness.

2. Lack of glucagon response in type 1—For unexplained reasons, patients with type 1 lose their glucagon responses to hypoglycemia (but not to amino acids in protein-containing meals) within a year or so after developing diabetes. These patients then rely predominantly on the sympathetic nervous system to counterregulate hypoglycemia and are at special risk in later years when aging, autonomic neuropathy, or frequent hypoglycemic episodes blunt their sympathetic responses.

3. Prevention and treatment of hypoglycemia— Because of the potential danger of insulin-induced reactions, the diabetic patient should carry packets of table sugar or a candy roll at all times for use at the onset of hypoglycemic symptoms. Tablets containing 3 g of glucose are available (Dextrosol). The educated patient soon learns to take the amount of glucose needed and avoids the excess that may occur with eating candy or drinking orange juice, causing very high hyperglycemia. A glucagon emergency kit (1 mg) should be provided to every diabetic receiving insulin therapy, and family or friends should be instructed how to inject it intramuscularly in the event that the patient is unconscious or refuses food. An identification Medic-Alert bracelet, necklace, or card in the wallet or purse should be carried by every diabetic receiving hypoglycemic drug therapy. The telephone number for the MedicAlert Foundation International in Turlock, California, is 800-ID-ALERT and the Internet address is www.medicalert.org.

All of the manifestations of hypoglycemia are rapidly relieved by glucose administration. If more severe hypoglycemia has produced unconsciousness or stupor, the treatment is 50 mL of 50% glucose solution by rapid intravenous infusion. If intravenous therapy is not available, 1 mg of glucagon injected intramuscularly will usually restore the patient to consciousness within 15 minutes to permit ingestion of sugar. If the patient is stuporous and glucagon is not available, small amounts of honey or syrup or glucose gel (15 g) can be inserted within the buccal pouch, but, in general, oral feeding is contraindicated in unconscious patients. Rectal administration of syrup or honey (30 mL per 500 mL of warm water) has been effective.

B. IMMUNOPATHOLOGY OF INSULIN THERAPY

At least five molecular classes of insulin antibodies are produced during the course of insulin therapy in diabetes, including IgA, IgD, IgE, IgG, and IgM. With the increased therapeutic use of purified pork and especially human insulin, the various immunopathologic syndromes such as insulin allergy, immune insulin resistance, and lipoatrophy have become quite rare since the titers and avidity of these induced antibodies are generally quite low. However, in parts of the world where less purified forms of beef insulin are still used, these disorders remain a clinical concern among some insulin-treated patients.

1. Insulin allergy—Insulin allergy, or immediate-type hypersensitivity, is a rare condition in which local or systemic urticaria is due to histamine release from tissue mast cells sensitized by adherence of anti-insulin IgE antibodies. In severe cases, anaphylaxis results. When only human insulin has been used from the onset of insulin therapy, insulin allergy is exceedingly rare. Antihistamines, corticosteroids, and even desensitization may be required, especially for systemic hypersensitivity. There have been case reports of successful use of insulin lispro in those rare patients who have a generalized allergy to human insulin or insulin resistance due to a high titer of insulin antibodies.

2. Immune insulin resistance—Most insulin-treated patients develop a low titer of circulating IgG anti-insulin antibodies that neutralize to a small extent the action of insulin. With the old animal insulins, a high titer of circulating antibodies sometimes developed, resulting in extremely high insulin requirements—often more than 200 units daily. This is now rarely seen with the switch to highly purified pork or human insulins and has not been reported with the analogs.

C. LIPODYSTROPHY AT INJECTION SITES

Atrophy of subcutaneous fatty tissue leading to disfiguring excavations and depressed areas may rarely occur at the site of injection. This complication results from an immune reaction, and it has become rarer with the development of pure insulin preparations. Injection of these preparations directly into the atrophic area often results in restoration of normal contours. Lipohypertrophy, on the other hand, is a consequence of the pharmacologic effects of insulin being deposited in the same location repeatedly. It can occur with purified insulins and as well. Rotation of injection sites will prevent lipohypertrophy. There is a case report of a patient who had intractable lipohypertrophy with human insulin but no longer had the problem when he switched to insulin lispro.

Chronic Complications of Diabetes

Late clinical manifestations of diabetes mellitus include a number of pathologic changes that involve small and large blood vessels, cranial and peripheral nerves, the skin, and the lens of the eye. These lesions lead to hypertension, renal failure, blindness, autonomic and peripheral neuropathy, amputations of the lower extremities, myocardial infarction, and cerebrovascular accidents. These late manifestations correlate with the duration of the diabetic state subsequent to the onset of puberty. In type 1 diabetes, end-stage renal disease develops in up to 40% of patients, compared with less than 20% of patients with type 2 diabetes. As regards proliferative retinopathy, it ultimately develops in both types of diabetes but has a slightly higher prevalence in type 1 patients (25% after 15 years' duration). In patients with type 1 diabetes, complications from end-stage renal disease are a major cause of death, whereas patients with type 2 diabetes are more likely to have macrovascular diseases leading to myocardial infarction and stroke as the main causes of death. Cigarette use adds significantly to the risk of both microvascular and macrovascular complications in diabetic patients.

A. OCULAR COMPLICATIONS

1. Diabetic cataracts—Premature cataracts occur in diabetic patients and seem to correlate with both the duration of diabetes and the severity of chronic hyperglycemia. Nonenzymatic glycosylation of lens protein is twice as high in diabetic patients as in age-matched nondiabetic persons and may contribute to the premature occurrence of cataracts.

2. Diabetic retinopathy—Three main categories exist: background, or "simple," retinopathy, consisting of microaneurysms, hemorrhages, exudates, and retinal edema; preproliferative retinopathy with arteriolar ischemia manifested as cotton-wool spots (small infarcted areas of retina); and proliferative, or "malignant," retinopathy, consisting of newly formed vessels. Proliferative retinopathy is a leading cause of blindness in the United States, particularly since it increases the risk of retinal detachment. Vision-threatening retinopathy virtually never appears in type 1 patients in the first 3–5 years of diabetes or before puberty. Up to 20% of patients with type 2 diabetes have retinopathy at the time of diagnosis. Annual consultation with an ophthalmologist should be arranged for patients who have had type 1 diabetes for more than 3–5 years and for all patients with type 2 diabetes, because many were probably diabetic for an extensive period of time before diagnosis. Patients with any macular edema, severe nonproliferative retinopathy, or any proliferative retinopathy require the care of an ophthalmologist. Extensive "scatter" xenon or argon photocoagulation and focal treatment of new vessels reduce severe visual loss in those cases in which proliferative retinopathy is associated with recent vitreous hemorrhages or in which extensive new vessels are located on or near the optic disk. Macular edema, which is more common than proliferative retinopathy in patients with type 2 diabetes (up to 20% prevalence), has a guarded prognosis, but it has also responded to scatter therapy with improvement in visual acuity if detected early. Avoiding tobacco use and correction of associated hypertension are important therapeutic measures in the management of diabetic retinopathy. There is no contraindication to using aspirin in patients with proliferative retinopathy.

3. Glaucoma—Glaucoma occurs in approximately 6% of persons with diabetes. It is responsive to the usual therapy for open-angle disease. Neovascularization of the iris in diabetics can predispose to closed-angle glaucoma, but this is relatively uncommon except after cataract extraction, when growth of new vessels has been known to progress rapidly, involving the angle of the iris and obstructing outflow.

B. DIABETIC NEPHROPATHY

As many as 4000 cases of end-stage renal disease occur each year among diabetic people in the United States. This is about one-third of all patients being treated for end-stage renal disease and represents a considerable national health expense.

The cumulative incidence of nephropathy differs between the two major types of diabetes. Patients with type 1 diabetes have a 30–40% chance of having nephropathy after 20 years—in contrast to the much lower frequency in type 2 diabetes patients, in whom only about 15–20% develop clinical renal disease. However, since there are many more individuals affected with type 2 diabetes, end-stage renal disease is much more prevalent in type 2 than in type 1 diabetes in the United States and especially throughout the rest of the world. Improved glycemic control and more effective therapeutic measures to correct hypertension—and with the beneficial effects of ACE inhibitors—can reduce the development of end-stage renal disease among diabetics.

Diabetic nephropathy is initially manifested by proteinuria; subsequently, as kidney function declines, urea and creatinine accumulate in the blood.

1. Microalbuminuria—Sensitive radioimmunoassay methods of detecting small amounts of urinary albumin have permitted detection of microgram concentrations—in contrast to the less sensitive dipstick strips, whose minimal detection limit is 0.3–0.5%. Conventional 24-hour urine collections, in addition to being inconvenient for patients, also show wide variability of albumin excretion, since several factors such as sustained erect posture, dietary protein, and exercise tend to increase albumin excretion rates. For these reasons, a timed overnight urine collection or albumin-creatinine ratio in an early morning spot urine collected upon awakening is preferable. Normal subjects excrete less than 15 mcg/min during overnight urine collections; values of 20 mcg/min or higher are considered to represent abnormal microalbuminuria. In the early morning spot urine, a ratio of albumin (mcg/L) to creatinine (mg/L) of < 30 mcg/mg creatinine is normal, and a ratio of 30–300 mcg/mg creatinine suggests abnormal microalbuminuria. At least two of three timed overnight or early morning spot urine collections over a 3- to 6-month period should be abnormal before a diagnosis of microalbuminuria is justified.

Subsequent renal failure can be predicted by persistent urinary albumin excretion rates exceeding 30 mcg/min. Increased microalbuminuria correlates with increased levels of blood pressure and increased LDL cholesterol, and this may explain why increased proteinuria in diabetic patients is associated with an increase in cardiovascular deaths even in the absence of renal failure. Glycemic control as well as a low-protein diet (0.8 g/kg/d) may reduce both the hyperfiltration and the elevated microalbuminuria in patients in the early stages of diabetes and those with incipient diabetic nephropathy. Antihypertensive therapy also decreases microalbuminuria. Evidence from some studies—but not the UKPDS—supports a specific role for ACE inhibitors in reducing intraglomerular pressure in addition to their lowering of systemic hypertension. An ACE inhibitor (captopril, 50 mg twice daily) in normotensive diabetics impedes progression to proteinuria and prevents the increase in albumin excretion rate. Since microalbuminuria has been shown to correlate with elevated *nocturnal* systolic blood pressure, it is possible that "normotensive" diabetic patients with microalbuminuria have slightly elevated systolic blood pressure during sleep, which is lowered during antihypertensive therapy. This action may contribute to the reported efficacy of ACE inhibitor drugs in reducing microalbuminuria in "normotensive" patients.

2. Progressive diabetic nephropathy—Progressive diabetic nephropathy consists of proteinuria of varying severity occasionally leading to nephrotic syndrome with hypoalbuminemia, edema, and an increase in circulating LDL cholesterol as well as progressive azotemia. In contrast to all other renal disorders, the proteinuria associated with diabetic nephropathy does not diminish with progressive renal failure (patients continue to excrete 10–11 g daily as creatinine clearance diminishes). As renal failure progresses, there is an elevation in the renal threshold at which glycosuria appears.

Hypertension develops with progressive renal involvement, and coronary and cerebral atherosclerosis seems to be accelerated. Approximately two-thirds of adult patients with diabetes have hypertension. Once diabetic nephropathy has progressed to the stage of hypertension, proteinuria, or early renal failure, glycemic control is not beneficial in influencing its course. In this circumstance, antihypertensive medications, including ACE inhibitors, and restriction of dietary protein to 0.8 g/kg body weight per day are recommended. ACE inhibitors have been shown to protect against deterioration in renal function in type 1 diabetic patients with clinical nephropathy. This beneficial effect appears to be due to improved glomerular hemodynamics that cannot be explained only by the antihypertensive action of these drugs. Captopril (25 mg three times daily) has shown a 50% reduction in the risk of the combined end points of death, dialysis, and transplantation in type 1 subjects with diabetic nephropathy and clinical proteinuria. During initiation of ACE inhibitor therapy, an increment in serum creatinine greater than 2 mg/dL due to a rapid fall in intraglomerular pressure—or the occurrence of persistent hyperkalemia (above 6 mEq/L) due to hyporeninemic hypoaldosteronism—is an indication to stop this medication.

Dialysis has been of limited value in the long-term treatment of renal failure due to diabetic nephropathy. At present, experience in renal transplantation—especially from related donors—is more promising and is the treatment of choice in cases where there are no contraindications such as severe cardiovascular disease.

C. DIABETIC NEUROPATHY

Diabetic neuropathies are the most common complications of diabetes affecting up to 50% of older patients with type 2 diabetes.

1. Peripheral neuropathy—

a. Distal symmetric polyneuropathy—This is the most common form of diabetic peripheral neuropathy where loss of function appears in a stocking-glove pattern and is due to an axonal neuropathic process. Longer nerves are especially vulnerable, hence the impact on the foot. Both motor and sensory nerve conduction is delayed in the peripheral nerves, and ankle jerks may be absent.

Sensory involvement usually occurs first and is generally bilateral, symmetric, and associated with dulled perception of vibration, pain, and temperature. The pain can range from mild discomfort to severe incapacitating symptoms (see below). The sensory deficit may eventually be of sufficient degree to prevent patients from feeling pain. Patients who have a sensory neuropathy should therefore be examined with a 5.07 Semmes Weinstein filament and those who cannot feel the filament must be considered at risk for unperceived neuropathic injury.

The denervation of the small muscles of the foot result in clawing of the toes and displacement of the submetatarsal fat pads anteriorly. These changes, together with the joint and connective tissue changes, alter the biomechanics of the foot and increase plantar pressures. This combination of decreased pain threshold, abnormally high foot pressures, and repetitive stress (such as from walking) can lead to calluses and ulcerations in the high-pressure areas such as over the metatarsal heads. Peripheral neuropathy, autonomic neuropathy, and trauma also predisposes to the development of Charcot's arthropathy. An acute case of Charcot's foot arthropathy presents with pain and swelling, and if left untreated, leads to a "rocker bottom" deformity and ulceration. The early radiologic changes show joint subluxation and periarticular fractures. As the process progresses, there is frank osteoclastic destruction leading to deranged and unstable joints particularly in the midfoot. Not surprisingly, the key issue for the healing of neuropathic ulcers in a foot with good vascular supply is mechanical unloading. In addition, any infection should be treated with debridement and appropriate antibiotics; healing duration of 8–10 weeks is typical. Occasionally, when healing appears refractory, platelet-derived growth factor (Regranex) should be considered for local application. Once ulcers are healed, therapeutic footwear is key to preventing recurrences. Custom molded shoes are reserved for patients with significant foot deformities. Other patients with neuropathy may require accommodative insoles that distribute the load over as wide an area as possible. Patients with foot deformities and loss of their protective threshold should get regular care from a podiatrist. Patients should be educated on appropriate footwear and those with loss of their protective threshold should be instructed to inspect their feet daily for reddened areas, blisters, abrasions, or lacerations.

b. Isolated peripheral neuropathy—Involvement of the distribution of only one nerve ("mononeuropathy") or of several nerves ("mononeuropathy multiplex") is characterized by sudden onset with subsequent recovery of all or most of the function. This neuropathology has been attributed to vascular ischemia or traumatic damage. Cranial and femoral nerves are commonly involved, and motor abnormalities predominate. The patient with cranial nerve involvement usually has diplopia and single third, fourth, or sixth nerve weakness on examination but the pupil is spared. A full recovery of function occurs in 6–12 weeks. Diabetic amyotrophy presents with onset of severe pain in the front of the thigh. Within a few days or weeks of the onset of pain, weakness and wasting of the quadriceps develops. As the weakness appears, the pain tends to improve. Management includes analgesia and improved diabetes controls. The symptoms improve over 6–18 months.

c. Painful diabetic neuropathy—Hypersensitivity to light touch and occasionally severe "burning" pain, particularly at night, can become physically and emotionally disabling. Amitriptyline, 25–75 mg at bedtime, has been recommended for pain associated with diabetic neuropathy. Dramatic relief has often resulted within 48–72 hours. This rapid response is in contrast to the 2 or 3 weeks required for an antidepressive effect. Patients often attribute the benefit to having a full night's sleep. Mild to moderate morning drowsiness is a side effect that generally improves with time or can be lessened by giving the medication several hours before bedtime. This drug should not be continued if improvement has not occurred after 5 days of therapy. If amitriptyline's anticholinergic effects are too troublesome, then nortriptyline can be used. Desipramine in doses of 25–150 mg/d seems to have the same efficacy as amitriptyline. Tricyclic antidepressants in combination with the phenothiazine, fluphenazine have been shown in two studies to be efficacious in painful neuropathy, with benefits unrelated to relief of depression. Gabapentin (900–1800 mg/d in three divided doses) has also been shown to be effective in the treatment of painful neuropathy and should be tried if the tricyclic drugs prove ineffective. Pregabalin, a congener of gabapentin, has been shown in an 8-week study to be more effective than placebo in treating painful diabetic peripheral neuropathy. However, this drug was not compared with an active control. Also because of its abuse potential, it has been categorized as a schedule V controlled substance. Duloxetine a serotonin and norepinephrine reuptake inhibitor, has been approved for the treatment of painful diabetic neuropathy. In clinical trials, this drug reduced the pain sensitivity score by 40–50%. Capsaicin, a topical irritant, has been found to be effective in reducing local nerve pain; it is dispensed as a cream (Zostrix 0.025%, Zostrix-HP 0.075%) to be rubbed into the skin over the painful region two to four times daily. Gloves should be used for application since hand contamination could result in discomfort if the cream comes in contact with eyes or sensitive areas such as the genitalia.

Diabetic neuropathic cachexia is a syndrome characterized by a symmetric peripheral neuropathy associated with profound weight loss (up to 60% of total body weight) and painful dysesthesias affecting the proximal lower limbs, the hands, or the lower trunk. Treatment is usually with insulin and analgesics. The prognosis is generally good, and patients typically recover their baseline weight with resolution of the painful sensory symptoms within 1 year.

2. Autonomic neuropathy—With autonomic neuropathy, there is evidence of postural hypotension, decreased cardiovascular response to Valsalva's maneuver, gastroparesis, alternating bouts of diarrhea (particularly nocturnal) and constipation, inability to empty the bladder, and impotence. Gastroparesis should be considered in type 1 diabetic patients in whom unexpected fluctuations and variability in their blood glucose levels develops after meals. Impotence due to neuropathy differs from psychogenic impotence in that the latter may be intermittent (erections occur under special circumstances), whereas diabetic impotence is usually persistent; aortoiliac occlusive disease may contribute to this problem.

a. Management of autonomic neuropathy—There is no consistently effective treatment for diabetic autonomic neuropathy. Metoclopramide has been of some help in treating diabetic gastroparesis over the short term, but its effectiveness seems to diminish over time. It is a dopamine antagonist that has central antiemetic effects as well as a cholinergic action to facilitate gastric emptying. It can be given intravenously (10 mg three or four times a day, 30 minutes before meals and at bedtime) or orally (20 mg of liquid metoclopramide) before breakfast and dinner. Drowsiness, restlessness, fatigue, and lassitude are common adverse effects. Tardive dyskinesia and extrapyramidal effects also occur. Because cisapride has caused life-threatening cardiac arrhythmias, including 80 deaths, it has been withdrawn from the market in the United States. Erythromycin appears to bind to motilin receptors in the stomach and has been found to improve gastric emptying in doses of 250 mg three times daily. Gastric electrical stimulation has been reported to improve symptoms and quality of life indices in patients with gastroparesis refractory to pharmacologic therapy. Diarrhea associated with autonomic neuropathy has occasionally responded to broad-spectrum antibiotic therapy, although it often undergoes spontaneous remission. Refractory diabetic diarrhea is often associated with impaired sphincter control and fecal incontinence. Therapy with loperamide, 4–8 mg daily, or diphenoxylate with atropine, two tablets up to four times a day, may provide relief. In more severe cases, tincture of paregoric or codeine (60-mg tablets) may be required to reduce the frequency of diarrhea and improve the consistency of the stools. Clonidine has been reported to lessen diabetic diarrhea; however, its usefulness is limited by its tendency to lower blood pressure in these patients who already have autonomic neuropathy, resulting in orthostatic hypotension. Constipation usually responds to stimulant laxatives such as senna. Bethanechol in doses of 10–50 mg three times a day has occasionally improved emptying of the atonic urinary bladder. Catheter decompression of the distended bladder has been reported to improve its function, and considerable benefit has been reported after surgical severing of the internal vesicle sphincter. Mineralocorticoid therapy with fludrocortisone, 0.2–0.3 mg/d, and elastic stockings or pressure suits have reportedly been of some help in patients with orthostatic hypotension occurring as a result of loss of postural reflexes.

b. Management of erectile dysfunction—There are medical, mechanical, and surgical treatments available for treatment of erectile dysfunction. Penile erection depends on relaxation of the smooth muscle in the arteries of the corpus cavernosum, and this is mediated by nitric oxide-induced cyclic 3′,5′-guanosine monophosphate (cGMP) formation. cGMP-specific phosphodiesterase type 5 (PDE5) inhibitors impair the breakdown of cGMP and improve the ability to attain and maintain an erection. Sildenafil (Viagra), vardenafil (Levitra), and tadalafil (Cialis) have been shown in placebo-controlled clinical trials to improve erections in response to sexual stimulation. The recommended dose of sildenafil for most patients is one 50-mg tablet taken approximately 1 hour before sexual activity. The peak effect is at 1.5–2 hours, with some effect persisting for 4 hours. Patients with diabetes mellitus using sildenafil reported 50–60% improvement in erectile function. The maximum recommended dose is 100 mg. The recommended doses of both vardenafil and tadalafil is 10 mg. The doses may be increased to 20 mg or decreased to 5 mg based on efficacy and side effects. Tadalafil has been shown to improve erectile function for up to 36 hours after dosing. In clinical trials, only a few adverse effects have been reported—transient mild headache, flushing, dyspepsia, and some altered color vision. Priapism can occur with these drugs and patients should be advised to seek immediate medical attention if an erection persists for longer than 4 hours. The PDE5 inhibitors potentiate the hypotensive effects of nitrates and their use is contraindicated in patients who are concurrently using organic nitrates in any form. Caution is advised for men who have suffered a heart attack, stroke, or life-threatening arrhythmia within the previous 6 months; men who have resting hypotension or hypertension; and men who have a history of cardiac failure or have unstable angina. Rarely, a decrease in vision or permanent visual loss has been reported after PDE5 inhibitor use.

Intracorporeal injection of vasoactive drugs causes penile engorgement and erection. Drugs most commonly used include papaverine alone, papaverine with phentolamine, and alprostadil (prostaglandin E$_1$). Alprostadil injections are relatively painless, but careful instruction is essential to prevent local trauma, priapism, and fibrosis. Intraurethral pellets of alprostadil avoid the problem of injection of the drug.

External vacuum therapy (Erec-Aid System) is a nonsurgical treatment consisting of a suction chamber operated by a hand pump that creates a vacuum around the penis. This draws blood into the penis to produce an erection which is maintained by a specially designed tension ring inserted around the base of the penis and which can be kept in place for up to 20–30 minutes. While this method is generally effective, its cumbersome nature limits its appeal.

In view of the recent development of nonsurgical approaches to therapy of erectile dysfunction, resort to surgical implants of penile prostheses is becoming less common.

D. Cardiovascular Complications

1. Heart disease—Microangiopathy occurs in the heart and may explain the etiology of congestive cardiomyopathies in diabetic patients who do not have demonstrable coronary artery disease. More commonly, however, heart disease in patients with diabetes is due to coronary atherosclerosis. Myocardial infarction is three to five times more common in diabetic patients and is the leading cause of death in patients with type 2 diabetes. Cardiovascular disease risk is increased in patients with type 1 diabetes as well, although the absolute risk is lower than in patients with type 2 diabetes. Premenopausal women who normally have lower rates of coronary artery disease lose this protection once diabetes develops. The increased risk in patients with type 2 diabetes reflects the combination of hyperglycemia, hyperlipidemia, abnormalities of platelet adhesiveness, coagulation factors, hypertension, oxidative stress, and inflammation. Large intervention studies of risk factor reduction in diabetes are lacking, but it is reasonable to assume that reducing these risk factors would have a beneficial effect. Lowering LDL cholesterol reduces first events in patients without known coronary disease and secondary events in patients with known coronary disease. These intervention studies included some patients with diabetes, and the benefits of LDL cholesterol lowering was apparent in this group. The National Cholesterol Education Program clinical practice guidelines have designated diabetes as a coronary risk equivalent and have recommended that patients with diabetes should have an LDL cholesterol goal of < 100 mg/dL.

The ADA also recommends lowering blood pressure to 130/80 mm Hg or less. The Heart Outcomes Prevention Evaluation (HOPE) study randomized 9297 high-risk patients who had evidence of vascular disease or diabetes plus one other cardiovascular risk factor to receive ramipril or placebo for a mean of 5 years. Treatment with ramipril resulted in a 25% reduction of the risk of myocardial infarction, stroke, or death from cardiovascular disease. The mean difference between the placebo and ramipril group was 2.2 mm Hg systolic and 1.4 mm Hg diastolic blood pressure. The reduction in cardiovascular event rate remained significant after adjustment for this small difference in blood pressure. The mechanism underlying this protective effect of ramipril is unknown. Patients with type 2 diabetes who already have cardiovascular disease or microalbuminuria should therefore be considered for treatment with an ACE inhibitor. More clinical studies are needed to address the question of whether patients with type 2 diabetes who do not have cardiovascular disease or microalbuminuria would specifically benefit from ACE inhibitor treatment.

Aspirin at a dose of 81–325 mg daily has been shown to effectively inhibit thromboxane synthesis by platelets and reduce the risk of diabetic atherothrombosis without increasing risks of gastrointestinal hemorrhage. Use of low-dose enteric-coated aspirin is recommended in diabetic adults with evident macrovascular disease or in those with increased cardiovascular risk factors or those older than 30 years. Contraindications for aspirin therapy are patients with aspirin allergy, bleeding tendency, recent gastrointestinal bleeding, or active hepatic disease. The Early Treatment Diabetic Retinopathy Study (ETDRS) showed that aspirin does not influence the course of proliferative retinopathy. There was no statistically significant difference in the severity of vitreous/preretinal hemorrhages or their rate of resolution between the aspirin and placebo groups. Thus, it appears that there is no contraindication to aspirin use to achieve cardiovascular benefit in diabetic patients who have proliferative retinopathy.

2. Peripheral vascular disease—Atherosclerosis is markedly accelerated in the larger arteries. It is often diffuse, with localized enhancement in certain areas of turbulent blood flow, such as at the bifurcation of the aorta or other large vessels. Clinical manifestations of peripheral vascular disease include ischemia of the lower extremities, impotence, and intestinal angina.

The incidence of **gangrene of the feet** in diabetics is 30 times that in age-matched controls. The factors responsible for its development, in addition to peripheral vascular disease, are small vessel disease, peripheral neuropathy with loss of both pain sensation and neurogenic inflammatory responses, and secondary infection. In two-thirds of patients with ischemic gangrene, pedal pulses are not palpable. In the remaining one-third who have palpable pulses, reduced blood flow through these vessels can be demonstrated by plethysmographic or Doppler ultrasound examination. Prevention of foot injury is imperative. Agents that reduce peripheral blood flow such as tobacco and propranolol should be avoided. Control of other risk factors such as hypertension is essential. Cholesterol-lowering agents are useful as adjunctive therapy when early ischemic signs are detected and when dyslipidemia is present. Patients should be advised to seek immediate medical care if a diabetic foot ulcer develops. Improvement in peripheral blood flow with endarterectomy and bypass operations is possible in certain patients.

E. SKIN AND MUCOUS MEMBRANE COMPLICATIONS

Chronic pyogenic infections of the skin may occur, especially in poorly controlled diabetic patients. Erup-

tive xanthomas can result from hypertriglyceridemia, associated with poor glycemic control. An unusual lesion termed **necrobiosis lipoidica diabeticorum** is usually located over the anterior surfaces of the legs or the dorsal surfaces of the ankles. They are oval or irregularly shaped plaques with demarcated borders and a glistening yellow surface and occur in women two to four times more frequently than in men.

"Shin spots" are not uncommon in adult diabetics. They are brownish, rounded, painless atrophic lesions of the skin in the pretibial area. Candidal infection can produce erythema and edema of intertriginous areas below the breasts, in the axillas, and between the fingers. It causes vulvovaginitis in most chronically uncontrolled diabetic women with persistent glucosuria and is a frequent cause of pruritus.

While antifungal creams containing miconazole or clotrimazole offer immediate relief of vulvovaginitis, recurrence is frequent unless glucosuria is reduced.

F. SPECIAL SITUATIONS

1. Insulin replacement during surgery—A prospective trial in surgical ICU patients reported that aggressive treatment of hyperglycemia (blood glucose > 110 mg/dL) reduced mortality and morbidity. Only a small number of persons in this study (204 of 1548) had a diagnosis of diabetes preoperatively, and so it seems that hyperglycemia per se (and not complications of diabetes) was an important cause of postoperative complications. Keeping blood glucose values as close to normal as possible is therefore the goal in the postsurgical patient *in the ICU*. When surgical patients leave the ICU, target glucose values between 100 mg/dL and 200 mg/dL may be appropriate, although this view is based on clinical observations rather than conclusive evidence. The same investigators performed a similar prospective trial in 1200 medical ICU patients and reported that aggressive treatment of hyperglycemia reduced morbidity (decreased acquired renal injury and increased early weaning from mechanical ventilation) but not mortality. Again, as in the surgical ICU study, only a small number of persons (16.9%) had a diagnosis of diabetes at admission. One of the inclusion criteria for the study was that patients would only be enrolled if they were likely to stay in the ICU for 3 days or longer. Some patients stayed in the ICU less than 3 days, and in that subgroup, intensive insulin therapy was associated with *increased* mortality. On the other hand, patients who stayed in the ICU for 3 days or longer had *reduced* mortality (and morbidity). Clearly, further studies are needed to address this observation.

During major surgery and in the immediate recovery period in patients with type 1 diabetes—and in most patients with type 2 diabetes—5% dextrose in physiologic saline containing 20 mEq of potassium chloride should be infused intravenously at a rate of 100–200 mL/h with regular human insulin (25 units/250 mL 0.9% saline) into the intravenous tubing at a rate of 1–3 units/h. The patient's blood glucose should be monitored every hour initially and the rates of insulin or dextrose adjusted to maintain blood glucose values between 80 mg/dL and 110 mg/dL in the ICU and 100–200 mg/dL on the wards.

Type 2 patients facing minor surgical procedures not requiring general anesthesia who have previously been controlled on oral agents or diet alone do not generally require insulin infusions. Glucose-containing solutions should be avoided during surgery in these patients, and blood glucose levels should be monitored every 4 hours. Regular human insulin or one of the rapid-acting insulin analogs should be administered subcutaneously if needed to maintain blood glucose below 200 mg/dL (see Chapter 3).

2. Pregnancy and the diabetic patient—Several features distinguish the management of diabetics during pregnancy from the general therapy of diabetes. These include the following: (1) Oral hypoglycemic agents are contraindicated. (2) Weight reduction is not advised, since fetal nutrition can be adversely affected. (3) Intensive insulin therapy with frequent self-monitoring of blood glucose is generally recommended to improve the likelihood of having healthy normal babies. Every effort should be made, utilizing multiple injections of insulin or a continuous infusion of insulin by pump, to maintain near-normalization of fasting and preprandial blood glucose values while avoiding hypoglycemia. Glycohemoglobin should be maintained in the normal range.

Since many diabetic pregnancies persist beyond the expected term—or because the infants are usually large and hydramnios may be present—it has been suggested that the baby should be delivered early (at 37–38 weeks), especially if glycemic control during pregnancy has been inadequate (eg, glycohemoglobin > 10%). There is a present trend away from elective cesarean section and toward induction of labor. See Chapter 18 for further details.

Prognosis

The DCCT showed that the previously poor prognosis for as many as 40% of patients with type 1 diabetes is markedly improved by optimal care. DCCT participants were generally young and highly motivated and were cared for in academic centers by skilled diabetes educators and endocrinologists who were able to provide more attention and services than are usually available. Improved training of primary care providers may be beneficial.

For type 2 diabetes, the UKPDS documented a reduction in microvascular disease with glycemic control, although this was not apparent in the obese subgroup. Cardiovascular outcomes were not improved by glycemic control, although antihypertensive therapy showed benefit in reducing the number of adverse cardiovascular complications as well as in reducing the occurrence of microvascular disease among hypertensive patients. In patients with visceral obesity, successful management of type 2 diabetes remains a major challenge in the attempt to achieve appropriate control of hyperglycemia,

hypertension, and dyslipidemia. Once safe and effective methods are devised to prevent or manage obesity, the prognosis of type 2 diabetes with its high cardiovascular risks should improve considerably.

In addition to poorly understood genetic factors relating to differences in individual susceptibility to development of long-term complications of hyperglycemia, it is clear that in both types of diabetes, the diabetic patient's intelligence, motivation, and awareness of the potential complications of the disease contribute significantly to the ultimate outcome.

American Association of Diabetes Educators http://www.aadenet.org/

American Diabetes Association http://www.diabetes.org/home

American Dietetic Association http://www.eatright.org

Abraira C et al: Intensive insulin therapy in patients with type 2 diabetes: implications of the Veterans Affairs (VA CSDM) feasibility trial. Am Heart J 1999;138:S360. [PMID: 10539798]

American Diabetes Association Position Statement: Diabetes nephropathy. Diabetes Care 2004;27(Suppl 1):S79. [PMID: 14693434]

American Diabetes Association Position Statement: Preventive foot care in people with diabetes. Diabetes Care 2004;27 (Suppl 1):S63. [PMID: 14693928]

American Diabetes Association: Standards of Medical Care in Diabetes. Diabetes Care 2006;29:476. [PMID: 16482699]

Atkinson MA et al: Type 1 diabetes: new perspectives on disease pathogenesis and treatment. Lancet 2001;358:221. [PMID: 11476858]

DeFronzo RA et al: Effects of exenatide (exendin-4) on glycemic control and weight over 30 weeks in metformin-treated patients with type 2 diabetes. Diabetes Care 2005;28:1092. [PMID: 15855572]

Diabetes Prevention Trial - Type 1 Diabetes Study Group: Effects of insulin in relatives of patients with type 1 diabetes mellitus. N Engl J Med 2002;346:1685. [PMID: 12037147]

Effect of intensive blood-glucose control with metformin on complications in overweight patients with type 2 diabetes (UKPDS 34). UK Prospective Diabetes Study (UKPDS) Group. Lancet 1998;352:854. [PMID: 9742977]

Efficacy of atenolol and captopril in reducing risk of macrovascular and microvascular complications in type 2 diabetes: UKPDS 39. UK Prospective Diabetes Study Group. BMJ 1998;317: 713. [PMID: 9732338]

Frank RN: Diabetic retinopathy. N Engl J Med 2004;350:48. [PMID: 14702427]

Gaede P et al: Multifactorial intervention and cardiovascular disease in patients with type 2 diabetes. N Engl J Med 2003; 348:383. [PMID: 12556541]

Genuth S et al: Expert Committee on the Diagnosis and Classification of Diabetes Mellitus: Follow-up report on the diagnosis of diabetes mellitus. Diabetes Care 2003;26:3160. [PMID: 14578255]

Harris R et al: Screening adults for type 2 diabetes: a review of the evidence for the U.S. Preventive Services Task Force. Ann Intern Med 2003;138:215. [PMID: 12558362]

Hebel G et al: Hypoglycemia: pathophysiology and treatment. Endocrinol Metab Clin North Am 2000;29:725. [PMID: 11149159]

Holst JJ et al: Role of incretin hormones in the regulation of insulin secretion in diabetic and nondiabetic humans. Am J Physiol Endocrinol Metab 2004;287:E199. [PMID: 15271645]

Intensive blood-glucose control with sulphonylureas or insulin compared with conventional treatment and risk of complications in patients with type 2 diabetes (UKPDS 33). UK Prospective Diabetes Study (UKPDS) Group. Lancet 1998;352: 837. [PMID: 9742976]

Juvenile Diabetes Foundation http://www.jdf.org/index.html

Knowler WC et al: Reduction in the incidence of type 2 diabetes with lifestyle intervention or metformin. N Engl J Med 2002;346:393. [PMID: 11832527]

Lipshultz LI et al: Treatment of erectile dysfunction in men with diabetes. JAMA 1999;281:465. [PMID: 9952210]

Ohkubo Y et al: Intensive insulin therapy prevents the progression of diabetic microvascular complications in Japanese patients with non-insulin-dependent diabetes mellitus: a randomized prospective 6-year study. Diabetes Res Clin Pract 1995;28:103. [PMID: 7587918]

Owens DR et al: Insulins today and beyond. Lancet 2001;358: 739. [PMID: 11551598]

Poncelet AN: Diabetic polyneuropathy. Risk factors, patterns of presentation, diagnosis, and treatment. Geriatrics 2003;58: 16. [PMID: 12813869]

Rosenstock J et al: Inhaled insulin improves glycemic control when substituted for or added to oral combination therapy in type 2 diabetes: a randomized, controlled trial. Ann Intern Med 2005;143:549. Summary for patients in: Ann Intern Med 2005;143:I28. [PMID: 16230721]

Screening for type 2 diabetes mellitus in adults: recommendations and rationale. Ann Intern Med 2003;138:212. [PMID: 12558361]

Setter SM et al: Metformin hydrochloride in the treatment of type 2 diabetes mellitus: a clinical review with a focus on dual therapy. Clin Ther 2003;25:2991. [PMID: 14749143]

Shichiri M et al: Long-term results of the Kumamoto Study on optimal diabetes control in type 2 diabetic patients. Diabetes Care 2000;23(Suppl 2):B21. [PMID: 10860187]

Snow V et al: The evidence base for tight blood pressure control in the management of type 2 diabetes mellitus. Ann Intern Med 2003;138:587. [PMID: 12667031]

Stumvoll M et al: Clinical features of insulin resistance and beta cell dysfunction and the relationship to type 2 diabetes. Clin Lab Med 2001;21:31. [PMID: 11211936]

Tight blood pressure control and risk of macrovascular and microvascular complications in type 2 diabetes: UKPDS 38. UK Prospective Diabetes Study Group. BMJ 1998;317: 703. [PMID: 9732337]

Van den Berghe G et al: Intensive insulin therapy in the critically ill patient. N Engl J Med 2001;345:1359. [PMID: 11794168]

Van den Berghe G et al: Intensive insulin therapy in the medical ICU. N Engl J Med 2006;354:449. [PMID: 16452557]

Vijan S et al: Treatment of hypertension in type 2 diabetes mellitus: blood pressure goals, choice of agents, and setting priorities in diabetes care. Ann Intern Med 2003;138:593. [PMID: 12667032]

Yki-Jarvinen H: Thiazolidinediones. N Engl J Med 2004;351: 1106. [PMID:15356308]

Yusuf S et al: Effects of an angiotensin-converting-enzyme inhibitor, ramipril, on cardiovascular events in high-risk patients. The Heart Outcomes Prevention Evaluation Study Investigators. N Engl J Med 2000;342:145. Erratum in: 2000;342:1376. N Engl J Med 2000;342:748. [PMID: 10639539]

Wajchenberg BL: Subcutaneous and visceral adipose tissue: their relation to the metabolic syndrome. Endocr Rev 2000;21: 697. [PMID: 11133069]

Weissberg-Benchell J et al: Insulin pump therapy: a meta-analysis. Diabetes Care 2003;26:1079. [PMID: 12663577]

Zinman B et al: American Diabetes Association: Physical activity/ exercise and diabetes. Diabetes Care 2004;27(Suppl 1):S58. [PMID: 14693927]

■ DIABETIC COMA

Coma may be due to a variety of causes not directly related to diabetes. Certain causes directly related to diabetes require differentiation: (1) Hypoglycemic coma resulting from excessive doses of insulin or oral hypoglycemic agents. (2) Hyperglycemic coma associated with either severe insulin deficiency (diabetic ketoacidosis) or mild to moderate insulin deficiency (hyperglycemic hyperosmolar state). (3) Lactic acidosis associated with diabetes, particularly in diabetics stricken with severe infections or with cardiovascular collapse.

DIABETIC KETOACIDOSIS

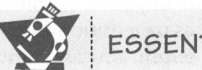 **ESSENTIALS OF DIAGNOSIS**

- *Hyperglycemia > 250 mg/dL.*
- *Acidosis with blood pH < 7.3.*
- *Serum bicarbonate < 15 mEq/L.*
- *Serum positive for ketones.*

General Considerations

Diabetic ketoacidosis may be the initial manifestation of type 1 diabetes or may result from increased insulin requirements in type 1 diabetes patients during the course of infection, trauma, myocardial infarction, or surgery. It is a life-threatening medical emergency with a mortality rate just under 5% in individuals under 40 years of age, but with a more serious prognosis in the elderly, who have mortality rates over 20%. The National Data Group report an annual incidence of five to eight episodes of diabetic ketoacidosis per 1000 diabetic persons. Ketoacidosis may develop in patients with type 2 diabetes when severe stress such as sepsis or trauma is present. Diabetic ketoacidosis has been found to be one of the more common serious complications of insulin pump therapy, occurring in approximately 1 per 80 patient-months of treatment. Many patients who monitor capillary blood glucose regularly ignore urine ketone measurements, which would signal the possibility of insulin leakage or pump failure before serious illness develops. Poor compliance is one of the most common causes of diabetic ketoacidosis, particularly when episodes are recurrent.

Clinical Findings

A. SYMPTOMS AND SIGNS

The appearance of diabetic ketoacidotic coma is usually preceded by a day or more of polyuria and polydipsia associated with marked fatigue, nausea and vomiting, and, finally, mental stupor that can progress to coma. On physical examination, evidence of dehydration in a stuporous patient with rapid deep breathing and a "fruity" breath odor of acetone would strongly suggest the diagnosis. Hypotension with tachycardia indicates profound fluid and electrolyte depletion, and mild hypothermia is usually present. Abdominal pain and even tenderness may be present in the absence of abdominal disease. Conversely, cholecystitis or pancreatitis may occur with minimal symptoms and signs.

B. LABORATORY FINDINGS

(Table 27–12.) Glycosuria of 4+ and strong ketonuria with hyperglycemia, ketonemia, low arterial blood pH, and low plasma bicarbonate are typical of diabetic ketoacidosis. Serum potassium is often elevated despite total body potassium depletion resulting from protracted polyuria or vomiting. Elevation of serum amylase is common but often represents salivary as well as pancreatic amylase. Thus, in this setting, an elevated serum amylase is not specific for acute pancreatitis. Serum lipase may be useful if the diagnosis of acute pancreatitis is being seriously considered. Azotemia may be a better indicator of renal status than serum creatinine, since multichannel chemical analysis of serum creatinine (SMA-6) is falsely elevated by nonspecific chromogenicity of keto acids and glucose. Most laboratories, however, now routinely eliminate this interference. Leukocytosis as high as 25,000/mcL with a left shift may occur with or without associated infection. The presence of an elevated or even a normal temperature would suggest the presence of an infection, since patients with diabetic ketoacidosis are generally hypothermic if uninfected.

Complications

Hyperglycemia and ketoacidemia are due to insulin lack, hyperglucagonemia, and elevated levels of the stress hormones catecholamines, cortisol, and growth hormone.

A. HYPERGLYCEMIA

Hyperglycemia results from increased hepatic production of glucose as well as diminished glucose uptake by peripheral tissues. Hepatic glucose output is a consequence of increased gluconeogenesis resulting from insulinopenia as well as from an associated hyperglucagonemia.

B. KETOACIDEMIA

Ketoacidemia represents the effect of insulin lack at multiple enzyme loci. Insulin lack associated with elevated levels of growth hormone, catecholamines, and glucagon contributes to an increase in lipolysis from adipose tissue and in hepatic ketogenesis. In addition, there is evidence that reduced ketolysis by insulin-deficient peripheral tissues contributes to the ketoacidemia. The only true "keto" acid present is acetoacetic acid, which, along with its by-product acetone, is measured by nitroprusside reagents (Acetest and Ketostix).

The sensitivity for acetone, however, is poor, requiring over 10 mmol, which is seldom reached in the plasma of ketoacidotic subjects—although this detectable concentration is readily achieved in urine. Thus, in the plasma of ketotic patients, only acetoacetate is measured by these reagents. The more prevalent β-hydroxybutyric acid has no ketone group and is therefore not detected by conventional nitroprusside tests. This takes on special importance in the presence of circulatory collapse during diabetic ketoacidosis, wherein an increase in lactic acid can shift the redox state to increase β-hydroxybutyric acid at the expense of the readily detectable acetoacetic acid. Bedside diagnostic reagents would then be unreliable, suggesting no ketonemia in cases where β-hydroxybutyric acid is a major factor in producing the acidosis. A combined glucose and ketone meter (Precision, Medisense) that is able to measure blood β-hydroxyubtyrate concentration on capillary blood is available.

C. FLUID AND ELECTROLYTE DEPLETION

Hyperglycemia results in an osmotic diuresis and dehydration and secondary loss of electrolytes. Ketonuria similarly causes loss of water and electrolytes. Balance studies during withdrawal of insulin and treatment in patients with type 1 diabetes show that on average the water depletion is about 5 L; sodium, 300–500 mmol; potassium, 270–400 mmol; chloride, 100–400 mmol.

Drowsiness is fairly common but frank coma only occurs in about 10% of patients. There is a correlation between the degree of depression of the sensorium and extracellular osmolarity. When serum hyperosmolality exceeds 320–330 mosm/L, central nervous system depression or coma may ensue. Coma in a diabetic patient with a lower osmolality should prompt a search for cause of coma other than hyperosmolality.

Treatment

A. PREVENTION

Education of diabetic patients to recognize the early symptoms and signs of ketoacidosis has done a great deal to prevent severe acidosis. Urine ketones should be measured in patients with signs of infection or in insulin pump-treated patients when capillary blood glucose is unexpectedly and persistently high. When heavy ketonuria and glycosuria persist on several successive examinations, supplemental regular insulin should be administered and liquid foods such as lightly salted tomato juice and broth should be ingested to replenish fluids and electrolytes. The patient should be instructed to contact the physician if ketonuria persists, and especially if vomiting develops or if appropriate adjustment of the infusion rate on an insulin pump does not correct the hyperglycemia and ketonuria. In juvenile-onset diabetics, particularly in the teen years, recurrent episodes of severe ketoacidosis often indicate poor compliance with the insulin regimen, and these patients will require intensive family counseling.

B. EMERGENCY MEASURES

If ketosis is severe, the patient should be placed in the hospital for correction of the hyperosmolality as well as the ketoacidemia. An ICU or, at the least, a step-down unit is preferable for more severe cases.

1. Therapeutic flow sheet—One of the most important steps in initiating therapy is to start a flow sheet listing vital signs and the time sequence of diagnostic laboratory values in relation to therapeutic maneuvers. Indices of the metabolic defects include urine glucose and ketones as well as arterial pH, plasma glucose, acetone, bicarbonate, serum urea nitrogen, and electrolytes. Serum osmolality should be measured or estimated and tabulated during the course of therapy.

A convenient method of estimating effective serum osmolality is as follows (normal values in humans are 280–300 mosm/kg):

$$mosm/kg = 2[Na^+] + \frac{Glucose \ (mg/dL)}{18}$$

These calculated estimates are usually 10–20 mosm/kg lower than values measured by standard cryoscopic techniques in patients with diabetic coma. Urea is freely permeable across cell membranes and therefore not included in calculations of effective serum osmolality. One physician should be responsible for maintaining this therapeutic flow sheet and prescribing therapy. An indwelling urinary catheter is required in all comatose patients but should be avoided if possible in a fully cooperative diabetic because of the risk of introducing bladder infection. Fluid intake and output should be recorded. Gastric intubation is recommended in the comatose patient to correct the commonly associated gastric dilatation that may lead to vomiting and aspiration. The patient should not receive sedatives or narcotics.

2. Insulin replacement—Only regular insulin should be used initially in all cases of severe ketoacidosis, and it should be given immediately after the diagnosis is established. Regular insulin can be given in a loading dose of 0.15 unit/kg as an intravenous bolus to prime the tissue insulin receptors. Following the initial bolus, doses of insulin as low as 0.1 unit/kg/h are continuously infused or given hourly as an intramuscular injection; this is sufficient to replace the insulin deficit in most patients. Replacement of insulin deficiency helps correct the acidosis by reducing the flux of fatty acids to the liver, reducing ketone production by the liver, and also improving removal of ketones from the blood. Insulin treatment reduces the hyperosmolality by reducing the hyperglycemia. It accomplishes this by increasing removal of glucose through peripheral utilization as well as by decreasing production of glucose by the liver. This latter effect is accomplished by direct inhibition of gluconeogenesis and glycogenolysis, as well as by lowered amino acid flux from muscle to liver and reduced hyperglucagonemia.

The insulin dose should be "piggy-backed" into the fluid line so the rate of fluid replacement can be changed without altering the insulin delivery rate. If the plasma glucose level fails to fall at least 10% in the first hour, a repeat loading dose is recommended. The availability of bedside glucometers and of laboratory instruments for rapid and accurate glucose analysis (Beckman or Yellow Springs glucose analyzer) has contributed much to achieving optimal insulin replacement. Rarely, a patient with immune insulin resistance is encountered, and this requires doubling the insulin dose every 2–4 hours if hyperglycemia does not improve after the first two doses of insulin.

3. Fluid replacement—In most patients, the fluid deficit is 4–5 L. Initially, 0.9% saline solution is the solution of choice to help reexpand the contracted vascular volume and should be started in the emergency department as soon as the diagnosis is established. The saline should be infused rapidly to provide 1 L/h over the first 1–2 hours. After the first 2 L of fluid have been given, the intravenous infusion should be at the rate of 300–400 mL/h. Use 0.9 % ("normal") saline unless the serum sodium is greater than 150 mEq/L, when 0.45% ("half normal") saline solution should be used. The volume status should be very carefully monitored. Failure to give enough volume replacement (at least 3–4 L in 8 hours) to restore normal perfusion is one of the most serious therapeutic shortcomings adversely influencing satisfactory recovery. Excessive fluid replacement (more than 5 L in 8 hours) may contribute to acute respiratory distress syndrome or cerebral edema. When blood glucose falls to approximately 250 mg/dL, the fluids should be changed to a 5% glucose solution to maintain serum glucose in the range of 250–300 mg/dL. This will prevent the development of hypoglycemia and will also reduce the likelihood of cerebral edema, which could result from too rapid decline of blood glucose. Intensive insulin therapy should be continued until the ketoacidosis is corrected.

4. Sodium bicarbonate—The use of sodium bicarbonate in management of diabetic ketoacidosis has been questioned since clinical benefit was not demonstrated in one prospective randomized trial and because of the following potentially harmful consequences: (1) development of hypokalemia from rapid shift of potassium into cells if the acidosis is overcorrected, (2) tissue anoxia from reduced dissociation of oxygen from hemoglobin when acidosis is rapidly reversed (leftward shift of the oxygen dissociation curve), and (3) cerebral acidosis resulting from lowering of cerebrospinal fluid pH. It must be emphasized, however, that these considerations are less important when severe acidosis exists. It is therefore recommended that bicarbonate be administered to diabetic patients in ketoacidosis if the arterial blood pH is 7.0 or less, with careful monitoring to prevent overcorrection. One or two ampules of sodium bicarbonate (one ampule contains 44 mEq/50 mL) should be added to 1 L of 0.45% saline. (**Note:** Addition of sodium bicarbonate to 0.9% saline would produce a markedly hypertonic solution that could aggravate the hyperosmolar state already present.) This should be administered rapidly (over the first hour). It can be repeated until the arterial pH reaches 7.1, but *it should not be given if the pH is 7.1 or greater* since additional bicarbonate would increase the risk of rebound metabolic alkalosis as ketones are metabolized. Alkalosis shifts potassium from serum into cells, which could precipitate a fatal cardiac arrhythmia.

5. Potassium—Total body potassium loss from polyuria and vomiting may be as high as 200 mEq. However, because of shifts of potassium from cells into the extracellular space as a consequence of acidosis, serum potassium is usually normal to slightly elevated prior to institution of treatment. As the acidosis is corrected, potassium flows back into the cells, and hypokalemia can develop if potassium replacement is not instituted. If the patient is not uremic and has an adequate urinary output, potassium chloride in doses of 10–30 mEq/h should be infused during the second and third hours after beginning therapy as soon as the acidosis starts to resolve. Replacement should be started sooner if the initial serum potassium is inappropriately normal or low and should be delayed if serum potassium fails to respond to initial therapy and remains above 5 mEq/L, as in cases of renal insufficiency. An ECG can be of help in monitoring the patient's potassium status: High peaked T waves are a sign of hyperkalemia, and flattened T waves with U waves are a sign of hypokalemia. Foods high in potassium content should be prescribed when the patient has recovered sufficiently to take food orally. Tomato juice has 14 mEq of potassium per 240 mL, and a medium-sized banana provides about 10 mEq.

6. Phosphate—Phosphate replacement is seldom required in treating diabetic ketoacidosis. However, if severe hypophosphatemia of less than 1 mg/dL (< 0.32 mmol/L) develops during insulin therapy, a small amount of phosphate can be replaced per hour as the potassium salt. Correction of hypophosphatemia helps restore the buffering capacity of the plasma, thereby facilitating renal excretion of hydrogen. It also corrects the impaired oxygen dissociation from hemoglobin by regenerating 2,3-diphosphoglycerate. However, three randomized studies in which phosphate was replaced in only half of a group of patients with diabetic ketoacidosis did not show any apparent clinical benefit from phosphate administration. Moreover, attempts to use the phosphate salt of potassium as the sole means of replacing potassium have led to a number of reported cases of severe hypocalcemia with tetany. To minimize the risk of inducing tetany from too-rapid replacement of phosphate, the average deficit of 40–50 mmol of phosphate should be replaced intravenously at a rate *no greater than 3–4 mmol/h* in a 60–70-kg person. A stock solution (Abbott) provides a mixture of 1.12 g KH_2PO_4 and 1.18 g K_2HPO_4 in a 5-mL single-dose vial (this equals 22 mmol of potas-

sium and 15 mmol of phosphate). One-half of this vial (2.5 mL) should be added to 1 L of either 0.45% saline or 5% dextrose in water. Two liters of this solution, infused at a rate of 400 mL/h, will correct the phosphate deficit at the optimal rate of 3 mmol/h while providing 4.4 mEq of potassium per hour. (Additional potassium should be administered as potassium chloride to provide a total of 10–30 mEq of potassium per hour, as noted above.) If the serum phosphate remains below 2.5 mg/dL after this infusion, a repeat 5-hour infusion can be given.

7. Hyperchloremic acidosis during therapy—Because of the considerable loss of keto acids in the urine during the initial phase of therapy, substrate for subsequent regeneration of bicarbonate is lost and correction of the total bicarbonate deficit is hampered. A portion of the bicarbonate deficit is replaced with chloride ions infused in large amounts as saline to correct the dehydration. In most patients, as the ketoacidosis clears during insulin replacement, a hyperchloremic, low-bicarbonate pattern emerges with a normal anion gap. This is a relatively benign condition that reverses itself over the subsequent 12–24 hours once intravenous saline is no longer being administered.

8. Treatment of associated infection—Antibiotics are prescribed as indicated. Cholecystitis and pyelonephritis may be particularly severe in these patients.

Prognosis

The frequency of deaths due to diabetic ketoacidosis has been dramatically reduced by improved therapy of young diabetics, but this complication remains a significant risk in the aged and in patients in profound coma in whom treatment has been delayed. Acute myocardial infarction and infarction of the bowel following prolonged hypotension worsen the outlook. A serious prognostic sign is renal failure, and prior kidney dysfunction worsens the prognosis considerably because the kidney plays a key role in compensating for massive pH and electrolyte abnormalities. Cerebral edema has been reported to occur rarely as metabolic deficits return to normal. This is best prevented by avoiding sudden reversal of marked hyperglycemia. Maintaining glycemic levels of 200–300 mg/dL for the initial 24 hours after correction of severe hyperglycemia reduces this risk.

Kitabchi AE et al: Management of hyperglycemic crises in patients with diabetes. Diabetes Care 2001;24:131. [PMID: 11194218]

HYPERGLYCEMIC HYPEROSMOLAR STATE

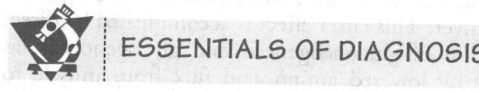

ESSENTIALS OF DIAGNOSIS

• *Hyperglycemia > 600 mg/dL.*

- *Serum osmolality > 310 mosm/kg.*
- *No acidosis; blood pH above 7.3.*
- *Serum bicarbonate > 15 mEq/L.*
- *Normal anion gap (< 14 mEq/L).*

General Considerations

This second most common form of hyperglycemic coma is characterized by severe hyperglycemia in the absence of significant ketosis, with hyperosmolality and dehydration. It occurs in patients with mild or occult diabetes, and most patients are at least middle-aged to elderly. Accurate figures are not available as to its true incidence, but from data on hospital discharges it is rarer than diabetic ketoacidosis even in older age groups. Lethargy and confusion develop as serum osmolality exceeds 310 mosm/kg, and coma can occur if osmolality exceeds 320–330 mosm/kg. A committee of the ADA has recommended replacing the previous name of this disorder (hyperglycemic, hyperosmolar, nonketotic coma) with the consensus term "hyperglycemic hyperosmolar state." Underlying renal insufficiency or congestive heart failure is common, and the presence of either worsens the prognosis. A precipitating event such as infection, myocardial infarction, stroke, or recent operation is often present. Certain drugs such as phenytoin, diazoxide, corticosteroids, and diuretics have been implicated in its pathogenesis, as have procedures associated with glucose loading such as peritoneal dialysis.

Pathogenesis

A partial or relative insulin deficiency may initiate the syndrome by reducing glucose utilization of muscle, fat, and liver while inducing hyperglucagonemia and increasing hepatic glucose output. With massive glycosuria, obligatory water loss ensues. If a patient is unable to maintain adequate fluid intake because of an associated acute or chronic illness or has suffered excessive fluid loss, marked dehydration results. As plasma volume contracts, renal insufficiency develops, and the resultant limitation of renal glucose loss leads to increasingly higher blood glucose concentrations. Severe hyperosmolality develops that causes mental confusion and finally coma. It is not clear why ketosis is virtually absent under these conditions of insulin insufficiency, although reduced levels of growth hormone may be a factor, along with portal vein insulin concentrations sufficient to restrain ketogenesis.

Clinical Findings

A. SYMPTOMS AND SIGNS

Onset may be insidious over a period of days or weeks, with weakness, polyuria, and polydipsia. The lack of features of ketoacidosis may retard recognition of the syndrome and delay therapy until dehydration becomes more profound than in ketoacidosis. Reduced intake of fluid is not an uncommon historical feature, due to either inappropriate lack of thirst, nausea, or inaccessibility of fluids to elderly, bedridden patients. Lethargy and confusion develop, progressing to convulsions and deep coma. Physical examination confirms the presence of profound dehydration in a lethargic or comatose patient without Kussmaul respirations.

B. LABORATORY FINDINGS

(Table 27–12.) Severe hyperglycemia is present, with blood glucose values ranging from 600 mg/dL to 2400 mg/dL. In mild cases, where dehydration is less severe, dilutional hyponatremia as well as urinary sodium losses may reduce serum sodium to 120–125 mEq/L, which

Table 27–12. Laboratory diagnosis of coma in diabetic patients.

	Urine		Plasma		
	Glucose	Acetone	Glucose	Bicarbonate	Acetone
Related to diabetes					
Hypoglycemia	0[1]	0 or +	Low	Normal	0
Diabetic ketoacidosis	++++	++++	High	Low	++++
Nonketotic hyperglycemic coma	++++	0	High	Normal or slightly low	0
Lactic acidosis	0 or +	0 or +	Normal or low or high	Low	0 or +
Unrelated to diabetes					
Alcohol or other toxic drugs	0 or +	0 or +	May be low	Normal or low[2]	0 or +
Cerebrovascular accident or head trauma	+ or 0	0	Often high	Normal	0
Uremia	0 or +	0	High or normal	Low	0 or +

[1]Leftover urine in bladder might still contain glucose from earlier hyperglycemia.
[2]Alcohol can elevate plasma lactate as well as keto acids to reduce pH.

protects to some extent against extreme hyperosmolality. However, as dehydration progresses, serum sodium can exceed 140 mEq/L, producing serum osmolality readings of 330–440 mosm/kg. Ketosis and acidosis are usually absent or mild. Prerenal azotemia is the rule, with serum urea nitrogen elevations over 100 mg/dL being typical.

Treatment

A. SALINE

Fluid replacement is of paramount importance in treating nonketotic hyperglycemic coma. The onset of hyperosmolarity is more insidious in elderly people without ketosis than in younger individuals with high serum ketone levels, which provide earlier indicators of severe illness (vomiting, rapid deep breathing, acetone odor, etc). Consequently, diagnosis and treatment are often delayed until fluid deficit has reached levels of 6–10 L.

If hypovolemia is present as evidenced by hypotension and oliguria, fluid therapy should be initiated with 0.9% saline. In all other cases, 0.45% saline appears to be preferable as the initial replacement solution because the body fluids of these patients are markedly hyperosmolar. As much as 4–6 L of fluid may be required in the first 8–10 hours. Careful monitoring of the patient is required for proper sodium and water replacement. Once blood glucose reaches 250 mg/dL, fluid replacement should include 5% dextrose in either water, 0.45% saline solution, or 0.9% saline solution. The rate of dextrose infusion should be adjusted to maintain glycemic levels of 250–300 mg/dL in order to reduce the risk of cerebral edema. An important end point of fluid therapy is to restore urinary output to 50 mL/h or more.

B. INSULIN

Less insulin may be required to reduce the hyperglycemia in nonketotic patients as compared to those with diabetic ketoacidotic coma. In fact, fluid replacement alone can reduce hyperglycemia considerably by correcting the hypovolemia, which then increases both glomerular filtration and renal excretion of glucose. An initial dose of 0.15 unit/kg is followed by an insulin infusion of 1–2 units/h, which is titrated to lower blood glucose levels by 50–70 mg/dL per hour.

C. POTASSIUM

With the absence of acidosis, there may be no initial hyperkalemia unless associated renal failure is present. This results in less severe total potassium depletion than in diabetic ketoacidosis, and less potassium replacement is therefore needed. However, because initial serum potassium is usually not elevated and because it declines rapidly as a result of insulin's effect on driving potassium intracellularly, it has been recommended that potassium replacement be initiated earlier than in ketotic patients, assuming that no renal in-

sufficiency or oliguria is present. Potassium chloride (10 mEq/L) can be added to the initial bottle of fluids administered if the patient's serum potassium is not elevated.

D. PHOSPHATE

If severe hypophosphatemia (serum phosphate < 1 mg/dL [< 0.32 mmol/L]) develops during insulin therapy, phosphate replacement can be given as described for ketoacidotic patients (at 3 mmol/h).

Prognosis

The overall mortality rate of hyperglycemic, hyperosmolar, nonketotic coma is more than ten times that of diabetic ketoacidosis, chiefly because of its higher incidence in older patients, who may have compromised cardiovascular systems or associated major illnesses and whose dehydration is often excessive because of delays in recognition and treatment. (When patients are matched for age, the prognoses of these two hyperglycemic emergencies are reasonably comparable.) When prompt therapy is instituted, the mortality rate can be reduced from nearly 50% to that related to the severity of coexistent disorders.

Hyperglycemic crises in patients with diabetes mellitus. Diabetes Care 2001;24:154. [PMID: 11221603]

Trence DL et al: Hyperglycemic crisis in diabetes mellitus type 2. Endocrinol Metab Clin North Am 2001;30:817. [PMID: 11727401]

LACTIC ACIDOSIS

 ESSENTIALS OF DIAGNOSIS

- Severe acidosis with hyperventilation.
- Blood pH below 7.30.
- Serum bicarbonate < 15 mEq/L.
- Anion gap > 15 mEq/L.
- Absent serum ketones.
- Serum lactate > 5 mmol/L.

General Considerations

Lactic acidosis is characterized by accumulation of excess lactic acid in the blood. Normally, the principal sources of this acid are the erythrocytes (which lack enzymes for aerobic oxidation), skeletal muscle, skin, and brain. Conversion of lactic acid to glucose and its oxidation principally by the liver but also by the kidneys represent the chief pathways for its removal. Overproduction of lactic acid (tissue hypoxia), deficient removal (hepatic failure), or both (circulatory collapse) can cause accumulation. Lactic acidosis is not uncommon in any severely ill patient suffering from cardiac decompensation, respiratory or hepatic failure, septicemia, or infarction of bowel or extremities. With the discontinuance of phenformin therapy in the United States, lactic acidosis in patients with diabetes mellitus has become uncommon but occasionally occurs in metformin-treated patients (see above) and it still must be considered in the acidotic diabetic, especially if the patient is seriously ill.

Clinical Findings

A. Symptoms and Signs

The main clinical feature of lactic acidosis is marked hyperventilation. When lactic acidosis is secondary to tissue hypoxia or vascular collapse, the clinical presentation is variable, being that of the prevailing catastrophic illness. However, in the idiopathic, or spontaneous, variety, the onset is rapid (usually over a few hours), blood pressure is normal, peripheral circulation is good, and there is no cyanosis.

B. Laboratory Findings

Plasma bicarbonate and blood pH are quite low, indicating the presence of severe metabolic acidosis. Ketones are usually absent from plasma and urine or at least not prominent. The first clue may be a high anion gap (serum sodium minus the sum of chloride and bicarbonate anions [in mEq/L] should be no greater than 15). A higher value indicates the existence of an abnormal compartment of anions. If this cannot be clinically explained by an excess of keto acids (diabetes), inorganic acids (uremia), or anions from drug overdosage (salicylates, methyl alcohol, ethylene glycol), then lactic acidosis is probably the correct diagnosis. (See Chapter 21 also.) In the absence of azotemia, hyperphosphatemia may be a clue to the presence of lactic acidosis for reasons that are not clear. The diagnosis is confirmed by demonstrating, in a sample of blood that is promptly chilled and separated, a plasma lactic acid concentration of 5 mmol/L or higher (values as high as 30 mmol/L have been reported). Normal plasma values average 1 mmol/L, with a normal lactate/pyruvate ratio of 10:1. This ratio is greatly exceeded in lactic acidosis.[1]

Treatment

Aggressive treatment of the precipitating cause of lactic acidosis is the main component of therapy, such as ensuring adequate oxygenation and vascular perfusion of tissues. Empiric antibiotic coverage for sepsis should be given after culture samples are obtained in any patient in whom the cause of the lactic acidosis is not apparent.

Alkalinization with intravenous sodium bicarbonate to keep the pH above 7.2 has been recommended by some in the emergency treatment of lactic acidosis; as much as 2000 mEq in 24 hours has been used. However, there is no evidence that the mortality rate is favorably affected by administering bicarbonate, and its use remains controversial. Hemodialysis may be useful in cases where large sodium loads are poorly tolerated.

Prognosis

The mortality rate of spontaneous lactic acidosis is high. The prognosis in most cases is that of the primary disorder that produced the lactic acidosis.

Forsythe SM et al: Sodium bicarbonate for the treatment of lactic acidosis. Chest 2000;117:260. [PMID: 10631227]

Salpeter S et al: Risk of fatal and nonfatal lactic acidosis with metformin use in type 2 diabetes mellitus. Cochrane Database Syst Rev 2003:CD002967. [PMID: 12804446]

■ THE HYPOGLYCEMIC STATES

Spontaneous hypoglycemia in adults is of two principal types: fasting and postprandial. Symptoms begin at plasma glucose levels in the range of 60 mg/dL and impairment of brain function at approximately 50 mg/dL. Fasting hypoglycemia is often subacute or chronic and usually presents with neuroglycopenia as its principal manifestation; postprandial hypoglycemia is relatively acute and is often heralded by symptoms of neurogenic autonomic discharge (sweating, palpitations, anxiety, tremulousness).

Differential Diagnosis (Table 27–13)

Fasting **hypoglycemia** may occur in certain endocrine disorders, such as hypopituitarism, Addison's disease, or myxedema; in disorders related to liver malfunction, such as acute alcoholism or liver failure; and in instances of renal failure, particularly in patients requiring dialysis. These conditions are usually obvious, with hypoglycemia being only a secondary feature. When fasting hypoglycemia is a primary manifestation developing in adults without apparent endocrine disorders or inborn metabolic diseases from childhood, the principal diagnostic possibilities include (1) hyperinsulinism, due to either pancreatic B cell tumors or islet hyperplasia or surreptitious administration of insulin (or sulfonylureas), and (2) hypoglycemia due to non–insulin-producing extrapancreatic tumors.

Postprandial (reactive) hypoglycemia may be classified as early (within 2–3 hours after a meal) or late (3–5 hours after eating). Early, or alimentary, hypoglycemia occurs when there is a rapid discharge of ingested carbohydrate into the small bowel followed

---

[1]In collecting samples, it is essential to rapidly chill and separate the blood in order to remove red cells, whose continued glycolysis at room temperature is a common source of error in reports of high plasma lactate. Frozen plasma remains stable for subsequent assay.

Table 27–13. Common causes of hypoglycemia in adults.[1]

Fasting hypoglycemia
  Hyperinsulinism
    Pancreatic B cell tumor
    Surreptitious administration of insulin or sulfonylureas
  Extrapancreatic tumors
Postprandial (reactive) hypoglycemia
  Early hypoglycemia (alimentary)
Postgastrectomy
Functional (increased vagal tone)
  Late hypoglycemia (occult diabetes)
Delayed insulin release due to B cell dysfunction
  Counterregulatory deficiency
  Idiopathic
Alcohol-related hypoglycemia
Immunopathologic hypoglycemia
  Idiopathic anti-insulin antibodies (which release their
    bound insulin)
  Antibodies to insulin receptors (which act as agonists)
Drug -induced hypoglycemia

[1]In the absence of clinically obvious endocrine, renal, or hepatic disorders and exclusive of diabetes treated with hypoglycemic agents.

by rapid glucose absorption and hyperinsulinism. It may be seen after gastrointestinal surgery and is particularly associated with the dumping syndrome after gastrectomy. In some cases, it is functional and may represent overactivity of the parasympathetic nervous system mediated via the vagus nerve. Rarely, it results from defective counterregulatory responses such as deficiencies of growth hormone, glucagon, cortisol, or autonomic responses.

Alcohol-related hypoglycemia is due to hepatic glycogen depletion combined with alcohol-mediated inhibition of gluconeogenesis. It is most common in malnourished alcohol abusers but can occur in anyone who is unable to ingest food after an acute alcoholic episode followed by gastritis and vomiting.

Immunopathologic hypoglycemia is an extremely rare condition in which anti-insulin antibodies or antibodies to insulin receptors develop spontaneously. In the former case, the mechanism appears to relate to increasing dissociation of insulin from circulating pools of bound insulin. When antibodies to insulin receptors are found, most patients do not have hypoglycemia but rather severe insulin-resistant diabetes and acanthosis nigricans. However, during the course of the disease in these patients, certain anti-insulin receptor antibodies with agonist activity mimicking insulin action may develop, producing severe hypoglycemia.

Factitious hypoglycemia is self-induced hypoglycemia due to surreptitious administration of insulin or sulfonylureas.

HYPOGLYCEMIA DUE TO PANCREATIC B CELL TUMORS

 ESSENTIALS OF DIAGNOSIS

- *Hypoglycemic symptoms—frequently neuroglycopenic (confusion, blurred vision, diplopia, anxiety, convulsions).*
- *Immediate recovery upon administration of glucose.*
- *Blood glucose < 40 mg/dL with a serum insulin level of 6 microunit/mL or more.*

General Considerations

Fasting hypoglycemia in an otherwise healthy, well-nourished adult is rare and is most commonly due to an adenoma of the islets of Langerhans. Ninety percent of such tumors are single and benign, but multiple adenomas can occur as well as malignant tumors with functional metastases. Adenomas may be familial, and multiple adenomas have been found in conjunction with tumors of the parathyroids and pituitary (multiple endocrine neoplasia type 1 [MEN 1]).

Clinical Findings

A. SYMPTOMS AND SIGNS

The most important prerequisite to diagnosing an insulinoma is simply to consider it, particularly in relatively healthy-appearing persons who have fasting hypoglycemia associated with some degree of central nervous system dysfunction such as confusion or abnormal behavior. A delay in diagnosis can result in unnecessary treatment for psychomotor epilepsy or psychiatric disorders and may cause irreversible brain damage. In longstanding cases, obesity can result as a consequence of overeating to relieve symptoms.

Whipple's triad is characteristic of hypoglycemia regardless of the cause. It consists of (1) a history of hypoglycemic symptoms, (2) an associated fasting blood glucose of 40 mg/dL or less, and (3) immediate recovery upon administration of glucose. The hypoglycemic symptoms in insulinoma often develop in the early morning or after missing a meal. Occasionally, they occur after exercise. They typically begin with evidence of central nervous system glucose lack and can include blurred vision or diplopia, headache, feelings of detachment, slurred speech, and weakness. Personality and mental changes vary from anxiety to psychotic behavior, and neurologic deterioration can result in convulsions or coma. Sweating and palpitations may not occur.

Hypoglycemic unawareness is very common in patients with insulinoma. They adapt to chronic hypoglycemia by increasing their efficiency in transporting glucose across the blood-brain barrier, which masks awareness that their blood glucose is approaching critically low levels. Counterregulatory hormonal responses as well as neurogenic symptoms such as tremor, sweating, and palpitations are therefore blunted during hypoglycemia. If lack of these warning symptoms prevents recognition of the need to eat to correct the problem, patients can lapse into severe hypoglycemic coma. However, symptoms and normal hormone responses during experimental insulin-induced hypoglycemia have been shown to be restored after successful surgical removal of the insulinoma. Presumably with return of euglycemia, adaptive effects on glucose transport into the brain are corrected, and thresholds of counterregulatory responses and neurogenic autonomic symptoms are therefore restored to normal.

B. Laboratory Findings

B cell adenomas do not reduce secretion in the presence of hypoglycemia, and the critical diagnostic test is to demonstrate inappropriately elevated serum insulin levels at a time when hypoglycemia is present. A reliable serum insulin level (radioimmunoassay) of 6 microunit/mL or more in the presence of blood glucose values below 40 mg/dL is diagnostic of inappropriate hyperinsulinism. Immunochemiluminometric assays (ICMA) have sensitivities of less than 1 microunit/mL, and with these assays, the cutoffs for insulinomas is insulin level 3 microunit/mL or higher. Other causes of hyperinsulinemic hypoglycemia must be considered, including factitious administration of insulin or sulfonylureas. Factitious use of insulin will result in suppression of endogenous insulin secretion and a low C-peptide levels. An elevated circulating proinsulin level in the presence of fasting hypoglycemia is characteristic of most B cell adenomas and does not occur in factitious hyperinsulinism. Thus, C-peptide and proinsulin levels (by ICMA) of > 200 pmol/L and > 5 pmol/L, respectively, are characteristic of insulinomas.

In patients with epigastric distress, a history of renal stones, or menstrual or erectile dysfunction, a serum calcium, gastrin, or prolactin level may be useful in screening for MEN 1 associated with insulinoma.

C. Diagnostic Tests

1. **Prolonged fasting**—Prolonged fasting under hospital supervision until hypoglycemia is documented is probably the most dependable means of establishing the diagnosis, especially in men. In 30% of patients with insulinoma, the blood glucose levels often drop below 40 mg/dL after an overnight fast, but some patients require up to 72 hours to develop symptomatic hypoglycemia. However, the term "72-hour fast" is actually a misnomer in most cases since the fast should be immediately terminated as soon as symptoms appear and laboratory confirmation of hypoglycemia is available. In normal male subjects, the blood glucose does not fall below 55–60 mg/dL during a 3-day fast. In contrast, in normal premenopausal women who have fasted for only 24 hours, the plasma glucose may fall normally to such an extent that it can reach values as low as 35 mg/dL. In

these cases, however, the women are not symptomatic, presumably owing to the development of sufficient ketonemia to supply energy needs to the brain. Insulinoma patients, on the other hand, become symptomatic when plasma glucose drops to subnormal levels, since inappropriate insulin secretion restricts ketone formation. Moreover, the demonstration of a nonsuppressed insulin level ≥ 6 microunit/mL using a RIA assay (> 3 microunit/mL using an ICMA assay) in the presence of hypoglycemia suggests the diagnosis of insulinoma. If hypoglycemia does not develop in a male patient after fasting for up to 72 hours—and particularly when this prolonged fast is terminated with a period of moderate exercise—insulinoma must be considered an unlikely diagnosis. A suggested protocol for the supervised fast is shown in Table 27–14.

2. **Stimulation tests**—Stimulation with pancreatic B cell secretagogues such as tolbutamide, glucagon, or leucine is generally not needed in most cases if basal insulin is found to be nonsuppressible and therefore inappropriately elevated during fasting hypoglycemia.

Intravenous glucagon (1 mg over 1 minute) can be useful in patients with "borderline" fasting inappropriate hyperinsulinism. A serum insulin rise above baseline of 200 microunit/mL or more at 5 and 10 minutes strongly suggests insulinoma, although poorly differentiated tumors may not respond. Glucagon has the advantage over tolbutamide of correcting rather than provoking hy-

Table 27–14. Suggested hospital protocol for supervised fast in diagnosis of insulinoma.

(1) Obtain baseline serum glucose, insulin, proinsulin, and C-peptide measurements at onset of fast and place intravenous cannula.

(2) Permit only calorie-free and caffeine-free fluids and encourage supervised activity (such as walking).

(3) Measure urine for ketones at the beginning and every 12 hours and at end of fast.

(4) Obtain capillary glucose measurements with a reflectance meter every 4 hours until values < 60 mg/dL are obtained. Then increase the frequency of fingersticks to each hour, and when capillary glucose value is < 49 mg/dL send a venous blood sample to the laboratory for serum glucose, insulin, proinsulin, and C-peptide measurements. Check frequently for manifestations of neuroglycopenia.

(5) If symptoms of hypoglycemia occur or if a laboratory value of serum glucose is < 45 mg/dL, or if 72 hours have elapsed then conclude the fast with a final blood sample for serum glucose, insulin, proinsulin, C-peptide, β-hydroxybutyrate or acetone and sulfonylurea measurements. Then give oral fast-acting carbohydrate followed by a meal. If the patient is confused or unable to take oral agents, then administer 50 mL of 50% dextrose intravenously over 3 to 5 minutes. Do not conclude a fast based simply on a capillary blood glucose measurement—wait for the laboratory glucose value --unless the patient is very symptomatic and it would be dangerous to wait.

poglycemia during stimulation testing and is diagnostic in 60–70% of patients with insulinoma. False-negative results can occur if the tumor is poorly differentiated and agranular.

D. PREOPERATIVE LOCALIZATION OF B CELL TUMORS

After the diagnosis of insulinoma has been unequivocally made by clinical and laboratory findings, studies to localize the tumor should be initiated. The focus of attention should be directed to the pancreas since that is where virtually all insulinomas originate.

A spiral CT angiography of the pancreas should be performed to rule out a large tumor of the pancreas or hepatic metastases from a malignant islet cell tumor. Endoscopic ultrasonographic examination of the pancreas can also be helpful in identifying the pancreatic lesions. Because of the small size of these tumors (averaging 1.5 cm in diameter in one large series), imaging studies do not necessarily identify all the tumors. Patients who do not have an obvious tumor on imaging (but have a definite biochemical diagnosis) should undergo selective calcium-stimulated angiography. In this test, angiography is combined with injections of calcium gluconate into the gastroduodenal, splenic, and superior mesenteric arteries and insulin levels are measured in the hepatic vein effluent. Calcium stimulates insulin release from insulinomas but not normal islets, and so a step-up of insulin levels regionalizes the hyperinsulinism to the head of the pancreas for the gastroduodenal artery, to the uncinate process for the superior mesenteric artery, and to the body and tail of the pancreas for the splenic artery. This technique may also provide data that are particularly helpful when multiple insulinomas are suspected (MEN 1) and it has become a major tool in confirming the diagnosis of diffuse islet hyperplasia in the recently described noninsulinoma pancreatogenous hypoglycemia syndrome (NIPHS) (see below). Since diazoxide might interfere with this test, it should be discontinued for at least 48–72 hours before sampling. An infusion of dextrose may be required, therefore, and patients should be closely monitored during the procedure to avoid hypoglycemia (as well as hyperglycemia, which could affect insulin gradients). These studies combined with careful intraoperative ultrasonography and palpation by a surgeon experienced in insulinoma surgery identifies up to 98% of tumors.

Treatment

A. SURGICAL MEASURES

It is imperative that the surgeon be convinced that the diagnosis of insulinoma has been unequivocally made by clinical and laboratory findings. Only then should surgery be considered, as there is no justification for exploratory operation—just as there is none for the use of current localization techniques as a preoperative diagnostic tool. Resection by a surgeon with previous experience in removing pancreatic B cell tumors is the treatment of choice. In patients with a single benign adenoma, 90–95% have a successful cure at the first surgical attempt

when intraoperative ultrasound is used by a skilled surgeon. Blood glucose should be monitored throughout surgery, and 10% dextrose in water should be infused at a rate of 100 mL/h or faster. In cases where the diagnosis has been established but no adenoma is located after careful palpation and use of intraoperative ultrasound, it is no longer advisable to blindly resect the body and tail of the pancreas, since a nonpalpable tumor missed by ultrasound is most likely embedded within the fleshy head of the pancreas that is left behind with subtotal resections. Most surgeons prefer to close the incision and schedule a selective arterial calcium stimulation with hepatic venous sampling to locate the tumor site prior to a repeat operation. Laparoscopy using ultrasound and enucleation has been successful with a single tumor of the body or tail of the pancreas, but open surgery remains necessary for tumors in the head of the pancreas.

B. DIET AND MEDICAL THERAPY

In patients with inoperable functioning islet cell carcinoma and in approximately 5–10% of MEN 1 cases when subtotal removal of the pancreas has failed to produce cure, reliance on frequent feedings is necessary. Since most tumors are not responsive to glucose, carbohydrate feedings every 2–3 hours are usually effective in preventing hypoglycemia, although obesity may become a problem. Diazoxide, 300–600 mg (or 3 mg to 8 mg/kg; 50 mg/mL oral suspension) daily orally in two or three divided doses, is the treatment of choice. Hydrochlorothiazide, 25–50 mg daily, should also be prescribed to counteract the sodium retention and edema secondary to diazoxide therapy as well as to potentiate its hyperglycemic effect. If patients are unable to tolerate diazoxide because of gastrointestinal upset, hirsutism, or edema, the calcium channel blocker verapamil may be beneficial in view of its inhibitory effect on insulin release from insulinoma cells. Octreotide, a potent long-acting synthetic octapeptide analog of somatostatin, has been used to inhibit release of hormones from a number of endocrine tumors. A dose of 50 mcg of octreotide injected subcutaneously twice daily has been tried in cases where surgery failed to remove the source of hyperinsulinism. However, its effectiveness is limited since its affinity for somatostatin receptors of the pancreatic B cell is very much less than for those of the anterior pituitary somatotrophs for which it was originally designed as treatment for acromegaly. When hypoglycemia persists after attempted surgical removal of the insulinoma and if diazoxide or verapamil is poorly tolerated or ineffective, multiple small feedings may be the only recourse until more selective somatostatin receptor agonists are available. Streptozocin can decrease insulin secretion in islet cell carcinomas, and effective doses have been delivered via selective arterial catheter so that the undue renal toxicity that characterized early experience is less of a problem.

Prognosis

When insulinoma is diagnosed early and cured surgically, complete recovery is likely, although brain damage following prolonged severe hypoglycemia is not reversible. A significant increase in survival rate has been shown in streptozocin-treated patients with islet cell carcinoma, with reduction in tumor mass as well as decreased hyperinsulinism.

Grant CS: Surgical aspects of hyperinsulinemic hypoglycemia. Endocrinol Metab Clin North Am 1999;28:533. [PMID: 10500930]

Hirshberg B et al: Forty-eight-hour fast: the diagnostic test for insulinoma. J Clin Endocrinol Metab 2000;85:3222. [PMID: 10999812]

Service FJ: Diagnostic approach to adults with hypoglycemic disorders. Endocrinol Metab Clin North Am 1999;28: 519. [PMID: 10500929]

Tucker ON et al: The management of insulinoma. Br J Surg 2006;93:264. [PMID: 16498592]

PERSISTENT ISLET HYPERPLASIA (Noninsulinoma Pancreatogenous Hypoglycemia Syndrome)

In a very small number of patients with organic hyperinsulinism, islet hyperplasia rather than an adenoma is present. These patients typically have documented hyperinsulinemic hypoglycemia after meals but not with fasting up to 72 hours. The patients have a positive response to calcium-stimulated angiography. A gradient-guided partial pancreatectomy leads to clinical remission, and the pathology of the pancreas shows evidence of islet hyperplasia and nesidioblastosis. These patients do not have mutations in the *Kir 6.2* and *SUR1* genes, which has been reported in children with familial hyperinsulinemic hypoglycemia.

HYPOGLYCEMIA DUE TO EXTRAPANCREATIC TUMORS

These rare causes of hypoglycemia include mesenchymal tumors such as retroperitoneal sarcomas, hepatocellular carcinomas, adrenocortical carcinomas, and miscellaneous epithelial-type tumors. The tumors are frequently large and readily palpated or visualized on CT scans or MRI.

The expression and release of an incompletely processed insulin-like growth factor-2 (IGF-2) has provided the best explanation for the clinical manifestations of hypoglycemia in these cases. A larger immature form of the IGF-2 molecule is released which binds to a carrier protein but not to an acid-labile component of serum which inactivates normal IGF-2. This immature IGF-2 complex therefore remains active and binds to insulin receptors in muscle to promote glucose transport and to insulin receptors in liver and kidney to reduce glucose output. It also binds to receptors for IGF-1 in the pancreatic B cell to inhibit insulin secretion. Serum levels of IGF-2 may be increased but often are "normal" in quantity, despite the presence of the immature, higher-molecular-weight form of IGF-2, which can only be detected by special laboratory techniques.

Laboratory diagnosis depends on documenting fasting hypoglycemia associated with undetectable serum insulin levels.

The prognosis for these tumors is generally poor, and surgical removal should be attempted when feasible. Dietary management of the hypoglycemia is the mainstay of medical treatment, since diazoxide is usually ineffective.

Le Roith D: Tumor-induced hypoglycemia. N Engl J Med 1999; 341:757. [PMID: 10471466]

POSTPRANDIAL HYPOGLYCEMIA (Reactive Hypoglycemia)

Postgastrectomy Alimentary Hypoglycemia

Reactive hypoglycemia following gastrectomy is a consequence of hyperinsulinism resulting from rapid gastric emptying of ingested food. Symptoms result from adrenergic hyperactivity in response to the hypoglycemia. Treatment consists of more frequent feedings with smaller portions of less rapidly assimilated carbohydrate combined with more slowly absorbed fat and protein. Cases of hypoglycemia have been reported in patients who have undergone Roux-en-Y gastric bypass surgery for the treatment of obesity. The hypoglycemia occurs after meals and can be severe. Some of these patients are found to have islet cell hyperplasia.

Functional Alimentary Hypoglycemia

This syndrome is classified as functional when no postsurgical explanation exists for the presence of early alimentary type reactive hypoglycemia. It is most often associated with chronic fatigue, anxiety, irritability, weakness, poor concentration, decreased libido, headaches, hunger after meals, and tremulousness. However, most patients with these symptoms do not have hypoglycemia after a mixed meal. (See Chronic Fatigue Syndrome in Chapter 2.)

Indiscriminate use and overinterpretation of glucose tolerance tests have led to an unfortunate tendency to overdiagnose functional hypoglycemia. As many as one-third or more of normal subjects have blood glucose levels as low as 40–50 mg/dL with or without symptoms during a 4-hour glucose tolerance test. Accordingly, to increase diagnostic reliability, hypoglycemia should preferably be documented during a spontaneous symptomatic episode accompanying routine daily activity, with clinical improvement following feeding. Oral glucose tolerance tests are overly sensitive and mixed meals are relatively insensitive in detecting postprandial reactive hypoglycemia. It has been shown that a high-carbohydrate breakfast has proved useful in differentiating persons with postprandial reactive hypoglycemia from normal controls. The test resulted in reactive hypoglycemia to levels below 59 mg/dL in 47% of 38 subjects, in contrast to only 2.2% of the 43 controls. This test was found to be much more sensitive than a standard mixed meal, which was also given to these two groups.

In patients with documented postprandial hypoglycemia on a functional basis, there is no harm and occasional benefit in reducing the proportion of carbohydrate in the diet while increasing the frequency and reducing the size of meals. Support and mild sedation should be the mainstays of therapy, with dietary manipulation only an adjunct.

Late Hypoglycemia (Occult Diabetes)

This condition is characterized by a delay in early insulin release from pancreatic B cells, resulting in initial exaggeration of hyperglycemia during a glucose tolerance test. In response to this hyperglycemia, an exaggerated insulin release produces a late hypoglycemia 4–5 hours after ingestion of glucose. These patients are usually quite different from those with early hypoglycemia occurring 2–3 hours after glucose ingestion, often being obese and frequently having a family history of diabetes mellitus.

In obese patients, treatment is directed at weight reduction to achieve ideal weight. Like all patients with postprandial hypoglycemia, regardless of cause, these patients often respond to reduced carbohydrate intake with multiple, spaced, small feedings. They should be considered potential diabetics and advised to have periodic medical evaluations.

Service GJ et al: Hyperinsulinemic hypoglycemia with nesidioblastosis after gastric-bypass surgery. N Engl J Med 2005; 353:249. [PMID: 16034010]

ALCOHOL-RELATED HYPOGLYCEMIA

Fasting Hypoglycemia after Ethanol

During the postabsorptive state, normal plasma glucose is maintained by hepatic glucose output derived from both glycogenolysis and gluconeogenesis. With prolonged starvation, glycogen reserves become depleted within 18–24 hours and hepatic glucose output becomes totally dependent on gluconeogenesis. Under these circumstances, a blood concentration of ethanol as low as 45 mg/dL can induce profound hypoglycemia by blocking gluconeogenesis. Neuroglycopenia in a patient whose breath smells of alcohol may be mistaken for alcoholic stupor. Prevention consists of adequate food intake during ethanol ingestion. Therapy consists of glucose administration to replenish glycogen stores until gluconeogenesis resumes.

Postethanol Reactive Hypoglycemia

When sugar-containing soft drinks are used as mixers to dilute alcohol in beverages (gin and tonic, rum and cola), there seems to be a greater insulin release than when the soft drink alone is ingested and a tendency for more of a late hypoglycemic overswing to occur 3–4 hours later. Prevention would consist of avoiding sugar mixers while ingesting alcohol and ensuring supplementary food intake to provide sustained absorption.

FACTITIOUS HYPOGLYCEMIA

Factitious hypoglycemia may be difficult to document. A suspicion of self-induced hypoglycemia is supported when the patient is associated with the health professions or has access to insulin or sulfonylurea drugs taken by a diabetic member of the family. The triad of hypoglycemia, high immunoreactive insulin, and suppressed plasma C peptide immunoreactivity is pathognomonic of exogenous insulin administration. Demonstration of circulating insulin antibodies supports this diagnosis in suspected cases. When sulfonylureas are suspected as a cause of factitious hypoglycemia, a plasma level of these drugs to detect their presence may be required to distinguish laboratory findings from those of insulinoma. Unfortunately, the newer sulfonylurea, glimepiride, and other insulinotropic hypoglycemic drugs like repaglinide and nateglinide are not detected in the standard assays for sulfonylureas.

IMMUNOPATHOLOGIC HYPOGLYCEMIA

This rare cause of hypoglycemia, documented in isolated case reports, may occur as two distinct disorders: one associated with spontaneous development of circulating anti-insulin antibodies and another associated with antibodies to insulin receptors, in which the antibodies apparently have agonist capabilities. This latter disorder is extremely rare, having been documented in no more than five cases. However, development of anti-insulin antibodies has been reported in over 200 patients most of whom were being treated with methimazole for thyrotoxicosis. In Western countries, 23 cases have been reported and include patients with a lupus-like syndrome or with various paraproteinemias. The hypoglycemia occurs 3–4 hours after meals following an initial postprandial hyperglycemic phase that is due to the antibodies interfering with the exit of insulin from the plasma to reach its target tissues. Later, after most of the meal is absorbed, inappropriate high levels of insulin dissociate from this antibody-bound compartment, resulting in hypoglycemia. Insulin levels in excess of 1000 pmol/L are observed at time of hypoglycemia, and these persons have high titers of insulin autoantibodies.

Redmon JB et al: Autoimmune hypoglycemia. Endocrinol Metab Clin North Am 1999;28:603. [PMID: 10500933]

DRUG-INDUCED HYPOGLYCEMIA

A number of drugs apart from the sulfonylureas can occasionally cause hypoglycemia, especially when ingested in large amounts. These include quinine, quinidine, disopyramide, and salicylates. ACE inhibitors, when taken with antidiabetic drugs, can cause hypoglycemia possibly by improving insulin sensitivity. Recently, it has been reported that the use of gatifloxacin in diabetic patients is associated with serious hypoglycemic and hyperglycemic reactions.

Ten to 20 percent of patients receiving pentamidine for *Pneumocystis jiroveci* pneumonia develop symptomatic hypoglycemia, particularly when the drug is administered intravenously. This apparently is due to lytic destruction of pancreatic B cells, causing acute hyperinsulinemia and hypoglycemia. It is later followed by insulinopenia and hyperglycemia, which occasionally is persistent. Since other drugs have been found to be as effective in treating *Pneumocystis* pneumonia, pentamidine administration and its hypoglycemic sequelae are less frequently encountered.

Lipid Abnormalities

28

Robert B. Baron, MD, MS

For patients with known cardiovascular disease (secondary prevention), cholesterol lowering leads to a consistent reduction in total mortality and recurrent cardiovascular events in men and women and in middle-aged and older patients. Among patients without cardiovascular disease (primary prevention), the data are less conclusive, with rates of cardiovascular events, heart disease mortality, and all-cause mortality differing among studies. Nonetheless, treatment algorithms have been designed to assist clinicians in selecting patients for cholesterol-lowering therapy based on their lipid levels and their overall risk of developing cardiovascular disease.

LIPIDS & LIPOPROTEINS

The two main lipids in blood are cholesterol and triglyceride. They are carried in lipoproteins, globular particles that also contain proteins known as apoproteins. Cholesterol is an essential element of all animal cell membranes and forms the backbone of steroid hormones and bile acids; triglycerides are important in transferring energy from food into cells. Why lipids are deposited into the walls of large and medium-sized arteries—an event with potentially lethal consequences—is not known.

Lipoproteins are usually classified on the basis of density, which is determined by the amounts of triglyceride (which makes them less dense) and apoproteins (which makes them more dense). The least dense particles, known as chylomicrons, are normally found in the blood only after fat-containing foods have been eaten. They rise as a creamy layer when nonfasting serum is allowed to stand. The other lipoproteins are suspended in serum and must be separated using a centrifuge. The densest (and smallest) family of particles consists mainly of apoproteins and cholesterol and is called high-density lipoproteins (HDL). Somewhat less dense are the low-density lipoproteins (LDL). Least dense are the large, very-low-density lipoproteins (VLDL), consisting mainly of triglyceride. In fasting serum, most of the cholesterol is carried on LDL particles and is therefore referred to as LDL cholesterol; most of the triglyceride is found in VLDL particles. Specific apoproteins are associated with each lipoprotein class.

Chylomicrons are made in the gut and travel via the portal vein into the liver and via the thoracic duct into the circulation. They are normally completely metabolized, transferring energy from food into muscle and fat cells. The liver manufactures VLDL particles from its own stores of fat and carbohydrate. VLDL particles transfer triglyceride to cells; after losing enough, they eventually become LDL particles, which provide cholesterol for cellular needs. Excess LDL particles are taken up by the liver, and the cholesterol they contain is then excreted into the bile. HDL particles are made in the liver and intestine and appear to facilitate the transfer of apoproteins among lipoproteins. They also participate in reverse cholesterol transport, either by transferring cholesterol into other lipoproteins or directly into the liver.

LIPOPROTEINS & ATHEROGENESIS

The plaques in the arterial walls of patients with atherosclerosis contain large amounts of cholesterol. The higher the level of LDL cholesterol, the greater the risk of atherosclerotic heart disease; conversely, the higher the HDL cholesterol, the lower the risk of coronary heart disease (CHD). This is true in men and women, in different racial and ethnic groups, and at all ages up to age 75 years. Because most cholesterol in serum is LDL, high total cholesterol levels are also associated with an increased risk of CHD. Middle-aged men whose serum cholesterol levels are in the highest quintile for age (above about 230 mg/dL) have a risk of coronary death before age 65 years of about 10%; men in the lowest quintile (below about 170 mg/dL) have a 3% risk. Death from CHD before age 65 years is less common in women, with equivalent risks one-third those of men. In men, each 10-mg/dL increase in cholesterol (or LDL cholesterol) increases the risk of CHD by about 10%; each 5-mg/dL increase in HDL reduces the risk by about 10%. The effect of HDL cholesterol is greater in women, whereas the effects of total and LDL cholesterol are smaller. All of these relationships diminish with age.

The exact mechanism by which LDL particles result in the formation of atherosclerotic plaques—or the means whereby HDL particles protect against their formation—is not known. The model of LDL carrying cholesterol into the walls of arteries with HDL removing it is simple but not established. The natural oxidation of LDL particles may be particularly atherogenic. Receptors on the surface of macrophages within atherosclerotic plaques bind and accumulate oxidized LDL. The formation of antibodies to oxidized LDL may also be important in plaque formation. The size of the LDL molecule may also influence atherogenesis; at the same LDL concentrations, individuals with large numbers of smaller particles appear to be at higher risk for CHD.

The relationship of VLDL cholesterol to atherogenesis is less certain. The number, size, or subtype of VLDL particles—in addition to the total amount in serum—may be important. In addition, HDL and VLDL levels are inversely related. Patients with a high VLDL level are likely to have a low HDL level and thus be at increased risk for CHD for that reason alone.

There are several genetic disorders that provide insight into the pathogenesis of lipid-related diseases. **Familial hypercholesterolemia**, rare in the homozygous state (about one per million) is a condition in which the cell-surface receptors for the LDL molecule are absent or defective, resulting in unregulated synthesis of LDL. Patients with two abnormal genes (homozygotes) have extremely high levels—up to eight times normal—and present with atherosclerotic disease in childhood. Homozygotes may require liver transplantation to correct their severe lipid abnormalities. Those with one defective gene (heterozygotes) have LDL concentrations twice normal; persons with this condition may develop CHD in their 30s or 40s.

Another rare condition is caused by an abnormality of lipoprotein lipase, the enzyme that enables peripheral tissues to take up triglyceride from chylomicrons and VLDL particles. Patients with this condition, one cause of **familial hyperchylomicronemia**, have marked hypertriglyceridemia with recurrent pancreatitis and hepatosplenomegaly in childhood.

Numerous other genetic abnormalities of lipid metabolism are named for the abnormality noted when serum is electrophoresed (eg, dysbetalipoproteinemia) or from combinations of lipid abnormalities in families (eg, familial combined hyperlipidemia). Thus, family members of patients with severe lipid disorders are appropriately studied. Other patients have abnormalities in the production of apoproteins, such as increased apoprotein B and its affiliated lipoproteins, LDL and VLDL; reduced apoprotein AII and its affiliated particle; or excess lipoprotein(a). Other mutations occur in lipoprotein lipase and in the gene encoding for cholesterol efflux regulatory protein.

Berneis K et al: Low-density lipoprotein size and subclasses are markers of clinically apparent and non-apparent atherosclerosis in type 2 diabetes. Metabolism 2005;54:227. [PMID: 15690318]

Carmena R et al: Atherogenic lipoprotein particles in atherosclerosis. Circulation 2004;109:III2. [PMID: 15198959]

Deb A et al: Lipoprotein(a): new insights into mechanisms of atherogenesis and thrombosis. Clin Cardiol 2004;27:258. [PMID: 15188938]

Drexel H et al: Is atherosclerosis in diabetes and impaired fasting glucose driven by elevated LDL cholesterol or by decreased HDL cholesterol? Diabetes Care 2005;28:101. [PMID: 15616241]

Marks D et al: A review on the diagnosis, natural history, and treatment of familial hypercholesterolaemia. Atherosclerosis 2003;168:1. [PMID: 12732381]

Moreno PR et al: New aspects in the pathogenesis of diabetic atherothrombosis. J Am Coll Cardiol 2004;44:2293. [PMID: 15607389]

Nam BH et al: Search for the optimal atherogenic lipid risk profile: from the Framingham study. Am J Cardiol 2006;97:372. [PMID: 16442398]

Rader DJ: Regulation of reverse cholesterol transport and clinical implications. Am J Cardiol 2003;92:42J. [PMID: 12957326]

LIPID FRACTIONS & THE RISK OF CORONARY HEART DISEASE

In fasting serum, cholesterol is carried primarily on three different lipoproteins—the VLDL, LDL, and HDL molecules. Total cholesterol equals the sum of these three components:

$$\text{Total cholesterol} = \text{HDL cholesterol} + \text{VLDL cholesterol} + \text{LDL cholesterol}$$

Most clinical laboratories measure the total cholesterol, the total triglycerides, and the amount of cholesterol found in the HDL fraction, which is easily precipitated from serum. Most triglyceride is found in VLDL particles, which contain five times as much triglyceride by weight as cholesterol. The amount of cholesterol found in the VLDL fraction can be estimated by dividing the triglyceride by 5:

$$\text{VLDL cholesterol} = \frac{\text{Triglycerides}}{5}$$

Because the triglyceride level is used as a proxy for the amount of VLDL, this formula works only in fasting samples and when the triglyceride level is less than 400 mg/dL. At higher triglyceride levels, LDL and VLDL cholesterol levels can be determined after ultracentrifugation or by direct chemical measurement.

The total cholesterol is reasonably stable over time; however, measurements of HDL and especially triglycerides may vary considerably because of analytic error in the laboratory and biologic variation in a patient's lipid level. Thus, the LDL should always be estimated as the mean of at least two determinations; if those two estimates differ by more than 10%, a third lipid profile is obtained and is estimated as follows:

$$\text{LDL cholesterol} = \frac{\text{Total cholesterol}}{(\text{mg/dL})} - \frac{\text{HDL cholesterol}}{(\text{mg/dL})} - \frac{\text{Triglycerides (mg/dL)}}{5}$$

When using SI units, the formula becomes

$$\text{LDL cholesterol} = \frac{\text{Total cholesterol}}{(\text{mmol/L})} - \frac{\text{HDL cholesterol}}{(\text{mmol/L})} - \frac{\text{Triglycerides (mmol/L)}}{2.2}$$

Understanding the relationships of the different lipid fractions leads to a more accurate understanding of a patient's lipid-related coronary risk than the total cholesterol. Two persons with the same total cholesterol of 275 mg/dL may have very different lipid profiles. One may have an HDL cholesterol of 110 mg/dL with a triglyceride of 150 mg/dL, giving an estimated LDL cholesterol of 135 mg/dL; the other may have an HDL cholesterol of 25 mg/dL with a triglyceride of 200 mg/dL and an LDL cholesterol of 210 mg/dL. The second would have more than a tenfold higher CHD risk than the first, assuming no differences in other factors. Because of high HDL cholesterol levels in women, many with apparently high total cholesterol levels have favorable lipid profiles. Thus, evaluation of the lipid fractions is essential before therapy is initiated.

Some authorities use the ratio of the total to HDL cholesterol as an indicator of lipid-related coronary risk: the lower this ratio is, the better. (In the example above, the first person would have a ratio of 275 ÷ 110 = 2.5, while the second would have a much less favorable ratio of 275 ÷ 25 = 11.) Although ratios are useful predictors within populations of patients, they may obscure important information in individual patients. (A total cholesterol of 300 mg/dL and an HDL of 60 mg/dL result in the same ratio of 5 as a total cholesterol of 150 mg/dL with an HDL of 30 mg/dL.) Moreover, errors in the measurement of HDL cholesterol are common in many laboratories, and the total cholesterol-to-HDL cholesterol ratio magnifies their importance.

There is no true "normal" range for serum lipids. In Western populations, cholesterol values are about 20% higher than in Asian populations and exceed 300 mg/dL in nearly 5% of adults. About 10% of adults have LDL cholesterol levels above 200 mg/dL. Total and LDL cholesterol levels tend to rise with age in persons who are otherwise in good health.

Declines are seen in acute illness, and lipid studies in such patients are of little value with the exception of the serum triglyceride level in a patient with pancreatitis. Cholesterol levels (even when expressed as an age-matched percentile rank, such as the highest 20%) do not remain constant over time, especially from childhood through adolescence and young adulthood. Thus, children and young adults with relatively high cholesterol may have lower levels later in life, whereas those with low cholesterol may show increases.

THERAPEUTIC EFFECTS OF LOWERING CHOLESTEROL

Most studies of the effect of cholesterol lowering have distinguished between primary and secondary prevention. Primary prevention trials enroll healthy subjects who have relatively low rates of coronary disease but in whom other causes of morbidity and mortality are proportionately more common. Secondary prevention trials, on the other hand, follow patients who have a high rate of subsequent coronary disease; other causes of mortality are relatively less important.

Reducing cholesterol levels in healthy middle-aged men without CHD (primary prevention) reduces their risk in proportion to the reduction in LDL cholesterol and the increase in HDL cholesterol. Treated patients have statistically significant and clinically important reductions in the rates of myocardial infarctions, new cases of angina, and need for coronary artery bypass procedures. The West of Scotland Study showed a 31% decrease in myocardial infarctions in middle-aged men treated with pravastatin compared with placebo. The Air Force/Texas Coronary Atherosclerosis Prevention Study (AFCAPS/TexCAPS) study showed similar results with lovastatin. As with any primary prevention interventions, large numbers of healthy patients need to be treated to prevent a single event. The numbers of patients needed to treat (NNT) to prevent a nonfatal myocardial infarction or a coronary artery disease death in these two studies were 46 and 50, respectively. The Anglo-Scandinavian Cardiac Outcomes Trial (ASCOT) study of atorvastatin in subjects with hypertension and other risk factors but without CHD also demonstrated a convincing 36% reduction in CHD events.

Primary prevention studies have found a less consistent effect on total mortality. The West of Scotland study found a 20% decrease in total mortality, tending toward statistical significance. The AFCAPS/TexCAPS study with lovastatin showed no difference in total mortality. The Antihypertensive and Lipid-Lowering Treatment to Prevent Heart Attack Trial (ALLHAT-LLT) also showed no reduction either in all-cause mortality or in CHD events when pravastatin was compared with usual care. Subjects treated with atorvastatin in the ASCOT study had a 13% reduction in mortality, but the result was not statistically significant. This study, however, was stopped early due to the marked reduction in CHD events.

In patients with CHD, the benefits of cholesterol lowering are more clear. Major studies with statins have shown significant reductions in cardiovascular events, cardiovascular deaths, and all-cause mortality in men and women with coronary artery disease. The NNT to prevent a nonfatal myocardial infarction or a coronary artery disease death in these three studies were between 12 and 34. Aggressive cholesterol lowering with these agents causes regression of atherosclerotic plaques in some patients, reduces the progression of atherosclerosis in saphenous vein grafts, and can slow or reverse carotid artery atherosclerosis. Meta-analysis suggests that this latter effect results in a significant decrease in strokes. Results with other classes of medications have been less consistent. For example, gemfibrozil treatment subjects had fewer cardiovascular events, but there was no benefit in all-cause mortality when compared with placebo.

The disparities in results between primary and secondary prevention studies highlight several important points. The benefits and adverse effects of cholesterol lowering may be specific to each type of drug; the clinician cannot assume that the effects will generalize to other classes of medication. Second, the net benefits from cholesterol lowering depend on the underlying risk of CHD and of other disease. In patients with atherosclerosis, morbidity and mortality rates associated with CHD are high, and measures that reduce it are more likely to be beneficial even if they have no effect—or even slightly harmful effects—on other diseases.

Ashen MD et al: Low HDL cholesterol levels. N Engl J Med 2005;353:1252. [PMID: 16177251]

Baigent C et al: Efficacy and safety of cholesterol-lowering treatment: prospective meta-analysis of data from 90,056 participants in 14 randomised trials. Lancet 2005;366:1267. [PMID: 16214597]

Cannon CP et al: Intensive versus moderate lipid lowering with statins after acute coronary syndromes. N Engl J Med 2004; 350:1495. [PMID: 15007110]

Corvol JC et al: Differential effects of lipid-lowering therapies on stroke prevention: a meta-analysis of randomized trials. Arch Intern Med 2003;163:669. [PMID: 12639199]

de Lemos JA et al: Early intensive vs. a delayed conservative simvastatin strategy in patients with acute coronary syndromes: phase Z of the A to Z trial. JAMA 2004;292:1307. [PMID: 15337732]

Grundy SM et al for the Coordinating Committee of the NCEP: Implications of recent clinical trials for the national cholesterol education program adult treatment panel III guidelines. Circulation 2004;110:227. [PMID: 15249516]

Larosa JC et al: Intensive lipid lowering with atorvastatin in patients with stable coronary disease. N Engl J Med 2005; 352:1425. [PMID: 15755765]

Sever PS et al: Prevention of coronary and stroke events with atorvastatin in hypertensive patients who have average or lower-than-average cholesterol concentrations, in the Anglo-Scandinavian Cardiac Outcomes Trial-Lipid Lowering Arm (ASCOT-LLA): a multicentre randomized controlled trial. Lancet 2003; 361:1149. [PMID: 12686036]

Whitney EJ et al: A randomized trial of a strategy for increasing high-density lipoprotein cholesterol levels: effects of progression of coronary heart disease and clinical events. Ann Intern Med 2005;142:95. [PMID: 15657157]

SECONDARY CONDITIONS THAT AFFECT LIPID METABOLISM

Several factors, including drugs, can influence serum lipids (Table 28–1). These are important for two reasons: Abnormal lipid levels (or changes in lipid levels) may be the presenting sign of some of these conditions, and correction of the underlying condition may obviate the need to treat an apparent lipid disorder. Diabetes and alcohol use, in particular, are commonly associated with high triglyceride levels that decline with improvements in glycemic control or reduction in alcohol use, respectively. Thus, secondary causes of high blood lipids should be considered in each patient with a lipid disorder before lipid-lowering therapy is started. In most instances, special testing is not needed: a history and physical examination are sufficient. However, screening for hypothyroidism in patients with hyperlipidemia is cost effective.

CLINICAL PRESENTATIONS

Most patients with high cholesterol levels have no specific symptoms or signs. The vast majority of patients

Table 28–1. Secondary causes of lipid abnormalities.

Cause	Associated Lipid Abnormality
Obesity	Increased triglycerides, decreased HDL cholesterol
Sedentary lifestyle	Decreased HDL cholesterol
Diabetes mellitus	Increased triglycerides, increased total cholesterol
Alcohol use	Increased triglycerides, increased HDL cholesterol
Hypothyroidism	Increased total cholesterol
Hyperthyroidism	Decreased total cholesterol
Nephrotic syndrome	Increased total cholesterol
Chronic renal insufficiency	Increased total cholesterol, increased triglycerides
Hepatic disease (cirrhosis)	Decreased total cholesterol
Obstructive liver disease	Increased total cholesterol
Malignancy	Decreased total cholesterol
Cushing's disease (or corticosteroid use)	Increased total cholesterol
Oral contraceptives	Increased triglycerides, increased total cholesterol
Diuretics[1]	Increased total cholesterol, increased triglycerides
β-Blockers[1,2]	Increased total cholesterol, decreased HDL

[1]Short-term effects only.
[2]β-Blockers with intrinsic sympathomimetic activity, such as pindolol and acebutolol, do not affect lipid levels.

with lipid abnormalities are detected by the laboratory, either as part of the workup of a patient with cardiovascular disease or as part of a preventive screening strategy. Extremely high levels of chylomicrons or VLDL particles (triglyceride level above 1000 mg/dL) result in the formation of **eruptive xanthomas** (red-yellow papules, especially on the buttocks). High LDL concentrations result in **tendinous xanthomas** on certain tendons (Achilles, patella, back of the hand). Such xanthomas usually indicate one of the underlying genetic hyperlipidemias. **Lipemia retinalis** (cream-colored blood vessels in the fundus) is seen with extremely high triglyceride levels (above 2000 mg/dL).

SCREENING FOR HIGH BLOOD CHOLESTEROL

All patients with CHD or CHD risk equivalents (other clinical forms of atherosclerosis such as peripheral artery disease, abdominal aortic aneurysm, and symptomatic carotid artery disease; patients with diabetes mellitus; and patients with multiple risk factors that confer a greater than 20% 10-year risk for developing CHD) should be screened for elevated lipids. The only exceptions are patients in whom lipid lowering is not indicated or desirable for other reasons. Patients who already have evidence of atherosclerosis are the group at highest risk of suffering additional manifestations in the near term and thus have the most to gain from reduction of blood lipids. Additional risk reduction measures for atherosclerosis are discussed in Chapter 10; lipid lowering should be just one aspect of a program to reduce the progression and effects of the disease.

In patients with cardiovascular disease, a complete lipid profile (total cholesterol, HDL cholesterol, and triglyceride levels) after an overnight fast should be obtained as a screening test. Those whose estimated LDL cholesterol level is high should have at least one repeat measurement. Specific treatments for high LDL cholesterol levels are discussed below. The goal of therapy should be to reduce the LDL cholesterol to below 100 mg/dL or optimally to below 70 mg/dL. Recent evidence suggests that treatment with a statin is effective even if the starting LDL cholesterol is below 100 mg/dL. These data suggest that most patients with CHD or CHD risk equivalents should be treated with statin therapy.

The best screening and treatment strategy for adults who do not have atherosclerotic cardiovascular disease is less clear. Several algorithms have been developed to guide the clinician in treatment decisions, but management decisions are individualized based on the patient's risk.

Although the National Cholesterol Education Program (NCEP) recommends screening of all adults aged 20 years or older for high blood cholesterol, the United States Preventive Services Task Force (USPSTF) suggests beginning at age 35 years in men and age 45 years in women unless there are other risk factors for CHD. This strategy focuses cholesterol screening on those at most immediate risk of coronary artery disease and increases the cost effectiveness of cholesterol screening.

Individuals without cardiovascular disease can then be stratified according to risk factors as defined by the NCEP. Those with two or more risk factors are considered to be at intermediate risk of coronary artery disease, and those with less than two are at low risk. These include age and gender (men aged 45 years or older, women aged 55 years or older), a family history of premature CHD (myocardial infarction or sudden cardiac death before age 55 years in a first-degree male relative or before age 65 years in a first-degree female relative), hypertension (whether treated or not), current cigarette smoking (10 or more cigarettes per day), and low HDL cholesterol (< 40 mg/dL). Because HDL cholesterol is protective against CHD, a risk factor is subtracted if the level is greater than 60 mg/dL. Patients with two or more risk factors are then further stratified by evaluating their 10-year risk of developing CHD using Framingham projections of 10-year risk (Table 28–2). Because risk factors alone are an imprecise measure of CHD risk, estimating the 10-year risk using Framingham data is likely to be helpful even in patients with one or no risk factors.

Several strategies for obtaining the initial cholesterol measurement have been proposed, including

(1) measuring total cholesterol alone, (2) measuring total cholesterol and HDL cholesterol, or (3) measuring LDL and HDL cholesterol. Each is acceptable, but treatment decisions are based on the LDL and HDL cholesterol levels. Measurement of the total cholesterol alone is the least expensive strategy and is adequate for low-risk individuals; those with total cholesterol greater than 200 mg/dL should then be reevaluated with a fasting LDL and HDL cholesterol measurement. Measurement of the total cholesterol and HDL cholesterol allows for better characterization of the risk factor profile but also requires reevaluation if the total cholesterol is greater than 200 mg/dL as recommended by the USPSTF. Initial measurement of the LDL and HDL cholesterol is least likely to lead to patient misinformation and misclassification and is the strategy recommended by the NCEP.

Treatment decisions are based on the LDL cholesterol, and the patient's risk factor profile (including the HDL cholesterol level) and estimated 10-year risk. Patients in the intermediate-risk group (two or more risk factors) are selected for diet therapy (therapeutic lifestyle changes) if LDL cholesterol is greater than 130 mg/dL. If the 10-year risk of CHD is < 10%, drug treatment is recommended if LDL is > 160 mg/dL; if the 10-year CHD risk is between 10% and 20%, drug treatment is recommended if LDL is > 130 mg/dL. Low-risk individuals with one or no risk factors and estimated 10-year CHD risk less than 10% are selected for diet therapy if LDL cholesterol is greater than 160 mg/dL and for drug therapy if it is greater than 190 mg/dL (Table 28–3).

Screening in Women

The foregoing screening and treatment guidelines, based largely on LDL cholesterol levels, are designed for both men and women. Yet several observational studies suggest that a low HDL cholesterol is a more important risk factor for CHD in women than a high LDL cholesterol. Meta-analysis of studies including women with known heart disease, however, has found that medications that primarily lower LDL cholesterol do prevent recurrent myocardial infarctions in women. There is insufficient evidence to be certain of a similar effect from LDL-lowering therapy in women without evidence of CHD. Although most experts recommend application of the same primary prevention guidelines for women as for men, clinicians should be aware of the uncertainty in this area. Using estimates of 10-year CHD risk may be particularly helpful in women since a larger percentage of women than men will have estimated 10-year CHD risks below 10% per year and thus women are less likely to benefit from therapy unless their LDL cholesterol is extremely high (greater than 190 mg/dL).

Screening in Older Patients

Meta-analysis of evidence relating cholesterol to CHD in the elderly suggests that cholesterol is not a risk fac-

Table 28–2. Framingham 10-year coronary heart disease risk projections. Calculate the number of points for each risk factor. Sum the total risk score and estimate the 10-year risk.

MEN		WOMEN	
Age	Points	Age	Points
20–34	–9	20–34	–7
35–39	–4	35–39	–3
40–44	0	40–44	0
45–49	3	45–49	3
50–54	6	50–54	6
55–59	8	55–59	8
60–64	10	60–64	10
65–69	11	65–69	12
70–74	12	70–74	14
75–79	13	75–79	16

MEN

Total Cholesterol	Points				
	Age 20–39	Age 40–49	Age 50–59	Age 60–69	Age 70–79
< 160	0	0	0	0	0
160–199	4	3	2	1	0
200–239	7	5	3	1	0
240–279	9	6	4	2	1
≥ 280	11	8	5	3	1

WOMEN

Total Cholesterol	Points				
	Age 20–39	Age 40–49	Age 50–59	Age 60–69	Age 70–79
< 160	0	0	0	0	0
160–199	4	3	2	1	1
200–239	8	6	4	2	1
240–279	11	8	5	3	2
≥ 280	13	10	7	4	2

MEN

Age	Points				
	20–39	40–49	50–59	60–69	70–79
Nonsmoker	0	0	0	0	0
Smoker	8	5	3	1	1

WOMEN

Age	Points				
	20–39	40–49	50–59	60–69	70–79
Nonsmoker	0	0	0	0	0
Smoker	9	7	4	2	1

MEN

HDL (mg/dL)	Points
≥ 60	–1
50–59	0
40–49	1
< 40	2

WOMEN

HDL (mg/dL)	Points
≥ 60	–1
50–59	0
40–49	1
< 40	2

MEN

Systolic BP (mm Hg)	Points if Untreated	Points if Treated
< 120	0	0
120–129	0	1
130–139	1	2
140–159	1	2
≥ 160	2	3

WOMEN

Systolic BP (mm Hg)	Points if Untreated	Points if Treated
< 120	0	0
120–129	1	3
130–139	2	4
140–159	3	5
≥ 160	4	6

(continued)

Table 28–2. Framingham 10-year coronary heart disease risk projections. Calculate the number of points for each risk factor. Sum the total risk score and estimate the 10-year risk. (continued)

MEN			WOMEN		
Point Total	10-Year Risk %		Point Total	10-Year Risk %	
< 0	< 1		< 9	< 1	
0	1		9	1	
1	1		10	1	
2	1		11	1	
3	1		12	1	
4	1		13	2	
5	2		14	2	
6	2		15	3	
7	3		16	4	
8	4		17	5	
9	5		18	6	
10	6		19	8	
11	8		20	11	
12	10		21	14	
13	12	Ten-Year Risk	22	17	Ten-Year Risk
14	16		23	22	
15	20		24	27	
16	25		≥ 25	≥ 30	
≥ 17	≥ 30	%			%

Reproduced, with permission, from Executive Summary of the Third Report of The National Cholesterol Education Program (NCEP) Expert Panel on Detection, Evaluation, and Treatment of High Blood Cholesterol In Adults (Adult Treatment Panel III). JAMA 2001; 285:2486. http://www.nhlbi.nih.gov/guidelines/cholesterol/index.htm.

tor for CHD for persons over age 75 years. Clinical trials have rarely included such individuals. One exception is the Prospective Study of Pravastatin in the Elderly at Risk (PROSPER). In this study, elderly patients with cardiovascular disease (secondary prevention) benefited from statin therapy, whereas those without cardiovascular disease (primary prevention) did not. Although the NCEP recommends continuing treatment in the elderly, many clinicians will prefer to stop screening and treatment in patients age 75 years or older who do not have CHD. In patients age 75 years or older who have CHD, LDL-lowering therapy can be continued as recommended for younger patients with the disease. Decisions to discontinue therapy should be based on overall functional status and life expectancy, comorbidities, and patient preference and should be made in context with overall therapeutic goals and end-of-life decisions.

Ballantyne CM et al: Role of lipid and lipoprotein profiles in risk assessment and therapy. Am Heart J 2003;146:227. [PMID: 12891189]

Grundy SM et al, for the Coordinating Committee of the NCEP: Implications of recent clinical trials for the national cholesterol education program adult treatment panel III guidelines. Circulation 2004;110:227. [PMID: 15249516]

Mora S et al: Justification for the use of statins in primary prevention: An intervention trial evaluating rosuvastatin (JUPITER)-Can C-reactive protein be used to target statin therapy in primary prevention? Am J Cardiol 2006;97:33. [PMID: 16442935]

Mosca L et al: Evidence-based guidelines for cardiovascular disease in women. Circulation 2004;109:672. [PMID: 14761900]

Nissen SE: Halting the progression of atherosclerosis with intensive lipid lowering: results from the reversal of atherosclerosis with aggressive lipid lowering (REVERSAL) trial. Am J Med 2005;118 Suppl 12A:22. [PMID: 16356804]

O'Keefe JH Jr et al: Optimal low-density lipoprotein is 50 to 70 mg/dl: lower is better and physiologically normal. J Am Coll Cardiol 2004;43:2142. [PMID: 15172426]

Pletcher M et al: Primary prevention of cardiovascular disease in women: New guidelines and emerging strategies. Adv Studies in Medicine 2005;5:412.

Sabharwal AK et al: Low-density lipoprotein reduction: Is the risk worth the benefit? Curr Atheroscleros Rep 2006;8:19. [PMID: 16455010]

Sepulveda JL et al: C-reactive protein and cardiovascular disease: a critical appraisal. Curr Opin Cardiol 2005;20:407. [PMID: 16093760]

Walsh JM et al: Drug treatment of hyperlipidemia in women. JAMA 2004;291:2243. [PMID: 15138247]

TREATMENT OF HIGH LOW-DENSITY LIPOPROTEIN CHOLESTEROL

Reduction of LDL cholesterol is just one part of a program to reduce the risk of cardiovascular disease. Other measures—including smoking cessation, hypertension

Table 28–3. LDL goals and treatment cutpoints: recommendations of the NCEP Adult Treatment Panel III.

Risk Category	LDL Goal (mg/dL)	LDL Level at Which to Initiate Lifestyle Changes (mg/dL)	LDL Level at Which to Consider Drug Therapy[1] (mg/dL)
High risk: CHD[2] or CHD risk equivalents[3] (10-year risk > 20%)	< 100 (optional goal: < 70 mg/dL)[4]	≥ 100[5]	≥ 100[6] (< 100: consider drug options)[1]
Moderately high risk: 2+ risk factors[7] (10-year risk 10% to 20%)[8]	< 130[9]	≥ 130[5]	≥ 130 (100–129; consider drug options)[10]
Moderate risk: 2+ risk factors[7] (10-year risk < 10%)[8]	< 130	≥ 130	≥ 160
Low risk: 0–1 risk factors[11]	< 160	≥ 160	≥ 190 (160–189: LDL-lowering drug optional)

[1]When LDL-lowering drug therapy is used, it is advised that intensity of therapy be sufficient to achieve at least a 30–40% reduction in LDL cholesterol levels.

[2]CHD includes history of myocardial infarction, unstable angina, coronary artery procedures (angioplasty or bypass surgery), or evidence of clinically significant myocardial ischemia.

[3]CHD risk equivalents include clinical manifestations of noncoronary forms of atherosclerotic disease (peripheral arterial disease, abdominal aortic aneurysm, and carotid artery disease [transient ischemic attacks or stroke of carotid origin with > 50% obstruction of a carotid artery]), diabetes mellitus, and ≥ 2 risk factors with 10-year risk for CHD > 20%.

[4]Very high risk favors the optional LDL cholesterol goal of < 70 mg/dL, or in patients with high triglycerides, non-high density lipoprotein (HDL) cholesterol < 100 mg/dL.

[5]Any person at high risk or moderately high risk who has lifestyle-related risk factors (eg, obesity, physical inactivity, elevated triglyceride, low HDL cholesterol, or metabolic syndrome) is a candidate for therapeutic lifestyle changes to modify these risk factors regardless of LDL cholesterol.

[6]If baseline LDL cholesterol is < 100 mg/dL, institution of an LDL-lowering drug is a therapeutic option on the basis of available clinical trial results. If a high-risk person has high triglycerides or low HDL cholesterol, combining a fibrate or nicotinic acid with an LDL-lowering drug can be considered.

[7]Risk factors include cigarette smoking, hypertension (blood pressure ≥ 140/90 mm Hg or on antihypertensive medication), low HDL cholesterol (< 40 mg/dL), family history of premature CHD (CHD in male first-degree relative < 55 years of age; CHD in female first-degree relative < 65 years of age), and age (men ≥ 45 years; women ≥ 55 years).

[8]Electronic 10-year risk calculators are available at www.nhlbi.nih.gov/guidelines/cholesterol.

[9]Optional LDL cholesterol goal < 100 mg/dL.

[10]For moderately high-risk persons, when the LDL cholesterol level is 100–129 mg/dL at baseline or on lifestyle therapy, initiation of an LDL-lowering drug to achieve an LDL cholesterol level < 100 mg/dL is a therapeutic option on the basis of available clinical trial results.

[11]Almost all people with zero or one risk factor have a 10-year CHD risk < 10%, and 10-year risk assessment in these people is thus not necessary.

LDL = low-density lipoprotein; NCEP = National Cholesterol Education Program; CHD = coronary heart disease.

Reproduced, with permission, from Grundy SM et al: Implications of recent clinical trials for the National Cholesterol Education Program Adult Treatment Panel III guidelines. Circulation 2004;110:227.

control, and aspirin—are also of central importance. Less well studied but of potential value is raising the HDL cholesterol level. Quitting smoking reduces the effect of other cardiovascular risk factors (such as a high cholesterol level); it may also increase the HDL cholesterol level. Exercise (and weight loss) may reduce the LDL cholesterol and increase the HDL. Modest alcohol use (1–2 ounces a day) also raises HDL levels and appears to have a salutary effect on CHD rates. Although the clinician may not wish to recommend alcohol use to patients, its use in moderation need not be discouraged.

Diet Therapy

Studies of nonhospitalized adults have reported only modest cholesterol-lowering benefits of dietary therapy, typically in the range of a 5–10% decrease in LDL cholesterol, with even less in the long term. The effect of diet therapy, however, varies considerably among individuals, as some patients will have striking reductions in LDL cholesterol—up to a 25–30% decrease—whereas others will have clinically important increases. Thus, the results of diet therapy should be assessed about 4 weeks after initiation.

Cholesterol-lowering diets may also have a variable effect on lipid fractions. Diets very low in total fat or in saturated fat may lower HDL cholesterol as much as LDL cholesterol. It is not known how these diet-induced changes affect coronary risk.

Several nutritional approaches to diet therapy are available. Most Americans currently eat over 35% of calories as fat, of which 15% is saturated fat. Dietary cholesterol intake averages 400 mg/d. A cholesterol-lowering diet recommends reducing total fat to 25–30% and saturated fat to less than 7% of calories. Dietary cholesterol should be limited to less than 200 mg/d. These diets replace fat, particularly saturated fat, with carbohydrate. In most instances, this approach will also result in fewer total calories consumed and will facilitate weight loss in overweight patients. Other diet plans, including the Dean Ornish Diet, the Pritikin Diet, and most vegetarian diets, restrict fat even further. Low-fat, high-carbohydrate diets may, however, result in reductions in HDL cholesterol.

An alternative strategy is the "Mediterranean diet," which maintains total fat at approximately 35–40% of total calories but replaces saturated fat with monounsaturated fat such as that found in canola oil and in olives, peanuts, avocados, and their oils. This diet is equally effective at lowering LDL cholesterol but is less likely to lead to reductions in HDL cholesterol. Recent studies have demonstrated that this approach may also be associated with reductions in endothelial dysfunction, insulin resistance, and markers of vascular inflammation and may result in better resolution of the metabolic syndrome than traditional cholesterol-lowering diets.

Other dietary changes may also result in beneficial changes in blood lipids. Soluble fiber, such as that found in oat bran or psyllium, may reduce LDL cholesterol by 5–10%. Garlic, soy protein, vitamin C, pecans, and plant sterols may also result in reduction of LDL cholesterol. Because oxidation of LDL cholesterol is a potential initiating event in atherogenesis, diets rich in antioxidant vitamins, found primarily in fruits and vegetables, may be helpful (see Chapter 29). Studies have suggested that when all of these elements are combined into a single dietary prescription, the impact of diet on LDL cholesterol may approach that of statin medications, lowering LDL cholesterol by close to 30%.

Anderson JW: Diet first, then medication for hypercholesterolemia. JAMA 2003;290:531. [PMID: 12876098]

Brunner E et al: Dietary advice for reducing cardiovascular risk. Cochrane Database Syst Rev 2005;(4):CD002128. [PMID: 16235299]

Ding EL et al: Chocolate and prevention of cardiovascular disease: A systematic review. Nutr Metab 2006;3:2. [PMID: 16390538]

Gardner CD et al: The effect of a plant-based diet on plasma lipids in hypercholesterolemic adults: a randomized trial. Ann Intern Med 2005;142:725. [PMID: 15867404]

Jenkins DJ et al: Direct comparison of a dietary portfolio of cholesterol-lowering foods with a statin in hypercholesterolemic participants. Am J Clin Nutr 2005;81:380. [PMID: 15699225]

Kelley GA et al: Exercise, lipids, and lipoproteins in older adults: a meta-analysis. Prev Cardiol 2005;8:206. [PMID: 16230875]

Maron DJ et al: Cholesterol-lowering effect of a theaflavin enriched green tea extract: a randomized controlled trial. Arch Intern Med 2003;163:1448. [PMID: 12824094]

Miettinen TA et al: Plant stanol and sterol esters in prevention of cardiovascular diseases. Ann Med 2004;36:126. [PMID: 15119832]

Moreyra AE et al: Effect of combining psyllium fiber with simvastatin in lowering cholesterol. Arch Intern Med 2005;165:1161. [PMID: 15911730]

Mukuddem-Petersen J et al: A systematic review of the effects of nuts on blood lipid profiles in humans. J Nutr 2005;135:2082. [PMID: 16140880]

Pignone MP et al: Counseling to promote a healthy diet in adults: a summary of the evidence for the U.S. Preventive Services Task Force. Am J Prev Med 2003;24:75. [PMID: 12554027]

Sacks FM et al: Soy protein, isoflavones, and cardiovascular health. An American Heart Association Science Advisory for professionals from the Nutrition Committee. Circulation 2006;113:1034. [PMID: 16418439]

Pharmacologic Therapy

All patients whose risk from CHD is considered high enough to warrant pharmacologic therapy of an elevated LDL cholesterol should be given aspirin prophylaxis at a dose of 81 mg/d unless there are contraindications such as aspirin sensitivity, bleeding diatheses, or active peptic ulcer disease. The benefit of aspirin in reducing the risk of CHD is equivalent to that of cholesterol lowering. Other CHD risk factors, such as hypertension and smoking, should also be controlled.

If the decision to treat a patient with an LDL-lowering drug is made, a goal for treatment is set. The National Cholesterol Education Program's Adult Treatment Panel III (NCEP ATP III) published revised, more intensive LDL treatment goals in 2004. For patients with CHD or CHD risk equivalents, the goal is LDL < 100 mg/dL, but for patients with very high risk, a goal of LDL < 70 mg/dL is a therapeutic option (see Table 28–3). This goal may also be appropriate for patients with very high risk who have a baseline LDL < 100 mg/dL. For patients with two or more risk factors and a 10-year CHD risk of 10–20%, the recommended goal is LDL < 130 mg/dL, but a goal of < 100 mg/dL is optional. For those with two or more risk factors and a 10-year CHD risk of < 10%, the goal is < 130 mg/dL. For those with zero or one risk factor, the goal is LDL < 160 mg/dL (see Table 28–3). In each instance, the therapeutic goal is approached slowly, watching for side effects and encouraging continued adherence to nonpharmacologic therapies. In most instances, intensity of therapy should be sufficient to achieve a 30–40% reduction in LDL cholesterol. Combinations of drugs may be necessary. Once the goal is reached, the lipid profile should be monitored periodically (every 6–12 months), with consideration given to periodic reductions in drug dose. Most lipid-lowering agents are expensive and may need to be given for decades. Thus, their cost effectiveness is low for some groups of patients, especially in primary prevention.

A. NIACIN (NICOTINIC ACID)

Niacin was the first lipid-lowering agent that was associated with a reduction in total mortality. Long-term follow-up of a secondary prevention trial of middle-aged men with previous myocardial infarction disclosed that about half of those who had been previously treated with niacin had died, compared with nearly 60% of the placebo group. This favorable effect on mortality was not seen during the trial itself, though there was a reduction in the incidence of recurrent coronary events.

Niacin reduces the production of VLDL particles, with secondary reduction in LDL and increases in HDL cholesterol levels. Studies have identified a niacin receptor in both adipocytes and hepatocytes. Niacin binding leads to reduction of lipolysis of triglycerides in adipocytes, reduced synthesis of triglycerides in the liver, and reduced hepatic production of VLDL. The average effect of full-dose niacin therapy, 3–4.5 g/d, is a 15–25% reduction in LDL cholesterol and a 25–35% increase in HDL cholesterol. Full doses are required to obtain the LDL effect, but the HDL effect is observed at lower doses, eg, 1 g/d. Niacin will also reduce triglycerides by half and will lower lipoprotein(a) (Lp[a]) levels and will increase plasma homocysteine levels. Thus, its effect on blood lipids and CHD risk is nearly optimal. Intolerance to niacin is common; only 50–60% of patients can take full doses. Niacin causes a prostaglandin-mediated flushing that patients may describe as "hot flashes" or pruritus and that can be decreased with aspirin (81–325 mg/d) or other nonsteroidal anti-inflammatory agents taken during the same day. Flushing may also be decreased by initiating niacin therapy with a very small dose, eg, 100 mg with the evening meal. The dose can be doubled each week until 1.5 g/d is tolerated. After rechecking blood lipids, the dose is divided and increased until the goal of 3–4.5 g/d is reached. Extended-release niacin is also available and is better tolerated by most patients. It is not known whether routine monitoring of liver enzymes results in early detection and thus reduced severity of this side effect. Niacin can also exacerbate gout and peptic ulcer disease. Although niacin may increase blood sugar in some patients, clinical trials have shown that niacin can be safely used in diabetics.

B. BILE ACID–BINDING RESINS

The bile acid–binding resins include cholestyramine, colesevelam, and colestipol. Treatment with these agents reduces the incidence of coronary events in middle-aged men by about 20%, with no significant effect on total mortality. The resins work by binding bile acids in the intestine. The resultant reduction in the enterohepatic circulation causes the liver to increase its production of bile acids, using hepatic cholesterol to do so. Thus, hepatic LDL receptor activity increases, with a decline in plasma LDL levels. The triglyceride level tends to increase slightly in some patients treated with bile acid–binding resins; they should be used with caution in those with elevated triglycerides and probably not at all in patients who have triglyceride levels above 500 mg/dL. The clinician can anticipate a reduction of 15–25% in the LDL cholesterol level, with insignificant effects on the HDL level.

The usual dose of cholestyramine is 12–36 g of resin per day in divided doses with meals, mixed in water or, more palatably, juice. Doses of colestipol are

20% higher (each packet contains 5 g of resin). The dose of colesevelam is 625 mg, 6–7 tablets per day.

These agents often cause gastrointestinal symptoms, such as constipation and gas. They may interfere with the absorption of fat-soluble vitamins (thereby complicating the management of patients receiving warfarin) and may bind other drugs in the intestine. Concurrent use of psyllium may ameliorate the gastrointestinal side effects.

C. HYDROXYMETHYLGLUTARYL-COENZYME A (HMG-CoA) REDUCTASE INHIBITORS (STATINS)

The HMG-CoA reductase inhibitors include atorvastatin, fluvastatin, lovastatin, pravastatin, rosuvastatin, and simvastatin. These agents work by inhibiting the rate-limiting enzyme in the formation of cholesterol. They reduce myocardial infarctions and total mortality in secondary prevention, as well as in older middle-aged men free of CHD. A meta-analysis has demonstrated significant reduction in risk of stroke. Cholesterol synthesis in the liver is reduced, with a compensatory increase in hepatic LDL receptors (presumably so that the liver can take more of the cholesterol that it needs from the blood) and a reduction in the circulating LDL cholesterol level by up to 35%. There are also modest increases in HDL levels and decreases in triglyceride levels.

Oral doses are as follows: atorvastatin, 10–80 mg/d; fluvastatin, 20–40 mg/d; lovastatin, 10–80 mg/d; pravastatin, 10–40 mg/d; rosuvastatin, 5–40 mg/d; and simvastatin, 5–40 mg/d. These agents are usually given once a day in the evening (most cholesterol synthesis takes place overnight); at the high end of the dose ranges, twice-a-day dosing may be used. Side effects include myositis, whose incidence may be higher in patients concurrently taking fibrates or niacin. Manufacturers recommend monitoring liver and muscle enzymes. Several agents (notably erythromycin, cyclosporine, and azole antifungals) reduce the metabolism of these agents.

D. FIBRIC ACID DERIVATIVES

The fibric acid derivatives or fibrates approved for use in the United States are gemfibrozil and fenofibrate. Ciprofibrate and bezafibrate are also available for use internationally. Gemfibrozil reduced CHD rates in hypercholesterolemic middle-aged men free of coronary disease in the Helsinki Heart Study. The effect was observed only among those who also had lower HDL cholesterol levels and high triglyceride levels. In a recent VA study, gemfibrozil was also shown to reduce cardiovascular events in men with existing CHD whose primary lipid abnormality was a low HDL cholesterol. There was no effect on all-cause mortality.

The fibrates are peroxisome proliferator-activated receptor-alpha (PPAR-alpha) agonists that result in potent reductions of plasma triglycerides and increases in HDL cholesterol. They reduce LDL levels by about 10–15%, although the result is quite variable, and triglyceride levels by about 40% and raise HDL levels by about 15–20%. The usual dose of gemfibrozil is 600 mg once or twice a day. Side effects include cholelithiasis, hepatitis, and myositis. The incidence of the latter two conditions may be higher among patients also taking other lipid-lowering agents. In the largest clinical trial that used clofibrate, there were significantly more deaths—especially due to cancer—in the treatment group; it should not be used.

E. EZETIMIBE

Ezetimibe is a lipid-lowering drug that inhibits the intestinal absorption of dietary and biliary cholesterol by blocking passage across the intestinal wall by inhibiting a newly discovered cholesterol transporter. Ezetimibe reduces LDL cholesterol between 15% and 20% when used as monotherapy and can further reduce LDL in patients taking statins who are not yet at therapeutic goal. The effects of ezetimide on CHD and its long-term safety are not yet known. The usual dose of ezetimibe is 10 mg/d orally.

Initial Selection of Medication

At present there are no absolute guidelines for selection of available lipid-modifying medications in particular patients. Nonetheless, clinical trials provide guidance (Table 28–4). For most patients who require a lipid-modifying medication, an HMG-CoA reductase inhibitor is preferred. Although niacin will also have beneficial effects on lipids in both men and women with CHD, there is less evidence demonstrating the desired effects on CHD and all-cause mortality. Resins are the only lipid-modifying medication considered safe in pregnancy.

Combinations of lipid-modifying medications may be more cost-effective than high doses of a single medication (usually an HMG-CoA reductase inhibitor) and may have beneficial effects on lipids. Combination therapy may also be needed to meet lower NCEP targets in some patients or to achieve other therapeutic goals. Low-dose niacin (0.5–1 g/d), for example, will substantially increase the HDL cholesterol when added to an HMG-CoA reductase inhibitor. Combinations, however, may increase the risk of complications of drug therapy. The combination of gemfibrozil and HMG-CoA reductase inhibitors increases the risk of myopathy more than either drug alone.

Birjmohun RS et al: Efficacy and safety of high-density lipoprotein cholesterol-increasing compounds: a meta-analysis of randomized controlled trials. J Am Coll Cardiol 2005;45: 185. [PMID: 15653014]

Brewer HB Jr: Increasing HDL cholesterol levels. N Engl J Med 2004;350:1491. [PMID: 15071124]

Brousseau ME et al: Effects of an inhibitor of cholesteryl ester transfer protein on HDL cholesterol. N Engl J Med 2004; 350:1505. [PMID: 15071125]

Bruckert E et al: Perspectives in cholesterol-lowering therapy: the role of ezetimibe, a new selective inhibitor of intestinal cholesterol absorption. Circulation 2003;107:3124. [PMID: 12835406]

Chapman MJ et al: Raising high-density lipoprotein cholesterol with reduction of cardiovascular risk: the role of nicotinic acid—a position paper developed by the European Consensus Panel on HDL-C. Curr Med Res Opin 2004;20:1253. [PMID: 15324528]

Dale KM et al: Statins and cancer risk: a meta-analysis. JAMA 2006;295:74. [PMID: 16391219]

Ferdinand KC: The importance of aggressive lipid management in patients at risk: evidence from recent clinical trials. Clin Cardiol 2004;27(6 Suppl 3):III12. [PMID: 15239486]

Grundy SM et al: Implications of recent clinical trials for the National Cholesterol Education Program Adult Treatment Panel III Guidelines. J Am Coll Cardiol 2004;44:720. [PMID: 15358046]

Kwiterovich PO: A review of lipid-modifying drugs used alone or in combination. Adv Stud Med 2005;5:475.

Miller M: Intensive versus moderate lipid lowering with statins after acute coronary syndromes. N Engl J Med 2004;351:714. [PMID: 15309746]

Mozaffarian D et al: Statin therapy is associated with lower mortality among patients with severe heart failure. Am J Cardiol 2004;93:1124. [PMID: 15110204]

Nissen SE et al: Effect of intensive compared with moderate lipid-lowering therapy on progression of coronary atherosclerosis: a randomized controlled trial. JAMA 2004;291:1071. [PMID: 14996776]

Thompson PD et al: Statin-associated myopathy. JAMA 2003; 289:1681. [PMID: 12672737]

Whitney EJ et al: A randomized trial of a strategy for increasing high-density lipoprotein cholesterol levels: effects on progression of coronary heart disease and clinical events. Ann Intern Med 2005;142:95. [PMID: 15657157]

Wilt TJ et al: Effectiveness of statin therapy in adults with coronary heart disease. Arch Intern Med 2004;164:1427. [PMID: 15249352]

HIGH BLOOD TRIGLYCERIDES

Patients with very high levels of serum triglycerides are at risk for pancreatitis. The pathophysiology is not certain, since pancreatitis never develops in some patients with very high triglyceride levels. Most patients with congenital abnormalities in triglyceride metabolism present in childhood; hypertriglyceridemia-induced pancreatitis first presenting in adults is more commonly due to an acquired problem in lipid metabolism.

Although there are no clear triglyceride levels that predict pancreatitis, most clinicians are uncomfortable with fasting levels above 500 mg/dL. The risk of pancreatitis may be more related to the triglyceride level following consumption of a fatty meal. Because postprandial increases in triglyceride are inevitable if fat-containing foods are eaten, fasting triglyceride levels in persons prone to pancreatitis should be kept well below that level.

The primary therapy for high triglyceride levels is dietary, avoiding alcohol, simple sugars, refined starches, saturated and trans fatty acids, and restricting total calories. Control of secondary causes of high triglyceride levels (see Table 28–1) may also be helpful. In patients with fasting triglycerides ≥ 500 mg/dL despite adequate dietary compliance—and certainly in those with a pre-

Table 28–4. Effects of selected lipid-modifying drugs.

Drug	Lipid-Modifying Effects			Initial Daily Dose	Maximum Daily Dose	Cost for 30 Days Treatment with Dose Listed[1]
	LDL	HDL	Triglyceride			
Atorvastatin (Lipitor)	–25 to –40%	+5 to 10%	↓↓	10 mg once	80 mg once	$118.70 (20 mg once)
Cholestyramine (Questran, others)	–15 to –25%	+5%	±	4 g twice a day	24 g divided	$126.68 (8 g divided)
Colesevelam (WelChol)	–10 to –20%	+10%	±	625 mg, 6–7 tablets once	625 mg, 6–7 tablets once	$181.44 (6 tablets once)
Colestipol (Colestid)	–15 to –25%	+5%	±	5 g twice a day	30 g divided	$120.92 (10 g divided)
Ezetimibe (Zetia)	–20%	+5%	±	10 mg once	10 mg once	$86.56 (10 mg once)
Fluvastatin (Lescol)	–20 to –30%	+5 to 10%	↓	20 mg once	40 mg once	$68.10 (20 mg once)
Gemfibrozil (Lopid)	–10 to –15%	+15 to 20%	↓↓	600 mg once	1200 mg divided	$74.80 (600 mg twice a day)
Lovastatin (Mevacor)	–25 to –40%	+5 to 10%	↓	10 mg once	80 mg divided	$71.15 (20 mg once)
Niacin (OTC, Niaspan)	–15 to –25%	+25 to 35%	↓↓	100 mg once	3–4.5 g divided	$7.20 (1.5 g twice a day, OTC) $201.60 (2 g Niaspan)
Pravastatin (Pravachol)	–25 to –40%	+5 to 10%	↓	20 mg once	40 mg once	$104.55 (20 mg once)
Rosuvastatin (Crestor)	–40 to –50%	+10 to 15%	↓↓	10 mg once	40 mg once	$94.54 (20 mg once)
Simvastatin (Zocor)	–25 to –40%	+5 to 10%	↓↓	5 mg once	80 mg once	$90.30 (10 mg once)

[1]Average wholesale price (AWP, for AB-rated generic when available) for quantity listed. Source: *Red Book Update*, Vol. 25, No. 5, May 2006. AWP may not accurately represent the actual pharmacy cost because wide contractual variations exist among institutions. LDL = low-density lipoprotein; HDL = high-density lipoprotein; ± = variable, if any; OTC = over the counter.

vious episode of pancreatitis—therapy with a triglyceride-lowering drug (eg, niacin, a fibric acid derivative, or an HMG-CoA reductase inhibitor) is indicated.

Whether patients with elevated triglycerides (> 150 mg/dL) should be treated to prevent CHD is not known. Meta-analysis of 17 observational studies suggests that after adjustment for other risk factors, elevated triglycerides increased CHD risk in men by 14% and in women by 37%. Triglyceride-rich lipoproteins (partially degraded VLDL, commonly called remnant lipoproteins) have been found in human atheromas, and elevated triglycerides are associated with small dense LDL in most instances. Elevated triglycerides are also an important feature of the **metabolic syndrome**, found in an estimated 25% of Americans—defined by three or more of the following five abnormalities: waist circumference > 102 cm in men or > 88 cm in women, serum triglyceride level of at

least 150 mg/dL, HDL level of < 40 mg/dL in men or < 50 mg/dL in women, blood pressure of at least 130/85 mm Hg, and serum glucose level of at least 110 mg/dL. Other data, however, suggest that triglyceride measurements do not improve discrimination between those with and without CHD events, and clinical trial data are not available to support the routine treatment of high triglycerides in all patients.

The NCEP ATP III guidelines, however, recommend an aggressive approach to triglyceride management. For those with borderline levels (150–199 mg/dL), emphasis is placed on calorie restriction and exercise. For patients with high triglycerides (> 200 mg/dL), the non-HDL cholesterol should be measured (total cholesterol – HDL cholesterol). The ATP III report recommends that non-HDL cholesterol should be treated with diet and medications to result in levels 30 mg/dL higher than the LDL goal. The ATP III report does not differentiate between primary and secondary prevention. It is reasonable to use this approach for patients with CHD and risk equivalents for that disease but not for lower-risk patients.

Garber AJ: The metabolic syndrome. Med Clin North Am 2004; 88:837. [PMID: 15308381]

Katzmarzyk PT et al: Metabolic syndrome, obesity, and mortality: impact of cardiorespiratory fitness. Diabetes Care 2005; 28:391. [PMID: 15677798]

Moller DE et al: Metabolic syndrome: a clinical and molecular perspective. Annu Rev Med 2005;56:45. [PMID: 15660501]

Park Y et al: The metabolic syndrome: prevalence and associated risk factor findings in the US population from the Third National Health and Nutrition Examination Survey, 1988-1994. Arch Intern Med 2003;163:427. [PMID: 12588201]

Szapary PO et al: The triglyceride-high-density lipoprotein axis: an important target of therapy? Am Heart J 2004;148:211. [PMID: 15308990]

Nutrition

29

Robert B. Baron, MD, MS

■ NUTRITIONAL REQUIREMENTS

Approximately 40 nutrients are required by the human body. Nutrients are essential if they cannot be synthesized by the body and if a deficiency causes recognizable abnormalities that disappear when the deficit is corrected. Required nutrients include the essential amino acids, water-soluble vitamins, fat-soluble vitamins, minerals, and the essential fatty acids. The body also requires an adequate energy substrate, a small amount of metabolizable carbohydrate, indigestible carbohydrate (fiber), additional nitrogen, and water.

Nutritional requirements have been most commonly expressed by recommended dietary allowances (RDAs). Published and periodically reviewed by the Food and Nutrition Board of the National Academy of Sciences, the RDAs were initially designed to meet the known nutritional needs of practically all healthy persons. RDAs have been established for carbohydrate and protein; the water-soluble vitamins thiamine, riboflavin, niacin, vitamin B_6, folate, vitamin B_{12}, and vitamin C; the fat-soluble vitamins A, D, and E; and the minerals copper, phosphorus, magnesium, iron, zinc, iodine, molybdenum, and selenium.

The Food and Nutrition Board has since developed a broader approach to defining nutritional adequacy. Known as dietary reference intakes (DRIs), these new guidelines go beyond the prevention of classic nutritional deficiency diseases and address the role of nutrients and other food components in long-term health and the reduction of risk of chronic diseases. The DRIs consist of four reference intakes: the RDA, the estimated average requirement (EAR), the tolerable upper intake level (UL), and the adequate intake (AI). The RDA remains the dietary intake that is sufficient to meet the nutritional requirements of nearly all individuals in an age- and gender-specific group. RDAs are intended as goals for individuals. The EAR is the intake value that is estimated to meet the requirements of 50% of individuals in an age- and gender-specific group. The UL is the maximum level of daily nutrient intake that is unlikely to pose health risks to most individuals. The AI is determined when insufficient data are available to establish the EAR and RDA for a given nutrient. It is based on fewer data and more expert opinion but is also intended as goals for individuals. The DRIs for vitamins, elements, and macronutrients are shown in Tables 29–1, 29–2 and 29–3.

ENERGY

The body requires energy to support normal functions and physical activity, growth, and repair of damaged tissues. Energy is provided by oxidation of dietary protein, fat, carbohydrate, and alcohol. Oxidation of 1 g of each provides 4 kcal of energy from protein and carbohydrate, 9 kcal from fat, and 7 kcal from alcohol.

In healthy adults, energy expenditure is primarily determined by three factors: basal energy expenditure (BEE), thermic effect of food (TEF), and physical activity.

The BEE is the amount of energy required to maintain basic physiologic functions. It is measured while the subject is resting in a warm room, not having eaten for 12 hours. In healthy persons, the BEE (in kcal/24 h) can be estimated by the Harris–Benedict equation, which will correctly predict measured BEE in 90% ± 10% of healthy subjects (See Nutritional Support, below). In clinical practice, patients rarely meet the strict criteria for BEE measurement. Instead, energy expenditure is measured in individuals at rest without food for 2 hours. This measurement, the resting energy expenditure (REE), is about 10% greater than BEE.

TEF, the amount of energy expended during and following the ingestion of food, averages approximately 10% of the BEE.

Physical activity has a major impact on energy expenditure. The average energy expenditure per hour by adults engaged in typical activities is shown in Table 29–4.

PROTEIN

Protein is required for growth and for maintenance of body structure and function. Although the nutritional requirement is commonly stated in grams of protein, the true requirement is for nine **essential amino acids** plus additional nitrogen for protein synthesis. The essential amino acids are leucine, isoleucine, lysine, methionine, phenylalanine, threonine, tryptophan, valine, and histidine.

Adequate protein must be consumed each day to replace essential amino acids lost through protein turnover. On a protein-free diet, the average male loses 3.8 g of ni-

Table 29–1. Dietary reference intakes: recommended intakes for individuals, vitamins.[1]

Life Stage Group	Vitamin A (mcg/d)[2]	Vitamin C (mg/d)	Vitamin D (mcg/d)[3,4]	Vitamin E (mg/d)[5]	Vitamin K (mcg/d)	Thiamin (mg/d)	Riboflavin (mg/d)	Niacin (mg/d)[6]	Vitamin B6 (mg/d)	Folate (mcg/d)[7]	Vitamin B12 (mcg/d)	Pantothenic Acid (mg/d)	Biotin (mcg/d)	Choline (mg/d)[8]
Infants														
0–6 months	400*	40*	5*	4*	2.0*	0.2*	0.3*	2*	0.1*	65*	0.4*	1.7*	5*	125*
7–12 months	500*	50*	5*	5*	2.5*	0.3*	0.4*	4*	0.3*	80*	0.5*	1.8*	6*	150*
Children														
1–3 years	300	15	5*	6	30*	0.5	0.5	6	0.5	150	0.9	2*	8*	200*
4–8 years	400	25	5*	7	55*	0.6	0.6	8	0.6	200	1.2	3*	12*	250*
Males														
9–13 years	600	45	5*	11	60*	0.9	0.9	12	1.0	300	1.8	4*	20*	375*
14–18 years	900	75	5*	15	75*	1.2	1.3	16	1.3	400	2.4	5*	25*	550*
19–30 years	900	90	5*	15	120*	1.2	1.3	16	1.3	400	2.4	5*	30*	550*
31–50 years	900	90	5*	15	120*	1.2	1.3	16	1.3	400	2.4	5*	30*	550*
51–70 years	900	90	10*	15	120*	1.2	1.3	16	1.7	400	2.4[9]	5*	30*	550*
>70 years	900	90	15*	15	120*	1.2	1.3	16	1.7	400	2.4[9]	5*	30*	550*
Females														
9–13 years	600	45	5*	11	60*	0.9	0.9	12	1.0	300	1.8	4*	20*	375*
14–18 years	700	65	5*	15	75*	1.0	1.0	14	1.2	400[10]	2.4	5*	25*	400*
19–30 years	700	75	5*	15	90*	1.1	1.1	14	1.3	400[10]	2.4	5*	30*	425*
31–50 years	700	75	5*	15	90*	1.1	1.1	14	1.3	400[10]	2.4	5*	30*	425*
51–70 years	700	75	10*	15	90*	1.1	1.1	14	1.5	400	2.4[9]	5*	30*	425*
>70 years	700	75	15*	15	90*	1.1	1.1	14	1.5	400	2.4[9]	5*	30*	425*
Pregnancy														
14–18 years	750	80	5*	15	75*	1.4	1.4	18	1.9	600[11]	2.6	6*	30*	450*
19–30 years	770	85	5*	15	90*	1.4	1.4	18	1.9	600[11]	2.6	6*	30*	450*
31–50 years	770	85	5*	15	90*	1.4	1.4	18	1.9	600[11]	2.6	6*	30*	450*
Lactation														
14–18 years	1200	115	5*	19	75*	1.4	1.6	17	2.0	500	2.8	7*	35*	550*
19–30 years	1300	120	5*	19	90*	1.4	1.6	17	2.0	500	2.8	7*	35*	550*
31–50 years	1300	120	5*	19	90*	1.4	1.6	17	2.0	500	2.8	7*	35*	550*

[1]Taken from the DRI reports, see www.nap.edu. Recommended dietary allowances (RDAs) are in **bold type** and adequate intakes (AIs) in ordinary type followed by an asterisk (*). RDAs and AIs may both be used as goals for individual intake. RDAs are set to meet the needs of 97–98% of individuals in a group. AIs are believed to cover the needs of all individuals in a group, though lack of or uncertainty in data prevents specification of the percentage of individuals covered by this intake.

[2]As retinol activity equivalents (RAEs); 1 RAE = 1 mcg retinol, 12 mcg β-carotene, 24 mcg α-carotene, or 24 mcg β-cryptoxanthin. To calculate RAEs from REs of provitamin A carotenoids in foods, divide the REs by 2. For preformed vitamin A in foods or supplements and for provitamin A carotenoids in supplements, 1 RE = 1 RAE.

[3]As calciferol: 1 mcg calciferol = 40 international units vitamin D.

[4]In the absence of adequate exposure to sunlight.

[5]As α-tocopherol. α-Tocopherol includes RRR-α-tocopherol that occurs naturally in foods, and the $2R$-stereoisomeric forms of α-tocopherol (RRR-, RSR-, RRS-, and RSS-α-tocopherol) that occur in fortified foods and supplements. It does not include the $2S$-stereoisomeric forms of α-tocopherol (SRR-, SSR-, SRS-, and SSS-α-tocopherol), also found in fortified foods and supplements.

[6]As niacin equivalents (NE): 1 mg of niacin = 60 mg of tryptophan; 0–6 months = preformed niacin (not NE).

[7]As dietary folate equivalents (DFE): 1 DFE = 1 mcg food folate = 0.6 mcg of folic acid from fortified food or as a supplement consumed with food = 0.5 mcg of a supplement taken on an empty stomach.

[8]AIs have been set for choline, but there are few data to assess whether dietary choline is needed at all life stages; endogenous synthesis may suffice at some life stages.

[9]Because 10–30% of older people may malabsorb food-bound B_{12}, patients older than age 50 years should meet their RDA mainly by consuming foods fortified with B_{12} or a B_{12} supplement.

[10]Because evidence links deficient folate intake with neural tube defects in the fetus, it is recommended that all women capable of becoming pregnant consume 400 mcg of folate from supplements or fortified foods in addition to intake of food folate.

[11]Women must continue to consume 400 mcg of folate from supplements or fortified food until pregnancy is confirmed and prenatal care begins, ordinarily after the end of the periconceptional period—the critical time for formation of the neural tube.

Reproduced, with permission, from Institute of Medicine: Committee on Use of Dietary Reference Intakes in Nutrition Labeling. Dietary reference intakes: guiding principles for nutrition labeling and fortification. National Academy of Sciences, Washington, D.C., 2003, Table C-2.

Table 29–2. Dietary reference intakes: recommended intakes for individuals, elements.[1]

Life Stage Group	Calcium (mg/d)	Chromium (mcg/d)	Copper (mcg/d)	Fluoride (mg/d)	Iodine (mcg/d)	Iron (mg/d)	Magnesium (mg/d)	Manganese (mg/d)	Molybdenum (mcg/d)	Phosphorus (mg/d)	Selenium (mcg/d)	Zinc (mg/d)
Infants												
0–6 months	210*	0.2*	200*	0.01*	110*	0.27*	30*	0.003*	2*	100*	15*	2*
7–12 months	270*	5.5*	220*	0.5*	130*	11	75*	0.6*	3*	275*	20*	3
Children												
1–3 years	500*	11*	340	0.7*	90	7	80	1.2*	17	460	20	3
4–8 years	800*	15*	440	1*	90	10	130	1.5*	22	500	30	5
Males												
9–13 years	1300*	25*	700	2*	120	8	240	1.9*	34	1250	40	8
14–18 years	1300*	35*	890	3*	150	11	410	2.2*	43	1250	55	11
19–30 years	1000*	35*	900	4*	150	8	400	2.3*	45	700	55	11
31–50 years	1000*	35*	900	4*	150	8	420	2.3*	45	700	55	11
51–70 years	1200*	30*	900	4*	150	8	420	2.3*	45	700	55	11
>70 years	1200*	30*	900	4*	150	8	420	2.3*	45	700	55	11
Females												
9–13 years	1300*	21*	700	2*	120	8	240	1.6*	34	1250	40	8
14–18 years	1300*	24*	890	3*	150	15	360	1.6*	43	1250	55	9
19–30 years	1000*	25*	900	3*	150	18	310	1.8*	45	700	55	8
31–50 years	1000*	25*	900	3*	150	18	320	1.8*	45	700	55	8
51–70 years	1200*	20*	900	3*	150	8	320	1.8*	45	700	55	8
>70 years	1200*	20*	900	3*	150	8	320	1.8*	45	700	55	8
Pregnancy												
14–18 years	1300*	29*	1000	3*	220	27	400	2.0*	50	1250	60	12
19–30 years	1000*	30*	1000	3*	220	27	350	2.0*	50	700	60	11
31–50 years	1000*	30*	1000	3*	220	27	360	2.0*	50	700	60	11
Lactation												
14–18 years	1300*	44*	1300	3*	290	10	360	2.6*	50	1250	70	13
19–30 years	1000*	45*	1300	3*	290	9	310	2.6*	50	700	70	12
31–50 years	1000*	45*	1300	3*	290	9	320	2.6*	50	700	70	12

[1]Recommended dietary allowances (RDAs) are in **bold type** and adequate intakes (AIs) in ordinary type followed by an asterisk (*). RDAs and AIs may both be used as goals for individual intake. RDAs are set to meet the needs of 97–98% of individuals in a group. AIs are believed to cover the needs of all individuals in a group, though lack of or uncertainty in data prevents specification of the percentage of individuals covered by this intake.

Reproduced, with permission, from Institute of Medicine: Committee on Use of Dietary Reference Intakes in Nutrition Labeling. Dietary reference intakes: guiding principles for nutrition labeling and fortification. National Academy of Sciences, Washington, D.C., 2003, Table C-3.

Table 29–3. Dietary reference intakes: recommended intakes for individuals, macronutrients.[1]

Life Stage Group	Carbohydrate (g/d)	Total Fiber (g/d)	Fat (g/d)	Linoleic Acid (g/d)	α-Linolenic Acid (g/d)	Protein[2] (g/d)
Infants						
0–6 months	60*	ND	31*	4.4*	0.5*	9.1*
7–12 months	95*	ND	30*	4.6*	0.5*	**13.5**
Children						
1–3 years	**130**	19*	ND	7*	0.7*	**13**
4–8 years	**130**	25*	ND	10*	0.9*	**19**
Males						
9–13 years	**130**	26*	ND	12*	1.2*	**34**
14–18 years	**130**	38*	ND	16*	1.6*	**52**
19–30 years	**130**	38*	ND	17*	1.6*	**56**
31–50 years	**130**	38*	ND	17*	1.6*	**56**
51–70 years	**130**	30*	ND	14*	1.6*	**56**
> 70 years	**130**	30*	ND	14*	1.6*	**56**
Females						
9–13 years	**130**	31*	ND	10*	1.0*	**34**
14–18 years	**130**	26*	ND	11*	1.1*	**46**
19–30 years	**130**	25*	ND	12*	1.1*	**46**
31–50 years	**130**	25*	ND	12*	1.1*	**46**
51–70 years	**130**	21*	ND	11*	1.1*	**46**
> 70 years	**130**	21*	ND	11*	1.1*	**46**
Pregnancy						
14–18 years	**175**	28*	ND	13*	1.4*	**71**
19–30 years	**175**	28*	ND	13*	1.4*	**71**
31–50 years	**175**	28*	ND	13*	1.4*	**71**
Lactation						
14–18 years	**210**	29*	ND	13*	1.3*	**71**
19–30 years	**210**	29*	ND	13*	1.3*	**71**
31–50 years	**210**	29*	ND	13*	1.3*	**71**

[1]Recommended dietary allowances (RDAs) are in **bold type** and adequate intakes (AIs) in ordinary type followed by an asterisk (*). RDAs and AIs may both be used as goals for individual intake. RDAs are set to meet the needs of 97–98% of individuals in a group. AIs are believed to cover the needs of all individuals in a group, though lack of or uncertainty in data prevents specification of the percentage of individuals covered by this intake.

[2]Based on 0.8 g protein/kg body weight for reference body weight.

Reproduced, with permission, from Institute of Medicine. Committee on Use of Dietary Reference Intakes in Nutrition Labeling: Dietary reference intakes: guiding principles for nutrition labeling and fortification. National Academy of Sciences, Washington, D.C., 2003, Table C-4.

trogen per day—equivalent to 24 g of protein. Allowing for differences in protein quality and utilization and for individual variability, the RDA for protein is 56 g/d for men and 45 g/d for women.

Protein and energy requirements are closely related. Diets that provide insufficient energy will require additional protein to maintain nitrogen equilibrium.

CARBOHYDRATE

A small amount of carbohydrate—approximately 100 g/d—is necessary to prevent ketosis. In practice, however, a substantial portion of dietary energy should be provided by carbohydrate. The average American diet contains 45% of calories as carbohydrate. Dietary carbohydrates include simple sugars, complex carbohydrates (starches), and indigestible carbohydrates (dietary fiber). The bulk of dietary carbohydrates should be derived from starches as found in whole grains and from sugars as found in fruits and vegetables. Sucrose and other forms of added sugar such as high fructose corn syrup are concentrated sources of calories without other sources of essential nutrients and contribute to excess calorie consumption. Sucrose consumption is also thought to be an important factor in the development of tooth decay. Starches, when unrefined, provide carbohydrate calories and vitamins, minerals, and dietary fiber.

Table 29–4. Average energy kilocalories expended per hour by adults at selected weights engaged in various activities.

Activity	54 kg (120 lb)	64 kg (140 lb)	73 kg (160 lb)	82 kg (180 lb)	91 kg (200 lb)	100 kg (220 lb)
Sleeping: Reclining	50	58	69	78	86	99
Very light: Sitting	73	83	103	115	127	150
Light: Walking on level, shopping, light housekeeping	143	166	200	225	250	290
Moderate: Cycling, dancing, skiing, tennis	226	262	307	345	382	430
Heavy: Walking uphill, shoveling, swimming, playing basketball or football	440	512	598	670	746	840

Data from McArdle WD, Katch FI, Katch VL: *Exercise Physiology: Energy, Nutrition and Human Performance.* Lea & Febiger, 1981.
Note: Range of rate of expenditure of calories per minute of activity (for a 70-kg man or a 58-kg woman): Sleeping, 0.9–1.2; very light, 1.5–2.5; light, 2–4.9; moderate, 5–7.4; and heavy, 6–12.

Dietary fiber is that portion of plant foods that cannot be digested by the human intestine. Fiber increases the bulk of the stool and facilitates excretion. Diets high in dietary fiber are associated with a lower incidence of digestive and cardiovascular diseases. The more insoluble fibers, such as those found in wheat bran, have the greatest effect on colonic function. Soluble fibers such as those found in legumes, oats, and fruit result in lower blood sugar levels in diabetics and lower blood cholesterol.

FAT

Dietary fat is the most concentrated source of food energy. Like energy from dietary carbohydrate, energy derived from fat can support protein synthesis. Dietary fat also provides the essential fatty acid linoleic acid. Other than the need for adequate quantities of linoleic acid, there is no specific requirement for dietary fat as long as the diet provides adequate nutrients oxidizable for energy. Although the average American diet contains 35–40% of calories as fat, current recommendations are to limit dietary fat to 20–35% of total calories. Diets containing as little as 5–10% of total calories as fat appear to be safe and well tolerated.

Dietary fats are composed primarily of fatty acids and dietary cholesterol. Fatty acids contain either no double bonds (saturated), one double bond (monounsaturated), or more than one double bond (polyunsaturated). Saturated fatty acids are associated with increased serum cholesterol, whereas polyunsaturated and monounsaturated fatty acids lower serum cholesterol. Trans-fatty acids, a particular form of unsaturated fat found in partially hydrogenated vegetable oils, also raise serum cholesterol levels. Saturated fats are solid at room temperature and in general are derived from animal foods; unsaturated fats are liquid at room temperature and in general are derived from plant foods.

The polyunsaturated fatty acid **linoleic acid** is an essential nutrient, required by the body for the synthesis of arachidonic acid, the major precursor of prostaglan-

dins. Deficiency of linoleic acid results in dermatitis, hair loss, and impaired wound healing. For individuals with average energy requirements, approximately 5 g of linoleic acid per day—1–2% of total calories—is required to prevent essential fatty acid deficiency.

Cholesterol is a major constituent of cell membranes. It is synthesized by the body and is not an essential nutrient. Diets that contain large amounts of cholesterol partially inhibit endogenous cholesterol synthesis but result in a net increase in serum cholesterol concentrations because of suppression of synthesis of low-density lipoprotein receptors. Average American diets contain approximately 450 mg/d of cholesterol, but 300 mg or less per day is recommended.

VITAMINS

Vitamins are a heterogeneous group of organic molecules required by the body for a variety of essential metabolic functions. They are grouped as **water-soluble vitamins:** thiamine, riboflavin, niacin, vitamin B_6 (pyridoxine), vitamin B_{12} (cobalamin), folate, pantothenic acid, biotin, and vitamin C (ascorbic acid); and **fat-soluble vitamins:** A, D, E, and K. Disorders of vitamin metabolism are discussed below.

MINERALS

The body also requires a number of inorganic minerals, commonly grouped as the **major minerals** calcium, magnesium, and phosphorus; the **electrolytes** sodium, potassium, and chloride; and the **trace elements** iron, zinc, copper, manganese, molybdenum, fluoride, iodine, cobalt, chromium, and selenium. Important characteristics of major minerals and electrolytes are summarized in Table 29–5.

DRUG-NUTRIENT INTERACTIONS

Many medications affect nutritional requirements. A variety of drugs induce nutrient deficiencies by appe-

Table 29–5. Essential macrominerals: summary of major characteristics.

Elements	Functions	Deficiency Disease or Symptoms	Toxicity Disease or Symptoms[1]
Calcium	Constituent of bones, teeth; regulation of nerve, muscle function.	Children: rickets. Adults: osteomalacia. May contribute to osteoporosis.	Occurs with excess absorption due to hypervitaminosis D or hypercalcemia due to hyperparathyroidism or other causes of hypercalcemia.
Phosphorus	Constituent of bones, teeth, adenosine triphosphate, phosphorylated metabolic intermediates. Nucleic acids.	Children: rickets. Adults: osteomalacia.	Low serum Ca^{2+}:P_i ratio stimulates secondary hyperparathyroidism; may lead to bone loss.
Sodium	Principal cation in extracellular fluid. Regulates plasma volume, acid-base balance, nerve and muscle function, Na^+-K^+-ATPase.	Unknown on normal diet, secondary to injury or illness.	Hypertension (in susceptible individuals).
Potassium	Principal cation in intracellular fluid; nerve and muscle function, Na^+-K^+-ATPase.	Occurs secondary to illness, injury, or diuretic therapy; muscular weakness, paralysis, mental confusion.	Cardiac arrest, small bowel ulcers.
Chloride	Fluid and electrolyte balance; gastric fluid.	Infants fed salt-free formula. Secondary to vomiting, diuretic therapy, renal disease.	Cardiac arrest, small bowel ulcers.
Magnesium	Constituent of bones, teeth; enzyme cofactor (kinases, etc.).	Secondary to malabsorption or diarrhea, alcoholism.	Depressed deep tendon reflexes and respiration.

[1]Excess mineral intake produces toxic symptoms. Unless otherwise specified, symptoms include nonspecific nausea, diarrhea, and irritability.
Modified from Murray RK et al: *Harper's Biochemistry*, 25th ed. Appleton & Lange, 1998.

tite suppression, intestinal malabsorption, and alterations in nutrient metabolism or excretion. The effects of selected drugs on nutrient absorption and metabolism are summarized in Table 29–6.

DIETARY GUIDELINES

Over the past two and a half decades, numerous authorities have published dietary guidelines that make specific nutritional recommendations. Dietary Guidelines for Americans were published by the U.S. Department of Health and Human Services and the U.S. Department of Agriculture in January 2005. These guidelines reinforce many long-standing nutritional principles while also placing greater emphasis on several recent observations. Key recommendations in the new guidelines include the following: limit the intake of saturated fat, trans fat, cholesterol, added sugars, salt, and alcohol; balance calories from food and beverages with calories expended; engage in regular physical activity at least 30–60 minutes most days of the week; consume greater quantities (up to 9 servings per day) and more varieties of fruits and vegetables per day; consume at least half of the daily grains as whole grains; consume 3 cups per day of low fat milk or milk products; consume less than 10% of calories as saturated fat, less than 300 mg/d of cholesterol, and as little trans-fatty acids as possible; consume fiber-rich fruits, vegetables, and whole grains; use little added sugars or caloric sweeteners; consume less than 2300

mg of sodium per day; use alcohol sensibly and in moderation; and prepare food safely. The guidelines also provide detailed suggestions of foods to consume to meet recommended nutrient intakes for 12 different calorie levels (Table 29–7).

Butte NF et al: Energy requirements of women of reproductive age. Am J Clin Nutr 2003;77:630. [PMID: 12600853]

Department of Health and Human Services and Department of Agriculture: Dietary Guidelines for Americans 2005. www.healthierus.gov.

Dwyer J et al: National Health and Nutrition Examination Survey. Estimation of usual intakes: What We Eat in America—NHANES. J Nutr 2003;133: 609S. [PMID: 12566511]

Howard BV et al: Low-fat dietary pattern and risk of cardiovascular disease: the Women's Health Initiative Randomized Controlled Dietary Modification Trial. JAMA 2006;295: 655. [PMID: 16467234]

Institute of Medicine: Committee on Use of Dietary Reference Intakes in Nutrition Labeling. Dietary reference intakes: guiding principles for nutrition labeling and fortification. National Academy of Sciences, Washington, D.C., 2003.

Niedert KC; American Dietetic Association: Position of the American Dietetic Association: Liberalization of the diet prescription improves quality of life for older adults in long-term care. J Am Diet Assoc 2005;105:1955. [PMID: 16402447]

Nicklas TA et al: The 2005 Dietary Guidelines Advisory Committee: developing a key message. J Am Diet Assoc 2005;105: 1418. [PMID: 16129084]

Rand WM et al: Meta-analysis of nitrogen balance studies for estimating protein requirements in healthy adults. Am J Clin Nutr 2003;77:109. [PMID: 12499330]

Table 29–6. Effect of drugs on nutrient absorption and metabolism.

Drug	Effect
Analgesics and anti-inflammatories	
Salicylates	Decrease serum ascorbic acid; increase urinary loss of ascorbic acid, potassium, and amino acids.
Sulfasalazine	Impairs folate absorption and antagonizes folate supplementation.
Antacids	
Aluminum antacids	Decrease absorption of phosphate and vitamin A.
H_2 blockers	Decrease iron and vitamin B_{12} absorption.
Octreotide acetate	Hypoglycemia and hyperglycemia; decreases fat and carotene absorption.
Anticonvulsants	
Phenobarbital	Decreases serum folate; increases vitamin D and vitamin K turnover and may cause deficiency.
Phenytoin	Decreases serum folate; increases vitamin D and vitamin K turnover and may cause deficiency.
Primidone	Decreases serum folate and vitamins B_6 and B_{12}; decreases calcium absorption; increases vitamin D and vitamin K turnover and may cause anxiety.
Antimicrobials	
Neomycin	Binds bile acids. Decreases absorption of fat and carotene; of vitamins A, D, K, and B_{12}; and of potassium, sodium, calcium, and nitrogen.
Amphotericin B	Decreases serum magnesium and potassium.
Aminosalicylic acid	Increases absorption of folate, vitamin B_{12}, iron, cholesterol, and fat.
Chloramphenicol	Increases need for vitamins B_2, B_6, B_{12}; increases serum iron.
Penicillin	Hypokalemia; renal potassium wasting.
Tetracycline	Calcium, iron, magnesium inhibit drug absorption; decreases vitamin K synthesis.
Cycloserine	May decrease absorption of calcium, magnesium; may decrease serum folate and vitamins B_6 and B_{12}; decreases protein synthesis.
Isoniazid	Vitamin B_6 antagonist; may cause deficiency.
Sulfonamide	Decreases absorption of folate; decreases serum folate, iron.
Nitrofurantoin	Decreases serum folate.
Pyrimethamine	Decreases serum B_{12} and folate.
Antimitotics	
Methotrexate	Decreases activation of folate.
Colchicine	Decreases absorption of vitamin B_{12}, carotene, fat, sodium, potassium, cholesterol, lactose, nitrogen.
Cathartics	
Phenolphthalein	Malabsorption, hypokalemia; deficiency of vitamin D, calcium.
Mineral oil	Malabsorption; decreased absorption of vitamins A, D, K.
Diuretics	Some cause hypokalemia, hypomagnesemia; may increase urinary excretion of vitamins B_1 and B_6; calcium, magnesium, potassium.
Hypocholesterolemics	
Cholestyramine	Binds bile acids; decreases absorption of fat, carotene; vitamins A, D, K, and B_{12}; folate, iron.
Clofibrate	Decreases absorption of carotene, vitamin B_{12}, iron, glucose.
Hypotensives	
Hydralazine	Vitamin B_6 deficiency.
Captopril	May cause hyponatremia, hyperkalemia; decreases taste acuity.
Oral contraceptives	Vitamin B_6, folate deficiency; may increase the need for other nutrients.

Table 29-7. USDA food guide.

Daily Amount of Food from Each Group (vegetable subgroup amounts are per week)												
Calorie level	1000	1200	1400	1600	1800	2000	2200	2400	2600	2800	3000	3200
Food group[2]	Food group amounts shown in cup (c) or ounce-equivalents (oz-eq), with number of servings (srv) in parentheses when it differs from the other units. See note for quantity equivalents for foods in each group.[3] Oils are shown in grams (g).											
Fruits	1 c (2 srv)	1 c (2 srv)	1.5 c (3 srv)	1.5 c (3 srv)	1.5 c (3 srv)	2 c (4 srv)	2 c (4 srv)	2 c (4 srv)	2 c (4 srv)	2.5 c (5 srv)	2.5 c (5 srv)	2.5 c (5 srv)
Vegetables[4]												
Dark green veg.	1 c/wk	1.5 c/wk	1.5 c/wk	2 c/wk	3 c/wk	3 c/wk	3 c/wk	3 c/wk	3 c/wk	3 c/wk	3 c/wk	3 c/wk
Orange veg.	.5 c/wk	1 c/wk	1 c/wk	1.5 c/wk	2 c/wk	2 c/wk	2 c/wk	2 c/wk	2.5 c/wk	2.5 c/wk	2.5 c/wk	2.5 c/wk
Legumes	.5 c/wk	1 c/wk	1 c/wk	2.5 c/wk	3 c/wk	3 c/wk	3 c/wk	3 c/wk	3.5 c/wk	3.5 c/wk	3.5 c/wk	3.5 c/wk
Starchy veg.	1.5 c/wk	2.5 c/wk	2.5 c/wk	2.5 c/wk	3 c/wk	3 c/wk	6 c/wk	6 c/wk	7 c/wk	7 c/wk	9 c/wk	9 c/wk
Other veg.	4 c/wk	4.5 c/wk	4.5 c/wk	5.5 c/wk	6.5 c/wk	6.5 c/wk	7 c/wk	7 c/wk	8.5 c/wk	8.5 c/wk	10 c/wk	10 c/wk
Grains[5]	3 oz-eq	4 oz-eq	5 oz-eq	5 oz-eq	6 oz-eq	6 oz-eq	7 oz-eq	8 oz-eq	9 oz-eq	10 oz-eq	10 oz-eq	10 oz-eq
Whole grains	1.5	2	2.5	3	3	3	3.5	4	4.5	5	5	5
Other grains	1.5	2	2.5	2	3	3	3.5	4	4.5	5	5	5
Lean meats and beans	2 oz-eq	3 oz-eq	4 oz-eq	5 oz-eq	5 oz-eq	5.5 oz-eq	6 oz-eq	6.5 oz-eq	6.5 oz-eq	7 oz-eq	7 oz-eq	7 oz-eq
Milk	2 c	2 c	2 c	3 c	3 c	3 c	3 c	3 c	3 c	3 c	3 c	3 c
Oils[6]	15 g	17 g	17 g	22 g	24 g	27 g	29 g	31 g	34 g	36 g	44 g	51 g
Discretionary calorie allowance[7]	165	171	171	132	195	267	290	362	410	426	512	648

[1]The suggested amounts of food to consume from the basic food groups, subgroups, and oils to meet recommended nutrient intakes at 12 different calorie levels. Nutrient and energy contributions from each group are calculated according to the nutrient-dense forms of foods in each group (eg, lean meats and fat-free milk). The table also shows the discretionary calorie allowance that can be accommodated within each calorie level, in addition to the suggested amounts of nutrient-dense forms of foods in each group.

[2]Food items included in each group and subgroup:

Fruits: All fresh, frozen, canned, and dried fruits and fruit juices: for example, oranges and orange juice, apples and apple juice, bananas, grapes, melons, berries, raisins. Only fruits and juices with no added sugars or fats are included (see note 7).

Vegetables: Only vegetables with no added fats or sugars are included (see note 7).

 • Dark green vegetables: Fresh, frozen, and canned dark green vegetables, cooked or raw: eg, broccoli; spinach; romaine; collard, turnip, and mustard greens.
 • Orange vegetables: All fresh, frozen and canned orange and deep yellow vegetables, cooked or raw: eg, carrots, sweet potatoes, winter squash, and pumpkin.
 • Legumes: All cooked dry beans and peas and soybean products: eg, pinto beans, kidney beans, lentils, chickpeas, tofu.
 • Starchy vegetables: All fresh, frozen, and canned starchy vegetables: eg, white potatoes, corn, green peas.
 • Other vegetables: All fresh, frozen, and canned other vegetables, cooked or raw: eg, tomatoes, tomato juice, lettuce, green beans, onions.

(continued)

1287

Table 29-7. USDA food guide. (continued)

Grains: Only grains in low-fat and low-sugar forms are included (see note 7).
- Whole grains: Whole-grain products and ingredients: eg, whole-wheat and rye breads, whole-grain cereals and crackers, oatmeal, and brown rice.
- Other grains: Refined grain products and ingredients: eg, white breads, enriched grain cereals and crackers, enriched pasta, white rice.

Meat, poultry, fish, dry beans, eggs, and nuts (meat and beans): Lean or low-fat meat, poultry, fish, dry beans and peas, eggs, nuts, seeds (see note 7). Dry beans and peas and soybean products are considered part of this group as well as the vegetable group, but should be counted in one group only.

Milk, yogurt, and cheese (milk): Fat-free or low-fat milks, yogurts, frozen yogurts, dairy desserts, cheeses (except cream cheese), including lactose-free and lactose-reduced products (see note 7). Calcium-fortified soy beverages are an option for those who want a nondairy calcium source.

[3]Quantity equivalents:

Grains: 1 ounce-equivalent (1 serving) of grains = $^1/_2$ cup cooked rice, pasta, or cooked cereal; 1 oz dry pasta or rice; 1 slice bread; 1 small muffin (1 oz); 1 cup ready-to-eat cereal flakes.

Fruits and vegetables: 1 cup (2 servings) of fruits or vegetables = 1 cup cut-up raw or cooked fruit or vegetable, 1 cup fruit or vegetable juice, 2 cups leafy salad greens.

Meat and beans: 1 ounce-equivalent = 1 oz lean meat, poultry, or fish; 1 egg; $^1/_4$ cup cooked dry beans or tofu; 1 Tbsp peanut butter; $^1/_2$ oz nuts or seeds.

Milk: The following each counts as 1 cup (1 serving) of milk: 1 cup milk or yogurt, 1.5 oz natural cheese such as Cheddar cheese or 2 oz processed cheese. Discretionary calories must be counted for all choices, except fat-free milk.

[4]Vegetable subgroup amounts are shown as weekly amounts, because it would be difficult for consumers to select foods from each subgroup daily. A daily amount that is one-seventh of the weekly amount listed is used in calculations of nutrient and energy levels in each pattern.

[5]The whole grain subgroup amounts shown represent at least three 1-oz servings and one-half of the total amount as whole grains for all calorie levels of 1600 and above. This is the minimum suggested amount of whole grains to consume as part of the food patterns. More whole grains up to all the grains recommended may be selected, with offsetting decreases in the amounts of other (enriched) grains. In patterns designed for younger children (1000, 1200, and 1400 calories), one-half of the total amount of grains is shown as whole grains.

[6]Oils shown represent the amounts that are added to foods during processing, cooking, or at the table. Oils and soft margarines include vegetable oils and soft vegetable oil table spreads that have no trans fats. The oils listed are a major source of dietary vitamin E and polyunsaturated fatty acids, including the essential fatty acids. In contrast, solid fats are listed separately in the discretionary calorie category. The amounts of each type of fat in the food intake pattern were based on 60% oils and/or soft margarines with no trans fats and 40% solid fat. The typical American diet contains about 42% oils or soft margarines and about 58% solid fats.

[7]The discretionary calorie allowance is the remaining amount of calories in each food pattern after selecting the specified number of nutrient-dense forms of foods in each food group. The number of discretionary calories assumes that food items in each food group are selected in nutrient-dense forms (that is, forms that are fat free or low fat and that contain no added sugars). Solid fat and sugar calories always need to be counted as discretionary calories:
- The fat in low-fat, reduced fat, or whole milk or milk products or cheese and the sugar and fat in chocolate milk, ice cream, pudding, etc.
- The fat in higher fat meats (eg, ground beef with more than 5% fat by weight; poultry with skin, higher fat luncheon meats, sausages).
- The sugars added to fruits and fruit juices with added sugars or fruits canned in syrup.
- The added fat and/or sugars in vegetables prepared with added fat or sugars.
- The added fats and/or sugars in grain products containing higher levels of fats and/or sugars (eg, sweetened cereals, higher fat crackers, pies and other pastries, cakes, cookies).

Total discretionary calories should be limited to the amounts shown in the table at each calorie level. The nutrient goals for the 1600-calorie pattern are set to meet the needs of adult women, which are higher and require that more calories be used in selections from the basic food groups.

Reprinted, with permission, from U.S. Department of Agriculture. Dietary Guidelines for Americans 2005, Appendix A-2, USDA Food Guide.

■ ASSESSMENT OF NUTRITIONAL STATUS

No single biochemical test or clinical technique is sufficiently accurate to serve as a reliable test for malnutrition. Techniques of nutritional assessment utilize a combination of methods, including evaluation of dietary intake, anthropometric measurements, clinical examination, and laboratory tests.

DIETARY HISTORY

Patients undergoing a history and physical examination should be asked questions to help identify those high-risk patients who require further evaluation for malnutrition. Of particular importance are the regularity and availability of meals; who does the shopping and food preparation; recent changes in appetite, intake, or body weight; use of special diets or dietary supplements; use of alcohol, drugs, or medications; food preferences and food allergies; and the presence of illnesses affecting nutritional intakes, losses, or requirements. Elderly and adolescent patients, pregnant or lactating women, and the poor and socially isolated are at particular risk for nutritional problems.

Further quantification of dietary intake can be performed using a variety of techniques. **Twenty-four-hour diet recalls** provide rough estimates of nutrient intakes. Patients are asked to describe their dietary intake over the preceding day, including snacks, beverages, and alcohol. Problems with this technique include poor patient recall, difficulties in estimating serving sizes, and the inaccuracy associated with generalizing from a single day's intake. More accurate information can be obtained by asking patients to complete a **3- to 5-day diet record**. Nutrient composition can then be analyzed with the aid of standard handbooks or computer software. Although prospective and less likely to be invalidated by memory lapses, omissions are still common, and the usual difficulties in estimating serving sizes persist.

CLINICAL EXAMINATION

A nutritionally focused physical examination should be performed on each patient at risk for nutritional problems. The examination targets body weight, muscle wasting, fat stores, volume status, and signs of micronutrient deficiencies (Table 29–8).

Evaluation of body weight is particularly useful. Body weight in relation to height can be assessed as the **body mass index (BMI)**—weight (in kilograms)/height (in meters)^2 (Table 29–9). In adult patients, however, a recent unintentional change in body weight is usually a better index of undernutrition than a low BMI. This change is best expressed as a percentage of usual weight lost per unit of time. A weight loss of 10% or more of usual weight within a period of 1–2 months is generally considered to be predictive of a poor clinical outcome.

Evaluation of body composition—particularly fat stores and skeletal muscle—can be performed by visual inspection or, more quantitatively, by using **anthropometric measurements**. The most commonly used are the triceps skin fold and mid arm muscle circumference. Because of variations in measurement, they have limited clinical utility.

A number of more sophisticated techniques are available for assessment of body composition. Most have little role in patient care. These include bioelectrical impedance, dual-energy x-ray absorptiometry, air-displacement plethysmography, hydrodensitometry, spectroscopy and mass spectrometry, neutron activation analysis, and MRI and body line scanners.

LABORATORY TESTS

Serum albumin is the most important laboratory test for the diagnosis of protein–calorie undernutrition. Most patients with severe protein depletion will have low serum albumin levels. Many nonnutritional conditions can also reduce serum albumin—particularly liver disease and severe illness in general. Other serum proteins with shorter half-lives (such as transferrin, transthyretin, and prealbumin) may reflect short-term changes in nutritional status but suffer from similar shortcomings.

Tests of cellular immunity are also abnormal in many patients with protein–calorie undernutrition. Measurements of the **total lymphocyte count** and **delayed hypersensitivity reactions** to common skin test antigens are nonspecific; abnormalities may be due to nonnutritional factors.

Despite their poor specificity, these tests are useful prognostically. Patients with abnormal nutritional assessment parameters have a markedly increased risk of poor clinical outcomes.

Blanck HM et al: Laboratory issues: use of nutritional biomarkers. J Nutr 2003;133(Suppl 3):888S. [PMID: 12612175]

Cupisti A et al: Skeletal muscle and nutritional assessment in chronic renal failure patients on a protein-restricted diet. J Intern Med 2004;255:115. [PMID: 14687247]

Kotler D: Challenges to diagnosis of HIV-associated wasting. J Acquir Immune Defic Syndr 2004;37:S280. [PMID: 15722871]

Mackerras D et al: 24-hour national dietary survey data: how do we interpret them most effectively? Public Health Nutr 2005; 8:657. [PMID: 16236196]

Muhlberg W et al: Low total protein increases injury risk in the elderly. J Am Geriatr Soc 2004;52:324. [PMID: 14728654]

Sahyoun NR et al: Nutritional status of the older adult is associated with dentition status. J Am Diet Assoc 2003;103: 61. [PMID: 12525795]

Singh H et al: Malnutrition is prevalent in hospitalized medical patients: Are housestaff identifying the malnourished patient? Nutrition 2006; January 31 Epub. [PMID: 16457988]

Yeh SS et al: Risk factors relating blood markers of inflammation and nutritional status to survival in cachectic geriatric patients in a randomized clinical trial. J Am Geriatr Soc 2004;52:1708. [PMID: 15450049]

Table 29–8. Clinical signs that may be due to nutrient deficiency.

Clinical Sign	Nutrient Deficiency	Clinical Sign	Nutrient Deficiency
Hair		**Neck**	
Transverse depigmentation	Protein, copper	Goiter	Iodine
Easily pluckable	Protein	**Chest**	
Sparse and thin	Protein, zinc, biotin	Thoracic rosary	Vitamin D
Skin		**Heart**	
Dry, scaling	Zinc, vitamin A, essential fatty acids	High-output failure	Thiamine
		Decreased output	Protein-calorie
Flaky paint dermatitis	Protein, niacin, riboflavin	**Abdomen**	
Follicular hyperkeratosis	Vitamins A and C	Hepatosplenomegaly	Protein–calorie
Perifollicular petechiae	Vitamin C	Distention	Protein–calorie
Petechiae, purpura	Vitamins C and K	Diarrhea	Niacin, folate, vitamin B_{12}
Pigmentation, desquamation	Niacin	**Extremities**	
		Muscle tenderness, pain	Thiamine, vitamin C
Nasolabial seborrhea	Niacin, riboflavin, pyridoxine	Muscle wasting	Protein–calorie
Pallor	Iron, folate, vitamin B_{12}, copper	Edema	Protein, thiamine
Scrotal/vulvar dermatoses	Riboflavin	Bone tenderness	Vitamin C, vitamin D, calcium, phosphorus
Subcutaneous fat loss	Calories		
Nails		**Neurologic**	
Spooning	Iron	Hyporeflexia	Thiamine
Transverse lines, ridging	Protein–calorie	Decreased position and vibratory sense	Vitamin B_{12}, thiamine
Head			
Temporal muscle wasting	Protein–calorie	Paresthesias	Vitamin B_{12}, thiamine, niacin
Parotid enlargement	Protein	Confabulation, disorientation	Thiamine
Eyes			
Night blindness	Vitamin A, zinc	Dementia	Niacin
Corneal vascularization	Riboflavin	Ophthalmoplegia	Thiamine, phosphorus
Xerosis, Bitot's spots, keratomalacia	Vitamin A	Tetany	Calcium, magnesium
		Other	
Conjunctival inflammation	Riboflavin	Delayed wound healing	Zinc, protein–calorie, vitamin C
Mouth			
Glossitis (scarlet, raw)	Niacin, pyridoxine, riboflavin, vitamin B_{12}, folate		
Bleeding gums	Vitamin C, riboflavin		
Cheilosis, angular stomatitis	Riboflavin		
Atrophic lingual papillae	Niacin, iron, riboflavin, folate, vitamin B_{12}		
Hypogeusia	Zinc, vitamin A		
Tongue fissuring	Niacin		

■ NUTRITIONAL DISORDERS

PROTEIN–ENERGY MALNUTRITION

ESSENTIALS OF DIAGNOSIS

- *History of decreased intake of energy or protein, increased nutrient losses, or increased nutrient requirements.*

- *Manifestations range from weight loss and growth failure to distinct syndromes, kwashiorkor, and marasmus.*

- *In severe cases, virtually all organ systems are affected.*

- *Protein loss correlates with weight loss: 35–40% total body weight loss is usually fatal.*

General Considerations

Protein–energy malnutrition occurs as a result of a relative or absolute deficiency of energy and protein. It may

Table 29–9. Body mass index chart.[1]

	Body Mass Index																
	19	20	21	22	23	24	25	26	27	28	29	30	31	32	33	34	35
Height (inches)	Body Weight (pounds)																
58	91	96	100	105	110	115	119	124	129	134	138	143	148	153	158	162	167
59	94	99	104	109	114	119	124	128	133	138	143	148	153	158	163	168	173
60	97	102	107	112	118	123	128	133	138	143	148	153	158	163	168	174	179
61	100	106	111	116	122	127	132	137	143	148	153	158	164	169	174	180	185
62	104	109	115	120	126	131	136	142	147	153	158	164	169	175	180	186	191
63	107	113	118	124	130	135	141	146	152	158	163	169	175	180	186	191	197
64	110	116	122	128	134	140	145	151	157	163	169	174	180	186	192	197	204
65	114	120	126	132	138	144	150	156	162	168	174	180	186	192	198	204	210
66	118	124	130	136	142	148	155	161	167	173	179	186	192	198	204	210	216
67	121	127	134	140	146	153	159	166	172	178	185	191	198	204	211	217	223
68	125	131	138	144	151	158	164	171	177	184	190	197	203	210	216	223	230
69	128	135	142	149	155	162	169	176	182	189	196	203	209	216	223	230	236
70	132	139	146	153	160	167	174	181	188	195	202	209	216	222	229	236	243
71	136	143	150	157	165	172	179	186	193	200	208	215	222	229	236	243	250
72	140	147	154	162	169	177	184	191	199	206	213	221	228	235	242	250	258
73	144	151	159	166	174	182	189	197	204	212	219	227	235	242	250	257	265
74	148	155	163	171	179	186	194	202	210	218	225	233	241	249	256	264	272
75	152	160	168	176	184	192	200	208	216	224	232	240	248	256	264	272	279
76	156	164	172	180	189	197	205	213	221	230	238	246	254	263	271	279	287

[1]To use this table, find the appropriate height in the left-hand column. Move across to a given weight. The number at the top of the column is the BMI at that height and weight. Pounds have been rounded off. A normal BMI is 18.5–24.9. Overweight is defined as a BMI of 25–29.9. Class I obesity is 30–34.9; class II obesity is a BMI of 35–39.9; and class III (extreme) obesity is a BMI of > 40.

be primary, due to inadequate food intake, or secondary, as a result of other illness. For most developing nations, primary protein–energy malnutrition remains among the most significant health problems. Protein–energy malnutrition has been described as two distinct syndromes. **Kwashiorkor**, caused by a deficiency of protein in the presence of adequate energy, is typically seen in weaning infants at the birth of a sibling in areas where foods containing protein are insufficiently abundant. **Marasmus**, caused by combined protein and energy deficiency, is most commonly seen where adequate quantities of food are not available.

In industrialized societies, protein–energy malnutrition is most often secondary to other diseases. **Kwashiorkor-like secondary protein–energy malnutrition** occurs primarily in association with hypermetabolic acute illnesses such as trauma, burns, and sepsis. **Marasmus-like secondary protein–energy malnutrition** typically results from chronic diseases such as chronic obstructive pulmonary disease (COPD), congestive heart failure, cancer, or AIDS. These syndromes have been estimated to be present in at least 20% of hospitalized patients. A substantially greater number of patients have risk factors that could result in these syndromes. In both syndromes, protein–energy malnutrition is caused either by decreased intake of energy and protein, increased nutrient losses, or increased nutrient requirements dictated by the underlying illness. For example, diminished oral intake may result from poor dentition or various gastrointestinal disorders. Loss of nutrients results from malabsorption and diarrhea as well as from glycosuria. Nutrient requirements are increased by fever, surgery, neoplasia, and burns.

Pathophysiology

Protein–energy malnutrition affects every organ system. The most obvious results are loss of body weight, adipose stores, and skeletal muscle mass. Weight losses of 5–10% are usually tolerated without loss of physiologic function; losses of 35–40% of body weight usually result in death. Loss of protein from skeletal muscle and internal organs is usually proportionate to weight loss. Protein mass is lost from the liver, gastrointestinal tract, kidneys, and heart.

As protein–energy malnutrition progresses, organ dysfunction develops. Hepatic synthesis of serum proteins decreases, and depressed levels of circulating proteins are observed. Cardiac output and contractility are decreased, and the electrocardiogram (ECG) may show decreased voltage and a rightward axis shift. Autopsies of patients who die with severe undernutrition show myofibrillar atrophy and interstitial edema of the heart.

Respiratory function is affected primarily by weakness and atrophy of the muscles of respiration. Vital capacity and tidal volume are depressed, and mucociliary clearance is abnormal. The gastrointestinal tract is affected by mucosal atrophy and loss of villi of small intestine, resulting in malabsorption. Intestinal disaccharidase deficiency and mild pancreatic insufficiency also occur.

Changes in immunologic function are among the most important changes seen in protein–calorie undernutrition. T lymphocyte number and function are depressed. Changes in B cell function are more variable. Impaired complement activity, granulocyte function, and anatomic barriers to infection are noted, and wound healing is poor.

Clinical Findings

The clinical manifestations of protein–energy malnutrition range from mild growth retardation and weight loss to a number of distinct clinical syndromes. Children in the developing world manifest marasmus and kwashiorkor. In secondary protein–energy malnutrition as seen in industrialized nations, clinical manifestations are affected by the degree of protein and energy deficiency, the underlying illness that resulted in the deficiency, and the patient's nutritional status prior to illness.

In marasmus-like secondary protein–energy malnutrition, most patients typically develop progressive wasting that begins with weight loss and proceeds to more severe cachexia. In the most severe form of this disorder, most body fat stores disappear and muscle mass decreases, most noticeably in the temporalis and interosseus muscles. Laboratory studies may be unremarkable—serum albumin, for example, may be normal or slightly decreased, rarely decreasing to < 2.8 g/dL. In contrast, owing to its rapidity of onset, kwashiorkor-like secondary protein–energy malnutrition may develop in patients with normal subcutaneous fat and muscle mass or, if the patient is obese, in patients with excess fat and muscle. The serum protein level, however, typically declines and the serum albumin is often < 2.8 g/dL. Dependent edema, ascites, or anasarca may develop. As with primary protein–energy malnutrition, combinations of the marasmus-like and kwashiorkor-like syndromes can occur simultaneously, typically in patients with progressive chronic disease in whom a superimposed acute illness develops.

Treatment

The treatment of severe protein–energy malnutrition is a slow process requiring great care. Initial efforts should be directed at correcting fluid and electrolyte abnormalities and infections. Of particular concern are depletion of potassium, magnesium, and calcium and acid–base abnormalities. The second phase of treatment is directed at repletion of protein, energy, and micronutrients. Treatment is started with modest quantities of protein and calories calculated according to the patient's actual body weight. Adult patients are given 1 g of protein and 30 kcal/kg. Concomitant administration of vitamins and minerals is obligatory. Either the enteral or parenteral route can be used, although the former is preferable. Enteral fat and lactose are withheld initially. Patients with less severe protein–calorie undernutrition can be given calories and protein simultaneously with the correction of fluid and electrolyte abnormalities. Similar quantities of protein and calories are recommended for initial treatment.

Patients treated for protein–energy malnutrition require close follow-up. In adults, both calories and protein are advanced as tolerated, adults to 1.5 g/kg/d of protein and 40 kcal/kg/d of calories.

Patients who are refed too rapidly may develop a number of untoward clinical sequelae. During refeeding, circulating potassium, magnesium, phosphorus, and glucose move intracellularly and can result in low serum levels of each. The administration of water and sodium with carbohydrate refeeding can overload hearts with depressed cardiac function and result in congestive heart failure. Enteral refeeding can lead to malabsorption and diarrhea due to abnormalities in the gastrointestinal tract.

Refeeding edema is a benign condition to be differentiated from congestive heart failure. Changes in renal sodium reabsorption and poor skin and blood vessel integrity result in the development of dependent edema without other signs of heart disease. Treatment includes reassurance, elevation of the dependent area, and modest sodium restriction. Diuretics are usually ineffective, may aggravate electrolyte deficiencies, and should not be used.

The prevention and early detection of protein–energy malnutrition in hospitalized patients require awareness of its risk factors and early symptoms and signs. Patients at risk require formal assessment of nutritional status and close observation of dietary intake, body weight, and nutritional requirements during the hospital stay.

Cooper BA et al: Protein malnutrition and hypoalbuminemia as predictors of vascular events and mortality in ESRD. Am J Kidney Dis 2004;43:61. [PMID: 14712428]

Delano MJ et al: The origins of cachexia in acute and chronic inflammatory diseases. Nutr Clin Pract 2006;21:68. [PMID: 16439772]

Faintuch J et al: Severe protein-calorie malnutrition after bariatric procedures. Obes Surg 2004;14:175. [PMID: 15018745]

Wanke C: Pathogenesis and consequences of HIV-associated wasting. J Acquir Immune Defic Syndr 2004;37(Suppl 4):S277. [PMID: 15722870]

OBESITY

 ESSENTIALS OF DIAGNOSIS

- *Excess adipose tissue, resulting in BMI > 30.*
- *Upper body obesity (abdomen and flank) of greater health consequence than lower body obesity (buttocks and thighs).*

- *Associated with multiple metabolic and structural disorders, including diabetes mellitus, hypertension, and hyperlipidemia.*

General Considerations

Obesity is one of the most common disorders in medical practice and among the most frustrating and difficult to manage. Little progress has been made in prevention or treatment, yet major changes have occurred in our understanding of its causes and its implications for health.

Definition & Measurement

Obesity is defined as an excess of adipose tissue. Accurate quantification of body fat requires sophisticated techniques not usually available in clinical practice. Physical examination is usually sufficient to detect excess body fat. More quantitative evaluation is performed by calculating the BMI.

The **BMI** closely correlates with excess adipose tissue. It is calculated by dividing measured body weight in kilograms by the height in meters squared (Table 29–9).

The National Institutes of Health (NIH) define a normal BMI as 18.5–24.9. Overweight is defined as BMI = 25–29.9. Class I obesity is 30–34.9, class II obesity is 35–39.9, and class III (extreme) obesity is BMI > 40. Factors other than total weight, however, are also important. Upper body obesity (excess fat around the waist and flank) is a greater health hazard than lower body obesity (fat in the thighs and buttocks). Obese patients with increased abdominal circumference (> 102 cm in men and 88 cm in women) or with high waist–hip ratios (> 1.0 in men and > 0.85 in women) have a greater risk of diabetes mellitus, stroke, coronary artery disease, and early death than equally obese patients with lower ratios. Further differentiation of the location of excess fat suggests that visceral fat within the abdominal cavity is more hazardous to health than subcutaneous fat around the abdomen.

Current U.S. survey data demonstrate that 65% of Americans are overweight and 30.4% are obese. Women in the United States are more apt to be obese than men, and African-American and Mexican-American women are more obese than whites. The poor are more obese than the rich regardless of race.

Health Consequences of Obesity

Obesity is associated with significant increases in both morbidity and mortality. A great many disorders occur with greater frequency in obese people. The most important and common of these are hypertension, type 2 diabetes mellitus, hyperlipidemia, coronary artery disease, degenerative joint disease, and psychosocial disability. Approximately 60% of individuals with obesity in the United States have the metabolic syndrome (including three or more of the following factors: elevated abdominal circumference, blood pressure, blood triglycerides, and fasting blood sugar, and low high-density lipoprotein [HDL] cholesterol). Certain cancers (colon, rectum, and prostate in men; uterus, biliary tract, breast, and ovary in women), thromboembolic disorders, digestive tract diseases (gallstones, reflux esophagitis), and skin disorders are also more prevalent in the obese. Surgical and obstetric risks are greater. Obese patients also have a greater risk of pulmonary functional impairment, endocrine abnormalities, proteinuria, and increased hemoglobin concentration.

In young and middle-aged adults, mortality from all causes and mortality from cardiovascular disease increase in proportion to the degree of obesity. The relative risk associated with obesity, however, decreases with age, and weight is no longer a risk factor in adults over age 75 years.

Etiology

Until recently, obesity was considered to be the direct result of a sedentary lifestyle plus chronic ingestion of excess calories. Although these factors are undoubtedly the principal cause in some cases, there is now evidence for strong genetic influences on the development of obesity. Adopted children demonstrate a close relationship between their body mass index and that of their biologic parents. No such relationship is found between the children and their adoptive parents. Twin studies also demonstrate substantial genetic influences on BMI with little influence from the childhood environment. As much as 40–70% of obesity may be explained by genetic influences.

Genetic determinants of some types of obesity have now been established. Five genes affecting control of appetite have been identified in mice. Mutations of each gene result in obesity, and each has a human homolog. One gene codes for a protein expressed by adipose tissue—leptin—and another for the leptin receptor in the brain. The other three genes affect brain pathways downstream from the leptin receptor. Numerous other candidate genes for human obesity have been identified. Only a small percentage (4–6%) of human obesity is thought to be due to single gene mutations. Most human obesity undoubtedly develops from the interactions of multiple genes, environmental factors, and behavior.

Medical Evaluation of the Obese Patient

Historical information should be obtained about age at onset, recent weight changes, family history of obesity, occupational history, eating and exercise behavior, cigarette and alcohol use, previous weight loss experience, and psychosocial factors including assessment for depression and eating disorders. Particular attention should be directed at use of laxatives, diuretics, hormones, nutritional supplements, and over-the-counter medications.

Physical examination should assess the degree and distribution of body fat, overall nutritional status, and signs of secondary causes of obesity.

Less than 1% of obese patients have an identifiable secondary, nonpsychiatric, cause of obesity. Hypothyroidism and Cushing's syndrome are important examples that can usually be diagnosed by physical examination in patients with unexplained recent weight gain. Such patients require further endocrinologic evaluation, including serum thyroid-stimulating hormone (TSH) determination and dexamethasone suppression testing (see Chapter 26).

All obese patients should be assessed for medical consequences of their obesity by screening for the metabolic syndrome. Blood pressure, waist circumference, fasting glucose, low-density lipoprotein (LDL) and HDL cholesterol, and triglycerides should be measured.

Treatment

Using conventional techniques, only 20% of patients will lose 20 lb and maintain the loss for over 2 years; 5% will maintain a 40-lb loss. Continued close provider–patient contact appears to be more important for success of treatment than the specific features of any given treatment regimen. Careful patient selection will improve success rates and decrease frustration of both patients and therapists. Only sufficiently motivated patients should enter active treatment programs. Specific attempts to identify motivated patients—eg, requesting a 3-day diet record—are often useful.

Most successful programs employ a multidisciplinary approach to weight loss, with hypocaloric diets, behavior modification to change eating behavior, aerobic exercise, and social support. Emphasis must be on *maintenance* of weight loss.

Dietary instructions for most patients incorporate the same principles that apply to healthy people who are not obese, ie, a low-fat, high-complex carbohydrate, high-fiber diet. This is achieved by emphasizing intake of a wide variety of predominantly "unprocessed" foods. Special attention is usually paid to limiting foods that provide large amounts of calories without other nutrients, ie, fat, sucrose, and alcohol. There is no special advantage to diets that restrict carbohydrates, advocate relatively larger amounts of protein or fats, or recommend ingestion of foods one at a time. In some instances, however, diets that are restricted in carbohydrates can be effective in achieving a lower total calorie intake. Several studies have demonstrated that low-carbohydrate diets can be used safely for weight loss for up to 1 year without adverse effects on lipids or other metabolic parameters. Meal replacement diets can also be used effectively and safely to achieve weight loss.

Long-term changes in eating behavior are required to maintain weight loss. Although formal **behavior modification** programs are available to which patients can be referred, the clinician caring for obese patients can teach a number of useful behavioral techniques. The most important technique is to emphasize planning and record keeping. Patients can be taught to plan menus and exercise sessions and to record their actual behavior. Record keeping not only aids in behavioral change, but also helps the provider to make specific suggestions for problem solving. Patients can be taught to recognize "eating cues" (emotional, situational, etc) and how to avoid or control them. Reward systems and refundable financial contracts are also useful for many patients. Regular self-monitoring of weight is also associated with improved long-term weight maintenance.

Exercise offers a number of advantages to patients trying to lose weight and keep it off. Aerobic exercise directly increases the daily energy expenditure and is particularly useful for long-term weight maintenance. Exercise will also preserve lean body mass and partially prevent the decrease in BEE seen with semistarvation. Up to 1 hour of moderate exercise per day is associated with long-term weight maintenance in individuals who have successfully lost weight. **Social support** is essential for a successful weight loss program. Continued close contact with clinicians and involvement of the family and peer group are useful techniques for reinforcing behavioral change and preventing social isolation.

Patients with severe obesity may require more aggressive treatment regimens. **Very-low-calorie diets** ($\leq$ 800 kcal/d) result in rapid weight loss and marked initial improvement in obesity-related metabolic complications. Patients are commonly maintained on such programs for 4–6 months and lose an average of 2–4 lb per week. Most programs use meal replacement diets to achieve the very-low-calorie intake. Long-term weight maintenance is less predictable and requires concurrent behavior modification, long-term use of low-calorie diets, careful self-monitoring, and regular exercise. Side effects such as fatigue, orthostatic hypotension, cold intolerance, and fluid and electrolyte disorders are observed in proportion to the degree of calorie reduction and require regular supervision by a physician. Other less common complications include gout, gallbladder disease, and cardiac arrhythmias. Although weight loss is more rapidly achieved with very-low-calorie diets as compared with traditional diets, long-term outcomes are equivalent.

Medications for the treatment of obesity are available both over the counter and by prescription. Considerable controversy exists as to the appropriate use of medications for obesity. NIH clinical obesity guidelines state that obesity drugs may be used as part of a comprehensive weight loss program for patients with BMI > 30 or those with BMI > 27 with obesity-related risk factors. Nonetheless, use of medications has decreased in the United States since dexfenfluramine and fenfluramine were withdrawn from the market in 1997 after multiple reports of medication-associated valvular heart disease. Although studies have since estimated the risk of valvular heart disease to be substantially less than the 30% prevalence first reported, this experience has led to considerable caution in the use of anorectic medications.

Anorectic medications can be classified as catecholaminergic or serotonergic. Catecholaminergic medications include amphetamines (with high abuse potential) and the nonamphetamine schedule IV appetite suppressants phentermine, diethylpropion, and mazindol. The selective serotonin reuptake inhibitor (SSRI) antidepressants, eg, fluoxetine and sertraline, have serotonergic activity but are not approved by the Food and Drug Administration (FDA) for weight loss.

Several medications remain available for treatment of obesity. Older catecholaminergic medications (eg, phentermine, diethylpropion, mazindol) are approved for short-term use only and have limited utility. Two newer medications are approved for weight loss: sibutramine and orlistat. Sibutramine blocks uptake of both serotonin and norepinephrine in the central nervous system. Orlistat reduces fat absorption in the gastrointestinal tract.

Sibutramine, typically at doses of 10 mg/d, results in average weight losses of 3–5 kg more than placebo in studies extending over 6–12 months. Sibutramine also appears to improve 1-year outcomes in patients on very-low-calorie diets. Side effects include dry mouth, anorexia, constipation, insomnia, and dizziness. In some patients (< 5%), sibutramine may substantially increase blood pressure.

Orlistat is the first approved medication for obesity that works in the gastrointestinal tract rather than the central nervous system. By inhibiting intestinal lipase, orlistat reduces fat absorption. As expected, orlistat may result in diarrhea, gas, and cramping and perhaps also reduced absorption of fat-soluble vitamins. In randomized trials with up to 2 years of follow-up, orlistat has resulted in 2–4 kg greater weight loss than placebo. The recommended dose of orlistat is 120 mg three times daily with meals. Despite FDA approval of sibutramine and orlistat and NIH guidelines supporting their use, long-term clinical benefits have not been demonstrated. Although these medications result in some additional weight loss at the end of 1- and 2-year clinical trials and, in some studies, improved obesity-related metabolic parameters, the impact of these medications on obesity-related clinical outcomes is unknown.

Bariatric surgery is an increasingly prevalent treatment option for patients with severe obesity. In the United States, gastric operations are considered the procedures of choice. Most popular is the roux-en-Y gastric bypass (GBP). In most centers, the operation can be done laparoscopically. GBP typically results in substantial amounts of weight loss—close to 50% of initial body weight in some studies. Complications occur in up to 40% of subjects undergoing bariatric surgery and include peritonitis due to anastomotic leak, abdominal wall hernias, staple line disruption, gallstones, neuropathy, marginal ulcers, stomal stenosis, wound infections, thromboembolic disease, and

various nutritional deficiencies and gastrointestinal symptoms. Within 30 days operative mortality rates are nil to 1% in low-risk populations but have been reported to be substantially higher in Medicare beneficiaries. One-year mortality rates have been reported as high as 7.5% in men with Medicare. The surgical volume (the number of cases performed by the surgeon or hospital) has been demonstrated to be an important predictor of outcome. NIH consensus panel recommendations are to limit obesity surgery to patients with BMIs over 40, or over 35 if obesity-related comorbidities are present. Recent studies suggest that the procedure is cost-effective for patients with severe obesity and some third-party payers now cover the procedure.

American Medical Association: Assessment and Management of Adult Obesity: A Primer for Physicians, 2003. http://www.ama-assn.org/ama/pub/category/10931.html.

Avenell A et al: What are the long-term benefits of weight reducing diets in adults? A systematic review of randomized controlled trials. J Hum Nutr Diet 2004;17:317. [PMID: 15250842]

Buchwald H et al: Bariatric surgery: a systematic review and meta-analysis. JAMA 2004;292:1724. [PMID: 15479938]

Dansinger ML et al: Comparison of the Atkins, Ornish, Weight Watchers, and Zone diets for weight loss and heart disease risk reduction: a randomized trial. JAMA 2005;293:43. [PMID: 15632335]

Flegal KM et al: Excess deaths associated with underweight, overweight, and obesity. JAMA 2005;293:1861. [PMID: 15840860]

Flum DR et al: Early mortality among Medicare beneficiaries undergoing bariatric surgical procedures. JAMA 2005;294:1903. [PMID: 16234496]

Hedley AA et al: Prevalence of overweight and obesity among US children, adolescents, and adults, 1999–2002. JAMA 2004;291:2847. [PMID: 15199035]

Howard BV et al: Low-fat dietary pattern and weight change over 7 years: the Women's Health Initiative Dietary Modification Trial. JAMA 2006;295:39. [PMID: 16391215]

Hu FB et al: Adiposity as compared with physical activity in predicting mortality among women. N Engl J Med 2004;351:2694. [PMID: 15616204]

Mathus-Vliegen EM et al: Health-related quality-of-life in patients with morbid obesity after gastric banding for surgically induced weight loss. Surgery 2004;135:489. [PMID: 15118585]

Noakes M et al: Meal replacements are as effective as structured weight-loss diets for treating obesity in adults with features of metabolic syndrome. J Nutr 2004;134:1894. [PMID: 15284372]

Norris S et al: Pharmacotherapy for weight loss in adults with type 2 diabetes mellitus. Cochrane Database Syst Rev 2005;(1):CD004096.

Pi-Sunyer FX et al; RIO-North America Study Group: Effect of rimonabant, a cannabinoid-1 receptor blocker, on weight and cardiometabolic risk factors in overweight or obese patients: RIO-North America: a randomized controlled trial. JAMA 2006;295:761. [PMID: 16478899]

Sjostrom L et al and the Swedish Obese Subjects Study Scientific Group: Lifestyle, diabetes, and cardiovascular risk factors 10 years after bariatric surgery. N Engl J Med 2004;351:2683. [PMID: 15616203]

Tsai AG et al: Systematic review: an evaluation of major commercial weight loss programs in the United States. Ann Intern Med 2005;142:56. [PMID: 15630109]

Wadden RA et al: Randomized trial of lifestyle modification and pharmacotherapy for obesity. N Engl J Med 2005;353:2111. [PMID: 16291981]

■ EATING DISORDERS

ANOREXIA NERVOSA

ESSENTIALS OF DIAGNOSIS

- Disturbance of body image and intense fear of becoming fat.
- Weight loss leading to body weight 15% below expected.
- In females, absence of three consecutive menstrual cycles.

General Considerations

Anorexia nervosa typically begins in the years between adolescence and young adulthood. Ninety percent of patients are females, most from the middle and upper socioeconomic strata. The diagnosis is based on weight loss leading to body weight 15% below expected, a distorted body image, fear of weight gain or of loss of control over food intake, and, in females, the absence of at least three consecutive menstrual cycles. Other medical or psychiatric illnesses that can account for anorexia and weight loss must be excluded.

The prevalence of anorexia nervosa is greater than previously suggested. In Rochester, Minnesota, for example, the prevalence per 100,000 population is estimated to be 270 for females and 22 for males. Many other adolescent girls have features of the disorder without the severe weight loss.

The cause of anorexia nervosa is not known. Although multiple endocrinologic abnormalities exist in these patients, most authorities believe they are secondary to malnutrition and not primary disorders. Most experts favor a primary psychiatric origin, but no hypothesis explains all cases. The patient characteristically comes from a family whose members are highly goal and achievement oriented. Interpersonal relationships may be inadequate or destructive. The parents are usually overly directive and concerned with slimness and physical fitness, and much of the family conversation centers around dietary matters. One theory holds that the patient's refusal to eat is an attempt to regain control of her body in defiance of parental control. The patient's unwillingness to inhabit an "adult body" may also represent a rejection of adult responsibilities and the implications of adult interpersonal relationships. Patients are commonly perfectionistic in

behavior and exhibit obsessional personality characteristics. Marked depression or anxiety may be present.

Clinical Findings

A. SYMPTOMS AND SIGNS

Patients with anorexia nervosa may exhibit severe emaciation and may complain of cold intolerance or constipation. Amenorrhea is almost always present. Bradycardia, hypotension, and hypothermia may be present in severe cases. Examination demonstrates loss of body fat, dry and scaly skin, and increased lanugo body hair. Parotid enlargement and edema may also occur.

B. LABORATORY FINDINGS

Laboratory findings are variable but may include anemia, leukopenia, electrolyte abnormalities, and elevations of blood urea nitrogen (BUN) and serum creatinine. Serum cholesterol levels are often increased. Endocrine abnormalities include depressed levels of luteinizing and follicle-stimulating hormones and impaired response of luteinizing hormone to luteinizing hormone-releasing hormone.

Diagnosis & Differential Diagnosis

The diagnosis can be difficult, since many common social and cultural factors promote and maintain anorexic behavior. The diagnosis depends on identification of the common behavioral features and exclusion of medical disorders that would account for weight loss.

Behavioral features required for the diagnosis include intense fear of becoming obese, disturbance of body image, weight loss of at least 15%, and refusal to exceed a minimal normal weight.

The differential diagnosis includes endocrine and metabolic disorders such as panhypopituitarism, Addison's disease, hyperthyroidism, and diabetes mellitus; gastrointestinal disorders such as Crohn's disease and celiac sprue; chronic infections and cancers such as tuberculosis and lymphoma; and rare central nervous system disorders such as hypothalamic tumors.

Treatment

The goal of treatment is restoration of normal body weight and resolution of psychological difficulties. Hospitalization may be necessary. Treatment programs conducted by experienced teams are successful in about two-thirds of cases, restoring normal weight and menstruation. One-half continue to experience difficulties with eating behavior and psychiatric problems. Occasional patients with anorexia develop obesity after treatment. Two to 6% of patients die from the complications of the disorder or commit suicide.

Various treatment methods have been used without clear evidence of superiority of one over another. Supportive care by physicians and nurses is probably the most important feature of therapy. Structured behavioral therapy, intensive psychotherapy, and family therapy may be tried. A variety of medications including tricyclic antidepressants, SSRIs, and lithium carbonate are effective in some cases; overall, however, clinical trial results have been disappointing. Patients with severe malnutrition must be hemodynamically stabilized and may require enteral or parenteral feeding. Forced feedings should be reserved for life-threatening situations, since the goal of treatment is to reestablish normal eating behavior.

American Dietetic Association: Position of the American Dietetic Association: Nutrition intervention in the treatment of anorexia nervosa, bulimia nervosa, and eating disorder not otherwise specified (EDNOS). http://www.eatright.org/adap0701.html.

Birch K: Female athlete triad. BMJ 2005;330:244. [PMID: 15677660]

Claudino A et al: Antidepressants for anorexia nervosa. Cochrane Database Syst rev 2006;(1):CD004365. [PMID: 16437485]

Fairburn CG et al: Eating disorders. Lancet 2003;361:407. [PMID: 12573387]

Fisher M: The course and outcome of eating disorders in adults and in adolescents: a review. Adolesc Med 2003;14:149. [PMID: 12529198]

McIntosh VV et al: Three psychotherapies for anorexia nervosa: a randomized, controlled trial. Am J Psychiatry 2005;162:741. [PMID: 15800147]

Pompili M et al: Suicide in anorexia nervosa: a meta-analysis. Int J Eat Disord 2004;36:99. [PMID: 15185278]

Rome ES: Eating disorders. Obstet Gynecol Clin North Am 2003;30:353. [PMID: 12836725]

Wadden TA et al: Dieting and the development of eating disorders in obese women: results of a randomized controlled trial. Am J Clin Nutr 2004;80:560. [PMID: 15321793]

Wilson GT et al: Eating disorders guidelines from NICE. Lancet 2005;365:79. [PMID: 15639682]

Yager J et al: Clinical practice. Anorexia nervosa. N Engl J Med 2005;353:1481. [PMID: 16207850]

BULIMIA NERVOSA

 ESSENTIALS OF DIAGNOSIS

- *Uncontrolled episodes of binge eating at least twice weekly for 3 months.*
- *Recurrent inappropriate compensation to prevent weight gain such as self-induced vomiting, laxatives, diuretics, fasting, or excessive exercise.*
- *Overconcern with weight and body shape.*

General Considerations

Bulimia nervosa is the episodic uncontrolled ingestion of large quantities of food followed by recurrent inappropriate compensatory behavior to prevent weight gain such as self-induced vomiting, diuretic or cathartic use, or strict dieting or vigorous exercise.

Like anorexia nervosa, bulimia nervosa is predominantly a disorder of young, white, middle- and upper-class women. It is more difficult to detect than anorexia, and some studies have estimated that the prevalence may be as high as 19% in college-aged women.

Clinical Findings

Patients with bulimia nervosa typically consume large quantities of easily ingested high-calorie foods, usually in secrecy. Some patients may have several such episodes a day for a few days; others report regular and persistent patterns of binge eating. Binging is usually followed by vomiting, cathartics, or diuretics and is usually accompanied by feelings of guilt or depression. Periods of binging may be followed by intervals of self-imposed starvation. Body weights may fluctuate but generally are within 20% of desirable weights.

Some patients with bulimia nervosa also have a cryptic form of anorexia nervosa with significant weight loss and amenorrhea. Family and psychological issues are generally similar to those encountered among patients with anorexia nervosa. Bulimics, however, have a higher incidence of premorbid obesity, greater use of cathartics and diuretics, and more impulsive or antisocial behavior. Menstruation is usually preserved.

Medical complications are numerous. Gastric dilatation and pancreatitis have been reported after binges. Vomiting can result in poor dentition, pharyngitis, esophagitis, aspiration, and electrolyte abnormalities. Cathartic and diuretic abuse also cause electrolyte abnormalities or dehydration. Constipation and hemorrhoids are common.

Treatment

Treatment of bulimia nervosa and bulimarexia requires supportive care and psychotherapy. Individual, group, family, and behavioral therapy have all been utilized. Antidepressant medications may be helpful. The best results have been with fluoxetine hydrochloride and other SSRIs. Although death from bulimia is rare, the long-term psychiatric prognosis in severe bulimia is worse than that in anorexia nervosa.

Duncan AE et al: Are there subgroups of bulimia nervosa based on comorbid psychiatric disorders? Int J Eat Disord 2005;37:19. [PMID: 15690461]

Hay PJ et al: Psychotherapy for bulimia nervosa and binging. Cochrane Database Syst Rev 2003;(1):CD000562. [PMID: 12535397]

Palmer R: Bulimia nervosa: 25 years on. Br J Psychiatry 2004;185:447. [PMID: 15572732]

Schneider M: Bulimia nervosa and binge-eating disorder in adolescents. Adolesc Med 2003;14:119. [PMID: 12529196]

Walsh BT et al: Treatment of bulimia nervosa in a primary care setting. Am J Psychiatry 2004;161:556. [PMID: 14992983]

■ DISORDERS OF VITAMIN METABOLISM

Deficiencies of single vitamins are less often encountered than those of multiple vitamins. Although any cause of protein–calorie undernutrition can result in concurrent vitamin deficiency, most deficiencies are associated with malabsorption, alcoholism, medications, hemodialysis, total parenteral nutrition, food faddism, or inborn errors of metabolism.

Vitamin deficiency syndromes develop gradually. Symptoms are commonly nonspecific, and the physical examination is rarely helpful in early diagnosis. Most characteristic physical findings are seen late in the course of the syndrome. Other characteristic physical findings, such as glossitis and cheilosis, are seen with deficiencies of many B vitamins. Such abnormalities suggest the presence of a nutritional deficiency but do not indicate which nutrient is deficient.

Despite the relative ease of meeting the recommended daily allowances with a mixed diet, many adults in the United States take vitamin supplements. In fact, syndromes of vitamin excess may be more common than deficiency syndromes, particularly those due to excess of vitamins A, D, and B_6. Most claims for significant health benefits of such supplements, particularly those taken in megadoses, remain unsubstantiated.

Some vitamins can be used efficaciously as drugs. Derivatives of vitamin A are used to treat cystic acne and, more recently, skin wrinkles. Niacin is an effective medication for hyperlipidemia. Vitamin-responsive inborn errors of metabolism also commonly require pharmacologic doses of vitamins.

Millen AE et al: Use of vitamin, mineral, nonvitamin, and non-mineral supplements in the United States: The 1987, 1992, and 2000 National Health Interview Survey results. J Am Diet Assoc 2004;104:942. [PMID: 15175592]

Radimer K et al: Dietary supplement use by US adults: data from the National Health and Nutrition Examination Survey, 1999-2000. Am J Epidemiol 2004;160:339. [PMID: 15286019]

THIAMINE (B_1) DEFICIENCY

ESSENTIALS OF DIAGNOSIS

- *Most common in patients with chronic alcoholism.*
- *Early symptoms of anorexia, muscle cramps, paresthesias, irritability.*
- *Advanced syndromes of high output heart failure ("wet beriberi"), peripheral nerve disorders, and Wernicke-Korsakoff syndrome ("dry beriberi").*

Clinical Findings

Most thiamine deficiency in the United States is due to alcoholism. Patients with chronic alcoholism may have poor dietary intakes of thiamine and impaired thiamine absorption, metabolism, and storage. Thiamine deficiency is also associated with malabsorption, dialysis, and other causes of chronic protein–calorie undernutrition. Thiamine deficiency can be precipitated in patients with marginal thiamine status with intravenous dextrose solutions.

Early manifestations of thiamine deficiency include anorexia, muscle cramps, paresthesias, and irritability. Advanced deficiency primarily affects the cardiovascular system ("wet beriberi") or the nervous system ("dry beriberi"). Wet beriberi occurs in thiamine deficiency accompanied by severe physical exertion and high carbohydrate intakes. Dry beriberi occurs in thiamine deficiency accompanied by inactivity and low calorie intake.

Wet beriberi is characterized by marked peripheral vasodilation resulting in high-output heart failure with dyspnea, tachycardia, cardiomegaly, and pulmonary and peripheral edema, with warm extremities mimicking cellulitis.

Dry beriberi involves both the peripheral and the central nervous systems. Peripheral nerve involvement is typically a symmetric motor and sensory neuropathy with pain, paresthesias, and loss of reflexes. The legs are affected more than the arms. Central nervous system involvement results in Wernicke–Korsakoff syndrome. Wernicke's encephalopathy consists of nystagmus progressing to ophthalmoplegia, truncal ataxia, and confusion. Korsakoff's syndrome includes amnesia, confabulation, and impaired learning.

Diagnosis

A variety of biochemical tests are available to assess thiamine deficiency. In most instances, however, the clinical response to empiric thiamine therapy is used to support a diagnosis of thiamine deficiency. The most commonly used and widely available biochemical tests are measurement of erythrocyte transketolase activity and urinary thiamine excretion. A transketolase activity coefficient greater than 15–20% suggests thiamine deficiency.

Treatment

Thiamine deficiency is treated with large parenteral doses of thiamine. Fifty to 100 mg/d is administered for the first few days, followed by daily oral doses of 5–10 mg/d. All patients should simultaneously receive therapeutic doses of other water-soluble vitamins. Although treatment results in complete resolution in half of patients (one-fourth immediately and another one-fourth over days), the other half obtain only partial resolution or no benefit.

THIAMINE TOXICITY

There is no known toxicity of thiamine.

Day E et al: Thiamine for Wernicke-Korsakoff Syndrome in people at risk from alcohol abuse. Cochrane Database Syst Rev 2004;(1):CD004033. [PMID: 14974055]

Klein M et al: Fatal metabolic acidosis caused by thiamine deficiency. J Emerg Med 2004;26:301. [PMID: 15028327]

Loh Y et al: Acute Wernicke's encephalopathy following bariatric surgery: clinical course and MRI correlation. Obes Surg 2004;14:129. [PMID: 14980048]

Morcos Z et al: Wernicke encephalopathy. Arch Neurol 2004;61:775. [PMID: 15148159]

Selitsky T et al: Wernicke's encephalopathy with hyperemesis and ketoacidosis. Obstet Gynecol 2006;107:486. [PMID: 16449159]

Sgouros X et al: Evaluation of a clinical screening instrument to identify states of thiamine deficiency in inpatients with severe alcohol dependence syndrome. Alcohol Alcoholism 2004;39:227. [PMID: 15082460]

RIBOFLAVIN (B$_2$) DEFICIENCY

Clinical Findings

Riboflavin deficiency almost always occurs in combination with deficiencies of other vitamins. Dietary inadequacy, interactions with a variety of medications, alcoholism, and other causes of protein–calorie undernutrition are the most common causes of riboflavin deficiency.

Manifestations of riboflavin deficiency include cheilosis, angular stomatitis, glossitis, seborrheic dermatitis, weakness, corneal vascularization, and anemia.

Diagnosis

Riboflavin deficiency is usually treated empirically when the diagnosis is suspected. Deficiency can be confirmed by measuring the riboflavin-dependent enzyme erythrocyte glutathione reductase. Activity coefficients greater than 1.2–1.3 are suggestive of riboflavin deficiency. Urinary riboflavin excretion and serum levels of plasma and red cell flavins can also be measured.

Treatment

Riboflavin deficiency is easily treated with foods such as meat, fish, and dairy products or with oral preparations of the vitamin. Administration of 5–15 mg/d until clinical findings are resolved is usually adequate. Riboflavin can also be given parenterally, but it is poorly soluble in aqueous solutions.

RIBOFLAVIN TOXICITY

There is no known toxicity of riboflavin.

Friedli A et al: Images in clinical medicine. Oculo-orogenital syndrome—a deficiency of vitamins B$_2$ and B$_6$. N Engl J Med 2004;350:1130. [PMID: 15014186]

McKinley MC et al: Effect of riboflavin supplementation on plasma homocysteine in elderly people with low riboflavin status. Eur J Clin Nutr 2002;56:850. [PMID: 12209373]

Powers HJ: Riboflavin (vitamin B-2) and health. Am J Clin Nutr 2003;77:1352. [PMID: 12791609]

NIACIN DEFICIENCY

General Considerations

Niacin is a generic term for nicotinic acid and other derivatives with similar nutritional activity. Unlike most other vitamins, niacin can be synthesized from the amino acid tryptophan. Niacin is an essential component of the coenzymes nicotinamide adenine dinucleotide (NAD) and nicotinamide adenine dinucleotide phosphate (NADP), which are involved in many oxidation-reduction reactions. The major food sources of niacin are protein foods containing tryptophan and numerous cereals, vegetables, and dairy products.

Niacin in the form of nicotinic acid is used therapeutically for the treatment of hypercholesterolemia and hypertriglyceridemia. Daily doses of 3–6 g can result in significant reductions in levels of LDL and very-low-density lipoproteins (VLDL) and in elevation of HDL. Niacinamide (the form of niacin usually used to treat niacin deficiency) does not exhibit the lipid-lowering effects of nicotinic acid.

Clinical Findings

Historically, niacin deficiency occurred when corn, which is relatively deficient in both tryptophan and niacin, was the major source of calories. Currently, niacin deficiency is more commonly due to alcoholism and nutrient–drug interactions. Niacin deficiency can also occur in inborn errors of metabolism.

As with other B vitamins, the early manifestations of niacin deficiency are nonspecific. Common complaints include anorexia, weakness, irritability, mouth soreness, glossitis, stomatitis, and weight loss. More advanced deficiency results in the classic triad of pellagra: dermatitis, diarrhea, and dementia. The dermatitis is symmetric, involving sun-exposed areas. Skin lesions are dark, dry, and scaling. The dementia begins with insomnia, irritability, and apathy and progresses to confusion, memory loss, hallucinations, and psychosis. The diarrhea can be severe and may result in malabsorption due to atrophy of the intestinal villi. Advanced pellagra can result in death.

Diagnosis

In advanced cases, the diagnosis of pellagra can be made on clinical grounds. In early deficiency, diagnosis requires a high index of suspicion and attempts at confirmation of niacin deficiency. Niacin metabolites, particularly N-methylnicotinamide, can be measured in the urine. Low levels suggest niacin deficiency but may also be found in patients with generalized undernutrition. Serum and red cell levels of NAD and NADP are also low but are similarly nonspecific.

Treatment

Niacin deficiency can be effectively treated with oral niacin, usually given as nicotinamide. Doses ranging from 10 mg/d to 150 mg/d have been used without difficulty.

NIACIN TOXICITY

At the high doses of niacin used to treat hyperlipidemia, side effects are common. These include cutaneous flushing (partially prevented by pretreatment with aspirin, 325 mg/d, and use of extended-release preparations) and gastric irritation. Elevation of liver enzymes, hyperglycemia, and gout are less common untoward effects.

Canner PL et al: Benefits of niacin in patients with versus without the metabolic syndrome and healed myocardial infarction (from the Coronary Drug Project). Am J Cardiol 2006; 97:477. [PMID: 16461040]

Krapels IP et al: Maternal dietary B vitamin intake, other than folate, and the association with orofacial cleft in the offspring. Eur J Nutr 2004;43:7. [PMID: 14991264]

Miller M: Niacin as a component of combination therapy for dyslipidemia. Mayo Clin Proc 2003;78:735. [PMID: 12934785]

Pitsavas S et al: Pellagra encephalopathy following B-complex vitamin treatment without niacin. Int J Psychiatry Med 2004;34:91. [PMID: 15242145]

Whitney EJ et al: A randomized trial of a strategy for increasing high-density lipoprotein cholesterol levels: effects on progression of coronary heart disease and clinical events. Ann Intern Med 2005;142:95. [PMID: 15657157]

VITAMIN B$_6$ DEFICIENCY

Clinical Findings

Vitamin B$_6$ deficiency most commonly occurs as a result of interactions with medications—especially isoniazid, cycloserine, penicillamine, and oral contraceptives—or of alcoholism. A number of inborn errors of metabolism and other pyridoxine-responsive syndromes, particularly pyridoxine-responsive anemia, are not clearly due to vitamin deficiency but commonly respond to high doses of the vitamin.

Vitamin B$_6$ deficiency results in a clinical syndrome similar to that seen with deficiencies of other B vitamins, including mouth soreness, glossitis, cheilosis, weakness, and irritability. Severe deficiency can result in peripheral neuropathy, anemia, and seizures. Recent studies have suggested a potential relationship of low vitamin B$_6$ levels and a variety of clinical conditions including cardiovascular diseases, inflammatory diseases, and certain cancers.

Diagnosis

The diagnosis of vitamin B$_6$ deficiency can be confirmed by measurement of pyridoxal phosphate in blood. Normal levels are greater than 50 ng/mL.

Treatment

Vitamin B$_6$ deficiency can be effectively treated with oral vitamin B$_6$ supplements. Doses of 10–20 mg/d are usually adequate, though some patients taking medications that interfere with pyridoxine metabolism may need doses as high as 100 mg/d. Inborn errors of metabolism and the pyridoxine-responsive syndromes often require doses up to 600 mg/d.

Vitamin B$_6$ should be routinely prescribed for patients receiving medications (such as isoniazid) that interfere with pyridoxine metabolism to prevent vitamin B$_6$ deficiency. This is particularly true for elderly patients, the urban poor, and alcoholics, who are more likely to have diets marginally adequate in vitamin B$_6$.

VITAMIN B$_6$ TOXICITY

A sensory neuropathy, at times irreversible, occurs in patients receiving large doses of vitamin B$_6$. Although most patients have taken 2 g or more per day, some patients have taken only 200 mg/d.

Chiang EP et al: Abnormal vitamin B$_6$ status is associated with severity of symptoms in patients with rheumatoid arthritis. Am J Med 2003;114:283. [PMID: 12681455]

Friso S et al: Low plasma vitamin B$_6$ concentrations and modulation of coronary artery disease risk. Am J Clin Nutr 2004; 79:992. [PMID: 15159228]

Stott DJ et al: Randomized controlled trial of homocysteine-lowering vitamin treatment in elderly patients with vascular disease. Am J Clin Nutr 2005;82:1320. [PMID: 16332666]

Toole JF et al: Lowering homocysteine in patients with ischemic stroke to prevent recurrent stroke, myocardial infarction, and death: the Vitamin Intervention for Stroke prevention (VISP) randomized controlled trial. JAMA 2004;291:565. [PMID: 14762035]

VITAMIN B$_{12}$ & FOLATE

Vitamin B$_{12}$ (cobalamin) and folate are discussed in Chapter 13. Vitamin B$_{12}$ is abundant in meat and dairy products; fresh fruits and vegetables supply folic acid.

Hvas AM et al: Vitamin B$_{12}$ treatment has limited effect on health-related quality of life among individuals with elevated plasma methylmalonic acid: a randomized placebo-controlled study. J Intern Med 2003;253:146. [PMID: 12542554]

Lange H et al: Folate therapy and in-stent restenosis after coronary stenting. N Engl J Med 2004;350:2673. [PMID: 15215483]

Nakamura K et al: Vitamin B$_{12}$ deficiency. Arch Neurol 2004;61:960. [PMID: 15210541]

Quadri P et al: Homocysteine, folate, and vitamin B$_{12}$ in mild cognitive impairment, Alzheimer disease, and vascular dementia. Am J Clin Nutr 2004;80:114. [PMID: 15213037]

Roth M et al: Oral vitamin B$_{12}$ therapy in vitamin B$_{12}$ deficiency. Am J Med 2004;116:358. [PMID: 14984828]

van Oijen MG et al: Association of aspirin use with vitamin B$_{12}$ deficiency (results of the BACH study). Am J Cardiol 2004; 94:975. [PMID: 15464695]

VITAMIN C (Ascorbic Acid) DEFICIENCY

Clinical Findings

Most cases of vitamin C deficiency seen in the United States are due to dietary inadequacy in the urban poor, the elderly, and chronic alcoholics. Patients with chronic illnesses such as cancer and chronic renal failure and individuals who smoke cigarettes are also at risk.

Early manifestations of vitamin C deficiency are nonspecific and include malaise and weakness. In more advanced stages, the typical features of scurvy develop. Manifestations include perifollicular hemorrhages, perifollicular hyperkeratotic papules, petechiae and purpura, splinter hemorrhages, bleeding gums, hemarthroses, and subperiosteal hemorrhages. Periodontal signs do not occur in edentulous patients. Anemia is common, and wound healing is impaired. The late stages of scurvy are characterized by edema, oliguria, neuropathy, intracerebral hemorrhage, and death.

Diagnosis

The diagnosis of advanced scurvy can be made clinically on the basis of the skin lesions in the proper clinical situation. Atraumatic hemarthrosis is also highly suggestive. The diagnosis can be confirmed with decreased plasma ascorbic acid levels, typically below 0.1 mg/dL.

Treatment

Adult scurvy can be treated with 300–1000 mg of ascorbic acid per day. Improvement typically occurs within days. Some studies have suggested that high intakes of vitamin C are associated with a decreased risk of cancer. Vitamin C may also protect against coronary heart disease by modifying blood cholesterol levels and preventing LDL cholesterol from oxidation. A decrease in all-cause and coronary heart disease mortality in individuals with high intakes (approximately 300–400 mg/d) of vitamin C has been reported.

VITAMIN C TOXICITY

Very large doses of vitamin C can cause gastric irritation, flatulence, or diarrhea. Oxalate kidney stones are of theoretic concern because ascorbic acid is metabolized to oxalate, but stone formation has not been frequently reported. Vitamin C can also confound common diagnostic tests by causing false-negative tests for fecal occult blood and both false-negative and false-positive tests for urine glucose.

Hampl JS et al: Vitamin C deficiency and depletion in the United States: the Third National Health and Nutrition Examination Survey, 1988 to 1994. Am J Public Health 2004;94: 870. [PMID: 15117714]

Salonen RM et al: Antioxidant Supplementation in Atherosclerosis Prevention Study. Six-year effect of combined vitamin C and E supplementation on atherosclerotic progression: the Antioxidant Supplementation in Atherosclerosis Prevention (ASAP) Study. Circulation 2003;107:947. [PMID: 12600905]

Shekelle P et al: Effect of supplemental antioxidants vitamin C, vitamin E, and coenzyme Q for the prevention and treatment of cardiovascular disease. Evid Rep Technol Assess (sum). 2003;1-3. http://www.ahrq.gov

Traxer O et al: Effect of ascorbic acid consumption on urinary stone risk factors. J Urol 2003;170(2 Pt 1):397. [PMID: 12853784]

VITAMIN A DEFICIENCY

Clinical Findings

Vitamin A deficiency is one of the most common vitamin deficiency syndromes, particularly in developing countries. In many such regions, it is the most common cause of blindness. In the United States, vitamin A deficiency is usually due to fat malabsorption syndromes or mineral oil laxative abuse and occurs most commonly in the elderly and urban poor.

Night blindness is the earliest symptom. Dryness of the conjunctiva (xerosis) and the development of small white patches on the conjunctiva (Bitot's spots) are early signs. Ulceration and necrosis of the cornea (keratomalacia), perforation, endophthalmitis, and blindness are late manifestations. Xerosis and hyperkeratinization of the skin and loss of taste may also occur.

Diagnosis

Abnormalities of dark adaptation are strongly suggestive of vitamin A deficiency. Serum levels below the normal range of 30–65 mg/dL are commonly seen in advanced deficiency.

Treatment

Night blindness, poor wound healing, and other signs of early deficiency can be effectively treated with 30,000 international units of vitamin A daily for 1 week. Advanced deficiency with corneal damage calls for administration of 20,000 units/kg for at least 5 days. The potential antioxidant effects of β-carotene can be achieved with supplements of 25,000–50,000 international units of β-carotene.

VITAMIN A TOXICITY

Excess intake of β-carotenes (hypercarotenosis) results in staining of the skin a yellow-orange color but is otherwise benign. Skin changes are most marked on the palms and soles, while the scleras remain white, clearly distinguishing hypercarotenosis from jaundice.

Excessive vitamin A (hypervitaminosis A), on the other hand, can be quite toxic. Chronic toxicity usually occurs after ingestion of daily doses of over 50,000 units/d for more than 3 months. Early manifestations include dry, scaly skin, hair loss, mouth sores, painful hyperostoses, anorexia, and vomiting. More serious findings include hypercalcemia; increased intracranial pressure, with papilledema, headaches, and decreased cognition; and hepatomegaly, occasionally progressing to cirrhosis. Excessive vitamin A has also recently been related to increased risk of hip fracture. Acute toxicity can result from ingestion of massive doses of vitamin A, such as in drug overdoses or consumption of polar bear liver. Manifestations include nausea, vomiting, abdominal pain, headache, papilledema, and lethargy.

The diagnosis can be confirmed by elevations of serum vitamin A levels. The only treatment is withdrawal of vitamin A from the diet. Most symptoms and signs improve rapidly.

Baeten JM et al: Use of serum retinol-binding protein for prediction of vitamin A deficiency: effects of HIV-1 infection, protein malnutrition, and the acute phase response. Am J Clin Nutr 2004;79:218. [PMID: 14749226]

Michaelsson K et al: Serum retinol levels and the risk of fracture. N Engl J Med 2003;348:287. [PMID: 12540641]

Wiysonge CS et al: Vitamin A supplementation for reducing the risk of mother-to-child transmission of HIV infection. Cochrane Database Syst Rev 2005;(4):CD003648. [PMID: 16235332]

VITAMIN D

Vitamin D is discussed in Chapter 26. The major food source of vitamin D is fortified milk, but sunlight on the skin is a prime resource as well.

Gartner LM et al: Prevention of rickets and vitamin D deficiency: new guidelines for vitamin D intake. Pediatrics 2003;111(4 Pt 1):908. [PMID: 12671133]

Jackson RD et al; Women's Health Initiative Investigators: Calcium plus vitamin D supplementation and the risk of fractures. N Engl J Med 2006;354:669. [PMID: 16481635]

Tajika M et al: Risk factors for vitamin D deficiency in patients with Crohn's disease. J Gastroenterol 2004;39:527. [PMID: 15235869]

Wactawski-Wende J et al; Women's Health Initiative Investigators: Calcium plus vitamin D supplementation and the risk of colorectal cancer. N Engl J Med 2006;354:684. [PMID: 16481636]

VITAMIN E DEFICIENCY

Clinical Findings

Clinical deficiency of vitamin E is most commonly due to severe malabsorption, the genetic disorder abetalipoproteinemia, or, in children with chronic cholestatic liver disease, biliary atresia or cystic fibrosis. Manifestations of deficiency include areflexia, disturbances of gait, decreased proprioception and vibration, and ophthalmoplegia.

Diagnosis

Plasma vitamin E levels can be measured; normal levels are 0.5–0.7 mg/dL or higher. Since vitamin E is normally transported in lipoproteins, the serum level should be interpreted in relation to circulating lipids.

Treatment

The optimum therapeutic dose of vitamin E has not been clearly defined. Large doses, often administered parenterally, can be used to improve the neurologic complications seen in abetalipoproteinemia and cholestatic liver disease. The potential antioxidant benefits of vitamin E can be achieved with supplements of 100–400 units/d. Clinical trials of supplemental vitamin E to prevent cardiovascular disease, however, have shown no beneficial effects.

VITAMIN E TOXICITY

Vitamin E is the least toxic of the fat-soluble vitamins. Large doses—many times the recommended daily requirement—have been taken for extended periods of time without apparent harm, though nausea, flatulence, and diarrhea have been reported. Large doses of vitamin E can increase the vitamin K requirement and can result in bleeding in patients taking oral anticoagulants.

Eidelman RS et al: Randomized trials of vitamin E in the treatment and prevention of cardiovascular disease. Arch Intern Med 2004;164:1552. [PMID: 15277288]

Lee IM et al: Vitamin E in the primary prevention of cardiovascular disease and cancer: the Women's Health Study: a randomized controlled trial. JAMA 2005;294:56. [PMID: 15998891]

Maras JE et al: Intake of alpha-tocopherol is limited among US adults. J Am Diet Assoc 2004;104:567. [PMID: 15054342]

Meydani SN et al: Vitamin E and respiratory tract infections in elderly nursing home residents: a randomized controlled trial. JAMA 2004;292:828. [PMID: 15315997]

Miller ER 3rd et al: Meta-analysis: high-dosage vitamin E supplementation may increase all-cause mortality. Ann Intern Med 2005;142:37. [PMID: 15537682]

VITAMIN K

Vitamin K is discussed in Chapter 13. Vitamin K is synthesized by intestinal bacteria.

■ DIET THERAPY

Specific therapeutic diets can be designed to facilitate the medical management of most common illnesses. In most cases, consultation with a registered dietitian is necessary in order to design and implement major dietary changes. Physicians should be familiar with the indications for special diets and their basic composition to facilitate patient referrals and to maximize patient compliance. Diet therapy is a difficult process, and not all patients are able to cooperate fully. Requesting the patient to record dietary intake for 3–5 days may provide useful insight into the patient's motivation.

Therapeutic diets can be divided into three groups: (1) diets that alter the consistency of food, (2) diets that restrict or otherwise modify dietary components, and (3) diets that supplement dietary components.

DIETS THAT ALTER CONSISTENCY

Clear Liquid Diet

This diet provides adequate water, 500–1000 kcal as simple sugar, and some electrolytes. It is fiber free and requires minimal digestion or intestinal motility.

A clear liquid diet is useful for patients with resolving postoperative ileus, acute gastroenteritis, partial intestinal obstruction, and as preparation for diagnostic gastrointestinal procedures. It is commonly used as the first diet for patients who have been taking nothing by mouth for long periods. Because of the low calorie and minimal protein content of the clear liquid diet, it is used only for short periods.

Full Liquid Diet

The full liquid diet provides adequate water and can be designed to provide adequate calories and protein. Vitamins and minerals—especially folic acid, iron, and vitamin B_6—may be inadequate and should be provided in the form of supplements. Dairy products, soups, eggs, and soft cereals are used to supplement clear liquids. Commercial oral supplements can also be incorporated into the diet or used alone.

This diet is low in residue and can be used in many instances instead of the clear liquid diet described above—especially in patients with difficulty in chewing or swallowing, with partial obstructions, or in preparation for some diagnostic procedures. Full liquid diets are commonly used following clear liquid diets to advance diets in patients who have been taking nothing by mouth for long periods.

Soft Diets

Soft diets are designed for patients unable to chew or swallow hard or coarse food. Tender foods are used, and most raw fruits and vegetables and coarse breads and cereals are eliminated. Soft diets are commonly used to assist in progression from full liquid diets to regular diets in postoperative patients, in patients who are too weak or those whose dentition is too poor to handle a general diet, in head and neck surgical patients, in patients with esophageal strictures, and in other patients who have difficulty with chewing or swallowing.

The soft diet can be designed to meet all nutritional requirements.

DIETS THAT RESTRICT NUTRIENTS

Diets can be designed to restrict (or eliminate) virtually any nutrient or food component. The most commonly used restricted diets are those that limit sodium, fat, and protein. Other restrictive diets include gluten restriction in sprue, potassium and phosphate reduction in renal insufficiency, and various elimination diets for food allergies.

Sodium-Restricted Diets

Low-sodium diets are useful in the management of hypertension and in conditions in which sodium retention and edema are prominent features, particularly congestive heart failure, chronic liver disease, and chronic renal failure. Sodium restriction is beneficial with or without diuretic therapy. When used in conjunction with diuretics, sodium restriction allows lower dosage of the diuretic medication and may prevent side effects. Potassium excretion, in particular, is directly related to distal renal tubule sodium delivery, and sodium restriction will decrease diuretic-related potassium losses.

Typical American diets contain a minimum of 4–6 g (175–260 mEq) of sodium per day. A no-added-salt diet contains approximately 3 g (132 mEq) of sodium per day. Further restriction can be achieved with sodium diets of 2 or 1 g/d. Diets with more severe restriction are poorly accepted by patients and are rarely used.

Dietary sodium includes sodium naturally occurring in foods, sodium added during food processing, and sodium added by the consumer during cooking and at the table. About a third of current dietary intake is derived from each. Diets that allow 2000 mg of sodium daily are easiest to design and implement. Such diets generally eliminate added salt, most processed foods, and selected foods with particularly high sodium content. Patients who follow such diets for 2–3 months lose their craving for salty foods and can often continue to restrict their sodium intake indefinitely. Many patients with mild hypertension will achieve significant reductions in blood pressure (approximately 5 mm Hg diastolic) with this degree of sodium restriction. Other patients require more severe sodium restriction (approximately 1000 mg of sodium per day) for reduction in blood pressure.

Diets allowing 1000 mg of sodium require further restriction of commonly eaten foods. Special "low-sodium" products are now available to facilitate such diets. These diets are difficult for most people to follow and are generally reserved for hospitalized patients and highly motivated outpatients—most commonly those with severe liver disease and ascites.

Fat-Restricted Diets

Traditional fat-restricted diets are useful in the treatment of fat malabsorption syndromes. Such diets will improve the symptoms of diarrhea with steatorrhea independently of the primary physiologic abnormality by limiting the quantity of fatty acids that reach the colon. The degree of fat restriction necessary to control symptoms must be individualized. Patients with severe malabsorption can be limited to 40–60 g of fat per day. Diets containing 60–80 g of fat per day can be designed for patients with less severe abnormalities.

In general, fat-restricted diets require broiling, baking, or boiling meat and fish; discarding the skin of poultry and fish and using those foods as the main protein source; using nonfat dairy products; and avoiding desserts, sauces, and gravies.

Low-Cholesterol, Low-Saturated-Fat Diets

Fat-restricted diets that specifically restrict saturated fats and dietary cholesterol are the mainstay of dietary treatment of hyperlipidemia (see Chapter 28). Similar diets are recommended also for diabetes (see Chapter 27) and for the prevention of coronary artery disease (see Chapter 10). Current recommendations for the prevention of cancer by dietary modification also include fat restriction. The large Women's Health Initiative Dietary Modification Trial, however, did not show any significant benefit of a low-fat diet on weight control or prevention of cardiovascular disease or cancer.

The aim of these diets is to restrict total fat to less than 30% of calories and to achieve a normal body weight by caloric restriction and increased physical activity. Saturated fat is restricted to 7% of calories and dietary cholesterol to 200 mg/d. Saturated fat can be replaced either with complex carbohydrates or, if energy balance permits, with monounsaturated fats. Saturated fat, total fat, and dietary cholesterol can be restricted further, but studies suggest that more extreme restriction offers little further advantage in overall modification of serum lipids. Cholesterol-lowering diets can be further augmented with the addition of plant stanols and sterols and with soluble dietary fiber.

Protein-Restricted Diets

Protein-restricted diets are most commonly used in patients with hepatic encephalopathy due to chronic liver disease and in patients with renal failure to slow the progression of early disease and to decrease symptoms of uremia in more severe disease. Patients with selected inborn errors of amino acid metabolism and other abnormalities resulting in hyperammonemia also require restriction of protein or of specific amino acids.

Protein restriction is intended to limit the production of nitrogenous waste products. Energy intake must be adequate to facilitate the efficient use of dietary protein. Proteins must be of high biologic value and be provided in sufficient quantity to meet minimal requirements. For most patients, the diet should contain at least 0.6 g/kg/d of protein. Patients with encephalopathy who do not respond to this degree of restriction are unlikely to respond to more severe restriction.

DIETS THAT SUPPLEMENT NUTRIENTS

High-Fiber Diet

Dietary fiber is a diverse group of plant constituents that is resistant to digestion by the human digestive tract. Typical American diets contain about 5–10 g of dietary fiber per day. Epidemiologic evidence has suggested that populations consuming greater quantities of fiber have a lower incidence of certain gastrointestinal disorders, including diverticulitis and colon cancer. Most authorities currently recommend higher intakes of dietary fiber for health maintenance.

Diets high in dietary fiber (20–35 g/d) are also commonly used in the management of a variety of gastrointestinal disorders, particularly irritable bowel syndrome and recurrent diverticulitis. Diets high in fiber may also be useful to reduce blood sugar in patients with diabetes and to reduce cholesterol levels in patients with hypercholesterolemia. Such diets include greater intakes of fresh fruits and vegetables, whole grains, legumes and seeds, and bran products. For some patients, the addition of psyllium seed (2 tsp per day) or natural bran (one-half cup per day) may be preferable.

High-Potassium Diets

Potassium-supplemented diets are used most commonly to compensate for potassium losses caused by diuretics. Although potassium losses can be partially prevented by using lower doses of diuretics, concurrent sodium restriction, and potassium-sparing diuretics, some patients require additional potassium to prevent hypokalemia. High-potassium diets may also have a direct antihypertensive effect. Typical American diets contain about 3 g (80 mEq) of potassium per day. High-potassium diets commonly contain 4.5–7 g (120–180 mEq) of potassium per day.

Most fruits, vegetables, and their juices contain high concentrations of potassium. Supplemental potassium can also be provided with potassium-containing salt substitutes (up to 20 mEq in one-quarter tsp) or as potassium chloride in solution or capsules, but this is rarely necessary if the above measures are followed to prevent potassium losses and supplement dietary potassium.

High-Calcium Diets

Additional intakes of dietary calcium have recently been recommended for the prevention of postmenopausal osteoporosis, the prevention and treatment of hypertension, and the prevention of colon cancer. Although the evidence in each case is preliminary, authorities recommend intakes of 1 g of calcium per day for most adults and 1.5 g/d for postmenopausal women. Average American daily intakes are approximately 700 mg/d.

Low-fat and nonfat dairy products are the mainstay of supplemental calcium intakes. Patients with lactose intolerance who cannot tolerate liquid dairy products may be able to tolerate nonliquid products such as cheese and yogurt. Leafy green vegetables and canned fish with bones also contain high concentrations of calcium, although the latter is also very high in sodium.

Chao A et al: Meat consumption and risk of colorectal cancer. JAMA 2005;293:172. [PMID: 15644544]

Esposito K et al: Effect of a Mediterranean-style diet on endothelial dysfunction and markers of vascular inflammation in the metabolic syndrome: a randomized trial. JAMA 2004;292:1440. [PMID: 15383514]

Gannon MC et al: Effect of a high-protein, low-carbohydrate diet on blood glucose control in people with type 2 diabetes. Diabetes 2004;53:2375. [PMID: 15331548]

Gardner CD et al: The effect of a plant-based diet on plasma lipids in hypercholesterolemic adults: a randomized trial. Ann Intern Med 2005;142:725. [PMID: 15867404]

Gerhard GT et al: Effects of a low-fat diet compared with those of a high-monounsaturated fat diet on body weight, plasma lipids and lipoproteins, and glycemic control in type 2 diabetes. Am J Clin Nutr 2004;80:668. [PMID: 15321807]

Howard BV et al: Low-fat dietary pattern and weight change over 7 years: the Women's Health Initiative Dietary Modification Trial. JAMA 2006;295:39. [PMID: 16391215]

Howard BV et al: Low-fat dietary pattern and risk of cardiovascular disease: the Women's Health Initiative Randomized Controlled Dietary Modification Trial. JAMA 2006;295:655. [PMID: 16467234]

Jackson RD et al: Calcium plus vitamin D supplementation and the risk of fractures. N Engl J Med 2006;354:669. [PMID: 16481635]

Little P et al: Randomized controlled factorial trial of dietary advice for patients with a single high blood pressure reading in primary care. BMJ 2004;328:1054. [PMID: 15082472]

MacLean et al: Effects of omega-3 fatty acids on cancer risk: A systematic review. JAMA 2006;295:403.[PMID: 16434631]

Moore H et al: Dietary advice for treatment of type 2 diabetes mellitus in adults. Cochrane Database Syst Rev 2004;(3):CD004097. [PMID: 15266517]

Park Y et al: Dietary fiber intake and risk of colorectal cancer: A pooled analysis of prospective cohort studies. JAMA 2005;294:2849. [PMID: 16352792]

Whelton SP et al: Meta-analysis of observational studies on fish intake and coronary heart disease. Am J Cardiol 2004;93:1119. [PMID: 15110203]

■ NUTRITIONAL SUPPORT

Nutritional support is the provision of nutrients to patients who cannot meet their nutritional requirements by eating standard diets. Nutrients may be delivered enterally, using oral nutritional supplements, nasogastric and nasoduodenal feeding tubes, and tube enterostomies, or parenterally, using lines or catheters placed in peripheral or central veins, respectively. Current nutritional support techniques permit adequate nutrient delivery to most patients. Nutrition support should be utilized, however, only if it is likely to improve the patient's clinical outcome. The financial costs and risks of side effects must be balanced against the potential advantages of improved nutritional status in each clinical situation.

INDICATIONS FOR NUTRITIONAL SUPPORT

The precise indications for nutritional support remain controversial. Most authorities agree that nutritional support is indicated for at least four groups of adult patients: (1) those with inadequate bowel syndromes, (2) those with severe prolonged hypercatabolic states (eg, due to extensive burns, multiple trauma, mechanical ventilation), (3) those requiring prolonged therapeutic bowel rest, and (4) those with severe protein–calorie undernutrition with a treatable disease who have sustained a loss of over 25% of body weight.

It has been difficult to prove the efficacy of nutritional support in the treatment of most other conditions. In most cases it has not been possible to show a clear advantage of treatment by means of nutritional support over treatment without such support.

The American Society for Parenteral and Enteral Nutrition (ASPEN) has published recommendations for the rational use of nutritional support. The recommendations emphasize the need to individualize the decision to begin nutritional support, weighing the risks and costs against the benefits to each patient. They also reinforce the need to identify high-risk malnourished patients by nutritional assessment.

NUTRITIONAL SUPPORT METHODS

Selection of the most appropriate nutritional support method involves consideration of gastrointestinal function, the anticipated duration of nutritional support, and the ability of each method to meet the patient's nutritional requirements. The method chosen should meet the patient's nutritional needs with the lowest risk and lowest cost possible. For most patients, enteral feeding is safer and cheaper and offers significant physiologic advantages. An algorithm for selection of the most appropriate nutritional support method is presented in Figure 29–1.

Prior to initiating specialized enteral nutritional support, efforts should be made to supplement food intake. Attention to patient preferences, timing of meals and diagnostic procedures and use of medications, and the use of foods brought to the hospital by family and friends can often increase oral intake. Patients unable to eat enough at regular mealtimes to meet nutritional requirements can be given **oral supplements** as snacks or to replace low-calorie beverages. Oral supplements of differing nutritional composition are available for the purpose of individualizing the diet in accordance with specific clinical requirements (see below). Fiber and lactose content, caloric density, protein level, and amino acid profiles can all be modified as necessary.

Patients unable to take adequate oral nutrients who have functioning gastrointestinal tracts and who meet the criteria for nutritional support are candidates for **tube feedings**. Small-bore feeding tubes are placed via the nose into the stomach or duodenum. Patients able to sit up in bed who can protect their airways can be fed into the stomach. Because of the increased risk of aspiration, patients who cannot adequately protect their airways should be fed nasoduodenally. Feeding tubes can usually be passed into the duodenum by

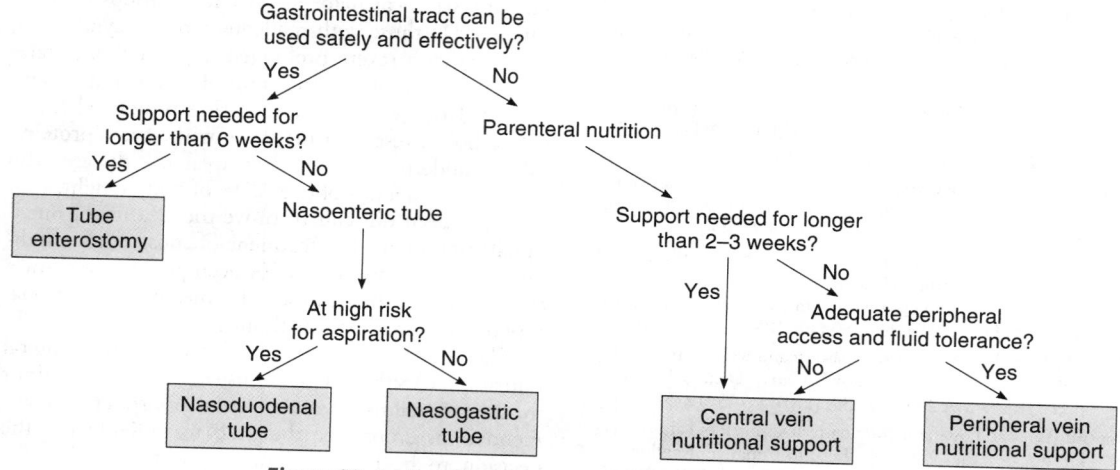

Figure 29–1. Nutritional support method decision tree.

leaving an extra length of tubing in the stomach and placing the patient in the right decubitus position. Metoclopramide, 10 mg intravenously, can be given 20 minutes prior to insertion and continued every 6 hours thereafter to facilitate passage through the pylorus. Occasionally patients will require fluoroscopic or endoscopic guidance to insert the tube distal to the pylorus. Placement of nasogastric and, particularly, nasoduodenal tubes should be confirmed radiographically before delivery of feeding solutions.

Feeding tubes can also be placed directly into the gastrointestinal tract using **tube enterostomies**. Most tube enterostomies are placed in patients who require long-term enteral nutritional support. Gastrostomies have the advantage of allowing bolus feedings, while jejunostomies require continuous infusions. Gastrostomies—like nasogastric feeding—should be used only in patients at low risk for aspiration. Gastrostomies can also be placed percutaneously with the aid of endoscopy. These tubes can then be advanced to jejunostomies. Tube enterostomies can also be placed surgically.

Patients who require nutritional support but whose gastrointestinal tracts are nonfunctional should receive **parenteral nutritional support**. Most patients receive parenteral feedings via a central vein—most commonly the subclavian vein. Peripheral veins can be used in some patients, but because of the high osmolality of parenteral solutions this is rarely tolerated for more than a few weeks.

Peripheral vein nutritional support is most commonly used in patients with nonfunctioning gastrointestinal tracts who require immediate support but whose clinical status is expected to improve within 1–2 weeks, allowing enteral feeding. Peripheral vein nutritional support is administered via standard intravenous lines. Solutions should always include lipid and dextrose in combination with amino acids to provide adequate nonprotein calories. Serious side effects are infrequent, but there is a high incidence of phlebitis and infiltration of intravenous lines.

Central vein nutritional support is delivered via intravenous catheters placed percutaneously using aseptic technique. Proper placement in the superior vena cava is documented radiographically before the solution is infused. Catheters must be carefully maintained by experienced nursing personnel and used solely for nutritional support to prevent infection and other catheter-related complications.

NUTRITIONAL REQUIREMENTS

Each patient's nutritional requirements should be determined independently of the method of nutritional support. In most situations, solutions of equal nutrient value can be designed for delivery via enteral and parenteral routes, but differences in absorption must be considered. A complete nutritional support solution must contain water, energy, amino acids, electrolytes, vitamins, minerals, and essential fatty acids.

Water

For most patients, water requirements can be calculated by allowing 1500 mL for the first 20 kg of body weight plus 20 mL for every kilogram over 20. Additional losses should be replaced as they occur. For average-sized adult patients, fluid needs are about 30–35 mL/kg, or approximately 1 mL/kcal of energy required (see below).

Energy

Energy requirements can be estimated by one of three methods: (1) by using standard equations to calculate BEE plus additional calories for activity and illness, (2) by applying a simple calculation based on calories per kilogram of body weight, or (3) by measuring energy expenditure with indirect calorimetry.

BEE can be estimated by the **Harris–Benedict equation**: for men, BEE = 666 + (13.7 × weight in kg) + (5 × height in cm) − (6.8 × age in years). For women, BEE = 655 + (9.5 × weight in kg) + (1.8 × height in cm) − (4.7 × age in years). For undernourished patients, actual body weight should be used; for obese patients, ideal body weight should be used. For most patients, an additional 20–50% of BEE is administered as nonprotein calories to accommodate energy expenditures during activity or relating to the illness. Occasional patients are noted to have energy expenditures greater than 150% of BEE.

Energy requirements can be estimated also by multiplying actual body weight in kilograms (for obese patients, ideal body weight) by 30–35 kcal.

Both of these methods provide imprecise estimates of actual energy expenditures, especially for the markedly underweight, overweight, and critically ill patient. Studies using indirect calorimetry have demonstrated that as many as 30–40% of patients will have measured expenditures 10% above or below estimated values. For accurate determination of energy expenditure, indirect calorimetry should be used.

Protein

Protein and energy requirements are closely related. If adequate calories are provided, most patients can be given 0.8–1.2 g of protein per kilogram per day. Patients undergoing moderate to severe stress should receive up to 1.5 g/kg/d. As in the case of energy requirements, actual weights should be used for normal and underweight patients and ideal weights for patients with significant obesity.

Patients who are receiving protein without adequate calories will catabolize protein for energy rather than utilizing it for protein synthesis. Thus, when energy intake is low, excess protein is needed for nitrogen balance. If both energy and protein intakes are low, extra energy will have a more significant positive effect on nitrogen balance than extra protein.

Electrolytes & Minerals

Requirements for sodium, potassium, and chloride vary widely. Most patients require 45–145 mEq/d of each. The actual requirement in individual patients will depend on the patient's cardiovascular, renal, endocrine, and gastrointestinal status as well as measurements of serum concentration.

Patients receiving enteral nutritional support should receive adequate vitamins and minerals according to the recommended daily allowances. Most premixed enteral solutions provide adequate vitamins and minerals as long as adequate calories are administered.

Patients receiving parenteral nutritional support require smaller amounts of minerals: calcium, 10–15 mEq/d; phosphorus, 15–20 mEq per 1000 nonprotein calories; and magnesium, 16–24 mEq/d. Most patients receiving nutritional support do not require supplemental iron because body stores are adequate. Iron nutrition should be monitored closely by following the hemoglobin concentration, mean corpuscular volume, and iron studies. Parenteral administration of iron is associated with a number of adverse effects and should be reserved for iron-deficient patients unable to take oral iron.

Patients receiving parenteral nutritional support should be given the trace elements zinc (about 5 mg/d) and copper (about 2 mg/d). Patients with diarrhea will require additional zinc to replace fecal losses. Additional trace elements—especially chromium, manganese, and selenium—are provided to patients receiving long-term parenteral nutrition.

Parenteral vitamins are provided daily. Standardized multivitamin solutions are currently available to provide adequate quantities of vitamins A, B_{12}, C, D, E, thiamine, riboflavin, niacin, pantothenic acid, pyridoxine, folic acid, and biotin. Vitamin K is not given routinely but administered when the prothrombin time becomes abnormal.

Essential Fatty Acids

Patients receiving nutritional support should be given 2–4% of their total calories as linoleic acid to prevent essential fatty acid deficiency. Most prepared enteral solutions contain adequate linoleic acid. Patients receiving parenteral nutrition should be given at least 250 mL of a 20% intravenous fat (emulsified soybean or safflower oil) about two or three times a week. Intravenous fat can also be used as an energy source in place of dextrose.

ENTERAL NUTRITIONAL SUPPORT SOLUTIONS

Most patients who require enteral nutritional support can be given commercially prepared enteral solutions (Table 29–10). Nutritionally complete solutions have been designed to provide adequate proportions of water, energy, protein, and micronutrients. Nutritionally incomplete solutions are also available to provide specific macronutrients (eg, protein, carbohydrate, and fat) to supplement complete solutions for patients with unusual requirements or to design solutions that are not available commercially.

Nutritionally complete solutions are characterized as follows: (1) by osmolality (isotonic or hypertonic), (2) by lactose content (present or absent), (3) by the molecular form of the protein component (intact proteins; peptides or amino acids), (4) by the quantity of protein and calories provided, and (5) by fiber content (present or absent). For most patients, isotonic solutions containing no lactose or fiber are preferable. Such solutions generally contain moderate amounts of fat and intact protein. Most commercial isotonic solutions contain 1000 kcal and about 37–45 g of protein per liter.

Solutions containing hydrolyzed proteins or crystalline amino acids and with no significant fat content

Table 29–10. Enteral solutions.

Complete

Blenderized (eg, Compleat Regular, Compleat Modified,[1] Vitaneed[1])

Whole protein, lactose-containing (eg, Mentene, Carnation and Delmark Instant Breakfast, Forta Shake)

Whole protein, lactose-free, low-residue:

   1 kcal/mL (eg, Ensure, Isocal, Osmolite, Nutren 1.0,[1] Nutrilan, Isolan,[1] Sustacal, Resource)

   1.5 kcal/mL (eg, Ensure Plus, Sustacal HC, Comply, Nutren 1.5, Resource Plus)

   2 kcal/mL (eg, Isocal HCN, Magnacal, TwoCal HN)

   High-nitrogen: > 15% total calories from protein (eg, Ensure HN, Attain,[1] Osmolite HN,[1] Replete, Entrition HN,[1] Isolan,[1] Isocal HN,[1] Sustacal HC, Isosource HN,[1] Ultralan)

Whole protein, lactose-free, high-residue:

   1 kcal/mL (eg, Jevity,[1] Profiber,[1] Nutren 1.0 with fiber,[1] Fiberian,[1] Sustacal with fiber, Ultracal,[1] Ensure with fiber, Fibersource)

   Chemically defined peptide- or amino acid-based (eg, Accupep HPF, Criticare HN, Peptamen,[1] Reabfin, Vital HN, AlitraQ, Tolerex, Vivonex TEN)

"Disease-specific" formulas

Renal failure: with essential amino acids (eg, Amin-Aid, Travasorb Renal, Aminess)

Malabsorption: with medium-chain triglycerides (eg, Portagen,[1] Travasorb MCT)

Respiratory failure: with > 50% calories from fat (eg, Pulmocare, NutriVent)

Hepatic encephalopathy: with high amounts of branched-chain amino acids (eg, Hepatic-Acid II, Travasorb Hepatic)

Incomplete (modular)

Protein (eg, Nutrisource Protein, Promed, Propac)

Carbohydrate (eg, Nutrisource Carbohydrate, Polycose, Sumacal)

Fat (eg, MCT Oil, Microlipid, Nutrisource Lipid)

Vitamins (eg, Nutrisource Vitamins)

Minerals (eg, Nutrisource Minerals)

[1]Isotonic.

are called elemental solutions, since macronutrients are provided in their most "elemental" form. These solutions have been designed for patients with malabsorption, particularly pancreatic insufficiency and limited fat absorption. Elemental diets are extremely hypertonic and often result in more severe diarrhea. Their use should be limited to patients who cannot tolerate isotonic solutions.

Although formulas have been designed for specific clinical situations—solutions containing primarily essential amino acids (for renal failure), medium-chain triglycerides (for fat malabsorption), more fat (for respiratory failure and CO_2 retention), and more branched-chain amino acids (for hepatic encephalopathy and severe trauma)—they have not been shown to be superior to standard formulas for most patients.

Enteral solutions should be administered via continuous infusion, preferably with an infusion pump. Isotonic feedings should be started at full strength at about 25–33% of the estimated final infusion rate. Feedings can be advanced by similar amounts every 12 hours as tolerated. Hypertonic feedings should be started at half strength. The strength and the rate can then be advanced every 6 hours as tolerated.

COMPLICATIONS OF ENTERAL NUTRITIONAL SUPPORT

Minor complications of tube feedings occur in 10–15% of patients. Gastrointestinal complications include diarrhea (most common), inadequate gastric emptying, emesis, esophagitis, and occasionally gastrointestinal bleeding. Diarrhea associated with tube feeding may be due to intolerance to the osmotic load or to one of the macronutrients (eg, fat, lactose) in the solution. Patients being fed in this way may also have diarrhea from other causes (as side effects of antibiotics or other drugs, associated with infection, etc), and these possibilities should always be investigated in appropriate circumstances.

Mechanical complications of tube feedings are potentially the most serious. Of particular importance is aspiration. All patients receiving nasogastric tube feedings are at risk for this life-threatening complication. Limiting nasogastric feedings to those patients who can adequately protect their airway and careful monitoring of patients being fed by tube should limit these serious complications to 1–2% of cases. Minor mechanical complications are common and include tube obstruction and dislodgment.

Metabolic complications during enteral nutritional support are common but in most cases are easily managed. The most important problem is hypernatremic dehydration, most commonly seen in elderly patients given excessive protein intake who are unable to respond to thirst. Abnormalities of potassium, glucose, and acid–base balance may also occur.

PARENTERAL NUTRITIONAL SUPPORT SOLUTIONS

Parenteral nutritional support solutions can be designed to deliver adequate nutrients to most patients. The basic parenteral solution is composed of dextrose, amino acids, and water. Electrolytes, minerals, trace elements, vitamins, and medications can also be added. Most commercial solutions contain the monohydrate form of dextrose that provides 3.4 kcal/g. Crystalline amino acids are available in a variety of concentrations, so that a broad range of solutions can be made up that will contain specific amounts of dextrose and amino acids as required.

Typical solutions for central vein nutritional support contain 25–35% dextrose and 2.75–6% amino acids depending upon the patient's estimated nutrient and water requirements. These solutions typically have

Table 29–11. Typical parenteral nutrition solution (for stable patients without organ failure).

Dextrose (3.4 kcal/g)	25%
Amino acids (4 kcal/g)	6%
Na^+	50 mEq/L
K^+	40 mEq/L
Ca^{2+}	5 mEq/L
Mg^{2+}	8 mEq/L
Cl^-	60 mEq/L
P	12 mEq/L
Acetate	Balance
MVI-12 (vitamins)	10 mL/d
MTE (trace elements)	5 mL/d
Fat emulsion 20%	250 mL 5 times a week
Typical rate	Day 1: 30 mL/h
	Day 2: 60 mL/h
By day 2, solution provides:	Calories: 1925 kcal total
	Protein: 86 g
	Fat: 19% of total kcal
	Fluid: 1690 mL

osmolalities in excess of 1800 mosm/L and require infusion into a central vein. A typical formula for patients without organ failure is shown in Table 29–11.

Solutions with lower osmolalities can also be designed for infusion into peripheral veins. Typical solutions for peripheral infusion contain 5–10% dextrose and 2.75–4.25% amino acids. These solutions have osmolalities between 800 and 1200 mosm/L and result in a high incidence of thrombophlebitis and line infiltration. These solutions will provide adequate protein for most patients but inadequate energy. Additional energy must be provided in the form of emulsified soybean or safflower oil. Such intravenous fat solutions are currently available in 10% and 25% solutions providing 1.1 and 2.2 kcal/mL, respectively. Intravenous fat solutions are isosmotic and well tolerated by peripheral veins. Typical patients are given 200–500 mL of a 20% solution each day. As much as 60% of total calories can be administered in this manner.

Intravenous fat can also be provided to patients receiving central vein nutritional support. In this instance, dextrose concentrations should be decreased to provide a fixed concentration of energy. Intravenous fat has been shown to be equivalent to intravenous dextrose in providing energy to spare protein. Intravenous fat is associated with less glucose intolerance, less production of carbon dioxide, and less fatty infiltration of the liver and has been increasingly utilized in patients with hyperglycemia, respiratory failure, and liver disease. Intravenous fat has also been increasingly used in patients with large estimated energy requirements. Recent studies suggest that the maximum glucose utilization rate is approximately 5–7 mg/min/kg.

Patients who require additional calories can be given them as fat to prevent excess administration of dextrose. Intravenous fat can also be used to prevent essential fatty acid deficiency. The optimal ratio of carbohydrate and fat in parenteral nutritional support has not been determined.

Infusion of parenteral solutions should be started slowly to prevent hyperglycemia and other metabolic complications. Typical solutions are given initially at a rate of 50 mL/h and advanced by about the same amount every 24 hours until the desired final rate is reached.

COMPLICATIONS OF PARENTERAL NUTRITIONAL SUPPORT

Complications of central vein nutritional support occur in up to 50% of patients. Although most are minor and easily managed, significant complications will develop in about 5% of patients. Complications of central vein nutritional support can be divided into catheter-related complications and metabolic complications.

Catheter-related complications can occur during insertion or while the catheter is in place. Pneumothorax, hemothorax, arterial laceration, air emboli, and brachial plexus injury can occur during catheter placement. The incidence of these complications is inversely related to the experience of the physician performing the procedure but will occur in at least 1–2% of cases even in major medical centers. Each catheter placement should be documented by chest radiograph prior to initiation of nutritional support.

Catheter thrombosis and catheter-related sepsis are the most important complications of indwelling catheters. Patients with indwelling central vein catheters in whom fever develops without an apparent source should have their lines changed over a wire or removed immediately, the tip quantitatively cultured, and antibiotics begun empirically. Quantitative tip cultures and blood cultures will help guide further antibiotic therapy. Catheter-related sepsis occurs in 2–3% of patients even if maximal efforts are made to prevent infection.

Metabolic complications of central vein nutritional support occur in over 50% of patients (Table 29–12). Most are minor and easily managed, and termination of support is seldom necessary.

PATIENT MONITORING DURING NUTRITIONAL SUPPORT

Every patient receiving enteral or parenteral nutritional support should be monitored closely. Formal nutritional support teams composed of a physician, a nurse, a dietitian, and a pharmacist have been shown to decrease the rate of complications.

Patients should be monitored both for the adequacy of treatment and to prevent complications or detect them early when they occur. Because estimates

Table 29–12. Metabolic complications of parenteral nutritional support.

Complication	Common Causes	Possible Solutions
Hyperglycemia	Too rapid infusion of dextrose, "stress," corticosteroids	Decrease glucose infusion; insulin; replacement of dextrose with fat
Hyperosmolar nonketotic dehydration	Severe, undetected hyperglycemia	Insulin, hydration, potassium
Hyperchloremic metabolic acidosis	High chloride administration	Decrease chloride
Azotemia	Excessive protein administration	Decrease amino acid concentration
Hyperphosphatemia, hypokalemia, hypomagnesemia	Extracellular to intracellular shifting with refeeding	Increase solution concentration
Liver enzyme abnormalities	Lipid trapping in hepatocytes, fatty liver	Decrease dextrose
Acalculous cholecystitis	Biliary stasis	Oral fat
Zinc deficiency	Diarrhea, small bowel fistulas	Increase concentration
Copper deficiency	Biliary fistulas	Increase concentration

of nutritional requirements are imprecise, frequent reassessment is necessary. Daily intakes should be recorded and compared with estimated requirements. Body weight, hydration status, and overall clinical status should be followed. Patients who do not appear to be responding as anticipated can be evaluated for nitrogen balance by means of the following equation:

$$\text{Nitrogen balance} = \frac{\text{24-hour protein intake (g)}}{6.25} - \left(\frac{\text{25-hour urinary nitrogen (g)}}{} + 4\right)$$

Patients with positive nitrogen balances can be continued on their current regimens; patients with negative balances should receive moderate increases in calorie and protein intake and then be reassessed. Monitoring for metabolic complications includes daily measurements of electrolytes; serum glucose, phosphorus, magnesium, calcium, and creatinine; and BUN until the patient is stabilized. Once the patient is stabilized, electrolytes, phosphorus, calcium, magnesium, and glucose should be obtained at least twice weekly. Red blood cell folate, zinc, and copper should be checked at least once a month.

August D et al: An evidence-based approach to optimal management of vascular and enteral access for home parenteral and enteral nutrition support. JPEN J Parenter Enteral Nutr 2006;30(1 Suppl):S5. [PMID: 16387911]

Braga JM et al: Implementation of dietician recommendations for enteral nutrition results in improved outcomes. J Am Diet Assoc 2006;106:281. [PMID: 16442879]

Edington J et al: A prospective randomized controlled trial of nutritional supplementation in malnourished elderly in the community: clinical and health economic outcomes. Clin Nutr 2004;23:195. [PMID: 15030959]

Farber MS et al: Reducing costs and patient morbidity in the enterally fed intensive care unit patient. J Parenter Enteral Nutr 2005;29(1 Suppl):S62. [PMID: 15709547]

Fiaccadori E et al: Enteral nutrition in patients with acute renal failure. Kidney Int 2004;65:999. [PMID: 14871420]

Forbes A: Parenteral nutrition. Curr Opin Gastroenterol 2006; 22:160. [PMID: 16462173]

Howard L et al: Nutrition in the perioperative patient. Annu Rev Nutr 2003;23:263. [PMID: 14527336]

Ireton-Jones C et al: Home parenteral nutrition registry: a five-year retrospective evaluation of outcomes of patients receiving home parenteral nutrition support. Nutrition 2005;21:156. [PMID: 15723743]

Jeejeebhoy KN: Enteral feeding. Curr Opin Gastroenterol 2005; 21:187. [PMID: 15711211]

Martin CM et al: Southwestern Ontario Critical Care Research Network: Multicentre, cluster-randomized clinical trial of algorithms for critical-care enteral and parenteral therapy (ACCEPT). CMAJ 2004;170:197. [PMID: 14734433]

McMahon MM et al: Medical and ethical aspects of long-term enteral tube feeding. Mayo Clin Proc 2005;80:1461. [PMID: 16295026]

Messing B et al: Guidelines for management of home parenteral support in adult chronic intestinal failure patients. Gastroenterology 2006;130(2 Suppl 1):S43. [PMID: 16473071]

Sayers GM et al: Parenteral nutrition: ethical and legal considerations. Postgrad Med J 2006;82:79. [PMID: 16461468]

Soop M et al: Randomized clinical trial of the effects of immediate enteral nutrition on metabolic responses to major colorectal surgery in an enhanced recovery protocol. Br J Surg 2004;91:1138. [PMID: 15449264]

Tappenden KA: Mechanisms of enteral nutrient-enhanced intestinal adaptation. Gastroenterology 2006;130(2 Suppl): S93. [PMID: 16473079]

General Problems in Infectious Diseases

30

Richard A. Jacobs, MD, PhD, & Peter V. Chin-Hong, MD

Most infections are confined to specific organ systems, and many of the important infectious disease pathogens are discussed in chapters dealing with the relevant anatomic areas. This chapter discusses some important general problems related to infectious diseases.

FEVER OF UNKNOWN ORIGIN (FUO)

ESSENTIALS OF DIAGNOSIS

- *Illness of at least 3 weeks duration.*
- *Fever over 38.3 °C on several occasions.*
- *Diagnosis has not been made after three outpatient visits or 3 days of hospitalization.*

General Considerations

The intervals specified in the criteria for the diagnosis of FUO are arbitrary ones intended to exclude patients with protracted but self-limited viral illnesses and to allow time for the usual radiographic, serologic, and cultural studies to be performed. Because of costs of hospitalization and the availability of most screening tests on an outpatient basis, the original criterion requiring 1 week of hospitalization has been modified to accept patients in whom a diagnosis has not been made after three outpatient visits or 3 days of hospitalization.

Several additional categories of FUO have been added: (1) Nosocomial FUO refers to the hospitalized patient with fever of 38.3 °C or higher on several occasions, due to a process not present or incubating at the time of admission, in whom initial cultures are negative and the diagnosis remains unknown after 3 days of investigation (see Nosocomial Infections, below). (2) Neutropenic FUO includes patients with fever of 38.3 °C or higher on several occasions with less than 500 neutrophils per microliter in whom initial cultures are negative and the diagnosis remains uncertain after 3 days (see Chapter 2 and Infections in the Immunocompromised Patient, below). (3) HIV-associated FUO pertains to HIV-positive patients with fever of 38.3 °C or higher who have been febrile for 4 weeks or more as an outpatient or 3 days as an inpatient, in whom the diagnosis remains uncertain after 3 days of investigation with at least 2 days for cultures to incubate (see Chapter 31). Although not usually considered separately, FUO in solid organ transplant recipients is a common scenario with a unique differential diagnosis and is discussed below.

For a general discussion of fever, see the section on fever and hyperthermia in Chapter 2.

A. COMMON CAUSES

Most cases represent unusual manifestations of common diseases and not rare or exotic diseases—eg, tuberculosis, endocarditis, gallbladder disease, and HIV (primary infection or opportunistic infection) are more common causes of FUO than Whipple's disease or familial Mediterranean fever.

B. AGE OF PATIENT

In adults, infections (25–40% of cases) and cancer (25–40% of cases) account for the majority of FUOs. In children, infections are the most common cause of FUO (30–50% of cases) and cancer a rare cause (5–10% of cases). Autoimmune disorders occur with equal frequency in adults and children (10–20% of cases), but the diseases differ. Juvenile rheumatoid arthritis is particularly common in children, whereas systemic lupus erythematosus, Wegener's granulomatosis, and polyarteritis nodosa are more common in adults. Adult Still's disease, giant cell arteritis, and polymyalgia rheumatica occur exclusively in adults. In the elderly (over 65 years of age), multisystem immune-mediated diseases such as temporal arteritis, polymyalgia rheumatica, sarcoidosis, rheumatoid arthritis, and Wegener's granulomatosis account for 25–30% of all FUOs.

C. DURATION OF FEVER

The cause of FUO changes dramatically in patients who have been febrile for 6 months or longer. Infection, cancer, and autoimmune disorders combined account for only 20% of FUOs in these patients. Instead, other entities such as granulomatous diseases (granulomatous hepatitis, Crohn's disease, ulcerative colitis) and factitious fever become important causes. One-fourth of patients who say they have been febrile for 6 months or longer actually have no true fever or underlying disease. Instead, the usual normal circadian variation in temperature (temperature 0.5–1 °C higher in the afternoon than in the morning) is interpreted as abnormal. Patients with episodic or recurrent fever (ie, those who meet the criteria for FUO but have fever-free periods of 2 weeks or longer) are similar to those with prolonged fever. Infection, malignancy, and autoimmune disorders account for only 20–25% of such fevers, whereas various miscellaneous diseases (Crohn's disease, familial Mediterranean fever, allergic alveolitis) account for another 25%. Approximately 50% of cases remain undiagnosed but have a benign course with eventual resolution of symptoms.

D. Immunologic Status

In the neutropenic patient, fungal infections and occult bacterial infection are important causes of FUO. In the patient taking immunosuppressive medications (particularly organ transplant patients), cytomegalovirus (CMV) infections are a frequent cause of fever, as are fungal infections, nocardiosis, *Pneumocystis jiroveci* (formerly *Pneumocystis carinii*) pneumonia, and mycobacterial infections.

E. Classification of Causes of FUO

Most patients with FUO will fit into one of five categories.

1. Infection—Both systemic and localized infections can cause FUO. Tuberculosis and endocarditis are the most common systemic infections, but mycoses, viral diseases (particularly infection with Epstein-Barr virus and CMV), toxoplasmosis, brucellosis, Q fever, cat-scratch disease, salmonellosis, malaria, and many other less common infections have been implicated. Primary infection with HIV or opportunistic infections associated with the AIDS—particularly mycobacterial infections—can also present as FUO. The most common form of localized infection causing FUO is an occult abscess. Liver, spleen, kidney, brain, and bone are organs in which abscess may be difficult to find. A collection of pus may form in the peritoneal cavity or in the subdiaphragmatic, subhepatic, paracolic, or other areas. Cholangitis, osteomyelitis, urinary tract infection, dental abscess, or paranasal sinusitis may cause prolonged fever.

2. Neoplasms—Many cancers can present as FUO. The most common are lymphoma (both Hodgkin's and non-Hodgkin's) and leukemia. Other diseases of lymph nodes, such as angioimmunoblastic lymphoma and Castleman's disease, can also cause FUO. Primary and metastatic tumors of the liver are frequently associated with fever, as are renal cell carcinomas. Atrial myxoma is an often forgotten neoplasm that can result in fever. Chronic lymphocytic leukemia and multiple myeloma are rarely associated with fever, and the presence of fever in patients with these diseases should prompt a search for infection.

3. Autoimmune disorders—Still's disease, systemic lupus erythematosus, cryoglobulinemia, and polyarteritis nodosa are the most common autoimmune causes of FUO. Giant cell arteritis and polymyalgia rheumatica are seen almost exclusively in patients over 50 years of age and are nearly always associated with an elevated erythrocyte sedimentation rate (> 40 mm/h).

4. Miscellaneous causes—Many other conditions have been associated with FUO but less commonly than the foregoing types of illness. Examples include thyroiditis, sarcoidosis, Whipple's disease, familial Mediterranean fever, recurrent pulmonary emboli, alcoholic hepatitis, drug fever, and factitious fever.

5. Undiagnosed FUO—Despite extensive evaluation, the diagnosis remains elusive in 10–15% of patients. Of these patients, the fever abates spontaneously in about 75%, and the clinician never knows the cause; in the remainder, more classic manifestations of the underlying disease appear over time.

Clinical Findings

Because the evaluation of a patient with FUO is costly and time-consuming, it is imperative to first document the presence of fever. This is done by observing the patient while the temperature is being taken to ascertain that fever is not factitious (self-induced). Associated findings that accompany fever include tachycardia, chills, and piloerection. A thorough history—including family, occupational, social (sexual practices, use of injection drugs), dietary (unpasteurized products, raw meat), exposures (animals, chemicals), and travel—may give clues to the diagnosis. Repeated physical examination may reveal subtle, evanescent clinical findings essential to diagnosis.

A. Laboratory Tests

In addition to routine laboratory studies, blood cultures should always be obtained, preferably when the patient has not taken antibiotics for several days, and should be held by the laboratory for 2 weeks to detect slow-growing organisms. Cultures on special media are requested if *Legionella, Bartonella,* or nutritionally deficient streptococci are considered possible pathogens. "Screening tests" with immunologic or microbiologic serologies ("febrile agglutinins") are of low yield and should not be done. Specific serologic tests are helpful if the history or physical examination suggests a specific diagnosis. A single elevated titer rarely allows one to make a diagnosis of infection; instead, one must demonstrate a fourfold rise or fall in titer to confirm a specific infectious cause. Because infection is the most common cause of FUO, other body fluids are usually cultured, ie, urine, sputum, stool, cerebrospinal fluid, and morning gastric aspirates (if one suspects tuberculosis). Direct examination of blood smears may establish a diagnosis of malaria or relapsing fever (*Borrelia*).

B. Imaging

All patients with FUO should have a chest radiograph. Studies such as sinus films, upper gastrointestinal series with small bowel follow-through, barium enema, proctosigmoidoscopy, and evaluation of gallbladder function are reserved for patients who have symptoms, signs, or a history that suggest disease in these body regions. CT scan of the abdomen and pelvis is also frequently performed and is particularly useful for looking at the liver, spleen, and retroperitoneum. When the CT scan is abnormal, the findings often lead to a specific diagnosis. A normal CT scan is not quite as useful; more invasive procedures such as biopsy or exploratory laparotomy may be needed. The role of MRI in the investigation of FUO has not been evaluated. In general, however, MRI is better than CT for detecting lesions of the nervous system and is useful in diagnosing various vasculitides. Ultrasound is sensitive for detecting lesions of the kidney, pancreas, and biliary tree. Echocardiography should be used if one is considering endocarditis or atrial myxoma. Transesophageal echocardiography is more sensitive than surface echocardiography for detecting valvular lesions, but even a negative transesophageal study does not exclude endocarditis (10% false-negative rate). The usefulness of radionuclide studies in diagnosing FUO is variable. Theoretically, a gallium or positron emission tomography (PET) scan would be more helpful than an indium-labeled white blood cell scan, because gallium and fluorodeoxy-glucose may be useful for detecting infection, inflammation, and neoplasm whereas the indium scan is useful only for detecting infection. Indium-labeled immunoglobulin may prove to be useful in detecting infection and neoplasm and can be used in the neutropenic patient. It is not sensitive for lesions of the liver, kidney, and heart because of high background activity. In general, radionuclide scans are plagued by high rates of false-positive and false-negative results that are not useful when used as screening tests and, if done at all, are limited to those patients whose history or examination suggests local inflammation or infection.

C. Biopsy

Invasive procedures are often required for diagnosis. Any abnormal finding should be aggressively evaluated: Headache calls for lumbar puncture to rule out meningitis; skin from a rash should be biopsied to look for cutaneous manifestations of collagen vascular disease or infection; and enlarged lymph nodes should be aspirated or biopsied and examined for cytologic features to rule out neoplasm and sent for culture. Bone marrow aspiration with biopsy is a relatively low-yield procedure (except in HIV-positive patients, in whom mycobacterial infection is a common cause of FUO), but the risk is low and the procedure should be done if other less invasive tests have not yielded a diagnosis. Liver biopsy will yield a specific diagnosis in 10–15% of patients with FUO and should be considered in any patient with abnormal liver function tests even if the liver is normal in size. The role of exploratory laparotomy is debatable since the advent of CT scanning and MRI. Laparotomy or laparoscopy should be considered when the patient continues to deteriorate and the diagnosis is elusive despite extensive evaluation.

Treatment

Therapeutic trials are indicated if a diagnosis is strongly suspected—eg, it is reasonable to give antituberculous drugs if tuberculosis is suspected, or tetracycline if brucellosis is suspected. However, if there is no clinical response in several weeks, it is imperative to stop therapy and reevaluate the patient. In the seriously ill or rapidly deteriorating patient, empiric therapy is often given. Antituberculosis medications (particularly in the elderly or foreign-born) and broad-spectrum antibiotics are reasonable in this setting.

Empiric administration of corticosteroids should be discouraged; they can suppress fever if given in high enough doses, but they can also exacerbate many infections, and infection remains a leading cause of FUO.

Crispin JC et al: Adult-onset Still disease as the cause of fever of unknown origin. Medicine (Baltimore) 2005;84:331. [PMID: 16267408]

Knockaert DC et al: Fever of unknown origin in adults: 40 years on. J Intern Med 2003;253:263. [PMID: 12603493]

Mourad O et al: A comprehensive evidence-based approach to fever of unknown origin. Arch Intern Med 2003;163:545. [PMID: 12622601]

Ozaras R et al: Is laparotomy necessary in the diagnosis of fever of unknown origin? Acta Chir Belg 2005;105:89. [PMID: 15790210]

Tal S et al: Fever of unknown origin in the elderly. J Intern Med 2002;242:295. [PMID: 12366602]

Vanderschueren S et al: From prolonged febrile illness to fever of unknown origin. Arch Intern Med 2003;163:1033. [PMID: 12742800]

Woolery WA et al: Fever of unknown origin: keys to determining the etiology in older patients. Geriatrics 2004;59:41. [PMID: 15508555]

INFECTIONS IN THE IMMUNOCOMPROMISED PATIENT

 ESSENTIALS OF DIAGNOSIS

- *Fever and other symptoms may be blunted because of immunosuppression; early diagnosis may be difficult.*
- *A contaminating organism in an immunocompetent individual may be a pathogen in an immunocompromised one.*
- *The interval since transplantation and the degree of immunosuppression can narrow the differential diagnosis.*

• Empiric broad-spectrum antibiotics may be appropriate in high-risk patients whether or not symptoms are localized because of high infection-related morbidity and mortality.

General Considerations

Immunocompromised patients have one or more defects in their natural defense mechanisms that put them at an increased risk for infections. Not only is the risk of infection greater in these individuals, but once established it is often severe, rapidly progressive, and life-threatening. Organisms that are not usually pathogens in the immunocompetent person may cause life-threatening infection in the compromised patient (eg, *Staphylococcus epidermidis*, *Corynebacterium jeikeium*, *Propionibacterium acnes*, *Bacillus* species). Therefore, culture results must be interpreted with caution, and isolates should not be disregarded as merely contaminants. Although the type of immunodeficiency is associated with specific infectious disease syndromes, any pathogen can cause infection in any immunosuppressed patient at any time. Thus, a systematic evaluation is required to identify a specific organism.

A. IMPAIRED HUMORAL IMMUNITY

Defects in humoral immunity are often congenital, although hypogammaglobulinemia can occur in multiple myeloma, chronic lymphocytic leukemia, and in patients who have undergone splenectomy. Patients with ineffective humoral immunity lack opsonizing antibodies and are at particular risk for infection with encapsulated organisms, such as *Haemophilus influenzae*, *Neisseria meningitidis* and *Streptococcus pneumoniae*.

B. GRANULOCYTOPENIA (NEUTROPENIA)

Granulocytopenia is common following hematopoietic cell transplantation ("bone marrow transplantation") and among patients with solid tumors—as a result of myelosuppressive chemotherapy—and in acute leukemias. The risk of infection begins to increase when the absolute granulocyte count falls below 1000/mcL, with a dramatic increase in frequency and severity when the granulocyte count falls below 100/mcL. The infection risk is also increased when there is a rapid rate of decline of neutrophils and in those with a prolonged period of neutropenia. The granulocytopenic patient is particularly susceptible to infections with gram-negative enteric organisms, *Pseudomonas*, gram-positive cocci (particularly *Staphylococcus aureus*, *S epidermidis*, and viridans streptococci), *Candida*, *Aspergillus*, and other fungi that have recently emerged as pathogens such as *Trichosporon*, *Scedosporium*, *Fusarium*, and *Pseudallescheria*. The methods used for detection of deficiencies in the immune system can be found in Chapter 19.

C. IMPAIRED CELLULAR IMMUNITY

Patients with cellular immune deficiency encompass a large and heterogeneous group, including patients with HIV infection (see Chapter 31); patients with lymphoreticular malignancies, such as Hodgkin's disease; and patients receiving immunosuppressive medications, such as corticosteroids, cyclosporine, tacrolimus, and other cytotoxic drugs. This latter group—those who are immunosuppressed as a result of medications—includes patients who have undergone transplantation, many patients receiving therapy for solid tumors, and patients receiving prolonged high-dose corticosteroid treatment (eg, for asthma, temporal arteritis, systemic lupus). Patients with cellular immune dysfunction are susceptible to infections by a large number of organisms, particularly ones that replicate intracellularly. Examples include bacteria, such as *Listeria*, *Legionella*, *Salmonella*, and *Mycobacterium*; viruses, such as herpes simplex, varicella, and CMV; fungi, such as *Cryptococcus*, *Coccidioides*, *Histoplasma*, and *Pneumocystis*; and protozoa, such as *Toxoplasma*.

D. HEMATOPOIETIC CELL TRANSPLANT RECIPIENTS

The length of time it takes for complications to occur in hematopoietic cell transplant recipients can be helpful in determining the etiologic agent. In the early (preengraftment) posttransplant period (day 1–21), almost all patients will become severely neutropenic for 7–21 days depending on whether growth factors are used and the source of stem cells. Patients are at risk for gram-positive (particularly catheter-related) and gram-negative bacterial infections as well as herpes simplex virus, respiratory syncytial virus, and candidal infections; mucositis is also a risk factor. In contrast to solid organ transplant recipients, the source of fever during this period cannot be found in 60–70% of hematopoietic cell transplant patients. Between 3 weeks and 3 months posttransplant, infections with CMV, adenovirus, *Aspergillus*, and *Candida* are most common. *P jiroveci* pneumonia can also be seen during this period, particularly in patients in whom graft-versus-host disease (GVHD) has developed and require immunosuppression. Patients continue to be at risk for infectious complications beyond 3 months following transplantation, particularly those who have received allogeneic transplantation and those who are taking immunosuppressive therapy for chronic GVHD. Varicella-zoster is common, and *Aspergillus* and CMV infections are increasingly seen in this period as well.

E. SOLID ORGAN TRANSPLANT RECIPIENTS

The length of time it takes for infection to occur following solid organ transplantation can also be helpful in determining the infectious origin. Immediate postoperative infections often involve the transplanted organ. Following lung transplantation, pneumonia and mediastinitis are particularly common; following liver transplantation, intra-abdominal abscess, cholangitis, and peritonitis may be seen; after renal transplantation, urinary tract infections, perinephric abscesses, and infected lymphoceles can occur.

Most infections that occur in the first 2–4 weeks posttransplant are related to the operative procedure and to hospitalization itself (wound infection, intravenous catheter infection, urinary tract infection from a Foley catheter) or are related to the transplanted organ. Infections that occur between the first and sixth months are often related to immunosuppression. During this period, reactivation of viruses occurs, and herpes simplex, varicella-zoster, and CMV infections are quite common. Opportunistic infections with fungi (eg, *Candida, Aspergillus, Cryptococcus, Pneumocystis*), *Listeria monocytogenes, Nocardia,* and *Toxoplasma* are also common. After 6 months, if immunosuppression has been reduced to maintenance levels, infections that are found in any population occur. Patients with poorly functioning allografts who receive long-term immunosuppression therapy continue to be at risk for opportunistic infections.

F. OTHER IMMUNOCOMPROMISED STATES

A large group of patients who are not specifically immunodeficient are at increased risk for infection because of debilitating injury (eg, burns or severe trauma), invasive procedures (eg, hyperalimentation lines, Foley catheters, dialysis catheters), central nervous system dysfunction (which predisposes patients to aspiration pneumonia and decubitus ulcers), obstructing lesions (eg, pneumonia due to an obstructed bronchus, pyelonephritis due to nephrolithiasis, cholangitis secondary to cholelithiasis), and use of broad-spectrum antibiotics. Patients with diabetes mellitus have alterations in cellular immunity that make them disproportionately susceptible to some diseases (eg, mucormycosis, emphysematous pyelonephritis, and foot infections).

Clinical Findings

A. LABORATORY FINDINGS

Routine evaluation includes complete blood count with differential, chest radiograph, and blood cultures; urine and sputum cultures should be obtained if indicated clinically or radiographically. Any focal complaints (localized pain, headache, rash) should prompt imaging and cultures appropriate to the site.

Patients who remain febrile without an obvious source should be evaluated for viral infection (CMV blood cultures or antigen test), abscesses (which usually occur near previous operative sites), candidiasis involving the liver or spleen, or aspergillosis. Serologic evaluation may be helpful if toxoplasmosis, aspergillosis (detected by galactomannan level in serum), or an endemic fungal infection (coccidioidomycosis, histoplasmosis) is a possible cause.

B. SPECIAL DIAGNOSTIC PROCEDURES

Special diagnostic procedures should also be considered. The cause of pulmonary infiltrates can be easily determined with simple techniques in some situations—eg, induced sputum yields a diagnosis of *Pneumocystis* pneumonia in 50–80% of AIDS patients with this infection. In other situations, more invasive procedures may be required (bronchoalveolar lavage, transbronchial biopsy, or even open lung biopsy). Other investigations such as skin, liver, or bone marrow biopsy may be helpful in establishing a diagnosis.

Differential Diagnosis

Transplant rejection, organ ischemia and necrosis, thrombophlebitis, and lymphoma (posttransplant lymphoproliferative disease) may all present as fever and must be considered in the differential diagnosis.

Prevention

There is great interest in preventing infection with prophylactic antimicrobial regimens but no uniformity of opinion about optimal drugs or dosage regimens. Hand washing is the simplest and most effective means of decreasing nosocomial infections in all patients, especially the compromised patient. Invasive devices such as central and peripheral lines and Foley catheters are a potential source of infection. Some centers use laminar airflow isolation or high-efficiency particulate air (HEPA) filtering in hematopoietic cell transplant patients during the neutropenic phase.

A. *PNEUMOCYSTIS* & HERPES SIMPLEX INFECTIONS

Trimethoprim-sulfamethoxazole (TMP-SMZ), one double-strength tablet orally three times a week, one double-strength tablet twice daily on weekends, or one single-strength tablet daily for 3–6 months, is frequently used to prevent *Pneumocystis* infections in transplant patients. It may also decrease the incidence of bacterial pneumonia, urinary tract infections, *Nocardia* infections, and toxoplasmosis. In patients allergic to TMP-SMZ, aerosolized pentamidine is used in a dosage of 300 mg once a month, as is dapsone, 50 mg orally daily or 100 mg three times weekly. (Glucose-6-phosphate dehydrogenase (G6PD) levels should be determined before therapy when the latter is instituted.) Acyclovir prevents herpes simplex infections in bone marrow and solid organ transplant recipients and is given to seropositive patients who are not receiving acyclovir or ganciclovir for CMV prophylaxis. The usual dose is 200 mg orally three times daily for 4 weeks (hematopoietic cell transplants) to 12 weeks (other solid organ transplants).

B. CMV

Prevention of CMV is more difficult, and no uniformly accepted approach has been adopted. Prevention strategies often depend on the serologic status of the donor and recipient and the organ transplanted, which determines the level of immunosuppression after transplant. In solid organ transplants (liver, kidney, heart, lung), the greatest risk of developing CMV disease is in seronegative patients who receive organs from seropositive donors. These high-risk patients usually receive ganciclovir, 2.5–5 mg/kg intravenously twice daily, during hospitalization (usually about 10 days) and then are given oral valganciclovir, 900 mg twice daily, or oral ganciclovir, 1 g three times daily, for 3 months; of note, oral ganciclovir is not absorbed as well as oral valganciclovir. Other solid organ transplant recipients (seropositive recipients) are at lower risk for developing CMV disease and usually receive intravenous ganciclovir while in the hospital followed by either high-dose oral acyclovir at a dosage of 800 mg four times daily or oral ganciclovir for 3 months. Ganciclovir, valganciclovir, and acyclovir prevent herpes virus reactivation. Because immunosuppression is increased during periods of rejection, patients treated for rejection usually receive intravenous ganciclovir during rejection therapy.

Recipients of hematopoietic cell transplants are more severely immunosuppressed than recipients of solid organ transplants, are at greater risk for developing serious CMV infection, and thus usually receive more aggressive prophylaxis. Two approaches have been used: universal prophylaxis or preemptive therapy. In the former, all high-risk patients (seropositive patients who receive allogeneic transplants) receive 5 mg/kg of intravenous ganciclovir every 12 hours for a week, followed by oral valganciclovir, 900 mg twice daily, or oral ganciclovir (which is not absorbed as well as valganciclovir), 1 g three times daily to day 100. This method is costly and associated with significant toxicity and is therefore being used less frequently. Alternatively, patients can be monitored without specific therapy and have blood sampled weekly for the presence of CMV. If CMV is detected by an antigenemia assay, preemptive therapy with ganciclovir is given (5 mg/kg intravenously twice daily for 7–14 days, followed by oral valganciclovir, 900 mg twice daily for a minimum of 3 weeks or until day 100, whichever is longer). This approach is effective but does miss a small number of patients in whom CMV disease subsequently develops. Other preventive strategies include use of CMV-negative or leukocyte-depleted blood products for CMV-seronegative recipients.

C. OTHER ORGANISMS

Routine decontamination of the gastrointestinal tract to prevent bacteremia in the neutropenic patient is not recommended. Prophylactic administration of antibiotics in the afebrile, asymptomatic neutropenic patient is controversial, although many centers have adopted this strategy. Rates of bacteremia are decreased, but overall mortality is not affected and emergence of resistant organisms is a common problem. Use of intravenous immunoglobulin is reserved for the small number of patients with severe hypogammaglobulinemia following bone marrow transplantation and should not be routinely administered to all transplant patients.

Prophylaxis with antifungal agents to prevent invasive mold (primarily *Aspergillus*) and yeast (primarily *Candida*) infections is routinely used, but the optimal agent, dose, and duration have not been standardized. Moderate-dose (0.5 mg/kg/d) and low-dose (0.1–0.25

mg/kg/d) amphotericin B, lipid-based preparations of amphotericin B, aerosolized amphotericin B, and itraconazole (capsules and solution) have all been used with varying success in the neutropenic patient. Because voriconazole appears to be more effective than amphotericin for documented *Aspergillus* infections, one approach to prophylaxis is to use oral fluconazole (400 mg/d) for patients at low risk for developing fungal infections (those who receive autologous bone marrow transplants) and oral voriconazole (200 mg twice daily) for those at high risk (allogeneic transplants) at least until engraftment (usually 30 days). In solid organ transplant recipients, the risk of invasive fungal infection varies considerably (1–2% in liver, pancreas, and kidney transplants and 6–8% in heart and lung transplants). Whether universal prophylaxis or observation with preemptive therapy is the best approach has not been determined. Although fluconazole is effective in preventing yeast infections, emergence of resistant strains of *Candida krusei*, other *Candida* species, and molds (*Fusarium, Aspergillus, Mucor*) has raised concerns about its routine use as a prophylactic agent.

Treatment

A. GENERAL MEASURES

Because infections in the immunocompromised patient can be rapidly progressive and life-threatening, diagnostic procedures must be done promptly, and empiric therapy is usually instituted before a specific pathogenic organism has been isolated.

Reduction or discontinuation of immunosuppressive medication may jeopardize the viability of the transplanted organ, but in life-threatening infections, it is necessary as an adjunct to effective antimicrobial therapy. Hematopoietic growth factors (granulocyte and granulocyte-macrophage colony-stimulating factors) stimulate proliferation of bone marrow stem cells, resulting in an increase in peripheral leukocytes. These agents shorten the period of neutropenia and have been associated with fewer infections. Use of growth factors in patients with prolonged neutropenia (> 7 days) is an effective means of reversing immunosuppression.

B. SPECIFIC MEASURES

Antimicrobial drug therapy is rationally based on culture results (see Chapter 37). Therapy should be specific for isolated pathogens, and bactericidal agents should be used. Combinations of antimicrobials are often required to provide synergy, to prevent resistance, or to serve as broad-spectrum coverage of multiple pathogens (since infections in these patients are often polymicrobial).

Empiric therapy is often instituted at the earliest sign of infection in the immunosuppressed patient because prompt therapy favorably affects outcome. The antibiotic or combination of antibiotics used depends on the type of immunocompromise and the site of infection.

For example, in the febrile neutropenic patient, the primary concern is bacterial and fungal infections. In this patient population, an algorithmic approach to therapy is often used, with initial treatment directed at gram-positive and gram-negative organisms. If the patient does not respond, broader-spectrum antibiotics and antifungal drugs are added. Although a number of different agents can be used, choices should be based on local microbiologic trends. One example would be to initiate therapy with a fluoroquinolone active against gram-positive organisms (such as levofloxacin, gatifloxacin, or moxifloxacin) when the absolute neutrophil count falls below 500/mcL. If fever develops, cultures are obtained, and vancomycin, 10–15 mg/kg intravenously every 12 hours, is given to cover methicillin-resistant *S aureus, S epidermidis*, and enterococcus. If fever continues after 48–72 hours, antifungal coverage can be increased by changing to either caspofungin, 50 mg daily intravenously, or voriconazole, 200 mg intravenously or orally twice daily (if the patient was receiving fluconazole prophylaxis); broader-spectrum antibiotics can be added sequentially. For example, to better cover *Acinetobacter, Citrobacter,* and *Pseudomonas,* the fluoroquinolone may be switched to cefepime, 2 g every 8 hours intravenously; with continued fever, imipenem, 500 mg intravenously every 6 hours (or meropenem, 1 g intravenously every 8 hours), with or without tobramycin, 1.8 mg/kg intravenously every 8 hours, may be used in place of cefepime. If fevers persist, TMP-SMZ at 10 mg/kg/d (of trimethoprim) intravenously in three divided doses can be added to cover *Stenotrophomonas.* Regardless of whether the patient becomes afebrile, therapy is continued until resolution of neutropenia. Failure to continue antibiotics through the period of neutropenia is associated with a high incidence of relapse that can be associated with septic shock.

Patients with fever and neutropenia who are at low risk for developing complications (neutropenia expected to persist for less than 10 days, no comorbid complications requiring hospitalization, and cancer adequately treated) can be treated with oral antibiotic regimens, such as ciprofloxacin, 750 mg every 12 hours, plus amoxicillin-clavulanic acid, 500 mg every 8 hours. In the organ transplant patient with interstitial infiltrates, the main concern is infection with *Pneumocystis* or *Legionella* species, so that empiric treatment with a macrolide and TMP-SMZ would be reasonable. If the patient does not respond to empiric treatment, a decision must be made to add more antimicrobial agents or perform invasive procedures (see above) to make a specific diagnosis. By making a specific diagnosis, therapy can be specific and polypharmacy with multiple potentially toxic agents can be avoided.

Bucaneve G et al: Levofloxacin to prevent bacterial infection in patients with cancer and neutropenia. N Engl J Med 2005; 353:977. [PMID: 16148283]

Kalil AC et al: Meta-analysis: the efficacy of strategies to prevent organ disease by cytomegalovirus in solid organ transplant recipients. Ann Intern Med 2005;143:870. [PMID: 16365468]

Rubin RH: The direct and indirect effects of infection in liver transplantation: pathogenesis, impact, and clinical management. Curr Clin Top Infect Dis 2002;22:125. [PMID: 12520651]

Viscoli C et al: Treatment of febrile neutropenia: what is new? Curr Opin Infect Dis 2002;15:377. [PMID: 12130933]

Walsh TJ et al: Caspofungin versus liposomal amphotericin B for empirical antifungal therapy in patients with persistent fever and neutropenia. N Engl J Med 2004;351:1391. [PMID: 15459300]

NOSOCOMIAL INFECTIONS

 ESSENTIALS OF DIAGNOSIS

- *Nosocomial infections are defined as those not present or incubating at the time of hospital admission and developing 48–72 hours after admission.*
- *Hand washing is the easiest and most effective means of preventing nosocomial infections and should be done routinely even when gloves are worn.*

General Considerations

In the United States, approximately 5% of patients who enter the hospital free of infection acquire a nosocomial infection, resulting in prolongation of the hospital stay, increase in cost of care, significant morbidity, and a 5% mortality rate. The most common infections are urinary tract infections, usually associated with Foley catheters or urologic procedures; bloodstream infections, most commonly from indwelling catheters but also from secondary sites, such as surgical wounds, abscesses, pneumonia, the genitourinary tract, and the gastrointestinal tract; pneumonia in intubated patients or those with altered levels of consciousness; surgical wound infections; and *Clostridium difficile* colitis.

Some general principles are helpful in preventing, diagnosing, and treating nosocomial infections:

1. Many infections are a direct result of the use of invasive devices for monitoring or therapy, such as intravenous catheters, Foley catheters, shunts, surgical drains, catheters placed by interventional radiology for drainage, nasogastric tubes, and orotracheal or nasotracheal tubes for ventilatory support. Early removal of such devices reduces the possibility of infection.

2. Patients in whom nosocomial infections develop are often critically ill, have been hospitalized for extended periods, and have received several courses of broad-spectrum antibiotic therapy. As a result, nosocomial infections are often caused by organisms that are multidrug resistant and are different from those encountered in community-acquired

infections. Examples are *S aureus* and *S epidermidis* (a frequent cause of prosthetic device infection) that may be resistant to nafcillin and cephalosporins and require vancomycin for therapy; *Enterococcus faecium* resistant to ampicillin and vancomycin; gram-negative infections caused by *Pseudomonas, Citrobacter, Enterobacter, Acinetobacter,* and *Stenotrophomonas,* which may be sensitive only to fluoroquinolones, carbapenems, aminoglycosides, or TMP-SMZ. When choosing antibiotics to treat the seriously ill patient with a nosocomial infection, the previous antimicrobial the patient has received as well as the "local ecology" must be considered. It is often necessary to institute therapy with vancomycin and a carbapenem or aminoglycoside until a specific agent is isolated and sensitivities are known, at which time the least toxic and most cost-effective drug can be used.

One promising approach to preventing the development of multidrug-resistant organisms is antibiotic cycling. By changing the class of antibiotic primarily used every 6–12 months (eg, a cephalosporin, then fluoroquinolones, then carbapenems), selection pressure is decreased and less resistance emerges.

Because widespread use of antimicrobial drugs contributes to the selection of drug-resistant organisms that cause nosocomial infections, every effort should be made to limit the use of antibiotics to treat documented infections. All too often, unreliable or uninterpretable specimens are obtained for culture that result in unnecessary use of antibiotics. The best example of this principle is the diagnosis of line-related or bloodstream infection in the febrile patient (see below). To avoid unnecessary use of antibiotics, thoughtful consideration of culture results is mandatory. A positive wound culture without signs of inflammation or infection, a positive sputum culture without pulmonary infiltrates on chest x-ray, or a positive urine culture in a catheterized patient without symptoms or signs of pyelonephritis are all likely to represent colonization, not infection.

Clinical Findings

A. SYMPTOMS AND SIGNS

Catheter-associated infections have a variable presentation, depending on the type of catheter used (peripheral or central venous catheters, nontunneled or tunneled). Local signs of infection may be present at the insertion site, with pain, erythema, and purulence. Fever is often absent in uncomplicated infections and if present, may indicate more disseminated disease such as bacteremia, cellulitis and septic thrombophlebitis. Often signs of infection at the insertion site are absent.

1. Fever in an intensive care unit patient—Fever complicates up to 70% of patients in intensive care units, and the etiology of the fever may be infectious or noninfectious. Common infectious causes include catheter-associated infections, hospital-acquired and ventilator-associated pneumonia (see Chapter 9), surgical site infections, urinary tract infections, and sepsis. Clinically relevant sinusitis is relatively uncommon in the patient in the intensive care unit.

An important noninfectious cause is thromboembolic disease. Fever in conjunction with refractory hypotension and shock may suggest sepsis; however, adrenal insufficiency, thyroid storm, and transfusion reaction may have a similar clinical presentation. Drug fever is difficult to diagnose and is usually a diagnosis of exclusion unless there are other signs of hypersensitivity, such as a typical maculopapular rash.

2. Fever in the postoperative patient—Postoperative fever is very common and in many cases resolves spontaneously. Etiologies are both infectious and noninfectious. Timing of the fever in relation to the surgery and the nature of the surgical procedure may help diagnostically.

a. Immediate fever (in the first few hours after surgery)—Immediate fever can be due to medications that were given perioperatively, to the trauma of surgery itself, or to infections that were present before surgery. Necrotizing fasciitis due to group A streptococci or mixed organisms may present in this period. Malignant hyperthermia is rare and presents 30 minutes to several hours following inhalational anesthesia (succinylcholine or halothane commonly) and is characterized by extreme hyperthermia, muscle rigidity, rhabdomyolysis, electrolyte abnormalities, and hypotension. Aggressive cooling and dantrolene are the mainstays of therapy. Fever due to the trauma of surgery itself usually resolves in 2–3 days, longer in more complicated operative cases and in patients with head trauma.

b. Acute fever (within 1 week of surgery)—Acute fever is usually due to common causes of nosocomial infections, such as ventilator-associated pneumonia (including aspiration pneumonia in patients with decreased gag reflex) and line infections. Noninfectious causes include alcohol withdrawal, gout, pulmonary embolism, and pancreatitis.

c. Subacute fever (at least 1 week after surgery)—Surgical site infections commonly present at least 1 week after surgery. The type of surgery that was performed may be related to specific infectious etiologies. Patients undergoing cardiothoracic surgery may be at higher risk for pneumonia and deep and superficial sternal wound infections. Meningitis without typical signs of meningismus may complicate neurosurgical procedures. Abdominal surgery may result in deep abdominal abscesses that require drainage.

B. LABORATORY FINDINGS

Blood cultures are universally recommended, and chest radiographs are frequently obtained. Sputum Gram stain and semi-quantitative sputum cultures are useful in selected patients where there is a high pretest probability of pneumonia. Other diagnostic strategies will be dictated by the clinical context (eg, transesophageal echocardiogram in a patient with *S aureus* bacteremia).

Any fever in a patient with a central venous catheter should prompt the collection of blood. The best method to evaluate bacteremia is to gather at least two peripherally obtained blood cultures. Blood cultures from unidentified sites, a single blood culture from any site, or a blood culture through an existing line will often be positive for *S epidermidis* and may lead to therapy with vancomycin. Yet, the likelihood that such a culture represents a true bacteremia is 10–20%. Unless two separate venipuncture cultures are obtained—not through catheters—interpretation of results is impossible and unnecessary therapy is given. Every such "pseudobacteremia" increases laboratory costs, antibiotic use, and length of stay, increasing costs of hospitalization by about $4500. Microbiologic evaluation of the removed catheter can sometimes be helpful, but only in addition to (not instead of) blood cultures drawn from peripheral sites. Semiquantitative cultures of the catheter is performed by rolling the distal 2 cm tip of the catheter on an agar plate. The presence of > 15 colony-forming units (CFU) of organisms on the catheter tip together with identical organisms on peripherally drawn blood cultures establishes the diagnosis of a catheter-associated bloodstream infection. Other methods may permit catheters to remain in place while infection is being ruled out. The differential time to positivity measures the difference in time that cultures simultaneously drawn through a catheter and a peripheral site become positive. A positive test (about 120 minutes difference in time) supports a catheter-related bloodstream infection, and a negative test may permit catheters to be retained.

Complications

Patients who have persistent bacteremia and continue to be febrile despite removal of the infected catheter may have complications such as septic thrombophlebitis, endocarditis, or metastatic foci of infection (particularly with *S aureus*). Additional studies such as venous Doppler studies, transesophageal echocardiogram, and chest radiographs may be indicated. Duration of therapy is longer, usually 4–6 weeks. In the case of septic thrombophlebitis, anticoagulation with heparin is also recommended if there are no contraindications.

Differential Diagnosis

Although most fevers are due to infections, about 25% of patients will have fever of noninfectious origin. These include drug fever, nonspecific postoperative fevers (atelectasis, tissue damage or necrosis), hematoma, pancreatitis, pulmonary embolism, myocardial infarction, and ischemic bowel disease.

Prevention

Prevention is of paramount importance in controlling nosocomial infections. The concept of universal precau-

tions emphasizes that all patients are treated as though they have a potential blood-borne transmissible disease, and thus all body secretions are handled with care to prevent spread of disease. Almost all hospitals have implemented body substance isolation, which requires use of gloves whenever a health care worker anticipates contact with blood or other body secretions. By wearing gloves, health care workers prevent contamination of their hands with infected secretions and subsequent spread of infection to other patients by direct contact. Even though gloves are worn, health care workers should routinely wash their hands, since it is the easiest and most effective means of preventing nosocomial infections. Application of a rapid drying, alcohol-based antiseptic is easy to do, takes less time than traditional hand washing with soap and water, is more effective at reducing hand colonization, promotes compliance with hand decontamination, and is rapidly becoming the method of choice for hand disinfection.

Peripheral intravenous lines should be replaced every 3 days, and arterial lines should be replaced every 4 days. Lines in the central venous circulation (including those placed peripherally) can be left in place indefinitely and are changed or removed when they are clinically suspected of being infected, when they are nonfunctional, or when they are no longer needed. Silver alloy–impregnated Foley catheters reduce the incidence of catheter-associated bacteriuria, and antibiotic-impregnated (minocycline plus rifampin or chlorhexidine plus silver sulfadiazine) venous catheters reduce line infections and bacteremia. Whether the increased cost of these devices justifies their routine use should be determined by individual institutions based on local infection rates. Selective decontamination of the digestive tract with nonabsorbable antibiotics to prevent nosocomial pneumonia is widely used in Europe, but the therapeutic efficacy of this expensive intervention is controversial.

Attentive nursing care (positioning to prevent decubitus ulcers, wound care, elevating the head during tube feedings to prevent aspiration) is critical in preventing nosocomial infections. In addition, monitoring of high-risk areas by hospital epidemiologists detects increases in infection rates early and is a key factor in prevention of these types of infections.

Several highly effective vaccines have been approved by the US Food and Drug Administration (FDA) that add to the armamentarium for preventing certain nosocomial infections. Hepatitis A, hepatitis B, and the varicella vaccine should be considered in the appropriate setting. (See section below on Immunization Against Infectious Diseases.)

Treatment

A. Fever in an Intensive Care Unit patient

Unless the patient has a central neurologic injury with elevated intracranial pressure or has a temperature > 41 °C, there is less physiologic need to maintain euthermia. Empiric broad-spectrum antibiotics (as noted above) are recommended for neutropenic and other immunocompromised patients and in patients who are clinically unstable.

B. CATHETER-ASSOCIATED INFECTIONS

Factors that inform treatment decisions include the type of catheter that is affected, the type of organism, the availability of alternate catheter access sites, the need for ongoing intravascular access, and the extent of disease involved.

In general, catheters should be removed if there is purulence at the exit site; if the organism is *S aureus*, gram-negative rods, or *Candida* species; if there is persistent bacteremia (> 48 hours while receiving antibiotics); or if complications, such as septic thrombophlebitis, endocarditis, or other metastatic disease exist. Central venous catheters may be exchanged over a guidewire and the tip sent for semiquantitative cultures if a catheter infection is suspected, provided there is no erythema or purulence at the exit site and the patient does not appear to be septic. If the catheter tip cultures return with > 15 CFU, replacement of the catheter at a new site is recommended. Given that coagulase-negative staphylococci are the most common organisms isolated and most are resistant to nafcillin, empiric therapy with vancomycin, 15 mg/kg IV twice daily, should be given to patients in whom a bloodstream infection is suspected and who have normal renal function. Empiric gram-negative coverage may be considered in patients who are immunocompromised or who are critically ill.

Antibiotic treatment duration depends on the organism identified and the extent of disease. For uncomplicated bacteremia, 5–7 days of therapy is usually sufficient for coagulase-negative staphylococci, even if the original catheter is retained. Fourteen days of therapy is generally recommended for uncomplicated bacteremia caused by gram-negative rods, *Candida* species, and *S aureus*.

Kollef MH: Prevention of hospital-associated pneumonia and ventilator-associated pneumonia. Crit Care Med 2004;32: 1396. [PMID: 15187525]

Lorente C et al: Prevention of infection in the intensive care unit: current advances and opportunities for the future. Curr Opin Crit Care 2002;8:461. [PMID: 12357116]

Raad I et al: Differential time to positivity: a useful method for diagnosing catheter-related bloodstream infections. Ann Intern Med 2004;140:18. [PMID: 14706968]

Vermeulen H et al: Diagnostic accuracy of routine postoperative body temperature measurements. Clin Infect Dis 2005;40: 1404. [PMID: 15844061]

Vincent JL: Nosocomial infections in adult intensive-care units. Lancet 2003;361:2068. [PMID: 12814731]

INFECTIONS OF THE CENTRAL NERVOUS SYSTEM

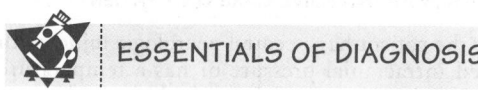

ESSENTIALS OF DIAGNOSIS

- Central nervous system infection is a medical emergency.

- Symptoms and signs common to all types of central nervous system infection include headache, fever, sensorial disturbances, neck and back stiffness, positive Kernig and Brudzinski signs, and cerebrospinal fluid abnormalities.

General Considerations

Infections of the central nervous system can be caused by almost any infectious agent, including bacteria, mycobacteria, fungi, spirochetes, protozoa, helminths, and viruses. The classic triad of fever, stiff neck and altered mental status has a low sensitivity (44%) for bacterial meningitis. However, nearly all patients with bacterial meningitis have at least two of the following symptoms—fever, headache, stiff neck, or altered mental status.

Etiologic Classification

Central nervous system infections can be divided into several categories that usually can be readily distinguished from each other by cerebrospinal fluid examination as the first step toward etiologic diagnosis (Table 30–1).

A. PURULENT MENINGITIS

Patients with bacterial meningitis usually seek medical attention within hours or 1–2 days after onset of symptoms. The organisms responsible depend primarily on the age of the patient as summarized in Table 30–2. The diagnosis is usually based on the Gram-stained smear (positive in 60–90%) or culture (positive in over 90%).

B. CHRONIC MENINGITIS

The presentation of chronic meningitis is less acute than purulent meningitis. Patients with chronic meningitis usually have a history of symptoms lasting weeks to months. The most common pathogens are *Mycobacterium tuberculosis*, atypical mycobacteria, fungi (*Cryptococcus, Coccidioides, Histoplasma*), and spirochetes (*Treponema pallidum* and *Borrelia burgdorferi*, the cause of Lyme disease). The diagnosis is made by culture or in some cases by serologic tests (cryptococcosis, coccidioidomycosis, syphilis, Lyme disease).

C. ASEPTIC MENINGITIS

Aseptic meningitis—a much more benign and self-limited syndrome than purulent meningitis—is caused principally by viruses, especially mumps virus and the enterovirus group (including coxsackieviruses and echoviruses). Infectious mononucleosis may be accompanied by aseptic meningitis. Leptospiral infection is also usually placed in the aseptic group because of the lymphocytic cellular response and its relatively benign course. This type of meningitis also occurs during secondary syphilis and disseminated Lyme disease.

Table 30–1. Typical cerebrospinal fluid findings in various central nervous system diseases.

Diagnosis	Cells/mcL	Glucose (mg/dL)	Protein (mg/dL)	Opening Pressure
Normal	0–5 lymphocytes	45–85[1]	15–45	70–180 mm H$_2$O
Purulent meningitis (bacterial)[2] community-acquired	200–20,000 polymorpho-nuclear neutrophils	Low (< 45)	High (> 50)	Markedly elevated
Granulomatous meningitis (my-cobacterial, fungal)[3]	100–1000, mostly lymphocytes[3]	Low (< 45)	High (> 50)	Moderately elevated
Spirochetal meningitis	100–1000, mostly lymphocytes[3]	Normal	Moderately high (> 50)	Normal to slightly ele-vated
Aseptic meningitis, viral or meningoencephalitis[4]	25–2000, mostly lymphocytes[3]	Normal or low	High (> 50)	Slightly elevated
"Neighborhood reaction"[5]	Variably increased	Normal	Normal or high	Variable

[1]Cerebrospinal fluid glucose must be considered in relation to blood glucose level. Normally, cerebrospinal fluid glucose is 20–30 mg/dL lower than blood glucose, or 50–70% of the normal value of blood glucose.
[2]Organisms in smear or culture of cerebrospinal fluid; counterimmunoelectrophoresis or latex agglutination may be diagnostic.
[3]Polymorphonuclear neutrophils may predominate early.
[4]Viral isolation from cerebrospinal fluid early; antibody titer rise in paired specimens of serum; polymerase chain reaction for her-pesvirus.
[5]May occur in mastoiditis, brain abscess, epidural abscess, sinusitis, septic thrombus, brain tumor. Cerebrospinal fluid culture results usually negative.

D. ENCEPHALITIS

Encephalitis (due to herpesviruses, arboviruses, rabies virus, flaviviruses [West Nile encephalitis, Japanese en-cephalitis], and many others) produces disturbances of the sensorium, seizures, and many other manifesta-tions. Patients are more ill than those with aseptic meningitis. Cerebrospinal fluid may be entirely nor-mal or may show some lymphocytes and in some in-stances (eg, herpes simplex) red cells as well.

E. PARTIALLY TREATED BACTERIAL MENINGITIS

Previous effective antibiotic therapy given for 12–24 hours will decrease the rate of positive Gram stain re-sults by 20% and culture by 30–40% but will have little effect on cell count, protein, or glucose. Occasionally, previous antibiotic therapy will change a predominantly polymorphonuclear response to a lymphocytic pleocy-tosis, and some of the cerebrospinal fluid findings may be similar to those seen in aseptic meningitis.

Table 30–2. Initial antimicrobial therapy for purulent meningitis of unknown cause.

Population	Common Microorganisms	Standard Therapy
18–50 years	Streptococcus pneumoniae, Neisseria meningitidis	Vancomycin[1] **plus** cefotaxime or ceftriaxone[2]
Over 50 years	S pneumoniae, N meningitidis, Listeria monocytogenes, gram-negative bacilli	Vancomycin[1] **plus** ampicillin,[3] **plus** cefotaxime or ceftriaxone[2]
Impaired cellular immunity	L monocytogenes, gram-negative bacilli, S pneumoniae	Vancomycin[1] **plus** ampicillin[3] **plus** ceftazidime[4]
Postsurgical or posttraumatic	Staphylococcus aureus, S pneumoniae, gram-negative bacilli	Vancomycin[1] **plus** ceftazidime[4]

[1]The dose of vancomycin is 10–15 mg/kg IV every 6 hours.
[2]The usual dose of cefotaxime is 2 g IV every 6 hours and that of ceftriaxone is 2 g IV every 12 hours. If the organism is sensitive to pen-icillin, 3–4 million units IV every 4 hours is given.
[3]The dose of ampicillin is usually 2 g IV every 4 hours.
[4]Ceftazidime is given in a dose of 50–100 mg/kg IV every 8 hours up to 2 g every 8 hours.

F. Neighborhood Reaction

As noted in Table 30–1, this term denotes a purulent infectious process in close proximity to the central nervous system that spills some of the products of the inflammatory process—white blood cells or protein—into the cerebrospinal fluid. Such an infection might be a brain abscess, osteomyelitis of the vertebrae, epidural abscess, subdural empyema, or bacterial sinusitis or mastoiditis.

G. Noninfectious Meningeal Irritation

Carcinomatous meningitis, sarcoidosis, systemic lupus erythematosus, chemical meningitis, and certain drugs—nonsteroidal anti-inflammatory drugs, muromonab-CD3 (OKT3), TMP-SMZ, and others—can also produce symptoms and signs of meningeal irritation with associated cerebrospinal fluid pleocytosis, increased protein, and low or normal glucose. Meningismus with normal cerebrospinal fluid findings occurs in the presence of other infections such as pneumonia and shigellosis.

H. Brain Abscess

Brain abscess presents as a space-occupying lesion; symptoms may include vomiting, fever, change of mental status, or focal neurologic manifestations. When brain abscess is suspected, a CT scan should be performed. If positive, lumbar puncture should *not* be performed since results rarely provide clinically useful information and herniation can occur. The bacteriology of brain abscess is usually polymicrobial and includes *S aureus*, gram-negative bacilli, streptococci, and anaerobes (including anaerobic streptococci and *Prevotella* species).

I. Amebic Meningoencephalitis

These infections are caused by free-living amebas and present as two distinct syndromes. The diagnosis is confirmed by culture (*Acanthamoeba* spp. and *Balamuthia mandrillaris*) or identification of the organism in a wet mount of cerebrospinal fluid (*Naegleria fowleri*) or on biopsy specimens. No effective therapy is available.

Primary amebic meningoencephalitis is caused by *N fowleri* and is an acute fulminant disease, usually seen in children and young adults with recent fresh water exposure, and is characterized by signs of meningeal irritation that rapidly progresses to encephalitis and death. Rare cures have been reported with intravenous and intraventricular administration of amphotericin B.

Granulomatous amebic encephalitis is caused by *Acanthamoeba* species. It is an indolent disease, frequently seen in immunocompromised patients and associated with cutaneous lesions. Central nervous system disease is characterized by headache, nausea, vomiting, cranial neuropathies, seizures, and hemiparesis. Infections with *Balamuthia* are similar to *Acanthamoeba* in that the course is subacute to chronic, but unlike *Acanthamoeba* both immunocompromised and immunocompetent persons can be affected.

Clinical Findings

A. Laboratory Tests

Evaluation of a patient with suspected meningitis includes a history, physical examination, blood count, blood culture, lumbar puncture followed by careful study and culture of the cerebrospinal fluid, and a chest film. The fluid must be examined for cell count, glucose, and protein, and a smear stained for bacteria (and acid-fast organisms when appropriate) and cultured for pyogenic organisms and for mycobacteria and fungi when indicated. Latex agglutination tests can detect antigens of encapsulated organisms (*S pneumoniae*, *H influenzae*, *N meningitidis*, and *Cryptococcus neoformans*) but are rarely used except for detection of *Cryptococcus* or in partially treated patients. Polymerase chain reaction (PCR) testing of cerebrospinal fluid has been used to detect bacteria (*S pneumoniae*, *H influenzae*, *N meningitidis*, *M tuberculosis*, *B burgdorferi*, and *Tropheryma whippelii*) and viruses (herpes simplex, varicella-zoster, CMV, Epstein-Barr virus, and enteroviruses) in patients with meningitis. The greatest experience is with PCR for herpes simplex and varicella-zoster, and the tests are very sensitive (> 95%) and specific. Tests to detect the other organisms may not be any more sensitive than culture, but the real value is the rapidity with which results are available, ie, hours compared with days or weeks. At present, with the exception of PCR for herpes simplex, these tests are performed only in reference laboratories. Although it is difficult to prove with existing clinical data that early antibiotic therapy improves outcome in bacterial meningitis, prompt therapy is still recommended.

B. Lumbar Puncture and Imaging

Since performing a lumbar puncture in the presence of a space-occupying lesion (brain abscess, subdural hematoma, subdural empyema, necrotic temporal lobe from herpes encephalitis) may result in brainstem herniation, a CT scan is performed prior to lumbar puncture if a space-occupying lesion is suspected on the basis of papilledema, seizures, or focal neurologic findings. Other indications for CT scan are an immunocompromised patient or moderate to severely impaired level of consciousness. If delays are encountered in obtaining a CT scan and bacterial meningitis is suspected, blood cultures should be drawn and antibiotics and corticosteroids administered even before cerebrospinal fluid is obtained for culture to avoid delay in treatment (Table 30–1). Antibiotics given within 4 hours before obtaining cerebrospinal fluid probably do not affect culture results.

Treatment

Increased intracranial pressure due to brain edema often requires therapeutic attention. Hyperventilation, mannitol (25–50 g as a bolus intravenous infusion), and even drainage of cerebrospinal fluid by repeated lumbar punctures or by placement of ventricular catheters have been used to control cerebral edema and increased intracranial pressure. Dexamethasone (4 mg intravenously every 4–6 hours) may also decrease cerebral edema. In purulent meningitis, the identity of the causative microorganism may remain unknown or doubtful for a few days and initial antibiotic treatment as set forth in Table 30–2 should be directed against the microorganisms most common for each age group.

The duration of therapy for bacterial meningitis varies depending on the etiologic agent: *H influenzae,* 7 days; *N meningitidis,* 3–7 days; *S pneumoniae,* 10–14 days; *L monocytogenes,* 14–21 days; and gram-negative bacilli, 21 days.

Dexamethasone therapy is recommended for adults with pneumococcal meningitis. Ten milligrams of dexamethasone administered intravenously 15–20 minutes before or simultaneously with the first dose of antibiotics and continued every 6 hours for 4 days decreases morbidity and mortality. The number of patients with meningitis due to *N meningitidis* and other bacterial pathogens studied does not support similar conclusions. However, because adverse effects of dexamethasone for short periods are few and because potential benefits are great, many clinicians would advocate dexamethasone even if *N meningitidis* is the causative agent.

Therapy of brain abscess consists of drainage (excision or aspiration) in addition to 3–4 weeks of systemic antibiotics directed against organisms isolated. A regimen often used includes metronidazole, 500 mg intravenously or orally every 8 hours, plus ceftizoxime, 2 g intravenously every 8 hours, or ceftriaxone, 2 g every 12 hours. In cases where abscesses are less than 2 cm in size, where there are multiple abscesses that cannot be drained, or if an abscess is located in an area where significant neurologic sequelae would result from drainage, antibiotics for 6–8 weeks without drainage can be used.

Therapy of other types of meningitis is discussed elsewhere in this book (fungal meningitis, Chapter 36; syphilis and Lyme borreliosis, Chapter 34; tuberculous meningitis, Chapter 33; herpes encephalitis, Chapter 32).

Bernardini GL: Diagnosis and management of brain abscess and subdural empyema. Curr Neurol Neurosci Rep 2004;4:448. [PMID: 15509445]

De Gans J et al: Dexamethasone in adults with bacterial meningitis. N Engl J Med 2002;347:1549. [PMID: 11144034]

Sinner SW et al: Antimicrobial agents in the treatment of bacterial meningitis. Infect Dis Clin North Am 2004;18:581. [PMID: 15308277]

van de Beek D et al: Community-acquired bacterial meningitis in adults. N Engl J Med 2006;354:44. [PMID: 16394301]

ANIMAL & HUMAN BITE WOUNDS

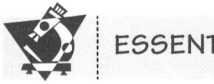

ESSENTIALS OF DIAGNOSIS

- Cat and human bites are more likely to become infected than dog bites.

- Bites to the hand are of special concern because of the possibility of closed-space infection.

- Antibiotic prophylaxis indicated for noninfected bites of the hand and hospitalization required for infected hand bites.

- All infected wounds need to be cultured to direct therapy.

General Considerations

About 1000 dog bite injuries require emergency department attention each day, most often in urban areas. Dog bites occur most commonly in the summer months. Biting animals are usually known by their victims, and most biting incidents are provoked (ie, bites occur while playing with the animal or after surprising the animal or waking it abruptly from sleep). Failure to elicit a history of provocation is important, because an unprovoked attack raises the possibility of rabies. Human bites are usually inflicted by children while playing or fighting; in adults, bites are associated with alcohol use and closed-fist injuries that occur during fights.

The animal inflicting the bite, the location of the bite, and the type of injury inflicted are all important determinants of whether they become infected. Cat bites are more likely to become infected than human bites—between 30% and 50% of all cat bites become infected. Infections following human bites are variable: Those inflicted by children rarely become infected because they are superficial, and bites by adults become infected in 15–30% of cases, with a particularly high rate of infection in closed-fist injuries. "Through and through" bites (eg involving the mucosa and the skin) have an infection rate similar to closed-fist injuries. Dog bites, for unclear reasons, become infected only 5% of the time. Bites of the head, face, and neck are less likely to become infected than bites on the extremities. Puncture wounds become infected more frequently than lacerations, probably because the latter are easier to irrigate and debride.

The bacteriology of bite infections is polymicrobial. Following dog and cat bites, over 50% of infections are caused by aerobes and anaerobes and 36% are due to aerobes alone. Pure anaerobic infections are rare. *Pasteurella* species are the single most common isolate (75% of cat bites and 50% of dog bites). Other common aerobic isolates include streptococci, staphylococci, *Moraxella,* and *Neisseria;* the most common anaerobes are *Fusobacterium, Bacteroides, Porphyromonas,* and *Prevotella.* The median number of isolates following human bites is four (three aerobes and one anaerobe). Like dog and cat bites, most human bites are a mixture of aerobes and anaerobes (54%) or are due to aerobes alone (44%). *Streptococcus, Staphylococcus,* and *Eikenella corrodens* (found in 30% of patients) are the most common aerobes. *Prevotella* and *Fusobac-*

terium are the most common anaerobes. Although the organisms noted are the most common, innumerable others have been isolated—including *Capnocytophagia* (dog and cats), *Pseudomonas,* and *Haemophilus*—emphasizing the point that all infected bites should be cultured to define the microbiology.

HIV can be transmitted from bites (either from biting or receiving a bite from an HIV-infected patient) but has rarely been reported.

Treatment

A. LOCAL CARE

Vigorous cleansing and irrigation of the wound as well as debridement of necrotic material are the most important factors in decreasing the incidence of infections. Radiographs should be obtained to look for fractures and the presence of foreign bodies. Careful examination to assess the extent of the injury (tendon laceration, joint space penetration) is critical to appropriate care.

B. SUTURING

If wounds require closure for cosmetic or mechanical reasons, suturing can be done. However, one should never suture an infected wound, and wounds of the hand should generally not be sutured since a closed-space infection of the hand can result in loss of function.

C. PROPHYLACTIC ANTIBIOTICS

Prophylaxis is indicated in high-risk bites, eg, cat bites in any location (dicloxacillin, 0.5 g orally four times a day for 3–5 days) and hand bites by any animal or by humans (penicillin V, 0.5 g orally four times a day for 3–5 days). Although dicloxacillin and penicillin have been specifically studied, there is concern about their use because of their narrow spectrum of activity. Based on the microbiology of bite wounds, other agents less adequately studied but that have broader spectrums of activity may be better as prophylactic agents. Examples include cefuroxime, amoxicillin-clavulanic acid and, in the penicillin-allergic patient, clindamycin plus a fluoroquinolone. Immunocompromised patients and especially individuals without functional spleens are at risk for developing overwhelming bacteremia (primarily with *Capnocytophagia* spp.) and sepsis following animal bites and should also receive prophylaxis, even for low-risk bites.

Because the risk of HIV transmission is so low following a bite, routine postexposure prophylaxis is not recommended. Each case should be evaluated individually and consideration for prophylaxis should be given to those who present within 72 hours of the incident, the source is known to be HIV infected, and the exposure is high risk.

D. ANTIBIOTICS

For wounds that are infected, antibiotics are clearly indicated. How they are given (orally or intravenously)

and the need for hospitalization are individualized clinical decisions. In general, *Pasteurella multocida* is best treated with penicillin or a tetracycline. Other active agents include second- and third-generation cephalosporins, fluoroquinolones, or azithromycin and clarithromycin. Response to therapy is slow, and therapy should be continued for at least 2–3 weeks. Human bites frequently require intravenous therapy with a β-lactam plus a β-lactamase inhibitor combination (Unasyn, Timentin, Zosyn), a second-generation cephalosporin with anaerobic activity (cefoxitin, cefotetan, cefmetazole) or, in the penicillin-allergic patient, clindamycin plus a fluoroquinolone. Because the bacteriology of these infections is so variable, infected wounds should always be cultured.

E. TETANUS AND RABIES

All patients must be evaluated for the need for tetanus (see Chapter 33) and rabies (see Chapter 32) prophylaxis.

Brook I: Microbiology and management of human and animal bite wound infections. Prim Care 2003;30:25. [PMID: 12825249]

Talan DA et al: Clinical presentation and bacteriologic analysis of infected human bites in patients presenting to emergency departments. Clin Infect Dis 2003;37:1481. [PMID: 14614671]

Taplitz RA: Managing bite wounds. Currently recommended antibiotics for treatment and prophylaxis. Postgrad Med 2004; 116:49. [PMID: 15323154]

SEXUALLY TRANSMITTED DISEASES

Some infectious diseases are transmitted most commonly—or most efficiently—by sexual contact. Most of the infectious agents that cause sexually transmitted diseases are fairly easily inactivated when exposed to a harsh environment. They are thus particularly suited to transmission by contact with mucous membranes. They may be bacteria, spirochetes, chlamydiae, viruses, or protozoa. In most infections caused by these agents, early lesions occur on genitalia or other sexually exposed mucous membranes; however, wide dissemination may occur, and involvement of nongenital tissues and organs may mimic many noninfectious disorders. All sexually transmitted diseases have subclinical or latent phases that play an important role in long-term persistence of the infection or in its transmission from infected (but largely asymptomatic) persons to other contacts. Laboratory examinations are of particular importance in the diagnosis of such asymptomatic patients. Simultaneous infection by several different agents is common, and any person with a sexually transmitted disease should be tested for syphilis; a repeat study should be done in 3 months if negative, since seroconversion is delayed after primary infection.

For each patient, there are one or more sexual contacts who require diagnosis and treatment. Prompt treatment of contacts by giving antibiotics to the index case to distribute all sexual contacts is an important strategy for preventing further transmission. The most common sexually transmitted diseases are gonorrhea,* syphilis,* condyloma acuminatum, chlamydial genital infections,* herpesvirus genital infections, trichomonas vaginitis, chancroid,* granuloma inguinale, scabies, louse infestation, and bacterial vaginosis (among lesbians). However, shigellosis,* hepatitis A, B, and C,* amebiasis, giardiasis,* cryptosporidiosis,* salmonellosis,* and campylobacteriosis may also be transmitted by sexual (oral-anal) contact, especially in homosexual males. Homosexual contact is a typical method of transmission of HIV, although bidirectional heterosexual transmission is occurring more commonly (see Chapter 31).

The risk of developing a sexually transmitted disease following a sexual assault has not been established. Victims of assault have a high baseline rate of infection (*Neisseria gonorrhoeae*, 6%; *Chlamydia trachomatis*, 10%; *Trichomonas vaginalis*, 15%; and bacterial vaginosis, 34%), and the risk of acquiring infection as a result of the assault is significant but is often lower than the preexisting rate (*N gonorrhoeae*, 6–12%; *C trachomatis*, 4–17%; *T vaginalis*, 12%; syphilis, 0.5–3%; and bacterial vaginosis, 19%). Victims should be evaluated within 24 hours after the assault, and cultures for *N gonorrhoeae* and *C trachomatis* should be obtained. (If culture is not available, nonculture tests, such as nucleic acid amplification tests, are acceptable. If the test is positive, it must be confirmed with a second test using a different target sequence.) Vaginal secretions are cultured and examined for *Trichomonas*. If a discharge is present, if there is itching, or if secretions are malodorous, a wet mount should be examined for *Candida* and bacterial vaginosis. In addition, a blood sample should be obtained for immediate serologic testing for syphilis, hepatitis B, and HIV. Follow-up examination for sexually transmitted disease should be repeated within 1–2 weeks, since concentrations of infecting organisms may not have been sufficient to produce a positive culture at the time of initial examination. If prophylactic treatment was given (see below), tests should be repeated only if the victim has symptoms. If prophylaxis was not administered, the individual should be seen in 1 week so that any positive tests can be treated. Follow-up serologic testing for syphilis and HIV infection should be performed in 6, 12, and 24 weeks if the initial tests are negative. The usefulness of presumptive therapy is controversial, some feeling that all patients should receive it and others that it should be limited to those in whom follow-up cannot be ensured or to patients who request it. If therapy is given, a reasonable regimen would be hepatitis B vaccination (without hepatitis B immune globulin, the first dose given at the initial evaluation and follow-up doses at 1–2 months and 4–6 months) and one dose of ceftriaxone, 125 mg intramuscularly, plus metronidazole, 2 g orally as a single dose, plus doxycycline, 100 mg orally

twice daily for 7 days, or azithromycin, 1 g orally as a single dose, instead of doxycycline. In premenopausal women, azithromycin should be used instead of doxycycline until the pregnancy status is determined; if the pregnancy test is positive, metronidazole should be given only after the first trimester.

Although seroconversion to HIV has been reported following sexual assault when this was the only known risk, this risk is believed to be low. The likelihood of HIV transmission from vaginal or anal receptive intercourse when the source is known to be HIV positive is 1 per 1000 and 5 per 1000, respectively. Although prophylactic antiretroviral therapy has not been studied in this setting, the Department of Health and Human Services recommends the prompt institution of postexposure prophylaxis with highly active antiretroviral therapy if the person seeks care within 72 hours of the assault, the source is known to be HIV positive, and the exposure presents a substantial risk of transmission.

Golden MR et al: Effect of expedited treatment of sex partners on recurrent or persistent gonorrhea or chlamydial infection. N Engl J Med 2005;352:676. [PMID: 15716561]

Sexually transmitted diseases treatment guidelines 2002. Centers for Disease Control and Prevention. MMWR Recomm Rep 2002;51(RR-6):1. [PMID: 12184549]

Smith DK et al: Antiretroviral postexposure prophylaxis after sexual, injection-drug use, or other nonoccupational exposure to HIV in the United States: recommendations from the U.S. Department of Health and Human Services. MMWR Recomm Rep 2005;54(RR-2):1. [PMID: 15660015]

INFECTIONS IN DRUG USERS

 ESSENTIALS OF DIAGNOSIS

- *Common infections that occur with greater frequency in drug users include the following: skin infections; hepatitis A, B, C, D; aspiration pneumonia; tuberculosis; pulmonary septic emboli; sexually transmitted diseases; AIDS; infective endocarditis; osteomyelitis; and septic arthritis.*

- *Rare infections in the United States include tetanus, malaria, and melioidosis.*

General Considerations

The use of parenterally administered recreational drugs has increased enormously in recent years. There are now an estimated 300,000 or more injection drug users in the United States.

Common Infections That Occur with Greater Frequency in Drug Users

Skin infections are associated with poor hygiene and use of nonsterile technique when injecting drugs. *S*

---

*Reportable to public health authorities.

aureus (including methicillin-resistant strains) and oral flora (streptococci, *Eikenella, Fusobacterium, Peptostreptococcus*) are the most common organisms, with enteric gram-negatives less common and seen in those who inject into the groin. Cellulitis and subcutaneous abscesses occur most commonly, particularly in association with subcutaneous ("skin-popping") or intramuscular injections and the use of cocaine and heroin mixtures (probably due to ischemia). Myositis, clostridial myonecrosis, and necrotizing fasciitis occur infrequently but are life-threatening. Wound botulism in association with black tar heroin occurs sporadically but often in clusters.

Hepatitis is very common among habitual drug users and is transmissible both by the parenteral (hepatitis B, C, and D) and by the fecal-oral route (hepatitis A). Multiple episodes of hepatitis with different agents can occur.

Aspiration pneumonia and its complications (lung abscess, empyema, brain abscess) result from altered consciousness associated with drug use. Mixed aerobic and anaerobic mouth flora are usually involved.

Tuberculosis also occurs in drug users, and infection with HIV has fostered the spread of tuberculosis in this population. Morbidity and mortality rates are increased in HIV-infected individuals with tuberculosis. Classic radiographic findings are often absent; tuberculosis is suspected in any patient with infiltrates who does not respond to antibiotics.

Pulmonary septic emboli may originate from venous thrombi or right-sided endocarditis.

Sexually transmitted diseases are not directly related to drug use, but the practice of exchanging sex for drugs has resulted in an increased frequency of sexually transmitted diseases. Syphilis, gonorrhea, and chancroid are the most common.

AIDS has a high incidence among injection drug users and their sexual contacts and among the offspring of infected women (see Chapter 31).

Infective endocarditis. The organisms that cause infective endocarditis in those who use drugs intravenously are most commonly *S aureus, Candida* (especially *Candida parapsilosis*), *Enterococcus faecalis*, other streptococci, and gram-negative bacteria (especially *Pseudomonas* and *Serratia marcescens*). A number of complications of endocarditis can occur, including splenic abscesses, central nervous system infections (meningitis, brain abscess, subdural empyema, epidural abscess), and endophthalmitis. Involvement of the right side of the heart is common, and infection of more than one valve is not infrequent. Right-sided involvement, especially in the absence of murmurs, is often suggested by the presence of septic pulmonary emboli. The diagnosis must be established by blood culture. Therapy, including empiric treatment, is discussed in Chapter 33.

Other vascular infections include septic thrombophlebitis and mycotic aneurysms. Mycotic aneurysms resulting from direct trauma to a vessel with secondary infection most commonly occur in femoral arteries and less commonly in arteries of the neck. Aneurysms resulting from hematogenous spread of organisms frequently involve intracerebral vessels and thus are seen in association with endocarditis.

Osteomyelitis and septic arthritis. Osteomyelitis involving vertebral bodies, sternoclavicular joints, the pubic symphysis, the sacroiliac joints, and other sites usually results from hematogenous distribution of injected organisms or septic venous thrombi. Pain and fever precede radiographic changes, sometimes by several weeks. While staphylococci—often methicillin-resistant—are common organisms, *Serratia, Pseudomonas, Candida* (usually not *Candida albicans*), and other pathogens rarely encountered in spontaneous bone or joint disease are found in injection drug users.

Infections Rare in United States

A. TETANUS

In the 1950s and 1960s, tetanus was commonly seen in drug users, especially in unimmunized women who injected drugs subcutaneously ("skin-popping"). Increased tetanus immunization among drug users has resulted in a decline in this disease, although cases are still reported.

B. MALARIA

Needle transmission occurs from injection drug users who acquired the infection in malaria-endemic areas outside the United States.

C. MELIOIDOSIS

This chronic pulmonary infection caused by *Burkholderia pseudomallei* occurs occasionally in debilitated drug users, but most cases are reported in Asia and Australia.

Treatment

A common and difficult clinical problem is management of the parenteral drug user who presents with fever. In general, after obtaining appropriate cultures (blood, urine, and sputum if the chest radiograph is abnormal), empiric therapy is begun. If the chest radiograph is suggestive of a community-acquired pneumonia (consolidation), therapy for outpatient pneumonia is begun with a third-generation cephalosporin, such as ceftriaxone, 1–2 g intravenously every 24 hours (many clinicians would add azithromycin, 500 mg orally or intravenously every 24 hours, or doxycycline, 100 mg orally or intravenously twice daily, to this regimen). If the chest radiograph is suggestive of septic emboli (nodular infiltrates), therapy for presumed endocarditis is initiated, usually with a combination of vancomycin 15 mg/kg every 12 hours intravenously (due to the high prevalence of methicillin-resistant *S aureus* and the possibility of enterococcus) and gentamicin, 1 mg/kg every 8 hours intravenously. If the chest radiograph is normal and no focal site of infection can be found, endocarditis is presumed. While awaiting the results of blood cultures, empiric treatment with vancomycin and gentamicin is started. If blood cultures are positive for organisms that frequently cause endocarditis in drug users (see above), endocarditis is presumed to be present and treated accordingly. If blood cultures are positive for an organism that is an unusual cause of endocarditis, evaluation for an occult source of infection should go forward. In this setting, a transesophageal echocardiogram may be quite helpful since it is 90% sensitive in detecting vegetations and a negative study is strong evidence against endocarditis. If blood cultures are negative and the patient responds to antibiotics, therapy should be continued for 7–14 days (oral therapy can be given once an initial response has occurred). In every patient, careful examination for an occult source of infection (eg, genitourinary, dental, sinus, gallbladder) should be done.

Gordon RJ et al: Bacterial infections in drug users. N Engl J Med 2005;353:1945. [PMID: 16267325]

Infections in injection drug users (entire issue). Infect Dis Clin North Am 2002;16:3.

ACUTE INFECTIOUS DIARRHEA

ESSENTIALS OF DIAGNOSIS

- *Arbitrarily divided into acute and chronic and mild, moderate, and severe.*
- *Diarrhea is acute if lasts < 2 weeks and chronic if lasts > 2 weeks.*
- *Disease is mild if there are three or fewer stools per day, moderate if there are four or more stools in association with local symptoms (abdominal cramps, nausea, tenesmus), and severe if there are four or more stools per day with systemic symptoms (fevers, chills, dehydration).*

General Considerations

Acute diarrhea can be caused by a number of different factors, including emotional stress, food intolerance, inorganic agents (eg, sodium nitrite), organic substances (eg, mushrooms, shellfish), drugs, and infectious agents (including viruses, bacteria, and protozoa). From a diagnostic and therapeutic standpoint, it is helpful to classify infectious diarrhea into syndromes that produce inflammatory or bloody diarrhea and those that are noninflammatory, nonbloody, or watery. In general, the term "inflammatory diarrhea" suggests colonic involvement by invasive bacteria or parasites or by toxin production. Patients complain of frequent bloody, small-volume stools, often associated with fever, abdominal cramps, tenesmus, and fecal ur-

gency. Common causes of this syndrome include *Shigella, Salmonella, Campylobacter, Yersinia,* invasive strains of *Escherichia coli, E coli* O157:H7, *Entamoeba histolytica,* and *C difficile.* Tests for fecal leukocytes or the neutrophil marker lactoferrin are frequently positive, and definitive etiologic diagnosis requires stool culture. Noninflammatory diarrhea is generally milder and is caused by viruses or toxins that affect the small intestine and interfere with salt and water balance, resulting in large-volume watery diarrhea, often with nausea, vomiting, and cramps. Common causes of this syndrome include viruses (eg, rotavirus, Norwalk virus, enteric adenoviruses, astrovirus, coronavirus), vibriones *(Vibrio cholerae, Vibrio parahaemolyticus),* enterotoxin-producing *E coli, Giardia lamblia,* cryptosporidia, and agents that can cause food-borne gastroenteritis.

The term "food poisoning" denotes diseases caused by toxins present in consumed foods. When the incubation period is short (1–6 hours after consumption), the toxin is usually preformed. Vomiting is usually a major complaint, and fever is usually absent. Examples include intoxication from *S aureus* or *Bacillus cereus,* and toxin can be detected in the food. When the incubation period is longer—between 8 hours and 16 hours—the organism is present in the food and produces toxin after being ingested. Vomiting is less prominent, abdominal cramping is frequent, and fever is often absent. The best example of this disease is that due to *Clostridium perfringens.* Toxin can be detected in food or stool specimens.

The inflammatory and noninflammatory diarrheas discussed above can also be transmitted by food and water and usually have incubation periods between 12 and 72 hours. *Cyclospora,* cryptosporidia, and *Isospora* are protozoans capable of causing disease in both immunocompetent and immunocompromised patients. Characteristics of disease include profuse watery diarrhea that is prolonged but usually self-limited (1–2 weeks) in the immunocompetent patient but can be chronic in the compromised host. Epidemiologic features may be helpful in determining etiology. Recent hospitalization or antibiotic use suggests *C difficile;* recent foreign travel suggests *Salmonella, Shigella, Campylobacter, E coli,* or *V cholerae;* undercooked hamburger suggests *E coli,* especially O157:H7; and fried rice consumption is associated with *B cereus* toxin. Prominent features of some of these causes of diarrhea are listed in Table 30–3.

Treatment

Treatment usually consists of replacement of fluids and electrolytes and, very rarely, management of hypovolemic shock and respiratory compromise. In mild diarrhea, increasing ingestion of juices and clear soups is adequate. In more severe cases of dehydration (postural lightheadedness, decreased urination), oral glucose-based rehydration solutions can be used (Ceralyte, Pedialyte). In general, most cases of acute

Table 30–3. Acute bacterial diarrheas and "food poisoning."

Organism	Incubation Period	Vomiting	Diarrhea	Fever	Associated Foods	Diagnosis	Clinical Features and Treatment
Staphylococcus (pre-formed toxin)	1–8 hours	+++	±	±	Staphylococci grow in meats, dairy, and bakery products and produce enterotoxin.	Clinical. Food and stool can be tested for toxin.	Abrupt onset, intense nausea and vomiting for up to 24 hours, recovery in 24–48 hours. Supportive care.
Bacillus cereus (pre-formed toxin)	1–8 hours	+++	±	–	Reheated fried rice causes vomiting or diarrhea.	Clinical. Food and stool can be tested for toxin.	Acute onset, severe nausea and vomiting lasting 24 hours. Supportive care.
B cereus (diarrheal toxin)	10–16 hours	±	+++	–	Toxin in meats, stews, and gravy.	Clinical. Food and stool can be tested for toxin.	Abdominal cramps, watery diarrhea, and nausea lasting 24–48 hours. Supportive care.
Clostridium perfringens	8–16 hours	±	+++	–	Clostridia grow in re-warmed meat and poultry dishes and produce an enterotoxin.	Stools can be tested for enterotoxin or cultured.	Abrupt onset of profuse diarrhea, abdominal cramps, nausea; vomiting occasionally. Recovery usual without treatment in 24–48 hours. Supportive care; antibiotics not needed.
Clostridium botulinum	12–72 hours	±	–	–	Clostridia grow in anaerobic acidic environment eg, canned foods, fermented fish, foods held warm for extended periods.	Stool, serum, and food can be tested for toxin. Stool and food can be cultured.	Diplopia, dysphagia, dysphonia, respiratory embarrassment. Treatment requires clear airway, ventilation, and intravenous polyvalent antitoxin (see text). Symptoms can last for days to months.
Clostridium difficile	Usually occurs after 7–10 days of antibiotics. Can occur after a single dose or several weeks after completion of antibiotics.	–	+++	++	Associated with antimicrobial drugs; clindamycin and cephalosporins most commonly implicated.	Stool tested for toxin.	Abrupt onset of diarrhea that may be bloody; fever. Oral metronidazole first-line therapy. If no response, oral vancomycin can be given.
Enterohemorrhagic Escherichia coli, including E coli O157:H7 and other Shiga-toxin producing strains (STEC)	1–8 days	+	+++	–	Undercooked beef, especially hamburger; unpasteurized milk and juice; raw fruits and vegetables.	E coli O157:H7 can be cultured on special medium. Other toxins can be detected in stool.	Usually abrupt onset of diarrhea, often bloody; abdominal pain. In adults, it is usually self-limited to 5–10 days. In children, it is associated with hemolytic-uremic syndrome (HUS). Antibiotic therapy may increase risk of HUS.
Enterotoxigenic E coli (ETEC)	1–3 days	±	+++	±	Water, food contaminated with feces.	Stool culture. Special tests required to identify toxin-producing strains.	Watery diarrhea and abdominal cramps, usually lasting 3–7 days. In travelers, fluoroquinolones shorten disease.

1328

Organism	Incubation period				Source	Diagnosis	Clinical features
Vibrio parahaemolyticus	2–48 hours	+	+	±	Undercooked or raw seafood.	Stool culture on special medium.	Abrupt onset of watery diarrhea, abdominal cramps, nausea and vomiting. Recovery usually complete in 2–5 days.
Vibrio cholerae	24–72 hours	+	+++	–	Contaminated water, fish, shellfish, street vendor food.	Stool culture on special medium.	Abrupt onset of liquid diarrhea in endemic area. Needs prompt intravenous or oral replacement of fluids and electrolytes. Tetracyclines shorten excretion of vibrios.
Campylobacter jejuni	2–5 days	±	+++	+	Raw or undercooked poultry, unpasteurized milk, water.	Stool culture on special medium.	Fever, diarrhea that can be bloody, cramps. Usually self-limited in 2–10 days. Early treatment (erythromycin) shortens course. May be associated with Guillain-Barré syndrome.
Shigella species (mild cases)	24–48 hours	±	+	+	Food or water contaminated with human feces. Person to person spread.	Routine stool culture.	Abrupt onset of diarrhea, often with blood and pus in stools, cramps, tenesmus, and lethargy. Stool cultures are positive. Therapy depends on sensitivity testing, but the fluoroquinolones are most effective. Do not give opioids. Often mild and self-limited.
Salmonella species	1–3 days	–	++	+	Eggs, poultry, unpasteurized milk, cheese, juices, raw fruits and vegetables.	Routine stool culture.	Gradual or abrupt onset of diarrhea and low-grade fever. No antimicrobials unless high risk (see text) or systemic dissemination is suspected, in which case give a fluoroquinolone. Prolonged carriage can occur.
Yersinia enterocolitica	24–48 hours	±	+	+	Undercooked pork, contaminated water, unpasteurized milk, tofu.	Stool culture on special medium.	Severe abdominal pain, (appendicitis-like symptoms) diarrhea, fever. Polyarthritis, erythema nodosum in children. If severe, give tetracycline or fluoroquinolone. Without treatment, self-limited in 1–3 weeks.
Rotavirus	1–3 days	++	+++	+	Fecally contaminated foods touched by infected food handlers.	Immunoassay on stool.	Acute onset, vomiting, watery diarrhea that lasts 4–8 days. Supportive care.
Noroviruses and other caliciviruses	12–48 hours	++	+++	+	Shell fish and fecally contaminated foods touched by infected food handlers.	Clinical diagnosis with negative stool cultures. PCR available on stool.	Nausea, vomiting (more common in children) diarrhea (more common in adults), fever, myalgias, abdominal cramps. Lasts 12–60 hours. Supportive care.

PCR = polymerase chain reaction.

gastroenteritis are self-limited and do not require therapy other than supportive measures. When symptoms persist beyond 3–4 days, initial presentation is accompanied by fever or bloody diarrhea, or if the patient is immunocompromised, cultures of stool are usually obtained. Symptoms have often resolved by the time cultures are completed. In this case, even if a pathogen is isolated, therapy is not needed (except for *Shigella*, since the infecting dose is so small that therapy to eradicate organisms from the stool is indicated for epidemiologic reasons). If symptoms persist and a pathogen is isolated, it is reasonable to institute specific treatment even though therapy has not been conclusively shown to alter the natural history of disease for most pathogens. Exceptions include infection with *Shigella* where antibiotic therapy has been shown to shorten the duration of symptoms by 2–3 days, infections with *E coli* O157:H7 (antibiotic therapy does not ameliorate symptoms and may increase the risk of developing hemolytic-uremic syndrome), and *Campylobacter* infections (early therapy, within 4 days of onset of symptoms, shortens the course of disease). Uncomplicated gastroenteritis due to *Salmonella* does not require therapy because the disease is usually self-limited and therapy may prolong carriage and perhaps increase relapses. Because bacteremia with complications can occur in high-risk patients, some experts have recommended therapy for *Salmonella* in patients over the age of 50, in organ transplant recipients, in those with HIV, in patients taking corticosteroids, in those with lymphoproliferative diseases, and in those with vascular grafts. Ciprofloxacin, 500 mg every 12 hours for 5 days, is effective in shortening the course of illness compared with placebo in patients presenting with diarrhea, whether a pathogen is isolated or not. However, because of concerns about selecting for resistant organisms (especially *Campylobacter,* where increasing resistance to fluoroquinolones has been documented and erythromycin is the drug of choice) coupled with the fact that most infectious diarrhea is self-limited, routine use of antibiotics for all patients with diarrhea is not recommended. Antibiotics should be considered in patients with evidence of invasive disease (white cells in stool, dysentery), with symptoms 3–4 days or more in duration, with multiple stools (eight to ten or more per day), and in those with impaired immune responses. Antimotility drugs may relieve cramping and decrease diarrhea in mild cases. Their use should be limited to patients without fever and without dysentery (bloody stools), and they should be used in low doses because of the risk of producing toxic megacolon.

Therapeutic recommendations for specific agents can be found elsewhere in this book.

Diagnosis and management of foodborne illnesses: a primer for physicians and other health care professionals. MMWR Recomm Rep 2004;53(RR-4):1. [PMID: 15123984]

Musher DM et al: Contagious acute gastrointestinal infections N Engl J Med 2004;351:2417. [PMID: 15575058]

Thielman NM et al: Clinical practice. Acute infectious diarrhea. N Engl J Med 2004;350:38. [PMID: 14702426]

INFECTIOUS DISEASES IN THE RETURNING TRAVELER

 ESSENTIALS OF DIAGNOSIS

- *Identify patients with acute, potentially life-threatening and treatable diseases, or those with transmissible diseases that require isolation.*
- *The incubation period may be helpful in diagnosis.*
- *Less than 3 weeks following exposure may suggest dengue, leptospirosis and yellow fever; greater than 3 weeks suggest typhoid fever, malaria, and tuberculosis.*

General Considerations

The differential diagnosis of fever in the returning traveler is broad, ranging from self-limited viral infections to life-threatening illness. The evaluation is best done by identifying whether a particular syndrome is present, then refining the differential diagnosis based on an exposure history. The travel history should include directed questions regarding geography (rural versus urban), animal or arthropod contact, unprotected sexual intercourse, ingestion of untreated water or raw foods, historical or pretravel immunizations, and adherence to malaria prophylaxis.

Etiologies

The most common infectious causes of fever—excluding simple causes such as upper respiratory infections, bacterial pneumonia and urinary tract infections—in returning travelers are malaria (see Chapter 35), diarrhea (see next section), and dengue (see Chapter 32). Others include respiratory infections, leptospirosis (see Chapter 34), typhoid fever (see Chapter 33), and rickettsial infections (see Chapter 32). Systemic febrile illnesses without a diagnosis also occurs commonly, particularly in travelers returning from sub-Saharan Africa or Southeast Asia.

A. FEVER AND RASH

Potential etiologies include dengue, viral hemorrhagic fever, leptospirosis, meningococcemia, yellow fever, typhus, *Salmonella typhi,* and acute HIV infection.

B. PULMONARY INFILTRATES

Tuberculosis, ascaris, *Paragonimus,* and *Strongyloides* can all cause pulmonary infiltrates.

C. MENINGOENCEPHALITIS

Etiologies include *N meningitidis,* leptospirosis, arboviruses, rabies, and (cerebral) malaria.

D. JAUNDICE

Consider hepatitis A, yellow fever, hemorrhagic fever, leptospirosis, and malaria.

E. FEVER WITHOUT LOCALIZING SYMPTOMS OR SIGNS

Malaria, typhoid fever, acute HIV infection, rickettsial illness, visceral leishmaniasis, trypanosomiasis, and dengue are possible etiologies.

F. TRAVELER'S DIARRHEA

See next section.

Clinical Findings

Fever and rash in the returning traveler should prompt blood cultures and various serologic tests based on the exposure history. The work-up of a pulmonary infiltrate should include the placement of a PPD, examination of sputum for acid-fast bacilli and possibly for ova and parasites. Patients with evidence of meningoencephalitis should receive lumbar puncture, blood cultures, thick/thin smears of peripheral blood, history-guided serologies, and a nape biopsy (if rabies is suspected). Jaundice in a returning traveler should be evaluated for hemolysis, and the following tests should be performed: liver function tests, thick/thin smears of peripheral blood, and directed serologic testing. The work-up of traveler's diarrhea is presented in the following section. Finally, patients with fever but no localizing signs or symptoms should have blood cultures performed. Routine laboratory studies usually include complete blood count with differential, electrolytes, liver function tests, urine analysis, and blood cultures. Thick and thin peripheral blood smears should be done (and repeated in 12–24 hours if clinical suspicion remains high) for malaria if there has been travel to endemic areas. Other studies are directed by the results of history, physical examination, and initial laboratory tests. They may include stool for ova and parasites, chest radiograph, HIV test, and specific serologies (eg, dengue, leptospirosis, rickettsial disease, schistosomiasis). Bone marrow biopsy to diagnose typhoid fever could be helpful in the appropriate patient.

Freedman DO et al; GeoSentinel Surveillance Network: Spectrum of disease and relation to place of exposure among ill returned travelers. N Engl J Med 2006;354:119. [PMID: 16407507]

Ryan ET et al: Illness after international travel. N Engl J Med 2002;347:505. [PMID: 12181406]

Stienlauf S et al: Epidemiology of travel-related hospitalization. J Travel Med 2005;12:136. [PMID: 15996442]

TRAVELER'S DIARRHEA

ESSENTIALS OF DIAGNOSIS

- *Usually a benign, self-limited disease occurring about 1 week into travel.*

- *Prophylaxis not recommended unless there is a comorbid disease (inflammatory bowel syndrome, HIV, immunosuppressive medication).*
- *Single-dose therapy of a fluoroquinolone usually effective if symptoms develop.*

General Considerations

Whenever a person travels from one country to another—particularly if the change involves a marked difference in climate, social conditions, or sanitation standards and facilities—diarrhea is likely to develop within 2–10 days. Bacteria cause 80% of cases of traveler's diarrhea, with enterotoxigenic *E coli*, *Shigella* species, and *Campylobacter jejuni* being the most common pathogens. Less common are *Aeromonas*, *Salmonella*, noncholera vibriones, *E histolytica*, and *G lamblia*. Contributory causes include unusual food and drink, change in living habits, occasional viral infections (adenoviruses or rotaviruses), and change in bowel flora. Chronic watery diarrhea may be due to amebiasis or giardiasis or, rarely, tropical sprue.

Clinical Findings

A. SYMPTOMS AND SIGNS

There may be up to ten or even more loose stools per day, often accompanied by abdominal cramps and nausea, occasionally by vomiting, and rarely by fever. The stools do not usually contain mucus or blood, and aside from weakness and dehydration, there are no systemic manifestations of infection. The illness usually subsides spontaneously within 1–5 days, although 10% remain symptomatic for 1 week or longer, and symptoms persist for longer than 1 month in 2%.

B. LABORATORY FINDINGS

In patients with fever and bloody diarrhea, stool culture may be indicated, but in most cases, cultures are reserved for those who do not respond to antibiotics.

Prevention

A. GENERAL MEASURES

Avoidance of fresh foods and water sources that are likely to be contaminated is recommended for travelers to developing countries, where infectious diarrheal illnesses are endemic.

B. SPECIFIC MEASURES

Prophylaxis is recommended for those with significant underlying disease (inflammatory bowel disease, AIDS, diabetes, heart disease in the elderly, conditions requiring immunosuppressive medications) and for those whose full activity status during the trip is so essential that even short periods of diarrhea would be unacceptable. Prophylaxis is started upon entry into the destination country and is continued for 1 or 2 days after leaving. For stays of more than 3 weeks, prophylaxis is not recommended because of the cost and increased toxicity. For prophylaxis, bismuth subsalicylate is effective but turns the tongue and the stools black and can interfere with doxycycline absorption, which may be needed for malaria prophylaxis; it is rarely used. Numerous antimicrobial regimens for once-daily oral prophylaxis are effective, such as norfloxacin, 400 mg, ciprofloxacin, 500 mg, ofloxacin, 300 mg, or TMP-SMZ, 160/800 mg. Because not all travelers will have diarrhea and because most episodes are brief and self-limited, an alternative approach currently recommended is to provide the traveler with a supply of antimicrobials to be taken if significant diarrhea occurs during the trip. Loperamide (4 mg oral loading dose, then 2 mg after each loose stool to a maximum of 16 mg/d) with a single oral dose of ciprofloxacin (750 mg), levofloxacin (500 mg), ofloxacin (300 mg), or azithromycin (1000 mg) cures most cases of traveler's diarrhea. In pregnant women and in areas with a high prevalence of fluoroquinolone-resistant *Campylobacter* (such as Thailand), azithromycin is the drug of choice. If diarrhea is severe, associated with fever or bloody stools, or persists despite single-dose ciprofloxacin treatment, then 3–5 days of ciprofloxacin, 500 mg orally twice daily; levofloxacin, 500 mg orally once daily; norfloxacin, 400 mg orally twice daily; ofloxacin, 300 mg orally twice daily; or azithromycin, 500 mg orally once daily (for pregnant women) can be given. TMP-SMZ, 160/800 mg orally twice daily, can be used as an alternative, but resistance is common in many areas. Rifaximin, a nonabsorbable, rifampin-like drug, is also approved for therapy of traveler's diarrhea at a dose of 200 mg orally three times per day or 400 mg twice a day for 3 days. Because luminal concentrations are high, but tissue level are quite low, it should not be used in situations where there is a high likelihood of invasive disease (eg, fever, systemic toxicity, or bloody stools).

Treatment

For most individuals, the affliction is short-lived, and symptomatic therapy with opioids or loperamide is all that is required, provided the patient is not systemically ill (fever ≥ 39 °C) and does not have dysentery (bloody stools), in which case antimotility agents should be avoided. Packages of oral rehydration salts to treat dehydration are available over the counter in the United States (Infalyte, Pedialyte, others) and in many foreign countries.

Guerrant RL et al; Infectious Diseases Society of America: Practice guidelines for the management of infectious diarrhea. Clin Infect Dis 2001;32:331. [PMID: 11170940]

Ramzan NN: Traveler's diarrhea. Gastroenterol Clin North Am 2001;30:665. [PMID: 11586551]

Rendi-Wagner P et al: Drug prophylaxis for travelers' diarrhea. Clin Infect Dis 2002;34:628. [PMID: 11803509]

Thielman NM et al: Clinical practice. Acute infectious diarrhea. N Engl J Med 2004;350:38. [PMID: 14702426]

■ ACTIVE IMMUNIZATION AGAINST INFECTIOUS DISEASES

RECOMMENDED IMMUNIZATION OF INFANTS, CHILDREN, & ADOLESCENTS

The recommended schedules and dosages of vaccination change often, so the manufacturer's package inserts should always be consulted.

The schedule for active immunizations in children is presented in Table 30–4 (see also www.cdc.gov/nip). All adolescents should see a health care provider to ensure vaccination of those who have not received varicella or hepatitis B vaccine, to make certain that a second dose of measles-mumps-rubella (MMR) has been given, to receive a booster of tetanus toxoid, reduced diphtheria toxoid and acellular pertussis vaccine (Tdap adolescent preparation), to receive meningococcal vaccine conjugate vaccine, and to receive immunizations (influenza and pneumococcal vaccines) that may be indicated for certain high-risk individuals.

RECOMMENDED IMMUNIZATION OF ADULTS

Several vaccines are recommended for adults depending on the individual's previous vaccination status and the risks of exposure to certain diseases. Recommendations are summarized in Table 30–5.

Tetanus, Diphtheria, and Pertussis

A tetanus toxoid, reduced diphtheria toxoid and acellular pertussis vaccine (Tdap) has been approved for use in persons 11–64 years of age, resulting in several changes in previous recommendations for adult immunization. All should receive a primary series of immunizations against tetanus, diphtheria, and pertussis (Table 30–4). Adults who have not previously been immunized should receive a dose of Tdap followed by a dose Td 4 weeks later and a booster with Td 6–12 months after the second dose. For adults previously immunized with a pertussis-containing vaccine, a single dose of Tdap should be administered instead of Td as a routine booster if the previous dose of Td was greater than 10 years ago. To prevent pertussis among infants younger than 12 months of age, a single dose of Tdap is recommended for adults anticipating close contact with these infants (eg, parents, grandparents younger than age 65, child care givers). In addition, a single dose of Tdap is also recommended for health care personnel with direct patient care. For wound management, adults between the ages of 19 and 64 should receive Tdap instead of Td if they have not previously received Tdap. Use of Tdap in pregnancy is under consideration, but in most cases, women should receive Tdap after delivery to comply with the above recommendations of immunizing

Table 30–4. Recommended childhood immunization schedule—United States, 2006.[1]

Vaccine ▼ \ Age ►	Birth	1 month	2 months	4 months	6 months	12 months	15 months	18 months	24 months	4–6 years	11–12 years	13–14 years	15 years	16–18 years
Hepatitis B[1]	HepB	HepB	HepB[1]		HepB						HepB Series			
Diphtheria, Tetanus, Pertussis[2]			DTaP	DTaP	DTaP		DTaP			DTaP	Tdap		Tdap	
Haemophilus influenzae type b[3]			Hib	Hib	Hib[3]	Hib								
Inactivated Poliovirus			IPV	IPV		IPV				IPV				
Measles, Mumps, Rubella[4]						MMR				MMR		MMR		
Varicella[5]						Varicella					Varicella			
Meningococcal[6]							Vaccines within broken line are for selected populations			MPSV4	MCV4		MCV4	MCV4
Pneumococcal[7]			PCV	PCV	PCV	PCV				PCV	PPV			
Influenza[8]					Influenza (yearly)						Influenza (yearly)			
Hepatitis A[9]						HepA series					HepA series			

This schedule indicates the recommended ages for routine administration of currently licensed childhood vaccines, as of December 1, 2005, for children through age 18 years. Any dose not administered at the recommended age should be administered at any subsequent visit, when indicated and feasible. ▨ Indicates age groups that warrant special effort to administer those vaccines not previously administered. Additional vaccines might be licensed and recommended during the year. Licensed combination vaccines may be used whenever any components of the combination are indicated and other components of the vaccine are not contraindicated and if approved by the Food and Drug Administration for that dose of the series. Providers should consult respective Advisory Committee on Immunization Practices (ACIP) statements for detailed recommendations. Clinically significant adverse events that follow vaccination should be reported through the Vaccine Adverse Event Reporting System (VAERS). Guidance about how to obtain and complete a VAERS form is available at http://www.vaers.hhs.gov or by telephone, 800-822-7967.

▨ Range of recommended ages   ▨ Catch-up immunization   ▨ Assessment at age 11–12 years

1. **Hepatitis B vaccine (HepB).** *AT BIRTH:* All newborns should receive monovalent HepB soon after birth and before hospital discharge. **Infants born to mothers who are hepatitis B surface antigen (HBsAg)-positive** should receive HepB and 0.5 mL of hepatitis B immune globulin (HBIG) within 12 hours of birth. **Infants born to mothers whose HBsAg status is unknown** should receive HepB within 12 hours of birth. The mother should have blood drawn as soon as possible to determine her HBsAg status; if HBsAg-positive, the infant should receive HBIG as soon as possible (no later than age 1 week). **For infants born to HBsAg-negative mothers,** the birth dose can be delayed in rare circumstances but only if a physician's order to withhold the vaccine and a copy of the mother's original HBsAg-negative laboratory report are documented in the infant's medical record. *FOLLOWING THE BIRTH DOSE:* The HepB series should be completed with either monovalent HepB or a combination vaccine containing HepB. The second dose should be administered at age 1–2 months. The final dose should be administered at age ≥24 weeks. Administering four doses of HepB is permissible (e.g., when combination vaccines are administered after the birth dose); however, if monovalent HepB is used, a dose at age 4 months is not needed. **Infants born to HBsAg-positive mothers** should be tested for HBsAg and antibody to HBsAg after completion of the HepB series at age 9–18 months (generally at the next well-child visit after completion of the vaccine series).

2. **Diphtheria and tetanus toxoids and acellular pertussis vaccine (DTaP).** The fourth dose of DTaP may be administered as early as age 12 months, provided 6 months have elapsed since the third dose and the child is unlikely to return at age 15–18 months. The final dose in the series should be administered at age ≥4 years. **Tetanus toxoid, reduced diphtheria toxoid, and acellular pertussis vaccine (Tdap adolescent preparation)** is recommended at age 11–12 years for those who have completed the recommended childhood DTP/DTaP vaccination series and have not received a tetanus and diphtheria toxoids (Td) booster dose. Adolescents aged 13–18 years who missed the age 11–12-year Td/Tdap booster dose should also receive a single dose of Tdap if they have completed the recommended childhood DTP/DTaP vaccination series. **Subsequent Td** boosters are recommended every 10 years.

3. *Haemophilus influenzae* **type b conjugate vaccine (Hib).** Three Hib conjugate vaccines are licensed for infant use. If PRP-OMP (PedvaxHIB® or ComVax® [Merck]) is administered at ages 2 and 4 months, a dose at age 6 months is not required. DTaP/Hib combination products should not be used for primary immunization in infants at ages 2, 4, or 6 months but may be used as boosters after any Hib vaccine. The final dose in the series should be administered at age ≥12 months.

4. **Measles, mumps, and rubella vaccine (MMR).** The second dose of MMR is recommended routinely at age 4–6 years but may be administered during any visit, provided at least 4 weeks have elapsed since the first dose and both doses are administered at or after age 12 months. Children who have not previously received the second dose should complete the schedule by age 11–12 years.

5. **Varicella vaccine.** Varicella vaccine is recommended at any visit at or after age 12 months for susceptible children (i.e., those who lack a reliable history of varicella). Susceptible persons aged ≥13 years should receive 2 doses administered at least 4 weeks apart.

6. **Meningococcal vaccine (MCV4).** Meningococcal conjugate vaccine (MCV4) should be administered to all children at age 11–12 years as well as to unvaccinated adolescents at high school entry (age 15 years). Other adolescents who wish to decrease their risk for meningococcal disease may also be vaccinated. All college freshmen living in dormitories should also be vaccinated, preferably with MCV4, although **meningococcal polysaccharide vaccine (MPSV4)** is an acceptable alternative. Vaccination against invasive meningococcal disease is recommended for children and adolescents aged ≥2 years with terminal complement deficiencies or anatomic or functional asplenia and for certain other high risk groups (see *MMWR* 2005;54[No. RR-7]); use MPSV4 for children aged 2–10 years and MCV4 for older children, although MPSV4 is an acceptable alternative.

7. **Pneumococcal vaccine.** The heptavalent **pneumococcal conjugate vaccine (PCV)** is recommended for all children aged 2–23 months and for certain children aged 24–59 months. The final dose in the series should be administered at age ≥12 months. **Pneumococcal polysaccharide vaccine (PPV)** is recommended in addition to PCV for certain high-risk groups. See *MMWR* 2000;49(No. RR-9).

8. **Influenza vaccine.** Influenza vaccine is recommended annually for children aged ≥6 months with certain risk factors (including, but not limited to, asthma, cardiac disease, sickle cell disease, human immunodeficiency virus infection, diabetes, and conditions that can compromise respiratory function or handling of respiratory secretions or that can increase the risk for aspiration), health-care workers, and other persons (including household members) in close contact with persons in groups at high risk (see *MMWR* 2005;54[No. RR-8]). In addition, healthy children aged 6–23 months and close contacts of healthy children aged 0–5 months are recommended to receive influenza vaccine because children in this age group are at substantially increased risk for influenza-related hospitalizations. For healthy, nonpregnant persons aged 5–49 years, the intranasally administered, live, attenuated influenza vaccine (LAIV) is an acceptable alternative to the intramuscular trivalent inactivated influenza vaccine (TIV). See *MMWR* 2005;54(No. RR-8). Children receiving TIV should be administered an age-appropriate dosage (0.25 mL for children aged 6–35 months or 0.5 mL for children aged ≥3 years). Children aged ≤8 years who are receiving influenza vaccine for the first time should receive 2 doses (separated by at least 4 weeks for TIV and at least 6 weeks for LAIV).

9. **Hepatitis A vaccine (HepA).** HepA is recommended for all children at age 1 year (i.e., 12–23 months). The 2 doses in the series should be administered at least 6 months apart. States, counties, and communities with existing HepA vaccination programs for children aged 2–18 years are encouraged to maintain these programs. In these areas, new efforts focused on routine vaccination of children aged 1 year should enhance, not replace, ongoing programs directed at a broader population of children. HepA is also recommended for certain high risk groups (see *MMWR* 1999;48[No. RR-12]).

The Childhood and Adolescent Immunization Schedule is approved by the Advisory Committee on Immunization Practices (http://www.cdc.gov/nip/acip), the American Academy of Pediatrics (http://www.aap.org), and the American Academy of Family Physicians (http://www.aafp.org).

(continued)

Table 30–4. Recommended childhood immunization schedule—United States, 2006.[1] (continued)

CATCH-UP SCHEDULE FOR CHILDREN AGED 4 MONTHS–6 YEARS					
Vaccine	Minimum age for dose 1	Minimum interval between doses			
		Dose 1 to Dose 2	Dose 2 to Dose 3	Dose 3 to Dose 4	Dose 4 to Dose 5
Diphtheria, Tetanus, Pertussis	6 weeks	4 weeks	4 weeks	6 months	6 months[1]
Inactivated Poliovirus	6 weeks	4 weeks	4 weeks	4 weeks[2]	
Hepatitis B[3]	Birth	4 weeks	8 weeks (and 16 weeks after first dose)		
Measles, Mumps, Rubella	12 months	4 weeks[4]			
Varicella	12 months				
Haemophilus influenza type b[5]	6 weeks	4 weeks if first dose administered at age <12 months 8 weeks (as final dose) if first dose administered at age 12–14 months No further doses needed if first dose administered at age ≥15 months	4 weeks[6] if current age <12 months 8 weeks (as final dose)[6] if current age ≥12 months and second dose administered at age <15 months No further doses needed if previous dose administered at age ≥15 months	8 weeks (as final dose) This dose only necessary for children aged 12 months–5 years who received 3 doses before age 12 months	
Pneumococcal[7]	6 weeks	4 weeks if first dose administered at age <12 months and current age <24 months 8 weeks (as final dose) if first dose administered at age ≥12 months or current age 24–59 months No further doses needed for healthy children if first dose administered at age ≥24 months	4 weeks if current age <12 months 8 weeks (as final dose) if current age ≥12 months No further doses needed for healthy children if previous dose administered at age ≥24 months	8 weeks (as final dose) This dose only necessary for children aged 12 months–5 years who received 3 doses before age 12 months	

CATCH-UP SCHEDULE FOR CHILDREN AGED 7–18 YEARS			
Vaccine	Minimum interval between doses		
	Dose 1 to Dose 2	Dose 2 to Dose 3	Dose 3 to Booster Dose
Tetanus, Diphtheria[8]	4 weeks	6 months	6 months if first dose administered at age <12 months and current age <11 years; otherwise 5 years
Inactivated Poliovirus[9]	4 weeks	4 weeks	IPV[2,9]
Hepatitis B	4 weeks	8 weeks (and 16 weeks after first dose)	
Measles, Mumps, Rubella	4 weeks		
Varicella[10]	4 weeks		

1. **DTaP.** The fifth dose is not necessary if the fourth dose was administered after the fourth birthday.
2. **IPV.** For children who received an all-IPV or all-oral poliovirus (OPV) series, a fourth dose is not necessary if the third dose was administered at age ≥4 years. If both OPV and IPV were administered as part of a series, a total of 4 doses should be administered, regardless of the child's current age.
3. **HepB.** Administer the 3-dose series to all persons aged <19 years if they were not previously vaccinated.
4. **MMR.** The second dose of MMR is recommended routinely at age 4–6 years but may be administered earlier if desired.
5. **Hib.** Vaccine is not generally recommended for children aged ≥5 years.
6. **Hib.** If current age is <12 months and the first 2 doses were PRP-OMP (PedvaxHIB® or ComVax® [Merck]), the third (and final) dose should be administered at age 12–15 months and at least 8 weeks after the second dose.
7. **PCV.** Vaccine is not generally recommended for children aged ≥5 years.
8. **Td.** Tdap adolescent preparation may be substituted for any dose in a primary catch-up series or as a booster if age appropriate for Tdap. A 5-year interval from the last Td dose is encouraged when Tdap is used as a booster dose. See ACIP recommendations for additional information.
9. **IPV.** Vaccine is not generally recommended for persons aged ≥18 years.
10. **Varicella.** Administer the 2-dose series to all susceptible adolescents aged ≥13 years.

Adverse reactions to vaccines should be reported through VAERS. Information on reporting reactions after vaccination is available at http://www.vaers.hhs.gov or by telephone, 800-822-7967. Suspected cases of vaccine-preventable diseases should be reported to the state or local health department.

Additional information about vaccines, including precautions and contraindications for vaccination and vaccine shortages, is available in English and Spanish from the National Immunization Program at http://www.cdc.gov/nip or by telephone, 800-CDC-INFO (800-232-4636).

adults with close contact with infants younger than 12 months of age. Tdap is contraindicated if there is a history of anaphylaxis to vaccine components or if there is a history of unexplained encephalitis within 7days of administration of a pertussis-containing vaccine.

The recommendations for use of Tdap are under review and will become official when published in the Centers for Disease Control and Prevention's

Morbidity and Mortality Weekly Report (MMWR) (www.cdc.gov/mmwr/).

Measles

Adults born before 1957 are considered immune to measles. Adults born in 1957 or later who lack documentation of immunization after age 1 or who do not

Table 30–5. Recommended adult immunization schedule—United States, 2006.

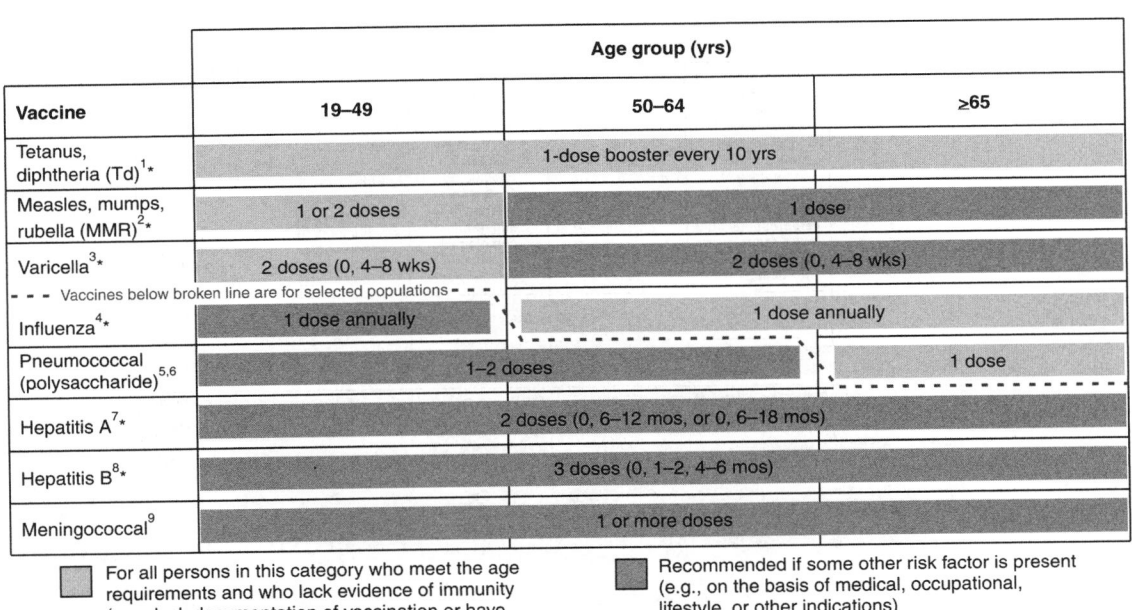

Vaccine	Age group (yrs) 19–49	50–64	≥65
Tetanus, diphtheria (Td)[1]*	1-dose booster every 10 yrs		
Measles, mumps, rubella (MMR)[2]*	1 or 2 doses	1 dose	
Varicella[3]*	2 doses (0, 4–8 wks)	2 doses (0, 4–8 wks)	
Influenza[4]*	— — — Vaccines below broken line are for selected populations — — — 1 dose annually	1 dose annually	
Pneumococcal (polysaccharide)[5,6]	1–2 doses		1 dose
Hepatitis A[7]*	2 doses (0, 6–12 mos, or 0, 6–18 mos)		
Hepatitis B[8]*	3 doses (0, 1–2, 4–6 mos)		
Meningococcal[9]	1 or more doses		

☐ For all persons in this category who meet the age requirements and who lack evidence of immunity (e.g., lack documentation of vaccination or have no evidence of prior infection)

■ Recommended if some other risk factor is present (e.g., on the basis of medical, occupational, lifestyle, or other indications)

* Covered by the Vaccine Injury Compensation Program.
Centers for Disease Control and Prevention. Recommended adult immunization schedule—United States, October 2005–September 2006. MMWR 2005;54:Q1–Q4.

Approved by the Advisory Committee on Immunization Practices, the American College of Obstetricians and Gynecologists, and the American Academy of Family Physicians

1. Tetanus and diphtheria (Td) vaccination. Adults with uncertain histories of a complete primary vaccination series with diphtheria and tetanus toxoid–containing vaccines should receive a primary series using combined Td toxoid. A primary series for adults is 3 doses; administer the first 2 doses at least 4 weeks apart and the third dose 6–12 months after the second. Administer 1 dose if the person received the primary series and if the last vaccination was received ≥10 years previously. Consult the ACIP statement for recommendations for administering Td as prophylaxis in wound management (http://www.cdc.gov/mmwr/preview/mmwrhtml/00041645.htm). The American College of Physicians Task Force on Adult Immunization supports a second option for Td use in adults: a single Td booster at age 50 years for persons who have completed the full pediatric series, including the teenage/young adult booster. A newly licensed tetanus-diphtheria-acellular–pertussis vaccine is available for adults. ACIP recommendations for its use will be published.

2. Measles, mumps, rubella (MMR) vaccination. *Measles component:* adults born before 1957 can be considered immune to measles. Adults born during or after 1957 should receive ≥1 dose of MMR unless they have a medical contraindication, documentation of ≥1 dose, history of measles based on health-care provider diagnosis, or laboratory evidence of immunity. A second dose of MMR is recommended for adults who 1) were

recently exposed to measles or in an outbreak setting; 2) were previously vaccinated with killed measles vaccine; 3) were vaccinated with an unknown type of measles vaccine during 1963–1967; 4) are students in postsecondary educational institutions; 5) work in a health-care facility; or 6) plan to travel internationally. Withhold MMR or other measles-containing vaccines from HIV-infected persons with severe immunosuppression. *Mumps component:* 1 dose of MMR vaccine should be adequate for protection for those born during or after 1957 who lack a history of mumps based on health-care provider diagnosis or who lack laboratory evidence of immunity. *Rubella component:* administer 1 dose of MMR vaccine to women whose rubella vaccination history is unreliable or who lack laboratory evidence of immunity. For women of childbearing age, regardless of birth year, routinely determine rubella immunity and counsel women regarding congenital rubella syndrome. Do not vaccinate women who are pregnant or who might become pregnant within 4 weeks of receiving vaccine. Women who do not have evidence of immunity should receive MMR vaccine upon completion or termination of pregnancy and before discharge from the health-care facility.

3. Varicella vaccination. Varicella vaccination is recommended for all adults without evidence of immunity to varicella. Special consideration should be given to those who 1) have close contact

(continued)

Table 30–5. Recommended adult immunization schedule—United States, 2006. (continued)

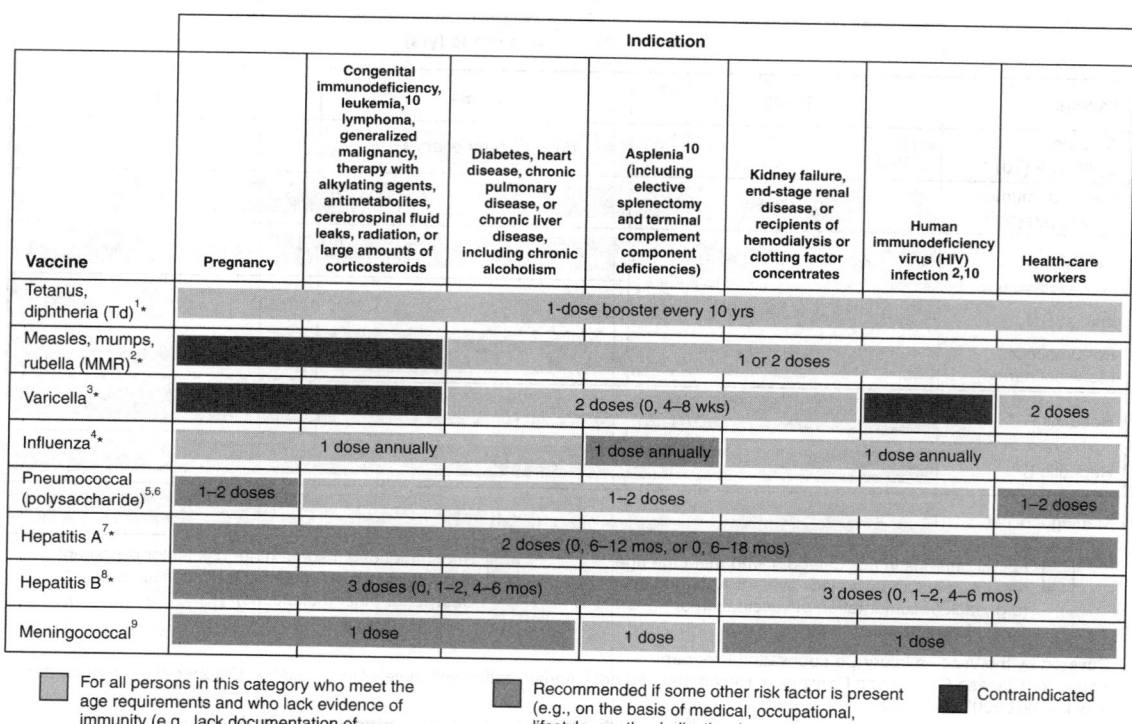

Vaccine	Pregnancy	Congenital immunodeficiency, leukemia,[10] lymphoma, generalized malignancy, therapy with alkylating agents, antimetabolites, cerebrospinal fluid leaks, radiation, or large amounts of corticosteroids	Diabetes, heart disease, chronic pulmonary disease, or chronic liver disease, including chronic alcoholism	Asplenia[10] (including elective splenectomy and terminal complement component deficiencies)	Kidney failure, end-stage renal disease, or recipients of hemodialysis or clotting factor concentrates	Human immunodeficiency virus (HIV) infection [2,10]	Health-care workers
			Indication				
Tetanus, diphtheria (Td)[1]*	1-dose booster every 10 yrs						
Measles, mumps, rubella (MMR)[2]*	Contraindicated		1 or 2 doses				
Varicella[3]*	Contraindicated		2 doses (0, 4–8 wks)			Contraindicated	2 doses
Influenza[4]*	1 dose annually			1 dose annually	1 dose annually		
Pneumococcal (polysaccharide)[5,6]	1–2 doses	1–2 doses					1–2 doses
Hepatitis A[7]*	2 doses (0, 6–12 mos, or 0, 6–18 mos)						
Hepatitis B[8]*	3 doses (0, 1–2, 4–6 mos)				3 doses (0, 1–2, 4–6 mos)		
Meningococcal[9]	1 dose			1 dose	1 dose		

For all persons in this category who meet the age requirements and who lack evidence of immunity (e.g., lack documentation of vaccination or have no evidence of prior infection)

Recommended if some other risk factor is present (e.g., on the basis of medical, occupational, lifestyle, or other indications)

Contraindicated

* Covered by the Vaccine Injury Compensation Program.

with persons at high risk for severe disease (health-care workers and family contacts of immunocompromised persons) or 2) are at high risk for exposure or transmission (e.g., teachers of young children; child care employees; residents and staff members of institutional settings, including correctional institutions; college students; military personnel; adolescents and adults living in households with children; nonpregnant women of childbearing age; and international travelers). Evidence of immunity to varicella in adults includes any of the following: 1) documented age-appropriate varicella vaccination (i.e., receipt of 1 dose before age 13 years or receipt of 2 doses [administered at least 4 weeks apart] after age 13 years); 2) U.S.-born before 1966 or history of varicella disease before 1966 for non-U.S.–born persons; 3) history of varicella based on health-care provider diagnosis or parental or self-report of typical varicella disease for persons born during 1966–1997 (for a patient reporting a history of an atypical, mild case, health-care providers should seek either an epidemiologic link with a typical varicella case or evidence of laboratory confirmation, if it was performed at the time of acute disease); 4) history of herpes zoster based on health-care provider diagnosis; or 5) laboratory evidence of immunity. Do not vaccinate women who are pregnant or who might become pregnant within 4 weeks of receiving the vaccine. Assess

pregnant women for evidence of varicella immunity. Women who do not have evidence of immunity should receive dose 1 of varicella vaccine upon completion or termination of pregnancy and before discharge from the health-care facility. Dose 2 should be administered 4–8 weeks after dose 1.

4. **Influenza vaccination.** *Medical indications:* chronic disorders of the cardiovascular or pulmonary systems, including asthma; chronic metabolic diseases, including diabetes mellitus, renal dysfunction, hemoglobinopathies, or immunosuppression (including immunosuppression caused by medications or HIV); any condition (e.g., cognitive dysfunction, spinal cord injury, seizure disorder, or other neuromuscular disorder) that compromises respiratory function or the handling of respiratory secretions or that can increase the risk for aspiration; and pregnancy during the influenza season. No data exist on the risk for severe or complicated influenza disease among persons with asplenia; however, influenza is a risk factor for secondary bacterial infections that can cause severe disease among persons with asplenia. *Occupational indications:* health-care workers and employees of long-term–care and assisted living facilities. *Other indications:* residents of nursing homes and other long-term–care and assisted living facilities; persons likely to transmit influenza to persons at high risk (i.e., in-home household

(continued)

have a provider-documented history or laboratory evidence of previous infection should receive at least one dose of vaccine. Persons born between 1963 and 1967—a period when inactivated measles vaccine was the only product available—should also receive one dose of live attenuated vaccine. Persons vaccinated before their first birthday should also receive a single dose of vaccine. Because most adults do not have de-

tailed information about childhood immunization or illnesses, a practical approach is to administer a single dose of MMR to all healthy adults born after 1956. Because outbreaks of measles have occurred in young adults who have received a single dose of measles vaccine, revaccination is recommended, particularly before going to college, entering a health care profession, or embarking on foreign travel to areas where contacts and caregivers of children aged 0–23 months, or persons of all ages with high-risk conditions), and anyone who wishes to be vaccinated. For healthy, nonpregnant persons aged 5–49 years without high-risk conditions who are not contacts of severely immunocompromised persons in special care units, intranasally administered influenza vaccine (FluMist®) may be administered in lieu of inactivated vaccine.

5. Pneumococcal polysaccharide vaccination. *Medical indications*: chronic disorders of the pulmonary system (excluding asthma); cardiovascular diseases; diabetes mellitus; chronic liver diseases, including liver disease as a result of alcohol abuse (e.g., cirrhosis); chronic renal failure or nephrotic syndrome; functional or anatomic asplenia (e.g., sickle cell disease or splenectomy [if elective splenectomy is planned, vaccinate at least 2 weeks before surgery]); immunosuppressive conditions (e.g., congenital immunodeficiency, HIV infection [vaccinate as close to diagnosis as possible when CD4 cell counts are highest], leukemia, lymphoma, multiple myeloma, Hodgkin disease, generalized malignancy, or organ or bone marrow transplantation); chemotherapy with alkylating agents, antimetabolites, or long-term systemic corticosteroids; and cochlear implants. *Other indications*: Alaska Natives and certain American Indian populations; residents of nursing homes and other long-term–care facilities.

6. Revaccination with pneumococcal polysaccharide vaccine. One-time revaccination after 5 years for persons with chronic renal failure or nephrotic syndrome; functional or anatomic asplenia (e.g., sickle cell disease or splenectomy); immunosuppressive conditions (e.g., congenital immunodeficiency, HIV infection, leukemia, lymphoma, multiple myeloma, Hodgkin disease, generalized malignancy, or organ or bone marrow transplantation); or chemotherapy with alkylating agents, antimetabolites, or long-term systemic corticosteroids. For persons aged ≥65 years, one-time revaccination if they were vaccinated ≥5 years previously and were aged <65 years at the time of primary vaccination.

7. Hepatitis A vaccination. *Medical indications*: persons with clotting-factor disorders or chronic liver disease. *Behavioral indications*: men who have sex with men or users of illegal drugs. *Occupational indications*: Persons working with hepatitis A virus (HAV)–infected primates or with HAV in a research laboratory setting. *Other indications*: persons traveling to or working in countries that have high or intermediate endemicity of hepatitis A (for list of countries, see http://www.cdc.gov/travel/diseases.htm#hepa) as well as any person wishing to obtain immunity. Current vaccines should be administered in a 2-dose series at either 0 and 6–12 months, or 0 and 6–18 months. If the

combined hepatitis A and hepatitis B vaccine is used, administer 3 doses at 0, 1, and 6 months.

8. Hepatitis B vaccination. *Medical indications*: hemodialysis patients (use special formulation [40 μg/mL] or two 20-μg/mL doses) or patients who receive clotting-factor concentrates. *Occupational indications*: health-care workers and public-safety workers who have exposure to blood in the workplace and persons in training in schools of medicine, dentistry, nursing, laboratory technology, and other allied health professions. *Behavioral indications*: injection-drug users; persons with more than one sex partner during the previous 6 months; persons with a recently acquired sexually transmitted disease (STD); and men who have sex with men. *Other indications*: household contacts and sex partners of persons with chronic hepatitis B virus (HBV) infection; clients and staff members of institutions for developmentally disabled persons; all clients of STD clinics; inmates of correctional facilities; and international travelers who will be in countries with high or intermediate prevalence of chronic HBV infection for more than 6 months (for list of countries, see http://www.cdc.gov/travel/diseases.htm#hepa).

9. Meningococcal vaccination. *Medical indications*: adults with anatomic or functional asplenia or terminal complement component deficiencies. *Other indications*: first-year college students living in dormitories; microbiologists who are routinely exposed to isolates of *Neisseria meningitidis*; military recruits; and persons who travel to or reside in countries in which meningococcal disease is hyperendemic or epidemic (e.g., the "meningitis belt" of sub-Saharan Africa during the dry season [December–June]), particularly if contact with local populations will be prolonged. Vaccination is required by the government of Saudi Arabia for all travelers to Mecca during the annual Hajj. Meningococcal conjugate vaccine is preferred for adults meeting any of the above indications who are aged ≤55 years, although meningococcal polysaccharide vaccine (MPSV4) is an acceptable alternative. Revaccination after 5 years might be indicated for adults previously vaccinated with MPSV4 who remain at high risk for infection (e.g., persons residing in areas in which disease is epidemic).

10. Selected conditions for which *Haemophilus influenzae* type b (Hib) vaccine may be used. Hib conjugate vaccines are licensed for children aged 6–71 months. No efficacy data are available on which to base a recommendation concerning use of Hib vaccine for older children and adults with the chronic conditions associated with an increased risk for Hib disease. However, studies suggest good immunogenicity in patients who have sickle cell disease, leukemia, or HIV infection or who have had splenectomies; administering vaccine to these patients is not contraindicated.

measles is endemic. Even though birth before 1957 implies immunity, unvaccinated health care workers (especially women of childbearing age) who do not have a history of measles or laboratory evidence of immunity should be vaccinated. Entrants to colleges and universities and employees of health care institutions who have not previously been vaccinated should receive two doses of vaccine at least 1 month apart. Revaccination of an immune person is not associated with adverse effects—if the vaccination status is unknown and an indication for vaccination exists, it can be safely done. Vaccination of susceptible adults within 72 hours after exposure to an active case of measles is protective.

Fever will develop in about 5–15% of unimmunized individuals, and a mild rash will develop in about 5% 5–12 days after vaccination. Fever and rash are self-limiting, lasting only 2–3 days. Local swelling and induration are particularly common in individuals previously vaccinated with inactivated vaccine. Pregnant women and immunosuppressed persons should not be vaccinated (with the exception of asymptom-

atic HIV-infected individuals whose CD4 count is > 200/mcL). It is believed that MMR vaccine can be safely given to patients with a history of egg allergy even when severe. A single 0.5 mL dose can be given without prior skin testing or desensitization as long as postvaccination observation for 90 minutes is possible.

Rubella

The purpose of rubella vaccination is to prevent transmission to the fetus. Immunization is recommended for all adults but particularly for women of childbearing age not previously immunized. Although persons born before 1957 are considered immune, this is not an acceptable criterion of immunity for women who could become pregnant. Thus, women of childbearing age, regardless of birth year, should have rubella immunity checked and should be vaccinated if they lack evidence of antibody. They should be counseled not to become pregnant within 4 weeks of immunization. Women who are already pregnant and lack immunity should be vaccinated in the postpartum period. In addition, both male and female hospital workers who may be exposed to patients with rubella or who might have contact with pregnant patients should be immunized. A single immunization is given. MMR trivalent vaccine is recommended, but if immunity to one or more of the components can be demonstrated, monovalent or bivalent vaccines can be used.

Adverse effects are usually mild. Up to 40% of unvaccinated adults (usually women) experience joint pain, often worse than that associated with natural infection. Symptoms begin 1–3 weeks after vaccination and are self-limited, lasting 3–10 days. Frank arthritis is rare. Although vaccination of pregnant women is *not* recommended, with the currently available RA27/3 vaccine strain the congenital rubella syndrome does not occur in the offspring of those inadvertently vaccinated during pregnancy or within 3 months before conception. Persons who are immunosuppressed by virtue of disease or medication should not receive vaccine. HIV infection is an exception—it should be given to asymptomatic individuals who do not have evidence of severe immunosuppression (CD4 count > 200/mcL; severe immunosuppression, CD4 count < 200/mcL) and may be considered in symptomatic patients. Since the vaccine contains trace amounts of neomycin, a history of anaphylaxis to this agent is a contraindication.

Mumps

Mumps vaccine is recommended for all adults thought to be susceptible. Persons born before 1957 are considered to be naturally immune. Those born in 1957 or later are believed to be susceptible unless they can document infection, prove vaccination, or have laboratory evidence of immunity. Vaccination in those already immune is not associated with an increased incidence of adverse effects.

Mumps vaccine is generally safe. It should not be given to those who are immunosuppressed (except HIV-infected individuals) or who have a history of anaphylaxis to neomycin.

Influenza

Influenza vaccination is recommended yearly. Those at greatest risk for severe complications of influenza should have priority in vaccination programs: (1) Adults and children with chronic cardiopulmonary disease, including asthmatics. (2) Residents, health care workers, and employees of long-term care facilities. (3) Healthy adults 50 years of age or older. (4) Adults and children who have required either regular medical follow-up or hospitalization in the last year for chronic metabolic disorders (including diabetes) or renal disease, those with hemoglobinopathies, and those receiving immunosuppressive drugs. (5) Children and teenagers (age 6 months to 18 years) who are on long-term aspirin therapy and would be at increased risk for developing Reye's syndrome following influenza.

(6) Women who will become pregnant during the influenza season. (7) Persons who are likely to transmit influenza to persons of high risk as defined above, such as in-home or out-of-home caregivers or household and close contacts of persons at high risk.

Certain high-risk groups of patients (the elderly, persons with AIDS, transplant patients) may have a poor antibody response to vaccine, but they should still be vaccinated. Concern that vaccination of HIV-positive patients may result in a brief (2- to 4-week) period of increased HIV viremia and viral replication has been raised. The clinical significance is probably minimal, as progression of disease after vaccination has not been observed. Thus, the potential benefit of vaccination of HIV-positive individuals outweighs any theoretic risks. To prevent disease in high-risk patients, vaccination is advised for household members and health care providers who have contact with these high-risk patients. Vaccination is recommended also for otherwise healthy adults who provide essential community services and for any individual who wishes to decrease the risk of becoming ill with influenza.

Local reactions (erythema and tenderness) at the site of injection are common, but fevers, chills, and malaise (which last in any case only 2–3 days) are rare. Like measles, mumps, and yellow fever vaccines, influenza vaccine is prepared using embryonated chicken eggs, and persons with a history of anaphylaxis to eggs should not be vaccinated. The risk of Guillain-Barré syndrome is not increased following vaccination. Influenza vaccination may be associated with multiple false-positive serologic tests to HIV, HTLV-1, and hepatitis C, but it is self-limited, lasting 2–5 months.

A trivalent live attenuated influenza vaccine administered as a single-dose intranasal spray is as effective as inactivated vaccine in preventing disease. It is approved for use in otherwise healthy individuals between the ages of 5 and 49 years (the group studied in clinical trials). Because the risk of transmission of the live attenuated vaccine virus to immunocompromised individuals is unknown, it should NOT be used in household members of immunosuppressed individuals, health care workers, or others with close contact with immunosuppressed persons. It is not recommended for those with reactive airway disease; chronic underlying metabolic, pulmonary, or cardiovascular diseases; children or adolescents receiving long-term aspirin therapy (because of the risk of Reye's syndrome); those with a history of Guillain-Barré syndrome; pregnant women; or those with a history of egg allergy. Two neuraminidase inhibitors (zanamivir and oseltamivir) are available for prevention and therapy of influenza A and B. The dose of oseltamivir is 75 mg/d for prophylaxis and 75 mg twice daily for 5 days for therapy. Zanamivir is administered by inhaler (10 mg dose) and is given twice daily for therapy and once daily for prophylaxis. The duration of prophylaxis depends on the clinical setting. Amantadine and rimantadine are also effective but only against influenza A, but increasing resistance has limited their usefulness.

Pneumococcal Pneumonia

Pneumococcal vaccine contains purified polysaccharide from 23 of the most common strains of *S pneumoniae*, which cause 90% of bacteremic episodes in the United States. Antibody response following vaccination depends on the patient's immune status and the presence of concomitant disease. Healthy adults have an excellent antibody response, as do patients who are postsplenectomy and those with sickle cell disease. Elderly individuals and those with chronic diseases (diabetes mellitus, alcoholic cirrhosis, chronic obstructive pulmonary disease, chronic renal insufficiency, lupus erythematosus, rheumatoid arthritis) have less vigorous response than young healthy adults. Patients with Hodgkin's disease respond to vaccination if it is given before splenectomy, radiation, or chemotherapy, whereas patients with leukemia, lymphoma, and HIV infection respond sluggishly.

Although the efficacy of pneumococcal vaccine has been questioned, most authorities believe that vaccination is about 60–70% effective in preventing bacteremic disease in immunocompetent persons, but less effective at preventing pneumonia. Fifty percent efficacy is observed in patients with underlying diseases (not severely immunocompromised), and less in immunocompromised patients (10%), largely because of inability to mount an antibody response in this population. It is presently recommended for patients at increased risk for developing severe pneumococcal disease, especially asplenic patients and those with sickle cell disease. It is also indicated for adults at increased risk for developing pneumococcal disease, including those with chronic illnesses (eg, cardiopulmonary disease, alcoholism, cirrhosis, chronic renal failure, nephrotic syndrome, cerebrospinal fluid leaks), those who are immunocompromised (eg, patients with Hodgkin's disease, lymphoma, chronic lymphocytic leukemia, multiple myeloma, congenital immunodeficiency, asymptomatic or symptomatic HIV infection, organ or bone marrow transplant recipients), those receiving immunosuppressive therapy (eg, long-term systemic corticosteroids, alkylating agents, and antimetabolites) and Alaskan Natives. Because of the increased risk of developing pneumococcal meningitis following cochlear implants, patients receiving these implants should be given age-appropriate vaccination. Although not currently recommended for smokers and black adults, some feel that these groups should be routinely immunized because of an increased risk of developing invasive disease. In addition, it is recommended for all individuals over 65 years of age. Whether 65 is the appropriate age to vaccinate healthy adults is unclear. Antibody response declines with age, and some have suggested routine immunization at age 50 similar to the recommendation for tetanus (see above). A single dose of vaccine usually confers lifelong immunity. One-time revaccination 5 years after initial vaccination is recommended for those at highest risk (see list above). In addition, a single revaccination is recommended for those 65 or more years of age who received the vaccine 5 years or more previously and were under age 65 at the time of primary vaccination. Elderly individuals with unknown vaccination status should be immunized once. Revaccination should also be considered for high-risk individuals previously immunized with the older 14-valent vaccine. Since immunocompetent patients respond best to the vaccine, it should be given 2 weeks before splenectomy or before starting chemotherapy if that can be anticipated.

A protein-conjugated heptavalent pneumococcal vaccine used in children under 2 years of age is very effective at preventing meningitis and pneumonia but only modestly effective at preventing otitis media. Unlike the adult polysaccharide vaccine, the pediatric conjugated vaccine decreases nasopharyngeal colonization, which results in less transmission to nonimmunized children and adults (herd immunity). Limited information about use of this vaccine in adults suggests that those with poor antibody response to the 23-valent vaccine (such as renal transplant recipients) also have poor antibody response to the protein-conjugated vaccine despite its higher immunogenicity.

Mild reactions (erythema and tenderness) to pneumococcal vaccine occur in up to 50% of recipients, but systemic reactions are uncommon. Similarly, revaccination at least 5 years after initial vaccination is associated with mild self-limited local but not systemic reactions.

Hepatitis B

Recombinant hepatitis B vaccine is given intramuscularly in the deltoid (gluteal injection often results in deposition of vaccine in fat rather than muscle, with fewer serologic conversions) on three separate occasions: the first two doses 1 month apart and the last dose 5 months after the second one. It is recommended for all individuals at increased risk for developing hepatitis B. These include injection drug users, men who have sex with men, individuals who have had more than one sex partner in the last 6 months, and persons with sexually transmitted diseases or who attend sexually transmitted disease clinics. Family (household and sexual contacts of hepatitis B carriers) or occupational factors (frequent exposure to blood and blood products, hemodialysis patients and staff, residents, medical students, laboratory technicians, morticians) also serve as indications. Others who should be considered for vaccination are those who work at or inhabit institutions for the developmentally disabled, travelers spending more than 6 months in high-risk areas, and inmates of correctional institutions. For immunosuppressed patients, those being maintained on hemodialysis, and chronic alcoholics, seroresponse to standard doses of vaccine is low, and for that reason preparations delivering a higher vaccine dose (40 mcg/mL) are administered. In addition to higher vaccine doses, these patients may require more frequent immunizations, and some authorities recommend annual screening to determine whether booster doses are needed. Although most often used for preexposure prophylaxis, the vaccine is also given as postexposure prophylaxis along with hepatitis B immunoglobulin following needlestick injury or mucous membrane exposure to blood from an individual who is HBsAg-positive. It is also given along with hepatitis B immunoglobulin to infants of mothers who are HBsAg-positive (Table 30–4). Immunity wanes with time, but protection against infection lasts at least 20 years, making periodic serologic monitoring and routine administration of booster doses unnecessary. Adverse reactions are minor and limited to local soreness.

Following vaccination, 90–95% of healthy young individuals develop protective antibodies. A number of factors decrease serologic response, including increasing age over 30, renal failure, HIV infection, diabetes, chronic liver disease, obesity, and smoking. Postvaccination serologic testing is not routinely performed. It is reserved for those whose clinical management would be influenced by their immune status (eg, health care workers, infants born to HBsAg-positive mothers, dialysis patients), and those who may have an impaired response. Those who do not respond should receive a second three-dose vaccine series with serologic testing 1–2 months after completion. Those who do not respond are unlikely to respond to further vaccination even with a different recombinant vaccine and should be considered susceptible; if exposed, they should receive hepatitis B immune globulin.

Varicella

A live attenuated varicella virus vaccine is currently recommended as part of routine childhood immunization (Table 30–4) and its use has been associated with decreased mortality due to varicella across all age ranges. Although only 10% of adults remain susceptible, varicella in adolescents and adults is a more serious disease. Only about 2% of all cases of varicella occur in adults, but almost 50% of all deaths are in adults. Thus, susceptible adolescents and adults should be immunized, with special emphasis on certain high-risk groups, ie, health care workers; household contacts of immunosuppressed individuals; persons who live or work in environments where transmission can occur, eg, teachers in day care centers or elementary schools, residents and workers in institutional settings such as military and correctional institutions, college students; nonpregnant women of childbearing age; and international travelers. The role of the present vaccine in postexposure prophylaxis has not been widely studied, but it has

been suggested that it is 90% effective in preventing varicella in an outbreak, particularly when given within 3–5 days after exposure. The Advisory Committee on Immunization Practices (ACIP) recommends vaccination in susceptible persons following exposure. The vaccine is very immunogenic. Seroconversion occurs in 95% of children after a single dose. In adolescents (older than 12 years of age) and adults, seroconversion is seen in 78% after one dose and 99% after two doses. For this reason, two doses given 4–8 weeks apart are recommended in persons 12 years of age and older. The duration of immunity is not known but is probably 10 years. Although the vaccine is very effective in preventing disease, breakthrough infections do occur—but are much milder than in unvaccinated individuals (usually less than 50 lesions, with milder systemic symptoms). Although the vaccine is very safe, adverse reactions can occur as late as 4–6 weeks after vaccination. Tenderness and erythema at the injection site are seen in 25%, fever in 10–15%, and a localized maculopapular or vesicular rash in 5%; a smaller percentage develop a diffuse rash, usually with five or fewer vesicular lesions. Spread of virus from vaccinees to susceptible individuals is possible, but the risk of such transmission even to immunocompromised patients is small and disease, when it develops, is mild and treatable with acyclovir. Nonetheless, the vaccine, being a live attenuated virus, should not be given to immunocompromised individuals, including HIV-positive children and adults, or pregnant women. It is contraindicated in persons allergic to neomycin. For theoretic reasons, it is recommended that following vaccination salicylates should be avoided for 6 weeks (to prevent Reye's syndrome). Several unresolved issues remain, including the need for booster doses, whether universal childhood vaccination will shift the incidence of disease to adolescence or adulthood with the possibility of more severe disease, and whether vaccination might prevent development of herpes zoster.

A varicella-zoster vaccine with higher potency than the existing varicella vaccine discussed above, named Oka/Merck VZV vaccine or "zoster vaccine" has been shown in clinical trials to decrease the incidence of zoster and its major complication, postherpetic neuralgia, in individuals older than 60. This vaccine is investigational but is likely to receive approval soon.

Hepatitis A

Two inactivated hepatitis A vaccines (Havrix, VAQTA) are approved for use in the United States. They are indicated for individuals 1 (Havrix) or 2 (VAQTA) years of age or older who are at an increased risk for developing hepatitis A. Potential vaccinees include travelers to areas where hepatitis is endemic (Africa, Asia, Central and South America, Mexico, parts of the Caribbean); certain populations that experience outbreaks (such as indigenous Alaskans, certain American Indian reservations, various religious communities and states where the risk of hepatitis A is high among children); employees of day care centers, caretakers for developmentally impaired institutionalized individuals, and laboratory workers who handle live hepatitis A virus or work closely with nonhuman primates; men who have sex with men; illicit drug users; persons who receive clotting factor concentrates; and those with chronic liver disease. The role of hepatitis A vaccine in controlling outbreaks in day care centers, hospitals, and institutions for the disabled has not been investigated, and immune globulin is used in those settings. A single intramuscular injection of vaccine in adults elicits antibodies in 55–60% of individuals at 2 weeks and 95% by 1 month, although rates of seroconversion may be lower in immunocompromised individuals. The different formulations come in different strengths, and dosage depends on the age of the vaccine and the preparation used (see package insert). In general, two doses are required, the second 6–18 months after the first. The duration of immunity may be lifelong, and at present repeat vaccination is not recommended. Adverse effects are minimal and consist mainly of pain at the injection site. If vaccine is not available, temporary passive immunity may be induced by the intramuscular injection of immune globulin, 0.02 mL/kg every 2–3 months or 0.1 mL/kg every 6 months. Protection with immune globulin is recommended for persons traveling to areas where sanitation is poor and the risk of exposure to hepatitis A high because of contaminated food and water supplies and contact with infected persons. Preparation of immunoglobulin from plasma involves steps that inactivate HIV, thus making it incapable of transmitting HIV infection.

Combined Hepatitis A & B Vaccine

A combined hepatitis A and B vaccine is approved for use in individuals 18 years of age and older. The components are identical to individual vaccines. It is highly immunogenic and should be used in individuals who have an indication for both hepatitis A and B vaccination, as noted above. The product is safe, and adverse effects are similar to those of the individual components. It is administered in three doses at 0, 1 and 6 months.

Smallpox

Smallpox vaccination, discontinued in the United States in the early 1970s, has been reinstituted because of concerns about bioterrorism. The vaccine is a live vaccinia virus derived through serial passage of cowpox and does not contain the actual smallpox virus. Vaccine is administered with a bifurcated needle, making 15 puncture wounds in a small area of the skin (5 mm) just deep enough to cause bleeding. Because the inoculation site is contagious, it should be covered with gauze or a semipermeable dressing such as OpSite. If vaccination is successful, the site goes through a characteristic evolution: In 3–4 days the site becomes red, itchy, and indurated; a vesicle umbilicates and evolves into a well-formed pustule by day 6–11; the pustule scabs over between week 2 and week 3; and by the end of the third week the scab falls off, leaving a scar. At the end of the first week, fever for several days, tenderness at the vaccination site, and localized axillary adenopathy occur in 10–20% of first-time vaccinees, but these reactions are less common in those who have been previously vaccinated within the last 10 years. Successful vaccination is indicated by the presence of a pustular lesion at day 7 in a nonimmune individual and by the presence of a pustule or area of induration in a previously vaccinated person. Failure to see these reactions is an indication for revaccination.

In general, adverse effects are more common in children under 5 years of age and in first-time vaccinees. Other than the local reactions, the most common adverse effect (estimated at 1:2000) is autoinoculation to another site, most commonly the face, eyelid, mouth, and genitalia. These lesions usually are self-limited and heal without specific therapy. Generalized vaccinia occurs in 1:5000 vaccinees and is characterized by widespread lesions appearing 6–9 days after vaccination, the result of hematogenous spread. The lesions usually heal without therapy in immunocompetent individuals but can be life-threatening in the immunosuppressed. Eczema vaccinatum occurs in patients with active or healed eczema and can progress to involve all areas of the skin involved with the skin disorder. Although uncommon (1:25,000), this is a potentially fatal complication. Progressive vaccinia or vaccinia necrosum is seen in immunocompromised individuals. The vaccination site fails to heal and the virus spreads to surrounding areas with progressive necrosis and gangrene, a serious complication with a high mortality. Postvaccination encephalitis occurs 1–2 weeks after vaccination, is usually seen in those under 1 year of age, occurs in 1:300,000 vaccinations, and is associated with death in 25% and severe disability in another 25%. Following mass vaccination of military personnel, two additional adverse events have been described—local and generalized folliculitis and myopericarditis. Folliculitis occurred 8–10 days following vaccination, was concentrated in hair-bearing areas (face, extremities, back), resolved spontaneously in 3–5 days, and was not associated with scarring. Myopericarditis was seen in first-time vaccine recipients, occurred 7–19 days after vaccination, and was self-limited. In brief follow-up, permanent sequelae have not been described.

Vaccinia immune globulin is available from the Centers of Disease Control and Prevention (CDC) but is in limited supply. It is recommended for severe adverse reactions such as eczema vaccinatum, progressive vaccinia, severe generalized vaccinia, and inadvertent inoculation of the eye or eyelid without vaccinia keratitis. It is not recommended for postvaccination encephalitis. Cidofovir, a nucleotide analog used to treat CMV infections, has activity against variola virus and has been effective in animal models for the therapy of vaccinia infections. It should be considered for those with serious adverse effects.

Routine vaccination—in the absence of a case of smallpox—is not recommended for those under 18 years of age. It is also not recommended for those with a history of or active eczema or household associates of such individuals. Those with other skin diseases (atopic dermatitis, impetigo) may also be at risk for complications and should not be vaccinated until skin lesions have healed. Pregnancy, altered immune states as described above, and allergy to vaccine components (neomycin, streptomycin, polymyxin, chlortetracycline) are contraindications to smallpox vaccination. Household contacts of individuals with altered immunity should also not be vaccinated.

Meningococcal Disease

Two vaccines are currently available, a polysaccharide vaccine (MPSV4) and the newer protein conjugated vaccine (MCV4). Both are highly immunogenic to serogroups A,C,Y and W-135 and well tolerated. Whereas the polysaccharide vaccine requires revaccination of at-risk groups every 3–5 years due to waning immunity, the protein conjugated vaccine likely will provide longer protection, although data on need for revaccination with MCV4 is not currently available. MCV4 is licensed for use in individuals 11–55 years of age, and MPSV4 is licensed for ages 2 years and above.

Vaccination with MCV4 is routinely recommended for adolescents aged 11–12. For those who miss that vaccination, "catch up " is recommended at high school entry (approximately age 15). MCV4 is also recommended for certain high-risk groups, including college freshman living in dormitories (the risk to nonfreshman and freshman not living in dormitories is the same as the general population and vaccination of these groups is elective), microbiologists who are routinely exposed to *N meningitidis,* military recruits, persons who travel to or reside in areas in which *N meningitides* is hyperendemic or epidemic (see below), those with terminal complement deficiencies, and persons with anatomic or functional asplenia. HIV-infected patients may be at increased risk for meningococcal disease, and vaccination should be considered elective in that group. MCV4 is the preferred preparation, but if availability is an issue, MPSV4 can be substituted. MCV4 is administered as a single 0.5-mL dose intramuscularly and MPSV4 as a single 0.5-mL dose subcutaneously. Both can be administered with other vaccines, but at different sites and both produce an antibody response in 7–10 days. Both are inactivated vaccines and can be administered to immunocompromised patients. MPSV4 is

safe in pregnancy, but there are no safety or efficacy data for MCV4 in pregnancy.

Minor reactions (fever, redness, swelling, erythema, pain) occur slightly more commonly with MCV4. Major reactions are rare. The protein conjugate used in MCV4 is diphtheria toxoid, so individuals with a history of adverse reaction to that component should not receive MCV4.

RECOMMENDED IMMUNIZATIONS FOR TRAVELERS

Individuals traveling to other countries frequently require immunizations in addition to those listed above and may benefit from chemoprophylaxis against various diseases. These are listed in *Health Information for International Travel,* published by the CDC. An updated version is published yearly and is available from the Superintendent of Documents, United States Government Printing Office, Washington, DC 20402, or on the Internet: http://www.cdc.gov/nip

Various vaccines can be given simultaneously at different sites. Some, such as cholera, plague, and typhoid vaccine, cause significant discomfort and are best given at different times. In general, live attenuated vaccines (measles, mumps, rubella, yellow fever, and oral typhoid vaccine) should not be given to immunosuppressed individuals or household members of immunosuppressed people or to pregnant women. Immunoglobulin should not be given for 3 months before or at least 2 weeks after live virus vaccines, because it may attenuate the antibody response.

Chemoprophylaxis of malaria is discussed in Chapter 35.

Cholera

Because cholera among travelers is rare and the vaccine marginally effective, the World Health Organization (WHO) does not require immunization for persons traveling to endemic areas. The only cholera vaccine licensed in the United States is no longer manufactured. Two oral vaccines are available in other countries and appear to be slightly more immunogenic than previous vaccines. However, the CDC does not recommend either of these two vaccines, and they are not available in the United States. No country requires vaccination for entry, but some local authorities may require documentation for entry. In such cases, a medical waiver will suffice or a single dose of the oral vaccine is usually sufficient. Information is available at http://www.bernaproducts.com.

Hepatitis B

Persons traveling to and spending more than 6 months in endemic areas of hepatitis B virus infection who will have close contact with the local population should be considered for vaccination. Short-term travelers to areas of moderate or high endemic infection (Southeast Asia, China, most of the Middle East, Haiti, the Dominican Republic, and most of Africa) who will be in contact with potentially infected body secretions of residents should be vaccinated. Vaccination should begin at least 6 months before travel to allow for completion of the series.

Hepatitis A

As indicated above, susceptible individuals traveling to areas of high or intermediate endemicity for hepatitis A (eg, anywhere except Canada, western Europe, Japan, Australia, and New Zealand) should be vaccinated. The vaccine is given at least 4 weeks prior to travel, as protective antibodies develop in 95% of vaccinees by that time. If given 2 weeks before travel, up to 45% will not have protective antibodies, and if the person is traveling to a high-risk area, intramuscular immune globulin (0.02 mL/kg) should be administered at a separate site.

Meningococcal Meningitis

If travel is contemplated to an area where meningococcal meningitis is epidemic (Nepal, sub-Saharan Africa, the "meningitis belt" from Senegal in the west to Ethiopia in the east, northern India) or highly endemic, vaccination with MCV4 is indicated for those 11–55 years of age, otherwise MPSV should be used. (Saudi Arabia requires immunization for pilgrims to Mecca.)

Plague

The risk of plague is so small to travelers that vaccine is no longer commercially available and vaccination is not required for entry into any country. Travelers at unavoidable high risk of exposure to rodents should consider chemoprophylaxis with doxycyline or TMP-SMZ.

Poliomyelitis

Polio remains endemic in six countries (Afghanistan, India, Pakistan, Nigeria, Niger, and Egypt) and outbreaks occur sporadically, mainly in Africa, the Middle East, and Asia. Adults traveling to endemic or epidemic areas who have not previously been immunized against poliomyelitis should receive a primary series of three doses of inactivated enhanced-potency poliovaccine (IPV), as follows: two doses of 0.5 mL subcutaneously 4–8 weeks apart and then a third dose 6–12 months after the second dose. If more than 8 weeks will elapse before travel, three doses of IPV can be given 4 weeks apart. If 4–8 weeks will elapse before travel, two doses are given 4 weeks apart, and if less than 4 weeks will elapse, a single dose is given. Vaccination can be completed upon return if continued or future exposure to polio is anticipated. Travelers who have previously been fully immunized with OPV or IPV should receive a one-time booster dose with IPV. Data do not indicate the need for more than one adult booster. Live attenuated poliovaccine is no longer recommended because of the risk of vaccine-associated disease and is no longer available in the United States, although it continues to be used in many other countries.

Rabies

For travelers to areas where rabies is common in domestic animals (eg, India, Asia, Mexico), with extensive outdoor activities or certain professional activities (veterinarians, animal handlers, field biologists), preexposure prophylaxis with human diploid cell vaccine (HDCV), rabies vaccine adsorbed (RVA), or purified chick embryo cell culture (PCEC) vaccine should be considered. It usually consists of two intramuscular (deltoid area) injections of 1 mL given 1 week apart with a booster dose 2–3 weeks later. Alternatively, two intradermal injections of 0.1 mL of HDCV are given 1 week apart, with a booster dose given 2–3 weeks later. Chloroquine can blunt the immunologic response to rabies vaccine. If malaria prophylaxis with chloroquine is required, vaccination should be given intramuscularly (*not* intradermally) to ensure adequate antibody response. Until further studies are done, interaction between mefloquine and rabies vaccine, while not established, makes intramuscular administration prudent if mefloquine is to be given.

Typhoid

Typhoid vaccination is recommended for travelers to developing countries (especially the Indian subcontinent, Asia, Africa, Central and South America, and the Caribbean) who will have prolonged exposure to contaminated food and water. Two preparations of approximately equal efficacy (50–75% effective) are available in the United States: (1) an oral live-attenuated Ty21a vaccine supplied as enteric-coated capsules, and (2) a Vi capsular polysaccharide (Vi CPS) vaccine for parenteral use. The Ty21a vaccine is given as one capsule every other day for four doses. The capsules must be refrigerated and taken with cool liquids (37 °C or less) at least 1 hour before meals. All four doses must be taken for maximum protection and should be completed 1 week before travel. It is not recommended for infants or children younger than 6 years. Adverse effects are minimal and consist primarily of gastrointestinal upset. The Vi CPS vaccine is given as a single intramuscular injection at least 2 weeks prior to travel. It is not recommended for infants younger than 2 years. Adverse effects consist mainly of local irritation at the site of injection, but fever and headache occur. If continued or repeated exposures are anticipated, boosters are recommended every 2 years for the ViCPS and every 5 years for the Ty21a. The live attenuated vaccine should not be used in immunosuppressed patients, including those with HIV infection.

Yellow Fever

The live attenuated yellow fever virus vaccine is administered once subcutaneously. Although the risk of yellow fever is low for most travelers, a number of countries require vaccination for all visitors and others require it for travelers to or from endemic areas (mainly equatorial Africa and parts of South and Central America). The WHO certificate requires registration of the manufacturer and the batch number of the vaccine. Vaccination is available in the United States only at approved centers; the local health department should be contacted for available resources. Reimmunization is recommended at 10-year intervals if continued risk exists.

Because it is a live attenuated vaccine prepared in embryonated eggs, the yellow fever vaccine should not be given to immunosuppressed individuals or those with a history of anaphylaxis to eggs. Pregnancy is a relative contraindication to vaccination.

Since 1996, nine cases of fever, jaundice, and multiple organ system failure following yellow fever vaccination were reported (yellow fever vaccine–associated viscerotropic disease) in the United States and an additional 17 cases have been reported worldwide. Clinically and histopathologically, the illness is identical to yellow fever and the death rate in the United States has been 67%. In addition, neurologic disease in the form of encephalitis, encephalomyelitis, and Guillain-Barré disease has been reported (yellow fever vaccine–associated neurotropic disease). Because yellow fever is a severe disease and deaths have been reported in travelers, and these serious adverse reactions are rare (3–5 cases of viscerotropic disease and 4–6 cases of neurotropic disease per 1,000,000 doses of vaccine distributed), vaccination is still recommended but limited to those traveling to areas reporting epidemic or endemic yellow fever. (Current information about the vaccine and yellow fever activity can be found at http://www2.ncid.cdc.gov/travel/yb/utils/ybGet.asp?section=dis&obj=yellowfever.htm.) The risk for serious adverse reactions are age-related (infants < 9 months; age > 60 years) and is greater in those with a history of thymus disease.

Japanese B Encephalitis

Japanese B encephalitis is a mosquito-borne viral encephalitis that affects primarily children and older adults (65 years and older) and usually occurs from May to September. It is the leading cause of encephalitis in Asia. Because the risk of infection is low and because adverse effects of the vaccine can be serious, not all travelers to Asia should be vaccinated. Vaccine should be given to travelers to endemic areas who will be staying at least 30 days and who are traveling during the transmission season, particularly if they are visiting rural areas. Travelers who spend less than 30 days in the region should be considered for vaccination if they intend to visit areas of epidemic transmission or if extensive outdoor activities are planned in rural rice-growing areas. The recommended primary immunization schedule is 1 mL of vaccine administered subcutaneously on days 0, 7, and 30. If time constraints are compelling, the last dose can be given on day 14. The last dose should be given at least 10 days before embarkation because urticaria and angioedema have been described, occurring from minutes up to 10 days after vaccination. Following vaccination, patients should be observed for 30 minutes and advised of the possibility of delayed reactions of angioedema and urticaria. In addition, local reactions have been reported in 20% of vaccinees and systemic reactions (fever, chills, malaise, headache) in 10%.

Bilukha OO et al; National Center for Infectious Diseases, Centers for Disease Control and Prevention (CDC): Prevention and control of meningococcal disease. Recommendations of the Advisory Committee on Immunization Practices (ACIP). MMWR Recomm Rep 2005;54(RR-7):1. [PMID: 15917737]

Casey CG et al: Adverse events associated with smallpox vaccination in the United States, January-October 2003. JAMA 2005;294:2734. [PMID: 16333009]

Centers for Disease Control and Prevention. Health Information for International Travel 2005–2006. http://www.cdc.gov/travel/yb/

Craig AS et al: Prevention of hepatitis A with hepatitis A vaccine. N Engl J Med 2004;350:476. [PMID: 14749456]

Mutsch M et al: Hepatitis A virus infections in travelers, 1988–2004. Clin Infect Dis 2006;42:490. [PMID: 16421793]

Poland GA et al: Clinical practice: prevention of hepatitis B with the hepatitis B vaccine. N Engl J Med 2004;351:2832. [PMID: 15625334]

Steinberg EB et al: Typhoid fever in travelers: who should be targeted for prevention? Clin Infect Dis 2004;39:186. [PMID: 15307027]

Vaccine-preventable hepatitis, a step toward elimination: reevaluating hepatitis A and B prevention (entire issue). Am J Med 2005;118(Suppl 10A).

Ward JI et al; APERT Study Group: Efficacy of an acellular pertussis vaccine among adolescents and adults. N Engl J Med 2005;353:1555. [PMID: 16221778]

HYPERSENSITIVITY TESTS & DESENSITIZATION

One should test for hypersensitivity before injecting antitoxin, materials derived from animal sources, or drugs (eg, penicillin) to which a patient has had a severe reaction in the past. If the test described below is negative, desensitization is not necessary, and a full dose of the material may be given. If the test is positive, alternative drugs should be strongly considered. If that is not feasible, desensitization is necessary.

Intradermal Test for Hypersensitivity

Penicillin is the drug that most frequently serves as an indication for sensitivity testing and desensitization. A clinical history of penicillin allergy has a positive predictive value of only 15%. In determining whether allergy testing should be performed, its nature should be determined. Immunoglobulin G-mediated delayed reactions such as erythematous or maculopapular skin rash or serum sickness should be distinguished from immediate-type immunoglobulin E-mediated reactions such as urticaria, angioedema, and anaphylaxis. Only patients with the latter history who require penicillin or a cephalosporin should undergo hypersensitivity testing. Skin testing requires two preparations: PPL (penicilloyl-polylysine) and a minor determinant mixture. Several points should be emphasized in performing and interpreting these tests. Whenever possible, both PPL and a minor determinant should be used, since 85% of skin test reactors are positive to PPL but 15% react only to the minor determinant mixture. In addition, if penicillin G is used instead of the minor determinant mixture, some allergic patients will be missed. About 25% of individuals who react to minor determinant mixture may not react to penicillin G, and such patients may still have an anaphylactic or accelerated reaction to penicillin. A pinprick test is performed with each solution at different sites by placing a small drop of solution on the skin and making small indentations of the skin with a needle. If there is no reaction within 10 minutes, 0.01–0.02 mL is injected intradermally, raising a small bleb. Development of a wheal greater than 5 mm in diameter is considered a positive test and an indication for desensitization. Even if the test is negative, about 1–2% of patients will have an immediate or accelerated reaction, but an anaphylactic reaction is rare. Thus, if the test is negative, the drug can be administered with relative safety, but the first dose should be medically supervised and the patient observed for 1 hour (serious reactions after 1 hour are rare).

Patients with a history of allergy to penicillin are also at an increased risk for having a reaction to cephalosporins. Since the specific immunogens responsible for anaphylaxis are not known for drugs other than penicillin, skin testing with cephalosporins is not recommended. A common approach to these patients is to assess the severity of the reaction. If an IgE-mediated reaction to penicillin can be excluded by history, a cephalosporin can be administered. When the history justifies concern about an immediate-type reaction, penicillin skin testing should be performed. If the test is negative, a cephalosporin can be given. If the test is positive, there is a 5–10% chance of cross reactivity, and cephalosporin desensitization should be performed.

Desensitization

A. Precautions

1. The desensitization procedure is not innocuous—deaths from anaphylaxis have been reported. If extreme hypersensitivity is suspected, it is advisable to use an alternative structurally unrelated drug and to reserve desensitization for situations when treatment cannot be withheld and no alternative drug is available.

2. An antihistaminic drug (25–50 mg of hydroxyzine or diphenhydramine intramuscularly or orally) should be administered before desensitization is begun in order to lessen any reaction that occurs.

3. Desensitization should be conducted in an intensive care unit where cardiac monitoring and emergency endotracheal intubation can be performed.

4. Epinephrine, 1 mL of 1:1000 solution, must be ready for immediate administration.

B. Desensitization Method

Several methods of desensitization have been described for penicillin, including use of both oral and intravenous preparations. All methods start with very small doses of drug and gradually increase the dose until therapeutic doses are achieved. For penicillin, 1 unit of drug is given intravenously and the patient observed for 15–30 minutes. If there is no reaction, some recommend doubling the dose while others recommend increasing it tenfold every 15–30 minutes until a dosage of 2 million units is reached; then give the remainder of the desired dose.

For recommendations on skin testing and desensitization for other preparations (botulism antitoxin, diphtheria antitoxin, etc), one should consult the manufacturer's package inserts.

Treatment of Reactions

A. Mild Reactions

If a mild reaction occurs, drop back to the next lower dose and continue with desensitization. If a severe reaction occurs, administer epinephrine (see below) and discontinue the drug unless treatment is urgently needed. If desensitization is imperative, continue slowly, increasing the dosage of the drug more gradually.

B. Severe Reactions

If bronchospasm occurs, epinephrine, 0.3–0.5 mL of 1:1000 dilution, should be given subcutaneously every 10–20 minutes. The following can also be given if symptoms persist: inhaled metaproterenol (0.3 mL of a 5% solution in 2.5 mL of saline), intravenous aminophylline (0.3–0.9 mL/kg/h maintenance after a 6 mg/kg loading dose over 30 minutes), or corticosteroids (250 mg of hydrocortisone or 50 mg of methylprednisolone intravenously every 6 hours for two to four doses). Hypotension should be treated with intravenous fluids (saline or colloid), epinephrine (1 mL of 1:1000 dilution in 500 mL of D$_5$W intravenously at a rate of 0.5–5 mcg/min), and antihistamines (25–50 mg of hydroxyzine or diphenhydramine intramuscularly or orally every 6–8 hours as needed). Cutaneous reactions, manifested as urticaria or angioedema, respond to epinephrine subcutaneously and antihistamines in the doses set forth above.

Arroliga ME et al: Penicillin allergy: consider trying penicillin again. Cleve Clin J Med 2003;70:313. [PMID: 12701985]

Gruchalla RS et al: Clinical practice. Antibiotic allergy. N Engl J Med 2006;354:601. [PMID: 16467547]

Robinson JL et al: Practical aspects of choosing an antibiotic for patients with a reported allergy to an antibiotic. Clin Infect Dis 2002;35:26. [PMID: 12060871]

Sexually transmitted diseases treatment guidelines 2002. MMWR Recomm Rep 2002;51(RR-6):1 [PMID: 12184549]

HIV Infection

31

Andrew R. Zolopa, MD, & Mitchell H. Katz, MD

ESSENTIALS OF DIAGNOSIS

- Risk factors: sexual contact with an infected person, parenteral exposure to infected blood by transfusion or needle sharing, perinatal exposure.
- Prominent systemic complaints such as sweats, diarrhea, weight loss, and wasting.
- Opportunistic infections due to diminished cellular immunity—often life-threatening.
- Aggressive cancers, particularly Kaposi's sarcoma and extranodal lymphoma.
- Neurologic manifestations, including dementia, aseptic meningitis, and neuropathy.

General Considerations

When AIDS was first recognized in the United States in 1981, cases were identified by finding severe opportunistic infections such as *Pneumocystis* pneumonia that indicated profound defects in cellular immunity in the absence of other causes of immunodeficiency. When the syndrome was found to be caused by HIV, it became obvious that severe opportunistic infections and unusual neoplasms were at one end of a spectrum of disease, while healthy seropositive individuals were at the other end.

The Centers for Disease Control and Prevention (CDC) AIDS case definition (Table 31–1) includes opportunistic infections and malignancies that rarely occur in the absence of severe immunodeficiency (eg, *Pneumocystis* pneumonia, central nervous system lymphoma). It also classifies persons as having AIDS if they have positive HIV serology and certain infections and malignancies that can occur in immunocompetent hosts but that are more common among persons infected with HIV (pulmonary tuberculosis, invasive cervical cancer). Several nonspecific conditions, including dementia and wasting (documented weight loss)—in the presence of a positive HIV serology—are considered AIDS. The definition includes criteria for both definitive and presumptive diagnoses of certain infections and malignancies. Finally, persons with positive HIV serology who have ever had a CD4 lymphocyte count below 200 cells/mcL or a CD4 lymphocyte percentage below 14% are considered to have AIDS. Inclusion of persons with low CD4 counts as AIDS cases reflects the recognition that immunodeficiency is the defining characteristic of AIDS. The choice of a cutoff point at 200 cells/mcL is supported by several cohort studies showing that over 80% of persons with counts below this level will develop AIDS within 3 years in the absence of effective antiretroviral therapy. The 1993 definition was also expanded to include persons with positive HIV serology and pulmonary tuberculosis, recurrent pneumonia, and invasive cervical cancer. Dramatic increases in the efficacy of antiretroviral treatments—especially those regimens that include protease inhibitors or nonnucleoside reverse transcriptase inhibitors—have improved the prognosis of persons with HIV/AIDS. One consequence is that fewer persons with HIV ever develop an infection or malignancy or have a low enough CD4 count to classify them as having AIDS, which means that the CDC definition has become a less useful measure of the impact of HIV/AIDS in the United States. Conversely, persons in whom AIDS had been diagnosed based on a serious opportunistic infection, malignancy, or immunodeficiency may now be markedly healthier, with high CD4 counts, due to the use of highly active antiretroviral therapy (HAART). Therefore, the Social Security Administration as well as most social service agencies focus on functional assessment for determining eligibility for benefits rather than the simple presence or absence of an AIDS-defined illness.

Clinicians with limited experience in HIV/AIDS should refer HIV-infected patients to specialists with experience, given the increasing number and complexity of treatment regimens available. Extra efforts should be made to obtain specialty consultation for those patients not responding to their current regimens; those intolerant of standard antiviral drugs; those in need of systemic chemotherapy; and those with complicated opportunistic infections, particularly when invasive procedures or experimental therapies are needed. Resources are available to help clinicians care for HIV-infected persons. Clinicians should call their state medical associations for a list of local resources.

Epidemiology

The modes of transmission of HIV are similar to those of hepatitis B, in particular with respect to sexual, parenteral, and vertical transmission. Although certain

Table 31–1. CDC AIDS case definition for surveillance of adults and adolescents.

Definitive AIDS diagnoses (with or without laboratory evidence of HIV infection)

1. Candidiasis of the esophagus, trachea, bronchi, or lungs.
2. Cryptococcosis, extrapulmonary.
3. Cryptosporidiosis with diarrhea persisting > 1 month.
4. Cytomegalovirus disease of an organ other than liver, spleen, or lymph nodes.
5. Herpes simplex virus infection causing a mucocutaneous ulcer that persists longer than 1 month; or bronchitis, pneumonitis, or esophagitis of any duration.
6. Kaposi's sarcoma in a patient < 60 years of age.
7. Lymphoma of the brain (primary) in a patient < 60 years of age.
8. *Mycobacterium avium* complex or *Mycobacterium kansasii* disease, disseminated (at a site other than or in addition to lungs, skin, or cervical or hilar lymph nodes).
9. *Pneumocystis jiroveci* pneumonia.
10. Progressive multifocal leukoencephalopathy.
11. Toxoplasmosis of the brain.

Definitive AIDS diagnoses (with laboratory evidence of HIV infection)

1. Coccidioidomycosis, disseminated (at a site other than or in addition to lungs or cervical or hilar lymph nodes).
2. HIV encephalopathy.
3. Histoplasmosis, disseminated (at a site other than or in addition to lungs or cervical or hilar lymph nodes).
4. Isosporiasis with diarrhea persisting > 1 month.
5. Kaposi's sarcoma at any age.
6. Lymphoma of the brain (primary) at any age.
7. Other non-Hodgkin's lymphoma of B cell or unknown immunologic phenotype.
8. Any mycobacterial disease caused by mycobacteria other than *Mycobacterium tuberculosis,* disseminated (at a site other than or in addition to lungs, skin, or cervical or hilar lymph nodes).
9. Disease caused by extrapulmonary *M tuberculosis.*
10. *Salmonella* (nontyphoid) septicemia, recurrent.
11. HIV wasting syndrome.
12. CD4 lymphocyte count below 200 cells/mcL or a CD4 lymphocyte percentage below 14%.
13. Pulmonary tuberculosis.
14. Recurrent pneumonia.
15. Invasive cervical cancer.

Presumptive AIDS diagnoses (with laboratory evidence of HIV infection)

1. Candidiasis of esophagus: (a) recent onset of retrosternal pain on swallowing; and (b) oral candidiasis.
2. Cytomegalovirus retinitis. A characteristic appearance on serial ophthalmoscopic examinations.
3. Mycobacteriosis. Specimen from stool or normally sterile body fluids or tissue from a site other than lungs, skin, or cervical or hilar lymph nodes, showing acid-fast bacilli of a species not identified by culture.
4. Kaposi's sarcoma. Erythematous or violaceous plaque-like lesion on skin or mucous membrane.
5. *Pneumocystis jiroveci* pneumonia: (a) a history of dyspnea on exertion or nonproductive cough of recent onset (within the past 3 months); and (b) chest x-ray evidence of diffuse bilateral interstitial infiltrates or gallium scan evidence of diffuse bilateral pulmonary disease; and (c) arterial blood gas analysis showing an arterial oxygen partial pressure of < 70 mm Hg or a low respiratory diffusing capacity of < 80% of predicted values or an increase in the alveolar-arterial oxygen tension gradient; and (d) no evidence of a bacterial pneumonia.
6. Toxoplasmosis of the brain: (a) recent onset of a focal neurologic abnormality consistent with intracranial disease or a reduced level of consciousness; and (b) brain imaging evidence of a lesion having a mass effect or the radiographic appearance of which is enhanced by injection of contrast medium; and (c) serum antibody to toxoplasmosis or successful response to therapy for toxoplasmosis.
7. Recurrent pneumonia: (a) more than one episode in a 1-year period; and (b) acute pneumonia (new symptoms, signs, or radiologic evidence not present earlier) diagnosed on clinical or radiologic grounds by the patient's physician.
8. Pulmonary tuberculosis: (a) apical or miliary infiltrates and (b) radiographic and clinical response to antituberculous therapy.

sexual practices (eg, receptive anal intercourse) are significantly riskier than other sexual practices (eg, oral sex), it is difficult to quantify per-contact risks. The reason is that studies of sexual transmission of HIV show that most people at risk for HIV infection engage in a variety of sexual practices and have sex with multiple persons, only some of whom may actually be HIV infected. Thus, it is difficult to determine which practice with which person actually resulted in HIV transmission.

Nonetheless, the best available estimates indicate that the risk of HIV transmission with receptive anal intercourse is between 1:100 and 1:30, with insertive anal intercourse 1:1000, with receptive vaginal intercourse 1:1000, with insertive vaginal intercourse 1:10,000, and with receptive fellatio with ejaculation 1:1000. The per-contact risk of HIV transmission with other behaviors, including receptive fellatio without ejaculation, insertive fellatio, and cunnilingus, is not known.

All per-contact risk estimates assume that the source is HIV infected. If the HIV status of the source is unknown, the risk of transmission is the risk of transmission multiplied by the probability that the source is HIV infected. This would vary by risk practices, age, and geographic area. A number of cofactors are known to increase the risk of HIV transmission during a given encounter, including the presence of ulcerative or inflammatory sexually transmitted diseases, trauma, menses, and lack of male circumcision.

The risk of acquiring HIV infection from a needlestick with infected blood is approximately 1:300. Factors known to increase the risk of transmission include depth of penetration, hollow bore needles, visible blood on the needle, and advanced stage of disease in the source. The risk of HIV transmission from a mucosal splash with infected blood is unknown but is assumed to be significantly lower.

The risk of acquiring HIV infection from illicit drug use with sharing of needles from an HIV-infected source is estimated to be 1:150. Use of clean needles markedly decreases the chance of HIV transmission but does not eliminate it if other drug paraphernalia are shared (eg, cookers).

When blood transfusion from an HIV-infected donor occurs, the risk of transmission is 95%. Fortunately, since 1985, blood donor screening using the HIV enzyme-linked immunosorbent assay (ELISA) has been universally practiced in the United States. Also, persons who have recently engaged in unsafe behaviors (eg, sex with a person at risk for HIV, injection drug use) are not allowed to donate. This eliminates donations from persons who are HIV infected but have not yet developed antibodies (ie, persons in the "window" period). In recent years, HIV antigen and viral load testing have been added to the screening of blood to further lower the chance of HIV transmission. With these precautions, the chance of HIV transmission with receipt of blood transfusion is about 1:1,000,000.

In the absence of perinatal HIV prophylaxis, between 13% and 40% of children born to HIV-infected mothers contract HIV infection. The risk is higher with vaginal than with cesarean delivery, higher among mothers with high viral loads, and higher among those who breast-feed their children. The risk can be decreased by administering antiretroviral treatment to the mother during pregnancy and to the infant immediately after birth (see below).

HIV has not been shown to be transmitted by respiratory droplet spread, by vectors such as mosquitoes, or by casual nonsexual contact.

Current estimates are that about 950,000 Americans are infected with HIV. At the end of 2004, there were approximately 415,193 persons in the United States living with AIDS. Fifty-one percent of those are gay or bisexual men, 16% are heterosexual male injection drug users, and 9% are heterosexual male nonin-jection drug users. Women account for 22% of living persons, of whom 64% were infected through heterosexual contact with an infected partner and 34% were infected through injection drug use.

The rapid increase of AIDS cases among women is of great concern. In 1985, women represented only 7% of new AIDS cases; in 2004, women represented 27% of new cases. African Americans have been disproportionately hard hit by the epidemic. The estimated rate in 2004 of new AIDS cases in the United States per 100,000 population was 56.4 among African Americans, 18.0 among Latinos, 7.9 among American Indians and Alaska Natives, 5.9 among whites, and 3.7 among Asian and Pacific Islanders.

In general, the progression of HIV-related illness is similar in men and women. However, there are some important differences. Women seek medical attention later than men. They are at risk for gynecologic complications of HIV, including recurrent candidal vaginitis, pelvic inflammatory disease, and cervical dysplasia. Violence directed against women, pregnancy, and frequent occurrence of drug use and poverty all complicate the treatment of HIV-infected women. Although "safer sex" campaigns dramatically decreased the rates of seroconversions among gay men living in metropolitan areas in the United States by the mid-1980s, there is concern that relapse to unsafe sexual practices will result in an increase in the number of new seroconversions. Several studies have reported recent increases in the rates of unsafe sexual behaviors and sexually transmitted diseases among gay men in several large cities in the United States and in western Europe. The higher rates of unsafe sex appear to be related to decreased concern about acquiring HIV due to the availability of HAART. Decreased interest in following safe sex recommendations and increasing use of crystal methamphetamine among certain risk groups also appears to be playing a role in the increased unsafe sex rates.

Worldwide there are nearly 40 million persons infected with HIV. In Central and East Africa in some urban areas, as many as one-third of sexually active adults are infected. HIV infection began to spread in Asia in the late 1980s. The most common mode of transmission is bidirectional heterosexual spread. The reason for the greater risk for transmission with heterosexual intercourse in Africa and Asia than in the United States may relate to cofactors such as general health status, the presence of genital ulcers, relative lack of male circumcision, the number of sexual partners, and different HIV serotypes.

Centers for Disease Control and Prevention: HIV/AIDS Surveillance Reports. Available at http://www.cdc.gov/hiv/topics/surveillance/resources/reports/index.htm.

Katz MH et al: Impact of highly active antiretroviral treatment on HIV seroincidence among men who have sex with men: San Francisco. Am J Public Health 2002;93:388. [PMID: 11867317]

Kleinman SH et al: The risks of transfusion-transmitted infection. Baillieres Best Pract Clin Haematol 2000;13:631. [PMID: 11102281]

Mofenson LM: U.S. Public Health Service Task Force recommendations for use of antiretroviral drugs in pregnant HIV-1 infected women for maternal health and interventions to reduce perinatal HIV-1 transmission in the United States. MMWR Recomm Rep 2002;51(RR-18):1. [PMID: 12489844]

Taha TE et al: Nevirapine and zidovudine at birth to reduce perinatal transmission of HIV in an African setting: a randomized controlled trial. JAMA 2004;292:202. [PMID: 15249569]

Vittinghoff E: Per-contact risk of human immunodeficiency virus transmission between male sexual partners. Am J Epidemiol 1999;150:306. [PMID: 10430236]

Etiology

HIV, like other retroviruses, depends on a unique enzyme, reverse transcriptase (RNA-dependent DNA polymerase), to replicate within host cells. The other major pathogenic human retrovirus, human T cell lymphotropic/leukemia virus (HTLV)-I, is associated with lymphoma, while HIV is not known to be directly oncogenic. The HIV genomes contain genes for three basic structural proteins and at least five other regulatory proteins; *gag* codes for group antigen proteins, *pol* codes for polymerase, and *env* codes for the external envelope protein. The greatest variability in strains of HIV occurs in the viral envelope. Since neutralizing activity is found in antibodies directed against the envelope, this variability presents problems for vaccine development.

In addition to the classic AIDS virus (HIV-1), a group of related viruses, HIV-2, has been isolated in West African patients. HIV-2 has the same genetic organization as HIV-1, but there are significant differences in the envelope glycoproteins. Some infected individuals exhibit AIDS-like illnesses, but most West Africans infected with HIV-2 are currently asymptomatic. HIV-2 has been found in several people in the United States. Thus, this variant may be less pathogenic or have a longer period of latency preceding disease. Cases have been documented in which AIDS-like illnesses have occurred in the absence of HIV infection or other known infectious causes of immunodeficiency.

Pathogenesis

The hallmark of symptomatic HIV infection is immunodeficiency caused by continuing viral replication. The virus can infect all cells expressing the T4 (CD4) antigen, which HIV uses to attach to the cell. Chemokine receptors (CCR5 and CXCR4) are important for virus entry, and individuals with CCR5 deletions are less likely to become infected, and, once infected, the disease is more likely to progress slowly. Once it enters a cell, HIV can replicate and cause cell fusion or death. A latent state is also established, with integration of the HIV genome into the cell's genome. The cell principally infected is the CD4 (helper-inducer) lymphocyte, which directs many other cells in the immune network. With increasing duration of infection, the number of CD4 lymphocytes falls. Some of the immunologic defects, however, are explained not by *quantitative* abnormalities of lymphocyte subsets but by *qualitative* defects in CD4 responsiveness induced by HIV.

Other cells in the immune network that are infected by HIV include B lymphocytes and macrophages. The defect in B cells is partly due to disordered CD4 lymphocyte function. These direct and indirect effects can lead to generalized hypergammaglobulinemia and can also depress B cell responses to new antigen challenges. Because of these defects, the immunodeficiency of HIV is mixed. Elements of humoral and cellular immunodeficiency are present, especially in children. Macrophages act as a reservoir for HIV and serve to disseminate it to other organ systems (eg, the central nervous system).

Apart from the immunologic effects of HIV, the virus can also directly cause a variety of neurologic effects. Neuropathology largely results from the release of cytokines and other neurotoxins by infected macrophages. Perturbations of excitatory neurotransmitters and calcium flux may contribute to neurologic dysfunction. Direct HIV infection of renal tubular cells and gastrointestinal epithelium may contribute to these organ system manifestations of infection.

Pathophysiology

Clinically, the syndromes caused by HIV infection are usually explicable by one of three known mechanisms: immunodeficiency, autoimmunity, and allergic and hypersensitivity reactions.

A. Immunodeficiency

Immunodeficiency is a direct result of the effects of HIV upon immune cells. A spectrum of infections and neoplasms is seen, as in other congenital or acquired immunodeficiency states. Two remarkable features of HIV immunodeficiency are the low incidence of certain infections such as listeriosis and aspergillosis and the frequent occurrence of certain neoplasms such as lymphoma or Kaposi's sarcoma. This latter complication has been seen primarily in gay or bisexual men, and its incidence has steadily declined through the first 15 years of the epidemic. A herpesvirus (KSHV or HHV-8) is the cause of Kaposi's sarcoma.

B. Autoimmunity/Allergic & Hypersensitivity Reactions

Autoimmunity can occur as a result of disordered cellular immune function or B lymphocyte dysfunction. Examples of both lymphocytic infiltration of organs (eg, lymphocytic interstitial pneumonitis) and autoantibody production (eg, immunologic thrombocytopenia) occur. These phenomena may be the only clinically apparent disease or may coexist with obvious immunodeficiency. Moreover, HIV-infected individuals appear to have higher rates of allergic reactions to unknown allergens as seen with eosinophilic pustular folliculitis ("itchy red bump syndrome") as well as increased rates of hypersensitivity reactions to medications (for example, the fever and sunburn-like rash seen with trimethoprim-sulfamethoxazole reactions).

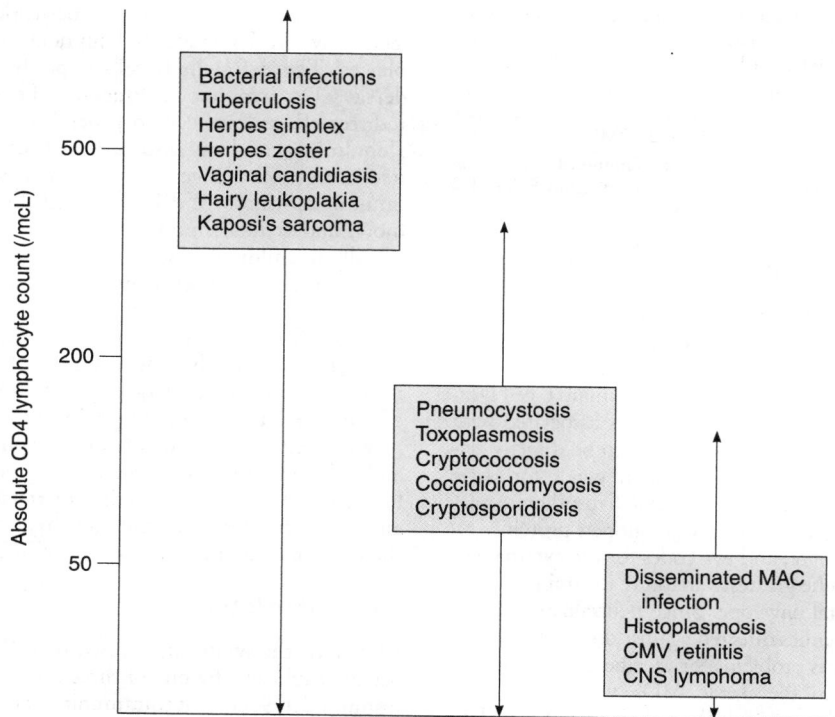

Figure 31–1. Relationship of CD4 count to development of opportunistic infections. MAC = *Mycobacterium avium* complex; CMV = cytomegalovirus; CNS = central nervous system.

Clinical Findings

The complications of HIV-related infections and neoplasms affect virtually every organ. The general approach to the HIV-infected person with symptoms is to evaluate the organ systems involved, aiming to diagnose treatable conditions rapidly. As can be seen in Figure 31–1, the CD4 lymphocyte count provides very important prognostic information. Certain infections may occur at any CD4 count, while others rarely occur unless the CD4 lymphocyte count has dropped below a certain level. For example, a patient with a CD4 count of 600 cells/mcL, cough, and fever may have a bacterial pneumonia but would be very unlikely to have *Pneumocystis* pneumonia.

A. Symptoms and Signs

Many individuals with HIV infection remain asymptomatic for years even without antiretroviral therapy, with a mean time of approximately 10 years between exposure and development of AIDS. When symptoms occur, they may be remarkably protean and nonspecific. Since virtually all the findings may be seen with other diseases, a combination of complaints is more suggestive of HIV infection than any one symptom.

Physical examination may be entirely normal. Abnormal findings range from completely nonspecific to highly specific for HIV infection. Those that are specific for HIV infection include hairy leukoplakia of the tongue, disseminated Kaposi's sarcoma, and cutaneous bacillary angiomatosis. Generalized lymphadenopathy is common early in infection.

1. Systemic complaints—Fever, night sweats, and weight loss are common symptoms in HIV-infected patients and may occur without a complicating opportunistic infection. Patients with persistent **fever** and no localizing symptoms should nonetheless be carefully examined, and evaluated with a chest radiograph (*Pneumocystis* pneumonia can present without respiratory symptoms), bacterial blood cultures if the fever is greater than 38.5 °C, serum cryptococcal antigen, and mycobacterial cultures of the blood. Sinus CT scans or sinus radiographs should be considered to evaluate occult sinusitis. If these studies are normal, patients should be observed closely. Antipyretics are useful to prevent dehydration.

Weight loss is a particularly distressing complication of long-standing HIV infection. Patients typically have disproportionate loss of muscle mass, with maintenance or less substantial loss of fat stores. The mechanism of HIV-related weight loss is not completely understood but appears to be multifactorial.

AIDS patients frequently suffer from anorexia, nausea, and vomiting, all of which contribute to weight loss by decreasing caloric intake. In some cases, these symptoms are secondary to a specific infection, such as viral hepatitis. In other cases, however, evaluation of the symptoms yields no specific pathogen, and it is assumed to be due to a primary effect of HIV. Malabsorption also plays a role in decreased caloric intake. Patients may suffer diarrhea from infections with bacterial, viral, or parasitic agents.

Exacerbating the decrease in caloric intake, many AIDS patients have an increased metabolic rate. This increased rate has been shown to exist even among asymptomatic HIV-infected persons, but it accelerates with disease progression and secondary infection. AIDS patients with secondary infections also have decreased protein synthesis, which makes maintaining muscle mass difficult.

Several strategies have been developed to slow AIDS wasting. Effective fever control decreases the metabolic rate and may slow the pace of weight loss, as does treating the underlying opportunistic infection. Food supplementation with high-calorie drinks may enable patients with not much appetite to maintain their intake. Selected patients with otherwise good functional status and weight loss due to unrelenting nausea, vomiting, or diarrhea may benefit from total parenteral nutrition (TPN). It should be noted, however, that TPN is more likely to increase fat stores than to reverse the muscle wasting process.

Two pharmacologic approaches for increasing appetite and weight gain are the progestational agent megestrol acetate (80 mg four times a day) and the antiemetic agent dronabinol (2.5–5 mg three times a day). Side effects from megestrol acetate are rare, but thromboembolic phenomena, edema, nausea, vomiting, and rash have been reported. Euphoria, dizziness, paranoia, and somnolence and even nausea and vomiting have been reported in 3–10% of patients using dronabinol. Dronabinol contains only one of the active ingredients in smoked marijuana, and many patients report better relief of nausea and improvement of appetite with smoking marijuana. Several states allow physicians to recommend the use of smoked marijuana to their patients. However, it is still illegal in the United States to sell marijuana. Thus, a physician's recommendation may at best decrease the chance that patients will be prosecuted for use of marijuana. Unfortunately, neither megestrol acetate nor dronabinol increases lean body mass.

Two regimens that have resulted in increases in lean body mass are growth hormone and anabolic steroids. Growth hormone at a dose of 0.1 mg/kg/d (up to 6 mg) subcutaneously for 12 weeks has resulted in modest increases in lean body mass. Treatment with growth hormone can cost as much as $10,000 per month. Anabolic steroids also increase lean body mass among HIV-infected patients. They seem to work best for patients who are able to do weight training. The most commonly used regimens are testosterone enanthate or testosterone cypionate (100–200 mg intramuscularly every 2–4 weeks). Testosterone transdermal system (apply 5 mg system each evening) and testosterone gel (1%; apply a 5-g packet [50 mg testosterone] to clean, dry skin daily) are also available. The anabolic steroid oxandrolone (20 mg orally in two divided doses) has also been found to increase lean body mass.

Nausea leading to weight loss is sometimes due to esophageal candidiasis. Patients with oral candidiasis and nausea should be empirically treated with an oral antifungal agent. Patients with weight loss due to nausea of unclear origin may benefit from use of antiemetics prior to meals (prochlorperazine, 10 mg three times daily; metoclopramide, 10 mg three times daily; or ondansetron, 8 mg three times daily). Dronabinol (5 mg three times daily) can also be used to increase appetite. Depression and adrenal insufficiency are two potentially treatable causes of weight loss.

2. Sinopulmonary disease—

a. *Pneumocystis* pneumonia—(See also discussions in Chapter 36.) *Pneumocystis jiroveci* pneumonia is the most common opportunistic infection associated with AIDS. *Pneumocystis* pneumonia may be difficult to diagnose because the symptoms—fever, cough, and shortness of breath—are nonspecific. Furthermore, the severity of symptoms ranges from fever and no respiratory symptoms through mild cough or dyspnea to frank respiratory distress.

Hypoxemia may be severe, with a PO_2 less than 60 mm Hg. The cornerstone of diagnosis is the chest radiograph. Diffuse or perihilar infiltrates are most characteristic, but only two-thirds of patients with *Pneumocystis* pneumonia have this finding. Normal chest radiographs are seen in 5–10% of patients with *Pneumocystis* pneumonia, while the remainder have atypical infiltrates. Apical infiltrates are commonly seen among patients with *Pneumocystis* pneumonia who have been receiving aerosolized pentamidine prophylaxis. Large pleural effusions are uncommon with *Pneumocystis* pneumonia; their presence suggests bacterial pneumonia, other infections such as tuberculosis, or pleural Kaposi's sarcoma.

Definitive diagnosis can be obtained in 50–80% of cases by Wright-Giemsa stain or direct fluorescence antibody (DFA) test of induced sputum. Sputum induction is performed by having patients inhale an aerosolized solution of 3% saline produced by an ultrasonic nebulizer. Patients should not eat for at least 8 hours and should not use toothpaste or mouthwash prior to the procedure since they can interfere with test interpretation. The next step for patients with negative sputum examinations still suspected of having *Pneumocystis* pneumonia should be bronchoalveolar lavage. This technique establishes the diagnosis in over 95% of cases.

In patients with symptoms suggestive of *Pneumocystis* pneumonia but with negative or atypical chest radiographs and negative sputum examinations, other diagnostic tests may provide additional information in deciding whether to proceed to bronchoalveolar lavage. Elevation of serum lactate dehydrogenase occurs in 95% of cases of *Pneumocystis* pneumonia, but the specificity of this finding is at best 75%. Either a normal diffusing capacity of carbon monoxide (DL_{CO}) or a high-resolution CT scan of the chest that demonstrates no interstitial lung disease makes the diagnosis of *Pneumocystis* pneumonia very unlikely. In addition, a CD4 count above 250 cells/mcL within 2 months prior to evaluation of respiratory symptoms makes a diagnosis of *Pneumocystis* pneumonia unlikely; only 1–5% of cases occur above this CD4 count level (Figure 31–1). This is true even if the patient previously had a CD4 count lower than 200 cells/mcL but has had an increase with antiretroviral therapy. Pneumothoraces can be seen in HIV-infected patients with a history of *Pneumocystis* pneumonia, especially if they have received aerosolized pentamidine treatment.

b. Other infectious pulmonary diseases—Other infectious causes of pulmonary disease in AIDS patients include bacterial, mycobacterial, and viral pneumonias. Community-acquired pneumonia is the most common cause of pulmonary disease in HIV-infected persons. An increased incidence of pneumococcal pneumonia with septicemia and *Haemophilus influenzae* pneumonia has been reported. *Pseudomonas aeruginosa* is an important respiratory pathogen in advanced disease. The incidence of infection with *Mycobacterium tuberculosis* has markedly increased in metropolitan areas because of HIV infection as well as homelessness. Tuberculosis occurs in an estimated 4% of persons in the United States who have AIDS. Apical infiltrates and disseminated disease occur more commonly than among immunocompetent hosts. Although a purified protein derivative (PPD) test should be performed on all HIV-infected persons in whom a diagnosis of tuberculosis is being considered, the lower the CD4 cell count, the greater the likelihood of anergy. Because "anergy" skin test panels do not accurately classify those patients who are infected with tuberculosis but unreactive to the PPD, they are not recommended. Treatment of HIV-infected persons with active tuberculosis is similar to treatment of HIV-uninfected tubercular individuals (see Figure 31–1). However, rifampin should not be given to patients receiving indinavir, nelfinavir, amprenavir, lopinavir, or delavirdine. In these cases, rifabutin may be substituted, but it may require dosing modifications depending on the antiretroviral regimen. Multidrug-resistant tuberculosis is a major problem in several metropolitan areas. Noncompliance with prescribed antituberculous drugs is a major risk factor. Several of the reported outbreaks appear to implicate nosocomial spread. The emergence of drug resistance makes it essential that antibiotic sensitivities be performed on all positive cultures. Drug therapy should be individualized. Patients with multidrug-resistant *M tuberculosis* infection should receive at least three drugs to which their organism is sensitive. Atypical mycobacteria can cause pulmonary disease in AIDS patients with or without preexisting lung disease and responds variably to treatment. Making a distinction between *M tuberculosis* and atypical mycobacteria requires culture of sputum specimens. If culture of the sputum produces acid-fast bacilli, definitive identification may take several weeks using traditional techniques. DNA probes allow for presumptive identification usually within days of a positive culture. While awaiting definitive diagnosis, clinicians should err on the side of treating patients as if they have *M tuberculosis* infection. In cases in which the risk of atypical mycobacteria is very high (eg, a person without risk for tuberculosis exposure with a CD4 count under 50 cells/mcL—see Figure 31–1), clinicians may wait for definitive diagnosis if the person is smear-negative for acid-fast bacilli, clinically stable, and not living in a communal setting. Isolation of cytomegalovirus (CMV) from bronchoalveolar lavage fluid occurs commonly in AIDS patients but does not establish a definitive diagnosis. Diagnosis of CMV pneumonia requires biopsy; response to treatment is poor. Histoplasmosis, coccidioidomycosis, and cryptococcal disease should also be considered in the differential diagnosis of unexplained pulmonary infiltrates.

c. Noninfectious pulmonary diseases—Noninfectious causes of lung disease include Kaposi's sarcoma, non-Hodgkin's lymphoma, and interstitial pneumonitis. In patients with known Kaposi's sarcoma, pulmonary involvement complicates the course in approximately one-third of cases. However, pulmonary involvement is rarely the presenting manifestation of Kaposi's sarcoma. Non-Hodgkin's lymphoma may involve the lung as the sole site of disease but more commonly involves other organs as well, especially the brain, liver, and gastrointestinal tract. Both of these processes may show nodular or diffuse parenchymal involvement, pleural effusions, and mediastinal adenopathy on chest radiographs.

Nonspecific interstitial pneumonitis may mimic *Pneumocystis* pneumonia. Lymphocytic interstitial pneumonitis seen in lung biopsies has a variable clinical course. Typically, these patients present with several months of mild cough and dyspnea; chest radiographs show interstitial infiltrates. Many patients with this entity undergo transbronchial biopsies in an attempt to diagnose *Pneumocystis* pneumonia. Instead, the tissue shows interstitial inflammation ranging from an intense lymphocytic infiltration (consistent with lymphoid interstitial pneumonitis) to a mild mononuclear inflammation. Corticosteroids may be helpful in some cases refractory to antiretroviral therapy.

d. Sinusitis—Chronic sinusitis can be a frustrating problem for HIV-infected patients even in those on adequate antiretroviral therapy. Symptoms include sinus congestion and discharge, headache, and fever. Some patients may have radiographic evidence of sinus disease on sinus CT scan or sinus x-ray in the absence of significant symptoms. Nonsmoking patients with purulent drainage should be treated with amoxicillin (500 mg orally three times a day). Patients who smoke should be treated with amoxicillin-potassium clavulanate (500 mg orally three times a day) to cover

H influenzae. Prolonged treatment (3–6 weeks) with an antibiotic and guaifenesin (600 mg orally twice daily) to decrease sinus congestion may be required. For patients not responding to amoxicillin-potassium clavulanate, levofloxacin should be tried (400 mg orally daily). Some patients may require referral to an otolaryngologist for sinus drainage.

3. Central nervous system disease—Central nervous system disease in HIV-infected patients can be divided into intracerebral space-occupying lesions, encephalopathy, meningitis, and spinal cord processes. Many of these complications have declined markedly in prevalence in the era of HAART.

a. Toxoplasmosis—Toxoplasmosis is the most common space-occupying lesion in HIV-infected patients. Headache, focal neurologic deficits, seizures, or altered mental status may be presenting symptoms. The diagnosis is usually made presumptively based on the characteristic appearance of cerebral imaging studies in an individual known to be seropositive for *Toxoplasma*. Typically, toxoplasmosis appears as multiple contrast-enhancing lesions on CT scan. Lesions tend to be peripheral, with a predilection for the basal ganglia.

Single lesions are atypical of toxoplasmosis. When a single lesion has been detected by CT scanning, MRI scanning may reveal multiple lesions because of its greater sensitivity. If a patient has a single lesion on MRI and is neurologically stable, clinicians may pursue a 2-week empiric trial of toxoplasmosis therapy. A repeat scan should be performed at 2 weeks. If the lesion has not diminished in size, biopsy of the lesion should be performed. Since many HIV-infected patients will have detectable titers, a positive *Toxoplasma* serologic test does not confirm the diagnosis. Conversely, less than 3% of patients with toxoplasmosis have negative titers. Therefore, negative *Toxoplasma* titers in an HIV-infected patient with a space-occupying lesion should be a cause for aggressively pursuing an alternative diagnosis.

b. Central nervous system lymphoma—Primary non-Hodgkin's lymphoma is the second most common space-occupying lesion in HIV-infected patients. Symptoms are similar to those with toxoplasmosis. While imaging techniques cannot distinguish these two diseases with certainty, lymphoma more often is solitary. Other less common lesions should be suspected if there is preceding bacteremia, positive tuberculin test, fungemia, or injection drug use. These include bacterial abscesses, cryptococcomas, tuberculomas, and *Nocardia* lesions.

Because techniques for stereotactic brain biopsy have improved, this procedure plays an increasing role in diagnosing cerebral lesions. Biopsy should be strongly considered if lesions are solitary or do not respond to toxoplasmosis treatment, especially if they are easily accessible. Diagnosis of lymphoma is important because many patients benefit from treatment (radiation therapy). In the future, it may be possible to avoid brain biopsy by utilizing polymerase chain reaction (PCR) assay of cerebrospinal fluid for Epstein–Barr virus DNA, which is present in 90% of cases.

c. AIDS dementia complex—The diagnosis of AIDS dementia complex (HIV-associated cognitive-motor complex) is one of exclusion based on a brain imaging study and on spinal fluid analysis that excludes other pathogens. Neuropsychiatric testing is helpful in distinguishing patients with dementia from those with depression. Patients with AIDS dementia complex typically have difficulty with cognitive tasks and exhibit diminished motor speed. Patients may first notice a deterioration in their handwriting. The manifestations of dementia may wax and wane, with persons exhibiting periods of lucidity and confusion over the course of a day. Many patients improve with effective antiretroviral treatment. Metabolic abnormalities may also cause changes in mental status: hypoglycemia, hyponatremia, hypoxia, and drug overdose are important considerations in this population. Other less common infectious causes of encephalopathy include progressive multifocal leukoencephalopathy (discussed below), CMV, syphilis, and herpes simplex encephalitis.

d. Cryptococcal meningitis—Cryptococcal meningitis typically presents with fever and headache. Less than 20% of patients have meningismus. Diagnosis is based on a positive latex agglutination test that detects cryptococcal antigen (or "CRAG") or positive culture of spinal fluid for *Cryptococcus*. Seventy to 90% of patients with cryptococcal meningitis have a positive serum CRAG. Thus, a negative serum CRAG test makes a diagnosis of cryptococcal meningitis unlikely and can be useful in the initial evaluation of a patient with headache, fever, and normal mental status. HIV meningitis, characterized by lymphocytic pleocytosis of the spinal fluid with negative culture, is common early in HIV infection.

e. HIV myelopathy—Spinal cord function may also be impaired in HIV-infected individuals. HIV myelopathy presents with leg weakness and incontinence. Spastic paraparesis and sensory ataxia are seen on neurologic examination. Myelopathy is usually a late manifestation of HIV disease, and most patients will have concomitant HIV encephalopathy. Pathologic evaluation of the spinal cord reveals vacuolation of white matter. Because HIV myelopathy is a diagnosis of exclusion, symptoms suggestive of myelopathy should be evaluated by lumbar puncture to rule out CMV polyradiculopathy (described below) and an MRI or CT scan to exclude epidural lymphoma.

f. Progressive multifocal leukoencephalopathy (PML)—PML is a viral infection of the white matter of the brain seen in patients with very advanced HIV infection. It typically results in focal neurologic deficits such as aphasia, hemiparesis, and cortical blindness. Imaging studies are strongly suggestive of the diagnosis if they show nonenhancing white matter lesions without mass effect. Extensive lesions may be difficult to differentiate from the changes caused by HIV. Several patients have stabilized or improved after the institution of combination antiretroviral therapy or cidofovir.

4. Peripheral nervous system—Peripheral nervous system syndromes include inflammatory polyneuropathies, sensory neuropathies, and mononeuropathies.

An inflammatory demyelinating polyneuropathy similar to Guillain-Barré syndrome occurs in HIV-infected patients, usually prior to frank immunodeficiency. The syndrome in many cases improves with plasmapheresis, supporting an autoimmune basis of the disease. CMV can cause an ascending polyradiculopathy characterized by lower extremity weakness and a neutrophilic pleocytosis on spinal fluid analysis with a negative bacterial culture. Transverse myelitis can be seen with herpes zoster or CMV.

Peripheral neuropathy is common among HIV-infected persons. Patients typically complain of numbness, tingling, and pain in the lower extremities. Symptoms are disproportionate to findings on gross sensory and motor evaluation. Beyond HIV infection itself, the most common cause is prior antiretroviral therapy with stavudine or didanosine. Patients who report these symptoms should be switched to an alternative agent if possible. Caution should be used when administering these agents to patients with a history of peripheral neuropathy. Unfortunately, drug-induced neuropathy is not always reversed when the offending agent is discontinued. Patients with advanced disease may also develop peripheral neuropathy even if they have never taken antiretroviral therapy. Evaluation should rule out other causes of sensory neuropathy such as alcoholism, thyroid disease, vitamin B_{12} deficiency, and syphilis.

Treatment of peripheral neuropathy is aimed at symptomatic relief. Patients should be initially treated with gabapentin (start at 300 mg at bedtime and increase to 300–900 mg orally three times a day). Although many clinicians initiate a trial of amitriptyline (10–25 mg orally at bedtime), responses to this agent are uncommon.

5. Rheumatologic manifestations—Arthritis, involving single or multiple joints, with or without effusion, has been commonly noted in HIV-infected patients. Involvement of large joints is most common. Although the cause of HIV-related arthritis is unknown, most patients will respond to nonsteroidal anti-inflammatory agents. Patients with a sizable effusion, especially if the joint is warm or erythematous, should have the joint tapped, followed by culture of the fluid to rule out suppurative arthritis as well as fungal and mycobacterial disease.

Several rheumatologic syndromes, including reactive arthritis (Reiter's syndrome), psoriatic arthritis, sicca syndrome, and systemic lupus erythematosus, have been reported in HIV-infected patients (see Chapter 20). However, it is unclear if the prevalence is greater than in the general population. Cases of avascular necrosis of the femoral heads have been reported sporad-

ically, generally in the setting of advanced disease with long-standing infection and in patients receiving long-term antiretroviral therapy. The etiology is not clear but is probably multifactoral in nature.

6. Myopathy—Myopathies are increasingly noted in HIV-infected patients. Proximal muscle weakness is typical, and patients may have varying degrees of muscle tenderness. The most important clinical distinction is between myopathy due to the primary effect of HIV and that due to zidovudine. Patients with symptomatic myopathy, especially with creatine kinase levels greater than 1000 units/L, should have their dose of zidovudine decreased or stopped and should be considered for alternative antiviral therapy. A muscle biopsy can distinguish HIV myopathy from zidovudine myopathy and should be considered in patients for whom continuation of zidovudine is essential.

7. Retinitis—Complaints of visual changes must be evaluated immediately in HIV-infected patients. CMV retinitis, characterized by perivascular hemorrhages and white fluffy exudates, is the most common retinal infection in AIDS patients and can be rapidly progressive. In contrast, cotton wool spots, which are also common in HIV-infected people, are benign, remit spontaneously, and appear as small indistinct white spots without exudation or hemorrhage. This distinction may be difficult at times for the nonspecialist, and patients with visual changes should be seen by an ophthalmologist. Other rare retinal processes include other herpesvirus infections or toxoplasmosis.

8. Oral lesions—The presence of oral candidiasis or hairy leukoplakia is significant for several reasons. First, these lesions are highly suggestive of HIV infection in patients who have no other obvious cause of immunodeficiency. Second, several studies have indicated that patients with candidiasis have a high rate of progression to AIDS even with statistical adjustment for CD4 count.

Hairy leukoplakia is caused by the Epstein-Barr virus. The lesion is not usually troubling to patients and sometimes regresses spontaneously. Hairy leukoplakia is commonly seen as a white lesion on the lateral aspect of the tongue. It may be flat or slightly raised, is usually corrugated, and has vertical parallel lines with fine or thick ("hairy") projections. Oral candidiasis can be bothersome to patients, many of whom report an unpleasant taste or mouth dryness. There are two major types of oral candidiasis: pseudomembranous (removable white plaques) and erythematous (red friable plaques). Treatment is with topical agents such as clotrimazole 10-mg troches (one troche four or five times a day). Patients with candidiasis who do not respond to topical antifungals can be treated with fluconazole (50–100 mg orally once a day for 3–7 days). Chronic suppression of oral candidiasis with fluconazole has been associated with development of candidiasis resistant to all available azoles and thus should be avoided except in frequently recurring cases.

Angular cheilitis—fissures at the sides of the mouth—is usually due to *Candida* as well and can be treated topically with ketoconazole cream (2%) twice a day.

Gingival disease is common in HIV-infected patients and is thought to be due to an overgrowth of microorganisms. It usually responds to professional dental cleaning and chlorhexidine rinses. A particularly aggressive gingivitis or periodontitis will develop in some HIV-infected patients; these patients should be given antibiotics that cover anaerobic oral flora (eg, metronidazole, 250 mg four times a day for 4 or 5 days) and referred to oral surgeons with experience with these entities.

Aphthous ulcers are painful and may interfere with eating. They can be treated with fluocinonide (0.05% ointment mixed 1:1 with plain Orabase and applied six times a day to the ulcer). For lesions that are difficult to reach, patients should use dexamethasone swishes (0.5 mg in 5 mL elixir three times a day). The pain of the ulcers can be relieved with use of an anesthetic spray (10% lidocaine). For patients with refractory ulcers, thalidomide, starting at a dose of 50 mg orally daily and increasing to 100–200 mg daily, has proved useful. It should be administered only to patients at zero risk of procreation. The most common side effects are sedation and peripheral neuropathy. Other lesions seen in the mouths of HIV-infected patients include Kaposi's sarcoma (usually on the hard palate) and warts.

9. Gastrointestinal manifestations—

a. Candidal esophagitis—(See also discussion in Chapter 14.) Esophageal candidiasis is a common AIDS infection. In a patient with characteristic symptoms, empiric antifungal treatment is begun with fluconazole (200 mg daily for 10–14 days). Further evaluation to identify other causes of esophagitis (herpes simplex, CMV) is reserved for patients who do not improve with treatment.

b. Hepatic disease—Autopsy studies have demonstrated that the liver is a frequent site of infections and neoplasms in HIV-infected patients. However, many of these infections are not clinically symptomatic. Clinicians may note elevations of alkaline phosphatase and aminotransferases on routine chemistry panels. Mycobacterial disease, CMV, hepatitis B virus, hepatitis C virus, and lymphoma cause liver disease and can present with varying degrees of nausea, vomiting, right upper quadrant abdominal pain, and jaundice. Sulfonamides, imidazole drugs, antituberculous medications, pentamidine, clarithromycin, and didanosine have also been associated with hepatitis. HIV-infected patients with chronic hepatitis may have more rapid progression of liver disease because of the concomitant immunodeficiency or hepatotoxicity of antiretroviral therapy. Percutaneous liver biopsy may be helpful in diagnosing liver disease, but some common causes of liver disease (eg, *Mycobacterium avium* complex, lymphoma) can be determined by less invasive measures (eg, blood culture, biopsy of a more accessible site). With patients living longer as a result of advances in antiretroviral therapy, advanced liver disease and hepatic failure due to chronic active hepatitis B and or C are increasing causes of morbidity and mortality. Treatment of HIV-infected persons with hepatitis B and C with peginterferon has been shown to be efficacious, although less so than in HIV-uninfected persons. HIV-infected persons are also more likely to have difficulty tolerating treatment with peginterferon than uninfected persons. Liver transplants have been performed successfully in HIV-infected patients. This strategy is most likely to be successful in persons who have CD4 counts above 100 cells/mcL and nondetectable viral loads.

c. Biliary disease—Cholecystitis presents with manifestations similar to those seen in immunocompetent hosts but is more likely to be acalculous. Sclerosing cholangitis and papillary stenosis have also been reported in HIV-infected patients. Typically, the syndrome presents with severe nausea, vomiting, and right upper quadrant pain. Liver function tests generally show alkaline phosphatase elevations disproportionate to elevation of the aminotransferases. Although dilated ducts can be seen on ultrasound, the diagnosis is made by endoscopic retrograde cholangiopancreatography, which reveals intraluminal irregularities of the proximal intrahepatic ducts with "pruning" of the terminal ductal branches. Stenosis of the distal common bile duct at the papilla is commonly seen with this syndrome. CMV, *Cryptosporidium*, and microsporidia are thought to play inciting roles in this syndrome.

d. Enterocolitis—Enterocolitis is a common problem in HIV-infected individuals. Organisms known to cause enterocolitis include bacteria (*Campylobacter, Salmonella, Shigella*), viruses (CMV, adenovirus), and protozoans (*Cryptosporidium, Entamoeba histolytica, Giardia, Isospora*, microsporidia). HIV itself may cause enterocolitis. Several of the organisms causing enterocolitis in HIV-infected individuals also cause diarrhea in immunocompetent hosts. However, HIV-infected patients tend to have more severe and more chronic symptoms, including high fevers and severe abdominal pain that can mimic acute abdominal catastrophes. Bacteremia and concomitant biliary involvement are also more common with enterocolitis in HIV-infected patients. Relapses of enterocolitis following adequate therapy have been reported with both *Salmonella* and *Shigella* infections.

Because of the wide range of agents known to cause enterocolitis, a stool culture and multiple stool examinations for ova and parasites (including modified acid-fast staining for *Cryptosporidium*) should be performed. Those patients who have *Cryptosporidium* in one stool with improvement in symptoms in less than 1 month should not be considered to have AIDS, as *Cryptosporidium* is a cause of self-limited diarrhea in HIV-negative persons. More commonly, HIV-infected patients with *Cryptosporidium* have persistent enterocolitis with profuse watery diarrhea.

To date, no consistently effective treatments have been developed for *Cryptosporidium* infection. The most effective treatment of cryptosporidiosis is to improve immune function through the use of effective antiretroviral treatment. The diarrhea can be treated symptomatically with diphenoxylate with atropine (one or two tablets orally three or four times a day). Those who do not respond may be given paregoric with bismuth (5–10 mL orally three or four times a day). Octreotide in escalating doses (starting at 0.05 mg subcutaneously every 8 hours for 48 hours) has been found to ameliorate symptoms in approximately 40% of patients with cryptosporidia or idiopathic HIV-associated diarrhea.

Patients with a negative stool examination and persistent symptoms should be evaluated with colonoscopy and biopsy. Patients whose symptoms last longer than 1 month with no identified cause of diarrhea are considered to have a presumptive diagnosis of AIDS enteropathy. Patients may respond to institution of effective antiretroviral treatment. Upper endoscopy with small bowel biopsy is not recommended as a routine part of the evaluation.

e. Other disorders—Two other important gastrointestinal abnormalities in HIV-infected patients are gastropathy and malabsorption. It has been documented that some HIV-infected patients do not produce normal levels of stomach acid and therefore are unable to absorb drugs that require an acid medium. This decreased acid production may explain, in part, the susceptibility of HIV-infected patients to *Campylobacter*, *Salmonella*, and *Shigella*, all of which are sensitive to acid concentration. There is no evidence that *Helicobacter pylori* is more common in HIV-infected persons.

A malabsorption syndrome occurs commonly in HIV-infected patients. It can be due to infection of the small bowel with *M avium* complex, *Cryptosporidium*, or microsporidia.

10. Endocrinologic manifestations—Hypogonadism is probably the most common endocrinologic abnormality in HIV-infected men. The adrenal gland is also a commonly afflicted endocrine gland in patients with AIDS. Abnormalities demonstrated on autopsy include infection (especially with CMV and *M avium* complex), infiltration with Kaposi's sarcoma, and injury from hemorrhage and presumed autoimmunity. The prevalence of clinically significant adrenal insufficiency is low. Patients with suggestive symptoms should undergo a cosyntropin stimulation test.

Although frank deficiency of cortisol is rare, an isolated defect in mineralocorticoid metabolism may lead to salt-wasting and hyperkalemia. Such patients should be treated with fludrocortisone (0.1–0.2 mg daily).

AIDS patients appear to have abnormalities of thyroid function tests different from those of patients with other chronic diseases. AIDS patients have been shown to have high levels of triiodothyronine (T_3), thyroxine (T_4), and thyroid-binding globulin and low levels of reverse triiodothyronine (rT_3). The causes and clinical significance of these abnormalities are unknown.

11. Skin manifestations—HIV-infected patients commonly develop skin manifestations that can be grouped into viral, bacterial, fungal, neoplastic, and nonspecific dermatitides.

Herpes simplex infections occur more frequently, tend to be more severe, and are more likely to disseminate in AIDS patients than in immunocompetent persons. Because of the risk of progressive local disease, all herpes simplex attacks should be treated with acyclovir (400 mg orally three times a day until healed, usually 7 days), famciclovir (500 mg orally twice daily until healed), or valacyclovir (500 mg orally twice daily until healed). To avoid the complications of attacks, many clinicians recommend suppressive therapy for HIV-infected patients with a history of recurrent herpes. Options for suppressive therapy include acyclovir (400 mg orally twice daily), famciclovir (250 mg orally twice daily), and valacyclovir (500 mg orally daily).

Herpes zoster is a common manifestation of HIV infection. As with herpes simplex infections, patients with zoster should be treated with acyclovir to prevent dissemination (800 mg orally four or five times per day for 7 days). Alternatively, famciclovir (500 mg orally three times a day) or valacyclovir (500 mg three times a day) may be used. Vesicular lesions should be cultured if there is any question about their origin, since herpes simplex responds to much lower doses of acyclovir. Disseminated zoster and cases with ocular involvement should be treated with intravenous (10 mg/kg every 8 hours for 7–10 days) rather than oral acyclovir.

Molluscum contagiosum caused by a pox virus is seen in HIV-infected patients, as in other immunocompromised patients. The characteristic umbilicated fleshy papular lesions have a propensity for spreading widely over the patient's face and neck and should be treated with topical liquid nitrogen.

Staphylococcus is the most common bacterial cause of skin disease in HIV-infected patients; it usually presents as **folliculitis, superficial abscesses (furuncles)**, or **bullous impetigo**. Because dissemination with sepsis has been reported, attempts should be made to treat these lesions aggressively. Folliculitis is initially treated with topical clindamycin or mupirocin, and patients may benefit from regular washing with an antibacterial soap such as chlorhexidine. Intranasal mupirocin has been used successfully for staphylococcal decolonization in other settings. In HIV-infected patients with recurrent staphylococcal infections, weekly intranasal mupirocin should be considered in addition to topical care and systemic antibiotics. Abscesses often require incision and drainage. Patients may need antistaphylococcal antibiotics as well. Due to high frequency of methicillin-resistant *Staphylococcus aureus* (MRSA) skin infections in HIV-infected populations, lesions should be cultured prior to initiating empiric antistaphylococcal therapy. Although there is limited experience treating MRSA with oral antibiotics, current recommendations for empiric treatment are trimethoprim-sulfamethoxazole (one double-strength tablet orally twice daily) or doxycycline (100 mg orally twice daily) with close follow-up.

Bacillary angiomatosis is a well-described entity in HIV-infected patients. It is caused by two closely related organisms: *Bartonella henselae* and *Bartonella quintana*. The epidemiology of these infections suggests zoonotic transmission from fleas of infected domestic cats. The most common manifestation is raised, reddish, highly vascular skin lesions that can mimic the lesions of Kaposi's sarcoma. Fever is a common manifestation of this infection; involvement of bone, lymph nodes, and liver has also been reported. The infection responds to doxycycline, 100 mg orally twice daily, or erythromycin, 250 mg orally four times daily. Therapy is continued for at least 14 days, and patients who are seriously ill with visceral involvement may require months of therapy.

The majority of **fungal rashes** afflicting AIDS patients are due to dermatophytes and *Candida*. These are particularly common in the inguinal region but may occur anywhere on the body. Fungal rashes generally respond well to topical clotrimazole (1% twice a day) or ketoconazole (2% twice a day).

Seborrheic dermatitis is more common in HIV-infected patients. Scrapings of seborrhea have revealed *Malassezia furfur (Pityrosporum ovale)*, implying that the seborrhea is caused by this fungus. Consistent with the isolation of this fungus is the clinical finding that seborrhea responds well to topical clotrimazole (1% cream) as well as hydrocortisone (1% cream).

Xerosis presents in HIV-infected patients with severe pruritus. The patient may have no rash, or nonspecific excoriations from scratching. Treatment is with emollients (eg, absorption base cream) and antipruritic lotions (eg, camphor 9.5% and menthol 0.5%).

Psoriasis can be very severe in HIV-infected patients. Phototherapy and etretinate (0.25–9.75 mg/kg/d orally in divided doses) may be used for recalcitrant cases in consultation with a dermatologist. Because of the underlying immunodeficiency, methotrexate should be avoided.

12. HIV-related malignancies—Four cancers are currently included in the CDC classification of AIDS: Kaposi's sarcoma, non-Hodgkin's lymphoma, primary lymphoma of the brain, and invasive cervical carcinoma. Epidemiologic studies have shown that between 1973 and 1987 among single men in San Francisco, the risk of Kaposi's sarcoma increased more than 5000-fold and the risk of non-Hodgkin's lymphoma more than tenfold. The increase in incidence of malignancies is probably a function of impaired cell-mediated immunity.

Kaposi's sarcoma lesions may appear anywhere; careful examination of the eyelids, conjunctiva, pinnae, palate, and toe webs is mandatory to locate potentially occult lesions. In light-skinned individuals, Kaposi's lesions usually appear as purplish, nonblanching lesions that can be papular or nodular. In dark-skinned individuals, the lesions may appear more brown. In the mouth, lesions are most often palatal papules, though exophytic lesions of the tongue and gingivae may also be seen. Kaposi's lesions may be confused with other vascular lesions such as angiomas and pyogenic granulomas. Visceral disease (eg, gastrointestinal, pulmonary) will develop in about 40% of patients with dermatologic Kaposi's sarcoma. Rapidly progressive dermatologic or visceral disease is best treated with systemic chemotherapy. Liposomally encapsulated doxorubicin given intravenously every 3 weeks has a response rate of approximately 70%. α-Interferon (10 million units subcutaneously three times a week) also has activity against Kaposi's sarcoma. However, symptoms such as malaise and anorexia limit the utility of this therapy. Patients with milder forms of Kaposi's sarcoma do not require specific treatment as the lesions usually improve and can completely resolve with antiretroviral therapy. However, it should be noted that the lesions may flare when antiretroviral therapy is first initiated—probably as a result of an immune reconstitution process (see Inflammatory reactions below).

Non-Hodgkin's lymphoma in HIV-infected persons tends to be very aggressive. The malignancies are usually of B cell origin and characterized as diffuse large-cell tumors. Over 70% of the malignancies are extranodal.

The prognosis of patients with systemic non-Hodgkin's lymphoma depends primarily on the degree of immunodeficiency at the time of diagnosis. Patients with high CD4 counts do markedly better than those diagnosed at a late stage of illness. Patients with primary central nervous system lymphoma are treated with radiation. Response to treatment is good, but prior to the availability of HAART, most patients died within a few months after diagnosis due to their underlying disease. Systemic disease is treated with chemotherapy. Common regimens are CHOP (cyclophosphamide, doxorubicin, vincristine, and prednisone) and modified M-BACOD (methotrexate, bleomycin, doxorubicin, cyclophosphamide, vincristine, and dexamethasone). Granulocyte colony-stimulating factor (G-CSF; filgrastim) is used to maintain white blood counts with this latter regimen. Intrathecal chemotherapy is administered to prevent or treat meningeal involvement.

Although **Hodgkin's disease** is not included as part of the CDC definition of AIDS, studies have found that HIV infection is associated with a fivefold increase in the incidence of Hodgkin's disease. HIV-infected persons with Hodgkin's disease are more likely to have mixed cellularity and lymphocyte depletion subtypes of Hodgkin's disease and to seek medical attention at an advanced stage of disease.

Anal dysplasia and squamous cell carcinoma have been noted in HIV-infected homosexual men.

These lesions have been strongly correlated with previous infection by human papillomavirus (HPV). Although many of the infected men report a history of anal warts or have visible warts, a significant percentage have silent papillomavirus infection. Cytologic (using Papanicolaou smears) and papillomavirus DNA studies can easily be performed on specimens obtained by anal swab. The growing frequency of these problems and the risk of progression from dysplasia to cancer in immunocompromised patients suggest that annual anal swabs for cytologic examination should be done in all HIV-infected persons who have engaged in receptive anal intercourse. An anal Papanicolaou smear is performed by rotating a moistened Dacron swab about 2 cm into the anal canal. The swab is immediately inserted into a cytology bottle.

HPV also appears to play a causative role in **cervical dysplasia and neoplasia**. The incidence and clinical course of cervical disease in HIV-infected women are discussed below.

13. Gynecologic manifestations—Vaginal candidiasis, cervical dysplasia and neoplasia, and pelvic inflammatory disease are more common in HIV-infected women than in uninfected women. These manifestations also tend to be more severe when they occur in association with HIV infection. Therefore, HIV-infected women need frequent gynecologic care. Vaginal candidiasis may be treated with topical agents (see Chapter 36). However, HIV-infected women with recurrent or severe vaginal candidiasis may need systemic therapy.

The incidence of cervical dysplasia in HIV-infected women is 40%. Because of this finding, HIV-infected women should have Papanicolaou smears every 6 months (as opposed to the Agency for Healthcare Research and Quality [AHRQ] Guideline recommendation for every 12 months). Some clinicians recommend routine colposcopy or cervicography because cervical intraepithelial neoplasia has occurred in women with negative Papanicolaou smears. Cone biopsy is indicated in cases of serious cervical dysplasia.

Cervical neoplasia appears to be more aggressive among HIV-infected women. Most HIV-infected women with cervical cancer die of that disease rather than of AIDS. Because of its frequency and severity, cervical neoplasia was added to the CDC definition of AIDS in 1993.

While pelvic inflammatory disease appears to be more common in HIV-infected women, the bacteriology of this condition appears to be the same as among HIV-uninfected women. At present, HIV-infected women with pelvic inflammatory disease should be treated with the same regimens as uninfected women (see Chapter 17). However, inpatient therapy is generally recommended.

14. Inflammatory reactions (immune reconstitution syndromes or "IRIS")—With initiation of HAART, some patients experience inflammatory reactions that appear to be associated with immune reconstitution as indicated by a rapid increase in CD4 count.

These inflammatory reactions may present with generalized signs of fevers, sweats, and malaise with or without more localized manifestations that usually represent unusual presentations of opportunistic infections. For example, vitreitis has developed in patients with CMV retinitis after they have been treated with HAART. *M avium* can present as focal lymphadenitis or granulomatous masses in patients receiving HAART. Tuberculosis may paradoxically worsen with new or evolving pulmonary infiltrates and lymphadenopathy. PML and cryptococcal meningitis may also behave atypically. Clinicians should be alert to these syndromes, which are most often seen in patients who have initiated antiretroviral therapy in the setting of advanced disease and who show rapid increases in CD4 counts with treatment. The diagnosis of IRIS is one of exclusion and can be made only after recurrence or new opportunistic infection has been ruled out as the cause of the clinical deterioration. Management of IRIS is conservative and supportive with use of corticosteroids only for severe reactions. Most authorities recommend that antiretroviral therapy be continued unless the reaction is life-threatening.

B. LABORATORY FINDINGS

Specific tests for HIV include antibody and antigen detection (Table 31–2). Conventional HIV antibody testing is done by ELISA. Positive specimens are then confirmed by a different method (eg, Western blot). The sensitivity of screening serologic tests is greater than 99.5%. The specificity of positive results by two different techniques approaches 100% even in low-risk populations. False-positive screening tests may occur as normal biologic variants or in association with recent influenza vaccination or other disease states, such as connective tissue disease. These are usually detected by negative confirmatory tests. Molecular biology techniques (PCR) show a small incidence of individuals (< 1%) who are infected with HIV for up to 36 months without generating an antibody response. However, antibodies that are detectable by screening serologic tests will develop in 95% of persons within 6 weeks after infection.

Rapid HIV antibody tests are now available. They provide results within 10–20 minutes and can be performed in physician offices, including by personnel without laboratory training and without a Clinical Laboratory Improvement Amendment (CLIA) approved laboratory. Persons who test positive on a rapid test should be told that they may be HIV-infected or their test may be falsely reactive. Standard testing (ELISA with Western blot confirmation) should be performed to distinguish these two possibilities. Rapid testing is particularly helpful in settings where a result is needed immediately (eg, a woman in labor who has not recently been tested for HIV) or when the patient is unlikely to return for a result.

Nonspecific laboratory findings with HIV infection may include anemia, leukopenia (particularly lymphopenia), and thrombocytopenia in any combi-

Table 31–2. Laboratory findings with HIV infection.

Test	Significance
HIV enzyme-linked immunosorbent assay (ELISA)	Screening test for HIV infection. Of ELISA tests 50% are positive within 22 days after HIV transmission; 95% are positive within 6 weeks after transmission. Sensitivity > 99.9%; to avoid false-positive results, repeatedly reactive results must be confirmed with Western blot.
Western blot	Confirmatory test for HIV. Specificity when combined with ELISA > 99.99%. Indeterminate results with early HIV infection, HIV-2 infection, autoimmune disease, pregnancy, and recent tetanus toxoid administration.
HIV rapid antibody test	Screening test for HIV. Produces results in 10–20 minutes. Can be performed by personnel with limited training. Positive results must be confirmed with standard HIV test (ELISA and Western blot).
Complete blood count	Anemia, neutropenia, and thrombocytopenia common with advanced HIV infection.
Absolute CD4 lymphocyte count	Most widely used predictor of HIV progression. Risk of progression to an AIDS opportunistic infection or malignancy is high with CD4 < 200 cells/mcL in the absence of treatment.
CD4 lymphocyte percentage	Percentage may be more reliable than the CD4 count. Risk of progression to an AIDS opportunistic infection or malignancy is high with percentage < 20% in the absence of treatment.
HIV viral load tests	These tests measure the amount of actively replicating HIV virus. Correlate with disease progression and response to antiretroviral drugs. Best tests available for diagnosis of acute HIV infection (prior to seroconversion); however, caution is warranted when the test result shows low-level viremia (ie, <500 copies) as this may represent a false-positive test.

nation, elevation of the erythrocyte sedimentation rate, polyclonal hypergammaglobulinemia, and hypocholesterolemia. Cutaneous anergy is common.

Several laboratory markers are available to provide prognostic information and guide therapy decisions (Table 31–2). The most widely used marker is the absolute CD4 lymphocyte count. As counts decrease, the risk of serious opportunistic infection over the subsequent 3–5 years increases (Figure 31–1).

There are many limitations to using the CD4 count, including diurnal variation, depression with intercurrent illness, and intralaboratory and interlaboratory variability. Therefore, the trend is more important than a single determination. The frequency of performance of counts depends on the patient's health status. Patients whose CD4 counts are substantially above the threshold for initiation of antiviral therapy (350 cells/mcL) should have counts performed every 6 months. Those who have counts near or below 350 cells/mcL should have counts performed every 3 months. This is necessary for evaluating the efficacy of antiviral therapy and for initiating *P jiroveci* prophylactic therapy when the CD4 count drops below 200 cells/mcL. Some studies suggest that the percentage of CD4 lymphocytes is a more reliable indicator of prognosis than the absolute counts because the percentage does not depend on calculating a manual differential. While the CD4 count measures immune dysfunction, it does not provide a measure of how actively HIV is replicating in the body. HIV viral load tests (discussed below) assess the level of viral replication and provide useful prognostic information that is independent of the information provided by CD4 counts.

Chung RT et al: Peginterferon alfa-2a plus ribavirin versus interferon alfa-2a plus ribavirin for chronic hepatitis C in HIV-coinfected persons. N Engl J Med 2004;351:451. [PMID: 15282352]

DeSimone JA et al: Inflammatory reactions in HIV-1-infected persons after initiation of highly active antiretroviral therapy. Ann Intern Med 2000;133:447. [PMID: 10975963]

Ellis E et al: Eosinophilic pustular folliculitis: a comprehensive review of treatment options. Am J Clin Dermatol 2004;5:189. [PMID: 15186198]

Grinspoon S et al: Effects of testosterone and progressive resistance training in eugonadal men with AIDS wasting. A randomized, controlled trial. Ann Intern Med 2000;133:348. [PMID: 10979879]

Keenan PA et al: Rapid HIV testing. Wait time reduced from days to minutes. Postgrad Med 2005;117:47. [PMID: 15782674]

Kovacs JA et al: New insights into the transmission, diagnosis, and drug treatment of *Pneumocystis carinii* pneumonia. JAMA 2001;286:2450. [PMID: 11712941]

Little RF et al: HIV-associated non-Hodgkin lymphoma: incidence, presentation, and prognosis. JAMA 2001;285:1880. [PMID: 11308402]

Marcellin P et al: Peginterferon alfa-2a alone, lamivudine alone, and the two in combination in patients with HbeAg-negative chronic hepatitis B. N Engl J Med 2004;351:1206. [PMID: 15371578]

Norris S: Outcomes of liver transplantation in HIV-infected individuals: the impact of HCV and HBV infection. Liver Transpl 2004;10:1271. [PMID: 15376307]

Sacktor N: The epidemiology of human immunodeficiency virus-associated neurological disease in the era of highly active antiretroviral therapy. J Neurovirol 2002;8(Suppl 2):115. [PMID: 12491162]

Stevens DL et al: Practice guidelines for the diagnosis and management of skin and soft-tissue infections. Clin Infect Dis 2005;41:1373. [PMID: 16231249]

Wyen C: Progressive multifocal leukoencephalopathy in patients on highly active antiretroviral therapy: survival and risk factors of death. J Acquir Immune Defic Syndr 2004;37:1263. [PMID: 15385733]

Differential Diagnosis

HIV infection may mimic a variety of other medical illnesses. Specific differential diagnosis depends on the mode of presentation. In patients presenting with constitutional symptoms such as weight loss and fevers, differential considerations include cancer, chronic infections such as tuberculosis and endocarditis, and endocrinologic diseases such as hyperthyroidism. When pulmonary processes dominate the presentation, acute and chronic lung infections must be considered as well as other causes of diffuse interstitial pulmonary infiltrates. When neurologic disease is the mode of presentation, conditions that cause mental status changes or neuropathy—eg, alcoholism, liver disease, renal dysfunction, thyroid disease, and vitamin deficiency—should be considered. If a patient presents with headache and a cerebrospinal fluid pleocytosis, other causes of chronic meningitis enter the differential. When diarrhea is a prominent complaint, infectious enterocolitis, antibiotic-associated colitis, inflammatory bowel disease, and malabsorptive symptoms must be considered.

Prevention

A. Primary Prevention

Until vaccination is a reality, prevention of HIV infection will depend on effective precautions regarding sexual practices and injection drug use, use of perinatal HIV prophylaxis, screening of blood products, and infection control practices in the health care setting. Primary care clinicians should routinely obtain a sexual history and provide risk factor assessment of their patients and, when appropriate, screening for HIV infection with pretest and posttest counseling. Pretest counseling should include review of risk factors for HIV infection, discussion of safe sex and safe needle use, and the meaning of a positive test. Posttest counseling should include a review of the importance of safe sex and needle use practices. For persons who test positive, information on available medical and mental health services should be provided as well as guidance for contacting sexual or needle-sharing partners. It is the duty of clinicians to counsel HIV-negative patients on how to avoid exposure to HIV. Patients should be counseled not to exchange bodily fluids unless they are in a long-term mutually monogamous relationship with someone who has tested HIV antibody-negative and has not engaged in unsafe sex, injection drug use, or other HIV risk behaviors for at least 6 months prior to or at any time since the negative test.

Only latex condoms should be used, along with a water-soluble lubricant. Although nonoxynol-9, a spermicide, kills HIV, it is contraindicated because in some patients it may cause genital ulcers that could facilitate HIV transmission. Patients should be counseled that condoms are not 100% effective. They should be made familiar with the use of condoms, including, specifically, the advice that condoms must be used every time, that space should be left at the tip of the condom as a receptacle for semen, that intercourse with a condom should not be attempted if the penis is only partially erect, that men should hold on to the base of the condom when withdrawing the penis to prevent slippage, and that condoms should not be reused. Although anal intercourse remains the sexual practice at highest risk of transmitting HIV, seroconversions have been documented with vaginal and oral intercourse as well. Therefore, condoms should be used when engaging in these activities. Women as well as men should understand how to use condoms so as to be sure that their partners are using them correctly.

Persons using injection drugs should be cautioned never to exchange needles or other drug paraphernalia. When sterile needles are not available, bleach does appear to inactivate HIV and should be used to clean needles.

Current efforts to screen blood and blood products have lowered the risk of HIV transmission with transfusion of a unit of blood to 1:1,000,000.

In the hospital, concerns about nosocomial infection have led to the recommendation for universal body fluid precautions. This involves the rigorous use of gloves when handling any body fluid and the addition of gown, mask, and goggles for procedures that may result in splash or droplet spread as well as the use of specially designed needles with sheath devices to decrease the risk of needle sticks. Reports of transmission of drug-resistant tuberculosis in health care settings also have had infection control implications. All patients with cough in outpatient settings should be encouraged to wear masks. Hospitalized HIV-infected patients with cough should be placed in respiratory isolation until tuberculosis can be excluded by chest radiograph and sputum smear examination.

Primate model data have suggested that development of a protective vaccine may be possible, but clinical trials in humans using gp120 or its precursor gp160 have shown development of neutralizing antibodies to laboratory but not field isolates of HIV and may not be protective of infection. Many scientists have abandoned the quest for a fully protective HIV vaccine and are focusing on developing a vaccine that would reduce the chances of HIV transmission given a particular exposure.

B. Secondary Prevention

In the era prior to the development of highly effective antiretroviral treatment, cohort studies of individuals with documented dates of seroconversion demonstrate that AIDS develops within 10 years in approximately 50% of untreated seropositive persons. Recent improvements in treatment would be expected to substantially improve this prognosis. Too few persons have been treated with these regimens prior to the development of AIDS to pro-

Table 31–3. Health care maintenance of HIV-infected individuals.

For all HIV-infected individuals:
  CD4 counts every 3–6 months
  Viral load tests every 3–6 months and 1 month following a
    change in therapy
  PPD
  INH for those with positive PPD and normal chest x-ray
  RPR or VDRL
  Toxoplasma IgG serology
  CMV IgG serology
  Pneumococcal vaccine
  Influenza vaccine in season
  Hepatitis B vaccine for those who are HBsAb-negative
  Haemophilus influenzae type b vaccination
  Papanicolaou smears every 6 months for women
  Consider anal swabs for cytologic evaluation yearly for pa-
    tients with history of receptive anal intercourse
For HIV-infected individuals with CD4 < 200 cells/mcL:
  Pneumocystis jiroveci[1] prophylaxis (see Table 31–6)
For HIV-infected individuals with CD4 < 75 cells/mcL:
  Mycobacterium avium complex prophylaxis
For HIV-infected individuals with CD4 < 50 cells/mcL:
  Consider CMV prophylaxis

---

[1]Formerly known as *Pneumocystis carinii*.
PPD = purified protein derivative; INH = isonicotinic acid hydrazide (isoniazid); RPR = rapid plasma reagin; VDRL = Venereal Disease Research Laboratories; IgG = immunoglobulin G; HBsAb = antibody to the hepatitis B surface antigen; CMV = cytomegalovirus.

---

vide good data on progression of disease with these new regimens. Nevertheless, decreases in the incidence of AIDS reflecting successful treatment of HIV and successful HIV prevention efforts have been reported in the United States and western Europe.

There is substantial evidence that prophylactic regimens can prevent opportunistic infections and improve survival. Prophylaxis and early intervention prevent several infectious diseases, including tuberculosis and syphilis, which are transmissible to others. Recommendations are listed in Table 31–3.

Because of the increased occurrence of tuberculosis among HIV-infected patients, all such individuals should undergo PPD testing. Although anergy is common among AIDS patients, the likelihood of a false-negative result is much lower when the test is done early in infection. Those with positive tests (defined for HIV-infected patients as > 5 mm of induration) need a chest radiograph. Patients with an infiltrate in any location, especially if accompanied by mediastinal adenopathy, should have sputum sent for acid-fast staining. Patients with a positive PPD but negative evaluations for active disease should receive isoniazid (300 mg daily) with pyridoxine (50 mg daily) for 9 months to a year. An alternative regimen of rifampin plus pyrazinamide for 2 months is no longer recommended because of the high associated incidence of hepatotoxicity. Recent analysis suggests also that HIV-infected individuals at high risk for tuberculosis

should receive a course of isoniazid prophylaxis regardless of the PPD status. This may include homeless individuals and injection drug users.

Because of recent increases in the number of cases of syphilis among men who have sex with men, including those who are HIV infected, all such men should be screened for syphilis by rapid plasma reagin (RPR) or Venereal Disease Research Laboratories (VDRL) test every 6 months. Increases of syphilis cases among HIV-infected persons are of particular concern because these individuals are at increased risk for reactivation of syphilis and progression to tertiary syphilis despite standard treatment. Because the only widely available tests for syphilis are serologic and because HIV-infected individuals are known to have disordered antibody production, there is concern about the interpretation of these titers. This concern has been fueled by a report of an HIV-infected patient with secondary syphilis and negative syphilis serologic testing. Furthermore, HIV-infected individuals may lose fluorescent treponemal antibody absorption (FTA-ABS) reactivity after treatment for syphilis, particularly if they have low CD4 counts. Thus, in this population, a nonreactive treponemal test does not rule out a past history of syphilis. In addition, persistence of treponemes in the spinal fluid after one dose of benzathine penicillin has been demonstrated in HIV-infected patients with primary and secondary syphilis. Therefore, the CDC has recommended an aggressive diagnostic approach to HIV-infected patients with reactive RPR or VDRL tests of greater than 1 year or unknown duration. All such patients should have a lumbar puncture with cerebrospinal fluid cell count and cerebrospinal fluid VDRL. Those with a normal cerebrospinal fluid evaluation are treated as having late latent syphilis (benzathine penicillin G, 2.4 million units intramuscularly weekly for 3 weeks) with follow-up titers. Those with a pleocytosis or a positive cerebrospinal fluid VDRL test are treated as having neurosyphilis (aqueous penicillin G, 2–4 million units intravenously every 4 hours, or procaine penicillin G, 2.4 million units intramuscularly daily, with probenecid, 500 mg four times daily, for 10 days). Some clinicians take a less aggressive approach to patients who have low titers (less than 1:8), a history of having been treated for syphilis, and a normal neurologic examination. Close follow-up of titers is mandatory if such a course is taken. For a more detailed discussion of this topic, see Chapter 34.

The efficacy of pneumococcal vaccine is debated, but since it is safe, HIV-infected individuals should receive it. Patients without evidence of hepatitis B surface antigen or surface antibody should receive hepatitis B vaccination. Live vaccines, such as yellow fever vaccine, should be avoided. Measles vaccination, while a live virus vaccine, appears relatively safe when administered to HIV-infected individuals and should be given if the patient has never had measles or been adequately vaccinated.

A randomized study found that multivitamin supplementation decreased HIV disease progression and mortality in HIV-infected women in Africa. However, supplementation is unlikely to be as effective in well-nourished populations.

HIV-infected individuals should be counseled with regard to safe sex. Because of the risk of transmission, they should be warned to use condoms with sexual intercourse, including oral intercourse. Partners of HIV-infected women should use latex barriers such as dental dams (available at dental supply stores) to prevent direct oral contact with vaginal secretions. Substance abuse treatment should be recommended for persons who are using recreational drugs. They should be warned to avoid consuming raw meat or eggs to avoid infections with *Toxoplasma, Campylobacter,* and *Salmonella.* HIV-infected patients should wash their hands thoroughly after cleaning cat litter or should forgo this household chore to avoid possible exposure to toxoplasmosis. To reduce the likelihood of infection with *Bartonella* species, patients should avoid activities that might result in cat scratches or bites. Although the data are not conclusive, many clinicians recommend that HIV-infected persons—especially those with low CD4 counts—drink bottled water instead of tap water to prevent cryptosporidia infection.

Because of the emotional impact of HIV infection and subsequent illness, many patients will benefit from supportive counseling.

C. HIV Risk for Health Care Professionals

Epidemiologic studies show that needle sticks occur commonly among health care professionals, especially among surgeons performing invasive procedures, inexperienced hospital house staff, and medical students. Efforts to reduce needle sticks should focus on avoiding recapping needles and use of safety needles whenever doing invasive procedures under controlled circumstances. The risk of HIV transmission from a needle stick with blood from an HIV-infected patient is about 1:300. The risk is higher with deep punctures, large inocula, and source patients with high viral loads. The risk from mucous membrane contact is too low to quantitate.

Health care professionals who sustain needle sticks should be counseled and offered HIV testing as soon as possible. HIV testing is done to establish a negative baseline for worker's compensation claims in case there is a subsequent conversion. Follow-up testing is usually performed at 6 weeks, 3 months, and 6 months.

A case-control study by the CDC indicates that administration of zidovudine following a needle stick decreases the rate of HIV seroconversion by 79%. Therefore, providers should be offered therapy with Combivir (zidovudine 300 mg plus lamivudine 150 mg orally twice daily). Providers who have exposures to persons who are likely to have antiretroviral drug resistance (eg, persons receiving therapy who have detectable viral loads) should have their therapy individualized, using at least two drugs to which the source is unlikely to be resistant. Some clinicians recommend triple combination regimens, including a protease inhibitor for all occupational exposures, because of uncertainty about drug resistance. Others save these more aggressive regimens for the higher-risk exposures listed above. Because reports have noted hepatotoxicity due to nevirapine in this setting, this agent should be avoided. Therapy should be started as soon as possible after exposure and continued for 4 weeks. Unfortunately, there have been documented cases of seroconversion following potential parenteral exposure to HIV despite prompt use of zidovudine prophylaxis. Counseling of the provider should include "safe sex" guidelines.

D. Postexposure Prophylaxis for Sexual and Drug Use Exposures to HIV

Following publication of a case-control study indicating that antiretroviral therapy decreased the odds of seroconversion among health care workers who had occupational exposure, some experts have recommended offering antiretroviral therapy following potential exposure to HIV through sexual activity or drug use. Although there are no efficacy data to support this practice, there are similarities between the immune response following transcutaneous and transmucosal exposures. The goal of postexposure prophylaxis is to reduce or prevent local viral replication prior to dissemination such that the infection can be aborted.

The choice of antiretroviral agents and the duration of treatment are the same as those for exposures that occur through the occupational route (see above). In contrast to those with occupational exposures, some individuals may present very late after exposure. Because the likelihood of success declines with length of time from HIV exposure, it is not recommended that treatment be offered after 72 hours. In addition, because the psychosocial issues involved with postexposure prophylaxis for sexual and drug use exposures are complex, it should be offered only in the context of prevention counseling. Counseling should focus on how to prevent future exposures.

E. Preventing Perinatal Transmission of HIV

A multicenter trial showed that when zidovudine is administered to women during pregnancy, labor, and delivery and to their newborns, the rate of HIV transmission is decreased by two-thirds. An observational trial demonstrated that zidovudine treatment is almost as effective when begun during labor or when administered only to the infant, as long as treatment is begun within 48 hours after birth. Nonetheless, treatment begun by at least the second trimester is still recommended. Many women are currently being offered combination antiretroviral treatment to further lower the risk of transmission. The availability of treatment makes it essential that all women who are pregnant or considering pregnancy be offered HIV counseling and testing. Many obstetricians recommend combination antiretroviral treatment, especially if zidovudine resistance is suspected. HIV-infected women receiving antiretroviral therapy in whom pregnancy is recognized during the first trimester should be counseled about the benefits and potential risks to the fetus of treatment during the first trimester. Because healthy mothers make healthy babies, continuation of therapy should be strongly considered. Because about half of fetal infections in non-breast-feeding women occur shortly before or during the birth process, antiretroviral therapy should be administered whenever a woman initiates perinatal care even if she did not begin therapy in the second trimester. Breast-feeding is thought to increase the rate of transmission by 10–20% and should be avoided.

Aragon TJ et al: Endemic cryptosporidiosis and exposure to municipal tap water in persons with acquired immunodeficiency syndrome (AIDS): a case-control study. BMC Public Health 2003;3:2. [PMID: 12515584]

Fawzi WW et al: A randomized trial of multivitamin supplements and HIV disease progression and mortality. N Engl J Med 2004;351:23. [PMID: 15229304]

Hammer SM: Management of newly diagnosed HIV infection. N Engl J Med 2005;353:1702. [PMID: 16236741]

Johnson WD et al: HIV prevention research for men who have sex with men: a systematic review and meta-analysis. J Acquir Immune Defic Syndr 2002;30(Suppl 1):S118. [PMID: 12107365]

Katz MH et al: Management of occupational and nonoccupational postexposure HIV prophylaxis. Curr HIV/AIDS Rep 2004;1:159. [PMID: 16091237]

Smith DK: Antiretroviral postexposure prophylaxis after sexual, injection-drug use, or other nonoccupational exposure to HIV in the United States: recommendations from the U.S. Department of Health and Human Services. MMWR Recomm Rep 2005;54(RR-2):1. [PMID: 15660015]

Treatment

Treatment for HIV infection can be divided into four categories: therapy for opportunistic infections and malignancies, antiretroviral treatment, hematopoietic stimulating factors, and prophylaxis of opportunistic infections.

Experimental treatment regimens for HIV infection are constantly changing. Clinicians may obtain up-to-date information on experimental treatments by calling the AIDS Clinical Trials Information Service (ACTIS), 800-TRIALS-A (English and Spanish), and the National AIDS Hot Line, 800-342-AIDS (English), 800-344-SIDA (Spanish), and 800-AIDS-TTY (hearing-impaired).

A. THERAPY FOR OPPORTUNISTIC INFECTIONS AND MALIGNANCIES

Treatment of common HIV infections and malignancies is detailed in Table 31–4. In the era prior to the use of HAART, patients required lifelong treatment for many infections, including CMV retinitis, toxoplasmosis, and cryptococcal meningitis. However, among patients who have a good response to HAART, maintenance therapy for some opportunistic infections can be terminated. For example, in consultation with an ophthalmologist, maintenance treatment for CMV infection can be discontinued in persons with durable suppression of viral load on HAART who have a CD4 count > 100–150 cells/mcL. Similar results have been observed in patients with *M avium* complex bacteremia.

The emergence of resistance is more common for some infections of HIV-infected people (eg, acyclovir-resistant herpes simplex) than among immunocompetent individuals. In addition, HIV-infected patients have an increased incidence of side effects to standard drugs such as trimethoprim-sulfamethoxazole.

Treating patients with repeated episodes of the same opportunistic infection can pose difficult therapeutic challenges. For example, patients with second or third episodes of *Pneumocystis* pneumonia may have developed allergic reactions to standard treatments with a prior episode. Fortunately, there are several alternatives available for the treatment of *Pneumocystis* infection. Trimethoprim with dapsone and primaquine with clindamycin are two combinations that often are tolerated in patients with a prior allergic reaction to trimethoprim-sulfamethoxazole and intravenous pentamidine. On the positive side, patients in whom second episodes of *Pneumocystis* pneumonia develop while taking prophylaxis tend to have milder courses.

Well-established alternative regimens now also exist for most AIDS-related opportunistic infections: amphotericin B or fluconazole for cryptococcal meningitis; ganciclovir, cidofovir, or foscarnet for CMV infection; and sulfadiazine or clindamycin with pyrimethamine for toxoplasmosis.

Although conceptually it would seem that **corticosteroid** therapy should be avoided in HIV-infected patients, corticosteroid use has been shown to improve the course of patients with moderate to severe pneumocystosis (oxygen saturation < 90%, P_{O_2} < 65 mm Hg) when administered within 72 hours after diagnosis. The mechanism of action is presumed to be a decrease in alveolar inflammation.

B. ANTIRETROVIRAL THERAPY

The availability of agents that in combination suppress HIV replication (Table 31–5) has had a profound impact on the natural history of HIV infection. Patients who achieve excellent suppression of HIV generally have stabilization or improvement of their clinical course that results from partial immunologic reconstitution and a subsequent decrease in complications of immunosuppression. The best time to initiate antiretroviral treatment remains controversial. It is best to weigh the benefits of viral suppression against the side effects of the drugs for each patient. In general, treatment for asymptomatic HIV disease should be initiated when the CD4 cell count drops below 350 cells/mcL or symptomatic HIV disease. Patients with rapidly dropping CD4 counts or very high viral loads (> 100,000/mcL) should be considered for earlier treatment. For those patients who might have difficulty adhering to treatment or who are at higher risk for toxicity (eg, underlying liver disease), waiting until the CD4 count nears 200 cells/mcL may be a better strategy. Although emerging data suggest that every effort should be made to initiate antiretroviral therapy at CD4 counts below 350 cells/mcL, patients who started treatment at higher CD4 levels than

Table 31–4. Treatment of AIDS-related opportunistic infections and malignancies.[1]

Infection or Malignancy	Treatment	Complications
Pneumocystis jiroveci infection[2]	Trimethoprim-sulfamethoxazole, 15 mg/kg/d (based on trimethoprim component) orally or intravenously for 14–21 days.	Nausea, neutropenia, anemia, hepatitis, drug rash, Stevens-Johnson syndrome.
	Pentamidine, 3–4 mg/kg/d IV for 14–21 days.	Hypotension, hypoglycemia, anemia, neutropenia, pancreatitis, hepatitis.
	Trimethoprim, 15 mg/kg/d orally, with dapsone, 100 mg/d orally, for 14–21 days.[3]	Nausea, rash, hemolytic anemia in G6PD[3]-deficient patients. Methemoglobinemia (weekly levels should be < 10% of total hemoglobin).
	Primaquine, 15–30 mg/d orally, and clindamycin, 600 mg every 8 hours orally, for 14–21 days.	Hemolytic anemia in G6PD-deficient patients. Methemoglobinemia, neutropenia, colitis.
	Atovaquone, 750 mg orally three times daily for 14–21 days.	Rash, elevated aminotransferases, anemia, neutropenia.
	Trimetrexate, 45 mg/m² intravenously for 21 days (given with leucovorin calcium) if intolerant of all other regimens.	Leukopenia, rash, mucositis.
Mycobacterium avium complex infection	Clarithromycin, 500 mg orally twice daily with ethambutol, 15 mg/kg/d orally (maximum, 1 g). May also add:	Clarithromycin: hepatitis, nausea, diarrhea; ethambutol: hepatitis, optic neuritis.
	Rifabutin, 300 mg orally daily.	Rash, hepatitis, uveitis.
Toxoplasmosis	Pyrimethamine, 100–200 mg orally as loading dose, followed by 50–75 mg/d, combined with sulfadiazine, 4–6 g orally daily in four divided doses, and folinic acid, 10 mg daily for 4–8 weeks; then pyrimethamine, 25–50 mg/d, with clindamycin, 2–2.7 g/d in three or four divided doses, and folinic acid, 5 mg/d, until clinical and radiographic resolution is achieved.	Leukopenia, rash.
Lymphoma	Combination chemotherapy (eg, modified CHOP, M-BACOD, with or without G-CSF or GM-CSF). Central nervous system disease: radiation treatment with dexamethasone for edema.	Nausea, vomiting, anemia, leukopenia, cardiac toxicity (with doxorubicin).
Cryptococcal meningitis	Amphotericin B, 0.6 mg/kg/d intravenously, with or without flucytosine, 100 mg/kg/d orally in four divided doses for 2 weeks, followed by:	Fever, anemia, hypokalemia, azotemia.
	Fluconazole, 400 mg orally daily for 6 weeks, then 200 mg orally daily.	Hepatitis.
Cytomegalovirus infection	Valganciclovir, 900 mg orally twice a day for 21 days with food (induction), followed by 900 mg daily with food (maintenance).	Neutropenia, anemia, thrombocytopenia.
	Ganciclovir, 10 mg/kg/d intravenously in two divided doses for 10 days, followed by 6 mg/kg 5 days a week indefinitely. (Decrease dose for renal impairment.) May use ganciclovir as maintenance therapy (1 g orally with fatty foods three times a day).	Neutropenia (especially when used concurrently with zidovudine), anemia, thrombocytopenia.
	Foscarnet, 60 mg/kg intravenously every 8 hours for 10–14 days (induction), followed by 90 mg/kg once daily. (Adjust for changes in renal function.)	Nausea, hypokalemia, hypocalcemia, hyperphosphatemia, azotemia.

(continued)

Table 31–4. Treatment of AIDS-related opportunistic infections and malignancies.[1] (continued)

Infection or Malignancy	Treatment	Complications
Esophageal candidiasis or recurrent vaginal candidiasis	Fluconazole, 100–200 mg daily for 10–14 days.	Hepatitis, development of imidazole resistance.
Herpes simplex infection	Acyclovir, 400 mg three times daily until healed; or acyclovir, 5 mg/kg intravenously every 8 hours for severe cases.	Resistant herpes simplex with chronic therapy.
	Famciclovir, 500 mg orally twice daily until healed.	Nausea.
	Valacyclovir, 500 mg orally twice daily until healed.	Nausea.
	Foscarnet, 40 mg/kg intravenously every 8 hours, for acyclovir-resistant cases. (Adjust for changes in renal function.)	See above.
Herpes zoster	Acyclovir, 800 mg orally four or five times daily for 7 days. Intravenous therapy at 10 mg/kg every 8 hours for ocular involvement, disseminated disease.	See above.
	Famciclovir, 500 mg orally three times daily for 7 days.	Nausea.
	Valacyclovir, 500 mg orally three times daily for 7 days.	Nausea.
	Foscarnet, 40 mg/kg intravenously every 8 hours for acyclovir-resistant cases. (Adjust for changes in renal function.)	See above.
Kaposi's sarcoma Limited cutaneous disease	Observation, intralesional vinblastine.	Inflammation, pain at site of injection.
Extensive or aggressive cutaneous disease	Systemic chemotherapy (eg, liposomal doxorubicin). Interferon-α (for patients with CD4 > 200 cells/mcL and no constitutional symptoms). Radiation (amelioration of edema).	Bone marrow suppression, peripheral neuritis, flu-like syndrome.
Visceral disease (eg, pulmonary)	Combination chemotherapy (eg, daunorubicin, bleomycin, vinblastine).	Bone marrow suppression, cardiac toxicity, fever.

[1]For treatment of *Mycobacterium tuberculosis* infection, see Chapter 9.
[2]For moderate to severe *P jiroveci* infection (oxygen saturation < 90%), corticosteroids should be given with specific treatment. The dose of prednisone is 40 mg twice daily for 5 days, then 40 mg daily for 5 days, and then 20 mg daily until therapy is complete.
[3]When considering use of dapsone, check glucose-6-phosphate dehydrogenase (G6PD) level in African-American patients and those of Mediterranean origin.
CHOP = cyclophosphamide, doxorubicin (hydroxydaunomycin), vincristine (Oncovin), and prednisone; modified M-BACOD = methotrexate, bleomycin, doxorubicin (Adriamycin), cyclophosphamide, vincristine (Oncovin), and dexamethasone; G-CSF = granulocyte-colony stimulating factor (filgrastim); GM-CSF = granulocyte-macrophage colony-stimulating factor (sargramostim).

are currently recommended for initiation of treatment are usually maintained on their regimens if they are doing well and are not suffering side effects from the treatment. When medication is stopped in this population, most patients drop back to their pretreatment nadir CD4 count in a matter of months. Some patients whose counts rise dramatically and who are fully suppressed (ie, plasma viral load < 50 copies/mcL) may be successfully transitioned from a high potency regimen to a lower potency regimen with fewer side effects; however, this "induction-maintenance" strategy is still being evaluated in clinical trials.

Once a decision to initiate therapy has been made, several important principles should guide therapy. First, because drug resistance to antiretroviral agents develops in HIV-infected patients, a major goal of

therapy should be total suppression of viral replication as measured by the serum viral load. Therapy that achieves a plasma viral load of < 50 or < 75 copies/mcL (depending on the test used) has been shown to correlate with antiviral effect in other compartments. To achieve this and maintain virologic control over time, aggressive combination therapy is essential, and partially suppressive combinations such as dual nucleoside therapy should be avoided. Similarly, if toxicity develops, it is preferable to either interrupt the entire regimen or change the offending drug rather than reduce individual doses. The current standard is to use at least three agents simultaneously. Because the number of drugs and potential combinations is finite and the development of drug resistance may severely compromise the efficacy of treatment, patients must be

Table 31–5. Antiretroviral therapy.

Drug	Dose	Common Side Effects	Special Monitoring[1]	Cost[2]	Cost/Month
Nucleoside reverse transcriptase inhibitors					
Zidovudine (AZT) (Retrovir)	600 mg orally daily in two divided doses	Anemia, neutropenia, nausea, malaise, headache, insomnia, myopathy	No special monitoring	$6.49/300 mg	$389.36
Didanosine (ddI) (Videx)	400 mg orally daily (enteric-coated capsule) for persons ≥ 60 kg	Peripheral neuropathy, pancreatitis, dry mouth, hepatitis	Bimonthly neurologic questionnaire for neuropathy, K⁺, amylase, bilirubin, triglycerides	$11.07/400 mg capsules	$332.20
Zalcitabine (ddC) (Hivid)	0.375–0.75 mg orally three times daily	Peripheral neuropathy, aphthous ulcers, hepatitis	Monthly neurologic questionnaire for neuropathy	$2.73/0.75 mg	$245.70
Stavudine (d4T) (Zerit)	40 mg orally twice daily for persons ≥ 60 kg	Peripheral neuropathy, hepatitis, pancreatitis	Monthly neurologic questionnaire for neuropathy, amylase	$6.17/40 mg	$370.44
Lamivudine (3TC) (Epivir)	150 mg orally twice daily	Rash, peripheral neuropathy	No special monitoring	$5.55/150 mg	$333.23
Emtricitabine (Emtriva)	300 mg orally once daily	Skin discoloration palms/soles (mild)	No special monitoring	$10.60/300 mg	$318.26
Abacavir (Ziagen)	300 mg orally twice daily	Rash, fever—if occur, rechallenge may be fatal	No special monitoring	$7.46/300 mg	$447.78
Nucleotide reverse transcriptase inhibitors					
Tenofovir (Viread)	300 mg orally once daily	Gastrointestinal distress	Renal function	$16.69/300 mg	$500.05
Protease inhibitors (PIs)					
Saquinavir hard gel (Invirase)	1000 mg twice daily with 100 mg ritonavir orally twice daily	Gastrointestinal distress	Cholesterol, triglycerides	$5.99/500 mg	$718.56 (plus cost of ritonavir)
Saquinavir soft gel (Fortovase)	1200 mg three times daily	Gastrointestinal distress	Cholesterol, triglycerides	$1.40/200 mg	$758.46
Ritonavir (Norvir)	600 mg orally twice daily or in lower doses (eg, 100 mg orally once or twice daily) for boosting other PIs	Gastrointestinal distress, peripheral paresthesias	Cholesterol, triglycerides	$10.29/100 mg	$3,704.40 ($617.40 in lower doses)
Indinavir (Crixivan)	800 mg orally three times daily	Kidney stones	Cholesterol, triglycerides, bilirubin level	$3.05/400 mg	$548.12

Drug	Dosage	Adverse effects	Monitoring[1]	Price	AWP cost[2]
Nelfinavir (Viracept)	750 mg orally three times daily or 1250 mg twice daily	Diarrhea	Cholesterol, triglycerides	$2.52/250 mg $6.05/625 mg	$680.99 $726.40
Amprenavir (Agenerase)	1200 mg orally twice daily	Gastrointestinal, rash	Cholesterol, triglycerides	$1.54/150 mg	$740.74
Fosamprenavir (Lexiva)	1400 mg orally twice daily or 1400 mg orally once daily with ritonavir 200 mg orally once daily	Same as amprenavir	Same as amprenavir	$10.54/700 mg	$632.63–$1265.26
Lopinavir/ritonavir (Kaletra)	400 mg/100 mg orally twice daily	Diarrhea	Cholesterol, triglycerides	$6.37/200 mg (lopinavir)	$764.41
Atazanavir (Reyataz)	400 mg orally once daily	Hyperbilirubinemia	Bilirubin level	$14.20/200 mg	$857.20
Tipranavir/ritonavir (Aptivus/Norvir)	500 mg of tipranavir and 200 mg of ritonavir orally twice daily	Gastrointestinal, rash	Cholesterol, triglycerides	$8.94/250 mg (tipranavir) $10.29/100 mg (ritonavir)	$2307.60 (for combination)
Nonnucleoside reverse transcriptase inhibitors (NNRTIs)					
Nevirapine (Viramune)	200 mg orally daily for 2 weeks, then 200 mg orally twice daily	Rash	No special monitoring	$7.08/200 mg	$424.75
Delavirdine (Rescriptor)	400 mg orally three times daily	Rash	No special monitoring	$1.76/200 mg	$316.35
Efavirenz (Sustiva)	600 mg orally daily	Neurologic disturbances	No special monitoring	$16.62/600 mg	$498.62
Entry inhibitor					
Enfuvirtide (Fuzeon)	90 mg subcutaneously twice daily	Injection site pain and allergic reaction	No special monitoring	$35.28/90 mg	$2116.93

[1]Standard monitoring is complete blood count (CBC) and differential, and amino transferases.
[2]Average wholesale price (AWP, for AB-rated generic when available) for quantity listed. Source: *Red Book Update, Vol. 25, No.5, May 2006.* AWP may not accurately represent the actual pharmacy cost because wide contractual variations exist among institutions.

able to adhere to these regimens. Patients who may miss many doses of treatment should be counseled to defer starting therapy until they are able to adhere to the regimen. Adherence can be promoted through the use of medication boxes with compartments (eg, Medisets), supportive counseling, or daily supervision of therapy. Therefore, decisions to withhold treatment should not be based on a patient's circumstances (eg, active drug use or housing status) alone. Often, a trial intervention such as offering *Pneumocystis* pneumonia prophylaxis may be helpful in determining the likelihood of adherence to a more complex antiretroviral regimen.

Monitoring of antiretroviral therapy has two goals. Laboratory evaluation for toxicity depends on the specific drugs in the combination but generally should be done approximately every 3 months once a patient is on a stable regimen. The second aspect of monitoring is to regularly measure objective markers of efficacy. The CD4 cell count and HIV viral load should be repeated 1–2 months after the initiation or change of antiretroviral regimen and every 3–4 months thereafter in clinically stable patients. Reasons for changing antiretroviral regimens include intolerable adverse reactions, rising or persistently detectable viral loads, the clinical progression of disease, and continued immunologic deterioration as reflected by a declining CD4 cell count. Although a rebound in HIV viral load is cited as an indication to change therapy, exact parameters have not been established, and many patients appear to have continued clinical benefit in the face of rising viral load measurements. When therapy is modified, clinicians should attempt to start at least two agents to which an individual has not been exposed or to which there is minimal or no resistance at the same time. Conversely, there is a risk to stopping a single medication because of the possibility of its causing a side effect if the remaining regimen contains too few medications to prevent rapid development of resistance.

Drug resistance testing is recommended for patients who are experiencing treatment failure (persistent or rising viral load despite adherence to an efficacious regimen).

Although the ideal combination of drugs has not yet been defined for all possible clinical situations, possible choices can be better understood after a review of the available agents. These drugs can be grouped into four major categories: nucleoside and nucleotide reverse transcriptase inhibitors (NRTI), protease inhibitors (PI), nonnucleoside reverse transcriptase inhibitors (NNRTI), and entry inhibitors.

1. Nucleoside and nucleotide reverse transcriptase inhibitors—

a. Zidovudine—Zidovudine (azidothymidine; AZT) was the first approved antiviral drug for HIV infection and remains an important agent. It is administered at a dose of 300 mg orally twice daily. A combination of zidovudine 300 mg and lamivudine 150 mg (Combivir) allows more convenient dosing of medication for individu-

als taking both of these agents. Side effects seen with zidovudine are listed in Table 31–5. Approximately 40% of patients experience subjective side effects that usually remit within 6 weeks. The common dose-limiting side effects are anemia and neutropenia, which can be exacerbated by other drugs such as ganciclovir that cause bone marrow suppression. A minority of patients have the more rapid onset of red cell aplasia. Bone marrow toxicity is generally reversible with cessation of the drug.

In monitoring patients receiving zidovudine, complete blood counts—with platelet and differential counts—should be done monthly for the first 2 months of therapy and then every 3 months. Creatine phosphokinase (CPK) levels should be checked every 6 months.

b. Didanosine—The most convenient formulation of didanosine (ddI) is the enteric-coated capsule. For adults weighing at least 60 kg, the dose is one 400-mg enteric-coated capsule orally daily; for those 30–59 kg, the dose is one 250-mg enteric-coated capsule orally daily. Didanosine should be taken on an empty stomach; if taken with indinavir, the two medications should be taken at least 1 hour apart. Didanosine levels are increased when it is administered with tenofovir, potentially resulting in increased side effects. Therefore, this combination should be used very cautiously.

Unlike zidovudine, didanosine does not cause anemia but may cause neutropenia. It has also been associated with pancreatitis. The incidence of pancreatitis with didanosine is 5–10%—of fatal pancreatitis, less than 0.4%. Patients with a history of pancreatitis, as well as those taking other medications associated with pancreatitis (including trimethoprim-sulfamethoxazole and intravenous pentamidine) are at higher risk for this complication. Patients should be warned to use alcohol judiciously while taking didanosine. Clinicians should also teach patients to watch for the symptoms of pancreatitis and to stop treatment if abdominal pain, nausea, or vomiting develops while taking didanosine until it can be determined if they have pancreatitis. Other common side effects with didanosine include a dose-related, reversible, painful peripheral neuropathy, which occurs in about 15% of patients, and dry mouth. Fulminant hepatic failure and electrolyte abnormalities, including hypokalemia, hypocalcemia, and hypomagnesemia, have been reported in patients taking didanosine.

c. Stavudine—Stavudine (d4T) has shown good activity as an antiretroviral drug. The dose is 40 mg orally twice daily for individuals weighing 60 kg or more. However, because of its side effects including lipoatrophy, lipodystrophy, peripheral neuropathy and, rarely, lactic acidosis and hepatitis, this drug should no longer be used except when there is no alternative. Patients taking stavudine should be routinely changed to abacavir or tenofovir, both of which are less likely to cause lipoatrophy and lipodystrophy.

d. Lamivudine—Lamivudine (3TC) is a safe and well-tolerated agent. The dosage is 150 mg orally twice daily or 300 mg orally once a day. There are no significant side effects with this agent, and it has activity also against hepatitis B. The dose should be reduced with renal insufficiency.

e. Emtricitabine—Emtricitabine is a nucleoside analog that is dosed at 200 mg orally. It was developed primarily as a once a day alternative to lamivudine. However, lamivudine can be dosed daily, eliminating the special indication for emtricitabine. As is true of lamivudine, emtricitabine has activity against hepatitis B and its dosage should be reduced in patients with renal insufficiency.

f. Abacavir—A daily dose of 300 mg orally twice daily results in potent antiretroviral activity. Abacavir retains activity against some HIV strains that have become resistant to other nucleoside drugs. Abacavir is formulated with zidovudine and lamivudine in a single pill (Trizivir, one tablet orally twice daily). Although it is a triple-drug regimen, it is not as efficacious as combining two nucleoside/nucleotide analogs with a PI or an NNRTI and should be used only for patients who cannot comply with other regimens. Abacavir is also available as a fixed dose combination pill with lamivudine for use as a once daily pill (Epzicom). The main toxicity of abacavir is a hypersensitivity syndrome in about 5% of patients, characterized by a flu-like syndrome with rash and fever that worsens with successive doses; individuals in whom this syndrome develops *should not* be rechallenged with this agent as reactions with rechallenge can be **fatal**.

g. Zalcitabine—Zalcitabine (ddC) is thought to be one of the least effective antiretroviral agents and is therefore not commonly used. Its advantages are that it is inexpensive, easy to administer, and has no known hematologic side effects. The usual dosage of zalcitabine is approximately 0.005–0.01 mg/kg orally every 8 hours. This drug is formulated in 0.375-mg and 0.75-mg tablets.

Zalcitabine, like didanosine, may cause peripheral neuropathy. It is also associated with aphthous ulcers, rash, and rare cases of pancreatitis.

h. Tenofovir—Tenofovir is the only licensed nucleotide analog. It is given as a single daily oral dose of 300 mg and is generally well tolerated. As is true of lamivudine, tenofovir is active against hepatitis B. Because HIV variants that are resistant to other nucleoside analogs are often sensitive to tenofovir, it is often included in second- and third-line treatment regimens. It is also available in a fixed dose combination pill with emtricitibine (Truvada) for daily dosing. A once a day single fixed dose combination pill that contains tenofovir, emtricitabine, and efavirenz should be available in 2006.

2. Protease inhibitors—Nine PIs—indinavir, nelfinavir, ritonavir, saquinavir, amprenavir, fosamprenavir, lopinavir (in combination with ritonavir), atazanavir, and tipranavir are currently available. PIs have been shown to potently suppress HIV replication in vitro and in vivo and are administered as part of a combination regimen.

All the PIs—to differing degrees—are metabolized by the cytochrome P-450 system, and each can inhibit and induce various P-450 isoenzymes. Therefore, drug interactions are common and difficult to predict. Clinicians should consult the product inserts before prescribing PIs with other medications. Drugs such as rifampin that are known to induce the P-450 system should be avoided.

The fact that the PIs are dependent on metabolism through the cytochrome P-450 system has led to some innovative dosing strategies. In particular, ritonavir has been used to boost the drug levels of saquinavir, lopinavir, indinavir, atazanivir, tipranavir, and amprenavir, allowing use of lower doses and simpler dosing schedules of these PIs.

PIs and NRTIs have been linked to a constellation of metabolic abnormalities, including elevated cholesterol levels, elevated triglyceride levels, insulin resistance, diabetes mellitus, and changes in body fat composition (eg, buffalo hump, abdominal obesity). The lipid abnormalities and body habitus changes are referred to as lipodystrophy. Its prevalence is known to be increased among persons treated with certain NRTIs (especially stavudine) and most of the PIs, but it has been seen also in HIV-infected persons who have never been treated with these agents.

Of the different manifestations of lipodystrophy, the dyslipidemias that occur are of particular concern because of the likelihood that increased levels of cholesterol and triglycerides will result in increased prevalence of heart disease. All patients taking PIs or NRTIs should have a fasting cholesterol, low-density lipoprotein cholesterol, and triglyceride level performed every 3–6 months. Until there is longer follow-up of HIV-infected persons with elevated cholesterol levels, treatment decisions should be the same as those for uninfected persons (see Chapter 28). HIV-infected persons who do not respond to dietary interventions should be started on pravastatin (20 mg daily orally) or atorvastatin (10 mg daily orally). Lovastatin and simvastatin should be avoided because of their interactions with PIs. Patients with persistently elevated fasting serum triglyceride levels of 500 mg/dL or more who do not respond to dietary intervention should be treated with gemfibrozil (600 mg twice daily prior to the morning and evening meals).

a. Indinavir—The standard dose of indinavir is 800 mg orally three times a day. Twice-daily dosing of indinavir is feasible in combination with ritonavir. It is recommended that indinavir be taken without food (if not boosted with ritonavir) but with water 1 hour before or 2 hours after a meal. Nausea and headache are common complaints with this drug. Indinavir crystals are present in the urine in approximately 40% of patients; this results in clinically apparent nephrolithiasis in about 15% of patients receiving indinavir. Lower urinary tract symptoms and renal failure have been increasingly reported. Patients taking this drug should be instructed to drink at least 48 ounces of fluid a day to ensure adequate hydration in an attempt to avoid these complications, but if stones occur repeatedly, an alternative PI may be needed. Mild indirect hyperbilirubinemia is also commonly observed in patients taking indinavir but is not an indication for discontinuation of the drug.

b. Nelfinavir—This agent appears to have slightly less potent antiviral activity than either indinavir or ritonavir but has shown short-term benefit in combination regimens. The dose of nelfinavir is 750 mg orally three times daily or 1250 mg orally twice daily. Diarrhea is a side effect in 25% of patients taking nelfinavir, and this symptom may be controlled in the majority of patients with over-the-counter antidiarrheal agents.

c. Ritonavir—Use of this potent PI has been limited by its inhibition of the cytochrome P-450 pathway causing a large number of drug–drug interactions and by its frequent side effects of fatigue, nausea, and paresthesias when the full dose of 600 mg orally twice daily is given. One of the major benefits of ritonavir is that it increases the bioavailability of other PIs (eg, saquinavir, lopinavir) and it is widely used in lower dose (eg, 100 mg daily to 100 mg twice daily) as a booster of other PIs.

d. Saquinavir—Saquinavir has two different formulations: a hard-gel capsule (Invirase) and a soft-gel capsule (Fortovase). The two are not bioequivalent and cannot be used interchangeably. The hard-gel capsule can be used only when boosted by ritonavir (1000 mg of hard-gel saquinavir with 100 mg of ritonavir orally twice daily). The soft-gel capsule (Fortovase) can be used as the sole PI (ie, without ritonavir boosting) at a dosage of 1200 mg three times daily with food. However, because of the large pill burden and because of the necessity for three-times-daily dosing with food, soft-gel saquinavir is not commonly used. The most common side effects with saquinavir are diarrhea, nausea, dyspepsia, and abdominal pain.

e. Amprenavir—Amprenavir has efficacy and side effects similar to those of other PIs. Common side effects are nausea, vomiting, diarrhea, rash, and perioral paresthesia. The dose is 1200 mg orally twice daily. This requires that the patient take 16 capsules a day. When used in combination with ritonavir, the recommended doses are amprenavir 1200 mg with ritonavir 200 mg daily or amprenavir 600 mg with ritonavir 100 mg twice daily.

f. Fosamprenavir—Fosamprenavir is a prodrug of amprenavir. Its major advantage over using amprenavir is a much lower pill burden. It can be dosed at 1400 mg orally twice daily (four capsules a day) or at 1400 mg orally daily (two capsules) with ritonavir 200 mg orally daily (two capsules). Side effects are similar to those with amprenavir.

g. Lopinavir/r—Lopinavir/r is lopinavir formulated with a low dose of ritonavir to maximize the bioavailability of lopinavir. It has been shown to be more effective than nelfinavir when used in combination with stavudine and lamivudine. The usual dose is 400

mg lopinavir with 100 mg of nelfinavir (two tablets) orally twice daily with food. When given along with efavirenz or nevirapine, a higher dose (600 mg/150 mg—three tablets) is usually prescribed. The most common side effect is diarrhea, and lipid abnormalities are frequent.

h. Atazanavir—Atazanavir has two major advantages compared to other PIs. It needs to be dosed only once daily (two 200-mg capsules with food) and has only minimal impact on cholesterol and triglyceride levels. The most common side effect is mild hyperbilirubinemia that resolves with discontinuation of the drug. Because ritonavir increases the serum concentrations of atazanavir, when these drugs are used together, atazanavir is dosed at 300 mg orally daily and ritonavir is dosed at 100 mg orally daily. Both tenofovir and efavirenz lower the serum concentration of atazanavir. Therefore, when either of these two drugs is used with atazanavir, it should be boosted by administering ritonavir. Proton pump inhibitors are contraindicated in patients taking atazanavir because atazanavir requires an acidic pH to remain in solution.

i. Tipranavir—Tipranavir is the first approved nonpeptidic PI. Because of its unique structure, it is active against some strains of the virus that are resistant to other available PIs. It is dosed with ritonavir (two 250 mg capsules of tipranavir with two 100 mg capsules of ritonavir orally twice daily with food). The most common side effects are nausea, vomiting, diarrhea, fatigue, and headache. Tipranavir/ritonavir has been also associated with liver damage and should be used very cautiously in patients with underlying liver disease. Because it is a sulfa-containing drug, its use should be closely monitored in patients with sulfa allergy.

3. Nonnucleoside reverse transcriptase inhibitors—NNRTIs inhibit reverse transcriptase at a site different from that of the nucleoside and nucleotide agents described above. All three have shown antiviral activity as measured by HIV viral load and CD4 responses. The major advantage of the NNRTIs is that two of them (nevirapine and efavirenz) have potencies comparable to that of PIs—with lower pill burden. In particular, they do not appear to cause lipodystrophy; patients with cholesterol and triglyceride elevations who are switched from a PI to an NNRTI may have improvement in their symptoms. The resistance patterns of the NNRTIs are distinct from those of the PIs, so their use still leaves open the option for future PI use.

The NNRTIs can be used with PIs in patients who are difficult to suppress on simpler regimens or when it is difficult to identify at least two agents to which the patient is not resistant. Because these agents may cause alterations in the clearance of PIs, dose modifications may be necessary when these two classes of medications are administered concomitantly. Resistance to one drug in this class uniformly predicts resistance to other drugs in the class, though second-generation drugs are being developed. There is no therapeutic reason for using more than one NNRTI at the same time.

a. Nevirapine—The target dose of nevirapine is 200 mg orally twice daily, but it is initiated at a dose of 200 mg once a day to decrease the incidence of rash, which is as high as 40% when full doses are begun immediately. If rash develops while the patient is taking 200 mg a day, liver enzymes should be checked and the dose should not be increased until the rash resolves. Patients with mild rash and no evidence of hepatotoxicity can continue to be treated with nevirapine. The hepatotoxicity of the drug can be fatal, particularly in women and those patients with high CD4 counts (> 250 mcL), which limits its role as a first-line agent.

b. Efavirenz—The major advantage of efavirenz is that it can be given once daily in a single dose (600 mg orally). The side effects are neurologic, with patients reporting symptoms ranging from lack of concentration and strange dreams to delusions and mania. Fortunately, the neurologic side effects of efavirenz subside over time, usually within a month. Due to teratogenicity, efavirenz should be avoided in women who wish to conceive or are already pregnant. A once-daily fixed dose combination of efavirenz, tenofovir, and emtricitabine in a single pill should be available in 2006.

c. Delavirdine—Of the three available NNRTIs, delavirdine is least used largely as a result of its less convenient dosing and pill burden compared to the other available NNRTIs. Unlike nevirapine and efavirenz, delavirdine inhibits P-450 cytochromes rather than inducing these enzymes. This means that delavirdine can act like ritonavir and boost other antiretrovirals, although delavirdine is not as potent as ritonavir in this capacity. The dosage is 400 mg orally three times a day, which makes it less convenient for patients than the other two medications in this class. As with nevirapine, the major side effect is rash, but the incidence of rash is lower with delavirdine.

4. Novel agents—

a. Entry inhibitors—Peptide T-20 (enfuvirtide) is the first drug in the new class of fusion inhibitors, which block the entry of HIV into cells. The addition of enfuvirtide to an optimized antiretroviral regimen improved CD4 counts and lowered viral loads in heavily pretreated patients with multidrug-resistant HIV. The dose is 90 mg by subcutaneous injection twice daily.

b. CCR5 antagonists—There are currently 2 CCR5 inhibitors in phase II/III clinical trials in humans. Although the exact role and level of activity of this new class of drugs have not been fully defined, it is clear that there is good antiviral activity and when combined with other active drugs can result in excellent virologic responses.

c. Integrase inhibitors—HIV integrase inhibitors are currently in phase II clinical trials and early reports suggest excellent antiviral activity. Because these drugs target a different enzyme of the HIV virus, there is great optimism that they will be helpful for patients who are resistant to other classes of medications and that they might help prevent resistance by use with available medications that target the reverse transcriptase and protease enzymes.

d. Maturation inhibitors—Recently, a drug has been tested in humans that appears to interfere with the maturation of HIV virions. This represents a promising new potential target for HIV drug development.

5. Constructing regimens—There is now little debate about the necessity for combining drugs to achieve long-term suppression of HIV and its associated clinical benefit. Only combinations of three or more drugs have been able to decrease HIV viral load by 2–3 logs and allow suppression of HIV RNA to below the threshold of detection for longer than 10 years in some individuals. However, there have been few studies directly comparing one triple combination therapy regimen to another. Therefore, clinicians and patients face difficult decisions in selecting therapy.

Current evidence supports the use of Truvada (tenofovir and emtricitabine) as the "nucleoside/nucleotide backbone" combined with efavirenz as the initial regimen. This regimen has been shown to be more effective and better tolerated than Combivir (zidovudine and lamivudine). It has the advantages of once daily dosing and low pill burden (two pills per day). This recommendation is likely to grow stronger with the availability of a single pill that contains efavirenz, tenofovir, and emtricitabine and that can be dosed once daily. Because 8–10% of newly infected persons in some urban areas of the United States have NNRTI resistance, resistance testing should be performed prior to initiating efavirenz in this population.

There are increasing data to suggest the virologic and clinical inferiority of regimens that include only nucleoside and nucleotide analogs without nonnucleoside agents or PIs. Thus, triple nucleoside/nucleotide regimens should be avoided when other options exist. Studies of "quad-nucs" in which four nucleosides or nucleotides are used in combination are currently ongoing but cannot be recommended at this time.

In the absence of head-to-head comparisons of different regimens in different situations, several general principles should guide the choice of combinations. The most important determinant of treatment efficacy is adherence to the regimen. Therefore, it is vitally important that the regimen chosen be one to which the patient can easily adhere. In general, patients are more compliant with medication regimens that are once or twice a day only, do not require special timing with regard to meals, can be taken at the same time as other medications, do not require refrigeration or special preparation, and do not have bothersome side effects. Second, it is desirable to prescribe combinations that have demonstrated clinical benefit; because these data do not exist for many combinations, it is reassuring to know that the combination under consideration has shown beneficial effects on HIV viral load levels in

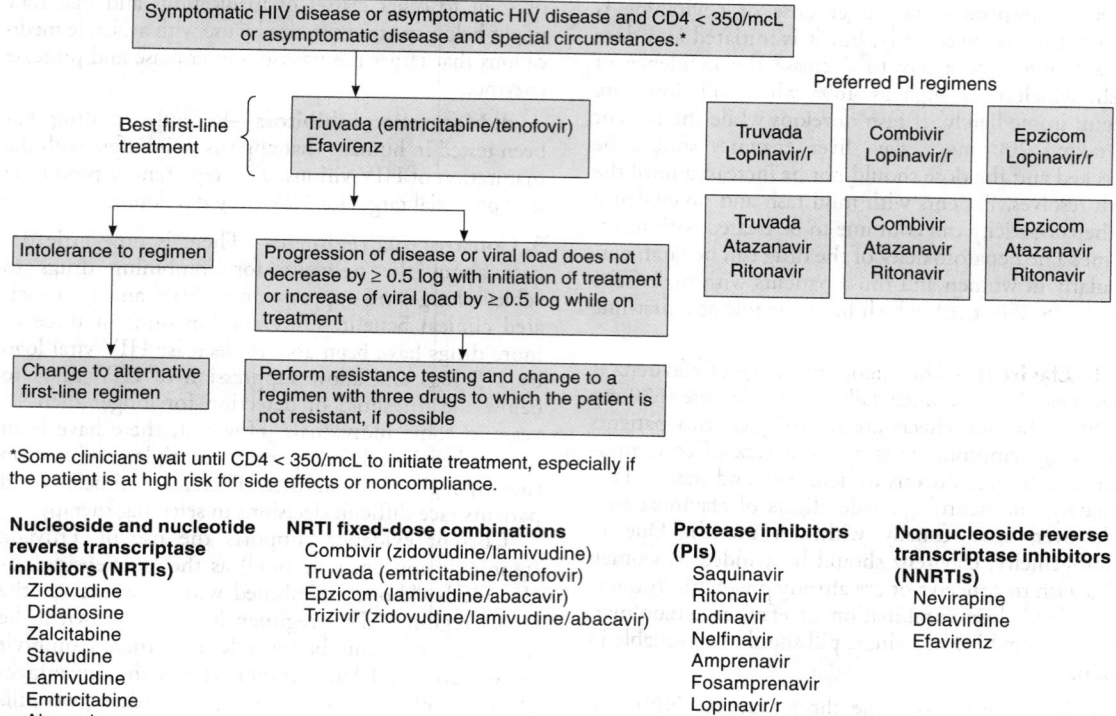

Figure 31–2. Approach to antiretroviral therapy.

short-term studies. To the extent possible, agents to which the patient has not been exposed are preferable to drugs for which resistance mutations may have already occurred. Toxicities should ideally be nonoverlapping. An individual's relative contraindications to a given drug or drugs should be considered. The regimen should not include agents that are either virologically antagonistic or incompatible in terms of drug–drug interactions. Compatible dosing schedules—prescribing medications that can be taken at the same time—improve adherence to treatment. Finally, highly complex therapeutic regimens should be reserved for individuals who are capable of adhering to the rigorous demands of taking multiple medications and having this therapy closely monitored. Conversely, simplified regimens that deliver the lowest number of pills given at the longest possible dosing intervals are desirable for patients who have difficulty taking multiple medications.

Possible ways of incorporating nonnucleoside agents and PIs into combinations are displayed in Figure 31–2.

A number of points about the "nucleoside/nucleotide backbone" of regimens have become clearer. The combination of stavudine plus didanosine should be avoided as there is increased risk of toxicities, in particular in pregnant women because of the increased risk of lactic acidosis. Also notable is the fact that the addition of lamivudine to didanosine does not appear

to result in the same level of viral suppression as when lamivudine is combined with zidovudine or stavudine. Moreover, the nucleoside pair of zidovudine and stavudine should be avoided because of increased toxicity and the potential for antagonism that results from intracellular competition for phosphorylation. Finally, the combination of didanosine with tenofovir can cause declines in CD4 counts despite excellent virologic response and appropriate dose adjustment of didanosine; the reason for this is unknown.

In choosing which agents to include in an initial antiretroviral regimen, ease of administration, minimization of side effects, drug resistance pattern, and future treatment options should all be considered. For some patients who have been heavily treated with antiretroviral agents, it may be difficult to design second-line regimens when they are showing evidence of progression of disease on their existing regimen. In designing second-line regimens (sometimes called salvage regimens—a term that some patients may find offensive), the goal is to identify drugs with at least some degree of antiviral activity. This can be quite complicated because of the problem of cross-resistance between drugs within a class. For example, the resistance patterns of lopinavir/ritonavir and indinavir are overlapping, and patients with virus resistant to these agents are unlikely to respond to nelfinavir or saquinavir even though they have never received treatment with these agents. Similarly, the resistance patterns of nevirapine and efavirenz are overlapping. Ideally, at least two drugs to which the patient's virus is susceptible should be added at the same time.

In addition to taking a careful history of what antiretroviral agents a patient has taken and for how long, genotypic and phenotypic resistance testing can provide useful information in designing second-line regimens (see below).

Whatever regimen is chosen, patients should be coached in ways to improve adherence. This should include taking medicines on an established schedule (eg, first thing in the morning), keeping a medication diary, and keeping medications in a variety of places the patient is likely to be (eg, car, workplace). For certain populations (eg, unstably housed individuals), specially tailored programs that include drug dispensing are needed.

For some patients, it is impossible to construct a tolerable regimen that fully suppresses HIV. In such cases, clinicians and patients should consider their goals. Patients maintained on effective antiretroviral agents often benefit from these regimens (eg, higher CD4 counts, fewer opportunistic infections) even if their virus is detectable. In some cases, patients may request a drug holiday during which they are taken off all medications. Patients often immediately feel better because of the absence of drug side effects. Unfortunately, structured treatment interruptions generally result in viral rebound and CD4 decline, and patients who interrupt their treatment fare poorly compared with patients who continue their regimens without interruption.

6. The challenge of drug resistance—HIV-1 drug resistance limits the ability to fully control HIV replication and is a leading cause for antiretroviral regimen failure. Resistance has been documented for all currently available antiretrovirals including the new class of fusion inhibitors. The problem of drug resistance is widespread in HIV-infected patients undergoing treatment in countries where antiretroviral therapy is widely available. A recent prevalence study of a representative sample of patients being treated in U.S. clinics revealed that nearly 80% of patients with detectable viremia had at least some degree of drug resistance. Patients who have been on various antiretroviral regimens and who now have resistant HIV-1 represent a major challenge for the treating clinician. However, the issue of resistant virus does not just concern the treatment-experienced patient. Resistance is now also documented in patients who are antiretroviral treatment naive, but who have been infected with a drug resistant strain—"primary resistance." Cohort studies of antiretroviral treatment–naive patients entering care in North America and Western Europe show that roughly 10–12% of recently infected individuals have been infected with a drug-resistant strain of HIV-1.

Current expert guidelines recommend resistance testing for patients who are recently infected and for pregnant women. Resistance testing is also recommended for patients who are on an antiretroviral regimen and

have suboptimal viral suppression (ie, viral loads > 1000 copies/mcL). Both genotypic and phenotypic tests are commercially available and in randomized controlled studies their use has been shown to result in improved short-term virologic outcomes compared to making treatment choices without resistance testing. Furthermore, multiple retrospective studies have conclusively demonstrated that resistance tests provide prognostic information about virologic response to newly initiated therapy that cannot be gleaned from standard clinical information (ie, treatment history, examination, CD4 count, and viral load tests).

Because of the complexity of resistance tests, many clinicians require expert interpretation of results. In the case of genotypic assays, results may show that the mutations that are selected for during antiretroviral therapy are drug-specific or contribute to broad cross-resistance to multiple drugs within a therapeutic class. An example of a drug-specific mutation for the reverse transcriptase inhibitors would be the M184V mutation that is selected for by lamivudine or emtricitabine therapy—this mutation causes resistance only to those two drugs. Conversely, the thymidine analog mutations ("TAMs") of M41L, D67N, K70R, L210W, T215Y/F, and T219Q/K/E are selected for by either zidovudine or stavudine therapy, but cause resistance to all the drugs in the class and often extend to the nucleotide inhibitor tenofovir when three or more of these TAMs are present. Further complicating the interpretation of genotypic tests is the fact that some mutations that cause resistance to one drug can actually make the virus that contains this mutation more sensitive to another drug. The M184V mutation, for example, is associated with increased sensitivity to zidovudine, stavudine and tenofovir. Figures 31–3, 31–4, and 31–5 show the most common mutations associated with drug resistance and cross-resistance patterns for NRTIs, NNRTIs, and PIs. Phenotypic tests also require interpretation in that the distinction between a resistant virus and sensitive one is not fully defined for all available drugs.

Both methods of resistance testing are limited by the fact that they may measure resistance in only some of the viral strains present in an individual. Resistance results may also be misleading if a patient is not taking antiretroviral medications at the time of testing. Thus, resistance results must be viewed cumulatively—ie, if resistance is reported to an agent on one test, it should be presumed to be present thereafter even if subsequent tests do not give the same result.

C. HEMATOPOIETIC STIMULATING FACTORS

Epoetin alfa (erythropoietin) is approved for use in HIV-infected patients with anemia, including those with anemia secondary to zidovudine use. It has been shown to decrease the need for blood transfusions. The drug is expensive, and an endogenous erythropoietin level < 500 mU/mL should be demonstrated before starting therapy. The starting dose is 8000 units

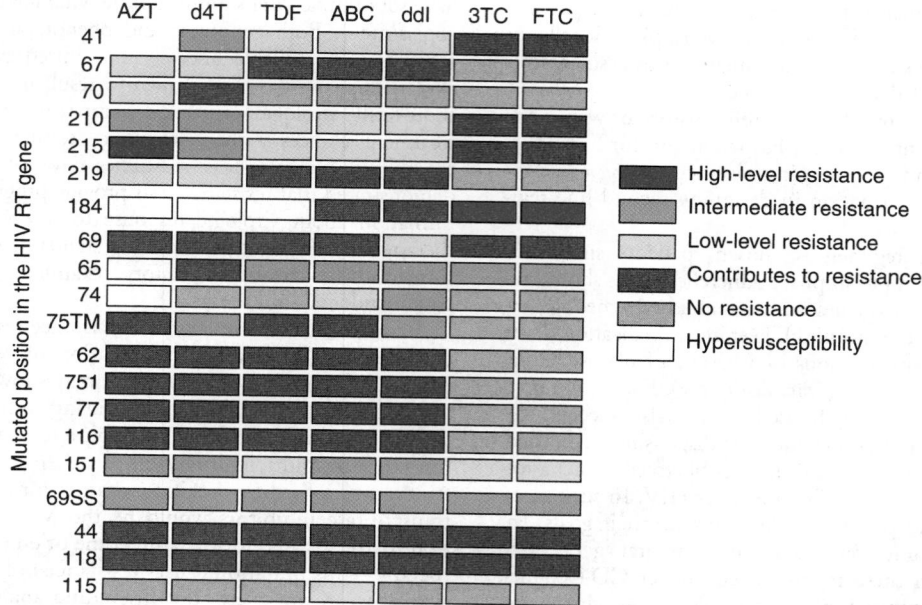

Figure 31–3. Most common mutations associated with drug resistance and cross-resistance with nucleotide reverse transcriptase inhibitors. AZT = zidovudine; d4T = stavudine; TDF = tenofovir; ABC = abacavir; ddI = didanosine; 3TC = lamivudine; FTC = emtricitabine. (Reproduced, with permission, from Stanford HIV Drug Resistance Database, http://hivdb.stanford.edu.)

subcutaneously three times a week. The target hematocrit is 35–40%. The dose may be increased by 12,000 units every 4–6 weeks as needed to a maximum dose of 48,000 units per week. Hypertension is the most common side effect.

Human G-CSF (filgrastim) and granulocyte-macrophage colony-stimulating factor (GM-CSF [sargramostim]) have been shown to increase the neutrophil counts of HIV-infected patients. G-CSF is preferred because of the theoretical concern of GM-CSF-stimulating HIV replication in infected monocytes. In patients receiving cytotoxic chemotherapy for lymphoma or Kaposi's sarcoma, daily subcutaneous doses of G-CSF at approximately 5 mcg/kg (a 300 mcg or 480 mcg vial, depending on weight) are given beginning 5–7 days after chemotherapy until the neutrophil count has rebounded to above 1000/mcL. G-CSF may also have a role in ameliorating neutropenia caused by

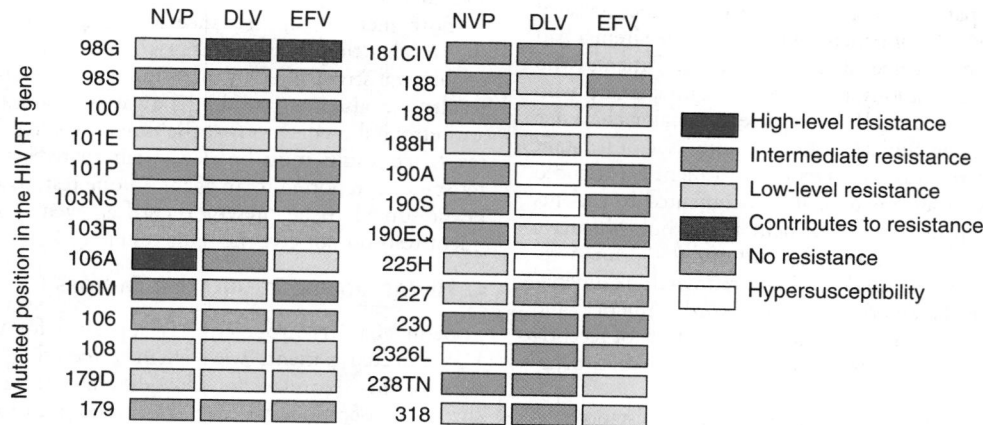

Figure 31–4. Most common mutations associated with drug resistance and cross-resistance patterns for nonnucleoside reverse transcriptase inhibitors. NVP = nevirapine; DLV = delavirdine; EFV = efavirenz. (Reproduced, with permission, from Stanford HIV Drug Resistance Database, http://hivdb.stanford.edu.)

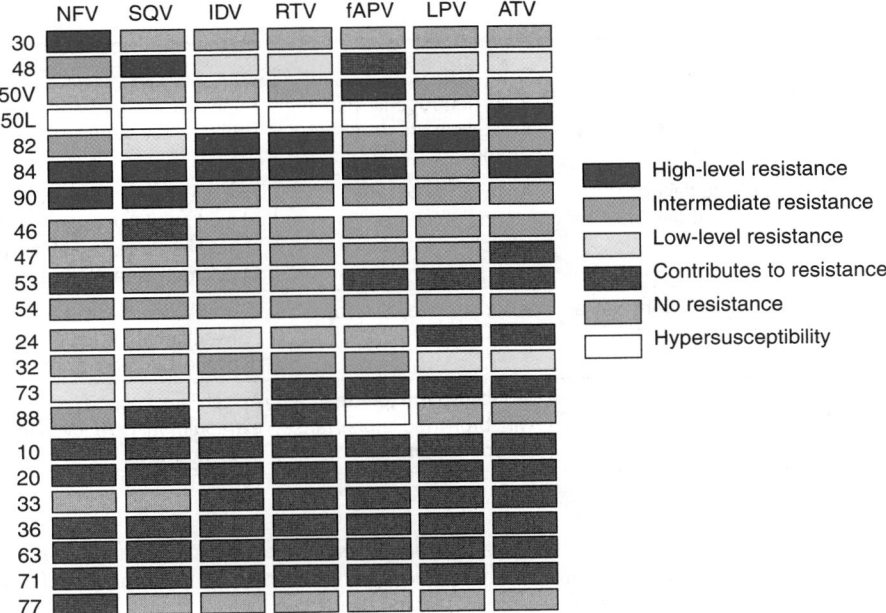

Figure 31–5. Most common mutations associated with drug resistance and cross-resistance patterns for protease inhibitors. NFV = nelfinavir; SQV = saquinavir; IDV = indinavir; RTV = ritonavir; fAPV = fosamprenavir; LPV = lopinavir; ATV = atazanavir. (Reproduced, with permission, from Stanford HIV Drug Resistance Database, http://hivdb.stanford.edu.)

other drugs such as zidovudine or ganciclovir, when other therapeutic alternatives are not possible. Because the cost of this therapy is approximately $150 per vial, dosage should be closely monitored and minimized, aiming for a neutrophil count of 1000/mcL. When the drug is used for indications other than cytotoxic chemotherapy, one or two doses at 5 mcg/kg per week are usually sufficient.

D. PROPHYLAXIS OF OPPORTUNISTIC INFECTIONS

In general, decisions about prophylaxis of opportunistic infections are based on the CD4 count, other evidence of severe immune suppression (eg, oral candidiasis), and a history of having had the infection in the past. In the era prior to HAART, patients started on prophylactic regimens were maintained on them indefinitely. However, studies have shown that in patients with robust improvements in immune function—as measured by increases in CD4 counts above the levels that are used to initiate treatment—prophylactic regimens can safely be discontinued.

Primary prophylaxis for *Pneumocystis* pneumonia should be offered to patients with CD4 counts below 200 cells/mcL, a CD4 lymphocyte percentage below 14%, or weight loss or oral candidiasis. Patients with a history of *Pneumocystis* pneumonia should receive secondary prophylaxis until they have had a durable virologic response to HAART for at least 3–6 months and maintain a CD4 count of > 250 cells/mcL.

Regimens for prophylaxis are trimethoprim-sulfamethoxazole, dapsone, atovaquone, and aerosolized pentamidine (see Table 31–6). Trimethoprim-sulfamethoxazole is inexpensive, widely available, and the most effective agent for prophylaxis. In two studies comparing once-daily double-strength trimethoprim-sulfamethoxazole with aerosolized pentamidine for primary and secondary prophylaxis of *Pneumocystis* pneumonia, patients randomized to trimethoprim-sulfamethoxazole were significantly less likely to develop *Pneumocystis* pneumonia. Bacterial infections (eg, pneumonia, sinusitis) are also less likely to develop in patients who receive trimethoprim-sulfamethoxazole. Common side effects with trimethoprim-sulfamethoxazole are primarily fever, rash, and nausea and vomiting. Trimethoprim-sulfamethoxazole is dosed as one double-strength tablet three times a week to once daily. Patients in whom mild rashes develop on this regimen may be treated with diphenhydramine (25–50 mg every 4 hours). However, clinicians and patients must watch carefully for signs of Stevens-Johnson syndrome. Some clinicians are also using desensitization regimens to overcome allergic reactions. Reports suggest that desensitization may be successful in 40% of cases. Dapsone is a second-line prophylactic agent with minimal side effects. As is the case with trimethoprim-sulfamethoxazole, it is inexpensive and widely available. It may be used in patients with an allergic reaction to trimethoprim-sulfamethoxazole. Before prescribing dapsone, cli-

Table 31–6. Pneumocystis jiroveci prophylaxis.

Drug	Dose	Side Effects	Limitations
Trimethoprim-sul-famethoxazole	One double-strength tablet three times a week to one tablet daily	Rash, neutropenia, hepatitis, Stevens-Johnson syndrome	Hypersensitivity reaction is common but, if mild, it may be possible to treat through.
Dapsone	50–100 mg daily or 100 mg two or three times per week	Anemia, nausea, methemoglobinemia, hemolytic anemia	Less effective than above. Glucose-6-phosphate dehydrogenase (G6PD) level should be checked prior to therapy. Check methemoglobin level at 1 month.
Atovaquone	1500 mg daily with a meal	Rash, diarrhea, nausea	Less effective than suspension trimethoprim-sulfamethoxazole; equal efficacy to dapsone, but more expensive.
Aerosolized penta-midine	300 mg monthly	Bronchospasm (pretreat with bronchodilators); rare reports of pancreatitis	Apical *Pneumocystis jiroveci* pneumonia, extrapulmonary *P jiroveci* infections, pneumothorax.

nicians should make certain that the patient is not glucose-6-phosphate dehydrogenase deficient, since such patients are at high risk for developing hemolytic anemia with dapsone therapy. Patients taking dapsone concomitantly with didanosine should take the dapsone at least 2 hours prior to the didanosine since dapsone is not absorbed well in the neutral pH stomach environment created by the didanosine buffering agent. Finally, atovaquone may be an option for individuals intolerant of other systemic therapies, but it appears to be less effective. It is available only as an oral suspension (1500 mg daily) and must be taken with food to promote absorption.

Finally, aerosolized pentamidine can be used if no systemic agents can be tolerated. Its disadvantages are expense (approximately $100 for one treatment per month) and decreased effectiveness in the apical and peripheral areas of the lung. Cases of extrapulmonary *Pneumocystis* infections in patients receiving aerosolized pentamidine have also been reported.

Aerosolized pentamidine may also increase the incidence of pneumothorax in patients with a history of *Pneumocystis* infection, although this complication is rarely seen in the current treatment era.

Patients who develop *Pneumocystis* infection on a particular prophylactic regimen should be switched to a different one.

Prophylaxis against *M avium* complex infection should be given to patients whose CD4 counts fall below 75–100 cells/mcL. Clarithromycin (500 mg orally twice daily) and azithromycin (1200 mg orally weekly) have both been shown to decrease the incidence of disseminated disease by approximately 75%, with a low rate of breakthrough of resistant disease. The latter regimen is generally preferred on the basis of ease of compliance and cost. Adding rifabutin increases the toxicity of the regimen but does not significantly increase its efficacy and is therefore not recommended. As sole therapy, rifabutin (300 mg orally daily) is less effective and more toxic than clarithromycin or azithromycin. Clinicians

should make certain that patients do not have active *M tuberculosis* infection by examination of a chest radiograph prior to starting rifabutin because of concern about the development of resistance to rifabutin with cross-resistance to rifampin. Similarly, before initiating prophylaxis, clinicians should establish with a blood culture that the patient does not have disseminated *M avium* complex infection. Common side effects of both azithromycin and clarithromycin are nausea and diarrhea. Two common side effects with rifabutin are rash and hepatic dysfunction. Rifabutin may induce hepatic enzymes, thereby decreasing the activity of some drugs metabolized by the liver.

Prophylaxis against *M avium* complex infection may be discontinued among patients whose CD4 counts go above 100 cells/mcL in response to HAART and whose plasma viral load has been optimally suppressed to < 50–75 copies/mL.

Prophylaxis against *M tuberculosis* infection—isoniazid 300 mg daily plus pyridoxine 50 mg orally daily for 9 months to a year—should be given to all HIV-infected patients with positive PPD reactions (defined for HIV-infected patients as > 5 mm of induration).

Toxoplasmosis prophylaxis is desirable in patients with positive IgG toxoplasma serology and CD4 counts below 100 cells/mcL. Trimethoprim-sulfamethoxazole (one double-strength tablet daily) offers good protection against toxoplasmosis, as does a combination of pyrimethamine, 25 mg orally once a week, plus dapsone, 50 mg orally daily, plus leucovorin, 25 mg orally once a week.

CMV infection is also common in late HIV disease. Oral ganciclovir (1000 mg orally three times daily with food) is approved for CMV prophylaxis among HIV-infected persons with advanced disease (eg, CD4 counts below 50 cells/mcL). However, because the drug causes neutropenia, it is not widely used. Clinicians should consider performing serum CMV IgG antibody testing. Persons who are CMV IgG-negative are not at risk for development of CMV disease. Importantly, patients who are CMV IgG-negative should receive CMV-negative blood if they require a transfusion. Because over 99% of gay men are positive for CMV IgG, it is appropriate to reserve testing for heterosexuals with HIV.

Cryptococcosis, candidiasis, and endemic fungal diseases are also candidates for prophylaxis. One prophylactic trial showed a decreased incidence of cryptococcal disease with the use of fluconazole, 200 mg orally daily, but the treated group had no benefit in terms of mortality. Fluconazole (200 mg orally once a week) was found to prevent oral and vaginal candidiasis in women with CD4 counts below 300 cells/mcL. In areas of the world where histoplasmosis and coccidioidomycosis are endemic and are frequent complications of HIV infection, prophylactic use of fluconazole or itraconazole may prove to be useful strategies. However, the problem of identifying individuals at highest risk makes the targeting of prophylaxis difficult.

Because individuals with advanced HIV infection are susceptible to a number of opportunistic pathogens, the use of agents with activity against more than one pathogen is preferable. It has been shown, for example, that trimethoprim-sulfamethoxazole confers some protection against toxoplasmosis in individuals receiving this drug for *Pneumocystis* prophylaxis.

Course & Prognosis

With improvements in therapy, patients are living longer after the diagnosis of AIDS. This has resulted in dramatic decreases in AIDS deaths nationally. In 2004 in the United States there were 15,798 deaths due to AIDS, compared with 50,610 deaths in 1995. It remains to be seen whether the decreases in number of deaths can be sustained over the long term. Maintaining access to quality care and treatment is one key element. Unfortunately, studies continue to show less access to treatment for some underserved groups, especially blacks, the homeless, and injection drug users. Another key element in sustaining lower mortality is developing new treatments for patients who have been heavily treated with existing agents. Despite new therapeutic options, people continue to die of HIV infection. For patients whose disease progresses even though they are receiving appropriate treatment, meticulous palliative care must be provided (see Chapter 5), with attention to pain control, spiritual needs, and family (biologic and chosen) dynamics.

Bamberger JD et al: Helping the urban poor stay with antiretroviral HIV drug therapy. Am J Pub Health 2000;90:699. [PMID: 10800416]

Benson CA: Treating opportunistic infections among HIV-infected adults and adolescents: recommendations from CDC, the National Institutes of Health, and the HIV Medicine Association/Infectious Diseases Society of America. MMWR Recomm Rep 2004;53(RR-1):1.

El-Sadr WM et al: Discontinuation of prophylaxis for *Mycobacterium avium* complex disease in HIV-infected patients who have a response to antiretroviral therapy. N Engl J Med 2000;342:1085. [PMID: 10766581]

Gallant JE et al; Study 934 Group: Tenofovir DF, emtricitabine, and efavirenz vs.zidovudine, lamivudine, and efavirenz for HIV. N Engl J Med 2006;354:251. [PMID: 16421366]

Gallant JE et al; 903 Study Group: Efficacy and safety of tenofovir DF vs stavudine in combination therapy in antiretroviral-naïve patients: a 3-year randomized trial. JAMA 2004; 292:191. [PMID: 15249568]

Grinspoon S et al: Cardiovascular risk and body-fat abnormalities in HIV-infected adults. N Engl J Med 2005;352:48. [PMID: 15635112]

Hirsch MS et al: Antiretroviral drug resistance testing in adults infected with human immunodeficiency virus type 1: 2003 recommendations of an International AIDS Society-USA panel. Clin Infect Dis 2003;37:113. [PMID: 12830416]

Lazzarin A et al: Efficacy of enfuvirtide in patients infected with drug-resistant HIV-1 in Europe and Australia. N Engl J Med 2003;348:2186. [PMID: 12773645]

Levine AM et al: Evaluation and management of HIV-infected women. Ann Intern Med 2002;136:228. [PMID: 11827499]

Martin DF et al: A controlled trial of valganciclovir as induction therapy for cytomegalovirus retinitis. N Engl J Med 2002; 346:1119. [PMID: 11948271]

Robbins GK et al: Comparison of sequential three-drug regimens as initial therapy for HIV-1 infection. N Engl J Med 2003; 349:2293. [PMID: 14668456]

Shafran SD et al: Successful discontinuation of therapy for disseminated *Mycobacterium avium* complex infection after effective antiretroviral therapy. Ann Intern Med 2002;137: 734. [PMID: 12416943]

Stringer JR et al: A new name (*Pneumocystis jiroveci*) for Pneumocystis from humans. Emerg Infect Dis 2002;8:891. [PMID: 12416943]

Vincent I et al: Modalities of palliative care in hospitalized patients with advanced AIDS. AIDS Care 2000;12:211. [PMID: 10827862]

Yeni PG et al: Treatment for adult HIV infection: 2004 recommendations of the International AIDS Society-USA Panel. JAMA 2004;292:251. [PMID: 15249575]

Infectious Diseases: Viral & Rickettsial

32

Wayne X. Shandera, MD, & Hoonmo Koo, MD

■ VIRAL DISEASES

This section discusses viral diseases caused by herpesviruses, those preventable by vaccines, and others causing distinct syndromes. Rickettsial illnesses and Kawasaki disease are also included. Disorders caused by hepatotropic viruses (see Chapter 15), papillomaviruses (see Chapters 6 and 17), and HIV (see Chapters 17 and 31) are dealt with elsewhere.

Clinical Diagnosis

Some viral illnesses present with typical syndromes (measles, mumps, and chickenpox). In others, the clinical picture suggests any of a number of viruses. For example, aseptic meningitis can be caused by the mumps virus, lymphocytic choriomeningitis virus, and several enteroviruses, among others. Symptoms of respiratory disease with many viruses are indistinguishable. Some viral diseases have a characteristic rash, although in most cases, the rash associated with viral syndromes is not pathognomonic.

Identification of a virus is useful for confirmation of atypical cases, help with outbreak investigation, elucidation of confusing syndromes, and increasingly to support the need for specific antiviral therapy. The frequency with which certain pathogens cause certain diseases allows for educated guesses, eg, respiratory syncytial virus (RSV) for bronchiolitis or parainfluenza virus for croup. Instances in which rapid diagnosis assists in patient management are noted.

Laboratory Diagnosis

Several techniques are used for diagnosis, including stain (the nonspecific Tzanck smear for herpesviruses), cell culture (coxsackievirus in suckling mice), immunologic detection (seroconversion with arboviruses, rabies virus on skin biopsy, detection of secretory immunoglobulin A [IgA]), or molecular techniques such as polymerase chain reaction (PCR) (for herpes simplex virus [HSV]) or antigen assays (for cytomegalovirus [CMV]).

Isolation of virus from a normally sterile site (cerebrospinal fluid, lung) or from a lesion (vesicles) in an immunocompetent individual is diagnostically significant. Isolation from nonsterile sites (nasopharynx, stool) may represent a carrier state, and seroconversion and pathologic change are needed to establish a diagnosis.

A. MICROSCOPIC METHODS

Microscopic techniques are used to examine cells, body fluids, or biopsy material in search of virus or cytopathic changes specific for one virus or a group of viruses (eg, multinucleated giant cells at the base of herpes lesions, rotavirus structures on electron micrographs of diarrheal stools).

Immunofluorescent methods, often with monoclonal antibodies, can rapidly identify some antigens (rabies, varicella, herpes simplex, RSV) in desquamated or scraped cells.

B. IMMUNOLOGIC STUDIES OF SERA

Specific antibodies to viruses rise during the course of illness, though the rise and persistence of titer depend on both the virus and the host response. A fourfold or greater rise in antibody titer during illness is considered evidence of disease.

Single determinations are seldom helpful, and laboratories require paired sera (acute and convalescent, typically 2–3 weeks apart). Antigenic detection is used for certain viruses (hepatitis B surface antigen [HBsAg], CMV, HIV), with viral presence detected independently of disease duration or host response. As more is learned of the natural history of HSV-1 and HSV-2 infections, these viruses are increasingly managed clinically with support from serologic data. Quantification of viral antigen titer is useful in the management of HIV disease and is becoming a standard of care for other chronic viral infections (eg, hepatitis B and C virus [HBV, HCV]).

C. MOLECULAR TECHNIQUES

Molecular technology has provided techniques such as PCR and nucleic acid probes that have proved useful in the identification of new pathogens (eg, HCV and

Kaposi's sarcoma herpesvirus) as well as for the management of patients in whom quantification of viral activity, as with immunologic techniques, assists in following the course of clinical illness or the response to therapy. Results vary among laboratories.

Treatment

The armamentarium of antiviral therapy has expanded greatly with the advent of the HIV outbreak (Table 31–5), though for many viruses there remains no definitive antiviral therapy.

The mainstay of controlling viral diseases is vaccination. Currently available live vaccines include those against measles, mumps, rubella, poliovirus (Sabin vaccine), yellow fever, and varicella. The inactivated vaccines protect against the agents implicated in poliovirus (Salk vaccine), hepatitis A, hepatitis B, influenza A and B, rabies, RSV, and Japanese B encephalitis. Passive immunoprophylaxis remains important in prevention of hepatitis A and B, RSV infection and, among the immunosuppressed, varicella. There is now a trend favoring the combination of vaccines, with the sacrifice in immunogenicity compensated for by the increased compliance with vaccinations by the vaccinated patient and their families.

Fletcher MA et al: Vaccines administered simultaneously: directions for new combination vaccines based on an historical review of the literature. Int J Infect Dis 2004;8:328. [PMID: 15494254]

HUMAN HERPESVIRUSES

Herpesviruses cause a wide spectrum of human disease. Eight identified human herpesviruses (HHV) include HSV (type 1), HSV (type 2), varicella-zoster virus (VZV) (type 3), Epstein–Barr infectious mononucleosis virus (type 4), and CMV (type 5). A sixth type (HHV-6) has been identified as a causative agent of roseola (exanthema subitum), and a seventh (HHV-7) is serologically associated with several syndromes. Another herpesvirus (HHV-8) is linked with Kaposi's sarcoma (see Chapter 31).

Subclinical primary infection with the herpesviruses is more common than clinically manifest illness. Each persists in a latent state for the remainder of the person's life. With HSV and VZV, virus remains latent in sensory ganglia; upon reactivation, lesions appear in the distal sensory nerve distribution. As a result of disease-, drug-, or radiation-induced immunosuppression, virus reactivation may lead to widespread lesions in affected organs such as the viscera or the central nervous system (CNS). Severe or fatal illness may occur in infants and the immunodeficient. Herpesviruses can transform cells in tissue culture. Associations with malignancies include Epstein–Barr virus (EBV) with Burkitt's lymphoma and nasopharyngeal carcinoma and HHV-8 with primary effusion lymphoma and Kaposi's sarcoma.

1. Herpesviruses 1 & 2

ESSENTIALS OF DIAGNOSIS

- Spectrum of illness from stomatitis and urogenital lesions to facial nerve paralysis (Bell's palsy) and encephalitis.
- Variable intervals between exposure and clinical disease, since HSV causes both primary (which may be subclinical) and reactivation disease.
- Successful management with acyclovir or related acyclic compounds (valacyclovir, famciclovir).

General Considerations

Herpesviruses 1 and 2 affect primarily the oral and genital areas, respectively. Seroprevalence to both viruses increases with age; seroprevalence to HSV-2 increases with sexual activity. Disease is typically a manifestation of reactivation, and the triggers for clinical reactivation are not well understood. Although HSV-1 is increasingly recognized as causing primary urogenital infections (> 65–70% in series from Israel and the United States), genital recurrences are much more frequent with HSV-2. Following the first year after infection, HSV-1 recurrences are rare, while HSV-2 reactivations gradually decrease.

Clinical Findings

A. MUCOCUTANEOUS DISEASE

HSV-1 mucocutaneous disease largely involves the mouth and oral cavity ("herpes labialis"). HSV-2 is the most common cause of genital ulcers in the developing world. Digital lesions (**whitlows**) are an occupational hazard in medicine, nursing, and dentistry.

Vesicles form moist ulcers after several days and epithelialize over 1–2 weeks if left untreated. Primary infection is usually more severe than recurrences but may be asymptomatic. Recurrences often involve fewer lesions, tend to be labial, heal faster, and are induced by stress, fever, infection, sunlight, chemotherapy (eg, fludarabine), or other undetermined factors.

HSV-2 lesions largely involve the genital tract. Virus remains latent in presacral ganglia. Typical lesions are multiple, painful, small, grouped, and vesicular. A manifestation of primary infection, predominantly in women, may be aseptic meningitis. Asymptomatic HSV-2 occurs frequently in the CNS. Urinary retention and chronic neuropathic pelvic pain may occur. Risk factors for HSV transmission include black race, female gender, a history of sexually transmitted infections (STIs), an increased number of partners, contact with commercial sex workers, lower socioeconomic status, young age of onset of sexual activity, and total duration of sexual activity. Asymptomatic shedding of either HSV-1 or HSV-2 is common, especially following primary infection or symptomatic recurrences, and appears to be responsible for transmission. HSV-2 increases the risk of HIV acquisition, and in advanced HIV infection, HSV reactivates more frequently.

Diagnosis is usually made clinically, but viral cultures of vesicular fluid or direct fluorescent antibody staining of scraped lesions remain the standard of diagnosis. HSV can be identified using PCR, and its presence correlates with clinical reactivation. The presence of intranuclear inclusion bodies and multinucleated giant cells on a Tzanck preparation or Calcofluor stain is supportive of a diagnosis of herpetic viral infection.

In STI, perinatal, and HIV clinics, type-specific serologies are useful for counseling HIV-infected individuals, pregnant women, and those with an uncertain clinical history, high-risk behavior, or increased number of sexual partners.

B. OCULAR DISEASE

HSV can cause keratitis, blepharitis, and keratoconjunctivitis. Keratitis is usually unilateral, is suggested by impaired visual acuity, and is diagnosed by branching (dendritic) ulcers that stain with fluorescein. It may be difficult to differentiate HSV conjunctivitis clinically from adenoviral conjunctivitis in the acute stage. Recurrences are frequent.

C. NEONATAL AND CONGENITAL INFECTION

Both herpesviruses can infect the fetus and induce congenital malformations (organomegaly, bleeding, and CNS abnormalities). Neonatal transmission during delivery is more common than intrauterine infection. Maternal infection during the third trimester is associated with the highest risk of neonatal transmission; about 70% of these infections are asymptomatic or unrecognized. Invasive fetal monitoring and vacuum or forceps delivery can facilitate the risk of transmitting herpes.

D. ENCEPHALITIS AND RECURRENT MENINGITIS

Herpes simplex encephalitis presents with nonspecific symptoms: a flu-like prodrome, followed by headache, fever, behavioral and speech disturbances, and seizures that may be focal or generalized. There is a propensity to involve the temporal lobe, with mass effect on imaging studies and temporal lobe seizure foci on electroencephalograms (EEGs). Cerebrospinal fluid pleocytosis is common, with roughly equal numbers of red cells. MRI scanning is often a useful adjunct showing increased signal in the temporal and frontal lobes.

HSV DNA PCR of the cerebrospinal fluid is a rapid, sensitive, and specific tool for early diagnosis. Cerebrospinal fluid findings of antibodies to HSV can confirm the diagnosis. Viral cultures show temperature dependence, with lower rates of recovery in the summer. Untreated disease and presentation with coma carry a high mortality rate, with many survivors suffering neurologic sequelae. HSV-1 predominantly causes herpes simplex encephalitis. However, HSV-1 and HSV-2 are both associated with benign recurrent lymphocytic (Mollaret's) meningitis.

E. DISSEMINATED INFECTION

Disseminated HSV infection occurs in the setting of immunosuppression, either primary or iatrogenic, including corticosteroid usage, or rarely with pregnancy. Skin lesions are a particular complication in patients with atopic eczema (eczema herpeticum). In disseminated disease, skin lesions are not always present.

F. BELL'S PALSY

An association between HSV-1 and Bell's palsy is established.

G. ESOPHAGITIS

Esophagitis from HSV-1 in AIDS and other immunocompromised patients is diagnosed by endoscopic biopsy and cultures. CMV esophagitis is distinguished by the size and depth of the lesion (smaller and deeper for HSV). HSV-1 is also postulated to activate mononuclear cells in the pathogenesis of achalasia.

H. ERYTHEMA MULTIFORME

Herpes simplex viruses remain, with drugs, the leading association with erythema multiforme and with the more severe, mucosally involved Stevens–Johnson syndrome.

I. OTHER

Recent studies suggest an association between HSV-1 and atrial myxoma.

Treatment & Prevention

Drugs that inhibit replication of HSV-1 and HSV-2 include trifluridine (for keratitis), acyclovir and related compounds (for urogenital, encephalitic, or disseminated disease), and foscarnet (for resistant strains in immunocompromised persons) (Table 32–1).

A. MUCOCUTANEOUS DISEASE

While treatment is often not necessary in immunocompetent patients, it can ameliorate and shorten the duration of symptoms if initiated early. Immunocompromised patients are treated with oral or topical acyclic derivatives, with intravenous acyclovir reserved for severe or recalcitrant disease. Lesions heal faster with topical penciclovir than with topical acyclovir. Oral agents are generally superior to topical ones and include (for primary infection) acyclovir, 200 mg five times a day for 10 days, valacyclovir, 1 g twice daily for 7–10 days, or famciclovir, 250 mg three times daily for 7–10 days. Reactivation disease is treated with half the dose of the oral agents used against primary infection.

Acyclovir-resistant isolates associated with mucocutaneous lesions in the HIV-positive population are treated with foscarnet (phosphonoformic acid), 40–60

Table 32–1. Agents for viral infections.[1]

Drug	Dosing	Spectrum	Renal Clearance/ Hemodialysis	CNS/CSF Penetration	Toxicities
Acyclovir	200–800 mg orally five times daily; 250–500 mg/ m² intravenously every 8 hours for 7 days	HSV, VZV	Yes/Yes	Yes	Neurotoxic reactions, reversible renal dysfunction, local reactions
Adefovir	10 mg daily orally	HBV	Yes/Yes	NA	Gastrointestinal symptoms, transaminitis, lactic acidosis, nephrotoxicity
Amantadine	100 mg orally twice daily (100 mg/d in elderly) for 10 days	Influenza A, not avian flu	Yes/No	Yes	Confusion, gastrointestinal symptoms
Cidofovir	5 mg/kg intravenously weekly for 2 weeks, then every other week	CMV	Yes/NA	NA	Neutropenia, renal failure, ocular hypotonia
Entecavir	0.5 mg orally daily, increase to 1 mg orally daily in lamivudine-resistant patients	HBV	Yes/NA	NA	Lactic acidosis, rare exacerbation of HBV infection
Famciclovir	500 mg orally three times daily for 7 days for acute VZV; 250 mg three times daily for 7–10 days for genital or cutaneous HSV-1/HSV-2 infection; 125 mg twice daily for 5 days for recurrences (500 mg twice daily for 7 days if HIV-infected)	HSV, VZV	Yes/NA	NA	NA
Fomivirsen	165 mcg by intravitreal injection once weekly for 3 weeks, then every other week	CMV	NA	NA	Ocular inflammation, retinal detachment
Foscarnet	20 mg/kg intravenous bolus, then 120 mg/kg intravenously every 8 hours for 2 weeks; maintain with 60 mg/kg/d intravenously for 5 days each week	CMV, HSV resistant to acyclovir, VZV, HIV-1	Yes/Yes	Variable	Nephrotoxicity, genital ulcerations, calcium disturbances
Ganciclovir	5 mg/kg intravenous bolus every 12 hours for 14–21 days; maintain with 3.75 mg/kg/d intravenously for 5 days each week	CMV	Yes/Yes	Yes	Neutropenia, thrombocytopenia, CNS side effects
Idoxuridine	Topical, 0.1% every 1–2 hours for 3–5 days	HSV keratitis	—	—	Local reactions
Interferon α-2b	3–5 million IU subcutaneously 3 times weekly to daily. Intralesionally: 1 million IU per 0.1 mL in up to 5 warts three times weekly for 3 weeks	HBV, HCV, HPV	Yes/Yes	—	Influenza-like syndrome, myelosuppression, neurotoxicity

(continued)

Table 32–1. Agents for viral infections.[1] (continued)

Drug	Dosing	Spectrum	Renal Clearance/ Hemodialysis	CNS/CSF Penetration	Toxicities
Interferon α-n3	0.05 mL/wart biweekly up to 8 weeks	HPV	NA/NA	NA	Local reactions
	3 mU intravenously three times per week	? HCV	NA/NA	NA	Influenza-like syndrome, myelosuppression, neurotoxicity
Lamivudine (3TC)	12 mg/kg/d	HIV-1, ?HIV-2, HBV	Yes/NA	Yes	Skin rash, headache, insomnia
Oseltamivir	75 mg twice daily for 5 days beginning 48 hours after onset of symptoms	Influenza A and B	Yes/NA	NA	Few
Penciclovir	Topical, 1% cream every 2 hours for 4 days	HSV	No/No	No	Local reactions
Palivizumab	15 mg/kg intramuscularly every month in RSV season	RSV	No/No	No	Upper respiratory infection symptoms
Ribavirin	Aerosol: 1.1 g/d as 20 mg/ mL dilution over 12–18 hours for 3–7 days (See text for Lassa fever doses.)	RSV, severe influenza A or B, Lassa fever	Yes/No	Yes	Wheezing
Rimantadine	100 mg orally twice daily	Influenza A	Yes/No	Yes	Same as amantadine, but less severe
Trifluridine	Topical, 1% drops every 2 hours to 9 drops/d	HSV keratitis	—	—	Local reactions
Valacyclovir	1 g orally three times daily for 7 days for acute VZV; 1 g twice daily for primary genital HSV-1/HSV-2 infection with 500 mg three times daily for recurrences	VZV, HSV	Yes/Poorly	NA	Thrombotic thrombocytopenic purpura or hemolytic-uremic syndrome in AIDS
Valganciclovir	900 mg orally twice daily for 3 weeks; 900 mg daily as maintenance	CMV	Yes/Yes	Yes	See ganciclovir
Vidarabine	15 mg/kg/d intravenously for 10 days	HSV, VZV	Yes/Yes	Yes	Teratogenic, megaloblastosis, neurotoxicity
Zanamivir	2–5 mg inhalations twice daily for 5 days	Influenza A and B	Yes/NA	NA	Few

[1]Agents used exclusively in the management of HIV infection and AIDS are found in Chapter 31.
CNS = central nervous system; CSF = cerebrospinal fluid; HSV = herpes simplex virus; VZV = varicella-zoster virus; HBV = hepatitis B virus; CMV = cytomegalovirus; HPV = human papillomavirus; HCV = hepatitis C virus; RSV = respiratory syncytial virus.

mg/kg intravenously every 8 hours, adjusting for renal function. The acyclic nucleotide analog cidofovir is used against HSV and CMV in rare cases of infection resistant to both acyclovir and foscarnet.

Acyclovir and related compounds are effective in secondary prevention. Patients with recurrent genital infections may be placed on maintenance acyclovir at a dosage of 400 mg twice a day. Prophylaxis for herpes labialis and mucocutaneous HSV infections may be especially useful for patients exposed to ultraviolet radia-

tion such as during skiing or sailing trips when topical sun-blocking agents cannot be used or for wrestlers at risk for herpes gladiatorum. Famciclovir (250 mg twice daily or 500 mg once daily) and valacyclovir (500 mg to 1 g—if the lower dose results in breakthrough lesions—once daily) are more costly alternatives for preventing recurrent disease. Studies with valacyclovir show a reduction in subclinical shedding and in the risk of transmission among HSV-2 discordant heterosexual partners. The advantages of these two agents include higher serum levels and less frequent administration. AIDS patients with a history of mucocutaneous disease should receive lifelong suppressive therapy. Acyclovir resistance occurs often among immunodeficient persons. Counseling, barrier protection or, in the future, microbicides, are useful to decrease the rate of transmission among sexual partners of infected persons.

HIV-infected individuals should be assayed for HSV-2 serologies and counseled if seropositive. In addition, among HIV-infected persons, the use of highly active antiretroviral therapy (HAART) is associated with fewer days of HSV-1 or -2 lesions.

B. KERATITIS

Ophthalmic trifluridine, vidarabine, and acyclovir given as drops for 10 days (without corticosteroids) are the available alternatives. Long-term (greater than 1 year) treatment with acyclovir at a dosage of 800 mg/d orally decreases recurrence rates.

C. NEONATAL DISEASE

Acyclovir intravenously is effective for disseminated lesions in neonatal disease. The dosage is 20 mg/kg intravenously every 8 hours for 14–21 days. The use of maternal antenatal suppressive therapy with acyclovir (typically, 800 mg/day) beginning at 36 weeks gestation decreases rates of HSV detection, asymptomatic shedding, and recurrence at delivery or need for cesarean section. However, cesarean section is recommended for pregnant women with active genital lesions or typical prodromal symptoms.

D. ENCEPHALITIS

Because of the need for rapid treatment and the difficulties associated with brain biopsy, patients with suspected HSV encephalitis are given intravenous acyclovir (10 mg/kg every 8 hours for 10 days or more, adjusting for renal impairment), starting upon suspicion of diagnosis, and stopping if another diagnosis is established. If the PCR is negative and clinical suspicion remains high in the absence of a biopsy, treatment should be continued for 10 days because of the relatively nontoxic nature of acyclovir. Long-term neurologic sequelae are common.

E. DISSEMINATED DISEASE

Disseminated disease responds best to parenteral acyclovir (see the preceding paragraph for dosages) when treatment is initiated early.

F. BELL'S PALSY

The efficacy of treating Bell's palsy with acyclovir or corticosteroids is not fully established although a number of studies suggest that a combination of acyclovir or valacyclovir and prednisone, if given in the first 3 days of disease, is associated with improved rates of recovery.

G. ESOPHAGITIS

Patients with esophagitis should receive either intravenous acyclovir at a dosage of 5–10 mg/kg every 8

hours or oral acyclovir, 400 mg five times daily. AIDS patients are maintained on acyclovir at a dosage of 400 mg three to five times daily.

H. ERYTHEMA MULTIFORME

Acyclovir may decrease the recurrence rate of HSV-associated erythema multiforme.

Prevention

Besides antiviral suppressive therapy, prevention also requires use of barrier precautions during sexual activity. Preventing spread to hospital staff and other patients from cases with mucocutaneous, disseminated, or genital disease requires isolation and the use of handwashing and gloving–gowning precautions. Staff with active lesions (eg, whitlows) should not have contact with patients. Asymptomatic transmission occurs, especially with HSV-2. A glycoprotein vaccine, preliminarily effective among female HSV-2 seronegative women, is under investigation.

Brown ZA et al: Genital herpes complicating pregnancy. Obstet Gynecol 2005;106:845. [PMID: 16199646]

Corey L et al; Valacyclovir HSV Transmission Study Group: Once-daily valacyclovir to reduce the risk of transmission of genital herpes. N Engl J Med 2004;350:11. [PMID: 14702423]

Holland NJ et al: Recent developments in Bell's palsy. BMJ 2004; 329:553. [PMID: 15345630]

Roberts CM et al: Increasing proportion of herpes simplex virus type 1 as a cause of genital herpes infection in college students. Sex Transm Dis 2003;30:797. [PMID: 14520181]

Sheffield JS et al: Acyclovir prophylaxis to prevent herpes simplex virus recurrence at delivery: a systematic review. Obstet Gynecol 2003;102:1396. [PMID: 14662233]

Tyler KL: Herpes simplex virus infections of the central nervous system: encephalitis and meningitis, including Mollaret's. Herpes 2004;11(Suppl 2):57A. [PMID: 15319091]

Whitley R: Neonatal herpes simplex virus infection. Curr Opin Infect Dis 2004;17:243. [PMID: 15166828]

2. Varicella (Chickenpox) & Herpes Zoster (Shingles)

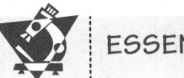 ESSENTIALS OF DIAGNOSIS

- Exposure 14–21 days before onset.
- Fever and malaise just before or with eruption.
- Rash: pruritic, centrifugal, papular, changing to vesicular ("dewdrops on a rose petal"), pustular, and finally crusting.

General Considerations

Varicella-zoster virus (VZV) is HHV-3. Disease manifestations are either chickenpox (varicella) or shingles (herpes zoster). Chickenpox is highly contagious and is generally a disease of childhood, with spread by inhalation of infective droplets or contact with lesions after an incubation of 10–20 days (average, 14–15 days).

The incidence and severity of herpes zoster ("shingles") increases with age (although cases are reported among infants and children) due to an age-related decline in immunity against VZV. More than half of all patients in whom herpes zoster develops are older than 60 years. The annual incidence of zoster in the United States is at least 1 million cases, which is expected to increase as the population ages. Other persons at risk include those who are immunosuppressed (eg, patients receiving cancer treatment, patients with AIDS, and organ transplant recipients) and occasionally infants after intrauterine infection.

Clinical Findings

A. VARICELLA

1. Symptoms and signs—(Table 32–2.) Fever and malaise are mild in children and more marked in adults. Vesicular lesions, quickly rupturing to form small ulcers, may appear first in the oropharynx. The pruritic rash begins prominently on the face, scalp, and trunk, and later involves the extremities. Maculopapules change in a few hours to vesicles that become pustular and eventually form crusts. New lesions may erupt for 1–5 days, so that different stages of the eruption are usually present simultaneously, unlike smallpox in which all lesions tend to evolve simultaneously. The crusts slough in 7–14 days. The vesicles and pustules are superficial and elliptical, with slightly serrated borders.

After the primary infection, the virus remains dormant in cranial nerves sensory ganglia and spinal dorsal root ganglia. Latent VZV will reactivate as herpes zoster in about 10–30% of persons (see below). Widespread dissemination can occur in the immunosuppressed, sometimes in the absence of cutaneous lesions. CNS complications, in particular cerebellar ataxia, vasculopathy, and encephalitis, occur rarely.

2. Laboratory findings—Diagnosis is usually made clinically, with confirmation by direct immunofluorescent antibody (DFA) staining or PCR of scrapings from lesions. Multinucleated giant cells are usually apparent on a Tzanck smear or Calcofluor stain of material from the vesicle bases. Leukopenia is often present.

B. HERPES ZOSTER

Herpes zoster (**"shingles"**) usually occurs among adults, but cases are reported among infants and children. Pain is often severe and may precede the appearance of rash. Lesions follow any nerve root distribution, with thoracic and lumbar roots being the most common; cervical or trigeminal involvement is typical. In most cases, a single unilateral dermatome is involved. The occurrence of zoster does not correlate with progression to AIDS in HIV-infected patients, but recurrent and in particular multidermatomal zoster indicates a poorer prognosis in established AIDS.

Skin lesions resemble those of chickenpox, developing as maculopapules and evolving into vesicles and pustules. Lesions on the tip of the nose indicate involvement of the nasociliary nerve, a branch of the ophthalmic division of the trigeminal nerve, which also serves the cornea. Facial palsy, lesions of the external ear with or without tympanic membrane involvement, vertigo and tinnitus, and deafness signify geniculate ganglion involvement (Ramsay Hunt syndrome). In either, treatment is indicated (see below).

Complications

A. VARICELLA

Interstitial pneumonia is more common in adults (especially smokers, HIV-infected patients, and pregnant women) than in children and may result in acute respiratory distress syndrome (ARDS). After healing, numerous densely calcified lesions are seen throughout the lung fields on chest radiographs. Ischemic strokes have been recognized in the wake of acute varicella and may be due to an associated vasculitis. Hepatitis is suggested by aminotransferase elevations and occurs in a small percentage of patients with varicella-zoster infection. Encephalitis is infrequent (1:1000) and is characterized by ataxia and nystagmus and may be life-threatening. Cerebellar ataxia occurs among younger people at a lower frequency than encephalitis (1:4000).

Secondary bacterial infections, particularly with group A β-hemolytic streptococci and *Staphylococcus aureus*, are common. Cellulitis, erysipelas, epiglottitis, osteomyelitis, scarlet fever and, rarely, meningitis are observed. Pitted scars are frequent sequelae.

Reye's syndrome (fatty liver with encephalopathy) also complicates varicella (and other viral infections, especially influenza B), usually in childhood, and is associated with aspirin therapy (see Influenza, below). The many manifestations of VZV infection that occur in HIV infection include multifocal encephalitis, ventriculitis, myeloradiculitis, and arteritis.

When contracted during the first or second trimesters of pregnancy, varicella carries a very small risk of congenital malformations, including cicatricial lesions of an extremity, growth retardation, microphthalmia, cataracts, chorioretinitis, deafness, and cerebrocortical atrophy. If a mother develops varicella within 5 days after delivery, the newborn is at risk for disseminated disease and should receive varicella-zoster immune globulin (VZIG). (See below for dosage.)

VZV is a major etiologic agent of Bell's palsy in patients lacking antibodies to HSV.

VZV is the major virus associated with **acute retinal necrosis (ARN)** and **progressive outer retinal necrosis (PORN)**, both of which occur with increased frequency among AIDS patients. Another AIDS-associated manifestation with VZV is immune restitution disease, among patients who have recently started HAART.

Table 32–2. Diagnostic features of some acute exanthems.

Disease	Prodromal Signs and Symptoms	Nature of Eruption	Other Diagnostic Features	Laboratory Tests
Eczema herpeticum	None.	Vesiculopustular lesions in area of eczema.		Herpes simplex virus isolated in cell culture. Multinucleate giant cells in smear of lesion.
Varicella (chickenpox)	0–1 day of fever, anorexia, headache.	Rapid evolution of macules to papules, vesicles, crusts; all stages simultaneously present; lesions superficial, distribution centripetal.	Lesions on scalp and mucous membranes.	Specialized complement fixation and virus neutralization in cell culture. Fluorescent antibody test of smear of lesions.
Infectious mononucleosis (EBV)	Fever, adenopathy, sore throat.	Maculopapular rash resembling rubella, rarely papulovesicular.	Splenomegaly, tonsillar exudate.	Atypical lymphocytes in blood smears; heterophil agglutination (Monospot test).
Exanthema subitum (HHV-6, 7; roseola)	3–4 days of high fever.	As fever falls by crisis, pink maculopapules appear on chest and trunk; fade in 1–3 days.		White blood count low.
Measles (rubeola)	3–4 days of fever, coryza, conjunctivitis, and cough.	Maculopapular, brick-red; begins on head and neck; spreads downward and outward, in 5–6 days rash brownish, desquamating. See atypical measles, below.	Koplik's spots on buccal mucosa.	White blood count low. Virus isolation in cell culture. Antibody tests by hemagglutination inhibition or neutralization.
Atypical measles	Same as measles.	Maculopapular centripetal rash, becoming confluent.	History of measles vaccination.	Measles antibody present in past, with titer rise during illness.
Rubella	Little or no prodrome.	Maculopapular, pink; begins on head and neck, spreads downward, fades in 3 days. No desquamation.	Lymphadenopathy, postauricular or occipital.	White blood count normal or low. Serologic tests for immunity and definitive diagnosis (hemagglutination inhibition).
Erythema infectiosum (parvovirus B19)	None. Usually in epidemics.	Red, flushed cheeks; circumoral pallor; maculopapules on extremities.	"Slapped face" appearance.	White blood count normal.
Enterovirus infections	1–2 days of fever, malaise.	Maculopapular rash resembling rubella, rarely papulovesicular or petechial.	Aseptic meningitis.	Virus isolation from stool or cerebrospinal fluid; complement fixation titer rise.
Typhus	3–4 days of fever, chills, severe headaches.	Maculopapules, petechiae, initial distribution centrifugal (trunk to extremities).	Endemic area, lice.	Complement fixation.
Rocky Mountain spotted fever	3–4 days of fever, vomiting.	Maculopapules, petechiae, initial distribution centripetal (extremities to trunk, including palms).	History of tick bite.	Indirect fluorescent antibody; complement fixation.
Ehrlichiosis	Headache, malaise.	Rash in one-third, similar to Rocky Mountain spotted fever.	Pancytopenia, elevated liver function tests.	Polymerase chain reaction, immunofluorescent antibody.
Scarlet fever	One-half to 2 days of malaise, sore throat, fever, vomiting.	Generalized, punctate, red; prominent on neck, in axillae, groin, skin folds; circumoral pallor; fine desquamation involves hands and feet.	Strawberry tongue, exudative tonsillitis.	Group A β-hemolytic streptococci in cultures from throat; antistreptolysin O titer rise.

(continued)

Table 32–2. Diagnostic features of some acute exanthems. (continued)

Disease	Prodromal Signs and Symptoms	Nature of Eruption	Other Diagnostic Features	Laboratory Tests
Meningococ-cemia	Hours of fever, vomiting.	Maculopapules, petechiae, purpura.	Meningeal signs, toxicity, shock.	Cultures of blood, cerebrospinal fluid. High white blood count.
Kawasaki disease	Fever, adenopa-thy, conjunctivitis.	Cracked lips, strawberry tongue, maculopapular polymorphous rash, peeling skin on fingers and toes.	Edema of extremi-ties. Angiitis of coronary arteries.	Thrombocytosis, electrocardiographic changes.
Smallpox (based on prior experience)	Fever, malaise, prostration.	Maculopapules to vesicles to pustules to scars (lesions develop at the same pace).	Centrifugal rash; fulminant sepsis in small percentage of patients, gastrointestinal and skin hemorrhages.	Contact CDC[1] for suspicious rash; EM and gel diffusion assays.

[1]http://www.bt.cdc.gov/agent/smallpox/response-plan/.
EBV = Epstein–Barr virus; HHV = human herpesvirus.

B. HERPES ZOSTER

In immunosuppressed and HIV-infected patients, herpes zoster may produce skin lesions beyond the dermatome, visceral lesions, and encephalitis. Postherpetic neuralgia occurs in 60–70% of zoster patients over age 60 years. The pain can be prolonged and debilitating. Risk factors for postherpetic neuralgia include age, female sex prodrome, and severity of rash or pain. There may also be an immunogenetic determinant to the development of postherpetic neuralgia.

Prevention

Patients with active varicella or zoster are separated from seronegative patients. Respiratory isolation is needed in varicella pneumonia. Health care workers should be screened for varicella and vaccinated if seronegative. They should stay away from work when active vesicles are present, typically from the tenth day after onset through the twenty-first day. VZIG is effective in preventing chickenpox in exposed susceptible—particularly immunosuppressed—individuals. These include (1) susceptible persons receiving immunosuppressive therapy; (2) persons with congenital cellular immunodeficiency; (3) persons with an acquired immunodeficiency, including AIDS; (4) susceptible and exposed persons, in particular pregnant females; (5) newborns; and (6) premature infants of low birth weight.

A. VARICELLA

A live attenuated vaccine, administered as one dose, or two doses 3 months apart, is safe and currently recommended for all children between 12 and 18 months of age who have not had chickenpox. Patients with impaired cellular immunity should not be immunized, although the vaccine appears to be safe and effective when given to asymptomatic or mildly symptomatic HIV-infected children or to patients with chronic kidney disease. Susceptible, nonimmunocompromised household contacts with no prior history of varicella should also be vaccinated. Under such conditions, the vaccine is 85% effective in preventing illness and 95% effective in preventing serious disease. Vaccine effectiveness decreases significantly within a year after administration and is lower when vaccination occurs at age 15 months or younger, although breakthrough cases are usually mild. Vaccination during early pregnancy (weeks 13–20), however, is associated with congenital malformations. Children receiving the vaccine should not take aspirin for at least 6 weeks, because of the possibility of hepatic encephalopathy (Reye's syndrome). Rashes occur after vaccination in up to 5% of healthy children and 50% of leukemic children. Concomitant administration with other childhood vaccinations, including the measles–mumps–rubella, *Haemophilus influenza*, or hepatitis B virus vaccines, appears to be safe with no significant loss of immunogenicity. Adults should receive a second dose of the vaccine, typically 1–3 months after the first dose.

Universal childhood vaccination in the United States has been very successful in reducing the incidence, mortality rate, and health care expenditures secondary to varicella. Preliminary results of quadrivalent measles, mumps, rubella, and varicella vaccine are favorable and may eventually replace separate vaccinations. There is a concern that varicella vaccination will increase reactivation of herpes zoster as a result of lack of reexposures in adults to varicella, which boosts their immunity to latent VZV, but this has not occurred thus far. The incidence of herpes zoster has not changed significantly between 1992 and 2002.

If given within 4 days of exposure to an active varicella case, VZIG is effective in preventing chickenpox in exposed susceptible—particularly immunosuppressed—individuals. It is given by intramuscular injection in a dosage of 12.5 units/kg up to a maximum of 625 units, with a repeat dose in 3 weeks if a high-risk patient remains exposed. VZIG has no place in therapy of established disease. Further information may be obtained by calling the Centers for Disease Control and Prevention's Immunization Information Hotline (800-232-2522). Because VZIG appears to bind the varicella vaccine, the two should not be given concomitantly.

B. ZOSTER

A recent trial investigating a new live attenuated herpes zoster vaccine among adults age 60 years and older, designed to boost their cell-mediated immunity to VZV, demonstrated dramatic decreases in incidence of herpes zoster and postherpetic neuralgia. Future studies are awaited.

Treatment

A. GENERAL MEASURES

Patients should be isolated until primary crusts have disappeared and kept at bed rest until afebrile. Hospitalized patients with VZV infections should be isolated, and caregivers should wear gowns, gloves, and masks when in contact with them. The skin is kept clean. Pruritus can be relieved with antihistamines, calamine lotion, and colloidal oatmeal baths. As an antipyretic, acetaminophen is used. Gabapentin is used for postherpetic neuralgia.

B. ANTIVIRAL THERAPY

For the infrequent varicella infection for which antiviral therapy is indicated, the mainstay of therapy is acyclovir; its analogs (the prodrug valacyclovir and the related drug famciclovir) are approved only for immunocompetent individuals. These agents reduce the severity and shorten the duration of chickenpox and zoster in adults and in children. These antiviral agents, however, do not prevent the development of postherpetic neuralgia.

In immunocompromised patients, in pregnant women during the third trimester, and in patients with extracutaneous disease (encephalitis, pneumonitis), antiviral therapy with high-dose acyclovir (30 mg/kg/d in three divided doses intravenously for at least 7 days) should be started once the diagnosis is suspected. Acyclovir-resistant varicella has been observed in AIDS patients receiving long-term acyclovir therapy. Foscarnet may be used for acyclovir-resistant virus, although resistance to foscarnet is also recognized. Acyclovir is useful but not fully effective for retinal disease in AIDS (ARN, PORN [above]).

C. TREATMENT OF COMPLICATIONS

The most troublesome issue with VZV infection is postherpetic neuralgia, especially in older patients. Initial treatment with antivirals and corticosteroids does not clearly reduce the incidence or severity of postherpetic neuralgia. Once established, pain may respond to tricyclic antidepressants, lidocaine patches, gabapentin, or analgesics. Secondary bacterial infections of lesions are treated with antibiotics providing coverage for staphylococci.

Prognosis

The total duration of varicella from onset of symptoms to disappearance of crusts rarely exceeds 2 weeks. Fatalities are rare except in immunosuppressed patients.

Zoster resolves in 2–6 weeks. Antibodies persist longer and at higher levels than with primary varicella.

Johnson RW et al: Management of herpes zoster (shingles) and postherpetic neuralgia. Expert Opin Pharmacother 2004;5:551. [PMID: 15013924]

Jumaan AO et al: Incidence of herpes zoster, before and after varicella-vaccination–associated decreases in the incidence of varicella, 1992–2002. J Infect Dis 2005;191:2002. [PMID: 15897984]

Klassen TP et al: Acyclovir for treating varicella in otherwise healthy children and adolescents. Cochrane Database Syst Rev 2004;(2):CD002980. [PMID: 15106185]

Nguyen HQ et al: Decline in mortality due to varicella after implementation of varicella vaccination in the United States. N Engl J Med 2005;352:450. [PMID: 15689583]

Oxman MN et al; Shingles Prevention Study Group: A vaccine to prevent herpes zoster and postherpetic neuralgia in older adults. N Engl J Med 2005;352:2271. [PMID: 15930418]

Shinefield H et al; Dose Selection Study Group for Proquod: Dose-response study of a quadrivalent measles, mumps, rubella and varicella vaccine in healthy children. Ped Infect Dis J 2005;24:670. [PMID: 16094218]

Sorensen HT et al: The risk and prognosis of cancer after hospitalisation for herpes zoster: a population-based follow-up study. Br J Cancer 2004;91:1275. [PMID: 15328522]

Zhou F et al: Impact of varicella vaccination on health care utilization. JAMA 2005;294:797. [PMID: 16106004]

3. Epstein–Barr Virus & Infectious Mononucleosis

 ESSENTIALS OF DIAGNOSIS

- *Malaise, fever, and sore throat, sometimes with exudates.*
- *Palatal petechiae, lymphadenopathy, splenomegaly, and, occasionally, a maculopapular rash.*
- *Positive heterophil agglutination test (Monospot).*
- *Atypical large lymphocytes in blood smear; lymphocytosis.*
- *Possible complications: hepatitis, myocarditis, neuropathy, encephalitis, airway obstruction secondary to lymph node enlargement, anti-i hemolytic anemia, thrombocytopenia.*

General Considerations

Infectious mononucleosis is usually due to the EBV (HHV-4, found as two variants, EBV-1 and EBV-2, with multiple strains present in disease). It is universal in distribution and may be seen at any age but usually occurs in the United States in persons between the ages of 10 and 35 years, sporadically or in epidemic distribution. In the developing world, acute infections occur at much younger ages and tend to be less symptomatic. Rare cases occur in the elderly, usually without the full complex of symptoms. Its mode of transmission is probably by saliva. Saliva may remain infectious during convalescence for 6 months or longer from symptom onset. The incubation period probably lasts several weeks.

Clinical Findings

A. SYMPTOMS AND SIGNS

The protean manifestations reflect the pathogenesis of infection with viruses disseminating in the oral cavity, peripheral blood lymphocytes, and cell-free plasma. Symptoms typically include fever, sore throat, fatigue and toxic symptoms (malaise, anorexia, and myalgia) in the early phase of the illness. Physical findings include lymphadenopathy (discrete, nonsuppurative, slightly painful, especially along the posterior cervical chain) and splenomegaly (in up to 50% of patients). A maculopapular or occasionally petechial rash occurs in less than 15% of patients unless ampicillin has been given (when rash is seen in > 90%). Exudative pharyngitis, tonsillitis, or gingivitis may occur and soft palatal petechiae may be noted.

Other manifestations include hepatitis, nervous system involvement (mononeuropathies and occasionally aseptic meningitis, encephalitis, or Guillain–Barré syndrome), renal failure (interstitial nephritis), pulmonary involvement (dyspnea and cough, and in severe forms, "pseudocroup"), and myocarditis. Airway obstruction from lymph node enlargement is an indication for hospitalization or close observation.

B. LABORATORY FINDINGS

Initially, EBV infection is associated with granulocytopenia followed within 1 week by a lymphocytic leukocytosis. Many lymphocytes are atypical; specifically, they are larger than normal mature lymphocytes, stain more darkly, and show vacuolated, foamy cytoplasm and dark chromatin in the nucleus. Hemolytic anemia, usually secondary to anti-i antibodies, is occasionally encountered, as is thrombocytopenia (at times marked).

Heterophil (sheep cell agglutination) antibody tests and the correlated mononucleosis spot (Monospot) test usually become positive within 4 weeks after onset of illness. Titer rises in antibodies directed at several EBV antigens can be detected. During acute illness, there is a rise and fall in immunoglobulin M (IgM) antibody to EB virus capsid antigen (VCA) and a rise in IgG antibody to VCA, which persists for life. Antibodies to EBV nuclear antigen (EBNA) appear at 3–4 weeks after onset and also persist. A false-positive rapid plasma reagin (RPR) occurs in 10%. PCR for EBV DNA is useful in immunocompromised patients in the differential diagnosis of CNS processes and perhaps in monitoring disease. Hepatic aminotransferases and bilirubin are commonly elevated. In aseptic meningitis, the cerebrospinal fluid may show increased opening pressure, lymphocytosis with abnormal morphology, and increased protein concentration.

Differential Diagnosis

CMV infection, toxoplasmosis, acute HIV infection, HHV-6, rubella, and drug hypersensitivity reactions may be indistinguishable from infectious mononucleosis due to EBV, but exudative pharyngitis is usually absent and the heterophil antibody tests are negative; false-positive heterophil antibody tests can occur with CMV and toxoplasmosis. With acute HIV infection, a rash is sometimes seen but lymphocytic atypia is much less common. Mycoplasmal infection may also present as pharyngitis, though lower respiratory symptoms usually predominate. A hypersensitivity syndrome induced by carbamazepine may mimic infectious mononucleosis.

The differential diagnosis of acute exudative pharyngitis includes diphtheria, gonococcal and streptococcal infections, and infections with adenovirus and herpes simplex. Head and neck soft tissue infections (pharyngeal and tonsillar abscesses) may occasionally be mistaken for the lymphadenopathy of mononucleosis.

Complications

Secondary bacterial pharyngitis can occur and is often streptococcal. Splenic rupture is a rare but dramatic complication, and a history of preceding trauma can be elicited in 50% of the cases. Fulminant hepatitis with massive necrosis is a reported complication. Pericarditis and myocarditis are also infrequent complications, although nonspecific electrocardiographic changes are seen in about 5% of all EBV-infected patients. Neurologic involvement—including transverse myelitis, encephalitis, and Guillain–Barré syndrome—is infrequent.

Treatment

A. GENERAL MEASURES

Given that over 95% of patients recover without specific antiviral therapy, treatment is largely symptomatic. Acyclovir decreases viral shedding but does not have verified clinical benefit. Efforts to sensitize the virus to nucleoside analogs have yet to be proved beneficial. Symptomatic relief can be achieved with acetaminophen or other nonsteroidal anti-inflammatory drugs and warm saline throat irrigations or gargles three or four times daily. Corticosteroid therapy, although widespread, is not recommended in uncomplicated cases; its use is reserved for impending airway obstruction from enlarged lymph nodes, hemolytic anemia, and severe thrombocytopenia. The value of corticosteroid therapy in impending splenic rupture, pericarditis, myocarditis, and nervous system involvement is less well defined. If a throat culture grows β-hemolytic streptococci, a 10-day course of penicillin or erythromycin is indicated. Ampicillin and amoxicillin are avoided because of the frequent association with rash.

B. TREATMENT OF COMPLICATIONS

Hepatitis, myocarditis, and encephalitis are treated symptomatically. Rupture of the spleen requires splenectomy and is most often caused by deep palpation of the spleen or vigorous activity. Patients should avoid contact or collision sports for at least 4 weeks to decrease the risk of splenic rupture (even if splenomegaly is not detected by physical examination which can be insensitive).

Prognosis

In cases without complications, fever disappears in 10 days and lymphadenopathy and splenomegaly in 4 weeks. The debility sometimes lingers for 2–3 months.

Death is uncommon and is usually due to splenic rupture, hypersplenic phenomena (severe hemolytic anemia, thrombocytopenic purpura), or encephalitis.

4. Other Epstein–Barr Virus Syndromes

EBV viral antigens have been found in over 90% of patients with African Burkitt's lymphoma or nasopharyngeal carcinoma (among whom quantified EBV DNA can be used to follow disease). A causative role for EBV has been postulated with both neoplasms. Chronic EBV infection is associated with aberrant cellular immunity (a low frequency of EBV-specific CD8 cells), an X-linked lymphoproliferative syndrome (Duncan's disease), and a fatal T cell lymphoproliferative disorder in children. EBV-induced lymphoproliferation gives rise to B cell lymphomas among immunodeficient patients, such as the HIV-infected individuals (HIV-infected patients, even on HAART, show higher EBV DNA loads than HIV-noninfected patients) or after transplantation ("posttransplant lymphoproliferative disorder"). Immunologically privileged areas such as the CNS are particularly susceptible. The prophylactic use of EBV-specific cytotoxic T cell lymphocytes may prevent the development of EBV-associated lymphoproliferative disease. Rituximab is useful before viral burdens become excessive.

EBV has also been associated with leiomyomas in children with AIDS and with nasal T cell lymphomas. There is no persuasive evidence that chronic fatigue syndrome is caused by EBV infection. Oral hairy leukoplakia (associated with EBV) is discussed in Chapter 8.

EBV is also implicated in the pathogenesis of a proportion of Hodgkin's disease (a subset with diminished cellular immunity) as well as a variety of solid neoplasms, including oral tumors, and of systemic lupus erythematosus, pediatric multiple sclerosis, encephalitis, rheumatoid arthritis, drug-induced hypersensitivity reactions, and Sézary's and Sjögren's syndromes.

Carpentier L et al: Epstein–Barr virus (EBV) early-antigen serologic testing in conjunction with peripheral blood EBV DNA load as a marker for risk of post transplantation lymphoproliferative disease. J Infect Dis 2003;188:1853. [PMID: 14673764]

Fafi-Kremer S et al: Long-term shedding of infectious Epstein–Barr virus after infectious mononucleosis. J Infect Dis 2005; 191:985. [PMID: 15717276]

Hjalgrim H et al: Characteristics of Hodgkin's lymphoma after infectious mononucleosis. N Engl J Med 2003;349:1324. [PMID: 14523140]

Lin JC et al: Quantification of plasma Epstein–Barr virus DNA in patients with advanced nasopharyngeal carcinoma. N Engl J Med 2004;350:2461. [PMID: 15190138]

Macsween KF et al: Epstein–Barr virus—recent advances. Lancet Infect Dis 2003;3:131. [PMID: 12614729]

Sitki-Green DL et al: Biology of Epstein–Barr virus during infectious mononucleosis. J Infect Dis 2004;189:483. [PMID: 14745706]

Thompson MP et al: Epstein–Barr virus and cancer. Clin Cancer Res 2004;10:803. [PMID: 14871955]

5. Cytomegalovirus Disease

Most CMV infections are asymptomatic, with the virus remaining latent. It can be isolated from a variety of tissues under nonpathogenic conditions including up to 25% of salivary glands and 10% of uterine cervices. The cells of latency include vascular endothelial cells, monocytes, macrophages, polymorphonuclear neutrophils, and renal and pulmonary epithelial cells. Seroprevalence increases with age and with the number of sexual partners. Detectable antibody is present in the serum of most homosexual men. Transmission is sexual, congenital, through breast-feeding, blood products or transplantation, and person-to-person (eg, day care centers). Serious disease occurs primarily in immunocompromised persons, especially those with AIDS and transplant recipients.

Clinical Findings

A. CLASSIFICATION

There are three recognizable clinical syndromes.

1. Perinatal disease and CMV inclusion disease—Congenital CMV infection is the most common congenital infection in developed countries, affecting about 1% of all neonates. About 10% of infected newborns born to mothers with primary CMV infection during pregnancy will be symptomatic with **CMV inclusion disease.** It is characterized by jaundice, hepatosplenomegaly, thrombocytopenia, purpura, microcephaly, periventricular CNS calcifications, mental retardation, and motor disability. Hearing loss develops in greater than 50% of infants who are symptomatic at birth. Most patients with congenital CMV infection are asymptomatic, but neurologic deficits may ensue later in life. Perinatal infection acquired through breast-feeding or blood products typically has a benign clinical course.

2. Disease in immunocompetent hosts—

a. Acute acquired CMV infection—Akin to EBV-associated infectious mononucleosis, this syndrome is characterized by fever, malaise, myalgias and arthralgias (but rarely exudative pharyngitis or cervical lymphadenopathy), splenomegaly, atypical lymphocytes, and abnormal liver function tests. The mean duration of symptoms is 7–8 weeks. Typically, leukopenia is followed by leukocytosis. Heterophil antibody is absent. Transmission occurs by sexual contact, in breast milk, via respiratory droplets among nursery or day care center attendants, and by transfusions of blood. Complications include mucosal gastrointestinal damage, encephalitis, Guillain–Barré syndrome, pericarditis, and myocarditis.

b. Other associations with CMV—Other clinical syndromes that are reported to be associated with CMV and whose role in pathogenesis requires further elucidation include inflammatory bowel disease, atherosclerosis and myocardial infarction, and breast cancer (the last of these is associated with a higher risk of late CMV disease in life).

3. Disease in immunocompromised hosts—Tissue and bone marrow transplant patients are mainly at risk in the first 100 days after allograft transplantation and in particular when graft-versus-host disease or CMV seropositivity is present. HIV-infected patients may show numerous manifestations, described below, and these occur most prominently when the CD4 count is < 100 cell/mcL or when the HIV viral load is > 10,000 copies/mcL. CMV is itself immunosuppressive and promotes other infections such as *Pneumocystis* and *Aspergillus* pneumonia. It may contribute to transplanted organ dysfunction, in particular, hepatitis, which can mimic organ rejection. The so-called "CMV syndrome" in renal transplant patients is a mononucleosis-like syndrome among new transplant recipients.

a. CMV retinitis—Retinitis occurs in AIDS patients with CD4 counts less than 50 cells/mcL and on occasion among the immunocompetent (among whom the rate of retinal detachment is lower). Ophthalmologic documentation of neovascular, proliferative lesions ("pizza-pie" retinopathy) is required for diagnosis. With HAART, the frequency of retinitis is reduced, CD4 counts are less predictive, and active disease may be reversible. Immune restoration with HAART is associated with CMV vitreitis and CMV-associated cystoid macular edema. Infants with CMV retinitis tend to have more macular than peripheral disease. CMV retinitis may also develop in persons who have undergone heart transplantation; it is usually asymptomatic.

b. Gastrointestinal and hepatobiliary CMV—Serious gastrointestinal CMV disease occurs in AIDS (usually with CD4 counts < 100 cells/mcL) and after organ transplantation, cancer chemotherapy, or corticosteroid therapy. Esophagitis presents with odynophagia; small

bowel disease may mimic inflammatory bowel disease or may present as ulceration or perforation. Colonic CMV disease causes diarrhea, hematochezia, abdominal pain, fever, and weight loss. CMV has been identified—often with other pathogens such as *Cryptosporidium*—in up to 15% of patients with AIDS cholangiopathy. Diagnosis is made by mucosal biopsy showing characteristic CMV histopathologic findings of intranuclear ("owl's eye") and intracytoplasmic inclusions.

c. Pulmonary CMV—CMV pneumonitis—characterized by cough, dyspnea, relatively little sputum production, and chest radiograph findings consistent with interstitial pneumonia—occurs in transplant recipients with a mortality rate up to 60–80%, and less commonly in AIDS patients. In AIDS patients, the significant morbidity and mortality appear to be diminished by the use of antiretroviral therapy. High-titer CMV immunoglobulin may be effective in preventing CMV pneumonia in seronegative recipients.

d. Neurologic CMV—Neurologic syndromes associated with CMV include polyradiculopathy, transverse myelitis, ventriculoencephalitis, and focal encephalitis. The encephalitis has a subacute onset in patients with advanced AIDS and is usually associated with disseminated CMV infection. CMV can be isolated in the cerebrospinal fluid in cases of transverse myelitis or disseminated disease.

B. Laboratory Findings

Virus isolation should be combined with pathologic findings to distinguish viral shedding from tissue invasion. Cultures alone are of little use in diagnosing AIDS-related CMV infections, but when positive have been associated with a risk of progressive retinitis. Tissue confirmation is especially useful in establishing a diagnosis of CMV pneumonitis and CMV gastrointestinal or neurologic disease.

The acute mononucleosis-like syndrome is associated with lymphocytosis, often 2 weeks after the fever, but absolute leukopenia may also be noted. Serologic tests are useful primarily in seroepidemiologic studies and occasionally in confirming acute infection (with IgM) in nonimmunosuppressed patients. Antigen detection in blood components, urine, or cerebrospinal fluid by virus technology (including the PCR technique) should be interpreted in the context of clinical and pathologic findings but is increasingly being used to guide both treatment and prevention. Among transplant recipients, PCR appears to be more useful than CMV antigenemia in predicting clinical disease.

A variety of false-positive immunologic assays occur in the setting of acute CMV infections, including positive rheumatoid factor, direct Coombs' test, cryoglobulins, and speckled antinuclear antibody.

Prevention

No vaccine is currently available. Strategies for prevention in transplant recipients include use of leukocyte-depleted blood products, antiviral agents, and CMV immune globulin. The risk for CMV disease is proportionate to the intensity of immunosuppression, which depends in part on the organ being transplanted. PCR and antigen assays increase the ability to detect CMV disease prior to clinical expression. Oral ganciclovir is being replaced by oral valganciclovir in prevention because of its greater bioavailability. The optimal method of monitoring and preventing CMV disease among transplant patients remains to be elucidated. HAART is effective in preventing CMV infections in HIV-infected patients.

The virus is so ubiquitous that it is not recommended that children with known CMV infection be withdrawn from day care centers or that health care workers restrict their patient contact beyond intensifying handwashing. Screening programs are not recommended for women of childbearing age and breastfeeding should not be restricted.

Treatment

First-line therapy against CMV infections is ganciclovir, 5 mg/kg intravenously every 12 hours for 14–21 days. Due to potential toxicities, foscarnet (loading with 90 mg/kg intravenously, followed by 60 mg/kg every 8 hours over weeks) and cidofovir (5 mg/kg intravenously every week for 2 weeks) are usually reserved for CMV infections that are resistant to ganciclovir. A daily maintenance regimen using both ganciclovir (3.75 mg/kg intravenously) and foscarnet (60 mg/kg intravenously), each over 1 hour, has been shown to be safe and effective in inhibiting CMV replication. Cidofovir is given only every 2 weeks, 375 mg intravenously, for maintenance. Oral valganciclovir (900 mg daily) is replacing oral ganciclovir for maintenance and for prophylactic therapy among persons who have undergone solid organ or bone marrow transplantation. Transplant recipients do not benefit from combined foscarnet and ganciclovir preemptive therapy. Dosage adjustments of all medications are needed for renal impairment. Adoptive immunotherapy with polyclonal CMV-specific T cells is a new modality of therapy for infections in the allogeneic bone marrow transplant population that may obviate the need for antivirals in the future.

In pregnant women with primary CMV infection, passive immunization with hyperimmune globulin appears preliminarily to be efficacious in both treatment and prevention of fetal infection, but controlled clinical trials are needed for confirmation.

A sustained-release ganciclovir implant controls disease in the implanted eye (but not elsewhere) more effectively than intravenous ganciclovir. Again, the role of HAART in reducing the need for CMV antivirals is primary. Fomivirsen is an intravitreal agent active against CMV strains that are resistant to ganciclovir, foscarnet, and cidofovir. Adjuvant filgrastim may be useful in managing the neutropenia associated with ganciclovir and its analogues.

Erice A et al: Cytomegalovirus (CMV) and human immunodeficiency virus (HIV) burden, CMV end-organ disease, and survival in subjects with advanced HIV infection (AIDS Clinical Trials Group Protocol 360). Clin Infect Dis 2003; 37:567. [PMID: 12905142]

Griffiths P: Cytomegalovirus infection of the central nervous system. Herpes 2004;11(Suppl 2):95A. [PMID: 15319096]

Kuo IC et al: Clinical characteristics and outcomes of cytomegalovirus retinitis in persons without human immunodeficiency virus infection. Am J Ophthalmol 2004;138:338. [PMID: 15364214]

Nigro G et al; Congenital Cytomegalovirus Collaborating Group: Passive immunization during pregnancy for congenital cytomegalovirus infection. N Engl J Med 2005;353:1350. [PMID: 16192480]

Peggs KS et al: Adoptive cellular therapy for early cytomegalovirus infection after allogeneic stem-cell transplantation with virus-specific T-cell lines. Lancet 2003;362:1375. [PMID: 14585640]

Whitley RJ: Congenital cytomegalovirus infection: epidemiology and treatment. Adv Exp Med Biol 2004;549:155. [PMID: 15250528]

Wreghitt TG et al: Cytomegalovirus infection in immunocompetent patients. Clin Infect Dis 2003;37:1603. [PMID: 14689339]

6. Human Herpesviruses 6, 7, & 8

HHV-6 is a B cell lymphotropic virus that is the principal cause of exanthema subitum (roseola infantum, sixth disease). Primary HHV-6 infection occurs most commonly in children under 2 years of age and is the most common cause of infantile febrile seizures. Reactivation of HHV-6 in adults is associated with immunocompromised states such as HIV and lymphoma. It is associated with graft rejection and bone marrow suppression in transplant patients and with encephalitis and pneumonitis in AIDS patients. Possible roles of HHV-6 in the evolution of multiple sclerosis and progressive multifocal leukoencephalopathy remain unproven.

Two variants (A and B) of HHV-6 have been identified. HHV-6B is the predominant strain found in both normal and immunocompromised persons. In vitro data suggest susceptibility to ganciclovir and foscarnet but not acyclovir. HHV-7 is a T cell lymphotropic virus that is associated with roseola (serologically), seizures and, rarely, encephalitis. Infection with HHV-7 appears to be synergistic with CMV in renal transplant recipients. The membrane glycoprotein CD4 is involved in HHV-7 recognition, and an antagonistic interaction between HHV-7 and HIV is established.

HHV-8 is associated with Kaposi's sarcoma in AIDS patients. It has also been implicated in multicentric Castleman's disease and primary effusion lymphoma (body cavity lymphoma). See Chapter 31 for pathogenesis and management.

Caserta MT et al: Human herpesvirus 6. Clin Infect Dis 2001;33: 829. [PMID: 11512088]

De Bolle L et al: Update on human herpesvirus 6 biology, clinical features, and therapy. Clin Microbiol Rev 2005;18:217. [PMID: 15653828]

Dewhurst S: Human herpesvirus type 6 and human herpesvirus type 7 infections of the central nervous system. Herpes 2004;11(Suppl 2):105A. [PMID: 15319097]

MAJOR VACCINE-PREVENTABLE VIRAL INFECTIONS

1. Measles

 ESSENTIALS OF DIAGNOSIS

- Exposure 10–14 days before onset in an unvaccinated patient.
- Prodrome of fever, coryza, cough, conjunctivitis, malaise, irritability, photophobia, Koplik's spots.
- Rash: brick-red, irregular, maculopapular; onset 3–4 days after onset of prodrome; begins on the face and proceeds "downward and outward," affecting the palms and soles last.
- Leukopenia.

General Considerations

Measles is an acute systemic paramyxoviral infection transmitted by inhalation of infective droplets. It is a major worldwide cause of pediatric morbidity and mortality, with nearly 800,000 estimated deaths annually. Illness confers permanent immunity. It is highly contagious and communicability is greatest during the preeruptive and catarrhal stages but continues as long as the rash remains. The largest recent outbreak in the Americas was in São Paulo, Brazil, in 1997, with over 42,000 cases among largely unvaccinated young adults. This and other sporadic recent outbreaks of the disease in adults, adolescents, and unvaccinated preschool children in dense urban areas emphasize the need for specific recommendations concerning prevention (see below).

In the United States, with largely imported cases and few geographically dispersed cases whose isolates fail to show a recurrent strain, measles is no longer considered endemic.

Clinical Findings

A. Symptoms and Signs

(Table 32–2.) Fever is often as high as 40–40.6 °C. It persists through the prodrome and early rash (about 5–7 days). Malaise may be marked. Coryza (nasal obstruction, sneezing, and sore throat) resembles that seen with upper respiratory infections. Cough is persistent and nonproductive. Conjunctivitis manifests as redness, swelling, photophobia, and discharge. These symptoms intensify over the 2–4 days before the onset of the rash and peak on the first day of the rash.

Koplik's spots are pathognomonic of measles. They appear about 2 days before the rash and last 1–4 days as tiny "table salt crystals" most often in the buccal mucosa opposite the second molars and vaginal mucous membranes. Other findings include pharyngeal erythema, a yellowish exudate on the tonsils, coating of the tongue in the center with a red tip and margins, moderate generalized lymphadenopathy and, in occasional cases, splenomegaly.

The rash usually appears first on the face and behind the ears 4 days after the onset of symptoms. The initial lesions are pinhead-sized papules that coalesce to form a brick-red, irregular, blotchy maculopapular rash. In severe cases, the rash may coalesce to form a nearly uniform erythema on some body areas. The rash next appears on the trunk, followed by the extremities, including the palms (25–50% of those infected) and soles. The rash lasts for 3–7 days and then it fades in the same manner it appeared. Hyperpigmentation remains in fair-skinned individuals and severe cases. Slight desquamation may follow.

Atypical measles is a syndrome occurring in adults who received inactivated measles vaccine (available 1963–1968) or who received live measles vaccine before age 12 months and as a result developed hypersensitivity rather than protective immunity. When persons are infected later with wild measles virus, a potentially fatal illness may develop, with high fever; unusual rashes (papular, hemorrhagic), most prominent on the extremities, without Koplik's spots; headache; arthralgias; hepatitis; and a high rate of pneumonitis, occasionally with pleural effusions; followed by the appearance of extremely high measles antibody titers.

Measles may occur in HIV-infected individuals in an uncharacteristic fashion, with higher rates of pneumonitis and higher mortality. Vaccine failure rates, both primary and secondary, are higher in HIV-infected children. The frequent difficulty in establishing a diagnosis suggests that measles may be more prevalent in epidemics than heretofore recognized.

Measles during pregnancy is not known to cause congenital abnormalities of the fetus. However, it is associated with spontaneous abortion and premature delivery. Measles in the offspring of mothers with measles ranges from mild to severe; therefore, it is recommended that infants born to such mothers be passively immunized with immunoglobulin at birth.

B. Laboratory Findings

Leukopenia is usually present unless secondary bacterial complications exist. A lymphocyte count under 2000/mcL is a poor prognostic sign. Proteinuria is often observed. Although technically difficult, virus can be cultured from nasopharyngeal washings and from blood. A fourfold rise in serum hemagglutination inhibition antibody supports the diagnosis. Fluorescent antibody staining of respiratory or urinary epithelial cells can also confirm the diagnosis.

Differential Diagnosis

Measles is usually diagnosed clinically but may be mistaken for other exanthematous infections (see Table 32–2).

Complications

A. CENTRAL NERVOUS SYSTEM

Postinfectious encephalomyelitis occurs in approximately 0.05–0.1% of cases. Higher rates of encephalitis occur in adolescents and adults than in school-aged children. Its onset is usually 3–7 days after the rash. Vomiting, convulsions, coma, and a variety of severe neurologic symptoms and signs may develop. Treatment is symptomatic and supportive. Virus is usually not found in the CNS, though demyelination is prominent. There is an appreciable mortality rate (10–20%), and 33% of survivors are left with neurologic morbidity.

A similar form, "inclusion body encephalitis," is also reported to occur after measles vaccination but is associated with isolation of the measles virus.

Subacute sclerosing panencephalitis (SSPE) is a very late CNS complication, the measles virus acting as a "slow virus" to produce degenerative CNS disease years after the initial infection. SSPE is rare (1: 100,000 cases of measles) and occurs more often when measles develops early in life among males who live in rural environments. SSPE very rarely develops in adults.

An acute progressive encephalitis (subacute measles encephalitis), characterized by seizures, neurologic deficits, and often progressive stupor and death, can occur among immunosuppressed patients. Measles virus opportunistically invades the CNS. Treatment is supportive, withholding immunosuppressive chemotherapy when feasible. Interferon and ribavirin are variably successful.

B. RESPIRATORY TRACT DISEASE

Early in the course of the disease, bronchopneumonia or bronchiolitis due to the measles virus may occur in up to 5% of patients and result in serious respiratory difficulties. Pneumonia occurring with or without an evanescent rash is seen in atypical measles.

C. SECONDARY BACTERIAL INFECTIONS

Immediately following measles, secondary bacterial infection, particularly cervical adenitis, otitis media (the most common complication), and pneumonia, occurs in about 15% of patients.

D. IMMUNE REACTIVITY

Measles produces temporary anergy to cell-mediated (eg, tuberculin) skin tests.

E. GASTROENTERITIS

Diarrhea and protein-losing enteropathy (prodromal rectal Koplik spots may be seen) are significant complications when measles affects malnourished children.

F. OTHER COMPLICATIONS

Ocular complications such as conjunctivitis and keratitis are common.

Prevention

In the United States, it is recommended that children receive their first vaccine dose at 12–15 months and a second at age 4–6 years prior to entry into school (see Table 30–4).

Students beyond high school and medical staff starting employment must have the above vaccination schedule documented or must have serologic evidence of immunity if they were born after 1956. For individuals born before 1957, herd immunity can be assumed. Health care workers should be screened and vaccinated if necessary regardless of date of birth.

Outbreak control in the United States is similar. If outbreaks are occurring in preschool children under 1 year of age, initial vaccination may be given at 6 months, with repeat at 15 months. When outbreaks take place in day care centers, K–12 institutions, or colleges and universities, revaccination is probably indicated for all, in particular for students and their siblings born after 1956 who do not have documentation of immunity as defined above. Susceptible personnel who have been exposed should be isolated from patient contact between the fifth and the twenty-first day after exposure regardless of whether they have been vaccinated or have received immune globulin. If measles develop in these persons, they should be isolated from patient contact until 7 days after the rash develops.

When susceptible individuals are exposed to measles, the live virus vaccine can prevent disease if given within 5 days of exposure. This is rarely feasible within a household. Later, immune globulin (0.25 mL/kg [0.11 mL/lb] body weight) can be injected intramuscularly for prevention or modification of clinical illness if given within 6 days after exposure. This must be followed by active immunization with live measles vaccine 3 months later. Vaccination of all immunocompetent persons born after 1956 who travel to the developing world is important. In the developing world, the use of the second vaccine dose is an important aspect of achieving control of measles in the community-at-large.

Pregnant women and immunosuppressed persons should *not* receive this vaccine. There are two exceptions: asymptomatic HIV-infected patients, who have not shown adverse effects from measles vaccination, and HIV-infected children, in whom exposure to vaccines improves survival after measles (and among whom HAART therapy is associated with an improved vaccine response). Immune globulin should be considered for postexposure prophylaxis in any high-risk person exposed to measles. This group includes children with malignant disease and patients with AIDS, who are more likely to develop severe disease or fatal measles. To be effective, immune globulin should be administered within 6 days after an exposure.

Severe allergic reactions to the measles, mumps, and rubella (MMR) vaccine are rare, though fever and rash appear to occur slightly more often among female recipients. Future vaccines for a variety of infectious agents may utilize measles vectors, thereby augmenting immunity to measles.

Treatment

A. GENERAL MEASURES

The patient should be isolated for the week following onset of rash and kept at bed rest until afebrile. Treatment is symptomatic including antipyretics and fluids as needed. Vitamin A, 200,000 units/d orally for 2 days (the beneficial effects of which include maintenance of gastrointestinal and respiratory epithelial mucosa and perhaps immune enhancement), reduces pediatric morbidity rates although high-dose vitamin A exposure increases the severity and risk of antibiotic failure in nonmeasles pneumonia.

B. TREATMENT OF COMPLICATIONS

Secondary bacterial infections are treated with appropriate antimicrobial drugs. Pneumonia is managed with antibacterial antibiotics when clinical signs suggest sepsis or significant pulmonary findings. Postmeasles encephalitis, including SSPE, can be managed only symptomatically.

Prognosis

During the past 13 years in the United States, the case-fatality rate stayed around 3 per 1000 reported measles cases; the mortality rate may be as high as 10% in developing nations. Deaths in the United States are due principally to encephalitis (15% mortality rate) and secondary bacterial pneumonia. Deaths in the developing world are mainly related to diarrhea and protein-losing enteropathy. Higher case-fatality rates in developing countries are related to young age at infection, crowding, and underlying immune deficiency, among other factors.

D'Souza RM et al: Vitamin A for preventing secondary infections in children with measles—a systematic review. J Trop Pediatr 2002;48:72. [PMID: 12521271]

Elliman D et al: Measles. Curr Opin Infect Dis 2005;18:229. [PMID: 15864100]

Ni J et al: Vitamin A for non-measles pneumonia in children. Cochrane Database Syst Rev 2005;(3):CD003700. [PMID: 16034908]

Ota MO et al: Emerging diseases: measles. J Neurovirol 2005;11: 447. [PMID: 16287686]

Tangy F et al: Live attenuated measles vaccine as a potential multivalent pediatric vaccination vector. Viral Immunol 2005; 18:317. [PMID: 16035943]

Wood DL: American Academy of Pediatrics Committee on Community Health Services; American Academy of Pediatrics Committee on Practice and Ambulatory Medicine: increasing immunization coverage. Pediatrics 2003;112:993. [PMID: 14523201]

2. Mumps

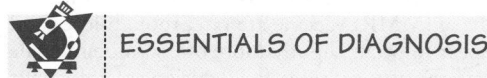

ESSENTIALS OF DIAGNOSIS

- *Exposure 14–21 days before onset.*
- *Painful, swollen salivary glands, usually parotid.*

- *Frequent involvement of other tissues, including testes, pancreas, and meninges, in unvaccinated individuals.*

General Considerations

Mumps is a paramyxoviral disease spread by respiratory droplets that usually produces inflammation of the salivary glands and, less commonly, orchitis, aseptic meningitis, encephalomyelitis, pancreatitis, and oophoritis. Most patients are children, and the incidence is highest in spring. The incubation period is 14–21 days (average, 18 days). Infectivity occurs via saliva and urine and precedes the symptoms by about 1 day and is maximal for 3 days but may last a week. Up to one-third of affected individuals have subclinical infection.

Clinical Findings

A. SYMPTOMS AND SIGNS

Parotid tenderness and overlying facial edema are the most common physical findings. Usually, one parotid gland enlarges a couple of days before the other, but unilateral parotitis alone occurs in 25% of patients. Swelling and tenderness of the submaxillary and sublingual glands are variable. The orifice of Stensen's duct may be red and swollen. Trismus may result from the parotitis. The parotid glands return to normal size within a week. Involvement of other salivary glands in conjunction with the parotids occurs in 10% of cases.

Fever and malaise are variable and are often minimal in young children. High fever usually accompanies meningitis or orchitis. Neck stiffness, headache, and lethargy suggest meningitis. Testicular swelling and tenderness (unilateral in 75% of cases) denote orchitis, which is the most common extrasalivary gland manifestation of mumps in adults. Orchitis, which develops typically 7–10 days after the onset of parotitis, occurs in about 25–40% of postpubertal men, but sterility is rare. Upper abdominal pain, nausea, and vomiting suggest pancreatitis. Mumps is the leading cause of pancreatitis in children. Lower abdominal pain and ovarian enlargement suggest oophoritis (which occurs in 5% of postpubertal women, usually unilateral), but the diagnosis may be difficult to make.

B. LABORATORY FINDINGS

Mild leukopenia with relative lymphocytosis may be present. Serum amylase is commonly elevated with or without pancreatitis because of salivary gland involvement. Lymphocytic pleocytosis (and normal to low glucose) of the cerebrospinal fluid is present in meningitis, which may be asymptomatic. Mild renal function abnormalities are the presenting finding in up to 60% of patients. The diagnosis of mumps is confirmed by isolating the virus from saliva, cerebrospinal fluid, or urine or demonstrating a fourfold rise in complement-fixing antibodies to mumps virus in paired sera.

Differential Diagnosis

Swelling of the parotid gland may be due to calculi in the parotid ducts, tumors or cysts, or to a reaction to iodides. Other causes include starch ingestion, sarcoidosis, cirrhosis, diabetes, bulimia, pilocarpine use for dry mouth, and Sjögren's syndrome. Parotitis may also be produced by pyogenic organisms (eg, *S aureus*, gram-negative organisms), particularly in debilitated individuals with poor oral intake, drug reaction (phenothiazines, propylthiouracil), and other viruses (influenza A, parainfluenza, EBV infection, coxsackieviruses, adenoviruses, HHV-6). Swelling of the parotid gland must be differentiated from inflammation of the lymph nodes located more posteriorly and inferiorly than the parotid gland.

Complications

Other manifestations of the disease are less common than inflammation of the salivary glands. These usually follow the parotitis but may precede it or occur without salivary gland involvement and include meningitis (30%), orchitis (on rare occasion leads to priapism or testicular infarction), pancreatitis (usually mild), oophoritis, thyroiditis, neuritis, hepatitis, myocarditis, thrombocytopenia, migratory arthralgias (noted infrequently among adults and rarely in children), and nephritis. Mumps has also been associated with cases of endocardial fibroelastosis.

Rare neurologic complications include encephalitis, Guillain–Barré syndrome, cerebellar ataxia, facial palsy, and transverse myelitis. Encephalitis is associated with cerebral edema, serious neurologic manifestations, and sometimes death. Deafness develops from eighth nerve neuritis and recent surveillance from Japan suggests it occurs in about 0.3% of patients.

Prevention

Mumps live virus vaccine is safe and highly effective. It is recommended for routine immunization for children over age 1 year, either alone or in combination with other virus vaccines (eg, in MMR vaccine or as a quadrivalent vaccine with varicella). A second dose is recommended for children prior to starting school. Reactions are reviewed in the measles section. It should not be given to pregnant women or to immunocompromised individuals, though the vaccine has been given to asymptomatic HIV-infected individuals without adverse sequelae. Mumps vaccine markedly decreased the incidence of mumps in the United States and in the United Kingdom. Persons in whom mumps develops are less likely to have received a second vaccine dose. The mumps skin tests are less reliable than serum neutralization titers in determining immunity.

Treatment

A. GENERAL MEASURES

The patient should be isolated until swelling subsides and kept at bed rest during the febrile period. Treatment is symptomatic as needed. Topical application of warm or cold compresses may relieve parotid discomfort.

B. MANAGEMENT OF COMPLICATIONS

1. Meningitis—The treatment of aseptic meningitis is purely symptomatic. The management of encephalitis requires attention to cerebral edema, the airway, and vital functions.

2. Orchitis—The scrotum should be supported using a suspensory or toweling "bridge" and ice bags applied. Incision of the tunica may be necessary in severe cases. Codeine or meperidine may be given as necessary for pain. Pain can also be relieved by injection of the spermatic cord at the external inguinal ring with 10–20 mL of 1% procaine solution. The merit of hydrocortisone sodium succinate (100 mg intravenously, followed by 20 mg orally every 6 hours for 2 or 3 days) to reduce the inflammatory reaction is not firmly established.

3. Pancreatitis—Symptomatic treatment should be provided, with emphasis on parenteral hydration.

Prognosis

The entire course of mumps rarely exceeds 2 weeks. Fatalities (usually from encephalitis) are rare.

Davidkin I et al: Etiology of mumps-like illnesses in children and adolescents vaccinated for measles, mumps, and rubella. J Infect Dis 2005;191:719. [PMID: 15688285]

Harling R et al: The effectiveness of the mumps component of the MMR vaccine: a case control study Vaccine 2005;23:4070. [PMID: 15950329]

Kawashima Y et al: Epidemiological study of mumps deafness in Japan. Auris Nasus Larynx 2005;32:125. [PMID: 15917168]

Shinefield H et al: Evaluation of a quadrivalent measles, mumps, rubella and varicella vaccine in healthy children. Pediatr Infect Dis J 2005;24:665. [PMID: 16094217]

3. Poliomyelitis

 ESSENTIALS OF DIAGNOSIS

- *Incubation period 9–12 days from exposure.*
- *Muscle weakness, headache, stiff neck, fever, nausea and vomiting, sore throat.*
- *Lower motor neuron lesion (flaccid paralysis) with decreased deep tendon reflexes and muscle wasting.*
- *Cerebrospinal fluid shows excess leukocytes, with lymphocytic predominance; count is rarely more than 500/mcL.*

General Considerations

Poliomyelitis virus, an enterovirus, is present in throat washings and stools (where it can be excreted for several weeks after infection). Infection is most commonly acquired by the fecal–oral route. Since the introduction of an effective vaccine, poliomyelitis has become a rare disease in developed areas of the world, and globally, between 1988 and 2001, the number of cases decreased by 99%. The global poliomyelitis eradication initiative was launched in 1988 and has led to elimination of wild poliovirus from the Western hemisphere. The Pacific Rim, Europe, and most of Central Asia also appear to be polio free. However, at the end of 2004, six countries had endemic polio (Afghanistan, Egypt, India, Niger, Nigeria, and Pakistan), and transmission was reestablished in six countries (Burkina Faso, Central African Republic, Chad, Côte d'Ivoire, Mali, and Sudan). An imported vaccine-associated case occurred in the United States in 2005.

Three antigenically distinct types of poliomyelitis virus are recognized, with little cross-immunity between them. Disease with type 2 (of the three types) in particular is on the verge of extinction. Infectivity is maximal during the first week.

Clinical Findings

A. SYMPTOMS AND SIGNS

At least 95% of infections are asymptomatic, but in those who become ill, manifestations include abortive poliomyelitis (minor illness), nonparalytic poliomyelitis, and paralytic poliomyelitis.

1. Abortive poliomyelitis (minor illness)—Minor illness occurs in 4–8% of infections and the symptoms are fever, headache, vomiting, diarrhea, constipation, and sore throat lasting 2–3 days. This entity can be suspected clinically only during an epidemic.

2. Nonparalytic poliomyelitis—In addition to the above symptoms, signs of meningeal irritation and muscle spasm occur in the absence of frank paralysis. This disease is indistinguishable from aseptic meningitis caused by other enteroviruses.

3. Paralytic poliomyelitis—Paralytic poliomyelitis represents 0.1% of all poliomyelitis cases (the incidence is higher when infections are acquired later in life). Paralysis may occur at any time during the febrile period. Tremors, muscle weakness, constipation, and ileus may appear. Paralytic poliomyelitis is divided into two forms, which may coexist: (1) **spinal poliomyelitis**, with involvement of the muscles innervated by the spinal nerves, and (2) **bulbar poliomyelitis**, with weakness of the muscles supplied by the cranial nerves (especially nerves IX and X) and of the respiratory and vasomotor centers.

In spinal poliomyelitis, paralysis of the shoulder girdle often precedes intercostal and diaphragmatic paralysis, which leads to diminished chest expansion and decreased vital capacity. The paralysis occurs over 2–3 days, is flaccid, has an asymmetric distribution, and affects the proximal muscles of the extremities more frequently. Sensory loss is very rare.

In bulbar poliomyelitis, symptoms include diplopia (uncommonly), facial weakness, dysphagia, dysphonia, nasal voice, weakness of the sternocleidomastoid and trapezius muscles, difficulty in chewing, inability to swallow or expel saliva, and regurgitation of fluids through the nose. The most life-threatening aspect of bulbar poliomyelitis is respiratory paralysis. Lethargy or coma may be due to hypoxia, most often from hypoventilation. Alterations in blood pressure and heart rate may occur. Convulsions are rare. Bulbar poliomyelitis is more common in adults.

B. LABORATORY FINDINGS

The peripheral white blood cell count may be normal or mildly elevated. Cerebrospinal fluid pressure and protein are normal or slightly increased. Glucose is not decreased. White blood cells usually number fewer than 500/mcL and are principally lymphocytes after the first 24 hours. Cerebrospinal fluid is normal in 5% of patients. The virus may be recovered from throat washings (early) and stools (early and late). Neutralizing and complement-fixing antibodies appear during the first or second week of illness. Serologic testing cannot distinguish between wild-type and vaccine-related virus infections.

Differential Diagnosis

Nonparalytic poliomyelitis is similar to other forms of enteroviral meningitis; the distinction is made serologically. Acute flaccid paralysis is the term used in the developing world for the variety of neurologic illnesses that both include and mimic poliomyelitis. Acute flaccid paralysis due to poliomyelitis is distinguished by the greater frequency of fever and asymmetric neurologic signs. Acute inflammatory polyneuritis (Guillain–Barré syndrome) and tick paralysis may initially resemble poliomyelitis. In Guillain–Barré syndrome (see Chapter 24), the weakness is more symmetric and ascending in most cases, but the Miller–Fisher variant is quite similar to bulbar polio. Paresthesias are uncommon in poliomyelitis but common in Guillain–Barré syndrome. The cerebrospinal fluid usually has a high protein content but normal cell count in Guillain–Barré syndrome.

Complications

Urinary tract infection, atelectasis, pneumonia, myocarditis, paralytic ileus, gastric dilation, and pulmonary edema may occur. Respiratory failure may be a result of paralysis of respiratory muscles, airway obstruction from involvement of cranial nerve nuclei, or lesions of the respiratory center.

Prevention

Given the epidemiologic distribution of poliomyelitis and the continued concern about vaccine-associated disease with the oral live vaccine, recommendations for prevention were modified. Currently in the United States, the inactive (Salk) parenteral vaccination is used for all four doses (at ages 2 months, 4 months, and 6–18 months and at 4–6 years). Inactivated vaccine is also routinely used elsewhere in the developed world. Oral vaccines are limited to usage for outbreak control, travel to endemic areas within the ensuing month, and protection of children whose parents do not comply with the recommended number of immunizations. The advantages of oral vaccination are the ease of administration, effective local gastrointestinal and circulating immunity, and herd immunity.

Routine immunization of adults in the United States is no longer recommended because of the low incidence of the disease. Exceptions include adults not vaccinated within the prior decade who are exposed to poliomyelitis or who plan to travel to endemic areas (mentioned above). These adults should be given inactivated poliomyelitis vaccine (Salk) as should immunodeficient or immunosuppressed individuals and members of their households.

In the developing world, the interval between oral polio vaccine doses should probably be longer than 1 month (because of interference from enteric pathogens). Intramuscular injections should be routinely avoided during the month following oral poliomyelitis vaccination to prevent provocation paralysis. Ancillary useful control measures in polio-endemic countries include national immunization days (mass campaigns in which all children are vaccinated twice, 4–6 weeks apart, regardless of vaccine history); cross-border vaccination activities; surveillance for acute flaccid paralysis, an indicator for poliomyelitis; and aggressive outbreak responses as well as intensified immunization activities in countries recently affected by armed conflicts. Recent outbreaks of vaccine-derived poliomyelitis occurred in Hispaniola (both Haiti and the Dominican Republic) with type 1 isolates and Madagascar with type 2 isolates. Both followed the administration of oral vaccine (Sabin). These incidents serve as a reminder of the need to maintain high levels of immunization coverage even in the absence of overt disease. The risks associated with oral vaccination and the importance of continued surveillance for disease are continuing public health concerns.

Recent success has been reported with a monovalent type 1 oral vaccine in India and Egypt.

Treatment

In the acute phase of paralytic poliomyelitis patients should be hospitalized. Strict bed rest in the first few days of illness reduces the rate of paralysis. Cranial nerve involvement must be vigilantly sought. Comfortable but rotating positions should be maintained in a "polio bed": firm mattress, footboard, sponge rubber pads or rolls, sandbags, and light splints. Fecal impaction and urinary retention (especially with paraplegia) are managed appropriately. In cases of respiratory weakness or paralysis, intensive care is needed.

Prognosis

During the febrile period, paralysis may develop or progress. Mild weakness of small muscles is more likely to regress than is severe weakness of large muscles. Bulbar poliomyelitis carries a mortality rate of up to 50%. New muscle weakness may develop and progress slowly years after recovery from acute paralytic poliomyelitis. This entity, postpoliomyelitis syndrome, presents with signs of chronic and new denervation, is not infectious in origin, and is associated with increasing dysfunction of surviving motor neurons. Series that report increased incidences of multiple sclerosis or other motor neuron diseases among poliomyelitis survivors need to be evaluated in the context of what is known about the postpoliomyelitis syndrome. Although bulbar poliomyelitis causes the greatest threat to life, it is rarely responsible for permanent damage among surviving patients.

Alexander LN et al: Vaccine policy changes and epidemiology of poliomyelitis in the United States. JAMA 2004;292: 1696. [PMID: 15479934]

Centers for Disease Control and Prevention (CDC): Brief report: Conclusions and recommendations of the Advisory Committee on Poliomyelitis Eradication—Geneva, Switzerland, October 2005. MMWR Morb Mortal Wkly Rep 2005;54: 1186. [PMID: 16323363]

Centers for Disease Control and Prevention (CDC): Progress toward interruption of wild poliovirus transmission—worldwide, January 2004–March 2005. MMWR Morb Mortal Wkly Rep 2005;54:408. [PMID: 15858461]

Duintjer Tebbens RJ et al: A dynamic model of poliomyelitis outbreaks: learning from the past to help inform the future. Am J Epidemiol 2005;162:358. [PMID: 16014773]

Nielsen NM et al: Long-term mortality after poliomyelitis. Epidemiology 2003;14:355. [PMID: 12859038]

Philip DM: Polio eradication, cessation of vaccination and reemergence of disease. Nat Rev Microbiol 2004;2:473. [PMID: 15152203]

Silver JK et al: What internists need to know about postpolio syndrome. Cleve Clin J Med 2002;69:704. [PMID: 12222974]

4. Rubella

 ESSENTIALS OF DIAGNOSIS

- *Exposure 14–21 days before onset.*
- *Arthralgia, particularly in young women.*
- *No prodrome in children, mild prodrome in adults; mild symptoms (fever, malaise, coryza) coinciding with eruption.*
- *Posterior cervical and postauricular lymphadenopathy 5–10 days before rash.*
- *Fine maculopapular rash of 3 days duration; face to trunk to extremities.*
- *Leukopenia, thrombocytopenia.*

General Considerations

Rubella is a systemic disease caused by a togavirus transmitted by inhalation of infective droplets. It is only moderately communicable. One attack usually confers permanent immunity. The incubation period is 14–21 days (average, 16 days). The disease is transmissible from 1 week before the rash appears until 15 days afterward.

The clinical picture of rubella is difficult to distinguish from other viral illnesses such as infectious mononucleosis, echovirus infections, and coxsackievirus infections, though arthritis is more prominent in rubella. Definitive diagnosis can be made only by isolating the virus or serologically.

In the United States, rubella is no longer endemic and congenital rubella syndrome is on the verge of elimination. Surveillance of female military recruits suggests, however, that serologic protection against rubella as well as measles and mumps are inadequate.

The principal importance of rubella lies in its devastating effects on the fetus in utero, producing teratogenic effects and a continuing congenital infection. Congenital rubella syndrome continues to occur in parts of the developing world at rates equivalent to those reported from the industrialized world during the prevaccine era. More than 100,000 cases occur annually in the developing world. Recent outbreaks occurred in Italy and Brazil, with Recife, Brazil reporting 49 cases of congenital rubella syndrome between 1998 and 2001. The majority of recent cases of congenital rubella syndrome in the United States occurred among immigrants; between 2001 and 2004 only four cases were reported to the Centers for Disease Control and Prevention (CDC) (three among immigrants).

Clinical Findings (Table 32–2)

A. Symptoms and Signs

Age is the most important determinant of the severity of rubella. Postnatally acquired rubella is usually innocuous, whereas fetal rubella can be devastating. In the postnatally acquired infection, fever and malaise, usually mild, accompanied by tender suboccipital adenitis, may precede the eruption by 1 week. Mild coryza may be present. Polyarticular arthritis occurs in about 25% of adult cases and involves the fingers, wrists, and knees. Rarely does chronic arthritis develop. The polyarthritis usually subsides within 7 days but may persist for weeks. Early posterior cervical and postauricular lymphadenopathy is very common. Erythema of the palate and throat, sometimes patchy, may be noted.

A fine, pink maculopapular rash appears on the face, trunk, and extremities in rapid progression (2–3 days) and fades quickly, usually lasting 1 day in each area. Rubella without rash may be at least as common as the exanthematous disease. Diagnosis, when suspected because of disease in the community, requires serologic confirmation.

B. Laboratory Findings

Leukopenia may be present early and may be followed by an increase in plasma cells. Virus isolation and serologic tests of immunity (rubella virus hemagglutination inhibition and fluorescent antibody tests) are available. Definitive diagnosis is based on a fourfold or greater rise in antibody titers.

Complications

A. Exposure during Pregnancy

Rubella antibodies are sought at the beginning of pregnancy, since fetal infection during the first trimester leads to congenital rubella in at least 80% of fetuses.

When a pregnant woman is exposed to a possible case of rubella, an immediate hemagglutination-inhibiting rubella antibody level should be obtained. There is no reason for concern with positive tests since these indicate immunity. If no antibodies are found, clinical observation and serologic follow-up are essential although an isolated IgM-positive test needs to be interpreted with caution because it does not necessarily imply acute infection. Confirmation of rubella in the expectant mother raises the question of therapeutic abortion, an alternative to be considered in light of personal, religious, legal, and other factors. The risk to the fetus is highest for maternal infection in the first trimester but continues into the second trimester.

B. Congenital Rubella

An infant acquiring the infection in utero may be normal at birth but probably—50% in a series of nearly 70 pregnant women with rubella in Mexico—will have a wide variety of manifestations, including early-onset cataracts, microphthalmia, glaucoma, hearing deficits, psychomotor retardation, congenital heart defects, organomegaly, and maculopapular rash. In general, the younger the fetus when infected, the more severe the illness. Viral excretion in the throat and urine persists for many months despite high antibody levels. The diagnosis is confirmed by isolation of the virus. A specific test for IgM rubella antibody is useful for diagnosis in the newborn. Treatment is directed toward the many anomalies.

C. Postinfectious Encephalopathy

In 1:6000 cases, postinfectious encephalopathy develops 1–6 days after the rash; the virus cannot always be isolated. The mortality rate is 20%, but residual deficits are rare among the recovered. The mechanism is unknown.

Other unusual complications of rubella include hemorrhagic manifestations due to thrombocytopenia and vascular damage, and mild hepatitis.

Prevention

Live attenuated rubella virus vaccine should be given to all infants and to susceptible girls before the menarche. When women are immunized, they should not be pregnant, and the absence of antibodies should be established. (In the United States, about 80% of 20-year-old women are immune to rubella.) Postpartum administration to susceptible female hospital employees is recommended, though many hospitals fail to comply. It is recommended that women not become pregnant for at least 1 month after vaccine administration. Nonetheless, there are no reports of congenital rubella syndrome after rubella immunization, and inadvertent immunization of a pregnant woman is not considered an indication for therapeutic abortion. Arthritis is more marked after rubella vaccination than in native disease and appears to be immunologically mediated. The association between chronic arthropathies and rubella vaccination is controversial. MMR may be given in conjunction with diphtheria–pertussis–tetanus (DPT) boosters as adequate serologic responses are documented. The administration of two or more doses appears to overcome an immunogenetic risk for vaccine failure in some vaccinees.

Treatment

Acetaminophen provides symptomatic relief. Encephalitis and non–life-threatening thrombocytopenia should be treated symptomatically.

Prognosis

Rubella is a mild illness and rarely lasts more than 3–4 days. Congenital rubella, on the other hand, has a high mortality rate, and the associated congenital defects are largely permanent.

Centers for Disease Control and Prevention (CDC): Elimination of rubella and congenital rubella syndrome—United States, 1969–2004. MMWR Morb Mortal Wkly Rep 2005;54: 279. [PMID: 15788995]

Centers for Disease Control and Prevention (CDC): Global Measles and Rubella Laboratory Network, January 2004–June 2005. MMWR Morb Mortal Wkly Rep 2005;54:1100. [PMID: 16267497]

Haas DM et al: Rubella, rubeola, and mumps in pregnant women: susceptibilities and strategies for testing and vaccinating. Obstet Gynecol 2005;106:295. [PMID: 16055578]

Lanzieri TM et al: Incidence, clinical features and estimated costs of congenital rubella syndrome after a large rubella outbreak in Recife, Brazil, 1999–2000. Pediatr Infect Dis J 2004;23: 1116. [PMID: 15626948]

Sheridan E: Congenital rubella syndrome: a risk in immigrant populations. Lancet 2002;359:675. [PMID: 11879866]

OTHER NEUROTROPIC VIRUSES

1. Rabies

ESSENTIALS OF DIAGNOSIS

- *History of animal bite.*
- *Paresthesia, hydrophobia, rage alternating with calm.*
- *Convulsions, paralysis, thick tenacious saliva.*

General Considerations

Rabies is a viral (rhabdovirus) encephalitis transmitted by infected saliva that gains entry into the body by an animal bite or an open wound. Globally, an estimated 30,000–70,000 deaths occur annually from rabies, and as a cause of disability, it is roughly equivalent in its public health impact to trachoma or onchocerciasis. In the United States domestically acquired rabies cases are rare but probably underreported; eight human cases were reported in 2004. Raccoons, skunks, bats, and foxes are common wildlife reservoirs. Biting species that cause rabies in the United States are geographically determined and include raccoons in the East, including New England; skunks in the Midwest, Southwest, and in California; coyotes in Texas; and foxes in the Southwest and in Alaska. The contribution of bats (particularly the eastern pipistrelle bat and the silver-haired bat) to the rabid wild animal population is increasing, and bats are distributed throughout the United States. As a result, most cases in the United States since 1990 until late 2005 (34 of 47 total) are associated with bat rabies virus variants. Greater than 90% of human cases acquired in developing countries, where rabid dogs are the major reservoirs of the rabies virus, are due to infected dog bites. Dogs and cats are rarely infected in the United States because of successful rabies vaccination campaigns. Rodents and lagomorphs (eg, rabbits) are unlikely to spread rabies because they cannot survive the disease long enough to transmit it, although woodchucks and groundhogs can become infected and transmit the virus. The virus gains entry into the salivary glands of dogs 5–7 days before their death from rabies, thus limiting their period of infectivity. Less common routes of transmission include contamination of mucous membranes with saliva or brain tissue, aerosol transmission, and corneal transplantation. Most recently, the rabies virus was transmitted to three persons who underwent solid organ transplant and one person who received a vascular segment from an infected donor with unrecognized rabies.

The incubation period may range from 10 days to many years but is usually 3–7 weeks. The interval is dependent in part on distance of the wound from the CNS. The virus travels in the nerves to the brain, multiplies there, and then migrates along the efferent nerves to the salivary glands.

Rabies is almost uniformly fatal, with only six documented surviving cases to date. Five received either preexposure or postexposure prophylaxis. Recently, a teenager survived with only naturally acquired immunity, but received intense antiviral treatment. The most common clinical problem confronting the physician is the management of a patient bitten by an animal (see Prevention).

Clinical Findings

A. SYMPTOMS AND SIGNS

There is usually a history of animal bite, though bat bites may not be recognized. The prodromal syndrome consists of pain at the site of the bite in association with fever, malaise, headache, nausea, and vomiting. The skin is sensitive to changes of temperature, especially air currents. About 10 days later, the CNS stage begins, which may be either encephalitic ("furious") or paralytic ("dumb"). The encephalitic form produces the classic rabies manifestations of delirium alternating with periods of calm, when attempts at drinking cause extremely painful laryngeal spasms (hydrophobia). In the less common paralytic form, an acute ascending paralysis resembling Guillain–Barré syndrome predominates with relative sparing of higher cortical functions initially. Both forms progress relentlessly to coma, autonomic nervous system dysfunction, and death despite intensive support.

B. LABORATORY FINDINGS

Biting animals that appear well should be quarantined under observation for 10 days. Sick or dead animals should be tested for rabies. A wild animal, if captured, should be sacrificed and the head shipped on ice to the nearest laboratory qualified to examine the brain for evidence of rabies virus; the diagnosis is made by the direct fluorescent antibody technique or immunohistochemistry testing. When the animal cannot be examined, raccoons, skunks, bats, and foxes should be presumed to be rabid.

Direct fluorescent antibody testing of skin biopsy material from the posterior neck (where hair follicles are highly innervated) has a sensitivity of 60–80%.

Reverse transcriptase PCR, nucleic acid sequence-based amplification, and viral isolation from the cerebrospinal fluid or saliva are being advocated as definitive diagnostic assays. Antibodies can be detected in the serum and the cerebrospinal fluid. Pathologic specimens often demonstrate round or oval eosinophilic inclusion bodies (Negri bodies) in the cytoplasm of neuronal cells, although their presence is neither sensitive nor specific. MRI signs include non-enhancing, ill-defined, mild hyperintense changes in the brainstem, hypothalamus, and multiple deep and subcortical white and gray matter zones and potential enhancement along the nerve course from the site of bites.

Prevention

Because rabies is almost always fatal, prevention is the only reasonable approach, and all exposures must be evaluated individually. Immunization of household dogs and cats and active immunization of persons with significant animal exposure (eg, veterinarians) are important. The most important common decisions, however, concern animal bites.

In the developing world, education, surveillance, and animal (particularly dog) vaccination programs are preferred over mass destruction of dogs, which is followed typically by invasion of susceptible feral animals into urban areas.

A. LOCAL TREATMENT OF ANIMAL BITES AND SCRATCHES

Thorough cleansing, debridement, and repeated flushing of wounds with soap and water are important. Rabies immune globulin or antiserum should be given as stated below. Wounds caused by animal bites should not be sutured.

B. POSTEXPOSURE IMMUNIZATION

Therapy is indicated when the disease is seriously under consideration. The decision to treat should be based on the circumstances of the bite, including the extent and location of the wound, the biting animal, the history of prior vaccination, and the local endemicity of rabies. Any contact or suspect contact with a bat is usually deemed a sufficient indication to warrant prophylaxis. Consultation with state and local health departments is recommended. Postexposure treatment including both immune globulin and vaccination, should be administered as promptly as possible when indicated.

The optimal form of passive immunization is rabies immune globulin (20 IU/kg). As much as possible of the full dose should be infiltrated around the wound, with any remaining injected intramuscularly at a site distant from the wound. If immune globulin (human) is not available, equine rabies antiserum (20–40 IU/kg) can be used if available (it was last produced in 2001) after appropriate tests for horse serum sensitivity. An inactivated human diploid cell rabies vaccine (HDCV) is given as five injections of 1 mL intramuscularly (in the deltoid rather than the gluteal muscle) on days 0, 3, 7, 14, and 28 after exposure.

Several cell culture vaccines are available and are preferable to embryonated tissue vaccine (eg, duck embryo vaccine; DEV) because of better antigenic response and fewer systemic reactions. HDCV availability and cost limit its use in the developing world.

Rabies immune globulin and rabies vaccine (HDCV) should never be given in the same syringe or at the same site. Allergic reactions to the vaccine are rare, though local reactions (pruritus, erythema, tenderness) occur in about 25% and mild systemic reactions (headaches, myalgias, nausea) in about 20% of recipients. The vaccine is commercially available or can be obtained through health departments. For patients who previously received preexposure or postexposure vaccine, rabies immune globulin should not be given; vaccine, 1 mL in the deltoid, should be given twice (on days 0 and 3).

In other countries, the less costly inactivated DEV or mouse brain vaccine may be available, but the method of administration is more complex, the rate of allergic reactions—including ascending paralysis—is higher, and the efficacy is lower.

Exposure to rabies still requires postexposure vaccination, even if preexposure vaccination was received, but the need for immune globulin is eliminated (rabies immune globulin is in short supply worldwide).

Neither the passive nor the active form or postexposure prophylaxis is associated with fetal abnormalities and thus pregnancy is not considered a contraindication to vaccination.

C. PREEXPOSURE IMMUNIZATION

Preexposure prophylaxis with three injections of HDCV intramuscularly (1 mL on days 0, 7, and 21 or 28) or intradermally (0.1 mL on days 0, 7, and 28, over the deltoid) is recommended for persons at high risk of exposure: veterinarians (who should have rabies antibody titers checked every 2 years and be boosted with 1 mL intramuscularly or 0.1 mL intradermally if seronegative); animal handlers; laboratory workers; Peace Corps workers; and travelers to remote areas in endemic countries in Africa, Asia, and Latin America. An intradermal route is available for preexposure prophylaxis only. Immunosuppressive illnesses and agents including corticosteroids as well as antimalarials—in particular chloroquine—may diminish the antibody response.

Treatment

This very severe illness with an almost universally fatal outcome requires intensive care with attention to the airway, maintenance of oxygenation, and control of seizures. Universal precautions are essential. Other modalities of therapy that may be beneficial include a combination of rabies vaccine, rabies immune globulin, monoclonal antibodies (investigational), ribavirin, interferon-α, amantadine, and ketamine. Corticosteroids are of no use.

Prognosis

If postexposure prophylaxis is given expediently, before clinical signs develop, it is nearly 100% successful in prevention of disease. Once the symptoms have appeared, death almost inevitably occurs after 7 days, usually from respiratory failure. Most deaths occur in persons with unrecognized disease who do not seek medical care.

CDC National Center for Infectious Diseases—Rabies http://www.cdc.gov/ncidod/dvrd/rabies

Coleman PG et al: Estimating the public health impact of rabies. Emerg Infect Dis 2004;10:140. [PMID: 15078611]

Hankins DG et al: Overview, prevention, and treatment of rabies. Mayo Clin Proc 2004;79:671. [PMID: 15132411]

Jerrard DA: The use of rabies immune globulin by emergency physicians. J Emerg Med 2004;27:15. [PMID: 15219298]

Krebs JW et al: Rabies surveillance in the United States during 2004. J Am Vet Med Assoc 2005;227:1912. [PMID: 16379626]

Rupprecht CE et al: Prophylaxis against rabies. N Engl J Med 2004;351:2626. [PMID: 15602023]

Srinivasan A et al; Rabies in Transplant Recipients Investigation Team: Transmission of rabies virus from an organ donor to four transplant recipients. N Engl J Med 2005;352:1103. [PMID: 15784663]

Willoughby RE Jr et al: Survival after treatment of rabies with induction of coma. N Engl J Med 2005;353:2508. [PMID: 15958806]

2. Arbovirus Encephalitides

 ESSENTIALS OF DIAGNOSIS

- Fever, malaise, stiff neck, sore throat, and nausea and vomiting, progressing to stupor, coma, and convulsions.
- Signs of an upper motor neuron lesion (exaggerated deep tendon reflexes, absent superficial reflexes, pathologic reflexes, and spastic paralysis).
- Cerebrospinal fluid protein and opening pressure often increased, with lymphocytic pleocytosis.

General Considerations

The arboviruses are arthropod-borne pathogens that produce clinical manifestations in humans. The mosquito-borne pathogens include three alphaviruses (causing Western, Eastern, and Venezuelan equine encephalitis), five flaviviruses (causing West Nile fever, St. Louis encephalitis, Japanese B encephalitis, dengue, and yellow fever), bunyaviruses (the California serogroup of viruses [in particular, California encephalitis caused by the Lacrosse agent]), and some causes of viral hemorrhagic fever (Rift Valley fever). The tick-borne causes of encephalitis include the flavivirus Powassan (northeastern United States and Canada) and tick-borne encephalitides of Europe. Pathogens associated with viral hemorrhagic fever are discussed below, and only those viruses causing primarily encephalitis in the United States will be discussed here.

Infection with West Nile virus was first identified in the United States in the New York City area in 1999. The virus spread rapidly, with initial cases reported along the Atlantic seaboard. Current cases are reported throughout the continental United States. Earlier outbreaks occurred in France in the early 1960s and in Romania in 1996.

Along with West Nile fever, the leading causes of arbovirus encephalitis in the United States are St. Louis encephalitis and California encephalitis. Pathogen-specific reservoirs (typically small mammals or birds) are responsible for maintaining the encephalitis-producing viruses in nature. Birds are the main reservoir for West Nile virus and substantial avian mortality accompanies West Nile fever outbreaks, a fact that is used to monitor disease patterns. Outbreaks tend to occur in late summer and early fall.

Transplacental transmission is documented for the viruses that cause Western and Venezuelan equine encephalitis and West Nile fever. The virus that causes West Nile fever is also transmissible via blood donation, organ transplantation, breast-feeding, and laboratory and possibly aerosol exposures. The human incubation period is 2–14 days. The proportion of patients in whom the disease develops after acquiring the virus is unknown. Estimates were reported from serologic surveillance from the New York epidemic; fever developed in 1 of 5 infected patients and severe neurologic disease developed in 1 of 150.

Clinical Findings

A. Symptoms and Signs

The symptoms of arboviral encephalitis include fever, malaise, sore throat, headache, gastrointestinal upset, lethargy, and stupor progressing to coma. Stiff neck and mental status changes are the most common neurologic signs. Seizures are present in 5% of patients and flaccid paralysis is seen in 10%. Other signs include tremors, convulsions, cranial nerve palsies, paralysis of extremities, and pathologic reflexes. About 50% of patients in the United States with West Nile virus infection with symptoms severe enough to warrant hospitalization had significant muscle weakness. This weakness can cause diagnostic confusion with the Guillain–Barré syndrome and may evolve into a poliomyelitis-like syndrome. Rash is reported in fewer than one-third of cases.

Among cases of encephalitis reported in 2003 in the United States, 70% were reported as West Nile fever (milder disease) and about 30% were reported as West Nile meningitis or encephalitis. Age older than 70 years seems to be the main risk factor for severe meningoencephalitis and death. The role of immunosuppression as a risk factor remains uncertain. The outcome of encephalitis is also age-dependent with residual damage principally in older patients. St. Louis encephalitis occurs among adults; Western and Venezuelan encephalitides occur primarily among children while the Eastern encephalitis is a disease of both children and the elderly. The disease manifestations associated with West Nile fever are strongly age-dependent with the acute febrile syndrome and mild neurologic symptoms more common in the young, aseptic meningitis and poliomyelitis-like syndromes in the middle aged, and frank encephalopathy in the elderly.

B. Laboratory Findings

The peripheral white blood cell count is variable. Cerebrospinal fluid protein is elevated; cerebrospinal fluid glucose is normal; there is usually a lymphocytic pleocytosis; and polymorphonuclear cells may predominate early. The diagnosis of arboviral encephalitides—including West Nile fever—depends on serologic tests. For West Nile virus, an IgM capture enzyme-linked immunosorbent assay (ELISA) can be done on either serum or cerebrospinal fluid and is almost always positive by the time the disease is clinically evident. The virus is also detectable in urine and blood using PCR but only during limited intervals, thus limiting PCR as a diagnostic assay. There is cross-reaction among the different flaviviruses, so a plaque reduction assay may be needed to definitively distinguish between West Nile fever and St. Louis encephalitis. Serum IgM may be positive for many months after acute infection, so an in-

crease in antibody titer between acute and convalescent samples is necessary to confirm acute infection when cerebrospinal fluid samples are unavailable. CT scans of the brain usually show no acute disease, but MRI may reveal leptomeningeal, basal ganglia, thalamic, or periventricular enhancement.

Differential Diagnosis

Mild forms of encephalitis must be differentiated from aseptic meningitis, lymphocytic choriomeningitis, and nonparalytic poliomyelitis.

Severe forms of arbovirus encephalitides (Table 32–2) are to be differentiated from other causes of viral encephalitis (HSV, mumps virus, poliovirus or other enteroviruses, HIV), encephalitis accompanying exanthematous diseases of childhood (measles, varicella, infectious mononucleosis, rubella), encephalitis following vaccination (a demyelinating type following rabies, measles, pertussis), toxic encephalitis (from drugs, poisons, or bacterial toxins such as *Shigella dysenteriae* type 1), Reye's syndrome, and severe forms of stroke, brain tumors, brain abscess, autoimmune processes such as lupus cerebritis, and intoxications. In the California Encephalitis Project, the cause for most cases of encephalitis was not identified.

Complications

Bronchial pneumonia, urinary retention and infection, prolonged weakness, and decubitus ulcers may occur. Late sequelae are mental deterioration, parkinsonism, and epilepsy.

Prevention

No human arbovirus vaccine is currently available (two equine encephalitis vaccines are available). Mosquito control (repellents, protective clothing, and insecticides) is effective in prevention. Because the virus that causes West Nile fever is transmissible via both organ donation and blood transfusion, all potential blood donors should be screened for neurologic symptoms and all donated blood should be assayed with nucleic acid amplification tests for West Nile virus during periods of maximum transmission (summer and fall for the continental United States). Laboratory precautions are indicated for handling all pathogens, in particular the West Nile virus.

A vaccine against Japanese B encephalitis is recommended for travelers to rural areas of East Asia, though the risk of disease acquisition among the exposed is estimated at only 1:1,000,000. This vaccination appears to provide protection against the West Nile pathogen (since both agents are related flaviviruses) in certain settings such as among laboratory workers.

Treatment

Although specific antiviral therapy is not available for most causative entities, vigorous supportive measures can be helpful. Such measures include reduction of intracranial pressure (mannitol) and monitoring of intraventricular pressure. The efficacy of corticosteroids in these infections is not established. Preliminary evidence that ribavirin was useful in West Nile encephalitis has now been substantiated. Other therapeutic options such as interferon-α and immunoglobulin are not proven to be effective.

Prognosis

The prognosis is always guarded, especially at the extremes of age. Sequelae may become apparent late in the course of what appears to be a successful recovery. The prognosis is generally better for Western equine than for Eastern equine or St. Louis encephalitis. St. Louis encephalitis is reportedly associated with a postinfectious encephalomyelitis. As of 2002, the case fatality rate for recognized cases of arboviral encephalitis was 5%. Many infections result in seroconversion only and do not result in clinical illness.

Centers for Disease Control and Prevention (CDC): West Nile virus activity—United States, January 1–December 1, 2005. MMWR Morb Mortal Wkly Rep 2005;54:1253. [PMID: 16357821]

Gea-Banacloche J et al: West Nile virus: pathogenesis and therapeutic options. Ann Intern Med 2004;140:545. [PMID: 15068983]

Hayes EB et al: Epidemiology and ecology of West Nile virus. Emerg Infect Dis 2005;11:1167. [PMID: 16102302]

Hayes EB et al: Virology, pathology, and clinical manifestations of West Nile virus disease. Emerg Infect Dis 2005;11:1174. [PMID: 16102303]

Mackenzie JS et al: Emerging flaviviruses: the spread and resurgence of Japanese encephalitis, West Nile and dengue viruses. Nat Med 2004;10(12 Suppl):S98. [PMID: 15577938]

Watson JT et al: Clinical characteristics and functional outcomes of West Nile fever. Ann Intern Med 2004;141:360. [PMID: 15353427]

Yamshchikov G et al: The suitability of yellow fever and Japanese encephalitis vaccines for immunization against West Nile virus. Vaccine 2005;23:4785. [PMID: 15939510]

3. Lymphocytic Choriomeningitis

ESSENTIALS OF DIAGNOSIS

- "Influenza-like" prodrome of fever, chills, malaise, and cough, followed by meningitis with associated stiff neck.
- Aseptic meningitis with positive Kernig's sign, headache, nausea, vomiting, and lethargy.
- Cerebrospinal fluid: slight increase of protein, lymphocytic pleocytosis (500–3000/mcL); low glucose in 25% of patients.
- Complement-fixing antibodies within 2 weeks.

General Considerations

Lymphocytic choriomeningitis is an arenaviral infection of the CNS (related to the pathogen causing Argentinian hemorrhagic fever, discussed below). The main reservoir of infection is the infected house mouse, though other reservoirs include guinea pigs, monkeys, dogs, swine, and even pet hamsters. The virus is shed by the infected animal via nasal secretions, urine, and feces, with transmission to humans probably through exposure to animal droppings via contaminated food and dust. Human cases of lymphocytic choriomeningitis are most common in autumn. The virus is not spread person to person, though vertical transmission occurs and lymphocytic choriomeningitis is a potential fetal teratogen. Rare cases related to solid organ transplantation are reported. The incubation period is 8–13 days to the appearance of systemic manifestations and 15–21 days to the appearance of meningeal symptoms. CD4 cells may be involved in pathogenesis. Lymphocytic choriomeningitis is considered a model of cell-mediated immunity in vaccine development.

Outbreaks occur among persons with rodent exposure. Complications of clinical disease are rare.

This disease is principally confined to the eastern seaboard and northeastern states of the United States, and serologic evidence of infection is increased among women, the elderly, and members of lower socioeconomic groups.

Clinical Findings

A. Symptoms and Signs

Symptoms are biphasic. The prodromal illness is characterized by fever, chills, headache, myalgia, cough, and vomiting, occasionally with lymphadenopathy and maculopapular rash. Signs of pneumonia are occasionally present during the prodromal phase. After 3–5 days, the fever subsides and recurs in 2–4 days with the meningeal phase, characterized by headache, nausea and vomiting, and lethargy. During the meningeal phase, there may be neck and back stiffness with a positive Kernig's sign. Obstructive hydrocephalus is a rare complication. Arthralgias can develop late.

Chorioretinitis also appears to be a sequela of lymphocytic choriomeningitis. Lymphocytic choriomeningitis is an underrecognized neuroteratogen.

B. Laboratory Findings

Leukocytosis or leukopenia and thrombocytopenia may be present. Cerebrospinal fluid lymphocytic pleocytosis (total count is often 500–3000/mcL) may occur, with a slight increase in protein and normal to low glucose in at least 25%. Complement-fixing antibodies appear during or after the second week. The virus may be recovered from the blood and cerebrospinal fluid by mouse inoculation. A PCR technique for the detection of lymphocytic choriomeningitis virus in the cerebrospinal fluid is described.

Differential Diagnosis

The influenza-like prodrome and latent period help distinguish this from other aseptic meningitides, and bacterial and granulomatous meningitis. A history of exposure to mice or other potential vectors is an important diagnostic clue.

Prevention

Pregnant women should be advised of the dangers to their unborn children inherent in exposure to rodents.

Treatment

Treatment is supportive as for encephalitis or aseptic meningitis. The membrane protein α-dystroglycan interacts with lymphocytic choriomeningitis and Lassa fever virus (both arenaviruses), and this interaction provides a potential avenue for future interventions.

Prognosis

Fatalities are rare. The illness usually lasts 1–2 weeks, though convalescence may be prolonged.

Barton LL et al: Lymphocytic choriomeningitis virus: emerging fetal teratogen. Am J Obstet Gynecol 2002;187:1715. [PMID: 12501090]

Centers for Disease Control and Prevention (CDC): Lymphocytic choriomeningitis virus infection in organ transplant recipients—Massachusetts, Rhode Island, 2005. MMWR Morb Mortal Wkly Rep 2005;54:537. [PMID: 15931158]

Riera L et al: Serological study of the lymphochoriomeningitis virus (LCMV) in an inner city of Argentina. J Med Virol 2005;76:285. [PMID: 15834871]

Sevilla N et al: Infection of dendritic cells by lymphocytic choriomeningitis virus. Curr Top Microbiol Immunol 2003;276:125. [PMID: 12797446]

4. Prion Disease

Several neurologic diseases are caused by communicable pathogens with slow replicative capacity and long latent intervals in the host. Such pathogens are called *proteinaceous infectious particles*, or "prions," and are resistant to most procedures that modify nucleic acid. The transmissible pathogens induce conversion of a normal brain protein (PrP^C) to an abnormal isoform (PrP^{Sc}), a process that appears to be both genetically determined and in need of the infectious organism. The accumulated abnormal isoform proteins are associated with disease, though the pathogenesis of spongiform changes and the accumulation in some cases of amyloid plaque are poorly understood. There is evidence of lymphoreticular involvement (spleen, lymph nodes, tonsils), but the significance of this is unclear. A variety of animal diseases exhibit these properties, including visna and scrapie in sheep and goats, chronic wasting disease of mule deer and elk, and transmissible encephalopathy of mink. The pathogens or related pathogens that cause human disease are discussed here.

Kuru and **Creutzfeldt–Jakob disease** are transmissible in brain or eye tissue to primates, including humans. After an incubation period measured in years, disease ensues, characterized by an inexorably progressive neurologic decline. Kuru—once prevalent in central New Guinea but no longer seen since abandonment of cannibalism—was characterized by cerebellar ataxia, tremors, dysarthria, and emotional lability.

The four forms of Creutzfeldt–Jakob disease (CJD) are sporadic (80–85%), familial (15%), iatrogenic (< 1%), and variant (vCJD), described below. Sporadic, familial, and iatrogenic are classified as classic CJD (cCJD). There are no definitive risk factors for cCJD, which occurs worldwide with an incidence of 1 per million, although data show that butchers and medical office staff may be at increased occupational risk. Classic CJD usually presents in the sixth or seventh decade with dementia progressive over several months, myoclonic fasciculations, ataxia, and somnolence. The characteristic electroencephalographic pattern shows paroxysms with high voltages and slow waves. MRI typically shows bilateral areas of increased signal intensity, predominantly in the caudate and putamen. Assays of the cerebrospinal fluid for 14-3-3 protein and neuron-specific enolase may help with the diagnosis. Familial cases are inherited in an autosomal dominant pattern with variable penetrance. Iatrogenic cases have occurred in patients who receive tissue, such as cadaveric growth hormone and dural grafts from the CNS of patients with CJD.

There is no specific treatment, and the only known means of prevention is avoidance of contamination by affected brain tissue, electrodes, or neurosurgical tools or by transplants of cornea, dura, or cadaveric growth hormone from infected donors. Disinfection of equipment requires autoclaving at 15 psi for 1 hour, and disinfection of contaminated surfaces requires 5% hypochlorite or 0.1 N sodium hydroxide solution. Predictors for survival are younger age at onset of illness, female sex, a particular codon heterozygosity of the prion protein (129), the presence in the cerebrospinal fluid of protein 14-3-3, and the 2a prion protein type.

New vCJD was originally described in an outbreak from Great Britain that spread to involve several countries in Western Europe. Rare cases in the United States and Canada are reported among former UK residents. Compared with patients who have cCJD, patients with vCJD are younger, the duration of disease is longer, the clinical symptoms are unique (psychiatric and sensory symptoms and cerebellar signs are more common), and the MRI characteristically demonstrates hyperintensity of the posterior thalamus ("pulvinar sign"). All patients with vCJD have been homozygous for methionine at codon 129. vCJD probably results from ingestion of beefsteak contaminated with neural tissue (brain, spinal cord) from livestock infected with **bovine spongiform encephalopathy (BSE)** ("mad cow disease"). Most cases of BSE to date are reported from Europe, particularly Great Britain. Over the past 12 years two cases of BSE occurred in Canada and two were recently reported from Texas and Washington State. BSE is a product of livestock contaminated by ingesting material rendered from infected ruminants (deer, cattle, bison, sheep, and goats). Such feeding practices are now forbidden in many countries including the United States and Canada. There is no animal-to-animal spread of BSE and milk and its derived products are not infected. The risk for vCJD associated with the ingestion of beef products in the United States and Canada is deemed very small. Nonetheless, the US Food and Drug Administration (FDA) is currently embarking on a set of restrictive measures that will prevent the use of potentially infected beef and other ruminant offal in food and cosmetic products. A case of vCJD attributed to blood transfusion was reported from the United Kingdom. Patients with vCJD studied to date show a unique PrP phenotype.

Another animal disease that causes slow neurologic deterioration is **chronic wasting disease** of elk. It is caused by a prion that is distinctive from the causative pathogen of BSE. Thus far, there is no evidence of transmission of chronic wasting disease to humans.

Other prion diseases include fatal familial insomnia (rarely sporadic) and Gerstmann-Sträussler-Scheinker disease (with dementia and spastic paraparesis).

Aguzzi A et al: Progress and problems in the biology, diagnostics, and therapeutics of prion diseases. J Clin Invest 2004;114: 153. [PMID: 15254579]

CDC National Center for Infectious Diseases—Variant Creutzfeldt-Jakob Disease http://www.cdc.gov/ncidod/dvrd/vcjd

Demaerel P et al: Accuracy of diffusion-weighted MR imaging in the diagnosis of sporadic Creutzfeldt-Jakob disease. J Neurol 2003;250:222. [PMID: 12574955]

Glatzel M et al: Extraneural pathologic prion protein in sporadic Creutzfeldt-Jakob disease. N Engl J Med 2003;349: 1812. [PMID: 14602879]

Llewelyn CA et al: Possible transmission of variant Creutzfeldt-Jakob disease by blood transfusion. Lancet 2004;363:417. [PMID: 14962520]

Pocchiari M et al: Predictors of survival in sporadic Creutzfeldt-Jakob disease and other human transmissible spongiform encephalopathies. Brain 2004;127:2348. [PMID: 15361416]

Wadsworth JDF et al: Human prion protein with valine 129 prevents expression of variant CJD phenotype. Science 2004; 306:1793. [PMID: 15539564]

5. Progressive Multifocal Leukoencephalopathy

Progressive multifocal leukoencephalopathy is a demyelinating CNS disorder with a propensity for affliction of immunosuppressed adults with impaired cell-mediated immunity, especially AIDS patients. Recently, natalizumab, a monoclonal antibody, against 4 integrins, with potential therapeutic roles in multiple sclerosis and inflammatory bowel disease, was withdrawn from the market after case reports of progressive multifocal leukoencephalopathy in patients receiving this medication.

The cause of all progressive multifocal leukoencephalopathy is reactivation of JC virus (JCV), a widespread papovavirus that initially infects children, leading to latent infection in the kidneys and lymphoid organs. JCV targets myelinating oligodendrocytes of the CNS. PCR of the cerebrospinal fluid for JCV is used for diagnosis in patients with compatible clinical and radiologic findings. HAART for HIV infection is effective when CD4 counts improve to > 100 cells/mcL in improving survival as well as the clinical and radiographic features associated with this disease, although a small number of cases appear to worsen with immune restoration. Other agents used include cidofovir, not routinely recommended, and topotecan, which appears to be of some benefit.

Berenguer J et al: Clinical course and prognostic factors of progressive multifocal leukoencephalopathy in patients treated with highly active antiretroviral therapy. Clin Infect Dis 2003;36:1047. [PMID: 12684918]

Cinque P et al: The effect of highly active antiretroviral therapy-induced immune reconstitution on development and outcome of progressive multifocal leukoencephalopathy: study of 43 cases with review of the literature. J Neurovirol 2003; 9(Suppl 1):73. [PMID: 12709876]

Langer-Gould A et al: Progressive multifocal leukoencephalopathy in a patient treated with natalizumab. N Engl J Med 2005;353:375. [PMID: 15947078]

Tyler KL: The uninvited guest: JC virus infection of neurons in PML. Neurology 2003;61:734. [PMID: 14504312]

6. Human T Cell Lymphotropic Virus (HTLV)

Retroviruses include both the lympholytic HIV agents and the lymphotropic oncoviruses, human T cell leukemia viruses types 1 and 2 (HTLV-1 and -2). The isolation of HTLV-1 from a young man with T cell lymphoma established an association of the virus with adult T cell lymphoma/leukemia (ATL)—an association that has been confirmed from endemic areas throughout the world, including the Caribbean, southern Japan, sub-Saharan Africa (where over 10% of the population of Gabon and Cameroon are seropositive), Latin America (an ancient HTLV-1 provirus has been detected in an Andean mummy), Eastern Europe, and the southeastern United States (where seroprevalence is most common among injection drug users). The viruses are transmitted horizontally, vertically, and parenterally (injection drug use and blood transfusion).

The lifetime risk of developing ATL among seropositive persons is estimated to be 3% among women and 7% among men, with an incubation period of at least 15 years.

ATL clinical syndromes may be classified as chronic, smoldering, lymphomatous, or leukemic. Common clinical features of ATL include diffuse lymphadenopathy, maculopapular skin lesions that may evolve into erythroderma, organomegaly, lytic bone lesions, and hypercalcemia. Increased amounts of seborrheic dermatitis, eczema, and lower extremity hyperreflexia are also seen. A bronchiolitis associated with HTLV may mimic that of diffuse panbronchiolitis although the response of the latter to antibiotics, typically macrolide, can differentiate the two.

ATL patients show a predisposition toward opportunistic infections such as *Pneumocystis jiroveci* pneumonia and cryptococcal meningitis. A large percentage of patients are infected with *Strongyloides stercoralis*. Diagnosis is supported by identification of HTLV-1 antibodies. Confirmatory evidence for clonal integration of the proviral DNA genome into tumor cells is the current diagnostic standard.

HTLV-1 also causes HTLV-associated myelopathy (HAM; tropical spastic paraparesis). It is characterized by progressive motor weakness, especially of the lower extremities, with spastic paraparesis or paraplegia with hyperreflexia. Sensory disturbances, peripheral neuropathy, and urinary incontinence may also be seen. Much of the pathology appears to be a product of HTLV-1-induced cytokine production and associated inflammation. The disease may resemble multiple sclerosis but does not remit. Cutaneous manifestations of HAM include xerosis, cutaneous candidiasis, and palmar erythema. Cranial nerve abnormalities are rare, and cognitive function is usually preserved. HAM develops in less than 1% of HTLV-1 seropositive individuals. Studies among seropositive blood donors suggest there is a spectrum of illness of HTLV-1-associated neurologic disease, which includes myopathy and neuropathy.

HTLV-2 was initially implicated in hairy cell leukemia, but this association has not been confirmed. HTLV-2 seropositivity is common in some American populations, especially injection drug users. The virus infects primarily CD8 cells, whereas HTLV-1 infects primarily CD4 cells. HTLV-2 appears to also cause a form of myelopathy that is milder and slower to progress. Coinfection with HTLV-2 and HIV appears to be associated with increased risk of peripheral neuropathy.

A viral load assay is under development that shows that viremia with HTLV-1 is higher than with HTLV-2 and that transfusion-acquired infections are associated with greater viremia than sexually acquired infections.

Management of ATL is similar to that for non-Hodgkin's lymphoma and includes combination chemotherapy and radiation of particular sites (weight-bearing bony lesions, paraspinal masses, intracerebral lesions). HTLV-associated myelopathy is treated with a variety of immune-modulating agents without consistent results. Antiretrovirals have not shown clear benefit for ATL- or HTLV-associated myelopathy, although in vitro sensitivity to several antiretrovirals is recognized. Interferon-α may be of some efficacy.

Screening of the blood supply for HTLV-1 is required in the United States, since transfusion is a recognized mode of transmission along with sexual contact and vertical transfer. There is significant cross-reactivity between HTLV-1 and HTLV-2 by serologic studies, but PCR can distinguish the two.

Kashiwagi K et al: A decrease in mother-to-child transmission of human T lymphotropic virus type I (HTLV-I) in Okinawa, Japan. Am J Trop Med Hyg 2004;70:158. [PMID: 14993627]

Mahieux R et al: HTLV-1 and associated adult T-cell leukemia/lymphoma. Rev Clin Exp Hematol 2003;7:336. [PMID: 15129647]

Murphy EL et al: Higher human T lymphotropic virus (HTLV) provirus load is associated with HTLV-I versus HTLV-II, with HTLV-II subtype A versus B, and with male sex and a history of blood transfusion. J Infect Dis 2004;190:504. [PMID: 15243924]

Orland JR et al: HTLV Outcomes Study. Prevalence and clinical features of HTLV neurologic disease in the HTLV Outcomes Study. Neurology 2003;61:1588. [PMID: 14663047]

Saito M et al: Decreased human T lymphotropic virus type I (HTLV-I) provirus load and alteration in T cell phenotype after interferon-alpha therapy for HTLV-I-associated myelopathy/tropical spastic paraparesis. J Infect Dis 2004; 189:29. [PMID: 14702150]

OTHER SYSTEMIC VIRAL DISEASES

1. Hemorrhagic Fevers

This diverse group of illnesses results from infection with one of several single-stranded RNA viruses (members of the families Arenaviridae, Bunyaviridae, Filoviridae, and Flaviviridae). Flaviviruses, such as the West Nile pathogen, are discussed above under arboviruses; dengue and yellow fever, both with occasional hemorrhagic complications, are discussed in the following sections alongside the immunologic responses to them. The clinical symptoms in the early phase of a viral hemorrhagic fever are very similar, irrespective of the causative virus, and resemble a flu-like illness or gastroenteritis. Headache, myalgia, gastrointestinal symptoms, and symptoms of upper respiratory tract infection dominate the clinical picture and hepatitis is common. Laboratory features usually include thrombocytopenia, leukopenia, (although with Lassa fever leukocytosis is noted), anemia, and often elevated liver function tests as well as findings consistent with disseminated intravascular coagulation (except in Lassa fever).

The late phase is more specific and is characterized by organ failure, persistent leukopenia, altered mental status, and hemorrhage. The case-fatality rate ranges from 5% to 30% and may be as high as 90% in Ebola fever. There is no evidence of chronic infection among survivors.

Modes of transmission are similarly diverse. Dengue and yellow fever are due to flaviviruses transmitted by mosquitoes, while Omsk hemorrhagic fever and Kyasanur Forest disease are due to tick-borne flaviviruses. Lassa fever is rodent associated, as are Junin hemorrhagic fever and other diseases due to New World Arenaviridae. Ebola fever and Marburg fever are due to filoviruses with unknown vectors. The bunyaviruses include the tick-borne Crimean-Congo hemorrhagic fever and the mosquito-borne Rift Valley fever (a major outbreak in Saudi Arabia in 2000–2001 involved over 800 persons), while infections due to the hantaviruses (discussed separately below) are associated with rodent exposure.

The Nipah virus in Malaysia is a zoonotic paramyxovirus that does not cause hemorrhagic fever but instead causes a primarily encephalitic infection. Most cases are associated with a history of contact with pigs. Flying foxes appear to be the natural host.

Persons with symptoms compatible with those of any hemorrhagic fever and who have traveled from a possible endemic area should be isolated for diagnosis and symptomatic treatment. Diagnosis may be made by growing the virus from blood obtained early in the disease, by reverse transcriptase PCR, or by demonstration of a significant specific fourfold or greater rise in antibody titer. These tests are generally available only through the CDC. Isolation is particularly important because diseases due to some of these agents, such as Ebola virus, are highly transmissible and carry a mortality rate of 50–90%.

The pathophysiology of these infections includes infection of a wide variety of cell types, but in particular lymphoid tissues, tissues involved in the coagulation cascade, and the immune system. Many of the symptoms are due to the effect of inflammatory mediators such as cytokines and chemokines. Adrenal dysfunction is a common sequela and a cause for the development of the late-stage shock associated with viral hemorrhagic fevers.

The differential diagnosis for hemorrhagic fever includes meningococcemia or other septicemias, Rocky Mountain spotted fever, dengue, and malaria. The likelihood of acquiring hemorrhagic fevers among travelers is low.

Certain arenaviruses (the Lassa pathogen, Junin virus in its viscerotropic phase, Machupo virus) and bunyaviruses (provisionally, the Congo-Crimean Hemorrhagic Fever and Rift Valley Fever pathogens) respond to ribavrin if it is started promptly: 30 mg/kg as loading dose, followed by 16 mg/kg every 6 hours for 4 days and then 8 mg/kg every 8 hours for 3 days (see Chapter 37). The filoviruses and the flaviviruses do not respond to ribavirin. Vaccines are needed for these pathogens. The successful yellow fever vaccine is discussed below. A live attenuated Junin vaccine is undergoing trials. A formalin-inactivated vaccine against the Rift Valley Fever pathogen is in use and a live-attenuated vaccine is under development. Therapeutic interventions that target the hematologic system are either ineffective or only marginally effective. Future studies will target combining antivirals with immune mediators.

Bray M: Pathogenesis of viral hemorrhagic fever. Curr Opin Immunol 2005;17:399. [PMID: 15955687]

Feldmann H et al: Therapy and prophylaxis of Ebola virus infections. Curr Opin Investig Drugs 2005;6:823. [PMID: 16121689]

Ferguson NE et al: Bioterrorism web site resources for infectious disease clinicians and epidemiologists. Clin Infect Dis 2003; 36:1458. [PMID: 12766842]

Geisbert TW et al: Exotic emerging viral diseases: progress and challenges. Nat Med 2004;10(12 Suppl):S110. [PMID: 15577929]

Jones SM et al: Live attenuated recombinant vaccine protects nonhuman primates against Ebola and Marburg viruses. Nat Med 2005;11:786. [PMID: 15937495]

Mardani M et al: The efficacy of oral ribavirin in the treatment of Crimean-Congo hemorrhagic fever in Iran. Clin Infect Dis 2003;36:1613. [PMID: 12802764]

2. Dengue

ESSENTIALS OF DIAGNOSIS

- *Exposure 7–10 days before onset.*
- *Sudden onset of high fever, chills, severe myalgias, headache, sore throat, prostration, and depression.*
- *Biphasic fever curve: initial phase, 3–7 days; remission, few hours to 2 days; second phase, 1–2 days.*
- *Biphasic rash: evanescent, then maculopapular, scarlatiniform, morbilliform, or petechial changes from extremities to torso.*
- *Leukopenia and thrombocytopenia in the hemorrhagic form.*

General Considerations

Dengue is due to a flavivirus transmitted by the bite of the *Aedes* mosquito. It may be caused by one of four serotypes widely distributed between the tropics of Capricorn and Cancer. An estimated 50–100 million cases of dengue fever and several hundred thousand cases of dengue hemorrhagic fever occur each year. The incubation period is 3–15 days (usually 7–10 days). When the virus is introduced into susceptible populations, usually by viremic travelers, epidemic attack rates range from 50% to 70%. Transmission occurred in the United States in southern Texas and nearby Mexican border towns in 1986 and 1999. In 2001, a large outbreak in Hawaii was traced to a traveler returning from French Polynesia. Severe epidemics of dengue hemorrhagic fever (serotype 3) occurred over the past 20 years in East Africa, Sri Lanka, and Latin America.

Clinical Findings

A. SYMPTOMS AND SIGNS

Dengue fever is usually a nonspecific, self-limited biphasic febrile illness, but its presentation may range from asymptomatic to severe hemorrhagic fever and fatal shock (**dengue shock syndrome**). Infection is asymptomatic in 80% of infants and children. The illness is more severe and begins more suddenly in adults. After an incubation period of 4–5 days, there is a sudden onset of high fever, chills, and "break bone" aching of the head, back, and extremities accompanied by sore throat, prostration, and malaise. There may be conjunctival redness and flushing or blotching of the skin. Initially, the skin appears flushed, but 3–4 days after the lysis of the fever, a maculopapular rash, which spares palms and soles, appears in over 50% of cases. As the rash fades, localized clusters of petechiae on the extensor surface of the limbs become apparent. Hepatitis frequently complicates dengue fever.

Dengue hemorrhagic fever usually affects children living in endemic areas and is most likely to occur in secondary infections with serotype 2. A few days into the illness, signs of hemorrhage such as ecchymoses, gastrointestinal bleeding, and epistaxis appear. Symptoms found more often among the hemorrhagic fever subset of patients include restlessness, epistaxis, and abdominal pain.

Some dengue virus envelope glycoproteins are homologous with segments of clotting factors, including plasminogen, and thus the hemorrhagic fever may represent an autoimmune reaction. A subset of patients progresses to dengue shock syndrome in which acute fever, hemorrhagic manifestations, and marked capillary leak are prominent, the latter manifesting as pleural effusions, ascites, and a tendency to develop shock.

Before the rash of dengue appears, the infection is difficult to distinguish from malaria, yellow fever, or influenza; the rash makes dengue far more likely. Continuous abdominal pain with vomiting, a decrease in the level of consciousness, and hypothermia should raise concern about dengue shock syndrome.

B. LABORATORY FINDINGS

Leukopenia is characteristic and elevated transaminases are found frequently in dengue fever. Thrombocytopenia, increased fibrinolysis, and hemoconcentration occur more often in the hemorrhagic form of the disease. Liver function abnormalities are nearly universal. The nonspecific nature of the illness mandates laboratory verification for diagnosis, usually with IgM and IgG ELISAs. Virus may be recovered from the blood during the acute phase, and several PCR protocols are being developed. Immunohistochemistry for antigen detection in tissue samples can also be used.

Complications

Usual complications include depression, chronic fatigue, pneumonia, bone marrow failure, hepatitis, iritis, orchitis, and oophoritis. Neurologic complications such as encephalitis and transverse myelitis are less often reported. Dengue hemorrhagic fever or shock with concomitant bacterial infection is associated with advanced age, higher fever, gastrointestinal bleeding, renal impairment, and altered consciousness.

Prevention

Available prophylactic measures include control of mosquitoes by screening and insect repellents, particularly during early morning and late afternoon exposures. A screening program at an airport for persons with fever facilitated the diagnosis of dengue and the implementation of public health measures in Taipei, Taiwan.

A variety of vaccines, involving attenuated or genetically modified virus, are under study including combinations of attenuated dengue strains.

Treatment

Treatment entails the appropriate use of volume support (with Ringer's lactate the preferred agent in moderately severe shock), blood products, and pressor agents, and acetaminophen rather than nonsteroidal anti-inflammatory drugs for analgesia. Activities are gradually restored during prolonged convalescences. Endoscopic therapy is useful in evaluating and managing gastrointestinal hemorrhage although injection therapy with sclerosing agents is not beneficial in most dengue hemorrhagic states. Monitoring platelet counts does not usefully predict clinically significant bleeding. Monitoring for hemoconcentration, however, may help in anticipating the complications of dengue hemorrhagic fever or shock syndrome.

Prognosis

Fatalities are rare but do occur, especially during epidemic outbreaks, with occasional patients dying from fulminant hepatitis. Convalescence for most patients is slow.

Centers for Disease Control and Prevention (CDC): Travel-associated dengue infections—United States, 2001–2004. MMWR Morb Mortal Wkly Rep 2005;54:556. [PMID: 15944525]

Lee IK: Clinical characteristics and risk factors for concurrent bacteremia in adults with dengue hemorrhagic fever. Am J Trop Med Hyg 2005;72:221. [PMID: 15741560]

Shu PY: Fever screening at airports and imported dengue. Emerg Infect Dis 2005;11:460. [PMID: 15757566]

Stephenson JR: Understanding dengue pathogenesis: implications for vaccine design. Bull World Health Organ 2005;83:308. [PMID: 15868023]

Wills BA et al: Comparison of three fluid solutions for resuscitation in dengue shock syndrome. N Engl J Med 2005;353:877. [PMID: 16135832]

3. Hantaviruses

Hantaviruses are rodent-borne enveloped RNA bunyaviruses with several distinct serotypes. These differ in rodent hosts, geographic distribution, and degree of pathogenicity for humans. They cause two major clinical syndromes: hemorrhagic fever (discussed above) and the hantavirus pulmonary syndrome. Aerosols of virus-contaminated rodent urine and perhaps feces are thought to be the main vehicle for transmission to humans. The ubiquity of hantaviruses is becoming recognized, with descriptions of infections from North and South America and additional infections from Europe and Asia. The Hantaan serotype viruses cause severe hemorrhagic fever with renal syndrome and are found primarily in Korea, China, and eastern Russia. The Seoul viruses produce a less severe form and are found primarily in Korea and China. The Puumala and Dobrava viruses are found in Scandinavia and Europe and are associated with a milder form of the syndrome, nephropathia epidemica, which usually presents with fever, headache, gastrointestinal symptoms, and impaired renal function.

The Sin Nombre (Muerto Canyon, Four Corners) virus is one of the viruses responsible for the **hantavirus pulmonary syndrome**, most cases of which have been seen in the southwestern United States. Approximately 300 cases have been reported from 31 states since 1993. Outbreaks are currently being reported from Central and South America. Hantavirus pulmonary syndrome begins as a nonspecific febrile illness followed by a severe increase in pulmonary vascular permeability, leading to respiratory failure, and rapid progression to a shock-like state. Hematologic features include thrombocytopenia, hemoconcentration, and leukocytosis, with abnormal lymphocytes and immature myeloid cells in the peripheral smear. Clinical similarities, including a propensity toward renal involvement exist between the New World hantaviruses and their Old World counterparts.

Diagnosis can be made serologically, with most patients having both IgM and IgG antibodies at the time of presentation; by immunohistochemical staining; or by PCR amplification of viral tissue DNA. Because infection is thought to occur by inhalation of rodent wastes, prevention is aimed toward eradication of rodents in houses and avoidance of exposure to rodent excreta in rural settings.

No treatment has been established as definitely effective for hantavirus pulmonary syndrome. Intravenous ribavirin has been used with some success in hemorrhagic fever with renal syndrome, and studies are currently ongoing for its use in hantavirus pulmonary syndrome.

Boroja M et al: Radiographic findings in 20 patients with hantavirus pulmonary syndrome correlated with clinical outcome. AJR Am J Roentgenol 2002;178:159. [PMID: 11756112]

Hujakka H et al: Diagnostic rapid tests for acute hantavirus infections: specific tests for Hantaan, Dobrava and Puumala viruses versus a hantavirus combination test. J Virol Methods 2003;108:117. [PMID: 12565162]

Olsson G et al: Human hantavirus infections, Sweden. Emerg Infect Dis 2003;9:1395. [PMID: 14718081]

Peters CJ et al: Hantavirus pulmonary syndrome: the new American hemorrhagic fever. Clin Infect Dis 2002;34:1224. [PMID: 11941549]

4. Yellow Fever

ESSENTIALS OF DIAGNOSIS

- *Endemic area exposure (tropical South and Central America, Africa, but not Asia).*
- *Sudden onset of severe headache, aching in legs, and tachycardia.*
- *Brief (1 day) remission, followed by bradycardia, hypotension, jaundice, hemorrhagic tendency.*
- *Proteinuria, leukopenia, bilirubinemia, bilirubinuria.*
- *Rare and potentially fatal reactions to vaccination.*

General Considerations

Yellow fever is a zoonotic flavivirus infection transmitted by *Aedes* and jungle mosquitoes. It occurs in an urban and jungle cycle in Africa and in a jungle cycle in South America. Epidemics have extended far into the temperate zone during warm seasons. The role of yellow fever in preventing economic development in tropical areas is devastating.

The mosquito transmits the infection by first biting an individual having the disease and then biting a susceptible individual after the virus has multiplied within the mosquito's body. The incubation period in humans is 3–6 days. Adults and children are equally susceptible, though attack rates are highest among adult males because of their work habits. Between 5% and 50% of infections are asymptomatic.

Clinical Findings

A. SYMPTOMS AND SIGNS

1. Mild form—Symptoms are malaise, headache, fever, retroorbital pain, nausea, vomiting, and photophobia. Relative bradycardia, conjunctival injection, and facial flushing may be present.

2. Severe form—Severe illness develops in about 15% of those infected with yellow fever. Initial symptoms are similar to the mild form, but a brief fever remission lasting hours to a few days is followed by a "period of intoxication" manifested by fever and relative bradycardia (Faget's sign), hypotension, jaundice, hemorrhage (gastrointestinal, nasal, oral), and delirium that may progress to coma.

B. LABORATORY FINDINGS

Leukopenia occurs, although it may not be present at the onset. Proteinuria is present, sometimes as high as 5–6 g/L, and disappears completely with recovery. Abnormal liver function tests are seen, and prothrombin time may be elevated. Serologic diagnosis is primarily by measurement of IgM by a capture ELISA. Other serologic tests include hemagglutination-inhibition and neutralization. PCR protocols are becoming more widely available.

Differential Diagnosis

It may be difficult to distinguish yellow fever from hepatitis, malaria, leptospirosis, louse-borne relapsing fever, dengue, and other hemorrhagic fevers on clinical evidence alone. Albuminuria is a constant feature in yellow fever patients and its presence helps differentiate yellow fever from other viral hepatitides. Serologic confirmation is often needed.

Prevention

Transmission is prevented through mosquito control. Live virus vaccine is highly effective and should be provided for immunocompetent persons over 9 months of age living in or traveling to endemic areas. Vaccine-induced reactions, including viscerotropic and hepatotropic diseases that resemble yellow fever, are reported (particularly among elderly patients). Mass campaigns with the vaccine were carried out without significant complications in Cote d'Ivoire. The safety of the vaccine in pregnant patients is not verified, and pregnant women should, if possible, defer travel to endemic areas (see Chapter 30). Eradication is difficult because of the sylvatic cycle, with forest rodents serving as a reservoir. Discrete enzootic foci of transmission appear to be more important than wandering epizootic foci as formerly thought. (See Chapter 30.)

Treatment

No specific antiviral therapy is available. Treatment is directed toward symptomatic relief and management of complications. If not in an endemic area, the patient should be isolated from mosquitoes to prevent transmission, since blood in the acute phase is potentially infectious.

Prognosis

The mortality rate of the severe form is 20–50%, with death occurring most commonly between the sixth and the tenth days. In survivors, the temperature returns to normal by the seventh or eighth day. The prognosis in any individual case is guarded at the onset, since sudden changes for the worse are common. Intractable hiccups, copious black vomitus, melena, and anuria are unfavorable signs. Convalescence is prolonged, including 1–2 weeks of asthenia. Infection confers lifelong immunity.

Gubler DJ: The changing epidemiology of yellow fever and dengue, 1900 to 2003: full circle? Comp Immunol Microbiol Infect Dis 2004;27:319. [PMID: 15225982]

Khromaava AY et al: Yellow fever vaccine: an updated assessment of advanced age as a risk factor for serious adverse events. Vaccine 2005;23:3256. [PMID: 15837230]

Pugachev KV et al: New developments in flavivirus vaccines with special attention to yellow fever. Curr Opin Infect Dis 2005;18:387. [PMID: 16148524]

Tattevin P et al: Yellow fever vaccine is safe and effective in HIV-infected patients. AIDS 2004;18:825. [PMID: 15075524]

Weir E at al: Yellow fever: readily prevented but difficult to treat. CMAJ 2004;170:1909. [PMID: 15210636]

5. Tick-Borne Encephalitis

 ESSENTIALS OF DIAGNOSIS

- *Flaviviral encephalitis found in Eastern, Central, and occasionally Northern Europe.*
- *Transmitted via ticks or ingestion of unpasteurized milk.*
- *Long-term neurologic sequelae occur in 2–25% of cases.*
- *Therapy is largely supportive.*
- *Prevention is based on avoiding tick exposure, pasteurization of milk, and vaccination.*

General Considerations

Tick-borne encephalitis (TBE) is a flaviviral infection caused by TBE virus that is endemic in Russia and in eastern and central Europe. In parts of Europe and the Baltic, attack rates exceed 100 cases per 100,0000 population and 10,000 to 12,000 cases are estimated to occur annually. TBE occurs predominantly in the late spring through fall. It is usually a consequence of exposure to infected ticks, although unpasteurized cow's, sheep's, and goat's milk are recognized forms of transmission. The incubation period is 7–14 days for tick-borne exposures but only 3–4 days for milk ingestion. The principal reservoirs for TBE virus are small rodents; humans are an accidental host. The vectors for most cases are *Ixodes persulcatus* and *Ixodes ricinus*.

Clinical Findings

A. SYMPTOMS AND SIGNS

Although the majority of cases are subclinical and many resemble a flu-like syndrome, symptomatic and severe disease occurs in all age groups. There are two variants, a Western and an Eastern subtype. Disease with the Western subtype occurs mainly in the fall and is most severe among the elderly, whereas disease with the Eastern subtype is associated with more severe disease among children.

Western subtype disease is biphasic; after a 2–10 day asymptomatic interval, a febrile period of 2–7 days is followed by neurologic symptoms. Eastern subtype disease is progressive without an asymptomatic interval. The leading neurologic symptom is a febrile headache, the clinical presentation accounting for up to 50% of Eastern subtype TBE cases. Aseptic meningitis is a significant clinical manifestation of disease. A greater degree of encephalitic symptoms presents in some patients, and a myelitis with severe extremity pain develops 5–10 days after the fever remits in a small percentage of patients. Mortality is usually a consequence of brain edema or bulbar involvement.

B. Diagnosis

Diagnosis is established clinically. Abnormal cerebrospinal fluid findings include a pleocytosis that may persist for up to 4 months. Leukocytosis and neutrophilia are common. PCR of infected tissue, such as brain, may be useful. Neuroimaging studies show hyperintense lesions in the thalamus, brainstem, and basal ganglia.

Complications

The main sequela of disease is paresis, which occurs in up to 10% of Western and up to 25% of Eastern subtype disease. Among those with encephalitis, about 25% recover within 2 months. In the remaining 40%, either protracted, cognitive dysfunction or persistent spinal nerve paralysis with or without other postencephalitic symptoms develops. The postencephalitic syndrome, characterized by headache, difficulties concentrating, balance disorders, dysphasia, hearing defects, and chronic fatigue, occurs with both subtypes. A progressive motor neuron disease may occur with the Eastern subtype.

Differential Diagnosis

The differential diagnosis includes other causes of aseptic meningitis such as enteroviral infections, herpes simplex encephalitis, and a variety of tick-borne pathogens including tularemia, the rickettsial diseases, babesiosis, Lyme disease, and other flaviviral infections.

Therapy

Therapy is largely supportive. Some clinicians believe corticosteroids or other nonsteroidal anti-inflammatory drugs may be useful, although no controlled clinical trials exist.

Prevention

Prevention is based on vaccination. Although a vaccine has not been approved in the United States, a variety of vaccines are in current use, with the most popular and most effective being a formaldehyde-inactivated whole virus vaccine from Austria. Alternative effective vaccines have been developed in Germany and Russia. The initial vaccination schedule requires 1 year with boosters every 3 years. Other prevention recommendations include avoidance of tick exposure, pasteurization of milk, and passive immunization with immunoglobulin within 4 days of exposure (disease exacerbation from exposure to immunoglobulin is not substantiated).

Charrel RN: Tick-borne virus diseases of human interest in Europe. Clin Microbiol Infect 2004;10:1040. [PMID: 15606630]

Kunze U et al: Tick-borne encephalitis in childhood—consensus 2004. Wien Med Wochenschr 2004;154:242. [PMID: 15244050]

Rendi-Wagner P et al: Persistence of protective immunity following vaccination against tick-borne encephalitis—longer than expected? Vaccine 2004;22:2743. [PMID: 15246606]

6. Colorado Tick Fever

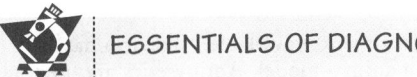

ESSENTIALS OF DIAGNOSIS

- Onset 1–19 days (average, 4 days) following tick bite.
- Fever, chills, myalgia, headache, prostration.
- Leukopenia.
- Second attack of fever after remission lasting 2–3 days.

General Considerations

Colorado tick fever is an acute coltivirus infection transmitted by *Dermacentor andersoni* bites. The disease is limited to the western United States and Canada and is most prevalent during the tick season (March to November). There is a discrete history of tick bite or exposure in 90% of cases. The virus infects the marrow erythrocyte precursors, leading to viremia lasting the life span of the infected red cells.

Clinical Findings

A. Symptoms and Signs

The incubation period is 3–6 days. The onset is usually abrupt with fever (to 38.9–40.6 °C), sometimes with chills. Severe myalgia, headache, photophobia, anorexia, nausea and vomiting, and generalized weakness are prominent symptoms. Physical findings are limited to an occasional faint rash. The acute symptoms resolve within a week. The remission is followed in 50% of cases by recurrent fever and a full recrudescence lasting 2–4 days. In an occasional case there may be three bouts of fever.

The differential diagnosis includes influenza, Rocky Mountain spotted fever, numerous other viral infections and, in the right setting, relapsing fevers.

B. Laboratory Findings

Leukopenia (2000–3000/mcL) with a shift to the left and atypical lymphocytes occurs, reaching a nadir 5–6 days after the onset of illness. Viremia may be demonstrated by inoculation of blood into mice or by fluorescent antibody staining of the patient's red cells (with adsorbed virus). Complement-fixing antibodies do not appear until the third week of disease but are the most frequently used tool to document an infection. A reverse transcriptase PCR assay may be used to detect viremia.

Complications

Aseptic meningitis (particularly in children), encephalitis, and hemorrhagic fever occur rarely. Malaise may ensue, but fatalities are very rare.

Treatment

No specific treatment is available. Ribavirin has shown efficacy in an animal model. Antipyretics are used, although aspirin should be avoided. Codeine or hydrocodone may be given for pain. Tick-avoidance measures may be effective in preventing the disease.

Prognosis

The disease is usually self-limited and benign.

Bratton RL et al: Tick-borne disease. Am Fam Physician 2005;71: 2323. [PMID: 15999870]

Klasco R: Colorado tick fever. Med Clin North Am 2002;86:435. [PMID: 11982311]

COMMON VIRAL RESPIRATORY INFECTIONS

Infections of the respiratory tract are perhaps the most common human ailments. Specific associations of some groups of viruses with certain disease syndromes are established. In young infants and in the elderly, or in persons with impaired respiratory tract reserve, bacterial superinfection increases morbidity and mortality. Croup, epiglottitis, and the common cold are discussed in Chapter 8.

Leder K et al: Respiratory tract infections in travelers: a review of the GeoSentinel surveillance network. Clin Infect Dis 2003; 36:399. [PMID: 12567296]

Muether PS: Variant effect of first- and second-generation antihistamines as clues to their mechanism of action on the sneeze reflex in the common cold. Clin Infect Dis 2001;33: 1483. [PMID: 11588693]

1. Respiratory Syncytial Virus & Other Paramyxoviruses

RSV is a paramyxovirus that causes annual outbreaks of pneumonia, bronchiolitis, and tracheobronchitis, with the majority of cases occurring in the very young. Premature infants with bronchopulmonary dysplasia are at highest risk. Other risk factors in children include male gender, age less than 6 months, and day care exposure. Incomplete immunity commonly leads to reinfection manifested typically as an upper respiratory tract infection and tracheobronchitis in older children or adults. Serious pulmonary RSV infections have been described in elderly and immunocompromised adults. Outbreaks with a high mortality rate in bone marrow transplant and pediatric liver transplant patients are reported.

Annual epidemics occur in winter and spring. The average incubation period is 5 days. Inoculation may occur through the nose or the eyes. RSV is an increasingly recognized as contributing to recurrent otitis media in children and upper respiratory tract infections. Among hematologic adult cancer patients with upper respiratory tract infections, the isolation of RSV is a significant marker for progression to pneumonia.

Other paramyxoviruses important in human disease include human metapneumovirus and parainfluenza viruses. **Human metapneumovirus** is less common and less pathogenic than RSV. Like RSV, it appears to cause bronchiolitis; croup; exacerbation of pneumonia; and pneumonia during the winter and spring among infants, with highest rates in the 3–24 month age range; and lower respiratory tract infections among elderly adults. **Parainfluenza viruses** that most commonly cause disease are types 1, 2, and 3. They tend to cause respiratory tract infections in the very young, the elderly, the immunocompromised, and those with chronic illnesses.

In RSV bronchiolitis, proliferation and necrosis of bronchiolar epithelium develop, producing obstruction from sloughed epithelium and increased mucus secretion. Signs include low-grade fever, tachypnea, and wheezes. Hyperinflated lungs, decreased gas exchange, and increased work of breathing are present. Otitis media is a frequent complication often with concomitant *Streptococcus pneumoniae* infection.

RSV is the only respiratory pathogen that produces its most serious illness at a time when specific maternal antibody is generally present. Most mothers report a recent infection. This—combined with the observation that infants who received a particular past live RSV vaccine had more severe disease—suggests an immune-mediated component to the disease. The complexity of the relationship between immunity and RSV is shown by the fact that among adults, low levels of RSV-specific nasal IgA are a risk factor for infection, and among infants, antibody levels appear to be lower during episodes of RSV reinfection. RSV infections are not thought to be a strong predictor for the later development of asthma.

Rapid diagnosis may be made by viral antigen identification of nasal washings using an ELISA or immunofluorescent assay. Culture of nasopharyngeal secretions remains the standard of diagnosis, although the usefulness of PCR methods for diagnosis is increasingly appreciated. Human metapneumovirus is diagnosed only using PCR.

Treatment of RSV consists of hydration, humidification of inspired air, and ventilatory support as needed. Although bronchodilating agents and ribavirin are widely used, evidence supporting their effectiveness in populations not at high risk is lacking. The effectiveness of corticosteroid therapy is also controversial. Pregnant women should avoid ribavirin exposure—and indeed, patients with upper RSV infections probably do not need ribavirin. Hyperimmune RSV immunoglobulin G (1500 mg/kg) is no longer available in the United States. RSV immune globulin is now replaced with palivizumab, a monoclonal RSV antibody, given safely at 15 mg/kg. The FDA recommends the administration of palivizumab prophylactically (parenterally at 15 mg/kg monthly during the season of high transmission) to infants with high-risk factors, such as congenital heart disease. Infants with acute RSV bronchiolitis may not always show severe prognostic criteria for RSV respiratory tract disease.

The search for an effective RSV vaccine, originally disheartened by early formalin-inactivated vaccine candidates which enhanced RSV disease, is encouraged now by studies showing that a live-attenuated vaccine is well tolerated and shows protection in challenge studies. Because nosocomial RSV infections disseminate rapidly, prevention in hospitals entails rapid diagnosis, handwashing, contact isolation, and perhaps passive immunization. Therapeutic modalities for human metapneumovirus and parainfluenzavirus infections are under investigation, including trials of ribavirin.

Bader MS et al: Viral infections in the elderly. The challenges of managing herpes zoster, influenza, and RSV. Postgrad Med 2005;118:45,51. [PMID: 16329530]

Bentur L et al: Dexamethasone inhalations in RSV bronchiolitis: a double-blind, placebo-controlled study. Acta Paediatr 2005;94:1866. [PMID: 16188807]

Ebbert JO et al: Respiratory syncytial virus pneumonitis in immunocompromised adults: clinical features and outcome. Respiration 2005;72:263. [PMID: 15942295]

Englund J: In search of a vaccine for respiratory syncytial virus: the saga continues. J Infect Dis 2005;191:1036. [PMID: 15747236]

Prais D et al: Impact of palivizumab on admission to the ICU for respiratory syncytial virus bronchiolitis: a national survey. Chest 2005;128:2765. [PMID: 16236953]

Williams JV et al: Human metapneumovirus and lower respiratory tract disease in otherwise healthy infants and children. N Engl J Med 2004;350:443. [PMID: 14749452]

2. Influenza

ESSENTIALS OF DIAGNOSIS

- *Cases usually in epidemic pattern.*
- *Abrupt onset with fever, chills, malaise, cough, coryza, and myalgias.*
- *Aching, fever, and prostration out of proportion to catarrhal symptoms.*
- *Leukopenia.*

General Considerations

Influenza (an orthomyxovirus) is a highly contagious disease transmitted by the respiratory route. In contrast to RSV and rhinoviruses, transmission occurs by droplet nuclei rather than fomites or large particle aerosols. Epidemics and pandemics appear at varying intervals, usually in the fall or winter (although sporadic cases occur as do summer outbreaks in northern areas such as Alaska) affecting 10–20% of the global population on average each year. Antigenic types A and B produce clinically indistinguishable infections, whereas type C is usually a minor illness. Annual influenza epidemics are the result of frequent and significant antigenic variation of the virus, or antigenic drift, which is more common in influenza A virus. Pandemics—associated with higher mortality—typically are associated with type A infections in which significant genetic recombination of the virus (antigenic shift) has taken place. The incubation period is 1–4 days.

Avian influenza is discussed in the next section.

Clinical Findings

A. SYMPTOMS AND SIGNS

Typical uncomplicated influenza often begins abruptly. Symptoms include fever, chills, malaise, myalgias, substernal soreness, headache, nasal stuffiness, and occasionally nausea. Fever lasts 1–7 days (usually 3–5). Coryza, nonproductive cough, and sore throat are present. Elderly patients may present with only lassitude and confusion, often without fever or respiratory symptoms. Signs include mild pharyngeal injection, flushed face, and conjunctival redness. Moderate enlargement of the cervical lymph nodes may be observed.

B. LABORATORY FINDINGS

Leukopenia is common. Proteinuria may be present. The virus may be isolated from throat washings by inoculation of embryonated eggs or cell cultures. Rapid laboratory tests for influenza antigens from nasal or throat swabs are becoming widely available. Complement-fixing and hemagglutination-inhibiting antibodies appear during the second week.

Complications

Influenza causes necrosis of the respiratory epithelium, which predisposes to secondary bacterial infections. Bacterial enzymes in turn (eg, proteases, trypsin-like compounds, streptokinase, and plasminogen) activate influenza viruses. Frequent complications are acute sinusitis, otitis media, purulent bronchitis, and pneumonia. The elderly and the chronically ill, including HIV-infected individuals, are at high risk for complications. Rhabdomyolysis is a rare late complication.

Pneumonia is commonly due to bacterial infection with pneumococci or, less often, staphylococci or *Haemophilus*. Primary viral pneumonia (caused by the influenza virus itself) may occur, particularly in patients with cardiovascular disease and pregnant women and has a high mortality. Pericarditis, myocarditis, toxic shock syndrome, and thrombophlebitis sometimes occur.

Reye's syndrome (fatty liver with encephalopathy) is a rare and severe complication of influenza (usually B type) and other viral diseases (eg, varicella), particularly in young children. It consists of rapidly progressive hepatic failure and encephalopathy, and there is a 30% fatality rate. The pathogenesis is unknown, but the syndrome is associated with aspirin use in a variety of viral infections. Hypoglycemia, elevation of serum aminotransferases and blood ammonia, prolonged prothrombin time, and change in mental status all occur within 2–3 weeks after onset of the viral infection. Histologically, the periphery of liver lobules shows striking fatty infiltration and glycogen depletion. Treatment is supportive and directed toward the management of cerebral edema.

Prevention

Trivalent influenza virus vaccine provides partial immunity (about 85% efficacy) for a few months to 1 year. The vaccine's antigenic configuration changes yearly and is based on prevalent strains of the preceding year. Vaccination in October or November each year is recommended for persons over 50 years of age (a substantial portion of the older population suffers from at least one chronic medical condition), children (over 6 months of age) and teenagers receiving long-term aspirin therapy, nursing home residents, patients with chronic lung or heart disease or other debilitating illnesses (including pregnant women during the second and third trimesters), health care workers, service personnel, and contacts of < 2-year-old children. The breadth of these recommendations includes much of the adult population.

The vaccine is contraindicated in persons with well-substantiated hypersensitivity to chicken eggs (based on dietary history) or other components of the vaccine (skin testing can be performed by an allergist), persons with Guillain–Barré syndrome, an acute febrile illness, or thrombocytopenia. Concomitant warfarin or corticosteroid therapy is not a contraindication. Side effects are infrequent and include tenderness, redness, or induration at the site of the injection and, rarely, myalgias, fever, or the oculorespiratory syndrome (conjunctivitis, facial edema, and respiratory symptoms within 2–48 hours of vaccination).

Adequate immunity is achieved about 2 weeks after vaccination. In healthy subjects, the antibody level remains sufficiently high throughout the season. Levels wane quickly, however, in elderly nursing home patients. Therefore, the time of administration of the vaccine should be based on surveillance data. The vaccination effectively reduces both morbidity (preventing 35–60% of hospital admissions in the elderly) and mortality (preventing 35–80% of hospital deaths). A new live-attenuated, nasally administered, vaccine is now licensed for use in the United States, while a nasally administered inactivated vaccine is under development.

HIV-infected persons can be safely vaccinated, and concerns about activating replication of the HIV virus by the immunogen appear to be exaggerated and may be less severe than the increase in HIV viral load associated with a full influenza infection. Vaccination is less effective when CD4 counts are less than 100/mcL.

False-positive assays for HIV, HTLV-1, and HCV antibodies have been reported in the wake of influenza vaccination.

Chemoprophylaxis can be accomplished with either amantadine or rimantadine or the newer neuraminidase inhibitors, zanamivir and oseltamivir. Amantadine (200 mg/d orally in two divided doses—or 100 mg/d in the elderly, who are susceptible to CNS side effects) and rimantadine (200 mg/d in two divided doses) are ineffective against influenza B and many avian strains. Oseltamivir (75 mg/d) and zanamivir (10 mg inhaled daily) are effective against influenza A and B. All the above medications will reduce the attack rate among unvaccinated individuals if begun within 48 hours after exposure, although a nursing home outbreak in 2004 documented the presence of amantadine resistance in 12 of 16 residents assayed.

Treatment

Many patients with influenza prefer to rest in bed. Analgesics and a cough mixture may be used. Amantadine or rimantadine, in the same doses as are used for prophylaxis, appreciably decrease the duration of symptoms and signs. Rimantadine is preferred in patients with renal failure. Resistance to amantadine and rimantadine develops in > 50% of children, typically after 3–5 days of exposure, and this resistance is reported in a majority of the influenza isolates from the 2005–2006 season. The clinical significance of resistance to antiviral agents is controversial. Ribavirin (1.1 g/d, diluted to 20 mg/mL and delivered as particulate aerosol with oxygen over 12–18 hours a day for 3–7 days [see Table 32–1]) helps severely ill patients with influenza A or B. The new neuraminidase inhibitors, either inhaled zanamivir (two 5-mg inhalations twice daily for 5 days) or oral oseltamivir (75 mg twice daily for 5 days), are equally helpful in the treatment of influenza but are more costly. Clinical trials have shown a reduction in the duration of symptoms, but not in the rate of hospitalizations or mortality when using these agents. All agents are most effective when given within 48 hours after symptom onset and are shown to be effective mainly in high-risk patients over age 12 years.

Antibacterial antibiotics should be reserved for treatment of bacterial complications. Acetaminophen rather than aspirin should be used for fever in children.

Prognosis

The duration of the uncomplicated illness is 1–7 days, and the prognosis is excellent in healthy, nonelderly adults. Purulent bronchitis and bronchiectasis may result in chronic pulmonary disease and fibrosis that persist throughout life. Most fatalities are due to bacterial pneumonia. Influenza pneumonia has a high mortality rate among pregnant women and persons with a history of rheumatic heart disease. In recent epidemics, the mortality rate has been low except in debilitated individuals.

If the fever persists for more than 4 days with productive cough and white cell count over 10,000/mcL, secondary bacterial infection should be suspected. Pneumococcal pneumonia is the most common such infection, and staphylococcal pneumonia is the most serious.

Armstrong BG et al: Effect of influenza vaccination on excess deaths occurring during periods of high circulation of influenza: cohort study in elderly people. BMJ 2004;329:660. [PMID: 15313884]

Fagan HB et al: What is the best agent for influenza infection? Am Fam Physician 2004;70:1331. [PMID: 15508545]

Schilling M et al: Emergence and transmission of amantadine-resistant influenza A in a nursing home. J Am Geriatr Soc 2004;52:2069. [PMID: 15571544]

Schmidt AC: Antiviral therapy for influenza: a clinical and economic comparative review. Drugs 2004;64:2031. [PMID: 15341496]

Thompson WW et al: Influenza-associated hospitalizations in the United States. JAMA 2004;292:1333. [PMID: 15367555]

3. Avian Influenza

ESSENTIALS OF DIAGNOSIS

- *Rare cases to date in humans, mostly from Southeast Asia.*
- *Clinically indistinguishable from influenza.*
- *Epidemiologic factors assist in diagnosis.*
- *Rapid antigen assays are the means of confirming diagnosis.*

General Considerations

The normal hosts for avian influenza viruses are birds and occasionally pigs. Recently, a highly pathogenic influenza A subtype (H5N1) was found in poultry in East and Southeast Asian countries. In 1997, an outbreak of H5N1 influenza occurred in poultry in Hong Kong, resulting in the first recognized human cases. A massive slaughter of poultry was attempted to contain the disease. New outbreaks of H5N1 influenza in poultry emerged, however, in 2003 and continue to spread to different nations. At least 20 countries reported poultry outbreaks as of early 2006, largely in Asia but also recently in Nigeria, Greece, Turkey, and Italy. There are, as of July 26, 2006, 232 confirmed human cases with 134 deaths (from Azerbaijan, Cambodia, China, Djibouti, Egypt, Iraq, Indonesia, Thailand, Turkey, and Vietnam).

Although the H5N1 strain of avian influenza is highly contagious from one bird to another, the transmission from human to human is relatively inefficient and not sustained. The result is only rare cases of person-to-person infection. Most human cases occur after exposure to infected poultry or surfaces contaminated with poultry droppings. Because infection in humans is associated with a mortality rate greater than 50% (most patients die of respiratory failure), there exists considerable concern that H5N1 strains might widely disseminate and initiate a pandemic. Current commercial rapid antigen tests are not optimally sensitive or specific for detection of H5N1 influenza, but are still first-line diagnostic tests because of their widespread availability. Diagnostic yield can be improved by earlier collection of samples. More sensitive tests such as reverse-transcription PCR are of limited availability. Throat or lower respiratory swabs may provide higher yield of detection than nasal swabs for H5N1 strains. Epidemiologic risk factors (travel to Southeast Asia, contact with known cases) should guide testing strategies.

Most Asian H5N1 influenza strains are resistant to amantadine and rimantadine, but this is not an inherent property of all H5N1 strains. Sensitivity to rimantadine and amantadine can also be possibly reacquired through genetic reassortment. The current recommendations for the neuraminidase inhibitors oseltamivir and zanamivir include administration within 48 hours from onset of illness. These medications should still be considered for patients with severe avian influenza disease even after several days of onset. Recent evidence of resistance to oseltamivir is reported.

The worldwide concern that the avian H5N1 subtype of influenza may transform by genetic reassortment and mutation, developing greater human-human transmissibility, is the basis for fear of a global avian influenza pandemic. The risk of these events appears more realistic as avian influenza continues to spread among birds, with many parts of Southeast Asia now considered endemic for the virus. Careful surveillance of new human cases and continued development of a commercially available vaccine are important aspects of influenza control. Only partial protection can be achieved using conventional tricomponent inactivated influenza vaccines because of major differences in the major components, particularly the hemagglutinin.

Prevention of exposure to avian influenza strains also includes hygienic practices during handling of poultry products, including handwashing and prevention of cross-contamination, as well as thorough cooking of poultry products (to 70 °C). Nonetheless, the risk of acquiring avian influenza through the consumption of poultry products is very small.

Beigel JH et al; Writing Committee of the World Health Organization (WHO) Consultation on Human Influenza A/H5. Avian influenza (H5N1) in humans. N Engl J Med 2005; 353:1374. [PMID: 16192482]

CDC Key Facts About Avian Influenza (Bird Flu) and Avian Influenza A (H5N1) Virus.
http://www.cdc.gov/flu/avian/gen-info/facts.htm

Ungchusak K et al: Probable person-to-person transmission of avian influenza A (H5N1). N Engl J Med 2005;352:333. [PMID: 15668219]

World Health Organization: Avian influenza frequently asked questions.
http://www.who.int/csr/disease/avian_influenza/avian_faqs/en/print.html

Yuen KY et al: Human infection by avian influenza A H5N1. Hong Kong J 2005;11:189. [PMID: 15951584]

4. Severe Acute Respiratory Syndrome (SARS)

ESSENTIALS OF DIAGNOSIS

- Mild, moderate, or severe respiratory illness.
- Travel to endemic area within 10 days before symptom onset, including mainland China, Hong Kong, Singapore, Taiwan, Vietnam, and Toronto.
- Persistent fever; dry cough, dyspnea in most.
- Diagnosis confirmed by antibody testing or isolation of virus.
- No specific treatment; mortality as high as 10% in clinically diagnosed cases.

General Considerations

SARS is a respiratory syndrome of varying severity but capable of causing death in as many as 10% of clinically established cases. It is caused by an apparently unique coronavirus. The earliest cases were traced to a health care worker in Guangdong Province in China in late 2002, with rapid spread thereafter to Hong Kong, Singapore, Vietnam, Taiwan, and Toronto. The primary mode of transmission appears to be through direct or indirect contact of mucous membranes (eyes, nose, or mouth) with infectious respiratory droplets or fomites. The use of aerosol-generating procedures (endotracheal intubation, bronchoscopy, nebulization treatments) in hospitals may amplify the transmission of the SARS coronavirus. The role of fecal–oral transmission is unknown. The natural reservoir appears to be the horseshoe bat (which eats and drops fruits ingested by civets, the earlier presumed reservoir).

The variable distribution of cases throughout Asia and Canada is considered a consequence of spread through travel. The virus is sufficiently virulent that it may be transmitted and acquired by patients during brief stops in airports. As a result, sporadic confirmed and suspected cases have appeared throughout the United States. As of September 2003, about 8098 cases were reported to the World Health Organization from about 30 countries, with 774 fatalities to that date.

Clinical Findings

A. SYMPTOMS AND SIGNS

SARS is considered an atypical pneumonia that affects persons in all age groups. The CDC recognizes asymptomatic or mild cases, moderate disease, and severe respiratory illness. The incubation period is 2–7 days, and it can be spread to contacts of affected patients for 10 days. The mean time from onset of clinical symptoms to hospital admission is 3–5 days. In all clinical cases, persistent fever is present; chills and/or rigor, cough, shortness of breath, rales, and rhonchi are the rule. Many patients report headache, myalgias, and sore throat as well. A watery diarrhea occurs in some patients late in the course of the illness. Elderly patients may report malaise and delirium, without the typical febrile response. No single symptom or sign is diagnostic or highly suggestive, and the history and physical examination of a patient in whom SARS in suspected are to be interpreted in this context.

B. LABORATORY FINDINGS AND IMAGING

Leukopenia and especially lymphopenia are observed commonly. A low-grade disseminated intravascular coagulation (thrombocytopenia, prolonged activated thromboplastin time, and elevated D-dimer level) is present in many patients. Other abnormalities include modest elevations of alanine aminotransferase and creatine kinase. Arterial oxygen saturation is less than 95% in 80% of affected individuals, and pulmonary infiltrates are noted in all. The roentgenographic pattern is not specific, and severe cases may progress to ARDS, with extensive bilateral consolidation. A high-resolution CT scan is abnormal (ground-glass opacifications or focal consolidation) in 67% of patients with initially normal chest radiographs. Serum serologies, including enzyme immunoassays and fluorescent antibody assays, are available through public health departments at the state level, although seroconversion may not occur until 3 weeks after the onset of symptoms.

The detection rates for the virus using conventional reverse transcriptase-PCR are generally low in the first week of illness. Urine, nasopharyngeal aspirate, and stool specimens are positive in 42%, 68%, and 97%, respectively, on day 14 of illness. Although viral isolation is possible, it is a technically laborious and time-consuming procedure.

Complications

To date, the principal complications are confined to the lung. As with any viral pneumonia, pulmonary decompensation is the most feared problem. About 20–30% of patients experience refractory hypoxemia requiring intubation and mechanical ventilation. Sequelae of intensive care include infection with nosocomial pathogens, tension pneumothorax from ventilation at high peak pressures, and noncardiogenic pulmonary edema.

Treatment

The benefit of ribavirin in the treatment of SARS is controversial. There is only one randomized study in which the drug was used at a low dose (400–600 mg/d) and was shown to be ineffective. Other nonrandomized studies used higher doses (4 g/d) and showed some benefit but a very high rate of side effects, mainly hemolysis. The limited data suggest that doses of 2 g/d may be effective and not produce adverse reactions. The use of high-dose pulse methylprednisolone during the clinical progression phase (with development of radiologic evidence of pneumonia and hypoxemia) is associated with a more favorable clinical improvement. The role of corticosteroids, alone or in combination with ribavirin, is also controversial. The synthetic form of interferon, alfacon-1, in combination with corticosteroids may be beneficial in reducing disease-associated hypoxemia and in promoting a more rapid resolution of radiographic abnormalities. Reports from one center in Hong Kong suggest that the addition of lopinavir/ritonavir as initial therapy is associated with an overall lower mortality. Recovery in severe cases requires intensive support.

Prognosis

The overall mortality rate of identified cases is about 14%. Mortality is age-related, ranging from less than 1% in persons under 24 years of age to greater than 50% in persons over 65 years of age. Poor prognostic factors include advanced age, chronic hepatitis B infection treated with lamivudine, high initial or high peak lactate dehydrogenase concentration, high neutrophil count on presentation, diabetes mellitus, and low counts of CD4 and CD8 on presentation. Many subclinical cases probably go undiagnosed. Seasonality, as with influenza, is not established. Although the overall case incidence diminishes in areas in which appropriate preventive measures are taken, sporadic outbreaks, including one near Toronto, were reported through summer 2003.

Prevention

Because the known modalities of transmission for the SARS agent include intubation, suctioning, and nebulization, health care workers engaged in procedures that involve these activities are at high risk for acquiring the virus. Transmission may occur shortly after the development of symptoms and perhaps before the appearance of fever, cough, and dyspnea. Thus, an increased level of suspicion is critical, and isolation of high-risk patients is essential. For health care workers exposed to presumptive cases of SARS, simple hygienic measures such as handwashing after touching patients, use of appropriate and well-fitted face masks, and early introduction of infection control measures, including quarantine, may help reduce transmission.

Measures enacted for air travelers have included screening for fever and compatible symptoms and quarantining in the home for high-risk exposed persons. Continual reporting of suspected cases is crucial, as is awareness of restrictions on international travel. The most cautious modalities include monitoring for 10 days after the last potential exposure and confinement of recovering patients for a similar interval. Use of face masks, adopted by many in endemic areas, is not harmful but its efficacy is not substantiated.

Chau T et al: Value of initial chest radiographs for predicting clinical outcomes in patients with severe acute respiratory syndrome. Am J Med 2004;117:249. [PMID: 15308434]

Cheng VC et al: Medical treatment of viral pneumonia including SARS in immunocompetent adults. J Infect 2004;29:262. [PMID: 15474623]

Jiang S et al: SARS vaccine development. Emerg Infect Dis 2005;11:1016. [PMID: 16022774]

Leung GM et al: The epidemiology of severe acute respiratory syndrome in the 2003 Hong Kong epidemic: an analysis of all 1755 patients. Ann Intern Med 2004;141:662. [PMID: 15520422]

Li W et al: Bats are natural reservoirs of SARS-like coronaviruses. Science 2005;310:676. [PMID: 16195424]

Perlman S et al: Immunopathogenesis of coronavirus infections: implications for SARS. Nat Rev Immunol 2005;5:917. [PMID: 16322745]

ADENOVIRUS INFECTIONS

Adenoviruses (there are over at least 51 serotypes) produce a variety of clinical syndromes. These infections are usually self-limited or clinically inapparent and most common among infants, young children, and military recruits. Adenoviruses, however, may cause significant morbidity and mortality in immunocompromised persons, such as HIV-infected persons and liver, renal, and stem cell transplant patients (risk factors for severe infection include immunosuppressive therapy, graft-versus-host disease and lymphocytopenia). The incubation period is 4–9 days. Adenoviruses, although a common cause of human disease, also receive particular recognition through their role in gene therapy.

Clinical syndromes of adenovirus infection, often overlapping, include the following. The common cold (see Chapter 8) is characterized by rhinitis, pharyngitis, and mild malaise without fever. Nonstreptococcal exudative pharyngitis is characterized by fever lasting 2–12 days and accompanied by malaise and myalgia. Conjunctivitis is often present. Lower respiratory tract infection may occur, including bronchiolitis, suggested by cough and rales, or pneumonia (type 3 and type 7 commonly cause acute respiratory disease and pneumonia). Pharyngoconjunctival fever is manifested by fever and malaise, conjunctivitis (often unilateral), and mild pharyngitis. Epidemic keratoconjunctivitis (transmissible person to person) occurs in adults and is manifested by unilateral conjunctival redness, pain, tearing, and an enlarged preauricular lymph node (multiple types may be involved in a single outbreak). Keratitis may lead to subepithelial opacities (especially with types 8, 19, or 37). Acute hemorrhagic cystitis is a disorder of children often associated with adenovirus type 11. Sexually transmitted genitourinary ulcers and urethritis may be caused by types 2, 8, and 37 in particular. Adenoviruses also cause acute gastroenteritis (types 40 and 41), leading to intussusception, and are rarely associated with encephalitis, acute flaccid paralysis, and pericarditis. In a recent review of viruses causing dilated cardiomyopathy, adenoviruses were the most common isolates, found in 12% of samples. Severity of systemic adenoviral disease correlates with the concentration of lactate dehydrogenase and with oxygen saturation on admission.

Hepatitis (type 5 adenovirus) tends to develop in infected liver transplant recipients, whereas pneumonia or hemorrhagic cystitis (types 11 and 34) tend to develop in bone marrow and renal transplant recipients.

A rapid diagnostic direct fluorescence assay may assist with directing appropriate therapy and a rapid-cycle PCR is currently available.

Treatment is symptomatic. Ribavirin and cidofovir are used in immunocompromised individuals with occasional success, although the use of cidofovir, especially in the immunocompromised, is attendant with significant renal toxicity. Immunosuppression should be reduced if possible. Adoptive immunotherapy with transfusion of adenovirus-specific T cells is currently being investigated.

Vaccines are not available for general use. Live oral vaccines containing attenuated type 4 and type 7 are used in military personnel.

Bowles NE et al: Detection of viruses in myocardial tissues by polymerase chain reaction. Evidence of adenovirus as a common cause of myocarditis in children and adults. J Am Coll Cardiol 2003;42:466. [PMID: 12906974]

Faix DJ et al: Evaluation of a rapid quantitative diagnostic test for adenovirus type 4. Clin Infect Dis 2004;38:391. [PMID: 14727210]

Guarner J et al: Intestinal intussusception associated with adenovirus infection in Mexican children. Am J Clin Pathol 2003; 120:845. [PMID: 14671973]

Leen AM et al: Adenovirus as an emerging pathogen in immunocompromised patients. Br J Haematol 2005;128:135. [PMID: 15638847]

Peled N et al: Adenovirus infection in hospitalized immunocompetent children. Clin Pediatr 2004;43:223. [PMID: 15094946]

OTHER EXANTHEMATOUS VIRAL INFECTIONS

1. Parvovirus Infections

Parvovirus B19 is quite widespread (by age 15 years about 50% of children have detectable IgG) and causes several syndromes. In children, an exanthematous illness ("fifth disease," erythema infectiosum) is characterized by a fiery red "slapped cheek" appearance, circumoral pallor, and a subsequent lacy, maculopapular, evanescent rash on the trunk and limbs. Malaise, headache, and pruritus (especially on the palms and soles) occur, but little fever. In immunosuppressed patients, including those with HIV infection, or posttransplantation, or with hematologic conditions such as sickle cell disease, transient aplastic crisis and pure red blood cell aplasia may occur. The pathophysiologic mechanism of red cell invasion is thought to be binding of the virus to the erythrocyte P

antigen (globoside). Middle-aged persons (especially women) develop a limited symmetric polyarthritis that mimics lupus erythematosus and rheumatoid arthritis, preferentially involving the proximal interphalangeal joints of the hands and the wrists and knees. Arthralgias are uncommon in children. Rashes, especially facial, are uncommon in adults. In pregnancy, fetal loss and hydrops fetalis are reported sequelae. An association with Henoch–Schönlein purpura has also been noted. Rare reported presentations include myocarditis with infarction, constrictive pericarditis, a lupus-like syndrome, CNS vasculitis, and a chronic fatigue syndrome. Less accepted associations with parvovirus infection include hepatitis, myositis, rheumatoid arthritis (the arthralgias of parvovirus infection tend to be transient) and systemic lupus erythematosus. Subclinical infection is documented among patients with sickle cell disease.

The diagnosis is clinical (Table 32–2) but may be confirmed by an elevated titer of IgM anti-parvovirus antibodies in serum or with PCR. Scarlet fever is the most similar disorder. Arthritis with hypocomplementemia is a common complication in some outbreaks. Uncommon complications of infection include encephalitis, chronic hemolytic anemia, thrombotic thrombocytopenic purpuric syndrome, acute postinfectious glomerulonephritis, and hepatitis.

Treatment in healthy persons is symptomatic. Nonsteroidal anti-inflammatory drugs can be used to treat arthralgias and transfusions to treat transient aplastic crises. In immunosuppressed patients, intravenous immunoglobulin aids in the reduction of anemia.

Screening of donated blood could potentially prevent transfusion-related infection. Several nosocomial outbreaks have been documented, and hospital infection control personnel should administer standard containment guidelines, including handwashing after patient exposure and avoiding contact with pregnant women.

The prognosis is generally excellent in immunocompetent individuals. In immunosuppressed patients, persistent anemia may require prolonged transfusion dependence. Remission of parvovirus infection in AIDS patients may occur with HAART, though the immune restoration syndrome is also reported with parvovirus.

Gilberte NL et al: Seroprevalence of parvovirus B19 infection in daycare educators. Epidemiol Infect 2005;133:299. [PMID: 15816155]

Mishra B et al: Human parvovirus B19 in patients with aplastic anemia. Am J Hematol 2005;79:166. [PMID: 15929106]

Young NS et al: Parvovirus B19. N Engl J Med 2004;350:586. [PMID: 14762186]

2. Poxvirus Infections

Among the nine poxviruses causing disease in humans, the following are clinically important.

1. **Variola/vaccinia:** Smallpox was a highly contagious disease characterized by severe headache, fever, and prostration and accompanied by a centrifugal rash

developing uniformly in order of progression from macules to papules to vesicles to pustules over 1–2 weeks. An international consensus among the scientific community in the 1990s resulted in a recommendation to destroy the virus since elimination of the disease was achieved. As long as this recommendation is not implemented, risk remains for unauthorized access to the remaining samples and potential misuse for military or terrorist purposes, resulting in exposure of large unvaccinated civilian populations.

In the wake of the recent international terrorism incidents, concern exists about the potential use of smallpox and other agents as biologic weapons.

Vaccination with vaccinia was historically crucial for smallpox eradication. Any form of immunosuppression is an absolute contraindication to smallpox vaccination. Eczema (or a history of it) in a patient or family member, other forms of dermatitis, and burns also contraindicate vaccination. Dilution of existing stores of vaccinia by fivefold to tenfold does not significantly reduce its effectiveness in stimulating an immune response and, of course, greatly increases availability. The current Department of Defense Smallpox Vaccination Program began on December 2002. Through April 2004, 615,000 persons were vaccinated. Potential side effects such as dermatologic, neurologic, and cardiac complications raise concerns among clinicians. Reported cardiac complications include myocarditis, cardiac arrhythmias, and pericarditis. A total of 67 cases of myopericarditis were reported between December 2002 and December 2003. Most of these cases presented with the prodromal symptoms of fever, myalgias, arthralgias, headache, and fatigue. The clinical, electrocardiographic, and biochemical presentation of smallpox vaccine-induced myopericarditis may mimic myocardial infarction.

Most physicians in practice today have not seen a case of clinical smallpox. The disseminated lesions of smallpox in the past were often confused with those of varicella, though the synchronous progression in smallpox readily distinguishes these lesions from those of varicella, wherein lesions of several stages are usually present simultaneously. (See also Chapter 6.)

A recent outbreak of a vaccinia virus (the Passatempo virus) was reported from Brazil. Exanthematous lesions were reported among both the dairy cattle and the cow milkers.

2. **Molluscum contagiosum** may be transmitted sexually or by other close contact. It is manifested by pearly, raised, umbilicated skin nodules sparing the palms and soles. Marked and persistent lesions in AIDS patients appear to respond readily to combination antiretroviral therapy. The many anecdotal agents reported to hasten resolution include cimetidine and CO_2 laser therapy combined with natural interferon-β gel. Imiquimod cream (5%) appears to be effective in curing molluscum lesions.

3. **Orf** (contagious pustular dermatitis, or ecthyma contagiosa) and **paravaccinia** (milker's nodules) are occupational diseases acquired by contact with sheep and cattle, respectively.

4. **Monkeypox**, first identified in 1970, is enzootic in the rain forests of equatorial Africa and presents in humans as a syndrome similar to smallpox. The incubation period is about 12 days, and limited person-to-person spread occurs. African mortality rates vary from 3% to 11% depending on the immune status of the patient. Secondary attack rates, which are hard to determine because of diagnostic confusion with varicella in older series, appear to be about 10%. The first community-acquired outbreak in the United States of monkeypox occurred in 2003 in Wisconsin and other states of the upper Midwest. The source appeared to be imported Gambian giant rats via consequent exposure of prairie dogs. Clinical findings included a prodrome of fever and chills, headaches, myalgias, and sweats. About one-third of patients reported a nonproductive cough. After 1–10 days, a papular rash appeared that progressed through stages of vesiculation, pustulation, umbilication, and crusting—and in some cases ulceration. The rash started on the head, trunk, and extremities, with occasional satellite lesions on the palms, soles, and extremities, and in some cases became generalized.

Susceptible animals include nonhuman primates, rabbits, and rodents. Contact with these species is the primary means of transmission to humans. General precautions that should be taken are avoidance of contact with prairie dogs and Gambian giant rats (whose illness is manifested by alopecia, rash, and ocular or nasal discharge), appropriate care and isolation of those who are ill and those exposed within 3 prior weeks to such animals, and veterinary examination and investigation of suspect animals through health departments.

Primary prevention entails the use of vaccinia immunization, a procedure accompanied by a risk of dissemination in HIV-infected persons—a real concern considering the coincident areas of endemicity of HIV-1 and monkeypox.

The CDC recommends smallpox vaccination to individuals if their exposure to infected animals is sufficient and if the candidate vaccinee has no contraindications (outlined above). Cidofovir is under current study as an agent for treatment. Submission of specimens and case reporting can be conducted using the Association of Public Health Laboratories' Web site listed below.

Association of Public Health Laboratories:
http://www.aphl.org/

CDC Bioterrorism Public Health Emergency Preparedness and Response—Smallpox: Laboratory Testing:
http://www.bt.cdc.gov/agent/smallpox/lab-testing.

Leite A et al: Passatempo virus, a vaccinia virus strain, Brazil. Emerg Infect Dis 2005;11:1935. [PMID: 16485483]

Ligon BL: Monkeypox: a review of the history and emergence in the Western hemisphere. Semin Pediatr Infect Dis 2004;15:280. [PMID: 15494953]

Seward JF et al: Development and experience with an algorithm to evaluate suspected smallpox cases in the United States, 2002–2004. Clin Infect Dis 2004;39:1477. [PMID: 15546084]

Weiss MM et al: Rethinking smallpox. Clin Infect Dis 2004;39:1668. [PMID: 15578369]

VIRUSES & GASTROENTERITIS

Viruses are responsible for at least 30–40% of cases of infectious diarrhea in the United States, and rotaviruses are a leading worldwide cause of dehydrating gastroenteritis in young children. The agents that can cause disease include groups A, B and C rotaviruses, caliciviruses such as Norwalk and Norwalk-like viruses (which cause epidemics of vomiting and diarrhea in contained environments), and other caliciviruses, astroviruses, enteric adenoviruses and, less often, toroviruses, coronaviruses, picobirnaviruses, and pestiviruses.

Rotaviruses (G1–G4 and G9 are the most common serotypes) are a major cause of diarrheal morbidity worldwide (nearly 600,000 die yearly, mainly due to dehydration), can also cause infections in adults exposed to infected infants, and are ubiquitous in the environment of an outbreak. (Secondary rates are between 16% and 30%.) Most rotavirus infections occur in children aged 6 months–2 years, and the incidence peaks during the winter. The disease is usually mild, and cases also occur among travelers, in epidemic fashion, and after waterborne exposure. The method of choice for diagnosis is PCR of the stool. Treatment is symptomatic, with fluid and electrolyte replacement. Local intestinal immunity gives protection against successive infection. Vaccine administration was discontinued because of a probable association with intussusception. New vaccines are under development (one was licensed recently in Mexico). Future administration of these vaccines may concentrate on the ages when the risk of intussusception is least likely (avoiding ages 3–9 months).

The **Norwalk virus** was first identified using electron microscopy on infectious stool infiltrate derived from an outbreak of gastroenteritis at a school in Norwalk, Ohio. This virus and the related **Norwalk-like viruses** are responsible for over 40% of cases of group-related and institutional outbreaks of diarrhea. There have been several recent reports of gastroenteritis outbreaks induced by Norwalk-like viruses on cruise ships.

Norwalk virus is also often responsible for military outbreaks. Although transmission is usually fecal–oral, airborne and waterborne (recently among snowmobilers in Wyoming) transmission is also documented. Infections appear to be more common during cold weather intervals. Reverse transcriptase-PCR of stool samples is used for epidemiologic purposes. Treatment is largely symptomatic. The presence of antibodies is not associated with protection against reinfection.

Bresee JS et al: Rotavirus in Asia: the value of surveillance for informing decisions about the introduction of new vaccines. J Infect Dis 2005;192(Suppl 1):S1. [PMID: 16088790]

Hutson AM et al: Norovirus disease: changing epidemiology and host susceptibility factors. Trends Microbiol 2004;12:279. [PMID: 15165606]

Kapikian AZ et al: A hexavalent human rotavirus-bovine rotavirus (UK) reassortant vaccine designed for use in developing countries and delivered in a schedule with the potential to eliminate the risk of intussusception. J Infect Dis 2005; 192(Suppl 1):S22. [PMID: 16088801]

Ruiz-Palacios GM et al; Human Rotavirus Vaccine Study Group: Safety and efficacy of an attenuated vaccine against severe rotavirus gastroenteritis. N Engl J Med 2006;354:11. [PMID: 16394298]

Walter JE et al: Astrovirus infection in children. Curr Opin Infect Dis 2003;16:247. [PMID: 12821816]

Ward RL: Rotavirus vaccines: is the second time the charm? Curr Opin Investig Drugs 2005;6:798. [PMID: 16121686]

ENTEROVIRUSES THAT PRODUCE SEVERAL SYNDROMES

1. Coxsackievirus Infections

Coxsackievirus infections cause several clinical syndromes. As with other enteroviruses, infections are most common during the summer. Two groups, A and B, are defined either serologically or by mouse bioassay. There are more than 50 serotypes.

Clinical Findings

A. SYMPTOMS AND SIGNS

The clinical syndromes associated with coxsackievirus infection may be described briefly as follows.

1. Summer grippe (A and B)—A febrile illness, principally of children, lasting 1–4 days. Minor symptoms and respiratory tract infection are often present.

2. Herpangina (A2–6, 10)—Sudden onset of fever, which may be as high as 40.6 °C, sometimes with febrile convulsions; headache, myalgia, and vomiting; and sore throat, characterized early by petechiae or papules on the soft palate that become shallow ulcers in about 3 days and then heal. Treatment is symptomatic.

3. Epidemic pleurodynia (Bornholm disease) (B1–5)—Pleuritic pain is prominent, and tenderness, hyperesthesia, and muscle swelling are present over the area of diaphragmatic attachment. Other findings include headache, sore throat, malaise, nausea, and fever. Orchitis and aseptic meningitis occur in less than 10% of patients. Most patients are ill for 4–6 days.

4. Aseptic meningitis (A and B) and other neurologic syndromes—Fever, headache, nausea, vomiting, stiff neck, drowsiness, and cerebrospinal fluid lymphocytosis without chemical abnormalities may occur, and pediatric clusters of group B meningitis are reported. Focal encephalitis, transverse myelitis, and acute flaccid paralysis are reported with coxsackievirus group A, and a disseminated encephalitis after group B infection.

5. Acute nonspecific pericarditis (B types)—Sudden onset of anterior chest pain, often worse with inspiration and in the supine position, is typical. Fever, myalgia, headache, and pericardial friction rub appear early and these symptoms are often transient. Evidence for pericardial effusion on imaging studies is often present, and the occasional patient has a paradoxic pulse. Electrocardiographic evidence of pericarditis is often present. Relapses may occur.

6. Myocarditis (B1–5)—Heart failure in the neonatal period secondary to in utero myocarditis and over 20% of adult cases of myocarditis and dilated cardiomyopathy are possibly associated with group B infections. Upregulation of mast cells through inducing the innate immune system (Toll-like receptors) may be the means by which coxsackieviruses induce myocarditis.

7. Hand, foot, and mouth disease (A5, 10, 16)— This disease is sometimes epidemic and is characterized by stomatitis and a vesicular rash on hands and feet. Enterovirus 71 is also a causative agent.

8. Hepatitis (B1)—Fulminant neonatal hepatitis with thrombocytopenia and coagulopathy occurs rarely.

9. Type 1 diabetes mellitus (B types)—An association purportedly exists between coxsackievirus B infections and subsequent development of type 1 diabetes mellitus, but results of different studies fail to definitively prove a causal association.

10. Glomerulopathy and tubular injury—Renal damage has been reported with several group B infections.

11. Sjögren's syndrome—Coxsackieviruses are theorized to initiate an autoimmune process in exocrine gland epithelial cells that results in Sjögren's syndrome,

12. Epidemic conjunctivitis—As with enterovirus 70 (see below), the A24 variant of coxsackievirus is associated with acute epidemic hemorrhagic conjunctivitis.

B. LABORATORY FINDINGS

Routine laboratory studies show no characteristic abnormalities. Neutralizing antibodies appear during convalescence. The virus may be isolated from throat washings or stools inoculated into suckling mice.

Treatment & Prognosis

Treatment is symptomatic. With the exception of myocarditis, pericarditis, perhaps diabetes, and rare illnesses such as pancreatitis or polio-like syndrome, the syndromes caused by coxsackieviruses are benign and self-limited. There are anecdotal reports of success with pleconaril as well as with intravenous immunoglobulin in severe disease.

Fairweather D et al: Viruses as adjuvants for autoimmunity: evidence from Coxsackievirus-induced myocarditis. Rev Med Virol 2005;15:17. [PMID: 15386590]

Traintafyllopoulou A et al: Autoimmunity and coxsackievirus infection in primary Sjogren's syndrome. Ann N Y Acad Sci 2005;1050:389. [PMID: 16014556]

2. Echovirus Infections

Echoviruses are enteroviruses that produce several clinical syndromes, particularly in children. Infection is most common during summer.

Over 30 serotypes have been demonstrated. Most cause aseptic meningitis, which may be associated with a rubelliform rash. Type 30 outbreaks have been reported from Canada (Saskatchewan), France, Germany, Italy, Japan, and Turkey. An increased number of type 13 cases, including five epidemics, occurred in the United States and cases are increasingly reported globally. Transmission is primarily fecal-oral. Handwashing is an effective control measure in outbreaks of aseptic meningitis. Outbreaks related to fecal contamination of water sources, including drinking water and swimming and bathing pools, were reported in the past.

Diseases associated with echoviruses range from common respiratory diseases and epidemic diarrhea (including type 22) to myocarditis, a hemorrhagic obstetric syndrome, keratoconjunctivitis, hepatitis with coagulopathy, leukocytoclastic vasculitis, and neonatal as well as adult cases of encephalitis and sepsis, interstitial pneumonitis, sudden deafness, encephalitis, optic neuritis, uveitis, and septic shock.

As with other enterovirus infections, diagnosis is best established by correlation of clinical, epidemiologic, and laboratory evidence. Cytopathic effects are produced in tissue culture after recovery of virus from throat washings, blood, or cerebrospinal fluid. PCR of the cerebrospinal fluid may be diagnostic. Fourfold or greater rises in antibody titer signify systemic infection.

Treatment is usually symptomatic, and the prognosis is excellent, though there are reports of mild paralysis after CNS infection. Trials are underway with pleconaril.

From a public health standpoint, the prevention of fecal-oral contamination and the maintenance of pool hygiene through chlorination and pH control are important.

Abzug MJ: Presentation, diagnosis, and management of enterovirus infections in neonates. Paediatr Drugs 2004;6:1. [PMID: 14969566]

Bernit E et al: Prospective investigation of a large outbreak of meningitis due to echovirus 30 during summer 2000 in Marseilles, France. Medicine (Baltimore) 2004;83:245. [PMID: 15232312]

Hauri AM et al: An outbreak of viral meningitis associated with a public swimming pond. Epidemiol Infect 2005;133:291. [PMID: 15816154]

Mullins JA et al: Emergence of echovirus type 13 as a prominent enterovirus. Clin Infect Dis 2004;38:70. [PMID: 14679450]

3. Enteroviruses 70 & 71

Several clinical syndromes are being described in association with newer enteroviruses. The most common of these are **enterovirus 70**, associated with **acute hemorrhagic conjunctivitis**, a ubiquitous agent first identified in 1969 and responsible for abrupt bilateral eye discharge and occasional systemic symptoms, but in most cases subconjunctival hemorrhage, and **enterovirus 71**, associated with **hand, foot, and mouth disease** as well as a form of **epidemic encephalitis** (genogroups B and C in the Western Pacific region) associated on occasion with pulmonary edema, and **acute flaccid paralysis**. Hand, foot, and mouth disease tends to infect the very young (under age 5) in nonendemic areas because of lower herd immunity. Sequelae include central hypoventilation, dysphagia, and limb weakness, all of which are minimized by stage-based treatment, dividing the illness into four classical stages (HFMD/herpangina, CNS disease, cardiopulmonary failure, and convalescence). Diagnosis of both entities is facilitated by the clinical and epidemiologic findings with the isolation of the suspect agent from either conjunctival scraping for enterovirus 70 or vesicle swabs, body secretions, or cerebrospinal fluid for enterovirus 71. An IgM capture ELISA is being developed for the latter agent.

Treatment of both entities remains largely symptomatic, though there are increasing reports of the successful use of pleconaril, an agent available in some countries but not the United States. The major complication associated with enterovirus 70 is the development in a small percentage of cases of an acute neurologic illness with motor paralysis akin to poliomyelitis. Household contacts, especially children under 6 months of age, are at particular risk for enterovirus 71 acquisition.

Enterovirus 72 is another term for hepatitis A virus (see Chapter 15).

Chang LY et al: Transmission and clinical features of enterovirus 71 infections in household contacts in Taiwan. JAMA 2004;291:222. [PMID: 14722149]

Kao SJ et al: Mechanism of fulminant pulmonary edema caused by enterovirus 71. Clin Infect Dis 2004;38:1784. [PMID: 15227628]

Palacios G et al: Enteroviruses as agents of emerging infectious diseases. J Neurovirol 2005;11:424. [PMID: 16287683]

Wang SY et al: Early and rapid detection of enterovirus 71 infection by an IgM-capture ELISA. J Virol Methods 2004;119: 37. [PMID: 15109819]

■ RICKETTSIAL DISEASES

The rickettsioses are febrile exanthematous diseases caused by rickettsiae, small gram-negative obligate intracellular bacteria. In arthropods, rickettsiae grow in the gut lining, often without harming the host. Human infection results from either an arthropod bite or contamination with its feces. In humans, rickettsiae grow principally in endothelial cells of small blood vessels, producing vasculitis, cell necrosis, thrombosis of vessels, skin rashes, and organ dysfunctions. Rickettsiae are also capable of growing in human macrophages and hepatocytes.

Different rickettsiae and their vectors are endemic in different parts of the world, but two or more types may coexist in the same geographic area. New organisms are identified regularly. Travel-associated cases occur with selected species. A summary of epidemiologic features is given in Table 32–3. The clinical picture is variable but usually includes a prodromal stage followed by fever, rash, and prostration. Isolation of rickettsiae from the patient is difficult and potentially hazardous to laboratory workers. Diagnosis is usually based on clinical examination and epidemiologic evidence. Laboratory diagnosis relies on the development of specific antibodies detected by complement fixation (for diagnosis), immunofluorescence, or hemagglutination (for species identification) tests. Other newer means of isolation are the centrifugation shell-vial technique and PCR.

Prevention & Treatment

Preventive measures are directed at control of the vector and avoidance of exposure by use of repellents and protective clothing. A search of body surfaces should be conducted after potential exposure and the vector (louse, tick, or mite) gently removed. Many patients do not recall exposure to a vector.

Rickettsiae can be inhibited by tetracyclines or chloramphenicol. All early infections respond to treatment with these drugs. Dosage schedules are listed in the sections below.

Fournier PE et al: Gene sequence-based criteria for identification of new rickettsia isolates and description of *Rickettsia heilongjiangensis* sp. nov. J Clin Microbiol 2003;41:5456. [PMID: 14662925]

Jensenius M et al: Rickettsiosis and the international traveler. Clin Infect Dis 2004;39:1493. [PMID: 15546086]

Walker D et al: Pathogenic mechanisms of diseases caused by rickettsiae. Ann NY Acad Sci 2003;990:1. (Whole volume dedicated to rickettsial disease.) [PMID: 12860594]

TYPHUS GROUP

1. Epidemic Louse-Borne Typhus

 ESSENTIALS OF DIAGNOSIS

- *Prodrome of headache, then chills and fever.*
- *Severe, intractable headaches, prostration, persisting high fever.*
- *Macular rash appearing on the fourth to seventh days on the trunk and in the axillae, spreading to the rest of the body but sparing the face, palms, and soles.*
- *Diagnosis confirmed by specific antibodies using complement fixation, microagglutination, or immunofluorescence.*

General Considerations

Epidemic louse-borne typhus is due to infection with *Rickettsia prowazekii*, a parasite of the body louse. Transmission is favored by crowded, unsanitary living conditions, famine, war, or any circumstances that predispose to heavy infestation with lice. When the louse sucks the blood of a person infected with *R prowazekii*, the organism becomes established in the

Table 32–3. Rickettsial diseases.

Disease	Rickettsial Pathogen	Geographic Areas of Prevalence	Insect Vector	Mammalian Reservoir	Travel Association
Typhus group					
Epidemic (louse-borne) typhus	*Rickettsia prowazekii*	South America, Central Africa	Louse	Humans, flying squirrels	Rare
Endemic (murine) typhus	*Rickettsia typhi*	Worldwide; small foci (United States: southeastern Gulf Coast)	Flea	Rodents	Often
Scrub typhus group					
Scrub typhus	*Orientia tsutsuga-mushi*	Southeast Asia, Japan, Australia, Western Siberia	Mite[1]	Rodents	Often
Spotted fever group					
Rocky Mountain spotted fever	*Rickettsia rickettsii*	Western Hemisphere; United States (especially mid-Atlantic coast region)	Tick[1]	Rodents, dogs	Rare
California flea rickettsiosis	*Rickettsia felis*	Worldwide?	Flea	Cats, opossums	
Mediterranean spotted fever, Boutonneuse fever, Kenya tick typhus, South African tick fever, Indian tick typhus	*Rickettsia conorii*	Africa, India, Mediterranean regions	Tick[1]	Rodents, dogs	Often
Queensland tick typhus	*Rickettsia australis*	Eastern Australia	Tick[1]	Rodents, marsupials	Rare
Siberian Asian tick typhus	*Rickettsia sibirica*	Siberia, Mongolia	Tick[1]	Rodents	Rare
African tick bite fever	*Rickettsia africae*	Rural sub-Saharan Africa Eastern Caribbean	Tick[1]	Cattle	Often
Rickettsialpox	*Rickettsia akari*	United States, Korea, former USSR	Mite[1]	Mice	
Other					
Ehrlichiosis and anaplasmosis, human Monocytic	*Ehrlichia chaffeensis, Anaplasma equi, Ehrlichia canis*	Southeastern United States	Tick[1]	Dogs	
Granulocytic	*Anaplasma phagocytophilum, Ehrlichia ewingii*	Northeastern United States	Tick[1]	Rodents, deer, sheep	
Q fever	*Coxiella burnetii*	Worldwide	None[2]	Cattle, sheep, goats	

[1]Also serve as arthropod reservoir by maintaining rickettsiae through transovarian transmission.
[2]Human infection results from inhalation of dust.

gut of the louse and grows there. When the louse is transmitted to another person (through contact or clothing) and has a blood meal, it defecates simultaneously, and the infected feces are rubbed into the itching bite wound. Dry, infectious louse feces may also enter the respiratory tract.

In a person who recovers from clinical or subclinical typhus infection, *R prowazekii* may survive in lymphoid tissues. Years later, there may be a recrudescence of disease (Brill-Zinsser disease) without exposure to infected lice, which can serve as a point source for future outbreaks.

Mild and atypical cases of *R prowazekii* infection have rarely occurred in the United States after contact with flying squirrels or their ectoparasites or decades following exposure (eg, among concentration camp victims of World War II). Cases can be acquired by travel to pockets of infection (eg, central and northeastern Africa, Central and South America). Recent outbreaks were reported from Peru, Burundi, and Russia.

Clinical Findings

A. SYMPTOMS AND SIGNS

(Table 32–3.) Prodromal malaise, cough, headache, backache, arthralgia, and chest pain begin after an incubation period of 10–14 days, followed by an abrupt onset of chills, high fever, and prostration, with flu-like symptoms progressing to delirium and stupor. The headache is severe and the fever is prolonged.

Other findings consist of conjunctivitis, hearing loss from neuropathy of the eighth cranial nerve, flushed facies, rales at the lung bases, and often splenomegaly. A macular rash (that may become confluent) appears first in the axillae and then over the trunk, spreading to the extremities but rarely involving the face, palms, or soles. In severely ill patients, the rash becomes hemorrhagic, and hypotension becomes marked. There may be renal insufficiency, stupor, and delirium. In spontaneous recovery, improvement begins 13–16 days after onset with a rapid drop of fever.

B. LABORATORY FINDINGS

The white blood cell count is variable. Thrombocytopenia, elevated liver enzymes, proteinuria and hematuria commonly occur. Serum obtained 5–12 days after onset of symptoms usually shows specific antibodies for *R prowazekii* antigens as demonstrated by complement fixation, microagglutination, or immunofluorescence. In primary rickettsial infection, early antibodies are IgM; in recrudescence (Brill's disease), early antibodies are predominantly IgG.

C. IMAGING

Radiographs of the chest may show patchy consolidation.

Differential Diagnosis

The prodromal symptoms and the early febrile stage are not specific enough to permit diagnosis in nonepidemic situations. The rash is usually sufficiently distinctive for diagnosis, but it may be absent in up to 50% of cases or may be difficult to observe in dark-skinned persons. A variety of other acute febrile diseases should be considered, including typhoid fever, meningococcemia, and measles.

Brill-Zinsser disease (recrudescent epidemic typhus) has a more gradual onset than primary *R prowazekii* infection, fever and rash are of shorter duration, and the disease is milder and rarely fatal.

Complications

Pneumonia, thromboses, vasculitis with major vessel obstruction and gangrene, circulatory collapse, myocarditis, and uremia may occur.

Prevention

Prevention consists of louse control with insecticides, particularly by applying chemicals to clothing or treating it with heat, and frequent bathing. A deloused and bathed typhus patient is not infectious. The disease is not transmitted from person to person. Patients are infectious for the lice during the febrile period and perhaps 2–3 days after the fever returns to normal. Infected lice pass rickettsiae in their feces within 2–6 days after the blood meal and can be infectious earlier if crushed. Rickettsiae remain viable in a dead louse for weeks.

Immunization with vaccines consisting of inactivated egg-grown *R prowazekii* gives some protection to laboratory personnel, physicians, or field workers who are exposed to the parasite. This vaccine is not currently commercially available in the United States or Canada. An improved cell culture vaccine is being developed.

Treatment

Treatment consists of either doxycycline (200 mg/d) or chloramphenicol (50–100 mg/kg/d in four divided doses) for 4–10 days.

Prognosis

The prognosis depends greatly on the patient's age and immunization status. In children under age 10 years, the disease is usually mild. The mortality rate is 10% in the second and third decades but in the past reached 60% in the sixth decade. Effective vaccination can convert a potentially serious disease into a mild one.

Reynolds MG et al: Flying squirrel-associated typhus, United States. Emerg Infect Dis 2003;9:1341. [PMID: 14609478]

Woodward T et al: The history of epidemic typhus. Infect Dis Clin N Am 2004;18:127. [PMID: 15081509]

2. Endemic Flea-Borne Typhus (Murine Typhus)

Rickettsia typhi, a ubiquitous pathogen, is transmitted from rat to rat through the rat flea. Humans usually acquire the infection in an urban or suburban setting when bitten by an infected flea, which releases infected feces while sucking blood. Rare human cases in the developed world follow travel, usually to Southeast Asia. A recent surge in cases was reported from Hawaii.

Endemic typhus resembles recrudescent epidemic typhus in that it has a gradual onset, less severe symptoms, and a shorter duration of illness than epidemic typhus (7–10 days versus 14–21 days). The presentation is nonspecific, including fever, headache, and chills. The rash is maculopapular and concentrated on the trunk and fades fairly rapidly. Peripheral facial paralysis is reported to occur. Fatalities are uncommon but up to 4% may occur, especially in the elderly.

The most common entity in the differential diagnosis is Rocky Mountain spotted fever, usually occurring after a rural exposure and with a different rash (centripetal versus centrifugal for endemic typhus). Serologic confirmation may be necessary for differentiation, with complement-fixing or immunofluorescent antibodies detectable within 15 days after onset, with specific *R typhi* antigens.

Preventive measures are directed at control of rats and ectoparasites (rat fleas) with insecticides, rat poisons, and rat-proofing of buildings. Antibiotic treatment with doxycycline (100 mg twice daily for adults and children weighing > 45 kg, and 2 mg/kg twice daily for children weighing < 45 kg) or chloramphenicol (50–75 mg/kg/d in four divided doses) is indicated through 3 full days of defervescence. Ciprofloxacin (500–750 mg twice a day) may be an acceptable alternative.

Centers for Disease Control and Prevention (CDC): Murine typhus—Hawaii,2002. MMWR Morb Mortal Wkly Rep 2003;52:1224. [PMID: 14681594]

Chen MI et al: Epidemiological, clinical and laboratory characteristics of 19 serologically confirmed rickettsial disease in Singapore. Singapore Med J 2001;42:553. [PMID: 11989575]

Gikas A et al: Comparison of the effectiveness of five different antibiotic regimens on infection with Rickettsia typhi: therapeutic data from 87 cases. Am J Trop Med Hyg 2004;70:576. [PMID: 15155995]

3. Scrub Typhus (Tsutsugamushi Fever)

ESSENTIALS OF DIAGNOSIS

- *Exposure to mites in endemic area of Southeast Asia, the western Pacific (including Korea), and Australia.*
- *Black eschar at site of the bite, with regional and generalized lymphadenopathy.*
- *Conjunctivitis and a short-lived macular rash.*
- *Frequent pneumonitis, encephalitis, and cardiac failure.*

General Considerations

Scrub typhus is caused by *Orientia tsutsugamushi*, which is principally a parasite of rodents transmitted by mites in the endemic areas listed above. The mites live on vegetation but complete their maturation cycle by biting humans who come in contact with infested vegetation. Vertical transmission occurs, and blood transfusions may transmit the pathogen. Serosurveys from Bangkok show prevalences over 20% for blood donors and nearly 60% for febrile malaria clinic pa-

tients. Rare occupational transmission via inhalation is documented among laboratory workers.

Clinical Findings

A. SYMPTOMS AND SIGNS

After a 1- to 3-week incubation period, malaise, chills, severe headache, and backache develop. At the site of the bite, a papule evolves into a flat black eschar. The regional lymph nodes are enlarged and tender, and there may be generalized adenopathy. Fever rises gradually, and a macular rash appears primarily on the trunk after a week of fever and may be fleeting or may last a week. The patient may become obtunded. During the second or third week, pneumonitis, myocarditis and cardiac failure, encephalitis or meningitis, acute abdominal pain, granulomatous hepatitis, disseminated intravascular coagulation, or acute renal failure may develop. Gastrointestinal symptoms including nausea, vomiting, and diarrhea occur in nearly two-thirds of patients and correspond to the presence of superficial mucosal hemorrhage, multiple erosions, or ulcers in the gastrointestinal tract. An attack confers prolonged immunity against homologous strains and transient immunity against heterologous strains. Heterologous strains produce mild disease if infection occurs within a year after the first episode.

B. LABORATORY FINDINGS

Blood obtained during the first few days of illness may permit isolation of the rickettsial organism by mouse inoculation. Fluorescein-labeled antirickettsial antibodies and indirect immunoperoxidase assays or commercial dot-blot ELISA dipstick assays are convenient means of establishing the diagnosis, though PCR may be the most sensitive test. A reticulonodular infiltrate is the most common finding on chest radiograph.

Differential Diagnosis

Leptospirosis, typhoid, dengue, malaria, and other rickettsial infections should be considered. Scrub typhus is a recognized cause of obscure tropical fevers, especially in children. When the rash is fleeting and the eschar is not evident, laboratory results are required for diagnosis, including a conventional indirect fluorescent assay or a more sensitive rapid immunochromatographic flow assay that is under development. Upper tract endoscopy may help with gastrointestinal lesions.

Prevention

Repeated application of long-acting miticides can make endemic areas safe. Insect repellents on clothing and skin provide some protection. For short exposure, chemoprophylaxis with doxycycline (200 mg weekly) can prevent the disease but permits infection. No effective vaccines are available.

Treatment & Prognosis

Without treatment, fever subsides spontaneously after 2 weeks, but the mortality rate may be 10–30%. Treatment for 3 days with doxycycline, 100 mg twice daily, or for 7 days with chloramphenicol, 25 mg/kg/d in four divided doses, eliminates most deaths and relapses. Chloramphenicol- and tetracycline-resistant strains have been reported from Southeast Asia, where azithromycin or roxythromycin may become the drug of choice for children, pregnant women, and patients with refractory disease. Rifampin also appears to be effective. HIV infection does not appear to influence the severity of scrub typhus.

Aung-Thu et al: Gastrointestinal manifestations of septic patients with scrub typhus in Maharat Nakhon Ratchasima Hospital. Southeast Asian J Trop Med Public Health 2004;35: 845. [PMID: 15916079]

Jiang J et al: Development of a quantitative real-time PCR assay specific for *Orientia tsutsugamushi*. Am J Trop Med Hyg 2004;70:351. [PMID: 15100446]

Sharma A et al: Investigation of an outbreak of scrub typhus in the Himalayan region of India. Jpn J Infect Dis 2005;58: 208. [PMID: 16116251]

Silpapojakul K et al: Paediatric scrub typhus in Thailand: a study of 73 confirmed cases. Trans R Soc Trop Med Hyg 2004; 98:354. [PMID: 15099991]

SPOTTED FEVERS

1. Rocky Mountain Spotted Fever

ESSENTIALS OF DIAGNOSIS

- *Exposure to tick bite in an endemic area.*
- *An influenza-like prodrome followed by chills, fever, severe headache, myalgias, restlessness, and prostration; occasionally, delirium and coma.*
- *Red macular rash appears between the second and sixth days of fever, first on the wrists and ankles and then spreading centrally; it may become petechial.*
- *Serial serologic examinations by indirect fluorescent antibody (IFA) confirm the diagnosis retrospectively.*

General Considerations

Despite its name, most cases occur outside the Rocky Mountain area, with cases in the United States concentrated along the Middle and Southern Atlantic seaboard and in the central Mississippi valley. The causative agent, *R rickettsii*, is transmitted to humans by the bite of ticks, including the Rocky Mountain wood tick, *Dermacentor andersoni*, in the western United States, and by the bite of the American dog tick, *Dermacentor variabilis*, in the eastern United States. The brown dog tick, *Rhipicephalus sanguineus*, recently was identifed as a vector in eastern Arizona.

Other hard ticks transmit the organism in the southern United States and in Central and South America and are responsible for transmitting it among rodents, dogs, porcupines, and other animals. Most human cases occur in late spring and summer. In the United States, most cases occur in the eastern third of the country, with about 1000 cases reported per year, primarily from April through September, and with a higher incidence among children and men.

Clinical Findings

A. SYMPTOMS AND SIGNS

Two to 14 days (mean, 7 days) after the bite of an infectious tick, symptoms begin with fever, chills, headache, nausea and vomiting, myalgias, restlessness, insomnia, and irritability. Cough and pneumonitis may develop. Delirium, lethargy, seizures, stupor, and coma may appear. The face is flushed and the conjunctiva injected. The rash (faint macules that progress to maculopapules and then petechiae) appears between days 2 and 6 of fever, first on the wrists and ankles, spreading centrally to the arms, legs, and trunk for 2–3 days; involvement of the palms and soles is characteristic. About 10% of cases, however, occur without rash or with minimal rash. In some cases there is splenomegaly, hepatomegaly, jaundice, myocarditis, or uremia. ARDS and necrotizing vasculitis are of greatest concern. About 3–5% of cases reported in the United States in recent years were fatal. Advanced age, underlying chronic diseases, and delay of appropriate treatment are predictors of poor prognosis.

B. LABORATORY FINDINGS

Thrombocytopenia, hyponatremia, elevated aminotransferases, and hyperbilirubinemia are common. Cerebrospinal fluid may show hypoglycorrhachia and mild pleocytosis. Disseminated intravascular coagulation is observed in severe cases. Diagnosis during the acute phase of the illness can be made by immunohistologic demonstration of *R rickettsiae* in skin biopsy specimens, but this must be performed as soon as skin lesions become apparent to achieve maximum sensitivity. Isolation of the organism using the shell-vial technique is available in some laboratories but is hazardous.

Serologic studies confirm the diagnosis, but most patients do not mount an antibody response until the second week of illness. The indirect fluorescent antibody test is most commonly used.

Differential Diagnosis

The diagnosis is challenging. Up to 40% of patients do not recall a tick bite, and initial diagnosis is made clinically. The early symptoms and signs of Rocky Mountain spotted fever resemble those of many other infections. The rash may be confused with that of measles, typhoid, and ehrlichiosis, or—most importantly—meningococcemia. Blood cultures and examination of cerebrospinal fluid establish the latter.

Prevention

Protective clothing, tick-repellent chemicals, and the removal of ticks at frequent intervals are helpful measures. Prophylactic therapy after a tick bite is not currently recommended.

Treatment & Prognosis

Doxycycline (200 mg/d) either orally or intravenously is the drug of choice even in the pediatric population. Chloramphenicol (50 mg/kg/d in four divided doses) is reserved for pregnant women. Patients usually defervesce within 48–72 hours. Mild cases in low-risk individuals may be observed without treatment.

The mortality rate for Rocky Mountain spotted fever varies strikingly with age. In the untreated elderly, it may be 70%, but it is usually less than 20% in children. Other risk factors for a fatal outcome include advanced age, atypical clinical features (absence of headache, no history of tick attachment, gastrointestinal symptoms), and a delay in initiation of appropriate antibiotic therapy. The usual cause of death is pneumonitis with respiratory or cardiac failure. Sequelae, more common than formerly recognized, may include seizures, encephalopathy, peripheral neuropathy, paraparesis, bowel and bladder incontinence, cerebellar and vestibular dysfunction, hearing loss, and motor deficits.

Demma LJ et al: Rocky Mountain spotted fever from an unexpected tick vector in Arizona. N Engl J Med 2005;353:587. [PMID: 16093467]

Paddock CD et al: *Rickettsia parkeri*: a newly recognized cause of spotted fever rickettsiosis in the United States. Clin Infect Dis 2004;38:805. [PMID: 14999622]

Sexton DJ et al: Rocky mountain spotted fever. Med Clin North Am 2002;86:351. [PMID: 11982306]

2. Rickettsialpox

Rickettsia akari is a parasite of mice, transmitted by mites *Liponyssoides sanguineus*. Rickettsialpox occurs in humans when crowded conditions and mouse-infested housing allow transmission of the pathogen to humans. Pathologic findings include dermal edema, subepidermal vesicles, and at times a lymphocytic vasculitis. The incubation period is 7–12 days. Onset is sudden, with chills, fever, headache, photophobia, and disseminated aches and pains. The primary lesion is a painless red papule that vesiculates and forms a black eschar. Two to 4 days after onset of symptoms, a widespread papular eruption appears that becomes vesicular and forms crusts that are shed in about 10 days. Early lesions may resemble those of chickenpox (typically vesicular versus papulovesicular in rickettsialpox).

Leukopenia and a rise in antibody titer to rickettsial antigen with complement fixation or indirect fluorescent assays using a conjugated antirickettsial globulin can identify antigen in punch biopsies of skin lesions.

Treatment includes doxycycline (200 mg/d) for 7 days.

The disease is usually mild and self-limited without treatment, but occasionally severe symptoms may require hospitalization. Control requires the elimination of mice from human habitations and insecticide applications to suppress the mite vectors.

Koss T et al: Increased detection of rickettsialpox in a New York City hospital following the anthrax outbreak of 2001: use of immunohistochemistry for the rapid confirmation of cases in an era of bioterrorism. Arch Dermatol 2003;139:1545. [PMID: 14676069]

3. Tick Typhus (Rickettsial Fever)

The term "tick typhus" denotes a variety of spotted rickettsial fevers. They are often named by geography, eg, Mediterranean spotted fever, Queensland tick typhus, Oriental spotted fever, African tick bite fever, Siberian tick typhus, or by morphology, eg, boutonneuse fever. These illnesses are transmitted by tick vectors of the rickettsial organisms *R conorii, R australis, R japonica, R africae,* and *R sibirica.* Dogs and wild animals, usually rodents but even reptiles, may serve as reservoirs. The pathogens usually produce an eschar or black spot (tache noire) at the site of the tick bite that may be useful in diagnosis, though spotless boutonneuse fever occurs. Symptoms include fever, headache, myalgias, and rash. Rarely, papulovesicular lesions may resemble rickettsialpox. Endothelial injury produces perivascular edema and dermal necrosis. Regional adenopathy, disseminated lesions, renal failure, and focal hepatic necrosis may occur. Diabetes, dehydration, and uremia were risk factors for mortality in one series. The disease occurs among travelers, the most common travel-associated rickettsiosis being African tick bite fever. Diagnosis is clinical, with serologic or PCR confirmation. Prevention entails protective clothing, repellents, and inspection for and removal of ticks. Treatment is with the following drugs given for 7–10 days: doxycycline (200 mg/d), chloramphenicol (50–75 mg/kg/d in four divided doses), or ciprofloxacin (500 mg twice daily). The combination of erythromycin and rifampin is effective and safe in pregnancy.

Another rickettsial infection, formerly classified as an endemic or murine typhus, is more properly classified as a spotted fever. The causative agent, *R felis,* is an organism that has been linked to the cat flea and opossum exposures. Most cases in the United States are reported from southern Texas and California and are treated as above.

de Sousa R et al: Mediterranean spotted fever in Portugal: risk factors for fatal outcome in 105 patients. Ann NY Acad Sci 2003;990:285. [PMID: 12860641]

Graves S et al: *Rickettsia honei*: a spotted fever Rickettsia group on three continents. Ann NY Acad Sci 2004;990:62. [PMID: 12860601]

Lewin MR et al: *Rickettsia sibirica* infection in members of scientific expeditions to northern Asia. Lancet 2003;362: 1201. [PMID: 14568744]

OTHER RICKETTSIAL & RICKETTSIAL-LIKE DISEASES

1. Ehrlichiosis & Anaplasmosis

 ESSENTIALS OF DIAGNOSIS

- *Infection of monocyte or granulocyte by tick-borne gram-negative bacteria.*
- *Nine-day incubation period, with variable clinical illness, ranging from asymptomatic to persistent or life-threatening.*
- *Common symptoms are malaise, nausea, fever, and headaches.*
- *Excellent response to therapy with tetracyclines.*

General Considerations & Clinical Findings

Ehrlichiosis and its analogous disease anaplasmosis present as two clinical entities involving either the monocyte or the granulocyte. Human monocytic ehrlichiosis (or when caused by its analog, anaplasma, anaplasmosis) is caused by *Ehrlichia chaffeensis* and by *Ehrlichia canis*. Human granulocytic ehrlichiosis (anaplasmosis) is caused by *Anasplasma phagocytophilium* and *Ehrlichia ewingii*. Another rickettsia-like organism, *Neorickettsia sennetsu,* is the etiologic agent of sennetsu fever, which appears to be confined to western Japan.

Ehrlichiae and anaplasmae are small tick-borne gram-negative obligate intracellular bacteria. The major nonhuman hosts include mice, dogs, and horses. These organisms grow as microcolonies in phagosomes of hematopoietic cells and form characteristic inclusions seen with Giemsa stain. Human monocytic ehrlichiosis (or its analog, anaplasmosis) is seen primarily in the Southeast, mid-Atlantic, and South Central states of the United States, though serologic evidence now documents a much more global endemicity (Israel, Japan, Mexico, Europe). Its major vector is the Lone Star tick (*Amblyomma americanus*). Reported incidences of both human monocytic and granulocytic ehrlichiosis are about 0.6 and 1.4 per million, respectively, with the highest attack rate in men over 60 years of age. Clinical disease ranges from mild to life-threatening. Typically, after about a 9-day incubation period and a prodrome consisting of malaise, rigors, and nausea, worsening fever and headache develop. A pleomorphic rash may occur. Infections among HIV-positive persons are more apt to be symptomatic. Disease is more severe among the elderly. Leukopenia, absolute lymphopenia, and thrombocytopenia occur often. Serious sequelae include acute respiratory failure and ARDS, encephalopathy, and acute renal failure, which may mimic thrombotic thrombocytopenic purpura. An indirect fluorescent antibody assay is available through the CDC and requires acute and convalescent sera. A PCR assay applied to whole blood samples is a rapid diagnostic tool, if available.

Human granulocytic ehrlichiosis (anaplasmosis) has an increasingly recognized ubiquitous geographic area of distribution with clinically consistent cases now reported from the United States (where it is tends to be present in the same geographic area as *Borrelia burgdorferi*, the causative agent of Lyme disease), Brazil, Israel, and Europe. The vectors are ticks of the *Ixodes* genus, and the reservoirs include woodrats, deer mice, chipmunks, deer, and perhaps horses. The incidence peaks in summer, but cases are seen year-round in warmer areas where ticks remain viable. The symptoms are similar to those seen with human monocytic ehrlichiosis. Persistent fever and malaise are reported to occur for 2 or more years. Coinfection with Lyme disease may occur, though patients with granulocytic ehrlichiosis appear to be older and sicker than those with acute Lyme disease.

Diagnosis & Treatment

Diagnosis is made by the history of tick exposure followed by a clinical illness with the characteristic symptoms and signs. Further laboratory evaluation is similar to that described for human monocytic ehrlichiosis.

Treatment for both forms of ehrlichiosis is with doxycycline, 200 mg orally or intravenously for at least 7 days or until 3 days of defervescence. Treatment should not be withheld while awaiting confirmatory serology when suspicion is high.

Demma LJ et al: Epidemiology of human ehrlichiosis and anaplasmosis in the United States, 2001–2002. Am J Trop Med Hyg 2005;73:400. [PMID: 16103612]

Dumler JS et al: Reorganization of genera in the families Rickettsiaceae and Anaplasmataceae in the order Rickettsiales: unification of some species of Ehrlichia with Anaplasma, Cowdria with Ehrlichia and Ehrlichia with Neorickettsia, descriptions of six new species combinations and designation of *Ehrlichia equi* and 'HE agent' as subjective synonyms of *Ehrlichia phagocytophila*. Int J Syst Evol Microbiol 2001;51:2145. [PMID: 11760958]

Stone JH et al: Human monocytic ehrlichiosis. JAMA 2004;292: 2263. [PMID: 15536115]

Talbot TR et al: *Ehrlichia chaffeensis* infections among HIV-infected patients in a human monocytic ehrlichiosis-endemic area. Emerg Infect Dis 2003;98:1123. [PMID: 14519250]

2. Q Fever

 ESSENTIALS OF DIAGNOSIS

- *Exposure to sheep, goats, cattle, or their products is common; some infections are laboratory acquired.*

- An acute or chronic febrile illness with severe headache, cough, prostration, and abdominal pain.
- Extensive pneumonitis, hepatitis, or encephalopathy; rarely, endocarditis or chronic fatigue syndrome.

General Considerations

Coxiella burnetii is unique among rickettsiae in that it is usually transmitted to humans not by arthropods but by inhalation or ingestion. It is distributed worldwide with few exceptions. *Coxiella* infections occur mostly in cattle, sheep, and goats, in which they cause mild or subclinical disease. Transmission by cows and goats is principally through the milk and placenta and by sheep through feces, placenta, and milk. Dry feces and milk, dust contaminated with them, and the tissues of these animals contain large numbers of infectious organisms that are spread by the airborne route. Inhalation of contaminated dust and of droplets from infected animal tissues is the main source of human infection. Outbreaks have been described in association with parturient cats. There is an occupational risk for animal handlers, slaughterhouse workers, veterinarians, and laboratory workers.

The route of acquisition appears to determine the main clinical syndrome. Endocarditis is an uncommon but serious form of *Coxiella* infection and has been linked with preexisting valvular conditions, immunocompromise, urban residence, and raw milk ingestion. *Coxiella* is resistant to heat and drying, perhaps because the organism forms endospore-like structures. Thus, it survives in dust, on the fleece of infected animals, or in inadequately pasteurized milk. Spread from one human to another does not seem to occur even in the presence of florid pneumonitis, but maternal–fetal infection can occur.

Clinical Findings

A. Symptoms and Signs

After an incubation period of 1–3 weeks, a febrile illness develops with headache, prostration, and muscle pains, often with a nonproductive cough. Pneumonia is the predominant manifestation of acute Q fever, although granulomatous hepatitis and CNS manifestations may occur. The most common manifestation of chronic Q fever is culture-negative endocarditis, which occurs in less than 1% of infected individuals. It is found mainly in the setting of preexisting valve disease. Uncommon manifestations of *Coxiella* infection include myocarditis, encephalitis, aortic aneurysm, hemolytic anemia, orchitis, acute renal failure, and mediastinal lymphadenopathy. The clinical course may be acute or may be chronic and relapsing. A Q fever chronic fatigue syndrome is thought by some experts to involve bacteremic shedding from bone marrow reservoirs and to be immunogenetically determined.

B. Laboratory Findings

Laboratory examination during the acute phase may show elevated liver function tests and occasionally leukocytosis. Patients with acute Q fever usually produce antibodies to *C burnetii* phase II antigen. A fourfold rise between acute and convalescent sera is diagnostic.

The diagnosis of Q fever endocarditis is made serologically. The IgG titer is usually 1:200 or greater and is directed against phase I antigen. Sometimes the diagnosis is not made until the time of valve replacement. Isolation of *C burnetii* from affected valves is possible using the shell-vial technique, but the organism is highly transmissible to laboratory workers. A nested PCR assay is most useful early in infection, typically during the first month.

C. Imaging

Radiographs of the chest show patchy pulmonary infiltrates, often more prominent than the physical signs would suggest.

Differential Diagnosis

Viral, mycoplasmal, and bacterial pneumonias, viral hepatitis, brucellosis, tuberculosis, psittacosis, and other animal-borne diseases must be considered. The history of exposure to animals or animal dusts or tissues (eg, in slaughterhouses) should lead to appropriate specific serologic tests. Unexplained fevers with negative blood cultures in association with embolic or cardiac disease should make one consider Q fever. Q fever is also one of the most common causes of culture-negative endocarditis.

Prevention

Prevention is based on detection of the infection in livestock, reduction of contact with infected animals or dusts contaminated by them, special care when working with animal tissues, and effective pasteurization of milk. A vaccine of formalin-inactivated phase 1 *Coxiella* is being developed for persons at high risk of infection and appears to be protective. A vaccine is available in some countries for persons with high-risk exposures.

Treatment & Prognosis

For acute infection, treatment with tetracycline (25 mg/kg/d in four divided doses) or doxycycline (100 mg twice daily) can suppress symptoms and shorten the clinical course but does not always eradicate the infection. The newer macrolides are an alternative. Treatment should continue through 3 full days of defervescence, which usually occurs within 72 hours. Even in untreated patients, the mortality rate is usually low, except when endocarditis develops (see below).

Although the optimal regimen for the treatment of endocarditis is not known, most experts recommend a combination of doxycycline (200 mg/d) plus hydroxy-chloroquine (600 mg/d), usually for at least 2 years. Se-rologic responses can be followed to determine cessation of therapy. Doxycycline levels correlate with declines in phase 1 antibody levels. Heart valve replacement may be necessary in refractory disease. Given the difficulty in treating endocarditis, the same combination therapy for 1 year is recommended for patients with acute disease and underlying valvular heart disease.

Arashima Y et al: Improvement of chronic nonspecific symptoms by long-term minocycline treatment in Japanese patients with *Coxiella burnetii* infection considered to have post-Q fever fatigue syndrome. Intern Med 2004;43:49. [PMID: 14964579]

Houpikian P et al: Blood culture-negative endocarditis in a reference center: etiologic diagnosis of 348 cases. Medicine (Baltimore) 2005;84:162. [PMID: 15879906]

Marmion BP et al: Long-term persistence of *Coxiella burnetii* after acute primary Q fever. QJM 2005;98:7. [PMID: 15625349]

Raoult D et al: Natural history and pathophysiology of Q fever. Lancet Infect Dis 2005;5:219. [PMID: 15792739]

Tissot-Dupont H et al: Wind in November, Q fever in December. Emerg Infect Dis 2004;10:1264. [PMID: 15324547]

■ KAWASAKI DISEASE

Kawasaki disease is a worldwide multisystemic disease initially described by Tomisaku Kawasaki in 1967. It is also known as the "mucocutaneous lymph node syndrome." It occurs mainly in children under age 5 years but occasionally in adults, at times in epidemic fashion. The higher risk among Asian children may be explained by receptor polymorphisms. A leading current theory for Kawasaki disease is an aberrant reaction to common infectious agents among genetically susceptible persons. IgA plasma cell infiltration is noted in the visceral organs, lungs, and coronary arteries of patients with Kawasaki disease.

The disease is characterized by fever and four of the following for at least 5 days: bilateral nonexudative conjunctivitis, mucous membrane changes of at least one type (injected pharynx, erythema, swelling and fissuring of the lips, strawberry tongue), peripheral extremity changes of at least one type (edema, desquamation, erythema of the palms and soles, induration of the hands and feet, Beau's lines [transverse grooves of the nails]), a polymorphous rash, and cervical lymphadenopathy greater than 1.5 cm.

A major complication is arteritis of the coronary vessels, occurring in about 25% of untreated patients, on occasion causing myocardial infarction, and more common among patients over 6 years of age. Its frequency is reduced by the use of intravenous immune globulin to about 10%. Noninvasive diagnosis can be made with magnetic resonance angiography or transthoracic ultrasound. Factors associated with the development of coro-nary artery aneurysms are leukocytosis and elevated C-reactive protein. Pericardial effusions occur in 30% of cases. Myocarditis is common in the acute phase of the disease, and mitral regurgitation may be present in 30% of patients but is usually mild. Arteritis of extremity vessels, peripheral gangrene, syndrome of inappropriate secretion of antidiuretic hormone (SIADH), and the hemophagocytic syndrome are also reported. Cerebrospinal fluid pleocytosis is reported in one-third of cases. The cause of these complications is also unknown. Differentiation from disseminated adenovirus infection is important and may be facilitated in the future with rapid adenovirus assays.

Management is with intravenous immune globulin, 2 g/kg over 10 hours, with repeat dosing appearing to prevent cardiac complications. The use of plasmapheresis in up to 10% of patients who are unresponsive to immune globulin is controversial. Corticosteroids, which are also used by some in disease refractory to two or more episodes of intravenous immunoglobulin, appear to be associated with a hastened resolution of fever and inflammatory markers and a shortened duration of hospitalization. Their role in increasing the likelihood of the development of coronary aneurysms is controversial. Aspirin, traditionally recommended in a high dose, does not appear to lower the risk of the development of coronary abnormalities. Its use (80–100 mg/kg/d in divided doses with subsequent tapering) is recommended indefinitely for patients with persisting coronary abnormalities. Warfarin is indicated in addition for aneurysms larger than 8 mm in diameter. Regular follow-up by a cardiologist is recommended for patients with coronary artery disease or aneurysms. Success is reported with interventional catheter treatment, including stent implantation in patients with long-term cardiac complications. Rare patients with irreversible myocardial dysfunction have successfully undergone cardiac transplantation.

Bergner D et al: Kawasaki disease: what is the epidemiology telling us about the etiology? Int J Infect Dis 2005;9:185. [PMID: 15936970]

Burns JC et al: Genetic variations in the receptor-ligand pair CCR5 and CCL3L1 are important determinants of susceptibility to Kawasaki disease. J Infect Dis 2005;192:344. [PMID: 15962231]

Hsieh KS et al: Treatment of acute Kawasaki disease: aspirin's role in the febrile stage revisited. Pediatrics 2004;114:e689. [PMID: 15545617]

Newburger JW et al: Diagnosis, treatment, and long-term management of Kawasaki disease: a statement for health professionals from the Committee on Rheumatic Fever, Endocarditis, and Kawasaki Disease, Council on Cardiovascular Disease in the Young, American Heart Association. Pediatrics 2004;114:1708. [PMID: 15574639]

Seve P et al: Adult Kawasaki disease: report of two cases and literature review. Semin Arthritis Rheum 2005;34:785. [PMID: 15942913]

Weiss JE et al: Infliximab as a novel therapy for refractory Kawasaki disease. J Rheumatol 2004;31:808. [PMID: 15088313]

Infectious Diseases: Bacterial & Chlamydial

33

Henry F. Chambers, MD

INFECTIONS CAUSED BY GRAM-POSITIVE BACTERIA

STREPTOCOCCAL INFECTIONS

1. Pharyngitis

 ESSENTIALS OF DIAGNOSIS

- *Abrupt onset of sore throat, fever, malaise, nausea, and headache.*
- *Throat red and edematous, with or without exudate; cervical nodes tender.*
- *Diagnosis confirmed by culture of throat.*

General Considerations

Group A β-hemolytic streptococci (*Streptococcus pyogenes*) are the most common bacterial cause of pharyngitis. Transmission occurs by droplets of infected secretions. Group A streptococci producing erythrogenic toxin may cause scarlet fever in susceptible persons.

Clinical Findings

A. SYMPTOMS AND SIGNS

"Strep throat" is characterized by a sudden onset of fever, sore throat, pain on swallowing, tender cervical adenopathy, malaise, and nausea. The pharynx, soft palate, and tonsils are red and edematous. There may be a purulent exudate. The Centor clinical criteria for the diagnosis of streptococcal pharyngitis are temperature > 38 °C, tender anterior cervical adenopathy, lack of a cough, and pharyngotonsillar exudate.

The rash of scarlet fever is diffusely erythematous, resembling a sunburn, with superimposed fine red papules, and is most intense in the groin and axillas. It blanches on pressure, may become petechial, and fades

in 2–5 days, leaving a fine desquamation. The face is flushed, with circumoral pallor, and the tongue is coated with enlarged red papillae (strawberry tongue).

B. LABORATORY FINDINGS

Leukocytosis with neutrophil predominance is common. Throat culture onto a single blood agar plate has a sensitivity of 80–90%. Rapid diagnostic tests based on detection of streptococcal antigen are slightly less sensitive than culture.

Complications

Suppurative complications include sinusitis, otitis media, mastoiditis, peritonsillar abscess, and suppuration of cervical lymph nodes.

Nonsuppurative complications are rheumatic fever and glomerulonephritis. Rheumatic fever may follow recurrent episodes of pharyngitis beginning 1–4 weeks after the onset of symptoms. Glomerulonephritis follows a single infection with a nephritogenic strain of streptococcus group A (eg, types 4, 12, 2, 49, and 60), more commonly on the skin than in the throat, and begins 1–3 weeks after the onset of the infection.

Differential Diagnosis

Streptococcal sore throat resembles (and cannot be reliably distinguished clinically from) pharyngitis caused by adenoviruses, Epstein-Barr virus, *Arcanobacterium haemolyticus* (which also may cause a rash), and other agents. Pharyngitis and lymphadenopathy are common findings in primary HIV infection. Generalized lymphadenopathy, splenomegaly, atypical lymphocytosis, and a positive serologic test distinguish mononucleosis from streptococcal pharyngitis. Diphtheria is characterized by a pseudomembrane; candidiasis shows white patches of exudate and less erythema; and necrotizing ulcerative gingivostomatitis (Vincent's fusospirochetal disease) presents with shallow ulcers in the mouth. Retropharyngeal abscess or bacterial epiglottitis should be considered when odynophagia and difficulty in handling secretions are present and when the severity of symptoms is disproportionate to findings on examination of the pharynx.

Treatment

Antimicrobial therapy has a modest effect on resolution of symptoms and primarily is administered for prevention of complications. Antibiotic therapy can be safely delayed until the diagnosis is established on the basis of a positive antigen test or culture. Empiric therapy usually is not a cost-effective approach to the management of most adults with pharyngitis because in typical clinical settings, the prevalence of streptococcal pharyngitis is likely to be no more than 10–20% and the positive predictive value of clinical criteria is low. Clinical criteria, such as the Centor criteria, are useful for identifying patients in whom a rapid antigen test or throat culture is indicated. Patients who meet two or more of these criteria merit further testing. When three of the four are present, laboratory sensitivity of rapid antigen testing exceeds 90%. When only one criterion is present, streptococcal pharyngitis is unlikely. In high-prevalence settings or if clinical suspicion for streptococcal pharyngitis is high, a negative antigen test or culture should be confirmed by a follow-up culture.

Gerber MA et al: Rapid diagnosis of pharyngitis caused by group A streptococci. Clin Microbiol Rev 2004;17:571. [PMID: 15258094]

McIsaac WJ et al: Empirical validation of guidelines for the management of pharyngitis in children and adults. JAMA 2004; 291:1587. [PMID: 15069046]

A. Benzathine Penicillin G

Benzathine penicillin G, 1.2 million units intramuscularly as a single dose, is optimal therapy.

B. Penicillin VK

Penicillin VK, 500 mg orally four times a day (or amoxicillin, 750 mg orally twice daily), is effective, but compliance may be poor after the patient becomes asymptomatic in 2–4 days.

C. Macrolides

Erythromycin, 500 mg orally four times a day, or azithromycin, 500 mg orally once daily for 3 days, is an alternative for the penicillin-allergic patient. Macrolides are less effective than penicillins and are considered second-line agents. Macrolide-resistant strains almost always are susceptible to clindamycin, an alternative for serious infections; a 10-day course of 300 mg orally three times a day should be effective.

Prevention of Recurrent Rheumatic Fever

Effectively controlling rheumatic fever depends on identification and treatment of primary streptococcal infection and secondary prevention of recurrences. Patients who have had rheumatic fever should be treated with a continuous course of antimicrobial prophylaxis for at least 5 years. Effective regimens are erythromycin, 250 mg orally twice daily, or penicillin G, 500 mg orally daily.

Neuner J et al: Diagnosis and management of adults with pharyngitis. A cost-effectiveness analysis. Ann Intern Med 2003; 139:113. [PMID: 12859161]

2. Streptococcal Skin Infections

Group A β-hemolytic streptococci are not normal skin flora. Streptococcal skin infections result from colonization of normal skin by contact with other infected individuals or by preceding streptococcal respiratory infection.

Clinical Findings

A. Symptoms and Signs

Impetigo is a focal, vesicular, pustular lesion with a thick, amber-colored crust with a "stuck-on" appearance.

Erysipelas is a painful superficial cellulitis that frequently involves the face. It is well demarcated from the surrounding normal skin. It affects skin with impaired lymphatic drainage, such as edematous lower extremities or wounds.

B. Laboratory Findings

Cultures obtained from a wound or pustule are likely to grow group A streptococci. Blood cultures are occasionally positive.

Treatment

Parenteral antibiotics are indicated for patients with facial erysipelas or evidence of systemic infection. Penicillin, 2 million units intravenously every 4 hours, is the drug of choice. However, staphylococci infections may at times be difficult to differentiate from streptococcal infections. In practice, initial therapy for patients with risk factors for *Staphylococcus aureus* (eg, injection drug use, diabetes, wound infection) should cover this organism. Nafcillin, 1.5 g every 6 hours intravenously, and cefazolin, 1 g intravenously or intramuscularly every 8 hours, are reasonable choices. In the patient with a serious penicillin allergy (ie, anaphylaxis), vancomycin, 1000 mg intravenously every 12 hours, should be used.

Patients who do not require parenteral therapy may be treated with amoxicillin, 750 mg twice daily for 7–10 days. A first-generation oral cephalosporin, eg, cephalexin, 500 mg four times daily, or clindamycin, 300 mg orally three times daily, is an alternative to amoxicillin.

3. Other Group A Streptococcal Infections

Arthritis, pneumonia, empyema, endocarditis, and necrotizing fasciitis are relatively uncommon infections that may be caused by group A streptococci. Toxic shock-like syndrome also occurs.

Arthritis generally occurs in association with cellulitis. In addition to intravenous therapy with penicillin G, 2 million units every 4 hours (or cefazolin or vancomycin in doses recommended above for penicillin-allergic patients), frequent percutaneous needle aspiration should be performed to remove joint effusions. Open surgical drainage may be necessary when the hip or shoulder is infected.

Pneumonia and **empyema** often are characterized by extensive tissue destruction and an aggressive, rapidly progressive clinical course associated with significant morbidity and mortality. High-dose penicillin and chest tube drainage are indicated for treatment of empyema. Vancomycin is an acceptable substitute in penicillin-allergic patients.

Group A streptococci can cause **endocarditis.** Endocarditis should be treated with 4 million units of penicillin G intravenously every 4 hours for 4–6 weeks. Vancomycin, 1 g intravenously every 12 hours, is recommended for persons allergic to penicillin.

Necrotizing fasciitis is a rapidly spreading infection involving the fascia of deep muscle. The clinical findings at presentation may be those of severe cellulitis, but the presence of systemic toxicity and severe pain, which may be followed by anesthesia of the involved area due to destruction of nerves as infection advances through the fascial planes, is a clue to the diagnosis. Surgical exploration is mandatory when the diagnosis is suspected. Early and extensive debridement is essential for survival.

Any streptococcal infection—and necrotizing fasciitis in particular—can be associated with **streptococcal toxic shock syndrome,** typified by invasion of skin or soft tissues, acute respiratory distress syndrome, and renal failure. The very young, the elderly, and those with underlying medical conditions are at particularly high risk for invasive disease. Bacteremia occurs in most cases. Skin rash and desquamation may not be present. Mortality rates can be up to 80%. The syndrome is due to elaboration of pyrogenic erythrotoxin (which also causes **scarlet fever**), a superantigen that stimulates massive release of inflammatory cytokines believed to mediate the shock. A β-lactam remains the drug of choice for treatment of serious streptococcal infections, but clindamycin, which is a potent inhibitor of toxin production, should also be administered at a dose of 600 mg every 8 hours intravenously for invasive disease, especially in the presence of shock. Intravenous immune globulin has also been recommended for streptococcal toxic shock syndrome for presumed, although unproven, therapeutic benefit from specific antibody to streptococcal exotoxins in immune globulin preparations. Two dosage regimens have been used: 450 mg/kg once daily for 5 days or a single dose of 2 g/kg with a repeat dose at 48 hours if the patient remains unstable.

Outbreaks of invasive disease have been associated with colonization by invasive clones that can be transmitted to close contacts who, though asymptomatic, may be a reservoir for disease. Tracing contacts of patients with invasive disease is controversial.

Stevens DL et al: Practice guidelines for the diagnosis and management of skin and soft-tissue infections. Clin Infect Dis 2005;41:1373. [PMID: 16231249]

Vinh DC et al: Rapidly progressive soft tissue infections. Lancet Infect Dis 2005;5:501. [PMID: 16048719]

4. Non-Group A Streptococcal Infections

Non-group A hemolytic streptococci (eg, groups B, C, and G) produce a spectrum of disease similar to that of group A streptococci. The treatment of infections caused by these strains is the same as for group A streptococci.

Group B streptococci are an important cause of sepsis, bacteremia, and meningitis in the neonate. Antepartum screening to identify carriers and peripartum antimicrobial prophylaxis are recommended in pregnancy. This organism, part of the normal vaginal flora, may cause septic abortion, endometritis, or peripartum infections and, less commonly, cellulitis, bacteremia, and endocarditis in adults. Treatment of infections caused by group B streptococci is with either penicillin or vancomycin in doses recommended for group A streptococci. Because of in vitro synergism, some experts recommend the addition of low-dose gentamicin, 1 mg/kg every 8 hours.

Viridans streptococci, which are nonhemolytic or α-hemolytic (ie, producing a green zone of hemolysis on blood agar), are part of the normal oral flora. Although these strains may produce focal pyogenic infection, they are most notable as the leading cause of native valve endocarditis (see below).

Group D streptococci include *Streptococcus bovis* and the enterococci. *S bovis* is a cause of endocarditis in association with bowel neoplasia or cirrhosis and is treated like viridans streptococci.

ENTEROCOCCAL INFECTIONS

Two species, *Enterococcus faecalis* and *Enterococcus faecium,* are responsible for most human enterococcal infections. Enterococci cause wound infections, urinary tract infections, bacteremia, and endocarditis. Infections caused by penicillin-susceptible strains should be treated with penicillin 3–4 million units every 4 hours; ampicillin 3 g every 6 hours; or if the patient is penicillin-allergic, vancomycin 15 mg/kg every 12 hours intravenously. If the patient has endocarditis, meningitis, or osteomyelitis, gentamicin 1 mg/kg every 8 hours intravenously should be added to the regimen in order to achieve the bactericidal activity that is required to cure these infections.

Resistance to vancomycin, penicillin, and gentamicin is common among enterococcal isolates, especially *E faecium;* it is essential to determine antimicrobial susceptibility of isolates. Infection control measures that may be indicated to limit their spread include isolation, barrier precautions, and avoidance of overuse of vancomycin and gentamicin. Consultation with an infectious diseases specialist is strongly advised when treating infections caused by resistant strains of enterococci. Quinupristin/dalfopristin and linezolid are approved by the US Food and Drug Administration

(FDA) for treatment of infections caused by vancomycin-resistant strains of enterococci. Quinupristin/dalfopristin is not active against strains of *E faecalis* and should be used only for infections caused by *E faecium*. The dose is 7.5 mg/kg intravenously every 8–12 hours. Phlebitis and irritation at the infusion site (often requiring a central line) and an arthralgia-myalgia syndrome are relatively common side effects. Quinupristin/dalfopristin is an inhibitor of cytochrome P450 enzyme 3A4 and has numerous, important drug interactions. Linezolid, an oxazolidinone, is active against both *E faecalis* and *E faecium*. The dose is 600 mg twice daily, and both intravenous and oral preparations are available. Its two principal side effects are thrombocytopenia and bone marrow suppression. Emergence of resistance has occurred during therapy with either quinupristin/dalfopristin or linezolid.

McDonald JR et al: Enterococcal endocarditis: 107 cases from the international collaboration on endocarditis merged database. Am J Med 2005;118:759. [PMID: 15989910]

Raad I et al: Prospective, randomized study comparing quinupristin-dalfopristin with linezolid in the treatment of vancomycin-resistant *Enterococcus faecium* infections. J Antimicrob Chemother 2004;53:646. [PMID: 14998986]

PNEUMOCOCCAL INFECTIONS

1. Pneumococcal Pneumonia

ESSENTIALS OF DIAGNOSIS

- *Productive cough, fever, rigors, dyspnea, early pleuritic chest pain.*
- *Consolidating lobar pneumonia on chest radiograph.*
- *Gram-positive diplococci on Gram stain of sputum.*

General Considerations

The pneumococcus is the most common cause of community-acquired pyogenic bacterial pneumonia. Alcoholism, asthma, HIV infection, sickle cell disease, splenectomy, and hematologic disorders are predisposing factors. The mortality rate remains high in the setting of advanced age, multilobar disease, severe hypoxemia, extrapulmonary complications, and bacteremia.

Clinical Findings

A. SYMPTOMS AND SIGNS

Presenting symptoms and signs include high fever, productive cough, occasionally hemoptysis, and pleuritic chest pain. Rigors occur within the first few hours of infection but are uncommon thereafter. Bronchial breath sounds are an early sign.

B. LABORATORY FINDINGS

Pneumococcal pneumonia classically is a lobar pneumonia with radiographic findings of consolidation and occasionally effusion. However, differentiating it from other pneumonias is not possible radiographically or clinically because of significant overlap in presentations. Diagnosis requires isolation of the organism in culture, although the Gram stain appearance of sputum can be suggestive. Sputum and blood cultures, positive in 60% and 25% of cases of pneumococcal pneumonia, respectively, should be obtained prior to initiation of antimicrobial therapy in patients who are admitted to the hospital. A good-quality sputum sample (less than 10 epithelial cells and more than 25 polymorphonuclear leukocytes per high-power field) shows gram-positive diplococci in 80–90% of cases.

Complications

Parapneumonic (sympathetic) effusion is common and may cause recurrence or persistence of fever. These sterile fluid accumulations need no specific therapy. Empyema occurs in 5% or less of cases and is differentiated from sympathetic effusion by the presence of organisms on Gram-stained fluid or positive pleural fluid cultures.

Pneumococcal pericarditis is a rare complication that can cause tamponade. Pneumococcal arthritis also is uncommon. Pneumococcal endocarditis usually involves the aortic valve and often occurs in association with meningitis and pneumonia (sometimes referred to as Austrian's or Osler's triad). Early heart failure and multiple embolic events are typical.

Treatment

A. SPECIFIC MEASURES

Initial antimicrobial therapy for pneumonia is empiric (see Chapter 9 for specific recommendations) pending isolation and identification of the causative agent. Once the pneumonia is determined to be caused by *Streptococcus pneumoniae*, any of several antimicrobial agents may be used depending on the clinical setting, community patterns of penicillin resistance, and susceptibility of the particular isolate. Uncomplicated pneumococcal pneumonia (ie, arterial PO_2 > 60 mm Hg, no coexisting medical problems, and single-lobe disease without signs of extrapulmonary infection) caused by penicillin-susceptible strains of pneumococcus may be treated on an outpatient basis with amoxicillin, 750 mg orally twice daily for 7–10 days. For penicillin-allergic patients, alternatives are azithromycin, one 500-mg dose orally on the first day and 250 mg for the next 4 days; clarithromycin, 500 mg orally twice daily for 10 days; doxycycline, 100 mg orally twice daily for 10 days; or levofloxacin, 750 mg orally for 5 days. Patients should be monitored for clinical response (eg, less cough, defervescence within 2–3 days) because pneumococci have become increasingly resistant to penicillin and the second-line agents.

Parenteral therapy is generally recommended for the hospitalized patient at least until there has been clinical improvement. Aqueous penicillin G, 2 million units intravenously every 4 hours, or ceftriaxone, 1 g intravenously every 24 hours, is effective for strains that are not highly penicillin-resistant (ie, strains for which the minimum inhibitory concentration [MIC] of penicillin is ≤ 1 mcg/mL). For serious penicillin allergy or infection caused by a highly penicillin-resistant strain, vancomycin, 1 g intravenously every 12 hours, is effective. Alternatively, a fluoroquinolone (eg, levofloxacin, 500 mg, or a comparable dose of any one of several newer fluoroquinolones now on the market, orally or intravenously) can be used. The total duration of therapy is not well defined but 10–14 days is standard.

B. TREATMENT OF COMPLICATIONS

Pleural effusions developing after initiation of antimicrobial therapy usually are sterile, and thoracentesis need not be performed if the patient is otherwise improving. Thoracentesis is indicated for an effusion present prior to initiation of therapy and in the patient who has not responded to antibiotics after 3–4 days. Chest tube drainage may be required if pneumococci are identified by culture or Gram stain, especially if aspiration of the fluid is difficult.

Echocardiography should be done if pericardial effusion is suspected. Patients with pericardial effusion who are responding to therapy and have no signs of tamponade may be monitored and treated with indomethacin, 50 mg orally three times daily, for pain. In patients with increasing effusion, unsatisfactory clinical response, or evidence of tamponade, pericardiocentesis will determine whether the pericardial space is infected. Infected fluid must be drained either percutaneously (by tube placement or needle aspiration), by placement of a pericardial window, or by pericardiectomy. Pericardiectomy eventually may be required to prevent or treat constrictive pericarditis, a common sequela of bacterial pericarditis.

Endocarditis should be treated for 4 weeks with 3–4 million units of penicillin G every 4 hours intravenously; ceftriaxone, 2 g once daily intravenously; or vancomycin, 15 mg/kg every 12 hours intravenously. Mild heart failure may respond to medical therapy, but moderate to severe heart failure is an indication for prosthetic valve implantation, as are systemic emboli or large friable vegetations as determined by echocardiography.

C. PENICILLIN-RESISTANT PNEUMOCOCCI

The prevalence of penicillin-resistant pneumococci (MIC > 0.1 mcg/mL) in the United States is approximately 20%, although there is considerable regional variability. All blood and cerebrospinal fluid isolates should now be tested for resistance to penicillin. Pneumonia caused by intermediately resistant strains (penicillin MIC > 0.1 mcg/mL but ≤ 1 mcg/mL) generally will respond to high-dose penicillin therapy. High-dose penicillin is likely to be effective for infections other than meningitis caused by highly penicillin-resistant strains (MIC > 1 mcg/mL). However, ceftriaxone, 1 g intravenously once daily, or vancomycin, 1 g intravenously every 12 hours, results in a more favorable ratio between serum drug concentration and MIC and may be preferred, especially for immunocompromised patients. Fluoroquinolones with enhanced gram-positive activity (eg, levofloxacin 500 mg once daily or moxifloxacin 400 mg once daily) are effective oral alternatives. Penicillin-resistant strains of pneumococci often are resistant to multiple antibiotics, including macrolides, trimethoprim-sulfamethoxazole, and chloramphenicol, and susceptibility must be documented prior to their use.

Aspa J et al; Pneumococcal Pneumonia in Spain Study Group: Drug-resistant pneumococcal pneumonia: clinical relevance and related factors. Clin Infect Dis 2004;38:787. [PMID: 14999620]

Lexau CA et al; Active Bacterial Core Surveillance Team: Changing epidemiology of invasive pneumococcal disease among older adults in the era of pediatric pneumococcal conjugate vaccine. JAMA 2005;294:2043. [PMID: 16249418]

Talbot TR et al: Asthma as a risk factor for invasive pneumococcal disease. N Engl J Med 2005;352:2082. [PMID: 15901861]

2. Pneumococcal Meningitis

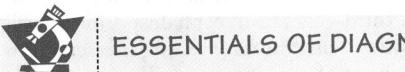 ESSENTIALS OF DIAGNOSIS

- *Fever, headache, altered mental status.*
- *Meningismus.*
- *Gram-positive diplococci on Gram stain of cerebrospinal fluid.*

General Considerations

S pneumoniae is the most common cause of meningitis in adults. Head trauma, with cerebrospinal fluid leaks, sinusitis, and pneumonia may precede it.

Clinical Findings

A. SYMPTOMS AND SIGNS

The onset is rapid, with fever, headache, meningismus, and altered mentation. Pneumonia may be present. Compared with meningitis caused by the meningococcus, pneumococcal meningitis lacks a rash, and focal neurologic deficits, cranial nerve palsies, and obtundation are more prominent features.

B. LABORATORY FINDINGS

The cerebrospinal fluid typically has more than 1000 white blood cells per microliter, over 60% of which are polymorphonuclear leukocytes; the glucose concentration is less than 40 mg/dL, or less than 50% of the simultaneous serum concentration; and the protein usually exceeds 150 mg/dL. Not all cases of meningitis will have these typical findings, and alterations in cerebrospinal fluid cell counts and chemistries may be surprisingly minimal, overlapping with those of aseptic meningitis.

Gram stain of cerebrospinal fluid shows gram-positive cocci in 80–90% of cases, and in untreated cases, blood or cerebrospinal fluid cultures are almost always positive.

Treatment

Antibiotics should be given as soon as the diagnosis is suspected. If lumbar puncture must be delayed (eg, while awaiting results of an imaging study to exclude a mass lesion), the patient should be treated empirically for presumed meningitis with intravenous ceftriaxone, 2 g, plus vancomycin, 15 mg/kg, plus dexamethasone, 0.15 mg/kg administered concomitantly after blood cultures (positive in 50% of cases) have been obtained. Once susceptibility to penicillin has been confirmed, penicillin, 24 million units intravenously daily in six divided doses, or ceftriaxone, 2 g every 12 hours intravenously, is continued for 10–14 days in documented cases.

The best therapy for penicillin-resistant strains is not known. Penicillin-resistant strains often are cross-resistant to the third-generation cephalosporins as well as other antibiotics. Susceptibility testing is essential to proper management of this infection. Treatment failures have been reported with ceftriaxone or cefotaxime for meningitis caused by strains with penicillin MICs ≥ 2 mcg/mL. If the MIC of ceftriaxone or cefotaxime is ≤ 0.5 mcg/mL, single-drug therapy with either of these cephalosporins is likely to be effective; when the MIC is ≥ 1 mcg/mL, treatment with a combination of ceftriaxone, 2 g intravenously every 12 hours, plus vancomycin, 30 mg/kg/d intravenously in two or three divided doses, is recommended. If a patient with a penicillin-resistant organism is slow to respond clinically, repeat lumbar puncture may be indicated to assess bacteriologic response.

Dexamethasone administered with antibiotic to adults has been associated with a 60% reduction in mortality and a 50% reduction in unfavorable outcomes. It is recommended that adults with acute bacterial meningitis be given 10 mg of dexamethasone intravenously immediately prior to or concomitantly with the first dose of appropriate antibiotic and every 6 hours thereafter for a total of 4 days. The effect of dexamethasone on outcome of meningitis caused by penicillin-resistant organisms is not known. Because its anti-inflammatory activity could impair penetration of some drugs into the cerebrospinal fluid, patients infected with highly penicillin-resistant organisms may be a risk for treatment failure.

van de Beek D et al: Clinical features and prognostic factors in adults with bacterial meningitis. N Engl J Med 2004;351: 1849. [PMID: 15509818]

van de Beek D et al: Steroids in adults with acute bacterial meningitis: a systematic review. Lancet Infect Dis 2004;4:139. [PMID: 14998499]

STAPHYLOCOCCUS AUREUS INFECTIONS

1. Skin & Soft Tissue Infections

ESSENTIALS OF DIAGNOSIS

- *Localized erythema with induration.*
- *Tendency toward abscess formation.*
- *Folliculitis commonly observed.*
- *Gram stain of pus with gram-positive cocci in clusters; cultures usually positive.*

General Considerations

Approximately one-quarter of people are asymptomatic nasal carriers of *S aureus*, which is spread by direct contact. Carriage often precedes infection, which occurs as a consequence of disruption of the cutaneous barrier or impairment of host defenses. *S aureus* tends to cause more localized skin infections than streptococci, and abscess formation is common. The prevalence of methicillin-resistant strains in community settings is increasing, and these strains have been associated with recurrent and severe skin and soft tissue infections, including necrotizing fasciitis.

Clinical Findings

A. SYMPTOMS AND SIGNS

S aureus skin infections may begin around one or more hair follicles, causing folliculitis; may become localized to form boils (or furuncles); or may spread to adjacent skin and deeper subcutaneous tissue (ie, a carbuncle). Deep abscesses involving muscle or fascia may occur, often in association with a deep wound or other inoculation or injection. Necrotizing fasciitis, a rare form of *S aureus* skin and soft tissues infection, has been reported with community strains of methicillin-resistant *S aureus*.

B. LABORATORY FINDINGS

Cultures of the wound or abscess material will almost always yield the organism. In patients with systemic signs of infection, blood cultures should be obtained because of potential endocarditis, osteomyelitis, or metastatic seeding of other sites. Patients who are bacteremic should have blood cultures taken early during therapy to exclude persistent bacteremia, an indicator of severe or complicated infection.

Treatment

Proper drainage of abscess fluid or other focal infections is the mainstay of therapy. Incision and drainage alone may sufficient for cutaneous abscess. For uncomplicated skin infections, oral antimicrobial therapy is satisfactory. Until recently, an oral penicillinase-resistant penicillin or cephalosporin, such as dicloxacillin or cephalexin, 500 mg four times a day for 7–10 days, has been the drug of choice for empiric therapy. Increasing prevalence of methicillin-resistant strains of *S aureus* among community isolates may necessitate use of other oral agents to which the isolate is susceptible in vitro, such as clindamycin, 300 mg three times daily; doxycycline, 100 mg twice daily; or trimethoprim-sulfamethoxazole, given in two or three divided doses based on 5–10 mg/kg/d of the trimethoprim component. Unfortunately, the efficacy of these agents is not well defined and not evidence based. Because of the high prevalence of macrolide resistance among *S aureus* strains, these agents should not be used unless susceptibility is documented.

For more complicated infections with extensive cutaneous or deep tissue involvement or fever, parenteral therapy is indicated initially. A penicillinase-resistant penicillin such as nafcillin or oxacillin in a dosage of 1.5 g every 6 hours intravenously or cefazolin 1 g intravenously or intramuscularly is preferred for infections caused by methicillin-susceptible isolates. In patients with a serious allergy to β-lactam antibiotics or if the strain is methicillin-resistant, vancomycin, 1 g intravenously every 12 hours, is the drug of choice. If the local prevalence of methicillin-resistance is high (eg, 10% or more), and particularly if the patient is seriously ill, vancomycin is indicated pending strain isolation and determination of susceptibility.

Linezolid is FDA-approved for treatment of skin and skin-structure infections as well as nosocomial pneumonia caused by methicillin-resistant strains of *S aureus* and is as effective as vancomycin according to clinical trial results. The dose is 600 mg orally (bioavailability of 100%) or intravenously twice a day for 10–14 days. Its considerable cost makes it an unattractive choice for most routine outpatient infections, and its safety in treatment courses lasting longer than 2–3 weeks is not well characterized; nevertheless, it is the only proven effective oral alternative to vancomycin.

King MD et al: Emergence of community-acquired methicillin-resistant staphylococcus aureus USA 300 clone as the predominant cause of skin and soft-tissue Infections. Ann Intern Med 2006;144:309. [PMID: 16520471]

Miller LG et al: Necrotizing fasciitis caused by community-associated methicillin-resistant *Staphylococcus aureus* in Los Angeles. N Engl J Med 2005;352:1445. [PMID: 15814880]

Zetola N et al: Community-acquired methicillin-resistant *Staphylococcus aureus*: an emerging threat. Lancet Infect Dis 2005; 5:275. [PMID: 15854883]

2. Osteomyelitis

S aureus causes of approximately 60% of all cases of osteomyelitis. Osteomyelitis may be caused by direct inoculation, eg, from an open fracture or as a result of surgery; by extension from a contiguous focus of infection or open wound; or by hematogenous spread. Long bones and vertebrae are the usual sites. Epidural abscess is a common complication of vertebral osteomyelitis and should be suspected if fever and severe back or neck pain are accompanied by radicular pain or symptoms or signs indicative of spinal cord compression (eg, incontinence, extremity weakness, pathologic reflexes).

Clinical Findings

A. Symptoms and Signs

The infection may be acute, with abrupt development of local symptoms and systemic toxicity, or indolent, with insidious onset of vague pain over the site of infection, progressing to local tenderness. Fever is absent in one-third or more of cases. Abscess formation is a late and unusual manifestation. Draining sinus tracts occur in chronic infections or infections of foreign body implants.

B. Laboratory Findings

The diagnosis is established by isolation of *S aureus* from the blood, bone, or a contiguous focus of a patient with signs and symptoms of focal bone infection. Blood culture will be positive in approximately 60% of untreated cases. Bone biopsy and culture are indicated if blood cultures are sterile.

C. Imaging

Bone scan and gallium scan, each with a sensitivity of approximately 95% and a specificity of 60–70%, are useful in identifying or confirming the site of bone infection. Plain bone films early in the course of infection are often normal but will become abnormal in most cases even with effective therapy. Spinal infection (unlike malignancy) traverses the disk space to involve the contiguous vertebral body. CT is more sensitive than plain films and helps localize associated abscesses. MRI is slightly less sensitive than bone scan but has a specificity of 90%. It is indicated when epidural abscess is suspected in association with vertebral osteomyelitis.

Treatment

Prolonged therapy is required to cure staphylococcal osteomyelitis. Durations of 4–6 weeks or longer are recommended. Although oral regimens can be effective, parenteral therapy is preferred, particularly during the acute phase of the infection for patients with systemic toxicity. Nafcillin or oxacillin, 9–12 g/d in six divided doses, is the drug of choice. Cefazolin, 1 g every 6–8 hours, also is effective. Vancomycin, 1 g every 12 hours, may be used for the penicillin-allergic patient, although the risk of relapse is higher than with β-lactam regimens. Addition of rifampin, 300 mg twice daily, to the regimen may prevent late relapse and should be strongly considered.

3. Staphylococcal Bacteremia

S aureus readily invades the bloodstream and infects sites distant from the primary site of infection, which may be relatively minor or even inapparent. Whenever *S aureus* is recovered from blood cultures, the possibility of endocarditis, osteomyelitis, or other metastatic deep infection must be considered. Bacteremia that persists for more than 48 to 96 hours after initiation of therapy is strongly predictive of worse outcome and complicated infection. The appropriate duration of therapy for uncomplicated bacteremia arising from a removable source (eg, intravenous device) or drainable focus (eg, skin abscess) has not been well defined, but a 10- to 14-day course of therapy appears to be the minimum. However, 5% or more of patients may relapse, usually with endocarditis or osteomyelitis, even if treated for 2 weeks.

Nafcillin or oxacillin, 1.5 g intravenously every 4–6 hours; cefazolin, 1 g every 8 hours; or vancomycin, 1 g every 12 hours, is recommended for uncomplicated staphylococcal bacteremia. Vancomycin as definitive therapy should be reserved for patients with serious penicillin allergy or with infections caused by methicillin-resistant strains because it is less active than β-lactam antibiotics and treatment failures are more common than with β-lactams. Transesophageal echocardiography (TEE) is a sensitive and cost-effective method for excluding underlying endocarditis. It is considered for patients for whom the pretest probability of endocarditis is 5% or higher—and for all patients with unexplained *S aureus* bacteremia.

Vancomycin treatment failures are relatively common, particularly for complicated bacteremia, in foreign body infection, or when the MIC of the isolate is > 2 mcg/mL. Consultation should be sought with an infectious diseases specialist when vancomycin treatment failure is encountered. Cases of vancomycin treatment failures in which the staphylococcal isolate exhibits a vancomycin MIC ≥ 4 mcg/mL should be reported to the Centers for Disease Control and Prevention (CDC) to help track this potentially serious and emerging problem of vancomycin resistance.

Empiric therapy of suspected staphylococcal infection, whether of community or hospital onset, depends on the severity of the infection and the likelihood that it is caused by methicillin-resistant strains. If the prevalence exceeds 5–10% for more seriously ill patients, initial therapy should include vancomycin, 1 g intravenously every 12 hours, until results of susceptibility tests are known. Resistance to vancomycin fortunately remains rare and should not affect the choice of empiric therapy; although with continuing use, emergence of staphylococci resistant to this drug and its relatively high rate of treatment failure merits concern.

Fowler VG Jr et al: Risk factors for hematogenous complications of intravascular catheter-associated *Staphylococcus aureus* bacteremia. Clin Infect Dis 2005;40:695. [PMID: 15714415]

Kuehnert MJ et al: Methicillin-resistant-*Staphylococcus aureus* hospitalizations, United States. Emerg Infect Dis 2005;11:868. [PMID: 15963281]

4. Toxic Shock Syndrome

S aureus produces toxins that cause three important entities: "scalded skin syndrome" in children, toxic shock syndrome in adults, and enterotoxin food poisoning. Toxic shock syndrome is characterized by abrupt onset of high fever, vomiting, and watery diarrhea. Sore throat, myalgias, and headache are common. Hypotension with renal and cardiac failure is associated with a poor outcome. A diffuse macular erythematous rash and nonpurulent conjunctivitis are common, and desquamation, especially of palms and soles, is typical during recovery. Fatality rates may be as high as 15%. Although originally associated with tampon use, any focus (eg, nasopharynx, bone, vagina, rectum, abscess, or wound) harboring a toxin-producing *S aureus* strain can cause toxic shock syndrome and nonmenstrual cases of toxic shock syndrome are common. Classically, blood cultures are negative because symptoms are due to the effects of the toxin and not systemic infection.

Important aspects of treatment include rapid rehydration, antistaphylococcal drugs, management of renal or cardiac failure, and addressing sources of toxin, eg, removal of tampon or drainage of abscess.

5. Infections Caused by Coagulase-Negative Staphylococci

Coagulase-negative staphylococci are an important cause of infections of intravascular and prosthetic devices and of wound infection following cardiothoracic surgery. These organisms may infrequently cause infections such as osteomyelitis and endocarditis in the absence of a prosthesis. Most human infections are caused by *Staphylococcus epidermidis*, *Staphylococcus haemolyticus*, *Staphylococcus hominis*, *Staphylococcus warnerii*, *Staphylococcus saprophyticus*, *Staphylococcus saccharolyticus*, and *Staphylococcus cohnii*. These common nosocomial pathogens are less virulent than *S aureus*, and infections caused by them tend to be more indolent.

Because coagulase-negative staphylococci are normal inhabitants of human skin, it is difficult to distinguish infection from contamination, the latter perhaps accounting for three-fourths of blood culture isolates. Infection is more likely if the patient has a foreign body (eg, sternal wires, prosthetic joint, prosthetic cardiac valve, pacemaker, intracranial pressure monitor, cerebrospinal fluid shunt, peritoneal dialysis catheter) or an intravascular device in place. Purulent or serosanguineous drainage, erythema, pain, or tenderness at the site of the foreign body or device suggests infection. Instability and pain are signs of prosthetic joint infection. Fever, a new murmur, instability of the prosthesis, or signs of systemic embolization are evidence of prosthetic valve endocarditis. Immunosuppression and recent antimicrobial therapy are risk factors.

Infection is also more likely if the same strain is consistently isolated from two or more blood cultures (particularly if samples were obtained at different times) and from the foreign body site. Contamination is more likely when a single blood culture is positive or if more than one strain is isolated from blood cultures. The antimicrobial susceptibility pattern and speciation are used to determine whether one or more strains have been isolated. More sophisticated typing methods, eg, pulse-field gel electrophoresis of restriction enzyme digested chromosomal DNA, may be required to identify distinct strains.

Whenever possible, the intravascular device or foreign body suspected of being infected by coagulase-negative staphylococci should be removed. However, removal and replacement of some devices (eg, prosthetic joint, prosthetic valve, cerebrospinal fluid shunt) can be a difficult or risky procedure, and it may sometimes be preferable to treat with antibiotics alone with the understanding that the probability of cure is reduced and that surgical management may eventually be necessary.

Coagulase-negative staphylococci are commonly resistant to β-lactams and multiple other antibiotics. For patients with normal renal function, vancomycin, 1 g intravenously every 12 hours, is the treatment of choice for suspected or confirmed infection caused by these organisms until susceptibility to penicillinase-resistant penicillins or other agents has been confirmed. Duration of therapy has not been established for relatively uncomplicated infections, such as those secondary to intravenous devices, which may be eliminated by simply removing the infected device. Infection involving bone or a prosthetic valve should be treated for 6 weeks. A combination regimen of vancomycin plus rifampin, 300 mg orally twice daily, and gentamicin, 1 mg/kg intravenously every 8 hours, is recommended for treatment of prosthetic valve endocarditis caused by methicillin-resistant strains.

Tokars JI: Predictive value of blood cultures positive for coagulase-negative staphylococci: implications for patient care and health care quality assurance. Clin Infect Dis 2004;39: 333. [PMID: 15306999]

Wisplinghoff H et al: Nosocomial bloodstream infections in US hospitals: analysis of 24,179 cases from a prospective nationwide surveillance study. Clin Infect Dis 2004;39:309. [PMID: 15306996]

CLOSTRIDIAL DISEASES

1. Clostridial Myonecrosis (Gas Gangrene)

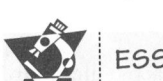

ESSENTIALS OF DIAGNOSIS

- Sudden onset of pain and edema in an area of wound contamination.
- Prostration and systemic toxicity.
- Brown to blood-tinged watery exudate, with skin discoloration of surrounding area.
- Gas in the tissue by palpation or radiograph.
- Gram-positive rods in culture or smear of exudate.

General Considerations

Gas gangrene or clostridial myonecrosis is produced by any one of several clostridia (*Clostridium perfringens, Clostridium ramosum, Clostridium bifermentans, Clostridium histolyticum, Clostridium novyi,* etc). Trauma and injection drug use are common predisposing conditions. Toxins produced in devitalized tissues under anaerobic conditions result in shock, hemolysis, and myonecrosis.

Clinical Findings

A. SYMPTOMS AND SIGNS

The onset is usually sudden, with rapidly increasing pain in the affected area, hypotension, and tachycardia. Fever is present but is not proportionate to the severity of the infection. In the last stages of the disease, severe prostration, stupor, delirium, and coma occur.

The wound becomes swollen, and the surrounding skin is pale. There is a foul-smelling brown, blood-tinged serous discharge. As the disease advances, the surrounding tissue changes from pale to dusky and finally becomes deeply discolored, with coalescent, red, fluid-filled vesicles. Gas may be palpable in the tissues.

B. LABORATORY FINDINGS

Gas gangrene is a clinical diagnosis, and empiric therapy is indicated if the diagnosis is suspected. Radiographic studies may show gas within the soft tissues, but this finding is not specific. The smear shows absence of neutrophils and the presence of gram-positive rods. Anaerobic culture confirms the diagnosis.

Differential Diagnosis

Other bacteria can produce gas in infected tissue, eg, enteric gram-negative organisms, or anaerobes.

Treatment

Penicillin, 2 million units every 3 hours intravenously, is effective. Other agents (eg, tetracycline, clindamycin, metronidazole, chloramphenicol, cefoxitin) are active against *Clostridium* species in vitro and probably in vivo as well. Adequate surgical debridement and exposure of infected areas are essential, with radical surgical excision often necessary. Hyperbaric oxygen therapy has been used empirically but must be used in conjunction with administration of an appropriate antibiotic and surgical debridement.

2. Clostridium sordellii Toxic Shock Syndrome

ESSENTIALS OF DIAGNOSIS

- Sudden onset after medical abortion.
- Abdominal pain.
- Absence of fever.
- Tachycardia, severe hypotension, capillary leak syndrome with edema.
- Profound leukocytosis, hemoconcentration.

General Considerations & Clinical Findings

C sordellii is a rare cause of endometritis and toxic shock syndrome following childbirth. Four cases, all fatal, of uterine infection following medically induced abortion with mefipristone have been recently reported. Onset of illness was within 4–5 days of ingestion of mefipristone and the clinical course fulminant. Infection appeared to be limited to the uterus, which showed necrosis, edema, hemorrhage, and acute inflammatory changes.

Treatment

Early recognition, aggressive resuscitation from shock, immediate surgical debridement with hysterectomy, and administration of an antimicrobial that is active against C sordellii are essential to survival. Based on in vitro susceptibility data, any of several agents should be active, including penicillin, ampicillin, a macrolide, clindamycin, a tetracycline, or metronidazole. Whether a protein synthesis inhibitor to block further toxin production offers any advantage over a β-lactam is unknown.

Fischer M et al: Fatal toxic shock syndrome associated with *Clostridium sordellii* after medical abortion. N Engl J Med 2005; 353:2352. [PMID: 16319384]

3. Tetanus

ESSENTIALS OF DIAGNOSIS

- History of wound and possible contamination.
- Jaw stiffness followed by spasms of jaw muscles (trismus).
- Stiffness of the neck and other muscles, dysphagia, irritability, hyperreflexia.
- Finally, painful convulsions precipitated by minimal stimuli.

General Considerations

Tetanus is caused by the neurotoxin tetanospasmin, elaborated by *Clostridium tetani*. Spores of this organism are ubiquitous in soil and may germinate when introduced into a wound. The vegetative bacteria produce tetanospasmin, a zinc metalloprotease that cleaves synaptobrevin, a protein essential for neurotransmitter release. Tetanospasmin interferes with neurotransmission at spinal synapses of inhibitory neurons. As a result, minor stimuli result in uncontrolled spasms, and reflexes are exaggerated. The incubation period is 5 days to 15 weeks, with the average being 8–12 days.

Most cases occur in unvaccinated individuals. Persons at risk are the elderly, migrant workers, newborns, and injection drug users. While puncture wounds are particularly prone to causing tetanus, any wound, including bites or decubiti, may become colonized and infected by *C tetani*.

Clinical Findings

A. SYMPTOMS AND SIGNS

The first symptom may be pain and tingling at the site of inoculation, followed by spasticity of the muscles nearby. Stiffness of the jaw, neck stiffness, dysphagia, and irritability are other early signs. Hyperreflexia develops later, with spasms of the jaw muscles (trismus) or facial muscles and rigidity and spasm of the muscles of the abdomen, neck, and back. Painful tonic convulsions precipitated by minor stimuli are common. Spasms of the glottis and respiratory muscles may cause acute asphyxia. The patient is awake and alert throughout the illness. The sensory examination is normal. The temperature is normal or only slightly elevated.

B. LABORATORY FINDINGS

The diagnosis of tetanus is made clinically.

Differential Diagnosis

Tetanus must be differentiated from various acute central nervous system infections such as meningitis. Trismus may occasionally develop with the use of phenothiazines. Strychnine poisoning should also be considered.

Complications

Airway obstruction is common. Urinary retention and constipation may result from spasm of the sphincters. Respiratory arrest and cardiac failure are late, life-threatening events.

Prevention

Tetanus is completely preventable by active immunization. Immunizations for children include tetanus toxoid, usually as DTP (see Table 30–4 for schedule). For primary immunization of adults, tetanus toxoid is administered as two doses 4–6 weeks apart, with a

Table 33–1. Guide to tetanus prophylaxis in wound management.

History of Absorbed Tetanus Toxoid	Clean, Minor Wounds		All Other Wounds[1]	
	Tdap or Td[2]	TIG[3]	Tdap or Td[2]	TIG[3]
Unknown or < 3 doses	Yes	No	Yes	Yes
3 or more doses	No[4]	No	No[5]	No

[1]Such as, but not limited to, wounds contaminated with dirt, feces, soil, saliva, etc; puncture wounds; avulsions; and wounds resulting from missiles, crushing, burns, and frostbite.
[2]Td indicates tetanus toxoid and diphtheria toxoid, adult form. Tdap indicates tetanous toxoid, reduced diphtheria toxoid, and acellular pertussis vaccine, which may be substituted as a single dose for Td. Unvaccinated individuals should receive a complete series of three doses, once of which is Tdap.
[3]Human tetanus immune globulin, 250 units intramuscularly.
[4]Yes if more than 10 years have elapsed since last dose.
[5]Yes if more than 5 years have elapsed since last dose. (More frequent boosters are not needed and can enhance side effects.) Tdap has been safely administered within 2 years of Td vaccination, although local reactions to the vaccine may be increased.

third dose 6–12 months later. Booster doses are given every 10 years or at the time of major injury if it occurs more than 5 years after a dose.

Passive immunization should be used in nonimmunized individuals and those whose immunization status is uncertain whenever a wound is contaminated or likely to have devitalized tissue. Tetanus immune globulin, 250 units, is given intramuscularly. Active immunization with tetanus toxoid is started concurrently. Table 33–1 provides a guide to prophylactic management.

Treatment

A. SPECIFIC MEASURES

Human tetanus immune globulin, 500 units, should be administered intramuscularly within the first 24 hours of presentation. Whether intrathecal administration has any additional benefit is controversial. A recent, but unblinded, randomized trial comparing intramuscular tetanus immune globulin to intramuscular plus intrathecal tetanus immune globulin found more rapid resolution of spasms, fewer days of ventilatory support, and a shorter hospital stay in the intrathecal group. However, the exact immunoglobulin preparation that was used was not specified and the total dose was 4000 units. Tetanus does not produce natural immunity, and a full course of immunization with tetanus toxoid should be administered once the patient has recovered.

B. GENERAL MEASURES

Minimal stimuli can provoke spasms, so the patient should be placed at bed rest and monitored under the qui-

etest conditions possible. Sedation, paralysis with curare-like agents, and mechanical ventilation are often necessary to control tetanic spasms. Penicillin, 20 million units intravenously daily, is given to all patients—even those with mild illness—to eradicate toxin-producing organisms.

Prognosis

High mortality rates are associated with a short incubation period, early onset of convulsions, and delay in treatment. Contaminated lesions about the head and face are more dangerous than wounds on other parts of the body.

Attygalle D et al: New trends in the management of tetanus. Expert Rev Anti Infect Ther 2004;2:73. [PMID: 15482173]

Miranda-Filho Dde B et al: Randomised controlled trial of tetanus treatment with antitetanus immunoglobulin by the intrathecal or intramuscular route. BMJ 2004;328:615. [PMID: 15003976]

4. Botulism

 ESSENTIALS OF DIAGNOSIS

- *History of recent ingestion of home-canned or smoked foods or of injection drug use and demonstration of toxin in serum or food.*
- *Sudden onset of diplopia, dry mouth, dysphagia, dysphonia, and muscle weakness progressing to respiratory paralysis.*
- *Pupils are fixed and dilated in most cases.*

General Considerations

Botulism is a paralytic disease caused by botulinum toxin, which is produced by *Clostridium botulinum*, a ubiquitous, strictly anaerobic, spore-forming bacillus found in soil. Four toxin types—A, B, E, and F—cause human disease. Botulinum toxin is a zinc metalloprotease that cleaves a specific component of the synaptic vesicle membrane docking and fusion complex at the neuromuscular junction blocking release of the neurotransmitter acetylcholine. Botulinum toxin is extremely potent and is classified by the CDC as a high-priority agent because of its potential for use as an agent of bioterrorism. Naturally occurring botulism occurs in one of three forms: food-borne botulism, infant botulism, or wound botulism. Food-borne botulism is caused by ingestion of preformed toxin present in canned, smoked, or vacuum-packed foods such as home-canned vegetables, smoked meats, and vacuum-packed fish. Commercial foods have also been associated with outbreaks of botulism. Infant botulism (associated with ingestion of honey) and wound botulism (which typically occurs in association with injection drug use) result from organisms present in the gut or wound that elaborate toxin in vivo.

Clinical Findings

A. SYMPTOMS AND SIGNS

Twelve to 36 hours after ingestion of the toxin, visual disturbances appear, particularly diplopia and loss of accommodation. Ptosis, cranial nerve palsies with impairment of extraocular muscles, and fixed dilated pupils are characteristic signs. The sensory examination is normal. Other symptoms are dry mouth, dysphagia, and dysphonia. Nausea and vomiting may be present, particularly with type E toxin. The sensorium remains clear and the temperature normal. Paralysis progressing to respiratory failure and death may occur unless mechanical assistance is provided.

B. LABORATORY FINDINGS

Toxin in patients' serum and in suspected foods can be demonstrated by mouse inoculation and identified with specific antiserum.

Differential Diagnosis

Cranial nerve involvement may be seen with vertebrobasilar insufficiency, the C. Miller Fisher variant of Guillain-Barré syndrome, myasthenia gravis, or any basilar meningitis (infectious or carcinomatous). Intestinal obstruction or other types of food poisoning are considered when nausea and vomiting are present.

Treatment

If botulism is suspected, the practitioner should contact the state health authorities or the CDC for advice and help with procurement of botulinus antitoxin and for assistance in obtaining assays for toxin in serum, stool, or food.

Respiratory failure is managed with intubation and mechanical ventilation. Parenteral fluids or alimentation should be given while swallowing difficulty persists.

The removal of unabsorbed toxin from the gut may be attempted. Any remnants of suspected foods should be assayed for toxin. Persons who might have eaten the suspected food must be located and observed.

Sobel J et al: Foodborne botulism in the United States, 1990–2000. Emerg Infect Dis 2004;10:1606. [PMID: 15498163]

ANTHRAX

ESSENTIALS OF DIAGNOSIS

- *Appropriate epidemiologic setting, eg, exposure to animals or animal hides, or potential exposure resulting from an act of bioterrorism.*
- *A painless cutaneous black eschar on exposed areas of the skin, with marked surrounding edema and vesicles.*

- *Nonspecific flu-like symptoms that rapidly progress to extreme dyspnea and shock in association with mediastinal widening and pleural effusions on chest radiograph.*

General Considerations

The death of a Florida photo editor from inhalational anthrax acquired from a letter deliberately contaminated with spores of *Bacillus anthracis* thrust this extremely rare infection into the public awareness. Between September 18 and November 21 of 2001, there were 13 cases of cutaneous anthrax and 11 cases of inhalational anthrax associated with exposure to anthrax spores in contaminated mail.

Naturally occurring anthrax is a disease of sheep, cattle, horses, goats, and swine. *B anthracis* is a gram-positive spore-forming aerobic rod. Spores—not vegetative bacteria—are the infectious form of the organism. These are transmitted to humans from contact with contaminated animals, animal products, or animal hides, or from soil by inoculation of broken skin or mucous membranes; by inhalation of aerosolized spores; or, rarely, by ingestion resulting in cutaneous, inhalational, or gastrointestinal forms of anthrax, respectively. Spores germinate into vegetative bacteria that multiply locally in cutaneous and gastrointestinal anthrax but may also disseminate to cause systemic infection. Inhaled spores are ingested by pulmonary macrophages and carried via lymphatics to regional lymph nodes, where they germinate. The bacteria rapidly multiply within the lymphatics, causing a hemorrhagic lymphadenitis. Invasion of the bloodstream leads to overwhelming sepsis, killing the host. Virulence is determined by two plasmids, pXO1 and pXO2, which encode, respectively, genes for two toxins, lethal toxin and edema toxin, and genes for capsule production. Loss of either plasmid attenuates strain virulence. Edema toxin impairs neutrophil function and probably is responsible for the striking edema present in cutaneous anthrax. Lethal factor provokes a cytokine-mediated shock syndrome. The capsule allows the bacteria to evade host immune defenses.

Clinical Findings

A. SYMPTOMS AND SIGNS

1. Cutaneous anthrax—This occurs within 2 weeks after exposure to spores; there is no latency period for cutaneous disease. The initial lesion is an erythematous papule, often on an exposed area of skin that vesiculates and then ulcerates and undergoes necrosis, ultimately progressing to a purple to black eschar. The eschar typically is painless; pain indicates secondary staphylococcal or streptococcal infection. The surrounding area is edematous and vesicular but not purulent. Regional adenopathy, fever, malaise, headache, and nausea and vomiting may be present. The infection is self-limited in most cases, but hematogenous spread with sepsis or meningitis may occur.

2. Inhalational anthrax—Illness occurs in two stages, beginning on average 10 days after exposure, but may begin up to 6 weeks after exposure. Nonspecific viral-like symptoms such as fever, malaise, headache, dyspnea, cough, and congestion of the nose, throat, and larynx are characteristic of the initial stage. Anterior chest pain is an early symptom of mediastinitis. Within hours to a few days, progression to the fulminant stage of infection occurs in which signs and symptoms of overwhelming sepsis predominate. Delirium, obtundation, or findings of meningeal irritation suggest an accompanying hemorrhagic meningitis.

3. Gastrointestinal anthrax—This form has not been reported in the United States. Fever, diffuse abdominal pain, rebound abdominal tenderness, vomiting, constipation, and diarrhea occur 2–5 days after ingestion of meat contaminated with anthrax spores. The primary lesion is ulcerative, producing emesis that may be blood-tinged or coffee-grounds and stool that may be blood-tinged or melenic. Bowel perforation can occur. The oropharyngeal form of the disease is characterized by local lymphadenopathy, cervical edema, dysphagia, and upper respiratory tract obstruction.

B. Laboratory Findings

Laboratory findings are nonspecific. The white blood cell count initially may be normal or modestly elevated, with polymorphonuclear predominance and an increase in early forms. Pleural fluid from patients with inhalational anthrax is typically hemorrhagic with few white cells. Cerebrospinal fluid from meningitis cases is also hemorrhagic. Gram stain of pleural fluid, cerebrospinal fluid, unspun blood, blood culture, or fluid from a cutaneous lesion may show the characteristic boxcar-shaped encapsulated rods in chains.

The diagnosis is established by isolation of the organism from culture of the skin lesion (or fluid expressed from it), blood, or pleural fluid—or cerebrospinal fluid in cases of meningitis. In the absence of prior antimicrobial therapy, cultures are invariably positive. Cultures obtained after initiation of antimicrobial therapy may be negative. If anthrax is suspected on clinical or epidemiologic grounds, immunohistochemical tests (eg, to detect capsular antigen), polymerase chain reaction assays, and serologic tests (useful for documenting past cutaneous infection) are available through the CDC and should be used to establish the diagnosis. Any suspected case of anthrax should be immediately reported to the CDC so that a complete investigation can be conducted.

C. Imaging Studies

The chest radiograph is the most sensitive test for inhalational disease, being abnormal (though the findings can be subtle) initially in every case of bioterrorism-associated disease. Mediastinal widening due to hemorrhagic lymphadenitis, a hallmark feature of the disease, has been present in 70% of the bioterrorism-related cases. Pleural effusions were present initially or occurred over the course of illness in all cases, and approximately three-fourths had pulmonary infiltrates or signs of consolidation.

Differential Diagnosis

Cutaneous anthrax, despite its characteristic appearance, can be confused with a variety of other also uncommon or rare conditions such as ecthyma gangrenosum, rat-bite fever, ulceroglandular tularemia, plague, glanders, rickettsialpox, orf (parapoxvirus infection), or cutaneous mycobacterial infection. Inhalational anthrax must be differentiated from mediastinitis due to other bacterial causes, fibrous mediastinitis due to histoplasmosis, coccidioidomycosis, atypical or viral pneumonia, silicosis, sarcoidosis, and other causes of mediastinal widening (eg, superior vena cava syndrome or aortic aneurysm or dissection). Gastrointestinal anthrax shares clinical features with a variety of common intra-abdominal disorders, including bowel obstruction, perforated viscus, peritonitis, gastroenteritis, and peptic ulcer disease.

Treatment

Strains of *B anthracis* (including the strain isolated in the bioterrorism cases) are susceptible in vitro to penicillin, amoxicillin, chloramphenicol, clindamycin, imipenem, doxycycline, ciprofloxacin (as well as other fluoroquinolones), macrolides, rifampin, and vancomycin. Susceptibility to cephalosporins is variable. *B anthracis* may express β-lactamases that confer resistance to cephalosporins and penicillins. For this reason, penicillin or amoxicillin is no longer recommended for use as a single agent in treatment of disseminated disease. Based on results of animal experiments and because of concern for engineered drug resistance in strains of *B anthracis* used in bioterrorism or weaponized, ciprofloxacin is considered the drug of choice (Table 33–2) for treat-

Table 33–2. Antimicrobial agents for treatment of or for prophylaxis against anthrax.

First-line agents and recommended doses
Ciprofloxacin, 500 mg twice daily orally or 400 mg every 12 hours intravenously
Doxycycline, 100 mg every 12 hours orally or intravenously
Second-line agents and recommended doses
Amoxicillin, 500 mg three times daily orally
Penicillin G, 2 mU every 4 hours intravenously
Alternative agents with in vitro activity and suggested doses
Rifampin, 10 mg/kg/d orally or intravenously
Clindamycin, 450–600 mg every 8 hours orally or intravenously
Clarithromycin, 500 mg orally twice daily
Erythromycin, 500 mg every 6 hours intravenously
Vancomycin, 1 g every 12 hours intravenously
Imipenem, 500 mg every 6 hours intravenously

ment and for prophylaxis following exposure to anthrax spores. Other fluoroquinolones activity against gram-positive bacteria (eg, levofloxacin, moxifloxacin) are likely to be just as effective as ciprofloxacin. Doxycycline is an alternative first-line agent. Combination therapy with at least one additional agent is recommended for inhalational or disseminated disease and in cutaneous infection involving the face, head, and neck or associated with extensive local edema or systemic signs of infection, eg, fever, tachycardia and elevated white blood cell count. Anecdotally, four of the six survivors of the 2001 inhalational cases were treated with combinations that included both a fluoroquinolone and rifampin. Single-drug therapy is recommended for prophylaxis following exposure to spores.

The required duration of therapy is poorly defined. In naturally occurring disease, treatment for 7–10 days for cutaneous disease and for at least 2 weeks following clinical response for disseminated, inhalational, or gastrointestinal infection have been standard recommendations. Because of concern about relapse from latent spores acquired by inhalation of aerosol in bioterrorism-associated cases, the initial recommendation was treatment for 60 days. In 2001, the CDC offered one of two options for postal workers receiving prophylaxis for exposure to contaminated mail: (1) antibiotics for 100 days (fearing that even with 60 days of treatment late relapses might occur) or (2) vaccination with an investigative agent (three doses administered over a 1-month period) in conjunction with 40 days of antibiotic administration to cover the time required for a protective antibody response to develop. Insufficient information exists to favor one recommendation over the other.

There is also an FDA-approved vaccine for persons at high risk for exposure to anthrax spores. The vaccine is cell-free antigen prepared from an attenuated strain of *B anthracis*. Multiple injections over 18 months and an annual booster dose are required to achieve and maintain protection. Existing supplies have been reserved for vaccination of military personnel.

The prognosis in cutaneous infection is excellent. Death is unlikely if the infection has remained localized, and lesions heal without complications in most cases. The reported mortality rate for gastrointestinal and inhalational infections is up to 85%. The experience with bioterrorism-associated inhalational cases in which six of eleven victims survived suggests a somewhat better outcome with modern supportive care and antibiotics provided that treatment is initiated before the patient has progressed to the fulminant stage of disease. No cases of anthrax have occurred among the several thousand individuals receiving antimicrobial prophylaxis following exposure to spores.

Fennelly KP et al: Airborne infection with *Bacillus anthracis*—from mills to mail. Emerg Infect Dis 2004;10:996. [PMID: 15207048]

Holty JE et al: Systematic Review: A century of inhalational anthrax cases from 1900 to 2005. Ann Intern Med 2006;144:270. [PMID: 16490913]

DIPHTHERIA

 ESSENTIALS OF DIAGNOSIS

- Tenacious gray membrane at portal of entry in pharynx.
- Sore throat, nasal discharge, hoarseness, malaise, fever.
- Myocarditis, neuropathy.
- Culture confirms the diagnosis.

General Considerations

Diphtheria is an acute infection caused by *Corynebacterium diphtheriae* that usually attacks the respiratory tract but may involve any mucous membrane or skin wound. The organism is spread chiefly by respiratory secretions. Exotoxin produced by the organism is responsible for myocarditis and neuropathy. This exotoxin inhibits elongation factor, which is required for protein synthesis.

Clinical Findings

A. Symptoms and Signs

Nasal, laryngeal, pharyngeal, and cutaneous forms of diphtheria occur. Nasal infection produces few symptoms other than a nasal discharge. Laryngeal infection may lead to upper airway and bronchial obstruction. In pharyngeal diphtheria, the most common form, a tenacious gray membrane covers the tonsils and pharynx. Mild sore throat, fever, and malaise are followed by toxemia and prostration.

Myocarditis and neuropathy are the most common and most serious complications. Myocarditis causes cardiac arrhythmias, heart block, and heart failure. The neuropathy usually involves the cranial nerves first, producing diplopia, slurred speech, and difficulty in swallowing.

B. Laboratory Findings

The diagnosis is made clinically but can be confirmed by culture of the organism.

Differential Diagnosis

Diphtheria must be differentiated from streptococcal pharyngitis, infectious mononucleosis, adenovirus or herpes simplex infection, Vincent's angina, pharyngitis due to *Arcanobacterium haemolyticum*, and candidiasis. A presumptive diagnosis of diphtheria should be made on clinical grounds without waiting for laboratory verification, since emergency treatment is needed.

Prevention

Active immunization with diphtheria toxoid is part of routine childhood immunization with appropriate booster injections. The immunization schedule for adults is the same as for tetanus.

Susceptible persons exposed to diphtheria should receive a booster dose of diphtheria toxoid (or a complete series if previously unimmunized), as well as a course of penicillin or erythromycin.

Treatment

Antitoxin, which is prepared from horse serum, must be given in all cases when diphtheria is suspected. For mild early pharyngeal or laryngeal disease, the dose is 20,000–40,000 units; for moderate nasopharyngeal disease, 40,000–60,000 units; for severe, extensive, or late (3 days or more) disease, 80,000–100,000 units. Diphtheria equine antitoxin can be obtained from the CDC.

Removal of membrane by direct laryngoscopy or bronchoscopy may be necessary to prevent or alleviate airway obstruction.

Either penicillin, 250 mg orally four times daily, or erythromycin, 500 mg orally four times daily, for 14 days is effective therapy, although erythromycin is slightly more effective in eliminating the carrier state. Azithromycin or clarithromycin is probably as effective as erythromycin. The patient should be isolated until three consecutive cultures at the completion of therapy have documented elimination of the organism from the oropharynx. Contacts to a case should receive erythromycin, 500 mg orally four times daily for 7 days, to eradicate carriage.

Centers for Disease Control and Prevention (CDC): Fatal respiratory diphtheria in a U.S. traveler to Haiti—Pennsylvania, 2003. MMWR Morb Mortal Wkly Rep 2004;52:1285. [PMID: 14712177]

LISTERIOSIS

Listeria monocytogenes is a facultative, motile, gram-positive rod that is capable of invading several cell types and causes intracellular infection. Most cases of infection caused by *L monocytogenes* are sporadic, but outbreaks have been traced to eating contaminated food, including unpasteurized dairy products, hot dogs, and delicatessen meats. Five types of infection are recognized:

(1) **Infection during pregnancy,** usually in the last trimester, is a mild febrile illness without an apparent primary focus. This relatively benign disease for both mother and fetus may resolve without specific therapy.

(2) **Granulomatosis infantisepticum** is a neonatal infection acquired in utero, characterized by disseminated abscesses, granulomas, and a high mortality rate.

(3) **Bacteremia** with or without sepsis syndrome is an infection of neonates or immunocompromised adults. The presentation is of a febrile illness without a recognized source.

(4) **Meningitis** caused by *L monocytogenes* affects infants under 2 months of age as well as older adults, ranking third after the meningococcus and pneumococcus among the common causes of bacterial meningitis. Cerebrospinal fluid shows a *neutrophilic* pleocytosis. Adults with meningitis are often immunocompromised, and cases have been associated with HIV infection and therapy with tumor necrosis factor-α (TNF-α) inhibitors such as infliximab.

(5) Finally, **focal infections**, including adenitis, brain abscess, endocarditis, osteomyelitis, and arthritis, occur rarely.

Ampicillin, 8–12 g/d intravenously in four to six divided doses (the higher dose for meningitis) is considered the treatment of choice. It penetrates well into cerebrospinal fluid, and clinical response is better than with penicillin, erythromycin, or chloramphenicol. Gentamicin is synergistic with ampicillin against *Listeria* in vitro and in animal models, and the use of combination therapy may be considered during the first few days of treatment to enhance eradication of organisms. Mortality and morbidity rates still are high, and relapses occur, perhaps related to poor intracellular penetration of ampicillin. Trimethoprim-sulfamethoxazole with its excellent intracellular and cerebrospinal fluid penetration may be more efficacious. The dose is 10–20 mg/kg/d intravenously of the trimethoprim component. Therapy should be administered for at least 2–3 weeks. Longer durations—between 3 and 6 weeks—have been recommended for treatment of meningitis, especially in immunocompromised persons.

Drevets DA et al: Invasion of the central nervous system by intracellular bacteria. Clin Microbiol Rev 2004;17:323. [PMID: 15084504]

Gerner-Smidt P et al: Invasive listeriosis in Denmark 1994–2003: a review of 299 cases with special emphasis on risk factors for mortality. Clin Microbiol Infect 2005;11:618. [PMID: 16008613]

■ INFECTIVE ENDOCARDITIS

 ESSENTIALS OF DIAGNOSIS

- *Fever*
- *Preexisting organic heart lesion.*
- *Positive blood cultures.*
- *Evidence of vegetation on echocardiography.*
- *New or changing heart murmur.*
- *Evidence of systemic emboli.*

General Considerations

Endocarditis is a bacterial or fungal infection of the valvular or endocardial surface of the heart. The clinical presentation depends on the infecting organism and the valve or valves that are infected. More virulent organisms—*S aureus* in particular—tend to produce a more rapidly progressive and destructive infection. Endocarditis caused by more virulent organisms often presents as an acute febrile illnesses and is complicated by early embolization, acute valvular regurgitation, and myocardial abscess formation. Viridans strains of streptococci, enterococci, other bacteria, yeasts, and fungi tend to cause a more subacute picture.

Underlying valvular disease, less common than in the past, is present in about 50% of cases. Valvular disease alters blood flow and produces jet effects that disrupt the endothelial surface, providing a nidus for attachment and infection of microorganisms that enter the bloodstream. Predisposing valvular abnormalities include rheumatic involvement of any valve, bicuspid aortic valves, calcific or sclerotic aortic valves, hypertrophic subaortic stenosis, mitral valve prolapse, and a variety of congenital disorders such as ventricular septal defect, tetralogy of Fallot, coarctation of the aorta, or patent ductus arteriosus. Rheumatic disease is no longer the major predisposing factor in developed countries. Regurgitation lesions are more susceptible than stenotic ones.

The initiating event in native valve endocarditis is colonization of the valve by bacteria or yeast that gain access to the bloodstream. Transient bacteremia is common during dental, upper respiratory, urologic, and lower gastrointestinal diagnostic and surgical procedures. It is less common during upper gastrointestinal and gynecologic procedures. Intravascular devices are increasingly implicated as a portal of access of microorganisms into the bloodstream. A large proportion of cases of *S aureus* endocarditis is attributable to healthcare-associated bacteremia.

Native valve endocarditis is usually caused by viridans streptococci, group D streptococci, *S aureus,* enterococci, or HACEK organisms (an acronym for *Haemophilus aphrophilus, Haemophilus parainfluenzae, Actinobacillus actinomycetemcomitans, Cardiobacterium hominis, Eikenella corrodens,* and *Kingella kingae).* Streptococcal species formerly accounted for the majority of native valve endocarditis cases, but the proportion of cases caused by *S aureus* has been increasing, and this organism is now the leading cause. Gram-negative organisms and fungi account for a small percentage.

In injection drug users, *S aureus* accounts for over 60% of all endocarditis cases and for 80–90% of cases in which the tricuspid valve is infected. Enterococci and streptococci comprise the balance in about equal proportions. Gram-negative aerobic bacilli, fungi, and unusual organisms may cause endocarditis in injection drug users.

The microbiology of prosthetic valve endocarditis also is distinctive. Early infections (ie, those occurring within 2 months after valve implantation) are commonly caused by staphylococci—both coagulase-positive and coagulase-negative—gram-negative organisms, and fungi. In late prosthetic valve endocarditis, streptococci are commonly identified, although coagulase-negative and coagulase-positive staphylococci still cause many cases.

Clinical Findings

A. Symptoms and Signs

Virtually all patients have fever at some point in the illness, although it may be very low grade (less than 38 °C) in elderly individuals and in patients with heart failure or renal failure. Rarely, there may be no fever at all.

The duration of illness typically is a few days to a few weeks. Nonspecific symptoms are common. The initial symptoms and signs of endocarditis may be caused by direct arterial, valvular, or cardiac damage. Although a changing regurgitant murmur is significant diagnostically, it is the exception rather than the rule. Symptoms also may occur as a result of embolization, metastatic infection or immunologically mediated phenomena. These include cough; dyspnea; arthralgias or arthritis; diarrhea; and abdominal, back, or flank pain.

The characteristic peripheral lesions—petechiae (on the palate or conjunctiva or beneath the fingernails), subungual ("splinter") hemorrhages, Osler nodes (painful, violaceous raised lesions of the fingers, toes, or feet), Janeway lesions (painless erythematous lesions of the palms or soles), and Roth spots (exudative lesions in the retina)—occur in about 25% of patients. Strokes and major systemic embolic events are present in about 25% of patients, and tend to occur before or within the first week of antimicrobial therapy. Hematuria and proteinuria may result from emboli or immunologically mediated glomerulonephritis, which can cause renal dysfunction.

B. Diagnostic Studies

Blood cultures establish the diagnosis. Three sets of blood cultures at least 1 hour apart before starting antibiotics are recommended to maximize the opportunity for a microbiologic diagnosis. Approximately 5% of cases will be culture-negative, usually attributable to administration of antimicrobials prior to obtaining cultures. If antimicrobial therapy has been administered prior to obtaining cultures and the patient is clinically stable, it is reasonable to withhold further antimicrobial therapy for 2–3 days so that appropriate cultures can be obtained. Culture-negative endocarditis may also be due to a fungus, organisms that require special media for growth (eg, *Legionella, Bartonella, Abiotrophia* species, formerly referred to as nutritionally deficient streptococci), organisms that do not grow on artificial media (*Tropheryma whippelii,* or pathogens of Q fever or psittacosis), or those that are slow-growing and may require prolonged incubation (eg, *Brucella,* anaerobes, HACEK). *Bartonella quintana* has emerged as an important cause of culture-negative endocarditis.

Chest radiograph may show evidence for the underlying cardiac abnormality and, in right-sided endocarditis, pulmonary infiltrates. The electrocardiogram is nondiagnostic, but new conduction abnormalities suggest myocardial abscess formation. Echocardiography is useful in identifying vegetations and other characteristic features suspicious for endocarditis and may provide adjunctive information about the specific valve or valves that are infected. The sensitivity of transthoracic echocardiography is between 55% and 65%; it cannot reliably rule out endocarditis but may confirm a clinical suspicion. TEE is 90% sensitive in detecting vegetations and is particularly useful for identifying valve ring abscesses as well as prosthetic valve endocarditis.

Clinical criteria, referred to as the **Modified Duke criteria,** for the diagnosis of endocarditis have been proposed. Major criteria include (1) two positive blood cultures for a microorganism that typically causes infective endocarditis or persistent bacteremia, (2) evidence of endocardial involvement documented by echocardiography (eg, definite vegetation, myocardial abscess, or new partial dehiscence of a prosthetic valve), or (3) development of a new regurgitant murmur. Minor criteria include the presence of a predisposing condition; fever $\geq$ 38 °C; vascular phenomena, such as cutaneous hemorrhages, aneurysm, systemic emboli, pulmonary infarction; immunologic phenomena, such as glomerulonephritis, Osler nodes, Roth spots, rheumatoid factor; and positive blood cultures not meeting the major criteria or serologic evidence of an active infection. A definite diagnosis can be made with 80% accuracy if two major criteria, one major criterion and three minor criteria, or five minor criteria are fulfilled. A possible diagnosis of endocarditis is made if one major and one minor criterion or three minor criteria are met. If fewer criteria are found, or a sound alternative explanation for illness is identified, or the endocarditis syndrome has resolved and the patient has defervesced within 4 days, endocarditis is unlikely.

Complications

The course of infective endocarditis is determined by the degree of damage to the heart, by the site of infection (right- versus left-sided, aortic versus mitral valve), by the presence of metastatic foci of infection, by the occurrence of embolization, and by immunologically mediated processes. Destruction of infected heart valves is especially common and precipitous with S aureus but can occur with any organism and can progress even after bacteriologic cure. The infection can also extend into the myocardium, resulting in abscesses leading to conduction disturbances, and involving the wall of the aorta, creating sinus of Valsalva aneurysms.

Peripheral embolization to the brain and myocardium may result in infarctions. Embolization to the spleen and kidneys is also common. Peripheral emboli may initiate metastatic infections or may become established in vessel walls, leading to mycotic aneurysms. Right-sided endocarditis, which usually involves the tricuspid valve, causes septic pulmonary emboli, occasionally with infarction and lung abscesses.

Prevention

Some cases of endocarditis occur after dental procedures or operations involving the upper respiratory, genitourinary, or intestinal tract. Prophylactic antibiotics are given to patients with predisposing congenital or valvular anomalies who are to have any of these procedures (Tables 33–3 and 33–4). Current recommendations are given in Table 33–5.

Table 33–3. Risk of bacterial endocarditis with underlying cardiac conditions.[1]

High Risk

Prosthetic cardiac valves, mechanical, bioprosthetic, or homograft

Previous bacterial endocarditis

Complex cyanotic congenital heart disease (eg, single ventricle states, transposition of the great arteries, tetralogy of Fallot)

Surgically constructed systemic pulmonary shunts or conduits

Moderate Risk

Most congenital cardiac malformations (other than those listed above and below)

Rheumatic heart disease

Hypertrophic cardiomyopathy

Mitral valve prolapse with valvular regurgitation[2]

Negligible Risk[3]

Isolated secundum septal defect

Surgical repair of atrial septal defect, ventricular septal defect, or patent ductus arteriosus (without residua beyond 6 months)

Previous coronary artery bypass graft surgery

Mitral valve prolapse without valvular regurgitation

Physiologic, functional, or innocent heart murmurs

Previous Kawasaki disease without valvular dysfunction

Rheumatic fever without valvular dysfunction

Cardiac pacemakers (intravascular and epicardial) and implanted defibrillators

[1]This table lists selected conditions and is not meant to be all-inclusive.

[2]Mitral regurgitation determined by the presence of a murmur or by echo-Doppler. Men older than 45 years may warrant prophylaxis even without a consistent systolic murmur. Mitral valve prolapse associated with thickening or redundancy of the valve leaflets may be associated with an increased risk for bacterial endocarditis.

[3]Risk no greater than in the general population; endocarditis prophylaxis not recommended.

Table 33–4. Recommendations for administration of bacterial endocarditis prophylaxis for high and moderate risk patients according to type of procedure.[1]

Prophylaxis recommended	Prophylaxis not recommended

1. Dental procedures
    Dental extractions
    Periodontal procedures
    Dental implantation
    Endodontic (root canal) instrumentation or surgery beyond the apex
    Subgingival placement of antibiotic fibers or strips
    Initial placement of orthodontic bands but not brackets
    Intraligamentary local anesthetic injections
    Cleaning of teeth or implants where bleeding is anticipated
2. Respiratory tract procedures
    Tonsillectomy, adenoidectomy
    Surgical operations of intestinal or respiratory mucosa
    Rigid bronchoscopy
3. Gastrointestinal tract procedures[4]
    Sclerotherapy for esophageal varices
    Esophageal stricture dilation
    Endoscopic retrograde cholangiography with biliary obstruction
    Biliary tract surgery
    Surgical operations that involve intestinal mucosa
4. Genitourinary tract
    Prostatic surgery
    Cystoscopy
    Urethral dilation
	1. Dental procedures
	    Restorative dentistry (filling cavities, operative and prosthodontic) with or without retraction cord[2]
	    Nonintraligamentary local anesthetic injections
	    Intracanal endodontic treatment; post placement and buildup
	    Placement of rubber dams, removable prosthodontic, or orthodontic appliances
	    Postoperative suture removal
	    Taking of oral impression
	    Fluoride treatments
	    Orthodontic appliance adjustment
	2. Respiratory tract procedures
	    Endotracheal intubation
	    Flexible bronchoscopy, with or without biopsy[3]
	    Tympanostomy (insertion)
	3. Gastrointestinal tract procedures
	    Transesophageal echocardiography[3]
	    Endoscopy with or without gastrointestinal biopsy[3]
	4. Genitourinary tract
	    Vaginal hysterectomy[3]
	    Vaginal delivery[3]
	    Cesarean section
	    In the absence of infection: urethral catheterization, uterine dilation and curettage, therapeutic abortion, sterilization procedures, insertion or removal of intrauterine devices
	5. Other
	    Cardiac catheterization, including balloon angioplasty; implanting cardiac pacemakers or defibrillators and coronary stents; incision or biopsy of surgically scrubbed skin; circumcision

[1] Based on recommendations by the American Heart Association. JAMA 1997;277:1794. The procedures listed are not meant to be all-inclusive.
[2] Clinical judgement may indicate antibiotic use in selected circumstances that may create significant bleeding.
[3] Prophylaxis is optional for high-risk patients, not recommended for moderate-risk patients.
[4] Prophylaxis is recommended for high-risk patients, optional for moderate-risk patients.

Treatment

Empiric regimens for endocarditis while culture results are pending should include agents active against staphylococci, streptococci, and enterococci. Vancomycin 1 g every 12 hours intravenously plus ceftriaxone 2 g every 24 hours provides appropriate coverage pending definitive diagnosis.

A. VIRIDANS STREPTOCOCCI

For penicillin-susceptible viridans streptococcal endocarditis (ie, MIC ≤ 0.1 mcg/mL), penicillin G, 2–3 million units intravenously every 4 hours for 4 weeks, is recommended. The duration of therapy can be shortened to 2 weeks if gentamicin, 1 mg/kg intrave-

nously every 8 hours, is used with penicillin. Ceftriaxone, 2 g once daily intravenously or intramuscularly for 4 weeks, is also effective therapy for penicillin-susceptible strains and is a convenient regimen for home therapy. For the penicillin-allergic patient, vancomycin, 15 mg/kg intravenously every 12 hours for 4 weeks, is given. The 2-week regimen is not recommended for patients with symptoms of more than 3 months' duration or with complications such as myocardial abscess or extracardiac infection. Prosthetic valve endocarditis is treated with a 6-week course of penicillin with at least 2 weeks of gentamicin.

Viridans streptococci relatively resistant to penicillin (ie, MIC > 0.1 mcg/mL but ≤ 0.5 mcg/mL) should be treated for 4 weeks. Penicillin G, 3 million units in-

Table 33–5. American Heart Association recommendations for endocarditis prophylaxis in high- and moderate-risk patients.[1]

DENTAL, RESPIRATORY, OR ESOPHAGEAL PROCEDURES		
Oral Penicillin allergy	Amoxicillin Clindamycin or	2 g 1 hour before procedure 600 mg 1 hour before procedure
	Cephalexin or cefadroxil or	2 g 1 hour before procedure (contraindicated if there is history of a β-lactam immediate hypersensitivity reaction)
	Azithromycin or clarithromycin	500 mg 1 hour before procedure
Parenteral Penicillin allergy	Ampicillin Clindamycin or	2 g IM or IV 30 minutes before procedure 600 mg IV 1 hour before procedure
	Cefazolin	1 g IM or IV 30 minutes before procedure (contraindicated if there is history of a β-lactam immediate hypersensitivity reaction)
GASTROINTESTINAL (EXCEPT ESOPHAGEAL) OR GENITOURINARY PROCEDURES		
High-risk patient (Table 33–3)	Ampicillin plus gentamicin or vancomycin plus gentamicin (for penicillin allergy)	Ampicillin, 2 g IM or IV, plus gentamicin, 1.5 mg/kg IV or IM (120 mg maximum) 30 minutes before procedure; 6 hours later, ampicillin, 1 g IM or IV, or amoxicillin, 1 g orally
		For the penicillin-allergic patient, instead of ampicillin, use a single dose of vancomycin, 1 g IV over 1–2 hours with completion of infusion 30 minutes before procedure
Moderate-risk patient	Amoxicillin or ampicillin or vancomycin (for penicillin allergy)	Amoxicillin, 2 g orally 1 hour before procedure, or ampicillin, 2 g IM or IV 30 minutes before starting procedure
		For the penicillin allergic patient instead of ampicillin use vancomycin, 1 g IV over 1–2 hours with completion of infusion 30 minutes before procedure; complete infusion 30 minutes before procedure

[1]See JAMA 1997;277:1794 for details.

travenously every 4 hours, is combined with gentamicin, 1 mg/kg intravenously every 8 hours for the first 2 weeks. In the patient with IgE-mediated allergy to penicillin, vancomycin alone, 15 mg/kg intravenously every 12 hours for 4 weeks, should be administered.

Endocarditis caused by viridans streptococci with an MIC > 0.5 mcg/mL or by nutritionally deficient streptococci should be treated the same as enterococcal endocarditis (see below).

B. OTHER STREPTOCOCCI

Endocarditis caused by *S pneumoniae*, *S pyogenes* (group A streptococcus), or groups B, C, and G streptococci is unusual. *S pneumoniae* sensitive to penicillin (MIC < 0.1 mcg/mL) can be treated with penicillin alone, 2–3 million units intravenously every 4 hours for 4–6 weeks. Vancomycin should be effective for endocarditis caused by strains resistant to penicillin. Group A streptococcal infection can be treated with penicillin, ceftriaxone, or vancomycin for 4–6 weeks. Groups B, C, and G streptococci tend to be more resistant to penicillin than group A streptococci, and some have recommended adding gentamicin, 1 mg/kg

intravenously every 8 hours, to penicillin for the first 2 weeks of a 4- to 6-week course. Endocarditis caused by *S bovis* is associated with liver disease and gastrointestinal abnormalities, especially colon cancer. Colonoscopy should be performed to exclude the latter.

C. ENTEROCOCCI

For enterococcal endocarditis, penicillin alone is inadequate; either streptomycin or gentamicin must be included in the regimen. Because aminoglycoside resistance occurs in enterococci, susceptibility should be documented. Gentamicin is the aminoglycoside of choice, because streptomycin resistance is more common and the nephrotoxicity of gentamicin is generally more easily managed than the vestibular toxicity of streptomycin. Ampicillin, 2 g intravenously every 4 hours, or penicillin G, 3–4 million units intravenously every 4 hours (or, in the penicillin-allergic patient, vancomycin, 15 mg/kg intravenously every 12 hours), plus gentamicin, 1 mg/kg intravenously every 8 hours, are recommended. The recommended duration of combination therapy is 4–6 weeks (the longer duration for patients with symptoms for more than 3 months, relapse, or prosthetic valve endocarditis), although a study from Sweden found that discontinuing the aminoglycoside before 4 weeks did not reduce efficacy. Experience is more extensive with penicillin and ampicillin than with vancomycin for treatment of enterococcal endocarditis, and penicillin and ampicillin are superior to vancomycin in vitro. Thus, whenever possible, either ampicillin or penicillin should be used.

Endocarditis caused by strains resistant to penicillin, vancomycin, or aminoglycosides is particularly difficult to treat. Such cases should be treated according to recent American Heart Association guidelines (see reference below) and managed in consultation with an infectious diseases specialist.

D. STAPHYLOCOCCI

For methicillin-susceptible *S aureus*, nafcillin or oxacillin, 1.5–2 g intravenously every 4 hours for 6 weeks, is the preferred therapy. Uncomplicated tricuspid valve endocarditis probably can be treated for 2 weeks with nafcillin or oxacillin alone. For penicillin-allergic patients, cefazolin, 2 g intravenously every 8 hours, or vancomycin, 15 mg/kg intravenously every 12 hours, may be used. For methicillin-resistant strains, vancomycin remains the preferred agent. Aminoglycoside combination regimens are probably of no benefit and in general should be avoided. The effect of rifampin with antistaphylococcal drugs is variable, and its routine use is not recommended.

Because coagulase-negative staphylococci—a common cause of prosthetic valve endocarditis—are routinely resistant to methicillin, β-lactam antibiotics should not be used for this infection unless the isolate is demonstrated to be susceptible. A combination of vancomycin 1 g intravenously every 12 hours for 6 weeks, rifampin, 300 mg every 8 hours for 6 weeks, and gentamicin, 1 mg/kg intravenously every 8 hours for the first 2 weeks, is recommended for prosthetic valve infection. If the organism is sensitive to methicillin, either nafcillin or oxacillin or cefazolin can be used in combination with rifampin and gentamicin. Combination therapy with nafcillin or oxacillin (vancomycin for methicillin-resistant strains or patients allergic to β-lactams), rifampin, and gentamicin is also recommended for treatment of *S aureus* prosthetic valve infection.

E. HACEK ORGANISMS

HACEK organisms are slow-growing, fastidious gram-negative coccobacilli or bacilli that are normal oral flora and cause less than 5% of all cases of endocarditis. They may produce β-lactamase, and thus the treatment of choice is ceftriaxone (or some other third-generation cephalosporin), 2 g intravenously once daily for 4 weeks. Prosthetic valve endocarditis should be treated for 6 weeks. In the penicillin-allergic patient, experience is limited, but trimethoprim-sulfamethoxazole, quinolones, and aztreonam have in vitro activity and should be considered; desensitization may be preferable.

F. ROLE OF SURGERY

While many cases can be successfully treated medically, operative management is frequently required. Acute heart failure unresponsive to medical therapy is an indication for valve replacement even if active infection is present, especially for aortic valve infection. Infections unresponsive to appropriate antimicrobial therapy after 7–10 days (ie, persistent fevers, positive blood cultures despite therapy) are more likely to be eradicated if the valve is replaced. Surgery is nearly always required for cure of fungal endocarditis and is more often necessary with gram-negative bacilli. It is also indicated when the infection involves the sinus of Valsalva or produces septal abscesses. Recurrent infection with the same organism prompts an operative approach, especially with infected prosthetic valves. Continuing embolization presents a difficult problem when the infection is otherwise responding; surgery may be the proper approach. Particularly challenging is a large and fragile vegetation demonstrated by echo in the absence of embolization. Most clinicians favor an operative approach, vegetectomy with valve repair if the patient is a good candidate. Embolization after bacteriologic cure does not necessarily imply recurrence of endocarditis.

G. ROLE OF ANTICOAGULATION

Anticoagulation is contraindicated in native valve endocarditis because of an increased risk of intracerebral hemorrhage. The role of anticoagulant therapy during active prosthetic valve endocarditis is more controversial. Reversal of anticoagulation may result in thrombosis of the mechanical prosthesis, particularly in the mitral position. On the other hand, anticoagulation during active prosthetic valve endocarditis caused by *S aureus* has been associated with fatal intracerebral hemorrhage. One approach is to discontinue anticoagulation during the septic phase of *S aureus* prosthetic valve endocarditis. In patients with *S aureus* prosthetic valve endocarditis complicated by a central nervous system embolic event, anticoagulation should be discontinued for the first 2 weeks of therapy. Indications for anticoagulation following prosthetic valve implantation for endocarditis are the same as for patients with prosthetic valves without endocarditis (eg, nonporcine mechanical valves and valves in the mitral position).

Response to Therapy

If infection is caused by viridans streptococci, enterococci, or coagulase-negative staphylococci, defervescence occurs in 3–4 days on average; with *S aureus* or *Pseudomonas aeruginosa*, fever commonly persists for 9–12 days. Blood cultures should be obtained to document sterilization of the blood. Other causes of persistent fever are myocardial or metastatic abscess, sterile embolization, superimposed nosocomial infection, and drug reaction. Most relapses occur within 1–2 months after completion of therapy. Obtaining one or two blood cultures during this period is prudent.

Baddour LM et al: Infective endocarditis: diagnosis, antimicrobial therapy, and management of complications: a statement for healthcare professionals from the Committee on Rheumatic Fever, Endocarditis, and Kawasaki Disease, Council on Cardiovascular Disease in the Young, and the Councils on Clinical Cardiology, Stroke, and Cardiovascular Surgery and Anesthesia, American Heart Association: endorsed by the Infectious Diseases Society of America. Circulation 2005;111:e394. [PMID: 15956145]

Fowler VG Jr et al: *Staphylococcus aureus* endocarditis: a consequence of medical progress. JAMA 2005;293:3012. [PMID: 15972563]

Le T et al: Combination antibiotic therapy for infective endocarditis. Clin Infect Dis 2003;36:615. [PMID: 12594643]

■ INFECTIONS CAUSED BY GRAM-NEGATIVE BACTERIA

BORDETELLA PERTUSSIS INFECTION (Whooping Cough)

 ESSENTIALS OF DIAGNOSIS

- *Predominantly in infants under age 2 years. Adolescents and adults are an important reservoir of infection.*
- *Two-week prodromal catarrhal stage of malaise, cough, coryza, and anorexia.*
- *Paroxysmal cough ending in a high-pitched inspiratory "whoop."*
- *Absolute lymphocytosis, often striking; culture confirms diagnosis.*

General Considerations

Pertussis is an acute infection of the respiratory tract caused by *B pertussis* that is transmitted by respiratory droplets. The incubation period is 7–17 days. Half of all cases occur before age 2 years. Neither immunization nor disease confers lasting immunity to pertussis. Consequently, adults are an important reservoir of the disease.

Clinical Findings

The symptoms of classic pertussis last about 6 weeks and are divided into three consecutive stages. The catarrhal stage is characterized by its insidious onset, with lacrimation, sneezing, and coryza, anorexia and malaise, and a hacking night cough that becomes diurnal. The paroxysmal stage is characterized by bursts of rapid, consecutive coughs followed by a deep, high-pitched inspiration (whoop). The convalescent stage begins 4 weeks after onset of the illness with a decrease in the frequency and severity of paroxysms of cough. The diagnosis often is not considered in adults, who may not have a typical presentation. Cough persisting more than 2 weeks is suggestive. Infection may also be asymptomatic.

The white blood cell count is usually 15,000–20,000/mcL (rarely, as high as 50,000/mcL or more), 60–80% of which are lymphocytes. The diagnosis is established by isolating the organism from nasopharyngeal culture. A special medium (eg, Bordet-Gengou agar) must be requested. Polymerase chain reaction assays for diagnosis of pertussis may be available in some clinical or health department laboratories.

Prevention

Acellular pertussis vaccine is recommended for all infants, combined with diphtheria and tetanus toxoids (DTaP). Infants and susceptible adults with significant exposure should receive prophylaxis with an oral macrolide (see below). In recognition of their importance as a reservoir of disease, vaccination of adolescents and adults against pertussis is now recommended. The FDA licensed two tetanus toxoid, reduced diphtheria toxoid and acellular pertussis vaccine (Tdap) products (BOOSTRIX, GlaxoSmithKline and ADACEL, Sanofi Pasteur) in 2005. Adolescents aged 11–18 years who have completed the DTP or DTaP vaccination series should receive a single dose of either Tdap product instead of Td (tetanus and diphtheria toxoids vaccine) for booster immunization against tetanus, diphtheria, and pertussis. Either vaccine may be used in place of Td for prophylaxis of tetanus in wound management. The ADACEL vaccine is indicated as a one-time dose for booster immunization for pertussis in children and adults (ages 11 through 64 years). It may be used as a replacement dose for one of the Td doses when completing a primary immunization series or in place of Td for tetanus wound prophylaxis. Postpartum women and adults who have not been previously vaccinated with Tdap and who have close contact to an infant younger than 12 months should receive a single dose of Tdap. Women of childbearing age are also candidates for one dose of Tdap.

Treatment

Erythromycin, 500 mg four times a day orally for 7 days, shortens the duration of carriage. It also may diminish the severity of coughing paroxysms. Azithromycin, 500 mg orally on day 1 and 250 mg for 4 more days; or clarithromycin, 500 mg orally twice daily for 7 days, is probably as effective as erythromycin and likely to be better tolerated. Trimethoprim-sulfamethoxazole 160 mg-800 mg orally twice a day for 7 days also is effective. These same regimens are indicated for prophylaxis of contacts to an active case of pertussis who are exposed within 3 weeks of the onset of cough in the index case.

Broder KR et al; Advisory Committee on Immunization (ACIP): Preventing tetanus, diphtheria, and pertussis among adolescents: use of tetanus toxoid, reduced diphtheria toxoid, and acellular pertussis vaccines recommendations of the Advisory Committee on Immunization (ACIP). MMWR Recomm Rep 2006;55(RR-3):1. [PMID: 16557217]

Hewlett EL et al: Clinical Practice. Pertussis—Not just for kids. N Engl J Med 2005;352:1215. [PMID: 15788498]

Mitka M: Age range widens for pertussis vaccine: boosters advised for adolescents and adults. JAMA 2006;295:871. [PMID: 16493092]

OTHER BORDETELLA INFECTIONS

Bordetella bronchiseptica is a pleomorphic gram-negative coccobacillus causing kennel cough in dogs. On occasion it causes upper and lower respiratory infection in humans, principally HIV-infected patients. Infection has been associated with contact with dogs and cats, suggesting animal-to-human transmission. Treatment of *B bronchiseptica* infection is guided by results of in vitro susceptibility tests.

MENINGOCOCCAL MENINGITIS

ESSENTIALS OF DIAGNOSIS

- *Fever, headache, vomiting, confusion, delirium, convulsions.*
- *Petechial rash of skin and mucous membranes in many.*
- *Neck and back stiffness with positive Kernig and Brudzinski signs is characteristic.*
- *Purulent spinal fluid with gram-negative intracellular and extracellular diplococci.*
- *Culture of cerebrospinal fluid, blood, or petechial aspiration confirms the diagnosis.*

General Considerations

Meningococcal meningitis is caused by *Neisseria meningitidis* of groups A, B, C, Y, and W-135, among others. Meningitis due to serogroup A is uncommon in the United States. Serogroup B generally causes sporadic cases. The frequency of outbreaks of meningitis caused by group C meningococcus has increased, and this serotype is the most common cause of epidemic disease in the United States. Up to 40% of persons are nasopharyngeal carriers of meningococci, but disease develops in relatively few of these persons. Infection is transmitted by droplets. The clinical illness may take the form of meningococcemia (a fulminant form of septicemia without meningitis), meningococcemia with meningitis, or meningitis. Recurrent meningococcemia with fever, rash, and arthritis is seen rarely in patients with certain terminal complement deficiencies.

Clinical Findings

A. SYMPTOMS AND SIGNS

High fever, chills, and headache; back, abdominal, and extremity pains; and nausea and vomiting are typical. Rapidly developing confusion, delirium, seizures, and coma occur in some.

On examination, nuchal and back rigidity are typical, with positive Kernig and Brudzinski signs. (Kernig's sign is pain in the hamstrings upon extension of the knee with the hip at 90-degree flexion; Brudzinski's sign is flexion of the knee in response to flexion of the neck.) A petechial rash appearing in the lower extremities and at pressure points is found in most cases. Petechiae may vary in size from pinpoint lesions to large ecchymoses or even skin gangrene that may later slough if the patient survives.

B. LABORATORY FINDINGS

Lumbar puncture typically reveals a cloudy or purulent cerebrospinal fluid, with elevated pressure, increased protein, and decreased glucose content. The fluid usually contains more than 1000 cells/mcL, with polymorphonuclear cells predominating and containing gram-negative intracellular diplococci. The absence of organisms in a Gram-stained smear of the cerebrospinal fluid sediment does not rule out the diagnosis. The capsular polysaccharide can be demonstrated in cerebrospinal fluid or urine by latex agglutination; this is useful in partially treated patients, though sensitivity is 60–80%. The organism is usually demonstrated by smear and culture of the cerebrospinal fluid, oropharynx, blood, or aspirated petechiae.

Disseminated intravascular coagulation is an important complication of meningococcal infection and is typically present in toxic patients with ecchymotic skin lesions.

Differential Diagnosis

Meningococcal meningitis must be differentiated from other meningitides. In small infants and in the elderly, fever or stiff neck is often missing, and altered mental status may dominate the picture.

Rickettsial, echovirus and, rarely, other bacterial infections (eg, staphylococcal infections, scarlet fever) also cause petechial rash.

Prevention

Two vaccines, meningococcal polysaccharide vaccine (MPSV4, indicated for vaccination of persons aged 2–10 years and over age 55) and a conjugate vaccine (MCV4, indicated for persons aged 11–55 years) are effective for meningococcal groups A, C, Y, and W-135. The Advisory Committee on Immunization Practices recommends immunization with a single dose of MCV4 for preadolescents ages 11–12, and for those not previously vaccinated, upon entry into high school. MCV4 is also recommended for college freshmen—particularly those living in dormitories (see Tables 30–4 and 30–5). Vaccine is also recommended for military recruits, asplenic individuals, those with deficiencies in terminal component of complement, and exposed persons during outbreaks.

Eliminating nasopharyngeal carriage of meningococci is an effective prevention strategy in closed populations and to prevent secondary cases in household or otherwise close contacts. Rifampin, 600 mg orally twice a day for 2 days, ciprofloxacin, 500 mg orally, or one intramuscular 250-mg dose of ceftriaxone is effective. School and work contacts ordinarily need not be treated. Hospital contacts receive therapy only if intense exposure has occurred (eg, mouth-to-mouth resuscitation). Accidentally discovered carriers without known close contact with meningococcal disease do not require prophylactic antimicrobials.

Treatment

Blood cultures must be obtained and intravenous antimicrobial therapy started immediately. This may be done prior to lumbar puncture in patients in whom the diagnosis is not straightforward and for those in whom MR or CT imaging is indicated to exclude mass lesions. Aqueous penicillin G is the antibiotic of choice (24 million units/24 h intravenously in divided doses every 4 hours). The prevalence of strains of *N meningitidis* with intermediate resistance to penicillin in vitro (MICs 0.1 to 1 mcg/mL) is increasing, particularly in Europe. At what level of resistance penicillin treatment failure can occur is not known. Penicillin-intermediate strains thus far remain fully susceptible to ceftriaxone and other third-generation cephalosporins used to treat meninigitis, and these should be effective alternatives to penicillin. In penicillin-allergic patients or those in whom *Haemophilus influenzae* or gram-negative meningitis is a consideration, ceftriaxone, 2 g intravenously every 12 hours, should be used. Treatment should be continued in full doses by the intravenous route until the patient is afebrile for 5 days. Shorter courses—as few as 4 days if ceftriaxone is used—are also effective.

Kimmel SR: Prevention of meningococcal diseases. Am Fam Physician 2005;72:2049. [PMID: 16342836]

Van de Beek D et al: Clinical features and prognostic factors in adults with bacterial meningitis. N Engl J Med 2004;351:1849. [PMID: 1550981]

Van de Beek D et al: Current concepts: community-acquired bacterial meningitis in adults. N Engl J Med 2006;354:44. [PMID: 16394301]

INFECTIONS CAUSED BY *HAEMOPHILUS* SPECIES

H influenzae and other *Haemophilus* species may cause sinusitis, otitis, bronchitis, epiglottitis, pneumonitis, cellulitis, arthritis, meningitis, and endocarditis. Nontypeable strains are responsible for most disease in adults. Alcoholism, smoking, chronic lung disease, advanced age, and HIV infection are risk factors. *Haemophilus* species colonize the upper respiratory tract in patients with chronic obstructive pulmonary disease and frequently cause purulent bronchitis.

β-Lactamase-producing strains are less common in adults than in children. For adults with sinusitis, otitis, or respiratory tract infection, oral amoxicillin, 750 mg twice daily for 10–14 days, is adequate. For β-lactamase-producing strains, use of the oral fixed drug combination of amoxicillin, 875 mg, with clavulanate, 125 mg, is indicated. For the penicillin-allergic patient, oral cefuroxime axetil, 250 mg twice daily, or trimethoprim-sulfamethoxazole, 800/160 mg orally twice daily, for 10 days is effective. Azithromycin and clarithromycin are less effective.

In the more seriously ill patient (eg, the toxic patient with multilobar pneumonia) ceftriaxone, 1 g/d intravenously is recommended pending determination of whether the infecting strain is a β-lactamase producer. Trimethoprim-sulfamethoxazole administered intravenously based on a dose of 10 mg/kg/d of trimethoprim, can be used for the penicillin-allergic patient. A 10- to 14-day course of therapy is adequate for most cases.

Epiglottitis is characterized by an abrupt onset of high fever, drooling, and inability to handle secretions. An important clue to the diagnosis is complaint of a severe sore throat despite an unimpressive examination of the pharynx. Stridor and respiratory distress result from laryngeal obstruction. The diagnosis is best made by direct visualization of the cherry-red, swollen epiglottis at laryngoscopy. Because laryngoscopy may provoke laryngospasm and obstruction, especially in children, it should be performed in an intensive care unit or similar setting, and only at a time when intubation can be performed promptly. Ceftriaxone, 1 g intravenously every 24 hours for 7–10 days, is the drug of choice. Trimethoprim-sulfamethoxazole (see above for dosage) may be used in the patient with serious penicillin allergy.

Meningitis, rare in adults, is a consideration in the patient who has meningitis associated with sinusitis or otitis. Initial therapy for suspected *H influenzae* meningitis should be with ceftriaxone, 4 g/d two divided doses, until the strain is proved not to produce β-lactamase. Meningitis is treated for 10–14 days. Dexamethasone, 0.15 mg/kg intravenously every 6 hours may reduce the incidence of long-term sequelae, principally hearing loss.

INFECTIONS CAUSED BY *MORAXELLA CATARRHALIS*

M catarrhalis is a gram-negative aerobic coccus morphologically and biochemically similar to *Neisseria*. It causes sinusitis, bronchitis, and pneumonia. Bacteremia and meningitis have also been reported in immunocompromised patients. The organism frequently colonizes the respiratory tract, making differentiation of colonization from infection difficult. If *M catarrhalis* is the predominant isolate, therapy is directed against it. *M catarrhalis* typically produces β-lactamase and therefore is usually resistant to ampicillin and amoxicillin. It is susceptible to amoxicillin-clavulanate, ampicillin-sulbactam, trimethoprim-sulfamethoxazole, ciprofloxacin, and second- and third-generation cephalosporins.

Murphy TF et al: *Moraxella catarrhalis* in chronic obstructive pulmonary disease: burden of disease and immune response. Am J Respir Crit Care Med 2005;172:195. [PMID: 15805178]

LEGIONNAIRE'S DISEASE

ESSENTIALS OF DIAGNOSIS

- *Patients are often immunocompromised, smokers, or have chronic lung disease.*
- *Scant sputum production, pleuritic chest pain, toxic appearance.*
- *Chest radiograph shows focal patchy infiltrates or consolidation.*
- *Gram stain of sputum shows polymorphonuclear leukocytes and no organisms.*

General Considerations

Legionella infection ranks among the three or four most common causes of community-acquired pneumonia and is considered whenever the etiology of a pneumonia is in question. Legionnaire's disease is more common in immunocompromised persons, in smokers, and in those with chronic lung disease. Outbreaks have been associated with contaminated water sources, such as shower heads and faucets in patient rooms and air conditioning cooling towers.

Clinical Findings

A. SYMPTOMS AND SIGNS

Legionnaire's disease is one of the atypical pneumonias, so called because a Gram-stained smear of sputum does not show organisms. However, many features of Legionnaire's disease are more like typical pneumonia, with high fevers, a toxic patient, pleurisy, and grossly purulent sputum. Classically, this pneumonia is caused by *Legionella pneumophila*, though other species can cause identical disease.

B. LABORATORY FINDINGS

Culture onto charcoal-yeast extract agar or similar enriched medium is the most sensitive method (80–90% sensitivity) for diagnosis and permits identification of infections caused by species and serotypes other than *L pneumophila* serotype 1. Dieterle's silver staining of tissue, pleural fluid, or other infected material is also a reliable method for detecting *Legionella* species. Direct fluorescent antibody stains and serologic testing are less sensitive because these will detect only *L pneumophila* serotype 1. In addition, making a serologic diagnosis requires that the host respond with sufficient specific antibody production. Urinary antigen tests, which are targeted for detection of *L pneumophila* serotype 1, are also less sensitive than culture.

Treatment

Azithromycin (500 mg orally once daily), clarithromycin (500 mg orally twice daily), or a fluoroquinolone (eg, levofloxacin 500 mg orally once daily), and not erythromycin, is the drug of choice for treatment of legionellosis because of their excellent intracellular penetration and in vitro activity, as well as desirable pharmacokinetic properties that permit oral administration and once or twice daily dosing. Duration of therapy is 10–14 days, although a 21-day course of therapy is recommended for immunocompromised patients.

Plouffe JF et al: Azithromycin in the treatment of Legionella pneumonia requiring hospitalization. Clin Infect Dis 2003; 37:1475. Epub 2003 Oct 29. [PMID: 14614670]

Sabria M et al: Fluoroquinolones vs macrolides in the treatment of Legionnaires' disease. Chest 2005;128:1401. [PMID: 16162735]

GRAM-NEGATIVE BACTEREMIA & SEPSIS

Gram-negative bacteremia can originate in a number of sites, the most common being the genitourinary system, hepatobiliary tract, gastrointestinal tract, and lungs. Less common sources include intravenous lines, infusion fluids, surgical wounds, drains, and decubitus ulcers.

Patients with potentially fatal underlying conditions in the short term such as neutropenia or immunoparesis have a mortality rate of 40–60%; those with serious underlying diseases likely to be fatal in 5 years, such as solid tumors, cirrhosis, and aplastic anemia, die in 15–20% of cases; and individuals with no underlying diseases have a mortality rate of 5% or less.

Clinical Findings

A. SYMPTOMS AND SIGNS

Most patients have fevers and chills, often with abrupt onset. However, 15% of patients are hypothermic (temperature ≤ 36.4 °C) at presentation, and 5% never develop a temperature above 37.5 °C. Hyperventilation with respiratory alkalosis and changes in mental status are important early manifestations. Hypotension and shock, which occur in 20–50% of patients, are unfavorable prognostic signs.

B. LABORATORY FINDINGS

Neutropenia or neutrophilia, often with increased numbers of immature forms of polymorphonuclear leukocytes, is the most common laboratory abnormality in septic patients. Thrombocytopenia occurs in 50% of patients, laboratory evidence of coagulation abnormalities in 10%, and overt disseminated intravascular coagulation in 2–3%. Both clinical manifestations and the laboratory abnormalities are nonspecific and insensitive, which accounts for the relatively low rate of blood culture positivity (approximately 20–40%). If possible, three blood cultures from separate sites should be obtained in rapid succession before starting antimicrobial therapy. The chance of recovering the organism in at least one of the three blood cultures is greater than 95%. The false-negative rate for a single culture of 5–10 mL of blood is 30%. This may be reduced to 5–10% (albeit with a slight false-positive rate due to isolation of contaminants) if a single volume of 30 mL is inoculated into several blood culture bottles. Because blood cultures may be falsely negative, when a patient with presumed septic shock, negative blood cultures, and inadequate explanation for the clinical course responds to antimicrobials, therapy should be continued for 10–14 days.

Treatment

Several factors are important in the management of patients with sepsis.

A. REMOVAL OF PREDISPOSING FACTORS

This usually means decreasing or stopping immunosuppressive medications and in certain circumstances (eg, positive blood cultures) giving granulocyte colony-stimulating factor (filgrastim; G-CSF) to the neutropenic patient.

B. IDENTIFYING THE SOURCE OF BACTEREMIA

By simply finding the source of bacteremia and removing it (intravenous line) or draining it (abscess), a fatal disease becomes easily treatable.

C. SUPPORTIVE MEASURES

The use of fluids and pressors for maintaining blood pressure is discussed in Chapter 12; management of disseminated intravascular coagulation is discussed in Chapter 13.

D. ANTIBIOTICS

Antibiotics are given as soon as the diagnosis is suspected, since delays in therapy have been associated with increased mortality rates. In general, bactericidal antibiotics should be used and given intravenously to ensure therapeutic serum levels. Penetration of antibiotics into the site of primary infection is critical for successful therapy—ie, if the infection originates in the central nervous system, antibiotics that penetrate the blood-brain barrier should be used—eg, penicillin, ampicillin, chloramphenicol, and third-generation cephalosporins—but not first-generation cephalosporins or aminoglycosides, which penetrate poorly. Sepsis caused by gram-positive organisms cannot be differentiated on clinical grounds from that due to gram-negative bacteria. Therefore, initial therapy should include antibiotics active against both types of organisms.

The number of antibiotics necessary remains controversial and depends on the cause. Table 37–2 provides a guide for empiric therapy. Most authorities believe that for patients with rapidly fatal underlying diseases, a synergistic combination of antibiotics, including an aminoglycoside, should be used. For patients with nonfatal or ultimately fatal diseases and who are not in shock, a single-drug regimen with any of several broad-spectrum antibiotics (eg, a third-generation cephalosporin, ticarcillin-clavulanate, imipenem) is adequate. Therapy can be altered once results of culture and sensitivity are known.

E. CORTICOSTEROIDS

The role of corticosteroids in treatment of septic shock is still quite controversial. Clinical data have suggested an association between mortality in patients with septic shock and poor adrenal reserve to cosyntropin (Cortrosyn) stimulation testing. Administration of "stress doses" of hydrocortisone, for example 100 mg intravenously three times a day for 5 days followed by a 6-day tapering-dose regimen, to patients with relative adrenal insufficiency and pressor-dependent septic shock may reduce mortality. However, the usefulness of cosyntropin stimulation testing and use of stress-dose hydrocortisone in patients with septic shock are not so well defined as to be standard of care.

F. ADJUNCTIVE THERAPY

Expanded knowledge of the pathophysiology of sepsis and septic shock and recognition that cytokines play a critical role suggest novel approaches to therapy. Strategies include blocking the effects of endotoxin with anti-endotoxin monoclonal antibodies; blockade of TNF-α, a potent cytokine mediator of septic shock, with anti-TNF monoclonal antibody or soluble TNF receptor; use of IL-1 receptor antagonists to inhibit the proinflammatory effects of IL-1 binding to its receptor; use of corticosteroids; and blocking platelet or thrombin activation. None of these strategies have been met with improved survival. However, a single randomized placebo-controlled trial showed that recombinant human activated protein C (drotrecogin alfa) reduced mortality septic patients with APACHE II scores ≥ 25. This drug should be used cautiously because of the risk of bleeding. Drotrecogin alfa is not beneficial for patients with severe sepsis and low risk of death (eg, APACHE score < 25 or single organ failure), and it is associated with serious bleeding complications; it should not be used in these patients. Patients considered to have an infectious cause of severe sepsis (defined as three or more signs of systemic inflammation—eg, fever or hypothermia, tachycardia, tachypnea—plus sepsis-induced dysfunction of at least one organ system) of less than 24 hours' duration are the best candidates. Platelet counts less than 30,000/mcL, conditions associated with an increased risk of bleeding (eg, recent trauma, surgery, or bleeding episode; anticoagulation), or hypercoagulable states have not been investigated. These criteria should be followed when selecting candidates for treatment with drotrecogin alfa (activated). The agent is administered intravenously by constant infusion at a dosage of 24 mcg/kg/h for 96 hours.

Abraham E et al; Administration of Drotrecogin Alfa (Activated) in Early Stage Severe Sepsis (ADDRESS) Study Group. Drotrecogin alfa (activated) for adults with severe sepsis and a low risk of death. N Engl J Med 2005;353:1332. [PMID: 16192478]

Annane D et al: Septic shock. Lancet 2005;365:63. [PMID: 15639681]

Minneci PC et al: Meta-analysis: the effect of steroids on survival and shock during sepsis depends on the dose. Ann Intern Med 2004;141:47. [PMID: 15238370]

SALMONELLOSIS

Salmonellosis includes infection by any of approximately 2000 serotypes of salmonellae. The taxonomy of *Salmonella* species has been confusing. All salmonella serotypes are members of a single species, *Salmonella enterica*. Human infections are caused almost exclusively by *S enterica* subsp *enterica*, of which three serotypes—typhi, typhimurium, and choleraesuis—are predominantly isolated. Three clinical patterns of infection are recognized: (1) enteric fever, the best example of which is typhoid fever, due to serotype typhi; (2) acute enterocolitis, caused by serotype typhimurium, among others; and (3) the "septicemic" type, characterized by bacteremia and focal lesions, exemplified by infection with serotype choleraesuis. All types are transmitted by ingestion of the organism, usually from contaminated food or drink.

1. Enteric Fever (Typhoid Fever)

ESSENTIALS OF DIAGNOSIS

- Gradual onset of malaise, headache, nausea, vomiting, abdominal pain.
- Rose spots, relative bradycardia, splenomegaly, and abdominal distention and tenderness.
- Slow (stepladder) rise of fever to maximum and then slow return to normal.
- Leukopenia; blood, stool, and urine culture positive for salmonella.

General Considerations

Enteric fever is a clinical syndrome characterized by constitutional and gastrointestinal symptoms and by headache. It can be caused by any *Salmonella* species. The term "typhoid fever" applies when serotype typhi is the cause. Infection is transmitted by consumption of contaminated food or drink. The incubation period is 5–14 days. Salmonella is an intracellular pathogen. Infection begins when organisms breach the mucosal epithelium of the intestines by transcytosis, an organism-mediated transport process through the cell via an endocytic vesicle. Having crossed the epithelial barrier, organisms invade and replicate in macrophages in Peyer's patches, mesenteric lymph nodes, and the spleen. Serotypes other than typhi usually do not cause invasive disease, presumably because they lack the necessary human-specific virulence factors. Bacteremia occurs, and the infection then localizes principally in the lymphoid tissue of the small intestine (particularly within 60 cm of the ileocecal valve). Peyer's patches become inflamed and may ulcerate, with involvement greatest during the third week of disease. The organism may disseminate to the lungs, gallbladder, kidneys, or central nervous system.

Clinical Findings

A. SYMPTOMS AND SIGNS

During the prodromal stage, there is increasing malaise, headache, cough, and sore throat, often with abdominal pain and constipation, while the fever ascends in a stepwise fashion. After about 7–10 days, it reaches a plateau and the patient is much more ill, appearing exhausted and often prostrated. There may be marked constipation, especially early, or "pea soup" diarrhea; marked abdominal distention occurs as well. If there are no complications, the patient's condition will gradually improve over 7–10 days. However, relapse may occur for up to 2 weeks after defervescence.

During the early prodrome, physical findings are few. Later, splenomegaly, abdominal distention and tenderness, relative bradycardia, and occasionally meningismus appear. The rash (rose spots) commonly appears during the second week of disease. The individual spot, found principally on the trunk, is a pink papule 2–3 mm in diameter that fades on pressure. It disappears in 3–4 days.

B. LABORATORY FINDINGS

Typhoid fever is best diagnosed by blood culture, which is positive in the first week of illness in 80% of patients who have not taken antimicrobials. The rate of positivity declines thereafter, but one-fourth or more of patients still have positive blood cultures in the third week. Cultures of bone marrow occasionally are positive when blood cultures are not. Stool culture is unreliable because it may be positive in gastroenteritis without typhoid fever. Relative bradycardia and leukopenia are typical.

Differential Diagnosis

Enteric fever must be distinguished from other gastrointestinal illnesses and from other infections that have few localizing findings. Examples include tuberculosis, infective endocarditis, brucellosis, lymphoma, and Q fever. Often there is a history of recent travel to endemic areas, and viral hepatitis, malaria, or amebiasis may be in the differential as well.

Complications

Complications occur in about 30% of untreated cases and account for 75% of deaths. Intestinal hemorrhage, manifested by a sudden drop in temperature and signs of shock followed by dark or fresh blood in the stool, or intestinal perforation, accompanied by abdominal pain and tenderness, is most likely to occur during the third week. Appearance of leukocytosis and tachycardia should suggest these complications. Urinary retention, pneumonia, thrombophlebitis, myocarditis, psychosis, cholecystitis, nephritis, osteomyelitis, and meningitis are less often observed.

Prevention

Immunization is not always effective but should be considered for household contacts of a typhoid carrier, for travelers to endemic areas, and during epidemic outbreaks. A multiple-dose oral vaccine and a single-dose parenteral vaccine are available. Their efficacies are similar, but oral vaccine causes fewer side effects. Boosters, when indicated, should be given every 5 years and 3 years for oral and parenteral preparations, respectively.

Adequate waste disposal and protection of food and water supplies from contamination are important public health measures to prevent salmonellosis. Carriers cannot work as food handlers.

Treatment

A. SPECIFIC MEASURES

Several antibiotics, including ampicillin, azithromycin, chloramphenicol, third-generation cephalosporins, and trimethoprim-sulfamethoxazole all are effective for treatment of enteric fever caused by drug-susceptible strains. These drugs can be given orally or intravenously depending on the patient's condition. Because many salmonella strains are resistant to ampicillin, chloramphenicol, and trimethoprim-sulfamethoxazole, a fluoroquinolone—such as ciprofloxacin 750 mg orally twice daily or levofloxacin 500 mg orally once daily, 5–7 days for uncomplicated enteric fever and 10–14 days for severe infection—is the agent of choice for treatment of salmonella infections. Ceftriaxone 2 g intravenously for 7 days is also effective. Resistance to fluoroquinolones or cephalosporins occurs rarely. Infection caused by a drug-resistant strain is treated by using an antibiotic to which the isolate is susceptible (eg, azithromycin), or in severe cases by increasing the dose of ceftriaxone to 4 g/d and treating for 10–14 days.

B. TREATMENT OF CARRIERS

Chemotherapy often is unsuccessful in eradicating the carrier state. While treatment of carriage with ampicillin, trimethoprim-sulfamethoxazole, or chloramphenicol may be successful, ciprofloxacin, 750 mg orally twice a day for 4 weeks, has proved to be highly effective. Cholecystectomy may also achieve this goal.

Prognosis

The mortality rate of typhoid fever is about 2% in treated cases. Elderly or debilitated persons are likely to do poorly. With complications, the prognosis is poor. Relapses occur in up to 15% of cases. A residual carrier state frequently persists in spite of chemotherapy.

Bhan MK et al: Typhoid and paratyphoid fever. Lancet 2005; 366:749. [PMID: 16125594]

Steinberg EB et al: Typhoid fever in travelers: who should be targeted for prevention? Clin Infect Dis 2004;39:186. [PMID: 15307027]

2. Salmonella Gastroenteritis

By far the most common form of salmonellosis is acute enterocolitis caused by numerous salmonella serotypes. The incubation period is 8–48 hours after ingestion of contaminated food or liquid.

Symptoms and signs consist of fever (often with chills), nausea and vomiting, cramping abdominal pain, and diarrhea, which may be grossly bloody, lasting 3–5 days. Differentiation must be made from viral gastroenteritis, food poisoning, shigellosis, amebic dysentery, and acute ulcerative colitis. The diagnosis is made by culturing the organism from the stool.

The disease is usually self-limited, but bacteremia with localization in joints or bones may occur, especially in patients with sickle cell disease.

Treatment of uncomplicated enterocolitis is symptomatic only. Malnourished or severely ill patients, those with sickle cell disease, and those with suspected bacteremia should be treated for 3–5 days with trimethoprim-sulfamethoxazole (one double-strength tablet twice a day), ampicillin (100 mg/kg intravenously or orally), or ciprofloxacin (750 mg orally twice a day).

Patrick ME et al: Salmonella enteritidis infections, United States, 1985–1999. Emerg Infect Dis 2004;10:1. [PMID: 15078589]

3. Salmonella Bacteremia

Salmonella infection may be manifested by prolonged or recurrent fevers accompanied by bacteremia and local infection in bone, joints, pleura, pericardium, lungs, or other sites. Mycotic abdominal aortic aneurysms may also occur. Serotypes other than typhi usually are isolated. This complication tends to occur in immunocompromised persons and is seen in HIV-infected individuals, who typically have bacteremia without an obvious source. Treatment is the same as for typhoid fever, plus drainage of any abscesses. In HIV-infected patients, relapse is common, and lifelong suppressive therapy may be needed. Ciprofloxacin, 750 mg orally twice a day, is effective both for therapy of acute infection and for suppression of recurrence. Incidence of infections caused by drug-resistant strains may be on the rise.

Varma JK et al: Antimicrobial-resistant nontyphoidal Salmonella is associated with excess bloodstream infections and hospitalizations. J Infect Dis 2005;191:554. [PMID: 15655779]

SHIGELLOSIS

 ESSENTIALS OF DIAGNOSIS

- Diarrhea, often with blood and mucus.
- Crampy abdominal pain and systemic toxicity.
- White blood cells in stools; organism isolated on stool culture.

General Considerations

Shigella dysentery is a common disease, often self-limited and mild but occasionally serious. *Shigella sonnei* is the leading cause in the United States, followed by *Shigella flexneri*. *Shigella dysenteriae* causes the most serious form of the illness. Shigellae are invasive organisms. The infective dose is 10^2–10^3 organisms. There has been a rise in strains resistant to multiple antibiotics.

Clinical Findings

A. SYMPTOMS AND SIGNS

The illness usually starts abruptly, with diarrhea, lower abdominal cramps, and tenesmus. The diarrheal stool often is mixed with blood and mucus. Systemic symptoms are fever, chills, anorexia and malaise, and headache. The abdomen is tender. Sigmoidoscopic examination reveals an inflamed, engorged mucosa with punctate and sometimes large areas of ulceration.

B. LABORATORY FINDINGS

The stool shows many leukocytes and red cells. Stool culture is positive for shigellae in most cases, but blood cultures grow the organism in less than 5% of cases.

Differential Diagnosis

Bacillary dysentery must be distinguished from salmonella enterocolitis and from disease due to enterotoxigenic *Escherichia coli*, *Campylobacter*, and *Yersinia enterocolitica*. Amebic dysentery may be similar clinically and is diagnosed by finding amebas in the fresh stool specimen. Ulcerative colitis is also an important cause of bloody diarrhea.

Complications

Temporary disaccharidase deficiency may follow the diarrhea. Reactive arthritis is an uncommon complication, usually occurring in HLA-B27 individuals infected by *Shigella*.

Treatment

Treatment of dehydration and hypotension is lifesaving in severe cases. The antimicrobial treatments of choice are trimethoprim-sulfamethoxazole, one double-strength tablet twice a day for 7–10 days, or a fluoroquinolone (ciprofloxacin 750 mg orally twice daily for 7–10 days, or levofloxacin, 500 mg orally once daily) for 3 days. Fluoroquinolones are contraindicated in pregnancy. Shigellae resistant to ampicillin are common, but if the isolate is susceptible, a dose of 500 mg orally four times a day is also effective. Amoxicillin, which is less effective, should not be used.

Gupta A et al: Laboratory-confirmed shigellosis in the United States, 1989–2002: epidemiologic trends and patterns. Clin Infect Dis 2004;38:1372. [PMID: 15156473]

Thielman NM et al: Clinical practice. Acute infectious diarrhea. N Engl J Med 2004;350:38. [PMID: 14702426]

GASTROENTERITIS CAUSED BY *ESCHERICHIA COLI*

E coli causes gastroenteritis by a variety of mechanisms. Enterotoxigenic *E coli* (ETEC) elaborates either a heat-stable or heat-labile toxin that mediates the disease. ETEC is an important cause of traveler's diarrhea. Enteroinvasive *E coli* (EIEC) differs from other *E coli* bowel pathogens in that these strains invade cells, causing bloody diarrhea and dysentery similar to infection with *Shigella* species. EIEC is uncommon in the United States. Neither ETEC nor EIEC strains are routinely isolated and identified from stool cultures because there is no selective medium. Antimicrobial therapy directed against *Salmonella* and *Shigella* shortens the clinical course, but the disease is self-limited.

Enterohemorrhagic *E coli* (EHEC) produces two shiga-like toxins that mediate the clinical manifestations, which include an asymptomatic carriage stage, nonbloody diarrhea, hemorrhagic colitis, hemolytic-uremic syndrome, and thrombotic thrombocytopenic purpura. Although there are several serotypes of EHEC, O157:H7 is responsible for most cases in the United States. *E coli* O157:H7 has caused several outbreaks of diarrhea and hemolytic-uremic syndrome related to consumption of undercooked hamburger and unpasteurized apple juice. Older individuals and young children are most affected, with hemolytic-uremic syndrome being more common in the latter group. *E coli* O157:H7 is not identified by routine stool cultures. Isolation requires identification of sorbitol-negative colonies of *E coli* on sorbitol-MacConkey agar followed by serologic testing to confirm the serotype. Antimicrobial therapy does not alter the course of the disease, and may increase the risk of hemolytic-uremic syndrome. Treatment is primarily supportive. Hemolytic-uremic syndrome or thrombotic thrombocytopenic purpura occurring in association with a diarrheal illness suggests the diagnosis and should prompt evaluation for EHEC. Confirmed infections should be reported to public health officials.

Thielman NM et al: Clinical practice. Acute infectious diarrhea. N Engl J Med 2004;350:38. [PMID: 14702426]

CHOLERA

ESSENTIALS OF DIAGNOSIS

- *History of travel in endemic area or contact with infected person.*
- *Voluminous diarrhea.*
- *Stool is liquid, gray, turbid, and without fecal odor, blood, or pus ("rice water stool").*
- *Rapid development of marked dehydration.*
- *Positive stool cultures and agglutination of vibrios with specific sera.*

General Considerations

Cholera is an acute diarrheal illness caused by certain serotypes of *Vibrio cholerae*. The disease is toxin-mediated, and fever is unusual. The toxin activates adenylyl cyclase in intestinal epithelial cells of the small intestines, producing hypersecretion of water and chloride ion and a massive diarrhea of up to 15 L/d. Death results from profound hypovolemia.

Cholera occurs in epidemics under conditions of crowding, war, and famine (eg, in refugee camps) and where sanitation is inadequate. Infection is acquired by ingestion of contaminated food or water. Cholera was rarely seen in the United States until 1991, when epidemic cholera returned to the Western Hemisphere, originating as an outbreak in coastal cities of Peru. The epidemic spread to involve several countries in South and Central America as well as Mexico, and cases have been imported into the United States. Cholera should be considered in the differential diagnosis of severe watery diarrhea, especially in those who have traveled to affected countries.

Clinical Findings

Cholera is characterized by a sudden onset of severe, frequent watery diarrhea (up to 1 L/h). The liquid stool is gray; turbid; and without fecal odor, blood, or pus ("rice water stool"). Dehydration and hypotension develop rapidly. Stool cultures are positive, and agglutination of vibrios with specific sera can be demonstrated.

Prevention

A vaccine is available that confers short-lived, limited protection and may be required for entry into or reentry after travel to some countries. It is administered in two doses 1–4 weeks apart. A booster dose every 6 months is recommended for persons remaining in areas where cholera is a hazard.

Vaccination programs are expensive and not particularly effective in managing outbreaks of cholera. When outbreaks occur, efforts should be directed toward establishing clean water and food sources and proper waste disposal.

Treatment

Treatment is by replacement of fluids. In mild or moderate illness, oral rehydration usually is adequate. A simple oral replacement fluid can be made from 1 teaspoon of table salt and 4 heaping teaspoons of sugar added to 1 L of water. Intravenous fluids are indicated for persons with signs of severe hypovolemia and those who cannot take adequate fluids orally. Lactated Ringer's infusion is satisfactory.

Antimicrobial therapy will shorten the course of illness. Several antimicrobials are active against *V cholerae*, including tetracycline, ampicillin, chloramphenicol, trimethoprim-sulfamethoxazole, and fluoroquinolones. Multiple antibiotic resistance does occur, so susceptibility testing, if available, is advisable.

Sack DA et al: Cholera. Lancet 2004;363:223. [PMID: 14738797]

INFECTIONS CAUSED BY OTHER VIBRIO SPECIES

Vibrios other than *V cholerae* that cause human disease are *Vibrio parahaemolyticus*, *Vibrio vulnificus*, and *Vibrio alginolyticus*. All are halophilic marine organisms. Infection is acquired by exposure to organisms in contaminated, undercooked, or raw crustaceans or shellfish and warm (> 20 °C) ocean waters and estuaries. Infections are more common during the summer months from regions along the Atlantic coast and the Gulf of Mexico in the United States and from tropical waters around the world. Oysters are implicated in up to 90% of food-related cases. *V parahaemolyticus* causes an acute watery diarrhea with crampy abdominal pain and fever, typically occurring within 24 hours after ingestion of contaminated shellfish. The disease is self-limited, and antimicrobial therapy is usually not necessary. *V parahaemolyticus* may also cause cellulitis and sepsis, though these findings are more characteristic of *V vulnificus* infection.

V vulnificus and *V alginolyticus*—neither of which is associated with diarrheal illness—are important causes of cellulitis and primary bacteremia following ingestion of contaminated shellfish or exposure to sea water. Cellulitis with or without sepsis may be accompanied by bulla formation and necrosis with extensive soft tissue destruction, at times requiring debridement and amputation. The infection can be rapidly progressive and is particularly severe in immunocompromised individuals—especially those with cirrhosis—with death rates as high as 50%. Patients with chronic liver disease and those who are immunocompromised should be cautioned to avoid eating raw oysters.

Tetracycline at a dose of 500 mg orally four times a day for 7–10 days is the drug of choice for treatment of suspected or documented primary bacteremia or cellulitis caused by *Vibrio* species. *V vulnificus* is susceptible in vitro to penicillin, ampicillin, cephalosporins, chloramphenicol, aminoglycosides, and fluoro-quinolones, and these agents may also be effective. *V parahaemolyticus* and *V alginolyticus* produce β-lacta-mase and therefore are resistant to penicillin and ampicillin, but susceptibilities otherwise are similar to those listed for *V vulnificus*.

Centers for Disease Control and Prevention: Vibrio illnesses after Hurricane Katrina—multiple states, August–September 2005. MMWR 2005;54:928. [PMID: 16177685]

INFECTIONS CAUSED BY *CAMPYLOBACTER* SPECIES

Campylobacters are microaerophilic, motile, gram-negative rods. Two species infect humans: *Campylobacter jejuni*, an important cause of diarrheal disease, and *Campylobacter fetus* subsp *fetus*, which typically causes systemic infection and not diarrhea. Dairy cattle and poultry are an important reservoir for campylobacters. Outbreaks of enteritis have been associated with consumption of raw milk. Campylobacter gastroenteritis is associated with fever, abdominal pain, and diarrhea characterized by loose, watery, or bloody stools. The differential diagnosis includes shigellosis, salmonella gastroenteritis, and enteritis caused by *Yersinia enterocolitica* or invasive *E coli*. The disease is self-limited, but its duration can be shortened with antimicrobial therapy. Both erythromycin, 250–500 mg orally four times daily for 5–7 days, and ciprofloxacin, 500 mg orally twice daily for 3 days, are effective regimens. Pending identification of the causative agent of suspected bacterial gastroenteritis, ciprofloxacin is a rational choice for empiric therapy, although the prevalence of fluoroquinolone-resistant *Campylobacter* has been increasing with approximately 20% resistance reported for US isolates in 2001.

C fetus causes systemic infections that can be fatal, including primary bacteremia, endocarditis, meningitis, and focal abscesses. It infrequently causes gastroenteritis. Patients infected with *C fetus* are often older, debilitated, or immunocompromised. Closely related species, collectively termed "campylobacter-like organisms," cause bacteremia in HIV-infected individuals. Systemic infections respond to therapy with gentamicin, chloramphenicol, ceftriaxone, or ciprofloxacin. Ceftriaxone or chloramphenicol should be used to treat infections of the central nervous system because of their ability to penetrate the blood-brain barrier.

Lecuit M et al: Immunoproliferative small intestinal disease associated with *Campylobacter jejuni*. N Engl J Med 2004;350: 239. [PMID: 14724303]

BRUCELLOSIS

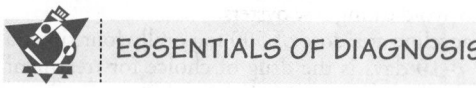

ESSENTIALS OF DIAGNOSIS

- *History of animal exposure, ingestion of unpasteurized milk or cheese.*
- *Insidious onset: easy fatigability, headache, arthralgia, anorexia, sweating, irritability.*
- *Intermittent and persistent fever.*
- *Cervical and axillary lymphadenopathy; hepatosplenomegaly.*
- *Lymphocytosis, positive blood culture, positive serologic test.*

General Considerations

The infection is transmitted from animals to humans. *Brucella abortus* (cattle), *Brucella suis* (hogs), and *Brucella melitensis* (goats) are the main agents. Transmission to humans occurs by contact with infected meat (slaughterhouse workers), placentae of infected animals (farmers, veterinarians), or ingestion of infected unpasteurized milk or cheese. The incubation period varies from a few days to several weeks. Brucellosis is a systemic infection that may become chronic. In the United States, brucellosis is very rare. Almost all US cases are imported from countries where brucellosis is endemic (eg, Mexico, Mediterranean Europe, Spain, South American countries).

Clinical Findings

A. SYMPTOMS AND SIGNS

The onset may be acute, with fever, chills, and sweats, but more often is insidious with symptoms of weakness, weight loss, low-grade fevers, sweats, and exhaustion upon minimal activity. Headache, abdominal or back pain with anorexia and constipation, and arthralgias are also common. The chronic form may assume an undulant nature, with periods of normal temperature between acute attacks; symptoms may persist for years, either continuously or intermittently.

Fever, hepatosplenomegaly, and lymphadenopathy are the most common physical findings. Infection may present with or be complicated by specific organ involvement with signs of endocarditis, meningitis, epididymitis, orchitis, arthritis (especially sacroiliitis), spondylitis, or osteomyelitis.

B. LABORATORY FINDINGS

The organism can be recovered from cultures of blood, cerebrospinal fluid, urine, bone marrow, or other sites. Modern automated systems have shortened the time to detection of the organism in blood culture. Cultures are more likely to be negative in chronic cases. The diagnosis often is made by serologic testing. Rising serologic titers or an absolute agglutination titer of greater than 1:160 supports the diagnosis.

Differential Diagnosis

Brucellosis must be differentiated from any other acute febrile disease, especially influenza, tularemia, Q fever, mononucleosis, and enteric fever. In its chronic form it resembles Hodgkin's disease, tuberculosis, HIV infection, malaria, and disseminated fungal infections such as histoplasmosis and coccidioidomycosis.

Complications

The most frequent complications are bone and joint lesions such as spondylitis and suppurative arthritis (usually of a single joint), endocarditis, and meningoencephalitis. Less common complications are pneumonitis with pleural effusion, hepatitis, and cholecystitis.

Treatment

Single-drug regimens are not recommended because the relapse rate may be as high as 50%. Combination regimens of two or three drugs are most effective. Regimens of doxycycline (200 mg/d orally for 6 weeks) plus rifampin (600 mg/d orally for 6 weeks) or streptomycin (1 g/d intramuscularly for 2–3 weeks) or gentamicin (240 mg intramuscularly once daily for 7 days) have the lowest recurrence rates. Longer courses of therapy may be required to prevent relapse of meningitis, osteomyelitis, or endocarditis.

Pappas G et al: New approaches to the antibiotic treatment of brucellosis. Int J Antimicrob Agents 2005;26:101. [PMID: 16039098]

Troy SB et al: Brucellosis in San Diego: epidemiology and species-related differences in acute clinical presentations. Medicine (Baltimore) 2005;84:1747. [PMID: 15879907]

TULAREMIA

 ESSENTIALS OF DIAGNOSIS

- *History of contact with rabbits, other rodents, and biting arthropods (eg, ticks in summer) in endemic area.*
- *Fever, headache, nausea, and prostration.*
- *Papule progressing to ulcer at site of inoculation.*
- *Enlarged regional lymph nodes.*
- *Serologic tests or culture of ulcer, lymph node aspirate, or blood confirm the diagnosis.*

General Considerations

Tularemia is a zoonotic infection of wild rodents and rabbits caused by *Francisella tularensis.* Humans usually acquire the infection by contact with animal tissues (eg, trapping muskrats, skinning rabbits) or from a tick or insect bite. Hamsters and prairie dogs also may carry the organism. An investigation of an outbreak of pneumonic tularemia on Martha's Vineyard in Massachusetts implicated lawn-mowing and brush-cutting as risk factors for infection, underscoring the

potential for probable aerosol transmission of the organism. *F tularensis* has been classified as a high-priority agent for potential bioterrorism use because of its virulence and relative ease of dissemination. Infection in humans often produces a local lesion and widespread organ involvement but may be entirely asymptomatic. The incubation period is 2–10 days.

Clinical Findings

A. SYMPTOMS AND SIGNS

Fever, headache, and nausea begin suddenly, and a local lesion—a papule at the site of inoculation—develops and soon ulcerates. Regional lymph nodes may become enlarged and tender and may suppurate. The local lesion may be on the skin of an extremity or in the eye. Pneumonia may develop from hematogenous spread of the organism or may be primary after inhalation of infected aerosols, which are responsible for human-to-human transmission. Following ingestion of infected meat or water, an enteric form may be manifested by gastrointestinal symptoms, stupor, and delirium. In any type of involvement, the spleen may be enlarged and tender and there may be nonspecific rashes, myalgias, and prostration.

B. LABORATORY FINDINGS

Culturing the organism from blood or infected tissue requires special media. For this reason and because cultures of *F tularensis* may be hazardous to laboratory personnel, the diagnosis is usually made serologically. A positive agglutination test (> 1:80) develops in the second week after infection and may persist for several years.

Differential Diagnosis

Tularemia must be differentiated from rickettsial and meningococcal infections, cat-scratch disease, infectious mononucleosis, and various bacterial and fungal diseases.

Complications

Hematogenous spread may produce meningitis, perisplenitis, pericarditis, pneumonia, and osteomyelitis.

Treatment

Streptomycin is drug of choice for treatment of tularemia. The recommended dose is 7.5 mg/kg intramuscularly every 12 hours for 7–14 days. Doxycycline (200 mg/d orally) is also effective but has a higher relapse rate. A variety of other agents (eg, fluoroquinolones) are active in vitro but their clinical effectiveness is less well established.

Centers for Disease Control and Prevention (CDC): Tularemia associated with a hamster bite—Colorado, 2004. MMWR Morb Mortal Wkly Rep 2005;53:1202. [PMID: 15635290]

PLAGUE

 ESSENTIALS OF DIAGNOSIS

- *History of exposure to rodents in endemic area.*
- *Sudden onset of high fever, malaise, muscular pains, and prostration.*
- *Axillary or inguinal lymphadenitis (bubo).*
- *Bacteremia, pneumonitis, and meningitis may occur.*
- *Positive smear and culture from bubo and positive blood culture.*

General Considerations

Plague is an infection of wild rodents with *Yersinia pestis*, a small bipolar-staining gram-negative rod. It is endemic in California, Arizona, Nevada, and New Mexico. It is transmitted among rodents and to humans by the bites of fleas or from contact with infected animals. Following a fleabite, the organisms spread through the lymphatics to the lymph nodes, which become greatly enlarged (bubo). They may then reach the bloodstream to involve all organs. When pneumonia or meningitis develops, the outcome is often fatal. The patient with pneumonia can transmit the infection to other individuals by droplets. The incubation period is 2–10 days. Because of its extreme virulence, its potential for dissemination and person-to-person transmission, and efforts to develop the organism as an agent of biowarfare, plague bacillus is considered a high-priority agent for bioterrorism.

Clinical Findings

A. SYMPTOMS AND SIGNS

The onset is sudden, with high fever, malaise, tachycardia, intense headache, delirium, and severe myalgias. The patient appears profoundly ill. If pneumonia develops, tachypnea, productive cough, blood-tinged sputum, and cyanosis also occur. There may be signs of meningitis. A pustule or ulcer at the site of inoculation and lymphangitis may be observed. Axillary, inguinal, or cervical lymph nodes become enlarged and tender and may suppurate and drain. With hematogenous spread, the patient may rapidly become toxic and comatose, with purpuric spots (black plague) appearing on the skin.

Primary plague pneumonia is a fulminant pneumonitis with bloody, frothy sputum and sepsis. It is usually fatal unless treatment is started within a few hours after onset.

B. LABORATORY FINDINGS

The plague bacillus may be found in smears from aspirates of buboes examined with Gram stain. Cultures from bubo aspirate or pus and blood are positive but may grow slowly. In convalescing patients, an antibody titer rise may be demonstrated by agglutination tests.

Differential Diagnosis

The lymphadenitis of plague is most commonly mistaken for the lymphadenitis accompanying staphylococcal or streptococcal infections of an extremity, sexually transmitted diseases such as lymphogranuloma venereum or syphilis, and tularemia. The systemic manifestations resemble those of enteric or rickettsial fevers, malaria, or influenza. The pneumonia resembles other bacterial pneumonias, and the meningitis is similar to those caused by other bacteria.

Prevention

Drug prophylaxis may provide temporary protection for persons exposed to the risk of plague infection, particularly by the respiratory route. Tetracycline hydrochloride, 500 mg orally once or twice daily for 5 days, is effective.

Plague vaccines—both live and killed—have been used for many years, but their efficacy is not clearly established.

Treatment

Therapy should be started immediately once plague is suspected. Either streptomycin (the agent with which there is greatest experience), 1 g every 12 hours intravenously, or gentamicin, administered as a 2-mg/kg loading dose, then 1.7 mg/kg every 8 hours intravenously, is effective. Alternatively, doxycycline, 100 mg orally or intravenously, may be used. The duration of therapy is 10 days. Patients with plague pneumonia are placed in strict respiratory isolation.

Boulanger LL et al: Gentamicin and tetracyclines for the treatment of human plague: review of 75 cases in New Mexico, 1985–1999. Clin Infect Dis 2004;38:663. [PMID: 14986250]

GONOCOCCAL INFECTIONS

 ESSENTIALS OF DIAGNOSIS

- *Purulent and profuse urethral discharge, especially in men, with dysuria, yielding positive smear.*
- *Epididymitis, prostatitis, periurethral inflammation, proctitis in men.*
- *Cervicitis in women with purulent discharge, or asymptomatic, yielding positive culture; vaginitis, salpingitis, proctitis also occur.*
- *Fever, rash, tenosynovitis, and arthritis with disseminated disease.*
- *Gram-negative intracellular diplococci seen in a smear or cultured from any site, particularly the urethra, cervix, pharynx, and rectum.*

General Considerations

Gonorrhea is caused by *Neisseria gonorrhoeae*, a gram-negative diplococcus typically found inside polymorphonuclear cells. It is transmitted during sexual activity and has its greatest incidence in the 15- to 29-year-old age group. The incubation period is usually 2–8 days.

Classification

A. Urethritis and Cervicitis

In men, there is initially burning on urination and a serous or milky discharge. One to 3 days later, the urethral pain is more pronounced and the discharge becomes yellow, creamy, and profuse, sometimes blood-tinged. The disorder may regress and become chronic or progress to involve the prostate, epididymis, and periurethral glands with painful inflammation. Chronic infection leads to prostatitis and urethral strictures. Rectal infection is common in homosexual men. Atypical sites of primary infection (eg, the pharynx) must always be considered. Asymptomatic infection is common and occurs in both sexes.

Gonococcal infection in women often becomes symptomatic during menses. Women may have dysuria, urinary frequency, and urgency, with a purulent urethral discharge. Vaginitis and cervicitis with inflammation of Bartholin's glands are common. Infection may be asymptomatic, with only slightly increased vaginal discharge and moderate cervicitis on examination. Infection may remain as a chronic cervicitis—an important reservoir of gonococci. It can progress to involve the uterus and tubes with acute and chronic salpingitis, with scarring of tubes and sterility. In pelvic inflammatory disease, anaerobes and chlamydiae often accompany gonococci. Rectal infection may result from spread of the organism from the genital tract or from anal coitus.

Gram stain of urethral discharge in men, especially during the first week after onset, shows gram-negative diplococci in polymorphonuclear leukocytes. Gram stain is less often positive in women. Culture has been the gold standard for diagnosis, particularly when the Gram stain is negative. Nucleic acid amplification tests that detect both *N gonorrhoeae* and *Chlamydia trachomatis* in cervical and urethral swab specimens and urine permit rapid diagnosis, have excellent sensitivity and specificity, and have largely replaced culture. Identification of *N gonorrhoeae* from rectal or pharyngeal sites, blood, and in joint fluid still requires culture.

B. Disseminated Disease

Systemic complications follow the dissemination of gonococci from the primary site via the bloodstream. Gonococcal bacteremia is associated with intermittent fever, arthralgia, and skin lesions ranging from maculopapular to pustular or hemorrhagic, which tend to be few in number and peripherally located. Rarely, gonococcal endocarditis or meningitis develops. Arthritis and tenosynovitis are common complications, particularly involving the knees, ankles, and wrists. One or occasionally a few joints usually are involved. Gonococci are isolated by culture from less than half of patients with gonococcal arthritis.

C. Conjunctivitis

The most common form of eye involvement is direct inoculation of gonococci into the conjunctival sac. In adults, this occurs by autoinoculation of a person with genital infection. The purulent conjunctivitis may rapidly progress to panophthalmitis and loss of the eye unless treated promptly. A single 1-g dose of ceftriaxone is effective.

Differential Diagnosis

Gonococcal urethritis or cervicitis must be differentiated from nongonococcal urethritis; cervicitis or vaginitis due to *C trachomatis, Gardnerella vaginalis, Trichomonas, Candida,* and many other pathogens associated with sexually transmitted diseases; and pelvic inflammatory disease, arthritis, proctitis, and skin lesions. Often, several such pathogens coexist in a patient. Reactive arthritis (urethritis, conjunctivitis, arthritis) may mimic gonorrhea or coexist with it.

Prevention

Prevention is based on education and mechanical or chemical prophylaxis. The condom, if properly used, can reduce the risk of infection. Effective drugs taken in therapeutic doses within 24 hours of exposure can abort an infection. Partner notification and referral of contacts for treatment has been the standard method used to control sexually transmitted diseases. Expedited treatment of sex partners by patient-delivered partner therapy is more effective than partner notification in reducing persistence and recurrence rates of gonorrhea and chlamydia. This strategy is being increasingly adopted as a means of disease control.

Treatment

Therapy typically is administered before antimicrobial susceptibilities are known. The choice of which regimen to use should be based on the prevalence of penicillin-resistant organisms. Nationwide, penicillin- and tetracycline-resistant gonococci have been increasingly observed. Consequently, penicillin should no longer be considered first-line therapy. All sexual partners should be treated and tested for HIV infection and syphilis, as should the patient as well.

A. Uncomplicated Gonorrhea

For urethritis or cervicitis, either ceftriaxone, 125 r intramuscularly, or cefpodoxime, 400 mg orally single dose, is the treatment of choice. Fluoroc lones are no longer recommended as first-line especially for treatment of gonorrhea in men ,ri- sex with men, because of emerging resistarfor nomycin, 1 g intramuscularly once, may the penicillin-allergic patient. Anal gonorrhea in women responds to the same drugs, but in males ceftriaxone is most effective. Pharyngeal gonorrhea is treated by ceftriaxone in the same dosage and by trimethoprim-sulfamethoxazole, nine regular-strength tablets orally daily for 5 days. Since coexistent chlamydial infection is common, doxycycline, 100 mg orally twice daily orally for 7 days, or a single 1 g oral dose of azithromycin, concurrently, should be given; women should be tested for pregnancy before any tetracycline is prescribed (see also below).

B. TREATMENT OF OTHER INFECTIONS

Salpingitis, prostatitis, bacteremia, arthritis, and other complications due to susceptible strains in adults should be treated with penicillin G, 10 million units intravenously daily, for 5 days. Ceftriaxone, 1 g intravenously daily for 5 days, or an oral fluoroquinolone (ciprofloxacin, 500 mg twice daily, or levofloxacin, 500 mg once daily) for 5 days also is effective, provided the isolate is susceptible. Endocarditis should be treated with ceftriaxone, 2 g every 24 hours intravenously, for at least 3 weeks. Postgonococcal urethritis and cervicitis, which are usually caused by chlamydia, are treated with a regimen of erythromycin, doxycycline, or azithromycin as described above.

Pelvic inflammatory disease requires cefoxitin, 2 g parenterally every 6 hours, or cefotetan, 2 g intravenously every 12 hours. Clindamycin, 900 mg intravenously every 8 hours, plus gentamicin, administered intravenously as a 2-mg/kg loading dose followed by 1.5 mg/kg every 8 hours, is also effective. Cefoxitin, 2 g intramuscularly, plus probenecid, 1 g orally as a single dose, followed by a 14-day oral regimen of doxycycline, 100 mg twice a day, is an effective outpatient regimen. Concurrent treatment for chlamydial infection also is indicated.

Centers for Disease Control and Prevention (CDC): Increases in fluoroquinolone-resistant *Neisseria gonorrhoeae* among men who have sex with men—United States, 2003, and revised recommendations for gonorrhea treatment, 2004. MMWR Morb Mortal Wkly Rep 2004;53:335. [PMID: 15123985]

Cook RL et al: Systematic review: noninvasive testing for *Chlamydia trachomatis* and *Neisseria gonorrhoeae*. Ann Intern Med 2005;142:914. [PMID: 15941699]

Golden MR et al: Effect of expedited treatment of sex partners on recurrent or persistent gonorrhea or chlamydial infection. N Engl J Med 2005;352:676. [PMID: 15716561]

Miller WC et al: Prevalence of chlamydial and gonococcal infections among young adults in the United States. JAMA 2004;291:2229. [PMID: 15138245]

CHANCROID

Chancroid is a sexually transmitted disease caused by the short gram-negative bacillus *Haemophilus ducreyi*. The incubation period is 3–5 days. At the site of inoculation, a vesicopustule develops that breaks down to a painful, soft ulcer with a necrotic base, surrounding erythema, and undermined edges. There

may be multiple lesions due to autoinoculation. The adenitis is usually unilateral and consists of tender, matted nodes of moderate size with overlying erythema. These may become fluctuant and rupture spontaneously. With lymph node involvement, fever, chills, and malaise may develop. Balanitis and phimosis are frequent complications in men. Women may have no external signs of infection. The diagnosis is established by culturing a swab of the lesion onto a special medium.

Chancroid must be differentiated from other genital ulcers. The chancre of syphilis is clean and painless, with a hard base. Mixed sexually transmitted disease is very common (including syphilis, herpes simplex, and HIV infection), as is infection of the ulcer with fusiforms, spirochetes, and other organisms.

A single dose of either azithromycin, 1 g orally, or ceftriaxone, 250 mg intramuscularly, is effective treatment. Effective multiple-dose regimens are amoxicillin-potassium clavulanate (500/125 mg) three times a day orally for 7 days, erythromycin, 500 mg orally four times a day for 7 days, or ciprofloxacin, 500 mg orally twice a day for 3 days.

GRANULOMA INGUINALE

Granuloma inguinale is a chronic, relapsing granulomatous anogenital infection due to *Calymmatobacterium (Donovania) granulomatis*. The pathognomonic cell, found in tissue scrapings or secretions, is large (25–90 mcm) and contains intracytoplasmic cysts filled with bodies (Donovan bodies) that stain deeply with Wright's stain.

The incubation period is 8 days to 12 weeks. The onset is insidious. The lesions occur on the skin or mucous membranes of the genitalia or perineal area. They are relatively painless infiltrated nodules that soon slough. A shallow, sharply demarcated ulcer forms, with a beefy-red friable base of granulation tissue. The lesion spreads by contiguity. The advancing border has a characteristic rolled edge of granulation tissue. Large ulcerations may advance onto the lower abdomen and thighs. Scar formation and healing occur along one border while the opposite border advances.

Superinfection with spirochete-fusiform organisms is common. The ulcer then becomes purulent, painful, foul-smelling, and extremely difficult to treat.

Several therapies are available. Because of the indolent nature of the disease, duration of therapy is relatively long. Erythromycin or tetracycline, 500 mg orally four times a day for 21 days, is effective. Ampicillin, 500 mg orally four times a day, is an alternative, but up to 12 weeks of therapy may be necessary.

BARTONELLA SPECIES

A revised classification of the α_2 subdivision of proteobacteria has grouped the species previously known as Rochalimaea as members of the Bartonellae based on ribosomal RNA. These organisms are responsible for a wide variety of clinical syndromes. **Bacillary angiomatosis**, an important manifestation of bartonellosis, is discussed in Chapter 31. A variety of atypical infections, including retinitis, encephalitis, osteomyelitis, and persistent bacteremia and endocarditis have been described.

Trench fever is a self-limited, louse-borne relapsing febrile disease caused by *B quintana*. The disease has occurred epidemically in louse-infested troops and civilians during wars and endemically in residents of scattered geographic areas (eg, Central America). An urban equivalent of trench fever has been described among the homeless. Humans acquire infection when infected lice feces enter sites of skin breakdown. Onset of symptoms is abrupt and fever lasts 3–5 days, with relapses. The patient complains of weakness and severe pain behind the eyes and typically in the back and legs. Lymphadenopathy, splenomegaly, and a transient maculopapular rash may appear. Subclinical infection is frequent, and a carrier state is recognized. The differential diagnosis includes other febrile, self-limited states such as dengue, leptospirosis, malaria, relapsing fever, and typhus. Recovery occurs regularly even in the absence of treatment.

Cat-scratch disease is an acute infection of children and young adults caused by *Bartonella henselae*. It is transmitted from cats to humans as the result of a scratch or bite. Within a few days, a papule or ulcer will develop at the inoculation site in one-third of patients. One to 3 weeks later, fever, headache, and malaise occur. Regional lymph nodes become enlarged, often tender, and may suppurate. Lymphadenopathy from cat scratches resembles that due to neoplasm, tuberculosis, lymphogranuloma venereum, and bacterial lymphadenitis. The diagnosis is usually made clinically. Special cultures for bartonellae, serology, or excisional biopsy, though rarely necessary, confirm the diagnosis. The biopsy reveals necrotizing lymphadenitis and is itself not specific for cat-scratch disease. Cat-scratch disease is usually self-limited, requiring no specific therapy. Encephalitis occurs rarely.

Disseminated forms of the disease—bacillary angiomatosis and peliosis hepatis—occur in HIV-infected persons. The lesions are vasculoproliferative and histopathologically distinct from those of cat-scratch disease. Unexplained fever in patients with late stages of HIV infection is not uncommonly due to bartonellosis. *B quintana*, the agent of trench fever, can also cause bacillary angiomatosis and persistent bacteremia or endocarditis (which will be "culture-negative" unless specifically sought), the latter two entities being associated with homelessness. Bacillary angiomatosis responds to treatment with a macrolide or doxycycline administered in standard doses for 4–8 weeks. Bacteremia and endocarditis can be effectively treated with a 4-week course of doxycycline (200 mg orally per day) for 4 weeks plus gentamicin 3 mg/kg/d intravenously for the first 2 weeks. Survival may be improved by the addition of gentamicin to the regimen. Relapse may occur.

Foucault C et al: Randomized open trial of gentamicin and doxycycline for eradication of *Bartonella quintana* from blood in patients with chronic bacteremia. Antimicrob Agents Chemother 2003;47:2204. [PMID: 12821469]

Koehler JE et al: Prevalence of *Bartonella* infection among human immunodeficiency virus-infected patients with fever. Clin Infect Dis 2003;37:559. [PMID: 12905141]

ANAEROBIC INFECTIONS

Anaerobic bacteria comprise the majority of normal human flora. Normal microbial flora of the mouth (anaerobic spirochetes, prevotella, fusobacteria), the skin (anaerobic diphtheroids), the large bowel (bacteroides, anaerobic streptococci, clostridia), and the female tract (bacteroides, anaerobic streptococci, fusobacteria) produce disease when displaced from their normal sites into tissues or closed body spaces.

Anaerobic infections tend to be polymicrobial and abscesses are common. Pus and infected tissue often are malodorous. Septic thrombophlebitis and metastatic infection are frequent and may require incision and drainage. Diminished blood supply that favors proliferation of anaerobes because of reduced tissue oxygenation may interfere with the delivery of antimicrobials to the site of anaerobic infection. Cultures unless carefully collected under anaerobic conditions may yield negative results.

Important types of infections that are most commonly caused by anaerobic organisms are listed below. Treatment of all these infections consists of surgical exploration and judicious excision in conjunction with administration of antimicrobial drugs.

Upper Respiratory Tract

Prevotella melaninogenica (formerly *Bacteroides melaninogenicus*) and anaerobic spirochetes are commonly involved in periodontal infections. These organisms, fusobacteria, and peptostreptococci may cause chronic sinusitis, peritonsillar abscess, chronic otitis media, and mastoiditis. Hygiene, drainage, and surgical debridement are as important in treatment as antimicrobials. Oral anaerobic organisms have been uniformly susceptible to penicillin, but there has been a recent trend of increasing penicillin resistance, usually due to β-lactamase production. Penicillin, 1–2 million units intravenously every 4 hours (if parenteral therapy is required) or 0.5 g orally four times daily for less severe infections, or clindamycin can be used (600 mg intravenously every 8 hours or 300 mg orally every 6 hours). Antimicrobial treatment is continued for a few days after signs and symptoms of infection have resolved. Indolent, established infections (eg, mastoiditis or osteomyelitis) may require prolonged courses of therapy, eg, 4–6 weeks or longer.

Chest Infections

Usually in the setting of poor oral hygiene and periodontal disease, aspiration of saliva (which contains

10^8 anaerobic organisms per milliliter in addition to aerobes) may lead to necrotizing pneumonia, lung abscess, and empyema. While polymicrobial infection is the rule, anaerobes—particularly *P melaninogenica*, fusobacteria, and peptostreptococci—are common etiologic agents. Most pulmonary infections respond to antimicrobial therapy alone. Percutaneous chest tube or surgical drainage is indicated for empyema.

Penicillin-resistant *Bacteroides fragilis* and *P melaninogenica* are commonly isolated and have been associated with clinical failures. Clindamycin, 600 mg intravenously once, followed by 300 mg orally every 6–8 hours, is the treatment of choice for these infections. Penicillin, 2 million units intravenously every 4 hours, followed by amoxicillin, 500 mg every 8 hours orally, is a reasonable alternative. Metronidazole does not cover facultative streptococci, which often are present. These infections respond slowly. A duration of 3–4 weeks or more of antimicrobial therapy is typical. The second-generation cephalosporins cefoxitin, cefotetan, and cefmetazole are active in vitro against anaerobes, including those that are penicillin-resistant.

Central Nervous System

Anaerobes are a common cause of brain abscess, subdural empyema, or septic central nervous system thrombophlebitis. The organisms reach the central nervous system by direct extension from sinusitis, otitis, or mastoiditis or by hematogenous spread from chronic lung infections. Antimicrobial therapy—eg, penicillin, 20 million units intravenously, in combination with metronidazole, 750 mg intravenously, every 8 hours—is an important adjunct to surgical drainage. Duration of therapy is 6–8 weeks. Some small multiple brain abscesses can be treated with antibiotics alone without surgical drainage. Alternatively, septic internal jugular thrombophlebitis (Lemierre's syndrome) originates from mouth anaerobes and may cause septic pulmonary embolization. Severe sore throat is a concomitant.

Intra-abdominal Infections

In the colon there are up to 10^{11} anaerobes per gram of content—predominantly *B fragilis*, clostridia, and peptostreptococci. These organisms play a central role in most intra-abdominal abscesses following trauma to the colon, diverticulitis, appendicitis, or perirectal abscess and may also participate in hepatic abscess and cholecystitis, often in association with aerobic coliform bacteria. The gallbladder wall can be infected with clostridia as well. The bacteriology includes anaerobes as well as enteric gram-negative rods and on occasion enterococci. Therapy should be directed both against anaerobes and gram-negative aerobes. Agents that are reliably active against *B fragilis* include metronidazole, chloramphenicol, imipenem, ampicillin-sulbactam, ticarcillin-clavulanic acid, and piperacillin-tazobactam. Resistance to cefoxitin, cefotetan, and

Table 33–6. Treatment of anaerobic intra-abdominal infections.

Oral therapy
Moxifloxacin 400 mg every 24 hours
Intravenous therapy
Moderate to moderately severe infections:
Ertapenem 1 g every 24 hours
or—
Cefotetan, 2 g every 12 hours
or—
Moxifloxacin 400 mg every 24 hours
Severe infections:
Imipenem, 0.5 g every 6–8 hours; or ceftriaxone, 1 g every 24 hours, plus metronidazole, 500 mg every 8 hours; or piperacillin/tazobactam 4.5 g every 8 hours.

clindamycin is increasingly encountered. Most third-generation cephalosporins have poor efficacy. Non-fragilis species of bacteroides may be less susceptible to the cephalosporins.

Table 33–6 summarizes the antibiotic regimens for management of moderate to moderately severe infections (eg, patient hemodynamically stable, good surgical drainage possible or established, low APACHE score, no multiple organ failure) and severe infections (eg, major peritoneal soilage, large or multiple abscesses, patient hemodynamically unstable), particularly if drug-resistant organisms are suspected. An effective oral regimen for patients able to take it is presented also.

Female Genital Tract & Pelvic Infections

The normal flora of the vagina and cervix includes several species of bacteroides, peptostreptococci, group B streptococci, lactobacilli, coliform bacteria, and, occasionally, spirochetes and clostridia. These organisms commonly cause genital tract infections and may disseminate from there.

While salpingitis is often caused by gonococci and chlamydiae, tubo-ovarian and pelvic abscesses are associated with anaerobes in most cases. Postpartum infections may be caused by aerobic streptococci or staphylococci, but anaerobes are often found, and the worst cases of postpartum or postabortion sepsis are associated with clostridia and bacteroides. These have a high mortality rate, and treatment requires both antimicrobials directed against anaerobes and coliforms (see above) and abscess drainage or early hysterectomy.

Bacteremia & Endocarditis

Anaerobic bacteremia usually originates from the gastrointestinal tract, the oropharynx, decubitus ulcers, or the female genital tract. Endocarditis due to anaerobic and microaerophilic streptococci and bacteroides originates from the same sites. Most cases of anaerobic or microaerophilic streptococcal endocarditis can be effectively treated with 12–20 million units of penicillin G daily for 4–6 weeks, but optimal therapy of other types of anaerobic bacterial endocarditis must rely on laboratory guidance. Anaerobic corynebacteria (propionibacteria), clostridia, and bacteroides occasionally cause endocarditis.

Skin & Soft Tissue Infections

Anaerobic infections in the skin and soft tissue usually follow trauma, inadequate blood supply, or surgery and are most common in areas that are contaminated by oral or fecal flora. These infections also occur in injection drug users and persons sustaining animal to human bites. There may be progressive tissue necrosis and a putrid odor.

Several terms, such as bacterial synergistic gangrene, synergistic necrotizing cellulitis, necrotizing fasciitis, and nonclostridial crepitant cellulitis, have been used to classify these infections. Although there are some differences in microbiology among them, their differentiation on clinical grounds alone is difficult. All are mixed infections caused by aerobic and anaerobic organisms and require aggressive surgical debridement of necrotic tissue for cure. Surgical consultation is obligatory to assist in diagnosis and treatment.

Broad-spectrum antibiotics active against both anaerobes and gram-positive and gram-negative aerobes (eg, vancomycin plus piperacillin-tazobactam or ceftriaxone plus metronidazole) should be instituted empirically and modified by culture results (see Table 37–2). They are given for about a week after progressive tissue destruction has been controlled and the margins of the wound remain free of inflammation.

Talan DA et al: Clinical presentation and bacteriologic analysis of infected human bites in patients presenting to emergency departments. Clin Infect Dis 2003;37:1481. [PMID: 14614671]

■ ACTINOMYCOSIS

 ESSENTIALS OF DIAGNOSIS

- *History of recent dental infection or abdominal trauma.*
- *Chronic pneumonia or indolent intra-abdominal or cervicofacial abscess.*
- *Sinus tract formation.*

General Considerations

Actinomyces israelii and other species of *Actinomyces* occur in the normal flora of the mouth and tonsillar crypts. They are anaerobic, gram-positive, branching filamentous bacteria (1 mcm in diameter) that may fragment into bacillary forms. When introduced into traumatized tissue and associated with other anaerobic bacteria, these actinomycetes become pathogens.

The most common site of infection is the cervicofacial area (about 60% of cases). Infection typically follows extraction of a tooth or other trauma. Lesions may develop in the gastrointestinal tract or lungs following ingestion or aspiration of the organism from its endogenous source in the mouth. Interestingly, *T whippelii*, the causative agent of Whipple's disease, is an actinomycete and therefore is related to the species that cause actinomycosis.

Clinical Findings

A. SYMPTOMS AND SIGNS

1. Cervicofacial actinomycosis—Cervicofacial actinomycosis develops slowly. The area becomes markedly indurated, and the overlying skin becomes reddish or cyanotic. Abscesses eventually draining to the surface persist for long periods. Sulfur granules—masses of filamentous organisms—may be found in the pus. There is usually little pain unless there is secondary infection. Trismus indicates that the muscles of mastication are involved. Radiography may reveal bony involvement.

2. Thoracic actinomycosis—Thoracic involvement begins with fever, cough, and sputum production with night sweats and weight loss. Pleuritic pain may be present. Multiple sinuses may extend through the chest wall, to the heart, or into the abdominal cavity. Ribs may be involved. Radiography shows areas of consolidation and in many cases pleural effusion. Cervicofacial or thoracic disease may occasionally involve the central nervous system, most commonly brain abscess or meningitis.

3. Abdominal actinomycosis—Abdominal actinomycosis usually causes pain in the ileocecal region, spiking fever and chills, vomiting, and weight loss; it may be confused with Crohn's disease. Irregular abdominal masses may be palpated. Pelvic inflammatory disease caused by actinomycetes has been associated with prolonged use of an intrauterine contraceptive device. Sinuses draining to the exterior may develop. CT scanning reveals an inflammatory mass extended to involve bone.

B. LABORATORY FINDINGS

The anaerobic, gram-positive organism may be demonstrated as a granule or as scattered branching gram-positive filaments in the pus. Anaerobic culture is necessary to distinguish actinomycetes from nocardiae because specific therapy differs for the two infections.

Treatment

Penicillin G is the drug of choice. Ten to 20 million units are given via a parenteral route for 4–6 weeks, followed by oral penicillin V, 500 mg four times daily. Alternatives include ampicillin, 12 g/d intravenously for 4–6 weeks followed by oral amoxicillin 500 mg three times daily. Response to therapy is slow. Therapy should be continued for weeks to months after clinical manifestations have disappeared in order to ensure cure. Surgical procedures such as drainage and resection may be beneficial.

With penicillin and surgery, the prognosis is good. The difficulties of diagnosis, however, may permit extensive destruction of tissue before the diagnosis is identified and therapy is started.

Sudhakar SS et al: Short-term treatment of actinomycosis: two cases and a review. Clin Infect Dis 2004;38:444. [PMID: 14727221]

Wagenlehner FM et al: Abdominal actinomycosis. Clin Microbiol Infect 2003;9:881. [PMID: 14616714]

■ NOCARDIOSIS

Nocardia asteroides, an aerobic filamentous soil bacterium, causes pulmonary and systemic nocardiosis. Bronchopulmonary abnormalities (eg, alveolar proteinosis) predispose to colonization, but infection is unusual unless the patient is also receiving systemic corticosteroids or is otherwise immunosuppressed.

Pulmonary involvement usually begins with malaise, loss of weight, fever, and night sweats. Cough and production of purulent sputum are the chief complaints. Radiography may show infiltrates accompanied by pleural effusion. The lesions may penetrate to the exterior through the chest wall, invading the ribs.

Dissemination involves any organ. Brain abscesses and subcutaneous nodules are most frequent. This is seen exclusively in immunocompromised patients.

N asteroides is usually found as delicate, branching, gram-positive filaments. It may be weakly acid-fast, occasionally causing diagnostic confusion with tuberculosis. Identification is made by culture.

Therapy is initiated with intravenous trimethoprim-sulfamethoxazole administered at a dosage of 5–10 mg/kg/d (trimethoprim) and continued with oral trimethoprim-sulfamethoxazole, one double-strength tablet twice a day. Surgical procedures such as drainage and resection may be needed as adjunctive therapy.

Response may be slow, and therapy must be continued for at least 6 months. The prognosis in systemic nocardiosis is poor when diagnosis and therapy are delayed.

Nocardia brasiliensis typically causes a digital lesion—resembling herpetic whitlow—and ascending lymphangitis in normal hosts. Antimicrobial treatment is as for *N asteroides* infection, and the prognosis is excellent.

Lederman ER et al: A case series and focused review of nocardiosis: clinical and microbiologic aspects. Medicine (Baltimore) 2004;83:300. [PMID: 15342974]

■ INFECTIONS CAUSED BY MYCOBACTERIA

NONTUBERCULOUS ATYPICAL MYCOBACTERIAL DISEASES

About 10% of mycobacterial infections are caused by atypical mycobacteria. Atypical mycobacterial infections are among the most common opportunistic infections in advanced HIV disease. These organisms have distinctive laboratory characteristics, occur ubiquitously in the environment, are not communicable from person to person, and are often resistant to standard antituberculous drugs.

Disseminated *Mycobacterium avium* Infection

Mycobacterium avium complex (MAC) produces asymptomatic colonization or a wide spectrum of diseases, including coin lesions, bronchitis in patients with chronic lung disease, and invasive pulmonary disease that is often cavitary and occurs in patients with underlying lung disease. MAC causes disseminated disease in the late stages of HIV infection, when the CD4 cell count is less than 50/mcL. Persistent fever and weight loss are the most common symptoms. The organism can usually be cultured from multiple sites, including blood, liver, lymph node, or bone marrow. Blood culture is the preferred means of establishing the diagnosis and has a sensitivity of 98%.

Agents with proved activity against MAC are rifabutin, azithromycin, clarithromycin, and ethambutol. Amikacin and ciprofloxacin work in vitro, but clinical results are inconsistent. A combination of two or more active agents should be used to prevent rapid emergence of secondary resistance. Clarithromycin, 500 mg orally twice daily, plus ethambutol, 15 mg/kg/d orally as a single dose, with or without rifabutin, 300 mg/d orally, is the treatment of choice. Azithromycin, 500 mg orally once daily, may be used instead of clarithromycin. Insufficient data are available to permit specific recommendations about second-line regimens for patients intolerant of macrolides or those with macrolide-resistant organisms. MAC therapy may be discontinued in patients who have been treated with 12 months of therapy for disseminated MAC, who have no evidence of active disease, and whose CD4 counts exceed 100 cells/mcL while receiving highly active antiretroviral therapy (HAART). Antimicrobial prophylaxis of MAC prevents disseminated disease and prolongs survival. It is the standard of care to offer it to all HIV-infected patients with CD4 counts ≤ 50/mcL. In contrast to active infection, single-drug oral regimens of clarithromycin, 500 mg twice daily, azithromycin, 1200 mg once weekly, or rifabutin, 300 mg once daily, are appropriate. Clarithromycin or azithromycin is more effective and better tolerated than rifabutin, and therefore preferred. Primary prophylaxis for MAC infection can be stopped in patients who have responded to antiretroviral combination therapy with elevation of CD4 counts above 100 cells/mcL for 3 months.

Pulmonary Infections

MAC causes a chronic, slowly progressive pulmonary infection resembling tuberculosis in immunocompetent patients, who typically have underlying pulmonary disease.

Treatment of immunocompetent patients with pulmonary infection is empiric and based entirely on anecdotal data. A combination of agents is probably best. Rifampin, 600 mg orally once daily, plus ethambutol, 15–25 mg/kg/d orally, plus streptomycin, 1 g intramuscularly three to five times a week for the first 4–6 months, have been used. The role of rifabutin, fluoroquinolones, and the macrolides is not known, but based on their excellent efficacy in immunocompromised AIDS patients, they may actually be more effective than the relatively weak agents traditionally used in immunocompetent patients. Clarithromycin is a very potent drug in the treatment of MAC in AIDS patients. Based on this, inclusion of clarithromycin in the initial treatment regimen of immunocompetent patients is prudent. Therapy is continued for a total of 18–24 months.

Mycobacterium kansasii can produce clinical disease resembling tuberculosis, but the illness progresses more slowly. Most such infections occur in patients with preexisting lung disease, though 40% of patients have no known pulmonary disease. Microbiologically, *M kansasii* is similar to *Mycobacterium tuberculosis* and is sensitive to the same drugs except pyrazinamide, to which it is resistant. Therapy with isoniazid, ethambutol, and rifampin for 2 years (or 1 year after sputum conversion) has been successful.

Less common causes of pulmonary disease include *Mycobacterium xenopi*, *Mycobacterium szulgai*, and *Mycobacterium gordonae*. These organisms have variable sensitivities, and treatment is based on results of sensitivity tests. *Mycobacterium fortuitum* and *Mycobacterium chelonei* also can cause pneumonia in the occasional patient.

Lymphadenitis

Most cases of lymphadenitis (scrofula) in adults are caused by *M tuberculosis* and can be a manifestation of disseminated disease. In children, the majority of cases are due to nontuberculous mycobacterial species, with *Mycobacterium scrofulaceum* and MAC being the most common. *M kansasii*, *Mycobacterium bovis*, *M chelonei*, and *M fortuitum* are less commonly observed. Unlike disease caused by *M tuberculosis*, which requires systemic therapy for 6 months, infection with nontuberculous mycobacteria can be successfully treated by surgical excision without antituberculous therapy.

Skin & Soft Tissue Infections

Skin and soft tissue infections such as abscesses, septic arthritis, and osteomyelitis can result from direct inoculation or hematogenous dissemination or may occur as a complication of surgery.

M chelonei and *M fortuitum* are frequent causes of this type of infection. Most cases occur in the extremities and initially present as nodules. Ulceration with abscess formation often follows. The organisms are resistant to the usual antituberculous drugs but may be sensitive to a variety of antibiotics, including erythromycin, doxycycline, amikacin, cefoxitin, sulfonamides, imipenem, and ciprofloxacin. Therapy includes surgical debridement along with drug therapy. Initially, parenteral drugs are given for several weeks, and this is followed by an oral regimen to which the organism is sensitive. The duration of therapy is variable but usually continues for several months after the soft tissue lesions have healed.

Mycobacterium marinum infection ("swimming pool granuloma") presents as a nodular skin lesion following exposure to nonchlorinated water. The lesions respond to therapy with doxycycline, minocycline, or trimethoprim-sulfamethoxazole.

Mycobacterium ulcerans infection (Buruli ulcer) is seen mainly in Africa and Australia and produces a large ulcerative lesion. Therapy consists of surgical excision and skin grafting.

Kaplan JE et al: Guidelines for preventing opportunistic infections among HIV-infected persons—2002. Recommendations of the U.S. Public Health Service and the Infectious Diseases Society of America. MMWR Recomm Rep 2002; 51(RR-8):1. [PMID: 12081007]

Karakousis PC et al: *Mycobacterium avium* complex in patients with HIV infection in the era of highly active antiretroviral therapy. Lancet Infect Dis 2004;4:557. [PMID: 15336223]

MYCOBACTERIUM TUBERCULOSIS INFECTIONS

Tuberculosis is discussed in Chapter 9. Further information and expert consultation can be obtained from the Francis J. Curry National Tuberculosis Center at the Web site http://www.nationaltbcenter.edu or, by phone, 415-502-4600, or fax, 415-502-4620.

TUBERCULOUS MENINGITIS

 ESSENTIALS OF DIAGNOSIS

- *Gradual onset of listlessness, irritability, and anorexia.*
- *Headache, vomiting, and seizures common.*
- *Cranial nerve abnormalities typical.*
- *Tuberculosis focus may be evident elsewhere.*
- *Cerebrospinal fluid shows several hundred lymphocytes, low glucose, and high protein.*

General Considerations

Tuberculous meningitis is caused by rupture of a meningeal tuberculoma resulting from earlier hematogenous seeding of tubercle bacilli from a pulmonary focus, or it may be a consequence of miliary spread.

Clinical Findings

A. SYMPTOMS AND SIGNS

The onset is usually gradual, with listlessness, irritability, anorexia, and fever, followed by headache, vomiting, convulsions, and coma. In older patients, headache and behavioral changes are prominent early symptoms. Nuchal rigidity and cranial nerve palsies occur as the meningitis progresses. Evidence of active tuberculosis elsewhere or a history of prior tuberculosis is present in up to 75% of patients.

B. LABORATORY FINDINGS

The spinal fluid is frequently yellowish, with increased pressure, 100–500 cells/mcL (predominantly lymphocytes, though neutrophils may be present early during infection), increased protein, and decreased glucose. Acid-fast stains of cerebrospinal fluid usually are negative, and cultures also may be negative in 15–25% of cases. Nucleic acid amplification tests for rapid diagnosis of tuberculosis have variable sensitivity and specificity and none are FDA-approved for use in meningitis. Chest x-ray often reveals abnormalities compatible with tuberculosis but may be normal.

Differential Diagnosis

Tuberculous meningitis may be confused with any other type of meningitis, but the gradual onset, the predominantly lymphocytic pleocytosis of the spinal fluid, and evidence of tuberculosis elsewhere often point to the diagnosis. The tuberculin skin test is usually (not always) positive. Fungal and other granulomatous meningitides, syphilis, and carcinomatous meningitis are in the differential diagnosis.

Complications

Complications of tuberculous meningitis include seizure disorders, cranial nerve palsies, stroke, and obstructive hydrocephalus with impaired cognitive function. These result from inflammatory exudate primarily involving the basilar meninges and arteries.

Treatment

Presumptive diagnosis followed by early, empiric antituberculous therapy is essential for survival and to minimize sequelae. Even if cultures are not positive, a full course of therapy is warranted if the clinical setting is suggestive of tuberculous meningitis.

Regimens that are effective for pulmonary tuberculosis are effective also for tuberculous meningitis (see Table 9–14). Rifampin, isoniazid, and pyrazinamide all penetrate into cerebrospinal fluid well. The penetration of ethambutol is more variable, but therapeutic concentrations can be achieved, and the drug has been successfully used for meningitis. Aminoglycosides penetrate less well. Regimens that do not include both isoniazid and rifampin may be effective but are less reliable and generally must be given for longer periods.

Some authorities recommend the addition of corticosteroids for patients with focal deficits or altered mental status. Dexamethasone, 0.15 mg/kg intravenously or orally four times daily for 1–2 weeks, then discontinued in a tapering regimen over 4 weeks, may be used.

Johansen IS et al: Improved sensitivity of nucleic acid amplification for rapid diagnosis of tuberculous meningitis. J Clin Microbiol 2004;42:3036. [PMID: 15243056]

Thwaites GE et al: Diagnosis of adult tuberculous meningitis by use of clinical and laboratory features. Lancet 2002;360: 1287. [PMID: 12414204]

LEPROSY

 ESSENTIALS OF DIAGNOSIS

- Pale, anesthetic macular—or nodular and erythematous—skin lesions.
- Superficial nerve thickening with associated anesthesia.
- History of residence in endemic area in childhood.
- Acid-fast bacilli in skin lesions or nasal scrapings, or characteristic histologic nerve changes.

General Considerations

Leprosy is a chronic infectious disease caused by the acid-fast rod *Mycobacterium leprae*. The mode of transmission probably is respiratory and involves prolonged exposure in childhood. The disease is endemic in tropical and subtropical Asia, Africa, Central and South America, and the Pacific regions, and rarely seen sporadically in the southern United States.

Clinical Findings

A. SYMPTOMS AND SIGNS

The onset is insidious. The lesions involve the cooler body tissues: skin, superficial nerves, nose, pharynx, larynx, eyes, and testicles. Skin lesions may occur as pale, anesthetic macular lesions 1–10 cm in diameter; discrete erythematous, infiltrated nodules 1–5 cm in diameter; or diffuse skin infiltration. Neurologic disturbances are caused by nerve infiltration and thickening, with resultant anesthesia, and motor abnormalities. Bilateral ulnar neuropathy is highly suggestive. In untreated cases, disfigurement due to the skin infiltration and nerve involvement may be extreme, leading to trophic ulcers, bone resorption, and loss of digits.

The disease is divided clinically and by laboratory tests into two distinct types: lepromatous and tuberculoid. The **lepromatous** type occurs in persons with defective cellular immunity. The course is progressive and malignant, with nodular skin lesions; slow, symmetric nerve involvement; abundant acid-fast bacilli in the skin lesions; and a negative lepromin skin test. In the **tuberculoid** type, cellular immunity is intact and the course is more benign and less progressive, with macular skin lesions, severe asymmetric nerve involvement of sudden onset with few bacilli present in the lesions, and a positive lepromin skin test. Intermediate ("borderline") cases are frequent. Eye involvement (keratitis and iridocyclitis), nasal ulcers, epistaxis, anemia, and lymphadenopathy may occur.

B. LABORATORY FINDINGS

Laboratory confirmation of leprosy requires the demonstration of acid-fast bacilli in a skin biopsy. Biopsy of skin or of a thickened involved nerve also gives a typical histologic picture. *M leprae* does not grow in artificial media but does grow in the foot pads of armadillos.

Differential Diagnosis

The skin lesions of leprosy often resemble those of lupus erythematosus, sarcoidosis, syphilis, erythema nodosum, erythema multiforme, cutaneous tuberculosis, and vitiligo.

Complications

Renal failure and hepatomegaly from secondary amyloidosis may occur with longstanding disease.

Treatment

Combination therapy is recommended for treatment of all types of leprosy. Single-drug treatment is accompanied by emergence of resistance, and primary resistance to dapsone also occurs. For borderline and lepromatous cases, a three-drug regimen such as dapsone, 50–100 mg/d, clofazimine, 50 mg/d, and rifampin, 10 mg/kg/d (up to 600 mg/d), all given orally, should be used. The triple-drug combination should be administered for a minimum of 2–3 years and, ideally, until all biopsies are negative for acid-fast bacilli. For indeterminate and tuberculoid leprosy, the dapsone-rifampin combination is recommended for 6–12 months, often followed by a course of dapsone alone for 2 or more years.

Two reactional states—erythema nodosum leprosum and reversal reactions—may occur as a consequence of therapy. The reversal reaction, typical of borderline lepromatous leprosy, probably results from enhanced host immunity. Skin lesions and nerves become swollen and tender, but systemic manifestations are not seen. Erythema nodosum leprosum, typical of lepromatous leprosy, is a consequence of immune injury from antigen-antibody complex deposition in skin and other tissues; in addition to skin and nerve manifestations, fever and systemic involvement may be seen. Prednisone, 60 mg/d orally, or thalidomide, 300 mg/d orally (in the nonpregnant patient only), is effective for erythema nodosum leprosum. Improvement is expected within a few days after initiating prednisone, and thereafter the dose may be tapered over several weeks to avoid recurrence. Thalidomide is also tapered over several weeks to a 100-mg bedtime dose. Erythema nodosum leprosum is usually confined to the first year of therapy, and prednisone or thalidomide can be discontinued. Thalidomide is ineffective for reversal reactions, and prednisone, 60 mg/d, is indicated. Reversal reactions tend to recur, and the dose of prednisone should be slowly tapered over weeks to months. Therapy for leprosy should not be discontinued during treatment of reactional states.

Britton WJ et al: Leprosy. Lancet 2004;363:1209. [PMID: 15081655]

■ INFECTIONS CAUSED BY CHLAMYDIAE

Chlamydiae are a large group of obligate intracellular parasites closely related to gram-negative bacteria. They are assigned to three species—*C trachomatis, Chlamydia psittaci*, and *Chlamydia pneumoniae*—on the basis of intracellular inclusions, sulfonamide susceptibility, antigenic composition, and disease production. *C trachomatis* causes many different human infections involving the eye (trachoma, inclusion conjunctivitis), the genital tract (lymphogranuloma venereum, nongonococcal urethritis, cervicitis, salpingitis), or the respiratory tract (pneumonitis). *C psittaci* causes psittacosis in humans and many animal diseases. *C pneumoniae* has recently been recognized as a cause of respiratory tract infections.

CHLAMYDIA TRACHOMATIS INFECTIONS

1. Lymphogranuloma Venereum

 ESSENTIALS OF DIAGNOSIS

- *Evanescent primary genital lesion.*
- *Lymph node enlargement, softening, and suppuration, with draining sinuses.*
- *Proctitis and rectal stricture in women or homosexual men.*
- *Positive complement fixation test.*

General Considerations

Lymphogranuloma venereum is an acute and chronic sexually transmitted disease caused by *C trachomatis* types L1–L3. The disease is acquired during intercourse or through contact with contaminated exudate from active lesions. The incubation period is 5–21 days. After the genital lesion disappears, the infection spreads to lymph channels and lymph nodes of the genital and rectal areas. Inapparent infections and latent disease are not uncommon.

Clinical Findings

A. SYMPTOMS AND SIGNS

In men, the initial vesicular or ulcerative lesion (on the external genitalia) is evanescent and often goes unnoticed. Inguinal buboes appear 1–4 weeks after exposure, are often bilateral, and have a tendency to fuse, soften, and break down to form multiple draining sinuses, with extensive scarring. In women, the genital lymph drainage is to the perirectal glands. Early anorectal manifestations are proctitis with tenesmus and bloody purulent discharge; late manifestations are chronic cicatrizing inflammation of the rectal and perirectal tissue. These changes lead to obstipation and rectal stricture and, occasionally, rectovaginal and perianal fistulas. They are also seen in homosexual men.

B. LABORATORY FINDINGS

The complement fixation test may be positive, but cross-reaction with other chlamydiae occurs. Although a positive reaction may reflect remote infection, high titers usually indicate active disease. Specific immunofluorescence tests for IgM are more specific for acute infection.

Differential Diagnosis

The early lesion of lymphogranuloma venereum must be differentiated from the lesions of syphilis, genital herpes, and chancroid; lymph node involvement must be distinguished from that due to tularemia, tuberculosis, plague, neoplasm, or pyogenic infection; and rectal stricture must be distinguished from that due to neoplasm and ulcerative colitis.

Treatment

The antibiotic of choice is doxycycline (contraindicated in pregnancy), 100 mg orally twice daily for 21 days. Erythromycin, 500 mg four times a day for 21 days, is also effective.

2. Chlamydial Urethritis & Cervicitis

C trachomatis immunotypes D–K are isolated in about 50% of cases of nongonococcal urethritis and cervicitis by appropriate techniques. In other cases, *Ureaplasma urealyticum* can be grown as a possible etiologic agent. *C*

trachomatis is an important cause of postgonococcal urethritis. Coinfection with gonococci and chlamydiae is common, and postgonococcal (ie, chlamydial) urethritis may persist after successful treatment of the gonococcal component. Occasionally, epididymitis, prostatitis, or proctitis is caused by chlamydial infection.

Females infected with chlamydiae may be asymptomatic or may have signs and symptoms of cervicitis, salpingitis, or pelvic inflammatory disease. Chlamydiae are a leading cause of infertility in females in the United States.

The diagnosis of chlamydial infection has been clinical because *C trachomatis* is difficult and expensive to culture. The urethral or cervical discharge tends to be less painful, less purulent, and watery in chlamydial versus gonococcal infection. A patient with urethritis or cervicitis and absence of gram-negative diplococci on Gram stain and of *N gonorrhoeae* on culture is assumed to have chlamydial infection. Direct immunofluorescence assay, enzyme-linked immunoassay, and a DNA probe test, although less sensitive than culture, are sometimes used to confirm the diagnosis and for screening. The ligase chain reaction (LCR) test for *C trachomatis* has superior sensitivity compared with all other methods (eg, sensitivity of 60–70% for DNA probe versus 90–95% for LCR). LCR also has excellent specificity, approaching 100%, and it can be performed on urine. For these reasons, it will probably replace all other methods for diagnosis of chlamydial urethritis and cervicitis.

Therapy often must be given presumptively. Sexual partners of infected patients should also be treated. Recommended regimens are a single oral 1-g dose of azithromycin or 100 mg of doxycycline orally for 7 days (contraindicated in pregnancy). Erythromycin, 500 mg (not the estolate form, which is contraindicated) orally four times a day for 7 days, is recommended for the pregnant patient, although the 1-g dose of azithromycin is also safe and appears to be effective. As for all sexually transmitted diseases, studies for HIV and syphilis should be performed.

Sexually transmitted diseases treatment guidelines 2002. Centers for Disease Control and Prevention. MMWR Recomm Rep 2002;51(RR-6):1. [PMID: 12184549]

CHLAMYDIA PSITTACI & PSITTACOSIS (Ornithosis)

 ESSENTIALS OF DIAGNOSIS

- *Fever, chills, and cough; headache common.*
- *Atypical pneumonia with slightly delayed appearance of signs of pneumonitis.*
- *Contact with infected bird (psittacine, pigeons, many others) 7–15 days previously.*
- *Isolation of chlamydiae or rising titer of complement-fixing antibodies.*

General Considerations

Psittacosis is acquired from contact with birds (parrots, parakeets, pigeons, chickens, ducks, and many others), which may or may not be ill. The history may be difficult to obtain if the patient acquired infection from an illegally imported bird.

Clinical Findings

The onset is usually rapid, with fever, chills, myalgia, dry cough, and headache. Signs include temperature-pulse dissociation, dullness to percussion, and rales. Pulmonary findings may be absent early. Dyspnea and cyanosis may occur later. Endocarditis, which is culture-negative, may occur. The radiographic findings in typical psittacosis are those of atypical pneumonia, which tends to be interstitial and diffuse in appearance, though consolidation can occur. Psittacosis is indistinguishable from other bacterial or viral pneumonias by radiography.

The organism is rarely isolated from cultures. The diagnosis is usually made serologically; antibodies appear during the second week and can be demonstrated by complement fixation or immunofluorescence. Antibody response may be suppressed by early chemotherapy.

Differential Diagnosis

The illness is indistinguishable from viral, mycoplasmal, or other atypical pneumonias except for the history of contact with birds. Psittacosis is in the differential diagnosis of culture-negative endocarditis.

Treatment

Treatment consists of giving tetracycline, 0.5 g orally every 6 hours or 0.5 g intravenously every 12 hours, for 14–21 days. Erythromycin may be effective as well.

CHLAMYDIA PNEUMONIAE INFECTION

C pneumoniae causes pneumonia and bronchitis and has been associated seroepidemiologically with coronary artery disease. The clinical presentation of pneumonia is that of an atypical pneumonia. The organism accounts for approximately 10% of community-acquired pneumonias, ranking second to mycoplasma as an agent of atypical pneumonia. Its putative role in coronary artery disease remains to be defined.

Like *C psittaci*, strains of *C pneumoniae* are resistant to sulfonamides. Erythromycin or tetracycline, 500 mg orally four times a day for 10–14 days, appears to be effective therapy. Fluoroquinolones such as levofloxacin or trovafloxacin are active in vitro against *C pneumoniae* and probably are effective clinically. The oral dose of levofloxacin is 500 mg once a day for 10–14 days.

Kalayoglu MV et al: *Chlamydia pneumoniae* as an emerging risk factor in cardiovascular disease. JAMA 2002;288:2724. [PMID: 12460096]

Infectious Diseases: Spirochetal

Richard A. Jacobs, MD, PhD

34

■ SYPHILIS

NATURAL HISTORY & PRINCIPLES OF DIAGNOSIS & TREATMENT

Syphilis is a complex infectious disease caused by *Treponema pallidum*, a spirochete capable of infecting almost any organ or tissue in the body and causing protean clinical manifestations (Table 34–1). Transmission occurs most frequently during sexual contact (including oral sex), through minor skin or mucosal lesions; sites of inoculation are usually genital but may be extragenital. The risk of developing syphilis after unprotected sex with an individual with early syphilis is approximately 30–50%. The organism is extremely sensitive to heat and drying but can survive for days in fluids; therefore, it can be transmitted in blood from infected persons. Syphilis can be transferred via the placenta from mother to fetus after the tenth week of pregnancy (congenital syphilis).

The immunologic response to infection is complex, but it provides the basis for most clinical diagnoses. The infection induces the synthesis of a number of antibodies, some of which react specifically with pathogenic treponemes and some with components of normal tissues (see below). If the disease is untreated, in most cases these immune reactions fail to eradicate existing infection and may contribute to tissue destruction in the late stages. Patients treated early in the disease are fully susceptible to reinfection.

The natural history of acquired syphilis is generally divided into two major clinical stages: early (infectious) syphilis and late syphilis. The two stages are separated by a symptom-free latent phase during the first part of which (early latency) the infectious stage is liable to recur. Infectious syphilis includes the primary lesions (chancre and regional lymphadenopathy), the secondary lesions (commonly involving skin and mucous membranes, occasionally bone, central nervous system, or liver), relapsing lesions during early latency, and congenital lesions. The hallmark of these lesions is an abundance of spirochetes; tissue reaction is usually minimal. Late syphilis consists of so-called benign (gummatous) lesions involving skin, bones, and viscera; cardiovascular disease (principally aortitis); and a

variety of central nervous system and ocular syndromes. These forms of syphilis are not contagious. The lesions contain few demonstrable spirochetes, but tissue reactivity (vasculitis, necrosis) is severe and suggestive of hypersensitivity phenomena.

As a result of intensive public health efforts and the introduction of penicillin during and after World War II, there was a reduction in the incidence of infectious syphilis. There was a resurgence of disease in the 1960s and 1970s, but the incidence never reached that of the pre-penicillin era. In the early 1980s, the incidence of infectious syphilis increased, with a particularly high rate among homosexual men. In the mid-1980s, there was a slight decrease, primarily a result of changes in sexual practices in response to the AIDS epidemic. Between 1985 and 1990, there was again a dramatic increase in infectious syphilis, with more than 50,000 cases of primary and secondary syphilis reported in 1990. This increase was broad based, affecting both men and women in inner city, urban, and rural areas, particularly in the southern regions of the United States. Although adolescent and young adult blacks were primarily affected, increases were seen in other ethnic groups also, as well as adults over 60 years of age. Limited access to health care, decreases in health department clinical services, increased use of illicit drugs (especially "crack cocaine"), the exchange of sex for drugs or money to buy drugs, and the difficulty of contact tracing when multiple sexual partners are involved all contributed to the dramatic increase. Concomitantly with the increase in acquired syphilis, there has also been an increase in congenital syphilis, particularly in urban areas. In response to this increase in infectious syphilis in 1998, the United States Congress allocated funds for a syphilis elimination program. This included intensive syphilis control programs targeting high-risk populations (women of childbearing age, sexually active teens, drug users, inmates of penal institutions, persons with multiple sexual partners or those who have sex with prostitutes) emphasizing screening, early treatment, contact tracing, and condom use. The effort was initially successful, as evidenced by a decrease in the number of primary and secondary cases reported in 2000 (5979 cases) compared with 1998 (7035 cases). However, in 2003, the number of cases was 7,177, the highest since 1997. These increases occurred mainly among men (suggesting that the increase is

Table 34–1. Stages of syphilis and common clinical manifestations.

Primary syphilis
  Genital ulcer: painless ulcer with clean base and firm indu-
    rated borders
  Regional lymphadenopathy
Secondary syphilis
  Skin and mucous membranes
    Rash: diffuse (including palms and soles), macular,
      papular, pustular, and combinations
    Condylomata lata
    Mucous patches: painless, silvery ulcerations of mu-
      cous membrane with surrounding erythema
  Generalized lymphadenopathy
  Constitutional symptoms
    Fever, usually low-grade
    Malaise
    Anorexia
    Arthralgias and myalgias
  Central nervous system
    Asymptomatic
    Symptomatic
    Headache
    Meningitis
    Cranial neuropathies (II–VIII)
  Ocular
    Iritis
    Iridocyclitis
  Other
    Renal: glomerulonephritis, nephrotic syndrome
    Liver: hepatitis
    Bone and joint: arthritis, periostitis
Late syphilis
  Late benign (gummatous): granulomatous lesion usually
    involving skin, mucous membranes and bones, but any
    organ can be involved
  Cardiovascular
    Aortic insufficiency
    Coronary ostial stenosis
    Aortic aneurysm
  Neurosyphilis
    Asymptomatic
    Meningovascular
      Seizures
      Hemiparesis or hemiplegia
    Tabes dorsalis
      Impaired proprioception and vibratory sensation
      Argyll Robertson pupil
      Shooting pains
      Ataxia
      Romberg's sign
      Urinary and fecal incontinence
      Charcot joint
      Cranial nerve involvement (II–VIII)
    General paresis
      Personality changes
      Hyperactive reflexes
      Argyll Robertson pupil
      Decreased memory
      Slurred speech
      Optic atrophy

likely in the group of men having sex with men and is due to disinhibition with availability of highly active antiretroviral therapy and the nonuse of condoms in partners who are HIV positive), whereas the number of cases actually declined among women and non-Hispanic blacks. Most cases are still reported from the South, but urban outbreaks (New York City, San Francisco) are being reported with increasing frequency, primarily among men having sex with men. Despite the increase in primary and secondary syphilis in men who have sex with men, there has not been a concomitant increase in the number of HIV cases.

Laboratory Diagnosis

Because the infectious agent of syphilis cannot be cultured in vitro, diagnostic measures must rely mainly on serologic testing, microscopic detection of *T pallidum* in lesions, and other examinations (biopsies, lumbar puncture, radiographs) for evidence of tissue damage.

A. SEROLOGIC TESTS FOR SYPHILIS

(Table 34–2.) There are two general categories of serologic tests for syphilis: (1) Nontreponemal tests detect antibodies to lipoidal antigens present in either the host or in *T pallidum*. The original antigens used to measure these nonspecific antibodies (reagin) were crude extracts of beef heart or liver and resulted in significant numbers of false-positive reactions. The cardiolipin–cholesterol–lecithin preparation presently used is much purer and gives fewer false-positive reactions. (2) Treponemal tests use live or killed *T pallidum* as antigen to detect antibodies specific for pathogenic treponemes.

1. Nontreponemal antigen tests—The most commonly used nontreponemal antigen tests are the Venereal Disease Research Laboratory (VDRL) and rapid plasma reagin (RPR), which measure the ability of heated serum to flocculate a suspension of cardiolipin–cholesterol–lecithin. The flocculation tests are inexpensive, rapid, and easy to perform and are therefore used primarily for routine screening. Quantitative expression of the reactivity of the serum, based on titration of dilutions of serum, is valuable in establishing the diagnosis and in evaluating the efficacy of treatment, since titers usually correlate with disease activity.

Table 34–2. Percentage of patients with positive serologic tests for syphilis.[1]

	Stage		
Test	**Primary**	**Secondary**	**Tertiary**
VDRL	75–85%	99%	95%
FTA-ABS	85–95%	100%	98%

[1]Based on untreated cases.
VDRL = Venereal Disease Research Laboratory test; FTA-ABS = fluorescent treponemal antibody absorption test.

Nontreponemal tests generally become positive 4–6 weeks after infection, or 1–3 weeks after the appearance of a primary lesion; they are almost invariably positive in the secondary stage, with titers ≥ 1:32. In the late stages, titers tend to be lower (< 1:4). These serologic tests are not highly specific and must be closely correlated with other clinical and laboratory findings. The tests are positive in patients with non-sexually transmitted treponematoses (see below). More importantly, "false-positive" serologic reactions are frequently encountered in a wide variety of nontreponemal states, including connective tissue diseases, infectious mononucleosis, malaria, febrile diseases, leprosy, injection drug use, infective endocarditis, old age, hepatitis C viral infection, and pregnancy. False-positive tests also occur more commonly in HIV-seropositive patients (4%) than in HIV-seronegative patients (0.8%). False-positive reactions are usually of low titer and transient and may be distinguished from true positives by specific treponemal antibody tests. False-negative results can be seen when very high antibody titers are present (the prozone phenomenon). If syphilis is strongly suspected and the nontreponemal test is negative, the laboratory should be instructed to dilute the specimen to detect a positive reaction. The RPR and VDRL tests are equally reliable, but titers of RPR tend to be higher than the VDRL. Thus, when these tests are used to follow disease activity, the same testing method should be used and preferably should be performed at the same laboratory.

Nontreponemal antibody titers are used to assess adequacy of therapy. The time required for the VDRL or RPR to become negative depends on the stage of the disease, the height of the initial titer, and whether the infection is an initial or repeat episode. In general, individuals with repeat infections, higher initial titers, and more advanced stages of disease at the time of treatment have a slower seroconversion rate and are more likely to remain serofast (ie, titers do not become negative). Older data derived from more intensive treatment regimens than are presently used indicate that in primary and secondary syphilis, the VDRL usually decreases fourfold by 3 months and eightfold by 6 months. Furthermore, seronegativity was seen in 97% of those with primary syphilis and 76% of those with secondary syphilis at 2 years. More recent data based on currently recommended treatment regimens (see below) suggest that decreases in titer may be slower—ie, in primary and secondary syphilis it may take 6 months to see a fourfold decrease in titer and 12 months to see an eightfold drop. In patients with early latent syphilis, response is even slower, with a fourfold drop in titer taking 12–24 months. Seronegativity was seen in 72% of patients with primary syphilis and only 56% of those with secondary syphilis after 3 years. Additional studies support a slower decline in titers with currently recommended treatment regimens.

2. Treponemal antibody tests—The fluorescent treponemal antibody absorption (FTA-ABS) test measures antibodies capable of reacting with killed *T pallidum* after absorption of the patient's serum with extracts of nonpathogenic treponemes. The FTA-ABS test is of value principally in determining whether a positive nontreponemal antigen test is false-positive or is indicative of syphilis. Because of its great sensitivity, particularly in the late stages of the disease, the FTA-ABS test is also of value when there is clinical evidence of syphilis but the nontreponemal serologic test for syphilis is negative. The test is positive in most patients with primary syphilis and in almost all patients with secondary syphilis. Like nontreponemal antigen tests, the specific treponemal antibody test may revert to negative with adequate therapy. This is seen almost exclusively in initial infections in individuals with primary syphilis. In one study, 11% of individuals with a first episode of primary syphilis were seronegative by the FTA-ABS test at 1 year posttreatment, and 24% were negative by 3 years. Immunologic status may also affect antibody titers. Seven percent of asymptomatic HIV-infected patients became seronegative after treatment, as opposed to 38% of symptomatic HIV-infected individuals. The long-held belief that a positive FTA-ABS persists indefinitely is clearly not valid, and this test therefore cannot be used as a reliable marker of previous infection. False-positive FTA-ABS tests occur rarely in systemic lupus erythematosus and in other disorders associated with increased levels of γ-globulins, malaria, leprosy, and other spirochetal infections. It is noteworthy that Lyme disease may cause a false-positive FTA-ABS test but rarely causes a false-positive reaginic test. The *T pallidum* hemagglutination (TPHA) test and the *T pallidum* particle agglutination (TPPA) test are comparable in specificity and sensitivity to the FTA-ABS. The TPPA test, because of ease of performance, has supplanted the FTA-ABS test as the means of confirming the diagnosis of syphilis.

Final decisions about the significance of the results of serologic tests for syphilis must be based on a total clinical appraisal.

B. MICROSCOPIC EXAMINATION

In infectious syphilis, *T pallidum* may be shown by darkfield microscopic examination of fresh exudate from lesions or material aspirated from regional lymph nodes. The darkfield examination requires considerable experience and care in the proper collection of specimens and in the identification of pathogenic spirochetes by observing characteristic features of morphology and motility. Repeated examinations may be necessary. Spirochetes usually are not found in late syphilitic lesions by this technique.

An immunofluorescent staining technique for demonstrating *T pallidum* in dried smears of fluid taken from early syphilitic lesions is available. Slides are fixed and treated with fluorescein-labeled antitreponemal antibody that has been preabsorbed with nonpathogenic treponemes. The slides are then examined for fluorescing spirochetes in an ultraviolet microscope. Because of its simplicity and convenience to clinicians (slides can be mailed), this technique has replaced darkfield microscopy in most health departments and medical center laboratories.

C. Spinal Fluid Examination

Cerebrospinal fluid findings in neurosyphilis are variable. In "classic" cases, there is an elevation of total protein, lymphocytic pleocytosis, and a positive cerebrospinal fluid reagin test (VDRL). However, cerebrospinal fluid may be completely normal in neurosyphilis, and the VDRL may be negative. In one study, 25% of patients with primary or secondary syphilis in whom *T pallidum* was isolated from cerebrospinal fluid had a normal cerebrospinal fluid examination. In later stages of syphilis, normal cerebrospinal fluid analysis in the presence of infection can occur, but it is unusual. Because false-positive reagin tests rarely occur in the cerebrospinal fluid, a positive test confirms the presence of neurosyphilis. Because the cerebrospinal fluid VDRL may be negative in 30–70% of cases of neurosyphilis, *a negative test does not exclude neurosyphilis.* The use of cerebrospinal fluid FTA-ABS in the diagnosis of neurosyphilis is controversial. It is a highly sensitive test but lacks specificity, and a high serum titer of FTA-ABS may result in a positive cerebrospinal fluid titer in the absence of neurosyphilis. However, because the test is so sensitive, a negative cerebrospinal fluid FTA-ABS is strong evidence against the diagnosis of neurosyphilis.

Cerebrospinal fluid examination is recommended depending on the clinical manifestations and the stage of disease, as discussed below. Asymptomatic neurosyphilis (ie, positive cerebrospinal fluid findings without symptoms) requires prolonged penicillin treatment as given for symptomatic neurosyphilis. Adequate treatment is indicated by gradual decrease in cerebrospinal fluid cell count, protein concentration, and VDRL titer. Rarely, serologic tests of cerebrospinal fluid may remain positive for years after adequate treatment of neurosyphilis even though all other parameters have returned to normal.

Treatment

A. Specific Measures

1. Penicillin—Penicillin, as benzathine penicillin G or aqueous procaine penicillin G, is the drug of choice for all forms of syphilis and other spirochetal infections. Effective tissue levels must be maintained for several days or weeks because of the spirochete's long generation time (about 30 hours). Penicillin is highly effective in early infections and variably effective in the late stages. The principal contraindication is hypersensitivity to the penicillins. The recommended treatment schedules are included below in the discussion of the various forms of syphilis.

2. Other antibiotic therapy—Oral tetracyclines are effective in the treatment of syphilis for patients who are allergic to penicillin. Tetracycline, 500 mg orally four times daily for 14 days, or doxycycline, 100 mg orally twice daily for 14 days, is given for primary, secondary, and early latent syphilis. In syphilis of more than 1 year's duration or of unknown duration, treatment is continued for 28 days in the same doses.

Preliminary data suggest that both ceftriaxone and azithromycin are effective for the therapy of early syphilis and are now accepted alternative regimens to penicillin after doxycycline and tetracycline. The recommended dose of ceftriaxone is 1 g daily either intramuscularly or intravenously for 8–10 days. Azithromycin can be administered as a single oral dose of 2 g. However, azithromycin resistance has been documented from several geographic areas (reported to be 56% in San Francisco in 2004 compared with 0% in 2000). Azithromycin should be used only if no alternatives are available, and the patient can be monitored closely. Ceftriaxone at a higher dose of 2 g daily intramuscularly or intravenously for 10–14 days can also be used as alternative therapy for neurosyphilis in patients with non-immunoglobulin E (IgE)-mediated hypersensitivity to penicillin.

B. Local Measures (Mucocutaneous Lesions)

Local treatment is usually not necessary. No local antiseptics or other chemicals should be applied to a suspected syphilitic lesion until specimens for microscopy have been obtained.

C. Public Health Measures

Patients with infectious syphilis must abstain from sexual activity until rendered noninfectious by antibiotic therapy. All cases of syphilis must be reported to the appropriate public health agency for assistance in identifying and treating contacts. In addition, all patients with syphilis should have an HIV test at the time of diagnosis. In areas of high HIV prevalence, a repeat HIV test should be performed in 3 months if the initial test was negative.

D. Empiric Postexposure Treatment

Patients who have been exposed to infectious syphilis within the preceding 3 months may be infected but seronegative and thus should be treated as for early syphilis. Persons exposed more than 90 days previously should be treated based on serologic results. If their partners are unavailable for testing or unreliable for follow-up, empiric therapy is indicated. Others at high risk either for infection (ie, those with other sexually transmitted diseases and those infected with HIV) or its consequences (ie, pregnant women) should undergo serologic tests for syphilis. The present recommended therapy for gonorrhea (single-dose ceftriaxone or cefpodoxime) may not be effective in treating incubating syphilis. Therefore, patients with gonorrhea and a known exposure to syphilis should be treated with separate regimens effective against both diseases.

Complications of Specific Therapy

The Jarisch–Herxheimer reaction is ascribed to the sudden massive destruction of spirochetes by drugs and release of toxic products and is manifested by fever and aggravation of the existing clinical picture. It is most likely to occur in early syphilis. It usually begins within the first 24 hours and subsides spontaneously within the next 24 hours of penicillin treatment. Treatment should not be discontinued unless the symptoms become severe or threaten to be fatal or unless syphilitic laryngitis, auditory neuritis, or labyrinthitis is present, where the reaction may cause irreversible damage.

The reaction may be prevented or modified by simultaneous administration of antipyretics or corticosteroids, though no proved method of prevention exists.

Follow-Up Care

Because treatment failures can occur and reinfection is always a possibility, patients treated for syphilis should be monitored clinically and serologically. Response to therapy is difficult to assess, and no definite criteria exist for cure in patients with primary or secondary syphilis. In primary and secondary syphilis, failure of nontreponemal antibody titers to decrease fourfold by 6 months may identify a group at high risk for treatment failure. Optimal management of these patients is unclear, but at a minimum, close clinical and serologic follow-up is indicated. If titers fail to decrease fourfold by 6 months, an HIV test should be repeated (all patients with syphilis should have an HIV test at the time of diagnosis); a lumbar puncture should be considered since unrecognized neurosyphilis can be a cause of treatment failure; and, if careful follow-up cannot be ensured (3-month intervals for HIV-positive individuals and 6-month intervals for HIV-negative patients), treatment should be repeated with 2.4 million units of benzathine penicillin intramuscularly weekly for 3 weeks. If symptoms or signs persist or recur after initial therapy or there is a fourfold or greater increase in nontreponemal titers, therapy has either failed or the patient has been reinfected. In those individuals, an HIV test should be performed, a lumbar puncture done (unless reinfection is a certainty), and re-treatment given as indicated above. In patients with latent syphilis, nontreponemal serologic tests should be repeated at 6, 12, and 24 months. If titers increase fourfold or if initially high titers ($\geq$ 1:32) fail to decrease fourfold by 12–24 months—or if symptoms or signs consistent with syphilis develop—an HIV test and lumbar puncture should be performed and re-treatment given according to the stage of the disease.

Prevention

Avoidance of sexual contact is the only completely reliable method of prophylaxis but is an impractical public health measure for obvious reasons. Annual screening for syphilis among men who have sex with men has been recommended based on preliminary data suggesting that this may decrease the rate of transmission. High-risk individuals (those who have multiple encounters with anonymous partners or who have sex in conjunction with the use of drugs) should be screened every 3–6 months.

A. MECHANICAL

The standard latex condom is effective but protects covered parts only. The exposed parts should be washed with soap and water as soon after contact as possible. This applies to both sexes.

B. ANTIBIOTIC

If there is known exposure to infectious syphilis, abortive penicillin therapy may be used. Give 2.4 million units of procaine penicillin G intramuscularly. Azithromycin administered as a single 1 g dose is also effective as preventive therapy in individuals exposed to infected partners, and in some areas Public Health Departments are giving azithromycin packets to persons with syphilis to give to sexual contacts whom they meet in high-risk venues. Treatment of gonococcal (and chlamydial) infection with tetracyclines and ceftriaxone is probably effective against incubating syphilis in most cases. However, other antimicrobial agents (eg, spectinomycin, quinolones) may be ineffective in aborting preclinical syphilis. Because of concerns about treating incubating syphilis with nonpenicillin regimens, patients treated for gonorrhea should have a serologic test for syphilis 3–6 months after treatment.

Course & Prognosis

The lesions associated with primary and secondary syphilis are self-limiting and resolve with few or no residua. Late syphilis may be highly destructive and permanently disabling and may lead to death. In broad terms, if no treatment is given, about one-third of people infected with syphilis will undergo spontaneous cure, about one-third will remain in the latent phase throughout life, and about one-third will develop serious late lesions. (See Table 34–3.)

CLINICAL STAGES OF SYPHILIS

1. Primary Syphilis

 ESSENTIALS OF DIAGNOSIS

- *History of sexual contact (often unreliable).*
- *Painless ulcer on genitalia, perianal area, rectum, pharynx, tongue, lip, or elsewhere 2–6 weeks after exposure.*
- *Nontender enlargement of regional lymph nodes.*
- *Fluid expressed from lesion contains T pallidum by immunofluorescence or darkfield microscopy.*
- *Serologic test for syphilis often positive.*

General Considerations

This is the stage of invasion and may pass unrecognized. The typical lesion is the chancre at the site or

Table 34–3. Natural course of untreated syphilis in immunocompetent individuals.

Stage of Disease	Likelihood of Developing Clinical Manifestations	Comment
Latent	24%	90% of relapses occur in first year after infection.
Late		
Benign (gummatous)	15%	Seen 1–46 years postinfection. Many patients have more than one late manifestation.
Cardiovascular	10%	Seen only in persons in whom syphilis develops after 15 years of age. Onset 20–30 years postinfection.
Neurosyphilis	6.5%	Asymptomatic neurosyphilis has been reported in 8–40%.
Early symptomatic	5%	Occurs weeks to years after infection; can coexist with primary and secondary disease; manifests as meningitis, cranial neuritis, ocular involvement, meningovascular disease (stroke).
Late (tertiary)	5–10%	2–50 years after primary infection; tabes or general paresis.

sites of inoculation, most frequently located on the penis, labia, cervix, or anorectal region. Anorectal lesions are especially common among men who have sex with men. The primary lesion occurs occasionally in the oropharynx (lip, tongue, or tonsil) and rarely on the breast or finger. The chancre starts as a small erosion 10–90 days (average, 3–4 weeks) after inoculation that rapidly develops into a painless superficial ulcer with a clean base and firm, indurated margins, associated with enlargement of regional lymph nodes, which are rubbery, discrete, and nontender. Bacterial infection of the chancre may occur and may lead to pain. Healing occurs without treatment, but a scar may form, especially with secondary bacterial infection. Although the "classic" ulcer of syphilis has been described as nontender, nonpurulent, and indurated, only 31% of patients have this triad.

Laboratory Findings

The serologic test for syphilis is usually positive 1–2 weeks after the primary lesion is noted; rising titers are especially significant when there is a history of previous infection. Immunofluorescence or darkfield microscopy shows treponemes in at least 95% of chancres. Cerebrospinal fluid pleocytosis has been reported in 10–20% of patients with primary syphilis.

Differential Diagnosis

The syphilitic chancre may be confused with chancroid (usually painful), lymphogranuloma venereum (uncommon in the United States), genital herpes, or neoplasm. Any lesion on the genitalia should be considered a possible primary syphilitic lesion.

Treatment

Benzathine penicillin G, 2.4 million units intramuscularly in the gluteal area, is given once. For the nonpreg-

nant penicillin-allergic patient, doxycycline, 100 mg orally twice daily for 2 weeks, or tetracycline, 500 mg orally four times a day for 2 weeks, can be used. There is more clinical experience with tetracycline, but compliance is probably better with doxycycline. As noted above, ceftriaxone and azithromycin can be used in the penicillin-allergic patient, although increasing resistance to azithromycin has limited its usefulness (see preceding section on "Other antibiotic therapy").

2. Secondary Syphilis

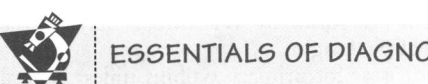 ESSENTIALS OF DIAGNOSIS

- *Generalized maculopapular skin rash.*
- *Mucous membrane lesions, including patches and ulcers.*
- *Weeping papules (condylomas) in moist skin areas.*
- *Generalized nontender lymphadenopathy.*
- *Fever.*
- *Meningitis, hepatitis, osteitis, arthritis, iritis.*
- *Many treponemes in scrapings of mucous membrane or skin lesions by immunofluorescence or darkfield microscopy.*
- *Serologic tests for syphilis always positive.*

General Considerations & Treatment

The secondary stage of syphilis usually appears a few weeks (or up to 6 months) after development of the chancre, when sufficient dissemination of *T pallidum* has occurred to produce systemic signs (fever, lymphadenopathy) or infectious lesions at sites distant from the site of inoculation. The most common manifestations are skin and mucosal lesions. The skin lesions are nonpruritic, macular, papular, pustular, or follicular (or combinations of any of these types, but *not* vesicular), though the maculopapular rash is the most common. The skin lesions usually are generalized; involvement of the palms and soles is especially suspicious. Annular lesions simulating ringworm are observed in dark-skinned individuals. Mucous membrane lesions range from ulcers and papules of the lips, mouth, throat, genitalia, and anus ("mucous patches") to a diffuse redness of the pharynx. Both skin and mucous membrane lesions are highly infectious at this stage. Specific lesions—**condylomata lata**—are fused, weeping papules on the moist areas of the skin and mucous membranes.

Meningeal (aseptic meningitis or acute basilar meningitis), hepatic, renal, bone, and joint invasion may occur, with resulting cranial nerve palsies, jaundice, nephrotic syndrome, and periostitis. Alopecia (moth-eaten appearance) and uveitis may also occur.

The serologic tests for syphilis are positive in most cases. The cutaneous and mucous membrane lesions often show *T pallidum* on darkfield microscopic examination. A transient cerebrospinal fluid pleocytosis is seen in 30–70% of patients with secondary syphilis, though only 5% have positive serologic cerebrospinal fluid reactions. There may be evidence of hepatitis or nephritis (immune complex type). Circulating immune complexes exist in the blood and are deposited in blood vessel walls.

Skin lesions may be confused with the infectious exanthems, pityriasis rosea, and drug eruptions. Visceral lesions may suggest nephritis or hepatitis due to other causes. The diffusely red throat may mimic other forms of pharyngitis.

Treatment is as for primary syphilis unless central nervous system or ocular disease is present, in which case a lumbar puncture should be performed and, if positive, treatment is as for neurosyphilis (see below). Isolation of the patient is important.

3. Relapsing Syphilis (Early Latent Syphilis)

The essentials of diagnosis are the same as in secondary syphilis.

The lesions of secondary syphilis heal spontaneously, but secondary syphilis may relapse if undiagnosed or inadequately treated. These relapses may include any of the findings noted under secondary syphilis: skin and mucous membrane, neurologic, ocular, bone, or visceral. Unlike the usual asymptomatic neurologic involvement of secondary syphilis, neurologic relapses may be fulminating, leading to death. Relapse is almost always accompanied by a rising titer in quantitative serologic tests; indeed, a rising titer may be the first or only evidence of relapse. About 90% of relapses occur during the first year after infection.

Treatment is as for primary syphilis unless central nervous system disease is present.

4. Late Latent ("Hidden") Syphilis

 ESSENTIALS OF DIAGNOSIS

- No physical signs.
- History of syphilis with inadequate treatment.
- Positive serologic tests for syphilis.

General Considerations & Treatment

Latent syphilis is the clinically quiescent phase during the interval after the disappearance of secondary lesions and before the appearance of tertiary symptoms. Early latency is defined as the first year after infection, during which time most infectious lesions recur ("relapsing syphilis"); after the first year, the patient is said to be in the late latent phase. Transmission to the fetus, however, can probably occur in any phase. There are (by definition) no clinical manifestations during the latent phase, and the only significant laboratory findings are positive serologic tests. A diagnosis of latent syphilis is justified only when the cerebrospinal fluid is entirely negative, radiographic studies and physical examination show no evidence of cardiovascular involvement, and false-positive tests for syphilis have been ruled out. The latent phase may last from months to a lifetime.

It is important to differentiate latent syphilis from a false-positive serologic test for syphilis, which can be due to the many causes listed above.

Treatment of late latent syphilis or latent syphilis of unknown duration is with benzathine penicillin G, 2.4 million units intramuscularly three times at 7-day intervals (total dose: 7.2 million units). The only alternative to penicillin for therapy of late latent syphilis is doxycycline, 100 mg orally twice daily, or tetracycline, 500 mg orally four times a day, both for 28 days. If there is evidence of central nervous system involvement, a lumbar puncture should be performed and, if positive, the patient should receive treatment as for neurosyphilis. Only a small percentage of serologic tests will be appreciably altered by treatment with penicillin. The treatment of this stage of the disease is intended to prevent the late sequelae.

5. Late (Tertiary) Syphilis

 ESSENTIALS OF DIAGNOSIS

- Infiltrative tumors of skin, bones, liver (gummas).
- Aortitis, aneurysms, aortic regurgitation.
- Central nervous system disorders, including meningovascular and degenerative changes, paresthesias, shooting pains, abnormal reflexes, dementia, or psychosis.

General Considerations

This stage may occur at any time after secondary syphilis, even after years of latency, and is seen in about one-third of untreated patients (Table 34–3). Late lesions probably represent, at least in part, a delayed hypersensitivity reaction of the tissue to the organism and are usually divided into two types: (1) a localized gummatous reaction, with a relatively rapid onset and generally prompt response to therapy ("benign late syphilis") and (2) diffuse inflammation of a more insidious onset that characteristically involves the central nervous system and large arteries, is often fatal if untreated, and is at best arrested by treatment. Gummas may involve any area or organ of the body but most often affect the skin or long bones. Cardiovascular disease is usually manifested by aortic aneurysm, aortic regurgitation, or aortitis. Various forms of diffuse or localized central nervous system involvement may occur.

Late syphilis must be differentiated from neoplasms of the skin, liver, lung, stomach, or brain; other forms of meningitis; and primary neurologic lesions.

Although almost any tissue and organ may be involved in late syphilis, the following are the most common types of involvement: skin, mucous membranes, skeletal system, eyes, respiratory system, gastrointestinal system, cardiovascular system, and nervous system.

Skin

Cutaneous lesions of late syphilis are of two varieties: (1) multiple nodular lesions that eventually ulcerate (lues maligna) or resolve by forming atrophic, pigmented scars and (2) solitary gummas that start as painless subcutaneous nodules, then enlarge, attach to the overlying skin, and eventually ulcerate.

Mucous Membranes

Late lesions of the mucous membranes are nodular gummas or leukoplakia, highly destructive to the involved tissue.

Skeletal System

Bone lesions are destructive, causing periostitis, osteitis, and arthritis with little or no associated redness or swelling but often marked myalgia and myositis of the neighboring muscles. The pain is especially severe at night.

Eyes

Late ocular lesions are gummatous iritis, chorioretinitis, optic atrophy, and cranial nerve palsies, in addition to the lesions of central nervous system syphilis.

Respiratory System

Respiratory involvement by late syphilis is caused by gummatous infiltrates into the larynx, trachea, and pulmonary parenchyma, producing discrete pulmonary densities. There may be hoarseness, respiratory distress, and wheezing secondary to the gummatous lesion itself or to subsequent stenosis occurring with healing.

Gastrointestinal System

Gummas involving the liver produce the usually benign, asymptomatic hepar lobatum. A picture resembling Laennec's cirrhosis is occasionally produced by liver involvement. Gastric involvement can consist of diffuse infiltration into the stomach wall or focal lesions that endoscopically and microscopically can be confused with lymphoma or carcinoma. Epigastric pain, early satiety, regurgitation, belching, and weight loss are common symptoms.

Cardiovascular System

Cardiovascular lesions (10–15% of late syphilitic lesions) are often progressive, disabling, and life-threatening. Central nervous system lesions are often present concomitantly. Involvement usually starts as an arteritis in the supracardiac portion of the aorta and progresses to one or more of the following: (1) narrowing of the coronary ostia, with resulting decreased coronary circulation, angina, and acute myocardial infarction; (2) scarring of the aortic valves, producing aortic regurgitation, and eventually congestive heart failure; and (3) weakness of the wall of the aorta, with saccular aneurysm formation and associated pressure symptoms of dysphagia, hoarseness, brassy cough, back pain (vertebral erosion), and occasionally rupture of the aneurysm. Recurrent respiratory infections are common as a result of pressure on the trachea and bronchi.

Treatment of tertiary syphilis (excluding neurosyphilis; see following section) is as for late latent syphilis. Reversal of positive serologic tests does not usually occur. A second course of penicillin therapy may be given if necessary. There is no known method for reliable eradication of the treponeme from humans in the late stages of syphilis. Viable spirochetes are occasionally found in the eyes, in cerebrospinal fluid, and elsewhere in patients with "adequately" treated syphilis, but claims for their capacity to cause progressive disease are speculative.

Nervous System (Neurosyphilis)

Neurosyphilis (15–20% of late syphilitic lesions; often present with cardiovascular syphilis) is also a progressive, disabling, and life-threatening complication. It develops more commonly in men than in women and in whites than in blacks. Asymptomatic and meningovascular syphilis occur earlier (months to years after infection, sometimes coexisting with primary and secondary syphilis) than tabes dorsalis and general paresis (2–50 years after infection).

A. CLASSIFICATION

There are four clinical types.

1. Asymptomatic neurosyphilis—This form is characterized by spinal fluid abnormalities (positive spinal fluid serology, increased cell count, occasionally increased protein) without symptoms or signs of neurologic involvement.

2. Meningovascular syphilis—This form is characterized by meningeal involvement or changes in the vascular structures of the brain (or both), producing symptoms of chronic meningitis (headache, irritability), cranial nerve palsies (basilar meningitis), unequal reflexes, irregular pupils with poor light and accommodation reflexes, and, when large vessels are involved, cerebrovascular accidents. The cerebrospinal fluid shows increased cells (100–1000/mcL), elevated protein, and usually a positive serologic test for syphilis. The symptoms of acute meningitis are rare in late syphilis.

3. Tabes dorsalis—This form is a chronic progressive degeneration of the parenchyma of the posterior columns of the spinal cord and of the posterior sensory ganglia and nerve roots. The symptoms and signs are impairment of proprioception and vibration sense, Argyll Robertson pupils (which react poorly to light but well to accommodation), and muscular hypotonia and hyporeflexia. Impairment of proprioception results in a wide-based gait and inability to walk in the dark. Paresthesias, analgesia, or sharp recurrent pains in the muscles of the leg ("shooting" or "lightning" pains) may occur. Crises are also common in tabes: gastric crises, consisting of sharp abdominal pains with nausea and vomiting (simulating an acute abdomen); laryngeal crises, with paroxysmal cough and dyspnea; urethral crises, with painful bladder spasms; and rectal and anal crises. Crises may begin suddenly, last for hours to days, and cease abruptly. Neurogenic bladder with overflow incontinence is also seen. Painless trophic ulcers may develop over pressure points on the feet. Joint damage may occur as a result of lack of sensory innervation (Charcot joint). The cerebrospinal fluid may have a normal or increased cell count (3–200/mcL), elevated protein, and variable results of serologic tests.

4. General paresis—This is generalized involvement of the cerebral cortex with insidious onset of symptoms. There is usually a decrease in concentrating power, memory loss, dysarthria, tremor of the fingers and lips, irritability, and mild headaches. Most striking is the change of personality; the patient becomes slovenly, irresponsible, confused, and psychotic. The cerebrospinal fluid findings resemble those of tabes dorsalis. Combinations of the various forms of neurosyphilis (especially tabes and paresis) are not uncommon.

B. Special Considerations in Treatment of Neurosyphilis

It is most important to prevent neurosyphilis by prompt diagnosis, adequate treatment, and follow-up of early syphilis. Indications for lumbar puncture vary depending on the stage of the disease and the host's immune status. In early syphilis (primary and secondary syphilis and early latent syphilis of less than 1 year's duration),

invasion of the central nervous system by *T pallidum* with cerebrospinal fluid abnormalities occurs commonly, but neurosyphilis rarely develops in patients who have received the standard therapy outlined above. Thus, unless clinical symptoms and signs of neurosyphilis or ophthalmologic involvement (uveitis, neuroretinitis, optic neuritis, iritis) are present, a lumbar puncture in early syphilis is not recommended as part of the routine evaluation. In latent syphilis, the decision to perform a lumbar puncture should be individualized. Routine lumbar puncture for all patients is not indicated since the yield is low and findings rarely influence therapeutic decisions. Cerebrospinal fluid evaluation is recommended, however, in the later stages of syphilis if neurologic or ophthalmologic symptoms and signs are present, if therapy other than with penicillin is to be given, if the patient is HIV positive (see next section), if there is evidence of treatment failure (see earlier discussion), or if there is evidence of active tertiary syphilis (eg, aortitis, iritis, optic atrophy, the presence of a gumma). Some experts also routinely recommend lumbar puncture for all individuals with latent syphilis if the serum nontreponemal antibody titer is ≥ 1:32. In the presence of definite cerebrospinal fluid or neurologic abnormalities, one should treat for neurosyphilis. The pretreatment clinical and laboratory evaluation should include neurologic, ocular, cardiovascular, psychiatric, and cerebrospinal fluid examinations.

The regimen of 2.4 million units of benzathine penicillin intramuscularly weekly for 3 consecutive weeks results in low to undetectable cerebrospinal fluid levels of penicillin, and treatment failures have been described when this regimen has been used to treat neurosyphilis. For these reasons, current recommendations for the therapy of neurosyphilis include higher doses of short-acting penicillin to achieve better penetration and higher levels of drug in the cerebrospinal fluid. Recommended regimens include 18–24 million units per day of aqueous crystalline penicillin G given as 3–4 million units intravenously every 4 hours or as a continuous infusion for 10–14 days. Alternatively, 2.4 million units of procaine penicillin can be given intramuscularly once daily along with 500 mg of probenecid orally four times daily, both for 10–14 days. Because of concerns about slowly dividing organisms that may persist after only 10–14 days of therapy, many experts recommend subsequent administration of 2.4 million units of benzathine penicillin intramuscularly once weekly for 3 weeks as additional therapy. Ceftriaxone, 2 g intramuscularly or intravenously once daily for 10–14 days, can be used as an alternative to penicillin. Because other regimens for neurosyphilis have not been adequately studied, patients with a history of an IgE-mediated reaction to penicillin should be skin tested for allergy to penicillin and, if positive, desensitized.

All patients should have spinal fluid examinations at 6-month intervals until the cell count is normal. Response may be gauged by clinical improvement and reversal of cerebrospinal fluid changes. In general, cerebrospinal fluid white blood cell count and cerebrospinal fluid VDRL normalize more quickly (usually in 12 months) than cerebrospinal fluid protein concentration, which can remain abnormal for extended periods, making it less useful as an indicator of success or failure of therapy. A second course of penicillin therapy may be given if the cell count has not decreased at 6 months or is not normal at 2 years. Not infrequently, there is progression of neurologic symptoms and signs despite high and prolonged doses of penicillin. These treatment failures may be related to the unexplained persistence of viable *T pallidum* in central nervous system or ocular lesions in at least some cases.

6. Syphilis in HIV-Infected Patients

Interpretation of serologic tests should be the same for HIV-positive and HIV-negative individuals. Because syphilis has variable clinical manifestations and an unpredictable course, evaluation of case reports of unusual clinical or laboratory manifestations of syphilis in HIV-infected patients is difficult. Although unusual serologic responses have been reported in HIV-positive patients, including high titers of nontreponemal tests, delayed appearance of positive titers, and false-negative tests, most HIV-positive patients respond serologically in somewhat the same way as noninfected patients. Some recommend that all HIV-positive men be screened twice a year by RPR or VDRL to identify latent disease and to appropriately identify the stage of the syphilis. By establishing a serologic history, unnecessary lumbar punctures required for latent syphilis of unknown duration can be avoided. Because of concerns about false-negative serologic tests or a delayed immunologic response, if the diagnosis of syphilis is suggested on clinical grounds but reagin tests are negative, alternative tests should be performed. These tests include darkfield examination of lesions and direct fluorescent antibody staining for *T pallidum* of lesion exudate or biopsy specimens.

The diagnosis of neurosyphilis in HIV-infected patients is complicated by the fact that cerebrospinal fluid abnormalities are frequently seen and may be due to neurosyphilis or HIV infection itself. The significance of these abnormalities is unknown, and similar abnormalities are frequently seen in non–HIV-infected patients with primary or secondary syphilis. Despite occasional reports of neurosyphilis developing in HIV-infected patients despite appropriate therapy for early disease, most HIV-infected patients with primary or secondary syphilis respond appropriately to currently recommended regimens. Thus, although some recommend a cerebrospinal fluid examination for all HIV-positive patients with syphilis, such testing is probably not needed in those with early disease. In contrast, a lumbar puncture should be performed in HIV-positive patients if they have late latent syphilis or syphilis of unknown duration, if neurologic signs are present, or if therapy has failed. A recent study found that HIV-positive patients with a nontreponemal antibody titer ≥ 1:32 had a sixfold increased risk of having neurosyphilis, and if the CD4 count was ≤ 350/mcL, there was a threefold

increased risk of neurosyphilis, suggesting that these subgroups should also undergo lumbar puncture. Following treatment, cerebrospinal fluid white blood cell counts normalize within 12 months regardless of HIV status, while the cerebrospinal fluid VDRL is slower to normalize in HIV-infected individuals, especially those with CD4 counts < 200 cells/mcL. As discussed above, the same criteria for failure apply to HIV-positive and HIV-negative patients, and re-treatment regimens are the same.

Treatment of HIV-positive patients with primary and secondary syphilis is the same as for HIV-negative patients. Because of concerns about the adequacy of this therapy, some experts recommend additional therapy with 2.4 million units of benzathine penicillin intramuscularly weekly for 3 weeks instead of single-dose therapy. Because of ongoing concerns about adequacy of therapy, careful clinical and serologic follow-up should be done at 3, 6, 9, 12, and 24 months.

HIV-infected patients with late latent syphilis, syphilis of unknown duration, and neurosyphilis should be treated like HIV-negative individuals, with follow-up at 6, 12, 18, and 24 months.

Because clinical experience in treating HIV-infected patients with syphilis is based on penicillin regimens, few options exist for treating the penicillin-allergic patient. For primary, secondary, and early latent syphilis, doxycycline or tetracycline regimens can be used. For late latent syphilis, latent syphilis of unknown duration, and neurosyphilis, penicillin regimens should be used even if this requires skin testing and desensitization.

7. Syphilis in Pregnancy

All pregnant women should have a nontreponemal serologic test for syphilis at the time of the first prenatal visit. In women suspected of being at increased risk for syphilis or for populations in which there is a high prevalence of syphilis, additional nontreponemal tests should be performed during the third trimester at 28 weeks and again at delivery. The serologic status of all women who have delivered should be known before discharge from the hospital. Seropositive women should be considered infected and should be treated unless prior treatment with fall in antibody titer is medically documented.

The preferred treatment is with penicillin in dosage schedules appropriate for the stage of syphilis (see above). Penicillin prevents congenital syphilis in 90% of cases, even when treatment is given late in pregnancy. Tetracycline and doxycycline are contraindicated in pregnancy. Erythromycin should not be used because of failure to eradicate infection in the fetus, and insufficient data are available to justify a recommendation for ceftriaxone or azithromycin. Thus, women with a history of penicillin allergy should be skin tested and desensitized if necessary.

The infant should be evaluated immediately, as noted below, and at 6–8 weeks of age.

8. Congenital Syphilis

Congenital syphilis is a transplacentally transmitted infection that occurs in infants of untreated or inadequately treated mothers. The physical findings at birth are quite variable: The infant may have many or minimal signs or even no signs until 6–8 weeks of life (delayed form). The most common findings are on the mucous membranes and skin—maculopapular rash, condylomas, mucous membrane patches, and serous nasal discharge (snuffles). These lesions are infectious; *T pallidum* can easily be found microscopically, and the infant must be isolated. Other common findings are hepatosplenomegaly, anemia, or osteochondritis. These early active lesions subsequently heal, and if the disease is left untreated it produces the characteristic stigmas of syphilis—interstitial keratitis, Hutchinson's teeth, saddle nose, saber shins, deafness, and central nervous system involvement.

The presence of negative serologic tests at birth in both the mother and the infant usually means that the newborn is free of infection. However, recent infection near the time of delivery may result in negative tests because there has been insufficient time to develop a serologic response. Thus, it is necessary to maintain a high index of suspicion in infants with delayed onset of symptoms despite negative serologic tests at birth, especially in infants born to high-risk mothers (HIV-positive, illicit drug users). All infants born to mothers with positive nontreponemal and treponemal antibody titers should have blood drawn for an RPR or VDRL test and, if positive, be referred to a pediatrician for further evaluation and therapy.

Gilleece Y et al: Management of sexually transmitted infections in HIV positive individuals. Curr Opin Infect Dis 2005;18:43. [PMID: 15647699]

Goh BT: Syphilis in adults. Sex Transm Infect 2005;81:448. [PMID: 16326843]

Golden MR et al: Update on syphilis: resurgence of an old problem. JAMA 2003;290:1510. [PMID: 13129993]

Hall CS et al: Managing syphilis in the HIV-infected patient. Curr Infect Dis Rep 2004;6:72. [PMID: 14733852]

Marra CM. Neurosyphilis. Curr Neurol Neurosci Rep 2004;4:435. [PMID: 15509443]

Marra CM et al: Normalization of cerebrospinal fluid abnormalities after neurosyphilis treatment: does HIV status matter? Clin Infect Dis 2004;38:1001. [PMID: 14745693]

O'donnell JA et al: Neurosyphilis:A current review. Clin Infect Dis Rep 2005;7:277. [PMID: 15963329]

Sexually transmitted diseases treatment guidelines 2002. MMWR Recomm Rep 2002;51(RR-6):1. [PMID: 12184549]

■ NON–SEXUALLY TRANSMITTED TREPONEMATOSES

A variety of treponemal diseases other than syphilis occur endemically in many tropical areas of the world. They are distinguished from disease caused by *T palli-dum* by their nonsexual transmission, their relatively high incidence in certain geographic areas and among children, and their tendency to produce less severe visceral manifestations. As in syphilis, organisms can be demonstrated in infectious lesions with darkfield microscopy or immunofluorescence but cannot be cultured in artificial media; the serologic tests for syphilis are positive, including the newer tests such as CAP-TIA Syph G; the diseases have primary, secondary, and sometimes tertiary stages; and penicillin is the drug of choice. There is evidence that infection with these agents may provide partial resistance to syphilis and vice versa. Treatment with penicillin in doses appropriate to primary syphilis (eg, 2.4 million units of benzathine penicillin G intramuscularly) is generally curative in any stage of the non–sexually transmitted treponematoses. In cases of penicillin hypersensitivity, tetracycline, 500 mg orally four times a day for 10–14 days, is usually the recommended alternative.

YAWS (Frambesia)

Yaws is a contagious disease largely limited to tropical regions that is caused by *T pallidum* subsp *pertenue*. It is characterized by granulomatous lesions of the skin, mucous membranes, and bone. Yaws is rarely fatal, though if untreated it may lead to chronic disability and disfigurement. Yaws is acquired by direct nonsexual contact, usually in childhood, although it may occur at any age. The "mother yaw," a painless papule that later ulcerates, appears 3–4 weeks after exposure. There is usually associated regional lymphadenopathy. Six to 12 weeks later, secondary lesions that are raised papillomas and papules that weep highly infectious material appear and last for several months or years. Painful ulcerated lesions on the soles are frequent and are called "crab yaws." Late gummatous lesions may occur, with associated tissue destruction involving large areas of skin and subcutaneous tissues. The late effects of yaws, with bone change, shortening of digits, and contractions, may be confused with similar changes occurring in leprosy. Central nervous system, cardiac, or other visceral involvement is rare. See above for therapy.

PINTA

Pinta is a non–sexually transmitted spirochetal infection caused by *Treponema carateum*. It occurs endemically in rural areas of Latin America, especially in Mexico, Colombia, and Cuba, and in some areas of the Pacific. A nonulcerative, erythematous primary papule spreads slowly into a papulosquamous plaque showing a variety of color changes (slate, lilac, black). Secondary lesions resemble the primary one and appear within a year after it. These appear successively, new lesions together with older ones; are most common on the extremities; and later show atrophy and depigmentation. Some cases show pigmentary changes and atrophic patches on the soles and palms, with or without hyperkeratosis, that are indistinguishable from "crab yaws." Very rarely, central nervous system or cardiovascular disease is observed late in the course of infection. See above for therapy.

ENDEMIC SYPHILIS

Endemic syphilis is an acute or chronic infection caused by an organism indistinguishable from *T pallidum* subsp *endemicum*. It has been reported in a number of countries, particularly in the eastern Mediterranean area, often with local names: bejel in Syria, Saudi Arabia, and Iraq, and dichuchwa, njovera, and siti in Africa. It also occurs in Southeast Asia. The local forms have distinctive features. Moist ulcerated lesions of the skin or oral or nasopharyngeal mucosa are the most common manifestations. Generalized lymphadenopathy and secondary and tertiary bone and skin lesions are also common. Deep leg pain points to periostitis or osteomyelitis. In the late stages of disease, destructive gummatous lesions similar to those seen in yaws can develop, resulting in loss of cartilage and saber shin deformity. Cardiovascular and central nervous system involvement are rare. See above for therapy.

Antal GM et al: The endemic treponematoses. Microbes Infect 2002;4:83. [PMID: 11825779]

Nnoruka EN: Skin diseases in south-east Nigeria: a current perspective. Int J Dermatol 2005;44:29. [PMID: 15663655]

■ MISCELLANEOUS SPIROCHETAL DISEASES

RELAPSING FEVER

Relapsing fever is endemic in many parts of the world. The main reservoir is rodents, which serve as the source of infection for ticks (eg, ornithodoros). The distribution and seasonal incidence of the disease are determined by the ecology of the ticks in different areas. In the United States, infected ticks are found throughout the West, especially in mountainous areas, but clinical cases are uncommon in humans.

The infectious organism is a spirochete, *Borrelia recurrentis*, though other poorly characterized *Borrelia*-like organisms can cause similar disease. It may be transmitted transovarially from one generation of ticks to the next. The spirochetes occur in all tissues of the tick, and humans can be infected by tick bites or by rubbing crushed tick tissues or feces into the bite wound. Tick-borne relapsing fever is endemic but is not transmitted from person to person. Different species (or strain) names have been given to *Borrelia* in different parts of the world where the organisms are transmitted by different ticks.

When an infected person harbors lice, the lice become infected with *Borrelia* by sucking blood. A few days later, the lice serve as a source of infection for other persons. Large epidemics may occur in louse-infested populations, and transmission is favored by crowding, malnutrition, and cold climate.

Clinical Findings

A. SYMPTOMS AND SIGNS

There is an abrupt onset of fever, chills, tachycardia, nausea and vomiting, arthralgia, and severe headache. Hepatomegaly and splenomegaly may develop, as well as various types (macular, popular, petechial) of rashes that usually occur at the end of a febrile episode. Delirium occurs with high fever, and there may be various neurologic and psychic abnormalities. The attack terminates, usually abruptly, after 3–10 days. After an interval of 1–2 weeks, relapse occurs, but often it is somewhat milder. Three to ten relapses may occur before recovery in tick-borne disease, whereas louse-borne disease is associated with only one or two relapses.

B. LABORATORY FINDINGS

During episodes of fever, large spirochetes are seen in blood smears stained with Wright's or Giemsa stain. The organisms can be cultured in special media but rapidly lose pathogenicity. The spirochetes can multiply in injected rats or mice and can be seen in their blood.

A variety of anti-borrelia antibodies develop during the illness; sometimes the Weil–Felix test for rickettsioses and nontreponemal serologic tests for syphilis may also be falsely positive. Infection with *B recurrentis* can cause false-positive indirect fluorescent antibody and Western blot tests for *Borrelia burgdorferi*, and some cases may be misdiagnosed as Lyme disease. Cerebrospinal fluid abnormalities occur in patients with meningeal involvement. Mild anemia and thrombocytopenia are common, but the white blood cell count tends to be normal.

Differential Diagnosis

The manifestations of relapsing fever may be confused with malaria, leptospirosis, meningococcemia, yellow fever, typhus, or rat-bite fever.

Prevention

Prevention of tick bites (as described for rickettsial diseases) and delousing procedures applicable to large groups can prevent illness. Arthropod vectors should be controlled if possible.

An effective means of chemoprophylaxis has not been developed.

Treatment

A single dose of tetracycline or erythromycin, 0.5 g orally, or a single dose of procaine penicillin G, 400,000–600,000 units intramuscularly, probably constitutes adequate treatment for louse-borne relapsing fevers. Because of higher relapse rates, tick-borne disease is treated with 0.5 g of tetracycline or erythromycin given orally four times daily for 5–10 days. Jarisch–Herxheimer reactions occur commonly following treatment and may be life-threatening. Treatment with aspirin—but not hydrocortisone—may ameliorate this reaction. The Jarisch–Herxheimer reaction is mediated in part by tumor necrosis factor, and administration of antibody to this cytokine prior to antibiotic therapy is effective in preventing the reaction.

Prognosis

The overall mortality rate is usually about 5%. Fatalities are most common in old, debilitated, or very young patients. With treatment, the initial attack is shortened and relapses are largely prevented.

Dworkin MS et al: Tick-borne relapsing fever in North America. Med Clin North Am 2002;86:417. [PMID: 11982310]

Roscoe C et al: Tick-borne relapsing fever. Am Fam Physician 2005;72:2039. [PMID: 16342834]

RAT-BITE FEVER (Spirillary Rat-Bite Fever, Sodoku)

Rat-bite fever is an uncommon acute infectious disease caused by *Spirillum minus*. It is transmitted to humans by the bite of a rat. Inhabitants of rat-infested slum dwellings and laboratory workers are at greatest risk.

Clinical Findings

A. SYMPTOMS AND SIGNS

The original rat bite, unless secondarily infected, heals promptly, but 1 to several weeks later the site becomes swollen, indurated, and painful; assumes a dusky purplish hue; and may ulcerate. Regional lymphangitis and lymphadenitis, fever, chills, malaise, myalgia, arthralgia, and headache are present. Splenomegaly may occur. A sparse, dusky-red maculopapular rash appears on the trunk and extremities in many cases, and there may be frank arthritis.

After a few days, both the local and systemic symptoms subside, only to reappear again in a few more days. This relapsing pattern of fever for 3–4 days alternating with afebrile periods lasting 3–9 days may persist for weeks. The other features, however, usually recur only during the first few relapses.

B. LABORATORY FINDINGS

Leukocytosis is often present, and the nontreponemal test for syphilis is often falsely positive. The organism may be identified in darkfield examination of the ulcer exudate or aspirated lymph node material; more commonly, it is observed after inoculation of a laboratory animal with the patient's exudate or blood. It has not been cultured in artificial media.

Differential Diagnosis

Rat-bite fever must be distinguished from the rat-bite–induced lymphadenitis and rash of streptobacillary fever. Clinically, the severe arthritis and myalgias seen in streptobacillary disease are rarely seen in disease caused by *S minus*. Reliable differentiation requires an increasing titer of agglutinins against *Streptobacillus moniliformis* or isolation of the causative organism in culture. Rat-bite fever must also be distinguished from tularemia, rickettsial disease, *Pasteurella multocida* infections, and relapsing fever by identification of the causative organism.

Treatment

Penicillin is given for 10–14 days. During the acute phase of illness, the intravenous route is used (1–2 million units every 4–6 hours) and once improvement has occurred, therapy is completed with oral medication, penicillin V 500 mg four times daily to complete 10–14 days of therapy. For the penicillin-allergic patient, tetracycline 500 mg orally four times daily or doxycycline 100 mg twice a day can be used.

Prognosis

The reported mortality rate of about 10% should be markedly reduced by prompt diagnosis and antimicrobial treatment.

Freels LK et al: Rat bite fever: three case reports and a literature review. Clin Pediatr 2004;43:291. [PMID: 15094956]

Ojukwu IC et al: Rat-bite fever in children: case report and review. Scand J Infect Dis 2002;34:474. [PMID: 12160180]

LEPTOSPIROSIS

 ESSENTIALS OF DIAGNOSIS

- *Clinical illness can vary from asymptomatic to fatal liver and kidney disease.*
- *Anicteric leptospirosis is the more common and milder form of the disease.*
- *Icteric leptospirosis (Weil's syndrome) is characterized by impaired renal and hepatic function, abnormal mental status, and hemorrhagic pneumonia and has a 5–40% mortality rate.*

General Considerations

Leptospirosis is an acute and often severe infection that frequently affects the liver or other organs and is caused by *Leptospira interrogans*, which is a diverse organism consisting of 24 serogroups and over 200 serovars. The three most common serovars of infection are *Leptospira icterohaemorrhagiae* of rats, *Leptospira cani-*

cola of dogs, and *Leptospira pomona* of cattle and swine, but no specific serovars have been linked to severity of illness. The disease is worldwide in distribution, and the incidence is higher than usually supposed. The leptospires are often transmitted to humans by the ingestion of food and drink contaminated by the urine of the reservoir animal. The organism may also enter through minor skin lesions and probably via the conjunctiva. Recreational cases have followed swimming or rafting in contaminated water, and occupational cases occur among sewer workers, rice planters, abattoir workers, and farmers. Sporadic urban cases have been seen in the homeless exposed to rat urine. The incubation period is 2–20 days.

Clinical Findings

A. SYMPTOMS AND SIGNS

Anicteric leptospirosis, the more common and milder form of the disease, is often biphasic. The initial or "septicemic" phase begins with abrupt fever to 39–40 °C, chills, abdominal pain, severe headache, and myalgias, especially of the calf muscles. There may be marked conjunctival suffusion. Leptospires can be isolated from blood, cerebrospinal fluid, and tissues. Following a 1- to 3-day period of improvement in symptoms and absence of fever, the second or "immune" phase begins. Leptospires are absent from blood and cerebrospinal fluid but are still present in the kidney, and specific antibodies appear. A recurrence of symptoms is seen as in the first phase of disease with the onset of meningitis. Uveitis (which can be unilateral or bilateral and usually involves the entire uveal tract), rash, and adenopathy may occur. A rare but severe manifestation is hemorrhagic pneumonia. The illness is usually self-limited, lasting 4–30 days, and complete recovery is the rule.

Icteric leptospirosis (Weil's syndrome) is the most severe form of the disease, characterized by impaired renal and hepatic function, abnormal mental status, hemorrhagic pneumonia, hypotension, and a 5–40% mortality rate. Symptoms and signs often are continuous and not biphasic.

Pretibial fever, a mild form of leptospirosis caused by *Leptospira autumnalis*, occurred during World War II at Fort Bragg. In pretibial fever, there is patchy erythema on the skin of the lower legs or generalized rash occurring with fever.

Leptospirosis with jaundice must be distinguished from hepatitis, yellow fever, and relapsing fever.

B. LABORATORY FINDINGS

The leukocyte count may be normal or as high as 50,000/mcL, with neutrophils predominating. The urine may contain bile, protein, casts, and red cells. Oliguria is common, and in severe cases uremia may occur. Elevated bilirubin and aminotransferases are seen in 75%, and elevated creatinine (> 1.5 mg/dL) is seen in 50% of cases. In cases with meningeal involve-

ment, organisms may be found in the cerebrospinal fluid during the first 10 days of illness. Early in the disease, the organism may be identified by darkfield examination of the patient's blood (a test requiring expertise since false-positives are frequent in inexperienced hands) or by culture on a semisolid medium (eg, Fletcher's EMJH). Cultures take 1–6 weeks to become positive. The organism may also be grown from the urine from the tenth day to the sixth week. Diagnosis is usually made by means of serologic tests, of which several are available. Agglutination tests (microscopic, using live organisms, and macroscopic, using killed antigen) become positive after 7–10 days of illness, peak at 3–4 weeks, and may persist at high levels for many years. Thus, to make a diagnosis, a fourfold or greater rise in titer must be documented. The agglutination tests are cumbersome to perform and require trained personnel. Indirect hemagglutination, enzyme immunosorbent assay (EIA), and enzyme-linked immunosorbent assay (ELISA) tests are also available. The IgM EIA is particularly useful in making an early diagnosis, since it is positive as early as 2 days into illness, a time when the clinical manifestations may be nonspecific, and it is extremely sensitive and specific (93%). Polymerase chain reaction (PCR) methods (presently investigational) appear to be sensitive, specific, positive early in disease, and able to detect leptospiral DNA in blood, urine, cerebrospinal fluid, and aqueous humor. Serum creatine kinase (CK) is usually elevated in persons with leptospirosis and normal in persons with hepatitis.

Complications

Myocarditis, aseptic meningitis, renal failure, and pulmonary infiltrates with hemorrhage are not common but are the usual causes of death. Iridocyclitis may occur.

Treatment

Various antimicrobial drugs, including penicillin, ceftriaxone, and tetracyclines, show antileptospiral activity. Penicillin (eg, 1.5 million units every 6 hours intravenously) or ceftriaxone (1 g daily intravenously) is the drug of choice in severe leptospirosis and is especially effective if started within the first 4 days of illness. Jarisch–Herxheimer reactions may occur. Doxycycline, 100 mg orally twice daily for 7 days, is also effective as therapy if started early, but this agent is most often used in mild to moderate disease. Although therapy for mild disease is controversial, most clinicians treat with oral penicillin, 500 mg four times daily, or doxycycline, 100 mg orally twice daily, for 7 days. Effective prophylaxis consists of doxycycline, 200 mg orally once weekly during the risk of exposure.

Prognosis

Without jaundice, the disease is almost never fatal. With jaundice, the mortality rate is 5% for those under age 30 years and 30% for those over age 60 years.

Ahmad SN et al: Laboratory diagnosis of leptospirosis. J Postgrad Med 2005;51:195. [PMID: 16333192]

Bharti AR et al: Leptospirosis: a zoonotic disease of global importance. Lancet Infect Dis 2003;3:757. [PMID: 14652202]

Edwards CN et al: Prevention and treatment of leptospirosis. Expert Rev Anti Infect Ther 2004;2:293. [PMID: 15482194]

Faucher JF et al: The management of leptospirosis. Expert Opin Pharmacother 2004;5:819. [PMID: 15102566]

Kobayashi Y: Human leptospirosis: Management and prognosis. J Postgrad Med 2005;51:201. [PMID: 16333193]

Ricaldi JN et al: Leptospirosis in the tropics and in travelers. Curr Infect Dis Rep 2006;8:51. [PMID: 16448601]

LYME DISEASE (Lyme Borreliosis)

 ESSENTIALS OF DIAGNOSIS

- Erythema migrans, a flat or slightly raised red lesion that expands with central clearing.
- Headache or stiff neck.
- Arthralgias, arthritis, and myalgias; arthritis is often chronic and recurrent.
- Wide geographic distribution, with most United States cases in the Northeast, mid-Atlantic, upper Midwest, and Pacific coastal regions.

General Considerations

This illness, named after the town of Old Lyme, Connecticut, is caused by the spirochete B burgdorferi and is transmitted to humans by ixodid ticks that are part of the Ixodes ricinus complex. Four genomic groups of the B burgdorferi sensu lato group have been identified: B burgdorferi sensu stricto, which causes disease in North America and less commonly in Europe and Asia; Borrelia garinii and Borrelia afzelii, which are the predominant etiologic agents of Lyme disease in Europe and Asia; and Borrelia bissettii sp nov found in California. Lyme disease is the most common vector-borne disease in the United States and is being reported with increasing frequency, but the true incidence is not known as overreporting remains a problem. In 2003, there were 21,273 cases reported from 45 states and the District of Columbia, an increase of 10% over 2002. Most cases (90%) were reported from the mid-Atlantic, northeastern, and north central regions of the country. As in years past, cases were reported from states without known enzootic cycles of B burgdorferi, raising questions about the accuracy of diagnosis. Because clinical manifestations are nonspecific and because laboratory diagnosis is insensitive early in the illness (see below), many patients are diagnosed with Lyme disease who do not have it. In a Lyme disease clinic at a major teaching hospital in an endemic area, only 23% of patients referred for active disease were found to have it. The consequences of overdiagnosis and overtreatment of Lyme disease are substantial. Individuals previously treated for Lyme disease, whether they actually had the disease or not, were avid users of the health care system, with multiple office visits to several different physicians resulting in numerous prescriptions for unnecessary antibiotics and frequent days of missed work.

The overreporting and overdiagnosis of Lyme disease are in part explained by the discovery of a noncultural spirochete in the Lone Star tick (Amblyomma americanum). This organism produces a Lyme disease-like illness referred to as STARI (Southern tick-associated rash illness) with a skin lesion indistinguishable from erythema migrans. As the Lone Star tick is found in the midwest and southern areas where enzootic cycles for B burgdorferi have not been reported, cases of Lyme disease reported from these areas are probably due to this newly discovered organism.

The vector of Lyme disease varies geographically and is Ixodes scapularis (also known as Ixodes dammini) in the northeastern, north central, and mid-Atlantic regions of the United States; Ixodes pacificus on the West Coast; I ricinus in Europe; and Ixodes persulcatus in Asia. The disease also occurs in Australia. Mice and deer make up the major animal reservoir of B burgdorferi, but other rodents and birds may also be infected. Domestic animals such as dogs, cattle, and horses can also develop clinical illness, usually manifested as arthritis.

Ticks feed once during each of their three stages of life. Larval ticks feed in late summer, nymphs in the following spring and early summer, and adults during the fall. In the northeastern United States and the mid-Atlantic states, the preferred host for the nymphs and larvae is the white-footed mouse (the black-striped mouse in Europe). This animal is tolerant of infection—a fact that is critical in maintaining infection, since the mouse can remain spirochetemic and transmit the agent to the larvae the following spring after being infected by the nymphal form in early summer. Adult ticks prefer the white-tailed deer as host. Although only 20–25% of nymphs harbor spirochetes compared with 50–65% of adults, most infections occur in the spring and summer (when nymphs are active), and fewer cases occur in the cooler months (October to April), when adults feed. This is probably due to the greater abundance of nymphs; greater human outdoor activity in spring and summer, when nymphs feed; and the fact that adult ticks are larger, easier to detect by the human host, and thus can be removed before disease is transmitted. Less than 1% of larvae are infected with spirochetes, and transmission of the disease through contact with larvae is unlikely. In the western United States, the I pacificus nymph prefers to feed on lizards, which are not susceptible to infection. It is only the few nymph and larval ticks that feed on wood rats, which can be infected, that are capable of transmitting disease.

The increased incidence of Lyme disease is due in part to the resurgence of the once-decimated deer population, the spread of tick vectors to new areas (infected Ixodes ticks have been isolated from migratory birds), and the encroachment of suburbs on once rural areas, bringing humans and ticks into closer proximity. Factors contributing to increased reporting include enhanced provider awareness and better laboratory surveillance.

Under experimental conditions, ticks must feed for 24–36 hours or longer to transmit infections. Human epidemiologic studies have indicated that the incidence of disease is significantly higher when tick attachment is for longer than 72 hours than if it is less than 72 hours, though rare cases have been documented with attachment of less than 24 hours. In addition, the percentage of ticks infected varies on a regional basis. In the northeastern and midwestern regions, 15–65% of *I scapularis* ticks are infected with the spirochete; in the western United States, only 2% of *I pacificus* are infected. These are important epidemiologic features in assessing the likelihood that tick exposure will result in disease. Exposure to *I pacificus* is unlikely to result in disease, since so few ticks are infected, but this is not true of exposure to *I scapularis*. Eliciting a history of brushing a tick off the skin (ie, the tick was not feeding) or removing a tick on the same day as exposure (ie, the tick did not feed long enough) decreases the likelihood that infection will develop, since the vast majority of cases occur when ticks feed for at least 24 hours.

Ixodes ticks are smaller than the more common dog ticks (*Dermacentor variabilis*). Larvae are less than 1 mm in size, and the adult female is 2–3 mm in size, with a red body and black legs. After a blood meal, ticks can reach two to three times their unengorged size. Because the tick is so small, the bite is usually painless and goes unnoticed. After feeding, the tick drops off in 2–4 days. If a tick is found, it should be removed immediately. The best way to accomplish this is to use a fine-tipped tweezers to pull firmly and repeatedly on the tick's mouth part—not the tick's body—until the tick releases its hold. Saving the tick in a bottle of alcohol for future identification may be useful, especially if symptoms develop.

Congenital infection has been documented, but the exact frequency and manifestations have not been clearly defined. Similarly, because the organism can be latent, it is not known if women infected prior to becoming pregnant can activate the disease and transmit infection to the fetus. In one retrospective study, 5 of 19 pregnancies complicated by Lyme disease resulted in an adverse outcome, but all of the outcomes were different and could not be conclusively linked to infection. Several serosurveys involving over 2000 pregnant women in endemic areas have not found any association between seropositivity in prospective mothers and the prevalence of congenital malformations, fetal death, and prematurity. Thus, if *B burgdorferi* causes a congenital syndrome like some other spirochetal illnesses, it must be extremely uncommon.

Clinical Findings

The typical clinical description of Lyme disease divides the illness into three stages: stage 1, flu-like

symptoms and a typical skin rash (**erythema migrans**); stage 2, weeks to months later, Bell's palsy or meningitis; and stage 3, months to years later, arthritis. The problem with this simplified scheme is that there is a great deal of overlap, and the skin, central nervous system, and musculoskeletal system can be involved early or late. A more accurate classification divides disease into early and late manifestations and specifies whether disease is localized or disseminated.

A. Symptoms and Signs

1. Stage 1, early localized infection—Stage 1 infection is characterized by erythema migrans. About 1 week after the tick bite (range, 3–30 days; median 7–10 days), a flat or slightly raised red lesion appears at the site, which is commonly seen in areas of tight clothing such as the groin, thigh, or axilla. This lesion expands over several days. Although originally described as a lesion that progresses with central clearing ("bulls-eye" lesion), often there is a more homogeneous appearance or even central intensification. About 10–20% of patients either do not have typical skin lesions or the lesions go unnoticed. A flu-like illness with fever, chills, and myalgia occurs in about 50% of patients. Even without treatment, the symptoms and signs of erythema migrans resolve in 3–4 weeks. Although the classic lesion of erythema migrans is not difficult to recognize, atypical forms can occur that may lead to misdiagnosis. Vesicular, urticarial, and evanescent erythema migrans have all been reported. Similarly, chemical reactions to tick and spider bites, drug eruptions, urticaria, and staphylococcal and streptococcal cellulitis have been mistaken for erythema migrans.

Completely asymptomatic disease, without erythema migrans or flu-like symptoms, can occur, but is very uncommon in the United States. Serosurveys done as part of vaccination trials found asymptomatic seroconversion in 7% or less of the population.

2. Stage 2, early disseminated infection—Up to 44% of patients with erythema migrans are bacteremic (especially if multiple lesions are present) leading to dissemination of the spirochete resulting in a wide variety of symptoms and signs. This usually occurs within days to weeks after inoculation of the organism. The most common manifestations involve the skin, central nervous system, and musculoskeletal system. In about 50% of patients, secondary lesions develop that are not associated with a tick bite. These lesions are similar in appearance to the primary lesion but are usually smaller. A rare skin lesion (1% of patients) seen primarily in Europe is *Borrelia lymphocytoma*. This presents as a small reddish nodule or plaque on the ear in children and on the nipple in adults. Headache and stiff neck can occur, as well as migratory pains in joints, muscles, and tendons. Fatigue and malaise are common. Generally, the neurologic and musculoskeletal symptoms are intermittent and last only hours to a few days, whereas fatigue is persistent. After hematogenous spread, the organism sequesters itself in certain areas and produces focal symptoms. Some patients experience cardiac (4–10% of patients) or neurologic (10–20% of patients) manifestations. Involvement of the heart includes myopericarditis, with atrial or ventricular arrhythmias and heart block. Neurologic disease is most commonly manifested as aseptic meningitis with mild headache and neck stiffness, Bell's palsy, or encephalitis with irritability, personality change, and forgetfulness that can wax and wane. Even in the absence of symptoms, seeding of the central nervous system can occur. Peripheral neuropathy (sensory or motor), transverse myelitis, and mononeuritis multiplex have also been described. Conjunctivitis, keratitis, and, rarely, panophthalmitis can occur.

3. Stage 3, late persistent infection—Stage 3 infection occurs months to years after the initial infection and again primarily manifests itself as musculoskeletal, neurologic, and skin disease. Musculoskeletal complaints develop in up to 60% of patients. Clinical manifestations are quite variable and include (1) joint and periarticular pain without objective findings (perhaps a manifestation of fibromyalgia that may be triggered by Lyme disease); (2) frank arthritis, mainly of large joints, that is chronic or recurrent over years (recurrences become less severe, less frequent, and shorter with time); and (3) chronic synovitis, which may result in permanent disability. The pathogenesis of chronic Lyme arthritis may be an immunologic phenomenon rather than persistence of infection. The observations that individuals with chronic arthritis have an increased frequency of HLA-DR4 gene expression, antibodies to OspA and OspB protein in joint fluid (major outer surface proteins of *B burgdorferi*), lack *B burgdorferi* DNA in synovial fluid as detected by PCR, and often fail to respond to antibiotics—all support the inference of an immunologic mechanism.

Both the central and the peripheral nervous systems may be involved. Subacute encephalopathy, characterized by memory loss, mood changes, and sleep disturbance, is the most common chronic neurologic manifestation. An axonal polyneuropathy, manifested as distal sensory paresthesias or radicular pain, can occur either alone or, more commonly, in association with encephalopathy. Most of these patients have objective signs of disease when tested by electromyography. A rare form of chronic neurologic dysfunction—leukoencephalitis—presents with cognitive dysfunction, spastic paraparesis, ataxia, and bladder dysfunction. This form of the disease is seen more commonly in Europe than in the United States.

The cutaneous manifestation of late infection, which can occur up to 10 years after infection, is **acrodermatitis chronicum atrophicans**. It has been described mainly in Europe and is due to infection with *B afzelii*, a species that commonly causes disease in Europe but not the United States. There is usually bluish-red discoloration of a distal extremity with associated swelling. These lesions become atrophic and sclerotic with time and eventually resemble localized scleroderma. At least two cases of diffuse fasciitis with eosinophilia, a rare entity that resembles scleroderma, have been associated with infection with *B burgdorferi*.

B. LABORATORY FINDINGS

The diagnosis of Lyme disease is based on both clinical manifestations and laboratory findings. The National Surveillance Case Definition specifies a person with exposure to a potential tick habitat (within the 30 days just prior to developing erythema migrans) with (1) erythema migrans diagnosed by a physician or (2) at least one late manifestation of the disease and (3) laboratory confirmation as fulfilling the criteria for Lyme disease.

Laboratory confirmation requires detection of specific antibodies to *B burgdorferi* in serum, either by indirect immunofluorescence assay (IFA) or ELISA; the latter is now preferred, because it is more sensitive and specific. A Western blot assay that can detect both IgM and IgG antibodies is used as a confirmatory test. IgM antibody appears first 2–4 weeks after onset of erythema migrans, peaks at 6–8 weeks, and then declines to low levels after 4–6 months of illness. The presence of IgM antibody in patients with prolonged symptoms persisting for several months is likely to be a false-positive result. IgG occurs later (6–8 weeks after onset of disease), peaks at 4–6 months, and may remain elevated at low levels indefinitely despite appropriate therapy and resolution of symptoms. A two-test approach is now recommended for the diagnosis of active Lyme disease. All specimens positive or equivocal by ELISA or IFA should be tested by Western immunoblot. When Western immunoblot is done during the first 4 weeks of illness, both IgM and IgG should be tested. If a patient with suspected early Lyme disease has negative serologic studies, acute and convalescent titers should be obtained since up to 50% of patients with early disease can be antibody negative in the first several weeks of illness. A fourfold rise in antibody titer would be diagnostic of recent infection. In patients with later stages of disease, almost all are antibody positive. False-positive reactions in the ELISA and IFA have been reported in juvenile rheumatoid arthritis, rheumatoid arthritis, systemic lupus erythematosus, infectious mononucleosis, subacute infective endocarditis, syphilis, relapsing fever, leptospirosis, enteroviral and other viral illnesses, and patients with gingival disease (presumably because of cross-reactivity with oral treponemes). False-negative serologic reactions occur early in illness, and antibiotic therapy early in disease can abort subsequent seroconversion.

VlsE is an outer surface lipoprotein of *B burgdorferi*. A new ELISA measuring antibodies against a peptide that is in the invariant region of this lipoprotein has been studied in a number of different clinical scenarios. The test is done in a single step (as opposed to the current two-step test recommended by the Centers for Disease Control and Prevention), is easy to standardize, and is less expensive than two-step testing. The ELISA appears to be as sensitive and specific as the current two-step test in the diagnosis of late stage disease and it is more sensitive for early disease.

Caution should be exercised in interpreting serologic tests. Serologic tests are not subject to national standards, and interlaboratory variation of results is a major problem. In addition, some laboratories perform tests that are entirely unreliable and should never be used to support the diagnosis of Lyme disease (eg, the Lyme urinary antigen test, immunofluorescent staining for cell wall-deficient forms of *B burgdorferi,* lymphocyte transformation tests, using PCR on inappropriate specimens such as blood or urine). In addition, testing is often done in patients with nonspecific symptoms such as headache, arthralgia, myalgia, fatigue, and palpitations. Even in endemic areas, the pretest probability of having Lyme disease is low in these patients, and the probability of a false-positive test result is greater than that of a true-positive result. For these reasons, the American College of Physicians has established guidelines for laboratory evaluation of patients with suspected Lyme disease:

1. The diagnosis of early Lyme disease is clinical (ie, exposure in an endemic area, with physician-documented erythema migrans), and does *not* require laboratory confirmation. (Tests are often negative at this stage.)

2. Late disease requires objective evidence of clinical manifestations (recurrent brief attacks of monoarticular or oligoarticular arthritis of the large joints; lymphocytic meningitis, cranial neuritis [Bell's palsy], peripheral neuropathy or, rarely, encephalomyelitis—but *not* headache, fatigue, paresthesias, or stiff neck alone; atrioventricular conduction defects with or without myocarditis) and laboratory evidence of disease (two-stage testing with ELISA and Western blot, as described above).

3. Patients with nonspecific symptoms without objective signs of Lyme disease should *not* have serologic testing done. It is in this setting that false-positive tests occur more commonly than true-positive tests.

4. The role of serologic testing in neuroborreliosis is unclear, as sensitivity and specificity of cerebrospinal fluid serologic tests have not been determined. However, it is rare for a patient with neuroborreliosis to have positive serologic tests on cerebrospinal fluid without positive tests on serum (see below).

5. Other tests such as the T cell proliferative assay, PCR testing, and urinary antigen detection have not yet been studied well enough to be routinely used (see discussion below).

Positive cultures for *B burgdorferi* can be obtained early in the course of disease. Aspiration of erythema migrans lesions has yielded positive cultures in up to 30% of cases, whereas culture of a 2-mm punch biopsy is positive in 50–70%. PCR of a skin biopsy is even more sensitive, with positivity rates of 80%. In early disease, blood cultures are positive in up to 50% if large volumes (9 mL) are used, but cerebrospinal fluid is rarely culture positive. The ability to culture organisms from skin lesions is greatly influenced by antibiotic therapy. Even a brief course of several days will result in negative cultures. Special silver staining of chronically inflamed synovial tissue demonstrates spirochetes in one-third of patients.

PCR is very specific for detecting the presence of *Borrelia* DNA, but sensitivity is variable and depends on which body fluid is tested and the stage of the disease. In general, PCR is more sensitive than culture, especially in chronic disease. Up to 85% of synovial fluid samples are positive in active arthritis. In contrast, 38% of cerebrospinal fluid samples in acute neuroborreliosis are PCR positive, and only 25% are positive in chronic neuroborreliosis. The significance of a positive reaction is unclear. Whether a positive PCR indicates persistence of viable organisms that will respond to further treatment or is a marker for residual DNA (not active infection) has not been clarified. In chronic Lyme arthritis, some have suggested that a positive PCR indicates active infection that requires further therapy, while others have found a positive reaction despite months of therapy, suggesting that the presence of DNA is indicative of an autoimmune arthritis.

The diagnosis of neuroborreliosis is often difficult since clinical manifestations, such as subtle memory impairment, may be difficult to document. Most patients with neuroborreliosis have a history of previous erythema migrans or monoarticular or polyarticular arthritis, and the vast majority have antibody present in serum. When cerebrospinal fluid is sampled, there may not be evidence of an inflammation (pleocytosis, elevated protein), but localized antibody production, ie, a ratio of cerebrospinal fluid to serum antibody of > 1.0, can often be demonstrated. The role of other tests such as PCR in detection of DNA or ELISA in detecting the presence of outer surface protein A (OspA) antigen is unclear, but in difficult cases these tests can be performed and, if positive, help establish the diagnosis. In addition, many patients with neuroborreliosis will have a peripheral neuropathy that may be detected by electromyography. In the absence of any of the above findings, it is difficult to make the diagnosis of central nervous system *Borrelia* infection.

Nonspecific laboratory abnormalities can be seen, particularly in early disease. The most common are an elevated sedimentation rate of > 20 mm/h seen in 50% of cases and mildly abnormal liver function tests present in 30%. The abnormal liver function tests are transient and return to normal within a few weeks of treatment. A mild anemia, leukocytosis (11,000–18,000/mcL), and microscopic hematuria have been reported in 10% or less of patients.

Prevention

Simple preventive measures such as avoiding tick-infested areas, covering exposed skin with long-sleeved shirts and wearing long trousers tucked into socks, wearing light-colored clothing, using repellents, and inspecting for ticks after exposure will greatly reduce the number of tick bites. Environmental controls directed at limiting ticks on residential property would be helpful, but trying to limit the deer, tick, or white-footed mouse populations over large areas is not feasible.

Routine use of prophylactic antibiotics following tick bites is not recommended. Analysis of the cost-effectiveness of prophylactic therapy suggests that antibiotics administered for 2 weeks would be beneficial in preventing illness in endemic areas, where the risk of acquiring disease following a tick bite is 3.6% or greater. However, prospective studies designed to examine the effect of prophylaxis have shown conflicting results. Two studies have shown no benefit of prophylaxis, but one study resulted in a decrease in erythema migrans from 3.2% in patients given placebo to 0.4% in those given a single 200-mg dose of doxycycline following a documented tick bite from *I scapularis*. Because most patients in whom Lyme disease develops are symptomatic and since treatment of early disease prevents late sequelae, it is reasonable to reserve treatment for patients in whom symptoms develop rather than to routinely administer prophylactic antibiotics unless the risk is extremely high (endemic area, documented *Ixodes* tick bite, feeding at least 40 hours). Exceptions might include situations in which the follow-up is uncertain, the patient is extremely anxious, the patient is a pregnant woman, or the tick was engorged when removed.

A highly effective (75% efficacy) recombinant vaccine (LYMErix, SmithKline Beecham) using a conserved region of *B burgdorferi* known as OspA has been removed from the market. Low sales were cited as the reason for withdrawal. However, initial controversy surrounding the vaccine concerned the theoretical possibility of inducing an autoimmune arthritis in recipients. Despite the fact that no cases of vaccine-induced arthritis had been documented, concerns about potential legal actions probably contributed to the decision to withdraw the product.

Treatment

Antibiotic sensitivity of *B burgdorferi* has been established in vitro. Tetracycline is effective against the spirochete, but penicillin is only moderately so. Erythromycin is effective in vitro but has been disappointing in clinical trials. Ampicillin, ceftriaxone, azithromycin, cefuroxime, and imipenem are also effective in vitro, but aminoglycosides, ciprofloxacin, and rifampin are not.

Present recommendations for therapy are outlined in Table 34–4. In general, infection confined to skin is treated for 2–3 weeks, although courses of doxycycline as short as 10 days have been shown to be effective. For central nervous system disease (with the exception of Bell's palsy), intravenous therapy is used. Other organ system involvement usually responds to oral medication. For erythema migrans, antibiotic therapy shortens the duration of rash and prevents late sequelae. Doxycycline, is most commonly used and has the advantage of being active against *Anaplasma phagocytophilum* (formerly *Ehrlichia*). Amoxicillin is also effective and is recommended for pregnant or lactating women and for those who cannot tolerate doxycycline. Cefuroxime axetil, is as effective as doxycycline, but because of its cost it should be considered an alternative choice for those who cannot tolerate doxycycline or amoxicillin or for those in whom the drugs are contraindicated. Erythromycin and azithromycin are less effective, associated with higher rates of re-

Table 34–4. Treatment of Lyme disease.

Manifestation	Drug and Dosage
Tick bite	No treatment in most circumstances (see text); observe
Erythema migrans	Doxycycline, 100 mg orally twice daily, or amoxicillin, 500 mg orally three times daily, or cefuroxime axetil, 500 mg twice daily—all for 2–3 weeks
Neurologic disease	
Bell's palsy	Doxycycline, or amoxicillin as above for 2–3 weeks
Other central nervous system disease	Ceftriaxone, 2 g intravenously once daily, or penicillin G, 18–24 million units daily intravenously in 6 divided doses, or cefotaxime, 2 g intravenously every 8 hours—all for 2–4 weeks
Cardiac disease	
First-degree block (P-R < 0.3 seconds)	Doxycycline or amoxicillin as above for 2–3 weeks
High-degree atrioventricular block	Ceftriaxone or penicillin G as above for 30–60 days (see text)
Arthritis	
Oral dosage	Doxycycline or amoxicillin as above for 30–60 days (see text)
Parenteral dosage	Ceftriaxone or penicillin G as above for 2–4 weeks
Acrodermatitis chronicum atrophicans	Doxycycline or amoxicillin as above for 4 weeks
"Chronic Lyme disease" or "post-Lyme disease syndrome"	Symptomatic therapy

lapse, and are not recommended as first-line therapy. Isolated Bell's palsy (without meningitis or peripheral neuropathy) can be treated with doxycycline or amoxicillin for 2–3 weeks. Although therapy does not affect the rate of resolution of the cranial neuropathy, it does prevent development of late manifestations of disease.

The need for a lumbar puncture in patients with seventh nerve palsy is controversial. Some perform lumbar puncture on all patients with Bell's palsy and others only if there are symptoms or signs of meningitis. If meningitis is present, therapy with a parenteral antibiotic is indicated. Ceftriaxone is most commonly used, but penicillin is equally efficacious. In European countries, doxycycline 400 mg/d for 14 days is frequently used and is comparable in efficacy to ceftriaxone. First- and second-degree heart block can be treated with oral agents, but third-degree block should be treated with ceftriaxone or penicillin, and the patient should be admitted to the hospital for monitoring.

Therapy of arthritis is difficult because some patients do not respond to any therapy, and those who do respond may do so slowly. Oral agents (doxycycline or amoxicillin) are as effective as intravenous regimens (ceftriaxone or penicillin). A reasonable approach to the patient with Lyme arthritis is to start with oral therapy for 30 days, and if this fails (persistent or recurrent joint swelling), to re-treat with an oral regimen for 60 days or switch to an intravenous regimen for 2–4 weeks. Re-treatment should be delayed for several months because of the slow resolution of joint symptoms. If arthritis persists after re-treatment, symptomatic therapy with nonsteroidal anti-inflammatory drugs is recommended. For severe refractory pain, synovectomy may be required.

Based on the limited published data, therapy of Lyme disease in pregnancy should be the same as therapy in other patients with the exception that doxycycline should not be used.

Clinicians are often confronted with patients with nonspecific symptoms (such as fatigue and myalgias) and positive serologic tests for Lyme disease who request (or demand) therapy for their illness. It is important in managing these patients to remember (1) that the diagnosis of Lyme disease is primarily a clinical one, and nonspecific symptoms alone are not diagnostic; (2) that serologic tests are fraught with difficulty (as noted above), and in areas where disease prevalence is low, false-positive serologic tests are much more common than true-positive tests; and (3) that parenteral therapy with ceftriaxone for 2–4 weeks is costly (approximately $5000) and has been associated with significant adverse effects (cholelithiasis). Parenteral therapy should be reserved for those most likely to benefit, ie, those with cutaneous, neurologic, cardiac, or rheumatic manifestations that are characteristic of Lyme disease.

Coinfections

Lyme disease, babesiosis (see Chapter 35), and human granulocytic ehrlichiosis (see Chapter 32) are endemic in similar areas of the country and are transmitted by the same tick, *I scapularis*. Coinfection with two or even all three of these organisms can occur, causing a clinical picture that is not "classic" for any of these diseases. The presence of erythema migrans is highly suggestive of Lyme disease, whereas flu-like symptoms without rash are more suggestive of babesiosis or ehrlichiosis. The complete blood count is usually normal in Lyme disease, but in patients with Lyme disease and babesiosis, anemia and thrombocytopenia are more common. Patients with Lyme disease and ehrlichiosis are more likely to have leukopenia. Patients with Lyme disease and babesiosis may have longer-lasting and more severe symptoms. Thus, persistent symptoms after what appears to be appropriate therapy for Lyme disease should raise the possibility of coexisting babesiosis.

Even in patients with documented Lyme disease, immunity is not complete. Individuals who live in endemic areas are subject to reinfection.

Prognosis

Most patients respond to appropriate therapy with prompt resolution of symptoms within 4 weeks. With adequate therapy, only a small percentage of patients will not respond or will develop a late relapse. True treatment failures are thus uncommon, and in most cases re-treatment or prolonged treatment of Lyme disease is instituted because of misdiagnosis or misinterpretation of serologic results (both IgG and IgM antibodies can persist for prolonged periods despite adequate therapy) rather than inadequate therapy. The terms "chronic Lyme disease" or "post-Lyme disease syndrome" have been applied to patients with documented Lyme disease who have been adequately treated but have persistent nonspecific symptoms such as fatigue, arthralgias, myalgias, and neurocognitive complaints. These entities are poorly defined, and the patients comprise a heterogeneous group. Although there is a tendency to treat these patients with multiple or prolonged courses of oral or intravenous antibiotics, there are no data suggesting that this is efficacious, and the prolonged use of antibiotics in this setting is emphatically discouraged.

The long-term outcome of adult patients with Lyme disease is generally favorable, but some patients have chronic complaints. Joint pain, memory impairment, and poor functional status secondary to pain are common subjective complaints in patients with Lyme disease, but physical examination and neurocognitive testing fail to document the presence of these symptoms as objective sequelae. Similarly, in highly endemic areas, patients with a diagnosis of Lyme disease commonly complain of pain, fatigue, and an inability to perform certain physical activities when followed for several years. However, these complaints occur just as commonly in age-matched controls without a history of Lyme disease. Attempts to document chronic cardiac disease in patients treated for Lyme disease also have been unsuccessful. The long-term outcome of treated neuroborelliosis is favorable, with complete recovery in 75% of patients. Of the remaining individuals, only 12% had sequelae that affected their daily activities.

Aguero-Rosenfeld ME et al: Diagnosis of Lyme borreliosis. Clin Microbiol Rev 2005;18:484. [PMID: 16020686]

Bunikis J et al: Laboratory testing for suspected Lyme disease. Med Clin North Am 2002;86:311. [PMID: 11982304]

Coyle PK et al: Neurologic aspects of Lyme disease. Med Clin North Am 2002;86:261. [PMID: 11982301]

Depietropaolo DL et al: Diagnosis of Lyme disease. Am Fam Physician 2005;72:297. [PMID: 16050454]

Halperin JJ: Central nervous system Lyme disease. Curr Infect Dis Rep 2004;6:298. [PMID: 15265459]

Hayes EB et al: How can we prevent Lyme disease? N Engl J Med 2003;348:2424. [PMID: 12802029]

Hengge UR et al: Lyme borreliosis. Lancet Infect Dis 2003;3:489. [PMID: 12901891]

Massarotti EM: Lyme arthritis. Med Clin North Am 2002;86:297. [PMID: 11982303]

Pinto DS: Cardiac manifestations of Lyme disease. Med Clin North Am 2002;86:285.[PMID: 11982302]

Stanek G et al: Lyme borreliosis. Lancet 2003;362:1639. [PMID: 14630446]

Infectious Diseases: Protozoal & Helminthic

35

Robert S. Goldsmith, MD, MPH, DTM&H

■ PROTOZOAL INFECTIONS

AFRICAN TRYPANOSOMIASIS (Sleeping Sickness)

ESSENTIALS OF DIAGNOSIS

- *History of exposure to tsetse flies, with subsequent bite lesion.*

Hemolymphatic stage:
- *Irregular fevers, headaches, joint pains, malaise, pruritus, papular skin rash, edemas.*
- *Posterior cervical or generalized lymphadenopathy; hepatosplenomegaly.*
- *Anemia, weight loss.*
- *Trypanosomes in blood or lymph node aspirates; positive serology.*

Meningoencephalitic stage:
- *Insomnia, motor and sensory disorders, abnormal reflexes, somnolence to coma.*
- *Trypanosomes and increased white cells and protein in cerebrospinal fluid.*

General Considerations

African trypanosomiasis is caused by *Trypanosoma brucei rhodesiense* and *Trypanosoma brucei gambiense*, both hemoflagellates. The organisms are transmitted by bites of tsetse flies (*Glossina* species), which inhabit shaded areas along streams and rivers. Trypanosomes ingested in a blood meal undergo a developmental period of 18–35 days in the fly; when the fly feeds again on a new mammalian host, the infective stage is injected. Human disease occurs locally (but strictly in rural areas) throughout tropical Africa from south of the Sahara to about 20 degrees south latitude. *T b gambiense* infections are in the moist sub-Saharan sa-

vanna and riverine forests of west and central Africa up to the eastern Rift Valley. *T b rhodesiense* infections occur to the east of the Rift Valley in the savannah of east and southeast Africa and along the shores of Lake Victoria (up to 18% in some areas of Uganda).

T b rhodesiense infection is primarily a zoonosis of game animals but also infects cattle; humans are infected sporadically. Humans are the principal mammalian host for *T b gambiense;* it is uncertain whether there is an animal reservoir, but domestic animals can be infected. A third trypanosome, *Trypanosoma brucei*, infects only wild and domestic animals.

Although African trypanosomiasis was largely controlled through the 1960s, the disease has reemerged as an increasing threat in west, central, and east Africa. Yearly, an estimated 30,000 new cases occur that result in a total prevalence of 300,000–500,000 infections (local prevalence in some foci exceeds 5%) and 100,000 deaths (most due to *T b gambiense* infection). Among visitors to the East African game parks, infections are rare, with about one case a year appearing in the United States.

Clinical Findings

A. Symptoms and Signs

Infections go through three stages: chancre, hemolymphatic, and encephalitic. The hemolymphatic period, which usually begins within 3–10 days after appearance of the chancre, is diagnosed by detecting the circulating parasite. Rhodesian trypanosomiasis is much more virulent, and untreated patients die within weeks to months. Gambian trypanosomiasis, however, usually goes through a long asymptomatic period in which a chancre is rare, the hemolytic stage may be absent or go unnoticed, and parasites are much more difficult to find. When Gambian symptoms do become manifest in weeks to months, they are often initially mild and nonspecific and are ignored by the patient; unless treated, however, death occurs within months to several years. There have been some reports of variations in severity.

1. The trypanosomal chancre—In *T b rhodesiense* infections, this is a local pruritic, painful inflammatory reaction (3–10 cm) with regional lymphadenopathy that appears about 48 hours after the tsetse fly bite and lasts 2–4 weeks.

2. The hemolymphatic (early) stage—High fever, severe headache, joint pains, and malaise recur at irregular intervals corresponding to waves of parasitemia. Between febrile episodes there are symptom-free periods that last up to 2 weeks. Transient rashes may appear, often pruritic and papular or circinate. Examination reveals mild enlargement of the liver and spleen, and edema (peripheral, pleural, ascites, etc). Enlarged, rubbery, and painless lymph nodes occur in 75% of patients. In Gambian trypanosomiasis, there may be lymphadenopathy, particularly of the posterior cervical group (Winterbottom's sign). With progression of the disease, there is weight loss and debilitation. Myocardial involvement may appear early in Rhodesian trypanosomiasis, and the patient may die of myocarditis before meningoencephalitic signs appear.

3. The meningoencephalitic (late) stage—This stage appears within a few weeks or months of onset of Rhodesian trypanosomiasis, but in Gambian trypanosomiasis, sleeping sickness develops more insidiously, starting 6 months to several years after onset. Insomnia, anorexia, personality changes, apathy, and headaches are the early findings. A variety of motor or tonus disorders may develop, including tremors; seizures; and disturbances of speech, gait, and reflexes. Sensory involvement includes hyperesthesia and pruritus. Somnolence appears late. The patient becomes severely emaciated and, finally, comatose. Death often results from secondary infection.

B. LABORATORY FINDINGS

Definitive diagnosis requires finding the organism. Detection in the blood is usually possible in Rhodesian trypanosomiasis but is very difficult in Gambian trypanosomiasis. The diagnosis of early-stage Gambian trypanosomiasis is by screening with a field-adapted card agglutination test (CATT) (sensitivity about 96%, specificity high), which is then followed by confirmatory microscopy to detect the parasite in the blood, cerebrospinal fluid, or other tissues. Circulating IgM antibody, which becomes positive about 12 days after infection, is sometimes useful; its titers may fluctuate or be undetectable during brief periods of antigen excess, and a negative test does not rule out infection. Several other antibody tests are used epidemiologically for Gambian trypanosomiasis. In late central nervous system disease, though both circulating antibody and parasitemia may fall below detectable levels, serologic tests of the cerebrospinal fluid (especially IgM) may prove useful. Polymerase chain reaction (PCR) testing is highly sensitive but is not commercially available.

Motile parasites are found in wet films and after Giemsa or Wright's staining of thin and thick blood films; of aspirates of bite lesions, lymph nodes, or bone marrow; or of cerebrospinal fluid. The two species, morphologically identical, are differentiated by molecular techniques. Because the number of trypanosomes in blood fluctuates (they may be undetectable 3 out of 5 days but are more common during febrile periods), multiple anticoagulated specimens should be examined daily for as many as 15 days using 10–15 mL for centrifugation; the trypanosomes are concentrated in the buffy coat. Other diagnostic tests with blood are intraperitoneal inoculation of rodents (sensitive but only effective for *T b rhodesiense*), culture, Millipore filtration, and DEAE-cellulose anion exchange centrifugation. Only soft lymph nodes should be selected for aspiration (25-gauge needle); after the node is gently kneaded, the aspirate is examined immediately for motile organisms.

Cerebrospinal fluid is clear and shows an increase in pressure, lymphocytes ($\geq$ 5 cells/mcL), and protein (> 35 mg/dL). Large eosinophilic plasma cells (Mott cells) are rarely seen but are considered pathognomonic by some experts. With progression of the disease, the parasite is more likely to be found in cerebrospinal fluid than in blood or lymph nodes. To detect the organism, the fluid should be examined within 20 minutes (to avoid parasitic lysis) and centrifuged twice (doubles sensitivity), inoculated into an experimental animal, and cultured.

Anemia, increased sedimentation rate, thrombocytopenia, and increased globulin are common. Eosinophilia is not seen. Electroencephalograms, MRI, and CT scans are nonspecific.

Differential Diagnosis

Trypanosomiasis may be mistaken for a variety of other diseases, including malaria, influenza, pneumonia, tuberculosis, infectious mononucleosis, leukemia, lymphoma, HIV infection, the arbovirus encephalitides, and psychosis. Serologic tests for syphilis may be falsely positive in trypanosomiasis.

Treatment

Because all of the drugs used are toxic, specific detection of the organism is a prerequisite for treatment; immunoassays are insufficient to make the diagnosis. A key issue in choice of drugs is to distinguish early- from late-stage disease. Treatment is also complicated by drug resistance (pentamidine and melarsoprol) and by the need for prolonged follow-up.

Suramin and pentamidine do not adequately cross the blood-brain barrier and cannot be used when the central nervous system is involved; melarsoprol and eflornithine, however, do pass the barrier. Melarsoprol causes a reactive encephalopathy in 5–10% of patients (corticosteroids are partially protective) and the mortality rate from that complication is 50% or higher. Side effects of pentamidine, although usually well-tolerated, can include hypotension, dizziness, vomiting, and sterile abscess; those of suramin include gastrointestinal symptoms and rarely nephrotoxicity, hypotension, and pancytopenia. Eflornithine, used only for *T b gambiense* infections, has side effects that include pancytopenia, diarrhea, hallucinations, and seizures. The drug is expensive and its continued availability (from the World Health Organization [WHO]) is uncertain. Suramin side effects, which may be severe, include vomiting, pruritus, paresthesias, and peripheral neuropathy. Suramin and melarsoprol are available only from the CDC Drug Service, Centers for Disease Control and Prevention, Atlanta, GA 30333. Telephone: 404-639-3670. Nifurtimox use continues to be under evaluation.

A. EARLY DISEASE, THE HEMOLYMPHATIC STAGE

The drug of choice for Gambian trypanosomiasis is pentamidine (4 mg/kg intramuscularly every day or every other day for 7–10 days; cure rare 93%). An alternate drug is intravenous eflornithine (400 mg/kg/d in four divided doses for 14 days). The treatment of Rhodesian trypanosomiasis is with intravenous suramin (100–200 mg [test dose], then 20 mg/kg [maximum 1 g] every 7 days for seven doses).

B. LATE DISEASE WITH CENTRAL NERVOUS SYSTEM INVOLVEMENT

Drugs of choice for both parasitic infections are intravenous melarsoprol, 2–3.6 mg/kg/d for 3 days; after 1 week, 3.6 mg/kg/d for 3 days; repeat after 10–21 days. Relapse rates for Gambian trypanosomiasis, formerly low (5–8%), have markedly increased as melarsoprol drug resistance has risen sharply in some areas of Africa, where failure rates approach 30%. A new shortened melarsoprol treatment schedule (2.2 mg/kg/d for 10 days by slow intravenous injection plus coadministration of a corticosteroid) has been evaluated in a multinational study and is now advocated for treatment of *T b gambiense* infections only. An alternative treatment only against *T b gambiense* is eflornithine (as above).

Proper follow-up to ensure detection of the encephalitic stage requires initial cerebrospinal fluid examination, repeat studies at intervals during treatment, 3 months after treatment, and then at 6-month intervals for 2 years.

Prevention

Individual prevention in endemic areas should include wearing long sleeves and trousers, avoiding dark-colored clothing, and using mosquito nets while sleeping. Repellents have no effect. Chemoprophylaxis with pentamidine is no longer in use. For *T b gambiense* infection, performing serologic tests every 6 months during exposure and for 3 years afterward is the safest method for detecting the disease at an early stage. Gambian control depends on detecting and treating the largely asymptomatic human reservoir.

Prognosis

Most patients—even those with advanced disease—recover following treatment. Relapses are uncommon (about 2%). If untreated or if therapy is started late, irreversible brain damage or death follows.

Burchmore RJ et al: Chemotherapy of human African trypanosomiasis. Curr Pharm Des 2002;8:256. [PMID: 11860365]

Chappuis F et al: Options for field diagnosis of human Africa trypanosomiasis. Clin Microbiol Rev 2005;18:133. [PMID: 15653823]

Kennedy PG: Human African trypanosomiasis of the CNS: current issues and challenges. J Clin Invest 2004;113:496. [PMID: 14966556]

Lejon V et al: Review Article: cerebrospinal fluid in human African trypanosomiasis: a key to diagnosis, therapeutic decision and post-treatment follow-up. Trop Med Int Health 2005; 10:395. [PMID: 15860085]

Schmid C et al: Effectiveness of a 10-day melarsoprol schedule for the treatment of late-stage human African trypanosomiasis: confirmation from a multinational study (IMPAMEL II). J Infect Dis 2005;191:1922. [PMID: 15871127]

Stich A et al: Human African trypanosomiasis. BMJ 2002;325: 203. [PMID: 12142311]

AMERICAN TRYPANOSOMIASIS (Chagas' Disease)

 ESSENTIALS OF DIAGNOSIS

Acute stage:

- *Inflammatory lesion at site of inoculation; prolonged fever, tachycardia, hepatosplenomegaly, lymphadenopathy, signs of myocarditis.*
- *Parasites in peripheral blood, positive serologic tests.*

Chronic stage:

- *Heart failure with cardiac arrhythmias; decreased intensity of heart sounds; episodes of thromboembolism.*
- *In some regions, dysphagia, severe constipation, and radiologic evidence of megaesophagus or megacolon.*
- *Positive xenodiagnosis or hemoculture, positive serologic tests; abnormal ECG.*

General Considerations

Chagas' disease is caused by *Trypanosoma cruzi*, a protozoan parasite of humans and wild and domestic animals. *T cruzi* occurs only in the Americas; it is found in wild animals and to a lesser extent in humans from southern South America to southern United States. An estimated 13 million people are infected, mostly in rural areas, resulting in about 45,000 deaths yearly due to cardiac disease. The disease is often acquired in childhood; the proportion of infected persons increases with age. In many countries in South America, Chagas' disease is the most important cause of heart disease. In southern United States, although the organism has been found in triatomine bugs and wild and domestic animals, only a few confirmed instances of local transmission have been reported. In the United States, a large number of immigrants from endemic areas of Latin America (particularly Central America) are infected (estimated 50,000–100,000); a handful of infections following blood transfusion have been reported.

T cruzi is transmitted by reduviid (triatomine) bugs infected by ingesting blood from animals or humans who have circulating trypanosomes. Multiplication occurs in the digestive tract of the bug; infective forms are eliminated in feces. Infection in humans occurs through "contamination" with bug feces; the parasite penetrates the skin (generally through the bite wound), mucous membranes, or the conjunctiva. Transmission can also occur by blood transfusion or in utero.

The trypanosomes first multiply close to the point of entry. They then enter the bloodstream as trypanosomes and later invade cells and assume the leishmanial form. The organism has a predilection for myocardium, smooth muscle, and central nervous system glial cells. Multiplication causes cellular destruction, inflammation, and fibrosis.

In South America, a major eradication program based on improved housing, use of residual pyrethroid insecticides and pyrethroid-impregnated bed curtains (under evaluation), and screening of blood donors has achieved striking reductions in new infections; Uruguay, Chile, and parts of Brazil and Argentina are now free of transmission.

Clinical Findings

A. SYMPTOMS AND SIGNS

Although infection continues for many years—probably for life—as many as 70% of persons remain asymptomatic. The **acute stage**, seen principally in children, lasts 2–4 months and leads to death in up to 10% of cases. The earliest findings are at the site of inoculation either in the eye—Romaña's sign (unilateral bipalpebral edema, conjunctivitis, local lymphadenopathy)—or in the skin—a chagoma (furuncle-like lesion with local lymphadenopathy). Subsequent findings include fever, malaise, headache, hepatomegaly, mild splenomegaly, and generalized lymphadenopathy. Acute myocarditis may lead to biventricular failure, but arrhythmias are rare. Meningoencephalitis is limited to young children and is often fatal.

A **latent period** (indeterminate phase) may last from 10 to 30 years in which the patient is without symptoms and signs of the disease but in which serologic tests and sometimes parasitologic examination confirm the presence of the infection.

The **chronic stage** is usually manifested by cardiac disease in the third and fourth decades of life, characterized by arrhythmias, congestive heart failure (often with prominent right-sided findings), ventricular aneurysms, and systemic or pulmonary embolization originating from mural thrombi. Valvular lesions are absent. Sudden cardiac arrest in young persons may occur and is attributed to ventricular fibrillation. Megacolon and mega-

esophagus, caused by damage to nerve plexuses in the bowel or esophageal wall, occur in some areas of Chile, Argentina, and Brazil; findings include dysphagia, regurgitation, constipation, sigmoid volvulus, bacterial overgrowth in the small intestine, and parotid gland hypertrophy. Megasyndromes can also affect the urinary tract.

In immunosuppressed persons—including infrequently in AIDS patients and transplant recipients—latent Chagas' disease may reactivate. Common findings are cardiomyopathy and brain lesions indistinguishable from cerebral toxoplasmosis.

B. LABORATORY FINDINGS

Diagnosis is by parasitologic and serologic methods. Trypanosomes can be detected in most acute and congenital cases and in up to 40% of chronic infections. In the *acute stage,* the organism may be found (1) as motile trypanosomes in anticoagulated blood, (2) as Giemsa-stained trypanosomes in anticoagulated blood used to prepare thin and thick or buffy coat films, or (3) by blood culture or animal inoculation. Occasionally, amastigotes can be found in tissue aspirates or biopsies of chagomas or lymph nodes by direct examination, staining, or culture. In the *chronic stage,* however, the organism is rarely found directly but may be detected by culture, animal inoculation, or xenodiagnosis. The latter consists of permitting uninfected laboratory-reared bugs of the local major vector to feed on the patients and then examining their intestinal contents for trypanosomes. Culture in appropriate media is kept for 30 days; animal inoculation is in 3-day-old to 10-day-old laboratory mice or rats. *Trypanosoma rangeli*, a nonpathogenic blood trypanosome also found in humans in Central America and northern South America, must not be mistaken for *T cruzi* trypomastigotes.

Several highly sensitive IgG serologic tests (hemagglutination inhibition, complement fixation, enzyme-linked immunosorbent assay [ELISA], immunofluorescence, Western blot, others) are routinely used and are of presumptive value when positive. However, two or three of these tests should be done because both false-negative (including some cases of depressed immune response) and false-positive tests are common. The latter may occur in other infections—including leishmaniasis, malaria, syphilis, and *T rangeli* infection—and in autoimmune diseases. For the ELISA and immunofluorescence tests, sensitivity is 93–98% and specificity (excluding leishmaniasis) is 99%. Antibodies of the IgM class are elevated early in the acute stage but are replaced by IgG antibodies as the disease progresses. Maximum titers are reached in 3–4 months; thereafter, titers can remain positive at a low level for life. In chronic infections, when serologic tests are negative, PCR and DNA methods sometimes make the diagnosis. These tests may also prove useful in assessing effectiveness of therapy (clearance of parasites), whereas serologic tests do not. Immunoassays are being evaluated to detect urine and blood antigens. The most important electrocardiographic abnormalities are right bundle branch block and arrhythmias. In certain regions of South America, radiologic examination may show megaesophagus, mega-colon, or cardiac enlargement with characteristic apical aneurysms.

Treatment

Treatment of Chagas' disease is inadequate because the two drugs used, nifurtimox and benznidazole, often cause severe side effects, must be used for long periods, and are ineffective against chronic infection. In acute disease and congenital infections, the drugs are effective in reducing the duration and severity of infection, but cure is achieved in only about 70% of patients. In the chronic phase, although parasitemia may disappear in up to 70% of patients, treatment does not alter the serologic reaction, cardiac function, or progression of the disease. Nevertheless, most experts concur that treatment should be attempted in all *T cruzi*-infected persons regardless of clinical status or time since infection.

Nifurtimox is given orally in daily doses of 8–10 mg/kg in four divided doses after meals for 90–120 days. It generally produces gastrointestinal complaints, weight loss, tremors, and peripheral neuropathy. Hallucinations, pulmonary infiltrates, and convulsions are rare. In the United States, nifurtimox is available only from the Parasitic Disease Drug Service, Centers for Disease Control and Prevention, Atlanta, GA 30333 (404-639-3670). Benznidazole—usually available only in Brazil—is given at a dosage of 5 mg/kg/d in divided doses for 60 days. Its side effects include granulocytopenia, rash, and peripheral neuropathy. The drug is better tolerated by children.

In the chronic stage, digoxin is not well tolerated and is used as a last resort. The most effective antiarrhythmic drug is amiodarone. Cardiac pacemakers are used for atrioventricular block. Amiodarone and angiotensin-converting enzyme inhibitors may result in better survival in selected patients. Surgery is important in the treatment of megaesophagus and megacolon. In endemic areas, blood should not be used for transfusion unless at least two serologic tests are negative; otherwise, blood can be treated with gentian violet to kill the parasites. Immigrants from endemic areas should be tested for the infection.

Prognosis

Acute infections in infants and young children are often fatal, particularly when the central nervous system is involved. Adults with chronic heart disease also may ultimately die of the disease.

Andrade AL et al: Short report: benznidazole efficacy among *Trypanosoma cruzi*-infected a six-year follow-up. Am J Trop Med Hyg 2004;71:594. [PMID: 15569790]

Lury KM et al: Chagas' disease involving the brain and spinal cord: MRI findings. AJR Am J Roentgenol 2005;185:550. [PMID: 16037535]

Meneghelli UG: Chagasic enteropathy. Rev Soc Bras Med Trop 2004;37:252. [PMID: 15330067]

Paulinoa M et al: The chemotherapy of Chagas' disease: an overview. Mini Rev Med Chem 2005;5:499. [PMID: 15892691]

Salomone OA et al: *Trypanosoma cruzi* in persons without serologic evidence of disease, Argentina. Emerg Infect Dis 2003; 9:1558. [PMID: 14720396]

AMEBIASIS

ESSENTIALS OF DIAGNOSIS

- *Mild to moderate colitis: recurrent diarrhea and abdominal cramps, sometimes alternating with constipation; mucus may be present; blood is usually absent.*
- *Severe colitis: semiformed to liquid stools streaked with blood and mucus, fever, colic, prostration; ileus, perforation with peritonitis, and hemorrhage occur.*
- *Hepatic amebiasis: fever, hepatomegaly, pain, localized tenderness.*
- *Laboratory findings: amebas or antigen in stools or in abscess aspirate followed by differentiation, when possible, of Entamoeba histolytica from Entamoeba dispar; positive serologic tests with severe colitis or hepatic abscess; ultrasound or CT scan showing hepatic abscess.*

General Considerations

Though the causative protozoan parasite *Entamoeba histolytica* was once considered a single species with varying virulence, it is now recognized that the *Entamoeba* complex contains two morphologically identical species: (1) *Entamoeba dispar* (about 90% of the complex), which remains in the colon as a stable commensal that is avirulent and produces an asymptomatic carrier state; and (2) *E histolytica*, which shows varying degrees of virulence ranging from a commensal state in the colon—in which it does not cause disease, yet is potentially invasive—to being invasive of the intestinal wall, resulting in acute diarrhea or dysentery or chronic diarrhea. *E histolytica* may also be carried by the blood to the liver where it may produce hepatic abscess. Rarely, the lungs, brain, other organs, or perianal skin may be infected. About 10% of asymptomatic carriers of *E histolytica* develop invasive disease; the others clear the infection within 1 year.

Both *E histolytica* and *E dispar* exist as two forms in the lumen and mucosal crypts of the large bowel: identical-appearing cysts (10–14 mcm) and motile trophozoites (12–50 mcm). In the absence of diarrhea, trophozoites encyst in the large bowel. Trophozoites passed into the environment die rapidly, but cysts remain viable in soil and water for several weeks to months at appropriate temperature and humidity.

The infections are present worldwide but are most prevalent and severe in subtropical and tropical areas under conditions of crowding, poor sanitation, and poor nutrition. Using the new taxonomy, prevalence estimates have changed. Of 500 million persons worldwide infected with entamoeba, most are infected with *E dispar* and an estimated 10% (50 million) with *E histolytica*. Invasive *E histolytica* may constitute 5 million cases, with mortality in the range of 100,000 per year. In the United States, infections are most common in immigrants from—and travelers to—developing countries.

Humans are the only established host and are universally susceptible. Only cysts are infectious, since after ingestion they survive gastric acidity, which destroys trophozoites. Transmission occurs through ingestion of cysts from fecally contaminated food or water. Flies and other arthropods also serve as mechanical vectors; to an undetermined degree, transmission results from contamination of food by the hands of food handlers. Where human excrement is used as fertilizer, it is often a source of food and water contamination. Person-to-person contact is also important in transmission; therefore, all household members as well as an infected person's sexual partner should have their stools examined. In communal settings such as mental hospitals, prevalence rates as high as 50% have been reported. Amebiasis is rarely epidemic, but urban outbreaks have occurred because of common-source water contamination. Although entamoeba infections occur frequently among homosexuals, in the developed countries these infections are usually due to the *E dispar* and do not require treatment. In AIDS, *E histolytica* infection does not become an opportunistic infection, except for reports from Taiwan.

Fulminant infections may occur in pregnancy and in young children. Corticosteroids and other immunosuppressive drugs given in error for inflammatory bowel disease may convert a commensal infection into an invasive one.

The characteristic intestinal lesion is the amebic ulcer, which can occur anywhere in the large bowel (including the appendix) and sometimes in the terminal ileum but predominates in the cecum, descending colon, and the rectosigmoid colon—areas of greatest fecal stasis. Trophozoites invade the colonic mucosa by means of their ameboid movement and proteolytic secretions and induce necrosis to form the characteristic flask-shaped ulcers. Ulcers are usually limited to the muscularis, but if penetration to the serous layer occurs, bowel perforation, local abscess, or generalized peritonitis may result. In fulminating cases, ulceration may be extensive, and the bowel becomes thin and friable. Hepatic abscesses range from a few millimeters to 15 cm or larger, usually are single, occur more often in the right lobe (particularly the upper portion), and are more common in men.

Clinical Findings

A. SYMPTOMS AND SIGNS

Amebiasis is classified into intestinal and extraintestinal disease and further subdivided into the clinical syndromes described below. Some patients have an acute onset of severe diarrhea as early as 8 days (commonly 2–4 weeks) after infection. Others may be asymptomatic or have mild intestinal infection for months to several years before either intestinal symptoms or liver abscess appears. Transition may occur from one type of intestinal infection to another, and each may give rise to hepatic abscess, or the intestinal infection may clear spontaneously.

1. Intestinal amebiasis—

   a. Asymptomatic infection—In most infected persons, the organism lives as a commensal, and the carrier is without symptoms.

   b. Mild to moderate colitis (nondysenteric colitis)—A few stools a day are passed that are semiformed and have no blood. There may be abdominal cramps, flatulence, fatigue, and weight loss; fever is uncommon. Periods of remission and recurrence may last days to weeks or longer; during remissions, the patient may have constipation. Abdominal examination may show distention, hyperperistalsis, and tenderness. In some patients with chronic infection, the colon is thick and palpable, particularly over the cecum and descending colon. Toxic products released as a result of the bowel infection may induce periportal inflammation, mild hepatomegaly, and low-grade liver enzyme abnormalities but without demonstrable trophozoites in the liver.

   c. Severe colitis (dysenteric colitis)—As the severity of intestinal infection increases, the number of stools increases, and they change from semiformed to liquid with streaks of blood beginning to appear. With larger numbers of stools, 10–20 or more, little fecal material is present, but blood (fresh or dark) and bits of necrotic tissue become increasingly evident. With increasing severity, the patient may become prostrate and toxic, with fever up to 40.5°C, and have colic, tenesmus, vomiting, generalized abdominal tenderness, and nonspecific hepatic enlargement and tenderness. Rare complications include appendicitis, bowel perforation, fulminating colitis, massive mucosal sloughing, and hemorrhage. Death may follow.

   d. Localized ulcerative lesions of the colon—Bowel ulcerations limited to the rectal area may result in passage of formed stools with bloody exudate. Ulcerations limited to the cecum may induce mild diarrhea and simulate appendicitis. Amebic appendicitis, in which the appendix is extensively involved but not the remainder of the large bowel, is rare.

   e. Localized granulomatous lesions of the colon (ameboma)—This occurs as a result of excessive production of granulation tissue in response to amebic infection, either in the course of dysentery or slowly in chronic intestinal infection. These masses may present as an irregular tumor (single or multiple) projecting into the bowel or as an annular constricting mass up to several centimeters in length. Clinical findings (pain, obstructive symptoms, and hemorrhage) and x-ray findings may simulate colonic carcinoma, tuberculosis, or lymphogranuloma venereum. At endoscopy, the mass is deep red and bleeds easily, and biopsy specimens show granulation tissue and *E histolytica;* the number of organisms may be relatively few. Antiamebic drugs are usually adequate treatment; surgical removal of the lesion without prior or immediate postoperative drug therapy is likely to result in death from disseminated disease.

2. Extraintestinal amebiasis—

a. Hepatic amebiasis—Amebic liver abscess, although a relatively infrequent (3–9%) consequence of intestinal amebiasis, is not uncommon given the large number of intestinal infections. A large proportion of patients with liver abscess do not have concurrent intestinal symptoms, nor can they recall having had chronic intestinal symptoms. The onset of symptoms can be sudden or gradual, ranging from a few days to many months. Cardinal manifestations are fever (often high), pain (continuous, stabbing, or pleuritic, and sometimes severe), and an enlarged and tender liver. Patients may also experience malaise or prostration, sweating, chills, anorexia, and weight loss. The liver enlargement may present subcostally, in the epigastrium, as a localized bulging of the rib cage, or, as a result of enlargement against the dome of the diaphragm, it may produce coughing and findings at the right lung base (dullness to percussion, rales, and diminished breath sounds). Intercostal tenderness is common. Localizing signs on the skin may be an area of edema or a point of maximum tenderness. Without prompt treatment, the abscess may rupture into the pleural, peritoneal, or pericardial space or other contiguous organs, and death may follow.

b. Other extraintestinal infections—Skin infections may develop in the perianal area. Metastatic infection may rarely occur throughout the body, particularly the lungs, brain, and genitalia.

B. LABORATORY FINDINGS

Diagnosis is by finding *E histolytica* or its antigen or by serologic tests. However, each method has limitations.

1. Intestinal amebiasis—A standard approach is to examine three stool specimens microscopically (preserved or fresh) and to test one for antigen. In microscopic examinations, trophozoites and cysts of *E histolytica* and *E dispar* cannot be distinguished from each other but can be distinguished from the other intestinal protozoa. Methods to differentiate between *E histolytica* and *E dispar* continue under evaluation. A sensitive and specific ELISA method is available to detect *E histolytica-specific* antigen in stool. The techLab *Entamoeba* test (sensitivity 93%, specificity 97%) is considered able to differentiate the organisms, but requires fresh or frozen stool specimens; preserved stool cannot be used.

Microscopic examination of stools. Microscopic examination is relatively insensitive and does not differentiate the two *Entamoeba* species or the free-living ameba, *Entamoeba moshkovskii*, which is now recognized in stool with an undetermined frequency. Testing

three specimens obtained under optimal conditions followed by concentration and staining methods will generally detect only 80% of entamoeba complex infections; three additional tests will raise the diagnostic rate to 90%. Trophozoites predominate in liquid stools, cysts in formed stools. A standard procedure is to collect three specimens at 2-day intervals or longer, with one of the three obtained after a laxative such as (1) sodium sulfate or phosphate (Fleet's Phospho-Soda), 30–60 g in a glass of water; or (2) bisacodyl 5–15 mL. Oil laxatives should not be used. Because trophozoites rapidly autolyze, stools should be examined within 30 minutes or immediately mixed with a preservative. If the patient has received specific therapy, antibiotics, antimalarials, antidiarrheal preparations (containing bismuth, kaolin, or magnesium hydroxide), barium, or mineral oil, specimen collection should be delayed.

Bowel examination. Colonoscopy is preferred over sigmoidoscopy. The bowel should not be cleansed by laxative or enema as this washes exudate from the ulcers and destroys trophozoites. Typically, there are no findings in mild intestinal disease; in severe disease, ulcers may be found that are 1 mm to 2 cm across, with intact intervening mucosa. If present, exudate should be collected with a glass pipette (not with cotton, to which trophozoites may adhere) or by scraping with a metal curette and examined immediately for motile trophozoites and for *E histolytica* antigen. In some centers, rectal biopsy (from the edge of the ulcer) has enhanced diagnosis; biopsy specimens are best examined by immunofluorescence methods.

Serology. Serologic tests for antibody are positive only in the case of *E histolytica* infection. Testing is usually not recommended in mild to moderate intestinal infection as it lacks sensitivity and does not differentiate present from past infection. The indirect hemagglutination and immunofluorescent tests have been replaced by the ELISA and enzyme immunoassays, which are positive in about 70% of patients with active intestinal disease (the frequency is lower in mild colitis, higher in dysentery) and in about 10% of asymptomatic *E histolytica* cyst passers; false-positive results are rare. The tests remain positive for months to 10 years after successful treatment, varying by the test used. The agar gel immunodiffusion test, though less sensitive, is rapidly conducted and may detect current infection because it becomes negative 3–6 months after eradication of the organism.

Other tests. Detection of trophozoites that contain ingested red blood cells is nearly diagnostic for invasive *E histolytica* but may be confused with the occasional *E dispar* or macrophage that also contains the red blood cells. Many patients with amebic colitis test positive for occult blood, whereas findings for fecal leukocytes are noncontributory. The white blood cell count can reach 20,000/mcL or higher in amebic dysentery but is not elevated in mild colitis. A low-grade eosinophilia is occasionally present.

2. Hepatic abscess—Elevation of the right dome of the diaphragm and the size and location of the abscess can be determined by ultrasonography (usually round or oval nonhomogeneous lesions, abrupt transition from normal liver to the lesion, hypoechoic center with diffuse echoes throughout the abscess), CT (well-defined, round, low-density lesions with an internal, non-homogeneous structure), MRI, and radioisotope scanning. After intravenous injection of contrast material, CT may show a hyperdense halo around the periphery of the abscess. Gallium scans, only infrequently useful, show a cold spot (sometimes with a bright rim) as opposed to the increased gallium uptake in the center of pyogenic abscesses. More than one abscess may be present. Serologic tests are almost always positive (except early in the infection). Examination of stools for antigen and the organism is frequently negative. The white count ranges from 15,000 to 25,000/mcL. Eosinophilia is not present. Liver function test abnormalities, when present, are usually minimal. As CT, MRI, and sonography do not distinguish amebic and pyogenic abscesses, percutaneous aspiration may be indicated; this is best done by an image-guided needle (risks described below). The aspirate is divided into serial 30- to 50-mL aliquots, but only the last sample is examined for amebas, as the organisms are found at the edge of the cyst. Detection of amebic antigen in aspirate appears to be very sensitive; studies are under way to evaluate tests for circulating antigen.

Differential Diagnosis

Amebiasis should be considered in patients with acute or chronic diarrhea (including cases associated with only mild changes in bowel habits; in patients who have an exposure history, including travel or household or sexual exposure); liver abscess; and annular lesions of the colon. All patients with presumed inflammatory bowel disease should be tested for antibodies, by multiple stool examinations for antigen and the organism, and by colonoscopy with biopsy because of the risk of overwhelming amebic disease if corticosteroid therapy were to be given in the presence of amebiasis. The differential diagnosis of amebic liver abscess includes pyogenic abscess, echinococcal cyst, benign cyst, and hepatocellular carcinoma.

Treatment

The decision to treat is based on a composite of data including (1) finding *Entamoeba* cysts or trophozoites, (2) differentiating *E histolytica* from *E dispar;* (3) testing for *E histolytica* antigen in stool or hepatic abscess aspirate; and (4) testing for serum antibody, which, if positive, could represent old infection. Asymptomatic infections should generally not be treated if differentiation between *E histolytica* and *E dispar* has not achieved; whereas, cases with a definitive diagnosis of *E histolytica* should be treated whether symptomatic or not.

The choice of drug depends on the clinical presentation and the site of drug action. Treatment may require the concurrent or sequential use of several drugs. Table 35–1 outlines a preferred and an alternative method of treatment for each clinical type of amebiasis.

The **tissue amebicides** dehydroemetine and emetine act on organisms in the bowel wall and in other tissues but not on amebas in the bowel lumen. Chloroquine is active principally against amebas in the liver. The **luminal amebicides** diloxanide furoate (not available in the United States), iodoquinol, and paromomycin act on organisms in the bowel lumen but are ineffective against amebas in the bowel wall or other tissues. Oral tetracycline inhibits the bacterial associates of *E histolytica* and thus has an indirect effect on amebas in the bowel lumen and bowel wall but not in other tissues; parenteral antibiotics have little efficacy at any site. Tinidazole and metronidazole are unique in that they are effective both in the bowel lumen and in the bowel wall and other tissues, including the central nervous system. Although, the two drugs are equally effective, tinidazole has a shorter course and may be better tolerated but is more expensive than metronidazole. When the drugs are used alone, they often fail to eradicate luminal organisms.

A. ASYMPTOMATIC INTESTINAL INFECTION

In asymptomatic cyst-passers, if stool antigen and serum antibody tests are negative, it can be presumed that the patient has an *E dispar* infection, which should not be treated. Nevertheless, an unrecognized commensal *E histolytica* infection could be present. Documented *E histolytica* infections should be treated. Cure rates for *E histolytica* infection with a single course of diloxanide furoate or iodoquinol are 80–85%. Within endemic areas, asymptomatic carriers generally are not treated because of the frequency of reinfection.

B. MILD TO MODERATE INTESTINAL DISEASE

In patients with intestinal symptoms and entamoeba in the stool in whom *E dispar* and *E histolytica* cannot be differentiated, if both stool antigen and serum antibody tests are negative it is possible that the latter tests are false negatives and that an *E histolytica* infection is present. In such cases, it is often best to proceed with anti-*E histolytica* treatment. Tinidazole or metronidazole plus a luminal amebicide is the treatment of choice. Alternatives are set forth in Table 35–1. The minimum dose of chloroquine needed to destroy trophozoites carried to the liver or to eradicate an undetected early-stage liver abscess is not established.

C. SEVERE INTESTINAL DISEASE

Fluid and electrolyte therapy and opioids to control bowel motility are necessary adjuncts. Opioids are used cautiously because of the risk of toxic megacolon. In fulminant disease, it may be prudent to add broad-spectrum antibiotics to treat intestinal bacteria that enter the peritoneum.

D. HEPATIC ABSCESS

There is no clinical evidence of tinidazole or metronidazole-resistant *E histolytica*, though it can be induced experimentally. Chloroquine has been included in treatment to

Table 35–1. Treatment of amebiasis.

Clinical Presentation	Drug(s) of Choice	Alternative Drug(s)
Asymptomatic intestinal infection	Diloxanide furoate[1,2]	Iodoquinol (diiodohydroxyquin)[3] or paromomycin[4]
Mild to moderate intestinal disease (nondysenteric colitis)	(1) Tinidazole[5] or metronidazole[5] plus (2) Diloxanide furoate,[1,2] iodoquinol,[3] or paromomycin[4]	(1) Diloxanide furoate[1,2] or iodoquinol[3] plus (2) A tetracycline[6] followed by (3) Chloroquine[7] or (1) Paromomycin[4] followed by (2) Chloroquine[7]
Severe intestinal disease (dysentery)	(1) Tinidazole[5] or metronidazole[5] plus (2) Diloxanide furoate[1,2] or iodoquinol[3] **or, if parenteral therapy is needed initially:** (1) Intravenous metronidazole[8] until oral therapy can be started; (2) Then give oral metronidazole[5] plus diloxanide furoate[1,2] or iodoquinol[3]	(1) A tetracycline[6] plus (2) Diloxanide furoate[1,2] or iodoquinol[3] followed by (3) Chloroquine[9] **or, if parenteral therapy is needed initially:** (1) Dehydroemetine[11] or emetine[1,10] followed by (2) A tetracycline[6] plus diloxanide furoate[1,2] or iodoquinol[3] followed by (3) Chloroquine[9]
Hepatic abscess	(1) Tinidazole[5] or metronidazole[5,8,] plus (2) Diloxanide furoate[1,2] or iodoquinol[3] followed by (3) Chloroquine[9]	(1) Dehydroemetine[11] or emetine[1,11] followed by (2) Chloroquine[12] plus (3) Diloxanide furoate[1,2] or iodoquinol[3]
Ameboma or extra-intestinal disease	As for hepatic abscess, but not including chloroquine	As for hepatic abscess, but not including chloroquine

[1]Not available in the United States.

[2]Diloxanide furoate, 500 mg orally three times daily with meals for 10 days.

[3]Iodoquinol (diiodohydroxyquin), 650 mg orally three times daily for 21 days. Available in the United States by calling 800-247-9767.

[4]Paromomycin, 25–35 mg/kg (base) (maximum 3 g) orally in three divided doses after meals daily for 7 days.

[5]Although tinidazole and metronidazole are equally effective, tinidazole is given in a shorter course and is better tolerated. The tinidazole dosage in asymptomatic and mild intestinal infection is 2 g orally daily for 3 days; in severe intestinal infection and hepatic abscess, the dosage is 2 g once daily for 5 days. The metronidazole dosage is 750 mg orally three times daily for 10 days. The drugs should be taken with food.

[6]Tetracycline, 250 mg orally four times daily for 10 days; in severe dysentery, give 500 mg four times daily for the first 5 days, then 250 mg four times daily for 5 days. Tetracycline should not be used during pregnancy.

[7]Chloroquine, 500 mg (salt) orally daily for 7 days.

[8]An intravenous metronidazole formulation is available; change to oral medication as soon as possible. See manufacturer's recommendation for dosage and cautions.

[9]Chloroquine, 500 mg (salt) daily for 14 days.

[10]Dehydroemetine or emetine, 1 mg/kg subcutaneously (preferred) or intramuscularly daily for the least number of days necessary to control severe symptoms (usually 3–5 days) (maximum daily dose for dehydroemetine is 90 mg; for emetine, 65 mg). Both drugs can be severely toxic.

[11]Use dosage recommended in footnote 10 for 8–10 days.

[12]Chloroquine, 500 mg (salt) orally twice daily for 2 days and then 500 mg orally daily for 19 days.

avoid rare long-term failures, although many sources do not include its use. Regarding rare short-term drug failures, if a satisfactory clinical response does not occur in 3–5 days, the abscess should be drained for therapeutic purposes and to exclude pyogenic abscess. Continued failure to achieve an adequate clinical response requires changing to the potentially toxic alternative drug dehydroemetine (or emetine) plus chloroquine. Treatment also requires a luminal amebicide (diloxanide furoate or iodoquinol), whether or not the organism is found in the stool. Antibiotics are added for concomitant bacterial liver abscess, although metronidazole itself is highly effective against anaerobic bacteria, a major cause of bacterial liver abscesses. Imaging defects in the liver disappear slowly (range: 3–13 months) after treatment; some calcify.

Most patients treated with tinidazole or metronidazole for an amebic liver cyst do not require therapeutic percutaneous drainage; when needed, the catheter method is preferred using image guiding. Indications are a large abscess (> 5–10 cm); threatening rupture; the presence of a left lobe abscess (due to the risk of perforation into the peritoneum); and the absence of medical response after 3–5 days of metronidazole therapy. The risks of aspiration or catheter drainage are bacterial superinfection, bleeding, peritoneal spillage, and inadvertent puncture of an infected hydatid cyst. In the absence of a rapid response to treatment, it is prudent to add antibiotics for the infrequent bacterial coinfection.

E. Adverse Drug Reactions

Metronidazole often induces transient nausea, vomiting, epigastric discomfort, headache, or a metallic taste in the mouth; if alcohol is taken during or shortly after treatment, a disulfiram-like reaction may occur. Drug interactions with some commonly used drugs (cimetidine, some anticoagulants, phenytoin, phenobarbital, cholestyramine, fluorouracil, cyclosporine, lithium) have been reported. Metronidazole increases the rate of naturally occurring tumors in mice but not in nonrodent species. Prudence dictates that metronidazole be given to pregnant or nursing mothers only if other drugs cannot be used. Probably, the same precautions for usage and drug interactions apply to tinidazole.

Dehydroemetine and emetine cause nausea, vomiting, and pain at the injection site. They are also cardiotoxic, with a narrow range between therapeutic and toxic effects; dehydroemetine may be the safer of the two drugs. The tetracyclines should not be used in pregnancy; erythromycin stearate and paromomycin are alternatives. Paromomycin may cause mild gastrointestinal symptoms, infrequently intense diarrhea, and rarely overgrowth of nonsusceptible organisms. Paromomycin should be used with caution in ulcerated bowel conditions and is not used in the presence of significant renal disease. Iodoquinol produces a mild, transient diarrhea. It should be taken with meals; used with caution in patients with optic neuropathy, renal, or thyroid disease; and discontinued in the event of iodine toxicity (dermatitis, fever). The neurotoxicity seen with extended treatment does not occur at the standard 3-week dosage. Diloxanide usage commonly results in flatulence.

Follow-Up Care

In follow-up, examine at least three stools at 2- to 3-day intervals, starting 2–4 weeks after the end of treatment. For some patients, colonoscopy and reexamination of stools within 3 months may be indicated.

Postdysenteric colitis is an uncommon sequela of severe amebic colitis. Following adequate treatment, diarrhea continues and the mucosa may be reddened and edematous, but no ulcers or organisms are found. Most such cases are self-limited, with permanent remission in weeks to months. Uncommonly, severe and unremitting diarrhea may represent ulcerative colitis triggered by the amebic infection.

Prevention & Control

Prevention requires safe water supplies, sanitary disposal of human feces, adequate cooking of foods, protection of foods from fly contamination, washing hands after defecation and before preparing or eating foods and, in endemic areas, avoidance of foods that cannot be cooked or peeled. Water supplies can be boiled (briefly) or treated with iodine (0.5 mL tincture of iodine per liter for 20 minutes, or longer if the water is cold); cysts are resistant to standard concentrations of chlorine. Filters are also available to purify drinking water. Disinfection dips for fruits and vegetables are not advised, and no drug is safe or effective in prophylaxis.

Prognosis

The mortality rate from untreated amebic dysentery, hepatic abscess, or ameboma may be high. With chemotherapy instituted early in the course of the disease, the prognosis is good.

Haque R et al: Amebiasis. N Engl J Med 2003;348:1565. [PMID: 12700377]

Lebbad M et al: PCR differentiation of *Entamoeba histolytica* and *Entamoeba dispar* from patients with amoeba infection initially diagnosed by microscopy. Scand J Infect Dis 2005;37:680. [PMID: 16126570]

Moran P et al: Infection by human immunodeficiency virus-1 is not a risk factor for amebiasis. Am J Trop Med Hyg 2005;73:296. [PMID: 16103593]

Stanley SL Jr: Amoebiasis. Lancet 2003;361:1025. [PMID: 12660071]

Tinidazole (Tindamax)—a new anti-protozoal drug. Med Lett Drugs Ther 2004;46:70. [PMID: 15375353]

INFECTIONS WITH PATHOGENIC FREE-LIVING AMEBAS

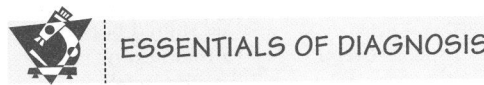

ESSENTIALS OF DIAGNOSIS

- *Meningoencephalitis.*

- *Granulomatous encephalitis and other granulomatous lesions.*
- *Keratitis.*

The free-living amebas that cause disease in humans are mainly of these genera: *Acanthamoeba*, *Naegleria*, and *Balamuthia*. The organisms are widely distributed in soil and fresh and brackish water. *Acanthamoeba* and *Naegleria* species have been found to harbor *Legionella*, *Vibrio cholerae*, and other endosymbiotic bacteria and may serve as a reservoir for these organisms.

1. Primary Amebic Meningoencephalitis

Primary amebic meningoencephalitis is a fulminating, hemorrhagic, necrotizing meningoencephalitis that occurs in healthy children and young adults and is rapidly fatal. It is caused by free-living amebas, most commonly by *Naegleria fowleri*. Other causes are *Balamuthia mandrillaris* and the *Acanthamoeba* species (see below).

N fowleri is a thermophilic organism found in fresh and polluted warm lake water, domestic water supplies, swimming pools, thermal water, and sewers. Most patients give a history of exposure to fresh water; dust is also a possible source. The organism apparently invades along the olfactory nerve to enter the central nervous system. Nasal and throat swabs have shown a carrier state, and serologic surveys suggest that inapparent infections occur.

Clinical Findings

A. SYMPTOMS AND SIGNS

The incubation period varies from 2 to 15 days. Early symptoms include headache, fever, and lethargy, often associated with rhinitis and pharyngitis. Vomiting, disorientation, and other signs of meningoencephalitis develop within 1 or 2 days, followed by coma and then death within 7–10 days. No distinctive clinical features distinguish the infection from acute bacterial meningoencephalitis. At autopsy, some victims have a nonspecific myocarditis.

B. LABORATORY TESTS

Lumbar or ventricular cerebrospinal fluid contains several hundred to 25,000 leukocytes/mcL (50–100% neutrophils) and erythrocytes (up to several thousand per microliter). Protein is usually somewhat elevated, and glucose is normal or moderately reduced. If conventional examinations for bacteria and fungi are negative, the fluid is examined for free-living amebas. Phase contrast is preferred. A wet mount examined by an ordinary optical microscope with the aperture restricted or condenser down will enhance contrast and refractility; a warm stage is not needed. The fluid should not be centrifuged at speeds over 150 × *g* (5 minutes) or refrigerated, as this tends to immobilize the amebas (7–14 mcm). Their brisk motility and lack of a large granular

nucleus distinguishes them from leukocytes of various types, which they closely resemble. Staining, culture, and mouse inoculation should be performed. Serologic testing is only useful epidemiologically; patients die before antibodies are detectable.

Precise species identification is based on morphology, demonstration of flagellate transformation (*Naegleria* only), and various immunologic methods.

Treatment

Seven well-documented survivors of *N fowleri* infection have been reported based on treatment with intravenous and intrathecal amphotericin B, intravenous miconazole, and oral rifampin.

B mandrillaris meningoencephalitis occurs in both immunocompetent and immunocompromised persons and runs a subacute course that can last months to 2 years. Multiple hypodense lesions are seen with imaging studies. Diagnosis is based on brain biopsy; culture is not effective. Several cases have been successfully treated with combination therapy using flucytosine, pentamidine, fluconazole, sulfadiazine, and azithromycin.

2. Acanthamoeba Infections

Granulomatous Lesions

Free-living amebas of the genus *Acanthamoeba* are ubiquitous, being found in soil and in fresh, brackish, thermal water, and chlorinated swimming pools as trophozoites (15–35 mcm) or cysts (10–15 mcm). Several species, including *Acanthamoeba culbertsoni*, cause a number of poorly defined syndromes, especially in debilitated or immunosuppressed patients, including those with AIDS: (1) subacute and chronic multifocal granulomatous necrotizing encephalitis leading to death in weeks to months, (2) skin lesions (ulcers or hard nodules in which ameba may be detected), (3) granulomatous dissemination to many tissues, and (4) keratitis. Portals of entry may include the skin, eyes, or respiratory tract. A commensal nasal carrier state occurs. Eighty percent of immunocompetent persons have antibodies against *Acanthamoeba* antigens.

The encephalitis presents with mental status abnormalities, meningismus, and neurologic features of a space-occupying lesion. Focal consolidation on chest films and cerebrospinal fluid lymphocytosis may be present. Antemortem diagnosis has been made by culture, brain biopsy, or cerebrospinal fluid wet mounts and by using specific fluorescent stains. PCR and DNA analysis are also used where available. No treatment has been effective, but ketoconazole, miconazole, itraconazole, sulfonamides, clotrimazole, pentamidine, paromomycin, propamidine, neomycin, amphotericin B, alkylphosphocholine, cotrimoxazole, or flucytosine can be tried.

Keratitis

Hundreds of cases of acanthamoeba keratitis and some of uveitis have been documented; most were associated with wearing contact lenses, others with penetrating corneal trauma or exposure to contaminated water. Suggestive features include (1) a waxing and waning clinical course over several months with severe ocular pain, photophobia, tearing, blurred vision, and conjunctival injection; (2) partial or 360-degree paracentral stromal ring infiltrate on ophthalmologic examination; (3) recurrent corneal epithelial breakdown; and (4) a corneal lesion refractory to the usual medications. Typically, the keratitis progresses slowly over months and can lead to blindness. The diagnosis can be confirmed by vigorously scraping the cornea with a swab or platinum-tipped spatula. The material is microscopically examined (1) as a wet preparation for cysts and motile trophozoites, (2) after staining, (3) by immunofluorescent techniques, and (4) after being cultured using various media. Isolates can be identified by isoenzyme analysis and DNA profiles. Because of variable drug sensitivities, each isolate should be tested for its drug susceptibility. Serologic tests have not been shown to be useful. Many cases of acanthamoeba keratitis are misdiagnosed as viral keratitis.

With early treatment, many patients can expect cure and a good visual result. Topical propamidine isethionate (0.1%) with either chlorhexidine digluconate (0.02%), polyhexamethylene biguanide, or neomycin-polymyxin B-gramicidin has been used successfully. Topical miconazole has also been used. Oral itraconazole or ketoconazole can be added for deep keratitis. Drug resistance has been reported. Use of corticosteroid therapy is controversial. In spite of medical treatment, penetrating keratoplasty is often necessary to excise diseased tissue; corneal grafting can be done after the amebic infection has been eradicated.

Prevention requires immersion of contact lenses in disinfectant solutions or by heat sterilization. The lens should not be cleaned in homemade saline solutions nor worn while swimming.

Bloch KC et al: Inability to make a premortem diagnosis of *Acanthamoeba* species infection in a patient with fatal granulomatous amebic encephalitis. J Clin Microbiol 2005;43:3003. [PMID: 15956445]

Driebe WT Jr: Present status of contact lens-induced corneal infections. Ophthalmol Clin North Am 2003;16:485. [PMID: 14564769]

Marciano-Cabral F et al: *Acanthamoeba* spp. as agents of disease in humans. Clin Microbiol Rev 2003;16:273. [PMID: 12692099]

Paltiel M et al: Disseminated cutaneous acanthamebiasis: a case report and review of the literature. Cutis 2004;73:241. [PMID: 15134324]

Vargas-Zepeda J et al: Successful treatment of *Naegleria fowleri* meningoencephalitis by using intravenous amphotericin B, fluconazole and rifampicin. Arch Med Res 2005;36:83. [PMID: 15900627]

BABESIOSIS

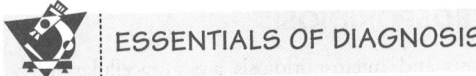

ESSENTIALS OF DIAGNOSIS

- *History of tick bite or exposure to ticks.*
- *Fever, other flu-like symptoms, anemia.*
- *Small intraerythrocytic protozoa on Giemsa-stained blood smears.*
- *Positive serologic tests.*

General Considerations

Babesiae are tick-borne protozoal parasites of wild and domestic animals worldwide. Babesiosis in humans is an uncommon intraerythrocytic infection caused mainly by two *Babesia* species. In Europe, infection is caused by *Babesia divergens*, and more than 30 cases have been reported. In the United States, infection is caused by *Babesia microti*, and hundreds of cases have been reported from coastal and island areas of northeastern and mid-Atlantic states as well as from Wisconsin, Minnesota, Missouri, Washington, and California. Antibody prevalence of 3–8% in serosurveys indicates a high level of subclinical infection. New *Babesia* species or strains (WA1 and others) have been described in humans in California, Washington, Georgia, and Kentucky. Gene sequencing of these isolates suggests that three are similar to *B divergens*. Serosurveys and limited confirmation of isolates suggest infection with *B microti* or other species in Taiwan, China, Japan, Egypt, South Africa, Mexico, Switzerland, and South America.

Natural hosts for *B microti* are various wild and domestic animals, particularly the white-footed mouse and white-tailed deer. With extension of the deer's habitat, the range of human infection is increasing as well. Humans are infected as a result of *Ixodes scapularis* (also called *Ixodes dammini*) tick bites (mainly nymphal) but also by blood transfusion and perinatally. Severe infections are most common in the elderly and immunosuppressed and in persons lacking a spleen. Coinfections with Lyme disease and ehrlichiosis occur because of cotransmission from the same tick. Without passing through an exoerythrocytic stage, *B microti* enters the red blood cell and multiplies, resulting in cell rupture followed by infection of other red blood cells.

Clinical Findings

A. SYMPTOMS AND SIGNS

The incubation period is 1 week to several months; parasitemia is evident in 2–4 weeks. Patients usually do not recall the tick bite. The flu-like illness is characterized by irregular fever, chills, headache, diaphoresis, cough, arthralgia, myalgia, and fatigue but is without malaria-like periodicity of symptoms. Other findings may include nausea, vomiting, jaundice, arthralgia, emotional lability, and splenomegaly. Although parasitemia may continue for months to years, with or without symptoms, the disease is usually self-limited; after several weeks to months (rarely to 18 months), most patients recover without sequelae. Severe complications, including acute respiratory, cardiac, and renal failure, are most likely to occur in older or splenectomized persons; mortality can reach 5–9% among those hospitalized.

All *B divergens* infections (in Europe, transmitted by *Ixodes ricinus*) have been in splenectomized patients. These infections progress rapidly with high fever, severe hemolytic anemia, jaundice, hemoglobinuria, and renal failure; death rates are over 40%.

B. LABORATORY FINDINGS

Diagnosis is established by identification of the intraerythrocytic parasite (2–3 mcm) on Giemsa-stained thick and thin blood smears; no gametocytes and no intracellular pigment are seen. A single red cell may contain different stages of the parasite, and parasitemia can exceed 10%. Repeated smears are often necessary because less than 1% of erythrocytes may be infected, especially early in infection. The organism must be differentiated from malarial parasites, particularly *Plasmodium falciparum*. As low-level *Babesia* parasitemia is easily missed, isolation can be attempted by intraperitoneal inoculation of blood into hamsters or gerbils. Antibody in humans is detectable within 2–4 weeks after onset of symptoms and persists for 6–12 months. Testing with specific antigens in the immunofluorescent test is relatively species-specific, with a titer of 1:1024 or greater considered diagnostic; antibody titers against *Plasmodium* are generally low or absent. An ELISA also has high sensitivity and specificity. The PCR method, where available, is more sensitive for low parasitemias but is of equal specificity. Immunoblot testing for IgM and IgG antibody is investigational; a positive IgM must be confirmed by a follow-up positive IgG. Other findings include hemolytic anemia, thrombocytopenia, low-grade leukocytosis or leukopenia, and abnormal liver and renal function tests. Imaging studies may detect morphologic changes in the spleen.

Treatment

No drug treatment is fully satisfactory. Although *B microti* infections in patients with intact spleens are usually self-limiting and can be treated asymptomatically, it is now recommended that all patients—even those mildly ill—should be treated with a 7- to 10-day course of oral atovaquone (750 mg every 12 hours) plus azithromycin (600 mg orally once daily). The alternative treatment is a 7-day course of quinine (650 mg three times daily) plus clindamycin (600 mg orally three times daily orally or 1200 mg twice daily intravenously). Following treatment of chronically infected persons, parasitemia can continue for several months. Exchange transfusion plus the antibiotics has been successful in several severely ill asplenic patients and in patients with parasitemia greater than 10%. Management of *B divergens* infection can be attempted with exchange transfusion and clindamycin-quinine plus atovaquone therapy or trimethoprim-sulfamethoxazole (TMP-SMZ) plus pentamidine.

Della-Giustina D et al: Transfusion-acquired babesiosis in a non-endemic area. Mil Med 2005;170:295. [PMID: 15916297]

Froberg MK et al: Babesiosis and HIV. Lancet 2004;363:704. [PMID: 15001329]

Herwaldt BL et al: Babesia divergens-like infection, Washington State. Emerg Infect Dis 2004;10:622. [PMID: 15200851]

Kogut SJ et al: *Babesia microti,* upstate New York. Emerg Infect Dis 2005;11:476. [PMID: 15757571]

BALANTIDIASIS

Balantidium coli is a large ciliated intestinal protozoan found worldwide, but particularly in the tropics. Pigs are considered the reservoir host, but the agent has been found in other animals and in insects. The disease is rare in humans, occurring as an acute or chronic infection resulting from ingestion of cysts passed in stools of humans or swine. Outbreaks have been reported. In the new host, the cyst wall dissolves and the trophozoite may invade the mucosa and submucosa of the terminal ileum, appendix, and large bowel, causing abscesses and irregularly rounded ulcerations. Many infections are asymptomatic and need not be treated. Chronic recurrent diarrhea, alternating with constipation, is most common, but mild to moderate diarrhea to severe dysentery with bloody mucoid stools, tenesmus, and colic may occur. Rare instances of infection in the lung, liver, and vagina have been reported in immunocompromised, including AIDS, patients.

Diagnosis is established by finding trophozoites in liquid stools, cysts in formed stools, or the trophozoite in scrapings or biopsy of ulcers of the large bowel. Specimens must be examined rapidly or placed in preservative.

The treatment of choice is tetracycline hydrochloride, 500 mg orally four times daily for 10 days. The alternative drug is iodoquinol (diiodohydroxyquin), 650 mg orally three times daily for 21 days. Occasional success has also been reported with metronidazole (750 mg orally three times daily for 5 days) or paromomycin (25–30 mg/kg [base] orally in three divided doses for 5–10 days).

In properly treated mild to moderate symptomatic cases, the prognosis is good, but in spite of treatment, fatalities have occurred in severe infections as a result of intestinal perforation or hemorrhage.

Ferry T et al: Severe peritonitis due to *Balantidium coli* acquired In France. Eur J Clin Microbiol Infect Dis 2004;23:393. [PMID: 15112068]

Vasilakopoulou A et al: *Balantidium coli* pneumonia in an immunocompromised patient. Scand J Infect Dis 2003;35: 144. [PMID: 12693570]

COCCIDIOSIS (Cryptosporidiosis, Isosporiasis, Cyclosporiasis) & MICROSPORIDIOSIS

Coccidiosis and microsporidiosis are intracellular infections of intestinal epithelial cells by spore-forming protozoa. The causes of coccidiosis are *Cryptosporidium* spp, particularly *Cryptosporidium parvum* and *Cryptosporidium hominis*; *Isospora belli*; *Cyclospora cayetanensis*; and *Sarcocystis bovihominis* and *Sarcocystis suihominis*. Various species are the etiologic agents of microsporidiosis (see below). Many of these infections occur worldwide, particularly in the tropics and in regions where hygiene is poor. They are causes of traveler's diarrhea; endemic childhood gastroenteritis (particularly in malnourished children in developing countries); institutional and community outbreaks of diarrhea; and acute and chronic diarrhea in immunosuppressed patients, including those with AIDS, in whom infection can be life-threatening. Clustering occurs in households, day care centers, and among sexual partners. Diarrhea in non-AIDS patients—sporadic, epidemic, and traveler's—is more likely to be due to cryptosporidia and less often to cyclospora or microsporidia. Diarrhea in AIDS is more commonly due to the microsporidia, *Enterocytozoon bieneusi*, and *Encephalitozoon* (formerly *Septata*) *intestinalis*, but *Cryptosporidium, Isospora,* and *Cyclospora* are also important causes.

The infectious agents are oocysts (spores) transmitted directly from person to person or by contaminated drinking or swimming water or food. Ingested oocysts release sporozoites that invade and multiply in enterocytes, primarily in the small bowel. Liberated merozoites reinvade other cells in the process of asexual intracellular multiplication. Eventually, sexual stages are released; following fertilization, immature oocysts form which are then shed in feces. The oocysts mature on exposure to air and can remain viable in a moist environment for months to years. All but the *Sarcocystis* species complete their life cycle in a single host.

The *Isospora* and *Cyclospora* species found in humans appear to be distinct to humans only. Cryptosporidiosis is a zoonosis in which infections in farm animals (cattle, goats, turkeys, and others) can be transmitted to humans; however, most human infections are acquired from humans. *Cyclospora* and probably *Isospora* require time outside the host to sporulate and become infectious. The oocysts of cryptosporidiosis, however, are infectious on excretion, thus permitting immediate human fecal-oral transmission.

Although the small bowel is the usual location of infection, other sites can be involved. Colon infection is common in cryptosporidiosis and has been reported with microsporidiosis. In AIDS patients, biliary tract infections may occur in cryptosporidiosis, cyclosporiasis, microsporidiosis, and isosporiasis and may result in either a sclerosing, cholangitis-like syndrome or an acalculous cholecystitis. Disseminated disease and corneal infections occur with several microsporidial species.

The pathogenesis of these diarrheas is not well understood. No enterotoxin has been identified. Voluminous secretory or malabsorption diarrhea (including vitamin B_{12}, D-xylose, and fat absorption dysfunction) can result. Although histologic examination of the small bowel can be normal, with intense infection there may be dense inflammatory infiltration accompanied by blunting to atrophy of the villi and crypt hyperplasia. The infections are nonulcerative and noninvasive except for *E intestinalis*, which can be invasive.

Clinical Findings

A. SYMPTOMS AND SIGNS

Generally, the forms of diarrhea caused by the coccidial and microsporidial organisms are clinically indistinguishable from each other. In immunocompetent persons, infection varies from no symptoms, to a mild diarrhea with flatulence and bloating, to severe and frequent watery diarrhea in which the onset may be explosive. Mucus may be present in stools but no microscopic or gross blood. Other findings may include low-grade fever, malaise, anorexia, abdominal cramps, vomiting, dehydration, and myalgia. These symptoms are generally self-limited, lasting a few days to several weeks (sometimes longer for isosporiasis). Weight loss can be marked. Parasitologic clearance, however, may take several months.

In immunologically deficient patients, the diarrhea can be profuse (up to 15 L daily has been reported), with cholera-like watery movements, accompanied by severe malabsorption, electrolyte imbalance, and marked weight loss; fever is uncommon. Mucus is seen in the stools, but blood and leukocytes are seldom present. The diarrhea may recur or persist, and passage of organisms continues for months to indefinitely.

B. LABORATORY FINDINGS

In diagnosis, three stool specimens should be obtained fresh and in preservative over 5–7 days and processed by a variety of flotation or concentration methods to detect the distinctive oocysts (differences are based on size and intracellular location). A modified acid-fast stain is used for cryptosporidia, cyclospora, and isospora; in microsporidiosis, a modified trichrome or Weber stain is used. *Clinicians should realize when ordering ova and parasite examinations that laboratories—unless specifically requested to do so—do not normally include the specialized tests needed to detect coccidia and microsporidia.* The organisms can sometimes also be detected by duodenal aspiration or biopsy. For diagnosis of biliary disease, ultrasonography is used initially followed by endoscopic retrograde cholangiopancreatography when necessary.

Specific Diseases

A. CRYPTOSPORIDIOSIS

The organism is found worldwide. Its fecal-oral mode of transmission is human-to-human (sometimes from asymptomatic persons) and animal-to-human from many vertebrate species, including chickens, birds, rodents, dogs, cats, sheep, and cattle. *C hominis* naturally infects humans; *C parvum* infects cattle (important reservoir) and humans. The organism is highly infectious (relatively few parasites can induce infection), is readily transmitted in day care settings and households, and can be transmitted by contaminated food and water.

The organism is the leading cause of recreational water–associated outbreaks of gastroenteritis. The incubation period appears to be 1–12 days. In immunocompetent persons, the illness is usually self-limited and lasts fewer than 30 days. Oocysts passed in stools are fully sporulated and infectious; therefore, hospitalized patients should be isolated and stool precautions strictly observed. The prevalence of asymptomatic human carriers in the United States is estimated to be about 1.5%. Outbreaks are of particular concern, as exemplified by the 1993 epidemic in Milwaukee in which 400,000 persons became ill. Since chlorine disinfection of water is not effective, adequate filtration is required. However, because of the oocysts' small size (2–5 mcm), filtration is difficult and unreliable (the < 1 mcm filters used frequently become obstructed).

Cryptosporidiosis develops in 10–20% of AIDS patients some time during their illness. Cryptosporidiosis may involve any part of the gastrointestinal tract, including the biliary tract (sclerosing cholangitis has been described); respiratory tract infection, hepatitis, pancreatitis, lymphadenopathy, and hepatosplenomegaly may occur, as well as multisystem involvement.

Diagnosis is by detecting the organism by the modified acid-fast and other staining methods; a minimum of two concentrated specimens should be tested. Using stool specimens, commercially available antigen detection kits improve on the diagnosis: direct fluorescent antibody methods have sensitivities and specificities of 99–100%; enzyme immunoassays have sensitivities and specificities of 93–100%. Immunochromatographic lateral-flow assays have also become available. Some of the kits can be used with both fresh and frozen specimens; others, however, can only be used if the specimen is fresh. Where available, the PCR test offers an alternative mode of diagnosis. Tests for serum antibody are useful epidemiologically but not for patient diagnosis.

Stools rarely show white or red blood cells. Blood leukocytosis and eosinophilia are uncommon. Radiologic changes have been reported in the stomach, intestines, and bile ducts in severe disease. Oocysts can be visualized in stained biopsy sections of intestinal mucosa. In AIDS patients with unexplained diarrhea, the organism should also be looked for in sputum and bronchoalveolar lavage fluid; specimens obtained from lung tissue have sometimes been positive.

B. ISOSPORIASIS

I belli oocysts in feces are 20–30 × 10–20 mcm. Opinion differs about whether the oocyst can be transmitted directly from person to person by anal-oral sexual contact or if it must pass into the environment and mature to its infectious stage. Outbreaks have occurred in day care centers and mental institutions. The incubation period is 7–11 days. The watery diarrhea can last for weeks to months, but is usually self-limited in immunocompetent persons; in immunocompromised patients, the severity of diarrhea can resemble

that in cryptosporidiosis. A hemorrhagic ulcerative colitis has been described.

Diagnosis by stool examination is often difficult, for the organisms may be scanty even in the presence of significant symptoms. Because of their buoyancy, oocysts must be looked for just beneath the coverslip using direct smears or concentrated specimens. Confirmation is by acid-fast staining. Frequently, diagnosis can be made only after duodenal aspiration or duodenal biopsy of multiple specimens. Serologic tests are available. Eosinophilia and eosinophils in stools are sometimes present.

C. CYCLOSPORIASIS

C cayetanensis oocysts (8–10 mcm) must undergo a period of sporulation in the environment before they become infectious. Although humans appear to be the only species that are carriers of *C cayetanensis,* this is an unsettled question. Transmission is by fecally contaminated food and water, generally in tropical and subtropical areas; large outbreaks have occurred. In the United States, outbreaks have been attributed to imported fresh fruit and leafy vegetables. Children, HIV-AIDS patients, and travelers are the more commonly recognized hosts. Diarrhea begins after an incubation period of 2–11 days. The illness can be self-limited or persist with weight loss. Rarely, the organisms invade the biliary tree, and Reiter's syndrome has been attributed to the infection. Oocysts can be identified in concentrated stool specimens by examination of wet mounts under phase microscopy, by use of modified acid-fast stains (oocysts are variably acid-fast), by the modified safranin stain, or by autofluorescence with ultraviolet light microscopy. Antibodies have been detected, and titers increase during convalescence.

D. MICROSPORIDIOSIS

Microsporidia are obligate intracellular protozoans (0.5–2 mcm × 1–4 mcm) that are pathogens of arthropods, fish, and vertebrates. Many human infections are of zoonotic origin from domestic and wild animals, but human-to-human transmission has been documented. Infection is mainly by ingestion of the spores but also by inhalation or finger contamination of the eyes. At least 14 species are known to infect humans; disease is seen mainly in immunocompromised persons, particularly those with AIDS. In chronic AIDS diarrhea, the two most common intestinal parasites are *Enterocytozoon bieneusi* and *Encephalitozoon intestinalis.* These parasites can also cause biliary infection (cholangitis, cholecystitis). In immunocompetent persons, the diarrhea due to these parasites (including traveler's diarrhea) is self-limited. *E intestinalis,* other *Encephalitozoon* species, *Enterocytozoon cuniculi, Enterocytozoon hellem, Brachiola connori,* and *Vittaforma corneae* can disseminate to many tissues, including the sinuses, lungs, liver, urinary tract, and brain. In *E cuniculi* infection, MRI has shown contrast-enhancing brain lesions. Most of the above parasites and others have been found as a nonpathogenic carrier state or as a cause of keratoconjunctivitis. *Pleistophora* species and *Trachipleistophora hominis* cause a myositis associated with high elevations of creatine phosphokinase, lactate dehydrogenase, and myoglobin. Thus, microsporidia should be considered in infections in immunocompromised persons in whom no other infectious agent can be found.

Microsporidia are detected in feces, body fluids (including duodenal fluid), and tissue biopsies (intestinal epithelium, cornea, conjunctiva, bronchi, and others) by light microscopy using various staining methods, particularly trichrome and Weber's chromotrope-based stains, followed by confirmatory fluorescence staining. In conducting stool examinations, after concentration, slide preparations should be very thin, stained for 90 minutes, and examined at × 1000 (or higher) magnification. In specialized laboratories, culture, molecular assays, and electron microscopic confirmation of histologic findings may be available. Although specific antibodies have been detected for some species, serologic diagnosis is controversial and of limited use. PCR is a research method.

Treatment

Most acute infections in immunocompetent persons are self-limited and do not require treatment. Supportive treatment for severe or chronic diarrhea includes fluid and electrolyte replacement and, in chronic cases, parenteral nutrition.

In **isosporiasis**, effective treatment in immunosuppressed persons has been described using (1) trimethoprim (160 mg) and sulfamethoxazole (800 mg) four times orally daily for 10 days and then twice daily for 3 weeks; or (2) sulfadiazine, 4 g orally, and pyrimethamine, 35–75 mg orally, in four divided doses daily, plus leucovorin calcium, 10–25 mg orally daily, for 3–7 weeks. In immunocompromised patients, it may be necessary to continue a maintenance dose indefinitely with TMP-SMZ three times weekly or Fansidar once weekly. Efficacy in primary infection has also been reported for furazolidone (400 mg/d orally for 10 days), roxithromycin, ciprofloxacin, nitrofurantoin, metronidazole, quinacrine, pyrimethamine, albendazole with ornidazole, and diclazuril.

In the treatment of **cyclosporiasis**, TMP (160 mg)-SMZ (800 mg) orally twice daily for 7 days is effective; in HIV infections, higher doses (four times daily for 10 days) and long-term maintenance (three times weekly) are needed. For patients intolerant of TMP-SMZ, ciprofloxacin (500 mg orally twice daily for 7 days) can be tried. In **microsporidiosis**, the *Encephalitozoon* species often respond to albendazole (400 mg two times daily for 3 weeks up to 3 months). In *E bieneusi* infection and in the various causes of disseminated disease, albendazole, octreotide, fumagillin (60 mg/d orally for 14 days), atovaquone, azithromycin, metronidazole, and nitazoxanide can be tried. For

ocular lesions, some infections respond to oral albendazole plus fumagillin eyedrops.

No treatment has been successful for **sarcocystosis** or **cryptosporidiosis**. However, for cryptosporidiosis, nitazoxanide is approved in the United States for use in children; evaluation in adults (500 mg orally twice daily for 3 days) continues. In this disease, vigorous treatment of underlying AIDS may relieve the parasitic diarrhea; other drugs that have been tried are roxithromycin (300 mg orally twice daily for 4 weeks), spiramycin (1 g orally three times daily for 2 weeks or longer), paromomycin (25–35 mg/kg/d orally in three or four divided doses; duration uncertain), zidovudine (AZT), azithromycin (600 mg daily), octreotide, eflornithine, letrazuril, hyperimmune bovine colostrum, and lactobacillus.

Prevention

Measures to reduce exposure to these organisms are recommended for immunocompromised patients. These include reduced exposure to swimming in fresh water and boiling of drinking water (1 minute) or use of a filter that removes particles over 1 mcm in size.

Didier ES: Microsporidiosis: an emerging and opportunistic infection in humans and animals. Acta Trop 2005;94:61. [PMID: 15777637]

Johnston SP et al: Evaluation of three commercial assays for detection of *Giardia* and *Cryptosporidium* organisms in fecal specimens. J Clin Microb 2003;41:623. [PMID: 12574257]

Palmieri F et al: Pulmonary cryptosporidiosis in an AIDS patient: successful treatment with paromomycin plus azithromycin. Int J STD AIDS 2005;16:515. [PMID: 16004637]

Sasaki M et al: A case of malabsorption syndrome caused by isosporiasis in an immunocompetent patient. J Gastroenterol 2004;39:88. [PMID: 14767744]

Smith HV et al: New drugs and treatment for cryptosporidiosis. Curr Opin Infect Dis 2004;17:557. [PMID: 15640710]

Wichro E et al: Microsporidiosis in travel-associated chronic diarrhea in immune-competent patients. Am J Trop Med Hyg 2005;73:285. [PMID: 16103591]

Zardi EM et al: Treatment of cryptosporidiosis in immunocompromised hosts. Chemotherapy 2005;51:193. [PMID: 16006765]

GIARDIASIS

 ESSENTIALS OF DIAGNOSIS

- *Most infections are asymptomatic.*
- *In some cases, acute or chronic diarrhea, mild to severe, with bulky, greasy, frothy, malodorous stools, free of blood and pus.*
- *Upper abdominal discomfort, cramps, distention, excessive flatus, and lassitude.*
- *Cysts and occasionally trophozoites in stools.*
- *Trophozoites in duodenal fluid.*

General Considerations

Giardiasis is a protozoal infection of the upper small intestine caused by the flagellate *Giardia lamblia* (also called *G intestinalis* and *G duodenalis*). The parasite occurs worldwide, most abundantly in areas with poor sanitation. In the United States and Europe, the infection is the most common intestinal protozoal pathogen; the US estimate is of 100,000 to 2.5 million new infections yearly and 5000 hospital admissions. Occurrence is particularly high among children.

The organism occurs in feces as a symmetric, heart-shaped flagellated trophozoite measuring $10–25 \times 6–12$ mcm and as a cyst measuring $11–14 \times 7–10$ mcm. Only the cyst form is infectious by the oral route; trophozoites are destroyed by gastric acidity. Humans are a reservoir for the infection; animals, including dogs, cats, beavers, and other mammals, have been implicated but not confirmed as reservoirs or zoonotic sources of infection. Under suitable moist, cool conditions, cysts can survive in the environment for weeks to months. The infectious dose is low, requiring as few as ten cysts.

Cysts are transmitted as a result of fecal contamination of water or food, by person-to-person contact, or by anal-oral sexual contact. Multiple cases are common in households, children's day care centers (often the nidus for spread of organisms to the community), and mental institutions. Outbreaks occur as a result of contamination of water supplies. Giardiasis is a well-recognized problem in special groups including travelers to *Giardia*-endemic areas, persons who swallow contaminated recreational water, male homosexuals, and persons with impaired immune states.

After the cysts are ingested, trophozoites emerge in the duodenum and jejunum. Infrequently, they cause epithelial damage, atrophy of villi, hypertrophic crypts, and extensive cellular infiltration of the lamina propria; mucosal invasion is rare; hematogenous dissemination does not occur. Hypogammaglobulinemia, low secretory IgA levels in the gut, achlorhydria, and malnutrition favor the development of infection. Gastric giardiasis may represent reflux from the duodenum or localized infection.

Clinical Findings

A. Symptoms and Signs

A large proportion of infected persons (especially children) remain asymptomatic cyst carriers, and their infection clears spontaneously. Giardia should be considered in most cases of diarrhea, especially where it is prolonged and associated with marked weight loss. Syndromes include (1) acute diarrhea, (2) chronic diarrhea, and (3) malabsorption. The incubation period is usually 1–3 weeks but may be longer. The illness may begin gradually or suddenly. The acute phase may last days or weeks, but it is usually self-limited, although cyst excretion may be prolonged. In a few patients, the disorder may become chronic and last for years. The disease can become life-threatening in infants, the aged, and immunosuppressed persons; in AIDS, it may be more frequent and severe than previously thought.

In both the acute and chronic forms, diarrhea ranges from mild to severe; most often it is mild. There may be no complaints other than of one bulky, loose bowel movement a day, often after breakfast. With larger numbers of movements, the stools become increasingly watery but are usually free of blood and pus; they are copious, frothy, malodorous, and greasy. The diarrhea may be daily or recurrent; if recurrent, stools may be normal to mushy during intervening days, or the patient may be constipated. Weight loss is frequent; weakness may occur. Infants and young children may show impaired growth and cognitive development. Less common are anorexia, nausea and vomiting, midepigastric discomfort and cramps (often after meals), belching, flatulence, borborygmi, and abdominal distention. In atypical presentations, gastrointestinal symptoms can appear without diarrhea.

Malabsorption occasionally develops in the acute or chronic stage. Findings may include fat- and protein-losing enteropathy and vitamin A, vitamin B_{12}, and disaccharidase deficiencies and marked weight loss. Certain extraintestinal manifestations (arthritis, anterior uveitis, urticaria) have been attributed to giardiasis infections, but a pathophysiologic relationship has not been established.

B. Laboratory Tests

Using stool specimens, diagnosis is (1) by standard microscopy to detect cysts and trophozoites or (2) by immunoassay by two methods: one is to detect coproantigen by an enzyme immunoassay (sensitivity 94–97%, specificity 100%), and the other to detect cysts by the direct fluorescent antibody assay (sensitivity and specificity, 96–100%). Although the coproantigen immunoassay is as sensitive and specific as microscopy and easier to perform, three stool specimens should be examined for ova and parasites if other organisms are being sought in addition to *Giardia*. Some immunoassays require fresh or frozen stool and cannot be used with preserved specimens; additionally, some assays detect only cysts or only trophozoites. With cure, the immunoassay normally reverts to negative, but excretion of antigen continues for several days after intact organisms are no longer excreted. Sometimes warranted is a search for trophozoites in the duodenum by (1) the duodenal string test (Entero-Test), (2) duodenal aspiration, (3) endoscopic brush cytology, or (4) duodenal biopsy (a mucosal imprint for staining should be made before sectioning). Tests for serum antibody are not recommended because of lack of sensitivity and specificity.

Detection of the parasite in feces can be difficult because the number of organisms passed varies considerably from day to day. At the onset of infection, patients may have symptoms for about a week before organisms can be detected; in chronic diarrhea, stool examinations can be persistently negative. Three stool specimens collected at intervals of 2 days or longer should be examined by concentration methods. One specimen will detect 50–75% of cases and three specimens about 90%. Unless the specimens can be submitted within an hour, they should be preserved immediately in a fixative. Purges do not increase the likelihood of finding the organism. Use of barium, antibiotics, antacids, kaolin products, or oily laxatives may temporarily (about 10 days) reduce the number of parasites or interfere with detection.

There is no eosinophilia, and the white blood cell count is normal. Radiologic examination of the small bowel is usually normal.

Treatment

Although controversial, treatment of asymptomatic patients should be considered since they can transmit the infection to others and may occasionally become symptomatic themselves. In selected cases, it may be best to wait a few weeks before starting treatment, as some infections will clear spontaneously. In the presence of a presumptive diagnosis but negative stool specimens and negative coproantigen tests, an empiric course of treatment is sometimes indicated. All persons in a household with an index case should be tested for infection; this also applies to children exposed in day care.

Treatment of adults is effective (> 90%) with tinidazole and metronidazole. A single dose of tinidazole, though more expensive, is the drug of choice because it provides the shorter course and is better tolerated. Retreatment with an alternative drug is sometimes needed, for which albendazole or paromomycin can be used. Furazolidone and nitazoxanide are available to treat children. In follow-up, two or more stools are analyzed weekly starting 2 weeks after therapy.

All of these drugs occasionally have unpleasant side effects. The potential for carcinogenicity of furazolidone, metronidazole, and tinidazole appears to be negligible based on over 2 decades of use. Because of its limited availability and rare potential for severe toxicity, quinacrine is no longer recommended.

A. TINIDAZOLE

An oral dose of 2 g given once has had reported cure rates of 90–100%. Adverse reactions consist of a metallic taste and mild gastrointestinal side effects in about 10% of patients; headache and vertigo are less common. The drug should not be taken with alcohol because of the potential for an antabuse-like reaction.

B. METRONIDAZOLE

The dose is 250 mg orally three times daily for 5–7 days. Metronidazole may cause gastrointestinal symptoms, headache, dizziness, a metallic taste, and candidal overgrowth, in addition to an antabuse-like reaction in alcohol users. In the United States, metronidazole for giardiasis treatment is only available for off-label use.

C. FURAZOLIDONE

The dose is 100 mg (in a palatable suspension) four times daily for 7–10 days. Gastrointestinal symptoms, fever, headache, rash, and a disulfiram-like reaction with alcohol occur. Furazolidone can cause mild hemolysis in glucose-6-phosphate dehydrogenase-deficient persons.

D. OTHERS

Albendazole (400 mg orally daily for 5 or more days) has shown cure rates that range from 10% to 95%. Reports with **paromomycin** (25–35 mg/kg/d orally in three divided doses for 7 days) have been mixed; because the drug is not absorbed, it has been proposed for use in pregnancy. **Nitazoxanide**, approved in the United States for children under 11 years of age (500 mg twice daily for 3 days), continues under study for adult treatment. Mild side effects include abdominal pain, vomiting, diarrhea, and headache.

Prevention

There is no effective chemoprophylaxis for giardiasis. Since community chlorination (0.4 mg/L) of water is relatively ineffective for inactivating cysts, filtration is required. For hikers, bringing water to a boil for 1 minute is adequate; filtration with a pore size less than 1 mcm can also be used. Relying on iodine halogenation is no longer recommended by the Centers for Disease Control and Prevention. In day care centers, appropriate disposal of diapers and frequent hand washing are essential.

Prognosis

With treatment and successful eradication of the infection, there are no sequelae. Without treatment, severe malabsorption may rarely contribute to death from other causes.

Ali SA et al: Giardia intestinalis. Curr Opin Infect Dis 2003;16: 453. [PMID: 14501998]

Bailey JM et al: Nitazoxanide treatment for giardiasis and cryptosporidiosis in children. Ann Pharmacother 2004;38:634. [PMID: 14990779]

Karabay O et al: Albendazole versus metronidazole treatment of adult giardiasis: An open randomized clinical study. World J Gastroenterol 2004;10:1215. [PMID: 15069729]

Lebwohl B et al: Giardiasis. Gastrointest Endosc 2003;57:906. [PMID: 12776040]

LEISHMANIASIS

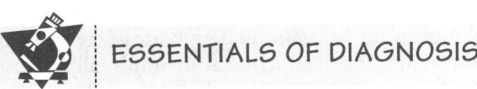

ESSENTIALS OF DIAGNOSIS

- *Exposure in an endemic area.*

- *Amastigotes demonstrable in macrophages in aspirate or biopsy smears.*

- *Promastigotes in cultures of aspirates or biopsy.*
- *Positive serologic tests, PCR, and skin test.*

Visceral leishmaniasis

- *Irregular fever, progressive hepatosplenomegaly, pancytopenia.*
- *Elevated total proteins with great increase in IgG.*

Old World cutaneous leishmaniasis

- *Chronic, painless, moist ulcers or dry nodules.*
- *Frequently self-healing.*

New World cutaneous leishmaniasis

- *Circular open ulcers; sometimes vegetative, verrucous, or nodular lesions.*

Mucocutaneous leishmaniasis (espundia)

- *Initial cutaneous ulcer.*
- *Followed in months to years by destructive nasopharyngeal lesions.*

Diffuse cutaneous leishmaniasis

- *Chronic, painless, fleshy nonulcerating nodules, spreading locally and metastatically.*
- *Skin test is negative.*

Leishmaniasis is infection by species of the genus *Leishmania*. The disease is a zoonosis transmitted by bites of female sand flies (2 mm) (phlebotomus [Old World leishmaniasis] and lutzomyia [New World leishmaniasis] species) from wild animal reservoirs (eg, rodents, Canidae, sloths, marsupials) and from domestic dogs (they can die of *Leishmania infantum* infections) to humans; however, kala azar is transmitted directly from humans to humans. Leishmaniae have two distinct forms in their life cycle: (1) In mammalian hosts, the parasite is found in its amastigote form (Leishman-Donovan bodies, 2–5 mcm) within mononuclear phagocytes. When sand flies feed on an infected host, the parasitized cells are ingested with the blood meal. (2) In the sand fly vector, the parasite converts to, multiplies, and is then transmitted during feeding as a flagellated extracellular promastigote (10–15 mcm).

In tropical and temperate zones, an estimated 12 million persons are infected with leishmaniasis; 1.5–2 million new cases occur yearly, of which more than 1 million are cutaneous and 500,000 are visceral disease. Approximately 50% are in children. An estimated 60,000 deaths occur each year. The incidence of disease is increasing in many endemic areas. Severity of infection ranges from subclinical or minimally pathologic (self-curing or easily treated cutaneous lesions) to persistent, disfiguring cutaneous and mucocutaneous lesions to potentially fatal visceral disease. Imported infections into the United States each year include about 40 cutaneous infections and several cases of visceral leishmaniasis. Several hundred cutaneous and a few visceral leishmaniasis infections have been found in US military personnel after exposure in Afghanistan and Iraq.

Four clinical syndromes occur, with overlap between them, and each syndrome is caused by more than one species. The speciation of leishmaniasis is complex (about 20 species are known to infect humans) and unsettled, and some species can cause more than one syndrome.

Visceral leishmaniasis (kala azar) is caused mainly by the *Leishmania donovani* complex: (1) *L donovani* (northeastern India, Bangladesh, Nepal, Southwest Asia, Sudan, Ethiopia, Kenya, Uganda scattered foci in sub-Saharan Africa, and northern and eastern China); (2) *L infantum* (Mediterranean littoral, Middle East, China, central and southwestern Asia, Ethiopia, Sudan, Afghanistan, Pakistan); and (3) *Leishmania chagasi* (South America, Central America, Mexico). More than 500,000 cases occur yearly. The number of cases is increasing, particularly in Sudan, Bangladesh, Brazil, northeastern India, and Nepal. In each locale, the disease has its own peculiar clinical and epidemiologic features and outbreaks have occurred. Three other species—*Leishmania tropica* in the Middle East, the Mediterranean littoral, Kenya, India, and western Asia, and *Leishmania mexicana* and *Leishmania amazonensis* in the New World—cause visceral leishmaniasis in a few patients, generally in a milder form. Although humans are the major reservoir, animal reservoirs such as the dog, other canids, and rodents are important. In the United States and Canada, foxhounds and other breeds of dogs and wild canids have been found to be serologically positive; *L infantum* has been isolated. There have been no findings in humans. The incubation period is usually 4–6 months (range: 10 days to 24 months). Without treatment, the fatality rate reaches 90%. Early diagnosis and treatment reduces mortality to 2–5%. Relapses (up to 10% in India and 30% in Kenya) are most likely to occur within 6 months after completion of treatment.

Old World cutaneous leishmaniasis is caused mainly by *L tropica*, *Leishmania major*, and *Leishmania aethiopica*. *L tropica* is the agent responsible for an urban infection of dogs and humans. It is found in the Middle East, northwestern India, East Africa, central Asian area of the former Soviet Union, Afghanistan, Pakistan, Turkey, Armenia, Greece, and southern France and Italy. *L major* infection causes lesions in dry or desert rural areas and is primarily a disease of desert rodents. Human disease occurs in the Middle East, central Asian area of the former Soviet Union, Arabian peninsula, Afghanistan, and Africa (North, East, and sub-Saharan Africa from Senegal to Sudan and Kenya). *L aethiopica* infection occurs in the Ethiopian and Kenyan highlands. Ulceration is rare; spontaneous healing is slow over several years. An uncommon complication is diffuse cutaneous leishmaniasis, an anergic form with nodular lesions and high parasite count. Treatment has sometimes been successful with sodium stibogluconate plus recombinant interferon gamma.

L donovani sometimes causes cutaneous disease with visceral manifestations.

In Afghanistan, Iraq, and Kuwait, the common agents are *L tropica* and *L major,* but *L infantum* has also been isolated in Iraq. From 2002 to 2004, more than 600 cases of cutaneous leishmaniasis were confirmed in military personnel and 176 isolations of *L major* were made. In the United States, for advice on treating such cases call 202-782-1663/8691.

New World cutaneous leishmaniasis is caused by *L mexicana* and *L amazonensis.* The *L mexicana* complex consists of *L mexicana* (Texas, Oklahoma, Arizona, Mexico, Central America—about 20 locally acquired human infections have been reported), *L amazonensis* (Amazonian basin, Venezuela, Panama, Trinidad), *L chagasi* (Central and South America), and other species (Venezuela and Dominican Republic). The *Leishmania (viannia)* group consists of *L (V) braziliensis* (Central and South America), *L (V) panamensis* (Central America and northeastern South America), and *Leishmania guyanensis* (South America). *L mexicana* and *L braziliensis* infections generally result from forest-related activities or from residence in dwellings situated near forests. *L panamensis* is also found in drier habitats. In parts of South America, several *Leishmania* species are now transmitted in domestic environments.

Mucocutaneous leishmaniasis (espundia) occurs in lowland forest areas and is caused by the *Leishmania (viannia)* group of organisms, usually by *L (V) braziliensis* (Central and South America; most cases are in Brazil, Bolivia, and Peru) and rarely by *L (V) panamensis* (Central and northeastern South America) or *L (V) peruviana* (Peru).

Diffuse cutaneous leishmaniasis, caused by the *L mexicana* complex in the New World and *L aethiopica* in the Old World, is a state of deficient cell-mediated immunity in which widespread leprosy-like skin lesions are generally progressive and refractory to treatment. The skin test is negative but amastigotes are abundant.

Leishmaniasis results in lifelong latent infection. If immunoparesis supervenes, leishmaniae can become opportunistic pathogens through reactivation or new infection; the latter may occur from sharing needles or syringes. Coinfections with HIV-visceral leishmaniasis (usually due to *L infantum* or *L donovani*) have been reported in many countries (eg, eastern Africa, India, Brazil), but the problem is worse in southwestern Europe (France, Italy, Spain, Portugal), where coinfections will develop in 2–9% of people with AIDS. Coinfections are being increasingly reported with other *Leishmania* species elsewhere in the world. In such cases, diagnostic criteria and clinical manifestations may be altered (*Leishmania* antibodies become undetectable and, in visceral disease, hepatosplenomegaly and fever may not occur). In leishmaniasis treatment, drug side effects may be greater, there may be a low rate of clinical and parasitologic response, and parasitic relapse may be more frequent. Antiviral treatment may prevent exacerbation of latent *Leishmania* infections and may also reduce findings in active leishmaniasis.

Clinical Findings

A. SYMPTOMS AND SIGNS

1. Visceral leishmaniasis (kala azar)—A local nonulcerating nodule at the site of the bite may precede systemic manifestations but usually is inapparent. The onset may be acute (as early as 2 weeks after infection) or insidious. Fever often peaks twice daily, with chills and sweats, weakness, weight loss, cough, and diarrhea. The spleen progressively becomes huge, hard, and nontender. The liver is somewhat enlarged, and generalized lymphadenopathy is common. Hyperpigmentation of skin, especially on the hands, feet, abdomen, and forehead, is marked in light-skinned patients. In blacks, there may be warty eruptions or skin ulcers. Petechiae, bleeding from the nose and gums, jaundice, edema, and ascites may occur. Wasting is progressive; death, often due to intercurrent infection, occurs within months to 1–2 years. In some regions, oral and nasopharyngeal or cutaneous manifestations occur with or without visceral involvement. **Post-kala azar dermal leishmaniasis** may appear after apparent cure in the Indian subcontinent and Sudan. It may simulate leprosy, as multiple hypopigmented macules or nodules develop on preexisting lesions. Erythematous patches may appear on the face. Leishmaniae are present in the skin. Although serologic tests are of limited value, the PCR test usually detects the parasite. Antimony treatment should be tried but is often ineffective.

In HIV-infected persons—with or without AIDS—visceral leishmaniasis can be an opportunistic infection (see above).

2. Cutaneous leishmaniasis—Cutaneous swellings appear 2 weeks to several months after sand fly bites and can be single or multiple. Depending on the leishmanial species and host immune response, lesions begin as small papules and develop into nonulcerated dry plaques or large encrusted ulcers with well-demarcated raised and indurated margins. Satellite lesions may be present. The lesions are painless unless secondarily infected. Local lymph nodes may be enlarged. Systemic symptoms are rare, but a low-grade fever of short duration may be present at the onset. For most species, healing usually occurs spontaneously in months to 1–3 years, starting with central granulation tissue that spreads peripherally. Pyogenic complications may be followed by lymphangitis or erysipelas. Contraction of scars can cause deformities and disfigurement, especially if lesions are on the face.

a. Old World cutaneous leishmaniasis—The incubation period is 2 months or longer, and healing is complete in 1–2 years. The lesions of *L tropica* infection tend to be single and dry, to ulcerate slowly or not at all, and to persist for a year or longer. *L major* lesions are characterized by multiple, wet, rapidly ulcerating sores with crusting. Spontaneous healing is generally complete in 6–12 months. **Leishmaniasis recidivans** is a relapsing form of *L tropica* infection in which the primary lesion nearly heals, lateral spread with central healing follows, and scarring can be extensive; it is associated with hypersensitivity and a strongly positive skin test but scarce amastigotes. Visceral involvement by *L tropica* has been reported rarely (including after troop exposure in Operation Desert Storm) and is relatively resistant to antimony treatment.

b. New World cutaneous leishmaniasis—Most New World cutaneous lesions are ulcers, but vegetative, verrucous, or nodular lesions may occur also. *L mexicana* ("chiclero's ulcer") in the Yucatan and Central America produces destructive lesions on the ear cartilage. Up to 80% of *L braziliensis* cutaneous lesions progress to espundia (see below); some *L braziliensis* complex strains also show a chain of palpable local lymph nodes, and some *L mexicana* and South American strains can cause diffuse cutaneous leishmaniasis.

c. Mucocutaneous leishmaniasis (espundia)—The initial lesion, single or multiple, is on exposed skin; at first, it is papular (can be pruriginous or painful), then nodular, and later may ulcerate or become wart-like or papillomatous. Local healing follows, with scarring within several months to a year. Subsequent naso-oral involvement occurs in a small proportion of patients either by direct extension or, more often, metastatically to the mucosa. It may appear concurrently with the initial lesion, shortly after healing, or after many years. The mucosa of the anterior part of the nasal septum is generally the first area to be involved. Extensive destruction of the soft tissues and cartilage of the nose, oral cavity, and lips may follow and may extend to the larynx and pharynx. Secondary bacterial infection is common. Regional lymphangitis, lymphadenitis, fever, weight loss, keratitis, and anemia may be present.

B. Laboratory Findings

Definitive diagnosis is by finding (1) the intracellular nonflagellated amastigote in Giemsa-stained biopsies from skin, mucosal lesions, liver, or lymph nodes; or from aspirates from spleen (the most sensitive site, but also a risky procedure), bone marrow, or lymph nodes; or (2) the flagellated promastigote state in culture of these tissues (requires up to 21 days). Occasionally, the organisms are seen in mononuclear cells of Giemsa-stained smears of the buffy coat. Golden hamster or Balb/c mouse inoculation of the nose, footpad, or tail base may also be used (2–12 weeks). PCR testing has up to 100% specificity and sensitivity and can be performed on any type of biologic specimen. Where available, species identification is by molecular, isoenzyme, and monoclonal antibody methods. Serologic tests (ELISA, indirect fluorescent antibody, direct agglutination, immunoblotting, dipstick, others) and the leishmanin (Montenegro) skin test (not licensed in the United States) may facilitate diagnosis, but none are sufficiently sensitive or specific to be used alone or for speciation purposes or to distinguish current from past

infection. Cross-reactions occur with Chagas' disease. No satisfactory antigen detection system is available.

Specimens from skin lesions should be obtained through intact skin (cleansed with 70% alcohol) at a raised edge of an ulcer margin. Local anesthesia can be used. To obtain tissue fluid for staining, press blood out of the site with two fingers, incise a 3-mm slit, and then scrape with the blade. When doing a biopsy, an impression smear is made, a portion is macerated for culture, and the remainder is reserved for pathologic sections. For needle aspiration, sterile preservative-free saline is inserted with a 23- to 27-gauge needle; the aspirate is then cytospun at 800 *g* for 5 minutes.

The diagnosis **of visceral leishmaniasis** can sometimes be made by demonstrating the organism in buffy coat preparations of blood, preferably obtained at night. More commonly, definitive diagnosis depends on Giemsa-stained smears, touch preparations, culture, or animal inoculation of aspirates of sternal marrow or iliac crest, liver, enlarged lymph nodes, or spleen. Although splenic aspiration is the most sensitive test, because of its hazard (intra-abdominal bleeding and death), it should be reserved for last and should be performed only by experienced persons; contraindications are a soft spleen in the acute phase, a prolonged prothrombin time, severe anemia, and platelet counts under 40,000/mcL. In immunocompetent persons, serologic tests are sensitive (> 90%) but false-positives may occur, especially in malaria and typhoid fever. The direct agglutination IgM test and the ELISA become positive early; the immunofluorescent IgG test becomes positive in most persons at a titer of 1:256 or higher. After treatment, the tests remain positive for months, though in immunocompromised persons, titers may be low or undetectable. The leishmanin skin test is always negative during active disease and becomes positive months to years after recovery. The PCR test has excellent sensitivity and specificity. Other characteristic findings are progressive leukopenia (seldom over 3000/mcL after the first 1–2 months), with lymphocytosis and monocytosis, normochromic anemia, thrombocytopenia, and eosinopenia. There is a marked increase in total protein up to or greater than 10 g/dL owing to an elevated IgG fraction; serum albumin is 3 g/dL or less. Liver function tests show hepatocellular damage. Proteinuria may be present.

Definitive diagnosis of **diffuse cutaneous leishmaniasis** is made by identification of the organisms (see above). Microscopic examination of skin scrapings has limited sensitivity, particularly in chronic infections. Where available after culture, species identification should be done by molecular methods. The skin test becomes positive within 3 months and remains positive for life; false-positives occur. Serologic tests are unreliable. Antibody may be undetectable or may appear only at low levels after 4–6 weeks; cross-reactions occur, including with leprosy.

Although they are difficult to find in **mucocutaneous leishmaniasis (espundia)**, diagnosis is by detecting amastigotes in scrapings, biopsy impressions or histologic sections, or aspirated tissue fluid. The organism grows with difficulty in culture or after inoculation of hamsters; if positive, speciation should be attempted. The leishmanin skin test is useful if it produces a fully developed papule in 2–3 days that disappears after a week. Standard serologic tests are often not useful; a direct agglutination for IgM antibodies may become positive in 4–6 weeks and subsequently an IgG test, but at low titer. PCR test is promising.

Differential Diagnosis

The differential diagnosis of **visceral leishmaniasis** includes leukemia, lymphoma, tuberculosis, histoplasmosis, infectious mononucleosis, brucellosis, malaria, typhoid, schistosomiasis, African trypanosomiasis, tropical splenomegaly syndrome, and cirrhosis. The differential diagnosis of **cutaneous leishmaniasis** includes tuberculosis, leprosy, fungal infections, yaws, syphilis, neoplasms, and sarcoidosis. Main considerations in the differential of **mucocutaneous leishmaniasis** diagnosis are paracoccidioidomycosis and other fungal infections, rhinoscleroma, polymorphic reticulosis, Wegener's granulomatosis, lymphoma, and nasopharyngeal carcinoma, yaws, syphilis, leprosy, and sarcoidosis.

Treatment

Treatment is less than adequate because of drug toxicity, long courses required, and frequent need for hospitalization. The drug of choice is a pentavalent antimonial, either sodium stibogluconate or meglumine antimoniate; resistance and treatment failures are increasing in frequency. Second-line drugs used in cases unresponsive to the antimonials—but potentially more toxic—are the deoxycholate formulation of amphotericin B and pentamidine. Three lipid-formulated amphotericins permit a shorter course of treatment with less toxicity and high effectiveness. AmBisome, recently approved for use in the United States, is considered by some workers to be the drug of choice for the treatment of visceral leishmaniasis but is very expensive. Miltefosine, an oral drug, has recently been approved in India for the treatment of visceral leishmaniasis.

A. Sodium Stibogluconate

Sodium stibogluconate is provided as a solution that contains 100 mg of antimony (Sb) per milliliter; only fresh solutions should be used. A generic formulation of sodium stibogluconate—at one-fourteenth the cost—has been shown to be equivalent in efficacy and safety to Pentostam. Treatment is started with a 200-mg Sb test dose followed by 20 mg Sb/kg/d; although dosages greater than 20 mg/kg should not be given, there is no upper limit to the total daily dose. The drug can be administered as a 5% solution intramuscularly (may be locally painful), but intravenous administration is preferred (cough may occur) when the volume is high, as is the case for most adults. Meglumine antimoniate (85 mg Sb/mL) is equal in efficacy and toxicity when used in equivalent Sb doses (20 mg Sb/kg/d). The appropri-

ate volume of drug is mixed with 50 mL of 5% dextrose in water and infused over at least a 10-minute interval. The selected drug is given on consecutive days: 28 days for visceral and mucocutaneous leishmaniasis and 20 days for cutaneous leishmaniasis. In certain regions of the world (especially with visceral leishmaniasis), because of resistance, longer courses are indicated.

Although few side effects occur initially, they are more likely to appear with cumulative doses. Most common are gastrointestinal symptoms, fatigue, fever, myalgia, arthralgia, phlebitis, and rash; hemolytic anemia, hepatitis, renal and heart damage, and pancreatitis are rare. The side effects are reversible. Patients should be monitored weekly for the first 3 weeks and twice weekly thereafter by serum chemistries, complete blood counts, and electrocardiography.

Therapy is discontinued if the following occur: aminotransferases three to four times normal levels or significant arrhythmias, corrected QT intervals greater than 0.50 s, or concave ST segments. Relapses should be treated at the same dosage level for at least twice the previous duration. In the United States, the only drug available is stibogluconate, obtainable from the Parasitic Drug Service, Centers for Disease Control and Prevention, Atlanta, GA 30333 (404-639-3670).

B. Amphotericin B

For the treatment of visceral leishmaniasis, the parenteral dosage of AmBisome (a liposomal formulation now approved for use in the United States) is 3 mg/kg/d on days 1–5, 14, and 21 and may be repeated; the dosage for immunocompromised persons is 4 mg/kg/d on days 1–5, 10, 17, 24, 31, and 38. A report indicated that comparable effectiveness could be achieved with lower doses over a shorter period; cumulative doses of 3.75 or 7.5 mg/kg were given in five divided doses over 5 days. Single-dose treatment is under evaluation. Infusion-related side effects include gastrointestinal symptoms, fever, chills, dyspnea, hypotension, and hepatic and renal toxicity. The dosage for the liposomal formulations for cutaneous and mucosal leishmaniasis has not been established. Conventional amphotericin B deoxycholate, as given in India, is slow infusion (4–6 hours) of 1 mg/kg daily for 20 days; this dosage achieved 99% cure rates but with side effects as above; an alternative dosage is 0.5–1 mg/kg/d or every second day intravenously for up to 8 weeks.

C. Pentamidine Isethionate

Pentamidine isethionate, 2–4 mg/kg intramuscularly (preferable) or intravenously, is given daily or on alternate days (fifteen doses for visceral and four doses for cutaneous leishmaniasis). For some forms of visceral leishmaniasis, it may be necessary to repeat treatment using up to twice the dose, but resistance may persist.

D. Paromomycin (Aminosidine)

When this drug was applied topically in various formulations in cutaneous leishmaniasis, it had variable success that differed by region. One ointment preparation is paromomycin 15% and methylbenzethonium chloride 12% in soft paraffin, applied twice daily for 15 days; skin reactions may occur. The ointment cannot be used in regions of mucocutaneous leishmaniasis as it does not prevent metastatic disease. In parenteral treatment of refractory visceral leishmaniasis, paromomycin is showing promise but has the potential for causing renal or otic toxicity.

E. MILTEFOSINE

Miltefosine, an alkyl phospholipid, is the first oral drug for the treatment of leishmaniasis. Approved for use in India for visceral leishmaniasis at a daily dose of 2.5 mg/kg in two divided doses for 3–4 weeks, it has resulted in 95% cure rates. Side effects included vomiting (40%), diarrhea (20%), and occasional transient and reversible elevations of aminotransferases, blood urea nitrogen (BUN), and creatinine. Owing to its teratogenic potential, the drug cannot be used in pregnancy. Preliminary reports have also shown efficacy in cutaneous leishmaniasis in Columbia but not in Guatemala. The drug is not available in the United States.

1. Visceral leishmaniasis—The drugs of choice (see above for doses) are liposomal amphotericin B and sodium stibogluconate. The liposomal formulation (AmBisome, available in the United States) replaces amphotericin B because of its reduced side effects but at a much higher cost. Whereas Mediterranean kala azar may respond to 10–15 doses of stibogluconate (one per day), the disease in Kenya, Sudan, and India requires at least 30 days of treatment. With incomplete response or relapse, the treatment should be repeated for 60 days. Drug resistance is now so high in parts of Bihar state, India, that cure rates are only 10–35%. In India, reported cure rates were 95% for liposomal amphotericin B (total dosage 15 mg/kg) and 89% for paromomycin (16 mg/kg/d for 21 days). Miltefosine, an oral treatment (approved for use in India; not available in the United States) has shown cure rates to 95% (see above for dosage, side effects, and contraindications). A fifth alternative drug is pentamidine; its efficacy has so declined in India that the drug is seldom used there.

2. Old World leishmaniasis—Especially in the Middle East, this type of leishmaniasis is generally self-healing in about 6 months and does not metastasize to the mucosa. Thus, it may be justified to withhold treatment if the lesions are small, in an unobtrusive place, and appear to be healing. Intralesional antimony is sometimes used in therapy. Parenteral sodium stibogluconate (20–28 days) should be used to treat patients with large or multiple lesions or if the lesions are on cosmetically or functionally important areas (eg, the wrist). Complete healing may not be evident until weeks after the first or second course of treatment. Amphotericin B desoxycholate and pentamidine are used for failures. Pentamidine is often effective against *L aethiopica* lesions and ketoconazole (400–600 mg/d for 4–6 weeks) against *L major* and *L (V) panamensis*. Miltefosine (2.5 mg/kg/d for 4 weeks), fluconazole (200 mg/kg/d for 6 weeks),

and ketoconazole (600 mg/kg/d for 4 weeks) continue under evaluation. Other treatments for less severe disease are physical measures (local cryotherapy or heat therapy, electrocoagulation, surgical removal). Paromomycin ointment may also be effective against *L tropica*.

3. New World leishmaniasis—In New World cutaneous *L mexicana* infections from Mexico and Central America, solitary nodules or ulcers in inconspicuous sites generally will heal spontaneously. Variable success has been had with paromomycin ointment (see above), ketoconazole, heat application, or metronidazole (750 mg three times daily for 10 days). Preliminary trials with oral miltefosine (150 mg/d for 3–4 weeks) had reported cure rates of 94%. Other drugs continue under evaluation. Lesions on the ear, face, or hands should be treated with sodium stibogluconate. Cutaneous lesions acquired in regions of mucocutaneous leishmaniasis may be due to *L braziliensis, L guyanesis,* or *L panamensis* and should be treated with a full course of sodium stibogluconate. Cure rates for *L braziliensis* and *L guyanesis* have been as low as 60% and 30%, respectively.

4. Mucocutaneous leishmaniasis (espundia)—This group of parasites should be treated because of their potential for developing into mucocutaneous disease. However, failure rates are high, even when a full course (28 days) of sodium stibogluconate treatment is used (see above). If repeated and extended antimony treatment fails, amphotericin B desoxycholate or pentamidine is used. Under evaluation are the liposomal formulations of amphotericin B and combined antimony and gamma interferon treatment. Corticosteroids may be needed to control local inflammation due to release of antigens. Antibiotics are usually needed to treat associated bacterial or fungal infections.

5. Diffuse cutaneous leishmaniasis—In spite of repeated doses of antimony, pentamidine, or amphotericin, cures are rare.

Prevention & Control

Infection occurs when humans encroach on sand fly habitats—warm, humid, dark microclimates, including rodent burrows, rock piles, or tree holes; these are often in sylvatic areas near forests or semiarid ecosystems. Peridomestic sandflies are found on debris close to buildings. Biting is generally at twilight or at night but may occur in shaded areas during the day. Personal protection may fail but is partially accomplished by clothing (pants, long sleeves) that covers exposed skin, permethrin applied to clothing, DEET repellent (see under Malaria), avoidance of endemic areas (especially at night), use of mosquito coils, and use of fine-mesh sand fly netting and screens for sleeping (may be too warm in tropical areas). Although sand flies can traverse the mesh of standard mosquito nets, permethrin-impregnated nets may prevent this. Often useful in control are destruction of animal reservoir hosts, mass treatment of humans in kala azar-prevalent areas, residual insecticide spraying in domestic and peridomestic areas, keeping dogs and other domesticated animals out of the house, particularly at night, and use of permethrin-impregnated collars for dogs.

Davis AJ et al: Recent advances in antileishmanial drug development. Curr Opin Investig Drugs 2005;6:163. [PMID: 15751739]

Magill AJ: Cutaneous leishmaniasis in the returning traveler. Infect Dis Clin North Am 2005;19:241. [PMID: 15701556]

Markle WH et al: Cutaneous leishmaniasis: recognition and treatment. Am Fam Physician 2004;69:1455. [PMID: 15053410]

Murray HW: Treatment of visceral leishmaniasis in 2004. Am J Trop Med Hyg 2004;71:787. [PMID: 15642973]

Shazad B et al: Comparison of topical paromomycin sulfate (twice/day) with intralesional meglumine antimoniate for the treatment of cutaneous leishmaniasis caused by *L. major*. Eur J Dermatol 2005;15:85. [PMID: 15757817]

Sinha PK et al: Diagnosis & management of leishmania/HIV co-infection. Indian J Med Res 2005;121:407. [PMID: 15817953]

Weina PJ et al: Old world leishmaniasis: an emerging infection among deployed US military and civilian workers. Clin Infect Dis 2004;39:1674. [PMID: 15578370]

MALARIA

ESSENTIALS OF DIAGNOSIS

- *History of exposure in a malaria-endemic area.*
- *Periodic attacks (every 2–3 days) of sequential chills, fever, and sweating.*
- *Malaise, headache, myalgia, nausea, vomiting, splenomegaly; anemia, leukopenia.*
- *Characteristic parasites in erythrocytes, identified in thick or thin blood films.*
- *Complications of falciparum malaria: Cerebral findings (mental disturbances, neurologic signs, convulsions, coma), prostration, hemolytic anemia, hyperpyrexia, hypotension, bleeding, secretory diarrhea or dysentery, hypoglycemia, metabolic acidosis, noncardiogenic pulmonary edema, hepatic or renal failure.*

General Considerations

Four species of the genus *Plasmodium* are responsible for human malaria: *P vivax, P malariae, P ovale,* and *P falciparum*. Although the disease has been eradicated from most temperate zone countries, it continues to be endemic in many parts of the tropics and subtropics, and imported cases occur in the United States and other countries free of transmission. Malaria is present in parts of Mexico, Haiti, Dominican Republic, Central and South America, Africa, the Middle East, the Indian subcontinent, Southeast Asia, China, and Oceania. *P vivax* and *P falciparum* are responsible for most infections and are found throughout the malarious regions. *P falciparum* is the predominant species in Africa and the only one in Haiti and the Dominican Republic. *P malariae* is

also widely distributed but is less common. *P vivax* is uncommon in much of Africa (except North Africa); in West Africa, it is replaced mainly by *P ovale,* which otherwise is rare. *P vivax* infection is uncommon among blacks because their red blood cells do not have the Duffy factor surface antigen. Annually worldwide, there are an estimated 500 million clinical cases of malaria that result in 1–3 million deaths; these deaths mainly occur among young children who live in sub-Saharan Africa. An estimated 30,000 travelers from the developed world are infected yearly with malaria, and several hundred die. Each year the United States experiences more than 1000 imported infections (44% due to *P falciparum*) and few cases of locally acquired, mosquito-transmitted cases from an imported case. An average of six deaths occur each year, almost all due to falciparum malaria. About 60% of the imported cases were acquired in tropical Africa; most of these cases were in persons who had failed to take malaria prophylaxis or had taken an inappropriate drug for the region of exposure.

Malaria is transmitted from human to human by the bite of infected female anopheles mosquitoes. Resistance of the vector to insecticides continues to increase. Congenital transmission and acquisition by blood transfusion also occurs. There are no animal reservoirs for human malaria.

The mosquito becomes infected by ingesting human blood containing the sexual forms of the parasite (microgametocytes and macrogametocytes). In the mosquito salivary glands, the gametocytes develop into sporozoites. When the mosquito next feeds on humans, inoculated sporozoites go to the liver (**exoerythrocytic stage**) where they transform within hepatic cells (hepatic schizogomy) into merozoites. The **erythrocytic stage** follows when merozoites released into the blood stream infect red blood cells. Subsequent parasitic transformation in the red blood cells (blood schizogomy) results in the following parasitic forms: the asexual forms (immature [trophozoites] and mature [merozoites]) and the two sexual gametocytes; lysis and release of these forms initiate the primary attack. The merozoites immediately invade new red cells to repeat the cycle many times over weeks. However, for *P vivax* and *P ovale* infections only, some sporozoites become a dormant form, the hypnozoite, upon invading hepatic cells. Reactivation of the hypnozoites can occur up to 6–8 months later initiating either a delayed primary infection or a **relapse**; the latter is due to failure of early treatment to adequately eradicate the hypnozoites. A different form of recurrent malaria is **recrudescence**, which can occur for all four malarial parasites; it is due to failure of early treatment to eliminate all infected red blood cells.

In *P falciparum* and *P malariae* malaria, the liver infection ceases spontaneously in less than 4 weeks; thereafter, multiplication is confined to the red cells. Thus, 4 weeks after departure from an endemic area, treatment that eliminates these species from the red cells will cure the infection. Cure of *P vivax* and *P ovale* malaria, however, requires treatment to eradicate infection from both red cells and liver hypnozoites.

The incubation period after exposure or after stopping chemoprophylaxis is, for *P falciparum*, approximately 12 days (range: 9–60 days); for *P vivax* and *P ovale*, 14 days (range: 8–27 days [initial attacks for some temperate strains may not occur for up to 8 months]); and for *P malariae*, 30 days (range: 16–60 days). Untreated infections can continue: *P falciparum* persists for up to 1.5 years but usually ends in 6–8 months; *P vivax* and *P ovale* infections persist for as long as 5 years; and *P malariae* infections have lasted for as long as 50 years. Protective immunity results from infection but decays after several years if reinfection does not occur.

Clinical Findings

A. SYMPTOMS AND SIGNS

Typical malarial attacks show sequentially, over 4–6 hours, shaking chills (the cold stage); fever (the hot stage) to 41 °C or higher; and marked diaphoresis (the sweating stage). Associated symptoms may include malaise, headache, dizziness, gastrointestinal symptoms (anorexia, nausea, slight diarrhea, vomiting, abdominal cramps), myalgia, arthralgia, backache, and dry cough.

Either from the onset or with progression of the disease, the attacks may show an every-other-day (tertian) periodicity in vivax, ovale, or falciparum malaria or an every-third-day (quartan) periodicity in malariae malaria. Splenomegaly usually appears when acute symptoms have continued for 4 or more days; the liver is frequently mildly enlarged. The presence of a rash or lymphadenopathy suggests an additional or other diagnosis. The patient may be tired between attacks but otherwise feels well. After this primary attack, recurrences are common, each separated by a latent period.

Because of its frequent and severe complications, *P falciparum* is the more serious infection and causes the most deaths, rarely within 24 hours. Severe disease results in part from intense sequestration and cytoadherence of parasitized red cells in capillaries and postcapillary venules. The severely ill patient may present with hyperpyrexia, prostration, impaired consciousness, agitation, hyperventilation, and bleeding. Other complications include (1) hypotension or shock; (2) cerebral malaria (headache, mental disturbances, neurologic signs, retinal hemorrhages, convulsions, delirium, coma); (3) hemolytic anemia; (4) noncardiogenic pulmonary edema or acute respiratory distress syndrome; (5) acute tubular necrosis and renal failure—rarely, this is associated with blackwater fever (dark urine), which most commonly is due to severe hemolysis following quinine treatment; (6) acute hepatopathy, with centrilobular necrosis and jaundice; (7) hypoglycemia; (8) cardiac dysrhythmias; (9) gastrointestinal syndromes (including secretory diarrhea and dysentery); (10) lactic acidosis; (11) water and other electrolyte imbalance; and (12) disseminated intravascular coagulation. The prognosis is poor if more than 20% of infected red cells contain mature parasites, if more than 5% of neutrophils contain pigment, or if parasitemia is > 500,000/mcL. Gram-negative bacteremia may contribute to death.

Immunologic disorders resulting from chronic infection are tropical splenomegaly and nephrotic syndrome (the latter due to *P malariae* only). Malaria infections do not appear to act as an opportunistic infection in AIDS patients, with the possible exception of malaria infection in pregnancy.

B. LABORATORY FINDINGS

Thick and thin peripheral blood films, Giemsa-stained, are the mainstay of diagnosis but require a high level of expertise to read; clinical diagnosis is only 20–60% reliable compared with microscopy. Blood from finger sticks or from the earlobe are preferred sources but should be free-flowing and uncontaminated by alcohol; if venipuncture blood is used, it should be examined shortly after it is drawn to avoid changes in morphology. Specimens should be obtained at about 8-hour intervals for 3 days, including during and between febrile periods. Patients need to stop their malarial prophylaxis during the diagnostic period because inadequate prophylaxis may have suppressed detectable parasitemia. The level of parasitemia should be quantified.

Because antibody becomes detectable only 8–10 days after onset of symptoms, serologic tests are not useful in diagnosis of acute attacks. The tests may be useful, however, after repeated attacks, especially if multiple blood films are negative. As antibody persists for 10 or more years, serologic tests are rarely useful in distinguishing current and past infection.

Alternative diagnostic tests—some commercially available and applicable in particular settings and others still under evaluation—have variable disadvantages of cost, of needing expert interpretation or specialized equipment, or of lacking the ability to differentiate the malarial species; the tests are not satisfactory for field use or for establishing cure. The tests include a variety of rapid antigen detection methods (including a dipstick format), fluorescent antibody methods, and PCR.

During paroxysms, there may be transient leukocytosis. Leukopenia develops subsequently, with a relative increase in large mononuclear cells. A marked anemia (normochromic, normocytic with reticulocytosis) may gradually develop.

Differential Diagnosis

It is imperative to consider malaria in every febrile patient who has a history of travel to an area where malaria is endemic. Uncomplicated malaria must be distinguished from a variety of other causes of splenomegaly, anemia, or hepatomegaly. Often considered are influenza, urinary tract infections, typhoid fever, infectious hepatitis, dengue, kala azar, amebic liver abscess, leptospirosis, and relapsing fever. Malaria complications can mimic many diseases.

Prevention

Prevention is based on evaluating the risk of exposure to infection, preventing mosquito bites, and chemoprophylaxis. Advice should also be given regarding medical care if malaria-like symptoms occur while traveling. All persons who will be exposed should receive chemoprophylaxis. Travelers should be advised that in spite of all precautions, no prophylactic regimen gives complete protection. Fever or other symptoms can develop in malaria as early as 6 days (range: 6–60 days) after exposure or stopping prophylaxis; for *P vivax* infections, however, the delay may be up to 8–12 months. To protect indigenous people in endemic areas, insecticide-treated bed nets are effective and are becoming more affordable.

A. Consultative Resources Regarding Risks, Chemoprophylaxis, and Treatment

Consultation with a center working on malaria may be necessary to obtain up-to-date information on risk and prophylaxis by country and on malarial treatment. A World Health internet source is http://www.who.int/ith/en/. A source of information and advice in the United States is the Malarial Branch, Centers for Disease Control and Prevention (CDC), Atlanta, Georgia. Recorded prophylaxis information for the public and health care professionals is available by telephone, 877-394-8747; fax, 888-232-3299; and Internet, http://www.cdc.gov (choose the Travelers' Health category). Additional information for professionals on prophylaxis or for management of acute attacks, phone 770-488-7788; after business hours, 770-488-7100 or 404-639-2888; additional guidelines for recommended treatment are at www.cdc.gov/malaria. Also, see references below.

B. Risk of Exposure

The risk of exposure to mosquitoes may be difficult to estimate since it varies by climate, rainy season, altitude, degree of mosquito control in urban versus rural areas, and according to whether exposure will occur during the time malaria mosquitoes are biting. Malaria transmission occurs in large parts of Central and South America, Hispaniola, Africa, Asia, the Middle East, Eastern Europe, and the South Pacific. Travel to urban areas of Central and South America and Southeast Asia entails minimal risk, and chemoprophylaxis is often not recommended for travelers to these areas.

C. Preventing Mosquito Bites

If being out of doors between dusk and dawn (the primary feeding time for anopheles mosquitoes) is necessary, protective measures should be used: Clothing should cover most of the body, and DEET (*N,N*-diethyl-3-methylbenzamide) mosquito repellent should be applied to exposed areas every 3–4 hours. To minimize the slight risk of toxic encephalopathy from DEET, use 30–50% concentrations (not higher; lower concentrations are shorter lasting) and apply sparingly and only to exposed skin and outer clothing; avoid inhalation and contamination of eyes, mouth, wounds, or irritated skin; and wash skin after coming indoors. The Ultrathon formulation provides a 33% DEET concentration with extended protection (12 hours). Picaridin has been in use in Europe as

an insect repellent as a 20% formulation. It has recently been approved for use in the United States as a 7% formulation but needs further evaluation for its comparative effectiveness to DEET. Living quarters should preferably be air-conditioned or be well screened. If screening is not available, mosquito bed nets should be used at night, preferably ones impregnated every 6 months with permethrin ($0.2 \, g/m^2$; Permanone) or deltamethrin. To kill mosquitoes in living quarters, use an antimosquito pyrethrum-containing spray or a powdered insecticide dispenser of pyrethroid tablets or burn pyrethroid mosquito coils. Garments can also be impregnated (sprayed or soaked) with permethrin, which repels for several weeks.

D. Advice Regarding Treatment of Malaria-Like Febrile Symptoms Occur While Traveling

The traveler should insist that blood smears be done and, if negative, repeated at intervals. If malaria is suspected but blood smears cannot be done, malaria treatment should be started empirically.

Emergency ("standby") presumptive self-treatment is a recognized resource for individuals who may be exposed to malaria and for whom medical attention cannot be provided within 24 hours. Such persons are advised beforehand to carry medication for self-treatment if fever or flu-like symptoms develop. However, *it is imperative that medical follow-up be sought promptly.* Patients should be given written instructions. The choice among available drugs depends on the malarial species to which the patient may be exposed and anticipated drug resistance (see above). In chloroquine-sensitive areas, for persons who have taken no prophylaxis, use the chloroquine 3-day course of treatment (see Table 35–3). In chloroquine-resistant areas, use Malarone (atovaquone 250 mg/proguanil 100 mg) tablets taking four tablets daily for 3 days; the patient should not have been taking Malarone for prophylaxis. Mefloquine, halofantrine, and quinine are not recommended because of their potential for toxicity.

Drugs Used in Chemoprophylaxis & Treatment (Tables 35–2 and 35–3)

A. Drug Classification

By chemical groups, some of the major antimalarial drugs are as follows: **4-aminoquinolines**—chloroquine, hydroxychloroquine, amodiaquine;* **diaminopyrimidines**—pyrimethamine, trimethoprim; **biguanides**—proguanil[†] (chlorguanide,* chlorproguanil*); **8-aminoquinolines**—primaquine; **cinchona alkaloids**—quinine, quinidine; **sulfonamides**—sulfadoxine, sulfadiazine, sulfamethoxazole; **sulfones**—dapsone; **4-quinoline-carbinolamines**—mefloquine; and **antibiotics**—tet-

---

*Not available in the United States.

[†]Available in the United States but approved for antimalarial use only as the combination drug atovaquone/proguanil (Malarone).

Table 35–2. Prevention of malaria in nonimmune adult travelers.[1]

TO PREVENT ATTACKS OF ALL FORMS OF MALARIA
    AND TO ERADICATE *P falciparum* **AND** *P malariae* **INFECTIONS**[2,3]

REGIONS WITH CHLOROQUINE-SENSITIVE *P falciparum* **MALARIA:** Central America west of the Panama Canal, the Caribbean, Mexico, and parts of the Middle East and China.

   Chloroquine[4,5]

      Dose: Chloroquine phosphate, 500 mg salt (300 mg base) orally weekly. Give a single dose of chloroquine weekly starting 1–2 weeks before entering the endemic area, while there, and for 4 weeks after leaving.

REGIONS WITH CHLOROQUINE-RESISTANT *P falciparum* **MALARIA:** All other regions of the world; the frequency and intensity of resistance vary by region.

   Malarone (atovaquone [250 mg] combined with proguanil [100 mg] [preferred method])[4,6]

      Dose: One tablet orally daily at the same time each day. Give one tablet the day before entering the endemic area, daily while there, and daily for 1 week after leaving.

   Mefloquine (alternative method)[4,7]

      Dose: One 250-mg tablet salt (228 mg base) orally weekly. Give a single dose of mefloquine weekly starting 2–3 weeks before entering the endemic area, while there, and for 4 weeks after leaving.

   Doxycycline (alternative method)[4,8]

      Dose: 100 mg orally daily. Give the daily dose for 2 days before entering the endemic area, while there, and for 4 weeks after leaving.

               TO ERADICATE *P vivax* **AND** *P ovale* **INFECTIONS**[2]

   Primaquine[9]

      Start primaquine only after returning home, during the last 2 weeks of chemoprophylaxis. Dose: 52.6 mg salt (30 mg base) daily for 14 days. An alternative regimen in regions where chloroquine is effective in prophylaxis is chloroquine phosphate, 500 mg (salt), plus primaquine phosphate, 78.9 mg (salt), weekly for 8 weeks.

---

[1]See text for additional information on drug cautions, contraindications, and side effects. For additional information on prophylaxis for specific countries, see the references or call the Centers for Disease Control and Prevention, Atlanta, GA at 770-488-7788 (for fax response: 888-232-3299). The information is also available on the Internet at http://www.cdc.gov (choose the Traveler's Health category).

[2]The blood schizonticides (chloroquine, mefloquine, Malarone, and doxycycline), when taken for 4 weeks (7 days for Malarone) after leaving the endemic area, are curative for sensitive *P falciparum* and *P malariae* infections; primaquine, however, is needed to eradicate the persistent liver stages of *P vivax* and *P ovale*.

[3]See text for a standby drug for emergency self-treatment of presumptive malaria; the drug should be used only when a physician is not immediately available. It is imperative, however, that medical follow-up be sought promptly.

[4]A test dose of the selected prophylactic drug should be given before departure to allow for changing to an alternative drug in the event of significant side effects: chloroquine (once weekly for 2 weeks), Malarone (daily for 2 days), doxycycline (daily for 2 days), mefloquine (weekly for 3 weeks); side effects from mefloquine sometimes do not appear until after the third or later doses.

[5]Chloroquine and proguanil can be used by pregnant women.

[6]Malarone is available in the United States. It eradicates falciparum infections after 1 week of postexposure treatment; its efficacy against *P malariae*, however, is undetermined. To eradicate *P vivax* and *P ovale* infections, a course of primaquine is needed, which should be started early in the final week of Malarone treatment. Malarone has not been shown to be safe in pregnancy. Malarone is more expensive than mefloquine.

[7]Because of the high frequency of resistance, mefloquine should not be used in Thailand or adjacent countries. Mefloquine is generally not recommended in the first trimester of pregnancy or under some other conditions (see text).

[8]Doxycycline is used in Thailand and adjacent countries and in other regions by persons who cannot tolerate mefloquine or Malarone. It is contraindicated in pregnant women. Take with evening meals. See text for side effects.

[9]Primaquine is indicated only for persons who have had a high probability of exposure to *P vivax* or *P ovale* (see text), and who have not taken the drug for daily prophylaxis. The drug should be taken with food and is contraindicated in pregnancy. Before use, patients must be screened for glucose-6-phosphate dehydrogenase deficiency. Note that the dosage recommended by CDC has increased.

---

racycline, doxycycline, clindamycin; and **others**—halofantrine,* artemisinin (qinghaosu)* and its derivatives, and atovaquone.† Pyrimethamine and proguanil are known as **antifolates**, since they inhibit dihydrofolate reductase of plasmodia. **Drug combinations** used to treat chloroquine-resistant *P falciparum* malaria include Fansidar (pyrimethamine plus sulfadoxine), Maloprim (pyrimethamine plus dapsone), Lapdap (proguanil plus dapsone), and Malarone (atovaquone plus proguanil). Chloroquine combined with proguanil has been used in prophylaxis in sub-Saharan Africa but is no longer recommended by the Centers for Disease Control and Prevention. Artemisinin and its derivatives are being used in treatment and continue under evaluation in fixed-dose combinations with other drugs: eg, artemether-lumefantrine (co-artemether), artesunate-Fansidar, artesunate-mefloquine, and artesunate-proguanil-dapsone.

The effectiveness of antimalarial drugs differs with different species of the parasite and with different stages of the life cycle. Drugs that act in the liver to eliminate developing exoerythrocytic schizonts or latent hypnozoites are called **tissue schizonticides** (primaquine). Those that act on blood schizonts are **blood schizonticides** or **suppressive agents** (eg, chloroquine, amodiaquine, proguanil, pyrimethamine, mefloquine, quinine, quinidine, halofan-

Table 35–3. Treatment of malaria in nonimmune adult populations.

Treatment[1] of Infection with All Species (Except Chloroquine-Resistant *P falciparum* or *P vivax*)	Treatment[1] of Infection with Chloroquine-Resistant *P falciparum* or *P vivax* Strains
Oral treatment of uncomplicated *P falciparum*[2] or *P malariae* infection Chloroquine phosphate, 1 g (salt)[3,4] as initial dose, then 0.5 g at 6, 24, and 48 hours.	**Oral treatment of uncomplicated *P falciparum* resistant to chloroquine** Malarone[10] two tablets twice daily with food for 3 days (each tablet contains atovaquone [250 mg] and proguanil [100 mg]).
Oral treatment of *P vivax*,[5] *P ovale* infection, or species not identified Chloroquine[3,4] as above followed by 0.5 g on days 10 and 17 plus primaquine phosphate, 52.6 mg (salt)[3–5] daily for 14 days starting about day 4.	*or* Quinine sulfate, 10 mg/kg 3 times daily for 3–7 days,[11] plus one of the following: (1) doxycycline,[10] 100 mg twice daily for 7 days; (2) clindamycin,[10] 7 mg/kg mg 3 times daily for 7 days; (3) tetracycline,[10] 250–500 mg 4 times daily for 7 days.
Treatment of severe attacks Parenteral quinine dihydrochloride[6] or quinidine gluconate.[7] Start oral chloroquine therapy as soon as possible; follow with primaquine if needed.[4]	*or* Artesunate,[8] 4 mg/kg/d orally for 3 days plus mefloquine[12] (750 mg followed by 500 mg 12 hours later)
or	*or* Mefloquine,[12] 750 mg (salt) followed after 6–12 hours by 500 mg.
Parenteral artesunate,[8] artemether,[8] or chloroquine[9] until the patient can take oral chloroquine. Follow with primaquine if needed.[4]	*or* Atovaquone/doxycycline, 500 mg/100 mg, twice daily for 3 days.
	Oral treatment of *P vivax* resistant to chloroquine Malarone or mefloquine (dosages above).
	or Quinine plus doxycycline, or tetracycline plus primaquine (dosages above).
	Parenteral treatment of severe attacks[13] Artemether,[8] or artesunate[8]; followed by oral mefloquine[12] (750 mg followed by 500 mg 12 hours later)
	or Quinine dihydrochloride[6] or quinidine gluconate[7] plus intravenous doxycycline, tetracycline, or clindamycin. Start oral therapy with quinine sulfate plus the second drug as soon as possible to complete the course[11] of treatment.

[1]See text for cautions, contraindications, and side effects of each drug. For advice on management, call the Centers for Disease Control and Prevention (CDC), Atlanta, GA 770-488-7788; after business hours, 770-488-7100, or go to its website http://www.cdc.gov/malaria.

[2]In falciparum malaria, if the patient has not shown a clinical response to chloroquine (48–72 hours for mild infections, 24 hours for severe ones), parasitic resistance to chloroquine should be considered. Chloroquine should be stopped and treatment started with an oral drug used for chloroquine-resistant strains.

[3]500 mg chloroquine phosphate = 300 mg base; 52.6 mg of primaquine salt = 30 mg base.

[4]Chloroquine alone is curative for infection with sensitive strains of *P falciparum* and *P malariae*, but primaquine is needed to eradicate the persistent liver stages of *P vivax* and *P ovale*. Start primaquine after the patient has recovered from the acute illness; continue chloroquine weekly during primaquine therapy. Patients should be screened for glucose-6-phosphate dehydrogenase deficiency before use of primaquine. An alternative mode for primaquine therapy is combined primaquine, 78.9 mg (salt), and chloroquine, 0.5 g (salt), weekly for 8 weeks.

[5]Strains of *P vivax* partially resistant to primaquine have appeared in some regions (see text). This is being dealt with by an increase in the primaquine dosage to 52.6 mg (salt) daily for 14 days.

(continued)

Continuing footnotes (Table 35–3)

[6]Parenteral quinine dihydrochloride. As a loading dose, give 20 mg/kg (salt) in 500 mL of 5% glucose solution intravenously slowly over 4 hours; repeat using 10 mg/kg every 8 hours until oral therapy is possible (maximum, 1800 mg/d). If more than 48 hours of parenteral treatment is required, some authorities reduce the quinine dose by one-third to one-half. Total plasma concentrations of 8–15 mg/mL is effective and does not cause serious toxicity. Blood pressure and ECG should be monitored constantly to detect arrhythmias or hypotension. As severe hypoglycemia may occur, blood glucose levels should be monitored. Extreme caution is required in treating patients with quinine who previously have been taking mefloquine in prophylaxis. In the United States, quinine dihydrochloride is no longer available.

[7]When parenteral quinine is unavailable (as in the United States), quinidine gluconate can be used, administered as a continuous infusion. A loading dose of 10 mg/kg (salt) (maximum, 600 mg) is diluted in 300 mL of normal saline and administered over 1–2 hours, followed by 0.02 mg/kg/min (maximum, 10 mg/kg every 8 hours) by infusion pump until oral quinine therapy is possible. If more than 48 hours of parenteral treatment is required, some authorities reduce the quinidine dose by one-third to one-half. Total plasma concentrations of 3.5–7 mg/mL is effective and does not cause serious toxicity. Fluid status, glucose, blood pressure, and ECG should be monitored closely; widening of the QRS interval or lengthening of the QT interval requires discontinuation.

[8]Not available in the United States. Give artesunate intravenously (2.4 mg/kg on the first day, followed by 1.2 mg/kg daily) or artemether intramuscularly (3.2 mg/kg on the first day, followed by 1.6 mg/kg daily); continue the drug for a minimum of 3 days until the patient can start oral artesunate. If parenteral treatment is not available, artemisinin rectal suppositories are being evaluated (40 mg/kg loading dose, then 20 mg/kg at 24, 48, and 72 hours) followed by oral medication. With all preparations of the artemisinin drugs, as soon as oral medication can be tolerated, treat concurrently with another effective blood schizonticide (Malarone preferred).

[9]Give parenteral chloroquine (1) preferably intravenously, 10 mg base/kg in isotonic fluid by constant rate of infusion over 8 hours, followed by 15 mg/kg over the next 24 hours; or (2) intramuscularly or subcutaneously, 3.5 mg base/kg every 6 hours.

[10]Contraindicated in pregnant women.

[11]Although oral quinine sulfate is usually given for 3 days, it should be continued for 7 days in patients who acquired infections in Southeast Asia and South America, where diminished responsiveness to quinine has been noted.

[12]Serious side effects are rare. See text for cautions and contraindications. In the United States, a 250-mg tablet of mefloquine contains 228 mg of base; outside the United States, each 275-mg tablet contains 250 mg of base. Mefloquine is hazardous with quinine, quinidine, or halofantrine.

[13]All of the drugs given intravenously should be administered slowly.

trine, artemisinin and its derivatives, and atovaquone). **Gametocides** are drugs that prevent infection of mosquitoes by destroying gametocytes in the blood (eg, primaquine for *P falciparum* and chloroquine for *P vivax, P malariae*, and *P ovale*). **Sporonticidal** agents are drugs that render gametocytes noninfective in the mosquito (eg, pyrimethamine, proguanil).

None of the drugs prevent infection (ie, are true **causal prophylactic drugs**). However, proguanil, chlorproguanil, atovaquone, and primaquine—and to some extent the antibiotics—prevent maturation of the early *P falciparum*. Blood schizonticides destroy circulating plasmodia and thus prevent malarial attacks (**suppressive prophylaxis**) and, when given weekly for 4 weeks after departure from the endemic area, result in cure of *P falciparum* and *P malariae* infections. Only primaquine destroys the hypnozoites of *P vivax* and *P ovale* and, when given with a blood schizonticide, prevents relapse from infection with these parasites and thus effects **radical cure (terminal prophylaxis)**.

B. PARASITE RESISTANCE TO DRUGS

Resistance has developed to all classes of antimalarial drugs except the artemisinins. To slow the development of resistance, the antimalarial drugs are increasingly being evaluated in combinations with an artemisinin derivative.

1. *P falciparum* resistance—

a. Chloroquine—P falciparum* resistance to chloroquine has been confirmed or is probably present in all malarious areas *except* Haiti, the Dominican Republic,

Mexico, Central America north and west of the Panama Canal, Argentina, North Africa, most of the Middle East, including Iraq, (resistance is present, however, in Oman, Yemen, Saudi Arabia, United Arab Emirates, Afghanistan, and Iran) and the Koreas. In some regions, some strains of *P falciparum* are only partially resistant to the drug, as manifested by temporary subsidence of symptoms and transient decrease or disappearance in asexual parasitemia, followed by return of both after several days to weeks.

b. Pyrimethamine-sulfadoxine (Fansidar)—Fansidar resistance is present at high levels in Southeast Asia, southern China, and the Amazon basin. Lower degrees are reported in sub-Saharan Africa (more in the east [20–40%] than the west), western Oceania, and parts of the Indian subcontinent and the Pacific coast of South America.

c. Pyrimethamine or proguanil—Resistance to either of these drugs when used alone is common in most endemic areas, but the degree and distribution are not accurately known.

d. Mefloquine—Along the border of Thailand with Myanmar and Cambodia and within parts of these countries and Laos and Vietnam, the frequency of *P falciparum* resistance to mefloquine reaches 30–60%. Sporadic or low levels of resistance have also been reported from southern Asia and parts of Africa, South America, the Middle East, and Oceania.

e. Quinine and quinidine—Variable degrees of decreased responsiveness have been reported sporadically in Southeast Asia (particularly in the border regions of Thailand) and western Oceania and rarely in sub-Saharan Africa and South America.

f. Halofantrine—A high degree of resistance has been reported in eastern Thailand. Strains resistant to halofantrine are sometimes resistant to mefloquine as well.

g. Malarone—Rare instances of *P falciparum* resistance to Malarone have been reported documented in Africa and reported elsewhere.

h. Artemisinin derivatives—There are no known artemisinin-resistant *P falciparum* strains.

2. *P vivax* resistance—

a. Antifolates—Resistance of *P vivax* blood schizonts to pyrimethamine and proguanil, including the pyrimethamine-containing drugs Fansidar and Maloprim, has been reported in many areas of the world, particularly Southeast Asia.

b. Chloroquine—There are frequent reports from Indonesia, Irian Jaya, and Papua New Guinea of *P vivax* blood schizonts resistant to chloroquine. Decreased susceptibility is also appearing in the Solomon Islands, Myanmar, India, Thailand, and from Central and South America.

c. Primaquine—Partial resistance of some strains of *P vivax* hepatic schizonts and hypnozoites to primaquine has been reported in areas of Southeast Asia, (17% failure rate in Thailand), Papua New Guinea (30%), the Amazon Basin, Central America, Somalia (43% in American military personnel), and Guyana. Treatment is usually successful with a higher dose (30 mg of base daily for 14 days) or a longer course (15 mg of base daily for 28 days).

3. *P ovale* and *P malariae*—*P ovale* has not shown resistance but strains of *P malariae* resistant to chloroquine have been reported from Indonesia.

C. Selected Drugs: Indications, Limitations, and Adverse Side Effects

1. Chloroquine phosphate—Chloroquine is the drug of choice in chemoprophylaxis and in treatment for all forms of malaria except for infections due to resistant strains of *P falciparum* and *P vivax* (see above). However, in *P vivax* and *P ovale* infections, primaquine is needed to eradicate the persistent liver phases and thus prevent relapse.

Oral chloroquine is usually well tolerated when used for malaria prophylaxis or treatment and is safe to use in pregnancy. Transient gastrointestinal symptoms, mild headache, pruritus (especially in blacks), dizziness, blurred vision, anorexia, malaise, and urticaria may occur; taking the drug after meals or in divided twice-weekly doses may reduce these side effects.

In parenteral treatment of severely ill patients, quinine, quinidine, or the parenteral artemisinin derivatives are the preferred drugs. If none are available, chloroquine can be given intramuscularly or intravenously. However, parenteral chloroquine can be severely toxic unless it is given in small amounts (3.5 mg [base]/kg) intramuscularly every 6 hours or by slow intravenous infusion.

Rare reactions from oral chloroquine include impaired hearing, psychosis, convulsions, blood dyscrasias, skin reactions, hypotension, and hemolysis in G6PD-deficient persons. When given in large doses for prolonged periods as an anti-inflammatory agent in autoimmune diseases, chloroquine has caused ocular damage. Theoretically, a total cumulative dosage of 100 g (base) may be critical in the development of ocular, ototoxic, and myopathic effects. However, with weekly long-term administration of chloroquine, serious eye damage has not been confirmed; therefore, periodic eye examinations may no longer be indicated. Chloroquine should be used with caution in patients who have histories of liver damage, alcoholism, or neurologic or hematologic disorders. It is contraindicated in patients with psoriasis. Chloroquine suppresses the immune response to the rabies vaccine.

Certain antacids and antidiarrheal agents (kaolin, calcium carbonate, and magnesium trisilicate) should not be taken within about 4 hours before or after chloroquine administration, since they interfere with its absorption.

2. Mefloquine hydrochloride—Mefloquine is used for oral prophylaxis and treatment of chloroquine-resistant and multidrug-resistant *P falciparum* malaria. In treatment, it is used only for mildly to moderately ill patients; severely ill patients require parenteral treatment with an alternative drug. Mefloquine has strong blood schizonticidal activity against the four malarial parasites (except for some *P falciparum* strains resistant to it)—but it is not active against *P falciparum* gametocytes or the hepatic stages of *P vivax* or *P ovale,* which require a course of primaquine. With weekly doses of mefloquine, the steady state drug level is reached in about 7 weeks, and adverse reactions thus may not appear for 3–7 weeks. The steady state interval can be reduced to 4 days, revealing adverse reactions within a week, by giving an initial course of 250 mg daily for 3 days followed by the standard weekly dose; this, however, is not standard practice.

With the lower doses used in prophylaxis, frequent (25–50%) minor and transient side effects are nausea, vomiting, epigastric pain, diarrhea, headache, dizziness, syncope, and extrasystoles. A small proportion of patients (up to 4%) experience anxiety, mood changes, insomnia, and nightmares. Severe neuropsychiatric symptoms are rare (estimated 1:1500 to 1:10,000). If prophylaxis is continued for more than a year, periodic liver function and ophthalmologic tests should be done. With treatment doses—particularly over 1000 mg—gastrointestinal symptoms and fatigue are more likely to occur, and the frequency of severe neuropsychiatric symptoms (visual disturbances, vertigo, tinnitus, insomnia, restlessness, anxiety, depression, confusion, disorientation, acute psychosis, or seizures) may be of the order of 1:1200. In experimental animals, the drug affects fertility and is teratogenic; it also causes degenerative changes in the epididymis in rats and in the lens and retina of some species. In human males, however, no deleterious effects on spermatozoa were found, and no effects have been noted in the human retina or lens. Because the drug may affect fine motor coordination and spatial orientation, caution in its use is recommended for pilots, drivers, and machinery operators.

Mefloquine is contraindicated in the presence of a cardiac conduction abnormality, liver impairment, or a history of a psychiatric or neurologic disorder, including epilepsy. Also contraindicated is concurrent administration of mefloquine with quinine, quinidine, chloroquine, or halofantrine. If these drugs precede use of mefloquine, 12 hours should elapse before mefloquine is started; however, because of the long elimination half-life of mefloquine (13–26 days), extreme caution is required because of arrhythmias if one of these drugs is used to treat malaria after mefloquine has been taken. Concurrent administration with tetracyclines or ampicillin results in increased mefloquine blood levels.

The development of neuropsychiatric symptoms during prophylaxis is an indication for stopping the drug. Patients taking anticonvulsant drugs may have breakthrough seizures. Mefloquine is no longer contraindicated when β-blockers and calcium channel blockers are taken. CDC has advised that mefloquine can be used throughout pregnancy; nevertheless, its use during the first trimester should be based on risk-benefit assessment. Women of childbearing potential who take mefloquine for antimalarial prophylaxis should preferably avoid conception for the duration of mefloquine usage and for 2 months after the last dose.

Note: The tablet formulation in the United States contains 250 mg of the salt (= 228 mg of base). However, in Canada and many other countries, the tablets contain 274 mg of the salt (= 250 mg of base). Mefloquine should not be taken on an empty stomach and should be taken with 8 oz of water.

3. Malarone—Malarone—atovaquone 250 mg and proguanil 100 mg—is a fixed-combination oral medication recently approved in the United States for prophylaxis and treatment of multidrug-resistant falciparum malaria, *P vivax,* and *P ovale;* effectiveness against *P malariae* has not been determined. In a limited number of studies in nonimmune adults, Malarone's prophylactic efficacy was 98% against *P falciparum* and 84% against *P vivax.* In treatment, its use is currently limited to uncomplicated malaria (cure rates 87–100%); data on effectiveness in treatment of severe malaria and in *P malariae* and *P ovale* infections are limited.

Malarone's components, proguanil and atovaquone, used together, are synergistic, but failures are frequent to either component used alone. Because the agents are effective against the liver and blood stages of *P falciparum,* only 7 days of treatment is needed after

leaving an endemic area, and primaquine is not required to eradicate a falciparum infection. Cross-resistance between Malarone and other antimalarials has not been noted. In *P vivax* and *P ovale* infections, however, in which the Malarone components are effective only against the erythrocytic stages, primaquine must be used to eradicate the liver form (hypnozoites). Malarone supersedes Fansidar as the preferred drug for standby treatment (see above).

Malarone appears to be better tolerated than chloroquine and causes significantly fewer neuropsychiatric side effects than mefloquine. The drug is taken orally with food to increase absorption of atovaquone and to reduce gastrointestinal side effects (10%: nausea, vomiting, diarrhea, abdominal pain, epigastric discomfort). These symptoms may also be reduced by giving the drug in divided doses twice daily. Other side effects include headache, rash, dizziness, and mild reversible elevations of liver aminotransferases. One case of anaphylaxis has been reported, and the drug has been associated with the Stevens-Johnson syndrome. There are insufficient data on fetal risks to allow Malarone to be used in pregnancy. Concomitant administration of Malarone with rifampin, tetracycline, or metoclopramide is associated with 40–50% reductions in atovaquone plasma levels. The drug is contraindicated in patients with severe renal impairment.

4. Primaquine phosphate—Primaquine is used to prevent relapse by eliminating persistent liver forms of *P vivax* or *P ovale* in patients who have had an acute attack and for individuals returning from an endemic area who have probably been exposed to malaria. However, in persons with a low probability of exposure, it may be preferable to avoid primaquine's potential toxicity by not giving the drug. Instead, such patients are advised to seek medical evaluation in the event of malaria-like symptoms, which usually occur within 2 years after infection but can occur up to 4 years after. Because primaquine is effective against the liver stages of all malarial parasites, including chloroquine-resistant *P falciparum,* it has been reevaluated recently for chemoprophylaxis when taken daily (30 mg base). A prophylactic efficacy of 85–95% has been shown against *P falciparum* and *P vivax* with apparent safety in long-term use, though the drug is not licensed for this indication. Primaquine is sometimes given as a single 45 mg (base) dose to eliminate *P falciparum* gametocytes.

Primaquine is generally well tolerated. Occasional side effects of the drug are gastrointestinal disturbances (minimized if taken with food), headache, dizziness, or neutropenia. Primaquine should not be used in pregnancy (risk of hemolytic disease in the fetus), in autoimmune disorders, or concurrently with quinine.

All patients should be tested for glucose-6-phosphate dehydrogenase (G6PD) deficiency before therapy is begun. They should be monitored carefully during treatment because primaquine may cause mild, self-limited hemolysis or marked hemolysis (pallor, weakness, abdominal pain, dark urine) or methemoglobinemia. G6PD deficiency is most common among persons of Mediterranean, African, or certain East Asian extractions. Patients with severe G6PD deficiency (< 10% residual enzyme activity) should not receive primaquine. For individuals with 10–60% residual activity, it is generally safe to give combined primaquine phosphate, 78.9 mg (45 mg base), and chloroquine phosphate, 0.5 g (0.3 g base), weekly for 8 weeks. However, for persons suspected of having the Mediterranean or Canton forms of G6PD deficiency, it may be preferable not to give primaquine but to treat attacks of malaria with chloroquine as they occur. Under development is tafenoquine, a congener of primaquine; it is more slowly eliminated than primaquine and is probably less toxic.

5. Quinine—Oral quinine sulfate in conjunction with another drug (see Table 35–3) is used to treat malaria due to multidrug-resistant strains of *P falciparum;* however, compliance with the 7-day course is poor because of quinine side effects.

Quinine should be taken with food. Mild to moderate quinine toxicity (cinchonism) is manifested by headache, nausea, slight visual disturbances, dizziness, and mild tinnitus. These symptoms may abate as treatment continues and usually do not require discontinuation of treatment. Where available, quinine blood levels can be monitored; desired plasma levels are 5–10 mcg/mL. Severe side effects (cinchonism) requiring temporary or permanent discontinuation of therapy are rare and begin to appear at plasma levels greater than 7 mcg/mL; findings include fever, skin eruptions, deafness, marked visual abnormalities (scotomas, diplopia, contracted visual fields, retinal vessel spasticity, optic atrophy, blindness), other central nervous system abnormalities (vertigo, somnolence, confusion, seizures), disturbances in cardiac rhythm or conduction, massive intravascular hemolysis with renal failure (blackwater fever), agranulocytosis, and thrombocytopenia.

Parenteral quinine dihydrochloride is used in the treatment of severe attacks of malaria due to *P falciparum* strains sensitive or resistant to chloroquine. The drug is given intravenously at a slow rate (Table 35–3); rapid infusions may be severely toxic. The drug should be used with extreme caution and only for patients who cannot take the medication orally; appropriate oral therapy should be started as soon as possible. Infusions may cause thrombophlebitis and hypoglycemia (blood glucose levels should be monitored). In the United States, parenteral quinine is no longer available and parenteral quinidine gluconate is used instead.

Manufacturers' recommendations for drug interactions (including aluminum-containing antacids, digoxin, anticoagulants, cimetidine, and rifampin) should be consulted. Quinine is safe to use in pregnancy. Systemic clearance of quinine slows in proportion to the severity of the disease.

6. Quinidine gluconate—Quinidine is the dextrorotatory diastereoisomer of quinine. The two drugs are equally efficacious in parenteral treatment of severe malaria (Table 35–3). They are also similar with regard to toxicity and drug interactions, but quinidine has a greater cardiosuppressant effect. The principal adverse effect associated with quinine and quinidine use in severe malaria is hypoglycemia, which usually develops after 24 hours of treatment; it is a particular problem in pregnancy.

7. Pyrimethamine-sulfadoxine (Fansidar)—Fansidar is supplied as tablets that contain pyrimethamine (25 mg) and sulfadoxine (500 mg). Fansidar's limitations are that it is effective only against susceptible strains of *P falciparum* (see above); its low efficacy against *P vivax, P ovale,* or *P malariae;* and the fact that it is slow-acting. Fansidar is no longer used for weekly prophylaxis because of rare reports of severe cutaneous toxicity and death. However, in single-dose treatment, Fansidar is generally well tolerated. Fansidar is currently used by some clinicians for intermittent prophylaxis for pregnant women in Africa south of the Sahara. Cutaneous reactions to the drug are more common in persons who are HIV-positive.

Fansidar is contraindicated for persons with known sulfonamide sensitivity and those in the last month of pregnancy (the sulfadoxine component, which has a long half-life, can cause kernicterus in the newborn). The drug should be used with caution in the presence of impaired renal or hepatic function, in patients with G6PD deficiency (hemolysis occurs in some), and in those with severe allergic disorders or bronchial asthma. If folic acid is needed, ingestion should be delayed 1 week to avoid an inhibitory effect on the antimalarial action of Fansidar.

8. Antibiotics—

a. Doxycycline—Doxycycline is effective against chloroquine-sensitive and chloroquine-resistant *P falciparum, P vivax,* and (apparently) against *P ovale* and *P malariae.* It is used prophylactically against chloroquine-resistant and mefloquine-resistant falciparum malaria in Thailand and adjacent countries and elsewhere for patients who cannot tolerate mefloquine or Malarone (Table 35–2). Doxycycline is also used as an adjunct drug with quinine for the treatment of resistant falciparum malaria (Table 35–3). Side effects include infrequent gastrointestinal symptoms (take with meals—but not at bedtime—plus copious amounts of water to avoid esophageal irritation); candidal vaginitis (advise carrying a self-treatment antifungal regimen, either vaginal suppositories or cream); and rare photosensitivity (prevention may be achieved by use of sunscreens that absorb ultraviolet radiation (UVA) and by avoidance of exposure to direct sunlight as much as possible). Milk, which reduces absorption, should be avoided. The drug is contraindicated in pregnancy, in nursing mothers, in children under 8 years of age, and in persons with hepatic dysfunction. No data are available on the long-term use of the drug.

b. Clindamycin—Clindamycin is highly effective in treatment when combined with quinine (Table 35–3). It should not be used as monotherapy, however, because of its slow onset of action. Side effects (gastrointestinal symptoms, perioral rash) are self-limited and mild; *Clostridium difficile* diarrhea is rare. Safety in pregnancy needs further evaluation.

9. Artemisinin (qinghaosu) and its derivatives—Artemisinin and its derivatives are available in some countries but not in the United States. The drugs are rapid-acting and effective against all malarial parasites and are partially gametocidal, but they are not active against the persistent liver stages of *P vivax* and *P ovale*. Artesunate, considered the most rapid-acting form, is water-soluble and is given orally or by intravenous infusion. Other parenteral preparations are oil-soluble artemether (erratically absorbed orally) and the newly marketed artemotil. Rectal suppository formulations are sometimes available. Having shown no parasite resistance, the artemisinin drugs are the only agents that remain reliably active against multidrug-resistant *P falciparum*, including agents resistant to quinine. The drugs are used only to treat acute malaria, including severe malaria. Because of their short half-lives, they cannot be used in prophylaxis. Mild adverse events—symptoms that also occur in malaria—are headache, gastrointestinal symptoms, pruritus, and fever. Instances of allergic reactions have been described. Animal studies suggest a potential for embryotoxicity (opinions differ on the safety of the drug in pregnancy) and central nervous system toxicity (but this has not been demonstrated in human prospective studies, except in one study that reported ototoxicity with co-artemeter). As recrudescences are common after treatment (10%), the drugs should not be used alone but in combination with a long-acting drug (eg, mefloquine or Malarone). The combinations also reduce the transmissibility of malaria by preventing gametocyte development. A combination approved by WHO is Riamet (Coartem), which is lumefantrine (120 mg) combined with artemether (20 mg); its dosage in treatment is four tablets initially, again at 8 hours, and then twice daily for the next 2 days. Cure rates up to 98% have been reported.

10. Proguanil—Proguanil (chlorguanide, Paludrine; not available in the United States), 200 mg/d, is a blood schizonticide against three of the malaria parasites (unknown degree against *P malariae*) and has some causal prophylactic action. The drug is no longer used alone but only in combination therapy. Proguanil (100 mg) with atovaquone (250 mg) (Malarone) has recently been approved in the United States for prophylaxis and treatment of multidrug-resistant falciparum malaria. Proguanil (100 mg daily) in combination with chloroquine (0.5 g weekly) for prophylaxis for travelers going to areas with low-intensity chloroquine-resistant *P falciparum* is no longer recommended for travelers going to areas with chloroquine-resistant malaria. Rarely reported side effects are nausea, vomiting, hair loss, and mouth ulcers. The drug is safe to use in pregnancy; it should not be used in persons with hepatic or renal dysfunction.

Chemoprophylaxis for Nonimmune Populations

See Table 35–2 for methods and dosages and under the individual drugs (above) for details on cautions, contraindications, and toxicities.

Antimalarials should be taken with water at mealtime. The selected drug should be tested for side effects in advance of departure (to allow time for selection of an alternative drug if necessary) and started sufficiently in advance of exposure that a satisfactory prophylactic blood level is achieved. On returning home, primaquine is given to eradicate persistent liver stages of *P vivax* or *P ovale* if there has been significant exposure to these parasites (see above under Primaquine).

A. CHEMOPROPHYLAXIS IN REGIONS WHERE *P FALCIPARUM* IS SENSITIVE TO CHLOROQUINE

1. Drug of choice—Chloroquine prevents attacks for all forms of malaria and is curative for *P falciparum* and *P malariae* when taken for 4 weeks after leaving the endemic area. For persons who cannot tolerate chloroquine, reducing the dose to 250 mg twice weekly or switching to hydroxychloroquine sulfate (400 mg [salt]) can be tried.

2. Alternative drugs—Malarone, mefloquine, and doxycycline are alternatives to chloroquine. Schizonticides *not used for chemoprophylaxis* are halofantrine (erratic absorption and variable bioavailability), Fansidar (hypersensitivity reactions with rare deaths; frequent parasite resistance to the drug), amodiaquine (agranulocytosis and toxic hepatitis), pyrimethamine (widespread resistance of both *P falciparum* and *P vivax*), artemisinin and related drugs (short duration of action), proguanil by itself (high failure rate), and generally quinine (toxicity).

B. CHEMOPROPHYLAXIS IN REGIONS WHERE *P FALCIPARUM* IS RESISTANT TO CHLOROQUINE

1. Drugs of choice—Malarone is preferred but is more expensive. Alternative drugs are mefloquine (more side effects, sometimes severe) and doxycycline.

2. Second alternative drugs—There is continuing evaluation of primaquine (30 mg base) starting 1 day before entering the endemic area, daily while there, and for 7 days afterward. Although it is not licensed for this use in the United States, the drug is recommended for this use by the Centers for Diseases Control and Prevention under special circumstances. The drug is contraindicated in pregnancy and in persons with G6PD deficiency. Under evaluation is tafenoquine, an analog of primaquine that is more potent than the parent drug and will require only weekly doses. Under exceptional circumstances, the daily use of quinine can be considered.

C. CHEMOPROPHYLAXIS IN SOUTHEAST ASIA

Multidrug *P falciparum* resistance is extensive in Southeast Asia. The drugs of choice are doxycycline, Malarone, and artesunate-mefloquine. Chloroquine and Fansidar cannot be used throughout the region because of resistance, and resistance to mefloquine and halofantrine is widespread.

D. PROPHYLAXIS FOR PREGNANT WOMEN

Pregnant women should be protected; malaria infection during pregnancy may be particularly severe with high maternal mortality and fetal and perinatal loss. The safest drug, where it remains effective, is weekly chloroquine (or hydroxychloroquine). Drugs contraindicated in pregnancy are primaquine, doxycycline, mefloquine in the first trimester (increase in stillbirths), Fansidar (toxicity), and Malarone (safety data are limited). The artemisinin drugs are not effective for prophylaxis because of their short half-life, and their safety has not been established. Generally, therefore, travel by pregnant women to areas with *P falciparum* resistance to chloroquine and mefloquine is not recommended.

E. EMERGENCY SELF-TREATMENT

In selected instances, medication should be provided for emergency self-treatment of breakthrough attacks (see above).

Treatment of Acute Attacks in Nonimmune Adult Populations

See under individual drugs and Table 35–3 for dosages.

A. GENERAL CONSIDERATIONS

At times when parasitologic confirmation is not readily available, it may be necessary to start treatment immediately based only on clinical findings. Patients with falciparum infections should be hospitalized. It is important to determine whether a patient has been treated with antimalarials in the previous 1–2 days (3 weeks for mefloquine because of its slow excretion) to avoid the risk of overdose or adverse drug interactions. In the event of mefloquine treatment failure after its use in prophylaxis, it is hazardous—although it may be essential—to use quinine or quinidine (Table 35–3); under these circumstances, the safest drug to use is artemisinin or one of its derivatives (not available in the United States).

It is essential to determine the density of parasites on the blood smear (as a measure of severity of infection) and to recheck at least twice daily. Within 48–72 hours after start of treatment, patients usually become afebrile and improve clinically; within 48 hours, parasitemia is generally reduced by about 75% (though there may be an initial increase during the first 6–12 hours). In the presence of adequate drug ingestion and retention, if there is no improvement within 48–72 hours for mild infections or 24 hours for severe ones

or if there is increasing asexual parasitemia after 1–2 days, parasite resistance to the drug must be assumed and treatment changed.

B. DRUG TREATMENT OF ALL FORMS OF MALARIA EXCEPT *P FALCIPARUM* AND *P VIVAX* STRAINS RESISTANT TO CHLOROQUINE (TABLE 35–3)

1. Elimination of asexual erythrocytic parasites— Infection by all four species of malaria is treated with oral chloroquine. Alternative oral drugs if chloroquine cannot be tolerated are Malarone, mefloquine, quinine sulfate, plus doxycycline or clindamycin or atovaquone plus doxycycline.

If the patient is severely ill, treat with intravenous quinine dihydrochloride* or quinidine gluconate, parenteral preparations of artemisinin derivatives,* or parenteral chloroquine. Start oral therapy with chloroquine as soon as possible.

2. Eradication of *P vivax* or *P ovale* infections— This is accomplished with a course of primaquine.

3. Elimination of persistent gametocytemia—Gametocytes of *P vivax*, *P ovale*, and *P malariae* can be eliminated by chloroquine. Gametocytes of *P falciparum* are eliminated by a single dose of 26.3 mg of primaquine salt.

4. Treatment of semi-immunes—Treatment of attacks in semi-immune patients generally requires shorter courses of drug treatment.

C. DRUG TREATMENT OF FALCIPARUM MALARIA ACQUIRED IN AREAS WHERE *P FALCIPARUM* IS RESISTANT TO CHLOROQUINE

Start treatment with oral quinine sulfate and a second drug. Alternative drugs are Malarone, mefloquine, artesunate* followed by mefloquine, atovaquone plus doxycycline. In Southeast Asia, mefloquine (when used alone) may not be effective because of multidrug resistance.

If the patient is severely ill, treat with intravenous quinine or quinidine. A second drug (doxycycline, tetracycline, or clindamycin) should also be given parenterally. Oral treatment with quinine plus the antibiotic should be started as soon as possible. For intravenous use, quinine is safer than quinidine; in comparison, the alternative drugs, the parenteral artemisinin derivatives—artesunate* and artemether*—are the safest but are equally effective. Artesunate and artemether should be followed by oral mefloquine.

D. SPECIAL MEASURES FOR MANAGEMENT OF SEVERE *P FALCIPARUM* MALARIA

(See references for further details.) Patients with falciparum malaria, even with low peripheral parasitic counts, should be hospitalized. Deterioration can occur even after start of adequate treatment. Any pa-

---

*Not available in the United States.

tient with a falciparum parasitemia greater than 2% should be treated with parenteral antimalarials. Severe (complicated) falciparum malaria is a medical emergency that requires intensive care with monitoring of electrolytes and acid-base balance, and immediate antimalarial treatment without waiting for all laboratory results to become available. Indications for parenteral treatment are (1) failure to ingest or retain drugs, (2) cerebral malaria, (3) multiple complications, and (4) peripheral asexual parasitemia of 5% (250,000/mcL) or higher. When possible, parenteral treatment should be intravenous, but quinine, artesunate, and chloroquine can be given intramuscularly; chloroquine can also be given subcutaneously. Patients receiving intravenous quinine and quinidine require a continuous infusion of 5–10% glucose as well as continuous ECG monitoring (especially to detect widening of the QRS complex or lengthening of the QT interval). Black urine suggests hemoglobinuria. Renal failure, metabolic acidosis, pulmonary edema, gram-negative sepsis, jaundice, severe anemia, and shock may ensue. Rehydration of the patient should be done with great caution, particularly in the first 24 hours, since overhydration may precipitate noncardiogenic pulmonary edema. In general, 2–3 L of fluid is required the first day, followed by 10–20 mL/kg/d; intake and output should be carefully recorded. After rehydration, the central venous pressure should be maintained at approximately 5 cm of water (pulmonary artery occlusion pressure < 15 mm Hg). For renal failure, early hemofiltration (more rapid than peritoneal dialysis) may be necessary and need to be sustained for 4–7 days or longer. Mechanical ventilation may also be indicated. Blood glucose levels should be monitored every 6 hours during the acute and early convalescent period, since hypoglycemia may be severe, either as a result of the malaria infection or the use of quinine or quinidine. In cerebral malaria, maintain the airway and exclude other treatable causes of coma (hypoglycemia, bacterial meningoencephalitis). The presence of papilledema is a contraindication to lumbar puncture. With convulsions, maintain the airway and treat with diazepam (0.15 mg/kg intravenously or 0.5 mg/kg rectally) or with paraldehyde (0.1 ml/kg intramuscularly, preferably dispensed from a glass syringe). Keep the temperature below 38.5 °C using acetaminophen (paracetamol) plus tepid sponging and fanning. Patients with clinically significant disseminated intravascular coagulation should be treated with fresh whole blood, clotting factors, or platelets as needed. For hematocrits below 20% or hemoglobins below 7 g/dL, transfusion of fresh whole blood or packed cells is required. Bacterial infections are common (eg, pneumonia, cystitis, salmonellosis). Exchange transfusion (5–10 L) should be considered when more than 10% of red blood cells are parasitized (5% if severe dysfunction of other organs is present). Corticosteroids, aspirin, other anti-inflammatory agents, dextran, norepinephrine, deferoxamine, and anticoagulants should not be used.

Follow-Up for *P falciparum* Malaria

Blood films should be checked daily until parasitemia clears; check weekly thereafter for 4 weeks to observe for recrudescence of infection.

Prognosis

The uncomplicated and untreated primary attack of *P vivax*, *P ovale*, or *P falciparum* malaria usually lasts 2–4 weeks; that of *P malariae* lasts about twice as long. Attacks of each type of infection may subsequently recur (once or many times) before the infection terminates spontaneously. With prompt antimalarial therapy, the prognosis is generally good, but in *P falciparum* infections, when severe complications such as cerebral malaria develop, the prognosis is poor (14–17% mortality) even with treatment. After cerebral malaria, residual neurologic deficits may remain.

Baird JK: Effectiveness of antimalarial drugs. N Engl J Med 2005; 352:1565. [PMID: 15829537]

Chen LH et al: New strategies for the prevention of malaria in travelers. Infect Dis Clin North Am 2005;19:185. [PMID: 15701554]

Greenwood PM et al: Malaria. Lancet 2005;365:1487. [PMID: 15870634]

Health Information for International Travel 2005–2006. U.S. Department of Health and Human Services, Centers for Disease Control and Prevention, Atlanta, Georgia. Available from 877-252-1200 International Travel and Health: *Vaccination Certificate Requirements and Health Advice.* WHO, 2006.

Pasvol G: Management of severe malaria: interventions and controversies. Infect Dis Clinic North Am 2005;19:211. [PMID: 15701555]

Prevention of malaria. Med Lett Drug Ther 2005;47:100. [PMID: 16331244]

Woodrow CJ et al: Artemisinins. Postgrad Med J 2005;81:71. [PMID: 15701735]

TOXOPLASMOSIS

 ESSENTIALS OF DIAGNOSIS

Acute primary infection:

- *Fever, malaise, headache, lymphadenopathy (especially cervical), myalgia, arthralgia, stiff neck, sore throat; occasionally, rash, hepatosplenomegaly, retinochoroiditis, confusion; in various combinations.*
- *Positive serologic tests with high and rising IgG and IgM.*
- *Isolation of* Toxoplasma gondii *from blood or body fluids; tachyzoites in histologic sections of tissue or cytologic preparations of body fluids.*

Acute primary or recrudescent infection in immunocompromised patients:

- *Central nervous system mass lesions; retinochoroiditis, pneumonitis, myocarditis less common; sometimes other findings as above.*

- *Positive IgG titers moderately high; IgM antibody usually absent. Tissue diagnosis as above.*

General Considerations

Toxoplasma gondii, an obligate intracellular protozoan, is found worldwide in humans and in many species of animals and birds. The parasite is a coccidian of cats, the definitive host, and exists in three forms: The *trophozoite* (tachyzoite) (3 × 7 mcm) is the rapidly proliferating form in tissues and body fluids that causes acute disease. The trophozoites can enter and multiply in most mammalian nucleated cells. The *cyst*, containing viable bradyzoites, is the latent form that can persist indefinitely as a chronic infection and is found particularly in muscle and nerve tissue. The *oocyst* is the form passed only in the feces of the cat family. In the intestinal epithelium of cats, a sexual cycle occurs, with subsequent release of oocysts for 3–14 days; cats may, however, become reinfected and excrete oocysts multiple times. The oocysts, which contain infective sporozoites, are infectious within 12 hours to several days after passage and can remain infective in moist soil for weeks to years.

Human infection results (1) from ingestion of cysts in raw or undercooked meat; (2) from ingestion of oocysts in contaminated food or water, by careless handling of cat litter, or from soil by soil-eating children; (3) from transplacental transmission of trophozoites; or (4) rarely, from direct inoculation of trophozoites, as in blood transfusion and organ transplants. Reservoirs of human infection are rodents and birds eaten by cats, and infected domestic animals used for human food. Antibody prevalence rates range from less than 5% in some parts of the world (absence of cats and minimal ingestion of meat) to 23% overall in the United States (16% in women aged 12–49) and over 80% in France. This range is due, in part, to culture differences that determine whether meat is eaten raw or undercooked.

On ingestion, bradyzoites (from cysts) or sporozoites (from oocysts) invade multiple cells types and propagate as trophozoites; cell death and inflammation follow, but true granulomas do not form.

Clinical Findings

A. SYMPTOMS AND SIGNS

Over 80% of primary infections, including during pregnancy, are asymptomatic. The incubation period for symptomatic persons is 1–2 weeks. Generally, on recovery, both asymptomatic and symptomatic infections persist as chronic latent (cyst) infections. Reactivation occurs almost exclusively in severely immunocompromised patients.

The clinical manifestations of toxoplasmosis may be grouped into four syndromes.

1. Primary infection in the immunocompetent host—Most symptomatic infections are acute, mild, febrile multisystem illnesses that resemble infectious mononucleosis. Lymphadenopathy, usually nontender, particularly of the head and neck, is the most common finding. Other features in various combinations are malaise, myalgia, arthralgia, headache, sore throat, and maculopapular or urticarial rash. Hepatosplenomegaly may occur. Rarely, severe cases are complicated by pneumonitis, meningoencephalitis, hepatitis, myocarditis, polymyositis, and retinochoroiditis. Symptoms may fluctuate, but most patients recover spontaneously within a few months.

2. Congenital infection—Congenital transmission occurs only as a result of infection (generally asymptomatic) in a nonimmune woman during pregnancy. In the United States, an estimated 400 to 4000 congenital infections occur yearly. Following maternal infection, the frequency of transmission to the fetus varies by trimester: 15%, 30%, and 60%, respectively, in the first, second, and third trimesters. Fetal infection is more severe when maternal infection occurs in the first trimester. However, if maternal infection occurs in the third trimester, most of the infected fetuses will have a subclinical infection at birth but, if left untreated, 85% will later develop overt disease, particularly chorioretinitis or delays in development. Treatment of the mother reduces the congenital infection rate by about 60%. See specialized sources for clinical manifestations, approach to diagnosis, and treatment.

3. Retinochoroiditis—In most cases, this develops gradually weeks to years after congenital infection (the preponderant form, which is generally bilateral) or infrequently after an acquired infection in a young child (generally unilateral). Acquired or reactivated infections in older children and adults rarely progress to retinochoroiditis. The inflammatory process persists for weeks to months as focally necrotic retinal lesions (yellow or white patches with blurred margins). Visual defects, which include blurring, central defects, and scotomas, are accompanied by pain and photophobia. Rarely, progression may result in glaucoma and blindness. With healing, white or dark-pigmented scars may result. Panuveitis may accompany retinochoroiditis.

4. Reactivated disease in the immunologically compromised host—Reactivated toxoplasmosis occurs in patients with AIDS, cancer, or those given immunosuppressive drugs. The infection may present in specific organs (brain, lungs, and eye most commonly, but also heart, skin, gastrointestinal tract, and liver) or as disseminated disease. Encephalitis will develop in 30–50% of AIDS patients seropositive for past *Toxoplasma* infection and 10–30% will die of the infection. Brain lesions include meningitis (uncommon), mass lesions (single or multiple), or diffuse intracerebral *Toxoplasma* lesions, associated with clinical findings of fever, headache, altered mental status, seizures, and focal (or, infrequently, nonfocal) motor or sensory neurologic deficits (see also Chapter 31).

B. LABORATORY FINDINGS

Diagnosis depends principally on serologic tests, which are sensitive and reliable. However, diagnosis is occasionally made from tissue (blood, bone marrow aspirates, cerebrospinal fluid sediment, sputum, and other tissues or body fluids or placental tissue) either by (1) demonstration of trophozoites or characteristic histology, (2) isolation of the organism in mice (more sensitive) or in tissue culture (more rapid, 3–6 days), or (3) amplification of *T gondii* DNA by PCR. The latter has become particularly useful through testing of amniotic fluid for congenital infection and testing immunocompromised patients for recrudescence. Detection of circulating antigen or antigen in body fluids is infrequently used and controversial. Interpretation of the results and deciding which patients should be treated or when to advise termination of a pregnancy may require assistance from a reference or research laboratory with large experience in toxoplasmosis.

1. Histology—Cysts or trophozoites may be directly identified in blood (buffy coat from centrifuged heparinized blood), other tissues, or body fluids by staining with standard stains or with specific antibody marked with fluorescein. Demonstration of cysts in biopsied tissue does not establish a causal relationship to clinical illness, since cysts may be found in both acute and chronic infections. However, finding tachyzoites confirms active infection. In the placenta, fetus, or newborn, the presence of cysts does indicate congenital infection.

2. Serologic tests—Parallel testing of serial blood specimens collected 3–4 weeks apart is necessary because a single high titer does not confirm the diagnosis. The Sabin-Feldman dye test, indirect hemagglutination and immunofluorescent (IFA), ELISA, Western blot, PCR, IgG avidity, and other tests can be done on blood, cerebrospinal fluid, aqueous humor, and other body fluids. The dye test is the standard but is rarely used because of laboratory safety factors; though extremely sensitive and specific, it does not separate IgM from IgG antibody. The ELISA, immunosorbent, IFA, and Western blot tests do separate IgM and IgG. IgM antibody appears 1–2 weeks after start of infection, reaches a peak at 6–8 weeks, and then gradually declines over 18 months. However, since IgM antibody can persist at low titers for 5 years or longer, a positive finding does not necessarily represent recent infection; a negative finding does rule out acute infection acquired in recent months. False-positive tests for IgM antibodies are common and therefore the test should be confirmed. IgG antibody appears within 1–2 weeks after onset of infection, peaks in 1–2 months, and may persist at high titers for many years and then at low levels for life. When positive, it reliably indicates present or past infection; a negative result reliably rules out either time frame. IgA antibody appears during the first month, reaches a peak in the second and third months, and then declines. IgM and IgA antibodies, particularly IgA, can be important in diagnosing acute infection because they rarely are found in chronic infection. Normally, maternal IgM and IgA are unable to cross the intact placenta; antibody that does pass through during the birth process has a half-life of 2–4 days for IgM and 10 days for IgA.

The following are selected serologic and other findings in specific toxoplasmosis syndromes.

a. Acute infection in immunocompetent persons—In screening, test initially for IgG antibody, which reliably establishes the presence or absence of infection. In a few patients, antibody may not be detectable within 3 weeks of initial infection; if acute disease is suspected, test again in 3 weeks. The diagnosis is established by seroconversion from negative to positive or by a 16-fold rise in serologic titers by any test. Acute infection can also be diagnosed by detection of tachyzoites in tissue, isolation of organism, or amplification of its DNA in blood or body fluids. The presence of circulating ELISA-IgA also favors the diagnosis of acute infection. A presumptive diagnosis is based on a single IgM titer of over 1:64 and a very high IgG titer (> 1:1000). However, because of the relatively high frequency of false-positive IgM tests, confirmatory testing should always be done, preferably in a reference laboratory.

b. Recrudescent infection in immunosuppressed patients—In AIDS patients, *Toxoplasma* can sometimes be isolated from the blood. Alternatively, definitive diagnosis is by finding *Toxoplasma* organisms in cerebrospinal fluid (Wright-Giemsa stain or by PCR amplification) or by brain biopsy. To avoid the latter, empiric antibiotic treatment is generally started after presumptive evidence is obtained by MRI (the more sensitive test) or CT scan (typically: multiple, isodense or hypodense, ring-enhancing mass lesions). Single-photon emission CT is under evaluation as a highly specific diagnostic method. Antibody titers cannot be depended on, since most patients have IgG titers that reflect past infection, significant rises are infrequent, and IgM antibody is rare. Absence of IgG does not rule out the diagnosis of toxoplasmic retinochoroiditis or encephalitis. The cerebrospinal fluid may show mild pleocytosis (predominantly lymphocytes and monocytes), elevated protein, and normal glucose. (See also Chapter 31.)

c. Toxoplasmic retinochoroiditis—This is usually associated with stable, usually low IgG titers and no IgM antibody. If IgG antibody in aqueous humor is higher than in the serum, the diagnosis is supported.

3. Other laboratory findings—Leukocyte counts are normal or reduced, often with lymphocytosis or monocytosis with rare atypical cells, but there is no heterophil antibody. Chest radiographs may show interstitial pneumonia. In cerebral imaging studies in HIV-infected persons, toxoplasmosis typically appears as multiple lesions with a predilection for the basal ganglion.

Differential Diagnosis

In acute febrile disease, consider cytomegalovirus infection, infectious mononucleosis, and other causes of pneumonitis, myocarditis, myositis, hepatitis, and splenomegaly. With lymphadenopathy, possibilities include sarcoidosis, tuberculosis, tularemia, lymphoma, cat-scratch disease, and metastatic carcinoma. With brain lesions in the immunosuppressed host, consider lymphoma, tuberculoma, brain abscess, metastatic carcinoma, and fungal lesions.

Treatment

A. APPROACH TO TREATMENT

In immunocompetent hosts, the **lymphadenopathic** form of the disease is usually not treated unless findings are severe or persistent or there is overt visceral disease. If treatment is started, it should continue for 3–4 weeks and the patient reevaluated. Serologic tests are not useful for evaluating response to treatment.

Since most episodes of **retinochoroiditis** are self-limited, opinions vary on indications for, type of, and the practical benefits of treatment. (See specialized texts.)

Immunocompromised patients with active infection (primary or recrudescent) must be treated. See Chapter 31 for details. Therapy should continue for 4–6 weeks after cessation of symptoms, which may require up to a 6-month course, to be followed by drug prophylaxis as long as immunosuppression persists. In HIV-infected persons, acute toxoplasmosis must be treated followed by continued prophylaxis; in patients who have a positive IgG *Toxoplasma* serology but are asymptomatic, prophylaxis is desirable.

For details on management of maternal infection and congenitally infected newborns, see specialized sources.

B. CHOICE OF DRUGS

The treatment of choice in nonimmunocompromised patients is pyrimethamine, 25–100 mg orally once daily, plus sulfadiazine, 1–1.5 g orally four times daily; continue this treatment for 3–4 weeks. Add folic acid at a dosage of 10–15 mg/d to prevent bone marrow suppression. Patients should be screened for a history of sulfonamide sensitivity (skin rashes, gastrointestinal symptoms, hepatotoxicity). To prevent crystal-induced nephrotoxicity, good urinary output should be maintained; alkalinization with sodium bicarbonate may also be useful. Pyrimethamine side effects include headache and gastrointestinal symptoms. Platelet and white blood cell counts should be performed at least twice weekly. Clindamycin (600 mg orally four times daily) may be a useful alternative drug because it concentrates in the choroid. Atovaquone (750 mg orally three or four times daily), azithromycin (1200–1500 mg orally), dapsone, other macrolides, and immunotherapy are under evaluation.

For the treatment of central nervous system toxoplasmosis in HIV-infected and immunocompromised persons, see Chapter 31.

Prevention

Irradiated meat or meat cooked to 66 °C kills cysts in tissues; freezing meat decreases infectivity but does not eliminate it. Hands, kitchen surfaces, and cooking utensils must be thoroughly cleaned with soap and water after contact with raw meat. Under appropriate environmental conditions, oocysts passed in cat feces can remain infective for a year or more. Thus, children's play areas, including sandboxes, should be protected from cat (and dog) feces; hand washing is indicated after contact with soil potentially contaminated by animal feces. Indoor cats should be fed only dry, canned, or cooked meat. Litter boxes should be changed daily and scalded, as freshly deposited oocysts are not infective for 48 hours.

Although universal screening is conducted in some countries, authorities in the United States generally do not consider it warranted because of low prevalence. Pregnant women should have their serum examined for *Toxoplasma* IgG and IgM antibody. If the IgM test is negative but an IgG titer is present and less than 1:1000, no further evaluation is necessary. Those with negative titers should take measures to prevent infection—preferably by having no further contact with cats and cat litter, by thoroughly cooking meat (66 °C/150 °F), and by hand washing after handling raw meat and before eating. Gloves should be worn when gardening; fruits and vegetables should be thoroughly washed; ingestion of dried meat should be avoided. For seronegative women who continue to have significant environmental exposure, serologic screening should be conducted several times during pregnancy.

Prognosis

The outlook for acute toxoplasmosis in adults is excellent as long as the patient is immunocompetent. In immunosuppressed patients, the disease is usually fatal if untreated; improvement results if treatment is started early, but recrudescence is common. Chronic asymptomatic infection is usually benign.

Cold CJ et al: Diagnosis—disseminated toxoplasmosis. Clin Med Res 2005;3:186. [PMID: 16160073]

Collazos J: Opportunistic infections of the CNS in patients with AIDS: diagnosis and management. CNS Drugs 2003;17: 869. [PMID: 12962527]

Lopez A et al: Preventing congenital toxoplasmosis. MMWR Recomm Rep 2000;49:59. [PMID: 15580732]

Montoya JG et al: Diagnosis and management of toxoplasmosis. Clin Perinatol 2005;32:705. [PMID: 16085028]

Montoya JG et al: Toxoplasmosis. Lancet 2004;363:1965. [PMID: 15194258]

Remington JS et al: Recent developments for diagnosis of toxoplasmosis. J Clin Microbiol 2004;42:941. [PMID: 15004036]

Stanford MR et al: Antibiotics for toxoplasmic retinochoroiditis: an evidence-based systematic review. Ophthalmology 2003; 110:926. [PMID: 12750091]

■ HELMINTHIC INFECTIONS

TREMATODE (Fluke) INFECTIONS

SCHISTOSOMIASIS (Bilharziasis)

ESSENTIALS OF DIAGNOSIS

- History of fresh water exposure in an endemic area.
- Acute phase: Abrupt onset (2–8 weeks postexposure) of abdominal pain, weight loss, headache, malaise, chills, fever, urticaria, myalgia, diarrhea (sometimes bloody), dry cough, hepatomegaly, and eosinophilia.
- Chronic phase: Either (1) diarrhea, abdominal pain, blood in stool, hepatomegaly or hepatosplenomegaly, and bleeding from esophageal varices (Schistosoma mansoni or Schistosoma japonicum infection); or (2) terminal hematuria, urinary frequency, urethral and bladder pain, and pyelitis (Schistosoma haematobium infection).
- Depending on species, characteristic eggs in feces, urine, or scrapings or biopsy of rectal or bladder mucosa; positive serology.

General Considerations

Schistosomiasis, which infects more than 200 million persons worldwide, induces severe consequences in 20 million persons annually, resulting in over 200,000 deaths. The disease is caused mainly by three blood flukes (trematodes). *Schistosoma mansoni*, which causes intestinal schistosomiasis, is widespread in Africa and occurs in the Arabian peninsula, South America (Brazil, Venezuela, Suriname), and the Caribbean (including Puerto Rico but not Cuba). Vesical (urinary) schistosomiasis, caused by *Schistosoma haematobium*, is found throughout the Middle East and Africa. Asiatic intestinal schistosomiasis, due to *Schistosoma japonicum*, is important in China and the Philippines, and a small focus is present in Sulawesi, Indonesia, but transmission in Japan has been interrupted. A number of schistosome species of animals sometimes infect humans, including *Schistosoma intercalatum* in central Africa and *Schistosoma mekongi* in the Mekong delta in Thailand, Cambodia, and Laos. In the United States, an estimated 400,000 immigrants are infected, but transmission does not occur because appropriate snail intermediate hosts are absent.

Mammals are important reservoirs for *S japonicum*. Humans are the main reservoir for *S mansoni* and *S haematobium*; the few animal species infected with *S mansoni* are not epidemiologically important.

In the life cycle involving humans, the adult worms live in terminal venules of the bowel (*S mansoni, S japonicum, S intercalatum, S mekongi*) or bladder (*S haematobium*). When eggs passed in feces or urine reach fresh water, a larval form is released that subsequently infects snails, the intermediate host. After development, infective larvae (cercariae) leave the snails, enter water, and infect exposed persons through the skin or mucous membranes. After penetration, the cercariae become schistosomula larvae that reach the portal circulation in the liver, where they rapidly mature. After a few weeks, adult worms pair, mate, and migrate mainly to terminal venules of specific veins, where females deposit their eggs. By means of lytic secretions, some eggs reach the lumen of the bowel or bladder and are passed with feces or urine. Others are retained in the bowel or bladder wall, while still others are carried in the circulation to the liver, lung, and (less often) to other tissues.

Except for the allergic response in the acute syndrome (see below), disease is primarily due to delayed hypersensitivity. Antigens released by the eggs stimulate a local T cell-dependent granulomatous response, followed by a strong fibrotic reaction. Live worms, however, produce no lesions and rarely cause symptoms. The type or degree of tissue damage and symptoms varies with the intensity of infection (worm burden), host genetic factors, site of egg deposition, concurrent infection (eg, hepatitis B), and duration of infection.

S mansoni adults migrate to the inferior mesenteric veins of the large bowel and *S japonicum* to the superior and inferior mesenteric veins in the large and small bowel. Ulcers and polyps (common only in Egypt) result from granuloma formation and fibrosis in the bowel wall. Egg accumulation in the liver may result in periportal fibrosis and portal hypertension of the presinusoidal type, but liver function typically remains intact even in advanced disease. Portal-systemic collateralization due to portal hypertension can result in embolization of eggs to the lungs, with subsequent endarteritis, pulmonary hypertension, and cor pulmonale. Because greater numbers of eggs are produced by *S japonicum*, the resulting disease is often more severe.

Adult *S haematobium* mature in the venous plexus of the bladder, ureters, rectum, prostate, and uterus. Ulcers and polyps result from granuloma formation and fibrosis in the bladder wall, and eggshell remnants may calcify. Stricture or distortion of the ureteral orifices or terminal ureters may result in hydroureter, hydronephrosis, and ascending infection. Lesions in the pelvic organs rarely progress to extensive fibrosis and infection. Eggs are carried to the liver or lungs, but severe pathologic changes in these organs are less frequent than in *S mansoni* and *S japonicum* infections.

In size, adult *S mansoni* are 6–13 × 1 mm. The prepatent period—from cercarial penetration until appearance of eggs in feces—is about 50 days. The life span of the worms ranges from 5 to 30 years or more.

Clinical Findings

A. Symptoms and Signs

Although a large proportion of infected persons have light infections (< 100 eggs per gram of feces) and are asymptomatic, an estimated 50–60% have symptoms and 5–10% have advanced organ damage. In children, schistosomal infections may contribute to decreased nutritional status and growth retardation. Persons with concomitant AIDS and schistosomiasis should be treated for the latter infection. Some evidence shows that in coinfections, responsiveness to schistosomiasis treatment is reduced and susceptibility to schistosomiasis reinfection is increased.

1. Cercarial dermatitis—Following cercarial penetration, clinical findings progress from a localized itchy erythematous or petechial rash to macules and papules that last 2–6 days. Most cases occur in fresh or marine water (worldwide) and are due to skin invasion by bird schistosome cercariae, parasites that do not mature in humans and do not cause systemic symptoms. The syndrome is uncommon with human schistosome infections.

2. Acute schistosomiasis (Katayama syndrome)—This syndrome, primarily an allergic response to the developing schistosomes, may occur with the three schistosomes (rare with *S haematobium*). The syndrome is usually not seen in natives but does occur in travelers, especially to Africa. The incubation period is 2–8 weeks, with serology becoming positive some weeks later followed by ova appearing in the stools. The severity of illness ranges from mild to (rarely) life-threatening, when use of corticosteroid treatment can be considered. In addition to fever, malaise, urticaria, diarrhea (sometimes bloody), myalgia, dry cough, leukocytosis, and marked eosinophilia, the liver and spleen may be temporarily enlarged. Pulmonary infiltrates and prostration may be present. The patient again becomes asymptomatic in 2–8 weeks.

3. Chronic schistosomiasis—This stage begins 6 months to several years after infection. In *S mansoni* and *S japonicum* infections, findings include diarrhea, abdominal pain, irregular bowel movements, blood in the stool, a hard enlarged liver, and splenomegaly. With subsequent slow progression over 5–15 years or longer, the following may appear: anorexia, weight loss, weakness, polypoid intestinal tumors, and features of portal and pulmonary hypertension. Immune complex glomerulonephritis may also occur.

In *S haematobium* infection, early symptoms of urinary tract disease are frequency and dysuria, followed by terminal hematuria and proteinuria. Frank hematuria may be recurrent. Sequelae may include bladder polyp formation, cystitis, chronic salmonella infection, pyelitis, pyelonephritis, urolithiasis, hydronephrosis due to ureteral obstruction, renal failure, and death. Severe liver, lung, genital, or neurologic disease is rare. Squamous cell bladder cancer has been associated with vesicular schistosomiasis.

4. Other complications—Portal hypertension may result in a contracted liver, splenomegaly, pancytopenia, esophageal varices, and variceal bleeding. Abnormal liver function, jaundice, ascites, and hepatic coma are end-stage findings. Pulmonary hypertension with cor pulmonale and edema due to right heart failure may supervene. Large bowel complications include stricture, granulomatous masses, and persistent salmonella infection; colonic polyposis is manifested by bloody diarrhea, anemia, hypoalbuminemia, and clubbing. Central nervous system lesions, transverse myelitis, or optic neuritis may result from egg metastasis or ectopic worms.

B. Laboratory Findings

Screening and diagnosis require testing for eggs in feces and urine (which may be irregular in excretion and require repeated testing), for occult blood in feces and urine, for protein and leukocytes in urine, and serology. Ova collected in fresh, nonpreserved specimens should be examined for internal detail (flame cell activity or miracidial movement) or by the hatching test to determine that some are alive and that the infection therefore warrants treatment.

1. Eggs—Definitive diagnosis is by finding characteristic live eggs in excreta or mucosal biopsy.

In *S haematobium* infection, eggs may be found in the urine or, less frequently, in the stools. Eggs are sought in urine specimens collected between 9 AM and 2 PM or in 24-hour collections. They are processed either by examination of the sediment or preferably by membrane filtration. Occasionally, eggs are sought by vesical mucosa biopsy.

In *S mansoni* and *S japonicum* infections, eggs may be found in stool specimens by direct examination, but some form of concentration is usually necessary; the Kato-Katz quantitative method is preferred over formal ether concentration. One stool examination can reach 70% sensitivity and four, 92%. If results are negative, rectal mucosal biopsy of inflamed or granulomatous lesions or random biopsy specimens at two or three sites of normal mucosa may yield the diagnosis. Biopsy specimens should be examined both as crush preparations between two glass slides and histologically. If eggs are found, a quantitative test should be done after collecting a 24-hour urine or stool; heavy infections are those with counts over 400 eggs per gram.

2. Serologic tests—ELISA, immunoblot, and other tests are used in screening and may detect some egg-negative or ectopic infections. Deficiencies of the tests are that they are commonly negative early in infection and, as they remain positive for long periods of time, do not distinguish active from past infection. The Centers for Disease Control and Prevention uses a "fast ELISA" for screening (specificity 99%; sensitivity varies by parasite: *S mansoni* [99%], *S haematobium* [95%], *S japonicum* [> 50%]) and a Western blot (specificity [96%]) for confirmation and speciation.

Positive tests do not correlate with worm burden. Accumulating research evidence supports the view that detection of antigen in blood and urine is sensitive, correlates with intensity of infection, and can distinguish old from new infection—and that loss of circulating antigen 5–10 days after treatment is indicative of cure. Skin testing is no longer recommended.

3. Other tests—Anemia is common. Eosinophilia, common during the acute stage, usually is absent in the chronic stage. In *S mansoni* and *S japonicum* infections, barium swallow, esophagoscopy, barium enema or colonoscopy, chest x-ray, or an ECG may be indicated. Ultrasound examination of the liver may show the pathognomonic pattern of periportal fibrosis and replaces the need for liver biopsy. The clinical settings in which ultrasonography is most useful are (1) evaluation of portal hypertension, (2) distinguishing schistosomiasis from cirrhosis, and (3) documenting regression of lesions following treatment; in early infections, however, findings are inconsistently present.

In *S haematobium* infection, occult hematuria can often be detected either microscopically or by reagent strip test, particularly if the first portion of the urine specimen is evaluated. In advanced disease, cystoscopy may show "sandy patches," ulcers, and areas of squamous metaplasia; lower abdominal plain films may show calcification of the bladder wall or ureters. Sonography is considered the imaging technique of choice but may fail to show the calcification. CT—which may demonstrate pathognomonic "turtleback" calcifications—intravenous pyelography, and retrograde cystography and pyelography may be useful. Up to 20% of the time, *S mansoni* eggs are found in the urine.

Differential Diagnosis

Early intestinal schistosomiasis may be mistaken for amebiasis, bacillary dysentery, or other causes of diarrhea and dysentery. Later, malignancy or the various causes of portal hypertension or of bowel polyps must be considered. In endemic areas, vesical schistosomiasis must be differentiated from other causes of urinary symptoms such as genitourinary tract cancer, bacterial infections of the urinary tract, nephrolithiasis, and the like.

Treatment

A. Medical Treatment

Treatment should be given only if live ova are identified. The safety and effectiveness of current drugs make it possible to treat all active infections orally, including advanced disease, and without concern for serious side effects. Praziquantel can be used to treat all species; alternative drugs of choice are oxamniquine for *S mansoni* and metrifonate (withdrawn from the US market) for *S haematobium*. Praziquantel is active against immature schistosomes during the first 2 days after cercarial penetration and then is inactive for approximately the next 4 weeks. Artemisinin and its derivatives, recently found to be active against the immature and adult forms, are being evaluated for prophylaxis, treatment of early infection, and cotreatment with praziquantel. Instances of decreased sensitivity and treatment failure of both oxamniquine and praziquantel have been recognized in some localities. Schistosomal spinal cord infection has been successfully treated with combined praziquantel and corticosteroids.

After treatment, periodic laboratory follow-up for continued passage of eggs is essential, starting at 3 months and continuing at intervals for 1 year; if found, viability should be determined, since dead eggs are passed for some months. No specific treatment is indicated for bird cercarial dermatitis, except for topical applications to relieve itching.

1. Praziquantel—Cure rates of 63–85% and higher are achieved at 6 months for *S haematobium*, *S mansoni*, and *S japonicum* infections, with marked reduction in egg counts (> 90%) in those not cured.

The praziquantel dosage is 20 mg/kg orally—give twice in 1 day for *S haematobium* and *S mansoni* and three times in 1 day for *S japonicum* and *S mekongi*. The dosages should be given at 4- to 6-hour intervals with a meal; the tablets should not be chewed.

Mild and transient side effects persisting for hours to 1 day are common and include malaise, headache, dizziness, and anorexia. Less frequent are fatigue, drowsiness, nausea, vomiting, generalized abdominal pain, loose stools, pruritus, urticaria, arthralgia and myalgia, and low-grade fever. Minimal elevations of liver enzymes have occasionally been reported. Because of drug-induced dizziness, patients should not drive and should be cautioned if their work requires physical coordination or alertness. WHO has recommended using praziquantel in pregnancy. In areas where cysticercosis may coexist with a schistosomal infection being treated with praziquantel, treatment is best conducted in a hospital to monitor for death of cysticerci, which may be followed by neurologic complications. Recently reported for praziquantel are comutagenic effects with several mutagens and carcinogens; the authors conclude that the import of these findings needs further study.

2. Oxamniquine—Oxamniquine, not available in the United States, is highly effective only in *S mansoni* infections. For strains in the western hemisphere and western Africa, a dose of 15 mg/kg orally is given once. Some experts recommend 40–60 mg/kg/d in two or three divided doses for 2–3 days in all of Africa and in the Arabian peninsula. The drug is administered with food; when divided doses are needed, they are separated by 6–8 hours. Cure rates are 70–95%, with marked reduction in egg counts in those not cured. Side effects occur within hours: dizziness is most common; less frequent are drowsiness, nausea and vomiting, diarrhea, abdominal pain, and headache. An orange or red discoloration of the urine may occur. Rarely reported is central nervous system stimulation with behavioral changes, hallucinations, or seizures; patients should be observed for 2 hours after ingestion of the drug for appearance of these findings. Since the drug makes some patients dizzy or drowsy, it should be used with caution in patients whose work or activity requires mental alertness. Instances of parasite resistance to the drug have been reported. Because the drug has shown mutagenic and embryotoxic effects, it is contraindicated in pregnancy.

B. SURGICAL MEASURES

In selected instances, surgery may be indicated for removal of polyps and for obstructive uropathy. For bleeding esophageal varices, sclerotherapy is the treatment of choice; whether some patients may benefit from propranolol treatment is under evaluation. As a last resort in patients who have repeated bleeding, shunting procedures (esophagogastric devascularization with splenectomy or distal—but not proximal—splenorenal shunt) are used, though their effectiveness and relative usefulness are not well established. Severe pancytopenia is an indication for splenectomy.

Prevention

Travelers to endemic areas should avoid swimming and other fresh water exposure. Use of topical agents to prevent cercarial penetration or oral prophylaxis has not been established.

Prognosis

With treatment, the prognosis is excellent in early and light infections. There may be shrinkage or elimination of bladder and bowel ulcerations, granulomas, and polyps and reduction in fibrosis by sonography. In advanced disease with extensive involvement of the intestines, liver, bladder, or other organs, the outlook is poor even with treatment. In endemic areas, mass treatment of children diminishes the risk of developing severely diseased organs, even though reinfection may occur.

Da Silva LC et al: Schistosomiasis mansoni—clinical features. Gastroenterol Hepatol 2005;28:30. [PMID: 15691467]

Inyang-Etoh PC et al: Efficacy of artesunate in the treatment of urinary schistosomiasis, in an endemic community in Nigeria. Ann Trop Med Parasitol 2004;98:491. [PMID: 15257799]

Laosebikan AO et al: Schistosomal portal hypertension. J Am Coll Surg 2005;200:795. [PMID: 15848374]

Utzinger J et al: Schistosomiasis and soil-transmitted helminthiasis: common drugs for treatment and control. Expert Opin Pharmacother 2004;5:263. [PMID: 14996624]

Vennervald BJ et al: Morbidity in schistosomiasis: an update. Curr Opin Infect Dis 2004;17:439. [PMID: 15353964]

FASCIOLOPSIASIS

The large intestinal fluke, *Fasciolopsis buski*, is a common parasite of humans and pigs in central and southern China, Taiwan, Southeast Asia, Indonesia, eastern India, and Bangladesh. When eggs shed in stools reach water, they hatch to produce free-swimming larvae that penetrate and develop in the flesh of snails. Cercariae subsequently escape from the snails and encyst on various water plants. Humans are infected by eating these plants uncooked (usually water chestnuts, bamboo shoots, or caltrops). Adult flukes (length 2–7.5 cm) mature in about 3 months and live in the small intestine attached to the mucosa or buried in mucous secretions. The number of parasites ranges from a few to several thousand.

After an incubation period of 2–3 months, manifestations of gastrointestinal irritation appear in all but light infections. Symptoms in severe infections include nausea, anorexia, upper abdominal pain, and diarrhea, sometimes alternating with constipation. Ascites and edema of the face and lower extremities may occur later; the physiologic mechanism is not understood. Intestinal obstruction, ileus, cachexia, and extreme prostration have been described.

Diagnosis depends on finding characteristic eggs or, occasionally, flukes in the stools. Leukocytosis with moderate eosinophilia is common. No serologic test is available. Because the adult worms live for only 6 months, absence from the endemic area for a longer period makes the diagnosis unlikely.

The drug of first choice is praziquantel, 25 mg/kg three times in 1 day only. The alternative drug is niclosamide (not available in the United States), administered as for taeniasis but given every other day for three doses.

In light infections—even without treatment—the prognosis is good; generally, spontaneous cure occurs within 1 year. In rare cases—particularly in children—heavy infections with severe toxemia have resulted in death from cachexia or intercurrent infection.

Many other human intestinal fluke infections include *Metagonimus yokogawai* (Far East and Indonesia), *Heterophyes heterophyes* (Middle East and Sudan), and *Nanophyetus salmincola* (California); these infections are treated with praziquantel 25 mg/kg three times in 1 day.

Le TH et al: Case report: unusual presentation of *Fasciolopsis buski* in a Vietnamese child. Trans R Soc Trop Med Hyg 2004;98:193. [PMID: 15024930]

FASCIOLIASIS

Infection by *Fasciola hepatica*, the sheep liver fluke, results from ingestion of encysted metacercariae on watercress or other aquatic vegetables or in water. A wide range of herbivorous mammals are reservoir hosts. The disease in humans probably occurs worldwide but is most prevalent in sheep-raising countries, particularly where raw salads are eaten. The infection has been reported from Europe; mainland United States; Hawaii; the West Indies; the Middle East; China; Siberia; and North, East, and South Africa. Eggs of the worm, passed in host feces into fresh water, release a miracidium that infects snails; the snails subsequently release cercariae that in turn encyst as metacercariae on vegetation (some cercariae become metacercariae directly in the water) to complete their life cycle. The adult flukes are leaf-shaped and measure 3×1.5 cm.

In humans, metacercariae excyst, penetrate and migrate through the liver, and mature in the bile ducts, where they cause local parenchymal necrosis and abscess formation. Although the infection is usually mild, three clinical syndromes can develop: acute, chronic latent, and chronic obstructive. The acute illness, associated with migration of immature larvae through the liver, shows an enlarged and tender liver, high fever, leukocytosis, and marked eosinophilia (to 90%). Pain may be present in the epigastrium or right upper quadrant or referred to a shoulder, and the patient may experience headache, anorexia, vomiting, myalgia, urticaria, and other allergic reactions. Jaundice, cachexia, and prostration may appear in severe illness. Anemia and hypergammaglobulinemia are common; other liver function tests may be abnormal. Early diagnosis is difficult in the acute phase because eggs are not found in the feces for 3–4 months. The chronic latent phase may be asymptomatic or characterized by hepatomegaly and other acute findings. The chronic obstructive phase takes place if the extrahepatic bile ducts are occluded, producing a clinical picture similar to that of sclerosing cholangitis, biliary cirrhosis, or choledocholithiasis. Occasionally, adult flukes migrate and produce lesions and symptoms in ectopic sites.

Diagnosis is established by detecting characteristic eggs in the feces; repeated examinations may be necessary. Sometimes the diagnosis can only be made by finding eggs in biliary drainage and, in rare instances, only after liver biopsy or at surgical exploration. Exogenous transient fecal carriage can occur as a result of ingestion of egg-containing cow or sheep liver. Hepatobiliary imaging methods, which include ultrasonography and endoscopic retrograde cholangiopancreatography, may show adult parasites in the gallbladder or ducts. Eosinophilia is characteristic, and hypergammaglobulinemia and abnormal liver function tests may be present. Serologic tests are often useful in presumptive diagnosis, particularly in the acute phase (before eggs have appeared) or in ectopic infection. The "fast" ELISA and immunoblot tests are 95–100% sensitive and highly specific, though cross-reactions occur with schistosomiasis. Serum and coproantigen tests are promising. Successful treatment correlates with a decline in antibody titer.

Triclabendazole (Egatin—available in the United States from Novartis Agribusiness), a veterinary fasciolicide, is the drug of choice; 10 mg/kg orally given once with food achieves a cure rate of 80% with an absence of side effects. In severe infection, some workers recommend 20 mg/kg in divided doses for 1 day. The treatment may need to be repeated. Instances of *F hepatica* resistance to triclabendazole in domestic animals have been reported. Bithionol (given as for paragonimiasis) is the alternative drug of choice; its

deficiencies are its long course, failure rates of up to 50%, and frequent adverse reactions. Recent reports indicate some effectiveness for metronidazole (750 mg/d orally in divided doses for 3 weeks), but albendazole usage has shown high failure rates. Results with praziquantel have been variable; generally, it is ineffective even when used for up to 7 days at a dose of 25 mg/kg three times daily. For any of these drugs, the destruction of parasites followed by release of antigen in sensitized patients may evoke symptoms. Bithionol is available in the United States only from the Parasitic Disease Drug Service, Centers for Disease Control and Prevention, Atlanta, GA 30333. In biliary obstruction due to *Fasciola*, endoscopic biliary sphincterotomy with extraction of the flukes has been effective and safe.

In endemic areas, aquatic plants should not be eaten raw; washing does not destroy the metacercariae, but cooking will. Drinking water must be boiled or purified. *Fasciola gigantica* may be encountered in Asia and Africa and *Metorchis conjunctus* in Canada.

Cheung J et al: Biliary fascioliasis. Gastrointest Endosc 2005;61: 596. [PMID: 15812418]

Saba R et al: Human fascioliasis. Clin Microbiol Infect 2004;10: 385. [PMID: 15113313]

Sezgin O et al: Hepatobiliary fascioliasis: clinical and radiologic features and endoscopic management. J Clin Gastroenterol 2004;38:285. [PMID: 15128078]

Talaie H et al: Randomized trial of a single, double and triple dose of 10 mg/kg of a human formulation of tricladendazole in patients with fascioliasis. Clin Exp Pharmacol Physiol 2004;31:777. [PMID: 15566392]

CLONORCHIASIS & OPISTHORCHIASIS

Infection by *Clonorchis sinensis*, the Chinese liver fluke, is endemic in areas of Japan, Korea, China, Taiwan, Southeast Asia, and the far eastern part of Russia. Over 20 million people are affected and, in some communities, prevalence can reach over 80%. Opisthorchiasis is caused by worms of the genus *Opisthorchis*, generally either *O felineus* (central, eastern, and southern Europe, eastern Asia, Southeast Asia, India) or *O viverrini* (Thailand, Laos, Vietnam). Clinically and epidemiologically, opisthorchiasis and clonorchiasis are identical.

Certain snails are infected when they ingest eggs shed into water in human or animal feces. Larval forms escape from the snails, penetrate the flesh of various freshwater fish, and encyst as metacercariae. Fish-eating wild and domestic mammals—including dogs, cats, and pigs—and humans maintain the life cycle. Human infection results from eating such fish, either raw or undercooked. Pickling, smoking, or drying may not suffice to kill the metacercariae. In humans, the ingested parasites excyst in the duodenum and ascend the bile ducts into the medium and small biliary radicals, but also into the larger ducts and the gallbladder, where they mature and remain throughout their lives (15–25 years), shedding eggs in the bile. In size, the worms are $7-20 \times 1.5-3$ mm. In the chronic stage of infection, there is progressive bile duct thickening, periductal fibrosis, dilation, biliary stasis, and secondary infection. Little fibrosis occurs in the portal tracts.

Most patients harbor few parasites and are asymptomatic. Among symptomatic patients, an acute and chronic syndrome occurs. Acute symptoms follow entry of immature worms into the biliary ducts and may persist for several weeks. Findings include malaise, low-grade fever, an enlarged, tender liver, pain in the hepatic area or epigastrium, urticaria, arthralgia, leukocytosis, eosinophilia, an elevated serum alanine aminotransferase, and jaundice. The acute syndrome is difficult to diagnose, since ova may not appear in the feces until 3–4 weeks after onset of symptoms.

In chronic infections, findings include weakness, anorexia, epigastric pain, diarrhea, prolonged low-grade fever, intermittent episodes of right upper quadrant pain, localized hepatic area tenderness, and progressive hepatomegaly; liver function tests are normal except in severe cases.

Complications include intrahepatic bile duct calculi that may lead to recurrent pyogenic cholangitis, biliary abscess, or endophlebitis of the portal-venous branches. Although focal initially, this may gradually result in destruction of the liver parenchyma, fibrosis and, in a few patients, cirrhosis with jaundice and ascites. Chronic cholecystitis, cholelithiasis, and a nonfunctional, enlarged gallbladder may occur. Flukes may also enter the pancreatic duct, causing acute pancreatitis or cholelithiasis. Cholangiocarcinoma has been causally linked with prolonged clonorchis and opisthorchis infection.

Diagnosis is made by finding characteristic eggs in stools (repeated concentration tests may be necessary) or duodenal aspirate (sensitivity approaches 100%); endoscopic retrograde cholangiopancreatography may be indicated. In severe infection, the number of eggs per gram of feces may not reflect the heavy worm burden. In complete biliary obstruction, eggs can be detected in bile only by needle aspiration or at surgery. In advanced chronic disease, (1) liver function tests will indicate parenchymal damage; (2) CT and sonography may show diffuse dilation of small intrahepatic bile ducts with no or minimal dilation of the large intra- and extrahepatic ducts; and (3) transhepatic cholangiograms may show alternating stricture and dilation of the biliary tree, with worms visualized as filling defects. Where available, of the several evaluated serologic tests, the ELISA is preferred (sensitivity, 77%); however, unless a specific monoclonal antibody is used, cross-reactions are common with other trematode and cestode infections, tuberculosis, and liver cancer. During the chronic stage, leukocytosis varies according to the intensity of infection; eosinophilia may be present.

The drug of choice is praziquantel. With a dosage of 25 mg/kg orally three times daily for 2 days (with a 4- to 6-hour interval between doses), cure rates over 95% can be anticipated for clonorchis infections. One day of treatment may be sufficient for opisthorchis infections. (For side effects, see Schistosomiasis, above.) Albendazole, at a dosage of 400 mg orally twice daily for 7 days, appears to be less effective (cures, 40–65%). In severe disease, treatment may be facilitated by endoscopic nasobiliary drainage plus antiparasitic medication. In relapsing cholangitis, antibiotics are indicated to cover pathogens.

The disease is rarely fatal, but patients with advanced infections and impaired liver function may succumb more readily to other diseases. The prognosis is good for light to moderate infections.

Choi BI et al: Clonorchiasis and cholangiocarcinoma: etiologic relationship and imaging diagnosis. Clin Microbiol Rev 2004; 17:540. [PMID: 15258092]

Fry LC et al: Sclerosing cholangitis caused by *Clonorchis sinensis.* Gastrointest Endosc 2002;56:114. [PMID: 12085048]

Thomas NE et al: Small-cell carcinoma of the extrahepatic bile duct and concurrent clonorchiasis. Diagn Cytopathol 2005; 32:92. [PMID: 15637679]

Wang KX et al: Clinical and epidemiological features of patients with clonorchiasis. World J Gastroenterol 2004;10:446. [PMID: 14760777]

Zhi FC et al: Treatment of severe *Clonorchiasis sinensis* by endoscopic nasobiliary drainage and oral praziquantel. World J Gastroenterol 2004;10:21. [PMID: 15237457]

PARAGONIMIASIS

Paragonimus westermani, the lung fluke, commonly infects humans (estimated 20 million) throughout the Far East (prevalence in Korea has reached 4%); foci are also present in West Africa, South and Southeast Asia, the Pacific Islands, Indonesia, and New Guinea. Many carnivores and omnivores in addition to humans serve as reservoir hosts for the adult fluke (8–16 × 4–8 × 3–5 mm). About a dozen other paragonimus species also infect humans in China, Japan, Mexico, Central and South America, and Africa. *Paragonimus killicotti* is found in North America. Most of these parasites, which are not well adapted to humans, produce ectopic lesions in the brain, skin (larva migrans), and other organs but do not mature into adult flukes.

Eggs reaching water, either in sputum or feces, hatch in 3–6 weeks. Released miracidia penetrate and develop in snails. Emergent cercariae encyst as metacercariae in the tissues of crabs and crayfish. Human infection results if metacercariae are ingested when the crustaceans are eaten raw or pickled or food, vessels, drinking water, or fingers become contaminated. The metacercariae excyst in the small intestine and penetrate the peritoneal cavity. Most migrate through the diaphragm and enter the peripheral lung parenchyma; some may lodge in the brain (about 1% of all cases) or at other ectopic sites. In the lungs, the parasite becomes encapsulated by granulomatous fibrous tissue, reaching up to 2 cm in diameter. The lesion, which usually opens into a bronchiole, may subsequently rupture, resulting in expectoration of eggs, blood, and inflammatory cells. Rarely, the eggs may also enter the general circulation and produce ectopic lesions in any tissue. The prepatent period until appearance of expectorated eggs is about 6 weeks.

In pulmonary infections, most persons have light to moderate worm burdens and are asymptomatic. In symptomatic cases, low-grade fever and dry cough are present initially; subsequently, pleuritic pain is common, and a rusty, blood-flecked, viscous sputum or frank hemoptysis may occur. Following slow progression, complications of bronchitis, bronchiectasis, bronchopneumonia, lung abscess, fibrosis, and pleural thickening or effusion may appear.

Only a minority of patients with cerebral infections present with acute disease, usually manifested by meningitis. In chronic central nervous system disease, seizures, cranial neuropathies, findings of space-occupying lesions, or meningoencephalitis may occur; death can follow. Parasites in the peritoneal cavity or the intestinal wall may cause abdominal pain, diarrhea or dysentery, and a palpable tumor mass. Painless, migratory subcutaneous nodules (a few millimeters to 1 cm in diameter) occur with about 10% of *P westermani* infections.

Pulmonary disease is diagnosed by finding (1) characteristic eggs in sputum (rusty sputum is nearly pathognomonic), feces, gastric aspirates, bronchoscopic washings, biopsy specimens, or pleural fluid; or (2) adult flukes in subcutaneous nodules or other surgical specimens. If eggs are not found after multiple direct sputum examinations, they may be detectable in a 24-hour sputum collection processed by alkaline sodium hypochlorite concentration. Stool examination for eggs has low sensitivity. Serologic tests are conducted using serum, cerebrospinal fluid, and pleural effusion fluid; the sensitivity and specificity of the ELISA are 99% and 97% and of the immunoblot 96% and 99%. The tests do not differentiate active from prior infection; a newly reported IgM test may do so. Most treated and cured patients become seronegative. Antigen detection assays are promising. Eosinophilia (sometimes to a high level) and low-grade leukocytosis are common. Chest films may show infiltrates, segmental or lobar consolidation, small cysts (5–30 mm), cavitary lesions (1–4 cm), fibrosis, nodules, pleural thickening or effusion, or calcifications. By CT, round, low-attenuation cystic lesions (5–15 mm) filled with fluid or gas are seen within the consolidation.

In acute cerebral disease, CT shows multilocular, ring-like enhancement with surrounding low-density areas. In chronic cerebral disease, plain skull films often show round or oval-shaped calcifications, sometimes surrounded by low-density areas that are highly specific for the disease. Cerebrospinal fluid may be turgid or bloody, with numerous eosinophils, and eggs may be found. The EEG is almost always abnormal. It is rare for cerebral disease to occur in the absence of pulmonary disease.

Paragonimiasis and tuberculosis must be differentiated, though chest x-ray appearance alone does not make the distinction. Since paragonimus ova are destroyed by Ziehl-Neelsen stain for acid-fast bacilli, the sputum should first be examined for the eggs. The presence of a large number of eosinophils or Charcot-Leyden crystals in sputum suggests paragonimiasis.

In pulmonary paragonimiasis, praziquantel is the drug of choice (25 mg/kg orally after meals three times daily for 2 days, with a 4- to 6-hour interval between doses). (For side effects, see above under Schistosomiasis.) In regions where there may be concurrent cysticercosis, praziquantal should not be used. Bithionol is the alternative drug (30–50 mg/kg orally, given on alternate days for 10–15 doses; the daily dose should be divided into a morning and evening dose). Bithionol side effects are frequent but generally mild and transient. Gastrointestinal side effects, particularly diarrhea, occur in most patients. Liver function should be tested serially. Bithionol is available in the United States only from the Parasitic Disease Drug Service, Centers for Disease Control and Prevention, Atlanta, GA 30333. Antibiotics may be necessary for secondary pulmonary infection. Cure rates of over 90% can be anticipated for both praziquantel and bithionol. A second alternative drug for pulmonary disease is triclabendazole, a veterinary fasciolicide, which continues under clinical trials and is available from the manufacturer Novartis. Cure rates reach 91% with a dosage of 10 mg/kg daily for 2 days; if treatment is repeated in 3 months, 100% cure rates have been reported. Drug side effects of dizziness and diarrhea are mild and transient.

In the acute stage of cerebral paragonimiasis, particularly meningitis, praziquantel or bithionol may be effective. With death of parasites, severe local reactions may occur; corticosteroids should therefore be given as in cerebral cysticercosis. In the chronic stage, both surgical removal of the parasites and drug usage are likely to be ineffective in diminishing neurologic symptoms.

Calvopina M et al: Comparison of two single-day regimens of triclabendazole for the treatment of human pulmonary paragonimiasis. Trans R Soc Trop Med Hyg 2003;97:451. [PMID: 15259481]

Castilla EA et al: Cavitary mass lesion and recurrent pneumothoraces due to *Paragonimus kellicotti* infection: North American paragonimiasis. Am J Surg Pathol 2003;27:1157. [PMID: 12883250]

Jeon K et al: Clinical features of recently diagnosed pulmonary paragonimiasis in Korea. Chest 2005;128:1423. [PMID: 16162738]

Kim TS et al: Pleuropulmonary paragonimiasis: CT findings in 31 patients. AJR Am J Roentgenol 2005;185:616. [PMID: 16120908]

CESTODE INFECTIONS

TAPEWORM INFECTIONS (See Also Cysticercosis and Echinococcosis, Below)

Classification

Six tapeworms infect humans frequently. The large tapeworms are *Taenia saginata* (the beef tapeworm, up to 25 m in length), *Taenia solium* (the pork tapeworm, 7 m), and *Diphyllobothrium latum* (the fish tapeworm, 10 m). A fourth large tapeworm, *Taenia asiatica* recently differentiated by DNA methods, has been found in China, the Koreas, Indonesia, and Southeast Asia; although acquired by humans by ingestion of pig viscera, it apparently does not cause cysticercosis. The small tapeworms are *Hymenolepis nana* (the dwarf tapeworm, 25–40 mm), *Hymenolepis diminuta* (the rodent tapeworm, 20–60 cm), and *Dipylidium caninum* (the dog tapeworm, 10–70 cm). Four of the six tapeworms occur worldwide; the pork and fish tapeworms have more limited distribution.

An adult tapeworm consists of a head (scolex), a neck, and a chain of individual segments (proglottids) in which eggs form in mature segments. The scolex is the attachment organ and generally lodges in the upper part of the small intestine.

Multiple infections are the rule for small tapeworms and may occur for *D latum;* however, it is rare for a person to harbor more than one or two of the taeniae.

A. Beef Tapeworm

The infection occurs in most countries with beef husbandry but is highly endemic in parts of the Far East, central and eastern Africa, and the central Asian area of the former Soviet Union. Gravid segments of *T saginata* in the human intestine detach themselves from the chain and are passed in feces to soil. When proglottids or eggs are ingested by grazing cattle or other domesticated bovines, the eggs hatch to release embryos that encyst in muscle as cysticerci. Humans are infected by eating raw or undercooked beef containing viable cysticerci, *Cysticercus bovis*. Humans are the definitive host; in the human intestine, the cysticercus develops into the adult worm.

B. Pork Tapeworm

This tapeworm is particularly prevalent in Mexico, Latin America, the Iberian Peninsula, the Slavic countries, Africa, Southeast Asia, India, and China. In the United States and Canada, cysticercosis in hogs is uncommon and human infection is rare, usually encountered in persons infected abroad. The infection is no longer found in northwestern Europe. The life cycle of *T solium* is similar to that of *T saginata* except that pigs ingest human feces containing proglottids and eggs to become the host of the larval stage. Humans, the definitive host, become infected when they eat undercooked pork containing viable *Cysticercus cellulosae*. Humans are also the intermediate host when they become infected with the larval stage (see Cysticercosis, below) by accidentally ingesting eggs in human feces; the eggs are immediately infectious. Transmission of eggs may occur as a result of autoinfection (hand to mouth), direct person-to-person transfer, ingestion of food or drink contaminated by eggs, or (rarely) regurgitation of proglottids into the stomach.

C. Fish Tapeworm

D latum is found in temperate and subarctic lake regions in many areas of the world, including northern Europe, Canada, Alaska, the Pacific Coast of the United States, Japan, Taiwan, Siberia, Manchuria, Australia, southern South America, and southern Africa. Eggs passed in human feces that reach fresh water are taken up first by crustaceans that in turn are eaten by fish, both of which are intermediate hosts. Human infection results from eating raw or inadequately cooked brackish or freshwater fish, including salmon. Nonhuman reservoir hosts include dogs, bears, and other fish-eating mammals.

D. Dwarf Tapeworm

H nana is the most common cestode. It can reach high prevalence, particularly in children, in regions of the world with poor fecal hygiene and in closed institutions. Humans are the definitive host of the human strain of the parasite; rodent-adapted strains occur in rodents. The life cycle is unusual in that both larval and adult stages are found in the human intestine, internal autoinfection can occur, and generally there is no intermediate host. Transmission usually results from eggs transferred directly from human to human (the eggs are immediately infective) but sometimes involves fomites, water, or food or the swallowing of fleas or beetles infected with the larval stage. *H nana* infections in children are usually lost spontaneously in adolescence.

E. Rodent Tapeworm

H diminuta is a common parasite of rodents. Many arthropods (eg, rat fleas, beetles, and cockroaches) serve as intermediate hosts. Humans—most commonly young children—are infected by accidentally swallowing the infected arthropods, usually in cereals or stored products.

F. Dog Tapeworm

D caninum infection generally occurs in young children in close association with infected dogs or cats. Transmission results from swallowing the infected intermediate hosts, ie, fleas or lice.

Clinical Findings

A. Symptoms and Signs

1. Large tapeworms—Large tapeworm infections are generally asymptomatic. Occasionally, vague gastrointestinal symptoms (eg, nausea, diarrhea, abdominal pain) and systemic symptoms (eg, fatigue, hunger, dizziness) have been attributed to the infections. Vomiting of proglottid segments or obstruction of the bile duct, pancreatic duct, or appendix is rare.

Some persons (mostly Scandinavian residents) who harbor the fish tapeworm develop a macrocytic megaloblastic anemia accompanied by thrombocytopenia and mild leukopenia. Gastric acidity is normal. The anemia is a result of the worm's competing with the host for vitamin B_{12}. Clinical findings are indistinguishable from those of pernicious anemia and include glossitis, dyspnea, tachycardia, and neurologic findings (numbness, paresthesias, disturbances of coordination, impairment of vibration and position sense, and dementia).

2. Small tapeworms—Light infections are generally asymptomatic. Heavy infections, particularly with *H nana*, may cause diarrhea, abdominal pain, anorexia, vomiting, weight loss, and irritability.

B. LABORATORY FINDINGS

Infection by a beef or pork tapeworm is often discovered by the patient finding segments in stool, clothing, or bedding. To determine the species, proglottid segments are either flattened between glass slides and examined microscopically for anatomic detail or differentiated by enzyme electrophoresis of glucose phosphate isomerase. Eggs are only infrequently present in stools, but the perianal cellophane tape test, as used to diagnose pinworm, is sometimes useful in detecting *T saginata* eggs. However, *T solium* and *T saginata* eggs look alike and do not permit species differentiation except by specialized methods. Where available, the best method for diagnosing taeniasis and differentiating the species is the ELISA coproantigen test (sensitivity 95% and specificity 99%); it is 2–3 times as sensitive as detection of ova. The test is being evaluated for its ability to confirm cure.

Fish tapeworm is diagnosed by finding characteristic operculated eggs in stool; repeat examinations and concentration may be necessary. Proglottids are occasionally vomited or passed in feces; their internal morphology is diagnostic. The presence of hydrochloric acid in the stomach differentiates tapeworm anemia from pernicious anemia; in both conditions, the Schilling test is abnormal.

H nana and *H diminuta* infections are diagnosed by finding characteristic eggs in feces; proglottids are usually not seen. *D caninum* infection is diagnosed by detection of proglottids (the size of melon seeds) in feces or after their active migration through the anus.

Serologic tests are not available for tapeworm infections.

Treatment

A. SPECIFIC MEASURES

Although niclosamide (not available in the United States) and praziquantel are both drugs of choice for most tapeworm infections, praziquantel is more effective in hymenolepiasis, and some workers consider it to be somewhat more effective in taeniasis. In areas endemic for neurocysticercosis, a dose of praziquantel of 5 mg/kg or higher carries a small risk of activating these lesions. Niclosamide preferably should not be used in pregnancy.

1. *T saginata* and *D latum*—Praziquantel in a single oral dose of 10 mg/kg achieves cure rates of about 99%. At this dose, side effects (see under Schistosomiasis, above) are minimal. With a single dose of four tablets (2 g) of niclosamide, cure rates over 90% can

be anticipated. The drug is given in the morning before the patient has eaten. The tablets *must be chewed thoroughly* and swallowed with water. Eating may be resumed in 2 hours. Niclosamide usually produces no side effects.

Pretreatment and posttreatment purges are not used for either drug. The anemia and neurologic manifestations of *D latum* respond to vitamin B_{12} as used in treatment of pernicious anemia.

2. *T solium*—The choice of drugs and methods of treatment are as above. Neither drug kills eggs released from disintegrating segments; therefore, to avoid the theoretical possibility of cysticercosis from hatching eggs, give a moderate purgative 2–3 hours after treatment to rapidly eliminate segments and eggs from the bowel. The patient must be instructed about the need after defecation for careful washing of the hands and perianal area and for safe disposal of feces for 4 days following therapy.

3. *H nana*—Praziquantel, the drug of choice, produces 95% cure rates with a single 25-mg/kg dose. Niclosamide, the alternative drug, produces cure rates of 75% when given at the above dosage for 5–7 days; some workers repeat the course 5 days later. Another alternative drug is nitazoxanide (500 mg orally for 3 days).

4. *H diminuta* and *D caninum*—Treatment is with niclosamide or praziquantel in dosages as for *H nana*. Cure rates are not established.

B. FOLLOW-UP CARE

In treatment of large tapeworm infections, a disintegrating worm is usually passed within 24–48 hours of treatment. Since efforts are not generally made to recover and identify the scolex, cure can be presumed only if regenerated segments have not reappeared 3–5 months later. If it is preferred that parasitic cure be established immediately, the head (scolex) must be found in posttreatment stools; a laxative is given 2 hours after treatment, and stools must be collected in a preservative for 24 hours. To facilitate examination, toilet paper must be disposed of separately.

Prevention & Prognosis

C cellulosae in pork is killed by cooking at 65 °C or freezing at –20 °C for 12 hours; *C bovis* in beef at 56 °C or –10 °C for 5 days. Pickling is not adequate. Because the prognosis is often poor in cerebral cysticercosis (see below), *T solium* infections must be immediately eradicated.

Dick TA et al: Diphyllobothriasis: update on human cases, foci, patterns and sources of human infections and future considerations. Southeast Asian J Trop Med Public Health 2001; 32(Suppl 2):59. [PMID: 12041607]

Flisser A et al: Portrait of human tapeworms. J Parasitol 2004;90: 914. [PMID: 15357104]

Ito A et al: Cysticercosis/taeniasis in Asia and the Pacific. Vector Borne Zoonotic Dis 2004;4:95. [PMID: 15228810]

Juan JO et al: Comparative clinical studies of nitazoxanide, albendazole and praziquantel in the treatment of ascariasis, trichuriasis and hymenolepiasis in children from Peru. Trans R Soc Trop Med Hyg 2002;96:193. [PMID: 12055813]

CYSTICERCOSIS

ESSENTIALS OF DIAGNOSIS

- *History of exposure to a person infected with Taenia solium or ingestion of pork contaminated with cysticeri; concomitant or past intestinal tapeworm infection.*
- *Seizures, headache, and other findings of a focal space-occupying central nervous system lesion.*
- *Subcutaneous or muscular nodules (5–10 mm); calcified lesions on x-rays of soft tissues.*
- *Brain imaging shows calcified or uncalcified cysts by CT or MRI; positive serologic tests.*

General Considerations

Human cysticercosis is infection by the larval (cysticercus) stage of the pork tapeworm *T solium* (see above). Worldwide, an estimated 20 million persons are infected with the larval stage; yearly, about 400,000 persons have neurologic symptoms and 50,000 die of the disease. Antibody prevalence rates to 10% are recognized in some endemic areas. The infection is one of the most important causes of seizures in the developing world. In the United States in recent years, hundreds of cases annually have been recognized in immigrants and travelers.

The natural history of the infection is incompletely known. Cysticerci complete their development within 2–4 months after egg ingestion and larval entry and live for months to 20 years. Several factors give rise to symptoms: Initially, a live larva grows within a thin-walled 10–20 mm cyst (the vesicular cyst) but remains minimally antigenic, causes little or no perilesional inflammation, and does not enhance with contrast media on neuroimaging. Attached to the inner wall of the cyst is an invaginated protoscolex with four suckers and a crown of hooks. When host immune response or chemotherapy causes gradual death of the cyst, marked inflammation and pericyst edema can occur, producing a ring-like or nodular area of enhancement with contrast media (the granulomatous or enhancing cyst); concurrent events include cyst enlargement, mechanical compression, increased intracranial pressure, cerebrospinal fluid changes, and sometimes a vasculitis that results in small cerebral infarcts. The immune response is intense in many patients, but some show a remarkable tolerance. Later, as the cyst degenerates over 2–7 years, it may become undetectable with imaging or be replaced by fibrosis with calcification that is detectable; perile-sional edema may be present around these foci. Seizures are thought to occur both from parenchymal irritation at sites of active inflammation and from gliosis associated with end-stage calcified lesions.

Locations of cysts in order of frequency are the central nervous system (where cysts at different life cycle stages—live, transitional, dead—may be present at the same time), subcutaneous tissues, striated muscle, vitreous humor of the eye and, rarely, other tissues.

Clinical Findings

A. SYMPTOMS AND SIGNS

1. Neurocysticercosis—In many patients, cysts remain asymptomatic. When symptomatic, the incubation period is highly variable (usually from 1 to 5 years). Almost any neurologic symptoms can occur based on the number and location of cysts; manifestations are due to mass effect, inflammatory response, or obstruction of the brain foramina and ventricular systems.

a. Acute invasive stage (cysticercotic encephalitis)—This rare event, occurring shortly after invasion, results from extensive acute spread of cysticerci to the brain parenchyma. Fever, headache, myalgia, marked eosinophilia, and coma may occur.

b. Parenchymal cysts—Cysticerci can present singly or multiply and may be scattered or in clumps. Findings include epilepsy (focal or generalized), intracranial hypertension (intense headache, vomiting, papilledema, visual loss), sensory defects, movement disorders, and altered mental status. Vasculitis can lead to small- or large-vessel infarcts. Sometimes the neurologic deficits are transient.

c. Subarachnoid space cysts and meningeal cysts—Small to large cysts are generally located in the cortical sulci or basal cisterns. The arachnoid is the principal basal membrane affected. Adhesive arachnoiditis may result in obstructive hydrocephalus, intracranial hypertension, arterial thrombosis leading to transient ischemia or stroke, and cranial nerve dysfunction (most often of the optic nerve).

d. Ventricular cysts—Ventricular cysts (more common in the fourth ventricle) may float freely (usually singly) within the ventricles or cerebral aqueduct or may be attached to the ventricular wall. They are usually asymptomatic but can cause increased intracranial pressure as a result of intermittent or total blockage.

e. Racemose cysts—These are rare aberrant forms that are multiple-branched, nonencysted, and lack a scolex; they present as grape-like irregular clusters and may reach over 10 cm in diameter. They generally are found in the ventricular and basal subarachnoid spaces, where they cause marked adhesive arachnoiditis and often obstructive hydrocephalus.

f. Spinal cord cysts—Cysts can be extraspinal or intraspinal and can cause arachnoiditis (meningitis, radiculopathy) or pressure symptoms.

2. Ophthalmocysticercosis—Usually there is a single cyst, free-floating in the vitreous or under the retina. Presenting symptoms include periorbital pain, scotomas, and progressive deterioration of visual acuity. Findings may include disk hemorrhage and edema, retinal detachment, iridocyclitis, and chorioretinitis. MRI but not CT may assist in diagnosis; immunologic tests are negative.

3. Subcutaneous and striated muscle cysticercosis—Subcutaneous cysts are usually asymptomatic; they present as nodules that tend to appear and disappear, or they may die and calcify and be detected on plain radiographs.

B. DIAGNOSTIC CRITERIA AND LABORATORY TESTS

Definitive diagnosis of neurocysticercosis is (1) by CT or MRI detection of brain or spinal cord cystic lesions that show the scolex ("hole-with-dot") image; (2) by visualization of the parasite by ophthalmoscopic examination (subretinal or in the anterior chamber); or (3) by finding the parasite in histologic sections of brain or spinal cord tissue (not usually recommended). Ranging from highly suggestive to compatible with the diagnosis are various combinations of other major and minor findings (criteria): (1) lesions on neuroimaging studies, (2) positive immunologic tests with serum or cerebrospinal fluid, (3) resolution of intracranial cystic lesions either spontaneously or after treatment, (4) cysticercosis outside the central nervous system, (5) clinical history, and (6) epidemiologic findings (personal history of a tapeworm, tapeworm in a household contact, travel in an endemic area).

1. Imaging—Plain radiographs of muscle (especially of thigh and calf) may detect oval or linear calcified lesions ($4-10 \times 2-5$ mm). The lesions are usually multiple, sometimes in the hundreds, and the long axes of the cysts are nearly always in the plane of the surrounding muscle fibers. Plain skull films may demonstrate one or more cerebral calcifications (generally 5–10 mm; sometimes 1–2 mm when only the scolex is calcified).

The most useful procedures for examining the skull are imaging initially by nonenhanced CT and then by MRI and enhanced CT. CT patterns include (1) vesicular cysts (viable cysts with no host immune reaction), which are rounded areas of low density with little or no enhancement after contrast medium; (2) colloidal cysts (dead or dying cysts with host immune reaction), which are hypodense or isodense lesions surrounded by edema associated with ring-like or nodular enhancement; and (3) granuloma or calcifications (dead cysts), which are often several millimeters in diameter but variable in size. Signs of increased intracranial pressure and diffuse brain edema may also be seen. A combination of images is often found, owing to different developmental stages. As compared with CT, MRI has superior sensitivity and resolution for vesicular cysts (isodense, similar to cerebrospinal fluid) and for colloidal cysts (hyperdense). However, CT is superior for granulomas and calcifications, the most frequent presentations of cysticercosis, which MRI may miss. The MRI sometimes detects pathognomonic 2- to 4-mm nodules (protoscoleces) within cyst fluid. Intraventricular cysts (isodense) are not seen on noncontrast CT but require intraventricular contrast medium. Recently described are findings of old calcified lesions that show perilesional edema and contrast enhancement at the time of symptom relapse. Spinal cysticercosis is evaluated by CT myelography or MRI.

2. Immunologic tests—With serum, the enzyme-linked immunoelectrotransfer blot (EITB) assay has nearly 100% specificity and 94–98% sensitivity. Both parameters are paradoxically lower, however, when the test is performed on cerebrospinal fluid. However, the test's sensitivity drops to about 30% if only one live cyst is present and is also low in patients with only calcified cysts. Where the EITB assay is not available, the older ELISA has a 63% specificity and 65% sensitivity with serum; the ELISA with cerebrospinal fluid, however, has a high specificity (95%) and sensitivity (87%) for both IgM and IgG antibody. As antibodies persist after cyst death, neither the EITB nor ELISA distinguishes current from past infection, and these tests cannot be used to monitor therapy; however, another ELISA (under study) to detect circulating antigen may do so. It is unknown whether the EITB or ELISA can distinguish between intestinal infection and neurocysticercosis.

3. Other laboratory tests—Cerebrospinal fluid typically shows increased protein, decreased glucose, and a cellular reaction of mainly lymphocytes and eosinophils; eosinophilia that may be over 20% is diagnostically important. Lumbar puncture is contraindicated, however, in case of increased intracerebral pressure. The electroencephalogram may be abnormal. Though the patient usually no longer harbors a tapeworm, all family members should examine their stools over several days for passage of proglottids, and stool specimens should be examined for proglottids and eggs.

Differential Diagnosis

The differential diagnosis includes tuberculoma, primary or metastatic tumor, hydatid disease, vasculitis, chronic fungal disorders, pyogenic brain abscess, toxoplasmosis and other parasitic diseases, and neurosyphilis. CT and MRI findings of cystic lesions without a scolex, single or multiple ring or nodular enhancing lesions, or parenchymal round calcifications may also be found in some of these other diseases.

Treatment

Treatment should be individualized based on the number and location of cysts and their viability. Medical treatment, which is usually preferable to surgery, is most effective for parenchymal cysts; less effective for intraventricular, subarachnoid, or racemose cysts. When only one or a few live parenchymal cysts are present, the evidence is still insufficient to establish that medical treatment is preferable to symptomatic management followed by normal death of the parasites. Some clinicians wait 3 months with selected patients to see whether cysts will spontaneously disappear without treatment. Although single enhancing lesions are likely to do well when treated only with anticonvulsants, some experts add albendazole or praziquantel treatment; however, patients with only calcified cysts without enhancement do not need these drugs.

Albendazole and praziquantel are both effective in treatment. Albendazole is preferred because its course of treatment is shorter (1 week) than that of praziquantel (2 weeks); because albendazole is less expensive; and because coadminstration of albendazole and a corticosteroid (to treat inflammation) results in increased albendazole absorption, whereas combined use of praziquantel and a corticosteroid greatly decreases plasma levels of praziquantel. Both drugs are given with fatty meals, which increases absorption fourfold to fivefold. Treatment should be conducted in hospital. Between the second and fifth days after starting treatment, increased inflammatory reactions around dying parasites may be manifested by meningismus, headache (analgesics may be sufficient for mild symptoms), vomiting, hyperthermia, mental changes, and convulsions; decompensation with death is very rare. It remains controversial whether to give corticosteroids concomitantly to avoid or diminish this reaction or to use them only if marked symptoms appear or increase. Even when corticosteroids are given prospectively, the inflammatory reaction may occur. Prednisone, 1 mg/kg/d in two or three divided doses, starting 1–2 days before use of the drug and continuing at diminishing doses for about 14 days afterward, is one regimen. The reaction usually subsides in 48–72 hours, but continuing severity may require corticosteroids in higher dosage and mannitol. For patients with seizures, anticonvulsants should be given during drug treatment and probably for an indefinite time afterward. Antiparasitic drug use is controversial for ventricular cysts; for ocular cysts, only surgical resection is used.

Cure rates following treatment (disappearance of cysts and clearing of symptoms) ranged up to 85% for albendazole and 50–60% for praziquantel. Of the remaining patients, many have amelioration of symptoms, including intracranial hypertension and seizures.

A. MEDICAL MEASURES

1. Albendazole—The dosage is 15 mg/kg in divided doses daily with a fatty meal. The duration of treatment is unsettled. Seven to 14 days may be sufficient for some patients, but a longer course (up to 28 days) is used for some types of infection; it can be repeated as necessary. Up to 3 months of treatment may be needed for ventricular and subarachnoid cysts. For albendazole side effects, see below under Hydatid Disease.

2. Praziquantel—Give 50–100 mg/kg/d orally in three divided doses for 15–30 days. Shorter courses are being tried. Phenytoin, phenobarbital, carbamazepine, cimetidine, and corticosteroids, when administered with praziquantel, reduce serum levels of the latter; high doses of praziquantel have been tried in these circumstances. Ingestion with a high-carbohydrate meal enhances absorption.

B. OTHER MEASURES

Seizures are treated with anticonvulsant drugs. Surgery has successfully removed accessible orbital, cisternal, ventricular, cerebral, meningeal, and spinal cord cysts. During the acute phase of cysticercotic encephalitis, if intracranial hypertension is present, mannitol (2 g/kg/d intravenously) and corticosteroids are used but albendazole and praziquantel are withheld. Obstructive hydrocephalus requires ventricular shunting plus a corticosteroid. Subarachnoiditis and vasculitis are treated with albendazole or praziquantel plus a corticosteroid. Albendazole or praziquantel, when used with ocular or spinal medullary lesions, may cause irreversible damage even when corticosteroids are given; therefore, an ophthalmologic examination should always be done in advance of antiparasitic drug treatment.

Prognosis

The fatality rate for untreated neurocysticercosis is about 50%; survival time from onset of symptoms ranges from days to many years. Drug treatment has reduced the mortality rate to about 5–15%. Surgical procedures to relieve intracranial hypertension along with use of corticosteroids to reduce edema improve the prognosis for those not effectively treated with the drugs.

Prevention

Indiscriminate defecation, free roaming pigs, and ingestion of undercooked pork allow the maintenance of the life cycle and human disease.

Garcia HH et al; Cysticercosis Working Group in Peru: Neurocysticercosis: updated concepts about an old disease. Lancet Neurol 2005;4:653. [PMID: 16168934]

Garcia HH et al: New concepts in the diagnosis and management of neurocysticercosis (*Taenia solium*). Am J Trop Med Hyg 2005;72:3. [PMID: 15728858]

Hawk MW et al: Neurocysticercosis: a review. Surg Neurol 2005; 63:123. [PMID: 15680651]

Nash TE: Human case management and treatment of cysticercosis. Acta Trop 2003;87:61. [PMID: 12781379]

Yancey LS et al: Cysticercosis: recent advances in diagnosis and management of neurocysticercosis. Curr Infect Dis Rep 2005;7:39. [PMID: 15610670]

ECHINOCOCCOSIS
(Hydatid Disease, Hydatidosis)

Human echinococcosis results from parasitism by the larval stage of four *Echinococcus* species of which *E granulosus* (cystic hydatid disease) and *E multilocularis* (alveolar hydatid disease) are the most important. Minor species are the polycystic species *E vogeli* (polycystic hydatid disease) and *E oligarthrus*, both from Central and South America. Echinococcosis is a zoonosis in which humans are an intermediate host of the larval stage of the parasite. The definitive host is a carnivore (all Canidae, except for the lion,) that harbors the adult tapeworm in the small intestine; the carnivore becomes infected by ingesting the larval form in tissue of the intermediate host. The intermediate hosts, chiefly herbivorous mammals but also humans, become infected by ingesting tapeworm eggs passed in carnivore feces. The larval stage is referred to as a hydatid cyst.

1. Cystic Hydatid Disease (Unilocular Hydatid Disease)

ESSENTIALS OF DIAGNOSIS

- *History of exposure to dogs associated with livestock in a hydatid-endemic region.*
- *Avascular cystic tumor of liver, lung, or, infrequently, bone, brain, or other organs as detected by imaging procedures.*
- *Symptoms and signs of a space-occupying mass.*
- *Positive serologic tests.*

General Considerations

Human infection with *E granulosus* is common throughout southern South America, the Mediterranean littoral and the Middle East, central Asia, China, and East Africa. Endemic foci are in eastern Europe, Russia, Australia, New Zealand, India, and the United Kingdom. In North America, foci with low endemicity have been reported from the western United States and the lower Mississippi valley; higher endemicity occurs in Alaska and northwestern Canada.

The pastoral strain—which is more pathogenic to humans—has a transmission cycle in which dogs are the definitive host, and sheep (usually) but also cattle and other domestic livestock are intermediate hosts. However, the strain in horses, pigs, and camels may be of low or no infectivity for humans. A northern, sylvatic strain is maintained in wolves and wild ungulates (moose and reindeer) and has involved sled-dogs in northern Alaska, Canada, Scandinavia, and Eurasia. In Australia, a sylvatic strain (which overlaps with a sheep-dog cycle) is maintained between dingoes (and feral dogs) and macropod marsupials.

Human infection occurs when eggs passed in dog feces are accidentally swallowed. Liberated embryos penetrate the intestinal mucosa, enter the portal bloodstream, and are carried to the liver where they become one or more hydatid cysts (65% of all cysts). Some larvae reach the lung (25%) and develop into pulmonary hydatids. Infrequently, cysts form in the brain, bones, skeletal muscles, kidneys, spleen, or other tissues. Cysts may occur in multiple organs. Cysts of the sylvatic strain tend to localize in the lungs.

The cyst wall has three layers: an inner germinal layer that gives rise within the cyst to germinal elements, a supporting intermediate layer, and an outer layer produced by the host. In the liver, cysts may increase in size 1–30 mm in diameter per year and become enormous, but symptoms generally do not develop until they reach about 10 cm. Some cysts die spontaneously; others may persist unchanged for years. Part or all of the inner layer of hepatic and splenic cysts may calcify, which does not necessarily mean cyst death. All age groups may be infected and the case-fatality rate is estimated at 2.2%.

Clinical Findings

A. SYMPTOMS AND SIGNS

A liver cyst may remain silent for 10–20 or more years until it becomes large enough to be palpable, to be visible as an abdominal swelling, to produce pressure effects, or (rarely) to produce symptoms due to leakage or rupture. There may be right upper quadrant pain, nausea, and vomiting. The effects of pressure may result in biliary obstruction, with secondary bacterial cholangitis, cirrhosis, and portal hypertension. If a cyst ruptures suddenly, anaphylaxis and death may occur. If fluid and hydatid particles escape slowly, allergic manifestations may result, including a rise in the eosinophil count. Rupture can occur into the pleural, pericardial, or peritoneal space or into the duodenum, colon, or renal pelvis. Dissemination of germinal elements may be followed by the development of multiple secondary cysts. A characteristic clinical syndrome may follow intrabiliary extrusion of cyst contents—jaundice, biliary colic, and urticaria.

Pulmonary cysts cause no symptoms until they leak; become large enough to obstruct a bronchus, causing segmental collapse; or erode into a bronchus with rupture and expectoration of cyst contents. Brain cysts produce symptoms earlier and may cause seizures or symptoms of increased intracranial pressure. Cysts in the bone marrow or spongiosa do not have a host layer, are irregular in shape, erode osseous tissue, and present as pain or as spontaneous fracture. The bones most often affected are the vertebrae; many of these patients develop epidural extension with compression of the spinal cord and paraplegia. Because 20% of patients have multiple cysts, upon diagnosis each patient should be screened for cysts in the liver, spleen, kidneys, lungs, brain, bones, skin, tongue, vitreous, and other tissues.

B. IMAGING

Methods of choice for liver and splenic cysts are sonography (best for demonstrating hydatid sand, daughter cysts, and floating membranes) and CT (best for information about location, depth, and calcification). The MRI is best for detection of central nervous system cysts. Scintillation scan and angiography are rarely used. Cysts may present as solitary lesions with interior echoes or as multilocular cysts with daughter cysts. Nearly pathognomonic is the presence within a hydatid cyst of daughter cysts; they must be distinguished, however, from blood clots within the cavity of a simple cyst. Spotty calcified densities or a calcified cyst wall may be seen in the liver or spleen. Chest films may show an elevated diaphragm. Pulmonary cysts are best detected by chest films (calcification of the wall is rare); CT and MRI can also be done. An intravenous urogram or bone scan may detect cysts at other sites.

C. LABORATORY FINDINGS

The immunoblot test, where available, is the test of choice (95% specific and 91% sensitive for liver cysts); the arc 5 test is also highly diagnostic. In both tests, cross-reactions can occur in 5–25% of patients with *T solium* cysticercosis infections. Several other serologic tests (ELISA and indirect hemagglutination and immunofluorescence) are useful for screening, but both false-negative and false-positive results are common. Persons from whom cysts have been completely removed and carriers of calcified or dead cysts may become seronegative. False-negative tests occur with about 50% of solitary lung cysts, more often with bone cysts, and most often with brain or splenic cysts. Testing for antigen in serum or hydatid cyst fluid is now available but is less sensitive than serum antibody detection. Although hydatid cyst aspiration was contraindicated in the past, ultrasonic percutaneous aspiration followed by injection of a scolicidal agent with the use of oral albendazole is now being increasingly used in diagnosis. Eosinophilia is uncommon except after cyst rupture. The intracutaneous skin test has been abandoned because of poor specificity.

Differential Diagnosis

Noninfected hydatid cysts of the liver need to be differentiated from simple epithelial cysts and bacterial and amebic abscesses. Hydatid cysts in any site may be mistaken for a variety of malignant and nonmalignant tumors and cysts. In the lung, a cyst may be confused with cavitary tuberculosis. Allergic symptoms arising from cyst leakage may resemble those associated with many other diseases.

Treatment & Prevention

Surgery was formerly the definitive approach to therapy but has now been partially supplanted by anthelmintic treatment. Decision-making between the two modes of treatment must take into account current surgical mortality rates (up to 4%), postoperative complications (10–25%), recurrence rates after surgery (2–25%), and cure rates after albendazole treatment of about 30–40%. Other issues are whether the cyst(s) is single or multiple, surgically accessible, likely to rupture, infected, or exerting substantial mass effect. One therapeutic approach is to give a course of albendazole to selected asymptomatic patients whose cysts are small and not in danger of rupture. If, after 6–12 months, the cyst has not disappeared or clearly died, it can then be removed surgically.

A. SURGICAL TREATMENT

Operative treatment of liver cysts involves several problems: total removal of all infective components of the cyst, avoiding cyst content spillage, selection of a scolicidal agent to be placed within the cyst, management of communications between the cyst and biliary tract (if present), management of the residual cavity, and minimizing the risk of operation. The main surgical options available for liver cysts are partial hepatic resection, pericystectomy, and cystectomy. Surgery for pulmonary cysts includes extrusion of cysts (Barrett's technique), pericystectomy, and lobectomy. Interoperative use of scolicidal solutions, which include cetrimide (5%), hypertonic saline (20%), silver nitrate (0.5%), ethanol (70–95%), and sodium hypochlorite (3.75%), has come under criticism because of their potential for direct and indirect toxicity (an estimated 20% of cysts are thought to communicate with the biliary tract). Preoperatively, to reduce the risk of recurrence due to spillage, two drugs (taken with meals) are used for 1 month: albendazole, 10 mg/kg/d in two divided doses, and praziquantel, 25 mg/kg/d. Postoperatively, albendazole should be continued for 1 month; the additional use of praziquantel is under evaluation. Pulmonary cysts are treated by surgery plus chemotherapy. The treatment of bone cysts is by combined curettage, lavage, instillation of sterilization substances, and chemotherapy.

B. DRUG TREATMENT

Albendazole is the drug of choice; mebendazole is less effective and is no longer recommended.

1. Albendazole—Albendazole is more readily absorbed than mebendazole; this permits a lower dosage of albendazole to be used, yet its active metabolite, the sulfoxide, reaches effective concentrations in cyst wall and fluid. A current regimen is four tablets (800 mg) daily in divided doses with meals for 3 months; continue for up to 6 months (some clinicians continue for up to 1 year) if there is evidence of a response. In multiple studies, apparent cure (shrinkage or disappearance of cysts) was approximately 30–40%, with substantial reduction in size in another 24%. To be emphasized, however, is that some of these changes result from the natural history of the disease. Relapses occur and should be re-treated, but long-term follow-up results have not been determined. Bone cysts are more refractory and may require a year of treatment. In the 3-month courses, drug side effects include reversible low-grade aminotransferase elevations (15%), leukopenia to 2900/mcL (2%), rare gastrointestinal symptoms (including pain at cyst sites), dizziness or headache, alopecia, rash, and pruritus. Anaphylaxis has been reported once and eosinophilia rarely, probably related to cyst fluid leakage. Two deaths attributed to long-term albendazole use have been reported. Liver function tests and complete blood counts should be monitored weekly. The drug is contraindicated in pregnancy.

2. Praziquantel—Praziquantel kills protoscoleces within hydatid cysts but does not affect the germinal membrane. The drug is being evaluated as adjunctive therapy with albendazole both preoperatively and postoperatively to protect against cyst spillage.

C. PERCUTANEOUS ASPIRATION, INJECTION (OF A SCOLICIDAL AGENT), AND REASPIRATION (PAIR)

Under ultrasonic guidance, PAIR is indicated in the treatment of accessible cysts in patients who are inoperable or refuse surgery and are not candidates for a chemotherapeutic trial. The procedure is contraindicated for cysts that communicate with the biliary tree, those that are superficially loculated, or those that have thick internal septal divisions. Complications are infection or leakage at the aspiration site followed by an allergic reaction or dissemination of the infection. Several thousand patients have now had the procedure while covered by oral albendazole. One case of anaphylaxis has been reported. Follow-up has not been sufficiently long to permit assessment of therapeutic efficacy or risk of spillage.

D. PREVENTION

In endemic areas, prevention is by prophylactic treatment of pet dogs with 5 mg/kg of praziquantel at monthly intervals to remove adult tapeworms and by health education to prevent feeding of offal to dogs.

Prognosis

About 15% of untreated patients eventually die because of the disease or its complications.

2. Alveolar Hydatid Disease (Multilocular Hydatid Disease)

Alveolar hydatid disease results from infection by the larval form of *E multilocularis* and occurs only in the northern hemisphere. The life cycle involves foxes (sometimes wolves) as definitive host and microtine rodents as intermediate host. Domestic dogs and cats can also become infected with the adult tapeworm when they eat infected wild rodents. Human infection is by accidental ingestion of tapeworm eggs passed in fox or dog feces. The disease in humans has been reported in parts of central Europe, much of Siberia, northern Japan, northwestern Canada, and western Alaska. An increase in the fox population in Europe, particularly in urban areas, has been associated with an apparent increase in human cases. Recent information has extended the Old World range southward to

Iran and northern India and China. The highest prevalence (15%) has been reported from villages in China. Increasing numbers of cases have been reported from central North America (eleven US states and four Canadian provinces). The primary localization of alveolar cysts is in the liver, where they may extend locally or metastasize to other tissues. The larval mass has poorly defined borders and behaves like a neoplasm; it infiltrates and proliferates indefinitely by exogenous budding of the germinative membrane, producing an alveolus-like pattern of microvesicles. Pulmonary involvement is rare, usually occurring by direct extension from the liver. X-rays show hepatomegaly and characteristic scattered areas of radiolucency often outlined by 2- to 4-mm calcific rings. The serologic tests using affinity-purified antigen (ELISA and Western blot) are usually positive at high titer and differentiate *E granulosa* from *E multilocularis*. Treatment is by surgical removal of the entire larval mass when possible, accompanied by drug treatment. Ninety percent of patients with nonresectable masses die within 10 years. Long-term drug therapy (5 years to life) is with albendazole (800 mg/d in divided doses). Preoperative and long-term adjuvant chemotherapy has been associated with a 10-year survival of approximately 80%.

Brunetti E et al: Twenty years of percutaneous treatments for cystic echinococcosis: a preliminary assessment of their use and safety. Parassitologia 2004;46:367. [PMID: 16044692]

Kuzucu A et al: Complicated hydatid cysts of the lung: clinical and therapeutic issues. Ann Thorac Surg 2004;77:1200. [PMID: 15063234]

Sayek I et al: Cystic hydatid disease: current trends in diagnosis and management. Surg Today 2004;34:987. [PMID: 15580379]

Schipper HG et al: Diagnosis and treatment of hepatic echinococcosis: an overview. Scand J Gastroenterol Suppl 2004: 50. [PMID: 15696850]

Smego RA Jr et al: Treatment options for hepatic cystic echinococcosis. Int J Infect Dis 2005;9:69. [PMID: 15708321]

Yaghan R et al: Is fear of anaphylactic shock discouraging surgeons from more widely adopting percutaneous and laparoscopic techniques in the treatment of liver hydatid cyst? Am J Surg 2004;187:533. [PMID: 15041506]

NEMATODE (Roundworm) INFECTIONS

ANISAKIASIS

Anisakiasis is larval invasion of the stomach or intestinal wall by anisakid nematodes. In the acute form, the infection may mimic surgical abdomen; in the chronic form, mild symptoms may persist for weeks to years.

Definitive hosts are marine mammals, including sea lions, seals, and dolphins. Eggs discharged with feces are ingested by crustaceans, in which larvae develop that are infective for squids, mackerel, herring, cod, halibut, rockfish, salmon, tuna, and other marine fish. In fish, in which infection rates can reach 80%, the larvae pass to the musculature and are able to transfer from fish to fish along the food chain, eventually reaching a marine mammal, where they mature into the adult stage.

Humans are infected when they ingest larvae in marine fish or squid eaten raw, undercooked, salted, or lightly pickled. Larvae liberated in the stomach attach to or partially penetrate the gastric or intestinal mucosa (small bowel is more common; colon is rare), resulting in localized ulceration, edema, and eosinophilic granuloma formation; eventually, the parasite dies. Rarely, worms are coughed up and expectorated or penetrate the gut wall, enter the peritoneal cavity, and migrate. Most larvae, however, probably fail to cause infection and are passed in feces. Although the larvae sometimes develop to the adult stages, gravid females are not found in humans.

The infection occurs worldwide, but most cases have been reported in Japan and the Netherlands, with a few in the United States, Scandinavia, the Pacific coast of South America, and other fish-eating countries. Regional foods eaten raw such as sashimi in Japan, pickled herring in the Netherlands, and ceviche (seviche) in Latin America are common vehicles of infection.

Clinical Findings

A. Symptoms and Signs

The majority of acute cases present as gastric anisakiasis. Occasionally, acute infection is followed by a chronic course.

1. Acute gastric anisakiasis—Within hours after larval ingestion, the patient experiences nausea, vomiting, and epigastric pain that progressively becomes more severe. Allergic symptoms (urticaria, bronchospasm, angioedema, or anaphylaxis [rare]) can occur; chest pain and hematemesis are rare.

2. Acute intestinal anisakiasis—Within 1–7 days, colicky pain appears in the lower abdomen, often localized at the ileocecal region, accompanied by diarrhea, nausea, vomiting, diffuse abdominal tenderness, and mild fever.

3. Chronic disease—For weeks to several years, symptoms may continue that mimic gastric ulcer, gastritis, gastric tumor, bowel obstruction, or inflammatory bowel disease.

B. Laboratory Findings

Stools may show occult blood, but eggs are not produced. Mild leukocytosis and eosinophilia may be present. ELISA and radioallergosorbent test (RAST) serologic tests may be helpful but are not reliable in chronic disease.

C. Imaging and Endoscopy

In acute infection, gastroscopy is preferred because the larvae sometimes can be seen and removed from the stomach. X-rays of the stomach may show a localized edematous, ulcerated area with an irregularly thickened wall, decreased peristalsis, and rigidity. Double contrast technique may show the threadlike larvae. Small bowel x-rays may show thickened mucosa and segments of stenosis with proximal dilation. Ultrasound examination of gastric and intestinal lesions may also be useful.

In the chronic stage, x-rays and endoscopy of the stomach—but not of the bowel—may be helpful. The diagnosis is often made only at laparotomy with surgical removal of the parasite. A rise in IgE levels is consistent with the diagnosis.

Prevention & Treatment

Prevention is by avoidance of ingestion of raw or incompletely cooked squid or marine fish, especially salmon, rockfish, herring, mackerel and, in Spain, marinated anchovies. Early evisceration of fish is recommended. Larvae within fish may with difficulty be seen as colorless, tightly coiled or spiraled worms in 3-mm whorls or as reddish or pigmented larvae lying open in muscles or viscera. The larvae are killed by temperatures above 60 °C or by freezing at –23 °C for 7 days or at –35 °C for 15 hours. Smoking procedures that do not bring the temperature to 60 °C, marinating in vinegar, and salt-curing are not reliable.

There is no drug treatment, although a single report suggests efficacy for albendazole. Except where larvae can be removed by fiberoptic gastroscopy or colonoscopy, treatment of acute and chronic lesions is limited to symptomatic measures; symptoms generally improve in 1–2 weeks. Surgical excision of the worm may be necessary in severe cases.

Daschner A et al: Anisakis simplex: sensitization and clinical allergy. Curr Opin Allergy Clin Immunol 2005;5:281. [PMID: 15864089]

Montalto M et al: Anisakis infestation: a case of acute abdomen mimicking Crohn's disease and eosinophilic gastroenteritis. Dig Liver Dis 2005;37:62. [PMID: 15702862]

Moore DA et al: Treatment of anisakiasis with albendazole. Lancet 2002;360:54. [PMID: 12114042]

Pellegrini M et al: Acute abdomen due to small bowel anisakiasis. Dig Liver Dis 2005;37:65. [PMID: 15702863]

Weir E: Sushi, nemotodes and allergies. CMAJ 2005;172:329. [PMID: 15684113]

ANGIOSTRONGYLIASIS

1. Angiostrongyliasis Cantonensis (Eosinophilic Meningoencephalitis)

A nematode of rats, *Angiostrongylus cantonensis*, is the causative agent of a form of eosinophilic meningoencephalitis. It has been reported from Hawaii and other Pacific islands, Southeast Asia, Japan, China, Taiwan, Hong Kong, Australia, Egypt, Madagascar, Nigeria, Bombay, Cuba, Puerto Rico, Bahamas, Brazil, and New Orleans.

Human infection results from the ingestion of infective larvae contained in uncooked food—either the intermediate mollusk hosts (snails, slugs, planarians), transport hosts that have ingested mollusks (crabs, shrimp, fish), leafy vegetables contaminated by small mollusks or by mollusk slime, or from raw vegetable juice. Infection can also result from exposure to fingers contaminated during collection or preparation of snails for cooking. Human infection with this larval stage is as an intermediate host. The definitive host is rodents; mollusks become infected by ingesting larvae excreted in rodent feces.

In humans, ingested larvae (0.5 × 0.025 mm) invade the central nervous system, where, during migration, they may cause extensive tissue damage; at their death, a local inflammatory reaction ensues. The usual clinical findings (incubation period, 1–3 weeks) are those of meningoencephalitis, including severe headache, fever, neck stiffness, nausea and vomiting, and multiple neurologic findings, particularly asymmetric transient cranial neuropathies. Worms in the spinal cord may result in sensory abnormalities in the trunk or extremities; worms have also been seen in the eye.

The spinal fluid characteristically shows elevated protein, normal glucose, and eosinophilic pleocytosis (its absence does not exclude the diagnosis). Occasionally, the parasite can be recovered from spinal fluid. Peripheral eosinophilia with a low-grade leukocytosis is common. IgG antibodies can be detected by ELISA and immunoblot testing. CT and MRI may show central nervous system lesions.

The differential diagnosis includes tuberculosis, coccidioidal or aseptic meningitis, syphilis, lymphoma, gnathostomiasis, cysticercosis, paragonimiasis, echinococcosis, and schistosomiasis japonicum.

No specific treatment is available; however, some anthelmintics can be tried: albendazole (400 mg orally twice daily for 7 days), thiabendazole (25 mg/kg orally three times daily for 3 days; this dose may be toxic and need to be reduced), mebendazole (100 mg orally twice daily for 5 days), pyrantel, or ivermectin. Theoretically, parasite deaths may exacerbate central nervous system inflammatory lesions. Symptomatic treatment with analgesics or corticosteroids may be necessary. The illness usually persists for weeks to months, the parasite dies, and the patient then recovers spontaneously, usually without sequelae. However, fatalities have been recorded.

Prevention is by rat control; by cooking of snails, prawns, fish, and crabs for 3–5 minutes or by freezing them (−15 °C for 24 hours); and by examining vegetables for mollusks before eating. Washing contaminated vegetables to eliminate larvae contained in mollusk mucus is not always successful.

Jin E et al: MRI findings of eosinophilic myelomeningoencephalitis due to *Angiostrongylus cantonensis*. Clin Radiol 2005;60: 242. [PMID: 15664579]

Mentz MB et al: Drug trials for treatment of human angiostrongyliasis. Rev Inst Med Trop Sao Paulo 2003;45:179. [PMID: 14502343]

Tsai HC et al: Outbreak of eosinophilic meningitis associated with drinking raw vegetable juice in southern Taiwan. Am J Trop Med Hyg 2004;71:222. [PMID: 15306715]

2. Angiostrongyliasis Costaricensis

Angiostrongylus costaricensis, which causes an eosinophilic ileocolitis, has been identified in humans (predominantly children) in Mexico, Central America, Venezuela, Brazil, and the United States (Texas, California). The known geographic range of the parasite in rodents (the definitive host) extends from northern South America to Texas. Infection occurs from ingestion of the larvae in the intermediate host (slugs, snails) or from food contaminated by larvae in slug or snail mucus. In humans, the larvae mature in the mesenteric vessels. The inflammatory response to the combination of adult worms, larvae, and eggs can be severe, resulting in a marked eosinophilic granulomatous reaction and intestinal vasculitis and ischemic necrosis. Most cases involve the ileocecal region, appendix, ascending colon, and regional nodes, but other organs can be affected, including the liver and testes. Findings include fever, right lower quadrant abdominal pain and a mass, leukocytosis, and eosinophilia. Some patients have relapsing symptoms that can continue for months. Bowel complications include perforation, bleeding, incomplete or complete obstruction, and infarction. Neither eggs nor larvae are passed in stool; a latex agglutination serologic test has been devised. The intra-abdominal mass can mimic tumor. There is no specific treatment; albendazole, thiabendazole, or mebendazole can be tried (as above). Operative treatment is frequently necessary.

ASCARIASIS

ESSENTIALS OF DIAGNOSIS

- *Transient pulmonary phase: Cough, dyspnea, wheezing, urticaria, with eosinophilia and pulmonary infiltrates.*
- *Intestinal phase: Vague upper abdominal discomfort; occasional vomiting, abdominal distention.*
- *Eggs in stools; worms passed per rectum, nose, or mouth.*

General Considerations

Ascaris lumbricoides is the most common of the intestinal helminths. The infection is limited to humans and appears in all age groups, but morbidity is mainly in children. An estimated 1.3 billion people are infected worldwide, and yearly, 12 million acute cases occur with 10,000 deaths. High prevalence wherever there are low standards of hygiene and sanitation (including focally in southeastern United States) or where human feces are used as fertilizer.

Adult worms (20–40 cm × 3–6 mm) live for 1 year or more in the upper small intestine. After fertilization, the female produces enormous numbers of eggs that pass in feces. Direct transmission between humans does not occur, as the eggs must remain on the soil for 2–3 weeks before they become infective. Thereafter, they can survive for years. Infection occurs through ingestion of mature eggs in fecally contaminated food and drink. The eggs hatch in the small intestine, releasing motile larvae that penetrate the intestinal wall to reach the right heart via the mesenteric venules and lymphatics. From the heart they move to the lung, burrow through the alveolar walls, and migrate up the bronchial tree into the pharynx, down the esophagus, and back to the small intestine. Egg production begins 60–75 days after ingestion of infective eggs.

Clinical Findings

A. Symptoms and Signs

As a result of their migration and induction of hypersensitivity, larvae in the lung cause capillary and alveolar damage, which may result in low-grade fever, nonproductive cough, blood-tinged sputum, wheezing, dyspnea, and substernal pain. There may be urticaria and localized rales. Rarely, larvae lodge ectopically in the brain, kidney, eye, spinal cord, and other sites and may cause symptoms referable to those organs.

Small numbers of adult worms in the intestine usually produce no symptoms. With heavy infection, peptic ulcer-like symptoms or vague preprandial or postprandial abdominal discomfort may be seen. Adult worms may also migrate with heavy infections; they may be coughed up, vomited, or emerge through the nose or anus. They may also force themselves into the common bile duct, pancreatic duct, appendix, diverticula, and other sites, which may lead to cholangitis, cholecystitis, cholelithiasis, pyogenic liver abscess, pancreatitis, or obstructive jaundice. With very heavy infestations, masses of worms may cause intestinal obstruction, volvulus, intussusception, or death. During typhoid fever, worms may penetrate the weakened bowel wall. Rare cases of lung abscess or laryngeal obstruction with suffocation have been described. Moderate to high worm loads, in children, have been associated with reduced nitrogen, fat, and D-xylose absorption and stunting of growth. Periodic treatment of children with albendazole for multiple intestinal parasitism has resulted in improved nutrition.

B. Imaging

During the larval migratory phase, chest radiographs may show transitory, patchy, ill-defined asymmetric infiltrations. Intestinal infection is sometimes established by chance, when radiologic examination of the abdomen (with or without barium) shows the presence of worms. The diagnosis of biliary ascariasis can be made by endoscopic retrograde cholangiopancreatography, which has the therapeutic potential of removing the worms, and by ultrasonography. In intestinal obstruction, plain abdominal films show air-fluid levels and multiple linear images of ascarides in dilated bowel loops; ultrasonography can also demonstrate the dilated bowel and worm mass.

C. Laboratory Findings

During the pulmonary phase, eosinophils may reach 30–50% and remain high for about a month; larvae are occasionally found in sputum. During the intestinal phase, diagnosis usually depends on finding the characteristic eggs in feces. Occasionally, an adult worm spontaneously passed per rectum or orally reveals an unsuspected infection. Serologic tests are not useful; there is no eosinophilia in the intestinal phase.

Differential Diagnosis

Pulmonary ascariasis with eosinophilia must be differentiated from nonparasitic causes (asthma, eosinophilic pneumonia, allergic bronchopulmonary aspergillosis) and parasitic causes (tropical pulmonary eosinophilia, toxocariasis, strongyloidiasis, hookworm, paragonimiasis). Ascaris-induced pancreatitis, appendicitis, and diverticulitis must be differentiated from other causes of inflammation of these tissues. Postprandial dyspepsia may simulate duodenal ulcer, hiatal hernia, gallbladder disease, or pancreatic disease.

Treatment

Albendazole, pyrantel pamoate, and mebendazole are the treatments of choice. The drugs listed below do not require pretreatment or posttreatment purges. Stools should be rechecked at 2 weeks and patients retreated until all ascarids are removed. Ascariasis, hookworm, and trichuriasis infections, which often occur together, may be treated simultaneously by albendazole, mebendazole, or oxantel-pyrantel pamoate.

Treatment with these anthelmintics can cause worms to migrate before they die. Because anesthesia stimulates worms to hypermotility, they should be removed in advance in patients undergoing elective surgery. In pregnancy, ascariasis should be treated after the first trimester. Albendazole and mebendazole are contraindicated in pregnancy, but pyrantel and piperazine can be used.

Drug treatment should not be used in the migratory phase. In intestinal obstruction or biliary ascariasis, surgery may be avoided by nasogastric suction followed by a standard dose of an anthelmintic given via the tube. In biliary ascariasis, endoscopic removal of the worm under ultrasonographic guidance is often successful; treatment by injection of a solution of albendazole or piperazine into the common duct followed by systemic treatment has also been effective.

A. Albendazole

In light infections, a single oral dose of albendazole (400 mg) results in cure rates over 95%; in heavy infections, however, a 2- to 3-day course is indicated. Side effects, including migration of ascaris through the nose or mouth, are rare. Albendazole is available in the United States though not approved for this indication.

B. Pyrantel Pamoate

Pyrantel pamoate as a single oral dose of 10 mg base/kg (maximum, 1 g) results in 85–100% cure rates. It may be given before or after meals. Infrequent and mild side effects include vomiting, diarrhea, headache, dizziness, and drowsiness.

C. Mebendazole

Although mebendazole is highly effective when given in a dosage of 100 mg orally twice daily before or after meals for 3 days, a single 500 mg dose or less is often sufficient. Mild gastrointestinal side effects are infrequent.

D. Piperazine

The dosage for piperazine (as the hexahydrate) is 75 mg/kg body weight (maximum, 3.5 g) orally for 2 days in succession, giving the drug orally before or after breakfast. For heavy infestations, treatment should be continued for 4 days in succession or the 2-day course should be repeated after 1 week.

Gastrointestinal symptoms and headache occur occasionally; central nervous system symptoms (temporary ataxia and exacerbation of seizures) are rare. Allergic symptoms have been attributed to piperazine. The drug should not be used for patients with hepatic or renal insufficiency or in those with a history of seizures or chronic neurologic disease.

E. Other Drugs

Using ivermectin, one oral dose (200 mcg/kg) had a cure rate of 78%; with two doses given at a 10-day interval, the cure rate increased to 99%.

Prognosis

The complications caused by wandering adult worms require that all ascaris infections be treated and eradicated.

Heukelbach J et al: Efficacy of ivermectin in a patient population concomitantly infected with intestinal helminths and ectoparasites. Arzneimittelforschung 2004;54:416. [PMID: 15344847]

Koumanidou C et al: Sonographic features of intestinal and biliary ascariasis in childhood: case report and review of the literature. Ann Trop Paediatr 2004;24:329. [PMID: 15720890]

Parente F et al: An unusual cause of recurrent biliary colics. Dig Liver Dis 2004;36:763. [PMID: 15571008]

Schulze SM et al: Acute abdomen secondary to ascaris lumbricoides infestation of the small bowel. Am Surg 2005;71:505. [PMID: 16044931]

Sherman SC et al: The CT diagnosis of Ascariasis. J Emerg Med 2005;28:471. [PMID: 15837034]

CUTANEOUS LARVA MIGRANS (Creeping Eruption)

Cutaneous larva migrans, prevalent throughout the tropics and subtropics (including the southeastern and Gulf of Mexico coasts of the United States) is caused by larvae of the dog and cat hookworms, *Ancylostoma braziliense* and *Ancylostoma caninum*. Gnathostomiasis, strongyloidiasis, and a number of other animal hookworms can also be causes of parasitic migration in human skin. Moist sandy soil (eg, beaches, children's sand piles) contaminated by dog or cat feces is a common site of infection. The infection is also reported in travelers to tropical beaches, among whom delayed onset beyond several weeks has been described.

At the site of larval entry, particularly on the hands or feet, up to several hundred minute, intensely pruritic erythematous papules appear. Two to 3 days later, serpiginous eruptions appear as the larvae migrate at a rate of several millimeters a day; the parasite lies slightly ahead of the advancing border. The process may continue for weeks; the lesions may become severely pruritic, vesiculate, encrusted, or secondarily infected. Without treatment, the larvae eventually die and are absorbed.

The diagnosis is based on the characteristic appearance of the lesions and the frequent presence of eosinophilia. Biopsy is usually not indicated.

Mild transient cases may not require treatment. For mild cases, thiabendazole, if available, can be applied topically three times daily for 5 or more days as a 15% cream, which can be formulated in a hygroscopic base using crushed 500 mg tablets. For more severe cases, oral treatment is indicated. Highly effective and nearly free of side effects are ivermectin (200 mcg/kg given for 1 or 2 days) or albendazole (400 mg twice daily for 3–5 days or 400 mg daily for 7 days). Thiabendazole, given orally as for strongyloidiasis, is a less satisfactory alternative drug because it has toxic side effects in about one-third of patients. With treatment, progression of the lesions and itching are usually stopped within 48 hours. Antihistamines are helpful in controlling pruritus; an antibiotic topically or orally may be necessary to treat secondary infections.

Brenner MA et al: Cutaneous larva migrans: the creeping eruption. Cutis 2003;72:111. [PMID: 12953933]

Caumes E et al: From creeping eruption to hookworm-related cutaneous larva migrans. Lancet Infect Dis 2004;4:659. [PMID: 15522674]

Chen TM et al: An unpleasant memento. Am J Med 2005;118:604. [PMID: 15922689]

DRACUNCULIASIS (Guinea Worm Disease, Dracunculosis, Dracontiasis)

Dracunculiasis is an infection of connective and subcutaneous tissues by the nematode *Dracunculus medinensis*. It occurs only in humans and is a major cause of disability. Since the start of the WHO eradication program, the number of infected persons has declined about 99% from an estimated 3.5 million cases. Endemic areas have been the Indian subcontinent; West and Central Africa north of the equator; and Saudi Arabia, Iran, and Yemen. The two remaining endemic foci are southern Sudan and northern Ghana. The disease occurs almost exclusively in isolated rural areas; all ages are affected, and prevalence may reach 60%.

Infection occurs by swallowing water containing the infected intermediate host, the crustacean cyclops (copepods, water fleas). In the stomach, larvae escape from the crustacean and mature in subcutaneous connective tissue. After mating, the male worm dies and the gravid female (60–80 cm × 1.7–2.0 mm) moves to the surface of the body, where its head reaches the dermis and provokes a blister that ruptures on contact with water. Intermittently over 2–3 weeks, whenever the ulcer comes in contact with water, the uterus discharges great numbers of larvae, which are ingested by copepods. Most adult worms are gradually extruded; some worms retract and reemerge; and others die in the tissues, disintegrate, and may provoke a severe inflammatory reaction. Infection does not induce protective immunity.

Clinical Findings

A. SYMPTOMS AND SIGNS

Infection may be at several sites. Patients are asymptomatic during the 9- to 14-month incubation period except in the last 1–2 weeks, when the worm reaches and becomes palpable in the skin and a blister develops around its anterior end. Several hours before the head appears at the skin surface, local erythema, burning, pruritus, and tenderness often develop at the site of emergence. There may also be a 24-hour systemic allergic reaction (pruritus, fever, nausea and vomiting, dyspnea, periorbital edema, and urticaria). After rupture, the tissues surrounding the ulceration frequently become indurated, reddened, and tender. Because most lesions appear on the leg or foot, patients often must give up walking and working for days to several months. Uninfected ulcers heal in 4–6 weeks. The worm rarely reaches ectopic sites.

Secondary infections, including tetanus, are common. Deep "cold" abscesses may result at the sites of dying, nonemergent worms. Ankle and knee joint infections with resultant deformity are common complications.

B. LABORATORY FINDINGS

When an emerging adult worm is not visible in the ulcer or under the skin, the diagnosis may be made by detection of larvae in smears from discharging sinuses. Immersion of an ulcer in cold water stimulates larval expulsion. Eosinophilia is usually present. Skin and serologic tests are not useful. Calcified worms can be recognized on radiographs.

Treatment

All persons in an endemic area should be actively immunized against tetanus.

A. GENERAL MEASURES

The patient should be at bed rest with the affected part elevated. Cleanse the lesion, control secondary infection with topical antibiotics, and change dressings twice daily.

B. MANUAL EXTRACTION

Traditional extraction of emerging worms by gradually rolling them out a few centimeters each day on a small stick is still useful, especially when done along with chemotherapy and use of aseptic dressings. The process appears to be facilitated by placing the affected part in water several times a day. If the worm is broken during removal, however, secondary infection almost always results, leading to cellulitis, abscess formation, or septicemia.

C. ANTHELMINTIC THERAPY

The following drugs have an anti-inflammatory effect but do not kill the adults or the larvae. This effect may alleviate symptoms, reduce duration of infection, facilitate worm removal, or expedite their spontaneous extrusion.

1. Metronidazole, 250 mg orally three times daily for 10 days, causes only minimal toxicity. (See under Amebiasis.)

2. Mebendazole, 400–800 mg orally daily for 6 days, can be tried.

D. SURGICAL REMOVAL

Preemergent female worms can sometimes be surgically removed intact under local anesthesia if not firmly embedded in deep fascia or around tendons.

Prevention & Control

The disease is prevented by use of only noncontaminated drinking water. This can be accomplished either by (1) preventing contamination of community water supplies through use of tube wells, hand pumps, or cisterns or treating water sources with the larvicide temephos; or (2) filtering water through finely woven cloth (eg, nylon nets of 100-mcm pore size); or (3) boiling water.

Centers for Disease Control and Prevention (CDC): Progress toward global eradication of dracunculiasis, January 2004–July 2005. MMWR Morb Mortal Wkly Rep 2005;54:1075. [PMID: 16251863]

Greenaway C: Dracunculiasis (guinea worm disease). CMAJ 2004;170:495. [PMID: 14970098]

ENTEROBIASIS (Pinworm Infection)

ESSENTIALS OF DIAGNOSIS

- *Nocturnal perianal and vulvar pruritus, insomnia, irritability, restlessness.*
- *Vague gastrointestinal symptoms.*
- *Eggs demonstrable by cellulose tape test; worms visible on perianal skin or in stool.*

General Considerations

Enterobius vermicularis (8–13 × 0.5 mm) is common worldwide and is the most prevalent nematode infection in the United States. Humans, the only host, can harbor a few to hundreds of worms. Young children are affected more often than adults, and multiple infections occur in households and institutions with young children. High rates have been recorded in homosexual men, but the infection does not become opportunistic in HIV.

The adult worms inhabit the cecum and adjacent bowel areas, lying loosely attached to the mucosa. Gravid females migrate through the anus to the perianal skin and deposit eggs in large numbers. The eggs become infective in a few hours and may then infect others or be autoinfective if transferred to the mouth by contaminated food, drink, fomites, or hands. After being swallowed, the eggs hatch in the duodenum, and the larvae migrate down to the cecum. Retroinfection occasionally occurs when the eggs hatch on the perianal skin and the larvae migrate through the anus into the large intestine. The development of a mature ovipositing female from an ingested egg requires about 3–4 weeks. Eggs remain viable for 2–3 weeks outside the host. The life span of the worm is 30–45 days.

Clinical Findings

A. SYMPTOMS AND SIGNS

Many patients are asymptomatic. The most common and important symptom is perianal pruritus (particularly at night), due to the presence of the female worms or deposited eggs. Insomnia, restlessness, enuresis, and irritability are common symptoms, particularly in children. Many mild gastrointestinal symptoms have also been attributed to enterobiasis, but the association is difficult to prove. Perianal scratching may result in excoriation and impetigo. Adults sometimes report a "crawling" sensation in the anal area. Rarely, worm migration—including migration through the female genital tract or into the urethra—results in ectopic inflammation (vulvovaginitis, diverticulitis, appendicitis, cystitis) or granulomatous reactions (colon, genital tract, peritoneum, and elsewhere). Colonic ulceration and eosinophilic colitis have been reported.

B. LABORATORY FINDINGS

Diagnosis is made by finding eggs on the perianal skin (eggs are seldom found on stool examination). The most reliable method is by applying a short strip of sealing cellulose pressure-sensitive tape (eg, Scotch Tape) to the perianal skin and then spreading the tape on a slide for low-power microscopic study; toluene is used to clear the preparation. Three such preparations made on consecutive mornings before bathing or defecation will establish the diagnosis in about 90% of cases. Before the diagnosis can be ruled out, five to seven such examinations are necessary. Nocturnal examination of the perianal area or gross examination of

stools may reveal adult worms, which should be placed in preservative, alcohol, or saline for laboratory examination. The worms can sometimes be seen on anoscopy. Eosinophilia is rare.

Differential Diagnosis

Pinworm pruritus must be distinguished from similar pruritus due to mycotic infections, allergies, hemorrhoids, proctitis, fissures, strongyloidiasis, and other conditions.

Treatment

A. GENERAL MEASURES

Symptomatic patients should be treated, and in some situations all members of the patient's household should be treated concurrently, since for each overt case there are usually several inapparent cases. Careful washing of hands with soap and water after defecation and again before meals is important. Fingernails should be kept trimmed close and clean and scratching of the perianal area avoided. Ordinary washing of bedding will usually kill pinworm eggs; some workers recommend daily washing.

B. SPECIFIC MEASURES

Albendazole, mebendazole, and pyrantel pamoate are the drugs of choice and can be given with or without food. The dosage should be repeated at 2 and 4 weeks to avoid potential reinfection from infective eggs in the household environment. Albendazole and mebendazole should not be used in pregnancy. Piperazine, although effective, is not recommended because treatment requires 1 week.

1. Albendazole, available in the United States though not approved for this indication, is given as a single oral 400 mg dose. Abdominal pain and diarrhea are rare.

2. Mebendazole is given as a single 100 mg oral dose.

3. Pyrantel pamoate is administered as a 10 mg (base)/kg (maximum, 1 g) dose. Infrequent side effects include vomiting, diarrhea, headache, dizziness, and drowsiness. In the United States, pyrantel is available as self-medication for pinworm infection.

Prognosis

Although annoying, the infection is usually benign. Reinfection is common, especially in children, because of continued exposure outside the home.

Horton J: Albendazole: a broad spectrum anthelminthic for treatment of individuals and populations. Curr Opin Infect Dis 2002;15:5998. [PMID: 12821837]

Nackley AC et al: Appendiceal enterobius vermicularis infestation associated with right-sided chronic pelvic pain. JSLS 2004; 8:171. [PMID: 15119664]

Petro M et al: Unusual endoscopic and microscopic view of *Enterobius vermicularis:* a case report with a review of the literature. South Med J 2005;98:927. [PMID: 16217987]

Tandan T et al: Pelvic inflammatory disease associated with *Enterobius vermicularis*. Arch Dis Child 2002;86:439. [PMID: 12023182]

FILARIASIS

ESSENTIALS OF DIAGNOSIS

- *History of residence in an endemic area (much of the tropics and subtropics between 40 °N and 30 °S).*
- *Episodic attacks of lymphangitis, lymphadenitis, and fever.*
- *Hydrocele; chyluria; acute or chronic lymphedema; or elephantiasis of arms, legs, genitalia, or breasts.*
- *Microfilariae in blood, chyluria, or hydrocele fluid; positive serology; circulating antigens.*

More than 120 million people are infected with lymphatic filariasis in 83 tropical and subtropical countries, 40 million are disfigured, and an estimated 1 million new persons, mainly children, are infected yearly. The disease is caused by three filarial nematodes: *Wuchereria bancrofti*, *Brugia malayi*, and *Brugia timori*. The filarial diseases are among the most important infections worldwide that cause a high degree of disability. *W bancrofti* is widely distributed in the tropics and subtropics of both hemispheres and on Pacific islands and is transmitted by culex, aedes, and anopheles mosquitoes. *B malayi* is transmitted by mansonia and anopheles mosquitoes of South India, Sri Lanka, Southeast Asia, South China, the northern coastal areas of China, and South Korea. *B timori* is found on the southeastern islands of Indonesia.

No animal reservoir hosts are known for *W bancrofti* or *B timori*; cats, monkeys, and other animals may harbor *B malayi*. Mosquitoes become infected by ingesting microfilariae with a blood meal; at subsequent feedings, they can infect new susceptible hosts. Over months, adult worms (females, 8–9 cm × 0.2–0.3 mm) mature and live (up to 2 decades) in or near superficial and deep lymphatics and lymph nodes and produce large numbers of viviparous circulating microfilariae.

Pathologic changes in lymph vessels are due to host immunologic reactions to developing and mature worms; also implicated are bacterial and fungal superinfections. An abscess may form at the site of a dying worm. Living microfilariae generally cause no lesions, except in tropical pulmonary eosinophilia. Rapid death of microfilariae, however, does produce findings.

Dirofilariasis, infections by *Dirofilaria immitis* and *Dirofilaria repens* (from dogs) and *Dirofilaria tenuis* (from raccoons) have been reported in the United States, Japan, Australia, and elsewhere. Nodules have been found in the periphery of the lungs as solitary "coin" lesions (1–4.5 cm), in the skin, or in other tissues. The parasites die in the larval stage, cause few symptoms, and rarely calcify. The serologic test for filariasis is positive, but there is no microfilaremia. Eosinophilia is seen in 15% of patients.

Several **other species of filarial worms** infect humans but usually without causing important findings: microfilariae of *Mansonella ozzardi* and *Mansonella streptocerca* appear in the skin, *Mansonella perstans* appears in the blood.

Clinical Findings

A. SYMPTOMS AND SIGNS

Many infections remain symptomatic, with or without microfilariae; if they do appear, it is 6–12 months after infection. The incubation period for symptoms is generally 8–16 months in expatriates but may be longer in indigenous persons. Many infections remain asymptomatic, with or without microfilariae.

1. Acute disease—Episodes of fever (filarial fever), with or without inflammation of lymphatics and nodes, occur at irregular intervals and last for several days. Characteristically, the adenolymphangitis presents as retrograde extension from the affected node (unlike ascending bacterial lymphangitis). With disease progression, epididymitis and orchitis as well as involvement of pelvic, abdominal, or retroperitoneal lymphatics may also occur intermittently. Lymph node enlargement may persist. In travelers, allergic-like findings (hives, rashes, eosinophilia) as well as lymphangitis and lymphadenitis are likely to be present.

2. Chronic disease—Obstructive phenomena that occur as a result of interference with normal lymphatic flow include hydrocele; scrotal lymphedema; lymphatic varices; and elephantiasis, particularly of the extremities, genitals, and breasts. Chyluria may result from rupture of distended lymphatics into the urinary tract. Manifestations seen in some patients include lymphadenopathy or moderate hepatomegaly or splenomegaly.

3. Occult disease—A small proportion of infected persons develop occult disease, in which the classic clinical manifestations and microfilaremia are not present but microfilariae are present in the tissues.

In **tropical pulmonary eosinophilia**, microfilariae of *W bancrofti* or *B malayi* are sequestered in the lungs but are not found in the blood. The condition, usually in young males, is characterized by episodic nocturnal coughing or wheezing, dyspnea, low-grade fever, scant expectoration, hypereosinophilia, high filarial antibody titers and IgE levels, diffuse miliary lesions or increased bronchovascular markings on chest films, and a rapid response to diethylcarbamazine treatment (6 mg/kg daily for 21 days). Relapses (in 20%) require re-treatment with up to 12 mg/kg daily for up to 30 days. If untreated, the condition can progress to chronic pulmonary fibrosis.

B. LABORATORY FINDINGS

Diagnosis of active infection is made by finding microfilariae in blood (or hydrocele fluid), a positive antigen test (only available for *W bancrofti*), or by ultrasound. In indigenous persons, microfilariae are rare in the first 2–3 years, abundant as the disease progresses, and again rare in the obstructive stage. Thus, amicrofilaremia does not exclude presence of the infection. In addition, there is no correlation between microfilarial density and disease severity. In nonindigenous persons, inflammatory reactions may be prominent in the absence of microfilariae. Microfilariae of *W bancrofti* are found in the blood chiefly at night (nocturnal periodicity 10 PM to 2 AM), except for a nonperiodic variety in the South Pacific. *B malayi* microfilariae are usually nocturnal periodic but in Southeast Asia may be present at all times, with a slight nocturnal rise. Anticoagulated blood specimens are collected at times that relate to the periodicity of the local strain. Specimens may be stored at ambient temperatures until examined in the morning by wet film for motile larvae and by Giemsa-stained smears—thick for sensitivity and thin for specific morphology to distinguish species. A formalin-anionic detergent preservative can also be used. If these are negative, the blood specimens should be concentrated by the membrane filtration technique or Knott concentration. Where available, testing for antigens of *W bancrofti, which circulate throughout the day,* should be done and can replace microscopy. ELISA and a rapid (5 min) immunochromatographic card test are sensitive (96–100%) and specific (nearly 100%) and thus are particularly useful for amicrofilaremic persons and for daytime examination of blood. A rapid dipstick test has shown a 97% sensitivity and 99% specificity for *B malayi*, and a PCR assay has been developed for both *W bancrofti* and *B malayi*. Other serologic tests may also be helpful in screening; negative tests usually rule out present or past infection, but false-positive tests occur with other filarial and helminthic infections, including ascariasis. An indirect hemagglutination titer of 1:128 and a bentonite flocculation titer of 1:5 in combination are considered the minimum significant titers. Eosinophil counts may be elevated. Live adult worms can be detected by high-frequency ultrasound of the scrotum (up to 80% of infected men) and of the female breast. In differential diagnosis, lymphangiography (potentially damaging to the lymphatics) and radionuclide lymphoscintigraphy may be useful lymphatic imaging methods.

Treatment

A. DRUG TREATMENT

Diethylcarbamazine is the drug of choice for treatment of individual patients. A mass drug treatment program involving 83 countries is underway to reduce lymphatic filariasis disability and to achieve worldwide eradication by 2020. Infected persons are given five consecutive annual doses. In most of the world, diethylcarbamazine plus albendazole is used, but in Africa, where persons may have concurrent onchocerciasis or loiasis infections, ivermectin plus albendazole is used.

1. Diethylcarbamazine—Diethylcarbamazine rapidly kills blood microfilariae; however it kills adults worms slowly and incompletely (20%). Treatment requires multiple 14-day courses (2 mg/kg orally three times a day after meals, starting with small doses and gradually increasing over 3–4 days). At this dose, direct drug-induced toxicity is rare. However, adverse immunologic reactions—more common in bancroftian filariasis—occur due to dying parasites. Reactions to dying microfilariae are frequent, rapid, and sometimes severe and include fever, headache, myalgia, dizziness, malaise, and other allergic responses; reactions to dying adult worms are slow and local and include lymphadenitis and abscess. Antipyretics and analgesics may be helpful. In areas where onchocerciasis or loiasis is also prevalent, the use of diethylcarbamazine is commonly contraindicated because of the potential for severe reactions to dying microfilariae of those parasites; instead, in Africa, ivermectin plus albendazole can be used. Diethylcarbamazine availability in the United States is only from the Parasitic Diseases Drug Service, Centers for Disease Control and Prevention, Atlanta, GA 30333; phone 404-639-3670.

2. Ivermectin—Effective only as a microfilaricide, ivermectin is given as a single oral 200 mcg/kg dose and repeated at 6-month intervals. The side effects of ivermectin against microfilariae are rapid and similar to that of diethylcarbamazine. Ivermectin should not be used in early pregnancy, although specific fetal problems have not been recognized. To kill the adult worms, diethylcarbamazine must also be given.

3. Albendazole—Albendazole continues under evaluation as a microfilaricide (a single oral dose of 400 mg) and as a macrofilaricide (400 mg twice daily for 3 weeks) but increasing findings suggest poor efficacy. The drug is free of significant side effects but is generally contraindicated in pregnancy.

B. OTHER TREATMENTS

During acute inflammatory episodes, it is controversial whether to treat and whether drug usage will shorten the attack. General measures include rest, antipyretics, analgesics, antibiotics for secondary infections, use of postural drainage, elastic stockings and pressure bandages for leg edema, and suspensory bandaging for orchitis and epididymitis.

Hydroceles may benefit from repeated drainage, a locally injected sclerosing agent, or surgery. To manage elephantiasis, lymphovenous shunt procedures may be useful, combined with antibiotics to treat superinfections. Reconstructive surgery on limbs is controversial.

The search for an effective macrofilaricide continues. Under evaluation is the finding that *Wolbachia* bacteria are obligate intracellular infections of filarial parasites. Doxycycline treatment of patients (100–200 mg/d for 4–6 weeks) leads to bacterial death followed by the slow death of the adult parasites. The bacteria have also been implicated in some of the chronic morbidity of filariasis.

Prognosis

The prognosis is good with treatment of early and mild cases (including low-grade lymphedema, chyluria, small hydrocele), but in advanced infection the prognosis is poor.

Critchley J et al: Albendazole for the control and elimination of lymphatic filariasis: systematic review. Trop Med Int Health 2005;10:818. [PMID: 16135187]

Kvelem D et al: Short communication: Impact of long-term (14 years) bi-annual ivermectin treatment on *Wuchereria bancrofti* microfilaraemia. Trop Med Int Health 2005;10:1002. [PMID: 16185234]

Simonsen PE et al: The effect of eight half-yearly single-dose treatments with DEC on *Wuchereria bancrofti* circulating antigenaemia. Trans R Soc Trop Med Hyg 2005;99:541. [PMID: 15869771]

Theis JH: Public health aspects of dirofilariasis in the United States. Vet Parasitol 2005;133:157. [PMID: 16039780]

Tisch DJ et al: Mass chemotherapy options to control lymphatic filariasis: a systematic review. Lancet Infect Dis 2005;5:514. [PMID: 16048720]

GNATHOSTOMIASIS

Gnathostomiasis, due for the most part to infection by the larval stage of the nematode *Gnathostoma spinigerum*, is rarely caused by other *Gnathostoma* species. Infection is most common in Thailand and Japan but is also reported from Southeast Asia, China, India, Central and South America, Israel, and East Africa. In Mexico, where the *Gnathostoma* species has not been identified, the number of cases is increasing; more than 1000 have been reported in recent years, commonly associated with increased eating of raw freshwater fish, especially sushi, sashimi, and a preparation called ceviche. In the United States, though *G spinigerum* has rarely been seen in minks, it has not been reported in humans. Eggs passed in feces of the definitive hosts, wild and domestic dogs and cats, are infective for copepods (water fleas). Ingestion of copepods by secondary hosts results in encysted larvae in their tissues; humans are infected when these larvae are ingested in raw, marinated, or inadequately cooked freshwater fish, shrimp, crab, crayfish, chicken or other fowl, frogs, or pork. Infection has also been attributed to ingestion of infected copepods in water.

Within 24–48 hours, larval migration through the intestinal wall can cause acute epigastric pain, vomiting, urticaria, and eosinophilia. The worm then migrates to subcutaneous and other tissues but is unable to mature. Most common is a pruritic subcutaneous swelling up to 25 cm across, occasionally accompanied by stabbing pain. Over weeks to years, the swelling may remain in one area for days or weeks, move continuously, or there may be an absence of physical signs between episodes. Occasionally the worm becomes visible under the skin.

Internal organs and the eye (pain, anterior uveitis, increased intraocular pressure, vitreous hemorrhage, and eventually blindness) may also be invaded. Spontaneous pneumothorax, leukorrhea, hematemesis, hematuria, hemoptysis, paroxysmal coughing, and edema of the pharynx with dyspnea have been reported as complications. Invasion of the brain can result in an eosinophilic meningoencephalitis or subarachnoid hemorrhage. Spinal cord invasion can lead to myelitis or radiculopathy.

Definitive diagnosis is sometimes possible by surgical removal of the worm when it appears close to the skin. Although common, marked eosinophilia may be absent, especially for parasites in the central nervous system. Serodiagnosis is by immunoblot assay (high sensitivity and specificity) or ELISA of blood or cerebrospinal fluid. Skin and other serologic tests are unsatisfactory.

Treatment is with ivermectin (200 mcg/kg orally daily for 2 days) or with albendazole (400 mg orally twice daily for 21 days). Larval death appears to occur slowly and a second course of treatment may be necessary; cure rates may reach 95%. Courses of prednisolone have provided temporary relief of symptoms. Lesions in the eye or brain should probably not be treated with an anthelmintic because of the potential for edema resulting from release of antigens from the dying worm.

Kraivichian K et al: Treatment of cutaneous gnathostomiasis with ivermectin. Am J Trop Med Hyg 2004;71:623. [PMID: 15569795]

Lingon BL: Gnathostomiasis: a review of a previously localized zoonosis now crossing numerous geographical boundaries. Semin Pediatr Infec Dis 2005;16:137. [PMID: 15825144]

Magana M et al: Gnathostomiasis: clinicopathologic study. Am J Dermatopathol 2004;26:91. [PMID: 15024188]

Moore DA et al: Gnathostomiasis: an emerging imported disease. Emerg Infect Dis 2003;9:647. [PMID: 12781003]

HOOKWORM DISEASE

 ESSENTIALS OF DIAGNOSIS

Early findings (not commonly recognized):

- *Dermatitis: pruritic, erythematous, papulovesicular eruption at site of larval invasion, often of the feet.*
- *Pulmonary migration of larvae: transient episodes of coughing, asthma, fever, blood-tinged sputum, marked eosinophilia.*

Later findings:

- *Intestinal symptoms: anorexia, diarrhea, abdominal discomfort.*
- *Anemia (iron deficiency): fatigue, pallor, dyspnea on exertion, poikilonychia, heart failure.*
- *Characteristic eggs and occult blood in the stool.*

General Considerations

Hookworm disease, widespread in the moist tropics and subtropics and sporadically in southeastern United States, is caused by *Ancylostoma duodenale* and *Necator americanus.* Probably a quarter of the world's population is infected, and in many areas the infection is a major cause of debility, retardation of growth and development of children, and increased susceptibility to infection. Prevalence rates can reach 80% in the humid tropics under unsanitary conditions.

Although in the Western Hemisphere and tropical Africa, *Necator* was the prevailing species, and in the Far East, India, China, and the Mediterranean area, *Ancylostoma* was prevalent, both species have now become widely distributed. Infection is rare in regions with less than 40 inches of rainfall annually. Humans are the only host for both species.

The adult worms are approximately 1 cm long. Eggs produced by females are passed in the stool and must fall on warm, moist soil if hatching followed by larval development is to take place. Larvae remain infective for hours to about a week, depending on environmental conditions. Following skin penetration, often of the feet, the larvae migrate in the bloodstream to the pulmonary capillaries, break into alveoli, and then are carried by ciliary action upward to the bronchi, trachea, and mouth. After being swallowed, they reach and attach to the mucosa of the upper small bowel; maturation and release of eggs occur in 6–8 weeks. *Ancylostoma* infection can also be acquired by ingestion of the larvae in food or water. Adult ancylostoma worms survive about a year; necator, about 3–5 years.

The worms suck blood at their attachment sites. Blood loss is proportionate to the worm burden. A light infection is approximately 1000 eggs per gram of feces (equivalent to about 11 ancylostoma and 32 necator adults); a moderate worm load is 2000–8000 eggs per gram of feces. Iron loss with moderate infection is 1.1 mg/d for *N americanus* and 2.3 mg/d for *A duodenale*. Over years—and depending on the host's dietary intake of iron—iron reserves can be depleted and severe anemia can result from moderate infections with 30 or more ancylostoma or 100 or more necator worms. Accompanying the anemia is loss of protein that can lead to hypoalbuminemia.

Clinical Findings

A. Symptoms and Signs

The first manifestation of infection is a pruritic erythematous dermatitis, either maculopapular or vesicular, that follows skin penetration of the infective larvae. Severity is a function of the number of invading larvae and host sensitivity. Scratching may result in secondary infection. Strongyloidiasis and cutaneous larva migrans must be considered in the differential diagnosis at this stage.

The pulmonary stage, in which there is larval migration through the lungs, may show dry cough, wheezing, blood-tinged sputum, and low-grade fever. The pulmonary migration of ascaris and strongyloides larvae can produce similar findings.

After 2 or more weeks, maturing worms attach to the mucosa of the duodenum and upper jejunum. In heavy infections, worms may reach the ileum. Patients who have light infections and adequate iron intake often remain asymptomatic. In heavy infections, however, there may be anorexia, diarrhea, vague abdominal pain, and ulcer-like epigastric symptoms. Severe anemia may result in pallor, deformed nails, pica, and cardiac decompensation. Marked protein loss may also occur, resulting in hypoalbuminemia, with edema and ascites. There are conflicting reports of malabsorption in some severe infections.

Reduction in worm loads and symptoms after the first decade of life suggests that a moderate degree of immunity develops.

B. Laboratory Findings

Diagnosis depends on demonstration of characteristic eggs in feces; a concentration method may be needed. The two species cannot be differentiated by the appearance of their eggs. The stool usually contains occult blood. Hypochromic microcytic anemia can be severe, with hemoglobin levels as low as 2 g/dL, a low serum iron and a high iron-binding capacity, and low serum ferritin. Eosinophilia (as high as 30–60% of a total white blood count reaching 17,000/mcL) is usually present in the pulmonary migratory stage of infection but is not marked in the chronic intestinal stage.

Treatment

A. General Measures

The availability of safe anthelmintics makes it possible to treat all patients initially, irrespective of the intensity of infection; nevertheless, it may not be necessary or beneficial to treat light infections. Heavy infections may need re-treatment at 2-week intervals until the worm burden is reduced to a low level as estimated by semiquantitative egg counts. Eradication of infection is not essential, since light infections do not injure the well-nourished patient and iron loss is replaced if the patient is receiving adequate dietary iron.

If anemia is present, oral ferrous sulfate and a diet high in protein and vitamins are required for at least 3 months after the anemia has been corrected in order to replace iron stores. A dosage schedule for ferrous sulfate or gluconate tablets (200 mg) is one tablet three times daily for 2 months followed by one tablet daily for 4 months. Parenteral iron is rarely indicated. Folic acid (5 mg daily for 1 month) should also be given. Blood transfusion may be necessary if anemia is severe.

B. Specific Measures

Pyrantel, mebendazole, albendazole, and levamisole are highly effective drugs for treatment of both hookworm species; ivermectin is not effective. Mebendazole, pyrantel, or albendazole can be used to treat concurrent trichuriasis, and all of the drugs can be used to treat concurrent ascariasis. The drugs are given before or after meals, without purges. For these drugs, mild gastrointestinal side effects and headache may occur; none should be used in pregnancy. Albendazole (400 mg) or mebendazole (500 mg) is being used for repeated (up to 3 times yearly) mass treatment of children for intestinal parasites (hookworm, ascariasis, trichuriasis). Improvements have been seen in blood hemoglobin levels and improved growth, even in light infections in young children. However, drug resistance may be emerging.

1. Albendazole—Albendazole given orally once only at a dosage of 400 mg results in the cure of 85–95% of patients with *Ancylostoma* infection and markedly reduces the worm burden in those not cured. Because cure rates for single-dose treatments of *Necator* infection were 33–90%, treatment should be continued for 2–3 days, especially in heavy infections. Albendazole is available in the United States, though it is not FDA-approved for this indication.

2. Pyrantel pamoate—In *A duodenale* infections, pyrantel given as a single dose, 10 mg (base)/kg (maximum 1 g), produces cures in 76–98% of cases and a marked reduction in the worm burden in the remainder. Drug resistance has been reported from northwestern Australia. For *N americanus* infections, a single dose may give a satisfactory cure rate in light infection, but for moderate or heavy infection a 3-day course is necessary. If the species is unknown, treat as for necatoriasis. Mild and transient drowsiness and headache may occur.

3. Mebendazole—When mebendazole is given at a dosage of 100 mg twice daily for 3 days, reported cure rates for both hookworm species range from 35% to 95%. A single 500 mg dose may be sufficient for light infections. Mebendazole sometime stimulates ascarids to emerge from the nose or mouth.

4. Levamisole— Levamisole is given as a single dose of 150 mg. The drug is less effective against *N americanus.*

Prognosis

If the disease is recognized before serious secondary complications appear, complete recovery is the rule following treatment.

Eosinophilic Enteritis

In Australia, *A caninum*, the dog hookworm, has been found to cause abdominal pain, diarrhea, and peripheral eosinophilia. Pathologic findings may include iliac ulcerations and regional lymphandenitis. The diagnosis is made by finding an immature adult worm at endoscopy. Treatment with albendazole or mebendazole can be tried.

Brooker S et al: Human hookworm infection in the 21st century. Adv Parasitol 2004;58:197. [PMID: 15603764]

Bungiro R et al: Hookworm infection: new developments and prospects for control. Curr Opin Infect Dis 2004;17:421. [PMID: 15353961]

Crompton DW et al: Nutritional impact of intestinal helminthiasis during the human life cycle. Annu Rev Nutr 2002;22:35. [PMID: 12055337]

Hotez PJ et al: Hookworm infection. N Engl J Med 2004; 351:799. [PMID: 15317893]

LOIASIS

ESSENTIALS OF DIAGNOSIS

- History of residence in rain forests of tropical Africa.
- Transitory (Calabar) swellings on various parts of the body.
- Adult worms noted beneath the skin or under the conjunctival epithelium.
- Characteristic microfilariae in the blood showing diurnal periodicity; eosinophilia; positive serologic tests.

General Considerations

Loiasis is a chronic filarial disease caused by infection with *Loa loa*. The infection occurs in humans and monkeys in rain and swamp forest areas of West Africa from Nigeria to Angola and throughout the Congo river watershed of central Africa eastward to southwestern Sudan and western Uganda. An estimated 3–13 million persons are infected.

The adult worms live in the subcutaneous tissues for up to 12 years. Gravid females release microfilariae into the bloodstream, which subsequently are ingested in a blood meal by the vector-intermediate host, female chrysops species, which are day-biting flies. When the fly feeds again, the larval stage can infect a new host or cause superinfection. The time to worm maturity and detection of new microfilariae is 6 months to several years. Unlike the other filarial parasites of humans, *L loa* does not harbor endosymbiont bacteria.

Clinical Findings

A. SYMPTOMS AND SIGNS

Many infected persons are asymptomatic. In symptomatic persons, the worms (females, 4–7 cm × 0.5 mm) are evidenced by their temporary appearance beneath the skin or conjunctiva, by unilateral edema of an extremity, or by Calabar swellings. The latter are subcutaneous edematous reactions, 3–10 cm in diameter, nonpitting and nonerythematous, and at times associated with low-grade fever, local pain, and pruritus. The swellings or edema may migrate a few centimeters for 2–3 days or stay in place before they subside. At irregular intervals, they recur at the same or different sites, but only one appears at a time. When near joints, they may be temporarily disabling. Migration across the eye may be asymptomatic or produce pain, intense conjunctivitis, and eyelid edema. Dying adult worms may elicit small nodules or local sterile abscesses, and dead worms may result in radiologically detectable calcification.

Microfilariae in the blood do not induce symptoms. Rarely, however, they enter the central nervous system and may cause encephalitis, myelitis, or jacksonian seizures; the larvae can also induce lesions and complications in the retina, heart, lungs, kidneys, and other tissues.

Natives generally have a mild form of the infection or are asymptomatic but are microfilaremic and serologically positive. The disease among visitors, however, is often characterized by more pronounced immunologically mediated symptoms (frequent and debilitating Calabar swellings, elevated leukocyte and eosinophil counts, hypergammaglobulinemia, increased polyclonal IgE) and frequently a positive serologic test but nondetectable microfilaremia.

B. LABORATORY FINDINGS

Specific diagnosis is made by finding characteristic microfilariae in daytime (10 AM to 4 PM) blood specimens by concentration methods; in order of increasing sensitivity, they are (1) thick films, (2) Knott's concentration, and (3) Nuclepore filtration. Multiple daily samples may be needed. Presumptive diagnosis that permits treatment is based on Calabar swellings or eye migration, a history of residence in an endemic area, and marked eosinophilia (40% or greater). Serologic tests may be positive, but cross-reactions occur with other filarial diseases and sometimes with other nematode infections. A PCR test, highly sensitive and specific, can detect the organism in some amicrofilaremic persons. Expatriates are usually amicrofilaremic.

Treatment & Prognosis

See specialized sources and references for details on proper use of diethylcarbamazine (drug of choice both as a microfilaricide and macrofilaricide), since side effects to dying microfilariae may be severe, and life-threatening encephalitis can occur rarely. The dosage is 50 mg once (day 1), 50 mg three times daily (day 2), 100 mg three times daily (day 3), and 3 mg/kg three times daily (days 4–21). One course of treatment cures about 50% of patients; three courses, 90%. Reactions are more likely with pretreatment microfilaria counts greater than 25/mcL. Apheresis has been used to reduce parasite loads before starting diethylcarbamazine. Prednisone (40–60 mg/d) is sometimes indicated in heavily infected persons to minimize reactions. Albendazole (200 mg twice daily for 3 weeks) and ivermectin (multiple doses) continue to be evaluated for microfilariae reduction. Albendazole is preferred because of its lower risk of encephalitis. Surgical removal of adult worms from the eye or skin is not recommended.

In the United States, diethylcarbamazine is available only from the Parasitic Diseases Drug Service, Centers for Disease Control and Prevention, Atlanta, GA 30333, telephone 404-639-3670.

Individual protection is facilitated by daytime use of insect repellent and by wearing light-colored clothing with long sleeves and trousers. Diethylcarbamazine prophylaxis, 300 mg weekly, may be useful if the risk of exposure is high. It is not indicated, however, for the casual traveler or for persons who might previously have acquired any of the filarial infections.

Most infections run a benign course, but some are accompanied by severe and temporarily disabling symptoms. The prognosis is excellent with treatment, except for patients with high pretreatment microfilariae counts.

Blum J et al: Encephalopathy following *Loa loa* treatment with albendazole. Acta Trop 2001;78:63. [PMID: 11164753]

Pion SD et al: Loiasis: the individual factors associated with the presence of microfilaraemia. Ann Trop Med Parasitol 2005; 99:491. [PMID: 16004708]

Tabi TE et al: Human loiasis in a Cameroonian village: a double-blind, placebo-controlled, crossover clinical trial of a three-day albendazole regimen. Am J Trop Med Hyg 2004;71: 211. [PMID: 15306713]

ONCHOCERCIASIS

 ESSENTIALS OF DIAGNOSIS

- *Skin: pruritus, excoriations, pigmentary changes, papular eruptions, atrophy, licenoid thickening.*
- *Subcutaneous nodules.*
- *Eyes: itching, photophobia, conjunctivitis, punctate and sclerosing keratitis, iridocyclitis, posterior segment lesions; impaired vision to blindness.*
- *Microfilariae in skin snips and on slit-lamp examination of cornea or anterior chamber; adult worms in subcutaneous nodules.*
- *Positive serologic tests.*

General Considerations

Onchocerciasis is a chronic filarial disease caused by *Onchocerca volvulus*. An estimated 18 million persons are infected, of whom 3–4 million have skin disease, 0.3 million are blinded, and 0.5 million severely visually impaired. In hyperendemic areas, more than 40% of inhabitants over 40 years of age are blind. The infection, predominant in West Africa, also occurs in many other parts of tropical Africa and in localized areas of the southwestern Arabian peninsula, southern Mexico, Guatemala, Venezuela, Colombia, and northwestern Brazil. The West African savanna strain is especially associated with severe blinding eye lesions. In some areas of Africa where blindness is not a severe problem, cutaneous onchocerciasis can nevertheless be severe and disabling.

Humans are the only important host. The vector and intermediate host are simulium flies, day biters that breed in rivers and fast-flowing streams and become infected by ingesting microfilariae with a human blood meal; at subsequent feedings, they can infect new susceptible hosts.

The skin and eye changes are the result of dead or dying microfilariae. However, recent findings suggest that the predominant corneal changes may be due to endoxins from *Wolbachia* bacteria, which are obligate intracellular organisms in the worms.

The advent of the safe drug ivermectin has led to effective individual treatment and to mass control programs. In target communities, mass treatment yearly in Africa and twice yearly in the Americas combined with anti-vector measures has resulted in a dramatic decrease in the prevalence of skin and eye disease. The drug has been provided free by the manufacturer, Merck & Co.

Clinical Findings

A. Symptoms and Signs

Adult worms, which can live for up to 15 years, typically are contained in fibrous subcutaneous nodules that cause insignificant pathology and are painless, freely movable, and 0.5–1 cm in diameter. Many nodules, however, are deep in the connective and muscular tissues. The interval from exposure to onset of symptoms can be as long as 1–3 years. Female worms release motile microfilariae into the skin, subcutaneous tissues, lymphatics, and eyes; microfilariae are occasionally seen in the urine but rarely in blood or cerebrospinal fluid. Skin manifestations are localized or cover large areas. Pruritus may be severe, leading to skin excoriation and lichenification; other findings include pigmentary changes, papules, scaling, atrophy, pendulous skin, and acute inflammation. Pruritus may occur in the absence of skin lesions. There may be marked enlargement of femoral and inguinal nodes and generalized lymph node enlargement. Microfilariae in the eye may lead to visual impairment and blindness; findings include itching, photophobia, anterior segment changes (limbitis, punctate and sclerosing keratitis, iritis, secondary glaucoma, cataract), and posterior segment changes (optic neuritis, optic atrophy, chorioretinitis, and other retinal and choroidal findings). Infected expatriates, as compared with indigenous persons, may show more prominent dermatitis and eosinophilia but have a low to nondetectable microfiladerma or eosinophilia and an absence of nodules and eye disease.

B. Laboratory Findings

Diagnosis is by demonstrating microfilariae in skin snips (usually obtained with a punch biopsy instrument), identifying them in the cornea or anterior chamber by slit-lamp examination (after the patient has sat with head lowered between knees for 2 minutes), in nodule aspirates, or sometimes in the urine. The preferred site for skin snips is the iliac crest in Africa and the deltoid and scapula areas in the Americas. Skin snips placed in saline are incubated for 2–4 hours before examination, or overnight for low-intensity infections. Where available, the PCR test done on skin snips and urine has a high sensitivity and specificity; it is positive only in active infection. Adult worms may be recovered in excised nodules, whereas ultrasound has been used to detect nonpalpable onchocercomas and to distinguish them from other lesions (lipomas, fibromas, lymph nodes, foreign body granulomas). Traditional serologic tests are usually positive, but cross-reactions occur with other forms of filariasis, and the tests do not distinguish current from past infection. The use of recombinant antigens has resulted in the development of the highly sensitive and specific ELISA and rapid-format card tests. Methods to detect circulating antigen are being evaluated but appear less useful. Eosinophilia (15–50%), polyclonal hypergammaglobulinemia, and elevated IgE levels are common. The Mazzotti oral test, done only if the above tests are negative, is based on the ingestion of diethylcarbamazine (0.5 to 1.0 mg/kg); a skin reaction or pruritus within several hours is highly suggestive of the infection. The Mazzotti skin test is no longer recommended because of the potential for dangerous reactions.

Treatment & Prognosis

Drug treatment is with ivermectin (a microfilaricide) as a single oral dose of 150 mcg/kg given with water on an empty stomach; the patient should remain fasting for 2 more hours. The number of microfilariae in the skin diminishes markedly within 2–3 days, remains low for about 6 months, and then gradually increases; the number of microfilariae in the anterior chamber of the eye, however, decrease slowly over months, eventually disappear, and then gradually return. The optimum frequency of treatment to control symptoms and prevent disease progression remains to be determined. To initiate treatment, three schedules have been proposed: (1) an initial and repeat dose at 6 months, (2) repeated doses at 3-month intervals for a year, or (3) repeated doses at monthly intervals for a total of three doses. Treatment is repeated at intervals of 6 months for 2 years and yearly thereafter until the patient is asymptomatic or until the worms have died normally (12–15 years). Although ivermectin is not effective in killing adult worms, evidence suggests that the drug has a limited effect on intrauterine embryogenesis. Adverse reactions, which are more marked with the first dose, are mild in 9% of patients and severe in 0.2%; these include edema (face and limbs), fever, pruritus, lymphadenitis, malaise, and hypotension. Ivermectin does not, however, cause a severe reaction in the eyes or skin as occurs with diethylcarbamazine. With the initial treatment only, patients with microfilariae in the cornea or anterior chamber may benefit from several days of prednisone treatment (1 mg/kg/d) to avoid inflammatory eye reactions. Ivermectin should not be used in the presence of concurrent *L loa* infections, in early pregnancy (no adverse events have been reported), or in patients with central nervous system diseases in which increased penetration of ivermectin may occur into the central nervous system. Safety in children under 15 kg has not been established. The possibility of drug resistance is emerging. In Latin America only, nodulectomy continues to be used for nodules on or near the head.

Diethylcarbamazine is no longer recommended in onchocerciasis therapy because of its potential for severe reactions and because it was no more effective than ivermectin in reducing microfilariae loads. For selected patients in whom repeated ivermectin treatments do not control symptoms, suramin can be given for its macrofilaricidal action; however, because of suramin's toxicity and complex administration, it should only be administered by experts. Amocarzine is under evaluation for its macrofilaricidal and microfilaricidal actions. Albendazole does not kill microfilariae but interferes with early embryogenesis; the drug is not macrofilarialcidal. Doxycycline has potential as a chemotherapeutic agent based on findings that a 6–8 week course of treatment has a long-term sterilizing effect through the drug's action on *Wolbachia* bacteria, which are obligate intracellular organisms in onchocerca adults and microfilariae.

With treatment, some skin and ocular lesions improve and ocular progression is prevented. The prognosis is unfavorable only for those patients who are seen for the first time with already far-advanced ocular onchocerciasis.

Fobi G et al: A randomized, double-blind, controlled trial of the effects of ivermectin at normal and high doses, given annually or three-monthly, against *Onchocerca volvulus*: ophthalmological results. Trans R Soc Trop Med Hyg 2005;99: 279. [PMID: 15708387]

Hoerauf A et al: Onchocerciasis. BMJ 2003;326:207. [PMID: 12543839]

Hopkins DR et al: Whither onchocerciasis control in Africa? Am J Trop Med Hyg 2005;72:1. [PMID: 15728857]

Kamgno J et al: Adverse systemic reactions to treatment of onchocerciasis with ivermectin at normal and high doses given annually or three-monthly. Trans R Soc Trop Med Hyg 2004;98:496. [PMID: 15186939]

Tielsch JM et al: Impact of ivermectin on illness and disability associated with onchocerciasis. Trop Med Int Hlth 2004;9: A45. [PMID: 15078278]

Twum-Danso NA et al: Variation in incidence of serious adverse events after onchocerciasis treatment with ivermectin in areas of Cameroon co-endemic for loiasis. Trop Med Int Health 2003;8:820. [PMID: 12950668]

STRONGYLOIDIASIS

ESSENTIALS OF DIAGNOSIS

- Pruritic dermatitis at sites of larval penetration.
- Diarrhea, epigastric pain, nausea, malaise, weight loss.
- Cough, rales, transient pulmonary infiltrates.
- Hyperinfection syndrome: Severe diarrhea, bronchopneumonia, ileus, septicemia.
- Positive serology (useful for screening); eosinophilia; larvae detected in stool, especially by the agar plate culture method.

General Considerations

Strongyloidiasis is caused by infection with *Strongyloides stercoralis* (2–2.5 mm × 30–50 mcm). Major symptoms result from adult parasitism, principally in the duodenum and jejunum, or from larval migration through pulmonary and cutaneous tissues. The primary host is humans, but dogs, cats, and primates have been found infected with strains indistinguishable from those of humans. Human infections with *Strongyloides fulleborni* have been encountered in Papua New Guinea and parts of Africa.

Strongyloidiasis is endemic in tropical and subtropical regions. Although prevalence is generally low, in some areas disease rates exceed 25%. In temperate areas, the disease occurs sporadically. In the United States, highest infection rates are found in immigrants from endemic areas, in parts of Appalachia, and in the Southeast. Puerto Rico is also an endemic area. Multiple infections in households are common, and prevalence may be high in institutions, particularly mental institutions (2–4%). The infection is also prevalent among immunocompromised persons (see below).

The parasite is uniquely capable of maintaining its life cycle both within the human host and in soil. Infection occurs when filariform larvae in soil penetrate the skin, enter the bloodstream, and are carried to the lungs, where they escape from capillaries into alveoli and ascend the bronchial tree to the glottis. The larvae are then swallowed and carried to the duodenum and upper jejunum, where maturation to the adult stage takes place. The parasitic female, generally held to be parthenogenetic, matures and lives embedded in the muscosa for up to 5 years. Eggs hatch to free noninfectious larvae (rhabditform) that pass to the ground via the feces.

In moist soil, these larvae metamorphose into the infective (filariform) larvae. However, the parasite also has a free-living cycle in soil, in which some rhabditiform larvae develop into adults that produce eggs from which rhabditiform larvae emerge to continue the life cycle.

Autoinfection in humans, which probably occurs at a low rate in most infections, is an important factor in determining worm burden and is responsible for the persistence of infections up to decades. Autoinfection takes place in the lower bowel when some rhabditiform larvae develop into filariform larvae that can penetrate the intestinal mucosa, enter the intestinal lymphatic and portal circulation, are carried to the lungs, and return to the small bowel to complete the cycle. This process is accelerated by achlorhydria, constipation, diverticula, and other conditions that reduce bowel motility. In addition, an external autoinfection cycle can occur as a result of fecal contamination of the perianal area.

The hyperinfection syndrome occurs when autoinfection greatly increases; a marked rise in the worm burden occurs with massive dissemination of filariform larvae to the lungs and other tissues. Local inflammatory reactions may follow, and occasionally larvae metamorphose into adults. Hyperinfection—as well as recrudescence of chronic asymptomatic infection—is generally initiated as a result of depressed host cellular immunity, especially associated with use of an immunosuppressive drug, debilitation, malnourishment, radiotherapy, diabetic ketoacidosis, alcohol abuse, or malignancy. Although hyperinfection is infrequent in AIDS, recrudescence and a protracted, difficult-to-cure course may occur. Human T-cell lymphotropic virus, type 1 (HTLV1) infection is highly associated with strongyloidiasis, especially with hyperinfection.

Clinical Findings

A. Symptoms and Signs

Up to 30% of infected persons are asymptomatic. The time from larval penetration of the skin by filariform larvae until their appearance in the feces is 3–4 weeks. An acute syndrome can sometimes be recognized in which cutaneous symptoms, usually of the feet, are followed by pulmonary and then intestinal symptoms. Patients usually present, however, with chronic symptoms (continuous or with irregular exacerbations) that can persist for years or for life. Immigrants from endemic areas should be screened for *Strongyloides* infection if they are to be treated with an immunosuppressive drug.

1. **Cutaneous manifestations**—In acute infection in sensitized patients, there may be focal edema, inflammation, petechiae, serpiginous or urticarial tracts, and intense itching. In chronic infections, both stationary urticaria and larva currens occur, the latter characterized by transient eruptions that migrate in serpiginous tracts.

2. **Intestinal manifestations**—Symptoms range from mild to severe, the most common being diarrhea, abdominal pain, and flatulence. Anorexia, nausea, vomiting, epigastric tenderness, and pruritus ani may be present; with increasing severity, fever and malaise may appear. Diarrhea may alternate with constipation, and in severe cases the feces contain mucus and blood. The pain is often epigastric in location and may mimic a duodenal ulcer. Malabsorption or a protein-losing enteropathy can result from a large intestinal worm burden.

3. **Pulmonary manifestations**—With migration of larvae through the lungs, bronchi, and trachea, symptoms may be limited to a dry cough and throat irritation, or low-grade fever, dyspnea, wheezing, and hemoptysis may occur; asthma is rare. Bronchopneumonia, bronchitis, pleural effusion, progressive dyspnea, and miliary abscesses can develop; the cough may become productive of an odorless, mucopurulent sputum.

4. **Hyperinfection syndrome**—Intense dissemination of filariform larvae to the lungs and other tissues can result in additional complications, including pleural effusion, pericarditis and myocarditis, hepatic granulomas, cholecystitis, purpura, ulcerating lesions at all levels of the gastrointestinal tract, central nervous system involvement, paralytic ileus, perforation and peritonitis, polymicrobial sepsis, and meningitis (due to larval carriage of enterobacteria from the colon), cachexia, shock, and death. Nephrotic syndrome is encountered on rare occasions.

B. Laboratory Findings

1. **Detection of eggs and larvae**—Eggs are seldom found in feces. Diagnosis, which may be difficult, requires finding the larval stages in feces or duodenal fluid. Rhabditiform larvae may be found in recently passed stool specimens; filariform larvae, however, will be present in specimens held in the laboratory for some hours. Four to six specimens, some unpreserved, should be collected at 2-day intervals or longer (the number of larvae in feces varies from day to day). Since the sensitivity of direct microscopic examination of one specimen is about 30%, it is essential that half of the specimens be processed, unpreserved by a more sensitive method, either agar plate culture (the most sensitive, up to 90%), Baermann concentration, or Harda-Mori filtration.

The diagnosis can sometimes be made by finding rhabditiform larvae or ova in mucus obtained by means of the duodenal string test or by duodenal intubation and aspiration. Duodenal biopsy is seldom indicated but will confirm the diagnosis in most patients. Rarely, filariform or rhabditiform larvae can be detected in urine or in sputum or bronchial washings during the pulmonary phase of the disease.

2. **Serologic and hematologic findings**—For screening, the ELISA is sensitive (84–95%) and specific (84–92%), but cross-reactions can occur with filarial and other helminthic infections. A newly developed dot blot test appears to have fewer cross-reactions. A positive test indicates current or past infection. These IgG antibodies remain detectable in immunocompromised patients.

In chronic low-grade intestinal strongyloidiasis, the white blood cell count is often normal, with a normal or slightly elevated percentage of eosinophils. However, with increasing larval migration, eosinophilia may reach 50% and leukocytosis 20,000/mcL. In immunocompromised patients, eosinophilia may not be seen. Mild anemia may be present.

3. **Hyperinfection**—Findings may include hypoproteinemia, malabsorption, abnormal liver function, extensive pulmonary infiltrates, and multiple organ failures. Filariform larvae may appear in the urine. Eosinopenia, when present, is thought to be an unfavorable prognostic sign.

C. Imaging

Small bowel x-rays may show inflammation, irritability, and prominent mucosal folds; there may also be bowel dilation, delayed emptying, and ulcerative duodenitis. In chronic infections, the findings can resemble those in nontropical and tropical sprue, or there may be narrowing, rigidity, and diminished peristalsis. During pulmonary migration of larvae, chest films are normal or show fine miliary nodules or irregular changing patches of pneumonitis, abscess, or pleural effusion.

Differential Diagnosis

Because of varied signs and symptoms, the diagnosis of strongyloidiasis is often difficult. Eosinophilia plus one or more of the following factors should further enhance consideration of the diagnosis: endemic area exposure, duodenal ulcer-like pain, persistent or recurrent diarrhea, malabsorption, recurrent coughing or wheezing, and transient pulmonary infiltrates. The duodenitis and jejunitis of strongyloidiasis can also mimic giardiasis, cholecystitis, and pancreatitis. Transient pulmonary infiltrates must be differentiated from tropical pulmonary eosinophilia and Löffler's syndrome. The diagnosis should be considered among the many causes of malabsorption in the tropics; in the differential diagnosis of ulcerative colitis; and in immunocompromised persons, including HIV-infected patients.

Treatment

Since *Strongyloides* can multiply in humans, treatment should continue until the parasite is eradicated. In follow-up, multiple stool examinations should be done at weekly intervals, preferably by the agar plate culture method. Patients receiving immunosuppressive therapy should be examined for strongyloidiasis before and at intervals during that treatment. Patients with strongyloidiasis infections who are resistant to treatment should be evaluated for AIDS. In concurrent infection with strongyloidiasis and ascariasis or hookworm (which is common), eradicate the latter infections first.

The drug of choice in treatment is ivermectin, which appears to be equal in effectiveness to thiabendazole but has far fewer side effects.

A. IVERMECTIN

The dosage is 200 mcg/kg orally followed by a second dose within several days (cure rates range from 82% to 98%). An enema preparation is being evaluated for patients unable to take oral medication. A parenteral formulation of ivermectin is available in some countries but is licensed only for veterinary use. In the hyperinfection syndrome in immunocompromised patients with or without AIDS, it may be necessary to prolong treatment or change to thiabendazole.

B. ALBENDAZOLE

Albendazole is given at a dosage of 400 mg twice daily for 3–7 days and repeated in 1 week; cure rates in several studies ranged from 38% to 95%. In comparative studies, albendazole is less effective than ivermectin.

C. THIABENDAZOLE

An oral dose of 25 mg/kg (maximum, 1.5 g per dose) is given after meals twice daily for 2–3 days. Repeat the course in 2 weeks. A 7-day (or longer) course is needed for disseminated infections. Tablet and liquid formulations are available; tablets should be chewed. Side effects, including headache, weakness, vomiting, vertigo, and decreased mental alertness, occur in as many as 30% of patients and may be severe, particularly if given for more than 2 days. Other potentially serious side effects occur rarely. Erythema multiforme and the Stevens-Johnson syndrome have been associated with thiabendazole therapy; several fatalities have occurred in children. The drug is not available in the United States.

Prognosis

The prognosis is favorable except in the hyperinfection syndrome and in infections associated with malnutrition, advanced liver disease, immunologic disorders, or the use of immunosuppressive drugs. In selected instances, to control infections that cannot be eradicated, once-monthly treatments can be tried with a 1-day dose of ivermectin or 2-day course of thiabendazole.

Concha R et al: Intestinal strongyloidiasis: recognition, management, and determinants of outcome. J Clin Gastroenterol 2005;39:2031. [PMID: 15718861]

Lanzafam M et al: Strongyloidiasis in an HIV-1-infected patient after highly active antiretroviral therapy–induced immune restoration. J Infect Dis 2005;191:1027. [PMID: 15717283]

Lim S et al: Complicated and fatal *Strongyloides* infection in Canadians: risk factors, diagnosis and management. CMAJ 2004;171:479. [PMID: 15337730]

Nuesch R et al: Imported strongyloidosis: a longitudinal analysis of 31 cases. J Travel Med 2005;12:80. [PMID: 155996452]

Pacanowski J et al: Subcutaneous ivermectin as a safe salvage therapy in *Strongyloides stercoralis* hyperinfection syndrome: a case report. Am J Trop Med Hyg 2005;73:122. [PMID: 16014846]

Pornsuriyasak P et al: Disseminated stronglyloidiasis successfully treated with extended duration ivermectin combined with albendazole: a case report of intractable strongyloidiasis. Southeast Asian J Trop Med Public Health 2004;35:531. [PMID: 15689061]

TRICHINOSIS (Trichinelliosis, Trichinellosis)

 ESSENTIALS OF DIAGNOSIS

- *History of ingestion of raw or inadequately cooked pork, boar, or bear.*
- *First week: diarrhea, cramps, malaise.*
- *Second week to 1–2 months: muscle pain and tenderness, fever, periorbital and facial edema, conjunctivitis, systemic toxicity.*

- *Eosinophilia and elevated serum enzymes; positive serologic tests; larvae in muscle biopsy.*

General Considerations

Trichinosis is caused worldwide by *Trichinella spiralis*. The disease is present wherever pork is eaten but is a greater problem in many temperate areas than in the tropics. Four other species of *Trichinella* have been recognized in humans: *T nativa* appears to be restricted to Arctic and sub-Arctic regions (including Alaska) and *T nelsoni* to tropical Africa. *T pseudospiralis*, reported rarely worldwide, occurs as a persistent muscular infection accompanied by prolonged myalgia, muscular weakness and swelling, elevated muscle enzymes, and asthenia. *T britovi* occurs in palaearctic areas of Europe and Asia.

Human infections occur sporadically or in outbreaks. Infection is usually acquired by eating viable encysted larvae in raw or uncooked pork or pork products. Ground beef has also been a source of infection when adulterated with pork or inadvertently contaminated in a common meat grinder. In some cases, the source of infection is the flesh of dogs (East Asia), horses (France), or wild animals, particularly bears, walruses, bush pigs, foxes, or cougars. In the United States, there has been a marked reduction in prevalence in pigs (rates in commercial pork are nil to 0.007%). As a result, only about fifty human infections have been reported yearly, 60% in association with eating wild game, mainly bear.

Gastric juices liberate the encysted larvae. They rapidly mature and mate, and the adult female then burrows into the mucosa of the small intestine. Within 4–5 days, the female begins to discharge viviparous larvae (100 × 6 mcm) that are disseminated via the lymphatics and bloodstream to most body tissues. Larvae that reach striated muscle encyst and remain viable for months to years; those that reach other tissues are rapidly destroyed. The adult worms (2–3.6 mm × 75–90 mcm) survive for up to about 6 weeks.

In the natural cycle, larvae develop into adult worms in the intestines when a carnivore or omnivore ingests parasitized muscle. Pigs generally become infected by feeding on uncooked food scraps or, less often, by eating infected rats. Other reservoir hosts include swine, dogs, cats, rats, and many wild animals, including the wolf, bear, and boar; marine animals in the Arctic; and the hyena, jackal, and lion in the tropics.

Clinical Findings

A. SYMPTOMS AND SIGNS

The incubation period is 2–7 days (range: 12 hours to 28 days). Severity depends on intensity of infection, tissues invaded, immune status and age of the host (children have less severe infections), and perhaps the strain of the parasite. Findings range from asymptom-

atic to a mild febrile illness with short-lasting symptoms to a severe progressive illness with multiple system involvement that in rare cases is fatal.

1. Intestinal stage—When present, intestinal symptoms persist for 1–7 days: diarrhea, abdominal cramps, and malaise are the major findings; nausea and vomiting occur less frequently; and constipation is uncommon. Fever, eosinophilia, and leukocytosis are rare during the first week.

2. Muscle invasion stage—This begins at the end of the first week and lasts about 6 weeks. Parasitized muscles show an intense inflammatory reaction. Findings include fever (low-grade to marked); muscle pain and tenderness, edema, and spasm; periorbital and facial edema; sweating; photophobia and conjunctivitis; weakness or prostration; pain on swallowing; dyspnea, coughing, and hoarseness; subconjunctival, retinal, and nail splinter hemorrhages; and rashes and formication. The most frequently parasitized muscles and sites of findings are the masseters, tongue, diaphragm, intercostals, extraocular, laryngeal, paravertebral, nuchal, deltoid, pectoral, gluteus, biceps, and gastrocnemius. Inflammatory reactions around larvae that reach tissues other than muscle may result in a broad range of findings, including the development of meningitis, encephalitis, myocarditis, bronchopneumonia, nephritis, and peripheral and cranial nerve disorders.

3. Convalescent stage—This generally begins in the second month but in severe infections may not begin before 3 months or longer. Vague muscle pains and malaise may persist for several more months. Permanent muscular atrophy has been reported.

B. LABORATORY FINDINGS

The diagnosis is supported by findings of eosinophilia, elevated serum muscle enzymes (creatine kinase, lactate dehydrogenase, aspartate aminotransferase), and positive serologic tests. There may be a marked hypergammaglobulinemia with reversal of the albumin-globulin ratio. Absence of an elevated sedimentation rate is a useful diagnostic clue. Confirmation of the diagnosis is by detection of larvae in muscle biopsy specimens.

Leukocytosis and eosinophilia appear during the second week. The proportion of eosinophils rises to a maximum of 20–90% in the third or fourth week and then slowly declines to normal over the next few months.

Serologic tests can detect most clinically manifest cases but are not sufficiently sensitive to detect low-level infections (ie, a few larvae per gram of ingested muscle). More than one antibody test should be used and then repeated to observe for seroconversion or for a rising titer. Seropositivity may not appear for 3–5 weeks, peak in 2–3 months, and remain detectable for 2–3 years. The ELISA becomes positive in 80–100% of symptomatic persons. The bentonite flocculation (BF) test (positive titer > 1:5) is highly sensitive and specific. The immunofluorescent test (positive titer > 16) may become positive in the second week. IgM and IgE antibodies may also appear but are less sensitive indicators of infection than IgG. Testing by immunoblot is also available. Circulating antigen—now being evaluated—can be detected about 2 weeks after infection in heavily infected persons and in 3–4 weeks in light infections. The intradermal test is no longer recommended, as it may remain positive for years and batches of antigen vary in potency.

Adult worms may be looked for in feces, though they are seldom found. In the second week, there are occasional larvae in blood, duodenal washings, and, rarely, in centrifuged spinal fluid. In the third to fourth weeks, biopsy of skeletal muscle (approximately 1 cm³) may be definitive (particularly gastrocnemius and pectoralis), preferably at a site of swelling or tenderness or near tendinous insertions. Portions of the specimen should be examined microscopically by compression between glass slides, by digestion, and by preparation of multiple histologic sections. If the biopsy is done too early, larvae may not be detectable. Myositis even in the absence of larvae is a significant finding.

C. IMAGING

Chest films during the acute phase may show disseminated or localized infiltrates. Late calcification of muscle cysts cannot be detected radiologically.

Complications

The more important complications are granulomatous pneumonitis, encephalitis, and cardiac failure.

Differential Diagnosis

Because of its protean manifestations, trichinosis may resemble many other diseases. Eosinophilia, muscle pain and tenderness, and fever should lead the physician to consider collagen vascular disorders such as dermatomyositis or polyarteritis nodosa, which is generally accompanied by an elevated sedimentation rate.

Treatment

Treatment is principally supportive, since in most cases recovery is spontaneous without sequelae.

A. INTESTINAL PHASE

Though supporting evidence for efficacy is limited, albendazole, because of its relatively high absorption and freedom from adverse reactions, is proposed as the drug of choice in a dosage of 400 mg orally twice daily for 10–15 days. Mebendazole is an alternative drug at a dosage of 200–400 mg orally three times daily for 3 days, followed by 400–500 mg three times daily for 10–15 days. Corticosteroids are contraindicated in the intestinal phase.

B. MUSCLE INVASION PHASE

In this stage, severe infections require hospitalization and high doses of corticosteroids (40–60 mg/d for 1–2 days), followed by lower doses for several days or weeks to control symptoms. However, because corticosteroids may suppress the inflammatory response to adult worms, they should be used only when symptoms are severe. Although drug treatment has not been shown to be effective in the muscle invasion stage, albendazole or mebendazole can be tried.

Prevention

The frequency and intensity of infection in the United States and other countries have been significantly reduced by public health measures to prevent feeding of uncooked garbage to hogs and by animal inspection (not in the United States). The chief safeguard against trichinosis is adequate cooking of pork to 160 °F (71 °C) or by freezing meat at –17 °C for 20 days (longer if meat is over 15 cm thick). *T nativa* in game is often relatively resistant to freezing. Low doses of gamma irradiation are also effective in killing larvae.

Prognosis

Death is rare—sometimes within 2–3 weeks in overwhelming infections, more often in 4–8 weeks from a major complication such as cardiac failure or pneumonia.

Centers for Disease Control and Prevention (CDC): Trichinellosis associated with bear meat—New York and Tennessee, 2003. MMWR Morb Mortal Wkly Rep 2004;53:606. [PMID: 15254452]

Pozio E et al: Clinical aspects, diagnosis and treatment of trichinellosis. Expert Rev Anti Infect Ther 2003;1:471. [PMID: 15482143]

Puljiz I et al: Electrocardiographic changes and myocarditis in trichinellosis: a retrospective study of 154 patients. Ann Trop Med Parasitol 2005;99:403. [PMID: 15949188]

Watt G et al: Areas of uncertainty in the management of human trichinellosis: a clinical perspective. Expert Rev Anti Infect Ther 2004;2:649. [PMID: 15482227]

TRICHURIASIS
(Trichocephaliasis, Whipworm)

Trichuris trichiura is a common intestinal parasite of humans throughout the world, particularly in the subtropics and tropics. Persons of all ages are affected, but infection is heaviest and most frequent in children. The slender worms, 30–50 mm in length, attach by means of their anterior whip-like end to the mucosa of the large intestine, particularly to the cecum. Eggs are passed in the feces but require 2–4 weeks for larval development after reaching the soil before becoming infective; thus, person-to-person transmission is not possible. Infections are acquired by ingestion of the infective egg. The larvae hatch in the small intestine and mature in the large bowel but do not migrate through the tissues.

Clinical Findings

A. SYMPTOMS AND SIGNS

Light (fewer than 10,000 eggs per gram of feces) to moderate infections rarely cause symptoms. Heavy infections (30,000 or more eggs per gram of feces) may be accompanied by abdominal cramps, tenesmus, diarrhea, distention, flatulence, and nausea and vomiting. With persistent dysentery and blood loss into the stool, the trichuris dysentery syndrome can appear—particularly in malnourished young children—which is accompanied by anemia, rectal prolapse, clubbing of fingers, growth stunting, and possibly cognitive defects. Adult worms are sometimes seen in stools. Invasion of the appendix, with resulting appendicitis, is rare.

B. LABORATORY FINDINGS

Diagnosis is by identification of characteristic eggs and, sometimes, adult worms in stools. Eosinophilia (5–20%) is common with all but light infections. Charcot-Leyden crystals may be seen in stool. Severe iron deficiency anemia may be present with heavy infections. Adult worms are seen at colonoscopy.

Treatment

Patients with asymptomatic light infections do not require treatment. For those with heavier or symptomatic infections, give mebendazole or albendazole. Thiabendazole should *not* be used because it is not effective and because it is potentially toxic. Iron replacement may be needed for anemia.

A. ALBENDAZOLE

Albendazole, given orally at a single dose of 400 mg, has resulted in cure rates of 33–90%, with marked reduction in egg counts in those not cured. For persons with heavy infections, treatment should continue for 3 days. Albendazole should not be used in pregnancy.

B. MEBENDAZOLE

A dosage of 100 mg orally twice daily before or after meals for 3 days results in cure rates of 60–80%, with marked reduction in ovum counts in the remaining patients. It may be therapeutically advantageous for the tablets to be chewed before swallowing. In mild disease, a 500-mg dose may be sufficient, whereas in severe trichuriasis, a longer course of treatment (up to 6 days) or a repeat course will often be necessary. Gastrointestinal side effects from the drug are rare. The drug is contraindicated in pregnancy.

Adams VJ et al: Efficacy of albendazole against the whipworm *Trichuris trichiura*—a randomized, controlled trial. S Afr Med J 2004;94:972. [PMID: 15662995]

Elsayed S et al: *Trichuris trichiura* worm infection. Gastrointest Endosc 2004;60:990. [PMID: 15605023]

Nascimento-Carvalho CM et al: Prolonged treatment with albendazole for massive trichuriasis infection. Pediatr Infect Dis J 2004;23:1070. [PMID: 15545874]

Sirivichayakul C et al: The effectiveness of 3, 5 or 7 days of albendazole for the treatment of *Trichuris trichiura* infection. Ann Trop Med Parasitol 2003;97:847. [PMID: 14754497]

VISCERAL LARVA MIGRANS (Toxocariasis)

ESSENTIALS OF DIAGNOSIS

- Usually in children under age 5 with history of eating soil in association with puppies.
- Fever, hepatomegaly, transient pulmonary infiltrates.
- Moderate to high leukocytosis with persistent eosinophilia hypergammaglobulinemia, high titer anti-A and anti-B isehemagglutinins, positive serologic tests; larvae occasionally in liver biopsy.

General Considerations

Most visceral larva migrans cases are due to *Toxocara canis*, an ascarid of dogs and other canids; *Toxocara cati* in domestic cats has occasionally been implicated and rarely *Belascaris procyonis* of raccoons. The adult worms live in the intestinal tracts of their respective hosts and release large numbers of eggs in the stool.

The reservoir mechanism for *T canis* is latent infection in female dogs, which is reactivated during pregnancy. Transmission from mother to puppies is via the placenta and milk. Most eggs passed to the environment are from puppies (2 weeks to 6 months) and lactating bitches (up to 6 months after parturition). The life cycle of *T cati* is similar, but transplacental transmission does not occur.

Human infections are sporadic and probably occur worldwide. In the United States, antibody seroprevalence is 5–7%. Infection is generally in dirt-eating young children who ingest *T canis* or *T cati* eggs from soil or sand contaminated with animal feces, most often from puppies. Direct contact with infected animals does not produce infection, as the eggs require a 3- to 4-week extrinsic incubation period to become infective; thereafter, eggs in soil remain infective for months to years.

In humans, hatched larvae are unable to mature but continue to migrate through the tissues for up to 6 months. Eventually they lodge in various organs, particularly the lungs and liver and less often the brain, eyes, and other tissues, where they produce eosinophilic granulomas up to 1 cm in diameter.

Clinical & Laboratory Findings

A. ACUTE INFECTION

Migrating larvae may induce fever, cough, urticaria, wheezing, hepatosplenomegaly, and lymphadenopathy. A variety of other findings may occur when other organs are invaded, including myelitis, encephalitis, and carditis. The acute phase may last 2–3 weeks, but resolution of all physical and laboratory findings may take up to 18 months.

Leukocytosis is marked (may exceed 100,000/mcL), with 30–80% due to eosinophils. Hyperglobulinemia occurs when the liver is extensively invaded and is a useful clue in diagnosis. Nonspecific isohemagglutinin titers (anti-A and anti-B) are usually greater than 1:1024. Chest radiographs may show infiltrates. Ultrasonography may detect 1-cm hypoechoic lesions in the liver, each with a thread-like hyperechoic line. With central nervous system involvement, the cerebrospinal fluid may show a marked eosinophilic pleocytosis. No parasitic forms can be found by stool examination.

Antibody detection is generally the only way to confirm a clinical diagnosis. The ELISA, the most specific (92%) and sensitive (78%) test, may permit a presumptive diagnosis, though it does not distinguish acute from prior infection. However, rising or falling titers with twofold differences are consistent with acute disease. IgE levels are also increased. Definitive diagnosis is by percutaneous liver biopsy or by direct biopsy of a granuloma at laparoscopy (mixed inflammatory infiltrate with numerous eosinophils), but these procedures are seldom justified and may not yield larvae.

B. Ocular Toxocariasis

Most cases occur in children, most commonly 5–10 years old, who present with visual impairment in one eye and sometimes leukocoria, squint, and red eye. The principal pathologic entity is eosinophilic granuloma of the retina that resembles retinoblastoma. Until the recent development of the *Toxocara* ELISA test, this resulted in the enucleation of many eyes. Other common clinical findings are peripheral retinochoroiditis, a diffuse, painless endophthalmitis; posterior pole granuloma; and a peripheral inflammatory mass. Uncommonly seen are an iris nodule, optic nerve granuloma, uniocular pars planitis, and a migrating retinal nematode. Ocular toxocariasis, which is generally recognized years after the acute infection, is generally not associated with peripheral eosinophilia, hypergammaglobulinemia, or isohemagglutinin elevation. Serum ELISA tests may be positive, but a negative test does not rule out the diagnosis. If doubt exists about whether a patient with a positive serum ELISA

test has toxocariasis or retinoblastoma, the vitreous humor should be examined for ELISA antibody (specificity has been reported as greater than 90% at a titer of 1:32 or higher) and eosinophils. High-resolution CT scanning of the orbit should be done.

Prevention, Treatment, & Prognosis

Disease in humans is best prevented by preventing defecation by dogs and cats in areas where children play and by periodic treatment of puppies, kittens, and nursing dog and cat mothers, starting at 2 weeks postpartum, repeating at weekly intervals for 3 weeks and then every 6 months.

A. Acute Infection

Treatment of symptomatic persons is primarily supportive. Although there is no proved specific treatment, the following drugs can be tried: albendazole (400 mg orally twice daily for 21 days), mebendazole (200 mg orally twice daily for 21 days), or ivermectin. Theoretically, release of antigens from dying parasites may exacerbate clinical and laboratory findings. Corticosteroids, antibiotics, antihistamines, and analgesics may be needed to provide symptomatic relief. Symptoms may persist for months but generally clear within 1–2 years. The ultimate outcome is usually good, but permanent neuropsychological deficits have been seen.

B. Ocular Toxocariasis

Treatment includes oral and subconjunctival corticosteroids, an anthelmintic drug, vitrectomy for vitreous traction, and laser photocoagulation. Partial or total permanent visual impairment is rare.

Despommier D: Toxocariasis: clinical aspects, epidemiology, medical ecology, and molecular aspects. Clin Microbiol Rev 2003;16:265. [PMID: 12692098]

Eberhardt O et al: Eosinophilic meningomyelitis in toxocariasis: case report and review of the literature. Clin Neurol Neurosurg 2005;107:423. [PMID: 16023542]

Good B et al: Ocular toxocariasis in schoolchildren. Clin Infect Dis 2004;39:173. [PMID: 15307025]

Moreira-Silva SF et al: Toxocariasis of the central nervous system: with report of two cases. Rev Soc Bras Med Trop 2004;37:169. [PMID: 15094904]

Vidal JE et al: Eosinophilic meningoencephalitis due to *Toxocara canis*: case report and review of the literature. Am J Trop Med Hyg 2003;69:341. [PMID: 14628955]

Infectious Diseases: Mycotic

36

Samuel A. Shelburne, MD, & Richard J. Hamill, MD

Fungal infections have assumed an increasingly important role as use of broad-spectrum antimicrobial agents has increased and the number of immunodeficient patients has risen. Some pathogens (eg, *Cryptococcus, Candida, Pneumocystis, Fusarium*) rarely cause serious disease in normal hosts. Other endemic fungi (eg, *Histoplasma, Coccidioides, Paracoccidioides*) commonly cause disease in normal hosts but tend to be more aggressive in immunocompromised ones. Superficial mycoses are discussed in Chapter 6.

CANDIDIASIS

ESSENTIALS OF DIAGNOSIS

- *Common normal flora but opportunistic pathogen.*
- *Gastrointestinal mucosal disease, particularly esophagitis, most common; catheter-associated fungemia occurs in patients who have sustained mucosal injury or received broad-spectrum antibiotics.*
- *Diagnosis of invasive systemic disease requires tissue biopsy or evidence of retinal disease.*

General Considerations

Candida albicans can be cultured from the mouth, vagina, and feces of most people. Cutaneous and oral lesions are discussed in Chapters 6 and 8, respectively. The risk factors for invasive candidiasis include prolonged neutropenia, recent abdominal surgery, broad-spectrum antibiotic therapy, renal failure, the presence of intravascular catheters (especially when providing total parenteral nutrition), and injection drug use. Cellular immunodeficiency predisposes to mucocutaneous disease. When no other underlying cause is found, persistent oral or vaginal candidiasis should arouse a suspicion of HIV infection.

Clinical Findings & Treatment

A. MUCOSAL CANDIDIASIS

Esophageal involvement is the most frequent type of significant mucosal disease. Individuals present with substernal odynophagia, gastroesophageal reflux, or nausea without substernal pain. Oral candidiasis, though often associated, is not invariably present. Diagnosis is best confirmed by endoscopy with biopsy and culture; the condition may be difficult to distinguish from esophagitis caused by infection with cytomegalovirus or herpes simplex virus when barium swallow alone is used for diagnosis. Therapy depends on the severity of disease. If patients are able to swallow and take adequate amounts of fluid orally, fluconazole, 100 mg/d (or itraconazole solution, 10 mg/mL, 100 mg/d), for 10–14 days will usually suffice. In the individual who is more ill or in whom esophagitis has developed while taking fluconazole, options include oral or intravenous voriconazole, 200 mg/twice daily; intravenous amphotericin B, 0.3 mg/kg/d; or intravenous caspofungin, 50 mg/d; or intravenous micafungin, 150 mg/d. Relapse is common with all agents when there is underlying HIV infection without adequate immune reconstitution.

Vulvovaginal candidiasis occurs in an estimated 75% of women during their lifetime. Risk factors include pregnancy, uncontrolled diabetes mellitus, broad-spectrum antimicrobial treatment, corticosteroid use, and HIV infection. Symptoms include acute vulvar pruritus, burning vaginal discharge, and dyspareunia. Various topical azole preparations (eg, clotrimazole, 100 mg vaginal tablet for 7 days, or miconazole, 200 mg vaginal suppository for 3 days) are effective. One 150 mg oral dose of fluconazole has been shown to have equivalent efficacy with better patient acceptance. Disease recurrence is common but can be decreased with weekly fluconazole therapy (150 mg weekly).

B. CANDIDAL FUNGURIA

Candidal funguria frequently resolves with discontinuance of antibiotics or removal of bladder catheters. Clinical benefit from treatment of asymptomatic candiduria has not been demonstrated, but persistent funguria should raise the suspicion of disseminated infection. When symptomatic funguria persists, oral fluconazole, 200 mg/d for 7–14 days, can be used if renal function is normal. Bladder irrigation with amphotericin B (50–200 mg/mL) is rarely indicated, though it may transiently clear candiduria, especially if colonization is confined to the bladder. However, failure to clear the candiduria in this way suggests the presence of upper urinary tract infection. Rare complications of candidal urinary tract infections are ureteral obstruction and dissemination.

C. DISSEMINATED CANDIDIASIS

The diagnosis of disseminated *Candida* infection is problematic because *Candida* species are often isolated from mucosal sites in the absence of invasive disease while blood cultures are positive only 50% of the time in disseminated infection. Serologic tests have not proved useful for distinguishing colonization from invasive disease. Thus, the decision to treat for *Candida* when organisms are isolated from urine or sputum (or both) needs to be individualized for each patient. Disseminated candidiasis may represent a benign, self-limited process, but until proven otherwise it should be considered a sign of serious, complicated disease. If fungemia resolves with removal of intravascular catheters, there are often no further complications, but the incidence of endophthalmitis may be higher than previously recognized.

Important clinical findings in invasive candidiasis are fluffy white retinal infiltrates that extend into the vitreous and raised, erythematous skin lesions that may be painful. Though characteristic, these are seen in less than 50% of cases. Other organ system involvement in invasive disease may include the brain, meninges, and myocardium. Antifungal therapy for invasive candidiasis is rapidly evolving with the addition of new agents and the emergence of non-*albicans* species causing significant disease. Options for treatment include fluconazole, 400–800 mg daily; amphotericin B, 0.3–0.5 mg/kg/d; voriconazole, 200 mg twice a day; or caspofungin, 50 mg/d. Combination therapy with azoles and amphotericin B is an area being explored. Flucytosine, 150 mg/kg/d orally in four divided doses, is added if central nervous system involvement occurs. Therapy for disseminated candidiasis should be continued for 2 weeks after the last positive blood culture and resolution of symptoms and signs of infection. Once patients have become clinically stable, parenteral therapy can be discontinued and oral fluconazole, 200–800 mg orally given as one or two doses daily, is used to complete treatment. Although debated, removal or exchange of intravascular catheters is generally recommended and substantially decreases the duration of candidemia and overall mortality, which approaches 30%.

Another form of invasive disease is hepatosplenic candidiasis. This results from aggressive chemotherapy and prolonged neutropenia in patients with underlying hematologic cancers. Typically, fever and variable abdominal pain present weeks after chemotherapy, when neutrophil counts have recovered. Blood cultures are generally negative. Hepatic enzymes reveal an alkaline phosphatase elevation that may be marked. CT scanning of the abdomen shows hepatosplenomegaly, most often with multiple low-density defects in the liver and spleen. Diagnosis is established by liver biopsy, histopathology, and culture. Fluconazole, 400 mg daily, or a lipid formulation of amphotericin B is given until clinical and radiographic improvement occurs.

D. CANDIDAL ENDOCARDITIS

Candidal endocarditis rarely is a complication of transient fungemia. It usually results from direct inoculation at the time of valvular heart surgery or repeated inoculation with injection drug use. Candidal endocarditis occurs with increased frequency on prosthetic valves in the first few months following surgery. Splenomegaly and petechiae are common, and there is a predilection for large-vessel embolization. Non-*albicans* species such as *Candida parapsilosis* and *Candida tropicalis* are more often important etiologic agents in endocarditis than in fungemia, which is most often due to *C albicans*. The diagnosis is established definitively by culturing *Candida* from emboli or from vegetations at the time of valve replacement. Valve destruction (usually aortic or mitral) is common, and surgical therapy is necessary in addition to a prolonged course of amphotericin therapy, given in a dosage of 0.5–1 mg/kg/d intravenously, usually to a total dose of 1–1.5 g intravenously.

It is important to note that non-*albicans* species of *Candida* now account for over 50% of clinical bloodstream isolates and are often resistant to imidazole antibiotics such as fluconazole. The widespread use of these agents for prophylaxis in immunocompromised patients can lead to the emergence of pathogens such as *Candida krusei*. Dissemination of this organism has been reported in patients undergoing bone marrow transplantation for leukemia. Azole-resistant *C albicans* has increased in frequency in immunocompromised patients, particularly in patients with late-stage AIDS receiving long-term suppressive fluconazole.

In all forms of invasive candidiasis, an important element of therapy is reversal of the underlying predisposing factor when possible. In high-risk patients undergoing induction chemotherapy, bone marrow transplantation, or liver transplantation, prophylaxis with antifungal agents has been shown to prevent invasive fungal infections although the effect on mortality and the preferred agent remain debated.

Kulberg BJ et al: Voriconazole versus a regimen of amphotericin B followed by fluconazole for candidaemia in non-neutropenic patients: a randomised non-inferiority trial. Lancet 2005;366:1435. [PMID: 16243088]

Pappas PG et al: Guidelines for the treatment of candidiasis. Clin Infect Dis 2004;38:161. [PMID: 14699449]

Raad I et al: Management of central venous catheters in patients with cancer and candidemia. Clin Infect Dis 2004;38:1119. [PMID: 15095217]

Sobel JD et al: Maintenance fluconazole therapy for recurrent vulvovaginal candidiasis. N Engl J Med 2004;351:876. [PMID: 15329425]

HISTOPLASMOSIS

ESSENTIALS OF DIAGNOSIS

- *Epidemiologically linked to bird droppings and bat exposure; common along river valleys (especially the Ohio River and the Mississippi River valleys).*
- *Most patients asymptomatic; respiratory illness most common clinical problem.*
- *Rare patients with normal immune function develop dissemination, with hepatosplenomegaly, lymphadenopathy, and oral ulcers.*
- *Widespread disease especially common in AIDS or other immunosuppressed states, with poor prognosis.*
- *Skin test and serology seldom diagnostic; biopsy of affected organs with culture, or urinary polysaccharide antigen most useful in disseminated disease.*

General Considerations

Histoplasmosis is caused by *Histoplasma capsulatum,* a dimorphic fungus that has been isolated from soil contaminated with bird or bat droppings in endemic areas (central and eastern United States, eastern Canada, Mexico, Central America, South America, Africa, and southeast Asia). Infection presumably takes place by inhalation of conidia. These convert into small budding cells that are engulfed by phagocytic cells in the lungs. The organism proliferates and is carried hematogenously to other organs.

Clinical Findings

A. SYMPTOMS AND SIGNS

Most cases of histoplasmosis are asymptomatic or mild and thus go unrecognized. Past infection is recognized by the development of a positive histoplasmin skin test and occasionally by pulmonary and splenic calcification noted on incidental radiographs. Symptoms and signs of pulmonary involvement are usually absent even in patients who subsequently show areas of calcification on chest radiographs. Symptomatic infection may present with mild influenza-like illness, often lasting 1–4 days. Moderately severe infections are frequently diagnosed as atypical pneumonia. These patients have fever, cough, and mild central chest pain lasting 5–15 days.

Clinically evident infections occur in several forms: (1) **Acute histoplasmosis** frequently occurs in epidemics, often when soil containing infected bird or bat droppings is disturbed. It is a severe disease manifested by marked prostration, fever, and relatively few pulmonary complaints even when radiographs show diffuse pneumonia. The illness may last from 1 week to 6 months but is almost never fatal. (2) **Progressive disseminated histoplasmosis** is usually fatal within 6 weeks or less. Symptoms usually consist of fever, dyspnea, cough, loss of weight, and prostration. Ulcers of the mucous membranes of the oropharynx may be present. The liver and spleen are nearly always enlarged, and all the organs of the body are involved, particularly the adrenal glands, though this infrequently results in adrenal insufficiency. Gastrointestinal involvement may mimic inflammatory bowel disease. (3) **Chronic progressive pulmonary histoplasmosis** is usually seen in older patients with chronic obstructive lung disease. The lungs show chronic progressive changes, often with apical cavities. (4) **Disseminated disease in the profoundly immunocompromised host** often represents reactivation of prior infectious foci or may reflect acute infection. This form is commonly seen in patients with underlying HIV infection—with CD4 cell counts usually < 100 cells/mcL—and is characterized by fever and multiple organ system involvement. Chest radiographs may show a miliary pattern. Presentation may be fulminant, simulating septic shock, with death ensuing rapidly unless treatment is provided.

B. LABORATORY FINDINGS

Most patients with progressive pulmonary disease show anemia of chronic disease. Bone marrow involvement may be prominent in disseminated forms with occurrence of pancytopenia. Alkaline phosphatase and marked lactate dehydrogenase (LDH) and ferritin elevations are also common.

In pulmonary disease, sputum culture is rarely positive except in chronic disease; antigen testing of bronchoalveolar lavage fluid may be helpful in acute disease. Blood or bone marrow cultures from immunocompromised patients with acute disseminated disease are positive more than 80% of the time but may take several weeks. A urine antigen assay has a sensitivity of greater than 90% for disseminated disease in AIDS patients and can be used to follow response to therapy. The sensitivity of screening immunodiffusion is 70% in acute pulmonary histoplasmosis, and complement fixation titers are positive in about 80% of cases. A combination of these two methods yields a sensitivity of up to 80% in immunodeficient adults.

Treatment

For progressive localized disease and for mild to moderately severe nonmeningeal disseminated disease in immunocompetent or immunocompromised patients, itraconazole, 200–400 mg/d orally divided into two doses, is the treatment of choice with an overall response rate of approximately 80%. The oral solution is better absorbed than the capsule formulation. Duration of therapy ranges from weeks to several months depending on the severity of illness. Amphotericin B is reserved for individuals who cannot take oral medications; for those who have not responded to itraconazole therapy; for those with meningitis; and for management of severe disseminated disease in an immunocompromised person. Up to 2.5 g total may need to be given in the latter two situations, though this course of treatment can be abbreviated and oral itraconazole instituted once clinical stabilization has occurred. (See Amphotericin B, Chapter 37.) Liposomal amphotericin B in a dosage of 3 mg/kg/d intravenously may be more effective and safer than conventional amphotericin B in seriously ill individuals. Patients with AIDS-related histoplasmosis require lifelong suppressive therapy with itraconazole, 200–400 mg/d orally, although secondary prophylaxis may be discontinued if immune reconstitution occurs in response to antiretroviral therapy.

Couppie P et al: Histoplasmosis and acquired immunodeficiency syndrome: a study of prognostic factors. Clin Infect Dis 2004;38:134. [PMID: 14679459]

Kahi CJ et al: Gastrointestinal histoplasmosis. Am J Gastroenterol 2005;100:220. [PMID: 15654803]

COCCIDIOIDOMYCOSIS

ESSENTIALS OF DIAGNOSIS

- *Influenza-like illness with malaise, fever, backache, headache, and cough.*
- *Arthralgia and periarticular swelling of knees and ankles.*
- *Erythema nodosum common.*
- *Dissemination may result in meningitis, bony lesions, or skin and soft tissue abscesses.*
- *Chest radiograph findings vary widely from pneumonitis to cavitation.*
- *Serologic tests useful; spherules containing endospores demonstrable in sputum or tissues.*

General Considerations

Coccidioidomycosis should be considered in the diagnosis of any obscure illness in a patient who has lived in or visited an endemic area.

Infection results from the inhalation of arthroconidia of *Coccidioides immitis* or *Coccidioides posadasii*; both organisms are molds that grow in soil in certain arid regions of the southwestern United States, in Mexico, and in Central and South America.

Less than 1% of immunocompetent persons show dissemination, but among these patients, the mortality rate is high.

In HIV-infected people in endemic areas, coccidioidomycosis is a common opportunistic infection. In these patients, disease manifestations range from focal pulmonary infiltrates to widespread miliary disease with multiple organ involvement and meningitis.

Clinical Findings

A. SYMPTOMS AND SIGNS

Symptoms of primary coccidioidomycosis occur in about 40% of infections. Symptom onset (after an incubation period of 10–30 days) is usually that of a respiratory tract illness with fever and occasionally chills. Pleuritic pain is common. Nasopharyngitis may be followed by bronchitis accompanied by a dry or slightly productive cough.

Arthralgia accompanied by periarticular swelling, often of the knees and ankles, is common. Erythema nodosum may appear 2–20 days after onset of symptoms. Persistent pulmonary lesions, varying from cavities and abscesses to parenchymal nodular densities or bronchiectasis, occur in about 5% of diagnosed cases.

Disseminated disease occurs in about 0.1% of white and 1% of nonwhite patients. Filipinos and blacks are especially susceptible, as are pregnant women of all races. Symptoms depend on the site of dissemination. Any organ may be involved. Pulmonary findings usually become more pronounced, with mediastinal lymph node enlargement, cough, and increased sputum production. Lung abscesses may rupture into the pleural space, producing an empyema. These may also extend to bones and skin, and pericardial and myocardial involvement has been occasionally observed. Fungemia may occur and is characterized clinically by a diffuse miliary pattern on chest radiograph and by early death. The course may be particularly rapid in immunosuppressed patients.

Bone lesions most often occur at bony prominences. Meningitis occurs in 30–50% of cases of dissemination. Subcutaneous abscesses and verrucous skin lesions are especially common in fulminating cases. Lymphadenitis may occur and may progress to suppuration. Mediastinal and retroperitoneal abscesses are not uncommon. HIV-infected persons with disseminated disease have a higher incidence of miliary infiltrates, lymphadenopathy, and meningitis, but skin lesions are uncommon.

B. LABORATORY FINDINGS

In primary coccidioidomycosis, there may be moderate leukocytosis and eosinophilia. Serologic testing is useful for both diagnosis and prognosis. The tube precipitin test and an immunodiffusion test detect IgM antibodies and are useful for diagnosis early in the disease process. Historically, a persistent rising complement fixation titer ($\geq$ 1:16) has been considered suggestive of disseminated disease; in addition, complement fixation titers can be used to assess the adequacy of therapy. Serum complement fixation titer may be low when there is meningitis but no other disseminated disease. In patients with HIV-related coccidioidomycosis, the false-negative rate may be as high as 30%.

Demonstrable complement-fixing antibodies in spinal fluid are diagnostic of coccidioidal meningitis. These are found in over 90% of cases. Spinal fluid findings include increased cell count with lymphocytosis and reduced glucose. Spinal fluid culture is positive in approximately 30% of meningitis cases. Spherules filled with endospores may be found in biopsy specimens; though they are not infectious, they convert to the highly contagious arthroconidia when grown in culture media. Blood cultures in appropriate media are only rarely positive in disseminated disease.

C. IMAGING

Radiographic findings vary, but patchy, nodular pulmonary infiltrates and thin-walled cavities are most common. Hilar lymphadenopathy may be visible and is seen in localized disease; mediastinal lymphadenopathy suggests dissemination. There may be pleural effusions and lytic lesions in bone with accompanying complicated soft-tissue collections.

Treatment

General symptomatic therapy is given as needed for disease limited to the chest with no evidence of progression. For progressive pulmonary or extrapulmonary disease, amphotericin B intravenously is generally used although oral azoles may be used for mild cases (see Chapter 37). Therapy should be continued, with duration of therapy determined by a declining complement fixation titer and a favorable clinical response. For meningitis, treatment usually is with high-dose oral fluconazole (400–800 mg/d) although lumbar or cisternal intrathecal administration of amphotericin B daily in increasing doses up to 1–1.5 mg/d is used initially by some physicians or in cases refractory to fluconazole. Systemic therapy with amphotericin B, 0.6 mg/kg/d intravenously, is generally given concurrently with intrathecal therapy but is not sufficient alone for the treatment of meningeal disease. Voriconazole may be an alternative to intrathecal amphotericin B in patients who do not respond to fluconazole. Once the patient is clinically stable, oral therapy with an azole for an indefinite period is the recommended alternative to intrathecal amphotericin B therapy.

Fluconazole, 200–400 mg orally once daily, or itraconazole, 400 mg orally daily divided into two doses, may be given for disease in the chest, bones, and soft tissues; however, therapy must be continued for 6 months or longer after the disease is inactive to prevent relapse. Response to therapy should be monitored by following the progressive decrease in serum complement fixation titers.

Thoracic surgery is occasionally indicated for giant, infected, or ruptured cavities. Surgical drainage is necessary for management of soft tissue abscesses and bone disease. Amphotericin B, 1 mg/kg/d intravenously, is advisable following extensive surgical manipulation of infected tissue until the disease is inactive, whereupon therapy may be continued with an azole.

Prognosis

The prognosis for patients with limited disease is good, but persistent pulmonary cavities may cause complications such as hemoptysis or rupture producing pyopneumothorax. Nodules, cavities, and fibrotic residuals may rarely progress after long periods of stability or regression. Serial complement fixation titers should be performed after therapy for patients with coccidioidomycosis; rising titers warrant reinstitution of therapy because relapse is likely. Disseminated and meningeal forms still have mortality rates exceeding 50% in the absence of therapy.

Galgiani JN et al: Coccidioidomycosis. Clin Infect Dis 2005;41: 1217. [PMID: 16206093]

Johnson RH et al: Coccidioidal meningitis. Clin Infect Dis 2005; 42:103. [PMID: 16323099]

PNEUMOCYSTOSIS
(*Pneumocystis jiroveci* Pneumonia)

 ESSENTIALS OF DIAGNOSIS

- *Fever, dyspnea, nonproductive cough.*
- *Bilateral diffuse interstitial disease without hilar adenopathy by chest radiograph.*
- *Bibasilar crackles on auscultation in many cases; others have no findings.*
- *Reduced partial pressure of oxygen.*
- *P jiroveci in sputum, bronchoalveolar lavage fluid, or lung tissue.*

General Considerations

Pneumocystis jiroveci, the *Pneumocystis* species that affects humans, is distributed worldwide. Although symptomatic *P jiroveci* disease is rare in the general population, serologic evidence indicates that asymptomatic infections have occurred in most persons by a young age. The overt infection is an acute interstitial plasma cell pneumonia that occurs with high frequency among two groups: (1) as epidemics of primary infections among premature or debilitated or marasmic infants on hospital wards in underdeveloped parts of the world, and (2) as sporadic cases among older children and adults who have an abnormal or altered cellular immune status. Cases occur generally in patients with cancer or severe malnutrition and debility, in patients treated with immunosuppressive or cytotoxic drugs or irradiation for the management of organ transplants and cancer, and, most commonly, in patients with AIDS (see Chapter 31).

The mode of transmission in primary infection is unknown, but the evidence suggests airborne transmission. Following asymptomatic primary infection, latent and presumably inactive organisms are sparsely distributed in the alveoli. Whether acute infection in older children and adults results from de novo infection or from reactivation of latent infection is unknown.

Pneumocystis pneumonia occurs in up to 80% of AIDS patients not receiving prophylaxis and is a major cause of death. Its incidence increases in direct proportion to the fall in CD4 cells, with most cases occurring at CD4 cell counts below 200/mcL. Dissemination of the infection to tissues other than the lung is rare, except in those who have received prophylactic aerosolized pentamidine. In non-AIDS patients receiving immunosuppressive therapy, symptoms frequently begin after corticosteroids have been tapered or discontinued.

Clinical Findings

A. SYMPTOMS AND SIGNS

Findings are usually limited to the pulmonary parenchyma; extrapulmonary disease is reported rarely. In the sporadic form of the disease associated with deficient cell-mediated immunity, the onset is abrupt, with fever, tachypnea, shortness of breath, and usually nonproductive cough. Pulmonary physical findings may be slight and disproportionate to the degree of illness and the radiologic findings; many patients have bibasilar crackles, but others do not. Without treatment, the course is usually one of rapid deterioration and death. Adult patients may present with spontaneous pneumothorax, usually in patients with previous episodes or those receiving aerosolized pentamidine prophylaxis. Patients with AIDS will usually have other evidence of HIV-associated disease, including fever, fatigue, and weight loss, for weeks or months preceding the illness.

B. LABORATORY FINDINGS

Chest radiographs most often show diffuse "interstitial" infiltration, which may be heterogeneous, miliary, or patchy early in infection. There may also be diffuse or focal consolidation, cystic changes, nodules, or cavitation within nodules. Pleural effusions are not seen. About 5–10% of patients with *Pneumocystis* pneumonia have normal chest films. High-resolution chest CT scans may be quite suggestive of *P jiroveci* pneumonia, helping distinguish it from other causes of pneumonia.

Typically, there is reduction in vital and total lung capacity, and the single-breath diffusing capacity for carbon monoxide shows impaired diffusion. Arterial blood gas determinations usually show hypoxemia with hypocapnia but may be normal; however, rapid desaturation occurs if patients are exercised before samples are drawn. Isolated elevation or rising levels of serum LDH are very sensitive but not specific findings for *P jiroveci*. Lymphopenia with depleted CD4 lymphocytes is common. Serologic tests, including tests to detect antigenemia, are not helpful in diagnosis.

Specific diagnosis depends on morphologic demonstration of the organisms in clinical specimens using specific stains. The organism cannot be cultured. Although patients rarely spontaneously produce sufficient sputum for examination, adequate specimens can sometimes be obtained with induced sputum by having patients inhale an aerosol of hypertonic saline (3%) produced by an ultrasonic nebulizer. Specimens are then stained with Giemsa stain or methenamine silver, either of which allows detection of cysts. The use of monoclonal antibody with immunofluorescence has increased the sensitivity of diagnosis. If diagnostic results cannot be achieved with induced sputum specimens and the diagnosis of *P jiroveci* pneumonia is strongly suspected, alternative techniques for obtaining specimens include bronchoalveolar lavage (sensitivity 86–97%) followed by transbronchial lung biopsy (85–97%), if necessary. Open lung biopsy and needle lung biopsy are infrequently done. Although conclusions are still preliminary, the polymerase chain reaction (PCR) test for the detection of *P jiroveci* appears to be sensitive but does not provide more rapid diagnosis.

Treatment

See Table 31–4.

It is appropriate to start empiric therapy for *P jiroveci* pneumonia if the disease is suspected clinically; however, in both AIDS patients and non-AIDS patients with mild to moderately severe disease, continued treatment should be based on a proved diagnosis because of the toxicity of therapy and the possible coexistence of other infections. Both in AIDS patients and in non-AIDS patients with mild to moderately severe disease, oral trimethoprim-sulfamethoxazole (TMP-SMZ) is the preferred agent because of its low cost and excellent bioavailability. Patients suffering from nausea and vomiting or intractable diarrhea should be given intravenous TMP-SMZ until they can tolerate the oral formulation. Other options include clindamycin/primaquine, dapsone/trimethoprim, pentamidine, and atovaquone. Therapy should be continued with the selected drug for at least 5–10 days before considering changing agents, as fever, tachypnea, and pulmonary infiltrates persist for 4–6 days after starting treatment. Some patients have a transient worsening of their disease during the first 3–5 days, which may be related to an inflammatory response secondary to the presence of dead or dying organisms. Early addition of corticosteroids may attenuate this response (see Chapter 31). Some clinicians prefer to treat episodes of AIDS-associated *Pneumocystis* pneumonia for 21 days rather than the usual 14 days recommended for non-AIDS cases.

A. TRIMETHOPRIM-SULFAMETHOXAZOLE

The dosage is TMP 20 mg/kg (12–15 mg/kg may decrease side effects without decreasing efficacy) and SMZ 100 mg/kg given orally or intravenously daily in three or four divided doses for 14–21 days. Adverse reactions are generally those of the sulfonamide component. Patients with AIDS have a high frequency of hypersensitivity reactions (approaching 50%), which may include fever, rashes (sometimes severe), malaise, neutropenia, hepatitis, nephritis, thrombocytopenia, hyperkalemia, and hyperbilirubinemia.

B. PENTAMIDINE ISETHIONATE

This drug is administered intravenously (preferred) or intramuscularly as a single dose of 3 mg (salt)/kg/d for 14–21 days. To avoid injection site pain or sterile abscesses, most clinicians administer the drug only intravenously by diluting it in 250 mL of 5% dextrose in water and giving it slowly over 1 hour. Pentamidine causes side effects in nearly 50% of patients. Occasional reactions include rash, neutropenia, abnormal liver function tests, serum folate depression, hyperkalemia, and hypocalcemia. Hypoglycemia (often clinically inapparent), hyperglycemia, hyponatremia, and delayed nephrotoxicity with azotemia may occur. Rarely, a variety of other severe adverse reactions may occur, including anemia, thrombocytopenia, ventricular arrhythmias, and fatal pancreatitis. Blood glucose levels should be monitored. Inadvertent rapid intravenous infusion may cause precipitous hypotension.

C. ATOVAQUONE

Atovaquone has been approved by the US Food and Drug Administration (FDA) for patients with mild to moderate disease who cannot tolerate TMP-SMZ or pentamidine, but failure is reported in 15–30% of cases. Mild side effects are common, but no serious reactions have been reported. The dosage is 750 mg three times daily for 21 days. Because poor gastrointestinal absorption can lead to low serum concentrations and treatment failure, the drug should be taken with food, especially a fatty meal.

D. OTHER DRUGS

Clindamycin, 600 mg three times daily, plus primaquine, 15 mg/d; and dapsone, 100 mg/d, plus trimethoprim 15 mg/kg/d, in three divided doses daily, are alternative oral regimens for mild to moderate disease or for continuation of therapy after intravenous therapy is no longer needed. Trimetrexate, 45 mg/m²/d intravenously, plus high-dose leucovorin has been approved for salvage use in patients not responding to other therapies, but the success rate is less than 25%.

E. PREDNISONE

In conjunction with antimicrobials, prednisone is given for moderate to severe pneumonia (when PaO₂ on admission is < 70 mm Hg or oxygen saturation is < 90%); its use during the first 72 hours of therapy for severe *Pneumocystis* pneumonia prevents deterioration in oxygenation and improves survival. The dosage of prednisone is 40 mg twice daily for 5 days, then 40 mg daily for 5 days, and then 20 mg daily until therapy is completed.

F. SUPPORTIVE CARE

Oxygen therapy is indicated to maintain the oxygen saturation over 90% by pulse oximeter.

Prevention

Primary prophylaxis for *Pneumocystis* pneumonia in HIV-infected patients should be given to persons with CD4 counts < 200 cells/mcL, a CD4 percentage below 14%, or weight loss or oral candidiasis. Development of *P jiroveci* pneumonia while on prophylaxis may be associated with development of resistance to TMP-SMZ. Patients with a history of *Pneumocystis* pneumonia should receive secondary prophylaxis until they have had a durable virologic response to antiretroviral therapy for at least 3–6 months and maintain a CD4 count of > 250 cells/mcL.

Prognosis

In the absence of early and adequate treatment, the fatality rate for the endemic infantile form of *Pneumocystis* pneumonia is 20–50%; for the sporadic form in immunodeficient persons, the fatality rate is nearly 100%. Early treatment reduces the mortality rate to about 3% in the former and 10–20% in AIDS patients. The mortality rate in other immunodeficient patients is still 30–50%, probably because of failure to make a timely diagnosis. In immunodeficient patients who do not receive prophylaxis, recurrences are common (30% in AIDS).

Crothers K et al: Severity and outcome of HIV-associated Pneumocystis pneumonia containing *Pneumocystis jirovecii* dihydropteroate synthase gene mutations. AIDS 2005;19:801. [PMID: 15867494]

Festic E et al: Acute respiratory failure due to pneumocystis pneumonia in patients without human immunodeficiency virus infection: outcome and associated features. Chest 2005;128: 573. [PMID: 16100140]

CRYPTOCOCCOSIS

 ESSENTIALS OF DIAGNOSIS

- *Most common cause of fungal meningitis.*
- *Predisposing factors: Hodgkin's disease, corticosteroid therapy, HIV infection.*
- *Symptoms of headache, abnormal mental status; meningismus seen occasionally, though rarely in HIV-infected patients.*
- *Demonstration of capsular polysaccharide antigen in cerebrospinal fluid diagnostic; 95% of HIV-infected patients also have a positive serum antigen.*

General Considerations

Cryptococcosis is mainly caused by *Cryptococcus neoformans var neoformans,* an encapsulated budding yeast that has been found worldwide in soil and on dried pigeon dung. *Cryptococcus gattii* is a closely related species that also causes disease in humans although *C gattii* appears to affect more immunocompetent persons, usually outside of North America.

Infections are acquired by inhalation. In the lung, the infection may remain localized, heal, or disseminate. Clinically apparent cryptococcal pneumonia rarely develops in immunocompetent persons. Progressive lung disease and dissemination most often occur in the setting of cellular immunodeficiency, including underlying hematologic cancer under treatment, Hodgkin's disease, long-term corticosteroid therapy, or HIV infection.

Clinical Findings

A. Symptoms and Signs

Disseminated disease may involve any organ, but central nervous system disease predominates. Headache is usually the first symptom of meningitis. Confusion and other mental status changes as well as cranial nerve abnormalities, nausea, and vomiting may be seen as the disease progresses. Nuchal rigidity and meningeal signs occur about 50% of the time but are uncommon in HIV-infected patients. Intracerebral mass lesions (cryptococcomas) are rarely seen. Communicating hydrocephalus may complicate the course. Primary *C neoformans* infection of the skin may mimic bacterial cellulitis, especially in immunocompromised persons.

B. Laboratory Findings

For suspected meningeal disease, lumbar puncture is the preferred diagnostic procedure. A substantial proportion of individuals who have systemic disease without clinical signs of meningitis will have meningeal involvement, mandating examination of the cerebrospinal fluid. Spinal fluid findings include increased opening pressure, variable pleocytosis, increased protein, and decreased glucose, though as many as 50% of AIDS patients have no pleocytosis. India ink smear or Gram stain of the cerebrospinal fluid usually reveals budding, encapsulated fungal cells. Cryptococcal capsular antigen in cerebrospinal fluid and culture together establish the diagnosis over 90% of the time. Patients with AIDS often have the antigen in both cerebrospinal fluid and serum, and extrameningeal disease (lungs, blood, urinary tract) is common. In patients with AIDS, the serum cryptococcal antigen is a sensitive screening test for meningitis, being positive in over 95% of cases. CT or MRI scanning of the head should be performed if focal neurologic signs or papilledema are present to evaluate for mass lesions (eg, cryptococcoma) or hydrocephalus.

Treatment

In AIDS-related cryptococcal meningitis, oral fluconazole, 400 mg/d for a minimum of 10 weeks, has reasonable efficacy as immediate therapy in patients with mild disease. Candidates for initial fluconazole therapy are patients with an intact level of consciousness and a spinal fluid cryptococcal antigen titer of less than 1:128. Higher-risk patients should receive amphotericin B initially.

There has been a trend away from regimens based on prolonged amphotericin B therapy, particularly in HIV-infected patients. However, this agent remains important, especially in severe disease. Amphotericin B, 0.7–1 mg/kg/d intravenously for 14 days, followed by an additional 8 weeks of fluconazole, 400 mg/d orally, has been quite effective, achieving clinical responses and cerebrospinal fluid sterilization in about 70% of patients. Adding flucytosine initially does prevent late relapses but does not substantially contribute to improved cure rates. Flucytosine is administered orally at a dose of 100 mg/kg/d divided into four equal doses and given every 6 hours. Hematologic parameters should be closely monitored during flucytosine therapy. Repeated lumbar punctures or ventricular shunting should be performed to relieve high cerebrospinal fluid pressures or if hydrocephalus is a complication. Failure to adequately relieve raised intracranial pressure is a major cause of morbidity and mortality. The end points for amphotericin B therapy and for switching to oral fluconazole are a favorable clinical response (decrease in temperature; improvement in headache, nausea, vomiting, and mini-mental status scores), declining cerebrospinal fluid cryptococcal antigen titer, and, most importantly, conversion of cerebrospinal fluid culture to negative.

A similar approach is reasonable for patients with cryptococcal meningitis in the absence of AIDS, though the mortality rate is considerably higher. Because of serious underlying illnesses and generally greater age, this group of patients does not tolerate the higher doses of amphotericin B as well as patients with AIDS. Lipid amphotericin B preparations appear to have equivalent efficacy with reduced nephrotoxicity. Therapy is generally continued until cerebrospinal fluid cultures become negative and cerebrospinal fluid antigen titers are below 1:8.

Maintenance antifungal therapy is important after treatment of an acute episode in HIV-related cases, since otherwise the rate of relapse is greater than 50%. Fluconazole, 200 mg/d, is the maintenance therapy of choice, decreasing the relapse rate approximately tenfold compared with placebo and threefold compared with weekly amphotericin B in patients whose cerebrospinal fluid has been sterilized by the induction therapy. After successful therapy of cryptococcal meningitis, it is possible to discontinue secondary prophylaxis with fluconazole in individuals with AIDS who have had a satisfactory response to antiretroviral therapy (eg, CD4 cell count > 100–200 cells/mcL for at least 6 months). Among practitioners treating patients without AIDS, there has been a trend in recent years to prescribe a brief course (eg, 3 months) of fluconazole as maintenance therapy following successful therapy for acute illness; recently published guidelines suggest this as an option.

Prognosis

Factors that indicate a poor prognosis include the activity of the predisposing conditions, older age, organ failure, lack of spinal fluid pleocytosis, high initial antigen titer in either serum or cerebrospinal fluid, decreased mental status, increased intracranial pressure, and the presence of disease outside the nervous system.

Brouwer AE et al: Combination antifungal therapies for HIV-associated cryptococcal meningitis: a randomized trial. Lancet 2004;363:1764. [PMID: 15172774]

Kidd SE et al: A rare genotype of *Cryptococcus gattii* caused the cryptococcosis outbreak on Vancouver Island (British Columbia, Canada). Proc Natl Acad Sci U S A 2004;101: 17258. [PMID: 15572442]

Mussini C et al: Discontinuation of maintenance therapy for cryptococcal meningitis in patients with AIDS treated with highly active antiretroviral therapy: an international observational study. Clin Infect Dis 2004;38:565. [PMID: 14665493]

ASPERGILLOSIS

Aspergillus fumigatus is the usual cause of aspergillosis, though many species of *Aspergillus* may cause a wide spectrum of disease. Burn eschar and debris in the external ear canal are often colonized by these fungi. Clinical illness results either from an aberrant immunologic response or tissue invasion.

Allergic bronchopulmonary aspergillosis occurs in patients with preexisting asthma who develop worsening bronchospasm and fleeting pulmonary infiltrates accompanied by eosinophilia, high levels of IgE, and IgG *Aspergillus* precipitins in the blood. It also may complicate cystic fibrosis. The disease characteristically pursues a waxing and waning course with gradual improvement over time, but it may result in saccular bronchiectasis and end-stage fibrotic lung disease. For acute exacerbations, oral prednisone is begun at a dose of 1 mg/kg/d and then tapered slowly over several months. Itraconazole at a dose of 200 mg daily for 16 weeks appears to improve pulmonary function and decrease corticosteroid requirements in these patients.

Invasive manifestations may be seen in immunocompetent or only mildly immunocompromised adults. These include chronic **sinusitis**, colonization of preexisting pulmonary cavities (**aspergilloma**), and chronic necrotizing pulmonary aspergillosis. Sinus involvement is usually diagnosed histologically after patients with chronic sinus disease undergo surgery. These patients may require protracted courses of antifungals (itraconazole, 200 mg twice daily, for weeks to months) in addition to the surgical debridement. Aspergillomas of the lung occur when preexisting lung lesions become secondarily colonized with *Aspergillus* species. These may be found by incidental radiographic studies but may also present with significant hemoptysis. Intracavitary instillation of amphotericin B and bronchoscopic removal have been tried with little success; several uncontrolled trials have suggested some benefit from oral itraconazole. The most effective therapy for symptomatic aspergilloma remains surgical resection.

Chronic necrotizing aspergillosis is a relatively rare disease seen in patients with some degree of immunocompromise and presents with a protracted course compared with the more common acute invasive form of the disease. Fibrosis and cavity formation may be prominent and the response to antifungal therapy is not clear at present, although it would be reasonable to institute therapy targeting *Aspergillus*. Surgical intervention may be necessary but complications are common.

Life-threatening **invasive aspergillosis** most commonly occurs in profoundly immunodeficient patients, particularly those with prolonged, severe neutropenia. Patients with very advanced HIV disease may also be at risk for invasive aspergillosis, particularly if they have other risk factors for the disease. Pulmonary disease is most common, with patchy infiltration leading to a severe necrotizing pneumonia. There is often tissue infarction as the organism grows into blood vessels; clues to this are the development of pleuritic chest pain and elevation of serum LDH. AIDS patients are also predisposed to a unique ulcerative tracheobronchitis that may coexist with parenchymal pulmonary disease. At any time, there may be hematogenous dissemination to the central nervous system, skin, and other organs. Early diagnosis and reversal of any correctable immunosuppression are essential. Blood cultures have very low yield. In contrast to allergic aspergillosis, serologic tests have low sensitivities for invasive disease; detection of galactomannan by enzyme-linked immunosorbent assay (ELISA) has recently been demonstrated to have a sensitivity of 89% and a specificity of 98% for the diagnosis of invasive disease, though multiple determinations should be done. False-positive galactomannan tests have been reported in patients receiving β-lactam antibiotics. Isolation of *Aspergillus* from pulmonary secretions does not necessarily imply invasive disease. Therefore, the mainstay of diagnosis is demonstration of *Aspergillus* in tissue. Biopsy specimens may show branched septate hyphae but will not invariably grow the organism. CT scan of the chest may show characteristics quite suggestive of invasive aspergillosis.

When severe invasive aspergillosis is considered clinically likely or is demonstrable by laboratory testing, rapid institution of voriconazole, high doses of amphotericin B, or caspofungin may be life-saving (see Chapter 37). Voriconazole has been shown to be more effective, improve survival, and be associated with fewer severe side effects than conventional amphotericin B when used as initial therapy in invasive aspergillosis. The dosage of voriconazole is 6 mg/kg intravenously twice on the first day, followed by 4 mg/kg twice daily given either intravenously or by mouth. Some experts believe that lipid preparations of amphotericin B should be used preferentially in this setting because they are better tolerated and can be given at higher doses. Caspofungin acetate, an echinocandin antifungal, has been approved for the treatment of invasive aspergillosis in patients who are refractory to or intolerant of other treatments. The drug is given as a 70 mg intravenous loading dose followed by 50 mg intravenously daily. In critically ill patients who are not responding to conventional antifungal treatment, there may be a role for the addition of caspofungin to amphotericin B or voriconazole therapy, although randomized trials are lacking. Based on promising results in neutropenic patients with invasive pulmonary aspergillosis, surgical resection warrants further study. The mortality rate of pulmonary or disseminated disease in the immunocompromised patient remains well above 50%, particularly in patients with refractory neutropenia. This high mortality rate often leads clinicians to institute prophylactic therapy around the time of bone marrow transplantation with agents such as itraconazole.

Bart-Delabesse E et al: Detection of *Aspergillus galactomannan* antigenemia to determine biological and clinical implications of beta-lactam treatments. J Clin Microbiol 2005;43:5214. [PMID: 16207986]

Klont RR: Utility of *Aspergillus* antigen detection in specimens other than serum samples. Clin Infect Dis 2004;39:1467. [PMID: 15546083]

Marr KA et al: Itraconazole versus fluconazole for prevention of fungal infections in patients receiving allogenic stem cell transplants. Blood 2004;103:1527. [PMID: 14525770]

Singh N et al: *Aspergillus* infections in transplant recipients. Clin Micro Rev 2005;18:44. [PMID: 15653818]

MUCORMYCOSIS

The term mucormycosis (zygomycosis, phycomycosis) is applied to opportunistic infections caused by members of the genera *Rhizopus, Mucor, Absidia*, and *Cunninghamella*. Predisposing conditions include diabetic ketoacidosis, chronic renal failure, desferoxamine therapy, and treatment with corticosteroids or cytotoxic drugs. These organisms appear in tissues as broad, branching nonseptate hyphae. Biopsy with histologic examination is almost always required for diagnosis; cultures are frequently negative. Invasive disease of the sinuses, orbits, and the lungs may occur. Widely disseminated disease has been more commonly seen recently in patients who have received aggressive chemotherapy and broad-spectrum antifungal prophylaxis. The diagnosis should be considered in immunocompromised patients with black necrotic lesions of the nose or sinuses or with new cranial nerve abnormalities. Without treatment, cerebral invasion may ensue. A prolonged course of high-dosage amphotericin B (1–1.5 mg/kg/d intravenously) or a lipid preparation of amphotericin B should be started early. Based on in vitro susceptibility, there may be a role for posaconazole in the treatment of these infections, but other azoles are likely to be ineffective. Control of diabetes and other underlying conditions, along with extensive repeated surgical removal of necrotic, nonperfused tissue, is essential. Even when these measures are introduced in a timely fashion, the prognosis is poor, with a 30–50% mortality rate for localized disease and higher rates in disseminated cases.

Kontoyiannis DP et al: Zygomycosis in a tertiary-care cancer center in the era of *Aspergillus*-active antifungal therapy. A case-control observational study of 27 recent cases. J Infect Dis 2005;191:1350. [PMID: 15776383]

Prabhu RM et al: Mucormycosis and entomophthoramycocis: a review of the clinical manifestations, diagnosis, and treatment. Clin Microbiol Infect 2004;10(Suppl 1):31. [PMID: 14748801]

Spellberg B et al: Novel perspectives on mucormycosis: pathophysiology, presentation, and management. Clin Micro Rev 2005;18:556. [PMID: 16020690]

BLASTOMYCOSIS

Blastomycosis occurs most often in men infected during occupational or recreational activities out of doors and in a geographically limited area of the south central and midwestern United States and Canada. A few cases have been found in Mexico and Africa. Disease usually occurs in immunocompetent individuals.

Pulmonary infection is most common and may be asymptomatic. When dissemination takes place, lesions are most frequently seen in the skin, bones, and urogenital system.

Cough, moderate fever, dyspnea, and chest pain are common. These may resolve or progress, with bloody and purulent sputum production, pleurisy, fever, chills, loss of weight, and prostration. Radiologic studies, either chest radiographs or CT scans, usually reveal pulmonary infiltrates and enlarged regional lymph nodes, though less commonly than in histoplasmosis or coccidioidomycosis.

Raised, verrucous cutaneous lesions that have an abrupt downward sloping border are usually present in disseminated blastomycosis. The border extends slowly, leaving a central atrophic scar. If left untreated for long periods, they may mimic skin cancer. Bones—often the ribs and vertebrae—are frequently involved. Lesions appear to be both destructive and proliferative on radiography. Epididymitis, prostatitis, and other involvement of the male urogenital system may occur. Central nervous system involvement is uncommon. Although they do not appear to be at greater risk for acquisition of disease, infection in HIV-infected persons may progress rapidly, with dissemination common.

Laboratory findings usually include leukocytosis and anemia, though these are not specific. The organism is found in clinical specimens, such as expectorated sputum or tissue, as a thick-walled cell 5–20 mcm in diameter that may have a single broad-based bud. It grows readily on culture. Serologic tests are not well standardized.

Itraconazole, 100–200 mg/d orally for at least 2–3 months, is now the therapy of choice for nonmeningeal disease, with a response rate of over 80%. Amphotericin B, 0.3–0.6 mg/kg/d intravenously for a total dose of 1.5–2.5 g, is given for treatment failures or cases with central nervous system involvement.

Clinical follow-up for relapse should be regularly made for several years so that therapy may be resumed or another drug instituted.

Bradsher RW et al: Blastomycosis. Infect Dis Clin North Am 2003;17:21. [PMID: 12751259]

Martynowicz MA et al: Pulmonary blastomycosis. An appraisal of diagnostic techniques. Chest 2002;121:768. [PMID: 11888958]

PARACOCCIDIOIDOMYCOSIS (South American Blastomycosis)

Paracoccidioides brasiliensis infections have been found only in patients who have resided in South or Central America or Mexico. Long asymptomatic periods enable patients to travel far from the endemic areas before developing clinical problems. Ulceration of the nasopharynx and oropharynx is usually the first symptom. Papules ulcerate and enlarge both peripherally and deeper into the subcutaneous tissue. Differential diagnosis includes mucocutaneous leishmaniasis and syphilis. Extensive coalescent ulcerations may eventually result in destruction of the epiglottis, vocal cords, and uvula. Extension to the lips and face may occur. Eating and drinking are extremely painful. Skin lesions may occur, usually on the face. Variable in appearance, they may have a necrotic central crater with a hard hyperkeratotic border. Lymph node enlargement may follow mucocutaneous lesions, eventually ulcerating and forming draining sinuses; in some patients, it is the presenting symptom. Hepatosplenomegaly may be present as well. Cough, sometimes with sputum, indicates pulmonary involvement, but the symptoms and signs are often mild, even though radiographic findings indicate severe parenchymatous changes in the lungs. The extensive ulceration of the upper gastrointestinal tract may prevent caloric intake and result in cachexia.

Laboratory findings are nonspecific. Serology by immunodiffusion is positive in 98% of cases. Complement fixation titers correlate with progressive disease and fall with effective therapy. The fungus is found in clinical specimens as a spherical cell that may have many buds arising from it. If direct examination does not reveal the organism, biopsy with Gomori staining may be helpful.

Itraconazole, 100–200 mg orally daily, is the treatment of choice and generally results in a clinical response within 1 month and effective control after 2–6 months.

Tobon AM et al: Residual pulmonary abnormalities in adult patients with chronic paracoccidioidomycosis: prolonged follow-up after itraconazole therapy. Clin Infect Dis 2003;37:898. [PMID: 13130400]

SPOROTRICHOSIS

Sporotrichosis is a chronic fungal infection caused by *Sporothrix schenckii*. It is worldwide in distribution; most patients have had contact with soil, sphagnum moss, or decaying wood. Infection takes place when the organism is inoculated into the skin—usually on the hand, arm, or foot, especially during gardening.

The most common form of sporotrichosis begins with a hard, nontender subcutaneous nodule. This later becomes adherent to the overlying skin and ulcerates. Within a few days to weeks, similar nodules develop along the lymphatics draining this area, and these may ulcerate as well. The lymphatic vessels become indurated and are easily palpable.

Disseminated sporotrichosis is rare in the immunocompetent person but may present with widespread cutaneous, lung, bone, joint, and central nervous system involvement in immunocompromised patients, especially those with AIDS and alcohol abuse.

Cultures are needed to establish diagnosis. Antibody tests may be useful for diagnosis of disseminated disease, especially meningitis.

Itraconazole, 200–400 mg orally daily for several months, is now the treatment of choice for localized disease and some milder cases of disseminated disease. Terbinafine, 500 mg twice daily, also appears to have good efficacy in noninvasive disease. Amphotericin B intravenously, 1–2 g (see Chapter 37), is used for severe systemic infection. Surgery is usually contraindicated except for simple aspiration of secondary nodules. Joint involvement may require arthrodesis.

The prognosis is good for lymphocutaneous sporotrichosis; pulmonary, joint, and disseminated disease respond less favorably.

Chapman SW et al: Comparative evaluation of the efficacy and safety of two doses of terbinafine (500 mg and 1000 mg/day) in the treatment of cutaneous and lymphocutaneous sporotrichosis. Mycoses 2004;47:62. [PMID: 14998402]

Lyon GM et al: Population-based surveillance and a case-control study of risk factors for endemic lymphocutaneous sporotrichosis in Peru. Clin Infect Dis 2003;36:34. [PMID: 12491199]

PENICILLIUM MARNEFFEI INFECTIONS

Penicillium marneffei is a dimorphic fungus, endemic in southeast Asia, that causes systemic infection in both healthy and immunocompromised hosts. There have been reports of travelers with advanced AIDS returning from southeast Asia with disseminated infection. Clinical manifestations include fever, generalized umbilicated papular rash, lymphadenopathy, cough, and diarrhea. Diagnosis is made by identification of the organism on smears or histopathologic specimens or by culture, where the fungus produces a characteristic red pigment. The best sites for isolation of the fungus include the skin, blood, bone marrow, respiratory tract, and lymph nodes. Antigen and antibody tests have been developed in endemic regions. Patients with mild to moderate infection can be treated with itraconazole, 400 mg divided into two doses daily by mouth for 8 weeks. Amphotericin B, 0.5–0.7 mg/kg/d, is the drug of choice for severe disease and should be continued until patients have had a satisfactory clinical response, at which time they can be switched to itraconazole. Because the relapse rate after successful treatment is 30%, maintenance therapy with itraconazole, 200–400 mg daily, is indicated indefinitely.

Chariyalertsak S et al: A controlled trial of itraconazole as primary prophylaxis for systemic fungal infections in patients with advanced human immunodeficiency virus infection in Thailand. Clin Infect Dis 2002;34:277. [PMID: 11740718]

Wong SS et al: Differences in clinical and laboratory diagnostic characteristics of *Penicillium marneffei* in human immunodeficiency virus (HIV)- and non-HIV-infected patients. J Clin Microbiol 2001;39:4535. [PMID: 11724878]

CHROMOBLASTOMYCOSIS (Chromomycosis)

Chromoblastomycosis is a chronic, principally tropical cutaneous infection usually affecting young men who are agricultural workers and caused by several species of closely related black molds; *Cladophialophora carrionii* and *Fonsecaea pedrosoi* are the most common etiologic agents.

Lesions usually follow puncture wounds and are slowly progressive, occurring most frequently on a lower extremity. The lesion begins as a papule or ulcer. Over months to years, papules enlarge to become vegetating, papillomatous, verrucous elevated nodules. Satellite lesions may appear along the lymphatics. There may be secondary bacterial infection. Elephantiasis may result.

The fungus is seen as brown, thick-walled, spherical, sometimes septate cells in potassium hydroxide preparations of pus or skin scrapings, which are quite sensitive for diagnosis. The type of reproduction found in culture determines the species.

Itraconazole, 200–400 mg/d orally for 6–18 months, achieves a response rate of 65%. Response rates may be improved by the addition to itraconazole of flucytosine, 100–150 mg/kg/d by mouth divided into four doses. Terbinafine at 500 mg/d may have similar efficacy to itraconazole. Cryosurgery alone for smaller lesions or combined with itraconazole for larger lesions is beneficial.

Andrade TS et al: Susceptibility of sequential *Fonsecaea pedrosoi* isolates from chromoblastomycosis patients to anti-fungal agents. Mycoses 2004;47:216. [PMID: 15189187]

Queiroz-Telles F et al: Subcutaneous mycoses. Infect Dis Clin North Am 2003;17:59. [PMID: 12751261]

MYCETOMA (Maduromycosis & Actinomycetoma)

Mycetoma is a chronic local, slowly progressive destructive infection, usually involving the foot, that begins in subcutaneous tissues, frequently after localized trauma, and then spreads to contiguous structures. Maduromycosis (also known as eumycetoma) is the term used to describe mycetoma caused by the true fungi and by phylogenetically diverse organisms. Actinomycotic mycetoma is caused by *Nocardia* and *Actinomadura* species. The disease begins as a papule, nodule, or abscess that over months to years progresses slowly to form multiple abscesses and sinus tracts ramifying deep into the tissue. Secondary bacterial infection may result in large open ulcers. Radiographs may show destructive changes in the underlying bone. Tissue Gram stain reveals fine branching hyphae with actinomycotic mycetoma. Larger hyphae are seen with fungal mycetoma; the causative species can often be identified by the color of the characteristic grains within the infected tissues.

The prognosis is good for patients with actinomycetoma, since they usually respond well to sulfonamides and sulfones, especially if treated early. TMP-SMZ, 160/800 mg orally twice a day, or dapsone, 100 mg twice daily after meals, has been reported to be effective. Streptomycin, 14 mg/kg/d intramuscularly, may be useful during the first month of therapy. All oral medications must be taken for months and continued for several months after clinical cure to prevent relapse. Debridement assists healing.

The prognosis for maduromycosis is poor, though surgical debridement along with prolonged terbinafine or itraconazole therapy may result in a response rate of 70%. The various etiologic agents may respond differently to antifungal agents, so culture results are invaluable. Amputation is necessary in far advanced cases.

OTHER OPPORTUNISTIC MOLD INFECTIONS

Fungi previously considered to be harmless colonizers, including *Pseudallescheria boydii* (*Scedosporium apiospermum*), *Scedosporium prolificans*, *Fusarium*, *Paecilomyces*, *Trichoderma longibrachiatium*, and *Trichosporon*, are emerging as significant pathogens in immunocompromised patients. This occurs most often in patients being treated for hematopoietic malignancies. Infection may be localized in the skin, lungs, or sinuses, or widespread disease may appear with lesions in multiple organs. Colonization of old cavitary disease may cause minimal symptoms or may precede dissemination with meningitis or brain abscesses. Endocarditis occurs more commonly in injection drug users. Sinus infection may cause bony erosion. Infection in subcutaneous tissues following traumatic implantation may develop as a well-circumscribed cyst or as an ulcer.

Nonpigmented septate hyphae are seen in tissue and are indistinguishable from those of *Aspergillus* when infections are due to *S apiospermum* or species of *Fusarium*, *Paecilomyces*, *Penicillium*, or other hyaline molds. Spores or mycetoma-like granules are rarely present in tissue.

Infection by any of a number of black molds is designated as phaeohyphomycosis. These black molds (eg, *Exophiala*, *Bipolaris*, *Cladophialophora*, *Curvularia*, *Alternaria*) are common in the environment, especially on decaying vegetation. Human disease due to these agents is rarely encountered but may result in

Table 36–1. Agents for systemic mycoses.

Drug	Dosing	Renal Clearance?	CSF Penetration?	Toxicities	Spectrum of Activity
Amphotericin B	0.3–1.5 mg/kg/d intravenously	No	Poor	Rigors, fever, azotemia, hypokalemia, hypomagnesemia, renal tubular acidosis, anemia	All major pathogens except *scedosporium*
Amphotericin B lipid complex	5 mg/kg/d intravenously	No	Poor	Fever, rigors, nausea, hypotension, anemia, azotemia, tachypnea	Same as amphotericin B, above
Liposomal amphotericin B	3–6 mg/kg/d intravenously	No	Poor	Fever, rigors, nausea, hypotension, azotemia, anemia, tachypnea, chest tightness	Same as amphotericin B, above
Anidulafungin	100 mg intravenous loading dose, followed by 50 mg/d intravenously in one dose	< 1%	Poor	Headache, phlebitis	Mucosal and invasive candidiasis
Caspofungin acetate	70 mg IV loading dose, followed by 50 mg/d intravenously in one dose	< 50%[1]	Poor	Transient neutropenia; hepatic enzyme elevations when used with cyclosporine	Aspergillosis, candidiasis
Micafungin sodium	150 mg intravenously in one dose (treatment) 50 mg (prophylaxis)	No	Poor	Rash, rigors, headache, phlebitis	Esophageal candidiasis, prophylaxis of hematopoietic stem cell transplatation
Fluconazole	100–400 mg/d in one or two doses intravenously or orally	Yes	Yes	Nausea, rash, alopecia, headache, hepatic enzyme elevations	Mucosal candidiasis (including urinary tract), cryptococcosis, histoplasmosis, coccidioidomycosis
Flucytosine (5-FC)	100–150 mg/kg/d orally in four divided doses	Yes	Yes	Leukopenia,[2] rash, diarrhea, hepatitis, nausea, vomiting	Cryptococcosis,[3] candidiasis,[3] chromomycosis
Itraconazole	100–400 mg/d orally in one or two doses; 200–400 mg/d IV in one or two doses	No	Variable	Nausea, hypokalemia, edema, hypertension	Histoplasmosis, coccidioidomycosis, blastomycosis, paracoccidioidomycosis, mucosal candidiasis (except urinary), sporotrichosis, aspergillosis, chromomycosis
Ketoconazole	200–800 mg/d orally in one or two doses	No	Poor	Anorexia, nausea, suppression of testosterone and cortisol, rash, headache, hepatic enzyme elevations, hepatic failure	Nonmeningeal histoplasmosis and coccidioidomycosis, blastomycosis, paracoccidioidomycosis, mucosal candidiasis (except urinary)

(continued)

Table 36–1. Agents for systemic mycoses. (continued)

Drug	Dosing	Renal Clearance?	CSF Penetration?	Toxicities	Spectrum of Activity
Posaconazole	400–800 mg/d orally in one or two doses	No	Yes	Headache, somnolence, dizziness, fatigue	Limited data suggest broad range of activity including zygomycosis
Terbinafine	250 mg/d orally in one dose	Yes	Poor	Nausea, abdominal pain, taste disturbance, rash, diarrhea, and hepatic enzyme elevations	Dermatophytes, sporotrichosis
Voriconazole	200–400 mg/d orally in two doses or 12 mg/kg intravenously as loading dose for 2 days followed by 6 mg/kg/d intravenously in two doses	Yes	Yes	Transient visual disturbances, rash, hepatic enzyme elevations[4]	All major pathogens except zygomycetes and sporotrichosis

[1] No dosage adjustment required for renal insufficiency; dosage adjustment necessary with moderate to severe hepatic dysfunction.
[2] Use should be monitored with blood levels to prevent this or the dose adjusted according to creatinine clearance.
[3] In combination with amphotericin B.
[4] Administration with drugs that are metabolized by the cytochrome P-450 system is contraindicated or requires careful monitoring.

soft tissue abscesses due to traumatic inoculation or may occur as a sequela of chronic sinusitis or profound immunosuppression. In tissues of patients with phaeohyphomycosis, the mold is seen as black or faintly brown hyphae, yeast cells, or both. Culture on appropriate medium is needed to identify the agent. Histologic demonstration of these organisms is definitive evidence of invasive infection; positive cultures must be interpreted cautiously and not assumed to be contaminants in immunocompromised hosts. Some isolates are sensitive to antifungal agents. The differentiation of *S apiospermum* and *Aspergillus* is particularly important, since the former is uniformly resistant to amphotericin B but may be sensitive to azole antifungals (eg, voriconazole).

Husain S et al: Infections due to *Scedosporium apiospermum* and *Scedosporium prolificans* in transplant recipients: clinical characteristics and impact of antifungal agent therapy on outcome. Clin Infect Dis 2005;40:89. [PMID: 15614697]

Revankar SG et al: Primary central nervous system phaeohyphomycosis: a review of 101 cases. Clin Infect Dis 2004;38:206. [PMID: 14699452]

Walsh TJ et al: Infections due to emerging and uncommon medically important fungal pathogens. Clin Microbiol Infect 2004;10(Suppl 1):48. [PMID: 14748802]

ANTIFUNGAL THERAPY

Table 36–1 summarizes the major properties of currently available or soon to be available antifungal agents. A number of lipid-based amphotericin B formulations are available. These agents are used to treat systemic candidiasis, invasive aspergillosis and other disseminated mold infections, disseminated histoplasmosis, and cryptococcal meningitis. Their principal advantage appears to be substantially reduced nephrotoxicity, allowing administration of much higher doses. Because of their expense, use of these agents should be reserved for individuals in whom significant nephrotoxicity develops during amphotericin B therapy. Two agents of the echinocandin class, caspofungin acetate and micafungin sodium, are currently approved and a third, anidulafungin should be available soon. The echinocandins have relatively few adverse effects. Caspofungin acetate is approved for use in esophageal and invasive candidiasis, as empiric therapy in patients with neutropenic fever, and in refractory cases of invasive aspergillosis. Voriconazole has excellent activity against a broad range of fungal pathogens and has been FDA approved for use in invasive *Aspergillus* cases, *Fusarium* and *Scedosporium* infections, *Candida* esophagitis, deep *Candida* infections, and candidemia. Posaconazole, a new azole, is currently used on a compassionate basis in zygomycetes infections and likely will be widely available soon. Cytokine therapy (such as with interferon-γ) and use of growth factors such as granulocyte macrophage-colony-stimulating factor (GM-CSF) (sargramostim or molgramostim) have been shown in animal models to increase clearance of fungi and result in better clinical outcomes and are being evaluated in human disease.

Higashiyama Y et al: Micafungin: a therapeutic review. Expert Rev Anti Infect Ther 2004;2:345. [PMID: 15482200]

Torres HA et al: Posaconazole: a broad-spectrum triazole antifungal. Lancet Infect Dis 2005;5:775. [PMID: 16310149]

Vazquez JA: Anidulafungin: a new echinocandin with a novel profile. Clin Ther 2005;27:657. [PMID: 16117974]

Anti-Infective Chemotherapeutic & Antibiotic Agents

37

Richard A. Jacobs, MD, PhD, & B. Joseph Guglielmo, PharmD

Selected Principles of Antimicrobial Therapy

Specific steps (outlined below) are required when considering antibiotic therapy for patients. Drugs of first choice and alternative drugs are presented in Table 37–1.

A. ETIOLOGIC DIAGNOSIS

Based on the organ system involved, the organism causing infection can often be predicted. See Tables 37–2 and 37–3.

B. "BEST GUESS"

Select an empiric regimen that is likely to be effective against the suspected pathogens.

C. LABORATORY CONTROL

Specimens for laboratory examination should be obtained before institution of therapy to determine susceptibility.

D. CLINICAL RESPONSE

Based on clinical response and other data, the laboratory reports are evaluated and then the desirability of changing the regimen is considered. If the specimen was obtained from a normally sterile site (eg, blood, cerebrospinal fluid, pleural fluid, joint fluid), the recovery of a microorganism in significant amounts is meaningful even if the organism recovered is different from the clinically suspected agent, and this may force a change in treatment. Isolation of unexpected microorganisms from the respiratory tract, gastrointestinal tract, or surface lesions (sites that have a complex flora) may represent colonization or contamination, and cultures must be critically evaluated before drugs are abandoned that were judiciously selected on a "best guess" basis.

E. DRUG SUSCEPTIBILITY TESTS

Some microorganisms are predictably inhibited by certain drugs; if such organisms are isolated, they need not be tested for drug susceptibility. For example, most group A hemolytic streptococci are inhibited by penicillin. Other organisms (eg, enteric gram-negative rods) are variably susceptible and often require susceptibility testing whenever they are isolated. Organisms that once had predictable susceptibility patterns have now become resistant and require testing. Examples include the pneumococci, which may be resistant to multiple drugs (including penicillin, macrolides, and trimethoprim-sulfamethoxazole) and the enterococci, which may be resistant to penicillin, aminoglycosides, and vancomycin.

Over the past 10 years, pharmaceutical companies have shifted away from developing and producing antibacterial medications. Consequently, few new agents, particularly those active against gram-negative pathogens, are expected. The lack of new drugs and increasing bacterial resistance reinforce the need to use these drugs judiciously.

Antimicrobial drug susceptibility tests may be performed on solid media as "disk tests," in broth in tubes, in wells of microdilution plates, or as E-tests (strips with increasing concentration of antibiotic). The latter three methods yield results expressed as MIC (minimal inhibitory concentration), and the broth and microdilution techniques can be modified to give MBC (minimal bactericidal concentration) results. In most infections, the MIC is the appropriate in vitro test to guide selection of an antibacterial agent. When there appear to be marked discrepancies between susceptibility testing and clinical response, the following possibilities must be considered:

1. Selection of an inappropriate drug, drug dosage, or route of administration.
2. Failure to drain a collection of pus or to remove a foreign body.
3. Failure of a poorly diffusing drug to reach the site of infection (eg, central nervous system) or to reach intracellular phagocytosed bacteria.
4. Superinfection in the course of prolonged chemotherapy.
5. Emergence of drug-resistant organisms.
6. Participation of two or more microorganisms in the infectious process, of which only one was originally detected and used for drug selection.
7. Inadequate host defenses, including immunodeficiencies and diabetes.

Table 37–1. Drugs of choice for suspected or proved microbial pathogens, 2004.[1]

Suspected or Proved Etiologic Agent	Drug(s) of First Choice	Alternative Drug(s)
Gram-negative cocci		
Moraxella catarrhalis	TMP-SMZ,[2] a fluoroquinolone[3]	Cefuroxime, cefotaxime, ceftriaxone, cefuroxime axetil, an erythromycin,[4] a tetracycline,[5] azithromycin, amoxicillin-clavulanic acid, clarithromycin
Neisseria gonorrhoeae (gonococcus)	Ciprofloxacin or ofloxacin	Ceftriaxone, spectinomycin, cefpodoxime proxetil
Neisseria meningitidis (meningococcus)	Penicillin[6]	Cefotaxime, ceftriaxone, ampicillin
Gram-positive cocci		
Streptococcus pneumoniae[8] (pneumococcus)	Penicillin[6]	An erythromycin,[4] a cephalosporin,[7] vancomycin, TMP-SMZ,[2] clindamycin, azithromycin, clarithromycin, a tetracycline,[5] certain fluoroquinolones[3]
Streptococcus, hemolytic, groups A, B, C, G	Penicillin[6]	An erythromycin,[4] a cephalosporin,[7] vancomycin, clindamycin, azithromycin, clarithromycin
Viridans streptococci	Penicillin[6] ± gentamicin	Cephalosporin,[7] vancomycin
Staphylococcus, methicillin-resistant	Vancomycin ± gentamicin	TMP-SMZ,[2] doxycycline, minocycline, a fluoroquinolone,[3] linezolid, daptomycin, quinupristin-dalfopristin
Staphylococcus, non-penicillinase-producing	Penicillin[6]	A cephalosporin,[8] clindamycin
Staphylococcus, penicillinase-producing	Penicillinase-resistant penicillin[9]	Vancomycin, a cephalosporin,[7] clindamycin, amoxicillin-clavulanic acid, ticarcillin-clavulanic acid, ampicillin-sulbactam, piperacillin-tazobactam, TMP-SMZ[2]
Enterococcus faecalis	Ampicillin ± gentamicin[10]	Vancomycin ± gentamicin
Enterococcus faecium	Vancomycin ± gentamicin[10]	Linezolid, quinupristin-dalfopristin, daptomycin
Gram-negative rods		
Acinetobacter	Imipenem or meropenem	Tigecycline, minocycline, doxycycline, aminoglycosides,[11] colistin
Prevotella, oropharyngeal strains	Clindamycin	Penicillin,[6] metronidazole
Bacteroides, gastrointestinal strains	Metronidazole	Clindamycin, ticarcillin-clavulanic acid, ampicillin-sulbactam, piperacillin-tazobactam
Brucella	Tetracycline + rifampin[5]	TMP-SMZ[2] ± gentamicin; chloramphenicol ± gentamicin; doxycycline + gentamicin
Campylobacter jejuni	Erythromycin[4] or azithromycin	Tetracycline,[5] a fluoroquinolone[3]
Enterobacter	TMP-SMZ,[2] imipenem, meropenem	Aminoglycoside, a fluoroquinolone,[3] cefepime
Escherichia coli (sepsis)	Cefotaxime, ceftriaxone,	Imipenem or meropenem, aminoglycosides,[11] a fluoroquinolone[3]
Escherichia coli (uncomplicated urinary infection)	Fluoroquinolones,[3] nitrofurantoin	TMP-SMZ,[2] oral cephalosporin, fosfomycin
Haemophilus (meningitis and other serious infections)	Cefotaxime, ceftriaxone	Aztreonam
Haemophilus (respiratory infections, otitis)	TMP-SMZ[2]	Ampicillin, amoxicillin, doxycycline, azithromycin, clarithromycin, cefotaxime, ceftriaxone, cefuroxime, cefuroxime axetil, ampicillin-clavulanate

(continued)

Table 37–1. Drugs of choice for suspected or proved microbial pathogens, 2004.[1] (continued)

Suspected or Proved Etiologic Agent	Drug(s) of First Choice	Alternative Drug(s)
Gram-negative rods (continued)		
Helicobacter pylori	Amoxicillin + clarithromycin + proton pump inhibitor (PPI)	Bismuth subsalicylate + tetracycline + metronidazole + PPI
Klebsiella	A cephalosporin	TMP-SMZ,[2] aminoglycoside,[11] imipenem or meropenem, a fluoroquinolone,[3] aztreonam
Legionella species (pneumonia)	Erythromycin[4] or clarithromycin or azithromycin, or fluoroquinolones[3] ± rifampin	Doxycycline ± rifampin
Proteus mirabilis	Ampicillin	An aminoglycoside,[11] TMP-SMZ,[2] a fluoroquinolone,[3] a cephalosporin[7]
Proteus vulgaris and other species (*Morganella, Providencia*)	Cefotaxime, ceftriaxone,	Aminoglycoside,[11] imipenem, TMP-SMZ,[2] a fluoroquinolone[3]
Pseudomonas aeruginosa	Aminoglycoside[11] + antipseudomonal penicillin[12]	Ceftazidime ± aminoglycoside; imipenem or meropenem ± aminoglycoside; aztreonam ± aminoglycoside; ciprofloxacin (or levofloxacin) ± piperacillin; ciprofloxacin (or levofloxacin) ± ceftazidime; ciprofloxacin (or levofloxacin) ± cefepime
Burkholderia pseudomallei (melioidosis)	Ceftazidime	Tetracycline,[5] TMP-SMZ,[2] amoxicillin-clavulanic acid, imipenem or meropenem
Burkholderia mallei (glanders)	Streptomycin + tetracycline[5]	Chloramphenicol + streptomycin
Salmonella (bacteremia)	Ceftriaxone, a fluoroquinolone[3]	
Serratia	Cefotaxime, ceftriaxone	TMP-SMZ,[2] aminoglycosides,[11] imipenem or meropenem, a fluoroquinolone[3]
Shigella	A fluoroquinolone[3]	Ampicillin, TMP-SMZ,[2] ceftriaxone
Vibrio (cholera, sepsis)	Tetracycline[5]	TMP-SMZ,[2] a fluoroquinolone[3]
Yersinia pestis (plague, tularemia)	Streptomycin ± a tetracycline[5]	Chloramphenicol, TMP-SMZ[2]
Gram-positive rods		
Actinomyces	Penicillin[6]	Tetracycline,[5] clindamycin
Bacillus (including anthrax)	Penicillin[6] (ciprofloxacin or doxycycline for anthrax; see Table 33–2)	Erythromycin,[4] tetracycline,[5] a fluoroquinolone[3]
Clostridium (eg, gas gangrene, tetanus)	Penicillin[6]	Metronidazole, clindamycin, imipenem or meropenem
Corynebacterium diphtheriae	Erythromycin[4]	Penicillin[6]
Corynebacterium jeikeium	Vancomycin	Ciprofloxacin, penicillin + gentamicin
Listeria	Ampicillin ± aminoglycoside[11]	TMP-SMZ[2]
Acid-fast rods		
Mycobacterium tuberculosis[13]	Isoniazid (INH) + rifampin + pyrazinamide ± ethambutol (or streptomycin)	Other antituberculous drugs (see Tables 9–13 and 9–14)
Mycobacterium leprae	Dapsone + rifampin ± clofazimine	Minocycline, ofloxacin, clarithromycin
Mycobacterium kansasii	INH + rifampin ± ethambutol	Ethionamide, cycloserine

(continued)

Table 37–1. Drugs of choice for suspected or proved microbial pathogens, 2004.[1] (continued)

Suspected or Proved Etiologic Agent	Drug(s) of First Choice	Alternative Drug(s)
Acid-fast rods (continued)		
Mycobacterium avium complex	Clarithromycin or azithromycin + one or more of the following: ethambutol, rifampin or rifabutin, ciprofloxacin	Amikacin
Mycobacterium fortuitum-cheilonei	Amikacin + clarithromycin	Cefoxitin, sulfonamide, doxycycline, linezolid
Nocardia	TMP-SMZ[2]	Minocycline, imipenem or meropenem, sulfisoxazole, linezolid
Spirochetes		
Borrelia burgdorferi (Lyme disease)	Doxycycline, amoxicillin, cefuroxime axetil	Ceftriaxone, cefotaxime, penicillin, azithromycin, clarithromycin
Borrelia recurrentis (relapsing fever)	Doxycycline[5]	Penicillin[6]
Leptospira	Penicillin,[6] ceftriaxone	Doxycycline[5]
Treponema pallidum (syphilis)	Penicillin[6]	Doxycycline, ceftriaxone
Treponema pertenue (yaws)	Penicillin[6]	Doxycycline
Mycoplasmas	Erythromycin[4] or doxycycline	Clarithromycin, azithromycin, a fluoroquinolone[3]
Chlamydiae		
C psittaci	Doxycycline	Chloramphenicol
C trachomatis (urethritis or pelvic inflammatory disease)	Doxycycline or azithromycin	Ofloxacin
C pneumoniae	Doxycycline[5]	Erythromycin,[4] clarithromycin, azithromycin, a fluoroquinolone[3,14]
Rickettsiae	Doxycycline[5]	Chloramphenicol, a fluoroquinolone[3]

[1]Adapted from Med Lett Drugs Ther 2004;2:13.

[2]TMP-SMZ is a mixture of 1 part trimethoprim and 5 parts sulfamethoxazole.

[3]Fluoroquinolones include ciprofloxacin, ofloxacin, levofloxacin, moxifloxacin, gatifloxacin, and others (see text). Gatifloxacin, gemifloxacin, levofloxacin, and moxifloxacin have the best activity against gram-positive organisms, including penicillin-resistant *S pneumoniae* and methicillin-sensitive *S aureus*. Activity against enterococci and *S epidermidis* is variable.

[4]Erythromycin estolate is best absorbed orally but carries the highest risk of hepatitis; erythromycin stearate and erythromycin ethylsuccinate are also available.

[5]All tetracyclines have similar activity against most microorganisms. Minocycline and doxycycline have increased activity against *S aureus*.

[6]Penicillin G is preferred for parenteral injection; penicillin V for oral administration—to be used only in treating infections due to highly sensitive organisms.

[7]Most intravenous cephalosporins (with the exception of ceftazidime) have good activity against gram-positive cocci.

[8]Infections caused by isolates with intermediate resistance may respond to high doses of penicillin, cefotaxime, or ceftriaxone. Infections caused by highly resistant strains should be treated with vancomycin. Many strains of penicillin-resistant pneumococci are resistant to macrolides, cephalosporins, tetracyclines, and TMP-SMZ.

[9]Parenteral nafcillin or oxacillin; oral dicloxacillin, cloxacillin, or oxacillin.

[10]Addition of gentamicin indicated only for severe enterococcal infections (eg, endocarditis, meningitis).

[11]Aminoglycosides—gentamicin, tobramycin, amikacin, netilmicin—should be chosen on the basis of local patterns of susceptibility.

[12]Antipseudomonal penicillins: ticarcillin, piperacillin.

[13]Resistance is common and susceptibility testing should be done.

[14]Ciprofloxacin has inferior antichlamydial activity compared with newer fluoroquinolones.

Key: ± = alone or combined with.

Table 37–2. Examples of initial antimicrobial therapy for acutely ill, hospitalized adults pending identification of causative organism.

Suspected Clinical Diagnosis	Likely Etiologic Diagnosis	Drugs of Choice
(A) Meningitis, bacterial, community-acquired	Pneumococcus,[1] meningococcus	Cefotaxime,[2] 2–3 g IV every 6 hours; **or** ceftriaxone, 2 g IV every 12 hours plus vancomycin, 10 mg/kg IV every 8 hours
(B) Meningitis, bacterial, age > 50, community-acquired	Pneumococcus, meningococcus, *Listeria monocytogenes*,[3] gram-negative bacilli	Ampicillin, 2 g IV every 4 hours, plus cefotaxime or ceftriaxone and vancomycin as in (A)
(C) Meningitis, postoperative (or posttraumatic)	*S aureus*, gram-negative bacilli (pneumococcus, in posttraumatic)	Vancomycin, 10 mg/kg IV every 8 hours, plus ceftazidime, 3 g IV every 8 hours
(D) Brain abscess	Mixed anaerobes, pneumococci, streptococci	Penicillin G, 4 million units IV every 4 hours, plus metronidazole, 500 mg orally every 8 hours; **or** cefotaxime or ceftriaxone as in (A) plus metronidazole, 500 mg orally every 8 hours
(E) Pneumonia, acute, community-acquired, severe	Pneumococci, *M pneumoniae*, Legionella, *C pneumoniae*	Doxycycline, 100 mg IV or orally every 12 hours (or azithromycin), plus cefotaxime, 2 g IV every 8 hours (or ceftriaxone, 1 g IV every 24 hours); **or** a fluoroquinolone[5] alone
(F) Pneumonia, postoperative or nosocomial	*S aureus*, mixed anaerobes, gram-negative bacilli	Cefepime, 2 g IV every 8 hours; **or** ceftazidime, 2 g IV every 8 hours; **or** piperacillin-tazobactam, 4.5 g IV every 6 hours; **or** imipenem, 500 mg IV every 6 hours; **or** meropenem, 1 g IV every 8 hours plus tobramycin, 5 mg/kg IV every 24 hours; **or** ciprofloxacin, 400 mg IV every 12 hours; **or** levofloxacin, 500 mg IV every 24 hours plus vancomycin, 15 mg/kg IV every 12 hours
(G) Endocarditis, acute (including injection drug user)	*S aureus*, *E faecalis*, gram-negative aerobic bacteria, viridans streptococci	Vancomycin, 15 mg/kg IV every 12 hours, plus gentamicin, 1 mg/kg every 8 hours
(H) Septic thrombophlebitis (eg, IV tubing, IV shunts)	*S aureus*, gram-negative aerobic bacteria	Vancomycin, 15 mg/kg IV every 12 hours plus ciprofloxacin, 400 mg IV every 12 hours; **or** levofloxacin, 500 mg IV every 24 hours; **or** ceftriaxone, 1 g IV every 24 hours
(I) Osteomyelitis	*S aureus*	Nafcillin, 2 g IV every 4 hours; **or** cefazolin, 2 g IV every 8 hours
(J) Septic arthritis	*S aureus*, *N gonorrhoeae*	Ceftriaxone, 1–2 g IV every 24 hours
(K) Pyelonephritis with flank pain and fever (recurrent urinary tract infection)	*E coli*, Klebsiella, Enterobacter, Pseudomonas	Ceftriaxone, 1 g IV every 24 hours; **or** ciprofloxacin, 400 mg IV every 12 hours (500 mg orally); **or** levofloxacin, 500 mg once daily (IV/PO)
(L) Fever in neutropenic patient receiving cancer chemotherapy	*S aureus*, Pseudomonas, Klebsiella, *E coli*	Ceftazidime, 2 g IV every 8 hours; **or** cefepime, 2 g IV every 8 hours
(M) Intra-abdominal sepsis (eg, postoperative, peritonitis, cholecystitis)	Gram-negative bacteria, Bacteroides, anaerobic bacteria, streptococci, clostridia	Piperacillin-tazobactam as in (F) or ticarcillin-clavulanate, 3.1 g IV every 6 hours; **or** ertapenem, 1 g every 24 hours; **or** moxifloxacin, 400 mg IV every 24 hours

[1]Some strains may be resistant to penicillin. Vancomycin can be used with or without rifampin.
[2]Cefotaxime, ceftriaxone, ceftazidime, or ceftizoxime can be used. Most studies on meningitis have been with cefotaxime or ceftriaxone (see text).
[3]TMP-SMZ can be used to treat *Listeria monocytogenes* in patients allergic to penicillin in a dosage of 15–20 mg/kg of TMP in three or four divided doses.
[4]Depending on local drug susceptibility pattern, use tobramycin, 5 mg/kg/d, or amikacin, 15 mg/kg/d, in place of gentamicin.
[5]Gatifloxacin, levofloxacin, moxifloxacin.

Table 37–3. Examples of empiric choices of antimicrobials for adult outpatient infections.

Suspected Clinical Diagnosis	Likely Etiologic Agents	Drugs of Choice	Alternative Drugs
Erysipelas, impetigo, cellulitis, ascending lymphangitis	Group A streptococcus	Phenoxymethyl penicillin, 0.5 g orally four times daily for 7–10 days	Cephalexin, 0.5 g orally four times daily for 7–10 days; **or** azithromycin, 500 mg on day 1 and 250 mg on days 2–5; **or** erythromycin, 0.5 g orally four times daily for 7–10 days
Furuncle with surrounding cellulitis	*Staphylococcus aureus*	Dicloxacillin, 0.5 g orally four times daily for 7–10 days	Cephalexin, 0.5 g orally four times daily for 7–10 days
Pharyngitis	Group A streptococcus	Phenoxymethyl penicillin, 0.5 g orally four times daily for 10 days	Clindamycin, 300 mg orally four times daily for 10 days; **or** erythromycin, 0.5 g orally four times daily for 10 days; **or** azithromycin, 500 mg on day 1 and 250 mg on days 2–5; **or** clarithromycin, 500 mg twice daily for 10 days
Otitis media	*Streptococcus pneumoniae, Haemophilus influenzae, Moraxella catarrhalis*	Amoxicillin, 0.5 g orally three times daily for 10 days	Augmentin,[2] 0.875 g orally twice daily; **or** cefuroxime, 0.5 g orally twice daily; **or** cefpodoxime, 0.2–0.4 g daily; **or** doxycycline, 100 mg twice daily; **or** TMP-SMZ,[1] one double-strength tablet twice daily (all regimens for 10 days).
Acute sinusitis	*S pneumoniae, H influenzae, M catarrhalis*	Amoxicillin, 0.5 g orally three times daily; or TMP-SMZ, one double-strength tablet twice daily for 10 days	Augmentin,[2] 0.875 g orally twice daily; **or** cefuroxime, 0.5 g orally twice daily; **or** cefpodoxime, 0.2–0.4 g daily; **or** doxycycline, 100 mg twice daily (all regimens for 10 days)
Aspiration pneumonia	Mixed oropharyngeal flora, including anaerobes	Clindamycin, 0.3 g orally four times daily for 10–14 days	Phenoxymethyl penicillin, 0.5 g orally four times daily for 10–14 days
Pneumonia	*S pneumoniae, Mycoplasma pneumoniae, Legionella pneumophila, Chlamydia pneumoniae*	Doxycycline, 100 mg orally twice daily; **or** clarithromycin, 0.5 g orally twice daily, for 10–14 days; **or** azithromycin, 0.5 g orally on day 1 and 0.25 g on days 2–5	Amoxicillin, 0.5 g orally four times daily; **or** a fluoroquinolone[5] for 10–14 days
Cystitis	*Escherichia coli, Klebsiella pneumoniae, Proteus* species, *Staphylococcus saprophyticus*	Fluoroquinolones,[4] 3 days for uncomplicated cystitis, nitrofurantoin macrocrystals, 100 mg orally QID × 7 days; nitrofurantoin monohydrate macrocrystals, 100 mg BID × 7 days	TMP-SMZ,[1] one double-strength tablet twice daily for 3 days; **or** cephalexin, 0.5 g orally four times daily for 7 days
Pyelonephritis	*E coli, K pneumoniae, Proteus* species, *S saprophyticus*	Fluoroquinolones[4] for 7–14 days	TMP-SMZ,[1] one double-strength tablet twice daily for 7–14 days
Gastroenteritis	*Salmonella, Shigella, Campylobacter, Entamoeba histolytica*	See Note 3.	
Urethritis, epididymitis	*Neisseria gonorrhoeae, Chlamydia trachomatis*	Ciprofloxacin, 500 mg orally once, for *N gonorrhoeae*; plus doxycycline, 100 mg orally twice daily for 10 days, or ofloxacin, 300 mg orally twice daily for 10 days	Ceftriaxone, 250 mg IM once or cefpodoxime 200–400 mg orally once, for *N gonorrhoeae*; plus doxycycline, 100 mg orally twice daily for 10 days, for *C trachomatis*

(continued)

Table 37–3. Examples of empiric choices of antimicrobials for adult outpatient infections. (continued)

Suspected Clinical Diagnosis	Likely Etiologic Agents	Drugs of Choice	Alternative Drugs
Pelvic inflammatory disease	*N gonorrhoeae, C trachomatis,* anaerobes, gram-negative rods	Ofloxacin, 400 mg orally twice daily, for 14 days, plus metronidazole, 500 mg orally twice daily, for 14 days	Cefoxitin, 2 g IM, with probenecid, 1 g orally, followed by doxycycline, 100 mg orally twice daily for 14 days; **or** ceftriaxone, 250 mg IM once, followed by doxycycline, 100 mg orally twice daily for 14 days
Syphilis			
Early syphilis (primary, secondary, or latent of < 1 year's duration)	*Treponema pallidum*	Benzathine penicillin G, 2.4 million units IM once	Doxycycline, 100 mg orally twice daily for 2 weeks
Latent syphilis of > 1 year's duration or cardiovascular syphilis	*T pallidum*	Benzathine penicillin G, 2.4 million units IM once a week for 3 weeks (total: 7.2 million units)	Doxycycline, 100 mg orally twice daily, for 4 weeks
Neurosyphilis	*T pallidum*	Aqueous penicillin G, 12–24 million units/d IV for 10–14 days	Procaine penicillin G, 2–4 million units/d IM, plus probenecid, 500 mg orally four times daily, both for 10–14 days

[1]TMP-SMZ is a fixed combination of 1 part trimethoprim and 5 parts sulfamethoxazole. Single-strength tablets: 80 mg TMP, 400 mg SMZ; double-strength tablets: 160 mg TMP, 800 mg SMZ.

[2]Augmentin is a combination of amoxicillin, 250 mg, 500 mg, or 875 mg, plus 125 mg of clavulanic acid. Augmentin XR is a combination of amoxicillin 1 g and clavulanic acid 62.5 mg.

[3]The diagnosis should be confirmed by culture before therapy. Salmonella gastroenteritis does not require therapy. For susceptible *Shigella* isolates, give TMP-SMZ double-strength tablets twice daily for 5 days; or ampicillin, 0.5 g orally four times daily for 5 days; or ciprofloxacin, 0.5 g orally twice daily for 5 days. For *Campylobacter* infection, give erythromycin, 0.5 g orally four times daily for 5 days, or ciprofloxacin, 0.5 g orally twice daily for 5 days. For *E histolytica* infection, give metronidazole, 750 mg orally three times daily for 5–10 days, followed by diiodohydroxyquin, 600 mg orally three times daily for 3 weeks.

[4]Fluoroquinolones and dosages include ciprofloxacin, 500 mg orally twice daily; ofloxacin, 400 mg orally twice daily; levofloxacin, 500 mg orally daily. For others see text.

[5]Fluoroquinolones with activity against *S pneumoniae,* including penicillin-resistant isolates, include levofloxacin (500 mg orally once daily), gatifloxacin (400 mg orally once daily), gemifloxacin (320 mg orally once daily), and moxifloxacin (400 mg orally once daily).

8. Noninfectious causes, including drug fever, malignancy, and autoimmune disease.

F. Promptness of Response

Response depends on a number of factors, including the patient (immunocompromised patients respond slower than immunocompetent patients), the site of infection (deep-seated infections such as osteomyelitis and endocarditis respond more slowly than superficial infections such as cystitis or cellulitis), the pathogen (virulent organisms such as *Staphylococcus aureus* respond more slowly than viridans streptococci; mycobacterial and fungal infections respond slower than bacterial infections), and the duration of illness (in general, the longer the symptoms are present, the longer it takes to respond). Thus, depending on the clinical situation, persistent fever and leukocytosis several days after initiation of therapy may not indicate improper choice of antibiotics but may be due to the natural history of the disease being treated. In most infections, either a bacteriostatic or a bactericidal agent can be used. In some infections (eg, infective endocarditis and meningitis), a bactericidal agent should be used. When potentially toxic drugs (eg, aminoglycosides, flucytosine) are used, serum levels of the drug are measured to minimize toxicity and ensure appropriate dosage. In patients with altered clearance of drugs, the dosage or frequency of administration must be adjusted. Especially in elderly, morbidly obese patients or those with altered renal function, it is best to measure levels directly and adjust therapy accordingly.

In renal or hepatic failure, the dosage should be adjusted as shown in Table 37–4.

G. Duration of Antimicrobial Therapy

Generally, effective antimicrobial treatment results in reversal of the clinical and laboratory parameters of active infection and marked clinical improvement. However, varying periods of treatment may be required for cure. Key factors include (1) the type of infecting organism (bacterial infections generally can be cured more rapidly than fungal or mycobacterial

Table 37-4. Use of antimicrobials in patients with renal failure[1] and hepatic failure.

Drug	Principal Mode of Excretion or Detoxification	Approximate Half-Life in Serum — Normal	Approximate Half-Life in Serum — Renal Failure[2]	Proposed Dosage Regimen in End-Stage Renal Failure (all doses IV unless stated otherwise) — Initial Dose[3]	Proposed Dosage Regimen in End-Stage Renal Failure (all doses IV unless stated otherwise) — Maintenance Dose	Removal of Drug by Hemodialysis	Dose after Hemodialysis	Dosage in Hepatic Failure
Acyclovir	Renal	2.5–3.5 hours	20 hours	2.5 mg/kg	2.5 mg/kg q24h	Yes	2.5 mg/kg	No change
Amphotericin B	Unknown	360 hours	360 hours	No change	No change	No	None	No change
Ampicillin	Tubular secretion	0.5–1 hour	8–12 hours	1 g	1 g q8–12h	Yes	1 g	No change
Ampicillin-sulbactam	Renal	0.5–1 hour	8–12 hours	3 g	1.5 g q8–12h	Yes	1.5 g	No change
Azithromycin	Renal 20%; hepatic 35%	3–4 hours	Not known	500 mg	250 mg q24h	No	None	Not known[4]
Aztreonam	Renal	1.7 hours	6 hours	1–2 g	0.5–1 g q6–8h	Yes	0.5–1 g	No change
Caspofungin	Liver	9–10 hours	9–10 hours	70 mg	50 mg q24h	No	None	35 mg q24h
Chloramphenicol	Mainly liver	3 hours	4 hours	0.5 g	0.5 g q6h	Yes	0.5 g	0.25–0.5 g q12h
Clarithromycin	Renal 30%; hepatic > 50%	3–4 hours	15 hours	500 mg PO	250 mg q12h PO	No	None	Not known[4]
Clindamycin	Liver	2–4 hours	2–4 hours	0.6 g IV	0.6 g q8h	No	None	0.3–0.6 g q8h
Daptomycin	Renal	8–12 hours	>24 hours	4 mg/kg	4 mg/kg q48h	No	None	No change
Doxycycline	Renal	15–24 hours	15–24 hours	100 mg	100 mg q12h	No	None	Not known[4]
Ertapenem	Renal	4 hours	20 hours	1 g	0.5 g q24h	Yes	0.15 g	No change
Erythromycin	Mainly liver	1.5 hours	1.5 hours	0.5–1 g	0.5–1 g q6h	No	None	0.25–0.5 g q6h
Famciclovir[5]	Renal	2.5 hours	13–20 hours	500 mg PO	500 mg q24h PO	Yes	500 mg	No change
Fluconazole	Renal	30 hours	98 hours	0.2 g	0.1 g q24h	Yes	Give q24h dose	No change
Flucytosine	Renal	3–6 hours	30–250 hours	37.5 mg/kg PO	25 mg/kg q24h PO	Yes	25 mg/kg	No change
Foscarnet	Renal	3–8 hours	Not known	90–120 mg	Not known[6]	No	None	No change
Fosfomycin	Renal	6 hours	11–50 hours	NA	NA	NA	NA	No change
Ganciclovir[7]	Renal	3 hours	11–28 hours	1.25 mg/kg	1.25 mg/kg q24h	Yes	Give q24h dose	No change
Gemifloxacin	Renal and liver	7 hours	Not known	320 mg PO	160 mg q24h PO	Not known	Not known	Not known
Imipenem	Glomerular filtration	1 hour	3 hours	0.5 g	0.25–0.5 g q12h	Yes	0.25–0.5 g	No change
Isoniazid	Renal	1–5 hours	2.5 hours	300 mg PO	300 mg q24h PO	Yes	None	Not known[4]
Itraconazole	Hepatic	21 hours	25 hours	50–200 mg PO	50–200 mg q24h PO	No	None	Not known[4]

(continued)

Table 37–4. Use of antimicrobials in patients with renal failure[1] and hepatic failure. (continued)

Drug	Principal Mode of Excretion or Detoxification	Approximate Half-Life in Serum		Proposed Dosage Regimen in End-Stage Renal Failure (all doses IV unless stated otherwise)		Removal of Drug by Hemodialysis	Dose after Hemodialysis	Dosage in Hepatic Failure
		Normal	Renal Failure[2]	Initial Dose[3]	Maintenance Dose			
Ketoconazole	Hepatic	8 hours	8 hours	200 mg PO	200–400 mg q24h PO	No	None	Not known[4]
Meropenem	Renal	1 hour	5–10 hours	1 g	0.5–1 g q24h	Yes	0.5 g	No change
Metronidazole	Liver	6–10 hours	6–10 hours	0.5 g IV	0.5 g q8h	Yes	0.25 g	0.25 g q12h
Micafungin	Bilary/hepatic	15 hours	15 hours	150 mg	150 mg q24h	No	None	No change
Nafcillin	Liver 80%; kidney 20%	0.75 hour	1.5 hours	1.5 g	1.5 g q4h	No	None	2–3 g q12h
Penicillin G	Tubular secretion	0.5 hour	7–10 hours	1–2 million units	1 million units q8h	Yes	500,000 units	No change
Pentamidine	Not known	6–9 hours	6–9 hours	4 mg/kg	4 mg/kg q24h	No	None needed	No change
Piperacillin and piper-acillin + tazobactam	Renal 50–70%; biliary 20–30%	1 hour	3–6 hours	3 g	2 g q6–8h	Yes	1 g	1–2 g q8h
Rifampin	Hepatic	2–3 hours	3–5 hours	600 mg PO	600 mg q24h PO	No	None	Not known[4]
Telithromycin	Hepatic	7–10 hours	7–10 hours	800 mg PO	800 mg q24h PO	Not known	Not known	Not known
Ticarcillin	Tubular secretion	1.1 hours	15–20 hours	3 g	2 g q6–8h	Yes	1 g	No change
Tigecycline	Hepatic	25–40 hours	25–40 hours	100 mg	50 mg q12h	No	None	No change
Trimethoprim-sulfa-methoxazole	Some liver	TMP 10–12 hours; SMZ 8–10 hours	TMP 24–48 hours; SMZ 18–24 hours	320 mg TMP + 1600 mg SMZ	80 mg TMP + 400 mg SMZ q12h	Yes	80 mg TMP + 400 mg SMZ	No change
Trimetrexate	Hepatic	15 hours	Not known	45 mg/m²	40 mg/m² q24h	No	None	Not known
Vancomycin	Glomerular filtration	6 hours	6–10 days	1 g	1 g q6–10d based on serum levels[8]	No	None	No change
Voriconazole	Hepatic	6–24 hours; dose-dependent	6–24 hours	200 mg orally; avoid IV in renal failure	200 mg orally twice daily; avoid IV in renal failure	No	None	100 mg twice daily

[1]For cephalosporins, see text and Table 37–7; for aminoglycosides, see Table 37–8.
[2]Considered here to be marked by creatinine clearance of 10 mL/min or less.
[3]For a 70-kg adult with a serious systemic infection.
[4]Dose adjustment in hepatic failure has not been studied, but because clearance of the drug is principally hepatic, dose reduction may be required.
[5]Pharmacokinetics and dosing are in reference to the active agent, penciclovir.
[6]When creatinine clearance is 30 mL/min, a dose of 60 mg/kg is given once daily. For clearances less than 30 mL/min, the dose has not been established.
[7]Oral valganciclovir is same as IV ganciclovir except that the initial dose is 900 mg. maintenance dose is 450 mg twice weekly in patients with creatinine clearance 10–40 mL/min. Post doses not known.
[8]When serum levels reach 10–15 mcg/mL, another dose should be given.

ones), (2) the location of the process (eg, endocarditis and osteomyelitis require prolonged therapy), and (3) the immunocompetence of the patient. Recommendations about duration of therapy are often given based on clinical experience, not prospective controlled studies of large numbers of patients.

H. Adverse Reactions and Toxicity

These include hypersensitivity reactions, direct toxicity, superinfection by drug-resistant microorganisms, and drug interactions. If the infection is life-threatening and treatment cannot be stopped, the reactions are managed symptomatically or another drug is chosen that does not cross-react with the offending one (Table 37–1). If the infection is less serious, it may be possible to stop all antimicrobials and monitor the patient closely.

I. Route of Administration

Parenteral therapy is preferred for acutely ill patients with serious infections (eg, endocarditis, meningitis, sepsis, severe pneumonia) when dependable levels of antibiotics are required for successful therapy. Certain drugs (eg, fluconazole, voriconazole, rifampin, metronidazole, trimethoprim-sulfamethoxazole, and fluoroquinolones) are so well absorbed that they generally can be administered orally in seriously ill patients.

Food does not significantly influence the bioavailability of most oral antimicrobial agents. However, the tetracyclines and the quinolones chelate heavy metals resulting in decreased antibacterial absorption. Azithromycin capsules are associated with decreased bioavailability when taken with food and should be given 1 hour before or 2 hours after meals.

A major complication of intravenous antibiotic therapy is catheter infections. Peripheral catheters are changed every 48–72 hours to prevent phlebitis, and antimicrobial-coated central venous catheters (minocycline and rifampin, chlorhexidine and sulfadiazine) have been associated with a decreased incidence of catheter-related infections. Most of these infections present with local signs of infection (erythema, tenderness) at the insertion site. In a patient with fever who is receiving intravenous therapy, the catheter must always be considered a potential source. Small-gauge (20–23F) peripherally inserted silicone or polyurethane catheters (Per Q Cath, A-Cath, Ven-A-Cath, and others) are associated with a low infection rate and can be maintained for 3–6 months without replacement. Such catheters are ideal for long-term outpatient antibiotic therapy.

J. Cost of Antibiotics

The cost of these agents can be substantial. In addition to acquisition cost, monitoring costs, (drug levels, liver function tests, electrolytes, etc), the cost of treating adverse reactions, the cost of treatment failure, and the costs associated with drug administration must be considered. Table 37–5 lists the costs of commonly used antibiotics.

Drusano GL: Antimicrobial pharmacodynamics: critical interactions of 'bug and drug'. Nat Rev 2004;2:289. [PMID: 15031728]

Lampiris HW, Maddix DS: Clinical use of antimicrobial agents. In: *Basic & Clinical Pharmacology,* 9th ed. Katzung BG (editor). McGraw-Hill, 2004.

Spellberg B et al: Trends in antimicrobial drug development: implications for the future. Clin Infec Dis 2004;38:1279. [PMID: 15127341]

PENICILLINS

The penicillins share a common chemical nucleus (6-aminopenicillanic acid) that contains a β-lactam ring essential to their biologic activity.

Antimicrobial Action & Resistance

The initial step in penicillin action is the binding of the drug to receptors—penicillin-binding proteins. The proteins of different organisms vary in number and in affinity for a given drug. After penicillins have attached to receptors, peptidoglycan synthesis is inhibited because the activity of transpeptidation enzymes is blocked. The final bactericidal action is the removal of an inhibitor of the autolytic enzymes in the cell wall, which activates the enzymes and results in cell lysis. Organisms that produce β-lactamases (penicillinases) are resistant to some penicillins because the β-lactam ring is broken and the drug is inactivated. Only organisms actively synthesizing peptidoglycan (in the process of multiplication) are susceptible to β-lactam antibiotics. Nonmultiplying organisms or those lacking cell walls are not susceptible.

Microbial resistance to penicillins is caused by four factors: (1) Production of β-lactamases, eg, by staphylococci, gonococci, *Haemophilus* species, and coliform organisms; (2) lack of penicillin-binding proteins or decreased affinity of penicillin-binding protein for β-lactam antibiotic receptors (eg, resistant pneumococci, methicillin-resistant staphylococci, enterococci) or impermeability of cell envelope; (3) failure of activation of autolytic enzymes in the cell wall—"tolerance," eg, in staphylococci, group B streptococci; and (4) cell wall-deficient (L) forms or mycoplasmas, which do not synthesize peptidoglycans.

1. Natural Penicillins

The natural penicillins include penicillin G for parenteral administration (aqueous crystalline, procaine, and benzathine penicillin G) or for oral administration (penicillin G and phenoxymethyl penicillin [penicillin V]). They are most active against gram-positive organisms and are susceptible to hydrolysis by β-lactamases. They are used (1) for infections caused by susceptible and moderately susceptible pneumococci, depending on the site of infection (however, up to 30–35% of strains now demonstrate intermediate- or high-level resistance to penicillin); (2) streptococci (including anaerobic streptococci); (3) meningococci; (4) non–β-lactamase-

Table 37–5. Approximate costs of antimicrobials.

Drug	Dose per Day[1]	Cost per Unit[2]	Daily Cost of Therapy[3]
INTRAVENOUS PREPARATIONS			
Acyclovir	15 mg/kg (mucocutaneous herpes)	$19.20/1 g	$19.20
Acyclovir	30 mg/kg (CNS herpes)	$19.20/1 g	$38.40
Amikacin (Amikin, others)	15 mg/kg	$7.80/0.5 g	$15.60
Ampicillin	100 mg/kg	$16.75/2 g	$67.00
Ampicillin plus sulbactam (Unasyn)	3 g q8h	$15.50/3 g (IV)	$46.50
Aztreonam (Azactam)	50 mg/kg	$26.70/1 g	$106.80
Caspofungin (Cancidas)	50 mg	$395.00	$395.00
Cefazolin (Ancef, others)	50 mg/kg	$4.30/1 g (IV)	$12.90
Cefepime (Maxipime)	500 mg/kg	$19.40/1 g	$58.20
Cefoxitin (Mefoxin)	80 mg/kg	$11.25/1 g	$33.75
Ceftazidime (Fortaz, others)	50 mg/kg	$14.25/1 g	$42.75
Ceftizoxime (Cefizox)	50 mg/kg	$11.40/1 g	$34.20
Ceftriaxone (Rocephin)	30 mg/kg	$49.00/1 g	$49.00
Cefuroxime (Zinacef, others)	60 mg/kg	$23.90/1.5 g	$71.70
Ciprofloxacin (Cipro IV)	0.8 mg	$28.80/0.4 g	$57.60
Clindamycin (Cleocin, others)	2400 mg	$4.30/0.6 g	$17.20
Daptomycin (Cubicin)	4 mg/kg	$171.10/500 mg	$171.10
Fluconazole (Diflucan IV)	0.2–0.4 g	$116.50/0.2 g $170.30/0.4 g	$116.50–170.30
Foscarnet (Foscavir)	180 mg/kg (induction) 90–120 mg/kg (maintenance)	$83.25 (24 mg/mL × 250 mL = 6000 mg)	$166.50 $83.25–111.00
Ganciclovir (Cytovene IV)	10 mg/kg	$44.80/0.5 g	$89.60
Gatifloxacin (Tequin)	400 mg	$38.20/400 mg	$38.20
Gentamicin	5 mg/kg	$0.80/80 mg	$2.40
Imipenem (Primaxin IV)	50 mg/kg	$34.40/0.5 g	$137.60
Meropenem (Merrem IV)	500 mg/kg	$30.00/0.5 g	$90.00–120.00
Metronidazole (Flagyl, others)	1500 mg	$2.80/0.5 g	$8.40
Micafungin (Mycamine)	150 mg	$112.20/50 mg	$336.60
Nafcillin	100 mg/kg	$15.20/2 g	$60.80
Penicillin	12 million units	$8.00/1 million units	$96.00
Piperacillin (Pipracil)	250 mg/kg	$12.50/3 g	$60.00
Piperacillin plus tazobactam (Zosyn)	3.75 g q6–8h	$17.20/3.375 g	$68.80
Ticarcillin (Ticar)	250 mg/kg	$12.40/3 g	$49.60
Ticarcillin-potassium clavulanic acid (Timentin)	3.1 g q6h	$15.10/3.1 g	$60.40
Tigecycline (Tygacil)	50 mg q12h	$54.30/50 mg	$108.60
Tobramycin	5 mg/kg	$6.00/80 mg	$30.00
Trimethoprim-sulfamethoxazole (Bactrim, Septra)	15 mg/kg TMP	$19.50 (0.48 g TMP in 30 mL)	$39.00

(continued)

Table 37–5. Approximate costs of antimicrobials. (continued)

Drug	Dose per Day[1]	Cost per Unit[2]	Daily Cost of Therapy[3]
INTRAVENOUS PREPARATIONS (continued)			
Vancomycin	20–30 mg/kg	$6.00/1 g	$12.00
Voriconazole (VFend)	200 mg q12h	$110.30/200 mg	$220.60
ORAL PREPARATIONS			
Acyclovir	1000 mg (therapy of herpes)	$1.10/0.2 g	$5.50
Acyclovir	800 mg three times daily (herpes suppression for immunocompromised patient)	$4.20/0.8 g	$12.60
Amoxicillin	20–30 mg/kg	$0.40/0.5 g	$1.20
Ampicillin	20–30 mg/kg	$0.40/0.5 g	$1.60
Augmentin (0.5 g amoxicillin plus 0.125 g clavulanic acid)	30 mg/kg	$3.80/0.5 g	$7.60
Azithromycin (Zithromax)	500 mg as loading dose, then 250 mg/d for 4 days	$8.80/0.25 g	$17.60 load, then $8.80
Azithromycin (Zithromax)	1 g as single dose for *C trachomatis* infection	$25.80/1 g packet	$25.80/1 g packet
Cefaclor (Ceclor)	20–30 mg/kg	$3.90/0.5 g	$11.70
Cefditoren (Spectracef)	400 mg twice daily	$2.10/200 mg	$8.40
Cefpodoxime proxetil (Vantin)	400 mg	$6.60/0.2 g	$13.20
Cefprozil (0.5 g) (Cefzil)	15 mg/kg	$8.90/0.5 g	$17.80
Cefuroxime (0.5 g) (Ceftin)	0.5 g twice daily	$8.00/0.5 g	$16.00
Cephalexin (0.5 g) (Keflex, others)	30 mg/kg	$1.40/0.5 g	$5.60
Ciprofloxacin (0.5 g) (Cipro)	0.5–0.75 g twice daily	$5.20/0.5 g	$10.40
Ciprofloxacin (0.75 g) (Cipro)		$5.40/0.75 g	$10.80
Clarithromycin (0.25 or 0.5 g) (Biaxin)	250–500 mg twice daily	$4.80/0.5 g	$9.60
Clindamycin (0.3 g) (Cleocin, others)	15 mg/kg	$1.20/150 mg	$9.60
Doxycycline (0.1 g)	3 mg/kg	$1.35/0.1 g	$2.70
Erythromycin (0.5 g)	30 mg/kg	$0.30/0.5 g	$0.90
Famciclovir (0.5 g) (Famvir)	500 mg three times daily	$9.40/0.5 g	$28.20
Fluconazole (0.1 g)	0.1–0.2 g daily	$8.30/0.1 g	$8.30
Fluconazole (0.2 g) (Diflucan)		$13.60/0.2 g	$13.60
Flucytosine (0.5 g) (Ancobon)	150 mg/kg	$9.70/0.5 g	$194.00
Gatifloxacin (0.4 g) (Tequin)	400 mg	$10.20/0.4 g	$10.20
Gemifloxacin (.32 g) (Factiv)	320 mg	$18.65/320 mg	$18.65
Itraconazole (0.1 g) (Sporanox)	200–400 mg	$9.90/0.1 g	$19.80–39.60
Ketoconazole (0.2 g) (Nizoral)	0.2–0.4 g	$3.20/0.2 g	$3.20–6.40
Levofloxacin (0.5 g) (Levaquin)	0.5 g daily	$11.80/0.5 g	$11.80
Loracarbef (0.4 mg) (Lorabid)	800 mg	$6.40/0.4 g	$12.80
Metronidazole (0.5 g) (Flagyl)	20 mg/kg	$0.70/0.5 g	$2.10
Moxifloxacin (0.4 g) (Avelox)	400 mg	$11.20/0.4 g	$11.20

(continued)

Table 37–5. Approximate costs of antimicrobials. (continued)

Drug	Dose per Day[1]	Cost per Unit[2]	Daily Cost of Therapy[3]
ORAL PREPARATIONS (continued)			
Ofloxacin (0.4 g) (Floxin)	400 mg twice daily	$6.80/0.4 g	$13.60
Penicillin VK (0.5 g)	30 mg/kg	$0.40/0.5 g	$1.60
Telithromycin (Ketec)	800 mg	$5.80/400 mg	$11.60
Tetracycline (0.5 g)	30 mg/kg	$0.10/0.5 g	$0.40
Trimethoprim-sulfamethoxazole (Bactrim, Septra)	5 mg/kg TMP	$1.20/160 mg TMP and 800 mg SMZ	$2.40
Valacyclovir (0.5 g) (Valtrex)	0.5–1 g three times daily	$5.50/0.5 g	$15.50–29.70
Valganciclovir 450 mg (Valcyte)	0.9 g twice daily	$31.70/450 mg	$126.80
Vancomycin (Vancocin)	125 mg three times daily	$9.20/125 mg	$27.60
Voriconazole (VFend)	200 mg twice daily	$35.40/200 mg	$70.80

[1]Doses based on a 70-kg individual with normal renal function.
[2]Approximate average wholesale price to pharmacist (for AB-rated generic when available) for quantity listed.
Source: *Red Book* Update, Vol. 25, No. 5, May 2006. Average wholesale price may not accurately represent the actual pharmacy cost because wide contractual variations exist among institutions.
[3]Daily cost for intravenous antibiotics includes acquisition cost only and not preparation and administration costs.

producing staphylococci; (5) *Treponema pallidum* and other spirochetes; (6) *Propionibacterium acnes* and other gram-positive rods; (7) non-difficile clostridia; (8) actinomyces; and (9) most gram-positive anaerobes. See Table 37–1.

Pharmacokinetics & Administration

After parenteral administration, penicillin has wide extracellular distribution. Lower levels are present in the eye, prostate, and central nervous system. However, with inflammation of the meninges and with appropriate dosing, adequate penetration into the cerebrospinal fluid takes place.

Special dosage forms of penicillin permit delayed absorption to yield low blood and tissue levels for long periods, eg, benzathine penicillin G and procaine penicillin G.

Phenoxymethyl penicillin (penicillin V) is the oral penicillin of choice because of its superior bioavailability. Primarily renally eliminated, 90% is cleared by tubular secretion.

Clinical Uses

Most infections due to susceptible organisms respond to aqueous penicillin G in daily doses of 1–2 million units administered intravenously every 4–6 hours. For life-threatening infections (meningitis, endocarditis), larger daily doses (18–24 million units intravenously) are required.

Penicillin V is indicated in minor infections such as streptococcal pharyngitis and cellulitis. Syphilis is usu-

ally treated with weekly injections of benzathine penicillin, 2.4 million units intramuscularly for 1–3 weeks, depending on the stage of the disease (see Table 37–3).

Procaine penicillin is rarely used except as an alternative regimen for neurosyphilis.

2. Extended-Spectrum Penicillins

The extended-spectrum group of penicillins includes the aminopenicillins: ampicillin and amoxicillin, the carboxypenicillin ticarcillin, and the ureidopenicillin piperacillin. These drugs are all susceptible to destruction by staphylococcal (and other) β-lactamases. While this group of penicillins is more active against certain gram-negative rods, they have approximately the same activity as natural penicillins against gram-positive bacteria.

Antimicrobial Activity

Ampicillin and amoxicillin are active against most strains of *Proteus mirabilis*, *Listeria* organisms, and non–β-lactamase-producing strains of *Haemophilus influenzae* but are inactive against most gram-negative pathogens. Both drugs are effective against penicillin-susceptible pneumococcus and *Enterococcus faecalis*.

Ticarcillin extends the activity of ampicillin to include many strains of *Pseudomonas*, but it has poor activity against most strains of *Klebsiella* and enterococci and is less active than ampicillin against pneumococci.

Piperacillin is more active than ticarcillin against *Pseudomonas aeruginosa* and *Klebsiella*. Similar to ampicillin, piperacillin is active against *E faecalis* and is superior to ticarcillin against pneumococci. The extended-spectrum penicillins inhibit many but not all anaerobes. Ampicillin and amoxicillin are not active against β-lactamase-producing strains of *Bacteroides fragilis*—in contrast to piperacillin, which is active against most (not all) isolates.

Pharmacokinetics & Administration

Ampicillin can be given orally or parenterally. Amoxicillin is preferable to ampicillin in the oral treatment of infection because of its improved oral bioavailability and less frequent dosage frequency.

Ticarcillin and piperacillin are given intravenously and increased doses (200–300 mg/kg/d) are required for treatment of infections due to *P aeruginosa*.

Dosage adjustments are required in renal failure and are summarized in Table 37–4.

Clinical Uses

Amoxicillin is given orally for minor infections, such as exacerbations of chronic bronchitis, sinusitis, or otitis. Ampicillin is administered intravenously for pneumonia, meningitis, bacteremia, or endocarditis.

Amoxicillin is also used as prophylaxis for endocarditis. Because of the increased serum and respiratory secretion levels, this agent is valuable in the treatment of susceptible and moderately penicillin-susceptible pneumococcus. In general, if amoxicillin levels remain above the MIC of the pneumococcus for more than 40% of the dosing interval (which can be achieved with a dose of 40 mg/kg/d in adults), bacteriologic cure rates are optimal. Although ticarcillin and piperacillin can be used as monotherapy, they are more commonly administered in combination with other agents.

3. Penicillins Combined with β-Lactamase Inhibitors

The addition of β-lactamase inhibitors (clavulanic acid, sulbactam, tazobactam) prevents inactivation of the parent penicillin by bacterial β-lactamases. Products available are Augmentin (amoxicillin, 250 mg, 500 mg, or 875 mg, plus 125 mg of clavulanic acid); Augmentin XR (amoxicillin 1 g plus 62.5 mg of clavulanic acid); Timentin (ticarcillin 3 g plus 100 mg of clavulanic acid); Unasyn (ampicillin 1 g plus sulbactam 0.5 g, and ampicillin 3 g plus sulbactam 1 g); and Zosyn (piperacillin 3 g plus tazobactam 0.375 g, and piperacillin 4 g plus tazobactam 0.5 g). Augmentin is given orally and the others intravenously. In general, the β-lactamase inhibitors effectively inactivate β-lactamases produced by *S aureus*, *H influenzae*, *Moraxella catarrhalis*, and *B fragilis*. In contrast, the β-lactamase inhibitors are variably and unpredictably effective against β-lactamases produced by certain aerobic gram-negative bacilli, such as *Enterobacter*. Of the available parenteral drugs, Zosyn has the broadest spectrum of activity. Like Unasyn (in contrast to Ti-

mentin), Zosyn is active against ampicillin-susceptible enterococci. It has greater in vitro activity against *P aeruginosa* than Timentin and is more active than either Timentin or Unasyn against *Serratia* and *Klebsiella* species. While these agents are sometimes active in vitro, they generally should not be used in the treatment of extended-spectrum β-lactamase (ESBL)–producing organisms.

Augmentin, because of its high cost and gastrointestinal intolerance, is limited to the treatment of refractory cases of sinusitis and otitis and prophylaxis of infections resulting from animal and human bites. The roles of Timentin, Unasyn, and Zosyn include the treatment of polymicrobial infections such as peritonitis from a ruptured viscus, osteomyelitis in a diabetic patient, or traumatic osteomyelitis.

The dosage regimens of these drugs are the same as those of the parent drugs. When Timentin or Zosyn is used to treat *Pseudomonas* infections, dosages of 200–300 mg/kg/d of the penicillin component are used. Nonpseudomonal infection can be treated with lower doses (100–200 mg/kg/d).

4. Penicillinase-Resistant Penicillins

Oxacillin, cloxacillin, dicloxacillin, and nafcillin are relatively resistant to destruction by β-lactamases produced by staphylococci. They are less active than natural penicillins against nonstaphylococcal gram-positives; however, they are still adequate in certain streptococcal infections, including those due to group A streptococci in skin and soft tissue infections.

The primary route of clearance of the above agents is nonrenal—thus, no dosage adjustment is needed in renal insufficiency.

5. Adverse Effects of Penicillins

Allergy

All penicillins are cross-sensitizing and cross-reacting. The responsible antigenic determinants appear to be degradation products of penicillins, particularly penicilloic acid and products of alkaline hydrolysis (minor antigenic determinants) bound to host protein. Skin tests with penicilloyl-polylysine, with minor antigenic determinants, and with undegraded penicillin can identify most individuals with IgE-mediated reactions (hives, bronchospasm). Among positive reactors to skin tests, the incidence of subsequent immediate severe penicillin reactions is high. Although many persons develop IgG antibodies to antigenic determinants of penicillin, the presence of such antibodies is not correlated with allergic reactivity (except for rare instances of hemolytic anemia), and serologic tests have little predictive value. A history of a penicillin reaction in the past is not reliable. Only 15–20% of patients with a history of penicillin allergy have an adverse reaction when challenged with the drug. The decision to administer penicillin or related drugs (other β-lactams) to patients with an allergic history depends on the severity of the reported reaction, the severity of the infection being treated, and the availability of alternative drugs. For patients with a history of severe reaction (anaphylaxis), alternative drugs should be used. In the rare situations when there is a strong indication for using penicillin (eg, syphilis in pregnancy) in allergic patients, desensitization can be performed. If the reaction is mild (nonurticarial rash), the patient may be rechallenged with penicillin or may be given another β-lactam antibiotic. (See Chapter 30 for discussion of penicillin allergy and methods of desensitization.)

Allergic reactions include anaphylaxis, serum sickness (urticaria, fever, joint swelling, angioneurotic edema 7–12 days after exposure), skin rashes, fever, interstitial nephritis, eosinophilia, hemolytic anemia, other hematologic disturbances, and vasculitis. The incidence of hypersensitivity to penicillin is estimated to be 1–5% among adults in the United States. Life-threatening anaphylactic reactions are very rare (0.05%). Ampicillin produces maculopapular skin rashes more frequently than other penicillins, but many ampicillin (and other β-lactam) rashes are not allergic in origin. The nonallergic ampicillin rash usually occurs after 3–4 days of therapy, is maculopapular, is more common in patients with coexisting viral illness (especially Epstein-Barr infection), and resolves with continued therapy. The maculopapular rash may or may not reappear with rechallenge. Rarely, penicillins can induce nephritis with primary tubular lesions associated with anti-basement membrane antibodies.

Toxicity

All penicillins in excessive doses, particularly in renal insufficiency, have been associated with seizures.

Of the oral penicillins, Augmentin is most commonly associated with diarrhea. Nafcillin administered at high doses is associated with a modest leukopenia. Oxacillin may cause a higher incidence of liver and skin toxicity than other agents in this class. High doses of penicillins, particularly ticarcillin or piperacillin, inhibit platelet aggregation and produce hypokalemia due to binding of potassium in the kidney.

Peterson LR: Penicillins for treatment of pneumococcal pneumonia: does in vitro resistance really matter? Clin Infect Dis 2006;42:224. [PMID: 16355333]

Robinson JL et al: Practical aspects of choosing an antibiotic for patients with a reported allergy to an antibiotic. Clin Infect Dis 2002;35:26. [PMID: 12060871]

Samaha-Kfoury JN et al: Recent developments in beta lactamases and extended spectrum beta lactamases. BMJ 2003;327:1209. [PMID: 14630759]

CEPHALOSPORINS
(Tables 37–6 and 37–7)

The cephalosporins, structurally related to the penicillins, consist of a β-lactam ring attached to a dihydrothiazoline ring. Substitutions of chemical groups

Table 37–6. Major groups of cephalosporins.

First Generation	Second Generation	Third Generation	Fourth Generation
Cephalothin	Cefamandole	Cefotaxime	Cefepime
Cephapirin	Cefuroxime	Ceftizoxime	
Cefazolin	Cefonicid	Ceftriaxone	
Cephalexin[1]	Ceforanide	Ceftazidime	
Cephradine[1]	Cefaclor[1]	Cefoperazone	
Cefadroxil	Cefoxitin	Cefpodoxime	
	Cefotetan	proxetil[1]	
	Cefprozil[1]	Ceftibuten[1]	
	Cefuroxime	Cefdinir[1]	
	axetil[1]	Cefditoren	
		pivoxil[1]	

[1]Oral agents.

result in varying pharmacologic properties and antimicrobial activities.

The mechanism of action of cephalosporins is analogous to that of the penicillins: (1) binding to specific penicillin-binding proteins, (2) inhibition of cell wall synthesis, and (3) activation of autolytic enzymes in the cell wall. Resistance to cephalosporins may be due to poor permeability of the drug into bacteria, lack of penicillin-binding proteins, or degradation by β-lactamases.

Cephalosporins have been divided into four major groups or "generations" (Table 37–6) based mainly on their antibacterial activity: First-generation cephalosporins have good activity against aerobic gram-positive organisms and some community-acquired gram-negative organisms (*P mirabilis, Escherichia coli, Klebsiella* species); second-generation drugs have a slightly extended spectrum against gram-negative bacteria, and some are active against gram-negative anaerobes; and third-generation cephalosporins are active against many gram-negative bacteria. Not all cephalosporins fit neatly into this grouping, and there are exceptions to the general characterization of the drugs in the individual classes; however, the generational classification of cephalosporins is useful for discussion purposes. Cefepime is considered a fourth-generation agent because it is more stable against plasmid-mediated β-lactamase and has little or no β-lactamase-inducing capacity. Cefepime compares favorably with ceftazidime with respect to its gram-negative activity; however, its stability versus plasmid-mediated β-lactamase results in improved coverage against *Enterobacter* and *Citrobacter* species. The gram-positive coverage of cefepime approaches that of cefotaxime or ceftriaxone. None of the currently available agents are active against the enterococcus.

1. First-Generation Cephalosporins

Antimicrobial Activity

These drugs are very active against gram-positive cocci, including penicillin-susceptible pneumococci,

Table 37–7. Pharmacology of the cephalosporins.

Drug	Peak Serum Level (mcg/mL) after 1 g IV	Serum Half-Life (min)	Total Daily Dose (mg/kg)	Dosage Interval (hrs)	Dosage Adjustments in Renal Failure		
					Moderate (Cl$_{cr}$ 10–50 mL/min)	Severe (Cl$_{cr}$ < 10 mL/min)	Post-Hemodialysis Dose
Cephapirin	40–60	40	50–200	4–6	1–2 g q6–12h	1 g q12h	1 g
Cefazolin	90–120	90	25–100	8	0.5–1 g q6–12h	0.5 g daily	0.5 g
Cephalexin, cephradine[1]	15–20	50–60	15–30	6	0.25–0.5 g q8–12h	0.25–0.5 g daily	0.5 g
Cefadroxil[1]	15	75	15–30	12–24	1 g daily	0.5 g daily	0.5 g
Cefamandole	60–80	45	75–200	6–8	1 g q12h	1–2 g daily	0.5 g
Cefditoren pivoxil	2–3	90	6	12	0.2 g q12h	0.2 g q12h	None
Cefepime	60–70	120	50–75	8–12	1 g q12h	1 g q24h	1 g
Ceftibuten[1]	20	120	9	12–24	0.4 g daily	0.1–0.2 g daily	0.7 g
Cefuroxime	80–100	80	50	6–12	1 g q12h	1–2 g daily	0.5 g
Cefuroxime axetil[1]	6–8	75	5–15	12	0.5 g q24h	0.25 g daily	0.25 g
Cefonicid	200–250	240	15–30	24	0.5 g daily	1 g q72h	0.25 g
Ceforanide	125	180	15–30	12	1 g daily	1 g q48h	0.25 g
Cefaclor[1]	15–20	50	10–15	6–8	0.5 g q8–12h	0.25–0.5 g q12–24h	0.25–0.5 g
Cefpodoxime proxetil[1]	2	150	5	12	0.2 g q24h	0.2 g 3 times/ wk after dialysis	0.2 g
Cefprozil[1]	10	90	10–15	12	0.5 g q12–24h	0.25–0.5 g q12–24h	0.5 g
Cefotetan	60–80	150	50–100	8–12	1 g q8–12h	0.5–1 g daily	0.5 g
Cefotaxime	40–60	60	50–75	6–8	1–2 g q6–8h	1–2 g q24h	1–2 g
Cefoxitin	60–80	60	50–100	6–8	1 g q12h	1–2 g daily	0.5 g
Ceftizoxime	80–100	100	50–75	8–12	0.5–1 g q8–12h	0.25–0.5 g q12–24h	0.5 g
Ceftriaxone	150	480	30–50	12–24	1–2 g daily	1–2 g daily	None
Ceftazidime	100–120	120	50–75	8–12	1 g q12h	0.5–1 g daily	0.5 g
Cefoperazone	150	120	30–200	8–12	1–2 g q12h	1–2 g q12h	None
Loracarbef[1]	10	60	10–15	12	0.2 g q24h	0.2 g 3 times/ wk after dialysis	0.2 g

[1]Oral agents. Serum levels based on 0.5 g oral dose.

viridans streptococci, group A hemolytic streptococci, and *S aureus.* As with all cephalosporins, they are inactive against enterococci and methicillin-resistant staphylococci. Activity against *H influenzae* is poor, and penicillin-resistant streptococci (both intermediately and highly resistant) are resistant to first-generation cephalosporins. Among gram-negative bacteria, *E coli, Klebsiella pneumoniae,* and *P mirabilis* are usually susceptible except for some hospital-acquired strains.

Anaerobic gram-positive cocci are usually susceptible, but *B fragilis* is not.

Pharmacokinetics & Administration

A. ORAL

Cephalexin, cephradine, and cefadroxil are variably absorbed. Cefadroxil, because of its longer half-life, can be given twice daily instead of four times daily.

B. INTRAVENOUS

Cefazolin is preferred because its longer half-life allows for less frequent dosing. In renal insufficiency, it requires dosage adjustment.

C. INTRAMUSCULAR

Cefazolin can be given intramuscularly; however, the intravenous route is preferred because of the every 8-hour dosing schedule.

Clinical Uses

Oral drugs are sometimes used for treatment of urinary tract infections, and they can be used for minor staphylococcal infections (eg, cellulitis, soft tissue abscess).

Intravenous first-generation cephalosporins are the drugs of choice for surgical prophylaxis, particularly for clean procedures. Second- and third-generation cephalosporins offer no advantage over first-generation agents except where anaerobes play an important role, such as for colorectal surgery or for hysterectomy.

First-generation cephalosporins do not adequately penetrate into cerebrospinal fluid and cannot be used to treat meningitis.

2. Second-Generation Cephalosporins

Second-generation cephalosporins are a heterogeneous group with marked individual differences in activity, pharmacokinetics, and toxicity. In general, they are active against gram-negative organisms inhibited by first-generation drugs, but they have an extended gram-negative coverage. Indole-positive *Proteus* and *Klebsiella* (including first-generation cephalosporin-resistant strains) as well as *M catarrhalis* and *Neisseria* species are usually sensitive. Cefuroxime is active against *H influenzae*, including β-lactamase-producing strains, but has little activity against *Serratia* and *B fragilis*. In contrast, cefoxitin and cefotetan are active against many strains of *B fragilis* and some strains of *Serratia*. Against gram-positive organisms, these drugs are generally less active than the first-generation cephalosporins (cefuroxime is an exception). Second-generation agents have no activity against *P aeruginosa*. Of note, the manufacturer has abandoned the marketing of cefotetan; thus, this agent is unlikely to be available.

Pharmacokinetics & Administration

A. ORAL

Only cefaclor, cefuroxime axetil, and cefprozil can be given orally. Cefuroxime axetil is deesterified to cefuroxime after absorption. Its longer half-life permits twice-daily dosing, and absorption is enhanced when it is taken with food (as is not the case with many other oral antibiotics).

B. INTRAVENOUS AND INTRAMUSCULAR

Because of differences in drug half-life and protein binding, peak serum levels achieved and dosing intervals vary greatly for this group of drugs (Table 37–7). Drugs with shorter half-lives (cefoxitin) require higher doses and more frequent dosing than drugs with longer half-lives (eg, cefuroxime). Dosage adjustment is required with renal impairment.

Clinical Uses

Because of their activity against β-lactamase-producing *H influenzae* and *M catarrhalis*, cefprozil and cefuroxime axetil can occasionally be used to treat sinusitis and otitis media in patients unresponsive to more established agents.

Because of their activity against *B fragilis*, cefoxitin and cefotetan can be used to treat mixed anaerobic infections, eg, peritonitis and diverticulitis. However, since many *B fragilis* and enteric gram-negative organisms are resistant to these drugs, alternative agents are preferred for life-threatening intra-abdominal infections. Cefoxitin and cefotetan (if and when available) are useful as prophylaxis in colorectal surgery, vaginal or abdominal hysterectomy, and appendectomy because of their activity against *B fragilis*.

3. Third- & Fourth-Generation Cephalosporins

Antimicrobial Activity

Most of these drugs are active against staphylococci (not methicillin-resistant strains) but less so than first-generation cephalosporins. Ceftazidime, however, has notably weak activity against *S aureus* and pneumococci. While inactive against enterococci, third- and fourth-generation cephalosporins inhibit most streptococci. Ceftriaxone and cefotaxime offer the most reliable antipneumococcal coverage. A major advantage of these cephalosporins is their expanded gram-negative coverage. In addition to organisms inhibited by other cephalosporins, they are consistently active against *Serratia marcescens, Providencia, Haemophilus,* and *Neisseria,* including β-lactamase-producing strains. Ceftazidime is unique among all third-generation agents because it is active against *P aeruginosa. Acinetobacter, Citrobacter, Enterobacter.* Nonaeruginosa strains of *Pseudomonas* are variably sensitive to third-generation cephalosporins, and Listeria is uniformly resistant. Activity against *B fragilis* is variable. In contrast to the third-generation agents, cefepime—the only currently available fourth-generation cephalosporin—is active against *Enterobacter* and *Citrobacter,* has activity comparable to that of ceftazidime against *P aeruginosa,* and has gram-positive activity similar to that of ceftriaxone.

Cefpodoxime proxetil, cefdinir, cefditoren pivoxil, cefixime and ceftibuten, the only oral agents in this group, are more active than cefuroxime axetil but are not as active as parenteral third-generation cephalosporins against gram-negative organisms such as *Pseudomonas, Enterobacter, Morganella,* and *S marcescens.* While temporarily discontinued, cefixime is once again available as a suspension. All third- and fourth-generation cephalosporins are active against *Streptococcus pyogenes* (group A streptococcus). Cefpodoxime proxetil, cefditoren pivoxil, and cefdinir are active against methicillin-sensitive *S aureus*, whereas ceftibuten has little activity (none are active against methicillin-resistant strains). Cefdinir, cefditoren pivoxil, and cefpodoxime proxetil are active against penicillin-sensitive strains of *Streptococcus pneumoniae* (the pneumococcus), but ceftibuten has marginal activity. None of the oral cephalosporins are reliable against intermediately susceptible or penicillin-resistant *S pneumoniae*. Like other members of this class, these drugs are ineffective against enterococci and *Listeria monocytogenes*.

Pharmacokinetics & Administration

The intravenous agents distribute into extracellular fluid and reach levels in the cerebrospinal fluid that exceed those needed to inhibit susceptible pathogens. The half-lives of these drugs are variable, which accounts for the differences in dosing intervals (Table 37–7). Ceftriaxone is eliminated primarily by biliary excretion, and no dosage adjustment is required in renal insufficiency. The other drugs are eliminated primarily by the kidney and thus require dosage adjustment in renal insufficiency.

Clinical Uses

Because of their penetration into the cerebrospinal fluid and potent in vitro activity, intravenous third-generation cephalosporins can be used to treat meningitis due to susceptible pneumococci, meningococci, *H influenzae*, and susceptible enteric gram-negative rods. In meningitis in older patients, third-generation cephalosporins should be combined with ampicillin or trimethoprim-sulfamethoxazole until *L monocytogenes* has been excluded as the etiologic pathogen. Ceftazidime has been used to treat meningitis due to *Pseudomonas*. The dosage for meningitis should be at the upper limits of the recommended range, because cerebrospinal fluid levels of these drugs are only 10–20% of serum levels. Ceftazidime or cefepime is frequently administered empirically in the febrile neutropenic patient. Ceftriaxone is indicated for gonorrhea, chancroid, and more serious forms of Lyme disease (see Chapter 34). Because of its long half-life and once-daily dosing requirement, ceftriaxone is an attractive option for the outpatient parenteral therapy of infections due to susceptible organisms.

Cefepime is useful for third-generation cephalosporin–resistant isolates such as *Enterobacter* and *Citrobacter*.

Cefdinir, cefditoren pivoxil, and cefpodoxime proxetil are the best third-generation oral agents against pneumococci and *S aureus*. Single-dose cefixime or cefpodoxime proxetil is probably as effective as ceftriaxone for the therapy of genital, rectal, and pharyngeal gonorrhea.

4. Adverse Effects of Cephalosporins

Allergy

Cephalosporins are sensitizing, and a variety of hypersensitivity reactions occur, including anaphylaxis, fever, skin rashes, nephritis, and hemolytic anemia. The frequency of IgE cross-allergy between cephalosporins and penicillins approximates 5–10%. Persons with a history of anaphylaxis to penicillins should not receive cephalosporins. Allergies to a given agent may or may not extend to the entire cephalosporin class.

Toxicity

Ceftriaxone has been associated with a dose-dependent biliary sludging syndrome and cholelithiasis due to precipitation of drug when its solubility in bile is exceeded. Long-term administration of 2 g/d or more is a risk factor for this complication.

Casey JR et al: Meta-analysis of cephalosporins versus penicillin treatment of group A streptococcal tonsillopharyngitis in adults. Clin Infect Dis 2004;38:1526. [PMID: 15156437]

Chapman TM et al: Cefepime: a review of its use in the management of hospitalized patients with pneumonia. Am J Respir Med 2003;2:75. [PMID: 14720024]

Romano A et al: Cross-reactivity and tolerability of cephalosporins in patients with immediate hypersensitivity to penicillins. Ann Intern Med 2004;141:16. [PMID: 15238366]

OTHER β-LACTAM DRUGS

Monobactams

These are drugs with a monocyclic β-lactam ring that are resistant to many β-lactamases and active against gram-negative organisms (including *Pseudomonas*) but have no activity against gram-positive organisms or anaerobes. Aztreonam resembles ceftazidime in its gram-negative activity. Clinical uses of aztreonam are limited because of the availability of third-generation cephalosporins with a broader spectrum of activity and minimal toxicity. Despite the structural similarity of aztreonam to penicillin, cross-reactivity is limited, and it can therefore be used in most patients with IgE-mediated penicillin allergy.

Carbapenems

This class of drugs is structurally related to β-lactam antibiotics. Imipenem, the first drug of this type, has a wide spectrum of activity that includes most gram-negative rods (including *P aeruginosa*) and gram-positive organisms and anaerobes, with the exception of *Burkholderia cepacia*, *Stenotrophomonas maltophilia*, *Enterococcus faecium*, and methicillin-resistant *S aureus* and *Staphylococcus epidermidis*. The half-life of imipenem is 1 hour. Dosage adjustment is required in renal insufficiency.

Meropenem is similar to imipenem in spectrum of activity and pharmacology. It is less likely to cause seizures than imipenem, although the risk of seizures is low with imipenem if dosage is appropriately adjusted for renal insufficiency. Meropenem is associated with less nausea and vomiting than imipenem, a feature of importance when high doses must be used, as in the treatment of *Pseudomonas* infection in patients with cystic fibrosis. The usual dose is 1–2 g intravenously every 8 hours. Dosage adjustment in renal insufficiency is required.

Ertapenem is similar to imipenem and meropenem in its activity against aerobic gram-positive and anaerobic organisms but is less active against *Pseudomonas* and *Acinetobacter*. Because of its long half-life (4 hours), it can be administered once daily. The usual dose is 1 g intravenously every 24 hours and adjustments are needed for renal insufficiency.

The carbapenems should not be routinely used as first-line therapy unless the pathogen is multidrug-resistant and is known to be susceptible to these agents. In patients hospitalized for a prolonged period with presumed infection with a multidrug-resistant organism, empiric use of carbapenems is reasonable. (Ertapenem should not be used if *Pseudomonas* and *Enterobacter* are common nosocomial pathogens.) *Pseudomonas* may rapidly develop resistance to carbapenems. The use of imipenem or meropenem alone appears to be as effective as combination therapy in the febrile neutropenic patient, and the carbapenems are as effective as combination therapy in certain polymicrobial infections such as peritonitis and pelvic infections.

The most common adverse effects of imipenem and meropenem are nausea, vomiting, diarrhea, reactions at the infusion site, and skin rashes. Seizures are more commonly observed with imipenem. Patients allergic to penicillins may be allergic to imipenem and meropenem as well.

Edwards SJ et al: Systematic review comparing meropenem with imipenem plus cilastatin in the treatment of severe infection. Curr Med Res Opin 2005;21:785. [PMID: 15969878]

Lipsky BA et al: Ertapenem versus piperacillin/tazobactam for diabetic foot infections (SIDESTEP): prospective, randomised, controlled, double-blinded, multicentre trial. Lancet 2005;366:1695. [PMID: 16291062]

ERYTHROMYCIN GROUP (Macrolides)

The macrolides are a group of closely related compounds characterized by a macrocyclic lactone ring to which various sugars are attached.

Antimicrobial Activity

Erythromycins inhibit protein synthesis by binding to the 50S subunit of bacterial ribosomes. They generally are bacteriostatic and sometimes bactericidal for gram-positive organisms, including most streptococci and corynebacteria. Similar to penicillin, the rate of macrolide-resistant *S pneumoniae* has increased (15–50%), and recent reports demonstrate increased resistance in group A streptococci in some centers. Erythromycin-resistant pneumococci are azalide-resistant as well (azithromycin, clarithromycin). *Chlamydia, Mycoplasma, Legionella,* and *Campylobacter* organisms are susceptible.

Pharmacokinetics & Administration

Preparations for oral use include erythromycin base, erythromycin stearate, estolate, and ethyl succinate. Erythromycins are excreted primarily nonrenally; no adjustment is therefore required in renal failure.

Erythromycin and azithromycin are available for intravenous use, particularly in the treatment of Legionnaires' disease.

Clinical Uses

Macrolides are effective in the treatment of infection due to *Legionella, Mycoplasma, Ureaplasma, Corynebacterium* (including diphtheria), and *Chlamydia* (including ocular and respiratory infections) organisms. They are useful adjuncts in the treatment of streptococcal and pneumococcal disease in penicillin-allergic patients. Oral erythromycin base is used with neomycin as prophylaxis for colonic surgery. When administered early, erythromycin may shorten the course of *Campylobacter* enteritis. Erythromycins are effective against certain *Bartonella* species (bacillary angiomatosis) and *Rhodococcus* species. In vitro data suggest that macrolides have a direct effect on neutrophil function and the production of cytokines associated with inflammation. Thus, these agents are being evaluated for their anti-inflammatory effects in infectious diseases as well. The most well-documented anti-inflammatory benefit associated with the macrolides is in the prevention of cystic fibrosis exacerbation. Earlier studies suggested that macrolides reduced the incidence of cardiac events in patients with coronary artery disease. A potential link between chlamydia infection and coronary disease was identified, and it was hypothesized that the benefit of macrolides was due to the antichlamydial activity of these agents. However, more recent studies have not demonstrated this benefit.

Adverse Effects

Nausea, vomiting, and diarrhea may occur after oral or intravenous intake. Erythromycins—particularly the estolate—can produce acute cholestatic hepatitis (fever, jaundice, impaired liver function), probably as a hypersensitivity reaction. Hepatitis recurs if the drug is readministered. Reversible auditory impairment occurs with large erythromycin doses (4 g/d or more), particularly in patients with impaired renal or hepatic function. However, ototoxicity has been reported with high doses of all agents. Intravenous erythromycin has been associated with prolongation of the QT interval and torsades de pointes—more commonly in women. Erythromycins (and clarithromycin) can increase the effects of oral anticoagulants, digoxin, theophylline, and cyclosporine by inhibiting cytochrome P450. An increased risk of cardiac-associated death has been reported with erythromycin, particularly in patients receiving concomitant inhibitors of cytochrome P450 3A4.

Azalides (azithromycin, clarithromycin, and others) are closely related structurally to the macrolides. They are similar to erythromycin in activity against most organisms and are slightly more active in vitro than erythromycin against *H influenzae* (azithromycin > clarithromycin > erythromycin). They are also active against *Chlamydia trachomatis, Ureaplasma urealyticum,* and *Haemophilus ducreyi.* In addition, these drugs have in vitro activity against a number of unusual pathogens, including atypical mycobacteria *(Mycobacterium avium-intracellulare, Mycobacterium chelonei, Mycobacterium fortuitum, Mycobacterium marinum), Toxoplasma gondii, Campylobacter jejuni, Helicobacter pylori,* and *Borrelia burgdorferi.*

The azalides are more acid-stable than erythromycin, concentrate intracellularly and in tissues, and have a long terminal half-life, with high tissue concentrations that persist for days with azithromycin. The elevated tissue levels associated with azithromycin and clarithromycin has been proposed to overcome the high incidence of in vitro resistance seen with pneumococci (30%), but clinical observations suggest that the reported resistance can translate to clinical failure. Azithromycin and clarithromycin are approved for treatment of streptococcal pharyngitis, uncomplicated skin infections, and acute bacterial exacerbations of chronic bronchitis. Because of the long half-life, outpatient oral treatment with azithromycin is with once-daily dosing for a total of 5 days (500 mg on day 1 and then 250 mg on days 2–5). Clarithromycin is usually administered in a dosage of 250–500 mg orally twice daily, although an extended-release formulation that is given as a single daily 1000-mg dose is approved for acute sinusitis and acute exacerbation of chronic bronchitis. The azalides are more expensive than erythromycin. However, the less frequent dosing and better tolerability make them preferable choices in certain patients.

Azithromycin has also been approved as single-dose therapy (1 g) for chlamydial genital infections. While more expensive than 7 days of treatment with doxycycline (Table 37–5), the assurance of adequate supervised therapy makes azithromycin preferred therapy in many patients. Azithromycin can also be used as single-dose therapy (1 g) for chancroid, and a single dose of 1 g is as efficacious as 7 days of doxycycline for nongonococcal urethritis in men and incubating syphilis. While a 2-g dose of azithromycin is used for the treatment of gonorrhea, its efficacy is less than that observed with ceftriaxone. Furthermore, the incidence of upper gastrointestinal side effects is increased with this dose. A single dose of azithromycin (20 mg/kg, maximum dose of 1 g) is effective in treating trachoma and reducing disease burden in endemic areas. The spectrum of activity of the macrolides—particularly their atypical coverage—results in their usefulness in mild to moderate cases of community-acquired pneumonia; however, penicillin-resistant strains are often resistant

to these agents as well. Weekly 1200-mg doses of azithromycin are effective in preventing *Mycobacterium avium* complex infections in HIV-positive patients, and doses of 500 mg daily may be effective in *M avium* complex pulmonary infections in non–HIV-positive patients. Azithromycin may be considered for therapy of dysentery caused by multidrug-resistant *Shigella* organisms. Used as prophylaxis, azithromycin (500 mg weekly) is as effective as benzathine penicillin in preventing upper respiratory tract infections in military recruits, and at a dose of 250 mg daily it is adequate as prophylaxis for malaria (although inferior to doxycycline for multidrug-resistant *Plasmodium falciparum*). Clarithromycin has been used for the therapy of *M avium* complex infections, usually in combination with other drugs (eg, rifabutin and ethambutol), and can be given daily (500 mg twice daily) or three times weekly (1000 mg) as intermittent therapy. Oral clarithromycin (500 mg twice daily for 6 months), in combination with other agents, is effective therapy for disseminated *M chelonei* infections. Clarithromycin has also been used in combination regimens for the therapy of *H pylori* infections. When clarithromycin is given with omeprazole and amoxicillin, cure rates in excess of 80–90% have been achieved.

Adverse effects of these agents are similar to those of erythromycin, but upper gastrointestinal upset, the major side effect, occurs less often with the azalides. Hepatic enzyme elevations and reversible cochlear toxicity have been reported. Clarithromycin is similar to erythromycin in its effect on the cytochrome P450 system. Azithromycin is associated with minimal to no drug interactions.

Grayston JT et al; ACES Investigators: Azithromycin for the secondary prevention of coronary events. N Engl J Med 2005; 352:1637. [PMID: 15843666]

Nuermberger E et al: The clinical significance of macrolide-resistant *Streptococcus pneumoniae*: it's all relative. Clin Infect Dis 2004;38:99. [PMID: 14679455]

Vanderkooi OG et al; Toronto Invasive Bacterial Disease Network: Predicting macrolide resistance in invasive pneumococcal infections. Clin Infect Dis 2005;40:1288. [PMID: 15825031]

KETOLIDES

Ketolides (such as telithromycin) are similar in structure to macrolides, but they have a broader spectrum of activity and may offer additional benefit in the treatment of community-acquired respiratory infections. They are active against both penicillin-resistant and macrolide-resistant pneumococci and equal to azithromycin therapeutically against atypical pathogens and *H influenzae.* Upper gastrointestinal adverse events are the complications most commonly associated with these drugs. Visual disturbances are moderately common, occurring more frequently in women. The dose is 800 mg/d orally, and no adjustment is needed for renal or hepatic insufficiency. Cytochrome P450 inhibition with telithromycin approximates that of erythromycin, and increased serum levels of war-farin and other agents would be expected with con-comitant administration of telithromycin.

Telithromycin (Ketek) for respiratory infections. Med Lett Drugs Ther 2004;46:66. [PMID: 15314586]

TETRACYCLINE GROUP

The tetracyclines are a large group of drugs with com-mon basic chemical structures, antimicrobial activity, and pharmacologic properties.

Antimicrobial Activity

Tetracyclines are inhibitors of protein synthesis and are bacteriostatic for many gram-positive and gram-negative bacteria. They are strongly inhibitory for the growth of mycoplasmas, rickettsiae, chlamydiae, spiro-chetes, and some protozoa (eg, amebas). Their antip-neumococcal activity approaches that of the macrolides; almost all *H influenzae* are inhibited. Tetracyclines also have moderate activity against some vancomycin-resis-tant enterococci. Doxycycline and minocycline are po-tential options for therapy of staphylococcal infections, including infections with many methicillin-resistant strains. There are marked in vitro differences between tetracyclines with respect to staphylococci. Tetracyclines are not useful in the treatment of gram-negative aerobic infection.

Pharmacokinetics & Administration

Oral bioavailability varies depending on the drug. Ab-sorption is impaired by dairy products, aluminum hy-droxide gels (antacids), and chelation with divalent cat-ions, eg, Ca^{2+} or Fe^{2+}. Chelation is less problematic with doxycycline and minocycline when compared with tet-racycline. Consequently, doses of tetracyclines should be staggered at least 2 hours before or after receipt of multivalent cations. Oral bioavailability is moderate with tetracycline and highest with doxycycline and mi-nocycline (95% or more). Lipid solubility of minocy-cline and doxycycline accounts for their penetration into the cerebrospinal fluid, prostate, tears, and saliva.

Tetracyclines are primarily metabolized in the liver and excreted in bile. Doxycycline requires no dosage adjustment in renal failure; in contrast, other tetracy-clines should be avoided or given in reduced dosage.

For patients unable to take oral medication, some tetracyclines (doxycycline, minocycline) are formu-lated for parenteral administration in doses similar to the oral ones.

Clinical Uses

Tetracyclines are drugs of choice for infections with *Chlamydia, Mycoplasma, Rickettsia, Ehrlichia,* and *Vibrio* organisms and for some spirochetal infections. Sexually transmitted diseases in which chlamydiae often play a role—endocervicitis, urethritis, proctitis, and epididymitis—should be treated with doxycy-cline for 7–14 days. Pelvic inflammatory disease is often treated with doxycycline plus cefoxitin or cefote-tan. Other chlamydial infections (psittacosis, lym-phogranuloma venereum, trachoma) and sexually transmitted diseases (granuloma inguinale) also re-spond to doxycycline. Other uses include treatment of acne, respiratory infections, Lyme disease and relaps-ing fever, brucellosis, glanders, tularemia (often in combination with streptomycin), cholera, mycoplas-mal pneumonia, actinomycosis, nocardiosis, malaria, infections caused by *M marinum* and *Pasteurella* spe-cies (typically after an animal bite), and as malaria pro-phylaxis (including multidrug-resistant *P falciparum*). They also have been used in combination with other drugs for amebiasis, falciparum malaria, and recurrent ulcers due to *H pylori*. Because of generally good activ-ity against pneumococci; *H influenzae;* and *Chlamy-dia, Legionella,* and *Mycoplasma* organisms, doxycy-cline should be considered as a potential empiric therapy for mild to moderate outpatient pneumonia.

Minocycline is equally as efficacious as doxycycline for the therapy of nongonococcal urethritis and cervicitis.

Adverse Effects

A. ALLERGY

Hypersensitivity reactions with fever or skin rashes are uncommon.

B. GASTROINTESTINAL SIDE EFFECTS

Diarrhea, nausea, and anorexia are common. Tetracy-cline administration, particularly doxycycline, should be avoided at bedtime due to the risk of esophageal erosion.

C. BONES AND TEETH

Tetracyclines are bound to calcium deposited in grow-ing bones and teeth, causing fluorescence, discolora-tion, enamel dysplasia, deformity, or growth inhibi-tion. Therefore, tetracyclines should not be given to pregnant women or children under 6 years of age.

D. LIVER DAMAGE

Tetracyclines can impair hepatic function or even cause liver necrosis, particularly during pregnancy or in the presence of preexisting liver disease.

E. KIDNEY EFFECTS

Demeclocycline can cause nephrogenic diabetes insipi-dus and has been used therapeutically to treat inappro-priate antidiuretic hormone secretion. Tetracyclines, particularly tetracycline, may increase blood urea ni-trogen (BUN) due to their antianabolic activity.

F. OTHER

Tetracyclines—principally demeclocycline—may in-duce photosensitization, especially in fair-skinned in-dividuals. Minocycline induces vestibular reactions (dizziness, vertigo, nausea, vomiting), with a frequency of 35–70% after doses of 200 mg daily and has also been implicated as a cause of hypersensitivity pneumonitis.

GLYCYLCYCLINES

Tigecycline, a tetracycline derivative, is available as a parenteral antibacterial for the treatment of nosocomial infection. It is active against most gram-positive bacteria, including methicillin-resistant staphylococci and vancomycin-resistant enterococci. It is active against a number of multidrug resistant aerobic gram-negative bacilli, including *Acinetobacter, Enterobacter,* and *Citrobacter.* However, tigecycline has little to no activity against *Pseudomonas* and *Proteus* spp. In addition, tigecycline demonstrates excellent anaerobic activity against *B fragilis* and gram-positive anaerobes. A loading dose of 100 mg is administered intravenously with maintenance at 50 mg every 12 hours. The drug distributes into deep compartments with a large volume of distribution and low serum levels; tigecycline is primarily eliminated via biliary/fecal excretion with a half-life of 30–40 hours. Dose adjustment to 25 mg every 12 hours is recommended in Child-Turcotte-Pugh C liver disease. Tigecycline has similar adverse events as the tetracyclines; upper gastrointestinal side effects are common. While approved for complicated skin and soft-tissue infection and intra-abdominal infection, tigecycline likely will have a role in the treatment of certain resistant gram-negative pathogens.

Frampton JE et al: Tigecycline. Drugs 2005;65:2623. [PMID: 16392879]

Jones RN et al: Doxycycline use for community-acquired pneumonia: contemporary in vitro spectrum of activity against *Streptococcus pneumoniae* (1999-2002). Diagn Microbiol Infect Dis 2004;49:147. [PMID: 15183865]

Stein GE: Safety of newer parenteral antibiotics. Clin Infect Dis 2005;41(Suppl 5):S293. [PMID: 16080068]

CHLORAMPHENICOL

Antimicrobial Activity

Chloramphenicol is active against certain rickettsiae. It binds to the 50S subunit of ribosomes and inhibits protein synthesis. While active against *S pneumoniae, H influenzae,* and *Neisseria meningitidis,* it is used minimally because of its toxicity and the availability of alternative agents.

Pharmacokinetics & Administration

Chloramphenicol is widely distributed in tissues, including the eye and cerebrospinal fluid. Chloramphenicol is metabolized in the liver, and less than 10% is excreted unchanged in the urine. Thus, no dosage adjustment is needed in renal insufficiency. Patients with liver disease may accumulate the drug, and levels should be monitored.

Clinical Uses

Chloramphenicol is an occasional alternative to more standard therapy for (1) meningococcal, *H influenzae,* or pneumococcal infections of the central nervous system; (2) anaerobic or mixed infections in the central nervous system, eg, brain abscess; (3) as an alternative to tetracyclines in rickettsial infections, especially in pregnant women, in whom tetracycline is contraindicated.

Adverse Effects

Nausea, vomiting, and diarrhea are uncommon. The most serious adverse effects are hematologic. Chloramphenicol in excess of 50 mg/kg/d regularly causes reversible disturbances in red cell maturation within 1–2 weeks. In contrast, aplastic anemia is an irreversible consequence of chloramphenicol administration and represents a specific, probably genetically determined individual defect. It occurs in 1:40,000–1:25,000 courses of chloramphenicol treatment.

AMINOGLYCOSIDES

Aminoglycosides are a group of bactericidal drugs sharing chemical, antimicrobial, pharmacologic, and toxic characteristics. At present, the group includes streptomycin, neomycin, kanamycin, amikacin, gentamicin, tobramycin, sisomicin, netilmicin, paromomycin, and spectinomycin. All these agents inhibit protein synthesis in bacteria by inhibiting the function of the 30S subunit of the bacterial ribosome. Resistance is based on (1) a deficiency of the ribosomal receptor (chromosomal mutant); (2) the enzymatic destruction of the drug (plasmid-mediated transmissible resistance of clinical importance) by acetylation, phosphorylation, or adenylylation; or (3) a lack of permeability to the drug molecule or failure of active transport across cell membranes. Resistance can be chromosomal (eg, streptococci are relatively impermeable to aminoglycosides) or plasmid-mediated (eg, in gram-negative enteric bacteria.) Anaerobic bacteria are resistant to aminoglycosides because transport across the cell membrane is an oxygen-dependent energy-requiring process.

All aminoglycosides are more active at alkaline than at acid pH. All are potentially ototoxic (cochlear and vestibular) and nephrotoxic, although to different degrees. All can accumulate in renal insufficiency; therefore, dosage adjustments must be made in patients with renal dysfunction (see Table 37–8).

Because of their considerable toxicity and the availability of less toxic agents, (eg, cephalosporins, quinolones, carbapenems, β-lactamase inhibitor combinations), aminoglycosides have been used less often in recent years. They are most commonly used to treat resistant gram-negative organisms that are sensitive only to aminoglycosides, or in low doses in combination with β-lactam drugs or vancomycin for their synergistic effect (eg, enterococci, penicillin-resistant viridans streptococci, right-sided *S aureus* endocardi-

Table 37–8. Dosing of aminoglycosides.[1]

Drug (IV)	Creatinine Clearance (mL/min)				
	> 80	60–80	40–60	20–40	< 20
Gentamicin, tobramycin, netilmicin	5 mg/kg q24h	1.5–2.5 mg/kg q12h	1.2–1.5 mg/kg q24h	1.2–1.5 mg/kg q12–24h	2 mg/kg as loading dose and then 1–1.5 mg/kg q24–48h
Amikacin	15 mg/kg q24h	4.5–7.5 mg/kg q12h	3.5–4.5 mg/kg q12h	3.5–4.5 mg/kg q12–24h	7.5 mg/kg as loading dose and then 3–4.5 mg/kg q24–48h

[1]Traditional dosing should be guided by serum level measurements (peaks 30 minutes after the end of intravenous infusion and troughs ≤ 30 minutes before the next dose). When a single large daily dose is given, peak levels are not required. Trough levels should be undetectable with high-dose (5 mg/kg) once-daily gentamicin or amikacin. For those patients with creatinine clearances less than 80 mL/min, the dosage ranges in the table are used to treat gram-negative infections and are intended to achieve, for gentamicin, tobramycin, and netilmicin, peak levels of 6–10 mg/L and trough levels of ≤ 2 mg/L; for amikacin, peak levels of 20–30 mg/L and trough levels of ≤ 5 mg/L. (See text.)

tis, *S aureus* and *S epidermidis* prosthetic valve infection). Although aminoglycosides demonstrate in vitro activity against many gram-positive bacteria, they should never be used alone to treat infections caused by these organisms—both because there is minimal clinical experience with such infections and because less toxic alternatives are available. Aminoglycosides are inferior as monotherapy in the treatment of *Pseudomonas* infections.

General Properties of Aminoglycosides

Because of the similarities of the aminoglycosides, a summary of properties is presented briefly.

A. Absorption, Distribution, Metabolism, and Excretion

Aminoglycosides are not absorbed from the gastrointestinal tract. They diffuse poorly into the eye, prostate, bile, central nervous system, and spinal fluid after parenteral injection.

The serum half-life is 2–3 hours in patients with normal renal function. Excretion is almost entirely by glomerular filtration. Aminoglycosides are removed effectively by hemodialysis or continuous hemofiltration.

B. Dosage and Effect of Impaired Renal Function

In persons with normal renal function who have gram-negative infections, the dosage of amikacin is 15 mg/kg/d in a single daily dose; that for gentamicin, tobramycin, or netilmicin is 5 mg/kg injected once daily. A single large daily dose of gentamicin, tobramycin, netilmicin, or amikacin is as efficacious as—and no more nephrotoxic than—traditional dosing every 8–12 hours. When a single large daily dose is given, peak levels are not required. Trough aminoglycoside levels should be undetectable in patients with normal body composition and renal function receiving once-daily dosing. Some clinicians recommend serum

level monitoring 12–18 hours after the dose and extending the interval to every 48–72 hours for patients with elevated aminoglycoside levels. Others have suggested maintaining the dosage interval but decreasing the dose. Patients with renal failure, volume overload, or obesity have altered antibiotic clearance or volume of distribution. In patients with abnormal renal function or body composition, once-daily dosing is not recommended and aminoglycoside levels are recommended to guide dosing. For more traditional dosing, peak levels greater than 6 mcg/mL are desirable in the treatment of serious gram-negative infection, including pneumonia. Trough levels of more than 2 mcg/mL have been associated with an increased incidence of nephrotoxicity. In patients with normal body composition, once-daily dosing regimens as set forth in Table 37–8 should be followed. Reduced gentamicin doses (1 mg/kg every 8 hours) are recommended when used synergistically with β-lactams or vancomycin in the treatment of serious gram-positive infection (eg, enterococcal endocarditis).

C. Adverse Effects

All aminoglycosides can cause ototoxicity and nephrotoxicity. Ototoxicity can be irreversible and is cumulative, presenting as hearing loss (cochlear damage), noted first with high-frequency tones, or as vestibular damage, manifested by vertigo and ataxia. Amikacin appears to be more cochlear-toxic than gentamicin, tobramycin, or netilmicin. Nephrotoxicity, which is more common than ototoxicity, is accompanied by rising serum creatinine levels or reduced creatinine clearance. Nephrotoxicity is usually reversible and occurs with similar frequency with gentamicin, tobramycin, amikacin, and netilmicin.

In very high doses, usually associated with irrigation of an inflamed peritoneum, aminoglycosides can be neurotoxic, producing a curare-like effect with reversible neuromuscular blockade that results in respiratory paralysis.

1. Streptomycin

The usual dosage of streptomycin is 15–25 mg/kg/d (about 1 g/d) injected in one or two divided doses intramuscularly. If administered over 30–60 minutes, it can also be given intravenously. Streptomycin exhibits all the adverse effects typically associated with the aminoglycosides; however, it has greater vestibular toxicity and probably less nephrotoxicity when compared with gentamicin.

Resistance emerges so rapidly and has become so widespread that only a few specific indications for this drug remain: plague and tularemia; endocarditis caused by *E faecalis* or viridans streptococci (use in conjunction with penicillin or vancomycin) in strains that are susceptible to high levels of streptomycin (ie, ≤ 2000 mcg/mL)—gentamicin may be substituted for streptomycin in this setting; active tuberculosis when other less toxic drugs cannot be used; and acute brucellosis (in combination with tetracycline).

2. Neomycin, Kanamycin, & Paromomycin

These aminoglycosides are closely related, with similar activity and complete cross-resistance. Systemic use has been abandoned because of ototoxicity and nephrotoxicity.

Ointments containing neomycin, often combined with bacitracin and polymyxin, can be applied to infected superficial skin lesions. While the drug mixture covers most staphylococci, streptococci, and gram-negative bacteria likely to be present, the efficacy of topical application is questionable.

In preparation for elective bowel surgery, 1 g of neomycin is given orally every 6–8 hours for 1–2 days (combined with erythromycin, 1 g) to reduce aerobic bowel flora. Activity against gram-negative anaerobes is negligible. In hepatic encephalopathy, the coliform bacteria can be suppressed for prolonged periods by oral neomycin, 1 g every 6–8 hours, during reduced protein intake, resulting in diminished ammonia production. Lactulose is more widely used for this indication.

Neomycin or kanamycin can give rise to allergic reactions when applied topically to skin or eye.

Paromomycin, closely related to neomycin and kanamycin, is poorly absorbed after oral administration and has been used mainly to treat asymptomatic intestinal amebiasis and in doses of 25–30 mg/kg/d in three divided doses for 7 days to treat giardiasis in pregnancy. A dosage of 500 mg orally three or four times daily is marginally effective for cryptosporidiosis in AIDS.

3. Amikacin

Amikacin is a semisynthetic derivative of kanamycin. It is relatively resistant to several of the enzymes that inactivate gentamicin and tobramycin. Many gram-negative enteric bacteria—including many gentamicin-resistant strains of *Proteus, Enterobacter,* and *Serra-*tia organisms—are inhibited. After injection of 500 mg of amikacin every 12 hours (15 mg/kg/d), peak levels in serum are 10–30 mcg/mL. In addition to therapy for serious gram-negative infections, amikacin is sometimes included with other drugs for therapy of *M avium* complex and *M fortuitum* complex.

Like all aminoglycosides, amikacin is nephrotoxic and ototoxic (particularly for the auditory portion of the eighth nerve). Its levels should be monitored in patients with renal failure.

4. Gentamicin

With doses of 5 mg/kg/d of this aminoglycoside, serum levels are sufficient for bactericidal effect against most gram-negative organisms. Enterococci are resistant unless a penicillin or vancomycin is also given. Gentamicin may be synergistic with penicillins active against *Pseudomonas, Proteus, Enterobacter,* and *Klebsiella* organisms as well as other gram-negatives.

Indications, Dosages, & Routes of Administration

Gentamicin is used in serious infections caused by gram-negative bacteria. The usual dosage is 5 mg/kg/d intravenously administered once daily. In endocarditis due to viridans streptococci or *E faecalis*, gentamicin in lower synergistic doses (3 mg/kg/d) is combined with penicillin or ampicillin. A single daily dose of 3 mg/kg is just as effective as divided daily doses in the synergistic treatment of endocarditis due to viridans streptococci. In renal insufficiency, the dose should be adjusted as noted above.

5. Tobramycin

Tobramycin closely resembles gentamicin in antibacterial activity, toxicity, and pharmacologic properties and exhibits partial cross-resistance. It may be effective against some gentamicin-resistant pseudomonads but is not used synergistically with penicillin for enterococcal endocarditis. Dosing is the same as for gentamicin. Tobramycin is also given by aerosol (300 mg twice daily) to patients with cystic fibrosis and improves pulmonary function and decreases colonization with *Pseudomonas* without toxicity and without selecting for resistant strains.

Netilmicin shares many characteristics with gentamicin and tobramycin and can be given in a similar dosage. It may be less ototoxic and less nephrotoxic than the other aminoglycosides.

6. Spectinomycin

Spectinomycin is an aminocyclitol antibiotic (related to aminoglycosides) for intramuscular administration. Its sole application is in the treatment of uncomplicated urogenital and anorectal gonorrhea in persons who are hypersensitive to penicillin and who cannot tolerate fluoroquinolones. It is not effective for pharyngeal gonorrhea.

Bliziotis IA et al: Effect of aminoglycoside and beta-lactam combination therapy versus beta-lactam monotherapy on the emergence of antimicrobial resistance: a meta-analysis of randomized, controlled trials. Clin Infect Dis 2005;41:149. [PMID: 15983909]

POLYMYXINS

The polymyxins (colistin and polymixin B) are basic polypeptides that are bactericidal for certain gram-negative aerobic rods, including *Pseudomonas*. Because of poor distribution into tissues and substantial toxicity (primarily nephrotoxicity and neurotoxicity), systemic use of these agents is limited to infections caused by multidrug-resistant gram-negative organisms that are sensitive only to the polymyxins. Colistin has been used with increasing frequency in the treatment of pan-resistant *Acinetobacter baumanii* and *P aeruginosa*. The more recent experience suggests colistin to be associated with less nephrotoxicity and neurotoxicity than previously described. Dosage adjustments are required with renal insufficiency.

Murray CK et al: Treatment of multidrug resistant *Acinetobacter*. Curr Opin Infect Dis 2005;18:502. [PMID: 16258323]

ANTITUBERCULOUS DRUGS

Singular problems exist in the treatment of tuberculosis and other mycobacterial infections. The organisms are intracellular, have long periods of metabolic inactivity, and tend to develop resistance to any one drug. Therefore, combined drug therapy is used to delay the emergence of this resistance. First-line drugs, increasingly used together in all tuberculosis, are isoniazid, ethambutol, rifampin, and pyrazinamide.

See Chapter 9 for a discussion of these medications.

ALTERNATIVE DRUGS IN TUBERCULOSIS TREATMENT

The drugs listed alphabetically below are usually considered only in cases of drug resistance (clinical or laboratory) to first-line drugs.

Capreomycin is an injectable agent given intramuscularly in doses of 15–30 mg/kg/d (maximal dose 1 g). Major toxicities include ototoxicity (both vestibular and cochlear) and nephrotoxicity. If the drug must be used in older patients, the dose should not exceed 750 mg.

Clofazimine is a phenazine dye used in the treatment of leprosy and is active in vitro against *M avium* complex and *Mycobacterium tuberculosis*. It is given orally as a single daily dose of 100 mg for treatment of *M avium* complex disease. Its clinical efficacy for the therapy of tuberculosis has not been established. Adverse effects include nausea, vomiting, abdominal pain, and skin discoloration.

Cycloserine, a bacteriostatic agent, is given in doses of 15–20 mg/kg (not to exceed 1 g) orally and has been used in re-treatment regimens and for primary therapy of highly resistant *M tuberculosis*. It can induce a variety of central nervous system dysfunctions and psychotic reactions.

Ethionamide, like cycloserine, is bacteriostatic and is given orally in a dose of 15–20 mg/kg (maximal dose 1 g). It has been used in combination therapy but is poorly tolerated with marked gastric irritation.

The **fluoroquinolones** ofloxacin, levofloxacin, ciprofloxacin, and moxifloxacin are active in vitro against *M tuberculosis*, with MICs of 0.25–2 mcg/mL. These drugs have been demonstrated to be efficacious in treating tuberculosis in patients unable to take isoniazid, rifampin, and pyrazinamide; however, rapid emergence of resistance recently has been described. Doses include ciprofloxacin, 750 mg orally twice daily; ofloxacin, 400 mg orally twice daily; levofloxacin, 750 mg orally once daily.

Jasmer RM et al: Clinical practice. Latent tuberculosis infection. N Engl J Med 2002;347:1860. [PMID: 12466511]

RIFAMYCINS

Rifaximin, a derivative of rifamycin, is nonabsorbable, reaches very high levels in the stool, and has a broad spectrum of antibacterial activity, including aerobic and anaerobic gram-positive and gram-negative organisms. It is approved for use in nonpregnant women and for persons aged 12 years and older to treat noninvasive traveler's diarrhea (200 mg three times daily for 3 days) and should not be used if fever or bloody diarrhea is present. Other potential uses include prophylaxis of traveler's diarrhea (200 mg/d) and therapy of hepatic encephalopathy (400 mg twice daily). It is well tolerated and safe. Concerns for inducing cross-resistance to rifampin and rifabutin will require post-marketing surveillance.

Adachi JA et al: Rifaximin: a novel nonabsorbed rifamycin for gastrointestinal disorders. Clinical Infect Dis 2006;42:541. [PMID: 16421799]

SULFONAMIDES & ANTIFOLATE DRUGS

Antimicrobial Activity

Sulfonamides are structural analogs of *p*-aminobenzoic acid (PABA) and compete with PABA to block its conversion to dihydrofolic acid. Organisms that utilize PABA in the synthesis of folates and pyrimidines are inhibited. Animal cells and some resistant microorganisms (eg, enterococci) use exogenous folate and thus are not affected by sulfonamides.

Trimethoprim, pyrimethamine, and trimetrexate are compounds that inhibit the conversion of dihydrofolic acid to tetrahydrofolic acid by blocking the enzyme dihydrofolate reductase. These agents are generally used in combination with other drugs (usually sulfonamides) to prevent or treat a number of bacterial and parasitic infections. At high doses, all can inhibit mammalian dihydrofolate reductase, but clinically this is a problem only with pyrimethamine and trimetrexate. Folinic acid (leucovorin) is given concurrently with pyrimethamine and trimetrexate to prevent bone marrow suppression.

Sulfonamides alone are rarely used in the treatment of bacterial infection. When used in combination with other drugs, sulfonamides are useful in the treatment of toxoplasmosis and pneumocystosis.

The combination of trimethoprim (one part) plus sulfamethoxazole (five parts) is bactericidal for such gram-negative organisms as *E coli*, *Klebsiella*, *Enterobacter*, *Salmonella*, and *Shigella*, though substantial resistance has emerged. It is also active against many strains of *Serratia*, *Providencia*, *S maltophilia*, *B cepacia* (formerly *Pseudomonas cepacia*), and *Burkholderia pseudomallei*, but not against *P aeruginosa*. It is inactive against anaerobes and enterococci but inhibits most *Nocardia* and *S aureus* and about 50% *S epidermidis*. *M catarrhalis*, *H influenzae*, *H ducreyi*, *L monocytogenes*, and some atypical mycobacteria are also inhibited by this combination.

Pharmacokinetics & Administration

Trimethoprim-sulfamethoxazole is well absorbed from the gastrointestinal tract and widely distributed in tissues and fluids, including cerebrospinal fluid. For patients who are unable to take oral drugs, intravenous trimethoprim-sulfamethoxazole is available. Dosage adjustment is required for significant renal impairment (creatine clearance ≤ 50 mL/min).

Clinical Uses

Present indications for sulfonamides are outlined below.

A. URINARY TRACT INFECTIONS

Coliform bacteria, the most common cause of urinary tract infections, are moderately inhibited by sulfonamides, though widespread resistance of *E coli* has emerged. Short-course therapy (3 days) with oral double-strength trimethoprim-sulfamethoxazole (160 mg trimethoprim + 800 mg sulfamethoxazole) given twice daily is effective therapy for lower urinary tract infections in women who are symptomatic for less than 1 week. Since trimethoprim is concentrated in the prostate, trimethoprim-sulfamethoxazole, one double-strength tablet twice daily for 14–21 days, is effective in acute prostatitis. In chronic prostatitis, treatment for 6–12 weeks is indicated. Considering the above resistance trend, the routine use of trimethoprim-sulfamethoxazole for empiric therapy of urinary tract infections has been questioned. In those areas where resistance of *E coli* is greater than 10–20%, alternative agents should be used as empiric therapy.

B. PARASITIC INFECTIONS

Trimethoprim-sulfamethoxazole is effective for prophylaxis and treatment of *Pneumocystis* pneumonia,

Cyclospora infection, and *Isospora belli* infection. For therapy of *Pneumocystis* pneumonia, 15–20 mg/kg/d of trimethoprim and 75–100 mg/kg/d of sulfamethoxazole in three or four divided doses is administered intravenously or orally—depending on the severity of disease—for 3 weeks. The dose for prophylaxis is 160 mg trimethoprim + 800 mg sulfamethoxazole daily or three times per week. (When given daily, it is also effective prophylaxis against toxoplasmal encephalitis.) *I belli* infection in AIDS has been successfully treated with 160 mg trimethoprim + 800 mg sulfamethoxazole orally four times daily for 10 days followed by twice-daily administration for 3 weeks. Cyclosporiasis is successfully treated with 160 mg trimethoprim and 800 mg sulfamethoxazole twice daily for 7–10 days. Sulfadiazine with pyrimethamine is also used to treat and prevent recurrence of toxoplasmosis.

C. OTHER BACTERIAL INFECTIONS

Sulfonamides are the drugs of choice for *Nocardia* infections. Trimethoprim-sulfamethoxazole is widely distributed in tissues, penetrates into the cerebrospinal fluid, and has been used to treat meningitis caused by gram-negative rods, though third-generation cephalosporins are now preferred. While it is occasionally used for outpatient respiratory tract infections, the increasing pattern of resistance associated with *S pneumoniae* has decreased its utility.

Trimethoprim-sulfamethoxazole is effective also for infections with *Enterobacter*, *B pseudomallei* (melioidosis), *S maltophilia*, or *B cepacia*; in combination with rifampin, for eradication of nasopharyngeal carriage of staphylococci; for prophylaxis against meningococcal disease when susceptible strains predominate; for antibacterial prophylaxis in organ transplant recipients or patients with chronic granulomatous disease; for treatment of *L monocytogenes* meningitis; and perhaps also for management of pulmonary Wegener's granulomatosis.

D. LEPROSY

Certain sulfones are widely used (see below).

Adverse Effects

Adverse reactions to sulfonamides occur in 10–15% of non-AIDS patients (usually a minor rash or gastrointestinal disturbance) and in up to 50% of patients with AIDS (predominantly rash, fever, neutropenia, and thrombocytopenia, often severe enough to require discontinuation of therapy). These drugs have many side effects—due partly to hypersensitivity, partly to direct toxicity—that must be considered whenever unexplained symptoms or signs occur in a patient who may have received these drugs.

A. SYSTEMIC SIDE EFFECTS

Fever, skin rashes, urticaria; nausea, vomiting, or diarrhea; stomatitis, conjunctivitis, arthritis, aseptic meningitis, exfoliative dermatitis; bone marrow depression, thrombocytopenia, hemolytic (in G6PD deficiency) or aplastic anemia, granulocytopenia, leukemoid reactions; hepatitis, polyarteritis nodosa, vasculitis, Stevens-Johnson syndrome; reversible hyperkalemia; and many others have been reported. Because of the risk of Stevens-Johnson syndrome, patients with a previous rash after trimethoprim-sulfamethoxazole should not receive the drug again. Patients reporting an allergic reaction to sulfonamides have an increased risk of allergy to penicillin.

HIV-positive patients intolerant to trimethoprim-sulfamethoxazole can often be desensitized. A 70% success rate has been reported after giving 0.004 mg trimethoprim/0.02 mg sulfamethoxazole as oral suspension and increasing the dose tenfold each hour to achieve a final dose of 160 mg trimethoprim/500 mg sulfamethoxazole.

B. URINARY TRACT DISTURBANCES

Older sulfonamides were relatively insoluble and would precipitate in urine. The most commonly used sulfonamides presently (sulfamethoxazole) are quite soluble, and the old admonition to force fluids is no longer warranted. Sulfonamides have been implicated in interstitial nephritis. Patients with toxoplasmosis receiving high-dose sulfadiazine therapy are predisposed to crystalluria.

SULFONES USED IN THE TREATMENT OF LEPROSY

A number of drugs closely related to the sulfonamides (eg, dapsone) have been used effectively in the long-term treatment of leprosy. The clinical manifestations of both lepromatous and tuberculoid leprosy can often be suppressed by treatment extending over several years. At least 5–30% of *Mycobacterium leprae* organisms are resistant to dapsone, so initial combined treatment with rifampin is advocated. Dapsone, 100 mg daily, is effective therapy for mild to moderate *Pneumocystis* pneumonia in AIDS when combined with trimethoprim, 15–20 mg/kg/d in four divided doses. At a dose of 50–100 mg daily or 100 mg two or three times a week, it is effective prophylaxis for *Pneumocystis jiroveci* (formerly *Pneumocystis carinii*) infection and, when combined with pyrimethamine, 50 mg per week, also prevents *Toxoplasma* encephalitis in HIV-infected patients.

Absorption, Metabolism, & Excretion

All sulfones are well absorbed from the intestinal tract, are distributed widely in all tissues, and tend to be retained in skin, muscle, liver, and kidney. Leprous skin contains ten times more drug than normal skin. Sulfones are excreted into the bile and reabsorbed by the intestine, prolonging therapeutic blood levels. Excretion into the urine is variable, and the drug occurs in urine mostly as a glucuronic acid conjugate. Some persons acetylate sulfones slowly and others rapidly, potentially requiring dosage adjustment.

Dosages & Routes of Administration

See the section on Leprosy in Chapter 33 for recommendations.

Adverse Effects

The sulfones may cause any of the side effects listed above for sulfonamides. Anorexia, nausea, and vomiting are common. Hemolysis, methemoglobinemia, or agranulocytosis may occur. G6PD levels should be determined prior to initiation of dapsone therapy. If sulfones are not tolerated, clofazimine can be substituted.

SPECIALIZED DRUGS USED AGAINST BACTERIA

1. Bacitracin

This polypeptide is selectively active against gram-positive bacteria. Because of severe nephrotoxicity upon systemic administration, its use has been limited to topical application on surface lesions, usually in combination with polymyxin or neomycin.

2. Mupirocin

Mupirocin (formerly pseudomonic acid) is a naturally occurring antibiotic produced by *Pseudomonas fluorescens* active against most gram-positive cocci, including methicillin-sensitive and methicillin-resistant *S aureus* and most streptococci (but not enterococci). Used topically, it is effective in eliminating staphylococcal nasal carriage in the majority of patients for up to 3 months after application to the anterior nares twice daily for 5 days. However, recurrent colonization occurs (50% at the end of 1 year), and when mupirocin is used long-term over months, resistant organisms can emerge. Monthly application for 5 days each month for up to a year decreases staphylococcal colonization, which in turn lowers the risk of recurrent staphylococcal skin infections. Recent studies demonstrate an associated reduction in postoperative staphylococcal lung infections in colonized patients treated with mupirocin. Whether it is more effective than trimethoprim-sulfamethoxazole or dicloxacillin plus rifampin for eradication of staphylococcal nasal carriage is unknown. The other major use of mupirocin is for therapy of impetigo; it is useful in mild disease.

3. Clindamycin

Clindamycin is active against gram-positive organisms including *S pneumoniae*, viridans streptococci, group A streptococci, and *S aureus*, though resistance has been described in all of these organisms. Pneumococci with an efflux-based mechanism of resistance can be effectively treated with clindamycin. However, isolates with ribosomal methylase resistance (about 10% of isolates) are also resistant to clindamycin. Enterococci, most methicillin-resistant *S aureus*, and most *S epidermidis* also are resistant. A dosage of 0.15–0.3 g orally every 6 hours generally is used. It is widely distributed in tissues but not in cerebrospinal fluid. Excretion is primarily nonrenal. Clindamycin is currently recommended as an alternative drug for prophylaxis against endocarditis following oral procedures in patients allergic to amoxicillin. Clindamycin, 300 mg orally twice daily for 7 days, can be used as an alternative to metronidazole for the therapy of bacterial vaginosis. Topical application of a 2% vaginal cream once or twice daily for 7 days is also effective. Clindamycin is active against most anaerobes, including *Bacteroides, Prevotella, Clostridium, Peptococcus, Peptostreptococcus,* and *Fusobacterium* organisms. However, up to 25% of *Bacteroides* isolates are resistant, and alternative agents should be considered for life-threatening anaerobic infections due to these organisms. It is frequently used to treat less severe infections in which anaerobes are significant pathogens (eg, aspiration pneumonia, pelvic and abdominal infections), often in combination with other drugs (aminoglycosides, cephalosporins, fluoroquinolones). Seriously ill patients are given clindamycin, 600–900 mg (20–30 mg/kg/d) intravenously every 8 hours. It has also been of use in staphylococcal osteomyelitis. Because tissue models document that clindamycin significantly decreases toxin production, the addition of clindamycin to penicillin for therapy of group A streptococcus toxic shock syndrome has been suggested. In the sulfonamide-allergic patient, high-dose clindamycin therapy (600–1200 mg intravenously every 6 hours or 600 mg orally every 6 hours) in conjunction with pyrimethamine has been used to treat toxoplasmosis of the central nervous system and appears to be as effective as pyrimethamine and sulfadiazine. Clindamycin in combination with primaquine is effective in *Pneumocystis* pneumonia, and clindamycin with quinine is of value for falciparum malaria. While useful in brain abscess, clindamycin is ineffective in meningitis.

Common side effects are diarrhea, nausea, and skin rashes. Antibiotic-associated colitis has been associated with the administration of clindamycin and other antibiotics and is due to a necrotizing toxin produced by *Clostridium difficile.* The organism is resistant to the antimicrobial, is selected out by its presence, and is favored in its growth and toxin production. *C difficile* is usually susceptible to—and can be treated with—metronidazole or vancomycin given orally, though metronidazole is the drug of choice (see below).

4. Metronidazole

Metronidazole is an antiprotozoal drug (see Chapter 35) that also has striking antibacterial effects against most anaerobic gram-negative bacilli (*Bacteroides, Prevotella, Fusobacterium*) and *Clostridium* species but has minimal activity against many anaerobic gram-positive and microaerophilic organisms. It is well absorbed after oral administration and is widely distributed in tissues.

It penetrates well into the cerebrospinal fluid, yielding levels similar to those in serum. The drug is metabolized in the liver, and dosage reduction is required in severe hepatic insufficiency or biliary dysfunction.

Metronidazole is used to treat amebiasis and giardiasis (see Chapter 35) and in the following circumstances:

(1) Vaginitis caused by *Trichomonas vaginalis* responds to either a single dose (2 g) or to 250 mg orally three times daily for 7–10 days. Bacterial vaginosis responds to a single 2-g dose or to 500 mg twice daily for 7 days. Metronidazole vaginal cream (0.75%) applied twice daily for 5 days is also effective.

(2) In anaerobic infections, metronidazole can be given orally or intravenously, 500 mg three times daily (30 mg/kg/d). It is more predictable against *B fragilis* than clindamycin or second-generation cephalosporins.

(3) Metronidazole is less expensive and equally as efficacious as oral vancomycin for the therapy of *C difficile* colitis and is the drug of choice for the disease. A dosage of 500 mg orally three times daily is recommended. If oral medication cannot be tolerated, intravenous metronidazole can be tried at the same dose; however, this route is unproved and usually less effective than the oral one. Because of the emergence of vancomycin-resistant enterococci as a major pathogen and the role of oral vancomycin in selecting for these resistant organisms, metronidazole should be used as first-line therapy for *C difficile* disease.

(4) Preparation of the colon before bowel surgery.

(5) Therapy of brain abscess, often in combination with penicillin or a third-generation cephalosporin.

(6) In combination with clarithromycin and omeprazole for therapy of *H pylori* infections.

Adverse effects include stomatitis, nausea, and diarrhea. Ingestion of alcohol while taking metronidazole occasionally results in a disulfiram reaction. With prolonged use at high doses, reversible peripheral neuropathy can develop. Metronidazole can decrease the metabolism of warfarin, necessitating dosage adjustment of warfarin. Metronidazole is carcinogenic in certain animal models and mutagenic for certain bacteria, but to date an increased incidence of malignancy has not been confirmed in humans.

Fihn SD: Acute uncomplicated urinary tract infection in women. N Engl J Med 2003;349:259. [PMID: 12867610]

Masters PA et al: Trimethoprim-sulfamethoxazole revisited. Arch Intern Med 2003;163:402. [PMID: 12588198]

Raz R et al: Empiric use of trimethoprim-sulfamethoxazole (TMP-SMX) in the treatment of women with uncomplicated urinary tract infections, in a geographic area with a high prevalence of TMP-SMX-resistant uropathogens. Clin Infect Dis 2002;34:1165. [PMID: 11941541]

Strom BL et al: Absence of cross-reactivity between sulfonamide antibiotics and sulfonamide nonantibiotics. N Engl J Med 2003;349:1628. [PMID: 14573734]

5. Vancomycin

This drug is bactericidal for most gram-positive organisms, particularly staphylococci and streptococci, and is bacteriostatic for most enterococci. While active against staphylococci, vancomycin kills more slowly when compared with nafcillin. Although vancomycin has retained activity against staphylococci and streptococci, vancomycin-resistant strains of enterococci (particularly *E faecium*) have emerged. *S aureus* both intermediately sensitive and highly vancomycin-resistant has been observed in patients receiving long-term vancomycin therapy. Vancomycin is not absorbed from the gastrointestinal tract. It is given orally only for the treatment of antibiotic-associated enterocolitis. For systemic effect, the drug must be administered intravenously (20–30 mg/kg/d in two or three divided doses). Vancomycin is excreted mainly via the kidneys. In renal insufficiency, the half-life may be up to 8 days. Vancomycin is cleared via high-flux hemodialysis and continuous arteriovenous hemofiltration (CAVH) generally resulting in the need for increased dosing. In patients with impaired renal function, the dosing interval is determined by measuring trough serum levels. When trough serum levels decline to 10–15 mcg/mL, repeat dosing is required.

Indications for parenteral vancomycin include the following: (1) Severe staphylococcal infections in penicillin-allergic patients; for methicillin-resistant *S aureus* and *S epidermidis* infections and for serious infections (pneumonia, meningitis) due to highly resistant *S pneumoniae*. (2) Severe enterococcal infections in the penicillin-allergic patient or if the enterococcus is penicillin-resistant. (3) Other gram-positive infections in penicillin-allergic patients, eg, viridans streptococcal endocarditis. (4) Surgical prophylaxis in penicillin-allergic patients. (5) For gram-positive infections due to organisms that are multidrug-resistant, ie, *Corynebacterium jeikeium*. (6) Endocarditis prophylaxis in the penicillin-allergic patient undergoing certain genitourinary and gastrointestinal procedures (in combination with an aminoglycoside). (See Table 33–3.)

In antibiotic-associated enterocolitis, vancomycin, 0.125 g, is given orally four times daily.

Vancomycin is irritating to tissues; thrombophlebitis sometimes follows intravenous injection. The drug is infrequently ototoxic when given concomitantly with aminoglycosides or high-dose intravenous erythromycins; it is potentially nephrotoxic when administered with aminoglycosides. Rapid infusion or high doses (1 g or more) may induce diffuse hyperemia ("red man syndrome") and can be avoided by extending infusions over 1–2 hours, by reducing the dose, or by pretreating with a histamine antagonist such as hydroxyzine.

Bal AM et al: Antibiotic resistance in *Staphylococcus aureus* and its relevance in therapy. Expert Opin Pharmacother 2005;6: 2257. [PMID: 16218886]

STREPTOGRAMINS

Streptogramins are structurally similar to macrolides but do not share cross-resistance with that class. **Pristinamycin** is an oral streptogramin marketed in France for treatment of gram-positive infections. **Synercid** is a combination of two synthetic derivatives of pristinamycin—quinupristin and dalfopristin—in a 30:70 ratio that is administered intravenously. It is bactericidal and inhibits protein synthesis by binding to bacterial ribosomes. In vitro, it has activity against *M catarrhalis*, *H influenzae*, *Clostridium*, *Peptostreptococcus*, *Mycoplasma*, *Legionella*, and *Chlamydia*. It has no activity against enteric gram-negative bacilli. However, its major clinical use is in the therapy of gram-positive infections, including those due to streptococci (including penicillin-resistant pneumococci) staphylococci (including methicillin-sensitive and methicillin-resistant *S aureus* and *S epidermidis*) and enterococci, including vancomycin-resistant *E faecium*. The combination is not reliably active against *E faecalis*. The drug is generally bacteriostatic against the enterococci. The recommended dose is 7.5 mg/kg/dose intravenously every 8 hours. In addition to phlebitis with peripheral administration, the major adverse effect is arthralgias and myalgias that resolve with discontinuation of the drug. It is primarily cleared via the liver; streptogramins inhibit the cytochrome P450 system, resulting in increased levels of cyclosporine and other agents.

OXAZOLIDINONES

Oxazolidinones represent a class of antibacterials of which linezolid is the one available agent. Linezolid is primarily active against aerobic gram-positive pathogens, including penicillin-resistant pneumococci, methicillin-resistant staphylococci and enterococci (both *E faecalis* and vancomycin-sensitive and vancomycin-resistant *E faecium*). Linezolid is bacteriostatic against all of these pathogens. Linezolid-resistant and vancomycin-resistant enterococci and linezolid-resistant *S aureus* may be encountered, however. The oral bioavailability of linezolid is complete, with serum levels approaching those observed with intravenous administration. The drug is eliminated primarily by nonrenal mechanisms. The primary toxicity is bone marrow suppression with long-term therapy, particularly the platelet line. Other adverse effects include tongue discoloration and mild MAO inhibition. Studies suggest a more rapid response to therapy and reduction in length of hospitalization associated with linezolid when compared with vancomycin; however, these findings require confirmation by prospective controlled studies. Of particular concern are the increasing reports of linezolid-resistant enterococcus, which reinforce that this agent should be used judiciously.

DAPTOMYCIN

Daptomycin is a bactericidal lipopeptide with a spectrum of activity similar to that of linezolid or quinupristin-dalfopristin. This spectrum includes methicillin-resistant staphylococci and vancomycin-resistant enterococci. Daptomycin has poor oral bioavailability, thus is only available as a parenteral product. Its long pharmacologic half-life allows for once-daily dosing (4 mg/kg every 24 hours); dosage adjustment is necessary in the presence of renal failure. The primary adverse event associated with daptomycin is a reversible, dose-dependent myopathy observed with > 7 days of therapy. At the present time, daptomycin is only approved in the treatment of skin and soft tissue infection; however, the drug is being investigated at higher doses in the treatment of staphylococcal bacteremia and endocarditis. Daptomycin cannot be used in the treatment of respiratory tract infection. Pulmonary surfactant binds daptomycin, resulting in minimal free drug concentrations in pulmonary secretions.

Carpenter CF et al: Daptomycin: another novel agent for treating infections due to drug-resistant gram-positive pathgogens. Clinical Infect Dis 2004;38:994. [PMID: 15034832]

Eliopoulos GM: Quinupristin-dalfopristin and linezolid: evidence and opinion. Clin Infect Dis 2003;36:473. [PMID: 12567306]

Steenbergen JN et al: Daptomycin: a lipopeptide antibiotic for the treatment of serious Gram-positive infections. J Antimicrob Chemother 2005;55:283. [PMID: 15705644]

Tedesco KL et al: Daptomycin. Pharmacotherapy 2004;24:41. [PMID: 14740787]

Weigelt J et al: Linezolid versus vancomycin in treatment of complicated skin and soft tissue infections. Antimicrob Agents Chemother 2005;49:2260. [PMID: 15917519]

QUINOLONES

The quinolones are synthetic analogs of nalidixic acid that have an exceedingly broad spectrum of activity against many bacteria. The mode of action of all quinolones involves inhibition of bacterial DNA synthesis by blocking the enzyme DNA gyrase.

The earlier quinolones (nalidixic acid, oxolinic acid, cinoxacin) did not achieve systemic antibacterial levels after oral intake and thus were useful only as urinary antiseptics. The newer fluorinated derivatives (ciprofloxacin, ofloxacin, levofloxacin, gatifloxacin, gemifloxacin, and moxifloxacin) have more potent antibacterial activity, achieve clinically useful levels in blood and tissues, and have low toxicity.

Antimicrobial Activity

A number of fluoroquinolones are in use. Most have quite similar spectrums of activity. In general, these drugs have moderate to excellent activity against enterobacteriaceae but are also active against other gram-negative bacteria such as *Haemophilus, Neisseria, Moraxella, Brucella, Legionella, Salmonella, Shigella, Campylobacter, Yersinia, Vibrio,* and *Aeromonas* organisms. Resistance to *E coli* has significantly increased over the past decade, with some centers reporting up to 20–30% resistance. Ciprofloxacin and levofloxacin have slightly better activity against *P aeruginosa* than the other fluoroquinolones, but the increasing resistance of *P aeruginosa* to

fluoroquinolones limits their usefulness in the treatment of infections caused by that organism. None of these agents have reliable activity against *S maltophilia* or *B cepacia*—though the newer drugs are more active against *S maltophilia*—as they are for treating genital tract pathogens such as *Mycoplasma hominis, U urealyticum,* and *Chlamydia pneumoniae. M tuberculosis* is sensitive to the quinolones, as is *M fortuitum* and *Mycobacterium kansasii.* Although most *M avium* complex organisms are resistant to fluoroquinolones, when combined with other antibiotics (ethambutol, rifabutin, and amikacin), fluoroquinolones may have a role.

In general, the fluoroquinolones are less potent against gram-positive than against gram-negative organisms. Gatifloxacin, gemifloxacin, levofloxacin, and moxifloxacin have the best gram-positive activity, including against pneumococci and strains of *S aureus* and *S epidermidis,* including some methicillin-resistant strains. However, the emergence of resistant strains of staphylococci has limited the use of these drugs as monotherapy of infections caused by these organisms. Enterococci, including *E faecalis, S pneumoniae,* group A, B, and D streptococci, and viridans streptococci, are only moderately inhibited by the older quinolones. Anaerobic bacteria, *T pallidum,* and *Nocardia* are resistant to the earlier fluoroquinolones.

Moxifloxacin demonstrates activity against many of the significant anaerobic pathogens, including *B fragilis* and mouth anaerobes, and is approved for the treatment of intra-abdominal infection. However, increased rates of anaerobic resistance over time have been reported.

Pharmacokinetics & Administration

After oral administration, the fluoroquinolones are well absorbed and widely distributed in body fluids and tissues and are concentrated intracellularly. Fluoroquinolones bind some heavy metals; thus, absorption is inhibited when given with iron, calcium, and other multivalent cations. Optimal oral bioavailability is achieved if fluoroquinolones are taken 1 hour before or 2 hours after meals. The serum half-life ranges from 4 hours (ciprofloxacin) to 12 hours (moxifloxacin). After ingestion of 500 mg, the peak serum level of ciprofloxacin is 2.5 mcg/mL, which is lower than that of the other quinolones (4–6 mcg/mL), but this is offset by ciprofloxacin's slightly greater in vitro potency against most gram-negative organisms. A number of the fluoroquinolones can be administered intravenously, resulting in peak serum levels ranging from 4 mcg/mL to 9 mcg/mL (Table 37–9). Most are eliminated via mixed renal and nonrenal pathways. As a result, only modest accumulation takes place in the presence of renal insufficiency. Exceptions are ofloxacin, levofloxacin, and gatifloxacin, which are primarily dependent upon the kidney for elimination.

Clinical Uses

Urinary tract infections caused by trimethoprim-sulfamethoxazole–resistant gram-negative organisms have

Table 37–9. Pharmacology of the quinolones.

Drug	Peak Serum Levels (mcg/mL)	Serum Half-Life (h)	Total Daily Dose	Dosage Adjustments in Renal Failure			
				Dosage Interval (h)	Moderate (Cl_{cr} 10–50 mL/min)	Severe (Cl_{cr} < 10 mL/min)	Posthemo-dialysis Dose
Ciprofloxacin	3–4 (400 mg IV, 500–750 mg PO)	3–6	800–1200 mg (IV), 0.5–1.5 g (PO)	8–12	400 mg q12h	200 mg q12h	None
Gatifloxacin	4–5 (400 mg PO or IV)	7	400 mg (PO/IV)	24	200 mg q24h	200 mg q24h	200 mg
Gemifloxacin	2–4 (320 mg PO)	7	320 mg PO	Not known	Not known	Not known	Not known
Levofloxacin	5–7 (500 mg PO or IV)	6–8	250–750 mg (PO/IV)	24	250–500 mg q24–48h	250–500 mg q48h	None
Moxifloxacin	3–4 (400 mg PO)	12	400 mg (PO)	24	400 mg q24h	400 mg q24h	Not known
Ofloxacin	5–7 (400 mg PO or IV)	6–8	400–800 mg (PO/IV)	12	200–400 mg q24h	200 mg q24h	None

resulted in quinolones being recognized as one of the drugs of choice in areas with > 10–20% resistance of *E coli* to trimethoprim-sulfamethoxazole.

Because of good penetration into prostatic tissue, quinolones are effective in treating bacterial prostatitis and are alternatives to trimethoprim-sulfamethoxazole (doses for prostatitis are the same as for urinary tract infection, but the duration should be 6–12 weeks).

Quinolones are approved for treatment of certain sexually transmitted diseases. Ofloxacin, 300 mg orally twice daily for 7 days, is as effective as doxycycline, 100 mg orally twice daily for 7 days, for the therapy of *C trachomatis* cervicitis, urethritis, and proctitis. It is also effective for nongonococcal urethritis caused by *U urealyticum*. Ciprofloxacin is not effective for the therapy of chlamydial infections or nongonococcal urethritis. In general, the use of quinolones for the treatment of any sexually transmitted disease will be limited by their lack of efficacy with concomitant syphilis. Gonococcal urethritis, cervicitis, pharyngitis, and proctitis can be treated with a single oral dose of 500 mg of ciprofloxacin or 400 mg of oral ofloxacin. However, the increased prevalence of quinolone-resistant gonococci in California and Hawaii has resulted in the use of ceftriaxone and certain oral cephalosporins as the primary choices in those regions.

Pelvic inflammatory disease is usually caused by *C trachomatis, N gonorrhoeae*, enterobacteriaceae, or anaerobes. Oral outpatient treatment with ofloxacin, 400 mg twice daily for 14 days, in addition to clindamycin, 450 mg orally four times daily for 14 days, or metronidazole, 500 mg orally twice daily for 14 days, can be used. Epididymitis in young men (< 35 years of age) is caused most commonly by chlamydia and the gonococcus. Single-dose oral ciprofloxacin (500 mg) or oral ofloxacin (400 mg) followed by oral doxycycline,

100 mg twice daily for 10 days, is adequate therapy. Alternatively, ofloxacin, 300 mg orally twice daily for 10 days, can be used. *H ducreyi*, the pathogen that causes chancroid, is sensitive to quinolones, and ciprofloxacin, 500 mg orally twice daily, or enoxacin, 400 mg orally daily for 3 days, can be used as an alternative to erythromycin, azithromycin, or ceftriaxone as therapy for this disease.

Fluoroquinolones have been used successfully to treat complicated skin and soft tissue infections and osteomyelitis caused by gram-negative organisms. Ciprofloxacin, 500–750 mg orally twice daily for at least 6 weeks, has been effective therapy for malignant otitis externa.

Quinolones are among the few oral agents active against *Campylobacter* despite increasing resistance. In addition, they are active against the other major bacterial pathogens associated with diarrhea (*Salmonella, Shigella*, toxigenic *E coli*). Consequently, they have been used for the therapy of traveler's diarrhea as well as domestically acquired acute diarrhea. Norfloxacin, ciprofloxacin, and ofloxacin may be effective in eradicating the chronic carrier state of salmonella when therapy is continued for 4–6 weeks.

Ciprofloxacin has been used to eradicate meningococci from the nasopharynx of carriers.

Fluoroquinolones are effective for prophylaxis against gram-negative infections in the neutropenic patient, and intravenous ciprofloxacin in combination with β-lactam antibiotics has been used successfully to treat the febrile neutropenic patient.

Gatifloxacin, gemifloxacin, levofloxacin, and moxifloxacin are sometimes referred to as "respiratory fluoroquinolones" due to their activity against the pneumococci, including penicillin-resistant strains as well as atypical bacteria. However, their broad aerobic gram-negative spectrum suggests that they should be reserved for the treatment of refractory infections or high-risk patients, including those with comorbidities or recent receipt of β-lactam antibacterials. One setting in which ciprofloxacin is indicated for the therapy of lower respiratory tract infections is in cystic fibrosis, where *P aeruginosa* is the predominant pathogen. However, the increasing rate of resistance to ciprofloxacin has diminished the use of the drug for this indication.

Ciprofloxacin in combination with other agents has been used to treat *M avium* complex infections, and ciprofloxacin, levofloxacin, ofloxacin, and moxifloxacin may be efficacious in the therapy of multi-drug-resistant tuberculosis.

Adverse Effects

The most prominent adverse effects of the quinolones are nausea, vomiting, and diarrhea. Occasionally, headache, dizziness, seizures, insomnia, impaired liver function, and skin rashes have been observed as well as more serious reactions such as acute renal failure, hypoglycemia (especially with gatifloxacin), and anaphylaxis. Fluoroquinolones as a class prolong the QT interval; it is debated whether any one agent is implicated more than another. Quinolones should be used cautiously in patients receiving antiarrhythmics such as amiodarone or in persons with a history of prolonged QT. Prolongation of the prothrombin time has been observed in some patients receiving stable doses of warfarin after ciprofloxacin has been given, but this interaction is unpredictable and modest. Tendinitis and tendon rupture have been reported with quinolone agents. Risk factors include concomitant corticosteroid use and age > 60 years. Patients experiencing musculoskeletal symptoms while receiving fluoroquinolones should discontinue therapy.

Lautenbach E et al: Association between fluoroquinolone resistance and mortality in *Escherichia coli* and *Klebsiella pneumoniae* infections: the role of inadequate empirical antimicrobial therapy. Clin Infect Dis 2005;41:923. [PMID: 16142655]

Mohr JF et al: A retrospective, comparative evaluation of dysglycemias in hospitalized patients receiving gatifloxacin, levofloxacin, ciprofloxacin, or ceftriaxone. Pharmacotherapy 2005;25:1303. [PMID: 16185173]

Saravolatz LD et al: Gatifloxacin, gemifloxacin, and moxifloxacin: the role of 3 newer fluoroquinolones. Clin Infect Dis 2003; 37:1210. [PMID: 14557966]

PENTAMIDINE & ATOVAQUONE

Pentamidine and atovaquone are antiprotozoal agents that are primarily used to treat *Pneumocystis* pneumonia. Pentamidine is discussed in Chapters 31 and 35. Atovaquone inhibits mitochondrial electron transport and probably also folate metabolism. The solid dosage form is poorly absorbed and should be given with food to maximize bioavailability. The suspension is significantly better absorbed and preferred especially in high-risk patients (those with diarrhea, malabsorption). It has moderate activity against *P jiroveci*. In comparative trials with trimethoprim-sulfamethoxazole and pentamidine in the therapy of *Pneumocystis* pneumonia in AIDS, atovaquone, 750 mg orally three times daily for 3 weeks, is less effective than both agents but better tolerated. It has also been used as prophylaxis in AIDS patients at a dosage of 1500 mg daily. Major adverse effects include rash, nausea, vomiting, diarrhea, fever, and abnormal liver function tests. The use of atovaquone is limited to patients with mild to moderate *Pneumocystis* infections who have not responded to or cannot tolerate other therapies.

URINARY ANTISEPTICS

These drugs exert antimicrobial activity in the urine but have little or no systemic antibacterial effect. Their usefulness is limited to therapy and prevention of urinary tract infections.

1. Nitrofurantoin

Nitrofurantoin is active against the common gram-positive urinary pathogens *E faecalis* and *Staphylococcus saprophyticus*, but the drug inhibits only about 50% of *E faecium*. It is also used against *E coli* and *Citrobacter*, but activity against *Proteus, Serratia,* and *Pseudomonas* is poor. Following oral administration, about 50% of the drug is absorbed, but serum concentrations are very low and tissue levels are undetectable. Levels in the urine reach concentrations of 200–400 mcg/mL, which are well above the MICs of susceptible organisms. However, in renal failure, subtherapeutic urine levels are present and drug accumulation takes place in serum. Given low serum levels, poor tissue penetration, and renal elimination, the use of nitrofurantoin is limited to therapy or prophylaxis of cystitis in patients with normal renal function. Nitrofurantoin should not be used to treat pyelonephritis or prostatitis.

The average daily dose in urinary tract infections is 100 mg orally four times daily, taken with food. The macrocrystal preparation can be given at a dosage of 100 mg twice daily. A single daily dose of 50–100 mg can prevent recurrent urinary tract infections in women.

Oral nitrofurantoin often causes nausea and vomiting. The crystalline formulation is better tolerated than previous preparations. Hemolytic anemia may occur in G6PD deficiency. Other side effects are skin rashes and, uncommonly, peripheral neuropathy. Acute and chronic pulmonary hypersensitivity reactions may occur, and pulmonary fibrosis has occurred with prolonged use.

2. Fosfomycin

Fosfomycin tromethamine is a phosphonic acid derivative useful in the treatment of uncomplicated urinary tract infection. The spectrum of activity includes *E coli, E faecalis,* and other gram-negative aerobic urinary pathogens, but not *P aeruginosa*. Available as a 3-g sachet, fosfomycin may be useful for the single-dose treatment of the above organisms. Like nitrofurantoin, fosfomycin should not be used for systemic infection. However, the increased concentrations in urine allow for its use in uncomplicated bacteriuria. The most frequently reported adverse effects include diarrhea, headache, and nausea.

ANTIFUNGAL DRUGS

Empiric antifungal therapy is rarely instituted except for febrile neutropenic and other high-risk patients. Therapy is reserved for situations in which yeast or mold is seen on KOH preparation or when isolated organisms are thought to be pathogenic. Antifungal standardized susceptibility testing is available for *Candida* spp, and predict clinical outcome. In contrast, susceptibility testing for most other fungi is not generally available; in vitro results for these pathogens is less predictive of patient outcomes.

1. Amphotericin B

Amphotericin B in vitro inhibits several organisms producing systemic mycotic disease in humans, including *Aspergillus, Histoplasma, Cryptococcus, Coccidioides, Candida, Blastomyces, Sporothrix,* and others. This drug can be used for treatment of these systemic fungal infections. *Pseudallescheria boydii* and *Fusarium* are often resistant to amphotericin B.

There is no consensus on how conventional amphotericin B should be administered or on the dosage and the duration of therapy. A test dose is unnecessary, since anaphylaxis is extremely rare. The daily dose of amphotericin B for most fungal infections varies from 0.3 mg/kg to 0.7 mg/kg, though infections caused by *Aspergillus* and *Mucor* are often treated with 1–1.5 mg/kg daily.

Combined treatment with flucytosine is beneficial in cryptococcal meningitis and possibly systemic candidiasis. Amphotericin B may have some benefit in *Naegleria* meningoencephalitis.

Amphotericin B has been used prophylactically to prevent invasive fungal infections in bone marrow transplant recipients; however, other agents are less toxic and may be more efficacious. Whether prophylactic antifungal use is better than early empiric therapy in febrile patients who have not responded to broad-spectrum antibiotics has not been determined.

In patients with Foley catheters in place who have candiduria, amphotericin B bladder irrigations decrease colony counts; however, the efficacy of irrigation is marginal, and long-term eradication of candiduria following amphotericin B bladder irrigation rarely occurs.

Neither renal nor hepatic failure alters the pharmacokinetic disposition of amphotericin. The drug concentrates in the lung, liver, spleen, and kidney with minimal penetration into skin or adipose tissue. The drug is not removed by hemodialysis.

The intravenous administration of amphotericin B often produces chills, fever, vomiting, and headache. As a rule, infusions given over 1–2 hours are as well tolerated as those given over 4–6 hours. However, patients who experience infusion-related adverse effects may benefit from slowing the rate of administration. Tolerability may be enhanced by temporary lowering of the dose or premedication with acetaminophen and diphenhydramine. Addition of 25 mg of hydrocortisone to the infusion decreases the incidence of rigors, and meperidine, 25–50 mg, is effective in arresting rigors once they start. Central intravenous administration eliminates the likelihood of thrombophlebitis. Electrolyte disturbances (hypokalemia, hypomagnesemia, distal renal tubular acidosis) also commonly occur. Renal insufficiency can be reduced with sodium supplementation. As a result, administration of 0.5–1 L of 0.9% saline prior to infusion of amphotericin B is recommended.

The nephrotoxicity of amphotericin has resulted in the development of lipid-based amphotericin B products. Three such products are available: amphotericin B lipid complex (ABLC; Abelcet), amphotericin B colloidal dispersion (ABCD; Amphotec), and liposomal amphotericin B (L-AmB; AmBisome). Complexing amphotericin B with lipid allows larger doses to be administered (3–6 mg/kg, depending on the preparation and the fungal species). All three preparations are associated with less nephrotoxicity than conventional amphotericin B. Liposomal amphotericin is somewhat less nephrotoxic than ABLC. Infusion-related adverse effects are variable, with liposomal amphotericin the best tolerated. Liposomal amphotericin is equal to or better than that of conventional amphotericin B in febrile neutropenia, particularly in prevention of emergent *Candida* infections.

Drug acquisition costs for all three products are much higher than for conventional amphotericin B. The availability of echinocandins and triazoles has resulted in additional choices in the prevention and treatment of fungal infection. The lipid formulations are particularly effective for therapy of visceral leishmaniasis. Short courses (5–10 days) with low doses (2–4 mg/kg/d depending on which preparation is used) are very effective in eradicating the parasite, probably because of distribution of the drug to the reticuloendothelial system, the major site of parasite invasion.

Drew RH et al: Is it time to abandon the use of amphotericin B bladder irrigation? Clin Infect Dis 2005;40:1465. [PMID: 15844069]

Gibbs WJ et al: Liposomal amphotericin B: clinical experience and perspectives. Expert Rev Anti Infect Ther Infect Dis 2005;3:167. [PMID: 15918775]

Wong-Beringer A et al: Systemic antifungal therapy: new options, new challenges. Pharmacotherapy 2003;23:1441. [PMID: 14620391]

2. Nystatin

Nystatin has a wide spectrum of antifungal activity but is used almost exclusively to treat superficial candidal infections. It is too toxic for systemic administration, and the drug is not absorbed from mucous membranes or the gastrointestinal tract. Several preparations are available, including oral suspension (100,000 units/mL) and ointments, gels, and creams (100,000 units/g). For oral candidiasis, 500,000 units of suspension is used to rinse the mouth and is retained in the mouth as long as possible before it is swallowed. This is repeated four times a day for at least 2 days after resolution of the infection. Infections of skin are treated with cream or ointment, 100,000 units applied to the affected area twice daily until resolution of the infection. Nystatin is less effective than azoles for therapy of vaginal candidiasis.

3. Flucytosine

Flucytosine inhibits some strains of *Candida, Cryptococcus, Aspergillus,* and other fungi. Dosages of 3–8 g daily (75–150 mg/kg/d) orally produce therapeutic levels in serum, urine, and cerebrospinal fluid. Clinical remissions of meningitis or sepsis due to yeasts have occurred. However, resistant organisms are selected out rapidly, and flucytosine is therefore not used as a single drug except in urinary tract infections.

In renal insufficiency, flucytosine may accumulate to toxic levels, and dosage adjustments are needed. Because patients with HIV infection and normal renal function do not tolerate the previously used doses of flucytosine (150 mg/kg/d in four divided doses), 75–100 mg/kg/d is recommended. The drug is effectively removed by hemodialysis. Toxic effects include bone marrow depression, abnormal liver function, and nausea. Bone marrow suppression is caused by conversion of flucytosine to fluorouracil. Combined use of flucytosine and amphotericin B in cryptococcal meningitis and possibly systemic candidiasis has been shown to be of value.

4. Natamycin

Natamycin is a polyene antifungal drug effective against many different fungi in vitro. When it is combined with appropriate surgical measures, topical application of 5% ophthalmic suspension may be beneficial in the treatment of keratitis caused by *Fusarium, Acremonium* (cephalosporium), or other fungi. The toxicity after topical application appears to be low.

5. Terbinafine

Terbinafine, an allylamine, inhibits fungal cell membrane function by blocking ergosterol synthesis. Terbinafine is available topically as well as in 250-mg tablets for oral administration. The recommended dosage is 250 mg daily for 12 weeks for toenail infections and 250 mg daily for 6 weeks for fingernail infections (success rate about 70%). Pulse therapy (1 week on and 3 weeks off) is as effective as continuous therapy for 6–12 weeks. The drug also is active against many strains of *Candida* and *Aspergillus* organisms and has been used in combination with other antifungals to treat severe infections with these pathogens. Most adverse effects are minor (diar-

rhea, dyspepsia) or transient (taste disturbance). Rare cases of severe hepatic injury have occurred.

6. Antifungal Imidazoles & Triazoles

These antifungal drugs inhibit synthesis of ergosterol, resulting in inhibition of membrane-associated enzyme activity, cell wall growth, and replication.

Clotrimazole, taken orally in the form of 10-mg troches five times daily, can prevent and treat oral candidiasis. Vaginal azole tablets inserted daily for 1–7 days are effective for vaginal candidiasis. Topical preparations for treatment of cutaneous dermatophytes are also available.

Fluconazole, a bis-triazole with activity similar to that of ketoconazole, is water-soluble and can be given both orally and intravenously. Absorption of the drug after oral administration is not pH-dependent. It penetrates well into the cerebrospinal fluid and eye. The drug has been shown to be effective primarily in the treatment of *Candida, Cryptococcus,* and *Blastomyces* infections. *Candida albicans, Candida tropicalis,* and *Candida parapsilosus* are usually sensitive to fluconazole, but many other species of candida (*C krusei, C glabrata,* etc) are often resistant. Fluconazole-resistant strains of *C albicans* primarily have been observed in HIV-positive patients receiving long-term fluconazole therapy. With the advent of highly active antiretroviral therapy, the rate of fluconazole resistance in *C albicans* has decreased in this patient population. The drug is inactive against *Aspergillus, Mucor,* and *Pseudallescheria.* Fluconazole is effective in oropharyngeal candidiasis and candidal esophagitis in immunosuppressed patients. It is also valuable in vaginal candidiasis, where a single oral dose of 150 mg is 80–90% effective. Fluconazole, 400 mg intravenously and orally daily, is as effective as amphotericin B, 0.5–0.6 mg/kg/d, for candidemia in both neutropenic and nonneutropenic patients. Most of these infections are intravenous line–related, and removal of the line is critical to successful therapy. Fluconazole (200 mg/d) is effective as long-term suppressive therapy of cryptococcal meningitis in patients with AIDS and is the drug of choice in this setting. In the treatment of cryptococcal meningitis, response rates and overall mortality rates are the same in patients treated with oral fluconazole and with amphotericin B. However, the mortality rate in the first 2 weeks is higher with fluconazole and it takes longer to sterilize the cerebrospinal fluid among patients treated with fluconazole than among patients treated with amphotericin. Most clinicians would initiate therapy with amphotericin B for 2 weeks and then switch to oral fluconazole. A dosage of 400 mg of fluconazole daily is effective therapy for coccidioidal meningitis (80% response), but improvement is slow, taking as long as 4–8 months; efficacy has been observed in both non–HIV-infected and HIV-infected individuals. Higher doses (800–1200 mg/d) have been used; however, they have not been found to be superior to usual doses. Fluconazole, 400 mg daily, is effective prophylaxis against superficial and invasive fungal infections in bone marrow and liver transplant recipients, but concern has been raised about superinfection with resistant organisms (*C krusei, C glabrata, Aspergillus*). Because the overall incidence of invasive fungal disease in HIV infection is low, universal prophylaxis to prevent disease is discouraged, especially with the advent of more potent antiretroviral therapy. Fluconazole is also effective for the therapy of cutaneous leishmaniasis due to *Leishmania major* in a dose of 200 mg/d for 6 weeks.

Fluconazole is well absorbed after oral administration (> 90% bioavailability), and serum levels approach those seen after administering the same dose intravenously. Thus, unless the patient cannot take medication by mouth or is hemodynamically unstable, the preferred route of administration is by mouth. While generally well tolerated, fluconazole is associated with dose-dependent nausea and vomiting. Altered liver function tests (alanine aminotransferase [ALT], aspartate aminotransferase [AST]) and hepatitis have been reported. While less potent than other azoles (itraconazole, ketoconazole, voriconazole), fluconazole inhibits cytochrome P450 resulting in reduced elimination of certain agents. Rifampin and phenytoin increase metabolism of fluconazole necessitating increased fluconazole dosage.

Itraconazole is an oral triazole that has variable bioavailability. It is moderately well absorbed from the gastrointestinal tract (food increases absorption from 30% to 60%; antacids and H_2-receptor antagonists decrease absorption) and widely distributed in tissues with the notable exception of the central nervous system, where levels in spinal fluid are undetectable. Itraconazole solution is more predictably absorbed than the tablets. While the tablet formulation should be administered with food, the solution is best absorbed on an empty stomach. A parenteral formulation is available, but it is not approved for patients with renal insufficiency (creatinine clearance < 30 mL/min) because of the theoretic risk of pancreatic adenocarcinoma associated with accumulation of the cyclodextran vehicle. The drug is metabolized by the liver, and no dosage adjustment is needed in renal insufficiency. Itraconazole is very active against most strains of *Histoplasma capsulatum, Blastomyces dermatitidis, Cryptococcus neoformans, Sporotrichum schenkii*, and various dermatophytes. It is also active against *Aspergillus* species but inactive against *Fusarium* and *Zygomycetes*. Itraconazole in doses of 200–400 mg/d is effective and approved therapy for localized or disseminated histoplasmosis. It is also effective in sporotrichosis, dermatophytic infections (including those of the nails), and oral and esophageal candidiasis. Noncomparative clinical trials indicate efficacy in therapy of invasive aspergillosis (55–80%) and coccidioidomycosis (57–94%). Itraconazole is at least as effective as fluconazole in the treatment of nonmeningeal coccidioidomycosis and may be superior in the management of skeletal disease. At doses of 200 mg twice daily, itraconazole increases exercise tolerance

and decreases corticosteroid requirements in patients with allergic bronchopulmonary aspergillosis. Itraconazole has been shown to decrease superficial and invasive fungal infections when used as prophylaxis in neutropenic patients. Itraconazole has been approved for onychomycosis. Pulse therapy with 200 mg twice daily for 1 week each month, repeated for 4 consecutive months, is effective in 70% of cases.

Adverse effects are similar to those of ketoconazole and fluconazole, with anorexia, nausea, vomiting, and abdominal pain occurring most commonly. Skin rash has been reported in up to 8% of patients. Hepatitis and hypokalemia occur uncommonly. Exacerbation of heart failure occasionally occurs with itraconazole. Drugs that increase hepatic drug-metabolizing enzymes (isoniazid, rifampin, phenytoin, phenobarbital) may increase itraconazole metabolism, and higher doses may be needed when these drugs are administered concurrently with itraconazole. Itraconazole also impairs the metabolism of cyclosporine and can result in increased levels of certain agents, including digoxin and warfarin.

The usual dosage is 200 mg once or twice daily with meals.

Voriconazole is a triazole antifungal with broad in vitro activity against a number of pathogens, including most species of *Candida* and molds, *Aspergillus, Fusarium, Pseudallescheria*, and others. It is as efficacious as liposomal amphotericin in the therapy of documented and suspected fungal infections in febrile neutropenic patients, and it is superior to liposomal amphotericin in preventing breakthrough fungemias. Voriconazole is superior to conventional amphotericin in the treatment of disseminated aspergillosis. Animal data also suggest voriconazole to be the most effective agent against *Aspergillus*, particularly in combination with caspofungin or another echinocandin. Voriconazole is the drug of choice in the treatment of *Fusarium* and *Scedosporium* infections. Voriconazole is widely used in the treatment of neutropenic patients with suspected or documented fungal infection. Voriconazole has limited activity against zygomycete pathogens, and some centers have reported increased rates of infection due to *Rhizopus* and *Mucor* in this patient population. Similar to fluconazole, oral administration leads to predictable absorption. The primary toxicity associated with voriconazole is infusion-related, transient visual disturbances, particularly during the first week of therapy. In addition, voriconazole is associated with photosensitivity reactions. Similar to itraconazole, voriconazole is associated with numerous drug interactions. Enzyme inducers can decrease voriconazole plasma levels with possible reduction in efficacy. Voriconazole inhibits cytochrome P450 activity reducing the clearance of numerous agents, including cyclosporine and tacrolimus.

Ketoconazole, the first orally bioavailable azole, previously was used in the treatment of a variety of fungal infections. However, the improved spectrum of activity, reduced toxicity, and superior pharmacokinetics of newer azoles have reduced ketoconazole to a secondary role.

Kontoyiannus DP et al: Zygomycoses in a tertiary-care cancer center in the era of *Aspergillus*-active antifungal therapy: a case-control observational study of 27 recent cases. J Infect Dis 2005;191:1350. [PMID: 15776383]

Marr KA et al: Combination antifungal therapy for invasive aspergillosis. Clin Infect Dis 2004;39:797. [PMID: 15472810]

7. Echinocandins

The echinocandins (caspofungin, anidulafungin, micafungin) act by inhibiting fungal cell wall synthesis. They are active against *Candida,* including nonalbicans species, as well as *Aspergillus* species. They are not active against *Cryptococcus* or *Fusarium.* Their long pharmacologic half-life confers the advantage of once-daily dosing. No change in dose is necessary in patients with renal failure; however, moderate to severe hepatic disease necessitates a reduction in dosage for caspofungin. Because rifampin and phenytoin significantly increase the metabolism of caspofungin, increased doses of the antifungal are necessary when rifampin and phenytoin are given concomitantly. Animal data suggest that caspofungin is inferior to voriconazole in the treatment of *Aspergillus;* however, the addition of caspofungin to voriconazole has been associated with in vitro and in vivo additive or synergistic effects. Caspofungin is superior to conventional amphotericin B in the treatment of candidemia, primarily on the basis of greater patient tolerability. The echinocandins should be considered the drugs of choice in the treatment of infections due to *C glabrata* and *C krusei.* These agents are associated with minimal toxicity or adverse effects. Histamine release is common with basic polypeptide compounds, such as the echinocandins; thus infusion-related reactions have been reported. While increased liver function tests have been observed with the combination of caspofungin and cyclosporine, more recent analyses suggest that these two agents can be safely administered together. Considering the similarities in spectrum efficacy and safety between products, the choice of echinocandin likely will be based on cost differences.

Betts R et al: Efficacy of caspofungin against invasive *Candida* or *Aspergillus* infections in neutropenic patients. Cancer 2006; 106:466. [PMID: 16353208]

Denning DW: Echinocandin antifungal drugs. Lancet 2003;362: 1142. [PMID: 14550704]

ANTIVIRAL CHEMOTHERAPY

Several compounds can influence viral replication and the development of viral disease.

Amantadine is active against influenza A (but not influenza B) and has efficacy both in prophylaxis and therapy of this infection. Yearly immunization against influenza is recommended (see Chapter 30) for disease prevention, but in certain select situations amantadine can be used for this purpose. Amantadine prophylaxis for 6–8 weeks is 70–90% effective in patients who cannot be immunized and who are at increased risk for developing complications of influenza; in medical personnel who cannot receive vaccine but are capable of transmitting influenza to high-risk patients; if vaccine is not available; and if vaccine strains differ from the strain causing an epidemic. Short-term prophylaxis (2 weeks) is indicated if an outbreak occurs before vaccination has been given. In this setting, amantadine will protect against disease while antibody production is induced and will not interfere with antibody production. Because of its modest therapeutic benefit, high-risk patients and others with influenza A may benefit from treatment with amantadine if it is instituted within 48 hours after the onset of symptoms and continued for 1 week. The usual adult dosage is 200 mg orally per day (in persons over 65 years of age, 100 mg). Emergence of influenza A resistance to amantadine and rimantadine has been observed in patients receiving therapy. Efficacy of amantidine/rimantidine for prophylaxis depends on the sensitivity of the predominant circulating strain. Worldwide rates of amantadine/rimantadine resistance have significantly increased over the years. Considering this predisposition for resistance, neuraminidase inhibitors such as zanamivir or oseltamivir would be preferable if the circulating strain is resistant to amantadine/rimantidine. In preparation for a possible avian influenza pandemic, the Centers for Disease Control and Prevention recommend the neuraminidase inhibitors due to current resistance trends and documented past record of development of amantadine resistance while on therapy. The most marked untoward effects are insomnia, nightmares, and ataxia, especially in the elderly. Amantadine may accumulate and be more toxic in patients with renal insufficiency, and the dosage should be reduced. **Rimantadine**, an analog of amantadine, is as effective as amantadine and is associated with fewer central nervous system adverse effects.

Neuraminidase inhibitors, including zanamivir inhalation and oseltamivir tablets, are available for prevention and treatment of influenza A and B and are also active against the avian influenza virus. While no vaccine for avian influenza is currently available, future prevention will depend on immunization rather than on antivirals. As with amantadine and rimantadine, they must be administered soon (within 48 hours) after the onset of symptoms to be effective. Zanamivir inhalers are difficult to use for some patients, especially those with asthma and chronic obstructive pulmonary disease, in whom bronchospasm has been reported. Oseltamivir is somewhat limited because of its gastrointestinal side effects. Both drugs are administered twice daily (oseltamivir, 75 mg orally; zanamivir 10 mg inhalation) for 5 days when used for therapy. Both agents are significantly more expensive than amantadine and reduce the duration of symptoms by only 1 day and viral shedding by 2 days. The major advantages of neuraminidase inhibitors over amantadine or rimantadine include activity against both influenza A and B and a low likelihood of development of resistance, resulting in their preferential use in outbreak settings. Both agents also effectively prevent disease in household contacts when administered prophylactically (oseltamivir 75 mg orally once daily, zanamivir 10 mg inhaled once daily) for 10 days.

Acyclovir is active against herpes simplex virus and varicella-zoster virus. In herpes-infected cells, it is selectively active against viral DNA polymerase and thus inhibits virus proliferation. Given intravenously (15 mg/kg/d in three divided doses), it can promote healing of mucocutaneous herpes simplex in immunocompromised patients. It can reduce pain, accelerate healing, and prevent dissemination of herpes zoster and varicella in immunocompromised patients. The usual dosage for varicella-zoster infections is 30 mg/kg/d intravenously in three equal doses. The drug has no effect on establishment of latency, frequency of recurrence, or incidence of postherpetic neuralgia. Acyclovir (30 mg/kg/d intravenously in three equal doses) is the drug of choice for herpes encephalitis. Intravenous or oral acyclovir is effective prophylaxis against recurrent mucocutaneous and visceral herpes infections in transplant and other severely immunosuppressed patients. Prophylactic intravenous or oral acyclovir is effective in preventing cytomegalovirus (CMV) disease in some transplant settings (renal and perhaps bone marrow) but not in others (liver).

Oral acyclovir, 400 mg three times daily for 7–10 days, is effective in primary genital herpes simplex infections. Oral acyclovir at a dose of 800 mg three times a day for 2 days for recurrent genital herpes reduces viral shedding and symptoms. Suppressive therapy (400 mg twice daily) for 4–6 months reduces the frequency and severity of recurrent genital herpetic lesions. Acyclovir minimally affects symptoms or viral shedding in recurrent herpes labialis and is not generally used for this disease. However, in a dose of 400 mg twice daily, it is effective in preventing recurrent herpes labialis in those with frequent relapses and in preventing sun-induced relapses.

Other uses of oral acyclovir include (1) therapy of acute herpetic keratitis and prevention of recurrences, (2) prevention and treatment of herpetic whitlow, (3) acceleration of healing of herpes zoster in immunocompetent patients if initiated within 48 hours after onset (800 mg five times daily for 7 days), (4) more rapid healing of rash and lessened clinical symptoms of primary varicella in adults and children if instituted within 24 hours after onset of rash and continued for 5–7 days, (5) therapy of herpes proctitis (400 mg five times daily for 10 days), (6) prevention of herpes simplex and CMV infections in transplant recipients (in doses of 800 mg four or five times daily), (7) prevention of erythema multiforme that is herpes simplex–related, and (8) prophylaxis against varicella in susceptible household contacts.

Topical 5% acyclovir ointment can shorten the period of pain and viral shedding in herpes simplex mucocutaneous oral lesions in immunosuppressed pa-

tients but not in patients with normal immunity. In contrast, acyclovir cream or penciclovir ointment (see famciclovir, below) appears to reduce the duration of pain and viral shedding by approximately 1 day in immunocompetent patients. Oral acyclovir is significantly more efficacious than topical therapy.

The absolute oral bioavailability of acyclovir is 10–30%. Famciclovir and valacyclovir (see below) are significantly better absorbed than oral acyclovir and are administered less frequently. Dosage reduction in renal insufficiency is required. Since hemodialysis reduces serum levels significantly, the daily dose should be given after hemodialysis.

Acyclovir is relatively nontoxic. Precipitation of drug in renal tubules has been described with intravenous acyclovir and can best be avoided by maintaining adequate hydration and urine flow. Central nervous system toxicity manifested by confusion, agitation, tremors, and hallucinations has been reported. Resistance has been described, usually in immunosuppressed patients who have received multiple courses of therapy.

Famciclovir is a prodrug of penciclovir. After oral administration, 75–80% is absorbed and deacetylated in the intestinal wall to the active drug, penciclovir. Penciclovir, like acyclovir, inhibits viral replication by interfering with viral DNA polymerase. Acyclovir-resistant strains of herpes simplex and varicella-zoster virus are also resistant to famciclovir. Famciclovir in a dose of 500 mg three times daily for 7 days accelerates healing of lesions in acute herpes zoster if started within 72 hours after the onset of rash. At a dose of 125 mg twice daily for 5 days, famciclovir is effective therapy of recurrent genital herpes; at a dose of 500 mg twice daily, it is effective as chronic suppressive therapy.

Valacyclovir is a prodrug of acyclovir that has significantly increased oral bioavailability when compared with acyclovir. After absorption, it is converted to acyclovir and serum levels are three to five times higher than those achieved with acyclovir. Valacyclovir at a dosage of 1 g three times daily for 7–10 days is effective therapy for herpes zoster when started within 72 hours after onset of rash and is slightly more effective than acyclovir in relieving zoster-associated pain. It shortens the course of initial episodes of genital herpes (1 g twice daily for 7–10 days), can be used to treat recurrent genital herpes (500 mg twice daily for three days), and is effective prophylaxis for recurrent genital herpes when given as a single 1-g daily dose. Valacyclovir prophylaxis (500 mg daily) reduces the rate of viral shedding and transmission of herpes in discordant monogamous couples. At doses of 2 g four times daily, valacyclovir is more effective than placebo in preventing CMV infections in seronegative recipients of a kidney from a seropositive donor. The adverse effect profile of valacyclovir is comparable to that of acyclovir.

Foscarnet (trisodium phosphonoformate) is a pyrophosphate analog that inhibits viral DNA polymerase of human herpesviruses (CMV, herpes simplex, varicella-zoster) and the reverse transcriptase of HIV. The drug is less well tolerated than acyclovir and ganciclovir and more difficult to administer. Therefore, its use is limited to patients who do not respond to ganciclovir or acyclovir or cannot tolerate these drugs. Isolates of CMV resistant to ganciclovir and herpes simplex and varicella-zoster isolates resistant to acyclovir usually are susceptible to foscarnet. Foscarnet has been used to treat acyclovir-resistant mucocutaneous herpes simplex in AIDS patients as well as varicella cutaneous lesions in AIDS patients who did not respond to acyclovir. Oral absorption is poor, and the drug must be given intravenously. The half-life is 3–5 hours, and this is prolonged with renal insufficiency. The usual induction dose is 60 mg/kg/dose every 8 hours, and the dose for maintenance therapy is 120 mg/kg once daily. Adjustments are required for even minimal impairment in renal function (see package insert).

Foscarnet can cause severe phlebitis and generally necessitates central intravenous access unless substantially diluted. Nephrotoxicity, which is dose-dependent and reversible, is its major toxicity. Prehydration with 2.5 L of 0.9% saline reduces nephrotoxicity. Foscarnet binds divalent cations, and hypocalcemia with peripheral neuropathy, seizures and arrhythmias, hypomagnesemia, and hypophosphatemia can occur. Monitoring of electrolytes and renal function is required during therapy. Anemia (20–50%) and nausea and vomiting (20–30%) are other common adverse effects.

Cidofovir is a nucleotide analog that is active against all human herpesviruses and poxviruses. The drug has a prolonged pharmacokinetic intracellular half-life, allowing for administration every 1–2 weeks. Strains of CMV, herpes simplex virus, and herpes zoster virus that are resistant to ganciclovir or acyclovir often are susceptible to cidofovir. Cidofovir delays progression of CMV retinitis in newly diagnosed disease (5 mg/kg weekly for 2 weeks, followed by maintenance of 3–5 mg/kg every other week) and is effective therapy in relapsed disease or in patients who are intolerant of traditional therapy (5 mg/kg every other day). The drug is ineffective or only marginally effective in the treatment of AIDS-associated progressive multifocal leukoencephalopathy. Cidofovir is associated with a high incidence of nephrotoxicity, sometimes severe. To avoid this complication, probenecid and intravenous saline are administered with each dose. Ocular toxicity, including uveitis and iritis, is another complication reported with cidofovir.

Ribavirin aerosol is used in the treatment of respiratory syncytial virus infections in bone marrow transplant patients. It is not known whether the addition of immune globulin provides additional benefit. Intravenous ribavirin can significantly lower the fatality rate of Lassa fever and has been used as a therapeutic agent for hantavirus pneumonia. However, the benefit in hantavirus infection is unclear. While used in some patients in the treatment of severe acute respiratory syndrome (SARS), its value and tolerability has been debated. The drug is teratogenic in animals, and pregnant women should not take care of patients receiving the aerosol. Oral ribavirin is used in combination with interferons to treat chronic hepatitis C infections (see Chapter 15). The combination has been found to be superior to monotherapy with interferon.

Ganciclovir is an analog of acyclovir that has broad antiviral activity, including activity against CMV. The drug is efficacious in the therapy of CMV retinitis in AIDS patients, but once therapy is stopped, the relapse rate is high, and long-term maintenance suppressive therapy is required in patients not receiving highly active antiretroviral therapy. It has been suggested that the addition of intravenous immunoglobulin or CMV immune globulin to ganciclovir may improve outcomes associated with CMV pneumonitis. Since CMV viremia often predicts the presence of invasive disease, it should be treated when it occurs. Ganciclovir is frequently used in solid organ and stem cell transplant patients in the treatment and prevention of infection. However, there is no uniformity of opinion about the duration of therapy or the route of administration. Before the availability of oral valganciclovir (see below), which results in serum levels equivalent to those achieved with intravenous drug, ganciclovir was frequently administered intravenously and in the immediate posttransplant period for 1–2 weeks. Depending on the type of transplant (bone marrow transplant patients are at greater risk for developing CMV disease than solid organ transplant patients) and the serologic status of the donor and recipient (seronegative recipients who receive transplants from seropositive donors are at greatest risk for developing disease), various antiviral agents were used to prevent infection. Acyclovir, valacyclovir, ganciclovir, and valganciclovir have been used in the prevention of CMV in stem cell transplant patients. With the availability of oral valganciclovir, many transplant patients—especially those with the greatest risk of developing CMV infection—are placed on this drug as prophylaxis. In addition, because tests to detect early infection with CMV are very sensitive, the strategy for prevention has shifted from one of universal prophylaxis to one of preemptive therapy. At many institutions, high-risk patients are routinely screened for CMV DNA in blood by antigen detection or polymerase chain reaction. If the test is positive, only then are patients treated with either intravenous ganciclovir or oral valganciclovir.

The major adverse effect is neutropenia, which is reversible but may require the concomitant use of colony stimulating factors. Thrombocytopenia, disorientation, nausea, rash, and phlebitis occur less commonly.

Oral ganciclovir is no longer used because of its poor bioavailability, and it has been replaced by **valganciclovir**, an esterification product of ganciclovir that is significantly better absorbed. Administration of 900 mg of valganciclovir orally results in serum ganciclovir levels equal to that achieved with an intravenous 5 mg/kg dose of ganciclovir. In CMV retinitis in AIDS patients, the drug is as efficacious as intravenous therapy. Valganciclovir is widely used as prophylaxis in transplant patients; however, it was found to be inferior to oral ganciclovir in the prevention of CMV infection after liver transplant. Consequently, it has not been approved for that indication.

Lamivudine (3TC), a well-tolerated oral antiviral nucleoside analog used in treatment of HIV infection, is effective against hepatitis B. Once-daily therapy (100 mg) results in clinical, serologic, and histologic improvement in approximately 50% of patients. While lamivudine is useful, development of resistance is common with long-term therapy. Therapy post–liver transplantation is associated with a reduced risk of reinfection with hepatitis B. Unlike the combination of ribavirin and interferon, lamivudine does not improve the outcome seen with interferon monotherapy.

Adefovir is an antiviral agent with activity against hepatitis B. It is as effective against lamivudine-susceptible and lamivudine-resistant isolates. While previously used higher doses have been associated with substantial nephrotoxicity, this complication is rare with the lower doses (10 mg/d) used to treat hepatitis B. Twenty-five to 35 percent of patients experience marked increases in liver function tests associated with discontinuation of adefovir, presumably secondary to rebound viral replication. The drug is primarily eliminated by the kidney.

Human interferons have been prepared from stimulated lymphocytes and by DNA recombinant technology. These agents have antiviral, antitumor, and immunoregulatory properties. The most common uses of these agents include therapy of chronic hepatitis due to hepatitis B, C, and D (see Chapter 15). A long-acting preparation of interferon, peginterferon, in combination with oral ribavirin is superior to conventional interferon for therapy of hepatitis C. Relapse of the underlying disease after cessation of therapy is common but usually responds to reinstitution of drug. Adverse effects are common and include an influenza-like illness with fever, chills, nausea, vomiting, headache, arthralgia, and myalgias. Bone marrow suppression, especially with high-dose therapy, also occurs. Considering the poor tolerability of interferon, only a minority of patients infected with hepatitis C are actually candidates for therapy.

Entecavir tablets and oral solution have been approved in the treatment of chronic hepatitis B. The results of three studies confirm significant improvement in liver function tests and viral markers when compared with lamivudine. The primary side effects associated with entecavir were similar to those seen with previous hepatitis B treatments, including headache, abdominal pain, diarrhea, fatigue, dizziness, and a severe, brief worsening of hepatitis B after discontinuation of therapy.

Peters MG: Managing hepatitis B coinfection in HIV-infected patients. Curr HIV/AIDS Rep 2005;2:122. [PMID: 16091258]

Singh N: Cytomegalovirus infection in solid organ transplant recipients: New challenges and their implications for preventive strategies. J Virol 2006;35:474. [PMID: 16406798]

Ward P et al: Oseltamivir (Tamiflu) and its potential for use in the event of an influenza pandemic. J Antimicrob Chemother 2005;55(Suppl 1):i5. [PMID: 15709056]

Disorders Due to Physical Agents 38

Richard Cohen, MD, MPH, & Brent R.W. Moelleken, MD, FACS

■ COLD & HEAT

Cold tolerance varies considerably among individuals. Factors that increase the likelihood of injury from exposure to cold include poor general physical conditioning, nonacclimatization, advanced age, altered mental status, systemic illness, poor tissue oxygenation, wet or insufficient clothing, previous cold weather injury, smoking, and the use of alcohol or other sedative drugs. High wind velocity ("windchill factor") increases the severity of cold injury at low temperatures.

COLD URTICARIA

Some persons have a familial or acquired hypersensitivity to cold, and urticaria may develop upon even limited exposure to a cold (eg, wind, freezer compartments). The urticaria usually occurs only on exposed areas, but in markedly sensitive individuals the response can be generalized and fatal. Immersion in cold water may result in severe systemic reactions from histamine release, including shock. Familial cold urticaria is an autosomal dominant inflammatory disorder, manifested as a burning sensation of the skin occurring about 30 minutes after exposure to cold. Acquired cold urticaria may be associated with medication (eg, griseofulvin) or with infection. Cold urticaria may occur secondarily to cryoglobulinemia or as a complication of syphilis. Most cases of acquired cold urticaria are idiopathic. For diagnosis, an ice cube is usually applied to the skin of the forearm for 4–5 minutes, then removed, and the area is observed for 10 minutes. As the skin rewarms, an urticarial wheal appears at the site and may be accompanied by itching. Peltier effect-based temperature testing has also been recommended for diagnostic testing. It involves the use of thermoelectric elements to quantitatively measure skin temperature thresholds. Cyproheptadine, 16–32 mg/d orally in divided doses, is the drug of choice. Desloratadine, 5 mg/d orally, has been shown to reduce or prevent symptoms.

RAYNAUD'S PHENOMENON

See Chapter 12.

ACCIDENTAL SYSTEMIC HYPOTHERMIA

 ESSENTIALS OF DIAGNOSIS

- A reduction of core body temperature below 35 °C.
- An esophageal or rectal probe that measures as low as 25 °C is required; oral temperatures are inaccurate.

General Considerations

Systemic hypothermia may result from exposure (atmospheric or immersion) to prolonged or extreme cold. The condition may arise in healthy individuals in the course of occupational or recreational exposure or in victims of accidents.

Systemic hypothermia may follow exposure to cool but not cold temperatures when there is altered homeostasis due to debility or disease. In colder climates, elderly and inactive individuals living in inadequately heated housing are particularly susceptible. Patients with cardiovascular or cerebrovascular disease, mental retardation, acute alcoholism, malnutrition, myxedema, hypopituitarism, or use of sedating or tranquilizing drugs are more vulnerable to accidental hypothermia. Prolonged postoperative hypothermia or administration of large amounts of refrigerated stored blood (without rewarming) can cause systemic hypothermia.

Systemic hypothermia causes reduced physiologic function—with decreased oxygen consumption and slowed myocardial repolarization, peripheral nerve conduction, gastrointestinal motility, and respirations—as well as hemoconcentration and pancreatitis. Defenses against cold exposure are superficial blood vessel constriction and increased metabolic heat production.

Clinical Findings

Early manifestations of hypothermia include weakness, drowsiness, lethargy, irritability, confusion, shivering, and impaired coordination. A lowered body temperature may be the sole finding; the skin may ap-

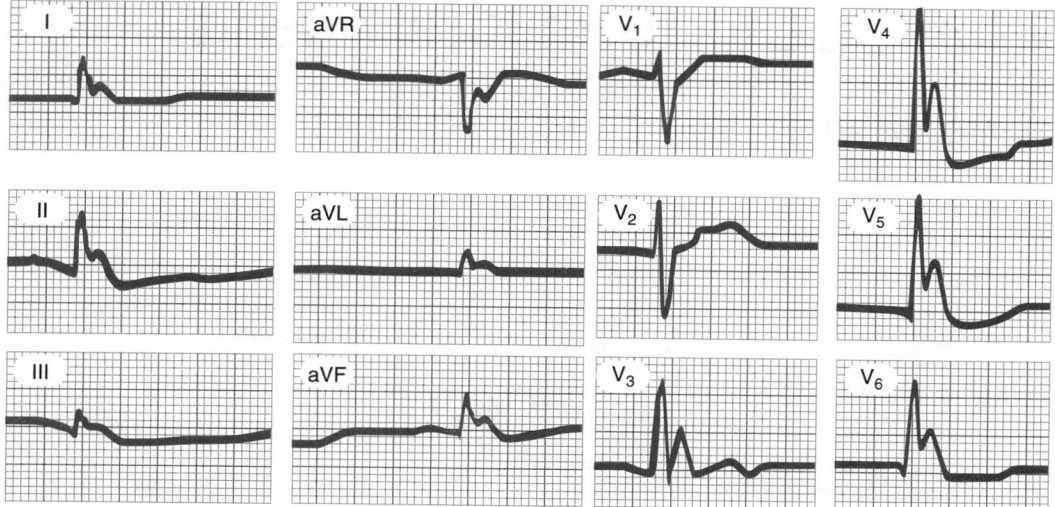

Figure 38–1. Hypothermia. The ventricular rate is 50/min. Atrial activity is not seen. The QRS complexes are narrow and are deformed at their terminal portions by a slurred wave occurring prior to the inscription of the ST–T waves; this is the J wave of Osborn. The QT interval is prolonged. (Courtesy of R Brindis. Reproduced, with permission from Goldschlager N, Goldman MJ: *Principles of Clinical Electrocardiography*, 13th ed. McGraw-Hill, 1989.)

pear blue or puffy. With extended exposure, apathy, impaired judgment, and ataxia appear.

The internal (core) body temperature in accidental hypothermia may range from 25 °C to 35 °C. At core temperatures below 35 °C, the patient may become delirious, drowsy, or comatose and may stop breathing. The pulse and blood pressure may be unobtainable, leading clinicians to believe the patient is dead. Metabolic acidosis, hyperkalemia, pneumonia, pancreatitis, ventricular fibrillation, hypoglycemia or hyperglycemia, coagulopathy, and renal failure may occur. Atrial and ventricular dysrhythmias, prolongation of the PR, QRS, and QT intervals, and the J wave of Osborn (positive deflection in the terminal portion of the QRS complex, most notable in leads II, V_5, and V_6) are directly related to the lowering of core temperature; cardiac arrhythmias may occur, especially during the rewarming process (Figure 38–1). Death in systemic hypothermia usually results from cardiac asystole or ventricular fibrillation.

Treatment

Aggressiveness of therapy should increase with the severity of hypothermia; a combination of external and core rewarming methods may be necessary. Patients with mild hypothermia (rectal temperature > 33 °C) who have been otherwise healthy usually respond well to a warm bed or to rapid passive rewarming with a warm bath or warm packs and blankets. A conservative approach is usually used in treating elderly or debilitated patients, using an electric blanket kept at 37 °C. Gentle handling and movement of the patient are essential to avoid triggering arrhythmias.

Patients with moderate or severe hypothermia (core temperatures of < 33 °C) do not have the thermoregulatory shivering mechanism and require active rewarming with supportive care. Cardiovascular support, acid-base balance, arterial oxygenation, and adequate intravascular volume should be established prior to rewarming to minimize the risk of organ infarction and "afterdrop" (recurrent hypothermia). *If CPR is initiated, it should be continued if the patient has not regained vital signs until the patient has been rewarmed to at least 32 °C.* The need for oxygen therapy, endotracheal intubation, controlled ventilation, warmed intravenous fluids, and treatment of metabolic acidosis should be dictated by clinical and laboratory monitoring during the rapid rewarming process. Essential laboratory tests include ECG, chest radiograph, complete blood count, prothrombin time, partial thromboplastin time, electrolytes, blood urea nitrogen (BUN), serum creatinine, liver function tests, amylase, glucose, pH, blood gases, urinalysis, and urine volume. Cardiac rhythm should be monitored, and cardiac, central vascular, or chest trauma or stimulation (catheter, cannulas, etc) should be avoided unless essential because of the risk of inducing ventricular fibrillation. However, patients who are comatose or in respiratory failure should be tracheally intubated. The patient should be evaluated for trauma and peripheral cold injury (eg, frostbite). Antibiotics are not routinely given and should be used only if indicated (neonate, elderly, or immunocompromised patient). Core temperature (esophageal preferred over rectal) should be monitored frequently during and after initial rewarming because of reports of recurrent hypothermia.

A. ACTIVE EXTERNAL REWARMING METHODS

Heated blankets, forced hot air, radiant heat, or warm baths may be used for active external rewarming. Rewarming by a warm bath is best done in a tub of moving water at 40–42 °C, with a rate of rewarming of about 1–2 °C/h. It is easier, however, to monitor the patient and to perform diagnostic and therapeutic procedures when heated blankets are used for active rewarming. Active external warming methods may predispose patients to ventricular fibrillation and hypovolemic shock and should be accompanied by core rewarming in moderate to severe hypothermia. Forced air rewarming (38–43 °C) is recommended for clinic or field use when extracorporeal blood rewarming is not available; heated blankets are recommended for transport.

B. ACTIVE INTERNAL (CORE) REWARMING METHODS

Internal rewarming is essential for patients with severe hypothermia; extracorporeal blood rewarming (cardiopulmonary, arteriovenous (femorofemoral), or venovenous bypass) is the treatment of choice, especially in the presence of cardiac arrest. Thoracic lavage and hemodialysis have also been recommended. Repeated peritoneal dialysis may be used with 2 L of warm (43 °C) potassium-free dialysate solution exchanged at intervals of 10–12 minutes until the core temperature is raised to about 35 °C. Parenteral fluids (D_5 normal saline) should be warmed to 43 °C prior to administration. Heated, humidified air warmed to 42 °C through a face mask or endotracheal tube may be administered. Warm colonic and gastrointestinal irrigations are of less value.

Prognosis

With proper early care, more than 75% of otherwise healthy patients may survive moderate or severe systemic hypothermia. Prognosis is directly related to the severity of metabolic acidosis; with low pH (≤ 6.6), elevated $PaCO_2$ (≥ 8.0 mm Hg), and/or elevated potassium (≥ 4.0 mEq/L), the prognosis is poor. The risk of aspiration pneumonia is great in comatose patients. The prognosis is grave if there are underlying predisposing causes or if treatment is delayed.

HYPOTHERMIA OF THE EXTREMITIES

Exposure of the extremities to cold produces immediate localized vasoconstriction followed by generalized vasoconstriction. When the skin temperature falls to 25 °C, tissue metabolism is slowed, but the demand for oxygen is greater than the slowed circulation can supply, and the area becomes cyanotic. At 15 °C, tissue metabolism is markedly decreased and the dissociation of oxyhemoglobin is reduced; this gives a deceptive pink, well-oxygenated appearance to the skin. Tissue damage occurs at this temperature. Tissue death may be caused by ischemia and thromboses in the smaller vessels or by actual freezing. Freezing (frostbite) does not occur until the skin temperature drops to −4 to −10 °C or even lower, depending on such factors as wind, mobility, venous stasis, malnutrition, and occlusive arterial disease. Neuropathic sequelae such as pain, numbness, tingling, hyperhidrosis, cold sensitivity of the extremities, and nerve conduction abnormalities may persist for many years after the cold injury.

Prevention

"Keep warm, keep moving, and keep dry." Individuals should wear warm, dry clothing, preferably several layers, with a windproof outer garment. Wet clothing, socks, and shoes should be replaced with dry ones. Extra socks, mittens, and insoles should always be carried in a pack in cold or icy areas. Cramped positions, constricting clothing, and prolonged dependency of the feet are to be avoided. Arms, legs, fingers, and toes should be exercised to maintain circulation. Wet and muddy ground and exposure to wind should be avoided. Tobacco and alcohol should be avoided when the danger of frostbite is present.

CHILBLAIN (Erythema Pernio)

Chilblains or erythema pernio are red, painful, burning, itching skin lesions, usually on the extremities, caused by exposure to cold without actual freezing of the tissues. They may be associated with edema or blistering and are aggravated by warmth. With continued exposure, ulcerative or hemorrhagic lesions may appear and progress to scarring, fibrosis, and atrophy. Chilblain lupus erythematosus, while clinically similar to ordinary chilblain, can be differentiated by an association with other lupus manifestations or by biopsy.

Treatment consists of elevating the affected part slightly and allowing it to warm gradually at room temperature. Do not rub or massage injured tissues or apply ice or heat. Protect the area from trauma and secondary infection. Prazosin, 1 mg orally daily, has been recommended for treatment and prevention of recurrence. Nifedipine (extended release 30–60 mg every 24 hours) has been recommended for pain.

FROSTBITE

Frostbite is injury due to freezing and formation of ice crystals within tissues. In mild cases, only the skin and subcutaneous tissues are involved; the symptoms are numbness, prickling, and itching. With increasing severity, deep frostbite involves deeper structures, and there may be paresthesia and stiffness. Thawing causes tenderness and burning pain. The skin is white or yellow, loses its elasticity, and becomes immobile. Edema, blisters, necrosis, and gangrene may appear. MRI with magnetic resonance angiography and triple-phase bone scanning have been used to assess the degree of involvement in severe frostbite and to distinguish viable from nonviable tissue.

Treatment

A. IMMEDIATE TREATMENT

Evaluate and treat the patient for associated systemic hypothermia.

1. Rewarming—Superficial frostbite (frostnip) of extremities in the field can be treated by firm steady pressure with the warm hand (without rubbing), by placing fingers in the armpits, and, in the case of the toes or heels, by removing footwear, drying feet, rewarming, and covering with adequate dry socks or other protective footwear.

For deep frostbite, rapid thawing at temperatures slightly above body heat may significantly decrease tissue necrosis. If there is any possibility of refreezing, the frostbitten part should not be thawed, even if this might mean prolonged walking on frozen feet. Refreezing results in increased tissue necrosis. Rewarming is best accomplished by immersing the frozen extremity for several minutes in a moving water bath heated to 40–42 °C until the distal tip of the part being thawed flushes. Water in this temperature range feels warm but not hot to the normal hand. Dry heat (eg, stove or open fire) is more difficult to regulate and is not recommended. After thawing has occurred and the part has returned to normal temperature (usually in about 30 minutes), discontinue external heat. Victims and rescue workers should be cautioned not to attempt rewarming by exercise or thawing of frozen tissues by rubbing with snow or ice water.

2. Protection of the part—Pressure or friction is avoided and physical therapy contraindicated in the early stage. The patient is kept at bed rest with the affected parts elevated and uncovered at room temperature. Casts, dressings, or bandages are not applied. A combination of ibuprofen, 200 mg four times daily, and aloe vera has been used to prevent dermal ischemia. Although white blisters may be debrided, hemorrhagic blisters should be left intact.

3. Anti-infective measures—Consider tetanus prophylaxis; frostbite increases susceptibility. Protect skin blebs from physical contact. Local infections may be treated with mild soaks of soapy water or povidone-iodine. Whirlpool therapy at 37–40 °C twice daily for 15–20 minutes for a period of 3 or more weeks helps cleanse the skin and debrides superficial sloughing tissue. Antibiotics may be required for deep infections.

4. Other therapy—Monitor fluid and electrolyte balance; administer tetanus prophylaxis if indicated. Other treatments used with varying results include platelet aggregation inhibition, hemodilution, peripheral vasodilation, fibrinolysis, and hyperbaric oxygen.

B. FOLLOW-UP CARE

Gentle, progressive physical therapy to promote circulation should be instituted as tolerated.

C. SURGERY

Early regional sympathetic blockade can reduce symptoms; sympathectomy (within 36–72 hours) is controversial. In general, other operative procedures are to be avoided. *Amputation should not be considered until it is definitely established that the tissues are dead.* Tissue necrosis (even with black eschar formation) may be quite superficial, and *the underlying skin may sometimes heal spontaneously even after a period of months.*

Prognosis

Recovery from frostbite is most often complete, but there may be increased susceptibility to discomfort in the involved extremity upon reexposure to cold.

IMMERSION SYNDROME (Immersion Foot or Trench Foot)

Immersion foot (or hand) is caused by prolonged immersion in cool or cold water or mud, usually less than 10 °C. The affected parts are first cold and anesthetic (prehyperemic stage). They become hot with intense burning and shooting pains during the hyperemic stage and pale or cyanotic with diminished pulsations during the vasospastic period (posthyperemic stage); blistering, swelling, redness, heat, ecchymoses, hemorrhage, necrosis, peripheral nerve injury, or gangrene and secondary complications such as lymphangitis, cellulitis, and thrombophlebitis can occur later.

Treatment is best instituted during the stage of reactive hyperemia. Treatment consists of air drying, protecting the extremities from trauma and secondary infection, and gradual rewarming by exposure to air at room temperature (not ice or heat) without massaging or moistening the skin or immersing it in water. Bed rest is required until all ulcers have healed. Affected parts are elevated to aid in removal of edema fluid, and pressure sites (eg, heels) are protected with pillows. Later treatment is as for Buerger's disease (see Chapter 12).

Kempainen RR et al: The evaluation and management of accidental hypothermia. Respir Care 2004;49:192. [PMID: 14744270]

Petrone P et al: Surgical management and strategies in the treatment of hypothermia and cold injury. Emerg Med Clin North Am 2003;21:1165. [PMID: 14708823]

Simon TD et al: Pernio in pediatrics. Pediatrics 2005;116:e472. [PMID:16140694]

Ulrich AS et al: Hypothermia and localized cold injuries. Emerg Med Clin North Am 2004;22:281. [PMID: 15163568]

DISORDERS DUE TO HEAT

 ESSENTIALS OF DIAGNOSIS

- *The four disorders that comprise the spectrum of illness due to heat exposure are heat syncope, heat cramps, heat exhaustion, and heat stroke.*

- *Heat disorders are caused by dehydration or electrolyte imbalance, or both.*

General Considerations

Conduction (convection)—the direct transfer of heat from the skin to the surrounding air—occurs with diminishing efficiency as ambient temperature rises. The passive transfer of heat from a warmer to a cooler object by radiation accounts for 65% of body heat loss under normal conditions. Radiant heat loss decreases as the temperature of the surrounding environment increases up to 37.2 °C, the point at which heat transfer reverses direction. At normal temperatures, evaporation accounts for approximately 20% of the body's heat loss, but at high temperatures it becomes the major mechanism for dissipation of heat; with vigorous exertion, sweat loss can be as much as 2.5 L/h. This mechanism diminishes as humidity rises.

Health conditions that inhibit sweat production or evaporation and increase susceptibility to heat disorders include obesity, skin disorders (miliaria), reduced cutaneous blood flow, dehydration, malnutrition, hypotension, and reduced cardiac output. Medications that impair sweating include anticholinergics, antihistamines, phenothiazines, tricyclic antidepressants, monoamine oxidase inhibitors, and diuretics; reduced cutaneous blood flow results from use of vasoconstrictors and β-adrenergic blocking agents; and dehydration results from use of alcohol. Illicit drugs—eg, phencyclidine, LSD, amphetamines, and cocaine—can cause increased muscle activity and thus generate increased body heat. Drug withdrawal syndromes or prolonged seizures may have the same effect. The risk of heat disorder increases with age, impaired cognition, concurrent illness, body mass index, reduced physical fitness, duration of exertion, and insufficient acclimatization.

Prevention

Medical evaluation and monitoring should be used to identify individuals at increased risk for heat disorders. The public should be made aware of the early symptoms and signs of heat disorders. It is not recommended to make salt tablets available for use without medical supervision; close monitoring of fluid and electrolyte intake and early intervention are recommended in situations necessitating exertion or activity in hot environments. Athletic events should be organized and managed with attention to thermoregulation: the wet bulb globe temperature (WBGT) index should be monitored, fluid consumption should be encouraged, and medical support should be immediately accessible. Competition is not recommended when the WBGT exceeds 26–28 °C. Workers should not begin work in hot temperatures without proper acclimatization and should be encouraged to drink water or balanced electrolyte fluids frequently. Guidance regarding heat hazard can be found in the National Weather Service's Heat Index that rates weather conditions based on humidity and temperature measurements (www.weather.gov/om/heat/index.shtml). The US Army provides guidance regarding activity levels according to WBGT levels (www.usariem.army.mil/heatill/appendc.htm).

Acclimatization is achieved by scheduled regulated exposure to hot environments and by gradually increasing the duration of exposure and the work load until the body adjusts by producing sweat of lower salt content in greater amounts at lower ambient temperatures. Acclimatization is accompanied by increased plasma volume, cardiac output, and cardiac stroke volume and a slower heart rate.

SPECIFIC SYNDROMES DUE TO HEAT EXPOSURE

1. Heat Syncope

Sudden unconsciousness can result from volume depletion and cutaneous vasodilation with consequent systemic and cerebral hypotension. Systolic blood pressure is usually less than 100 mm Hg, and there is typically a history of vigorous physical activity for 2 hours or more just preceding the episode. The skin is typically cool and moist, and the pulse is weak.

Treatment consists of rest and recumbency in a cool place and rehydration by mouth (or intravenously if necessary).

2. Heat Cramps

Fluid and electrolyte depletion can result in slow, painful skeletal muscle contractions ("cramps") and severe muscle spasms lasting 1–3 minutes, usually of the muscles most heavily used. Cramping results from dilutional hyponatremia as sweat losses are replaced with water alone. The skin is moist and cool, and the muscles are tender. There may be muscle twitching. The victim is alert, with stable vital signs, but may be agitated and complaining of pain. The body temperature may be normal or slightly increased. Involved muscle groups are hard and lumpy. There is almost always a history of vigorous activity just preceding the onset of symptoms. Laboratory evaluation may show low serum sodium, hemoconcentration, and elevated urea and creatinine.

The patient should be moved to a cool environment and given oral saline solution (4 tsp of salt per gallon of water) to replace both salt and water. *Because of their slower absorption, salt tablets are not recommended.* The victim may have to rest for 1–3 days with continued dietary salt supplementation before returning to work or resuming strenuous activity in the heat.

3. Heat Exhaustion

Heat exhaustion results from prolonged strenuous activity with inadequate water or salt intake in a hot environment and is characterized by dehydration, sodium depletion, or isotonic fluid loss with accompanying cardiovascular changes.

The diagnosis is based on prolonged symptoms and a rectal temperature over 37.8 °C, increased pulse (> 150% of the patient's normal) and moist skin. Symptoms associated with heat syncope and heat cramps may be present. Nausea, vomiting, malaise, and myalgia may occur. The patient may be quite thirsty and weak, with central nervous system symptoms such as headache, dizziness, fatigue, and, in cases due chiefly to water depletion, anxiety, paresthesias, impaired judgment, hysteria, and occasionally psychosis. Hyperventilation secondary to heat exhaustion can cause respiratory alkalosis; lactic acidosis may also occur due to poor tissue perfusion. Heat exhaustion may progress to heat stroke if sweating ceases.

Treatment consists of patient location in a shaded, cool environment, providing adequate hydration (1–2 L over 2–4 hours), salt replenishment—orally, if possible—and active cooling (fans, ice packs, etc) if necessary. Physiologic saline or isotonic glucose solution should be administered intravenously when oral administration is not appropriate. Intravenous 3% (hypertonic) saline may be necessary if sodium depletion is severe. At least 24 hours of rest is recommended.

4. Heat Stroke

Heat stroke is a life-threatening medical emergency resulting from failure of the thermoregulatory mechanism. Heat stroke is imminent when the core (rectal) temperature approaches 41 °C. It presents in one of two forms: **Classic heat stroke** occurs in patients with compromised homeostatic mechanisms; **exertional heat stroke** occurs in healthy persons undergoing strenuous exertion in a thermally stressful environment. Morbidity or even death can result from cerebral, cardiovascular, hepatic, or renal damage.

The hallmarks of heat stroke are cerebral dysfunction with impaired consciousness, high fever, and absence of sweating. Persons at greatest risk are the very young, the elderly (age > 65), chronically infirm, and patients receiving medications (eg, anticholinergics, antihistamines, phenothiazines) that interfere with heat-dissipating mechanisms.

Exertional heat stroke and exertion-related disorders such as rhabdomyolysis are appearing more frequently as complications of participation by unconditioned amateurs in strenuous athletic activities such as marathon and triathlon competition.

Clinical Findings

A. SYMPTOMS AND SIGNS

Heat stroke may present with dizziness, weakness, emotional lability, nausea and vomiting, diarrhea, confusion, delirium, blurred vision, convulsions, collapse, and unconsciousness. The skin is hot and initially covered with perspiration; later it dries. The pulse is strong initially. Tachycardia and hyperventilation (with subsequent respiratory alkalosis) occur. Blood pressure may be slightly elevated at first, but hypotension develops later. The core temperature is usually over 40 °C. Exertional heat stroke may present with sudden collapse and loss of consciousness followed by irrational behavior. Anhidrosis may not be present. Twenty-five percent of heat stroke victims have prodromal symptoms for minutes to hours that may include dizziness, weakness, nausea, confusion, disorientation, drowsiness, and irrational behavior. Multiorgan dysfunction or injury is a common and serious complication.

B. LABORATORY FINDINGS

Laboratory evaluation may reveal dehydration; leukocytosis; elevated BUN; hyperuricemia; hemoconcentration; acid-base abnormalities (eg, lactic acidosis, respiratory alkalosis); and decreased serum potassium, sodium, calcium, and phosphorus. Urine is concentrated, with elevated protein, tubular casts, and myoglobinuria. Thrombocytopenia, fibrinolysis, and disseminated intravascular coagulopathy (DIC) may occur; coagulopathy is likely. Rhabdomyolysis and myocardial, hepatic, or renal damage may be identified by elevated serum creatine kinase and aminotransferase levels and BUN and by the presence of anuria, proteinuria, and hematuria. Electrocardiographic findings may include ST–T changes consistent with myocardial ischemia. P_{CO_2} may be less than 20 mm Hg.

Treatment

Treatment is aimed at reducing the core temperature rapidly (within 1 hour) while supporting organ system function. Immersion in an ice-water bath (1–5 °C) is the most effective cooling method but may not be practical due to its physical requirements and patient access limitations. Evaporative cooling is a rapid and effective alternative and is easily performed in most emergency settings. The patient's clothing should be removed and the entire body sprayed with water (20 °C) while ambient or slightly warmed (45 °C) air is passed across the patient's body with large fans or other means at high velocity (100 ft/min). The patient should be in the lateral recumbent position or supported in a hands-and-knees position to expose as much skin surface as possible to the air. Also effective are use of cold wet sheets accompanied by fanning, immersion in chilled water, and localized ice or ice slush application. Skin massage is recommended to prevent cutaneous vasoconstriction. Intravascular heat exchange catheter systems as well as hemodialysis using cold dialysate (30–35 °C) have been successful in reducing core temperature. Other cooling alternatives include hand and forearm immersion in cold water, ice packs (groin, axillas, neck), and iced gastric lavage, although these are much less effective than evaporative cooling.

Treatment should be continued until the rectal temperature drops to 39 °C. The temperature remains stable in most cases, but it should continue to be monitored for 24 hours. Antipyretics (aspirin, acetaminophen) have no effect on environmentally induced hyperthermia and are contraindicated.

Hypovolemic and cardiogenic shock must be carefully distinguished, as either or both may occur. Central venous or pulmonary artery wedge pressure should be monitored. Five percent dextrose in half-normal or normal saline should be administered for fluid replacement.

The patient should also be observed for renal failure due to rhabdomyolysis, hypokalemia, cardiac arrhythmias, DIC, and hepatic failure. Creatine phosphokinase (CPK) >1000 units/L, metabolic acidosis, and elevated liver enzymes are predictive of multiorgan dysfunction, the usual cause of heat stroke–related death. Multiorgan dysfunction and inflammation may continue after temperature is normalized. Hypokalemia frequently accompanies heat stroke but may not appear until rehydration. Maintenance of extracellular hydration and electrolyte balance should reduce the risk of renal failure due to rhabdomyolysis. Fluid administration to ensure a high urinary output (> 50 mL/h), mannitol administration (0.25 mg/kg), and alkalinizing the urine (intravenous bicarbonate administration, 250 mL of 4%) are recommended. Fluid output should be monitored through the use of an indwelling urinary catheter.

Because sensitivity to high environmental temperature may persist for prolonged periods following an episode of heat stroke, immediate reexposure should be avoided.

Glazer JL: Management of heatstroke and heat exhaustion. Am Fam Physician 2005;71:2133. [PMID: 15952443]

Lugo-Amador NM et al: Heat-related illness. Emerg Med Clin North Am 2004;22:315. [PMID: 15163570]

■ BURNS

The incidence and severity of burn injuries has been declining, with both deaths and acute hospitalizations attributable to burns down about 50%. Over three-fourths of burns involve less than 10% of total body surface area. Aggressive, early excision (24–72 hours postburn) of deeply burned tissues and skin grafting, early enteral feeding, and improved infection control have contributed to significantly lower mortality rates and shorter hospitalizations. Nonetheless, an estimated 1.25 million burn injuries and 51,000 acute hospitalizations of burn victims occur each year in the United States. Severe burns cause problems in the initial phase from hemodynamic compromise, related injuries such as smoke inhalation or fractures, and associated microbacterial superinfection, sepsis and multiorgan failure. Later, secondary scarring and constrictive wounds occur.

Significant quality of life and social functionality can be expected even for severely burned patients.

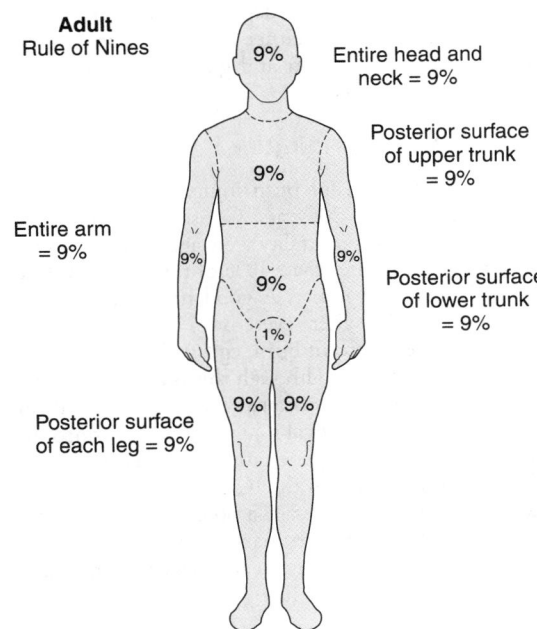

Figure 38–2. Estimation of body surface area in burns.

CLASSIFICATION

Burns are classified by extent, depth, patient age, and associated illness or injury. Accurate estimation of burn size and depth will determine the adequacy of resuscitation.

Extent

The "rule of nines" (Figure 38–2) is useful for rapidly assessing the extent of a burn. More detailed charts based on age are available when the patient reaches the burn unit. Therefore, it is important to view the entire patient after cleaning soot to make an accurate assessment, both initially and on subsequent examinations. Only second- and third-degree burns are included in calculating the total burn surface area, since first-degree burns usually do not represent significant injury in terms of prognosis or fluid and electrolyte management. However, first- or second-degree burns may convert to deeper burns, especially if treatment is delayed or bacterial colonization or superinfection occurs.

Depth

Judgment of depth of injury is difficult. The **first-degree burn** may be red or gray but will demonstrate excellent capillary refill. First-degree burns are not blistered initially. If the wound is blistered, this represents a partial-thickness injury to the dermis, or a **second-degree burn**. As the degree of burn is progressively deeper, there is a progressive loss of adnexal structures. Hairs can be easily extracted or are absent, sweat glands become less visible, and the skin appears smoother.

Deep second- and third-degree burns are treated in a similar fashion, since neither will heal appropriately without early debridement and grafting; the resultant skin is thin and scarred.

Survival after Burn Injury

The survival from major burn injury has dramatically increased in the last 20 years. Consistently, the three major risk factors for mortality were age greater than 60 years, burn area greater than 40% of total body surface area, and inhalation injury. A good rule of thumb for predicting mortality after severe burn injury is still the Baux Score (age + percent burn, eg, age 50 years + 20% burn = 70% mortality), although this is obviously quite variable depending on associated medical factors. Burn size, age, history of electrical injury, history of concomitant trauma (especially penetrating) and female sex as well as duration of stay in the ICU and the presence of mechanical ventilation presage a poorer outcome. Likewise, a base deficit during resuscitation of greater than -6 mmol/L predicts a far higher incidence of multiple organ dysfunction and death.

Associated Injuries or Illnesses

An injury commonly associated with burns is smoke inhalation (see Chapter 9). Suspicion of inhalation injury is aroused when the nasal hairs are singed, the mechanism of burn involves closed spaces, the sputum is carbonaceous, or the carboxyhemoglobin level exceeds 5% in nonsmokers. This suspicion should lead the clinician to institute early intubation before airway edema supervenes. The products of combustion, not heat, are responsible for lower airway injury. Electrical injury that causes burns may also produce cardiac arrhythmias that require immediate attention. Pancreatitis occurs in severe burns. Development of hyperamylasemia or hyperlipasemia may signal the development of pancreatic inflammation and subsequent pseudocyst or abscess formation. Prior alcohol exposure may exacerbate the pulmonary components of burn injury.

Toxic epidermal necrolysis (TEN) occasionally occurs following sulfonamide or phenytoin administration (see Chapter 6). If TEN is severe, patients are best transferred to a burn unit and treated as having severe burn injury. Corticosteroid therapy should be avoided.

SYSTEMIC REACTIONS TO BURN INJURY

The actual burn injury is only the incipient event in a cascade of deleterious local tissue and systemic inflammatory reactions leading to multiorgan system failure in the severely burned patient. Locally, substance P, serotonin, prostaglandins E_2 and $F_2\alpha$, histamine, platelet-activating factor, nitric oxide, bradykinin, and leukotrienes B_4 and D_4 play a role in the increased local capillary permeability and initiation of the systemic inflammatory cascade. Systemically, levels of interleukin-2, -4, -6, and interferon-gamma (IFN-γ) are elevated in proportion to the severity of the burn injury, perhaps as part of a gen-

eralized systemic release of inflammatory mediators and generalized macrophage dysfunction. There is often an altered CD4/CD8 (T helper/T suppressor) cell ratio. In addition, in the first 24 hours following a significant burn, there is production of tumor necrosis factor and IFN-γ, which in turn stimulate production of the enzyme nitric oxide synthetase in hepatocytes. After 24 hours, lipopolysaccharide plays a dominant role in its production. Nitric oxide has been proposed as a mediator of the acute inflammation. Transforming growth factor beta and IL-10 and a markedly elevated level of IL-6 serve as harbingers of a declining clinical course in severely burned patients.

INITIAL MANAGEMENT

Airway

The practitioner or emergency medical technician should proceed as with any other trauma using standard Advanced Trauma Life Support (ATLS) guidelines. The priorities are first to establish an airway, recognizing the frequent necessity to intubate a patient who may appear to be breathing normally but who has sustained an inhalation injury; next, to evaluate the cervical spine and head injuries; and finally, to stabilize fractures. Fluid resuscitation by the Parkland formula (see below) may be instituted simultaneously with initial resuscitation. Endotracheal intubation or tracheotomy should be considered for major burn cases regardless of the area of the body involved, because as fluid resuscitation proceeds generalized edema develops, including edema of the soft tissues of the upper airway and perhaps the lungs as well. Chest radiographs are typically normal initially but may develop an acute respiratory distress syndrome picture in 24–48 hours with severe inhalation injury. Supplemental oxygen should be administered. Inhalation injuries should be monitored with serial blood gas determination and bronchoscopy. The use of corticosteroids is contraindicated because of the potential for immunosuppression.

Vascular Access

All clothing and jewelry should be removed and an expedient physical examination performed to assess the extent of burn and associated injuries. Simultaneously with the above procedures, venous access must be sought, since the victim of a major burn may develop hypovolemic shock. A percutaneous large-bore (14- or 16-gauge) intravenous line through nonburned skin is preferred. Subclavian lines are avoided in the emergency setting because of the risk of pneumothorax and subclavian vein laceration when such a line is placed in a volume-depleted patient. Femoral lines provide good temporary access during resuscitation. *All lines—without exception—placed in the emergency department should be changed within 24 hours because of the high risk of nonsterile placement.* Distal saphenous cutdown is occasionally necessary. An arterial line is useful for monitoring mean arterial pressure and drawing blood.

FLUID RESUSCITATION

Crystalloids

Generalized capillary leak results from burn injury over more than 25% of total body surface area. This often necessitates replacement of a large volume of fluid.

There are many guidelines for fluid resuscitation. The **Parkland formula** relies on the use of lactated Ringer's injection. The fluid requirement in the first 24 hours is estimated as 4 mL/kg body weight per percent of body surface area burned. Half the calculated fluid is given in the first 8-hour period. The remaining fluid, divided into two equal parts, is delivered over the next 16 hours. An extremely large volume of fluid may be required. For example, an injury over 40% of the total body surface area in a 70-kg victim may require 11.2 L in the first 24 hours [4 mL $\times$ 40(%) $\times$ 70 (kg) = 11,200 mL]. The first 8-hour period is measured from the hour of injury. These guidelines may be inadequate, since crystalloid solutions alone may be insufficient to restore cardiac preload during the period of burn shock.

Deep electrical burns and inhalation injury increase the fluid requirement. Adequacy of resuscitation is determined by clinical parameters, including urinary output and specific gravity, blood pressure, and central venous catheter or, if necessary, Swan-Ganz catheter readings.

Colloids

Overly aggressive crystalloid administration must be avoided in patients with pulmonary injury, since significant pulmonary edema can develop in patients with normal pulmonary capillary wedge and central venous pressures. In addition, routine colloid administration, previously commonplace, is no longer warranted in routine burn resuscitation in view of its deleterious effect on glomerular filtration and its association with pulmonary edema.

Monitoring Fluid Resuscitation

A Foley catheter is essential for monitoring urinary output. Diuretics have no role in this phase of patient management unless fluid overload has occurred or mannitol diuresis is performed in the case of rhabdomyolysis.

Abdominal Compartment Syndrome

Abdominal compartment syndrome is emerging as a complication in severely burned patients. Increased intra-abdominal pressures can cause excessively high peak inspiratory pressures and increase fluid requirements considerably. Elevated intra-abdominal pressure can make pulmonary artery wedge pressure and urinary output unreliable indices of preload or intravascular volume, causing improper management of the patient's fluid status. Only 40% of patients with this severe form of increased intra-abdominal pressure sur-

vive. Bladder pressures over 30 mm Hg establish the diagnosis in at-risk patients. Surgical abdominal decompression may be indicated, and may improve ventilation and oxygen delivery.

Escharotomy

As edema fluid accumulates, ischemia may develop under any constricting eschar of an extremity, neck, or trunk if the full-thickness burn is circumferential. Escharotomy incisions through the anesthetic eschar can save life and limb and can be performed in the emergency department or operating room. Recent studies have shown efficacy of enzymatic debridement of wounds requiring escharotomy.

Fasciotomy in Electrical Burns or Crush Injuries

When high-voltage electrical injury occurs, extensive deep tissue necrosis should be suspected. Deep tissue necrosis leads to profound tissue swelling. Because deep tissue compartments in the arms and legs are contained by unyielding fascia, these compartments must be opened by surgical fasciotomy to prevent further soft tissue, vascular, and nerve death.

Electrical burn injuries remain the most devastating and underrecognized burn injuries, causing amputations (often because of unrecognized compartment syndromes) and acute renal failure, resulting in part from rhabdomyolysis. Creatine kinase levels are usually elevated in patients with severe electrical burns (and constitute a negative prognostic indicator). Severe (often underrecognized) muscle necrosis due to electrical burns may occur in the absence of significant skin burns.

THE BURN WOUND

In general, when burn wounds are seen in the emergency department, the causative agents have been eliminated. However, acute burns caused by hydrofluoric acid should be treated by water rinsing followed by application of topical calcium. Treatment of the burn wound is based on several principles. (1) Protection from desiccation and further injury of those burned areas that will spontaneously reepithelialize in 7–10 days by application of topical antibiotic such as silver sulfadiazine or mafenide acetate. Silver sulfadiazine is the most popular topical agent. It is painless, easy to apply, and effective against most strains of *Pseudomonas*. (2) Regular and thorough cleansing of burned areas is a critically important intervention in burn units. Early excision and grafting of burned areas as soon as 24 hours after burn injury or when the patient will hemodynamically tolerate the excision and grafting procedure. The tumescent technique (injection under the burn scar of dilute epinephrine and lidocaine prior to surgery) may reduce blood loss, though lidocaine toxicity must be considered.

Systemic infection remains a leading cause of morbidity among patients with major burn injuries, with nearly all severely burned patients having one or more septicemic episodes during the hospital course. Coagulase-negative staphylococci (63%) and *Staphylococcus aureus* (20%) are commonly cultured from burn wounds. Methicillin-resistant *S aureus* and *Pseudomonas aeruginosa* are also commonly cultured but usually later in the hospital course. Methicillin resistance in gram-positive organisms is becoming common, but vancomycin-resistant staphylococci are fortunately still rare in burn patients. Increasingly, sterile multiple organ failure is regarded as a leading cause of death among severely burned patients.

Wound Closure

The goal of therapy after fluid resuscitation is rapid and stable closure of the wound. Wounds that will not heal spontaneously in 7–10 days (ie, deep second-degree or third-degree burns) are best treated by excision and autograft; otherwise, granulation and infection may develop, and the quality of the skin in regenerated deep partial thickness burns is marginal because of the very thin dermis that emerges.

Biosynthetic skin replacements are now routinely used when autologous skin grafts are in short supply. Cultured allogeneic keratinocyte grafts, autologous/allogeneic composites, acellular biological matrices, and cellular matrices, including biological substances as fibrin sealant, various types of collagen, and hyaluronic acid, have provided alternatives. With severe burns, skin substitution with cultured grafts can be lifesaving. Research continues on the development of the completely engineered skin substitute, with especially promising results in the area of fetal cell constructs.

PATIENT SUPPORT

Burn patients require extensive support. An attempt must be made to maintain normal core body temperature (by maintaining environmental temperature at or above 30 °C) in patients with burns over more than 20% of total body surface area, since the hypermetabolic state of burns is exacerbated by subnormal temperatures. Respiratory injury, sepsis, and multiorgan failure are common. Enteral feedings may be started once the ileus of the resuscitation period has resolved, usually the day after the injury. There is often a markedly increased metabolic rate after burn injury, due in large part to whole body synthesis and increased fatty acid substrate cycles. If the patient does not tolerate low-residue tube feedings, total parenteral nutrition should be started without delay through a central venous catheter. As much as 4000–6000 kcal/d in high-carbohydrate, high-fat diet may be required in the postburn period. The metabolic demands are immense. A useful guide is to provide 25 kcal/kg body weight plus 40 kcal per percent of burn surface area. Early aggressive enteral nutrition reduces infections, noninfectious complications, length of hospital stay, impaired healing, and mortality. Anticatabolic treatments such as β-blockade, growth hormone, insulin, oxandrolone, and synthetic testosterone have been advocated. Occasionally, acute respiratory distress syndrome or respiratory failure unresponsive to maximal ventilatory support may develop in burn patients. In addition, the incidence of venous thromboembolism in the lower extremities is high among burn patients. Duplex ultrasonography is the best method for identifying venous thromboembolism. Early pulmonary dysfunction after severe burn injury is widely recognized. It is now apparent in children that late and permanent pulmonary dysfunction with later obstructive and restrictive lung disease can result from major burn injury. Growth hormone (0.05 mg/kg/d from hospital discharge to 1 year postdischarge) may reduce the long-term deleterious effects on hepatic acute phase and constitutive proteins.

Ophthalmologic consultation is indicated early when ocular or corneal injury is suspected.

Prevention of long-term scars remains a formidable problem in seriously burned patients. The V-beam laser (or long-pulsed dye laser) is emerging as adjunctive treatment to the usual regimen of corticosteroid injections, silicone patches, compression, and scar revision. Permanent sequelae can be avoided by prevention of infection, early aggressive rehabilitation, compressive garments, and early psychological support. Prefabricated flaps offer promise to severely burned patients. Facial transplantation has become a controversial but emerging treatment for those patients with devastating facial burns.

Complex reconstructions of severely burned structures such as the neck continue to benefit from advances in microsurgical plastic surgery techniques. After severe hand burns, function may be aided by expedient splinting or axial pin fixation to prevent flexion contractures and facilitate prompt skin grafting and physical therapy. Aggressive microsurgical reconstructions of hand injuries facilitate early motion and improved function of burn injuries to the hand.

Patients who have suffered severe burn injuries can recover to a general health status slightly lower than that of the general population but still have very significant vocational and psychological problems.

Atiyeh BS et al: State of the art in burn treatment. World J Surg 2005;29:131. [PMID: 15654666]

Herndon DN et al: Support of the metabolic response to burn injury. Lancet 2004;363:1895. [PMID: 15183630]

Hohlfeld J et al: Tissue engineered fetal skin constructs for paediatric burns: Lancet 2005;366:840. [PMID: 16139659]

Horch RE et al: Tissue engineering of cultured skin substitutes: J Cell Mol Med 2005;9:592. [PMID: 16202208]

Kono T et al: Treatment of hypertrophic scars using a long-pulsed dye laser with cryogen-spray cooling: Ann Plast Surg 2005; 54:487. [PMID: 15838209]

Krieger Y et al: Escharotomy using an enzymatic debridement agent for treating experimental burn-induced compartment syndrome in an animal model. J Trauma 2005;58:1259. [PMID: 15995479]

Lee JO et al: Nutrition support strategies for severely burned patients. Nutr Clin Pract 2005;20:325. [PMID: 16207671]

Nagasao T et al: Preliminary repair of eyelids for the treatment of opaque corneas caused by burns. Scand J Plast Reconstr Surg Hand Surg 2005;39:227. [PMID: 16208786]

Oda J et al: Effects of escharotomy as abdominal decompression on cardiopulmonary function and visceral perfusion in abdominal compartment syndrome with burn patients. J Trauma 2005;59:369. [PMID: 16294077]

Ulkur E et al: Comparison of silver-coated dressing (Acticoat), chlorhexidine acetate 0.5% (Bactigrass), and silver sulfadiazine 1% (Silvadine) for topical antibacterial effect in *Pseudomonas aeruginosa*-contaminated, full-thickness burn wounds in rats. J Burn Care Rehabil 2005;26:430. [PMID: 16151289]

■ ELECTRIC SHOCK

 ESSENTIALS OF DIAGNOSIS

- Injury is determined by quantity, duration, and type of current; area of exposure/contact; and pathway of current through the body.

General Considerations

Current passing through skeletal muscle can cause muscle necrosis and contractions severe enough to result in bone fracture. Current traversing peripheral nerves can cause acute or delayed neuropathy. Delayed effects can include damage to the eye, spinal cord, peripheral nerves, bone, kidneys, and gastrointestinal tract. If the current passes through the heart or brainstem, death may be immediate due to ventricular fibrillation, asystole, or apnea.

With alternating currents (AC) of 25–300 Hz, low voltages (< 220 Hz) tend to produce ventricular fibrillation; high voltages (> 1000 Hz) cause respiratory failure; intermediate voltages (220–1000 Hz) cause both. More than 100 mA of domestic house AC of 110 volts at 60 Hz is, accordingly, dangerous to the heart, since it can cause ventricular fibrillation. Direct current (DC) contact is more likely to cause asystole.

Lightning injuries differ from high-voltage electric shock injuries; lightning usually involves higher voltage, briefer duration of contact, asystole, nervous system injury, and multisystem pathologic involvement.

Electrical burns are of three distinct types: flash (arcing) burns, flame (clothing) burns, and the direct heating effect of tissues by the electric current. The latter lesions are usually sharply demarcated, round or oval, painless yellow-brown areas (Joule burn) with inflammatory reaction. Significant subcutaneous damage can be accompanied by little skin injury, particularly with larger skin surface area electrical contact.

Clinical Findings

Electric shock may produce loss of consciousness. With recovery there may be muscular pain, fatigue, headache, and nervous irritability. The physical signs vary according to the action of the current. Ventricular fibrillation or respiratory failure—or both—can occur; the patient may be unconscious, pulseless, hypotensive, cold and cyanotic, and without respirations.

Treatment

A. EMERGENCY MEASURES

The victim must be separated from the electric current prior to initiation of CPR or other treatment; the rescuer must be protected. Turn off the power, sever the wire with a dry wooden-handled ax, make a proper ground to divert the current, or separate the victim using nonconductive implements such as dry clothing.

B. HOSPITAL MEASURES

Lightning or unstable electric shock victims should be hospitalized when revived and observed for shock, arrhythmia, thrombosis, infarction, sudden cardiac dilation, hemorrhage, and myoglobinuria. A urinalysis, urine myoglobin, serum creatine kinase and creatine kinase-MB, and an ECG should be obtained immediately. Victims should also be evaluated for hidden injury (eg, ophthalmic, otologic, muscular, compartment syndromes), organ injury (myocardium, liver, kidney, pancreas), blunt trauma, dehydration, skin burns, hypertension, posttraumatic stress, acid-base disturbances, and neurologic damage. Indications for hospitalization include significant arrhythmia or electrocardiographic changes, large burn, loss of consciousness, pulmonary or cardiac symptoms, or evidence of significant deep tissue or organ damage. Extra caution is indicated when the electroshock current has followed a transthoracic route (hand to hand or hand to foot) and in patients with a cardiac history.

To counteract fluid losses and myoglobinuria due to electric shock (not lightning) burns, aggressive hydration with Ringer's lactate should seek to achieve a urinary output of 50–100 mL/h.

Prognosis

Complications may occur in almost any part of the body but most commonly include sepsis; gangrene requiring limb amputation; or neurologic, cardiac, cognitive, or psychiatric dysfunction. Psychiatric support may be necessary following lightning or severe electroshock exposures.

Edlich RF et al: Modern concepts of treatment and prevention of lightning injuries. J Long Term Eff Medical Implants 2005; 15:185. [PMID: 15777170]

O'Keefe Gatewood M et al: Lightning injuries. Emerg Med Clin North Am 2004;22:369. [PMID: 15163573]

Selvaggi G et al: Rehabilitation of burn injured patients following lightning and electrical trauma. NeuroRehabilitation 2005; 20:35. [PMID: 15798354]

■ IONIZING RADIATION REACTIONS

The extent of damage due to radiation exposure depends on the quantity of radiation delivered to the body, the dose rate, the organs exposed, the type of radiation (x-rays, neutrons, gamma rays, alpha or beta particles), the duration of exposure, and the energy transfer from the radioactive wave or particle to the exposed tissue. The Chernobyl experience suggests that the best biologic indicators of dose from an acute exposure are the duration of the asymptomatic latent period (particularly for nausea or emesis), the severity of early symptoms, the rate of decline of the lymphocyte count, and the number and distribution of dicentric chromosomes in peripheral lymphocytes.

The National Committee on Radiation Protection has established the maximum permissible radiation exposure for occupationally exposed workers over age 18 as 1 mSv (0.1 rem)* per week for the whole body (but not to exceed 50 mSv per year) and 15 mSv per week for the hands. (For purposes of comparison, routine chest radiographs deliver from 1 mSv to 2 mSv.) The FDA has recommended 1 Gy as a threshold for skin-absorbed dose from medical fluoroscopy.

Death after whole body acute lethal radiation exposure is usually due to hematopoietic failure, gastrointestinal mucosal damage, central nervous system damage, widespread vascular injury, or secondary infection. The acute radiation syndrome may be dominated by central nervous system, gastrointestinal, or hematologic manifestations depending on dose and survival. Fatigue, weakness, and anorexia can occur following exposures exceeding 50 cGy. Hematopoietic effects consisting of anemia, platelet loss, and bone marrow suppression can occur 1–3 weeks after exposures exceeding 100 cGy. Exposure to 400–600 cGy may be fatal within 60 days; death is usually due to hemorrhage, anemia, and infection secondary to hematopoietic injury. Whole body exposure levels of 1000–3000 cGy destroy gastrointestinal mucosa; this leads to toxemia and death within 2 weeks. Total body doses above 3000 cGy cause widespread vascular damage, cerebral anoxia, hypotensive shock, and death within 48 hours.

---

*In radiation terminology, a rad is the unit of absorbed dose and a rem is the unit of any radiation dose to body tissue in terms of its estimated biologic effect. Roentgen (R) refers to the amount of radiation dose delivered to the body. For x-ray or gamma ray radiation, rems, rads, and roentgens are virtually the same. For particulate radiation from radioactive materials, these terms may differ greatly (eg, for neutrons, 1 rad equals 10 rems). In the Système International (SI) nomenclature, the rad has been replaced by the gray (Gy), and 1 rad equals 0.01 Gy = 1 cGy. The SI replacement for the rem is the Sievert (Sv), and 1 rem equals 0.01 Sv.

ACUTE (Immediate) IONIZING RADIATION EFFECTS ON NORMAL TISSUES

Clinical Findings

A. INJURY TO SKIN AND MUCOUS MEMBRANES

Irradiation may cause erythema, epilation, destruction of fingernails, or epidermolysis. Ionizing radiation burns appear similar to thermal burns but usually have a slower onset and course.

B. INJURY TO DEEP STRUCTURES

1. Hematopoietic tissues—Injury to the bone marrow may cause diminished production of blood elements. Lymphocytes are most sensitive, polymorphonuclear leukocytes next most sensitive, and erythrocytes least sensitive. Damage to the blood-forming organs may vary from transient depression of one or more blood elements to complete destruction.

2. Cardiovascular system—Pericarditis with effusion or constrictive pericarditis may occur after a period of months or even years. Myocarditis is less common. Smaller vessels (the capillaries and arterioles) are more readily damaged than larger blood vessels.

3. Reproductive effects—In men, small single doses of radiation (200–300 cGy) cause temporary aspermatogenesis, and larger doses (600–800 cGy) may cause permanent sterility. In women, single doses of 200 cGy may cause temporary cessation of menses, and 500–800 cGy may cause permanent castration. Moderate to heavy irradiation of the embryo results in injury to the fetus (eg, mental retardation) or in embryonic death and abortion.

4. Respiratory tract—High or repeated moderate doses of radiation may cause pneumonitis, often delayed for weeks or months.

5. Mouth, pharynx, esophagus, and stomach—Mucositis with edema and painful swallowing of food may occur within hours or days after exposure. Gastric secretion may be inhibited by high doses of radiation.

6. Intestines—Inflammation and ulceration may follow moderately large doses of radiation.

7. Endocrine glands and viscera—Hepatitis and nephritis may be delayed effects of therapeutic radiation. The normal thyroid, pituitary, pancreas, adrenals, and bladder are relatively resistant to low or moderate doses of radiation; parathyroid glands are especially resistant.

8. Nervous system—The brain and spinal cord are much more sensitive to acute exposures than the peripheral nerves.

C. SYSTEMIC REACTION (RADIATION SICKNESS)

The basic mechanisms of radiation sickness are not known. Anorexia, nausea, vomiting, weakness, exhaustion, lassitude, and in some cases prostration may occur, singly or in combination. Dehydration, anemia, and infection may follow. Radiation sickness associated with x-ray therapy is most likely to occur when the therapy is given in large dosage to large areas over the abdomen, less often when given over the thorax, and rarely when therapy is given over the extremities.

Prevention

Persons handling radiation sources can minimize exposure to radiation by recognizing the importance of time, distance, and shielding. Areas housing x-ray and nuclear materials must be properly shielded. X-ray equipment should be periodically checked for reliability of output, and proper filters should be used. When feasible, it is advisable to shield the gonads, especially of young persons. Fluoroscopic procedures should be performed as rapidly as possible using an optimal combination of beam characteristics and filtration, and the beam size should be kept to a minimum required by the examination. Special protective clothing may be necessary to protect against contamination with radioisotopes. In the event of accidental contamination, all clothing should be removed and the body vigorously bathed with soap and water. This should be followed by careful instrument (Geiger counter) check to localize the ionizing radiation.

Nuclear Terrorism & Emergency Treatment for Radiation Accident Victims

The proliferation of radiation equipment and nuclear energy plants, terrorism, and the increasing need for transportation of radioactive materials have made necessary hospital plans for managing patients who are accidentally exposed to ionizing radiation or are contaminated with radioisotopes. The plans should provide for effective emergency care and disposition of victims and materials with the least possible risk of spreading radioactive contamination to health care personnel and facilities.

The threat of nuclear terrorism is raising the level of awareness about medical aspects of ionizing radiation exposure. The Gusev and Mettler references (see below) provide detailed guidance regarding decontamination, diagnosis, treatment, and isotope-specific postexposure prophylaxis. The Radiation Assistance Center provides 24-hour access to expert guidance regarding medical and safety aspects of ionizing radiation exposures and incidents (865-576-1005). The Centers for Disease Control and Prevention "Radiation Emergency" website (www.bt.cdc.gov/radiation/index.asp) is also helpful.

Treatment

The success of treatment of local radiation effects depends on the extent, degree, and location of tissue injury. Particulate or radioisotope exposures should be decontaminated in designated confined areas. Serial lymphocyte counts are useful for dose estimation and monitoring of the clinical impact of exposure. For some radioisotopes (eg, iodine), chelation, blocking, or dilution therapy may be indicated. Treatment of systemic reactions is symptomatic and supportive. Blood and platelet transfusions,

blood stem cell transplantation, bone marrow transplantation, antibiotics, fluid and electrolyte maintenance, and other supportive measures may be useful. Recombinant hematopoietic colony stimulating factors/cytokines (filgrastim, sargramostim, or pegfilgrastim) have been effective in accelerating hematopoietic recovery.

DELAYED EFFECTS OF IONIZING RADIATION

These disorders may occur following excessive ionizing radiation exposure: skin scarring, atrophy, and telangiectasis; cataract, dry eye syndrome, retinopathy; neuropathy, myelopathy, cerebral injury; obliterative endarteritis, coronary artery disease, pericarditis; thyroid disease; pulmonary fibrosis, hepatitis, intestinal stenosis, nephritis, and chromosomal aberrations. Neoplastic disease, including leukemia and cancers of the skin, breast, lung, and thyroid, is increased in persons exposed to radiation at relatively low doses (< 0.2 Gy). High-dose radon exposure is associated with an increased risk of lung cancer. Association of ionizing radiation with several other cancers has been reported but not well quantified (salivary glands, skin, stomach, colon, bladder, ovary, and central nervous system). Prenatal irradiation may increase the risk of childhood cancer.

Microcephaly and other congenital abnormalities may occur in children exposed in utero, especially if the fetus was exposed during early pregnancy. Carcinogenesis from low-dose (50–100 mSv/5–10 rem) exposure to adults probably occurs, but risk is proportional to total dose. Age-related differences in sensitivity to radiation have also resulted in carcinogenesis following childhood exposures (eg, Chernobyl and childhood thyroid cancer).

Brenner DJ et al: Cancer risks attributable to low doses of ionizing radiation: Assessing what we really know. Proc Natl Acad Sci U S A 2003;100:13761. [PMID: 14610281]

Burnham JW et al: Radiation. Crit Care Clin 2005;21:785. [PMID: 16168315]

Koenig KL et al: Medical treatment of radiological casualties: current concepts. Ann Emerg Med 2005;45:643. [PMID: 15940101]

Radiation Emergency Assistance Center/Training Site (REACTS): www.orau.gov/reacts.

Waselenko JK et al: Strategic National Stockpile Radiation Working Group: Medical management of the acute radiation syndrome: recommendations of the Strategic National Stockpile Radiation Working Group. Ann Intern Med 2004;140:1037. [PMID: 15197022]

■ DROWNING

ESSENTIALS OF DIAGNOSIS

- *Clinical manifestations of hypoxemia, pulmonary edema, and hypoventilation.*

General Considerations

The asphyxia of drowning is usually due to aspiration of fluid, but it may result from airway obstruction caused by laryngeal spasm while the victim is gasping under water. The rapid sequence of events after submersion—hypoxemia, laryngospasm, fluid aspiration, ineffective circulation, brain injury, and brain death—may take place within 5–10 minutes. This sequence may be delayed for longer periods if the victim, especially a child, has been submerged in very cold water or if the victim has ingested significant amounts of barbiturates. About 10% of victims develop laryngospasm after the first gulp and never aspirate water ("dry drowning"). Immersion in cold water can also cause a rapid fall in the victim's core temperature, so that systemic hypothermia and death may occur before actual drowning.

The primary effect is hypoxia due to perfusion of poorly ventilated alveoli, intrapulmonary shunting, and decreased compliance. *The first requirement of rescue is immediate CPR.*

A number of circumstances or primary events may precede near drowning and must be taken into consideration in management: (1) use of alcohol or other drugs (a contributing factor in an estimated 25% of adult drownings), (2) extreme fatigue, (3) intentional hyperventilation, (4) sudden acute illness (eg, seizure, arrhythmia, myocardial infarction), (5) head or spinal cord injury sustained in diving, (6) venomous stings by aquatic animals, and (7) decompression sickness in deep water diving.

Spontaneous return of consciousness often occurs in otherwise healthy individuals when submersion is very brief. Many other patients respond promptly to immediate ventilation. Other patients, with more severe degrees of near drowning, may have frank respiratory failure, pulmonary edema, shock, anoxic encephalopathy, cerebral edema, and cardiac arrest. A few patients may be deceptively asymptomatic during the recovery period—only to deteriorate or die as a result of acute respiratory failure within the following 12–24 hours.

Clinical Findings

A. Symptoms and Signs

The patient may be unconscious, semiconscious, or awake but apprehensive, restless, and complaining of headaches or chest pain. Vomiting is common. Examination may reveal cyanosis, trismus, apnea, tachypnea, and wheezing. A pink froth from the mouth and nose indicates pulmonary edema. Cardiovascular manifestations may include tachycardia, arrhythmias, hypotension, cardiac arrest, and circulatory shock. With prolonged or cold water immersion, hypothermia is likely.

B. Laboratory Findings

Urinalysis shows proteinuria, hemoglobinuria, and acetonuria. Leukocytosis is usually present. The PaO_2 is usually decreased and the $PaCO_2$ increased or decreased. The blood pH is decreased as a result of metabolic acidosis. Chest x-rays may show pneumonitis or pulmonary edema.

Prevention

Prevention consists of avoidance of alcohol during recreational swimming or boating, close supervision of toddlers, swimming lessons early in life, and use of personal flotation devices when boating. All swimming pools should be fenced.

Treatment

A. First Aid

Immediate measures to combat hypoxemia at the scene of the incident—sustained ventilation, oxygenation, and circulatory support—are critical to survival with complete recovery. Hypothermia and cervical spine injury should always be suspected.

1. Standard CPR is initiated if pulse and respirations are absent.

2. *Do not* attempt to drain water from the victim's lungs. The Heimlich maneuver (subdiaphragmatic pressure) should be used only if airway obstruction by a foreign body is suspected. The cervical spine should be immobilized if neck injury is possible.

3. *Do not* discontinue basic life support for seemingly "hopeless" patients until core temperature reaches 32 °C. Complete recovery has been reported after prolonged resuscitation of hypothermic patients.

B. Hospital Care

Requirements are careful observation of the patient; continuous monitoring of cardiorespiratory function; maintenance of cerebral oxygenation, serial determination of arterial blood gases, pH, renal function (serum creatinine), and electrolytes; and measurement of urinary output. Pulmonary edema may not appear for 24 hours.

1. Ensure optimal ventilation and oxygenation— The danger of hypoxemia exists even in the alert, conscious patient who appears to be breathing normally. Oxygen should be administered immediately at the highest available concentration. Endotracheal intubation and mechanical ventilation are necessary for patients unable to maintain an open airway or normal blood gases and pH. Nasogastric intubation will allow removal of swallowed water and prevention of aspiration. If the victim does not have spontaneous respirations, intubation is required. Oxygen saturation should be maintained at 90% or higher. Continuous positive airway pressure (CPAP) is the most effective means of reversing hypoxia in patients with spontaneous respirations and patent airways. Positive end-expiratory pressure (PEEP) is also effective for treating respiratory insufficiency. Assisted ventilation may be necessary with pulmonary edema, respiratory failure, aspiration, pneumonia, or severe central nervous system injury. Serial physical examinations and chest x-rays should be carried out to detect possible pneumonitis, atelectasis, and pulmonary edema. Bronchospasm due to aspirated material may require use of bronchodilators. Antibiotics should be given only when there is clinical evidence of infection—not prophylactically.

2. Cardiovascular support—Central venous pressure (or, preferably, pulmonary artery wedge pressure) may be monitored as a guide to determining whether vascular fluid replacement and pressors or diuretics are needed. If low cardiac output persists after adequate intravascular volume is achieved, pressors should be given. Otherwise, standard therapy for pulmonary edema is administered.

3. Correction of blood pH and electrolyte abnormalities—Metabolic acidosis is present in 70% of near-drowning victims, but it is usually of minor importance and corrected through adequate ventilation and oxygenation. Glycemic control improves outcome.

4. Cerebral injury—Some near-drowning patients may progress to irreversible central nervous system damage despite apparently adequate treatment of hypoxia and shock. Mild hyperventilation to achieve a $PaCO_2$ of approximately 30 mm Hg is recommended to lower intracranial pressure.

5. Hypothermia—Core temperature should be measured and managed as appropriate (see Systemic Hypothermia, above).

Course & Prognosis

Victims of near drowning who have had prolonged hypoxemia should remain under close hospital observation for 2–3 days after all supportive measures have been withdrawn and clinical and laboratory findings have been stable. Residual complications of near drowning may include intellectual impairment, convulsive disorders, and pulmonary or cardiac disease.

Olshaker JS: Submersion. Emerg Med Clin North Am 2004;22: 357. [PMID: 15163572]

Salomez F et al: Drowning: a review of epidemiology, pathophysiology, treatment and prevention. Resuscitation 2004;63: 261. [PMID: 15582760]

■ OTHER DISORDERS DUE TO PHYSICAL AGENTS

DECOMPRESSION SICKNESS & DYSBARIC ILLNESS

Decompression sickness and other disorders related to rapid changes in environmental pressure are hazards for fliers and for divers who are involved in recreational diving (eg, scuba diving), deep-water exploration, rescue or salvage operations, or construction.

At low depths the greatly increased pressure (eg, at 30 meters [100 feet] the pressure is four times greater than at the surface) compresses the respiratory gases into the blood and other tissues. During ascent from depths greater than 9 meters (30 feet), gases dissolved in the blood and other tissues escape as the external pressure decreases. The appearance of symptoms depends on the depth and duration of submersion; the degree of physical exertion; the age, weight, and physical condition of the diver; and the rate of ascent. The size and number of gas bubbles (notably nitrogen) escaping from the tissues depend on the difference between the atmospheric pressure and the partial pressure of the gas dissolved in the tissues. The release of gas bubbles and (particularly) the location of their release determine the symptoms. Predisposing factors include injury, right to left cardiac shunt, obesity, dehydration, alcoholic excess, hypoxia, some medications (eg, narcotics, antihistamines), and cold.

Decompression sickness also occurs among fliers during rapid ascent from sea level to high altitudes when there is no adequate pressurizing protection. Deep-sea and scuba divers may be vulnerable to air embolism if airplane travel is attempted too soon (within a few hours) after diving. Asthma, pneumothorax, reduced pulmonary function, lung cysts, or thoracic trauma may be contraindications to diving.

Clinical Findings

The range of clinical manifestations includes gas bubble formation in the joints ("bends"), cerebral or pulmonary decompression sickness, arterial gas embolism (cerebral, pulmonary), ear and sinus barotrauma, and dysbaric osteonecrosis. Reported sequelae include hemiparesis, neurologic dysfunction, and bone damage.

The onset of acute decompression symptoms occurs within 30 minutes in half of cases and almost invariably within 6 hours. Symptoms, which are highly variable, include pain (largely in the joints), headache, fatigue, numbness, confusion, pruritic rash, visual disturbances, nausea, vomiting, loss of hearing, weakness, paralysis, dizziness, vertigo, dyspnea, paresthesias, aphasia, and coma.

Pulmonary decompression sickness ("chokes") presents with burning, pleuritic substernal pain, cough, and dyspnea.

Treatment

Early recognition and prompt treatment are extremely important. Continuous administration of 100% oxygen is indicated as a first aid measure whether or not cyanosis is present. Aspirin may be given for pain, but narcotics should be used very cautiously, since they may obscure the patient's response to recompression. Rapid transportation to a treatment facility for recompression, hyperbaric oxygen, hydration treatment of plasma deficits, and supportive measures is necessary not only to relieve symptoms but also to prevent permanent impairment. It has been recommended, however, that decompression symptoms be treated whenever they are seen—even up to 2 weeks post injury—since it is still possible to reduce morbidity. The clinician should be familiar with the nearest compression center. The National Divers Alert Network at Duke University (DAN; 919-684-8111 or www.diversalertnetwork.org) provides assistance in the management of underwater diving accidents.

Bove AA, Davis J: *Diving Medicine,* 4th ed. WB Saunders, 2003.

DeGorordo A et al: Diving emergencies. Resuscitation 2003;59: 171. [PMID: 14625107]

Hamilton-Farrell M et al: Barotrauma. Injury 2004;35:359. [PMID: 15037370]

ALTITUDE ILLNESS

ESSENTIALS OF DIAGNOSIS

- *Five manifestations of altitude illness are: (1) acute mountain sickness, (2) high-altitude pulmonary edema, (3) high-altitude encephalopathy, (4) subacute mountain sickness, and (5) chronic mountain sickness (Monge's disease).*

General Considerations

Lack of sufficient time for acclimatization, increased physical activity, and varying degrees of health may be responsible for the acute, subacute, and chronic disturbances that result from (hypobaric) hypoxia at altitudes greater than 2000 meters (6560 feet). Acclimatization to altitudes above 5500 m (18,045 ft) is incomplete or physiologically impossible, although individual differences in tolerance to hypoxia exist. Altitude exacerbated conditions include cardiac and pulmonary dysfunction and disease, sickle cell, high-risk pregnancy, radial keratotomy, and others.

Acute Mountain Sickness

The severity of acute mountain sickness (AMS) correlates with altitude and rate of ascent. Initial manifestations include headache (most severe and persistent symptom), lassitude, drowsiness, dizziness, chilliness, nausea and vomiting, facial pallor, dyspnea, and cyanosis. Later, there is facial flushing, irritability, difficulty in concentrating, vertigo, tinnitus, visual disturbances, auditory disturbances, anorexia, insomnia, increased dyspnea and weakness on exertion, increased headaches (due to cerebral edema), palpitations, tachycardia, Cheyne-Stokes breathing, and weight loss. More severe manifestations include pulmonary edema and encephalopathy (see below). Voluntary periodic hyperventilation may relieve symptoms. In most individuals, symptoms clear within 24–48 hours, but in some instances, if the symptoms are sufficiently persistent or severe, the patient must be returned to lower altitudes. Definitive treatment is immediate descent, which is essential if reduced consciousness, ataxia, or pulmonary edema occurs. Administration of oxygen, 1–2 L/min, will often relieve acute symptoms. If immediate descent is not possible, portable hyperbaric chambers can provide symptomatic relief depending on altitude and severity. Acetazolamide, 250 mg orally every 8–12 hours, or dexamethasone, 8 mg orally initially followed by 4 mg every 6 hours, for as long as symptoms persist, is recommended therapy; they may be used together in severe cases.

Preventive measures include slow ascent—300 meters (984 feet) per day—adequate rest and sleep the day before travel, reduced food intake, and avoidance of alcohol, tobacco, and unnecessary physical activity during travel. Acetazolamide, 250 mg orally every 8–12 hours, beginning the day before ascent and continuing for 48–72 hours at altitude, may be used as prophylaxis. Dexamethasone, 4 mg orally every 12 hours beginning on the day of ascent, continuing for 3 days at the higher altitude, and then tapering over 5 days, is an alternative.

Acute High-Altitude Pulmonary Edema

This serious complication usually occurs at levels above 3000 meters (9840 feet). Early symptoms may appear within 6–36 hours after arrival at a high-altitude area: incessant dry cough, shortness of breath disproportionate to exertion, headache, decreased exercise performance, fatigue, dyspnea at rest, and chest tightness. Later, wheezing, orthopnea, and hemoptysis may occur. Recognition of the early symptoms may enable the patient to descend before incapacitating pulmonary edema develops, but strenuous exertion should be avoided. An early descent of even 500 or 1000 meters may result in improvement of symptoms. Physical findings include tachycardia, mild fever, tachypnea, cyanosis, prolonged respiration, and rales and rhonchi. The patient may become confused or comatose, and the clinical picture may resemble severe pneumonia. The white count is often slightly elevated, but the erythrocyte sedimentation rate is usually normal. Chest x-ray findings vary from irregular patchy infiltration in one lung to nodular densities bilaterally or with transient prominence of the central pulmonary arteries. Transient nonspecific electrocardiographic changes, occasionally showing right ventricular strain, may occur. Pulmonary arterial blood pressure is elevated, whereas wedge pressure is normal.

Treatment, which must often be given under field conditions, consists of rest in the semi-Fowler position (head raised) and administration of 100% oxygen by mask at a rate of 4–6 L/min for 15–30 minutes. *Immediate descent (at least 610 meters [2000 feet]) is essential.* Recompression in a portable hyperbaric bag will temporarily reduce symptoms if rapid or immediate descent is not possible. To conserve oxygen, lower flow rates (2–4 L/min) may be used until the victim recovers or can be evacuated to a lower altitude and $SaO_2 \geq 90\%$. Treatment for acute respiratory distress syndrome (see Chapter 9) may be required for some patients who have a prolonged course of pulmonary edema. Nifedipine, 10 mg initially followed by 30 mg slow-release tablets every 12 hours is recommended for symptomatic relief. Dexamethasone, 4 mg every 6 hours, has been recommended if central nervous system symptoms are present. Acetazolamide, 250 mg every 8–12 hours, should be administered if acute mountain sickness is suspected. If bacterial pneumonia occurs, appropriate antibiotic therapy should be given.

Preventive measures include education of prospective mountaineers regarding the possibility of serious pulmonary edema, optimal physical conditioning before travel, gradual ascent to permit acclimatization, and a period of rest and inactivity for 1–2 days after arrival at high altitudes. Salmeterol, 125 mcg by inhaler every 12 hours beginning 24 hours prior to ascent, has been shown to reduce the incidence of high-altitude pulmonary edema (HAPE) in susceptible patients. Prompt medical attention with rest and high-flow oxygen if respiratory symptoms develop may prevent progression to frank pulmonary edema. Persons with a history of HAPE should be hospitalized for further observation if possible. Pulmonary embolism and high-altitude bronchitis can also occur. Mountaineering parties at levels of 3000 meters (9840 feet) or higher should carry a supply of oxygen and equipment sufficient for several days. Persons with symptomatic cardiac or pulmonary disease should avoid high altitudes.

Acute High-Altitude Encephalopathy

High-altitude encephalopathy appears to be an extension of the central nervous system symptoms of AMS and results from cerebral vasogenic edema. It usually occurs at elevations above 2500 meters (8250 feet) and is more common in unacclimatized individuals. Clinical findings are due largely to hypoxemia and cerebral edema. Hallmarks are altered consciousness and ataxic gait; the patient appears "mildly drunk." Severe headaches, confusion, truncal ataxia, urinary retention or incontinence, focal deficits, papilledema, nausea, vomiting, and seizures may also occur and progress to obtundation and coma. High-altitude retinopathy is a separate but related effect of altitude. It can include dilated vessels, retinal hemorrhage, vitreous hemorrhage, and papilledema.

Treatment is immediate descent for at least 610 meters (2000 feet), continuing until symptoms improve. One-hundred percent oxygen (2–4 L/min) should be administered by mask. Dexamethasone, 4–8 mg orally every 6 hours, is recommended thereafter. If immediate descent is impossible, a portable hyperbaric chamber should be used until symptomatic improvement occurs.

Prophylaxis using acetazolimide as recommended for AMS is effective.

Subacute Mountain Sickness

This occurs most frequently in unacclimatized individuals and at altitudes above 4500 meters (14,764 feet). Symptoms—dyspnea and cough—are probably due to hypoxic pulmonary hypertension and secondary congestive heart failure. There are additional problems of dehydration, skin dryness, and pruritus. The hematocrit may be elevated, and there may be electrocardiographic and chest x-ray evidence of right ventricular hypertrophy. Treatment consists of rest, oxygen administration, diuretics, and return to lower altitudes.

Chronic Mountain Sickness (Monge's Disease)

This uncommon condition, consisting of chronic hypoxia, polycythemia and, in some cases, pulmonary hypertension in residents of high-altitude communities who have lost their acclimatization to such an environment, is difficult to differentiate from chronic pulmonary disease. The disorder is characterized by somnolence, mental depression, hypoxemia, cyanosis, clubbing of fingers, hemoglobin > 22 g/dL, polycythemia (hematocrit often > 75%), signs of right ventricular failure, electrocardiographic evidence of right axis deviation and right atrial and ventricular hypertrophy, and x-ray evidence of right heart enlargement and central pulmonary vessel prominence. There is no x-ray evidence of structural pulmonary disease. Pulmonary function tests usually disclose alveolar hypoventilation and elevated PCO_2 but fail to reveal defective oxygen transport. There is a diminished respiratory response to CO_2. Almost complete disappearance of all abnormalities eventually occurs when the patient returns to sea level.

Otherwise, phlebotomy, oxygen supplementation, respiratory training, medroxyprogesterone (20–60 mg/d orally for 10 weeks), acetazolamide (250 mg/d orally for 3 weeks) and enalapril (5 mg orally daily) have each been recommended for treatment.

Gallagher SA et al: High-altitude illness. Emerg Med Clin North Am 2004;22:329. [PMID: 15163571]

Hackett PH et al: High altitude cerebral edema. High Alt Med Biol 2004;5:136. [PMID: 15265335]

Leon-Velarde F et al: Consensus statement on chronic and subacute high altitude diseases. High Alt Med Biol 2005;6:147. [PMID: 16060849]

MEDICAL EFFECTS OF AIR TRAVEL & SELECTION OF PATIENTS FOR AIR TRAVEL

The medical safety of air travel depends not only on the nature and severity of the traveler's illness but also on such factors as the duration of flight, pressurization, the availability of supplementary oxygen and other medical supplies, the presence of health care professionals, and other special considerations. Airline policies, charges, and other details regarding on-board oxygen and medical supplies must be checked with each carrier. The medical hazard most likely to be realized is hypoxia.

Table 38–1. More frequent contraindications to air travel.

Congestive heart failure[1]

Uncomplicated myocardial infarction within 3 weeks; complicated myocardial infarction within 6 weeks

Post CABG within 2 weeks

CVA within 2 weeks

Uncontrolled hypertension

Uncontrolled ventricular or supraventricular tachycardia

Severe symptomatic valvular heart disease

New or unstable angina

Deep venous thrombosis unless the person is stable, receiving anticoagulant therapy, and has no pulmonary complications[2]

Nasal congestion unresponsive to therapy

Pulmonary cysts

Pneumothorax

Active communicable tuberculosis or other communicable virulent infection (eg, measles, chickenpox)

Breathlessness or hypoxemia

Anemia (hemoglobin < 8.5 g/dL), sickle cell disease

Postsurgery (eye, thorax, abdomen) within 2–3 weeks unless surgeon approves

Emotionally unstable, agitated, or psychotic

Pregnancy unless low risk, without complications, and less than 8 months

---

[1]Oxygen should be made available for persons with cardiovascular, respiratory, or hematologic illness.

[2]Susceptible patients should wear support hose, perform leg exercises, and walk during flight. Preflight low-molecular-weight heparin may also be indicated.

CABG = coronary artery bypass grafting; CVA = cerebrovascular accident.

The most common in-flight emergencies are cardiovascular, respiratory, syncopal, neuropsychiatric, metabolic, and substance related. The Air Transport Association of America defines an incapacitated passenger as "one who is suffering from a physical or mental disability and who, because of such disability or the effect of the flight on the disability, is incapable of self-care; would endanger the health or safety of such person or other passengers or airline employees; or would cause discomfort or annoyance of other passengers."

Pretravel clinician evaluation is advisable for patients with hospitalization, surgery, chronic disease, emergency care, or substantive medication change within the past 4 weeks.

Patients subject to motion sickness can be given sedatives or antihistamines (eg, dimenhydrinate, 50 mg orally every 4–6 hours; promethazine, 25 mg orally every 6 hours; or meclizine, 25–50 mg orally every 24 hours) before and during the flight. Small meals of easily digested food before and during the flight may reduce the tendency to nausea and vomiting. Table 38–1 lists the more common contraindications to air travel.

Pregnancy

Pregnant women may be permitted to fly during the first 8 months of pregnancy unless there is a history of complications of pregnancy or premature birth. During the ninth month of pregnancy, air travel is not recommended; if travel is essential, a physician's authorization is required. Infants less than 1 week old should not be flown at high altitudes or for long distances.

DeHart RL: Health issues of air travel. Annu Rev Public Health 2003;24:133. [PMID: 12428033]

Low JA et al: Air travel in older people. Age Ageing 2002;31: 17. [PMID: 11850303]

Poisoning

39

Kent R. Olson, MD

■ INITIAL EVALUATION: POISONING OR OVERDOSE

Patients with drug overdoses or poisoning may initially have no symptoms or they may have varying degrees of overt intoxication. The asymptomatic patient may have been exposed to or may have ingested a lethal dose of a poison but not yet exhibit any manifestations of toxicity. It is important to (1) quickly assess the potential danger, (2) consider gut decontamination to prevent absorption, and (3) observe the patient for an appropriate interval.

Assess the Danger

If the drug or poison is known, its danger can be assessed by consulting a text or computerized information resource (eg, Poisindex) or by calling a regional poison control center. (Dialing 800-222-1222 will direct the call to the appropriate United States regional poison control center.) Assessment will usually take into account the dose ingested (in milligrams per kilogram of body weight); the time interval since ingestion; the presence of any symptoms or clinical signs; preexisting cardiac, respiratory, renal, or liver disease; and, occasionally, specific serum drug or toxin levels. Be aware that the history given by the patient or family may be incomplete or unreliable.

The manufacturer or its local representative may be able to provide information over the phone concerning the toxic ingredients in question and can be contacted directly or via the regional poison control center (800-222-1222).

Gut Decontamination

The choice of gut decontamination procedure depends on the toxin and the circumstances. (See below for a more detailed discussion of methods.)

Observation of the Patient

Asymptomatic or mildly symptomatic patients should be observed for at least 4–6 hours. Longer observation is indicated if the ingested substance is a sustained-release preparation or is known to slow gastrointestinal motility or if there may have been exposure to a poison with delayed onset of symptoms (such as acetaminophen, colchicine, or hepatotoxic mushrooms). After that time, the patient may be discharged if no symptoms have developed and adequate gastric decontamination has been provided. Before discharge, psychiatric evaluation should be performed to assess suicidal risk. Intentional ingestions in adolescents should raise the possibility of unwanted pregnancy or sexual abuse.

■ THE SYMPTOMATIC PATIENT

In symptomatic patients, treatment of life-threatening complications takes precedence over in-depth diagnostic evaluation. Patients with mild symptoms may deteriorate rapidly, which is why all potentially significant exposures should be observed in an acute care facility. The following complications may occur, depending on the type of poisoning.

COMA

Assessment & Complications

Coma is commonly associated with ingestion of large doses of antihistamines, barbiturates, benzodiazepines and other sedative-hypnotic drugs, γ-hydroxybutyrate (GHB), ethanol, opioids, antipsychotic drugs, or antidepressants. The most common cause of death in comatose patients is respiratory failure, which may occur abruptly. Pulmonary aspiration of gastric contents may also occur, especially in victims who are deeply obtunded or convulsing. Hypoxia and hypoventilation may cause or aggravate hypotension, arrhythmias, and seizures. Thus, protection of the airway and assisted ventilation are the most important treatment measures for any poisoned patient.

Treatment

A. EMERGENCY MANAGEMENT

The initial emergency management of coma can be remembered by the mnemonic *ABCD*, for *A*irway, *B*reathing, *C*irculation, and *D*rugs (dextrose, thiamine, and naloxone or flumazenil), respectively (Table 39–1).

Table 39–1. Initial management of coma.

A	Airway control
B	Breathing
C	Circulation
D	Drugs (give all three): Dextrose 50%, 50–100 mL IV (unless bed-side glucose is normal) Thiamine, 100 mg IM or IV Naloxone, 0.45–2 mg IV[1] And consider flumazenil, 0.2–0.5 mg IV[2]

[1]Repeated doses, up to 5–10 mg, may be required.
[2]Do not give if patient has coingested a tricyclic antidepressant or other convulsant drug or has a seizure disorder.

1. Airway—Establish a patent airway by positioning, suction, or insertion of an artificial nasal or oropharyngeal airway. If the patient is deeply comatose or if there is no gag or cough reflex, perform endotracheal intubation. These airway interventions may not be necessary if the patient is intoxicated by an opioid or a benzodiazepine and responds rapidly to intravenous naloxone or flumazenil (see below).

2. Breathing—Clinically assess the quality and depth of respiration, and provide assistance if necessary with a bag-valve-mask device or mechanical ventilator. Provide supplemental oxygen. The arterial blood CO_2 tension is useful in determining the adequacy of ventilation. The arterial blood PO_2 determination may reveal hypoxemia, which may be caused by respiratory arrest, bronchospasm, pulmonary aspiration, or noncardiogenic pulmonary edema. Pulse oximetry provides an assessment of oxygenation but is not reliable in patients with methemoglobinemia or carbon monoxide poisoning.

3. Circulation—Measure the pulse and blood pressure and estimate tissue perfusion (eg, by measurement of urinary output, skin signs, arterial blood pH). Place the patient on continuous electrocardiographic monitoring. Insert an intravenous line, and draw blood for complete blood count, glucose, electrolytes, serum creatinine and liver tests, and possible quantitative toxicologic testing.

4. Drugs—

a. Dextrose and thiamine—Unless promptly treated, severe hypoglycemia can cause irreversible brain damage. Therefore, in all comatose or convulsing patients, give 50% dextrose, 50–100 mL by intravenous bolus, unless a rapid bedside blood sugar test is available and rules out hypoglycemia. In alcoholic or very malnourished patients who may have marginal thiamine stores, give thiamine, 100 mg intramuscularly or over 2–3 minutes intravenously.

b. Narcotic antagonists—Naloxone, 0.4–2 mg intravenously, may reverse opioid-induced respiratory de-

pression and coma. If opioid overdose is strongly suspected, give additional doses of naloxone (up to 5–10 mg may be required to reverse the effects of potent opioids or propoxyphene). **Caution:** Naloxone has a much shorter duration of action (2–3 hours) than most common opioids; repeated doses may be required, and continuous observation for at least 3–4 hours after the last dose is mandatory. Nalmefene, a newer opioid antagonist, has a duration of effect longer than that of naloxone but still shorter than that of the opioid methadone.

c. Flumazenil—Flumazenil, 0.2–0.5 mg intravenously, repeated every 30 seconds as needed up to a maximum of 3 mg, may reverse benzodiazepine-induced coma. **Caution:** Flumazenil has a short duration of effect (2–3 hours), and resedation requiring additional doses is common. Furthermore, flumazenil should **not** be given if the patient has coingested a tricyclic antidepressant, is a user of high-dose benzodiazepines, or has a seizure disorder—because its use in these circumstances may precipitate seizures. *In most circumstances, use of flumazenil is not advised as the potential risks outweigh its benefits.*

HYPOTHERMIA

Assessment & Complications

Hypothermia commonly accompanies coma due to opioids, ethanol, hypoglycemic agents, phenothiazines, barbiturates, benzodiazepines, and other sedative-hypnotics and depressants. Hypothermic patients may have a barely perceptible pulse and blood pressure and often appear to be dead. Hypothermia may cause or aggravate hypotension, which will not reverse until the temperature is normalized.

Treatment

Treatment of hypothermia is discussed in Chapter 38. Gradual rewarming is preferred unless the patient is in cardiac arrest.

HYPOTENSION

Assessment & Complications

Hypotension may be due to poisoning by many different drugs and poisons, including antihypertensive drugs, β-blockers, calcium channel blockers, disulfiram (ethanol interaction), iron, theophylline, phenothiazines and other antipsychotic agents, and antidepressants. Poisons causing hypotension include cyanide, carbon monoxide, hydrogen sulfide, arsenic, and certain mushrooms.

Hypotension in the poisoned or drug-overdosed patient may be caused by venous or arteriolar vasodilation, hypovolemia, depressed cardiac contractility, or a combination of these effects. The only certain way to determine the cause of hypotension in any individual patient is to insert a pulmonary artery catheter and calculate the cardiac output and peripheral vascular resistance. Alternatively, a central venous pressure (CVP) monitor may indicate a need for further fluid therapy.

Treatment

Most patients respond to empiric treatment with 200 mL intravenous boluses of 0.9% saline or other isotonic crystalloid up to a total of 1–2 L. If fluid therapy is not successful, give dopamine, 5–15 mcg/kg/min by intravenous infusion. Consider pulmonary artery catheterization if hypotension persists.

Hypotension caused by certain toxins may respond to specific treatment. For hypotension caused by overdoses of tricyclic antidepressants or related drugs, administer sodium bicarbonate, 50–100 mEq by intravenous bolus injection. Norepinephrine 4-8 mcg/min by intravenous infusion is more effective than dopamine in some patients with overdoses of tricyclic antidepressants or of drugs with predominantly vasodilating effects. For β-blocker overdose, glucagon (5–10 mg intravenously) may be of value. For calcium channel blocker overdose, administer calcium chloride, 1–2 g intravenously (repeated doses may be necessary; doses of 5–10 g and more have been given in some cases).

HYPERTENSION

Assessment & Complications

Hypertension may be due to poisoning with amphetamines, anticholinergics, cocaine, ephedrine-containing performance-enhancing products, monoamine oxidase (MAO) inhibitors, and other drugs.

Severe hypertension (eg, diastolic blood pressure > 105–110 mm Hg in a person who does not have chronic hypertension) can result in acute intracranial hemorrhage, myocardial infarction, or aortic dissection. Patients often present with headache, chest pain, or encephalopathy.

Treatment

Treat hypertension if the patient is symptomatic or if the diastolic pressure is greater than 105–110 mm Hg—especially if there is no prior history of hypertension.

Hypertensive patients who are agitated or anxious may benefit from a sedative such as lorazepam, 2–3 mg intravenously. For persistent hypertension, administer phentolamine, 2–5 mg intravenously, or nitroprusside sodium, 0.25–8 mcg/kg/min intravenously. If excessive tachycardia is present, add propranolol, 1–5 mg intravenously, or esmolol, 25–100 mcg/kg/min intravenously. **Caution:** Do not give β-blockers alone, since doing so may paradoxically worsen hypertension as a result of unopposed α-adrenergic stimulation.

ARRHYTHMIAS

Assessment & Complications

Arrhythmias may occur with a variety of drugs or toxins (Table 39–2). They may also occur as a result of hypoxia, metabolic acidosis, or electrolyte imbalance (eg, hyperkalemia or hypokalemia, hypocalcemia), or following ex-

Table 39–2. Common toxins or drugs causing arrhythmias.

Arrhythmia	Common Causes
Sinus bradycardia	β-Blockers, calcium channel blockers, clonidine, digitalis glycosides, organophosphates, opioids, sedative-hypnotics
Atrioventricular block	β-Blockers, calcium channel blockers, class Ia antiarrhythmics (including quinidine), clonidine, digitalis glycosides, lithium, tricyclic antidepressants
Sinus tachycardia	β-Agonists (eg, albuterol), amphetamines, anticholinergics, antihistamines, caffeine, cocaine, ephedrine, theophylline, tricyclic antidepressants
Wide QRS complex	Class Ia (including quinidine) and class Ic antiarrhythmics, phenothiazines (eg, thioridazine), potassium (hyperkalemia), tricyclic antidepressants
QT interval prolongation and torsade de pointes	Arsenic, cisapride, class Ia (including quinidine) and class III antiarrhythmics; droperidol, lithium, methadone, pentamidine, thioridazine, and many other drugs (see http://www.torsades.org/medical-pros/drug-lists/drug-lists.htm)

posure to chlorinated solvents or chloral hydrate overdose. Atypical ventricular tachycardia (torsade de pointes) is often associated with drugs that prolong the QT interval.

Treatment

Arrhythmias are often caused by hypoxia or electrolyte imbalance, and these conditions should be sought and treated. If ventricular arrhythmias persist, administer lidocaine at usual antiarrhythmic doses. **Caution:** Avoid class Ia agents (quinidine, procainamide, disopyramide), which may aggravate arrhythmias caused by tricyclic antidepressants, calcium channel blockers, or β-blockers. Wide QRS complex tachycardia in the setting of tricyclic antidepressant overdose (or quinidine and other class Ia drugs) should be treated with sodium bicarbonate, 50–100 mEq intravenously by bolus injection. (See discussion of tricyclic antidepressant poisoning.) Torsade de pointes associated with prolonged QT interval may respond to intravenous magnesium (2 g intravenously over 2 minutes) or overdrive pacing.

For tachyarrhythmias induced by chlorinated solvents, chloral hydrate, Freons, or sympathomimetic agents, use propranolol or esmolol (see doses given above in hypertension section).

SEIZURES

Assessment & Complications

Seizures may be due to poisoning with many drugs and poisons, including amphetamines, antidepressants (especially tricyclic antidepressants and bupropion), antihistamines, antipsychotics, cocaine, isoniazid, phencyclidine (PCP), and theophylline.

Seizures may also be caused by hypoxia, hypoglycemia, hypocalcemia, hyponatremia, withdrawal from alcohol or sedative-hypnotics, head trauma, central nervous system infection, or idiopathic epilepsy.

Prolonged or repeated seizures commonly lead to hypoxia, metabolic acidosis, hyperthermia, and rhabdomyolysis.

Treatment

Administer lorazepam, 2–3 mg, or diazepam, 5–10 mg, intravenously over 1–2 minutes, or—if intravenous access is not immediately available—midazolam, 5–10 mg intramuscularly. If convulsions continue, administer phenobarbital, 15–20 mg/kg slowly intravenously over no less than 30 minutes; or phenytoin, 15 mg/kg intravenously over no less than 30 minutes (maximum infusion rate, 50 mg/min). For drug-induced seizures, phenobarbital is preferred over phenytoin. The drugs may be used together if necessary. Maintenance doses may be required if drug toxicity is expected to last more than 18–24 hours.

Seizures due to a few drugs and toxins may require antidotes or other specific therapies (as listed in Table 39–3).

HYPERTHERMIA

Assessment & Complications

Hyperthermia may be associated with poisoning by amphetamines (especially ecstasy), atropine and other anticholinergic drugs, cocaine, dinitrophenol and pentachlorophenol, PCP, salicylates, strychnine, tricyclic

Table 39–3. Seizures related to toxins or drugs requiring special consideration.[1]

Toxin or Drug	Comments
Isoniazid	Administer pyridoxine.
Lithium	May indicate need for hemodialysis.
Organophosphates	Administer pralidoxime (2-PAM) and atropine.
Strychnine	"Seizures" are actually spinally mediated muscle spasms and usually require neuromuscular paralysis.
Theophylline	Seizures indicate need for hemodialysis.
Tricyclic antidepressants	Hyperthermia and cardiotoxicity are common complications of repeated seizures; paralyze early with neuromuscular blockers to reduce muscular hyperactivity.

[1]See text for dosages.

antidepressants, and various other medications. Overdoses of serotonin reuptake inhibitors (eg, fluoxetine, paroxetine, sertraline) or use in a patient taking an MAO inhibitor may cause agitation, hyperactivity, and hyperthermia ("serotonin syndrome"). Haloperidol and other antipsychotic agents can cause rigidity and hyperthermia (neuroleptic malignant syndrome [NMS]). (See section on schizophrenia and other psychotic disorders in Chapter 25.) Malignant hyperthermia is a rare disorder associated with general anesthetic agents.

Hyperthermia is a rapidly life-threatening complication. Severe hyperthermia (temperature > 40–41°C) may rapidly cause brain damage and multiorgan failure, including rhabdomyolysis, renal failure, and coagulopathy (see Chapter 38).

Treatment

Treat hyperthermia aggressively by removing all clothing, spraying the patient with tepid water, and fanning the patient. If this is not rapidly effective, as shown by a normal rectal temperature within 30–60 minutes, or if there is significant muscle rigidity or hyperactivity, induce neuromuscular paralysis with a nondepolarizing neuromuscular blocker (eg, pancuronium, vecuronium). Once paralyzed, the patient must be intubated and mechanically ventilated. In patients with seizures, absence of visible muscular convulsive movements may give the false impression that brain seizure activity has ceased; however, this must be confirmed by electroencephalography.

Dantrolene (2–5 mg/kg intravenously) may be effective for hyperthermia associated with muscle rigidity that does not respond to neuromuscular blockade (ie, malignant hyperthermia). Bromocriptine, 2.5–7.5 mg orally daily, has been recommended for neuroleptic malignant syndrome. Cyproheptadine, 4 mg orally every hour for three or four doses, has been used to treat serotonin syndrome.

■ ANTIDOTES & OTHER TREATMENT

ANTIDOTES

Give an antidote (if available) when there is reasonable certainty of a specific diagnosis (Table 39–4). Antidotes themselves may have serious side effects. The indications and dosages for specific antidotes are discussed in the respective sections for specific toxins.

DECONTAMINATION OF THE SKIN

Corrosive agents rapidly injure the skin and eyes and must be removed immediately. In addition, many toxins are readily absorbed through the skin, and systemic absorption can be prevented only by rapid action.

Table 39–4. Some toxic agents for which there are specific antidotes.[1]

Toxic Agent	Specific Antidote
Acetaminophen	N-Acetylcysteine
Anticholinergics (eg, atropine)	Physostigmine
Anticholinesterases (eg, organophosphate pesticides)	Atropine and pralidoxime (2-PAM)
Benzodiazepines	Flumazenil (rarely used; see warning in text)
Carbon monoxide	Oxygen, hyperbaric oxygen
Cyanide	Sodium nitrite, sodium thiosulfate
Digitalis glycosides	Digoxin-specific Fab antibodies
Heavy metals (eg, lead, mercury, iron) and arsenic	Specific chelating agents
Isoniazid	Pyridoxine (vitamin B_6)
Methanol, ethylene glycol	Ethanol (ethyl alcohol) or fomepizole (4-methylpyrazole)
Opioids	Naloxone, nalmefene
Snake venom	Specific antivenin

[1]See text for indications and dosages.

Wash the affected areas with copious quantities of lukewarm water or saline. Wash carefully behind the ears, under the nails, and in skin folds. For oily substances (eg, pesticides), wash the skin at least twice with plain soap and shampoo the hair. Specific decontaminating solutions or solvents (eg, alcohol) are rarely indicated and in some cases may paradoxically enhance absorption. For exposure to chemical warfare poisons such as nerve agents or vesicants, some authorities recommend use of a dilute hypochlorite solution (household bleach diluted 1:10 with water).

DECONTAMINATION OF THE EYES

Act quickly to prevent serious damage. Flush the eyes with copious amounts of saline (preferred) or water. (If available, instill local anesthetic drops in the eye before beginning irrigation.) Remove contact lenses if present. Direct the irrigating stream so that it will flow across both eyes after running off the nasal bridge. Lift the tarsal conjunctiva to look for undissolved particles and to facilitate irrigation. Continue irrigation for 15 minutes or until each eye has been irrigated with at least 1 L of solution. If the toxin is an acid or a base, check the pH of the tears after irrigation, and continue irrigation until the pH is between 6.5 and 7.5.

After irrigation is complete, perform a careful examination of the eye, using fluorescein and a slit lamp or Wood's lamp to identify areas of corneal injury. Patients with serious conjunctival or corneal injury should be immediately referred to an ophthalmologist.

GASTROINTESTINAL DECONTAMINATION

Removal of ingested poisons was a routine part of emergency treatment for decades. However, studies in volunteers indicate that if more than 60 minutes has passed, induced emesis and gastric lavage are relatively ineffective, and prospective clinical studies have failed to demonstrate improved outcome after gastric emptying. For small or moderate ingestions of most substances, toxicologists generally recommend oral activated charcoal alone without prior gastric emptying. Exceptions are large ingestions of anticholinergic compounds and salicylates, which often delay gastric emptying, and ingestion of sustained-release or enteric-coated tablets, which may remain intact for several hours.

Gastric emptying is not generally used for ingestion of corrosive agents or petroleum distillates, because further esophageal injury or pulmonary aspiration may result. However, in certain cases, removal of the toxin may be more important than concern over possible complications. Consult a medical toxicologist or regional poison control center (800-222-1222) for advice.

Emesis

Emesis using syrup of ipecac can partially evacuate gastric contents if given very soon after ingestion (eg, at work or at home). However, it may increase the risk of pulmonary aspiration and delay or prevent the use of oral activated charcoal. Therefore, it is no longer used in the routine management of ingestions.

Gastric Lavage

Gastric lavage is more effective for liquid poisons or small pill fragments than for intact tablets or pieces of mushroom. It is most useful when started within 60 minutes after ingestion. However, the lavage procedure may delay administration of activated charcoal and may stimulate vomiting and pulmonary aspiration in an obtunded patient. It is no longer used in the routine management of overdose.

A. INDICATIONS

Gastric lavage is sometimes used after very large ingestions (eg, massive aspirin overdose), for collection and examination of gastric contents for identification of poison, and for convenient administration of charcoal and antidotes.

B. CONTRAINDICATIONS

Do *not* use lavage for stuporous or comatose patients with absent gag reflexes unless they are endotracheally intubated beforehand. Some authorities advise against lavage when caustic material has been ingested; others regard it as essential to remove liquid corrosives from the stomach.

C. TECHNIQUE

In obtunded or comatose patients, the danger of aspiration pneumonia is reduced by performing endotracheal intubation with a cuffed tube before the procedure. Gently insert a lubricated, soft but noncollapsible stomach tube (at least 37–40°F) through the mouth or nose into the stomach. Aspirate and save the contents, and then lavage repeatedly with 50- to 100-mL aliquots of fluid until the return fluid is clear. Use lukewarm tap water or saline.

Activated Charcoal

Activated charcoal effectively adsorbs almost all drugs and poisons. Poorly adsorbed substances include iron, lithium, potassium, sodium, cyanide, mineral acids, and alcohols.

A. INDICATIONS

Activated charcoal should be used for prompt adsorption of drugs or toxins in the stomach and intestine. Studies in volunteers show that activated charcoal given alone may be as effective as or more effective than ipecac-induced emesis or gastric lavage. However, evidence of benefit in clinical studies is lacking. Administration of charcoal, especially if mixed with sorbitol, can provoke vomiting, which could lead to pulmonary aspiration in an obtunded patient.

B. CONTRAINDICATIONS

Activated charcoal should not be used for comatose or convulsing patients unless it can be given by gastric tube and the airway is first protected by a cuffed endotracheal tube. It is also contraindicated for patients with ileus or intestinal obstruction or those who have ingested corrosives for whom endoscopy is planned.

C. TECHNIQUE

Administer activated charcoal, 60–100 g orally or via gastric tube, mixed in aqueous slurry. Repeated doses may be given to ensure gastrointestinal adsorption or to enhance elimination of some drugs (see below).

Catharsis

A. INDICATIONS

Cathartics are used by some toxicologists for stimulation of peristalsis to hasten the elimination of unabsorbed drugs and poisons and the activated charcoal slurry. There is no clinical evidence to support their use, and some agents (eg, sorbitol) can provoke vomiting, increasing the risk of pulmonary aspiration.

B. CONTRAINDICATIONS AND CAUTIONS

Do not use mineral oil or other oil-based cathartics. Do not give a cathartic to patients with suspected intestinal obstruction. Avoid sodium-based cathartics in patients with hypertension, renal failure, and congestive heart failure and magnesium-based cathartics in patients with renal failure. Sorbitol (an osmotic cathartic found in some prepackaged activated charcoal slurry products) can cause hypotension and dehydration due to third-spacing and also causes intestinal cramping and vomiting.

C. TECHNIQUE

Magnesium sulfate 10%, 2–3 mL/kg, or other agents given orally or via gastric tube.

Whole Bowel Irrigation

Whole bowel irrigation uses large volumes of balanced polyethylene glycol-electrolyte solution to mechanically cleanse the entire intestinal tract. Because of the composition of the irrigating solution, there is no significant gain or loss of systemic fluids or electrolytes.

A. INDICATIONS

Whole bowel irrigation is particularly effective for massive iron ingestion in which intact tablets are visible on abdominal x-ray. It has also been used for ingestions of sustained-release and enteric-coated tablets as well as swallowed drug-filled packets.

B. CONTRAINDICATIONS

Do not use in patients with suspected intestinal obstruction. Use with caution in patients who are obtunded or have depressed airway protective reflexes.

C. TECHNIQUE

Administer a balanced polyethylene glycol-electrolyte solution (CoLyte, GoLYTELY) into the stomach via gastric tube at a rate of 1–2 L/h until the rectal effluent is clear. This may take several hours. It is most effective when patients are able to sit on a commode to pass the intestinal contents.

Increased Drug Removal

A. URINARY MANIPULATION

Forced diuresis is hazardous; the risk of complications (pulmonary edema, electrolyte imbalance) usually outweighs its benefits. Acidic drugs (eg, salicylates, phenobarbital) are more rapidly excreted with an alkaline urine. Acidification (sometimes promoted for amphetamines, phencyclidine) is *not* very effective and is contraindicated in the presence of rhabdomyolysis or myoglobinuria.

B. HEMODIALYSIS

The indications for dialysis are as follows: (1) Known or suspected potentially lethal amounts of a dialyzable drug (Table 39–5). (2) Poisoning with deep coma, apnea, severe hypotension, fluid and electro-

Table 39–5. Recommended use of hemodialysis in poisoning.[1]

Poison	Indications[1]
Carbamazepine	Seizures, severe cardiotoxicity
Ethylene glycol	Acidosis, serum level > 50 mg/dL
Lithium	Severe symptoms; level > 4 mEq/L more than 12 hours after last dose
Methanol	Acidosis, serum level > 50 mg/dL
Phenobarbital	Intractable hypotension, acidosis despite maximal supportive care
Salicylate	Severe acidosis, CNS symptoms, level > 100 mg/dL (acute overdose) or > 60 mg/dL (chronic intoxication)
Theophylline	Serum level > 90–100 mg/L (acute) or seizures and serum level > 40–60 mg/L (chronic)
Valproic acid	Serum level > 900–1000 mg/L or deep coma, severe acidosis

[1]See text for further discussion of indications.

lyte or acid-base disturbance, or extreme body temperature changes that cannot be corrected by conventional measures. (3) Poisoning in patients with severe renal, cardiac, pulmonary, or hepatic disease who will not be able to eliminate toxin by the usual mechanisms.

Peritoneal dialysis may rarely be used for acute poisonings when hemodialysis is not available, but it is very inefficient. Continuous renal replacement therapy (also known as continuous venovenous hemodiafiltration) is of uncertain benefit for elimination of most poisons but has been used successfully in the management of lithium intoxication.

C. REPEAT-DOSE CHARCOAL

Repeated doses of activated charcoal, 20–30 g orally or via gastric tube every 3–4 hours, may hasten elimination of some drugs (eg, theophylline, phenobarbital) by absorbing drugs excreted into the gut lumen ("gut dialysis"). However, clinical studies have failed to prove better outcome using multiple-dose charcoal. Sorbitol or other cathartics should *not* be used with each dose, or resulting large stool volumes may lead to dehydration or hypernatremia.

Bond GR: The role of activated charcoal and gastric emptying in gastrointestinal decontamination: a state-of-the-art review. Ann Emerg Med 2002;39:273. [PMID: 11867980]

Heard K: Gastrointestinal decontamination. Med Clin North Am 2005;89(6):1067. [PMID: 16227054]

Proudfoot AT et al: Position paper on urine alkalinization. J Toxicol Clin Toxicol 2004;42:1. [PMID: 15083932]

■ DIAGNOSIS OF POISONING

The identity of the ingested substance or substances is usually known, but occasionally a comatose patient is found with an unlabeled container or refuses or otherwise fails to give a coherent history. By performing a directed physical examination and ordering common clinical laboratory tests, the clinician can often make a tentative diagnosis that may allow empiric interventions or may suggest specific toxicologic tests.

PHYSICAL EXAMINATION

Important diagnostic variables in the physical examination include blood pressure, pulse rate, temperature, pupil size, sweating, and the presence or absence of peristaltic activity. Poisonings with many drugs fit into one of four common syndromes.

Sympathomimetic Syndrome

The blood pressure and pulse rate are elevated, though with severe hypertension reflex bradycardia may occur. The temperature is often elevated, pupils are dilated, and the skin is sweaty, though mucous membranes are dry. Patients are usually agitated, anxious, or frankly psychotic.

Examples: Amphetamines, cocaine, ephedrine and pseudoephedrine.

Sympatholytic Syndrome

The blood pressure and pulse rate are decreased and body temperature is low. The pupils are small or even pinpoint. Peristalsis is usually decreased. Patients are usually obtunded or comatose.

Examples: Barbiturates, benzodiazepines and other sedative hypnotics, GHB, clonidine and related antihypertensives, ethanol, opioids.

Cholinergic Syndrome

Stimulation of muscarinic receptors causes bradycardia, miosis, sweating, and hyperperistalsis as well as bronchorrhea, wheezing, excessive salivation, and urinary incontinence. Nicotinic receptor stimulation may produce initial hypertension and tachycardia as well as fasciculations and muscle weakness. Patients are usually agitated and anxious.

Examples: Carbamates, nicotine, organophosphates (including nerve agents), physostigmine.

Anticholinergic Syndrome

Tachycardia with mild hypertension is common, and the body temperature is often elevated. Pupils are widely dilated. The skin is flushed, hot, and dry. Peristalsis is decreased, and urinary retention is common. Patients may have myoclonic jerking or choreoathetoid movements. Agitated delirium is frequently seen, and severe hyperthermia may occur.

Examples: Atropine, scopolamine, other naturally occurring and pharmaceutical anticholinergics, antihistamines, tricyclic antidepressants.

■ LABORATORY TESTS

The following clinical laboratory tests are recommended for screening of the overdosed patient: measured serum osmolality and osmolar gap, electrolytes, glucose, creatinine, blood urea nitrogen (BUN), urinalysis (eg, oxalate crystals with ethylene glycol poisoning, myoglobinuria with rhabdomyolysis), and electrocardiography. Serum acetaminophen and ethanol quantitative levels should be determined in all patients with drug overdoses.

OSMOLAR GAP

The osmolar gap is defined and calculation of the gap is described in Table 39–6. It is increased in the presence of large quantities of low-molecular-weight substances, most commonly ethanol. Common poisons associated with increased osmolar gap are acetone, ethanol, ethylene glycol, isopropyl alcohol, methanol, and propylene glycol. **Note:** Severe alcoholic ketoacidosis and diabetic ketoacidosis can also cause an elevated osmolar gap resulting from the production of ketones and other low-molecular-weight substances.

ANION GAP

Metabolic acidosis associated with an elevated anion gap is usually due to an accumulation of lactic acid or other acids (see Chapter 21). Common causes of elevated anion gap in poisoning include carbon monoxide, cyanide, ethylene glycol, medicinal iron, isoniazid, methanol, metformin, ibuprofen and salicylates.

The osmolar gap should also be checked; combined elevated anion and osmolar gap suggests poisoning by methanol or ethylene glycol, though this may also occur in patients with diabetic ketoacidosis and alcoholic ketoacidosis.

TOXICOLOGY LABORATORY EXAMINATION

A comprehensive toxicology screen is of little value in the initial care of the poisoned patient—on the contrary, it is time-consuming and expensive. Specific quantitative levels of certain drugs may be extremely helpful (Table 39–7), however, especially if specific antidotes or interventions (eg, dialysis) would be indicated based on the results.

If a toxicology screen is required, urine is the best specimen. Many hospitals can perform a quick but

Table 39–6. Use of the osmolar gap in toxicology.

The osmolar gap (Δosm) is determined by subtracting the calculated serum osmolality from the measured serum osmolality.

$$\begin{array}{c} \text{Calculated} \\ \text{osmolality} \\ \text{(osm)} \end{array} = 2[Na^+(meq/L)] + \frac{\overset{\text{Glucose}}{(mg/dL)}}{18} + \frac{\overset{\text{BUN}}{(mg/dL)}}{2.8}$$

Δosm = Measured osmolality – Calculated osmolality

Serum osmolality may be increased by contributions of circulating alcohols and other low-molecular-weight substances. Since these are not included in the calculated osmolality, there will be a gap proportionate to their serum concentration and inversely proportionate to their molecular weight:

$$\begin{array}{c} \text{Serum concentration} \\ \text{(mg/dL)} \end{array} = \Delta osm \times \frac{\text{Molecular weight}}{10}$$

	Molecular Weight	Toxic Concentration	Approximate Corresponding Δosm (mosm/L)
Ethanol	46	300	65
Methanol	32	50	16
Ethylene glycol	60	100	16
Isopropanol	60	150	25

Modified from Saunders CE, Ho MT (editors): *Current Emergency Diagnosis & Treatment*, 4th ed. Originally published by Appleton & Lange. Copyright © 1992 by The McGraw-Hill Companies, Inc. **Note:** Most laboratories use the freezing point method for calculating osmolality. If the vaporization point method is used, alcohols are driven off and their contribution to osmolality is lost.

limited screen for "drugs of abuse" (typically these screens include only opioids, amphetamines, and cocaine, and some add benzodiazepines, barbiturates, and tetrahydrocannabinol [marijuana]). There are numerous false-positive and false-negative results. Blood samples may be saved for possible quantitative testing, but blood is not generally used for screening purposes since it is relatively insensitive for many common drugs, including psychotropic agents, opioids, and stimulants.

ABDOMINAL X-RAYS

A plain film of the abdomen may reveal radiopaque iron tablets, drug-filled condoms, or other toxic material. Studies suggest that few tablets are predictably visible (eg, ferrous sulfate, sodium chloride, calcium carbonate, and potassium chloride). Thus, the x-ray is useful only if positive.

Table 39–7. Specific quantitative levels and potential therapeutic interventions.[1]

Drug or Toxin	Treatment
Acetaminophen	Specific antidote (acetylcysteine) based on serum level
Carbon monoxide	High carboxyhemoglobin level indicates need for 100% oxygen, consideration of hyperbaric oxygen
Carbamazepine	High level may indicate need for hemodialysis
Digoxin	On basis of serum digoxin level and severity of clinical presentation, treatment with Fab antibody fragments (Digibind) may be indicated
Ethanol	Low serum level may suggest nonalcoholic cause of coma (eg, trauma, other drugs, other alcohols). Serum ethanol may also be useful in monitoring ethanol therapy for methanol or ethylene glycol poisoning.
Iron	Level may indicate need for chelation with deferoxamine
Lithium	Serum levels can guide decision to institute hemodialysis
Methanol, ethylene glycol	Acidosis, high levels indicate need for hemodialysis, therapy with ethanol or fomepizole
Methemoglobin	Methemoglobinemia can be treated with methylene blue intravenously
Salicylates	High level may indicate need for hemodialysis, alkaline diuresis
Theophylline	Immediate hemodialysis or hemoperfusion may be indicated based on serum level
Valproic acid	Elevated levels may indicate need to consider hemodialysis

[1]Some drugs or toxins may have profound and irreversible toxicity unless rapid and specific management is provided outside of routine supportive care. For these agents, laboratory testing may provide the serum level or other evidence required for administering a specific antidote or arranging for hemodialysis.

Bartlett D: Understanding the anion and osmolal gaps laboratory values: what they are and how to use them. J Emerg Nurs 2005;31:109.[PMID: 15682142]

Goldfrank LR (editor): *Goldfrank's Toxicologic Emergencies,* 8th ed. McGraw-Hill, 2004.

Hovda KE et al: Anion and osmolal gaps in the diagnosis of methanol poisoning: clinical study in 28 patients. Intensive Care Med 2004;30:1842. [PMID: 15241587]

Olson KR (editor): *Poisoning and Drug Overdose,* 4th ed. McGraw-Hill, 2004.

■ SELECTED POISONINGS

ACETAMINOPHEN

Acetaminophen (paracetamol in the UK, Europe) is a common analgesic found in many nonprescription and prescription products. After absorption, it is metabolized mainly by glucuronidation and sulfation, with a small fraction metabolized via the P450 mixed-function oxidase system (2E1) to a highly toxic reactive intermediate. This toxic intermediate is normally detoxified by cellular glutathione. With acute acetaminophen overdose (> 140 mg/kg, or 7 g in an average adult), hepatocellular glutathione is rapidly depleted and the reactive intermediate attacks other cell proteins, causing necrosis. Patients with enhanced P450 2E1 activity, such as chronic alcoholics and patients taking isoniazid, are at increased risk of developing hepatotoxicity. Hepatic toxicity may also occur after chronic accidental overuse of acetaminophen—eg, as a result of taking two or three acetaminophen-containing products concurrently or intentionally exceeding the recommended maximum dose of 4 g/d.

Clinical Findings

Shortly after ingestion, patients may have nausea or vomiting, but there are usually no other signs of toxicity until 24–48 hours after ingestion, when hepatic aminotransferase levels begin to increase. With severe poisoning, fulminant hepatic necrosis may occur, resulting in jaundice, hepatic encephalopathy, renal failure, and death. Rarely, massive ingestion (eg, serum levels over 500–1000 mg/L) can cause acute coma, hypotension, and metabolic acidosis unrelated to hepatic injury.

The diagnosis after acute overdose is based on measurement of the serum acetaminophen level. Plot the serum level versus the time since ingestion on the acetaminophen nomogram shown in Figure 39–1. Ingestion of sustained-release products or coingestion of an anticholinergic agent, salicylate, or opioid drug may cause delayed elevation of serum levels and may render the nomogram useless. The nomogram is not useful after chronic overdose.

Treatment

A. EMERGENCY AND SUPPORTIVE MEASURES

Administer activated charcoal (see p 1644) within 1–2 hours of the ingestion. Although charcoal may interfere with absorption of the oral antidote acetylcysteine, this is not considered clinically significant.

B. SPECIFIC TREATMENT

Although the general recommendation is to treat if the serum acetaminophen level is above the toxic line on the nomogram (Figure 39–1), many clinicians prefer to use the lower line as a guide to treatment, as it provides

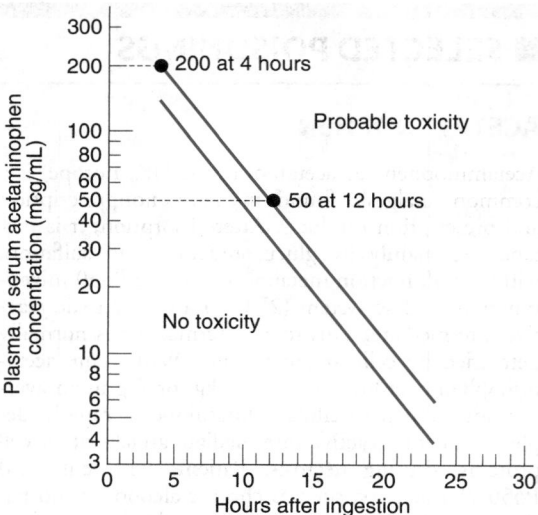

Figure 39–1. Nomogram for prediction of acetaminophen hepatotoxicity following acute overdosage. The upper line defines serum acetaminophen concentrations known to be associated with hepatotoxicity; the lower line defines serum levels 25% below those expected to cause hepatotoxicity. To give a margin for error in the estimation of the time of ingestion and for patients at higher risk for hepatotoxicity, the lower line is often used as a guide to treatment. (Modified and reproduced, with permission, from Rumack BH, Matthew H: Acetaminophen poisoning and toxicity. Pediatrics 1975;55:871.)

a 25% safety margin. Begin treatment with a loading dose of N-acetylcysteine, 140 mg/kg orally, followed by 70 mg/kg every 4 hours. Dilute the solution to 5% with water, juice, or soda. If vomiting interferes with oral N-acetylcysteine administration, consider giving the antidote intravenously (see below). The most widely used oral N-acetylcysteine protocol in the United States calls for 72 hours of treatment. However, other regimens have demonstrated equivalent success with 20–48 hours of treatment. A 20-hour intravenous regimen was recently approved by the FDA (Acetadote). Treatment with N-acetylcysteine is most effective if started within 8–10 hours after ingestion. If the precise time of ingestion is unknown or if the patient is at higher risk of hepatotoxicity (eg, alcoholic, liver disease, chronic use of P450-inducing drugs), then use a lower threshold for initiation of N-acetylcysteine (in some case reports, a level of 100 mg/L at 4 hours was suggested in very high-risk patients).

The conventional oral formulation may also be given intravenously using a micropore filter and a slow rate of infusion. Call a regional poison control center or medical toxicologist for assistance.

Lavonas EJ et al: Intravenous administration of N-acetylcysteine: oral and parenteral formulations are both acceptable. Ann Emerg Med 2005;45:223. [PMID: 15671984]

Sivilotti ML et al: A new predictor of toxicity following acetaminophen overdose based on pretreatment exposure. Clin Toxicol (Phila) 2005;43:229. [PMID: 16035198]

ACIDS, CORROSIVE (Table 39–8)

The strong mineral acids exert primarily a local corrosive effect on the skin and mucous membranes. Symptoms include severe pain in the throat and upper gastrointestinal tract; bloody vomitus; difficulty in swallowing, breathing, and speaking; discoloration and destruction of skin and mucous membranes in and around the mouth; and shock. Severe systemic metabolic acidosis may occur both as a result of cellular injury and from systemic absorption of the acid.

Severe deep destructive tissue damage may occur after exposure to hydrofluoric acid because of the penetrating and highly toxic fluoride ion. Systemic hypocalcemia and hyperkalemia may also occur after fluoride absorption, even following skin exposure.

Inhalation of volatile acids, fumes, or gases such as chlorine, fluorine, bromine, or iodine causes severe irritation of the throat and larynx and may cause upper airway obstruction and noncardiogenic pulmonary edema.

Treatment

A. INGESTION

Dilute immediately by giving a glass (4–8 oz) of milk or water to drink. Do *not* give bicarbonate or other neutralizing agents, and do *not* induce vomiting. Some experts recommend immediate placement of a small

Table 39–8. Common corrosive agents.

Category and Examples	Injury Caused
Concentrated alkalies Clinitest tablets Drain cleaners Industrial-strength ammonia Lye Oven cleaners	Penetrating liquefaction necrosis
Concentrated acids Pool disinfectants Toilet bowl cleaners	Coagulation necrosis
Weaker cleaning agents Cationic detergents (dishwasher detergents) Household ammonia Household bleach	Superficial burns and irritation; deep burns (rare)
Other Hydrofluoric acid	Penetrating, delayed, destructive injury

Reproduced, with permission, from Saunders CE, Ho MT (editors): *Current Emergency Diagnosis & Treatment,* 4th ed. McGraw-Hill, 1992.

flexible gastric tube and removal of stomach contents followed by lavage, particularly if the corrosive is a liquid or has important systemic toxicity.

Perform flexible endoscopic esophagoscopy promptly to determine the presence and extent of injury. X-rays of the chest and abdomen may reveal the presence of free air in patients with esophageal or gastric perforation. Perforation, peritonitis, and major bleeding are indications for surgery.

B. Skin Contact

Flood with water for 15 minutes. Use no chemical antidotes; the heat of the reaction may cause additional injury.

For hydrofluoric acid burns, soak the affected area in benzalkonium chloride solution or apply 2.5% calcium gluconate gel (prepared by adding 3.5 g calcium gluconate to 5 oz of water-soluble surgical lubricant, eg, K-Y Jelly); then arrange immediate consultation with a plastic surgeon or other specialist. Binding of the fluoride ion may be achieved by injecting 0.5 mL of 5% calcium gluconate per square centimeter under the burned area. (**Caution:** *Do not use calcium chloride.*) Intra-arterial infusion of calcium is sometimes required for extensive burns or those involving the nail bed; consult with a hand surgeon.

C. Eye Contact

Anesthetize the conjunctiva and corneal surfaces with topical local anesthetic drops (eg, proparacaine). Flood with water for 15 minutes, holding the eyelids open. Check pH with pH 6.0–8.0 test paper, and repeat irrigation, using 0.9% saline, until pH is near 7.0. Check for corneal damage with fluorescein and slit lamp examination; consult an ophthalmologist about further treatment.

D. Inhalation

Remove from further exposure to fumes or gas. Check skin and clothing. Treat pulmonary edema.

Dunser MW et al: Critical care management of major hydrofluoric acid burns: a case report, review of the literature, and recommendations for therapy. Burns 2004;30;391. [PMID: 15145201]

ALKALIES (Table 39–8)

The strong alkalies are common ingredients of some household cleaning compounds and may be suspected by their "soapy" texture. Those with alkalinity above pH 12.0 are particularly corrosive. Clinitest tablets and disk batteries are also a source. Alkalies cause liquefactive necrosis, which is deeply penetrating. Symptoms include burning pain in the upper gastrointestinal tract, nausea, vomiting, and difficulty in swallowing and breathing. Examination reveals destruction and edema of the affected skin and mucous membranes and bloody vomitus and stools. X-ray may reveal the presence of disk batteries in the esophagus or lower gastrointestinal tract.

Treatment

A. Ingestion

Dilute immediately with a glass of water. Do *not* induce emesis. Some gastroenterologists recommend immediate placement of a small flexible gastric tube and removal of stomach contents followed by gastric lavage after ingestion of liquid caustic substances to remove residual material.

Immediate endoscopy is recommended to evaluate the extent of damage. If x-ray reveals the location of ingested disk batteries in the esophagus, immediate endoscopic removal is mandatory.

The use of corticosteroids to prevent stricture formation is of no proved benefit and is definitely contraindicated if there is evidence of esophageal perforation.

B. Skin Contact

Wash with running water until the skin no longer feels soapy. Relieve pain and treat shock.

C. Eye Contact

Anesthetize the conjunctival and corneal surfaces with topical anesthetic (eg, proparacaine). Irrigate with water or saline continuously for 20–30 minutes, holding the lids open. Check pH with pH test paper, and repeat irrigation, using 0.9% saline, for additional 30-minute periods until the pH is near 7.0. Check for corneal damage with fluorescein and slit lamp examination; consult an ophthalmologist for further treatment.

Ramasamy K et al: Corrosive ingestion in adults. J Clin Gastroenterol 2003;37:119. [PMID: 12869880]

AMPHETAMINES & COCAINE

Amphetamines and cocaine are widely abused for their euphorigenic and stimulant properties. Both drugs may be smoked, snorted, ingested, or injected. Amphetamines and cocaine produce central nervous system stimulation and a generalized increase in central and peripheral sympathetic activity. The toxic dose of each drug is highly variable and depends on the route of administration and individual tolerance. The onset of effects is most rapid after intravenous injection or smoking. Amphetamine derivatives and related drugs include methamphetamine ("crystal meth," "crank"), methylenedioxymethamphetamine (MDMA, "ecstasy"), ephedrine ("herbal ecstasy"), and methcathinone ("cat"). Nonprescription medications and nutritional supplements may contain stimulant or sympathomimetic drugs such as ephedrine or caffeine (see Theophylline, below): Phenylpropanolamine was withdrawn from the market because of an increased incidence of hypertensive intracerebral hemorrhage in young women.

Clinical Findings

Presenting symptoms may include anxiety, tremulousness, tachycardia, hypertension, diaphoresis, dilated pupils, agitation, muscular hyperactivity, and psychosis. Metabolic acidosis may occur. In severe intoxication, seizures and hyperthermia may occur. Sustained or severe hypertension may result in intracranial hemorrhage, aortic dissection, or myocardial infarction. Hyponatremia has been reported after MDMA use; the mechanism is not known but may involve excessive water intake, syndrome of inappropriate antidiuretic hormone (SIADH), or both.

The diagnosis is supported by finding amphetamines, cocaine, or the cocaine metabolite benzoylecgonine in the urine. Blood screening is generally not sensitive enough to detect these drugs.

Treatment

A. EMERGENCY AND SUPPORTIVE MEASURES

Maintain a patent airway and assist ventilation, if necessary. Treat coma or seizures as described at the beginning of this chapter. Rapidly lower the body temperature (see hyperthermia, above) in patients who are hyperthermic (40°C).

For poisoning by ingestion, administer activated charcoal (p 1644). Do *not* induce emesis because of the risk of seizures.

B. SPECIFIC TREATMENT

Treat agitation, psychosis, or seizures with a benzodiazepine such as lorazepam, 2–3 mg intravenously. Add phenobarbital 15 mg/kg intravenously for persistent seizures. Treat hypertension with a vasodilator drug such as phentolamine (1–5 mg intravenously) or a combined α- and β-adrenergic blocker such as labetalol (10–20 mg intravenously). Do *not* administer a pure β-blocker such as propranolol alone, as this may result in paradoxic worsening of the hypertension as a result of unopposed α-adrenergic effects.

Treat tachycardia or tachyarrhythmias with a short-acting β-blocker such as esmolol (25–100 mcg/kg/min by intravenous infusion). Treat hyponatremia as outlined in Chapter 21.

Greene SL et al: Multiple toxicity from 3,4-methylene-dioxymethamphetamine ("ecstasy"). Am J Emerg Med 2003; 21:121. [PMID: 12671812]

Kashani J et al: Methamphetamine toxicity secondary to intra-vaginal body stuffing. J Toxicol Clin Toxicol 2004;42: 987. [PMID: 15641645]

ANTICOAGULANTS

Warfarin and related compounds (including ingredients of many commercial rodenticides) inhibit the clotting mechanism by blocking hepatic synthesis of vitamin K–dependent clotting factors.

Anticoagulants may cause hemoptysis, gross hematuria, bloody stools, hemorrhages into organs, widespread bruising, and bleeding into joint spaces. The prothrombin time is increased within 12–24 hours (peak 36–48 hours) after a single overdose. After in-gestion of brodifacoum and indanedione rodenticides (so-called "superwarfarins"), inhibition of clotting factor synthesis may persist for several weeks or even months after a single dose.

Treatment

A. EMERGENCY AND SUPPORTIVE MEASURES

Discontinue the drug at the first sign of gross bleeding, and determine the prothrombin time (international normalized ratio, INR). If the patient has ingested an acute overdose, administer activated charcoal (see p 1644).

B. SPECIFIC TREATMENT

Do not treat prophylactically with vitamin K—wait for evidence of anticoagulation (elevated prothrombin time). If the INR is elevated, give phytonadione (vitamin K_1), 10–25 mg orally, and additional doses as needed to restore the prothrombin time to normal. Doses as high as 200 mg/d have been required after ingestion of "superwarfarins." Give fresh-frozen plasma or activated Factor VII as needed to rapidly correct the coagulation factor deficit if there is serious bleeding. If the patient is chronically anticoagulated and has strong medical indications for being maintained in that status (eg, prosthetic heart valve), give much smaller doses of vitamin K (1 mg orally) and fresh-frozen plasma (or both) to titrate to the desired prothrombin time.

If the patient has ingested brodifacoum or a related superwarfarin, prolonged observation (over weeks) and repeated administration of large doses of vitamin K may be required.

Ingels M et al: A prospective study of acute, unintentional, pediatric superwarfarin ingestions managed without decontamination. Ann Emerg Med 2002;40:73. [PMID: 12085076]

Zupancic-Salek S et al: Successful reversal of anticoagulant effect of superwarfarin poisoning with recombinant activated factor VII. Blood Coagul Fibrinolysis 2005;16:239. [PMID: 15870542]

ANTICONVULSANTS

Anticonvulsants (carbamazepine, phenytoin, valproic acid) are widely used in the management of seizure disorders. In addition, carbamazepine and valproic acid are increasingly used for treatment of mood disorders.

Phenytoin can be given orally or intravenously. Rapid intravenous injection of phenytoin can cause acute myocardial depression and cardiac arrest owing to the solvent propylene glycol; a newer form of phenytoin (fosphenytoin) is available that does not contain this diluent. Chronic phenytoin intoxication can occur following only slightly increased doses because of zero-order kinetics and a small toxic-therapeutic window. Phenytoin intoxication can also occur following acute intentional or accidental overdose. The overdose syndrome is usually mild even with high serum levels. The most common manifestations are ataxia, nystagmus, and drowsiness. Choreoathetoid movements have been described.

Carbamazepine was first used for the treatment of trigeminal neuralgia. It has since become a first-line agent for temporal lobe epilepsy and other seizure disorders. Intoxication causes drowsiness, stupor, and, with high levels, coma and seizures. Dilated pupils and tachycardia are common. Toxicity may be seen with serum levels greater than 20 mg/L, though severe poisoning is usually associated with concentrations greater than 30–40 mg/L. Because of erratic and slow absorption, intoxication may progress over several hours to days.

Valproic acid intoxication produces a unique syndrome consisting of hypernatremia (from the sodium component of the salt), metabolic acidosis, hypocalcemia, elevated serum ammonia, and mild liver aminotransferase elevation. Hypoglycemia may occur as a result of hepatic metabolic dysfunction. Coma with small pupils may be seen and can mimic opioid poisoning. Encephalopathy and cerebral edema can occur.

The newer anticonvulsants **lamotrigine** and **tiagabine** have also been reported to cause seizures after overdose. **Topiramate** intoxication has caused acute agitation and confusion.

Treatment

A. EMERGENCY AND SUPPORTIVE MEASURES

For recent ingestions, give activated charcoal orally or by gastric tube. For large ingestions of carbamazepine or valproic acid—especially of sustained-release formulations—consider whole bowel irrigation (see p 1644). Multiple-dose activated charcoal may be beneficial in ensuring gut decontamination for large ingestions and might enhance elimination of absorbed drugs.

B. SPECIFIC TREATMENT

There are no antidotes. Naloxone was reported to have reversed valproic acid overdose in one anecdotal case. Consider hemodialysis for massive intoxication with valproic acid or carbamazepine (eg, carbamazepine levels > 100 mg/L or valproic acid levels > 1000 mg/L).

Lofton AL, Klien-Schwartz W: Evaluation of lamotrigine toxicity reported to poison centers. Ann Pharmacother 2004;38(11):1811. [PMID: 15353576]

Singh SM et al: Extracorporeal management of valproic acid overdose: a large regional experience. J Nephrol 2004;17:43. [PMID: 15151258]

ARSENIC

Arsenic is found in some pesticides and industrial chemicals, and arsenic trioxide has recently been reintroduced as a chemotherapeutic agent. A massive epidemic of chronic arsenic poisoning has occurred in Bangladesh due to naturally occurring arsenic in deep aquifers. Symptoms of acute poisoning usually appear within 1 hour after ingestion but may be delayed as long as 12 hours. They include abdominal pain, vomiting, watery diarrhea, and skeletal muscle cramps. Profound dehydration and shock may occur. In chronic poisoning, symptoms can be vague but often include pancytopenia, painful peripheral sensory neuropathy, and skin changes including melanosis, keratosis, and desquamating rash. Urinary arsenic levels may be falsely elevated after certain meals (eg, seafood) that contain large quantities of a nontoxic form of organic arsenic.

Treatment

A. EMERGENCY MEASURES

After recent ingestion (within 1–2 hours), perform gastric lavage and administer 60–100 g of activated charcoal (see p 1643–1644). Administer intravenous fluids to replace losses due to vomiting and diarrhea.

B. ANTIDOTE

For patients with severe acute intoxication, give dimercaprol injection (bronchoalveolar lavage, BAL), 10% solution in oil, 3–5 mg/kg intramuscularly every 4–6 hours for 2 days. The side effects include nausea, vomiting, headache, and hypertension. Follow dimercaprol with oral succimer (dimercaptosuccinic acid, DMSA), 10 mg/kg every 8 hours, for 1 week. Consult a medical toxicologist or regional poison control center (800-222-1222) for advice regarding chelation.

Kalia K et al: Strategies for safe and effective therapeutic measures for chronic arsenic and lead poisoning. J Occup Health 2005;47:1. [PMID: 15703449]

Yoshida T et al: Chronic health effects in people exposed to arsenic via the drinking water: dose-response relationships in review. Toxicol Appl Pharmacol 2004;198:243. [PMID: 15276403]

ATROPINE & ANTICHOLINERGICS

Atropine, scopolamine, belladonna, diphenoxylate with atropine, *Datura stramonium*, *Hyoscyamus niger*, some mushrooms, tricyclic antidepressants, and antihistamines are antimuscarinic agents with variable central nervous system effects. The patient complains of dryness of the mouth, thirst, difficulty in swallowing, and blurring of vision. The physical signs include dilated pupils, flushed skin, tachycardia, fever, delirium, myoclonus, ileus, and flushed appearance. Antidepressants and antihistamines may induce convulsions.

Antihistamines are commonly available with or without prescription. Diphenhydramine commonly causes delirium, tachycardia, and seizures. Massive overdose may mimic tricyclic antidepressant poisoning. The first-generation "nonsedating" agents terfenadine and astemizole caused QT interval prolongation and torsade de pointes (atypical ventricular tachycardia) and were removed from the United States market. Loratadine and fexofenadine have not caused this problem.

Treatment

A. EMERGENCY AND SUPPORTIVE MEASURES

Administer activated charcoal (see p 1644). Tepid sponge baths and sedation, or neuromuscular paralysis in rare cases, are indicated to control high temperatures (see p 1642).

B. SPECIFIC TREATMENT

For pure atropine or related anticholinergic syndrome, if symptoms are severe (eg, agitated delirium or excessively rapid tachycardia), give physostigmine salicylate, 0.5–1 mg slowly intravenously over 5 minutes, with electrocardiographic monitoring, until symptoms are controlled. Bradyarrhythmias and convulsions are a hazard with physostigmine administration, and it should be avoided in patients with tricyclic antidepressant overdose.

DeFrates LJ et al: Antimuscarinic intoxication resulting from the ingestion of moonflower seeds. Ann Pharmacother 2005;39: 173. Epub 2004 Nov 30. [PMID: 15572604]

Sharma AN et al: Diphenhydramine-induced wide complex dysrhythmia responds to treatment with sodium bicarbonate. Am J Emerg Med 2003;21:212. [PMID: 12811715]

β-ADRENERGIC BLOCKERS

There are a wide variety of β-adrenergic blocking drugs, with varying pharmacologic and pharmacokinetic properties (see Table 11–7). The most toxic β-blocker is propranolol. Propranolol competitively blocks β_1 and β_2 adrenoceptors and also has direct membrane-depressant and central nervous system effects.

Clinical Findings

The most common findings with mild or moderate intoxication are hypotension and bradycardia. Cardiac depression from more severe poisoning is often unresponsive to conventional therapy with β-adrenergic stimulants such as dopamine and norepinephrine. In addition, with propranolol and other lipid-soluble drugs, seizures and coma may occur.

The diagnosis is based on typical clinical findings. Routine toxicology screening does not usually include β-blockers.

Treatment

A. EMERGENCY AND SUPPORTIVE MEASURES

Initially, treat bradycardia or heart block with atropine (0.5–2 mg intravenously), isoproterenol (2–20 mcg/min by intravenous infusion, titrated to the desired heart rate), or an external transcutaneous cardiac pacemaker. However, these measures are often ineffective, and specific antidotal treatment may be necessary (see below).

For ingested drugs, administer activated charcoal (see p 1644).

B. SPECIFIC TREATMENT

If the above measures are not successful in reversing bradycardia and hypotension, give glucagon, 5–10 mg intravenously, followed by an infusion of 1–5 mg/h. Glucagon is an inotropic agent that acts at a different receptor site and is therefore not affected by β-blockade.

Bailey B: Glucagon in beta-blocker and calcium channel blocker overdoses: a systematic review. J Toxicol Clin Toxicol 2003; 41:595. [PMID: 14514004]

Wax PM et al: Beta-blocker ingestion: an evidence-based consensus guideline for out-of-hospital management. Clin Toxicol (Phila) 2005;43:131. [PMID: 15906457]

CALCIUM CHANNEL BLOCKERS

Calcium channel blockers used in the United States include verapamil, diltiazem, nifedipine, nicardipine, amlodipine, felodipine, isradipine, nisoldipine, and nimodipine. These drugs share the ability to cause arteriolar vasodilation and depression of cardiac contractility, especially after acute overdose. Patients may present with bradycardia, atrioventricular (AV) nodal block, hypotension, or a combination of these effects. With severe poisoning, cardiac arrest may occur.

Treatment

A. EMERGENCY AND SUPPORTIVE MEASURES

Maintain a patent airway and assist ventilation, if necessary. Treat coma, hypotension, and seizures as described at the beginning of this chapter. Treat bradycardia with atropine (0.5–2 mg intravenously), isoproterenol (2–20 mcg/min by intravenous infusion), or a transcutaneous or internal cardiac pacemaker.

For ingested drugs, administer activated charcoal (see p 1644). In addition, whole bowel irrigation should be initiated as soon as possible if the patient has ingested a sustained-release product.

B. SPECIFIC TREATMENT

If bradycardia and hypotension are not reversed with these measures, administer calcium chloride intravenously. Start with calcium chloride 10%, 10 mL, or calcium gluconate 10%, 20 mL. Repeat the dose every 3–5 minutes. The optimum (or maximum) dose has not been established, but there are reports of success after as much as 10–12 g of calcium chloride. Calcium is most useful in reversing negative inotropic effects and is less effective for AV nodal blockade and bradycardia. Epinephrine infusion (1–4 mcg/min initially) and glucagon (5–10 mg intravenously) have also been recommended. In addition, high doses of insulin (0.5–1 U/kg intravenous bolus followed by 0.5–1 U/kg/h infusion) along with sufficient dextrose to maintain euglycemia have been reported to be beneficial but there are no controlled studies.

DeWitt CR et al: Pharmacology, pathophysiology and management of calcium channel blocker and beta-blocker toxicity. Toxicol Rev 2004;23:223. [PMID: 15898828]

Marques M et al: Treatment of calcium channel blocker intoxication with insulin infusion: case report and literature review. Resuscitation 2003;57:211. [PMID: 12745190]

Shepherd G et al: High-dose insulin therapy for calcium-channel blocker overdose. Ann Pharmacother 2005;39:923. Epub 2005 Apr 5. [PMID: 15811898]

CARBON MONOXIDE

Carbon monoxide is a colorless, odorless gas produced by the combustion of carbon-containing materials. Poisoning may occur as a result of suicidal or accidental exposure to automobile exhaust, smoke inhalation in a fire, or accidental exposure to an improperly vented gas heater or other appliance. Carbon monoxide avidly binds to hemoglobin, with an affinity approximately 250 times that of oxygen. This results in reduced oxygen-carrying capacity and altered delivery of oxygen to cells (see also Smoke Inhalation in Chapter 9).

Clinical Findings

At low carbon monoxide levels (carboxyhemoglobin saturation 10–20%), victims may have headache, dizziness, abdominal pain, and nausea. With higher levels, confusion, dyspnea, and syncope may occur. Hypotension, coma, and seizures are common with levels greater than 50–60%. Survivors of acute severe poisoning may develop permanent obvious or subtle neurologic and neuropsychiatric deficits. The fetus and newborn may be more susceptible because of high carbon monoxide affinity for fetal hemoglobin.

Carbon monoxide poisoning should be suspected in any person with severe headache or acutely altered mental status, especially during cold weather, when improperly vented heating systems may have been used. Diagnosis depends on specific measurement of the arterial or venous carboxyhemoglobin saturation, although the level may have declined if high-flow oxygen therapy has already been administered, and levels do not always correlate with clinical symptoms. Routine arterial blood gas testing and pulse oximetry are not useful because they give falsely normal Po_2 and oxyhemoglobin saturation determinations, respectively.

Treatment

A. EMERGENCY AND SUPPORTIVE MEASURES

Maintain a patent airway and assist ventilation, if necessary. Remove the victim from exposure. Treat patients with coma, hypotension, or seizures as described at the beginning of this chapter.

B. SPECIFIC TREATMENT

The half-life of the carboxyhemoglobin (CoHb) complex is about 4–5 hours in room air but is reduced dramatically by high concentrations of oxygen. Administer 100% oxygen by tight-fitting high-flow reservoir face mask or endotracheal tube. Hyperbaric oxygen (HBO) can provide 100% oxygen under higher than atmospheric pressures, further shortening the half-life; it may also reduce the incidence of subtle neuropsychiatric sequelae. Recent studies disagree about the benefit of HBO, but recommended indications for HBO in patients with carbon monoxide poisoning include a history of loss of consciousness, CoHb greater than 25%, metabolic acidosis, age over 50 years, and cerebellar findings on neurologic examination.

Henry CR et al: Myocardial injury and long-term mortality following moderate to severe carbon monoxide poisoning. JAMA 2006;295:398. [PMID: 16434630]

Juurlink DN et al: Hyperbaric oxygen for carbon monoxide poisoning. Cochrane Database Syst Rev 2005;CD002041. [PMID: 15674890]

Weaver LK et al: Hyperbaric oxygen for acute carbon monoxide poisoning. N Engl J Med 2002;347:1057. [PMID: 12362006]

CHEMICAL WARFARE: NERVE AGENTS

Nerve agents used in chemical warfare work by cholinesterase inhibition and are most commonly organophosphorus compounds. Agents such as **tabun** (GA), **sarin** (GB), **soman** (GD), and **VX** are similar to insecticides such as malathion but are vastly more potent. They may be inhaled or absorbed through the skin. Systemic effects due to unopposed action of acetylcholine include miosis, salivation, abdominal cramps, diarrhea, and muscle paralysis producing respiratory arrest. Inhalation also produces severe bronchoconstriction and copious nasal and tracheobronchial secretions.

Treatment

A. EMERGENCY AND SUPPORTIVE MEASURES

Perform thorough decontamination of exposed areas with repeated soap and shampoo washing. Personnel caring for such patients must wear protective clothing and gloves, since cutaneous absorption may occur through normal skin.

B. SPECIFIC TREATMENT

Give atropine in an initial dose of 2 mg intravenously, and repeat as needed to reverse signs of acetylcholine excess. (Some victims have required several hundred milligrams.) Treat also with the cholinesterase-reactivating agent pralidoxime, 1–2 g intravenously initially followed by an infusion at a rate of 200–400 mg/h. United States military personnel in the Iraq invasion were equipped with autoinjectable units containing 2 mg of atropine plus 600 mg of the cholinesterase-reactivating agent pralidoxime.

Barthold CL et al: Organic phosphorus compounds—nerve agents. Crit Care Clin 2005;21:673. [PMID: 16168308]

Leikin JB et al: A review of nerve agent exposure for the critical care physician. Crit Care Med 2002;30:2346. [PMID: 12394966]

CHEMICAL WARFARE: RICIN

Ricin is a naturally occurring toxin found in minute quantities in the castor bean (*Ricinus communis*). It can cause toxicity if castor beans are thoroughly chewed or blenderized, although the quantity of ricin is small and it is poorly absorbed from the gastrointestinal tract, so symptoms following castor bean ingestion are usually limited to diarrhea and abdominal pain. Less commonly, severe gastroenteritis can lead to volume depletion and renal failure. On the other hand, purified ricin is extremely toxic if administered parenterally: the LD_{50} for injected ricin in animals is as low as 0.1 mcg/kg. A fatal case of suspected ricin poisoning by homicidal injection of an estimated 0.28 mg of ricin was associated with diffuse organ damage and death from cardiac failure after 2 days. Inhalation of ricin powder has not been reported in humans, but animal studies suggest it could cause hemorrhagic tracheobronchitis and pneumonia.

Treatment

A. EMERGENCY AND SUPPORTIVE MEASURES

After suspected ricin inhalation or exposure to powdered ricin, remove clothing and wash skin with water. Personnel caring for such patients should wear protective respiratory gear, clothing, and gloves.

B. SPECIFIC TREATMENT

There is no known antidote or other specific treatment. Provide supportive care for volume loss due to gastroenteritis and cardiac and respiratory support as needed.

Audi J et al: Ricin poisoning: a comprehensive review. JAMA 2005;294:2342. [PMID: 16278363]

Doan LG: Ricin: mechanism of toxicity, clinical manifestations, and vaccine development. A review. J Toxicol Clin Toxicol 2004;42:201. [PMID: 15214627]

CHLORINATED INSECTICIDES

Lindane (Kwell) and other chlorinated insecticides (chlorophenothane [DDT], lindane, toxaphene, chlordane, aldrin, endrin) are central nervous system stimulants that can cause poisoning by ingestion, inhalation, or direct contact. Most of these agents have been removed from the United States market because of their acute toxicity and their potential to accumulate in the food chain. The estimated lethal dose is about 20 g for DDT, 3 g for lindane, 2 g for toxaphene, 1 g for chlordane, and less than 1 g for endrin and aldrin. The manifestations of poisoning are nervous irritability, muscle twitching, seizures, and coma. Arrhythmias may occur. Hepatic and renal damage are reported.

Treatment

Give activated charcoal (see p 1644) and consider gastric lavage for large recent ingestions (see p 1643). Repeat-dose activated charcoal may be effective for large ingestions. For seizures, give diazepam, 5–10 mg slowly intravenously, or other anticonvulsants as described on p 1642.

Perform thorough decontamination of exposed areas with repeated soap and shampoo washing. Personnel caring for such patients must wear protective clothing and gloves, since cutaneous absorption may occur through normal skin.

Forrester MB et al: Epidemiology of lindane exposures for pediculosis reported to Poison Centers in Texas, 1998–2002. J Toxicol Clin Toxicol 2004;42:55. [PMID: 15083937]

CLONIDINE & OTHER SYMPATHOLYTIC ANTIHYPERTENSIVES

Overdosage with these agents (clonidine, guanabenz, guanfacine, methyldopa) causes bradycardia, hypotension, miosis, respiratory depression, and coma. (Transient hypertension occasionally occurs after clonidine overdosage, a result of peripheral α-adrenergic effects of this drug in high doses.) Symptoms are usually resolved in less than 24 hours, and deaths are rare. Similar symptoms may occur after ingestion of topical nasal decongestants chemically similar to clonidine (oxymetazoline, tetrahydrozoline, naphazoline). Brimonidine is used as an ophthalmic preparation for glaucoma. Tizanidine is a centrally acting muscle relaxant structurally related to clonidine; it produces similar toxicity in overdose.

Treatment

A. EMERGENCY AND SUPPORTIVE MEASURES

Give activated charcoal (see p 1644). Maintain the airway and support respiration if necessary. Symptomatic treatment is usually sufficient even in massive overdose. Maintain blood pressure with intravenous fluids. Dopamine can also be used. Atropine is usually effective for bradycardia.

B. SPECIFIC TREATMENT

There is no specific antidote. Although tolazoline has been recommended for clonidine overdose, its effects are unpredictable and it should not be used. Naloxone has been reported to be successful in a few anecdotal and poorly substantiated cases.

Spiller HA et al: Retrospective review of tizanidine (Zanaflex) overdose. J Toxicol Clin Toxicol 2004;42:593. [PMID: 15462150]

Spiller HA et al: Toxic clonidine ingestion in children. J Pediatr 2005;146:263. [PMID: 15689921]

COCAINE

See Amphetamines & Cocaine, above.

CYANIDE

Cyanide is a highly toxic chemical used widely in research and commercial laboratories and many industries. Its gaseous form, hydrogen cyanide, is an important component of smoke in fires. Cyanide-generating glycosides are also found in the pits of apricots and other related plants. Cyanide is generated by the breakdown of nitroprusside, and poisoning can result from rapid high-dose infusions. Cyanide is also formed by metabolism of acetonitrile, a solvent found in some over-the-counter fingernail glue removers. Cyanide is rapidly absorbed by inhalation, skin absorption, or ingestion. It disrupts cellular function by inhibiting cytochrome oxidase and preventing cellular oxygen utilization.

Clinical Findings

The onset of toxicity is nearly instantaneous after inhalation of hydrogen cyanide gas but may be delayed for minutes to hours after ingestion of cyanide salts or cyanogenic plants or chemicals. Effects include headache, dizziness, nausea, abdominal pain, and anxiety, followed by confusion, syncope, shock, seizures, coma, and death. The odor of "bitter almonds" may be detected on the victim's breath or in vomitus, though this is not a reliable finding. The venous oxygen saturation may be elevated (> 90%) in severe poisonings because tissues have failed to take up arterial oxygen.

Treatment

A. EMERGENCY AND SUPPORTIVE MEASURES

Remove the victim from exposure, taking care to avoid exposure to rescuers. For suspected cyanide poisoning due to nitroprusside infusion, stop or slow the rate of infusion. (Metabolic acidosis and other signs of cyanide poisoning usually clear rapidly.)

For cyanide ingestion, administer activated charcoal (see p 1644). Although charcoal has a low affinity for cyanide, the usual doses of 60–100 g are adequate to bind typically ingested lethal doses (100–200 mg).

B. SPECIFIC TREATMENT

In the United States, the cyanide antidote package (Taylor Pharmaceuticals) (Table 39–9) contains nitrites (to induce methemoglobinemia, which binds free cyanide) and thiosulfate (to promote conversion of cyanide to the less toxic thiocyanate). Administer amyl nitrite by crushing an ampule under the victim's nose or at the end of the endotracheal tube, and administer 3% sodium nitrite solution, 10 mL intravenously. **Caution:** Nitrites may induce hypotension and dangerous levels of methemoglobin. Also administer 25% sodium thiosulfate solution, 50 mL intravenously (12.5 g).

Gracia R et al: Cyanide poisoning and its treatment. Pharmacotherapy 2004;24:1358. [PMID: 15628833]

Mannaioni G et al: Acute cyanide intoxication treated with a combination of hydroxycobalamin, sodium nitrite, and sodium thiosulfate. J Toxicol Clin Toxicol 2002;40:181. [PMID: 12126191]

Table 39–9. Currently available (prepackaged) cyanide antidotes.

Antidote	How Supplied	Dose
Amyl nitrite[1]	0.3 mL (aspirol inhalant)	Break one or two aspirols under patient's nose.
Sodium nitrite[1]	3 g/dL (300 mg in 10 mL vials)	6 mg/kg IV (0.2 mL/kg)
Sodium thiosulfate[1]	25 g/dL (12.5 g in 50 mL vials)	250 mg/kg IV (1 mL/kg)

[1]In the United States, manufactured by Taylor Pharmaceuticals.

DIGITALIS & OTHER CARDIAC GLYCOSIDES

Cardiac glycosides are derived from a variety of plants and are widely used to treat heart failure and supraventricular arrhythmias. These drugs paralyze the Na^+-K^+-ATPase pump and have potent vagotonic effects. Intracellular effects include enhancement of calcium-dependent contractility and shortening of the action potential duration. Digoxin and ouabain are highly tissue-bound, but digitoxin has a volume of distribution of just 0.6 L/kg, making it the only cardiac glycoside accessible to enhanced removal procedures such as hemoperfusion or repeated doses of activated charcoal. There are a number of plants (eg, oleander, foxglove, lily-of-the-valley) that contain cardiac glycosides. Bufotenin, a cardiotoxic steroid found in certain toad secretions and used as an herbal medicine and a purported aphrodisiac, has pharmacologic properties similar to cardiac glycosides.

Clinical Findings

Intoxication may result from acute single exposure or chronic accidental overmedication. After acute overdosage, nausea and vomiting, bradycardia, hyperkalemia, and AV block frequently occur. Patients in whom toxicity develops gradually during long-term therapy are often hypokalemic and hypomagnesemic owing to concurrent diuretic treatment and more commonly present with ventricular arrhythmias (eg, ectopy, bidirectional ventricular tachycardia, or ventricular fibrillation). Digoxin levels may be only slightly elevated in patients with intoxication from cardiac glycosides other than digoxin because of limited cross-reactivity of immunologic tests.

Treatment

A. EMERGENCY AND SUPPORTIVE MEASURES

Maintain a patent airway and assist ventilation, if necessary. Monitor potassium levels and cardiac rhythm closely. Treat ventricular arrhythmias initially with lidocaine (2–3 mg/kg intravenously) or phenytoin (10–15 mg/kg intravenously slowly over 30 minutes) and treat bradycardia initially with atropine (0.5–2 mg intravenously) or a transcutaneous external cardiac pacemaker.

After acute ingestion, administer activated charcoal (see p 1644).

B. SPECIFIC TREATMENT

For patients with significant intoxication, administer digoxin-specific antibodies (digoxin immune Fab [ovine]; Digibind or DigiFab). Estimation of the Digibind dose is based on the body burden of digoxin calculated from the ingested dose or the steady-state serum digoxin concentration:

1. From the ingested dose—Number of vials = approximately 1.5 % ingested dose (mg).

2. From the serum concentration—Number of vials = serum digoxin (ng/mL) % body weight (kg) % 10^{-2}. **Note:** This is based on the equilibrium digoxin level; after acute overdose, serum levels are falsely high before tissue distribution is complete, and overestimation of the Digibind or DigiFab dose is likely.

3. Empiric dosing—Empiric dosing of Digibind or DigiFab may be used if the patient's condition is relatively stable and an underlying condition (eg, atrial fibrillation) suggests a residual level of digitalis activity. Start with one or two vials and reassess the clinical condition after 20–30 minutes. For cardiac glycosides other than digoxin or digitoxin, there is no formula for estimation of vials needed and treatment is empiric.

Note: After administration of digoxin-specific Fab antibody fragment, serum digoxin levels may be falsely elevated depending on the assay technique.

Barrueto F Jr et al: Cardioactive steroid poisoning from an herbal cleansing preparation. Ann Emerg Med 2003;41:396. [PMID: 12605208]

Bateman DN: Digoxin-specific antibody fragments: how much and when? Toxicol Rev 2004;23:135. [PMID: 15862081]

Husby P et al: Immediate control of life-threatening digoxin intoxication in a child by use of digoxin-specific antibody fragments (Fab). Paediatr Anaesth 2003;13:541. [PMID: 12846714]

ETHANOL, BARBITURATES, BENZODIAZEPINES, & OTHER SEDATIVE-HYPNOTIC AGENTS

The group of agents known as sedative-hypnotic drugs includes a variety of products used for the treatment of anxiety, depression, insomnia, and epilepsy. Ethanol and other selected agents are also popular recreational drugs. All of these drugs depress the central nervous system reticular activating system, cerebral cortex, and cerebellum.

Clinical Findings

Mild intoxication produces euphoria, slurred speech, and ataxia. Ethanol intoxication may produce hypoglycemia, even at relatively low concentrations. With more severe intoxication, stupor, coma, and respiratory arrest may occur. Carisoprodol commonly causes muscle jerking or myoclonus. Death or serious morbidity is usually the result of pulmonary aspiration of gastric contents. Bradycardia, hypotension, and hypothermia are common. Patients with massive intoxication may appear to be dead, with no reflex responses and even absent electroencephalographic activity. Diagnosis and assessment of severity of intoxication are usually based on clinical findings. Ethanol serum levels greater than 300 mg/dL (0.3 g/dL; 65 mmol/L) usually produce coma in persons who are not chronically abusing the drug, but regular users may remain awake at much higher levels. Phenobarbital levels greater than 100 mg/L usually cause coma.

Treatment

A. EMERGENCY AND SUPPORTIVE MEASURES

Administer activated charcoal (see p 1644). Repeat-dose charcoal may enhance elimination of phenobarbital, but it has not been proved to improve clinical outcome. Hemodialysis may be necessary for patients with severe phenobarbital intoxication.

B. SPECIFIC TREATMENT

Flumazenil is a benzodiazepine receptor-specific antagonist; it has no effect on ethanol, barbiturates, or other sedative-hypnotic agents. If used, flumazenil is given slowly intravenously, 0.2 mg over 30–60 seconds, repeated in 0.5 mg increments as needed up to a total dose of 3–5 mg. **Caution:** Flumazenil may induce seizures in patients with preexisting seizure disorder, benzodiazepine addiction, or concomitant tricyclic antidepressant overdose. If seizures occur, diazepam and other benzodiazepine anticonvulsants will not be effective. As with naloxone, the duration of action of flumazenil is short (2–3 hours) and resedation may occur, requiring repeated doses.

Isbister GK et al: Alprazolam is relatively more toxic than other benzodiazepines in overdose. Br J Clin Pharmacol 2004;58:88. [PMID: 15206998]

Olshaker JS et al: Flumazenil reversal of lorazepam-induced acute delirium. J Emerg Med 2003;24:181. [PMID: 12609649]

Seger DL: Flumazenil—treatment or toxin. J Toxicol Clin Toxicol 2004;42:209. [PMID: 15214628]

γ-HYDROXYBUTYRATE

GHB has become a popular drug of abuse. It originated as a short-acting general anesthetic and is occasionally used in the treatment of narcolepsy. It gained popularity among bodybuilders for its alleged growth hormone stimulation and found its way into social settings, where it is consumed as a liquid. It has been used to facilitate sexual assault ("date-rape" drug). Symptoms after ingestion include drowsiness and lethargy followed by coma with respiratory depression. Muscle twitching and seizures are sometimes observed. Recovery is usually rapid, with patients awakening within a few hours. Other related chemicals with similar effects include butanediol and γ-butyrolactone (GBL). A prolonged withdrawal syndrome has been described in some heavy users.

Treatment

For recent ingestions, give activated charcoal orally or by gastric tube (see p 1644). There is no specific treatment. Most patients recover rapidly with supportive care. GHB withdrawal syndrome may require very large doses of benzodiazepines.

Anderson IB et al: Trends in gamma-hydroxybutyrate (GHB) intoxication: 1999-2003. Ann Emerg Med 2006;47:177. [PMID: 16431231]

Lora-Tamayo C et al: Intoxication due to 1,4-butanediol. Forensic Sci Int 2003;133:256. [PMID: 12787662]

Mason PE et al: Gamma hydroxybutyric acid (GHB) intoxication. Acad Emerg Med 2002;9:730. [PMID: 12093716]

Tarabar AF et al: The gamma-hydroxybutyrate withdrawal syndrome. Toxicol Rev 2004;23:45. [PMID: 15298492]

IRON

Iron is widely used therapeutically for the treatment of anemia and as a daily supplement in multiple vitamin preparations. Most children's preparations contain about 12–15 mg of elemental iron (as sulfate, gluconate, or fumarate salt) per dose, compared with 60–90 mg in most adult-strength preparations. Iron is corrosive to the gastrointestinal tract and, once absorbed, has depressant effects on the myocardium and on peripheral vascular resistance. Intracellular toxic effects of iron include disruption of Krebs cycle enzymes.

Clinical Findings

Ingestion of less than 30 mg/kg of elemental iron usually produces only mild gastrointestinal upset. Ingestion of more than 40–60 mg/kg may cause vomiting (sometimes with hematemesis), diarrhea, hypotension, and acidosis. Death may occur as a result of profound hypotension due to massive fluid losses and bleeding, metabolic acidosis, peritonitis from intestinal perforation, or sepsis. Fulminant hepatic failure may occur. Survivors of the acute ingestion may suffer permanent gastrointestinal scarring.

Serum iron levels greater than 350–500 mcg/dL are considered potentially toxic, and levels over 1000 mcg/dL are usually associated with severe poisoning. A plain abdominal x-ray may reveal radiopaque tablets.

Treatment

A. EMERGENCY AND SUPPORTIVE MEASURES

Maintain a patent airway and assist ventilation if necessary. Treat hypotension aggressively with intravenous crystalloid solutions (0.9% saline or lactated Ringer's solution). Fluid losses may be massive owing to vomiting and diarrhea as well as third-spacing into injured intestine.

Perform whole bowel irrigation to remove unabsorbed pills from the intestinal tract (see p 1644). Activated charcoal is not effective but may be appropriate if other ingestants are suspected.

B. SPECIFIC TREATMENT

Deferoxamine is a selective iron chelator. It is not useful as an oral binding agent. For patients with established manifestations of toxicity—and particularly those with markedly elevated serum iron levels (eg, greater than 800–1000 mcg/dL)—administer 10–15 mg/kg/h by constant intravenous infusion; higher doses (up to 40–50 mg/kg/h) have been used in massive poisonings. Hypotension may occur. The presence of an iron-deferoxamine complex in the urine may give it a "vin rosé" appearance. Deferoxamine is safe for use in pregnant women with acute iron overdose. **Caution:** Prolonged infusion of deferoxamine (> 36–48 hours) has been associated with development of acute respiratory distress syndrome (ARDS)—the mechanism is not known.

Bar-Oz B et al: Medications that can be fatal for a toddler with one tablet or teaspoonful: a 2004 update. Paediatr Drugs 2004;6:123. [PMID: 15035652]

Manoguerra AS et al: Iron ingestion: an evidence-based consensus guideline for out-of-hospital management. Clin Toxicol (Phila) 2005;43:553. [PMID: 16255338]

ISONIAZID

Isoniazid (INH) is an antibacterial drug used mainly in the treatment and prevention of tuberculosis. It may cause hepatitis with long-term use, especially in alcoholic patients and elderly persons. It produces acute toxic effects by competing with pyridoxal 5-phosphate, resulting in lowered brain γ-aminobutyric acid (GABA) levels. Acute ingestion of as little as 1.5–2 g of INH can cause toxicity, and severe poisoning is likely to occur after ingestion of more than 80–100 mg/kg.

Clinical Findings

Confusion, slurred speech, and seizures may occur abruptly after acute overdose. Severe lactic acidosis—out of proportion to the severity of seizures—is probably due to inhibited metabolism of lactate. Peripheral neuropathy and acute hepatitis may occur with long-term use.

Diagnosis is based on a history of ingestion and the presence of severe acidosis associated with seizures. Isoniazid is not usually included in routine toxicologic screening, and serum levels are not readily available.

Treatment

A. EMERGENCY AND SUPPORTIVE MEASURES

Seizures may require higher than usual doses of benzodiazepines (eg, lorazepam, 3–5 mg intravenously) or administration of pyridoxine as an antidote (see below).

Administer activated charcoal (see p 1644). Do *not* induce emesis, because of the risk of abrupt onset of seizures.

B. Specific Treatment

Pyridoxine (vitamin B_6) is a specific antagonist of the acute toxic effects of INH and is usually successful in controlling convulsions that do not respond to benzodiazepines. Give 5 g intravenously over 1–2 minutes or, if the amount ingested is known, give a gram-for-gram equivalent amount of pyridoxine. Patients taking INH are usually given 10–20 mg of pyridoxine orally daily to help prevent neuropathy.

Huang YS et al: Cytochrome P450 2E1 genotype and the susceptibility to antituberculosis drug-induced hepatitis. Hepatology 2003;37:924. [PMID: 12668988]

Topcu I et al: Seizures, metabolic acidosis and coma resulting from acute isoniazid intoxication. Anaesth Intensive Care 2005;33:518. [PMID: 16119496]

LEAD

Lead is used in a variety of industrial and commercial products, such as storage batteries, solders, paints, pottery, plumbing, and gasoline and is found in some traditional Hispanic and Ayurvedic ethnic medicines. Lead toxicity usually results from chronic repeated exposure and is rare after a single ingestion. Lead produces a variety of adverse effects on cellular function and primarily affects the nervous system, gastrointestinal tract, and hematopoietic system.

Clinical Findings

Lead poisoning often goes undiagnosed initially because presenting symptoms and signs are nonspecific and exposure is not suspected. Common symptoms include colicky abdominal pain, constipation, headache, and irritability. Severe poisoning may cause coma and convulsions. Chronic intoxication can cause learning disorders (in children) and motor neuropathy (eg, wrist drop). Lead-containing bullet fragments in or near joint spaces can result in chronic lead toxicity.

Diagnosis is based on measurement of the blood lead level. Whole blood lead levels less than 10 mcg/dL are usually considered nontoxic. Levels between 10 and 25 mcg/dL have been associated with impaired neurobehavioral development in children. Levels of 25–50 mcg/dL may be associated with headache, irritability, and subclinical neuropathy. Levels of 50–70 mcg/dL are associated with moderate toxicity, and levels greater than 70–100 mcg/dL are often associated with severe poisoning. Other laboratory findings of lead poisoning include microcytic anemia with basophilic stippling and elevated free erythrocyte protoporphyrin.

Treatment

A. Emergency and Supportive Measures

For patients with encephalopathy, maintain a patent airway and treat coma and convulsions as described at the beginning of this chapter.

For recent acute ingestion, if a large lead-containing object (eg, fishing weight) is still visible in the stomach on abdominal x-ray, repeated cathartics (see p 1644), whole bowel irrigation (see p 1644), endoscopy, or even surgical removal may be necessary to prevent subacute lead poisoning. (The acidic gastric contents may corrode the metal surface, enhancing lead absorption. Once the object passes into the small intestine, the risk of toxicity declines.)

Conduct an investigation into the source of the lead exposure.

Workers with a single lead level greater than 60 mcg/dL (or three successive monthly levels greater than 50 mcg/dL) or construction workers with any single blood lead level greater than 50 mcg/dL must by federal law be removed from the site of exposure. Contact the regional office of the United States Occupational Safety and Health Administration (OSHA) for more information. Several states mandate reporting of cases of confirmed lead poisoning.

B. Specific Treatment

The indications for chelation depend on the blood lead level and the patient's clinical state. A medical toxicologist or regional poison control center (800-222-1222) should be consulted for advice about selection and use of these antidotes.

Note: It is impermissible under the law to treat asymptomatic workers with elevated blood lead levels in order to keep their levels under 50 mcg/dL rather than remove them from the exposure.

1. Severe toxicity—Patients with severe intoxication (encephalopathy or levels greater than 70–100 mcg/dL) should receive edetate calcium disodium (ethylenediaminetetraacetic acid, EDTA), 1500 mg/m^2/kg/d (approximately 50 mg/kg/d) in four to six divided doses or as a continuous intravenous infusion. Some clinicians also add dimercaprol (BAL), 4–5 mg/kg intramuscularly every 4 hours for 5 days.

2. Less severe toxicity—Patients with less severe symptoms and asymptomatic patients with blood lead levels between 55 and 69 mcg/dL may be treated with edetate calcium disodium alone in dosages as above. An oral chelator, succimer (DMSA), is available for use in patients with mild to moderate intoxication. The usual dose is 10 mg/kg orally every 8 hours for 5 days, then every 12 hours for 2 weeks.

Brewster UC et al: A review of chronic lead intoxication: an unrecognized cause of chronic kidney disease. Am J Med Sci 2004;327:341. [PMID: 15201648]

Needleman H: Lead poisoning. Annu Rev Med 2004;55:209. [PMID: 14746518]

Weide R et al: Severe lead poisoning due to Ayurvedic Indian plant medicine. Dtsch Med Wochenschr 2003;128:2418. [PMID: 14614655]

LSD & OTHER HALLUCINOGENS

A variety of substances—ranging from naturally occurring plants and mushrooms to synthetic substances such as PCP, toluene and other solvents, and lysergic acid diethylamide (LSD)—are abused for their hallucinogenic properties. The mechanism of toxicity and the clinical effects vary for each substance.

Many hallucinogenic plants and mushrooms produce anticholinergic delirium, characterized by flushed skin, dry mucous membranes, dilated pupils, tachycardia, and urinary retention. Other plants and mushrooms may contain hallucinogenic indoles such as mescaline and LSD, which typically cause marked visual hallucinations and perceptual distortion, widely dilated pupils, and mild tachycardia. PCP, a dissociative anesthetic agent similar to ketamine, can produce fluctuating delirium and coma, often associated with vertical and horizontal nystagmus. Toluene and other hydrocarbon solvents (butane, trichloroethylene, "chemo," etc) cause euphoria and delirium and may sensitize the myocardium to the effects of catecholamines, leading to fatal dysrhythmias.

Treatment

A. EMERGENCY AND SUPPORTIVE MEASURES

Maintain a patent airway and assist respirations if necessary. Treat coma, hyperthermia, and seizures as outlined at the beginning of this chapter. For recent large ingestions, consider giving activated charcoal orally or by gastric tube.

B. SPECIFIC TREATMENT

Patients with anticholinergic delirium may benefit from a dose of physostigmine, 0.5–1 mg intravenously, not to exceed 1 mg/min. Dysphoria, agitation, and psychosis associated with LSD or mescaline intoxication may respond to benzodiazepines (eg, lorazepam, 1–2 mg orally or intravenously) or haloperidol (2–5 mg intramuscularly or intravenously). Monitor patients who have sniffed solvents for cardiac dysrhythmias (most commonly premature ventricular contractions, ventricular tachycardia, ventricular fibrillation); treatment with β-blockers such as propranolol (1–5 mg intravenously) or esmolol (250–500 mcg/kg intravenously, then 50 mcg/kg/min by infusion) may be more effective than lidocaine.

Gertsch JH et al: Case report: an ingestion of Hawaiian Baby Woodrose seeds associated with acute psychosis. Hawaii Med J 2003;62:127. [PMID: 12886727]

Tang HL: Renal tubular acidosis and severe hypophosphataemia due to toluene inhalation. Hong Kong Med J 2005;11:1:50. [PMID: 15687517]

MERCURY

Acute mercury poisoning usually occurs by ingestion of inorganic mercuric salts or inhalation of metallic mercury vapor. Ingestion of the mercuric salts causes a burning sensation in the throat, discoloration and edema of oral mucous membranes, abdominal pain, vomiting, bloody diarrhea, and shock. Direct nephro-toxicity causes acute renal failure. Inhalation of high concentrations of metallic mercury vapor may cause acute fulminant chemical pneumonia. Chronic mercury poisoning causes weakness, ataxia, intention tremors, irritability, and depression. Exposure to alkyl (organic) mercury derivatives from contaminated fish or fungicides used on seeds has caused ataxia, tremors, convulsions, and catastrophic birth defects.

Treatment

A. ACUTE POISONING

There is no effective specific treatment for mercury vapor pneumonitis. Remove ingested mercuric salts by lavage, and administer activated charcoal (see p 1644). For acute ingestion of mercuric salts, give dimercaprol (BAL) at once, as for arsenic poisoning. Unless the patient has severe gastroenteritis, consider succimer (DMSA), 10 mg/kg orally every 8 hours for 5 days and then every 12 hours for 2 weeks. Unithiol is a chelator that can be given orally or parenterally, but is not commonly available In the United States. Maintain urinary output. Treat oliguria and anuria if they occur.

B. CHRONIC POISONING

Remove from exposure. Neurologic toxicity is not considered reversible with chelation, although some authors recommend a trial of succimer or uniothiol (contact a regional poison center or medical toxicologist for advice).

Johnson CL: Mercury in the environment: sources, toxicities, and prevention of exposure. Pediatr Ann 2004;33:437. [PMID: 15298308]

Saper RB et al: Heavy metal content of ayurvedic herbal medicine products. JAMA 2004;292:2868. [PMID: 15598918]

Weil M et al: Blood mercury levels and neurobehavioral function. JAMA 2005;293:1875. [PMID: 15840862]

Wilson JF: Balancing the risks and benefits of fish consumption. Ann Intern Med 2004;141:977. [PMID: 15611502]

METHANOL & ETHYLENE GLYCOL

Methanol (wood alcohol) is commonly found in a variety of products, including solvents, duplicating fluids, record cleaning solutions, and paint removers. It is sometimes ingested intentionally by alcoholic patients as a substitute for ethanol and may also be found as a contaminant in bootleg whiskey. Ethylene glycol is the major constituent in most antifreeze compounds. The toxicity of both agents is caused by metabolism to highly toxic organic acids—methanol to formic acid; ethylene glycol to glycolic and oxalic acids.

Clinical Findings

Shortly after ingestion of either of these agents, patients usually appear "drunk." The serum osmolality (measured with the freezing point device) is usually increased, but acidosis is often absent early. After several hours, metabolism to toxic organic acids leads to a severe anion gap metabolic acidosis, tachypnea, confusion, convulsions, and coma. Methanol intoxication frequently causes visual disturbances, while ethylene glycol often produces oxalate crystalluria and renal failure.

Treatment

A. EMERGENCY AND SUPPORTIVE MEASURES

For patients presenting within 30–60 minutes after ingestion, empty the stomach by gastric lavage (see p 1643). Charcoal is not very effective but should be administered if other poisons or drugs have also been ingested.

B. SPECIFIC TREATMENT

Patients with significant toxicity (manifested by severe metabolic acidosis, altered mental status, serum methanol or ethylene glycol level > 50 mg/dL, or osmolar gap > 10 mosm/L) should undergo hemodialysis as soon as possible to remove the parent compound and the toxic metabolites. Treatment with folic acid, thiamine, and pyridoxine may enhance the breakdown of toxic metabolites.

Ethanol blocks metabolism of the parent compounds by competing for the enzyme alcohol dehydrogenase. The desired serum ethanol concentration is 100 mg/dL. To achieve this, administer a loading dose of approximately 750 mg/kg orally or in a dilute intravenous solution (available from the pharmacy in 5% and 10% solution), and then provide a maintenance infusion of 100–150 mg/kg/h. The infusion will have to be increased to about 175–250 mg/kg/h during hemodialysis to replace dialysis elimination of ethanol. Fomepizole (4-methylpyrazole; Antizol) blocks alcohol dehydrogenase and can be used instead of ethanol. A regional poison control center (800-222-1222) should be contacted for indications and dosing.

Megarbane B et al: Current recommendations for treatment of severe toxic alcohol poisonings. Intensive Care Med 2005;31: 189. Epub 2004 Dec 31. [PMID: 15627163]

Mycyk MB et al: Antidote review: fomepizole for methanol poisoning. Am J Ther 2003;10:68. [PMID: 12522524]

METHEMOGLOBINEMIA-INDUCING AGENTS

A large number of chemical agents are capable of oxidizing ferrous hemoglobin to its ferric state (methemoglobin), a form that cannot carry oxygen. Drugs and chemicals known to cause methemoglobinemia include benzocaine (a local anesthetic found in some topical anesthetic sprays and a variety of nonprescription products), aniline, nitrites, nitrogen oxide gases, nitrobenzene, dapsone, phenazopyridine (Pyridium), and many others. Dapsone has a long elimination half-life and may produce prolonged or recurrent methemoglobinemia.

Clinical Findings

Methemoglobinemia reduces oxygen-carrying capacity and may cause dizziness, nausea, headache, dyspnea, confusion, seizures, and coma. The severity of symptoms depends on the percentage of hemoglobin oxidized to methemoglobin; severe poisoning is usually present when methemoglobin fractions are greater than 40–50%. Even at low levels (15–20%), victims appear cyanotic because of the "chocolate brown" color of methemoglobin, but they have normal P_{O_2} results on arterial blood gas determinations. Pulse oximetry gives inaccurate oxygen saturation measurements; the reading is often between 85% and 90%. Severe metabolic acidosis may be present. Hemolysis may occur, especially in patients susceptible to oxidant stress (ie, those with glucose-6-phosphate dehydrogenase deficiency).

Treatment

A. EMERGENCY AND SUPPORTIVE MEASURES

Administer high-flow oxygen. If the causative agent was recently ingested, administer activated charcoal (see p 1644). Repeat-dose activated charcoal may enhance dapsone elimination (see p 1645).

B. SPECIFIC TREATMENT

Methylene blue enhances the conversion of methemoglobin to hemoglobin by increasing the activity of the enzyme methemoglobin reductase. For symptomatic patients, administer 1–2 mg/kg (0.1–0.2 mL/kg of 1% solution) intravenously. The dose may be repeated once in 15–20 minutes if necessary. Patients with hereditary methemoglobin reductase deficiency or glucose-6-phosphate dehydrogenase deficiency may not respond to methylene blue treatment.

Armstrong C et al: Benzocaine-induced methemoglobinemia: a condition of which all endoscopists should be aware. Can J Gastroenterol 2004;18:625. [PMID: 15497003]

Bradberry SM: Occupational methaemoglobinaemia. Mechanisms of production, features, diagnosis and management including the use of methylene blue. Toxicol Rev 2003;22: 13. [PMID: 14579544]

MONOAMINE OXIDASE INHIBITORS

Overdoses of MAO inhibitors (isocarboxazid, phenelzine, selegiline, moclobemide) cause ataxia, excitement, hypertension, and tachycardia, followed several hours later by hypotension, convulsions, and hyperthermia.

Ingestion of tyramine-containing foods may cause a severe hypertensive reaction in patients taking MAO inhibitors. Foods containing tyramine include aged cheese and red wines. Hypertensive reactions may also occur with any sympathomimetic drug. Severe or fatal hyperthermia (serotonin syndrome) may occur if patients receiving MAO inhibitors are given meperidine, fluoxetine, paroxetine, fluvoxamine, venlafaxine, tryptophan, dextromethor-

Table 39–10. Poisonous mushrooms.

Toxin	Genus	Symptoms and Signs	Onset	Treatment
Amanitin	*Amanita (A phalloides, A verna, A virosa)*	Severe gastroenteritis followed by delayed hepatic and renal failure after 48–72 hours	6–24 hours	Supportive. Correct dehydration. Give repeated doses of activated charcoal orally. Consider silymarin (see text)
Muscarine	*Inocybe, Clitocybe*	Muscarinic (salivation, miosis, bradycardia, diarrhea)	30–60 minutes	Supportive. Give atropine, 0.5–2 mg intravenously, for severe cholinergic symptoms and signs.
Ibotenic acid, muscimol	*Amanita muscaria* ('fly agaric')	Anticholinergic (mydriasis, tachycardia, hyperpyrexia, delirium)	30–60 minutes	Supportive. Give physostigmine, 0.5–2 mg intravenously, for severe anticholinergic symptoms and signs.
Coprine	*Coprinus*	Disulfiram-like effect occurs with ingestion of ethanol	30–60 minutes	Supportive. Abstain from ethanol for 3–4 days.
Monomethyl-hydrazine	*Gyromitra*	Gastroenteritis; occasionally hemolysis, hepatic and renal failure	6–12 hours	Supportive. Correct dehydration. Pyridoxine, 2.5 mg/kg intravenously, may be helpful.
Orellanine	*Cortinarius*	Nausea, vomiting; renal failure after 1–3 weeks	2–14 days	Supportive.
Psilocybin	*Psilocybe*	Hallucinations	15–30 minutes	Supportive.
Gastrointestinal irritants	Many species	Nausea and vomiting, diarrhea	$1/2$–2 hours	Supportive. Correct dehydration.

phan, tramadol, or other serotonin-enhancing drugs. This reaction can also occur with the newer selective MAO inhibitor moclobemide, and the antibiotic linezolid, which has MAO-inhibiting properties. The serotonin syndrome has also been reported in patients taking selective serotonin reuptake inhibitors (SSRIs) in large doses or in combination with other SSRIs, even in the absence of an MAO inhibitor or meperidine.

Treatment

Administer activated charcoal (see p 1644). Treat severe hypertension with nitroprusside, phentolamine, or other rapid-acting vasodilators (see p 1641). Treat hypotension with fluids and positioning, but avoid use of pressor agents if possible. Observe patients for at least 24 hours, since hyperthermic reactions may be delayed. Treat hyperthermia with aggressive cooling; neuromuscular paralysis may be required (see p 1642). Cyproheptadine, 4 mg orally (or by gastric tube) every hour for three or four doses, has been reported to be effective against serotonin syndrome.

Boyer EW et al: The serotonin syndrome. N Engl J Med 2005; 352:1112. [PMID: 15784664]

Gillman PK: Monoamine oxidase inhibitors, opioid analgesics and serotonin toxicity. Br J Anaesth 2005;95:434. Epub 2005 Jul 28. [PMID: 16051647]

MUSHROOMS

There are thousands of mushroom species that cause a variety of toxic effects. The most dangerous species of mushrooms are *Amanita phalloides*, *Amanita verna*, *Amanita virosa*, *Gyromitra esculenta*, and the *Galerina* species, all of which contain amatoxin, a potent cytotoxin. Ingestion of even a portion of one mushroom of a dangerous species may be sufficient to cause death.

The characteristic pathologic finding in fatalities from amatoxin-containing mushroom poisoning is acute massive necrosis of the liver.

Clinical Findings (Table 39–10)

A. SYMPTOMS AND SIGNS

1. Amatoxin-type cyclopeptides—(*A phalloides, A verna, A virosa,* and *Galerina* species.) After a latent interval of 8–12 hours, severe abdominal cramps and vomiting begin and progress to profuse diarrhea, followed in 1–2 days by hepatic necrosis, hepatic encephalopathy, and frequently renal failure. The fatality rate is about 20%. Cooking the mushrooms does not prevent poisoning.

2. Gyromitrin type—(*Gyromitra* and *Helvella* species.) Toxicity is more common following ingestion of uncooked mushrooms. Vomiting, diarrhea, hepatic necrosis, convulsions, coma, and hemolysis may occur after a latent period of 8–12 hours. The fatality rate is probably less than 10%.

3. Muscarinic type—(*Inocybe* and *Clitocybe* species.) Vomiting, diarrhea, bradycardia, hypotension, salivation, miosis, bronchospasm, and lacrimation occur shortly after ingestion. Cardiac arrhythmias may occur. Fatalities are rare.

4. Anticholinergic type—(Eg, *Amanita muscaria, Amanita pantherina.*) This type causes a variety of symptoms that may be atropine-like, including excitement, delirium, flushed skin, dilated pupils, and muscular jerking tremors, beginning 1–2 hours after ingestion. Fatalities are rare.

5. Gastrointestinal irritant type—(Eg, *Boletus, Cantharellus.*) Nausea, vomiting, and diarrhea occur shortly after ingestion. Fatalities are rare.

6. Disulfiram type—(*Coprinus* species.) Disulfiram-like sensitivity to alcohol may persist for several days. Toxicity is characterized by flushing, hypotension, and vomiting after coingestion of alcohol.

7. Hallucinogenic—(*Psilocybe* and *Panaeolus* species.) Mydriasis, nausea and vomiting, and intense visual hallucinations occur 1–2 hours after ingestion. Fatalities are rare.

8. *Cortinarius orellanus*—This mushroom may cause acute renal failure due to tubulointerstitial nephritis. *Amanita smithiana* has also been reported to cause acute renal failure.

Treatment

A. EMERGENCY MEASURES

After the onset of symptoms, efforts to remove the toxic agent are probably useless, especially in cases of amatoxin or gyromitrin poisoning, where there is usually a delay of 12 hours or more before symptoms occur and patients seek medical attention. However, induction of vomiting or administration of activated charcoal is recommended for any recent ingestion of an unidentified or potentially toxic mushroom (see p 1644).

B. GENERAL MEASURES

1. Amatoxin-type cyclopeptides—A variety of antidotes (eg, thioctic acid, penicillin, corticosteroids) have been suggested for amatoxin-type mushroom poisoning, but controlled studies are lacking and experimental data in animals are equivocal. Aggressive fluid replacement for diarrhea and intensive supportive care for hepatic failure are the mainstays of treatment. Silymarin (a derivative of milk thistle) is commonly used in Europe (20 mg/kg over 24 hours given in four 2-hour infusions) and has recently become available in the United States (Apothecare, 1-800-969-6601).

Interruption of enterohepatic circulation of the amatoxin by the administration of activated charcoal and laxatives may be of value. However, by the time this method is used, most of the amatoxin has already caused cellular damage and has already been excreted. Charcoal hemoperfusion has been recommended but is of unproved value.

Liver transplant may be the only hope for survival in gravely ill patients—contact a liver transplant center early.

2. Gyromitrin type—For gyromitrin poisoning, give pyridoxine, 25 mg/kg intravenously.

3. Muscarinic type—For mushrooms producing predominantly muscarinic-cholinergic symptoms, give atropine, 0.005–0.01 mg/kg intravenously, and repeat as needed.

4. Anticholinergic type—For anticholinergic type, physostigmine, 0.5–1 mg intravenously, may calm extremely agitated patients and reverse peripheral anticholinergic manifestations, but it may also cause bradycardia, asystole, and seizures. Alternately, use a benzodiazepine such as lorazepam, 1–2 mg intravenously.

5. Gastrointestinal irritant type—Treat with antiemetics and intravenous or oral fluids.

6. Disulfiram type—For *Coprinus* ingestion, avoid alcohol. Treat alcohol reaction with fluids and supine position.

7. Hallucinogenic type—Provide a quiet, supportive atmosphere. Diazepam or haloperidol may be used for sedation.

8. *Cortinarius*—Provide supportive care and hemodialysis as needed for renal failure.

Diaz JH: Syndromic diagnosis and management of confirmed mushroom poisonings. Crit Care Med 2005;33:427. [PMID: 15699849]

Enjalbert F et al: Treatment of amatoxin poisoning: 20-year retrospective analysis. J Toxicol Clin Toxicol 2002;40:715. [PMID: 12475187]

Ganzert M et al: Indication of liver transplantation following amatoxin intoxication. J Hepatol 2005;42:202. [PMID: 15664245]

OPIOIDS

Prescription and illicit opioids (morphine, heroin, codeine, oxycodone, propoxyphene, etc) are popular drugs of abuse and the cause of frequent hospitalizations for overdose. These drugs have widely varying potencies and durations of action; for example, some of the illicit fentanyl derivatives are up to 2000 times more potent than morphine. All of these agents decrease central nervous system activity and sympathetic outflow by acting on opiate receptors in the brain. Tramadol is a newer analgesic that is unrelated chemically to the opioids but acts on opioid receptors. Buprenorphine is a partial agonist-antagonist opioid recently introduced for the outpatient treatment of opioid addiction.

Clinical Findings

Mild intoxication is characterized by euphoria, drowsiness, and constricted pupils. More severe intoxication may cause hypotension, bradycardia, hypothermia, coma, and respiratory arrest. Pulmonary edema may occur. Death is usually due to apnea or pulmonary aspiration of gastric contents. Propoxyphene may cause seizures and prolongation of the QRS interval. Methadone has been associated with QT interval prolongation and torsade de pointes. Tramadol, dextromethorphan, and meperidine also occasionally cause seizures. With meperidine, the metabolite normeperidine is probably the cause of seizures and is most likely to accumulate with repeated dosing in patients with renal insufficiency. While the duration of effect for heroin is usually 3–5 hours, methadone intoxication may last for 48–72 hours or longer. Most opioids, with the exception of illicit newer fentanyl derivatives, tramadol, oxycodone, and methadone, are usually detectable on routine urine toxicology screening. Wound botulism has been associated with skin-popping, especially involving "black tar" heroin. Buprenorphine added to an opioid regimen may produce acute narcotic withdrawal symptoms.

Treatment

A. Emergency and Supportive Measures

Protect the airway and assist ventilation. Administer activated charcoal (see p 1644).

B. Specific Treatment

Naloxone is a specific opioid antagonist that can rapidly reverse signs of narcotic intoxication. Although it is structurally related to the opioids, it has no agonist effects of its own. Administer 0.4–2 mg intravenously, and repeat as needed to awaken the patient and maintain airway protective reflexes and spontaneous breathing. Very large doses (10–20 mg) may be required for patients intoxicated by some opioids (eg, propoxyphene, codeine, fentanyl derivatives). **Caution:** The duration of effect of naloxone is only about 2–3 hours; repeated doses may be necessary for patients intoxicated by long-acting drugs such as methadone. Continuous observation for at least 3 hours after the last naloxone dose is mandatory.

Buajordet I et al: Adverse events after naloxone treatment of episodes of suspected acute opioid overdose. Eur J Emerg Med 2004;11:19. [PMID: 15167188]

Clarke SF et al: Naloxone in opioid poisoning: walking the tightrope. Emerg Med J 2005;22:612. [PMID: 16113176]

Sporer KA: Buprenorphine: a primer for emergency physicians. Ann Emerg Med 2004;43:580. [PMID: 15111917]

Tharp AM et al: Fatal intravenous fentanyl abuse: four cases involving extraction of fentanyl from transdermal patches. Am J Forensic Med Pathol 2004;25:178. [PMID: 15166776]

PARAQUAT

Paraquat is used as a herbicide. Concentrated solutions of paraquat are highly corrosive to the oropharynx, esophagus, and stomach. The fatal dose after ab-

sorption may be as small as 4 mg/kg. If ingestion of paraquat is not rapidly fatal because of its corrosive effects, the herbicide may cause progressive pulmonary fibrosis, with death ensuing after 2–3 weeks. Patients with plasma paraquat levels above 2 mg/L at 6 hours or 0.2 mg/L at 24 hours are likely to die.

Treatment

Remove ingested paraquat by immediate induced emesis, or by gastric lavage if the patient is already in a health care facility (see p 1643). Clay (bentonite or fuller's earth) and activated charcoal are effective adsorbents. Administer repeated doses of 60 g of activated charcoal by gastric tube every 2 hours for at least three or four doses. Charcoal hemoperfusion, 8 hours per day for 2–3 weeks, has been anecdotally reported to be lifesaving, but clinical and animal studies are equivocal. Supplemental oxygen should be withheld unless the PO_2 is less than 70 mm Hg because oxygen may contribute to the pulmonary damage, which is mediated through lipid peroxidation.

Eddleston M et al: Prospects for treatment of paraquat-induced lung fibrosis with immunosuppressive drugs and the need for better prediction of outcome: a systematic review. QJM 2003;96:809. [PMID: 14566036]

Sittipunt C: Paraquat poisoning. Respir Care 2005;50:383. [PMID: 15779152]

PESTICIDES: CHOLINESTERASE INHIBITORS

Organophosphorus and carbamate insecticides (organophosphates: parathion, malathion, etc; carbamates: carbaryl, aldicarb, etc) are widely used in commercial agriculture and home gardening and have largely replaced older, more environmentally persistent organochlorine compounds such as DDT and chlordane. The organophosphates and carbamates—also called anticholinesterases because they inhibit the enzyme acetylcholinesterase—cause an increase in acetylcholine activity at nicotinic and muscarinic receptors and in the central nervous system. There are a variety of chemical agents in this group, with widely varying potencies. Most of them are poorly water-soluble, are formulated with an aromatic hydrocarbon solvent such as xylene, and are well absorbed through intact skin. Most chemical warfare "nerve agents" (see above) are organophosphates.

Clinical Findings

Inhibition of cholinesterase results in abdominal cramps, diarrhea, vomiting, excessive salivation, sweating, lacrimation, miosis (constricted pupils), wheezing and bronchorrhea, seizures, and skeletal muscle weakness. Initial tachycardia is usually followed by bradycardia. Profound skeletal muscle weakness, aggravated by excessive bronchial secretions and wheezing, may result in respiratory arrest and death. Symptoms and signs of poisoning may persist or recur over several days, especially with highly lipid-soluble agents such as fenthion or dimethoate.

The diagnosis should be suspected in patients who present with miosis, sweating, and hyperperistalsis. Serum and red blood cell cholinesterase activity can be measured in the laboratory and is usually depressed at least 50% below baseline in those victims who have severe intoxication.

Treatment

A. EMERGENCY AND SUPPORTIVE MEASURES

If the agent was recently ingested, empty the stomach by gastric lavage and administer activated charcoal (see p 1643). If the agent is on the victim's skin or hair, wash repeatedly with soap or shampoo and water. Providers must take care to avoid skin exposure by wearing gloves and waterproof aprons. Dilute hypochlorite solution (eg, household bleach diluted 1:10) is reported to help break down organophosphate pesticides and nerve agents.

B. SPECIFIC TREATMENT

Atropine reverses excessive muscarinic stimulation and is effective for treatment of salivation, wheezing, abdominal cramping, and sweating. However, it does not interact with nicotinic receptors at autonomic ganglia and at the neuromuscular junction and has no effect on muscle weakness. Administer 2 mg intravenously, and give repeated doses as needed to dry bronchial secretions and decrease wheezing; as much as several hundred milligrams of atropine has been given to treat severe poisoning.

Pralidoxime (2-PAM, Protopam) is a specific antidote that reverses organophosphate binding to the cholinesterase enzyme; therefore, it is effective at the neuromuscular junction as well as other nicotinic and muscarinic sites. It should be started as soon as possible, to prevent permanent binding of the organophosphate to cholinesterase. Administer 1–2 g intravenously as a loading dose, and begin a continuous infusion (200–500 mg/h, titrated to clinical response). Constant infusion is more effective because of the short duration of action of single doses. Continue to give pralidoxime as long as there is any evidence of acetylcholine excess. Pralidoxime is of questionable benefit for carbamate poisoning, because carbamates have only a transitory effect on the cholinesterase enzyme. High-dose sodium bicarbonate (5 mEq/kg intravenously over 5 minutes) has been reported effective although the mechanism is unclear and the treatment has not been widely adopted.

Balali-Mood M et al: Effect of high doses of sodium bicarbonate in acute organophosphorous pesticide poisoning. Clin Toxicol (Phila) 2005;43:571. [PMID: 16255339]

Buckley NA et al: Oximes for acute organophosphate pesticide poisoning. Cochrane Database Syst Rev 2005;CD005085. [PMID: 15654704]

PETROLEUM DISTILLATES & SOLVENTS

Petroleum distillate toxicity may occur from inhalation of the vapor or as a result of pulmonary aspiration of the liquid during or after ingestion. Acute manifestations of aspiration pneumonitis are vomiting, coughing, and bronchopneumonia. Some hydrocarbons—ie, those with aromatic or halogenated subunits—can also cause severe systemic poisoning after oral ingestion (Table 39–11). Hydrocarbons can also cause systemic intoxication by inhalation. Vertigo, muscular incoordination, irregular pulse, myoclonus, and seizures occur with serious poisoning and may be due to hypoxemia or the systemic effects of the agents. Chlorinated and fluorinated hydrocarbons (trichloroethylene, freons, etc) and many other hydrocarbons can cause ventricular arrhythmias due to increased sensitivity of the myocardium to the effects of endogenous catecholamines.

Treatment (Table 39–11)

Remove the patient to fresh air. Since aspiration is the primary danger after ingestion of many common products, use of lavage or emesis is not recommended; administration of activated charcoal may be helpful if the preparation contains toxic solutes (eg, an insecticide) or is an aromatic or halogenated product. Observe the victim for 6–8 hours for signs of aspiration pneumonitis (cough, localized rales or rhonchi, tachypnea, and infiltrates on chest radiograph). Corticosteroids are not recommended. If fever occurs, give a specific antibiotic only after identification of bacterial pathogens by laboratory studies. Because of the risk of arrhythmias, use bronchodilators with caution in patients with chlorinated or fluorinated solvent intoxication.

Finch CK et al: Acute inhalant-induced neurotoxicity with delayed recovery. Ann Pharmacother 2005;39:169. Epub 2004 Dec 8. [PMID: 15590879]

Harris D et al: Butane encephalopathy. Emerg Med J 2005;22: 676. [PMID: 16113204]

PHENOTHIAZINES & OTHER ANTIPSYCHOTIC AGENTS

Promethazine, prochlorperazine, chlorpromazine, haloperidol, droperidol, risperidone, olanzapine, ziprasidone, quetiapine, and aripiprazole are used as antiemetics and antipsychotic agents and as potentiators of analgesic and hypnotic drugs.

Phenothiazines (particularly chlorpromazine) induce drowsiness and mild orthostatic hypotension in as many as 50% of patients. Larger doses can cause obtundation, miosis, severe hypotension, tachycardia, convulsions, and coma. Abnormal cardiac conduction may occur, resulting in prolongation of QRS or QT intervals (or both) and ventricular arrhythmias. Droperidol now has a "black box" warning about prolonged QT interval and the risk of torsade de pointes.

With therapeutic or toxic doses, an acute extrapyramidal dystonic reaction similar to Parkinson's dis-

Table 39-11. Clinical features of hydrocarbon poisoning.

Type	Examples	Risk of Pneumonia	Risk of Systemic Toxicity	Treatment
High-viscosity	Vaseline[1] Motor oil	Low	Low	None.
Low-viscosity, nontoxic	Furniture polish Mineral seal oil Kerosene Lighter fluid	High	Low	Observe for pneumonia. *Do not* induce emesis. *Do not* administer activated charcoal.
Low-viscosity, unknown systemic toxicity	Turpentine Pine oil	High	Variable	Observe for pneumonia. Consider activated charcoal.
Low-viscosity, known systemic toxicity	Camphor Phenol Chlorinated insecticides Aromatic hydrocarbons (benzene, toluene, etc)	High	High	Observe for pneumonia. Give activated charcoal.

[1]"Vaseline" is one of several proprietary names for petrolatum (petroleum jelly, paraffin jelly).

ease may develop in some patients, with spasmodic contractions of the face and neck muscles, extensor rigidity of the back muscles, carpopedal spasm, and motor restlessness. This reaction is more common with haloperidol and the butyrophenones and less common with newer atypical antipsychotics such as ziprasidone, olanzapine, and quetiapine. Severe rigidity accompanied by hyperthermia and metabolic acidosis ("neuroleptic malignant syndrome") may occasionally occur and is life-threatening (see Chapter 25).

Treatment

A. EMERGENCY AND SUPPORTIVE MEASURES

Administer activated charcoal. For severe hypotension, treatment with fluids and pressor agents may be necessary. Treat hyperthermia as outlined on p 1642. Maintain cardiac monitoring.

B. SPECIFIC TREATMENT

Hypotension and cardiac arrhythmias associated with widened QRS intervals on the ECG in a patient with thioridazine poisoning may respond to intravenous sodium bicarbonate as used for tricyclic antidepressants. Prolongation of the QT interval and torsade de pointes is usually treated with intravenous magnesium or overdrive pacing.

For extrapyramidal signs, give diphenhydramine, 0.5–1 mg/kg intravenously, or benztropine mesylate, 0.01–0.02 mg/kg intramuscularly. Treatment with oral doses of these agents should be continued for 24–48 hours.

Bromocriptine (2.5–7.5 mg orally daily) may be effective for mild or moderate neuroleptic malignant syndrome. Dantrolene (2–5 mg/kg intravenously) has also been used for muscle contractions but is not a true antidote.

Carstairs SD et al: Overdose of aripiprazole, a new type of antipsychotic. J Emerg Med 2005;28:311. [PMID: 15769575]

Palenzona S et al: The clinical picture of olanzapine poisoning with special reference to fluctuating mental status. J Toxicol Clin Toxicol 2004;42:27. [PMID: 15083933]

Strachan EM et al: Electrocardiogram and cardiovascular changes in thioridazine and chlorpromazine poisoning. Eur J Clin Pharmacol 2004;60:541. Epub 2004 Sep 15. [PMID: 15372128]

QUINIDINE & RELATED ANTIARRHYTHMICS

Quinidine, procainamide, and disopyramide are class Ia antiarrhythmic agents, and flecainide and propafenone are class Ic agents. These drugs have membrane-depressant effects on the sodium-dependent channel responsible for cardiac cell depolarization. Manifestations of cardiotoxicity include arrhythmias, syncope, hypotension, and widening of the QRS complex on the ECG (> 100–120 ms). With type Ia drugs, a lengthened QT interval and atypical or polymorphous ventricular tachycardia (torsade de pointes) may occur. The antimalarials chloroquine and hydroxychloroquine have similar effects in overdose.

Treatment

A. EMERGENCY AND SUPPORTIVE MEASURES

Administer activated charcoal (see p 1644); consider gastric lavage after large recent overdose. Assist ventilation if needed. Perform continuous cardiac monitoring.

B. Specific Treatment

Treat cardiotoxicity (hypotension, QRS interval widening) with intravenous boluses of sodium bicarbonate, 50–100 mEq. Ventricular tachycardia of the torsade de pointes variety may be treated with intravenous magnesium or overdrive pacing.

Clarot F et al: Fatal propafenone overdoses: case reports and a review of the literature. J Anal Toxicol 2003;27:595. [PMID: 14670140]

Messant I: Massive chloroquine intoxication: importance of early treatment and pre-hospital treatment. Resuscitation 2004; 60:343. [PMID: 15050768]

SALICYLATES

Salicylates (aspirin, methyl salicylate, etc) are found in a variety of over-the-counter and prescription medications. Salicylates uncouple cellular oxidative phosphorylation, resulting in anaerobic metabolism and excessive production of lactic acid and heat, and they also interfere with several Krebs cycle enzymes. A single ingestion of more than 200 mg/kg of salicylate is likely to produce significant acute intoxication. Poisoning may also occur as a result of chronic excessive dosing over several days. Although the half-life of salicylate is 2–3 hours after small doses, it may increase to 20 hours or more in patients with intoxication.

Clinical Findings

Acute ingestion often causes nausea and vomiting, occasionally with gastritis. Moderate intoxication is characterized by hyperpnea (deep and rapid breathing), tachycardia, tinnitus, and elevated anion gap metabolic acidosis. Serious intoxication may result in agitation, confusion, coma, seizures, cardiovascular collapse, pulmonary edema, hyperthermia, and death. The prothrombin time is often elevated owing to salicylate-induced hypoprothrombinemia.

Diagnosis is suspected in any patient with metabolic acidosis and is confirmed by measuring the serum salicylate level. Patients with levels greater than 100 mg/dL (1000 mg/L) after an acute overdose are more likely to have severe poisoning. On the other hand, patients with subacute or chronic intoxication may suffer severe symptoms with levels of only 60–70 mg/dL. The arterial blood gas typically reveals a respiratory alkalosis with an underlying metabolic acidosis.

Treatment

A. Emergency and Supportive Measures

Administer activated charcoal (see p 1644). Gastric lavage followed by administration of extra doses of activated charcoal may be needed in patients who ingest more than 10 g of aspirin (see p 1643). The desired ratio of charcoal to aspirin is about 10:1 by weight; while this cannot always be given as a single dose, it may be administered over the first 24 hours in divided doses every 2–4 hours.

Treat metabolic acidosis with intravenous sodium bicarbonate. This is critical because acidosis (especially acidemia, pH < 7.40) promotes greater entry of salicylate into cells, worsening toxicity. Brief hypoventilation during rapid sequence intubation may cause sudden and severe deterioration if the pH is allowed to fall.

B. Specific Treatment

Alkalinization of the urine enhances renal salicylate excretion by trapping the salicylate anion in the urine. Add 100 mEq (two ampules) of sodium bicarbonate to 1 L of 5% dextrose in 0.2% saline, and infuse this solution intravenously at a rate of about 150–200 mL/h. Unless the patient is oliguric, add 20–30 mEq of potassium chloride to each liter of intravenous fluid. Patients who are volume-depleted often fail to produce an alkaline urine (paradoxical aciduria) unless potassium is given.

Hemodialysis may be lifesaving and is indicated for patients with severe metabolic acidosis, markedly altered mental status, or significantly elevated salicylate levels (eg, > 100–120 mg/dL [1000–1200 mg/L] after acute overdose or > 60–70 mg/dL [600–700 mg/L] with subacute or chronic intoxication).

Parker D et al: The analysis of methyl salicylate and salicylic acid from Chinese herbal medicine ingestion. J Anal Toxicol 2004;28:214. [PMID: 15107154]

Rivera W et al: Delayed salicylate toxicity at 35 hours without early manifestations following a single salicylate ingestion. Ann Pharmacother 2004;38:1186. [PMID: 15173556]

SEAFOOD POISONINGS

A variety of intoxications may occur after eating certain types of fish or other seafood. These include scombroid, ciguatera, paralytic shellfish, and puffer fish poisoning. The mechanisms of toxicity and clinical presentations are described in Table 39–12. In the majority of cases, the seafood has a normal appearance and taste (scombroid may have a peppery taste).

Treatment

A. Emergency and Supportive Measures

Caution: Abrupt respiratory arrest may occur in patients with acute paralytic shellfish and puffer fish poisoning. Observe patients for at least 4–6 hours. Replace fluid and electrolyte losses from gastroenteritis with intravenous saline or other crystalloid solution.

For recent ingestions, it may be possible to adsorb residual toxin in the gut with activated charcoal, 50–60 g orally (see p 1644).

B. Specific Treatment

There is no specific antidote for paralytic shellfish or puffer fish poisoning.

1. Ciguatera—There are anecdotal reports of successful treatment of acute neurologic symptoms with mannitol, 1 g/kg intravenously.

Table 39–12. Common seafood poisonings.

Type of Poisoning	Mechanism	Clinical Presentation
Ciguatera	Reef fish ingest toxic dinoflagellates, whose toxins accumulate in fish meat. Commonly implicated fish in the United States are barracuda, jack, snapper, and grouper.	1–6 hours after ingestion, victims develop abdominal pain, vomiting, and diarrhea accompanied by a variety of neurologic symptoms, including paresthesias, reversal of hot and cold sensation, vertigo, headache, and intense itching. Autonomic disturbances, including hypotension and bradycardia, may occur.
Scombroid	Improper preservation of large fish results in bacterial degradation of histidine to histamine. Commonly implicated fish include tuna, mahimahi, bonita, mackerel, and kingfish.	Allergic-like (anaphylactoid) symptoms are due to histamine, usually begin within 15–90 minutes, and include skin flushing, itching, urticaria, angioedema, bronchospasm, and hypotension as well as abdominal pain, vomiting, and diarrhea.
Paralytic shellfish poisoning	Dinoflagellates produce saxitoxin, which is concentrated by filter-feeding mussels and clams. Saxitoxin blocks sodium conductance and neuronal transmission in skeletal muscles.	Onset is usually within 30–60 minutes. Initial symptoms include perioral and intraoral paresthesias. Other symptoms include nausea and vomiting, headache, dizziness, dysphagia, dysarthria, ataxia, and rapidly progressive muscle weakness that may result in respiratory arrest.
Puffer fish poisoning	Tetrodotoxin is concentrated in liver, gonads, intestine, and skin. Toxic effects are similar to those of saxitoxin. Tetrodotoxin is also found in some North American newts and Central American frogs.	Onset is usually within 30–40 minutes but may be as short as 10 minutes. Initial perioral paresthesias are followed by headache, diaphoresis, nausea, vomiting, ataxia, and rapidly progressive muscle weakness that may result in respiratory arrest.

2. Scombroid—Antihistamines such as diphenhydramine, 25–50 mg intravenously, and the H₂ blocker cimetidine, 300 mg intravenously, are usually effective. For severe reactions, give also epinephrine, 0.3–0.5 mL of a 1:1000 solution subcutaneously.

Isbister GK et al: Neurotoxic marine poisoning. Lancet Neurol 2005;4:219. [PMID: 15778101]

Kiernan MC et al: Acute tetrodotoxin-induced neurotoxicity after ingestion of puffer fish. Ann Neurol 2005;57:339. [PMID: 15732107]

SNAKE BITES

The venom of poisonous snakes and lizards may be predominantly neurotoxic (coral snake) or predominantly cytolytic (rattlesnakes, other pit vipers). Neurotoxins cause respiratory paralysis; cytolytic venoms cause tissue destruction by digestion and hemorrhage due to hemolysis and destruction of the endothelial lining of the blood vessels. The manifestations of rattlesnake envenomation are mostly local pain, redness, swelling, and extravasation of blood. Perioral tingling, metallic taste, nausea and vomiting, hypotension, and coagulopathy may also occur. Neurotoxic envenomation may cause ptosis, dysphagia, diplopia, and respiratory arrest.

Treatment

A. EMERGENCY MEASURES

Immobilize the patient and the bitten part in a neutral position. Avoid manipulation of the bitten area.

Transport the patient to a medical facility for definitive treatment. Do *not* give alcoholic beverages or stimulants; do *not* apply ice; do *not* apply a tourniquet. The trauma to underlying structures resulting from incision and suction performed by unskilled people is probably not justified in view of the small amount of venom that can be recovered.

B. SPECIFIC ANTIDOTE AND GENERAL MEASURES

1. Pit viper (eg, rattlesnake) envenomation—A new antivenin (CroFab) has replaced the Wyeth horse serum-based product. With local signs such as swelling, pain, and ecchymosis but no systemic symptoms, give 4–6 vials of crotalid antivenin (CroFab) by slow intravenous drip in 250–500 mL saline. Repeated doses of 2 vials every 6 hours for up to 18 hours has been recommended. For more serious envenomation with marked local effects and systemic toxicity (eg, hypotension, coagulopathy), higher doses and additional vials may be required. Monitor vital signs and the blood coagulation profile. Type and cross-match blood. The adequacy of venom neutralization is indicated by improvement in symptoms and signs, and the rate of swelling slows. Prophylactic antibiotics are not indicated after a rattlesnake bite.

2. Elapid (coral snake) envenomation—Give 1–2 vials of specific antivenom as soon as possible. To locate antisera for exotic snakes, call a regional poison control center (800-222-1222).

Camilleri C et al: Conservative management of delayed, multicomponent coagulopathy following rattlesnake envenomation. Clin Toxicol (Phila) 2005;43:201. [PMID: 15902796]

Gold BS et al: North American snake envenomation: diagnosis, treatment, and management. Emerg Med Clin North Am 2004;22:423. [PMID: 15163575]

SPIDER BITES & SCORPION STINGS

The toxin of most species of spiders in the United States causes only local pain, redness, and swelling. That of the more venomous black widow spiders (*Latrodectus mactans*) causes generalized muscular pains, muscle spasms, and rigidity. The brown recluse spider (*Loxosceles reclusa*) causes progressive local necrosis as well as hemolytic reactions (rare). Stings by most scorpions in the United States cause only local pain. Stings by the more toxic *Centruroides* species (found in the southwestern United States) may cause muscle cramps, twitching and jerking, and occasionally hypertension, convulsions, and pulmonary edema. Stings by scorpions from other parts of the world are not discussed here.

Treatment

A. BLACK WIDOW SPIDER BITES

Pain may be relieved with parenteral narcotics or muscle relaxants (eg, methocarbamol, 15 mg/kg). Calcium gluconate 10%, 0.1–0.2 mL/kg intravenously, may relieve muscle rigidity, though its effectiveness is questionable. Antivenin is available, but because of concerns about acute hypersensitivity reactions it is often reserved for very young or elderly patients or those who do not respond to the above measures. Horse serum sensitivity testing is required. (Instruction and testing materials are included in the antivenin kit.)

B. BROWN RECLUSE SPIDER BITES

Because bites occasionally progress to extensive local necrosis, some authorities recommend early excision of the bite site, whereas others use oral corticosteroids. Anecdotal reports have claimed success with dapsone and colchicine. All of these treatments remain of unproved value.

C. SCORPION STINGS

No specific treatment is available for envenomations by scorpions found in the United States. For *Centruroides* stings, some toxicologists use a specific antivenom developed in Arizona, but this is neither FDA-approved nor widely available.

Foex B et al: Best evidence topic report. Scorpion envenomation: does antivenom reduce serum venom concentrations? Emerg Med J 2005;22:195. [PMID: 15735271]

Isbister GK et al: Antivenom treatment in arachnidism. J Toxicol Clin Toxicol 2003;41:291. [PMID: 12807312]

LoVecchio F et al: Scorpion envenomations in young children in central Arizona. J Toxicol Clin Toxicol 2003;41:937. [PMID: 14705838]

Saucier JR: Arachnid envenomation. Emerg Med Clin North Am 2004;22:405. [PMID: 15163574]

THEOPHYLLINE & CAFFEINE

Theophylline toxicity may be caused by several of its pharmacologic effects, including inhibition of phosphodiesterase and adenosine and release of catecholamines. Theophylline may cause intoxication after an acute single overdose, or intoxication may occur as a result of chronic accidental repeated overmedication or reduced elimination resulting from hepatic dysfunction or interacting drug (eg, cimetidine, erythromycin). The usual serum half-life of theophylline is 4–6 hours, but this may increase to more than 20 hours after overdose. Caffeine and caffeine-containing herbal products can produce similar toxicity.

Clinical Findings

Mild intoxication causes nausea, vomiting, tachycardia, and tremulousness. Severe intoxication is characterized by ventricular and supraventricular tachyarrhythmias, hypotension, and seizures. Status epilepticus is common and often intractable to the usual anticonvulsants. After acute overdose (but not chronic intoxication), hypokalemia, hyperglycemia, and metabolic acidosis are common. Seizures and other manifestations of toxicity may be delayed for several hours after acute ingestion, especially if a sustained-release preparation such as Theo-Dur was taken.

Diagnosis is based on measurement of the serum theophylline concentration. Seizures and hypotension are likely to develop in acute overdose patients with serum levels greater than 100 mg/L. Serious toxicity may develop at lower levels (ie, 40–60 mg/L) in patients with chronic intoxication.

Treatment

A. EMERGENCY AND SUPPORTIVE MEASURES

After acute ingestion, administer activated charcoal (see p 1644). Repeated doses of activated charcoal may enhance theophylline elimination by "gut dialysis." Addition of whole bowel irrigation should be considered for large ingestions involving sustained-release preparations.

Hemodialysis is effective in removing theophylline and is indicated for patients with status epilepticus or markedly elevated serum theophylline levels (eg, > 100 mg/L after acute overdose or > 60 mg/L with chronic intoxication).

B. SPECIFIC TREATMENT

Treat seizures with benzodiazepines (lorazepam, 2–3 mg intravenously, or diazepam, 5–10 mg intravenously) or phenobarbital (10–15 mg/kg intravenously). Phenytoin is not effective. Hypotension and tachycardia—which are mediated through excessive β-adrenergic stimulation—may respond to β-blocker therapy even in low doses: Administer esmolol, 25–50 mcg/kg/min by intravenous infusion, or propranolol, 0.5–1 mg intravenously.

Barnes PJ: Theophylline: new perspectives for an old drug. Am J Respir Crit Care Med 2003;167:813. [PMID: 12623857]

Kerrigan S et al: Fatal caffeine overdose: two case reports. Forensic Sci Int 2005;153:67. [PMID: 15935584]

TRICYCLIC & OTHER ANTIDEPRESSANTS

Tricyclic and related cyclic antidepressants are among the most dangerous drugs involved in suicidal overdose. These drugs have anticholinergic and cardiac depressant properties ("quinidine-like" sodium channel blockade). Tricyclic antidepressants produce more marked membrane-depressant cardiotoxic effects than the phenothiazines.

Newer antidepressants such as trazodone, fluoxetine, citalopram, paroxetine, sertraline, bupropion, venlafaxine, and fluvoxamine are not chemically related to the tricyclic antidepressant agents and do not generally produce quinidine-like cardiotoxic effects. However, they may cause seizures in overdoses and they may cause serotonin syndrome (see Monoamine Oxidase Inhibitors, above). Seizures are also reported rarely after therapeutic doses of bupropion.

Clinical Findings

Signs of severe intoxication may occur abruptly and without warning within 30–60 minutes after acute tricyclic overdose. Anticholinergic effects include dilated pupils, tachycardia, dry mouth, flushed skin, muscle twitching, and decreased peristalsis. Quinidine-like cardiotoxic effects include QRS interval widening (> 0.12 s; see Figure 39–2), ventricular arrhythmias, AV block, and hypotension. Rightward-axis deviation of the terminal 40 ms of the QRS has also been described. Prolongation of the QT interval has been reported with citalopram and venlafaxine. Seizures and coma are common with severe intoxication. Life-threatening hyperthermia may result from status epilepticus and anticholinergic-induced impairment of sweating. Among newer agents, bupropion and venlafaxine have been associated with a greater risk of seizures.

The diagnosis should be suspected in any overdose patient with anticholinergic side effects, especially if there is widening of the QRS interval or seizures. For intoxication by most tricyclics, the QRS interval correlates with the severity of intoxication more reliably than the serum drug level.

Serotonin syndrome should be suspected if a patient taking serotonin reuptake inhibitors develops agitation, delirium, muscular hyperactivity, and fever.

Treatment

A. EMERGENCY AND SUPPORTIVE MEASURES

Observe patients for at least 6 hours, and admit all patients with evidence of anticholinergic effects (eg, delirium, dilated pupils, tachycardia) or signs of cardiotoxicity (see above).

Administer activated charcoal, and consider gastric lavage after recent large ingestions (see p 1644). All of

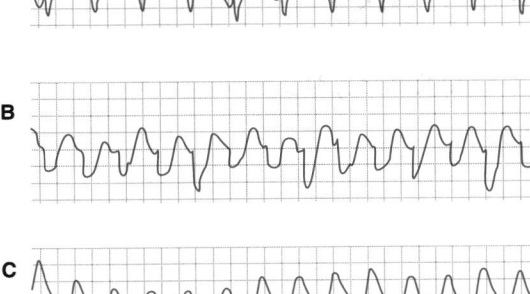

Figure 39–2. Cardiac arrhythmias resulting from tricyclic antidepressant overdose. **A:** Delayed intraventricular conduction results in prolonged QRS interval (0.18 s). **B** and **C:** Supraventricular tachycardia with progressive widening of QRS complexes mimics ventricular tachycardia. (Reproduced, with permission, from Benowitz NL, Goldschlager N: Cardiac disturbances in the toxicologic patient. In: *Clinical Management of Poisoning and Drug Overdose*, 3rd ed. Haddad LM, Winchester JF [editors]. Saunders, 1998.)

these drugs are highly tissue-bound and are not effectively removed by hemodialysis procedures.

B. SPECIFIC TREATMENT

Cardiotoxic sodium channel-depressant effects may respond to boluses of sodium bicarbonate (50–100 mEq intravenously). Sodium bicarbonate provides a large sodium load that alleviates depression of the sodium-dependent channel. Reversal of acidosis may also have beneficial effects at this site. Maintain the pH between 7.45 and 7.50. Alkalinization does not promote excretion of tricyclics. Prolongation of the QT interval or torsade de pointes is usually treated with intravenous magnesium or overdrive pacing.

Mild serotonin syndrome may be treated with benzodiazepines and withdrawal of the antidepressant. Moderate cases may respond to cyproheptadine (4 mg orally or via gastric tube hourly for three or four doses). Severe hyperthermia should be treated with neuromuscular paralysis and endotracheal intubation in addition to external cooling measures.

Bailey B et al: A meta-analysis of prognostic indicators to predict seizures, arrhythmias or death after tricyclic antidepressant overdose. J Toxicol Clin Toxicol 2004;42:877. [PMID: 15533027]

Isbister GK et al: Relative toxicity of selective serotonin reuptake inhibitors (SSRIs) in overdose. J Toxicol Clin Toxicol 2004; 42:277. [PMID: 15362595]

Kelly CA et al: Toxicity of citalopram and the newer antidepressants after overdose. J Toxicol Clin Toxicol 2004;42: 67. [PMID: 15083939]

Cancer

Hope S. Rugo, MD

40

This chapter mainly covers the clinical aspects of cancer: prevention, diagnosis, primary treatment, management of complications, and paraneoplastic syndromes. Further information may be obtained by calling the National Cancer Institute (NCI) Cancer Information Service at 1-800-4CANCER or accessing NCI's comprehensive cancer information database "Physician Data Query" (PDQ) via the Internet at www.cancer.gov/cancerinformation. PDQ is also available on CD-ROM. The CANCERLIT feature of Medline (PubMed) is a familiar resource for articles about cancer that can be accessed by author or by subject words. A series of oncology practice guidelines compiled by a panel of United States experts and encompassing diagnosis and treatment of a wide variety of cancers as well as pain management is now available free of charge at the National Comprehensive Cancer Network Web site (www.nccn.org) and is updated yearly. This site also provides a stepwise guide to diagnosis and to treatment options for patients as well as links to a variety of useful sites, including the American Cancer Society.

Many new Web sites are now available for both clinician and patient use, and are regularly updated with new drug approvals and prevention and treatment guidelines. Information includes statistics, treatment, and clinical trial information. Web sites can be found by searching for the words "cancer" or "oncology." The American Society of Clinical Oncology has an information Web site for patients and their families (www.PeopleLivingWithCancer.org) as well as patient guides on subjects such as follow-up care for breast and colorectal cancers, understanding tumor markers, treatment of nausea and vomiting, and advanced lung cancer. Two Web sites provide updated data as well as review articles on advances in oncology; these sites allow the user to search for specific areas of interest as well: PeerView Press (info@peerviewpress.com) and Medscape Hematology-Oncology (http://www.medscape.com/hematology-oncologyhome).

■ INCIDENCE & ETIOLOGY

Cancer is the second most common cause of death in the United States. The American Cancer Society esti-

mates that almost 1.4 million new cases of invasive cancer will be diagnosed in the year 2006, with over 570,000 deaths. Some type of invasive cancer will develop in slightly less than one of every two men and slightly more than one of every three women in the United States during their lifetime. Based on the SEER 2005 database, the lifetime probability of developing cancer is about 46% for men and 38% for women and varies by race, and age. Table 40–1 summarizes current U.S. incidence and mortality figures for the ten leading types of cancer. Women have an approximately 1:8 lifetime chance of developing breast cancer, and men have an approximately 1:6 chance of developing prostate cancer. Cancers of the lung, prostate, and breast and of the colon and rectum account for about 55% of all new cancer diagnoses and for over 50% of cancer deaths in the United States. Lung cancer is the leading cause of cancer death in the United States, accounting for almost one-third of deaths in men and women. Table 40–2 summarizes the lifetime risk of being diagnosed with or dying from the leading causes of cancer as well as from all types of cancer. Rates are age adjusted to the year 2000 standard million population based on the 2000 census data.

The single most important risk factor for developing cancer is age. About 76% of cancers are diagnosed in persons aged 75 years or older. As the United States population increases in numbers and grows older, it is estimated that the number of cancer cases will double, by the year 2050, from 1.3 million cases per year to 2.6 million cases per year. In the United States, the incidence of cancer stayed relatively stable and cancer-related mortality decreased an average of 1% per year from 1995 to 2002, although this progress has not been shared equally across all racial and ethnic populations. This now sustained decline is attributed to changes in lifestyle as well as improved prevention, early detection, and treatment that clearly needs to be generalized to include all populations. Interestingly, among men, the rate of cancers of the prostate and kidney, and melanoma increased; the same was true for cancers of the breast, lymphoma and melanoma in women. Colorectal cancers decreased in both sexes. Lung cancer incidence in women has stabilized since 1998, after increasing for the prior three decades.

Cancer incidence and mortality vary significantly among racial and ethnic groups, with blacks having

Table 40–1. Incidence of and mortality from the ten most common cancers in the United States in males and females (all races), 1998–2002.

Rank	Men	Incidence[1]	Mortality[1]	Women	Incidence[1]	Mortality[1]
1	Prostate	178	30	Breast	137	26
2	Lung	82	76	Lung	51	41
3	Colorectal	63	25	Colorectal	47	17
4	Bladder	38	8	Uterus[2]	33	7
5	Non-Hodgkin's lymphoma	24	10	Ovary	14	9
6	Melanoma	23	4	Non-Hodgkin's lymphoma	16	7
7	Oral cavity and pharynx[3]	16	4	Melanoma	15	2
8	Kidney	17	6	Thyroid	11	0.5
9	Leukemias[4]	16	10	Pancreas	10	9
10	Pancreas	13	12	Leukemia	10	6

[1]Rates are per 100,000, 1998–2002, and are age adjusted to the 2000 United States population by 5-year age groups.
[2]Uterus includes the cervix and corpus uteri.
[3]Both oropharynx and larynx are included.
[4]All subtypes of leukemia are included.
Data obtained from the NCI SEER Program. Ries LAG et al (editors): *SEER Cancer Statistics Review, 1975–2002*, National Cancer Institute, 2005. http://seer.cancer.gov.csr/1975_2002/2005.

the highest rates of mortality even in diseases for which the incidence of the specific cancer is lower than that seen in the white population. Stage for stage, 5-year survival rates are lower, even when the fact that cancers are less likely to be diagnosed in localized sites is taken into account. Recent data suggest that this difference is due in part to marked variations in the biology of the cancer itself, with a higher incidence of worse prognosis disease found in blacks compared to whites. In addition, differences in treatment and comorbid conditions play a significant role. Overall, cancer rates are higher for whites and blacks than for Asians/Pacific Islanders. Among the leading cancers, the incidence of prostate cancer among black men is about 1.5 times higher than among white men, and 2.7 times higher than among Asian/Pacific Islanders. In contrast, breast cancer among white women is about 1.2 times higher than among black women, and 1.7 times higher than among Asian/Pacific Islander women. Other racial differences include a higher rate of multiple myeloma in black men and women and a higher rate of liver, intrahepatic bile duct, and stomach cancers in Asian/Pacific Islander men and women. Data from the 2000 census confirm the existence of geographic variability in cancer incidence, although this is not as marked as previously thought; for example, breast cancer rates in Marin County in California and in Washington state appear to be among the highest in the United States. Interestingly, the increased incidence is similar to that seen in higher socioeconomic groups with higher attained education, delayed childbearing, a lower rate of breast-feeding, and higher

relative alcohol intake—and appears to primarily affect the white population. The contribution of environmental factors, exposure to toxins, and other dietary factors is not fully understood but clearly plays a

Table 40–2. Lifetime risks for the most common cancers, 2000–2002.

Cancer	Risk of Diagnosis (%)	Risk of Death (%)
Prostate	17.9 (1 in 6)	3.0
Breast (women)	13.2 (1 in 8)	3.0
Lung		
(men)	7.6	7.43
(women)	5.7	4.8
Colorectal		
(men)	5.8	2.4
(women)	5.5	2.3
Bladder (men)	3.6	0.7
Uterus[1]	3.4	0.8
Any cancer		
(men)	45.8 (1 in 2)	23.6
(women)	38.1 (1 in 3)	20.0

[1]Uterus includes the cervix and corpus uteri.
Data obtained from the NCI Seer Program. Ries LAG et al (editors): *SEER Cancer Statistics Review, 1975–2002*, National Cancer Institute, 2005. http://seer.cancer.gov/csr/1975_2002.

role. Current research is focusing on exposures and risks that occur in childhood and adolescence to better understand the factors that increase risk of cancer in adulthood.

The cause of most cancers remains unknown, although workers in the field of molecular biology have begun to unravel the complex pathways leading to cancer cell growth and metastases. Mutations in DNA sequences leading to abnormal or unregulated expression of protooncogenes or deletion of tumor suppressor genes—or both—have been linked to abnormal cellular proliferation. Oncogenes encode for cellular growth factor receptors, growth factors, or elements of the proliferative machinery of the cancer cell. Tumor suppressor genes either code for or control regulatory proteins that normally suppress cellular proliferation; loss of these genes leads to cell growth. Cancer results from these and other mutations, which may be due to environmental exposure, genetic susceptibility, infectious agents, and other factors.

Most tumors exhibit chromosomal abnormalities such as deletions, inversions, translocations, or duplications. Although usually nonspecific, certain genetic alterations are strongly associated with specific malignancies and in some cases can be used to assess prognosis. In Burkitt's lymphoma, the c-*myc* oncogene is activated by translocation of genetic material from chromosome 8 to chromosome 14. Chronic myelogenous leukemia (CML) is defined by a reciprocal translocation of the long arms of chromosomes 9 and 22, resulting in the generation of a fusion protein (BCR-ABL) with tyrosine kinase activity. In colon cancer, loss of the long arm of chromosome 18 (18q) predicts a poor outcome, whereas mutations in the gene for the type II receptor for transforming growth factor-β1 (TGF-β1) with microsatellite instability predict a favorable outcome. In one study, 5-year survival following adjuvant chemotherapy for stage III colon cancer was 74% in those who retained the 18q allele and 50% in those with loss of the allele. Five-year survival was 74% for patients whose cancers had both microsatellite instability and a mutated gene for the type II receptor for TGF-β1 and 46% if the tumor did not have the mutation. Genetic mutations in chronic lymphocytic leukemia (CLL) have been shown to occur in up to 82% of cases and strongly predict outcomes. For example, patients with deletions of the short arm of chromosome 17 had a survival of only 2.7 years, whereas those with deletions of the long arm of chromosome 13 had a survival of 11 years. Amplification of the HER-2/*neu* oncogene in breast cancer has been associated with more aggressive tumors, a higher stage at diagnosis, and a shorter survival. However, this gene has also been associated with marked chemotherapy responsiveness to specific agents, and has provided a successful target for a targeted biologic agent (trastuzumab) in the treatment of breast cancer. Treatment of HER-2/*neu*-positive early-stage breast cancer with the combination of chemotherapy and the targeted agent trastuzumab has resulted in striking improve-

ments in outcome—so much so that finding this gene not only predicts response to treatment but also a lower risk of recurrence.

The *p53* gene appears to trigger programmed cell death (apoptosis) as a way of regulating uncontrolled cellular proliferation in the setting of aberrant growth signals. Mutations in the *p53* gene result in loss of the ability of the gene product to bind to DNA, thereby removing its suppressive effect. *p53* can also be inactivated by overexpression of an oncogene whose protein product binds to normal *p53* and prevents its action. This occurs in many soft tissue sarcomas. The Bcl-2 family of proteins act as "arbiters of cell death" with a balance of both "antideath" and "prodeath" activity. Bcl-2 and Bcl-X$_L$ appear to function as "antideath" proteins to prevent programmed cell death of cancer cells; overexpression of these proteins in cancer confers resistance to chemotherapy and radiation therapy. Bcl-2 and Bcl-X$_L$ are overexpressed at a high level (50–100%) on common cancers, including cancers of the breast, colon, prostate, head and neck, and ovary. Agents that target the receptors to which these proteins bind or their production might work to overcome cancer resistance (see section on novel therapies at the end of this chapter).

Another control against abnormal cellular proliferation also contributes to cellular aging. As a cell divides and ages, there is progressive shortening of the ends of the chromosomes, or telomeres. A striking correlation between cancer and the overexpression of telomerase (an enzyme capable of preventing the shortening of telomeres) suggests that it might be partially responsible for tumor cell immortality. Telomerase activity is present in about 85% of malignant tumors but absent in most normal somatic tissues. The stage and severity of neuroblastoma, breast cancer, and other cancers have been found to correlate with levels of telomerase activity, indicating a prognostic role of enzyme activity. Normal human cells transfected with the telomerase gene in vitro exceed their normal life span and ability to divide, thereby establishing a causal relationship between telomere shortening and cellular senescence. This suggests important possibilities for targeting telomerase activity as part of cancer therapy.

The development of cancer is a complicated multistep process that appears to involve the acquisition of an increasing number of genetic mutations, eventually resulting in invasive disease. Clinical examples of this stepwise progression can be found in many common cancers, including breast, colon, and prostate cancers. A history of the benign finding of atypical ductal hyperplasia on breast biopsy is clearly associated with a two- to fourfold increase in the risk of subsequent invasive cancer. Noninvasive breast cancer (ductal carcinoma in situ) is a preinvasive lesion that can progress into invasive cancer if left untreated. Understanding the cascade of genetic changes associated with the progression of benign cells to invasive cancer is a critical step in developing therapies targeted to a specific cancer and appropriate preventive strategies.

These genetic changes can now be mapped by a process called comparative genomic hybridization; this is an intense area of research. DNA microarray studies can detect activation of thousands of genes in a single experiment. The resulting DNA expression profile can be used not only to understand the development of cancer but also to assess prognosis, predict response to therapy, and direct targeted therapies. Studies have recently associated certain DNA profiles with specific cancer phenotypes, an important first step in this exciting area of research. In non-small cell lung cancer, reduced expression of the adhesion molecule E-cadherin detected by tissue microarray analysis correlated with reduced survival as well as local invasion and regional metastases.

Defining chromosomal aberrations and their association with prognosis and response to treatment will help in designing targeted therapies as well as risk-adapted treatment strategies. Several recent studies suggest that clusters of genes may help both to define specific chemotherapy sensitivities of specific tumors and to more accurately estimate prognosis. **Gene expression analysis** using array technologies allows the simultaneous examination of the relative abundance of thousands of genes in a cell or tissue and avoids the need to identify each gene individually. Specific gene expression profiles have been associated with survival in breast cancer. In one study, frozen tissues from diagnostic biopsies of breast tumors were analyzed and the results then correlated with response to neoadjuvant chemotherapy administered before surgery. A specific clustering of genes was highly correlated to the complete disappearance of tumor at the time of surgery. There were very few patients in this pilot trial; ongoing studies are examining serial biopsies during chemotherapy in an attempt to further predict response to treatment. Ideally, these data will be used in the future to individualize treatment for specific cancers. Rapid progress is being made in the use of genetic analysis of tumors to more accurately predict prognosis and perhaps response to therapy in breast cancer. The Oncotype Dx assay is a test that evaluates sixteen cancer-related and five reference genes in fixed tumor tissue—as expressed in RNA—to assess the risk of metastatic breast cancer recurrence 10 years after diagnosis in women with estrogen- or progesterone-receptor-positive breast cancers and negative axillary node involvement. A recurrence score is calculated based on the relative expression of the cancer-related genes in a particular tumor. In a large study evaluating tumors from patients enrolled in a clinical trial more than 10 years ago, the recurrence score was found to be a more accurate predictor of risk of recurrence than standard prognostic indicators such as tumor grade or size. Subsequent studies have suggested that the recurrence score may also be able to predict benefit from chemotherapy, with the primary benefit being in women with high scores corresponding to rapidly proliferating tumors. A woman with a higher risk of recurrence might receive chemotherapy as well as hormonal therapy, whereas a woman with a low risk would receive hormonal therapy alone. Current studies are trying to further validate this interesting tool, which is now clinically available and covered by most insurers (www.genomichealth.com). The assay can be performed in fixed, paraffin-embedded tissue, which should be readily available in all patients with a cancer diagnosis. It is validated only in axillary-node negative, hormone receptor-positive breast cancer.

A second study evaluated gene expression in 86 patients with newly diagnosed stage I adenocarcinoma of the lung. Clustering of gene expression profiles with 4966 genes revealed three clusters of lung adenocarcinomas with a significant relationship between the specific cluster and tumor stage or differentiation. In addition, high-risk and low-risk groups were identified with very different survival statistics. Understanding differences in the behavior of early-stage cancers using gene expression profiling will in the future permit differential treatment directed toward maximizing outcome, choosing appropriate therapy, and accurately estimating prognosis.

Genetic analysis may help determine appropriate dosing of effective but toxic chemotherapeutic agents. Specific polymorphisms or variations in the *UGT1A1* gene have recently been shown to predict severe neutropenia resulting from the colorectal cancer drug irinotecan. The *UGT1A1* gene produces an enzyme that metabolizes the active metabolite of irinotecan; 10% of North Americans have an identified polymorphism of this gene resulting in reduced enzyme activity. Genotyping using a simple blood test can help identify patients at high risk for life-threatening side effects, allowing individualization of dosing to improve the therapeutic ratio for patients with colorectal cancer. This test is clinically available; specific recommendations for dosing alterations are being validated in clinical trials.

Another area of study is the field of **proteomics**. Genes encode proteins, and proteins may be easier to evaluate than genes. Identifying and analyzing individual proteins are both difficult and time consuming, but describing patterns or panels of proteins is more straightforward. The field of proteomics seeks to associate specific patterns of protein expression with disease states, prognosis, and response to treatment in both tissue and serum. Proteomics has already been used successfully to aid in early detection of cancer; a good example is the use of prostate-specific antigen for the detection of prostate cancer. A division of the NCI is devoted to the study of proteomics and serves as an important source of information for researchers.

Hereditary Factors

Hereditary predisposition to some cancers has been linked to genetic events and is manifested by a family history of a common cancer or cancers occurring frequently—in a younger than expected age group—or any history of a relatively rare cancer. Examples include familial retinoblastoma, familial adenomatous polyposis (FAP), multiple endocrine neoplasia (MEN) syndromes, and the hereditary breast and ovarian cancer syndromes. Although FAP is a rare syndrome, somatic mutations in the affected gene (adenomatous polyposis coli; *APC*) occur in more than 60% of patients with colonic carcinomas and in an equal proportion of patients with adenomas. Genetic mutations associated with an increased risk of developing breast and ovarian cancers appear to be much more common than previously thought and are strongly related to age at diagnosis of cancer. It is estimated that 5–10% of all breast cancers and more than 40% of breast cancers occurring in women under 30 years of age are due to inheritance of an abnormal gene. The risk of ovarian and other cancers is also significantly increased in carriers of these susceptibility genes.

A tumor suppressor gene termed *BRCA1* on chromosome 17 has been shown to be abnormal in some families with early onset and high frequencies of breast cancer and ovarian cancer. More than 100 mutations have been identified in the *BRCA1* gene, making identification of high-risk individuals difficult. Two population-based studies found that up to 20% of Jewish women with breast cancer diagnosed at or before the age of 40 years and approximately 10% of all women with breast cancer diagnosed before the age of 35 years harbor one of two mutations in the *BRCA1* gene. Inheritance of a mutated *BRCA1* gene confers a lifelong risk of approximately 85% for breast cancer and 50% for ovarian cancer. Inheritance of the *BRCA1* gene also appears to increase the risk of developing both colon and prostate cancers. Another susceptibility gene, *BRCA2*, has been associated with an increased risk for male in addition to female breast cancer as well as malignant melanoma and other cancers. There is clearly an association of phenotype and inheritance of susceptibility genes. Breast cancers in *BRCA1* carriers tend to be hormone receptor negative, whereas cancers in *BRCA2* carriers are generally hormone receptor positive. For a woman in whom breast cancer is diagnosed between the ages of 30 and 34 years, the likelihood of a *BRCA1* mutation is as high as 27% if her tumor is both hormone receptor negative and of high grade.

A new gene has been identified that appears to be linked to a significant percentage of familial as well as sporadic cancers. Mutations in this tumor suppressor gene, termed "ADP-ribosylation factor-like tumor suppressor 1 (*ARLTS1*)," increases the risk of cancer only a little but may represent the first in a set of genes that are important in cancer risk for large populations.

Risk Factors & Prevention

Carriers of *BRCA* mutations who have children appear to be at higher risk for developing breast cancer by age 40 years than carriers who are nulliparous—in contrast to the usual risk factors for sporadic breast cancer. Interestingly—and despite the association of *BRCA1* with an increased risk of hormone receptor-negative breast tumors—recent data confirm that oophorectomy in women with either mutation before the age of 40 years significantly reduces the risk of breast cancer (up to 75%) and ovarian cancer, presumably by decreasing exposure of breast tissue to estrogen. The use of oral contraceptives for more than 5 years appears to significantly reduce the risk of ovarian cancer as well, perhaps by regulating ovarian cycling. Compared with sporadic ovarian cancers, those associated with the *BRCA1* mutation appeared to have a better clinical course, with a median survival of 77 months in women carrying the mutation compared with 29 months in controls. Many other less common genes have been identified that increase the risk of breast and other cancers, although clearly there are many yet to be identified. One study found that women who have an identical twin sister with breast cancer are at least three times more likely than average to develop cancer. If the twin was diagnosed before age 40 years, 25% of the remaining siblings developed cancer over the next 20 years. Increased risk in this setting is probably due to a combination of genes that will be more difficult to discern.

Screening for Genetic Risk Factors

With the discovery and cloning of cancer susceptibility genes such as *BRCA1*, commercial testing has been developed for "screening" using linked genetic markers. Tests for genes linked to familial cancer have raised concerns about the impact of positive results on patients. One study has evaluated indications for testing of the *APC* gene. Of the patients tested, 85% were felt to have valid indications for testing. However, only 20% received genetic counseling before the test; only 15% gave informed consent; and in 30% of cases the clinicians misinterpreted the results. It is essential that clinicians recognize the limitations of these tests and that genetic testing be made available in the appropriate setting. Educational programs and publications are available to help educate patients regarding genetic testing. Many cancer centers now have genetic screening and counseling programs. Patients with a strong family history of cancer should be referred to such programs before testing is performed. Early and regular cancer screening is recommended for affected members of the family, and aggressive but relatively effective preventive measures such as prophylactic mastectomy and oophorectomy should also be discussed. Updated guidelines for testing—including indications for testing, counseling about medical management, confidentiality of results, insurance coverage, and protection from discrimination—have recently been published (see reference below) and are available without cost at www.asco.org (search under genetic testing).

Other Familial Cancers

Other familial clusterings of cancer have been described that have not yet been associated with inheritance of a particular gene. Evaluation of participants in a study of colonic polyps revealed an increased risk of colorectal cancer in the siblings and parents of patients with adenomatous polyps, particularly when the adenoma was diagnosed before age 60 years or (for a sibling) when a parent had colorectal cancer. This syndrome, referred to as a hereditary nonpolyposis colorectal cancer (HNPCC), has been associated with a germline mutation of DNA mismatch-repair genes. In one European cohort, at least 2% of patients with colorectal cancer had these mutations. Testing for replication errors should be considered in patients under age 50 years with colorectal cancer who have a family history of colorectal or endometrial cancer. Family members of patients with this syndrome may benefit from early screening.

In addition to the germline mutations found in HNPCC, up to 10–15% of sporadic colorectal cancers have somatic mutations in DNA repair genes resulting in microsatellite instability (MSI) or alterations in the size of repetitive nucleotide sequences. These cancers are usually in the right side of the colon and have been associated with both a better prognosis and a striking sensitivity to adjuvant chemotherapy. The HER-2/*neu* oncogene is a somatic (not inherited or germline) mutation that encodes a tyrosine kinase receptor in the epidermal growth factor receptor (EGFR) family and is amplified in about 20% of breast cancers. HER-2/*neu* receptor overexpression is associated with more aggressive cancers, a worse prognosis (until recently), and enhanced tumor sensitivity to anthracycline chemotherapy. An antibody that targets this receptor (trastuzumab) has been shown to improve survival when used with chemotherapy to treat HER-2/*neu* overexpressing metastatic breast cancer, and has recently been shown in four large international trials to markedly reduce recurrence and improve survival from early-stage disease. HER-2/*neu* overexpression in prostate cancer also appears to correlate with a poorer 5-year prognosis, though this result remains to be validated. Identifying genetic factors that are associated with specific cancer phenotypes has already resulted in effective tailoring of adjuvant chemotherapy in the limited situations described above and will hopefully lead to the development of additional targeted therapeutics to effectively treat the biologic pathways driving tumor growth.

Immune Factors

Autoimmune suppression may contribute to the development of cancer. Tumors are allowed to exist because of tolerance—the ability of the tumor to escape the host immune system. The host immune system cannot recognize the tumor as foreign because of an absence of critical immunostimulatory molecules on the tumor itself, resulting in a state of anergy (deletion of tumor-specific lymphocytes) toward the growing cancer. Novel therapies (such as vaccines) aimed at correcting this immunodeficient state and stimulating the host immune response against tumor cells are now being tested clinically. (See section on novel therapies at the end of this chapter.)

Environmental, Infectious, & Therapeutic Carcinogens

It is difficult to link exposures to specific carcinogens with the development of cancer, since latency is generally quite long and the nature of exposure is poorly documented. Environmental carcinogens include chemical carcinogens such as benzene and asbestos, oncogenic viruses such as the human papillomavirus and the Epstein–Barr virus, and physical agents such as ionizing radiation and ultraviolet light.

Certain viral infections may increase the risk of cancer and clearly have a pathogenetic role, such as the association between Epstein–Barr virus infection and endemic Burkitt's lymphoma and non-Hodgkin's lymphoma. Chronic infection with hepatitis B or C viruses increases the risk of hepatocellular carcinoma. Largely owing to the increase in chronic hepatitis, the incidence of hepatocellular carcinoma significantly increased during the 1990s compared with the 1970s. Interestingly, treatment with the antiviral agent interferon-α following resection of hepatitis C-related hepatocellular carcinoma in a randomized trial appeared to significantly reduce the risk of cancer recurrence. Screening for cancer with regular scans in patients with known persistent hepatitis B and C infection is now standard practice as early identification of hepatocellular carcinoma is critical to effective treatment. Infection with HIV has been associated with non-Hodgkin's lymphoma, Hodgkin's disease, Kaposi's sarcoma (KS), and cervical and anal cancers. The finding of human herpesvirus-8 (HHV-8) DNA sequences in both AIDS-associated and non–AIDS-associated KS supports a causative role of the herpesviruses in the development of some cancers. It appears that HHV-8 is sexually transmitted among men. Antibodies to HHV-8 correlate with the subsequent development of KS and it is now thought that infection is necessary for KS to develop. The sexually transmitted human papillomavirus (HPV) is a major risk factor for the development of cervical carcinoma and anal cancer; nearly 100% of women with cervical cancer have evidence of this infection. Fifteen HPV subtypes have been identified with an increased risk of cervical cancer; HPV 16 and 18 are the most common and are associated with a more than 200-fold increased risk of cancer. HPV is a common infection, and most infected women do not develop cancer. Progression is associated with persistent infection over a decade or more; additional genetic or systemic cofactors are required, although only partially understood. Understanding the infectious cause of cervical cancer has led to the development of two vaccines directed against HPV 16 and 18 as well as other subtypes; large-scale testing of this vaccine has demonstrated marked protection from infection. The first trial treated 755 healthy sexually active women with three injections over 6 months; none developed precancerous lesions in the cervix over 4 years of observation. Approval of this vaccine is currently under regulatory review. Chronic infection with bacteria has also been associated with an increased risk of malignancy. Infection with *Helicobacter pylori* is thought to increase the risk of cancer of the distal portion of the stomach approximately sixfold and also increases the risk for gastric lymphoma. Approximately 60% of gastric cancers are associated with *H pylori* infection. Geographic variations in the incidence of gastric cancer appear to be influenced by geographic variations in the strain of *H pylori*; strains that produce a specific protein are more likely to be associated with cancer than those that do not. Screening for and treatment of *H pylori* may be a cost-effective way to prevent gastric cancer in the United States.

An additional cause of cancer is chemotherapy or radiation therapy for a prior malignancy. More aggressive chemotherapeutic and radiation regimens—and especially those combining the two treatment modalities—have been associated with increased rates of both secondary leukemias and solid tumors. The latency period may be short (2–5 years for leukemia) or very long (10–20 years for solid tumors), but the prognosis is uniformly poor. Chemotherapeutic agents known to cause secondary malignancies include alkylating agents—busulfan, cyclophosphamide, mechlorethamine, etc—and topoisomerase II inhibitors, including epipodophyllotoxins (etoposide), anthracyclines, ie, doxorubicin and epirubicin, and anthracenediones (mitoxantrone). Secondary leukemias can be characterized to some degree by the causative agent. Alkylator-induced leukemias are usually associated with abnormalities involving chromosomes 5 and 7 and generally occur within 5–7 years after exposure. In contrast, topoisomerase II-induced leukemias occur within 2–3 years following exposure and involve aberrations in a specific gene within the long arm of chromosome 11 (11q23). Abnormalities of 11q23 often occur at a specific breakpoint region thought to be involved in DNA transcription. An increase in the rate of secondary acute leukemia has been reported in breast cancer patients treated with dose intensification of cyclophosphamide in combination with doxorubicin (a topoisomerase II active drug) from 1992 to 1994. The incidence is approximately 0.3% in a multicenter study involving over 2500 women with positive axillary nodes. Increased dosages and frequency of administration of anthracyclines, anthracenediones, and the alkylating agent cyclophosphamide have been reported to increase the risk of leukemia to as high as 3–4%. Prolonged oral exposure to etoposide or alkylator agents can result in a much higher risk of secondary leukemia as well. Platinum-based chemotherapy for ovarian cancer has been reported to increase the risk of leukemia twofold to eightfold, with larger doses and longer treatment courses associated with higher risks. This risk was significantly higher in women who had also received intravenous melphalan.

The risk of certain secondary cancers may be age dependent. Radiation therapy for Hodgkin's disease increases the risk of breast cancer (including bilateral disease), particularly if the radiation occurred in women under the age of 30 years. The relative risk of subsequent solid tumors and leukemias has been found to increase significantly with younger age at first chemotherapy treatment for Hodgkin's disease. This risk is especially high when chemotherapy and radiation are combined. Nevertheless, the risk of secondary malignancies in children surviving at least 5 years after diagnosis is relatively low at 3.2% 20 years postdiagnosis, with primary disease recurrence remaining the most common cause of mortality. The Childhood Cancer Survivor Study (CCSS) is a large prospective study of over 14,000 survivors of childhood cancer designed to characterize the late effects of therapy in this increasing population. Although the risk of complications is highest in the first 5 years after diagnosis and treatment, risks of additional sequelae persist for many years.

Estrogen & Progesterone

Retrospective data indicate that the combination of estrogen and progesterone given as long-term hormonal replacement to postmenopausal women may significantly increase the risk of breast cancer over estrogen therapy alone. The best evidence for the risks and benefits of postmenopausal hormone use comes from the Women's Health Initiative (WHI), a large randomized clinical trial of over 16,000 healthy women ages 50–79 years that compared the effects of combined estrogen and progesterone to placebo on a variety of health outcomes. The trial, sponsored by the National Institutes of Health (NIH), was halted early when, in July 2002, investigators reported that the overall risks of estrogen plus progestin—specifically Prempro—outweighed the benefits. The WHI found that use of Prempro increased the risk of breast cancer (by 24%, or an additional eight cases of breast cancer for every 10,000 women treated), heart disease, stroke, and blood clots, although there were fewer cases of hip fractures and colon cancer in the treatment arm. Follow-up is still short, and at this time there is no difference in mortality. However, recent data from this trial indicate that the breast cancers developing in women receiving combined hormonal therapy were significantly larger than those developing in women on placebo and were diagnosed at a more advanced stage. Hormonal therapy increases breast density, increasing the difficulty in diagnosing cancers at an early stage. The WHI study has also shown that almost twice the number of women receiving Prempro had abnormal mammograms at 1 year compared with women receiving placebo medication. The HABITS (hormonal replacement therapy after breast cancer) trial evaluated the safety of hormone replacement therapy (HRT) after a diagnosis of breast cancer. After a median follow-up of only 2.1 years, more than three times the number of women in the HRT group had developed a new breast cancer event compared to the women in the best treatment group. These dramatic differences led to early closing of the trial.

An update of the WHI study showed that in women aged 65 years and over, use of estrogen plus progestin doubled the risk of developing dementia. Additionally, an analysis of the quality of life of a subgroup of WHI participants aged 50–79 years found no change in general health, vitality, mental health, depressive symptoms, or sexual satisfaction associated with use of combined hormonal replacement.

Estrogen alone appears to be less risky, but does not protect against chronic disease. The estrogen alone component of the WHI study randomized over 10,700 postmenopausal women with prior hysterectomy to either conjugated equine estrogen (CEE) or placebo. At 6.8 years of follow-up, women treated with CEE had an increased risk of stroke, a decreased risk of hip fracture, and no difference in the rate of either coronary heart disease or breast cancer. The rate of incident disease events was equivalent in the placebo and CEE arms, indicating no overall benefit. However, a recent longer term follow-up of women treated with CEE compared with placebo found a fascinating and striking 35% relative decrease in the incidence of invasive breast cancers in women without prior exposure to postmenopausal hormones, indicating that estrogen has a protective effect against breast cancer. Women with a history of oophorectomy had a similar decrease in breast cancer risk. This marked contrast to the effects of combination hormone therapy is perhaps explained by the promoting effects of progesterone. In women aged 65 years and older, CEE had an adverse effect on cognition, although there was no apparent increase in dementia. An extension study is ongoing to continue to observe all women enrolled in the WHI study through 2010.

In an observational study of over 40,000 women, those who used estrogen alone for 10–19 years were twice as likely to develop ovarian cancer as women who did not use menopausal hormones. For women who used estrogen for 20 or more years, the risk of ovarian cancer increased to three times that of women who did not use menopausal hormones. Another study suggests that the increased risk appears to be limited to women who used estrogens for 10 or more years; longer follow-up from the WHI trial will be critical to understand this risk. To date, this study has not shown an increased risk of ovarian cancer in women taking CEE. There are insufficient data on which to base a conclusion about whether combined estrogen and progesterone use affects the risk of developing ovarian cancer.

It is clear that other dietary and lifestyle factors play a significant role in the risk of developing specific cancers, although much of the specifics still need to be elucidated (see section on Primary Prevention, below).

American Society of Clinical Oncology policy statement update: genetic testing for cancer susceptibility. Adopted on March 1, 2003. J Clin Oncol 2003;21:1. [PMID: 12692171]

Anderson GL et al: Effects of conjugated equine estrogen in postmenopausal women with hysterectomy: the Women's Health Initiative randomized controlled trial. JAMA 2004; 291:1701. [PMID: 15082697]

Beer DG et al: Gene-expression profiles predict survival of patients with lung adenocarcinoma. Nat Med 2002;8:816. [PMID: 12118244]

Buys CH: Telomeres, telomerase, and cancer. N Engl J Med 2000;342:1282. [PMID: 10781627]

Calin GA et al: Familial cancer associated with a polymorphism in ARLTS1. N Engl J Med 2005;352:1667. [PMID: 15843669]

Edwards BK et al: Annual report to the nation on the status of cancer, 1975-2002, featuring population-based trends in cancer treatment. J Natl Cancer Inst 2005;97:1407. [PMID: 16204691]

Hankinson SE et al: Towards an integrated model for breast cancer etiology: the lifelong interplay of genes, lifestyle, and hormones. Breast Cancer Res 2004;6:213. [PMID: 15318928]

Holmberg L et al: HABITS (hormonal replacement therapy after breast cancer—is it safe?), a randomised comparison: trial stopped. Lancet 2004;363:453. [PMID: 14962527]

Jemal A et al: Cancer statistics, 2005. CA Cancer J Clin 2005;55: 10. [PMID: 15661684]

McTiernan A et al; Women's Health Initiative Mammogram Density Study Investigators: Estrogen-plus-progestin use and mammographic density in postmenopausal women: women's health initiative randomized trial. J Natl Cancer Inst 2005;97:1366. [PMID: 16174858]

Modugno F et al: Ovarian cancer and high-risk women—implications for prevention, screening, and early detection. Gynecol Oncol 2003;91:15. [PMID: 14529658]

Nelson HD et al; U.S. Preventive Services Task Force: Genetic risk assessment and BRCA mutation testing for breast and ovarian cancer susceptibility: systematic evidence review for the U.S. Preventive Services Task Force. Ann Intern Med 2005;143:362. [PMID: 16144895]

Rossouw JE et al: Risks and benefits of combined estrogen and progestin in healthy menopausal women: principal results from the Women's Health Initiative randomized controlled trial. JAMA 2002;288:321. [PMID: 12117397]

Schiffman MH et al: Epidemiologic studies of a necessary causal risk factor: human papillomavirus infection and cervical neoplasia. J Natl Cancer Inst 2003;95:E2. [PMID: 12644550]

Soussi T: The p53 tumor suppressor gene: from molecular biology to clinical investigation. Ann NY Acad Sci 2000;910: 121. [PMID: 10911910]

van de Vijver MJ et al: A gene-expression signature as a predictor of survival in breast cancer. N Engl J Med 2002;347:1999. [PMID: 12490681]

Weir HK et al: Annual report to the nation on the status of cancer, 1975–2000, featuring the uses of surveillance data for cancer prevention and control. J Natl Cancer Inst 2003;95: 1276. [PMID: 12953083]

Wulfkuhle JD et al: Proteomic applications for the early detection of cancer. Nat Rev Cancer 2003;3:267. [PMID: 12671665]

■ PREVENTION OF CANCER

PRIMARY PREVENTION

1. Lifestyle Modifications

Population studies suggest that lifestyle—including tobacco use, diet, obesity, and alcohol consumption—accounts for a majority of avoidable cancer deaths in the United States. Other factors, including obesity, parity, and length of lactation, have also been associated with increased cancer risk. Although prostate and breast cancers are the most common malignancies in men and women, respectively, the most common cause of cancer-related death in both sexes is still lung cancer. Since 1973, there has been only a 10% increase in the incidence of lung cancer in men compared with a 124% increase in women, reflecting a marked increase in the number of women who smoke. In 2005, the American Cancer Society estimates that more than 175,000 cancer deaths will be caused by tobacco use, and smoking remains the most preventable cause of death in our society. Because tobacco-related cancers account for at least 30% of all fatal forms of cancer and 87% of lung cancer-related deaths, smoking cessation is an important area for continued education and prevention efforts. Starting in the mid 1990s, lung cancer rates in women leveled off and rates in men decreased by about 2% per year, a tribute to national efforts to curtail tobacco use. Unfortunately, mortality from this disease remains high. Strategies for helping patients stop smoking are described in Chapter 1. In several states, comprehensive tobacco control programs directed both at cessation of smoking and at reversing the social acceptability of cigarette smoking have resulted in a substantial decrease in the prevalence of adult smoking. In California, this program was responsible for halving of the per capita consumption of cigarettes and translated into a significant decline (almost five times greater than the rest of the United States) in the incidence of lung cancer in both men and women in the state from 1988 to 1997. The decline in women is even more striking when compared with the rest of the United States. For an excellent article (with graphics) on this topic, go to www.asco.org and search under Tobacco Control and Global Issues, or see Cancer Prevention and Early Detection Facts and Figures 2004, accessible at http://www.cancer.org/downloads/STT/CPED2005v5PWSecured.pdf.

The molecular targets for carcinogens such as alcohol and tobacco have not yet been identified. However, an evaluation of tumor samples from over 100 patients with squamous cell carcinoma of the head and neck found an association between smokers and genetic mutations in the *p53* gene, thought to result in the initiation or progression of this cancer. This supports epidemiologic evidence that abstinence from smoking is important in preventing head and neck cancer. Cigarette smoking has been linked to cancers of the lung, mouth, larynx, esophagus, pancreas, kidney, and bladder. In addition, a study by the American Cancer Society found a 30–40% increase in the risk of death from colorectal cancer in cigarette smokers, with the increased risk occurring after 20 years of smoking and increasing with the number of cigarettes smoked daily. The risk decreased each year after quitting smoking, indicating that change in this major lifestyle factor can still reduce risk of death from cancer. In addition, patients who stop smoking following a diagnosis of small cell lung cancer and who are treated with chemotherapy and radiation have a significantly longer 2-year and 5-year survival than those who continue smoking. A similar prolongation in survival occurs in patients with head and neck cancer who quit smoking following diagnosis. Although cigarette smoking has not been related to the incidence of breast cancer, early data suggest that mortality from established breast cancer is higher in smokers than in nonsmokers. This supports the hypothesis that ongoing toxicity even in patients already diagnosed with cancer contributes to mortality. However, up to 50% of all lung cancers occur in those who have stopped smoking for at least 1 year, indicating that at least some of the carcinogenic effect of cigarette smoking may be irreversible.

Diet is an important area of intervention for primary cancer prevention. Epidemiologic studies suggest an inverse relationship between fruit and vegetable intake and the risk of common carcinomas, indicating a potential protective role of these dietary components. A case-control study in South Asia found a small reduction in the risk of breast cancer associated with a diet rich in vegetables. High intakes of fat and specific fatty acids have been postulated to increase the risk of breast, colon, prostate, and lung cancer, although a recent study in Canada found no association between carbohydrate intake and risk of colorectal cancer in women. Linoleic acids in essential fatty acids are the food source for arachidonic acid—and this metabolic pathway has been postulated to play an important role in the development of cancer. However, the Nurses' Health Study, which followed more than 88,000 women for 14 years with food frequency questionnaires every 4 years beginning in 1980, found no evidence that a lower intake of total fat or specific major types of fat decreased the risk of breast cancer. A recent subset analysis of premenopausal women aged 26–46 years within the Nurses' Health Study found a slightly increased risk of breast cancer with intake of animal but not vegetable fat. A higher intake of animal fat was also associated with a larger body mass index as well as other known risk factors. Data from the Nurses' Health Study and other epidemiologic studies suggest that a high consumption of red meat and excess alcohol consumption (probably also in combination with a diet low in possible preventive vitamins such as folate) may increase the risk of colorectal cancer. A meta-analysis published in 1999 evaluated dietary fat intervention studies (published from 1966 through 1998) on serum estradiol levels and fat consumption. These findings did not rule out the possibility that reducing fat consumption below 20% of calories might reduce breast cancer risk by lowering serum estradiol levels. Another study compared the dietary intake of saturated fat of 1665 men with prostate cancer to the diet of an equal number of men without the disease. A high intake of saturated fat increased the risk of prostate cancer in all four major ethnic groups evaluated. There was no increase in prostate cancer among men with the lowest intake of saturated fats.

Phytoestrogens are plant estrogenic substances including isoflavones, coumestans, and lignans. There has been interest in the role of phytoestrogens in the prevention of breast cancer, due to the lower rates of breast cancer observed in women with a high consumption of phytoestrogens, such as in Asia. A variety of studies have evaluated epidemiologic data regarding intake, but are limited based on problems with dietary recall, or short duration of exposures in prospective designs. Ongoing trials are assessing the role of phytoestrogen supplementation on the reduction of breast density, a surrogate and short-term marker for breast cancer risk. Phytoestrogens clearly have the potential to affect estrogen-driven cell growth in either a positive or negative way. To date, there are no data to suggest that dietary plant phytoestrogens stimulate cancer growth.

Obesity or a high body mass index has been implicated as a risk factor for breast, colorectal, and lung cancers (in nonsmokers) as well as others. Body mass index and elevated blood pressure have been associated with an increased risk of renal cell cancer in men. Dietary factors may further increase risk in already high-risk populations. A high intake of saturated fat in 27,111 smokers participating in the Alpha-Tocopherol, Beta-Carotene (ATBC) Cancer Prevention study significantly increased the risk of developing pancreatic cancer, suggesting that diet may be a modifiable factor in the prevention of pancreatic cancer in this population.

Increased intake of dietary fiber has been thought to reduce the risk of colorectal cancer and adenomas. The Nurses' Health Study investigated the intake of dietary fiber in the same population specified above, and no association was found between the intake of dietary fiber and the risk of colorectal cancer or adenomas. A prospective study of over 10,000 men likewise did not find a significant association between fiber intake and the risk of developing adenomas. Two prospective, randomized trials tested the value of a high-fiber, low-fat diet or a high-fiber cereal supplement versus a standard diet in reducing the risk of recurrent colorectal adenomas in men and women with a recent prior diagnosis of adenoma and demonstrated no difference in the risk of recurrent adenoma based on dietary regimens. Other dietary factors such as folate, methionine, and vitamin D may reduce the risk of colorectal malignancy, but this too will require further investigation.

Various lifestyle and dietary factors have been associated with a reduced risk of breast cancer. Increased duration of lactation, particularly for at least 1 year and with more than one pregnancy, reduced the subsequent risk of breast cancer in one large meta-analysis. In another study, Korean women who breast-fed for less than a year had a 20% lower risk of developing breast cancer, and those who breast-fed for more than 24 months had a 40% reduced risk compared with those who had no history of lactation. The California Teachers Study is a prospective study of over 133,000 active and retired teachers and administrators that is evaluating a variety of factors related to the risk of developing cancer over time. At 2 years of follow-up, the only dietary factor associated with an increased risk of breast cancer was alcohol ingestion, with two or more

glasses of wine per day associated with a 50% increased risk (relative risk 1.5) compared with non-drinkers. It may be that women with a higher risk of breast cancer could modify their risk by reducing overall alcohol intake.

The WHI, begun in 1992, examined the effects of three distinct interventions—a low-fat eating pattern, hormone replacement therapy, and calcium and vitamin D supplementation—on the prevention of cancer, cardiovascular disease, and osteoporosis in 64,500 postmenopausal women of all races. An additional 100,000 women have been enrolled in an observational study. Both the estrogen–progesterone and estrogen-alone components of this study have been closed (see Incidence & Etiology, above). Information on the dietary and vitamin intervention component of this trial should be available in the next 2 years. Recent data from the WHI study found that postmenopausal women who exercised regularly and not necessarily strenuously had a lower risk of breast cancer than those who did not; those who reported the equivalent of 1.25–2.5 hours of brisk walking per week had an 18% lower risk of breast cancer compared with inactive women. This impact increased with duration and intensity of exercise. The Women's Intervention Nutrition Study (WINS) is a large, phase III trial that randomized over 2400 postmenopausal women within 1 year of a diagnosis of early-stage breast cancer to an intensive dietary fat reduction (15% of dietary calories from fat) or no dietary intervention. During the course of the trial, from1994 to 2001, approximately 56% of the dietary calories in the control group, and 35% in the treatment group were from fat. At 60 months of follow-up, there was a significant 24% relative improvement in relapse-free survival in the low-fat diet group. On multivariate analysis, this benefit was only seen in women with hormone receptor negative cancers. The treatment group had a 5 lb average weight loss compared with a 2 lb weight gain in the control group, raising the question of whether the observed reduction in relapse was due to the weight loss or to the dietary fat content. Other ongoing intervention trials include the Women's Healthy Eating and Living (WHEL) study, which targets women 1–3 years following a diagnosis of breast cancer to assess the effects of a low-fat, high-fiber diet on recurrence and death from cancer.

Given the general lack of specific information linking diet to the risk of cancer, what should we recommend to patients now? A diet low in saturated fat and rich in whole grains, fruits, and vegetables appears to improve health in a variety of ways—certainly in reducing cardiovascular disease and diabetes and, based on epidemiologic data, reducing the overall risk of developing cancer. Similarly, weight loss appears to be a prudent recommendation. For more specific diets—in particular, reducing the risk of recurrence of a known cancer or precancer—we will have to wait for more data. Regular physical exercise should be incorporated into all general health recommendations.

Another lifestyle factor with important implications for primary prevention is exposure to ultraviolet light. Chronic cumulative exposure to solar ultraviolet radiation is the major risk factor for nonmelanomatous skin cancer. Regular use of sunscreen prevents the development of precancerous solar keratoses and results in regression of existing keratoses, although the effect of sunscreens on the prevention of melanoma is not clear. Protection from sunlight and the regular use of sunscreens should be recommended for the primary prevention of skin cancers.

Campos FG et al: Diet and colorectal cancer: current evidence for etiology and prevention. Nutr Hosp 2005;20:18. [PMID: 15762416]

Cho E et al: Premenopausal fat intake and the risk of breast cancer. J Natl Cancer Inst 2003;95:1079. [PMID: 12865454]

Colditz GA et al: The Nurses' Health Study: lifestyle and health among women. Nat Rev Cancer 2005;5:388. [PMID: 15864280]

Correa Lima MP et al: Colorectal cancer: lifestyle and dietary factors. Nutr Hosp 2005;20:235. [PMID: 16045124]

Gerber B et al: Nutrition and lifestyle factors on the risk of developing breast cancer. Breast Cancer Res Treat 2003;79:265. [PMID: 12825861]

Gotay CC: Behavior and cancer prevention. J Clin Oncol 2005; 23:301. [PMID: 15637393]

Kotsopoulos J et al: Towards a dietary prevention of hereditary breast cancer. Cancer Causes Control 2005;16:125. [PMID: 15868454]

McTiernan A et al: Recreational physical activity and the risk of breast cancer in postmenopausal women: the Women's Health Initiative Cohort Study. JAMA 2003;290:1331. [PMID: 12966124]

Nishino H et al: Cancer prevention by phytochemicals. Oncology 2005;69 Suppl 1:38. [PMID: 16210876]

Riboli E et al: Epidemiologic evidence of the protective effect of fruit and vegetables on cancer risk. Am J Clin Nutr 2003; 78(3 Suppl):559S. [PMID: 12936950]

Taylor PR et al: Nutritional interventions in cancer prevention. J Clin Oncol 2005;23:333. [PMID: 15637396]

Westmaas JL et al: Altering risk in patients who smoke. Respir Care Clin North Am 2003;9:259. [PMID: 12911292]

2. Chemoprevention

Chemoprevention focuses on the prevention of cancer by administering chemical compounds that interfere with the multistaged carcinogenic process. Better understanding of the biochemical and molecular mechanisms of carcinogenesis has made possible the identification of potential chemopreventive agents. Four risk groups have been identified for intervention: (1) previous cancer patients (to prevent second malignancies), (2) patients with preneoplastic lesions, (3) patients at high risk for malignancy (family history, lifestyle, occupation), and (4) the general population.

Chemicals used in chemoprevention must be nontoxic and well tolerated by otherwise asymptomatic individuals. Because of the long natural history of carcinogenesis, there must also be a method of evaluating the efficacy of chemopreventive agents other than waiting for the development of tumors. Biomarkers, including the premalignant markers such as leukoplakia, colonic polyps, and aberrant crypt formation in the colon, are currently in clinical use. Other less specific surrogate markers for cancer risk such as breast density are also in use as primary end points in prevention studies. Molecular susceptibility markers may become useful; nuclear retinoic acid receptor agonists are under investigation in chemoprevention studies of patients with head and neck cancer.

Retinoids, the natural derivatives and synthetic analogs of vitamin A, are the best-studied chemopreventive agents. Nonsteroidal anti-inflammatory drugs (NSAIDs)—specifically, the selective cyclooxygenase (COX)-2 inhibitors—and hormonal agents such as tamoxifen, raloxifene, and finasteride appear to have an important role in prevention of some cancers. Numerous additional investigations include the role of specific dietary components such as vitamins and of pharmaceutical agents such as the statins. Ongoing research in this area is assessing the impact and appropriate use of selective NSAIDs, vitamins, hormonal agents, and, more recently, statins in cancer prevention.

Isotretinoin & Acyclic Retinoids

Retinoids are modulators of epithelial cell differentiation both in vivo and in vitro that are thought to act on nuclear receptors to regulate both cellular growth and differentiation and cell apoptosis.

Isotretinoin has been shown to suppress leukoplakia, a premalignant lesion of the aerodigestive tract. Effectiveness and tolerability of low doses of isotretinoin have been demonstrated. In a randomized maintenance trial, only patients with a demonstrated response to high-dose induction (1.5 mg/kg/d) were placed on low-dose maintenance therapy (0.5 mg/kg/d). The disease progression rate was only 8% compared with a rate of 55% in a separate group taking β-carotene.

High doses of isotretinoin may prevent the development of second primary tumors in patients with early squamous cell carcinoma of the head and neck. An initial phase III study showed a statistically significant reduction in the incidence of new aerodigestive cancers when isotretinoin versus placebo was given for 1 year following definitive local therapy (4% versus 24%). There were no significant differences in disease recurrence or survival at a median follow-up of 55 months, and 30–40% of patients required reduced dosages or discontinued therapy due to toxicity. A second randomized study using lower doses of a different and probably less active retinoid showed no differences in the incidence of second primary tumors. Based on these preliminary results, three large randomized trials were performed to assess the preventive effects of retinoids on second primary tumors.

The first trial (Euroscan) studied 2 years of treatment with retinyl palmitate and acetylcysteine in over 2500 patients with either lung cancer or head and neck cancer. No differences were found in the incidence of second primary tumors. A U.S. intergroup trial studied the use of isotretinoin to prevent second primary tumors following definitive therapy of stage I non-small cell lung cancer. Because of side effects seen with the higher (50- to 100-mg) dose, the drug was given at a dosage of 30 mg/d for 3 years. After a median follow-up of 3.5 years, there was no difference in time to second primary tumor, recurrence, or mortality. Subset analysis suggested that never-smokers might benefit from isotretinoin, whereas there was a higher risk of cancer recurrence and mortality in smokers in the isotretinoin arm. The major toxicity at higher doses includes skin dryness, cheilitis, hypertriglyceridemia, and conjunctivitis. These toxicities require dose reduction or temporary discontinuation of the drug. The third double-blind randomized study investigated the effect of low-dose isotretinoin for 3 years in the prevention of second primary tumors in 1200 patients definitively treated for stage I or stage II head and neck cancer, with 4 years of subsequent follow-up. The annual second primary tumor rate was 4.7% in both arms and was highest in current smokers, with the most common tumor being tumor of the lung. Although there was a transient protective effect on local recurrence in patients who received isotretinoin, this effect was lost after treatment was discontinued. A number of trials have confirmed a significantly higher rate of second primary tumor formation in smokers versus former smokers or never-smokers as well as a significant adverse effect on survival—prospectively proving the impact of active smoking on second primary tumor development. An interesting recent report suggests that nicotine may suppress the antigrowth effects of retinoids in lung cancer cells.

Retinoids have been synthesized that may be more potent chemopreventive agents with less side effects. The acyclic retinoid polyprenoic acid inhibits chemically induced hepatocarcinogenesis in rats and spontaneous hepatomas in mice. In patients with hepatocellular carcinoma, the rate of recurrent and second primary tumors is high despite curative therapy with surgical resection and ethanol injection therapy. In one study, 89 patients who were free of disease after either method of treatment were randomized to receive either 600 mg/d of polyprenoic acid or placebo for 12 months. After a median follow-up of 38 months, 27% of patients in the polyprenoic acid group versus 49% of the patients in the placebo group had recurrent or new hepatocellular carcinomas, a result that was statistically significant. The difference was even greater in the groups that had secondary hepatomas. Longer follow-up has also shown a survival advantage. At a median of 62 months of follow-up, 75% of the treatment group versus 45% of the placebo group are alive. Toxicity was quite modest (headache, nausea), with none of the side effects usually described with isotretinoin. Three strategies that have been proved to prevent liver carcinogenesis are vaccination against hepatitis B, treatment of chronic active hepatitis C with interferon, and deletion of premalignant and latent malignant cells in the remnant livers

of patients undergoing complete resection of hepatocellular carcinomas.

The retinamide fenretinide (4-HPR) is a potent apoptosis-inducing synthetic vitamin A analog with significant in vitro activity. Fenretinide appears to reduce the activity of telomerase, which is important in lung carcinogenesis. Expression of telomerase reverse transcriptase (TERT), the catalytic subunit of telomerase, was evaluated on bronchial biopsies in 57 heavy smokers before and after 6 months of treatment with fenretinide or placebo. A 25% reduction in expression of TERT was found in the fenretinide-treated patients. Although clinical follow-up is clearly critical, the hope is that this type of surrogate marker will improve our ability to assess the effectiveness of possible chemopreventive agents and perhaps also identify patients at higher risk for cancer development. A large randomized trial evaluated the effect of fenretinide versus placebo for 5 years to prevent contralateral breast cancer in women aged 30–70 years with a history of resected breast cancer and no other adjuvant therapy. Although no overall effect was observed, subset analysis found a reduction in contralateral and ipsilateral breast cancer rates in premenopausal women. Fenretinide is being studied in randomized trials as a chemopreventive agent in patients with superficial bladder cancer and in women at increased risk for ovarian cancer. Newer and more potent retinoids are being developed and tested for use in a variety of cancers.

Aspirin & Other NSAIDs

Aspirin and other NSAIDs inhibit tumor growth in experimental systems. In rats, prostaglandin inhibitors reduce the size and number of colon tumors induced by chemicals or radiation by inhibiting COX activity in the arachidonic acid pathway (COX-1 and COX-2). Regular aspirin administration at low doses (16 or more doses of 325 mg per month for at least 1 year) may reduce the risk of fatal colon cancer by as much as 40–50%. Low-dose aspirin may also protect against cancers of the esophagus, stomach, and rectum.

A study evaluating the use of sulindac versus placebo in patients with FAP showed reduction of both the number and the size of colorectal adenomas. The effect was incomplete, without complete regression of all polyps in any patient. After the sulindac was discontinued, both polyp size and polyp number increased. A large prospective cohort study was subsequently published evaluating aspirin use and the risk for both colorectal cancer and adenoma in 48,000 male health professionals over a 4-year period. The subsequent risk of developing colorectal cancer and adenomas was lower in men reporting regular use of aspirin (250 mg more than twice a week) on the study entry questionnaire even when multiple other variables were taken into account. In the Nurses' Health Study, 90,000 women were evaluated for the risk of colorectal cancer over a 12-year period according to the number of consecutive years of regular aspirin use (two or more 325-mg tablets per week) reported on three consecutive questionnaires. There was a statistically significant decrease in the risk of colorectal cancer after 20 years of consistent aspirin use, with the maximal reduction seen in women who took four to six tablets per week. A slight reduction in risk was seen in women who took aspirin for 10–19 years as well. Known risk factors such as diet did not influence this risk reduction. The Physicians Health Study is the only randomized prospective trial of aspirin (325 mg every other day for 5 years) versus placebo. At the end of the trial, no differences were seen in the frequency of self-reported new colorectal cancers.

The selective COX-2 enzyme inhibitors have been the subject of intense research in the area of prevention and treatment of cancer. COX-2 expression is inducible, unlike the constitutive expression of COX-1, and COX-2 up-regulation occurs in most epithelial tumors, including colorectal cancer and cancers of the lung and breast. This up-regulation is thought to be secondary to other initiating events, such as oncogene activation or mutation of a tumor suppressor gene. COX-2 levels increase throughout oncogenesis, and expression appears to promote angiogenesis (new blood vessel growth) and decrease apoptosis (programmed cell death). One selective COX-2 inhibitor, celecoxib, has been shown to induce regression of polyps in patients with FAP at a dosage of 400 mg twice a day for 6 months. Based on these data, celecoxib was approved by the Food and Drug Administration (FDA) for chemoprevention of polyps in patients with FAP. Up until recently, the primary known side effect of COX-2 inhibitors was thought to be gastrointestinal bleeding. However, in September 2004, a study evaluating rofecoxib found an increased incidence of cardiovascular events, including deaths, in patients taking the medication for 18 months or more. Subsequent data have confirmed an increase in cardiovascular risk for all the COX-2 inhibitors, including celecoxib and valdecoxib. Unfortunately, this apparent class effect of the selective COX-2 inhibitors markedly limits their possible use as chemopreventive agents; multiple national trials focusing on either prevention or treatment of cancer have been either closed or redesigned to eliminate the arms containing celecoxib. The gene for COX-2 is overexpressed in a number of common cancers, and overexpression correlates with worse outcomes including shorter remission durations and survival. Based on in vitro data suggesting antitumor activity of NSAIDs, including antiangiogenic effects, induction of apoptosis, and reduction of proliferation, it still appears that COX-2 inhibition is a reasonable target—but clearly new agents need to be tested that better fit the criteria for safe chemopreventive agents.

β-Carotene & Vitamin E

The carotenoids are plant pigments that protect plant cells from damage and were thought to have an antioxidant role in human tissues. β-Carotene is a carotenoid found in high concentrations in human tissues; its importance as an antioxidant is controversial. A role for β-carotene and another antioxidant, vitamin E, in the prevention of either premalignant or malignant disease has not been established.

Several randomized studies have evaluated the effect of β-carotene and vitamin E on the prevention of cancer in high-risk populations. The ATBC Cancer Prevention Study randomized 29,000 Finnish male smokers to receive β-carotene, vitamin E, both agents, or neither agent for an average of 6 years. A minimal (2%) and statistically insignificant reduction in the incidence of lung cancer was seen in the men who received vitamin E. In contrast, there was a statistically significant 18% higher incidence of lung cancer in the group taking β-carotene. Vitamin E supplementation reduced prostate cancer incidence by 34% and colorectal cancer by 16%, though only the reduction in prostate cancer incidence was statistically significant. Men in the control group with higher levels of vitamin E or β-carotene before the study was initiated developed fewer lung cancers, suggesting that other components of foods high in these vitamins may be responsible for the protective effects noted in epidemiologic studies.

The Beta-Carotene and Retinol Efficacy Trial (CARET), a lung cancer chemoprevention study targeting high-risk populations, randomized a total of 18,000 smokers, nonsmokers, and workers with extensive occupational exposure to asbestos to receive either a combination of 30 mg/d of β-carotene (as an antioxidant) and 25,000 international units/d of retinol (vitamin A—as a tumor suppressor) or placebo. With an average of 4 years and 73,000 person-years of follow-up, the combination of β-carotene and vitamin A had no benefit on the incidence of lung cancer. In fact, the active treatment group had a 28% higher incidence of lung cancer than the placebo group, and the mortality from all causes and the rate of death from cardiovascular disease were higher by 17% and 26%, respectively. On the basis of these results, this study was stopped early.

The Physician's Health Study randomized 22,000 U.S. male physicians to receive β-carotene (50 mg on alternate days) or placebo. The physicians were treated for an average of 12 years; 11% were current smokers and 39% were former smokers at the beginning of the study. In this trial, no evidence either of benefit or of increased risk for cancer was found, with a much longer follow-up than either of the two other studies. There were no differences in the overall incidence of malignant neoplasms, cardiovascular disease, or overall mortality in the group as a whole or in the smokers.

One additional randomized study that found a positive effect of β-carotene supplementation evaluated a poorly nourished population group rather than the well-nourished populations described above. Linxian, China, is an area with one of the world's highest rates of esophageal and stomach cancers and a habitually low intake of several nutrients. In nearly 30,000 participants from the general population, the mortality rates from cancer were substantially lower among those who received daily supplementation with a combination of β-carotene, α-tocopherol, and selenium over a 5-year period. A marked reduction in the cancer death rate (13%) was observed in the supplemented group, largely due to a 21% decrease in stomach cancer mortality. Over 85% of cancers arose in the esophagus or stomach, but 31 deaths were caused by lung cancer. The risk of death from lung cancer was reduced by 45% among those receiving supplements, though the numbers were very small (11 versus 20 lung cancer deaths), and only 30% were cigarette smokers. A second study evaluated the effect of supplements, including β-carotene, on prevention of esophageal and gastric cancers in over 3300 people with esophageal dysplasia. Although esophageal cancer mortality and total cancer mortality were not significantly lower in the supplemented group, the incidence of mortality due to stomach cancer was higher. On repeat endoscopy comparing results 2 and 6 years after randomization, dysplasia had resolved in about two-thirds of patients in both arms at 6 years. These findings emphasize the need for placebo-controlled trials in the area of cancer prevention. The NCI is currently collaborating with agencies in China to pursue further chemoprevention studies in this unique population.

In summary, there is no evidence to support the use of β-carotene in the primary prevention of cancer in well-nourished populations. The major criticism of the large studies conducted to date is that increasing one type of vitamin—even one stereoisomer of a vitamin—does not reflect the vitamin content of a diet high in vegetables. In addition, intake of β-carotene is a marker of increased fruit and vegetable consumption. The balanced mixture of antioxidants found in a diet rich in fruit and vegetables may be more important and more effective in reducing cancer risk than β-carotene supplementation. Other micronutrients such as vitamin E may prove more promising.

The Women's Health Study, begun in 1992, is a randomized, double-blind, placebo-controlled trial testing the risks and benefits of vitamin E, β-carotene, and aspirin in the primary prevention of cancer and cardiovascular disease in 40,000 healthy female health professionals in the United States. Results are expected in the next few years.

Calcium & Selenium

Dietary patterns continue to be associated with a risk of colorectal neoplasia. The changes in risk may be contributed to by alterations in bile acids. Calcium appears to bind bile acids in the bowel lumen, inhibiting bile-induced mucosal damage and perhaps carcinogenesis. A modest reduction in the incidence of adenomas in patients taking calcium supplementation has been shown in patients receiving it over a 4-year period. The Selenium and Vitamin E Cancer Prevention Trial (SELECT) is the largest chemoprevention study ever

to be undertaken and began in August 2001. This NCI-sponsored trial will randomize 32,400 men aged 50–55 years and older to selenium, vitamin E, both, or placebo for 7–12 years in 435 sites in the United States, Canada, and Puerto Rico. This study is based on the results of the ATBC Cancer Prevention Study, in which vitamin E reduced prostate cancer incidence by 32%, and the selenium and skin cancer trial, in which selenium reduced the incidence of prostate cancer by 63%. Results are not expected until 2012. Further information on the SELECT trial can be found at the following Web sites: www.crab.org/select and www.cancer.gov/select.

Tamoxifen

Tamoxifen is a selective estrogen receptor modulator (SERM) with both antiestrogen and proestrogen activity that has an important role in the treatment of both early and advanced breast cancer. Studies of women taking tamoxifen as adjuvant therapy for unilateral breast cancer have shown a 30–40% reduction in the risk of developing a second primary in the opposite breast. The Breast Cancer Prevention Trial (BCPT) is a nationwide trial that randomized 13,400 women at high risk for breast cancer to receive either tamoxifen (20 mg/d) or placebo for 5 years. The trial was stopped at a median follow-up of 4 years due to a striking 50% reduction in the risk of breast cancer in the women taking tamoxifen—89 women taking tamoxifen developed breast cancer, compared with 175 taking placebo. This benefit was restricted solely to the development of estrogen-receptor-positive cancers. In addition to invasive cancer, there was a similar reduction in the risk of noninvasive breast cancer such as ductal or lobular carcinoma in situ. Tamoxifen also decreased the number of bone fractures. Two much smaller European studies that used different parameters to determine risk (and study eligibility) did not show a significant reduction in cancers with the use of tamoxifen. It is likely that tamoxifen is not as effective in preventing breast cancer in very high-risk groups, ie, those with genetic predispositions. Side effects of tamoxifen include an age-dependent small increase in the risk of endometrial cancer (including sarcoma of the uterus), deep venous thrombosis, and pulmonary embolism. These side effects are seen primarily in women over age 50 years.

The use of tamoxifen for primary prevention of cancer is controversial because of its known secondary effects, mainly the increase in endometrial cancer. This risk is small when compared with the incidence of breast cancer in younger women on placebo in the trial. Even if the incidences of endometrial cancer and breast cancer are considered together, there was still a 30% reduction in the risk of cancer in the women receiving tamoxifen. Alternatives to tamoxifen (and raloxifene) are under study; these agents (aromatase inhibitors) are likely to be more effective and have a different side effect profile (see ongoing trials, below).

Raloxifene

Early results of the Multiple Outcomes of Raloxifene Evaluation (MORE) trial have provided more information regarding prevention of breast cancer. Raloxifene is a novel SERM with estrogenic effects on bone and lipids and estrogen antagonist effects on the breast and uterus. Two different doses of raloxifene or placebo were administered to 7700 postmenopausal women to test the hypothesis that raloxifene would reduce the risk of bone fractures. After 2.5 years, a 70% relative reduction in the risk of breast cancer was found in the women taking raloxifene compared with the women taking placebo. A suggestion of decreased risk of endometrial cancer was also found. The long-term safety and follow-up of raloxifene in these women are ongoing. The effects of raloxifene in women with breast cancer or in women at high risk for developing breast cancer have not been evaluated (see below). Raloxifene should not be combined with tamoxifen, or used for the treatment of osteoporosis in women on hormonal therapy for breast cancer.

Ongoing Trials in Breast Cancer

The Study of Tamoxifen and Raloxifene (STAR) is designed to determine whether raloxifene is as effective as tamoxifen at reducing the risk for breast cancer. The trial opened in 1999 and closed to enrollment in 2004 after randomizing 19,000 American and Canadian postmenopausal women who are at least 35 years of age and who are at increased risk of breast cancer to either daily tamoxifen (20 mg/d) or raloxifene (60 mg/d) for 5 years. Initial results will be presented in 2006. Additional information regarding the STAR trial as well as other studies on breast cancer can be found at the NCI clinical trials Web site (www.cancer.gov/clinical_trials) or by calling 800-4-CANCER. At the prevention Web site (www.breastcancerprevention.org), a link is provided to permit calculation of the risk for an individual patient of developing breast cancer.

A new class of hormonal agents is being tested in clinical trials for primary prevention of breast cancer. The aromatase inhibitors block the peripheral conversion of androstenedione and testosterone to estradiol in postmenopausal women and are highly effective as treatment of early- and late-stage breast cancer. There is significant variability in tissue estradiol levels in postmenopausal women, and the aromatase inhibitors block the tissue production of estrogen that plays an important role in the development of postmenopausal breast cancer. Data from a number of adjuvant hormonal therapy trials indicate that the aromatase inhibitors have a potent effect in the prevention of new breast cancers in women with previously diagnosed invasive cancer.

These agents do not cause either an increased risk of thrombosis or endometrial cancer, making them possibly more suitable agents for prevention in a healthy population. The primary side effects include accelerated loss of bone mineral density, joint and muscle aches, and an altered lipid profile. Aromatase inhibitors are effective only in postmenopausal women, as they stimulate ovarian follicle development and production of estradiol in premenopausal women making them useful agents for egg retrieval for in vitro fertilization. Ongoing trials targeting women at high risk for developing breast cancer, postmenopausal women with *BRCA* mutations, and women with a diagnosis of ductal carcinoma in situ are comparing the different aromatase inhibitors to each other, or to tamoxifen. Further follow-up and results from these trials will be needed to understand the impact of aromatase inhibitors in the area of prevention as well as their long-term side effects.

Isoflavones

Isoflavones are found in a variety of natural substances, including soy. Laboratory studies have shown that isoflavones such as those found in soy inhibit the growth of breast cancer cell lines; however, epidemiologic studies evaluating consumption of isoflavone-containing foods have shown inconsistent results. The Japan Public Health Center-based Prospective Study on Cancer and Cardiovascular Diseases enrolled almost 22,000 Japanese women between the ages of 40 and 59 years. The risk of breast cancer in women who consumed three or more bowls of miso soup daily containing over 25 mg of genistein was 50% less than the risk in women who consumed less than one bowl (about 7 mg genistein), and this effect was greatest among postmenopausal women. Interestingly, consumption of other foods containing soy—soybeans, tofus, etc—was not associated with a reduction in risk of breast cancer. Further trials, including trials in white women who have a higher baseline risk of breast cancer, are required to confirm this interesting observation.

Finasteride

Finasteride is a 5α-reductase inhibitor used to treat benign prostatic hyperplasia. This agent inhibits the enzyme responsible for converting testosterone to 5α-dihydrotestosterone, suppressing prostate cell and organ growth. In rats, finasteride prevented macroscopic but not microscopic prostate carcinogenesis—supporting the use of this agent in the prevention of conversion of latent prostate carcinoma to life-threatening disease. The Prostate Cancer Prevention Trial (PCPT) randomized 18,000 healthy men aged 55 years or older with normal digital rectal examinations and prostate-specific antigen (PSA) concentrations to finasteride or placebo. The trial was closed a year before its planned completion in response to the documented strength of the reduction in prostate cancer in the treatment arm. There was a 25% reduction in the incidence of prostate cancer in the treatment arm, with absolute rates of 18% versus 24% in the placebo arm. This corresponds to 15 less cancers in 1000 older men. Interestingly—and similar to results seen in prevention trials targeting breast cancer with tamoxifen—more high-grade tumors were seen in the finasteride group (37%) than in the placebo-treated men (22%). Although there was enthusiasm about these data—supporting manipulation of androgen levels as a way of preventing prostate cancer—caution was advised in the use of finasteride across the board. There are no survival data from the PCPT as yet, and it is not clear that the tumors prevented in this trial posed a significant threat to life or health. However, finasteride may be a reasonable preventive option for men with a high risk of prostate cancer until additional data are obtained. Side effects from finasteride, given at a dose of 5 mg by mouth every day, include reduced libido and improved ability to urinate in men with prostatic hyperplasia (the current approved use of this drug).

Other Current Trials

Additional trials are underway investigating the effect of both diet and pharmacologic agents in the prevention of cancer, including studies of folic acid, dietary fat and fish oils, vitamin supplementation, and others. Dietary agents such as polyprenols in green tea are thought to play a role in chemoprevention and are under investigation. There is great interest in moving the new biologic therapies that target specific pathways important in carcinogenesis into the prevention setting, such as farnesyl transferase inhibitors and agents that block the EGFR.

A recent case-control study of 300,000 residents in Europe found a 20% reduction in cancer risk in those taking cholesterol-lowering statin drugs. Data were adjusted for diabetes mellitus, hospitalizations, comorbidities, use of other medications, and sex hormone levels. When specific cancer rates were analyzed separately, reductions in risk were significant only for prostate cancer and renal carcinoma since the rates of other cancers were too low to show significance. Only people who took statins for more than 4 years had a significant 36% reduction in cancer risk, and an increase in cumulative dose also appeared to have a protective effect. The majority of patients took simvastatin as their cholesterol-lowering agent. A second prospective study evaluated the incidence of breast cancer in 7528 white women with a mean age of 77 years in the United States, 7.7% of whom reported using lipid-lowering drugs; patients were followed for almost 7 years. A marked reduction in the rate of breast cancers was found in women reporting statin use, with a 72% reduction in risk. Women taking any lipid-lowering drug had a 68% reduction in risk, even when results were adjusted for known breast cancer risk factors. Inhibition of 3-hydroxy-3-methylglutaryl coenzyme A (HMG-CoA) reductase reduces endogenous production of mevalonate, resulting eventually in decreased biologic activity of several oncogenes, including *ras*. These data are preliminary but intriguing; future studies must also control for important risk factors such as smoking and diet. Prevention studies are planned for the future to investigate the use of statins in the prevention of the most common malignancies, including breast cancer. Further information about ongoing chemoprevention trials can be obtained from the Chemoprevention Branch of the National Cancer Institute (301-496-8563) and at www.cancer.gov/prevention/index.html.

Brenner DE et al: Cancer chemoprevention: lessons learned and future directions. Br J Cancer 2005;93:735. [PMID: 16160697]

Ford LG et al: Prevention and early detection clinical trials: opportunities for primary care providers and their patients. CA Cancer J Clin 2003;53:82. [PMID: 12691266]

Hawk ET et al: Colorectal cancer chemoprevention—an overview of the science. Gastroenterology 2004;126:1423. [PMID: 15131803]

Jacobs EJ et al: A large cohort study of aspirin and other nonsteroidal anti-inflammatory drugs and prostate cancer incidence. J Natl Cancer Inst 2005;97:975. [PMID: 15998950]

Kalidas M et al: Aromatase inhibitors for the treatment and prevention of breast cancer. Clin Breast Cancer 2005;6:27. [PMID: 15899070]

Klein EA et al: SELECT: the selenium and vitamin E cancer prevention trial. Urol Oncol 2003;21:59. [PMID: 12684129]

Moyad MA: Heart healthy equals prostate healthy equals statins: the next cancer chemoprevention trial. Part I. Curr Opin Urol. 2005;15:1. [PMID: 15586021]

Rao CV et al: NSAIDs and chemoprevention. Curr Cancer Drug Targets 2004;4:29. [PMID: 14965265]

Rhee JC et al: Advances in chemoprevention of head and neck cancer. Oncologist 2004;9:302. [PMID: 15169985]

Samoha S et al: Cyclooxygenase-2 inhibition prevents colorectal cancer: from the bench to the bedside. Oncology 2005;69 (Suppl 1):33. [PMID: 16210875]

Serrano D et al: Progress in chemoprevention of breast cancer. Crit Rev Oncol Hematol 2004;49:109. [PMID: 15012972]

Thompson IM et al: The influence of finasteride on the development of prostate cancer. N Engl J Med 2003;349:213. [PMID: 12824459]

Tsao AS et al: Chemoprevention of cancer. CA Cancer J Clin 2004;54:150. [PMID: 15195789]

SECONDARY PREVENTION (Early Detection)

Given the inadequacy of current knowledge concerning the causes of cancer, effective prevention can be achieved for only a minority of malignancies. Other than primary prevention and perhaps chemoprevention, the most effective clinician intervention is early diagnosis. Screening is used for early detection of cancer in otherwise asymptomatic populations. Detection of cancer may be achieved through observation (eg, skin, mouth, external genitalia, cervix), palpation (eg, breast, mouth, thyroid, rectum and anus, prostate, testes, ovaries and uterus, lymph nodes), and laboratory tests and procedures (eg, Papanicolaou smear, sigmoidoscopy or colonoscopy, mammography). Effective screening requires a test that will specifically detect early cancers or premalignancies, be cost effective, and result in improved therapeutic outcomes. For most cancers, stage at presentation is related to curability, with the highest cure rates reported when the tumor is small and there is no evidence of metastasis. However, for some tumors (eg, lung or ovarian cancer), distant metastases tend to occur early, even from a small primary tumor. More sensitive detection methods such as tumor markers are being developed for many forms of cancer. Some tumor markers, such as PSA, are already a regular (though controversial) part of routine cancer screening (see section on tumor markers). Screening is not useful if a method of early detection does not exist (eg, cancer of the pancreas) or if there is no apparent localized stage (eg, leukemia). Current guidelines for cancer screening from the American Cancer Society can be found on line at http://caonline.amcancersoc.org in the January/February 2006 issue, and are updated regularly at http://www.cancer.org/docroot/PED/content/PED_2_3X_ACS_Cancer_Detection_Guidelines_36.asp. These recommendations include general cancer-related check-ups as well as screening for cancers of the prostate, breast, colorectum, and cervix.

Cancers for which screening or early detection has led to an improvement in outcome include cancers of the breast, cervix, colon, prostate, oral cavity, and skin. Ongoing trials are evaluating the use of newer screening methods for the most common malignancies, including cancers of the breast, lung, and prostate as well as colorectal and ovarian cancers.

It is critical that clinicians involve patients in decisions about whether to order tests for early detection of breast and prostate cancers so that patients will understand the risks and benefits. The rates of routine cancer screening in the United States remain low, with less than 50% having recent screening for colorectal cancer and less than 60% having recent mammography and clinical breast examination. Data from the WHI Observational Study cohort, which represents a large and diverse group of older women, indicate that health insurance is among the most important determinants of cancer screening independent of other factors. Improving insurance coverage of screening and access to health insurance for older adults in the United States may have an important role in improving early detection of cancer through screening. Screening is underutilized in minority groups in the United States, especially in inner city and rural areas. This results in the diagnosis of cancers at more advanced stages. Educational and outreach programs should be directed at these underserved areas.

Screening for Breast Cancer

Techniques for early detection of breast cancer include self-examination, clinical examination, and mammography. The benefits of screening mammography have been reviewed in two large meta-analyses and these results remain controversial based on a number of factors. First, several of the large published studies evaluating the value of mammography have serious flaws. Second, mammography increases the detection of the preinvasive ductal carcinoma in situ (DCIS), which has an extremely low 10-year mortality. Lastly, available data suggest that the most significant reduction in mortality obtained from mammographic screening may be in women over the age of 60 years (24–33% reduction), with smaller benefits in younger women. The Agency for Healthcare Research and Quality (AHRQ) conducted its own review of the meta-analysis and rated the included studies based on the quality of data and the inclusion of younger age groups as well as other factors. They concluded that there is a demonstrated 20% reduction in the number of deaths from breast cancer in women undergoing screening mammography both in the over-50 and under-50 year age groups, though the times required in follow-up to see these benefits may be quite different. The AHRQ—along with the American Cancer Society (ACS) and the NCI—have put forth the following recommendations for mammographic screening: Every 1–2 years for women between the ages of 40 and 49 years, then annually in women 50 years and older. The upper age limit for mammographic screening has not been established.

Both mammography and clinical examination of the breast are associated with a significant number of false-positive results, leading to further testing. Screening mammograms and clinical breast examinations in 2400 women over a 10-year period found that 24% and 13%, respectively, of women had at least one false-positive mammogram or false-positive clinical examination. The controversy regarding mammographic screening is thus far from resolved; however, it is the best screening method currently available. Women between the ages of 40 and 49 years should be active participants in decisions regarding screening and should have an understanding of known risks and benefits. Despite the sensitivity of mammography, between 15% and 25% of breast cancers are not visible by this radiographic technique; this is particularly true for young women with dense breasts. All clinically suspicious lesions should be biopsied regardless of a negative mammogram.

Digital mammography is a newer technique that uses computers and special detectors to produce a digital image displayed on high-resolution monitors. The NCI launched the Digital Mammographic Imaging Screening Trial (DMIST) in October 2001 to determine whether digital mammography is as good as or better than standard screen (x-ray) mammography with regard to sensitivity, specificity, and predictive values. Overall, 42,760 women in the United States and Canada entered this trial, and all women had both types of radiographic screening at study entry and at 1 year with 2 years of follow-up. Digital mammograms were 11% to 15% more accurate than standard mammograms in women under age 50, premenopausal women, and women with dense breasts. However, standard films were just as good as digital mammograms in all other women. Both types of mammogram missed about 30% of the breast cancers. At this time, digital mammograms account for only 8% of mammography equipment, largely because of cost. The majority of breast cancers will be diagnosed with equal accuracy regardless of the type of mammography technique.

MRI screening of the breast appears to be a useful technique in women at very high risk for developing breast cancer. This highly sensitive test is unfortunately not very specific, leading to unnecessary biopsies. It is currently of value only in very high-risk women when regular screening might not be sensitive enough to detect breast cancer.

The value of clinical breast examination for the early detection of breast cancer remains unclear. A large study in China found no benefit in survival in women trained to perform monthly examinations; however, these data may not apply to the U.S. population for a variety of reasons. At this time, screening guidelines include monthly breast self-examination as well as yearly mammography.

Screening for Lung Cancer

It is clear that current and former smokers are at high risk for developing lung cancer and that early detection of lung cancer may result in detection of lesions when they are still surgically resectable and, therefore, potentially curable. However, data available so far are inconclusive as to whether either chest x-rays or the more sensitive CT scan can reduce lung cancer mortality, although CT screening has been shown to identify tumors that are smaller and do not have lymph node metastases. The National Lung Screening Trial (NLST) is a large randomized trial designed to determine whether lung cancer mortality is reduced in long-term or heavy current and former smokers by screening with chest x-ray versus spiral CT. The trial, which opened in September 2002, enrolled 50,000 participants as of February 2004 and included men and women in good health between the ages of 55 and 74. Spiral CT or chest x-ray is performed once a year for 3 years. Interim results are hoped for in 2006; the study will continue until 2009. Further information regarding the NLST can be found at www.cancer.gov/nlst and at www.cancer.org.

Screening for Cervical Cancer

Regular screening for cervical cancer (every 3 years in standard risk groups) with Papanicolaou tests has been found to decrease the mortality rate in women who are sexually active or are 18 years of age or older. Testing for HPV DNA in high-risk populations may improve early detection and management of cervical cancer, helping to determine which women with low-grade cytologic abnormalities require colposcopic evaluation. Recent data indicate that screening every 2 years with both Papanicolaou and HPV testing is more cost effective than screening with either test alone. A large German study found that HPV testing was a highly sensitive method for detecting high-grade cervical intraepithelial neoplasia (CIN), suggesting that routine HPV testing might be of value in higher-risk women.

Self-collected vaginal swabs for DNA testing may improve screening in areas where cytologic study is not readily available or in populations in which women are hesitant to undergo regular examinations. The ACS has updated its screening guidelines to include HPV DNA testing in high-risk individuals. Routine screening with vaginal Papanicolaou smears in women who have previously undergone a hysterectomy for benign gynecologic disease is not useful because of the very low incidence of squamous cell cancers of the vagina. Two vaccines designed to prevent infection from the most oncogenic HPV strains are in clinical trials; one study has already been shown to be effective in preventing primary infection.

Screening for Colorectal Cancer

Annual fecal occult blood testing and screening with sigmoidoscopy every 5 years in people over age 50 years decreases the mortality rate from colorectal cancer. An evaluation of over 46,000 people aged 50–80 years in the Minnesota Colon Cancer Control study over an 18-year follow-up period showed that either annual or biennial screening of two stool samples significantly reduced the incidence of colorectal cancer when an abnormal fecal blood screen was followed by colonoscopy. Removing polyps detected by colonoscopy reduces the risk of colorectal cancer, and, following polypectomy, colonoscopy is superior to double-contrast barium enema for the detection of recurrent polyps. Even adenomatous polyps 5 mm or less in diameter detected in the rectosigmoid by sigmoidoscopy are markers for more advanced proximal neoplasms. These patients should undergo colonoscopy to evaluate the proximal bowel. However, colonoscopic screening can detect advanced colonic neoplasms in asymptomatic adults even in the absence of distal adenomas. Regular fecal occult blood testing and flexible sigmoidoscopy are still recommended for general screening because of the lower cost and facility of sigmoidoscopy compared with colonoscopy. Computed tomographic "virtual" colonoscopy is a new technique used to screen for colorectal neoplasia. A small rectal catheter is used to introduce air into the colon, then CT scanning is performed while the patient is supine and prone. Image processing allows image interpretation of the air-filled colon. This controversial imaging modality is nonetheless appealing to patients and less invasive; skilled interpretation and state of the art equipment are required. Further data will be required to fully validate the sensitivity and specificity of virtual colonoscopy. A novel test to examine stool for DNA alterations that might help to screen for colorectal cancer is in development.

The Prostate, Lung, Colorectal, & Ovarian (PLCO) Cancer Screening Trial

The PLCO Cancer Screening Trial is a large cancer screening study that was opened between 1992 and

2001 and randomized over 154,000 healthy men and women between the ages of 55 and 74 years to routine health care versus prescribed screening. The goal of this study is to determine the effect of cancer screening tests on site-specific cancer mortality. Screening will occur for a total of 6 years, with 10 years of follow-up. Screening tests include PSA annually for 6 years; digital rectal examination (DRE) annually for 4 years; chest x-ray annually for 4 years in smokers and for 3 years in never-smokers; sigmoidoscopy at entry and then after 3 or 5 years on study (see below); transvaginal ultrasound annually for 4 years; and CA 125 (an ovarian cancer tumor marker; see section on tumor markers) annually for 6 years. Preliminary results are available on the role of sigmoidoscopy repeated at a 3-year interval in 9317 participants. A polyp or growth was detected in 13.9%, with 3.1% having a distal colon advanced adenoma or cancer—in an area that had been carefully evaluated 3 years earlier. These data suggest that higher-risk patients might benefit from more frequent sigmoidoscopic screening, though there are no data on mortality at this time. Additional data on the role of the PSA test in prostate cancer screening is discussed below.

Screening for Other Cancers

Unfortunately, screening for ovarian cancer with serum markers (eg, CA 125), transvaginal ultrasound, or pelvic examinations has not been shown to decrease the mortality rate from this disease. The PLCO trial should help to assess the impact of combined markers and ultrasound on both detection and mortality for this difficult disease. Screening for prostate cancer and hepatocellular cancer is discussed in the section on tumor markers; prostate cancer is evaluated in the PLCO trial (see above).

Bach PB et al: Screening for lung cancer: the guidelines. Chest 2003;123(1 Suppl):83S. [PMID: 12527567]

Henschke CI et al; International Early Lung Cancer Action Program Investigators: Computed tomographic screening for lung cancer: the relationship of disease stage to tumor size. Arch Intern Med 2006;166:321. [PMID: 16476872]

Pickhardt PJ et al: Computed tomographic virtual colonoscopy to screen for colorectal neoplasia in asymptomatic adults. N Engl J Med 2003;349:2191. [PMID: 14657426]

Pisano ED et al; Digital Mammographic Imaging Screening Trial (DMIST) Investigators Group: Diagnostic performance of digital versus film mammography for breast-cancer screening. N Engl J Med 2005;353:1773. [PMID: 16169887]

Saslow D et al: American Cancer Society guidelines for the early detection of cervical neoplasia and cancer. CA Cancer J Clin 2003;52:342. [PMID: 12469763]

Schoen RE et al: Results of repeat sigmoidoscopy 3 years after a negative examination. JAMA 2003;290:41. [PMID: 12837710]

Segnan N et al: Randomized trial of different screening strategies for colorectal cancer: patient response and detection rates. J Natl Cancer Inst 2005;97:347. [PMID: 15741571]

Smith RA et al: American Cancer Society guidelines for breast cancer screening: Update 2003. CA Cancer J Clin 2003;54:141. [PMID: 1280948]

Smith RA et al: American Cancer Society guidelines for the early detection of cancer, 2006. CA Cancer J Clin 2006;56:11. [PMID: 16449183]

Subramanian S et al: Use of colonoscopy for colorectal cancer screening: evidence from the 2000 National Health Interview Survey. Cancer Epidemiol Biomarkers Prev 2005;14:409. [PMID: 15734966]

Winawer SJ: Screening of colorectal cancer. Surg Oncol Clin N Am 2005;14:699. [PMID: 16226687]

SPECIAL TOPICS IN PREVENTION

Patients with a family history of colorectal cancer are at increased risk to develop this disease and should undergo regular screening, which clearly reduces the incidence and mortality from invasive cancer. Guidelines for patients with a risk of hereditary nonpolyposis colon cancer are referenced below.

Approximately 10% of breast and ovarian cancers are due to inherited genetic mutations, occurring primarily in women with mutations of *BRCA1* and *BRCA2*. Patients with a family history of breast or ovarian cancer are at higher risk to develop these cancers and require frequent monitoring for early detection, though screening is inadequate to detect early ovarian cancer. Women with a family history of premenopausal or bilateral breast cancer—or any family history of ovarian cancer—should be referred for genetic counseling to better assess their risk of carrying one of the known mutations.

Prophylactic oophorectomy after completion of childbearing can significantly decrease the risk of ovarian cancer in women with *BRCA1* and *BRCA2* mutations; there is still a small risk of peritoneal cystadenocarcinoma. The actual risk reduction in a recent small prospective trial was 96%, similar to results from the Prevention and Observation of Surgical Endpoints (PROSE) study group and significantly higher than women electing intensive surveillance. In addition, bilateral prophylactic oophorectomy reduces the risk of subsequent breast cancer in high-risk women by 50–75%, presumably because of decreased exposure to ovarian estrogens. Oral contraceptive use for 6 years or more decreased the risk of ovarian cancer by as much as 60% in women with a family history of ovarian cancer. Prophylactic mastectomy has been used for decades to reduce the risk of breast cancer in high-risk women and is associated with a substantial reduction in breast cancer risk. In women at both high and moderate risk of breast cancer based on family history, the incidence of breast cancer (and death from breast cancer) is reduced by up to 99%. Decisions about such prophylactic surgery in high-risk women must be made taking full account of many other factors—breast or ovarian cancer will develop in most but not all women with *BRCA* mutations.

Any patient with a history of dysplasia or premalignant lesions is at high risk for development of invasive cancer and should undergo frequent and thorough screening for subsequent malignancy. Patients at a particularly high individual risk for cancer may require additional screening procedures. Enthusiasm about the ability of **spiral CT** to image early lung cancers has reawakened interest in screening high-risk individuals with the goal of reducing lung cancer mortality with detection of early, treatable lesions. Randomized trials are ongoing (see above) to investigate whether screening for lung cancer with this expensive test can actually reduce mortality rates. At present, general guidelines are to consider routine chest x-ray screening on an annual basis for heavy current or former smokers (more than 20 pack-years) over the age of 55 years.

Deligeoroglou E et al: Oral contraceptives and reproductive system cancer. Ann NY Acad Sci 2003;997:199. [PMID: 14644827]

Domcheck SM et al: Mortality after bilateral salpingo-oophorectomy in *BRCA1* and *BRCA2* mutation carriers: a prospective cohort study. Lancet Oncol 2006;7:223. [PMID: 16510331]

Hampel H et al: Referral for cancer genetics consultation: a review and compilation of risk assessment criteria. J Med Genet 2004;41:81. [PMID: 14757853]

Lostumbo L et al: Prophylactic mastectomy for the prevention of breast cancer. Cochrane Database Syst Rev. 2004;(4): CD002748. [PMID: 15495033]

■ STAGING OF CANCER

Standardized staging for tumor burden at the time of diagnosis is important both for determining prognosis and for making decisions about treatment. The American Joint Committee on Cancer (AJCC) has developed a simple classification scheme that can be incorporated into a form for staging and universally applied. This scheme is designed to encompass the life history of a tumor and is referred to as the TNM system. The untreated primary tumor (T) will gradually increase in size, leading to regional lymph node involvement (N) and, finally, distant metastases (M). The tumor is usually not clinically evident until local invasion or even spread to regional draining lymph nodes has occurred.

TNM staging is used clinically to indicate the extension of cancer before definitive therapy begins. The manner in which staging is accomplished—eg, by clinical examination or pathologic examination of a surgical specimen—must be carefully documented. Certain types of tumors, such as lymphomas and Hodgkin's disease, are usually staged by a different classification scheme that reflects the natural history of this type of tumor spread and helps to direct treatment decisions.

The TNM system allows a numerical assessment of the extent of primary tumor (T), the absence or presence and extent of regional lymph node metastases (N), and the absence or presence of distant metastases (M). The AJCC has just published a new version of the TNM staging criteria with major revisions directed toward providing a standardized method for classifying the extent of cancer at diagnosis and esti-

mating the risk of recurrence and death from cancer. Examples of changes in staging included in the new system are staging melanoma based on the thickness and ulceration of the lesion instead of the level of invasion and the stratification of breast cancer stage based on the number of involved axillary nodes. Based on data that indicate prolonged survival in breast cancer patients with a single involved ipsilateral supraclavicular node, this presentation is now staged as stage IIIb rather than stage IV. The new staging system took effect internationally in January 2003 and is a required part of medical records for all cancer patients. Details regarding these revisions may be found at the AJCC Web site: www.cancerstaging.net.

Traditional staging does not take into account the biology or aggressiveness of a particular tumor and may not allow differentiation of prognostic risk groups. For this reason, specific pathologic characteristics are added into the prognostic evaluation for certain tumors (eg, estrogen and progesterone receptors, grade and proliferative index for breast cancer; histologic grade for sarcomas and the majority of adenocarcinomas). Overexpression or underproduction of oncogene products (eg, HER-2/*neu* in breast cancer), infection of cancer cells with specific viral genomes (eg, HPV-18 in cervical cancer), and certain chromosomal translocations or deletions (eg, alteration of the retinoic acid receptor gene in acute promyelocytic leukemia) have important prognostic significance and may direct risk-adapted or cancer-specific therapy. As these characteristics become standardized and better understood, they may allow us to identify patients with a poorer prognosis early in the course of disease when the patient might benefit from more aggressive therapy. In addition, characterizing cancers with genetic profiling or proteomics may completely change our concept of cancer staging in the future.

Greene FL et al (editors): *AJCC Cancer Staging Manual*, 6th ed. Springer, 2002.

■ PRIMARY CANCER TREATMENT

The reader is referred to the National Comprehensive Cancer Network (NCCN) Oncology Practice Guidelines: www.cancernet.com. These guidelines are updated yearly.

SURGERY & RADIATION THERAPY

Most cancers present initially as localized tumor nodules and cause local symptoms. Depending on the type of cancer, initial therapy may be directed locally in the form of surgery or radiation therapy. Surgical excision or local radiation (or both) is the treatment of choice for a variety of potentially curable cancers, including most gastrointestinal and genitourinary cancers, central nervous system tumors, and cancers arising from the breast, thyroid, or skin as well as most sarcomas.

Surgery at presentation has both diagnostic and therapeutic effectiveness, since it permits pathologic staging of the extent of local and regional invasion as well as an opportunity for removal of the primary neoplasm. CT and MRI play an increasing role in noninvasive tumor staging. Based on results of a prospective clinical trial, **positron emission tomography (PET)** appears to be a more sensitive method than traditional imaging with CT scanning for detecting local and distant metastases in patients with non-small cell lung cancer. The effect on survival is unknown. One way to improve the specificity and sensitivity of these scans is to integrate the PET and CT images with computer technology rather than the traditional visual correlation. One study evaluated integrated PET-CT in 50 patients with non-small cell lung cancer. Additional information was obtained on 41% of patients compared with visual correlation; this included improved tumor staging, detection of involved nodes, and certainty of metastases. PET has also been shown to improve detection of recurrent disease for the purpose of second-look laparotomy and debulking in colon cancer patients with rising levels of carcinoembryonic antigen (CEA).

A **monoclonal antibody against CEA labeled with technetium-99m (arcitumomab, CEA-Scan)** can be used for imaging of cancers with increased levels of CEA and has been found to be more sensitive and specific than CT scans in the detection of both resectable and nonresectable disease. High-resolution MRI scanning with highly lymphotropic superparamagnetic nanoparticles may improve radiographic detection of occult lymph node metastases in patients with prostate cancer. The nanoparticles gain access to lymph nodes by means of interstitial-lymphatic fluid transport. Eighty patients with prostate cancer were evaluated before surgery; MRI with nanoparticles correctly identified all patients with nodal metastases, compared with a detection rate of only 30% using standard imaging. These newer, more sensitive (and much more expensive) scans may allow better assessment of resectability before surgery, sparing patients needless surgery but also providing appropriate surgery when cure with local treatment alone is possible. The best and most cost-effective use of these techniques remains to be determined.

Although standard surgery for breast cancer has included excision of axillary nodes, this can result in chronic lymphedema, pain, and decreased range of motion of the arm. Sentinel axillary nodes can be detected by injection of radioactive colloid or blue dye into the breast around the tumor or the biopsy cavity. "Hot spots" are then identified with a gamma probe and resected. **Biopsy of sentinel nodes** can predict the presence or absence of axillary node metastases and direct more aggressive surgery with up to 97% accu-

racy. However, the procedure is technically challenging and the success rate varies with surgeon experience. This technique is also used for staging of malignant melanoma and has been shown to markedly reduce morbidity associated with traditional node dissection. Cryosurgical ablation of localized prostate cancers has been used instead of radiotherapy by some investigators and appears to reduce postablation voiding dysfunction. Radiofrequency ablation (frictional heating) and cryosurgical ablation are being tested as primary treatment of small, localized breast cancers.

Surgery may also play an important role in the treatment of selected patients with limited metastatic cancer. Resection of isolated metastases has been used most commonly for breast cancer with single brain lesions or isolated liver or lung lesions. Removal of isolated liver metastases may result in long-term survival, with 20% of patients living more than 5 years. Additional surgery after subsequent limited recurrence may also result in long-term disease-free survival. Surgical resection of both hepatic and pulmonary metastases may improve survival in appropriately selected colon cancer patients.

For certain tumor sites, complete surgical removal of the tumor can be disfiguring, disabling, or unachievable. Under those circumstances, primary local therapy with ionizing radiation may prove to be the treatment of choice. In other instances, surgery and radiation therapy are used in sequence. For stage I and stage II breast cancer, local excision or "lumpectomy" with axillary or sentinel node sampling combined with radiation results in equivalent 10-year survival when compared with the more disfiguring mastectomy procedure. Despite these well-established data, breast-conserving therapy is still underused in patients with larger tumors, mainly because of surgeon bias and lack of technical skill. Preoperative or "neoadjuvant" chemotherapy and radiation therapy allow limb-sparing surgery in osteosarcoma and organ preservation in oropharyngeal cancer, among others. Laser surgery is used to minimize surgical resection in esophageal and non-small cell lung cancers.

Radiation therapy is usually delivered as brachytherapy or teletherapy. In **brachytherapy**, the radiation source is placed close to the tumor. This intracavitary approach is used for many gynecologic or oral neoplasms and occasionally for breast cancer. In **teletherapy**, supervoltage radiotherapy is usually delivered with a linear accelerator, as this instrument permits more precise beam localization and avoids the complication of skin radiation toxicity. Various beam-modifying wedges, rotational techniques, and other specific approaches are used to increase the radiation dosage to the tumor bed while minimizing toxicity to adjacent normal tissues. Changes in dosing schedules have been used to either improve response or minimize long-term toxicity, although few data exist on the effectiveness of these approaches. For example, twice-daily radiation to the breast over 2 weeks is being compared to the standard 6-week daily dosing schedule, and radiation to the whole brain is often given in smaller doses over 4 weeks rather than the standard 2-week schedule to reduce long-term cognitive effects. Examples of new approaches to minimize radiation to surrounding tissues while maximizing radiation to the cancer include **three-dimensional-conformal radiation therapy (3D CRT)** and intensity modulated radiation therapy (IMRT). Conventional radiation beams are of uniform intensity. In contrast, IMRT's beam intensity is modulated to produce maximum doses where desired and minimal radiation to sensitive surrounding normal tissues. Improved outcomes have been shown for prostate cancer patients receiving IMRT.

Novel modalities are occasionally used to enhance penetrance into large tumors or to specifically target the site of radiation. **Gamma knife radiosurgery** allows focused radiation for limited brain metastases and is associated with fewer long-term complications such as cognitive dysfunction compared with whole brain irradiation. It also extends treatment options for patients with isolated brain recurrences following whole brain radiation. **Cyberknife** is a newer radiosurgical technique designed to perform tumor ablation in any site in the body. This unique system combines robotics and advanced image guidance to deliver radiosurgery treatment to tumors along the spinal cord or at other critical locations previously considered untreatable with surgery or radiation. It can also be used to treat recurrences in a previously radiated site or to boost standard radiotherapy. Treatment to previously radiated sites in the spinal cord, even with localized methods such as cyberknife, can result in significant long-term toxicity to the treated organ. Treatment should be done at an experienced center with a full discussion of possible toxicities.

Well-oxygenated tumors are more radiosensitive than hypoxic ones. Hypoxic tumors are often bulky, implying a potential synergistic role of surgical debulking prior to radiotherapy. Radiation therapy is normally delivered in a fractionated fashion over 4–6 weeks, this method appearing to have radiobiologic superiority by permitting time for recovery of normal host tissues (but not the tumor) from sublethal damage during treatment. However, a more accelerated fraction radiation schedule improves local-regional control in patients with head and neck cancer compared with standard fractionated radiation. **Efaproxiral (RSR13)** binds to hemoglobin and reduces oxygen-binding affinity (allosteric modification), enhancing oxygen unloading from hemoglobin to hypoxic tissue, potentially enhancing the effectiveness of radiation therapy. Clinical trials have demonstrated a possible improvement in response and survival in patients with primary brain tumors when patients are given efaproxiral during whole brain radiation therapy, compared to historic controls. Ongoing randomized trials are testing the efficacy of efaproxiral in patients with primary and metastatic tumors to the brain. The primary toxicity of this agent is hypoxia; pa-

tients require close monitoring and supplemental oxygen following therapy.

For most tumor types, there is a sigmoid curve of increasing rate of control of the local tumor with increasing radiation dose. Radiosensitive tumors usually exhibit radiosensitivity over the dose range of 3500–5000 cGy.

Currently, more than 50% of all patients with cancer receive radiation therapy during the course of their illness. Radiation therapy is frequently the sole agent used with curative intent for tumors of the larynx (permitting cure without loss of the voice), oral cavity, pharynx, esophagus, uterine cervix, vagina, prostate, and skin, Hodgkin's disease, and some tumors of the brain and spinal cord. For more extensive cancers, radiation is combined with surgery (eg, cancer of the breast, ovary, uterus, cervix, urinary bladder, rectum, and lung, soft tissue sarcomas, and seminoma of the testis). Following mastectomy for breast cancer, radiation has been shown to reduce the risk of local recurrence from large or high-risk tumors and may increase overall survival by decreasing distant recurrence.

Radiation given in combination with chemotherapy may improve long-term disease control. The combination of chemotherapy and radiation therapy for the treatment of invasive carcinoma of the cervix is significantly superior to radiation therapy alone. There is at least a 10% improvement in 3-year survival and a 30–50% reduction in the risk of death from cervical cancer with combination therapy. Twice-daily radiation given concurrently with combination chemotherapy for the treatment of limited small cell lung cancer results in significantly improved 5-year survival rates compared with any prior treatment results. Twice-daily radiation also appears superior to once-daily treatment for this disease. Radiation combined with chemotherapy for cancer of the rectum or hormone therapy for cancer of the prostate improves survival over treatment with radiation alone, and concurrent radiation and chemotherapy for cancer of the head and neck reduces mortality from that disease compared with either treatment alone. Radiation can also improve disease control when given as an adjuvant to chemotherapy for bulky lymphomas, for non-small cell lung cancer, and for some cancers in children.

Occasionally, chemotherapy is used to sensitize tumor cells to the toxic effects of radiation. Radiation therapy for palliation of pain or dysfunction (eg, bone pain associated with advanced breast or other cancers) may improve the quality of life of patients suffering from incurable malignancies. Radiation therapy to lytic lesions of the bone can reduce the risk of fracture as well.

Various normal tissues (particularly skin, mucosa, myocardium, spinal cord, bone marrow, and lymphoid system) can exhibit early or late toxicity from radiation therapy. Acute toxicity may include generalized fatigue and malaise, anorexia, nausea and vomiting, local skin changes, diarrhea, and mucosal ulceration of the irradiated area. Radiation of large areas, especially the pelvis and proximal long bones, may result in bone marrow suppression. Radiation of the lungs, heart, and gastrointestinal tract must be approached with appropriate shielding to avoid toxicity such as radiation pneumonitis, congestive heart failure, or radiation gastroenteritis. Long-term toxicity from radiation therapy has significant long-term side effects that must be weighed against its possible benefits. Women under age 60 years treated with left-sided adjuvant radiation for breast cancer with 10–15 years of follow-up have a significant increase in risk of death from myocardial infarction. However, current radiation techniques use tangential beams that avoid significant radiation to adjacent organs such as the heart or lung. Increased cardiac mortality has also been seen in patients who received radiation at a young age for Hodgkin's disease. Secondary leukemias and solid tumors can be seen after radiation therapy for a wide variety of cancers. This risk is particularly high in patients receiving a combination of both radiation and chemotherapy that includes alkylating agents. Treatment programs now combine less toxic chemotherapy with limited field radiation therapy to limit these life-threatening side effects in long-term survivors from cancer. Other long-term toxicities include decreased function of the radiation organ (eg, decreased cognitive function after whole brain radiation), myelopathy, osteonecrosis, and hyperpigmentation of the involved skin.

Regional hyperthermia (40–42 °C) is an adjunct to ionizing irradiation for some tumor sites. The most useful application of hyperthermia to date has been in superficial or easily implantable tumors as well as in relatively bulky hypovascular tumors with some degree of hypoxia. **Electron beam therapy** has been used effectively to treat superficial tumors in the skin. **Radiolabeled antibodies** are currently under investigation as a means of delivering high levels of radiation locally to the tumor bed, thereby avoiding systemic toxicity. Ibritumomab tiuxetan and tositumomab are the first radiolabeled antibodies to be FDA approved for the treatment of cancer—specifically, relapsed low-grade non-Hodgkin's lymphoma (see section on novel therapies at the end of this chapter).

Increasingly, the primary local therapy of cancer is integrated with systemic therapy, an approach that has proved to be superior for apparently localized tumor types with a high propensity for early metastatic spread and for which anticancer drugs are available.

Bosset JF et al: Preoperative chemoradiotherapy versus preoperative radiotherapy in rectal cancer patients: assessment of acute toxicity and treatment compliance. Report of the 22921 randomised trial conducted by the EORTC radiotherapy group. Eur J Cancer 2004;40:219. [PMID: 14728936]

Chao C et al: Update on the use of the sentinel node biopsy in patients with melanoma: who and how. Curr Opin Oncol 2002;14:217. [PMID: 11880714]

Choti MA et al: Trends in long-term survival following liver resection for hepatic colorectal metastases. Ann Surg 2002;235:759. [PMID: 12035031]

Goyal A et al: Factors affecting failed localisation and false-negative rates of sentinel node biopsy in breast cancer—results of the ALMANAC validation phase. Breast Cancer Res Treat 2006 [Epub ahead of print]. [PMID: 16541308]

Harisingham MG et al: Noninvasive detection of clinically occult lymph-node metastases in prostate cancer. N Engl J Med 2003;348:2491. [PMID: 12815134]

Lardinois D et al: Staging of non-small-cell lung cancer with integrated positron-emission tomography and computed tomography. N Engl J Med 2003;348:2500. [PMID: 12815135]

Stauffer PR et al: Evolving technology for thermal therapy of cancer. Int J Hyperthermia 2005;21:731. [PMID: 16338856]

Steffan RP et al: Allosteric modification of hemoglobin by RSR13 as a therapeutic strategy. Adv Exp Med Biol 2003;530:249. [PMID: 14562722]

Welch WC et al: Accuray CyberKnife image-guided radiosurgical system. Expert Rev Med Devices 2005;2:141. [PMID: 16293050]

SYSTEMIC CANCER THERAPY

Use of cytotoxic drugs, hormones, antihormones, and biologic agents has become a highly specialized and increasingly effective means of treating cancer. Therapy should be administered by a medical oncologist. Selection of specific drugs or protocols for various types of cancer has traditionally been based on results of prior clinical trials. Many patients are treated on protocols to search for optimal therapy for refractory or poorly responsive malignancies. Treatment may be inadequate or ineffective because of drug resistance of the tumor cells. This has been attributed to spontaneous genetic mutations in subpopulations of cancer cells prior to exposure to chemotherapy. After chemotherapy has eliminated the sensitive cells, the resistant subpopulation grows to become the predominant cell type (Goldie–Coldman hypothesis). This has been the basis of alternating non-cross-resistant chemotherapy regimens.

Molecular mechanisms of drug resistance are now the subject of intense study. In many instances, specific drug resistance results from an amplification in the number of gene copies for an enzyme inhibited by a specific chemotherapeutic agent. A more general form of "multidrug resistance" (MDR) has been described in association with expression of a gene (MDR1) encoding a 170-kDa transmembrane glycoprotein (P-glycoprotein) on tumor cells. This protein is an energy-dependent transport pump that facilitates drug efflux from tumor cells and promotes resistance to a broad spectrum of unrelated cancer drugs. Although a variety of agents have been shown to at least partially and temporarily reverse acquired MDR in multiple myeloma and lymphoma, the doses of these agents required to overcome drug resistance are associated with serious side effects. MDR modulators will need to be both less toxic and more potent to be clinically useful. Both improved response rates and improved survival with a tolerable toxicity profile using novel therapy such as this will have to be demonstrated to prove the effectiveness of this approach.

Variation in drug metabolism due to gene polymorphisms is emerging as a cause of relative resistance or sensitivity to chemotherapeutic agents. In one study, women with breast cancer who had single-nucleotide polymorphisms in the *CYP3A4* and *CYP3A5* genes were not able to metabolize cyclophosphamide and had a significantly shorter survival than women without this polymorphism. Polymorphisms in *CYP* have also been shown to increase sensitivity to some environmental carcinogens. Genetic variations in the DNA repair genes *XPD* and *XRCC1* may predict response to the chemotherapy drugs cisplatin or carboplatin in lung cancer, with certain variations associated with a shortened survival. With an increased understanding of individual susceptibility or resistance factors, pretreatment evaluation of drug metabolism genes might allow individualization of therapy.

Chemotherapy is used primarily to cure a small percentage of malignancies, as adjuvant therapy to decrease the rate of relapse or improve the disease-free interval, and to palliate symptoms and prolong survival in some patients with incurable malignancies. In addition, chemotherapy is playing an increasing role as preoperative or "neoadjuvant" therapy to reduce the size and extent of the primary tumor, thereby allowing complete excision at the time of surgery. Neoadjuvant (preoperative) chemotherapy results in identical survival when compared with standard postsurgical chemotherapy for breast cancer and allows more limited or complete surgical excision of the primary tumor as well as giving important information about chemosensitivity. Randomized studies now suggest that neoadjuvant chemotherapy may improve survival in patients with esophageal cancer and bladder cancer. Combined neoadjuvant chemotherapy and radiation followed by surgery and additional chemotherapy has been shown to prolong survival in patients with non-small cell lung cancer that has metastasized to mediastinal nodes compared with those who received only chemotherapy and radiation. In addition, survival rates at 3 years exceeded those seen in prior studies. There are two additional benefits to the neoadjuvant approach. First, understanding the clinical response to specific chemotherapeutic agents may allow modification of this treatment in an individual patient to improve response. Second, serial biopsies during treatment along with improved imaging may help us to understand the genes responsible for chemotherapy resistance and sensitivity and hopefully allow for individualization of cancer treatment with combinations of chemotherapy and targeted agents in the future.

Chemotherapy was first shown to be curative in the treatment of advanced stages of choriocarcinoma in women. It is also curative in Hodgkin's disease, diffuse large cell and some high-grade lymphomas (including Burkitt's), carcinoma of the testis, some cases of acute leukemia, and embryonal rhabdomyosarcoma. When combined with initial surgery—and in some instances with irradiation—chemotherapy increases the rate of long-term control and cure of breast cancer, cervical cancer, small cell and non-small cell lung cancer, colon cancer, gastric cancer, esophageal cancer, rectal cancer, and osteogenic sarcomas. Combination chemotherapy provides palliation and prolongation of survival in adults with low-grade non-Hodgkin's lymphoma, mycosis fungoides, multiple myeloma and Waldenström's macroglobulinemia, acute and chronic leukemias, and breast, ovarian, cervical, and small cell lung carcinoma as well as carcinoid. Patients with incurable tumors who desire aggressive treatment should be referred for experimental therapy in well-designed clinical trials. (See section on novel therapies at the end of this chapter.)

High-dose chemotherapy followed by bone marrow transplantation is curative therapy for various types of leukemia, high-risk or relapsed lymphoma, and testicular cancer and occasionally multiple myeloma. Allogeneic or autologous bone marrow or peripheral blood stem cells with or without ex vivo purging are used depending on the disease. The use of growth factors and blood stem cells has decreased the toxicity and cost of bone marrow transplantation. Autologous transplantation may now be used with relatively low morbidity and mortality on selected patients up to age 70 years. Dose-intense chemotherapy with autologous bone marrow or peripheral blood stem cell rescue has been extensively studied for the treatment of both high-risk and metastatic breast cancer for the past decade and has shown no apparent benefit over standard therapy and significantly more toxicity and risk of mortality. Details of these studies are presented in the section on adjuvant therapy.

Nonmyeloablative allogeneic peripheral blood stem cell transplantation ("mini" transplant) is now being investigated as immunotherapy for some advanced cancers. This highly toxic and intensive therapy has been shown to result in sustained regression of chemotherapy-resistant metastatic renal cell carcinoma in ten out of nineteen treated patients, with three complete remissions. Tumor response was associated with acquisition of the donor immune system, resulting in a "graft-versus-tumor" effect. Further investigation is required to confirm sustained beneficial effects, reduce toxicity, improve efficacy, and better understand in which diseases this type of therapy can be effective. However, nonmyeloablative transplant is now an alternative to the much more toxic full allogeneic transplant for hematologic malignancies when the patient cannot tolerate a full transplant due to age or comorbidity, or as a second transplant following autologous transplantation. Although the initial treatment is less intensive, the late immune effects are still a significant problem, as is disease relapse.

Chemotherapeutic agents can now be given on a variety of schedules to reduce toxicity and enhance antitumor effects. "Dose-dense" chemotherapy can be given in two ways, either as standard doses of chemotherapy given more frequently with growth factor support or as smaller doses given on a weekly or more frequent schedule ("metronomic" dosing). Animal studies have suggested that these dosing regimens may reverse some types of chemotherapy resistance. A recent study found that standard doses of chemotherapy for breast cancer given every 2 weeks were superior to the same doses given at the standard 3-week interval. Both disease-free and overall survival were improved in this study. Somewhat surprisingly, toxicity was lower in the "dose-dense" arm, due to the routine use of myeloid growth factors to avoid neutropenia and its associated complications.

Although most anticancer drugs are used systemically, there are selected indications for local or regional administration. Regional administration involves direct infusion of active chemotherapeutic agents into the tumor site (eg, intravesical therapy for bladder cancer, intraperitoneal therapy for ovarian cancer, hepatic artery infusion with or without embolization of the main blood supply of the tumor for cancers metastatic to the liver or as primary therapy for hepatocellular carcinoma). These treatments can result in palliation and prolonged survival. A recent phase III trial compared intravenous paclitaxel and cisplatin to the intravenous paclitaxel combined with intraperitoneal paclitaxel and cisplatin in women with optimally debulked stage III epithelial ovarian cancer. Patients treated with the intraperitoneal therapy had a 25% relative prolongation of survival, despite the fact that 48% of patients received three or fewer treatment cycles. These striking results have led to a new treatment paradigm for selected patients with newly diagnosed, optimally debulked ovarian cancer.

A summary of the types of cancer responsive to chemotherapy and the current treatments of choice is offered in Table 40–3. In some instances (eg, Hodgkin's disease, breast cancer, ovarian and lung cancers), optimal therapy may require a combination of therapeutic resources, eg, radiation plus chemotherapy rather than either modality alone. Patients with stage I and II Hodgkin's disease are often treated with radiation alone, avoiding the potential toxicity of systemic chemotherapy. A small percentage of these patients may require chemotherapy later for disease recurrence.

Newer Anticancer Drugs

New drugs to treat cancer are under constant development and testing, with the aim of reducing toxicity to normal cells and increasing the toxicity to resistant cancer cells. Several of these newer agents developed over the past decade and now available are described in this section.

We have entered an exciting new era in the understanding and treatment of malignancies. Molecular techniques have allowed insight into the biologic events resulting in cancer, and these same techniques have resulted in identification of just the beginning of a cascade of biologic therapies directed toward specific molecular or cellular factors critical to the pathogenesis of cancer growth and survival. Rather than the traditional cytotoxic therapy, newer treatments are more specific and less globally cytotoxic, but are still associated with the potential for serious side effects. A number of biologic therapies are either approved or under investigation for use in the treatment of cancer. The time from development of a novel agent to clinical use and FDA approval has been markedly shortened; in the first 6 months of 2001, two biologic therapies, imatinib mesylate and alemtuzumab, were rapidly approved for use based on marked efficacy with low toxicity for the treatment of two different hematologic malignancies. In 2003 through the first quarter of 2004, seven new agents were approved by the FDA for the treatment of a variety of cancers, including novel cytotoxics, biologic therapy, and radioimmunoconjugates. Two agents to reduce chemotherapy-associated nausea and vomiting were also released for use. In the beginning of 2005, the first nanoparticle taxane, nab-paclitaxel was approved for the treatment of metastatic breast cancer. In the next decade we will probably see the development of a whole new class of agents and, consequently, a new paradigm for the treatment of cancer.

Newer Cytotoxics

Paclitaxel (Taxol) is a novel agent isolated from the pacific yew tree that has replaced cyclophosphamide as front-line therapy (combined with carboplatin) for the treatment of ovarian cancer. Intraperitoneal instillation may also be helpful for advanced disease. Paclitaxel (and docetaxel; see below) has also been shown to be one of the most effective agents available to treat early- and late-stage breast cancer; it is also effective in AIDS-associated KS and cancer of the lung among other cancers. The primary toxicities of paclitaxel are hematologic and neurologic. Both are dose dependent; the hematologic toxicity can be ameliorated by the use of myeloid growth factors. Recent data on breast cancer indicate that weekly or every-2-week dosing is the most effective way to give paclitaxel. **Nab-paclitaxel ABI-007** (abraxane) is a novel taxane that combines paclitaxel with albumin into a nanoparticle 1/100th the size of a red blood cell. This avoids the need for solvents, which result in a risk of serious allergic reactions to standard paclitaxel. A recent randomized, phase III trial compared paclitaxel to abraxane in the treatment of metastatic breast cancer. Treatment with abraxane significantly increased the response rate as well as time to tumor progression, and there were no allergic reactions seen—thereby avoiding the use of routine steroid premedications. The major toxicity of abraxane appears to be neuropathy, which can be ameliorated by giving lower doses on a weekly schedule. This drug was FDA approved for the treatment of metastatic breast cancer in early 2005. A number of novel taxanes (also called epothilones) are in clinical trials at this time.

Docetaxel is a synthetic analog of paclitaxel that has also been shown to be highly effective in the treatment of breast cancer as well as many other advanced malignancies, including non-small cell lung cancer and ovarian cancer. Its toxicities include bone marrow suppression and significant peripheral edema. The

Table 40–3. Treatment choices for cancers responsive to systemic agents.

Diagnosis	Current Treatment of Choice	Other Valuable Agents and Procedures
Acute lymphocytic leukemia	**Induction:** combination chemotherapy. *Adults:* Vincristine, prednisone, daunorubicin, and asparaginase (DVPLasp). **Consolidation:** multiagent alternating chemotherapy. Allogeneic bone marrow transplant for young adults or high-risk disease or second remission. Central nervous system prophylaxis with intrathecal methotrexate with or without whole brain radiation. **Remission maintenance:** methotrexate, thioguanine.	Doxorubicin, cytarabine, cyclophosphamide, etoposide, teniposide, clofarabine, allopurinol,[1] autologous bone marrow transplantation T cell disease: Nelarabine (relapsed or refractory)
Acute myelocytic and myelomonocytic leukemia	**Induction:** combination chemotherapy with cytarabine and an anthracycline (daunorubicin, idarubicin). Tretinoin with idarubicin for acute promyelocytic leukemia. **Consolidation:** high-dose cytarabine. Autologous (with or without purging) or allogeneic bone marrow transplantation for high-risk disease or second remission.	Gemtuzumab ozogamicin (Mylotarg), mitoxantrone, idarubicin, etoposide, mercaptopurine, thioguanine, azacitidine,[2] amsacrine,[2] methotrexate, doxorubicin, tretinoin, allopurinol,[1] leukapheresis, prednisone, arsenic trioxide for acute promyelocytic leukemia
Chronic myelocytic leukemia	Imatinib mesylate (Gleevec), hydroxyurea, interferon-α. Allogeneic bone marrow transplantation for younger patients.	Busulfan, mercaptopurine, thioguanine, cytarabine, plicamycin, melphalan, autologous bone marrow transplantation,[2] allopurinol[1]
Chronic lymphocytic leukemia	Fludarabine, chlorambucil, and prednisone (if treatment is indicated) rituximab with fludarabine or cyclophosphamide. Second-line therapy: alemtuzumab (Campath-1H).	Rituximab, vincristine, cyclophosphamide, doxorubicin, cladribine (2-chlorodeoxyadenosine; CdA), allogeneic bone marrow transplantation, androgens,[2] allopurinol[1]
Hairy cell leukemia	Cladribine (2-chlorodeoxyadenosine; CdA).	Pentostatin (deoxycoformycin), interferon-α
Hodgkin's disease (stages III and IV)	**Combination chemotherapy:** doxorubicin (Adriamycin), bleomycin, vinblastine, dacarbazine (ABVD) or alternative combination therapy without mechlorethamine. Autologous bone marrow transplantation for high-risk patients or relapsed disease.	Mechlorethamine, vincristine, prednisone, procarbazine (MOPP); carmustine, lomustine, etoposide, thiotepa, autologous bone marrow transplantation
Non-Hodgkin's lymphoma (intermediate to high grade)	**Combination therapy:** depending on histologic classification but usually including cyclophosphamide, vincristine, doxorubicin, and prednisone (CHOP) with or without rituximab in older patients. Autologous bone marrow transplantation in high-risk first remission or first relapse.	Bleomycin, methotrexate, etoposide, chlorambucil, fludarabine, lomustine, carmustine, cytarabine, thiotepa, amsacrine, mitoxantrone, allogeneic bone marrow transplantation
Non-Hodgkin's lymphoma (low grade)	Fludarabine, rituximab, if CD20 positive; ibritumomab tiuxetan or ^{131}I tositumomab for relapsed or refractory disease.	**Combination chemotherapy:** cyclophosphamide, prednisone, doxorubicin, vincristine; chlorambucil, autologous or allogeneic transplantation
Cutaneous T cell lymphoma (mycosis fungoides)	Topical carmustine, electron beam radiotherapy, photochemotherapy, targretin, denileukin diftitox (ONTAK) for refractory disease.	Interferon, combination chemotherapy, denileukin diftitox (ONTAK), targretin
Multiple myeloma	**Combination chemotherapy:** vincristine, doxorubicin, dexamethasone; melphalan and prednisone; melphalan, cyclophosphamide, carmustine, vincristine, doxorubicin, prednisone, thalidomide. Autologous transplantation in first complete or partial remission, miniallogeneic transplant for poor-prognosis disease. Bortezomib for relapsed or refractory disease.	Clarithromycin, etoposide, cytarabine, interferon-α, dexamethasone, autologous bone marrow transplantation

(continued)

Table 40–3. Treatment choices for cancers responsive to systemic agents. (continued)

Diagnosis	Current Treatment of Choice	Other Valuable Agents and Procedures
Waldenström's macro-globulinemia	Fludarabine **or** chlorambucil **or** cyclophosphamide, vincristine, prednisone. Allogeneic bone marrow transplantation for high-risk young patients.	Cladribine, etoposide, interferon-α, doxoru-bicin, dexamethasone, plasmapheresis, au-tologous bone marrow transplantation
Polycythemia vera, es-sential thrombocytosis	Hydroxyurea, phlebotomy for polycythemia. Anagrelide for thrombocytosis.	Busulfan, chlorambucil, cyclophospha-mide, interferon-α, radiophosphorus [32]P
Carcinoma of the lung Small cell	**Combination chemotherapy:** cisplatin and etoposide. Palliative radiation therapy.	Cyclophosphamide, doxorubicin, vincris-tine
Non-small cell[3]	**Localized disease:** cisplatin or carboplatin, docetaxel. **Advanced disease:** cisplatin or carboplatin, doce-taxel, gemcitabine, gefitinib, erlotinib, etoposide, vin-blastine, vinorelbine.	Doxorubicin, etoposide, pemetrexed, mito-mycin, ifosfamide, paclitaxel, capecitabine, radiation therapy
Malignant pleural me-sothelioma	Pemetrexed with cisplatin.	Doxorubicin, radiation, pleurectomy
Carcinoma of the head and neck[3]	**Combination chemotherapy:** cisplatin and fluoro-uracil, paclitaxel, cetuximab with radiation (locally ad-vanced) or alone (second-line metastatic).	Methotrexate, bleomycin, hydroxyurea, doxorubicin, vinblastine
Carcinoma of the esophagus[3]	**Combination chemotherapy:** fluorouracil, cisplatin, mitomycin.	Methotrexate, bleomycin, doxorubicin, mi-tomycin
Carcinoma of the stomach and pancreas[3]	**Stomach:** etoposide, leucovorin,[1] fluorouracil (ELF). **Pancreas:** fluorouracil or ELF, gemcitabine with or without erlotinib.	Carmustine, mitomycin, lomustine, doxoru-bicin, gemcitabine, methotrexate, cisplatin, combinations for stomach
Carcinoma of the colon and rectum[3]	**Colon:** oxaliplatin with infusional 5-fluorouracil (5-FU)/leucovorin (FOLFOX4) (adjuvant); bevacizumab with irinotecan, 5-FU/leucovorin with irinotecan, cetuximab, capecitabine (advanced). **Rectum:** fluorouracil with radiation therapy (adju-vant), advanced similar to colon cancer.	Methotrexate, mitomycin, carmustine, cis-platin, floxuridine
Carcinoma of the kidney[3]	Floxuridine, vinblastine, interleukin-2 (IL-2), inter-feron-α, sunitinib, sorafenib; consider miniallogeneic transplantation.[2]	Interferon-α, progestins, infusional fluoro-deoxyuridine, fluorouracil
Carcinoma of the bladder[3]	Intravesical bacillus Calmette-Guérin (BCG) or thiotepa. **Combination chemotherapy:** methotrexate, vinblas-tine, doxorubicin (Adriamycin), cisplatin (M-VAC) or CMV alone.	Cyclophosphamide, fluorouracil, intravesi-cal valrubicin, gemcitabine, cisplatin
Carcinoma of the testis[3]	**Combination chemotherapy:** etoposide and cis-platin. Autologous bone marrow transplantation for high-risk or relapsed disease.	Bleomycin, vinblastine, ifosfamide, mesna,[1] carmustine, carboplatin
Carcinoma of the prostate[3]	Estrogens or luteinizing hormone-releasing hor-mone analog (leuprolide, goserelin, or triptorelin) plus an antiandrogen (flutamide).	Ketoconazole, doxorubicin, aminoglutethi-mide, progestins, cyclophosphamide, cis-platin, vinblastine, etoposide, suramin[2]; PC-SPES; estramustine phosphate
Carcinoma of the uterus[3]	Progestins or tamoxifen.	Doxorubicin, cisplatin, fluorouracil, ifosfa-mide
Carcinoma of the ovary[3]	**Combination chemotherapy:** paclitaxel and cis-platin or carboplatin. Intraperitoneal chemotherapy with cisplatin and paclitaxel combined with intrave-nous paclitaxel.	Docetaxel, doxorubicin, topotecan, cyclo-phosphamide, etoposide, liposomal doxo-rubicin
Carcinoma of the cervix[3]	**Combination chemotherapy:** methotrexate, doxoru-bicin, cisplatin, and vinblastine; or mitomycin, bleomy-cin, vincristine, and cisplatin with radiation therapy.	Carboplatin, ifosfamide, lomustine

(continued)

Table 40–3. Treatment choices for cancers responsive to systemic agents. (continued)

Diagnosis	Current Treatment of Choice	Other Valuable Agents and Procedures
Carcinoma of the breast[3]	**Combination chemotherapy:** a variety of regimens are used for adjuvant therapy. For node-positive disease—combinations including doxorubicin or epirubicin and at least one of the following additional drugs: 5-FU, cyclophosphamide, docetaxel, paclitaxel. For node-negative disease—a combination of the drugs listed above or cyclophosphamide, methotrexate, and 5-FU (CMF). For HER2/*neu* positive disease, anthracycline-based chemotherapy followed by trastuzumab with paclitaxel or docetaxel. For estrogen- or progesterone-positive disease, tamoxifen with or without ovarian suppression of estrogen production (premenopausal women) or anastrozole/letrozole/exemestane following or instead of tamoxifen (postmenopausal women) is given for 5 years regardless of the use of adjuvant chemotherapy.	Trastuzumab (Herceptin) with chemotherapy, paclitaxel, docetaxel, nab-paclitaxel, epirubicin, mitoxantrone, pegylated doxorubicin, capecitabine, gemcitabine, vinorelbine, thiotepa, vincristine, vinblastine, carboplatin or cisplatin, anastrozole, letrozole, exemestane, fulvestrant, toremifine, progestins, goserelin, leuprolide, triptorelin
Choriocarcinoma (trophoblastic neoplasms)[3]	Methotrexate or dactinomycin (or both) plus chlorambucil.	Vinblastine, cisplatin, mercaptopurine, doxorubicin, bleomycin, etoposide
Carcinoma of the thyroid gland[3]	Radioiodine (^{131}I).	Doxorubicin, cisplatin, bleomycin, melphalan
Carcinoma of the adrenal gland[3]	Mitotane.	Doxorubicin, suramin[2]
Carcinoid[3]	Fluorouracil plus streptozocin with or without interferon-α.	Doxorubicin, cyclophosphamide, octreotide, cyproheptadine,[1] methysergide[1]
Osteogenic sarcoma[3]	High-dose methotrexate, doxorubicin, vincristine.	Cyclophosphamide, ifosfamide, bleomycin, dacarbazine, cisplatin, dactinomycin
Soft tissue sarcoma[3]	Doxorubicin, dacarbazine.	Ifosfamide, cyclosphosphamide, etoposide, cisplatin, high-dose methotrexate, vincristine
Melanoma[3]	Dacarbazine, interferon-α, interleukin-2.	Carmustine, lomustine, melphalan, thiotepa, cisplatin, paclitaxel, tamoxifen, vincristine, vaccine therapy (Melacine)[2]
Kaposi's sarcoma	Doxorubicin, vincristine alternating with vinblastine or vincristine alone. Palliative radiation therapy.	Interferon-α, bleomycin, etoposide, doxorubicin
Neuroblastoma[3]	**Combination chemotherapy:** variations of cyclophosphamide, cisplatin, vincristine, doxorubicin, dacarbazine.	Melphalan, ifosfamide, autologous or allogeneic bone marrow transplantation

[1]Supportive agent; not oncolytic.

[2]Investigational agent or procedure. Treatment is available through qualified investigators and centers authorized by the National Cancer Institute and Cooperative Oncology Groups.

[3]These tumors are generally managed initially with surgery with or without radiation therapy and with or without adjuvant chemotherapy. For metastatic disease, the role of palliative radiation therapy is as important as that of chemotherapy.

edema can be treated and generally prevented with steroids. Changing the schedule of administration appears to change toxicity. When docetaxel is given on a weekly schedule, it is associated with significantly less hematopoietic toxicity, but also with novel toxicities including lacrimal duct stenosis requiring stenting, and marked damage to the fingernails. A recent randomized trial compared every-3-week dosing of docetaxel to paclitaxel in women with metastatic breast cancer. Time to progression and survival were superior in patients treated with docetaxel. Weekly paclitaxel has been shown to be superior to every-3-week dosing, raising questions about the use of paclitaxel and appropriate dosing schedules.

Vinorelbine, a semisynthetic vinca alkaloid, has been shown to be effective in treating advanced non-small cell lung cancer. Response rates of 30% have been observed when vinorelbine is used as a single agent against this poorly responsive tumor. Vinorelbine is also used to treat metastatic breast cancer as well as other tumors. Toxicities include significant bone marrow suppression, neuropathy, and transient ileus.

Capecitabine is an oral 5-fluorouracil (5-FU) pro-drug that is approved to treat anthracycline- and tax-ane-resistant breast cancers as well as metastatic colo-rectal cancer. Response rates range from 25% to 35%. Treatment can be complicated by a painful, red, and sometimes blistering rash on the palms and soles and severe diarrhea that resolves upon withholding therapy and subsequent dose reduction. A variety of other 5-FU prodrugs are in clinical trials but are not yet approved for use. One study showed a 3-month improvement in survival using the combination of docetaxel and capecitabine versus docetaxel alone in the treatment of advanced metastatic breast cancer, though there were considerably more side effects in the combination arm. This combination is now FDA approved, al-though newer dosing schedules with reduced toxicity are being used. It is still not clear that the combination is better than sequential single agent chemotherapy, however; a substantial number of patients treated on the docetaxel alone arm were never able to receive capecitabine due to geographic location outside of the United States and Europe.

Gemcitabine, a pyrimidine analog for intravenous use, has been approved to treat pancreatic cancer and non-small cell lung cancer but is active in other ad-vanced malignancies, including breast cancer, particu-larly in combination with other chemotherapeutic or biologic agents. Toxicities are quite modest, and are primarily fatigue, myelosuppression, and an occasional rash. A recent trial combining gemcitabine and pacli-taxel in the treatment of metastatic breast cancer showed a short survival benefit compared to paclitaxel alone; however, less than 50% of patients received ad-ditional chemotherapy after study treatment similar to the capecitabine study outlined above. The primary toxicity was bone marrow suppression.

Topotecan was the first of a class of drugs called camptothecans that inhibits the enzyme topoisomerase I to be FDA approved for use. It is used to treat ad-vanced ovarian cancer and has shown some efficacy in the treatment of several other tumors.

Irinotecan is highly effective in the treatment of metastatic colorectal cancer. Two randomized studies compared the combination of irinotecan, fluoroura-cil, and leucovorin (IFL) to treatment with fluoroura-cil and leucovorin alone in patients with untreated metastatic colorectal cancer. The use of irinotecan re-sulted in a significantly higher response rate, delayed time to progression, and, in one study, improved sur-vival. Toxicity in the irinotecan arm was also signifi-cantly higher, and with longer follow-up mortality was concerningly high at 3.5%. With appropriate manage-ment, much of the toxicity appears to be reversible and includes severe diarrhea and neutropenia. It is now understood that genetic polymorphisms result-ing in delayed metabolism of irinotecan are largely re-sponsible for the severe toxicities that are occasionally seen. Studies are ongoing to better understand and test for these individual differences in drug metabolism. Guidelines are available to improve management and

reduce mortality from this regimen, which was due ei-ther to inflammation of the bowel, leading to sepsis, or to thrombosis. A newer agent, **oxaliplatin**, is now an alternative to irinotecan as first-line therapy for colo-rectal cancer (see below). Antitumor responses have been shown using irinotecan to treat non-small cell lung cancer, small cell lung cancer, ovarian cancer, gliomas, breast cancer, and others.

Results of a phase III randomized trial demonstrated a significant improvement in response rates, time to progression, and median survival using a new regimen to treat metastatic colorectal cancer consisting of the platinum derivative **oxaliplatin** combined with infu-sional fluorouracil and leucovorin (FOLFOX4) com-pared with the IFL regimen. Toxicity was also reduced, with less nausea, vomiting, diarrhea, and myelosuppres-sion but an increase in neuropathy. Oxaliplatin is now approved for use in the United States based on the re-sults of this trial. The primary toxicities of oxaliplatin are infusion reactions and reversible neuropathy. One of the challenges in the treatment of cancer is that few agents cross the blood–brain barrier, making it difficult to treat primary or metastatic cancers in the central ner-vous system. **Temozolamide** is an oral alkylating agent with the very unusual property of excellent central ner-vous system penetration. It is useful in the treatment of primary tumors of the brain, and is also being tested as a treatment for tumors metastatic to the brain. Temozola-mide has recently been found to be effective in the treatment of metastatic melanoma as well.

Inhibitors of Thymidylate Synthase

Novel inhibitors of thymidylate synthase are under study for the treatment of advanced colorectal cancer. Treatment of malignant mesothelioma with the multi-targeted antifolate agent **pemetrexed**—in combination with cisplatin—has been shown to significantly im-prove survival from this highly resistant disease when compared with treatment with cisplatin alone. This is the first chemotherapeutic agent that has been shown to alter survival from malignant mesothelioma, a cancer that is rising in incidence due to occupational exposure to asbestos. Pemetrexed, recently approved by the FDA, must be given with folic acid and vitamin B_{12} supple-mentation. **Raltitrexed** is currently being used in Eu-rope based on early data showing similar efficacy com-pared with fluorouracil and high-dose leucovorin.

Liposomal encapsulation of active chemotherapeu-tic agents may improve drug delivery and decrease sys-temic toxicity. Two liposomally encapsulated drugs, doxorubicin (**Doxil**) and daunorubicin (**Dauno-some**), are indicated in the treatment of KS and have shown efficacy in treating many other diseases, includ-ing breast cancer and lymphoma.

Monoclonal Antibodies

An increasing number of monoclonal antibodies are used in cancer chemotherapy. **Rituximab**, a chimeric antibody against the B lymphocyte antigen CD20, is effective therapy for relapsed or resistant low-grade lymphomas and has shown limited usefulness in higher-grade lymphomas as well. Almost 50% of patients with low-grade lymphoma respond with shrinkage of lymph nodes to once-weekly dosing for 4 weeks. Responses lasted a median of over 1 year. Rituximab has been shown to be effective in longer courses lasting 8 weeks and as retreatment following relapse. A randomized study compared standard cyclophosphamide, doxorubicin (hydroxydaunomycin; Adriamycin), vincristine (Oncovin), and prednisone (CHOP) chemotherapy with rituximab combined with CHOP as initial therapy for patients aged 60 years or older with diffuse large B cell lymphomas. Response rates, 12-month event-free survival, and overall survival were significantly improved in the combination arm. Rituximab has been effective in treating a wide range of B-lymphocyte-mediated disorders including benign autoimmune disease as well as lymphoid malignancies. Toxicities are generally quite mild, though anaphylaxis (resulting in death) and infusion-related side effects have been reported.

The HER-2/*neu* oncogene (also called c-*erb*B-2), a gene that encodes a receptor tyrosine kinase, is known to be overexpressed in many human cancers and is associated with tumors with poorer prognoses. In breast cancer, overexpression of HER-2/*neu* is seen in about 20% of women and is associated with a higher risk of metastatic disease and poorer survival. **Trastuzumab (Herceptin)** is a recombinant humanized monoclonal antibody directed against the HER-2/*neu* gene product (a cells surface receptor) that is indicated for the treatment of HER-2/*neu* overexpressing early-stage and metastatic breast cancer. When trastuzumab was used as a single agent to treat anthracycline-resistant metastatic breast cancer, the response rate was about 15%, with a median duration of response of over 8 months. However, when trastuzumab was added to first-line chemotherapy for metastatic breast cancer and compared with chemotherapy alone, patients receiving the combination therapy had a response rate of almost 50% with significant improvement in both duration of remission and survival. The most promising combination appears to be trastuzumab and paclitaxel (Taxol) or docetaxel (Taxotere) either with or without platinum salts (carboplatin or cisplatin); combinations with other agents, including vinorelbine and gemcitabine, also appear to be effective. Four recent international randomized trials have demonstrated remarkable improvements in disease-free and overall survival when trastuzumab is combined with standard adjuvant chemotherapy for early stage, HER2/*neu* overexpressing invasive breast cancer. Treatment is well tolerated, and trastuzumab is given for 1 year. This dramatic effect has revolutionized the treatment of a previously poor prognosis subgroup of early-stage breast cancer so much so that it is now a positive prognostic factor. The combination of trastuzumab and doxorubicin (Adriamycin) resulted in an increase in

subclinical and clinical cardiac toxicity; combinations with anthracyclines should be avoided. Other toxicities of trastuzumab appear to be primarily infusion related. In addition, trastuzumab is being tested for use in other HER-2/*neu*-expressing tumors such as prostate and ovarian cancers.

Alemtuzumab is a humanized monoclonal antibody that is approved to treat relapsed or resistant CLL. It targets the CD52 antigen, which is prevalent on the abnormal B lymphocytes found in this common leukemia. In clinical trials of patients with CLL refractory to fludarabine and with prior exposure to alkylating agents, response rates of 33% were seen with a median duration of response of 7 months. Early studies in untreated patients suggest a response rate of up to 87% with a high rate of complete responses. Alemtuzumab is given by subcutaneous injection, and side effects include infusion-related events, infections, and bone marrow suppression.

Cetuximab is a chimeric human/mouse recombinant monoclonal antibody, recently FDA approved to treat metastatic colorectal cancer that overexpresses the *EGFR*. *EGFR* is a gene that is also overexpressed in many human cancers and has been associated with a poorer prognosis and resistance to therapy. Similar to the HER-2/*neu* oncogene, *EGFR* encodes a receptor tyrosine kinase that is closely related to HER-2. In patients with cancers that are resistant to irinotecan with or without oxaliplatin, the addition of cetuximab has been shown to result in about a 25% response rate, suggesting reversal of resistance. Response rates to its use as a single agent are about 11–15%. The major toxicities are infusion reactions and a significant and often painful acneiform rash. Cetuximab is indicated in the treatment of *EGFR*-expressing metastatic colorectal cancer in patients who are refractory to irinotecan-based chemotherapy.

Bevacizumab is the first antiangiogenic agent to be approved for clinical use in the treatment of cancer. Bevacizumab is a monoclonal antibody that binds to vascular endothelial growth factor (VEGF), the ligand for the VEGF receptors—thereby inhibiting activation of this receptor on the surface of endothelial cells as well as resulting endothelial cell proliferation and new blood vessel formation. As first-line therapy for metastatic colorectal cancer, the combination of bevacizumab with IFL was found to result in improved response rates as well as a 25% improvement in survival compared to the chemotherapy regimen alone. Bevacizumab is indicated for use in combination with fluorouracil-based chemotherapy in the first-line treatment of metastatic colorectal cancer. Preliminary data indicate activity of bevacizumab against a variety of other malignancies, including renal cell cancer and breast cancer. As a single agent, bevacizumab resulted in tumor shrinkage in renal cell cancer, and about a 10–15% response rate in resistant breast cancer. Ongoing large randomized trials are assessing the effectiveness of bevacizumab combined with chemotherapy in a variety of tumor types. The primary toxicities of bevacizumab include hypertension and proteinuria. Delays in wound healing, fatal hemorrhage, and bowel perforation have been reported in patients with lung and colorectal cancers.

Antibodies Linked to Cytotoxic Agents or Radiation

Radiolabeled and toxin-linked antibodies have been used to treat lymphomas with very encouraging results and appear more effective than antibody therapy alone. **Ibritumomab tiuxetan** is an yttrium-90-labeled antibody to CD20 that is FDA approved for the treatment of low-grade non-Hodgkin's lymphoma refractory to rituximab or transformed B cell non-Hodgkin's lymphoma. This is the first targeted radioimmunotherapy to be FDA approved for clinical use. This unique drug consists of an antibody to CD20 bound to tiuxetan, a high-affinity chelator for yttrium-90 and indium-111. A recently published randomized controlled trial compared ibritumomab tiuxetan with rituximab in patients with relapsed or refractory low-grade non-Hodgkin's lymphoma or transformed non-Hodgkin's lymphoma. The overall response rate was 80% for the radiolabeled antibody versus 56% for rituximab alone, with a corresponding prolongation in duration of response and time to disease progression. Durable responses were significantly longer in the ibritumomab tiuxetan group. The primary toxicity is reversible but significant myelosuppression. This agent must not be used in patients with impaired marrow function or extensive involvement of marrow with lymphoma. Treatment is given in two steps. On day 1, a dose of rituximab is given followed by indium-111-labeled ibritumomab tiuxetan to determine biodistribution of antibody. One week later, a second dose of rituximab is followed by yttrium-90-labeled antibody. Yttrium-90 is a pure β emitter with a half-life of 64 hours and a short path length of 5 mm, making it relatively safe to use in clinical practice.

A second radiolabeled antibody, **tositumomab**, is linked to ^{131}I, which requires dosimetry and shielding, making clinical use more cumbersome. Tositumomab was recently approved by the FDA for the treatment of low-grade non-Hodgkin's lymphoma refractory to rituxan and chemotherapy and is given in two steps—the dosimetric and therapeutic steps. Each step includes an infusion of tositumomab followed by radiolabeled tositumomab. Toxicity is similar to that of ibritumomab tiuxetan. Many other antibody combinations are either under development or in preliminary clinical trials.

Another agent approved for the treatment of cutaneous T cell lymphomas (CTCL) such as mycosis fungoides resistant to standard therapy is **denileukin difti-tox (ONTAK)**, a recombinant DNA-derived cytotoxic protein composed of amino acid sequences for diphtheria toxin fragments followed by the sequences for interleukin-2 (IL-2). This fusion protein was designed to direct the cytocidal action of diphtheria toxin to cells that express the IL-2 receptor (CD25), such as the tumor cells in CTCL. Thirty percent of patients with advanced CTCL responded to denileukin diftitox in a phase III randomized trial. Toxicity is significant, including acute hypersensitivity reactions—requiring administration of this agent in a close-observation setting—and delayed pulmonary and peripheral edema.

Gemtuzumab ozogamicin is an antibody to CD33 linked to a potent antitumor antibiotic, calicheamicin, that is approved for the treatment of patients over the age of 60 years with relapsed or refractory acute myelogenous leukemia (AML). This is the first example of antibody-targeted chemotherapy used clinically. In clinical trials, gemtuzumab ozogamicin resulted in a 31% remission rate in elderly patients with AML in first relapse who could not tolerate standard chemotherapy. Side effects are primarily infusion-related events and bone marrow suppression.

Agents with Novel Mechanisms of Action

Thalidomide, approved for treatment of lepromatous leprosy, has been found to induce significant responses in advanced and relapsed multiple myeloma. It is now being tested in many clinical trials, and the combination of thalidomide with dexamethasone results in enhanced responses. Toxicities that limit the usefulness of thalidomide include rashes, somnolence, and constipation. **Revlimid** is the lead compound of a new class of more potent and less toxic immunomodulatory drugs or ImiDs, which are believed to affect multiple pathways within the cell and inhibit tumor necrosis factor-α (TNF-α), and is now approved for the treatment of transfusion-dependent myelodysplasia. Multiple ongoing studies are evaluating the effect of revlimid in a variety of malignancies. Preliminary data indicate effectiveness in multiple myeloma and myelodysplastic syndromes.

Bortezomib (Velcade) is the first of a new class of agents, termed proteasome inhibitors, to be approved for the treatment of cancer. Bortezomib is a reversible inhibitor of the chymotrypsin-like activity of the 26S proteasome that degrades ubiquitinated proteins. The ubiquitin-proteasome pathway plays an essential role in regulating the intracellular concentration of specific proteins, thereby maintaining homeostasis within cells. Inhibition of the 26S proteasome prevents targeted breakdown of proteins, which affects multiple signaling cascades within the cell. The disruption in these normal homeostatic mechanisms can lead to cell death. In an open-label study of bortezomib in patients with multiple myeloma who had failed at least two prior therapies, the overall response rate was 28%, with 18% obtaining a clinical remission. The median duration of response was long at about 1 year. Bortezomib is approved for the treatment of multiple myeloma that progresses despite at least two prior therapies. Significant responses have also been seen in patients with relapsed and refractory low-grade lymphomas. It is given intravenously twice weekly for 2 weeks followed by a 10-day rest, then repeated every 3 weeks. The major side effects are peripheral neuropathy, cytopenias, and hypersensitivity reactions.

Tretinoin is the first agent designed to target a specific fusion protein caused by a chromosome translocation. This oral agent induces differentiation and decreased proliferation without cytolysis of acute promyelocytic leukemia cells. Use of tretinoin combined with chemotherapy has been shown to improve disease-free and overall survival from this form of leukemia. **Arsenic trioxide** has been shown to induce remission in 70% of patients with relapsed or refractory acute promyelocytic leukemia (APL). It is indicated both for induction of remission and for consolidation in this high-risk group of patients.

Retinoids modulate the growth and differentiation of a variety of epithelial cells. **Bexarotene**, a retinoid that selectively activates the retinoid X receptor (RXR), is now FDA approved to treat cutaneous T cell lymphomas such as mycosis fungoides. Targretin is also in clinical trials for use in a variety of advanced solid tumors, but toxicity limits its usefulness.

A purine analog, **cladribine** (2-chlorodeoxyadenosine; 2-CdA), is used as the primary agent to treat hairy cell leukemia. A 1-week course of therapy results in high and durable remission rates with modest and short-lived toxicity. Repeated courses for disease recurrence are also effective. **Pentostatin** (2-deoxycoformycin, an adenosine deaminase inhibitor) is also used to treat hairy cell leukemia.

Fludarabine phosphate, another purine analog, has shown improved response rates and progression-free survival compared with oral chlorambucil or combination chemotherapy for CLL. Fludarabine is now indicated as first-line therapy for most patients with CLL. Side effects include an increased risk of opportunistic infections as well as very rare problems such as hemolytic anemia and severe bone marrow suppression. Fludarabine is also effective therapy for low-grade lymphomas and Waldenström's macroglobulinemia. Cladribine and pentostatin are also used to treat CLL and the above disorders.

Recombinant Growth Factors

Several recombinant growth factors have been shown to be effective in the treatment of malignancy. **Recombinant interferon-α** has marked antitumor effects in hairy cell leukemia and chronic myelogenous leukemia and moderate effects in lymphomas, in the epidemic (AIDS-associated) form of KS, in multiple myeloma, and as adjuvant therapy for malignant melanoma. Interferon-α has some utility also in metastatic melanoma, renal cell carcinoma, and carcinoid syndrome. Unfortunately, chronic use of interferon-α is associated with fatigue, cytopenias, and fluid retention.

High-dose interferon for about 1 year in patients with malignant melanoma and lymph node metastases has been shown to improve disease-free and overall survival. Combinations of interferon-α-2b and **interleukin-2** given with standard chemotherapy for metastatic melanoma prolongs time to progression and survival (by a median of 2.7 months) but is associated with a significant increase in toxicity. Interleukin-2 treatment is effective in a subset of patients with advanced renal cell carcinoma. Recent data indicate improved survival in patients with AL type amyloidosis treated with a combination of dexamethasone and interferon-α compared with standard treatment with oral melphalan and prednisone. The addition of interferon-α to systemic chemotherapy for multiple myeloma appears to enhance the degree of cytoreduction achieved as compared with chemotherapy alone; however, toxicity is additive. Use of interferon-α for myeloma following chemotherapy or autologous bone marrow transplant has prolonged remission duration, though overall survival is not altered.

Prior to the availability of imatinib, patients with CML were treated with interferon-α given with low doses of the chemotherapeutic agent cytarabine. About 30% of patients achieved a cytogenic response to this combination, which was associated with a significantly longer survival than that of patients treated with standard oral chemotherapy. CML is unusual in that almost all cases are associated with a specific reciprocal chromosomal translocation resulting in activation of a tyrosine kinase that is critical to the pathogenesis of the disease.

Oral Small Molecule Tyrosine Kinase Inhibitors

A novel and exciting oral agent, **imatinib mesylate (Gleevec)**, specifically blocks the active tyrosine kinase in CML and is now approved for clinical use in both early-stage and late-stage CML. The response in patients with chronic phase CML was striking, with a 94% hematologic and an 83% cytogenetic response rate. These responses appear to be durable; progression-free survival at 12 months was significantly longer with imatinib mesylate than with the combination of interferon and cytarabine at 97% versus 80% in a phase III trial. Lower but significant response rates are seen in more advanced disease. The effect of imatinib mesylate on long-term disease control will require further follow-up of treated patients, although relapses and resistance clearly occur. Imatinib mesylate also inhibits two other tyrosine kinases, receptors encoded by c-*kit* and platelet-derived growth factor (PDGF). Expression of the c-*kit* receptor is found in high frequency in a relatively uncommon tumor of the gastrointestinal tract, gastrointestinal stromal tumor (GIST). GISTs are highly resistant to chemotherapy, and there is no effective therapy for advanced disease. Imatinib mesylate has demonstrated significant activity in GISTs, with a 60% overall response rate. This drug is also being tested in conditions such as myelofibrosis, chronic myelomonocytic leukemia, prostate cancer, and glioblastoma that express PDGF.

Gefitinib (Iressa) is another small molecule tyrosine kinase inhibitor that has recently been approved to treat advanced lung cancer that progresses despite at least two prior chemotherapy regimens. Gefitinib blocks the intracellular component of the epidermal growth factor receptor (EGFR), which is overexpressed on a number of tumors and correlates with poorer prognosis. Response rates in a phase III trial were low at just over 10% overall, but no other treatments are available to this population of patients, and up to 43% of treated individuals experienced symptom relief. For patients who had failed up to two prior treatments, the response rate rose to about 19%. A similar agent, **erlotinib** (Tarceva), was FDA approved for the treatment of metastatic lung cancer in 2004 based on a study showing a 2 month improvement in survival in patients treated with erlotinib versus those treated with placebo. In separate trials, neither gefitinib nor erlotinib combined with first-line chemotherapy for advanced lung cancer offered any advantage over first-line chemotherapy alone. Toxicity from both agents is modest and consists primarily of skin rash and diarrhea. Specific mutations in tumor EGFR are associated with responsiveness to gefitinib and erlotinib. An unusual and resistant form of lung cancer, bronchoalveolar carcinoma (BAC), has demonstrated striking responsiveness to gefitinib and erlotinib therapy and is known to express high levels of EGFR. A number of other oral tyrosine kinase inhibitors that block multiple receptors or angiogenesis have been recently FDA approved or are in clinical trials, including two inhibitors of the VEGF receptor, sunitinib (approved for advanced renal cell cancer and GIST) and sorafenib (approved for advanced renal cell cancer).

Hormonal Therapy

Hormonal therapy plays a critical role in the management of specific cancers. Hormonal therapy or ablation is important in the treatment and palliation of breast and prostatic carcinoma, whereas added progestins are useful in the suppression of endometrial carcinoma. Women with metastatic breast cancer who show objective improvement with hormonal therapy have tumors that contain nuclear estrogen and progesterone receptors. The SERM **tamoxifen** has been shown to be effective in prolonging survival in both early-stage and late-stage breast cancer. Tamoxifen has both antiestrogen and proestrogen effects, resulting in side effects that include an increase in the risk of endometrial cancer and thrombosis. Newer SERMs without estrogen-like effects are being developed.

Aromatase inhibitors (eg, **anastrozole**, **letrozole**) and inactivators (**exemestane**) block the peripheral conversion of adrenal androgens into estrogens and have been shown to be at least as effective as or more effective than tamoxifen as first-line therapy for metastatic hormone receptor-expressing breast cancer. Aromatase inhibitors are effective only in postmenopausal women and have now been shown to be very effective in the adjuvant setting as well. The Arimidex and Tamoxifen Alone or in Combination (ATAC) trial is a

large randomized trial that compared 5 years of tamoxifen to either anastrozole or to the combination as adjuvant therapy in postmenopausal women with hormone receptor-positive early-stage breast cancer. The combination arm was no better than tamoxifen; this arm was closed at the first evaluation of the trial. At 5 years of follow-up, there was a significant decrease in both distant and local recurrence as well as new breast cancers in the opposite breast in the women treated with anastrozole, compared to treatment with tamoxifen. There was no difference in survival, probably due to the slow growth of hormone responsive cancers and variable poststudy therapy in patients depending on the treatment arm of the study. Preliminary data from a second trial, BIG I-98, that compared letrozole to tamoxifen was presented in early 2005 and indicated a similar improvement in disease-free survival favoring the letrozole treated patients. Further data from this trial, and from a subset of patients who were switched from one agent to the other 2 years into therapy, should be available in the next 2 years.

Three additional studies have reinforced the importance and efficacy of aromatase inhibitors in the treatment of early-stage breast cancer. Two trials randomized postmenopausal women who had received tamoxifen for 2–3 years to exemestane or continued tamoxifen (the EIS trial) or to anastrozole or continued tamoxifen (the ABSCG/ARNO trials). Women who switched to the aromatase inhibitor had significantly fewer relapses and new breast cancers than women who continued tamoxifen.

Hormone receptor-positive breast cancer is a relatively slow growing disease, with 50% of all relapses occurring after 5 years. For that reason, extending hormone therapy has long been of interest to researchers. However, the toxicity of continued tamoxifen has precluded its use after 5 years in the adjuvant setting. The MA.17 trial randomized women to letrozole or placebo following 5 years of tamoxifen. This trial was closed early due to results showing an unexpectedly large benefit from letrozole at 3 years. Women treated with letrozole had a significant reduction in the risk of recurrence as well as in the incidence of new cancers. Survival was improved in women with node-positive breast cancer who were randomized to letrozole.

Toxicities in all five trials were modest. The primary toxicities of the aromatase inhibitors are accelerated bone mineral density loss, altered lipid profiles, and temporary but bothersome joint aches and stiffness. Longer-term follow-up, survival, and toxicity data—in particular the impact of these new agents on non-cancer-related morbidity and mortality—should be available over the next few years. Women treated with aromatase inhibitors should have their bone mineral density monitored, with early institution of antiresorptive therapy.

Given the weight of this evidence, for postmenopausal women with early-stage breast cancer, aromatase inhibitors appear to be an important part of treatment. Whether treatment should be given at diagnosis, at 2–3 years into tamoxifen, or after 5 years of tamoxifen is not known. Ongoing trials are comparing different strategies and should help answer these questions in the future. New trials are exploring the use of ovarian suppression and aromatase inhibition or inactivation in the treatment of early-stage breast cancer in premenopausal women.

A new pure antiestrogen (estrogen receptor down regulator), **fulvestrant**, has now been FDA approved as second-line therapy for metastatic hormone receptor-positive breast cancer. This agent is unique in its class, does not have the estrogen-like effects of tamoxifen, and is given by intramuscular injection once a month. Hormonal approaches are also available to treat prostate cancer, though androgen receptors remain difficult to measure. These include the use of estrogen therapy, gonadotropin-releasing hormone agonists (eg, leuprolide, triptorelin, goserelin), and antiandrogens (eg, bicalutamide, flutamide). The use of leuprolide plus flutamide (total androgen blockade) can be considered as an alternative to orchiectomy but also causes erectile dysfunction. High-dose ketoconazole has been used to rapidly suppress adrenal production of steroids in crises such as cord compression. Use of this agent requires hydrocortisone supplementation.

Bisphosphonates

Bisphosphonates inhibit osteoclast activation and may also have antitumor and antiangiogenic effects. In addition to reducing bone pain, **pamidronate** reduces by approximately 50% the frequency of new skeletal events in breast cancer and prostatic cancer metastatic to bone and in multiple myeloma and delays the time to new bone events. Pamidronate must be given intravenously on a monthly basis, and is associated with bone and muscle pain as well as fever on the day following the first infusion. A new and significantly more potent intravenous bisphosphonate, **zoledronic acid**, was FDA approved in early 2002 for the treatment of metastatic bone lesions. Its advantage compared with pamidronate is a shorter infusion time (15 minutes compared with 2 hours or more) and improved efficacy in some situations. Faster-than-indicated infusion rates of this bisphosphonate can result in reversible renal insufficiency. Zoledronic acid or pamidronate is indicated for the treatment of patients with known bone metastases due to any type of malignancy. Once-yearly infusions of zoledronic acid have been shown to improve bone mineral density in osteopenic postmenopausal women. Ongoing trials are evaluating the ability of zoledronic acid to prevent bone loss associated with hormonal therapy and chemotherapy in breast and prostate cancers. Guidelines for the use of bisphosphonates in the treatment of cancer were recently published.

Clodronate is an oral bisphosphonate that has been shown to reduce the number of new bone metastases in women with breast cancer. A study of women with a primary diagnosis of breast cancer and microscopic evidence of tumor cells in bone marrow randomized to receive either clodronate, 1600 mg/d for 2 years, or placebo—in addition to standard adjuvant therapy—showed a significant reduction of both osseous metastases initially and a reduction in mortality out to 10 years of follow-up. Results of a larger study of women with operable breast cancer but no other specific high-risk features showed a reduction in the incidence of bone metastases during the study period only but no difference in visceral metastases. Surprisingly, this study also showed a survival advantage at 10 years in women treated with clodronate. These observations suggest that bisphosphonates may be a useful treatment in a subset of women with primary breast cancer to prevent recurrence. Clodronate is a less potent bisphosphonate than zoledronic acid and is currently available only in Europe. A clinical trial in the United States comparing the effect of clodronate in women with node-positive breast cancer has recently been completed. As a follow-on trial, a national study opening later in 2005 will evaluate the effects of adjuvant zoledronic acid, clodronate, or ibandronate, a new and potent oral bisphosphonate, for 3 years in 6000 women with early stage breast cancer.

Growth Factors

Hematologic or other toxicity may limit the therapeutic effectiveness of treatment. It is possible to avoid the need for dose reductions or delay in therapy by using granulocyte colony-stimulating factor (G-CSF; **filgrastim**) or granulocyte-macrophage colony-stimulating factor (GM-CSF; **sargramostim**) to stimulate white blood cell recovery. A long-acting pegylated G-CSF (**pegfilgrastim**) is now FDA approved to reduce the incidence of neutropenic fever associated with chemotherapy. This agent can be given as a single 6 mg dose subcutaneously on day 2 of each 3-week chemotherapy cycle and in randomized trials was equivalent to 11 doses of filgrastim. Pegfilgrastim is now being used to reduce neutropenia in chemotherapy regimens given every 2 weeks as well; preliminary data indicate that this is a safe and effective approach. Interleukin-11 (**oprelvekin**) can be used to reduce the need for delay or dose reductions due to thrombocytopenia; however, the usefulness of this cytokine is limited because of its ineffectiveness in severe thrombocytopenia and its toxicity, which includes significant edema. Guidelines are available to direct usage of these expensive but critical growth factors. Erythropoietic growth factors are a very important part of supportive care during cancer chemotherapy; these agents are covered under the section on supportive care.

Table 40–4 sets forth the dosage schedules and toxicities of the most commonly used cancer chemotherapeutic agents. The dosage schedules given are for single-agent therapy; combination therapy is used for most cancers. Newer experimental therapies are discussed briefly at the end of this chapter.

Table 40–4. Single-agent dosage and toxicity of anticancer drugs.[1]

Drug	Dosage	Acute Toxicity	Delayed Toxicity
Alkylating agents			
Mechlorethamine	6–10 mg/m² intravenously every 3 weeks	Severe vesicant; severe nausea and vomiting	Moderate suppression of blood counts. Melphalan effect may be delayed 4–6 weeks. High doses produce severe bone marrow suppression with leukopenia, thrombocytopenia, and bleeding. Alopecia and hemorrhagic cystitis occur with cyclophosphamide, while busulfan can cause hyperpigmentation, pulmonary fibrosis, and weakness (see text). Ifosfamide is always given with mesna to prevent cystitis. Acute leukemia may develop in 5–10% of patients receiving prolonged therapy with melphalan, mechlorethamine, or chlorambucil; all alkylators probably increase the risk of secondary malignancies with prolonged use. Most cause either temporary or permanent aspermia or amenorrhea.
Chlorambucil	0.1–0.2 mg/kg/d orally (6–12 mg/d) or 0.4 mg/kg pulse every 4 weeks	None	
Cyclophospha-mide	100 mg/m²/d orally for 14 days; 400 mg/m² orally for 5 days; 1–1.5 g/m² intravenously every 3–4 weeks	Nausea and vomiting with higher doses	
Melphalan	0.25 mg/kg/d orally for 4 days every 6 weeks	None	
Busulfan	2–8 mg/d orally; 150–250 mg/course	None	
Estramustine	14 mg/kg orally in three or four divided doses	Nausea, vomiting, diarrhea	Thrombosis, thrombocytopenia, hypertension, gynecomastia, glucose intolerance, edema.
Carmustine (BCNU)	200 mg/m² intravenously every 6 weeks	Local irritant	Prolonged leukopenia and thrombocytopenia. Rarely hepatitis. Acute leukemia has been observed to occur in some patients receiving nitrosoureas. Nitrosoureas can cause delayed pulmonary fibrosis with prolonged use.
Lomustine (CCNU)	100–130 mg orally every 6–8 weeks	Nausea and vomiting	
Procarbazine	100 mg/m²/d orally for 14 days every 4 weeks	Nausea and vomiting	Bone marrow suppression, mental suppression, MAO inhibition, disulfiram-like effect.
Dacarbazine	250 mg/m²/d intravenously for 5 days every 3 weeks; 1500 mg/m² intravenously as single dose	Severe nausea and vomiting; anorexia	Bone marrow suppression; flu-like syndrome.
Cisplatin	50–100 mg/m² intravenously every 3 weeks; 20 mg/m² intravenously for 5 days every 4 weeks	Severe nausea and vomiting	Nephrotoxicity, mild otic and bone marrow toxicity, neurotoxicity.
Carboplatin	360 mg/m² intravenously every 4 weeks	Severe nausea and vomiting	Bone marrow suppression, prolonged anemia; same as cisplatin but milder.
Oxaliplatin	85 mg/m² intravenously in 250–500 mL D₅W over 2 hours on day 1, with infusional 5-FU/leucovorin on days 1 and 2 every 2 weeks (FOLFOX4)	Nausea, vomiting, diarrhea, fatigue, rare anaphylactic reactions	Peripheral neuropathy, cytopenias, pulmonary toxicity (rare).
Structural analogs or antimetabolites			
Methotrexate	2.5–5 mg/d orally; 20–25 mg intramuscularly twice weekly; high-dose: 500–1000 mg/m² every 2–3 weeks; 12–15 mg intrathecally every week for 4–6 doses	None	Bone marrow suppression, oral and gastrointestinal ulceration, acute renal failure; hepatotoxicity, rash, increased toxicity when effusions are present. ***Note:*** Citrovorum factor (leucovorin) rescue for doses over 100 mg/m².
Pemetrexed (Alimta)	500 mg/m² intravenously every 3 weeks; given with cisplatin or alone; requires folate and vitamin B₁₂ supplementation	Skin rash, cytopenias, decreased clearance of agent if given with NSAIDs, nausea, diarrhea, mucositis, hypersensitivity reactions	Cytopenias, rash, neuropathy.

(continued)

Table 40–4. Single-agent dosage and toxicity of anticancer drugs.[1] (continued)

Drug	Dosage	Acute Toxicity	Delayed Toxicity
Mercaptopurine	2.5 mg/kg/d orally; 100 mg/m^2/d orally for 5 days for induction	None	Well tolerated. Larger doses cause bone marrow suppression.
Thioguanine	2 mg/kg/d orally; 100 mg/m^2/d intravenously for 7 days for induction	Mild nausea, diarrhea	Well tolerated. Larger doses cause bone marrow suppression.
Fluorouracil	15 mg/kg/d intravenously for 3–5 days every 3 weeks; 15 mg/kg weekly as tolerated; 500–1000 mg/m^2 intravenously every 4 weeks	None	Nausea, diarrhea, oral and gastrointestinal ulceration, bone marrow suppression, dacrocystitis.
Capecitabine	2500 mg/m^2 orally twice daily on days 1–14 every 3 weeks	Nausea, diarrhea	Hand and foot syndrome, mucositis.
Cytarabine	100–200 mg/m^2/d for 5–10 days by continuous intravenous infusion; 2–3 g/m^2 intravenously every 12 hours for 3–7 days; 20 mg/m^2 subcutaneously daily in divided doses	High-dose: nausea, vomiting, diarrhea, anorexia	Nausea and vomiting; cystitis; severe bone marrow suppression; megaloblastosis; CNS toxicity with high-dose cytarabine.
Temozolamide	150 mg/m^2 orally for 5 days; repeat every 4 weeks	Headache, nausea, vomiting	Unknown.
Clofarabine	52 mg/m^2 intravenously daily for 5 days every 2–6 weeks	Nausea, vomiting	Bone marrow suppression, hepatobiliary and renal toxicity, capillary leak syndrome
Androgens and androgen antagonists			
Testosterone propionate	100 mg intramuscularly three times weekly	None	Fluid retention, masculinization, leg cramps. Cholestatic jaundice in some patients receiving fluoxymesterone.
Fluoxymesterone	20–40 mg/d orally	None	
Flutamide	250 mg three times a day orally	None	Gynecomastia, hot flushes, decreased libido, mild gastrointestinal side effects, hepatotoxicity.
Bicalutamide	50 mg/d orally		
Nilutamide	300 mg/d orally for 30 days, then 150 mg/d		
Ethinyl estradiol	3 mg/d orally	None	Fluid retention, feminization, uterine bleeding, exacerbation of cardiovascular disease, painful gynecomastia, thromboembolic disease.
Selective estrogen receptor modulators			
Tamoxifen	20 mg/d orally	Hot flushes, joint aching, vaginal discharge or dryness, vaginal bleeding, reduced libido, acne, nausea, transient flare of bone pain (metastatic disease only)	Thromboembolic disease, anovulation, endometrial cancer, endometrial polyps, ovarian cysts, cataracts, weight gain.
Toremifene	60 mg/d orally		
Aromatase inhibitors			
Anastrozole	1 mg/d orally	Hot flushes, joint and muscle aching, joint stiffness, vaginal dryness, reduced libido	Accelerated bone mineral density loss, possible exacerbation of hyperlipidemia.
Letrozole	2.5 mg/d orally		
Exemestane	25 mg/d orally		

(continued)

Table 40–4. Single-agent dosage and toxicity of anticancer drugs.[1] (continued)

Drug	Dosage	Acute Toxicity	Delayed Toxicity
Pure estrogen receptor antagonist			
Fulvestrant	250 mg intramuscularly once a month	Transient injection site reactions, hot flushes	Nausea, vomiting, constipation, diarrhea, abdominal pain, headache, back pain.
Progestins			
Megestrol acetate	40 mg orally four times daily	Hot flushes	Fluid retention; rare thrombosis, weight gain.
Medroxyprogesterone	100–200 mg/d orally; 200–600 mg orally twice weekly	None	
GnRH analogs			
Leuprolide	7.5 mg intramuscularly (depot) once a month or 22.5 mg every 3 months as depot injection	Local irritation, transient flare of symptoms	Hot flushes, decreased libido, impotence, gynecomastia, mild gastrointestinal side effects, nausea, diarrhea, fatigue.
Goserelin acetate	3.6 mg subcutaneously monthly or 10.8 mg every 3 months as depot injection		
Triptorelin pamoate	3.75 mg intramuscularly once a month (a 3-month depot formulation also exists)		
Adrenocorticosteroids			
Prednisone	20–100 mg/d orally or 50–100 mg every other day orally with systemic chemotherapy	Alteration in mood	Fluid retention, hypertension, diabetes, increased susceptibility to infection, "moon facies," osteoporosis, electrolyte abnormalities, gastritis.
Dexamethasone	5–10 mg orally daily or twice daily		
Ketoconazole	400 mg orally three times daily	Acute nausea	Gynecomastia, hepatotoxicity.
Biologic response modifiers			
Interferon-α-2a Interferon-α-2b	3–5 million units subcutaneously three times weekly or daily	Fever, chills, fatigue, anorexia	General malaise, weight loss, confusion, hypothyroidism, retinopathy, autoimmune disease.
Aldesleukin (IL-2)	600,000 units/kg intravenously over 15 minutes every 8 hours for 14 doses, repeated after 9-day rest period. Some doses may be withheld or interrupted because of toxicity. ***Caution:*** High doses must be administered in an ICU setting by experienced personnel.	Hypotension, fever, chills, rigors, diarrhea, nausea, vomiting, pruritus; liver, kidney, and CNS toxicity; capillary leak (primarily at high doses), pruritic skin rash, infections (can be severe)	Hypoglycemia, anemia.
Peptide hormone inhibitor			
Octreotide acetate	100–600 mcg/d subcutaneously in two divided doses	Local irritant; nausea and vomiting	Diarrhea, abdominal pain, hypoglycemia.
Natural products and miscellaneous agents			
Vinblastine	0.1–0.2 mg/kg or 6 mg/m^2 intravenously weekly	Mild nausea and vomiting; severe vesicant	Alopecia, peripheral neuropathy, bone marrow suppression, constipation, SIADH, areflexia.
Vincristine	1.5 mg/m^2 (maximum: 2 mg weekly)	Severe vesicant	Areflexia, muscle weakness, peripheral neuropathy, paralytic ileus, alopecia (see text), SIADH.
Vinorelbine	25–30 mg/m^2 intravenously weekly	Mild nausea and vomiting, fatigue, severe vesicant	Granulocytopenia, constipation, peripheral neuropathy, alopecia.

(continued)

Table 40–4. Single-agent dosage and toxicity of anticancer drugs.[1] (continued)

Drug	Dosage	Acute Toxicity	Delayed Toxicity
Paclitaxel (Taxol)	175 mg/m² over 3 hours every 2 to 3 weeks or 80 mg/m² over 1 hour every week	Hypersensitivity reaction (premedicate with diphenhydramine and dexamethasone), mild nausea and vomiting	Peripheral neuropathy, bone marrow suppression, sensory neuropathy fluid retention, myalgia/arthralgias, asthenia alopecia.
Nab-paclitaxel (Abraxane)	260 mg/m² intravenously every 3 weeks		
Docetaxel (Taxotere)	60–100 mg/m² intravenously every 3 weeks		
Dactinomycin	0.04 mg/kg intravenously weekly	Nausea and vomiting; severe vesicant	Alopecia, stomatitis, diarrhea, bone marrow suppression.
Daunorubicin	30–60 mg/m² daily intravenously for 3 days, or 30–60 mg/m² intravenously weekly		Alopecia, stomatitis, bone marrow suppression, late cardiotoxicity. Risk of cardiotoxicity increases with radiation, cyclophosphamide.
Idarubicin	12 mg/m² daily intravenously for 3 days		
Doxorubicin	60 mg/m² intravenously every 3 weeks to a maximum total dose of 550 mg/m²		
Epirubicin	60–100 mg/m² intravenously every 3 weeks		
Liposomal doxorubicin (Doxil)	35–40 mg/m² intravenously every 4 weeks	Mild nausea	Hand and foot syndrome; alopecia, stomatitis, and bone marrow suppression uncommon.
Liposomal daunorubicin (DaunoXome)	40 mg/m² intravenously every 2 weeks		
Etoposide	100 mg/m²/d intravenously for 5 days or 50–150 mg/d orally	Nausea and vomiting; occasionally hypotension	Alopecia, bone marrow suppression, secondary leukemia.
Mitomycin	10–20 mg/m² every 6–8 weeks	Severe vesicant; nausea	Prolonged bone marrow suppression, rare hemolytic-uremic syndrome.
Mitoxantrone	12–15 mg/m²/d intravenously for 3 days with cytarabine; 8–12 mg/m² intravenously every 3 weeks	Mild nausea and vomiting	Alopecia, mild mucositis, bone marrow suppression.
Bleomycin	Up to 15 units/m² intramuscularly, intravenously, or subcutaneously twice weekly to a total dose of 200 units/m²	Allergic reactions, fever, hypotension	Fever, dermatitis, pulmonary fibrosis.
Hydroxyurea	500–1500 mg/d orally	Mild nausea and vomiting	Hyperpigmentation, bone marrow suppression.
Mitotane	6–12 g/d orally	Nausea and vomiting	Dermatitis, diarrhea, mental suppression, muscle tremors.
Fludarabine	25 mg/m²/d intravenously for 5 days every 4 weeks	Nausea and vomiting	Bone marrow suppression, diarrhea, mild hepatotoxicity, immune suppression.
Cladribine (CdA)	0.09 mg/kg/d by continuous intravenous infusion for 7 days	Mild nausea, rash, fatigue	Bone marrow suppression, fever, immune suppression.
Topotecan	1.5 mg/m² intravenously daily for 5 days every 3 weeks	Nausea, vomiting, diarrhea, headache, dyspnea	Alopecia, bone marrow suppression.

(continued)

Table 40–4. Single-agent dosage and toxicity of anticancer drugs.[1] (continued)

Drug	Dosage	Acute Toxicity	Delayed Toxicity
Gemcitabine	1000 mg/m^2 every week up to 7 weeks, then 1 week off, then weekly for 3 out of 4 weeks	Nausea, vomiting, diarrhea, fever, dyspnea	Bone marrow suppression, rash, fluid retention, mouth sores, flu-like symptoms, paresthesias.
Irinotecan	125 mg/m^2 weekly for 4 weeks, then a 2-week rest, then repeat; given with bevacizumab, 5-FU, and leucovorin Dose reduced for homozygous polymorphism in the *UGT1A1* gene	Flushing, salivation, lacrimation, bradycardia, abdominal cramps, diarrhea	Bone marrow suppression, diarrhea.
Azacitidine	75 mg/m^2 subcutaneously daily for 7 days, repeat every 4 weeks. May increase to 100 mg/m^2 after two cycles if no response	Nausea, fever, injection site infection	Neutropenia, thrombocytopenia, fatigue, anorexia, liver and renal toxicity (rare).
Novel therapeutic agents			
Imatinib mesylate (Gleevec)	400–600 mg/d orally	Mild nausea	Myalgias, edema, bone marrow suppression, abnormal liver function tests.
Gefitinib (Iressa)	250 mg by mouth daily	Nausea, vomiting	Diarrhea, rash, acne, dry skin, pruritus, anorexia, asthenia, interstitial lung disease (rare).
Erlotinib (Tarceva)	150 mg by mouth daily	Mild nausea	Rash, diarrhea, anorexia, fatigue, transaminitis, interstitial lung disease (rare).
Alemtuzumab (Campath-1H)	30 mg three times a week by subcutaneous injection for up to 12 weeks. (Use dose escalation to reduce infusion-related events.)	Severe infusion-related events, injection site irritation	Infections, short-term bone marrow suppression, autoimmune hemolytic anemia.
Gemtuzumab ozogamicin (Mylotarg)	9 mg/m^2 for two doses given 14 days apart	Infusion-related events	Profound bone marrow suppression.
Tretinoin	45 mg/m^2 by mouth daily until remission or for 90 days	Retinoic acid syndrome (fever, dyspnea, pleural or pericardial effusion) must be treated emergently with dexamethasone	Headache, dry skin, rash, flushing.
Arsenic trioxide	Induction: 0.15 mg/kg intravenously daily until remission; maximum 60 doses Consolidation: 0.15 mg/kg intravenously daily for 25 doses	Same as tretinoin	Nausea, vomiting, diarrhea, edema.
Trastuzumab (Herceptin)	Load: 4 mg/kg intravenously followed by 2 mg/kg weekly	Low-grade fever, chills, fatigue, constitutional symptoms with first infusion	Cardiac toxicity, especially when given with anthracyclines.
Denileukin diftitox (ONTAK)	9–10 mcg/kg/d intravenously for 5 days every 21 days	Hypersensitivity type reactions with first infusion	Vascular leak syndrome, low albumin, increased risk of infections, diarrhea, rash.

(continued)

Table 40–4. Single-agent dosage and toxicity of anticancer drugs.[1] (continued)

Drug	Dosage	Acute Toxicity	Delayed Toxicity
Rituximab	375 mg/m^2 intravenously weekly for 4–8 doses	Hypersensitivity type reactions with first infusion; fever, tumor lysis syndrome (can be life-threatening)	Mild cytopenias, rare red cell aplasia or aplastic anemia, severe mucocutaneous reactions.
Ibritumomab tiuxetan (Zevalin)	0.3–0.4 mCi/kg (not to exceed 32 mCi); dosing must follow rituximab	Rituximab infusion reaction symptom complex	Prolonged and severe myelosuppression, nausea, vomiting, abdominal pain, arthralgias.
Bortezomib (Velcade)	1.3 mg/m^2 by intravenous bolus twice a week for 2 weeks followed by a 10-day rest. Repeat every 3 weeks.	Low-grade nausea, diarrhea, low-grade fever, weakness	Peripheral neuropathy, thrombocytopenia, edema.
^{131}I Tositumomab (Bexxar)	^{131}I Tositumomab must be given with tositumomab (T). Dosimetric step: 450 mg T over 60 minutes followed by ^{131}I T containing 35 mg T with 5 mCi ^{131}I. Therapeutic step: Calculated to deliver 75 cGy total body irradiation with 35 mg T.	Hypersensitivity reactions	Prolonged and severe myelosuppression, nausea, vomiting, abdominal pains, arthralgias.
Targretin	300 mg/m^2/d orally	Nausea	Hyperlipidemia, dry mouth, dry skin, constipation, leukopenia, edema.
Bevacizumab (Avastin)	5 mg/kg intravenously every 2 weeks; given with irinotecan, 5-FU, and leucovorin (IFL)	Asthenia, hypertension, diarrhea, hypersensitivity reactions	Proteinuria, hypertension, thromboembolism, gastrointestinal perforation, wound dehiscence, hemoptysis (lung cancer).
Cetuximab (Erbitux)	400 mg/m^2 intravenous loading dose, then 250 mg/m^2 once a week; given alone or with irinotecan; requires special tubing	Rare severe infusion reactions, diarrhea, nausea, abdominal pain	Interstitial lung disease, acneiform rash, sun sensitivity.
Sunitinib (Sutent)	50 mg/day orally for 4 weeks, then 2 weeks off treatment. Adjust dose for patient tolerability	Fatigue, diarrhea, anorexia, nausea, mucositis, rash, skin discoloration	Bone marrow suppression, fall in left ventricular ejection fraction.
Sorafenib (Nexavar)	400 mg twice daily by mouth, dose reduce for toxicity to 400 mg/day	Diarrhea, rash, desquamation, fatigue, hand/foot syndrome, pruritus, skin erythema and blisters	Bone marrow suppression, bleeding, sensory neuropathy.
Supportive agents (antiemetics are covered in detail in the text, under chemotherapy-induced nausea and vomiting)			
Allopurinol (Prevent hyperuricemia from tumor lysis syndrome)	300–900 mg/d orally for prevention or relief of hyperuricemia	None	Rash, Stevens-Johnson syndrome; enhances effects and toxicity of mercaptopurine when used in combination.
Mesna (Prevent ifosfamide bladder toxicity)	20% of ifosfamide dosage at the time of ifosfamide administration, then 4 and 8 hours after each dose of chemotherapy to prevent hemorrhagic cystitis	Nausea, vomiting, diarrhea	None.

(continued)

Table 40–4. Single-agent dosage and toxicity of anticancer drugs.[1] (continued)

Drug	Dosage	Acute Toxicity	Delayed Toxicity
Leucovorin (Protect against methotrexate toxicity to normal cells)	10 mg/m² every 6 hours intravenously or orally until serum methotrexate levels are below 5×10^{-8} mol/L with hydration and urinary alkalinization (about 72 hours)	None	Enhances toxic effects of fluorouracil.
Amifostine (Prevent radiation toxicity)	910 mg/m² intravenously daily, 30 minutes prior to chemotherapy with cyclophosphamide or ifosphamide	Hypotension, nausea, vomiting, flushing	Decrease in serum calcium.
Dexrazoxane (Protect against anthracycline cardiac toxicity)	10:1 ratio of anthracycline intravenously, before (within 30 minutes of) chemotherapy infusion	Pain on injection	Increased bone marrow suppression.
Palifermin (Prevent mucositis)	60 mcg/kg/d intravenous bolus daily for 3 days before and 3 days after myelotoxic chemotherapy (total of six doses separated from chemotherapy by at least 24 hours)	None	Skin rash, skin erythema, edema, pruritus, oral dysesthesias.
Pilocarpine hydrochloride (Ameliorate dry mouth from radiation)	5–10 mg orally three times daily	Sweating, headache, flushing; nausea, chills, rhinitis, dizziness, and urinary frequency at high dosage.	
Pamidronate (Treat hypercalcemia, reduce effects of bone metastases)	90 mg intravenously every month	Symptomatic hypoglycemia (rare), flare of bone pain, local irritation	Osteonecrosis, renal insufficiency.
Zoledronic acid (Treat hypercalcemia, reduce effects of bone metastases)	4 mg intravenously every month		
Epoetin alfa (erythropoietin) (Treat cancer or chemotherapy-related anemia)	100–300 units/kg intravenously or subcutaneously 3 times a week	Skin irritation or pain at injection site	Hypertension, headache, seizures in patients on dialysis (rare).
Darbopoetin alfa (Long-acting erythropoietin)	200 mcg subcutaneously every other week or 300 mcg subcutaneously every 3 weeks[2]	Injection site pain	Hypertension, thromboses, headache, diarrhea.
Filgrastim (G-CSF) (Reduce severity and duration of chemotherapy-induced neutropenia)	5 mcg/kg/d subcutaneously or intravenously daily until neutrophils recover	Mild to moderate bone pain, mild hypotension (rare), irritation at injection sites (rare)	Bone pain, hypoxia.
Pegfilgrastim (Long-acting neupogen)	6 mg subcutaneously on day 2 of each 2- to 3-week chemotherapy cycle[2]	Injection site reactions	Bone pain, hypoxia.

(continued)

Table 40–4. Single-agent dosage and toxicity of anticancer drugs.[1] (continued)

Drug	Dosage	Acute Toxicity	Delayed Toxicity
Sargramostim (GM-CSF)	250 mcg/kg/d as a 2-hour intravenous infusion (can be given subcutaneously)	Fluid retention, dyspnea, capillary leak (rare), supraventricular tachycardia (rare), mild to moderate bone pain, irritation at injection sites	
Neumega (IL-11) (Treat chemotherapy-induced thrombocytopenia)	50 mcg/kg/d subcutaneously	Fluid retention, arrhythmias, headache, arthralgias, myalgias	Unknown.
Gallium nitrate (Treat hypercalcemia, bone pain from cancer)	200 mg/m^2 intravenously daily by continuous infusion for 5 days	Hypocalcemia, transient hypophosphatemia	Renal insufficiency, hypocalcemia.
Samarium-153 lexidronam (Sm-153 EDTMP) (Treat bone metastases)	1 mCi/kg intravenously as single dose	None	Hematopoietic suppression.
Strontium-89 (Treat bone metastases)	4 mCi every 3 months intravenously	None	Hematopoietic suppression.

[1]5-FU = 5-fluorouracil; NSAIDs = nonsteroidal anti-inflammatory drugs; MAO = monoamine oxidase; GnRH = gonadotropin-releasing hormone; CNS = central nervous system; IL = interleukin; SIADH = syndrome of inappropriate antidiuretic hormone; G-CSF = granulocyte colony-stimulating factor; GM-CSF = granulocyte-macrophage colony-stimulating factor.
[2]Off label.

Armstrong DK: Intraperitoneal cisplatin and paclitaxel in ovarian cancer. N Engl J Med 2006;354:34. [PMID: 16394300]

Baum M et al: The ATAC (Arimidex, Tamoxifen Alone or in Combination) Trialists' Group. Anastrozole alone or in combination with tamoxifen versus tamoxifen alone for adjuvant treatment of postmenopausal women with early-stage breast cancer: results of the ATAC (Arimidex, Tamoxifen Alone or in Combination) trial efficacy and safety update analyses. Cancer 2003;98:1802. [PMID: 14584060]

Coiffier B et al: CHOP chemotherapy plus rituximab compared with CHOP alone in elderly patients with diffuse large-B-cell lymphoma. N Engl J Med 2002;346:280. [PMID: 11807147]

Coombes RC et al: A randomized trial of exemestane after two to three years of tamoxifen therapy in postmenopausal women with primary breast cancer. N Engl J Med 2004;350:1081. [PMID: 15014181]

Eton O et al: Sequential biochemotherapy versus chemotherapy for metastatic melanoma: results from a phase III randomized trial. J Clin Oncol 2002;20:2045. [PMID: 11956264]

Folprecht G et al: The role of new agents in the treatment of colorectal cancer. Oncology 2004;66:1. [PMID: 15031593]

Goss PE et al: A randomized trial of letrozole in postmenopausal women after five years of tamoxifen therapy for early-stage breast cancer. N Engl J Med 2003;349:1793. [PMID: 14551341]

Grossman HB et al: Neoadjuvant chemotherapy plus cystectomy compared with cystectomy alone for locally advanced bladder cancer. N Engl J Med 2003;349:859. [PMID: 12944571]

Hilner BE et al: American Society of Clinical Oncology 2003 update on the role of bisphosphonates and bone health issues in women with breast cancer. J Clin Oncol 2003;21:4042. [PMID: 12963702]

Hussein MA: New treatment strategies for multiple myeloma. Semin Hematol 2004;41:2. [PMID: 15768473]

Johnston SR: Fulvestrant. Curr Opin Investig Drugs 2002;3:305. [PMID: 12020064]

Kris MG et al: Efficacy of gefitinib, an inhibitor of the epidermal growth factor receptor tyrosine kinase, in symptomatic patients with non-small cell lung cancer: a randomized trial. JAMA 2003;290:2149. [PMID: 14570950]

Neville-Webbe HL et al: The anti-tumour activity of bisphosphonates. Cancer Treat Rev 2002;28:305. [PMID: 12470981]

O'Brien SG et al: Imatinib compared with interferon and low-dose cytarabine for newly diagnosed chronic-phase chronic myeloid leukemia. N Engl J Med 2003;348:994. [PMID: 12637609]

Piccart-Gebhart MJ et al; Herceptin Adjuvant (HERA) Trial Study Team: Trastuzumab after adjuvant chemotherapy in HER2-positive breast cancer. N Engl J Med 2005;353:1659. [PMID: 16236737]

Romond EH et al: Trastuzumab plus adjuvant chemotherapy for operable HER2-positive breast cancer. N Engl J Med 2005;353:1673. [PMID: 16236738]

Rosen LS et al: Long-term efficacy and safety of zoledronic acid compared with pamidronate disodium in the treatment of skeletal complications in patients with advanced multiple myeloma or breast carcinoma: a randomized, double-blind, multicenter, comparative trial. Cancer 2003;98:1735. [PMID: 14534891]

Shigematsu H et al: Clinical and biological features associated with epidermal growth factor receptor gene mutations in lung cancers. J Natl Cancer Inst 2005;97:339. [PMID: 15741570]

Slamon DJ et al: Use of chemotherapy plus a monoclonal antibody against HER2 for metastatic breast cancer that overexpresses HER2. N Engl J Med 2001;344:783. [PMID: 11248153]

Takahashi Y et al: Nonmyeloablative transplantation: an allogeneic-based immunotherapy for renal cell carcinoma. Clin Cancer Res 2004;10(18 Pt 2):6353S. [PMID: 15448030]

ADJUVANT CHEMOTHERAPY FOR MICROMETASTASES

One of the most important roles of cancer chemotherapy is as adjuvant therapy to eradicate or suppress minimal residual disease after local treatment with surgery or irradiation. Failure of local therapy to eradicate tumor is due principally to occult micrometastases of tumor stem cells outside the primary field. These distant micrometastases are more likely to be present in patients with positive lymph nodes at the time of surgery (eg, breast and prostate cancer), in patients with tumors known to have a propensity for early hematogenous spread (eg, osteogenic sarcoma, Wilms' tumor), and in patients with certain pathologic or molecular risk factors (eg, high proliferative index, vascular invasion, oncogene amplification). Given specific risk factors, the risk of recurrent or metastatic disease can be extremely high (> 80%). Only systemic therapy can adequately eradicate micrometastases. Chemotherapeutic regimens that have been shown to be effective in inducing regression of advanced cancers may be curative when combined with surgery and/or radiation for high-risk "early" cancer.

More data are now available to support the use of adjuvant therapy in many common neoplasms. Prolongation of survival with combination chemotherapy has been shown for women with breast cancer and negative or positive axillary lymph nodes (stages I, II, and III) following surgical resection; several regimens are used. Anthracycline-based regimens (eg, doxorubicin, epirubicin) have been found to be superior to cyclophosphamide, methotrexate, and fluorouracil (CMF), particularly in node-positive patients. The addition of taxanes to anthracycline combinations appears to further reduce the risk of recurrence and improve survival. Patients with node-negative breast cancer are treated with chemotherapy depending on a variety of risk factors in the primary tumor. The SERM tamoxifen (blocks the estrogen receptor) and the aromatase inhibitors anastrozole, letrozole, and exemestane (block estrogen production) are used routinely either with or without antecedent chemotherapy if receptors for estrogen or progesterone are present (see preceding section on hormonal therapy). The main challenge in treating women with node-negative (stage I) hormone receptor-positive breast cancer is to identify prognostic

factors that distinguish patients at higher risk who are more likely to benefit from adjuvant therapy. A recent study evaluated the use of a 21 gene expression assay (Oncotype Dx Breast Cancer Assay) to predict a patient's individual risk of recurrent breast cancer 10 years after initial diagnosis. All of the women in the study had received 5 years of adjuvant tamoxifen; the test is performed on the original tumor block. A "recurrence score" from 0 to 100 is reported, and defines the level of risk of distant disease recurrence as low, intermediate, or high. This score could help in determining the appropriate treatment for these relatively good risk cancers. The assay has been validated in two studies, and specifically in women with cancers that are hormone receptor positive and in women who have received adjuvant tamoxifen. One additional trial suggested that the primary benefit of adjuvant chemotherapy with CMF was in the high-risk groups with rapidly proliferating disease, whereas the primary benefit of hormonal therapy was in the low-risk group with slow growing cells. Although the test is now approved for use, it is very expensive and is not routinely covered by most insurers. Amplification of the HER-2/*neu* oncogene in breast cancer clearly correlates with a poorer prognosis, and these patients appear to have a marked benefit from adjuvant chemotherapy containing anthracyclines and taxanes. The antibody trastuzumab, which blocks activation of this receptor and improves survival in metastatic breast cancer, is being tested in combination with chemotherapy as treatment for early-stage breast cancer that overexpresses HER-2/*neu*. Current research is focusing on the identification of additional and more specific risk factors early in diagnosis that can aid in prognosis and treatment decisions. A study using cytokeratin staining of bone marrow aspirates in women with newly diagnosed breast cancer found a 36% incidence of occult marrow metastases that correlated with a fourfold increased risk of death from breast cancer. A second study found that the presence of these cells 3 years after diagnosis was an even stronger prognostic factor for risk of recurrence and death from this disease. These results must be confirmed before they can be used in clinical practice to direct therapy. The goal is to identify patients with high-risk features at the time of diagnosis with localized disease and provide risk-directed (and effective) therapy.

Adjuvant chemotherapy with fluorouracil plus leucovorin is indicated in Dukes B and C (node-positive) colon cancer and has been shown to reduce the risk of cancer recurrence. Many other cancers may be cured with adjuvant chemotherapy, including cancers of the ovary and testes, malignant melanoma, and choriocarcinoma. Still other malignancies are cured when radiation and chemotherapy are used concurrently as described in the section on radiation therapy. Chemotherapy instilled into the peritoneum and combined with intravenous chemotherapy has been shown to improve survival and reduce the risk of recurrence from stage III ovarian cancer.

Other tumors that have been shown to respond to adjuvant therapy include gastric, esophageal, colorectal, and bladder cancers, prostate cancer, osteogenic sarcoma, stage I and II ovarian cancer, and malignant melanoma—and, recently, non-small cell cancer of the lung. Adjuvant therapy remains investigational for a number of common tumors, including pancreatic cancer. Chemotherapy is often given with curative intent after surgical remission in testicular cancer, non-Hodgkin's lymphoma, and Hodgkin's lymphoma.

Although adjuvant therapy has been shown to reduce the rate of recurrence for some cancers, there is still a high failure rate (up to 60–80% in some high-risk breast cancers despite adjuvant therapy). In most cases, tumor recurrence signifies incurability. The evidence for a dose-response effect of adjuvant chemotherapy for most cancers remains unclear. Although high-dose chemotherapy with either bone marrow or peripheral blood stem cell rescue is curative for some otherwise incurable patients with testicular cancer and lymphomas, efficacy data are lacking for other solid tumors. Research in the past focused on very high doses of chemotherapy for high-risk and metastatic breast cancer; this translated into thousands of transplants and several large randomized clinical trials. Phase II data suggested clinical benefit to this toxic and expensive procedure, but the studies were biased by inappropriate historical controls, rigorous selection criteria, and short follow-up. To date, all randomized studies have failed to show any benefit to high-dose chemotherapy with stem cell rescue compared with intermediate or standard-dose chemotherapy. Two studies performed in South Africa appeared encouraging; however, an on-site review revealed significant scientific misconduct that invalidated all results. At present, high-dose chemotherapy for breast cancer should be performed only in the setting of a properly designed clinical trial; it is experimental therapy. Bone marrow transplantation for other malignancies is covered in more detail in Chapter 13.

Citron ML et al: Randomized trial of dose-dense versus conventionally scheduled and sequential versus concurrent combination chemotherapy as postoperative adjuvant treatment of node-positive primary breast cancer: first report of Intergroup Trial C9741/Cancer and Leukemia Group B Trial 9741. J Clin Oncol 2003;21:1431. [PMID: 12668651]

Hobday TJ et al: Adjuvant therapy of colon cancer: a review. Clin Colorectal Cancer 2002;1:230. [PMID: 12450421]

Janni W et al: The persistence of isolated tumor cells in bone marrow from patients with breast carcinoma predicts an increased risk for recurrence. Cancer 2005;103:884. [PMID: 15666325]

Mariotto A et al: Trends in use of adjuvant multi-agent chemotherapy and tamoxifen for breast cancer in the United States: 1975–1999. J Natl Cancer Inst 2002;94:1626. [PMID: 12419789]

Scagliotti GV et al: Randomized study of adjuvant chemotherapy for completely resected stage I, II or IIIA non-small-cell lung cancer. J Natl Cancer Inst 2003;95:1453. [PMID: 14519751]

Sun W et al: Adjuvant therapy of colon cancer. Semin Oncol 2005;32:95. [PMID: 15726511]

Tallman MS et al: Conventional adjuvant chemotherapy with or without high-dose chemotherapy and autologous bone marrow transplantation in high-risk breast cancer. N Engl J Med 2003;349:17. [PMID: 12840088]

Trimbos JB et al: International Collaborative Ovarian Neoplasm trial 1 and Adjuvant ChemoTherapy In Ovarian Neoplasm trial: two parallel randomized phase III trials of adjuvant chemotherapy in patients with early-stage ovarian carcinoma. J Natl Cancer Inst 2003;95:105. [PMID: 12529343]

TOXICITY & DOSE MODIFICATION OF CHEMOTHERAPEUTIC AGENTS

A number of cancer chemotherapeutic agents have cytotoxic effects on rapidly proliferating normal cells in bone marrow, mucosa, and skin. Still other drugs such as the vinca alkaloids and taxanes produce neuropathy, and hormones often have psychological as well as physical effects. Acute and chronic toxicities of various drugs used to treat cancer are summarized in Table 40–4. Appropriate dose modification may minimize these side effects, so that therapy can be continued with relative safety. Dose modifications are usually considered in settings where treatment is given with palliative intent. Dose intensity and schedule should be maintained if at all possible in the adjuvant setting, when treatment is directed toward preventing recurrence or metastases of the cancer.

Bone Marrow Toxicity

Depression of bone marrow is usually the most serious limiting toxicity of cancer chemotherapy. Autologous bone marrow or peripheral blood stem cell transplantation or rescue can reduce the myelosuppressive toxicity of high-dose chemotherapy; however, cost and toxicity limit its general use. Growth factors that stimulate myeloid proliferation (eg, **G-CSF; filgrastim**, the longer acting **pegfilgrastim**, and **GM-CSF; sargramostim**) or erythroid proliferation (**epoetin alfa [erythropoietin]**) and the longer acting **darbepoetin alfa** are now used to ameliorate bone marrow toxicity. G-CSF and GM-CSF have been shown to shorten the period of neutropenia following both standard and high-dose chemotherapy as well as to allow dosing of chemotherapy at more frequent intervals. The risk of febrile neutropenia and mucosal toxicity is reduced as well. Myeloid growth factors are also used to stimulate circulation of stem cells in the peripheral blood either at steady state or during white blood cell recovery following myelosuppressive chemotherapy. These cells are then harvested using an apheresis machine and frozen for later use. When stimulated peripheral blood stem cells are used instead of or in conjunction with bone marrow for autologous transplantation following high-dose chemotherapy and radiotherapy, recovery of both neutrophils and platelets may be hastened by as much as 7–10 days as opposed to the use of bone marrow alone. Recombinant growth factors are expensive and must be used judiciously. Published standard practice guidelines are referenced at the end of this section.

Epoetin alfa (erythropoietin) and the newer **darbepoetin alfa** have been shown to improve anemia associated with malignancy or cancer chemotherapy. Patients must have adequate iron stores to respond to this agent, and even patients with marrow infiltration with tumor may benefit. Higher doses are necessary for patients with cancer than for patients with renal failure (40,000 units a week compared with about 10,000 units a week epoetin alfa). It is useful to check the level of erythropoietin before instituting therapy in patients with hematopoietic malignancies; this is not necessary in patients with solid tumors with either chemotherapy- or cancer-related anemia. Very high levels (≥ 500 ng/mL) predict a poor response. Epoetin alfa may be given as a subcutaneous injection once a week. This dosage schedule is as effective as the traditional three times a week dosing and is much more convenient. For anemia related to cancer chemotherapy or marrow infiltration, a dose of 40,000 units a week is used. **Novel erythropoiesis-stimulating protein (NESP; darbepoetin alfa)** is now approved to treat anemia associated with renal failure and cancer chemotherapy. Its main advantage over epoetin alfa is its longer half-life, which allows dosing every 2–3 weeks, usually on the same schedule as chemotherapy administration. Current dosing is 200 units every other week, or 300 units every 3 weeks. Clinical trials comparing the two agents suggest similar results in terms of red cell production and need for transfusions. Data from a variety of trials have shown that anemia during treatment for advanced cancer is associated with a poorer outcome. In addition, correction of anemia is associated with improvement across all aspects of quality of life. This has led to trials evaluating the effect of prophylactic epoetin alfa during treatment for early-stage cancers. Clearly, this approach results in improved quality of life in the short term; however, no long-term differences have been demonstrated. The cost as well as potential side effects such as cerebrovascular events associated with high hemoglobin levels have discouraged the routine use of erythroid growth factors as prophylaxis for anemia. However, erythropoietic growth factors should be instituted when the hemoglobin falls to 11 g/dL if continued chemotherapy is planned, or at higher levels in older patients with comorbidities.

Thrombocytopenia remains a problem with high doses of or prolonged exposure to chemotherapeutic agents and may limit therapy. **Oprelvekin (recombinant interleukin-11)** may be used in treating and preventing chemotherapy-induced thrombocytopenia. It is less effective in treating very severe thrombocytopenia, and its use can be associated with significant fluid retention, arrhythmias, and congestive heart failure.

Commonly used short-acting drugs that affect the bone marrow include the alkylating agents (eg, cyclophosphamide, melphalan, chlorambucil), procarbazine, mercaptopurine, methotrexate, irinotecan, vinorelbine, dactinomycin, anthracyclines, taxanes, and others. The standard dosage schedules for tumor response often induce bone marrow suppression. Continuing some drugs in the face of falling blood counts may result in serious infectious complications or

Table 40–5. A common scheme for dose modification of cancer chemotherapeutic agents.[1]

Granulocyte Count	Platelet Count	Suggested Dosage (% of Full Dose)
> 2000/mcL	> 100,000/mcL	100%
1000–2000/mcL	75,000–100,000/mcL	50%
< 1000/mcL	< 50,000/mcL	0%

[1]In general, dose modification should be avoided to maintain therapeutic efficacy. The use of myeloid growth factors or a delay in the start of the next cycle of chemotherapy is usually effective.

bleeding. Simple guidelines for treatment and follow-up can usually prevent this complication.

In patients with normal blood counts as well as normal liver and kidney function, drugs should be started in full dosages. Indeed, the effectiveness of many chemotherapeutic agents, particularly in the adjuvant setting, is dependent on maintaining dose and schedule for efficacy. Bone marrow toxicity is cumulative over time, and this must be anticipated during follow-up. Cumulative toxicity from long-term chemotherapy can require cessation of therapy or reduction in dose. Patients with bone marrow involvement may tolerate chemotherapy poorly initially, with improved counts on future cycles as the tumor burden is reduced.

Drug dosage may be modified as a function of the peripheral white blood cell count or platelet count (or both). These modifications assume that the blood counts are checked shortly before the next course of chemotherapy is to be administered. Dosage modifications should be avoided in the adjuvant setting when treatment is given with curative intent, and are used primarily for repeated courses of oral alkylator or antimetabolite therapy used to treat chronic, incurable disease. A scheme for dosage modification is presented in Table 40–5. Alternatively, the interval between drug courses can be lengthened, thereby permitting more complete hematologic recovery and repetition of full-dose chemotherapy. Both dosage modification and delay of chemotherapy limit the efficacy of treatment.

Dale D: Current management of chemotherapy-induced neutropenia: the role of colony stimulating factors. Semin Oncol 2003;30:3. [PMID: 14508714]

Lyman GH: Balancing the benefits and costs of colony-stimulating factors: a current perspective. Semin Oncol 2003;30:10. [PMID: 14508715]

Schwartzberg L et al: A multicenter retrospective cohort study of practice patterns and clinical outcomes of the use of darbepoetin alfa and epoetin alfa for chemotherapy-induced anemia. Clin Ther 2003;25:2781. [PMID: 14693304]

Chemotherapy-Induced Nausea & Vomiting

A number of cytotoxic anticancer drugs induce nausea and vomiting. In general, these symptoms are thought to originate in the central nervous system rather than peripherally. Parenteral administration of agents such as doxorubicin, etoposide, or cyclophosphamide is usually associated with mild to moderate nausea and vomiting, whereas nitrosoureas, dacarbazine, and particularly cisplatin cause more severe symptoms. Combination chemotherapy can also cause severe symptoms. Antiemetics clearly reduce and often eliminate nausea and vomiting associated with these drugs and are especially useful in conjunction with cisplatin.

5-Hydroxytryptamine-3 receptor antagonists (**ondansetron, granisetron, dolasetron**) have now replaced other drugs as the primary agents for the prevention and treatment of emesis from chemotherapy. These drugs are serotonin receptor-blocking agents with few side effects. They are also effective against radiation-induced and postanesthetic emesis and can be useful in the treatment of delayed and refractory nausea and vomiting following chemotherapy. **Ondansetron** is administered by the parenteral route as a single dose of 32 mg prior to chemotherapy and may be repeated every 24 hours, or it may be given orally at a dose of 8 mg every 8 hours. Lower parenteral doses may be just as effective. **Granisetron** is given as a single dose of 10 mcg/kg intravenously 30 minutes before chemotherapy, or orally at a dose of 1–2 mg/d. The dose of **dolasetron** is 1.8 mg/kg intravenously or 100–200 mg orally before chemotherapy. The serotonin receptor-blocking agents are more effective when given in conjunction with dexamethasone. **Palonosetron** is a new selective serotonin receptor antagonist with strong binding to the receptor, a long half-life, and little interaction with other medications. It is an effective antiemetic for both acute and delayed nausea and vomiting caused by cancer chemotherapy. It is given as a one-time dose of 0.25 mg intravenously 30 minutes before the start of chemotherapy, and can be repeated as often as once a week. **Dexamethasone** has antiemetic effects when administered at a dosage of 6–10 mg either as a single dose prior to—or both prior to and every 6 hours following—the administration of chemotherapy for two to four total doses.

Substance P appears to have a causative role in chemotherapy-induced nausea. Its biologic actions are mediated through the neurokinin-1 receptor. A novel oral agent, **aprepitant,** is a selective high-affinity neurokinin-1 receptor antagonist that is effective in preventing chemotherapy-induced nausea. Two randomized trials comparing granisetron and dexamethasone with or without this agent showed a significant reduction in acute emesis following chemotherapy with cisplatin with the three-drug combination. In addition, aprepitant was effective in preventing delayed emesis from cisplatin. Aprepitant is approved for the treatment of acute and delayed nausea and vomiting associated with initial and repeat courses of highly emetogenic cancer chemotherapy. It is given for 3 days beginning on the day chemotherapy starts.

Other active agents often used in combination as premedication for less emetogenic chemotherapy or as treatment for delayed nausea and vomiting include **prochlorperazine, metoclopramide, thiethylpera-**zine, and **lorazepam**. The phenothiazines (prochlorperazine, thiethylperazine) and metoclopramide can induce extrapyramidal side effects; their incidence is increased with prolonged use. **Prochlorperazine** is given at a dose of 10 mg orally or intravenously every 6–8 hours. The total dose given over 24 hours should not exceed 40 mg. A 25-mg suppository may be used for patients who are too nauseated to swallow pills without inducing further emesis. **Metoclopramide** is given at a dose of 10–20 mg orally or intravenously before and then every 6 hours after chemotherapy, usually in combination with dexamethasone. **Lorazepam** has both antiemetic and sedative effects and is administered at a dose of 0.5–1 mg every 4–6 hours by the sublingual or oral route, making it particularly useful in the outpatient setting. Older patients may experience intolerable psychological side effects.

Combinations of antiemetics are usually more effective than maximal doses of any one agent to block severe emesis. A typical antiemetic regimen might include ondansetron combined with sublingual lorazepam or prochlorperazine and dexamethasone with aprepitant for severely emetogenic regimens. For less emetogenic regimens, the serotonin antagonists can be reserved for failure to control nausea with less expensive regimens.

Dronabinol (Δ^9-tetrahydrocannabinol) is effective in some patients at a dose of 5 mg/m^2 prior to and then every 2–4 hours following chemotherapy for a total of four to six doses a day. Dronabinol may cause undesirable side effects such as dysphoria, and it is available only for oral administration.

A patient receiving antiemetics (eg, lorazepam, prochlorperazine, metoclopramide) along with chemotherapy on an outpatient basis must be escorted to and from the clinic, since the antiemetics often induce marked sedation and transient impairment of balance and reflexes. Antiemetics are more effective when given prophylactically. Therefore, regular dosing of an agent such as lorazepam or prochlorperazine is recommended after chemotherapy until the emetogenic effects have dissipated. This is dependent on the patient as well as on the type of chemotherapy administered. One problem with all combinations of antiemetic agents is the development of tachyphylaxis over 4–5 days with continuing highly emetogenic chemotherapy. This limits the effectiveness of any regimen. Acute mucosal injury to the upper gastrointestinal tract may complicate nausea associated with chemotherapy or delayed nausea and vomiting. Agents that reduce acid secretion (eg, omeprazole, ranitidine) can be useful adjunctive therapy to the antinausea regimen.

Aapro M: 5-HT(3)-receptor antagonists in the management of nausea and vomiting in cancer and cancer treatment. Oncology 2005;69:97. [PMID: 16131816]

Ezzo J et al: Acupuncture-point stimulation for chemotherapy-induced nausea and vomiting. J Clin Oncol 2005;23:7188. [PMID: 16192603]

Hesketh PJ: New treatment options for chemotherapy-induced nausea and vomiting. Support Care Cancer 2004;12:550. [PMID: 15232725]

Pendergrass K et al: Aprepitant: an oral NK1 antagonist for the prevention of nausea and vomiting induced by highly emetogenic chemotherapy. Drugs Today (Barc) 2004;40:853. [PMID: 15605119]

Wiser W et al: Practical management of chemotherapy-induced nausea and vomiting. Oncology (Williston Park) 2005;19: 637. [PMID: 15945344]

Gastrointestinal & Skin Toxicity

Chemotherapeutic agents generally act on rapidly proliferating cells, resulting in damage to the normal cells lining the gastrointestinal tract and mouth. This can result in mouth and throat sores, chronic nausea, and diarrhea. Erythema is an early sign of mucosal toxicity. Ulcerations in the mouth due to chemotherapy must be carefully evaluated for the presence of herpes simplex virus. Herpes ulcerations are common in immunosuppressed cancer patients and may be treated with acyclovir or other antiviral agents. Throat or esophageal pain may be due to either chemotherapy or infection from fungal or viral pathogens. These infections are more common in patients receiving steroids with their chemotherapy regimens. Chemotherapy should be delayed or withheld to allow healing or treatment of infection.

Adequate mouth care with antimicrobial mouthwashes and attention to dental hygiene are essential and may prevent severe toxicity. Common mouthwashes include the microbicidal oral rinse chlorhexidine and a mixture of salt and bicarbonate of soda in warm water, which aids in debridement of dead mucosa. A prophylactic antifungal mouthwash such as nystatin oral suspension may also be used. Certain chemotherapeutic agents can also cause toxicity to the skin, particularly the palms and soles and the skin in the axilla and groin. Common findings are erythema and hyperpigmentation, which may be painful or pruritic. Blistering is uncommon but can occur if chemotherapy is continued after the early signs of skin irritation occur. Toxicities to the gastrointestinal tract and skin may be more serious and harder to treat than bone marrow suppression. Patients receiving drugs that cause these side effects should be monitored closely.

Radiation therapy may cause xerostomia, which can lead to difficulty in swallowing, discomfort, and gum disease. **Pilocarpine hydrochloride**, 5–10 mg orally three times a day, can relieve symptoms of dry mouth but must be used regularly. **Amifostine**, a thiol-containing compound that reduces cisplatin-induced nephrotoxicity, has also been shown to reduce acute and chronic xerostomia in patients with head and neck cancers receiving radiation therapy. The dose of amifostine is 200 mg/m^2 intravenously daily 15–30 minutes before irradiation. Side effects include nausea and vomiting.

Radiation therapy to areas that include the gastrointestinal tract can cause diarrhea that resolves gradually with cessation of therapy and healing of normal cells. Topical butyrate appears to improve symptoms of acute radiation proctitis following radiation therapy for malignant pelvic disease. The **sodium butyrate** is given per rectum. Skin toxicity in the form of erythema and

occasionally blistering and exfoliation of the area receiving radiation can also occur. Severe skin toxicity requires holding the radiation doses; the affected area is treated with local application of emollients.

Miscellaneous Drug-Specific Toxicities

The toxicities of individual drugs have been summarized in Table 40–4. Several of these warrant additional mention, since they occur with commonly administered agents, and special preventive measures are often indicated.

A. Hemorrhagic Cystitis Induced by Cyclophosphamide or Ifosfamide

Metabolic products of cyclophosphamide that retain cytotoxic activity are excreted into the urine. Some patients appear to metabolize more of the drug to these active excretory products. If their urine is concentrated, the toxic metabolite may cause severe bladder damage. Patients receiving cyclophosphamide must be advised to maintain a high fluid intake. Early symptoms of bladder toxicity include dysuria and frequency despite the absence of bacteriuria. If microscopic hematuria develops, it is advisable to stop the drug temporarily or switch to a different alkylating agent, increase fluid intake, and administer a urinary analgesic such as phenazopyridine. With severe cystitis, large segments of bladder mucosa may be shed and the patient may have prolonged gross hematuria. Such patients should be observed for signs of urinary obstruction and may require cystoscopy for removal of obstructing blood clots. The risk of developing hemorrhagic cystitis is dose related and more common in patients who take the drug orally over a prolonged period of time. The cyclophosphamide analog ifosfamide or very high doses of cyclophosphamide can cause severe hemorrhagic cystitis when either is used alone. However, when they are used in conjunction with the neutralizing agent mesna, bladder toxicity can usually be prevented. Mesna is given with the chemotherapeutic agent and in a series of doses over the following 24 hours. Continuous bladder irrigation with 0.9% saline has been used with high-dose cyclophosphamide to prevent hemorrhagic cystitis. This appears to be less effective than mesna and may result in complications from Foley catheter trauma to the urethra, so it is used infrequently in high-risk situations—often in combination with mesna.

B. Neuropathy Induced by Vincristine and Other Agents

Neuropathy is a toxic side effect that is peculiar to the vinca alkaloid drugs, especially vincristine and vinorelbine. A primarily sensory peripheral neuropathy is also commonly caused by two of the newer anticancer therapeutic agents, paclitaxel and docetaxel, as well as cisplatin, carboplatin, and topotecan. The peripheral neuropathy associated with vincristine can be sensory, motor, autonomic, or a combination of these effects. In its mildest form, it consists of paresthesias of the fingers and toes. Occasional patients develop acute jaw or throat pain after vincristine therapy. This may be a form of trigeminal or glossopharyngeal neuralgia. With continued vincristine therapy, the paresthesias may extend to the proximal interphalangeal joints, hyporeflexia can appear in the lower extremities, and weakness may develop in the quadriceps muscle group. At this point, it is wise to discontinue vincristine therapy until the neuropathy has subsided. A useful means of judging whether peripheral motor neuropathy is severe enough to warrant stopping treatment is to have the patient attempt to do deep knee bends or rise from a chair without using the arm muscles. In general, the neuropathy associated with paclitaxel and vinorelbine is mild, well-tolerated, and both dose sensitive and schedule sensitive. More frequent dosing of smaller amounts of chemotherapy can reduce this side effect; the neuropathy significantly improves when the chemotherapy is stopped.

Constipation is the most common symptom of autonomic neuropathy associated with vincristine therapy. Patients receiving vincristine or vinorelbine should be started on stool softeners and mild cathartics when therapy is begun; otherwise, severe impaction may result as a consequence of an atonic bowel. More serious autonomic involvement can lead to acute intestinal ileus with signs indistinguishable from those of an acute abdomen.

Bladder neuropathies are uncommon but may be severe. Paralytic ileus and bladder atony are absolute contraindications to continued vincristine therapy. The majority of symptoms from vincristine are mild and resolve slowly although often not completely after therapy has been discontinued. Peripheral neuropathy associated with paclitaxel, docetaxel, vinorelbine, cisplatin, carboplatin, and topotecan worsens over time and can be painful and debilitating.

C. METHOTREXATE TOXICITY AND LEUCOVORIN RESCUE

In addition to standard uses of methotrexate for cancer chemotherapy, this drug is also used in very high doses that could lead to fatal bone marrow toxicity if given without an antidote. High-dose methotrexate therapy with leucovorin rescue is routinely used to treat osteogenic sarcoma, acute lymphocytic leukemia, and some cases of non-Hodgkin's lymphoma as well as primary lymphoma of the central nervous system.

The bone marrow and mucosal toxicity of methotrexate can be prevented by early administration of leucovorin (folinic acid). Serum levels of methotrexate are usually monitored and doses of leucovorin adjusted accordingly. Rescue is required for methotrexate doses over 80 mg/m^2 and is usually begun within 4 hours after completing treatment. Up to 100 mg/m^2 of leucovorin is given initially every 6 hours, with further doses adjusted for the serum methotrexate level.

Rescue is usually continued orally for 3 days or longer until the serum methotrexate level is below 0.05 mcmol/L. Asparaginase can be given as rescue for methotrexate in the treatment of lymphoblastic leukemia. If an overdose of methotrexate is administered accidentally, leucovorin therapy should be initiated as soon as possible, preferably within 1 hour. Intravenous infusion should be employed for larger overdosages to ensure adequate drug delivery. It is generally advisable to give leucovorin repeatedly in this situation. A new agent, carboxypeptidase G2, may be useful for the treatment of patients with methotrexate toxicity, and rapidly reduces high serum methotrexate levels. It is expected to obtain FDA approval in 2005.

Vigorous hydration and bicarbonate loading also appear to be important in preventing crystallization of high-dose methotrexate in the renal tubular epithelium. Serum creatinine is determined before beginning therapy and daily thereafter, since methotrexate excretion is slowed by renal insufficiency and toxicity will be enhanced. In high doses, methotrexate can itself cause renal injury. Methotrexate doses are reduced in renal insufficiency. Concomitant use of certain drugs will slow methotrexate excretion, and they are avoided during therapy. These drugs include aspirin, NSAIDs, penicillins, sulfonamides, and probenecid.

D. BUSULFAN TOXICITY

The alkylating agent busulfan, occasionally used for the treatment of myeloproliferative diseases, has curious delayed toxicities, including increased skin pigmentation, a wasting syndrome similar to that seen in adrenal insufficiency, and progressive pulmonary fibrosis. Patients in whom either of the latter two problems develop should be switched to a different drug (eg, melphalan) when further therapy is needed. The pigmentary changes are innocuous and will usually regress slowly after treatment is discontinued. Long-term treatment with busulfan also results in an increased risk of secondary leukemias.

E. BLEOMYCIN TOXICITY

Bleomycin is used to treat squamous cell carcinoma, Hodgkin's disease, non-Hodgkin's lymphoma, and testicular cancer. It can produce edema of the interphalangeal joints and hardening of the palmar and plantar skin. More serious toxicities include an anaphylactic or serum sickness-like reaction and a potentially fatal pulmonary fibrotic reaction (seen especially in elderly patients receiving a total dose of over 300 units). If a nonproductive cough, dyspnea, and pulmonary infiltrates develop, the drug is discontinued, and high-dose corticosteroids are instituted as well as empirical antibiotics pending cultures. Fever alone or with chills is an occasional complication of bleomycin and is not an absolute contraindication to continued treatment. The fever may be avoided by administration of hydrocortisone just prior to the injection. Fever alone is not predictive of pulmonary toxicity.

About 1% of patients (especially those with lymphoma) may have a severe or even fatal hypotensive reaction after the initial dose of bleomycin. To identify and treat such patients, it is wise to administer a test dose of 5 units of bleomycin first and to have adequate monitoring and emergency facilities available. Patients exhibiting a hypotensive reaction should not receive further bleomycin therapy.

F. ANTHRACYCLINE-INDUCED CARDIOMYOPATHY

The anthracycline antibiotics doxorubicin, daunomycin, and idarubicin and the similar drug mitoxantrone have both acute and delayed cardiac toxicity. The problem is greater with doxorubicin because it has a major role and is used in repeated doses in the treatment of sarcomas, breast cancer, lymphomas, acute leukemia, and certain other solid tumors. Studies of left ventricular function and endomyocardial biopsies indicate that changes in cardiac dynamics occur in most patients by the time they have received 300 mg/m^2 of doxorubicin. The *multiple-ga*ted ("MUGA") radionuclide cardiac scan is the most reproducible noninvasive test for assessing toxicity. Patients should not receive a total dose in excess of 450 mg/m^2, and 1–10% of patients who receive this dose develop cardiomyopathy. Doxorubicin should not be used in patients with intrinsic cardiac disease. Prior chest or mediastinal radiotherapy increases the risk of doxorubicin heart disease at lower total doses. The appearance of a high resting pulse may herald the appearance of cardiac toxicity. Unfortunately, the toxicity may be irreversible at dosage levels above 550 mg/m^2. At lower doses (eg, 350 mg/m^2), the symptoms and signs of cardiac failure generally respond well to medical therapy and cessation of doxorubicin.

Laboratory studies suggest that cardiac toxicity may be due to a mechanism involving the formation of intracellular free radicals in cardiac muscle. Pretreatment with **dexrazoxane**, an iron chelator that decreases free radical formation, appears to protect the myocardium from anthracycline-induced injury but may also reduce the anticancer efficacy of the anthracycline. Dexrazoxane is useful for the prevention of cardiomyopathy in women with metastatic breast cancer receiving cumulative doxorubicin doses > 300 mg/m^2. **Liposomally encapsulated doxorubicin** and **daunorubicin** have been FDA approved and appear to have minimal cardiac toxicity. Their main use to date has been to treat KS, but they are also effective in the treatment of other anthracycline-sensitive cancers. The anthracycline analog idarubicin has shown efficacy against acute nonlymphocytic leukemia and breast cancer when used in combination with other agents. Idarubicin appears to have a similar potential for causing cardiotoxicity when compared with other anthracyclines, though a maximum lifetime dosage recommendation has not been made. **Epirubicin**, an anthracycline with lower cardiac toxicity than doxorubicin (but similar gastrointestinal toxicity), is approved for the treatment of breast cancer. A dose of up to 900 mg/m^2 can be tolerated without significant cardiac toxicity. There are no data comparing the effects of doxorubicin with epirubicin, which has been studied primarily in Europe and Canada.

G. CISPLATIN NEPHROTOXICITY AND NEUROTOXICITY

Cisplatin is effective in the treatment of testicular, bladder, and ovarian cancer as well as in several other types of tumor. Nausea and vomiting are common, but nephrotoxicity and neurotoxicity are more serious. Vigorous hydration with or without mannitol diuresis may substantially reduce nephrotoxicity. Renal function must be carefully monitored during cisplatin therapy, as should serum magnesium, which may fall during therapy with this agent. Ototoxicity is a potentially serious neurotoxicity that can result in deafness. Other manifestations include peripheral neuropathy of mixed sensorimotor type that may be associated with painful paresthesias. The neurotoxicity of this drug is delayed and is more common after a total dose of 300 mg/m^2. The second-generation platinum analog carboplatin has been shown to be as effective as cisplatin in ovarian cancer. Carboplatin is less nephrotoxic and causes less severe nausea or vomiting, but it does induce significant myelosuppression along with neurotoxicity. **Amifostine**, an organic thiophosphate initially developed as a radioprotective agent, is effective in preventing renal toxicity from cisplatin. It is approved to reduce cumulative renal toxicity associated with repeat administration of cisplatin in advanced ovarian cancer. In addition, amifostine may reduce chemotherapy-induced hematologic toxicity and neurotoxicity. Glutathione also appears to be a promising agent in preventing cisplatin neurotoxicity. Glutathione has been given at a dose of 1.5 g/m^2 intravenously before cisplatin administration, then at a dose of 600 mg by intramuscular injection on days 2–5. These supportive measures do not appear to reduce the therapeutic effectiveness of platinum agents.

H. INTERFERON-α TOXICITIES

Although interferon-α is generally tolerated in the standard doses listed in Table 40–4, it has significant toxicity with the higher doses required to treat CML and malignant melanoma and is more toxic in elderly patients. Even standard doses may be intolerable to some patients. Fever and chills are initial side effects but are infrequent after continued treatment. These symptoms may be ameliorated or prevented by premedication with acetaminophen and bedtime dosing. However, anorexia, fatigue, and weight loss can be cumulative and with time may become severe. These symptoms may be dose or treatment limiting. Thirty percent or more of patients are intolerant of interferon therapy even at low doses. In some patients, central nervous system symptoms develop, usually manifested as confusion or somnolence. Interferon causes a reduction in blood counts, but this is usually not clinically important and is part of the desired effect in the treatment of CML. Interferon-induced side effects are sometimes confused with the symptoms of progressive cancer but usually clear within 1–2 weeks following cessation of interferon therapy.

Brizel DM et al: Phase III randomized trial of amifostine as a radioprotector in head and neck cancer. J Clin Oncol 2000; 18:3339. [PMID: 11013273]

Chu E et al (editors): *Physicians' Cancer Chemotherapy Drug Manual 2005*. Jones & Bartlett, 2005.

Kremer LC et al: Frequency and risk factors of subclinical cardiotoxicity after anthracycline therapy in children: a systematic review. Ann Oncol 2002;13:819. [PMID: 12123328]

■ EVALUATION OF TUMOR RESPONSE

Inasmuch as cancer chemotherapy can induce clinical improvement, serious toxicity, or both, it is important to critically assess the beneficial effects of treatment in patients with advanced cancer to determine that the net effect is favorable. The most valuable signs to follow during therapy include the following.

TUMOR SIZE

Shrinkage in tumor size can be demonstrated by physical examination, chest film or other x-ray, sonography, or a procedure such as radionuclide bone scanning (breast, lung, prostate cancer). CT scanning is important for the evaluation of tumor size and location and the extent of distant spread for a wide variety of tumors and sites. MRI is now the best noninvasive means of evaluating posterior fossa brain tumors, spinal cord tumors, spinal cord compression, and pelvic disease, but CT scanning remains useful and may provide additional information. Sonography is also helpful in the evaluation of pelvic neoplasms. Gallium scanning can be useful to detect residual disease in lymphomas, but some tumors are not gallium avid, which limits the usefulness of this test. PET scanning is an emerging radiographic detection method that depends on metabolic activity for visualization. It appears to be very useful in detection of residual disease in lymphomas and in assessing the extent of disease in several solid tumors. PET combined with CT scans may allow a more accurate determination of response to therapy, differentiating between metabolically active residual tumor and scar. It may also help in evaluating resectable versus nonresectable or early metastatic disease.

A partial response (PR) is defined as a 50% or greater reduction in the original tumor mass. A complete response (CR) refers to the complete disappearance of detectable tumor. Progression is an increase of more than 25% in the size of the tumor or the appearance of any new lesions. Criteria for measuring responses of solid tumors have been established by the World Health Organization to avoid conflicts and inconsistency in measurements that influence reporting of tumor responses and to lead to more uniform reporting of outcomes of clinical trials. The RECIST criteria are based on measuring the largest single diameter of any tumor mass and include a minimum diameter for measurable lesions. These criteria are now incorporated into cancer treatment protocols.

The effectiveness of any agent or combination of agents in the treatment of cancer is determined by the response rates (combination of CR, PR, and, for some aggressive neoplasms, stable disease), response duration, and survival. Treatment efficacy for metastatic or incurable disease is often measured by event-free survival (EFS) or time to progression (TTP). The usefulness of treatment given to prevent recurrence of potentially curable neoplasms is measured by relapse-free survival or disease-free survival as well as overall survival. The goal of effective palliative therapy for advanced incurable malignancy is to increase survival and improve quality of life. Newer agents and new delivery methods have expanded the treatment options and increased their tolerability for some common cancers. Generally, response to therapy is associated with palliation, but it often happens that just stabilization of disease will have the same effect. Tumor response in this setting must be measured against toxicity, and treatment decisions should be made after available options have been discussed with the patient and family. Because patients tend to have unrealistic expectations of the benefits of palliative chemotherapy, clinician–patient communication is critical.

TUMOR MARKERS

A decrease in the quantity of a tumor product or marker substance reflects a reduced amount of tumor in the body. Examples of such markers include paraproteins (abnormal immunoglobulins) in multiple myeloma and macroglobulinemia, human chorionic gonadotropin (hCG) in choriocarcinoma and testicular cancer, prostatic acid phosphatase and PSA in prostatic cancer, urinary steroids in adrenal carcinoma and paraneoplastic Cushing's syndrome, and 5-hydroxyindoleacetic acid (5-HIAA) in carcinoid syndrome.

Tumor-secreted fetal antigens are also used to follow the course and response to treatment of cancers. These include α_1-fetoprotein (AFP) in hepatocellular carcinoma, testicular cancer, teratoembryonal carcinoma, and in occasional cases of gastric carcinoma; ovarian tumor antigen (CA 125) in ovarian cancer; and CEA in carcinomas of the colon, lung, breast, and pancreas. CA 15-3 and CA 27.29 may become important in detecting early recurrence of breast cancer but are mainly used to follow response to therapy in metastatic disease. The CA 19-9 radioimmunoassay is used to monitor response to therapy of pancreatic cancer. Monoclonal antibodies are now used for measurement of a number of tumor markers and offer the potential of delineating a number of additional markers for diagnostic purposes.

Tumor markers may play an important role in the early detection of some common tumors when combined with good physical examinations. PSA, an immunogenic glycoprotein produced solely by the prostate, is currently the only tumor marker with widespread (and controversial) use in cancer screening. PSA was initially used to indicate tumor bulk and disease progression, but it is now commonly used as a screening tool when paired with the digital rectal examination. The American Cancer Society National Prostate Cancer Detection Project is a multi-center study evaluating the use of PSA, DRE, and trans-rectal ultrasound (TRUS) in a large cohort of healthy men. In this and other studies, the combination of a monoclonal PSA greater than 4 ng/mL and an abnormal DRE was felt to produce a highly sensitive and specific method for detecting prostate cancer. A large Canadian study showed a significant reduction in death from prostate cancer in men undergoing regular screening. This study randomized more than 46,000 men aged 45–80 years to screening, with PSA (using 3 ng/mL as the upper limit of normal) and DRE followed by TRUS for abnormal test results or for a 10% increase in PSA over 12 months. There was an almost threefold advantage of screening and early treatment to reduce mortality.

Annual screening for prostate cancer with DRE and PSA beginning at age 50 years should be offered to men with a life expectancy of at least 10 years. Data obtained from the PLCO Screening Trial suggest that the initial PSA level can be used as a guide to direct frequency of testing. Thirty thousand men aged 55–74 years qualified for inclusion in the trial, and over 90% had normal PSA levels of < 4 ng/mL at baseline. A PSA < 1 ng/mL was associated with only a 1.4% chance of rise over 5 years, and a high percentage of those with a level of 1–2 ng/mL were normal over a period of 2 years. In contrast, 83% of those with an initial screening level of 3–4 ng/mL became abnormal over 5 years. The recommendations are to screen men with an initial level of < 1 ng/mL every 5 years, 1–1.9 ng/mL every 2 years, and ≥ 2 ng/mL yearly. It is estimated that this schedule could reduce PSA testing by 55%, with only a 2.6% risk of missing a positive test. As always, patients need to be involved in the decision to obtain screening PSA testing and should understand the advantages and possible consequences of testing or not testing. A major concern is that PSA testing will detect tumors that would not have resulted in mortality—small, slow-growing tumors in older men.

An abnormal PSA or DRE requires further evaluation by TRUS and possible biopsy. The role of PSA screening must be carefully evaluated for each patient and the risks of screening (unnecessary biopsies and surgeries) discussed in detail. The PSA may be elevated in benign prostatic hypertrophy and in prostatitis. Levels in benign disease are usually between 4 and 10 ng/mL; a level greater than 10 ng/mL increases the likelihood of finding cancer. In addition, 25–45% of patients with localized prostate cancer may have a normal PSA value. The increase in screening for prostate cancer over the past few years has markedly increased the reported incidence of this disease, though prostate cancer-specific

mortality has been essentially stable. (See Table 40–1.) The PSA is also used to define early relapse following local treatment with surgery or radiotherapy. One recent study indicated that pelvic radiotherapy and adjuvant androgen deprivation initiated at the time when elevation of the PSA is detected significantly improve survival and decrease the death rate due to prostate cancer. This effect was most prominent in patients with more aggressive, high-grade disease.

Tumor markers may be useful to screen populations at high risk for a specific cancer. A recent study has shown that elevated and altered profiles of AFP can serve as predictive markers for the development of hepatocellular carcinoma in patients with cirrhosis. Most tumor markers are not specific or sensitive enough to be useful as screening tools owing to their frequent elevation in benign disease and their absence in some cases of malignancy. Although screening for ovarian cancer with CA 125 is still being investigated, a rapid fall in levels to normal (versus a slow fall or plateau) following surgery or chemotherapy has favorable prognostic significance.

In general, tumor markers are used to follow response to therapy of a specific cancer. In diseases where early treatment of recurrence can influence survival (eg, testicular cancer and now prostate cancer), tumor markers may be used to screen for recurrent disease before it becomes radiographically or clinically evident.

Andriole GL et al: Prostate cancer screening in the Prostate, Lung, Colorectal and Ovarian (PLCO) Cancer Screening Trial: findings from the initial screening round of a randomized trial. J Natl Cancer Inst 2005;97:433. [PMID: 15770007]

Aus G: Individualized screening interval for prostate cancer based on prostate-specific antigen level: results of a prospective, randomized, population-based study. Arch Intern Med 2005;165:1857. [PMID: 16157829]

Bast RC et al: 2000 update of recommendations for the use of tumor markers in breast and colorectal cancer: clinical practice guidelines of the American Society of Clinical Oncology. J Clin Oncol 2001;19:1865. [PMID: 11251019]

Bast RC Jr et al: New tumor markers: CA125 and beyond. Int J Gynecol Cancer 2005;15(Suppl 3):274. [PMID: 16343244]

Duffy MJ: Evidence for the clinical use of tumour markers. Ann Clin Biochem 2004;41:370. [PMID: 15333188]

Lieberman R: Evidence-based medical perspectives: the evolving role of PSA for early detection, monitoring of treatment response, and as a surrogate end point of efficacy for interventions in men with different clinical risk states for the prevention and progression of prostate cancer. Am J Ther 2004; 11:501. [PMID: 15543092]

Molina R et al: Tumor markers in breast cancer—European Group on Tumor Markers recommendations. Tumour Biol 2005;26:281. [PMID: 16254457]

GENERAL WELL-BEING, PERFORMANCE STATUS, & SUPPORTIVE CARE

The functional status of the cancer patient at diagnosis (or at the start of treatment) is a major prognostic factor and determinant of outcome with or without tumor-directed therapy. It is therefore important to assess functional status as well as tumor burden and symptoms before deciding on possible anticancer therapy. Functional status or performance status evaluates the patient's ability to perform activities of daily living and is clearly related to tumor burden, tumor site, and the patient's underlying physical condition.

Two scales are commonly used to measure performance status. The Eastern Cooperative Oncology Group (ECOG) scale is a five-point system that is simple and easy to apply to clinical practice. The ECOG scoring system ranges from 0 to 4 as follows: 0, entirely asymptomatic; 1, symptomatic but fully ambulatory; 2, symptomatic and in bed less than 50% of the day; 3, symptomatic and in bed more than 50% of the day but not bedridden; and 4, bedridden. The Karnofsky scale ranges from 100% (asymptomatic and fully functional) through 0% (dead) in steps of 10%. For example, a Karnofsky performance status of 40% implies a patient who is disabled and requires special care and assistance. This patient would be unable to work but would be able to live at home with special assistance. These two systems are often the basis for clinical decisions despite their obvious lack of precision. They are also useful in assessing the impact of therapy and disease progression.

The measures assessing functional status described above do not adequately assess quality of life, a major goal of cancer chemotherapy. Performance status is only one component of quality of life, which is a combination of subjective and objective factors. Factors included in the assessment of general well-being include improved appetite and weight gain and decreased pain as well as improved performance status. In general, cancer patients perceive that they receive inadequate analgesia and have impairment of function because of pain. The adequate use of pain medications is hampered by their sedating side effects (see Chapter 5). New guidelines for the management of pain and long-acting opioids delivered by a transdermal system may help (eg, fentanyl patch, changed every 3 days). In addition, a short-acting oral transmucosal fentanyl preparation is available that may allow easier titration of analgesia. Tramadol is a centrally acting synthetic opioid analgesic that is available alone or in combination with acetaminophen for management of acute pain.

Sedating effects can sometimes be avoided by adding NSAIDs or antidepressants to opioid therapy. Gabapentin or the newer agent pregabalin can be a useful adjunct to management of pain characterized by nerve compression-like symptoms and can also treat insomnia if given at bedtime. In general, depression is underdiagnosed and undertreated by clinicians; treatment of depression in patients with advanced cancer has been shown to improve functional status. Occasionally, opioids may be given epidurally to relieve severe pain. As with the use of antiemetics, pain medications work better when given prophylactically on a regular schedule rather than as needed for chronic or severe pain. It is only by completely evaluating all of the factors described above that the physi-

cian is able to judge whether the net effect of chemotherapy is worthwhile palliation. See Chapter 5 for further discussions of pain management and care at the end of life.

In addition to opioids, agents that inhibit bone resorption may decrease bone pain and protect against skeletal complications (thereby improving quality of life) in patients with cancer metastatic to bone. Either the bisphosphonate pamidronate or the more potent zoledronic acid is well tolerated; the indications for zoledronic acid are broader and include both lytic and blastic bone lesions in any type of cancer. Pamidronate is given at a dosage of 90 mg intravenously over 2 hours once a month; zoledronic acid is given at a dosage of 4 mg intravenously over 15 minutes once a month. Invasive dental procedures should be avoided; osteonecrosis of the jaw is a rare complication associated with dental procedures in cancer patients on potent bisphosphonates and can be very difficult to treat. In addition to spot radiation, two radioactive agents are available for the palliation of bone pain. Strontium-89 and samarium-153 lexidronam are both given intravenously and have been shown to be effective in reducing bone pain from osteoblastic lesions. The major toxicity is hematopoietic suppression, which may limit the ability to provide other palliative therapy. The use of agents such as pamidronate or zoledronic acid, growth factors such as epoetin alfa (erythropoietin) or darbopoetin, and appetite stimulants such as megestrol acetate (given in dosages ranging from 40 mg orally four times a day up to 800 mg once a day) or dronabinol can improve the quality of life for cancer patients. Mucositis can be a problem that is particularly severe in patients with hematologic malignancies receiving inpatient high dose chemotherapy. Palifermin is a human keratinocyte growth factor (KGF) with improved protein stability produced by recombinant DNA technology in *Escherichia coli* that was recently FDA approved for mucositis prevention in patients with hematologic malignancies. Palifermin binds to the KGF receptor to stimulate proliferation, differentiation, and migration of epithelial cells. In randomized, placebo-controlled clinical trials, palifermin reduced the duration and incidence of severe mucositis as well as the use of narcotics. The safety of palifermin in patients with nonhematologic malignancies has not yet been established.

As early detection of cancer increases and cancer therapy improves, a growing area of concern is the long-term care of cancer survivors. Careful attention must be paid to psychosocial as well as physical problems resulting from therapy. Chemotherapy often leads to early menopause, depression, sexual difficulties, and osteoporosis, among other problems. Long-term cognitive problems are related to intensity and type of therapy. Clinician awareness and referral to the appropriate resources are critical for maintaining quality of life in patients who are "survivors." Patient advocacy groups can play a very important role in patient education and support. Local groups can be located through cancer resource centers or at the local branch of the American Cancer Society.

Chang HM: Pain and its management in patients with cancer. Cancer Invest 2004;22:799. [PMID: 15581060]

Hilner BE et al: American Society of Clinical Oncology 2003 update on the role of bisphosphonates and bone health issues in women with breast cancer. J Clin Oncol 2003;21:4042. [PMID: 12963702]

Kattlove H et al: Ongoing care of patients after primary treatment for their cancer. CA Cancer J Clin 2003;54:172. [PMID: 12809410]

Kelman A et al: The management of secondary osteoporosis. Best Pract Res Clin Rheumatol 2005;19:1021. [PMID: 16301195]

Lewington VJ: Bone-seeking radionuclides for therapy. Nucl Med 2005;46(Suppl 1):38S. [PMID: 15653650]

Malin JL et al: Results of the National Initiative for Cancer Care Quality: how can we improve the quality of cancer care in the United States? J Clin Oncol 2006;24:626. [PMID: 16401682]

Stasi R et al: Cancer-related fatigue: evolving concepts in evaluation and treatment. Cancer 2003;98:1786. [PMID: 14584059]

■ CANCER COMPLICATIONS: DIAGNOSIS & MANAGEMENT

ONCOLOGIC EMERGENCIES

Cancer is a chronic disease, but acute emergencies may occur as a consequence of local involvement (spinal cord compression, superior vena cava syndrome, malignant effusions, etc) or generalized systemic effects (hypercalcemia, opportunistic infections, hypercoagulability, hyperuricemia, etc). These complications may be the presenting manifestation of cancer. Two relatively common complications covered elsewhere will not be discussed here: superior vena cava syndrome (see Chapter 12) and hypercoagulability (see Chapter 13).

Brigden ML: Hematologic and oncologic emergencies. Doing the most good in the least time. Postgrad Med 2001;109:143. [PMID: 11265352]

Krimsky WS et al: Oncologic emergencies for the internist. Cleve Clin J Med 2002;69:213. [PMID: 11890211]

Merrill P: Oncologic emergencies. Lippincotts Prim Care Pract 2000;4:400. [PMID: 11261116]

1. Spinal Cord Compression

Spinal cord compression by tumor mass is manifested by back pain, progressive weakness, and sensory loss (usually in the lower extremities). Less commonly, spinal cord disease may present as chest or abdominal pain or as signs of nerve root compression due to the epidural location of the tumor. Bowel and bladder dysfunction are late findings. Spinal cord compression may occur as a complication of metastatic solid tumor, lymphoma, or myeloma. Back pain at the level of the spinal cord lesion occurs in over 80% of cases and may be aggravated by lying down, weight-bearing, sneezing, or coughing. Because back pain may precede the development of neurologic symptoms or signs, it is important to investigate this complaint thoroughly in any patient with cancer.

If neurologic deficits are present at diagnosis, they are usually irreversible, though treatment immediately after symptoms develop may result in partial recovery. Neurologic impairment can progress rapidly. Treatment of early lesions may completely avoid significant compromise. Although patients who present with paralysis may not recover function, they should still be treated for pain relief and to limit the extent of progression. In addition, patients may respond to systemic therapy depending on the specific tumor type.

The diagnosis of spinal cord compression is made by MRI scan with contrast. With this noninvasive and sensitive test, it is possible to obtain detailed views of the area in question as well as sagittal images of the entire spinal cord and vertebral canal. With the increasing availability of MRI scanning to evaluate bony lesions of the spine, true spinal cord compression has become increasingly uncommon as radiation is used earlier in the course of disease for local control. A detailed examination is important for detection and treatment of multiple lesions. Bone radiographs and bone scans are useful for detecting vertebral metastases, but they do not aid in assessing spinal cord compromise.

Emergency Treatment

Classic treatment of spinal cord compression from tumor metastases has included corticosteroids and radiation therapy to the area of compression as well as two adjacent vertebrae above and below the lesion, with surgery reserved for progression following radiation. However, a recent randomized controlled trial in patients with spinal cord compression involving no more that two vertebral levels demonstrated a marked improvement in outcome in patients treated with surgery followed by radiation versus those treated with radiation alone—so dramatic that the trial was closed early. Patients receiving combined therapy were more likely to walk and regain mobility—and actually walked for more total time, with a trend toward longer survival compared with those who received radiation without surgery. Based on this observation, surgery followed by radiation has become the standard of care for patients presenting with limited spinal cord compression from metastatic cancer.

High doses of glucocorticoids (usually dexamethasone, 10–100 mg intravenously) are administered as soon as the diagnosis is suspected or confirmed. A lower dose (eg, 4–6 mg every 6 hours intravenously or orally) is continued throughout the course of radiation therapy and tapered at or near the end of treatment. Chemotherapy is useful in treating lymphomas and multiple myeloma in conjunction with or following completion of radiation therapy.

2. Leptomeningeal Disease

Leptomeningeal disease, or carcinomatous meningitis, is an uncommon complication occurring in about 3–8% of all cancer patients, though it is being diagnosed more frequently with improved imaging studies and increased longevity in patients with advanced cancer. The most common tumors involving the meninges are cancers of the breast and lung and malignant melanoma. Patients present with varied symptoms, including sequential cranial nerve abnormalities, stroke, and hydrocephalus. The diagnosis is made by finding malignant cells on cerebrospinal fluid cytologic examination or by enhancement of the meninges on gadolinium-enhanced MRI scans. The prognosis is poor, with median survival ranging from 3 to 6 months despite treatment.

Emergency Treatment

Treatment is by radiation to symptomatic areas (usually whole brain and spinal cord) or with intrathecal chemotherapeutic agents, most commonly methotrexate and cytarabine. For this purpose, an intraventricular reservoir system is recommended. Aggressive therapy (particularly the combination of intrathecal therapy and radiation) can be complicated by necrotizing leukoencephalopathy. Patients with chemotherapy-sensitive cancers and an excellent performance status have the best chance of benefiting from therapy. Temozolomide, a newer agent approved for treatment of primary brain tumors, is being tested as a treatment for recurrent metastatic disease to the brain as well as leptomeningeal disease with some preliminary success. Temozolomide is given orally for 5 days each month; its primary side effects are nausea and cytopenias.

Kesari S et al: Leptomeningeal metastases. Neurol Clin 2003;21: 25. [PMID: 12690644]

Quinn JA et al: Neurologic emergencies in the cancer patient. Semin Oncol 2000;27:311. [PMID: 10864219]

Schiff D: Spinal cord compression. Neurol Clin 2003;21:67. [PMID: 12690645]

Schmidt MH et al: Metastatic spinal cord compression. J Natl Compr Canc Netw 2005;3:711. [PMID: 16194459]

3. Hypercalcemia

Hypercalcemia occurs in 10–20% of patients with cancer. Common causes include breast, lung, kidney, and head and neck carcinomas as well as multiple myeloma and lymphoma. Although the majority of cancers associated with hypercalcemia metastasize to the bones, approximately 20% of cases are not associated with bony lesions. The identification of a novel protein called parathyroid hormone-related protein (PTHrP) has revised some previously held views about the pathogenesis of hypercalcemia. Radioimmunoassays have identified this peptide in the serum of approximately two-thirds of cancer patients with hypercalcemia. High levels have been found in patients with hypercalcemia that was previously thought to be due solely to local osteolysis. PTHrP may become a useful tumor marker in normocalcemic patients. In addition, antibodies to PTHrP may be useful as treatment.

The symptoms and signs of hypercalcemia include nausea, vomiting, constipation, polyuria, muscular weakness and hyporeflexia, confusion, psychosis, tremor, and lethargy. Some patients may be asymptomatic. Electrocardiography often shows a shortening of the QT interval. The presence of hypercalcemia does not invariably indicate a dismal prognosis, especially in breast or prostate cancer and multiple myeloma or lymphoma. In the absence of signs or symptoms of hypercalcemia, a laboratory finding of elevated serum calcium should be rechecked to exclude the possibility of laboratory error. The most common cause of hypercalcemia is hyperparathyroidism; caution should be exercised when evaluating a mildly elevated calcium in a patient with a history of localized cancer.

Emergency Treatment

A. HYDRATION

Emergency treatment consists of aggressive intravenous hydration with 3–4 L/d of 0.9% saline followed by diuresis with 10–40 mg of intravenous furosemide. It is essential that the patient be well hydrated before beginning diuretic therapy and that hydration be maintained after diuresis is initiated. Although hydration alone is effective at slowly reducing the calcium level, it is rarely sufficient treatment and can lead to problems with fluid overload.

B. DRUG THERAPY

There are several options for the emergent treatment of hypercalcemia used in conjunction with aggressive hydration.

1. Bisphosphonates—Bisphosphonates are potent inhibitors of osteoclast bone resorption and are currently the most important and least toxic agents for the treatment of cancer-related hypercalcemia. Zoledronic acid is the most potent bisphosphonate available and has replaced pamidronate disodium as the treatment of choice for malignant hypercalcemia. A single 15-minute intravenous infusion of 4 mg with adequate hydration produces complete normalization of serum calcium in less than 3 days in 80–100% of patients—with a more rapid onset and duration of effect than pamidronate. Zoledronic acid administration can be repeated as necessary to control hypercalcemia. The most commonly reported side effects have been transient fever, myalgias, and an infusion site reaction. Zoledronic acid has also been found to reduce the incidence of new skeletal lesions and decrease pain from bone disease in cancers with metastatic lesions to bone.

2. Gallium nitrate—Gallium nitrate exerts a hypocalcemic effect by inhibiting calcium resorption from bone. For treatment of hypercalcemia, gallium nitrate is given at a dose of 200 mg/m^2/d by continuous intravenous infusion for 5 days. Gallium nitrate is superior to calcitonin both in reducing calcium levels acutely and in keeping the levels low after treatment is completed. Renal function must be carefully monitored. It may take 3–4 days to see the maximum hypocalcemic effect from gallium nitrate; the effect lasts for about 5 days so other treatment must be instituted.

3. Calcitonin—Synthetic calcitonin-salmon works immediately to inhibit bone resorption, however, the effect is short-lived. The usual dose of 4 international units/kg intramuscularly, subcutaneously, or intranasally every 12 hours may be increased to 8 international units/kg every 12 hours after 1–2 days. Calcitonin-salmon alone is not effective at lowering serum calcium levels but can be added to zoledronic acid if necessary for resistant hypercalcemia. Repeated treatment with calcitonin is usually not as effective, and tachyphylaxis usually occurs after 1–3 days of treatment.

4. Other drugs—Prednisone has not been shown to be effective as a single agent to treat hypercalcemia, though it can be used in diseases that are responsive to steroids such as multiple myeloma or lymphoma. Refractory hypercalcemia may be treated with intravenous plicamycin, 25 mcg/kg/d for 3 or 4 days. Although often effective, its effect may be short-lived, and its use is often associated with hepatic, renal, and bone marrow toxicity.

C. CHEMOTHERAPY

Patients with breast cancer may develop hypercalcemia as a "flare" associated with bone pain after initiation of estrogen or antiestrogen therapy. These patients often achieve excellent tumor response with continued therapy. Tumors may respond to chemotherapy or radiation therapy, leading to resolution of hypercalcemia. If chronic hypercalcemia persists and is refractory to chemotherapy, pamidronate and aggressive oral hydration may be tried but are unfortunately rarely effective for long. When the more potent bisphosphonates become available in oral formulations, the management of chronic hypercalcemia may improve.

Body JJ: Hypercalcemia of malignancy. Semin Nephrol 2004;24: 48. [PMID: 14730509]

Conte P et al: Bisphosphonates in the treatment of skeletal metastases. Semin Oncol 2004;31:59. [PMID: 15490377]

Hubner RA et al: Bisphosphonates' use in metastatic bone disease. Hosp Med 2005;66:414. [PMID: 16025799]

Leyland-Jones B: Treatment of cancer-related hypercalcemia: the role of gallium nitrate. Semin Oncol 2003;30:13. [PMID: 12776255]

Major P: The use of zoledronic acid, a novel, highly potent bisphosphonate, for the treatment of hypercalcemia of malignancy. Oncologist 2002;7:481. [PMID: 12490736]

4. Hyperuricemia & Acute Urate Nephropathy

Hyperuricemia can occur both as a complication of rapidly proliferating malignancies or with treatment-associated tumor lysis of hematologic malignancies

such as leukemia, lymphoma, and multiple myeloma. Neoplasms with a high nucleic acid turnover such as acute leukemia and lymphoma may present with elevated serum uric acid and associated renal insufficiency. This problem may be compounded by use of thiazide diuretics, which decreases urate excretion. If a patient presents with hyperuricemia, care must be taken to reduce the uric acid before institution of cancer therapy. Patients at risk for tumor lysis syndrome should be followed with twice-daily measurements of uric acid, phosphate, calcium, and creatinine for the first 2–3 days following initiation of chemotherapy. Rapid elevation of serum uric acid can result in acute urate nephropathy caused by uric acid crystallization in the distal tubules, collecting ducts, and renal parenchyma. A serum urate concentration above 15 mg/dL is associated with a high risk of uric acid nephropathy. Gouty arthritis is usually a problem only in patients with a history of gout.

Prophylactic therapy consists of decreasing the production and increasing the renal excretion of uric acid. Allopurinol is a competitive inhibitor of xanthine oxidase and prevents conversion of highly soluble hypoxanthine and xanthine to the relatively insoluble uric acid. Twelve to 24 hours before beginning chemotherapy, a dose of 600 mg is given, followed by 300 mg/d during the period of high risk. Higher doses (up to 900–1200 mg/d) are used when severe hyperuricemia is anticipated following chemotherapy. Patients receiving the purine antagonists mercaptopurine or azathioprine should be given only 25–35% of the calculated dose of chemotherapy if they are also receiving allopurinol, since the latter drug will potentiate both the therapeutic effects and the toxicity of these agents. Renal excretion of uric acid is enhanced by maintaining a high urinary flow and by alkalinizing the urine to prevent uric acid crystallization, which occurs at acid pH. The urine can be alkalinized with 6–8 g of oral sodium bicarbonate per day or by adding two or three ampules of sodium bicarbonate to 1 L of D_5W by infusion. Alkaline diuresis to maintain a urine pH near 7.0 is required only for prophylaxis in patients expected to have a rapid tumor response with marked hyperuricemia.

A new option for the treatment of tumor-related hyperuricemia now exists. Rasburicase is a recombinant urate oxidase enzyme that converts uric acid to allantoin, which is more easily excreted in the urine due to enhanced solubility. A randomized trial in pediatric patients demonstrated that rasburicase was more effective than allopurinol in controlling uric acid. Rasburicase is given at a dose of 0.2 mg/kg by intravenous injection once a day.

Emergency Treatment

Emergency therapy for established severe hyperuricemia consists of (1) hydration with 2–4 L of fluid per day; (2) alkalinization of the urine with 6–8 g of sodium bicarbonate per day; (3) allopurinol, 900–1200 mg/d; and (4) in severe cases, emergency hemodialysis. When severe hyperuricemia is present, adequate therapy may be impossible because of associated renal insufficiency and inadequate urinary output. Intravenous allopurinol and rasburicase are available for use in patients unable to tolerate oral allopurinol. Even if renal failure occurs and dialysis is required, renal function may return to normal after the acute tumor lysis has resolved.

Cairo MS: Prevention and treatment of hyperuricemia in hematological malignancies. Clin Lymphoma 2002;3(Suppl 1): S26. [PMID: 12521386]

Davidson MB et al: Pathophysiology, clinical consequences, and treatment of tumor lysis syndrome. Am J Med 2004;116: 546. [PMID: 15063817]

Del Toro G et al: Tumor lysis syndrome: pathophysiology, definition, and alternative treatment approaches. Clin Adv Hematol Oncol 2005;3:54. [PMID: 16166968]

Goldman SC: Rasburicase: potential role in managing tumor lysis in patients with hematological malignancies. Expert Rev Anticancer Ther 2003;3:429. [PMID: 12934655]

5. Malignant Carcinoid Syndrome

Although tumors of argentaffin cells are uncommon, they are important because they secrete a variety of vasoactive materials. These include serotonin, histamine, catecholamines, prostaglandins, and vasoactive peptides. Carcinoid syndrome is usually associated with carcinoid tumors of the small bowel metastatic to the liver and, less commonly, with primary carcinoid tumors in other sites such as the lung or stomach. These tumors tend to metastasize early but have a relatively indolent course, making control of the syndrome important. Related syndromes occur in patients with pancreatic tumors secreting vasoactive peptides, which can cause severe watery diarrhea (pancreatic cholera).

The manifestations of carcinoid syndrome include facial flushing, edema of the head and neck (especially with bronchial carcinoid), abdominal cramps and diarrhea, bronchospasm, cardiac lesions (tricuspid or pulmonary stenosis or regurgitation), telangiectasias, and increased urinary 5-HIAA. The most common symptoms are flushing and diarrhea. The diagnosis is made by finding elevated levels of 5-HIAA in a 24-hour urine collection. Patients with symptomatic carcinoid usually excrete more than 25 mg of 5-HIAA per day in the urine. Ideally, all drugs and serotonin-rich foods such as bananas should be withheld for several days before beginning the urine collection.

Emergency Treatment

Emergency therapy for patients with symptomatic bronchial carcinoid includes prednisone, 15–30 mg/d. The associated abdominal cramping and diarrhea of intestinal carcinoids can often be managed by hydration and diphenoxylate with atropine. For severe diarrhea, the H_1-histamine receptor antagonist cyproheptadine (4 mg orally three times daily) or an antiserotonin agent such as methysergide maleate (2 mg orally three times daily until 16 mg has been given) may be effective. Other useful agents include cimetidine and the phenothiazines.

The synthetic peptide somatostatin agonist, octreotide acetate, is the most effective agent for reducing symptoms due to the carcinoid syndrome in association with achieving a reduction in levels of urinary 5-HIAA. The dosage of octreotide in carcinoid syndrome is 100–600 mcg/d in two to four divided doses by subcutaneous injection. Octreotide is also effective in the treatment of symptoms related to vasoactive intestinal peptide-secreting pancreatic tumors (VIPomas), markedly reducing the watery diarrhea syndrome associated with this neoplasm. The dose of octreotide used to treat patients with VIPomas is 200–300 mcg/d in two to four divided doses.

Surgery is important in the treatment of localized carcinoid. Chemotherapy is moderately effective for patients with progressive advanced-stage disease. Active agents include fluorouracil, streptozocin, dacarbazine, cisplatin, doxorubicin, and interferon-α.

Boudreaux JP et al: Surgical treatment of advanced-stage carcinoid tumors: lessons learned. Ann Surg 2005;241:839. [PMID: 15912033]

Comaru-Schally AM et al: A clinical overview of carcinoid tumors: perspectives for improvement in treatment using peptide analogs. Int J Oncol 2005;26:301. [PMID: 15645113]

Kulke MH: Neuroendocrine tumours: clinical presentation and management of localized disease. Cancer Treat Rev 2003; 29:363. [PMID: 12972355]

■ OTHER COMPLICATIONS

MALIGNANT EFFUSIONS

The development of effusions in the pleural, pericardial, and peritoneal spaces may be the presenting sign of some tumors or may cause diagnostic and therapeutic problems in patients with advanced neoplasms. Although the cause of an effusion can be elusive in a newly diagnosed asymptomatic patient, it is rarely difficult in the patient with advanced cancer. Approximately 50% of undiagnosed effusions in patients not known to have cancer will be malignant. The differential diagnosis includes congestive heart failure, pulmonary embolism, trauma, and infections such as tuberculosis. Direct involvement of the serous surface of the involved space with tumor appears to be the most frequent initiating factor, though many other mechanisms such as obstruction of lymphatic drainage that control the flow of fluid in the pleural space may play a role.

Most patients with pleural or pericardial effusions are symptomatic at presentation with chest pain, shortness of breath, or cough. The diagnosis is made by tapping the involved space. Pericardial effusions are aspirated under fluoroscopic guidance or direct vision through a subxiphoid incision. The fluid should be heparinized and sent for cell count and differential, protein content, lactate dehydrogenase level, and cytologic study. The gross appearance of the fluid is often helpful as well. Bloody effusions are usually due to cancer but occasionally are due to pulmonary embolism, tuberculosis, or trauma. Chylous effusions may be associated with thoracic duct obstruction or may result from enlarged mediastinal lymph nodes in lymphoma. If the cytologic smear is negative on two occasions but the suspicion of tumor is still high, closed pleural biopsy may be helpful.

Treatment

The management of effusions should be appropriate to the severity of involvement. Treatment of the underlying neoplasm would be ideal but is often not effective in controlling local effusions. Treatment may result in palliation and improve short-term survival when there is substantial pulmonary or cardiac compromise. Diuretics are used as initial treatment for small to moderate-sized peritoneal effusions and as an adjunct to drainage of large effusions to minimize the possibility of reexpansion pulmonary edema that can occur after thoracentesis. Small or loculated effusions may require ultrasonographic localization, but drainage of a large pleural or peritoneal effusion can be accomplished rapidly using an intravenous catheter and phlebotomy tubing connected to a vacuum bottle. Thoracentesis alone controls fewer than 10% of effusions but may be useful in conjunction with systemic chemotherapy for sensitive tumors (eg, lymphoma, small cell lung cancer, breast cancer). Pleural effusions may occasionally be managed by closed water-seal drainage with a chest tube for 3–4 days; this procedure is usually performed in conjunction with chemosclerosis (see below). The aim of pleural drainage is to allow the pleural surfaces to come into close contact and become adherent.

Recurrent symptomatic effusions can often be controlled by drainage followed by chemosclerosis. In this procedure, a chemotherapeutic or nonchemotherapeutic agent is instilled with or without lidocaine into the involved space. The intended effect is local inflammation and sclerosis to encourage adherence of the serosal surfaces. Several drugs used in the past for this purpose have been abandoned because of severe pain or systemic toxicity, including myelosuppression. The agent in primary use at present is talc; other agents include bleomycin and the anthracenedione compound mitoxantrone.

Five randomized trials have evaluated the efficacy and safety of talc poudrage compared with a control procedure. For the 89 evaluable patients, there was an 89% success rate, with a range of 75–100%. For these reasons as well as cost considerations, talc is now the sclerosing agent of choice for malignant pleural effusions, and is the only FDA-approved substance for this purpose. The primary side effects are fever and pain, with rare acute pneumonitis.

Bleomycin is also effective at controlling pleural effusions. The major side effects of bleomycin are pain, fever, and hypersensitivity reactions. Mitoxantrone has been reported to be effective in controlling malignant pleural effusions, causing minimal fever and local pain. However, one trial evaluated the effectiveness of mitoxantrone versus chest tube alone and found no differences in response or in duration of response. The instillation of sclerosing agents may best be reserved for patients who fail pleural tube drainage alone.

Sclerosis is generally less useful for the management of malignant ascites, but success has been reported using bleomycin, mitoxantrone, doxorubicin, thiotepa, and other agents.

Before instilling the sclerosing agent, it is important that the space be drained as thoroughly as possible. For pleural effusions, a small-bore chest tube or pigtail catheter is usually placed and fluid is removed by negative suction until the drainage is under 100 mL/d and the lung has expanded. Sclerotherapy is ineffective if there is a large residual effusion. Talc is insufflated into the pleural space via a thoracoscope or instilled in a 5-g slurry in sodium chloride via a chest tube. Talc instillation through a chest tube or via a thoracoscope can be done quickly, has minimal complications, and appears highly effective. To use chemotherapeutic agents, the patient is premedicated with an opioid, and 60 units of bleomycin or 30 mg of mitoxantrone in 50–100 mL of 0.9% saline is instilled directly into the chest tube. Regardless of whether talc or chemotherapy is instilled, the chest tube is then clamped, and the patient is placed in different positions every 15 minutes for 4 hours to distribute the agent equally within the pleural space. At the end of this period, the clamp is removed and the chest tube is allowed to drain with suction. After 24 hours, the chest tube is removed from suction, and when the drainage is minimal, the tube is removed. The whole process takes 3–5 days. Occasionally, repeated doses of the sclerosing agent may be required to stop persistent reaccumulation of the effusion.

In some situations, the daily drainage of the effusion is continuously greater than 100 mL/d, making sclerosis procedures impossible. One option for these patients is the placement of an indwelling pleural drainage catheter with a valve that allows intermittent home drainage of the effusion. This catheter is also being tested in the management of malignant ascites. Use of this catheter is reserved for patients with a limited life expectancy, as the risk of infection and blockage reduces long-term effectiveness. Pleuroperitoneal shunting may have limited value in selected patients with high performance status who can participate actively in pumping the shunt for 5–10 minutes four times a day while in a supine position. For the first 24 hours after shunt placement, the catheter must be pumped frequently to drain the accumulated fluid; this is usually done in the hospital. Pleurectomy has a high complication rate but offers excellent control of effusion in carefully selected patients. For malignant pericardial effusion, a pericardial window or stripping also offers good control with a lower complication rate and may also be performed for constrictive pericarditis following radiation therapy to the chest.

Bennett R et al: Management of malignant pleural effusions. Curr Opin Pulm Med 2005;11:296. [PMID: 15928495]

Dresler CM et al: Phase III intergroup study of talc poudrage vs talc slurry sclerosis for malignant pleural effusion. Chest 2005;127:909. [PMID: 15764775]

Kolschmann S et al: Clinical efficacy and safety of thoracoscopic talc pleurodesis in malignant pleural effusions. Chest 2005; 128:1431. [PMID: 16162739]

Lee YC et al: Management of malignant pleural effusions. Respirology 2004;9:148.[PMID: 15182263]

Link KH et al: Intraperitoneal chemotherapy with mitoxantrone in malignant ascites. Surg Oncol Clin North Am 2003;12: 865. [PMID: 14567037]

Marrazzo A et al: Video-thoracoscopic surgical pleurodesis in the management of malignant pleural effusion: the importance of an early intervention. J Pain Symptom Manage 2005;30: 75. [PMID: 16043010]

Ohm C et al: Use of an indwelling pleural catheter compared with thorascopic talc pleurodesis in the management of malignant pleural effusions. Am Surg 2003;69:198. [PMID: 12678474]

INFECTIOUS COMPLICATIONS

The reader is referred also to the section on infections in the immunocompromised patient in Chapter 30.

Many patients with cancer have increased susceptibility to both bacterial and opportunistic infections. This may result from impaired host defense mechanisms (eg, Hodgkin's or non-Hodgkin's lymphoma, CLL, multiple myeloma, acute leukemia or preleukemia) or from the myelosuppressive and immunosuppressive effects of cancer chemotherapy. Impaired host defense mechanisms include defects in neutrophil function, abnormalities in antibody production, depressed cell-mediated immune function, impairment of mechanical barriers by indwelling intravenous catheters, and impairment of mucosal integrity. At least half of the infections seen in neutropenic patients are believed to be endogenous.

The bacterial organisms accounting for the majority of infections in cancer patients include Enterobacteriaceae (*Klebsiella, Enterobacter, Serratia, E coli*), *Pseudomonas, Staphylococcus,* and *Streptococcus.* Other important pathogens include *Corynebacterium, Clostridium difficile, Mycobacterium,* and *Legionella.* Patients with prolonged neutropenia or those who have undergone bone marrow transplantation are at risk for infections with fungi such as *Candida, Aspergillus,* and *Pneumocystis* and with viruses such as herpes zoster, cytomegalovirus, respiratory syncytial virus, and influenza virus. Infections with resistant bacteria, such as vancomycin-resistant *Enterococcus,* are being seen with increasing frequency. The incidence of bacteremia rises dramatically when the white count is less than 1000/mcL or when there are fewer than 200 granulocytes per microliter. In patients with neutropenia, hematologic malignancies, or following bone marrow transplantation, infection must be treated emergently

and empirically. Although fever may be due to multiple causes, including mucositis, drugs, and the malignancy itself, infection must be the first consideration and may be present even in the absence of fever, especially in patients who are receiving glucocorticoids. Negative cultures in febrile neutropenic patients do not rule out infection, and treatment should be instituted immediately without waiting for culture results to become available. If an indwelling line is present, blood cultures should be drawn from the periphery as well as through the line itself.

Prevention

Details of prevention in immunocompromised hosts are outlined in Chapter 30.

Prophylaxis of infections in high-risk or neutropenic patients can prevent the complications of sepsis. Two randomized clinical trials tested oral versus intravenous antibiotic therapy for hospitalized low-risk febrile patients with neutropenia during cancer chemotherapy. Oral ciprofloxacin plus amoxicillin and potassium clavulanate appeared as effective as intravenous ceftazidime or ceftriaxone and amikacin, indicating that for low-risk patients, outpatient therapy is feasible and safe.

In patients who are severely immunocompromised, some bacterial infections may be prevented with intravenous immune globulin. This is important in patients with chronic lymphocytic leukemia, multiple myeloma, and following bone marrow transplantation if associated immunoglobulin deficiencies are observed.

The availability of recombinant bone marrow growth factors has helped to reduce the morbidity and mortality of infections in immunocompromised hosts. G-CSF (filgrastim and pegfilgrastim) and GM-CSF (sargramostim) have been shown to be effective at reducing the duration of neutropenia and the frequency and severity of infection after myelosuppressive chemotherapy or autologous bone marrow transplantation for nonmyeloid malignancies. These growth factors improve bone marrow tolerance of escalating doses of chemotherapy, allowing higher doses to be given at shorter intervals. The availability of the long-acting pegfilgrastim (filgrastim with polyethylene glycol) now allows a single dose of myeloid growth factor for each 3-week chemotherapy dose. G-CSF and GM-CSF have been used to stimulate bone marrow stem cell production in both the circulating blood and in bone marrow cell populations collected for autologous transplantation. Administration of growth factors may improve survival after the failure of autologous or allogeneic bone marrow grafts.

Treatment

Infection management has been aimed at treatment of gram-negative bacterial sepsis, the most rapidly lethal infection. Current concepts have been broadened to include prophylaxis and prevention of the most common infections, including those caused by gram-negative, gram-positive, and fungal pathogens. Until recently, empiric therapy of fever consisted of two- or three-drug combinations, including an aminoglycoside and an antipseudomonal penicillin, with resolution of fever and bacteremia in about 70% of patients. Current results using initial monotherapy with a third-generation cephalosporin such as ceftazidime or cefepime or a combination β-lactam appear to yield similar results. Vancomycin or antifungal therapy with fluconazole, intraconazole, or voriconazole may be added on the basis of clinical suspicion, culture results, or prolonged fever in the absence of positive cultures. Multiple alternatives to the more toxic antifungal amphotericin B now exist. These include caspofungin and liposomal encapsulated formulations of amphotericin B. A recent study found that the newer antifungal agent, voriconazole, was as effective as and less toxic than amphotericin B in the empiric treatment of neutropenic patients with persistent fever. For persistent fevers or clinical deterioration, gram-negative rod coverage should be changed to an agent with a broader spectrum (eg, ciprofloxacin or imipenem). If stenotrophomonas is suspected, trimethoprim-sulfamethoxazole should be added.

Garcia-Carbonero R et al: Antibiotics and growth factors in the management of fever and neutropenia in cancer patients. Curr Opin Hematol 2002;9:215. [PMID: 11953667]

Garcia-Carbonero R et al: Granulocyte colony-stimulating factor in the treatment of high-risk febrile neutropenia: a multicenter randomized trial. J Natl Cancer Inst 2001;93:31. [PMID: 11136839]

Walsh TJ et al: Voriconazole compared with liposomal amphotericin B for empirical antifungal therapy in patients with neutropenia and persistent fever. N Engl J Med 2002;346:225. [PMID: 11807146]

Wong-Beringer A et al: Systemic antifungal therapy: new options, new challenges. Pharmacotherapy 2003;23:1441. [PMID: 14620391]

■ THE PARANEOPLASTIC SYNDROMES (Table 40–6)

The clinical manifestations of cancer are usually nonspecific—eg, anorexia, malaise, weight loss, fever—or are due to local effects of tumor growth, either in the primary site or at a distant site. The term "paraneoplasia" has been coined to denote the remote effects of malignancy that cannot be attributed either to direct invasion or metastatic lesions. These syndromes may be the first sign of a malignancy and may affect up to 15% of patients with cancer.

The paraneoplastic syndromes are of considerable clinical importance for the following reasons:

1. They may accompany relatively limited neoplastic growth and provide an early clue to the presence of certain types of cancer.

2. The course of the paraneoplastic syndrome usually parallels the course of the tumor. Therefore, effective treatment should be accompanied by resolution of the syndrome, and, conversely, recurrence of the cancer may be heralded by the return of systemic symptoms.

3. The metabolic or toxic effects of the syndrome may constitute a more urgent hazard to life than the underlying cancer (eg, hypercalcemia, hyponatremia).

The paraneoplastic syndromes are usually caused by the secretion of proteins not normally associated with a cancer's normal tissue equivalent. Clinical findings may resemble those of primary endocrine, metabolic, hematologic, or neuromuscular disorders. The mechanisms for such remote effects can be classified into three groups: (1) effects initiated by a tumor product (eg, carcinoid syndrome), (2) effects due to the destruction of normal tissues by tumor products (eg, hypercalcemia due to local secretion of cytokines), and (3) effects due to unknown mechanisms such as unidentified tumor products or circulating immune complexes stimulated by the tumor (eg, osteoarthropathy due to bronchogenic carcinoma and some neurologic syndromes). Even such nonspecific symptoms as fever and weight loss are truly paraneoplastic and are due to the production of specific factors (eg, tumor necrosis factor) by tumor cells or by normal cells in response to the tumor.

Paraneoplastic syndromes associated with ectopic hormone production are the best-characterized entities. Tumor cells secrete a hormone or prohormone that may be of a higher or lower molecular weight than hormones secreted by the more differentiated normal endocrine cell (eg, parathyroid hormone-related peptide in hypercalcemia, ACTH in Cushing's syndrome, antidiuretic hormone in the syndrome of inappropriate antidiuretic hormone [SIADH] secretion). This ectopic hormone production by cancer cells is believed to result from activation of genes in malignant cells that are normally suppressed in most somatic cells. A single syndrome such as hypercalcemia may be due to more than one of a variety of causes. Effective antitumor treatment usually results in return of the serum calcium to normal, though additional therapy may be required (see Hypercalcemia, above). In some cases, a rapid response to cytotoxic chemotherapy may briefly increase the severity of the paraneoplastic syndrome in association with tumor lysis (eg, hyponatremia with SIADH). Several neurologic paraneoplastic syndromes have been found to be caused by the production of antineuronal antibodies that circulate in the serum and spinal fluid. It is thought that the underlying tumor expresses a similar antigen, resulting in production of a cross-reactive antibody. Treatment of the underlying tumor usually results in only modest improvement of the neurologic deficit. Examples of antineuronal antibodies include the anti-Hu antibody causing sensory neuropathy or encephalitis, associated with small cell cancer of the lung; the

Table 40–6. Paraneoplastic syndromes associated with common cancers.[1]

Syndromes; Hormone Excess	Small Cell Lung Cancer	Non-Small Cell Lung Cancer	Breast Cancer	Multiple Myeloma	Gastrointestinal Cancers	Hepatocellular Cancer	Gestational Trophoblastic Disease	Lymphoma	Renal Cell Cancer	Carcinoid	Thymoma	Ovarian Cancer	Prostate Cancer	Myeloproliferative Disease	Adrenocortical Tumors	Cerebellar Hemangioblastomas
Endocrine																
Cushing's syndrome	XX	X														
SIADH	XX	X														
Hypercalcemia	XX	X	X	X				X	X			X				
Hypoglycemia					X	X										
Gonadotropin excess	XX	X			X		X		X	X						
Hyperthyroidism							X									
Neuromuscular																
Subacute cerebellar degeneration	XX	X			X			X				X				
Sensorimotor peripheral neuropathy	XX	X														
Lambert-Eaton syndrome	XX		X		X							X				
Stiff man syndrome	XX		X									X				
Dermatomyositis/polymyositis	XX		X		XX							X		X		
Skin																
Dermatomyositis	XX	X	X		XX							X		X		

(continued)

Table 40–6. Paraneoplastic syndromes associated with common cancers.[1] (continued)

Syndromes; Hormone Excess	Small Cell Lung Cancer	Non-Small Cell Lung Cancer	Breast Cancer	Multiple Myeloma	Gastro-intestinal Cancers	Hepato-cellular Cancer	Gestational Tropho-blastic Disease	Lym-phoma	Renal Cell Cancer	Carci-noid	Thy-moma	Ovarian Cancer	Prostate Cancer	Myelo-prolifer-ative Disease	Adreno-cortical Tumors	Cerebellar Heman-gioblasto-mas
Acanthosis nigricans	X	X	X		X					X			X	X		
Sweet's syndrome	X	X	X		X			XX	X			X	X	XX	X	
Hematologic																
Erythrocytosis						X			X			X			X	X
Pure red cell aplasia		X	X		X			X			XX					
Eosinophilia								XX								
Thrombocytosis	X	X	X		X	X	X	X	X	X	X	X	X	X	X	
Coagulopathy			X		X			X	X				X	X		
Fever	X	X	X		X	X	X	X	X	X	X	X	X	X	X	X
Amyloidosis				X	X			X	X						X	

[1]XX = strong association; X = reported association.
SIADH = syndrome of inappropriate antidiuretic hormone.

anti-Yo antibody causing cerebellar degeneration, associated most often with breast or gynecologic malignancies; the stiff man syndrome, associated with breast cancer; and anti-Purkinje cell antibodies causing cerebellar ataxia, associated with Hodgkin's disease as well as gynecologic, breast, and lung cancers.

Other well-described paraneoplastic syndromes include those involving the skin with or without other organ involvement (eg, dermatomyositis, Sweet's syndrome), hematologic syndromes (eg, polycythemia, thrombocytosis), and those involving the kidneys, the gastrointestinal tract, and the joints.

The most common cancer associated with paraneoplastic syndromes is small cell cancer of the lung. This is thought to be due to its neuroectodermal origin.

Bataller L et al: Paraneoplastic neurologic syndromes. Neurol Clin 2003;21:221. [PMID: 12690651]

Briemberg HR et al: Neuromuscular complications of cancer. Neurol Clin 2003;21:141. [PMID: 12690648]

Dropcho EJ: Update on paraneoplastic syndromes. Curr Opin Neurol 2005;18:331. [PMID: 15891421]

Falah M et al: Neuromuscular complications of cancer diagnosis and treatment. J Support Oncol 2005;3:271. [PMID: 16092597]

Mareska M et al: Lambert-Eaton myasthenic syndrome. Semin Neurol 2004;24:149. [PMID: 15257511]

Mazzone PJ et al: Endocrine paraneoplastic syndromes in lung cancer. Curr Opin Pulmon Med 2003;9:313. [PMID: 12806246]

Posner JB: Immunology of paraneoplastic syndromes: overview. Ann NY Acad Sci 2003;998:178. [PMID: 14592873]

Stone SP et al: Life-threatening paraneoplastic cutaneous syndromes. Clin Dermatol 2005;23:301. [PMID: 15896545]

Sutton I et al: The immunopathogenesis of paraneoplastic neurological syndromes. Clin Sci 2002;102:475. [PMID: 11980564]

■ NOVEL THERAPIES FOR CANCER TREATMENT

The use of cytotoxic drugs against cancer is limited by a number of factors, including toxicity, tumor resistance, and lack of targeted cell death. New strategies are based on increasing and improved knowledge of the molecular events responsible for disordered cellular growth and include antibodies to block receptors, small molecules that inhibit receptor tyrosine kinase-mediated cell signaling, agents directed at suppressing growth of blood vessels that feed cancer growth, vaccines to stimulate immune recognition of cancer cells, cell cycle inhibitors, and gene therapy to turn off signaling pathways or provide a missing tumor suppressor.

One way to block cellular growth is to block growth factor receptors. These receptors cross the cell membrane; the extracellular portion is the ligand-binding site, and the intracellular portion is the receptor tyrosine kinase. Activation of the receptor with ligand phosphorylates the tyrosine kinase and results in cell signaling through a complex series of events.

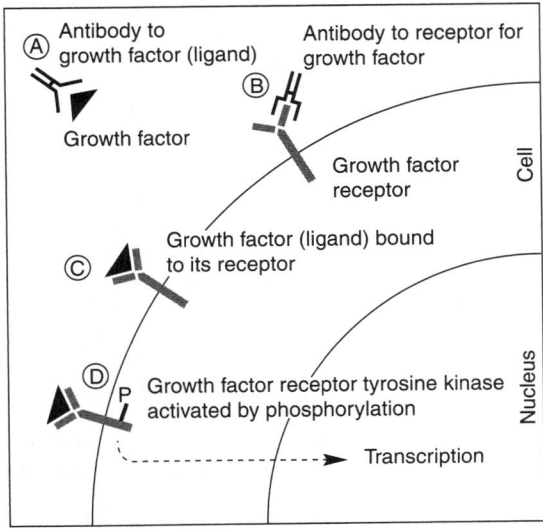

Figure 40–1. Signaling through growth factor receptors can be blocked by antibodies to either the growth factor (ligand) **(A)** (eg, antibody to vascular endothelial growth factor; bevacizumab) or to the extracellular portion of the receptor for the growth factor (tyrosine kinase receptor) **(B)** (eg, trastuzumab, cetuximab). The binding of growth factors to their receptors **(C)** leads to phosphorylation of the intracellular portion of the receptor or the receptor tyrosine kinase **(D)**. Phosphorylation activates the receptor and results in many downstream signals in the cell that activate gene transcription, and consequently proliferation. Blockade of receptor phosphorylation—eg, by erlotinib (Tarceva) or gefitinib (Iressa) (oral small molecule tyrosine kinase inhibitors)—interrupts this pathway, with the hoped-for result of blocking tumor growth.

The growth factor receptors and various methods to block their activation are presented in Figure 40–1. EGFR is expressed on most epithelial cells, and activation of the receptor has been shown to promote tumor cell growth, proliferation, and survival. Preclinical models have shown that blockade of this receptor results in tumor growth delay or regression and can potentiate radiation and chemotherapy effects. **Trastuzumab (Herceptin)** is a monoclonal antibody directed against the HER-2/*neu* receptor, one of the EGF family of receptors, and was the first growth factor receptor inhibitor approved for clinical use.

Agents that block the EGFR are directed against the HER-1 receptor. Two agents targeting the EGFR are in clinical trials with encouraging results. **Cetuximab (IMC-C225)** is a monoclonal antibody that binds to the extracellular domain of the EGFR, resulting in inhibition of the receptor tyrosine kinase and is now approved for the treatment of advanced colorectal cancer that is resistant to irinotecan and oxaliplatin. In addition to reversing chemotherapy resistance, cetuximab appears to potentiate the effect of radiation therapy in head and neck cancer. This is now being studied in the setting of an ongoing phase III clinical trial.

Erlotinib and **gefitinib** are oral small molecule tyrosine kinase inhibitors that blocks the EGFR by directly blocking phosphorylation of the intracellular receptor tyrosine kinase. One recent study evaluated the effect of erlotinib in patients with bronchoalveolar carcinoma (BAC), a form of non-small cell lung cancer. Twenty-seven percent of patients responded to this novel agent, which was quite striking given that this form of cancer does not usually respond to treatment. Erlotinib given with the chemotherapy drug gemcitabine has recently been approved for advanced pancreatic cancer, based on data from a clinical trial showing prolonged progression-free and overall survival compared with gemcitabine alone. Ongoing trials are evaluating the effect of these agents in combination with standard chemotherapy or hormonal therapy. Gefitinib and erlotinib have also been shown to inhibit the HER-2/*neu* receptor tyrosine kinase in preclinical models; trials are now evaluating the effects of these agents in advanced breast cancers in combination with trastuzumab. The primary toxicity of gefitinib and erlotinib is a potentially severe follicular rash. **Lapatanib** (GW572016) is an oral dual kinase inhibitor that blocks both HER-1 and HER-2. Early phase clinical trials suggest significant activity against multiply pretreated HER-2-positive metastatic breast cancers. Multiple trials are ongoing in this and other malignancies. Other small molecule tyrosine kinase inhibitors that block multiple receptors within the EGF family are also in clinical trials. These oral agents block receptor combinations of EGF, HER-1, and HER-4.

Angiogenesis (the growth of new blood vessels) is thought to be an essential component of the ability of tumors to invade locally and to metastasize from the primary tumor site. Tumor angiogenesis is regulated by angiogenic stimulators such as VEGF (the ligand for the VEGF receptor) and the newly described inhibitors of angiogenesis: angiostatin and endostatin. There is now intense interest in using inhibitors of angiogenesis to suppress tumor growth and metastases. This type of therapy might avoid the development of chemotherapy resistance and have less toxicity than standard cytotoxic therapy.

A recombinant humanized antibody to VEGF (anti-VEGF, rhuMAb VEGF, **bevacizumab**) was the first antiangiogenic agent to be FDA approved for the treatment of cancer. Bevacizumab is now available for the first-line treatment of metastatic colorectal cancer, where its use in combination with standard chemotherapy demonstrated improvement in survival as well as response rates. A study evaluating the use of bevacizumab in the treatment of early-stage colorectal cancer was recently closed due to unanticipated toxicity from the combination chemotherapy plus bevacizumab regimen used in that study. Although a dose-finding phase II trial in advanced refractory breast cancer with bevacizumab found an overall response rate of 11–

20%, a phase III randomized trial using bevacizumab in combination with capecitabine in the treatment of chemotherapy-resistant breast cancer showed an improvement in response rate without an improvement in time to disease progression compared with capecitabine alone. However, recent results from a second phase III study evaluating the combination of bevacizumab in combination with paclitaxel compared with paclitaxel alone as first-line therapy for metastatic breast cancer showed a doubling of response rate and time to tumor progression in the bevacizumab-treated patients, although there is no significant difference in survival as yet. It is likely that data from this trial will lead to approval of bevacizumab for the treatment of metastatic breast cancer, and bevacizumab has already been incorporated into a number of clinical trials treating early-stage disease. Treatment with bevacizumab in patients with renal cell cancer resulted in significant slowing of cancer cell growth, with a 2.5-fold prolongation in time to progression from 2 to 5 months. Tumor regression was rare, with three partial responses. The antibody was well tolerated in this trial, and a confirmatory multi-institution trial is ongoing. Side effects of bevacizumab include hypertension, proteinuria, and headache; in colorectal and ovarian cancers, rare cases of bowel dehiscence have been observed. Use of bevacizumab in the perioperative period should be avoided. Combinations of bevacizumab with the EGF inhibitor erlotinib are being tested in a variety of cancers; effectiveness has been demonstrated in resistant non-small cell lung cancer and glioblastoma multiforme, among others.

Endostatin and **angiostatin** are potent inhibitors of angiogenesis that may be promising. A preclinical study showed that transfer of cells engineered to produce angiostatin into mice inhibited the growth of both the primary tumor and lung metastases from fibrosarcoma. Trials using endostatin to treat patients with advanced malignancy began in late 1999. Two phase I dose-escalation trials using recombinant human endostatin (rHE) or angiostatin (rHA) in patients with advanced solid tumors showed few tumor responses, although both agents were associated with minimal side effects at the doses used. Tumor blood flow decreased with both agents. Phase II trials are ongoing to assess the antitumor effects of endostatin and angiostatin.

Another novel way to suppress angiogenesis is with oral small molecules that inhibit receptor tyrosine kinases and block VEGF-mediated receptor signaling. Striking responses have been seen in traditionally chemotherapy-resistant tumors, including renal cell cancer and GIST. Sunitinib inhibits multiple receptor tyrosine kinases, including platelet-derived growth factor (PDGF) as well as the VEGF receptors among others. This unique agent was recently approved for the treatment of cytokine-resistant renal cell cancer, where response rates were between 26% and 37% in two phase II trials, and of GIST, where treatment increased time to tumor progression from 6 weeks on placebo to 27 weeks with sunitinib. Sunitinib has also demonstrated efficacy in advanced breast cancer as well as other malignancies; a number of combination clinical trials are in progress. Sorafenib is another multikinase inhibitor that was recently approved to treat advanced renal cell carcinoma. Compared with placebo, treatment with sorafenib significantly prolonged progression-free survival but did not improve response rates. A third agent, AG013736, has shown significant activity in the treatment of renal cell as well as lung cancers and other solid tumors. Clinical trials with these agents in various settings and in combination with chemotherapy are ongoing. **Thalidomide** has been shown to have antiangiogenic properties as well as other antitumor effects. Responses have been seen in advanced and resistant multiple myeloma. Clinical trials using thalidomide in combination with chemotherapy in multiple myeloma, prostate cancer, and other malignancies are ongoing. **Lenalidomide** is a novel 4-aminoglutarimide oral analog of thalidomide that is more potent but does not have the neurotoxic and teratogenic effects of thalidomide. A recent study treated 148 patients with transfusion dependent anemia due to low- or intermediate-risk myelodysplasia with lenalidomide at either 10 mg daily or 10 mg for 21 days in a 28-day cycle. Two thirds (67%) of patients participating in this trial became transfusion-independent; 90% responded within 3 months of starting therapy for a median 44-week duration of response. The major side effects of this agent are bone marrow suppression, diarrhea, and a pruritic rash. Lenalidomide is now approved for the treatment of transfusion-dependent myelodysplasia with restricted distribution due to its teratogenic effects. One interesting therapy targets matrix metalloproteases that are thought to be important in the ability of cancer cells to metastasize. Unfortunately, phase III results in small cell lung cancer have been disappointing, indicating at least that the current products are not active enough for clinical use.

Immunotherapy is an exciting area of investigation of the treatment of cancer. The most extensively treated disease with immunotherapeutic modalities is malignant melanoma—for a variety of reasons, including easily identified immunogenic antigens, easy access to tumor cells, and the ability to grow these cells in vitro. Active specific immunotherapy with melanoma vaccines has been evaluated in phase II trials for advanced melanoma as well as in the adjuvant setting with encouraging results. A phase III trial testing the **allogeneic melanoma cell lysate vaccine Melacine** in 689 patients with intermediate-thickness and clinically node-negative melanoma showed no evidence of improvement in disease-free survival at a median follow-up of 5.6 years among patients receiving the vaccine. Criticisms of the trial include the lack of sentinel node biopsy and lack of ability to detect small differences in recurrence. However, when patients expressing two or more specific HLA class I antigens were evaluated separately, a highly significant benefit was seen in patients receiving adjuvant treatment with Melacine. This suggests that specific HLA types can determine the immune response and disease impact of vaccine strategies. Further studies are ongoing. Identification of a suitable target is critical for the development of any vaccine. Interesting agents in clinical trials include a vaccine directed against HPV to prevent cervical cancer and individualized vaccines directed toward the unique set of B cell tumor antigens that comprises each participating patient's low-grade lymphoma. This type of vaccine has been demonstrated to induce an immune response as well as either stable disease or actual tumor shrinkage in preliminary trials. Other interesting vaccines include monoclonal antibodies directed toward tumor products such as CA 125 for ovarian cancer, CEA for colon cancer, and HER-2/*neu* for breast cancer.

The field of cancer vaccines is growing rapidly. One type of tumor vaccine in many clinical trials capitalizes on dendritic cells, which are antigen-presenting cells that enhance the response of the immune system to foreign antigens. Dendritic cells may be loaded with a particular abnormal protein to stimulate the immune response to a specific cancer. Early clinical trials in melanoma, multiple myeloma, and other cancers are in progress. One interesting strategy is to target the dendritic cells to a known growth factor present on the tumor cell. A clinical trial using dendritic cells loaded with HER-2/*neu* for the treatment of metastatic breast cancer is evaluating the ability of this type of vaccine to stimulate a specific immune response in women with advanced breast cancer. Preliminary results indicate stability of disease, with an immune response generated in all treated patients. In one study, patients with late-stage colorectal cancer were treated with a growth factor, FLT-3 ligand, to expand the number of circulating dendritic cells in vivo. The cells were then harvested, loaded with CEA antigen, and reinfused as a cellular vaccine. Early results in all four patients include tumor response or disease stabilization. A larger trial is planned. This type of therapy might also be useful early in the disease course of an aggressive tumor. **Dendritic cell vaccines** can be used in conjunction with autologous stem cell transplantation; cells are removed at the time of stem cell harvesting, undergo in vitro stimulation, and are then returned to the patient after completion of chemotherapy and radiation therapy to eradicate bulk tumor.

Several problems with vaccine therapy exist, including the difficulty of generating an immune response in an immunosuppressed cancer patient and the fact that an immune response does not necessarily correlate with tumor response. To enhance the immune response to vaccines, growth factors such as GM-CSF are given with the treatment. A GM-CSF gene-modified vaccine is in clinical trials that produces GM-CSF locally to enhance the immune response. Early results show some evidence of tumor response in non-small cell lung cancer.

The arachidonic acid metabolic pathway is thought to be important in the pathogenesis of cancer. COX-2 is overexpressed in many solid tumors, including tumors of the lung, colon, and breast. Higher levels are thought to increase angiogenesis and decrease apoptosis. However, due to the concern regarding an increase in cardiovascular events in patients on COX-2 inhibitors, trials utilizing celecoxib in treatment or prevention of cancer have largely been halted—it will remain to be seen which studies, if any, are allowed to continue.

The goal of gene therapy for cancer is to inhibit the constitutive signals that drive tumor growth. Expanding knowledge about signal transduction has provided multiple possible attack points within this complicated multistep process involving a variety of somatic gene alterations. Although at present it is impossible to deliver therapeutic genes to every cancer cell, bystander effects or the cytotoxic effects produced by engineered cells on nonengineered cells may allow broad effects from a limited number of transduced cells. A variety of approaches are being investigated. These include enhancing the ability of the host immune system to respond to a specific tumor, sensitizing tumor cells to relatively nontoxic drugs or prodrugs, and selective replacement of altered or missing tumor suppressor genes or inactivation of oncogenes. Selective targeting of cells would allow either cell death or return of normal growth patterns without toxicity to nonneoplastic cells. **Oblimersen sodium** is an antisense oligonucleotide that inhibits the production of Bcl-2. Bcl-2 confers resistance to apoptosis, is overexpressed, and is a negative prognostic indicator in a number of malignancies. Oblimersen sodium binds to Bcl-2 messenger RNA, causing fragmentation of the protein message. Ongoing studies are evaluating the role of oblimersen sodium in combination with chemotherapy in CLL, hormone refractory prostate cancer (HRPC), metastatic malignant melanoma, and other cancers. Encouraging results have been seen in both CLL and HRPC.

One area of research in active clinical trial is replacement of the missing function of the mutated tumor suppressor gene, *p53*, or inhibition of the function of a dominant oncogene such as *ras*. One approach is to create a vaccine directed against cells with mutant *p53* to generate a cytotoxic T cell response to tumor cells expressing the p53 protein. A vaccine made from a disabled adenovirus (the vector or carrier) and the *p53* gene and injected into the arterial circulation is delivered to tumors that have metastasized to the liver with subsequent expression of the *p53* gene.

Another unique approach to tumor killing is the use of an adenovirus engineered to selectively kill tumor cells that are lacking *p53* but leave normal cells alone. This agent, ONYX-015, is also in clinical trials both with and without chemotherapy. It appears to be more effective when injected directly into tumors. Results from this and other agents are limited by a variety of problems, including difficulty in delivering the agent, identifying tumors that lack *p53*, and production of the novel agent. The Bcl-2 protein, overexpressed in many common solid tumors, is thought to be responsible for blocking apoptosis or natural cell death and appears to confer tumor cell resistance to chemotherapy and radiation therapy. Gene therapy is also being investigated in autologous stem cell transplantation for a variety of malignancies. In this setting, antitumor genes are added to cells that have been removed for transplantation following myeloablative chemotherapy. Trials are ongoing to study this form of therapy in chronic myelogenous leukemia. Multiple other trials, including the introduction of new genes that encode inhibitors of oncogene products or enhance tumor cell immunogenicity, are in progress.

Motexafin gadolinium is the first of an investigational class of drugs called **texaphyrins**, which are rationally designed small molecules that target reactive oxygen species (ROS) and selectively accumulate inside cancer cells to disrupt cellular metabolism and increase sensitivity to oxidative stress caused by radiation and chemotherapy and to induce apoptosis (programmed cell death). This novel agent is a paramagnetic compound so that its presence is visible with MRI. Motexafin is being investigated as a potential therapeutic agent in combination with radiation therapy and/or chemotherapy, monoclonal antibody therapy, and as a single agent for various types of cancers with promising early results.

Tesmilifene (BMS-217380-01) is an intracellular histamine antagonist that is being developed as a chemopotentiator for the treatment of malignant solid tumors. Results of one phase III trial in breast cancer have shown an improvement in response and survival in patients treated with the combination of tesmilifene and doxorubicin, compared with those treated with doxorubicin alone. In animal models, tesmilifene has been shown to augment the activity of numerous cytotoxic drugs including doxorubicin, cyclophosphamide, 5-fluorouracil, cisplatin, and mitoxantrone. A number of trials are ongoing in breast cancer, head and neck cancer, and prostate cancer.

TLK286 is a novel small molecule that is activated by glutathione *S*-transferase P1-1 (GST P1-1), an enzyme that is overexpressed in many human cancers and that correlates with resistance to chemotherapy. When activated, TLK286 initiates apoptosis, or programmed cell death. TLK286 has shown activity in advanced ovarian, non-small cell lung, and colorectal cancers, and a phase III trial is ongoing in ovarian cancer.

Advexin supplies p53 protein in very high concentrations in cancer tissue, selectively killing cancer cells. This interesting agent has shown activity in head and neck cancer, among other tumors. Two phase III trials are ongoing.

A number of other small molecules are in clinical trials to treat cancer. **T67** is a novel small molecule agent that binds irreversibly to B-tubulin, an anticancer drug target. T67 has shown clinical activity against hepatocellular carcinoma; early phase clinical trials are investigating its activity compared with doxorubicin. A similar agent, T607, is being tested in esophageal cancer. **Tipifarnib** (R115777) is a small molecule that blocks activation or farnesylation of the ras protein by suppressing the activity of farnesyl protein transferase. This agent has shown activity in primary brain tumors and in breast cancer. A multicenter trial comparing tipifarnib with hormonal therapy for metastatic breast cancer with hormonal therapy alone is ongoing, along with earlier studies in glioma.

Other areas of investigation include discovery of novel agents that induce apoptosis, stimulate differentiation, prevent tumor invasion or metastases, and specifically target hormone pathways that stimulate tumor growth. In addition, new antiproliferative agents with improved toxicity profiles and less cross-resistance to known agents are being evaluated or are already in use. These include novel taxanes that cross the blood–brain barrier, with encouraging results in phase II trials. Ongoing research is focusing on the identification of new growth factor receptors associated with malignant behavior that can be targeted to suppress cancer growth, such as the HER-2/*neu* receptor targeted by the antibody trastuzumab. The current proliferation of clinical trials targeting various pathways of tumor growth as well as ongoing research to identify antigenic targets should lead to a new paradigm for cancer therapy in the coming decades.

Bitton RJ: Cancer vaccines: a critical review on clinical impact. Curr Opin Mol Ther 2004;6:17. [PMID: 15011777]

Blay JY et al: Targeted cancer therapies. Bull Cancer 2005;92:E13. [PMID: 15749638]

Cao Y: Antiangiogenic cancer therapy. Semin Cancer Biol 2004;14:139. [PMID: 15018898]

Ferrari M: Cancer nanotechnology: opportunities and challenges. Nat Rev Cancer 2005;5:161. [PMID: 15738981]

Gianni L: The future of targeted therapy: combining novel agents. Oncology 2002;63:47. [PMID: 12422055]

Knox SJ et al: Clinical radioimmunotherapy. Semin Radiat Oncol 2000;10:73. [PMID: 10727597]

Mazieres J et al: Perspectives on farnesyl transferase inhibitors in cancer therapy. Cancer Lett 2004;206:159. [PMID: 15013521]

Reyno L et al: Phase III study of N,N-diethyl-2-[4-(phenylmethyl) phenoxy]ethanamine (BMS-217380-01) combined with doxorubicin versus doxorubicin alone in metastatic/recurrent breast cancer: National Cancer Institute of Canada Clinical Trials Group Study MA.19. J Clin Oncol 2004;22: 269. [PMID: 14722035]

Scappaticci FA: Mechanisms and future directions for angiogenesis-based cancer therapies. J Clin Oncol 2002;20:3906. [PMID: 12228212]

Sondak VK et al: Adjuvant immunotherapy of resected, intermediate-thickness, node-negative melanoma with an allogeneic tumor vaccine: overall results of a randomized trial of the Southwest Oncology Group. J Clin Oncol 2002;20:2058. [PMID: 11956266]

Sosman JA et al: Adjuvant immunotherapy of resected, intermediate-thickness, node-negative melanoma with an allogeneic tumor vaccine: impact of HLA class I antigen expression on outcome. J Clin Oncol 2002;20:2067. [PMID: 11956267]

Witzig TE et al: Randomized controlled trial of yttrium-90-labeled ibritumomab tiuxetan radioimmunotherapy versus rituximab immunotherapy for patients with relapsed or refractory low-grade follicular, or transformed B-cell non-Hodgkin's lymphoma. J Clin Oncol 2002;20:2453. [PMID: 12011122]

■ ALTERNATIVE & COMPLEMENTARY THERAPIES FOR CANCER TREATMENT

New areas of cancer therapy are rapidly expanding, and the next decade could bring important changes in the treatment of common malignancies. Many alternatives to traditional cancer therapy exist (one well-known example is shark cartilage, which is widely available and purported to have completely unproven antiangiogenic properties), but there is little evidence to support their efficacy or assess their potential toxicity, and at present there is no federal regulation of these products. Agents that are commonly used include green tea, echinacea, essiac tea, flaxseed, mistletoe, and coenzyme Q as well as others.

It is critical that herbs be tested with the same rigorous standards as chemotherapeutic agents in scientifically based clinical trials. Most herbal preparations are available over the counter, and no information exists regarding the interaction of these herbs with other medications. Many interactions have been described between St. John's wort and critical medications such as antiretrovirals, cyclosporine, chemotherapeutic agents, and hormonal agents, among others, that resulted in decreased drug levels due to enhanced metabolism.

A dietary supplement containing a combination of eight Chinese herbs with potent estrogenic activity, PC-SPES, has been tested in prostate cancer. All patients with hormone-sensitive and about 60% of patients with hormone-refractory prostate cancer responded with a decline in PSA; some patients also had improvement in bone scans. Toxicity was modest, including allergic reactions and thromboembolic events in about 4% of patients. Unfortunately, laboratory analysis of PC-SPES by the California Department of Health Services found significant contamination of this product with undeclared prescription drugs such as warfarin and alprazolam as well as hormonal agents. Based on these data, the manufacturer of PC-SPES and SPES voluntarily recalled the products nationwide. Investigations will need to be repeated if a noncontaminated product is produced, as the finding of hormonal agents in the herbal preparation suggests that the responses seen in published studies could have been due to contaminants instead of the herbs themselves.

Ongoing research is evaluating the effects of herbal combinations on side effects of adjuvant chemotherapy for breast cancer. The NCI is actively supporting research in the field of alternative therapies for cancer through the National Center for Complementary and Alternative Medicine (NCCAM). Additional information on alternative treatment modalities can be found in Chapter 42.

There are now many Web sites devoted to providing information on alternative cancer therapies.

NCCAM lists new research and research trials as well as an introduction to alternative medicine. There is also an extensive bibliography. This Web site may be reached at nccam.nih.gov. Additional resources can be found at the Cancer Guide Material on Alternative Medicine Web site www.cancerguide.org/alternative.html. The Center for Alternative Medicine Research in Cancer at the University of Texas-Houston Health Science Center (UT-CAM) maintains an excellent Web site with data pertaining to a wide variety of alternative medications and therapies. The site can be reached at www.nccam.nih.gov.

Buchanan DR et al: Research-design issues in cancer-symptom-management trials using complementary and alternative medicine: lessons from the National Cancer Institute Community Clinical Oncology Program experience. J Clin Oncol 2005;23:6682. [PMID: 16170176]

Deng G et al: Complementary therapies for cancer-related symptoms. J Support Oncol 2004;2:419. [PMID: 15524070]

Ernst E: The current position of complementary/alternative medicine in cancer. Eur J Cancer 2003;39:2273. [PMID: 14556917]

Ezzo J et al: Acupuncture-point stimulation for chemotherapy-induced nausea and vomiting. J Clin Oncol 2005;23:7188. [PMID: 16192603]

Kronenberg F et al: The future of complementary and alternative medicine for cancer. Cancer Invest 2005;23:420. [PMID: 16193642]

Richardson MA et al: Complementary and alternative medicine: opportunities and challenges for cancer management and research. Semin Oncol 2002;29:531. [PMID: 12516036]

Wilkinson S: Critical review of complementary therapies for prostate cancer. J Clin Oncol 2003;21:2199. [PMID: 12775747]

Genetic Disorders

41

Reed E. Pyeritz, MD, PhD

ACUTE INTERMITTENT PORPHYRIA

ESSENTIALS OF DIAGNOSIS

- Unexplained abdominal crisis, generally in young women.
- Acute peripheral or central nervous system dysfunction.
- Recurrent psychiatric illnesses.
- Hyponatremia.
- Porphobilinogen in the urine during an attack.

General Considerations

Though there are several different types of porphyrias, the one with the most serious consequences and the one that usually presents in adulthood is acute intermittent porphyria, which is inherited as an autosomal dominant, though it remains clinically silent in the majority of patients who carry the trait. Clinical illness usually develops in women. Symptoms begin in the teens or 20s, but onset can begin after menopause in rare cases. The disorder is caused by partial deficiency of porphobilinogen deaminase activity, leading to increased excretion of aminolevulinic acid and porphobilinogen in the urine. The diagnosis may be elusive if not specifically considered. The characteristic abdominal pain may be due to abnormalities in autonomic innervation in the gut. In contrast to other forms of porphyria, cutaneous photosensitivity is absent in acute intermittent porphyria. Attacks are precipitated by numerous factors, including drugs and intercurrent infections. Harmful and relatively safe drugs for use in treatment are listed in Table 41–1. Hyponatremia may be seen, due in part to inappropriate release of antidiuretic hormone, though gastrointestinal loss of sodium in some patients may be a contributing factor.

Clinical Findings

A. SYMPTOMS AND SIGNS

Patients show intermittent abdominal pain of varying severity, and in some instances it may so simulate acute abdomen as to lead to exploratory laparotomy. Because the origin of the abdominal pain is neurologic, there is an absence of fever and leukocytosis. Complete recovery between attacks is usual. Any part of the nervous system may be involved, with evidence for autonomic and peripheral neuropathy. Peripheral neuropathy may be symmetric or asymmetric and mild or profound; in the latter instance, it can even lead to quadriplegia with respiratory paralysis. Other central nervous system manifestations include seizures, psychosis, and abnormalities of the basal ganglia. Hyponatremia may further cause or exacerbate central nervous system manifestations.

B. LABORATORY FINDINGS

Often there is profound hyponatremia. The diagnosis can be confirmed by demonstrating an increased amount of porphobilinogen in the urine during an acute attack. Freshly voided urine is of normal color but may turn dark upon standing in light and air.

Most families have a different mutation in the porphobilinogen deaminase gene causing acute intermittent porphyria. Mutations can be detected and used for presymptomatic and prenatal diagnosis.

Prevention

Avoidance of factors known to precipitate attacks of acute intermittent porphyria—especially drugs (sulfonamides and barbiturates, or drugs listed in Table 41–1)—can reduce morbidity. Starvation diets also cause attacks and so must be avoided.

Treatment

Treatment with a high-carbohydrate diet diminishes the number of attacks in some patients and is a reasonable empiric gesture considering its benignity. Acute attacks may be life-threatening and require prompt diagnosis, withdrawal of the inciting agent (if possible), and treatment with analgesics and intravenous glucose and hematin. A minimum of 300 g of carbohydrate per day should be provided orally or intravenously. Electrolyte balance requires close attention. Hematin therapy is still evolving and should be undertaken with full recognition of adverse consequences, especially phlebitis and coagulopathy. The intravenous dosage is up to 4 mg/kg once or twice daily. Liver

Table 41–1. Some of the "unsafe" and "probably safe" drugs used in the treatment of acute porphyrias.

Unsafe	Probably Safe
Alcohol	Acetaminophen
Alkylating agents	β-Adrenergic blockers
Barbiturates	Amitriptyline
Carbamazepine	Aspirin
Chloroquine	Atropine
Chlorpropamide	Chloral hydrate
Clonidine	Chlordiazepoxide
Dapsone	Corticosteroids
Ergots	Diazepam
Erythromycin	Digoxin
Estrogens, synthetic	Diphenhydramine
Food additives	Guanethidine
Glutethimide	Hyoscine
Griseofulvin	Ibuprofen
Hydralazine	Imipramine
Ketamine	Insulin
Meprobamate	Lithium
Methyldopa	Naproxen
Metoclopramide	Nitrofurantoin
Nortriptyline	Opioid analgesics
Pentazocine	Penicillamine
Phenytoin	Penicillin and derivatives
Progestins	Phenothiazines
Pyrazinamide	Procaine
Rifampin	Streptomycin
Spironolactone	Succinylcholine
Succinimides	Tetracycline
Sulfonamides	Thiouracil
Theophylline	
Tolazamide	
Tolbutamide	
Valproic acid	

transplantation may provide an option for patients with disease poorly controlled by medical therapy.

Desnick RJ et al: Inherited porphyrias. In: *Emery and Rimoin's Principles and Practice of Medical Genetics*, 5th ed. Rimoin DL et al (editors). Churchill Livingstone, 2006.

Foran SE et al: Guide to porphyrias. A historical and clinical perspective. Am J Clin Pathol 2003;119(Suppl):S86. [PMID: 12951846]

Kauppinen R: Molecular diagnostics of acute intermittent porphyria. Expert Rev Mol Diagn 2004;4:243. [PMID: 14995910]

Norman RA: Past and future: porphyria and porphyrins. Skinmed 2005;4:287. [PMID: 16282750]

Soonawalla ZF et al: Liver transplantation as a cure for acute intermittent porphyria. Lancet 2004;363:705. [PMID: 15001330]

ALKAPTONURIA

Alkaptonuria is caused by a recessively inherited deficiency of the enzyme homogentisic acid oxidase. This acid derives from metabolism of both phenylalanine and tyrosine and is present in large amounts in the urine throughout the patient's life. An oxidation product accumulates slowly in cartilage throughout the body, leading to degenerative joint disease of the spine and peripheral joints. Indeed, examination of patients in the third and fourth decades shows a slight darkish blue color below the skin in areas overlying cartilage, such as in the ears, a phenomenon called "ochronosis." In some patients, a more severe hyperpigmentation can be seen in the sclera, conjunctiva, and cornea. Accumulation of metabolites in heart valves can lead to aortic or mitral stenosis. A predisposition to coronary artery disease may also be present. Although the syndrome causes considerable morbidity, life expectancy is reduced only modestly. Symptoms are more often attributable to spondylitis with back pain, leading to a clinical picture difficult to distinguish from that of ankylosing spondylitis, though on radiographic assessment the sacroiliac joints are not fused in alkaptonuria.

The diagnosis is established by demonstrating homogentisic acid in the urine, which turns black spontaneously on exposure to the air; this reaction is particularly noteworthy if the urine is alkaline or when alkali is added to a specimen. Molecular analysis of the homogentisic acid oxidase gene, recently mapped to chromosome 3, is available but not necessary for diagnosis.

Treatment of the arthritis is similar to that for other arthropathies. Though in theory rigid dietary restriction might reduce accumulation of the pigment, this has not proved to be of practical benefit.

Keller JM et al: New developments in ochronosis: review of the literature. Rheumatol Int 2005;25:81. [PMID: 15322814]

La Du BN: Alkaptonuria. In: *The Metabolic and Molecular Bases of Inherited Disease*, 8th ed. Scriver CR et al (editors). McGraw-Hill, 2001.

Mannoni A et al: Alkaptonuria, ochronosis, and ochronotic arthropathy. Semin Arthritis Rheum 2004;33:239. [PMID: 14978662]

Phornphutkul C et al: Natural history of alkaptonuria. N Engl J Med 2002;347:2111. [PMID: 12501223]

DOWN SYNDROME

Down syndrome is usually diagnosed at birth on the basis of the typical facial features, hypotonia, and single palmar crease. Several serious problems that may be evident at birth or may develop early in childhood include duodenal atresia, congenital heart disease (especially atrioventricular canal defects), and leukemia. The intestinal and cardiac anomalies usually respond to surgery, and the leukemia generally responds to conservative management. Intelligence varies across a wide spectrum. Many people with Down syndrome do well in sheltered workshops and group homes, but few achieve full independence in adulthood. An Alzheimer-like dementia usually becomes evident in the fourth or fifth decade and, for those who survive childhood, accounts for a reduced life expectancy. Studies addressing the risk and severity of dementia in relation to the apolipoprotein E genotype have had conflicting results. Cytogenetic analysis should always be performed—even though most patients will have simple trisomy for chromosome 21—to detect unbalanced translocations; such patients may have a parent with a balanced translocation, and there will be a substantial recurrence risk of Down syndrome in future offspring.

The presence of a fetus with Down syndrome can be detected in many pregnancies in the early second trimester through screening maternal serum for α-fetoprotein and certain hormones ("multiple marker screening") and by detecting increased nuchal thickness on fetal ultrasound.

The risk of bearing a child with Down syndrome increases exponentially with the age of the mother at conception and begins a marked rise after age 35. By age 45 years, a mother has one chance in 40 of having an affected child. The risk of other conditions associated with trisomy also increases, because of the increased predisposition of older oocytes to nondisjunction during meiosis. There is little risk of trisomy associated with increased paternal age. However, older men do have an increased risk of fathering a child with a new autosomal dominant condition. But because there are so many distinct conditions, the chance of fathering an offspring with any given one is extremely small.

Andriolo RB et al: Aerobic exercise training programmes for improving physical and psychosocial health in adults with Down syndrome. Cochrane Database Syst Rev 2005;(5): CD005176. [PMID: 16034968]

Baliff JP et al: New developments in prenatal screening for Down syndrome. Am J Clin Pathol 2003;120(Suppl):S14. [PMID: 15298140]

Galley R: Medical management of the adult patient with Down syndrome. JAAPA 2005;18:45. [PMID: 15859488]

Roizen NJ: Down's syndrome. Lancet 2003;12:1281. [PMID: 12699967]

Tolmie JL: Down syndrome and other autosomal trisomies. In: *Emery and Rimoin's Principles and Practice of Medical Genetics*, 5th ed. Rimoin DL et al (editors). Churchill Livingstone, 2006.

Tyler C et al: Down syndrome, Turner syndrome, and Klinefelter syndrome: primary care throughout the life span. Prim Care 2004;31:627. [PMID: 15331252]

FRAGILE X MENTAL RETARDATION

This X-linked condition accounts for more cases of mental retardation in males than any condition except Down syndrome; about one in 4000 to 6000 males is affected; the condition also affects intellectual function in females about 50% less frequently than in males. The first marker for this condition was a small gap, or fragile site, evident near the tip of the long arm of the X chromosome. Subsequently, the condition was found to be due to expansion of a trinucleotide repeat (CGG) near a gene called *FMR1*. All individuals have some CGG repeats in this location, but as the number increases beyond 52, the chances of further expansion during spermatogenesis or oogenesis increase. Being born with one *FMR1* allele with 200 or more repeats results in mental retardation in most men and in about 60% of women. The more repeats, the greater

the likelihood that further expansion will occur during gametogenesis; this results in **anticipation**, in which the disorder can worsen from one generation to the next. Affected (heterozygous) women show no physical signs other than early menopause, but they may have learning difficulties or frank retardation. Affected males show macroorchidism (enlarged testes) after puberty, large ears and a prominent jaw, a high-pitched voice, and mental retardation. Some show evidence of a mild connective tissue defect, with joint hypermobility and mitral valve prolapse.

Men who are not retarded but carry an increased number of CGG repeats in the *FMR1* locus (premutation carriers) are at increased risk for developing intention tremor, ataxia, or both. Likewise, women who are premutation carriers (55–200 CGG repeats) are at increased risk for premature ovarian failure and mild cognitive or behavioral abnormalities. Male and female premutation carriers are at risk for developing tremor and ataxia beyond middle age. Because of the relatively high prevalence of premutation carriers in the general population, older people in whom any of these problems develop should undergo testing of the *FMR1* locus.

DNA diagnosis for the number of repeats has supplanted cytogenetic analysis for both clinical and prenatal diagnosis. This should be done on any male or female who has unexplained mental retardation.

Hagerman PJ et al: The fragile-X premutation: a maturing perspective. Am J Hum Genet 2004;74:805. [PMID: 15052536]

Hatton DD et al: Problem behavior in boys with fragile X syndrome. Am J Med Genet 2002;108:105. [PMID: 11857559]

Jacquemont S et al: Penetrance of the fragile X-associated tremor/ataxia syndrome in a premutation carrier population. JAMA 2004;291:460. [PMID: 14747503]

Kenneson A et al: The female and the fragile X reviewed. Semin Reprod Med 2001;19:159. [PMID: 11480913]

Sutherland GR et al: Fragile X syndrome and other causes of X-linked mental handicap. In: *Emery and Rimoin's Principles and Practice of Medical Genetics*, 5th ed. Rimoin DL et al (editors). Churchill Livingstone, 2006.

Terracciano A et al: Fragile X syndrome. Am J Med Genet C Semin Med Genet 2005;137:32. [PMID: 16010677]

GAUCHER DISEASE

Gaucher disease has an autosomal recessive pattern of inheritance. A deficiency of β-glucocerebrosidase causes an accumulation of sphingolipid within phagocytic cells throughout the body. Anemia and thrombocytopenia are common and may be symptomatic; both are due primarily to hypersplenism, but marrow infiltration with Gaucher cells may be a contributing factor. Cortical erosions of bones, especially the vertebrae and femur, are due to local infarctions, but the mechanism is unclear. Episodes of bone pain (termed "crises") are reminiscent of those in sickle cell disease. A hip fracture in a patient with a palpable spleen—especially in a Jewish person of Eastern European origin—suggests the possibility of Gaucher disease. Bone marrow aspirates reveal typical Gaucher cells, which have an eccentric nucleus and periodic acid–Schiff (PAS)-positive inclusions, along with wrinkled cytoplasm and inclusion bodies of a fibrillar type. In addition, the serum acid phosphatase is elevated. Definitive diagnosis requires the demonstration of deficient glucocerebrosidase activity in leukocytes.

Two uncommon forms of Gaucher disease, called type II and type III, involve neurologic accumulation of sphingolipid and a variety of neurologic problems. Type II is of infantile onset and has a poor prognosis.

Over 200 mutations have been found to cause Gaucher disease, and some are highly predictive of the neuronopathic forms. Thus, mutation detection, especially in a young person, is of potential value. Only four mutations in glucocerebrosidase account for more than 90% of the disease among Ashkenazic Jews, in whom the carrier frequency is 1:15.

Heterozygotes for Gaucher disease may be at increased risk for developing Parkinson disease.

For many years, treatment was supportive and included splenectomy for thrombocytopenia secondary to platelet sequestration. A recombinant form of the enzyme glucocerebrosidase (imiglucerase) for intravenous administration on a regular basis now permits a reduction in total body stores of glycolipid and improvement in orthopedic and hematologic manifestations. Unfortunately, the neurologic manifestations of types II and III have not improved with enzyme replacement therapy. The major drawback is the exceptional cost of imiglucerase, which can exceed $350,000 per year for a severely affected patient. Administration of less enzyme (30 units/kg per month) is effective for most adults and reduces the cost to about $100,000–150,000 annually.

Aharon-Peretz J et al: Mutations in the glucocerebrosidase gene and Parkinson's disease in Ashkenazi Jews. N Engl J Med 2004;351:1972. [PMID: 15525722]

Beutler E et al: Gaucher disease. In: *The Metabolic Basis of Inherited Disease*, 8th ed. Scriver CR et al (editors). McGraw-Hill, 2001.

Charrow J et al: The Gaucher registry: demographics and disease characteristics of 1698 patients with Gaucher disease. Arch Intern Med 2000;160:2835. [PMID: 11025794]

Germain DP: Gaucher's disease: a paradigm for interventional genetics. Clin Genet 2004;65:77. [PMID: 14984463]

Hollak CE et al: Clinically relevant therapeutic endpoints in type I Gaucher disease. J Inherit Metab Dis 2001;24(Suppl 2): 97. [PMID: 11758685]

Wenstrup RJ et al: Skeletal aspects of Gaucher disease: a review. Br J Radiol 2002;75(Suppl 1)A2. [PMID: 12036828]

DISORDERS OF HOMOCYSTEINE METABOLISM

Homocystinuria in its classic form is caused by cystathionine β-synthase deficiency and exhibits an autosomal recessive pattern of inheritance. This results in extreme elevations of plasma and urinary homocystine levels, a basis for diagnosis of this disorder. Homocystinuria is similar in certain superficial aspects to Marfan's syndrome, since patients may show a similar body habitus and ectopia lentis is almost always present. However, mental retardation is often present, and the cardiovascular events are those of repeated venous and arterial thromboses whose precise cause remains obscure. Life expectancy is reduced, especially in untreated and pyridoxine-unresponsive patients; myocardial infarction, stroke, and pulmonary embolism are the most common causes of death. This condition is diagnosed in some states by newborn screening for hypermethioninemia; however, pyridoxine-responsive infants may not be detected. The diagnosis should be suspected in patients in the second and third decades of life who show evidence of arterial or venous thromboses and have no other risk factors. Although many mutations have been identified in the cystathionine β-synthase gene, amino acid analysis of plasma remains the most appropriate diagnostic test. Patients should be studied after they have been off folate or pyridoxine supplementation for at least 1 week. The plasma should be separated promptly from the fresh venous blood specimen.

About 50% of patients have a form of cystathionine β-synthase deficiency that improves biochemically and clinically through pharmacologic doses of pyridoxine and folate. For these patients, treatment from infancy can prevent retardation and the other clinical problems. Patients who are pyridoxine nonresponders must be treated with a dietary reduction in methionine and supplementation of cysteine, also from infancy. The vitamin betaine is also useful in reducing plasma methionine levels by facilitating a metabolic pathway that bypasses the defective enzyme. Patients who have suffered venous thrombosis receive anticoagulation therapy, but there are no studies to support prophylactic use of warfarin or antiplatelet agents.

Over the past 5 years, considerable evidence has accumulated to support the 20-year-old observation that patients with clinical and angiographic evidence of coronary artery disease tend to have higher levels of plasma homocysteine than controls without coronary artery disease. The relationship has been extended to cerebrovascular and peripheral vascular diseases. Although this effect was initially thought to be due at least in part to heterozygotes for cystathionine β-synthase deficiency (see above), there is little evidence for this. Rather, the major factor leading to hyperhomocysteinemia is folate deficiency. Pyridoxine (vitamin B_6) and vitamin B_{12} are also important in the metabolism of methionine, and deficiency of any of these vitamins can lead to accumulation of homocysteine. A number of genes influence utilization of these vitamins and can predispose to deficiency. For example, having one—and especially two—copies of an allele that causes thermolability of methylene tetrahydrofolate reductase predisposes patients to elevated fasting homocysteine levels. However, both nutritional and most genetic deficiencies of these vitamins can be corrected by dietary supplementation of folic acid and, if serum levels are low, vitamins B_6 and B_{12}. In the United States, cereal grains are now fortified with folic acid. Studies are ongoing to determine the long-term utility of routine vitamin supplementation in people at risk for arterial occlusive disease, but many workers in this field recommend, at a minimum, taking 1 mg of folic acid per day. Because patients with end-stage renal disease tend to have marked hyperhomocysteinemia and low serum folate, 5 mg of folic acid per day seems warranted.

Relatively few laboratories currently provide highly reliable assays for homocysteine. Processing of the specimen is crucial to obtain accurate results. The plasma must be separated within 30 minutes; otherwise, blood cells release the amino acid and the measurement will then be artificially elevated.

Carmel R et al (editors): *Homocysteine in Health and Disease.* Cambridge University Press, 2001.

Kelly PJ et al: Stroke in young patients with hyperhomocysteinemia due to cystathionine beta-synthase deficiency. Neurology 2003;28:275. [PMID: 12552044]

Knekt P et al: Hyperhomocystinemia: a risk factor or a consequence of coronary heart disease? Arch Intern Med 2001; 161:1589. [PMID: 11434790]

Mudd H et al: Disorders of transsulfuration. In: *The Metabolic and Molecular Bases of Inherited Disease*, 8th ed. Scriver CR et al (editors). McGraw-Hill, 2001.

Refsum H et al: Birth prevalence of homocystinuria. J Pediatr 2004; 144:830. [PMID: 15192637]

Schnyder G et al: Decreased rate of coronary restenosis after lowering of plasma homocysteine levels. N Engl J Med 2001; 345:1593. [PMID: 11757505]

Soinio M et al: Elevated plasma homocysteine level is an independent predictor of coronary heart disease events in patients with type 2 diabetes mellitus. Ann Intern Med 2004;140: 94. [PMID: 14734331]

Undas A et al: Homocysteine and thrombosis: from basic science to clinical evidence. Thromb Haemost 2005;94:907. [PMID: 16363230]

Yap S et al: Vascular outcome in patients with homocystinuria due to cystathionine beta-synthase deficiency treated chronically: a multicenter observational study. Arterioscler Thromb Vasc Biol 2001;21:2080. [PMID: 11742888]

KLINEFELTER SYNDROME

Boys with an extra X chromosome are normal in appearance before puberty; thereafter, they have disproportionately long legs and arms, a female escutcheon, gynecomastia, and small testes. Infertility is due to azoospermia; the seminiferous tubules are hyalinized. The diagnosis is often not made until a couple is evaluated for inability to conceive. Mental retardation is somewhat more common than in the general population. Many men with Klinefelter syndrome have learning problems. However, their intelligence usually tests within the broad range of normal. As adults, detailed psychometric testing may reveal a deficiency in executive skills. The risk of breast cancer is much higher in men with Klinefelter syndrome than in 46,XY men, as is the risk of diabetes mellitus.

Treatment with testosterone after puberty is advisable but will not restore fertility. However, men with Klinefelter syndrome have had mature sperm aspirated

from their testes and injected into oocytes, resulting in fertilization. After the blastocysts were implanted into the uterus of a partner, "natural" children resulted. However, men with Klinefelter syndrome do have an increased risk for aneuploidy in sperm, and chromosome analysis of a blastocyst before implantation should be considered.

Allanson J et al: Sex chromosome abnormalities. In: *Emery and Rimoin's Principles and Practice of Medical Genetics*, 5th ed. Rimoin DL et al (editors). Churchill Livingstone, 2006.

Ferlin A et al: Chromosome abnormalities in sperm of individuals with constitutional sex chromosomal abnormalities. Cytogenet Genome Res 2005;111:310. [PMID: 16192710]

Lanfranco F et al: Klinefelter's syndrome. Lancet 2004;364:273. [PMID: 15262106]

Swerdlow AJ et al: Mortality and cancer incidence in persons with numerical sex chromosome abnormalities. Ann Hum Genet 2001;65:177. [PMID: 11427177]

Temple CM et al: Executive skills in Klinefelter's syndrome. Neuropsychologia 2003;41:1547. [PMID: 12849773]

Wattendorf DJ et al: Klinefelter syndrome. Am Fam Physician 2005;72:2259. [PMID: 16342850]

MARFAN SYNDROME

ESSENTIALS OF DIAGNOSIS

- *Disproportionately tall stature, thoracic deformity, and joint laxity or contractures.*
- *Ectopia lentis and myopia.*
- *Aortic dilation and dissection.*
- *Mitral valve prolapse.*

General Considerations

Marfan syndrome, a systemic connective tissue disease, has an autosomal dominant pattern of inheritance. It is characterized by abnormalities of the skeletal system, ocular system, and cardiovascular system. Spontaneous pneumothorax, dural ectasia, and striae atrophicae can also occur. Of most concern is disease of the ascending aorta, which is associated with a dilated aortic root. Histology of the aorta shows diffuse medial abnormalities. Aortic and mitral valve leaflets are also abnormal and mitral regurgitation may be present as well, often with elongated chordae tendineae, which on occasion may rupture.

Clinical Findings

A. SYMPTOMS AND SIGNS

Affected patients are typically tall, with particularly long arms, legs, and digits (arachnodactyly). However, there can be wide variability in the clinical presentation. Commonly, joint dislocations and pectus excavatum are found. Ectopia lentis may lead to severe myopia and retinal detachment. Mitral valve prolapse is seen in about 85% of patients. Aortic root dilation with aortic regurgitation or dissection with rupture can occur. To diagnose Marfan syndrome, people with an affected relative need features in at least two systems. People with no family history need features in the skeletal system, two other systems, and one of the major criteria of ectopia lentis, dilation of the aortic root, or aortic dissection. Patients with homocystinuria due to cystathionine synthase deficiency also have dislocated lenses; tall, disproportionate stature; and thoracic deformity. They tend to have below normal intelligence, stiff joints, and a predisposition to arterial and venous occlusive disease. Males with Klinefelter syndrome do not show the typical ocular or cardiovascular features of Marfan syndrome and are generally sporadic occurrences in the family.

B. LABORATORY FINDINGS

Mutations in the fibrillin gene on chromosome 15 cause Marfan syndrome. Nonetheless, no simple laboratory test is available to support the diagnosis in questionable cases because related conditions may also be due to defects in fibrillin. The pathogenesis of Marfan syndrome involves aberrant regulation of transforming growth factor (TGF)b activity. Mutations in either of two receptors for TGFb can cause conditions that resemble Marfan syndrome in terms of aortic aneurysm and dissection and autosomal dominant inheritance.

Prevention

There is prenatal and presymptomatic diagnosis for patients in whom the molecular defect in fibrillin has been found and for large enough families in whom linkage analysis using polymorphic markers around the fibrillin gene can be performed.

Treatment

Children with Marfan syndrome require regular ophthalmologic surveillance to correct visual acuity and thus prevent amblyopia, and annual orthopedic consultation for diagnosis of scoliosis at an early enough stage so that bracing might delay progression. Patients of all ages require echocardiography at least annually to monitor aortic diameter and mitral valve function. All patients should use standard endocarditis prophylaxis. Chronic β-adrenergic blockade, titrated to individual tolerance but enough to produce a negative inotropic effect (atenolol, 1–2 mg/kg), retards the rate of aortic dilation. Restriction from vigorous physical exertion protects from aortic dissection. Prophylactic replacement of the aortic root with a composite graft when the diameter reaches 50–55 mm (normal: < 40 mm) prolongs life. A procedure to reimplant the patient's native aortic valve and replace just the aneurysmal sinuses of Valsalva shows promise and also avoids the need for lifelong anticoagulation.

Prognosis

People with Marfan syndrome who are untreated commonly die in the fourth or fifth decade from aortic dissection or congestive heart failure secondary to aortic regurgitation. However, because of earlier diagnosis, lifestyle modifications, β-adrenergic blockade, and prophylactic aortic surgery, life expectancy has increased by several decades in the past 25 years.

de Oliveira NC et al: Results of surgery for aortic root aneurysm in patients with Marfan syndrome. J Thorac Cardiovasc Surg 2003;125:789. [PMID: 12698141]

Dietz HC et al: Marfan syndrome and related disorders. In: *The Metabolic and Molecular Bases of Inherited Disease*, 8th ed. Scriver CR et al (editors). McGraw-Hill, 2001.

Erkula G et al: Growth and maturation in Marfan syndrome. Am J Med Genet 2002;109:100. [PMID: 11977157]

Judge DP et al: Marfan's syndrome. Lancet 2005;366:1965. [PMID: 16325700]

Miller DC: Valve-sparing aortic root replacement in patients with Marfan syndrome. J Thorac Cardiovasc Surg 2003;125:773. [PMID: 12698136]

Pyeritz RE: The Marfan syndrome. Annu Rev Med 2000;51:481. [PMID: 10774478]

Complementary & Alternative Medicine

42

Ellen F. Hughes, MD, PhD, Bradly P. Jacobs, MD, MPH, & Brian M. Berman, MD

The use of complementary and alternative medicine (CAM) has become common in the United States. To maintain effective clinician-patient communication and ensure responsible clinical practice, it is important that clinicians learn the theory, practice, and scientific evidence associated with these therapies. This chapter provides an overview of four alternative medicine therapies: herbal medicine, nonherbal dietary supplements, acupuncture, and homeopathy.

Background

CAM is defined by the National Institutes of Health (NIH) as a group of diverse health care systems, practices, and products that are not presently considered to be part of conventional medicine. CAM therapies may be used alone as an alternative to conventional therapies or in addition to conventional, mainstream medicine to treat conditions and promote well being.

CAM modalities have been classified by NIH into five major categories:

1. **Biologically based practices** use substances found in nature, such as herbs, special diets, or vitamins (in doses outside those used in conventional medicine).
2. **Energy medicine** involves the use of energy fields, such as magnetic fields or biofields (energy fields that some believe surround and penetrate the human body). Examples include Reiki, external qigong, and therapeutic touch.
3. **Manipulative and body-based practices** use manipulation or movement of one or more body parts (massage, chiropractic, Feldenkrais method and other "body work" systems).
4. **Mind-body medicine** uses a variety of techniques designed to enhance the mind's ability to affect bodily function and symptoms, such as meditation, prayer, art and music healing, and imagery.
5. **Whole medical systems** are built on complete systems of theory and practice that have evolved apart from—and often earlier than—the conventional medical approach used in the United States. Systems such as traditional Oriental medicine, acupuncture, homeopathy, naturopathy, Ayurveda,

and Tibetan medicine often use one or more of the methods listed above.

The Centers for Disease Control and Prevention conducted the National Health Interview Survey (NHIS) in 2002; 31,000 American adults from diverse populations were asked about their use of CAM. Thirty-eight percent reported using some form of CAM in the previous 12 months. When prayer (used specifically for health reasons) and megavitamins were included in the definition of CAM, this percentage increased to 62%.

The most commonly reported CAM therapy was prayer. When prayer was excluded from the definition of CAM, biologically based therapies, such as herbs and other dietary supplements, were most popular (22%).

The most common conditions for which adults used CAM were similar to those seen in most primary care offices: musculoskeletal complaints, such as back, neck, and joint pain; colds; anxiety or depression; gastrointestinal disorders; and sleeping problems. Most of the respondents in this survey used CAM on their own, with only 12% seeking care from a licensed CAM practitioner.

Most people who use CAM combine it with conventional medicine because they perceive the combination to be superior to either alone. Half of the NHIS respondents also thought that CAM would be interesting to try. One quarter sought CAM because a conventional medical professional suggested they try it and 13% because they felt that conventional medicine was too expensive. Dissatisfaction with conventional medicine has not previously been found to predict greater CAM use, but more than 25% of US adults said they used CAM because they believed conventional medicine could not help them. No questions on health care spending were asked during NHIS interviews, but a smaller national phone survey conducted in 1997 estimated that the US public paid $36 billion on CAM therapies, much of it out-of-pocket.

In January 2005, the Institute of Medicine of the National Academies released a report on the use of CAM in the United States. They recommended "health profession schools incorporate sufficient information about complementary and alternative medicine (CAM) into the standard curriculum at all levels to enable licensed professionals to competently advise their patients about CAM." Indeed, despite the growing numbers of patients seeking CAM, less than 40% of alternative therapies used are disclosed to physicians. A lack of communication may be dangerous because some CAM therapies can interact adversely with conventional treatments.

Funding for biomedical research in this field has increased dramatically. The NIH established the Office of Alternative Medicine in 1992 with an annual budget of $2 million; in 1998, its role was expanded as the National Center for Complementary and Alternative Medicine (NCCAM). NCCAM's budget for fiscal year 2005 is $123 million. Although some CAM modalities are not easily evaluated using randomized control trial methodology, the 2005 Institute of Medicine report recommends that conventional and CAM treatments both be held to similar standards of safety and efficacy.

Astin JA: Why patients use alternative medicine: results of a national study. JAMA 1998;279:1548. [PMID: 9605899]

Barnes PM et al: Complementary and alternative medicine use among adults: United States, 2002. Adv Data 2004;(343):1. [PMID: 15188733]

Eisenberg DM et al: Perceptions about complementary therapies relative to conventional therapies among adults who use both: results from a national survey. Ann Intern Med 2001; 135:344. [PMID: 11529698]

Eisenberg DM et al: Trends in alternative medicine use in the United States, 1990–1997: results of a follow-up national survey. JAMA 1998;280:1569. [PMID: 9820257]

Institute of Medicine. Complementary and Alternative Medicine in the United States 2005.
http://www.nap.edu/books/0309092701/html/

■ HERBAL MEDICINES

Epidemiology

The use of herbs for medicinal purposes has increased dramatically over the past decade, although sales have leveled off over the past several years. Herbal products are used by one of three Americans at an annual total cost of more than $4 billion, but fewer than half of those individuals discuss the matter with a conventional health care provider. Consumers hold strong views about the efficacy of the supplements they take. Seventy percent state that they would continue to take their favorite supplement even if a government study claimed it was not effective.

In the 1850s, 80% of medicines in the *United States Pharmacopeia* were derived from plants. Today, approximately 20–30% of the drugs listed in *USP Dictionary* are plant-derived—important examples include atropine, colchicine, digoxin, and many antineoplastic agents.

Herbal medicines have been dispensed for centuries by traditional herbalists who have been involved with their cultivation and preparation as well as assessment of their potency. At present, most herbal products are commercially cultivated, processed in unregulated environments, and purchased over-the-counter without the counseling of a qualified health practitioner.

Regulatory Issues

In 1994, the United States Congress passed the Dietary Supplement and Health Education Act (DSHEA). DSHEA classifies vitamins, minerals, herbs, and amino acids as nutritional or dietary supplements. Under DSHEA, supplements can be marketed without proof of safety or efficacy as long as no claim is made for their use in the diagnosis, treatment or cure, or prevention of disease. Manufacturers can, however, make "structure and function" claims that a product enhances a normal body function or state such as thinking, mood, or immune function. For example, saw palmetto can be marketed to support urinary tract health but not to treat benign prostatic hyperplasia. In contrast to prescription drugs, the US Food and Drug Administration (FDA) must first prove that a herbal preparation is *unsafe* before it can order that a product be taken off the market.

Quality Assurance

In March 2003, the FDA proposed new labeling and manufacturing standards for all dietary supplements. Prior to this, consumers had no guarantee of the quality of the products they purchased. They could not be certain that the plant was accurately identified; that the product was free of microbial, pesticide, and heavy metal contamination; or that all batches contained the same ingredients in the same strengths. Indeed, a 17-fold difference in the amount of active ingredient was found when six national brands of St. John's wort were tested off the shelf. Only 12 of 81 randomized controlled trials of five popular herbs published between 2000–2004 performed tests to quantify the actual contents of the products being evaluated.

Such lack of consistency prompted the Institute of Medicine to call on the government to amend DSHEA to implement improved quality-control manufacturing standards for supplements, more accurate labeling requirements, and greater consumer protections.

Patients should be advised to follow certain guidelines when considering whether to use herbal medicines (Table 42–1).

Product Formulations & Standardization

Herbal formulations include liquids (extracts, tinctures, infusions, and decoctions) and fresh, dried, and powdered preparations. The potency of herbs varies widely depending on which part of the plant is used, where it is cultivated, and what variations there may be in growing conditions and methods of preparation.

To ensure a consistent percentage of the primary active ingredients across batches and brand names, standardized extracts have been developed. Since multiple constituents may have pharmacologic activity, determining the active ingredients for standardization purposes can be a difficult task. The European scientific community has played a significant role in producing and investigating high-quality standardized extracts that contain consistent quantities of marker compounds (ideally, the active

Table 42–1. Advice to patients using herbal medicines.

Communication

Discuss use of all therapies with your health care provider.

Product Quality

Manufacturers are not required to submit evidence to the FDA or any regulatory body to demonstrate product safety, effectiveness, or product quality.

Ask your primary care provider, a pharmacist, or a trained herbalist regarding the specific herbs you are using.

Use herbs that are standardized to contain a specific quantity of the active ingredients.

Select formulations that have been studied in clinical trials.

Select formulations produced by larger companies. They are more likely to ensure product quality in order to protect their reputation.

Labeling

Look for a seal of approval from an independent testing agency such as NNFA, NSF, or ConsumerLab.

It should state the common and scientific names of herb(s).

It should state the concentration or dose of the herb(s) and provide instructions on dose and frequency.

It should state that the product is "standardized" to contain a certain amount of the active ingredient(s).

It should state the methods used to ensure product quality.

It should state the name and address of the manufacturer.

It should state the batch or lot number and the expiration date.

It should list potential side effects and interactions.

Pregnancy

Few herbs have been studied for safety during pregnancy.

Seek advice from your primary care provider before using herbs during pregnancy.

Interactions

Discuss with your health care provider the safety profile and interactions that may occur when combining herbs and when taking herbs plus drugs.

Reporting

Report any adverse reactions to your state poison control program or the FDA.

---

ingredients). This work has laid the foundation for conducting phase 2 and phase 3 clinical trials. The quality of research in the field is improving, but most herbal remedies have not been evaluated in controlled clinical trials.

Safety of Herbal Medicines

Although many medicinal herbs are relatively safe, some have significant toxicity. Herbs themselves can have unanticipated effects such as hepatotoxicity as seen with chaparral and germander. Ten of twenty patients with fulminant hepatic failure referred to a liver transplant service over a 21-month period were recent or active users of potentially hepatotoxic supplements. Ma-huang contains ephedrine and was sold as a component of many weight loss products and in a banned euphoriant called

"herbal ecstasy." Over 800 adverse events associated with Ma-huang have been reported, including the widely publicized death of a US major league baseball player in 2003, causing the FDA to ban ephedra-containing products from the market. (See Ephedra in the specific herbs section for details.) Herbal products may also be intentionally adulterated with prescription drugs or contaminated with harmful substances such as pesticides or heavy metals. Prescription drugs such as prednisone, nonsteroidal anti-inflammatory drugs (NSAIDs), antibiotics, and testosterone have been detected in imported Chinese patent medicines. In January 2006, the FDA issued a warning that two weight loss products available over the Internet contained chlordiazepoxide, fluoxetine, and a stimulant that is converted in the body to amphetamines. An estimated 15 million adults in 1997 took herbal medicines concurrently with prescription medications, creating a potential risk for adverse drug-herb or drug-supplement interactions. Patients taking St. John's wort along with the drugs indinavir or cyclosporine have lower blood levels of these prescription medicines. St. John's wort has the capacity to induce the cytochrome P450 system, which can lead to increased metabolism (ie, lower blood levels) of almost 50% of all prescription medicines that are processed by this system such as warfarin, theophylline, and birth control pills. Proving that a side effect experienced by a patient taking a dietary supplement is caused by that supplement is often difficult. Practitioners should take a detailed history from the patient and, if possible, obtain a sample of the product to facilitate further analysis if needed. All suspected adverse events should be reported to the FDA's Medwatch Program (http://www.fda.gov/medwatch), although it is estimated that less than 1% are actually reported.

Basch EM et al: *Natural Standard Herb and Supplement Handbook:* The Clinical Bottom Line. Elsevier Mosby, 2005.

Bent S et al: Commonly used herbal medicines in the United States: a review. Am J Med 2004;116:478. [PMID: 15047038]

Blendon RJ et al: Americans' views on the use and regulation of dietary supplements. Arch Intern Med 2001;161:805. [PMID: 11268222]

Bruno JJ et al: Herbal use among US elderly: 2002 National Health Interview Study. Ann Pharmacother 2005;39:643. [PMID: 15741417]

Estes JD et al: High prevalence of potentially hepatotoxic herbal supplement use in patients with fulminant hepatic failure. Arch Surg 2003;138:852. [PMID: 12912743]

Hu Z et al: Herb-drug interactions: a literature review. Drugs 2005;65:1239. [PMID: 15916450]

Kelly JP et al: Recent trends in use of herbal and other natural products. Arch Intern Med 2005;165:281. [PMID: 15710790]

Wolsko PM et al: Lack of herbal supplement characterization in published randomized controlled trials. Am J Med 2005; 118:1087. [PMID:16194636]

REVIEW OF THE EVIDENCE FOR SELECTED HERBAL MEDICINES

Table 42–2 provides an overview of selected herbal medicines.

Table 42–2. Overview of selected herbal medicines.

	Leading Indications	Active Constituents	Mechanism of Action	Standardized Complex	Dosage	Level of Evidence[1] and Effect Size[2]	Safety[3]	Interaction; Side Effects	Comments
Echinacea (purple coneflower)	1. Treatment of URIs 2. Prevention of URIs	Isobutyl-amides, chicoric acid, polyenes, alkaloids, and alkylamides	Immunostimulant, phagocytosis, cytokines (IL-1, TNF, IFN)	Above-the-ground preparations of *E purpurea*	300 mg, or 3 mL q3–4h	1. B: small 2. C	I	None known: rash, pruritus, nausea	Avoid in immuno-compromised patients; avoid use > 4 weeks
Ephedra	1. Weight loss 2. Stimulant	Ephedrine alkaloids	Sympathomimetic		Max: 8 mg/dose; 24 mg/d	1. A: small 2. B: dose-dependent	V (especially at high doses)	Agitation, arrhythmias, stroke, MI, death	Banned by FDA
Garlic (*Allium sativum*)	1. Cholesterol 2. Hypertension 3. Coronary artery disease	Allicin	1. HMG CoA-reductase, 14α-demethylase 2. Unclear 3. Antiplatelet effects	Allicin 0.6–1.3%	600–900 mg qd	1. B: small 2. C: small 3. C	I	1. Odor, flatulence 2. May have antiplatelet activity	
Ginkgo biloba (EGb 761, GBE)	1. Dementia 2. Claudication	Flavonoid glycosides, terpenes such as ginkgolide B	PAF inhibition, antioxidant, membrane stabilization	24% flavonoid glycoside	60 mg tid	1. A: small 2. A: small	II	May have anticoagulant effect	Do not use in patients on anticoagulants and use caution if allergic to urushiols (mango rind, sumac, poison ivy, cashew nuts)
Asian ginseng (*Panax ginseng*)	Stamina, aphrodisiac, fertility, "tonic," "energy-booster," "adaptogen"	Ginsenosides	Unclear	> 2% ginsenosides	200–600 mg qd extract;1–2g crude drug	C: multiple studies but few for any given indication	I	Previous reports of toxicity have been attributed to adulterants	
Kava (*Piper methysticum*)	Anxiety	Kava lactones	May modulate GABA binding	30–55% kava lactones in the United States	70 mg bid-tid kava lactones	A: moderate	II–IV (with recent concerns about liver toxicity)	With excess use, possible yellow scaling of skin; sedation	Avoid combining with sedatives and alcohol

St. John's wort (Hypericum perforatum)	1. Depression: mild to moderate 2. Depression: major	Napthodianthrones (such as hypericum or hyperforin), flavonoids, and xanthones	May modulate neurotransmitters (serotonin, NE, GABA)	Hypericin 0.3% or hyperforin 3%	300 mg tid	1. A: moderate 2. B: no better than placebo	I (but significant drug-herb interaction)	Induces cytochrome P450, leading to lower serum levels of certain drugs	Cyclosporine, protease inhibitors, oral contraceptives, warfarin, digoxin levels reduced
Saw palmetto (Serenoa repens)	Benign prostatic hyperplasia	Sterols, free fatty acids	5[α]-Reductase inhibition; inhibition of DHT binding to androgen receptor	85–95% sterols and fatty acids	160 mg bid	B: small or none	I	Mild GI upset and headaches (rare)	Does not effect PSA levels or prostate size

[1] Level of evidence: A, good evidence; B, some evidence; C, insufficient evidence.

[2] Effect size: none, small, moderate, large.

[3] Safety: I, generally safe; II, relatively safe; III, insufficient evidence; IV, may be harmful; V, clear evidence of harm.

URI = upper respiratory infection; IL = interleukin; IFN = interferon; TNF = tumor necrosis factor; HMG = hydroxymethylglutaric acid; PAF = platelet-activating factor; MI = myocardial infarction; NE = norepinephrine; DHT = dihydrotestosterone; PSA = prostate-specific antigen.

St. John's Wort (*Hypericum perforatum*)

St. John's wort is used in the treatment of mild to moderate depression. Most preparations are standardized to hypericin or hyperforin. The precise mechanisms of action are not known. Irreversible monoamine oxidase inhibitory activity noted in vitro has not been observed in vivo. Other postulated mechanisms include selective inhibition of serotonin, γ-aminobutyrate, norepinephrine, and dopamine reuptake in the central nervous system.

Over the past two decades, St. John's wort has been studied in thousands of patients with mild to moderate depression. Most of the 60-plus randomized controlled clinical trials, systematic reviews, and meta-analyses have shown that it is more effective than placebo and as effective as tricyclic agents for the treatment of mild to moderate depression. Several recent placebo-controlled studies lasting 4–12 weeks have also shown that St. John's wort has efficacy similar to the selective serotonin reuptake inhibitors (SSRIs) sertraline, fluoxetine, and paroxetine. Pooled analyses of six recent, large trials restricted to patients with major depression, however, showed only minimal effects of St. John's wort compared with placebo. A 4-year NIH study of 300 patients with mild symptoms of depression began in 2003. Patients are being randomized to St. John's wort, placebo, or citalopram for 12 weeks.

St. John's wort is generally well tolerated. Side effects are not common and include mild headache, photosensitivity, gastrointestinal upset, and restlessness. Data from 35 double-blind randomized trials show that drop out and adverse event rates in patients receiving *Hypericum* extracts were similar to placebo, lower than with older antidepressants, and slightly lower than with SSRIs. Patients are advised to avoid taking St. John's wort in addition to prescription antidepressants, as there have been case reports of serotonin syndrome. St. John's wort also induces the cytochrome P450 system (isozyme CYP3A4), which may lower the blood levels of other drugs that are metabolized by this system (eg, ethinyl estradiol, warfarin, cyclosporine, and indinavir). At least 50% of all medications currently on the market are at least partially metabolized by this isozyme. Several cases of cardiac and renal organ rejection have been reported in patients whose previously stable level of cyclosporine was lowered after initiation of St. John's wort. Of further concern is that this herb-drug interaction may persist even after St. John's wort is discontinued. A 40% decrease in serum levels of the chemotherapeutic agent irinotecan noted in five patients taking concurrent St. John's wort persisted for 3 weeks after St. John's wort was discontinued.

Bjerkenstedt L et al: Hypericum extract LI-160 and fluoxetine in mild to moderate depression: a randomized, placebo-controlled, multicenter study in outpatients. Eur Arch Psychiatry Clin Neurosci 2005;255:40. [PMID: 15538592]

Fava M et al: A double-blind, randomized trial of St. John's wort, fluoxetine and placebo in major depressive disorder. J Clin Psychopharmacol 2005;25:441. [PMID: 16160619]

Hypericum Depression Trial Study Group: Effect of *Hypericum perforatum* (St John's wort) in major depressive disorder: a randomized controlled trial. JAMA 2002;287:1807. [PMID: 11939866]

Knuppel L et al: Adverse effects of St. John's wort: a systematic review. J Clin Psychiatry 2004;65:1470. [PMID: 15554758]

Linde K et al: St. John's wort for depression: meta-analysis of randomized controlled trials. Br J Psychiatry 2005;186:99. [PMID: 15684231]

Madabushi R et al: Hyperforin in St. John's wort drug interactions. Eur J Clin Pharmacol 2006;14:1. [PMID: 16477470]

Szegedi A et al: Acute treatment of moderate to severe depression with hypericum extract WS5570 (St. John's wort): randomized controlled double blind non-inferiority trial versus paroxetine. BMJ 2005;330:503. [PMID: 15708844]

Garlic

Garlic was the top-selling herb in 2004 with greater than $27 million in sales. The German Federal Health Agency Commission E and the European Scientific Cooperative on Phytotherapy have approved garlic for the treatment of hyperlipidemia and atherosclerosis. Allicin, the ingredient believed responsible for garlic's therapeutic benefit and odor, is highly unstable. Both heat and acid destroy the enzyme allinase, which is necessary to produce allicin, and for that reason garlic is best ingested raw. Garlic is also available over-the-counter in multiple formulations (dried, powdered, oils). The best-studied form is an enteric-coated capsule of dehydrated garlic. Freeze-drying helps retain most of the active ingredients found in raw garlic. Enteric coating permits allicin to be released in the small intestine, thereby enhancing absorption and reducing the breath odor. Over-the-counter preparations are frequently standardized to yield 0.6% allicin, but allicin yield among powdered preparations varies as much as 230-fold in brands used in trials. This lack of standardization may contribute to inconsistent results in dozens of clinical trials.

Doses of 600–900 mg of freeze-dried herb (equivalent to one-half to one clove of raw garlic) appear to have small effects on cholesterol (4–12% reduction when taken for 4–6 weeks), minimal effect on blood pressure (< 10 mm Hg), and none on glucose levels. A small study of 15 men with coronary artery disease suggests that short-term treatment with an aged garlic extract may improve impaired endothelial function in men taking aspirin and a statin. Numerous observational studies have suggested that regular consumption of garlic might reduce the risk of developing certain malignancies, but no prospective controlled trials have been performed.

Garlic is well tolerated and apparently safe for long-term use. In addition to the well-known breath and body odor, common side effects include gastrointestinal upset, nausea, and flatulence.

A more than 50% reduction in blood levels of saquinavir after garlic supplementation has been reported. Although the induction of the cytochrome P450 system was hypothesized as the mechanism of action of this significant herb-drug interaction, a recent study of healthy volunteers did not reveal an effect of garlic on isozymes CYPP2D6 or CYP3A4. Garlic has been shown to have some antiplatelet activation activity, so there is a theoretical risk of increased bleeding, especially if taken with aspirin, anticoagulants, or NSAIDs. Although there is insufficient evidence to determine a causal association, some physicians recommend stopping garlic 1–2 weeks prior to undergoing elective surgery.

Markowitz JS et al: Effects of garlic (*Allium sativum L.*) supplementation on cytochrome P450 2D6 and 3A4 activity in healthy volunteers. Clin Pharmacol Ther 2003;74:170. [PMID: 12891227]

Mulrow C et al: Garlic: Effects on cardiovascular risks and disease, protective effects against cancer, and clinical adverse effects. Rockville, MD: Agency for Healthcare Research and Quality; 2003. AHRQ publication 01-E023.

Piscitelli SC et al: The effect of garlic supplements on the pharmacokinetics of saquinavir. Clin Infect Dis 2002;34:234. [PMID: 8875379]

Stevinson C et al: Garlic for treating hypercholesterolemia. A meta-analysis of randomized clinical trials. Ann Intern Med 2000;133:420. [PMID: 10975959]

Tattelman E: Health effects of garlic. Am Fam Physician 2005; 72:103. [PMID: 16035690]

Williams MJ et al: Aged garlic extract improves endothelial function in men with coronary artery disease. Phytother Res 2005;19:314. [PMID: 16041725]

Ginkgo

The dried leaf of the ginkgo tree has been used medicinally for thousands of years. More than 400 studies over the past 30 years have investigated ginkgo's ability to improve blood flow in a variety of conditions, including memory impairment, dementia, peripheral vascular disease, vertigo, tinnitus, asthma, SSRI-induced sexual dysfunction, and acute mountain sickness. The German Commission E has approved a standardized form of ginkgo leaf extract (EGb 761) for the treatment of cognitive impairment and intermittent claudication. Multiple pharmacologically active compounds have been isolated from ginkgo, including flavonoid glycosides and terpene lactones (ginkgolides). The flavonoids have antioxidant and free radical scavenging ability. The terpene lactones (especially ginkgolide B) have platelet-activating factor antagonist activity. In addition, ginkgo extracts increase the production of nitric oxide and activate certain central neurotransmitters, including the cholinergic system, which may contribute to their beneficial effects on memory and cognition. EGb 761—the formulation that has been studied most extensively—is standardized to contain 24% flavonoid glycosides and 6% terpene lactones.

Early studies that assessed ginkgo's efficacy on cognitive function in the elderly showed a modest improvement when compared to placebo. The longest of these studies (1 year) showed stabilization of cognitive and functional abilities in 309 demented patients treated with EGb 761 compared with placebo, with no differences in adverse outcomes. In contrast, EGb 761 was no more effective than placebo in 214 elderly Dutch patients with dementia or age-associated memory impairment. There is conflicting evidence about ginkgo's ability to enhance memory in healthy individuals. The NIH has funded investigators at the University of Pittsburgh to determine whether ginkgo taken over 5 years can prevent or delay the development of dementia in 3000 patients 75 years of age or older.

In general, ginkgo is well tolerated in healthy adults at recommended doses for up to 6 months. Allergic skin reactions, gastrointestinal disturbances, and headache occur in less than 2% of patients. There are theoretical concerns about a risk of increased bleeding because antiplatelet activating factor activity has been demonstrated in vitro. Nearly 20 cases of increased bleeding in patients taking ginkgo have been reported, but establishing a causal relationship is challenging because many of these patients had other risk factors including age and use of medications, such as warfarin, aspirin, or NSAIDs. Of note, no excess bleeding complications have been reported in clinical trials and no differences in coagulation, platelet function, or pharmacokinetics of warfarin have been noted in healthy male volunteers. Caution should still be exercised in patients with bleeding disorders or who are taking anticoagulants, aspirin, or other herbs that may increase the risk of bleeding.

Gingko has also been evaluated for its effect on intermittent claudication. A meta-analysis of nine randomized, placebo-controlled, double-blinded trials of patients treated with EGb 761 showed a modest treatment effect in the increase of pain-free walking distance in favor of ginkgo over placebo. There is insufficient evidence to support ginkgo's efficacy in treating tinnitus, acute mountain sickness, vertigo, or SSRI-associated sexual dysfunction.

Bent S et al: Spontaneous bleeding associated with *Ginkgo biloba.* A case report and systematic review of the literature. J Gen Intern Med 2005;20:657. [PMID: 16050865]

Birks J: *Ginkgo biloba* for cognitive impairment and dementia. Cochrane Database Syst Rev 2002;(4):CD003120. [PMID: 12519586]

Elsabagh S et al: Differential cognitive effects of *Ginkgo biloba* after acute and chronic treatment in healthy young volunteers. Psychopharmacology (Berl) 2005;179:437. [PMID: 15739076]

Jiang X et al: Effect of ginkgo and ginger on the pharmacokinetics and pharmacodynamics of warfarin in healthy subjects. Br J Clin Pharmacol 2005;59:425. [PMID: 15801937]

Kohler S et al: Influence of a 7-day treatment with *Ginkgo biloba* special extract EGb 761 on bleeding time and coagulation: a randomized, placebo-controlled, double-blind study in healthy volunteers. Blood Coagul Fibrinolysis 2004;15:303. [PMID: 15166915]

Pittler MH et al: Complementary therapies for peripheral arterial disease: systematic review. Atherosclerosis 2005;181:1. [PMID: 15939048]

Soloman PR et al: Ginkgo for memory enhancement: a randomized controlled trial. JAMA 2002;288:835. [PMID: 12186600]

van Dongen M et al: Ginkgo for elderly people with dementia and age-associated memory impairment: a randomized clinical trial. J Clin Epidemiol 2003;56:367. [PMID: 12767414]

Echinacea

Echinacea ranks second among the top-selling herbs in the United States, accounting for more than $300 million in sales annually. Three of nine *Echinacea* species are currently used for the treatment and prevention of upper respiratory infections. Preparations are made from roots (*Echinacea pallida* and *Echinacea angustifolia*), above-ground parts (stems, leaves, and flowers of *Echinacea purpurea*), or a combination of both. Multiple forms are available over-the-counter, including capsules, fresh pressed juice, tinctures, and teas. Differences in species, growing conditions, plant parts used, and extraction procedures can result in differences in chemical composition and biologic activity. Several active ingredients have been identified, including polysaccharides, glycoproteins, alkaloids, and flavonoids. In vitro, animal, and human studies suggest that these ingredients cause stimulation of the immune system (natural killer cells, macrophages, and cytokine activity) and that they possess anti-inflammatory, free radical-scavenging, and antiviral activity.

The quality of most clinical trials has been limited by use of multiple products and doses (including formulations containing multiple herbs) and the lack of rigorous methodology.

The majority of early trials reported that echinacea is effective in reducing the duration and severity of colds if started within several days of the onset of symptoms but no more effective when taken to prevent infection. A well-designed, 2005 trial studied three different *E angustifolia* root preparations for the prevention and treatment of laboratory-induced rhinovirus infections. Four hundred thirty-seven volunteers were randomized to receive either prophylaxis (beginning 7 days before a challenge with rhinovirus) or treatment (beginning at the time of viral challenge), with one of the three different echinacea preparations. No statistically significant effects were seen on rates of infection or severity of symptoms in patients taking the herb. The echinacea used in this trial was well characterized and of high quality, but some clinicians feel that the dose used was lower than that used in routine practice. In contrast, an updated meta-analysis of echinacea monopreparations found that 10 out of 16 trials showed the herb to be more effective than placebo for the treatment of colds. Enough data were available for preparations made of the above-the-ground parts of *E purpurea* that the authors concluded that there is some evidence that these specific formulations may be effective for the early treatment of colds in adults. Data for other echinacea formulations and for prevention of colds were less consistent.

In general, echinacea is well tolerated, with few reported adverse events. Rare allergic reactions including rash have been reported (especially in patients with ragweed allergies), and there was a single case of recurrent erythema nodosum. The German Commission E recommends that patients who are pregnant, have autoimmune disease, or who are immunocompromised

not take echinacea because of its immune-stimulating effects. The Commission also recommends that its use be limited in others to less than 4 weeks. The data supporting these recommendations are not clear.

Barrett B et al: Treatment of the common cold with unrefined echinacea. A randomized, double-blind, placebo-controlled trial. Ann Intern Med 2002;137:939. [PMID: 12484708]

Goel V et al: A proprietary extract from the echinacea plant (*Echinacea purpurea*) enhances systemic immune response during a common cold. Phytother Res 2005;19:689. [PMID: 16177972]

Linde K et al: Echinacea for preventing and treating the common cold. Cochrane Database Syst Rev 2006;(1):CD000530. [PMID: 16437427]

Sperber SJ: *Echinacea purpurea* for prevention of experimental rhinovirus colds. Clin Infect Dis 2004;38:1367. [PMID: 15156472]

Turner RB et al: An evaluation of *Echinacea angustifolia* in experimental rhinovirus infections. N Engl J Med 2005;353:341. [PMID: 16049208]

Yale SH et al: *Echinacea purpurea* therapy for the treatment of the common cold: a randomized, double-blind, placebo-controlled clinical trial. Arch Intern Med 2004;164:1237. [PMID: 15197051]

Kava

Kava beverages prepared from the dried rhizome of the *Piper methysticum* plant have been consumed for centuries as ceremonial drinks in the South Pacific islands. Its present-day uses include the treatment of anxiety, stress, and insomnia. The active ingredients (kavapyrones) have central muscle-relaxing properties and anticonvulsant activity. The precise anxiolytic mechanism of action is not fully understood.

A systematic review and meta-analysis of eleven randomized, double-blind, placebo-controlled trials concluded that kava was more effective than placebo in relieving anxiety, with effects observed after as few as 1–2 doses and with progressive improvement over 1–4 weeks. The longest study involved 101 German outpatients randomized to kava or placebo for 6 months. Compared with placebo, kava-treated patients had progressively lower Hamilton anxiety scale scores at 3 and 6 months. In two shorter trials, kava also relieved acute anxiety more effectively than placebo. A recent meta-analysis of six clinical trials that used a standardized kava preparation (WS1490) also concluded that the herb is more effective than placebo in treating anxiety, with greatest benefit seen in women and patients younger than 53 years.

Kava has been well tolerated in clinical trials. Less than 2.3% of patients report gastrointestinal complaints, drowsiness, tremor, headache, or allergic skin reactions. There are several case reports of patients feeling sedated, disoriented, or ataxic after consuming high doses of kava (or kava in combination with alcohol or prescription drugs that act on the central nervous system). These include two "driving under the influence" arrests of patients who had consumed 8–16 cups of a kava beverage. Kava may have dopamine antagonist properties. Three patients using European kava preparations developed extrapyramidal dystonic reactions or worsening Parkinson's disease. A reversible kava toxic syndrome with dermopathy (dry, flaky, yellow skin), ataxia, partial hearing loss, and weight loss has been reported in South Pacific Islanders who consume kava at doses 100 times higher than recommended.

In 2001, the German government reported 29 cases of hepatitis, cirrhosis, and liver failure possibly associated with the use of kava. Although 18 of these reports were in patients who were also taking medications with known or potential liver toxicity, one case involved a previously healthy 50-year-old man who was not taking prescription medications or alcohol who required a liver transplant. As a result of almost 80 case reports, kava products have been taken off the market in the European Union, Australia and Canada. Warnings about possible hepatic toxicity have been issued to patients with acute or chronic liver disease. How kava causes hepatic toxicity is not clear, but possible mechanisms of action include idiosyncratic reactions, differences in preparation (commercial kava is prepared in acetone, methanol, or ethanol while traditional kava is aqueous), inhibition of the cytochrome P450, or reduction in liver glutathione levels.

Clouatre DL: Kava Kava: examining new reports of toxicity. Toxicol Lett 2004;150:85. [PMID: 15068826]

Cote CS et al: Composition and biological activity of traditional and commercial kava extracts. Biochem Biophys Res Commun 2004;322:147. [PMID: 15313185]

Ernst E: Herbal remedies for anxiety—a systematic review of controlled clinical trials. Phytomedicine 2006;13:205. [PMID: 16428031]

From the Centers for Disease Control and Prevention. Hepatic toxicity possibly associated with kava-containing products—United States, Germany, and Switzerland, 1999–2002. JAMA 2003;289:36. [PMID: 12515265]

Perez J et al: Altered mental status and ataxia secondary to acute Kava ingestion. J Emerg Med 2005;28:49. [PMID: 15657005]

Witte S et al: Meta-analysis of the efficacy of the acetonic kava-kava extract WS1490 in patients with non-psychotic anxiety disorders. Phytother Res 2005;19:183. [PMID: 15934028]

Ginseng

Ginseng root has been used for medicinal purposes in Asia for over 2000 years. There are three major forms of ginseng in use today: Asian ginseng (*Panax ginseng*); American ginseng (*Panax quinquefolius*); and Siberian ginseng (*Eleutherococcus senticosus*), which is not a member of the *Panax* genus. The German Commission E monograph on ginseng root approves its use as "a tonic to counteract weakness and fatigue, as a restorative for declining stamina and impaired concentration, and as an aid to convalescence." Extracts are made from dried roots and contain ginsenosides. Over 25 ginsenosides have been isolated, each with unique and sometimes oppositional effects on the cardiovascular, central nervous, and immune systems. The mechanisms of action have not been clearly delineated.

There is an extensive body of scientific literature on this subject, with over 4000 books and papers published. Multiple indications have been studied using different ginseng species, often with poor methodologic rigor. One European study identified 57 randomized controlled trials of ginseng in the world's literature, but only 16 studies were of good enough quality to be included in their systematic review. Insufficient evidence was available to support or refute the use of ginseng for any of the purported indications, including improvement of physical performance, cognitive functioning, and quality of life. Two small 2004 clinical trials suggest ginseng may improve cognitive performance in healthy persons and prevent acute respiratory illness in institutionalized older adults. A larger Canadian trial examined the efficacy of a proprietary North American ginseng extract, previously shown to stimulate the immune system in vitro, in preventing colds. Three hundred twenty-three healthy subjects who had at least two colds in the previous year were randomized to daily ginseng or placebo for 4 months, beginning just after the onset of influenza season. The mean number of colds per person and the severity and duration of symptoms were less in the ginseng-treated group. A study done in 2000 suggested that one form of American ginseng may attenuate postprandial glycemia in both normal and diabetic persons, but follow-up reports from the same researchers showed no or variable effects of ginsengs with different ginsenoside composition.

Ginseng is well tolerated at recommended doses, with few adverse effects. A recent systematic review of adverse reactions reports that the incidence is similar in ginseng monopreparations and placebo. Possible drug interactions have been reported between *P ginseng* and warfarin, phenelzine, calcium channel blockers, digoxin, and alcohol. Earlier reports of "ginseng abuse syndrome" and other toxicities are now attributed to adulterants found in earlier unregulated over-the-counter ginseng products. Indeed, 13 of 21 ginseng products recently evaluated for quality and purity failed because they contained unacceptable levels of pesticides or heavy metals or inadequate concentrations of ginsenosides.

Coon JT et al: *Panax ginseng*: a systematic review of adverse effects and drug interactions. Drug Safety 2002;25:323. [PMID: 12020172]

McElhaney JE et al: A placebo-controlled trial of a proprietary extract of North American ginseng (CVT-E002) to prevent acute respiratory illness in institutionalized older adults. J Am Geriatr Soc 2004;52:13. [PMID: 14687309]

Predy GN et al: Efficacy of an extract of North American ginseng containing poly-furanosyl-pyranosyl-saccharides for preventing upper respiratory tract infections: a randomized trial. CMAJ 2005;173:1043. [PMID: 16247099]

Sievenpiper JL et al: Decreasing, null and increasing effects of eight popular types of ginseng on acute postprandial glycemic indices in healthy humans: the role of ginsenosides. J Am Coll Nutr 2004;23:248. [PMID: 15190050]

Sievenpiper JL et al: Null and opposing effects of Asian ginseng (*Panax ginseng* C.A. Meyer) on acute glycemia: results of two acute dose escalation studies. J Am Coll Nutr 2003;22:524. [PMID: 14684758]

Vogler BK et al: The efficacy of ginseng. A systematic review of randomised clinical trials. Eur J Clin Pharmacol 1999;55: 567. [PMID: 10541774]

Yuan CS et al: Brief communication: American ginseng reduces warfarin's effect in healthy patients: a randomized, controlled trial. Ann Intern Med 2004;141:23. [PMID: 15238367]

Saw Palmetto

Saw palmetto is used by over 2 million men in the United States to treat benign prostatic hyperplasia, and in Europe, it is often the first-line therapy for lower urinary tract symptoms. Lipophilic extracts are prepared from the berries of the dwarf palm tree (*Serenoa repens*) and are standardized to sterols and free fatty acids. Several mechanisms of action have been proposed, including inhibition of 5α-reductase activity, as well as antiandrogenic, anti-inflammatory, and antiproliferative activity. The most studied brand of saw palmetto (Permixon) is not available in the United States.

A 2004 meta-analysis of 17 trials (14 randomized) using Permixon in 4280 patients showed significant improvement in peak flow rate, reduction in nocturia relative to placebo, and a 5-point reduction in the International Prostate Symptom Score. These clinical data are comparable to effects of some α-blockers. In contrast, a well-designed 2006 trial showed no difference in symptom scores, flow rates, prostate size, postvoid residual volume, quality of life, or prostate-specific antigen in 225 men with moderate to severe benign prostatic hyperplasia treated with saw palmetto (160 mg twice daily) or placebo for 1 year.

Saw palmetto is very well tolerated by most patients for up to 3–5 years, with only mild and rare gastrointestinal symptoms being reported. Saw palmetto has not been shown to reduce prostate size or lower the serum level of prostate-specific antigen. No herb-drug interactions have been reported. In a 2003 study, the herb did not alter cytochrome P450 activity in healthy volunteers. Saw palmetto was one of eight ingredients in PC-SPES, a popular herbal product used by many men with prostate cancer. PC-SPES was withdrawn from the market when it was found to be contaminated with the prescription drugs diethylstilbestrol and warfarin.

Bent S et al: Saw palmetto for benign prostate hyperplasia. N Engl J Med 2006;354:557. [PMID: 16467543]

Boyle P et al: Updated meta-analysis of clinical trials of *Serenoa repens* extract in the treatment of symptomatic benign prostatic hyperplasia. BJU Int 2004;93:751. [PMID: 15049985]

Buck AC: Is there a scientific basis for the therapeutic effects of *Serenoa repens* in benign prostatic hyperplasia? Mechanisms of action. J Urol 2004;172:1792. [PMID: 15540722]

Fong YK et al: Role of phytotherapy in men with lower urinary tract symptoms. Curr Opin Urol 2005;15:45. [PMID: 15586030]

Markowitz JS et al: Multiple doses of saw palmetto (*Serenoa repens*) did not alter cytochrome P450 2D6 and 3A4 activity in normal volunteers. Clin Pharmacol Ther 2003;74:536. [PMID: 14663456]

Ephedra (Ma-huang)

The dried young stems of *Ephedra sinica* have been used for thousands of years in traditional Oriental medicine to treat respiratory disorders, especially bronchospasm and congestion. Ephedra has also been widely marketed for its stimulant and appetite suppressant effects (alone or in combination with caffeine-like herbs). Ephedra's alkaloids are structurally similar to amphetamines. A meta-analysis concluded that patients taking ephedra or ephedra plus caffeine products lost 1.3 or 2.2 more pounds per month respectively than those taking placebo. These products were associated with a twofold to threefold risk of psychiatric, autonomic, gastrointestinal symptoms, and heart palpitations. Of all the adverse effects caused by ingestion of herbs reported to US poison control centers, 64% were due to products containing ephedra, even though they represented only 0.82% of herbal product sales. Over 800 cases of adverse events, including more than 20 deaths, have been reported to the FDA, which prohibited the sales of ephedra-containing dietary supplements in February 2004. This ban was challenged in April 2005 when a supplement manufacturer argued in the Utah Federal District Court that the FDA had not demonstrated that ephedra was dangerous when used at lower doses. Many "Ephedra-free" weight loss products contain bitter orange (citrus aurantium), which could pose similar risks because it contains synepherine, which has sympathomimetic activity.

Bent S et al: The relative safety of ephedra compared with other herbal products. Ann Intern Med 2003;138:468. [PMID: 12639079]

Bent S et al: Safety and efficacy of citrus aurantium for weight loss. Am J Cardiol 2004;94:1359. [PMID: 15541270]

Haller CA et al: Hemodynamic effects of ephedra-free weight loss supplements in humans. Am J Med 2005;118:998. [PMID: 16164886]

McBride BF et al: Electrocardiographic and hemodynamic effects of a multicomponent dietary supplement containing ephedra and caffeine: a randomized controlled trial. JAMA 2004;291:216. [PMID: 14722148]

Shekelle PG et al: Efficacy and safety of ephedra and ephedrine for weight loss and athletic performance: a meta-analysis. JAMA 2003;289:1537. [PMID: 12672771]

■ DIETARY SUPPLEMENTS

Sales of dietary supplements have increased dramatically over the past decade. The Dietary Supplement Health Education Act of 1994 has made it possible for manufacturers to sell dietary supplements directly to the public without FDA approval or oversight. Reports of adulteration and contamination are available, but the magnitude of this problem remains unknown. Furthermore, there have been several reports of the dose printed on the label being different from the actual dose provided. (See section on herbal medicines, above, for further details on regulatory and quality assurance issues and advice for patients to follow when purchasing these products.) Table 42–3 provides an overview of selected dietary supplements commonly used in the United States today.

S-Adenosylmethionine

S-Adenosylmethionine (SAMe) is an endogenous compound that serves as a methyl group donor for hundreds of compounds, including neurotransmitters, fatty acids, nucleic acids, proteins, and membrane phospholipids. Endogenous production is dependent on vitamin B_{12} and folic acid metabolism. Primary uses of the drug are the treatment of depression, osteoarthritis, alcoholic liver disease, and migraine headaches. Originally discovered in the 1950s, SAMe was not synthesized as a stable compound that could be made commercially available until the 1970s. It is available by prescription throughout Europe. The mechanism of action is unclear for most conditions. Based on clinical trial data from over 22,000 patients, SAMe is well-tolerated and safe. Side effects include nausea, flatulence, headache, and anxiety. A phase 4 open-label clinical trial involving over 20,000 patients observed for 8 weeks found that 87% of the cohort reported good to very good tolerance with SAMe. There are no significant drug-herb interactions, although a case of serotonin syndrome in a patient taking SAMe with clomipramine has been reported.

A 2002 Evidence Report and Technology Assessment by the Agency for Healthcare Research and Quality concluded that SAMe is more effective than placebo for relief of symptoms of depression, pain of osteoarthritis, and pruritus in cholestasis of pregnancy, and in intrahepatic cholestasis. Furthermore, the authors concluded that SAMe was equivalent to standard therapy for depression and osteoarthritis but not for cholestasis of pregnancy. Early studies suggesting that SAMe may be helpful in treating depression were limited by short duration and poor methodology. SAMe may affect multiple neurotransmitters; increased levels of serotonin, 5-hydroxyindoleacetic acid, and dopamine as well as inhibition of norepinephrine reuptake have been noted after SAMe administration. An electroencephalogram mapping study of SAMe showed significant central effects of SAMe compared with placebo typical of activating antidepressants. Two recent multicenter trials of SAMe versus imipramine report that both oral and intramuscular preparations of SAMe are as effective as the tricyclic agent in reducing depression and with fewer side effects, though neither study was placebo-controlled. No head-to-head trials have compared SAMe with SSRIs. SAMe appears to have analgesic and anti-inflammatory properties and was studied extensively in the 1980s for the treatment of osteoarthritis. The mechanism of action for these effects is unknown. Although

many early studies used a parenteral form of SAMe, only an oral formulation is available in the United States, and it is expensive ($50–$150 per month) and has poor bioavailability. A review of 11 randomized controlled trials (1418 patients) comparing SAMe with placebo or NSAIDs for osteoarthritis concluded that SAMe was as effective as NSAIDs in reducing pain and functional limitation and better-tolerated. Compared with placebo, SAMe was more effective in improving functional limitations and did not differ in adverse events.

Studies of alcohol-fed baboons suggest that SAMe increases glutathione levels and attenuates liver injury. There is some evidence that SAMe increases glutathione levels in humans as well. Investigators performed a multicenter clinical randomized, double-blind, placebo-controlled trial involving 123 patients with alcoholic liver cirrhosis treated with SAMe or placebo for 2 years. Combined mortality and liver transplantation rate was 30% in the placebo group compared with 16% in the SAMe group ($P = .08$). When Child-Turcotte-Pugh class C subjects (n = 8) were excluded, respective rates were 29% and 12% ($P = .03$). This study provides support for SAMe supplementation in alcoholic liver disease.

Arnold O et al: Double-blind, placebo-controlled pharmacodynamic studies with a nutraceutical and a pharmaceutical dose of ademetionine (SAMe) in elderly subjects, utilizing EEG mapping and psychometry. Eur Neuropsychopharmacol 2005;15:533. [PMID: 16046102]

Chiaie R et al: Efficacy and tolerability of oral and intramuscular S-adenosyl-L-methionine 1,4-butanedisulfonate (SAMe) in the treatment of major depression: comparison with imipramine in 2 multicenter studies. Am J Clin Nutr 2002;76: 1172S. [PMID: 12418499]

Hardy M et al: S-adenosyl-L-methoionine for treatment of depression, osteoarthritis, and liver disease. Agency for Healthcare Research and Quality (AHRQ) 2002; (Evidence Report/Technology Assessment 64):1.

Mato JM et al: S-Adenosylmethionine in alcoholic liver cirrhosis: a randomized, placebo-controlled, double-blind, multicenter clinical trial. J Hepatol 1999;30:1081. [PMID: 10406187]

Soeken KL et al: Safety and efficacy of S-adenosylmethionine (SAMe) for osteoarthritis. J Fam Pract 2002;51:425. [PMID: 12019049]

Dehydroepiandrosterone

Dehydroepiandroesterone (DHEA) and its sulfate ester, DHEAS, are secreted by the adrenal cortex and serve as precursors for the synthesis of male and female sex hormones. In healthy individuals there is a 25% decrease in serum DHEA levels per decade until age 70, when levels are at 20–30% of lifetime peak levels. In addition, low DHEA levels have been reported in people who suffer from a wide variety of chronic illness, including depression, cancer, type 2 diabetes, HIV, Alzheimer's disease, renal failure, anorexia, and atherosclerosis. DHEA levels may be depleted by certain prescription medications, including insulin, corticosteroids, and opiates. Low levels of DHEA associ-

Table 42-3. Overview of selected dietary supplements.

	Leading Indications	Mechanism of Action	Dosage	Level of Evidence[1] and Effect Size[2]	Safety[3]	Interactions; Side Effects	Comments
S-Adenosylmethionine (SAMe, SAM)	1. Depression 2. Osteoarthritis 3. Alcohol-related liver disease	Universal methyl donor	200–800 mg bid	1. B: moderate 2. B: moderate 3. C	I	None; may precipitate mania in persons with bipolar affective disorder	
Dehydroepiandrosterone (DHEA, DHEAS)	1. Depression, dysthymia 2. Lupus 3. Insulin sensitivity 4. Adrenal insufficiency	1. Unknown 2. Possibly IL-10 3. Unknown 4. Replacement	50 mg qd	1. C: small 2. B: moderate 3. B: small 4. C: small	IV (with long-term use)	None reported; androgenic effects	Theoretical concerns that long-term use may result in hormone-dependent malignancies
Glucosamine sulfate and chondroitin	Osteoarthritis (knee)	Proteoglycan production	Glucosamine 500 mg tid; chondroitin 400 mg tid	A: moderate	I	None reported; rare reports of constipation, diarrhea, drowsiness	Insulin resistance not seen in clinical trials
Coenzyme Q$_{10}$ (ubiquinone, ubidecarenone, Co-Q$_{10}$)	Congestive heart failure, cardiac arrest, angina, acute myocardial infarction, migraine prophylaxis	ATP production, membrane stabilization	50 qd–150 mg tid; goal is to achieve serum level of 2.1 mcg/mL	C	I	Patients taking statins noted to have lower serum levels of Co-Q$_{10}$	Fat-soluble, so absorption improved when taken with meals

[1]Level of evidence: A, good evidence; B, some evidence; C, insufficient evidence.
[2]Effect size: none, small, moderate, large.
[3]Safety: I, generally safe; II, relatively safe; III, insufficient evidence; IV, may be harmful; V, clear evidence of harm.

ated with aging and medical illness have been cited in the popular press as evidence that DHEA supplementation would be beneficial.

The mechanism of action of DHEA remains unknown. Preliminary evidence suggests that DHEA supplementation might be useful in depression, dysthymia, systemic lupus erythematosus (SLE), insulin sensitivity, and adrenal insufficiency.

Animal studies suggest that DHEA and DHEAS have excitatory effects on the central nervous system, which may account for their influence on mood and sense of well-being. A 6-week clinical trial randomized 52 subjects with major or minor depression to monotherapy with DHEA or placebo and found DHEA to be superior as measured by multiple well-validated depression scales.

Low DHEA levels in men and women with SLE and reduction in interleukin-10 levels after supplementation compared with placebo suggest that DHEA may play a causative role. One hundred women with active, mild to moderate SLE were randomized to receive 200 mg/d of oral DHEA or placebo for 24 weeks. DHEA was well tolerated, significantly reduced the number of SLE flares, and improved patients' global assessment of disease activity. DHEA supplementation has been shown to reduce abdominal visceral fat and insulin resistance. Villareal and colleagues randomized 56 adults to DHEA (50 mg/d) or placebo for 6 months and found reductions in visceral fat, subcutaneous fat, and insulin sensitivity. Women with adrenal insufficiency have unmeasurable DHEA serum levels. Treatment with DHEA in a 3-month randomized, double-blinded, placebo-controlled crossover study was associated with improvements in insulin sensitivity in this population. Using a similar design, a 4-month study of DHEA was associated with improvements in mood, well-being, and libido. In contrast, a 9-month randomized, placebo-controlled study of 39 women with adrenal failure failed to find a beneficial effect of DHEA supplementation on subjective health status or sexuality.

Side effects of DHEA include acne, deepening of the voice, and facial hair growth. No serious adverse events have been reported. The long-term effects of DHEA supplementation remain unknown. The safety issue of most concern is that DHEA—as a potent precursor of sex steroids—may increase the risk of estrogen- or androgen-dependent malignancies. Therefore, if supplementation is used, patients should be monitored closely. Furthermore, patients at high-risk for prostate, ovarian, breast, or uterine cancer should be counseled against DHEA supplementation.

Arlt W et al: Dehydroepiandrosterone replacement in women with adrenal insufficiency. N Engl J Med 1999;341:1013. [PMID: 10502590]

Chang D-M et al: Dehydroepiandrosterone treatment of women with mild-to-moderate systemic lupus erythematosus: a multicenter randomized, double-blind, placebo-controlled trial. Arthritis Rheum 2002;46:2924. [PMID: 12428233]

Dhatariya K et al: Effect of dehydroepiandrosterone replacement on insulin sensitivity and lipids in hypoadrenal women. Diabetes 2005;54:765. [PMID: 15734854]

Schmidt PJ et al: Dehydroepiandrosterone monotherapy in midlife-onset major and minor depression. Arch Gen Psychiatry 2005;62:154. [PMID 15699292]

Villareal DT et al: Effect of DHEA on abdominal fat and insulin action in elderly women and men: a randomized controlled trial. JAMA 2004;292:2243. [PMID: 15536111]

Glucosamine & Chondroitin

Glucosamine and chondroitin have been used in Europe alone and in combination to treat osteoarthritis since the 1980s. These compounds are substrates for the production of articular cartilage. Glucosamine stimulates the production of glycosaminoglycans, leading to increased synthesis of cartilage. Chondroitin may help maintain articular fluid viscosity, inhibit enzymes that break down cartilage, and stimulate cartilage repair. Glucosamine is prepared commercially from crustacean shells. Chondroitin is extracted from bovine tissues such as cow trachea.

Two meta-analyses and a Cochrane Review of twenty randomized, double-blind, placebo-controlled trials involving more than 2570 patients with osteoarthritis support the use of glucosamine (or glucosamine and chondroitin) in the treatment of osteoarthritis of the knee. The Cochrane Review identified efficacy only for trials using preparations manufactured by Rotta Pharmaceuticals. GAIT is a multicenter randomized double-blind placebo- and celecoxib-controlled clinical trial involving 1583 persons randomized to glucosamine, chondroitin, glucosamine and chondroitin, celecoxib, or placebo. Investigators found no difference overall between the supplements alone and in combination and placebo. In a predefined subgroup of patients with moderate to severe pain, combined therapy with glucosamine and chondroitin sulfate provided greater pain relief than placebo, which in that subgroup was not different than celecoxib.

Glucosamine not only reduces the symptoms of osteoarthritis but may also slow the progression of the disease. Reginster and coworkers randomized 212 patients with osteoarthritis of the knee to receive either 1500 mg/d of glucosamine or placebo. After 3 years, patients taking glucosamine reported a 24% reduction in symptoms versus a 10% increase in the placebo group. X-rays revealed that the treatment patients experienced a loss of only 0.06 mm joint space versus 0.31 mm in the placebo group after 3 years. Glucosamine was very well-tolerated and did not elevate serum glucose levels. Similar results were found in 200 patients with mild to moderate knee osteoarthritis who were randomized to glucosamine sulfate or placebo for 3 years. Patients in the glucosamine group had greater pain relief and less joint space narrowing on radiographs. Several negative trials have been reported in patients with more severe arthritis and in those taking forms of glucosamine other than those made by the European manufacturer Rotta Pharmaceuticals. No drug-herb interactions have been reported. In contrast to NSAIDs, glucosamine is not an analgesic and may take weeks to months before improvement is noticed. In summary, clinical trial literature suggests that glucosamine with or without chondroitin is well tolerated, safe, and effective in the treatment of osteoarthritis, with fewer side effects than NSAIDs.

Clegg DO et al: Glucosamine, chondroitin sulfate, and the two in combination for painful knee osteoarthritis. N Engl J Med 2006;354:795. [PMID: 16495392]

Hughes R et al: A randomized, double-blind, placebo-controlled trial of glucosamine sulphate as an analgesic in osteoarthritis of the knee. Rheumatology (Oxford) 2002;41:279. [PMID: 11934964]

Pavelka K et al: Glucosamine sulfate use and delay of progression of knee osteoarthritis: a 3-year, randomized, placebo-controlled, double-blind study. Arch Intern Med 2002;162:2113. [PMID: 12374520]

Reginster JY et al: Long-term effects of glucosamine sulphate on osteoarthritis progression: a randomized, placebo-controlled clinical trial. Lancet 2001;357:251. [PMID: 11214126]

Richy F et al: Structural and symptomatic efficacy of glucosamine and chondroitin in knee osteoarthritis: a comprehensive meta-analysis. Arch Intern Med 2003;163:1514. [PMID: 12860572]

Towheed TE et al: Glucosamine therapy for treating osteoarthritis. Cochrane Database Syst Rev 2005;(2):CD002946. [PMID: 15846645]

Coenzyme Q$_{10}$

Coenzyme Q$_{10}$ (Ubidecarenon; also known as ubiquinone-10) is an endogenous provitamin that resides in the lipid layer of the mitochondria. It plays a crucial role in oxidative phosphorylation for adenosine triphosphate (ATP) production and is necessary for the basic functioning of all cells. It has also been observed to have effects on membrane stabilization, free radical scavenging, and calcium-dependent slow channels. Coenzyme Q$_{10}$ levels decrease with age. Deficiencies have been observed among patients with certain chronic medical conditions, including cardiovascular disease (hypertension, acute coronary syndromes, congestive heart failure), renal failure, male infertility, periodontal disease, cancer, HIV/AIDS, muscular dystrophies, Parkinson's disease, and Alzheimer's disease. Certain prescription medications may also lower coenzyme Q$_{10}$ levels, including HMG-CoA reductase inhibitors, diabetes medications, β-blockers, diuretics, and antidepressants. Serum levels of coenzyme Q$_{10}$ are increased by taking supplements, but whether this results in clinical benefit remains unproven.

Studies of coenzyme Q$_{10}$ for the prevention and treatment of cardiovascular disease have had mixed results. A 2005 study of 121 patients undergoing elective cardiac surgery showed enhanced myocardial tolerance to in vitro hypoxia-reoxygenation stress among persons receiving coenzyme Q$_{10}$ (300 mg daily) for 2 weeks preoperatively, compared with placebo. A preliminary study showed that combining coenzyme Q$_{10}$ with mild hypothermia after cardiac arrest improved 3-month survival (17/25 vs 7/24; P = .04) and may improve neurologic outcomes. In parts of Russia, Europe, and Japan, coenzyme Q$_{10}$ is part of standard therapy for congestive heart failure. Earlier trials in patients with congestive heart failure demonstrated fewer disease exacerbations,

reduced hospitalizations, improved ejection fraction, and more favorable quality-of-life measurements. However, a 1999 study showed that coenzyme Q$_{10}$ had no effect on ejection fraction, hemodynamic parameters, or quality of life. A study of 55 patients with class III and class IV congestive heart failure receiving standard medical therapy also showed no benefit of coenzyme Q$_{10}$ on ejection fraction, peak oxygen consumption, or exercise duration. Other studies have evaluated coenzyme Q$_{10}$ for acute myocardial infarction, angina, diabetes, hypertension, migraine prophylaxis, and periodontal disease. A year-long study of 144 patients who suffered an acute myocardial infarction had fewer nonfatal myocardial infarctions and cardiac deaths. A randomized, placebo-controlled trial of 74 subjects with uncomplicated type 2 diabetes and dyslipidemia showed that coenzyme Q$_{10}$ supplementation may improve blood pressure control and long-term glycemic control. Although other medical conditions are also associated with low levels of coenzyme Q$_{10}$, additional randomized controlled clinical trials are needed before supplementation with coenzyme Q$_{10}$ can be routinely recommended to improve outcomes for any particular condition.

Because coenzyme Q$_{10}$ is lipophilic, it is often formulated with vegetable oil or vitamin E to enhance its absorption. Its bioavailability is also enhanced when it is taken with meals, especially fat-rich foods. Insomnia, elevated liver enzymes, rash, and abdominal complaints are among the mild adverse reactions reported in clinical trials. No serious adverse events have been noted with coenzyme Q$_{10}$ use, and it is generally well tolerated. No significant drug-herb interactions have been reported, but coenzyme Q$_{10}$ is chemically similar to vitamin K and so theoretically may reduce the effectiveness of warfarin.

Berman M et al: Coenzyme Q$_{10}$ in patients with end-stage heart failure awaiting cardiac transplantation: a randomized, placebo-controlled study. Clin Cardiol 2004;27:295. [PMID: 15188947]

Damian MS et al: Coenzyme Q$_{10}$ combined with mild hypothermia after cardiac arrest: a preliminary study. Circulation 2004;110:3011. [PMID: 15520321]

Hodgson JM et al: Coenzyme Q$_{10}$ improves blood pressure and glycaemic control: a controlled trial in subjects with type 2 diabetes. Eur J Clin Nutr 2002;56:1137. [PMID: 12428181]

Rosenfeldt F et al: Coenzyme Q$_{10}$ therapy before cardiac surgery improves mitochondrial function and in vitro contractility of myocardial tissue. J Thorac Cardiovasc Surg 2005;129:25. [PMID: 15632821]

Singh RB et al: Effect of coenzyme Q$_{10}$ on risk of atherosclerosis in patients with recent myocardial infarction. Mol Cell Biochem 2003;246:75. [PMID: 12841346]

■ ACUPUNCTURE

In acupuncture, certain locations on the surface of the body are stimulated, often with needles, to treat illness and promote health. Practitioners trained in Oriental medicine believe that a vital energy called chi (pronounced "chee") circulates in the body through 12 main pathways called meridians. Each meridian is named after a particular organ or "official," but the term actually relates to the energetic function more than the structure or anatomy of the organ. There are both surface and internal projections for each meridian. The surface projections contain sites called acupuncture points. Oriental medicine practitioners insert needles into these points to influence the body's chi to restore health.

History

The earliest reference to acupuncture can be traced to a text on Chinese medicine called *The Yellow Emperor's Classic of Internal Medicine* (the *Huang Ti Nei Ching*), which dates from the second century BC. This text is often referenced to support the authenticity of a particular practice or theory and is used as part of the curriculum in training colleges. Acupuncture spread through much of Asia and by the sixteenth century Jesuit missionaries had brought the practice to Europe. As early as 1912, William Osler described its use in the first edition of *The Principles and Practice of Medicine.* "For lumbago," he wrote, "acupuncture is, in acute cases, the most efficient treatment." Research and enthusiasm in the United States grew dramatically in 1971 when James Reston wrote an article describing his experience with acupuncture for postoperative analgesia after undergoing an appendectomy while in China.

Mechanism of Action

Acupuncture for analgesia stimulates the nerve fibers that enter the dorsal horn of the spinal cord. An impulse is then sent to other levels within the spinal cord, the midbrain, and the hypothalamic-pituitary system, which then release neurotransmitters that cause analgesia. Therefore, when practitioners place a needle in the region of pain, all three centers are activated to provide an analgesic effect. When practitioners place needles in locations distant from the pain site, only the midbrain and hypothalamic-pituitary systems are activated. Although this theory implies that sham acupuncture may be as effective as real acupuncture, experimentally induced acute pain studies in animals and humans have consistently shown that real point stimulation is far superior to sham. These conflicting findings have prevented sham acupuncture from being widely accepted as an appropriate control. The 1998 NIH Consensus Statement on Acupuncture strongly recommends that future acupuncture research focus on finding such a control. A study of functional brain MRI imaging of healthy volunteers identified preferential activation of the hypothalamus and nucleus accumbens and deactivation of the rostral part of the anterior cingulate cortex, amygdala, and hippocampal complex among patients receiving active needling compared with minimally stimulated controls. Chronic pain studies, however, have shown less consistent results.

Yet, in 2003, Han found that acupuncture or electrical stimulation in specific frequencies can facilitate the release of certain neuropeptides in the central nervous system. Peripheral stimulation of the skin or deeper structures showed activation of specific brain structures and the spinal cord via neural pathways, producing profound physiologic effects and stimulating self-healing mechanisms.

Han JS: Acupuncture: neuropeptide release produced by electrical stimulation of different frequencies. Trends Neurosci 2003; 26:17. [PMID: 12495858]

Stux G, Berman B, Pomeranz B (editors): *Basics of Acupuncture.* 5th ed. Springer, 2003.

Wu MT et al: Central nervous pathways for acupuncture stimulation: localization of processing with functional MR imaging of the brain—preliminary experience. Radiology 1999;212: 133. [PMID: 10405732]

Training, Licensure, & Regulation

Acupuncture educational programs are accredited by the Accreditation Commission for Acupuncture and Oriental Medicine (ACAOM). Typical acupuncture training for nonphysicians in the United States requires completion of an accredited 4-year (2500 hours) master's degree training program. In order to become a licensed acupuncturist (LAc), a national and, frequently, state board examination must be passed. Although many states do not require physicians to obtain additional training, most states require a minimum of 200 hours of training in an accredited program. There are currently over 10,000 licensed acupuncture practitioners and 3000 physician acupuncturists in the United States. In 22 of the 42 states that license, register, or certify acupuncturists, these practitioners are permitted to work independently.

Clinical Practice

In the United States and Europe, Oriental medicine-trained practitioners conduct a comprehensive multisystem history, observation, and physical examination during the initial consultation. Examination consists of palpation of the abdomen and selected acupuncture points; examination of the tongue to assess color, shape, and coating; and palpation of the pulse along the wrist at three locations on both arms to assess its quality, rhythm, and strength. Treatment by the **classic acupuncture method** is based on the belief that each patient presents with a unique constellation of symptoms and signs. What this means is that ten patients presenting with migraine headaches may receive ten different treatments. Western-style practitioners will conduct a conventional examination and include variable components of the Oriental medicine approach depending on the individual's depth of training. Treatment is based on the **formula acupuncture method**, which utilizes a fixed combination of acupuncture points for a given medical diagnosis such that a cohort of migraine sufferers will be treated in the same way.

Treatment involves inserting four to fifteen needles at selected acupuncture points for 10–30 minutes—though certain schools leave the needles in place for only a few seconds to minutes. Needles are approximately 37-gauge, stainless steel, and disposable. Needles are stimulated with electricity, heat, or manually. Follow-up consultations last from 20 minutes to 45 minutes.

Patients can expect to see the practitioner weekly or biweekly for 4–10 weeks, followed by less frequent visits as the condition improves.

Adverse Events

In current practice in the United States and Europe, acupuncture is generally considered safe, associated with a very low incidence of adverse events. Precautions useful for avoiding serious adverse events are listed in Table 42–4. The most frequent problems are vasovagal or sedating reactions such as presyncope, syncope, and drowsiness. These are easily prevented by having the patient lie flat on the table, monitoring patients during the initial visit, and permitting the patient to remain in the office until a normal state of awareness is achieved. Serious complications in the literature over the past 30 years have been due to the reuse of needles between patients, leading to transmission of infection such as hepatitis B and C or HIV, and needling the thorax in patients with emphysema, leading to pneumothorax. There have also been case reports of unusual serious adverse events, including endocarditis in patients with prosthetic heart valves who had small indwelling needles in place for several days, cardiac tamponade after needling directly over the heart, spinal cord trauma from deep insertion or migration of cut or broken retained needles, and pacemaker malfunction during acupuncture with electrical stimulation.

Table 42–4. How to avoid preventable adverse events associated with acupuncture.

Make certain that only sterile disposable needles are used.
When press-in needles are used, make certain that sterile technique is used.
Make certain that the patient is lying flat during the treatment.
Make certain that the practitioner counts the number of needles used before and after treatment.
Exert caution when patients are taking anticoagulants.
Avoid electrical stimulation in patients with pacemakers.
Exert caution when needling the thorax in patients with emphysema.

Modified, with permission, from Rampes H: Adverse reactions to acupuncture. In: *Medical Acupuncture: A Western Scientific Approach.* Filshie J, White A (editors). Churchill Livingstone, 1998.

Most surveys estimate that the frequency of adverse events is 1:100,000 to 1:10,000. A 14-year review of the world literature identified 193 complications and concluded that acupuncture is generally safe except for patients with emphysema, in whom the risk of pneumothorax is significant. Another review identified 300 complications reported in the literature over a 30-year period.

CLINICAL USES OF ACUPUNCTURE

In the United States, acupuncture is frequently used to treat acute non–life-threatening conditions or chronic conditions that conventional medicine is unable to treat effectively (Table 42–5). What follows is a survey of some conditions for which patients frequently seek acupuncture care.

Stroke Rehabilitation

A 2001 systematic review of randomized controlled trials of acupuncture for stroke rehabilitation identified nine trials, including 538 persons meeting study entry criteria. Six of nine trials found acupuncture superior to control interventions, but study quality was poor. These findings suggest that acupuncture appears promising for the treatment of stroke, but studies of high quality are needed to confirm these preliminary findings.

Sze et al performed a meta-analysis assessing the efficacy of acupuncture with and without stroke rehabilitation. Fourteen trials with 1213 patients met the study inclusion criteria. The pooled random-effects estimates of change in motor impairment and disability were 0.06 (95% CI, −0.12 to 0.24) and 0.49 (95% CI, 0.03 to 0.96) for acupuncture and no acupuncture in addition to stroke rehabilitation, respectively. For the comparison of real acupuncture with sham acupuncture, the pooled random-effects estimate of the change in disability was 0.07 (95% CI, −0.34 to 0.48). This study suggests that in conjunction with stroke rehabilitation, acupuncture has no additional effect on motor recovery but has a small positive effect on disability. This may be due to a true placebo effect or to the wide variation in study quality. More high-quality studies are needed to assess the efficacy of acupuncture as an adjunct for stroke rehabilitation.

Park J et al: Effectiveness of acupuncture for stroke: a systematic review. J Neurol 2001;248:558. [PMID: 11517996]

Sze FK et al: Does acupuncture improve motor recovery after stroke? A meta-analysis of randomized controlled trials. Stroke 2002;33:2604. [PMID: 12411650]

Chronic Pain

A criterion-based review of 51 controlled trials of acupuncture for the treatment of chronic pain found 24 trials reporting results favoring acupuncture. Using a 100-point quality scale, only 11 trials scored at least 50 points. The investigators concluded that poor study quality made it impossible to arrive at definitive

Table 42-5. Overview of acupuncture literature for selected medical conditions.

	Condition	Study	Inclusion Criteria	No. of Studies	No. of Patients	Measures	Results
Park, 2001	Stroke rehabilitation	Systematic review	RCTs, all types of stroke.	9	538	Scandinavian and Chinese stroke scales, Barthel Index, Nottingham Health Profile, motor function, balance, and days in hospital.	Overall, acupuncture appears promising for stroke rehabilitation. 6 of 9 trials favor acupuncture compared with control. Future studies require higher study quality to confirm findings.
Sze et al, 2002	Stroke rehabilitation	Meta-analysis	RCTs, intervention within 6 months of stroke.	14	1213	Scandinavian and Chinese stroke scales, Rivermead Mobility Index, Brunnstrom Stages, Fugl-Meyer motor scale, Barthel Index Functional Independence Measure, Sunnaas ADL Index	No additional effect on motor recovery, but small positive effect on disability; future studies require higher qualities to ascertain whether effect on disability is due to placebo effect.
Ezzo, 2000	Chronic pain	Systematic review	RCTs published in English. Pain > 3 months.	47	N/A	Positive report of pain relief; otherwise, not specified.	Inconclusive.
Manheimer, 2005	Low back pain	Meta-analysis	RCTs, acute or chronic low back pain.	33	2138	Pain relief.	Acupuncture is significantly more effective than sham treatment for short-term relief of chronic pain, but it is not more effective than other active therapies for chronic low back pain. The data were sparse and inconclusive for acute low back pain.
Furlan, 2005	Low back pain	Systematic review	RCTs, acute and chronic low back pain.	35	2861	Pain and function.	Acupuncture is better than sham or no treatment for short-term relief and improvement of function in chronic low back pain. The data suggest it is a useful adjunct to other therapies.
Ezzo et al, 2001	Osteoarthritis of the knee	Systematic review	RCTs, quasi-RCTs of all languages.	7	393	Pain, function, global improvement, imaging.	For pain and functioning, limited evidence of acupuncture efficacy over control. For pain, real acupuncture is more effective than sham. For functioning, inconclusive evidence that real acupuncture is better than sham.

(continued)

Table 42–5. Overview of acupuncture literature for selected medical conditions. (continued)

	Condition	Study	Inclusion Criteria	No. of Studies	No. of Patients	Measures	Results
Ernst, 1998	Acute dental pain	Systematic review	Controlled trials.	16	941	Pain relief.	Definitive conclusion that acupuncture is superior to sham and placebo-controlled acupuncture. Evidence for use as adjunctive therapy.
Melchart, 2002	Recurrent headache	Systematic review	RCTs, quasi-RCTs.	26	1151	Any one clinical outcome related to headache, eg, pain intensity, global assessment.	Overall, the data support acupuncture for the treatment of recurrent headaches. 8/16 found real acupuncture superior to sham acupuncture; 4/16 found a trend favoring real acupuncture.
Linde, 2000	Asthma	Systematic review	Randomized and quasi-randomized trials.	7	174	All subjective and objective outcomes.	There is insufficient evidence to make recommendations about the value of acupuncture for chronic asthma.
Martin et al, 2002	Asthma	Systematic review and meta-analysis	RCTs.	11	N/A	Peak expiratory flow rate, FEV_1, and FVC.	Inconclusive. Did not find evidence for value of acupuncture in reducing asthma. However, methodologic limitations of trials were present.
Lee, 1999	Postoperative nausea and vomiting	Meta-analysis	RCTs, trials stimulating P6 acupuncture point by needling, manual pressure, or electricity.	19	N/A	Number of episodes of nausea, vomiting or both 0–6 h or 0–48 h after surgery.	Equal benefit compared with first-line antiemetics. Clear benefit compared with placebo.
White, 2002	Tobacco addiction	Meta-analysis	RCTs.	22	4608	Abstinence	No better than sham acupuncture at 6 weeks, 6 months, 12 months.

RCT = randomized controlled trial; N/A = not applicable; FEV_1 = forced expiratory volume in 1 second; FVC = forced vital capacity.

conclusions. Preliminary results from studies of auricular acupuncture for cancer pain and acupuncture for chronic epicondylitis and chronic neck pain show that acupuncture may be beneficial.

Overall, there is some evidence suggesting benefit of acupuncture for persons with chronic pain when compared with placebo and insufficient evidence to suggest acupuncture is superior to standard medical care or sham acupuncture. The ability to make definitive recommendations regarding efficacy for chronic pain is hampered by poor methodologic study quality.

Alimi D et al: Analgesic effect of auricular acupuncture for cancer pain: A randomized, blinded, controlled trial. J Clin Oncol 2003;15:4120. [PMID: 14615440]

Ezzo J et al: Is acupuncture effective for the treatment of chronic pain? A systematic review. Pain 2000;86:217. [PMID: 10812251]

Green S et al: Acupuncture for lateral elbow pain. Cochrane Database Syst Rev 2002;(1):CD003527. [PMID: 11869671]

Lewith et al: Acupuncture versus placebo for the treatment of chronic mechanical neck pain. A randomized, controlled trial. Ann Intern Med 2004;141:911. [PMID: 15611488]

Low Back Pain

Manheimer and colleagues published a meta-analysis in 2005 on acupuncture in the treatment of low back pain that included 33 randomized, controlled trials that met inclusion criteria, involving a total of 2138 patients. For the primary outcome of short-term relief of chronic pain, the meta-analysis showed that acupuncture is significantly more effective than sham treatment and no additional treatment. Similar conclusions were reached in a Cochrane systematic review of 35 randomized controlled trials (involving 2861 patients) published by Furlan and coworkers. Furlan et al also concluded that acupuncture improved function in patients with chronic low back pain. Neither review found that acupuncture was more effective than other active therapies for chronic low back pain. However, when acupuncture was added to other conventional therapies, it relieved pain and improved function more than the conventional therapies alone. Effect sizes tended to be small. The data was sparse and inconclusive for acute low back pain.

Furlan AD et al: Acupuncture and dry-needling for low back pain: an updated systematic review within the framework of the cochrane collaboration. Spine 2005;30:944. [PMID: 15834340]

Manheimer E et al: Meta analysis: acupuncture for low back pain. Ann Intern Med 2005;142:651. [PMID: 15838072]

Osteoarthritis

In 2001, Ezzo and colleagues performed a systematic review of acupuncture for osteoarthritis of the knee. Seven trials assessed 393 patients on the outcomes of pain, function, global improvement, and imaging. For pain and function, limited support was found for the efficacy of acupuncture over a wait list control or treatment as usual. For pain, real acupuncture was more effective than sham acupuncture. For level of

function, however, real acupuncture was not found to be more effective than sham acupuncture.

Vas and colleagues performed a randomized, controlled trial of 97 patients suffering from osteoarthritis of the knee. The patients were separated into two groups: one received acupuncture in conjunction with diclofenac and the other received placebo acupuncture with diclofenac. The study concluded that acupuncture, as an adjunctive therapy to pharmacologic treatment for osteoarthritis of the knee, was more effective than pharmacologic treatment alone.

In a larger and more extensive trial, the NIH funded a multicenter randomized controlled trial based at the University of Maryland; 570 patients were tested to see whether acupuncture provides greater pain relief and improved function compared with sham acupuncture or education in patients with osteoarthritis of the knee. The 570 patients were separated into three groups: 190 patients received true acupuncture, 191 received sham acupuncture, and 189 received educational treatment. Over a period of 26 weeks the two acupuncture groups received a total of 23 sessions. After 8 weeks, optimal acupuncture effects were observed in the experimental, true acupuncture group compared with the sham acupuncture. Overall, Berman and colleagues concluded that acupuncture may have an important role in adjunctive therapy as a part of a multidisciplinary integrative approach to treating symptoms related to knee osteoarthritis.

An additional randomized controlled trial of 300 patients with osteoarthritis of the knee was published in 2005 by Witt et al, comparing acupuncture with sham and no acupuncture. The acupuncture and sham acupuncture groups received twelve treatments over 8 weeks. Sham acupuncture involved superficial needling at nonacupuncture points not at the knee, whereas in the Vas and Berman studies there was no needle penetration. There was greater improvement in the acupuncture group than both the sham and waiting list groups in both pain and function at end of treatment. However, the benefit appeared to decrease over time and was no longer significant at 26 weeks.

Berman BM et al: Effectiveness of acupuncture as adjunctive therapy in osteoarthritis of the knee. Ann Intern Med 2004; 141:901. [PMID: 15611487]

Ezzo J et al: Acupuncture for osteoarthritis of the knee: A systematic review. Arthritis Rheum 2001;44:819. [PMID: 11315921]

Vas J et al: Acupuncture as a complementary therapy to the pharmacological treatment of osteoarthritis of the knee: randomised controlled trial. BMJ 2004;329:1216. [PMID: 15494348]

Witt C et al: Acupuncture in patients with osteoarthritis of the knee: a randomised trial. Lancet 2005;366:136. [PMID: 16005336]

Acute Dental Pain

The NIH consensus development statement on acupuncture states, "There is evidence of efficacy for postoperative dental pain." A review in 1998 identified 16 controlled trials of acupuncture for the treatment of acute dental pain. Among the eight randomized and at least partially blinded trials, seven showed benefit. Among the seven trials using sham control, six showed benefit. Subsequent to this review, a randomized, double-blind, placebo acupuncture-controlled trial involving 39 patients evaluated acupuncture for the treatment of postsurgical dental pain. Controls experienced a similar tap sensation next to the acupuncture sites to produce a noticeable sensation; however, needle insertion was not performed. Patients receiving acupuncture scored more favorably than controls on multiple outcomes. There is thus sufficient evidence to recommend the use of acupuncture as effective adjunctive treatment for the treatment of acute dental pain. Multiple studies have demonstrated its efficacy when compared with sham acupuncture.

Ernst E et al: The effectiveness of acupuncture in treating acute dental pain: a systematic review. Br Dent J 1998; 184:443. [PMID: 9617000]

Lao L et al: Evaluation of acupuncture for pain control after oral surgery: a placebo-controlled trial. Arch Otolaryngol Head Neck Surg 1999;125:567. [PMID: 10326816]

Headache

Melchart et al performed a systematic review in 2002 to evaluate the treatment of acupuncture for recurrent headaches. That group identified 26 randomized and quasi-randomized trials involving 1151 subjects in which 16 trials studied migraine headaches, 6 studied tension headaches, and 4 studied mixed headaches. Of the 16 trials that used sham acupuncture, 8 found real acupuncture superior to sham acupuncture and 4 found a trend in favor of real acupuncture. Two trials found no difference between groups, and 2 trials were uninterpretable. In the remaining 10 trials, conflicting results were reported. Overall, investigators believed there was evidence that acupuncture is effective in the treatment of recurrent headaches.

In a 2004 trial performed by Vickers and colleagues, 401 patients with chronic headache, predominantly migraine, received up to 12 acupuncture treatments and the results showed that the experimental group experienced 22 fewer days of headache per year, used 15% less medication, made 25% fewer visits to general practitioners, and took 15% fewer sick days, in comparison to the group that received no acupuncture in addition to medication. Overall, the study showed that acupuncture leads to persisting, clinically relevant benefits for primary care patients with chronic headache, particularly migraine.

Melchart D et al: Acupuncture for idiopathic headache. Cochrane Database Syst Rev 2002;(1):CD001218. [PMID: 11279710]

Vickers AJ et al: Acupuncture for chronic headache in primary care: large, pragmatic, randomised trial. BMJ 2004;328: 744. [PMID: 15023828]

Asthma

Linde performed a systematic review of randomized and possibly randomized clinical trials that evaluated the effects of acupuncture for the treatment of asthma. Seven trials met study entry criteria, including 174 participants. All trials compared real acupuncture with sham acupuncture. Among the three trials that measured postexpiratory flow rates, there was no difference between the real and sham acupuncture groups. The authors conclude that there is insufficient evidence that acupuncture has a significant treatment effect for people with asthma. No research has evaluated the efficacy of acupuncture as part of a comprehensive treatment program. Among trials reporting positive results, benefit was primarily identified in subjective rather than objective measures. Because asthma can be a life-threatening condition for which effective standard medical therapy exists, acupuncture should be used only as an adjunct to conventional therapy.

Martin performed a systematic review and meta-analysis from 11 randomized controlled trials. Trials compared acupuncture at real and placebo points with outcome measures consisting of at least one of the following: peak expiratory flow rate, forced expiratory volume in 1 second (FEV_1), and vital capacity. Studies in which bronchoconstriction was experimentally induced showed a significant effect favoring real acupuncture. Overall, no evidence for an effect of acupuncture in reducing asthma was found; however, methodologic shortcomings such as small sample size may have precluded identifying statistically significant differences between groups.

Linde K et al: Acupuncture for chronic asthma. Cochrane Database Syst Rev 2000;(2):CD000008. [PMID: 10796465]

Martin J et al: Efficacy of acupuncture in asthma: systematic review and meta-analysis of published data from 11 randomised controlled trials. Eur Respir J 2002;20:846. [PMID: 12412674]

Nausea & Vomiting

Based on multiple randomized controlled trials, there is strong evidence demonstrating effectiveness of acupuncture in the treatment of pregnancy-induced, chemotherapy-induced, and postoperative nausea and vomiting. One review identified 33 trials using a particular acupuncture point (P6) for treatment of nausea and vomiting. None of the four trials in which acupuncture was given while the patient was under general anesthesia demonstrated a positive effect. Among the remaining 29 trials, 27 identified real acupuncture as being more effective than sham acupuncture or placebo control. In subgroup analyses, all five studies evaluating acupuncture for cancer chemotherapy-induced nausea and vomiting were positive. Six of the seven studies for pregnancy-induced symptoms were positive. Among trials in which acupuncture was performed while the subjects were not under general anesthesia, 16 of 17 studies of treatment for postoperative nausea and vomiting were positive. In sensitivity analyses, 11 of the 12 high-quality trials involving over 2000 patients identified acupuncture as superior to control. A subsequent review on studies of treatment for postoperative nausea and vomiting reported acupuncture to be equivalent to first-line antiemetics in preventing early and late vomiting. The NIH consensus development panel on acupuncture stated, "There is clear evidence that needle acupuncture is efficacious for adult postoperative and chemotherapy induced nausea and vomiting and probably for the nausea of pregnancy."

Lee A et al: The use of nonpharmacologic techniques to prevent postoperative nausea and vomiting: a meta-analysis. Anesth Analg 1999;88:1362. [PMID: 10357346]

Shen J et al: Electroacupuncture for control of myeloablative chemotherapy-induced emesis. JAMA 2000;284:2755. [PMID: 11105182]

Vickers AJ: Can acupuncture have specific effects on health? A systematic review of acupuncture antiemesis trials. J R Soc Med 1996;89:303. [PMID: 8758186]

Nicotine, Heroin, Cocaine, & Alcohol Addiction

There is good evidence suggesting that acupuncture is not effective in maintaining abstinence from nicotine addiction. Systematic reviews have identified multiple trials of sufficient quality to determine that there is no evidence to support its use. In a randomized trial comparing electroacupuncture and sham control for nicotine withdrawal symptoms, there was no difference in nicotine withdrawal symptoms or abstinence rates at day 14. The NIH consensus development statement acupuncture states, "There is evidence that acupuncture does not demonstrate efficacy for cessation of smoking."

Despite insufficient evidence to support its use, auricular acupuncture is in widespread use throughout American drug treatment facilities. Although heroin, alcohol, and cocaine addiction studies have frequently reported positive outcomes, serious methodologic flaws are present. For example, an 8-week clinical trial showed patients assigned to acupuncture were significantly more likely to remain abstinent from cocaine use. However, analyses did not adjust for the 50% versus 20% dropout rate in the acupuncture and relaxation groups, respectively. A randomized controlled, single-blind trial conducted in six community-based ___ in the United States found that acupuncture ___ ___ive than needle insertion control or ___ ___ucing cocaine use. Until scien___ ___s can demonstrate efficacy, acu___ ___e used as monotherapy in the ___ctions.

___ized controlled trial of auricular acu___ dependence. Arch Intern Med 2000; ___)927727]

___re for the treatment of cocaine addition: ___led trial. JAMA 2002;287:55. [PMID: ___

___e for smoking cessation. Cochrane Da___ ;(2):CD000009. [PMID: 12076375]

■ HOMEOPATHY

Christian F.S. Hahnemann is credited with devising the system of homeopathy in 1790. Three main principles of homeopathy include the "law of similars," the use of dilute concentrations of medicines, and "potentization." The second and third principles remain the most controversial for many scientists and conventionally trained physicians.

The law of similars is also known as the principle of "like cures like"; it is derived from the observation that a homeopathic medicine when given to a healthy volunteer will produce a constellation of symptoms similar to those it will cure in an ill patient. Since the 1800s, the process of testing medicines on healthy volunteers to record the symptoms provoked (known as "provings") has been recorded and compiled to create several materia medicas. A randomized double-blind crossover trial was performed to evaluate whether homeopathic substances can bring about symptoms different from observation and placebo. Investigators report an insignificant tendency to report more symptoms when taking belladonna 30CH compared with control arms. However, there was no indication that symptoms were different between groups or compared with baseline presentations.

The second principle—the use of dilute concentrations of medicine—entails serially diluting and "succussing" (shaking) a substance to concentrations in which there is little probability of any molecules remaining in solution. Homeopathic physicians assert that these remedies remain pharmacologically active and allude to allergy desensitization and immunization as sharing similar approaches to homeopathy in that both use low doses of potentially toxic substances to achieve beneficial clinical effects.

Potentization is based on the claim that once a medicine is at low concentration, the more dilute the solute the more potent the effect.

The World Health Organization states that homeopathy is the second most used medical system internationally, with over $1 billion in expenditures for such therapy. Twenty to 30 percent of French and German physicians use homeopathy in clinical practice. In Great Britain, five homeopathic hospitals are part of the National Health System, and over 30% of generalists use homeopathy. In the United States, there are more than 500 physicians and 5000 nonphysicians using homeopathy in clinical practice, and 2.5 million Americans currently use homeopathic medicines—of which two-thirds are self-prescribed—spending more than $250 million annually.

Mechanisms of Action

Although there are several mechanisms under investigation, none are well validated. One of the more interesting findings in the chemistry literature reports the presence of the solute clusters in highly diluted water. This report requires independent replication and if confirmed requires demonstration of the clinical effects in living organisms.

Adverse Events & Interactions

Given the low concentration of homeopathic medicines, the probability of adverse events is remote. However, adverse events have been reported from ingestion of large quantities of remedies containing heavy metals. Some patients report an exacerbation of symptoms initially. Homeopaths explain this reaction as the initial phase of the healing response. Homeopathic remedies are not known to have interaction with conventional medicines.

Training, Licensure, & Regulation

In Europe, practitioners usually enroll in a 3–6 year professional degree program or physicians enroll in postgraduate training. In the United States, homeopathic educational programs are accredited by the Council for Homeopathic Education, which was founded in 1982 as an independent agency to assess homeopathic training in the United States and Canada. There are two levels of training for homeopaths. The Primary Care Certificate in Homeotherapeutics requires 60–100 hours of course work and passage of a written examination. The more advanced level, the Diplomate in Homeotherapeutics (DHt), requires an additional 3 years of clinical practice. There is comprehensive homeopathic training that involves 3 or more years of part-time to full-time study. Nonphysicians may practice homeopathy within the scope of practice of their specific profession. The American Board of Homeotherapeutics governs certification for physicians; the Homeopathic Association of Naturopathic Physicians governs naturopaths; and the Council for Homeopathic Certification governs all other practitioners. Physicians are licensed to practice homeopathy in three states (Connecticut, Arizona, and Nevada).

The *Homeopathic Pharmacopoeia of the United States* was included in the original Food and Drug Act of 1938, which declared that homeopathic remedies may be purchased without a physician prescription, in the same manner as over-the-counter, nonprescription compounds. Unlike over-the-counter drugs in the United States, there is no requirement for testing for safety and effectiveness. However, the FDA does require the products to meet good manufacturing practices for quality, purity, packaging, and strength. In addition, the FDA requires companies to include on the label indications for use, dilutions, and ingredients.

Clinical Encounter

The initial consultation takes about 1–1.5 hours, with significant time spent on obtaining a detailed history. Attention is given to the physical, mental, and emotional symptoms, overall personality type, and any internal or external factors that influence the presenting symptoms, such as emotions, wind, season of the year, and reactions to different foods. The symptom inventory is then matched to an appropriate remedy taken from the materia medica. Follow-up visits may last for a few minutes to 40 minutes. During the follow-up visit, the practitioner determines if there has been improvement in symptoms, no change, or aggravation of symptoms. The latter scenario, if transient, is viewed as the first sign of recovery.

Clinical Uses

Homeopathic physicians are trained to treat a broad range of conditions in the primary care and specialty setting. In clinical practice, however, practitioners frequently treat patients with chronic conditions that conventional medicine cannot adequately address, including arthritis, allergies, autoimmune diseases, or non–life-threatening acute conditions such as viral infections or minor trauma. Parents may take their children to homeopathic physicians for recurrent conditions such as otitis media and allergies with the goal of avoiding repetitive antibiotic, corticosteroid, or long-term conventional medications.

Research

The findings for individual randomized controlled trials on homeopathy have been contradictory. Over 180 controlled trials and over 10 reviews have been published on the effects of homeopathy compared with placebo. The majority of trials are published in non-English language journals and are frequently not listed in Medline. A few methodologically rigorous reviews have been published in English (Table 42–6). The majority of systematic reviews have pooled trials on homeopathy regardless of the medical condition being treated. Many reviews have found that patient outcomes in homeopathic treatment groups were superior to placebo group outcomes. Since many of the trials do not provide in-depth reports on the treatment encounter, it remains unclear whether these positive effects are specific to the homeopathic remedy itself or to nonspecific effects that occur as part of the treatment encounter. Since few trials have been replicated by independent investigators, there is insufficient evidence to determine whether treatment effects found for a single medical condition are reproducible. Conditions with the best evidence for a positive clinical effect include acute childhood diarrhea, influenza, and postoperative ileus; whereas, the homeopathic remedy arnica frequently used to reduce tissue trauma appears to have no clinical benefit over placebo (Table 42–6).

A 1997 systematic review identified 89 double-blind or randomized placebo-controlled trials and found the overall combined odds ratio was 2.45 (95% CI, 2.0–2.9) favoring patients in the homeopathy-treated group. Analyses restricted to high-quality stud-

Table 42–6. Overview of English language homeopathy systematic reviews.

	Condition or Remedy	Inclusion Criteria	No. of Studies	Measures	Results	Conclusions
Linde, 1997	No limitation	RBTs or RCTs	89	Pooled summary estimates	Overall: OR = 2.45 (95% CI 2.0–2.9) High-quality: OR = 1.7 (95% CI 1.3–2.1) Publication-bias correction: OR = 1.8 (95% CI 1.0–3.1) Seasonal allergies[1]: OR = 2.0 (95% CI 1.5–2.7) Postoperative ileus[2]: effect-size difference = −0.22 SD (95% CI −0.33 to −0.03)	Positive findings. Unable to determine whether homeopathy is effective for any single clinical condition under prior defined criteria.
Cucherat, 2000	No limitation	RCTs with clearly defined primary outcome	16	Pooled summary estimates	Overall: $P = 0.000036$ High-quality trials: $P = .08$	Positive findings overall. Study quality is inversely associated with probability of obtaining a statistically significant result.
Barnes, 1997	Postoperative ileus/no limitations	RCTs	6	Pooled summary estimates	Time to first flatus: 7.4 hours earlier favoring homeopathy ($P < .05$). Effect remained after adjustment for study quality.	Clinically meaningful effect with reservation due to variable study quality of trials.
Ernst, 1998	No limitation/Arnica	RCTs	8	Descriptive analysis	6 of 8 trials showed no statistically significant benefit over placebo.	Arnica appears no more effective than placebo. Most studies evaluated Arnica for tissue trauma and bruising.
Vickers, 2004	Influenza/Oscillococcinum	RBTs	7	Pooled summary estimates	Length of illness: 0.28 days reduction (95% CI 0.50–0.06). Prevention of influenza: RR = 0.64 (95% CI 0.28–1.43)	Reduction in length of illness promising; however, not sufficient to recommend as first-line therapy. Current evidence does not support Oscillococcinum for influenza prevention.
Jacobs, 2003	Childhood diarrhea/individualized treatment	Convenient sample of RBTs	3	Pooled summary estimate	Duration of diarrhea: 0.66 day reduction ($P = .008$)	Individualized homeopathic treatment decreases duration of childhood diarrhea.
McCarney, 2004	Chronic asthma/no limitation	RCTs	6	Descriptive analysis	Conflicting results for lung function between studies. No trial reported significant difference on validated symptom scales.	Insufficient evidence to assess effectiveness.

[1]Not independent investigators.
[2]Different remedies used.
RBT = randomized double-blind trial; RCT = randomized controlled trial; OR = odds ratio; CI = confidence interval.

ies found similar statistically significant results with an odds ratio of 1.66 (95% CI, 1.3–2.1); this effect persisted after adjustment for publication bias. Pooled analysis of four multicenter trials by the same investigator evaluating the effects of *Galphimia glauca* for seasonal allergies found an odds ratio of 2.0 (95% CI, 1.5–2.7) for improvement in ocular and nasal symptoms at 4 weeks.

A meta-analysis conducted in 2000 identified 118 randomized controlled clinical trials of which 16 satisfied inclusion criteria. Investigators reported that patients receiving homeopathic remedies compared with placebo were significantly more likely to have improved treatment outcomes (P = .00003); however, analyses limited to the five high-quality studies revealed only a trend for improvement (P = .08). Overall, there is some evidence that homeopathy is more effective than placebo; however, multiple high-quality studies of individual conditions are needed to validate these findings.

Cucherat M et al: Evidence of clinical efficacy of homeopathy: a meta-analysis of clinical trials. Eur J Clin Pharmacol 2000; 56:27. [PMID: 10853874]

Jacobs J et al: Homeopathy for childhood diarrhea: combined results and meta-analysis from three randomized, controlled clinical trials. Pediatr Infect Dis J 2003:22:229. [PMID: 12634583]

Jonas W: Neuroprotection from glutamate toxicity with ultra-low dose glutamate. Neuroreport 2001;12:335. [PMID: 11209946]

Linde K et al: Are the clinical effects of homeopathy placebo effects? A meta-analysis of placebo-controlled trials. Lancet 1997;350:834. [PMID: 9310601]

McCarney R et al: Homeopathy for chronic asthma. Cochrane Database Syst Rev 2004;1:CD000353. [PMID: 14973954]

Reilly D et al: Is evidence for homoeopathy reproducible? Lancet 1994;344:1601. [PMID: 7983994]

Samal S et al: Unexpected solute aggregation in water on dilution. Chem Commun (Camb) 2001;(21):2224. [PMID: 12240122]

Vickers AJ: Homoeopathic Oscillococcinum for preventing and treating influenza and influenza-like syndromes. Cochrane Database Syst Rev 2004;(1):CD001957. [PMID: 14973976]

Appendix: Therapeutic Drug Monitoring & Laboratory Reference Ranges

C. Diana Nicoll, MD, PhD, MPA

Table 1. Therapeutic drug monitoring.[1]

Drug	Effective Concentrations	Half-Life (hours)	Dosage Adjustment	Comments
Amikacin	Peak: 20–30 mg/L; trough: < 10 mg/L	2–3 ↑ in uremia	↓ in renal dysfunction	Concomitant kanamycin or tobramycin therapy may give falsely elevated amikacin results by immunoassay.
Amitriptyline	95–250 ng/mL	9–46		Drug is highly protein-bound. Patient-specific decrease in protein binding may invalidate quoted range of effective concentration.
Carbamazepine	4–12 mg/L	10–15		Induces its own metabolism. Metabolite 10,11-epoxide exhibits 13% cross-reactivity by immunoassay. Toxicity: diplopia, drowsiness, nausea, vomiting, and ataxia.
Cyclosporine	100–300 mcg/L (ng/mL) whole blood	6–12	Need to know specimen and methodology used	Cyclosporine is lipid-soluble (20% bound to leukocytes; 40% to erythrocytes; 40% in plasma, highly bound to lipoproteins). Binding is temperature-dependent, so whole blood is preferred to plasma or serum as specimen. High-performance liquid chromatography (HPLC) or monoclonal fluorescence polarization immunoassay measures cyclosporine reliably; polyclonal fluorescence polarization immunoassays cross-react with metabolites, so the therapeutic range used with those assays is higher. Anticonvulsants and rifampin increase metabolism. Erythromycin, ketoconazole, and calcium channel blockers decrease metabolism.
Desipramine	100–250 ng/mL	13–23		Drug is highly protein-bound. Patient-specific decrease in protein binding may invalidate quoted range of effective concentration.
Digoxin	0.8–2 ng/mL	42; ↑ in uremia, CHF	↓ in renal dysfunction, CHF, hypothyroidism ↑ in hyperthyroidism	Bioavailability of digoxin tablets is 50–90%. Specimen must not be drawn within 6 hours of dose. Dialysis does not remove a significant amount. Hypokalemia potentiates toxicity. Digitalis toxicity is a clinical and *not* a laboratory diagnosis. Digibind (digoxin-specific antibody) therapy of digoxin overdose can interfere with measurement of digoxin levels depending on the digoxin assay. Elimination reduced by quinidine, verapamil, and amiodarone.
Ethosuximide	40–100 mg/L	Child: 30 Adult: 50		Levels used primarily to assess compliance. Toxicity is rare and does not correlate well with plasma concentrations.

(continued)

Table 1. Therapeutic drug monitoring.[1] (continued)

Drug	Effective Concentrations	Half-Life (hours)	Dosage Adjustment	Comments
Gentamicin	Peak: 4–8 mg/L; trough: < 2 mg/L	2–5 ↑ in uremia (7.3 on dialysis)	↓ in renal dysfunction	Draw peak specimen 30 minutes after end of infusion. Draw trough just before next dose. In uremic patients, carbenicillin may decrease gentamicin half-life from 46 hours to 22 hours.
Imipramine	180–350 ng/mL	10–16		Drug is highly protein-bound. Patient-specific decrease in protein binding may invalidate quoted range of effective concentration.
Lidocaine	1–5 mg/L	1.8 ↔ in uremia, CHF; ↑ in cirrhosis	↓ in CHF, liver disease	Levels increased with cimetidine therapy. Central nervous system toxicity common in the elderly.
Lithium	0.7–1.5 mmol/L	22 ↑ in uremia	↓ in renal dysfunction	Thiazides and loop diuretics may increase serum lithium levels.
Methotrexate		8.4 ↑ in uremia	↓ in renal dysfunction	7-Hydroxymethotrexate cross-reacts 1.5% in immunoassay. To minimize toxicity, leucovorin should be continued if methotrexate level is > 0.1 mcmol/L at 48 hours after start of therapy. Methotrexate > 1 mcmol/L at > 48 hours requires an increase in leucovorin rescue therapy.
Nortriptyline	50–140 ng/mL	18–44		Drug is highly protein-bound. Patient-specific decrease in protein binding may invalidate quoted range of effective concentration.
Phenobarbital	10–40 mg/L	86 ↑ in cirrhosis	↓ in liver disease	Metabolized primarily by the hepatic microsomal enzyme system. Many drug-drug interactions.
Phenytoin	10–20 mg/L; 5–10 mg/L in uremia, hypoalbuminemia	Dose-dependent		Metabolite cross-reacts 10% in immunoassay. Metabolism is capacity-limited. Increase dose cautiously when level approaches therapeutic range, since new steady-state level may be disproportionately higher. Drug is very highly protein-bound; protein binding is decreased in uremia and hypoalbuminemia.
Primidone	5–10 mg/L	8		Phenobarbital cross-reacts 0.5%. Metabolized to phenobarbital. Primidone/phenobarbital ratio > 1:2 suggests poor compliance.
Procainamide	4–8 mg/L	3 ↑ in uremia	↓ in renal dysfunction	30% of patients with plasma levels of 12–16 mcg/mL have electrocardiographic changes; 40% of patients with plasma levels of > 16 mcg/mL have severe toxicity. Metabolite *N*-acetylprocainamide is active.
Quinidine	1–4 mg/L	7 ↔ in CHF; ↑ in liver disease	↓ in liver disease, CHF	Effective concentration is lower in chronic liver disease and nephrosis, where binding is decreased.
Salicylate	150–300 mg/L	Dose-dependent		
Theophylline	5–20 mg/L	9	↓ in CHF, cirrhosis, and with cimetidine	Caffeine cross-reacts 10%. Elimination is increased 1.5–2 times in smokers. 1,3-Dimethyl uric acid metabolite increased in uremia and, because of cross-reactivity, may cause an apparent slight increase in serum theophylline.

(continued)

Table 1. Therapeutic drug monitoring.[1] (continued)

Drug	Effective Concentrations	Half-Life (hours)	Dosage Adjustment	Comments
Tobramycin	Peak: 5–10 mg/L; trough: < 2 mg/L	2–3 ↑ in uremia	↓ in renal dysfunction	Tobramycin, kanamycin, and amikacin may cross-react in immunoassay.
Valproic acid	55–100 mg/L	13–19		95% protein-bound. Decreased binding in uremia and cirrhosis.
Vancomycin	Trough: 5–15 mg/L	6 ↑ in uremia	↓ in renal dysfunction	Toxicity in uremic patients leads to irreversible deafness. Keep peak level < 30–40 mg/L to avoid toxicity.

[1]Use red-topped tube (not marbled) for therapeutic drug monitoring. In general, the specimen should be drawn just before the next dose (trough).
× = unchanged; ↑ = increase(d); ↓ = decrease(d); CHF = congestive heart failure.
Modified and reproduced, with permission, from Nicoll D et al: *Pocket Guide to Diagnostic Tests*, 4th ed. McGraw-Hill, 2004.

Table 2. Reference ranges for commonly used tests.[1,2]

		Current metric units × Conversion factor = SI units SI units ÷ Conversion factor = Current metric units			
Test	Specimen	Conventional Units	Conversion Factor	SI Units[2]	Collection
Acetaminophen	Serum	10–20 mg/L **Panic: > 50 mg/L**	66.16	66–132 mcmol/L	Serum separator tube (SST)
Acetoacetate	Serum or urine	Negative		Negative	SST or urine container
Adrenocorticotropic hormone (ACTH)	Plasma	9–52 pg/mL (laboratory-specific)	0.22	2–11 pmol/L	Siliconized glass or plastic lavender
Alanine aminotransferase (ALT, SGPT, GPT)	Serum	7–56 units/L (laboratory-specific)	0.02	0.14–1.12 mckat/L (laboratory-specific)	SST
Albumin	Serum	3.4–4.7 g/dL	10.00	34–47 g/L	SST
Aldosterone	Serum	Salt-loaded (120 mEq Na^+/d): Supine: 3–10 ng/dL Upright: 5–30 ng/dL Salt-depleted (20 mEq Na^+/d): Supine: 12–36 ng/dL Upright: 17–137 ng/dL	27.74	83–277 pmol/L 139–831 pmol/L 332–997 pmol/L 471–3795 pmol/L	SST
	Urine	Salt-loaded (120 mEq Na^+/d for 3–4 days): 1.5–12.5 mcg/24 h Salt-depleted (20 mEq Na^+/d for 3–4 days): 18–85 mcg/24 h	2.77	4.2–34.6 nmol/d 49.9–235.5 nmol/d	Boric acid
Alkaline phosphatase	Serum	41–133 units/L (method- and age-dependent)	0.02	0.7–2.2 mckat/L (method- and age-dependent)	SST
Ammonia (NH_3)	Plasma	18–60 mcg/dL	0.59	11–35 mcmol/L	Green (iced)
Amylase	Serum	20–110 units/L (laboratory-specific)	0.02	0.33–1.83 mckat/L (laboratory-specific)	SST

(continued)

Table 2. Reference ranges for commonly used tests.[1,2] (continued)

| | | **Current metric units × Conversion factor = SI units** | | | |
| | | **SI units ÷ Conversion factor = Current metric units** | | | |
Test	**Specimen**	**Conventional Units**	**Conversion Factor**	**SI Units[2]**	**Collection**
Angiotensin-converting enzyme (ACE)	Serum	12–35 units/L (method-dependent)	16.67	< 590 nkat/L (method-dependent)	SST
Antithrombin III (AT III)	Plasma	84–123% (qualitative) 22–39 mg/dL (quantitative)			Blue
α_1-Antitrypsin	Serum	110–270 mg/dL	0.01	1.1–2.7 g/L	SST
Aspartate aminotransferase (AST, SGOT, GOT)	Serum	0–35 units/L (laboratory-specific)	0.02	0–0.58 mckat/L (laboratory-specific)	SST
Basophil count	Whole blood	$0.01–0.12 \times 10^3$/mcL	1.00	$0.01–0.12 \times 10^9$/L	Lavender
Bilirubin	Serum	Total: 0.1–1.2 mg/dL Direct (conjugated to glucuronide): 0.1–0.5 mg/dL Indirect (unconjugated): 0.1–0.7 mg/dL	17.10	2–21 mcmol/L < 8 mcmol/L < 12 mcmol/L	SST
Blood urea nitrogen (BUN)	Serum	8–20 mg/dL	0.36	2.9–7.1 mmol/L	SST
β-Natriuretic peptide	Whole blood	< 50 pg/mL			Lavender
C-peptide	Serum	0.8–4.0 ng/mL	1.00	0.8–4.0 mcg/L	Iced (fasting) Gold SST
C-reactive protein	Serum	< 5 mg/L	1.00	< 5 mg/L	SST
Calcitonin	Plasma	Male: 0–11.5 pg/mL Female: 0–4.6 pg/mL	1.00	Male: 0–11.5 ng/L Female: 0–4.6 ng/L	Green Gold SST
Calcium (Ca^{2+})	Serum	8.5–10.5 mg/dL **Panic:** < 6.5 or > 13.5 mg/dL	0.25	2.1–2.6 mmol/L	SST
Calcium (ionized)	Serum	4.6–5.3 mg/dL	0.25	1.15–1.32 mmol/L	Green (anaerobic)
Calcium (U_{Ca})	Urine	100–300 mg/d	0.025	2.5–7.5 mmol/d	Urine bottle containing hydrochloric acid
Carbon dioxide, partial pressure (P_{CO_2})	Whole blood	32–48 mm Hg	0.13	4.26–6.38 kPa	Heparinized syringe (iced)
Carbon dioxide (CO_2), total (bicarbonate)	Serum	22–32 mEq/L **Panic:** < 15 or > 40 mEq/L	1.00	22–32 mmol/L **Panic:** < 15 or > 40 mmol/L	SST
Carboxyhemoglobin (HbCO)	Whole blood	< 9% of total hemoglobin (Hb)	0.01	< 0.09 fraction of total hemoglobin	Green
Carcinoembryonic antigen (CEA)	Serum	0–5 ng/mL	1.00	0–5 mcg/L	SST
CD4 T cell count	Whole blood	359–1725 cells/mcL			Lavender (complete blood count and differential and % CD4 required)
Ceruloplasmin	Serum	20–60 mg/dL (laboratory-specific)	10.00	200–600 mg/L	SST

(continued)

Table 2. Reference ranges for commonly used tests.[1,2] (continued)

		Current metric units × Conversion factor = SI units SI units ÷ Conversion factor = Current metric units			
Test	**Specimen**	**Conventional Units**	**Conversion Factor**	**SI Units[2]**	**Collection**
Chloride (Cl⁻)	Serum	101–112 mEq/L	1.00	101–112 mmol/L	SST
Cholesterol	Serum	Desirable: < 200 mg/dL Borderline: 200–239 mg/dL High risk: > 240 mg/dL	0.03	Desirable: < 5.2 mmol/L Borderline: 5.2–6.1 mmol/L High risk: > 6.2 mmol/L	SST
Chorionic gonadotropin, β-subunit (β-hCG), quantitative	Serum	Males and nonpregnant females: undetectable or < 5 mU/mL	1.00	Males and nonpregnant females: undetectable or < 5 units/L	SST
Complement C3	Serum	64–166 mg/dL	10.00	640–1660 mg/L	SST
Complement C4	Serum	15–45 mg/dL	10.00	150–450 mg/L	SST
Complement CH50	Serum	(Laboratory-specific)			Red
Cortisol	Serum	8:00 AM: 5–20 mcg/dL	27.59	140–550 nmol/L	SST
Cortisol (urinary free)	Urine	10–110 mcg/24 h	2.76	30–300 nmol/d	Urine bottle containing boric acid
Creatine kinase (CK)	Serum	32–267 units/L (method-dependent)	0.02	0.53–4.45 mckat/L (method-dependent)	SST
Creatine kinase MB (CKMB)	Serum	< 16 units/L or < 4% of total CK (laboratory-specific) Mass units: 0–7 mcg/L	0.04	< 0.27 mckat/L	SST
Creatinine (Cr)	Serum	0.6–1.2 mg/dL	83.3	50–100 mcmol/L	SST
Creatinine clearance (Cl$_{Cr}$)	See Collection column.	Adults: 90–140 mL/min/1.73 m² body surface area (BSA)	0.017	1.5–2.3 mL/s/1.73 m² BSA	Carefully timed 24-hour urine and simultaneous serum or plasma creatinine sample
Cryoglobulins	Serum	< 0.12 mg/dL			Red (at 37 °C)
Eosinophil count	Whole blood	0.04–0.5 × 10³/mcL	1.00	0.04–0.5 × 10⁹/L	Lavender
Erythrocyte count (RBC count)	Whole blood	4.7–6.1 × 10⁶/mcL	1.00	4.7–6.1 × 10¹²/L	Lavender
Erythrocyte sedimentation rate	Whole blood	Male: < 10 mm/h Female: < 15 mm/h (laboratory-specific)		Same	Lavender
Erythropoietin (EPO)	Serum	5–20 mU/mL	1.00	5–20 units/L	SST
Ethanol	Serum	mg/dL Legal "driving under the influence" in many states is defined as > 80 mg/dL (> 17 mmol/L) blood alcohol level; serum alcohol levels are 10–35% higher than blood alcohol levels	0.217	mmol/L	SST

(continued)

Table 2. Reference ranges for commonly used tests.[1,2] (continued)

		Current metric units × Conversion factor = SI units			
		SI units ÷ Conversion factor = Current metric units			
Test	**Specimen**	**Conventional Units**	**Conversion Factor**	**SI Units[2]**	**Collection**
Factor VIII assay	Plasma	40–150% of normal (varies with age)			Blue
Fecal fat	Stool	Random: < 60 droplets of fat per high-power field 72-hour: < 7 g/d			Qualitative: Random stool sample Quantitative: 72-hour collection following 2-day dietary fat regimen
Ferritin	Serum	Male: 16–300 ng/mL Female: 4–161 ng/mL	1.00	Male: 16–300 mcg/L Female: 4–161 mcg/L	SST
α-Fetoprotein (AFP)	Serum	0–15 ng/mL	1.00	0–15 mcg/L	SST
Fibrin D-dimers	Plasma	Negative			Blue
Fibrinogen (functional)	Plasma	175–433 mg/dL **Panic:** < 75 mg/dL	0.01	1.75–4.3 g/L	Blue
Folic acid (red cells)	Whole blood	165–760 ng/mL	2.27	370–1720 nmol/L	Lavender

Follicle-stimulating hormone (FSH)	Serum	Female:
		  Follicular phase 4–13 mU/mL
		  Luteal phase 2–13 mU/mL
		  Midcycle 5–22 mU/mL
		  Postmenopausal 30–138 mU/mL
		Male: 1–10 mU/mL (laboratory-specific)
			1.00	Female:
				4–13 units/L
				
				2–13 units/L
				
				5–22 units/L
				30–138 units/L
				
				Male: 1–10 units/L (laboratory-specific)
					SST

Free erythrocyte protoporphyrin (FEP)	Whole blood	< 35 mcg/dL (method-dependent)			Lavender
Fructosamine	Serum			190–270 mcmol/L	SST
γ-Glutamyltranspeptidase (GGT)	Serum	9–85 units/L (laboratory-specific)	0.02	0.15–1.42 mckat/L (laboratory-specific)	SST
Gastrin	Serum	< 100 pg/mL (laboratory-specific)	1.00	< 100 ng/L	SST
Glucose	Serum	60–110 mg/dL **Panic:** < 40 or > 500 mg/dL	0.055	3.3–6.1 mmol/L	(Fasting) SST
Glucose-6-phosphate dehydrogenase (G6PD) screen	Whole blood	5–14 units/g Hb	0.02	0.1–0.28 mckat/L	Lavender
Glutamine	Cerebrospinal fluid (CSF)	6–15 mg/dL **Panic:** > 40 mg/dL	68.5	411–1028 mcmol/L	Collect CSF in a plastic tube

(continued)

Table 2. Reference ranges for commonly used tests.[1,2] (continued)

		Current metric units × Conversion factor = SI units SI units ÷ Conversion factor = Current metric units			
Test	**Specimen**	**Conventional Units**	**Conversion Factor**	**SI Units**[2]	**Collection**
Glycated (glycosylated) hemoglobin (HbA$_{1c}$)	Serum	3.9–6.9% (method-dependent)			Lavender
Growth hormone (GH)	Serum	0–5 ng/mL	1.00	0–5 mcg/L	SST
Haptoglobin	Serum	46–316 mg/dL	0.01	0.5–3.2 g/L	SST
HDL cholesterol	Serum	Male: 27–67 mg/dL Female: 34–88 mg/dL	0.026	0.7–1.73 mmol/L 0.88–2.28 mmol/L	SST
Helicobacter pylori antibody	Serum	Negative			SST
Hematocrit (Hct)	Whole blood	Male: 39–49% Female: 35–45% (age-dependent)	0.01	Male: 0.39–0.49 Female: 0.35–0.45	Lavender
Hemoglobin A$_{1c}$ (See Glycated Hemoglobin)	Serum				
Hemoglobin A$_2$ (HbA$_2$)	Whole blood	1.5–3.5% of total hemoglobin	0.01	0.015–0.035	Lavender
Hemoglobin electrophoresis	Whole blood	HbA: > 95% HbA$_2$: 1.5–3.5%			Lavender
Hemoglobin, fetal (HbF)	Whole blood	Adult: < 2% (varies with age)			Lavender
Hemoglobin, total (Hb)	Whole blood	Male: 13.6–17.5 g/dL Female: 12.0–15.5 g/dL **Panic:** ≤ 7 g/dL (age-dependent)	10.00	Male: 136–175 g/L Female: 120–155 g/L	Lavender
Hemosiderin	Urine	Negative			Urine container
HIV viral load	Plasma	Negative			Lavender
Homocysteine	Plasma	4–12 mcmol/L	1.00	4–12 mcmol/L	Lavender
5-Hydroxyindoleacetic acid (5-HIAA)	Urine	2–8 mg/24 h	5.23	10–40 mcmol/d	Urine bottle containing hydrochloric acid
IgG index	Serum and CSF	0.29–0.59 ratio			SST and plastic tube for CSF
Immunoglobulins (Ig)	Serum	IgA: 78–367 mg/dL IgG: 583–1761 mg/dL IgM: 52–335 mg/dL	0.01	IgA: 0.78–3.67 g/L IgG: 5.83–17.6 g/L IgM: 0.52–3.35 g/L	SST
Insulin, immunoreactive	Serum	6–35 mcU/mL	7.18	42–243 pmol/L	SST
Insulin-like growth factor-1	Plasma	123–463 ng/mL (age- and sex-dependent)	1.0	123–463 mcg/L	SST
Iron (Fe^{2+})	Serum	50–175 mcg/dL	0.18	9–31 mcmol/L	SST
Iron-binding capacity, total (TIBC)	Serum	250–460 mcg/dL	0.18	45–82 mcmol/L	SST
Lactate dehydrogenase (LDH)	Serum	88–230 units/L (laboratory-specific)	0.02	1.46–3.82 mckat/L (laboratory-specific)	SST

(continued)

Table 2. Reference ranges for commonly used tests.[1,2] (continued)

Test	Specimen	Conventional Units	Conversion Factor	SI Units[2]	Collection
		Current metric units × Conversion factor = SI units			
		SI units ÷ Conversion factor = Current metric units			
Lactic acid (lactate)	Venous blood	0.5–2.0 mEq/L	1.00	0.5–2.0 mmol/L	Gray
LDL cholesterol	Serum	< 130 mg/dL	0.026	< 3.37 mmol/L	SST
Lead (Pb)	Whole blood	Child: < 25 mcg/dL Adult: < 40 mcg/dL	0.05	Child: < 1.21 mcmol/L Adult: < 1.93 mcmol/L	Navy
Lecithin/sphingomyelin (L/S) ratio	Amniotic fluid	> 2.0 (method-dependent)			Collect in a plastic tube
Leukocyte alkaline phosphatase (LAP)	Whole blood	40–130 Based on 0 to 4+ rating of 100 polymorphonuclear neutrophils stained for alkaline phosphatase			Green
Leukocyte (white blood cell) count, total (WBC count)	Whole blood	4.8–10.8 × 10³/mcL **Panic:** < 1.5 × 10³/mcL	1.00	4.8–10.8 × 10⁹/L	Lavender
Lipase	Serum	0–160 units/L (laboratory-specific)	0.02	0–2.66 mckat/L (laboratory-specific)	SST
Luteinizing hormone (LH)	Serum	Female: Follicular phase 1–18 mU/mL Luteal phase 0.4–20 mU/mL Midcycle 24–105 mU/mL Postmenopausal 15–62 mU/mL Male: 1–10 mU/mL (laboratory-specific)	1.00	1–18 units/L 0.4–20 units/L 24–105 units/L 15–62 units/L Male: 1–10 units/L (laboratory-specific)	SST
Lymphocyte count	Whole blood	0.8–3.5 × 10³/mcL	1.00	0.8–3.5 × 10⁹/L	Lavender
Magnesium (Mg²⁺)	Serum	1.8–3.0 mg/dL **Panic:** < 0.5 or > 4.5 mg/dL	0.41	0.75–1.25 mmol/L	SST
Mean corpuscular hemoglobin (MCH)	Whole blood	26–34 pg			Lavender
Mean corpuscular hemoglobin concentration (MCHC)	Whole blood	31–36 g/dL	10.00	310–360 g/L	Lavender
Mean corpuscular volume (MCV)	Whole blood	80–100 fL			Lavender
Metanephrines	Urine	0.3–0.9 mg/24 h	5.46	1.6–4.9 mcmol/d	Urine bottle containing hydrochloric acid

(continued)

Table 2. Reference ranges for commonly used tests.[1,2] (continued)

		Current metric units × Conversion factor = SI units SI units ÷ Conversion factor = Current metric units			
Test	**Specimen**	**Conventional Units**	**Conversion Factor**	**SI Units[2]**	**Collection**
Methemoglobin (MetHb)	Whole blood	< 1% of total hemoglobin	0.01	< 0.01 fraction of total hemoglobin	Green
Methylmalonic acid	Serum	0–0.05 mg/L	8.475	0–0.4 mcmol/L	SST
Monocyte count	Whole blood	$0.2–0.8 \times 10^3$/mcL	1.00	$0.2–0.8 \times 10^9$/L	Lavender
Neutrophil count	Whole blood	$2.2–8.6 \times 10^3$/mcL	1.00	$2.2–8.6 \times 10^9$/L	Lavender
Osmolality	Serum	275–293 mosm/kg H_2O **Panic:** < 240 or > 320 mosm/kg H_2O	1.00	275–293 mmol/kg H_2O	SST
	Urine	Random: 100–900 mosm/kg H_2O	1.00	Random: 100–900 mmol/kg H_2O	Urine container
Oxygen, partial pressure (Po_2)	Whole blood	83–108 mm Hg	0.13	11.04–14.36 kPa	Heparinized syringe (iced)
Parathyroid hormone (PTH)	Serum	Intact PTH: 11–54 pg/mL (laboratory-specific)	0.11	Intact PTH: 1.2–5.7 pmol/L (laboratory-specific)	Red
Partial thromboplastin time, activated (PTT)	Plasma	25–35 seconds (range varies) **Panic:** ≥ 60 seconds			Blue
pH	Whole blood	Arterial: 7.35–7.45 Venous: 7.31–7.41			Heparinized syringe (iced)
Phosphorus	Serum	2.5–4.5 mg/dL **Panic:** < 1.0 mg/dL	0.32	0.8–1.45 mmol/L	SST
Platelet count (Plt)	Whole blood	$150–450 \times 10^3$/mcL **Panic:** $< 25 \times 10^3$/mcL	1.0	$150–450 \times 10^9$/L **Panic:** $< 25 \times 10^9$/L	Lavender
Platelet-associated IgG	Whole blood	Negative			Lavender
Porphobilinogen (PBG)	Urine	Negative			Protect from light
Potassium (K^+)	Serum	3.5–5.0 mEq/L **Panic:** < 3.0 or > 6.0 mEq/L	1.00	3.5–5.0 mmol/L	SST
Prolactin (PRL)	Serum	< 20 ng/mL	1.00	< 20 mcg/L	SST
Prostate-specific antigen (PSA)	Serum	0–4 ng/mL	1.00	0–4 mcg/L	SST
Protein C	Plasma	71–176%			Blue
Protein electrophoresis	Serum	Adults: Albumin: 3.3–4.7 g/dL α_1: 0.1–0.4 g/dL α_2: 0.3–0.9 g/dL β_2: 0.7–1.5 g/dL γ: 0.5–1.4 g/dL	10.00	33–47 g/L 1–4 g/L 3–9 g/L 7–15 g/L 5–14 g/L	SST

(continued)

Table 2. Reference ranges for commonly used tests.[1,2] (continued)

Test	Specimen	Conventional Units	Conversion Factor	SI Units[2]	Collection
		Current metric units × Conversion factor = SI units			
		SI units ÷ Conversion factor = Current metric units			
Protein S (antigen)	Plasma	76–178%			Blue
Protein, total	Serum	6.0–8.0 g/dL	10.00	60–80 g/L	SST
Prothrombin time (PT)	Whole blood	11–15 seconds **Panic:** ≥ 30 seconds (laboratory-specific)			Blue
Red blood cell count	Whole blood	$4.7–6.1 \times 10^6$/mcL	1.00	$4.7–6.1 \times 10^{12}$/L	Lavender
Red cell volume	Whole blood	25–35 mL/kg			Green
Renin activity (PRA)	Plasma	High-sodium diet (75–150 mEq Na^+/d): Supine: 0.2–2.3 ng/mL/h Standing: 1.3–4.0 ng/mL/h) Low-sodium diet (30–75 mEq Na^+/d): Standing: 4.0–7.7 ng/mL/h)			Lavender
Reptilase clotting time	Plasma	13–19 seconds			Blue
Reticulocyte count	Whole blood	$33–137 \times 10^3$/mcL	1.00	$33–137 \times 10^9$/L	Lavender
Russell's viper venom clotting time (dilute) (RVVT)	Plasma	24–37 seconds			Blue
Salicylate (aspirin, others)	Serum	20–30 mg/dL **Panic:** > 35 mg/dL	10.00	200–300 mg/L	SST
Sodium (Na^+)	Serum	135–145 mEq/L **Panic:** < 125 or > 155 mEq/L	1.00	135–145 mmol/L	SST
Testosterone	Serum	Male: 175–781 ng/dL Female: 10–75 ng/dL	0.0347	Male: 6–27 nmol/L Female: 0.3–2.6 nmol/L	SST
Thrombin time	Plasma	8–12 seconds (laboratory-specific)			Blue
Thyroglobulin	Serum	3–42 ng/mL	1.00	3–42 mcg/L	SST
Thyroid-stimulating hormone (TSH)	Serum	0.4–6 mcU/mL	1.00	0.4–6 mU/L	SST
Thyroid-stimulating hormone receptor antibody (TSH-R Ab [stim])	Serum	< 130% of basal activity; based on cAMP generation in thyroid cell tissue culture			
Thyroxine, free (FT$_4$)	Serum	9–24 pmol/L (varies with method)			SST
Thyroxine (T$_4$), total	Serum	5–11 mcg/dL	12.80	64–142 nmol/L	SST

(continued)

Table 2. Reference ranges for commonly used tests.[1,2] (continued)

Test	Specimen	Conventional Units	Conversion Factor	SI Units[2]	Collection
		Current metric units × Conversion factor = SI units **SI units ÷ Conversion factor = Current metric units**			
Thyroxine index, free (FT$_4$I)	Serum	6.5–12.5			SST
Transferrin	Serum	190–375 mg/dL	0.01	1.9–3.75 g/L	SST
Triglycerides	Serum	< 165 mg/dL	0.01	< 1.8 mmol/L	SST (fasting)
Triiodothyronine (T$_3$), total	Serum	95–190 ng/dL	0.015	1.5–2.9 nmol/L	SST
Troponin-I (cTnI)	Serum	< 0.05 ng/mL			SST
Uric acid	Serum	Male: 2.4–7.4 mg/dL Female: 1.4–5.8 mg/dL	59.48	Male: 140–440 mcmol/L Female: 80–350 mcmol/L	SST
Vanillylmandelic acid (VMA)	Urine	2–7 mg/24 h	5.05	10–35 mcmol/d	Urine bottle containing hydrochloric acid
Vitamin B$_{12}$	Serum	140–820 pg/mL	0.74	100–600 pmol/L	SST
Vitamin B$_{12}$ absorption test (Schilling test)	24-hour urine	Excretion of > 8% of administered dose			Urine bottle
Vitamin D, 25-hydroxy (25[OH]D)	Serum	10–50 ng/mL	2.5	25–125 nmol/L	SST
Vitamin D, 1,25-dihydroxy (1,25[OH]$_2$D)	Serum	20–76 pg/mL	2.4	48–182 pmol/L	SST
White blood cell count	Whole blood	4.8–10.8 × 10^3/mcL	1.00	4.8–10.8 × 10^9/L	Lavender

[1]The reference ranges given here in conventional units and in SI units are from several large medical centers. Always use the reference ranges provided by your clinical laboratory, since ranges may be method-dependent.
[2]Reference: Young DS: Implementation of SI units for clinical laboratory data. Ann Intern Med 1987;106:114; JAMA Instructions for Authors, JAMA 1997;278:74.

Table 3. Commonly used specimen collection tubes.

Tube	Tube Contents	Typical Use
Lavender	EDTA	Complete blood count
SST	Serum separator	Serum chemistry tests
Red	None	Blood banking (serum); therapeutic drug monitoring
Blue	Citrate	Coagulation studies
Gray	Inhibitor of glycolysis (sodium fluoride)	Lactic acid
Green	Heparin	Plasma studies
Yellow	Acid citrate	HLA typing
Navy	Trace metal free	Trace metals (eg, lead)

EDTA = ethylenediaminetetraactic acid; SST = serum separator tube.

INDEX

NOTE: Page numbers in **boldface** type indicate a major discussion. A *t* following a page number indicates tabular material, an *f* following a page number indicates a figure, and a *b* following a page number indicates a boxed feature. Drugs are listed under their generic names. When a drug trade name is listed, the reader is referred to the generic name.

for endometriosis, 759–760
for hypogonadotropic hypogonadism, 1130
for ovarian ablation in breast cancer, 741
Gonadotropins
cancer-related production of, 1729t
deficiency of, 1128. *See also* Hypogonadism
in amenorrhea, 1207, 1208–1209
human chorionic (hCG). *See* Human chorionic gonadotropin
human menopausal (hMG), for ovulation induction, 769
Gonococcal infections/gonorrhea, **1462–1464**, 1583t
anorectal involvement and, 660, 1463, 1464
arthritis and, **878–879**, 1463, 1464
cervicitis, 1463, 1463–1464
chlamydial coinfection and, 1464, 1472
conjunctivitis, 157, 1463
disseminated, 1463
drug resistant, 879, 1463
epididymitis in, 966, 1463
pelvic inflammatory disease, 761, 1463, 1464
pharyngitis, 1463, 1464
during pregnancy, 799
rape/sexual assault in transmission of, 779, 1325
urethritis, 1463, 1463–1464
Goodpasture's syndrome, 297
alveolar hemorrhage in, 297
glomerulonephritis in, 297, 938f
HLA in, 820t
Gordon syndrome (pseudohypoaldosteronism type II), 896t
Goserelin, 1706t. *See also* Luteinizing hormone-releasing hormone (LHRH) analogs
for breast cancer, 740t
for prostate cancer, 1703
GOT. *See* Aspartate aminotransferase
Gottron's sign, 860
Gout/gouty arthritis, **829–833**, 830t, 832t
renal manifestations of, 830, **952**
rheumatoid arthritis differentiated from, 831, 848
saturnine, in lead poisoning, 831
in transplant patient, 833
gp120/160, HIV vaccine development and, 1360
GPI (glycosylphosphatidylinositol) anchor deficiency, in paroxysmal nocturnal hemoglobinuria, 503
GPT. *See* Alanine aminotransferase
GRACE Risk Score, 361, 373
Gradenigo's syndrome, 188
Graft-versus-host disease, in HPC transplantation, 822, 1314
Graft-versus-leukemia effect, 822
Graft-versus-tumor effect, 1693
Graham–Steel murmur, 344
Gram-negative infections, **1451–1467**, 1583t, 1584t. *See also specific causative agent*
bacteremia and sepsis, **1454–1456**
folliculitis, acne and, 116, 119, 120
Gram-positive infections, **1431–1445**, 1583t, 1584t. *See also specific causative agent*
Gram stain
ascitic fluid, 572
in pneumonia diagnosis, 255

Grand mal (tonic-clonic) seizures, 1005–1006, 1005t. *See also* Seizures
Grand mal (tonic-clonic) status epilepticus, 1010
Granisetron, 552, 552t, 1715. *See also* Antiemetics
Granular urinary casts, 919t, 958
Granulocyte colony-stimulating factor (G-CSF). *See* Filgrastim
Granulocyte macrophage colony-stimulating factor (GM-CSF). *See* Sargramostim
Granulocyte transfusion, 547
Granulocytic ehrlichiosis/anaplasmosis, 1423t, 1428
Granulocytopenia. *See also* Neutropenia
infections and, 1314
Granuloma. *See also* Granulomatosis; Granulomatous disorders
hepatic, drugs/toxins causing, 682
inguinale, **1464**
intubation, 214
lethal midline, 204
pulmonary, in sarcoidosis, 283
swimming pool, 1469
in toxocariasis (visceral larva migrans), 1565, 1566
Granulomatosis
allergic angiitis and. *See* Allergic angiitis and granulomatosis
infantisepticum, 1445
Wegener's. *See* Wegener's granulomatosis
Granulomatous disorders. *See also specific type and* Granuloma; Granulomatosis
acanthamoeba causing, 1322, 1504
gastritis in, 599
hypercalcemia in, 1176
neck involved in, 219
of nose and paranasal sinuses, **202–204**
Granulomatous thyroiditis. *See* Subacute (de Quervain's) thyroiditis
Granulosa cell tumor, 764t
Graves' dermopathy (pretibial myxedema), 1158, 1161, 1166
Graves' disease, 1158, 1162–1164. *See also* Graves' ophthalmopathy; Hyperthyroidism
HLA in, 820t, 1158
thyroid antibodies/TSH receptor antibody in, 1141, 1158
Graves' ophthalmopathy/exophthalmos (dysthyroid eye disease), 154, **172**, 1158, 1160, 1164–1165
Gray top tubes, 1777t
Great toe, in gout, 830
Green poultice, chronic pain disorders and, 1076
Green top tubes, 1777t
Grief reaction/grieving, 86, 1090
Grip (handgrip), heart murmurs affected by, 334t
Grippe, summer, 1420
Griseofulvin, 101
Group A beta-hemolytic streptococcal infection, **1432–1433**, 1583t
cellulitis, 125
endocarditis, 1433, 1449
erysipelas, **125**, 1432
glomerulonephritis and, 937, 1431
impetigo, 114, 1432
pharyngitis, 207–209, **1431–1432**
rapid antigen tests for, 207, 208
rheumatic fever and, 414, 1431, 1432

scarlet fever, 1431, 1433
skin infections, **1432**
Group B streptococcal infection, 1433, 1583t
endocarditis, 1449
in pregnancy, 785, 799, 1433
Group C streptococcal infection, 1433, 1583t
endocarditis, 1449
Group D streptococcal infection, 1433
endocarditis, 1433, 1446
Group G streptococcal infection, 1433, 1583t
endocarditis, 1449
Group therapy. *See also* Support groups
for anxiety disorders, 1072
for chronic pain disorders, 1076
for personality disorders, 1080
for somatoform disorders, 1074
Growth factors. *See also* Filgrastim; Sargramostim
in cancer chemotherapy, 1701, 1703
cancer vaccine modification and, 1733
for chemotherapy-induced toxicity, 1703, 1713
for HIV infection/AIDS, 1373–1375
for infection in cancer/immunocompromised host, 1316, 1727
for neutropenia, 511
platelet-derived, in myelofibrosis, 515
receptors for, blockade of in cancer treatment, 1731, 1731f
Growth hormone (GH)
deficiency of, 1129, 1130, 1131
excess of, acromegaly and gigantism caused by, 1134–1136
in phosphate metabolism, 903
replacement therapy with, 1131
for AIDS wasting, 1351
for burn patients, 1630
for Turner's syndrome, 1215
serum levels of
in acromegaly/gigantism, 1134
laboratory reference range for, 1773t
tumors secreting, 1216
Guaiac testing. *See* Fecal occult blood testing
Guanabenz, 449, 451t
overdose/toxicity of, 1654
Guanadrel, 452
Guanethidine, 452
antidepressant drug interactions and, 1099t
monoamine oxidase inhibitor interactions and, 1099t
Guanfacine, 449, 451t
overdose/toxicity of, 1654
Guargum. *See also* Fiber, dietary
for constipation, 556t
Guillain-Barré syndrome (acute idiopathic polyneuropathy), 1051, 1396
dysautonomia in, 1011, 1051
influenza vaccination and, 1339, 1414
yellow fever vaccination and, 1344
Guinea worm infection (dracunculiasis), **1550–1551**
Gum disease. *See* Gingivitis
Gummas, in syphilis, 1474, 1475t, 1479t, 1481
Guns. *See* Firearms
Gut. *See* Gastrointestinal system
Gut dialysis, (repeat-dose charcoal), 1645
Guttate psoriasis, 98. *See also* Psoriasis
GW572016. *See* Lapatinib